D1568690

Smolin and Thoft's

THE CORNEA
SCIENTIFIC FOUNDATIONS
AND CLINICAL PRACTICE

Smolin and Thoft's

THE CORNEA
SCIENTIFIC FOUNDATIONS
AND CLINICAL PRACTICE

FOURTH EDITION

Editors

C. STEPHEN FOSTER, M.D., F.A.C.S.

Director, Ocular Immunology and Uveitis Service
Professor of Ophthalmology
Massachusetts Eye and Ear Infirmary
Harvard Medical School
Boston, Massachusetts

DIMITRI T. AZAR, M.D.

Director, Corneal, External Disease, and Refractive Surgery Services
Professor of Ophthalmology
Massachusetts Eye and Ear Infirmary
Harvard Medical School
Boston, Massachusetts

CLAES H. DOHLMAN, M.D., Ph.D.

Professor of Ophthalmology
Massachusetts Eye and Ear Infirmary
Harvard Medical School
Boston, Massachusetts

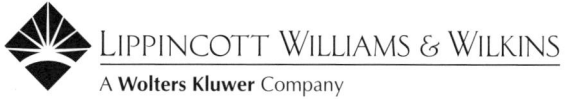
LIPPINCOTT WILLIAMS & WILKINS
A **Wolters Kluwer** Company
Philadelphia · Baltimore · New York · London
Buenos Aires · Hong Kong · Sydney · Tokyo

Acquisitions Editor: Jonathan Pine
Developmental Editor: Eileen Wolfberg
Production Service: Print Matters, Inc.
Manufacturing Manager: Benjamin Rivera
Project Manager: Nicole Walz
Marketing Manager: Kathleen Neely
Cover Designer: Andrew Gatto
Compositor: Compset, Inc.
Printer: Quebecor World-Kingsport

©2005 by LIPPINCOTT WILLIAMS & WILKINS
530 Walnut Street
Philadelphia, PA 19106 USA
LWW.com

Printed in the USA

Library of Congress Cataloging-in-Publication Data

Smolin and Thoft's the cornea : scientific foundations and clinical
    practice.—4th ed. / editors, C. Stephen Foster, Dimitri T. Azar, Claes H. Dohlman.
        p. ; cm.
    Rev. ed. of: Cornea. 3rd ed. c1994.
    Includes bibliographical references and index.
    ISBN 0-7817-4206-4 (HC)
    1. Cornea—Diseases. 2. Cornea. I. Title: Cornea. II. Smolin, Gilbert.
III. Foster, C. Stephen (Charles Stephen), 1942– IV. Azar, Dimitri T. V. Dohlman,
Claes H. VI. Cornea.
    [DNLM: 1. Corneal Diseases. WW 220 S666 2004]
RE336.C66 2004
616.7′19—dc22

                                                          2004057603

   Care has been taken to confirm the accuracy of the information presented and to describe generally accepted practices. However, the authors, editors, and publisher are not responsible for errors or omissions or for any consequences from application of the information in this book and make no warranty, expressed or implied, with respect to the currency, completeness, or accuracy of the contents of the publication. Application of this information in a particular situation remains the professional responsibility of the practitioner.
   The authors, editors, and publisher have exerted every effort to ensure that drug selection and dosage set forth in this text are in accordance with current recommendations and practice at the time of publication. However, in view of ongoing research, changes in government regulations, and the constant flow of information relating to drug therapy and drug reactions, the reader is urged to check the package insert for each drug for any change in indications and dosage and for added warnings and precautions. This is particularly important when the recommended agent is a new or infrequently employed drug.
   Some drugs and medical devices presented in this publication have Food and Drug Administration (FDA) clearance for limited use in restricted research settings. It is the responsibility of the health care provider to ascertain the FDA status of each drug or device planned for use in their clinical practice.

10 9 8 7 6 5 4 3 2 1

To my son, Marc David Foster, a wonderful son, husband, and father
—C. Stephen Foster

With gratitude to the 1986–88 Cornea Service physicians:
C. H. Dohlman, C. S. Foster, K. R. Kenyon, D. P. Langston, M. Wagoner,
M. B. Abelson, A. M. Bajart, S. A. Boruchoff, J. Gilbard, and R. F. Steinert.
—Dimitri T. Azar

To the memory of Richard A. Thoft
—Claes H. Dohlman

To the Memory of J. Wayne Streilein, M.D.
—C. Stephen Foster, Dimitri T. Azar, and Claes H. Dohlman

CONTRIBUTORS

Anthony P. Adamis, MD Chief Scientific Officer, Eyetech Pharmaceuticals, Eyetech Research Center, Woburn, MA

Esen Karamursel Akpek, MD Assistant Professor, Department of Ophthalmology, Johns Hopkins University School of Medicine, Staff Surgeon, Division of Cornea and External Disease, Wilmer Eye Institute, Baltimore, MD

Eduardo C. Alfonso, MD Professor, Department of Ophthalmology, University of Miami, Bascom Palmer Eye Institute, Miami, FL

Ali A. Al-Rajhi, MD, FRCS Director of Research, Assistant Supervisor General, King Khaled Eye Specialist Hospital, Riyadh, Saudi Arabia

Renato Ambrósio, Jr, MD Department of Ophthalmology, University of São Paulo, São Paulo, Brazil

William Ayliffe, FRCS, FRCOphth, PhD Consultant Ophthalmic Surgeon, Croydon Eye Unit, Mayday University Hospital, Surrey, United Kingdom

Dimitri T. Azar, MD Director, Corneal, External Disease, and Refractive Surgery Services; Professor of Ophthalmology, Massachusetts Eye and Ear Infirmary, Harvard Medical School, Boston, MA

Nathalie Azar, MD Harvard Medical School, Massachusetts Eye and Ear Infirmary, Boston, MA

Scott D. Barnes, MD Clinical Fellow, Ophthalmology Department, Cornea and Refractive Surgery Service, Massachusetts Eye and Ear Infirmary, Boston, MA

Neal P. Barney, MD Associate Professor, Department of Ophthalmology and Visual Sciences, University of Wisconsin Medical School, University of Wisconsin Hospital and Clinics, Madison, WI

Jules L. Baum, MD Boston Eye Associates, Chestnut Hill, MA

C. Robert Bernardino, MD Assistant Professor of Ophalmology, Oculoplastics and Orbital Surgery, Emory Eye Center, Atlanta, GA

Andra S. Bobart, BA, MBBCh LRCP & SI, MMedSci, FRCOphth(Irl), EBOD Registrar and Lecturer in Ophthalmology, Royal Victoria Eye and Ear Hospital and the Royal College of Surgeons, Dublin, Ireland

Helene Boisjoly, MD, MPH Professor and Chair, Département d'Ophtalmologie, Université de Montréal; Attending Physician, Maisonneuve-Rosemont Hopital, Montréal, Québec, Canada

Fina Cañas Barouch, MD Instructor, Department of Ophthalmology, Harvard Medical School; Director, Eye Trauma Service, Massachusetts Eye and Ear Infirmary, Boston, MA

H. Dwight Cavanagh, MD, PhD, FACS Professor and Vice Chairman, Department of Ophthalmology, University of Texas Southwestern Medical Center; Medical Director, Zale Lipshy University Hospital, Dallas, TX

Margaret Chang, MD Resident, The Wilmer Eye Institute, Johns Hopkins University, Baltimore, MD

Shu-Wen Chang, MD Department of Ophthalmology, Chang Gung Memorial Hospital, Taoyuan, Taiwan

Puwat Charukamnoetkanok, MD Assistant Professor, Department of Ophthalmology, University of Pittsburgh, University of Pittsburgh Medical Center Eye Center, Pittsburgh, PA

Henrique V. Chaves, MD Director of Cornea Service, Brazil Belo Horizonte, São Paolo, Brazil

Glenn C. Cockerham, MD Associate Professor, Department of Ophthalmology, Stanford University School of Medicine, Stanford, CA; Chief of Service, Department of Ophthalmology, Veteran's Affairs Palo Alto Health Care System, Palo Alto, CA

Kimberly P. Cockerham, MD, FACS Associate Professor, Department of Ophthalmology, University of California–San Francisco, San Francisco, CA

Kathryn Colby, MD, PhD Instructor, Department of Ophthalmology, Harvard Medical School; Director, Clinical Research Center, Department of Ophthalmology, Massachusetts Eye and Ear Infirmary, Boston, MA

Joseph Colin, MD Service Opthalmologie, Groupe Hospitalier Pellegrin, Bordeaux, France

Janis Cotter, OD Affiliated Clinical Professor of Optometry, New England College of Optometry, Boston, MA

Christopher B. Courville, BSc Research Associate, Department of Ophthalmology, Louisiana State University School of Medicine, Louisiana State University Eye Center, New Orleans, LA

Reza Dana, MD, MPH Associate Professor, Harvard Medical School; Senior Scientist, Schepens Eye Research Institute, Attending Physician, Cornea Service, Massachusetts Eye and Ear Infirmary, Boston, MA

Darlene A. Dartt, PhD Senior Scientist, Schepens Eye Research Institute, Harvard Medical School, Boston, MA

Elizabeth A. Davis, MD, FACS University of Minnesota, Minneapolis, MN, Minnesota Eye Consultants, P.A, Bloomington, MN

John F. Doane, MD, FACS Clinical Assistant Professor, Department of Ophthalmology, University of Kansas Medical Center, Kansas City, KS; Cornea and Refractive Surgeon, Discover Vision Centers, Kansas City, MO

Murat Dogru, MD Department of Ophthalmology, Tokyo Dental College, Ichikawa General Hospital, Tokyo, Japan

Claes H. Dohlman, MD, PhD Professor of Ophthalmology, Massachusetts Eye and Ear Infirmary, Harvard Medical School, Boston, MA

Peter C. Donshik, MD Clinical Professor, Departments of Surgery and Ophthalmology, University of Connecticut Health Center, Farmington, CT; Hartford Hospital, Hartford, CT

Marlene L. Durand, MD Assistant Professor, Department of Medicine, Harvard Medical School; Director, Infectious Disease Service, Massachusetts Eye and Ear Infirmary, Boston, MA

Kourosh Eghbali, MD Department of Ophthalmology, University of California–Irvine, Irvine, CA

Daniel Epstein, MD, PhD Professor and Doctor of Medicine, University Hospital, Zurich, Switzerland

Martin Filipec, MD General Teaching Hospital, Prague, Czech Republic

Nicoletta Fynn-Thompson, MD Harvard Medical School, Boston, MA

Richard K. Forster, MD Professor, Bascom Palmer Eye Institute, University of Miami School of Medicine, Miami, FL

C. Stephen Foster, MD, FACS Director, Ocular Immunology and Uveitis Service, Professor of Ophthalmology, Massachusetts Eye and Ear Infirmary, Harvard Medical School, Boston, MA

Gary N. Foulks, MD Professor and Chairman, Department of Ophthalmology, University of Pittsburgh School of Medicine, Pittsburgh, PA

Cláudia M. Francesconi, MD Instructor in Ophthalmology, Federal University of São Paulo, Paulista School of Medicine, Medical Assistant, Eye Clinic Day Hospital, São Paulo, Brazil

Beatrice E. Frueh, MD Associate Professor, Department of Ophthalmology, University of Bern; Chief, Anterior Segment Division, Department of Ophthalmology, Inselspital, Bern, Switzerland

Matthew Gardiner, MD Instructor, Department of Ophthalmology, Harvard Medical School; Director, Emergency Ophthalmology Services, Massachusetts Eye and Ear Infirmary, Boston, MA

Prashant Garg, MBBS L.V. Prasad Eye Institute, Hyderabad, India

Damien Gatinel, MD Foundation Rothschild, Hôpital Bichat-Claude Bernard, Paris, France

Emiliano Ghinelli, MD Schepens Eye Research Institute, Department of Ophthalmology, Harvard Medical School, Boston, MA

Ilene K. Gipson, PhD Professor, Department of Ophthalmology, Harvard Medical School, Ocular Surface Scholar and Senior Scientist, Schepens Eye Research Institute, Boston, MA

John D. Goosey, MD Adjunct Faculty, Corneal Specialist, University of Houston College of Optometry, Houston Eye Associates, Houston, TX

Abha Gulati, MD Postdoctoral Research Fellow, Department of Ophthalmology, Harvard Medical School, Schepens Eye Research Institute, Boston, MA

D. Rex Hamilton, MD, MS Assistant Professor of Ophthalmology, Department of Cornea–External Ocular Disease and Uveitis Division, University of California–Los Angeles; Medical Director, University of California–Los Angeles Laser Refractive Center, Jules Stein Eye Center, University of California–Los Angeles Medical Center, Los Angeles, CA

David R. Hardten, MD, FACS Associate Clinical Professor of Ophthalmology, University of Minnesota; Director of Refractive Surgery, Minnesota Eye Consultants, Minneapolis, MN

Mark P. Hatton, MD Director, Trauma Service, Massachusetts Eye and Ear Infirmary, Boston, MA

Ramzi K. Hemady, MD Associate Professor, Department of Ophthalmology, University of Maryland

School of Medicine; Program Director, Department of Ophthalmology, University of Maryland Medical Systems, Baltimore, MD

Thanh Hoang–Xuan, MD   Professor, Department of Ophthalmology, University of Paris–Bichat; Chief of Ophtholmology, Fondation Ophtalmologique Rothschild, Paris, France

Robin R. Hodges, MS   Scientific Associate III, Schepens Eye Research Institute, Boston, MA

Ozge Ilhan-Sarac, MD   Post-Doctoral Fellow, Department of Ophthalmology, Johns Hopkins University School of Medicine, Division of Cornea and External Disease, Wilmer Eye Institute, Johns Hopkins School of Medicine, Baltimore, MD

Sandeep Jain, MD   Instructor, Department of Ophthalmology, Harvard Medical School; Medical Director, Methuen and Stoneham Eye Center, Massachusetts Eye and Ear Infirmary, Boston, MA

Faisal Jehan, MD   Clinical Instructor, Department of Ophthalmology, University of California–Irvine, Irvine, CA, Clinical Instructor, Department of Ophthalmology, University of California–Irvine Medical Center, Orange, CA

James V. Jester, PhD   Department of Ophthalmology, University of Texas Southwestern Medical Center at Dallas, Dallas, TX

Nancy C. Joyce, PhD   Associate Professor, Department of Ophthalmology, Harvard Medical School; Senior Scientist, Schepens Eye Research Institute, Boston, MA

Tibor Juhasz, PhD   Professor, Departments of Ophthalmology and Biomedical Engineering, University of California–Irvine, Irvine, CA

Sajeev S. Kathuria, MD   Assistant Professor, Department of Ophthalmology, University of Maryland School of Medicine; Director, Oculoplastic Service, University of Maryland Medical Systems, Baltimore, MD

Kenneth R. Kenyon, MD   Associate Clinical Professor, Harvard Medical School, Senior Surgeon, Massachusetts Eye and Ear Infirmary, Senior Clinical Scientist, Schepens Eye Research Institute, Boston, MA

Shigeru Kinoshita, MD, PhD   Professor, Department of Ophthalmology, Kyoto Prefectural University of Medicine, Kyoto, Japan

Stephen D. Klyce, PhD   Professor of Ophthalmology and Cell Biology/Anatomy, Department of Ophthalmology, Louisiana State University School of Medicine, Louisiana State University Eye Center, New Orleans, LA

Douglas D. Koch, MD   Professor, Department of Ophthalmology, Baylor College of Medicine, Houston, TX

Aaleya F. Koreishi, MD   Wilmer Ophthalmological Institute, Johns Hopkins University School of Medicine, Baltimore, MD

Regis P. Kowalski, MS, [M]ASCP   Ophthalmic Microbiology, The Eye and Ear Institute, Pittsburgh, PA

Ronald M. Kurtz, MD   Associate Professor, Department of Ophthalmology, University of California–Irvine, Irvine, CA

George D. Kymionis, MD, PhD   Research Fellow, Vardinoyannion Eye Institute of Crete, University of Crete Medical School; Resident, Department of Ophthalmology, University Hospital of Crete, Crete, Greece

Patrick M. Ladage, PhD   Department of Ophthalmology, University of Texas Southwestern Medical Center at Dallas, Dallas, TX

Peter R. Laibson, MD   Department of Ophthalmology, Jefferson Medical College, Thomas Jefferson University; Cornea Service, Wills Eye Hospital, Philadelphia, PA

Michael A. Lemp, MD   Clinical Professor, Department of Ophthalmology, Georgetown University School of Medicine, Washington, DC

Erik Letko, MD   Harvard Medical School, Massachusetts Eye and Ear Infirmary, Boston, MA

Raymond S. Loh, MBBCh, FRCOphth   Department of Ophthalmology, The General Infirmary at Leeds, Leeds, United Kingdom

Joseph J. K. Ma, MD, FRCSC   Harvard Medical School, Cornea/Refractive/External Diseases, Massachusetts Eye and Ear Infirmary, Boston, MA

Michele Mabon, MD, FRCSC   Clinical Assistant Professor, Département d'Ophtalmologie, Université de Montréal, Hopital Marsonneuse–Rosemont, Montréal, Quebec, Canada

Gregory S. Makowski, PhD   Associate Professor, Department of Laboratory Medicine, University of Connecticut Health Center; Associate Director, Department of Laboratory Medicine, John Dempsey Hospital, Farmington, CT

Maite Sainz de la Maza, MD, PhD   Associate Professor, Department of Ophthalmology, Central University of Barcelona; Chief, Ocular Immunology and Uveitis Service, Department of Ophthalmology, Barcelona, Spain

Peter J. McDonnell, MD   Wilmer Ophthalmological Institute, Johns Hopkins University School of Medicine, Baltimore, MD

Lawrence M. Merin, RBP, FIMI FOPS, FBCA Assistant Professor of Opthalmology, Department of Ophthalmology and Visual Sciences, Vanderbilt University School of Medicine; Director, Vanderbilt Ophthalmic Imaging Center, Nashville, TN

Elisabeth M. Messmer, MD Department of Ophthalmology, Ludwig–Maximilians University, Munich, Germany

Parveen K. Nagra, MD   Department of Ophthalmology, Jefferson Medical College, Thomas Jefferson University; Cornea Service, Wills Eye Hospital, Philadelphia, PA

Marcelo Netto, MD   Clinical Instructor, Department of Ophthalmology, University of Washington, Seattle, WA

Anh T. Q. Nguyen, MD   Fellow, Department of Cornea and Refractive Surgery, Harvard Medical School, Massachusetts Eye and Ear Infirmary, Boston, MA

Mahnaz Nouri, MD   Associate Staff, Department of Ophthalmology, Harvard Medical School; Clinical Fellow, Department of Cornea and Refractive Surgery, Massachusetts Eye and Ear Infirmary, Boston, MA

Terrence P. O'Brien, MD   Director, Ocular Infectious Diseases, Ocular Microbiology Laboratorym Wilmer Ophthalmological Institute, Johns Hopkins University School of Medicine, Baltimore, MD

Ioannis G. Pallikaris, MD, PhD   Professor, Department of Ophthalmology, University of Crete Medical School; Chief, Department of Ophthalmology, University Hospital of Crete, Crete, Greece

Deborah Pavan-Langston, MD, FACS Associate Professor, Department of Ophthalmology, Harvard Medical School; Surgeon, Director of Clinical Virology, Department of Ophthalmology, Massachusetts Eye and Ear Infirmary, Boston, MA

W. Matthew Petroll, PhD   Department of Ophthalmology, University of Texas Southwestern Medical Center at Dallas, Dallas, TX

Roswell R. Pfister, MD   Clinical Professor, Department of Ophthalmology, University of Alabama School of Medicine; Consultant, Department of Ophthalmology, Brookwood Medical Center, Birmingham, AL

Roberto Pineda II, MD   Assistant Professor, Department of Ophthalmology, Harvard Medical School; Associate Surgeon, Active Staff, Massachusetts Eye and Ear Infirmary, Boston, MA

William J. Power, MCh, FRCOphth (Glas), FRCOphth, MRCPI   Consultant Ophthalmic Surgeon, Director of Research and Training, Royal Victoria Eye and Ear Hospital, St. Vincent's University Hospital, Dublin, Ireland

Jonathan D. Primack, MD   Assistant Professor of Ophthalmology and Visual Sciences, Albert Einstein College of Medicine; Director of Refractive Surgery, Department of Ophthalmology, North Shore–Long Island Jewish Hospital, Great Neck, NY

Yaron S. Rabinowitz, MD   Clinical Professor, Department of Ophthalmology, University of California–Los Angeles School of Medicine; Director of Ophthalmology Research, Cedars-Sinai Medical Center, Los Angeles, CA

Melinda L. Ramsby, MD, PhD   Assistant Professor, Department of Medicine, University of Connecticut Health Center; Attending Physician, John Dempsey Hospital, Farmington, CT

Azhar N. Rana, MD   Clinical Cornea Fellow, Massachusetts Eye and Ear Infirmary, Boston, MA; Consultant Ophthalmologist, Rana Eye Hospital, Quetta, Pakistan

Andre C. Romano, MD   Resident, Department of Ophthalmology, Federal University of São Paulo, Paulista School of Medicine, São Paulo, Brazil

Perry Rosenthal, MD   Assistant Clinical Professor, Department of Ophthalmology, Harvard Medical School, Boston, MA; President and Founder, Boston Foundation for Sight, Needham, MA

Peter A. D. Rubin, MD, FACS   Associate Professor of Ophthalmology, Harvard Medical School, Massachusetts Eye and Ear Infirmary, Ophthalmic Plastic, Orbital, and Cosmetic Surgery, Boston, MA

Maite Sainz de la Maza, MD   Associate Professor of Ophthalmology, Hospital Clinico of Barcelona, Barcelona, Spain

Melvin A. Sarayba, MD   Associate Specialist, Department of Ophthalmology, University of California–Irvine, Irvine, CA

Debra A. Schaumberg, ScD, OD, MPH Assistant Professor, Departments of Medicine and Ophthalmology, Harvard Medical School; Director, Ophthalmic Epidemiology, Division of Preventive Medicine, Brigham and Women's Hospital, Boston, MA

Oliver D. Schein, MD, MPH   Department of Ophthalmology, Wilmer Ophthalmological Institute, Johns Hopkins University School of Medicine, Baltimore, MD

Neda Shamie, MD Department of Ophthalmology, University of California–Irvinem Irvine, CA

Savitri Sharma, MD L.V. Prasad Eye Institute, Hyderabad, India

Carol L. Shields, MD Professor of Ophthalmology, Thomas Jefferson University, Associate Director, Ocular Oncology Service, Wills Eye Hospital, Philadelphia, PA

Jerry A. Shields, MD Professor of Ophthalmology, Thomas Jefferson University, Director, Ocular Oncology Service, Wills Eye Hospital, Philadelphia, PA

Gurinder Singh, MD, MHA Clinical Professor, Department of Ophthalmology, University of Kansas Medical Center, Chief, Department of Ophthalmology, Providence Medical Center, Kansas City, KS

Michael K. Smolek, PhD Assistant Research Professor, Department of Ophthalmology, Louisiana State University School of Medicine, Louisiana State University Eye Center, New Orleans, LA

Lee A. Snyder, MD Wilmer Ophthalmological Institute, Johns Hopkins University School of Medicine, Baltimore, MD

Walter J. Stark, MD Wilmer Ophthalmological Institute, Johns Hopkins University School of Medicine, Baltimore, MD

Christopher Starr, MD Clinical Assistant Professor, New York University School of Medicine, Manhattan Eye, Ear and Throat Hospital, New York Presbyterian Hospital, New York, NY

Stephen Stechschulte, MD Discover Vision Centers, Kansas City, MO

J. Wayne Steilein, MD* Schepens Eye Research Institute, Boston, MA

Roger F. Steinert, MD Professor of Ophthalmology, Professor of Biomedical Engineering, University of California–Irvine, Irvine, CA

Christopher W. Sturbaum, MD Staff Physician, Department of Surgery, Valley Hospital and Medical Center, Spokane Valley, WA

Jonathan H. Talamo, MD Assistant Clinical Professor, Department of Ophthalmology, Harvard Medical

School, Associate Surgeon, Massachusetts Eye and Ear Infirmary, Boston, MA

Joseph Tauber, MD Clinical Professor, Department of Ophthalmology, University of Kansas School of Medicine, Kansas City, KS; Tauber Eye Center, Kansas City, MO

Kazuo Tsubota, MD Department of Ophthalmology, Tokyo Dental College, Ichikawa General Hospital, Tokyo, Japan

Suhas Tuli, MD Clinical Instructor, Department of Ophthalmology, Doheny Eye Institute, Keck School of Medicine, Los Angeles, CA; Providence Sáint Joseph Medical Center, Burbank, CA

Michael D. Wagoner, MD Medical Director, King Khaled Eye Specialist Hospital, Riyadh, Saudi Arabia

Nadia K. Waheed, MD Fellow, Harvard Medical School, Department of Ophthalmology, Massachusetts Eye and Ear Infirmary, Boston, MA

Li Wang, MD, PhD Research Associate, Department of Ophthalmology, Baylor College of Medicine, Houston, TX

Steven E. Wilson, MD Director of Corneal Research, Cole Eye Institute, Cleveland Clinic Foundation, Cleveland, OH

Helen K. Wu, MD New England Eye Center, Tufts University School of Medicine, Boston, MA

Patrick C. Yeh, MD Harvard Medical School, Massachusetts Eye and Ear Infirmary, Schepens Eye Research Institute, Boston, MA

Norihiko Yokoi, MD, PhD Associate Professor, Department of Ophthalmology, Kyoto Prefectural University of Medicine, Kyoto, Japan

Sonia H. Yoo, MD Assistant Professor of Clinical Ophthalmology, University of Miami School of Medicine, Bascom Palmer Eye Institute, Miami, FL

James D. Zieske, PhD Associate Professor, Department of Ophthalmology, Harvard Medical School, Senior Scientist, Schepens Eye Research Institute, Harvard Medical School, Boston, MA

PREFACE

The original idea for this textbook was conceived by Drs. Richard A. Thoft at the Massachusetts Eye and Ear Infirmary and Gilbert Smolin of the University of California–San Francisco and the Proctor Foundation. The idea of a "bicoastal product" with cornea experts from two major academic institutions authoring the chapters was appealing, and the size of the text was designed to be user-friendly yet comprehensive enough to be a centerpiece in cornea fellowship training programs around the world. The success of the text resulted in three subsequent editions before the untimely death of Dr. Thoft and the retirement from active practice of Dr. Smolin.

Little, Brown and Company published the book originally. When Lippincott Williams & Wilkins acquired Little, Brown's line of medical books, Lippincott's executive editor, Jonathan Pine, approached me to create a fourth edition of this esteemed text. I agreed to take on the responsibility but only if my colleagues on the Cornea Service at the Massachusetts Eye and Ear Infirmary, Drs. Dimitri T. Azar and Claes H. Dohlman, would be part of the

effort. Happily, they enthusiastically joined me in this endeavor.

The book that you see here is an almost completely new product with expanded coverage of disease entities and their treatments, accompanied by greater use of illustrations, most particularly color illustrations. The authors we invited to participate in this effort are all internationally recognized cornea and external disease experts as well as cornea biochemists and physiologists. It has been an extraordinary pleasure to work with them in bringing forth this new edition. It has been especially pleasurable to have the wonderful collegiality and cooperation of Drs. Azar and Dohlman in accomplishing this task. We did not aim to make the text encyclopedic; instead, we strove for coverage extensive enough to be authoritative yet compact enough to be portable and truly usable. We hope that you will enjoy reading it as much as we enjoyed creating it.

C. Stephen Foster
Boston, Massachusetts

CONTENTS

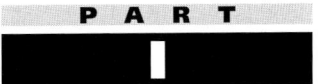

FUNDAMENTALS

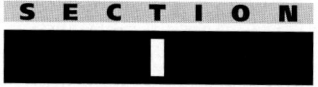

SECTION
I

BASIC SCIENCE

1

THE ANATOMY AND CELL BIOLOGY OF THE HUMAN CORNEA, LIMBUS, CONJUNCTIVA, AND ADNEXA

ILENE K. GIPSON, NANCY C. JOYCE,
AND JAMES D. ZIESKE

The cornea, conjunctiva, and intervening transition area known as the limbus comprise the tissues at the ocular surface. These three regions, shown diagrammatically and histologically in Figs. 1-1 and 1-2, have both structural and functional features in common. All three are covered by a stratified, squamous, nonkeratinizing epithelium at the surface of the eye that functions in innate defense at the ocular surface. These epithelia sit on a basement membrane and are connected through an identical anchoring complex to an underlying connective tissue stroma. Functionally, all three regions of the epithelium serve as the most important barrier to fluid loss and pathogen entrance, and they support the tear film by synthesizing membrane-associated and secreted mucins. The connective tissue of all three regions serves not only as a structural support but also as the conduit of fluids and nutrients, and it houses support cells that provide for maintenance of the matrix and overlying epithelium. The unique features of each region, however, indicate the special functional roles of the tissue zones. The cornea, because of its critically important functions of light refraction and transmittance, has accordingly received the most attention in studies of its structure, function, and pathology. Recently, more attention has been given to the surrounding limbal and conjunctival regions, which to some degree function as support tissues for the cornea.

Maintenance and support of the ocular surface are also provided by the adnexa (Figs. 1-1 and 1-3), which include the all-important eyelids that function to spread and mix the tear film and, thus, lubricate the ocular surface. Glands that secrete products for maintenance and defense of the ocular surface include the meibomian glands, the main lacrimal gland, the accessory lacrimal glands of Kraus and Wolfring, and the small glands of Zeiss and Moll, which empty into the space surrounding the eyelash cilia.

This chapter reviews aspects of anatomy and cell biology of, first, the cornea, followed by the limbus and the conjunctiva—highlighting the unique features of each—and, finally, major features of the anatomy and cell biology of the adnexa. More complete details of the gross anatomy of these ocular surface regions are available (1–3).

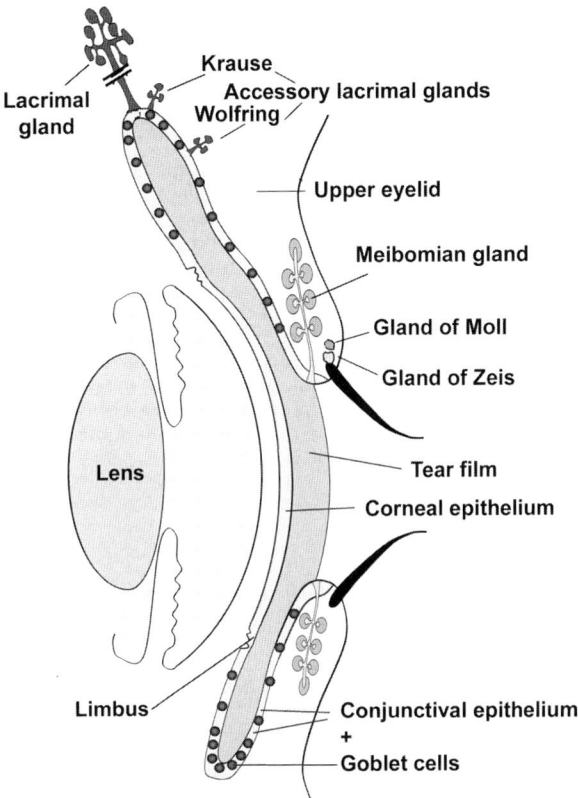

FIGURE 1-1. Diagram demonstrating the ocular surface and adnexal tissues described in this chapter. The ocular surface tissues include the cornea, limbus, and conjunctiva; and the adnexa include the lids with eyelash cilia, the meibomian gland, the main lacrimal gland, the accessory lacrimal glands of Krause and Wolfring and the small glands, that empty into the cilia sheath—the glands of Zeiss and Moll.

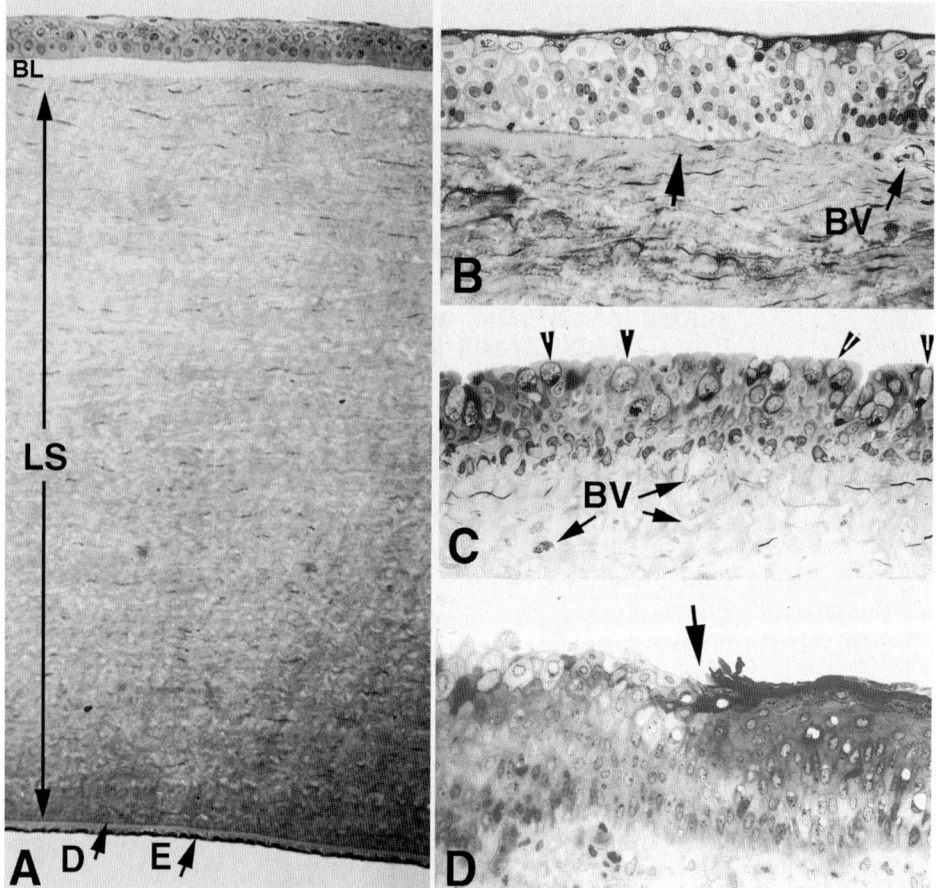

FIGURE 1-2. A: Histologic appearance of a full-thickness cross-section of human cornea shows the five- to seven-cell-layered epithelium, the three layers of the stroma, including Bowman's layer (BL), the lamellar stroma with its resident keratocytes, which occupies over 90% of the corneal tissue (LS), and Descemet's membrane (D), which is the thickened basement membrane of the corneal endothelium. The endothelium (E) is a low, cuboidal monolayer of cells that borders the anterior chamber. **B:** Light micrograph of anterior limbus showing the end of Bowman's layer (*arrow*) at the juncture between cornea to the left and the first limbal blood vessel (BV) directly beneath the area of corneal epithelial stem cells. **C:** Micrograph of bulbar conjunctiva. Note numerous goblet cells (*arrowheads*) intercalated within the stratified epithelium as well as numerous blood vessels (BV) in the connective tissue. **D:** The junction (*arrow*) between nonkeratinized (*left*) and keratinized (*right*) epithelium of the epidermal tarsal and palpebral conjunctiva. Note numerous cells with the substantia propria below the epithelium. (Original magnifications: **A,** ×180; **B, C, D,** ×250.)

CORNEA

The cornea is a tissue highly specialized to refract and transmit light. It is approximately 1 mm thick peripherally and 0.5 mm centrally. It comprises an outer stratified squamous nonkeratinized epithelium, an inner connective tissue stroma with resident keratocytes, and, bordering the anterior chamber, a low cuboidal endothelium (Fig. 1-2). Although this avascular tissue seems simple in composition, it is extraordinarily regular and precisely arranged. All three layers have a uniform and consistent arrangement throughout the tissue so that light is precisely bent and transmitted through to the lens and then to the retina.

Corneal Epithelium

The human corneal epithelium has five to seven cell layers and is 50 to 52 μg thick (1,4,5) (Fig. 1-4). It has several unique characteristics among other stratified squamous epithelia of the body. It is extraordinarily regular in thickness over the entire cornea and it has an absolutely smooth, wet, apical surface that serves as the major refractive surface of the eye. Its location on the surface of the translucent cornea requires that it be transparent. Unlike other epithelia of its class, it is specialized to exist over an avascular connective tissue. Protection of the vital refraction and "light passage" functions is provided by an extraordinarily dense sensory nerve system that can induce rapid response to

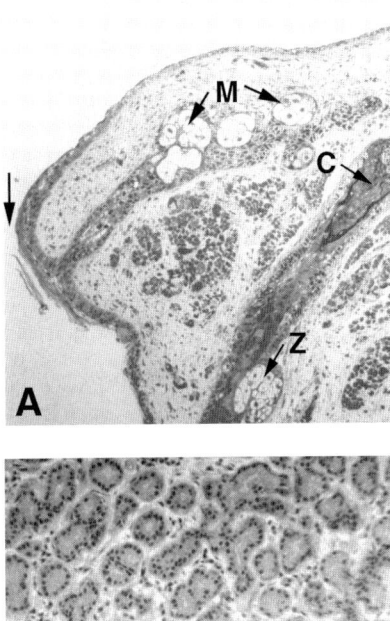

FIGURE 1-3. A: Low-power light micrographs of the lid margin showing the meibomian gland (M), a portion of the eyelash cilia (C), and its associated gland of Zeiss (Z). The juncture between conjunctival epithelium and epidermal epithelium is indicated by the *arrow*. **B:** Low-magnification micrograph of a section of human lacrimal gland. Acini are single cell layered. A duct (*arrow*) at D from the acini is shown running through connective tissue at lower left. (Original magnifications: **A,** ×120; **B,** ×220.)

recently, it was thought that after they undergo mitosis, one daughter cell remains on the basal lamina while the other moves into the suprabasal layers. More recent studies using bromodeoxyuridine to label dividing cells have shown that the two progeny of basal cell division move together toward the apical surface (7).

The basal cells of the epithelium adhere to their basement membrane and underlying stroma through an anchoring complex that is a series of linked structures, described later (8). The major component of the cytoplasm of the basal cells, as well as that of wing and squamous cells, is the intermediate filaments, composed of proteins known as *keratins* or *cytokeratins* (Fig. 1-5). Keratins are a complex family of approximately 30 proteins, each given designations of "K" plus a specific number. There are two classes of keratins—type I or acidic, and type II or neutral/basic. Intermediate filaments are formed by the pairing of type I and type II proteins. As cells of the corneal epithelium differentiate from the basal layer to the apical layer, two keratin pairs are sequentially expressed. K5 and K14 are expressed by basal cells, and K3 and K12 are expressed by all cells (9–11). One of these keratins, K12, a 64-kD protein, is cornea specific (12,13). Keratins in general constitute the major protein of the corneal epithelium.

The two other cytoskeletal filament types present in cells—actin filaments and microtubules—are also present in corneal epithelial cells. Actin filaments are distributed throughout the cytoplasm of cells of the corneal epithelium, but they are particularly prominent within and under the microplicae region of the apical cell membrane (14). Microtubules have not been studied extensively in human corneal epithelium, but they are prominent in mitotic cells, where they determine the plane of cell division and are involved in chromosome separation.

Perhaps in keeping with its requirement that the epithelium be transparent, all cell layers of the epithelium have, by comparison, a rather sparse accumulation of cytoplasmic organelles such as mitochondria, Golgi apparatus, and endoplasmic reticulum. In all cells, mitochondria and endoplasmic reticulum are sparsely distributed around the ectoplasm, and a prominent Golgi apparatus can usually be seen (Fig. 1-5). In basal cells, the apparatus is particularly obvious in the supranuclear position. In squamous cell layers, Golgi cisterna and small membrane-bound vesicles consistent in size and structure to Golgi-associated vesicles are prominent (Fig. 1-5). Also in keeping with maintenance of corneal epithelial transparency is the high expression level of transketolase, which has been proposed to be a corneal crystalline (15).

The apical membranes of basal cells and the entire membranes of wing and squamous cells are highly undulating and interdigitating (Fig. 1-5). Desmosomes are prominent cell–cell anchoring junctions along these cell borders (Fig. 1-5). Other cell–cell junctions in the corneal epithelium are gap junctions, which contain the gap junction protein connexin 43 (16), and, between lateral membranes of the apical cells,

potential danger. In addition to its unique functions over the translucent cornea, the epithelium carries out "routine" housekeeping functions common to any epithelium that borders the external environment. These include provision of a barrier to fluid loss and pathogen entrance, and resistance to abrasive pressure. A barrier to fluid loss is provided by tight junctions surrounding lateral membranes of apical cells, and a pathogen barrier is provided by membrane-spanning mucins at the apical surface. Resistance to abrasion requires that cells of the epithelium be specialized for tight adherence to one another and to their underlying extracellular matrix. Finally, its position adjacent to the outside world requires that the epithelium have a rapid and highly developed ability to respond to wounding.

The cell layers of the epithelium include three to four outer, flattened squamous cells (squames); one to three layers of mid-epithelial cells, termed *wing cells* because they have lateral, thin, winglike extensions from a more rounded cell body; and a single layer of columnar basal cells (Fig. 1-4). The corneal epithelium, like all stratified squamous epithelia, is self-renewing and, in the cornea, complete turnover occurs in approximately 5 to 7 days (6). The basal cells are the mitotically active cells of the epithelium, and until

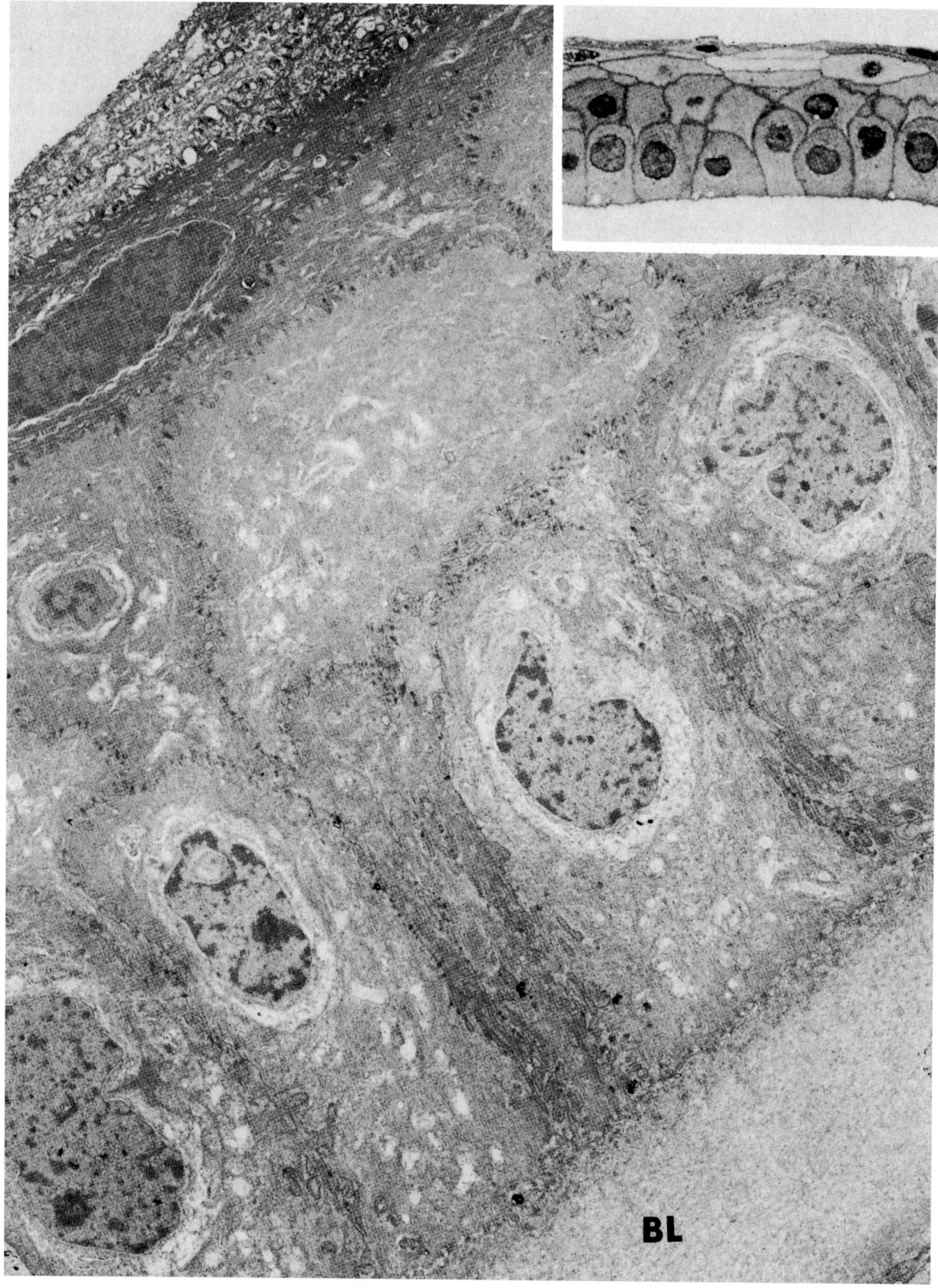

FIGURE 1-4. Low-magnification electron micrograph and light micrograph (*inset*) of the corneal epithelium and subjacent Bowman's layer (BL). Note single layer of columnar basal cells, one to two layers of wing cells, and two to three layers of flattened squamous cells. (Original magnifications: *main*, ×4800; *inset*, ×750.)

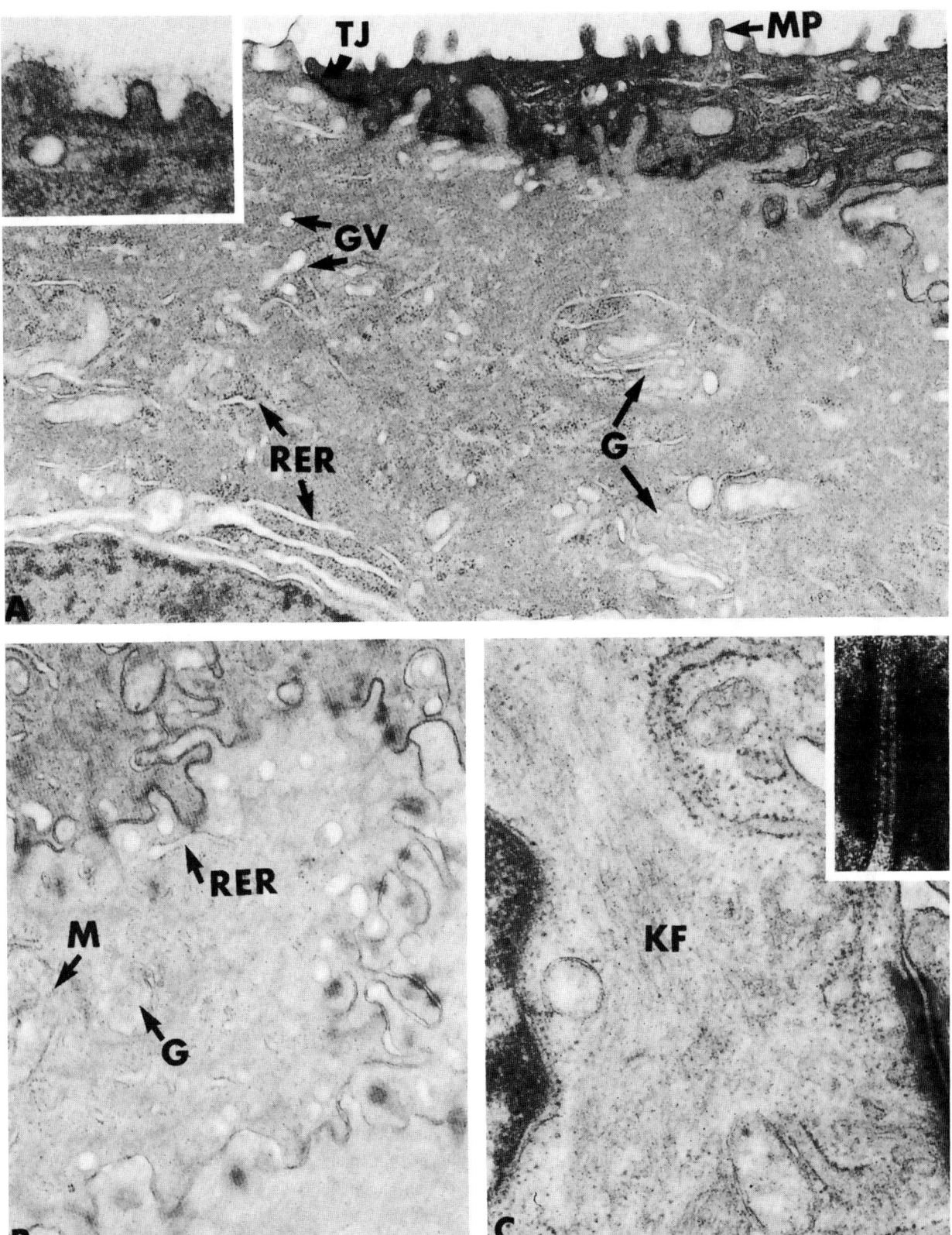

FIGURE 1-5. Electron micrographs demonstrating aspects of the ultrastructure of the corneal epithelium of apical cells (**A** plus *inset*) and wing cells (**B** and **C** plus *inset*). **A:** Apical and lateral borders of several adjacent apical cells are evident. Note microplicae (MP), region of tight junction (TJ), presence of Golgi apparatus (G), Golgi vesicles (GV), and rough endoplasmic reticulum (RER). The *inset* demonstrates a filamentous glycocalyx on the surface of the microplicae. **B:** Electron micrograph demonstrates the elaborate interdigitation of membranes of adjacent cells, characteristic of wing and squamous cells. A mitochondrion (M), Golgi apparatus (G), and rough endoplasmic reticulum (RER) are present. **C:** Higher-magnification electron micrograph demonstrates that the cytoplasm of epithelial cells is rich in keratin filaments (KF). **A, B,** and **C** all show the presence of the cell-cell anchoring junctions known as *desmosomes*, which are present along interdigitating cell membranes. A high-magnification section through a desmosome is shown in the *inset* of **C.** Desmosomes of corneal epithelia appear similar to those of all other stratified squamous epithelium. (Original magnifications: **A,** ×21,000, *inset,* ×51,000; **B,** ×21,000; **C,** ×42,000, *inset,* ×164,000.)

tight junctions containing Z01 protein (17) (Fig. 1-5). A more complete description of the cytoskeletal and molecular natures of cell–cell junctions in the corneal epithelium of humans and other species has been published (18).

Specializations of the Corneal Epithelium at Its Apical Tear Film Surface

The outermost apical cell layer has microplicae, ridgelike folds that form regular undulations of the membrane as viewed in cross-section (Fig. 1-5). Scanning electron microscopy of the surface of the cornea demonstrates that apical cells scatter electrons to varying degrees (19,20). Cells that scatter fewer electrons have been termed *dark cells*; those that do so to a greater degree are called *light cells*. The number of surface microplicae correlates with the degree of scatter, with dark cells having the fewest per unit area (19). It has been hypothesized that the dark cells are the "oldest" cells at the ocular surface, indicating that they are about to desquamate (19,20). This undulating, specialized apical membrane exhibits a prominent filamentous glycocalyx (Figs. 1-5 and 1-6), which has been studied most extensively

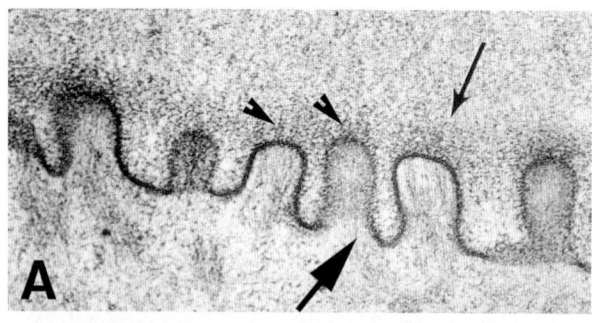

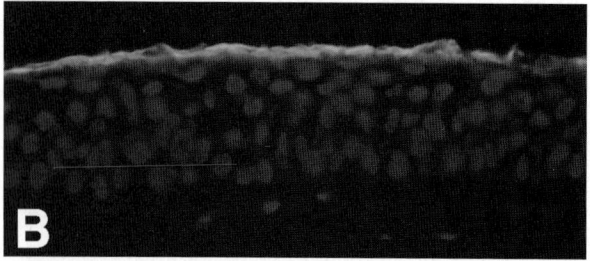

FIGURE 1-6. A: Electron micrograph of microplicae and glycocalyx (*small arrow*) on the surface of guinea pig conjunctiva. The membrane-associated mucins can be seen emanating from the tips of the microplicae (*arrowheads*) in the electron-dense glycocalyx. At least three different membrane-associated mucins are present in the human glycocalyx; these include MUC1, MUC4, and MUC16. The cytoplasmic domains of the mucins are believed to associate with actin filaments (*large arrow*), which extend toward the membrane where membrane-associated mucins insert. (From Nichols BA, Chiappino ML, Dawson CR. Demonstration of the mucous layer of the tear film by electron microscopy. *Invest Ophthalmol Vis Sci* 1985;26:464–473.) **B:** The immunohistochemical localization of one of the membrane-associated mucins, MUC16, is shown on a section of corneal epithelium. (Original magnifications: **A,** ×89,000; **B,** ×300.)

in guinea pig (21) and rat (22). The glycocalyx has been hypothesized to be intimately but loosely associated with the mucus of the tear film layer (21), and it has been further hypothesized to play a role in mucin and tear film spread over the surface of the eye (22,23).

Major components of the glycocalyx along the apical cell–tear film interface are membrane-associated mucins (Fig. 1-6). [For review, see Gipson and Argüeso (23) and Argüeso and Gipson (24).] Once thought to be secreted only from goblet cells, molecular techniques have demonstrated that mucins also are expressed by the surface cells of all wet-surfaced epithelia. On the corneal glycocalyx, at least three membrane-associated mucins are present, and they appear to be particularly prominent at the tips of the microplicae (Fig. 1-6). These mucins, designated MUC1, MUC4, and MUC16, have structural features in common, a short cytoplasmic domain, which may be associated with cytoskeletal proteins and the actin cytoskeleton in the cytoplasm of the microplicae, and an extended, 200- to 500-μm extracellular domain that is highly *O*-glycosylated. One of the membrane-spanning mucins, MUC16, carries carbohydrate recognized by an antibody designated H185, whose distribution at the ocular surface is altered in non-Sjögren's dry eye (25, 26). Current concepts of the function of the membrane-associated mucins is that these highly glycosylated hydrophilic glycoproteins in the glycocalyx are responsible for maintenance of the tear fluid on the ocular surface and that their alteration leads to dry spots as stained by rose bengal (23). Studies of regulation of expression and glycosylation of these mucins will yield information relevant to treatment of drying, keratinizing ocular surface disease. To date, two compounds, dexamethasone (27) and retinoic acid, are known to regulate the expression of membrane-associated mucins MUC1 and MUC4, respectively (28).

Epithelial Anchorage to the Stroma

Basal cells (Fig. 1-7) adhere to their basement membrane and underlying connective tissue stroma by a series of linked structures termed collectively the *anchoring complex* (8). These structures and basement membrane are products of the basal cells of the epithelium. Figure 1-7 ultrastructurally and diagrammatically shows the components of the anchoring complex and their molecular constituents. The structural components include, on the cytoplasmic face of the basal cell membrane, an electron-dense region into which keratin filaments insert. This dense region is termed the *hemidesmosome*, and approximately 28% of the basal cell membrane is occupied by these junctions in central cornea (29). An integral membrane protein, $\alpha6\beta4$-integrin, links the intracellular components of the hemidesmosome to the extracellular components of the basement membrane (30). On the opposite side of the basement membrane from the hemidesmosome, anchoring fibrils insert. These uniquely cross-banded anchoring fibrils have as a component type VII

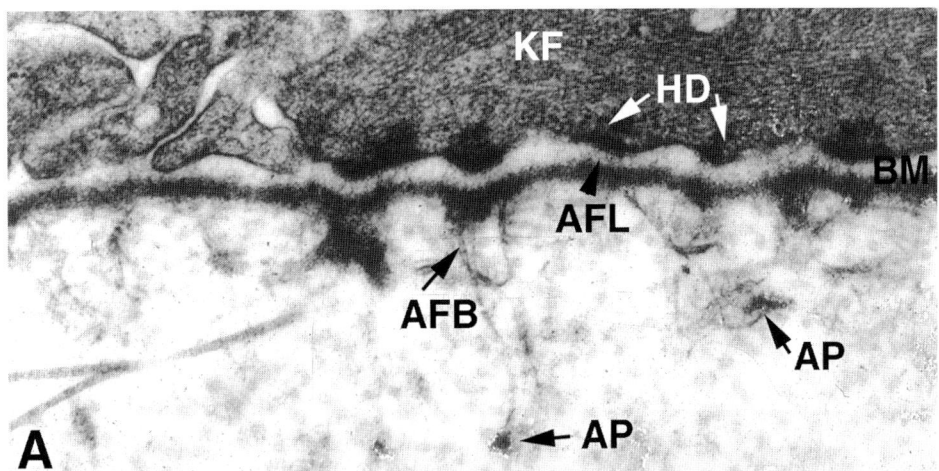

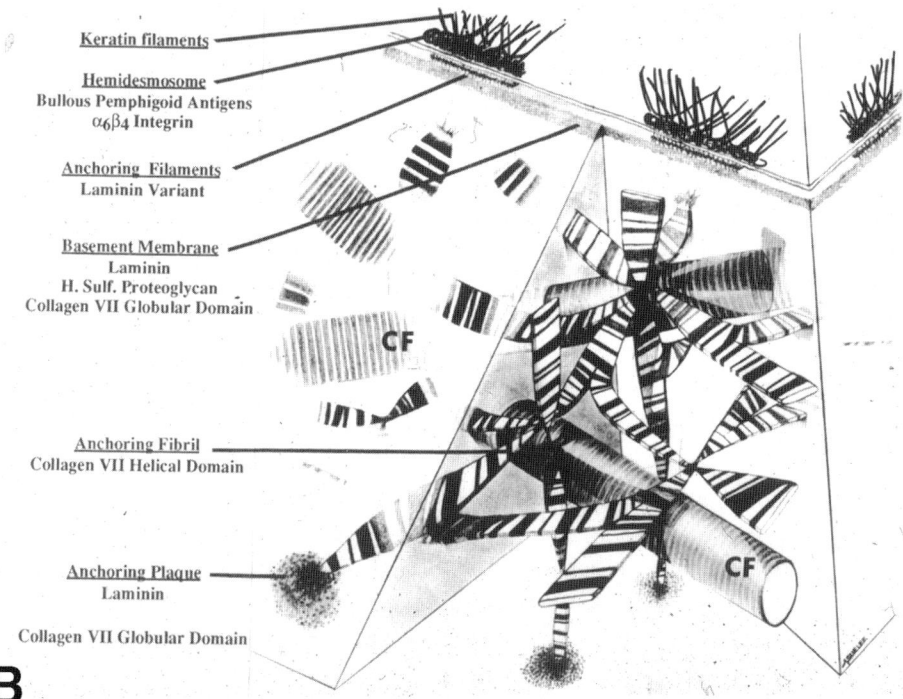

FIGURE 1-7. A: Electron micrograph of section through the epithelial-stromal junction region. The structures that are linked to form the epithelial anchoring complex can be seen. They include the hemidesmosome with keratin filaments (KF) inserting into the hemidesmosome plaque (HD). Extracellularly, anchoring filaments (AFL) can be seen in the lamina lucida zone of the basement membrane (BM). Anchoring fibrils (AFB) extend into the stroma at sites opposite the basement membrane from hemidesmosomes; anchoring fibrils insert into anchoring plaques (AP) distal from their insertion into the basement membrane. These plaques have the appearance of small bits of basement membrane. (Original magnification, ×65,000.) **B:** Diagram illustrating a three-dimensional view of the anchoring complex of the corneal epithelium. The column on the left lists the individual structures (*underlined*) of the linked complex with their known components underneath. The anchoring fibrils insert into the basement membrane opposite from hemidesmosomes. The cross-banded fibrils splay out among the collagen fibrils (CF), forming a three-dimensional network holding the epithelium tightly to the stroma. The anchoring fibrils terminate distally from the basement membrane in anchoring plaques.

collagen (31). Type VII collagen has a globular domain and a helical domain (32). Groups of helical domains of molecules associate to form the cross-banded fibril; globular domains of type VII collagen associate within the basement membrane at hemidesmosome sites as well as distal from the basement membrane in the anterior 1 to 2 μm of Bowman's layer, in small patches of basement membrane–appearing material termed *anchoring plaques*. Cross-banded anchoring fibrils thus extend from the basement membrane throughout the anterior 1 to 2 μg of Bowman's layer, forming a complex network that is interwoven with the conventionally cross-banded type I and type V collagen fibrils. The network serves to hold the epithelium and its basement membrane to the stroma; this is clearly demonstrated in the human blistering disease, epidermolysis bullosa acquisita, where a defect in the genetic expression of type VII collagen causes a lack of anchoring fibrils. In this disease, all stratified epithelia are disadherent (33). An example demonstrating the function of the anchoring fibril network in corneal epithelial anchoring comes from a study of diabetic eyes. Diabetic patients have duplicated and thickened basement membranes, including the corneal epithelial basement membrane. During vitrectomy surgery, if the corneal epithelium is removed, the thickened basement membrane, which has within it pockets of anchoring fibrils no longer extending into anterior stroma, comes off with the epithelium (34). This does not occur in normal individuals. A study of the depth of penetration of the anchoring fibril network in diabetic corneas showed a significant decrease in depth compared with age-matched control subjects (35). These data indicate the importance of anchoring fibril network penetration into the anterior stroma in anchorage of the basement membrane and its epithelium.

Corneal Stroma

Structural Zones

The human corneal stroma is the middle connective tissue layer, which, at a thickness of approximately 500 μm, forms the bulk of or approximately 90% of the thickness of the cornea (36) (Figs. 1-2, 1-8, and 1-9). It is unique among connective tissues in that it is the most highly organized and most transparent of any in the body. In addition to its function as a window to light passage, the stroma meshes with the surrounding scleral connective tissue to form a rigid framework for maintaining intraocular pressure and, thus, alignment of the optic pathway.

The stroma is arranged in three clearly defined layers of extracellular matrix (Fig. 1-2). These include, bordering the epithelium, the thin 8- to 10-μm Bowman's layer, the middle lamellar stroma, which comprises by far the major portion of the stroma, and, adjacent to the endothelium, the 8- to 12-μm Descemet's membrane, the thickened basement membrane secreted by the corneal endothelium.

Bowman's Layer

Bowman's layer is an acellular zone consisting of collagen fibrils and associated proteoglycans densely woven in a random manner into a felt-like matrix (Fig. 1-8). Individual collagen fibrils are approximately 20 to 30 μm in diameter (36). The layer stretches from limbus to limbus, tapering in thickness and ending at the limbus (Fig. 1-2). Based on ultrastructural criteria, Bowman's has been described embryonically as being derived from stromal cells (36), but at 13 weeks of gestation, one can also see palisades of collagen fibrils emanating from the epithelial basement membrane (37), indicative of a potential epithelial contribution to Bowman's assembly. The function of Bowman's layer is not clear; some have hypothesized that it functions to form a smooth, rigid base for maintaining epithelial uniformity and, thus, appropriate refractive power. Others have proposed that the acellular zone is necessary to prevent close contact between epithelial and stromal cells. Such proximity might induce stromal cell "activation" and an inappropriate extracellular matrix assembly. Still others (38) have proposed, however, that Bowman's layer is the result of the epithelial–stromal interactions, and that Bowman's layer has no critical function. Most species of mammals do not have a Bowman's layer and seemingly have appropriate refraction and no epithelial–stromal cell interaction problems. Thus, the question as to the function of Bowman's layer remains unanswered.

Lamellar Stroma

The lamellar stroma is the major layer of the stroma and comprises lamellae formed from flattened bundles of collagen fibrils oriented in a parallel manner. These bundles, shown ultrastructurally in Fig. 1-8, number approximately 200 to 250 in the human cornea (36). Each bundle extends the width of the cornea, is 2 μm thick, and 9 to 260 μm wide (1). The lamellae in the posterior part of the stroma have a regular orthogonal layering—that is, bundles are at right angles to one another. In the anterior third of the stroma, the lamellae have a more oblique layering, and branching of lamellae in this superficial region has been described (1). Individual collagen fibrils in the bundles have a diameter of 27 to 35 nm and therefore are larger than those of Bowman's layer (36). The fibril diameters of both Bowman's and the lamellar stroma are extraordinarily uniform compared with those in other connective tissues.

Within lamellae of the human or bovine cornea, small bundles of microfibrils can be observed. Individual fibers in these bundles are 10 nm in diameter. These microfibrils are composed of fibrillin (39) and are identical in composition to the microfibrils of the zonular fibers, which extend between the ciliary body and the lens. The function of these microfibrillar bundles is unknown, but they are characteristic of most connective tissue.

The lamellar stroma is secreted and maintained by the stromal fibroblasts, commonly termed *keratocytes*.

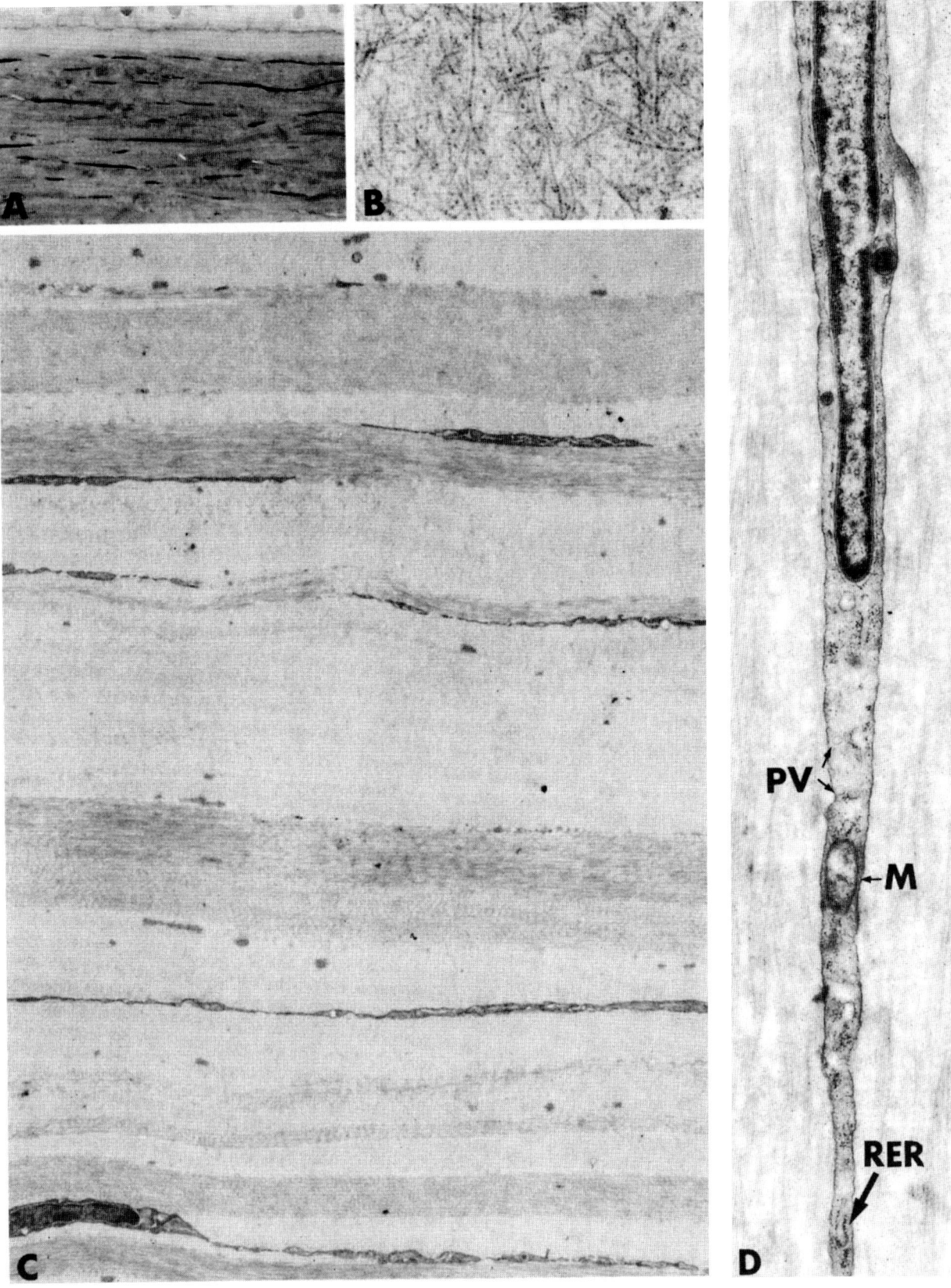

FIGURE 1-8. Micrographs depicting structural aspects of the corneal stroma. **A:** Light micrograph showing basal epithelial cells, subjacent Bowman's layer, and the anterior lamellar stroma with its flattened and attenuated stromal fibroblasts, termed *keratocytes*. **B:** Electron micrograph of a region in Bowman's layer demonstrating the random, felt-like interweaving of the collagen fibrils. **C:** Lower-power electron micrograph of the layered lamellar stroma. Note the presence of the keratocytes running between lamellae. **D:** Micrograph showing a segment of a flattened keratocyte. Rough endoplasmic reticulum (RER), a mitochondrion (M), and numerous pinocytic vesicles (PV) are present in the cytoplasm. (Original magnifications: **A,** ×300; **B,** ×31,000; **C,** ×4800; **D,** ×21,000.)

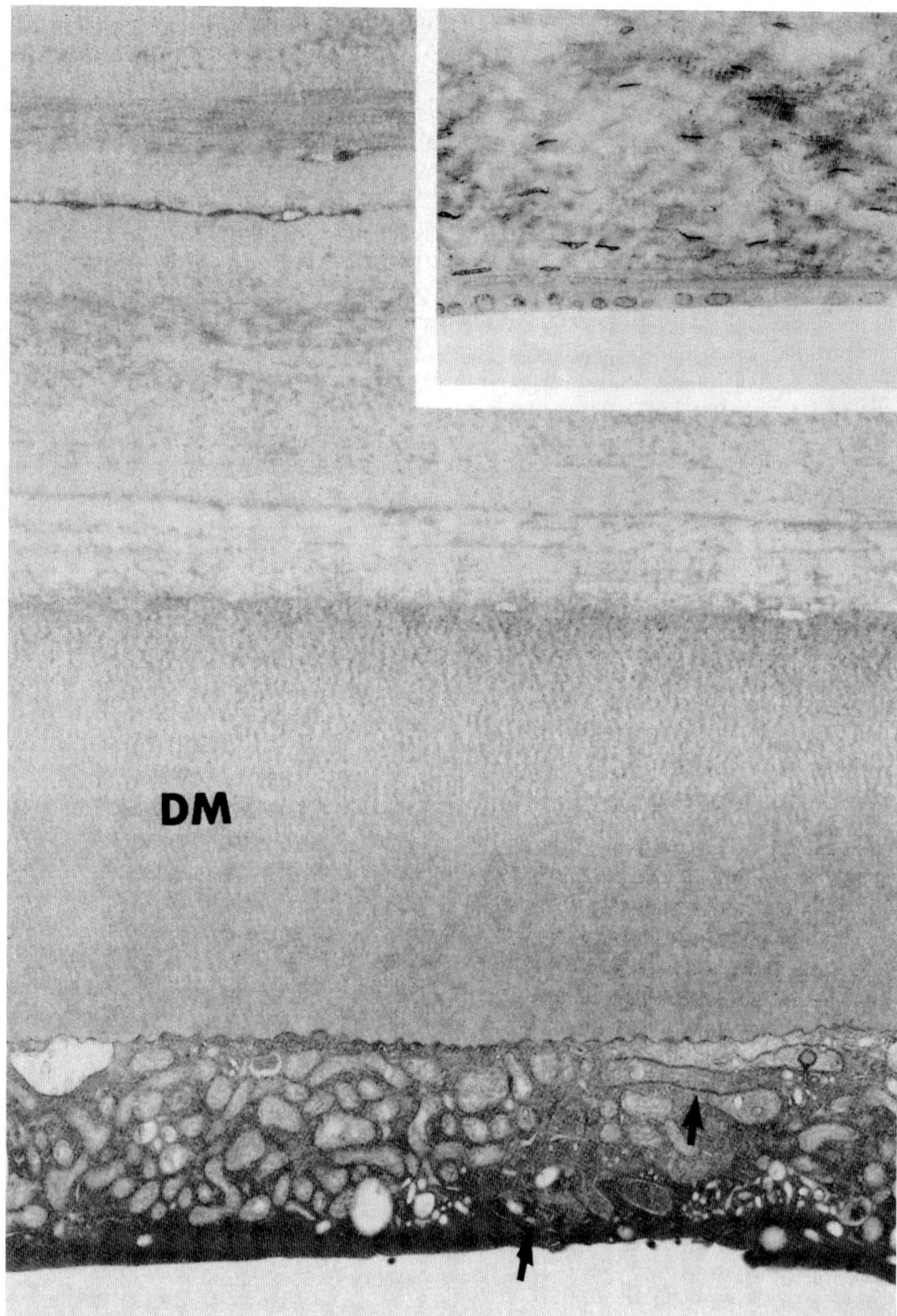

FIGURE 1-9. Micrographs of posterior corneal stroma, Descemet's membrane (DM), and the corneal endothelium. The *inset* is a light micrograph section from a newborn with its comparatively thin Descemet's membrane. The electron micrograph is of a section from an 18-year-old human. Note the two layers in Descemet's membrane. The inner-banded layer was deposited by the endothelium during fetal life. The portion of the endothelial cell visible in the micrograph shows the presence of numerous mitochondria and an interdigitating lateral membrane (*arrows*). (Original magnifications: *main*, ×10,000; *inset*, ×300.)

(*Keratinocytes* is the term classically given to individual cells of the stratified squamous epithelia, which occasionally leads to confusion in the literature.) These cells usually reside between lamellae (occasionally they are seen with processes in lamellae) and are very flat, with many long, attenuated processes extending from a central cell body in all directions. The tips of the processes touch processes of adjacent cells, forming gap junctions (40,41). Thus, cells of the stroma form a network of coupled cells. Segments of basement membrane can also be demonstrated along the keratocytes. The cytoplasm of the stromal fibroblast is rich in rough endoplasmic reticulum and Golgi apparatus, in keeping with its function as the synthesizer and maintenance cell of the stromal lamellae. Recent data suggest that the stroma also houses a relatively high number of bone marrow-derived cells (42).

The mechanism by which these cells initially lay down the lamellae in their orthogonal pattern has long been a subject of interest. In the developing chick, Birk and Trelstad (43) have demonstrated that surface compartments with bundles of parallel collagen fibrils are present in fibroblasts. These compartments are oriented along the fibroblast axes, and the orthogonality of the cells is in register with that of the extracellular matrix.

Descemet's Membrane

Descemet's membrane is the basement membrane of the corneal endothelium. It is synthesized by the endothelium and assembled at the basal surface of the cell layer. At birth, the human Descemet's membrane is approximately 3 μm wide, but, by late adulthood, it can measure up to 12 μm (36). Its accrual during life is comparable with the thickening of the other basement membranes of the body, including

that of the corneal epithelium (44). Two distinct regions can be discerned in electron micrographs of Descemet's membrane (Fig. 1-9). The anterior one half to one third, depending on the age of the individual, is the "fetal" or "oldest" layer of the membrane. This region displays 100- to 110-nm "long spacing" or a banded collagen pattern. The posterior layer is not banded and appears as amorphous matrix, like all other basement membranes. The mechanism by which this switch in synthesis and matrix organization takes place is not known. The gradual increase in thickness of the posterior layer with age suggests that either there is no degradation of its constituents or the rate of synthesis of constituents is greater than the degradation rate.

Descemet's membrane is composed of a number of proteins, including fibronectin (45), laminin (46), collagen types IV and VIII (47,48), and proteoglycans containing heparan sulfate, dermatan sulfate, or keratan sulfate (49).

Descemet's membrane is unique among basement membranes, not so much in its composition, but in its thickness and regional variation in structure. Why this basement membrane is so thick remains an unanswered question. Basement membranes in general are believed to serve as substrates of epithelial cell layers, functioning in the filtering of solutes passing to and from the epithelia and serving as substrates that induce polarity and differentiation of the overlying epithelium.

Corneal Stromal Components

The stroma consists of three main groups of proteins, which include collagens, associated proteoglycans, and other glycoproteins (Table 1-1). All three groups of proteins contain covalently attached carbohydrates and can thus be called

TABLE 1-1. CORNEAL EXTRACELLULAR MATRIX COMPONENTS

Component	Localization	
	Normal/Matrix	**Provisional Matrix**
Collagens I, V, VI, VII, VIII, XII, XVII, XVIII, XX	See Table 1-2	—
Collagen III	—	Scar
Collagen IV	Basement membrane	Anterior stroma
Decorin	Stroma	—
Keratocan	Stroma	—
Lumican	Stroma	Basement membrane
Mimecan	Stroma	—
Perlecan	Basement membrane	Anterior stroma
Entactin/nidogen	Basement membrane	Basement membrane
Laminin-1	Basement membrane	Basement membrane
Laminin-5	Basement membrane	Basement membrane
Laminin-10	Basement membrane	—
Amyloid precursor–like protein-2	—	Basement membrane
Fibrillin	Microfibrils	Anterior stroma
Fibrin	—	Anterior stroma
Fibronectin	Descemet's membrane	Anterior stroma
Tenascin-C	—	Anterior stroma

glycoproteins. However, any glycoprotein with a collagenous domain is generally referred to as collagen. The remaining noncollagenous proteins in the stroma are subdivided into two major groups, glycoproteins and proteoglycans. Proteoglycans are a special class of glycoproteins that have glycosaminoglycan (GAG) side chains.

Collagen

The most abundant group of proteins in the body is the collagens. In the cornea, collagen makes up 71% of the dry weight of the cornea (50,51). Collagen, along with proteoglycans, forms the scaffolding of many tissues, including cornea, cartilage, skin, and tendon. These two groups of proteins make up the majority of the extracellular matrix between the cells. In the cornea, collagen is present in the epithelial and endothelial basement membranes, the relatively unorganized fibrils of Bowman's layer, and the lamellae of the stroma.

Although collagens are expressed in a variety of locations and exhibit various functions, they are defined by the common feature of containing one or more domains having glycine in every third position of the polypeptide chain (52). This feature results in the collagenous domains of the protein, forming a helical structure. This helix in turn is assembled with two other collagen molecules to form a triple helix, resulting in a rod-shaped macromolecule. The triple helices, as well as the individual collagen chains, are cross-linked to each other, resulting in a structure with incredible strength and resiliency (53,54).

The collagen type is determined by the polypeptide chains (termed α chains) present in the triple helix. The various α chains are individual gene products and thus have differing amino acid sequences. Each collagen type consists of three α chains. These chains can be identical or different gene products. Based on α-chain composition, there are 21 types of collagen in human tissues (53,54). Type I collagen is the most abundant collagen in the body and is found in bone, tendon, cornea, and skin. It contains two $\alpha1$ type I chains and one $\alpha2$ chain. The amount of collagenous domain (the portion of the polypeptide chain having glycine in every third position) varies tremendously between the different α chains. This results in a wide variation in the structure and function of the resulting collagen. For example, collagen types I, II, III, V, and VI are almost entirely formed by collagenous domains. In electron micrographs of corneal stroma and other tissues, they appear as classic banded collagen fibrils. In contrast, collagen type IV has numerous small noncollagenous domains interspersed between relatively short collagenous domains. In electron micrographs, type IV collagen appears as an amorphous matrix. As another example, type VI collagen has a beaded appearance in electron micrographs. This results from a structure that includes a single, large, uninterrupted collagenous domain in the middle of the chain that is flanked by globular domains at the ends. Collagens can be divided

TABLE 1-2. COLLAGENS PRESENT IN CORNEA

Type	Localization
Type I	Stromal fibrils
Type III	Scars
Type IV	Basement membrane
Type V	Stromal fibrils
Type VI	Stroma
Type VII	Anchoring fibrils
Type VIII	Descemet's membrane
Type XII	Stroma, basement membrane
Type XIII	Stroma
Type XVII	Hemidesmosomes
Type XVIII	Basement membrane
Type XX	Basement membrane

into several subfamilies based on their structure and organization (53,55). Fibrillar collagens (types I to III, V, and XI) have the same general structure and participate in the formation of cross-banded fibrils. The other collagen subfamilies have interruptions in their collagenous domains and are classified as nonfibrillar collagens. These subfamilies include: (a) basement membrane (type IV) collagen, which forms networks; (b) type VI, which forms beaded filaments; (c) type VII, which forms anchoring fibrils and is involved in anchorage of the basement membrane; (d) short-chain collagens, types VIII and X; (e) fibril-associated collagens with interrupted triple helices (FACIT), which include types IX, XII, XIV, XX, and XXI; (f) FACIT-related collagens, types XVI and XIX; (g) membrane collagens (types XIII and XVII); and (h) multiplexins, derived from multiple triple-helical domains and interruptions (types XV and XVIII). Type XVII is also known as bullous pemphigoid antigen and is a component of hemidesmosomes, and type XVIII can be cleaved to form the angiogenesis inhibitor endostatin. Of the 21 collagens identified in human tissues, at least 11 are present in adult mammalian cornea, including types I, III, IV, V, VI, VII, VIII, XII, XVII, XVIII, and XX (55–57) (Table 1-2). Spliced variants of some of the collagens are also present.

Proteoglycans

The second major group of proteins found in the stroma is the proteoglycans (58). They consist of a core protein containing one or more GAG side chains. The size and percentage of GAG can vary considerably in different proteoglycans. At one extreme is aggrecan, the major proteoglycan of cartilage, which has a core protein of approximately 220 kD and 100 to 150 GAG side chains of approximately 25,000 kD. Thus, it is composed of at least 90% GAG and has a molecular weight of over one million daltons. At the other extreme is decorin, a major corneal proteoglycan, which has a 40-kD molecular weight core protein with one GAG side chain of approximately 50 kD. Thus, it is only 55% GAG and has a molecular weight of under 100 kD.

GAGs, also known as mucopolysaccharides or acid mucopolysaccharides, are characterized by linear polymers of repeating disaccharide units. The disaccharide typically consists of a hexosamine (D-glucosamine or D-galactosamine) plus an uronic acid (D-glucuronic acid or L-iduronic acid). As a result, the GAGs are highly charged, resulting from the presence of many carboxyl [—COOH] and sulfate [—SO$_4$] groups.

The proteoglycans were originally named based on their GAG side chains because these were characterized long before their core proteins were. For example, chondroitin sulfate proteoglycans contain the GAG chondroitin sulfate. At least 30 different proteoglycans have been cloned (58). To date, no relationship between the type of GAG side chain on the core and any particular structural domain on the core protein has been found. Also, in contrast to the collagens, there is no amino acid sequence that is common to all proteoglycan core proteins.

Corneal Proteoglycans. The presence of GAGs in the stroma was first demonstrated with metachromatic toluidine blue and periodic acid-Schiff (PAS) staining (59). Subsequent biochemical analysis of the stromal GAGs has shown that approximately 65% of the corneal GAG is keratan sulfate, whereas 30% is chondroitin/dermatan sulfate. The two major chondroitin/dermatan sulfate proteoglycans in the cornea have been identified as decorin and biglycan. The major keratan sulfate core proteins have been identified as lumican, keratocan, mimecan/osteoglycan, and fibromodulin. Of the known proteoglycans present in the stroma, most are present in other tissues. Only keratocan appears to be specific to the cornea (60). All of the stromal proteoglycans belong to the family of the small leucine-rich proteoglycans (SLRPs). This gene family is defined by the following characteristics: (a) a molecular mass of 32 to 39 kD; (b) a centrally located leucine-rich domain, repeated seven to nine times, with the sequence -L-X-X-LX-L-X-X-N-X-L/I, where L is leucine, N is asparagine, I is isoleucine, and X is any other amino acid; and (c) cysteine residues in the carboxyl- and amino-terminal domains. The spacing and position of the leucine-rich repeats and the cysteine residues are highly conserved in all members of this gene family. The SLRPs bind to the fibrillar collagens and are thought to regulate spacing of the collagens. The cornea also contains a heparan sulfate proteoglycan, perlecan, which is localized in the epithelial basement membrane.

Glycoproteins

The third group of proteins that make up the corneal stroma are the glycoproteins, not included in the collagen or proteoglycan categories (Table 1-1). Glycoproteins are proteins containing one or more sugars covalently bound to the polypeptide chain. The sugar side chains most commonly contain several sugars (oligosaccharides), but may also contain only one or two (disaccharides) sugars. Compared with proteoglycans or mucins, the amount of sugar is low compared with the amount of protein. Also, unlike proteoglycans, there is no serially repeating sugar unit. The carbohydrate side chains in glycoproteins contain certain characteristic sugars, including D-galactose, D-mannose, L-fucose, D-xylose, *N*-acetyl-D-glucosamine, *N*-acetyl-D-galactosamine, and sialic acid. Some of the corneal glycoproteins localized in the epithelium and/or Descemet's membrane are laminin, fibronectin, and entactin/nidogen (Table 1-1). Interestingly, over half of the total amount of soluble glycoproteins in bovine stroma consists of serum proteins (61), including albumin, gamma globulin, transferrin, and α-lipoprotein. This suggests that many of the corneal stromal glycoproteins are derived from other sources.

Corneal Collagen Fibrillogenesis

One of the unique features of the corneal stroma is the regular alignment of collagen fibrils. This alignment is crucial to the maintenance of transparency of the cornea as well as to the strength of the tissue. Another unique feature is the consistent diameter of the collagen fibrils (27 to 35 nm), with all other tissues exhibiting fibrils of a much larger and more heterogeneous diameter. Subsequently, the regulation of corneal fibril diameter has been of great interest to many corneal cell biologists. The synthesis of collagen molecules and their association into fibrils requires a series of events that are common to all fibrillar collagens. These events have been extensively reviewed elsewhere (53,54,62). These processes include hydroxylation and glycosylation of the individual molecules and then proteolytic processing and cross-linking. In part, the relatively small diameter of the corneal collagen fibers is the result of the elevated levels of type V collagen. In most other tissues, including tendon and sclera, type V collagen represents only 2% to 5% of the total collagen. However, in the cornea, type V makes up 15% to 20% of the total. In a series of elegant experiments, it has been demonstrated that type V and type I collagen form heterotypic fibrils in the cornea, and that the size of the fibril is regulated by the amount of type V collagen present. Experimental data suggested that type V collagen can lead to a reduction of the diameter of the fibril by over 50% compared with a fibril composed entirely of type I collagen [reviewed in Birk (62)]. The interaction of the two collagens does not completely explain the small size of the corneal fibrils, however. The size also depends on the association of the fibrils with proteoglycans. Decorin, lumican, keratocan, and fibromodulin are all known to associate with collagen fibrils. Studies using purified native collagen have shown that both decorin and lumican inhibit fibril diameter growth (63). This inhibition is due to properties of the core protein of these proteoglycans because enzymatic removal of the GAGs from the core protein does not alter the inhibitory activity. This suggests that the core proteins of lumican and decorin bind to collagen and limit the size of the fibril. The importance of proteoglycans in corneal stromal fibril formation is demonstrated in mice lacking lumican, which have corneal opacities as a result of irregular fibril size and spacing (64), and also in humans who have mutations in keratocan. This mutation results in corneal flattening (65).

Wound Repair

For many years, stromal and epithelial wound repair have been generally examined and discussed as separate events. However, since the early 1990s, it has become increasingly clear that even the simplest epithelial wound results in the death of the subjacent keratocytes. Loss of keratocytes has been observed in corneal debridements, incision wounds, penetrating keratoplasty, photorefractive keratectomy (PRK), and laser *in situ* keratomileusis (LASIK). It therefore appears that almost all corneal wound repair involves both an epithelial and a stromal component.

Because of the difficulty in the use of human corneas for experimental studies, there are few direct studies that have examined corneal epithelial wound repair in humans. It is assumed that human corneas respond in a manner similar to that in animal models, but this has not been substantiated to any great extent. In animal models, corneal epithelial wound healing is a complex process that can be roughly divided into three overlapping phases. In the first phase, the epithelial cells flatten, elongate, and migrate as an intact sheet to cover the wound. To migrate, the hemidesmosomes, which normally attach the epithelial cells to the basement membrane, are disrupted, and dynamic anchoring structures termed *focal contacts* are formed. In the second phase of epithelial healing, cells distal to the original wound, including the limbal and peripheral corneal epithelium, undergo cell proliferation to repopulate the wound area. Stratification and differentiation of the epithelium follow cell proliferation. In the third phase, the hemidesmosomes are reformed and, depending on the original wound, basement membrane and the extracellular matrix are resynthesized and reassembled. Numerous proteins and signaling pathways have been postulated to be involved in these processes in animal models, and readers are referred to a number of reviews (66–71). Two proteins, epidermal growth factor and fibronectin, found to promote epithelial healing in animal models, have been tested in human clinical trials for therapeutic effects. However, the results have been inconclusive, with some trials reporting a positive effect on healing rates, but others showing no beneficial effect.

Stromal wound healing can also be considered to occur in phases [reviewed in Zieske (71)]. In the first phase, the keratocytes adjacent to the area of epithelial damage undergo apoptosis, leaving a zone devoid of cells. This cell death has been postulated to be the result of the wounded epithelium, as well as due to unknown components in the tear film (72). In the second phase of stromal repair, the keratocytes immediately adjacent to the area of cell death enter the cell cycle and proliferate. This proliferation occurs 24 to 48 hours after wounding in both a rat and rabbit model (73,74). As part of the second phase, the keratocytes undergo a phenotype transformation (and are termed *fibroblasts*) and migrate into the wound area. This migration takes up to a week in animal models and may be even slower in human corneas. The third phase involves the transformation of fibroblasts into myofibroblasts. These cells express elevated levels of smooth muscle actin and are involved in contracting the wound. The extent of myofibroblast formation depends on the type of wound and the extent of interaction with the epithelium. In general, gaping wounds and wounds that destroy the basement membrane (e.g., PRK) result in greater myofibroblast formation than wounds that leave the basement membrane intact or disrupt it minimally (e.g., LASIK). In addition, larger wounds appear to generate a larger number of myofibroblasts than smaller ones. Myofibroblast formation in a rabbit model of PRK peaked at 1 month after wounding (74). The last phase of stromal healing involves the remodeling of the stroma and is also greatly dependent on the original wound. Wounds, such as those caused by PRK, that are horizontal to the corneal surface usually heal with minimal scarring. In this type of wound, the myofibroblasts regress and the basement membrane is reformed. However, in humans, this may require a year or more. In contrast, gaping or incisional wounds stimulate the synthesis of collagens not normally present in the cornea (type III) and other abnormal extracellular matrix materials. This results in improper collagen fibril formation and spacing, and corneal scarring. This type of wound can require many years of remodeling for the cornea to regain its normal optical quality. In humans, one of the complications after PRK is a resultant haze seen immediately subjacent to the ablated area. This appears to be the result of the deposition of extracellular matrix materials, and also to the wound-healing stromal cells themselves. It has recently been demonstrated that myofibroblasts localize beneath the area of laser ablation and that the reflectivity of these cells is a major cause of light scattering (75).

Recent studies suggest that the stroma contains a relatively high number of immature bone marrow–derived cells in addition to the keratocytes (42). To date, almost all studies of stromal wound healing have focused on the keratocytes and their wound-healing phenotypes. Thus, it is unknown if the immature bone marrow–derived cells play a role in the repair process.

Provisional Matrix

Although it is sometimes assumed that the corneal epithelium migrates over the basement membrane or underlying extracellular matrix component after a wound, this may not be correct. Indeed, a variety of matrix components are synthesized by the epithelium in response to a wound [reviewed in Zieske (71)] (Table 1-1). These include laminin-5, entactin, collagen IV, and perlecan, which are normally present in the basement membrane. In addition, components not normally present are synthesized and deposited, including lumican, fibrin, and an unprocessed form of laminin-5. These components appear to be present in all types of wounds and make up a wound-healing surface that has, in the past, been termed a *pseudomembrane*, but is more properly termed a *provisional matrix*. Epithelial cells actually migrate on this provisional matrix after wounding, and several lines of evidence in animal models suggest that the matrix influences wound healing [reviewed in Zieske (71)]. For example, corneal epithelial cells in culture migrate at a faster rate on unprocessed laminin-5 than on the processed form seen in unwounded corneas. Stromal wound healing also appears to involve a provisional matrix. A number of extracellular matrix components not normally seen in the stroma have been localized after wounding, including fibronectin, fibrin, tenascin, collagen types IV and VII, and laminin-1 (Table 1-1). In addition, keratan sulfate proteoglycan levels decrease whereas chondroitin sulfate levels increase in the wounded stroma. In an experimental model, fibronectin and chondroitin sulfate stimulate fibroblast migration into a matrix. Thus, the provisional matrix may promote migration of fibroblasts into the wound area.

Corneal Endothelium

Ultrastructure

Corneal endothelium is the single layer of cells forming a boundary between the corneal stroma and anterior chamber (Figs. 1-2 and 1-9). The endothelial monolayer from young individuals consists of polygonal cells, 4 to 6 μm thick, with a diameter of approximately 20 μm (76). The posterior (apical) cell surface contains numerous microvilli (77), whereas the lateral and basal plasma membranes are extensively interdigitated (78,79). Both of these types of membrane folding provide for increased surface area, and the interdigitations between neighboring cells provide a means for maintaining strong cell–cell contacts. A circumferential band of actin filaments, located toward the apical aspect of the cells, helps maintain cell shape (80,81). Ultrastructural studies of corneal endothelial cells reveal the presence of abundant mitochondria, indicating that these cells are highly metabolically active (Fig. 1-9). Extensive rough and smooth endoplasmic reticulum, as well as a distinct Golgi apparatus, provide evidence of significant protein synthesis. The apical aspect of the lateral membranes contain focal, rather than "beltlike," tight junctions (*maculae occludentes*) (82,83). Corneal endothelial cells express occludin, a tight junctional protein located in the lateral plasma membrane, and ZO-1, a member of a submembranous cytoplasmic complex associated with tight junctions

(84,85). Ultrastructurally, endothelial cells form gap junctions, with typical connexin structure between cells. These junctions are located on the lateral plasma membranes anterior to the tight junctions (78,86,87) and are sites of dye transfer and electrical coupling between cells (88). Corneal endothelial cells express the gap junction protein, connexin-43 (85). Anchoring junctions mediate close contact between the plasma membranes of adjacent cells and the underlying actin filament network, thereby strengthening cell–cell associations. N-cadherin and α-, β-, and γ-catenin (plakoglobin) are among the constituents of the anchoring junction complex in corneal endothelial cells (89,90). The basal (anteriormost) aspect of corneal endothelial cells rests on Descemet's membrane, the thick basement membrane that is secreted by the endothelium. The nature of structural specializations that anchor endothelial cells to Descemet's membrane is unclear, although focal areas of increased electron density suggest the presence of anchoring plaques (86). Proteins expressed in corneal endothelial cells that are known to facilitate normal cell–substrate anchoring include vinculin (91), talin (92), β3-integrin (85), and α-v, β5-integrin (93).

Functions of the Corneal Endothelium Related to Transparency

Transparency is essential for the function of the cornea as the primary lens of the eye and results from the uniformity of the corneal tissue and the spatial arrangement of the collagen lamellae in the stroma. A major function of the corneal endothelium is to maintain corneal transparency by regulating corneal hydration. Proteoglycans associated with stromal collagens bind water and produce a pressure gradient across the endothelium. Another function of the corneal endothelium is to permit the passage of nutrients from the aqueous humor into the avascular cornea. The endothelium forms a "leaky" barrier by permitting paracellular percolation of aqueous humor into the cornea, but preventing bulk fluid flow. This leaky barrier is formed structurally by the formation of focal, rather than "band-like" tight junctions, and by the sinuous interdigitation of lateral membranes. The endothelium counteracts the tendency of the corneal stroma to swell by removing excess stromal fluid through the activity of Na$^+$/K$^+$-adenosine triphosphatase (ATPase) (94) and bicarbonate-dependent Mg^{2+}-ATPase (95) ionic pumps, which are located mainly on the lateral plasma membranes. Both the barrier and pump functions of the endothelium are essential for maintaining the relatively dehydrated state of the stroma required for transparency (96,97). The "pump-leak hypothesis" was developed to explain how fluid flow is regulated in the cornea. This hypothesis states that normal corneal thickness is maintained by the relative balance between the rate of fluid flow into the cornea and the relative rate of pumping of excess fluid out of the cornea (96). This equilibrium

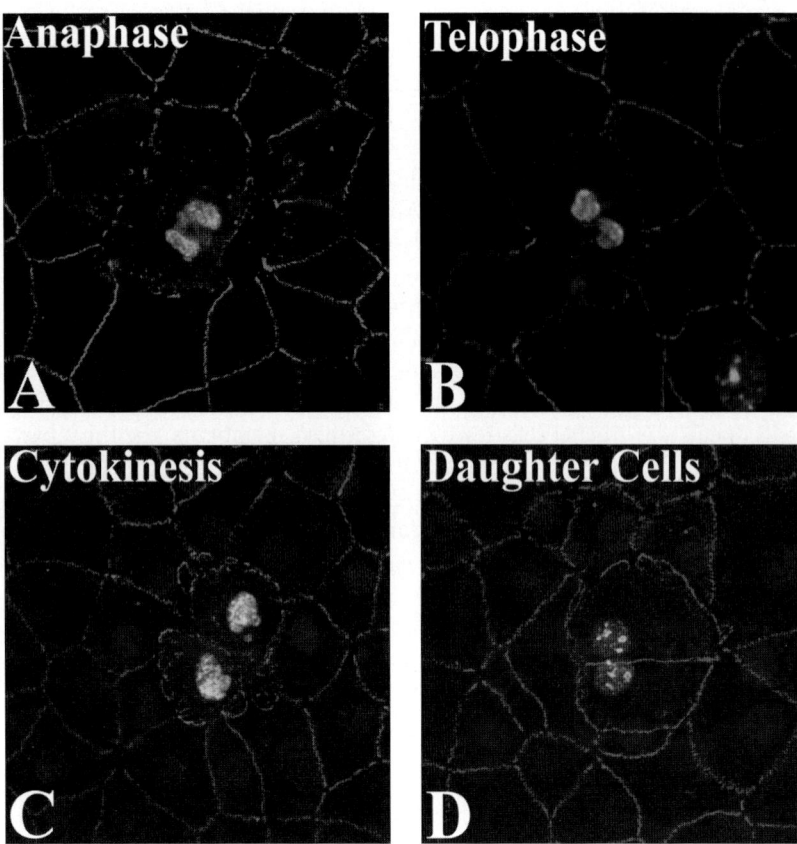

FIGURE 1-10. Final stages of mitosis and daughter cell formation in *ex vivo* human corneal endothelium [after Joyce (108)]. Cornea from a 52-year-old donor was treated with ethylenediamine tetraacetic acid to break cell–cell contacts, followed by incubation for 48 hours in the presence of 10% serum. (Original magnification, ×600.)

is maintained as long as the integrity of the endothelial monolayer is maintained. Recent studies suggest that, besides the sodium and bicarbonate pumps, aquaporins may also play a role in fluid movement across the endothelium. Aquaporins are integral membrane proteins that serve as water-selective channels. Several aquaporin isoforms have been identified and, of these, aquaporin-1 (AQP1) is expressed in corneal endothelial cells (98). In mice lacking AQP1, recovery of corneal transparency and thickness after hypotonic swelling was markedly delayed, indicating that AQP1 plays an active role in movement of fluid from the stroma across the endothelium (99).

Proliferative Capacity of Corneal Endothelial Cells

During eye development, both cell proliferation and migration contribute to the formation of the endothelium from neural crest–derived mesenchymal cells (100,101). There is ample evidence, however, to indicate that once the mature endothelial monolayer has formed, human corneal endothelium does not normally replicate *in vivo* at a rate sufficient to replace dead or injured cells (102). Immunocytochemical localization studies indicate that corneal endothelium *in vivo* has not exited the cell cycle, as have the

suprabasal cells of corneal epithelium, but is arrested in the G1 phase of the cell cycle (103). These cells retain proliferative capacity as indicated by extensive proliferation after expression of viral oncogenes (104) and by the completion of mitosis after *ex vivo* treatment to break cell–cell contacts, as illustrated in Fig. 1-10. The fact that endothelial cells *in vivo* do not normally replicate strongly suggests that they are actively maintained in a nonproliferative state. Several conditions appear to contribute to maintenance of the endothelium in G1 phase arrest, including age (105), transforming growth factor-β2 in the aqueous humor (106), and contact-dependent inhibition of proliferation (85,107). See Joyce (108) for a review of the current knowledge regarding corneal endothelial cell proliferation. Overall, the relative lack of proliferation in the endothelium results in an age-related decrease in cell density throughout life, with an average cell loss of 0.3% to 0.6% per year (109).

Innervation of the Cornea

The cornea is exceptional in its innervation, being one of the most densely innervated tissues of the body. Most corneal nerves are sensory, being derived from the trigeminal nerve. [For an excellent recent review of corneal nerves,

Human Corneal Innervation

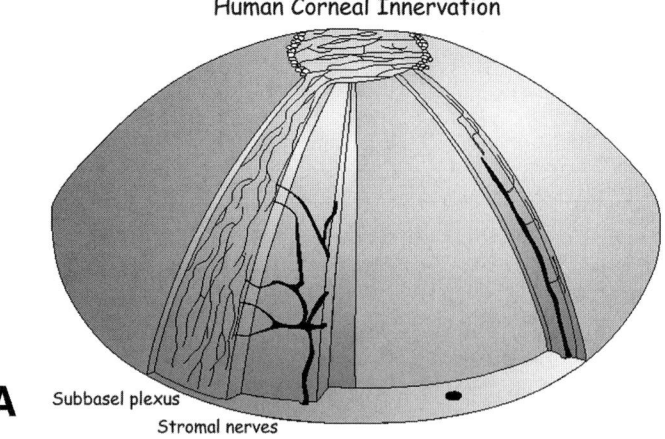

A   Subbasel plexus
Stromal nerves

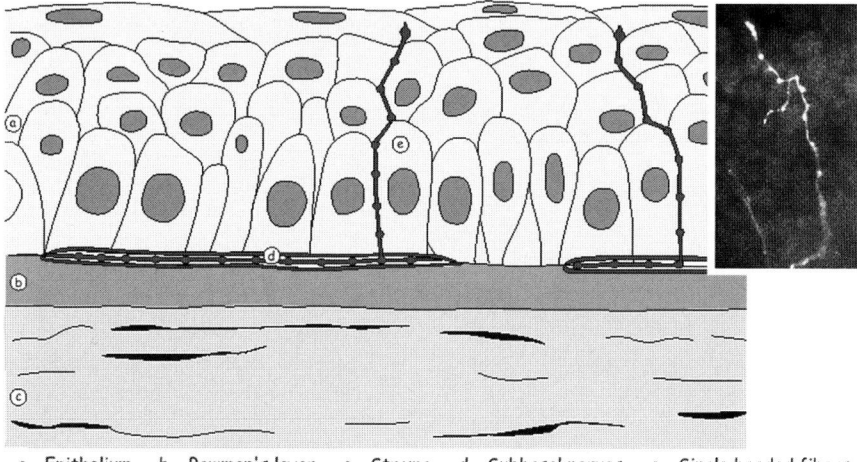

a - Epithelium   b - Bowman's layer   c - Stroma   d - Subbasal nerves   e - Single beaded fibers

B

FIGURE 1-11. A: Diagram of human cornea showing distribution of nerves in the stroma and subbasal plexus. At the apex of the cornea, the nerve fibers are oriented in the 6-to-12, 5-to-11, or 7-to-1 direction [From Müller LJ, Marfurt CF, Kruse F, et al. Corneal nerves: structure, contents and function. *Exp Eye Res* 2003; 76:521–542; as adapted from Maurice (4), after data from R. W. Beuerman.] **B:** Diagram adapted from Müller et al. (107) of the corneal epithelium showing the nerve bundles (leashes) in the subbasal plexus (d). The bundle contains both beaded and straight fibers, but as demonstrated in the micrograph at right, which has been labeled with antibodies to substance P, only the beaded nerves turn to enter the epithelium, where they terminate in the apical layers of cells (Adapted from Müller LJ, Marfurt CF, Kruse F, et al. Corneal nerves: structure, contents and function. *Exp Eye Res* 2003;76:521—542.)

see Müller et al. (110).] Bundles of nerves enter the cornea in a radial pattern and run parallel to the epithelium below the anterior third of the stroma (Fig. 1-11). Approximately 1 mm outside the limbus, the nerves lose their perineurium and myelin sheath, loss of which contributes to corneal transparency (110). Eventually nerve fibers turn 90 degrees, moving toward the epithelium and maintaining a Schwann cell sheath through Bowman's layer (1). After crossing Bowman's layer and the epithelial basement membrane, the bundles again turn 90 degrees and run parallel to the base of the epithelium. These sub-basal bundles are called *leashes* (Fig. 1-11). These epithelial leashes are oriented in a superior-to-inferior pattern and consist of straight and beaded fibers (Fig. 1-11). At the point of crossing the epithelial basement membrane, the Schwann cell sheath is lost. Beaded nerves of the leashes move obliquely into the epithelium between cell layers, terminating among the outer squamous cells (36) (Fig. 1-11B). The corneal epithelium is the most highly innervated of all epithelia, with

approximately 300 to 400 more nerve endings per unit area than epidermis (111).

A number of neurotransmitters and neuropeptides are expressed by corneal nerves [for review, see Müller et al. (110)]. In humans, these include substance P and calcitonin gene–related peptide (CGRP) expressed by sensory nerves, and norepinephrine expressed by sympathetic nerves. Numerous studies have also demonstrated that the corneal nerves provide trophic factors necessary for maintenance of a healthy cornea (110). Degeneration of corneal nerves from injury or disease leads to neurotrophic keratitis, characterized by epithelial sloughing and impaired healing.

LIMBUS

Anatomically, the limbus is a zone between the cornea and the conjunctiva and sclera (Figs. 1-1 and 1-2). It is a zone formed on the corneal side by a line drawn between

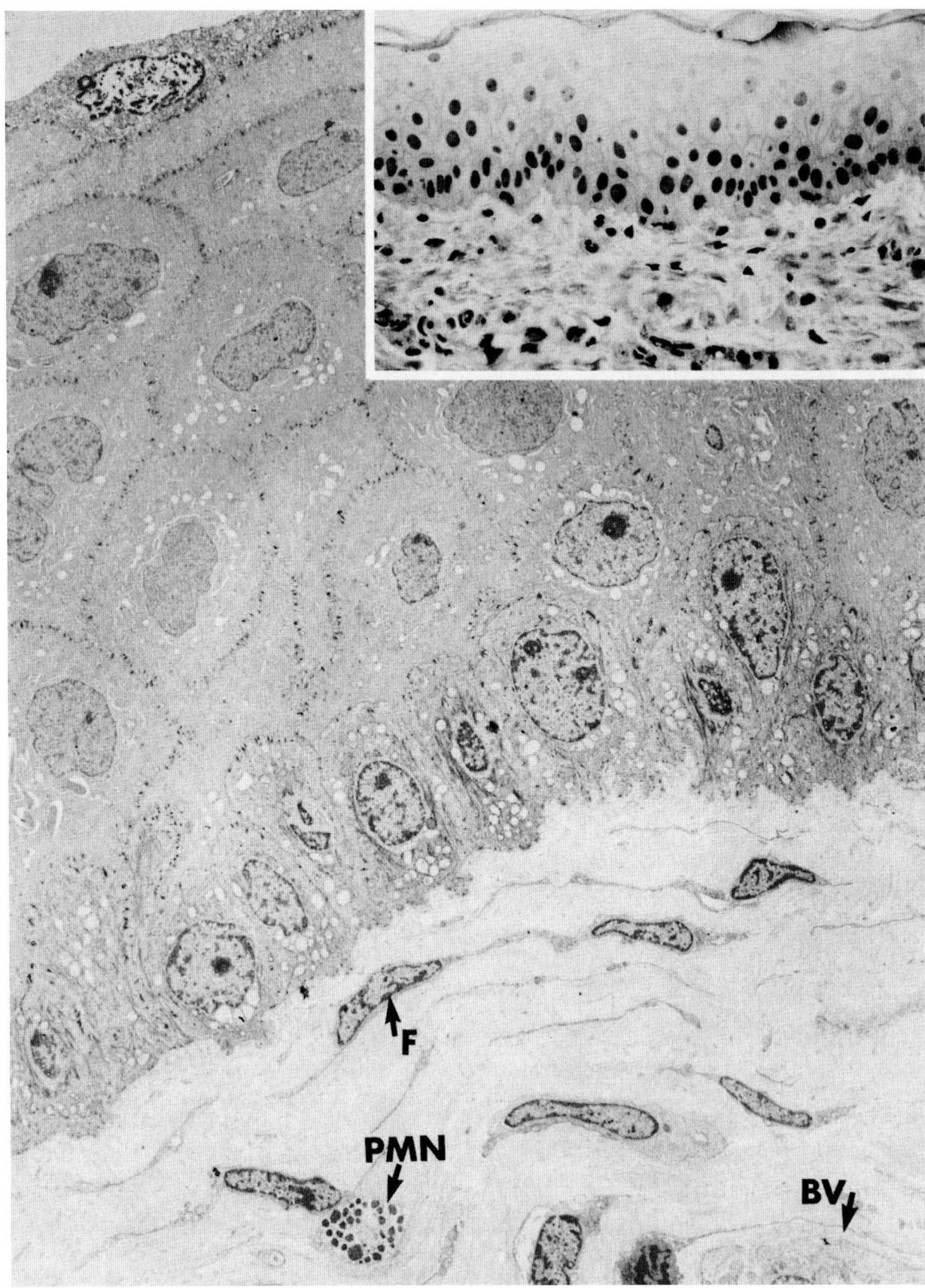

FIGURE 1-12. Light (*inset*) and electron micrographs of the limbal epithelium and adjacent connective tissue. The basal cells of the region are smaller and less columnar than those of the cornea. Note the absence of Bowman's layer, the presence of fibroblasts (F), blood vessels (BV), and a portion of a polymorphonuclear neutrophil (PMN). (Original magnifications: main, ×2700; *inset*, ×300.)

the termination of Bowman's layer and Descemet's membrane, and on the conjunctival/scleral side by a parallel line approximately 1 mm peripherally. This latter line runs just outside Schlemm's canal (1,112). Thus, the anatomic limbus includes both Schlemm's canal and the trabecular meshwork. More commonly, the limbus is considered to be the outer portion of that zone, including only the epithelium and underlying connective tissue down to the corneal-scleral collagen lamellae. It is this latter superficial region that is described here. Several functions have been ascribed to this zone; the basal cells of the epithelium are generally accepted to be the stem cells for the corneal epithelium, and the vascular elements, which loop into the stromal connective tissue, provide nutrients to the avascular cornea.

The limbal tissue includes the stratified-squamous, nonkeratinizing epithelium connecting the corneal and conjunctival epithelium and the subjacent vascularized, loose connective tissue. Each of these regions in the tissues has unique characteristics.

Limbal Epithelium

The limbal epithelium is structurally similar to the corneal epithelium (Fig. 1-12). Unlike the cornea, melanocytes or Langerhans cells can frequently be found interspersed between cells of the limbal epithelium (1,113). The epithelium has 7 to 10 cell layers, and the cell–cell and cell–substrate junctions appear similar to those of cornea. The apical cells of the region have microplicae or microvilli at their apical membrane, and at their lateral borders tight junctions are present. It is the basal cells of the region that appear unique. They appear smaller and less columnar than basal cells of the corneal epithelium and appear to have comparatively more mitochondria. Another difference is the undulating extensions of the basal surface of the basal cells into the underlying matrix (1) (Figs. 1-12 and 1-13; and see discussion later). The basal cells of the limbus have a significantly smaller amount of their basal surface covered by hemidesmosomes (29). The undulation of the basal membrane may provide additional adhesive strength for the epithelium and perhaps an increased basal surface area for absorbance of nutrients from the limbal vasculature.

Most experts now agree that a subpopulation of these basal cells comprises the stem cells for the corneal epithelium. Stem cells are defined as cells with the capacity for unlimited or prolonged self-renewal that can produce at least one type of highly differentiated descendent. To date, no single marker or group of markers has been identified that allows cells to be positively identified as stem cells. Therefore, these cells are usually defined by a group of common characteristics [for review, see Zieske and others (114–119)]. First, stem cells are the ultimate precursors for all other cells in the tissue. Second, stem cells are a self-maintaining population. The cells are capable of asymmetric cell division, allowing one daughter cell to remain a stem cell while the other enters the path of terminal differentiation. Third, stem cells make up a small proportion of the total cells in a tissue. This ranges from 2% to 4% of the total in small intestine and epidermis to as little as 0.01% of bone marrow cells. Fourth, stem cells are undifferentiated compared with the remainder of the tissue. Fifth, stem cells are slow cycling *in vivo* but highly clonogenic when placed into cell culture. This means that single stem cells in culture can give rise to many cells and have an almost unlimited ability to proliferate. In some tissues, such as gut epithelia and hematopoietic cells, one stem cell can give rise to several differentiated cell types, but in some stratified squamous epithelia, such as that of the epidermis and the corneal epithelium, the stem cells are believed to be unipotent and give rise to only one cell type. The daughter cells derived from stem cell division that are committed to the differentiation pathway have been called *transit cells* (120), *transit amplifying cells* (121), or *transient amplifying cells* (12). These cells are an intermediate population of committed progenitors with limited proliferative capacity and restricted differentiation potential. Their primary function is to increase the number of differentiated cells produced by each stem cell division (12). Because stem cells cycle less frequently than transient amplifying cells (120,121), they retain ^{3}H-thymidine and bromodeoxyuridine for longer time periods. Because the transient amplifying cells, compared with stem cells, have a shorter cell cycle and a limited self-renewal capacity, they are unlikely to be involved in carcinogenesis.

Several lines of evidence support the limbal localization of the corneal epithelial stem cells. The first suggestion of this localization was reported by Davenger and Evensen, who observed that pigmented cells migrate from the limbus to central cornea (122). This centripetal movement of cells has subsequently been confirmed in animal models (123,124). A second line of evidence is that the limbal cells are less differentiated than the other cells of the limbal and corneal epithelium. This was elegantly demonstrated by Schermer et al. (12), who found that the keratin, K3, was a differentiation marker of corneal epithelium and that it was localized in all cells except the limbal basal cells. Third, limbal basal cells are label retaining. This was first demonstrated by Lavker and coworkers (125), who found that mice injected with ^{3}H-thymidine retained the marker only in the limbal basal cells, thus indicating that these cells divide less frequently than the remainder of the epithelial cells. Fourth, in culture, limbal basal cells have a much higher proliferative potential than the remainder of the corneal epithelial cells (126,127). Fifth, limbal transplant surgery results in healing with corneal epithelium (128). Conversely, in animal models, surgical removal of the limbus results in healing with noncorneal epithelium (129). In addition to these lines of evidence, the preferential expression of a number of proteins in the limbal basal cells also supports the concept that the limbal epithelium differs

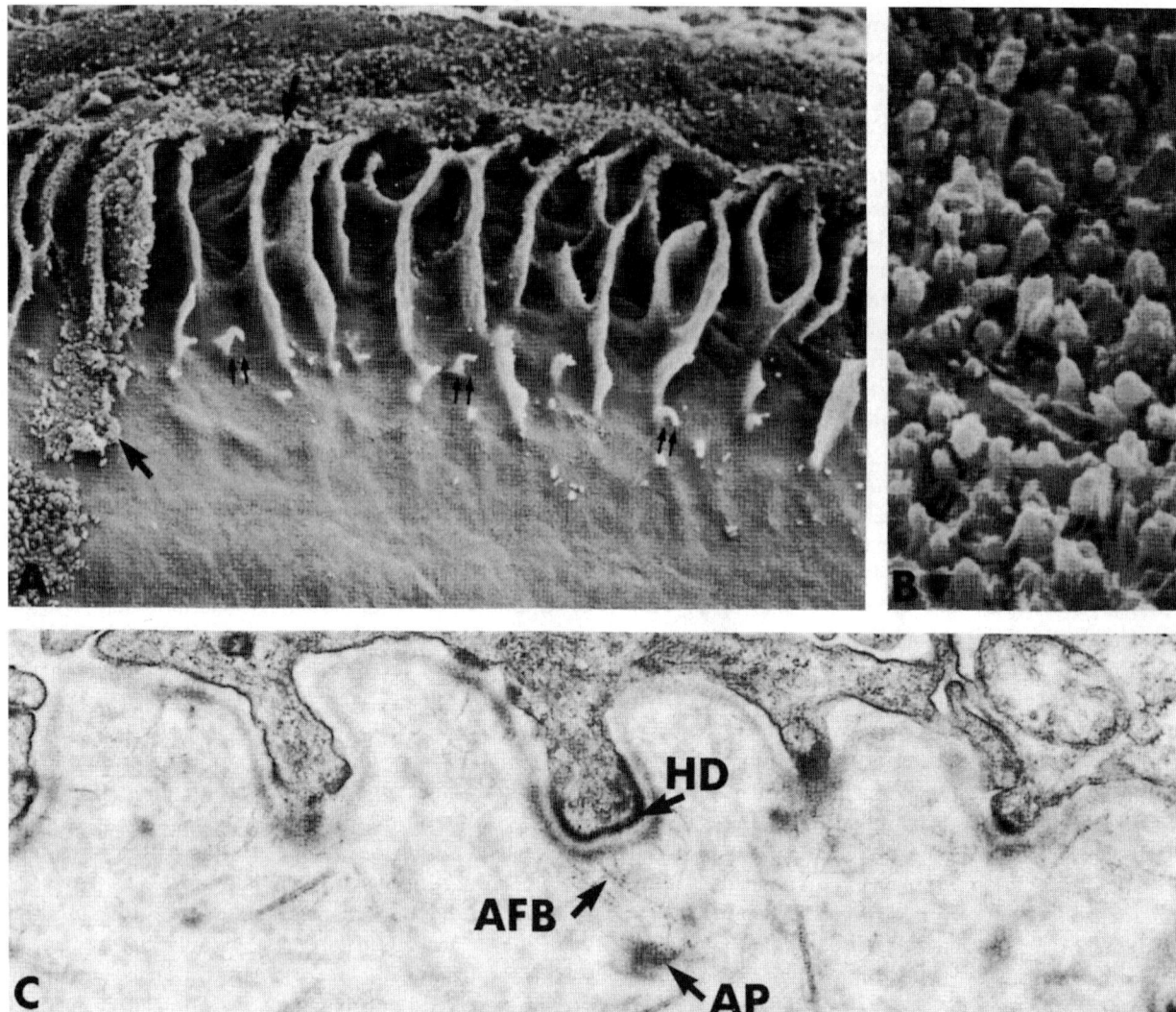

FIGURE 1-13. Electron micrographs demonstrating the surface modulations of the stroma in the limbal region. Scanning electron micrograph **(A)** of a cornea with its limbal epithelium partially removed after incubation in the presence of EDTA (29). *Arrows* indicate edges of remnant epithelium. The palisades appear to taper down toward the cornea, and at the tip of each fold, small villus-like projections occur (double arrows). Lateral folds emanate from or between individual palisades, and some of the palisades appear to branch. The scanning micrograph **(B)** and the transmission micrograph **(C)** show smaller scale peg-like projections from denuded stroma **(B)** or in cross section **(C)**. These peg-like projections of the stroma may provide increased surface area for basal cells to receive nutrients from the limbal vasculature or they may increase the adhesive strength of the cell since there is a smaller percent of these basal cell membranes occupied by hemidesmosomes (29). Hemidesmosomes (HD), associated anchoring fibrils (AFB), and anchoring plaques (AP) are visible in C. (Original magnifications: **A,** ×2000; **B,** ×5100; **C,** ×31,000.)

from the corneal epithelium (Table 1-3). These proteins include metabolic enzymes, growth factor receptors, cytoskeleton components, cell cycle regulators, transcription factors, and extracellular matrix components. Most of these proteins are expressed in a majority of the limbal basal cells. One exception is the ATP-binding cassette transporter G2 (ABCG2). This protein is expressed in a variety of stem cells (130), and preliminary reports (131,132) indicate that ABCG2 is present in less than 10% of the limbal basal cells.

Several proteins have also been found that are expressed in central corneal epithelium but are present at much lower levels in the limbal basal cells. These include the keratins K3 and K12, aldehyde dehydrogenase class 3, and connexin-43. The absence of connexin-43 in limbal basal cells suggests that they are not chemically linked to the remainder of the epithelium.

One popular misconception is that all limbal basal cells are stem cells. However, the best current data suggest that

TABLE 1-3. PROTEINS LOCALIZED TO LIMBAL BASAL CELLS

Metabolic Enzymes	Receptors	Cytoskeleton Components	Cell Cycle Components	Others
α-Enolase	Epithelial growth factor receptor	Keratin 19	Cyclin D	Melanin
Cytochrome oxidase	TGF-β receptor I	Vimentin	Cyclin E	p63
Na$^+$, K$^+$-ATPase	TGF-β receptor II	—	p107 (nuclear)	ATP-binding cassette transporter G2
Carbonic anhydrase	TrkA	—	—	—
Glucose transporter I	—	—	—	—

ATP, adenosine triphosphate; TGF, transforming growth factor; TrkA, nerve growth factor receptor.

only 5% to 15% of the cells in the limbus are stem cells. This is based on label retaining and clonal culture studies. This is somewhat at odds with the localization of most of the proteins in Table 1-3, which are present in most of the limbal basal cells. One possible explanation for this finding involves the niche hypothesis first proposed by Schofield (1983) (133) (Fig. 1-14). In this hypothesis, cells are influenced by their microenvironment to remain stem cells. The entire limbus may provide a microenvironment that maintains the limbal basal cells in a relatively undifferentiated state, and it is not until the cells leave the limbus that they become easily distinguishable from stem cells. This concept is supported by the findings that the extracellular matrix of the limbus varies from that of central cornea (Table 1-4).

These data, taken together, suggest that a subpopulation of basal cells of the limbus, which in humans are protected by pigmentation and their deeper position in the crypts between the palisades of Vogt (see later and Fig. 1-13), are stem cells of the corneal epithelium. The position of the stem cell population at the periphery of the cornea implies a centripetal movement of cells from the periphery toward central cornea (123,134) (Fig. 1-14). The concept of centripetal migration of the limbal stem cells is in large part based on the pioneering work of Richard Thoft and Judy Friend. Among their elegant studies were demonstrations that there is a gradual replacement of donor epithelium by host epithelium after corneal transplantation (135), and that limbal epithelium can heal a corneal wound with cornea-like epithelium (136). Based on their work, Thoft and Friend (134) proposed an "x, y, z hypothesis" in 1983 that stated that corneal epithelial mass depended on the centripetal movement of cells from the periphery. This hypothesis differs from the currently accepted hypothesis of centripetally migrating cells only in that Thoft and Friend did not specify the source of cells as corneal epithelial stem cells.

Limbal Connective Tissue

The connective tissue below the limbal epithelium can be classified by comparison with the corneal stroma as more loosely and irregularly arranged. Collagens, proteoglycans, and soluble glycoproteins in the region seemingly correspond to those found in the cornea, with the exception of the proteoglycan, keratocan, which is present only in the cornea (137). The cellular elements in it include fibroblasts, melanocytes, macrophages, mast cells, lymphocytes, and plasma cells, and the cells that make up the blood vessels and lymphatics, which loop into the region (113). These vessels include capillaries, small arterioles and venules, and large lymphatic vessels (Fig. 1-15). Bundles of unmyelinated nerves are also present (Fig. 1-15). The unique aspects of this connective tissue are the large radial folds or ridges that form the palisades of Vogt (Fig. 1-13). These outward folds of the limbal connective tissue are large enough to house small blood vessels, lymphatics, and nerves. Crypts of limbal epithelium reach down into the valleys between the palisades, and it is hypothesized that the deep housing of the basal cells protects this stem cell population. Another, less macroscopic feature of the limbal connective tissue is the tiny, rete, peglike outpocketings of stroma (1,29) (Fig. 1-13). These pegs begin in the peripheral cornea and extend throughout the limbal region into the conjunctival zone. These pegs with the concomitant extensions of basal cells between them may increase the adhesive strength of the epithelium because hemidesmosomes are not as extensive (29).

CONJUNCTIVA

The conjunctiva is a mucous membrane that covers the inner surface of the upper and lower lids and extends to the limbus on the surface of the globe. The major unique functions of this tissue are to provide the tear film mucous layer and to provide the immune tissue, as well as bactericidal/virucidal agents, to protect the ocular surface. Ducts of all the glands associated with tear and lipid components of the tear layer enter the conjunctival epithelium. The tissue comprises a surface epithelium that is unique among the nonkeratinizing squamous types in that goblet cells are

A

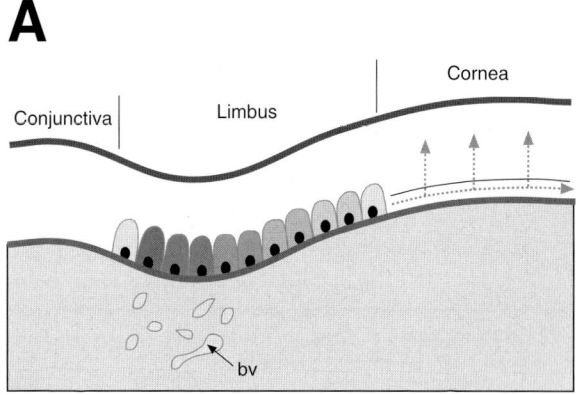

B

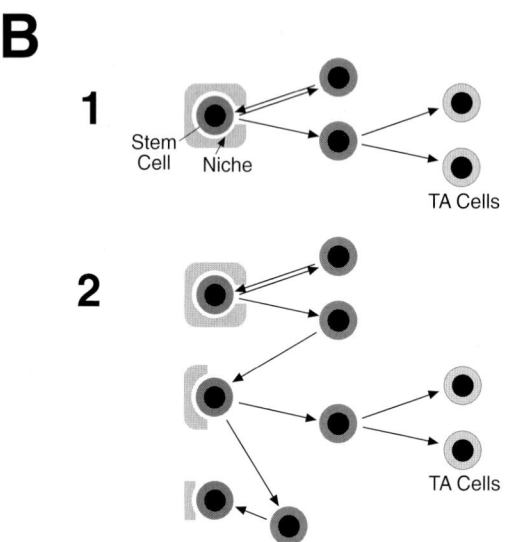

TABLE 1-4. UNIQUE PROPERTIES OF LIMBAL EXTRACELLULAR MATRIX

AE27*–patchwork staining in limbal basement membrane
Laminin $\alpha2$ and $\beta2$ chains
$\alpha2$ Chain of type IV collagen
$\alpha9$ Integrin
Type XII collagen absent

*Antigen for AE27 was never identified.

FIGURE 1-14. A: Diagram demonstrating corneal stem cells in the limbal zone. A stem cell is indicated, along with a gradient of undifferentiated cells with some stem cell-like characteristics. Blood vessels (bv) are localized directly subjacent to the limbal basal cells. (Adapted from Zieske JD, Gipson IK. Agents that affect corneal wound healing: Modulation of structure and function. In: Albert DM, Jakobiec FA, eds. *Principles and practice of ophthalmology: basic sciences.* Philadelphia: WB Saunders, 1994: 1093–1099, and Schermer A, Galvin S, Sun TT. Differentiation-related expression of a major 64K corneal keratin in vivo and in culture suggests limbal location of corneal epithelial stem cells. *J Cell Biol* 1986;103:49–62.) **B:** Diagrammatic representation of stem cell differentiation based on the niche hypothesis. (1) In this hypothesis, the stem cell is maintained in an optimal microenvironment termed the niche, which maintains the cell as a stem cell. Following cell proliferation, one daughter cell re-enters the niche, while the other becomes an early transient amplifying cell (TA cell) and enters the pathway of terminal differentiation. (2) In an alternate hypothesis, following stem cell proliferation the daughter cells can either re-enter the stem cell niche or enter a less advantageous niche that allows the cell to retain stem-like characteristics. This model allows for cells in a given tissue to exhibit a gradient of characteristics ranging from "true" stem cell to early TA to late TA to terminally differentiated cell. This model is in agreement with experimental data that suggests that most limbal basal cells are undifferentiated, but that only 5-15% are "true" stem cells. (Adapted from Zieske JD, Gipson IK. Agents that affect corneal wound healing: Modulation of structure and function. In: Albert DM, Jakobiec FA, eds. *Principles and practice of ophthalmology: basic sciences.* Philadelphia: WB Saunders, 1994:1093–1099.)

intercalated within it (113,138) (Fig. 1-16). A substantia propria, which is highly vascularized, supplies not only connective tissue support, but sensory nerves as well as much lymphoid tissue.

Three regions of conjunctiva are recognized (113,139). These include the palpebral or tarsal conjunctiva, which lines the inner region of the lids, the forniceal conjunctiva, which lines the upper and lower forniceal recesses, and the bulbar conjunctiva, which is the region between the fornix and limbus, overlying the sclera.

Conjunctival Epithelium

The stratified nonkeratinizing squamous epithelium of the conjunctiva does not appear to vary dramatically in the three conjunctival regions except that the epithelium at the lid margin appears thicker and has few, if any goblet cells. There are varying accounts of the number of cell layers in the conjunctival epithelium, particularly that of the bulbar and forniceal areas. It is the authors' opinion that these variations are a result of the degree of stretch on the mucous membrane at the time of fixation of the tissue for histologic study. For example, when the globe moves downward, stretching the superior bulbar region, the epithelium may appear to be two to three cell layers, whereas a globe in the medial position may have a bulbar epithelium covered with five to seven cell layers. In any event, reports of the number of cell layers vary from 2 to 3 to 10 to 12 at the lid margin, where the number of cell layers is probably constant because the tarsal substantia propria is not as loose and pliable as that over forniceal and bulbar regions.

The site of the stem cells of the conjunctival epithelium is debated. Clonal cultures of human conjunctival epithelium suggest that the stem cells are dispersed throughout the epithelium (140). In mice, epithelial stem cells appear to be concentrated in the forniceal region (141).

The major differences between cells of the conjunctival epithelium and those of the cornea appear to be an increase in cytoplasmic organelles (notably mitochondria) and distinct clumping of keratin filaments into bundles. In other aspects, particularly in the anchoring complex (hemidesmosome–anchoring fibril complex), the desmosome, and the apical tight junctions, the conjunctival epithelium

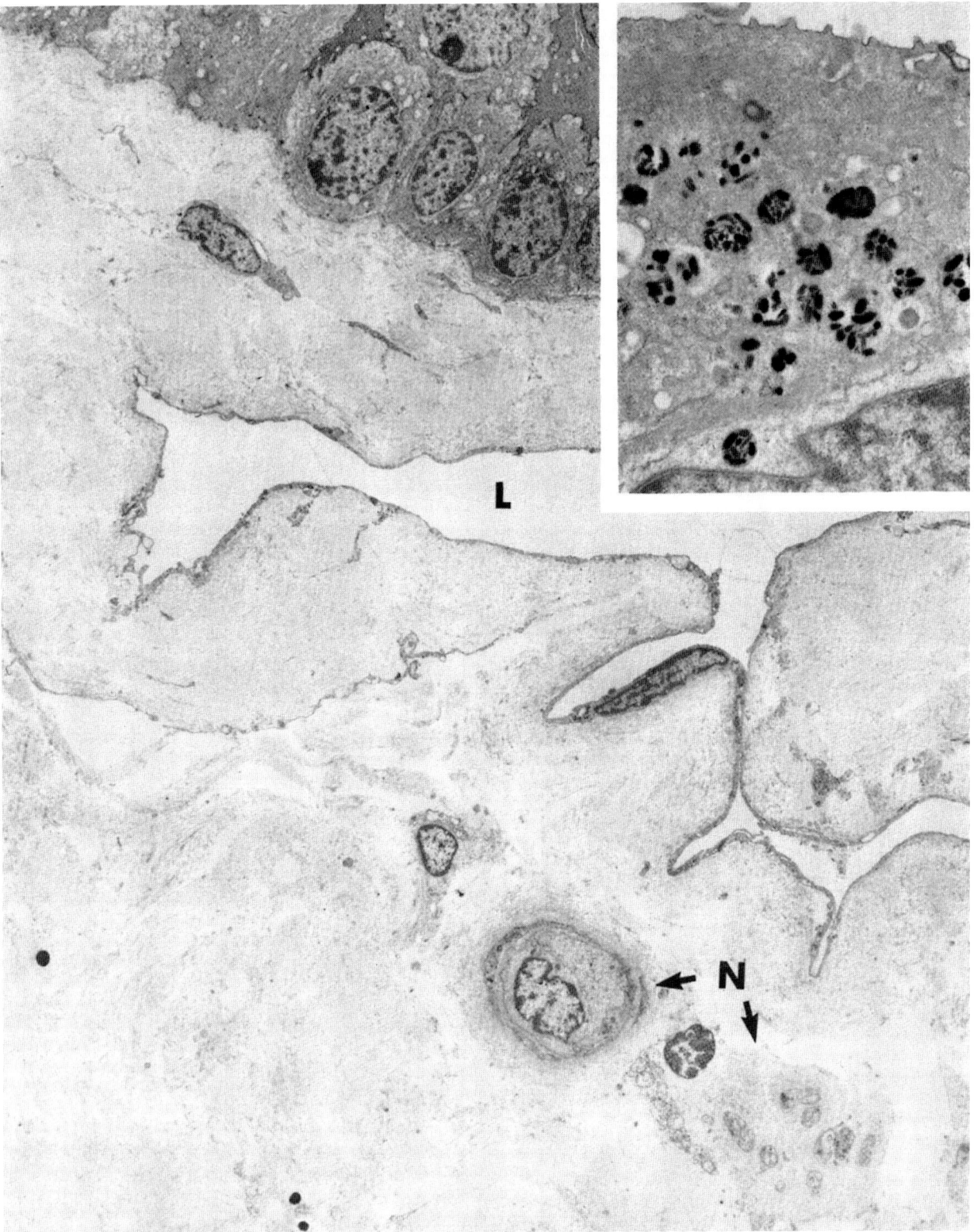

FIGURE 1-15. Micrographs of limbal region demonstrating presence of a large lymphatic (L), and bundles of unmyelinated nerves (N). The *inset* shows presence of packets of melanin granules derived from basally located melanocytes in an apical cell of the limbal epithelium. Presence of these pigment granules is believed to protect limbal basal cells, the purported stem cells of the corneal epithelium. (Original magnifications: main, ×2700; *inset*, ×13,000.)

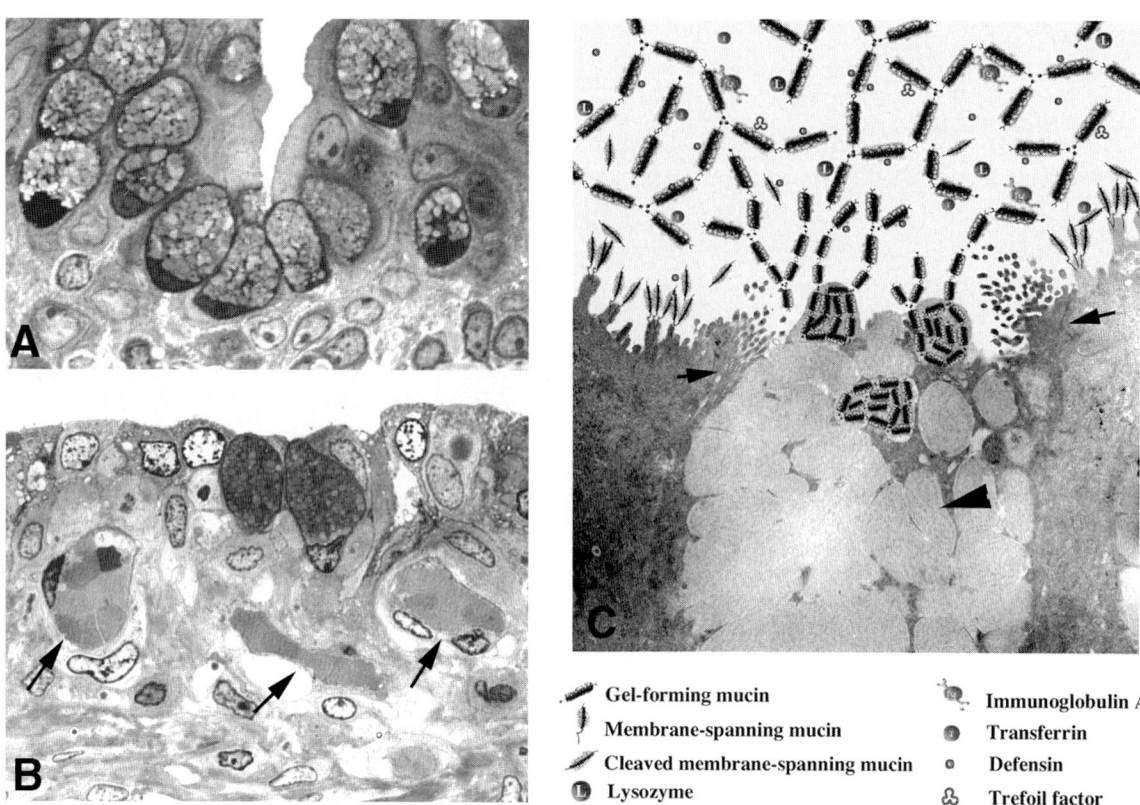

Gel-forming mucin		*Immunoglobulin A*	
Membrane-spanning mucin		*Transferrin*	
Cleaved membrane-spanning mucin		*Defensin*	
Lysozyme		*Trefoil factor*	

FIGURE 1-16. Micrographs demonstrating regions of bulbar **(A)** and palpebral conjunctiva **(B, C)**. In the bulbar region, particularly in the nasal zone, goblet cells are very dense. **A:** As shown in this micrograph, they can occur in crypts or groups which have the appearance of acini. [For review, see Kessing (139).] **B:** The palpebral conjunctiva section demonstrates fewer goblet cells and the highly vascularized stroma (arrows) characteristic of conjunctival substantia propria. This is a section from a newborn and the lymphoid zone that develops several months after birth (113) is not yet present under the epithelium. **C:** This electron micrograph shows the apical region of a goblet cell secreting mucin. Superimposed on the micrograph is a diagram illustrating how the gel-forming mucin MUC5AC is packaged within the mucin packets of the goblet cell and how it expands to form a mucin network upon hydration after secretion. The mucin packets of the goblet cells have a filamentous interweaving substructure (*arrowhead*). Housed within the mucin network are bactericidal and other defense molecules of the tear film that are secreted by the adnexal glands and/or the conjunctival epithelium. Several of these components of the tear film are shown in the diagram and listed below part **C**. The two cells adjacent to the goblet cell have numerous microvilli that have membrane-associated mucins emanating from their tips. At the lateral borders of the cells near the apical membrane, junctional complexes can be seen (*arrows*). (Original magnifications: **A, B,** ×900; **C,** ×7500.)

appears similar to the rest of the ocular surface epithelium. Unlike the cornea, the basal aspect of basal cells undulates along with the undulation of the underlying substantia propria.

The apical cells of the epithelium do not have the flattened appearance of those of the corneal epithelium, and they have numerous vesicles in their cytoplasm (Fig. 1-16). Apparent fusion between these vesicles and the apical plasmalemma (142,143) has led to the question as to whether these vesicular fusions result from phagocytosis or exocytosis. Both are possible. The conjunctival epithelia of several species have been shown to be capable of phagocytosing

bacteria (144) and experimental particles (145). Conversely, it has been proposed that these vesicles in the apical cells, based on PAS staining, provide a second source of mucin for the mucin layer of the tear film. Data from the rat indicate that these vesicles, as well as similar ones in apical cells of human corneal and limbal epithelium, provide a high–molecular-weight, highly glycosylated glycoprotein to the apical cell glycocalyx and tear film (22). These vesicles in humans may well be delivering membrane-associated mucins to the tear film surface of the apical cells.

As in corneal epithelium, the stratified squamous epithelial cells of the conjunctival epithelium produce at least three different membrane-associated mucins for their glycocalyx at the tear film interface. The membrane-associated mucins, MUC1, MUC4, and MUC16, are expressed by apical and subapical cells of the conjunctival epithelium (23,24). As in the cornea, these mucins provide a hydrophilic, highly negatively charged barrier at the epithelial surface that prevents pathogen penetrance, allows goblet cell mucus movement over the surface, and lubricates the epithelial surface, preventing adherence of epithelial surfaces during eye blink and sleep.

Conjunctival Goblet Cells

Unlike any other ocular tissue, or even any other stratified squamous epithelia, the conjunctival epithelium has goblet cells intercalated between the epithelial cells. There is a regional variation in their distribution and density per unit area [for review, see Kessing (139)]. The highest density of the cells is in the medial forniceal and palpebral regions near the tear drainage apparatus. In some regions of the conjunctiva, notably the temporal bulbar region, goblet cell density is so great that the cells appear clustered (Fig. 1-16A).

The structure of the goblet cells is similar to that of those found in other simple epithelia (Fig. 1-16). The mucin packets accumulate supranuclearly, and at the lateral membrane at the apical region of the cell, there appear to be tight junctions with neighboring epithelial cells. The cell's nucleus plus cytoplasmic organelles are displaced toward the basal aspect of the cell. The mucin packets appear electron lucent; however, a filamentous network can be discerned. The conjunctival goblet cells produce the large gel-forming mucin designated MUC5AC (146) (Fig. 1-16C). Gel-forming mucins are some of the largest genes/glycoproteins known [for review, see Gipson and Argüeso (23)]. During their transit through the synthetic machinery of the cell, they form homopolymers through cysteine-rich domains in their amino- and carboxyl-termini. They are heavily glycosylated in the Golgi and as a result are negatively charged. To package these charged hydrophilic molecules efficiently, the storage packets in goblet cells sequester large amounts of Ca^{2+} ions to shield negatively charged mucins, thus allowing compaction (147). The mucin multimers, when secreted, lose their shielding Ca^{2+} ions and become fully hydrated, which expands their size dramatically. These mucin networks move about over the surface of the eye as a result of the blink, cleaning debris and pathogens from the ocular surface. Because they are highly negatively charged, they can move smoothly over the highly glycosylated, hydrophilic, and negatively charged membrane-associated mucins of the glycocalyx through "wet-repulsive interactions." In the Sjögren's form of dry eye, the amount of MUC5AC in the tears has been shown to be decreased (148).

Little is known regarding the life cycle of the human conjunctival goblet cell. It is not known if the goblet cell and the conjunctival stratified epithelial cell have the same stem cell population, as appears to be the case with rabbits (149). In culture of human conjunctival epithelium, Pelligrini et al. (140) found that goblet cells differentiated from the cultures every 45 to 50 cell divisions and underwent approximately 15 cell doublings before senescence. Stimuli or factors controlling goblet cell differentiation or secretion in the human are relatively unknown, and little is known regarding regulation of MUC5AC expression by these cells.

Conjunctival Substantia Propria

The substantia propria of the conjunctiva consists of highly vascularized, loose connective tissue that, compared with the limbus and cornea, is rich in immune cells (Fig. 1-16). In addition to resident fibroblasts, large numbers of lymphocytes plus mast cells, plasma cells, and neutrophils are present in its matrix (113). Indeed, the substantia propria has been described as having two layers, an outer lymphoid layer (not present at birth but present several months later) and an inner fibrous layer (113). Within the lymphoid layer, dense accumulations of lymphocytes occur, although they do not form classic lymph nodules. The accumulation of lymphoid tissue plus the phagocytic capabilities of the conjunctival epithelium demonstrate the enormous potential this tissue has of dealing with infectious agents (150).

ADNEXA

Eyelids

The first and outermost adnexal tissue involved in the maintenance of the cornea is the eyelid. The eyelids provide protection from the environment, air, and light, and also serve as a mechanical barrier. Other functions of the eyelids include the spreading of the tear film and assisting in the removal of particulates. The gross anatomy of the eyelid has been described extensively by Maus (3), and the reader is directed there for further details. In brief, the eyelid consists of several layers. These layers include the skin, subcutaneous tissue, the striated orbicular muscle of the eye, the septum and tarsal plate, the smooth muscle of Müller, and, finally, the conjunctiva. The eyelids also contain a number of secretory glands described in following sections.

In the human, eyelid development occurs at the 7th week of gestation. The upper lid is formed by the fusion of the medial and lateral aspect of the frontonasal processes. The lower lid is formed by the maxillary process. Eyelid fusion occurs at 9 weeks of gestation and differentiation of the lids continues while they are fused. The meibomian glands develop during this time. Eyelid opening occurs in the 6th month. In animal models, eyelid opening triggers corneal development, but it is not clear if this also occurs in the human.

Glands

The adnexal structures, including the meibomian glands, lacrimal gland, and the accessory lacrimal glands of Krause and Wolfring, are of great importance in maintaining the health of the ocular surface. Secretions from each gland contribute specific constituents of the tear film. The sebaceous glands of Zeiss and the sweat glands of Moll, which are associated with the hair follicles of the eyelashes (Figs. 1-1 and 1-3), may also contribute a minor amount of fluid to the tear film. The meibomian glands lie in a parallel row in the tarsal plate of the upper and lower eyelids, perpendicular to the lid margin (Fig. 1-1). These glands secrete the lipid component of the tear film. The lacrimal gland is an almond-shaped, branched structure located beneath the conjunctiva at the anterior, lateral roof of the orbit. The accessory lacrimal glands of Krause and Wolfring are smaller, branched structures located on the upper and lower conjunctiva close to the conjunctival fornix. The lacrimal and accessory lacrimal glands contribute the aqueous portion of the tear film, which is composed of proteins, electrolytes, and water.

Meibomian Gland

Morphology and Ultrastructure

Meibomian glands are sebaceous tubular glands and are the major contributors to the lipid layer of the tear film. Excellent descriptions of meibomian gland physiology and ultrastructure can be found in reviews by Tiffany (151) and Jester, et al. (152), respectively. (See also Chapter 27 for an additional discussion of the meibomian gland.) As illustrated in Fig. 1-1, the main duct of each gland opens directly onto the inner margin of the eyelid near the mucocutaneous junction. This duct is located centrally within the gland and is lined with stratified squamous epithelial cells. The duct epithelium consists of a basal cell layer, an intermediate layer, and superficial horny cell layer. The basal cell layer rests on a basal lamina and consists of a single layer of cuboidal to columnar-shaped cells. These cells are characterized by a high nucleus/cytoplasm ratio with numerous cytoplasmic tonofilaments, as well as membrane-associated desmosomes, and hemidesmosomes. Overlying the basal cells are one or two layers of intermediate cells with a somewhat less electron-dense cytoplasm containing fewer filamentous structures. The superficial horny cells are anuclear and contain a homogeneous, finely granular cytoplasm. Large, electron-dense inclusions with the appearance of keratohyaline granules are also present in this layer. Indirect immunofluorescence studies of keratin expression in ductal epithelium of the human meibomian gland (153) indicate that keratins recognized by antibodies AE1 and AE3 are expressed in all duct epithelial cells. The keratin recognized by antibody AE2, which acts as a marker for fully keratinized epithelia, binds the suprabasal,

but not basal, cells of the central duct, suggesting that the ductal epithelium comprising the suprabasal layers is keratinized.

The large central duct branches multiple times, forming short ductules, which terminate in grapelike acini. Cells comprising the meibomian gland acini are organized into several distinct layers. Figure 1-17A illustrates the organization of epithelial cells comprising the meibomian gland acinus. Basal epithelial cells form the generative layer and do not contain lipid droplets. As these cells migrate toward the luminal surface, they begin to differentiate. Ultrastructural studies (153,154) have documented acinar cell differentiation in which the smooth endoplasmic reticulum and Golgi membranes become prominent and the first clear lipid droplets appear in the cytoplasm. These droplets have an onion-like structure consisting of membranous material organized in irregularly shaped, concentric lamellae, thus forming secretory granules (154,155). As the cells move toward the luminal surface, the number of lipid-containing secretory granules increases. Secretion occurs in a holocrine fashion in which mature cells at the luminal surface rupture, releasing both lipid and cell debris. Lipid secretions are stored in the ducts until blinking induces spreading of the lipid over the tear film (156). The composition of the lipid secretion of the meibomian gland has been described in detail by Nicolaides (157) and Tiffany (158). The major constituents of the lipid secretion are wax monoesters and sterol esters. Also present are diesters, diglycerides, free alcohols, free fatty acids, free sterols, hydrocarbons, monoglycerides, and polar lipids, including phospholipids and triglycerides (159).

Secretion Stimuli

It is suggested that secretion from the meibomian gland could be controlled by two methods (159). One is by regulating the rate of synthesis of lipid within the endoplasmic reticulum and Golgi apparatus, and the second is by regulating fusion of the secretory granules in the superficial acinar cells with the apical surface plasma membrane, thus releasing the lipid contents into the duct. Increasing evidence suggests that androgen sex steroids play an important role in regulating meibomian gland lipid synthesis and secretion. A review by Sullivan et al. (160) provides a strong argument that androgens play an important role in meibomian gland function and regulation of lipid secretion. Evidence implicating androgens in this regulation includes the finding that strong enzymatic activity of 3α-hydroxysteroid dehydrogenase, 3β-hydroxysteroid dehydrogenase, and 17β-hydroxysteroid dehydrogenase has been detected histochemically in the suprabasal acinar cells of the meibomian gland, indicating that these cells can metabolize androgens in a manner characteristic of target tissues (161). Human meibomian gland cells express messenger RNA (mRNA) for types 1 and 2 5α-reductase, an enzyme that converts testosterone and dehydroepiandrosterone to

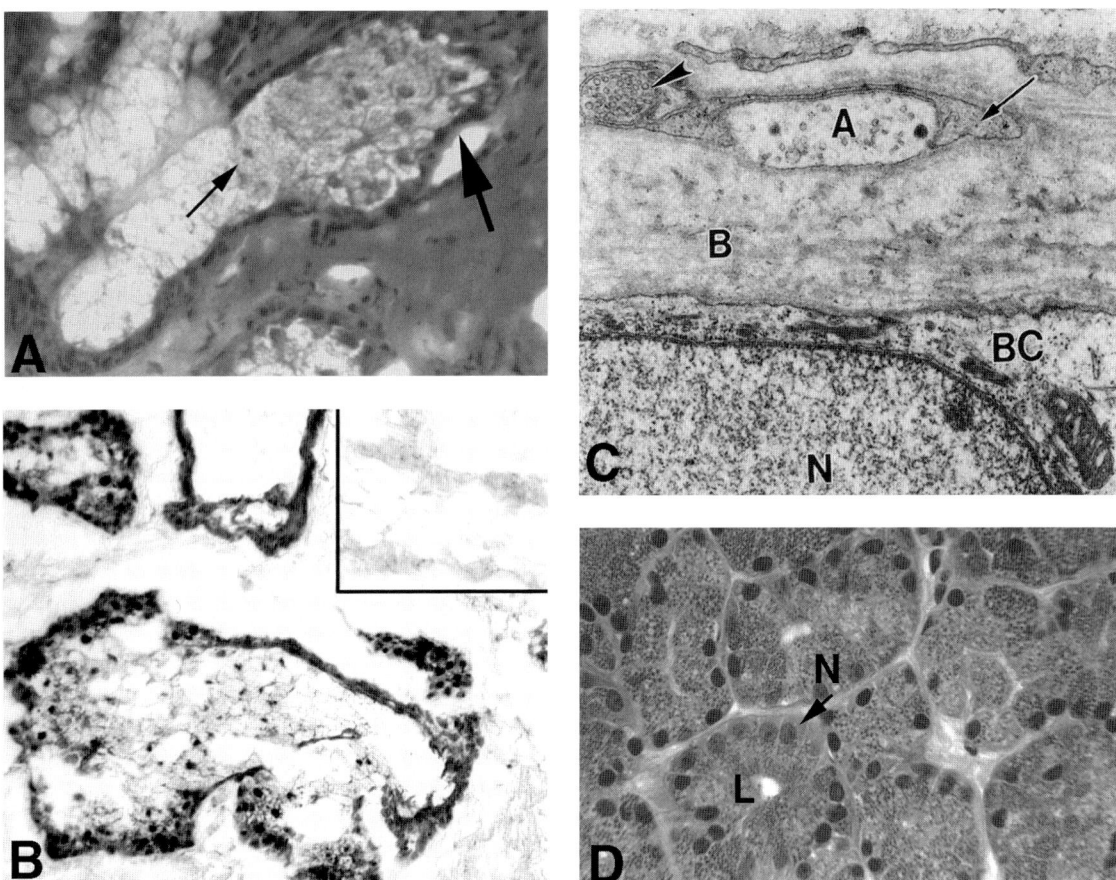

FIGURE 1-17. A: Section through the acinus of a human meibomian gland stained with hematoxylin-eosin. A single layer of basal epithelial cells (*large arrow*) gives rise to more differentiated suprabasal cells containing lipid droplets. The superficial, inner layer of cells (*small arrow*) ruptures in a holocrine fashion releasing both the lipid secretion and cell debris. (Original magnification, ×350.) **B:** Immunoperoxidase localization of androgen receptor protein in the nuclei of acinar cells of human meibomian gland. Tissue was obtained from a 70-year-old female donor. Tissue section in inset was preincubated with a peptide derived from a sequence of the androgen receptor not reactive with the primary anti-androgen receptor antibody. The *inset* shows an antibody specificity control. (Original magnification, ×240.) (From Rocha EM, Wickham LA, da Silveira LA, et al. Identification of androgen receptor protein and 5alpha-reductase mRNA in human ocular tissues. *Br J Ophthalmol* 2000;84:76–84.) **C:** Electron micrograph reveals the presence of axons within the basal lamina (B) associated with an acinar basal epithelial cell (BC) of the human meibomian gland. The axon (A) contains dense vesicles, while the axon indicated by the arrowhead contains clear vesicles, suggesting different types of neurotransmitters. *Arrow* indicates Schwann cell. N, nucleus. (Original magnification, ×30,000; Bar = 0.5 μm.) [From Seifert P, Spitznas M. Vasoactive intestinal polypeptide (VIP) innervation of the human eyelid glands. *Exp Eye Res* 1999;68:685–692.] **D:** Light micrograph of a section of human lacrimal gland showing acinar morphology. Epithelial cells are arranged concentrically with the apical aspect of the plasma membrane toward the lumen (L) of the secretory tubule. Secretory granules fill the cell and displace the nucleus (N) basally. (Original magnification, ×350.)

the potent metabolite, 5α-dihydrotestosterone. These glands also synthesize androgen receptor mRNA and, as shown in Fig. 1-17B, express androgen receptor protein within acinar cell nuclei (162). Androgens are known to regulate pathways of lipid metabolism in other sebaceous glands, providing additional evidence that they could play a role in regulating lipid secretion in the meibomian gland. In addition, studies indicate that treatment with topical androgens can alter the quality of meibomian lipids and stimulate the production and release of meibomian fluid (163), whereas androgen deficiency appears to be associated with meibomian gland dysfunction (160,164).

Neural stimulation may also help regulate lipid secretion from the meibomian gland. Ultrastructural analysis of human meibomian glands has revealed the presence of unmyelinated nerves and axons with both clear and dense core vesicles. As shown in Fig. 1-17C, these nerves are in direct contact with the multilamellar basal laminae of acinar epithelial cells, but are not internal to the basal lamina (165–167). Similar association of nerve fibers was observed by immunohistochemistry of neuron-specific enolase (168). Several types of nerves appear to innervate the meibomian gland, as indicated by the expression of a number of neuropeptides and neuronal enzymes. Nervelike structures in close apposition to the basement membrane of acinar basal epithelial cells are immunoreactive for vasoactive intestinal polypeptide (VIP) (165–167), neuropeptide Y (NPY) (165,167), and substance P (SP) (165). In addition, acetylcholinesterase reaction product has been detected in the nerve fibers surrounding acinar and ductal tissues (168). The abundant nerves associated with meibomian gland acini are probably parasympathetic because these nerves usually contain both VIP and acetylcholine (159). Sympathetic and sensory nerves appear to be more sparsely distributed and mainly located in association with the gland vasculature. For example, tyrosine hydroxylase, a marker for sympathetic nerves, has been localized mainly in vessels associated with the gland (165). NPY, which is usually contained in sympathetic nerves, appears to be distributed differently from tyrosine hydroxylase, suggesting that, in the meibomian gland, NPY-containing nerves are of parasympathetic origin (159). Exactly how neuronal stimulation would lead to lipid secretion is still under investigation.

Effects of Normal Aging on Meibomian Gland Morphology

A number of studies have been conducted to characterize age-related changes in the meibomian gland, thereby making it possible to distinguish normal from disease-related morphologic changes (169,170). Among the identified age-related changes are an increase in the frequency of narrowing of the duct orifice, atrophy of acini, thickening of the basement membrane associated with the acini, an increase in granulation tissue, and development of lipogranulomatous inflammation. There also appears to be an age-related change in the relative expressibility of lipid secretion (171). The ability to express lipid from meibomian glands appears to correlate with the relative thickness of the lipid layer of the tear film. Expressibility was negatively correlated with retraction of meibomian orifices, but not with elevated orifices, foam formation, tarsal cysts, or casts around the eyelashes. Together, hyperkeratinization of the ductal epithelium and atrophy of acinar cells is considered to play a role in the development of meibomian gland dysfunction (172,173).

Main Lacrimal Gland

Excellent descriptions of lacrimal gland structure can be found in reviews by Dartt and Sullivan (159) and Walcott (174). The main lacrimal gland in humans is the relative size and shape of an almond and forms a multilobar, tubuloacinar structure. As shown in the schematic in Fig. 1-1,

each lobe contains many branched tubules, forming a tree-like structure. When transversely sectioned across the tubule (Figs. 1-3 and 1-17D), the single layer of acinar cells is arranged circularly, surrounding a small lumen. The apical aspect of the acinar cells faces the lumen of the secretory tubule, whereas the basal side rests on basement membrane. Secretions from the acinar cells empty directly into the secretory tubules. These tubules converge to form an intralobular duct, which is lined by a single layer of cuboidal epithelial cells. The intralobular ducts drain secretions into larger interlobular ducts. These ducts have larger lumens and are lined by two layers of epithelial cells. The interlobular ducts form the 6 to 12 secretory ducts, which deliver the lacrimal gland secretions onto the ocular surface on the upper and lateral surfaces of the superior conjunctival fornix.

Acinar and Duct Epithelial Cell Structure and Function

The apical aspect of the plasma membrane is much narrower than the basal aspect and contains numerous microvilli to increase the surface area. The apical portion of the acinar cell cytoplasm is filled with membrane-bound secretory granules, which appear clear or dense depending on their specific contents. Because of the secretory nature of the acinar cells, there is a prominent endoplasmic reticulum and Golgi apparatus. These are located below the secretory granules, whereas the nucleus is displaced basally. Lateral membranes are highly folded to increase surface area. Individual cells comprising the acinus are polarized, and it is this polarity that forms the basis for the unidirectional delivery of secretory products into the lumen of the acinus. Polarity is achieved by the formation of tight junctions (*zonula occludens*) between adjacent cells. These junctions form a "belt" around the apical aspect of the lateral membranes, effectively separating the apical and basolateral surfaces and acting as a barrier to the free diffusion of molecules between the apical and basolateral surfaces. The specific nature and protein composition of tight junctional complexes in the acinar cells remain to be elucidated. Of interest is the discovery of a novel peripheral membrane protein, called junction-enriched and -associated protein. This protein colocalizes with the tight junction–associated protein, ZO-1, in acinar cells of mouse lacrimal gland, as well as in a number of other exocrine glands (175). What the specific function of this protein is and whether it is also expressed in human lacrimal gland is still to be determined. Anchoring junctions (*zonula adherens*) and desmosomes in the lateral membranes help strengthen cell–cell contacts (174). E-cadherin is a major component of the anchoring junction complex in these cells (176). Gap junctions facilitate cell–cell communication by permitting diffusion of small molecules, including ions, between cells. Various connexin isoforms are integral to the formation of gap junctions. Lacrimal gland acinar cells in both rat (177,178) and mouse (179) express connexin-32 and connexin-26; however, the specific isoforms expressed in human acinar cells is unknown. Functional gap junctions appear to be required for optimal fluid secretion of the lacrimal gland, possibly by facilitating a coordinated burst of secretion (179). Acinar cells in the lacrimal gland secrete a variety of proteins required for normal health and maintenance of the ocular surface. A list of proteins secreted by cells in the lacrimal gland can be found in Dartt and Sullivan (159). Recent data indicate that the small soluble mucin MUC7 is expressed by the lacrimal gland (180). Of note are the number of growth factors (including basic fibroblast growth factor, epidermal growth factor, hepatocyte growth factor, transforming growth factors-α, -$\beta1$, and -$\beta2$) and antibacterials contributed to the tear film by cells of the lacrimal gland.

The cuboidal epithelial cells of the ducts are polarized in a manner similar to that of the acinar cells, with the endoplasmic reticulum, Golgi apparatus, and mitochondria located apically and the nucleus in a more basal position (138). These cells contain fewer secretory granules than the acinar cells. Although they synthesize and secrete some protein components of the tears, their major contribution to tears is secretion of electrolytes and water.

Myoepithelial Cell Structure and Function

A dense basement membrane surrounds the acinar cells and consists of a loose assembly of collagen fibers. Myoepithelial cells are flat, stellate cells located in the basement membrane of both the acinar cells and cells of the intralobular ducts (181). Multiple processes from these cells surround the basal aspect of the acinar cells and the epithelial cells of the intralobular ducts. Particularly striking is the fact that myoepithelial cells cover approximately 80% of the basal surface of the intralobular ducts (174). Myoepithelial cells are considered to have a contractile function because they contain many microfilament bundles and express α-smooth muscle actin (182). They may be able to respond to neuronal stimulation because electron microscopy demonstrates the presence of nerve terminals, with the morphology expected for cholinergic, parasympathetic nerves, adjacent to myoepithelial cells in the ducts and basal regions of the acinar cells (181). Myoepithelial cells in monkey synthesize endothelin, a potent vasoconstrictor peptide with autocrine and paracrine function. They also express endothelin-A receptors (183). The specific function of myoepithelial cells is not currently understood. Their anatomy relative to the acinar cells and ducts suggests that their contraction might aide in the expulsion of fluid out of the secretory tubules or help maintain the patency of acinar and ductal lumens (183,184).

Immunomodulatory Cells

In the lacrimal gland, scattered among the secretory tubules, are small groups of immunomodulatory cells (185,186).

Plasma cells represent greater than 50% of immunomodulatory cells in the lacrimal gland. The major secretion of these cells is immunoglobulin A (IgA). IgA is secreted into the interstitial space and then transported across the acinar and ductal epithelium to become a component of tears. In addition to IgA, plasma cells secrete IgG, IgM, IgE, and IgD. Among the other immunomodulatory cells located in the interstitial space of the lacrimal gland are lymphocytes, helper and suppressor T cells, B cells, dendritic cells, macrophages, and mast cells.

Innervation

Nerves appear to play an important role in the stimulation of regulated protein secretion. Details regarding neuronal stimulation and the specific transmembrane signaling pathways that lead to protein secretion can be found in reviews by Dartt and Sullivan (159), Walcott (174), and Dartt (187), and in Chapter 27 in this volume. Studies of lacrimal gland in humans, as well as in other species, indicate that the gland receives parasympathetic, sympathetic, and sensory innervation (181). Parasympathetic nerves are predominant in the lacrimal gland and form a network of fibers associated with the acinar cells (188). Fiber density suggests that not every acinar cell is directly innervated; however, gap junctions between the cells could facilitate dissemination of the stimulatory signal throughout the acinus (159). Interlobular ducts and blood vessels in the lacrimal gland are also innervated by parasympathetic nerves (159,189). Immunohistochemical studies have demonstrated that parasympathetic nerves associated with acinar cells and in the interstitial connective tissue contain VIP (166,190) and/or acetylcholine (159,174,191). Nerve fibers containing enkephalins surround acini and ducts, but do not appear to be associated with blood vessels in the gland (192,193). The relative distribution of enkephalin-containing fibers suggests that they are also of parasympathetic origin (159). Sympathetic nerves are less frequent, but appear to be associated with acinar and ductal cells, as well as the vasculature in the lacrimal gland. These nerves contain the sympathetic neurotransmitter, norepinephrine (174). Nerves containing NPY have the same relative distribution as those containing norepinephrine (189), suggesting that sympathetic nerves in lacrimal gland contain both neurotransmitters (159). Sensory nerves are also present in the lacrimal gland, but are more sparsely distributed. CGRP and SP have been immunolocalized to blood vessels in the interlobular connective tissue (190,194). CGRP-containing fibers are also associated with interlobular duct epithelia (189). Studies using a rabbit model (195) have demonstrated that sensory denervation results in pronounced effects on the structure of the lacrimal gland, resulting in a massive accumulation of secretory granules in the acinar cells. In addition, pharmacologic responsiveness of the gland was altered. In the same study, similar effects were not observed with sympathetic denervation.

Hormonal Regulation

Hormones play an important role in stimulating the secretion of constitutive secretory proteins, as well as in the growth and differentiation of cells of the lacrimal gland (196,197). A number of hormones appear to contribute to the maintenance of normal lacrimal gland structure and secretory function. These include α-melanocyte–stimulating hormone, adrenocorticotropic hormone, luteinizing hormone, follicle-stimulating hormone, growth hormone, thyroid-stimulating hormone, prolactin, thyroxine, androgens, estrogens, and progestins (159). Of these, androgen appears to be among the most potent. This steroid hormone stimulates protein secretion and appears to be responsible for a number of sex-related differences observed in the lacrimal gland. Immunostaining has demonstrated the presence of androgen receptors in the nucleus and cytoplasm of epithelial cells of acinar and ductal cells in human lacrimal gland (162,198), as well as in the lacrimal glands of other species (162). Studies using a rabbit model indicate that a critical level of androgens is necessary for maintaining lacrimal gland structure and function (199). A decrease from this critical level results in necrosis of interstitial cells, as well as increased lymphocytic infiltration. Changes in hormone levels appear to correlate with certain sex- and age-related changes in the lacrimal gland. For example, the thickness and area of the lacrimal gland decrease with age in women, but a similar decrease is not found in men (200,201). A table of identified sex-related differences in lacrimal gland and tear film composition can be found in Dartt and Sullivan (159).

Accessory Lacrimal Glands (Glands of Kraus and Wolfring)

The accessory lacrimal glands of Kraus and Wolfring are located close to the conjunctival fornix and at the edge of the upper tarsus. The total mass of the accessory glands is approximately 10% of the mass of the main lacrimal gland (202). Each accessory gland is an individual "organ" with its own connective tissue coat and excretory duct (203). The single excretory duct branches to form intralobular ducts, which lead to the secretory epithelium. These glands are tubular glands and do not contain true acini. Cells of the tubules contain secretory granules. The secretory tubules and, to a lesser extent, the intralobular ducts are associated with myoepithelial cells. These glands appear to be innervated in that axons of nonmyelinated fibers make close contact with secretory cells, as well as with the blood vessels and other cells in the connective tissue. Axons with parasympathetic and sympathetic characteristics are associated with the secretory epithelium, myoepithelial cells, and vasculature in the gland. Most of the axons in the accessory lacrimal glands exhibit morphologic characteristics typical of parasympathetic nerves (204).

ACKNOWLEDGMENTS

The authors gratefully acknowledge Ann Tisdale, who did the light and electron microscopy, and Gale Unger, Sandra Spurr-Michaud, and Audrey Hutcheon for their assistance with the manuscript.

REFERENCES

1. Hogan MJ, Alvarado JA, Wedell JE. *Histology of the human eye*. Philadelphia: WB Saunders, 1971.
2. Jakobiec FA, Ozanics V. General topographic anatomy of the eye. In: Jakobiec FA, ed. *Ocular anatomy, embryology and teratology*. Philadelphia: Harper & Row, 1982:1–9.
3. Maus M. Basic eyelid anatomy. In: Albert DM, Jakobiec FA, eds. *Principles and practice of ophthalmology: clinical practice*. Philadelphia: WB Saunders, 1994:1689–1692.
4. Maurice DM. *The cornea and the sclera*. London: Academic Press, 1985.
5. Warwick R. *Eugene Wolff's anatomy of the eye and orbit*, 8th ed. London: Chapman & Hall Medical, 1997:235.
6. Hanna C, O'Brien JE. Cell production and migration in the epithelial layer of the cornea. *Arch Ophthalmol* 1960;64:536.
7. Beebe DC, Masters BR. Cell lineage and the differentiation of corneal epithelial cells. *Invest Ophthalmol Vis Sci* 1996;37:1815–1825.
8. Gipson IK, Spurr-Michaud SJ, Tisdale AS. Anchoring fibrils form a complex network in human and rabbit cornea. *Invest Ophthalmol Vis Sci* 1987;28:212–220.
9. Doran TI, Vidrich A, Sun T-T. Intrinsic and extrinsic regulation of the differentiation of skin, corneal and esophageal epithelial cells. *Cell* 1980;22:17–25.
10. Kurpakus MA, Stock EL, Jones JCR. Expression of the 55-kD/64-kD corneal keratins in ocular surface epithelium. *Invest Ophthalmol Vis Sci* 1990;31:448–456.
11. Sun T-T, Green H. Cultured epithelial cells of cornea, conjunctiva and skin: absence of marked intrinsic divergence of their differentiated states. *Nature* 1976;269:489.
12. Schermer A, Galvin S, Sun TT. Differentiation-related expression of a major 64K corneal keratin in vivo and in culture suggests limbal location of corneal epithelial stem cells. *J Cell Biol* 1986;103:49–62.
13. Shiraishi A, Converse RL, Liu CY, et al. Identification of the cornea-specific keratin 12 promoter by in vivo particle-mediated gene transfer. *Invest Ophthalmol Vis Sci* 1998;39:2554–2561.
14. Gipson IK, Anderson RA. Actin filaments in normal and migrating corneal epithelial cells. *Invest Ophthalmol Vis Sci* 1977;16:161–166.
15. Sax CM, Salamon C, Kays WT, et al. Transketolase is a major protein in the mouse cornea. *J Biol Chem* 1996;271:33568–33574.
16. Williams K, Watsky M. Gap junctional communication in the human corneal endothelium and epithelium. *Curr Eye Res* 2002;25:29–36.
17. Langbein L, Grund C, Kuhn C, et al. Tight junctions and compositionally related junctional structures in mammalian stratified epithelia and cell cultures derived therefrom. *Eur J Cell Biol* 2002;81:419–435.
18. Gipson IK, Sugrue SP. Cell biology of the corneal epithelium. In: Albert DM, Jakobiec FA, eds. *Principles and practice of ophthalmology: basic sciences*. Philadelphia: WB Saunders, 1994:3–16.

19. Lohman LE, Rao GN, Tripathi RC, et al. In vivo specular microscopy of edematous human corneal epithelium with light and scanning electron microscopic correlation. *Ophthalmology* 1982;89:621–629.
20. Pfister RR. The normal surface of corneal epithelium: a scanning electron microscopic study. *Invest Ophthalmol Vis Sci* 1973;12:656–658.
21. Nichols BA, Chiappino ML, Dawson CR. Demonstration of the mucous layer of the tear film by electron microscopy. *Invest Ophthalmol Vis Sci* 1985;26:464–473.
22. Gipson IK, Yankauckas M, Spurr-Michaud SJ, et al. Characteristics of a glycoprotein in the ocular surface glycocalyx. *Invest Ophthalmol Vis Sci* 1992;33:218-227.
23. Gipson IK, Argüeso P. Role of mucins in the function of the corneal and conjunctival epithelia. *Int Rev Cytol* 2003;231:1–49.
24. Argüeso P, Gipson IK. Epithelial mucins of the ocular surface: structure, biosynthesis and function. *Exp Eye Res* 2001;73:281–289.
25. Danjo Y, Watanabe H, Tisdale AS, et al. Alteration of mucin in human conjunctival epithelia in dry eye. *Invest Ophthalmol Vis Sci* 1998;39:2602–2609.
26. Argüeso P, Spurr-Michaud S, Russo CL, et al. MUC16 mucin is expressed by the human ocular surface epithelia and carries the H185 carbohydrate epitope. *Invest Ophthalmol Vis Sci* 2003;44:2487–2495.
27. Gipson IK, Spurr-Michaud S, Argüeso P, et al. Mucin gene expression in immortalized human corneal-limbal and conjunctival epithelial cell lines. *Invest Ophthalmol Vis Sci* 2003;44:2496–2506.
28. Hori Y, Spurr-Michaud S, Rheinwald JG, et al. Regulation of MUC4 gene expression in TERT-immortalized human conjunctival epithelial cells. *Invest Ophthalmol Vis Sci* 2002;E-Abstract, 3162.
29. Gipson IK. The epithelial basement membrane zone of the limbus. *Eye* 1989;3:132–140.
30. Stepp MA, Spurr-Michaud S, Tisdale A, et al. Alpha 6 beta 4 integrin heterodimer is a component of hemidesmosomes. *Proc Natl Acad Sci U S A* 1990;87:8970–8974.
31. Sakai LY, Keene DR, Morris NP, et al. Type VII collagen is a major structural component of anchoring fibrils. *J Cell Biol* 1986;103:1577–1586.
32. Lunstrum GP, Sakai LY, Keene DR, et al. Large complex globular domains of type VII procollagen contribute to the structure of anchoring fibrils. *J Biol Chem* 1986;261:9042–9048.
33. Woodley DT, Sarret Y, Briggaman RA. Autoimmunity to type VII collagen. *Semin Dermatol* 1991;10:232–239.
34. Foulks GN, Thoft RA, Perry HD, et al. Factors related to corneal epithelial complications after closed vitrectomy in diabetics. *Arch Ophthalmol* 1979;97:1076–1078.
35. Azar DT, Spurr-Michaud SJ, Tisdale AS, et al. Decreased penetration of anchoring fibrils into the diabetic stroma: a morphometric analysis. *Arch Ophthalmol* 1989;107:1520–1523.
36. Rodrigues MM, Waring G III, Hackett J, et al. Cornea. In: Jakobiec FA, ed. *Ocular anatomy, embryology, and teratology*. Philadelphia: Harper & Row, 1982.
37. Tisdale AS, Spurr-Michaud SJ, Rodrigues M, et al. Development of the anchoring structures of the epithelium in rabbit and human fetal corneas. *Invest Ophthalmol Vis Sci* 1988;29:727–736.
38. Wilson SE, Hong JW. Bowman's layer structure and function: critical or dispensable to corneal function? A hypothesis. *Cornea* 2000;19:417–420.
39. Sakai LY, Keene DR, Engvall E. Fibrillin, a new 350-kD glycoprotein, is a component of extracellular microfibrils. *J Cell Biol* 1986;103:2499–2509.
40. Kuwabara T. The corneal stromal cell. In: Yamada E, Mishima S, eds. *The structure of the eye: proceedings of the 3rd Symposium on the Structure of the Eye*. Yamanashi, Japan. 1975:39–47.
41. Ueda A, Nishida T, Otori T, et al. Electron-microscopic studies on the presence of gap junctions between corneal fibroblasts in rabbits. *Cell Tissue Res* 1987;249:473–475.
42. Hamrah P, Liu Y, Zhang Q, et al. The corneal stroma is endowed with a significant number of resident dendritic cells. *Invest Ophthalmol Vis Sci* 2003;44:581–589.
43. Birk DE, Trelstad RL. Extracellular compartments in matrix morphogenesis: collagen fibril, bundle, and lamellar formation by corneal fibroblasts. *J Cell Biol* 1984;99:2024–2033.
44. Alvarado J, Murphy C, Juster R. Age-related changes in the basement membrane of the human corneal epithelium. *Invest Ophthalmol Vis Sci* 1983;24:1015–1028.
45. Sabet MD, Gordon SR. Ultrastructural immunocytochemical localization of fibronectin deposition during corneal endothelial wound repair. evidence for cytoskeletal involvement. *Biol Cell* 1989;65:171–179.
46. Marshall GE, Konstas AG, Lee WR. Immunogold fine structural localization of extracellular matrix components in aged human cornea: I. types I–IV collagen and laminin. *Graefes Arch Clin Exp Ophthalmol* 1991;229:157–163.
47. Nakayasu K, Tanaka M, Konomi H, et al. Distribution of types I, II, III, IV and V collagen in normal and keratoconus corneas. *Ophthalmic Res* 1986;18:1–10.
48. Kapoor R, Sakai LY, Funk S, et al. Type VIII collagen has a restricted distribution in specialized extracellular matrices. *J Cell Biol* 1988;107:721–730.
49. Davies Y, Lewis D, Fullwood NJ, et al. Proteoglycans on normal and migrating human corneal endothelium. *Exp Eye Res* 1999;68:303–311.
50. Linsenmayer TF. Collagen. In: Hay ED, ed. *Cell biology of the extracellular matrix*. New York: Plenum Press, 1981:5–37.
51. Miller EJ, Gay S. Collagen: an overview. *Methods Enzymol* 1982;82:3–32.
52. van der Rest M, Garrone R. Collagen family of proteins. *FASEB J* 1991;5:2814–2823.
53. Exposito JY, Cluzel C, Garrone R, et al. Evolution of collagens. *Anat Rec* 2002;268:302–316.
54. Boot-Handford RP, Tuckwell DS. Fibrillar collagen: the key to vertebrate evolution? A tale of molecular incest. *Bioessays* 2003;25:142–151.
55. Robert L, Legeais JM, Robert AM, et al. Corneal collagens. *Pathol Biol (Paris)* 2001;49:353–363.
56. Lin HC, Chang JH, Jain S, et al. Matrilysin cleavage of corneal collagen type XVIII NC1 domain and generation of a 28-kDa fragment. *Invest Ophthalmol Vis Sci* 2001;42:2517–2524.
57. Kadrofske MM, Openo KP, Wang JL. The human LGALS3 (galectin-3) gene: determination of the gene structure and functional characterization of the promoter. *Arch Biochem Biophys* 1998;349:7–20.
58. Tanihara H, Inatani M, Koga T, et al. Proteoglycans in the eye. *Cornea* 2002;21:S62–S69.
59. Maurice DM, Riley MV. The cornea. In: Graymore CN, ed. *Biochemistry of the eye*. New York: Academic Press, 1970.
60. Corpuz LM, Funderburgh JL, Funderburgh ML, et al. Molecular cloning and tissue distribution of keratocan: bovine corneal keratan sulfate proteoglycan 37A. *J Biol Chem* 1996;271:9759–9763.
61. Holt WS, Kinoshita JH. The soluble proteins of the bovine cornea. *Invest Ophthalmol* 1973;12:114–126.
62. Birk DE. Type V collagen: heterotypic type I/V collagen interactions in the regulation of fibril assembly. *Micron* 2001;32:223–237.

63. Rada JA, Cornuet PK, Hassell JR. Regulation of corneal collagen fibrillogenesis in vitro by corneal proteoglycan (lumican and decorin) core proteins. *Exp Eye Res* 1993;56:635–648.

64. Chakravarti S, Petroll WM, Hassell JR, et al. Corneal opacity in lumican-null mice: defects in collagen fibril structure and packing in the posterior stroma. *Invest Ophthalmol Vis Sci* 2000;41:3365–3373.

65. Pellegata NS, Dieguez-Lucena JL, Joensuu T, et al. Mutations in KERA, encoding keratocan, cause cornea plana. *Nat Genet* 2000;25:91–95.

66. Suzuki K, Saito J, Yanai R, et al. Cell-matrix and cell-cell interactions during corneal epithelial wound healing. *Prog Retin Eye Res* 2003;22:113–133.

67. Lu L, Reinach PS, Kao WW. Corneal epithelial wound healing. *Exp Biol Med* 2001;226:653–664.

68. Wilson SE. Role of apoptosis in wound healing in the cornea. *Cornea* 2000;19:S7–S12.

69. Fini ME. Keratocyte and fibroblast phenotypes in the repairing cornea. *Prog Retin Eye Res* 1999;18:529–551.

70. Zieske JD, Gipson IK. Agents that affect corneal wound healing: modulation of structure and function. In: Albert DM, Jakobiec FA, eds. *Principles and practice of ophthalmology*, 2nd ed. Vol 1. Philadelphia: WB Saunders, 2000:364–372.

71. Zieske JD. Extracellular matrix and wound healing. *Curr Opin Ophthalmol* 2001;12:237–241.

72. Wilson SE, Mohan RR, Hutcheon AE, et al. Effect of ectopic epithelial tissue within the stroma on keratocyte apoptosis, mitosis, and myofibroblast transformation. *Exp Eye Res* 2003;76:193–201.

73. Zieske JD, Guimaraes SR, Hutcheon AE. Kinetics of keratocyte proliferation in response to epithelial debridement. *Exp Eye Res* 2001;72:33–39.

74. Mohan RR, Hutcheon AE, Choi R, et al. Apoptosis, necrosis, proliferation, and myofibroblast generation in the stroma following LASIK and PRK. *Exp Eye Res* 2003;76:71–87.

75. Jester JV, Petroll WM, Cavanagh HD. Corneal stromal wound healing in refractive surgery: the role of myofibroblasts. *Prog Retin Eye Res* 1999;18:311–356.

76. Waring GO, 3rd, Bourne WM, Edelhauser HF, et al. The corneal endothelium: normal and pathologic structure and function. *Ophthalmology* 1982;89:531–590.

77. Svedbergh B, Bill A. Scanning electron microscopic studies of the corneal endothelium in man and monkeys. *Acta Ophthalmol (Copenh)* 1972;50:321–336.

78. Kreutziger GO. Lateral membrane morphology and gap junction structure in rabbit corneal endothelium. *Exp Eye Res* 1976;23:285–293.

79. Montcourrier P, Hirsch M. Intercellular junctions in the developing rat corneal endothelium. *Ophthalmic Res* 1985;17:207–215.

80. Gordon SR, Essner E, Rothstein H. In situ demonstration of actin in normal and injured ocular tissues using 7-nitrobenz-2-oxa-1,3-diazole phallacidin. *Cell Motil* 1982;2:343–354.

81. Petroll WM, Jester JV, Barry-Lane P, et al. Assessment of f-actin organization and apical-basal polarity during in vivo cat endothelial wound healing. *Invest Ophthalmol Vis Sci* 1995;36:2492–2502.

82. Hirsch M, Renard G, Faure JP, et al. Study of the ultrastructure of the rabbit corneal endothelium by the freeze-fracture technique: apical and lateral junctions. *Exp Eye Res* 1977;25:277–288.

83. Stiemke MM, McCartney MD, Cantu-Crouch D, et al. Maturation of the corneal endothelial tight junction. *Invest Ophthalmol Vis Sci* 1991;32:2757–2765.

84. Barry PA, Petroll WM, Andrews PM, et al. The spatial organization of corneal endothelial cytoskeletal proteins and their relationship to the apical junctional complex. *Invest Ophthalmol Vis Sci* 1995;36:1115–1124.

85. Joyce NC, Harris DL, Zieske JD. Mitotic inhibition of corneal endothelium in neonatal rats. *Invest Ophthalmol Vis Sci* 1998;39:2572–2583.

86. Iwamoto T, Smelser GK. Electron microscopy of the human corneal endothelium with reference to transport mechanisms. *Invest Ophthalmol* 1965;4:270.

87. Leuenberger PM. Lanthanum hydroxide tracer studies on rat corneal endothelium. *Exp Eye Res* 1973;15:85–91.

88. Rae JL, Lewno AW, Cooper K, et al. Dye and electrical coupling between cells of the rabbit corneal endothelium. *Curr Eye Res* 1989;8:859–869.

89. Petroll WM, Hsu JK, Bean J, et al. The spatial organization of apical junctional complex-associated proteins in feline and human corneal endothelium. *Curr Eye Res* 1999;18:10–19.

90. Ickes R, Harris DL, Joyce NC. "Classical" cadherin expression in corneal endothelium. *Invest Ophthalmol Vis Sci* 2002;E-abstract, 3190.

91. Sakamoto T, Nakashima Y, Sueishi K. The effect of thrombin on actin filaments and vinculin of corneal endothelial cells. *Invest Ophthalmol Vis Sci* 1993;34:438–446.

92. Hamanaka T, Thornell LE, Bill A. Cytoskeleton and tissue origin in the anterior cynomolgus monkey eye. *Jpn J Ophthalmol* 1997;41:138–149.

93. Rayner SA, Gallop JL, George AJ, et al. Distribution of integrins alpha v beta 5, alpha v beta 3 and alpha v in normal human cornea: possible implications in clinical and therapeutic adenoviral infection. *Eye* 1998;12:273–277.

94. Maurice DM. The location of the fluid pump in the cornea. *J Physiol (Lond)* 1972;221:43–54.

95. Hodson S, Miller F. The bicarbonate ion pump in the endothelium which regulates the hydration of rabbit cornea. *J Physiol (Lond)* 1976;263:563–577.

96. Maurice DM. The structure and transparency of the cornea. *J Physiol (Lond)* 1957;136:263.

97. Dikstein S, Maurice D. The metabolic basis to the fluid pump in the cornea. *J Physiol (Lond)* 1972;221:29–41.

98. Hamann S, Zeuthen T, La Cour M, et al. Aquaporins in complex tissues: distribution of aquaporins 1-5 in human and rat eye. *Am J Physiol* 1998;274:C1332–C1345.

99. Thiagarajah JR, Verkman AS. Aquaporin deletion in mice reduces corneal water permeability and delays restoration of transparency after swelling. *J Biol Chem* 2002;277:19139–19144.

100. Johnston MC, Noden DM, Hazelton RD, et al. Origins of avian ocular and periocular tissues. *Exp Eye Res* 1979;29:27–43.

101. Adamis AP, Molnar ML, Tripathi BJ, et al. Neuronal-specific enolase in human corneal endothelium and posterior keratocytes. *Exp Eye Res* 1985;41:665–668.

102. Murphy C, Alvarado J, Juster R, et al. Prenatal and postnatal cellularity of the human corneal endothelium: a quantitative histologic study. *Invest Ophthalmol Vis Sci* 1984;25:312–322.

103. Joyce NC, Meklir B, Joyce SJ, et al. Cell cycle protein expression and proliferative status in human corneal cells. *Invest Ophthalmol Vis Sci* 1996;37:645–655.

104. Wilson SE, Weng J, Blair S, et al. Expression of E6/E7 or SV40 large T antigen-coding oncogenes in human corneal endothelial cells indicates regulated high-proliferative capacity. *Invest Ophthalmol Vis Sci* 1995;36:32–40.

105. Senoo T, Joyce NC. Cell cycle kinetics in corneal endothelium from old and young donors. *Invest Ophthalmol Vis Sci* 2000;41:660–667.

106. Chen KH, Harris DL, Joyce NC. TGF-β2 in aqueous humor suppresses S-phase entry in cultured corneal endothelial cells. *Invest Ophthalmol Vis Sci* 1999;40:2513–2519.

107. Joyce NC, Harris DL, Mello DM. Mechanisms of mitotic inhibition in corneal endothelium: contact inhibition and TGF-β2. *Invest Ophthalmol Vis Sci* 2002;43:2152–2159.

108. Joyce NC. Proliferative capacity of the corneal endothelium. *Prog Retin Eye Res* 2003;22:359–389.

109. Bourne WM, Nelson LR, Hodge DO. Central corneal endothelial cell changes over a ten-year period. *Invest Ophthalmol Vis Sci* 1997;38:779–782.

110. Müller LJ, Marfurt CF, Kruse F, et al. Corneal nerves: structure, contents and function. *Exp Eye Res* 2003;76:521–542.

111. Rozsa AJ, Beuerman RW. Density and organization of free nerve endings in the corneal epithelium of the rabbit. *Pain* 1982;14:105–120.

112. Torczynski E. Sclera. In: Jakobiec FA, ed. *Ocular anatomy, embryology and teratology*. Philadelphia: Harper and Row, 1982:587–599.

113. Srinivasan BD, Jakobiec FA, Iwamoto T. Conjunctiva. In: Jakobiec FA, ed. *Ocular anatomy, embryology, and teratology*. Philadelphia: Harper & Row, 1982:733–766.

114. Zieske JD. Perpetuation of stem cells in the eye. *Eye* 1994;8 (Pt 2):163–169.

115. Daniels JT, Dart JK, Tuft SJ, et al. Corneal stem cells in review. *Wound Repair Regen* 2001;9:483–494.

116. Dua HS, Azuara-Blanco A. Limbal stem cells of the corneal epithelium. *Surv Ophthalmol* 2000;44:415–425.

117. Watt FM, Hogan BL. Out of Eden: stem cells and their niches. *Science* 2000;287:1427–1430.

118. Alison MR, Poulsom R, Forbes S, et al. An introduction to stem cells. *J Pathol* 2002;197:419–423.

119. Slack JM. Stem cells in epithelial tissues. *Science* 2000;287:1431–1433.

120. Potten CS, Morris RJ. Epithelial stem cells in vivo. *J Cell Sci* 1988;10[Suppl]:45–62.

121. Hall PA, Watt FM. Stem cells: the generation and maintenance of cellular diversity. *Development* 1989;106:619–633.

122. Davanger M, Evensen A. Role of the pericorneal papillary structure in renewal of corneal epithelium. *Nature* 1971;229:560–561.

123. Nagasaki T, Zhao J. Centripetal movement of corneal epithelial cells in the normal adult mouse. *Invest Ophthalmol Vis Sci* 2003;44:558–566.

124. Collinson JM, Morris L, Reid AI, et al. Clonal analysis of patterns of growth, stem cell activity, and cell movement during the development and maintenance of the murine corneal epithelium. *Dev Dyn* 2002;224:432–440.

125. Cotsarelis G, Cheng SZ, Dong G, et al. Existence of slow-cycling limbal epithelial basal cells that can be preferentially stimulated to proliferate: implications on epithelial stem cells. *Cell* 1989;57:201–209.

126. Ebato B, Friend J, Thoft RA. Comparison of limbal and peripheral human corneal epithelium in tissue culture. *Invest Ophthalmol Vis Sci* 1988;29:1533–1537.

127. Lindberg K, Brown ME, Chaves HV, et al. In vitro propagation of human ocular surface epithelial cells for transplantation. *Invest Ophthalmol Vis Sci* 1993;34:2672–2679.

128. Kenyon KR, Tseng SC. Limbal autograft transplantation for ocular surface disorders. *Ophthalmology* 1989;96:709–722; discussion 722–703.

129. Huang AJ, Tseng SC. Corneal epithelial wound healing in the absence of limbal epithelium. *Invest Ophthalmol Vis Sci* 1991;32:96–105.

130. Zhou S, Schuetz JD, Bunting KD, et al. The ABC transporter Bcrp1/ABCG2 is expressed in a wide variety of stem cells and is a molecular determinant of the side-population phenotype. *Nat Med* 2001;7:1028–1034.

131. Budak MT, Akinci MA, Wolosin JM. Ocular surface epithelial cells express the MDR transporter ABCG2 and thus can be iso-

lated as a side population following staining with bisbenzimide. *Invest Ophthalmol Vis Sci* 2003;E-abstract, 859.

132. de Paiva CS, Li D, Kim H, et al. ABCG2 transporter, a potential molecular marker to identify human corneal epithelial stem cells. *Invest Ophthalmol Vis Sci* 2003;E-abstract, 2032.

133. Schofield R. The stem cell system. *Biomed Pharmacother* 1983;37:375–380.

134. Thoft RA, Friend J. The X,Y,Z hypothesis of corneal epithelial maintenance. *Invest Ophthalmol Vis Sci* 1983;24:1442–1443.

135. Kinoshita S, Friend J, Thoft RA. Sex chromatin of donor corneal epithelium in rabbits. *Invest Ophthalmol Vis Sci* 1981;21:434–441.

136. Kinoshita S, Kiorpes TC, Friend J, et al. Limbal epithelium in ocular surface wound healing. *Invest Ophthalmol Vis Sci* 1982;23:73–80.

137. SundarRaj N, Chao J, Gregory JD, et al. Ocular distribution of keratan sulfates during pre- and post-natal development in rabbits. *J Histochem Cytochem* 1986;34:971–976.

138. Jakobiec FA, Iwamoto T. The ocular adnexa: lids, conjunctiva, and orbit. In: Fine BS, Yanoff M, eds. *Ocular histology*. Philadelphia: Harper & Row, 1979:290.

139. Kessing SV. Mucous gland system of the conjunctiva. *Acta Ophthalmol* 1968;95[Suppl]:9–131.

140. Pellegrini G, Golisano O, Paterna P, et al. Location and clonal analysis of stem cells and their differentiated progeny in the human ocular surface. *J Cell Biol* 1999;145:769–782.

141. Wei Z-B, Cotsarelis G, Sun T-T, et al. Label-retaining cells are preferentially located in fornical epithelium: Implications for conjunctival epithelial homeostasis. *Invest Ophthalmol Vis Sci* 1995;36:236–246.

142. Dilly PN. On the nature and the role of the subsurface vesicles in the outer epithelial cells of the conjunctiva. *Br J Ophthalmol* 1985;69:477–481.

143. Greiner JV, Weidman TA, Korb DR, et al. Histochemical analysis of secretory vesicles in nongoblet conjunctival epithelial cells. *Acta Ophthalmol (Copenh)* 1985;63:89–92.

144. Zimianski MC, Dawson CR, Togni B. Epithelial cell phagocytosis of *Listeria monocytogenes* in the conjunctiva. *Invest Ophthalmol* 1974;13:623–626.

145. Latkovic S, Nilsson SE. Phagocytosis of latex microspheres by the epithelial cells of the guinea pig conjunctiva. *Acta Ophthalmol (Copenh)* 1979;57:582–590.

146. Inatomi T, Spurr-Michaud S, Tisdale AS, et al. Expression of secretory mucin genes by human conjunctival epithelia. *Invest Ophthalmol Vis Sci* 1996;37:1684–1692.

147. Paz et al. The role of calcium in mucin packaging within goblet cells. *Exp Eye Res* 2003;77:69–75.

148. Argüeso P, Balaram M, Spurr-Michaud S, et al. Decreased levels of the goblet cell mucin MUC5AC in tears of patients with Sjögren's syndrome. *Invest Ophthalmol Vis Sci* 2002;43:1004–1011.

149. Wei Z-G, Lin T, Sun T-T, et al. Clonal analysis of the in vivo differentiation potential of keratinocytes. *Invest Ophthalmol Vis Sci* 1997;38:753–761.

150. Jakobiec FA, Iwamoto T. Ocular adnexa: introduction to lids, conjunctiva and orbit. In: Jakobiec FA, ed. *Ocular anatomy, embryology, and teratology*. Philadelphia: Harper & Row, 1982:677–731.

151. Tiffany JM. Physiological functions of the meibomian glands. *Prog Retin Eye Res* 1995;14:47.

152. Jester JV, Nicolaides N, Smith RE. Meibomian gland studies: histologic and ultrastructural investigations. *Invest Ophthalmol Vis Sci* 1981;20:537–547.

153. Jester JV, Nicolaides N, Smith RE. Meibomian gland dysfunction. I. Keratin protein expression in normal human and rabbit meibomian glands. *Invest Ophthalmol Vis Sci* 1989;30:927–935.

154. Sirigu P, Shen RL, Pinto da Silva P. Human meibomian glands: the ultrastructure of acinar cells as viewed by thin section and freeze-fracture transmission electron microscopies. *Invest Ophthalmol Vis Sci* 1992;33:2284–2292.

155. Niizuma K. Lipid droplet of sebaceous carcinoma: electron microscopic study utilizing glycol methacrylate-glutaraldehyde-urea procedure. *Arch Dermatol Res* 1977;260:111–119.

156. Linton RG. The meibomian glands: an investigation into the secretion and some aspects of the physiology. *Br J Ophthalmol* 1961;45:718.

157. Nicolaides N. Recent findings on the chemical composition of the lipids of steer and human meibomian glands. In: Holly FJ, ed. *The preocular tear film: in health, disease and contact lens wear.* Lubbock, TX: Dry Eye Institute. 1986:570–596.

158. Tiffany JM. The lipid secretion of the meibomian glands. *Adv Lipid Res* 1987;22:1–62.

159. Dartt DA, Sullivan DA. Wetting of the ocular surface. In: Albert DM, Jakobiec FA, eds. *Principles and practice of ophthalmology*, 2nd ed. Vol 2. Philadelphia: WB Saunders, 2000: 960–981.

160. Sullivan DA, Sullivan BD, Evans JE, et al. Androgen deficiency, meibomian gland dysfunction, and evaporative dry eye. *Ann NY Acad Sci* 2002;966:211–222.

161. Perra MT, Lantini MS, Serra A, et al. Human meibomian glands: a histochemical study for androgen metabolic enzymes. *Invest Ophthalmol Vis Sci* 1990;31:771–775.

162. Rocha EM, Wickham LA, da Silveira LA, et al. Identification of androgen receptor protein and 5alpha-reductase mRNA in human ocular tissues. *Br J Ophthalmol* 2000;84:76–84.

163. Sullivan DA, Rocha EM, Ullman MD, et al. Androgen regulation of the meibomian gland. *Adv Exp Med Biol* 1998;438: 327–331.

164. Sullivan BD, Evans JE, Dana MR, et al. Impact of androgen deficiency on the lipid profiles in human meibomian gland secretions. *Adv Exp Med Biol* 2002;506:449–458.

165. Kirch W, Horneber M, Tamm ER. Characterization of meibomian gland innervation in the cynomolgus monkey (*Macaca fascicularis*). *Anat Embryol (Berl)* 1996;193:365–375.

166. Seifert P, Spitznas M. Vasoactive intestinal polypeptide (VIP) innervation of the human eyelid glands. *Exp Eye Res* 1999;68: 685–692.

167. Chung CW, Tigges M, Stone RA. Peptidergic innervation of the primate meibomian gland. *Invest Ophthalmol Vis Sci* 1996; 37:238–245.

168. Perra MT, Serra A, Sirigu P, et al. Histochemical demonstration of acetylcholinesterase activity in human meibomian glands. *Eur J Histochem* 1996;40:39–44.

169. Hykin PG, Bron AJ. Age-related morphological changes in lid margin and meibomian gland anatomy. *Cornea* 1992;11: 334–342.

170. Obata H. Anatomy and histopathology of human meibomian gland. *Cornea* 2002;21:S70–S74.

171. Norn M. Expressibility of meibomian secretion: relation to age, lipid precorneal film, scales, foam, hair and pigmentation. *Acta Ophthalmol (Copenh)* 1987;65:137–142.

172. Obata H, Kaburaki T, Kato M, et al. Expression of TGF-beta type I and type II receptors in rat eyes. *Curr Eye Res* 1995;15: 335–340.

173. Jester JV, Nicolaides N, Kiss-Palvolgyi I, et al. Meibomian gland dysfunction: II. the role of keratinization in a rabbit model of MGD. *Invest Ophthalmol Vis Sci* 1989;30:936–945.

174. Walcott B. Anatomy and innervation of the human lacrimal gland. In: Albert DM, Jakobiec FA, eds. *Principles and practice of ophthalmology: clinical practice.* Philadelphia: WB Saunders, 1994:454.

175. Nishimura M, Kakizaki M, Ono Y, et al. JEAP, a novel component of tight junctions in exocrine cells. *J Biol Chem* 2002; 277:5583–5587.

176. Fujihara T, Fujita H, Tsubota K, et al. Preferential localization of CD8+ alpha E beta 7+ T cells around acinar epithelial cells with apoptosis in patients with Sjögren's syndrome. *J Immunol* 1999;163:2226–2235.

177. Meda P, Pepper MS, Traub O, et al. Differential expression of gap junction connexins in endocrine and exocrine glands. *Endocrinology* 1993;133:2371–2378.

178. Takayama T, Tatsukawa S, Kitamura H, et al. Characteristic distribution of gap junctions in rat lacrimal gland in vivo and reconstruction of a gap junction in an in vitro model. *J Electron Microsc (Tokyo)* 2002;51:35–44.

179. Walcott B, Moore LC, Birzgalis A, et al. Role of gap junctions in fluid secretion of lacrimal glands. *Am J Physiol* 2002;282: C501–C507.

180. Jumblatt MM, McKenzie RW, Steele PS, et al. MUC7 expression in the human lacrimal gland and conjunctiva. *Cornea* 2003;22:41–45.

181. Ruskell GL. Nerve terminals and epithelial cell variety in the human lacrimal gland. *Cell Tissue Res* 1975;158:121–136.

182. Leoncini P, Cintorino M, Vindigni C, et al. Distribution of cytoskeletal and contractile proteins in normal and tumour bearing salivary and lacrimal glands. *Virchows Arch A Pathol Anat Histopathol* 1988;412:329–337.

183. Matsumoto Y, Ishibashi T, Niiya A, et al. Distribution of endothelin and endothelin-A receptor in the lacrimal glands of the monkey (*Macaca fuscata*). *Exp Eye Res* 1997;64:127–132.

184. Satoh Y, Oomori Y, Ishikawa K, et al. Configuration of myoepithelial cells in various exocrine glands of guinea pigs. *Anat Embryol (Berl)* 1994;189:227–236.

185. Wieczorek R, Jakobiec FA, Sacks EH, et al. The immunoarchitecture of the normal human lacrimal gland: relevancy for understanding pathologic conditions. *Ophthalmology* 1988;95: 100–109.

186. Sullivan DA. Ocular mucosal immunity. In: Ogra PL, Mestecky J, Lamm ME, et al., eds. *Handbook of mucosal immunology*, 2nd ed. Orlando, FL: Academic Press, 1999:1241–1281.

187. Dartt DA. Regulation of lacrimal gland secretion by neurotransmitters and the EGF family of growth factors. *Exp Eye Res* 2001;73:741–752.

188. Ichikawa A, Nakajima T. Electron microscope study on the lacrimal gland of the rat. *Tohoku J Exp Med* 1962;77:136.

189. Seifert P, Stuppi S, Spitznas M, et al. Differential distribution of neuronal markers and neuropeptides in the human lacrimal gland. *Graefes Arch Clin Exp Ophthalmol* 1996;234:232–240.

190. Sibony PA, Walcott B, McKeon C, et al. Vasoactive intestinal polypeptide and the innervation of the human lacrimal gland. *Arch Ophthalmol* 1988;106:1085–1088.

191. Ehinger B. Cholinesterases in ocular and orbital tissues of some mammals. *Acta Univ Lund* 1966;2:1.

192. Frey WH, II, Ahern C, Gunderson BD, et al. Biochemical, behavioral and genetic aspects of psychogenic lacrimation: the unknown function of emotional tears. In: Holly FJ, ed. *The preocular tear film: in health, disease and contact lens wear.* Lubbock, TX: Dry Eye Institute. 1986:543–551.

193. Lehtosalo J, Uusitalo H, Mahrberg T, et al. Nerve fibers showing immunoreactivities for proenkephalin A–derived peptides in the lacrimal glands of the guinea pig. *Graefes Arch Clin Exp Ophthalmol* 1989;227:455–458.

194. Matsumoto Y, Tanabe T, Ueda S, et al. Immunohistochemical and enzymehistochemical studies of peptidergic, aminergic and cholinergic innervation of the lacrimal gland of the monkey (*Macaca fuscata*). *J Auton Nerv Syst* 1992;37:207–214.

195. Meneray MA, Bennett DJ, Nguyen DH, et al. Effect of sensory denervation on the structure and physiologic responsiveness of rabbit lacrimal gland. *Cornea* 1998;17:99–107.

196. Sullivan DA, Wickham LA, Rocha EM, et al. Influence of gender, sex steroid hormones, and the hypothalamic-pituitary axis on the structure and function of the lacrimal gland. *Adv Exp Med Biol* 1998;438:11–42.

197. Sullivan DA, Block L, Pena JD. Influence of androgens and pituitary hormones on the structural profile and secretory activity of the lacrimal gland. *Acta Ophthalmol Scand* 1996;74:421–435.

198. Smith RE, Taylor CR, Rao NA, et al. Immunohistochemical identification of androgen receptors in human lacrimal glands. *Curr Eye Res* 1999;18:300–309.

199. Azzarolo AM, Wood RL, Mircheff AK, et al. Androgen influence on lacrimal gland apoptosis, necrosis, and lymphocytic infiltration. *Invest Ophthalmol Vis Sci* 1999;40:592–602.

200. Cornell-Bell AH, Sullivan DA, Allansmith MR. Gender-related differences in the morphology of the lacrimal gland. *Invest Ophthalmol Vis Sci* 1985;26:1170–1175.

201. Ueno H, Ariji E, Izumi M, et al. MR imaging of the lacrimal gland: age-related and gender-dependent changes in size and structure. *Acta Radiol* 1996;37:714–719.

202. Allansmith MR, Kajiyama G, Abelson MB, et al. Plasma cell content of main and accessory lacrimal glands and conjunctiva. *Am J Ophthalmol* 1976;82:819–826.

203. Seifert P, Spitznas M, Koch F, et al. The architecture of human accessory lacrimal glands. *German J Ophthalmol* 1993;2:444–454.

204. Seifert P, Spitznas M, Koch F, et al. Light and electron microscopic morphology of accessory lacrimal glands. In: Sullivan DA, ed. *Lacrimal gland, tear film, and dry eye syndromes: basic science and clinical relevance.* New York: Plenum Press, 1994:19–23.

2

CORNEAL PHYSIOLOGY

STEPHEN D. KLYCE

The cornea forms the transparent anterior portion of the ocular tunic, serving as the major refractive element in the eye while protecting its contents through unique physical and physiologic properties. Tissue transparency is rarely found in the animal kingdom outside of the eye, and the cornea and lens have served as models for understanding the structural and functional requisites for this property that conveys images from the environment to the photoreceptor layers in the retina. The cornea evolved as an avascular tissue, relying on the atmosphere for the bulk of its oxygen requirements and on the aqueous humor for most of its other nutritional needs. Being privileged through the constant moistening action of the tears spread by the blinking of the eyelids, the corneal surface normally maintains an optically smooth surface. Components of the tears derived from specialized cells in the conjunctiva and from the lacrimal gland further serve to protect the corneal surface from disruption and infection. The mechanical strength needed by the corneal stroma is provided by collagen fibers whose structure and organization is different from that of skin or the contiguous sclera. All connective tissues in the body rely on membrane active ion transport processes for the prevention of edema; the cornea, in particular, must rely on the metabolic activity of its outer stratified epithelium and inner monocellular endothelium for the maintenance of its state of hydration, for edema can lead to opacification and loss of vision.

The principal layers of the cornea are the epithelium, Bowman's layer, stroma, Descemet's membrane, and the endothelium (Fig. 2-1). This chapter concentrates on the fundamentals of corneal physiology to provide a foundation for understanding the normal condition as well as how corneal disease and trauma can upset corneal homeostatic regulatory processes, requiring medical and, sometimes, surgical intervention.

CORNEAL THICKNESS

One of the most useful and direct measures of corneal health is pachymetry; thin corneal areas can indicate keratoconus or other ectatic disease, whereas a thickened cornea usually relates to endothelial dysfunction. The normal adult human cornea obtains a nearly uniform thickness in its central 3 mm and thickens considerably in the periphery. Hence, in profile the posterior surface overall has a shorter radius of curvature (it is steeper in units of diopter) than the anterior surface. It is important to differentiate this natural, global feature of corneal posterior surface shape from posterior keratoconus, which usually confines itself to a localized area of decreased radius of curvature and consequent corneal thinning. The early measures of corneal thickness using manual optical pachometers reported an average central corneal thickness of 520 μm (1–3). However, the manual methods, although capable of good accuracy, remain cumbersome in routine clinical use, and automatic acoustic pachometers became the gold standard despite calibration uncertainties. Although the speed of sound is not well established in the living cornea, modern ultrasound pachometers generally yield average central corneal thicknesses of approximately 560 μm. Still, the most careful and recent optical studies place normal central corneal thickness at approximately 520 μm (4). Accurate measurement of corneal thickness has become relevant to clinicians because screening criteria for refractive surgeries have been established based on the lower limit of the range for normal thickness. With calibration factors among pachometers at variance and producing errors in accuracy of 40 μm or more, caution is suggested in the comparison of data obtained from different instruments.

THE CORNEAL STROMA

The bulk of the cornea is formed by the fibrous stroma, which in the human adult is approximately 470 μm thick centrally. Collagen fibers approximately 22 to 32 nm (5,6) in diameter appear to run uninterrupted from limbus to limbus in flat sheathes or lamellae. The lamellae are stacked at angles to one another and number in the hundreds in the human cornea. Unlike collagen fibers in most other

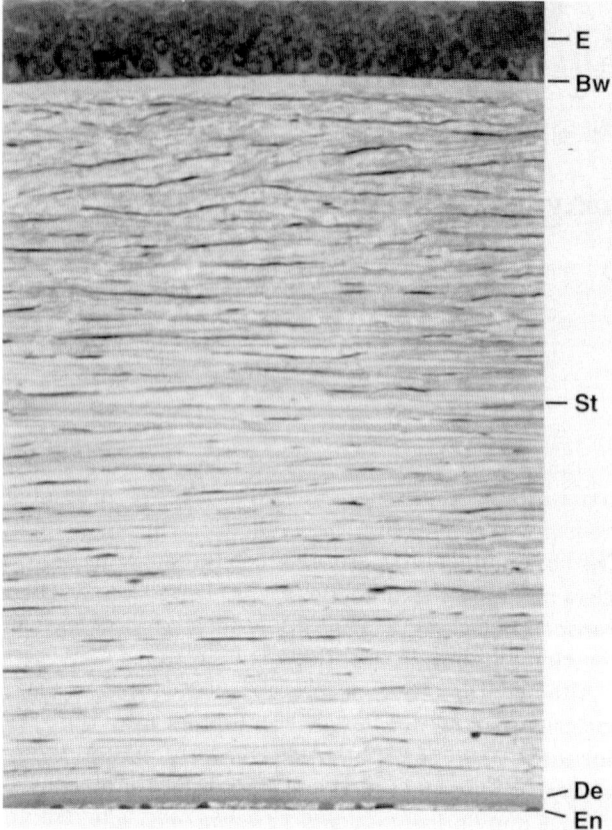

FIGURE 2-1. Histologic section of the cornea illustrating the epithelium (E), Bowman's layer (Bw), stroma (St), Descemet's membrane (De), and the endothelium (En). (From Klyce SD, Beuerman RW. Anatomy and physiology of the cornea. In: Kaufman HE, Barron BA, McDonald MB, eds. *The cornea*, 2nd ed. Boston: Butterworth-Heinemann, 1998:3–50, with permission.)

connective tissues, stromal collagen has a fairly uniform diameter, and in the bulk of the tissue does not branch at all. This is in contrast to collagen fibers in the sclera, which branch freely and whose diameters range from 25 to 480 nm. Corneal stromal fibers also exhibit a uniform center-to-center spacing of approximately 55 nm that is maintained by intramolecular forces in the surrounding extracellular matrix and by hydrational control mechanisms, which are discussed later.

This organization of collagen fibers in the stroma is important for its optical characteristics, but the lack of significant interweaving and branching enhances the ability of the corneal stroma to swell. The extracellular matrix has a high content of hydrophilic glycosaminoglycans, notably chondroitin and keratin sulfates, which provide connective tissue with a great capacity to imbibe fluid when provided free access to it. Although the corneal stroma can swell significantly before light scatter from within it causes significant problems with vision, the mechanism of its transparency was a matter of conjecture for a considerable period of time.

The uniform distribution of collagen fibers in the stroma (Fig. 2-2) led Maurice to propose that transparency was achieved by a perfect crystalline lattice arrangement. He proposed that light scattered by individual fibers is cancelled by destructive interference with scattered light from neighboring fibers (7). However, Goldman and Benedek (8) and others (9,10) recognized that refractive elements in tissues whose dimensions are small (<200 nm) compared with the wavelength of light (~500 nm) should not scatter as much light as might be predicted by the stringent requirements of the crystalline lattice theory. Consequently, the normal stroma scatters light minimally because its collagen fibers are uniformly small in diameter and closely spaced. Furthermore, even the quasiregular arrangement of stromal collagen fibers appears to be an unnecessary requirement for transparency. In the human, Bowman's layer is 8 to 12 μm thick and its constituent collagen fibers are arranged irregularly; nevertheless, it is relatively transparent. According to the Goldman-Benedek criterion, connective tissue should remain relatively transparent as long as the spatial dimensions of variations in refractive index remain less than 200 nm. As the stroma swells, fluid entry expands the ground substance, which increases the spacing between collagen fibers. As the spacing increases, the orderliness of the fibers decreases, and light scatter ensues when the fluctuations in refractive index exceed the Goldman-Benedek criterion. This criterion also applies to the origin of light scattering in the human corneal epithelium, where intracellular fluid collection causes large spatial fluctuations in refractive index (11). Although the physical basis for transparency of the stroma and epithelium is identical in this respect, stromal edema and epithelial

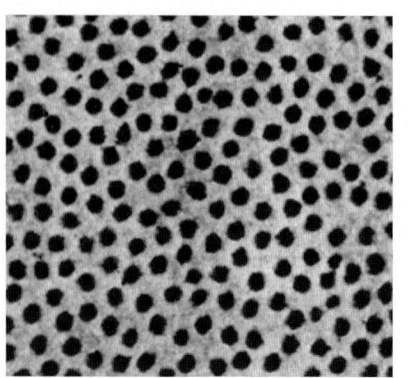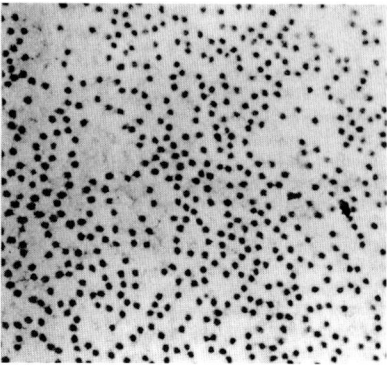

FIGURE 2-2. Transparency depends on the compactness of the corneal stroma. *Left*, Human corneal stromal fiber distribution in the normal (original magnification × 51,800). *Right*, Stromal fiber distribution in the edematous human cornea (original magnification × 46,700). (From Edelhauser HF, Geroski DH, Ubels JL: Physiology. In: Smolin G, Thoft RA, eds. *The cornea*, 2nd ed. Boston: Little, Brown, 1987:29, with permission.)

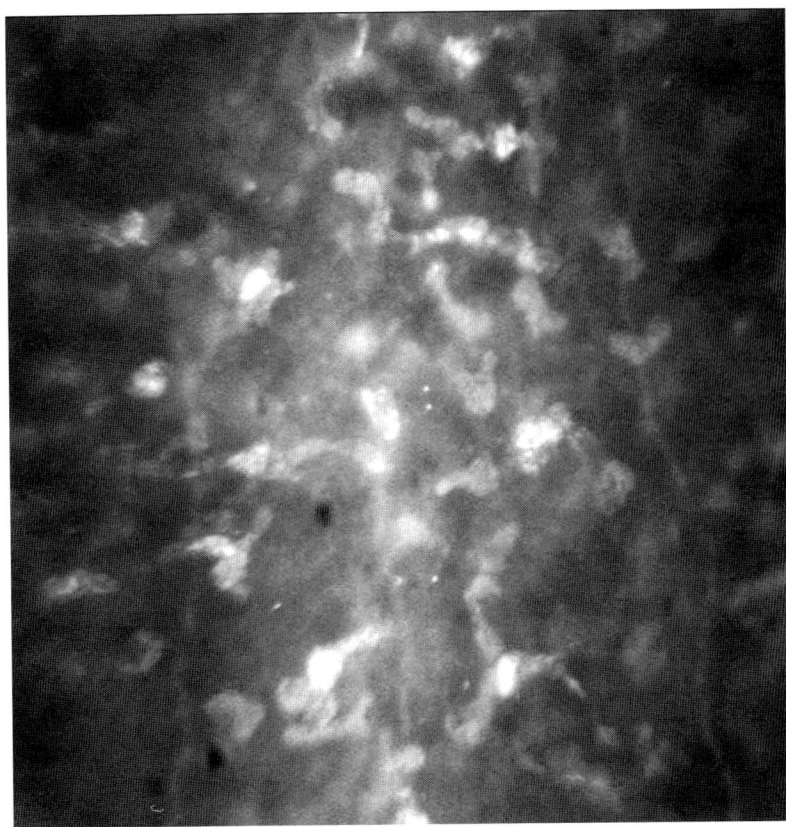

FIGURE 2-3. The keratocyte nuclei in Bowman's layer are highly refractile on confocal microscopy in this normal human cornea.

edema are considered separately later because the pathophysiologic processes and clinical effects are somewhat different.

The Cells of the Stroma

The cellular density in the stroma is low in keeping with the optical characteristics of this tissue. Each stromal cell scatters light, as slit-lamp or confocal microscopic examination reveals (Figs. 2-3 and 2-4), but the total light scattered by the stroma at normal hydration is small, permitting most light to be transmitted. The numerous keratocytes occupy 3% to 5% of the volume of the stroma and are distributed throughout the stroma, with their flattened cell bodies lying primarily between lamellae. Keratocytes extend processes outward from their cell bodies between the collagen lamellae, and the tips of these processes sometimes touch those of a neighboring keratocyte and form a tight junction. The tight junctions are a form of cell-to-cell communication and are thought to be important in the regulation of keratocyte function (12). Nerve axons and their associated Schwann cells are found in the anterior and middle thirds of the stroma. Each of these very different cell types plays important roles in maintaining the health and function of the cornea.

Role of the Keratocytes

Keratocytes maintain the collagen scaffold and extracellular matrix of the stroma. Collagen constitutes approximately 71% of the dry weight of the cornea (13,14), and in the quiescent cornea, both procollagen and collagen are secreted at a low basal rate. However, keratocytes can become activated by surgery or trauma, initiating a wound-healing response that invokes greatly increased collagen secretion (15).

Keratocytes undergo extensive cellular alteration in response to corneal injury, particularly in regions proximal to damaged epithelium. In response to an epithelial scrape, keratocytes are depleted rapidly from the subjacent corneal stroma (16). The mechanism of this response has been studied extensively (17,18). Injury to the corneal epithelium causes the release of cytokines to the stroma, which in turn stimulates programmed cell death (apoptosis) of the underlying anterior stromal keratocytes. It is hypothesized that proteolytic enzymes are also released during apoptosis, causing a local breakdown of stromal macromolecules that increases the stromal colloid osmotic pressure and leads to localized edema (19,20). It is thought that the localized edema that characterizes the acute phase of the injury response in all tissues provides an avenue of greater mobility for activated keratocytes and, in some cases, inflammatory cells in their migration to the wound site. When the stroma is repopulated with activated keratocytes, these cells can produce collagen and other components associated with stromal remodeling. In addition, activated keratocytes can secrete hepatocyte growth factor and keratinocyte growth factor, which can stimulate proliferation and inhibit differentiation of epithelial cells (21). When this occurs, epithelial

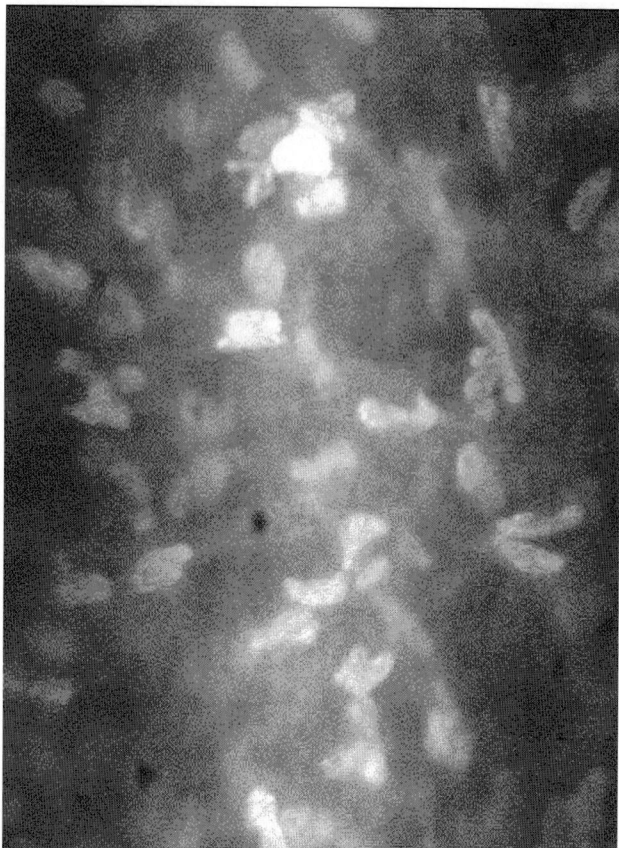

FIGURE 2-4. In the mid-stromal level, keratocyte nuclei are only occasionally refractile. Note that the stromal collagen fibers are perfectly transparent—the stromal light scatter is almost entirely derived from the keratocyte nuclei.

hyperplasia can result, with alteration of the corneal surface curvature and an associated change in refractive error that can cause a variable outcome after refractive surgical procedures.

Stromal Transport Properties

The corneal stroma is primarily an extracellular compartment, with keratocytes and nerves accounting for only 5% and 0.01% of its volume, respectively. Although the concentrations of K^+ and Na^+ are 35 mEq/L higher in the stroma than in the aqueous humor (22), their effective concentrations (activities) are reduced by physicochemical factors such as ion binding by anionic sites on stromal macromolecules. This makes the chemical activities of the major diffusible micro-ions (K^+, Na^+, and Cl^-) similar in the stroma and the aqueous humor. This feature is central to the concept of osmotic control of corneal stromal hydration, discussed later.

The negative charges of glycosaminoglycans (10 to 50 mEq/L) are primarily responsible for the abundance of Na^+ and K^+ in the stroma (23–25). When the stroma swells, the diameter of the collagen fibrils remains essentially constant; swelling takes place in the ground substance,

which is rich in glycosaminoglycans, and leads to an increased spatial separation of the collagen fibrils (26). Several factors influence the swelling force generated by the ground substance: long-range electrostatic repulsive forces between negative charges on the glycosaminoglycans, excess cations required to preserve ionic charge neutrality (Donnan effect), mechanical limitations in the corneal structure that prevent swelling beyond a certain limit (27), and chemical effects such as changes in pH and total ionic strength. For corneal stroma, the major forces normally involved in stromal swelling appear to be long-range electrostatic repulsion and the Donnan effect (14).

In addition to imparting the underlying force for stromal swelling, the glycosaminoglycan component of the stromal ground substance has other effects on the nature of stromal swelling. Glycosaminoglycans form polymeric macromolecules, which in turn associate with protein cores to form megamolecular complexes in the ground substance. These complexes increase the viscosity of the fluid in the ground substance in a stromal hydration–dependent fashion. Fatt and Goldstick (28) pointed out an important feature of fluid flow in tissues such as stroma: The ability of fluid to flow (to even out hydration gradients) is greatest in tissue that has near-normal hydration and less for swollen or dehydrated tissue, which helps preserve homeostasis in the internal environment. For example, as the stroma is dehydrated below normal conditions, the driving force for fluid flow (swelling pressure gradient) increases exponentially, whereas the stromal hydraulic fluid conductivity decreases as a power function of hydration. Because of these properties, normal corneal thickness is responsive to subtle changes in the environment, as demonstrated by the 5% thinning during waking hours, yet local dry spots or dellen can persist in the anterior stroma while the surrounding tissue is normally hydrated.

The stroma is normally maintained in a relatively dehydrated state compared with its ability to swell. The stroma consists of 78% water, which is equivalent to a ratio of 3.45 parts water (by weight) to 1 part solid material. Thus, the hydration is 3.45. The ability of the stroma to swell decreases as its hydration increases. This relationship has been carefully measured for corneal stroma by placing disks of stroma between layers of rigid, porous glass in a saline solution. The force necessary to prevent stromal swelling at various hydrations has been termed the *swelling pressure* (SP); these measurements show a near-exponential drop with increasing stromal hydration (Fig. 2-5). At normal hydration (3.45), the stromal SP is approximately 80 g/cm^2 or 55 mm Hg (29,30). This is the amount of force that corneal membranes must create to counterbalance stromal swelling in the living cornea, and is equivalent to a stromal osmotic deficit of 2 to 3 milliosmoles (mOsm).

It has been proposed that the SP of stroma as measured *in vitro* is not an adequate measure of the situation in the living cornea. It was suggested that measurements of SP

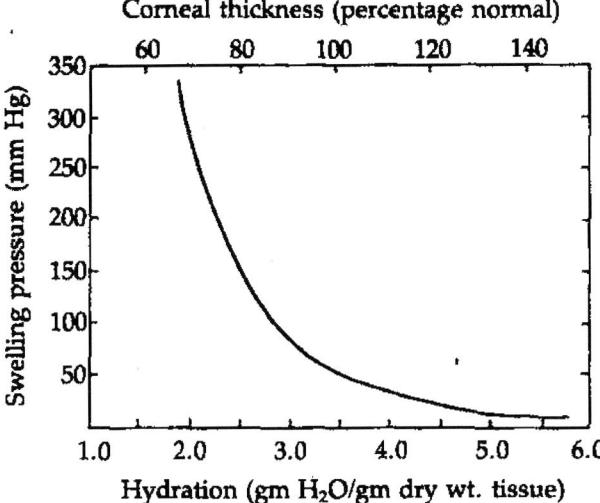

FIGURE 2-5. Swelling pressure, hydration, and thickness of the cornea. As corneal thickness and hydration increase, the tendency to swell decreases markedly. (From Dohlman CH: Physiology. In: Smolin G, Thoft RA, eds. *The cornea*. Boston: Little, Brown, 1983, with permission.)

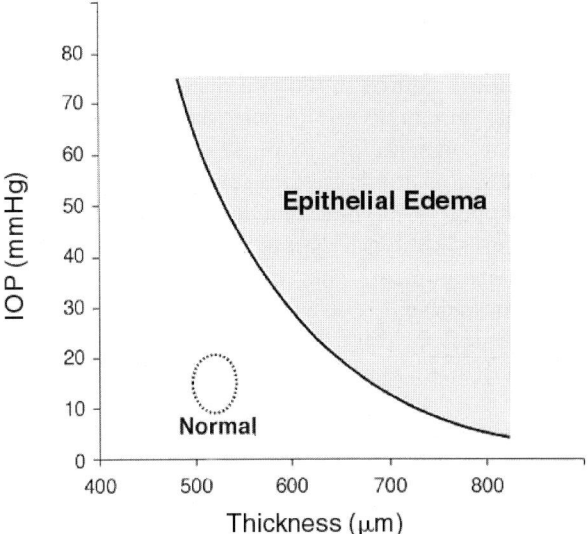

FIGURE 2-6. Corneal thickness and intraocular pressure (IOP) as they relate to epithelial edema. Such edema is expected to the right of the *solid line*. The *circle* encompasses normal values. (From Dohlman CH: Physiology. In: Smolin G, Thoft RA, eds. *The cornea*. Boston: Little, Brown, 1983, with permission.)

determined with excised stroma could be misleading because the conditions normally present in the living eye have been altered. However, Hedbys and coworkers (31) implanted fine saline-filled cannulas into the central stroma of living rabbits and showed that a negative pressure in the cannula was necessary to prevent the stroma from drawing fluid continuously from the tube. The equilibrium suction that prevented this fluid loss was termed the *stromal imbibition pressure* (IP) and was found to be related to the stromal SP by the simple relation:

$$IP = IOP - SP \qquad [1]$$

In the absence of intraocular pressure (IOP) effects, the IP measured *in vivo* was identical to the SP measured *in vitro*. Because the tension of the IOP is taken up principally by that anterior corneal lamellae, this hydrostatic pressure diminishes the measured IP.

The pressure of swelling in the normal cornea *in vivo* was confirmed by a second approach by Klyce and colleagues (32), who inserted thin, high–water-content hydrogel disks into intralamellar stromal pockets and found that, after the eyes stabilized, the disks were thinner by the amount previously predicted on the basis of stromal SP. The *in vivo* cannulation and gel implant experiments confirm the notion that the tendency of the stroma to swell *in vivo* is the same as was indicated by earlier *in vitro* experiments.

Ytteborg and Dohlman (33) explored the significance of equation [1], and showed that when the IOP exceeds the SP, the IP turns positive and subepithelial edema ensues. This dynamic relationship has clinical implications. Stromal SP is normally 50 to 60 mm Hg; the IOP in glaucoma rarely exceeds this value. However, as noted previously, stromal SP drops off exponentially with stromal edema, so

that mild stromal edema combined with mild IOP elevation can lead to positive stromal IP, which, because of the barrier properties of the epithelium, can lead to the collection of intraepithelial fluid. Figure 2-6 relates the appearance of epithelial edema to IOP and corneal thickness.

The stromal experiments led to another important topic in stromal physiology, which deals with how IOP distributes itself across corneal thickness in terms of stress factors on the structural tunic. This has an important bearing on current problems in refractive surgery (34). IOP normally commutes through the stroma and is dissipated by stress on the anteriormost stromal lamellae. Several implications of this concept are discussed later. It is, however, important to emphasize that when anterior stromal lamellae are cut, they can no longer bear the stress of IOP, which is then transferred to the deeper, intact lamellae (34).

There is a linear relationship between central corneal thickness (q), expressed in millimeters, and stromal hydration (H), expressed as the ratio of the weight of water in the tissue to the dry tissue weight:

$$H = 8q - 0.7 \qquad [2]$$

It has been shown experimentally that the hydration of the anterior stroma is less than that of the posterior stroma (35). This is usually taken to mean that there are differences in the types or concentrations of glycosaminoglycans at these different locations. However, such a gradient can be predicted by computer simulation on the basis of dissimilarities in the permeability properties between the epithelium and endothelium alone, even in the absence of tear film evaporation (36).

The stroma requires continuous maintenance by its keratocytes to sustain its macromolecular composition and consequent organization. Normally, keratocytes, while having all the anatomic features consistent with synthetic activity, appear to be quiescent in terms of mobility. In fact, however, keratocytes are quite responsive to changes in their environment. They can mobilize to repopulate stromal areas devoid of keratocytes, and may rapidly undergo apoptosis below areas where trauma to the epithelium has occurred, as noted previously.

THE CORNEAL LIMITING CELL LAYERS

The corneal stroma is bounded by two cell layers with distinctly different structural and functional characteristics. On the outer surface a stratified layer of epithelial cells isolates the cornea from tearborne pathogens, providing a high-resistance barrier. The epithelial cells also provide marked regenerative properties to heal surface injuries rapidly through mitotic activity and migration. By contrast, the inner surface of the stroma is lined with a monocellular layer of fragile, highly permeable cells that show extremely limited regenerative capability after birth. But the inner cell layer, the corneal endothelium, is critical for the maintenance of normal corneal thickness through its membrane active ion transport processes that provide a homoeostatic mechanism to prevent stromal edema.

CORNEAL EPITHELIUM

The epithelium of the cornea consists of four to six layers of cells and represents 10% or approximately 55 μm of the corneal thickness (37). The three layers (squamous cell, wing cell, and basal cell) are coupled tightly by junctional complexes forming a functional syncytium through which electrochemical cross-talk can occur. The basal cells are the only epithelial cells that undergo mitosis. The daughter cells move anteriorly to the surface, maintaining communication with neighboring cells until desquamating into the tear film.

Epithelial Cell Turnover

The epithelium turns over approximately every 7 days (38). Limbal stem cells also provide a constantly renewing source for the corneal epithelium as they continually divide and migrate centripetally toward the corneal center in a vortex pattern. They move inward at a rate of 20 to 30 μm/day, reaching the center in approximately 7 weeks in the mouse (39). The stem cells that arrive at the center

of the cornea are the progeny of those cells arising at the limbus. This constant renewal process is apparently necessary for homeostasis of the epithelium because limbal stem cell deficiency can cause reepithelialization by the neighboring conjunctival epithelium, vascularization, and recurring epithelial defects. Whether these limbal cells are true stem cells or "committed progenitors" is being debated (40); nevertheless, their contribution to the epithelium is essential.

Superficial Epithelial Cells

An important property of the superficial cell layer is the junctional complex formed with laterally adjacent cells. This complex consists of tight junctions that completely encircle the cell (41). The joining of adjacent superficial cells at their lateral borders in this manner prevents the movement of substances from the tear film into the intercellular spaces of the epithelium.

The apical tight junctional complex in combination with the very low permeability of the outermost membrane of the superficial squamous cell is the anatomic representation of the barrier property of the corneal epithelium, as demonstrated in electrophysiologic studies (42). Sensory nerve terminals in the epithelium help preserve the integrity of this important surface barrier structure by eliciting a severe pain response to injury. A clinical test to determine if this barrier is intact uses dyes, such as fluorescein, which are instilled into the conjunctival sac. The normal epithelial surface stains little or not at all. Rubbing the corneal surface under the closed eyelid damages the fragile surface cells, resulting in punctate staining (43). Diabetic patients have increased surface staining, which suggests that the barrier property of the epithelium is impaired (44). Several factors, such as rapid or abnormal epithelial cell loss or the inability to form tight junctions, could lead to surface staining in diabetes.

Wing Cells

The wing cell layer is formed by the transition and anterior migration from the basal cell layer. The wing cells interdigitate extensively and are interconnected by desmosomal junctions and gap junctions that serve as electrochemical conduits. This conductance extends to the squamous cells and to a lesser degree to the basal cells, and facilitates cell-to-cell communication. In this way, a pathway is provided for micro-ion transport in the commission of cell volume regulation.

Basal Cells

The cytoplasm of the basal cell has large numbers of glycogen granules, which represent a source of stored metabolic energy to be used in times of epithelial stress, such as hypoxia and wound healing. Actin filaments are seen along the cytoplasmic side of the membrane, and may be important for cell migration in the healing of abrasions, during which these cells may become motile (45).

CORNEAL TRANSPORT PROPERTIES

At the heart of corneal homeostasis are the membrane transport and permeability properties of the epithelium and endothelium as well as the fluid flow characteristics of the corneal stroma. The individual properties of these three layers are presented, followed by a discussion of a holistic model for the control of corneal hydration and transparency.

Epithelial Transport Properties

The primary function of the corneal epithelium with respect to corneal homeostasis is that of a barrier restricting both the entry of fluid as well as pathogens. Nevertheless, the corneal epithelium possesses active ion transport systems under neural control that also play a role in maintaining corneal function.

Active Na^+ Transport in the Epithelium

Corneal ion transport systems have been intensely studied since it was shown that cooling the tissue, which slows down metabolism, produces edema. A tears-to-stroma transport of Na^+ has been demonstrated in the rabbit and frog (46–52). This absorptive transport of Na^+ presents somewhat of an anomaly inasmuch as an inward solute transport to the stroma would increase its osmotic pressure and presumably favor stromal edema. It has been proposed (53,54) that an increase in the stromal content of Na^+ might neutralize the anionic groups of the glycosaminoglycans and reduce or prevent their ability to swell. However, in both rabbits (51) and humans (55), when factors such as corneal resting potential and other ion transport systems are taken into account, the net flow of Na^+ (and Cl^-) across the epithelium is from stroma to tears (56).

Nevertheless, the active Na^+ transport system in the epithelium is powered by the specific energy-supplying enzyme for Na^+ transport, Na^+/K^+-adenosine triphosphatase (ATPase), which has been demonstrated histochemically (57). The activity of this enzyme can be enhanced severalfold by reacting the superficial epithelial cell membrane with amphotericin B or Ag^+ (58,59). Normally, the superficial epithelial cell membrane restricts the entry of Na^+. However, both amphotericin B and Ag^+ create cation channels in this membrane, which greatly increases intracellular Na^+ concentration and the rate of absorptive Na^+ transport. In this situation, the stroma swells in accord with the added osmotic load (59). The epithelial

Na^+ transport system is inhibited by ouabain, a specific inhibitor of Na^+/K^+-ATPase.

The transepithelial transport of Na^+ is most likely secondary to the K^+/Na^+ exchange activity of the deeper epithelial membrane, which maintains the high K^+ and low Na^+ characteristic of the cells. The Na^+/K^+-ATPase activity of the epithelial surface is less than that of the basolateral membranes, which accounts for the directionality of transepithelial Na^+ transport. The small amount of Na^+ that leaks into the cells across the apical membrane is more efficiently removed by the basolateral membrane K^+/Na^+ exchange mechanism.

Active Cl^- Transport in the Epithelium

The corneal epithelium also transports Cl^- in a secretory direction, that is, from stroma to tears (49,60,61). Corneal epithelial transport of Cl^- is regulated by the β-adrenergic receptor/adenylate cyclase complex. Stimulation of Cl^- transport is accompanied by an elevation of intracellular cyclic adenosine monophosphate (cAMP) and can be accomplished by the addition of membrane-permeable forms of cAMP (49). Catecholamines, such as epinephrine, stimulate Cl^- secretion, unless blocked by β-adrenoreceptor antagonists, such as propranolol or timolol. This stimulation is enhanced by theophylline, which is a compound that inhibits phosphodiesterase and slows the breakdown of cAMP.

Net Na^+ absorptive transport and net Cl^- secretory transport can occur simultaneously only under special experimental conditions, such as are found with the short-circuit current technique. In the living eye, the epithelium generates an electrical potential of approximately 30 mV, tear side negative, and in this situation the net movement of NaCl across the epithelium appears to be in the stroma-to-tears direction (51).

Microelectrodes have been used to analyze the site of action of epinephrine in the stimulation of Cl^- transport. In the transport of ions across epithelial cells, there is an energy-consuming translocation of the transported ion at one epithelial surface and a passive diffusional translocation of the same ion at the opposite surface. In the rabbit cornea, the active step in Cl^- transport appears to be Cl^- uptake by the epithelial cells from the stroma in conjunction with a passive diffusional barrier at the corneal surface, which limits the exit of Cl^- from the superficial epithelial cells to the tear film. The action of epinephrine in the regulation of the overall net secretion of Cl^- appears to be the formation of functional Cl^- conductance channels in the apical membrane of the superficial epithelial cells (62).

The presence of active Cl^- secretory transport in the epithelium raises the possibility that the epithelium might participate in the regulation of stromal hydration in addition to its role as a diffusion barrier. In the frog, Cl^- secretion by the epithelium produces significant stromal dehydration

(63,64). Epithelial fluid secretion has also been identified in the rabbit (65), where stromal thinning at a rate of 1.3 μm/hour is observed. Epithelial fluid transport in the primate has not been reported, although, as mentioned previously, Cl$^-$ secretion has been demonstrated.

The presence of catecholamine-activated β-adrenergic receptors as a control mechanism for epithelial function has been confirmed in a number of studies. The population of these receptors is dynamic; their density decreases after topical administration of epinephrine (66) and increases after superior cervical ganglionectomy (67), a manipulation that would be expected to deplete the normal supply of corneal catecholamines. Other sources of catecholamines, such as the tears and the aqueous humor, that might activate corneal β-adrenergic receptors have been considered, but concentrations of epinephrine in these compartments are minute, owing in part to the cellular activity of monoamine oxidase, the principal enzyme responsible for the catabolism of catecholamines. In addition, anatomic evidence presented earlier underscores the role of sympathetic fibers as the likely physiologic source of catecholamines in the cornea.

Other epithelial regulatory receptors have been identified, again using Cl$^-$ transport as a measure of functional response. Both serotonin (68) and dopamine (69) stimulate Cl$^-$ secretion in the rabbit cornea through mechanisms inhibited by specific receptor antagonists. Serotonin increases cAMP in the epithelium (70) and evokes membrane conductance changes similar to those of epinephrine, including increased Cl$^-$ conductance in the outer membrane of the superficial cells (71). The specificity of the serotonin and dopamine responses became suspect when it was found that timolol blocks their activity, especially because timolol has been found to cross-react with other receptor types, although it is nonselective, and blocks both β_1- and β_2-adrenoreceptors. In addition, it was shown that the corneas of animals that had undergone superior cervical ganglionectomy (67) and pure subcultures of corneal epithelium (72) lack responsiveness to serotonin. On this basis, it was suggested that the serotonin receptors and, potentially, the dopamine receptors are located on the sympathetic fibers themselves. In this scheme, activation of serotonin or dopamine receptors located on the sympathetic fibers causes the release of catecholamines (presumably norepinephrine), which, in turn, activates epithelial β-adrenoreceptors. Such a mechanism explains the apparent anomalous timolol antagonism to the serotonin response, as well as the disappearance of serotonin receptors in epithelial subculture. It does not alter the earlier notion that the β-adrenoreceptors are located on the epithelial membranes themselves, in that the responses to catecholamines in cultured cells remain intact (72). A summary of membrane ion transport in the corneal epithelium and its putative neural control is presented in Fig. 2-7.

This section has emphasized the neuropharmacology of specific corneal membrane receptors to detail a model for a sequence of events linked to epithelial Cl$^-$ transport, which, on its own merit, provides some understanding of epithelial function. However, activation of the β-adrenoreceptor increases cell levels of cAMP, which is a rather common second messenger in terms of cell signaling, and the assay of one specific function (Cl$^-$ transport) may reveal only one aspect of receptor activation in this tissue. Other functional modalities are likely to be controlled by this receptor, such as cell proliferation (72) during epithelial repair, corneal immunologic response, and recurrence of herpes simplex viral disease (73,74).

Barrier Function

One of the most useful clinical tools in the assessment of the barrier properties of the corneal epithelium is the topical application of fluorescein. Normally, the corneal epithelium is impermeable to this anionic molecule. As a result, normal areas stain little or not at all, whereas areas with epithelial defects stain intensely. The location of this barrier and the membrane events associated with the corneal epithelial transport systems have been examined by means of intracellular measurements of electrical potential and ion activities with microelectrodes.

Intracellular microelectrode recordings in the corneal epithelium have been reported in frogs, rabbits, and cats (37,42,59,62,75–81). Such work has led to several general conclusions, which are summarized in Fig. 2-8. As with other cells, corneal epithelial cells have negative intracellular potentials, which are an expression of the fact that most cells maintain a high ratio of K$^+$ to Na$^+$ by means of the ubiquitous K$^+$/Na$^+$ exchange pump, which assists in the regulation of individual cell volume. The negative intracellular potential is also related to the relatively high K$^+$ permeability of most cell membranes. In such a situation, K$^+$, which is favored to diffuse out of the cell, creates a Nernst diffusion potential across the cell membrane oriented so that the cell interior remains electrically negative.

Measurement of the electrical potential profile across the epithelial cell membranes reveals three major steps (Fig. 2-8). Starting on the tear side, the microelectrode records a negative potential of 30 mV as the superficial epithelial cell is penetrated. No additional change in potential is recorded until the microelectrode penetrates the basal cell layer, whereupon the potential becomes 5 to 10 mV more negative. Normally, the superficial epithelial cells have the same intracellular potential as the deeper wing cells because of the presence of numerous ion-conducting desmosomes between these cells. The small step in potential between the deep wing and the basal cell layers indicates less electrical coupling between cells at this site. As the microelectrode penetrates the posterior membrane of the basal cell, the potential becomes more positive. The level of this potential is similar to the electrical potential in

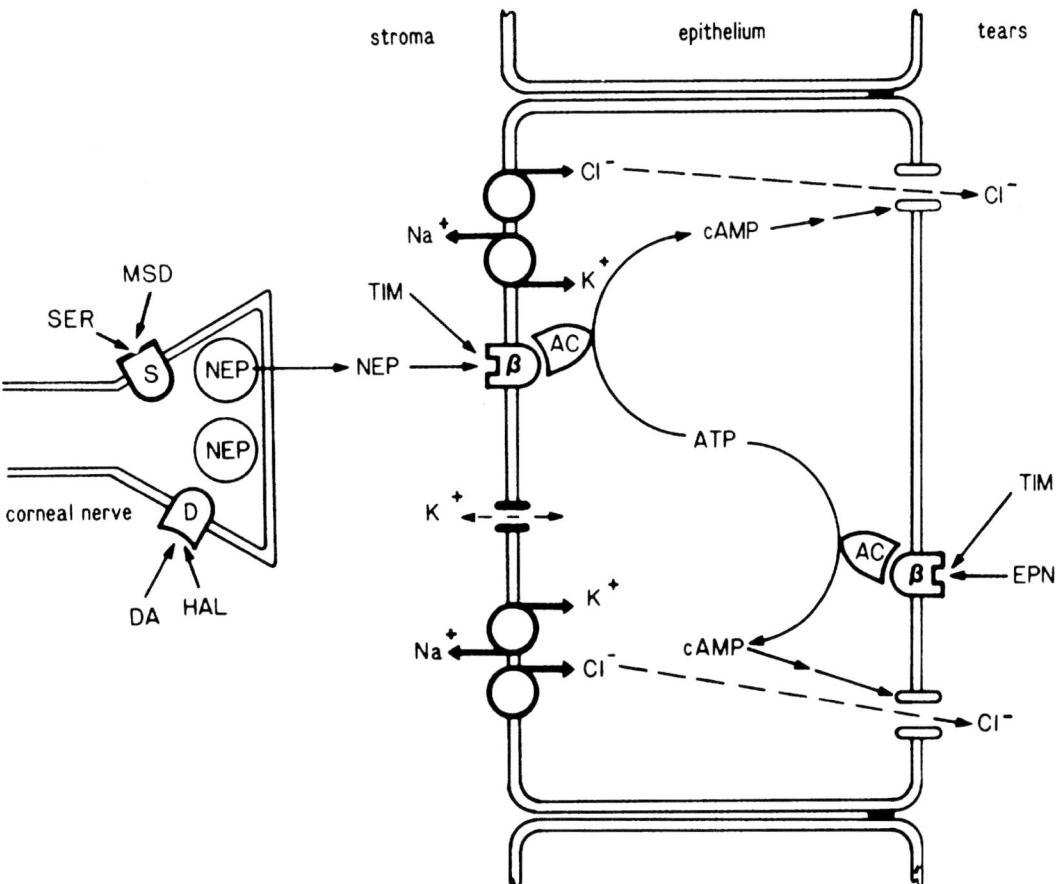

FIGURE 2-7. Cl⁻ transport in the corneal epithelium is under neural control. Serotonin and dopamine may evoke the release of norepinephrine from the sympathetic nerve fibers in the cornea. In turn, norepinephrine may activate adenylate cyclase through β-adrenoreceptors to increase cell levels of cyclic adenosine monophosphate (AMP), and finally, to increase the chloride conductance of the apical epithelial membrane. EPN, epinephrine; NEP, norepinephrine; TIM, timolol; SER, serotonin; MSD, methysergide; DA, dopamine; HAL, haloperidol; β, β-adrenoreceptor; S, serotonin receptor; D, dopamine receptor; AC, adenylate cyclase. (From Klyce SD, Crosson CE: Transport processes across the rabbit corneal epithelium: a review. Curr Eye Res 1985;4:323, with permission.)

the aqueous humor inasmuch as transendothelial potential is small. The difference between stromal potential and tear potential is equal to transepithelial potential, and is similar in magnitude to values measured *in vivo* (10 to 35 mV) (42,82).

During the measurement of the electrical potential profile of the epithelium, it is possible to measure the resistance of the cell membranes (Fig. 2-8). Sixty percent of total corneal resistance to ion flow is ascribed to the outer membranes of the superficial epithelial cells. This places the major barrier to corneal permeation of polar (charged) substances at the superficial epithelial cells, a site that is vulnerable to trauma. The measurement also implies that the parallel route for epithelial ion permeation, the paracellular pathway, is of low permeability. The site of the resistive barrier in the paracellular pathway is thought to be the continuous tight junctions present between the superficial

epithelial cells. Despite the fact that the epithelial cell layer is continually regenerated, the barrier remains intact; before a superficial cell desquamates, the underlying cells reorganize to establish tight junctions with adjacent cells to maintain the electrical potential.

The effectiveness of the tight junctions as an ionic diffusion barrier can be measured with microelectrode experiments, and estimates of the cellular pathway resistance to ion permeation can be made (81). The outer membrane of the superficial cell, in the absence of factors that stimulate ion transport, is twice as good a barrier to ion flow as the tight junction. Considered on the basis of actual surface areas represented by membranes and by junctions, this ratio increases by at least two orders of magnitude. Hence, the tight junctions in the corneal epithelium offer a significant barrier to ion diffusion across the epithelium, but,

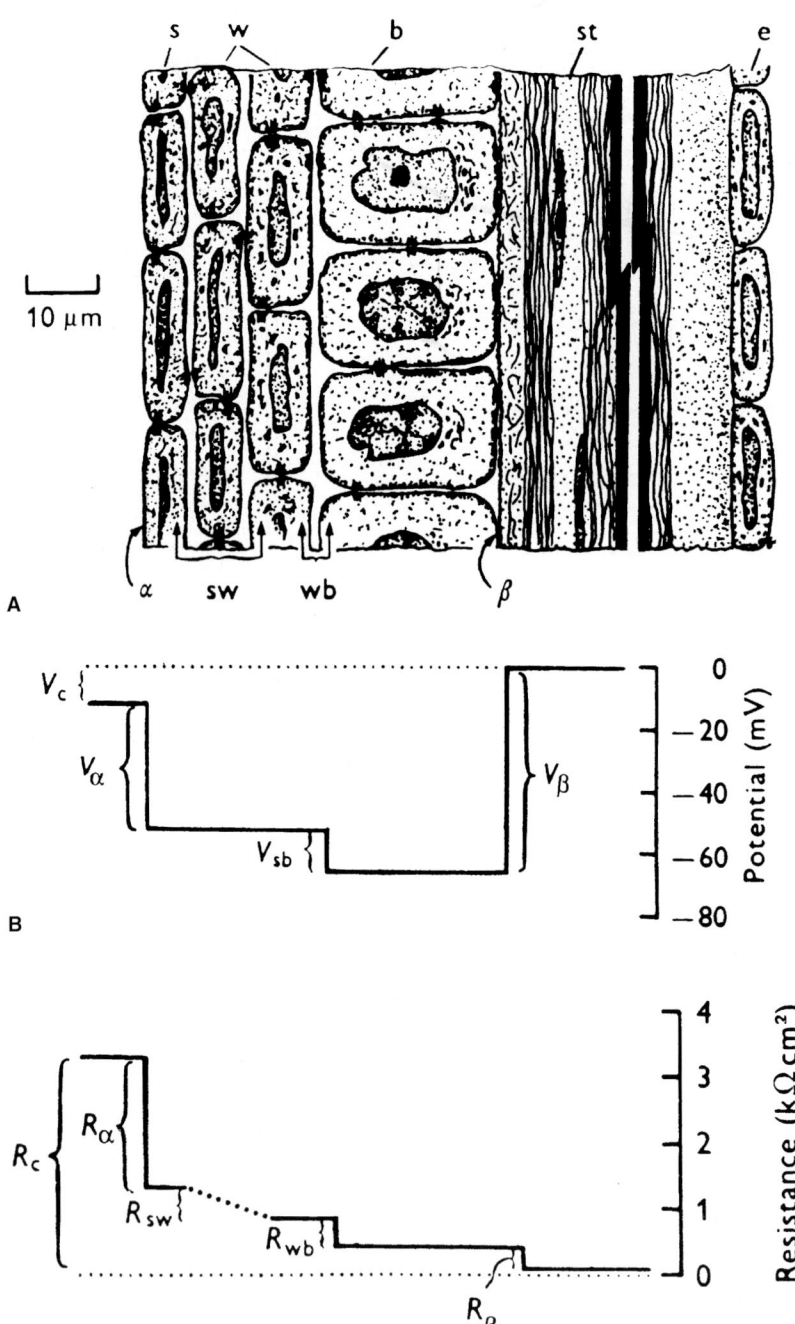

FIGURE 2-8. Membrane electrical profiles measured across the rabbit corneal epithelium. **A:** Diagram of cornea showing the epithelium, a portion of stroma (st), and the endothelium (e). With intracellular dye injections, several regions of the epithelium were identified in the electrical profiles: α, the outer membrane of the superficial (s) cells; β the inner membrane of the basal (b) cells; sw, the region between the superficial and wing (w) cells; wb, the transition region between the wing and basal cells. **B:** Average potential profile for the corneal epithelium. **C:** Average resistance profile for the corneal epithelium. Note the large resistance of the outer membrane of the superficial cell—the site of the major barrier property. Whereas the epithelium generates a potential, V_c, of 20 to 30 mV, by contrast, the low-resistance corneal endothelium (not shown) generates a little more than 1 mV. [From Klyce SD: Electrical profiles in the corneal epithelium. *J Physiol (Lond)* 1972;226: 407, with permission.]

area for area, the tight junctions are more permeable than the cell membranes they surround.

CORNEAL ENDOTHELIUM

The corneal endothelium forms a single layer of approximately 400,000 cells, 4 to 6 μm thick, on the posterior corneal surface. Viewed from their posterior surface, these cells are predominantly hexagonal and approximately 20 μm wide (83) (Fig. 2-9). Their outline at the level of

Descemet's membrane is irregular because of the marked infolding and interdigitation between adjacent cells. The posterior cell membrane is thought by some to be coated with a viscous substance (84,85), possibly of endothelial origin, which, like the glycocalyx on the epithelial surface, may reduce lipid membrane surface tension to promote wettability. A single primary cilium has been demonstrated in many endothelial cells, but its function is unclear (86,87). The cilium is apparently not motile and is structurally associated with the cell's centriole pair. This association may be related to the inability of these cells to undergo mitosis in

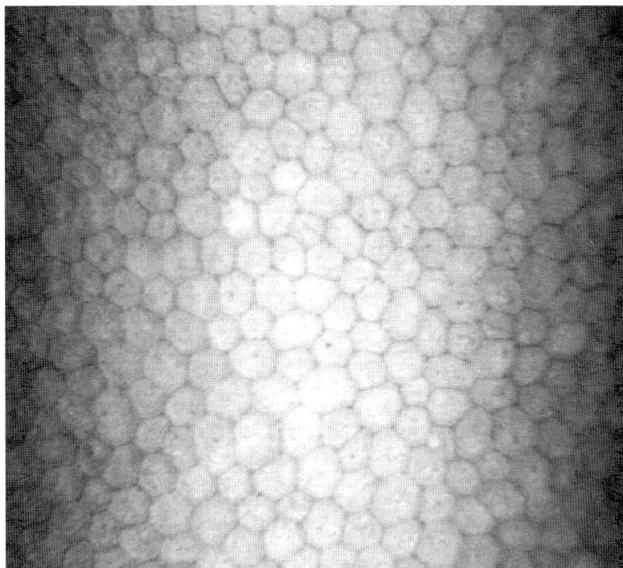

FIGURE 2-9. Normal, predominantly hexagonal human corneal endothelia. The dark spot near the center of many cells may represent the endothelial cilium (see text for details).

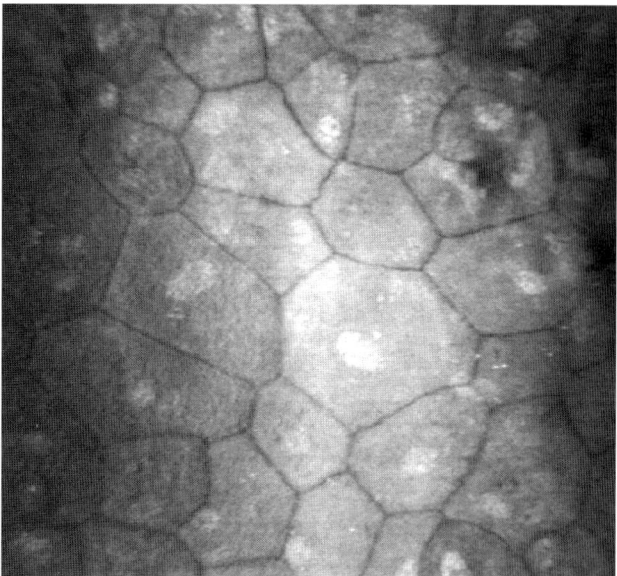

FIGURE 2-10. After penetrating keratoplasty, cell numbers decrease markedly, but the endothelium has a remarkable ability to expand in area. Note the apparent membrane features and the internal nuclei. A distinct bleb is seen in one cell in the upper right.

the adult. However, the cells do have the ability to enlarge and to maintain tight apposition with neighboring cells, preventing excessive seepage of aqueous humor into the stroma. Endothelial cells, almost without regard for specific cell density or cell size, abut one another with elaborate interdigitations. Additional resistance to paracellular flow is provided by specific junctional complexes located between endothelial cell membranes near the apical membranes close to the anterior chamber. Although these intermembranous specializations do not form continuous occluding zones around each cell, thereby permitting the penetration of relatively large probing ions such as lanthanum (88), they do help reduce fluid flow between endothelial cells.

A large nucleus dominates the cell interior, and in transverse view it may appear circular or lobate, depending on the species examined. The cytoplasm has numerous mitochondria and elaborate smooth and rough endoplasmic reticulum, as well as a Golgi complex, all of which are characteristic of cells actively involved in metabolic energy production and molecular synthetic processes. Pinocytotic vesicles near the posterior cell membrane have been identified, and may be related to the maintenance of the layer of viscous substance noted previously.

At the light and transmission electron microscopic level, endothelial cell cross-sections suggest a relatively homogeneous population of cells despite the fact that certain metabolic stresses, such as anterior corneal hypoxia (89), appear to alter the status of some cells before others.

From a clinical point of view, the corneal endothelium is functionally essential to the cornea. Normally, the endothelium

enjoys a privileged and protected environment in the anterior chamber, but it remains a fragile cell layer whose integrity and viability must be guarded to ensure the success of any intraocular procedure.

Similar to central nervous tissue, the cells of the human corneal endothelium essentially do not undergo cell division after birth. However, corneal endothelial cells have a remarkable ability to enlarge and to maintain normal function in the face of cellular inadequacies or deficiencies, as are seen during the postnatal growth of the cornea, during normal cell loss in the aging process, and after cell loss caused by intraocular surgery and trauma. At birth, cell densities range from 3500 to 4000 cells/mm^2, whereas the adult cornea normally has densities of 1400 to 2500 cells/mm^2. Corneal transplants may have fewer than 1000 cells/mm^2 and remain clear. It would appear that as long as endothelial cells can enlarge to provide a confluent monolayer on Descemet's membrane, normal corneal function is maintained. A lower limit to this ability occurs at densities of 400 to 700 cells/mm^2, below which endothelial function falters and corneal edema and loss of vision ensue.

The clinical specular microscope has been a useful tool for noninvasive evaluation of endothelial cell densities (90). Advances in confocal microscopy have also allowed *in situ* automatic endothelial cell counting. An extreme in cell size (or density) is shown in Fig. 2-10; a normal cell density (Fig. 2-9) is in marked contrast to that of a patient with a marginal cell density after having undergone clinically successful penetrating keratoplasty. Confocal microscopy has been useful for evaluating prospective corneal donor material, for predicting preoperatively the ability of a patient's cornea to tolerate cell loss, and for detecting posterior corneal lesions such as the alterations seen after contact lens wear or grafting (91) (Fig. 2-10). However, given the wide range of cell densities found in normal adult corneas, precise estimates of cell densities are of limited clinical value; endothelial function correlates poorly with this measurement.

As endothelial cells enlarge to compensate for losses, one might anticipate a gradual decrease in endothelial stromal dehydration function. Such is the case in early Fuchs' dystrophy, in which stromal edema is associated with decreased cell density and increased endothelial fluorescein permeability (92). However, in patients with cell densities as low as 615 cells/mm² after penetrating keratoplasty, stromal edema was absent and endothelial fluorescein permeability was reduced compared with normal cornea (93). Fluorescein traverses cell layers predominantly through paracellular pathways. The density of ATPase pump sites, located in the lateral membranes of endothelial cells and quantified by binding to radioactive ligands, is significantly decreased in dystrophic compared with normal corneas (94). One can conclude from these findings that a reduction in endothelial cell density alone is not sufficient to cause stromal edema. However, when the barrier property of the endothelium is compromised, as occurs with cornea guttata, the corneal dehydrating mechanism is overwhelmed by ion and water leakage into the stroma through damaged paracellular pathways.

In summary, there is a critical density of endothelial cells (400 to 700 cells/mm²) below which endothelial decompensation occurs, with progressive stromal edema and eventual epithelial edema. Stromal edema, which is associated with endothelial pathologic states, can occur with higher cell densities, and is the probable result of disruption of the paracellular pathways, as in early Fuchs' dystrophy.

When endothelial cells are subjected to stress, and especially when some cells are lost, the remaining cells may lose their regular hexagonal shape and become irregular in shape (pleomorphism) and size (polymegethism). These changes can occur with age, after trauma, and in long-term contact lens wearers. The significance of pleomorphism and polymegethism is unclear, but there is evidence that a cornea with these changes cannot withstand additional trauma as well as a normal cornea. In contact lens wearers, small blebs can develop in the endothelium shortly after a contact lens is inserted. These blebs are transient and are probably caused by the osmotic effect or low pH from lactic acid accumulation.

ENDOTHELIAL TRANSPORT PROPERTIES

In a number of early exploratory experiments, it was recognized that stromal edema ensued when the corneal endothelium was subjected to trauma, cold, or metabolic inhibitors.

Initial studies reported that ouabain inhibits fluid transport by the rabbit corneal endothelium *in vitro* (95). Ouabain inhibits Na^+/K^+-ATPase and is normally associated with the regulation of cell volume; this suggested that active Na^+ transport is intimately involved in the endothelial fluid transport function. However, whether Na^+ transport is simply a necessary prerequisite for normal cell function or whether it is the primary mechanism for endothelial fluid transport awaited further experimental demonstration. In keeping with its high ionic permeability, the corneal endothelium has a low electrical resistance (96). This leaky property made classic tracer experiments to demonstrate net ion transport mechanisms (97) technically difficult. Nevertheless, clear demonstrations showed that the endothelium transports bicarbonate from the stroma to the aqueous humor in amounts sufficient to explain the simultaneous isotonic transport of fluid (98,99). Subsequently, the transport of sodium ions in the same direction was inferred (100). Although the specific details of these transport mechanisms are unclear, several different schemes appear in the literature (101–103), indicating involvement of several alternate anion pathways (104).

How the transport of solute by the endothelium brings about the transport of fluid across the endothelium is still not clear. It is generally agreed that the basic mechanism for the corneal endothelial fluid pump is the transport of solute(s) from some sequestered volume into the aqueous humor. On a theoretical basis, a model of corneal hydration dynamics that used the stroma as this sequestered volume was remarkably accurate in its ability to predict the corneal response to a variety of environmental and metabolic perturbations (36,105). However, it has been argued that the endothelial fluid pumping capability remains intact despite the removal of most (106–108) or all (109) of the corneal stroma (106–108). Hence, whether this sequestered volume may be the endothelial extracellular space, or the endothelial cells themselves, remains unclear (58,101–103,106–112).

Fischbarg and coworkers (113) promote the idea that endothelial fluid transport involves electroosmosis through the intercellular junctions as the primary process in a sequence of events secondary to active ion transport. Ruberti and Klyce (114) report that transendothelial fluid transport may be rapidly self-modulating to control stromal hydration in response to small osmotic stresses, and this may assist in the regulation of corneal hydration.

In summary, the corneal endothelium secretes solute into the aqueous humor, and this transport system creates an osmotic gradient that draws fluid out of the stroma to balance its swelling tendency.

Endothelial "Fluid Pump"—a Misnomer

The early experiments clearly showed that the endothelium spent metabolic energy to transfer fluid from the stroma to the aqueous humor, and Maurice coined the term *endothelial fluid pump* (106). However, he envisioned this "pump" not as a literal entity that packaged up fluid and removed it from the stroma, but as a consequence of an active ion transport process associated with the endothelium. This process would obey the laws of thermodynamics to move an ion and co-ion (to maintain electroneutrality) out of the stroma to lower the osmotic pressure of the connective tissue. The consequence of this process in the normal tissue would lead to a steady-state situation in which a constant solute gradient would be maintained across the corneal cell layers that would balance the SP and prevent the imbibition of water. However, the endothelial fluid pump terminology was adopted and was soon accompanied by the term *fluid leak*. This provides an easily understood concept—fluid leaks in and is pumped out. However, this concept confuses the underpinnings of corneal hydration control, for water is actually always close to equilibrium in living systems, obeying the osmotic force gradients across membranes developed and maintained by active ion transport processes.

It was clear that active ion transport was involved in the control of corneal hydration, particularly because the active transport of water had never been demonstrated. The model for the control of corneal hydration that held the most promise postulated that an ion pump or pumps located in the endothelium would transport solute out of the stroma to balance the solute that leaked in across the imperfect semipermeable corneal endothelium.

THE CONTROL OF CORNEAL HYDRATION

The control of corneal hydration has received considerable attention because failure of the corneal membranes leads to corneal edema, vascularization, and opacification. The driving force for this pathologic process is the stromal IP, which must be counteracted to prevent swelling. In the past, it was suggested that although the cornea is surrounded by fluid, it would not swell if the epithelium and endothelium were impermeable to either water (115) or salt (29,116). Although both these cell layers have defined barrier properties, neither membrane is impermeable to either water or electrolytes (117). The effect of evaporation from the tear film has also been suggested as a major source for the control of corneal hydration (118) and, in fact, the cornea is 5% thinner during waking hours than during sleep (119,120). However, an isolated rabbit cornea at body temperature and bathed by simulated aqueous humor on both surfaces can maintain nearly normal thickness for up to 30 hours (121), which argues against a major role for evaporation in the control of hydration. The IOP has also been considered as a force in the regulation of corneal hydration, but although the corneal thickness does vary with changes in IOP, these changes are not sufficient to explain the control of normal corneal

hydration. In addition, isolated corneas can maintain near-normal thickness in the absence of IOP.

Such external factors may not normally be paramount in the control of stromal hydration, but they can become clinically important. Disruption of the lipid layer of the tear film leads to evaporation from the epithelial surface, which can lead to dellen formation. High postoperative IOP can promote more rapid clearing of a corneal graft by accelerating the movement of fluid through the anterior corneal surface, thereby thinning the cornea. However, elevated IOP can also cause epithelial edema, as well as stromal swelling, in certain refractive surgical procedures (34).

Maurice (117), recognizing that the corneal membranes are not impermeable to solute or water, first proposed that corneal edema could be prevented if ions were actively transported out of the stroma as fast as they moved in by passive means (solvent drag, diffusion). Such a process would, in essence, lead to the sustaining of an osmotic gradient (2 to 3 mOsm) between the corneal stroma and the external solutions, which would balance the SP of the stroma. This stromal solute deficit is 1% or less of the aqueous humor osmolarity, and would be difficult to detect with freezing-point depression measurements (122). However, Davson (123) and Harris and Nordquist (124) convincingly demonstrated that corneal hydration is closely linked to the metabolic activity of corneal membranes: Corneas swelled when refrigerated at temperatures that slowed metabolic processes and returned to normal thickness when warmed to body temperature. The temperature reversal phenomenon, as it has come to be known, is mediated by the corneal endothelium and inhibited by ouabain (125). Studies involving the temperature reversal phenomenon have provided much information on the functional characteristics of the corneal endothelium in terms of the ability of the corneal endothelium to cause the transport fluid from the stroma into the aqueous humor. As noted, this fluid transport is accomplished by the active transport of one or more ions by the endothelium, causing osmotic gradients to occur and water to flow in accordance with the laws of thermodynamics.

Because corneal epithelial and endothelial ion transport processes have been fairly well described and because the water flow properties of the stroma have also been characterized, it has been possible to combine these properties into models that describe the dynamics of corneal hydration.

Fluid flow (J_v) across a membrane is equal to the difference between two forces—the hydrostatic pressure gradient ($\triangle P$) and the osmotic gradient ($\triangle \pi$)—multiplied by the membrane water permeability (Lp):

$$J_v = Lp \, (\triangle P - \triangle \pi) \qquad [3]$$

This equation states that an increase in hydrostatic pressure on one side of a membrane or an increase in osmotic pressure on the other side of the membrane will produce a flow rate controlled by the water permeability of the membrane. With regard to fluid flow into the cornea across the endothelium, equation [3] shows that stromal IP tending to drive fluid into the stroma is balanced by an osmotic force created by ion pumps that remove solute from the stroma. When the net fluid flow is zero, as is nearly the case for the healthy cornea, the hydrostatic pressure gradient across the endothelium (IOP − SP) is equal to the osmotic gradient (reduced stromal solute).

To complete this model, flows of solute must be considered. Solutes diffuse across membranes at a rate equal to their solute permeability (T) times their concentration gradient, $\overline{C}_s$. Solutes are also transported actively across corneal membranes and this may be expressed by the term J_a. Finally, it has been shown that in many membranes (such as the highly permeable corneal endothelium), the bulk flow of fluid carries solute with it, which adds a third term to net solute flow (J_s). This relationship can be written:

$$J_s = (1 - F)\overline{C}_s J_v + TRT)C_s + J_a \qquad [4]$$

net solvent active
solute = drag + diffusion + transport
flow

where F, the reflection coefficient, is a membrane property related to the extent that bulk fluid flow across a membrane can drag along solute, $\overline{C}_s$ is the average solute concentration on each side of the membrane, and RT is the product of the gas constant and the temperature. In the normal case, where the stroma is not changing in thickness, equation [4] would predict that $J_s = J_v = 0$, where the active transport of solute (J_a) out of the stroma just balances the diffusional leak [(TRT)C_s] of solute into the stroma, which is the basis of Maurice's original pump-leak hypothesis (106).

Equations [3] and [4] form the basis for our understanding of the contribution of various factors in corneal hydration control. As noted previously, it is easy to state that the endothelial pump controls normal hydration, but this simplification does not help us to understand the causes of edema, especially when factors other than endothelial decompensation are involved. These equations have been used in their simplest form to provide a quantitative method to help evaluate the cause of corneal stromal edema. Yet, in the model described, simplicity has been preserved in that the corneal membranes are considered to be homogeneous, which makes it possible to determine the unknowns experimentally without using indirect inference or best guesses. For this reason a more sophisticated approach would be required to evaluate the electroosmosis predictions of the Fischbarg model (113). The epithelial and endothelial

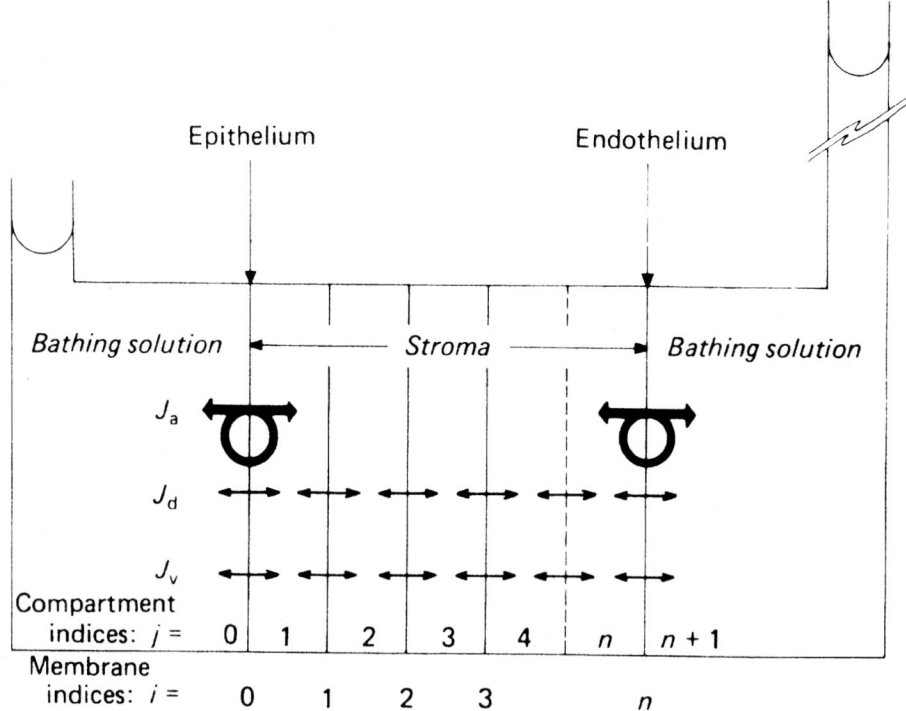

FIGURE 2-11. Numeric model simulation of corneal hydration dynamics. Flows of fluid volume (J_v), and solute, both active (J_a) and passive (J_d), can be calculated across the series of n + 1 membranes, where n is determined by stability criteria for a given calculation. The thicknesses of the stromal compartments, hence the relative positions of the membranes, are permitted to vary in time. By varying specific parameters in this model, several well-known corneal responses are duplicated. [From Klyce SD, Russell SR: Numerical solution of coupled transport equations applied to corneal hydration dynamics. J Physiol (Lond) 1979;292:107, with permission.]

TABLE 2-1. CORNEAL MEMBRANE PERMEABILITY

Epithelium				Endothelium				
σNaCL	Lp[a]	ωRT[b]	J_a^c	σNaCL	Lp[a]	ωRT[b]	J_a^c	Reference
—	—	0.016 (Na)	—	—	—	2 (Na)	—	Maurice (1953)[207]
1[d]	6.9	—	—	0.6	15.8	—	—	Mishima and Hedbys (1967)[208]
1[d]	6.5	—	—	0.6[d]	13.8	—	—	Stanley et al (1966)[209]
—	—	—	—	—	—	2.1 (urea)	—	Trenberth and Mishima (1968)[181]
0.8	0.4	—	—	0.4	1.4	—	—	Green and Green (1969)[210]
—	—	—	—	—	—	2.2 (Cl)	—	Kim et al (1971)[211]
—	—	0.014 (Cl)	<0.03[e]	—	—	—	—	Klyce (1975)[131]
—	—	—	—	—	—	—	3.9 (HCO₃)	Hodson and Miller (1976)[184]
—	0.9	—	—	—	3	—	—	Green and Downs (1976)[212]
—	—	—	—	0.6[d]	8	—	—	Fischbarg et al (1977)[213]
—	—	—	—	—	—	—	12.9 (HCO₃)	Hull et al (1977)[185]
0.79	6.1	0.019 (NaCl)	<0.08[e]	0.45	42	8 (NaCl)	4.7	Klyce and Russell (1979)[178]

[a] $\times 10^{-12}$ cm³/dyne · sec.
[b] $\times 10^{-5}$ cm/sec.
[c] $\times 10^{-10}$ mole/cm² · sec.
[d] Assumed values.
[e] Basal epithelial transport rate (Cl secretion unstimulated).
Source: Adapted from SD Klyce, SR Russell: Numerical solution of coupled transport equations applied to corneal hydration dynamics. J Physiol 292:107, 1979, with permission.

corneal membranes are characterized by equations [3] and [4], whereas the stroma is characterized by reduced forms of these equations. There is no active transport of solute within the stroma and no volume transport owing to osmotic gradients across the stroma. Whereas the concentration of solutes across the stroma is fairly uniform as a result of a relatively high stromal permeability (only two times less than free diffusion in aqueous medium), the flow of water is far more restricted. Hence, to allow for the steep gradients that can arise (corneal dellen are a good example), the corneal stroma is subdivided into layers in the model shown in Fig. 2-11.

In this approach, no assumptions were made as to the permeability coefficients (F, T, L$_p$) for the corneal epithelium or endothelium. These were determined by fit to experiments that measured the response of corneal thickness to small changes in the osmolarity of the tear-side bathing solution. Permeability coefficients for solute and water across the stroma were taken directly from the precise work of Fatt and Goldstick (28). Table 2-1 summarizes the results of these determinations and compares them with previous measurements and with solute permeabilities measured with tracers (36,51,95,98,99,114,126–132).

The model was tested rigorously against well-documented experimental observations. These included matching the temperature reversal thinning behavior of the cornea, the corneal swelling response to ouabain, osmotic perturbations applied to the endothelium, and several other reactions of the cornea to experimental manipulations (35,36). In addition, this model has been used to provide evidence supporting the thesis that stromal edema after hypoxia of the tear film is the result of stromal accumulation of lactate (133), an osmotically active byproduct of anaerobic respiration.

CORNEAL EDEMA

The model discussed in the previous section for the control of corneal hydration concerns itself with the normal healthy cornea with intact functioning membranes and avascular, compact corneal stroma. However, these normal properties are modified by disease and the reaction of the cornea can be complex. Although acute corneal edema, as can be seen in contact lens wear and in angle-closure glaucoma, is often reversible, chronic corneal edema is usually irreversible and treatment varies depending on the nature of the disorder.

Chronic corneal edema develops as a consequence of endothelial dysfunction, regardless of whether the original clinical condition was dystrophy, inflammation, or trauma. The increased permeability or decreased ion transport function, or both, of this cellular layer leads to the subsequent corneal changes. In mild cases only, increased stromal thickness occurs with initially little consequence to vision. In advanced cases, epithelial edema ensues, which rapidly decreases visual acuity. Late, painful bullous changes can develop—bullous keratopathy. If the natural clinical course is not interrupted by keratoplasty, a thick subepithelial pannus eventually develops, leading to the disappearance of the bullae and, with them, the discomfort. Vision at this stage is usually reduced to hand movement level because of both epithelial and stromal scar formation.

Endothelial Changes

The endothelium under stress changes in a few nonspecific, but characteristic ways. Thus, in acute inflammation or in trauma, rapid cell degeneration and death can occur in a focal manner that is then repaired by sliding and rearrangement of neighboring cells. The resulting endothelium is characterized by decreased cell number and enlarged and irregularly shaped cells (polymegathism and pleomorphism) (134).

In chronic inflammation, endothelial cells may undergo fibrous metaplasia (135); this can result in a fibrous membrane between Descemet's membrane and the endothelium. In Fuchs' dystrophy the cells exhibit a change in form and show vacuoles, phagocytized pigment, and periodic acid-Schiff–positive material that is eventually deposited on Descemet's membrane. These irregular depositions become visible as the characteristic warts (guttae) over which the endothelial cells eventually become quite attenuated. Even in advanced cases of Fuchs' dystrophy, however, the endothelial surface appears intact (136,137).

Stromal Edema

When the endothelial cell density falls below a critical level (200 to 400 cells/mm^2), the ability of the endothelium to maintain stromal hydration begins to falter and stromal edema develops gradually. The two opposing forces—the osmotic pressure developed by the endothelial ion transport on one hand and the stromal SP on the other—remain in balance, but the osmotic gradient established by the endothelial pump must diminish with reduced transport function and possibly greater ion leakage across the endothelium. Because the stroma can swell only in the posterior direction (corneal anterior curvature and diameter remain normal), its thickness increases, especially centrally because the peripheral corneal swelling appears to be limited to some extent by structural restriction imposed by the limbus. This flattening of the posterior surface can throw Descemet's membrane into multiple folds that become visible as striae on slit-lamp microscopy. There is little tissue reaction to the swelling as a rule, and it is only in massive, chronic edema that scarring of the tissue eventually develops, more markedly in the posterior layers and especially in the folds created by Descemet's membrane.

Epithelial Edema

Epithelial edema resulting from endothelial dysfunction or elevated IOP, or a combination of both, is predominantly extracellular (138). Thus, fluid begins to accumulate in the space between the basal epithelial cells, stretching the bridging desmosomes. Later in the process these fluid-filled spaces enlarge to form fine blisters, visible as microcystic edema by slit-lamp examination. Finally, larger bullae develop, characteristic of bullous keratopathy. Epithelial edema rarely involves the anteriormost squamous cells of the epithelium.

The underlying pathophysiologic mechanism seems to involve a forward movement of stromal fluid and aqueous, generated by the IOP. Thus, if the endothelial functional reserve falls below a certain level, leading to edema and a reduction in stromal SP to below the value of the IOP, fluid from the aqueous humor can collect (33). Because the otherwise healthy epithelium has such a high resistance to electrolytes and to the flow of water, the fluid can be trapped within the epithelium, resulting in the formation of cysts and bullae. The anteriormost wing cells usually are unaffected, suggesting that the resistance to this anterior fluid movement is situated primarily in this layer.

The situation of the IOP being higher than the stromal SP, thereby resulting in the epithelial edema, can exist in different clinical settings. On the one hand, poor endothelial function even with normal IOP is sufficient to cause epithelial edema (e.g., Fuchs' dystrophy, aphakic or pseudophakic edema). On the other hand, even with normal endothelium, very high IOP (such as occurs in angle-closure glaucoma) can also cause epithelial edema. In between these two extremes, edema may occur from various combinations of endothelial dysfunction and elevated IOP (33). The concept that the IOP is the driving force for the fluid movement in epithelial edema is particularly supported by the fact that in phthisis with marked hypotony, epithelial edema does not occur, no matter how damaged the endothelium is and how thick the stroma is. These cases are illustrated in Fig. 2-12.

Evaporation can be a balancing factor in borderline epithelial edema. It is a common occurrence in early edema that vision is blurred in the morning but clears as the day progresses. It is clearly the lack of evaporation when the lids are closed during the night that allows fluid to accumulate in the epithelium. After opening the eyes, evaporation results in slight hypertonicity of the tear film, which in turn extracts water from the epithelium, clearing the vision. This state can last for months, rarely years, but eventually the edema worsens.

Edema with Contact Lens Wear

The edema that can occasionally be seen as a result of contact lens wear differs in many respects from the forms of edema described earlier. The symptoms and signs are usually attributable to hypoxia or hypercapnia (elevated CO_2 tension), or both, under the lens. Therefore, gas permeability of the lens and tear fluid exchange are the most important parameters in maintaining normal fluid balance in the cornea.

Mild stromal edema is common in soft contact lens wear. Epithelial hypoxia causes lactic acid buildup in the

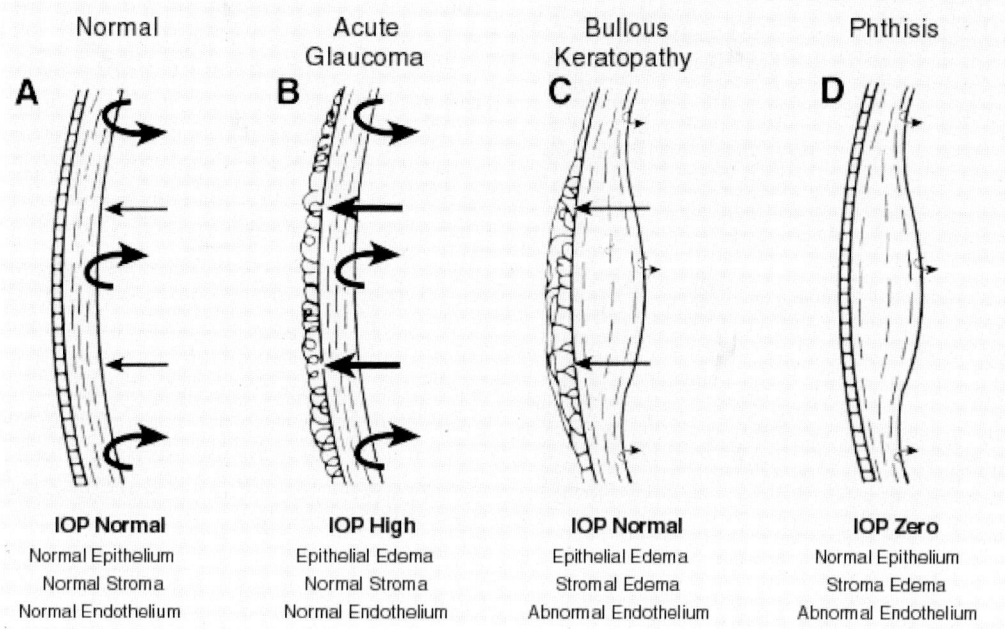

FIGURE 2-12. Development of epithelial edema. When the intraocular pressure overpowers the endothelial pump, fluid collects between the cells in the epithelium, behind the barrier of the outer membranes of the squamous cells. This can occur with a normal endothelium and very high pressure (acute glaucoma). In chronic edema, the intraocular pressure is normal, but the endothelium is severely dysfunctional.

stroma (105,139) and reduced pH (133), which in turn may affect endothelial performance. However, the lactic acid accumulation raises stromal osmotic pressure, drawing in water for osmotic reasons, as noted previously, and pH effects on the corneal endothelium may not occur under acute situations. This thickening of the stroma is usually clinically acceptable because it has little influence on visual acuity or contrast sensitivity (140).

Epithelial edema, on the other hand, resulting from hard contact lens overwear (Sattler's veil, epithelial bedewing) can be visually quite debilitating, although it is readily reversible on removal of the lens. Histologically, the location of the fluid collection is primarily *intra*cellular, in contrast to the primarily *extra*cellular edema in Fuchs' dystrophy or similar conditions, and may be related to induced abnormalities caused by hypoxia and lactate accumulation.

Visual Acuity in Edema

Because of its surface smoothness and its transparency, the cornea normally allows a remarkably sharp image to be focused on the retina. In general these optical qualities can be reduced by opacities within the tissue (stroma or epithelium) or by surface irregularities, either in the form of gross astigmatism (e.g., keratoconus) or from minute central irregularities (e.g., bullous keratopathy and basement membrane dystrophy).

As noted, normal stromal transparency can be explained by maintenance of average uniformity of its refractive index over distances of up to half the wavelength of light (approximately 2000 Å). In the normal corneal stroma, the collagen fibrils spaced some 600 Å from center to center are closer together than half the wavelength of light, explaining the optical qualities of the tissue. Transparency is still fairly well preserved in mild or moderate stromal edema, and backscattering toward the source is minimal (141). In more advanced and long-standing edema, however, irregular fluid accumulations occur in the stroma that can reduce transparency (11). Later stromal scarring and posterior irregular astigmatism from folds in Descemet's membrane reduce vision further.

In Sattler's veil, reduction in vision is usually minor, and is caused by a diffraction phenomenon that occurs in the slightly swollen epithelial cells (142) (Fig. 2-13). True epithelial edema, in contrast to Sattler's veil and stromal edema, can reduce vision early and often profoundly. The fluid accumulations between or within the epithelial cells markedly increase light scattering. Even more important are the minute surface irregularities from the edema that break up the smoothness normally provided by the corneal tears and consequently lead to blurring of the retinal image. In general, in a patient with vision reduced by corneal disease, there is often a tendency for the clinician to overestimate the contribution of opacities within the tissue and to underestimate the role of surface irregularities. A hard contact lens

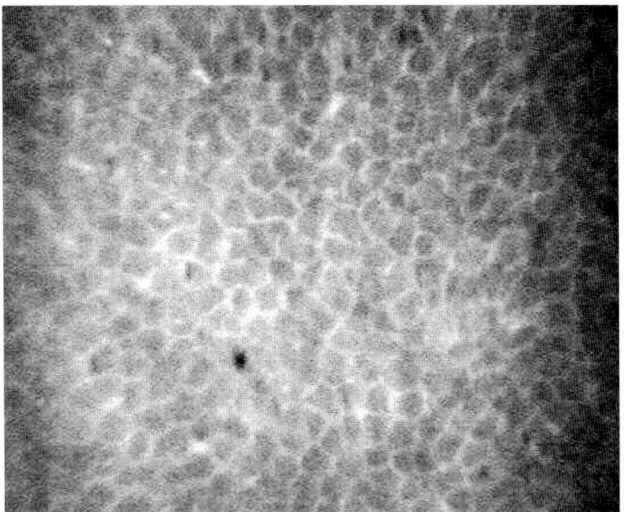

FIGURE 2-13. Outline of the basal cells in the corneal epithelium by confocal microscopy. The intracellular space, which is evident here, increases in brightness owing to light scatter during hypoxia, producing the diffraction phenomena of haloes around bright lights at night (Sattler's veil).

refraction or corneal topography analysis will settle the question of the influence of surface irregularities on visual acuity.

CORNEAL NUTRITION

The cells of the cornea are actively involved in the maintenance of the functions required for structural integrity and hydration control. Much of the energy for these processes is derived from the catabolism of glucose through both aerobic and anaerobic pathways. The bulk of the glucose used (105 μg/cm^2/hour) (143) is derived from the aqueous humor; negligible amounts enter the cornea from the tears and the limbus (144). Glucose reserves are present in the form of epithelial glycogen granules, which serve as a source of energy during periods of metabolic stress (hypoxia and trauma). In the short term, glycogenolysis provides a metabolic buffer, maintaining adequate cell glucose levels.

Utilization of glucose through the anaerobic glycolytic pathway results in the formation of pyruvate, which is converted either to CO_2 in the Krebs cycle or to lactate by lactic acid dehydrogenase. Elimination of CO_2 from the cornea is not a problem because corneal membranes are highly permeable to this metabolic byproduct. In contrast, the elimination of lactate is not as easily accomplished. The barrier properties of the superficial corneal epithelial cells preclude the diffusive transfer of significant amounts of corneal lactate to the tears (105,143). Instead, lactate must be removed by diffusion across the stroma and endothelium into the aqueous humor. As discussed previously, lactate buildup in the cornea can produce both epithelial and stromal edema.

The normal metabolism of the corneal cells also requires a constant supply of amino acids, vitamins, and other constituents. As with glucose, the principal source of these molecules is the aqueous humor. If these needs are not met or the supply is significantly reduced over a long time, such as by a large, nutrient-impermeable implant (145), anterior corneal necrosis can occur. Although the cornea has some tolerance for interruption of the normal nutrient supply, neither the limbus nor the tears can provide sufficient nutrients to maintain corneal function when the aqueous humor is deficient, as during ciliary body shutdown (146).

Oxygen is the single known corneal metabolic requirement not met by the aqueous humor. Normally, a substantial portion of the oxygen used by the cornea is derived by diffusion from the tear film. Tight-fitting contact lenses made from materials with a low oxygen permeability can reduce oxygen tension below critical levels, resulting in epithelial or stromal edema (147), as well as morphologic alterations in the corneal endothelium (89). The partial pressure of oxygen in the tears normally ranges from 155 mm Hg (with the eyelids open) to 55 mm Hg (with the eyelids closed) (148). The cornea can tolerate sustained exposure to oxygen levels down to 25 mm Hg in the tear film before edema is induced (149). During sleep, some oxygen is provided to the anterior cornea by diffusion from the eyelid vasculature, while during waking hours a surplus is available from the atmosphere.

CONCLUSION

The basic functional aspects of the maintenance of corneal hydration and transparency are well established and the major concepts are summarized in Fig. 2-14. Corneal homeostasis

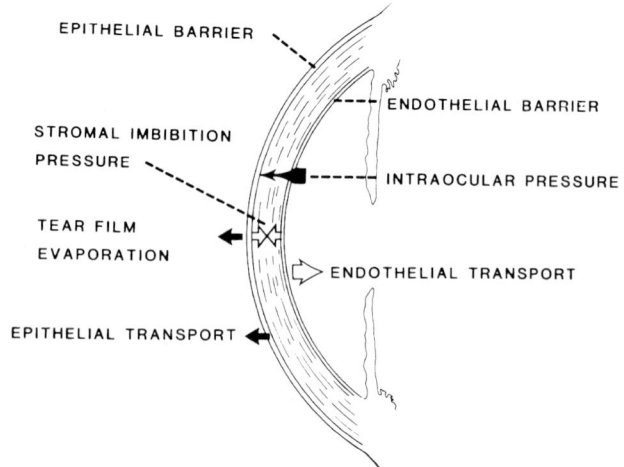

FIGURE 2-14. Factors and forces involved in the control of corneal stromal hydration. Intraocular pressure and stromal imbibition pressure are forces that promote water accumulation in the stroma. Ion transport pumps in the corneal membranes reduce the osmotic pressure of the stroma such that the semipermeable membrane properties of the epithelium and endothelium balance the forces promoting edema. (From Klyce SD, Beuerman RW: Anatomy and physiology of the cornea. In: Kaufman HE, Barron BA, McDonald MB, eds. *The cornea*, 2nd ed. Boston: Butterworth-Heinemann, 1998:3–50, with permission.)

can be understood on the basis of cell membrane transport systems regulating stromal hydration through the reduction of solute in that extracellular space, and the consequences of membrane osmotic forces balancing the swelling forces generated by the hydrophilic glycosaminoglycans contained within. This regulatory mechanism is exactly analogous to those membrane ion transport processes that are responsible for maintaining the normal volume of all cells in the body. Still, the cornea is a remarkable and unique tissue that provides the window on the world for all to see.

ACKNOWLEDGMENTS

This work was supported in part by USPHS grants EY03311 (SDK) and EY02377 (LSU Eye Center) from the National Eye Institute, National Institutes of Health, Bethesda, Maryland.

REFERENCES

1. Donaldson DD. A new instrument for the measurement of corneal thickness. *Arch Ophthalmol* 1966;76:25.
2. Mishima S, Hedbys BO. Measurement of corneal thickness with the Haag-Streit pachometer. *Arch Ophthalmol* 1968; 80:710.
3. Mishima S. Corneal thickness. *Surv Ophthalmol* 1968;13:57.
4. McLaren JW, Bourne WM. A new video pachometer. *Invest Ophthalmol Vis Sci* 1999;40:1593.
5. Giraud JP, Pouliquen Y, Offret G, et al. Statistical morphometric studies in normal human and rabbit corneal stroma. *Exp Eye Res* 1975;21:221.
6. Hogan MJ, Alvarado JA, Weddell E. *Histology of the human eye.* Philadelphia: WB Saunders, 1971.
7. Maurice DM. The structure and transparency of the cornea. *J Physiol (Lond)* 1957;136:263.
8. Goldman JN, Benedek GB. The relationship between morphology and transparency in the nonswelling corneal stroma of the shark. *Invest Ophthalmol* 1967;6:574.
9. Benedek GB. Theory of transparency of the eye. *Appl Optics* 1971;10:459.
10. Farrell RA, McCally RL, Tatham PER. Wavelength dependencies of light scattering in normal and cold swollen rabbit corneas and their structural implications. *J Physiol (Lond)* 1973;233:589.
11. Goldman JN, Benedek GB, Dohlman CH, et al. Structural alterations affecting transparency in swollen human corneas. *Invest Ophthalmol* 1968;7:501.
12. Assouline M, Chew SJ, Thompson HW, et al. Effect of growth factors on collagen lattice contraction by human keratocytes. *Invest Ophthalmol Vis Sci* 1992;33:1742.
13. Newsome DA, Foidart JM, Hassell JR, et al. Detection of specific collagen types in normal and keratoconus corneas. *Invest Ophthalmol Vis Sci* 1981;20:738.
14. Maurice DM. The cornea and sclera. In: Davson H (ed). *The eye*, vol 1B: *Vegetative physiology and biochemistry*, 3rd ed. New York, Academic Press, 1984:1.
15. Cintron C, Schneider H, Kublin C. Corneal scar formation. *Exp Eye Res* 1973;17:251.
16. Dohlman CH, Gasset AR, Rose J. The effect of the absence of corneal epithelium or endothelium on the stromal keratocytes. *Invest Ophthalmol* 1968;7:520.
17. Wilson SE, Mohan RR, Ambrosio R Jr, et al. The corneal wound healing response: cytokine-mediated interaction of the epithelium, stroma, and inflammatory cells. *Prog Retin Eye Res* 2001;20:625.
18. Wilson SE, Mohan RR, Hutcheon AE, et al. Effect of ectopic epithelial tissue within the stroma on keratocyte apoptosis, mitosis, and myofibroblast transformation. *Exp Eye Res* 2003; 76:193.
19. Ruberti JW, Klyce SD, Smolek MK, et al. Anomalous acute inflammatory response in rabbit corneal stroma. *Invest Ophthalmol Vis Sci* 2000;41:2523.
20. Karon MD, Klyce SD. Effect of inhibition of inflammatory mediators on trauma-induced stromal edema. *Invest Ophthalmol Vis Sci* 2003;44:2507.
21. Wilson SE. Molecular cell biology for the refractive corneal surgeon: programmed cell death and wound healing. *J Refract Surg* 1997;13:171.
22. Otori T. Electronic content of the rabbit corneal stroma. *Exp Eye Res* 1967;6:356.
23. Friedman MH, Green K. Swelling rate of corneal stroma. *Exp Eye Res* 1971;12:239.
24. Hodson S. Why the cornea swells. *J Theor Biol* 1971;33:419.
25. Elliot GF, Goodfellow JM, Woolgar AE. Swelling studies of bovine corneal stroma without bounding membranes. *J Physiol (Lond)* 1980;298:453.
26. Kanai A, Kaufman HE. Electron microscopic studies of swollen corneal stroma. *Ann Ophthalmol* 1973;5:178.
27. Ehlers N. Variations in hydration properties of the cornea. *Acta Ophthalmol (Copenh)* 1966;44:461.
28. Fatt I, Goldstick TK. Dynamics of water transport in swelling membranes. *J Colloid Sci* 1965;20:434.
29. Cogan DG, Kinsey VE. The cornea: V. Physiologic aspects. *Arch Ophthalmol* 1942;28:661.
30. Hedbys BO, Dohlman CH: A new method for the determination of the swelling pressure of the corneal stroma in vitro. *Exp Eye Res* 1963;2:122.
31. Hedbys BO, Mishima S, Maurice DM. The imbibition pressure of the corneal stroma. *Exp Eye Res* 1963;2:99.
32. Klyce SD, Dohlman CH, Tolpin DW. In vivo determination of corneal swelling pressure of the corneal stroma. *Exp Eye Res* 1971;11:220.
33. Ytteborg J, Dohlman CH. Corneal edema and intraocular pressure: II. Clinical results. *Arch Ophthalmol* 1965;74:477.
34. McPhee TJ, Bourne WM, Brubaker RF. Location of the stress-bearing layers of the cornea. *Invest Ophthalmol Vis Sci* 1985;26:869.
35. Wilson G, O'Leary DJ, Vaughn W. Differential swelling in the compartments of the corneal stroma. *Invest Ophthalmol Vis Sci* 1984;25:1105.
36. Klyce SD, Russell SR. Numerical solution of coupled transport equations applied to corneal hydration dynamics. *J Physiol (Lond)* 1979;292:107.
37. Ehlers N. Some comparative studies on the mammalian corneal epithelium. *Acta Ophthalmol (Copenh)* 1970;48:821.
38. Hanna C, Bicknell DS, O'Brien J. Cell turnover in the adult human eye. *Arch Ophthalmol* 1961;65:695.
39. Nagasaki T, Zhao J. Centripetal movement of corneal epithelial cells in the normal adult mouse. *Invest Ophthalmol Vis Sci* 2003;44:558.
40. Dua HS, Joseph A, Shanmuganathan VA, et al. Stem cell differentiation and the effects of deficiency. *Eye* 2003;17:877.
41. McLaughlin BJ, Caldwell RB, Sasaki Y, et al. Freeze-fracture quantitative comparison of rabbit corneal epithelial and endothelial membranes. *Curr Eye Res* 1985;4:951.

42. Klyce SD. Electrical profiles in the corneal epithelium. *J Physiol (Lond)* 1972;226:407.
43. Kikkawa Y. Normal corneal staining with fluorescein. *Exp Eye Res* 1972;14:13.
44. Schultz RO, Peters MA, Sobocinski K, et al. Diabetic keratopathy as a manifestation of peripheral neuropathy. *Am J Ophthalmol* 1983;96:368.
45. Gipson IK, Anderson RA. Actin filaments in normal and migrating corneal epithelial cells. *Invest Ophthalmol Vis Sci* 1977;16:161.
46. Donn A, Maurice DM, Mills NL. Studies on the living cornea in vitro: I. Method and physiologic measurements. *Arch Ophthalmol* 1959;62:741.
47. Donn A, Maurice DM, Mills NL. Studies on the living cornea in vitro: II. The active transport of sodium across the epithelium. *Arch Ophthalmol* 1959;62:748.
48. Green K. Ion transport in isolated cornea of the rabbit. *Am J Physiol* 1965;209:1311.
49. Klyce SD, Neufeld AH, Zadunaisky JA. The activation of chloride transport by epinephrine and Db cyclic-AMP in the cornea of the rabbit. *Invest Ophthalmol* 1973;12:127.
50. Van der Hayden C, Weekers JF, Schoffeniels E. Sodium and chloride transport across the isolated rabbit cornea. *Exp Eye Res* 1975;20:89.
51. Klyce SD. Transport of Na, Cl, and water by the rabbit corneal epithelium at resting potential. *Am J Physiol* 1975;228:1446.
52. Candia OA, Askew WA. Active sodium transport in the isolated bullfrog cornea. *Biochim Biophys Acta* 1968;163:262.
53. Langham ME, Hart RW, Cox J. The interaction of collagen and mucopolysaccharides. In: Langham M (ed). *The cornea: macromolecular organization of a connective tissue.* Baltimore: Johns Hopkins University Press, 1969:157.
54. Green K. Relation of epithelial ion transport to corneal thickness hydration. *Nature* 1968;217:1074.
55. Fischer FH, Schmitz L, Hoff W, et al. Sodium and chloride transport in the isolated rabbit cornea. *Pflugers Arch* 1978;373:179.
56. Friedman MH. Mathematical modeling of transport in structured tissues: corneal epithelium. *Am J Physiol* 1978;234:F215.
57. Kaye GI, Tice LW. Studies on the cornea: V. Electron microscopic localization of adenosine triphosphate activity in the rabbit cornea in relation to transport. *Invest Ophthalmol* 1968;5:22.
58. Shapiro MP, Candia OA. Corneal hydration and metabolically dependent transcellular passive transfer of water. *Exp Eye Res* 1973;15:659.
59. Klyce SD, Marshall WS. Effect of Ag+ on the electrophysiology of the rabbit corneal epithelium. *J Membr Biol* 1982;66:133.
60. Zadunaisky JA. Active transport of chloride in frog cornea. *Am J Physiol* 1966;211:506.
61. Wiederholt M. Physiology of epithelial transport in the human eye. *Klin Wochenschr* 1980;58:975.
62. Klyce SD, Wong RKS. Site and mode of adrenaline action of chloride transport across the rabbit corneal epithelium. *J Physiol (Lond)* 1977;266:777.
63. Zadunaisky JA, Lande MA. Active chloride transport and control of corneal transparency. *Am J Physiol* 1971;221:1837.
64. Candia OA. Fluid and Cl transport by the epithelium of the isolated frog cornea. ARVO Abstracts. *Invest Ophthalmol Vis Sci* 1976;15[4 Suppl]:12(abstr).
65. Klyce SD. Enhancing fluid secretion by the corneal epithelium. *Invest Ophthalmol Vis Sci* 1977;16:968.
66. Candia OA, Neufeld AH. Topical epinephrine causes a decrease in density of β-adrenergic receptors and catecholamine-stimulated chloride transport in rabbit cornea. *Biochim Biophys Acta* 1978;543:403.
67. Klyce SD, Beuerman RW, Crosson CE. Alteration of corneal epithelial transport by sympathectomy. *Invest Ophthalmol Vis Sci* 1985;26:434.
68. Klyce SD, Palkama KA, Neufeld AH, et al. Neural serotonin stimulates chloride transport in the rabbit corneal epithelium. *Invest Ophthalmol Vis Sci* 1982;23:181.
69. Crosson CE, Beuerman RW, Klyce SD. Dopamine modulation of active ion transport in rabbit corneal epithelium. *Invest Ophthalmol Vis Sci* 1984;25:1240.
70. Neufeld AH, Ledgard SE, Jumblatt MM, et al. Serotonin-stimulated cyclic AMP synthesis in the rabbit corneal epithelium. *Invest Ophthalmol Vis Sci* 1982;23:193.
71. Marshall WS, Klyce SD. Cellular mode of serotonin action on Cl− transport in the rabbit corneal epithelium. *Biochim Biophys Acta* 1984;778:139.
72. Jumblatt MM, Neufeld AH. β-Adrenergic and serotonergic responsiveness of rabbit corneal epithelial cells in culture. *Invest Ophthalmol Vis Sci* 1983;24:1139.
73. Hill JM, Shimomuera Y, Kwon BS, et al. Iontophoresis of epinephrine isomers to rabbit eyes induced HSV-1 ocular shedding. *Invest Ophthalmol Vis Sci* 1985;26:1299.
74. Hill JM, Shimomura Y, Dudley JB, et al. Timolol induces HSV-1 ocular shedding in the latently infected rabbit. *Invest Ophthalmol Vis Sci* 1987;28:585.
75. Kikkawa Y. The intracellular potential of the corneal epithelium. *Exp Eye Res* 1964;3:132.
76. Fee JP, Edelhauser HF. Intracellular electrical potentials in the rabbit corneal epithelium. *Exp Eye Res* 1970;9:233.
77. Akaike N, Hori M. Effect of anions and cations on membrane potential of rabbit corneal epithelium. *Am J Physiol* 1970;219:1811.
78. Akaike N. The origin of the basal cell potential in frog corneal epithelium. *J Physiol (Lond)* 1971;219:57.
79. Klyce SD. *Electrophysiology of the corneal epithelium.* PhD Thesis, Department of Physiology. New Haven, CT: Yale University, 1971.
80. Festen CMAW, Slegers JFG. The influence of ions, ouabain, propranolol and amiloride on the transepithelial potential and resistance of rabbit cornea. *Exp Eye Res* 1979;28:413.
81. Marshall WS, Klyce SD. Cellular and paracellular pathway resistances in the "tight" Cl−-secreting epithelium of the rabbit cornea. *J Membr Biol* 1983;73:275.
82. Maurice DM. Epithelial potential of the cornea. *Exp Eye Res* 1967;6:138.
83. Alaerts ML. Aspects de l'endothelium corneen au biomicroscope. *Bull Soc Belg Ophthalmol* 1959;122:320.
84. Wolf J. The secretory activity and the cuticle of the corneal endothelium. *Doc Ophthalmol* 1968;25:150.
85. Sperling S, Jacobsen SR. The surface coat on human corneal endothelium. *Acta Ophthalmol (Copenh)* 1980;58:96.
86. Svedbergh B, Bill A. Scanning electron microscopic studies of the corneal endothelium in man and monkeys. *Acta Ophthalmol (Copenh)* 1972;50:321.
87. Gallagher B. Primary cilia of the corneal endothelium. *Am J Anat* 1980;159:475.
88. Kreutziger GO. Lateral membrane morphology and gap junction structure in rabbit corneal endothelium. *Exp Eye Res* 1976;23:285.
89. Zantos SG, Holden BA. Transient endothelial changes soon after wearing soft contact lenses. *Am J Optom Physiol Optics* 1977;54:856.
90. Maurice DM. Cellular membrane activity in the corneal endothelium of the intact eye. *Experientia* 1968;24:1094.
91. Laing RA, Sandstrom MA, Liebowitz HM. In vivo photomicrography of corneal endothelium. *Arch Ophthalmol* 1975;93:143.

92. Burns RR, Bourne WM, Brubaker RF. Endothelial function in patients with cornea guttata. *Invest Ophthalmol Vis Sci* 1981; 20:77.

93. Bourne WM, Brubaker RF. Decreased endothelial permeability in transplanted corneas. *Am J Ophthalmol* 1983;96:362.

94. McCartney MD, Robertson DP, Wood TO, et al. ATPase pump site density in human dysfunctional corneal endothelium. *Invest Ophthalmol Vis Sci* 1987;28:1955.

95. Tenberth SM, Mishima S. The effect of ouabain on the rabbit corneal endothelium. *Invest Ophthalmol* 1968;7:44.

96. Lim JJ, Fischbarg J. Electrical profiles of rabbit corneal endothelium as determined from impedance measurements. *Biophys J* 1981;36:677.

97. Ussing HH. The distinction by means of tracers between active transport and diffusion. *Acta Physiol Scand* 1949;19:43.

98. Hodson S, Miller F. The bicarbonate ion pump in the endothelium which regulates the hydration of the rabbit cornea. *J Physiol (Lond)* 1976;263:563.

99. Hull DS, Green K, Boyd M, et al. Corneal endothelium bicarbonate transport and the effect of carbonic anhydrase inhibitors on endothelial permeability and fluxes and corneal thickness. *Invest Ophthalmol Vis Sci* 1977;16:883.

100. Lim JJ, Ussing HH. Analysis of presteady-state Na^+ fluxes across the rabbit corneal endothelium. *J Membr Biol* 1982; 65:197.

101. Fischbarg J, Hernandez J, Liebovitch LS, et al. The mechanism of fluid and electrolyte transport across corneal endothelium: critical revision and update of a model. *Curr Eye Res* 1985;4:351.

102. Wiederholt M, Jentsch TJ, Keller SK. Electrical sodium-bicarbonate symport in cultured corneal endothelial cells. *Pflugers Arch* 1985;405:S167.

103. Kuang KY, Xu M, Koniarek JP, et al. Effects of ambient bicarbonate, phosphate and carbonic anhydrase inhibitors on fluid transport across rabbit corneal endothelium. *Exp Eye Res* 1990; 50:487.

104. Bonanno JA. Identity and regulation of ion transport mechanisms in the corneal endothelium. *Prog Retin Eye Res* 2003; 22:69.

105. Klyce SD. Stromal lactate accumulation can account for corneal edema osmotically following epithelial hypoxia in the rabbit. *J Physiol (Lond)* 1981;321:49.

106. Maurice DM. The location of the fluid pump in the cornea. *J Physiol (Lond)* 1972;221:43.

107. Fischbarg J, Lim JJ, Bourget J. Adenosine stimulation of fluid transport across rabbit corneal endothelium. *J Membr Biol* 1977;35:95.

108. Hodson S, Miller F, Riley M. The electrogenic pump of rabbit corneal endothelium. *Exp Eye Res* 1977;24:249.

109. Narula P, Xu M, Kuang KY, et al. Fluid transport across cultured bovine corneal endothelial cell monolayers. *Am J Physiol* 1992;262:C98.

110. Fischbarg J, Montoreano R. Osmotic permeability across corneal endothelium and antidiuretic hormone-stimulated toad urinary bladder structures. *Biochim Biophys Acta* 1982; 690:207.

111. Liebovitch LS, Weinbaum S. A model of epithelial water transport: the corneal endothelium. *Biophys J* 1981;35:315.

112. Wigham C, Hodson S. The movement of sodium across short-circuited rabbit corneal endothelium. *Curr Eye Res* 1985; 4:1241.

113. Sanchez JM, Li Y, Rubashkin A, et al. Evidence for a central role for electro-osmosis in fluid transport by corneal endothelium. *J Membr Biol* 2002;187:37.

114. Ruberti JW, Klyce SD. NaCl osmotic perturbation can modulate hydration control in rabbit cornea. *Exp Eye Res* 2003; 76:349.

115. Leber T. Studies on fluid exchange in the eye. *Graefes Arch Ophthalmol* 1973;19:87.

116. von Bahr G. Measurements of the effect of solutions of different osmotic pressure on the thickness of the living cornea. *Trans Ophthalmol Soc UK* 1948;68:515.

117. Maurice DM. The permeability to sodium ions of the living rabbit cornea. *J Physiol (Lond)* 1951;112:367.

118. Friedman MH. Unsteady transport on hydration dynamics of the in vivo cornea. *Biophys J* 1973;13:890.

119. Mishima S, Maurice DM. The effect of normal evaporation on the eye. *Exp Eye Res* 1961;1:46.

120. Mandell RB, Fatt I. Thinning in the human cornea on awakening. *Nature* 1965;208:292.

121. Klyce SD, Maurice DM. Automatic recording of corneal thickness in vitro. *Invest Ophthalmol* 1976;15:550.

122. Brubaker RF, Kupfer C. Microcryoscopic determination of the osmolarity of interstitial fluid in the living rabbit cornea. *Invest Ophthalmol* 1962;1:653.

123. Davson H. The hydration of the cornea. *Biochem J* 1955; 59:24.

124. Harris JE, Nordquist LT. The hydration of the cornea: I. The transport of water from the cornea. *Am J Ophthalmol* 1955;40:100.

125. Mishima S, Trenberth SM. Permeability of the corneal endothelium to nonelectrolytes. *Invest Ophthalmol* 1968;7:34.

126. Maurice DM. The permeability of the cornea. *Ophthalmic Lit* 1953;7:3.

127. Mishima S, Hedbys BO. The permeability of the corneal epithelium and endothelium to water. *Exp Eye Res* 1967;6:10.

128. Stanley JA, Mishima S, Klyce SD. In vivo determination of endothelial permeability to water. *Invest Ophthalmol* 1966; 5:371.

129. Green K, Green MA. The permeability to water of rabbit corneal membranes. *Am J Physiol* 1969;217:635.

130. Kim JH, Green K, Martinez M, et al. Solute permeability of the corneal endothelium and Descemet's membrane. *Exp Eye Res* 1971;12:231.

131. Green K, Downs SJ. Corneal membrane water permeability as a function of temperature. *Invest Ophthalmol* 1976; 15:304.

132. Fischbarg J, Warshavsky CR, Limm JJ. Pathways for hydraulically and osmotically-induced water flows across epithelia. *Nature* 1977;266:71.

133. Bonanno JA, Polse KA. Corneal acidosis during contact lens wear: effects of hypoxia and CO_2. *Invest Ophthalmol Vis Sci* 1987;28:1514.

134. Spencer WH. *Ophthalmic pathology: an atlas and textbook*, vol 1. Philadelphia: WB Saunders, 1985:259.

135. Michels RG, Kenyon KR, Maumenee AE. Retrocorneal fibrous membrane. *Invest Ophthalmol* 1972;11:82.

136. Iwamoto T, DeVoe AG. Electron microscopic studies on Fuchs' combined dystrophy: I. Posterior portion of the cornea. *Invest Ophthalmol* 1971;10:9.

137. Waring GO, Bourne WM, Edelhauser HF, et al. The endothelium: normal and pathologic structure and function. *Ophthalmology* 1982;89:531.

138. Iwamoto T, DeVoe AG. Electron microscopic studies on Fuchs' combined dystrophy: II. Anterior portion of the cornea. *Invest Ophthalmol* 1971;10:29.

139. Smelser G, Chen D. Physiological changes in cornea induced by contact lenses. *Arch Ophthalmol* 1955;53:676.

140. Lancon M, Miller D. Corneal hydration, visual acuity and glare sensitivity. *Arch Ophthalmol* 1973;90:227.

141. Griffiths S, Drasdo N, Barnes D, et al. Effect of epithelial and stromal edema on the light scattering properties of the cornea. *Am J Optom Physiol Optics* 1986;63:888.

142. Lambert SR, Klyce SD. The origins of Sattler's veil. Am J Ophthalmol 1981;91:51.
143. Riley MV. Glucose and oxygen utilization by the rabbit cornea. *Exp Eye Res* 1969;8:193.
144. Turss R, Friend J, Dohlman CH. Effect of a corneal fluid barrier on the nutrition of the epithelium. *Exp Eye Res* 1970;9:254.
145. Brown SI, Dohlman CH. A buried corneal implant serving as a barrier to fluid. *Arch Ophthalmol* 1965;73:635.
146. Berkowitz RA, Klyce SD, Kaufman HE. Aqueous hyposecretion after penetrating keratoplasty. *Ophthalmic Surg* 1984;15:323.
147. Polse KA, Mandell RB. Critical tension at the corneal surface. *Arch Ophthalmol* 1970;84:505.
148. Efron N, Carney LG. Oxygen levels beneath the closed eyelid. *Invest Ophthalmol Vis Sci* 1979;18:93.
149. Mandell RB, Farrell R. Corneal swelling at low atmospheric oxygen pressures. *Invest Ophthalmol Vis Sci* 1980;19:697.

3

BASIC IMMUNOLOGY

C. STEPHEN FOSTER AND J. WAYNE STREILEIN

CELLS OF THE IMMUNE SYSTEM

The cellular components of the immune system include lymphocytes, macrophages, Langerhans cells, neutrophils, eosinophils, basophils and mast cells. Many of these cell types can be further subdivided into subtypes and sub-subsets. For example, lymphocytes include T lymphocytes, B lymphocytes, and non-T, non-B (null) lymphocytes. Each subtype can be further subcategorized, both by functional differences and by differences in cell surface glycoprotein specialization and uniqueness. The latter differentiating aspect of cell types and cell type subsets has been made possible through the development of hybridoma–monoclonal antibody technology (1,2) (Table 3-1).

Lymphocytes

Lymphocytes are mononuclear cells that are round, 7 to 8 μm in diameter, and found in lymphoid tissue (lymph node, spleen, thymus, gut-associated lymphoid tissue, mammary-associated lymphoid tissue, and conjunctiva-associated lymphoid tissue) and in blood. They ordinarily constitute approximately 30% of the total peripheral white blood cell count. The lymphocyte is the premier character in the immune drama; it is the primary recognition unit for foreign material, the principal specific effector cell type in immune reactions, and the cell exclusively responsible for immune memory.

T lymphocytes, or thymus-derived cells, comprise 65% to 80% of the peripheral blood lymphocyte population, 30% to 50% of the splenocyte population, and 70% to 85% of the lymph node cell population. B lymphocytes comprise 5% to 15% of peripheral blood lymphocytes, 20% to 30% of splenocytes, and 10% to 20% of lymph node cells.

T cells possess cell surface receptors for sheep erythrocytes and for the plant-derived mitogens concanavalin A and phytohemagglutinin. They do not possess surface immunoglobulin or surface membrane receptors for the Fc portion of antibody—two notable cell surface differences from B lymphocytes, which do possess these two

entities. B cells also exhibit cell surface receptors for the third component of complement, for the Epstein-Barr virus, and for the plant mitogen known as pokeweed mitogen, as well as for the purified protein derivative of *Mycobacterium tuberculosis* and for lipopolysaccharide.

Null cells are lymphocytes that possess none of the aforementioned cell surface antigens characteristic of T cells or B cells. This cell population is heterogeneous, and some authorities include natural killer (NK) cells among the null cell population, even though the origin of NK cells may be in monocytes/macrophage precursor lines rather than the lymphocyte lineage. Nonetheless, the morphologic characteristics and behaviors of NK cells, along with the ambiguity of their origin, enable their inclusion under the null cell rubric. NK cells are nonadherent (unlike macrophages, they do not stick to the surface of plastic tissue culture dishes) mononuclear cells present in peripheral blood, spleen, and lymph nodes. The most notable function of these cells is the killing of transformed (malignant) cells and virus-infected cells. Because they do this without prior sensitization, they are an important component of the early natural response in the immune system. The cytotoxicity of NK cells is not major histocompatibility complex (MHC)–restricted, a dramatic contrast with cytotoxic T cells. (More about the MHC and the products of those gene loci is provided later.) But they do have recognition structures that detect class I MHC molecules; when these receptors engage class I MHC molecules on target cells, the NK cell *fails* to trigger cytolysis of that target cell. The large granules present in NK cells (the cells are sometimes called *large granular lymphocytes*) contain perforin and perhaps other cell membrane–lysing enzymes; it is the enzymes in the granules that are responsible for the lethal-hit cytolysis for which NK cells are famous.

Killer cells are the other notable null cell subpopulation. These cells do have receptors for the Fc portion of immunoglobulin G (IgG) and thus can attach themselves to the Fc portion of IgG molecules. Through this receptor, they are a primary cell responsible for cytolysis in the so-called antibody-dependent, cell-mediated cytotoxicity reaction. These cells probably participate in type II Gell and Coombs

TABLE 3-1. CLUSTERS OF DIFFERENTIATION (CD) DESIGNATIONS

Clusters	Cell Specificity	Function
CD1	Thymocytes, Langerhans cells	
CD2	T cells, NK subset	CD58 receptor/sheep erythrocyte receptor; adhesion molecule—binds to LFA-3
CD3	T cells	T-cell antigen-complex receptor
CD4	Helper-inducer T cells	MHC class II immune recognition; human immunodeficiency virus receptor
CD5	T cells, B-cell subset	
CD6	T-cell subset	?
CD7	T cells, NK cells, platelets	?Fc receptor IgM
CD8	Cytotoxic and suppressor T cells	MHC class I immune recognition
CD9	Pre-B cells	?
CD10	Pre-B cells, neutrophils	Neutrophil endopeptidases
CD11a	Leukocytes	Adhesion molecule (LFA-1) binds to ICAM-1
CD11b	Monocytes, granulocytes, NK cells	α-Chain of complement receptor CR3
CD11c	Monocytes, granulocytes, NK cells	Adhesion
CD13	Monocytes, granulocytes	Aminopeptidase N
CD14	Macrophages	Lipopolysaccharide receptor
CD15	Neutrophils, activated T cells	
CD16	Granulocytes, macrophages, NK cells	Fc-receptor IgG (Fc-γ RIII); activation of NK cells
CD19	B cells	B-cell activation
CD20	B cells	B-cell activation
CD21	B cells	Complement receptor CR2—Epstein-Barr virus receptor
CD22	B cells	Adhesion; B-cell activation
CD23	Activated B cells, macrophages	Low-affinity Fc-ϵ receptor; induced by IL-4
CD25	Activated T cells, B cells	IL-2 receptor
CD28	T cells	Receptor for costimulator molecules B7-1 and B7-2
CD30	Activated B and T cells	?
CD31	Platelets, molecules and B cells	Role in leukocyte–endothelial adhesion
CD32	B lymphocytes, granulocytes, macrophages, eosinophils	Fc receptor IgG (Fc-γ RIII), ADCC
CD35	B cells, erythrocytes, neutrophils, mononuclear cells	Complement receptor CR1
CD37	B cells	
CD38	Activated T cells and plasma cells	?
CD40	B cells	B-cell activation by T-cell contact
CD41	Megakaryocytes, platelets	Gp11b/11a platelet aggregation; Fc receptor
CD42	Megakaryocytes, platelets	Gp1b-platelet adhesion
CD43	Leukocytes	T-cell activation
CD44	Leukocytes	Pgp1 (Hermes) receptor; homing receptor for matrix components (e.g., hyaluronate)
CD45	All leukocytes	Leukocyte common antigen—signal transduction (tyrosine phosphatase)
CD45RA	Naive cells	
CD45RO	Activated/memory T cells	
CD45RB	B cells	
CD49 (VLA)	T cells, monocytes	Adhesion to collagen, laminin, Fc, VCAM
CD54 (ICAM-1)	Activated cells	Adhesion to LFA-1 and Mac-1
CD56	NK	NCAM-adhesion
CD58 (LFA-3)	B cells, antigen-presenting cells	Binds to CD2
CD62E E-selectin, ELAM-1	Endothelial cells	Adhesion
CD62L L-selectin, LAM-1	T cells	Adhesion
CD62P P-selectin, PADGEM	Platelets, endothelial cells	Adhesion
CD64	Monocytes, macrophages	Adhesion, Fc-γ receptor; ADCC
CD69	Activated lymphocytes	
CD71	Proliferating cells	Transferrin receptor
CD72	B cells	Ligand for CD5; B-cell–T-cell interactions
CD80 (B7-1)	B cells; dendritic cells, macrophages	Ligand for CD28; costimulator for T-cell activation
CD81 (B7-2)		
CD89 (Fc-α receptor)	Neutrophils, monocytes	IgA-dependent cytotoxicity
CD95 (Fas)	Multiple cell types	Role in programmed cell death
CD102 (ICAM-2)	Endothelial cells, monotypes	Ligand for LFA-1 integrin
CD103 (HML-1)	T cells	Role in T-cell homing to mucosae
CD106 (VCAM-1)	Endothelial cells, macrophages	Receptor for VLA-4 integrin; adhesion

ADCC, antibody-dependent cell-mediated cytotoxicity; ELAM, endothelial leukocyte adhesion molecule; HML, human mucosal lymphocyte antigen; ICAM, intercellular adhesion molecule; Ig, immunoglobulin; IL, interleukin; LAM, leukocyte adhesion molecule; LFA, leukocyte functional antigen; Mac, macrophage antigen; MHC, major histocompatibility complex; NCAM. neural cell adhesion molecule; NK, natural killer; PADGEM, platelet activation–dependent granule external membrane protein; VCAM, vascular cell adhesion molecule; VLA, very late antigen.

hypersensitivity reactions and are involved in immune removal of cellular antigens when the target cell is too large to be phagocytosed.

It is clear that both B cells and T cells can be further divided into specialized subsets. B cells, for example, are subdivided into the B cells that synthesize the five separate classes of immunoglobulin (IgG, IgA, IgM, IgD, and IgE). All B cells initially produce IgM specific for an antigenic determinant (epitope) to which it has responded, but some subsequently switch from synthesis of IgM to synthesis of other immunoglobulin classes. The details of the control of antibody synthesis and class switching are discussed later in this chapter. Less known is the fact that functionally distinct subsets of B cells exist, in addition to the different B cells involved in antibody class synthesis. The field of B-cell diversity analysis is embryonic, but it is clear that the exploitation of monoclonal antibody technology will distinguish, with increasingly fine specificity, differences in B-cell subpopulations. It is clear, for example, that a subpopulation of B lymphocytes possess the CD5 glycoprotein on the cell surface plasma membrane (a CD glycoprotein not ordinarily present on B lymphocytes but rather on the cell surfaces of T cells) (3). These cells appear to be associated with autoantibody production (4).

It is also clear now that B cells are functionally important as antigen-presenting cells (APCs) for previously primed or memory (not naive) T cells, a fact that startles most physicians who studied immunology before 1991. T-cell receptors (TCRs) cannot react with native antigen; rather, they respond to processed antigenic determinants of that antigen. APCs phagocytose the antigen, process it, and display denatured, limited peptide sequences of the native antigen on the cell surface of the APC in association with cell surface class II MHC glycoproteins. B cells, as well as classic APCs, such as macrophages and Langerhans cells, can perform this function. The antigen is endocytosed by the B cell and processed in the B-cell endosome (possibly through involvement of cathepsin D) to generate short, denatured peptide fragments, which are then transported to the B-cell surface bound to class II glycoprotein peptides; here, the antigenic peptides are "presented" to CD4 helper T lymphocytes.

Finally, regarding B-cell heterogeneity, it is becoming apparent that some B lymphocytes also have suppressor or regulatory activity. The emerging data on B-cell functional and cell surface heterogeneity will be exciting to follow in the coming years.

Much more widely recognized, of course, is that subsets of T lymphocytes exist. Helper (CD4) T cells "help" in the induction of an immune response, in the generation of an antibody response, and in the generation of other, more specialized components of the immune response. Cytotoxic (CD8) T cells, as the name implies, are involved in cell killing or cytotoxic reactions. Delayed-type hypersensitivity (CD4) T cells are the classic participants in the chronic inflammatory responses characteristic of certain antigens such as mycobacteria. Regulatory T cells (CD8) are responsible for modulating immune responses, thereby preventing uncontrolled, host-damaging inflammatory responses. It is even likely that there are sub-subsets of these T cells. Excellent evidence exists, for example, that there are at least three subsets of regulatory T cells and at least two subsets of helper T cells.

Mosmann and Coffman (5) described two types of helper (CD4) T cells with differential cytokine production profiles. T_H1 cells secrete interleukin-2 (IL-2) and interferon-γ (IFN-γ) but do not secret IL-4 or IL-5, whereas T_H2 cells secrete IL-4, IL-5, IL-10, and IL-13, but not IL-2 or IFN-γ. Furthermore, T_H1 cells can by cytolytic and can assist B cells with IgG, IgM, and IgA synthesis but not IgE synthesis. T_H2 cells are not cytolytic but can help B cells with IgE synthesis, as well as with IgG, IgM, and IgA production (6). It is becoming clear that T_H1 CD4 or T_H2 CD4 cells are selected in infection and in autoimmune diseases. Thus, T_H1 cells accumulate in the thyroid of patients with autoimmune thyroiditis (7), whereas T_H2 cells accumulate in the conjunctiva of patients with vernal conjunctivitis (8). The T cells that respond to *M. tuberculosis* protein are primarily T_H1 cells, whereas those that respond to *Toxocara canis* antigens are T_H2 cells. Romagnani has proposed that T_H1 cells are preferentially "selected" as participants in inflammation associated with delayed-type hypersensitivity reactions and low antibody production (as in contact dermatitis or tuberculosis), and T_H2 cells are preferentially selected in inflammation associated with persistent antibody production, including allergic responses in which IgE production is prominent (9). Further, it is now clear that these two major CD4 T-lymphocyte subsets regulate each other through their cytokines. Thus, T_H2 CD4 lymphocyte cytokines (notably IL-10) inhibit T_H1 CD4 lymphocyte proliferation and cytokine secretion, and T_H1 CD4 lymphocyte cytokines (notably IFN-γ) inhibit T_H2 CD4 lymphocyte proliferation and cytokine production.

Macrophages

The macrophage ("large eater") and dendritic cells are the preeminent professional APCs. Macrophages are 12 to 15 μm in diameter, the largest of the lymphoid cells. They posses a high density of class II MHC glycoproteins on their cell surfaces, along with receptors for complement components, the Fc portion of immunoglobulin molecules, receptors for fibronectin, IFNs-α, β, and γ, IL-1, tumor necrosis factor (TNF), and macrophage colony-stimulating factor. These cells are widely distributed throughout the various tissues (when found in tissue, they are called *histiocytes*); the microenvironment of the tissue profoundly influences the extent of the expression of the various cell surface glycoproteins as well as the intracellular metabolic characteristics. It is clear that further compartmentalization of macrophage subtypes occurs in the spleen. Macrophages that express a high density of class II MHC glycoproteins are present in red pulp, and macrophages with significantly less surface class II MHC glycoprotein expression are in the marginal zone, where intimate contact with B cells exists. It is likely that, just as in the murine system (10), so too in humans, one subclass of macrophage preferentially presents antigen to one particular subset of helper T cells responsible for induction of regulatory T-cell activation, whereas a different subset of macrophage preferentially presents antigen to a different helper T-cell subset responsible for cytotoxic or delayed-type hypersensitivity effector functions.

Macrophages also participate more generally in inflammatory reactions. They are members of the natural (early defense) immune system and are incredibly potent in their capacity to synthesize and secrete a variety of powerful biologic molecules, including proteases, collagenase, angiotensin-converting enzyme, lysozyme, IFN-α, IFN-β, IL-6, TNF-α, fibronectin, transforming growth factor (TGF), macrophage colony-stimulating factor, granulocyte colony-stimulating factor, platelet-activating factor, arachidonic acid derivatives (prostaglandins and leukotrienes), and oxygen metabolites (oxygen free radicals, peroxide anion, and hydrogen peroxide). These cells are extremely important, even pivotal, participants in inflammatory reactions and are especially important in chronic inflammation. The epithelioid cell typical of so-called granulomatous inflammatory reactions evolves from the tissue histiocyte, and multinucleated giant cells form through fusion of many epithelioid cells.

Specialized macrophages exist in certain tissues and organs, including the Kupffer cells of the liver, dendritic histiocytes in lymphoid organs, interdigitating reticular cells in lymphoid organs, and Langerhans cells in skin, lymph nodes, conjunctiva, and cornea.

Langerhans Cells

Langerhans cells are particularly important to the ophthalmologist. They probably are the premier APC for the external eye. Derived from bone marrow macrophage precursors, like macrophages, their function is basically identical to that of the macrophage in antigen presentation. They are rich in cell surface class II MHC glycoproteins and have cell surface receptors for the third component of complement and for the Fc portion of IgG. Langerhans cells are abundant in the mucosal epithelium of the mouth, esophagus, vagina, and conjunctiva. They are also abundant at the corneoscleral limbus, less so in the peripheral cornea; they are normally absent from the central third of the cornea (11). If the center of the cornea is provoked through trauma or infection, the peripheral cornea Langerhans cells quickly "stream" into the center of the cornea (12). These CD1$^+$ dendritic cells possess a characteristic racket-shaped cytoplasmic granule on ultrastructural analysis, the Birbeck granule, whose function is unknown.

Polymorphonuclear Leukocytes

Polymorphonuclear leukocytes (PMNs) are part of the natural immune system. They are central to the host defense through phagocytosis, but if they accumulate in excessive numbers, persist, and are activated in an uncontrolled manner, the result may be deleterious to host tissues. As the name suggests, they contain a multilobed nucleus and many granules. PMNs are subcategorized as neutrophils, basophils, or eosinophils, depending on the differential staining of their granules.

Neutrophils

Neutrophils account for more than 90% of circulating granulocytes. They possess surface receptors for the Fc portion of IgG (CD16) and for complement components, including C5a (important in adhesion and phagocytosis). When appropriately stimulated by chemotactic agents (complement components, fibrinolytic and kinin system components, and products from other leukocytes, platelets, and certain bacteria), neutrophils move from blood to tissues through margination (adhesion to receptors or adhesion molecules on vascular endothelial cells) and diapedesis (movement through the capillary wall). Neutrophils release the contents of their primary (azurophilic) granules (lysosomes) and secondary (specific) granules (Table 3-2) into an endocytic vacuole, resulting in (a) phagocytosis of a microorganism or tissue injury, (b) type II antibody–dependent, cell-mediated cytotoxicity, or (c) type III hypersensitivity reactions (immune complex–mediated disease). Secondary granules release collagenase, which mediates collagen degradation. Aside from the products secreted by the granules, neutrophils produce arachidonic acid metabolites (prostaglandins and leukotrienes), as well as oxygen free radical derivatives.

Eosinophils

Eosinophils constitute 3% to 5% of the circulating PMNs. They possess surface receptors for the Fc portion of IgE (low affinity) and IgG (CD16) and for complement components, including C5a, CR1 (CD35), and CR3 (CD11b). Eosinophils play a special role in allergic conditions and parasitoses. They also participate in type III hypersensitivity reactions or immune complex–mediated disease, after attraction to the inflammatory area by products from mast cells (eosinophil chemotactic factor of anaphylaxis), complement, and other cytokines from other inflammatory cells. Eosinophils release the contents of their granules to the outside of the cell after fusion of the intracellular granules with the plasma membrane (degranulation). Table 3-3 shows the known secretory products of eosinophils; the role these products of inflammation play, even in nonallergic diseases (such as Wegener's granulomatosis), is underappreciated.

TABLE 3-2. NEUTROPHIL GRANULES AND THEIR CONTENTS

Azurophil Granules	Specific Granules	Other Granules
Myeloperoxidase	Alkaline phosphatase	Acid phosphatase
Acid phosphatase	Histaminase	Heparinase
5'-Nucleotidase	Collagenase	β-Glucosaminidase
Lysozyme	Lysozyme	α-Mannosidase
Elastase	Vitamin B_{12}–binding proteins	Acid proteinase
Cathepsins B, D, G	Plasminogen activator Lactoferrin	Elastase, gelatinase
Proteinase 3		Glycosaminoglycans
β-Glycophosphatase		
N-Acetyl-β-glucosaminidase	Cytochrome	
β-Glucuronidase		
α-Mannosidase		
Arylsulfatase		
α-Fucosidase		
Esterase		
Histonase		
Cationic proteins		
Defensins		
Bactericidal permeability–increasing protein (BPI)		
Glycosaminoglycans		

Basophils

Basophils account for les than 0.2% of circulating granulocytes. They possess surface receptors for the Fc portion of IgE (high affinity) and IgG (CD16) and for complement components, including C5a, CR1 (CD35), and CR2 (CD11b). Their role, other than perhaps as tissue mast cells, is unclear.

Mast Cells

The mast cell is indistinguishable from the basophil in many respects, particularly its contents. There are at least two classes of mast cells, based on their neutral protease composition, T-lymphocyte dependence, ultrastructural characteristics, and predominant arachidonic acid metabolites (Table 3-4). Mucosa-associated mast cells (MMC or MC-T) contain primarily tryptase as the major protease (hence, some authors designate these MC-T, or mast cells—tryptase) and prostaglandin D_2 as the primary product of arachidonic acid metabolism. MMCs are T-cell dependent for growth and development (specifically IL-3 dependent), and they are located predominantly in mucosal stroma (e.g., gut). MMCs are small and short-lived (<40 days). They contain chondroitin sulfate but not heparin, and

TABLE 3-3. GRANULAR CONTENT OF EOSINOPHILS

Lysosomal hydrolases	Cathepsin
Arylsulfatase	Histaminase
β-Glucuronidase	Peroxisomes
Acid phosphatase	Major basic proteins
β-Glycerophosphatase	Eosinophil cationic protein
Ribonuclease	Eosinophil peroxidases
Proteinases	Phospholipases
Collagenase	Lysophospholipases

their histamine content is modest (Table 3-5). MMCs degranulate in response to antigen–IgE triggering but not to exposure to compound 48/80, and they are not stabilized by disodium cromoglycate. They are formalin sensitive, so formalin fixation of tissue eliminates or greatly reduces our ability to find these cells using staining technique. With special fixation techniques, MMC granules stain with Alcian blue but not with safranin.

Connective tissue mast cells (CTMCs) contain both tryptase and chymase (so some authors designate them MC-TC), as well as leukotrienes B_4, C_4, and D_4, as the primary products of arachidonic acid metabolism. CTMCs are T-cell independent. They are larger than MMCs and are located principally in skin and at mucosal interfaces with the environment. They contain heparin and large amounts of histamine, and they degranulate in response to compound 48/80 in addition to antigen–IgE interactions. CTMCs are stabilized by disodium cromoglycate. They stain with alkaline Giemsa, toluidine blue, Alcian blue, safranin, and berberine sulfate.

The ultrastructural characteristics of MMCs and CTMCs are also different. Electron microscopy shows that the granules of CTMCs contain scroll-like structures. Mast cells play a special role in allergic reactions—they are the preeminent cell in the allergy drama. However, they also can participate in type II, III, and IV hypersensitivity reactions. Their role in these reactions, aside from notable vascular effects, is not well understood. Non–IgE-mediated mechanisms (e.g., C5a) can trigger mast cells to release histamine, platelet-activating factor, and other biologic molecules when antigen binds to two adjacent IgE molecules on the mast cell surface. Histamine and other vasoactive amines cause increased vascular permeability, allowing immune complexes to become trapped in the vessel wall.

TABLE 3-4. MAST CELL TYPES AND CHARACTERISTICS

Characteristics	Mucosal Mast Cell	Connective Tissue Mast Cell
Morphology		
Size	Small, pleomorphic	Large, uniform
Nucleus	Unilobed or bilobed	Unilobed
Granules	Few	Many
Location	Gut	Peritoneum
Histochemistry		
Protease	Tryptase	Tryptase and chymase
Proteoglycans	Chondroitin sulfate	Heparin
Histamine	<1 pg/cell	≥5 pg/cell
IgE	Surface and cytoplasmic	Heparin
Formalin-sensitive	Yes	No
***In Vitro* Effect of**		
Compound 48/80	Proliferation	Degranulation
Polymyxin	Proliferation	Degranulation
Secretagogues		
Antigen	Yes	Yes
Anti-IgE	Yes	Yes
Compound 48/80	No	Yes
Bee venom	No	Yes
Concanavalin A	Yes	Yes
Staining		
Alcian blue	Yes	Yes
Safranin	No	Yes
Berberine sulfate	No	Yes
Antiallergic compounds		
Cromoglycate	No	Yes
Theophylline	No	Yes
Doxanarile	Yes	Yes
Enhancement of secretion		
Phosphatidyl serine	No	Yes
Adenosine	Yes	Yes
Predominant arachidonic acid metabolite	Prostaglandin D_2	Leukotrienes B_4, C_4, D_4
Ultrastructural features of granules	Lattice	Scroll

IgE, immunoglobulin E.

Platelets

Blood platelets, cells well adapted for blood clotting, also are involved in the immune response to injury, which is a reflection of their evolutionary heritage as myeloid (inflammatory) cells. They possess surface receptors for the Fc portion of IgG (CD16) and IgE (low affinity), for class I histocompatibility glycoproteins [human leukocyte antigen (HLA)-A, -B, or –C], and for factor VIII. They also carry molecules such as Gp11b/111a (CDw41), which binds fibrinogen, and Gp1b (CDw42), which binds von Willebrand factor.

After endothelial injury, platelets adhere to and aggregate at the endothelial surface, releasing permeability-increasing molecules from their granules (Table 3-6). Endothelial injury may be caused by type III hypersensitivity. Platelet-activating factor released by mast cells after antigen–IgE antibody complex formation induces platelets to aggregate and release their vasoactive amines. These amines separate endothelial cell tight junctions and allow immune complexes to enter the vessel wall. Once the immune complexes are deposited, they initiate an inflammatory reaction through activation of complement components and neutrophil lysosomal enzyme release.

IMMUNE SYSTEM

Cells of the immune system are derived from primordial stem cell precursors of the bone marrow. They originate in

TABLE 3-5. MAST CELL CONTENTS

Histamine
Serotonin
Rat mast cell protease I and II
Heparin
Chondroitin sulfate
β-Hexosaminidase
β-Glucuronidase
β-D-Galactosidase
Arylsulfatase
Eosinophil chemotactic factor for anaphylaxis
Slow-reactive substance of anaphylaxis
High–molecular-weight neutrophil chemotactic factor
Arachidonic acid derivatives
Platelet-activating factor

the blood islands of the yolk sac (13), and populate embryonic liver and bone marrow (14). These stem cells are pluriopotential. Characteristics of the microenvironment in the bone marrow, particularly with respect to a stem cell's association with other resident cells in the bone marrow, contribute to or are responsible for the different pathways of maturation and differentiation. For example, specific cells in the bone marrow in the endosteal region promote the differentiation of hematopoietic stem cells into B lymphocytes (15). In birds, primordial pluripotential stem cells that migrate to a gland near the cloaca of the chicken known as the *bursa of Fabricius* (for reasons of probable stimuli in the bone marrow not yet understood) are influenced by the epithelial cells in that gland to differentiate terminally into B lymphocytes (16,17).

T-cell development results from stem cell migration from the bone marrow to the thymus. Thymic hormones (at least 20 have been preliminarily described) produced by the thymic epithelium initiate the complex series of events

TABLE 3-6. PLATELET GRANULES AND THEIR CONTENTS

α-Granules
 Fibronectin
 Fibrinogen
 Plasminogen
 Thrombospondin
 von Willebrand factor
 α_2-Plasmin inhibitor
 Platelet-derived growth factor
 Platelet factor 4
 Transforming growth factor-α and -β
 Thrombospondin
 β-Lysin
 Permeability factor
 Factors D and H
 Decay-accelerating factor
Dense granules
 Serotonin
 Adenosine diphosphate
Others
 Arachidonic acid derivatives

that results not only in differentiation of the stem cells into T lymphocytes but subdifferentiation of T lymphocytes into their various functional subsets: Helper function, killer function, and suppressor function are acquired while the T cells are still in the thymus. These hormones are also responsible for the induction of cell surface glycoprotein expression on the surfaces of T cells. The cell surface expression of the various glycoproteins changes during T-cell maturation in the thymus. For example, the CD2 glycoprotein is the first that can be identified on the differentiating T cell, but this is eventually joined by CD5; these are both eventually replaced (CD2 completely and CD5 partially) by CD1 glycoprotein, which in turn is lost and replaced by the mature CD3 marker. CD4 and CD8 glycoproteins are acquired before emigration from the thymus by helper and cytotoxic-regulatory T cells, respectively.

Monocytes, NK cells, and killer cells evolve from stem cells through influences that are incompletely understood. All three types of cells do arise from a common monocyte precursor and later subdifferentiate under unknown influences.

Lymphoid Traffic

Lymphatic vessels and blood vessels connect the central lymphoid organs (bone marrow, thymus, liver) and the peripheral lymphoid organs (spleen, lymph nodes, gut, bronchial- and conjunctival-associated lymphoid tissues) to one another and to the other organs of the body (18,19) (Table 3-7). Lymphatic vessels drain every organ except the nonconjuntival parts of the eye, internal ear, bone marrow, spleen, and cartilage, and some parts of the central nervous system. The interstitial fluid and cells entering the lymphatic system are propelled (predominantly by skeletal muscle contraction) to regional lymph nodes. Efferent lymphatics draining these regional nodes converge to form large lymph vessels that culminate in the thoracic duct and the right lymphatic duct. The thoracic duct empties into the left subclavian vein, carrying approximately three fourths of the lymph, whereas the right lymphatic duct empties into the right subclavian vein.

One or more homing receptors is present on the surface of all lymphoid cells. These receptors can be regulated, induced, and suppressed. Mature T cells emerging from the thymus cortex toward the medulla are rich either in cell surface or plasma membrane homing receptors, or adhesion molecules or "adhesomes," which are ligands for various addressins or adhesion molecules at other, remote foci. In the mouse, homing

TABLE 3-7. LYMPHOID ORGANS

Primary	Secondary
Thymus	Lymph nodes
Bone marrow	Spleen
	Mucosa-associated lymphoid tissue

receptors on the surface of mature T cells have been identified for the lymph node (MEL-14 or L-selectin [leukocyte functional antigen (LFA)-1]) and for Peyer's patch [leukocyte Peyer's patch adhesion molecule (LPAM)-1 $\alpha_4\beta_7$ integrin, CD44]. Equivalent homing receptors undoubtedly exist in humans, but work in this area is currently embryonic. A 90-kD glycoprotein designated Hermes-3, however, has been identified as a specific heterotypic recognition unit on lymphocytes (20). The Hermes glycoprotein has been shown to be identical to the CD44 molecule (21). Antibodies to this glycoprotein prevent binding of lymphocytes to mucosal lymph node high-endothelial venules (22,23).

Immune Response

Professional APCs phagocytose foreign material (antigens), process it through protease endosomal–lysosomal degradation, "package" it with MHC molecules, and transport the peptide–MHC complex to the cell surface. B cells and dendritic cells (including Langerhans cells) also perform this function, but differences in protease types and class II MHC molecules among these APCs may influence the type of T cell activated by an antigen. It is this unit of antigenic peptide determinant and self-MHC glycoproteins, along with the aid of adhesion molecules [intercellular adhesion molecule (ICAM)-1; (CD54) and LFA-3 (CD58)] and costimulatory molecules [B7 (CD80)], that forms the recognition unit for TCRs specific for the antigenic epitope of the foreign material. The TCR is composed of recognition units for the epitope and for the autologous MHC glycoprotein. Endogenous antigens, such as endogenously manufactured viral protein, typically collect in cytoplasm, associate with class I MHC molecules, and are transported to the surface of the APC, where the class I MHC–peptide complex preferentially associates with the TCR of CD8$^+$ cells. As described earlier, exogenous antigens that are phagocytosed typically associate, in the endosomal, endocytic, and exocytic pathways, with class II MHC molecules; this complex preferentially associates with CD4$^+$ TCRs.

The $\alpha\beta$ heterodimer of the TCR is associated with CD3 and $\zeta\eta$ proteins and (for CD4$^+$ cells) the CD4 molecule, thus forming the TCR complex. Antigen presentation can then occur as the TCR complex interacts with the antigenic determinant/MHC complex on the macrophage, with simultaneous CD28–CD80 interaction or "costimulation." Macrophage secretion of IL-1 during this cognitive "presentation" phase of the acquired immune response to CD4 T cells completes the requirements for successful antigen presentation to the helper T cell (Fig. 3-1).

The CD3 and $\zeta\eta$ proteins are the signal-transducing components of the TCR complex; transmembrane signaling by this pathway results in activation of several phosphotyrosine kinases, including those of the tyk/jak family, and other signal transduction and activation of transcription molecules and phosphorylation of tyrosine residues in the cytoplasmic

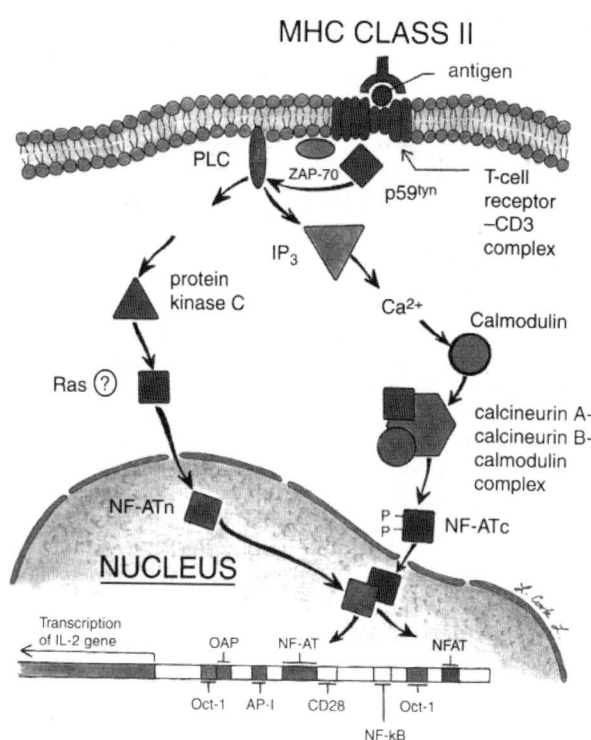

FIG. 3-1. Signal transduction: intracellular and intranuclear. With antigen-presenting cell presentation of antigen to the T cell [green peptide fragment in the major histocompatibility complex (MHC) class II groove of the macrophage], an extraordinary cascade of events occurs, through the cell membrane, into the cytoplasm, and subsequently into the nucleus, to the level of specific genes on the chromosomes of the nucleus. Specifically, tyrosine-rich phosphorylases catalyze phosphorylation of a series of intracellular proteins, with resultant liberation of calcium stores, and production of the calcineurin–calmodulin complex, which then facilitates the production of nuclear factor of activated T cells, cytoplasmic component capable of being transported through one of the nuclear pores into the nucleus, where interaction then with specific foci on the gene results in induction of gene transcription (in this instance, production of messenger RNA for ultimate synthesis of the protein interleukin-2). (Original drawing by Laurel Cook Lowe.)

tails of the CD3 and $\zeta\eta$ proteins, leading to the creation of multiple sites that bind proteins (enzymes), like phosphatidylinositol phospholipase C-γ1 (PI-PLC-γ1) with SH2-binding domain. PI-PLC-γ1 in turn is phosphorylated (and thereby activated), and it catalyzes hydrolysis of plasma membrane phosphatidylinositol 4,5-biphosphate into inositol 1,4,5-trisphosphate (IP$_3$), and diacylglycerol. IP$_3$ then provokes the release of calcium from its endoplasmic reticulum storage sites. The increased intracellular calcium concentration that results from the release from storage in turn results in increased binding of calcium to calmodulin; this then activates the phosphatase, calcineurin. Calcineurin catalyzes the conversion of phosphorylated nuclear factor of activated T cells, cytoplasmic component (NFATc) to free NFATc. This protein (and probably others) then enters the cell nucleus, where gene transcription of cellular protooncogene/transcription factor genes, cytokine receptor genes, and

TABLE 3-8. ADHESION MOLECULES

LFA-1α	(CD11a)
Macrophage antigen (Mac)-1	(CD11b)
Gp150,95	(CD11c)
LFA-1β	(CD18)
Integrin α-4	(CD49c)
TCRαβ	
TCRγ/δ	
LFA-2	(CD2)
CD22	
Neural cell adhesion molecule (NCAM)	(CD56)
Intercellular adhesion molecule (ICAM)-1	(CD54)
LFA-3	(CD58)
Leukocyte/endothelial cell adhesion molecule (LECAM)-1	
CD5	
Homing cell adhesion molecule (HCAM)	(CD44)
Human progenitor cell antigen (HPCA)-2	(CD34)
CD28	
88-1	
Platelet/endothelial cell adhesion molecule (PECAM)	(CD31)
CMP140	(CD62)
Human natural killer cell antigen (HNK)-1	(CD57)

LFA, leukocyte functional antigen; TCR, T-cell receptor.

cytokine genes is then activated and regulated by it (them). For example, NFATc translocates to the nucleus, where it combines with adaptor proteins (AP-1); this complex then binds to the NFAT-binding site of the IL-2 promoter. This, coupled with nuclear factor-kappa B binding by proteins *possibly* induced by the events stimulated by CD28–CD80 signal transduction, results in IL-2 gene transcription typical of T-cell activation (Fig. 3-1). Thus, this activation phase of the acquired immune response is characterized by lymphocyte proliferation and cytokine production.

Expression of Immunity

The emigration of hematopoietic cells from the vascular system typically occurs at the region of the postcapillary high-endothelial venule cells. These cells are rich in the constitutive expression of so-called addressins, which are tissue or organ specific endothelial cell molecules involved in lymphocyte homing. These adhesion molecules are lymphocyte-binding molecules for the homing receptors on lymphocytes (Table 3-8). Thus, the mucosal addressin (21) specifically binds to the Hermes 90-kD glycoprotein. In the murine system, a 90-kD glycoprotein (designated MECA-79) is a peripheral lymph node addressin specifically expressed by high-endothelial venules. Along with the constitutive expression of addressins or adhesion molecules, expression of additional adhesion molecules is induced by a panoply of proinflammatory cytokines (Table 3-9). The adhesion molecules

give the expression of an immune response its focus, its specifically directed, targeted expression.

Lymphocytes, monocytes, and neutrophils preferentially migrate or "home" to sites of inflammation because of this upregulation of cytokines and the induction of adhesion molecules promoted by them. Thus, L-selectin (CD62L) on the neutrophil cell surface membrane does not adhere to normal vascular endothelium, but ICAM and endothelial leukocyte adhesion molecule (CD62E) expression on the vascular endothelial surface induced by IFN-α, IFN-γ, IL-1, IL-17, or a combination thereof results in low-affinity binding of CD62L, with resultant slowing of neutrophil transit through the vessel, neutrophil "rolling" on the endothelial surface, and (with complement split product and IL-8–driven chemotaxis of increasing numbers of neutrophils) neutrophil margination in the vessels of inflamed tissue. Neutrophil LFA-1 (CD11a, CD18)–activated expression (stimulated by IL-6 and IL-8) then results in stronger adhesion of the neutrophil to endothelial cell ICAM molecules, with resultant neutrophil spreading and diapedesis into the subendothelial spaces and into the surrounding tissue.

Immunologic Memory

The anamnestic capacity of the acquired immune response system is one of its most extraordinary properties. Indeed, it is this remarkable property that was the first to be recognized by the Chinese ancients and (later) by Jenner. We take it as axiomatic that our immunization in childhood with killed or attenuated smallpox and poliovirus provokes not only a primary immune response, but the development of long-lived "memory" cells that immediately produce a rapid, vigorous secondary immune response whenever we might encounter smallpox or poliovirus, thereby resulting in specific antibody- and lymphocyte-mediated killing of the microbe and defending us from the harm the virus would otherwise have done.

Niels Jerne first hypothesized a clonal selection theory to explain at once the specificity and the diversity of the acquired immune response, and Frank Macfarlane Burnet expanded on Jerne's original hypothesis, clearly predicting the necessary features that would prove the theory; many subsequent studies have done so. Clones are derived from the development of antigen-specific clones of lymphocytes arising from single precursors before and independently of exposure to antigen. Approximately 10^9 such clones have been estimated to exist in an individual, allowing him or her to respond to all currently known or future antigens. Antigen contact results in preferential activation of the preexisting clone with the cell surface receptors specific for it, with resultant proliferation of the clone and differentiation into effector and memory cells. The secondary or anamnestic immune response is greater and more rapid in onset than is the primary immune response because of the large

TABLE 3-9. CYTOKINES AND TARGET CELLS

Cytokine	Source	Target Cells
IL-1	MΦ, T$_H$, FB, NK, B, NΦ, EC	Pluripotent stem cells, T$_C$T$_H$, B, MΦ, FB, NΦ
IL-2	T$_H$1	T$_C$T$_H$, B, NK
IL-3	BM, T$_H$, MC	T$_C$T$_H$, B, MC, stem cells
IL-4	T$_H$2, MC	T$_H$1, B, MΦ, MC, T$_H$2, NK, FC
IL-5	T$_H$2, MC, EΦ	T$_C$T$_H$, B, EΦ
IL-6	BM, MΦ, MC, EC, B, T$_H$2, FB	Pluripotent stem cells, T$_C$T$_H$, B, FB, NΦ
IL-7	FB, BM	Subcapsular thymocytes, T$_C$T$_H$, FB
IL-8	BM, FB, EC, MΦ, NΦ, EΦ	T$_C$T$_H$, MΦ, NΦ
IL-9	T$_H$2	Pluripotent stem cells, T$_C$T$_H$, B
IL-10	T$_H$2, B, MΦ	T$_{CD2}$, T$_C$, T$_H$1, MC
IL-11	BM	Pluripotent stem cells, T$_C$T$_H$, B
IL-12	MΦ, NΦ	NK, T$_H$-T$_H$1
IL-13	T$_H$2	T$_H$1, MΦ, B
IL-14	T	B
IL-15	MΦ, FB, BM	T, NK, B
IL-16	T, EΦ	T
IL-17	T$_H$	FB, T
IL-18	MΦ	T, NK
TNF-α	MΦ	T$_C$T$_H$, B, MΦ, FB
TNF-β	T$_C$, T$_H$1	EC, NΦ
GM-CSF	T$_H$, MΦ, MC, null cells, FB	T$_C$T$_H$, EΦ, NΦ
G-CSF	BM, MΦ, FB	T$_C$T$_H$, FB, NΦ
M-CSF	BM, MΦ, FB	
LIF	BM	Myeloid progenitor
SCF	BM	Myeloid progenitor, cortical thymocytes
IFN-γ	NK, T$_H$1	NK, T$_C$, T$_H$2,
IFN-α	MΦ	T$_C$H$_C$, B
IFN-β	FB	T$_C$H$_C$
TGF-β	MΦ	T$_C$H$_C$, B, MΦ, FB

B, B cell; BM, bone marrow; CSF, colony-stimulating factor; EΦ, eosinophil; EC, endothelial cell; FB, fibroblast; GM, granulocyte–macrophage; IFN, interferon; IL, interleukin; LIF, leukocyte inhibitory factor; MΦ, macrophage; MC, mast cell; NΦ, neutrophil; NK, natural killer cell; SCF, stem cell factor; T, T cell; T$_C$, cytotoxic T cell; TGF, transforming growth factor; T$_H$, helper T cell; TNF, tumor necrosis factor.

number of lymphocytes derived from the original clone of cells stimulated by primary contact with antigen, and because of the longevity of many of the cells (memory cells). The memory cells can survive for very long periods, even decades. They express cell surface proteins not expressed by nonmemory cells (CD45RO). In memory cells, the level of cell surface expression of peripheral lymph node homing receptors is low compared with the population of such receptors on the surfaces of nonmemory cells; in contrast, the population of other adhesion molecules includes CD11a, CD18 (LFA-1), CD44, and HLA molecules. Because of the constitutive expression of the cell surface adhesion molecules, memory T cells rapidly home to sites of inflammation, "looking" for antigen to which they might respond.

B-LYMPHOCYTE RESPONSES

When an antigen encounters cell surface IgM that has binding specificities for the antigen (e.g., self-antigens), tolerance to the antigen is the typical result if such an encounter precedes emigration of the B cell from the bone marrow.

Once the immature B cell has acquired its "exit visa" (complete surface IgM), it leaves the bone marrow, residing primarily in the peripheral lymphoid organs (and blood), where it further matures to express both IgM and IgD on its cell surface. It is now a mature B cell, responsive to antigen with proliferation and antibody synthesis.

The ability to generate a diverse immune response depends on the assembly of discontinuous genes that encode the antigen-binding sites of immunoglobulin and TCRs during lymphocyte development. Diversity is generated through the recombination of various germline gene segments, the imprecise joining of segments with insertion of additional nucleotides at the junctions, and somatic mutations occurring within the recombining gene segments.

Antibody Diversity

The paradox of an individual possessing a limited number of genes but the capability to generate an almost infinite number of different antibodies remained an enigma to immunologists for a considerable time. The discovery of distinct variable (V) and constant (C) regions in the light (L) and heavy (H) chains of immunoglobulin molecules (Fig. 3-2) raised the

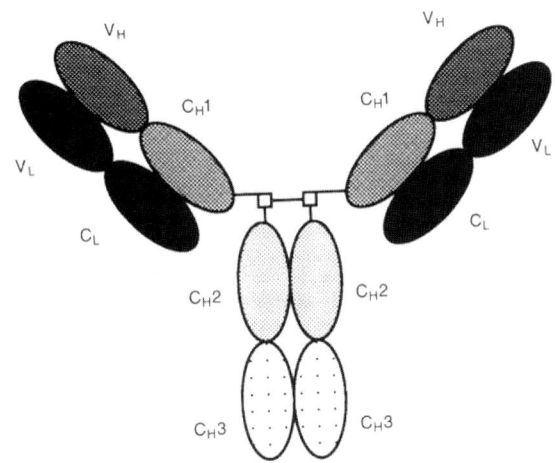

FIG. 3-2. Structure of immunoglobulin G showing the regions of similar sequence (domains). (From Albert DA, Jakobiec FA. *Principles and practice of ophthalmology*, 2nd ed. Philadelphia: WB Saunders, 2000:66.)

possibility that immunoglobulin genes possess an unusual architecture. In 1965, Dreyer and Bennett proposed that the V and C regions of an immunoglobulin chain are encoded by two separated genes in embryonic (germline) cells (germline gene diversity) (24). According to this model, one of several V genes becomes joined to the C gene during lymphocyte development. In 1976, Hozumi and Tonegawa discovered that V and C regions are encoded by separate, multiple genes far apart in germline DNA that become joined to form a complete immunoglobulin gene active in B lymphocytes (25). Immunoglobulin genes are thus translocated during the differentiation of antibody-producing cells (somatic recombination; Fig. 3-3).

Structure and Organization of Immunoglobulin Genes

The V regions of immunoglobulins contain three hypervariable segments that determine antibody specificity (26)

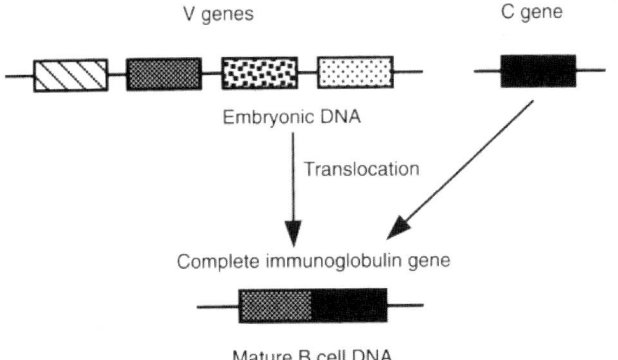

FIG. 3-3. Translocation of a V-segment gene to a C gene in the differentiation of an antibody-producing B cell. (From Albert DA, Jakobiec FA. *Principles and practice of ophthalmology*, 2nd ed. Philadelphia: WB Saunders, 2000:67.)

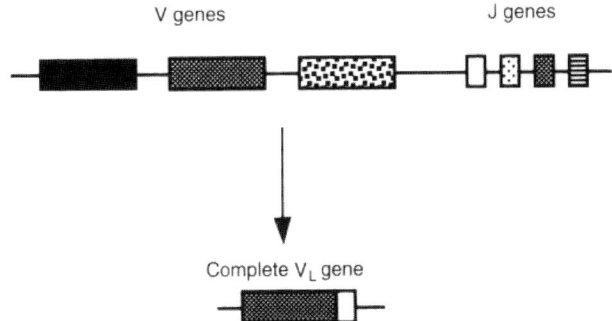

FIG. 3-4. Hypervariable or complementarity-determining regions (CDRs) on the antigen-binding site of the variable regions of immunoglobulin G. (From Albert DA, Jakobiec FA. *Principles and practice of ophthalmology*, 2nd ed. Philadelphia: WB Saunders, 2000:67.)

(Fig. 3-4). Hypervariable segments of both the L and H chains form the "antigen-binding" site. Hypervariable regions are also called *complementarity-determining regions* (CDRs). The V regions of L and H chains have several hundred gene segments in germline DNA; the exact number of segments is still being debated but is estimated to range between 250 and 1000 segments.

Light-Chain Genes

A complete gene for the V region of an L chain is formed by the splicing of an incomplete V-segment gene with one of several J (joining)-segment genes, which encodes part of the last hypervariable segment (27–29) (Fig. 3-5). Additional diversity is generated by V and J genes becoming spliced in different joining frames (junctional diversity) (28) (Fig. 3-6). There are at least three frames for the joining of V and J. Two forms of L chain exist: kappa (κ) and lambda (λ). For $\kappa\lambda$ chains, assume that there are approximately 250 V-segment genes and four J-segment genes. Therefore, a total of 250 × 4 × 3 (for junctional diversity), or 3000, kinds of complete VJ genes can be formed by combinations of V and J.

Heavy-Chain Genes

H-chain V region genes are formed by the somatic recombination of V, an additional segment called D (diversity), and J-segment genes (Fig. 3-7). The third CDR of the heavy chain is encoded mainly by a D segment. Approximately 15 D segments lie between hundreds of V_H and at least four J_H gene segments. A D segment joins a J_H segment; a V_H segment then becomes joined to the DJ_H to form the complete V_H gene. To diversify further the third CDR of the heavy chain, extra nucleotides are inserted between V and D, and between D and J (N-region addition) by the action of terminal deoxyribonucleotidyl transferase (30). Introns, which are noncoding intervening sequences, are removed from the primary RNA transcript.

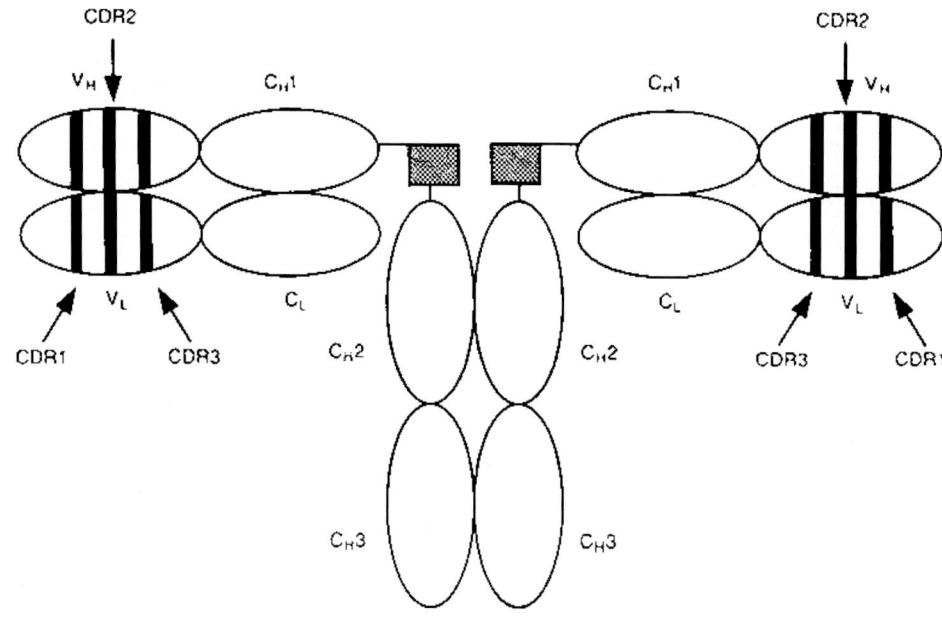

FIG. 3-5. A V gene is translocated near a J gene in forming a light-chain V region gene. (From Albert DA, Jakobiec FA. *Principles and practice of ophthalmology*, 2nd ed. Philadelphia: WB Saunders, 2000:67.)

The site-specific recombination of V, D, and J genes is mediated by enzymes (immunoglobulin recombinase) that recognize conserved nonamer and palindromic heptamer sequences flanking these gene segments (31,32). The nonamer and heptamer sequences are separated by either 12-base pair (bp) or 23-bp spacers (Fig. 3-8). Recombination can occur only between the 12- and 23-bp spacers, not between two 12-bp types or two 23-bp types (called the 12/23 rule of V gene-segment recombination). For example, V_H segments and J_H segments are flanked by 23-bp types on both their

5′ and 3′ ends. Consequently, they cannot recombine with each other or among themselves. Instead, they recombine with D segments, which are flanked on both 5′ and 3′ ends by recognition sequences of the 12-bp type.

Sources of Immunoglobulin Gene Diversity

For 250 V_H, 15 D_H, and 4 J_H gene segments that can be joined in 3 frames, at least 45,000 complete V_H genes can be formed. Therefore, more than 10^8 different specificities can

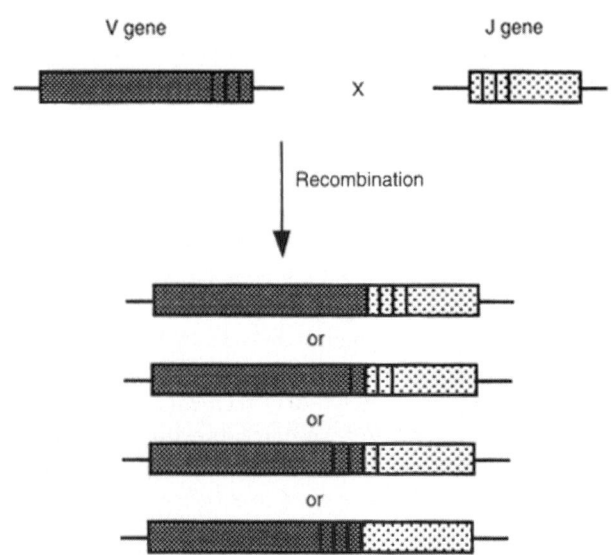

FIG. 3-6. Imprecision in the site of splicing of a V gene to a J gene (junctional diversity). (From Albert DA, Jakobiec FA. *Principles and practice of ophthalmology*, 2nd ed. Philadelphia: WB Saunders, 2000:68.)

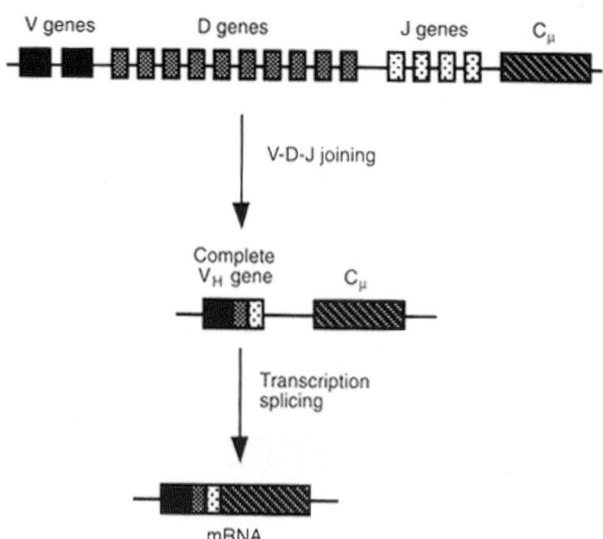

FIG. 3-7. The variable region of the heavy chain is encoded by V-, D-, and J-segment genes. (From Albert DA, Jakobiec FA. *Principles and practice of ophthalmology*, 2nd ed. Philadelphia: WB Saunders, 2000:68.)

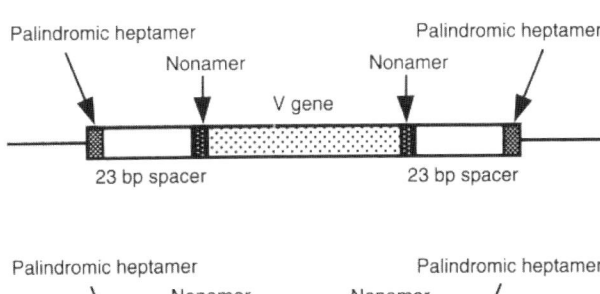

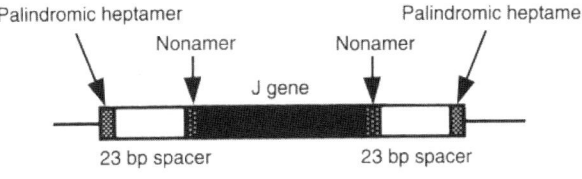

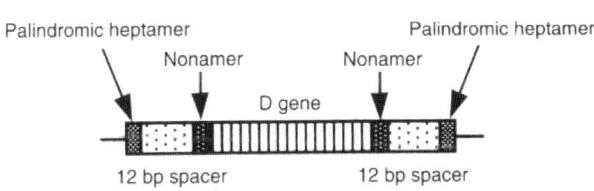

FIG. 3-8. Recognition sites for the recombination of V-, D-, and J-segment genes. V and J genes are flanked by sites containing 23-bp spacers, whereas D-segment genes possess 12-bp spacers. Recombination can occur only between sites with different classes of spacers. (From Albert DA, Jakobiec FA. *Principles and practice of ophthalmology*, 2nd ed. Philadelphia: WB Saunders, 2000:68.)

be generated by combining different V, D, and J gene segments and by combining more than 3000 L chains and 45,000 H chains. If the effects of N-region additional are included, more than 10^{11} different combinations can be formed. This is large enough to account for the immense range of antibodies that can be synthesized by an individual.

Far fewer V genes than Vκ genes encode L chains. However, many more V amino acid sequences are known (33–35). It is therefore likely that mutations introduced somatically give rise to much of the diversity of λ L chains (somatic hypermutation) (28). Likewise, somatic hypermutation further amplifies the diversity of H chains. To summarize, four sources of diversity are used to form the almost limitless array of antibodies that protect a host from foreign invasion: germline gene diversity, somatic recombination, junctional diversity, and somatic hypermutation.

Regulation of Immunoglobulin Gene Expression

An incomplete V gene becomes paired to a J gene on only one of a pair of homologous chromosomes. Successful rearrangement of one H-chain V region prevents the process from occurring on the other H-chain allele. Only the properly recombined immunoglobulin gene is expressed. Therefore, all of the V regions of immunoglobulins produced by a single lymphocyte are the same. This is called *allele exclusion* (36,37).

There are five classes of immunoglobulins. An antibody-producing cell first synthesizes IgM and then IgG, IgA, IgE, or IgD of the same specificity. Different

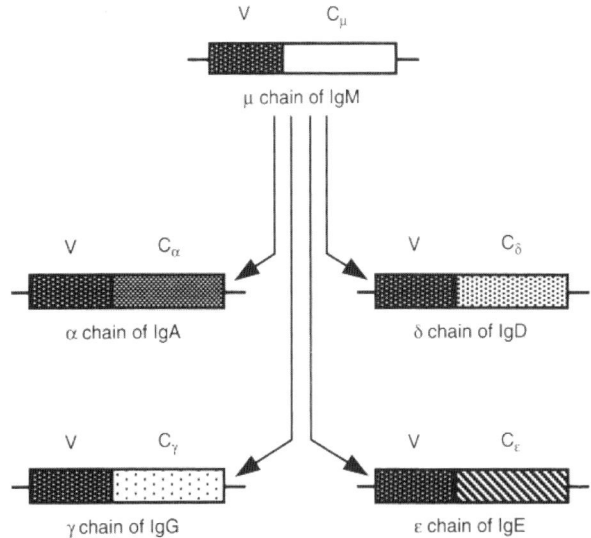

FIG. 3-9. The V$_H$ region is first associated with Cμ and then with another C region to form an H chain of a different class in the synthesis of different classes of immunoglobulins. (From Albert DA, Jakobiec FA. *Principles and practice of ophthalmology*, 2nd ed. Philadelphia: WB Saunders, 2000:69.)

classes of antibodies are formed by the translocation of a complete V$_H$ (V$_{HDH}$) gene from the C$_H$ gene of one class to that of another (38). Only the constant region of the H chain changes; the variable region of the H chain remains the same (Fig. 3-9). The L chain remains the same in this switch. This step in the differentiation of an antibody-producing cell is called *class switching* and is mediated by another DNA rearrangement called *single-stranded (SS) recombination* (39) (Fig. 3-10). This process is regulated by

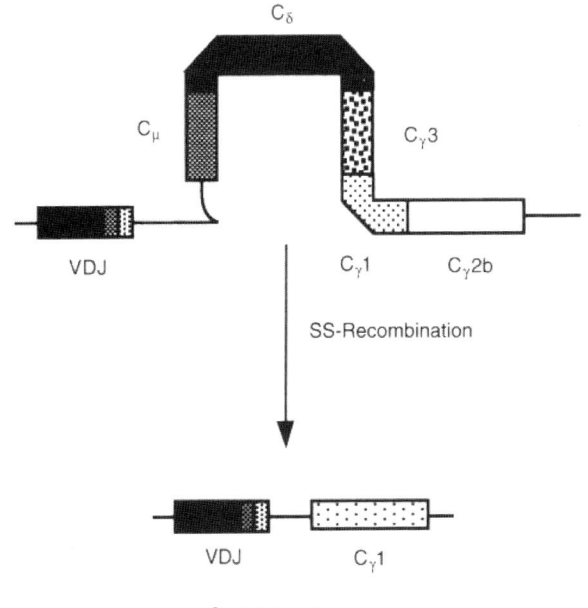

FIG. 3-10. The V$_H$DJ$_H$ gene moves from its position near Cμ to one near Cγ1 by SS recombination. (From Albert DA, Jakobiec FA. *Principles and practice of ophthalmology*, 2nd ed. Philadelphia: WB Saunders, 2000:69.)

cytokines produced by helper T cells (28). For example, switching to IgE class immunoglobulin production is provoked by the CD4 T_H2 cytokine, IL-4.

Determination of B-Cell Repertoire

V-segment genes can be grouped into families based on their DNA sequence homologies. In general, variable genes sharing greater than 80% nucleotide similarity are defined as a family (40). Currently, there are 11 known V_H gene families in the mouse (40–43) and 6 in humans (44–47). At least 29 families are known for the V segment of murine L-chain genes (48,49). In fetal pre-B cells, chromosomal position is a major determinant of V_H rearrangement frequency, resulting in a nonrandom repertoire that is biased toward use of V_H families closest to the J_H segments (50–55). In contrast, random use of V_H families based on the number of members in each family occurs in mature B cells without bias toward J_H proximal families (54–56). The preferential V_H gene rearrangement frequency seen in pre-B cells presumably becomes normalized when contact of the organism with a foreign antigen selects for the expression of the entire V_H gene repertoire. One can speculate that members of V_H families preferentially used in the pre-B cell encode antibody specificities that are needed in the early development of the immune system (57).

Immunoglobulin

Immunoglobulins are serum proteins that migrate with the globulin fractions by electrophoresis (25). Although they are glycoproteins, primary functions of the molecules are determined by their polypeptide sequence (26). At one end of the immunoglobulin is the amino terminus, a region that binds a site (epitope) on an antigen with great specificity. At the other end is the carboxyl terminus, a non–antigen-binding region responsible for various functions, including complement fixation and cellular stimulation through binding to cell surface immunoglobulin receptors.

IgG is composed of four polypeptide chains: two identical H chains and two identical L chains. H chains weigh approximately twice as much as L chains. The identical H chains are covalently linked by two disulfide bonds. One L chain is associated with each of the H chains by a disulfide bond and noncovalent forces. The two L chains are not linked. Asparagine residues on the H chains contain carbohydrate groups. The amino terminals of one L chain and its linked H chain compose the region for specific epitope binding. The carboxyl termini of the two H chains constitute the non–antigen-binding region.

Each polypeptide chain, whether L or H, is composed of regions that are called *constant* (C) or *variable* (V). A variable region on an L chain is called V_L, the constant region of a heavy chain is called C_H, and so forth. If the amino acid sequence of multiple L or H chains is compared, the constant regions vary little, whereas the variable regions differ greatly. The L chains are divided approximately equally into a constant (C_L) and a variable (V_L) region at the carboxyl and amino terminals, respectively. The H chains also contain a similar length of variable region (V_H) at the amino terminals, but the constant region (C_H) is three times the length of the variable region (V_H). The variable regions are responsible for antigen binding, and it is this variability that accounts for the ability to bind to millions of potential and real epitopes (27). Because each antibody molecule has two antigen-binding sites with variable regions, cross-linking of two identical antigens may be performed by an antibody. The constant regions carry out effector functions common to all antibodies of a given class (e.g., IgG) without the requirement of unique binding sites.

The functions of various regions of the immunoglobulin molecule were determined in part by the use of proteolytic enzymes that digest these molecules at specific locations. These enzymes have also been exploited for the development of laboratory reagents. The enzyme papain splits the molecule on the amino terminal side of the disulfide bonds that link the H chains, resulting in three fragments: two identical Fab fragments (each composed of the one entire H chain and a portion of the associated H chain) and one Fc fragment composed of the linked carboxyl terminal ends of the two H chains. In contrast, treatment with the enzyme pepsin results in one molecule composed of two linked Fab fragments know as F(ab') (25). The Fc fragment is degraded by pepsin treatment.

Within some classes of immunoglobulins, whole molecules may combine with other molecules of the same class to form polymers with additional functional capabilities. J chains facilitate the association of two or more immunoglobulins (Fig. 3-11), most notably IgA and IgM. Secretory component is a polypeptide synthesized by nonmotile epithelium found near mucosal surfaces. This polypeptide may bind noncovalently to IgA molecules, allowing their transport across mucosal surfaces to be elaborated in secretions.

Five immunoglobulin classes are recognized in humans: IgG, IgM, IgA, IgE, and IgD. Some classes are composed of subclasses as well. The class or subclass is determined by the structure of the H-chain constant region (C_H) (28). The H chains γ, μ, α, ϵ, and δ are found in IgG, IgM, IgA, IgE, and IgD, respectively. Four subclasses of IgG and two subclasses of both IgA and IgM exist. The two L chains on any immunoglobulin are identical and, depending on the structures of their constant regions, may be designated κ or λ. The κ chains tend to predominate in human immunoglobulins regardless of the H-chain–determined class. Whether an immunoglobulin is composed of two κ or two λ chains does not determine its functional capabilities. H-chain–determined class does not dictate important capacities (29).

limited by steric considerations.) IgM appears early in the immune response to antigen and is especially efficient at initiating agglutination, complement fixation, and cytolosis. IgM probably preceded IgG in the evolution of the immune response and is the most important antibody class in defending the circulation.

Immunoglobulin A

IgA is found in secretions of mucosal surfaces as well as in the serum. In secretions, it exists as a dimer coupled by J chain and stabilized by secretory component. IgA protects mucosal surfaces from infection but may also be responsible for immunologic surveillance at the site of first contact with antigen. IgA secretion is hardy, able to withstand the ravages of proteolytic degradation.

Immunoglobulin D

IgD is present in minute amounts in the serum and is the least stable of the immunoglobulins. Its function is not known, but it probably serves as a differentiation marker. IgD is found on the surfaces of B lymphocytes (along with IgM) and may have a role in class switching and tolerance.

Immunoglobulin E

IgE is notable for its ability to bind to mast cells; when cross-linked by antigen, it causes a variety of changes in the mast cell, including release of granular contents and membrane-derived mediators. Although IgE is recognized as a component of the allergic response, its role in protective immunity is speculative.

Immunoglobulin Intraclass Differences

Differences among the immunoglobulin classes are known as *isotypes* because all normal individuals in a species possess all of the classes. *Allotype* refers to antigenic structures on immunoglobulins that may differ from one individual to another within a species. *Idiotype* refers to differences among individual antibody molecules in a given individual, and is determined by the variable domain. Just as the variable domain allows for antibodies to recognize many antigens (epitopes), these differences also allow individual antibodies to be recognized on the basis of idiotype. In fact, antibodies directed against antibodies exist and are called *anti-idiotypic antibodies*. These anti-idiotypic antibodies are crucial to the regulation of the antibody response and constitute the basis for Jerne's idiotype network.

Complement

The complement system functions in the immune response by allowing animals to recognize foreign substances

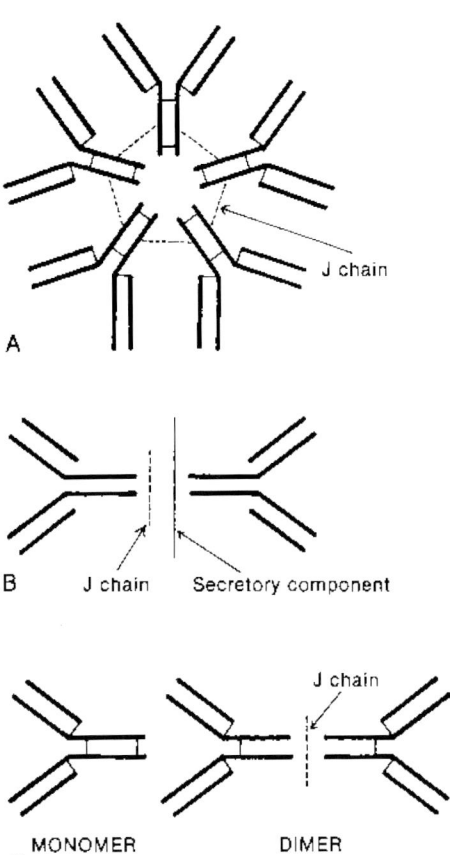

FIG. 3-11. Schematic diagram of polymeric human immunoglobulins. (From Albert DA, Jakobiec FA. *Principles and practice of ophthalmology*, 2nd ed. Philadelphia: WB Saunders, 2000:70.)

Immunoglobulin G

The most abundant of the human classes in serum, IgG constitutes approximately three fourths of the total serum immunoglobulins. Respectively, IgG$_1$ and IgG$_2$ make up approximately 60% and 20% of the total IgG. IgG$_3$ and IgG$_4$ are relatively minor components. IgG is the primary immunoglobulin providing immune protection in the extravascular compartments of the body. IgG is able to fix complement in the serum, an important function in inducing inflammation and controlling infection. IgG$_3$ and IgG$_1$ are most adept at complement fixation. IgG is the only immunoglobulin class to cross the placenta, an important aspect in fetal defense. Through their Fc portions, IgG molecules bind Fc receptors found on a host of inflammatory cells. Such binding activates cells such as macrophages and NK cells, enhancing cytotoxic activities important in the immune response.

Immunoglobulin M

Less abundant in the serum than IgG, IgM typically exists as a permanent form, stabilized by J chains, theoretically allowing the biding of 10 epitopes. (*In vivo*, this is usually

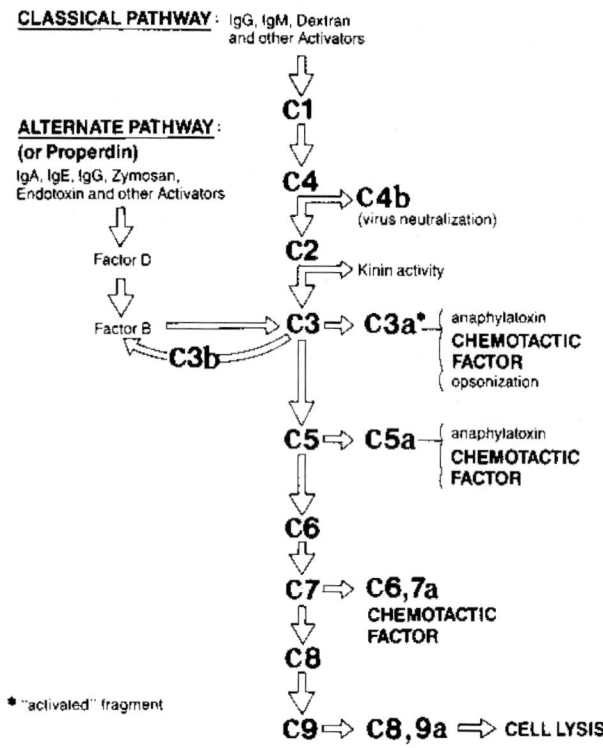

COMPLEMENT CASCADE

CLASSICAL PATHWAY: IgG, IgM, Dextran
and other Activators

C1

ALTERNATE PATHWAY:
(or Properdin)
IgA, IgE, IgG, Zymosan,
Endotoxin and other Activators

C4 → **C4b**
(virus neutralization)

Factor D

C2 → Kinin activity

Factor B → **C3** ⇒ **C3a*** anaphylatoxin
**CHEMOTACTIC
FACTOR**
opsonization

C3b

C5 ⇒ **C5a** anaphylatoxin
**CHEMOTACTIC
FACTOR**

C6

C7 ⇒ **C6,7a**
**CHEMOTACTIC
FACTOR**

C8

* "activated" fragment

C9 ⇒ **C8,9a** ⇒ CELL LYSIS

FIG. 3-12. Simplified schematic of steps in classic and alternate complement cascades. (From Albert DA, Jakobiec FA. *Principles and practice of ophthalmology*, 2nd ed. Philadelphia: WB Saunders, 2000:72.)

and defend themselves against infection (46). The pathways of complement activation are complex (47) (Fig. 3-12). Activation begins with the formation of antigen–antibody complexes and the ensuing generation of peptides that leads to a cascade of proteolytic events. The particle that activates the system accumulates a protein complex on its surface that often leads to cellular destruction through disruption of membranes.

Two independent pathways of complement activation are known. The classic pathway is initiated by IgG- and IgM-containing immune complexes. The alternative pathway is activated by aggravated IgA or complex polysaccharides from microbial cell walls (49). One component, C3, is crucial to both pathways and in its proactive form can be found circulating in plasma in large concentrations. Deficiency or absence of C3 results in increased susceptibility to infection (50). Cleavage of C3 may result in at least seven products (lettered *a* through *g*), each with biologic properties related to cellular activation and immune and nonimmune responses (51). C3a, for instance, causes the release of histamine from mast cells, neutrophil enzyme release, smooth muscle contraction, suppressor T-cell induction, and secretion of macrophage IL-1, prostaglandin, and leukotriene (52). C3e enhances vascular permeability. C3b binds to target cell surfaces and allows opsonization of biologic particles.

The alternative pathway probably is a first line of defense because, unlike the classic pathway, it may neutralize foreign material in the absence of antibody. The initiating enzyme of this pathway, factor D, circulates in an active form and may protect bystander cells from inadvertent destruction after activation of the pathway.

The final step of both pathways is membrane damage leading to cytolysis. Both pathways require the assembly of five precursor proteins to effect this damage: C5, C6, C7, C8, and C9. The mechanism of complement-mediated cell lysis is similar to that of cell-mediated cytotoxicity (as with NK cells). Membrane lesions result from insertion of tubular complexes into the membranes, leading to uptake of water with ion exchange disruption and eventual osmotic lysis.

The complement system interfaces with a variety of immune responses, as outlined earlier, and with the intrinsic coagulation pathways (53). Complement activity is usually measured by assessing the ability of serum to lyse sensitized sheep red blood cells (54). Values are expressed as 50% hemolytic complement units per millimeter. The function of an individual component may be studied by supplying excess quantities of all other components in a sheep red blood cell lysis assay (55). Components are quantitated by radical diffusion or immunoassay. Complement may be demonstrated in tissue sections by immunofluorescence or enzymatic techniques.

Complement plays a role in a number of human diseases. Complement-mediated cell lysis is the final common pathologic event in type II hypersensitivity reactions. Deficiencies of complement exist in recurrent gonococcal and meningococcal infections, hereditary angioedema, and others (50).

B-Cell Response to Antigen

Primary Response

Naive B cells respond to protein antigen in much the same way that T cells do, through the help of APCs and helper T cells. An APC (usually a macrophage or dendritic cell) processes the antigen and presents it to an antigen-specific helper (CD4) T cell, usually in the T-cell–rich zones of the required lymph node. The T cell is thus activated, expresses the membrane protein gp39, secretes cytokines (e.g., IL-2 and IL-6), and binds to similarly activated antigen-specific B cells (activated by the binding cross-linking of antigen to surface IgM- and IgD-binding sites). The T-cell/B-cell proliferation and a cascade of intracellular protein phosphorylation events, together with T-cell cytokine signals, results in production of IgM L and H chains with paratopes specific to the antigen epitopes that initiated this primary B-cell response. The proliferating B cells form germinal centers in the lymph node follicles, and somatic hypermutation of the IgM genes in some of these cells results in the evolution of a collection of B cells in the germinal center with surface IgM of even higher antigen-binding affinity. This phenomenon is called affinity

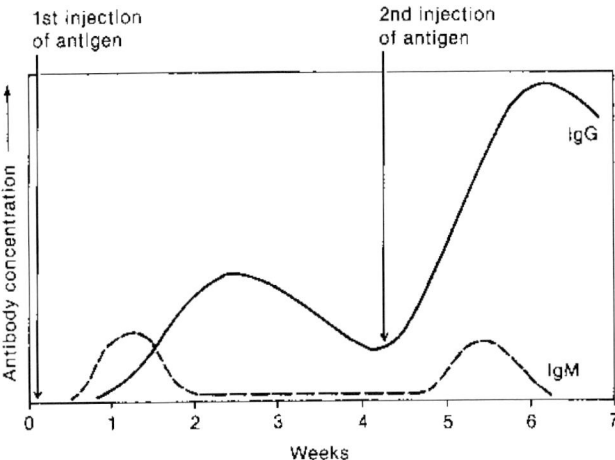

FIG. 3-13. Relative synthesis of immunoglobulin G (IgG) and IgM after initial and subsequent antigen injection. (From Albert DA, Jakobiec FA. *Principles and practice of ophthalmology*, 2nd ed. Philadelphia: WB Saunders, 2000:72.)

maturation of the primary antibody response. Those cells with the greatest antigen-binding affinity survive as this primary B-cell response subsides, persisting as long-lived memory cells responsible for the classic distinguishing characteristics of secondary humoral immune response.

Secondary Response

The development of the secondary humoral immune response is markedly accelerated compared with the primary response, and it is greatly amplified in terms of magnitude of antibody production (Fig. 3-13). The secondary response differs from the primary one in the isotype or isotypes of antibody produced, as well as in the avidity of the paratopes for the epitopes on the eliciting antigen. IgG, IgA, and IgE isotypes may now be seen in the effector phase of this secondary humoral immune response, and the binding affinities of these antibodies are usually greater than that of the IgM elicited in the primary response.

The cellular and molecular events of the secondary B-cell response are considerably different from those of the primary response. Memory B cells themselves become the preeminent antigen-binding, processing, and presenting cells, presenting peptide fragments (antigenic determinants) to CD4 helper T cells in typical MHC-restricted fashion, with "processed" peptide/HLA/DR motifs interacting with appropriate elements of the TCR for antigen at the same time that B-cell CD40 and T-cell gp39 signaling occurs (58). In addition, various T-cell cytokines induce the memory B cells to divide, proliferate, produce antibody, and switch the class of antibody being produced, depending on the sum-total message being received by the B cell, that is, the nature of the antigenic stimulus, the amount and the site of stimulation, and the sites of cells involved in the cognitive and activation phases of the secondary response. Memory

cells of each immunoglobulin isotype involved in the secondary response, of course, persist after devolution of the response.

T-LYMPHOCYTE RESPONSES

T lymphocytes stand at the center of the adaptive immune response (59). In the presence of T cells, the entire array of immune effector responses and tolerance are possible, but in the absence of T cells, only primitive antibody responses and no cell-mediated immune responses can be made. T cells are leukocytes that originate from lymphocyte precursors in the bone marrow. Most T cells undergo differentiation in the thymus gland and, on reaching maturity, disseminate through the blood to populate secondary lymphoid organs and to circulate among virtually all tissues of the body. A second population of T cells undergoes differentiation extrathymically; these cells have a somewhat different (and not yet completely defined) set of functional properties. T cells are exquisitely antigen specific, a property conferred on them by unique surface receptors that recognize antigenic material. Once activated, T cells initiate or participate in the various forms of cell-mediated immunity, humoral immunity, and tolerance.

T-Lymphocyte Development

From the pluripotent hematopoietic stem cell, a lineage of cells emerges that becomes the oligopotent lymphocyte progenitor (59). During fetal life, this lineage of cells is observed first in the liver, but as the fetus matures, the lymphocyte progenitors shift to the bone marrow. According to developmental signals not completely understood, lymphocyte progenitors in the bone marrow differentiate into (at least) three distinct lineages of committed precursor cells: prethymocytes, pre-B lymphocytes, and pre-NK lymphocytes. Prethymocytes, which give rise eventually to T lymphocytes, escape from the bone marrow (or fetal liver) and migrate through the blood primarily to the thymus, where cell adhesion molecules on microvascular endothelial cells direct them into the cortex. The differentiation process that thymocytes experience in the thymus accomplishes several critical goals in T-cell biology: (a) each cell acquires a unique surface receptor for antigen; (b) cells with receptors that recognize antigen molecules in the context of "self" class I or class II molecules [encoded b genes within the histocompatibility complex (MHCT)] are positively selected (60); (c) cells with receptors that recognize self-antigenic molecules in the context of self-MHC molecules are negatively selected (deleted or inactivated) (61); and (d) each mature cell acquires unique effector functions—the capacity to respond to antigen by secreting immunomodulatory cytokines or by delivering to a target cell a "lethal hit" (58).

Differentiation in the Thymic Cortex

In the thymic cortex, prethymocytes receive differentiation signals from resident thymic epithelial cells and thus initiate the process of maturation (59). A unique set of genes is activated, including (a) genes that commit the cells to proliferation, (b) genes that encode the TCRs for antigen, and (c) genes that code accessory molecules that developing and mature T cells use for antigen recognition and signal transduction. The genes that make it possible for T cells to create surface receptors for antigen are the structural genes that encode the four distinct polypeptide chains ($\alpha, \beta, \gamma, \delta$) from which the TCR for antigen is composed, as well as the genes that create genetic rearrangements that confer an extremely high degree of diversity on TCR molecules. Each TCR is a heterodimer of transmembrane polypeptides ($\alpha\beta$ or $\gamma\delta$). The portion of the TCR that is involved in antigen recognition resides at the ends of the peptide chains distal to the cell surface and is called the *combining site*. The accessory genes encode, on the one hand, the CD3 molecular complex ($\gamma, \delta, \epsilon, \zeta$), which enable a TCR that has engaged antigen to signal the T cells across the plasma membrane and, on the other hand, the CD4 and CD8 molecules that promote the affinity of the TCR for antigenic peptides in association with class I and II molecules, respectively, of the MHC. Thus, within the thymic cortex, individual prethymocytes proliferate, come to express a unique TCR, and simultaneously express CD3, CD4, and CD8 on the cell surface. Each day, a very large number of thymocytes is generated; therefore, an enormous diversity of TCR is also generated. Conservative estimates place the number of novel TCRs produced each day in excess of 10^9.

Nature of Antigen Recognition by T Cells

Thymocytes acquire one of two types of TCRs: $\alpha\beta$-TCRs are heterodimers composed of polypeptides encoded by the TCR-α and TCR-β chain genes; $\gamma\delta$-TCRs are heterodimers composed of polypeptides encoded by the TCR-γ and TCR-δ chain genes (62). Because much is known about the $\alpha\beta$-TCR, whereas much remains to be learned about the $\gamma\delta$-TCR, this discussion is limited to the former. The $\alpha\beta$-TCR for antigen does not recognize a protein antigen in its native configuration. Rather, the TCR recognizes peptides (ranging in size from 7 to 22 amino acids in length) derived from limited proteolysis of the antigen, and it recognizes these peptides when they are bound noncovalently to highly specialized regions of antigen-presenting molecules (63). Two types of antigen-presenting molecules exist, and both are encoded in the MHC (64). Class I molecules are transmembrane proteins expressed on APCs. These molecules possess on their most distal domains a platform of two parallel α-helices separated by a groove. This groove accommodates peptides (generated by regulated proteolysis of antigenic proteins), ranging from seven

to nine amino acids in length. Class II molecules are also transmembrane proteins expressed on APCs; the platforms on their distal domains contain similar grooves, which accept peptides of 15 to 22 amino acids in length. The "combining site" of an individual TCR possesses three contact points: a central point that interacts directly with an antigenic peptide in the groove, and two side points that interact directly with the platform (α-helices) of class I or class II molecules. Thus, the conditions that must be met for successful recognition of antigen by TCR are (a) a class I or II molecule must be available on an APC, and (b) a peptide must occupy the groove of the presenting molecule's platform.

CD4 molecules that are expressed on certain T cells and thymocytes have the ability to bind class II molecules at a site distinct from the antigen presentation platform. As a consequence, CD4-bearing T cells whose TCR has engaged a peptide-containing class II molecule are more likely to be stimulated than T cells with similar receptors that do not express CD4. Similarly, CD8-bearing T cells whose TCR has engaged a peptide-containing molecule are much more likely to be stimulated than T cells without CD8.

In the thymic cortex, epithelial cells express class I and II molecules encoded by the individual's own MCH genes (59,60). When TCR-bearing thymocytes are generated in the cortex, cells with TCR that recognize peptide-containing self-class I or -class II molecules are induced to undergo successive rounds of proliferation, leading to clonal expansion. By contrast, TCR-bearding thymocytes that fail to recognize peptide-containing class I or class II molecules are not activated in the cortex. In the absence of this cognate signal, all such cells enter a default pathway, which ends inevitably in cell death (apoptosis). This process is called *positive selection* because thymocytes with TCR that have an affinity for self-MHC molecules (plus peptide) are being selected for further clonal expansion. Unselected cells simply die by apoptosis. At the completion of their sojourn in the thymic cortex, large numbers of positively selected TCR$^+$, CD3$^+$, CD4$^+$, and CD8$^+$ thymocytes migrate into the thymic medulla.

Differentiation in the Thymic Medulla

In addition to epithelial cells, the thymic medulla contains a unique population of bone marrow-derived cells called *dendritic cells* (61,65). These nonphagocytic cells express large numbers of class I and class II molecules and actively endocytosed proteins in their environment. Peptides derived from these proteins by proteolysis are loaded into the grooves of MHC-encoded antigen presentation platforms. In the thymic medulla, the vast majority of such endocytosed proteins are self-proteins. As thymocytes enter the medulla from the cortex, a subpopulation expresses TCR that recognize peptides of self proteins expressed on self-class I or -class II molecules. By contrast, another sub-population fails to recognize self-class I or -class II molecules because the TCR is specific for a peptide not included among peptides from self-proteins. The former population, comprising cells that recognize self exclusively, engages self-derived peptides plus MHC molecules on medullary dendritic cells. This engagement delivers a "death" signal to the T cell, and all such cells undergo apoptosis. This process is called *negative selection* because thymocytes with TCR that have an affinity for self-peptides in self-MHC molecules are being eliminated. In part, this process plays a major role in eliminating autoreactive T cells that would be capable of causing autoimmunity if they should escape from the thymus. Many other thymocytes that enter the medulla express TCRs that are unable to engage self-class I or -class II molecules on dendritic cells because the relevant peptide does not occupy the antigen-presenting groove. T cells of this type proceed to downregulate expression of either CD4 or CD8 and acquire the properties of mature T cells. The T cells that are ready at this point to leave the thymus are TCR$^+$, CD3$^+$, and either CD4$^+$ or CD8$^+$ (but not both). Moreover, they are in G0 of the cell cycle, that is, resting. The number of such cells exported from the thymus per day is very large; in humans, it is estimated that more than 10^8 new mature T cells are produced daily. These cells are fully immunocompetent and are prepared to recognize and respond to a large diversity of foreign antigens that are degraded into peptides and presented on self-class I or -class II molecules on tissues outside the thymus. It is estimated that the number of different antigenic specificities that can be recognized by mature T cells (i.e., the T-cell repertoire for antigens) exceeds 10^9.

Properties and Functions of Mature T Lymphocytes

Mature, resting T cells with $\alpha\beta$-TCR migrate from the thymus to any and all tissues of the body, but there are vascular specializations (postcapillary venules) in secondary lymphoid organs (lymph nodes, Peyer's patches, tonsils) that promote the selective entry of T cells into these tissues (66). More than 99% of T cells in blood that traverse a lymph node are extracted into the parafollicular region of the cortex. This region of the nodal cortex is designed to encourage the interaction of T cells with APCs. Because of the encounter of any single, antigen-specific T cell with its antigen of interest on an APC is a rather rare event, most T cells that enter a secondary lymphoid organ fail to find their antigen of interest. In this case, the T cells disengage from resident APCs and migrate into the effluent of the node, passing through lymph ducts back into the general blood circulation. An individual T cell may make journeys such as this numerous times during a single day, and countless journeys are accomplished during its lifetime

(which may be measured in tens of years). This monotonous behavior changes dramatically if and when a mature T cells encounters its specific antigen through recognition of the relevant peptide in association with a class I or class II molecule on an APC in a secondary lymphoid organ. It is this critical encounter that initiates T-cell–dependent, antigen-specific immune responses.

T-Cell Activation by Antigen

There is a general rule regarding the minimal requirements for activation of lymphocytes, including T cells, which are in a resting state: Two different surface signals received simultaneously are required to arouse the cell out of G0 (67). One signal is delivered through CD3 and is triggered by successful engagement of the TCR with its peptide in association with an MHC molecule. The other signal is delivered through numerous cell surface molecules other than the TCR. Signals of this type are also referred to as *costimulation*, and costimulation is usually the result of receptor–ligand interactions in which the receptor is on the T cell and the ligand is expressed on the APC. For example, B7-1 (CD80) and B7-2 (CD81) are surface molecules expressed on APCs; these molecules engage the receptor CD28 on T cells, thus delivering a costimulatory activation signal to the recipient cells. Similarly, CD40 ligand on T cells and CD40 on APCs function in a costimulatory manner. Another example of costimulation occurs when a cytokine produced by an APC, such as IL-1 or IL-2, is presented to T cells expressing the IL-1 or IL-2 receptor, respectively. When both conditions are met—TCR binds to peptide plus MHC molecule and CD80 binds to CD28-the T cell receives coordinated signals across the plasma membrane, and these signals initiate a cascade of intracytoplasmic events that lead to dramatic changes.

Antigen-Activated T-Cell Responses

When a T cell encounters its antigen of interest along with satisfactory costimulation, it escapes from G0. *Proliferation* results in emergence of a "clone" of cells, all of the identical phenotype, including the TCR. This process, called clonal expansion, results from the elaboration of growth factor (e.g., IL-2), is one hallmark of the process of immunization or sensitization, and accounts for why the number of T cells able to recognize a particular antigen increases dramatically after sensitization has taken place. The signal that triggers proliferation arises first from the APC, but sustained T-cell proliferation takes place because the responding T cell activates its own IL-2 and IL-2 receptor (CD25) receptor genes (68,69). IL-2 is a potent growth factor for T cells, and T cells expressing CD25 respond to IL-2 by undergoing repetitive rounds of replication. IL-2 is not the only growth factor for T cells; IL-4, also made by T cells, adds the capacity of T cells to autocrine stimulate their own proliferation—so long as their TCRs remain engaged with the antigen (plus MHC) of interest.

In addition to proliferation, antigen-activated T cells proceed down pathways of further *differentiation*. The functional expressions of this differentiation include (a) secretion of lymphokines that promote inflammation or modify the functional properties of other lymphoreticular cells in their immediate environment; and (b) acquisition of the cytoplasmic machinery required for displaying cytotoxicity, that is, the ability to lyse target cells (70). The list of lymphokines that an activated mature T cell can make is long: IL-2, IL-3, IL-4, granulocyte–macrophage colony-stimulating factor, IL-5, IL-6, IL-10, IFN-γ, TNF-α, and TGF-β. The range of biologic activities attributable to these cytokines is extremely broad, and no single T cell produces all of these factors simultaneously. The pattern of cytokines produced by a T cell accounts in large measure for the functional phenotype of the cell (see later discussion).

The ability of antigen-activated T cells to lyse antigen-bearing target cells is embodied in specializations of the cell cytoplasm and cell surface. Cytotoxic T cells possess granules in their cytoplasm that contain a molecule, perforin, that can polymerize and insert into the plasma membrane of a target cell, creating large pores. The granules also contain a series of lytic enzymes (granzymes) that enter the target cell, perhaps through the perforin-created pores, and trigger programmed cell death. There is a second mechanism by which T cells can cause death of neighboring cells. Activated T cells express Fas or CD95, a cell surface glycoprotein. The coreceptor for Fas, Fas ligand or CD95L, is a member of the TNF receptor superfamily, and its cytoplasmic tail contains a "death domain." After sustained activation, T cells also express Fas ligand; when Fas interacts with Fas ligand, the cell bearing Fas undergoes programmed cell death. Thus, Fas ligand–positive T cells can trigger apoptotic death in adjacent cells that are Fas$^+$, including other T cells. In fact, the ability of antigen-activated T cells to elicit apoptosis among neighboring, similarly activated T cells may serve to downregulate the immune response to that particular antigen by eliminating responding T cells.

Imperfect Antigen-Activated T-Cell Responses

On occasion, T cells may encounter their antigen of interest (in association with an MHC molecule) under circumstances in which an appropriate costimulatory signal does not exist (71). This can be arranged *in vitro*, for example, by using paraformaldehyde-fixed APCs. Antigen–TCR binding alone fails to activate the T cells. However, if these same T cells are reexposed subsequently to the same antigen/MHC on viable APCs capable of costimulation, activation of the T cells *still fails*. The inability of T cells first activated by antigen–TCR binding in the absence of costimulatory signals to respond subsequently is referred to as

anergy. This phenomenon occurs *in vivo* and is important in regulating the immune response and some forms of tolerance.

T-Lymphocyte Heterogeneity

The adaptive immune response is separable into a cell-mediated immune arm and an antibody-mediated or humoral immune arm (58). T cells themselves initiate and mediate cell-mediated autoimmunity, and they play a dominant role in promoting antibody-mediated responses. There is heterogeneity among T cells that function in cell-mediated immunity, and there is heterogeneity among T cells that promote humoral immunity.

Cell-mediated immunity arises when effector T cells are generated in secondary lymphoid organs in response to antigen-induced activation. Two types of cell-mediated effector cells are recognized: (a) T cells that elicit delayed hypersensitivity, and (b) T cells that are cytotoxic for antigen-bearing target cells. T cells that elicit delayed hypersensitivity recognize their antigen of interest on cells in peripheral tissues and, on activation, they secrete proinflammatory cytokines such as IFN-γ and TNF-α. These cytokines act on microvascular endothelium, promoting edema formation and recruitment of monocytes, neutrophils, and other leukocytes to the site. In addition, monocytes and tissue macrophages exposed to these cytokines are activated to acquire phagocytic and cytotoxic functions. Because it takes hours for these inflammatory reactions to emerge, they are called "delayed." It is generally believed that the T cells that elicit delayed hypersensitivity reactions are CD4$^+$ and recognize antigens of interest in association with class II MHC molecules. However, ample evidence exists to implicate CD8$^+$ T cells in this process too (especially in reactions in the central nervous system). Although the elicitation of delayed hypersensitivity reactions is antigen specific, the inflammation that attends the response is itself nonspecific. This feature accounts for the high level of tissue injury and cell destruction that is found in delayed hypersensitivity responses. By contrast, effector responses elicited by cytotoxic T cells are characterized by much less nonspecific inflammation. Cytotoxic T cells interact directly with antigen-bearing target cells and deliver a "lethal hit" that is highly specific; there is virtually no innocent bystander injury in this response.

Humoral immunity arises when B cells produce antibodies in response to antigenic challenge (58). Although antigen alone may be sufficient to activate B cells to produced IgM antibodies, this response is amplified in the presence of helper T cells. Moreover, the ability of B cells to produce more differentiated autoantibody isotypes, such as IgG or IgE, depends on helper signals from T cells. T cells provide "help" in the form of lymphokines. The pattern of lymphokines produced by a helper T cell plays a key role in determining the nature of the B-cell antibody response. One helper T cell, called T_H1, responds to antigen stimulation by producing IL-2, IFN-γ, and TNF-α (72). These cytokines influence B-cell differentiation in the direction of producing complement-fixing antibodies. T_H2 cells respond to antigen stimulation by producing IL-4, IL-5, IL-6, and IL-10. These cytokines influence B-cell differentiation in the direction of producing non–complement-fixing IgG antibodies or IgA and IgE antibodies. A similar difference in cytokine profiles exists for subpopulations of $CD8^+$ T cells. T_H1-type cells mediated delayed hypersensitivity reactions and thus can function as helper cells. T_H2-type cells have been implicated in inflammatory reactions of both immediate and intermediate types.

T-Cell–Dependent Inflammation

Primarily by virtue of the lymphokines they produce, T cells can produce immunogenic inflammation if they encounter their antigens of interest in a peripheral tissue. If the responding T cell is of the T_H1 type, it produces IFN-γ along with other proinflammatory molecules. IFN-γ is a potent activator of microvascular endothelial cells and macrophages. Activated endothelial cells become "leaky," permitting edema fluid and plasma proteins to accumulate at the site. Activated endothelial cells also promote the immigration of blood-borne leukocytes, including monocytes, into the site; it is the activated macrophages (histiocytes, which may evolve in time to epithelioid cells and thence to multinucleated giant cells) that provide much of the "toxicity" at the inflammatory site. These cells respond to IFN-γ by upregulating the genes responsible for nitric oxide (NO) synthesis. NO, together with newly generated reactive oxygen intermediates, creates much of the local necrosis associated with immunogenic inflammation. T_H2 cells have been directly implicated in immune inflammation, including that found in the eye, particularly that associated with atopy (73). The offending lymphokine may be IL-10, although other cytokines may also participate.

T Cells in Disease: Infectious, Immunopathogenic, Autoimmune

The inflammation associated with the immune attack on pathogen can lead to injury of surrounding tissues (74). If the extent of this injury is of sufficient magnitude, disease may result from the inflammation itself, quite apart from the toxicity of the pathogen. The eye is particularly vulnerable to such injury. The immune response may prove to be more problematic than the triggering infection or event. And in some pathologic circumstances, T cells mistake "self" molecules as "foreign," producing an autoimmune response.

IMMUNE-MEDIATED TISSUE INJURY

The immune response of an organism to an antigen may be either helpful or harmful. If the response is excessive or inappropriate, the host may incur tissue damage. The term *hypersensitivity reaction* has been applied to such excessive or inappropriate immune responses. Four major types of hypersensitivity reactions are described, and all can occur in the eye (Table 3-10). The necessary constituents for these reactions are already present in, or can be readily recruited into, ocular tissues. Immunoglobulins, complement components, inflammatory cells, and inflammatory mediators can, under certain circumstances, be found in ocular fluids (i.e., tears, aqueous humor, and vitreous) and

TABLE 3-10. GELL, COOMBS, AND LACKMANN HYPERSENSITIVITY REACTIONS

Type	Participating Elements	Systemic Examples	Ocular Examples
Type I	Allergen, IgE, mast cells, eosinophils	Allergic rhinitis, allergic asthma, anaphylaxis	Seasonal allergic conjunctivitis, vernal keratoconjunctivitis, atopic keratoconjunctivitis, giant papillary conjunctivitis
Type II	Antigen, IgG1, IgG3, or IgM, complement, neutrophils (enzymes), macrophages (enzymes)	Goodpasture's syndrome, myasthenia gravis, cicatricial pemphigoid	Ocular cicatricial pemphigoid, pemphigus vulgaris, dermatitis herpetiformis
Type III	Antigen, IgG1, IgG3, or IgM, complement–immune complex, neutrophils (enzymes), macrophages (enzymes)	Stevens-Johnson syndrome, rheumatoid arthritis, systemic lupus erythematosus, polyarteritis nodosa, Behçet's disease, relapsing polychondritis	Ocular manifestations of diseases listed in systemic examples
Type IV	Antigen, T cells, neutrophils, macrophages	Transplant rejection, tuberculosis, sarcoidosis, Wegener's granulomatosis, stromal keratitis	Contact hypersensitivity (drug allergy), herpes disciform keratitis, phlyctenulosis, corneal transplant rejection, tuberculosis, sarcoidosis, Wegener's granulomatosis, uveitis, herpes simplex virus stromal keratitis, river blindness

Ig, immunoglobulin.

in the ocular tissues, adnexa, and orbit. Unfortunately, these tissues (especially the ocular tissues) can be rapidly damaged by inflammatory reactions that produce irreversible alterations in structure and function. Some authors have described a fifth type of hypersensitivity reaction, but this adds little to our real understanding of disease mechanisms and is unimportant to us as ophthalmologists in the study and care of patients with destructive ocular inflammatory diseases. For this reason, this discussion is confined to the classic four types of hypersensitivity reactions that were originally proposed by Gell, Coombs, and Lackmann.

Injury Mediated by Antibody

Type I Hypersensitivity Reactions

The antigens responsible for type I (immediate) hypersensitivity reactions are ubiquitous environmental allergens such as dust mites, pollens, danders, microbes, and drugs. Under ordinary circumstances, exposure of an individual to such materials is associated with no harmful inflammatory response. The occurrence of such a response is considered, therefore, "out of place" (Greek, *a topos*) or inappropriate; it is for this reason that Cocoa and Cooke coined the word *atopy* in 1923 to describe the predisposition of individuals who mount such inappropriate inflammatory or immune responses to ubiquitous environmental agents (75). The antibodies responsible for type I hypersensitivity reactions are homocytotropic antibodies, principally immunoglobulin E (IgE) but sometimes IgG4 as well. The mediators of the clinical manifestations of type I reactions include histamine, serotonin, leukotrienes (including slow-reacting substance of anaphylaxis), kinins, and other vasoactive amines. Examples of type I hypersensitivity reactions include anaphylactic reactions to insect bites or to penicillin injections, allergic asthma, hay fever, and seasonal allergic conjunctivitis. It should be emphasized that in real life, the four types of hypersensitivity reactions are rarely observed in pure form, in isolation from each other; it is typical for hypersensitivity reactions to have more than one of the classic Gell and Coombs responses as participants in the inflammatory problem. For example, eczema, atopic blepharoconjunctivitis, and vernal keratoconjunctivitis have hypersensitivity reaction mechanisms of both type I and type IV. The atopic individuals in whom such abnormal reactions to environmental materials develop are genetically predisposed to such responses. The details of the events responsible for allergy (a term coined in 1906 by von Pirquet, in Vienna, meaning "changed reactivity") are clearer now than they were even a decade ago.

Genetically predisposed allergic individuals have defects in the population of suppressor T lymphocytes responsible for modulating IgE responses to antigens. After the initial contact of an allergen with the mucosa of such an individual, abnormal amounts of allergen-specific IgE antibody are produced at the mucosal surface and at the regional lymph nodes. This IgE has high avidity, through its Fc portion, to Fc receptors on the surfaces of mast cells in the mucosa. The antigen-specific IgE antibodies, therefore, stick to the receptors on the surfaces of the tissue mast cells and remain there for unusually long periods. Excess locally produced IgE enters the circulation and binds to mast cells at other tissue locations, as well as to circulating basophils. A subsequent encounter of the allergic individual with the antigen to which he or she has become sensitized results in antigen binding by the antigen-specific IgE molecules affixed to the surfaces of the tissue mast cells. The simultaneous binding of the antigen to adjacent IgE molecules on the mast cell surface results in a change in the mast cell membrane and particularly in membrane-bound adenyl cyclase (Fig. 3-14). The feature common to all known mechanisms that trigger mast cell degranulation stimulated by pharmacologic agents or anaphylatoxins like C3a and C5a and antigen-specific IgE-mediated degranulation is an abrupt increase in cytoplasmic calcium concentrations, with subsequent aggregation of tubulin into microtubules, which then participate in the degranulation of vasoactive amines (Fig. 3-12). In addition to the degranulation of the preformed mediators such as histamine, induction of synthesis of newly formed mediators from arachidonic acid also occurs with triggering of mast cell degranulation (Table 3-11). The preformed and newly synthesized mediators then produce the classic clinical signs of a type I hypersensitivity reaction: wheal (edema), flare (erythema), itch, and, in many cases, the subsequent delayed appearance of the so-called late-phase reaction characterized by subacute signs of inflammation.

Control of Immunoglobulin E Synthesis

The T_H2 subset of helper T cells bearing Fc receptors produce, in addition to IL-4, IgE-binding factors after stimulation by interleukins produced by antigen-specific helper T cells activated by APCs and antigen. The two known types of IgE-binding factor that can be produced are IgE-potentiating factor and IgE-suppressor factor; both are encoded by the same codon, and the functional differences are created by post-translational glycosylation. The glycosylation is either enhanced or suppressed by cytokines derived from other T cells. For example, glycosylation-inhibiting factor (identical to migration inhibitory factor) is produced by antigen-specific suppressor T cells. Glycosylation-enhancing factor is produced by an Fc receptor helper T cell (Fig. 3-15). The relative levels of these factors control the production of IgE-potentiating factor and IgE-suppressor factor by the central helper T cell and, thus, ultimately control the amount of IgE produced (Fig. 3-15). They probably do so through regulation of IgE B-lymphocyte proliferation and synthesis of IgE by these cells.

Mast Cell Subpopulations

It has become increasingly clear that at least two subpopulations of mast cells exist. CTMCs contain heparin as the

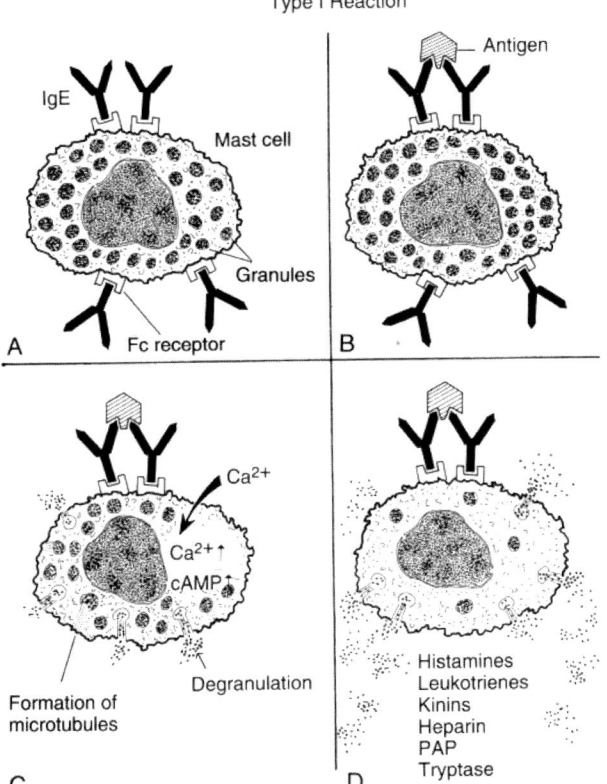

Type I Reaction

FIG. 3-14. Type I hypersensitivity reaction mechanism. **A:** Mast cell Fcε receptors have antigen-specific immunoglobulin E (IgE) affixed to them by virtue of the patient's being exposed to the antigen and mounting an inappropriate (atopic) immune response to that antigen, with resultant production of large amounts of antigen-specific IgE antibodies. The antibodies have found their way to the mucosal mast cell and have bound to the mast cells but have not provoked allergic symptoms because the patient is no longer exposed to the antigen. **B:** Second (or subsequent) exposure to the sensitizing antigen or allergen results in a "bridging" binding reaction of antigen to two adjacent IgE antibodies affixed to the mast cell plasma membrane. **C:** The antigen–antibody bridging reaction shown in **B** results in profound changes in the mast cell membrane, with alterations in membrane-bound adenyl cyclase, calcium influx, tubulin aggregation into microtubules, and the beginning of the degranulation of the preformed mast cell mediators from their storage granules. **D:** The degranulation reaction proceeds, and newly synthesized mediators, particularly those generated by the catabolism of membrane-associated arachidonic acid, begin. The array of liberated and synthesized proinflammatory mediators is impressive. (From Albert DA, Jakobiec FA. *Principles and practice of ophthalmology*, 2nd ed. Philadelphia: WB Saunders, 2000:75.)

major proteoglycan, produce large amounts of prostaglandin D_2 in response to stimulation, and are independent of T-cell–derived interleukins for their maturation, development, and function. These cells stain brilliantly with toluidine blue in formalin-fixed tissue sections.

MMCs do not stain well with toluidine blue. They are found primarily in the subepithelial mucosa in gut and lung; they contain chondroitin sulfate as the major proteoglycan; they manufacture leukotriene C_4 as the predominant arachidonic acid metabolite after stimulation; and

TABLE 3-11. MAST CELL MEDIATORS

Preformed in Granules	Newly Synthesized
Histamine	LTB_4
Heparin	LTC_4
Tryptase	LTD_4
Chymase	Prostaglandins
Kinins	Thromboxanes
Eosinophil chemotactic factor	Platelet-activating factor
Neutrophil chemotactic factor	
Serotonin	
Chondroitin sulfate	
Arylsulfatase	

LT, leukotriene.

they are dependent on IL-3 (and IL-4) for their maturation and proliferation. Interestingly, MMCs placed in culture with fibroblasts rather than T cells transform to cells with the characteristics of CTMCs. Disodium cromoglycate inhibits histamine release from CTMCs but not from MMCs. Steroids suppress the proliferation of MMCs, probably through inhibition of IL-3 production.

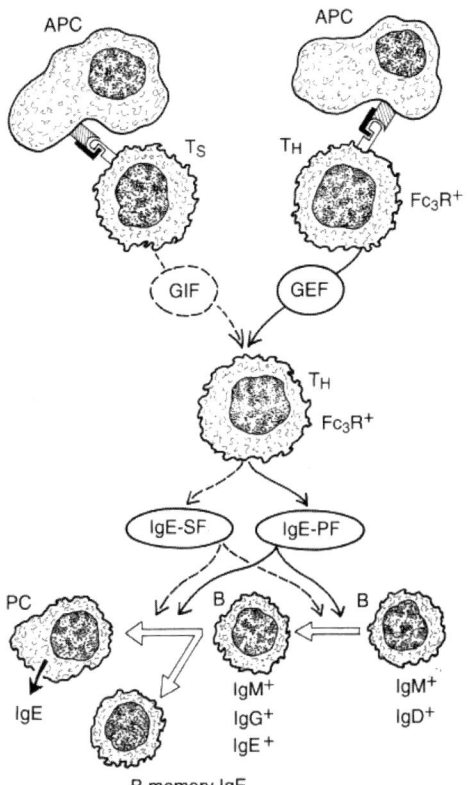

FIG. 3-15. Immunoglobulin E (IgE) synthesis. Glycosylation-enhancing factor, glycosylation-inhibiting factor, IgE-promoting factor, IgE-suppressor factor, and the helper and suppressor T lymphocytes specific for regulation of IgE synthesis are shown. (From Albert DA, Jakobiec FA. *Principles and practice of ophthalmology*, 2nd ed. Philadelphia: WB Saunders, 2000:76.)

Atopy Genetics and the Role of the Environment

Both genetic and environmental components are clearly involved in the allergic response. Offspring of marriages in which one parent is allergic have approximately a 30% risk of being allergic, and if both parents are allergic, the risk to each child is greater than 50%. At least three genetically linked mechanisms govern the development of atopy: (a) general hyperresponsiveness, (b) regulation of serum IgE levels, and (c) sensitivity to specific antigens. General hyperresponsiveness, defined as positive skin reactions to a broad range of environmental allergens, is associated with HLA-B8/HLA-DW3 phenotypy, and this general hyperresponsiveness appears not to be IgE class specific. Total serum IgE levels are also controlled genetically, and family studies indicate that total IgE production is under genetic control. Finally, experimental studies using low–molecular-weight allergenic determinants disclose a strong association between IgE responsiveness to such allergens and HLA-DR/DW2 type, whereas for at least some high–molecular-weight allergens, responsiveness is linked to HLA-DR/DW3. In mice at least, gene regulation of IgE production occurs at several levels, including (a) regulation of antigen-specific, IgE-specific suppressor T cells; (b) manufacture of glycosylation-inhibiting factor or of glycosylation-enhancing factor by helper T cells; (c) at the level of IL-4, regulation of class switching to IgE synthesis; and (d) at the level of IgE binding, factors such as IgE-potentiating factor and IgE-suppressor factor.

The environment plays a major role in whether a genetically predisposed individual expresses major clinical manifestations of atopy. The "dose" of allergens to which the individual is exposed is a critical determinant of whether clinical expression of an allergic response develops. Less well recognized, however, is the fact that the general overall quality of the air in an individual's environment plays a major role in whether clinical expression of allergic responses to allergens to which the individual is sensitive develops. It has become unmistakably clear that, as the general quality of air in urban environments has deteriorated and as the air has become more polluted, the prevalence in the population of overt atopic clinical manifestations has increased dramatically. On a global level, the immediate environment in which an individual finds himself much of the time, the home, plays an important part in the expression of allergic disease. Allergically predisposed persons whose household includes at least one member who smokes cigarettes have enhanced sensitivity to allergens such as house dust mites and molds, among others. It is probably also true that the overall health and nutritional status of an individual influence the likelihood of that person having a clinically obvious allergy.

Diagnosis of Type I Reactions

The definite diagnosis of type I hypersensitivity reactions requires the passive transfer of the reaction using a method known as the Prausnitz-Küstner reaction. Intradermal injection of serum of a patient suspected of having a type I hypersensitivity–mediated problem into the skin of a volunteer is followed by injection of varying dilutions of the presumed offending antigen at the same intradermal sites as the patient's serum injection. A positive Prausnitz-Küstner reaction occurs when local flare-and-wheal formation follows injection of the antigen. This method for proving type I reactions is not used clinically; therefore, diagnosis of type I mechanisms contributing to a patient's inflammatory disorder is always based on a collection of circumstantial evidence that strongly supports the hypothesis of a type I reaction. Such evidence includes a typical history (e.g., a family history of allergy or a personal history of eczema, hay fever, asthma, or urticaria), elicitation of allergic symptoms, especially itching, after exposure to suspected allergens, elevated IgE levels in serum or other body fluids, and blood or tissue eosinophilia.

Therapy for Type I Reactions

Therapy for type I reactions must include scrupulous avoidance of the offending antigen. This is not easy, and it is a component of proper treatment that is often neglected by the patient and the physician alike. It is crucial, however, for a patient with an incurable disease such as atopy, to recognize that, throughout a lifetime, he or she will slowly sustain cumulative permanent damage to structures affected by atopic responses (e.g., lung, eye) if he or she is subjected to repetitive triggering of the allergic response. Pharmacologic approaches to this disorder can never truly succeed for careless patients who neglect their responsibility to avoid allergens. A careful environmental history is, therefore, a critical ingredient in history taking, and convincing education of the patient and family alike is an essential and central ingredient in the care plan.

A careful environmental history and meticulous attention to environmental details can make the difference between relative stability and progressive inflammatory attacks that ultimately produce blindness. Elimination of pets, carpeting, feather pillows, quilts, and wool blankets and installation of air-conditioning and air-filtering systems are therapeutic strategies that should not be overlooked (76).

One of the most important advances in the care of patients with type I disease during the past two decades has been the development of mast cell–stabilizing agents. Disodium cromoglycate, sodium nedocromil, lodoxamide, and olopatedine are four such agents. Topical administration is both safe and effective in the care of patients with allergic eye disease (77,78). This therapeutic approach is to be strongly recommended and is very much favored over simply using competitive H$_1$ antihistamines. Clearly, if the mast cells can be prevented from degranulating, the therapeutic effect of such degranulation-inhibiting agents would be expected to be vastly superior to that of antihistamines, simply by virtue of preventing liberation of an entire panoply of mediators from the mast cell rather than competitive inhibition of one such mediator, histamine.

Histamine action inhibition by H$_1$ antihistamines is also helpful in patients with ocular allergy. The efficacy of such agents used topically is marginal in some atopic individuals, and long-term use can result in the development of sensitivity to ingredients in the preparations. The consistent use of systemic antihistamines can be helpful as well. In addition, slow escalation of the amount of hydroxyzine used in the care of atopic patients can help to interrupt the itch-scratch-itch psychoneurotic component that often accompanies eczema and atopic blepharoconjunctivitis.

Generalized suppression of inflammation through use of topical corticosteroids is commonly used for treatment of type I ocular hypersensitivity reactions, and this is appropriate for acute breakthrough attacks of inflammation. It is, however, completely inappropriate for long-term care. Corticosteroids have a direct effect on all inflammatory cells, including eosinophils, mast cells, and basophils. They are extremely effective, but the risks of long-term topical steroid use are considerable and unavoidable, and thus such use is discouraged.

Although desensitization immunotherapy can be an important additional component to the therapeutic plan for a patient with type I hypersensitivity, it is difficult to perform properly. The first task, of course, is to document to which allergens the patient is sensitive. The second task is to construct a "serum" containing ideal proportions of the allergens that induce the production of IgG-blocking antibody and stimulate the generation of antigen-specific suppressor T cells. For reasons that are not clear, the initial concentration of allergens in such a preparation for use in a patient with ocular manifestations of atopy must often be considerably lower than the initial concentrations usually used when caring for a person with extraocular allergy problems. If the typical starting concentrations for nonocular allergies are used, a dramatic exacerbation of ocular inflammation may immediately follow the first injection of the desensitizing preparation.

Plasmapheresis is an adjunctive therapeutic maneuver that can make a substantial difference in the care of patients with atopy, high levels of serum IgE, and documented *Staphylococcus*-binding antibodies (76). This therapeutic technique is expensive, is not curative, and must be performed at highly specialized centers, approximately three times each week, indefinitely. It is also clear, from our experience, that the aggressiveness of the plasmapheresis must be greater than that typically used by many pheresis centers. Three to four plasma exchanges per pheresis session typically are required to achieve therapeutic effect for an atopic person.

Intravenous or intramuscular gamma-globulin injections may also benefit selected atopic patients. It has been recognized that, through mechanisms that are not yet clear,

TABLE 3-12. THERAPY FOR THE ATOPIC PATIENT

Environmental control
Mast cell stabilizers
Systemic antihistamines
Topical steroids (for acute intervention only)
Desensitization monotherapy
Plasmapheresis
Intravenous gamma-globulin
Cyclosporine (systemic and topical)
Psychiatric intervention for patient and family

gamma-globulin therapy involves much more than simple passive "immunization" through adoptive transfer of antibody molecules. In fact, intravenous immunoglobulin therapy has a pronounced immunomodulatory effect, and it is because of this action that such therapy is now recognized and approved as effective therapy for idiopathic thrombocytopenic purpura (79). The use of gamma-globulin therapy is also being explored for other autoimmune diseases, including systemic lupus erythematosus, bullous and cicatricial pemphigoid, and atopic disease.

Cyclosporine and tacrolimus are being tested in patients with certain atopic diseases. Preliminary evidence suggests that topical cyclosporine can have some beneficial effect on patients with atopic keratoconjunctivitis and vernal keratoconjunctivitis (80). Furthermore, in selected desperate cases of blinding atopic keratoconjunctivitis, we have demonstrated that systemic cyclosporine can be a pivotal component of the multimodality approach to the care of this complex problem (76).

Finally, appropriate psychiatric care may be (and usually is) indicated in patients with severe atopy (and family members). It is not hyperbole to state that, in most cases, patients with severe atopic disease and the family members with whom they live demonstrate substantial psychopathology and destructive patterns of interpersonal behavior. The degree to which these families exhibit self-destructive, passive-aggressive, and sabotaging behaviors is often astonishing. Productive engagement in psychiatric care is often difficult to achieve, but it can be extremely rewarding when accomplished successfully. Table 3-12 summarizes the components of a multifactorial approach to the care of atopic patients.

Type II Hypersensitivity Reactions

Type II reactions require the participation of complement-fixing antibodies (IgG1, IgG3 or IgM) and complement. The antibodies are directed against antigens on tissue (i.e., endogenous antigens). The damage caused by type II hypersensitivity reactions, therefore, is localized to the particular target cell or tissue. The mediators of the tissue damage in type II reactions include complement as well as recruited macrophages and other leukocytes that liberate their enzymes. The mechanism of tissue damage involves antibody

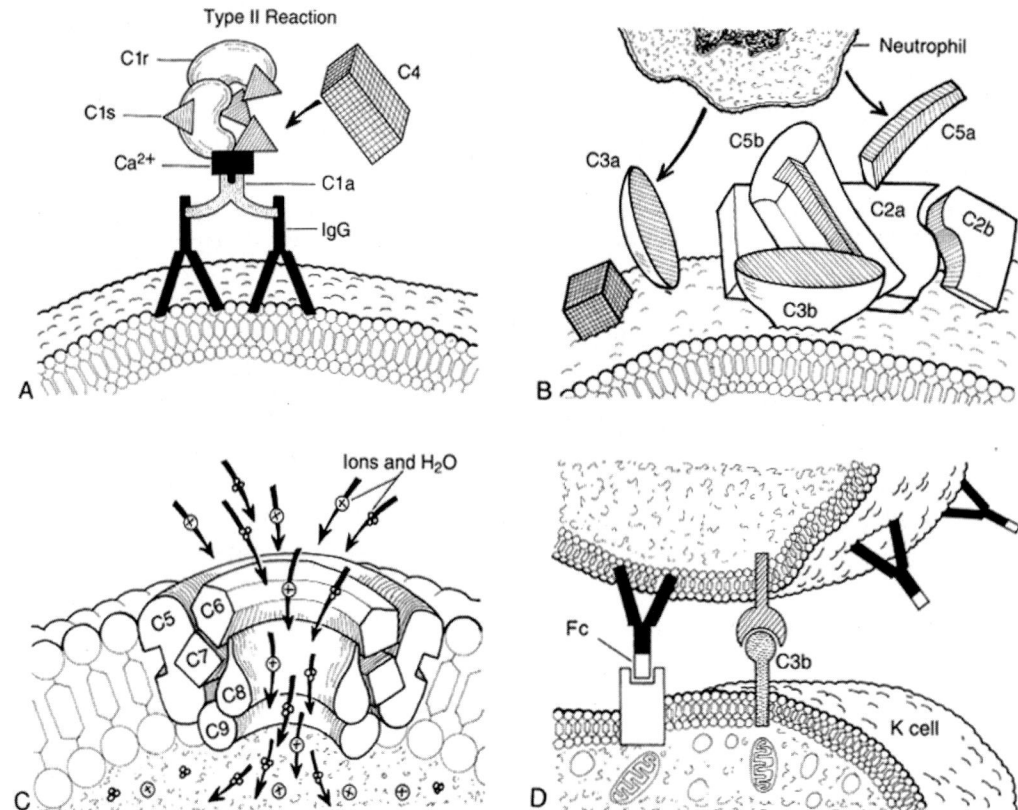

FIG. 3-16. Type II hypersensitivity. **A:** A "sensitized" cell with two antibodies specific for antigenic determinants on the cell surface has attached to the target cell. C1q, C1r, and C1s complement components have begun the sequence that will result in the classic cascade of complement factor binding. **B:** The complement cascade has progressed to the point of C5 binding. Note that two anaphylatoxin and chemotactic split products, C3a and C5a, have been generated, and a neutrophil is being attracted to the site by virtue of the generation of these two chemotactic moieties. **C:** The complement cascade is complete, with the result that a pore has been opened in the target cell membrane, and osmotic lysis is the nearly instantaneous result. **D:** A variant type II hypersensitivity reaction is the antibody-dependent cellular cytotoxicity (ADCC) reaction. Target-specific antibody has attached to the target cell membrane, and the Fc receptor on a neutrophil, a macrophage, or a killer (K) cell is attaching to that membrane-affixed antibody. The result is lysis of the target cell. (From Albert DA, Jakobiec FA. *Principles and practice of ophthalmology*, 2nd ed. Philadelphia: WB Saunders, 2000:78.)

binding to the cell membrane with resultant cell membrane lysis or facilitation of phagocytosis, macrophage and neutrophil cell-mediated damage (Fig. 3-16), and NK cell damage to target tissue through antibody-dependent cell-mediated cytotoxicity reactions (Fig. 3-16). It is important to remember (particularly in the case of type II hypersensitivity reactions that do not result in specific target cell lysis through the complement cascade with eventual osmotic lysis) that neutrophils are prominent effectors of target cell damage. Neutrophil adherence, oxygen metabolism, lysosomal enzyme release, and phagocytosis are tremendously "upregulated" by IgG–C3 complexes and by the activated split product of C5a. As mentioned in the description of type I hypersensitivity reactions, mast cells also participate in nonallergic inflammatory reactions, and type II hypersensitivity reactions provide an excellent example of this. The complement split products C3a and C5a both produce

mast cell activation and degranulation, with resultant liberation of preformed vasoactive amines and upregulation of membrane synthesis of leukotriene B_4 (and other cytokines, e.g., TNF-α, with known chemoattractant activity for neutrophils even more potent than IL-8/RANTES), eosinophil chemotactic factor, and other arachidonic acid metabolites. Neutrophils and macrophages attracted to this site of complement-fixing IgG or IgM in a type II hypersensitivity reaction cannot phagocytose entire cells and target tissues; they thus liberate their proteolytic and collagenolytic enzymes and cytokines in "frustrated phagocytosis." It is through this liberation of tissue-digestive enzymes that the target tissue is damaged. Direct target cell damage (as opposed to "innocent bystander" damage caused by liberation of neutrophil and macrophage enzymes) in type II hypersensitivity reactions may be mediated by NK cells through the antibody-dependent cytotoxicity reaction. In fact, definitive diagnosis of type II reactions requires the demonstration of fixed antitissue antibodies at the disease site, as well as demonstration of *in vitro* NK cell activity against the tissue. No ocular disease has been definitively proved to represent a type II reaction, but several candidates, including ocular cicatricial pemphigoid, exist.

Goodpasture's syndrome is the classic human autoimmune type II hypersensitivity disease. Many believe ocular cicatricial pemphigoid is analogous (in mechanism at least) to Goodpasture's syndrome, in which complement-fixing antibody directed against a glycoprotein of the glomerular basement membrane fixes to the glomerular basement membrane. This action causes subsequent damage to the membrane by proteolytic and collagenolytic enzymes liberated by phagocytic cells, including macrophages and neutrophils.

Therapy for Type II Reactions

Therapy for type II reactions is extremely difficult, and immunosuppressive chemotherapy has, in general, been the mainstay of treatment. Experience with ocular cicatricial pemphigoid has been especially gratifying in this regard (81–83). Progressive cicatricial pemphigoid affecting the conjunctiva was, eventually, almost universally blinding before the advent of systemic immunosuppressive chemotherapy for this condition. With such therapy available now, however, 90% of cases of the disease are arrested and vision is preserved (84).

Type III Hypersensitivity Reactions

Type III reactions, or immune complex diseases, require, like type II hypersensitivity reactions, participation of complement-fixing antibodies (IgG1, IgG3, or IgM). The antigens participating in such reactions may be soluble and diffusible antigens, microbes, drugs, or autologous antigens. Microbes that cause such diseases are usually those that cause persistent infection in which both the infected organ and the kidneys are affected by the immune complex–stimulated inflammation. Autoimmune–immune complex diseases are the best known of these hypersensitivity reactions—the classic collagen vascular diseases and Stevens-Johnson syndrome. Kidney, skin, joints, arteries, and eyes are frequently affected in these disorders. Mediators of tissue damage include antigen–antibody–complement complexes and the proteolytic and collagenolytic enzymes from phagocytes such as macrophages and neutrophils. As with type II reactions, the C3a and C5a split products of complement exert potent chemotactic activity for the phagocytes and also activate mast cells, which through degranulation of their vasoactive amines and TNF-α increase vascular permeability and enhance emigration of such phagocytic cells. It is again through frustrated phagocytosis that the neutrophils and macrophages liberate their tissue-damaging enzymes (Fig. 3-17).

Arthus reaction, a special form of type III hypersensitivity, is mentioned for completeness. Antigen injected into the skin of an animal or individual previously sensitized with the same antigen, and with circulating antibodies against that antigen, results in an edematous, hemorrhagic, and eventually necrotic lesion of the skin. A passive Arthus reaction can also be created if intravenous injection of antibody into a normal host recipient is followed by intradermal injection of the antigen. An accumulation of neutrophils develops in the capillaries and venule walls after deposition of antigen, antibody, and complement in the vessel walls.

Immune complexes form in all of us as a normal consequence of our "immunologic housekeeping." Usually, however, these immune complexes are continually removed from circulation. In humans, the preeminent immune complex–scavenging system is the red blood cells, which have a receptor (CR1) for the C3b and C4b components of complement. This receptor binds immune complexes that contain complement, and the membrane-bound complexes are removed by fixed tissue macrophages and Kupffer cells as the red blood cells pass through the liver. Other components of the reticuloendothelial system, including the spleen and the lung, also remove circulating immune complexes. Small immune complexes may escape binding and removal; not surprisingly, smaller immune complexes are principally responsible for immune complex–mediated hypersensitivity reactions. It is also true that IgA complexes (as opposed to IgG or IgM complexes) do not bind well to red blood cells. They are found in the lung, brain, and kidney rather than in the reticuloendothelial system.

The factors that govern whether immune complexes are deposited into tissue (and if so, where) are complex and

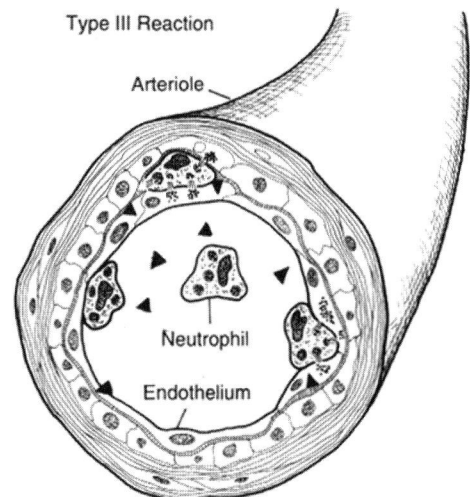

FIG. 3-17. Type III hypersensitivity reaction. Circulating immune complexes (shown here as triangle-shaped moieties in the vascular lumen) percolate between vascular endothelial cells but become trapped at the vascular endothelial basement membrane. Neutrophils and other phagocytic cells are attracted to this site of immune complex deposition. These phagocytic cells liberate their proteolytic and collagenolytic enzymes and damage not only the vessel but the surrounding tissue. (From Albert DA, Jakobiec FA. *Principles and practice of ophthalmology*, 2nd ed. Philadelphia: WB Saunders, 2000:79.)

incompletely understood. It is clear that the size of the immune complex plays a role in tissue deposition. It is also clear that increased vascular permeability at a site of immune system activity or inflammation is a major governor of whether immune complexes are deposited in that tissue. In addition, it is clear that immune complex deposition is more likely to occur at sites of vascular trauma; this includes trauma associated with the normal hemodynamics of a particular site, such as the relatively high pressure inside capillaries and kidneys, the turbulence associated with bifurcations of vessels, and, obviously, sites of artificial trauma as well. Excellent examples of the latter include the areas of trauma in the fingers, toes, and elbows of patients with rheumatoid arthritis, in which subsequent vasculitic lesions and rheumatoid nodules form, and the surgically traumatized eyes of patients with rheumatoid arthritis or Wegener's granulomatosis, wherein immune complexes are deposited subsequently and necrotizing scleritis develops (85). It is likely that addressins or other attachment factors in local tissue play a role in the "homing" of a particular immune complex. Antibody class and immune complex size are also important determinants of immune complex localization at a particular site, as is the type of basement membrane itself.

Therapy for Type III Reactions

Therapy for type III reactions consists predominantly of large doses of corticosteroids, of immunosuppressive chemotherapeutic agents, or both. Cytotoxic immunosuppressive chemotherapy may or may not be necessary to save both the sight and the life of a patient with Behçet's disease, but it is categorically required to save the life of a patient with either polyarteritis nodosa (86) or Wegener's granulomatosis (87). In the case of rheumatoid arthritis–associated vasculitis affecting the eye, it is likely that systemic immunosuppression will also be required if death from a lethal extraarticular, extraocular, vasculitic event is to be prevented (88).

Injury Mediated by Cells

Type IV Hypersensitivity Reactions: Immune-Mediated Injury Due to Effector T Cells

The original classification of immunopathogenic mechanisms arose in an era when considerably more was known about antibody molecules and serology than about T cells and cellular immunity. T-cell–mediated mechanisms were relegated to the "type IV" category, and all types of responses were grouped together (89) (Fig. 3-18). We now know that T cells capable of causing immune injury exist in at least three functionally distinct phenotypes: cytotoxic T cells (typically CD8$^+$) and two populations of helper T cells (typically CD4$^+$). Because cytotoxic T lymphocytes were discovered well after the original Gell and Coombs classification, they were never anticipated in that classification

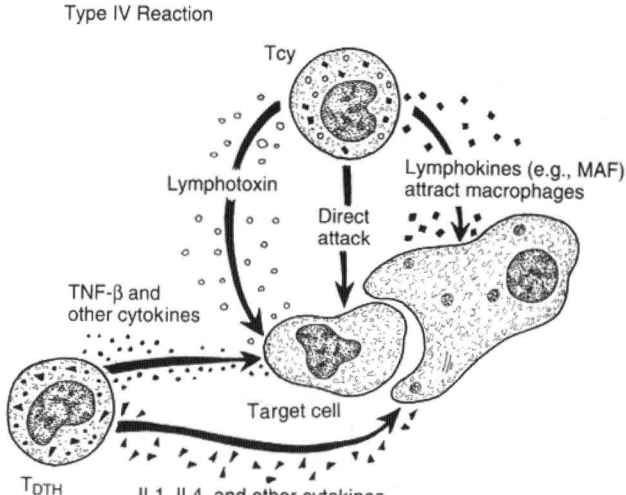

FIG. 3-18. Type IV hypersensitivity reaction. Delayed-type hypersensitivity [DTH(CD4)] T lymphocytes and cytotoxic (CD8 and CD4) T lymphocytes directly attack the target cell or the organism that is the target of the type IV hypersensitivity reaction. Surrogate effector cells are also recruited through the liberation of cytokines. The most notable surrogate or additional effector cell is the macrophage, or tissue histiocyte. If the reaction becomes chronic, certain cytokines or signals from mononuclear cells result in the typical transformation of some histiocytes into epithelioid cells, and the fusion of multiple epithelioid cells produces the classic multinucleated giant cell. (From Albert DA, Jakobiec FA. *Principles and practice of ophthalmology*, 2nd ed. Philadelphia: WB Saunders, 2000:80.)

system. As mentioned previously, CD4$^+$ T cells can adopt one of two polar positions with regard to their lymphokine secretions (72). T$_H$1 cells secrete IL-2, IFN-γ, and lymphotoxin, whereas T$_H$2 cells are the initiators of delayed hypersensitivity reaction. The latter cells, in addition to providing helper factors that promote IgE production, mediate tissue inflammation, albeit of a somewhat different type than that with T$_H$1 cells.

Immunopathogenic T Cells

Cytotoxic T lymphocytes exhibit exquisite antigen specificity in their recognition of target cells; the extent of injury that cytotoxic T cells effect is usually limited to target cells that bear the relevant instigating antigens. Therefore, if a cytotoxic T cell causes tissue injury, it is because host cells express an antigen encoded by an invading pathogen [e.g., herpes simplex virus (HSV)], an antigen for which the TCR on the cytotoxic T cell is highly specific. Delivery of a cytolytic signal eliminates host cells, and in so doing aborts the intracellular infection. Assuming that the infected host cell is not indispensible (e.g., epidermal keratinocytes), there may be few or no physiologic consequences of this cytotoxic T cell–mediated loss of host cells. However, if the infected cell is strategic, is limited in number, or cannot be replaced by regeneration (e.g., neurons, corneal endothelial cells), then the immunopathogenic consequences may be severe.

CD4$^+$ effector cells also exhibit exquisite specificity in recognition of target antigens. However, the extent of injury that these cells can effect is diffuse and is not limited to cells that bear the target antigen. CD4$^+$ effector cells secrete cytokines that possess no antigen specificity in their own right. Instead, these molecules indiscriminately recruit and activate macrophages, NK cells, eosinophils, and other mobile cells that form the nonspecific host defense network. It is this defense mechanism that leads to eradication and elimination of the offending pathogen. In other words, CD4$^+$ effector cells protect by identifying the pathogen antigenically, but they cause elimination of the pathogen by enlisting the aid of other cells. The ability of CD4$^+$ effector cells to orchestrate this multicellular response rests with the capacity of these cells to secrete proinflammatory cytokines to arm inflammatory cells with the ability to "kill." Once armed, these "mindless assassins" mediate inflammation in a nonspecific manner that leads often, if not inevitably, to innocent bystander injury to surrounding tissues. For an organ like the eye that can scarcely tolerate inflammation of even the lowest amount, innocent bystander injury is a formidable threat to vision.

Autoimmune T Cells

The foregoing discussion addresses immunopathogenic injury due to T cells that develop among host tissues invaded by pathogenic organisms. But T cells can sometimes make a mistake and mount an immune attack on host tissue simply because those tissue cells express self molecules (i.e., autoantigens). Although an enormous amount of experimental and clinical literature is devoted to autoimmunity and autoimmune diseases, very little is known in a factual sense that enables us to understand this curious phenomenon. What seems clear is that T cells with receptors that recognize "self" antigens, as well as B cells bearing surface antibody receptors that recognize self antigens, exist under normal conditions (89). Moreover, there are examples of T and B cells with self-recognizing receptors that become activated in putatively normal individuals. Thus, immunologists have learned to distinguish an autoimmune response (not necessarily pathologic) from an autoimmune disease. Whereas all autoimmune diseases arise in a setting in which an autoimmune response has been initiated, we understand little about what causes the latter to evolve into the former. Whatever the pathogenesis, autoimmune disease results when effector T cells (or antibodies) recognize autoantigens in a fashion that triggers a destructive immune response (90,91).

The eye comprises unique cells bearing unique molecules. Moreover, the internal compartments of the eye exist behind a blood–tissue barrier. The very uniqueness of ocular molecules and their presumed sequestration from the systemic immune system have provoked immunologists to speculate that ocular autoimmunity arises when, through trauma or infection, eye-specific antigens are "revealed" to

TABLE 3-13. TYPES OF DELAYED HYPERSENSITIVITY REACTIONS

Reaction Type	Example	Peak Reaction
Tuberculin contact	Tuberculin skin test	48–72 h
Contact	Drug contact hypersensitivity	48–72 h
Granulomatous	Leprosy	14 days
Jones-Mote	Cutaneous basophil hypersensitivity	24 h

the immune system. Sympathetic ophthalmia is a disease that fits this scenario almost perfectly. Trauma to one eye, with attendant disruption of the blood–ocular barrier and spillage of ocular tissues and molecules, leads to a systemic immune response that is specific to the eye. However, even in sympathetic ophthalmia, not every case of ocular trauma leads to this outcome; in fact, only in a few cases does this type of injury produce inflammation in the undamaged eye. Suspicion is high that polymorphic genetic factors may be responsible for determining who will, and who will not, acquire sympathetic ophthalmia after ocular injury. However, environmental factors may also participate.

Range of Hypersensitivity Reactions Mediated by T Cells

Because a wealth of new information about T-cell-mediated immunopathology has accrued within the past decade, our ideas about the range of hypersensitivity reactions that can be mediated by T cells have expanded. But, as yet, any attempt to classify these reactions must necessarily be incomplete. In the past, four types of delayed hypersensitivity reactions were described: (a) tuberculin, (b) contact hypersensitivity, (c) granulomatous, and (d) Jones-Mote (Table 3-13). Delayed hypersensitivity reactions of these types were believed to be caused by IFN-γ–producing CD4$^+$ T cells and to participate in numerous ocular inflammatory disorders, ranging from allergic keratoconjunctivitis, through Wegener's granulomatosis, to drug contact hypersensitivity. Based on recent knowledge concerning other types of effector T cells, this list must be expanded to include cytotoxic T cells and proinflammatory, but not IFN-γ–secreting, T$_H$2-type cells, such as the cells that are believed to cause corneal clouding in river blindness (92).

Herpes Simplex Keratitis as an Example of T-Cell-Mediated Ocular Inflammatory Disease

Infections of the eye with HSV are significant causes of morbidity and vision loss in developed countries. Although direct viral toxicity is damaging to the eye, the bulk of ocular damage from HSV infection appears to be immunopathogenic in origin. That is, the immune response to antigens expressed during a herpes infection leads to tissue injury, even though the virus itself is directly responsible for little of the pathologic process (93).

Numerous experimental models have been developed in an effort to understand the pathogenesis of herpes simplex keratitis (HSK). Perhaps the most informative studies have been conducted in laboratory mice. Evidence from these models indicates that T cells are central to the pathosis observed in HSK (84). At least four different pathogenic mechanisms have been discovered, each of which alone can generate stromal keratitis. Genetic factors of the host play a crucial role in dictating which mechanism will predominate. First, HSV-specific cytotoxic T cells can cause HSK and do so in several strains of mice. Second, HSV-specific T cells of the T_H1 type, which secrete IFN-γ and mediate delayed hypersensitivity, also cause HSK, but in other, genetically different strains of mice. Third, HSV-specific T cells of the T_H2 type, which secrete IL-4 and IL-10, correlate with HSK in yet another strain of mice. Fourth, in association with HSK, T cells have been found that recognize a corneal antigen that is "unmasked" during a corneal infection with HSV, and these T cells then mount an autoimmune response in which the cornea becomes the target of the attack.

Only time will tell whether similar immunopathogenic mechanisms will prove to be responsible for HSK in humans, but the likelihood is very great that this will be the case. Furthermore, it is instructive to emphasize that quite different pathologic T cells can be involved in ocular disease, which implies that it will be necessary to devise different therapies to meet the challenge of preventing immunopathogenic injury from proceeding to blindness.

Summary

Faced with a patient who is experiencing extraocular or intraocular inflammation, the thoughtful ophthalmologist will try, to the best of his or her ability, to diagnose the specific cause of the inflammation, or at the very least to investigate the problem so that the mechanisms responsible for the inflammation are understood as completely as possible. Armed with this knowledge, the ophthalmologist is then prepared to formulate an appropriate therapeutic plan rather than indiscriminately to prescribe corticosteroids. It is clear as we move into the 21st century that the past four decades of relative neglect of ocular immunology by mainstream ophthalmic practitioners are coming to an end. Most ophthalmologists are no longer satisfied to cultivate practices devoted exclusively to the "tissue carpentry" of cataract and keratorefractive surgery, or even to a broadbased ophthalmic practice that includes "medical ophthalmology" but is restricted to problems related exclusively to the eye (e.g., glaucoma) yet divorced from the eye as an organ in which systemic disease is often manifested. More ophthalmologists than ever before are demanding the

continuing education they need to satisfy intellectual curiosity and to prepare for modern care of the total patient when a patient presents with an ocular manifestation of a systemic disease. It is to these physicians that this chapter is directed. The eye can be affected by any of the immune hypersensitivity reactions; acquiring an understanding of the mechanism of a particular patient's inflammatory problem lays the ground work for correct treatment. In the course of the average ophthalmologist's working life, the diagnostic pursuit of mechanistic understanding will also result in a substantial number of instances when the ophthalmologist has been responsible for diagnosing a disease that, if left undiagnosed, would have been fatal.

REGULATION OF IMMUNE RESPONSES

Immunization with an antigen leads, under normal circumstances, to a robust immune response, in which effector T cells and antibodies are produced with specificity for the initiating antigen. Viewed teleologically, the purpose of these effectors is to recognize and combine with antigen (e.g., on an invading pathogen) in such a manner that the antigen and pathogen are eliminated. Once the antigen has been eliminated, there is little need for the persistence of high levels of effector cells and antibodies; what is regularly observed is that levels of these effectors in blood and peripheral tissues fall dramatically. Only the T cells and B cells that embody antigen-specific memory (anamnesis) are retained.

The ability of the immune system to respond to an antigenic challenge in a sufficient and yet measured manner such as this is a dramatic expression of the ability of the system to regulate itself. Examples abound of unregulated immune responses leading to tissue injury and disease; therefore, an understanding of the basis of immune regulation is an important goal.

Regulation by Antigen

Antigen itself is a critical factor in the regulation of an immune response (94). When nonreplicating antigens have been studied, it has been found that the high concentration of antigen required for initial sensitization begins to fall through time. In part, this occurs because antibodies produced by immunization interact with the antigen and cause its elimination. As the antigen concentration falls, the efficiency with which specific T and B cells are stimulated to proliferate and differentiate also falls; eventually, when antigen concentration slips below a critical threshold, further activation of specific lymphocytes stops. Thus, antigen proves to be a central player in determining the vigor and duration of the immune response. As a corollary, immune effectors (specific T cells and antibodies) also play a key role in terminating the immune response, in part by removing antigen from the system. The use of anti-Rh antibodies (RhoGAM) to prevent sensitization of Rh-negative women bearing Rh-positive fetuses is a clear, clinical example of the ability of antibodies to terminate (and in this particular case, even prevent) a specific (unwanted) immune response.

Regulation by T$_H$1 and T$_H$2 Cells

There are other, more subtle and more powerful, regulatory mechanisms that operate to control immune responses. More than 20 years ago, experimentalists discovered that certain antigen-specific T lymphocytes are capable of suppressing immune responses (95), and the mechanism of suppression was found to be unrelated to the simple act of clearing antigen from the system. Although immunologists first suspected that a functionally distinct population of T lymphocytes (analogous to helper and killer cells) was responsible for immune suppression, it is now clear that there is a broad range of T cells that, depending on the circumstances, can function as suppressor cells. Moreover, the mechanisms by which these different T cells suppress are also diverse.

The concept has previously been introduced that helper T cells exist, cells that are responsible for enabling other T and B cells to differentiate into effector cells and antibody-producing cells, respectively. And it is now evident that the effectors of immunity include functionally diverse T cells (delayed hypersensitivity, cytotoxic) and antibodies (IgM, IgG1, IgG2, IgG3, IgG4, IgA, IgE). Any particular immunizing event does not necessarily lead to the production of the entire array of effector modalities; one of the reasons for this is that helper T cells tend to polarize into one or the other of two distinct phenotypes (72). T$_H$1 cells provide a type of help that leads to the generation of T-cell effectors that mediate T-cell–dependent inflammatory responses (e.g., delayed hypersensitivity), as well as B cells that secrete complement-fixing antibodies. The ability of T$_H$1 cells to promote these types of immune response rests with their capacity to secrete a certain set of cytokines—IFN-γ, TNF-β, and large amounts of TNF-α and IL-2. It is these cytokines acting on other T cells, B cells, and macrophages that shape proinflammatory responses. By contrast, T$_H$2 cells provide a type of help that leads to the generation of B cells that secrete non–complement-fixing IgG antibodies, as well as IgA and IgE. Once again, the ability of T$_H$2 cells to promote these types of antibody response rests with their capacity to secrete a different set of cytokines—IL-4, IL-5, IL-6, and IL-10. These cytokines act on other antigen-specific B and T cells to promote the observed responses.

As it turns out, T$_H$1 and T$_H$2 cells can cross-regulate each other. Thus, T$_H$1 cells with specificity for a particular antigen secrete IFN-γ, and in the presence of this cytokine, T$_H$2 cells with specificity for the same antigen fail to become activated. Moreover, they are unable to provide the

type of help for which they are uniquely suited. Similarly, if T$_H$2 cells respond to a particular antigen by secreting their unique set of cytokines (especially IL-4 and IL-10), T$_H$1 cells in the same microenvironment are prevented from responding to the same antigen. Thus, precocious activation of T$_H$1 cells to an antigen, such as ragweed pollen, may prevent the activation of ragweed-specific T$_H$2 cells and thereby prevent the production of ragweed-specific IgE antibodies. Alternatively, precocious activation of T$_H$2 cells to an antigen (e.g., urushiol, the agent responsible for poison ivy dermatitis) may prevent the activation of urushiol-specific T$_H$1 cells and thus eliminate the threat of dermatitis when the skin is exposed to the leaf of the poison ivy plant.

The discovery of T$_H$1 and T$_H$2 cell diversity has led to a profound rethinking of immune regulation. It is still too early to know, on the one hand, whether the extent to which sensitization leads to polarization in the direction of T$_H$1- or T$_H$2-type responses is responsible for human inflammatory diseases and, on the other hand, whether the extent to which the ability to influence an immune response toward the T$_H$1 or T$_H$2 phenotype will have therapeutic value in humans.

Regulation by Suppressor T Cells

Suppressor T cells are defined operationally as cells that suppress an antigen-specific immune response. Cells of this functional property were described before the discovery of T$_H$1 and T$_H$2 cells. It is now apparent that at least some of the phenomena previously attributed to suppressor T cells initially are explained by the cross-regulating abilities of T$_H$1 and T$_H$2 cells. However, it is also abundantly clear that there remain forms and examples of suppression of immune responses that depend on T cells that are neither T$_H$1 nor T$_H$2 cells.

Various experimental maneuvers have been described that lead to the generation of suppressor T cells. The list includes, but is not limited to (a) injection of soluble heterologous protein antigen intravenously; (b) application of hapten to skin previously exposed to ultraviolet B radiation; (c) ingestion of antigen by mouth; (d) injection of allogeneic hematopoietic cells into neonatal mice; (e) injection of antigen-pulsed APCs that have been treated *in vitro* with TGF-β (or aqueous humor, cerebrospinal fluid, or amniotic fluid); and (f) engraftment of a solid tissue (e.g., heart, kidney) under cover of immunosuppressive agents (96,97). In each of these examples, T cells harvested from spleen or lymph nodes of experimentally manipulated animals induce antigen-specific unresponsiveness when injected into immunologically naive recipient animals. Cell transfers such as this have helped to define different types of suppressor cell activity. Because the immune response is functionally divided into its afferent phase (induction) and efferent phase (expression), it is no surprise that certain suppressor T cells suppress the afferent process by which antigen is first detected by specific lymphocytes, and other suppressor T cells inhibit the expression of immunity. Moreover, different suppressor cells inhibit the activation of CD4$^+$ helper or CD8$^+$ cytotoxic T cells, whereas other suppressor cells interfere with B-cell function. There are even suppressor cells that inhibit the activation and effector functions of macrophages and other APCs.

The mechanisms by which suppressor T cells function remain ill defined. Certain suppressor T cells secrete immunosuppressive cytokines, such as TGF-β, whereas other suppressor cells inhibit only when they make direct cell surface contact with target cells. The notion that suppressor cells act by secreting suppressive factors (other than known cytokines) has been challenged and is a controversial topic in immunology. There is convincing evidence that suppressor T cells play a key role in regulating the normal immune response. The decay in immune response that is typically observed after antigen has been successfully neutralized by specific immune effectors correlates with the emergence of antigen-specific suppressor T cells, and these cells have been found to be capable of secreting TGF-β.

Tolerance as an Expression of Immune Regulation

Immunologic tolerance is defined as the state in which immunization with a specific antigen fails to lead to a detectable immune response. In a sense, tolerance represents the ultimate expression of the effectiveness of immune regulation because active mechanisms are responsible for producing the tolerant state. In another sense, tolerance is the obverse of immunity; the fact that an antigen can induce either immunity or tolerance, depending on the conditions at the time of antigen exposure, indicates the vulnerability of the immune system to manipulation.

Originally described experimentally in the 1950s (98,99), but accurately predicted by Ehrlich and other immunologists at the end of the 19th century, immunologic tolerance has been the subject of considerable experimental study during the past 50 years. It has been learned that several distinct mechanisms contribute singly, or in unison, to creation of the state of tolerance. These mechanisms include clonal deletion, clonal anergy, suppression, and immune deviation.

Mechanisms Involved in Tolerance

The term *clonal* refers to a group of lymphocytes that all have identical receptors for a particular antigen. During regular immunization, a clone of antigen-specific lymphocytes responds by proliferating and undergoing differentiation. *Clonal deletion* refers to an aberration of this process, in which a clone of antigen-specific lymphocytes responds to antigen exposure by undergoing apoptosis (programmed cell death) (100). Deletion of a clone of cells in this manner

eliminates the ability of the immune system to respond to the antigen in question (i.e., the immune system is tolerant of that antigen). Subsequent exposures to the same antigen fail to produce the expected immune response (sensitized T cells and antibodies) because the relevant antigen-specific T and B cells are missing.

Clonal anergy resembles clonal deletion in that a particular clone of antigen-specific lymphocytes fails to respond to antigen exposure by proliferating and undergoing differentiation (101). However, in clonal anergy, the lymphocytes within the clone are not triggered to undergo apoptosis by exposure to antigen. What has been learned experimentally is that lymphocytes exposed to their specific antigen under specialized experimental conditions enter an altered state in which their ability to respond is suspended, but the cells are protected from programmed cell death. Even though these cells survive this encounter with antigen, subsequent encounters still fail to cause their expected activation; that is, the immune system is tolerant of that antigen, and the tolerant cell is said to be anergic.

Antigen-specific *immune suppression*, as described earlier, is another mechanism that has been shown to cause immunologic tolerance. As in clonal deletion and anergy, immune suppression creates a situation in which subsequent encounters with the antigen in question fail to lead to signs of sensitization. However, in suppression, the failure to respond is actively maintained. Thus, suppressor cells actively inhibit antigen-specific lymphocytes from responding, even though the antigen-specific cells are present at the time antigen is introduced into the system.

Immune deviation is a special form of immune suppression (102). Originally described in the 1960s, immune deviation refers to the situation wherein administration of a particular antigen in a particular manner fails to elicit the expected response. In the first such experiments, soluble heterologous protein antigens injected intravenously into naive experimental animals failed to induce delayed hypersensitivity responses. Moreover, subsequent immunization with the same antigens plus adjuvant injected subcutaneously also failed to induce delayed hypersensitivity. With respect to delayed hypersensitivity, one could say that the animals were tolerant. However, the sera of these animals contained unexpectedly large amounts of antibody to the same antigen, indicating the so-called tolerance was not global. Thus, in immune deviation, a preemptive exposure to antigen in a nonimmunizing mode prejudices the quality of subsequent immune responses to the same antigen. In other words, the immune response is deviated from the expected pattern, hence the term *immune deviation*.

Factors That Promote Tolerance Rather Than Immunity

Experimentalists have defined various factors that influence or promote the development of immunologic tolerances.

The earliest description of tolerance occurred when antigenic material was injected into newborn (and therefore developmentally immature) mice. This indicates that exposure of the developing immune system to antigens before the system has reached maturity leads to antigen-specific unresponsiveness. In large part, maturation of the thymus gland during ontogeny correlates positively with development of resistance to tolerance induction. Much evidence reveals that the mechanism responsible for tolerance in this situation is clonal deletion of immature, antigen-specific thymocytes. In large measure, because cells in the thymus gland are normally expressing self-antigens, the thymocytes that are deleted represent those cells with TCRs of high affinity for self-antigens. This mechanism undoubtedly contributes to the success with which the normal immune system is able to respond to all biologically relevant molecules, except those expressed on self-tissues, and therefore avoids autoimmunity.

However, tolerance can also be induced when the immune system is developmentally mature. The factors that are known to promote tolerance under these conditions include (a) the physical form of the antigen, (b) the dose of antigen, and (c) the route of antigen administration. More specifically, soluble antigens are more readily able to induce tolerance than particulate or insoluble antigens. Very large doses of antigens, as well as extremely small quantities of antigens, are also likely to induce tolerance. This indicates that the immune system is disposed normally to respond to antigens within a relatively broad, but nonetheless defined, range of concentrations or amounts. Antigen administered in quantities above or below the range can induce tolerance. Injection of antigen intravenously also favors tolerance induction, whereas injection of antigen intracutaneously favors conventional sensitization. In a similar, but not identical, manner, oral ingestion of antigen produces a kind of immune deviation in which, on the one hand, delayed hypersensitivity to the antigen is impaired (i.e., tolerance), but on the other hand, IgA antibody production to the antigen is exaggerated. [See the following discussion of ocular surface immunity (103).] In addition, antigens injected with adjuvants induce conventional immune responses, whereas antigens administered in the absence of adjuvants may either promote tolerance or elicit no response whatever.

Additional factors influencing whether tolerance is induced concern the status of the immune system itself. For example, antigen X may readily induce tolerance when injected intravenously into a normal, immunologically naive individual. However, if the same antigen is injected into an individual previously immunized to antigen X, then tolerance will not occur. Thus, a prior state of sensitization militates against tolerance induction. Alternatively, if a mature immune system has been assaulted by immunosuppressive drugs, by debilitating systemic diseases, or by particular types of pathogens (the human immunodeficiency virus is

a good example), it may display increased susceptibility to tolerance. Thus, when an antigen is introduced into an individual with a compromised immune response, tolerance may develop and be maintained, even if the immune system recovers.

Regional Immunity and the Eye

All tissues of the body require immune protection from invading or endogenous pathogens. Because pathogens with different virulence strategies threaten different types of tissues, the immune system consists of a diversity of immune effectors. The diversity includes at least two different populations of effector T cells (that mediate delayed hypersensitivity and kill target cells) and seven different types of antibody molecules (IgM, IgG1, IgG2, IgG3, IgG4, IgA, and IgE). Thus, evolution has had to meet the challenge of designing an immune system that is capable of responding to a particular pathogen or antigen in a particular tissue with a response that is effective in eliminating the threat, while at the same time not damaging the tissue itself. Different tissues and organs display markedly different susceptibilities to immune-mediated tissue injury (104,105). The eye is an excellent example. Because integrity of the microanatomy of the visual axis is absolutely required for accurate vision, the eye can tolerate inflammation to only a very limited degree. Vigorous immunogenic inflammation, such as that found in a typical delayed hypersensitivity reaction in the skin, wreaks havoc with vision, and it has been argued that the threat of blindness has dictated an evolutionary adaptation in the eye that limits the expression of inflammation.

The conventional type of immunity that is generated when antigens or pathogens enter through the skin is almost never seen in the normal eye. Therefore, almost by definition, any immune responses that take place in or on the eye are regulated. On the ocular surface, immunity resembles that observed on other mucosal surfaces, such as the gastrointestinal tract, the upper respiratory tract, and the urinary tract. Within the eye, an unusual form of immunity is observed; a description of this follows in the section on Intraocular Immunology: Ocular Immune Privilege.

Ocular Surface Immunity: Conjunctiva, Lacrimal Gland, Tear Film, Cornea, and Sclera

The normal human conjunctiva is an active participant in immune defense of the ocular surface against invasion of exogenous substances. The presence of blood vessels and lymphatic channels fosters transit of immune cells that can participate in the afferent and efferent arms of the immune response. The marginal and peripheral palpebral arteries and anterior ciliary arteries are the main blood suppliers of the conjunctiva. The superficial and deep lymphatic plexuses of the bulbar conjunctiva drain toward the palpebral commissures, where they join the lymphatics of the lids. Lymphatics of the palpebral conjunctiva on the medial side drain into the submandibular lymph nodes. Lymphatics draining the palpebral conjunctiva on the lateral side drain into the submandibular lymph nodes. Major immune cells found in the normal human conjunctiva are dendritic cells, T and B lymphocytes, mast cells, and neutrophils. Dendritic cells, Langerhans and non-Langerhans, have been detected in different regions of the conjunctiva (106). Dendritic cells act as APCs to T lymphocytes and may stimulate antigen-specific class II region–mediated T-lymphocyte proliferation (107). T lymphocytes, the predominant lymphocyte subpopulation in conjunctiva, are represented in the epithelium and in the substantia propria. T lymphocytes are the main effector cells in immune reactions such as delayed hypersensitivity or cytotoxic responses. B lymphocytes are absent except for rare scattered cells in the substantia propria of the fornices. Plasma cells are detected only in the conjunctival accessory lacrimal glands of Krause or in minor lacrimal glands (108). T and B lymphocytes and plasma cells are also present between the acini of the major lacrimal gland. Plasma cells from major and minor lacrimal glands synthesize immunoglobulins, mainly IgA (109,110). IgA is a dimer that is transported across the mucosal epithelium bound to a receptor complex. IgA dimers are released to the luminal surface of the ducts associated with a secretory component after cleavage of the receptor and are excreted with the tear film. Secretory IgA is a protectant of mucosal surface receptors that might otherwise be available for viral and bacterial fixation (111), and it may modulate the normal flora of the ocular surface (112). Foreign substances can be processed locally by the mucosal immune defense system. Somehow, after exposure to antigen, specific IgA helper T lymphocytes stimulate IgA B lymphocytes to differentiate into IgA-secreting plasma cells. Dispersed T and B lymphocytes and IgA-secreting plasma cells of the conjunctiva and lacrimal gland are referred to as the conjunctival and lacrimal gland–associated lymphoid tissue (CALT) (113). CALT is considered part of a widespread mucosa-associated lymphoid tissue (MALT) system, including the oral mucosa and salivary gland–associated lymphoid tissue, the gut-associated lymphoid tissue (GALT) (114), and the bronchus-associated lymphoid tissue (BALT) (115), CALT drains to the regional lymph nodes in an afferent arc; effector cells may return to the eye through an efferent arc.

The adaptive and the innate immune responses form part of an integrated system. Immunoglobulins and lymphokines produced by the lymphoid tissue of the conjunctiva help neutrophils and macrophages to destroy antigens. Macrophages in turn help the lymphocytes by transporting the antigens from the eye to the lymph nodes. Some immunoglobulins (e.g., IgE) bind to mast cells; others (IgG, IgM) bind complement. Mast cells and complement facilitate the arrival of neutrophils and macrophages.

Mast cells are located mainly perilimbally, although they can also be found in bulbar conjunctiva. Their degranulation in response to an allergen or an injury results in the release of vasoactive substances such as histamine, heparin, platelet-activating factor, and leukotrienes, which can cause blood vessel dilation and increased vascular permeability (116).

The tears contain several substances known to have antimicrobial properties. Lysozyme, immunoglobulins, and lactoferrin may be synthesized by the lacrimal gland. Lysozyme is an enzyme capable of lysing bacteria cell walls of certain gram-positive organisms (117). Lysozyme may also facilitate secretory IgA bacteriolysis in the presence of complement (118). The tear IgG has been shown to neutralize virus, lyse bacteria, and form immune complexes that bind complement and enhance bacterial opsonization and chemotaxis of phagocytes (119). The tear components of the complement system enhance the effects of binding lysozyme and immunoglobulins (120). Lactoferrin, an iron-binding protein, has both bacteriostatic and bactericidal properties (121,122). Lactoferrin may also regulate the production of granulocyte–macrophage colony-stimulating factor (123), may inhibit the formation of the complement system component C3 convertase (124), and may interact with specific antibody to produce an antibacterial effect more powerful than that of either lactoferrin or antibody alone (125).

Autoimmune disorders that involve the conjunctiva include cicatricial pemphigoid, pemphigus vulgaris, erythema multiforme, and collagen vascular diseases. Autoimmune disorders that involve the lacrimal gland include Sjögren's syndrome. The mechanisms by which immunopathologic damage occurs in these diseases vary, depending on whether they are organ specific. When the antigen is localized in a particular organ, type II hypersensitivity reactions appear to be the main mechanisms (e.g., cicatricial pemphigoid and pemphigus vulgaris). In non–organ-specific diseases, type III and type IV hypersensitivity reactions are more important (e.g., erythema multiforme, collagen vascular diseases).

The unique anatomic and physiologic characteristics of the human cornea explain, on the one hand, its predilection for involvement in various immune disorders and, on the other hand, its ability to express immune privilege. The peripheral cornea differs from the central cornea in several ways. The former is closer to the conjunctiva, in which blood vessels and lymphatic channels provide a mechanism for the afferent arc of corneal immune reactions. Blood vessels derived from the anterior conjunctival and deep episcleral arteries extend 0.5 mm into the clear cornea (126). Adjacent to these vessels, the subconjunctival lymphatics drain into regional lymph nodes. The presence of this vasculature allows diffusion of some molecules, such as immunoglobulins and complement components, into the cornea. IgG and IgA are found in similar concentrations in the peripheral and central cornea; however, more IgM is found in the periphery, probably because its high molecular weight restricts diffusion into the central area (127). Both classic and alternative pathway components of complement and their inhibitors have been demonstrated in normal human corneas. However, although most of the complement components have a peripheral-to-central cornea ratio of 1.2:1.0, C1 is denser in the periphery by a factor of five. The high molecular weight of C1, the recognition unit of the classic pathway, may also restrict its diffusion into the central area (128,129). Normal human corneal epithelium contains small number of Langerhans cells, which are distributed almost exclusively at the limbus; very few cells are detected in the central cornea (130). The peripheral cornea also contains a reservoir of inflammatory cells, including neutrophils, eosinophils, lymphocytes, plasma cells, and mast cells (126). The presence of antibodies, complement components, Langerhans cells, and inflammatory cells makes the peripheral cornea more susceptible than the central cornea to involvement in a wide variety of autoimmune and hypersensitivity disorders, such as Mooren's ulcer and collagen vascular diseases. A discussion of corneal antigens and immune privilege follows (131).

The sclera consists almost entirely of collagen and proteoglycans. It is traversed by the anterior and posterior ciliary vessels but retains a scanty vascular supply for its own use. Its nutrition is derived from the overlying episclera and underlying choroid (132); similarly, both classic and alternative pathway components of complement are derived from these sources (133). Normal human sclera has few, if any, lymphocytes, macrophages, Langerhans cells, or neutrophils (134). In response to an inflammatory stimulus in the sclera, the cells pass readily from blood vessels of the episclera and choroid. Because of the collagenous nature of the sclera, many systemic autoimmune disorders, such as the collagen vascular diseases, may affect it (134).

Intraocular Immunology: Ocular Immune Privilege

For more than 100 years, it has been known that foreign tissue grafts placed in the anterior chamber of an animal's eye can be accepted indefinitely (135). The designation of this phenomenon as immune privilege had to await the seminal work of Medawar and colleagues, who discovered the principles of transplantation immunology in the 1940s and 1950s. These investigators studied immune-privileged sites—the anterior chamber of the eye, the brain—as a method of exploring the possible ways to thwart immune rejection of solid tissue allografts (136–139). It had been learned that transplantation antigens on grafts were carried to the immune system by regional lymphatic vessels and that immunization leading to graft rejection took place in draining lymph nodes. Because the eye and brain were regarded at the time as having no lymphatic drainage, and because both tissues resided behind a blood–tissue barrier, Medawar and associates postulated

that immune privilege resulted from immunologic ignorance—although this was not a term that was used at the time. What these investigators meant was that foreign tissues placed in immune-privileged sites were isolated by physical vascular barriers from the immune system and that they never alerted the immune system to their existence. During the past 25 years, immunologists who have studied immune privilege at various sites in the body have learned that this original postulate is basically untrue (140–147). First, some privileged sites possess robust lymphatic drainage pathways; the testis is a good example. Second, antigens placed in privileged sites are known to escape and to be detected at distant sites, including lymphoid organs such as lymph nodes and the spleen. Third, antigens in privileged sites evoke antigen-specific, systemic immune responses, albeit of a unique nature. Thus, the modern view of immune privilege states that privilege is an actively acquired, dynamic state in which the immune system conspires with the privileged tissue or site in generating a response that is protective, rather than destructive. In a sense, immune privilege represents the most extreme form of the concept of regional immunity.

Immune-Privileged Tissues and Sites

Immune privilege has two different manifestations: privileged sites and privileged tissues (Table 3-14). Immune-privileged sites are regions of the body in which grafts of foreign tissue survive for an extended, even indefinite time, compared with nonprivileged or conventional sites. Immune-privileged tissues, compared with nonprivileged tissues, are able to avoid, or at least resist, immune rejection when grafted into conventional body sites. The eye contains examples of both privileged tissues and privileged sites, of which the best studied site is the anterior chamber, and the best studied tissue is the cornea.

Much has been learned about the phenomenon of immune privilege during the past two decades. The forces that confer immune privilege have been shown to act during both induction and expression of the immune response on antigens placed in, or expressed on, privileged sites and tissues. The forces that shape immune-privileged sites and tissues include an ever-expanding list of microanatomic,

TABLE 3-14. SITES OF IMMUNE PRIVILEGE

Site	Tissues
Eye	
Cornea, anterior chamber	Cornea
Vitreous cavity, subretinal space	Lens
Brain	Cartilage
Pregnant uterus	Placenta/fetus
Testis	Testis
Ovary	Ovary
Adrenal cortex	Liver
Hair follicles	
Tumors	Tumors

TABLE 3-15. FEATURES OF IMMUNE-PRIVILEGED SITES

Passive
  Blood–tissue barriers
  Deficient efferent lymphatics
  Tissue fluid that drains into blood vasculature
  Reduced expression of major histocompatibility complex
    class I and II molecules

Active
  Constitutive expression of inhibitory cell surface molecules:
    Fas ligand, decay-accelerating factor, CD59, CD46
  Immunosuppressive microenvironment: transforming
    growth factor-β, α-melanocyte–stimulating hormone,
    vasoactive intestinal peptide, calcitonin gene–related
    peptide, macrophage migration inhibitory factor, free cortisol

biochemical, and immunoregulatory features. A short list of privilege-promoting features is displayed in Table 3-15. The eye expresses virtually every one of these features. Although passive features such as blood–ocular barrier, lack of lymphatics, and low expression of MHC class I and II molecules are important, experimental attention has focused on immunomodulatory molecules expressed on ocular tissues and present in ocular fluids.

Regulation of Immune Expression in the Eye

As mentioned previously, activated T cells that express Fas on their surfaces are vulnerable to programmed cell death if they encounter other cells that express Fas ligand (148). Constitutive expression of Fas ligand on cells that surround the anterior chamber has been shown to induce apoptosis among T cells and other leukocytes exposed to this ocular surface (149). More important, Fas ligand expressed by cells of the cornea plays a key role in rendering the cornea resistant to immune attack and rejection (150,151). Similarly, constitutive expression on corneal endothelial cells, as well as iris ciliary body epithelium, of several membrane-bound inhibitors of complement activation is strategically located to prevent complement-dependent intraocular inflammation and injury (152).

The realization that the intraocular microenvironment is immunosuppressive arises chiefly from studies of aqueous humor and secretions of cultured iris and ciliary body. TGF-β_2, a normal constituent of aqueous humor (153–155), is a powerful immunosuppressant that inhibits various aspects of T-cell and macrophage activation. However, it is by no means the only (or perhaps even the most) important inhibitor present. Although the list is still incomplete, other relevant factors in aqueous humor include α-melanocyte–stimulating hormone (156), vasoactive intestinal peptide (157), calcitonin gene–related peptide (158), and macrophage migration inhibitory factor (159). These factors account in part for the immunosuppressive properties of aqueous humor: inhibition of T-cell activation

(proliferation) and differentiation (secretion of lymphokines such as IFN-γ) after ligation of the TCR for antigen; suppression of macrophage activation (phagocytosis, generation of nitric oxide) (160); and inhibition of NK cell lysis of target cells (161). Aqueous humor does not inhibit all immune reactivity, however. For example, antibody neutralization of virus infection of target cells in not prevented in the presence of aqueous humor (160). Moreover, cytotoxic T cells that are fully differentiated are fully able to lyse antigen-bearing target cells cultured in aqueous humor. The ability of the immune system to express itself in the eye is highly regulated by the factors just described; suppression of immune expression that leads to inflammation and damage is one important dimension of ocular immune privilege.

Regulation of Induction of Immunity to Eye-Derived Antigens

Another dimension to immune privilege is the ability of the eye to regulate the nature of the systemic immune response to antigens placed within it. It has been known for more than 20 years that injection of alloantigenic cells into the anterior chamber of rodent eyes evokes a distinctive type of immune deviation, now called *anterior chamber–associated immune deviation* (ACAID) (162–164). In ACAID, eye-derived antigens elicit an immune response that is selectively deficient in T cells that mediate delayed hypersensitivity and B cells that secrete complement-fixing antibodies. There is not, however, a global lack of response; animals with ACAID display a high level of antigen-specific serum antibodies of the non–complement-fixing varieties (165,166). In ACAID, regulatory T cells are also generated that, in an antigen-specific manner, suppress both induction and expression of delayed hypersensitivity to the antigen in question (167–172). ACAID can be elicited by diverse types of antigens, ranging from soluble protein to histocompatibility to virus-encoded antigens. A deviant systemic response similar to ACAID can even be evoked by antigen injected into the anterior chamber of the eye of an individual previously immunized to the same antigen.

Induction of ACAID by intraocular injection of antigen begins in the eye itself (172–177). After injection of antigen into the eye, local APCs capture the antigen, migrate across the trabecular meshwork into the canal of Schlemm, and then traffic through the blood to the spleen. In the splenic white pulp, the antigen is presented in a unique manner to T and B lymphocytes, resulting in the spectrum of functionally distinct antigen-specific T cells and antibodies found in ACAID. The ocular microenvironment sets the stage for this sequence of events by virtue of the immunoregulatory properties of aqueous humor. This ocular fluid or, more precisely, TGF-β, confers on conventional APCs the capacity to induce ACAID. Thus, the ocular microenvironment regulates not only the expression of immunity within the eye, but the functions of eye-derived APCs, and thus promotes a systemic immune response that is deficient in those immune effector modalities most capable of inducing immunogenic inflammation: delayed hypersensitivity T cells and complement-fixing antibodies.

Relationship Between Immune Privilege and Intraocular Inflammatory Diseases

The rationale of immune privilege is that all tissues, including the eye, require immune protection. Immune privilege represents the consequence of interactions between the immune system and the eye in which local protection is provided by immune effectors that do not disrupt the eye's primary vision. Because maintenance of a precise microanatomy is essential for vision, privilege allows for immune protection that is virtually devoid of immunogenic inflammation.

At the experimental level, ocular immune privilege has been implicated in (a) the extraordinary success of corneal allografts (178–181), (b) progressive growth of intraocular tumors (182), (c) resistance to herpes stromal keratitis (183), and (c) suppression of autoimmune uveoretinitis (184–186). When immune privilege prevails in the eye, corneal allografts succeed, trauma to the eye heals without incident, and ocular infections are cleared without inflammation. However, ocular tumors may grow relentlessly, and uveal tract infections may persist and recur.

The consequences of failed immune privilege have been explored experimentally and considered clinically. When privilege fails in the eye, blindness is a likely outcome. As examples, ocular trauma may result in sympathetic ophthalmia, ocular infections may produce sight-threatening inflammation, and corneal allografts may fail.

Corneal Transplantation Immunology

The cornea is an immune-privileged tissue and, in part, this attribute accounts for the extraordinary success of orthoptic corneal allografts in experimental animals and in humans. It is pertinent that the corneal graft forms the anterior surface of a site that is also typically immune privileged (the anterior chamber). Despite the advances that have been made in corneal tissue preservation and surgical techniques, a significant proportion of grafts eventually fail (187–190). The main cause of transplant failure now is immune-mediated graft rejection, which occurs in 16% to 30% of recipients in a large series after several years of follow-up. Certain recipients are at increased risk of graft rejection (191–193). Corneal vascularization, either preoperative from recipient herpetic, interstitial, or traumatic keratitis, or stimulated by silk or loose sutures, contact lenses, infections, persistent epithelial defects, and other disorders associated with inflammation, has been widely recognized as a clear risk factor for decreased graft survival.

It is estimated that the failure rate is 25% to 50% in vascularized corneas and 5% to 10% in avascular ones. Other factors that increase the risk of allograft rejection include a history of previous graft loss (194–196), eccentric and large grafts, and glaucoma. The reasons why corneal bed neovascularization is a dominant risk factor for cornea graft rejection remain to be elucidated. Evidence indicates that neovascularized corneas also contain neolymphatic vessels (197). Moreover, the graft bed is heavily infiltrated with APCs, especially Langerhans cells. These factors are probably important for increasing the immunogenic potential of the allogeneic corneal graft.

Transplantation Antigen Expression on Corneal Tissue

In outbred species, such as humans, transplants of solid tissue grafts usually fail unless the recipient is immunosuppressed; the reason for failure is the development of an immune response directed at so-called transplantation antigens displayed on cells of the graft. Immunologists have separated transplantation antigens into two categories, major and minor, primarily because major antigens induce more vigorous alloimmunity than do minor antigens (198). The genes that encode the major transplantation antigens in humans are located in the MHC, called HLA. Minor histocompatibility antigens are encoded at numerous loci spread throughout the genome. The HLA complex, which is a large genetic region, is situated on the short arm of the sixth human chromosome. HLA genes that encode class I and class II antigens are extremely polymorphic. Similarly, minor histocompatibility loci contain highly polymorphic genes. In the aggregate, polymorphisms at the major and minor histocompatibility loci account for the observation that solid tissue grafts exchanged between any two individuals selected at random within a species are acutely rejected.

The expression of HLA antigens on corneal cells is somewhat atypical (199–203). Class I MHC antigens are expressed strongly on the epithelial cells of the cornea, comparable in intensity with the expression of epidermal cells of the skin. Keratinocytes express less class I than conventional fibroblasts, and corneal endothelial cells express small amounts of class I antigen under normal circumstances. Except at the periphery near the limbus, the cornea contains no adventitial cells (i.e., cells of bone marrow origin) that express MHC class II molecules (204,205). In most solid tissues, class II HLA antigens are expressed primarily on these types of cells (206). Therefore, under normal conditions, the burden of class II MHC antigens on corneal grafts is minimal. Corneal epithelial cells and keratocytes resemble other cells of the body in responding to IFN-γ by upregulation of class I antigen expression. Among IFN-γ–treated epithelial cells, class II antigens are also expressed. However, corneal endothelial cells resist expression of class II antigens even in response to IFN-γ.

Because class II antigens, especially those expressed on bone marrow–derived cells, are extremely important in providing solid tissue grafts with their ability to evoke transplantation immunity, the deficit of these antigens on corneal cells offers a significant barrier to sensitization.

A major accomplishment of modern immunology is the ability of contemporary clinical pathology laboratories to tissue-type for HLA class I and class II antigens. With most solid tissue allografts, tissue typing that identifies HLA matching between a graft donor and a recipient correlates with improved graft survival (207). Thus, HLA-matched kidney grafts survive with fewer rejection episodes and with a reduced need for immunosuppressive therapy, compared with HLA-mismatched grafts. The evidence that HLA tissue typing similarly improves the fate of matched corneal allografts is conflicting (208–215). There seems to be no controversy regarding the influence of tissue typing on grafts placed in eyes of patients with low risk. In this situation, virtually no studies suggest a positive typing effect. The rate of graft success is so high in low-risk situations with unmatched grafts that there is little opportunity for a matching effect to be seen. However, in high-risk situations, the literature contains reports that claim (a) HLA matching, especially for class I antigens, has a powerful positive effect on graft outcome; (b) HLA matching has no effect on graft outcome; or (c) HLA matching may have a deleterious effect on graft outcome.

The reasons for confusion about the effects of HLA matching on corneal allograft success may relate to studies on orthoptic corneal allografts conducted in mice. It has been reported that minor transplantation antigens offer a significant barrier to graft success in rodents (216–218). In fact, corneal allografts that display minor, but not major, transplantation antigens are rejected more vigorously and with a higher frequency than grafts that display MHC, but not minor, transplantation antigens. Two factors seem to be important in this outcome. First, the reduced expression of MHC antigens on corneal grafts renders these grafts less immunogenic than other solid tissue grafts. Second, corneal antigens are detected by the recipient immune system largely when the recipient's own APCs infiltrate the graft and capture donor antigens. Therefore, the recipient mounts an immune response directed primarily at minor transplantation antigens. Because tissue typing is unable at present to match organs and donors for minor histocompatibility antigens, it is no surprise that current tissue typing has proved to be ineffectual at improving corneal allograft success.

Corneal Allograft Acceptance: When Immune Privilege Succeeds

The normal cornea is an immune-privileged tissue, and several features are known to contribute to this privileged status. First, as mentioned earlier, expression of MHC class I and II molecules is reduced and impaired, especially on the corneal endothelium. The net antigenic load of corneal tissue is thus reduced compared with other tissues, which has a mitigating effect on both induction and expression of alloimmunity. Second, the cornea lacks blood and lymph vessels. The absence of these vascular structures isolates the corneal graft in a manner that prevents antigenic information from escaping from the tissue while at the same time prevents immune effectors from gaining access to the tissue. Third, the cornea is deficient in MHC class II–positive, bone marrow–derived cells, especially Langerhans cells. Mobile cells of this type are one way in which antigenic information from a solid tissue graft alerts the immune system in regional lymph nodes to its presence. The absence of activated APCs from the cornea dramatically lengthens the time it takes for the recipient immune system to become aware of the graft's existence. An important recent discovery is the presence of significant numbers of bone marrow–derived dendritic cells and macrophages in the corneal stroma (219,220). Importantly, these cells are normally MHC class II negative, but a variety of stimuli, including the simple act of surgery associated with penetrating keratoplasty, induce the expression of MHC class II molecules. This induced expression account for the eventual development of donor MHC class II–specific T-cell immunity when grafts are placed in low-risk eyes. Fourth, cells of the cornea constitutively secrete molecules with immunosuppressive properties (221–225). Cells of all three corneal layers secrete TGF-β as well as yet-to-be-defined inhibitory molecules. In addition, corneal epithelial cells and keratinocytes constitutively produce an excess of IL-1 receptor antagonist, compared with the endogenous production of IL-1γ (223). These immunosuppressive molecules have powerful modulatory effects on APCs, T cells, B cells, NK cells, and macrophages and can act during induction and expression of alloimmunity to prevent or inhibit graft rejection. Fifth, cells of the cornea constitutively express surface molecules that inhibit immune effectors. Corneal endothelial cells display on their surfaces decay-accelerating factor (DAF), CD59, and CD46—molecules that inhibit complement effector functions (224). These inhibitors protect corneal endothelial cells from injury by complement molecules generated during an alloimmune response. Corneal cells have been found to express CD95L (Fas ligand), and expression of this molecule on mouse cornea grafts has been formally implicated in protecting the grafts from attack by Fas-positive T cells and other leukocytes (150,151,225). Finally, the corneal graft forms the anterior surface of the anterior chamber; antigens released from the graft endothelium escape into aqueous humor. Experimental evidence indicates that allogeneic corneal grafts induce donor-specific ACAID in recipients (216,226), and the inability of these recipients to acquire donor-specific delayed hypersensitivity plays a key role in maintaining the integrity of accepted grafts.

When placed in low-risk (normal) eyes of mice, a high proportion of corneal allografts with the features listed earlier experience prolonged, even indefinite, survival in the complete absence of any immunosuppressive therapy. This dramatic expression of immune privilege is mirrored by the success of keratoplasties performed in low-risk situations in humans. However, neither in mice nor in humans are all such grafts successful. This observation indicates that immune privilege is by no means absolute and irrevocable.

Pathogenesis of Corneal Allograft Rejection: When Immune Privilege Fails

The high rate of failure of corneal allografts in high-risk situations in humans resembles the high rate of failure of orthoptic corneal allografts placed in high-risk mouse eyes (227). Studies of the rejection process in experimental animals have begun to unravel the pathogenic mechanisms responsible. Sensitization develops in recipient animals with surprising rapidity when grafts are placed in high-risk eyes. Within 8 days of engraftment, immune donor-specific T cells can be detected in lymphoid tissues. Similar grafts placed in low-risk mouse eyes do not achieve T-cell sensitization until at least 3 weeks after engraftment. The reason for rapid sensitization when grafts are place in high-risk eyes appears to be the rapid conversion of resident MHC class II–negative dendritic cells in the donor cornea to the MHC class II–positive state, compounded by the migration of recipient MHC class II–bearing Langerhans cells from the limbus into the graft and its bed. Whereas detection of class II MHC–bearing Langerhans cells in allografts placed in low-risk eyes is detectable between 1 and 2 weeks after grafting, similar MHC class II–bearing cells can be detected in grafts in high-risk eyes within a few days of engraftment. It is very likely that the vulnerability to rejection of grafts is dictated by the efficiency with which resident APCs in the graft acquire MHC class II expression, and by the rate at which recipient APCs enter the graft, capture antigens, and migrate to the regional lymph nodes where recipient T cells are initially activated. Support for this view is provided by the observation that Langerhans cell detection in graft epithelium can be inhibited by topical application of IL-1 receptor antagonist (228). Experiments indicate that grafts that have been treated with IL-1 receptor antagonist take longer to induce donor-specific sensitization, and the majority of such grafts avoid immune rejections.

When normal corneal grafts are placed in high-risk eyes, they are typically rejected. In this case, the inherent immune-privileged status of the graft is clearly insufficient to overcome the fact that the graft site (a neovascularized eye) can no longer act as an immune-privileged site. It is also possible to show that grafts that have lost their immune-privileged status are vulnerable to rejection, even when placed in normal, low-risk eyes (which display immune privilege). Langerhans cells can be induced to migrate into the central corneal epithelium by several different experimental maneuvers. When grafts containing Langerhans cells are placed in low-risk eyes, rapid recipient sensitization occurs, and the grafts are rejected. The tempo and vigor of rejection of these grafts strongly resemble the fate of normal grafts placed in high-risk eyes. These results indicate that both the privileged tissue (the corneal graft) and the privileged site (the low-risk eye) make important contributions to the success of orthoptic corneal allografts.

Summary and Conclusion

The eye is defended against pathogens, just as is every other part of the body. Components of both the natural and the acquired immune systems respond to pathogens in the eye, but the responses are different from those following antigen encounter in most other places in the body, perhaps as a result of evolutionary pressures that have led to the survival of those species and members of species in which a blinding, exuberant inflammatory response was prevented by "regulation" of the response. In any event, we are left for the moment with an organ (the eye) in which special immunologic responsiveness allows us to enjoy a degree of "privileged" tolerance to transplanted tissue not experienced by other organs. It is clear now that this tolerance is an active process, not simply a passive one derived from the invisibility of the transplant to the recipient's immune system.

REFERENCES

1. Kohler J, Milstein C. Continuous cultures of fused cells secreting antibody of predefined specificity. *Nature* 1975;256:495.
2. Reinherz EL, Schlossman SF. The differentiation and function of human T lymphocytes. *Cell* 1980;19:821.
3. Hardy RR, Hayakawa K, Parks DR, et al Murine B cell differentiation lineages. *J Exp Med* 1984;1959:1969.
4. Hardy RR, Hayakawa K, Schimizu M, et al. Rheumatoid factor secretion from human Leu-1 B cells. *Science* 1987;236:81.
5. Mosmann TR, Coffman R. Two types of mouse helper T cell clones: implications from immune regulation. *Immunol Today* 1987;8:233.
6. Coffman R, O'Hara J, Bond MW, et al. B cell stimulatory factor-1 enhances the IgE response of lipopolysaccharide-activated B cells. *J Immunol* 1986;136:4538.
7. Mariotti S, del Prete GF, Mastromauro C, et al. The autoimmune infiltrates of Basedow's disease: analysis of clonal level and comparison with Hashimoto's thyroiditis. *Exp Clin Endocrinol* 1991;97:139.
8. Maggi E, Biswas P, del Prete GF, et al. Accumulation of TH2-like helper T cells in the conjunctiva of patients with vernal conjunctivitis. *J Immunol* 1991;146:1169.
9. Romagnani S. Human TH1 and TH2 subsets: doubt no more. *Immunol Today* 1991;12:256.
10. Murphy DB, Mamauchi K, Habu S, et al. T cells in a suppressor circuit and non-T:non-B cells bear different I-J determinants. *Immunogenetics* 1981;13:205.
11. Gillette TE, Chandler JW, Greiner JV. Langerhans cells of the ocular surface. *Ophthalmology* 1982;89:700.
12. Tagawa Y, Takeuchi T, Saga T, et al. Langerhans cells: role in ocular surface immunopathology. In: O'Connor GR, Chandler

JW, eds. *Advances in immunology and immunopathology of the eye.* New York: Masson, 1985:203–207.

13. Le Douarin NM. Ontogeny of hematopoietic organ studies in avian embryo interspecific chimeras. In: Clarkson D, Marks PA, Till JE, eds. *Cold Spring Harbor meeting on differentiation of normal and neoplastic hematopoietic cells.* Cold Spring Harbor, NY, Cold Spring Harbor Laboratory, 1978:5–32.

14. Metcalf D, Moore MAS. Hematopoietic cells. *Front Biol* 1971; 24:550.

15. Hermans MJA, Hartsuiker H, Opstelten D. An in situ study of B lymphocytopoiesis in rat bone marrow: topographical arrangement of terminal deoxynucleotidyl transferase positive cells and pre-B cells. *J Immunol* 1989;44:67.

16. Szengerg A, Warner ML. Association of immunologic responsiveness in fowls with a hormonally arrested development of lymphoid material. *Nature* 1962;194:146.

17. Cooper MD, Peterson RD, South MA, et al. The functions of the thymus system and the bursa system in the chicken. *J Exp Med* 1966;123:75.

18. Papiernik M. Lymphoid organs. In: Bach JF, ed. *Immunology,* 2nd ed. New York: John Wiley & Sons, 1982:15–37.

19. Butcher EC, Weissman IL. Lymphoid tissues and organs. In: Paul W, ed. *Fundamental immunology,* 2nd ed. New York: Raven Press, 1989:117–137.

20. Berg EL, Goldstein LA, Jutila MA, et al. Homing receptors and vascular addressins: cell adhesion molecules that direct lymphocyte traffic. *Immunol Rev* 1989;108:5.

21. Picker LJ, de los Toyos J, Tellen MJ, et al. Monoclonal antibodies against the CD 44 and Pgp-1 antigens in man recognize the Hermes class of lymphocyte homing receptors. *J Immunol* 1989; 142:2046.

22. Holzmann T, McIntyre BW, Weissman IC. Identification of a murine Peyer's patch-specific lymphocyte homing receptor as an integrin molecule with an alpha chain homologous to human VLA-4 alpha. *Cell* 1989;56:37.

23. Streeter PR, Rause ET, Butcher EC. Immunohistologic and functional characterization of a vascular addressin involved in lymphocyte homing into peripheral lymph nodes. *J Cell Biol* 1988;107:1853.

24. Dreyer WJ, Bennett JC. The molecular basis of antibody formation: a paradox. *Proc Natl Acad Sci U S A* 1965;54:864.

25. Hozumi N, Tonegawa S. Evidence for somatic rearrangement of immunoglobulin genes coding for variable and constant regions. *Proc Natl Acad Sci U S A* 1976;73:3628.

26. Wu TT, Kabat EA. An analysis of the sequences of the variable regions of Bence Jones proteins and myeloma light chains and their implications for antibody complementarity. *J Exp Med* 1970; 132:211.

27. Leder P. The genetics of antibody diversity. *Sci Am* 1982; 246:102.

28. Tonegawa S. Somatic generation of antibody diversity. *Nature* 1983;302:575.

29. Honjo T, Habu S. Origin of immune diversity: genetic variation and selection. *Annu Rev Biochem* 1985;54:803.

30. Alt FW, Baltimore D. Joining of immunoglobulin heavy chain gene segments: implications from a chromosome with evidence of three D-JH fusions. *Proc Natl Acad Sci U S A* 1982;79:4118.

31. Early P, Huang H, Davis M, et al. An immunoglobulin heavy chain variable region gene is generated from three segments of DNA: VH, D and JH. *Cell* 1980;12:981.

32. Sakano H, Huppi K, Heinrich G, et al. Sequences at the somatic recombination sites of immunoglobulin light chain genes. *Nature* 1979;280:288.

33. Weigert MG, Cesari IM, Yondovich SJ, et al. Variability in the lambda light chain sequences of mouse antibody. *Nature* 1970; 228:1045.

34. Brack C, Hirama M, Lenhard-Schuller R, et al. A complete immunoglobulin gene is created by somatic recombination. *Cell* 1978;15:1.

35. Bernard O, Hozumi N, Tonegawa S. Sequences of mouse immunoglobulin light chain genes before and after somatic changes. *Cell* 1978;15:1133.

36. Pernis BG, Chiappino G, Kelus AS, et al. Cellular localization of immunoglobulins with different allotypic specificities in rabbit lymphoid tissues. *J Exp Med* 1965;122:853.

37. Cebra J, Colberg JE, Dray S. Rabbit lymphoid cells differentiated with respect to alpha-, gamma-, and mu-heavy polypeptide chains and to allotypic markers for Aa1 and Aa2. *J Exp Med* 1966;123:547.

38. Kataoka T, Kawakami T, Takahshi N, et al. Rearrangement of immunoglobulin g1-chain gene and mechanism for heavy-chain class switch. *Proc Natl Acad Sci U S A* 1980;77:919.

39. Gritzmacher CA. Molecular aspects of heavy-chain class switching. *Crit Rev Immunol* 1989;9:173.

40. Broduer PH, Riblet T. The immunoglobulin heavy chain variable region (Igh-V) locus in the mouse: I. One hundred Igh-V genes comprise seven families of homologous genes. *Eur J Immunol* 1984;14:922.

41. Winter EA, Radbruch A, Krawinkel U. Members of novel VH gene families are found in VDJ regions of polyclonally activated B lymphocytes. *EMBO J* 1985;4:2861.

42. Kofler R. A new murine Ig VH family. *J Immunol* 1988; 140:4031.

43. Reininger L, Kaushik A, Jaton JC. A member of a new VH gene family encodes anti-bromelinised mouse red blood cell autoantibodies. *Eur J Immunol* 1988;18:1521.

44. Rechavi G, Bienz B, Ram D, et al. Organization and evolution of immunoglobulin VH gene subgroups. *Proc Natl Acad Sci U S A* 1982;79:4405.

45. Rechavi G, Ram D, Glazer R, et al. Evolutionary aspects of immunoglobulin heavy chain variable region (VH) gene subgroups. *Proc Natl Acad Sci U S A* 1983;80:855.

46. Matthysens G, Rabbitts TH. Structure and multiplicity of genes for the human immunoglobulin heavy chain variable region. *Proc Natl Acad Sci U S A* 1980;77:6561.

47. Berman JE, Mellis SJ, Pollock R, et al. Content and organization of the human Ig VH locus: definition of three new VH families and linkage to the Ig CH locus. *EMBO J* 1988;7:727.

48. Potter M, Newell JG, Rudikoff S, Haber E. Classification of mouse VK groups based on the partial amino acid sequence to the first invariant tryptophan: impact of 14 new sequences from IgG myeloma proteins. *Mol Immunol* 1982;12:1619.

49. D'Joostelaere LA, Huppi K, Mock B, et al. The immunoglobulin kappa light chain allelic groups among the Igk haplotypes and Igk crossover populations suggest a gene order. *J Immunol* 1988;141:652.

50. Yanacopoulos GD, Desiderio SV, Pasking M, et al. Preferential utilization of the most JH-proximal VH gene segments in pre-B cell lines. *Nature* 1984;311:727.

51. Perlmutter RM, Kearney JF, Chang SP, et al. Developmentally controlled expression of immunoglobulin VH genes. *Science* 1985;227:1597.

52. Reth M, Jackson N, Alt FW. VHDJH formation and DJH replacement during pre-B differentiation: non-random usage of gene segments. *EMBO J* 1986;5:2131.

53. Lawler AM, Lin PS, Gearhart PJ. Adult B-cell repertoire is biased toward two heavy-chain variable region genes that rearrange frequently in fetal pre-B cells. *Proc Natl Acad Sci U S A* 1987; 84:2454.

54. Yanacopoulos GD, Malynn B, Alt FW. Developmentally regulated and strain-specific expression of murine VH gene families. *J Exp Med* 1988;168:417.

55. Dildrop R, Krawinkel U, Winter E, et al. VH-gene expression in murine lipopolysaccharide blasts distributes over the nine known VH-gene groups and may be random. *Eur J Immunol* 1985;15:1154.

56. Schulze DH, Kelsoe G. Genotypic analysis of B cell colonies by in situ hybridization. Stoichiometric expression of the three VH families in adult C57BL/6 and BALB/c mice. *J Exp Med* 1987;166:163.

57. Krawkinkel U, Cristoph T, Blankenstein T. Organization of the Ig *VH* locus in mice and humans. *Immunol Today* 1989;10:339.

58. Janeway CA Jr, Travers P, eds. *Immunobiology: the immune system in health and disease*, 3rd ed. New York: Current Biology/Garland, 1997.

59. Von Boehmer H. The developmental biology of T lymphocytes. *Annu Rev Immunol* 1993;6:309.

60. Moller C, ed. Positive T cell selection in the thymus. *Immunol Rev* 1993;135:5.

61. Nossal CJV. Negative selection of lymphocytes. *Cell* 1994; 76:229.

62. Havran WL, Boismenu R. Activation and function of γδ T cells. *Curr Opin Immunol* 1994;6:442.

63. Germain RN. MHC-dependent antigen processing and peptide presentation: providing ligands for T lymphocyte activation. *Cell* 1994;76:287.

64. Fremont DH, Rees WA, Kozono H. Biophysical studies of T cell receptors and their ligands. *Curr Opin Immunol* 1996;8:93.

65. Sprent J, Webb SR. Intrathymic and extrathymic clonal deletion of T cells. *Curr Opin Immunol* 1995;7:196.

66. Picker LJ, Butcher EC. Physiological and molecular mechanisms of lymphocyte homing. *Annu Rev Immunol* 1993;10:561.

67. Janeway CA, Bottomly K. Signals and signs for lymphocyte responses. *Cell* 1994;76:275.

68. Jain J, Loh C, Rao A. Transcription regulation of the IL-2 gene. *Curr Opin Immunol* 1995;7:333.

69. Minami Y, Kono T, Miyazaki T, et al. The IL-2 receptor complex: its structure, function and target genes. *Annu Rev Immunol* 1993; 11:245.

70. Griffiths GM. The cell biology of CTL killing. *Curr Opin Immunol* 1995;7:343.

71. Mueller DL, Jenkins MK. Molecular mechanisms underlying functional T cell unresponsiveness. *Curr Opin Immunol* 1995; 7:325.

72. Mosmann TR, Coffman RL. Th1 and Th2 cells: different patterns of lymphokine secretion lead to different functional properties. *Annu Rev Immunol* 1989;7:145.

73. Maggi E, Romagnani S. Role of T cells and T cell-derived cytokines in the pathogenesis of allergic diseases. *Ann NY Acad Sci* 1994; 725:2.

74. von Pirquet C. Allergie. *Munch Med Wochenschr* 1906;53:1457.

75. Cocoa AF, Cooke RA. On the classification of the phenomena of hypersensitiveness. *J Immunol* 1923;8:163.

76. Foster CS, Calonge M. Atopic keratoconjunctivitis. *Ophthalmology* 1990;97:992.

77. Foster CS, Duncan J. Randomized clinical trial of disodium cromoglycate therapy in vernal keratoconjunctivitis. *Am J Ophthalmol* 1980;90:175.

78. Foster CS. Evaluation of topical cromolyn sodium in the treatment of vernal keratoconjunctivitis. *Ophthalmology* 1988;95:194.

79. Bussel JB, Kimberly RP, Inamen RD, et al. Intravenous gamma globulin treatment of chronic idiopathic cytopenic purpura. *Blood* 1983;62:480.

80. Bleik JH, Tabbara KS. Topical cyclosporine in vernal keratoconjunctivitis. *Ophthalmology* 1991;98:1679.

81. Foster CS. Cicatricial pemphigoid. Thesis of the American Ophthalmological Society. *Trans Am Ophthalmol Soc* 1986; 84:527.

82. Foster CS, Wilson LA, Ekins MB. Immunosuppressive therapy for progressive ocular cicatricial pemphigoid. *Ophthalmology* 1982;89:340.

83. Tauber J, Sainz de la Maza M, Foster CS. Systemic chemotherapy for ocular cicatricial pemphigoid. *Cornea* 1991;10:185.

84. Neumann R, Tauber J, Foster CS. Remission and recurrence after withdrawal of therapy for ocular cicatricial pemphigoid. *Ophthalmology* 1991;98:868.

85. Sainz de al Maza M, Foster CS. Necrotizing scleritis after ocular surgery: a clinical pathologic study. *Ophthalmology* 1991; 98:1720.

86. Leib ES, Restivo C, Paulus AT. Immunosuppressive and corticosteroid therapy of polyarteritis nodosa. *Am J Med* 1979; 67:941.

87. Wolf SM, Fauci AS, Horn RG, et al. Wegener's granulomatosis. *Ann Intern Med* 1974;81:513.

88. Foster CS, Forstot SL, Wilson LA. Mortality rate in rheumatoid arthritis patients developing necrotizing scleritis or peripheral ulcerative keratitis. *Ophthalmology* 1984;91:1253.

89. Janeway CA Jr, Travers P, eds. *Immunobiology: the immune system in health and disease*, 3rd ed. New York: Current Biology/Garland, 1997.

90. Steinman L. Escape from "horror autotoxicus": pathogenesis and treatment of autoimmune disease. *Cell* 1995;80:7.

91. Tan EM. Autoantibodies in pathology and cell biology. *Cell* 1991;67:841.

92. Pearlman E, Lass HJ, Bardenstein DS, et al. Interleukin 4 and T helper type 2 cells are required for development of experimental onchocercal keratitis (river blindness). *J Exp Med* 1995; 182:931.

93. Steilein JW, Dana MR, Ksander BR. Immunity causing blindness: five different paths to herpes stromal keratitis. *Immunol Today* 1997;18:443.

94. Janeway CA Jr, Travers P, eds. *Immunobiology: the immune system in health and disease*, 3rd ed. New York: Current Biology/Garland, 1997.

95. Qin S, Cobbold SP, Pope H, et al. Infectious transplantation tolerance. *Science* 1993;259:974.

96. Asherwon GL, Collizi V, Zembala M. An overview of T-suppressor cell circuits. *Annu Rev Immunol* 1986;4:37.

97. Groux H, O'Garra A, Bigler M, et al. A CD4⁺ T-cell subset inhibits antigen-specific T-cell responses and prevents colitis. *Nature* 1997;389:737.

98. Billingham RE, Brent L, Medawar PB. Actively acquired tolerance of foreign cells. *Nature* 1953;172:603.

99. Burnet FM. *The clonal selection theory of acquired immunity.* Cambridge, Cambridge University Press, 1959.

100. Kappler JW, Roehm N, Marrack P. T cell tolerance by clonal elimination in the thymus. *Cell* 1987;49:273.

101. Jenkins MK, Pardoll DM, Mizguchi J, et al. RH: molecular events in the induction of a non-responsive state in interleukin-2 producing helper lymphocyte clones. *Proc Natl Acad Sci USA* 1987;84:5409.

102. Asherson GL, Stone SH. Selective and specific inhibition of 24-hour skin reactions in the guinea-pig: I. Immune deviation: description of the phenomenon and the effect of splenectomy. *Immunology* 1965;9:205.

103. Khoury SJ, Hancock WW, Weiner HL. Oral tolerance to myelin basic protein and natural recovery from experimental autoimmune encephalomyelitis are associated with downregulation of inflammatory cytokines and differential upregulation of transforming growth factor β, interleukin 4 and prostaglandin E expression in the brain. *J Exp Med* 1992;176:1355.

104. Streilein JW. Regional immunology of the eye. In: Pepose JW, Holland GN, Wilhemus KR, eds. *Ocular infection and immunity*. St. Louis: Mosby-Year Book, 1996:19–33.

105. Streilein JW. Regional immunity. In: Dulbecco R, ed. *Encyclopedia of human biology*, 2nd ed, vol 4. San Diego, Academic Press, 1997:767–776.
106. Sacks E, Rutgers J, Jakobiec FA, et al. A comparison of conjunctival and nonocular dendritic cells utilizing new monoclonal antibodies. *Ophthalmology* 1986;93:1089.
107. Murphy GF. Cell membrane glycoproteins and Langerhans cells. *Hum Pathol* 1986;16:103.
108. Sacks E, Wieczorek R, Jakobiec FA, et al. Lymphocytic subpopulations in the normal human conjunctiva. *Ophthalmology* 1986;93:1276.
109. Franklin RM, Remus LE. Conjunctival-associated lymphoid tissue: evidence for a role in the secretory immune system. *Invest Ophthalmol Vis Sci* 1984;25:181.
110. Wieczorek R, Jakobiec FA, Sacks E, et al. The immunoarchitecture of the normal human lacrimal gland. *Ophthalmology* 1988;95:100.
111. Tomasi TB. *The immune system of secretion*. Englewood Cliffs, NJ, Prentice-Hall, 1976.
112. Gibbons RJ. Bacterial adherence to the mucosal surfaces and its inhibition by secretory antibodies. *Adv Exp Med Biol* 1974;45:315.
113. Jackson DE, Lally ET, Nakamura MC, et al. Migration of IgA-bearing lymphocytes into salivary glands. *Cell Immunol* 1981;63:203.
114. Parrot DM. The gut as a lymphoid organ. *Clin Gastroenterol* 1976;5:211.
115. Bienenstock J, Johnston N, Perey DYE. Bronchial lymphoid tissue: I. Morphological characteristics. *Lab Invest* 1973;28:686.
116. Allansmith MR. *The eye and immunology*. St. Louis: CV Mosby, 1982.
117. Allansmith MR. Defense of the ocular surface. *Int Ophthalmol Clin* 1979;12:93.
118. Fleming A. On a remarkable bacteriolytic element found in tissues and secretions. *Proc R Soc Lond (Biol)* 1922;93:306.
119. Strober W, Hague HE, Lum LG, et al. IgA-Fc receptors on mouse lymphoid cells. *J Immunol* 1978;121:2140.
120. Bluestone R. Lacrimal immunoglobulins and complement quantified by counterimmunoelectrophoresis. *Br J Ophthalmol* 1975;59:279.
121. Masson PL, Heremans JF, Prignot JJ, et al. Immunohistochemical localization and bacteriostatic properties of an iron-binding protein from bronchial mucus. *Thorax* 1966;21:358.
122. Arnold RR, Cole MF, McGhee JR. A bacteriocidal effect for human lactoferrin. *Science* 1977;197:263.
123. Badgy GC. Interaction of lactoferrin monocytes and lymphocyte subsets in the regulation of steady-state granulopoiesis in vitro. *J Clin Invest* 1981;68:56.
124. Kjilstra A, Jeurissen SHM. Modulation of classical C_3 convertase of complement by tear lactoferrin. *Immunology* 1982;47:263.
125. Bullen JJ, Rogers HJ, Leigh L. Iron-binding proteins in milk and resistance of *Escherichia coli* infection in infants. *BMJ* 1972;1:69.
126. Hogan MH, Alvarado JA, Weddell JE. The limbus. In: *Histology of the human eye: an atlas and textbook*. Philadelphia: WB Saunders, 1971:112–182.
127. Allansmith MR, McClellan BH. Immunoglobulins in the human cornea. *Am J Ophthalmol* 1975;80:123.
128. Mondino BJ, Ratajczak HV, Goldberg DB, et al. Alternate and classical pathway components of complement in the normal cornea. *Arch Ophthalmol* 1980;98:346.
129. Mondino BJ, Brady KJ. Distribution of hemolytic complement in the normal cornea. *Arch Ophthalmol* 1981;99:1430.
130. Klaresjkog L, Forsum U, Tjernlund VM, et al. Expression of Ia antigen-like molecules on cells in the corneal epithelium. *Invest Ophthalmol Vis Sci* 1979;18:310.
131. Mondino BJ. Inflammatory diseases of the peripheral cornea. *Ophthalmology* 1988;95:463.
132. Watson PG, Hazleman BL. *The sclera and systemic disorders*. Philadelphia: WB Saunders, 1976.
133. Brawman-Mintzer O, Mondino BJ, Mayer FJ. Distribution of complement in the sclera. *Invest Ophthalmol Vis Sci* 1989;30:2240.
134. Fong LP, Sainz de la Maza M, Rice BA, et al. Immunopathology of scleritis. *Ophthalmology* 1991;98:472.
135. van Dooremall JC. Die Entwickelung der in fremden Grund versetzten lebenden Gewebe. *Graefes Arch Clin Exp Ophthalmol* 1873;19:358.
136. Medawar P. Immunity to homologous grafted skin: III. The fate of skin homografts transplanted to the brain, to subcutaneous tissue and to the anterior chamber of the eye. *Br J Exp Pathol* 1948;29:58.
137. Barker CF, Billingham RE. Immunologically privileged sites. *Adv Immunol* 1977;25:1.
138. Streilein JW. Immune privilege as the result of local tissue barriers and immunosuppressive microenvironments. *Curr Opin Immunol* 1993;5:428.
139. Streilein JW. Perspective: unraveling immune privilege. *Science* 1995:270:1158.
140. Streilein JW. Immune regulation and the eye: a dangerous compromise. *FASEB J* 1987;1:199.
141. Niederkorn JY. Immune privilege and immune regulation in the eye. *Adv Immunol* 1990;48:191.
142. Tompsett E, Abi-Hanna D, Wakefield D. Immunological privilege in the eye: a review. *Curr Eye Res* 1990;9:114.
143. Ksander BR, Streilein JW. Regulation of the immune response within privileged sites. In: Granstein R, ed. *Mechanisms of regulation of immunity chemical immunology*. Basel, Karger, 1993:117–145.
144. Streilein JW. Ocular regulation of systemic immunity. *Reg Immunol* 1994;6:143.
145. Streilein JW. Ocular immune privilege and the Faustian dilemma. *Invest Ophthalmol Vis Sci* 1996;37:1940.
146. Streilein JW, Ksander BR, Taylor AW. Commentary: immune privilege, deviation and regulation in the eye. *J Immunol* 1997;158:3557.
147. Streilein JW, Takeuchi M, Taylor AW. Immune privilege, T cell tolerance, and tissue-restricted autoimmunity. *Hum Immunol* 1997;52:138.
148. Nagata S, Golstein P. The Fas death factor. *Science* 1995;267:1449.
149. Griffith TS, Brunner T, Fletcher SM, et al. Fas ligand-induced apoptosis as a mechanism of immune privilege. *Science* 1995;270:1189.
150. Stuart PM, Griffith TS, Usui N, et al. CD95 ligand (FasL)-induced apoptosis is necessary for corneal allograft survival. *J Clin Invest* 1997;99:396.
151. Yamagami S, Kawashima H, Tsuru T, et al. Role of Fas/Fas ligand interactions in the immunorejection of allogeneic mouse corneal transplantation. *Transplantation* 1997;64:1107.
152. Bora NS, Gobleman CL, Atkinson JP, et al. Differential expression of the complement regulatory proteins in the human eye. *Invest Ophthalmol Vis Sci* 1993;34:3579.
153. Granstein R, Stszewski R, Knisely T, et al. Aqueous humor contains transforming growth factor-β and a small (<3500 daltons) inhibitor of thymocytes proliferation. *J Immunol* 1990;144:302.
154. Cousins SW, McCabe MM, Danielpour D, et al. Identification of transforming growth factor-beta as an immunosuppressive factor in aqueous humor. *Invest Ophthalmol Vis Sci* 1991;32:2201.
155. Jampel HD, Roche N, Stark WJ, Roberts AB. Transforming growth factor-β in human aqueous humor. *Curr Eye Res* 1990;9:963.
156. Taylor AW, Streilein JW, Cousins SW. Identification of alpha-melanocyte stimulating hormone as a potential immunosuppressive factor in aqueous humor. *Curr Eye Res* 1992;11:1199.

157. Taylor AW, Streilein JW, Cousins SW. Vasoactive intestinal peptide (VIP) contributes to the immunosuppressive activity of normal aqueous humor. *J Immunol* 1994;153:1080.

158. Wahlstedt C, Beding N, Ekman R. Calcitonin gene-related peptide in the eye: release by sensory nerve stimulation and effects associated with neurogenic inflammation. *Regul Pept* 1986;16:107.

159. Apte RS, Niederkorn JY. MIF: a novel inhibitor of NK cell activity in the anterior chamber (AC) of the eye. *J Allergy Clin Immunol* 1997;99:S467.

160. Kaiser CJ, Ksander BR, Streilein JW. Inhibition of lymphocyte proliferation by aqueous humor. *Reg Immunol* 1989;2:42.

161. Apte RS, Niederkorn JY. Isolation and characterization of a unique natural killer cell inhibitory factor present in the anterior chamber of the eye. *J Immunol* 1996;156:2667.

162. Kaplan HJ, Streilein JW. Immune response to immunization via the anterior chamber of the eye: I. F_1 lymphocyte-induced immune deviation. *J Immunol* 1977;118:809.

163. Kaplan HJ, Streilein JW. Immune response to immunization via the anterior chamber of the eye: II. An analysis of F_1 lymphocyte induced immune deviation. *J Immunol* 1978;120:689.

164. Streilein JW, Niederkorn JY, Shadduck JA. Systemic immune unresponsiveness induced in adult mice by anterior chamber presentation of minor histocompatibility antigens. *J Exp Med* 1980;152:1121.

165. Niederkorn JY, Streilein JW. Analysis of antibody production induced by allogeneic tumor cells inoculated into the anterior chamber of the eye. *Transplantation* 1982;33:573.

166. Wilbanks GA, Streilein JW. Distinctive humoral responses following anterior chamber and intravenous administration of soluble antigen: evidence for active suppression of IgG2a-secreting B-cells. *Immunology* 1990;71:566.

167. Niederkorn JY, Streilein JW. Alloantigens placed into the anterior chamber of the eye induce specific suppression of delayed type hypersensitivity but normal cytotoxic T lymphocyte responses. *J Immunol* 1983;131:2670.

168. Ksander BR, Streilein JW. Analysis of cytotoxic T cell responses to intracameral allogeneic tumors: I. Quantitative and qualitative analysis of cytotoxic precursor and effector cells. *Invest Ophthalmol Vis Sci* 1989;30:323.

169. Waldrep JC, Kaplan HJ. Anterior chamber-associated immune deviation induced by TNP-splenocytes (TNP-ACAID): II. Suppressor T cell networks. *Invest Ophthalmol Vis Sci* 1983;24:1339.

170. Streilein JW, Niederkorn JY. Characterization of the suppressor cell(s) responsible for anterior chamber associated immune deviation (ACAID) induced BALB/c mice by P815 cells. *J Immunol* 1985;134:1381.

171. Ferguson TA, Kaplan HJ. The immune response and the eye: II. The nature of T suppressor cell induction of anterior chamber associated immune deviation (ACAID). *J Immunol* 1987;139:346.

172. Wilbanks GA, Streilein JW. Characterization of suppressor cells in anterior chamber-associated immune deviation (ACAID) induced by soluble antigen: evidence of two functionally and phenotypically distinct T-suppressor cell populations. *Immunology* 1990;71:383.

173. Kosiewicz MM, Okamoto S, Miki S, et al. Imposing deviant immunity on the presensitized state. *J Immunol* 1994;153:2962.

174. Wilbanks GA, Streilein JW. Studies on the induction of anterior chamber associated immune deviation (ACAID): I. Evidence that an antigen-specific, ACAID-inducing, cell-associated signal exists in the peripheral blood. *J Immunol* 1991;146:2610.

175. Wilbanks GA, Mammolenti MM, Streilein JW. Studies on the induction of anterior chamber associated immune deviation (ACAID): II. Eye-derived cells participate in generating blood borne signals that induce ACAID. *J Immunol* 1991;146:3018.

176. Wilbanks GA, Mammolenti MM, Streilein JW. Studies on the induction of anterior chamber associated immune deviation (ACAID): III. Induction of ACAID depends upon intraocular transforming growth factor-β. *Eur J Immunol* 1992;22:165.

177. Hara Y, Okamoto S, Rouse B, et al. Evidence that peritoneal exudate cells cultured with eye-derived fluids are the proximate antigen presenting cells in immune deviation of the ocular type. *J Immunol* 1993;151:5162.

178. Maumanee AE. The influence of donor-recipient sensitization on corneal grafts. *Am J Ophthalmol* 1951;34:142.

179. Sonoda Y, Streilein JW. Orthoptic corneal transplantation in mice: evidence that the immunogenetic rules of rejection do no apply. *Transplantation* 1992;54:694.

180. Streilein JW. Anterior chamber privilege in relation to keratoplasty. In: Zierhut M, ed. *Immunology of corneal transplantation*. Buren, the Netherlands: Aeolus Press, 1994:117–134.

181. Streilein JW. Immune privilege and the cornea. In: Pleye U, Hartmann C, Sterry W, eds. *Proceedings of symposium: Bullous ocular-muco-cutaneous disorders*. Buren, the Netherlands: Aeolus Press, 1997:43–52.

182. Niederkorn J, Streilein JW, Shadduck JA. Deviant immune responses to allogeneic tumors injected intracamerally and subcutaneously in mice. *Invest Ophthalmol Vis Sci* 1980;20:355.

183. McLeish W, Rubsamen P, Atherton SS, et al. Immunobiology of Langerhans cells on the ocular surface: II. Role of central corneal Langerhans cells in stromal keratitis following experimental HSV-I infection in mice. *Reg Immunol* 1989;2:236.

184. Mizuno K, Clark AF, Streilein JW. Induction of anterior chamber associated immune deviation in rats receiving intracameral injections of retinal S antigen. *Curr Eye Res* 1988;7:627.

185. Hara Y, Caspi RR, Wiggert B, et al. Suppression of experimental autoimmune uveitis in mice by induction of anterior chamber associated immune deviation with interphotoreceptor retinoid binding protein. *J Immunol* 1992;148:1685.

186. Gery I, Streilein JW. Autoimmunity in the eye and its regulation. *Curr Opin Immunol* 1994;6:938.

187. Khodadoust AA. The allograft rejection reaction: the leading cause of late failure of clinical corneal grafts. *Ciba Found Symp* 1973;15:151.

188. Stark WJ. Transplantation immunology of penetrating keratoplasty. *Trans Am Ophthalmol Soc* 1980;78:1079.

189. Epstein RJ, Seedor JA, Dreizen NG, et al. Penetrating keratoplasty for herpes simplex keratitis and keratoconus: allograft rejection and survival. *Ophthalmology* 1987;94:935.

190. Wilson SE, Kaufman JE. Graft failure after penetrating keratoplasty. *Surv Ophthalmol* 1990;34:325.

191. Paque J, Poirier RH. Corneal allograft reaction and its relationship to suture site neovascularization. *Ophthalmic Surg* 1977;8:71.

192. Volker-Dieben HJM, D'Amaro J, Kok-van Alphen CC. Hierarchy of prognostic factors for corneal allograft survival. *Aust N Z J Ophthalmol* 1987;15:11.

193. Boisjoly HM, Bernard P-M, Dube I, et al. Effect of factors unrelated to tissue etching on corneal transplant endothelial rejection. *Am J Ophthalmol* 1989;107:647.

194. Donshik PC, Cavanagh HD, Boruchoff SA, et al. Effect of bilateral and unilateral grafts on the incidence of rejections after keratoconus. *Am J Ophthalmol* 1979;87:823.

195. Khodadoust AA, Karnema Y. Corneal grafts in the second eye. *Cornea* 1984;3:17.

196. Meyer RF. Corneal allograft rejection in bilateral penetrating keratoplasty: clinical and laboratory studies. *Trans Am Ophthalmol Soc* 1986;84:664.

197. Dana MR, Streilein JW. Loss and restoration of immune privilege in eyes with corneal neovascularization. *Invest Ophthalmol Vis Sci* 1996;37:2485.

198. Klein J. *Natural history of the major histocompatibility complex.* New York: Wiley, 1986.

199. Fujikawa LS, Colvin RB, Bhan AK, et al. Expression of HLA-A/B/C and –DR locus antigens on epithelial, stromal and endothelial cells of the human cornea. *Cornea* 1982;1:213.

200. Mayer DL, Daar AS, Casey TA, et al. Localization of HLA-A, B, C and HLA-DR antigens in the human cornea: practical significance for grafting technique and HLA typing. *Transplant Proc* 1983; 15:126.

201. Whitsett CF, Stulting RD. The distribution of HLA antigens on human corneal tissue. *Invest Ophthalmol Vis Sci* 1984;25:519.

202. Treseler PA, Foulks GN, Sanfilippo F. The expression of HLA antigens by cells in the human cornea. *Am J Ophthalmol* 1984;98:763.

203. Abi-Hanna D, Wakefield D, Watkins S. HLA antigens in ocular tissues: I. In vivo expression in human eyes. *Transplantation* 1988; 45:610.

204. Streilein JW, Toews GB, Bergstresser PR. Corneal allografts fail to express Ia antigens. *Nature* 1979;282:326.

205. William KA, Ash JK, Coster DJ. Histocompatibility antigen and passenger cell content of normal and diseased human cornea. *Transplantation* 1985;39:265.

206. Austyn JM, Larsen CP. Migration patterns of dendritic leukocytes: implications for transplantation. *Transplantation* 1990;48:1.

207. Martin S, Dyer PA. The case for matching MHC genes in human organ transplantation. *Nat Genet* 1993;5:210.

208. Batchelor JR, Casey TA, Gibbs DC, et al. HLA matching and corneal grafting. *Lancet* 1976;1:551.

209. Kissmeyer-Nielsen F, Ehlers N. Corneal transplantation and matching for HLA-A and B. *Scand J Urol Nephrol* 1977;42 [Suppl]:44.

210. Foulks GN, Sanfilippo FP, Locascio JA, et al. Histocompatibility testing for keratoplasty in high-risk patients. *Ophthalmology* 1983;90:239.

211. Stark WJ, Taylor HR, Datiles M, et al. Transplantation antigens and keratoplasty. *Aust J Ophthalmol* 1983;11:333.

212. Sanfilippo F, MacQueen JM, Vaughn WK, et al. Reduced graft rejection with good HLA-A and B matching in high-risk corneal transplantation. *N Engl J Med* 1986;315:29.

213. Boisjoly HM, Bernard P-M, et al. Association between corneal allograft rejections and HLA compatibility. *Ophthalmology* 1990; 97:1689.

214. Stark W, Stulting D, Maguire M, et al. The Collaborative Corneal Transplantation Studies (CCTS): effectiveness of histocompatibility matching of donors and recipients in high risk corneal transplantation. *Arch Ophthalmol* 1992;110:1392.

215. Gore SM, Vail A, Bradley BA, et al. HLA-DR matching in corneal transplantation. *Transplantation* 1995;60:1033.

216. Sonoda Y, Streilein JW. Impaired cell mediated immunity in mice bearing healthy orthoptic corneal allografts. *J Immunol* 1993; 150:1727.

217. Sonoda Y, Sano Y, Ksander B, et al. Characterization of cell mediated immune responses elicited by orthoptic corneal allografts in mice. *Invest Ophthalmol Vis Sci* 1995;36:427.

218. Sano Y, Ksander BR, Streilein JW. Murine orthoptic corneal transplantation in "high-risk" eyes: rejection is dictated primarily by weak rather than strong alloantigens. *Invest Ophthalmol Vis Sci* 1991;38:1130.

219. Liu Y, Mamrah P, Zhang Q, Taylor AW, Dana MR. Draining lymph nodes of corneal transplant hosts exhibit evidence for donor major histocompatibility complex (MHC) class II-positive dendritic cells derived from MHC class II-negative grafts. *J Exp Med* 2002;195:259.

220. Hamrah P, Liu Y, Zhang Q, Dana MR. The corneal stroma is endowed with a significant number of resident dendritic cells. *Invest Ophthalmol Vis Sci* 2003;44:581.

221. Wilson SE, Lloyd SA. Epidermal growth factor and its receptor, basic fibroblast growth factor beta-1, and interleukin 1 alpha messenger RNA production in human corneal endothelial cells. *Invest Ophthalmol Vis Sci* 1991;32:2747.

222. Kawashima H, Prasad SA, Gregerson DS. Corneal endothelial cells inhibit T cell proliferation by blocking IL-2 production. *J Immunol* 1994;153:1982.

223. Kennedy MC, Rosenbaum JT, Brown J. Novel production of interleukin-1 receptor antagonist peptides in normal human cornea. *J Clin Invest* 1995;95:82.

224. Bora NS, Gobleman CL, Atkinson JP. Differential expression of the complement regulatory proteins in the human eye. *Invest Ophthalmol Vis Sci* 1993;34:3579.

225. Mohan RR, Liang Q, Kim WJ, et al. Apoptosis in the cornea: further characterization of Fas/Fas ligand system. *Exp Eye Res* 1997; 65:575.

226. Yamada J, Streilein JW. Induction of anterior chamber-associated immune deviation by corneal allografts placed in the anterior chamber. *Invest Ophthalmol Vis Sci* 1997;38:2833.

227. Sano Y, Ksander BR, Streilein JW. Fate of orthoptic corneal allografts in eyes that cannot support ACAID induction. *Invest Ophthalmol Vis Sci* 1995;36:2176.

228. Dana MR, Yamada J, Streilein JW. Topical IL-1 receptor antagonist promotes corneal transplant survival. *Transplantation* 1997; 63:1501.

4

MORPHOLOGY AND PATHOLOGIC RESPONSE IN CORNEAL AND CONJUNCTIVAL DISEASE

KENNETH R. KENYON, EMILIANO GHINELLI, AND HENRIQUE V. CHAVES

The cornea is composed of relatively few components and includes three different cell types (epithelium, keratocytes, and endothelium) plus an extracellular matrix of collagen and glycosaminoglycans. Thus it is appropriate to consider corneal morphology and pathology in terms of the three major anatomic and functional units formed by these cells and matrix: the epithelium and its basement membrane, the keratocytes and the stromal collagen, and the endothelium and Descemet's membrane (1,2).

Because normal corneal morphology is discussed elsewhere (Chapter 1), this chapter surveys the basic principles of normal wound healing, the response to specific insults (such as chemical injury, bacterial infection, and surgical procedures), and the response during selected diseases.

EPITHELIUM AND BASEMENT MEMBRANE

Normal Wound Healing

Subsequent to a full-thickness wound of the corneal epithelium, the damaged cells adjacent to the wound edge lose their surface microvilli (3–5). Within 1 hour, the basal cells begin to flatten as intermediate and superficial cells reduce their desmosomal junctions and glycogen storage, evidencing their impending movement.

Fibronectin, the glycoprotein widely involved in cell-to-cell and cell-to-substrate interactions, is deposited on the denuded corneal surface, along with fibrinogen and fibrin (6). Neutrophils arrive through the tear film, initiating the process of debriding cellular remnants. At 6 hours postwounding, the epithelial cells initiate wound closure by sliding into the area of defect at a rate of approximately 0.75 mm/min (7,8). At the same time, basal cells distant from the wound begin to undergo mitosis.

The epithelial sliding process is quite active for 15 hours, as the leading cells extend ruffled pseudopods whose motility depends on the actin filaments of the cytoskeleton (9).

The cytoskeletal filaments may also be involved in cell adhesion because they insert into the electron-dense inner aspect of the hemidesmosome attachment plaques.

The moment the defect is closed, a contact inhibition message evokes the cessation of cell movement and the alteration of cellular configuration, causing these migrating squamous cells to regain the cuboidal configuration of basal cells. At the same time, DNA synthesis begins. Between 24 and 48 hours after wounding, epithelial proliferation in the wound, now at its peak, forms an epithelial plug, and all neutrophils vanish. By 3 to 4 days after wounding, the epithelial plug regresses and mitotic figures first appear in the wound (10) (Fig. 4-1).

If the epithelial basement membrane remains healthy, the recovering epithelial cells are able to use it for tight adhesion to the underlying stroma, as is evidenced both morphologically by the reappearance of hemidesmosomes on day 2 after injury and clinically by tight adhesion shortly thereafter (11).

In the event of basement membrane damage, however, new basement membrane complexes, comprising short, discontinuous segments of basement membrane material with associated hemidesmosomes and anchoring fibrils, begin to reform within 5 to 7 days after injury (12). Depending on the severity of basement membrane damage, as long as 6 to 8 weeks may be required for complete basement membrane reconstruction. This process is closely paralleled by delayed epithelium-to-stroma adhesion until the intact basement membrane has been restored (13). After regression of the epithelial plug, mitoses appear in the wound base, and soon the overlying new epithelium becomes even with the adjacent old epithelium. The regenerating epithelium is important in activating the underlying keratocytes because they fail to transform into fibroblasts in the absence of overlying epithelium (14,15). The damaged epithelium may also be involved in the recruitment of neutrophils into the wound area. Moreover, neutrophils

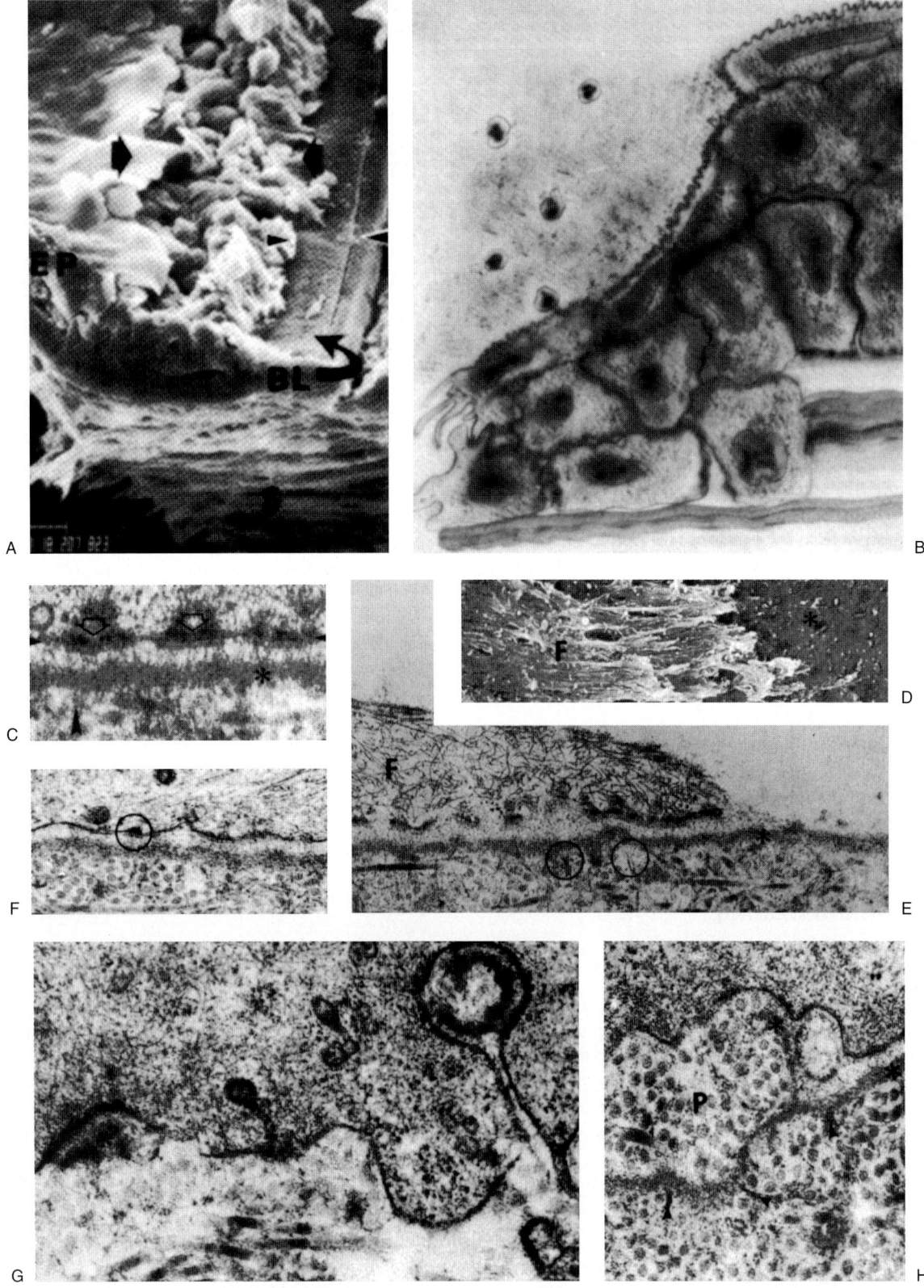

and mononuclear cells can delay the closure of the epithelial wound, such that continuing inflammation may foster the persistence of a corneal epithelial defect (16). A crucial role in corneal epithelial wound healing is also played by hormones, biochemical messengers, and pharmacologic agents. The classic studies of Friedenwald and Bushke (17) indicated that influences on corneal epithelial healing were adrenergically mediated because topically administered epinephrine reduced epithelial cell locomotion, mitosis, and wound healing. In addition, second messengers, including adenosine 3′,5′-cyclic adenosine monophosphate (cAMP) and guanosine 3′,5′-cyclic guanosine monophosphate (cGMP), have been implicated in corneal epithelial cell metabolic control (18). The proliferation of corneal epithelial cells is regulated by a bidirectional control process characterized by an adrenergic cAMP-dependent "off" response, and a cholinergic, muscarinic cGMP-dependent "on" response. Exogenous substances that raise intracellular cAMP levels such as isoproterenol or prostaglandin-E$_1$ shut off epithelial mitosis, and carbamylcholine and acetylcholine (ACh) raise intranuclear cGMP levels and increase mitosis by specific, regulatory stimulation of RNA polymerase II activity (19). This mechanism explains the transitory mitotic suppression induced by superficial corneal wounding (interruption of adrenergic fibers), as well as the permanent depression of epithelial mitosis associated with

decreased intracellular ACh levels after total corneal denervation, resulting in neurotrophic keratitis (20–23).

Another important modulator of mitotic rate in corneal epithelium is human epidermal growth factor (hEGF). Classic works performed by Frati and coworkers (24) and by Savage and Cohen (25) independently showed that hEGF applied to wounded rabbit corneas stimulates reepithelialization by a transient hyperplasia of epithelial cell layers. Soong and coworkers (26) found that acceleration of corneal wound healing by hEGF is entirely due to stimulation of cellular mitosis, not to increased cell motility. Also, Kitazawa and coworkers showed that topical application of hEGF in rabbits induces a dose-dependent high rate of epithelial replication, particularly near the limbal region, with a significant increase in the DNA content in regenerating epithelium over 24 to 48 hours.

Transforming growth factor-β (TGF-β) is a multifunctional peptide that modulates cell proliferation and differentiation in many cell types and accelerates tissue repair response (27,28). *In vivo* studies have shown that TGF-β present in fibroblasts, macrophages, and possibly the cell membrane may accelerate stromal wound healing, induce neovascularization, and decrease plasminogen activator (PA) activity, resulting in the prevention of degradation of extracellular matrix. However, in the absence of retinoic acid, the effect of TGF-β is more prominent, suggesting

FIGURE 4-1. Normal epithelial wound healing. **A:** Scanning electron micrograph immediately after trephine incision of epithelium and stroma, with the wound margin seen at the right. Immediately adjacent to the wound margin, an exposed zone of Bowman's layer (BL) appears intact (*between the arrowheads*) but is devoid of epithelial cells. Farther from the wound margin, an area of disrupted epithelial cells is evident (*between the arrows*), and more distant from the wound edge, the epithelium (EP) appears unaffected. S, stroma (×600). **B:** Diagram of the epithelium 15 to 72 hours after wounding. Epithelial sliding is active as filopodia extend from the crest and edges of ruffled epithelial cells into the defect area. Intracellular spaces are distended. As the base of the wound is covered, the cells increase in height and begin again to resemble basal cells. Cellular organelles increase in size and complexity, and villous specializations of the free surface membrane begin to reappear. (**A, B** from Binder PS, et al. Corneal anatomy and wound healing. In: *Transactions of the New Orleans Academy of Ophthalmology.* St. Louis: Mosby, 1980:1–35, with permission.) **C:** Transmission electron micrograph at high magnification shows basement membrane attachment complexes to comprise cytoplasmic filaments within basal epithelial cells, converging at hemidesmosomes (*arrows*), penetrating the plasma membrane (*small arrowheads*), bridging the lamina lucida between the plasma membrane and basement membrane (*asterisk*), and establishing continuity with anchoring fibrils (*large arrowhead*) in Bowman's layer (×100,000). **D:** Scanning electron micrograph of rabbit cornea immediately after surgery reveals filamentous cellular debris (F) adherent to exposed and intact basement membrane (*asterisk*; ×1500). **E:** Transmission electron micrograph of rabbit cornea corresponding to **D.** The basal cells have been ruptured transversely, leaving masses of filamentous debris (F) overlying an intact basement membrane (*asterisk*) with well-developed anchoring fibrils (*circled*; ×30,000). **F:** Transmission electron micrograph of rabbit cornea 3 days after mechanical scraping of the epithelium. Newly migrating epithelium has come to rest on the original basement membrane, and hemidesmosomal attachment sites (*circled*) have formed (×40,000). **G:** Transmission electron micrograph of rabbit cornea 7 days after superficial keratectomy illustrates the beginnings of the attachment complex reconstruction as short, discontinuous segments of basement membrane (*asterisk*) with attendant hemidesmosomes along infoldings of the basal cell membrane (×40,000). **H:** Transmission electron micrograph of rabbit cornea 30 days after superficial keratectomy shows areas of irregularity and duplication of basement membrane (*asterisks*), separated from basal cell membrane by fibrillar collagenous pannus (P), as evidence of probable epithelial erosion or edema. Numerous anchoring fibrils (*arrowheads*) are evident (×40,000).

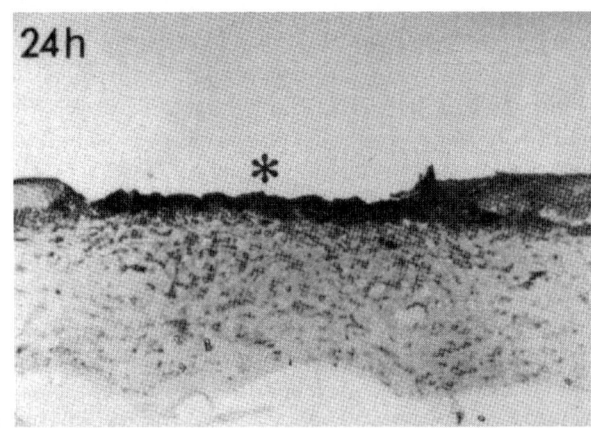
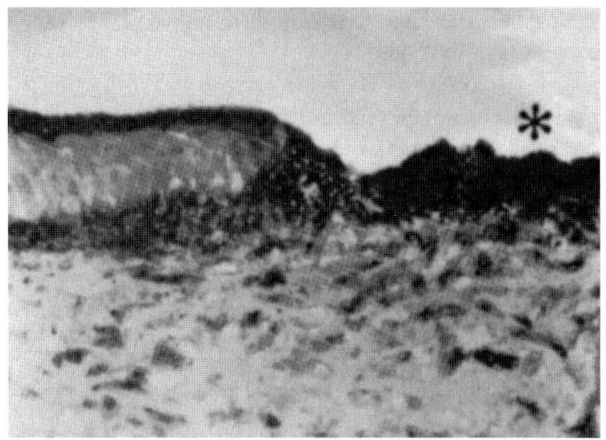

FIGURE 4-2. Immunohistochemical staining of transforming growth factor-beta (TGF-β) in the vitamin A–deficient rat cornea. At 24 hours after superficial mechanical injury **(A)** a positive reaction for TGF-β is evident as well as the formation of a pseudomembrane (*asterisks*) in the central epithelial defect and anterior stroma. At higher magnification **(B)** many infiltrating inflammatory cells and keratocytes show a positive reaction (**A** ×87; **B** ×220).

that TGF-β plays a more important role in the healing of vitamin A–deficient corneas than in normal corneas (29) (Fig. 4-2).

Nishida and coworkers (30) also showed that hyaluronan (hyaluronic acid) stimulates corneal epithelial migration by mechanisms different from those of fibronectin and hEGF. Further studies are necessary to prove that beyond its utility as a viscoelastic substance in ophthalmic surgeries, hyaluronan with its biologic signal to cells could be therapeutically promoting corneal epithelial wound healing.

Several studies have shown that fibronectin, a high–molecular-weight glycoprotein found in plasma, on cell surfaces, and in extracellular matrices, is an important factor in adhesion, chemotaxis, tissue repair, and phagocytic activity of keratocytes (31–39). After abrasion of the corneal epithelium, fibronectin is detected in the anterior margin of the denuded stroma in areas where the epithelium has not healed 18 hours after the injury, but not 40 hours later (40). Recent experimental studies suggest that fibronectin might be important in the healing of corneal epithelial wounds (6,41–46), although other investigators could not prove the clinical usefulness of fibronectin to promote wound healing of corneal epithelium (47,48).

The proteinases plasmin and PA have been detected in ocular tissues (49,50), and Berman and Wang suggest their involvement in ocular surface disorders involving sterile corneal ulceration (51,52).

Plasmin is able to degrade fibronectin and laminin (53–56), both of which are important in cell sliding during corneal wound healing.

Recent studies have shown that urokinase-like PA (uPA) but not tissue-type PA is present at the leading edge of migrating corneal epithelium both after abrasion and after alkali injuries (57–59). The abnormally prolonged presence

of enzymatically active uPA at the leading epithelium edge after burn results in a persistent corneal epithelial defect. Therefore, the regulation of uPA activity at the leading edge of corneal epithelium after injury might be useful therapeutically in the healing of epithelial defects and the prevention of stromal ulceration.

Recently, the mechanisms of action of EGF and other factors, molecules, and receptors have been summarized and a mechanism proposed for the different and specific moments of the corneal wound healing process (60). During the cell migration phase of the corneal wound repair, many different molecules are considered key actors that variously affect the early phase of epithelial renewal. They include fibroblast growth factor (FGF), TGF, keratinocyte growth factor, hepatocyte growth factor, platelet-derived growth factor, insulin-like growth factor, interleukin (IL)-1 and IL-6, tumor necrosis factor-α, endothelin-1, fibronectin, retinoids, CD44, hyaluronan receptor, cytokeratins 3 and 12 (K3 and K12), amyloid precursor protein, and chondroitin sulfate proteoglycans (60). Some peptides like nerve growth factor and substance P also play a role in the process, providing evidence that the corneal epithelium is richly innervated and responsive to neuropeptides (60,61).

Response to Limited Ocular Surface Injury

The healing rate of the ocular surface epithelium varies with the extent as well as the intensity of the injury (Fig. 4-3). Limited mechanical abrasion and mild chemical or thermal burns of the central cornea usually heal rapidly by the mechanism detailed in the previous section. In the rabbit, regenerated corneal epithelium shows restoration of its biochemical components, including glycogen and glycolytic enzymes, as soon as healing is completed, and this corresponds to a normal clinical and morphologic appearance as well (62,63). However, with more severe injury of the corneal surface, involving damage to the basement membrane complexes of the basal epithelial cells and the anterior stroma, recovery may be slower. For example, extreme chemical burns involving both the corneal and conjunctival epithelia heal slowly with recurrent epithelial erosions, scarring, and neovascularization; this pattern of healing is related in part to the intrinsically different regenerative capacities of the corneal and conjunctival epithelial cells, especially after widespread destruction of the limbal stem cells.

Compromise of the epithelial cells and their surface characteristics is clinically evident as surface irregularity and superficial punctate keratitis (corresponding to microscopic epithelial defects) and also as loss of cell surface microplicae. Although basement membrane damage can also contribute to the formation of persistent epithelial defects or recurrent erosions, as described later, these problems are fortunately unusual. Thus, for example, even after a relatively extensive acid burn of the human cornea and bulbar conjunctiva, epithelial recovery is rapid and secure (64). As shown in Fig. 4-3, the denatured corneal epithelium demonstrates nuclear pyknosis and cytoplasmic shrinkage. However, transmission electron microscopy fails to disclose any basement membrane material adherent to these devitalized basal epithelial cells, and the functional integrity of the original basement membrane is clinically attested by tight adhesion of the regenerated epithelium, which rapidly resurfaces the entire cornea and involved bulbar conjunctiva. Because of limited acid-induced denaturation of stromal collagen and ground substance, topical steroids can be liberally applied to inhibit inflammation.

Should, however, chemical penetration be more severe, then subepithelial fibroblastic proliferation may result in superficial stromal scarring in the form of a fibrocellular pannus with or without neovascularization. This pannus comprises randomly arrayed type II collagen fibrils of variable sizes and is the product of keratocytes that have been stimulated to transform into fibroblasts. Such a pannus may accumulate between the epithelium and Bowman's layer or, more commonly, may develop in the anterior stroma with minimal detriment to corneal clarity and vision (65–67).

Response to Extensive Ocular Surface Injury

When an injury involves a large area of the ocular surface, a different pattern of healing occurs (Fig. 4-4). Subsequent to Thoft's initial hypothesis of the conjunctiva's role in the maintenance of the normal corneal epithelial cell mass, studies have shown that the stem cells (cells with great potential for clonogenic cell division and with responsibility for cell replacement and tissue regeneration) of the

corneal epithelium are localized in the basal cell layer of the limbus (68–72) (Chapter 1). In fact, when the wound involves the entire cornea and extends beyond the limbus, thereby destroying the stem cells, the corneal surface must be recovered with epithelium of conjunctival origin, suggesting that the limbal epithelium also may be a barrier between corneal and conjunctival epithelia (73). Further experimental studies have also shown that total or partial surgical removal of limbal stem cells contributes to the triad of conjunctival epithelial ingrowth, corneal vascularization, and delayed healing with recurrent erosion (74,75). In this situation, the obligate transformation of conjunctival cells into corneal epithelium is prolonged functionally, morphologically, and biochemically (62–64). Such eyes face extended clinical morbidity because they are beset with chronic inflammation, persistent epithelial defects, recurrent erosions, stromal neovascularization, and sterile ulceration. Epithelial cells at the margin of persistent defects often display an elevated border, having undergone an arrest of both migratory and mitotic activity. Nor is there synthesis of the basement membrane material that may have been chemically denatured by the injury (76).

The overgrowth of conjunctival epithelium onto the cornea is also marked by the presence of goblet cells. Such retention of goblet cells on the cornea has been observed to correspond very closely to areas where the stroma has become vascularized, perhaps indicative of the persistently altered biochemical state and metabolic needs of conjunctivally derived epithelial cells (63,77). Somewhat paradoxically, as has been observed in chemically burned human eyes, not only are goblet cells numerous and morphologically normal (78), but non-goblet epithelial cells appear to be increasingly involved in mucus secretion (79). Hence, in contrast to previous interpretations, mucus deficiency need not be invoked as a significant contributor to the ocular surface abnormalities of the chemically burned eye (Fig. 4-5).

The conjunctiva-derived epithelium also has a dramatic effect on the response of the corneal stroma to subsequent injury; a rabbit cornea covered by epithelium of conjunctival origin demonstrates a marked stromal neovascular response to subsequent wounding (80). These findings explain why the response to major destruction of the limbal zone includes corneal vascularization and conjunctivalization, as well as why limbal transplantation is more effective than conjunctival transplantation in restoring a severely damaged corneal surface (81,82).

The whole anterior ocular surface is accessible to growth factors, especially neurotrophins, which are produced and released by the lacrimal gland into the tear film (83). These important growth factors can presumably be used by the conjunctival epithelium and possibly also the goblet cells because these cells show a plethora of neurotrophin receptors (84). Cell culture studies of human limbal epithelium have shown high rates of cell multiplication compared with the central cornea and conjunctiva, and have also demonstrated

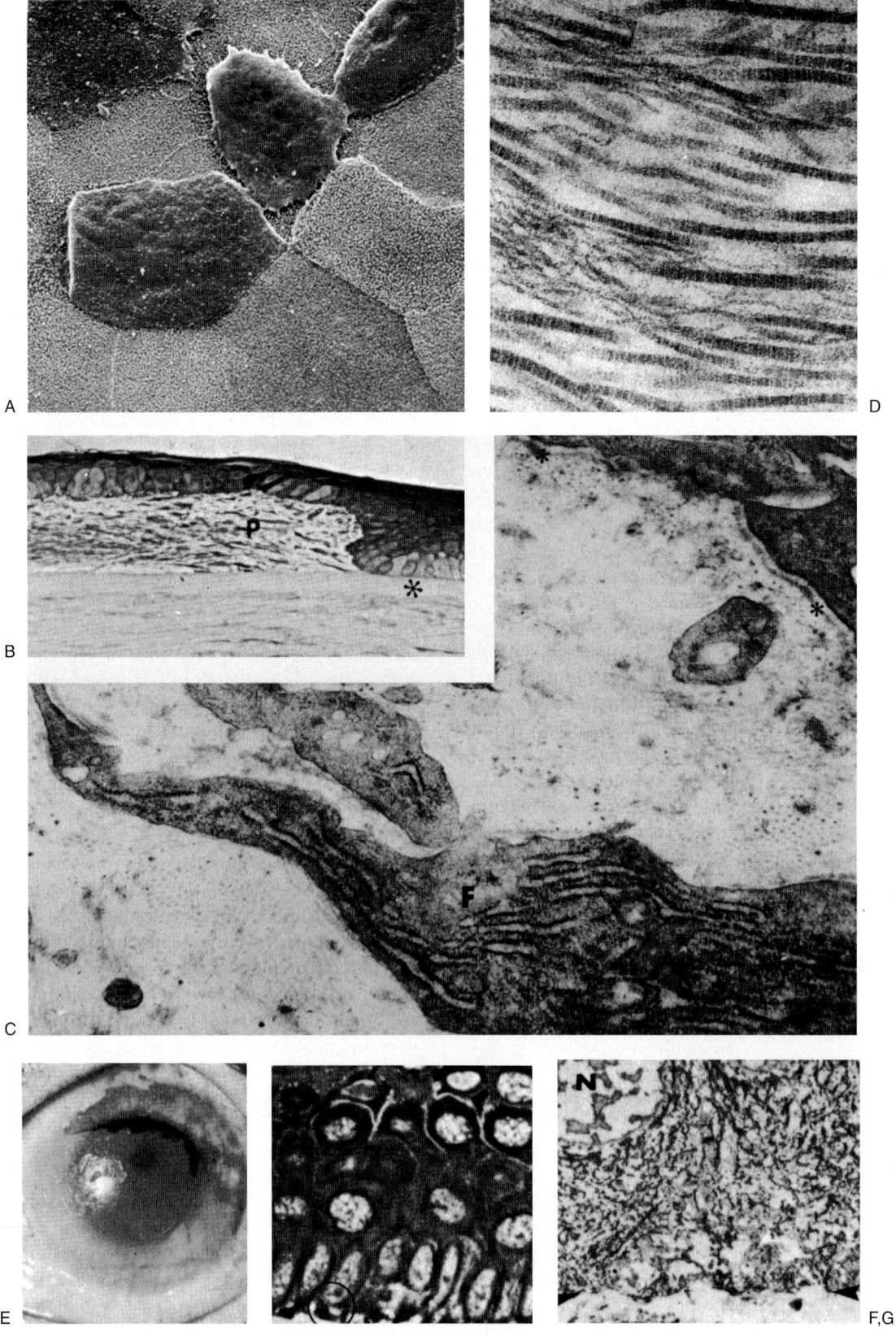

the ability of limbal cells to attach and form a stratified epithelium when suitably grafted (85) (Fig. 4-6). Recently, autologous fibrin-cultured limbal stem cells have been shown permanently to restore the corneal surface of patients with total limbal stem cell deficiency (86). These results again support the concept of limbal location of stem cells in the cornea, and suggest that monolayers of cultured epithelial cells may be useful as autografts for repair of a damaged ocular surface.

Keratinization: Xerophthalmia

Xerophthalmia is a highly clinically relevant example of ocular surface keratinization. Xerophthalmia is the term used to describe the irregular, lusterless, poorly wettable surface of the conjunctiva and cornea associated with vitamin A deficiency. Bitot's spots, the triangular, foamy, keratotic areas of interpalpebral bulbar conjunctiva adjacent to the limbus, are also sometimes correlated with vitamin A deficiency. In humans, biopsy specimens of xerotic conjunctiva and cornea show remarkable acanthosis and hyperkeratosis with a prominent granular cell layer containing keratofibrils and keratohyalin granules (87,88) (Fig. 4-7A–D). Frequently, pleomorphic gram-positive bacilli, presumably diphtheroids, are clustered about the superficial keratin debris. Electron microscopy shows that the superficial cell layers appear cornified and have lost almost all recognizable organelles except extremely compacted keratofibrils (Fig. 4-8). The surface plasma membrane has greatly reduced microplicae, as confirmed by scanning electron microscopy. If vitamin A therapy is effective, clinical and histologic normalization begins within 1 to 2 weeks, although conjunctival goblet cells are initially evident only at 1 month, and may require 2 to 3 months or longer for complete restoration (87). The effect of topical drugs and preservatives on the tears and the corneal epithelium during xerophthalmia due to dry eye represents a very important issue in the pathogenesis of this condition, because the same topical agent used to treat a compromised ocular surface epithelium can also impede the healing of a wounded corneal epithelium (89).

Cicatrization: Pemphigoid

Ocular cicatricial pemphigoid is a slowly progressive, chronic condition primarily affecting the mucosa of the mouth, nose, pharynx, and conjunctiva with formation of bullae, shrinkage, and scarring (Chapter 20). Cutaneous lesions may involve the face and scalp. These bullous lesions occur between the basal cells and basement membrane, and in a fully developed blister the basement membrane is usually destroyed. In many patients with clinically active disease, immunofluorescence studies show fixed immunoglobulins in the basement membrane zone (BMZ) of involved skin or mucosa as well as circulating basement membrane antibodies (90,91). The production of autoantibody reactive with a component in the lamina lucida of the conjunctival epithelial BMZ activates the complement pathway, leading to monocyte and mast cell recruitment and degranulation (immunoglobulin E–independent). This in turn amplifies the reaction with vascular damage, fibroblast proliferation, and collagen synthesis, plus increased basal epithelial cell mitosis and squamous metaplasia. These immune deposits are bound at sites where the earliest pathologic lesions are identified, and the circulating autoantibodies reactive with the lamina lucida of the BMZ play a central role in lesion production (92). With progression of conjunctival involvement, connective tissue proliferation and symblepharon result. In extreme cases, xerosis, keratinization of the conjunctiva, and epidermalization of the cornea develop (Fig. 4-7E–I).

FIGURE 4-3. Healing response to mild ocular surface injury. **A:** Scanning electron micrograph of monkey cornea after thermal cauterization illustrates the morphology of superficial punctate keratitis; individual epithelial cells have lost surface membrane infoldings and are desquamating. Underlying and surrounding normal-appearing epithelium exhibits surface microplicae (×1000). **B:** Phase-contrast photomicrograph of human cornea 1 year after penetrating injury demonstrates proliferation of fibrocellular pannus (P) between the epithelium and an intact Bowman's layer (*asterisk*; paraphenylenediamine, ×500). **C:** Transmission electron micrograph of a corresponding area reveals the basement membrane (*asterisks*) to be complete except for focal discontinuity. Multiple fibroblastic cells (F) in collagenous pannus appear synthetically active, as evidenced by abundant rough endoplasmic reticulum (×42,000). **D:** At higher magnification, a transmission electron micrograph reveals collagenous components of pannus to be randomly organized, banded fibrils of variable large diameter (up to 500 Å), with fine filaments interspersed (×62,000). **E:** A 33-year-old woman sustained an extensive burn by weak acid of nearly the total ocular surface epithelium. Anatomic and visual recovery was excellent after vigorous topical steroid and antibiotic therapy. **F:** Phase-contrast photomicrograph of debrided corneal epithelium (48 hours after injury) of the eye shown in **E** demonstrates preservation of the epithelial cell organization, despite cytoplasmic coagulation (paraphenylenediamine, ×1000). **G:** Transmission electron micrograph of the area circled in **F** shows nuclear (N) and cytoplasmic coagulation of basal epithelial cells. The basal plasma membrane (*between the arrowheads*) is notably devoid of basement membrane, which is presumed to have remained attached to Bowman's layer (×5000).

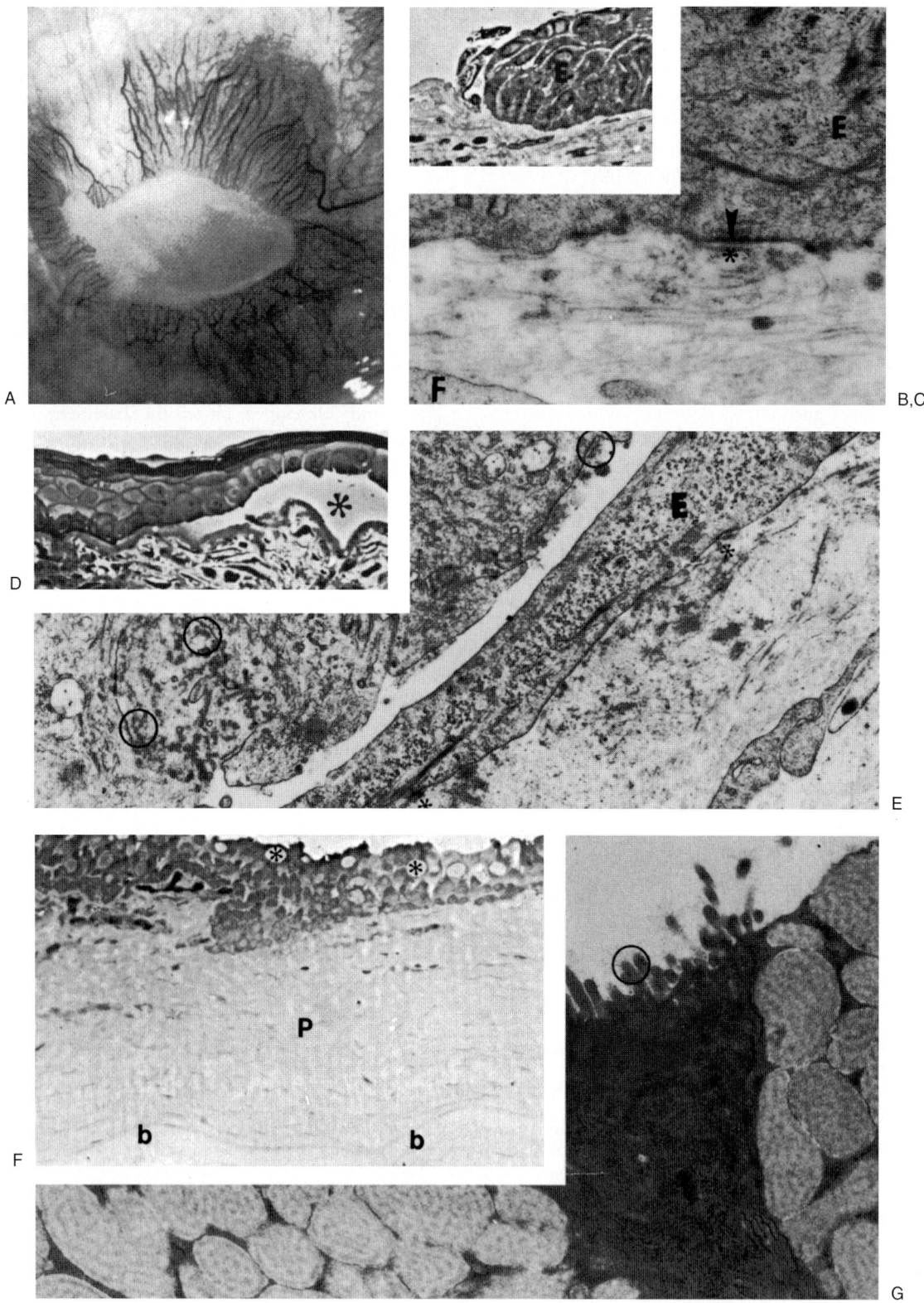

Histologically, the conjunctival and corneal epithelia demonstrate surface keratinization with acanthosis and spongiosis. By transmission electron microscopy, keratohyalin granules are particularly visible in the thickened granular cell layer, as are increased desmosomes (93). Although actual bullous lesions are not seen clinically in the conjunctiva, ultrastructural examination discloses duplications of multilaminar basement membrane in the bulbar conjunctival epithelium, which may be related to the reformation of basement membrane complexes after resolution of an epithelial separation.

Mast cells are prominent participants in the conjunctival inflammatory reaction with varying degrees of vasculopathy or true vasculitis (92). These histologic and immunopathologic findings are similar to those in bullous pemphigoid, a nonocular bullous disease in which circulating antibodies react with a specific antigen localized to the lamina lucida portion of the BMZ (94). Because of these similarities, it may be appropriate to consider cicatricial mucous membrane pemphigoid and bullous pemphigoid as representing the same pathologic process. Recently, detailed histomorphometric analysis of human conjunctiva has demonstrated that tissue remodeling of the extracellular matrix is an essential and dynamic process that coexists with conjunctival scarring in ocular cicatricial pemphigoid and is linked with an immunoinflammatory process mediated by cytokines released by activated conjunctival cells and infiltrating cells; the final effect is a remodeling of the matrix in the conjunctival stroma, potentially regulating the altered metabolism of matrix proteins (95).

Persistent Defects and Recurrent Erosion of the Corneal Epithelium: Basement Membrane Disorders

As previously emphasized, the basement membrane complexes are responsible for the maintenance of tight adhesions between the corneal epithelium and stroma. The components of these complexes include hemidesmosomes of the basal epithelial cell membrane, the underlying basement membrane, and the subjacent anchoring fibrils of Bowman's layer. Consequently, any traumatic, dystrophic, or degenerative disturbance at this level can predispose the epithelial cell layer to defective adhesion and repetitive breakdown, known as *recurrent erosion syndrome* (96). When the ocular surface is further compromised by extensive epithelial damage, inflammation, denervation, tear deficiency, or superficial stromal scarring, epithelial adhesion problems are compounded by a failure of epithelial mitosis or migration, or both, resulting in a persistent defect (96). In fact, when basement membrane is experimentally damaged by any technique, the consistent sequelae include irregularity and defects of the epithelial surface. Discontinuities and duplications of basement membrane complexes persist for 8 weeks or more, during which time the nonadherent epithelium is easily separable from the stroma (11,13). These same studies also emphasized the importance of the anterior stromal collagen of Bowman's layer to which the basement membrane adheres. Although abnormalities of basement membrane complexes alone may explain poor adhesion and recurrent erosions in some situations, in others, damage to Bowman's layer and anterior stroma with the accumulation of cellular and extracellular debris may also confound adhesion, despite the presence of basement membrane that appears morphologically normal (76).

Many clinical conditions that affect the corneal surface are manifested by recurrent erosions and persistent defects of the epithelium. These conditions can be considered as either primary or secondary causes of erosion, depending on whether the defect in the epithelial basement membrane is intrinsic or acquired. Among the primary disorders, epithelial basement membrane dystrophy (map-dot-fingerprint dystrophy, Cogan's epithelial microcystic corneal dystrophy) is most common (Fig. 4-9A–G). This designation is based on the

FIGURE 4-4. Healing response to severe ocular surface injury. **A:** A 43-year-old industrial worker is seen 1 year after acid and alkali injury to the entire ocular surface, with a central persistent epithelial defect surrounded by vascularized conjunctival overgrowth. **B:** Phase-contrast photomicrograph of monkey cornea 2 weeks after thermal cauterization shows multilayered, amitotic epithelium (E) at the edge of a persistent epithelial defect. Severe inflammatory and fibrocytic cells appear in the superficial stroma (paraphenylenediamine, ×900). **C:** Transmission electron micrograph of area in **B** shows slowly advancing epithelium (E) to have produced only rare basement membrane (*asterisk*) and hemidesmosomes (*arrowhead*). A fibroblast (F) has infiltrated Bowman's layer (×32,000). **D:** Phase-contrast photomicrograph at 10 weeks after a dilute sulfuric acid burn of a rhesus monkey cornea shows an irregular epithelial sheet separated (*at asterisk*) from the scarred Bowman's layer and anterior stroma (paraphenylenediamine, ×600). **E:** Transmission electron micrograph of the corresponding area shows the epithelium to have become elevated with adherent fragments of basement membrane material (*circled*), allowing insinuation of flattened epithelial cells (E) with limited basement membrane deposition (*asterisk*; ×17,500). **F:** Light photomicrograph of the human cornea shown in **A** demonstrates characteristics of conjunctival overgrowth. Disorganized epithelium containing goblet cells (*asterisks*) overlies a thick fibrovascular pannus (P) that has developed anterior to the relatively intact Bowman's layer (b; paraphenylenediamine, ×250). **G:** Transmission electron micrograph of an area shown in **F** shows that epithelial surface cells have normal microvillous surface membrane specialization (*circled*), and adjacent goblet cells have normal-appearing mucin globules (×18,700).

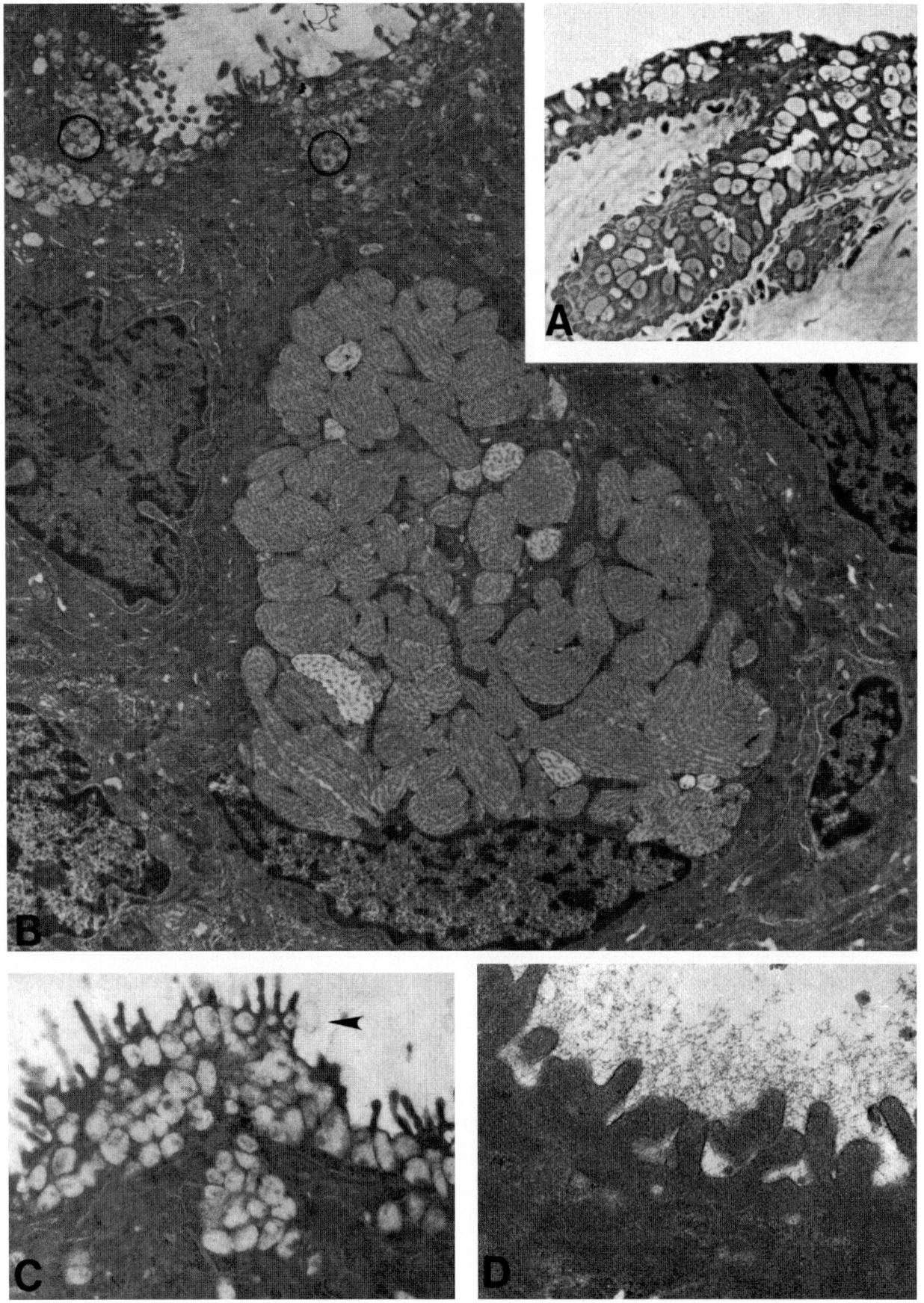

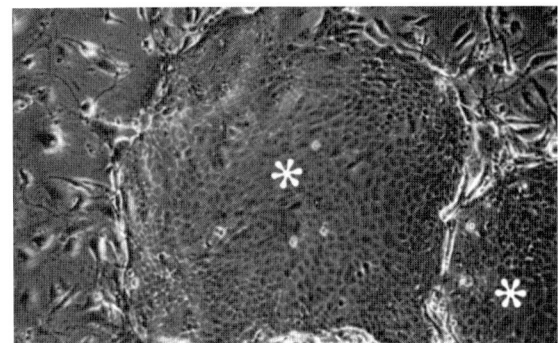

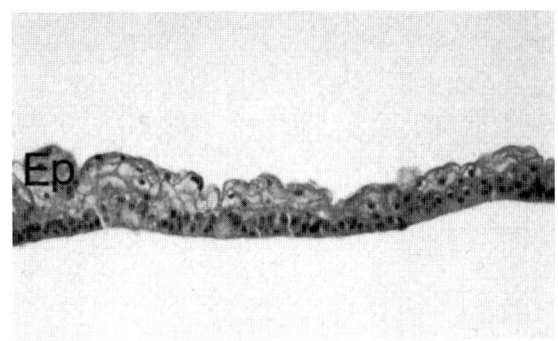

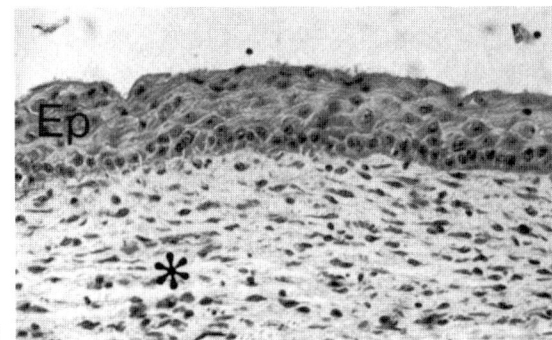

FIGURE 4-6. Xenograft transplantation of cultured human limbal cells. Phase-contrast microscopy (*top*) shows two colonies (*asterisks*) of cultured human limbal epithelial cells in culture surrounded by irradiated 3T3 fibroblasts (×100). Light microscopy (*middle*) of a confluent sheet of cultured limbal epithelial cells (Ep) displays considerable differentiation of compact basal cells and squamous superficial cells (hematoxylin-eosin, ×150). Light microscopy (*bottom*) of epithelium (Ep) formed from a sheet of cultured limbal epithelial cells grafted in the subdermal stroma (*asterisk*) of a nude mouse demonstrates cellular differentiation closely resembling corneal epithelium *in vivo* (hematoxylin-eosin, ×150). (Courtesy of Dr. Kristina Lindberg, with permission.)

clinical morphologic finding of opaque intraepithelial cysts (dots), maplike geographic patterns, and whorled fingerprint-like ridges at the level of the epithelial basement membrane (97,98). Such changes have been noted in many people who are clinically asymptomatic, and in some families an apparent autosomal dominant inheritance has been determined (99). In symptomatic persons, the epithelium shows loose adhesion, and it may detach either spontaneously or after minor trauma. Thus, in patients presenting with recurrent erosion, slit-lamp examination of the uninvolved eye and of asymptomatic family members may establish an etiologic diagnosis.

Recent application of *in vivo* confocal microscopy in patients with corneal recurrent erosion syndrome or epithelial basement membrane dystrophy showed deposits in basal epithelial cells, subbasal microfolds and streaks, damaged sub-basal nerves, or altered morphology of the anterior stroma, confirming clinically some observations achieved by other procedures (100). In fact, light and electron microscopic studies have also established that the microcystic areas correspond to the intraepithelial pseudocysts containing cellular debris. Geographic configurations represent thickened subepithelial plaques composed of abnormal multiple laminations of basement membrane and fibrillar collagens, whereas fingerprint lines consist of ridges of aberrant collagen and fibrous tissue (97,98,101). In these conditions, it is possible that dystrophic abnormalities of basement membrane complexes or adjacent structures permit the loosely adherent epithelium to shift, which would account for the accumulation of these abnormal configurations and for the predisposition to symptomatic erosions.

Although the effects can be variable, diabetes mellitus produces abnormalities of corneal epithelial adhesion. These corneal changes may also be considered a primary corneal basement membrane disorder. Ultrastructural studies of the human diabetic cornea have revealed an abnormality of the epithelial basement membrane that consists of thickening of the multilaminar basement membrane, duplication of anchoring fibrils, and decreased penetration of the anchoring fibrils from the deepest layer of the basal lamina into the stroma, which compromises the strength of the basement membrane complex at this level (96,102) (Fig. 4-9H–J). These changes are identical to those of the primary epithelial dystrophies.

FIGURE 4-5. Human conjunctiva after chemical burn. **A:** Phase-contrast micrograph of conjunctival epithelium shows abnormally numerous light-stained goblet cells (paraphenylenediamine, ×250). **B:** Transmission electron microscopy shows a normal-appearing goblet cell in bulbar conjunctival epithelium, plus mucin granules (*circles*) in superficial epithelial cells (×8800). **C:** Higher magnification of mucin granules in nongoblet epithelial cells. Apparent secretion is indicated at the *arrowhead* (×18,700). **D:** At high magnification, epithelial microvilli with surface glycocalyx appear normal (×50,000).

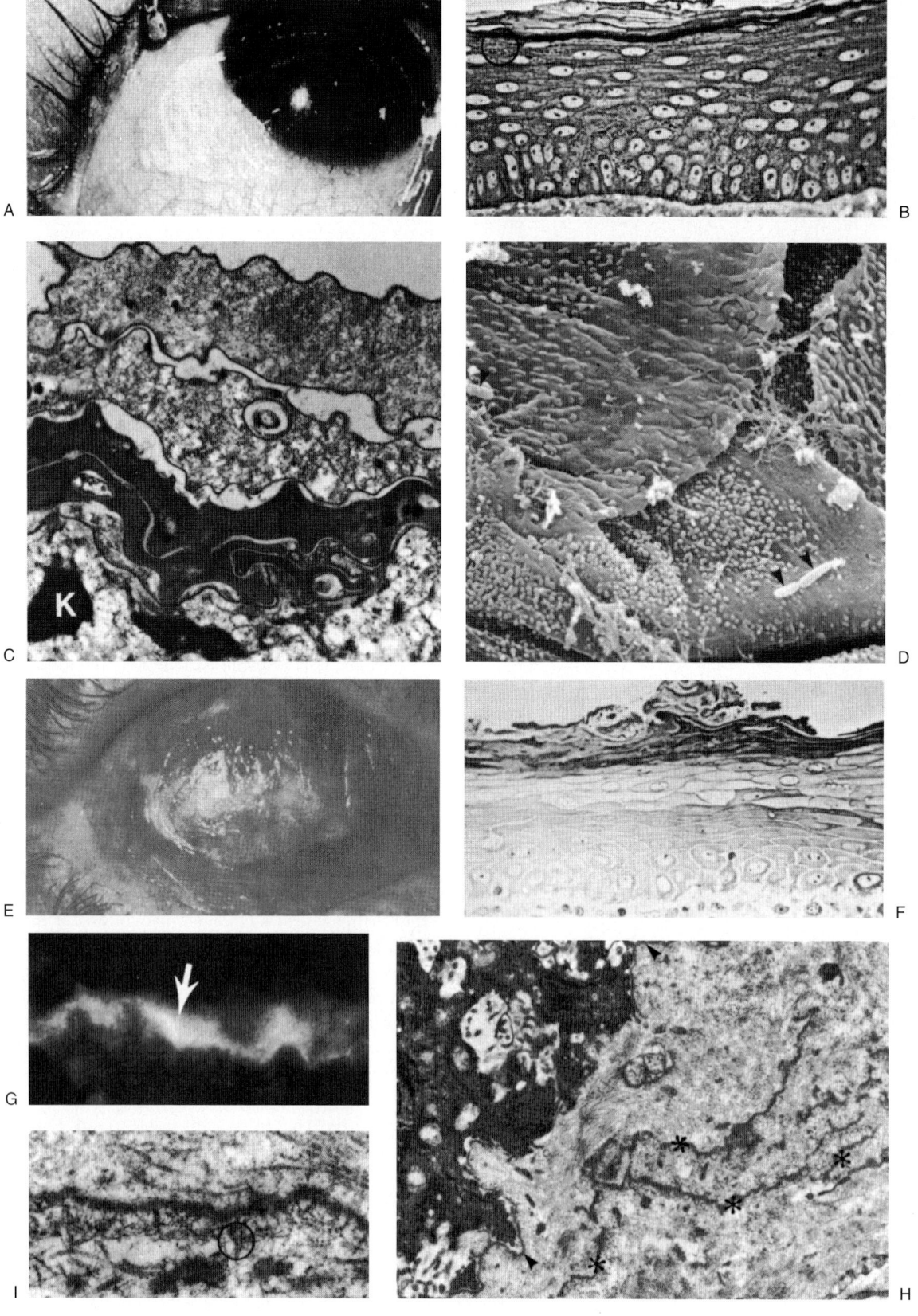

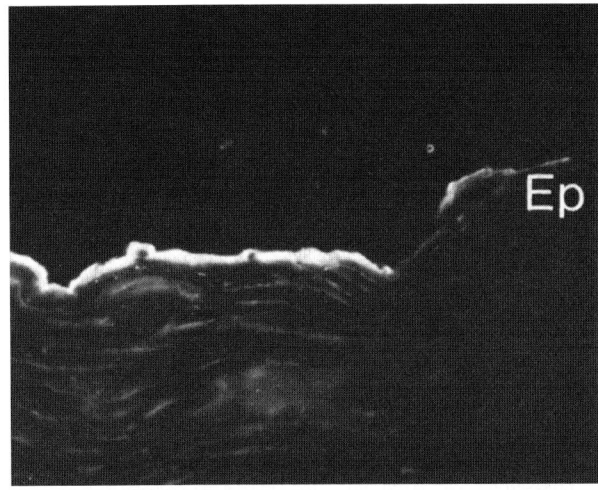

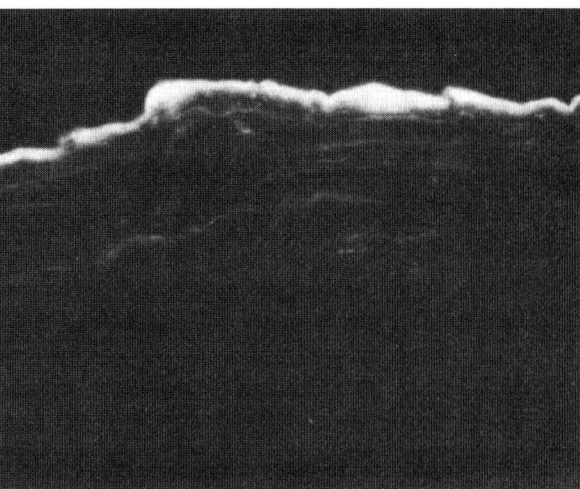

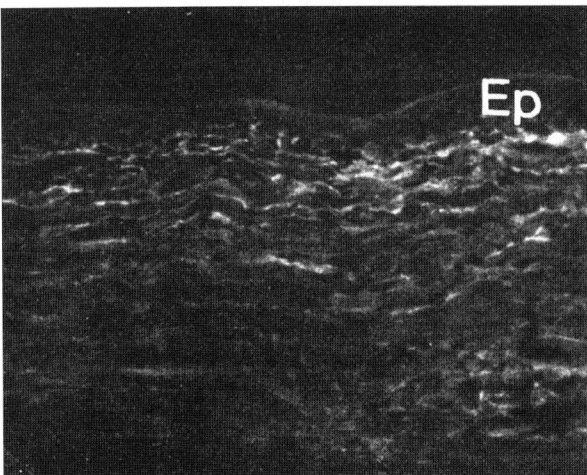

FIGURE 4-8. Fibronectin and corneal epithelial wound healing. Immunofluorescence staining for fibronectin in rat corneas after a central 3-mm epithelium abrasion. At 30 minutes after injury, fibronectin appeared as a bright band across the denuded stromal surface **(A)** and remained at 16 hours **(B)**, but had disappeared by 24 hours **(C)**. Epithelium (Ep) healed completely at 32 hours (goat antibody against rat fibronectin, ×300).

FIGURE 4-7. Keratinization and cicatrization. **A:** In this patient with vitamin A deficiency, corneal xerosis and conjunctival Bitot's spot are evident. **B:** Phase-contrast photomicrograph of conjunctival epithelium from Bitot's spot discloses surface keratinization, granulosa cell layer with numerous keratohyalin granules (*circled*), acanthosis, and disorganization of basal cells (paraphenylenediamine, ×700). **C:** Transmission electron micrograph of the area circled in **B** shows multiple cornified epithelial remnants, with granulosa cells containing keratohyalin (K; ×13,500). **D:** Scanning electron micrograph of this specimen shows multiple laminations of keratinized cellular remnants with bacilli (*arrowheads*) adherent (×5000). **E:** This advanced case of cicatricial mucous membrane pemphigoid shows total ankyloblepharon with an absolutely dry, vascularized, epidermalized corneal surface. **F:** Phase-contrast microscopy of bulbar conjunctiva of the eye in **E** shows surface keratinization, granulosa cell layer containing keratohyalin granules, and chronic inflammatory infiltrate of stroma (paraphenylenediamine, ×400). **G:** Normal human conjunctiva stained by indirect immunofluorescence technique after exposure to serum from a patient with pemphigoid demonstrates immunoglobulins localized along the basement membrane zone (*arrow*) of the epithelium (fluorescein-conjugated anti-human immunoglobulin G, ×400). (From Franklin RM, Fitzmorris CT. Antibodies against conjunctival basement membrane zone in cicatricial pemphigoid. *Am J Ophthalmol* 1983;101:1611. Published with permission from *The American Journal of Ophthalmology*. Copyright by the Ophthalmic Publishing Company.) **H:** Transmission electron microscopy of conjunctiva shows intracellular edema of basal cells and discontinuous basement membrane (*arrowheads*). Multiple laminations of basement membrane material (*asterisks*) are separated from the basal epithelium by scar collagen (×6000). **I:** Higher magnification of the area indicated by asterisks in **H** shows duplication of entire basement membrane complexes, complete with anchoring fibrils (*circled*) and random arrangement of fibrillar collagen intervening between laminations (×30,000).

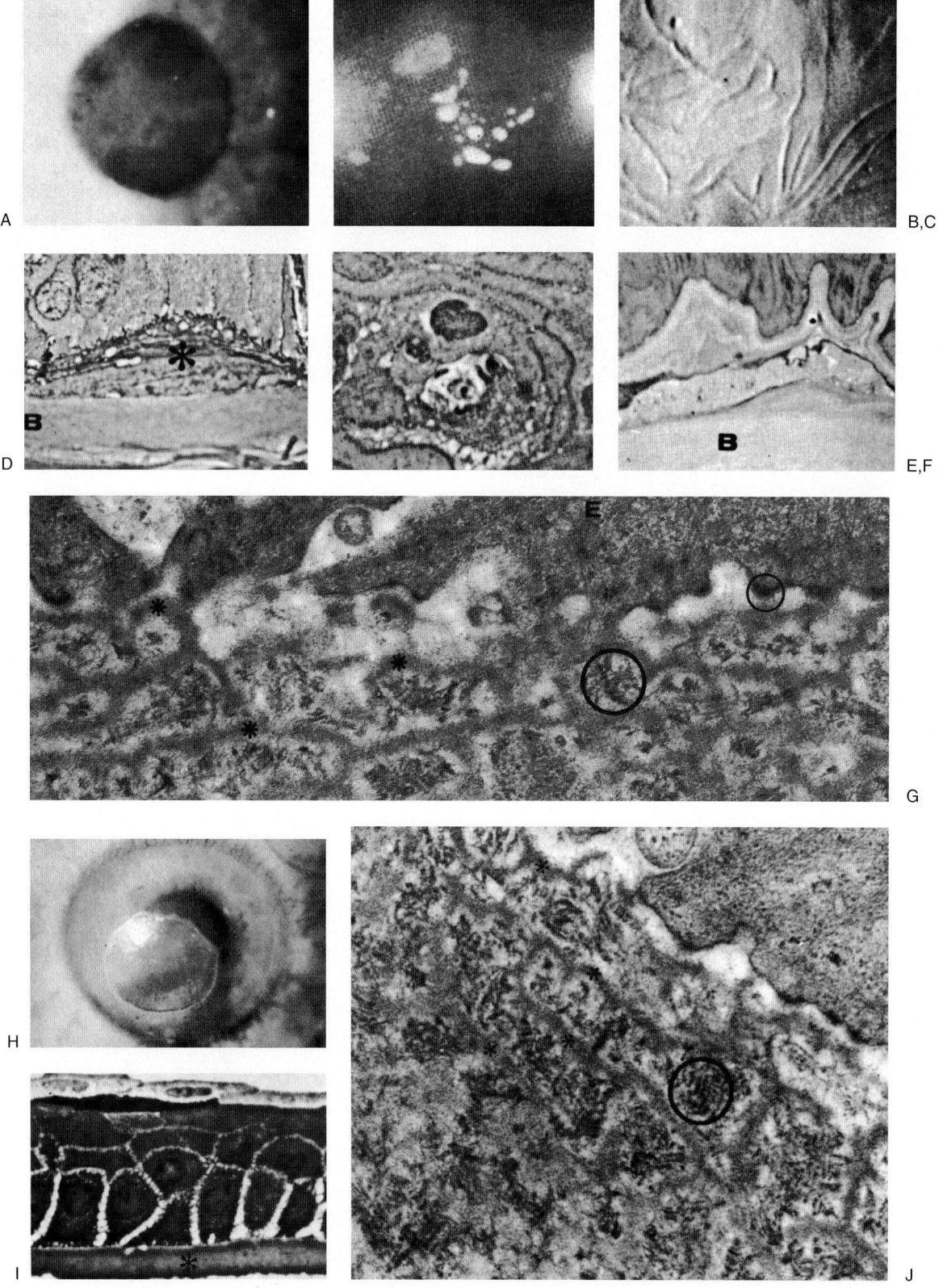

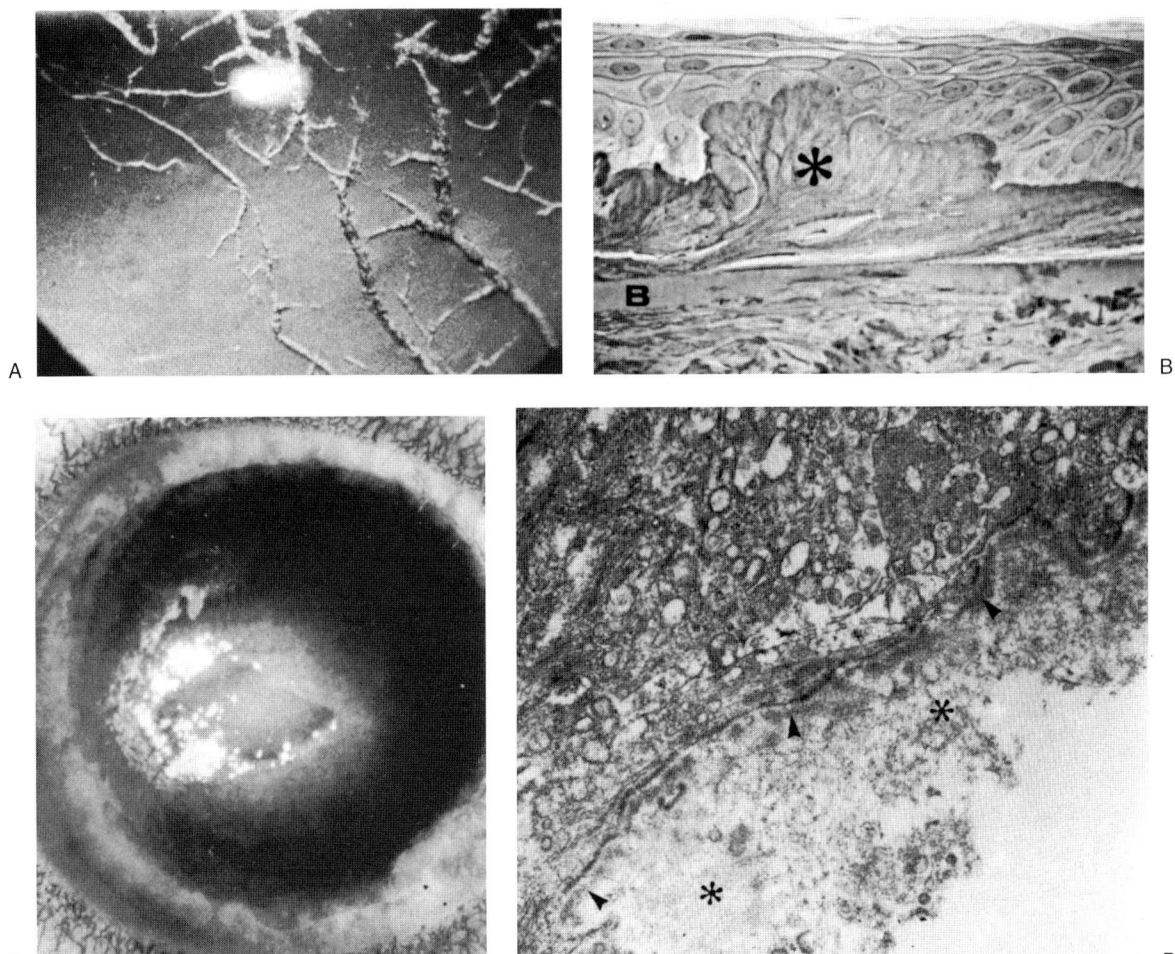

FIGURE 4-10. Secondary basement membrane disorder: recurrent corneal erosion. Lattice corneal dystrophy: **A:** Clinical appearance of typical branching stromal lesions. (Slit-lamp photograph courtesy of W. J. Stark, MD.) **B:** Phase-contrast photomicrograph shows subepithelial accumulation of fibrillar amyloid deposits (*asterisk*) causing distortion of basal epithelial contour. B, Bowman's layer (paraphenylenediamine, ×800). Metaherpetic keratitis: **C:** Persistent epithelial defect and superficial stromal scarring are evident. **D:** Transmission electron micrograph of debrided loosely adherent epithelium shows fragmented segments of basement membrane material (*arrowheads*) with attached fibrillar debris (*asterisks*) that interferes with epithelial stromal adhesion (×22,000).

FIGURE 4-9. Primary basement membrane disorder: recurrent corneal erosion. Map-dot-fingerprint dystrophy: **A:** Clinical photograph of a 37-year-old man with nontraumatic recurrent erosion shows characteristics of map dystrophy with superficial geographic haze interrupted by clear areas. **B:** In the dot form of microcystic dystrophy, superficial opaque cysts are evident in the epithelium. **C:** In fingerprint dystrophy, subepithelial ridges are particularly enhanced by retroillumination. (Slit-lamp photograph courtesy of Lawrence Hirst, M.D., with permission) **D:** Phase-contrast microscopy of map dystrophy shows fibrous tissue (*asterisk*) between epithelium and Bowman's layer (B; paraphenylenediamine, ×1000). **E:** Phase-contrast microscopy of dot dystrophy shows an intraepithelial pseudocyst evolving from the disintegration of desquamating cells (paraphenylenediamine, ×1200). **F:** Phase-contrast photomicrograph of fingerprint dystrophy illustrates intraepithelial extensions of abnormal fibrocellular material anterior to the normal-appearing Bowman's layer (B; paraphenylenediamine, ×800). **G:** Transmission electron micrograph of these disorders consistently shows multiple laminations of basement membrane material (*asterisks*) with reduced hemidesmosomes (*small circle*) and increased anchoring fibrils (*large circle*) beneath the epithelium (E; ×40,000). Diabetes mellitus: **H:** Trophic-appearing epithelial defect in a diabetic patient after vitreous surgery. **I:** Phase-contrast photomicrograph of nonadherent epithelium removed during vitreous surgery reveals extensively thickened basement membrane material (*asterisk*) adherent to the intact epithelial layer (paraphenylenediamine, ×1000). **J:** Transmission electron micrograph of this specimen shows remarkable multilaminar configuration of the basement membrane (*asterisks*) with aberrant anchoring fibrils (*circled*) interspersed (compare with **G**; ×40,000).

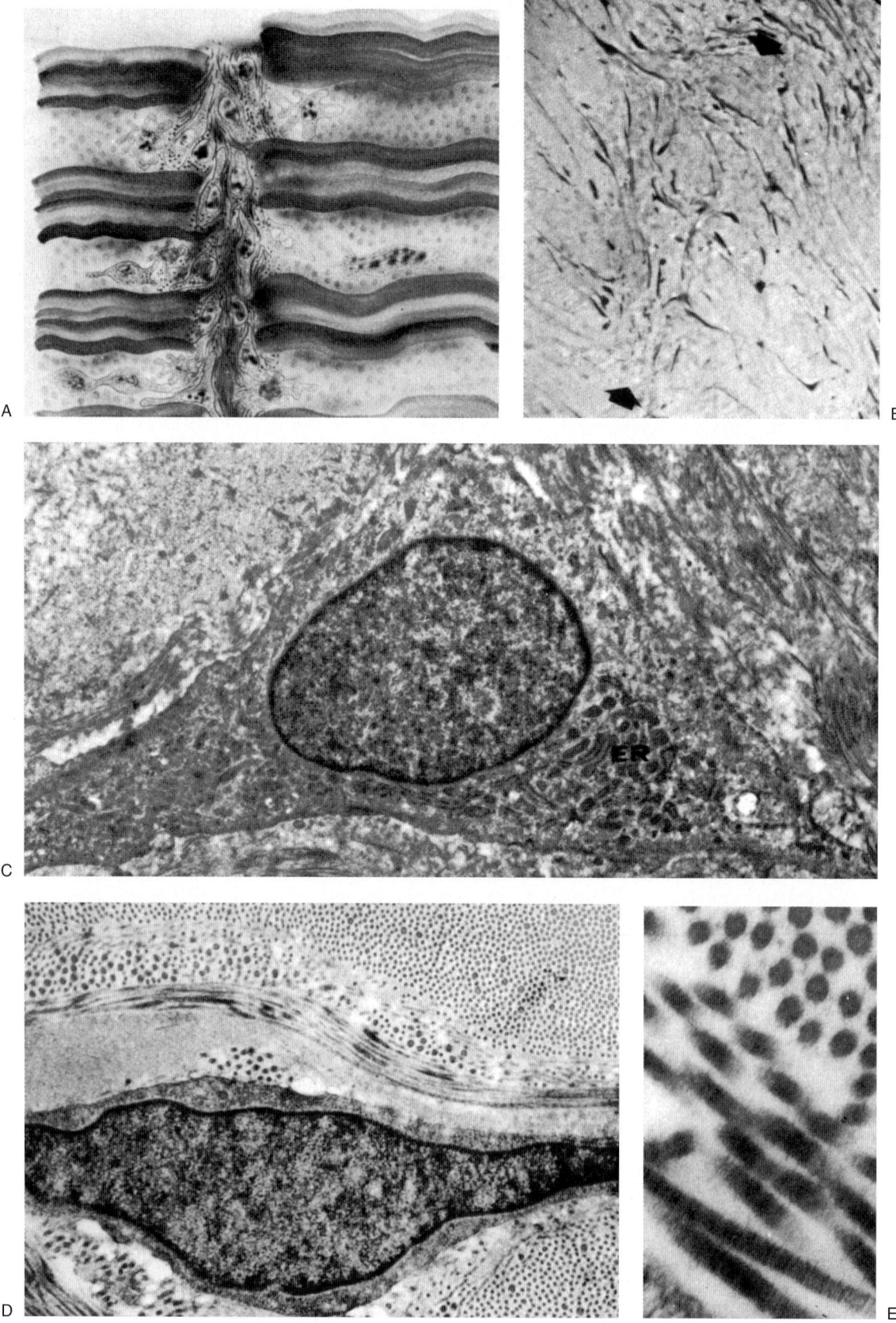

Although diabetic patients apparently do not experience an increased incidence of spontaneous epithelial erosions, vitreoretinal surgeons know that the diabetic corneal epithelium becomes clouded very early during surgery and often sloughs as an intact epithelial sheet. After surgery, these corneas are slow to reepithelialize, and persistent defects can develop in them (103). In nondiabetic humans and animals, corneal epithelial scraping results in rupture of basal cells with maintenance of basement membrane attached to Bowman's layer. In the diabetic cornea, on the other hand, the entire epithelium separates as an intact sheet, with the entire basement membrane remaining adherent to the basal cells (96). This observation suggests that a major component of this erosive disorder is the lack of adhesion between the basement membrane complex and the underlying stroma caused primarily by decreased penetration of the anchoring fibrils into the stroma.

Among secondary erosive disorders, stromal dystrophies of the cornea may also be clinically evident as surface problems, particularly in patients with lattice or granular dystrophy. Although lattice dystrophy, a dominantly inherited form of corneal amyloidosis, primarily involves the stroma, amyloid deposition also frequently occurs between the epithelium and Bowman's layer (104). The resultant irregularity of basement membrane complexes interferes with epithelial adhesion, and erosive episodes are frequently the initial visual symptom in the young patient with lattice dystrophy (Fig. 4-10A, B).

Although intraepithelial herpes simplex virus does not produce erosive problems, the corneal epithelium frequently does not adhere to the stroma in metaherpetic keratitis because of damage to basement membrane complexes and the anterior stroma (105). This may result from multiple recurrences of viral infection, from overly vigorous debridement using chemical cauterization, from toxic effects of antiviral drugs, or from collagenolytic enzymes. In metaherpetic keratitis, ultrastructural examination of debrided epithelium frequently discloses segmental basement membrane material remaining adherent to the cell along with other fine fibrillar debris (Fig. 4-10C, D). This finding again emphasizes the importance of the anterior stromal substrate in epithelial adhesion. Limited mechanical debridement of devitalized cellular and other remnants seems clinically appropriate as the means of providing a smooth substrate to which regenerating epithelium may better adhere.

KERATOCYTES AND STROMA

Normal Wound Healing

After penetrating injury of the stroma, keratocytes immediately adjacent to the wound margin are killed, and the defect soon fills with a fibrin clot (Fig. 4-11). The stromal lamellae become edematous, and the adjacent keratocytes withdraw their cytoplasmic processes (106). Within 2 hours, these cells increase their RNA content and endoplasmic reticulum cisternae, and they begin protein synthesis (107). Neutrophils appear in the wound within 2 to 6 hours and engage in the proteolytic debridement of necrotic cellular and extracellular debris. By 24 hours, DNA synthesis by the keratocytes is at a maximum. Within 3 days after wounding, these reactive keratocytes have reached the wound edge, are lined up parallel with the wound margins, and are secreting collagens, predominantly type II, plus glycosaminoglycans, particularly keratan sulfate (108–110). The first neutrophils reaching the stromal wound come from the limbal vasculature through the tear film; additional neutrophils reach the wound by migration through the stroma.

By the end of the first week, fibroblasts and neutrophils have invaded the fibrin plug. With increasing deposition of collagen, the tensile strength of the wound slowly improves. This collagen is randomly organized, large-diameter, extracellular fibrillar collagen. Subsequent wound healing largely involves additional collagen secretion. By the end of 8 weeks, there are virtually no inflammatory cellular components, but rather only numerous fibroblastic cells.

FIGURE 4-11. Normal stromal wound healing. **A:** Diagram of stroma 2 to 8 days after a penetrating wound. The transformation of fibrocytes into fibroblasts continues until day 6. Fibroblasts and neutrophils invade the fibrin plug. The fibroblasts continue to produce primitive collagen and glycosaminoglycan. Mononuclear cells that have migrated through the stroma from the limbus arrive at the wound and are transformed into macrophages. Fibroblasts adjacent to the wound are actively dividing. (From Binder PS, et al., Corneal anatomy and wound healing. In: *Transactions of the New Orleans Academy of Ophthalmology.* St. Louis: Mosby, 1980:1–35, with permission.) **B:** Phase-contrast photomicrograph of human cornea 1 year after perforating injury shows hypercellularity of the wound area with fibroblasts aligned along the wound axis (*arrows*; paraphenylenediamine, ×500). **C:** Transmission electron micrograph of the area shown in **B** depicts reactive keratocytes with extensive endoplasmic reticulum cisternae (ER). The extracellular collagen is markedly disarrayed (×9000). **D:** Transmission electron micrograph of stromal scar appearing several years after alkali injury shows collagen fibers with an abnormally large diameter. Amorphous granular material is adjacent to a quiescent-appearing keratocyte (×8000). **E:** Transmission electron micrograph at higher magnification resolves individual collagen fibrils of normal longitudinal macroperiodicity but with cross-sectional diameters more than twice normal (×80,000).

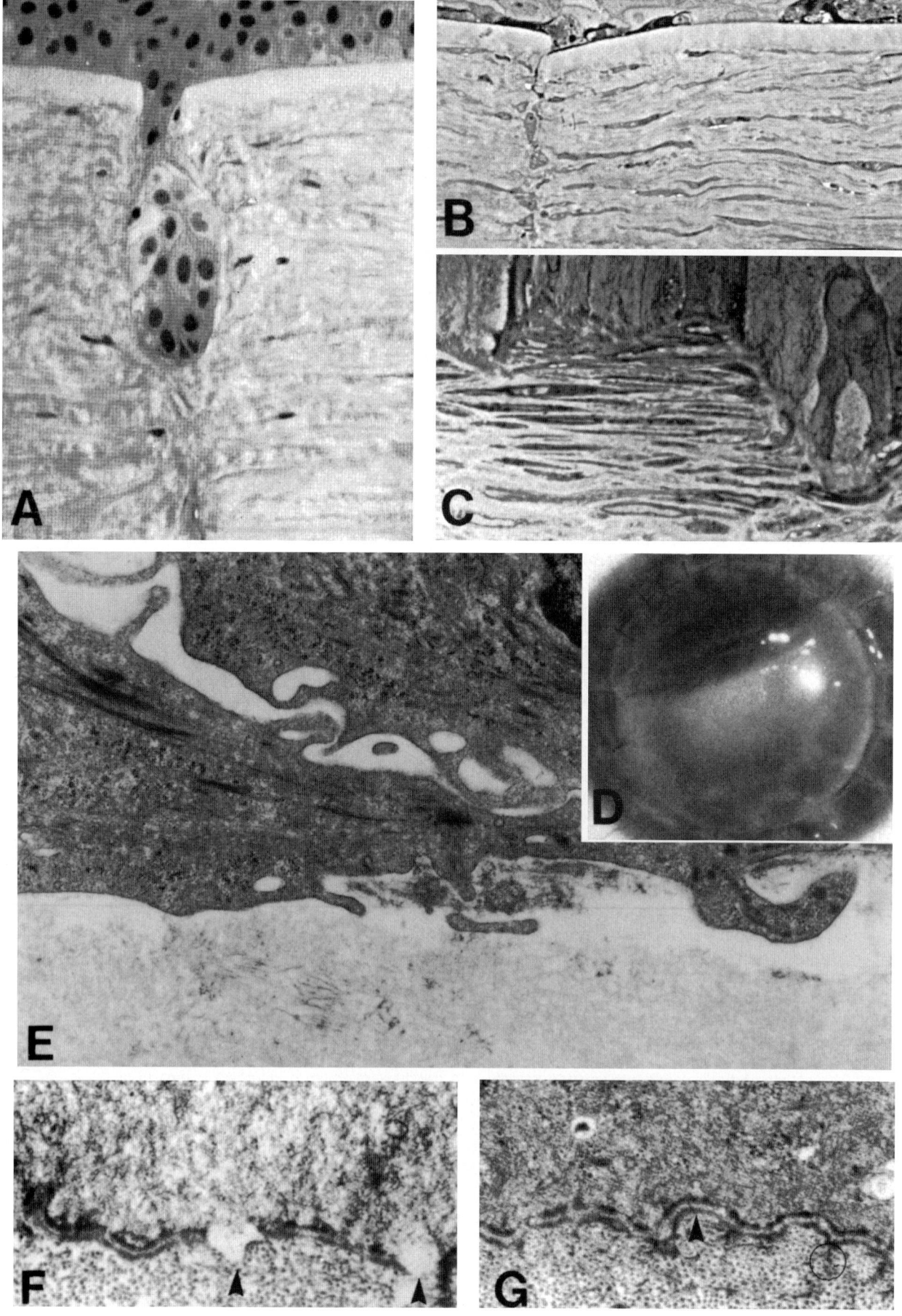

The wound strength continues to increase for 3 to 6 months. Cintron and coworkers (111) found that after injury, the adult rabbit cornea produces structural macromolecules and collagen cross-links similar to those in the developing cornea. Although the scar tissue becomes more compact and eventually blends into the adjacent stroma, uniformity of fibrillar organization is never restored; however, the pattern of macromolecules and cross-links becomes more similar to that in normal transparent tissue (112). Numerous factors and molecules have been identified as promoters or regulators of stromal and epithelial healing (113). Factors such as keratinocyte growth factor, hepatocyte growth factor, IL-1, and the Fas/Fas ligand system appear to offer the potential to regulate corneal wound healing and possibly to treat corneal diseases (113).

Response to Refractive Surgical Procedures

In the many new surgical procedures designed to alter corneal curvature and thereby correct refractive power, the corneal epithelial cells and their adhesion structures as well as Bowman's layer and the anterior stroma are disrupted. Hence, the reassembly of these structures and therapeutic efforts to modulate the reparative process represent clinically relevant variations of the wound healing response. Histopathologic studies of human epikeratoplasty lenticules removed after surgery because of suboptimal optical results have shown near-normal reformation of basement membrane and hemidesmosomes as early as 10 weeks, although in some specimens hemidesmosome and basement membrane irregularities persisted (114). In patients exhibiting delayed or arrested reepithelialization, folds and interruptions of Bowman's layer were found in the lenticules (115–117) or in the patient's excised cornea (118,119). In the extreme, such persistent epithelial abnormalities and defects can lead to sterile proteolytic degradation of the epikeratoplasty lenticules and even recipient stroma (120). Studies in rabbits have shown that in epikeratoplasty, the processes of reepithelialization, recovery of epithelial thickness, formation of differentiated desmosomes or hemidesmosomes, and normalization of ultrastructural abnormalities take longer than reepithelialization of usual epithelial defects (121). This may explain the reason for the chronic epithelial defects or failure of reepithelialization in epikeratoplasty. Similar alterations in keratomileusis lenticules (115,118) further support the importance of the integrity of epithelial cell adhesion (Fig. 4-12).

Animal studies have shown that healing of corneal incisions by wound fibrosis in radial keratotomy is effected by the transformation of adjacent keratocytes to contractile myofibroblasts (122,123) with consequent stromal wound contraction. A further consistent finding is the appearance of abnormal epithelial basement membrane synthesis, including both discontinuities and duplication over areas of extensive fibrosis (124). These findings are also consistent with previous histopathologic findings of delayed wound healing after radial keratotomy (122,124). Wound healing events after astigmatic keratotomy procedures appear similar to those in radial keratotomy, with the exception that tangential incisions appear to heal faster than radial incisions (125).

The excimer laser, which uses ultraviolet radiation (argon fluoride, 193 nm), is applicable to both photorefractive and phototherapeutic keratectomy. Although some studies have demonstrated that the healing response of the cornea after use of the excimer laser appears generally similar to that after incisional radial keratotomy (126,127), the wound healing process after excimer photoablation is characterized by reepithelialization within 24 to 48 hours, followed by subepithelial synthesis of new collagen fibrils, reorganization of the epithelium, and then hyperplasia of the reactive keratocytes with incipient reorganization of the collagen fibrils and an increase in biomicroscopically visible subepithelial haze that decreases after 6 months (128). By 8 months, corneal morphology is near normal except for the absence of Bowman's layer with disorder in the immediate subepithelial stromal fibers and variation of the regenerated basement membrane (129). After 6 to 15 months, the epithelium is thickened, Bowman's layer remains absent, and superficial stromal scarring has developed in the area of ablation (130). Ultrastructural studies have confirmed a reduction in the number of epithelial hemidesmosomes after photoablation, but this does not

FIGURE 4-12. Response to refractive surgical procedures. **A:** In a human cornea after radial keratotomy, phase-contrast microscopy demonstrates intrastromal epithelial cyst. Keratocytes surround the incision (paraphenylenediamine, ×300). **B:** Stromal scar after radial keratotomy. Bowman's layer is visibly disrupted (paraphenylenediamine, ×300). **C:** Phase-contrast microscopy of keratomileusis *in situ* specimen demonstrates extensive irregularity of the epithelial-stroma interface devoid of Bowman's layer, with remarkably reactive proliferation of fibroblastic cells and scar tissue (paraphenylenediamine, ×1000). **D:** Clinical appearance of stromal ulceration beneath persistent area of epithelial defect after epikeratophakia. **E:** Transmission electron microscopy of the epikeratophakia lenticule shows a dysplastic epithelium with complete absence of basement membrane and hemidesmosomes (×18,700). **F:** Transmission electron microscopy of human corneal specimen 6 months after excimer laser keratectomy exhibits a discontinuous basement membrane (*arrowheads*; ×31,200). **G:** Fifteen months after excimer laser keratectomy, the appearance of the basement membrane (*arrowhead*) and anchoring fibrils (*circled*) is normal (×31,200). (**F, G** courtesy Dimitri T. Azar, M.D., with permission.)

seem to compromise epithelial–stromal adhesion because there are only rare reports of corneal epithelial defects after laser keratectomy. Use of the excimer laser for anterior keratomileusis similarly is associated with a minimal healing response, but with alterations that persisted for 18 months after surgery (131).

Recent studies demonstrate that stromal injury induces activation and transformation of corneal keratocytes to myofibroblasts, which then regulate the deposition and organization of extracellular matrix in corneal wounds. Such myofibroblasts might be crucial in establishing an interconnected meshwork of cells with an extracellular matrix that deposits new matrix and contracts wounds using a novel and unexpected "shoestring-like" mechanism. The transformation of keratocytes into myofibroblasts has been studied in culture, as promoted by TGF-β and blocked *in vivo* by antibodies to TGF-β. Most important, the appearance of myofibroblasts in corneal wounds is associated with wound contraction and regression after incisional keratotomy, promoting in this way the development of the corneal "haze" or increased light scattering after laser photorefractive keratectomy. In contrast, the absence of myofibroblasts is often associated with continued widening of wound defect and progressive corneal flattening after incisional procedures. Based on these observations, the importance of further study of the complex molecular biology of this cell type is evident (132).

Specific Pathologic Reactions

Inflammation

The classic experiments of Cohnheim first provided the initial pathologic description of the recruitment of leukocytes from limbal vasculature into inflammatory corneal stromal lesions (133). From these observations evolved the general recognition of several aspects of the inflammatory response. As with other tissues, even corneal inflammation is a nonspecific result of tissue damage, whatever the cause. Corneal tissues, for example, can be directly damaged by foreign bodies and chemical or thermal burns. Among the several agents that can elicit an inflammatory response in the cornea, the two most common are microbial infections (bacterial, viral, parasitic, or fungal) and various immunologic conditions (134). Antigens initiate the immune response, with B and T lymphocytes responsible for antibody and cytotoxic components, respectively. Two other components are macrophages, which have an important role in processing antigens, and neutrophils, whose proteolytic enzymes have extensive destructive potential.

Vascularization

Neovascularization of the cornea is a sequela of numerous inflammatory diseases of the ocular anterior segment,

including trachoma, luetic and viral interstitial keratitis, microbial keratoconjunctivitis, and the immune reaction elicited by corneal transplantation.

This response is also caused by various noxious stimuli, including the application of alloxan, thermal and chemical cautery, and intrastromal implantation of tumor angiogenesis factor. The well-known sequence of limbal capillary and venule dilation is followed by diapedesis of leukocytes into the stroma with extravasation of fibrin and other serum proteins (Fig. 4-13). Subsequent vascular endothelial migration and proliferation occur in a pattern suggestive of directed growth toward the neovascular stimulus, possibly caused by a substance diffusing from the point of injury.

Although early studies incorrectly related the ingrowth of new blood vessels to stromal edema, Fromer and Klintworth observed that stromal neovascularization was preceded by inflammation, and postulated that the neutrophils producing a growth-stimulating substance were responsible for vascular proliferation (135,136). Further, they showed that neovascularization of the cornea did not develop in leukopenic rats after silver nitrate burns. However, Eliason reported corneal vascularization resulting from chemical cautery in leukopenic rats and suggested that the regenerating corneal epithelium was the source of vasostimulating substances (137). Sholley and associates similarly showed that corneal neovascularization in leukopenic rats does occur after thermal cautery, albeit at a slower rate than in non-leukopenic controls (138). Folkman and colleagues found the basement membranes of bovine corneas to contain an angiogenic endothelial cell mitogen, basic FGF (b-FGF) (139), whereas Adamis and coworkers further suggested that uninjured corneal epithelium contains b-FGF and that one mechanism for the release of the growth factor is passive leakage after the cell injury with secondary binding to heparan sulfate proteoglycan in Bowman's layer (140). Thus, stromal inflammation appears to provide a sufficient but not altogether necessary stimulus for new blood vessel formation.

Other investigators have attempted to alter or inhibit the ingrowth of new blood vessels by various agents. For example, intracorneal implantation of tumor angiogenesis factor, biogenic amines, ACh, prostaglandin E$_1$, histamine, serotonin, bradykinin, endotoxin (*Escherichia coli* lipopolysaccharide), and IL-1 has been shown to induce new blood vessel growth in the cornea (141–147). The role of prostaglandins in the sequence of neovascularization is further suggested by Deutsch and Hughes (148), who showed that topical indomethacin suppresses neovascularization after thermal cautery and that this suppression is associated with a decreased number of neutrophils. IL-2, which is known to stimulate vascular endothelial cells *in vitro*, is one of the potential agents in immune-mediated corneal neovascularization (149) that can be inhibited by cyclosporine (150). Inhibition of corneal

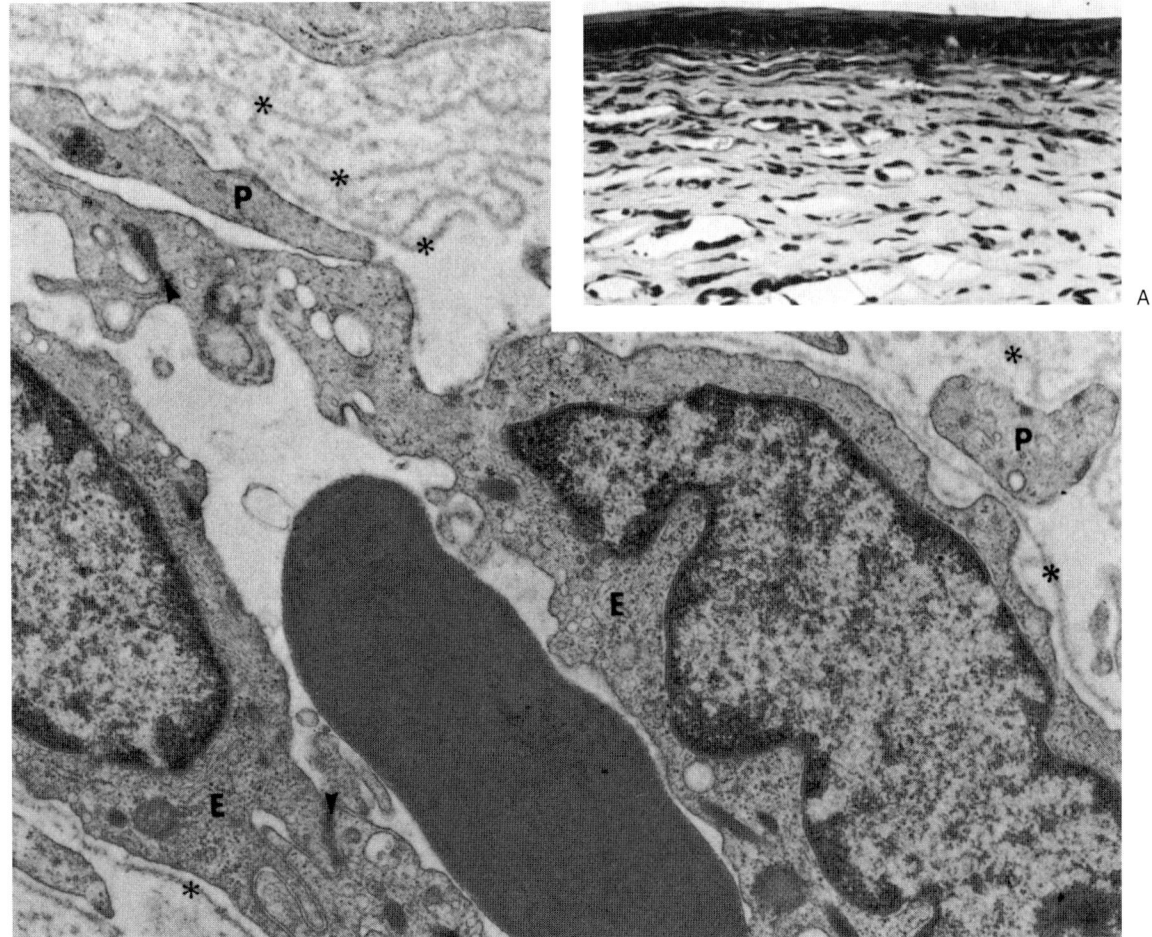

FIGURE 4-13. Stromal vascularization. **A:** Light photomicrograph of peripheral rabbit cornea 2 months after mild chemical injury shows hypercellular stroma with a few chronic inflammatory cells and numerous small-diameter blood vessels (hematoxylin-eosin, ×250). **B:** Transmission electron micrograph of the corresponding area demonstrates stromal vessels comprising mature-appearing endothelial cells (E) with well-developed intracellular junctions (*arrowheads*). Cytoplasmic processes of pericytes (P) are seen adjacent to the epithelium, and multiple laminations of basement material (*asterisks*) envelop both cell types. An erythrocyte is evident in the capillary lumen (×14,000).

vascularization was reported by Keutner and associates (151), who observed a proteinase inhibitor activity in the cornea, aorta, and cartilage. This led others to show that purified extract of bovine aorta or cartilage injected subconjunctivally inhibited neovascularization of the cornea after chemical cautery (152). Hydrocortisone administered together with heparin or betacyclodextrin tetradecasulfate has been noted to produce an antiangiogenic effect against endotoxin-induced corneal vascularization in rabbits (153).

Laser photocoagulation has been used with limited success to treat corneal neovascularization. Argon laser photocoagulation has been used to treat neovascularization experimentally (154–158), and in patients with lipid keratopathy and after penetrating keratoplasty (159,160). A 577-nm yellow-dye laser showed relative success in similar clinical circumstances (161); however, in patients with

neovascularization before keratoplasty, the change in vascular activity was insignificant. As laser technology continues to develop, laser photocoagulation could prove a useful adjunct in the treatment of corneal neovascularization in selected patients.

Interesting observations on corneal lymphangiogenesis point out the importance of certain molecules, including the lymphatic endothelial markers, vascular endothelial growth factor receptor-3, LYVE-1 (a lymphatic endothelium-specific hyaluronan receptor), Prox 1, and podoplanin, all of which are key actors in the phenomena of angiogenesis (162).

Scarring

Corneal scarring frequently is a consequence of external factors, including infectious diseases (e.g., trachoma), penetrating corneal injuries, and other cicatricial diseases (e.g., pemphigoid and erythema multiforme). As fibroblasts in the corneal and conjunctival tissues proliferate and elaborate collagens, their productive potential is greatly enhanced by the presence of inflammatory cells. The interaction and unfortunate synergism of primary inflammatory reactions and coincident bacterial infection are also known to enhance the cicatricial process.

Stromal transparency has been hypothesized to require two factors: individual stromal collagen fibers must be of small uniform diameter (approximately 240 Å), and the distances between adjacent fibrils must be less than half the wavelength of visible light (approximately 2,000 Å) so that fluctuations in the refractive index do not result in light scattering (163). Stromal scarring disturbs these important parameters in both respects because the collagen fibrils that are produced vary markedly in cross-sectional diameter, from 200 to 1,200 Å, and never become organized into the lattice-like array with elements less than 2,000 Å apart that is characteristic of normal lamellar architecture. Stromal scar tissue differs from normal cornea in containing unusually large chondroitin sulfate proteoglycans with glycosaminoglycan side chains of normal size, and it is thought that corneal stromal proteoglycans may be important determinants of collagen fibril spatial arrangement (164). Studies in rabbits showed that healing adult cornea partially recapitulates the chemical and cytochemical properties of proteoglycans in normal developing cornea (165). In contrast, in any condition causing stromal edema alone (e.g., compromised endothelial function), loss of stromal transparency occurs as the spaces among collagen fibrils become distended by fluid. No change, however, occurs in the individual fibril dimensions, and hence when the edema subsides, stromal transparency is restored, with return of the normal interfibrillar spatial relationships.

Ulceration

The development of corneal ulceration can be a disastrous sequela to bacterial, viral, or fungal infection, the concomitant of a systemic dermatologic or connective tissue disease, or the result of chemical or thermal injury (Figs. 4-14 and 4-15). Even if bacterial toxins themselves are not directly capable of collagenolytic activity, *Pseudomonas* species do produce a protease capable of glycosaminoglycan destruction (166). Thus, it is likely that host cellular responses, particularly those of acute inflammation, are responsible for corneal destruction in most infectious and sterile injuries. Indeed, the pathogenesis of noninfectious stromal ulceration, or "melting," is of particular concern because it is a frequent complication of chemical injury, herpetic keratitis, collagen vascular diseases, and nutritional deficiency (167).

Independent of the cause, stromal melting is almost invariably preceded by a corneal epithelial defect and appears to be associated with an inappropriate inflammatory response. As Berman stated (51), "Why the cornea ulcerates might be related to the trapping of wound healing in a phase of proteolytic debridement related to a persistent epithelial defect." Such ulceration is known to be secondary to the action of tissue collagenases, which perform the initial cleavage of stromal collagen fibrils, with further degradation of collagen and glycosaminoglycans involving proteases, peptidases, and cathepsins. The initiation of tissue collagen breakdown can potentially be controlled at the levels of collagenase concentration and activity by cellular and humoral activators and inhibitors (168) (Fig. 4-16).

The cellular constituents responsible for ulceration and their interactions are subjects of extensive research interest. Although substantial evidence has implicated the actions and interactions of injured corneal epithelium and keratocytes, other pathologic and experimental studies have emphasized the role of acute inflammatory cells, particularly neutrophils. These cells contain more than a dozen lytic enzymes (including collagenase, elastase, and cathepsin) in their primary lysosomes and are ubiquitous at the site of active ulceration and in the tear film of melting corneas (96). In herpes simplex interstitial keratitis, for example, current pathogenetic concepts implicate immune system efforts aimed at destroying stromal cells that have acquired herpes antigens, thereby resulting in an influx of neutrophils and phagocytes, which are effectors of tissue destruction.

On the reparative side, keratocytes and blood vessels are essential. Reactive fibroblasts with dilated cisternae of rough endoplasmic reticulum participate in the secretion of new collagen for wound healing, although their presence in the central ulcerative areas is somewhat delayed. Equally apparent from cell culture, however, is that such fibroblasts can simultaneously synthesize both collagen and collagenase, thereby allowing the same cells to participate both in ulceration and repair. Conn and coworkers demonstrated the ability of stromal neovascularization to inhibit ulceration; corneas prevascularized by tumor angiogenesis factor were less likely to ulcerate after experimental thermal burns (169). It is likely that both serum antiproteases (e.g., α_2-macroglobulin) and nutrients (including ascorbate) are delivered by vessels to the ulcerated area. Tissue adhesives used to strengthen or seal ulcerating and perforated corneas appear to decrease the number of inflammatory cells in the surrounding corneal stroma. It has been demonstrated that the application of tissue adhesive to sterile ulcers arrests further stromal loss in the same manner as does the glued-on hard contact lens, that is, by the exclusion of acute inflammatory cells from the involved stroma (170). This effect is undoubtedly due partly to denying neutrophils from the tears access to the ulcer site. The adhesive may also interrupt the further chemotaxis of intrastromal or tear-borne inflammatory cells. These findings have therefore prompted the earlier application of adhesive in either progressive stromal ulceration

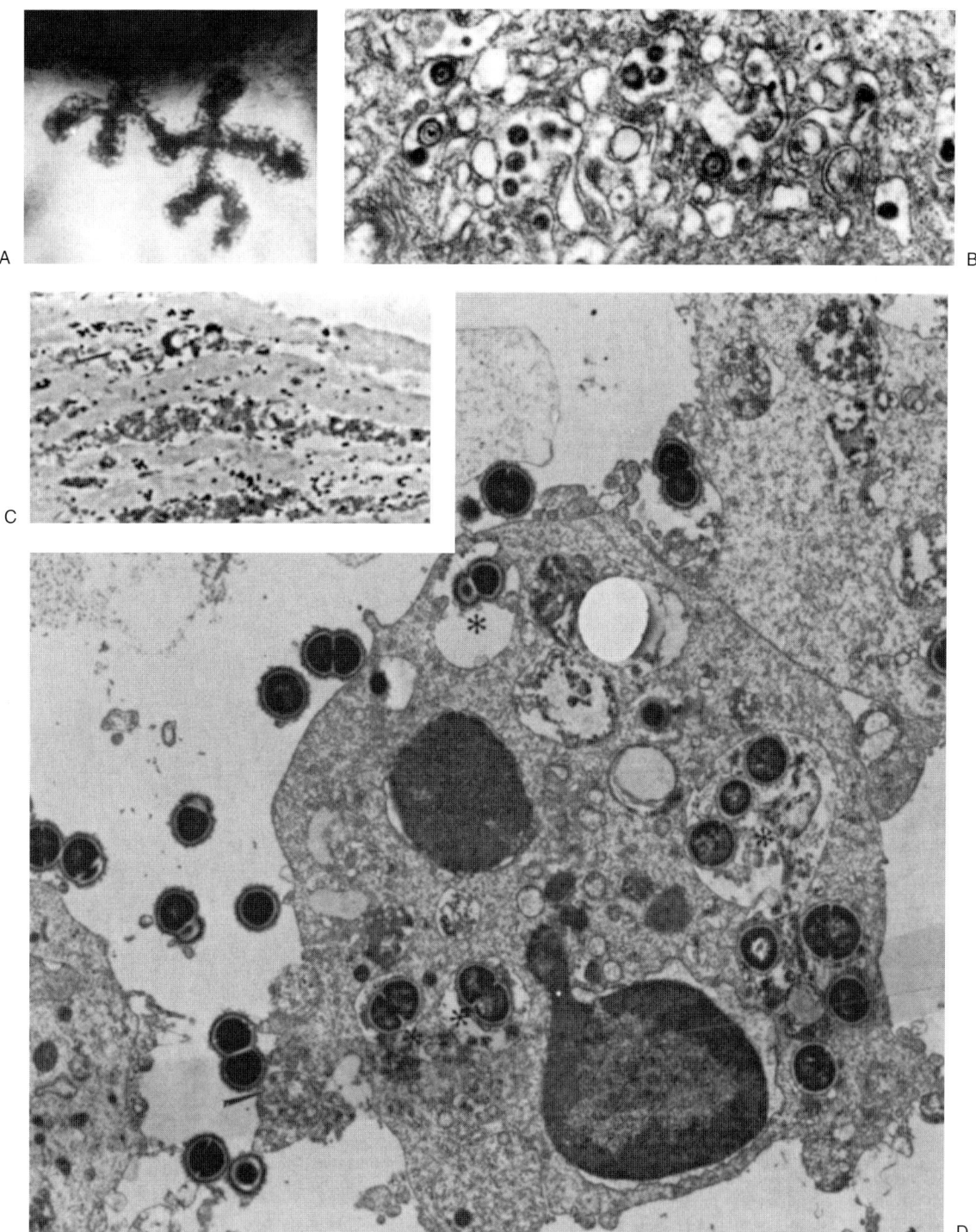

FIGURE 4-14. Infectious ulceration. **A:** Slit-lamp photograph with rose bengal staining shows a dendritic figure with balloon swelling of marginal epithelial cells in intraepithelial herpes simplex. (Courtesy of L. Hirst, M.D., with permission) **B:** Transmission electron micrograph of debrided epithelial cells shows numerous virus particles consisting of DNA-containing nucleoid surrounded by protein capsid (×30,000). **C:** Phase-contrast photomicrograph of bacterial corneal ulceration shows separation of disorganized stromal lamellae by inflammatory cell debris interspersed with a myriad of bacterial forms (paraphenylenediamine, ×700). **D:** Transmission electron micrograph of corresponding area shows a polymorphonuclear leukocyte containing several phagosomes (*asterisks*) with bacteria and extracellular debris content. The cell has discharged most of its primarily lysosomal granules. Extracellularly, many other diplococcal bacterial profiles are evident (×13,000).

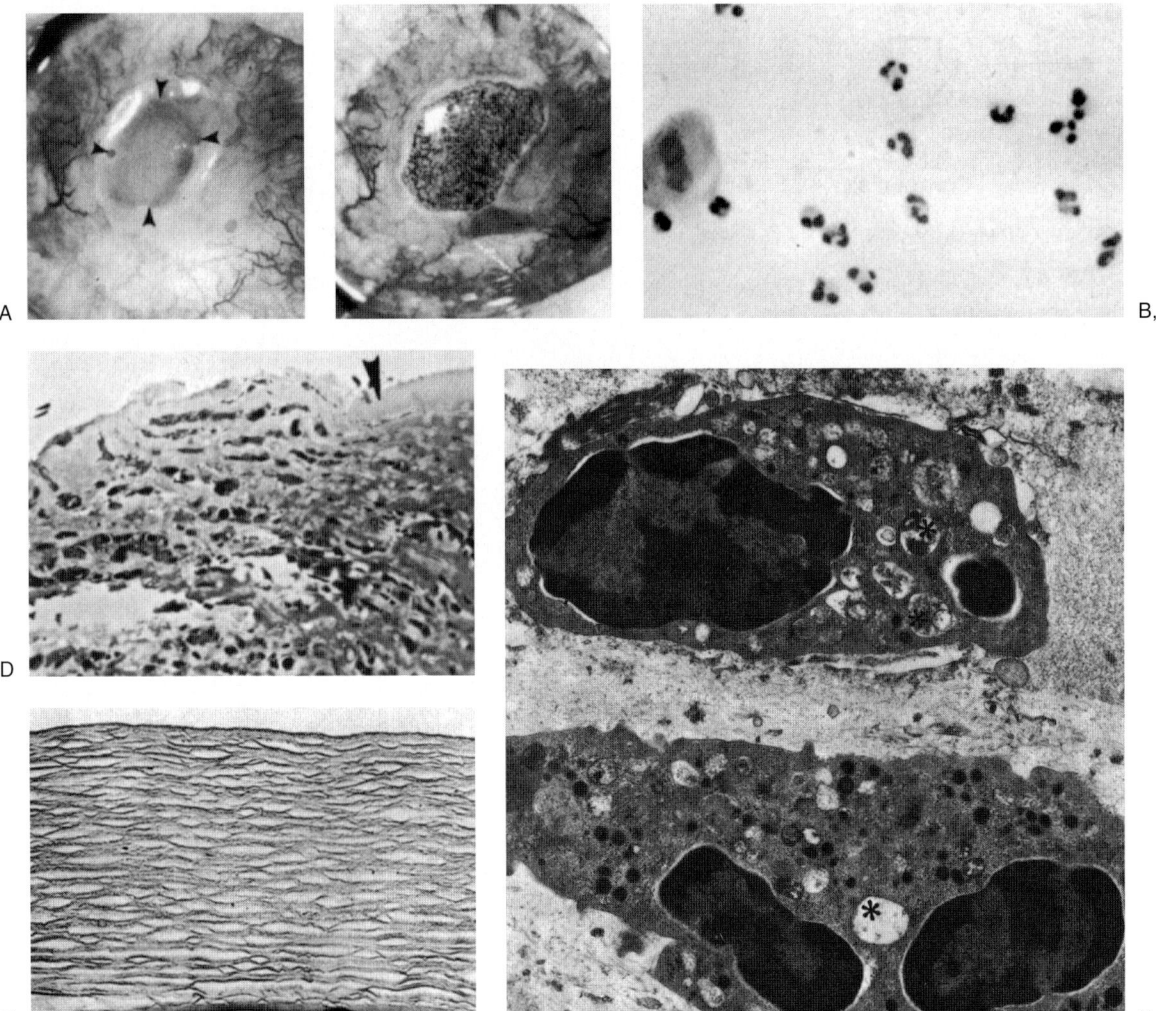

FIGURE 4-15. Noninfectious ulceration. **A:** In a patient with erythema multiforme who had undergone multiple penetrating keratoplasties, a central epithelial defect developed with extensive stromal melting to a descemetocele (*arrowheads*). **B:** Treatment of this eye with cyanoacrylate tissue adhesive and therapeutic soft contact lens resulted in arrest of the ulceration and stabilization of the cornea. **C:** Tear samples taken from the descemetocele disclosed numerous polymorphonuclear leukocytes (Giemsa, ×1000). **D:** In a patient with a severe alkali burn, two penetrating keratoplasties succumbed to sterile stromal melting. As shown by phase-contrast microscopy, the actively ulcerating stroma contained numerous polymorphonuclear leukocytes. Note termination of Bowman's layer at the *arrowhead* (paraphenylenediamine, ×450). **E:** Transmission electron micrograph of the stromal areas shown in **D** demonstrates polymorphonuclear leukocytes appearing actively engaged in degranulation and phagocytosis (*asterisks*), indicating their involvement in the degradation of the melting stroma (×9000). **F:** The effect of cyanoacrylate tissue adhesive is shown in the alkali-burned rabbit cornea several weeks after injury. The cornea has not undergone stromal degradation and maintains stromal acellularity after application of a glued-on contact lens (×100).

or impending perforation; the adhesive is easily applied at slit-lamp examination (171).

Although tetracycline has been shown to inhibit angiogenesis and collagenase activity in animal studies (172,173), the ideal pharmacologic agent for the treatment of sterile ulceration will have to be specific to the regulatory pathways favorable to repair, while at the same time controlling collagenase synthesis, activation, inhibition, and activity (168).

ENDOTHELIUM AND DESCEMET'S MEMBRANE

Normal Wound Healing

Because maintaining the continuity of the endothelial cell monolayer is critical to stromal deturgescence and hence optical clarity, endothelial repair processes after a variety of inflammatory and mechanical insults are of great clinical concern. Immediately after a posterior corneal wound, the cut edges of

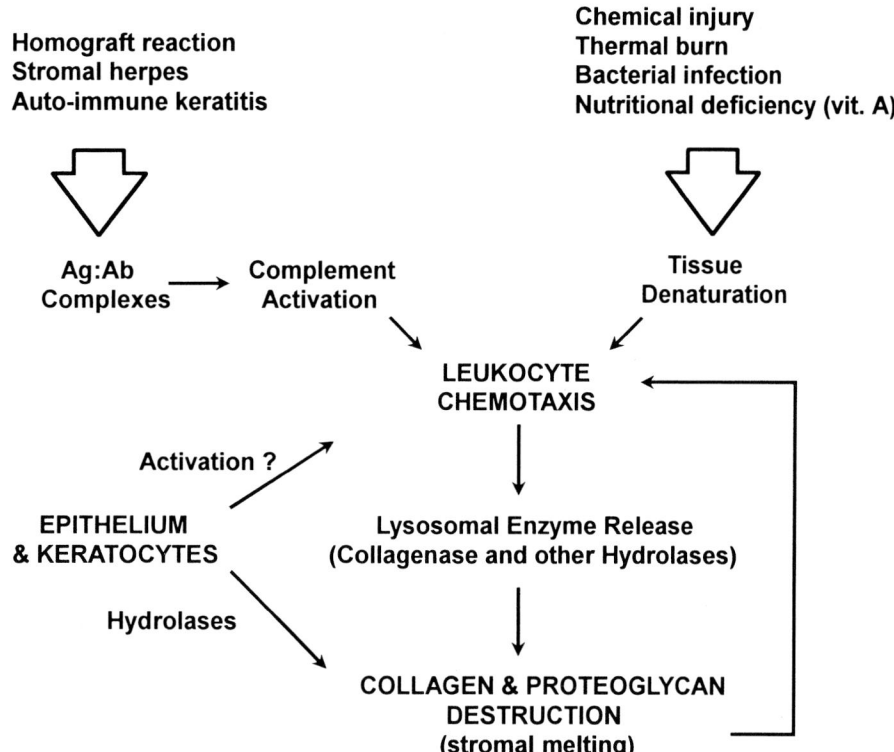

FIGURE 4-16. Pathogenesis of noninfected corneal ulceration. Immunologic mechanisms and direct tissue injury lead to chemotaxis of acute inflammatory cells. These inflammatory cells release proteolytic enzymes that digest stromal collagen and proteoglycans. Tissue destruction is itself chemotactic for the recruitment of additional inflammatory cells. Corneal epithelial cells and keratocytes may be directly involved in enzyme secretion and serve as activators of inflammatory cells. Ag:Ab, antigen–antibody.

Descemet's membrane retract and curl anteriorly toward the stroma (Fig. 4-17A–D). Adjacent endothelial cells are lost, and a fibrin clot is formed in the wound. Within hours, adjoining endothelial cells attenuate with extensive cytoplasmic processes and migrate into the wound (164,174,175). In the adult human, virtually the entire healing effort occurs by means of cellular reorganization, enlargement, and migration to reconstitute an intact monolayer, despite the evidences for mitosis (165). In rabbits, the endothelium is capable of mitotic division; in cats and primates, the mitotic capabilities of the endothelium are limited. After exposure to a variety of physical and chemical insults, the human corneal endothelium can repair itself either by limited mitotic division or by simple expansion and spreading of neighboring cells, or through an elaborate DNA repair system (176–183).

Depending on the size of the wound, the entire defect can be re-covered within 1 or more weeks. Extracellular matrix glycoproteins, EGF, and actin appear to be important in regulating the growth and formation of the corneal endothelium *in vivo* (184–186). Once Descemet's membrane has been resurfaced by a continuous endothelial monolayer, the cells become contact-inhibited and form contiguous cellular junctions. The cells that have been involved in the healing process are now much larger than those in uninvolved areas. Once the integrity of the endothelial cell layer has been restored, its pump and barrier functions soon begin to stabilize, as evidenced by stromal deturgescence, thinning, and increasing clarity.

As part of the wound healing response, and indeed as a nonspecific response to any form of endothelial trauma, the regenerating endothelium deposits new layers of Descemet's membrane material (187). This is clearly evident, for example, in keratoconus cases with acute hydrops, as the migrating endothelium that resurfaces the exposed posterior stroma secretes new Descemet's membrane (188) (Fig. 4-17E, F). Where the wound is well apposed, a single endothelial layer appears and functions normally. Where there is poor wound apposition, endothelial cells are multi-layered and undergo a fibroblastic transformation that results in posterior collagen layers comprising fibrillar banded collagen, basement membrane material, and fine filaments. In time, these cells also appear capable of reverting to a more normal endothelial morphology. However, the chronology of posterior wound healing is prolonged—months to years may be required for transformation into endothelium with new Descemet's membrane of normal morphology and thickness. As in other tissues, FGF and TGF-β1 have recently been described as key molecules

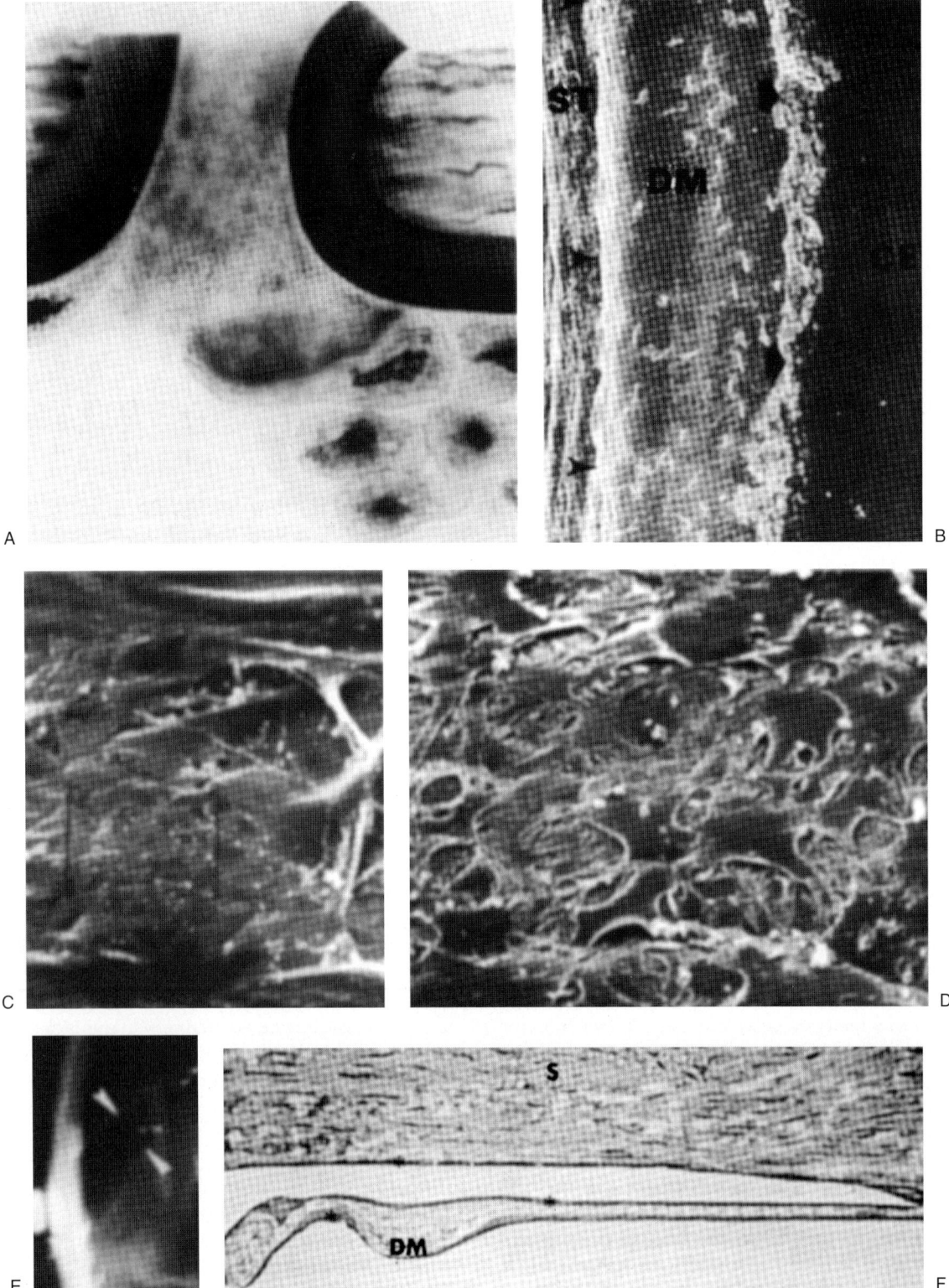

able to modulate the endothelial response to wounds and promote an efficient endothelial healing (189).

Dysgenesis: Peters' Anomaly and Congenital Hereditary Endothelial Dystrophy

Mesenchymal dysgeneses of the cornea are a spectrum of developmental disorders of the corneogenic mesenchyme, including posterior keratoconus, posterior central corneal opacity (Peters' anomaly), congenital hereditary endothelial dystrophy (CHED), sclerocornea, and the iridocorneal endothelial (ICE) syndromes (190).

Peters' anomaly is correctly described as a congenital central corneal opacity with corresponding defects in the posterior stroma, Descemet's membrane, and endothelium. In addition, strands of iris tissue frequently extend to the posterior border of the corneal leukoma, and central keratolenticular adherence sometimes occurs with shallowing of the anterior chamber. The peripheral cornea is usually clear but may be partially scleralized. Histopathologic changes are present in all layers of the cornea (Fig. 4-18A–E). Fibronectin, laminin, and collagen types I, IV, V, and VI have been detected in keratoplasty specimens from patients with Peters' anomaly with enhanced fibronectin staining, suggesting that this protein plays a role in the developmental process (191). Anterior changes, including disorganization of epithelium, pannus, and loss of Bowman's layer, are probably secondary to the primary posterior abnormalities. The stroma is edematous in the affected region; ultrastructural studies of stromal collagen have disclosed fibrils as large as 600 Å. In peripheral, unaffected areas, the endothelium is continuous, and Descemet's membrane is of normal uniform thickness. In the area of the defect, however, endothelium and Descemet's membrane can terminate abruptly or be severely attenuated. The lens may be involved, which suggests a primary incomplete separation of the lens vesicle or a secondary anterior displacement of normally developed lens causing apposition between the lens and the cornea. Etiologically, although there may be multiple causes of this clinical entity, incomplete central migration of mesenchymal cells destined to become keratocytes and endothelium probably accounts for concurrent posterior stromal and endothelial defects (192,193).

CHED is another dysgenesis appropriate for comparison with Peters' anomaly; this disorder is characterized clinically by diffuse, bilaterally symmetric corneal edema in the presence of normal intraocular pressure. The degree of edematous corneal clouding varies from a mild haze to a milky, ground-glass opacification (Fig. 4-18F–H). Histologic study reveals anterior and stromal changes consistent with long-standing secondary edema.

It may be important that in some cases greatly enlarged stromal collagen fibrils are evident ultrastructurally. Descemet's membrane is uniform, with no evidence of guttae. Although the thickness of Descemet's membrane is always uniform in a given specimen, it may range from less than 3 μm to more than 40 μm. In eyes with a thin Descemet's membrane, it appears that complete endothelial loss occurred *in utero*, so that only the fetal anterior portion of Descemet's membrane was secreted (194). In contrast, thickened Descemet's membrane is the result of dystrophic but persistent endothelium having secreted a hypertrophic collagen layer. With the exception of the lack of guttae, these Descemet's membrane findings are similar to those in adult endothelial dystrophy (Fuchs') and thus represent another example of posterior collagenous layer formation by either primarily or secondarily abnormal endothelium (191).

FIGURE 4-17. Endothelial wound healing. **A:** Diagram of endothelium 5 to 72 hours after wounding. The endothelial cells adjacent to the wound are flattened and begin to slide into the defect. As they do so, they take on fibroblast-like characteristics. The cut edges of Descemet's membrane retract and curl anteriorly. The wound is filled with fibrin and cell remnants. **B:** Scanning electron micrograph of posterior corneal surface after posterior trephination. The edge (*arrowheads*) of the cut stroma (ST) is some distance away from the edge (*arrows*) of the remaining endothelial cells (CE). The intervening area of bare Descemet's membrane (DM) shows endothelial debris (×130). (**A, B** from Binder PS, et al. Corneal anatomy and wound healing. In: *Transactions of the New Orleans Academy of Ophthalmology*. St. Louis: Mosby, 1980:1–35, with permission.) **C:** Scanning electron micrograph of posterior surface of human cornea 1 year after perforating injury shows areas of corrugated Descemet's membrane (*asterisk*) overlaid by fibrillar collagen strands. Distended and disorganized endothelial cells have recovered part of this surface (×100). **D:** Scanning electron micrograph of the area bracketed in **C** shows attenuated endothelial cells in multilayered configuration. These cells have extensive cytoplasmic processes interdigitating with the fibrillar posterior collagen layer (×500). **E:** In keratoconus with healed hydrops, a slit-lamp photograph reveals margins of Descemet's membrane rupture (*arrowheads*). **F:** Phase-contrast photomicrograph of posterior stroma in healed hydrops shows a ledge of Descemet's membrane (DM) with adherent collagen that has separated from the posterior stroma (S). Note that a continuous endothelial cell layer (*asterisks*) has migrated to resurface the anterior aspect of the ledge plus the entire denuded posterior surface of the stroma (paraphenylenediamine, ×250).

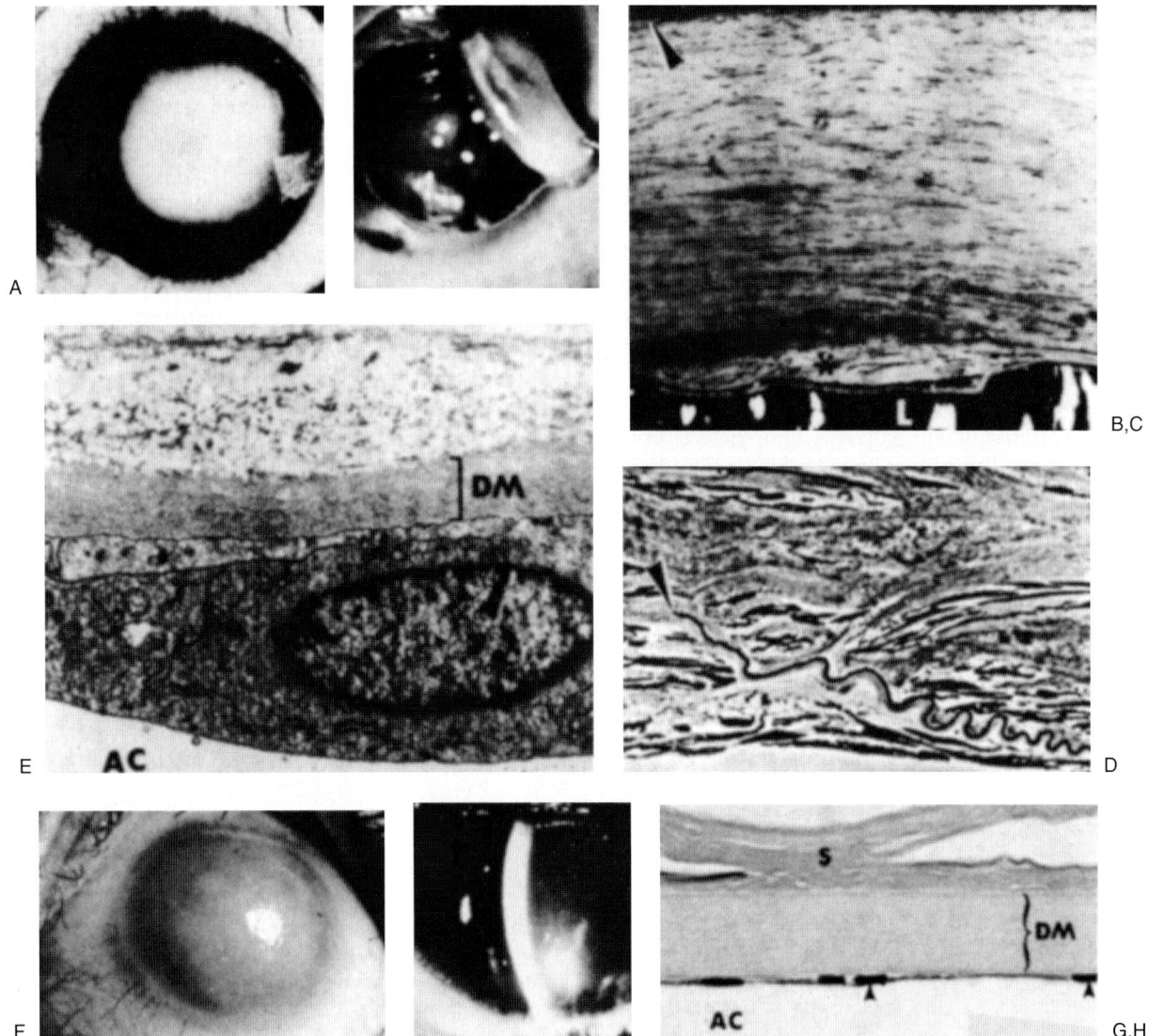

FIGURE 4-18. Dysgenesis. **A,** Clinical photograph of a large, dense central leukoma typical of Peters' anomaly. **B,** Intraoperative photograph of penetrating keratoplasty in Peters' anomaly shows adherence of the clear lens (centrally) to the thickened cornea (grasped by forceps.) **C,** Phase-contrast photomicrograph of the cornea illustrated in **B** shows thickened central stroma with the adherent lens (L). Bowman's layer terminates centrally (*arrowhead*). Descemet's membrane is present peripherally, but ends centrally in a layer of retrocorneal fibrous tissue (*asterisk*) approximately 75 μm thick between the lens and corneal stroma (paraphenylenediamine, ×60). **D,** Phase-contrast photomicrograph of the posterior cornea adjacent to a central stromal defect shows termination (*at the arrowhead*) of undulating Descemet's membrane in the posterior collagen layer (paraphenylenediamine, ×400). **E,** Transmission electron micrograph in Peters' anomaly shows an extremely thin, abnormally laminated Descemet's membrane (DM) with attenuated endothelium (E). AC, anterior chamber (×7700). **F,** Congenital hereditary endothelial dystrophy (CHED). In this severe case, there is a diffuse ground-glass opacification of the stroma with edematous stippling of the epithelium. **G,** In this more mildly affected patient, the cornea has only moderate haze that obscures the iris and lens but nonetheless permits 20/200 vision. Note the diffuse edematous thickening of the stroma revealed by the slit-lamp beam. **H,** Light photomicrograph of the cornea of a 6-year-old boy with CHED reveals enormous thickening of Descemet's membrane (DM) with dystrophic endothelial cells (*arrowheads*). AC, anterior chamber; S, posterior stroma (hematoxylin-eosin, ×600).

The ICE syndrome is a disease entity of unknown etiology comprising the spectrum of Chandler's syndrome, essential iris atrophy, and Cogan-Reese syndrome. The endothelial cells in this disease have the ability to migrate into the surrounding tissues as trabecular meshwork and anterior iris surface. Alvarado and coworkers showed that this migration could be promoted by a loss of contact inhibition and restricted motility that probably has a viral etiology (Fig. 4-19), but the complete mechanism of this disease is still unclear.

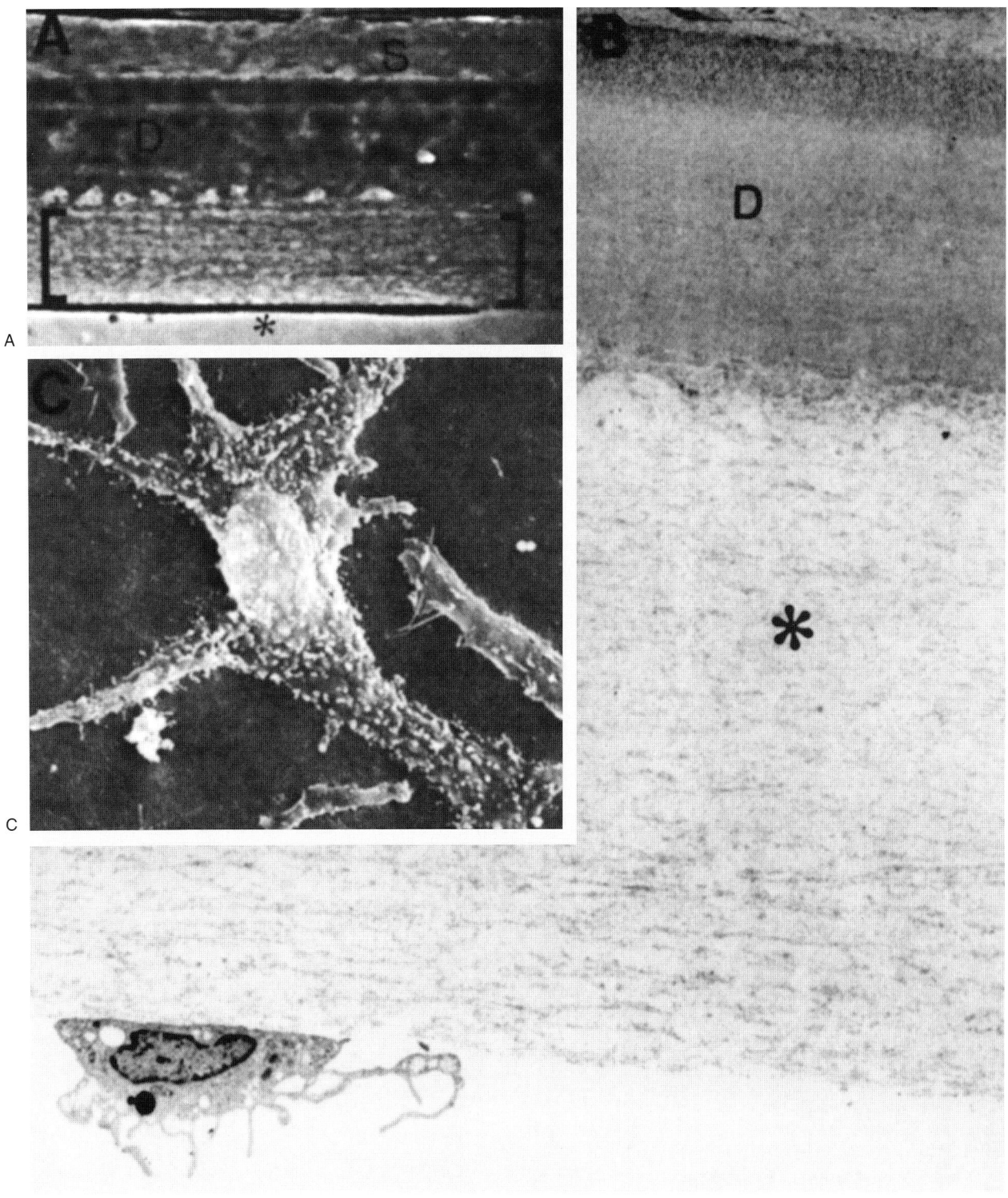

FIGURE 4-19. Iridocorneal endothelial syndrome. **A,** Phase-contrast photomicrograph illustrates uniformly thickened Descemet's membrane (D) covered posteriorly by an acellular fibrous layer (*bracketed*) approximately 20 μm thick. An extremely attenuated endothelial layer (*asterisk*) is evident. S, stroma (paraphenylenediamine, ×800). **B,** Transmission electron micrograph contrasts the normal ultrastructure of Descemet's membrane (D) with the loose fibrillar structure of the posterior collagen layer (*asterisk*). A single macrophage with phagocytosed pigment and extended cytoplasmic processes is present (×5000). **C,** Scanning electron microscopy of keratoplasty specimen shows unusual dendriform configuration of an attenuated endothelial cell that fails to cover completely the exposed posterior fibrous tissue layer (×2000).

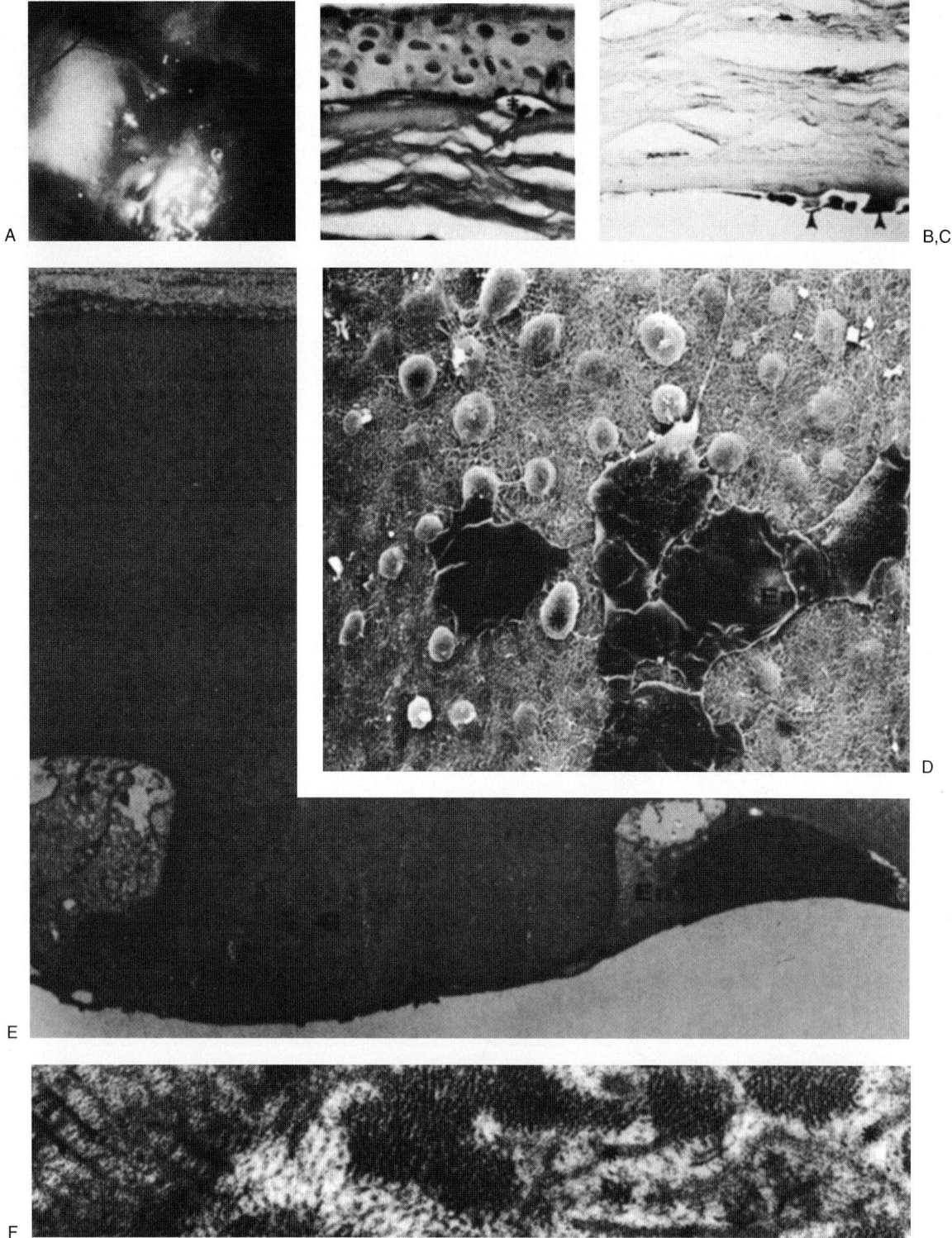

A

B,C

D

E

F

Dystrophy: Guttae and Fuchs' Dystrophy

A conventional slit-lamp examination of a patient with corneal guttae can reveal focal excrescences of Descemet's membrane that represent abnormal basement membrane elaboration by aging or otherwise distressed endothelial cells.

The guttae are often seen as a primary condition in patients of middle to older age. Progressive bilateral accumulation of guttae, usually seen in the fifth or sixth decade and somewhat more commonly in women, is typical of late hereditary endothelial dystrophy of Fuchs. As guttae become numerous and central, the endothelial cells are compromised to the extent that both their barrier and fluid transport functions become inefficient. Stromal edema then occurs, followed by bullous epithelial edema, and the condition may be termed Fuchs' dystrophy (195).

Another class of guttae is the secondary guttae, which are usually associated with degenerative corneal disease, trauma, or inflammation. The endothelial cells may be adversely affected by iritis, deep stromal inflammation (e.g., luetic interstitial keratitis), corneal ulcers, and anterior segment surgery. In severe inflammation, edema of the endothelial cells may resemble corneal guttae. However, on removal of the causative agent, the edema and guttae subside, whereas true cornea guttae are permanent (196).

With the aid of light microscopy, corneal guttae indent the underlying endothelial cells and display a mushroom-shaped configuration (Fig. 4-20). Descemet's membrane can become thickened to three or more times normal (20 to 40 μm). The endothelial cells undergo degeneration and alteration to fibroblast-like cells that become thin or focally absent beneath the excrescences. These abnormal cells produce the thickened Descemet's membrane in the form of guttae by laying down randomly organized collagen fibrils, small-diameter filaments (approximately 100 Å), and multiple laminations of basement membrane material on the posterior surface of the thickened Descemet's membrane (197).

Degeneration: Bullous Keratopathy

Bullous keratopathy is an endothelial degeneration with special clinical relevance. This condition of persistent corneal edema is a clinically important complication of cataract surgery and has become an increasingly common indication for penetrating keratoplasty, now accounting for nearly 50% of corneal grafts performed. As a functional disturbance of the corneal endothelium, postoperative bullous keratopathy most often develops in eyes with preexisting endothelial dystrophy, with surgical complications, or with persistent vitreo-ocorneal contact (vitreous touch syndrome). Pathologically, bullous keratopathy consistently involves endothelial cell degeneration and proliferation of a posterior collagen layer between Descemet's membrane and the endothelial cells (Fig. 4-21). By scanning electron microscopy, focal discontinuities of the endothelial cell layer are seen diffusely over the entire posterior corneal surface. The remaining endothelial cells become flat, attenuated, and enormously enlarged with numerous cytoplasmic extensions, often assuming elongated configurations in an apparent effort to recover the bare surface of Descemet's membrane.

The posterior collagen layer appears by light microscopy as a cellular fibrous band extending uniformly across the entire posterior aspect of Descemet's membrane. Transmission electron microscopy shows this layer to be composed of randomly arrayed collagen fibrils, approximately 200 to 300 Å in diameter, interspersed among multilaminar basement membrane segments and bundles of fine filaments. Similarly, on scanning electron microscopy, the exposed surface of the fibrous layer is a loosely fibrillar feltwork of a consistency different from that of the normally compact Descemet's membrane.

In some cases, another pattern characterized by a thicker fibrocellular layer is sometimes evident, presumably the result of fibrous ingrowth by stromal keratocytes (198). In many specimens, definite histologic evidence of preexisting endothelial disease is apparent: thickened Descemet's membrane, along with typical central corneal guttae.

The collagenous tissue lining the posterior aspect of Descemet's membrane is a typical response of distressed

FIGURE 4-20. Endothelial dystrophy: bullous keratopathy. **A,** Clinical photograph illustrates epithelial bullae, scarring, and neovascularization resulting from long-standing stromal edema. **B,** Light photomicrograph of early bullous keratopathy shows intracellular and extracellular hydropic changes of basal epithelial cells, with duplication and thickening of the basement membrane and subepithelial neovascularization (*asterisk*; hematoxylin-eosin, ×250). **C,** Light photomicrograph of the posterior cornea shows thickened Descemet's membrane with guttate excrescences (*arrowheads*) and dystrophic, attenuated endothelial cells (hematoxylin-eosin, ×250). **D,** Scanning electron micrograph of an area comparable with that shown in **C** reveals extensive areas of exposed Descemet's membrane with numerous guttae (*asterisks*). The remaining endothelial cells (En) are severely degenerated and attenuated. The exposed surface of the posterior collagen layer appears as a fibrous feltwork (×300). **E,** Transmission electron micrograph of the posterior cornea shows unremarkable stroma and anterior Descemet's membrane but thickening of posterior Descemet's membrane to 12 μm with additional superimposition of large guttae (G). The remaining endothelial cells (En) are extremely attenuated (×5000). **F,** High-magnification transmission electron micrograph of guttae resolves fine filaments, multiple segments of basement material (*asterisks*), and collagen in long-spacing configuration (*arrowheads*; ×50,000).

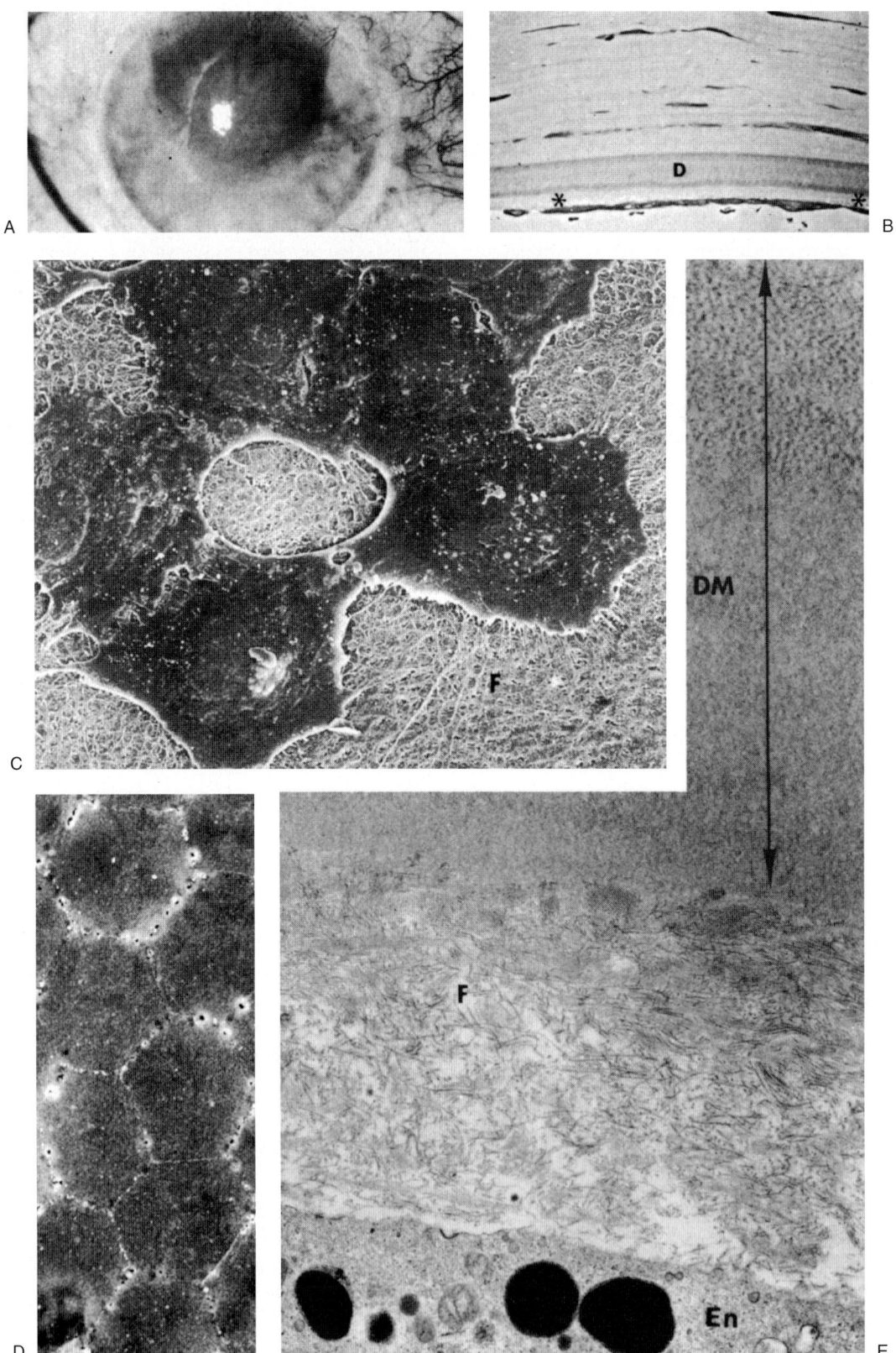

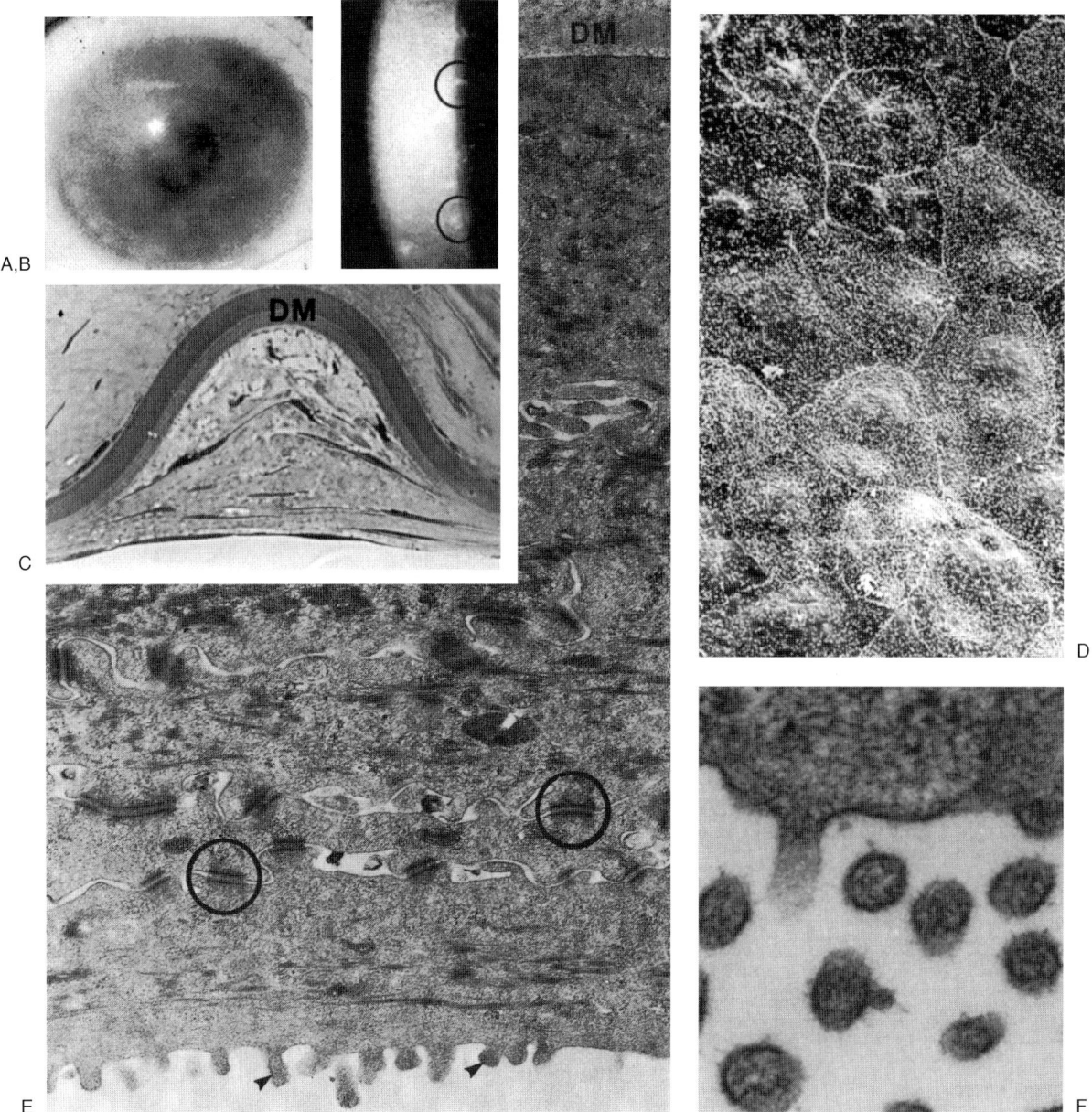

FIGURE 4-22. Posterior polymorphous dystrophy. **A,** Clinical photograph of an advanced case shows stromal edema plus irregular posterior geographic areas on Descemet's membrane. **B,** Slit-lamp biomicroscopy resolves additional polymorphic opacities (*circled*) at the level of Descemet's membrane. **C,** Phase-contrast microscopy of stroma and Descemet's membrane (DM) demonstrates the focal deposition of collagenous material causing infolding of Descemet's membrane, presumably corresponding to polymorphous lesions (paraphenylenediamine, ×600). **D,** Scanning electron micrograph demonstrates epithelium-like profiles and surface characteristics of transformed endothelial cells (×2000). **E,** Transmission electron micrograph shows transformed endothelial cells to have epithelial characteristics: Multiple cell layers have numerous desmosomes (*circled*) and individual cells show increased keratofibrils and microvillous surface projections (*arrowheads*; ×19,000). **F,** A higher-magnification transmission electron micrograph of the posterior cellular surface reveals an organization of filaments at the core of surface membrane microvilli (×80,000).

FIGURE 4-21. Endothelial degeneration: bullous keratopathy. **A.** Clinical photograph shows diffuse stromal edema. **B.** Phase-contrast photomicrograph shows normal Descemet's membrane (D) with an associated posterior collagen layer (*asterisks*) anterior to the degenerating endothelial cells (paraphenylenediamine, ×700). **C.** Scanning electron micrograph of the posterior corneal surface reveals remaining endothelial cells to be extremely flattened and attenuated. Note the exposed surface of the posterior collagenous layer (F) appearing as a randomly organized fibrous network (×1000). **D.** For direct comparison with **C,** normal adult human endothelium demonstrates uniformly hexagonal cells approximately 20 μm in diameter arranged in a continuous monolayered mosaic (×1000). **E.** Transmission electron micrograph of an eye with bullous keratopathy discloses the usual ultrastructure of banded and nonbanded portions of Descemet's membrane (DM) and loose fibrous composition of the posterior collagen layer (F). The remaining endothelial cell (En) contains phagocytosed melanin (×13,000).

endothelial cells. The ultrastructural composition of this posterior collagenous layer is identical to that found in many situations involving endothelial dysgenesis, dystrophy, trauma, or inflammation. In each of these "endothelial distress syndromes," the endothelial cells undergo transformation to fibroblast-like cells producing the observed collagenous tissue beneath Descemet's membrane (187,199).

Transformation: Posterior Polymorphous Dystrophy

Posterior polymorphous dystrophy (PPMD) is a bilateral, dominantly inherited corneal dystrophy, that may be unchanging or only slowly progressive, such that affected patients usually have normal visual acuity and no stromal edema.

This condition is characterized by polymorphous opacities, some of them vesicular, at the level of Descemet's membrane. The association of PPMD with other anterior segment abnormalities, particularly peripheral anterior synechiae and glaucoma, relates this dystrophy to the ICE syndromes specifically, and more broadly to the mesenchymal dysgeneses (200).

An interesting pathologic aspect of this dystrophy is the evidence of either focal transformation or mosaicism of the endothelium into epithelium-like cells. By transmission electron microscopy, these cells are morphologically identical to epithelium; they contain keratofibrils and assume a multilayered configuration, with adjacent cells connected by well-developed desmosomes (Fig. 4-22). Scanning electron microscopy reveals myriad microvilli along the posterior surface membrane, again suggestive of an epithelial cell. Adjacent endothelial cells have an altogether typical morphologic appearance of endothelium. Although the exact clinicopathologic correlation between the polymorphous opacities that are biomicroscopically visible and the morphologically evident transformation of endothelial cells is not entirely clear, it seems likely that localized posterior collagen layer formation, sometimes associated with infoldings of Descemet's membrane, may be responsible. Although the true pathogenesis of PPMD remains entirely unknown (201), recent genetic studies on inherited diseases affecting the cornea are now available. Interesting insights into some of these disorders at a basic molecular level are now emerging, with the knowledge that distinct clinicopathologic phenotypes can result from specific mutations in a particular gene, as well as from apparently different mutations in the same gene. This suggests that a molecular genetic study of inherited corneal diseases will give better insight into the pathogenesis of these conditions, and such insight will undoubtedly stimulate a revision of the classification of inherited corneal diseases (202).

REFERENCES

1. Jacobsen IE, Jensen OA, Prause JU. Structure and composition of Bowman's membrane. *Acta Ophthalmol (Copenh)* 1984;62:39.
2. Jakus MA. Further observations on the fine structure of the cornea. *Invest Ophthalmol* 1962;1:202.
3. Haik BG, Zimmy ML. Scanning electron microscopy of corneal wound healing in the rabbit. *Invest Ophthalmol Vis Sci* 1977;16:787.
4. Matsuda H, Smelser GK. Electron microscopy of corneal wound healing. *Exp Eye Res* 1973;16:427.
5. Sellheyer K, Spitznas M. Surface differentiation of the human corneal epithelium during prenatal development. *Graefes Arch Clin Exp Ophthalmol* 1988;226:482.
6. Fujikawa LS, et al. Fibronectin in healing rabbit corneal wounds. *Lab Invest* 1981;45:120.
7. Kuwabara T, Perkins DG, Cogan D. Sliding of the epithelium in experimental corneal wounds. *Invest Ophthalmol* 1976;15:4.
8. Pfister RR. The healing of corneal epithelial abrasions in the rabbit: a scanning electron microscopic study. *Invest Ophthalmol* 1975;14:468.
9. Gipson IK, Anderson RA. Actin filaments in normal and migrating corneal epithelial cells. *Invest Ophthalmol Vis Sci* 1977;16:161.
10. Binder PS, et al. Corneal anatomy and wound healing. In: *Transactions of the New Orleans Academy of Ophthalmology*. St. Louis: Mosby, 1980:1–35.
11. Khodadoust AA, et al. Adhesion of regenerating corneal epithelium: the role of basement membrane. *Am J Ophthalmol* 1968;65:339.
12. Keene DR, et al. Type VII collagen forms an extended network of anchoring fibrils. J Cell Biol 1987;104:611.
13. Kenyon KR, et al. Regeneration of corneal epithelial basement membrane following thermal cauterization. *Invest Ophthalmol Vis Sci* 1977;16:292.
14. Dohlman CH, Gasset AR, Rose J. The effect of the absence of corneal epithelium or endothelium on the stromal keratocytes. *Invest Ophthalmol* 1968;7:520.
15. Dunnington JH, Weimar V. Influence of the epithelium on the healing of corneal incisions. *Am J Ophthalmol* 1958;45:89.
16. Wagoner MD, et al. Polymorphonuclear neutrophils delay corneal epithelial wound healing in vitro. *Invest Ophthalmol Vis Sci* 1984;25:1217.
17. Friedenwald JS, Bushke W. The effects of excitement, of epinephrine, and of sympathectomy on the mitotic activity of the corneal epithelium in rats. *Am J Physiol* 1944;141:689.
18. Cavanagh HD. Herpetic ocular disease: therapy of persistent epithelial defects. *Int Ophthalmol Clin* 1975;15:67.
19. Fogle JA, et al. Defective epithelial adhesion in anterior corneal dystrophies. *Am J Ophthalmol* 1975;79:925.
20. Alper MG. The anesthetic eye: an investigation of changes in the anterior ocular segment of the monkey caused by interrupting the trigeminal nerve at various levels along its course. *Trans Am Ophthalmol Soc* 1976;73:323.
21. Butterfield LC, Neufeld AH. Cyclic nucleotides and mitosis in the rabbit cornea following superior cervical ganglionectomy. *Exp Eye Res* 1977;25:427.
22. Cavanagh HD, Colley AM. The molecular basis of neurotrophic keratitis. *Acta Ophthalmol (Copenh)* 1989;192:115.
23. Mishima S. The effects of the denervation and the stimulation of the sympathetic and trigeminal nerve on the mitotic rate of corneal epithelium in the rabbit. *Jpn J Ophthalmol* 1957;1:67.
24. Frati L, et al. Selective binding of the epidermal growth factor and its specific effects on the epithelial cells of the cornea. *Exp Eye Res* 1972;14:135.
25. Savage CR, Cohen S. Proliferations of corneal epithelium induced by epidermal growth factor. *Exp Eye Res* 1972;14:135.
26. Soong HK, et al. EGF does not enhance corneal epithelial cell motility. *Invest Ophthalmol Vis Sci* 1989;30:1808.

27. Girard MT, Matsubara M, Fini ME. Transforming growth factor-beta and interleukin-1 modulate metalloproteinase expression by corneal stromal cells. *Invest Ophthalmol Vis Sci* 1991;32:2441.
28. Sporn MB, et al. Transforming growth factor-β: biological function and chemical structure. *Science* 1986;233:532.
29. Hayashi K, et al. Expression of transforming growth factor-beta in wound healing of vitamin A-deficient rat corneas. *Invest Ophthalmol Vis Sci* 1989;30:239.
30. Nishida T, et al. Hyaluronan stimulates corneal epithelial migration. *Exp Eye Res* 1991;53:753.
31. Grinnell F, Feld MK. Initial adhesion of human fibroblasts in serum-free medium: possible role of secreted fibronectin. *Cell* 1979;17:117.
32. Grinnell F, Hays DG. Cell adhesion and spreading factor: similarity to cold-insoluble globulin in human serum. *Exp Cell Res* 1978;115:221.
33. Hedman K, Vaheri A, Wartiovaara J. External fibronectin on cultured human fibroblasts is predominantly a matrix protein. *J Cell Biol* 1978;76:748.
34. Hook M, et al. Cold-insoluble globulin mediates the adhesion of rat liver cells to plastic Petri dishes. *Biochem Biophys Res Commun* 1977;79:726.
35. Klebe RJ. Isolation of a collagen-dependent cell attachment factor. *Nature* 1974;250:248.
36. Mishima H, et al. Fibronectin enhances the phagocytic activity of cultured rabbit keratocytes. *Invest Ophthalmol Vis Sci* 1987;28:1521.
37. Niederkorn JY, Peeler JS, Mellon J. Phagocytosis of particulate antigens by corneal epithelial cells stimulates interleukin-1 secretion and migration of Langerhans cells into the central cornea. *Reg Immunol* 1989;2:83.
38. Perlstein E. Plasma membrane glycoprotein which mediates adhesion of fibroblasts to collagen. *Nature* 1976;262:497.
39. Stasko T, De Villez RL. Fibronectin. *Dermatology* 1982;21:68.
40. Tervo T, et al. Distribution of fibronectin in human and rabbit corneas. *Exp Eye Res* 1986;42:1986.
41. Frangieh GT, et al. Fibronectin and corneal epithelial wound healing in the vitamin A-deficient rat. *Arch Ophthalmol* 1989;107:567.
42. Nishida T, et al. Fibronectin: a new therapy for corneal trophic ulcer. *Arch Ophthalmol* 1983;101:1046.
43. Nishida T, et al. Fibronectin enhancement of corneal epithelial wound healing of rabbits *in vivo*. *Arch Ophthalmol* 1984;102:455.
44. Phan TMM, et al. Topical fibronectin in the treatment of persistent corneal epithelial defects and trophic ulcers. *Am J Ophthalmol* 1987;104:494.
45. Spigelman AV, Deutsch TA, Sugar J. Application of homologous fibronectin to persistent human corneal epithelial defects. *Cornea* 1987;6:128.
46. Watanabe K, et al. Effect of fibronectin on corneal epithelial wound healing in the vitamin A-deficient rat. *Invest Ophthalmol Vis Sci* 1991;32:2159.
47. Boisjoly HM, et al. Topical fibronectin and aprotinin for keratectomy wound healing in rabbits. *Arch Ophthalmol* 1990;108:1758.
48. Newton C, et al. Topical fibronectin and corneal epithelial wound healing in the rabbit. *Arch Ophthalmol* 1988;106:1277.
49. Lantz E, Anderson A. Release of fibrinolytic activators from cornea and conjunctiva. *Graefes Arch Clin Exp Ophthalmol* 1982;219:263.
50. Lantz E, Pandolfi M. Fibrinolysis in conjunctiva: evidence of two types of activators. *Graefes Arch Clin Exp Ophthalmol* 1986;224:393.
51. Berman M, Leary R, Gage J. Evidence for a role of the plasminogen activator-plasmin system in corneal ulceration. *Invest Ophthalmol Vis Sci* 1980;19:1204.
52. Wang HM, Berman M, Law M. Latent and active plasminogen activator in corneal ulceration. *Invest Ophthalmol Vis Sci* 1985;26:511.
53. Liotta LA, et al. Effect of plasminogen activator (urokinase), plasmin, and thrombin on glycoprotein and collagenous components of basement membrane. *Cancer Res* 1981;41:4629.
54. Pavilack MA, et al. Differential expression of human corneal and perilimbal ICAM-1 by inflammatory cytokines. *Invest Ophthalmol Vis Sci* 1992;33:564.
55. Vaheri A, et al. Fibronectin and proteinases in tumor invasion. In: Strauli P, Barret AJ, Baici A, eds. *Proteinases and tumor invasion.* New York: Raven Press, 1980:49–57.
56. Vaheri A, Salonen EM, Vartio T. Fibronectin in formation and degradation of the pericellular matrix. *Ciba Found Symp* 1985;114:111.
57. Hayashi K, et al. Pathogenesis of corneal epithelial defects: role of plasminogen activator. *Curr Eye Res* 1991;10:381.
58. Shams NB, Sigel MM, Davis RM. Interferon-gamma, *Staphylococcus aureus*, and lipopolysaccharide/silica enhance interleukin-1 beta production by human corneal cells. *Reg Immunol* 1989;2:136.
59. Shams NB, et al. Corneal epithelial cells produce thromboxane in response to interleukin 1 (IL-1). *Invest Ophthalmol Vis Sci* 1986;27:1543.
60. Lu L, Reinach PS, Kao WW. Corneal epithelial wound healing. *Exp Biol Med* 2001;226:653–664.
61. Lambiase A, Rama P, Bonini S, et al. Topical treatment with nerve growth factor for corneal neurotrophic ulcers. *N Engl J Med* 1998;23:1174.
62. Friend J, Thoft RA. Functional competence of regenerating ocular surface epithelium. *Invest Ophthalmol Vis Sci* 1978;17:134.
63. Thoft RA, Friend J. Biochemical transformation of regenerating ocular surface epithelium. *Invest Ophthalmol Vis Sci* 1977;16:1.
64. Thoft RA, Friend J, Kenyon KR. Ocular surface response to trauma. *Int Ophthalmol 6Clin* 1979;19:111.
65. Cintron C, Covington HI, Kublin CL. Morphologic analyses of proteoglycans in rabbit corneal scars. *Invest Ophthalmol Vis Sci* 1990;31:1789.
66. Hassell JR, et al. Proteoglycan changes during restoration of transparency in corneal scars. *Arch Biochem Biophys* 1983;222:362.
67. Nakayasu K, et al. Distribution of types I, II, III, IV and V collagen in normal and keratoconus corneas. *Ophthalmic Res* 1986;18:1.
68. Bukusoglu G, Zieske JD. Characterization of a monoclonal antibody that specifically binds basal cells in the limbal epithelium. *Invest Ophthalmol Vis Sci* 1988;29:192.
69. Cotsarelis G, et al. Existence of slow-cycling limbal epithelial basal cells that can be preferentially stimulated to proliferate: implications on epithelial stem cells. *Cell* 1989;57:201.
70. Schermer A, Galvin S, Sun TT. Differentiation-related expression of a major 64K corneal keratin in vivo, and in culture suggests limbal location of corneal epithelial stem cells. *J Cell Biol* 1986;103:49.
71. Tseng SCG. Concept and application of limbal stem cells. *Eye* 1989;3:141.
72. Zieske JD, Bukusoglu G, Yankauckas MA. Characterization of a potential marker of corneal epithelial stem cells. *Invest Ophthalmol Vis Sci* 1992;33:143.
73. Chen JJY, Tseng SCG. Corneal epithelial wound healing in partial limbal deficiency. *Invest Ophthalmol Vis Sci* 1990;31:1301.
74. Chen JJY, Tseng SCG. Abnormal corneal epithelial wound healing in partial-thickness removal of limbal epithelium. *Invest Ophthalmol Vis Sci* 1991;32:2219.
75. Kruse FE, et al. Conjunctival transdifferentiation is due to the incomplete removal of limbal basal epithelium. *Invest Ophthalmol Vis Sci* 1990;31:1903.
76. Hirst LW, et al. Comparative studies of corneal surface injury in the monkey and rabbit. *Arch Ophthalmol* 1981;99:1066.

77. Shapiro MS, Friend J, Thoft RA. Corneal reepithelization from the conjunctiva. *Invest Ophthalmol Vis Sci* 1981;21:135.

78. Faulkner W, et al. Chemical burns of the human ocular surface: clinicopathologic studies of 14 cases. *Invest Ophthalmol Vis Sci* 1981;20:8.

79. Greiner JV, et al. Mucus secretory vesicles in conjunctival epithelial cells of wearers of contact lenses. *Arch Ophthalmol* 1980; 98:1843.

80. Thoft RA, Friend J, Murphy H. Ocular surface epithelium and corneal vascularization in rabbits: I. The role of wounding. *Invest Ophthalmol Vis Sci* 1979;18:85.

81. Kenyon KR, Tseng SCG. Limbal autograft transplantation for ocular surface disorders. *Ophthalmology* 1989;96:709.

82. Tsai RJF, Sun TT, Tseng SCG. Comparison of limbal and conjunctival autograft transplantation in corneal surface reconstruction in rabbits. *Ophthalmology* 1990;97:446.

83. Ghinelli E, Johansson J, Rios JD, et al. Presence and localization of neurotrophins and neurotrophin receptors in rat lacrimal gland. *Invest Ophthalmol Vis Sci* 2003;44:3352.

84. Ghinelli E, Rios JD, Chen LL, et al. Neurotrophins and their receptors in rat conjunctiva: presence of mRNA and effects on p44/p42 the activation mitogen-activated protein kinase. ARVO Abstracts. *Invest Ophthalmol Vis Sci* 2003;44[4 Suppl]: E-Abstract 3773(abstr).

85. Lindberg K, et al. Serial propagation of human ocular surface epithelial cells and reconstitution of differentiated epithelia. *Invest Ophthalmol Vis Sci* 1992;33:2422.

86. Rama P, Bonini S, Lambiase A, et al. Autologous fibrin-cultured limbal stem cells permanently restore the corneal surface of patients with total limbal stem cell deficiency. *Transplantation* 2001;15;72:1478.

87. Sommer A, Green WR, Kenyon KR. Bitot's spots responsive and nonresponsive to vitamin A: clinicopathologic correlations. *Arch Ophthalmol* 1981;99:2014.

88. Sommer A, Green WR, Kenyon KR. Clinical histopathologic correlations in xerophthalmic ulceration and necrosis. *Arch Ophthalmol* 1982;100:593.

89. Burstein NL. The effects of topical drugs and preservatives on the tears and corneal epithelium in dry eye. *Trans Ophthalmol Soc UK* 1985;104:402.

90. Furey N, et al. Immunofluorescent studies of ocular cicatricial pemphigoid. *Am J Ophthalmol* 1975;80:825.

91. Mondino BJ, et al. Autoimmune phenomena in ocular cicatricial pemphigoid. *Am J Ophthalmol* 1977;83:443.

92. Foster CS. Cicatricial pemphigoid. *Trans Am Ophthalmol Soc* 1986;84:527.

93. Carroll J, Kuwabara T. Ocular pemphigus: an electron microscopic study of conjunctival and corneal epithelium. *Arch Ophthalmol* 1968;8:561.

94. Franklin RM, Fitzmorris CT. Antibodies against conjunctival basement membrane zone in cicatricial pemphigoid. *Am J Ophthalmol* 1983;101:1611.

95. Razzaque MS, Foster CS, Ahmed AR. Tissue and molecular events in human conjunctival scarring in ocular cicatricial pemphigoid. *Histol Histopathol* 2001;16:1203.

96. Kenyon KR. Recurrent corneal erosion: pathogenesis and therapy. *Int Ophthalmol Clin* 1979;19:169.

97. Cogan DG, Kuwabara T, Donaldson DD. Microcystic dystrophy of the cornea. *Arch Ophthalmol* 1974;92:470.

98. Rodrigues MM, Fine BS, Laibson PR. Disorders of the corneal epithelium: a clinicopathologic study of dot, geographic and fingerprint patterns. *Arch Ophthalmol* 1974;92:474.

99. Trobe JD, Laibson PR. Dystrophic changes in the anterior cornea. *Arch Ophthalmol* 1972;87:378.

100. Rosenberg ME, Tervo TM, Petroll WM, et al. *In vivo* confocal microscopy of patients with corneal recurrent erosion syndrome or epithelial basement membrane dystrophy. *Ophthalmology* 2000;107:565.

101. Fogle JA, Neufeld RH. The adrenergic and cholinergic corneal epithelium. *Invest Ophthalmol Vis Sci* 1979;18:1212.

102. Azar DT, et al. Decreased penetration of anchoring fibrils into the diabetic stroma: a morphologic analysis. *Arch Ophthalmol* 1989;107:1520.

103. Perry HD, et al. Corneal complications after closed vitrectomy through the pars plana. *Arch Ophthalmol* 1978;96:401.

104. Starck T, et al. Clinical and histopathologic studies of two families with lattice corneal dystrophy and familial systemic amyloidosis (Meretoja syndrome). *Ophthalmology* 1991;98:1197.

105. Kaufman HE. Epithelial erosion syndrome: metaherpetic keratitis. *Am J Ophthalmol* 1964;57:983.

106. Wolter JR. Reactions of the cellular elements of the corneal stroma. *Arch Ophthalmol* 1958;59:873.

107. Smelser GK, Ozanics V. Reaction of the cornea to injury and wound healing. In: *Transactions of the New Orleans Academy of Ophthalmology.* St. Louis: Mosby, 1972:239.

108. Baum JL. Source of the fibroblasts in central wound healing. *Arch Ophthalmol* 1971;85:473.

109. Dunnington JH, Smelser GK. Incorporation of S35 in healing wounds in normal and devitalized corneas. *Arch Ophthalmol* 1958;60:116.

110. Robb TM, Kuwabara T. Corneal wound healing: II. An autoradiographic study of the cellular components. *Arch Ophthalmol* 1964;72:401.

111. Cintron C, et al. Biochemical and ultrastructural changes in collagen during corneal wound healing. *J Ultrastruct Res* 1978; 65:13.

112. Marshall GE, Konstas AG, Lee WR. Immunogold fine structural localization of extracellular matrix components in aged human cornea: I. Types I-IV collagen and laminin. *Graefes Arch Clin Exp Ophthalmol* 1991;229:157.

113. Wilson SE, Liu JJ, Mohan RR. Stromal-epithelial interactions in the cornea. *Prog Retin Eye Res* 1999;18:293.

114. Azar DT, et al. Reassembly of the corneal endothelial adhesion structures following human epikeratoplasty. *Arch Ophthalmol* 1991;109:1279.

115. Baumgartner SD, Binder PS. Refractive keratoplasty: histopathology of clinical specimens. *Ophthalmology* 1985;92:1606.

116. Bechara SJ, Grossniklaus HE, Waring GO III. Subepithelial fibrosis after myopic epikeratoplasty: report of a case. *Arch Ophthalmol* 1992;110:228.

117. Mader P, et al. Histological study of 4 lenses from epikeratoplasty: anatomoclinical correlation. *J Fr Ophthalmol* 1988;11:143.

118. Pokorny KS, et al. Histopathology of human keratorefractive lenticules. *Cornea* 1990;9:223.

119. Price FW, Binder PS. Scarring of a recipient cornea following epikeratoplasty. *Arch Ophthalmol* 1987;105:1556.

120. Frangieh GT, et al. Epithelial abnormalities and sterile ulceration of epikeratoplasty grafts. *Ophthalmology* 1988;95:213.

121. Sahori A, et al. Reepithelization of keratolens in the wound healing process following epikeratoplasty in rabbits. *Nippon Ganka Gakkai Zasshi* 1989;93:747.

122. Gerana RM, et al. Cell biology of corneal wound fibroblasts' mechanism of wound contraction in radial keratotomy (RK). *Invest Ophthalmol Vis Sci* 1990;31:3.

123. Jester JV, et al. *In vivo* modulation of corneal curvature during wound healing in radial keratotomy. *Invest Ophthalmol Vis Sci* 1990;31:300.

124. Jester JV, et al. Variations in corneal wound healing after radial keratotomy: possible insights into mechanisms of clinical complications and refractive effects. *Cornea* 1992;11:191.

125. Deg JK, Binder PS. Wound healing after astigmatic keratotomy in human eyes. *Ophthalmology* 1987;94:1290.

126. Binder PS, et al. Ultrastructural and histochemical study of long-term wound healing after radial keratotomy. *Am J Ophthalmol* 1987;103:432.

127. Deg J, Zavala EY, Binder PS. Delayed corneal wound healing following radial keratotomy. *Ophthalmology* 1985;92:734.

128. Kahle G, et al. Wound healing of the cornea of New World monkeys after surface keratectomy: Er:YAG-excimer laser. *Fortschr Ophthalmol* 1991;88:380.

129. Marshall J, et al. Long-term healing of the central cornea after photorefractive keratectomy using an excimer laser. *Ophthalmology* 1988;95:1411.

130. Wu WC, Stark WJ, Green WR. Corneal wound healing after 193 nm excimer laser keratectomy. *Arch Ophthalmol* 1991; 109:1426.

131. SundarRaj N, et al. Healing of excimer laser ablated monkey corneas: an immunohistochemical evaluation. *Arch Ophthalmol* 1990;108:1604.

132. Jester JV, Petroll WM, Cavanagh HD. Corneal stromal wound healing in refractive surgery: the role of myofibroblasts. *Prog Retin Eye Res* 1999;18:311.

133. Cohnheim J. *Lectures on general pathology: I. The pathology of the circulation*. London: New Sydenham Society, 1889:284.

134. Coster DJ. Inflammatory disease of the outer eye. *Trans Ophthalmol Soc UK* 1979;99:463.

135. Fromer CH, Klintworth GK. An evaluation of the role of leukocytes in the pathogenesis of experimentally induced corneal vascularization: I. Comparison of experimental models of corneal vascularization. *Am J Pathol* 1975;79:537.

136. Fromer CH, Klintworth GK. An evaluation of the role of leukocytes and the pathogenesis of experimentally induced corneal vascularization: II. Studies on the effect of leukocyte elimination on corneal vascularization. *Am J Pathol* 1975;81:531.

137. Eliason JA. Leukocyte and experimental corneal vascularization. *Invest Ophthalmol Vis Sci* 1978;17:1087.

138. Sholley MM, Gimbrone MA, Cotran RA. The effects of leukocyte depletion on corneal neovascularization. *Lab Invest* 1978; 38:32.

139. Folkman J, et al. A heparin-binding angiogenic protein-basic fibroblast growth factor is stored within basement membrane. *Am J Pathol* 1988;130:393.

140. Adamis AP, Meklir B, Joyce NC. *In situ* injury-induced release of basic-fibroblast growth factor from corneal epithelial cells. *Am J Pathol* 1991;139:961.

141. BenEzra D. Neovasculogenic ability of prostaglandins, growth factors, and chemoattractants. *Am J Ophthalmol* 1978;86:455.

142. BenEzra D, Hemo I, Maftzir G. *In vivo* angiogenic activity of interleukins. *Arch Ophthalmol* 1990;108:573.

143. Folkman J. Tumor angiogenesis factor. *Cancer Res* 1974;34:2109.

144. Li WW, et al. Sustained-release endotoxin: a model for inducing corneal neovascularization. *Invest Ophthalmol Vis Sci* 1991; 32:2906.

145. Li WW, et al. Angiostatic steroids potentiated by sulfated cyclodextrins inhibit corneal neovascularization. *Invest Ophthalmol Vis Sci* 1991;32:2898.

146. Maurice DM, Zauberman H, Michaelson IC. The stimulus to neovascularization in the cornea. *Exp Eye Res* 1966;5:168.

147. Zauberman H, et al. Stimulation of neovascularization of the cornea by biogenic amines. *Exp Eye Res* 1969;8:77.

148. Deutsch TA, Hughes WF. Suppressive effects of indomethacin on thermally induced neovascularization of rabbit corneas. *Am J Ophthalmol* 1979;87:536.

149. Epstein RJ, Hendricks RL, Stulting RD. Interleukin-2 induces corneal neovascularization in A/J mice. *Cornea* 1990;9:318.

150. Lipman RM, Epstein RJ, Hendricks RL. Suppression of corneal neovascularization with cyclosporine. *Arch Ophthalmol* 1992;110:405.

151. Keutner KE, et al. Proteinase inhibitors activity in connective tissues. *Experientia* 1974;30:595.

152. Goren SB, Eisenstein R, Choromokos E. The inhibition of corneal neovascularization in rabbits. *Am J Ophthalmol* 1977; 84:305.

153. Folkman J, et al. Control of angiogenesis with synthetic heparin substitutes. *Science* 1989;243:1490.

154. Cherry PM, Garner A. Corneal neovascularization treated with argon laser. *Br J Ophthalmol* 1976;60:464.

155. Epstein RJ, Hendricks RL, Harris DM. Photodynamic therapy for corneal neovascularization. *Cornea* 1991;10:424.

156. Huang AJ, et al. Induction of conjunctival transdifferentiation on vascularized corneas by photothrombotic occlusion of corneal neovascularization. *Ophthalmology* 1988;95:228.

157. Huang AJ, et al. Photothrombosis of corneal neovascularization by intravenous rose bengal and argon laser irradiation. *Arch Ophthalmol* 1988;106:680.

158. Mendelsohn AD, et al. Laser photocoagulation of feeder vessels in lipid keratopathy. *Ophthalmic Surg* 1986;17:502.

159. Marsh RJ, Marshall J. Treatment of lipid keratopathy with the argon laser. *Br J Ophthalmol* 1982;66:127.

160. Nirankari VS, Baer JC. Corneal argon laser photocoagulation for neovascularization in penetrating keratoplasty. *Ophthalmology* 1986;93:1304.

161. Baer JC, Foster CS. Corneal laser photocoagulation for treatment of neovascularization: efficacy of 577 nm yellow dye laser. *Ophthalmology* 1992;99:173.

162. Cursiefen C, Chen L, Dana MR, et al. Corneal lymphangiogenesis: evidence, mechanisms, and implications for corneal transplant immunology. *Cornea* 2003;22:273.

163. Goldman JN, et al. Structural alterations affecting transparency in swollen human corneas. *Invest Ophthalmol* 1968;7:501.

164. Matsuda M, et al. Cellular migration and morphology in corneal endothelial wound repair. *Invest Ophthalmol Vis Sci* 1985;26:443.

165. Laing RA, et al. Evidence for mitosis in the adult corneal endothelium. *Ophthalmology* 1984;91:1129.

166. Kessler E, Mondino B, Brown SI. The corneal response to *Pseudomonas aeruginosa*: histopathological and enzymatic characterization. *Invest Ophthalmol Vis Sci* 1977;16:116.

167. Kenyon KR. Inflammatory mechanisms in corneal ulceration. *Trans Am Ophthalmol Soc* 1985;83:610.

168. Wagoner MD, Kenyon KR. Distribution of collagenase and cell types in sterile ulceration of human corneal grafts. *Acta Ophthalmol (Copenh)* 1989;67:65.

169. Conn H, et al. Stromal vascularization prevents corneal ulceration. *Invest Ophthalmol Vis Sci* 1980;19:362.

170. Kenyon KR, Berman MB, Hanninen LA. Tissue adhesive prevents ulceration and inhibits inflammation in the thermal burned rabbit cornea. *Invest Ophthalmol Vis Sci* 1979;18:1196.

171. Fogle JA, Kenyon KR, Foster CS. Tissue adhesive arrests stromal melting in the human cornea. *Am J Ophthalmol* 1980; 89:795.

172. Levy JH, Katz HR. Effect of systemic tetracycline on progression of *Pseudomonas aeruginosa* keratitis in the rabbit. *Ann Ophthalmol* 1990;22:179.

173. Tamargo RJ, Bok RA, Brem H. Angiogenesis inhibition by minocycline. *Cancer Res* 1991;51:672.

174. Chi HH, Teng CC, Katzen HH. Healing processes in the mechanical denudation of the corneal endothelium. *Am J Ophthalmol* 1960;49:693.

175. Van Horn DL, Hyndiuk RA. Endothelial wound repair in primate cornea. *Exp Eye Res* 1975;21:113.

176. Bahn CF, et al. Postnatal development of corneal endothelium. *Invest Ophthalmol Vis Sci* 1986;27:44.

177. Capella JA. Regeneration of endothelium in diseases and injured cornea. *Am J Ophthalmol* 1972;74:810.

178. Doughman DJ, et al. Human corneal endothelial layer repair during organ culture. *Arch Ophthalmol* 1976;4:1791.

179. Elner VM, et al. Intercellular adhesion molecule-1 in human corneal endothelium: modulation and function. *Am J Pathol* 1991;138:525.

180. Elner VM, et al. Human corneal interleukin-8, IL-1 and TNF-induced gene expression and secretion. *Am J Pathol* 1991;139:977.

181. Rahi AHS, Robins E. Human corneal endothelial cell repair in health and disease. *Trans Ophthalmol Soc UK* 1981;101:30.

182. Singh G. Mitosis and cell division in human corneal endothelium. *Ann Ophthalmol* 1986;18:88.

183. Van Horn DL, et al. Regenerative capacity of the corneal endothelium in rabbit and cat. *Invest Ophthalmol Vis Sci* 1977;16:597.

184. Couch JM, et al. Mitotic activity of corneal endothelial cells in organ culture with recombinant human epidermal growth factor. *Ophthalmology* 1987;94:1.

185. Gordon SR. Changes in extracellular matrix proteins and actin during corneal endothelial growth. *Invest Ophthalmol Vis Sci* 1990;31:94.

186. Samples JR, Binder PS, Nayak SK. Propagation of human corneal endothelium in vitro effect of growth factors. *Exp Eye Res* 1991;52:121.

187. Waring GO, Laibson PR, Rodrigues M. Clinical and pathologic alterations of Descemet's membrane: with emphasis on endothelial metaplasia. *Surv Ophthalmol* 1974;18:325.

188. Stone DL, Kenyon KR, Stark WJ. Ultrastructure of keratoconus with healed hydrops. *Am J Ophthalmol* 1976;82:450.

189. Petroll WM, Jester JV, Barry-Lane PA, et al. Effects of basic FGF and TGF beta 1 on F-actin and ZO-1 organization during cat endothelial wound healing. *Cornea* 1996;15:525.

190. Kenyon KR. Mesenchymal dysgenesis in Peters' anomaly, sclerocornea and congenital endothelial dystrophy. *Exp Eye Res* 1975;21:125.

191. Lee CF, et al. Immunohistochemical studies of Peters' anomaly. *Ophthalmology* 1989;96:958.

192. Nakanishi I, Brown SI. The histopathology and ultrastructure of congenital central corneal opacity (Peters' anomaly). *Am J Ophthalmol* 1971;72:801.

193. Stone DL, et al. Congenital central corneal leukoma (Peters' anomaly). *Am J Ophthalmol* 1976;81:173.

194. Kenyon KR, Maumenee AE. Further studies of congenital hereditary endothelial dystrophy. *Am J Ophthalmol* 1973;76:419.

195. Bergmanson JP, Sheldon TM, Goosey JD. Fuchs' endothelial dystrophy: a fresh look at an aging disease. *Ophthalmic Physiol Opt* 1999;19:210–222.

196. Krachmer JH, Schnitzer J, Fratkin J. Cornea pseudoguttata: a clinical and histopathologic description of endothelial cell edema. *Arch Ophthalmol* 1981;99:1377.

197. Hogan MJ, Wood I, Fine M. Fuchs' endothelial dystrophy of the cornea. *Am J Ophthalmol* 1974;78:363.

198. Kenyon KR, Van Horn DL, Edelhauser HF. Endothelial degeneration and posterior collagenous proliferation in aphakic bullous keratopathy. *Am J Ophthalmol* 1978;85:329.

199. Kenyon KR, Stark WJ, Stone DL. Corneal endothelial degeneration and fibrous proliferation after pars plana vitrectomy. *Am J Ophthalmol* 1976;81:486.

200. Grayson M. The nature of hereditary deep polymorphous dystrophy of the cornea: its association with iris and anterior chamber dysgenesis. *Trans Am Ophthalmol Soc* 1974;72:516.

201. Henriquez AS, et al. Morphologic characteristics of posterior polymorphous dystrophy: a study of nine corneas and review of the literature. *Surv Ophthalmol* 1984;29:139.

202. Klintworth G. The molecular genetics of the corneal dystrophies: current status. *Front Biosci* 2003;8:D687.

CORNEAL ANGIOGENESIS

JOSEPH J. K. MA AND ANTHONY P. ADAMIS

Angiogenesis is defined as the formation of new vessels from vascular endothelial cells derived from existing blood vessels. Aside from female reproductive cycles and wound healing, angiogenesis seldom occurs in the normal adult; only approximately 0.01% of vascular endothelial cells divide at any given time in the adult (1,2). Although much of the prior work in angiogenesis has focused on the role and interaction of vascular endothelium in angiogenesis, recent evidence has highlighted the importance of pericytes in competent vessel formation, the presence of bone marrow–derived endothelial precursor cells, and a clarification of the roles of the cytokines involved.

Corneal neovascularization is always pathologic, and represents an important cause of visual morbidity (3). It occurs in a significant proportion of corneal transplants (41%), and is an important risk factor for corneal transplant rejection and failure (4,5). There is animal model evidence that the presence of patent corneal vessels impairs transdifferentiation (6), the process by which proliferating and migrating epithelial limbal stem cells differentiate to assume a transparent corneal epithelium phenotype (7). These new, immature vessels are friable, have increased permeability, lack structural integrity, and can result in lipid deposition and corneal opacities. It is estimated that approximately 4.14% of patients in the United States may have some degree of corneal neovascularization (8). Of these patients, it is estimated that approximately 12% may have an associated decrease in visual acuity. Both diagnostically and therapeutically, it is often useful to distinguish between neovascularization that is located deep within the stroma of the cornea from that which is superficial or associated with a superficial pannus of fibrous tissue.

ETIOLOGY

The growth of new vessels in the cornea typically results from pathologic etiologies that cause acute or chronic inflammation, stem cell deficiency, or hypoxia. In the United States, herpes simplex and bacterial keratitis are the most

significant causes of neovascularization from inflammation resulting from infection. Infectious etiologies such as trachoma and onchocerciasis, however, are internationally important. Trachoma is estimated to affect 400 million people and to blind approximately 6 million people worldwide (9). Onchocerciasis affects 50 million and is estimated to blind 1 million people (10).

Stem cell deficiency leading to neovascularization of the cornea can result from trauma, alkali burns, or inflammation from diseases such Stevens-Johnson syndrome and cicatricial pemphigoid, or in association with congenital anomalies such as aniridia. Although contact lens wear is probably the most frequent cause of neovascularization from hypoxic injury to the cornea, the incidence of visual impairment from this is low. Contact lens–induced neovascularization depends on the oxygen permeability (Dk) of the contact lens material as well as duration of wear, and it often regresses with discontinuation of contact lens use (11–13). Recent advances with high-Dk lenses and daily-wear lenses are expected to decrease the incidence of corneal neovascularization secondary to contact lens wear.

THE "ANGIOGENIC SWITCH" AND STEPS INVOLVED IN ANGIOGENESIS

Angiogenesis is thought to be initiated by a disequilibrium in the balance between angiogenic and antiangiogenic factors. Collectively termed the *angiogenic switch* by Hanahan and Folkman (14), this theory arose from a study of tumor models and observations that certain tissues with constitutive expression of proangiogenic molecules [e.g., vascular endothelial growth factor (VEGF)] can remain without new blood vessel growth, whereas other tissues and assay systems could undergo steps in angiogenesis simply with the addition of these same molecules. In this latter group, however, angiogenesis could be blocked with increasing amounts of angiogenesis inhibitors (e.g., thrombospondin-1) (15,16). It is thought that this critical balance, which may be tissue specific (i.e., high inhibitory levels in some, low levels of both in others), may explain why different levels of angiogenic and antiangiogenic molecules are necessary to initiate the process in any given tissue (14). The metalloproteinases (MMPs), tissue-inhibitors of metalloproteinases (TIMPs), angiostatin, endostatin, prolactin, thrombospondin-1, arresten, tumstatin, canstatin, and pigment epithelium–derived factor are all thought to be involved, either in whole or in part, with the "angiogenic switch."

The paradigm of cryptic inhibitors of angiogenesis emerged with the discovery that certain ubiquitous extracellular matrix proteins (e.g., fibronectin, plasminogen, collagen) could be degraded by proteolytic enzymes (including MMPs) into fragments with potent antiangiogenic properties (e.g., angiostatin and endostatin-like molecules) (14). Coupled with the presence of angiogenic factors [e.g., basic fibroblast growth factor (bFGF), VEGF] nested within the extracellular matrix, a paracrine balance of factors in the angiogenic switch mechanism is also thought to play an important role in homeostasis and normal physiologic regulation (14). Matrilysin (MMP-7) may play such a role in the cornea, allowing for what some have termed the angiogenic "privilege" of the cornea (17,18).

When a disequilibrium in the angiogenic switch favors angiogenesis, the cascade of steps that follows includes (a) the disruption of the basement membrane, (b) endothelial cell migration, (c) endothelial cell proliferation, (d) endothelial cell differentiation and tube formation (19), (e) vascular pruning by leukocytes (20), and (f) maturation of the blood vessels with the recruitment of pericytes (21,22) (Fig. 5-1). There is evidence that circulating bone marrow–derived endothelial precursor cells are also involved and incorporated into new vessels (22,23) and that placental growth factor (PlGF) may play a role in recruiting them (24). VEGF-A plays a vital role in the switch mechanism and steps (a) through (e). The disruption of the basement membrane is titrated by a balance between urokinase-type plasminogen activator, MMPs, cysteine proteinase systems and plasminogen activator inhibitors, TIMPs, and cystatins (25). Endothelial cell migration is facilitated by the expression of integrins ($\alpha5\beta3$, $\alpha5\beta5$). The maturation of the blood vessels by pericytes/smooth muscle cells appears to be mediated by angiopoietins, platelet-derived growth factor (PDGF),

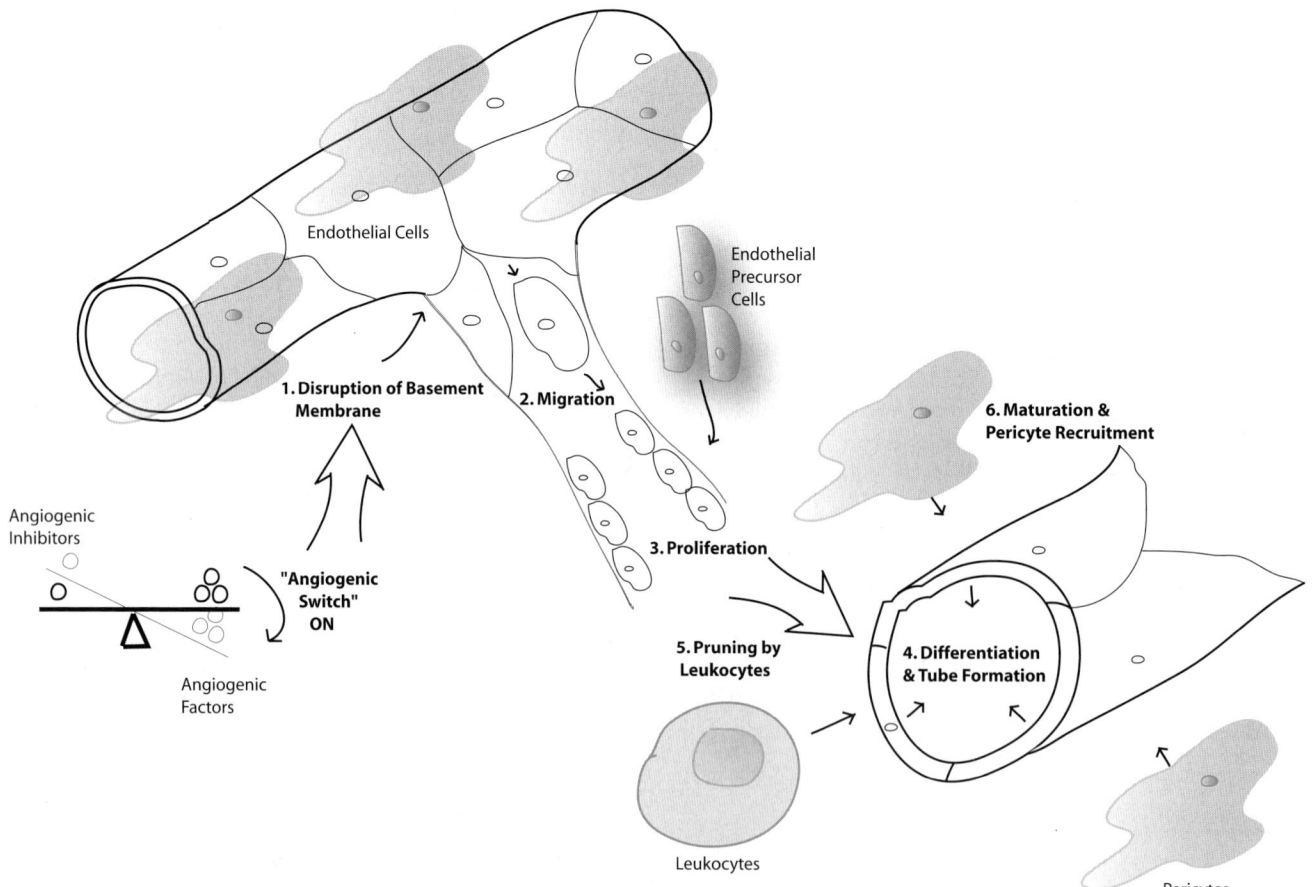

FIGURE 5-1. Steps involved in angiogenesis (described in detail in the accompanying text). Vascular endothelial growth factor-A (VEGF-A) is involved in steps 1 through 5. Placental growth factor (PlGF) is thought to be important in endothelial precursor cell recruitment. Platelet-derived growth factor (PDGF) plays a vital role in pericyte recruitment and the maturation of new vessels.

and transforming growth factor (TGF)-β, with PDGF playing a critical role in pericyte recruitment. Both *in vitro* and *in vivo* assays for angiogenesis have been developed to observe the effects of various factors on each of these crucial steps, and are briefly elaborated in the following section.

ASSAYS USED IN ANGIOGENESIS RESEARCH

In Vitro Methodologies

In vitro methods allow for the rapid screening and quantification of compounds purported to be involved in angiogenesis. However, because the endothelial cells used in these assays are usually either derived from bovine aorta or human umbilical vein, their results must be tempered by the knowledge that these cell lines may not necessarily represent those present in the *in vivo* situation. Assays for endothelial DNA synthesis (thymidine incorporation assays), endothelial cell proliferation, migration (modified Boyden chamber assays), and tube formation in extracellular matrices such as Matrigel (a product of Engelbreth-Holm-Swarm tumor cells consisting of extracellular matrix components) are available and have been useful in differentiating the specific effects of angiogenic factors on each of these critical steps in angiogenesis. Organ culture assays, which usually involve the placement of sections of rat aorta or chick aortic arch on an extracellular matrix such as Matrigel, allow for the influence of surrounding nonendothelial cells to be factored into assay responses (26).

In Vivo Methodologies

The avascular and easily accessible cornea is one of the most commonly studied *in vivo* models of angiogenesis. The corneal micropocket assay is the most widely used of these, and involves the stimulation of angiogenesis by the implantation of an angiogenic substance such as endotoxin, bFGF, or VEGF (13,27,28) in sustained-release polymers or sponge material. Originally described in rabbits (29), it has been adapted to rats and mice, allowing, in the latter, study in genetically altered models. Corneal injury models of neovascularization, involving mechanical scrape, cautery, xenograft transplants, alkali injury with NaOH, suture placement, and infection, have also been studied (30,31). Although much of the fundamentals of what we know about ocular angiogenesis has been garnered from cancer research, the classic proof of principle that tumor growth and metastasis require angiogenesis was first demonstrated in tumor cells placed on a rabbit cornea assay (32).

The earliest *in vivo* assays for angiogenesis consisted of diffusion chambers composed of Millipore filters designed to monitor neovascularization in implanted tumors (26). Chick chorioallantoic membrane (CAM) assays, which involve the study of a fertilized chick embryo that can be transferred and incubated in a culture dish (33), have become a useful tool for studying angiogenesis. Substances incorporated on membranes, gels, or coverslips are placed on the CAM, and their effect on neovascularization can be analyzed by quantifying either surface area or bifurcation points (34,35). Their results, however, can be confounded by the vessel development associated with normal embryologic development. Matrigel plug assays (36) involve the subcutaneous injection of Matrigel impregnated with test cells. A plug is formed and then harvested for the histologic analysis and quantification of neovascularization. The effect of endogenous substances administered by peritoneal pumps or similar devices can then be studied. A number of retinal and choroidal models of neovascularization have also been developed and are useful in the study of specific disease entities (37).

IMPORTANT MOLECULAR FACTORS IN ANGIOGENESIS

The Vascular Endothelial Growth Factors

The VEGFs appear to be key regulators in angiogenesis and lymphangiogenesis. VEGF, also known as VEGF-A, was first described as a vascular permeability factor isolated from tumor-induced ascitic fluid with a vessel permeability potency 50,000 times that of histamine (38,39). Since then, five related genes have been identified: PlGF, VEGF-B, VEGF-C, VEGF-D, and VEGF-E. In humans, VEGF-A has at least 3 isoforms (121, 165, and 189 amino acids in length) that result from differential splicing of a single gene.

VEGF-A is produced by a variety of cells, including macrophages, retinal pigment epithelial cells, Müller cells, astrocytes, smooth muscle cells, and T cells, and is the most extensively studied of these molecules. It is required for vascular development during embryogenesis and can stimulate endothelial cells to undergo crucial steps in angiogenesis, including basement membrane destruction, the release of MMPs and plasminogen activators, the expression of integrins, and the formation of tubes, as demonstrated by *in vitro* techniques (25,40–42). VEGF-A is temporally and spatially correlated with corneal neovascularization associated with inflammation in animal models and is increased in hypoxia (31,43–45). It is thought that the latter is mediated by hypoxia-inducible transcription factors (46,47). VEGF-A upregulation has also been demonstrated in the human cornea in inflammatory disease associated with neovascularization (48,49).

The functions of the related VEGFs are currently being characterized. VEGF-B is thought to have a significant role in nonangiogenic tumor progression. VEGF-C and VEGF-D are being investigated for their role in angiogenesis and lymphangiogenesis associated with cancer, and PlGF, for its role in vascular permeability, proliferation, chemotaxis, and angiogenesis (24,50,51).

The VEGFs interact with three receptor tyrosine kinases (RTKs) identified to date: Flt-1/VEGFR-1, Flk-1/KDR/VEGFR-2, and Flt-4/VEGFR-3. A soluble form of VEGFR-1 also exists *in vivo*. VEGF-A is thought to mediate its action on vascular endothelial cells primarily through VEGFR-2 and its effect on pericytes and smooth muscles cells through VEGFR-1. Neuropilin-1, which acts as a mediator of axonal repulsion in the nervous system, is a coreceptor for VEGF-A (165 isoform only), binds to VEGFR-2, and appears to play an important role in vascular development (52). VEGFR-1 is also expressed on goblet cells, and the inhibition of VEGF-A activity in an animal model of limbal stem cell deficiency suppressed VEGFR-1 in a pattern that was temporally and spatially related to the degree of corneal neovascularization. Thus, the suppression of neovascularization with VEGF-A may also inhibit the process of conjunctivalization of the cornea (53).

VEGF-C and VEGF-D can bind to VEGFR-2 and VEGFR-3, but with a higher affinity to the latter. VEGF-B and PlGF bind to VEGFR-1 and VEGF-E binds to VEGFR-2 (54–57). VEGF-C and VEGFR-3 are thought to be important in the process of lymphangiogenesis as well as angiogenesis (58–60). The receptors for these related compounds and their potential roles in angiogenesis are being investigated and characterized.

Angiopoietins

Angiopoietins are glycoproteins that appear to be crucial for vessel stabilization and remodeling by acting in concert with VEGF in angiogenesis and lymphangiogenesis (47,61,62). There are two known angiopoietins (Ang1 and Ang2). Angiopoietins mediate their actions through the endothelial cell–specific Tie 2 receptor through signaling that affects the regulation of PDGF-BB (63) and its effect on pericytes and smooth muscle cells.

In blood vessels, Ang1-Tie 2 signaling recruits pericytes and smooth muscle cells to stabilize vessels, whereas Ang2 inhibits this interaction. These interactions may allow for angiogenesis in the presence of VEGF and apoptosis in its absence (64,65). Ang2 appears to be important for the recruitment of smooth muscle cells and the maturation and proper functioning of lymphatic vessels (62).

Ephrins

Ephrins are the ligands for the Eph family of RTKs. There are 8 known ephrin ligands and 14 known Eph RTKs divided into two classes based on the anchoring structure of the ligand (66). Eph RTKs and ephrin ligands mediate their role through bidirectional and reciprocal interactions. Originally identified because of their critical roles in axon guidance in neuronal tissue, their importance in vascular

development during embryogenesis was subsequently appreciated when genetically altered animal models were studied. Disruption of ephrinB2 or EphB4 results in 100% embryo lethality, termination of vasculogenesis, and endothelial cell disorganization with disruption of mesenchymal support cells (67,68). Ephrins may play a vital role in distinguishing arteries and veins as well as initiating capillary development. EphrinB2 and EphB4 are excellent markers for arterial and venous endothelial cells in early embryologic development (68).

There is evidence that Eph RTKs (e.g., EphA2) have a negative effect on PDGF- and VEGF-induced endothelial cell proliferation (66,69), can mediate cell–cell repulsion (70,71), and can prevent communication between cells by reducing gap junctions (72). They also influence cellular dissociation and cadherin-induced cell attachment (73,74) and affect cellular migration and cell-to-extracellular matrix attachment by affecting integrin–receptor function (74). It is thought that the repulsion or restriction of arterial and venous endothelial cells stimulates new capillary sprout development.

Platelet-Derived Growth Factor and Pericytes

PDGF is composed of four polypeptide chains, A, B, C, and D, that form the homodimers AA, BB, CC, and DD and the heterodimer AB. There are two related RTKs: PDGFR-α (binds to AA, BB, AB, CC) and PDGFR-β (binds to BB and DD) (75). Animal models have shown that PDGF–BB and PDGFR-β are important in angiogenesis (76–79).

Mature vessel walls are composed of endothelial cells and either pericytes (arterioles, capillaries, and venules) or vascular smooth muscle cells (arteries and veins). PDGF-BB plays a critical paracrine role in vessel maturation by recruiting pericytes, which are thought to aid in basal lamina assembly and the prevention of endothelial cell apoptosis after VEGF withdrawal (80). Without pericytes, newly formed vessels consisting of endothelial capillary tubules have increased diameter, develop capillary aneurysms similar to those found in diabetic adults, are leaky, and regress in the absence of VEGF, such as occurs in retinal development (22,78,80–82). In normal retinal development, there is a critical time corresponding to the period before vessels are coated with pericytes, where endothelial cell apoptosis and vessel regression is prevented by the presence of VEGF (80). In mice, a reduction of pericyte density to 50% of normal can cause a retinopathy similar to that found in diabetic patients (81).

Although we do not yet know which is more significant, smooth muscle cells and pericytes can be derived either *de novo* from undifferentiated mesenchymal cells or through migration from a preexisting pool (83). Either way, it has been demonstrated that expression and release of PDGF-BB from endothelial cells both in angiogenesis and vasculogenesis (81,83–87) stimulates both the proliferation and migration of mesenchymal cells (88,89).

Recent evidence from tumor research has clearly demonstrated the importance of PDGFR-β in the maintenance of tumor blood vessels that have undergone some degree of maturation. Bergers et al. (21) have demonstrated in developing vessels in tumors that blocking PDGF and VEGF together can cause more regression of vessels both in early-stage (presumably before pericyte recruitment) and later-stage tumors (once pericyte attachment has occurred), than either VEGF inhibition or PDGF inhibition alone. However, because VEGF and PDGF inhibition had no purported effect on preexisting normal vessels, some other maturation process presumably occurs that prevents regression in these normal vessels (21). This indicates that there may be a therapeutic opportunity for treating relatively new vessels that have recently acquired pericytes.

TREATMENTS

Despite significant progress in the study of angiogenesis, our current clinical arsenal for treating corneal neovascularization is still limited. We wait in anticipation for the application of our newfound knowledge in angiogenesis to the clinical setting.

Preventing and arresting ongoing disease processes with antiinflammatory and antimicrobial therapy is the first line of treatment of neovascularization from infectious and inflammatory etiologies such as herpetic keratitis. Lid hygiene and doxycycline are useful in treating rosacea and meibomian gland dysfunction. Doxycycline may also exert an angiostatic effect by its inhibitory effects on collagenase (MMPs). Immunosuppressive treatment for autoimmune inflammatory disorders such as ocular cicatricial pemphigoid and peripheral ulcerative keratitis is often necessary. Clearly, the removal of local stimuli for inflammation such as sutures and foreign bodies, or hypoxic stimuli such as contact lenses, are important when these are contributing factors. Often, some of the new vessels derived from these causes regress. Nonfunctioning canalized vascular structures, known as ghost vessels, may remain. These may refill again when keratitis is reactivated, such as occurs in herpes simplex stromal keratitis.

Medical Therapy

Currently, our best medical therapy against neovascularization is the suppression of inflammation with the use of steroids (90–97). Beyond immunosuppression, steroids are also thought to exert their angiostatic activity by extracellular membrane alteration and basement membrane breakdown (98–100). Many steroids have angiostatic activity in the presence of heparin. Tetrahydrocortisol, a metabolite of cortisol, is considered one of the most potent (101). Intraocular triamcinolone acetonide has been used to inhibit retinal and subretinal neovascularization in animals with some success, and is currently being evaluated clinically (102,103).

A number of angiogenesis inhibitors have been tested in various animal models with variable efficacy, including nonsteroidal antiinflammatory drugs, cyclooxygenase-2 inhibitors (104–106), octreotide (107), cyclosporine (30), tacrolimus (108), interleukin-1 inhibitors (109), plasminogen fragments (110,111), spironolactone (112), amiloride (113), curumin (114), platelet-activating factor antagonist (115), TIMPs (116–118), and thalidomide (119,120), among others (121–126). However, the degree of vascular maturity and method for inducing neovascularization can significantly affect the assessed efficacy of therapies (122). Furthermore, most medical therapy to date has been effective in inhibiting, but not at reversing established neovascularization. In many clinical situations, it may be neither feasible nor desirable to treat patients prophylactically. Angiostatin, a cleavage product of plasminogen, has been demonstrated to regress 2-week-old vessels in an animal model (126). As mentioned earlier, the inhibition of VEGF and PDGF together in a tumor model was found to be efficacious even in advanced tumors with more mature vasculature, presumably by causing their regression (21).

Surgical Interventions

Laser treatment of corneal neovascularization has been used in animal models (127,128); its role remains uncertain in humans (129,130). Diathermy has also been used for this purpose (131). Photodynamic therapy, a method by which new vessels are labeled with a photoactivating dye, has had some success in the treatment of subretinal neovascularization in various retinal diseases. It has been attempted for the treatment of vessels in the cornea in animals, with temporary closure of new vessels (132–136).

Limbal stem cell grafting has been used with some success in ocular surface rehabilitation after the mechanical debridement of vascular pannus tissue (137). Conjunctival and amniotic membrane transplantation has also been used successfully in cases with lesser degrees of limbal stem cell deficiency, presumably by affecting epithelial transdifferentiation (138,139). Antiangiogenic molecules have also been isolated from amniotic membranes (140–142). The long-term maintenance of corneal clarity and the true efficacy of these approaches, however, have yet to be definitively validated.

CONCLUSION

The transparent, avascular cornea seems almost an anomaly in the context of otherwise vascular and opaque tissues in the body. Preserved under normal conditions, these properties have been central to its utility as an *in vivo* model of choice for fundamental studies in the identification of factors and processes in angiogenesis. This understanding has precipitated crucial research into the understanding of disease processes throughout the body, most notably in the realm of cancer, fueling exciting developments and potentially ground-breaking therapies. Because treatments with the potential for the inhibition, and perhaps even more promising, the regression of vessels, could have rippling effects in the treatment of both cancer and posterior segment disease, it would be highly desirable if such therapies could also be effectively applied to restore corneal clarity and vision in some of our most difficult-to-treat patients.

REFERENCES

1. Engerman RL, Pfaffenbach D, Davis MD. Cell turnover of capillaries. *Lab Invest* 1967;17:738–743.
2. Hobson B, Denekamp J. Endothelial proliferation in tumours and normal tissues: continuous labelling studies. *Br J Cancer* 1984;49:405–413.
3. Conn H, Berman M, Kenyon K, et al. Stromal vascularization prevents corneal ulceration. *Invest Ophthalmol Vis Sci* 1980;19:362–370.
4. Dana MR, Schaumberg DA, Kowal VO, et al. Corneal neovascularization after penetrating keratoplasty. *Cornea* 1995;14:604–609.
5. Volker-Dieben HJ, D'Amaro J, Kok-van Alphen CC. Hierarchy of prognostic factors for corneal allograft survival. *Aust N Z J Ophthalmol* 1987;15:11–18.
6. Huang AJ, Watson BD, Hernandez E, et al. Induction of conjunctival transdifferentiation on vascularized corneas by photothrombotic occlusion of corneal neovascularization. *Ophthalmology* 1988;95:228–235.
7. Kinoshita S, Kiorpes TC, Friend J, et al. Limbal epithelium in ocular surface wound healing. *Invest Ophthalmol Vis Sci* 1982;23:73–80.
8. Colby K, Adamis AP. Prevalence of corneal neovascularization in a general eye service population. ARVO Abstracts. *Invest Ophthalmol Vis Sci* 1996;37[4 Suppl]:S593.
9. World Health Organization. Methodology for trachoma control. *WHO Tech Rep Ser* 1970:703.
10. Lee P, Wang CC, Adamis AP. Ocular neovascularization: an epidemiologic review. *Surv Ophthalmol* 1998;43:245–269.
11. Binder PS. Complications associated with extended wear of soft contact lenses. *Ophthalmology* 1979;86:1093–1101.
12. Moses MA, Sudhalter J, Langer R. Identification of an inhibitor of neovascularization from cartilage. *Science* 1990;248:1408–1410.
13. Kenyon BM, Voest EE, Chen CC, et al. A model of angiogenesis in the mouse cornea. *Invest Ophthalmol Vis Sci* 1996;37:1625–1632.
14. Hanahan D, Folkman J. Patterns and emerging mechanisms of the angiogenic switch during tumorigenesis. *Cell* 1996;86:353–364.
15. Good DJ, Polverini PJ, Rastinejad F, et al. A tumor suppressor-dependent inhibitor of angiogenesis is immunologically and functionally indistinguishable from a fragment of thrombospondin. *Proc Natl Acad Sci U S A* 1990;87:6624–6628.
16. Rastinejad F, Polverini PJ, Bouck NP. Regulation of the activity of a new inhibitor of angiogenesis by a cancer suppressor gene. *Cell* 1989;56:345–355.
17. Lin HC, Chang JH, Jain S, et al. Matrilysin cleavage of corneal collagen type XVIII NC1 domain and generation of a 28-kDa fragment. *Invest Ophthalmol Vis Sci* 2001;42:2517–2524.
18. Kure T, Chang JH, Kato T, et al. Corneal neovascularization after excimer keratectomy wounds in matrilysin-deficient mice. *Invest Ophthalmol Vis Sci* 2003;44:137–144.
19. Folkman J. Tumor angiogenesis. In: Mendelsohn J, Howley PM, Israel MA, et al., (eds). *The molecular basis of cancer*. Philadelphia: WB Saunders, 1995:206–232.
20. Ishida S, Yamashiro K, Usui T, et al. Leukocytes mediate retinal vascular remodeling during development and vaso-obliteration in disease. *Nat Med* 2003;9:781–788.
21. Bergers G, Song S, Meyer-Morse N, et al. Benefits of targeting both pericytes and endothelial cells in the tumor vasculature with kinase inhibitors. *J Clin Invest* 2003;111:1287–1295.
22. Saharinen P, Alitalo K. Double target for tumor mass destruction. *J Clin Invest* 2003;111:1277–1280.
23. Asahara T, Murohara T, Sullivan A, et al. Isolation of putative progenitor endothelial cells for angiogenesis. *Science* 1997;275:964–967.
24. Luttun A, Tjwa M, Moons L, et al. Revascularization of ischemic tissues by PlGF treatment, and inhibition of tumor angiogenesis, arthritis and atherosclerosis by anti-Flt1. *Nat Med* 2002;8:831–840.
25. Witmer AN, Vrensen GF, Van Noorden CJ, et al. Vascular endothelial growth factors and angiogenesis in eye disease. *Prog Retin Eye Res* 2003;22:1–29.
26. Auerbach R, Lewis R, Shinners B, et al. Angiogenesis assays: a critical overview. *Clin Chem* 2003;49:32–40.
27. Li WW, Grayson G, Folkman J, et al. Sustained-release endotoxin: a model for inducing corneal neovascularization. *Invest Ophthalmol Vis Sci* 1991;32:2906–2911.
28. Loughman MS, Chatzistefanou K, Gonzalez EM, et al. Experimental corneal neovascularisation using sucralfate and basic fibroblast growth factor. *Aust N Z J Ophthalmol* 1996;24:289–295.
29. Gimbrone MA Jr, Cotran RS, Leapman SB, et al. Tumor growth and neovascularization: an experimental model using the rabbit cornea. *J Natl Cancer Inst* 1974;52:413–427.
30. Benelli U, Ross JR, Nardi M, et al. Corneal neovascularization induced by xenografts or chemical cautery: inhibition by cyclosporin A. *Invest Ophthalmol Vis Sci* 1997;38:274–282.
31. Amano S, Rohan R, Kuroki M, et al. Requirement for vascular endothelial growth factor in wound- and inflammation-related corneal neovascularization. *Invest Ophthalmol Vis Sci* 1998;39:18–22.
32. Gimbrone MA Jr, Leapman SB, Cotran RS, et al. Tumor dormancy in vivo by prevention of neovascularization. *J Exp Med* 1972;136:261–276.
33. Auerbach R, Kubai L, Knighton D, et al. A simple procedure for the long-term cultivation of chicken embryos. *Dev Biol* 1974;41:391–394.
34. Brooks PC, Montgomery AM, Cheresh DA. Use of the 10-day-old chick embryo model for studying angiogenesis. *Methods Mol Biol* 1999;129:257–269.
35. Nguyen M, Shing Y, Folkman J. Quantitation of angiogenesis and antiangiogenesis in the chick embryo chorioallantoic membrane. *Microvasc Res* 1994;47:31–40.
36. Passaniti A, Taylor RM, Pili R, et al. A simple, quantitative method for assessing angiogenesis and antiangiogenic agents using reconstituted basement membrane, heparin, and fibroblast growth factor. *Lab Invest* 1992;67:519–528.
37. Tolentino M, Adamis AP, Miller JW. Angiogenic factors and inhibitors. In: Albert D, Jakobiec FA (eds). *Principles and practice of ophthalmology*. Philadelphia: WB Saunders, 2000: CD ROM.

38. Senger DR, Galli SJ, Dvorak AM, et al. Tumor cells secrete a vascular permeability factor that promotes accumulation of ascites fluid. *Science* 1983;219:983–985.
39. Ribatti D, Vacca A, Presta M. The discovery of angiogenic factors: a historical review. *Gen Pharmacol* 2000;35:227–231.
40. Carmeliet P, Ferreira V, Breier G, et al. Abnormal blood vessel development and lethality in embryos lacking a single VEGF allele. *Nature* 1996;380:435–439.
41. Senger DR, Brown LF, Claffey KP, et al. Vascular permeability factor, tumor angiogenesis and stroma generation. *Invasion Metastasis* 1994;14:385–394.
42. Ferrara N. Vascular endothelial growth factor: molecular and biological aspects. *Curr Top Microbiol Immunol* 1999;237:1–30.
43. Shima DT, Adamis AP, Ferrara N, et al. Hypoxic induction of endothelial cell growth factors in retinal cells: identification and characterization of vascular endothelial growth factor (VEGF) as the mitogen. *Mol Med* 1995;1:182–193.
44. Hata Y, Nakagawa K, Ishibashi T, et al. Hypoxia-induced expression of vascular endothelial growth factor by retinal glial cells promotes in vitro angiogenesis. *Virchows Arch* 1995;426:479–486.
45. Aiello LP, Northrup JM, Keyt BA, et al. Hypoxic regulation of vascular endothelial growth factor in retinal cells. *Arch Ophthalmol* 1995;113:1538–1544.
46. Kaelin WG Jr. How oxygen makes its presence felt. *Genes Dev* 2002;16:1441–1445.
47. Veikkola T, Alitalo K. Dual role of Ang2 in postnatal angiogenesis and lymphangiogenesis. *Dev Cell* 2002;3:302–304.
48. Philipp W, Speicher L, Humpel C. Expression of vascular endothelial growth factor and its receptors in inflamed and vascularized human corneas. *Invest Ophthalmol Vis Sci* 2000;41: 2514–2522.
49. Cursiefen C, Rummelt C, Kuchle M. Immunohistochemical localization of vascular endothelial growth factor, transforming growth factor alpha, and transforming growth factor beta1 in human corneas with neovascularization. *Cornea* 2000;19:526–533.
50. Odorisio T, Schietroma C, Zaccaria ML, et al. Mice overexpressing placenta growth factor exhibit increased vascularization and vessel permeability. *J Cell Sci* 2002;115:2559–2567.
51. Ziche M, Maglione D, Ribatti D, et al. Placenta growth factor-1 is chemotactic, mitogenic, and angiogenic. *Lab Invest* 1997; 76:517–531.
52. Fuh G, Li B, Crowley C, et al. Requirements for binding and signaling of the kinase domain receptor for vascular endothelial growth factor. *J Biol Chem* 1998;273:11197–11204.
53. Joussen AM, Poulaki V, Mitsiades N, et al. VEGF-dependent conjunctivalization of the corneal surface. *Invest Ophthalmol Vis Sci* 2003;44:117–123.
54. Olofsson B, Korpelainen E, Pepper MS, et al. Vascular endothelial growth factor B (VEGF-B) binds to VEGF receptor-1 and regulates plasminogen activator activity in endothelial cells. *Proc Natl Acad Sci U S A* 1998;95:11709–11714.
55. Clauss M, Weich H, Breier G, et al. The vascular endothelial growth factor receptor Flt-1 mediates biological activities: implications for a functional role of placenta growth factor in monocyte activation and chemotaxis. *J Biol Chem* 1996;271: 17629–17634.
56. Eriksson U, Alitalo K. Structure, expression and receptor-binding properties of novel vascular endothelial growth factors. *Curr Top Microbiol Immunol* 1999;237:41–57.
57. Meyer M, Clauss M, Lepple-Wienhues A, et al. A novel vascular endothelial growth factor encoded by Orf virus, VEGF-E, mediates angiogenesis via signalling through VEGFR-2 (KDR) but not VEGFR-1 (Flt-1) receptor tyrosine kinases. *EMBO J* 1999;18:363–374.
58. Veikkola T, Jussila L, Makinen T, et al. Signalling via vascular endothelial growth factor receptor-3 is sufficient for lymphangiogenesis in transgenic mice. *EMBO J* 2001;20:1223–1231.
59. Skobe M, Hawighorst T, Jackson DG, et al. Induction of tumor lymphangiogenesis by VEGF-C promotes breast cancer metastasis. *Nat Med* 2001;7:192–198.
60. Makinen T, Veikkola T, Mustjoki S, et al. Isolated lymphatic endothelial cells transduce growth, survival and migratory signals via the VEGF-C/D receptor VEGFR-3. *EMBO J* 2001;20: 4762–4773.
61. Wong AL, Haroon ZA, Werner S, et al. Tie2 expression and phosphorylation in angiogenic and quiescent adult tissues. *Circ Res* 1997;81:567–574.
62. Gale NW, Thurston G, Hackett SF, et al. Angiopoietin-2 is required for postnatal angiogenesis and lymphatic patterning, and only the latter role is rescued by angiopoietin-1. *Dev Cell* 2002;3:411–423.
63. Folkman J, D'Amore PA. Blood vessel formation: what is its molecular basis? *Cell* 1996;87:1153–1155.
64. Maisonpierre PC, Suri C, Jones PF, et al. Angiopoietin-2, a natural antagonist for Tie2 that disrupts in vivo angiogenesis. *Science* 1997;277:55–60.
65. Holash J, Wiegand SJ, Yancopoulos GD. New model of tumor angiogenesis: dynamic balance between vessel regression and growth mediated by angiopoietins and VEGF. *Oncogene* 1999;18:5356–5362.
66. Cheng N, Brantley DM, Chen J. The ephrins and Eph receptors in angiogenesis. *Cytokine Growth Factor Rev* 2002;13:75–85.
67. Gerety SS, Wang HU, Chen ZF, et al. Symmetrical mutant phenotypes of the receptor EphB4 and its specific transmembrane ligand ephrin-B2 in cardiovascular development. *Mol Cell* 1999;4:403-414.
68. Wang HU, Chen ZF, Anderson DJ. Molecular distinction and angiogenic interaction between embryonic arteries and veins revealed by ephrin-B2 and its receptor Eph-B4. *Cell* 1998;93: 741–753.
69. Miao H, Wei BR, Peehl DM, et al. Activation of EphA receptor tyrosine kinase inhibits the Ras/MAPK pathway. *Nat Cell Biol* 2001;3:527–530.
70. Klein R. Excitatory Eph receptors and adhesive ephrin ligands. *Curr Opin Cell Biol* 2001;13:196–203.
71. Flanagan JG, Vanderhaeghen P. The ephrins and Eph receptors in neural development. *Annu Rev Neurosci* 1998;21:309–345.
72. Mellitzer G, Xu Q, Wilkinson DG. Eph receptors and ephrins restrict cell intermingling and communication. *Nature* 1999; 400:77–81.
73. Orsulic S, Kemler R. Expression of Eph receptors and ephrins is differentially regulated by E-cadherin. *J Cell Sci* 2000;113: 1793–1802.
74. Winning RS, Scales JB, Sargent TD. Disruption of cell adhesion in *Xenopus* embryos by Pagliaccio, an Eph-class receptor tyrosine kinase. *Dev Biol* 1996;179:309–319.
75. Betsholtz C, Karlsson L, Lindahl P. Developmental roles of platelet-derived growth factors. *Bioessays* 2001;23:494–507.
76. Leveen P, Pekny M, Gebre-Medhin S, et al. Mice deficient for PDGF B show renal, cardiovascular, and hematological abnormalities. *Genes Dev* 1994;8:1875–1887.
77. Lindahl P, Hellstrom M, Kalen M, et al. Endothelial-perivascular cell signaling in vascular development: lessons from knockout mice. *Curr Opin Lipidol* 1998;9:407–411.
78. Lindahl P, Johansson BR, Leveen P, et al. Pericyte loss and microaneurysm formation in PDGF-B-deficient mice. *Science* 1997;277:242–245.
79. Soriano P. Abnormal kidney development and hematological disorders in PDGF beta-receptor mutant mice. *Genes Dev* 1994;8:1888–1896.
80. Benjamin LE, Hemo I, Keshet E. A plasticity window for blood vessel remodelling is defined by pericyte coverage of the preformed endothelial network and is regulated by PDGF-B and VEGF. *Development* 1998;125:1591–1598.

81. Enge M, Bjarnegard M, Gerhardt H, et al. Endothelium-specific platelet-derived growth factor-B ablation mimics diabetic retinopathy. *EMBO J* 2002;21:4307–4316.

82. Benjamin LE, Golijanin D, Itin A, et al. Selective ablation of immature blood vessels in established human tumors follows vascular endothelial growth factor withdrawal. *J Clin Invest* 1999;103:159–165.

83. Hellstrom M, Kalen M, Lindahl P, et al. Role of PDGF-B and PDGFR-beta in recruitment of vascular smooth muscle cells and pericytes during embryonic blood vessel formation in the mouse. *Development* 1999;126:3047–3055.

84. Mudhar HS, Pollock RA, Wang C, et al. PDGF and its receptors in the developing rodent retina and optic nerve. *Development* 1993;118:539–552.

85. Barrett TB, Gajdusek CM, Schwartz SM, et al. Expression of the sis gene by endothelial cells in culture and in vivo. *Proc Natl Acad Sci U S A* 1984;81:6772–6774.

86. Collins T, Ginsburg D, Boss JM, et al. Cultured human endothelial cells express platelet-derived growth factor B chain: cDNA cloning and structural analysis. *Nature* 1985;316:748–750.

87. DiCorleto PE, Bowen-Pope DF. Cultured endothelial cells produce a platelet-derived growth factor-like protein. *Proc Natl Acad Sci U S A* 1983;80:1919–1923.

88. Hirschi KK, Rohovsky SA, D'Amore PA. PDGF, TGF-beta, and heterotypic cell-cell interactions mediate endothelial cell-induced recruitment of 10T1/2 cells and their differentiation to a smooth muscle fate. *J Cell Biol* 1998;141:805–814.

89. Hirschi KK, Rohovsky SA, Beck LH, et al. Endothelial cells modulate the proliferation of mural cell precursors via platelet-derived growth factor-BB and heterotypic cell contact. *Circ Res* 1999;84:298–305.

90. Mahoney JM, Waterbury LD. Drug effects on the neovascularization response to silver nitrate cauterization of the rat cornea. *Curr Eye Res* 1985;4:531–535.

91. Nikolic L, Friend J, Taylor S, et al. Inhibition of vascularization in rabbit corneas by heparin: cortisone pellets. *Invest Ophthalmol Vis Sci* 1986;27:449–456.

92. Phillips K, Arffa R, Cintron C, et al. Effects of prednisolone and medroxyprogesterone on corneal wound healing, ulceration, and neovascularization. *Arch Ophthalmol* 1983;101:640–643.

93. Suzuki T, Sano Y, Sotozono C, et al. Regulatory effects of 1alpha,25-dihydroxyvitamin D(3) on cytokine production by human corneal epithelial cells. *Curr Eye Res* 2000;20:127–130.

94. McNatt LG, Weimer L, Yanni J, et al. Angiostatic activity of steroids in the chick embryo CAM and rabbit cornea models of neovascularization. *J Ocul Pharmacol Ther* 1999;15:413–423.

95. Boneham GC, Collin HB. Steroid inhibition of limbal blood and lymphatic vascular cell growth. *Curr Eye Res* 1995;14:1–10.

96. BenEzra D, Griffin BW, Maftzir G, et al. Topical formulations of novel angiostatic steroids inhibit rabbit corneal neovascularization. *Invest Ophthalmol Vis Sci* 1997;38:1954–1962.

97. Chang JH, Gabison EE, Kato T, et al. Corneal neovascularization. *Curr Opin Ophthalmol* 2001;12:242–249.

98. Ingber DE, Madri JA, Folkman J. A possible mechanism for inhibition of angiogenesis by angiostatic steroids: induction of capillary basement membrane dissolution. *Endocrinology* 1986;119:1768–1775.

99. Ingber D, Folkman J. Inhibition of angiogenesis through modulation of collagen metabolism. *Lab Invest* 1988;59:44–51.

100. Maragoudakis ME, Sarmonika M, Panoutsacopoulou M. Antiangiogenic action of heparin plus cortisone is associated with decreased collagenous protein synthesis in the chick chorioallantoic membrane system. *J Pharmacol Exp Ther* 1989;251:679–682.

101. Crum R, Szabo S, Folkman J. A new class of steroids inhibits angiogenesis in the presence of heparin or a heparin fragment. *Science* 1985;230:1375–1378.

102. Danis RP, Bingaman DP, Yang Y, et al. Inhibition of preretinal and optic nerve head neovascularization in pigs by intravitreal triamcinolone acetonide. *Ophthalmology* 1996;103:2099–2104.

103. Ishibashi T, Miki K, Sorgente N, et al. Effects of intravitreal administration of steroids on experimental subretinal neovascularization in the subhuman primate. *Arch Ophthalmol* 1985;103:708–711.

104. Yamada M, Kawai M, Kawai Y, et al. The effect of selective cyclooxygenase-2 inhibitor on corneal angiogenesis in the rat. *Curr Eye Res* 1999;19:300–304.

105. Tsujii M, Kawano S, Tsuji S, et al. Cyclooxygenase regulates angiogenesis induced by colon cancer cells. *Cell* 1998;93:705–716.

106. Shen WY, Constable IJ, Chelva E, et al. Inhibition of diclofenac formulated in hyaluronan on angiogenesis in vitro and its intraocular tolerance in the rabbit eye. *Graefes Arch Clin Exp Ophthalmol* 2000;238:273–282.

107. Demir T, Celiker UO, Kukner A, et al. Effect of octreotide on experimental corneal neovascularization. *Acta Ophthalmol Scand* 1999;77:386–390.

108. Benelli U, Lepri A, Del Tacca M, et al. FK-506 delays corneal graft rejection in a model of corneal xenotransplantation. *J Ocul Pharmacol Ther* 1996;12:425–431.

109. Dana MR, Zhu SN, Yamada J. Topical modulation of interleukin-1 activity in corneal neovascularization. *Cornea* 1998;17:403–409.

110. Kim JH, Kim JC, Shin SH, et al. The inhibitory effects of recombinant plasminogen kringle 1-3 on the neovascularization of rabbit cornea induced by angiogenin, bFGF, and VEGF. *Exp Mol Med* 1999;31:203–209.

111. Cao R, Wu HL, Veitonmaki N, et al. Suppression of angiogenesis and tumor growth by the inhibitor K1-5 generated by plasmin-mediated proteolysis. *Proc Natl Acad Sci U S A* 1999;96:5728–5733.

112. Klauber N, Browne F, Anand-Apte B, et al. New activity of spironolactone: inhibition of angiogenesis in vitro and in vivo. *Circulation* 1996;94:2566–2571.

113. Sood AK, Gupta B, Chugh P. Topical amiloride accelerates healing and delays neovascularization in mechanically produced corneal ulcers in rabbits. *Methods Find Exp Clin Pharmacol* 1999;21:491–497.

114. Arbiser JL, Klauber N, Rohan R, et al. Curcumin is an in vivo inhibitor of angiogenesis. *Mol Med* 1998;4:376–383.

115. Cohen RA, Gebhardt BM, Bazan NG. A platelet-activating factor antagonist reduces corneal allograft inflammation and neovascularization. *Curr Eye Res* 1994;13:139–144.

116. Taraboletti G, Garofalo A, Belotti D, et al. Inhibition of angiogenesis and murine hemangioma growth by batimastat, a synthetic inhibitor of matrix metalloproteinases. *J Natl Cancer Inst* 1995;87:293–298.

117. Qi JH, Ebrahem Q, Moore N, et al. A novel function for tissue inhibitor of metalloproteinases-3 (TIMP3): inhibition of angiogenesis by blockage of VEGF binding to VEGF receptor-2. *Nat Med* 2003;9:407–415.

118. Hadeyama T, Ebihara N, Watanabe Y, et al. Inhibitory effects of matrix metalloproteinase inhibitor on corneal neovascularization [in Japanese]. *Nippon Ganka Gakkai Zasshi* 1998;102:270–275.

119. Kruse FE, Joussen AM, Rohrschneider K, et al. Thalidomide inhibits corneal angiogenesis induced by vascular endothelial growth factor. *Graefes Arch Clin Exp Ophthalmol* 1998;236:461–466.

120. Kenyon BM, Browne F, D'Amato RJ. Effects of thalidomide and related metabolites in a mouse corneal model of neovascularization. *Exp Eye Res* 1997;64:971–978.

121. Duenas Z, Torner L, Corbacho AM, et al. Inhibition of rat corneal angiogenesis by 16-kDa prolactin and by endogenous prolactin-like molecules. *Invest Ophthalmol Vis Sci* 1999;40: 2498–2505.

122. Klotz O, Park JK, Pleyer U, et al. Inhibition of corneal neovascularization by alpha(v)-integrin antagonists in the rat. *Graefes Arch Clin Exp Ophthalmol* 2000;238:88–93.

123. Joussen AM, Kruse FE, Volcker HE, et al. Topical application of methotrexate for inhibition of corneal angiogenesis. *Graefes Arch Clin Exp Ophthalmol* 1999;237:920–927.

124. Hepsen IF, Er H, Cekic O. Topically applied water extract of propolis to suppress corneal neovascularization in rabbits. *Ophthalmic Res* 1999;31:426–431.

125. Volpert OV, Tolsma SS, Pellerin S, et al. Inhibition of angiogenesis by thrombospondin-2. *Biochem Biophys Res Commun* 1995;217:326–332.

126. Ambati BK, Joussen AM, Ambati J, et al. Angiostatin inhibits and regresses corneal neovascularization. *Arch Ophthalmol* 2002;120:1063–1068.

127. Nirankari VS. Laser photocoagulation for corneal stromal vascularization. *Trans Am Ophthalmol Soc* 1992;90:595–669.

128. Nirankari VS, Dandona L, Rodrigues MM. Laser photocoagulation of experimental corneal stromal vascularization: efficacy and histopathology. *Ophthalmology* 1993;100:111–118.

129. Nirankari VS, Baer JC. Corneal argon laser photocoagulation for neovascularization in penetrating keratoplasty. *Ophthalmology* 1986;93:1304–1309.

130. Baer JC, Foster CS. Corneal laser photocoagulation for treatment of neovascularization: efficacy of 577 nm yellow dye laser. *Ophthalmology* 1992;99:173–179.

131. Pillai CT, Dua HS, Hossain P. Fine needle diathermy occlusion of corneal vessels. *Invest Ophthalmol Vis Sci* 2000;41:2148–2153.

132. Primbs GB, Casey R, Wamser K, et al. Photodynamic therapy for corneal neovascularization. *Ophthalmic Surg Lasers* 1998; 29:832–838.

133. Gohto Y, Obana A, Kanai M, et al. Treatment parameters for selective occlusion of experimental corneal neovascularization by photodynamic therapy using a water soluble photosensitizer, ATX-S10(Na). *Exp Eye Res* 2001;72:13–22.

134. Gohto Y, Obana A, Kanai M, et al. Photodynamic therapy for corneal neovascularization using topically administered ATX-S10 (Na). *Ophthalmic Surg Lasers* 2000;31:55–60.

135. Gohto Y, Obana A, Kaneda K, et al. Accumulation of photosensitizer ATX-S10 (Na) in experimental corneal neovascularization. *Jpn J Ophthalmol* 2000;44:348–353.

136. Gohto Y, Obana A, Kaneda K, et al. Photodynamic effect of a new photosensitizer ATX-S10 on corneal neovascularization. *Exp Eye Res* 1998;67:313–322.

137. Ma DH, Tsai RJ, Chu WK, et al. Inhibition of vascular endothelial cell morphogenesis in cultures by limbal epithelial cells. *Invest Ophthalmol Vis Sci* 1999;40:1822–1828.

138. Kwitko S, Marinho D, Barcaro S, et al. Allograft conjunctival transplantation for bilateral ocular surface disorders. *Ophthalmology* 1995;102:1020–1025.

139. Tseng SC, Prabhasawat P, Barton K, et al. Amniotic membrane transplantation with or without limbal allografts for corneal surface reconstruction in patients with limbal stem cell deficiency. *Arch Ophthalmol* 1998;116:431–441.

140. Hao Y, Ma DH, Hwang DG, et al. Identification of antiangiogenic and antiinflammatory proteins in human amniotic membrane. *Cornea* 2000;19:348–352.

141. Tsai RJ, Li LM, Chen JK. Reconstruction of damaged corneas by transplantation of autologous limbal epithelial cells. *N Engl J Med* 2000;343:86–93.

142. Burgos H. Angiogenic and growth factors in human amniochorion and placenta. *Eur J Clin Invest* 1983;13:289–296.

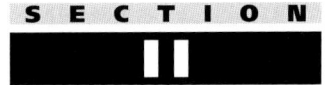

SECTION

II

EXAMINATION AND EVALUATION TECHNIQUES

6

SLIT-LAMP BIOMICROSCOPY AND PHOTOGRAPHY

MARK P. HATTON AND LAWRENCE M. MERIN

Slit-lamp biomicroscopy of the anterior segment provides the ability to view an illuminated tissue under high magnification. It is not one technique. Rather, various methods of examination are used by adjusting the illumination intensity, beam width, viewing angle, and magnification of the slit-lamp biomicroscope. Alone, each method offers a unique perspective into the normal or abnormal tissue under investigation. Together, the dynamic process of slit-lamp biomicroscopy provides the examiner a complete picture of the nature of the healthy and diseased anterior segment.

EXAMINATION TECHNIQUES

Diffuse Broad-Beam Illumination

Opening the aperture of the slit to its widest setting creates a full, broad illuminating beam. The intensity of this beam can be dampened by the introduction of the neutral density filter to reduce the discomfort experienced by the patient. The wide beam provides diffuse illumination such as would be obtained from the illumination provided by a penlight or muscle light.

This technique is used to perform a general inspection of the anterior segment and adnexal structures under low magnification. It offers the observer the "big picture," which might otherwise be missed if an area of interest is immediately isolated with high magnification. This technique is useful in assessing the overall degree of ocular erythema, identifying areas of corneal opacity or surface irregularity, localizing corneal and conjunctival foreign bodies, and determining patterns of normal and abnormal pigmentation (Fig. 6-1).

Examination with broad-beam illumination should also be performed while the light source is actively rotated from side to side. As the beam is applied tangentially at different angles, variations in elevation and depressions are emphasized and contrast is increased. This permits the observer to determine whether the lesion of interest is flat or if it has any degree of elevation (Fig. 6-2).

Focal Illumination

By narrowing the beam and shortening its height, the examiner can create a "spotlight" to permit viewing an object of interest in isolation without illuminating surrounding tissues. An essential derivative of this technique is the optical section. The slit-lamp biomicroscope provides the unique ability to view an optical cross section of the semitransparent (i.e., translucent) tissues of the eye (cornea, aqueous, lens) in vivo. Although the vast majority of light rays pass through the cornea unimpeded, slight irregularities in its substance result in reflection of light back to the examiner. This fact can be used to localize abnormalities to one or more layers of the cornea. Rotating the illumination arm allows the narrow slit beam to strike obliquely the lesion of regard. When angled at 45 degrees from the observation axis, maximal information about the internal structure of the cornea is revealed. At a lesser angle, the optical section collapses, whereas more than 45 degrees decreases brightness and gives a false impression of angular distance between the corneal layers.

The slit lamp is designed so that the slit beam and biomicroscope are focused at the same plane, thus allowing for movement of the illumination and viewing arms by the examiner to appreciate best the nature and depth of the lesion while remaining in focus. With this slit-beam technique, each layer of the cornea and tear film may be examined. Thus, the location of a lesion in the cornea may be determined by noting where it falls in the optical section. (Fig. 6-3).

The thin slit beam also permits the examiner to note the thickness and curvature of the cornea. Localized depressions result in the beam of light appearing to bend posteriorly. Similarly, elevated lesions within the cornea cause the light beam to appear to bend toward the observer (Fig. 6-4). This ability to detect changes in thickness may also be applied to the conjunctiva, where deviation in the appearance of the slit beam can detect elevations and depressions.

Focal illumination with a small, narrow slit beam also permits examination of the aqueous. The normal aqueous is transparent: Light rays pass through it unimpeded. White blood cells or increased protein content (flare) present during

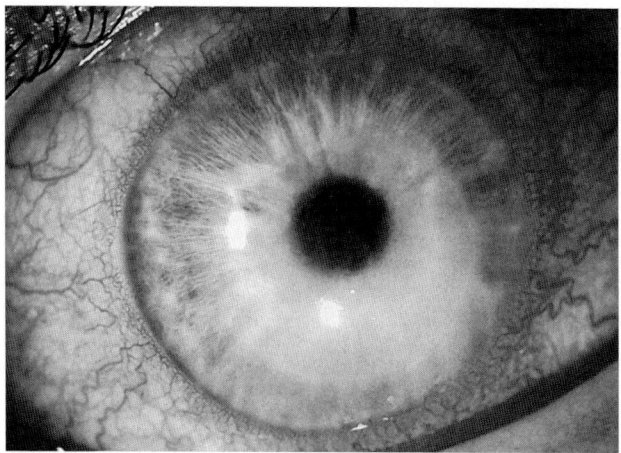

FIG. 6-1. Diffuse, broad-beam illumination of a patient with herpes simplex keratouveitis. The low magnification combined with diffuse illumination permits the examiner to comprehend the "big picture." In this case, this technique documents ciliary flush, keratic precipitates, and corneal edema.

inflammation result in reflection of light, or Tyndall's phenomenon. A 0.2 × 0.2 light beam is applied at an oblique angle. On Haag-Streit and similar instruments, the light tower should be tilted forward. This technique is enhanced by observing the findings in the light beam against the black background provided by the pupil. The degree of inflammation is graded using a standard system (Tables 6-1 and 6-2).

SPECULAR REFLECTION

Examination of the cornea with any light source results in the reflection of the light source back toward the examiner (e.g., corneal light reflex). This phenomenon obeys Snells's law stating that the angle of incidence is equal to the angle of reflection. To observe objects in the cornea by specular reflection, the examiner must align the angle of observation to be equal with the angle of light directed toward the cornea.

Specular reflection occurs both at the epithelium–tear interface as well as the endothelial–aqueous interface. The corneal light reflex, due to specular reflection from the epithelium–tear interface, is usually crisp and well defined. Any disruption in the surface of the cornea does not permit uniform reflection of light, which suggests areas of discontinuity or irregularity of the corneal surface.

Focusing the beam deeper into the cornea permits observation of specular reflection from the endothelial–aqueous interface. This method allows for visualization of the endothelial cells and can accentuate abnormalities, such as abnormal morphology characteristic of endothelial cell damage (Fig. 6-5).

The examination techniques discussed to this point rely on direct illumination of the object of interest by the light source. Additional information can be obtained by viewing the object of interest with light reflected from another location.

Sclerotic Scatter

Total internal reflection of light rays in the anterior segment requires the use of a gonioscopy lens to view the angle structures. Similarly, a portion of the light rays directed at the cornea undergoes total internal reflection between the anterior and posterior corneal surfaces. This can be maximized by directing the light beam at the corneoscleral junction. In the normal cornea, this technique results only in a faint glow at the limbus; the remainder of the cornea is not affected and remains clear. However, irregularities in the cornea, if present, cause the light being reflected in the stroma to be scattered and, in part, reflected toward the examiner (Fig. 6-6).

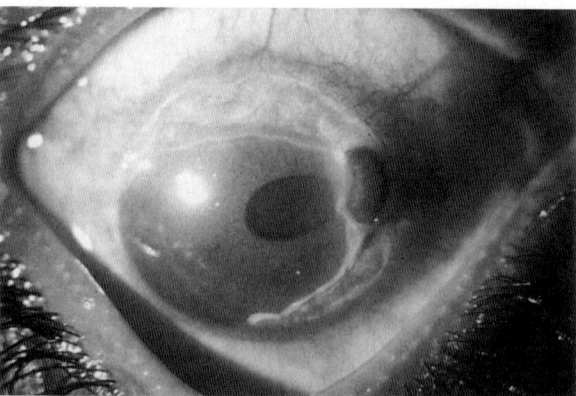

A

B

FIG. 6-2. A. Tangential illumination with a broad beam of a normal iris. The observed shadows result from elevations on the iris surface. This technique can permit the examiner to determine whether an observed lesion is flat or elevated. **B.** Tangential illumination of an eye with Mooren's ulcer with perforation. The protruding iris casts a shadow, suggesting it is elevated above the plane of the cornea.

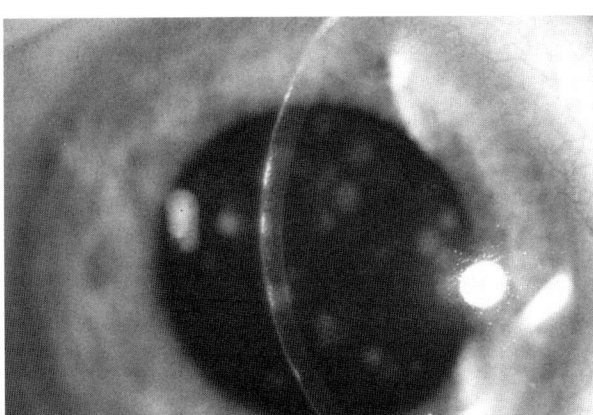

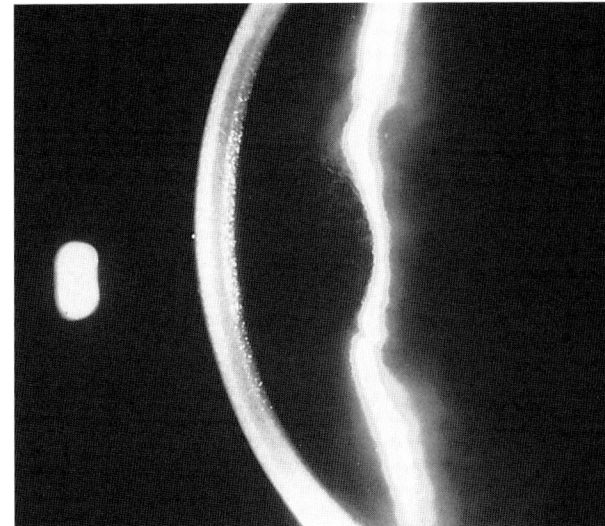

A
B

FIG. 6-3. A. In this photograph, the opacities that occurred during the course of adenoviral infection were located in the first part of the optical section, suggesting localization to the subepithelium or anterior stroma. **B.** Optical section of a cornea with Fuchs' dystrophy. In this photograph, the abnormality (guttata) exists in the most posterior aspect of the slit beam, consistent with the endothelial location of the lesion.

Sclerotic scatter is performed by directing the light beam tangentially toward the limbus until the entire limbal circumference appears to glow. Observation of the cornea is then performed. This technique is particularly useful for detecting subtle irregularities that might be missed with other examination techniques.

RETROILLUMINATION

Retroillumination is the technique of visualizing structures against an illuminated background. The beam of light, directed at a location more posterior than the object of interest, is reflected and viewed in its return pathway toward the

examiner. Objects in this returning beam's path block the transmission of light, thus permitting them to be visualized in silhouette. This is most frequently performed by directing light toward the pupil to create the familiar red reflex from the posterior segment (Fig. 6-7). However, retroillumination of the cornea can also be performed by directing the light beam at the iris (Fig. 6-8). Objects can appear different with each source of back-lighting (fundus or iris), and each can provide a different perspective to the examiner.

By aligning the junction between the illuminated and nonilluminated background with the subject, subtle corneal changes, such as basement membrane dystrophies, may be seen in the interface region.

DYES

Fluorescein, commercially available in solution or concentrated on filter paper strips, is nontoxic to corneal epithelium and is taken up in areas in which disruptions of cell–cell junctions exist or epithelium is absent completely. As such, it is useful in documenting the presence of corneal epithelial defects resulting, for example, from abrasion or

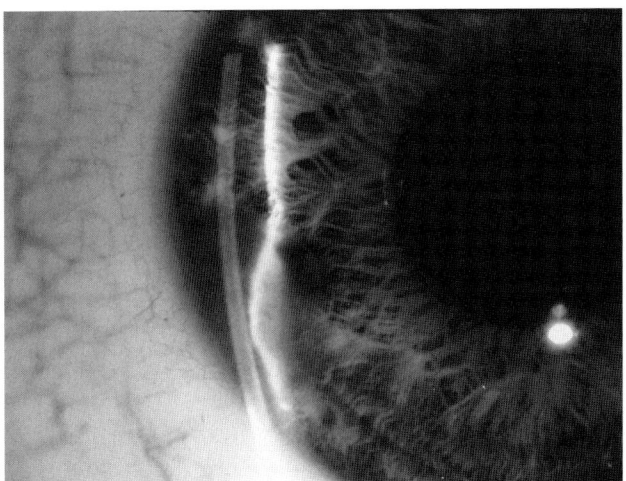

FIG. 6-4. Slit-beam examination of iris melanoma. The elevated lesion results in a light beam that appears to bend toward the examiner.

TABLE 6-1. GRADATION OF CELLS IN THE AQUEOUS

Grade	Cells
0	No cells
½+	1-5
1+	6-15
2+	16-25
3+	26-60

TABLE 6-2. GRADATION OF FLARE IN THE AQUEOUS

Grade	Flare
0	No flare
1+	Faint
2+	Slight obscuration of lens/iris
3+	Marked obscuration of lens/iris
4+	Fibrin present

active herpetic infection (Fig. 6-9). The fluorescein molecule emits green light (520 nm) when it is excited by light in the blue range (490 nm). As a result, observation of the pattern of fluorescein staining requires introduction of the cobalt blue excitation filter. The use of a wide-aperture beam permits the examiner to determine patterns of fluorescein staining across the entire cornea. The observed patterns can often provide clues toward determining the etiology of disease. For example, exposure keratopathy typically results in fluorescein uptake in the interpalpebral space, whereas a toxic keratopathy (such as after chemical exposure) most often results in diffuse uptake across the entire cornea.

True staining should be distinguished from pooling, in which the fluorescein collects in depressions on the ocular surface but is not taken up because of the presence of an intact epithelium. "Negative" staining can also occur and refers to the pattern of fluorescein collection around elevated lesions on the surface of the eye. In the Seidel test, fluorescein is also used to demonstrate wound leakage by providing a fluorescent background through which streams of aqueous are revealed.

Unlike fluorescein, rose bengal does exhibit toxicity *in vitro*, but is considered safe for clinical applications. It is

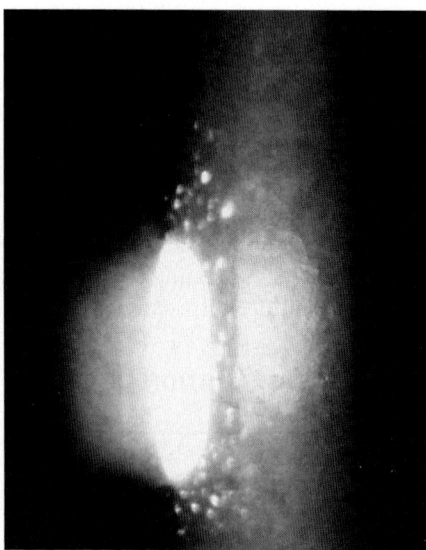

FIG. 6-5. Specular reflection demonstrating endothelial cells, seen in the region of moderate reflection to the left of the glaring epithelial reflex.

a derivative of the fluorescein molecule and stains devitalized epithelial cells even when the epithelium remains intact. Rose bengal is also taken up by healthy epithelial cells that lack an adequate mucin layer (1,2). Accordingly, severe tear film abnormalities result in rose bengal, but not fluorescein, staining (Fig. 6-10). The two dyes may be used consecutively to provide a more complete assessment of the integrity of the ocular surface. As with fluorescein, rose bengal comes concentrated on paper strips. Unlike fluorescein, however, it is nonfluorescent, and so can be viewed in direct light, and is irritating to the patient, usually requiring application of topical anesthetic.

Lissamine green offers many of the same applications as rose bengal, and its patterns of distribution are observed and recorded with white light.

PHOTOGRAPHY

Slit-lamp photography has become a standard component of ophthalmic practice. The benefits of obtaining photographs of the eye are myriad, and include documentation of normal and abnormal ocular structure, the ability to provide objective records and measurements of the progress of disease course, and the generation of images which can be shared (from lectures to telemedicine).

As with slit-lamp examination of the eye, slit-lamp biomicrography is not just one technique. One challenge of slit-lamp biomicrography is to use individual static photographs to convey the nature of a lesion that is appreciated during the dynamic slit-lamp examination (3). (Note that in the following discussion, *photo slit lamp* denotes a slit-lamp biomicroscope capable of recording images. *Film-based* and *digital* refer to specific recording media.)

Although variations do exist in the composition of the commercially available photographic slit lamps, each shares similar core components. These include lighting sources with adjustable intensity and direction, flash with variable intensity, and adjustable magnification. Most photo slit lamps are similar to the arrangement of the clinical slit-lamp biomicroscope with the addition of a beam splitter to divide the available light between the camera and the examiner. As a result, the image "seen" by the camera is identical to that observed by the examiner. This allows for accurate assessments of the subject to be made during photography, permitting the examiner to obtain accurate representations of the subject.

Film-based instruments may use either a dedicated 35-mm instrument camera incorporating a shutter and film chamber (but with no viewfinder), or a 35-mm single-lens reflex (SLR) camera, in which the viewfinder is not used to preview the image.

Color slide (transparency) film provides the highest color fidelity and is most often used for imaging. An ISO

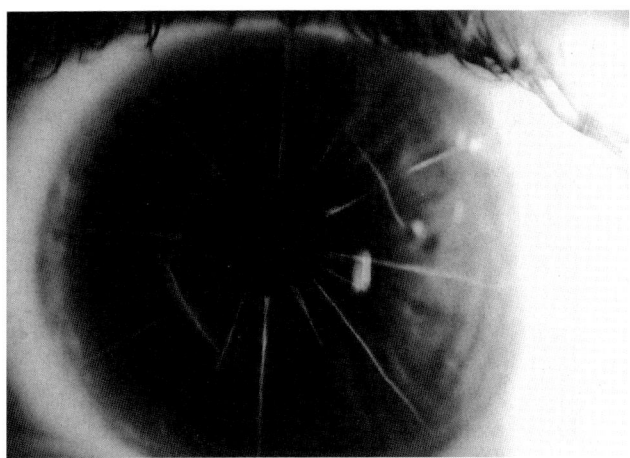
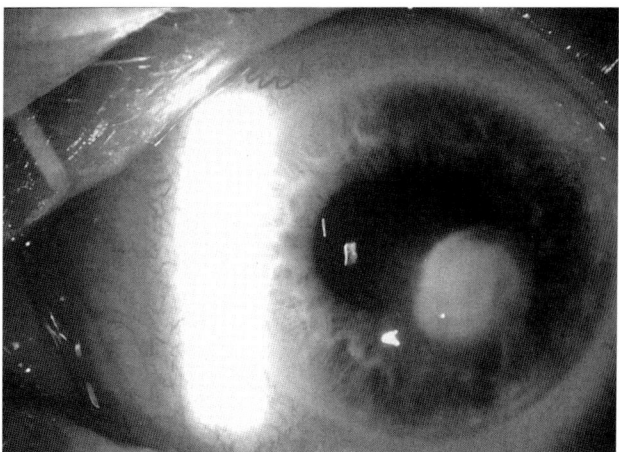

A

B

FIG. 6-6. A. Sclerotic scatter demonstrating stromal opacities after radial keratotomy. **B.** Sclerotic scatter reveals diffuse stromal infiltrate surrounding a bacterial corneal ulcer.

speed of at least 200 is needed to record typical corneal or anterior segment lesions.

Exposures are regulated by use of either a multistepped flash intensity switch, or through an aperture diaphragm that is interposed between the beamsplitter and the camera body.

The advent of digital photography has provided an alternative to traditional film-based slit-lamp photography. Digital imaging, unlike traditional film, does not rely on a light-sensitive emulsion. Instead, light is detected by a grid of sensors called *charge-coupled devices* (CCDs). Colored filters placed over the CCDs allow the sensors to detect not only the amount of light present, but the color. Images are then converted to numeric data. The detail obtainable by a digital camera depends on the available number of picture elements, or pixels. The higher the number of pixels, the

greater the resolution. Traditional 100 ASA 35-mm film is estimated to have 60 million light-sensitive grains (4). At present, high-end digital cameras can capture up to 6 megapixels. Despite this difference, the quality of images obtained by digital cameras is adequate for most slit-lamp photography applications.

Digital imaging has significant advantages over traditional film photography:

1. Data from digital cameras are collected and stored electronically, either on portable media or directly on a computer's hard drive. This reduces the storage space requirements of 35-mm slides. Digital storage media can also be erased and reused indefinitely.
2. Digital imaging offers the ability to determine immediately whether an accurate representation has been obtained.

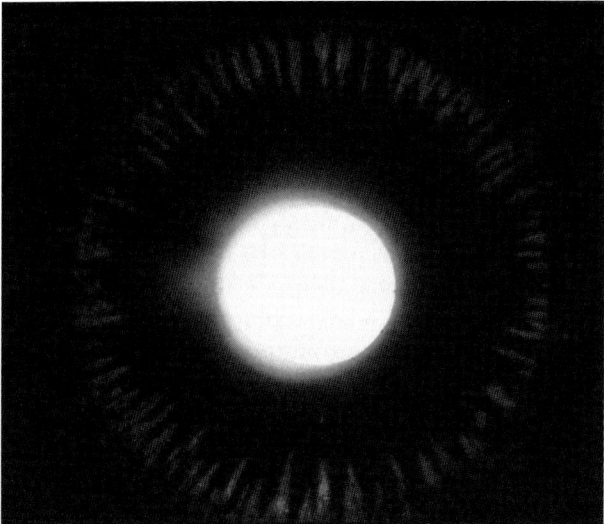

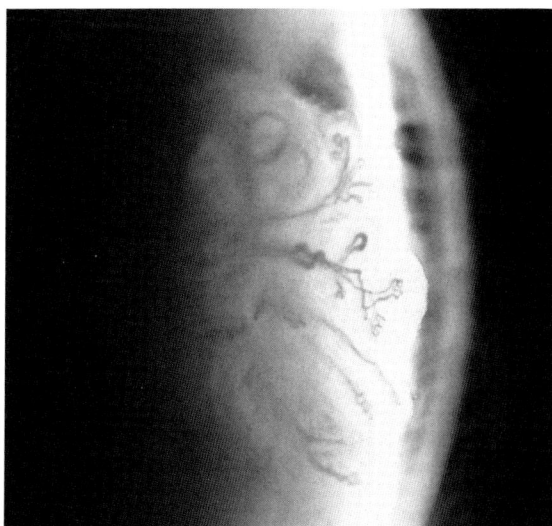

FIG. 6-7. Radial iris transillumination defects in pigment dispersion syndrome observed with retroillumination from the fundus.

FIG. 6-8. Retroillumination from the iris demonstrates the fibrovascular proliferation associated with conjunctival intraepithelial neoplasia.

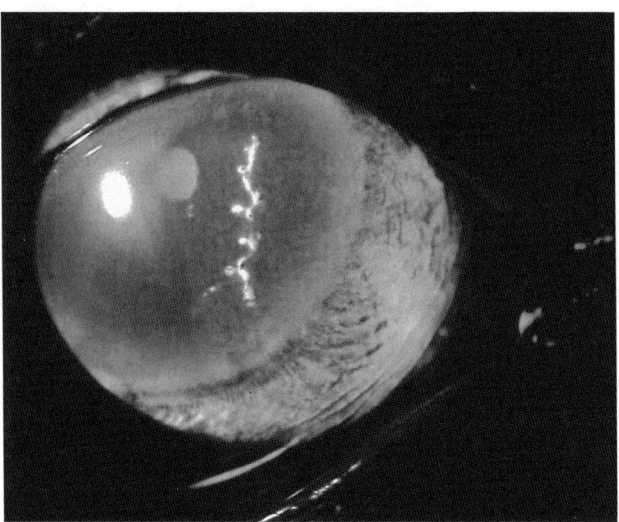

FIG. 6-9. Herpes simplex dendrite stained with fluorescein and observed with the cobalt blue filter. (See color figure.)

Images that are technically good (focus and exposure parameters are achieved) and also convey the desired information about the subject may be chosen and saved, whereas those that fail these criteria may be deleted from the set.

3. Digital photography eliminates the delay associated with film processing. Although some cameras have the ability to send the electronic information directly to a printer, so that paper prints can be quickly produced, the most significant benefit associated with digital technology is its ability to place images into an electronic medical record.

4. Digital photography is cost-effective. Digital camera prices are on par with traditional SLR cameras. However, unlike film cameras, digital imaging incurs no direct per-patient expenses for consumable items like film and processing costs, and it has been estimated that savings equal the initial equipment cost 1 year after purchase (5).

5. Software programs are readily available to help organize a collection of images and to provide an easy method of

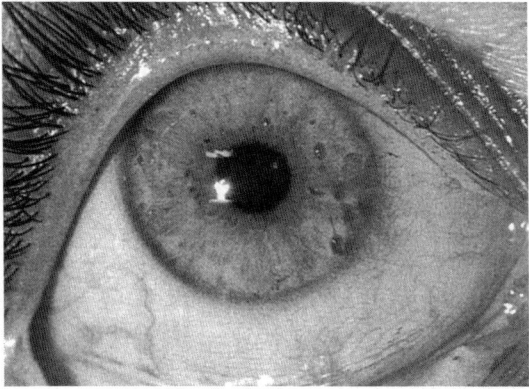

FIG. 6-10. Rose bengal staining of filamentary keratitis in severe dry eye. (See color figure.)

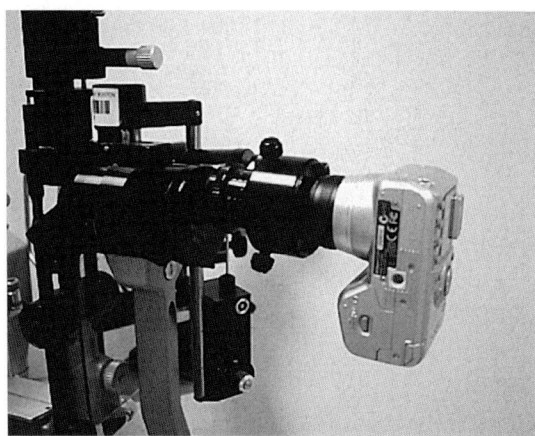

FIG. 6-11. Digital camera attached by an adapter to the eyepiece of the slit-lamp biomicroscope.

archiving according to patient identifiers as well as lesion characteristics. Other programs permit images to be adjusted for color balance, exposure, resolution, and the like (although the original digital file should be retained as well as the manipulated image, for medicolegal purposes).

Digital photography is quickly gaining acceptance. Digital photography of the external eye and adnexa, to illustrate ptosis, dermatochalasis, sulcus defects, and other preoperative and postoperative conditions is routine in ophthalmic plastic surgery practices and, for many, has replaced traditional film-based photography. A survey of ophthalmic plastic practices using digital imaging reported 92% were "very satisfied" or "completely satisfied" with their digital system, compared with 58% satisfaction among those using nondigital photography (5). Digital slit-lamp photography can also be performed without a dedicated photo slit lamp. Adapters can be purchased to connect digital cameras to the ocular of the slit lamp. These adapters have been designed for digital camera adaptation to optical instruments such as telescopes (e.g., www.scopetronix.com/digitalcam/html; www.lensadapter.com), but can be modified for attaching a digital camera to the ocular of a clinical slit lamp (Fig. 6-11) with good results (Fig. 6-12). Because of the lack of electronic flash illumination, images made with converted biomicroscopes may exhibit motion artifacts and may not produce results equal to those obtained with a traditional photo slit lamp. However, it does permit photography to be performed without a dedicated camera and is useful when only occasional photographs are taken.

Before embarking on slit-lamp imaging as a routine clinical activity, the camera and biomicroscope should be calibrated to produce optimal results. When centered, the fine slit beam should bisect the precise center of the observed field. If available, the biomicroscope should be fitted with an eyepiece reticle that provides an indication of the film plane; this is most helpful in finding where the scope

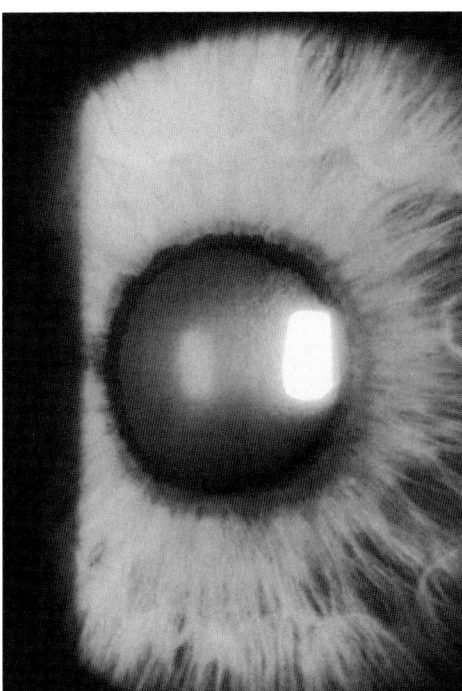

FIG. 6-12. Photograph taken with the apparatus depicted in Fig. 6-11.

should be focused. Experimentation with flash intensity and viewing lamp brightness control should be performed, with the goal of setting these controls to produce low-power images that successfully record good iris detail. Although many lesions of the anterior segment may be either quite bright or rather faint, with practice the biomicrographer becomes adept at changing illumination brightness to record the most important features.

In general, image recording mirrors the use of the biomicroscope for clinical applications. One exception to that rule is low-power views with broad, diffuse illumination. The illumination should provide information throughout the camera's recorded field. Thus, the biomicroscope should be provided with a "ground-glass" filter accessory to diffuse and broaden the beam. If such a manufacturer-provided device is unavailable, a substitute may be provided by placing a piece of frosted plastic (an old translucent plastic film canister works well) across the beam.

Regardless of the choice of recording medium, slit-lamp imaging should be based on the use of a routine methodology beginning with low-power, diffusely illuminated views, and progressing to more magnified images that reveal the most characteristic features of the lesion. Use special care when directing the light source toward the subject so that its specular reflection does not obscure important subject detail.

The initial images should be made with the patient in primary gaze. The lids should be opened maximally so that the entire cornea is visible. The next images should use higher magnification to record just the cornea from limbus to limbus. To illustrate the most accurate perspective, the lesion of interest should be centered in the image, and also positioned as the anterior-most aspect of the recorded field (achieved by repositioning the patient's gaze as needed).

Next, the slit lamp should be configured to project a very thin beam, positioned at a 45-degree angle from the observation axis to bisect the lesion. When focused critically, the beam should produce an optical section in which the epithelium, stroma, and endothelium are seen as bright lines of varying widths and intensities against a dark background (reminiscent of darkfield microscopy images). It is particularly useful to use a background illuminator for this type of work, although this may be missing when using a converted clinical biomicroscope. The background light provides low-intensity illumination to help understand where the slit beam is placed on the corneal surface.

Finally, the most emphatic lighting to accentuate the characteristic features of the lesions should be used. This may include tangential or sclerotic scatter illumination to reveal geographic information about the cornea; retroillumination from the iris or lens to produce a silhouette; repositioning the lesion at the light–dark interface to portray subtle basement membrane abnormalities; and Tyndall's phenomenon for significant amounts of cell and flare.

REFERENCES

1. Feenstra RPG, Tseng SCG. What is actually stained by rose bengal? *Arch Ophthalmol* 1992;110:984–983.
2. Feenstra RPG, Tseng SCG. Comparison of fluorescein and rose bengal staining. *Ophthalmology* 1992;99:605–617.
3. Martonyi CL, Bahn CF, Meyer RF. *Clinical slit lamp biomicroscopy and photo slit lamp biomicrography.* Ann Arbor, MI: Time One Ink, 1985:4.
4. Andrews P. *The digital photography manual.* London: Carlton Books, 2000:25.
5. Brown MS, Jindal V, Rubin PAD. Digital photography for the ophthalmic plastic surgeon. *Ophthalmic Plast Reconstr Surg* 2001;17:151–153.

CORNEAL PACHYMETRY

JOSEPH J. K. MA AND ANTHONY P. ADAMIS

The term *pachymetry* is a contraction of two Greek words, *pachos* ("thick") and *metry* ("measure"). Traditionally, the primary role of pachymetry in clinical practice was to act as a gauge of corneal endothelial cell layer function. The emergence of refractive surgery and the identification of corneal thickness as an important clinical variable in the assessment of intraocular pressure in glaucoma and glaucoma-suspect patients, has and will continue to redefine the importance of pachymetry not only for corneal and refractive surgeons, but in routine ophthalmic care.

Although optical slit-lamp pachymetry and specular microscopy have been available for decades, most clinicians rely on traditional ultrasonic pachymetry methods for determining corneal thickness primarily because of its simplicity and shallow learning curve for paramedical staff. However, the technological advances of the last decade have given birth to a cornucopia of new methodologies, as well as improved versions of existing techniques. The techniques can be divided into methodologies that are based on optical principles, such as traditional optical pachymetry, optical coherence tomography (OCT), optical low-coherence reflectometry (OLCR), confocal microscopy through-focusing (CMTF), specular microscopy, and laser Doppler interferometry, and on ultrasonic principles. We briefly describe the essentials of each, and Table 7-1 summarizes what we believe are the essential elements published at the time of writing. We refer the reader to the primary references listed at the end of the chapter for more detailed descriptions.

Although each technique is idiosyncratic in its own way, most methods have been touted as reliable in their own right. There are, however systematic differences in the values obtained by different methods. Because true corneal thickness cannot be verified, the accuracy of any given method is uncertain. From a practical standpoint, this means that although most methods are reliable enough for the longitudinal follow-up of patients, the values obtained cannot simply be substituted between modalities. Although the systematic deviation of pachymetry measurements is not consistent between studies and varies between model types, it is generally observed that the order of measurements, from the modality that provides the highest measurements on down, is as follows: contact specular, Orbscan, ultrasound, noncontact specular, OCT, OLCR, and optical pachymetry (1–18). Furthermore, in applications that require accurate corneal thickness measurements such as with lamellar or refractive techniques, a method-dependent safety margin of error must be factored into estimations of corneal thickness.

METHODS FOR PACHYMETRY

Ultrasound

Traditional ultrasound pachymetry is a simple dry contact technique that measures corneal thickness at 10 to 20 MHz with an estimated of velocity of sound through cornea of 1630 m/sec and has become the standard method used by most clinicians (19). It is generally thought to underestimate corneal thickness in edematous corneas (20,21). Ultrasound biomicroscopy (50 MHz) and very–high-frequency ultrasound (70 MHz) require a water bath and are able to discern sublayer detail and pachymetry (22–27).

Optical Pachymetry

Optical pachymetry is measured using a slit-lamp–mounted device that allows the observer to align the front and back surface of the cornea through image doubling, to attain an estimation of corneal thickness on a Vernier scale. This is an observer-dependent technique based on assumptions of the refractive index of the cornea and anterior radius of curvature (28–31).

Specular Microscopy

This method is based on recording the adjustment required in the focal plane of a specular microscope. The contact technique tends to overestimate corneal thickness compared with other methods (3,5,9,10,32,33).

Scanning Slit Based (Orbscan)

Orbscan is a noncontact technique that incorporates a scanning-slit–based method of pachymetry in the process

TABLE 7-1. COMPARISON OF PACHYMETRY METHODS

Method	Traditional Ultrasound	Ultrasound Biomicroscopy and Very-High-Frequency Ultrasound	Optical Slit-Lamp Pachymetry	Specular Microscopy Based: Contact and Noncontact	Scanning-Slit Based: Orbscan	Optical Coherence Tomography	Optical Low-Coherence Reflectometry	Confocal Microscopy Through-Focusing	Laser Doppler Interferometry
Operating principle	10- to 20-MHz frequency sound waves	50-MHz (ultrasound biomicroscopy) and 70-MHz sound waves	Image doubling, manual	Measures focus through front-back cornea	Scanning-slit: front-back corneal reflections	Infrared interferometry	Infrared interferometry (like OCT)	Focuses through planes with a confocal microscope	Dual-beam laser Doppler
Contact/noncontact	Contact	Contact with water bath	Noncontact	Both contact and noncontact	Noncontact	Noncontact	Noncontact	Contact	Noncontact
Resolution	No sublayer pachymetry	Sublayer pachymetry	No sublayer pachymetry	No sublayer pachymetry	No sublayer pachymetry	Sublayer pachymetry	Potential for sublayer pachymetry	High resolution with sublayer pachymetry and cellular details	No sublayer details
Dimensional sections (2D/3D)	Low resolution, NA	High-resolution 3D views possible	No	No	2D display of data	2D display of data	Not available, potential possible	3D views	No
Peripheral pachymetry	Not reliable	Easy to obtain, difficult to standardize	Not reliable	Not reliable	Standard	Easy to obtain, relatively easy to standardize	Not available, potential possible	Requires repositioning	Not reliable
Special applications	Most common method used clinically	Postrefractive surgery: lamellar thickness	Slit-lamp mounted	Simultaneous measurement of cell counts	Postrefractive surgery	Postrefractive surgery	Intraoperative measurement during laser ablations	Cellular morphology/detail; detects microbes	Can measure axial length
Advantages	Fast, simple, dry technique	Sublayer detail	Simple	Measure cell counts concurrently	Concurrent topography/elevation data	Measures through opacity, high resolution	Intraoperative measurements possible	High resolution, can quantify haze/light scatter	Purportedly good precision
Disadvantages	Not accurate in edematous corneas, difficult to reposition/standardize location with precision	Requires water bath, risk of corneal abrasion, complicated technique, difficult location standardization	Manual: observer-dependent precision	Contact method: risk for abrasion of corneas	May be less accurate post-laser in situ keratomileusis or in corneas with haze	Interinstrument variability, preliminary clinical experience to date	Currently not able to acquire 2D or 3D images, same as for OCT	Slow data acquisition, poor penetration of corneal opacity, contact method, minimal clinical experience	Minimal clinical experience reported to date

	1 sec	Setup complicated, acquisition quick	1–2 sec, manual	1 sec	2 sec	1–2 sec	18 Hz	10 sec	1 sec
Time per measurement/simplicity									
Average pachymetry (μm) of normal corneas[a] (n, number of eyes)	550, SD 33, n = 89 (22) 524, SD 39, n = 68 (4) 570, SD 42, n = 119 (32) 580, SD 43, n = 34 (9) 542, SD 33, n = 20 (11) 549, SD 44, n = 92 (15)	60 MHz: 515, SD 33, n = 20 (26)	543, SD 28, n = 62 (1) 531, SD 40, n = 68 (4) 518, SD 20, n = 40 (26) 539, SD 33, n = 20 (11)	Noncontact: 542, SD 46, n = 119 (32) 547, SD 49, n = 34 (9) 543, SD 46, n = 65 (33) Contact: 640, SD 43, n = 34 (9) 642, SD 42, n = 65 (33) 638, SD 43, n = 119 (32)	571, SD 44, n = 51 (12) 596, SD 40, n = 20 (11) 602, SD 59, n = 34 (9)	541, SD 43, n = 92 (15)	502, SD 42, n = 34 (14) Note: same study ultrasound values of 527, SD 40, n = 34	532, SD 19, n = 7 (16)	NA
Precision (repeatability)[a]	3.5-8.8 μm (26)	2 μm (64) 1.3-7.7 μm (26)	5.6-19 μm (26)	4.8-14 μm (9,26,32)	6.2-20 μm (11,12)	5.8 μm (15)	Not known	10 μm (16)	3.9 μm (17,18)

2D, two-dimensional; 3D, three-dimensional; NA, not available; OCT, optical coherence tomography; SD, standard deviation.
[a]Numbers in parentheses are reference citations.

of topography and elevation data acquisition. There has been concern that this method underestimates corneal thickness in hazy corneas and corneas that have undergone refractive surgery (7,11,34).

Optical Coherence Tomography and Optical Low-Coherence Reflectometry

OCT is a noncontact technique that acquires pachymetry measurements based on optical interferometry. It tends to produce measurements that are thinner than traditional ultrasound pachymetry, but can delineate sublayer pachymetry and detail, and is potentially more useful for repeat measurements on the same portion of a cornea. It has also been demonstrated to be able to acquire measurements not possible by traditional ultrasound techniques (2,13,23,35).

OLCR is a continuous version of OCT that can measure corneal thickness at the rate of 18 Hz using light in the infrared range. It has been incorporated into an excimer laser platform and can perform measurements during corneal ablation (14,36,37).

Confocal Microscopy Through-Focusing

CMTF is a contact technique that acquires pachymetry measurements by through-focusing a confocal microscope through the thickness of the cornea (38). It can measure and display detailed sublayer cellular structure (39) as well as corneal microbial pathologic processes, and has been used to correlate cellular gene expression (38,40,41). Its use clinically, however, is limited in the presence of corneal opacities and by its long acquisition times (16).

Laser Doppler Interferometry

Laser Doppler interferometry is a noncontact technique that uses dual-beam infrared laser Doppler interferometry to measure corneal thickness. To date, there have not been any extensive studies comparing it with other pachymetry methods (17,18).

PACHYMETRY AS A MEASURE OF ENDOTHELIAL FUNCTION

Although absolute pachymetry measurements are difficult to interpret given the wide range of normal values in the general population, serial pachymetry measurements are an excellent measure of corneal endothelial cell layer function. One study of 114 eyes demonstrated that 5-day postoperative pachymetry is an excellent marker of long-term endothelial function that correlates well with specular quantity and morphology as well as fluorophotometry endothelial permeability coefficients, which can be interpreted as an indirect measure of endothelial cell function in a physiologically

stressed cornea (42). Serial pachymetry measurements correlate well with corneal edema and endothelial function in Fuchs' dystrophy (43). Pachymetry can theoretically influence specular counts if image magnification secondary to increased corneal thickness is not factored into endothelial cell count measurements (42,43).

Many clinicians use clinically significant diurnal variation in corneal endothelial function as a surgical threshold for patients with Fuchs' endothelial dystrophy. However, even in normal corneas, a diurnal variation in pachymetry measurements has been documented, with the thickest measurements obtained immediately on waking. It is estimated that these measurements stabilize in approximately 2 to 3 hours and that the magnitude of this variation is approximately 10 μm centrally and 20 μm peripherally (44). The cornea can thin significantly simply by evaporative forces. In an OLCR study of photorefractive keratectomy, it was estimated that the cornea is thinned by up to approximately 6% within 5 minutes simply by exposure to air in a cornea with an intact epithelium (36). Approximately 9% thinning (50 μm) occurs within 5 minutes in a cornea that has had its epithelium removed (36). The quality of the tear film and ocular surface environment may also play a significant role in corneal pachymetry. One small study demonstrated that corneas in patients with dry eye were on average 37 μm thinner than in healthy patients (45).

DEMOGRAPHICS AND PACHYMETRY

The range of normal corneal pachymetry measurements is fairly wide and varies based on the method and instrumentation used; however, the average pachymetry of normal corneas is accepted as being approximately 540 to 560 μm with traditional ultrasound pachymetry.

There appears to be a racial variation in corneal pachymetry measurements. One small study found that pachymetry measurements were on average 27 μm thinner in African Americans than in the white population for both glaucomatous patients and healthy subjects (46).

Although central corneal pachymetry does not change significantly with age, there is evidence that paracentral and peripheral areas of the cornea are thinner with age (19,47). There is also evidence that steeper corneas tend to be thinner than flat corneas (1,19).

REFRACTIVE SURGERY, KERATOCONUS, ECTASIA, AND PACHYMETRY

Although topography is more useful in the diagnosis of keratoconus, pachymetry is a desirable adjunct and can be ascertained simultaneously with scanning-slit–based systems such as the Orbscan (48). Two- and three-dimensional systems are also useful for the diagnosis of postsurgical ectasia, as in patients who have undergone laser *in situ* keratomileusis

(LASIK) (49,50). However, there is evidence that Orbscan pachymetry measurements performed in hazy corneas or eyes that have undergone refractive surgery underestimate ultrasonic values because of light scattering due to haze or the intralamellar interface (7,34). Noncontact systems such as OLCR have been adapted for real-time intraoperative measurements, which are important because of differential interpatient variability in ablation rates that may be partially due to the state of corneal hydration during ablation (36). As stated earlier, OCT has also been demonstrated to be able to obtain measurements where ultrasound pachymetry has failed (13). After surgery, corneal sublayer pachymetry detail, which can be obtained by CMTF, OCT, and high-frequency ultrasound techniques, may be important.

GLAUCOMA AND PACHYMETRY

Pachymetry is becoming more important in general ophthalmology because of evidence from the Ocular Hypertension Study that has identified thin corneas as a significant variable in patients with high intraocular pressures, and that early intervention may prevent vision loss. Some studies have demonstrated that corneas in patients with normal-tension glaucoma are on average 39 μm thinner than normal corneas (51–53); others, however, have demonstrated conflicting results (20,54–56). Patients with ocular hypertension without evidence of glaucomatous damage have been shown to have corneas that are on average 30 to 40 μm thicker than in healthy patients (53,57–59). Furthermore, studies have shown that, post-LASIK, intraocular pressure decreases by approximately 4.3 mm Hg in 95.4% and 100% of patients when measured by applanation and noncontact methods, respectively (56). Intraocular pressure also decreases by approximately 3.4 mm Hg in patients who have undergone photorefractive keratectomy. Although the exact mechanism for this decrease is not known, corneal thickness is thought to play a role (60–62). Applanation tonometry is based on the Imbert-Fick law, which assumes that the cornea is perfectly spherical, flexible, dry, and infinitely thin. Therefore, thicker corneas that are less compliant owing to an increase in tissue tend to cause an overestimation of intraocular pressure; conversely, thinner corneas tend to lead to an underestimation of intraocular pressure. However, corneas with increased thickness due to edema are expected to lead to an underestimation of true intraocular pressure. The relationship is less clear for noncontact devices (63). It has been estimated that intraocular pressure measurements are affected by up to 4 mm Hg in 20% of patients (59).

DISCUSSION AND FUTURE SIGNIFICANCE OF PACHYMETRY

As the accuracy of laser subtraction techniques in the realm of refractive surgery improves, pachymetry measurements will become more important as clinicians attempt to refine algorithms for customized ablations in attempts to achieve maximal optical refractive corrections. Techniques that will allow for two- and three-dimensional assessments of corneal tissue volume such as OCT, optical slit techniques, ultrasound biomicroscopy, high-frequency ultrasonography, and CMFT will become increasingly important. Differential corneal ablation rates, such as are seen with stromal scarring and neovascular tissue, are another potential use for real-time accurate pachymetry in treating lesions. Furthermore, the refinement of these methods can be potentially helpful in the study of corneal ectatic disorders, both innate and iatrogenic. In addition, the recent availability of femtosecond intrastromal lasers introduces the possibility of removing intrastromal scars without the need for keratoplasty. With lamellar surgical techniques, these new modes of pachymetry presumably can eventually be used for the intraoperative monitoring of lamellar dissections in addition to quantifying and mapping corneal opacities to single-micron accuracy. Traditional point pachymetry techniques will likely continue to be important as manufacturers seek to integrate pachymetry with tonometry to obtain more accurate measurements of intraocular pressure.

As our sophistication and ability to improve the accuracy and precision of pachymetry increase, the art of deciphering the relevance of this information becomes crucial. In corneal and refractive clinical experience, it is not unusual to encounter strikingly low endothelial cell counts in normal or thin corneas, without evidence of a corneal thinning disease such as keratoconus. Conversely, it is not uncommon to see normal cell counts and endothelial cell morphology associated with supranormal corneal thickness. It is likely that in the near future, techniques for directly and accurately evaluating endothelial cell function, keratocyte cell density, and corneal hydration will be available to gauge corneal function and provide additional assistance to the assessment of both surgical and medical treatments.

REFERENCES

1. Giasson C, Forthomme D. Comparison of central corneal thickness measurements between optical and ultrasound pachometers. *Optom Vis Sci* 1992;69:236–241.
2. Bechmann M, Thiel MJ, Neubauer AS, et al. Central corneal thickness measurement with a retinal optical coherence tomography device versus standard ultrasonic pachymetry. *Cornea* 2001;20:50–54.
3. Sallet G. Comparison of optical and ultrasound central corneal pachymetry. *Bull Soc Belg Ophtalmol* 2001:35–38.
4. Nissen J, Hjortdal JO, Ehlers N, et al. A clinical comparison of optical and ultrasonic pachometry. *Acta Ophthalmol (Copenh)* 1991;69:659–663.
5. Tam ES, Rootman DS. Comparison of central corneal thickness measurements by specular microscopy, ultrasound pachymetry, and ultrasound biomicroscopy. *J Cataract Refract Surg* 2003;29:1179–1184.

6. Giraldez Fernandez MJ, Diaz Rey A, Cervino A, et al. A comparison of two pachymetric systems: slit-scanning and ultrasonic. *CLAO J* 2002;28:221–223.

7. Fakhry MA, Artola A, Belda JI, et al. Comparison of corneal pachymetry using ultrasound and Orbscan II. *J Cataract Refract Surg* 2002;28:248–252.

8. Chakrabarti HS, Craig JP, Brahma A, et al. Comparison of corneal thickness measurements using ultrasound and Orbscan slit-scanning topography in normal and post-LASIK eyes. *J Cataract Refract Surg* 2001;27:1823–1828.

9. Modis L Jr, Langenbucher A, Seitz B. Scanning-slit and specular microscopic pachymetry in comparison with ultrasonic determination of corneal thickness. *Cornea* 2001;20:711–714.

10. Bovelle R, Kaufman SC, Thompson HW, et al. Corneal thickness measurements with the Topcon SP-2000P specular microscope and an ultrasound pachymeter. *Arch Ophthalmol* 1999;117:868–870.

11. Marsich MW, Bullimore MA. The repeatability of corneal thickness measures. *Cornea* 2000;19:792–795.

12. Yaylali V, Kaufman SC, Thompson HW. Corneal thickness measurements with the Orbscan Topography System and ultrasonic pachymetry. *J Cataract Refract Surg* 1997;23:1345–1350.

13. Wang J, Fonn D, Simpson TL, et al. Relation between optical coherence tomography and optical pachymetry measurements of corneal swelling induced by hypoxia. *Am J Ophthalmol* 2002;134:93–98.

14. Genth U, Mrochen M, Walti R, et al. Optical low coherence reflectometry for noncontact measurements of flap thickness during laser in situ keratomileusis. *Ophthalmology* 2002;109:973–978.

15. Wirbelauer C, Scholz C, Hoerauf H, et al. Noncontact corneal pachymetry with slit lamp-adapted optical coherence tomography. *Am J Ophthalmol* 2002;133:444–450.

16. Li HF, Petroll WM, Moller-Pedersen T, et al. Epithelial and corneal thickness measurements by in vivo confocal microscopy through focusing (CMTF). *Curr Eye Res* 1997;16:214–221.

17. Hitzenberger CK, Drexler W, Fercher AF. Measurement of corneal thickness by laser Doppler interferometry. *Invest Ophthalmol Vis Sci* 1992;33:98–103.

18. Hitzenberger CK, Baumgartner A, Drexler W, et al. Interferometric measurement of corneal thickness with micrometer precision. *Am J Ophthalmol* 1994;118:468–476.

19. Rapuano CJ, Fishbaugh JA, Strike DJ. Nine point corneal thickness measurements and keratometry readings in normal corneas using ultrasound pachymetry. *Insight* 1993;18:16–22.

20. Arner RS, Rengstorff RH. Error analysis of corneal thickness measurements. *Am J Optom Arch Am Acad Optom* 1972;49:862–865.

21. Fatt I, Harris MG. Refractive index of the cornea as a function of its thickness. *Am J Optom Arch Am Acad Optom* 1973;50:383–386.

22. Price FW Jr, Koller DL, Price MO. Central corneal pachymetry in patients undergoing laser in situ keratomileusis. *Ophthalmology* 1999;106:2216–2220.

23. Maldonado MJ, Ruiz-Oblitas L, Munuera JM, et al. Optical coherence tomography evaluation of the corneal cap and stromal bed features after laser in situ keratomileusis for high myopia and astigmatism. *Ophthalmology* 2000;107:81–87, discussion 88.

24. Silverman RH, Reinstein DZ, Raevsky T, et al. Improved system for sonographic imaging and biometry of the cornea. *J Ultrasound Med* 1997;16:117–124.

25. Reinstein DZ, Silverman RH, Raevsky T, et al. Arc-scanning very high-frequency digital ultrasound for 3D pachymetric mapping of the corneal epithelium and stroma in laser in situ keratomileusis. *J Refract Surg* 2000;16:414–430.

26. Reinstein DZ, Silverman RH, Rondeau MJ, et al. Epithelial and corneal thickness measurements by high-frequency ultrasound digital signal processing. *Ophthalmology* 1994;101:140–146.

27. Reinstein DZ, Aslanides IM, Silverman RH, et al. High-frequency ultrasound corneal pachymetry in the assessment of corneal scars for therapeutic planning. *CLAO J* 1994;20:198–203.

28. Maurice D, Giardini A. A simple optical apparatus for measuring the corneal thickness and the average thickness of the human cornea. *Br J Ophthalmol* 1951;35:169–177.

29. Donaldson DD. A new instrument for the measurement of corneal thickness. *Arch Ophthalmol* 1966;76:25–31.

30. Mishima S, Hedbys BO. Measurement of corneal thickness with the Haag-Streit pachometer. *Arch Ophthalmol* 1968;80:710–713.

31. Mishima S. Corneal thickness. *Surv Ophthalmol* 1968;13:57–96.

32. Modis L Jr, Langenbucher A, Seitz B. Corneal thickness measurements with contact and noncontact specular microscopic and ultrasonic pachymetry. *Am J Ophthalmol* 2001;132:517–521.

33. Modis L Jr, Langenbucher A, Seitz B. Corneal endothelial cell density and pachymetry measured by contact and noncontact specular microscopy. *J Cataract Refract Surg* 2002;28:1763–1769.

34. Giessler S, Duncker GI. Orbscan pachymetry after LASIK is not reliable. *J Refract Surg* 2001;17:385–387.

35. Wong AC, Wong CC, Yuen NS, et al. Correlational study of central corneal thickness measurements on Hong Kong Chinese using optical coherence tomography, Orbscan and ultrasound pachymetry. *Eye* 2002;16:715–721.

36. Bohnke M, Widmer S, Walti R. Real-time pachymetry during photorefractive keratectomy using optical low-coherence reflectometry. *J Biomed Opt* 2001;6:412–417.

37. Wirbelauer C, Pham DT. Intraoperative optical coherence pachymetry during laser in situ keratomileusis: first clinical experience. *J Refract Surg* 2003;19:372–377.

38. Petroll WM, Yu A, Li J, et al. A prototype two-detector confocal microscope for in vivo corneal imaging. *Scanning* 2002;24:163–170.

39. Ivarsen A, Stultiens BA, Moller-Pedersen T. Validation of confocal microscopy through focusing for corneal sublayer pachymetry. *Cornea* 2002;21:700–704.

40. Jester JV, Moller-Pedersen T, Huang J, et al. The cellular basis of corneal transparency: evidence for "corneal crystallins." *J Cell Sci* 1999;112:613–622.

41. Jester JV, Li HF, Petroll WM, et al. Area and depth of surfactant-induced corneal injury correlates with cell death. *Invest Ophthalmol Vis Sci* 1998;39:922–936.

42. Beneyto P, Gutierrez R, Perez TM. Comparative study of three methods of evaluation of the corneal endothelium in pseudophakic patients: fluorophotometry, specular microscopy and pachymetry. *Graefes Arch Clin Exp Ophthalmol* 1996;234:623–627.

43. Oh KT, Weil LJ, Oh DM, et al. Corneal thickness in Fuchs' dystrophy with and without epithelial oedema. *Eye* 1998;12:282–284.

44. Lattimore MR Jr, Kaupp S, Schallhorn S, et al. Orbscan pachymetry: implications of a repeated measures and diurnal variation analysis. *Ophthalmology* 1999;106:977–981.

45. Liu Z, Pflugfelder SC. Corneal thickness is reduced in dry eye. *Cornea* 1999;18:403–407.

46. La Rosa FA, Gross RL, Orengo-Nania S. Central corneal thickness of Caucasians and African Americans in glaucomatous and nonglaucomatous populations. *Arch Ophthalmol* 2001;119:23–27.

47. Martola EL, Baum JL. Central and peripheral corneal thickness: a clinical study. *Arch Ophthalmol* 1968;79:28–30.

48. Rabinowitz YS, Rasheed K, Yang H, et al. Accuracy of ultrasonic pachymetry and videokeratography in detecting keratoconus. *J Cataract Refract Surg* 1998;24:196–201.

49. Wang Z, Chen J, Yang B. Posterior corneal surface topographic changes after laser in situ keratomileusis are related to residual corneal bed thickness. *Ophthalmology* 1999;106:406–409, discussion 409–410.

50. Lee DH, Seo S, Jeong KW, et al. Early spatial changes in the posterior corneal surface after laser in situ keratomileusis. *J Cataract Refract Surg* 2003;29:778–784.

51. Shah S, Chatterjee A, Mathai M, et al. Relationship between corneal thickness and measured intraocular pressure in a general ophthalmology clinic. *Ophthalmology* 1999;106:2154–2160.

52. Emara BY, Tingey DP, Probst LE, et al. Central corneal thickness in low-tension glaucoma. *Can J Ophthalmol* 1999;34:319–324.

53. Copt RP, Thomas R, Mermoud A. Corneal thickness in ocular hypertension, primary open-angle glaucoma, and normal tension glaucoma. *Arch Ophthalmol* 1999;117:14–16.

54. Kothy P, Vargha P, Hollo G. Ocuton-S self tonometry vs. Goldmann tonometry: a diurnal comparison study. *Acta Ophthalmol Scand* 2001;79:294–297.

55. Iskander NG, Anderson Penno E, Peters NT, et al. Accuracy of Orbscan pachymetry measurements and DHG ultrasound pachymetry in primary laser in situ keratomileusis and LASIK enhancement procedures. *J Cataract Refract Surg* 2001;27:681–685.

56. Faucher A, Gregoire J, Blondeau P. Accuracy of Goldmann tonometry after refractive surgery. *J Cataract Refract Surg* 1997;23:832–838.

57. Bron AM, Creuzot-Garcher C, Goudeau-Boutillon S, et al. Falsely elevated intraocular pressure due to increased central corneal thickness. *Graefes Arch Clin Exp Ophthalmol* 1999;237:220–224.

58. Stodtmeister R. Central corneal thickness on GAT (Goldman applanation tonometry accuracy). *J Glaucoma* 2002;11:543.

59. Stodtmeister R. Applanation tonometry and correction according to corneal thickness. *Acta Ophthalmol Scand* 1998;76:319–324.

60. Chatterjee A, Shah S, Bessant DA, et al. Reduction in intraocular pressure after excimer laser photorefractive keratectomy: correlation with pretreatment myopia. *Ophthalmology* 1997;104:355–359.

61. Emara B, Probst LE, Tingey DP, et al. Correlation of intraocular pressure and central corneal thickness in normal myopic eyes and after laser in situ keratomileusis. *J Cataract Refract Surg* 1998;24:1320–1325.

62. El Danasoury MA, El Maghraby A, Coorpender SJ. Change in intraocular pressure in myopic eyes measured with contact and non-contact tonometers after laser in situ keratomileusis. *J Refract Surg* 2001;17:97–104.

63. Recep OF, Hasiripi H, Cagil N, et al. Relation between corneal thickness and intraocular pressure measurement by noncontact and applanation tonometry. *J Cataract Refract Surg* 2001;27:1787–1791.

64. Reinstein DZ, Silverman RH, Sutton HF, et al. Very high-frequency ultrasound corneal analysis identifies anatomic correlates of optical complications of lamellar refractive surgery: anatomic diagnosis in lamellar surgery. *Ophthalmology* 1999;106:474–482.

KERATOMETRY

MICHAEL K. SMOLEK AND STEPHEN D. KLYCE

Keratometry is the optical process of determining the curvature of the central cornea. Typically, keratometry is expressed as dioptric power (D) or as dioptric curvature (Kd) of the cornea. Dioptric power measurements are useful for assessing the cornea's contribution to the overall refractive state of the eye and for the detection of corneal distortions that may be indicative of various diseases and disorders. On the other hand, keratometry can also be expressed as the radius of curvature of the cornea (the inverse of corneal curvature), which is mostly relevant for fitting contact lenses. Whereas curvature is normally expressed in inverse meters (m^{-1}), in accordance with the manner in which optical vergence is expressed, the radius of curvature is normally expressed in millimeters, which is a far more practical measurement for the base curves of contact lenses. Keratometry is one of the simplest and most informative clinical measurements than can be made of the eye, and so it will remain an important and relevant diagnostic tool to assess a patient's visual potential.

HISTORICAL BACKGROUND

Corneal curvature has been of interest to vision scientists for centuries. A description of corneal curvature was first reported in 1619 by Christoph Scheiner. He compared the apparent size of images of window panes viewed by reflection from the cornea with the relative size of the images seen in glass marbles of various size held next to the eye. By trial and error, Scheiner could find the ball that produced a similar-sized image to that seen in the cornea, and which was therefore equivalent in curvature. The first device built exclusively for keratometric measurements was constructed in 1796 by Jesse Ramsden, who used the device to study the possibility of corneal accommodation in aphakia (1). This instrument did not promote significant scientific interest until 1854, when Herman von Helmholtz improved on Ramsden's keratometer design to facilitate his work in the rapidly growing science of physiologic optics (2). Essentially the device was built around a low-power telescope that could magnify and permit measurement of the first surface corneal reflection located immediately behind the

cornea. The image is the reflection of a bright object (i.e., mire) of known size and distance. The ratio of the apparent size of the reflected mire image to the size of the actual mire allows corneal curvature to be determined precisely.

Helmholtz referred to his process of measuring corneal curvature as *ophthalmometry* and the device as an *ophthalmometer*. This terminology is still used today, but as Emsley pointed out, it is confusing because it implies measurement of the whole eye and not just the cornea (3). For this reason, *keratometry* and *keratometer* are the more commonly used terms today, although some manufacturers still use the term *ophthalmometer*. Although Helmholtz devised a successful experimental device, the first practical keratometer that was suited for clinical use was developed by Javal and Schiötz in 1881 (4). Many improvements have been made to keep the keratometer current with modern ophthalmic standards, but the basic optical design of these instruments has changed very little over the last century. In 1932, the Bausch & Lomb company introduced improved focusing, circular mires for better qualitative assessment of astigmatism, and simultaneous curvature measurement along orthogonal meridians, which significantly improved the ease of use of the keratometer.

DETERMINATION OF THE RADIUS OF CURVATURE

Strictly speaking, neither corneal curvature nor the radius of curvature are measured directly by a keratometer, but these values are calculated from the apparent size of the image of a bright object (the mire) viewed by reflection from the anterior corneal surface (actually from the tear film), which acts as a convex mirror. The formula for a convex mirror states that

the radius of curvature, r, of a spherical mirror is proportional to the ratio of image to object size:

$$r = 2 \times h'/h \qquad [1]$$

The ray trace diagram of Fig. 8-1 shows that the image h′ is formed behind the curved mirror surface as a minified, virtual, erect image of the mire object of height h. Because the

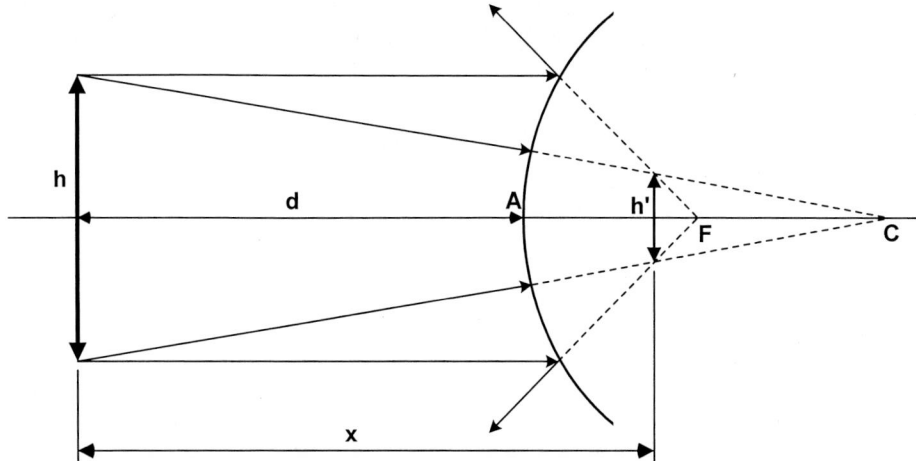

FIG. 8-1. Optical ray-trace construction of the virtual image of an object as seen by reflection from a convex mirror.

distance, x, from the mire to the principal focus of the convex mirror is never known precisely, the distance, d, from the mire to the convex surface (i.e., to the corneal apex, A) is used instead. As long as d is relatively large, the calculation is sufficiently accurate to allow a small error in working distance. When the formula is applied to the cornea, the radius of curvature is always expressed as a positive number in millimeters.

The size and distance of the mire from the cornea places the mire image typically within the central 3 to 4 mm of the cornea. This location encompasses the region of the normal cornea that tends to be most spherical. The location is also within the region of the cornea in front of the entrance pupil that is most useful for vision under normal daytime lighting (the average photopic entrance pupil is approximately 4 mm in diameter).

One of the difficulties that must be overcome when measuring the size of the virtual mire image is that eye movements make direct measurements relative to an eyepiece reticule scale impossible to perform with any degree of accuracy. Ramsden was an astronomer who understood that the doubling prism micrometers that were used with telescopes to measure the size of celestial objects like the sun could be adapted to measure mire images in the presence of normal eye movements. Essentially, a doubling prism allows the operator to see two images of the same mire image displaced with respect to one another. When the side of one image is aligned to just touch the side of the fellow image, the overall size of the image can be determined even when the image is constantly moving. The doubling prism method is still used in modern keratometers, although the mire targets are more refined and have fiducial marks to make alignment even easier.

DETERMINATION OF CORNEAL POWER

The convex mirror formula calculates the front surface radius of curvature, but keratometry was devised originally

to estimate the dioptric power of the entire cornea, front and back surfaces combined, as if it were a single refracting surface. Specifically, dioptric power, D, is calculated from the radius of curvature, r, by the equation:

$$D = (n' - n)/r \qquad [2]$$

where n' is the index of refraction of the medium into which light passes and n is the index of refraction of the medium from which the light originates. Thus, we see that corneal dioptric power as reported by keratometry is based on two independent factors. The first factor is that a change in refractivity from air to stroma exists at the cornea that causes light to slow and therefore bend toward a new direction (light always travels along the path of least time between two points in space). The second factor is the curvature of the interface separating air from stroma also causes a change in vergence for any rays striking the surface at a nonnormal angle. The refractivity factor is merely an estimated value and never actually measured during keratometry.

The index of refraction of air is 1.00 and that of corneal stroma is approximately 1.376. For a radius of curvature of 7.8 mm, this would produce a dioptric power of approximately 48.2 D for the front surface of the cornea (the total dioptric power of the eye is approximately 60 D). However, because keratometry was designed as a method to estimate the dioptric power of the total cornea (front plus back surfaces), the index of refraction of the stroma is not used in keratometry. Instead, an index of 1.3375 is used with most keratometers, which produces a dioptric power of approximately 43.27 D for a radius of curvature of 7.8 mm. The keratometric power in diopters (or dioptric curvature) is thus expressed by the keratometric equation as:

$$K = 337.5/r \qquad [3]$$

Note that this is merely a simplification of the basic dioptric power formula shown previously; the refractive index of 1.3375 has been subtracted from the index of air

(1.00) and multiplied by 1000 to allow r to be entered into the equation directly in millimeters. The unusual keratometric index of 337.5 can be explained on the basis of several factors. First, Helmholtz realized that the posterior corneal curvature had a dioptric value of approximately −5 D, which would place the total average corneal power (front plus back surfaces) very close to 43 D in a normal eye, which he knew to be true from independent measurements. Second, a small correction factor was needed to account for the thickness of the cornea and the fact that the measurement is made from the reflectance off the tear film (both very minor effects, considering that the instrument working distance is already inexact). Third, the earliest research keratometers did not use hand dials with calibrated reference marks, but instead required data tables to convert radius of curvature into dioptric power. To simplify the use of the keratometer in his laboratory, Helmholtz assigned the keratometric index to a value of 337.5 so that it produced a round number of 45 D when the radius of curvature was 7.5 mm.

Not all keratometers use the standard keratometric value of 337.5; American Optical and Haag-Streit instruments use 336.0 (the index of the tear film layer is 1.336), whereas Hoya keratometers use 338.0, and Zeiss and Topcon keratometers use 1.332. By inserting the appropriate value into the keratometric equation, the reader can see that slight differences in the index will produce a difference in K.

Use of the keratometric equation has led to some confusion as to whether *dioptric power* or *dioptric curvature* is the correct terminology for keratometry measurements. Helmholtz traditionally used the term *dioptric power* because the keratometric equation incorporates a term for refractivity of the tissue to estimate the dioptric power of the cornea, and he specifically wanted to know the dioptric power of the total cornea to simplify his calculations for the optical arrangement of the eye. However, some will point out that because only curvature is actually being assessed (albeit indirectly), it is not appropriate to label keratometry measurements as dioptric power, but only as dioptric curvature. The argument is moot and in fact neither term is strictly correct, but in practice either term is acceptable and understood.

CORNEAL SHAPE

In the simplest sense, the general shape of the cornea is spherical, in which case, the radius of curvature would be the same at any orientation of the surface. This is obviously a fiction simply because the radius of curvature of the cornea is seen to blend smoothly into the much larger radius of curvature of the scleral globe. A better description of corneal shape is that it is aspherical, where the central 4 mm of the cornea tends to be spherical, but then gradually flattens toward the periphery, much like the pointed (prolate)

end of an ellipsoid or an egg. It follows therefore that as the curvature decreases toward the corneal periphery, the radius of curvature must increase relative to the central cornea when measured with respect to the optic axis. However, even this description of shape is inaccurate. In reality, the corneal shape may be smooth overall in the normal cornea, but the radius of curvature nevertheless tends to vary along different meridians and with different distances from the central cornea. The shape is similar to the back of a teaspoon, with the handle held horizontally. The vertical meridian tends to be more curved and the horizontal meridian is less so. On the other hand, the corneal surface may be highly irregular, as is the case in many corneal diseases and disorders.

When performing keratometry, it does not matter whether corneal shape is simple or complex; the sole purpose of keratometry is simply to find the two meridians at which the central anterior corneal surface has the steepest and flattest spherical curvatures. In keratometry, we can largely ignore the complex topographic shape of the cornea, which is better assessed by a corneal topography device, and instead simplify the overall shape to only two curvature components. It should be understood that *steep* and *flat* are relative terms; a flat meridian in keratometry is not truly flat, but only relatively flatter than the other meridians of that surface. In fact, in instances where the cornea is severely distorted by disease or trauma, the flattest meridian may be much steeper than the steepest meridian of a normal cornea.

TYPICAL KERATOMETRY METHOD

All keratometers share the same basic principle of measuring curvature, but there are individual variations among systems. Therefore, it is best for users to standardize on one machine and avoid combining or comparing data from different keratometers; otherwise, small variations in corneal power will influence the data. Users should always refer to the manual for specific details about the operation of the keratometer.

The mire pattern when viewing the cornea in a typical keratometer is shown in Fig. 8-2A. Three ring images will be seen because of the two doubling prisms in the keratometer, with plus (+) and minus (−) fiducial marks located horizontally and vertically on each ring. The primary mire image is located in the corner of the pattern of three and may have a black alignment cross at the center (not shown). If the keratometer is out of focus, the primary mire image will itself be doubled vertically (Fig. 8-2B). Notice that horizontal bars of the plus marks for the horizontal pair of mire images should be aligned. If they are not, the orientation of the principal meridians of the cornea must be determined by rotating the optics of the keratometer about the instrument axis

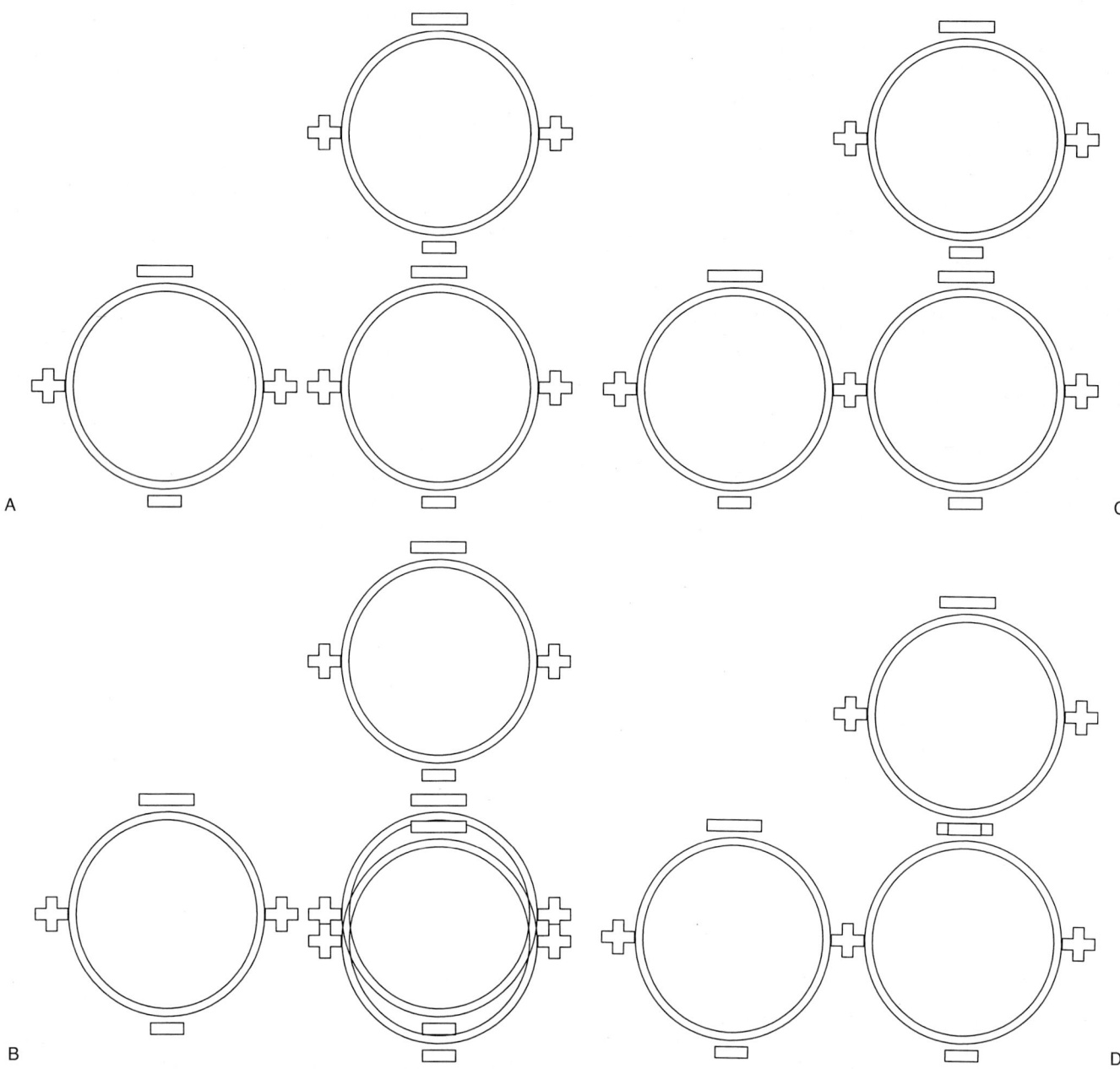

FIG. 8-2. Alignment of the mires during keratometry. **A,** A typical keratometer mire pattern. **B,** The image of the mire pattern when viewed with an unfocused keratometer. **C,** The image of the mire pattern with proper focus and when the first K-reading is determined. **D,** The image of the mire pattern when determining the second K-reading.

(i.e., rotation of the barrel of the instrument) until the horizontal bars of the plus signs are aligned (best focus may need to be readjusted after rotation of the keratometer). The axis reading is the axis of the cylinder component of astigmatism. Next, the horizontal measuring knob is turned until the + signs overlap along both their vertical and horizontal bars (Fig. 8-2C). The reading on the drum of the knob is the first K-reading. Finally, the vertical measuring knob is turned until the minus signs overlap (Fig. 8-2D). This is the second K-reading. The

dioptric difference in the drum readings is the astigmatism present in the cornea.

ASTIGMATISM AND K-READINGS

The steepest and flattest curvatures give rise to the concept of the principal meridians of the cornea, and the dioptric values associated with the principal meridians are called *K-readings*. In normal corneas, the K-readings for the two principal meridians are nearly the same magnitude, 43 D on average and usually within ±0.5 D of one another. However, a difference in K-readings is defined as astigmatism, and the greater the difference, the more corneal astigmatism is present. A difference of ±0.5 D is within the range of normal corneas and is generally well tolerated in terms of visual performance, but larger differences tend to indicate a significant amount of astigmatism that can greatly diminish visual performance.

It should be kept in mind that the astigmatism detected by keratometry is but a portion of the astigmatism found in the ocular refraction because the lens also has some amount of astigmatism to contribute to the refraction of the eye, and may add or subtract from the amount of corneal astigmatism that is present. In regular corneal astigmatism, the principal meridians tend to be oriented at 90 degrees to one another, or are said to be orthogonal. When the corneal astigmatism is clinically significant and the angle between the principal meridians is found to deviate from orthogonality, the condition is considered to be irregular corneal astigmatism. A deviation of more than a few degrees combined with atypical K-readings is often a sign of an abnormally shaped cornea due to corneal disease or warpage. Visually, the image of the mire circle is distorted so that it is neither perfectly round or oval. Nearly all keratometers are designed to measure curvature only at orthogonal meridians, so irregular astigmatism cannot be assessed perfectly with keratometry alone.

Typically, there are three forms of regular astigmatism: with-the-rule (by far the most common), against-the-rule (less common, except in older adults), and oblique (also less common). In with-the-rule astigmatism, the steepest meridian is within ±15 degrees of being vertical (i.e., with respect to the normal vertical orientation of the body). On the keratometer, the value of the horizontal meridian is flatter than that of the vertical meridian. In against-the-rule astigmatism, the steepest meridian is within ±15 degrees of being horizontal. In this case, the horizontal meridian value is more than the value found along the vertical meridian. Oblique astigmatism has an orientation somewhere between with- and against-the-rule. Meridional angles in keratometry are specified only from 0 to 180 degrees. It is important to note that to use the term *steep axis* is a misnomer because axis is used to denote the axis of the cylinder component, which by definition has no curvature and therefore no refractive power along the axis. Therefore the correct phrase is always *steep meridian*, and never *steep axis*. Always refer to the axis of astigmatism when referring to the cylinder axis, in which case the meridian at 90 degrees to the axis has the most curvature.

LIMITATIONS

Clearly, on normal corneas keratometry provides useful curvature data, but, as pointed out previously, the measurements are made only at points that are 3 to 4 mm apart along only two meridians. Distortion of the surface curvature between or beyond these points is not evaluated by the keratometer. When refractive surgery made its debut in the early 1980s, the performance of the keratometer in postoperative corneal curvature assessment was found to be inadequate. The relatively small diameter of the affected central zone of the cornea and occasional decentration of the procedure made keratometry measurements unreliable. The mires could lie within, outside, or even straddle the zone where curvature was changed by refractive surgery. Errors in the average corneal central curvature of ±1 D or more have been reported (4). Because keratometry measurements are often used for calculating the desired power for intraocular lens implants, for estimating contact lens base curves, as well as for excimer laser ablation profiles in keratorefractive surgery, such errors can lead to suboptimal visual results. Finally, keratometer measurements made on misshapen corneas such as those with keratoconus and those after penetrating keratoplasty will not be very useful, again for the same reason that measurements are not obtained from the bulk of the central cornea, but only at four points. For these applications, it is imperative to make measurements using a corneal topographer to obtain useful data.

CONCLUSION

The keratometer remains a useful clinical tool for inexpensive and rapid determination of corneal curvature in the normal, unoperated eye. When disease, surgery, or trauma produces irregularities in corneal shape, a corneal topographer is the preferred instrument for management of cornea-related visual problems.

REFERENCES

1. Mandell R. Jesse Ramsden: inventor of the ophthalmometer. *Am J Optom Arch Am Acad Optom* 1960;37:633-638.
2. Gullstrand A. The cornea. In: Southhall J, ed. *Helmholtz's treatise on physiological optics.* New York: Optical Society of America, 1924.
3. Emsley H. Keratometry. In: *Visual optics.* London: Hatton Press, 1946.
4. Maeda N, Klyce SD, Smolek MK, et al. Disparity of keratometry readings and corneal power within the pupil after refractive surgery for myopia. *Cornea* 1997;16:517-524.

CORNEAL TOPOGRAPHY

CHRISTOPHER B. COURVILLE AND STEPHEN D. KLYCE

Corneal surface topography plays a critical role in the performance of the visual system, accounting for two thirds of the eye's total refractive power. Irregularities in corneal shape and tear film distribution can lead to severe degradation in the optical quality of the cornea and, therefore, markedly reduce visual acuity. Hence, being able accurately to measure corneal shape is extremely important. Detection of surface distortions has been difficult because of often subtle nature and, thus, they have often gone undetected with traditional biomicroscope examination. Although retinoscopy can detect the presence of surface distortions, it is unable to pinpoint the source of the aberrations. The keratometer, measuring only four spots on the corneal surface, is not adequate to detect surface distortions over any great area. These limitations led to the application of the Placido disc. Projecting a series of mires onto the corneal surface and adding an instant film camera allowed a more complete surface area to be analyzed; this approach was embodied in the Photokeratoscope by Nidek (Nidek PKS-1000) (1) and in the Corneascope by Kera Corp. (2). This tool provided more details of the cornea's topography, but was limited to the management of relatively severe irregularities in the corneal surface such as occur in corneal grafts, moderately advanced keratoconus, and trauma.

It was the advent of refractive surgery—particularly radial keratotomy—into U.S. clinics in 1979 that drove the need for a more accurate analysis of corneal topography. With concurrent advances in digital computers, corneal topographers quickly evolved to serve the needs of refractive surgeons in preoperative screening and investigation of problematic outcomes such as halos, glare, and reduced contrast. This chapter reviews the current status of corneal topography and its association with wavefront analysis. The clinical applications of corneal topography are briefly introduced; these are covered in greater depth in the clinical sections of this text.

BASIC PRINCIPLES OF MEASUREMENT

As the number of commercial corneal topographers continues to grow, their optical principles and techniques have varied somewhat, but their common purpose has been to display corneal curvature. The corneal topographers that have found widespread use in the clinic are all based on Placido disc technology. The measurement of corneal curvature with the scanning slit, laser holographic interferometry, and rastersterography have not enjoyed productive clinical use, but it is instructive to view the different approaches that have been tried. Corneal topographers that have been developed are listed in Table 9-1.

Placido Disc

The first modern corneal topographer, the Corneal Modeling System (Computed Anatomy, Inc., New York, NY) (3), carried forward the concept of the Placido disc coupled with digital image processing and analysis to measure corneal power; this approach remains the only proven technology owing to its sensitivity, reproducibility, relative freedom from movement artifact, and noninvasiveness. The Placido disc consists of a circular target of alternating concentric light and dark rings that are reflected from the convex, mirror-like corneal surface. The resulting image is captured with a charge-coupled device (CCD)–equipped digital camera and is used automatically to transform mire shapes into the three-dimensional shape and power of the corneal surface. Several computer algorithms are available with which to reconstruct a model of the corneal surface, but because there is no exact solution, approximations can lead to inaccuracies. Fortunately, these are usually confined to the corneal periphery (4,5). Although these techniques can be very accurate (5), some have limitations that can lead to the false indication of keratoconus (6).

Two general types of Placido target are available (Fig. 9-1). The large-diameter target is less sensitive to magnification errors because of its long working distance, but these devices tend to lose data from the periphery because of shadows caused by the nose and the brow. The small-diameter, cone-shaped targets do not suffer from shadow-induced data loss and can project mires well out onto the sclera, but must rely on very accurate range compensation for

TABLE 9-1. LIST OF COMMERCIALLY AVAILABLE CORNEAL TOPOGRAPHERS

Manufacturer	Model(s)	Method
Alcon Surgical	EyeMap EH-290	Placido
Alliance Medical Mkts	Keratron CT; Scout	Placido
B & L Surgical	Orbscan II	Scanned slits and Placido
B & L Surgical	Orbshot	Placido
Dicon	CT-200	Placido
Euclid Systems	ET-800	Flurorescein profilometry
EyeSys/Premier	EyeSys 2000; Vista	Placido
Eyetek	CT2000	Placido
Humphrey Insruments	Atlas 991,992	Placido
Kera Metrics	CLAS-1000	Laser holography
Medmont	E300	Placido
Oculus	Keratograph	Placido
PAR Vision Systems	CTS, Accugrid	Flurorescein profilometry
PAR Vision Systems	Intraop. CTS	Flurorescein profilometry
Sun Contact Lens Co.	SK-2000	Placido
TechnoMed Technology	C-SCAN	Placido
Tomey Technology	AutoTopographer	Placido
Topcon America Corp.	CM-1000	Placido

accuracy. As a result, the small cone Placido devices may be a more amenable adjunct to accurate contact lens fitting.

Rasterstereography

An approach that avoids the uncertainties of the Placido approximation calculations is rasterstereography (7–9). A drop of fluorescein is instilled into the cul de sac and a grid or raster pattern of cobalt blue light is projected onto the anterior surface of the eye. The stereo images are captured and processed using triangulation to reconstruct the cornea's topography without approximating algorithms.

A limitation of this technique is that direct measurement of surface position does not yield the same sensitivity of measurement as does reflected image positions. This, along with the uncertain effects of fluorescein on tear film stability and structure, reduces rasterstereography's apparent usefulness in the clinic, and a commercial device may not be currently available.

Scanning Slit

Scanning slit technology allows the measurement of both anterior and posterior surfaces of the cornea. This was first implemented in the Corneal Modeling System (3). Because

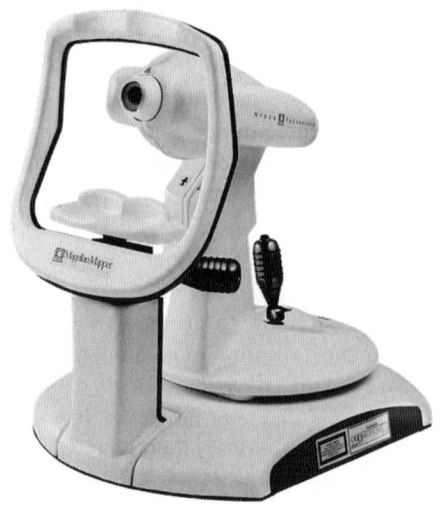

A

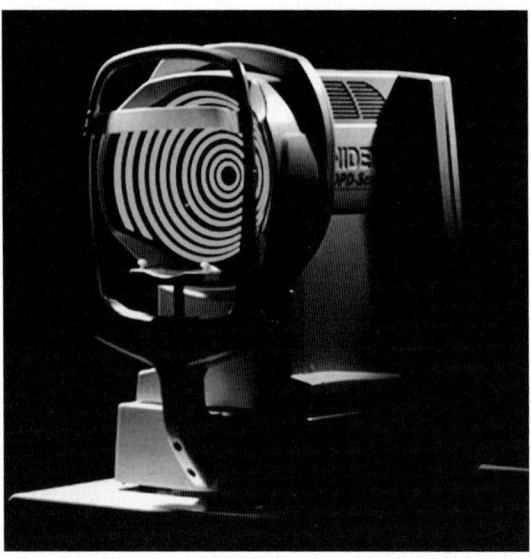

B

FIGURE 9-1. Two types of Placido target have been used in corneal topographers. **A:** The Nidek Magellan topographer uses the small, cone-shaped target. **B:** The Nidek OPD-Scan aberrometer/topographer uses the large-diameter target.

both surfaces, along with corneal thickness, are needed accurately to calculate total corneal power, directly measuring the relative positions of the surfaces would seem to be a major advantage. This technique not only eliminates the need for elevation or shape measurement approximations, it has the important ability to measure corneal thickness over a broad area. The scanning slit measurement does have its limitations, however. First, measurement requires over 1 second for completion, leaving the data replete with motion artifact from fixation drift, muscle tremor, pulse, and nystagmus, which occur when the data are not captured in less than 30 msec. This error can be reduced with a tracking system or postcapture registration techniques, but this adds great expense and registration has proved difficult because landmarks are absent on the normally transparent cornea. Lack of sensitivity when reconstructing corneal topography from direct surface measurement is also a problem. To overcome this problem, corneal topography is measured with the addition of a Placido target in the Orbscan II model (Bausch & Lomb, Rochester, NY). Thus, although the scanning slit alone is not useful for measuring topography, there appears to be some utility in the thickness profiles that can be generated with this method.

Interferometry

The method with potentially the highest sensitivity is interferometry (10–12). Such techniques have been used by the optical industry to detect lens and mirror aberrations with subwavelength accuracy. With this procedure a reference surface, or its hologram, and the measured corneal surface are optically compared and the resulting interference fringes are used to calculate the difference between the two shapes. However, there is such wide variation in corneal shapes (even among normal subjects) that it is difficult to represent all variations with a single interference device.

Trials have been underway with this technology, including laser holography–based devices (13,14) and acoustic holographic devices (15), although neither approach has enjoyed clinical acceptance.

PRESENTATION AND DISPLAY

Background

In 1981, Doss and coworkers (2,16) published a method for the automatic scanning of Corneascope photographs calculate corneal power. Klyce (17) took this a step further by devising a method for reconstructing corneal shape and power by digitally scanning the mires from Nidek photokeratoscope photographs and then displaying the data in a three-dimensional wire-mesh plot. Building on these advances, Maguire et al. (4) introduced the color-coded

contour map as a display format for corneal powers, and this method soon became the international standard. Other, more recent developments include the plotting of contour maps directly onto the video image of the eye to relate scale and position, the display of multiple examinations simultaneously to view the progression of a disease or postsurgical results, and the construction of difference maps that aid in such aspects as showing early postoperative effects of a surgical procedure or the evolution of specific topographic features.

Units of Measure

Corneal topographers measure corneal surface curvature by design and, when used in contact lens fitting, this curvature is most usefully expressed in units of millimeters. However, when a corneal topographer is used to evaluate a pathologic process, the optics of the eye, and refractive errors, it is more convenient for the clinician to evaluate corneal power in units of diopters (D). It is important to distinguish between corneal surface power and total corneal power. Corneal surface power should be calculated using Snell's law from the gradient in refractive index between air (1.000) and cornea (1.376). The curvature of the average corneal surface is 7.85 mm. The refractive power of that surface is $0.367/7.85 \times 1000$ mm/m or approximately 48 D. However, by convention from keratometry, clinicians have been accustomed to converting curvatures to the equivalent power of the whole cornea; this is done using the "keratometric index" (0.3375). Hence, the average corneal power becomes $0.3375/7.85 \times 1000$ mm/m or close to 43 D. This may seem confusing at first, but the latter calculation converts corneal topography measurements to the clinically familiar K reading values, and for this reason one of the first indexes that was derived for corneal topography data was the Simulated Keratometry (SimK) reading. One important caveat is that keratometry does not approximate well the power changes that occur with most refractive surgical procedures (18,19). The tissue subtraction procedures such as laser *in situ* keratomileusis change the anterior corneal curvature (but not the posterior surface) and corneal thickness. To calculate the refractive effect of changing corneal anterior surface curvature, one should use the refractive index, 1.376, whereas for general clinical use, the keratometric power with the index 1.3375 has been preferred.

Color-Coded Contour Map

With the introduction of the color-coded contour map, clinicians can now view topographic information through color association and pattern recognition (4). The palette of colors chosen was constructed so that powers near normal levels appear as green, lower powers as cool colors,

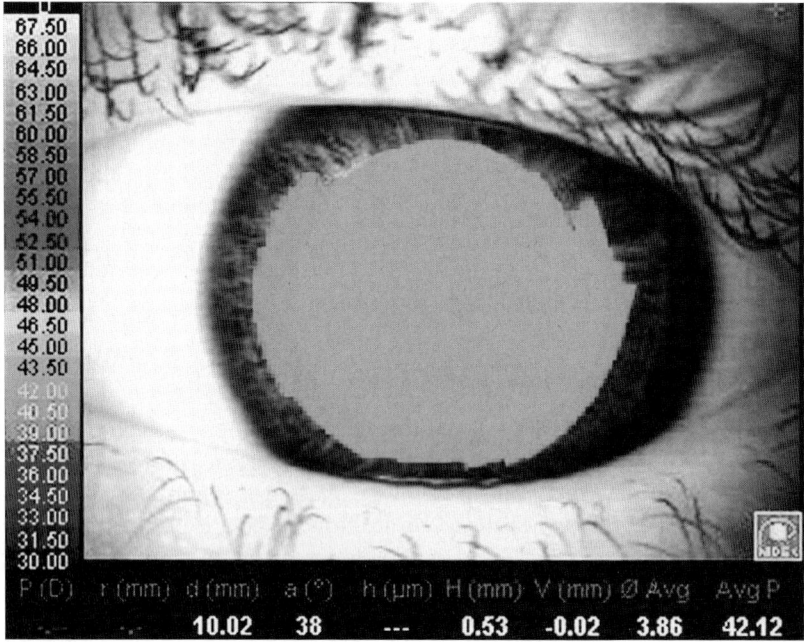

P (D)	r (mm)	d (mm)	a (°)	h (µm)	H (mm)	V (mm)	Ø Avg	Avg P
	10.02	38	---	0.53	-0.02	3.86		42.12

FIGURE 9-2. Topographic example of a normal cornea. Note the smooth power contours, uniform central power, and peripheral flattening.

and higher than normal powers as warm colors (Fig. 9-2). Furthermore, only a few identifiable colors are selected for the central range of corneal powers so that specific power intervals can be identified easily. This allows for the recognition of certain characteristic patterns in corneal topography such as a cylinder, which presents as a "bow-tie" pattern (Fig. 9-3); keratoconus, which is characterized by a local area of steepening (Fig. 9-4); and pellucid marginal degeneration (usually inferior arcuate steepening; Fig. 9-5), as well as characteristics associated with refractive surgery, including optical zone size, centration, and, occasionally, defects such as central islands (Fig. 9-6).

Standardized Scales

A study by Bogan and associates (20) has shown that, at high resolution, normal corneas (neither pathologic nor surgical) exhibit a variety of topographies—including

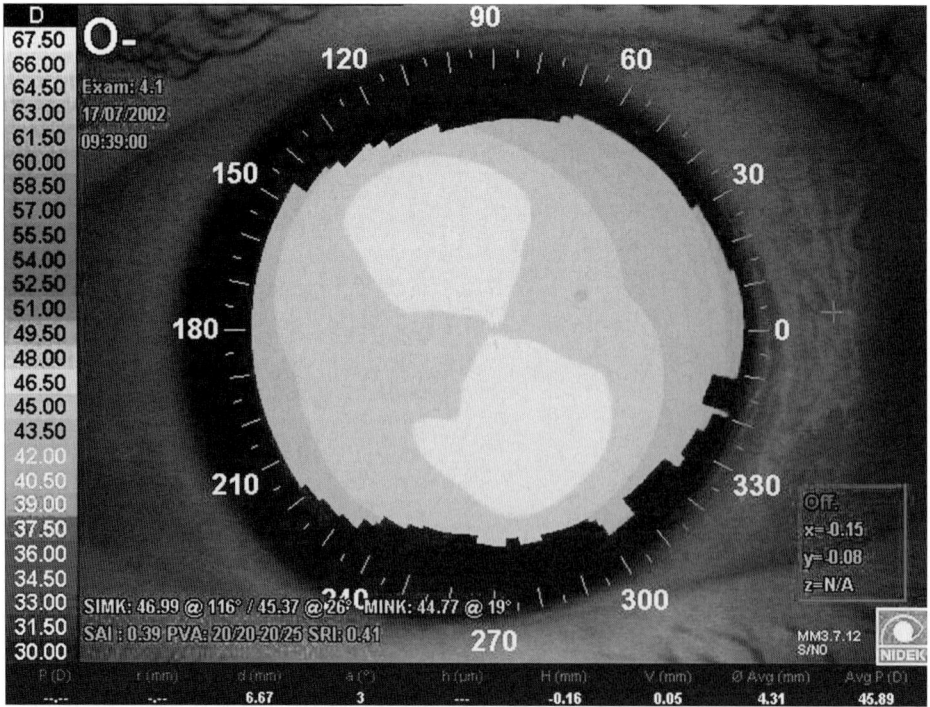

FIGURE 9-3. Topographic example of cylinder. Note the characteristic "bow-tie" pattern.

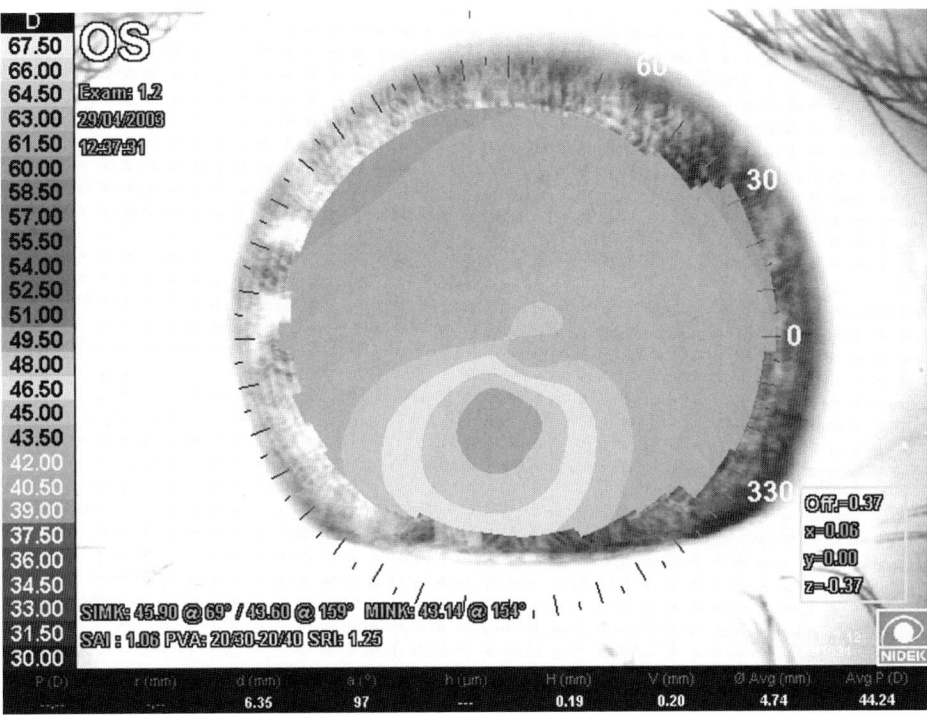

FIGURE 9-4. Topographic example of clinical keratoconus.

round, oval, and irregular patterns—making any attempt at developing a generalized classification scheme immaterial. We now know that examination of corneal topography at high-sensitivity levels reveals details of irregularity that are not often of clinical significance (21). This fact makes a fixed, universal standard scale essential to allow only features of clinical significance to be displayed. The set of colors and intervals originally proposed by Maguire and colleagues in 1987 (4) provided a range of 9 to 101.5 D, but has since been changed in numerous ways by manufacturers, and efforts to promote the adoption of single a standardized scale have failed. In 1993,

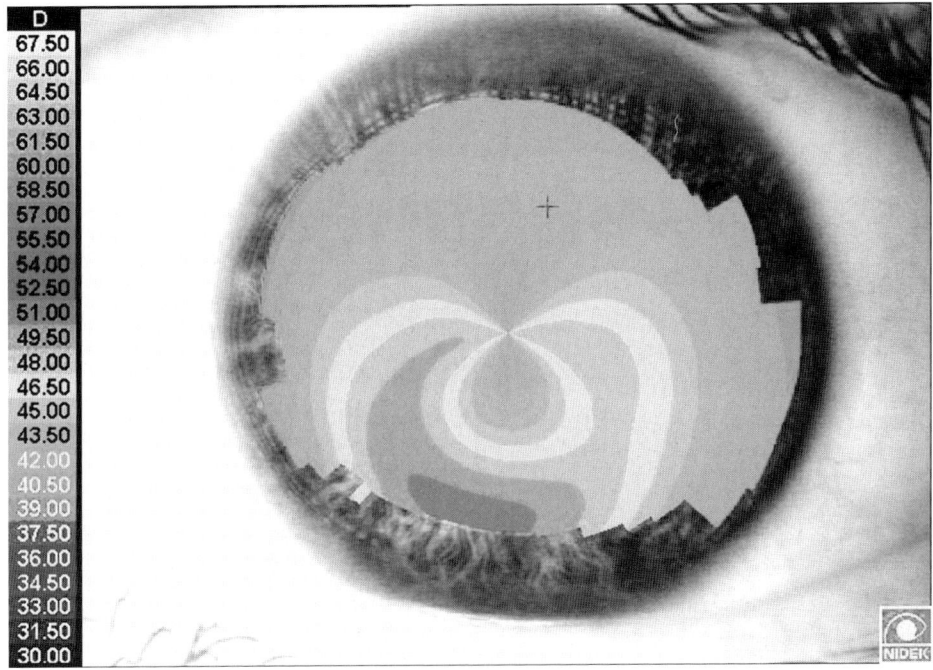

FIGURE 9-5. Topographic example of pellucid marginal degeneration. Note the characteristic inferior arcuate steepening.

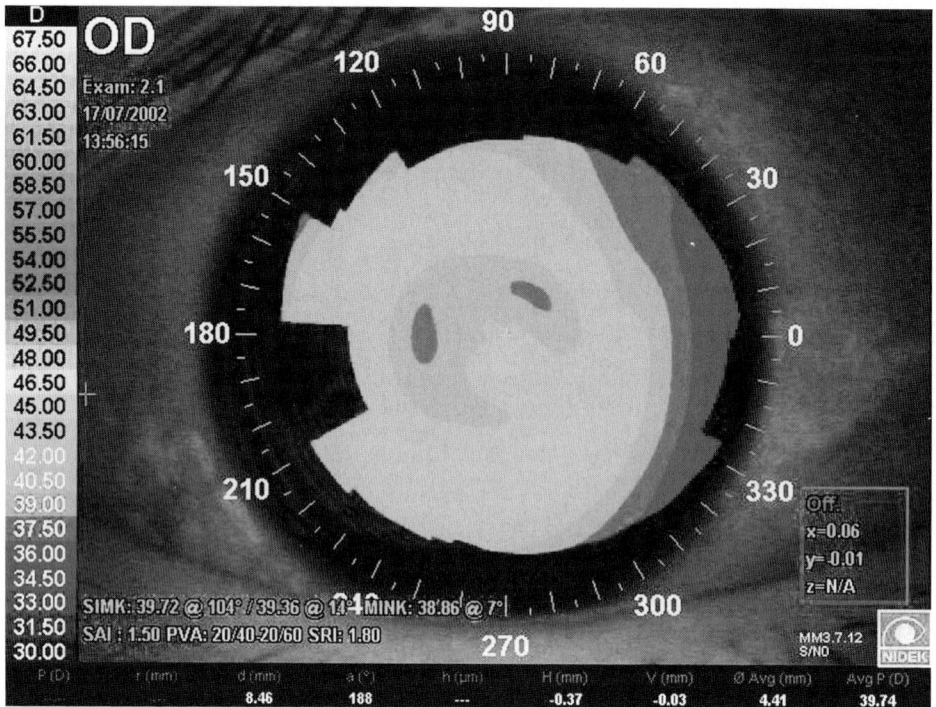

FIGURE 9-6. Topographic example of central island or peninsula after myopic refractive surgery.

Wilson et al. (21) introduced a more practical scale (the Klyce-Wilson scale) ranging from 28 to 65.5 D at uniform 1.5-D intervals. Although it has been argued that an interval of 1.5 D could be too wide to display all the important features in corneal topography, its adequacy has been proved sufficient for clinical use, at least with the higher-resolution corneal topographers. The adequacy of this scale was evaluated in a consecutive series of examinations that included normal corneas, contact lens–wearing corneas, different stages of keratoconus, penetrating keratoplasties, extracapsular cataract surgeries, excimer laser photorefractive keratectomies, radial keratotomies, aphakic epikeratoplasties, and myopic epikeratoplasties. It was found that a correct diagnosis could be made in all included cases with the 1.5-D scale without resorting to a more sensitive interval. The scale was also broad enough to cover the full range of powers present in the study (21).

Traditionally, corneal topographers have offered adaptable scales that automatically adjust to a given cornea's power range. Such scales can be disastrously misleading, making irregular corneas look normal and normal corneas look abnormal, and should be avoided except as a tool to examine specific topographic details (Fig. 9-7). The use of

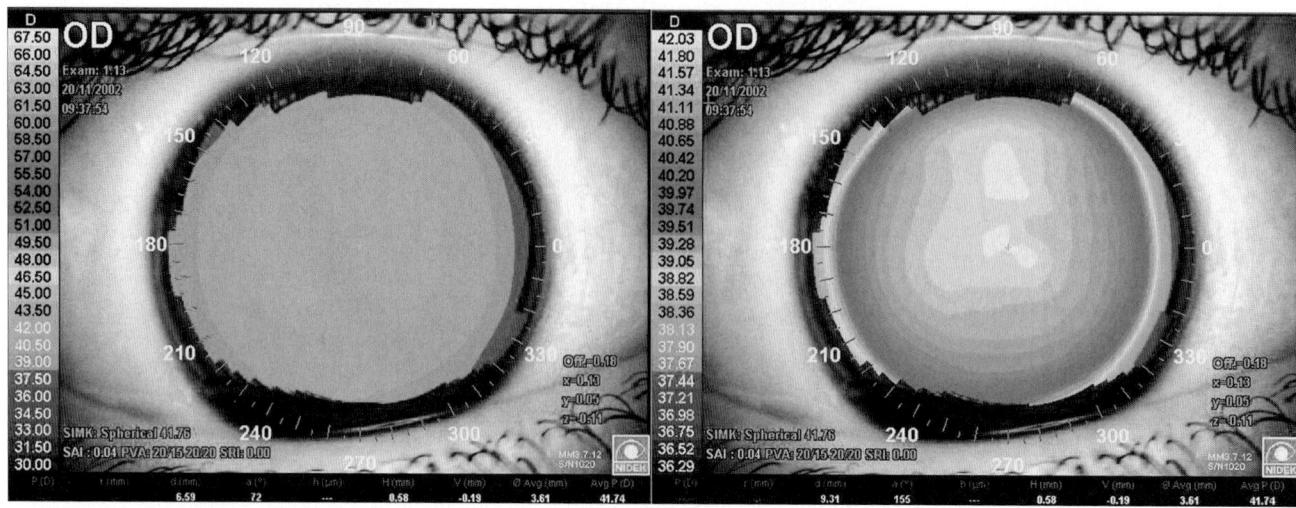

FIGURE 9-7. Example of clinical keratoconus and its detection by two different methods.

a fixed standard scale capable of displaying adequate detail without superfluous or extraneous information is essential for quick and accurate clinical use. Smolek and coworkers (22) have revisited this issue in depth and have proposed a universal standard scale for use in corneal topography.

QUANTITATIVE INDEXES

Although the color-coded contour maps by themselves are extremely useful, they alone cannot produce numeric values for use in clinical management. Therefore, quantitative indexes have been developed to complement corneal topography maps. Such indexes include the simulated keratometry values noted previously, optical-quality indicators, keratoconus detectors, and other indexes that can be used in artificial intelligence systems to interpret corneal topography patterns.

Power and Shape Indexes

SimK

SimK values, one of the first indexes made widely available, simulate the curvature measures given by the keratometer (23)—the powers and axes of the steepest and flattest meridians—which are designated SimK1 and SimK2, respectively. These numbers are computed using the mires that correspond to points on the cornea that would be used to determine keratometer readings. With these values, cylinder and spherical equivalent can be easily calculated and are often displayed alongside color maps. SimK values prove to be extremely useful in determining the amount and axis of astigmatism when refracting eyes with irregular corneas, can aid in the fitting of contact lenses, and can be helpful as well in refractive surgery and intraocular lens calculations.

Corneal Eccentricity Index

The corneal eccentricity index (CEI) indicates the eccentricity of the cornea (24) and is typically determined by fitting an ellipse to the elevation data provided by the topographer. In a study of 22 normal corneas, the CEI obtained was 0.33 ± 0.26 (mean $\pm$ 1 standard deviation), corresponding to the prolate shape of the normal central cornea. This index is helpful in contact lens fitting and to differentiate between normal prolate corneas and oblate corneas flattened by myopic refractive surgery.

Average Corneal Power

The average corneal power (ACP) is an area-corrected average of corneal power lying ahead of the entrance pupil (25). ACP is basically equal to the keratometric spherical equivalent except in cases of decentered refractive surgery.

In these cases, ACP may help to determine average central corneal curvature for intraocular lens power calculations.

Optical Quality Indexes

The advent of refractive surgery was really the driving force behind the development of the modern corneal topographer as a means to investigate complications and improve surgical techniques. This has led to a long search for methods that could be used for the evaluation of the optical quality of the corneal surface derived from corneal topography measurements. Although this journey is far from over, clinically useful progress has been made.

Surface Regularity Index

The first index developed to measure the impact of corneal irregularities on optical quality was the surface regularity index (SRI) (26). This index sums the meridional mire-to-mire power changes over the apparent entrance pupil, increasing as topographic irregularities increase. SRI was correlated to visual acuity for a group of normal subjects, patients with keratoconus, and corneal transplant recipients. This correlation allows the clinically useful prediction of the potential visual acuity in Snellen chart format.

A different approach was taken by Maloney et al. (27) and Holladay (28). They chose first to determine the best-fitting ellipsoid for the central cornea, then calculate the difference between this surface and corneal elevation. Correlating these distortions with clinical data, the results are displayed as color-coded maps of predicted regional Snellen acuity (28).

Fourier and Zernike Methods

Fourier series transformations, which prove useful in fitting and decomposing periodic functions, can provide average corneal power, amount and axis of regular astigmatism, and terms that can be summed to estimate irregularities in topography (29–31). More recently, investigators have turned to using the Zernike polynomial to dissect out components of aberrations (irregularities) in the optics of the eye, and this formalism is also amenable to application to corneal topography measurements. However, it has been shown that although Zernike polynomials are a powerful approach to extracting lower-order information from corneal topography (defocus, prism, cylinder, spherical aberration, and coma), the method lacks the ability faithfully to extract all the higher-order aberrations that affect vision (M. K. Smolek, S. D. Klyce, unpublished data.).

Ray Tracing

Ray tracing methods have been used by several groups as a means to measure and illustrate the impact of corneal aberrations on vision. Using this approach, for example, Seiler and coworkers developed an index they named *effective spherical aberration,* which showed a statistically significant correlation with best-corrected visual acuity in a cohort of patients undergoing photorefractive keratectomy (32). TechnoMed's C-Scan also uses ray tracing through a Gullstrand model eye to determine visual acuity from an index based on the smallest resolvable separation between points. As well, Camp et al. (33) and Maguire et al. (34) were among the first to use ray tracing to demonstrate how scenery (e.g., an eye chart) is modified by specific aberrations.

Aberration Structures and Wavefront Sensing

As a result of the major role the corneal surface plays in image formation, the measurement of aberrations resulting from corneal shape irregularities with corneal topographers has been the subject of much attention. *Wavefront analysis* is the generic term for analyzing a light ray's optical path length through an optical system. In early work, wavefront analysis took the form of subtracting the best-fitting sphere from the measured shape of the corneal surface; the result was called the *aberration structure.* Its components were evaluated with the Taylor polynomial series and the method applied to evaluate corneas before and after refractive surgery to determine the effects on visual function (35–37). Key elements of this analytic method were the

ability to quantify, for the first time, spherical-like and coma-like aberrations in the eye. This method can also be used to examine aberrations under different lighting conditions; a 3-mm pupil is used to evaluate photopic characteristics, whereas a 7-mm pupil is used to evaluate mesopic or night vision (37).

Indexes for Keratoconus Detection

Typically, keratoconus-suspect corneas are characterized in topography by a localized area of steepness, usually displaced inferiorly. Clinical keratoconus is associated with localized steepness along with the traditional signs such as thinning near the cone apex and Vogt's striae. The difficulty has been in establishing "cutoff" values to differentiate between normal variations in corneal steepness and asymmetry and true disease. Additional indexes calculated from topography maps have been created to accomplish this goal (Fig. 9-8).

Rabinowitz and McDonnell (38) were the first to use numeric methods to detect keratoconus systematically through corneal topography data. They developed indexes that measured power differences between the superior and inferior paracentral corneal regions (designated I-S values), the central corneal power (Max K), and the power differences between the left and right eye. Their analysis showed that a central corneal power greater than 47.2 D or an I-S value greater than 1.4 D is consistent with suspect keratoconus, whereas

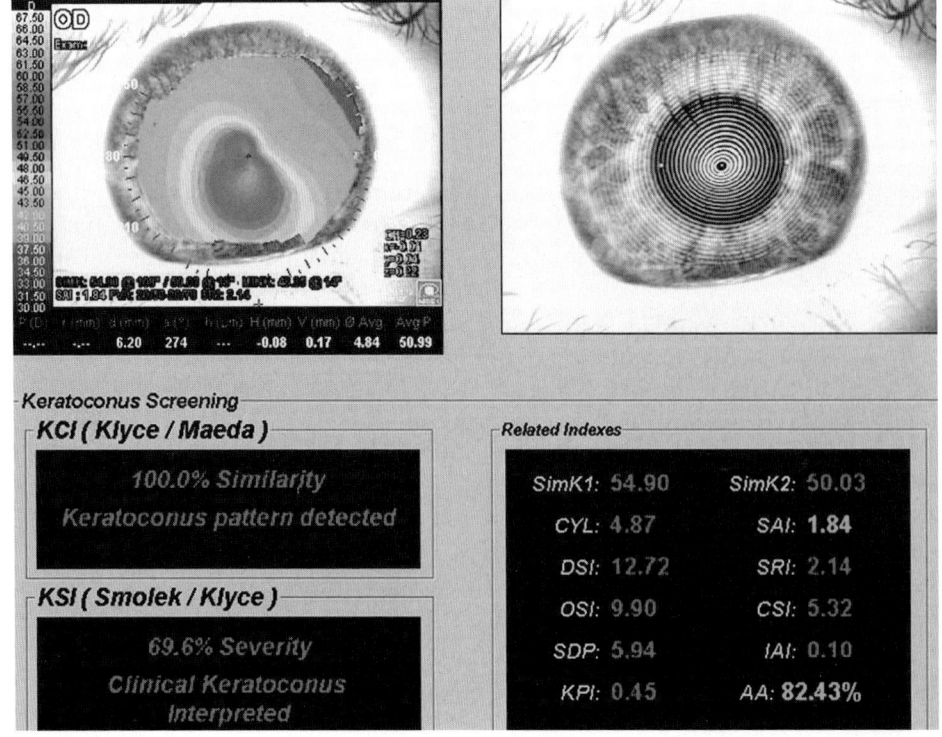

FIGURE 9-8. Example of the problems encountered when adaptable scales are used. *Left,* A normal cornea displayed with the Smolek/Klyce scale. *Right,* The same cornea displayed with an adaptable scale, which makes it look erroneously problematic.

central corneal powers greater than 48.7 D or I–S values greater than 1.9 D are consistent with clinical keratoconus. Although these criteria can distinguish the topography of keratoconus corneas from that of normal corneas, specificity of the method is not optimum. To address this need, Maeda and associates (39,40) developed an expert system classifier that, through discriminant analysis, yields the keratoconus prediction index. This value was derived from topographic indexes specifically designed to capture determining characteristics such as local abnormal elevations in corneal power. These include the differential sector index, the opposite sector index, the center/surround index, the surface asymmetry index, the irregular astigmatism index, and the percent analyzed area. The results of the discriminate analyzer were fed to a binary decision tree to enhance this method's performance.

Classification with Neural Networks

The search for a more sophisticated approach to corneal topography classification and topographic abnormality detection led to the development of artificial intelligence neural network models by Maeda and associates (41). This method performs automated pattern interpretation using a neural network program. Smolek and Klyce (42) improved on this approach by presenting a method capable of 100% accuracy, specificity, and sensitivity with both the original training set and, notably, a test set that the system had never seen.

CLINICAL APPLICATIONS

Although specific examples of clinical applications are provided elsewhere in this book, a few basic principles are set forth here.

Normal Corneas

The topography of normal corneas can vary considerably from one subject to another, as well as from one area of the cornea to another. It is important to have a sufficient understanding of the topography of normal corneas to distinguish them from those affected by trauma, surgery, or disease.

For over a century, it has been known that normal corneas are aspheric, with the central cornea being steeper than the periphery (Fig. 9-2). This characteristic compensates to some extent for the eye's spherical aberration. A 1989 study by Dingeldein and Klyce (43) of eyes with normal vision and no history of contact lens wear or corneal abnormalities found the average central corneal power to be 42.84 D. All corneas flattened progressively toward the limbus, although the degree and rate of flattening along with the location of the shortest radius of curvature varied extensively. Normal corneas flatten more quickly nasally

than temporally. With the color-coded map, the corneas of each person showed an individualized pattern, like a fingerprint. The topographies of fellow eyes were typically mirror images (enantiomorphs) of each other, an example of midline symmetry. Even with all of these variations, normal corneas were found to have smooth power map contours, in keeping with their optical performance requirements.

A normal corneal topography depends on the presence of an intact and normal tear film. Tear film breakup caused by dry eye, lagophthalmus, or the instillation of medications can modify the measured corneal topography dramatically. For this reason, it is standard procedure to perform corneal topography during clinical examination as a first test and before instillation of any medication (e.g., mydriatics). Tear film breakup usually causes mistracking of the mires, and, if this is a transient condition, the measured topography will contain artifact and not reflect the true corneal optical quality.

Corneal Topography and Astigmatism

Regular Astigmatism

In corneal topography, naturally occurring regular astigmatism is represented by a bow-tie pattern (Fig. 9-3). When examining the topography of normal corneas, Bogan and associates found 50% to have bow-tie patterns (20). Corneas with significant keratometric cylinder also possessed the bow-tie pattern, confirming corneal topography's efficacy in detecting cylinder.

Corneal topographers provide quantitative measures of astigmatism, as noted previously in the discussion of simulated keratometry. As expected, there is a strong correlation between the ACP measured with topography and average keratometric power ($r = 0.96$, $p < .001$) (44). Similarly, there is a strong correlation between simulated keratometry from corneal topography and keratometric measurements (26). One caveat: Refractive astigmatism does not always agree with corneal astigmatism because the lens or macula can be responsible for all or part of the refractive astigmatism, although this appears to be rare.

Irregular Astigmatism

"Irregular astigmatism" has been used as a catch-all phrase for any nonspherocylindrical aberration that diminishes vision. Although it may be difficult to eradicate long-standing terminology, it is now preferable to use more specific terms for separable components such as cylinder, prism, spherical aberrations, and coma, and to refer to all other components collectively as higher-order aberrations. Irregularities in the corneal surface after trauma or corneal transplantation often result in significant amounts of higher-order aberrations, although disease and other surgery can produce this situation as well. In judging the clinical significance of corneal topography aberrations of any type, it is critically important to use a fixed, standard 1.5-D interval scale, as noted earlier. With this approach, irregular contours become detectable only when there is an associated visual deficit; in such cases the degree of aberrations can be determined with a quantitative measure like the surface regularity index.

CONCLUSION

Since its introduction nearly two decades ago, corneal topography has been adopted as the standard of care in anterior segment practice. Originally appearing as a tool in refractive surgery clinical laboratories, modern corneal topographers have been developed into tools that permit the management of visual loss from ocular aberrations. Corneal topography analysis has enabled the accelerated development of refractive surgical techniques and raised the bar in terms of visual outcomes for our patients.

ACKNOWLEDGMENTS

This work was supported in part by U.S. Public Health Service grants R01EY03311 and P30EY002377 from the National Eye Institute, National Institutes of Health, Bethesda, Maryland. Dr. Klyce has been a paid consultant to Nidek Co., Ltd., manufacturer of the OPD-Scan topographer/aberrometer.

REFERENCES

1. Riss I, Hoyston P, Kuhne F, et al. Viabilite et reproductibilite de photokeratoanlyseur de Nidek. *J Fr Ophtalmol* 1991;14:451–454.
2. Rowsey JJ, Reynolds AE, Brown R. Corneal topography: corneascope. *Arch Ophthalmol* 1981;99:1093–1100.
3. Gormley DJ, Gersten M, Koplin RS, et al. Corneal modeling. *Cornea* 1988;7:30–35.
4. Maguire LJ, Singer DE, Klyce SD. Graphic presentation of computer analyzed keratoscope photographs. *Arch Ophthalmol* 1987;105:223–230.
5. Wilson SE, Kyce SD. Advances in the analysis of corneal topography. *Surv Ophthalmol* 1991;35:269–277.
6. Mandell RB, Chiang CS, Yee L. Asymmetric corneal torricity and pseudokeratoconus in videokeratography. *J Am Optom Assoc* 1996;67:540–547.
7. Arffa RC, Warnicki JW, Rehkopf PG. Corneal topography using rasterstereography. *J Refract Corneal Surg* 1989;5:414–417.
8. Naufal SC, Hess JS, Friedlander MH, et al. Rasterstereography-based classification of normal corneas. *J Cataract Refract Surg* 1997;23:222–230.
9. Warnicki JW, Rehkopf PG, Curtin DY, et al. Corneal topography using computer analyzed rasterstereographic images. *Appl Optics* 1998;27:1135.
10. MacRae S, Rich L, Phillips D, et al. Diurnal variation in vision after radial keratotomy. *Am J Ophthalmol* 1989;107:262–267.
11. Rottenkolber M, Podbielska H. High precision Twyman-Green interferometer for the measurement of ophthalmic surfaces. *Acta Ophthalmol Scand* 1996;74:348–353.
12. Smith TW. Corneal topography. *Doc Ophthalmol* 1997;43:249–276.
13. Burris TE, Baker PC, Ayer CT, et al. Flattening of central corneal curvature with intrastromal corneal rings of increasing thickness: an eye-bank eye study. *J Cataract Refract Surg* 1993;19[Suppl]:182–187.
14. Shack R, Barker R, Buchroeder R, et al. Ultrafast laser scanner microscope. *J Histochem Cytochem* 1979;27:153–159.
15. Smolek MK. Holographic interferometry of intact and radially incised human eye-bank corneas. *J Cataract Refract Surg* 1994;20:277–286.
16. Doss JD, Hutson RL, Rowsey JJ, et al. Method for calculation of corneal profile and power distribution. *Arch Ophthalmol* 1981;99:1261–1265.
17. Klyce SD. Computer-assisted corneal topography: high resolution graphical presentation and analysis of keratoscopy. *Invest Ophthalmol Vis Sci* 1984;25:1426–1435.
18. Arffa RC, Klyce SC, Busin M. Keratometry in epikeratophakia. *J Refract Corneal Surg* 1986;2:61–64.
19. Swinger CA, Barker BA. Prospective evaluation of myopic keratomileusis. *Ophthalmology* 1984;91:785–792.
20. Bogan SJ, Waring GO III, Ibrahim O, et al. Classification of normal corneal topography based computer-assisted videokeratography. *Arch Ophthalmol* 1990;108:945–949.
21. Wilson SE, Klyce SD, Husseini ZM. Standardized color-coded maps for corneal topography. *Ophthalmology* 1993;100:1723–1727.
22. Smolek MK, Klyce SD, Hovis JK. The universal standard scale: proposed improvements to the ANSI standard corneal topography map. *Ophthalmology* 2002;109:361–369.
23. Dingelein SA, Klyce SD, Wilson SE. Quantitative descriptors of corneal shape derived from computer assisted analysis of photokeratographs. *J Refract Corneal Surg* 1989;5:372–378.
24. Maeda N, Klyce SD, Hamano H. Alteration of corneal asphericity in rigid gas permeable contact lens induced warpage. *CLAO J* 1994;20:27–31.
25. Maeda N, Klyce SD, Smolek MK, et al. Disparity of keratometry-style readings and corneal power within the pupil after refractive surgery for myopia. *Cornea* 1997;16:517–524.
26. Wilson SE, Klyce SD. Quantitative descriptors of corneal topography: a clinical study. *Arch Ophthalmol* 1991;109:349–353.
27. Maloney RK, Bogan SJ, Waring GO. Determination of corneal image-forming properties from corneal topography. *Am J Ophthalmol* 1993;115:31–41.
28. Holladay JT. Corneal topography using the Holladay Diagnostic Summary. *J Cataract Refract Surg* 1997;23:209–221.
29. Hjortdal JO, Erdmann L, Bek T. Fourier analysis of videokeratographic data: a tool for separation of spherical, regular astigmatic and irregular astigmatic corneal power components. *Ophthalmic Physiol Opt* 1995;15:171–185.
30. Olsen T, Dam-Johansen M, Bek T. Evaluating surgically induced astigmatism by Fourier analysis of corneal topography data. *J Cataract Refract Surg* 1996;22:318–323.
31. Oshika T, Tomidokoro A, Maruo K, et al. Quantitative evaluation of irregular astigmatism by Fourier series harmonic analysis of videokeratography data. *Invest Ophthalmol Vis Sci* 1998;39:705–709.
32. Seiler T, Reckmann W, Maloney RK. Effective spherical aberration of the cornea as a quantitative descriptor in corneal topography. *J Cataract Refract Surg* 1993;19[Suppl]:155–165.
33. Camp JJ, Maguire LJ, Cameron BM, et al. A computer model for the evaluation of the effect of corneal topography on optical performance. *Am J Ophthalmol* 1990;109:379–386.

34. Maguire LJ, Zabel RW, Parker P, et al. Topography and ray tracing analysis of patients with excellent visual acuity 3 months after excimer laser photorefractive keratectomy for myopia. *J Refract Corneal Surg* 1991;7:122–128.

35. Applegate RA, Howland HC, Buettner L et al. Changes in the aberration structure of the RK cornea from videokeratographic measurements. ARVO Abstracts. *Invest Ophthalmol Vis Sci* 1994; 35[4 Suppl]:1740(abstr).

36. Applegate RA, Howland HC. Refractive surgery, optical aberrations, and visual performance. *J Refract Corneal Surg* 1997; 13: 295–299.

37. Martinez CE, Applegate RA, Klyce SD, et al. Effect of pupillary dilation on corneal optical aberrations after photorefractive keratectomy. *Arch Ophthalmol* 1998;116:1053–1062.

38. Rabinowitz YS, McDonnell PJ. Computer assisted corneal topography in keratoconus. *J Refract Corneal Surg* 1989;5:400–408.

39. Maeda N, Klyce SD, Smolek MK. Comparison of methods for detecting keratoconus using videokeratography. *Arch Ophthalmol* 1995;113:870–874.

40. Maeda N, Klyce SD, Smolek MK, et al. Automated keratoconus screening with corneal topography analysis. *Invest Ophthalmol Vis Sci* 1994;35:2749–2757.

41. Maeda N, Klyce SD, Smolek MK. Neural network classification of corneal topography: preliminary demonstration. *Invest Ophthalmol Vis Sci* 1995;36:1327–1335.

42. Smolek MK, Klyce SD. Current keratoconus detection methods compared with a neural network approach. *Invest Ophthalmol Vis Sci* 1997;38:2290–2299.

43. Dingeldein SA, Klyce SD. The topography of normal corneas. *Arch Ophthalmol* 1989;107:512–518.

44. Wilson SE, Klyce SD. Quantitative descriptors of corneal topography: a clinical study. *Arch Ophthalmol* 1991;109: 349–353.

CLINICAL CONFOCAL MICROSCOPY

**H. DWIGHT CAVANAGH, PATRICK M. LADAGE,
W. MATTHEW PETROLL, AND JAMES V. JESTER**

BACKGROUND

The basic concept of confocal microscopy is derived from a clinical need to look into living tissues noninvasively in a more dynamic way than is provided by conventional light and ultrastructural microscopy. Fixation and mechanical sectioning of *ex vivo* specimens not only introduce artifacts in interpreting the function of living cells in tissues, but most important, make conventional microscopy a static technique. In 1955, Marvin Minsky (1) developed the concept of the first confocal microscope for studying neural networks in the living brain. The Minsky microscope condenser focused the light source within a small area of neural tissue with concomitant focusing of the microscope objective lens on exactly the same area. Because both condenser and objective lens had the same focal point, the microscope was termed *confocal*.

Since Minsky's original concept, the optical theory of confocal microscopy has been formally developed by Wilson and Sheppard (2) and Sheppard and Cogswell (3). In the two modern confocal microscopes in general clinical or research use for corneal imaging, either a *point* or *slit* (i.e., optically diffraction-limited) light source is focused onto a small volume in the living cornea, and a simultaneously placed confocal point (pinhole) or slit detector is used to collect the resulting signal. This optical alignment excludes or reduces the out-of-focus reflected signal from above and below the focal plane (volume) defined by the objective lens, which contributes to the detected image, and the overall result is a marked increase in both lateral (x, y) and axial (z) resolution as well as contrast. Because only one tiny volume element of the cornea is observed by each point or slit source detector (trading field of view for enhanced resolution), a usefully wide field of view of the cornea as a whole must be regained by rapid mechanical scanning. This is achieved by a synchronous movement of the illuminator and detector. Therefore, the *time* resolution of the microscope is defined by the speed at which the single x, y field at a given depth can be scanned and recorded. Most important, however, by varying the plane of focus of *both* source and detector in the cornea along the z axis, the cornea can be optically sectioned noninvasively, traveling without moving. This remarkable property produces a true paradigm shift in the ability to image normal and pathophysiologic processes *in situ* at magnifications sufficient to resolve cellular and subcellular interactions over time (four-dimensional *in vivo* microscopy: x, y, z, time).

Because of concerns over retinal toxicity, the light source used to achieve either point or slit illumination for clinical confocal microscopy is restricted to white light in both currently U.S. Food and Drug Administration (FDA)–approved ophthalmic instruments.

The first practical application of confocal optical theory to the eye was the development in 1974 of the specular microscope by David Maurice (4), who demonstrated enhanced resolution and contrast in both endothelial and *in situ* keratocyte images that were obtained by narrowing a slit beam, thus reducing the volume of scattered light reaching the final image, an optical result identical to diffraction-limited pinhole or slit (source/detector) confocal imaging. Maurice's approach led to the further refinement of a usable clinical specular microscope by Bourne et al. (5) and later by Koester (6), who used a scanning mirror system to move a slit over the tissue, rather than moving the object (the cornea) over the slit as Maurice had done. This basic design, still in widespread clinical practice in outpatient clinics and eye banking, provides a useful wide field view of the corneal endothelium *in situ*. Unfortunately, because specular microscopes use wide (500 μm) scanning slit detectors in place of a diffraction-limited pinhole (20 μm) or slit source illumination, and because the objective lens splits the light into two paths (incidence/detector), thus reducing by *half* the available effective numerical aperture (NA) of the objective lens (e.g., from 0.75 to 0.38), this approach provides much less lateral and axial resolution than a confocal microscope using an objective lens of the same NA.

Koester and colleagues (7) redesigned the objective lens to improve the optical sectioning ability of the contact-specular microscope, thus allowing images to be obtained from all three cellular layers of the cornea. The redesigned system has several severe limitations, however. In addition to decreased optical resolution and contrast, use of the wide scan (500 μm) increases signal-to-noise background problems, which do not permit video recording of images viewed at a 1/20 scan (30 Hz) in real time. Instead, only static images are obtained, using a xenon-arc 35-mm flash camera with film pushed to grain resolution to improve contrast (8). Thus, the study of dynamic vision microphysiology is difficult to achieve with this method, and the high light levels achieved by the flash are toxic to the retina so that central corneal imaging is not possible past the pupillary edge, even when the pupil is constricted by topical pilocarpine to facilitate examination. For those clinicians who prefer this approach, however, a specular/confocal microscope is commercially available from Mission Research Associates (Laguna Beach, CA).

The design of the objective lens for *in vivo* confocal microscopy is also a critical element in the clinical usefulness of individual instruments. First, the *z*-axis spatial resolutions (actual volume element visualized) under confocal conditions is determined by the NA (light-gathering ability) and magnification of the objective lens (similar to reflecting telescopes of larger aperture). However, commercially available, high–numerical-aperture lenses usually possess short working distances, which limit the depth of tissue penetration (i.e., optical sectioning) that can be obtained. To solve this problem, two practical design approaches have been used: (a) a *contact* objective lens with an applanating tip that touches a drop of fluid on the cornea (eliminates a back-reflection "hot spot" in the center of the image); and (b) a *noncontact* objective lens not directly optically coupled to the cornea. As will be seen in a later discussion of the strengths and weaknesses of currently commercially available instruments, each of these approaches has significant functional consequences.

Proper orientation of the cornea during confocal viewing is an additional critical element in obtaining flat-field *x, y* plane images in which accurate three-dimensional epithelial keratocyte or endothelial cell shapes, areas, and interactions can be verified. Alignment of the objective lens in any orientation other than directly perpendicular to the corneal surface results in an oblique optical section through the cornea, which produces distorted three-dimensional views that cannot be quantified in the *x, y, z* volume. Thus, achievement of both perpendicularity and a *zero z*-axis reference point that does not shift and that allows true three-dimensional viewing and quantitation requires an optically coupled dipping-cone objective lens tip with either a concave or flat-front surface and a convex posterior surface that is concentric with the axial focal point. Such lenses "applanate" by riding on a coupling fluid cushion, and touch (if any) occurs only at the lateral edges of the field.

DESIGN AND FUNCTION OF THE PINHOLE DISK AND SCANNING SLIT CLINICAL CONFOCAL MICROSCOPE

The Pinhole Disk Microscope

In 1968, Petran and coworkers (9) developed the first scanning confocal microscope consisting of a single white light source and a modified Nipkow disk containing thousands of optical conjugate (source–detector), 20-μm (diffraction-limited) pinholes arranged in Archimedean spirals to permit maximum packing of holes without "cross-talk" signal between them (one hole leaking light into another). Rotation of the disk results in even "scanning" of the cornea by the source pinholes, whereas the conjugate pinholes prevent light from outside the optical volume, determined by the objective lens and pinhole diameter, from reaching a photodetector. Petran's original tandem scanning design was adapted for viewing ocular structures *in vivo* in 1988 (10), and was originally commercially produced by Tandem Scanning Corporation (Reston, VA) (11). More recently, however, this microscope became commercially available from Advanced Scanning, Ltd. (New Orleans, LA). The optical light path for the tandem-scanning confocal microscope (TSCM) is shown in Fig. 10.1-1, and routine clinical use is illustrated in Fig. 10.1-2.

TSCMs in current clinical use are horizontally configured on a standard slit-lamp table for routine clinical use (Advanced Scanning, Ltd.) and use two specially designed dipping-cone objectives: 24×, 0.6 NA, 0- to 1.5-mm working distance, and 16× 0.40 NA, 0- to 8-mm working distance; each objective provides an *x, y* frame of 400 × 400 or 640 × 640 μm, respectively. For the tandem-scanning instrument, the position of the focal plane relative to the objective tip is varied by moving the lens within the

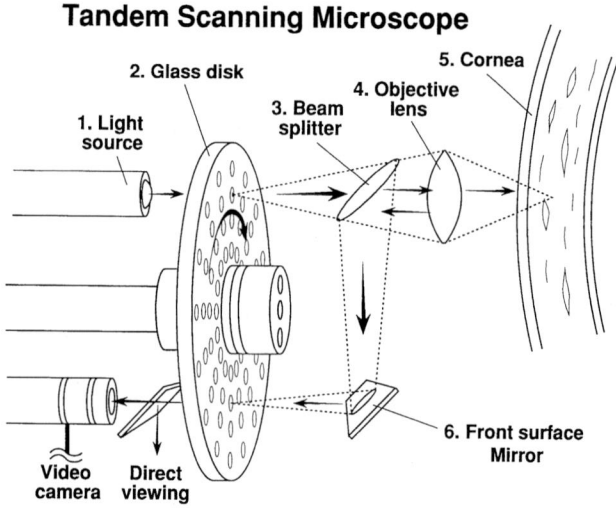

Tandem Scanning Microscope

FIG. 10.1-1. The optical sectioning light path of the tandem-scanning confocal microscope.

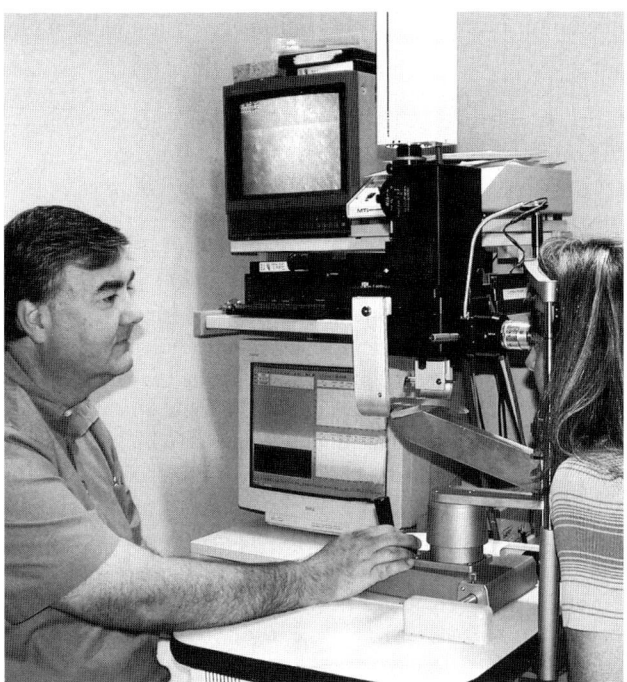

FIG. 10.1-2. Clinical examination with the tandem-scanning confocal microscope and video recording.

objective casing. Lens movement is controlled using an Oriel 18011 Encoder Mike Controller (Oriel Co., Stratford, CT) with a digital readout interfaced to a personal computer (PC) by a serial port. A program converts the encoder mike reading to the corresponding *z*-axis position (depth) to the focal plane in micrometers. This number is continuously updated and written into the user bit register of a time code generator (Fast Forward Model F30; Oriel

Co.) through an RS232 interface. The time code generator writes this number onto the audio track of a super VHS recording; the depth can also be displayed on the video monitor during recording or playback. Thus, the depth of the focal plane in the tissue can easily be calibrated, and accurate quantitative four-dimensional imaging is possible with this system (12) (Fig. 10.1-3). The glass disks contain 64,000 20- or 30-μm pinholes with total optical transmittances of 0.25% or 0.33%, respectively; disk rotation speed is 900 rotations per minute, which produces "streak-free" images. The light path is composed of prisms and mirrors with a stable and easily maintained alignment. The light source is a 100-W mercury lamp; the instrument is currently approved by the FDA for clinical use in examining the eye (11).

The axial response of the TSCM system was determined with the 0.6 NA, 24× objective and the 0.25% transmittance, 20-μm pinhole disk by focusing through a perfect planar reflector (mirror) and measuring the reflected intensity curve; this yields a *z*-axis resolution of 9 μm (13). Lateral *x, y* resolution *in vivo* ranges from 0.5 to 1 μm.

One important limitation in obtaining high-frame speeds with the TSCM is the dramatic loss of light reaching the tissue because Nipkow disks transmit only 0.25% to 1% of the available light. This loss of luminance limits the amount of light reflected from low-contrast structures in opaque tissue. Thus, a low–light-level camera is needed for image acquisition. An additional obstacle to *in vivo* imaging is that the field of view is often moving owing to pulse and respiration. Video frames generated while an object is in motion are often blurred, giving poor resolution of cellular detail. Single frames generated by low–light-level cameras also suffer from significant noise produced by the

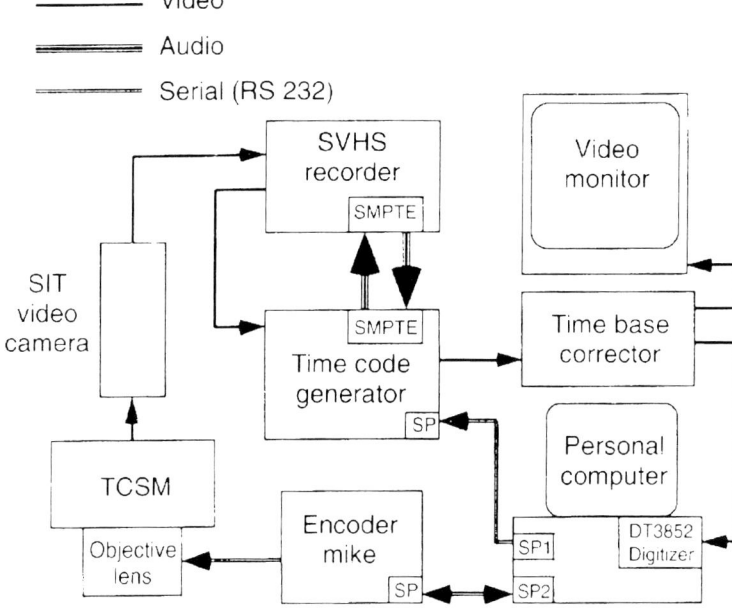

FIG. 10.1-3. Flow diagram of tandem-scanning confocal microscopy and image recording and analysis.

image intensifier. A standard technique for reducing the amount of random noise in a single image is to average several sequential frames. However, for image averaging to be successful, the sequential images must be perfectly registered, that is, there must be no positional changes between them. In many *in vivo* studies, there often is only a short pause between movements in which the frames are stationary and can be averaged successfully (12).

These problems have been addressed successfully through the development of a real-time digitizing system that allows the user to step through consecutive digitized frames easily and interactively to align and average sequential frames (to reduce noise) and to save the nonblurred, best-quality images. Current system design uses a Pentium PC platform with a high-speed peripheral computer interface (PCI) bus to digitize video signal sequences from either a DAGE-MTI VE camera (DAGE-MTI, Michigan City, IN) or a super VHS recorder (12) directly to the random access memory, with utilities for automatic registration, averaging, and shading correction of TSCM images. The

maximum number of sequential images is limited only by the amount of system random access memory on the PC.

This approach has allowed the development of a powerful new technique called *confocal microscopy through-focusing* (CMTF) (14,15). CMTF is the operation of rapidly moving the focal plane of the objective lens through the entire cornea at a high constant speed (5 to 8 seconds) while equally spaced *x, y* images at the focal plane are digitized, resulting in a stack of 400 to 500 two-dimensional images from which a *z*-axis intensity profile is generated by calculating the average pixel intensity in a central region of each image and plotting versus *z*-depth. This approach takes advantage of the mechanical advance mechanism for the internal lens elements, which can be set by the Oriel encoder to a specific speed to facilitate fast or slow focusing through the tissue. While advancing the internal lens elements and simultaneously video recording the images, the axial distance between consecutive video frames can be calculated based on the lens advance speed. For the current system, a lens advance speed of 80 μm/sec

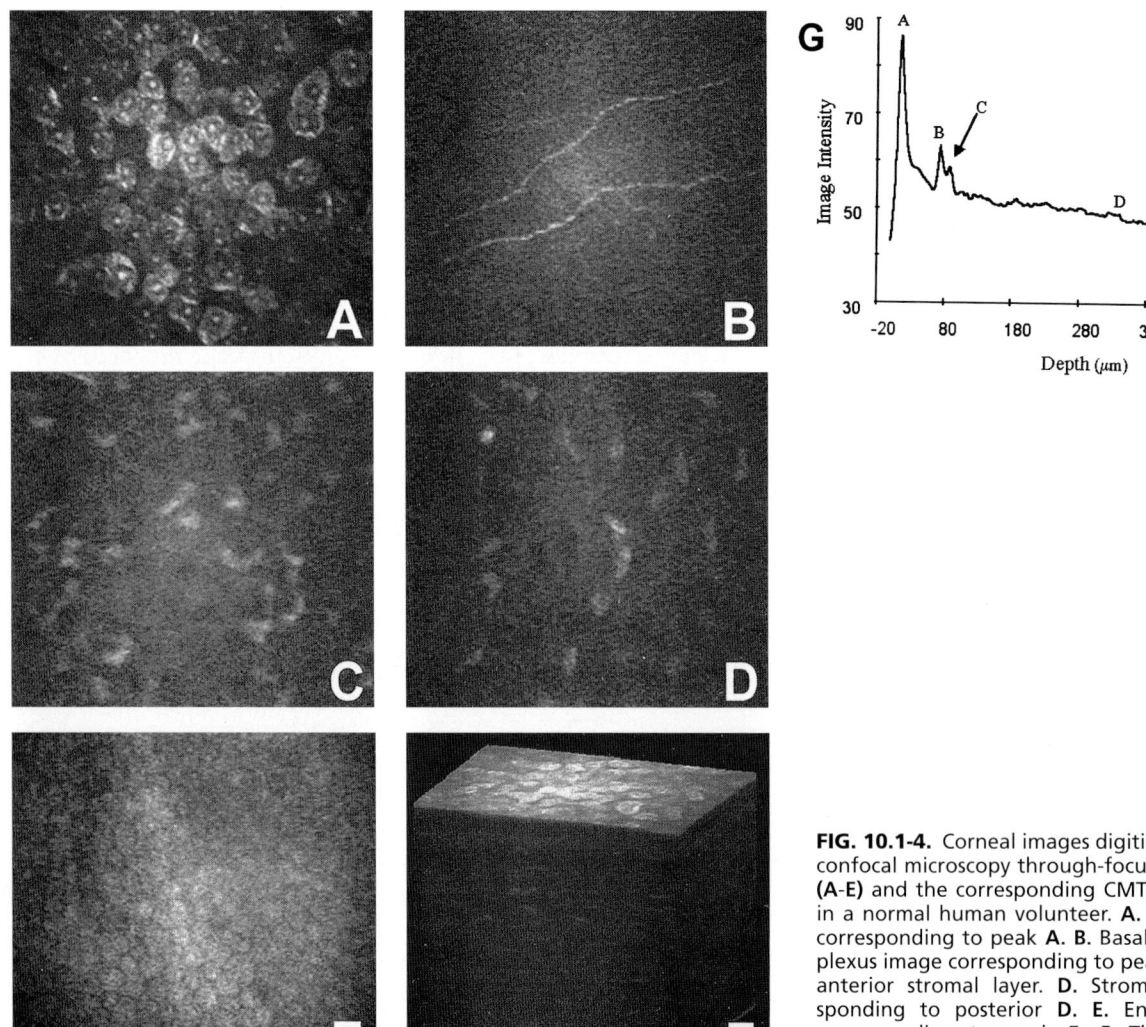

FIG. 10.1-4. Corneal images digitized directly from confocal microscopy through-focusing (CMTF) scan (**A-E**) and the corresponding CMTF intensity curve in a normal human volunteer. **A.** Epithelial image corresponding to peak **A. B.** Basal-epithelial nerve plexus image corresponding to peak **B. C.** Image of anterior stromal layer. **D.** Stromal image corresponding to posterior **D. E.** Endothelial image corresponding to peak **E. F.** Three-dimensional reconstruction. **G.** CMTF intensity curve.

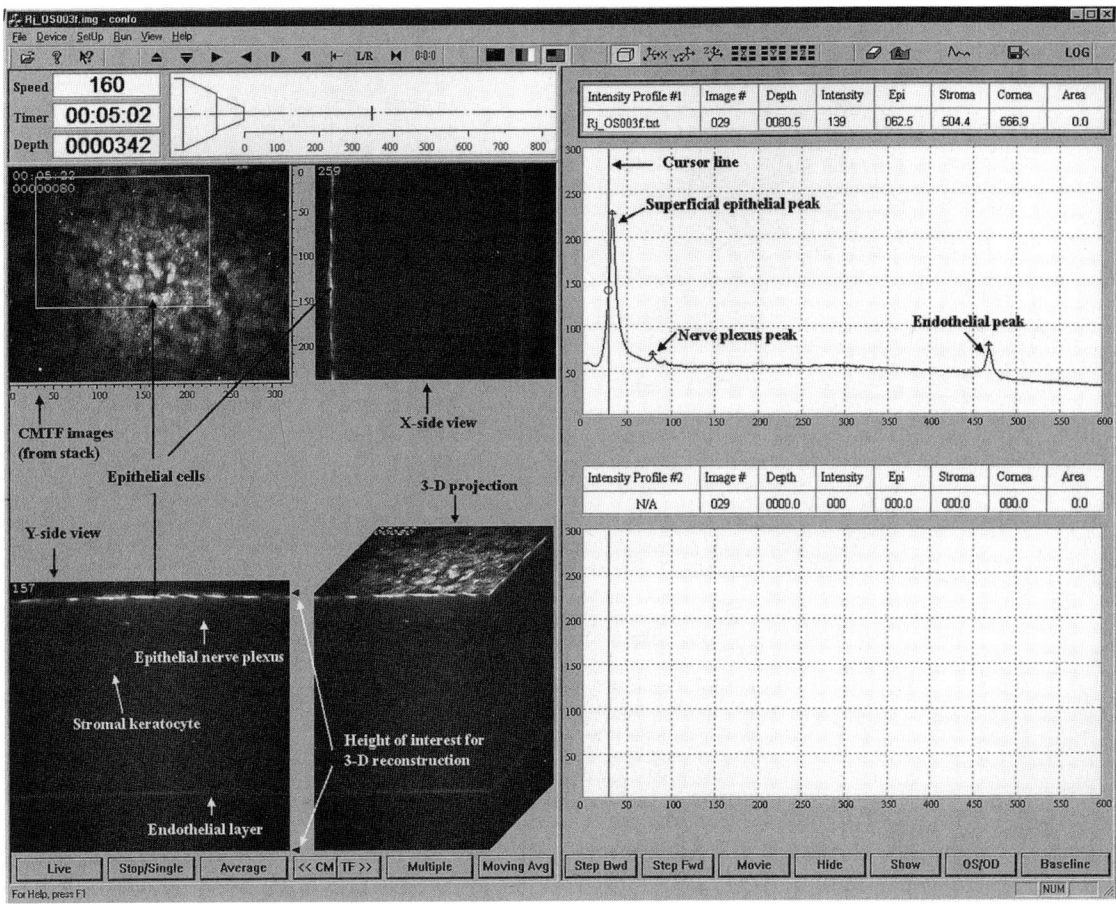

FIG. 10.1-5. On-line confocal microscopy through-focusing scan and data processing of a normal human cornea *in vivo*. The measured epithelial thickness, stromal thickness, and corneal thicknesses were 62.5, 504.4, and 599.0 μm, respectively; three-dimensional reconstruction is performed interactively on line.

translates to an axial distance of -1.06 μm between consecutive images. Using this approach, approximately 400 to 500 images or 15 seconds are required to focus through and capture the entire corneal thickness. This speed can be increased to 160 μm/sec without loss of axial resolution owing to the interlacing of video lines from the DAGE/MTI camera, albeit at the expense of horizontal resolution. At this higher speed, recording of the entire cornea takes only approximately 8 seconds, whereas the corneal epithelium can be captured in less than 1 second, substantially reducing the risk of axial drift interfering with thickness measurements. Furthermore, multiple scans through the cornea, or just the corneal epithelium, can be performed rapidly and easily for a more accurate measurement of tissue thickness.

Digitizing the through-focus scan and reconstructing the cornea three-dimensionally using a volume/surface projection generated from the ANALYZE software program (Mayo Medical Ventures, Rochester, MN) produces a cross-sectional (*x, y*) view of the living cornea that appears similar to that of histologic sections (Figs. 10.1-4 and 10.1-5). Fur-

thermore, the relative thickness of the corneal epithelial sheet and stroma as defined by the respective separation between the superficial epithelium (Epi) and basal lamina (BL) and the basal lamina and endothelium (Endo) appears equivalent to that observed histologically. Although thickness measurements from the surface projection are possible, an axial, light-scattering profile can be calculated by measuring the average pixel intensity of each image comprising the through-focus scan and plotting as a function of axial depth (Figs. 10.1-4 and 10.1-5). This representation identifies the major sublayer corneal structures that backscatter or reflect light as peaks in the depth–intensity profile. Interestingly, tissue interfaces between cells and matrix (epithelium and stroma) or tissues and fluid (tears or anterior chamber aqueous), where there are changes in the refractive index, appear to be the major source of backscatter.

Using the two-dimensional depth–intensity profile, tissue or sublayer thickness can be measured objectively, without operator bias, by measuring the distance between the intensity peaks. For the cornea, the corneal thickness

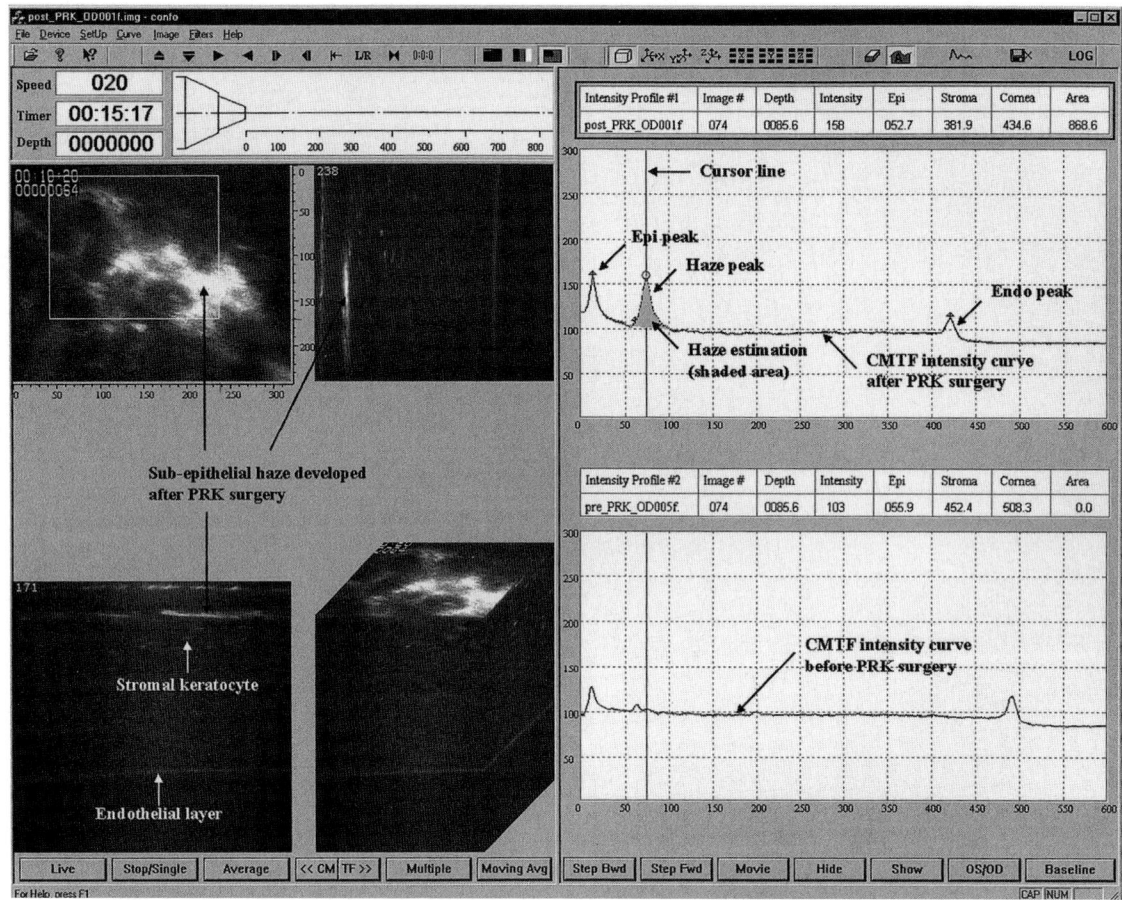

FIG. 10.1-6. Confocal microscopy through-focusing (CMTF) image acquisition and data analysis of a patient who had undergone photorefractive keratectomy (PRK), 1 month postsurgery. The CMTF intensity of the same cornea before surgery is shown for comparison. The measured epithelial thickness, stromal thickness, and corneal thickness were 53.9, 380.7, and 434.6 μm, respectively. The PRK-induced stromal thinning was 7.17 μm and the total thinning was 73.7 μm. The three-dimensional display shows subepithelial haze. The graphically shaded area on the CMTF curve was used to quantify a haze value of 934.8 units/μm² intensity).

(CT), epithelial thickness (ET), and stromal thickness (ST) can be calculated using the following equations:

$$CT = Z_{endo} - Z_{epi}$$
$$ET = Z_{bl} - Z_{epi}$$
$$ST = Z_{endo} - Z_{bl}$$

where Z_{epi}, Z_{bl}, and Z_{endo} are the axial depths of the intensity peaks for the superficial epithelium, basal lamina, and endothelium, respectively. For the corneal epithelium, the standard deviation of repeat scans ranges from 1.3 to 3.1, with a coefficient of variation of 2.5%, suggesting that CMTF is reproducible and accurate. For human patients, similar accuracy and repeatability have been reported, and intracorneal structures as small as 16 μm (Bowman's membrane) have been measured reproducibly.

In addition to measuring sublayer thickness, CMTF analysis also provides a simple and quantitative method of studying tissue responses in four dimensions (14–16). This has been demonstrated in studies of corneal wound healing after excimer laser keratorefractive surgery [laser *in situ* keratomileusis

(LASIK)] in which a portion of the anterior cornea is photoablated, changing the central corneal curvature (15). Using CMTF image data sets, the same cornea can be reconstructed three-dimensionally at various times before and after surgery (Fig. 10.1-6). By comparing the images from one time point to another, the immediate loss of corneal tissue can be quantified and the effects of laser ablation and later healing responses can be assessed. These three-dimensional images can then be represented as a pixel-intensity–depth profile and measurements of LASIK flap thickness, tissue loss, or regrowth determined, as well as other corneal responses quantified. Finally, CMTF profiles can also be used to estimate the amount of backscattering of light from the tissue. If the camera gain, Kilovolt setting (Kv), and the black level are set to constant levels, then the amount of light detected by the camera is principally related to changes in the reflectivity or backscattering of light by the tissue. Light backscattering can then be estimated by integrating the area under each peak or the entire curve; the unit of measurement (U) is defined as microns × pixel in-

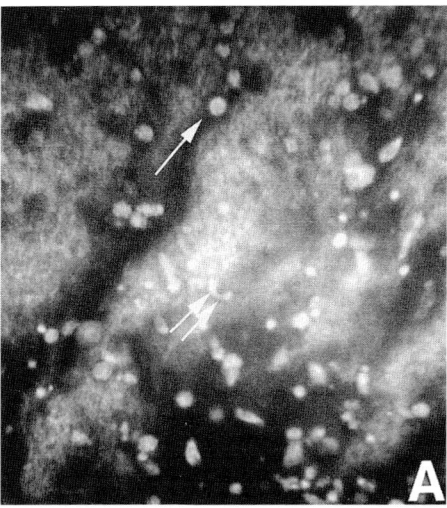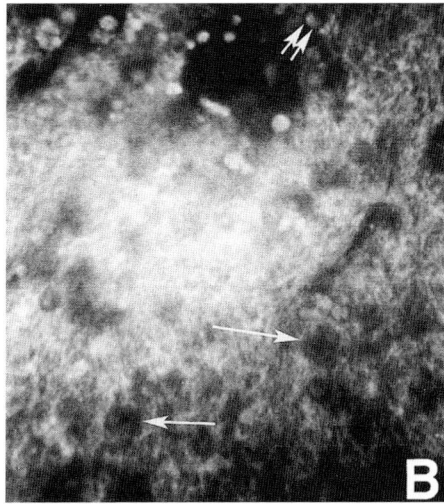

FIG. 10.1-7. Intracorneal tandem-scanning confocal microscopy imaging of *Acanthamoeba castellanii* in situ. **A.** *Single arrows* indicate cysts and *double arrows* show trophozoites. **B.** Deeper (subepithelial) image than in **A,** but note typical "honeycomb" cavities cleared by the protozoan parasite.

tensity. Using this method, a close correlation between the loss of corneal transparency, as measured by the clinical examination of the cornea, and the CMTF estimate of light backscattering can be shown (Fig. 10.1-6). Furthermore, integration of the CMTF intensity peak can also be used to evaluate ocular irrigation and to provide an objective, quantitative measure of the corneal response to injury, including inflammation, fibrosis, and repair. Although the pixel intensity values do not by themselves indicate any specific response, values can be correlated directly to actual images taken during scanning to identify unique pathologic processes underlying the elevated intensities. Integration of intensity values over a region of the cornea (i.e., stroma) then allows objective quantitative measurement of the area and depth of response occurring in the same tissue.

Currently, perhaps the most valuable clinical use of TSCM-CMTF is for the accurate and rapid diagnosis of *Acanthamoeba* corneal infections. Noninvasive, *in situ* TSCM-CMTF imaging permits quantitative counts and localization of both parasitic cysts and trophozoites in the living eye (11), and can be used for subsequent monitoring of the efficacy of medical treatment. Figure 10.1-7 shows the typical appearance of the intracorneal *Acanthamoeba castellanii* trophozoites and cysts (30 μm). Cysts appear as bright "headlights" and demonstrate a characteristic "double-wall" appearance. The invasive trophozoites often seem to follow along and attack basal epithelial plexus or anterior stromal nerves, which may explain the severe pain of most patients. Over time, the amoebae seem to "hollow out" a series of smaller cystic cavities which can become confluent and appear empty after successful therapeutic medication, and which resemble the results of termite activity inside solid wood. The three-dimensional nature (depth, width) of the infection can thus be determined and used to guide therapy and subsequent potential penetrating keratoplasty to guarantee

removal of all infected tissue if needed for visual restoration. Similarly, other eye infections, including microsporidium, fungal keratitis, or bacterial keratitis, can often be confirmed by TSCM-CMTF (11).

The ability to visualize cellular details of the cornea quantitatively *in vivo* also finds an increasingly important application in corneal research. Two classic examples of this are illustrated in Figs. 10.1-8 and 10.1-9.

Figure 10.1-8 demonstrates *in vivo* CMTF stromal images of control mice and transgenically altered littermates overexpressing transforming growth factor-β, which is known to control differentiation of normal keratocytes (optically transparent) into a myofibroblastic phenotype seen after virtually any form of corneal wounding that produces a decrease in corneal transparency (17). Figure 10.1-9 shows the result of such a transcorneal freeze injury to a rabbit, showing conversion of transparent normal keratocytes, which have been shown to contain high cytoplasmic concentrations of two novel crystallins [aldehyde dehydrogenase class 1 (ALDH1) and transketolase (TKT); 25% to 35% of total soluble cell protein] and activated keratocytes (fibroblasts and myofibroblasts), which express fewer crystallins associated with increased backscattered light (haze). Taken together, these findings suggest a *cellular* basis of corneal transparency as well as the classic structural basis arising from the extracellular matrix organization of collagen fibrils (matrix transparency).

Variable-Slit Scanning Confocal Microscopy

In 1994, use of a variable-slit, real-time, noncontact scanning confocal microscope (SSCM) was described in detail by Masters and Thaer (18). This system has evolved through several redesigns and is commercially available

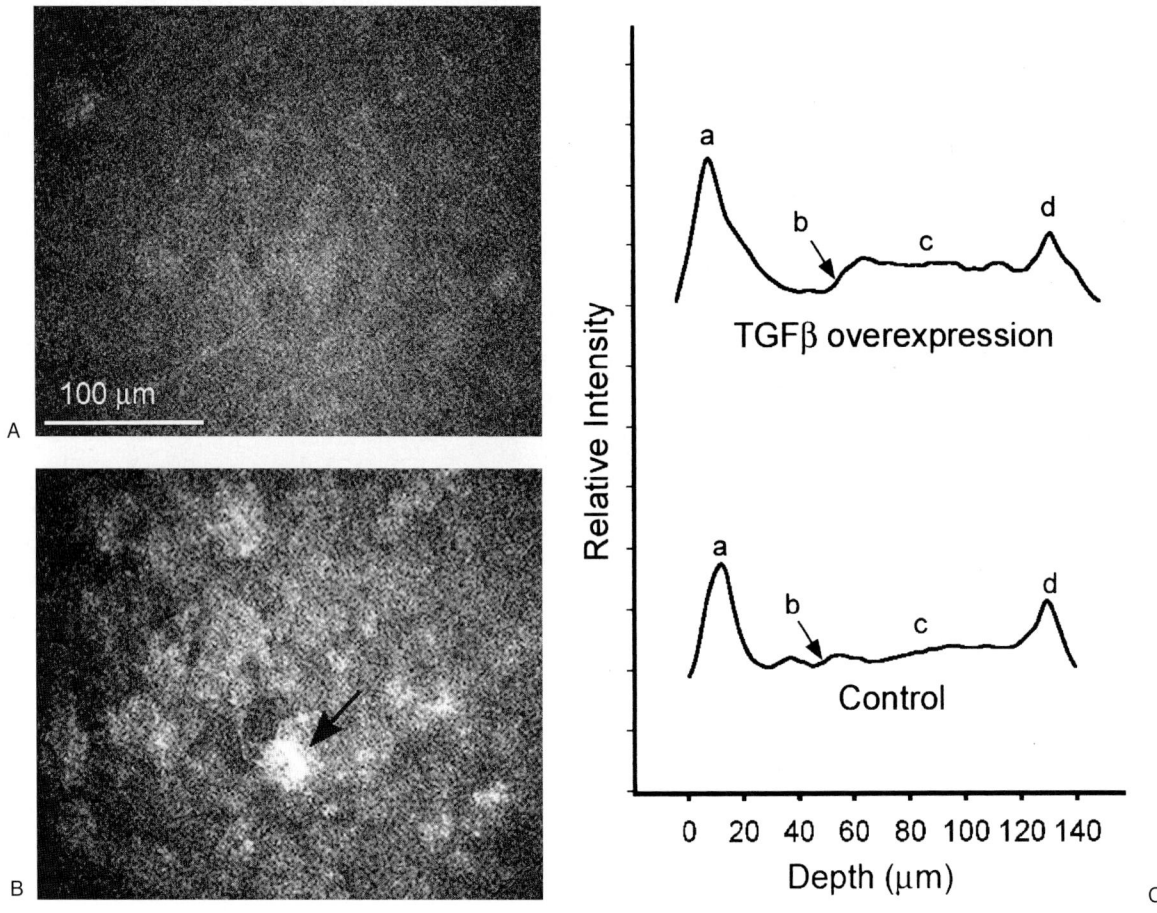

FIG. 10.1-8. *In vivo* confocal microscopy through-focusing (CMTF) stromal images **(A, B)** and CMTF profiles **(A′, B′)** of control mice and transforming growth factor-β–overexpressing mice **(B, B′)**. Note that stromal reflectivity is greatly increased in the transgenic mice **(B′, region C)**, which correlates with the prominent appearance of stromal keratocytes **(B, arrow)**. The pixel intensity curves have been offset in the corneal epithelial peak for demonstration.

from Nidek, USA (Fremont, CA) as the Confoscan. Mounted on a slit-lamp stand and using a 12-V halogen lamp for noncoherent illumination, the instrument can be used clinically in conjunction with a silicon-intensified target (SIT) or charge-coupled device (CCD) video camera to examine the living eye.

The optical design of this instrument is similar to the scanning double-sided mirror used in a real-time laser scanning slit confocal microscope previously developed by Brakenhoff and Visscher (19). In this design, two independently adjustable slits are located in conjugate optical planes; a rapidly oscillating two-sided mirror is used to scan the image of the slit over the plane of the cornea to produce optical sectioning in real time.

There are two apparent significant advantages inherent in the scanning slit design: (a) by continually adjusting the slit and hence depth of focus in the *z*-axis, the signal-to-noise ratio can be maximized, ensuring optical image contrast for increasing tissue depths of optical sectioning; and (b) the use of a slit provides for higher signal and, when

used with high-NA objective lenses, the constantly maintained confocality of the adjustable slits produces single video frames of high image clarity. There are also three drawbacks to the microscope as currently available: (a) the cost is high compared with the Nipkow, disk-based instruments; (b) it is not possible to achieve *z*-axis quantification with currently used standard objective lenses; and (c) despite production of a "clear image" for each video frame, the problem of potential geometric distortion induced by eye movement within the image scan times is unresolved. In the intensified DAGE/MIT VE 1-SIT camera used with TSCM at video rates, motion often induces blur in some *x, y* images through persistence of signal in the video camera phototube from frame to frame. Even when the SSCM slits are synchronously coupled to the camera (CCD or SIT) chip, and every second video frame generated (1/15 second) is "clear," eye movement, which is more rapid (1/30 second), induces geometric distortion in the acquired image (e.g., circles may become ellipses). Because this distortion occurs in three dimensions, the problem is compounded. In

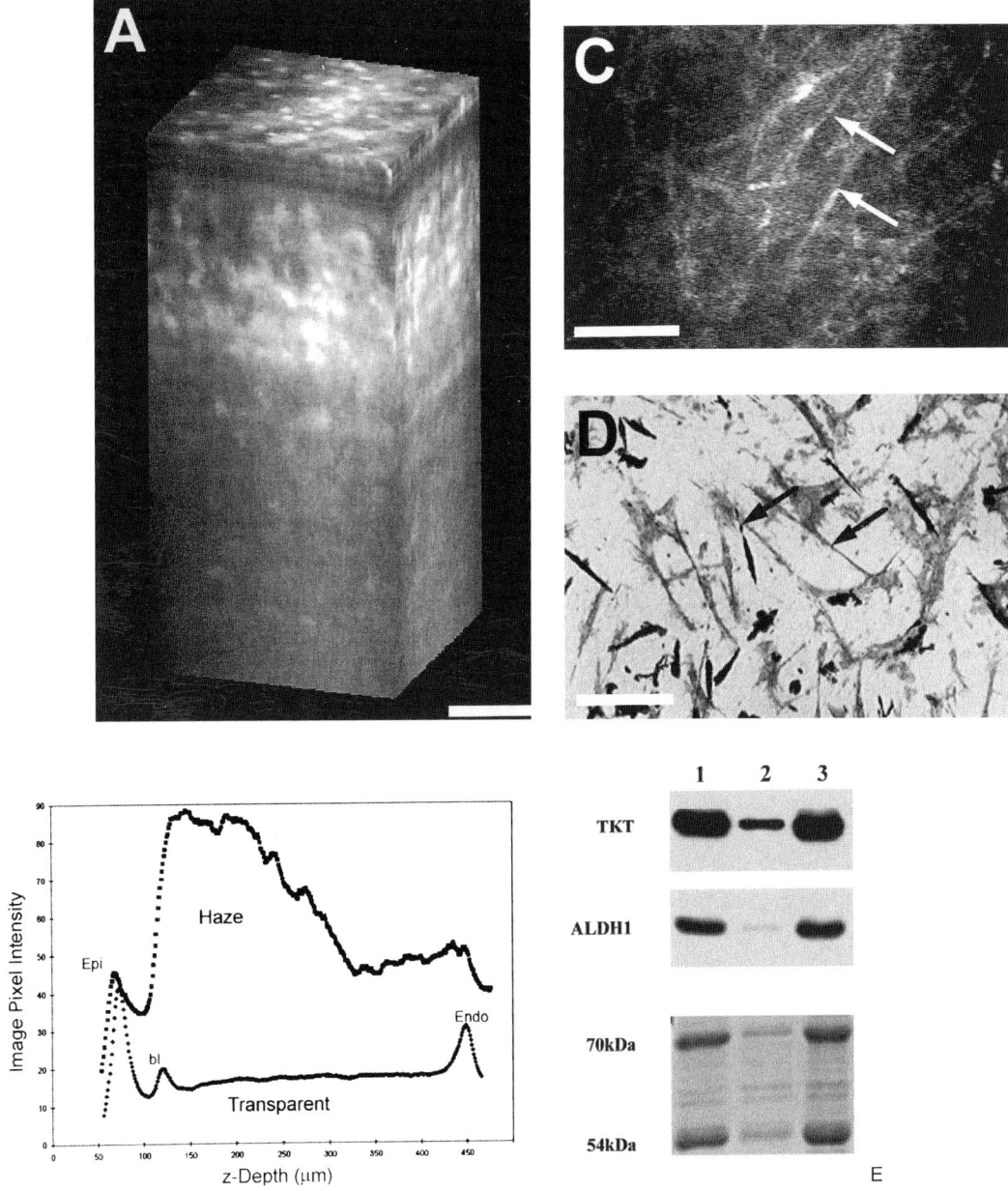

FIG. 10.1-9. Transcorneal freeze injury in the rabbit. **A.** Three-dimensional display of the living cornea 14 days after injury showing greatly enhanced scattering of light from the anterior cornea. **B.** Image intensity depth profile from cornea shown in **A** in region of freeze injury (haze) compared with transparent cornea (transparent) adjacent to the freeze injury in the same cornea (curves have been offset along the *y*-axis the better to demonstrate differences). Note the presence at baseline of peak intensities localized to the epithelial surface (Epi), basal lamina (bl), and endothelium (Endo). **C.** Two-dimensional *in vivo* confocal microscopy (CM) image taken from the three-dimensional stack shown in **A**. Note that the backscattering of light shown in **A** is from the highly reflective spindle-shaped structures. **D.** Light micrograph of gold chloride–stained tissue showing that migrating keratocytes assume a spindle-shaped morphology similar to that detected by *in vivo* CM and shown in **C**. **E.** Sodium dodecyl sulfate–polyacrylamide gel electrophoresis (SDS-PAGE) and immunoblots of water-soluble proteins extracted from keratocytes isolated from normal rabbit cornea (lane 1), wound cornea (lane 2), and the corneal rim adjacent to the wounded cornea (lane 3). Note the marked reduction in the ~70-kD and 54-kD proteins in the injured keratocytes (lane 2) and the decreased staining with antibodies to transketolase (TKT) and aldehyde dehydrogenase class 1 (ALDH1), whereas there is no change in the staining of keratocytes isolated from the adjacent corneal rim (lane 3). Bars = 100 μm.

this situation, when the presence and limits of movement cannot be visualized by eliminating blur sequences, clear images alone are insufficient to validate the actual quantitation localization of all image points observed in the four-dimensional space (x, y, z, time) recorded. Finally, it is important to realize that replacement of the point detector in a pinhole system with a slit always results in lower z-axis resolution (approximately 15 μm for the Nidek system vs. 9 μm for a TSCM).

The only layer of the cornea that can be examined noninvasively, *in vivo* by SSCM and not imaged routinely by TSCM is the epithelial wing cell layer (18). If imaging of this structure is critical for the research or clinical questions to be answered, the increased costs of an SSCM and lack of z-axis quantification could be justified. Currently available Nipkow disk–based TSCMs, however, provide quantitative routine clinical four-dimensional imaging in real time at generally less expense for all other routine clinical applications.

Currently, the manufacturer is in the process of remedying the unfortunate impossibility for the "noncontact" design to generate equally spaced x, y plane images that will allow a quantitative three-dimensional image of the cornea *in situ*. Owing to the lack of a suitable, fixed "zero" point on the z-axis in SSCM systems, which is the signal feature of the applanating-tip TSCM-CMTF systems, sublayer structures cannot be located accurately, such as the depth of a post-LASIK flap or a quantitative assessment of keratocyte numbers by corneal depth, other than by measuring cell numbers "somewhere" in the "anterior," "middle," and "posterior" stroma (20), as can be done using TSCM-CMTF (21). An optional add-on device that allows fluid coupling of the objective tip with the cornea is under development by the manufacturer, and may soon be available for trial clinical use. Thus, the prospective user who requires accurate three-dimensional numbers from confocal microscopy as well as crisp images for diagnostic use should monitor future SSCM developments carefully and compare their results with the TSCM-CMTF design.

CONCLUSIONS

Confocal microscopy is becoming an indispensable tool in clinical assessment of the cornea and for an ever-widening area of applications in research. *In vivo* TSCM or SSCM is particularly useful in the diagnosis of infectious keratitis and has important applications in future natural history studies of corneal dystrophies in both humans and genetically altered animals. TSCM-CMTF (and perhaps modified SSCM in the future) is uniquely valuable in the quantitative assessment of epithelial, flap, stromal, and total corneal thicknesses in the postsurgical cornea after photorefractive keratectomy or LASIK

procedures. Both TSCM-CMTF and SSCM, however, provide higher magnification and better spatial resolution in the cornea than current comparable, parallel-imaging technologies such as high-frequency digital ultrasonography or optical coherence tomography. With *in vivo* confocal microscopy, we have the ability to go where no one has gone before, and to image dynamic living processes in the cornea and other tissues that no one has been able to see. Thus, the future for this technology is truly immense.

ACKNOWLEDGMENTS

Supported in part by an unrestricted research grant from Research to Prevent Blindness, Inc., New York, New York.

None of the authors has any proprietary interest in the technology discussed.

REFERENCES

1. Minksy M. Memoir on inventing the confocal scanning microscope. *J Scanning* 1988;10:128–138.
2. Wilson T, Sheppard C. *Theory and practice of scanning optical microscopy.* London: Academic Press, 1984.
3. Sheppard CJR, Cogswell CJ. Optimization of the confocal microscopy system. *Trans R Microsc Soc* 1990;1:231–234.
4. Maurice DM. A scanning slit optical microscopy. *Invest Ophthalmol* 1974;13:1033–1037.
5. Bourne WM, McCarey BE, Kaufman HE. Clinical specular microscopy. *Trans Am Acad Ophthalmol Otolaryngol* 1976;81:743–753.
6. Koester CJ. Scanning mirror microscope with optical sectioning characteristics: applications in ophthalmology. *Appl Optics* 19890;19:1749–1757.
7. Koester CJ, Auran JD, Rosskother HD, et al. Clinical microscopy of the cornea using optical sectioning and a high numerical aperture objective. *J Opt Soc Am* 1993;10:1670–1679.
8. Koester CJ, Auran JD, Rapaport R, et al. Confocal scanning slit microscopy of normal human corneal basal epithelium centripetal slide and presumed Langerhans cell movement. ARVO Abstracts. *Invest Ophthalmol Vis Sci* 1993;34[4 Suppl]:1014(abstr).
9. Petran M, Hadravsky M, Egger MD, et al. Tandem-scanning reflected-light microscope. *J Opt Soc Am* 1968;58:661–664.
10. Cavanagh HD, Jester JV, Essepian J, et al. Confocal microscopy of the living eye. *CLAO J* 1990;16:65–73.
11. Cavanagh HD, Petroll WM, Alizadeh H, et al. Clinical and diagnostic use of in vivo confocal microscopy in patients with corneal disease. *Ophthalmology* 1993;100:1444–1454.
12. Petroll WM, Jester JV, Cavanagh HD. In vivo confocal imaging. *Int Rev Exp Pathol* 1996;36:93–129.
13. Petroll WM, Cavanagh HD, Jester JV. Three-dimensional imaging of corneal cells using in vivo confocal microscopy. *J Microsc* 1993;170:213–219.
14. Li HF, Petroll WM, Moller-Pedersen T, et al. Epithelial and corneal thickness measurements by in vivo confocal microscopy through focusing (CMTF). *Curr Eye Res* 1997;16:214–221.
15. Li J, Jester JV, Cavanagh HD, et al. On-line 3-dimensional confocal imaging in vivo. *Invest Ophthalmol Vis Sci* 2000;41:2945–2953.

16. Cavanagh HD, Petroll WM, Jester JV. Confocal microscopy: uses in measurement of cellular structure and function. *Prog Retinal Eye Res* 1995;14:527–565.
17. Jester JV, Lee YG, Li J, et al. Measurement of corneal sublayer thickness and transparency in transgenic mice with altered corneal clarity using in vivo confocal microscopy. *Vision Res* 2001;41:1283–1290.
18. Masters BR, Thaer AA. Real-time scanning slit confocal microscopy of the in vivo human cornea. *Appl Optics* 1994;33:695–701.
19. Brakenhoff GJ, Visscher K. Confocal imaging with bilateral scanning and away detectors. *J Microsc* 1992;165:139–146.
20. Mustonen RK, McDonald MB, Srivannaboon S, et al. Normal human cell populations evaluated by in vivo scanning slit confocal microscopy. *Cornea* 1998;17:485–492.
21. Patel SV, McLaren JW, Camp JJ, et al. Automated quantification of keratocyte density by using confocal microscopy in vivo. *Invest Ophthalmol Vis Sci* 1999;40;320–326.

CLINICAL SPECULAR MICROSCOPY

**H. DWIGHT CAVANAGH, PATRICK M. LADAGE,
W. MATTHEW PETROLL, AND JAMES V. JESTER**

BACKGROUND

The corneal endothelium plays a critical role in the maintenance of overall corneal transparency essential for normal visual function. Transparency is regulated, in part, by modulation of stromal water content, counterbalancing a steady inward "leak" of water and nutrients from the anterior chamber, which is driven both by intraocular pressure exogenously and by an endogenous stromal swelling pressure. The apical junctions between endothelial cells are "leaky," and water is "pumped" out of the stroma by a number of ion-specific independent pumps (H^+, Na^+/K^+, HCO_3^-) located around the circumference of each cell in the endothelial monolayer. Unfortunately, corneal endothelial cells in the adult human become growth downregulated and do not regenerate if damaged by eye surgery, external chemical or blunt trauma, or internal inflammatory diseases.

The noncontact specular microscope is a widely available clinical instrument that is ubiquitously used to evaluate the corneal endothelium of both the normal and diseased or injured cornea *in vivo*, or in *ex vivo* assessment of tissue viability for corneal transplantation in eye banking (Fig. 10.2-1). As is discussed in more detail in Chapter 10.1, the optical principles of specular microscopy represent a special case of general confocal microscopy, which may ultimately replace the specular microscope in general clinical use.

STRENGTHS AND LIMITATIONS OF CLINICAL SPECULAR MICROSCOPY

David Maurice (1) developed the first specular microscope in 1974 to visualize the corneal endothelium at high magnification and *x, y* plane resolution. This was successful because of two "tricks": (a) When the angle of the light passing into the cornea was placed exactly at the same angle as the observer's view (angle of incidence equals angle of reflection), all other backscattered light is out of phase and hence "not seen," producing an excellent view of the endothelial monolayer; and (b) endothelial cells are thin (3 to 6 μm), and thus focus on the apex of the cells provides an image of a flat *x, y* sheet of cells. If there are protuberances that prolapse individual cells or groups of cells forward (i.e., toward the aqueous), these are seen as black areas that represent no backscattering of light from the normal cell sheet focal plane. Such protuberances occur in Fuchs' endothelial corneal dystrophy as "warts" or guttata on the underlying basal limiting membrane (Descemet's), pushing forward the apex of endothelial cells, which are then out of focus and appear black on specular micrographs. Scattered areas of endothelial cell damage and cell swelling that may occur in the excision of scleral rim–corneal tissue in eye banking also are imaged as out-of-focus or black areas.

Unfortunately, there are important limitations of specular microscopy in providing useful clinical information. To obtain clear images, the overlying cornea must be transparent (i.e., no corneal edema, Descemet's folds, and the like) and the endothelial apical surface must be smooth and uniform. The second major disadvantage is that specular microscopy does not permit three-dimensional optical sectioning of the cornea; viewing is restricted to a thin, single-cell plane. Thus, views of the corneal epithelial surface obtained with specular microscopy show light and dark cells with overlapping borders, making quantitative assessment of surface cell areas or number infeasible, even when a contact lens is used to flatten the corneal surface. By contrast, as discussed in Chapter 10.1, confocal microscopy easily overcomes both of these limitations.

Despite these problems, noncontact specular microscopy is a low-cost technology that can provide a useful assessment of the corneal endothelium *in vivo* in many cases, and remains in widespread use in most clinics and eye banks (2).

IN VIVO SPECULAR MICROSCOPY

The most common use of clinical specular microscopy is for assessing the number of endothelial cells per square millimeter

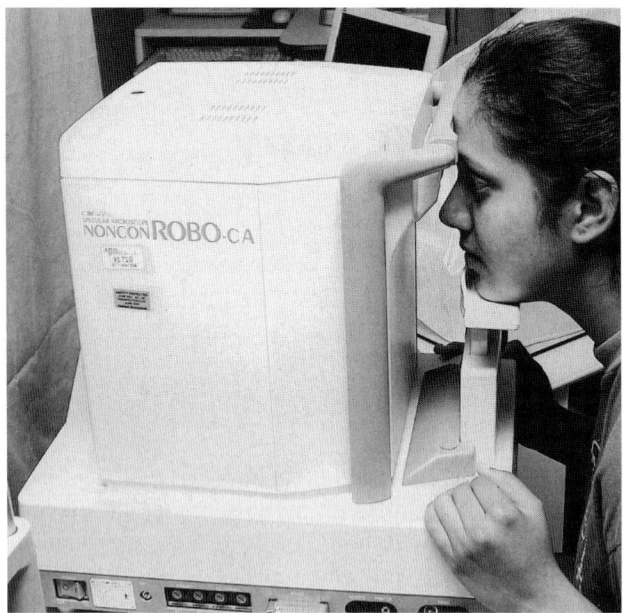

FIG. 10.2-1. Noncontact clinical specular microscopy.

in the central or peripheral cornea in patients being considered for cataract surgery. There are a wide variety of computer-assisted software approaches that provide automated morphometric analyses. In addition to cell number, the percentage of "normal" six-sided or hexagonal cells can also be determined. The latter measurement is believed to reflect endothelial health because the hexagon represents the lowest thermodynamic energy level for "tiling" a single cell layer on a flat surface (*x, y* plane), as is the corresponding dodecahedron for three-dimensional volumes. It is believed

that sharp deviations from hexagonality, such as those seen in long-standing diabetes mellitus (type 1 or 2), represent an abnormal state. As cell numbers decrease normally with age, or become more pleomorphic in shape, the "pump–leak" ratio may be altered unfavorably, allowing water accumulation first in the corneal stroma and then later in the epithelium, which collectively decreases corneal transparency. Typically, when a visually significant cataract is seen with the concomitant finding of central corneal guttata or an otherwise low endothelial cell count produced by long-standing glaucoma, past trauma, or endogenous inflammation, a decision must be made as to whether the corneal endothelium has enough healthy cells (pump function) to withstand the inevitable cell loss induced by cataract surgery without loss of preoperative transparency. Resolution of this dilemma is illustrated in Fig. 10.2-2, which shows specular micrographs of the left (Fig. 10.2-2A) and right (Fig. 10.2-2B) eyes of a 62-year-old white woman with central endothelial guttata visible on slit-lamp biomicroscopy. As can be seen, although the overlying cornea is clear, the endothelium in each eye demonstrates low cell counts as well as wide black areas that represent out-of-focus changes typical of advanced Fuchs' endothelial dystrophy.

Although there is continuing controversy among clinicians over the lowest number of viable endothelial cells acceptable for cataract extraction alone versus simultaneous corneal transplantation combined with cataract removal, most surgeons would agree that the values and clinical findings demonstrated in Fig. 10.2-2 require the combined surgical approach. Thus, in these cases, where the overlying cornea is not yet edematous, specular microscopy can provide data of great clinical value.

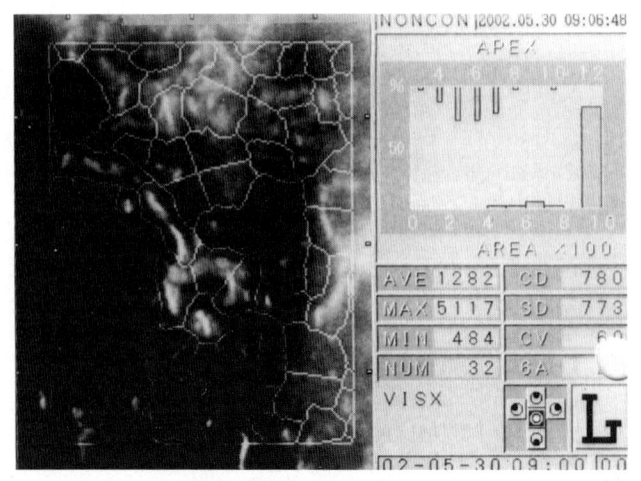
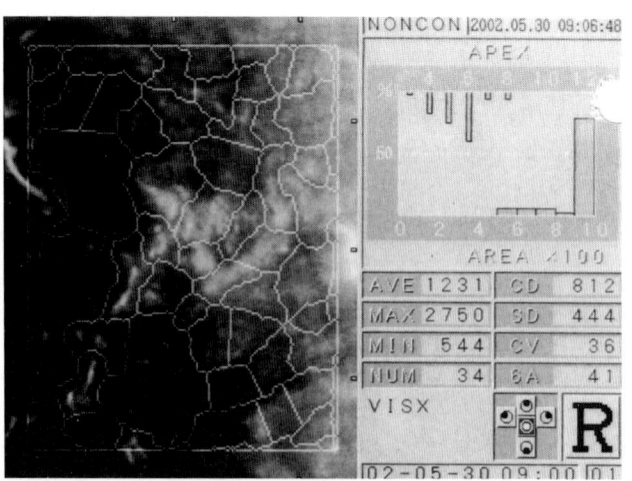

FIG. 10.2-2. Left eye (L) **(A)** and right eye (R) **(B)** central specular images of the corneal endothelium in a 62-year-old white woman (best corrected vision 20/70 R; 20/100 L) being assessed for removal of visually significant cataracts with concomitant intraocular lens implantation. On slit-lamp examination, the patient shows extensive central guttata characteristic of Fuchs' endothelial dystrophy (not shown). Both corneas are transparent. Note the extensive areas of dystrophy (black) and the marked pleomorphism of the remaining cells. Viable cell counts are clearly depressed.

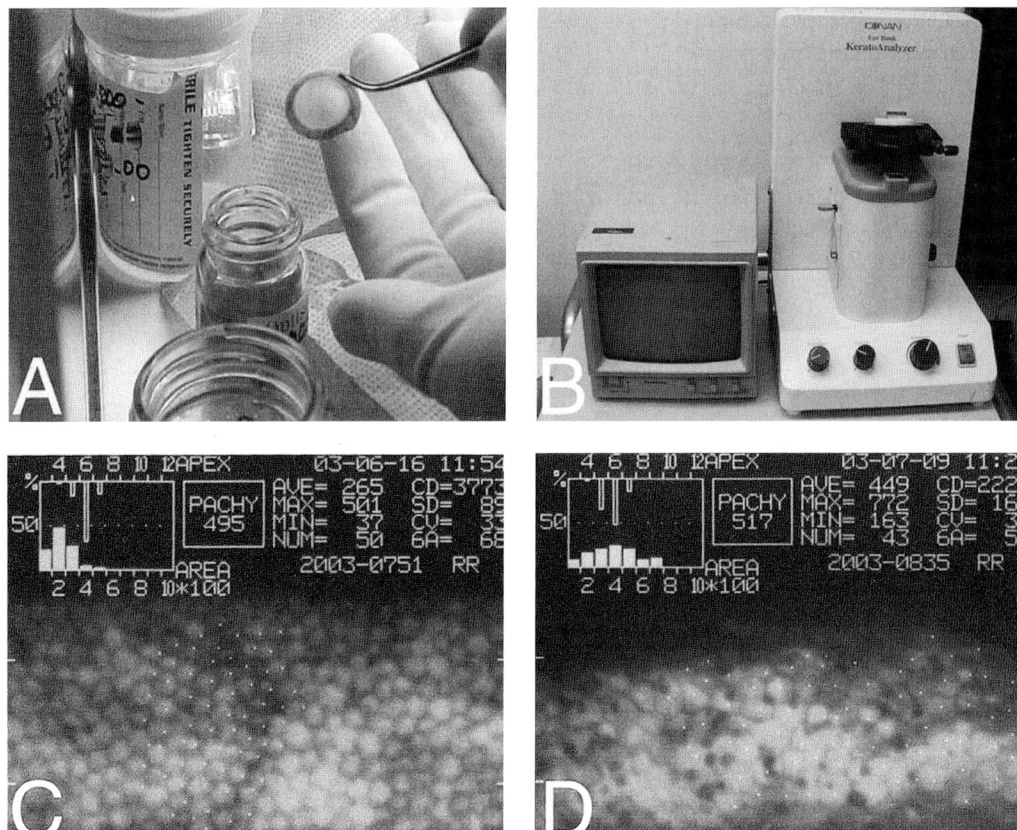

FIG. 10.2-3. A. Sterile excision of a corneal donor cap with attached scleral rim under sterile, laminar-flow hood conditions and placement of the donor into tissue culture medium for storage. **B.** Eye bank specular microscope. **C.** Specular microscopy of the corneal endothelium shows an exceptionally good donor with a high cell count (3773) and a healthy endothelium. **D.** This donor has lower cell counts (2227), yet still is in the acceptable range for surgical transplantation. The "dark" areas show some individual or group cell edema as "black" cell areas. These are usually transient or reversible after tissue culture storage at 4°C with rewarming to room temperature at the time of surgery.

EX VIVO SPECULAR MICROSCOPY IN EYE BANKING

It is well known that the normal corneal endothelium experiences a gradual decline in cell number with age; however, the need for corneal replacement for lack of transparency in normal aging is virtually nonexistent without an underlying, injury, disease, or dystrophic process. Because it is also widely appreciated that corneal endothelial cells are lost at a higher rate after penetrating keratoplasty, most corneal surgeons somewhat arbitrarily require donor corneas to contain at least 2,000 endothelial cells per square millimeter. The use of specular microscopy to obtain these data has now become widespread in virtually all modern eye banks. The process of donor cornea retrieval from an excised globe with transfer of the scleral rim–corneal button to a preservative tissue culture medium containing antibiotics is shown in Fig. 10.2-3A. Subsequent placement in a typical specular microscope is shown in Fig. 10.2-3B, and

the resulting endothelial images with cell counts are displayed in Fig. 10.2-3C and 10.2-3D. Using this method, corneas with preexisting damage (mechanical) or diseases such as Fuchs' dystrophy can be rejected for surgical transplantation.

CONCLUSIONS

A clinical comparison between *in vivo* noncontact specular and confocal microscopy has been published recently (3). As is seen in Chapter 10.1, both methods of noninvasive, *in vivo* examination can provide quantitative data concerning the shape, area, and number of endothelial cells in the normal cornea. However, confocal microscopy can supply the same data when the overlying cornea is edematous (nontransparent), whereas specular microscopy has preexisting transparency as a limiting requirement for adequate imaging. For these reasons, it is probable that confocal microscopy will gradually replace specular microscopy in coming years in routine clinical use and in eye banking applications.

ACKNOWLEDGMENTS

Supported in part by an unrestricted research grant from Research to Prevent Blindness, Inc., New York, New York.

None of the authors has any proprietary interest in the technology discussed.

REFERENCES

1. Maurice DM. A scanning slit optical microscopy. *Invest Ophthalmol* 1974;13:1033–1037.
2. Bourne WM, McCarey BE, Kaufman HE. Clinical specular microscopy. *Trans Am Acad Ophthalmol Otolaryngol* 1976;81: 743–753.
3. Hara M, Morishise N, Chikama T, et al. Comparison of confocal biomicroscopy and new cataract specular microscopy for evaluation of the corneal endothelium. *Cornea* 2003;22: 512–515.

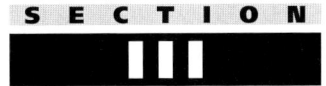

EPIDEMIOLOGY OF CORNEA
AND EXTERNAL DISEASES

11

EPIDEMIOLOGY OF MAJOR CORNEA AND EXTERNAL DISEASES

DEBRA A. SCHAUMBERG, MATTHEW GARDINER, AND OLIVER D. SCHEIN

The epidemiology of cornea and external eye disease is a very broad topic because there are a large number of conditions that can affect the health of the cornea, conjunctiva, and ocular adnexa. In this chapter, we attempt to summarize the literature on the epidemiology of some of the most common conditions affecting the ocular surface, including dry-eye syndrome (DES), ocular allergy, keratoconus, and infections. For many other conditions, such as bullous keratopathy and hereditary corneal dystrophies, epidemiologic data are lacking and the limited epidemiologic information is covered in the chapters on such conditions.

DRY-EYE SYNDROME

DES is characterized by inadequate lubrication of the ocular surface resulting from insufficient tear quantity or quality. Any number of possible alterations in the tear film could theoretically be responsible for the syndrome, including reduced tear production, excessive tear evaporation, or alterations in the molecular composition of the various tear secretions. DES is associated with debilitating symptoms of ocular dryness and discomfort (1), and it is perhaps for this reason that it appears to be one of the leading causes of patient visits to ophthalmologists and optometrists in the United States (2). When severe, DES may affect psychological health and ability to work (3).

A 1993–1994 workshop cosponsored by the National Eye Institute (NEI) and industry concluded that there had been very little study of the epidemiology of DES (4). Since that time, the NEI has identified a need for further study of the tear film, and DES and investigators have taken advantage of opportunities to collect information about the epidemiology of DES in a number of relatively large epidemiologic studies, including the Salisbury Eye Evaluation (5), the Beaver Dam Eye Study (6), the Melbourne Visual Impairment Project (7), the Physicians' Health Study (PHS) and the Women's Health Study (WHS) (8).

Four types of global tests for DES for use in research were proposed at the NEI/industry workshop, including (a) vali-

dated questionnaires of symptoms, (b) objective demonstration of ocular surface damage by vital dye staining, (c) demonstration of tear instability by decreased tear breakup time, and (d) demonstration of tear hyperosmolarity (4). However, diagnostic standardization of DES for clinical and epidemiologic studies has proven difficult largely because of inadequacies of currently available tests, as well as disease variability both across time and within persons. A report from the Salisbury study showed minimal overlap within individuals in the results of some commonly used clinical tests (9), but this must be interpreted in light of poor repeatability that would result in predictably poor correlations.

In the absence of a consensus definition of DES, studies have assessed dry eye in several ways. Assessment of dry-eye symptoms, used in all epidemiologic studies, has been shown to have very good reproducibility (10). Moreover, assessment of dry-eye symptoms is likely to provide the most useful information about the public health importance of DES because (a) clinically important degrees of ocular surface damage rarely occur in the absence of symptoms, (b) the presence of symptoms is likely to contribute to care-seeking behavior, and (c) a major goal of therapy for DES is the relief of symptoms. Assessment of dry-eye symptoms was also determined to be the single most important test for DES identified by clinicians in practice (11,12).

Epidemiologic Studies and Methods

The Salisbury Eye Evaluation was a population-based study of visual function in the elderly on the Eastern Shore of Maryland. The dry-eye component of this investigation studied 2420 men and women 65 years of age or older (5). Fifty-eight percent of the dry eye study cohort was female, and 26% was black. DES was assessed by a questionnaire that queried subjects about six symptoms including dryness, grittiness/sandiness, burning, redness, crusting on the eyelashes, and eyes being stuck shut in the morning. Each subject was asked to rate the frequency with which she or he experienced each symptom, with choices of all of the time, often, sometimes, or rarely. A subject was considered to have DES if she or he experienced a minimum of one of the six symptoms at least often.

The Melbourne Visual Impairment Project dry-eye study included a population-based sample of 926 men and women at least 40 years of age (mean, 59.2 years) (7). Forty-seven percent of subjects were male. Subjects were interviewed to rate the severity of six dry-eye symptoms: discomfort, foreign-body sensation, itching, tearing, dryness, and photophobia. Definitions were provided for the possible ratings of absent/none, mild, moderate, or severe. Severe symptoms generally had to present constantly. A subject was considered to have DES if at least one of the six symptoms was considered by the subject to be "severe," with the additional condition that the symptom was not attributable by the patient to hay fever.

DES was assessed during the second Beaver Dam Eye Study examination in 3722 men and women at least 48 years of age (mean, 65 years) (6). Ninety-nine percent of subjects were white, and 43% were male. DES was assessed by the question, "For the past 3 months or longer have you had dry eyes?" If needed, the subject was given a description of "foreign body sensation with itching, burning, sandy feeling, not related to allergy." Subjects who answered this question affirmatively were considered to have DES.

The WHS, a randomized trial to assess the benefits and risks of aspirin and vitamin E in the prevention of cardiovascular disease and cancer in healthy women, comprises 39,876 female health professionals (13), aged 49 years and older at the time of dry-eye assessment on the 4-year follow-up questionnaire (8). The PHS was a randomized trial of aspirin and beta-carotene in the prevention of cardiovascular disease and cancer conducted among 22,071 U.S. male physicians (14), who were aged 55 years and older at the time of dry-eye ascertainment at 14-years of follow-up (8). DES was ascertained by three questions pertaining to diagnosis or symptoms of DES: (a) "Have you ever been diagnosed by a clinician as having dry-eye syndrome?" (b) "How often do your eyes feel dry (not wet enough)?" and (c) "How often do your eyes feel irritated?" Possible answers to the latter two questions included "constantly," "often," "sometimes," or "never." These two questions were found to have a sensitivity of approximately 60% coupled with a specificity of 94% compared with clinical diagnosis of dry eye (15), and nearly the same predictability as a longer 14-item questionnaire. DES was defined as the presence of clinically diagnosed DES or severe dry-eye symptoms of both dryness and irritation either constantly or often.

Prevalence of Dry-Eye Syndrome

The Salisbury study was the first large-scale epidemiologic study to report an estimate of the prevalence of DES, finding that 14% of subjects reported one or more symptoms to be present at least often (5). In the Melbourne study, DES had been previously diagnosed in less than 1% of subjects. Overall, 5.5% of subjects reported at least one severe symp-

tom not attributable to hay fever (7). Of the 3703 subjects in the second Beaver Dam Eye Study examination with data on dry eye, the prevalence of dry-eye symptoms was 14.4% [95% confidence interval (CI), 13.3%–15.6%] (6).

In the WHS, the age-adjusted prevalence of DES was 7.8%, or 3.23 million women aged 50 years or older in the United States (16). The prevalence of diagnosed DES was 6.1%, and that of symptoms of both dryness and irritation constantly or often was 3.4%. In preliminary findings from the PHS, the age-standardized prevalence was 3.5% among men aged 55 years and older. Based on this estimate, 900,000 men in this age group are predicted to have DES.

Demographic Associations with Dry-Eye Syndrome

Clinicians have long suspected that DES becomes more common with aging, and there is some evidence of an age-related decrease in tear production (16,17). Until recently, however, epidemiologic data showing an age-related increase in DES were lacking. Figure 11-1 summarizes data on the relationship of the prevalence of DES according to age in the large epidemiologic studies described previously. Inspection of Fig. 11-1 suggests that the results of all studies taken together are most consistent with a trend toward a higher prevalence of DES in the older age groups. There is currently little information on the incidence of DES. Moss and colleagues have estimated the 5-year incidence of DES in the Beaver Dam Study as 13%, with a significantly higher incidence in older subjects (17.9% for those 80 years of age and older, vs. 10.7% for 48- to 59-year-olds) (18).

Basic research points to a possible role for sex steroid hormones in the pathogenesis of DES, including both androgens (as a protective factor) and estrogens (as a risk factor) (19–27). Apparently consistent with the basic research, clinical and epidemiologic observations have long suggested that DES is more common in women. In the Melbourne study, women were nearly two times more likely to report severe symptoms of dry-eye [odds ratio (OR), 1.85] (7). Similarly, in the Beaver Dam study, the prevalence of DES was significantly higher in women (17.0%) compared with men (11.1%) (6). Based on data from the WHS and PHS, the estimated age-standardized prevalence of DES in the United States appears to be higher in women than in men (Fig. 11-2). In contrast, investigators of the Salisbury study observed no significant sex-related difference in the prevalence of dry-eye symptoms among women (15.6%) and men (13.3%) aged 65 years and older (5).

Only two studies have been able to address the issue of potential racial/ethnic differences in DES. The Salisbury study included 650 blacks and 1832 whites from the same community in Maryland and observed a prevalence of DES symptoms of 13.5% among blacks and 15.0% among whites, with no statistically significant difference between these groups (5). In the WHS, 95% of the women indicated they were white, 2.2% black, 1.4% Asian/Pacific is-

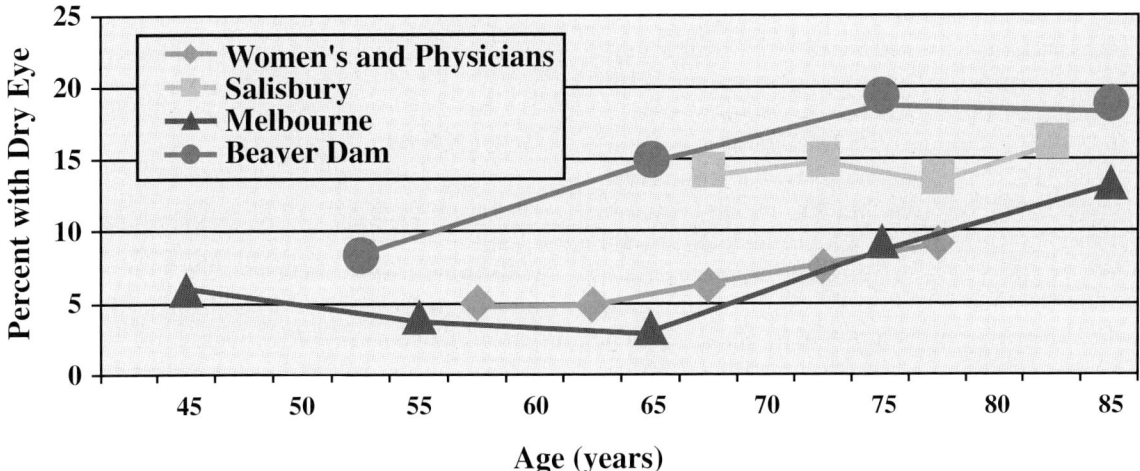

FIGURE 11-1. Prevalence of Dry Eye Syndrome by Age. Estimates are derived from Epidemiological studies including: the Salisbury Eye Evaluation (5), the Melbourne Visual Impairment Project (7), the Beaver Dam Eye Study (6), and combined data from the Women's Health Study (16) and the Physicians' Health Study (Schaumberg DA, unpublished).

lander, 1% Hispanic, and 0.3% Native American; 0.2% were of other or unknown race/ethnicity (13). The prevalence of DES was similar among these groups of women, and there were no significant differences in the prevalence DES among blacks and whites. However, both Hispanic and Asian women reported a higher prevalence of severe dry-eye symptoms compared with whites (16). The reasons for this are unclear but may be related to several factors. For example, some groups of women with DES may be getting less relief from dry-eye symptoms. In addition, the higher prevalence of dry-eye symptoms in some minority groups could be related to existence of a greater number of health problems in these women, which either themselves or by virtue of their treatments may be associated with a higher prevalence of dry-eye symptoms. There is also the possibility of underdiagnosis of DES among some minority groups. Further studies are needed to clarify these issues.

Other Risk Factors for Dry-Eye Syndrome

Current information on other risk factors for DES is limited. Future studies should examine compelling hypotheses in more detail. In the Melbourne study (7), investigators found no significant associations with the use of contact lenses, cigarette smoking, history of previous eye injury, definite symptoms of dry mouth, menopause, or the use of hormone therapy among postmenopausal women. Arthritis was found to be significantly associated with a higher prevalence of clinical signs of dry eye. However, the usefulness of these analyses was limited because some of these exposures were rare in the population (e.g., only 21 subjects wore contact lenses) and no estimates of the magnitude or confidence intervals for these relationships were provided. In the Salisbury study, dry-eye symptoms were reported to be significantly associated with self-reported poor health and with the number of medical comorbidities (5). Further, a combined end point of either dry-eye or dry-mouth symptoms was also associated with use of certain classes of systemic medications, including nonsteroidal antiinflammatory drugs (OR, 1.30), diuretics (OR, 1.25), vasodilators (OR, 1.37), analgesics and antipyretics (OR, 1.28), antiulcer agents (OR, 1.44), anxiolytics and benzodiazepines (OR, 2.35), antiinfectives (OR, 1.88), antidepressants and antipsychotics (OR, 2.54), antihypertensive

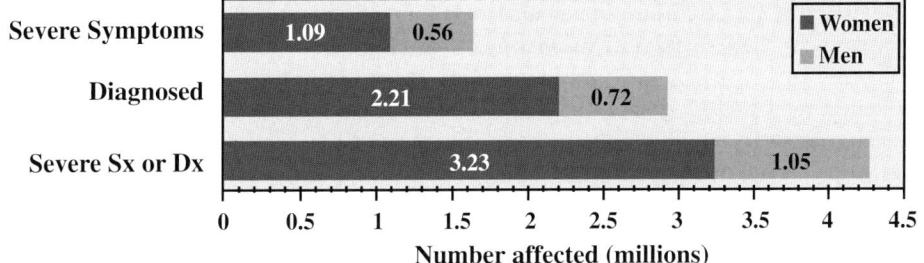

FIGURE 11-2. Prevalence of Dry Eye Syndrome in the United States, by Sex. Estimates are derived from the Women's Health Study (16) and the Physicians' Health Study (Schaumberg DA, unpublished) and standardized to the US population in 1999. Estimates are provided for three definitions of dry eye syndrome; severe symptoms, diagnosed dry eye (based on self-reported data), or either of these. Severe symptoms refers to a report of both dryness and irritation either constantly or often.

agents (OR, 1.98) and antihistamines (OR, 1.67). The number of medication classes associated with drying symptoms used was also associated with a monotonic increase in risk of dry-eye or dry-mouth symptoms (OR of 2.5 for use of three; and OR of 4.2 for use of six or more vs. none). On the other hand, no relationship was found for rheumatoid arthritis, smoking, alcohol consumption, use of estrogen, presence of anti-Ro/SS-A or La/SS-B autoantibodies, antinuclear antibody positivity of at least 1:320, or rheumatoid factor positivity (28). Investigators in the Beaver Dam study (6) performed a non–hypothesis-driven type of analysis of a long list of factors to determine whether any would show a statistical relationship with dry-eye. In these analyses, statistically significant independent associations were observed for arthritis history (OR, 1.91); past (OR, 1.22) and current (OR, 1.82) cigarette smoking; caffeine use (OR, 0.75); thyroid disease (OR, 1.41); history of gout (OR, 1.42); total/high-density lipoprotein cholesterol ratio (OR, 0.93); diabetes mellitus (OR, 1.38); and past (OR, 1.35) and current (OR, 1.41) use of multivitamins. These findings must be interpreted cautiously because many statistical tests were performed, increasing the probability of spurious findings.

Given the basic research supporting the hypothesis that sex steroid hormones modulate the production and release of tear components, the potential relationship of hormone therapy with DES is of particular interest. In the WHS, compared with women who never used hormone therapy, the multivariate-adjusted ORs for DES were 1.69 (95% CI, 1.49–1.91) for women who used estrogen alone and 1.29 (95% CI, 1.13–1.48) for women who used estrogen plus progesterone or progestins (29). Thus, use of estrogen replacement therapy appears to increase the risk of DES by approximately 70% if used alone, and by 30% if used in combination with progesterone or progestins. In this study, there was also a significant association with the duration of hormone therapy such that for each 3-year increase in the duration of hormone therapy, the risk of DES increased by 15% (95% CI, 11%–19%). There is also emerging clinical evidence that androgen deficiency in humans (e.g., in patients taking antiandrogen medication) is associated with meibomian gland dysfunction and DES (25).

Recent evidence from the WHS suggests that dietary factors may also play a role in the development of DES (30). In this study, 32,470 female health professionals aged between 45 and 84 years who provided information on diet and DES were studied. Intake of omega-3 fatty acids was assessed by a validated food frequency questionnaire. After adjusting for age, other demographic factors, hormone therapy, and total fat intake, there was a significant reduction in risk of DES of approximately 20% for the highest versus the lowest fifth of dietary intake of omega-3 fatty acids. In addition, consumption of two to four 4-ounce servings of tuna fish per week was association with a 20% reduction in risk of DES, whereas consumption of five to six 4-ounce servings was related to a nearly 70% reduction in risk of DES. However, there may be other factors associated with individuals habitually consuming tuna on an almost daily basis.

OCULAR ALLERGY

Ocular allergy is almost universally associated with systemic allergic conditions. Broadly speaking, allergic diseases of the ocular surface can be broken down into four categories: allergic conjunctivitis, giant papillary conjunctivitis (GPC), vernal keratoconjunctivitis (VKC), and atopic keratoconjunctivitis (AKC). To date, with the exception of allergic conjunctivitis in children, the epidemiology of these conditions has not received a great deal of attention in the literature.

Allergic Conjunctivitis

Allergic conjunctivitis comprises one of the most common forms of conjunctivitis and is a significant public health problem in the United States. Most reports consistently indicate that the syndrome is usually part of a larger complex related to seasonal allergy, with as much as 95% of sufferers having associated allergic conditions, particularly allergic rhinitis (31,32). Because of this tendency toward association with other disorders, which also include asthma and sinusitis, the overall economic burden of allergic rhinoconjunctivitis is large. Indeed, overall direct medical expenditures attributable to allergic rhinoconjunctivitis have been estimated at $5.9 billion for 1996, with 38% of these expenditures accounted for by care of children 12 years of age and younger (33).

Although the condition can affect those of any age, the prevalence of allergic rhinoconjunctivitis has been most extensively studied in children, though even for children there is a paucity of recently published data from the United States. The International Study of Asthma and Allergies in Childhood (ISAAC) is a large-scale, multinational, collaborative study to evaluate the epidemiology of allergic diseases in children around the world. An ISAAC protocol study of 27,507 children throughout the United Kingdom reported a prevalence of rhinoconjunctivitis of 18.2% (34). In 37,592 children studied in 6 ISAAC centers in New Zealand, the prevalence of allergic rhinoconjunctivitis was 10% among 6- to 7-year-olds and 19% among 12- to 13-year-olds (35), whereas among a random sample of 3058 children in Nigeria, the prevalence of rhinoconjunctivitis was 39.2% (36). A nationwide survey of a sample of 38,955 Korean children revealed a prevalence of approximately 10% for rhinoconjunctivitis (37). A study from Sweden reported that 7% of school children and 15% of adolescents have seasonal allergic conjunctivitis (38). The prevalence of allergic rhinoconjunctivitis was 20.8% among an unselected group of 1175 Italian school children (39). Studies in Turkey have estimated a prevalence of allergic conjunctivitis of between 4.6% and 7.1% in primary school children (40,41). The most recent estimates from Sweden indicate that approximately 17% of 12- and 13-year-olds suffer from allergic rhinoconjunctivitis (42). The suggestion has been made that the prevalence of allergic rhinoconjunctivitis has been rising in recent decades (43–45).

Family history appears to be a significant risk factor for allergic conjunctivitis. In one study of 445 patients with allergic conjunctivitis, 65% had a family history of allergy (31). Evidence for genetic linkage of allergic conjunctivitis has been identified in one study for chromosomes 5, 16, and 17, further supporting the idea that a genetic predisposition exists (46). Environmental factors are also likely to play a key role in the development of allergic conjunctivitis, and as with asthma there is some evidence suggesting that exposure to high antigen loads at a young age may offer a protective effect (42,47,48). Others have suggested that poorly ventilated homes, rather than outdoor pollution, may play a larger role in the incidence of allergic conjunctivitis (49). Early research suggests that diet may also play a role in allergic conjunctivitis, with one study demonstrating an increased risk with higher intake of n-6 polyunsaturated fatty acids (50). An ecological study of per capita dietary consumption and prevalence of allergic rhinoconjunctivitis in the ISAAC population identified a consistent inverse trend between the prevalence of allergic rhinoconjunctivitis and the intake of starch, cereals, and vegetables (51), and an increased risk associated with higher per capita consumption of *trans* fatty acids (52). However, these studies are far from conclusive, and further study of these issues is needed.

Giant Papillary Conjunctivitis

GPC was first described in 1974 (53). Since this early report, this entity has been shown to be closely associated with soft contact lenses, longer contact lens wearing times, and less frequent lens replacement. Nonetheless, there are no reliable estimates of the prevalence or incidence of GPC among the contact lens–wearing population. Although the syndrome is clearly associated with soft contact lenses, it also occurs in wearers of hard contact lenses (54). For example, in one study of 221 patients with GPC, 15.4% were wearers of hard contact lenses (55).

The possibility that the lens material itself is antigenic has been debated, but studies of potential lens antigenicity in animals dispute this theory (56). Nonetheless, different lens materials may be more prone to absorbing ocular proteins onto their surfaces, and this has been proposed as a potential cause of GPC-related allergy (57). Despite this, there is no convincing evidence to show that one type of soft lens is more prone to lead to the development of GPC than any other (58,59). The frequency of contact lens replacement appears to play a greater role than these factors in the pathogenesis of GPC, with one study showing that patients who replaced their lenses after 4 or more weeks had an incidence of GPC of 36%, versus 4.5% for those who replaced them after fewer than 4 weeks (60). Although there are few, if any additional data to support this theory, if it is true the recent shift toward more frequent replacement of contact lenses may reduce the impact of this condition.

Vernal Keratoconjunctivitis

The epidemiology of VKC has been little studied, though it appears clearly related to atopy (61,62). Case series reports demonstrate a higher frequency in children than adults, and the condition appears to show a male predilection (63,64). One recent publication of a series of 195 patients found the mean age to be 11 years and the male-to-female ratio to be 2.8:1.0, but it is not certain that this would reflect the overall demographic profile of VKC sufferers. Most patients in this study (77%) had seasonal disease (usually springtime), and 41% had a personal history of atopy. The overall prevalence of VKC is not known, although there are thought to be significant geographic variations in its frequency and severity, with it being potentially a greater problem in parts of the Middle East (65,66). Further study of the epidemiology of VKC, although perhaps somewhat difficult to conduct because of the (presumed) relatively low incidence of the condition, would be desirable.

Atopic Keratoconjunctivitis

Representing the most severe and clinically least encountered form of ocular allergy, AKC has been termed the adult variant of VKC and is often characterized by an association with dermatitis. The prevalence of AKC is unknown. It appears to affect predominantly men between 30 and 50 years of age and tends to be chronic (67). AKC is usually associated with systemic atopy, and a personal or family history of asthma or eczema is very common (68–70). One of the most damaging aspects of the disease is its tendency to cause corneal melting and severe vision loss. In one 9-year retrospective study of 45 patients with AKC, 34 had keratopathy and 21 had persistent epithelial defects causing severe visual compromise (69). Penetrating keratoplasty may be required for patients with permanent visual disability, but a very high rate of complications and graft rejection may occur (71,72).

Future studies of the incidence of these less frequent ocular allergic conditions might be most feasible in managed care or other settings with relatively large numbers of regularly followed patients.

KERATOCONUS

Keratoconus is a usually bilateral but often asymmetric noninflammatory disease of the cornea distinguished by deformation of the corneal tissue, specifically involving steepening, apical thinning, and anterior protrusion (73). This architectural distortion of the cornea results in myopia and irregular astigmatism that impair vision quality. Onset of keratoconus is gradual but is usually clinically apparent in the late teenage years to early adulthood. The disease typically progresses in severity for a number of years and then often seems to stabilize somewhat. Vision may initially be adequately correctable with spectacles or soft contact lenses, but a large proportion of patients eventually require rigid, gas-permeable contact lenses to achieve acceptable levels of visual performance (73,74). Penetrating keratoplasty may be recommended for those patients who cannot tolerate contact lenses or when visual acuity remains inadequate despite an appropriate contact lens fit. Although the likelihood of surgery has been shown to depend on the severity of the disease (75), survivorship without the performance of corneal transplantation has been reported to be greater than 80% after 20 years of follow-up among individuals with keratoconus (76).

Incidence, Prevalence, and Demographic Characteristics

A number of issues make study of the incidence and prevalence of keratoconus a difficult undertaking. The condition is relatively rare, making population-based prevalence surveys impractical. Furthermore, the gradual onset of the condition may delay clinical diagnosis, and relatively mild cases may go undetected. Given these limitations, the best population-based data on keratoconus incidence and prevalence in the United States have been published from records of patients in Olmsted County, Minnesota (76). Investigators reviewed medical information systems of the Mayo Clinic for all cases of newly diagnosed keratoconus identified from 1935 through 1982, supplemented with a questionnaire sent to local optometrists who were not covered in the database. Using U.S. census data to derive an appropriate denominator, the overall age-adjusted prevalence of keratoconus was estimated at 54.5 cases per 100,000 population. The age- and sex-adjusted incidence rate was estimated at 2.0 cases per 100,000 person-years of observation, with a rate of 2.4 per 100,000 among men and 1.6 per 100,000 among women. The higher incidence of keratoconus among men in this study was not statistically significant, although there was a statistically significantly higher prevalence among men in the study population (69.5 per 100,000 among men versus 39.2 per 100,000 among women). The incidence of keratoconus was observed to peak between the ages of 15 and 24 for men and 25 to 34 among women. Although the design of this study may have resulted in some underdetection of milder cases, it likely provides the best available estimate of the incidence and prevalence of clinically (and hence visually) important keratoconus. These data are further supported by a similar study in the United Kingdom, in which investigators conducted a retrospective review of ophthalmology records from a large hospital in Leicestershire with a catchment population of approximately 900,000 (77). In this study,

the incidence of keratoconus among whites was found to be nearly the same (2.2 per 100,000 person-years) as that in Olmstead County, Minnesota, with a similar finding of a higher prevalence among men. An incidence of 1.4 per 100,000 person-years was observed in a study based at the Oulu University Central Hospital in Finland, where two thirds of cases occurred among men (78). Given these findings, previous reports of larger numbers of female patients among keratoconus series are perhaps more likely to be due to a greater use of health care services among women or some other factor. Studies of racial differences in keratoconus are lacking in the United States, but some data are available from the Leicestershire study in the United Kingdom. The overall incidence of patients with keratoconus presenting to hospital for contact lens fitting or corneal grafting was 11.8 per 100,000 person-years among Asians (primarily of Indian origin), an incidence more than five-fold higher than that among whites.

Possible Risk Factors

Certain types of mechanical trauma have long been suspected as risk factors for keratoconus. In particular, studies have focused on the use of hard contact lenses and eye rubbing. Although the latter factor's association with the development of keratoconus is difficult to prove, some supportive evidence may be derived from animal models (79) and mechanistic research (80,81). In addition, a number of studies have reported a high prevalence of eye-rubbing behavior among individuals with keratoconus (82–84). Nonetheless, it has thus far not been possible to separate a possible effect of eye rubbing from other possibilities such as a genetic predisposition or other condition (e.g., atopy or use of hard contact lenses) that may be associated with both an increased tendency for eye rubbing as well as keratoconus. Unfortunately, although the theory is not entirely implausible, studies to date of the potential relationship of the use of hard contact lenses with the development of keratoconus suffer from possible biases introduced by flaws in study design that severely limit the usefulness of the findings.

As summarized by Rabinowitz, a number of systemic and ocular disorders have been reported in association with keratoconus (85). However, many of these may have been chance associations (74), and keratoconus purportedly occurs in isolation in as many as 99% of cases (74,85). Nonetheless, most reports based on ocular examinations of individuals with Down's syndrome are consistent with a higher risk of keratoconus in this group, in whom the prevalence of the condition may range from approximately 8% to 15% (86–88), orders of magnitude above that seen in the general population. It remains unclear whether this higher prevalence of keratoconus among individuals with Down's syndrome is due to increased occurrence of eye rubbing or some other cause.

An association between keratoconus and various connective tissue disorders has also been the subject of some investigation, given reports of associations with disorders of collagen metabolism, and hypothesis-generating reports suggesting that many patients with keratoconus exhibited joint hypermobility (89) and mitral valve prolapse (MVP) (90). More recent studies have provided mixed support for these hypotheses. Using two-dimensional echocardiography, Sharif and colleagues studied 50 patients with advanced keratoconus requiring penetrating keratoplasty (91). These investigators observed an overall prevalence of MVP of 38% among patients with keratoconus versus 7% among a group of age- and sex-matched control subjects. However, in a study of 95 consecutive patients with keratoconus identified at the Emory Eye Center by Street and colleagues and 96 age-, sex-, and race-matched control subjects, no significant difference was observed in the prevalence of MVP as detected by M-mode and two-dimensional echocardiography, although odds ratios were most consistent with a modestly increased risk of MVP, ranging between 1.27- and 1.77-fold higher among patients with keratoconus compared with control subjects, depending on the definition of MVP (92). Subsequently, Lichter and colleagues used videokeratography to examine 36 patients with an echocardiographic diagnosis of MVP and 25 individuals without MVP selected from the echocardiography unit in which the patients with MVP were diagnosed. In this study, unilateral asymptomatic keratoconus was found in 22.2% of patients with MVP versus 4% in the group without evidence of MVP ($p = .05$). A report from Moorfields Eye Hospital examined the prevalence of joint hypermobility among 84 patients with keratoconus and 84 sex-, age-, and race-matched control subjects. In this relatively small study, the exclusion of patients with myopia of more than 5D and astigmatic patients from the control group on the grounds that they might also be at increased risk of joint hypermobility may have introduced some bias. Nonetheless, the relative risk of joint hypermobility among the patients with keratoconus was found to be over five times higher than that among the control group (93). In contrast, no significant differences were observed by Street and colleagues in the prevalence of hypermobile joints in patients with keratoconus (11%) versus control subjects (13%) (92).

A possible relationship between atopy and keratoconus has also been the subject of a number of investigations. Early reports of studies conducted among large series of atopic individuals failed to detect many cases of keratoconus. Similarly, Lowell and Carroll found no significant difference in the prevalence of atopy among patients with keratoconus versus control subjects (94). On the contrary, a number of investigators report an increased risk of keratoconus associated with atopic diseases (84,95–98). More recently, Bawazeer and colleagues studied 49 incident cases of keratoconus and 71 control subjects from the University of Ottawa Eye Institute. In univariable analysis, there was a significantly higher prevalence of atopy among the keratoconus group than among control subjects. However, although the relative risk (RR) remained elevated (RR of 3.67 for complete atopy) after adjustment for other risk factors including eye rubbing, the association was no longer statistically significant ($p = .08$), whereas that for eye rubbing remained so (RR, 5.38; $p = .001$) (82). Zadnick and colleagues in a report of baseline findings from the prospective Collaborative Longitudinal Evaluation of Keratoconus (CLEK) study found a prevalence of atopic disease of 53%, contrasting with prevalence estimates of approximately 10% to 20% for the general population (74). Totan and colleagues used videokeratography to study the prevalence of keratoconus among a group of 82 consecutive subjects with vernal keratoconjunctivitis. The prevalence of keratoconus of 26.8% diagnosed by quantitative evaluation of videokeratographic findings is strikingly high, although no estimates using this definition of keratoconus were provided for comparison among subjects without vernal keratoconjunctivitis (83).

In addition to environmental risk factors, it appears likely that genetic susceptibility may also increase the risk of keratoconus in some individuals. A family history of keratoconus is present in approximately 6% to 23% of cases (76,78,99). Although case reports of both concordance (100,101) and discordance (102) for the disease among monozygotic twins have been published, it appears that concordance is more common. Segregation analysis has also suggested that genetics plays a role in the development of keratoconus (103). Furthermore, Tyynismaa and colleagues found evidence for linkage to 16q22.3-q23.1 in a sample of 20 Finnish families with autosomal dominant keratoconus (maximum LOD [log of the odds] score = 4.10). In a recent Japanese study, human leukocyte antigens A26, B40, and DR9 were found at a higher frequency among patients with keratoconus with onset before 20 years of age.

COMMON EXTERNAL OCULAR INFECTIONS

The frequencies of occurrence of infections commonly affecting the external ocular structures are difficult to determine because of the acute nature of most of these conditions, which precludes estimation from population-based surveys. Reports have been published based on clinical series from patients presenting to large ophthalmic centers, but such data must be viewed cautiously given the difficulty of determining an appropriate denominator. The estimated incidence of common infections is presented in Table 11-1.

Infectious Blepharitis

Blepharitis is thought to be one of the most common reasons for visiting an ophthalmologist. The posterior variety

TABLE 11-1. INCIDENCE OF COMMON EXTERNAL OCULAR INFECTIONS

Condition	Estimated Incidence[a]
Ocular herpes zoster	120–340 (104)
Epidemic keratoconjunctivitis	84–195[b]
Ocular herpes simplex	8.4 (105)
Bacterial keratitis	5.3 (106)
Acanthamoeba keratitis	1.8 (U.K. contact lens wearers) (107) 0.1 (U.K. overall) (107)
0.2 (U.S. contact lens wearers) (108)	
Fungal keratitis	Unknown but rare except in subtropical/tropical areas Perhaps 20% (of all keratitis cases in Florida) (109) Perhaps 44% (of all keratitis cases in southern India) (110)

[a]100, 000 person-years.
[b]Based on very rough estimate provided for comparison. Based on the estimated incidence of ocular herpes simplex infection and a rough estimate of the relative percentage of all cases of suspected viral keratitis due to herpes (4.3% to 10%).

is characterized by meibomian gland dysfunction and its epidemiology follows closely that of DES. Anterior blepharitis is more commonly associated with infection of the lid margins and the accumulation of crusted debris. Studies of the various bacterial causes of blepharitis have shown that the predominant organisms are *Staphylococcus* species, particularly *Staphylococcus epidermidis*, which was found in one series to be present in 95.8% of cases (111). Although arguably a significant drain on health care resources, the prevalence of anterior blepharitis remains unknown and no population-based data are available. Clinical series suggest that compared with posterior blepharitis and meibomian gland dysfunction, patients with anterior blepharitis are younger and more likely to be female (up to 80% of patients with *Staphylococcus* species) (112). Clinicians have also reported associations between anterior blepharitis and atopy (113) as well rosacea (114), but there are no supportive epidemiologic data to substantiate these reports.

Infectious Conjunctivitis

Although trachoma may be the most common cause of conjunctivitis worldwide, viral etiologies are most common in the developed world. The most common forms of infectious conjunctivitis in the United States present acutely and are of a time-limited nature, often occurring in outbreaks, and epidemiologic data are lacking as to the overall incidence of infectious conjunctivitis.

Adenovirus appears to be one of the most common causes of infectious conjunctivitis, being the cause of 75% of cases in a series of 965 patients in Japan with presumed viral conjunctivitis. A seasonal peak in July to August was apparent and the predominant age group was 30 to 39 years of age (115). The

disease, known as epidemic keratoconjunctivitis (EKC), is extremely infectious and is spread by direct contact. Many reports have demonstrated that the physician's office or hospital can be a major reservoir for the virus during outbreaks, perhaps owing to the ability of the virus to remain infectious on the hands of providers despite handwashing (116,117). For example, one study of 145 patients with adenoviral conjunctivitis found that 30% had visited their eye care specialist during the 2 weeks before diagnosis (118), and an ophthalmology clinic was determined to be the source of a recent outbreak of EKC in a neonatal intensive care unit (117). Adenovirus may also be spread in chronic care facilities where patients' hygiene is difficult to control (119).

Herpes simplex virus (HSV) is a less common cause of viral conjunctivitis and is better known for its ability to cause keratitis. A Japanese study of viral conjunctivitis found that, among 478 patients, 4.3% of cases diagnosed as EKC were actually HSV type 1 (HSV-1), and stated that it was very difficult to differentiate between adenovirus and HSV on clinical grounds alone (120). Another study showed that unlike adenovirus, there is no seasonal predilection for HSV (115). Most patients become infected as children and recurrence is common (25% patients over 2 years) (121), with some recurrences occurring only as conjunctivitis (122).

Bacterial etiologies of conjunctivitis are much less common than their viral counterparts. In children, *Streptococcus pneumoniae* and *Haemophilus influenzae* are the most common, whereas in adults *Staphylococcus aureus* is the usual offending agent (123). One report of outbreaks in a chronic care facility found bacterial pathogens in 21% and 38% of cultures in two episodes, with *S. aureus* predominating (124). Outbreaks can occur in patterns and settings more commonly associated with viral etiologies. An outbreak in 2002 in a New Hampshire college affecting 698 students was found to be caused by *S. pneumoniae* (125). Other bacterial pathogens, such as *Pseudomonas aeruginosa* and *Neisseria meningitidis*, can be associated with invasive disease and life-threatening bacteremia, with *N. meningitidis* infection having a reported mortality rate of 2.4% (126,127).

Disease caused by *Chlamydia trachomatis* is a major global public health problem and a serious cause of ocular morbidity in trachoma endemic areas. The subtypes causing adult inclusion conjunctivitis are D through K, whereas trachoma is caused by subtypes A through C. Adult inclusion conjunctivitis most commonly occurs in young, sexually active adults and is usually acquired from a preexisting genital infection due to hand–eye contact (121). In a study of 65 patients with chlamydial conjunctivitis, 54% of men had a positive urethral culture (70% of these were asymptomatic) and 74% of women had a positive urethral culture (60% of these were asymptomatic) (128). The overall prevalence of chlamydial conjunctivitis was estimated by one report to be 2% of patients with acute conjunctivitis in Australia (129). Of the 12 patients diagnosed with chlamydial conjunctivitis who were later tested, 10 were found to have genital infection, and all were asymptomatic.

Trachoma is endemic in parts of Africa, Asia, and Australia. It is associated with poor hygiene that leads to its spread through direct contact or through fomites. It is the most common infectious cause of blindness worldwide. According to World Health Organization data, it is responsible for 15.5% of cases of blindness in developing countries: more specifically, 9.7% in India, 19.4% in sub-Saharan Africa, and 25.7% in the Middle East (130). The prevalence of trachoma has been estimated by population-based studies to be 10.7% in Saudi Arabia (131), 49% in aboriginal Australia (132), and 51% in Ethiopia (133). It is more common in rural areas and in children and women (134). The main cause of visual compromise is corneal scarring, often secondary to trichiasis. Elimination of trachoma is almost invariably associated with improvements in the general economic and hygienic environments of underdeveloped regions. A major public health effort is underway by the World Health Organization to eradicate trachoma with the reinforcement of hygiene and use of antibiotics. Although much work has yet to be done, there is evidence that the use of oral azithromycin is significantly more effective than topical tetracycline in treating the disease (135). In response to these findings, Pfizer Pharmaceuticals has initiated a program (the International Trachoma Initiative) of donating their formulation of azithromycin toward the goal of elimination of trachoma.

Although coinfection with *C. trachomatis* and gonorrhea is common, the rarer infection with *Neisseria gonorrhoeae* is hyperacute and therefore more likely to bring the patient to medical attention. Like other sexually transmitted diseases, it tends to affect people in their second and third decades and is usually transferred to the eye by autoinoculation. Outbreaks are common (136–138), and in some cases there is no concomitant genitourinary infection, with the infection transferred from person to person by hand–eye contact (139).

N. gonorrhoeae is also important for its role in ophthalmia neonatorum. The prevalence of gonorrhea in pregnant women has been quoted as less than 1% in industrialized nations and as high as 3% to 15% in developing countries (140). In industrialized societies, *C. trachomatis* is more common than *N. gonorrhoeae* as an etiology of ophthalmia neonatorum, being reported in large surveys as causing between 6% and 8% of cases (141,142). Most studies have also shown that the most common pathogens overall are *S. aureus*, *H. influenzae*, and *Streptococcus* species (141–144). Routine prophylaxis with topical antibiotics has decreased the incidence of this serious cause of neonatal morbidity, but recent randomized trials have demonstrated the superior efficacy, tolerability, and cost savings of the use of 2.5% povidone–iodine over other treatments (145).

Bacterial Keratitis

In developed countries, the principal risk factor for bacterial keratitis is contact lens wear, whereas in developing settings, trauma or other ocular disease (e.g., trachoma or vitamin A deficiency) are major risk factors.

Contact lens wear significantly increases the risk of bacterial keratitis, the relative risk varying by lens type and wearing habits. In 1981, the U.S. Food and Drug Administration (FDA) approved certain soft contact lenses for up to 30 days of consecutive use. By the mid-1980s, there were many case reports indicating an apparent excess risk of ulcerative keratitis associated with this modality. The first controlled study examining this issue was performed by Schein and colleagues, and published in 1989 (146). This study reported approximately a fourfold excess risk for extended-wear compared with daily-wear soft contact lenses. However, once the investigators took actual lens wear into account (i.e., not everyone using a contact lens approved for overnight wear slept with the lens in, and some users of daily-wear lenses slept with their lenses in), the excess risk for actual overnight wear was approximately 10 times greater than for strict daily wear use. Moreover, a dose–response effect was observed, wherein risk of ulcerative keratitis increased with increasing nights of consecutive wear. A companion investigation reported the results of a population-based incidence study performed in New England that estimated the risks of ulcerative keratitis by lens type at 4.1/10,000 for daily-wear lenses and 20.9/10,000 for extended-wear lenses (147). These two studies resulted in the reduction of approval for overnight wear from 30 nights to 6 nights by the FDA. Subsequent case–control studies showed that the risk of keratitis associated with overnight wear persisted after the introduction of disposable soft contact lenses in the 1990s (148). Approximately 10 years after the original incidence study in New England, the study was repeated in the Netherlands by other investigators and showed a remarkably similar pattern of results indicating that risk varied by lens type, with a risk of 1.1 per 10,000 for gas-permeable lenses, 3.5 per 10,000 for daily-wear soft lenses, and 20 per 10,000 for extended-wear soft lenses (149).

Although there are few reliable data on the subject, other suggestive risk factors for contact lens–related keratitis have been reported to include smoking (146) and male sex (150). Contact lens hygiene may play only a minor role in the development of keratitis (146), but is commonly poor in soft contact lens wearers. One study found that only 10 of 27 patients using extended-wear lenses were fully compliant with ideal lens care, and only 5 of 14 daily wearers used surfactant cleaners regularly (151).

Although the incidence of contact lens–related keratitis might be decreasing, the numbers remain high. Dart et al. reported that contact lens wear was the most common cause of microbial keratitis at Moorfields Eye Hospital, and found that the relative risk for keratitis with contact lens wear was 80, but with trauma was 14 (compared with cases without predisposing risks) (152). One retrospective review of 320 patients with a corneal ulcer seen at an eye hospital found that 96 (30%) were secondary to contact lens use, with the predominant organism being *Pseudomonas* (153). As education regarding avoidance of overnight wear of conventional lenses improves and with the introduction of daily disposable lenses, the incidence may fall further. Recently, the FDA has approved a new generation of silicon hydrogel contact lenses for continuous wear up to 30 days. It is hoped that the greater oxygen permeability of these materials compared with the older extended-wear lenses will result in fewer cases of ulcerative keratitis. To date, there have been several case reports of bacterial keratitis associated with this lens type (154,155), although epidemiologic data are not yet available.

The best estimate of the overall incidence of bacterial conjunctivitis in the general population has been derived using population-based data from Olmstead County, Minnesota. The mean annual incidence of bacterial keratitis has been estimated to be 5.3/100,000 population with no statistically significant difference in risk between men and women, but a highly significant increase in risk with age (106). A 435% increase in the incidence of keratitis was observed from 1950 to 1980, in large part secondary to the increase in contact lens wear. Non–contact lens–related bacterial keratitis in developed countries is predominantly secondary to gram-positive organisms such as *S. aureus* (156), although there my be a trend shifting toward gram-negative organisms (157). Increasing resistance to the fluoroquinolones also is developing among some gram-positive organisms (157,158). Trauma and other means of epithelial loss are major risk factors for corneal infection. Atypical mycobacterial infections, previously rare, have become more common as a complication of laser *in situ* keratomileusis treatments (159). In tropical areas, *Pseudomonas* and *Streptococcus* may be more common (160–162), and fungus may be the predominant organism isolated (162,163). In these environments, trauma and low socioeconomic status are predisposing factors (160,164).

Herpes Simplex Keratitis

HSV is one of the most common viruses to infect humans. HSV-1 more commonly causes oral infections, whereas HSV-2 is more likely to cause genital infections, but either type may infect either site. Infection rates differ greatly by country, with 50% of the population in the United States having positive HSV-1 serology, compared with 80% in Africa. Socioeconomic status and age greatly affect seropositivity rates (165). Only limited epidemiologic data are available, but Liesegang et al. reported the incidence of first-episode ocular HSV infection to be 8.4 per 100,000 person-years, with an overall prevalence of a history of ocular HSV infection of 149 per 100,000 persons in 1980 (105).

The mean age of presentation was 37 years, and 36% of patients had a recurrence within 5 years. A study from Moorfields Eye Hospital in London followed patients for recurrence for up to 15 years. Similar rates of recurrence were reported as in other studies, but most involved the lids or conjunctiva, with only 9% showing corneal dendritic recurrence (166). Of those who present with corneal epithelial disease, however, up to 45% may have recurrent epithelial disease, and 25% may have stromal disease (167). Regarding other risk factors, Brandt et al. found no relationship between male sex, corticosteroid use, contact lens wear, or oral HSV infections (168). In addition, authors of one report observed that human immunodeficiency virus (HIV) infection predisposes to an increased risk of recurrent disease among patients with ocular HSV disease (169,170).

The Herpetic Eye Disease Study (HEDS) was important in establishing therapeutic guidelines for the treatment and prevention of recurrent ocular herpes (171–173). The study provided a number of important findings: (a) recurrence of ocular herpes is decreased by the administration of oral acyclovir; (b) oral acyclovir does not prevent the development of corneal stromal disease, nor does it help resolution of stromal disease in patients already on topical antivirals and steroids; and (c) topical steroids are beneficial for resolution of stromal keratitis.

Herpes Zoster Ophthalmicus

Herpes zoster ophthalmicus (HZO) represents reactivation of the varicella zoster virus in the V1 dermatome affecting the ocular structures. Its relatively high incidence represents the near-universal infection of the population with varicella. Of adults in their sixth decade, >99.8% are seropositive (174). The estimated incidence of HZO is 1.2 to 3.4 cases per 1000 person-years, with most cases occurring after age 65 years (104). Major risk factors include age, immunosuppression (including HIV disease), and chronic illness (175).

Keratitis is the most common cause of visual impairment in HZO, affecting two thirds of patients with the disease (176). Most patients have dendritic keratitis, but the disease may progress to nummular keratitis in 20% to 35% of patients (177) or disciform in 10% (176). Unlike HSV disease, HZO is strongly associated with HIV infection, and the increase in the rate of HZO in HIV infection is sufficient to consider it an opportunistic infection (178). In young adults, HZO can raise suspicion of HIV infection in the absence of other causes of immunosuppression. A recent review of the Olmsted County data has demonstrated that the use of systemic antivirals may have a benefit in the prevention of neurotrophic keratitis and the development of severe vision loss at 5 and 10 years after diagnosis of HZO (179).

Acanthamoeba Keratitis

Before the era of contact lenses, *Acanthamoeba* keratitis (AK) was exceedingly rare. The popularity of soft lenses in the

1980s led to an increase in the incidence of the disease. Although it is difficult to estimate the number of contact lens wearers from which to calculate the increased risk, the annual incidence has been estimated to have been between 1.65 and 2.01 per million contact lens wearers in the United States between 1985 and 1987 (108). Estimates for 1997 through 1999 have been published for the United Kingdom, with an annual incidence for the 2 years of 1.26 and 1.13 cases per million per year overall, and 21.14 and 17.53 cases per million per year for contact lens wearers (107). The higher incidence shown in this recent study from the United Kingdom may reflect greater recognition of the disease in contact lens wearers as knowledge regarding its pathogenesis has spread. Other important factors may include the use of chlorine-based disinfection systems (which have lower efficacy than systems used popularly in the United States), use of hard water in many households (the presence of lime scale may promote survival of *Acanthamoeba*), and swimming while wearing contact lenses (especially in the ocean or fresh water).

Risk factors for AK have been examined in a few studies, particularly in the United Kingdom. Radford et al. published a series of 243 cases diagnosed from 1992 to 1996 (180), showing that 93% were contact lens wearers, among whom 62% did not reliably disinfect their lenses and 34% often swam in their lenses. However, no comparison group was studied, so it is unclear how these contact lens hygiene practices compare with those of the contact lens–wearing population in general. Nonetheless, in a prior case–control study, these investigators demonstrated a significantly increased risk related to lack of disinfection (OR, 55.9), use of chlorine-based disinfection (OR, 14.6), and use of frequent replacement soft contact lenses (OR, 3.8). Of some interest, there did not appear to be an increased risk of AK associated with overnight wear, although power may have been extremely limited for this analysis (estimates were not provided) (181). In the more recent study, a poorer outcome was seen for non–contact lens wearers, perhaps secondary to delayed correct diagnosis (180).

Contamination of lenses and lens storage materials with nonsterile water has been thought to be a major risk factor for AK, and several lines of evidence support the connection. Mathers et al. found that levels of *Acanthamoeba* in ground water may correlate with cases of AK (182). Meier et al. reported on an outbreak of AK after a period of flooding in Iowa (183). The use of homemade saline has been definitively associated with risk of AK. The earliest reports implicating homemade saline emerged in the mid-1980s. In 1987, Stehr-Green et al. published a case–control study sponsored by the Centers for Disease Control wherein 78% of cases used homemade saline compared with 17% of control subjects (odds ratio approaching infinity) (184). Several additional studies directly examining contamination of contact lens solutions revealed that tap water was clearly the source of *Acanthamoeba* introduction (185,186).

Although there has been education to stop the use of homemade saline for the care of contact lenses and to reduce other risky behaviors, recent studies suggest that this effort has been less than entirely successful (180). Future estimates from previously studied populations would provide useful data to assess trends in AK incidence and risk factors.

Fungal Keratitis

Although a rare cause of keratitis in the United States, fungal infections are often suspected in cases of nonresolving ulceration. The actual incidence of the disease is difficult to ascertain, but geographic trends suggest a dramatically increased risk in warmer climates.

One U.S. study of 24 cases over an 8-year period found that the main risk factors were ocular surface disease, contact lens wear, atopy, topical steroid use, and, last, trauma (187). *Candida* was the most common organism isolated. Six of the 24 (25%) eventually underwent penetrating keratoplasty, and 13 (54.1%) achieved best-corrected vision of 20/100 or better.

Many groups have published data on fungal keratitis in tropical regions. One review of 1352 cases of fungal keratitis in southern India found that young men were predominantly represented, perhaps related to the finding that a preceding history of trauma (typically agricultural) was noted in 54.4% of cases (188). Cases were more likely to have occurred in the monsoon season. *Fusarium* was the most prevalent species found. A series of 29 patients in Singapore reported similar findings, with 23 of 29 being male, and ocular trauma reported in more than half of the patients (189). *Fusarium* was also the most commonly isolated species. A review of 211 cases of fungal keratitis in children in India reported a history of trauma in 55.3%, with *Aspergillus* and *Fusarium* being the most common pathogens (190). The overall prevalence of fungal keratitis as a percentage of all cases of suppurative keratitis was reported by one group as 35.9% in Bangladesh (vs. 53.5% bacterial) (191), but even higher in another study comparing Ghana (37.6%) with southern India (44%) (110). A further risk factor for fungal keratitis in Africa may be the high prevalence of HIV disease (192). The significance of the high incidence of fungal keratitis in the tropics is that these regions may not have the equipment needed to establish the microbiologic diagnosis; therefore, providers must maintain high suspicion and choose empirical treatment based on geographic trends.

REFERENCES

1. McMonnies CW, Ho H. Patient history in screening for dry eye conditions. *J Am Optom Assoc* 1987;58:296–301.
2. Lemp MA. Epidemiology and classification of dry eye. *Adv Exp Med Biol* 1998;438:791–803.
3. Nelson JD, Helms H, Fiscella R, et al. A new look at dry eye disease and its treatment. *Adv Ther* 2000;17:84–93.
4. Lemp MA. Report of the National Eye Institute/Industry Workshop on Clinical Trials in Dry Eyes. *CLAO J* 1995;21:221–232.
5. Schein OD, Munoz B, Tielsch JM, et al. Prevalence of dry eye among the elderly. *Am J Ophthalmol* 1997;124:723–728.

6. Moss SE, Klein R, Klein BE. Prevalence of and risk factors for dry eye syndrome. *Arch Ophthalmol* 2000;118:1264–1268.

7. McCarty CA, Bansal AK, Livingston PM, et al. The epidemiology of dry eye in Melbourne, Australia. *Ophthalmology* 1998; 105:1114–1119.

8. Schaumberg DA, Buring JE, Sullivan DA, et al. The epidemiology of dry eye syndrome. *Cornea* 2000;19:S120.

9. Schein OD, Tielsch JM, Munoz B, et al. Relation between signs and symptoms of dry eye in the elderly: a population-based perspective. *Ophthalmology* 1997;104:1395–1401.

10. Schaumberg DA, Sullivan DA, Buring JE, et al. Hormone replacement therapy and the prevalence of dry eye symptoms in women. *Invest Ophthalmol Vis Sci* 2000;41:S740.

11. Nichols KK, Nichols JJ, Zadnik K. Frequency of dry eye diagnostic test procedures used in various modes of ophthalmic practice. *Cornea* 2000;19:477–482.

12. Korb DR. Survey of preferred tests for diagnosis of the tear film and dry eye. *Cornea* 2000;19:483–486.

13. Rexrode KM, Lee I, Cook NR, et al. Baseline characteristic of participants in the Women's Health Study. *J Womens Health Gend Based Med* 2000;9:19–27.

14. Steering Committee of the Physicians' Health Study Research Group. Final report on the aspirin component of the ongoing Physicians' Health Study [see comments]. N Engl J Med 1989; 321:129–135.

15. Oden NL, Lilienfeld DE, Lemp MA, et al. Sensitivity and specificity of a screening questionnaire for dry eye. *Adv Exp Med Biol* 1998;438:807–820.

16. Schaumberg DA, Sullivan DA, Buring JE, et al. Prevalence of dry eye syndrome among US women. *Am J Ophthalmol* 2003 Aug;136(2):318–326.

17. Mathers WD, Lane JA, Zimmerman MB. Tear film changes associated with normal aging. *Cornea* 1996;15:229–234.

18. Henderson JW, Prough WA. Influence of age and sex on flow of tears. *Arch Ophthalmol* 1950;43:224–231.

19. Moss SE, Klein R, Klein BE. Incidence of dry eye in an older population. ARVO Abstracts. *Invest Ophthalmol Vis Sci* 2003; 44[4 Suppl]:810(abstr).

20. Sullivan DA, Wickham LA, et al. Influence of gender, sex steroid hormones, and the hypothalamic-pituitary axis on the structure and function of the lacrimal gland. *Adv Exp Med Biol* 1998;438:11–42.

21. Ahmed SA, Aufdemorte TB, et al. Estrogen induces the development of autoantibodies and promotes salivary gland lymphoid infiltrates in normal mice. *J Autoimmun* 1989;2:543–552.

22. Sato EH, Sullivan DA. Comparative influence of steroid hormones and immunosuppressive agents on autoimmune expression in lacrimal glands of a female mouse model of Sjögren's syndrome. *Invest Ophthalmol Vis Sci* 1994;35:2632–2642.

23. Sullivan DA, Wickham LA, et al. Androgens and dry eye in Sjögren's syndrome. *Ann NY Acad Sci* 1999;876:312–324.

24. Cutolo M, Sulli A, Seriolo B, et al. Estrogens, the immune response and autoimmunity. *Clin Exp Rheumatol* 1995;13:217–226.

25. Imperato-McGinley J, Gautier T, et al. The androgen control of sebum production: studies of subjects with dihydrotestosterone deficiency and complete androgen insensitivity. *J Clin Endocrinol Metab* 1993;76:524–528.

26. Sullivan DA, Rocha EM, et al. Androgen regulation of the meibomian gland. *Adv Exp Med Biol* 1998;438:327–31.

27. Bologna JL. Aging skin. *Am J Med* 1995;[Suppl 1A]:99S–102S.

28. Schein OD, Hochberg MC, et al. Dry eye and dry mouth in the elderly: a population-based assessment. *Arch Intern Med* 1999; 159:1359–1363.

29. Schaumberg DA, Buring JE, Sullivan DA, et al. Hormone replacement therapy and dry eye syndrome. *JAMA* 2001; 286:2114–2119.

30. Trivedi KA, Dana MR, Gilbard JP, et al. Omega-3 fatty acid intake and risk of clinically diagnosed dry eye syndrome in women. ARVO Abstracts. *Invest Ophthalmol Vis Sci* 2003;44[4 Suppl]: 811(abstr).

31. Kosrirukvongs P, Visitsunthorn N, Vichyanond P, et al. Allergic conjunctivitis. *Asian Pac J Allergy Immunol* 2001;19:237–244.

32. Wuthrich B, Brignoli R, Canevascini M, et al. Epidemiological survey in hay fever patients: symptom prevalence and severity and influence on patient management. *Schweiz Med Wochenschr* 1998;128:139–143.

33. Ray NF, Baraniuk JN, et al. Direct expenditures for the treatment of allergic rhinoconjunctivitis in 1996, including the contributions of related airway illnesses. *J Allergy Clin Immunol* 1999;103:401–407.

34. Austin JB, Kaur B, et al. Hay fever, eczema, and wheeze: a nationwide UK study (ISAAC, international study of asthma and allergies in childhood). *Arch Dis Child* 1999;81:225–230.

35. Asher MI, Barry D, et al. The burden of symptoms of asthma, allergic rhinoconjunctivitis and atopic eczema in children and adolescents in six New Zealand centres: ISAAC Phase One. *N Z Med J* 2001;114:114–120.

36. Falade AG, Olawuyi F, Osinusi K, et al. Prevalence and severity of symptoms of asthma, allergic rhino-conjunctivitis and atopic eczema in secondary school children in Ibadan, Nigeria. *East Afr Med J* 1998;75:695–698.

37. Lee S, Shin M, et al. Prevalences of symptoms of asthma and other allergic diseases in Korean children: a nationwide questionnaire survey. *J Korean Med Sci* 2001;16:155–164.

38. Norrman E, Rosenhall L, Nystrom L, et al. Prevalence of positive skin prick tests, allergic asthma, and rhinoconjunctivitis in teenagers in northern Sweden. *Allergy* 1994;49:808–815.

39. Novembre E, Cianferoni A, et al. Epidemiology of insect venom sensitivity in children and its correlation to clinical and atopic features. *Clin Exp Allergy* 1998;28:834–838.

40. Saraclar Y, Yigit S, Adalioglu G, et al. Prevalence of allergic diseases and influencing factors in primary-school children in the Ankara Region of Turkey. *J Asthma* 1997;34:23–30.

41. Kucukoduk S, Aydin M, et al. The prevalence of asthma and other allergic diseases in a province of Turkey. *Turk J Pediatr* 1996;38:149–153.

42. Hesselmar B, Aberg B, Eriksson B, et al. Allergic rhinoconjunctivitis, eczema, and sensitization in two areas with differing climates. *Pediatr Allergy Immunol* 2001;12:208–215.

43. Aberg N. Asthma and allergic rhinitis in Swedish conscripts. *Clin Exp Allergy* 1989;19:59–63.

44. Sly RM. Changing prevalence of allergic rhinitis and asthma. *Ann Allergy Asthma Immunol* 1999;82:233–248.

45. Davies RJ, Rusznak C, Devalia JL. Why is allergy increasing?— Environmental factors. *Clin Exp Allergy* 1998;28[Suppl 6]:8–14.

46. Nishimura A, Campbell-Meltzer RS, Chute K, et al. Genetics of allergic disease: evidence for organ-specific susceptibility genes. *Int Arch Allergy Immunol* 2001;124:197–200.

47. Kilpelainen M, Terho EO, Helenius H, et al. Farm environment in childhood prevents the development of allergies. *Clin Exp Allergy* 2000;30:201–208.

48. Kilpelainen M, Koskenvuo M, Helenius H, et al. Wood stove heating, asthma and allergies. *Respir Med* 2001;95:911–916.

49. Dotterud LK, Odland JO, Falk ES. Atopic diseases among adults in the two geographically related arctic areas Nikel, Russia and Sor-Varanger, Norway: possible effects of indoor and outdoor air pollution. *J Eur Acad Dermatol Venereol* 2000;14:107–111.

50. Wakai K, Okamoto K, et al. Seasonal allergic rhinoconjunctivitis and fatty acid intake: a cross-sectional study in Japan. *Ann Epidemiol* 2001;11:59–64.

51. Ellwood P, Asher MI, et al. Diet and asthma, allergic rhinoconjunctivitis and atopic eczema symptom prevalence: an ecological analysis of the International Study of Asthma and Allergies in

Childhood (ISAAC) data. ISAAC Phase One Study Group. *Eur Respir J* 2001;17:436–443.

52. Weiland SK, von Mutius E, Husing A, et al. Intake of trans fatty acids and prevalence of childhood asthma and allergies in Europe. ISAAC Steering Committee. *Lancet* 1999;353:2040–2041.

53. Spring TF. Reaction to hydrophilic lenses. *Med J Aust* 1974; 1:449–450.

54. Korb DR, Allansmith MR, et al. Prevalence of conjunctival changes in wearers of hard contact lenses. *Am J Ophthalmol* 1980; 90:336–341.

55. Donshik PC. Giant papillary conjunctivitis. *Trans Am Ophthalmol Soc* 1994;92:687–744.

56. Allansmith MR, Baird RS. Evidence for lack of antigenicity of polymacon contact lens material in guinea pigs. *Ophthalmic Res* 1980;12:192–198.

57. Refojo M, Holly F. Tear protein adsorption on hydrogels: a possible cause of contact lens allergy. *Contact Intraoc Lens Med J* 1977;3:23–25.

58. Kari O, Teir H, Huuskonen R, et al. Tolerance to different kinds of contact lenses in young atopic and non-atopic wearers. *CLAO J* 2001;27:151–154.

59. Hart DE, Schkolnick JA, Bernstein S, et al. Contact lens induced giant papillary conjunctivitis: a retrospective study. *J Am Optom Assoc* 1989;60:195–204.

60. Donshik PC, Porazinski AD. Giant papillary conjunctivitis in frequent-replacement contact lens wearers: a retrospective study. *Trans Am Ophthalmol Soc* 1999;97:205–216.

61. Montan PG, Ekstrom K, et al. Vernal keratoconjunctivitis in a Stockholm ophthalmic centre: epidemiological, functional, and immunologic investigations. *Acta Ophthalmol Scand* 1999; 77:559–563.

62. Frankland AW, Easty D. Vernal kerato-conjunctivitis: an atopic disease. *Trans Ophthalmol Soc U K* 1971;91:479–482.

63. Neumann E, Gutmann M, Blumenkrantz N, et al. A review of four hundred cases of vernal conjunctivitis. *Am J Ophthalmol* 1959;47:166–172.

64. Bonini S, Lambiase A, et al. Vernal keratoconjunctivitis revisited: a case series of 195 patients with long-term followup. *Ophthalmology* 2000;107:1157–1163.

65. O'Shea JG. A survey of vernal keratoconjunctivitis and other eosinophil-mediated external eye diseases amongst Palestinians. *Ophthalmic Epidemiol* 2000;7:149–157.

66. Tabbara KF. Ocular complications of vernal keratoconjunctivitis. *Can J Ophthalmol* 1999;34:88–92.

67. Trocme SD, Sra KK. Spectrum of ocular allergy. *Curr Opin Allergy Clin Immunol* 2002;2:423–427.

68. Bielory L. Allergic and immunologic disorders of the eye: Part II. Ocular allergy. *J Allergy Clin Immunol* 2000;106:1019–1032.

69. Foster CS, Calonge M. Atopic keratoconjunctivitis. *Ophthalmology* 1990;97:992–1000.

70. Garrity JA, Liesegang TJ. Ocular complications of atopic dermatitis. *Can J Ophthalmol* 1984;19:21–24.

71. Lyons CJ, Dart JK, Aclimandos WA, et al. Sclerokeratitis after keratoplasty in atopy. *Ophthalmology* 1990;97:729–733.

72. Ghoraishi M, Akova YA, Tugal-Tutkun I, et al. Penetrating keratoplasty in atopic keratoconjunctivitis. *Cornea* 1995;14: 610–613.

73. Krachmer JH, Feder RS, Belin MW. Keratoconus and related noninflammatory corneal thinning disorders. *Surv Ophthalmol* 1984;28:293–322.

74. Zadnik K, Barr JT, et al. Baseline findings in the Collaborative Longitudinal Evaluation of Keratoconus (CLEK) Study. *Invest Ophthalmol Vis Sci* 1998;39:2537–2546.

75. Tuft SJ, Moodaley LC, Gregory WM, et al. Prognostic factors for the progression of keratoconus. *Ophthalmology* 1994;101: 439–447.

76. Kennedy RH, Bourne WM, Dyer JA. A 48-year clinical and epidemiologic study of keratoconus. *Am J Ophthalmol* 1986; 101:267–273.

77. Pearson AR, Soneji B, Sarvananthan N, et al. Does ethnic origin influence the incidence or severity of keratoconus? *Eye* 2000; 14:625–628.

78. Ihalainen A. Clinical and epidemiological features of keratoconus genetic and external factors in the pathogenesis of the disease. *Acta Ophthalmol Suppl* 1986;178:1–64.

79. Greiner JV, Leahy CD, et al. Histopathology of the ocular surface after eye rubbing. *Cornea* 1997;16:327–332.

80. Kim WJ, Rabinowitz YS, Meisler DM, et al. Keratocyte apoptosis associated with keratoconus. *Exp Eye Res* 1999;69: 475–481.

81. Wilson SE, He YG, et al. Epithelial injury induces keratocyte apoptosis: hypothesized role for the interleukin-1 system in the modulation of corneal tissue organization and wound healing. *Exp Eye Res* 1996;62:325-7.

82. Bawazeer AM, Hodge WG, Lorimer B. Atopy and keratoconus: a multivariate analysis. *Br J Ophthalmol* 2000;84: 834–836.

83. Totan Y, Hepsen IF, Cekic O, et al. Incidence of keratoconus in subjects with vernal keratoconjunctivitis: a videokeratographic study. *Ophthalmology* 2001;108:824–827.

84. Gasset AR, Hinson WA, Frias JL. Keratoconus and atopic diseases. *Ann Ophthalmol* 1978;10:991–994.

85. Rabinowitz YS. Keratoconus. *Surv Ophthalmol* 1998;42:297-319.

86. Shapiro MB, France TD. The ocular features of Down's syndrome. *Am J Ophthalmol* 1985;99:659–663.

87. van Allen MI, Fung J, Jurenka SB. Health care concerns and guidelines for adults with Down syndrome. *Am J Med Genet* 1999; 89:100–110.

88. Walsh SZ. Keratoconus and blindness in 469 institutionalised subjects with Down syndrome and other causes of mental retardation. *J Ment Defic Res* 1981;25:243–251.

89. Robertson I. Keratoconus and the Ehlers-Danlos syndrome: a new aspect of keratoconus. *Med J Aust* 1975;1:571–573.

90. Beardsley TL, Foulks GN. An association of keratoconus and mitral valve prolapse. *Ophthalmology* 1982;89:35–37.

91. Sharif KW, Casey TA, Coltart J. Prevalence of mitral valve prolapse in keratoconus patients. *J R Soc Med* 1992;85:446–448.

92. Street DA, Vinokur ET, et al. Lack of association between keratoconus, mitral valve prolapse, and joint hypermobility. *Ophthalmology* 1991;98:170–176.

93. Woodward EG, Morris MT. Joint hypermobility in keratoconus. *Ophthalmic Physiol Opt* 1990;10:360–362.

94. Lowell FC, Carroll JM. A study of the occurrence of atopic traits in patients with keratoconus. *J Allergy* 1970;46:32–39.

95. Davies PD, Lobascher D, Menon JA, et al. Immunological studies in keratoconus. *Trans Ophthalmol Soc U K* 1976;96:173–178.

96. Rahi A, Davies P, Ruben M, et al. Keratoconus and coexisting atopic disease. *Br J Ophthalmol* 1977;61:761–764.

97. Harrison RJ, Klouda PT, et al. Association between keratoconus and atopy. *Br J Ophthalmol* 1989;73:816–822.

98. Khan MD, Kundi N, Saeed N, et al. Incidence of keratoconus in spring catarrh. *Br J Ophthalmol* 1988;72:41–43.

99. Owens H, Gamble G. A profile of keratoconus in New Zealand. *Cornea* 2003;22:122–125.

100. Bechara SJ, Waring GO III, Insler MS. Keratoconus in two pairs of identical twins. *Cornea* 1996;15:90–93.

101. Parker J, Ko WW, et al. Videokeratography of keratoconus in monozygotic twins. *J Refract Surg* 1996;12:180–183.

102. McMahon TT, Shin JA, et al. Discordance for keratoconus in two pairs of monozygotic twins. *Cornea* 1999;18:444–451.

103. Wang Y, Rabinowitz YS, Rotter JI, et al. Genetic epidemiological study of keratoconus: evidence for major gene determination. *Am J Med Genet* 2000;93:403–409.

104. Schmader KE. Epidemiology of herpes zoster. In: Arvin AM, Gershon AA, eds. *Varicella zoster virus: virology and clinical management.* Cambridge, United Kingdom: Cambridge University Press, 2000:220–245.

105. Liesegang TJ, Melton LJ III, Daly PJ, et al. Epidemiology of ocular herpes simplex: incidence in Rochester, Minn, 1950 through 1982. *Arch Ophthalmol* 1989;107:1155–1159.

106. Erie JC, Nevitt MP, Hodge DO, et al. Incidence of ulcerative keratitis in a defined population from 1950 through 1988. *Arch Ophthalmol* 1993;111:1665–1671.

107. Radford CF, Minassian DC, Dart JK. *Acanthamoeba* keratitis in England and Wales: incidence, outcome, and risk factors. *Br J Ophthalmol* 2002;86:536–542.

108. Schaumberg DA, Snow KK, Dana MR. The epidemic of *Acanthamoeba* keratitis: where do we stand? *Cornea* 1998;17: 3–10.

109. Liesegang TJ, Forster RK. Spectrum of microbial keratitis in South Florida. *Am J Ophthalmol* 1980;90:38–47.

110. Leck AK, Thomas PA, et al. Aetiology of suppurative corneal ulcers in Ghana and south India, and epidemiology of fungal keratitis. *Br J Ophthalmol* 2002;86:1211–1215.

111. Groden LR, Murphy B, Rodnite J, et al. Lid flora in blepharitis. *Cornea* 1991;10:50–53.

112. McCulley JP. Blepharoconjunctivitis. *Int Ophthalmol Clin* 1984; 24:65–77.

113. Smolin G, Okumoto M. Staphylococcal blepharitis. *Arch Ophthalmol* 1977;95:812–816.

114. Huber-Spitzy V, Baumgartner I, Bohler-Sommeregger K, et al. Blepharitis—a diagnostic and therapeutic challenge: a report on 407 consecutive cases. *Graefes Arch Clin Exp Ophthalmol* 1991; 229:224–227.

115. Saitoh-Inagawa W, Aoki K, Uchio E, et al. Ten years' surveillance of viral conjunctivitis in Sapporo, Japan. *Graefes Arch Clin Exp Ophthalmol* 1999;237:35–38.

116. Jernigan JA, Lowry BS, et al. Adenovirus type 8 epidemic keratoconjunctivitis in an eye clinic: risk factors and control. *J Infect Dis* 1993;167:1307–1313.

117. Chaberny IE, Schnitzler P, Geiss HK, et al. An outbreak of epidemic keratoconjunctivitis in a pediatric unit due to adenovirus type 8. *Infect Control Hosp Epidemiol* 2003;24:514–519.

118. Mueller AJ, Klauss V. Main sources of infection in 145 cases of epidemic keratoconjunctivitis. *German J Ophthalmol* 1993;2: 224–227.

119. Buffington J, Chapman LE, et al. Epidemic keratoconjunctivitis in a chronic care facility: risk factors and measures for control. *J Am Geriatr Soc* 1993;41:1177–1181.

120. Uchio E, Takeuchi S, et al. Clinical and epidemiological features of acute follicular conjunctivitis with special reference to that caused by herpes simplex virus type 1. *Br J Ophthalmol* 2000; 84:968–972.

121. Darougar S, Monnickendam MA, Woodland RM. Management and prevention of ocular viral and chlamydial infections. *Crit Rev Microbiol* 1989;16:369–418.

122. Jackson WB. Differentiating conjunctivitis of diverse origins. *Surv Ophthalmol* 1993;38:91–104.

123. Seal DV, Barrett SP, McGill JI. Aetiology and treatment of acute bacterial infection of the external eye. *Br J Ophthalmol* 1982; 66:357–360.

124. Boustcha E, Nicolle LE. Conjunctivitis in a long-term care facility. *Infect Control Hosp Epidemiol* 1995;16:210–216.

125. Martin M, Turco JH, et al. An outbreak of conjunctivitis due to atypical *Streptococcus pneumoniae. N Engl J Med* 2003;348: 1112–1121.

126. Shah SS, Gloor P, Gallagher PG. Bacteremia, meningitis, and brain abscesses in a hospitalized infant: complications of *Pseudomonas aeruginosa* conjunctivitis. *J Perinatol* 1999;19:462–465.

127. Santer DM, Myhre JA, Yogev R. Primary group Y meningococcal conjunctivitis and occult meningococcemia. *Pediatr Infect Dis J* 1992;11:54–55.

128. Postema EJ, Remeijer L, van der Meijden WI. Epidemiology of genital chlamydial infections in patients with chlamydial conjunctivitis: a retrospective study. *Genitourin Med* 1996;72: 203–205.

129. Garland SM, Malatt A, et al. *Chlamydia trachomatis* conjunctivitis: prevalence and association with genital tract infection. *Med J Aust* 1995;162:363–36.

130. Thylefors B, Negrel AD, Pararajasegaram R, et al. Global data on blindness. *Bull World Health Organ* 1995;73:115–121.

131. Tabbara KF, al-Omar OM. Trachoma in Saudi Arabia. *Ophthalmic Epidemiol* 1997;4:127–140.

132. Lansingh VC, Weih LM, Keeffe JE, et al. Assessment of trachoma prevalence in a mobile population in Central Australia. *Ophthalmic Epidemiol* 2001;8:97–108.

133. Bejiga A, Alemayehu W. Prevalence of trachoma and its determinants in Dalocha District, Central Ethiopia. *Ophthalmic Epidemiol* 2001;8:119–125.

134. Ezz al Arab G, Tawfik N, El Gendy R, et al. The burden of trachoma in the rural Nile Delta of Egypt: a survey of Menofiya governorate. *Br J Ophthalmol* 2001;85:1406–1410.

135. Schachter J, West SK, et al. Azithromycin in control of trachoma. *Lancet* 1999;354:630–635.

136. Mikru FS, Molla T, et al. Community-wide outbreak of *Neisseria gonorrhoeae* conjunctivitis in Konso district, North Omo administrative region. *Ethiop Med J* 1991;2:27–35.

137. Schwab L, Tizazu T. Destructive epidemic *Neisseria gonorrhoeae* keratoconjunctivitis in African adults. *Br J Ophthalmol* 1985;69: 525–528.

138. Alfonso E, Friedland B, et al. *Neisseria gonorrhoeae* conjunctivitis: an outbreak during an epidemic of acute hemorrhagic conjunctivitis. *JAMA* 1983;250:794–795.

139. Mak DB, Smith DW, Harnett GB, et al. A large outbreak of conjunctivitis caused by a single genotype of *Neisseria gonorrhoeae* distinct from those causing genital tract infections. *Epidemiol Infect* 2001;126:373–378.

140. Laga M, Meheus A, Piot P. Epidemiology and control of gonococcal ophthalmia neonatorum. *Bull World Health Organ* 1989; 67:471–477.

141. Dannevig L, Straume B, Melby K. Ophthalmia neonatorum in northern Norway: II. Microbiology with emphasis on *Chlamydia trachomatis. Acta Ophthalmol* 1992;70:19–25.

142. Di Bartolomeo S, Mirta DH, et al. Incidence of *Chlamydia trachomatis* and other potential pathogens in neonatal conjunctivitis. *Int J Infect Dis* 2001;5:139–143.

143. Mohile M, Deorari AK, Satpathy G, et al. Microbiological study of neonatal conjunctivitis with special reference to *Chlamydia trachomatis. Indian J Ophthalmol* 2002;50:295–299.

144. Nsanze H, Dawodu A, Usmani A, et al. Ophthalmia neonatorum in the United Arab Emirates. *Ann Trop Paediatr* 1996;16: 27–32.

145. Isenberg SJ, Apt L, Wood M. A controlled trial of povidone-iodine as prophylaxis against ophthalmia neonatorum. *N Engl J Med* 1995;332:562–566.

146. Schein OD, Glynn RJ, Poggio EC, et al. The relative risk of ulcerative keratitis among users of daily-wear and extended-wear soft contact lenses: a case-control study. Microbial Keratitis Study Group. *N Engl J Med* 1989;321:773–778.

147. Poggio EC, Glynn RJ, et al. The incidence of ulcerative keratitis among users of daily-wear and extended-wear soft contact lenses. *N Engl J Med* 1989;321:779–783.

148. Schein OD, Buehler PO, Stamler JF, et al. The impact of overnight wear on the risk of contact lens-associated ulcerative keratitis. *Arch Ophthalmol* 1994;112:186–190.

149. Cheng KH, Leung SL, et al. Incidence of contact-lens-associated microbial keratitis and its related morbidity. *Lancet* 1999;354: 181–185.

150. Liesegang TJ. Contact lens-related microbial keratitis: Part I. Epidemiology. *Cornea* 1997;16:125–131.

151. Matthews TD, Frazer DG, Minassian DC, Radford CF, Dart JK. Risks of keratitis and patterns of use with disposable contact lenses. *Arch Ophthalmol* 1992;110:1559–1562.

152. Dart JK, Stapleton F, Minassian D. Contact lenses and other risk factors in microbial keratitis. *Lancet* 1991;338:650–653.

153. Cohen EJ, Fulton JC, Hoffman CJ, et al. Trends in contact lens-associated corneal ulcers. *Cornea* 1996;15:566–570.

154. Dunn JP Jr, Mondino BJ, Weissman BA, et al. Corneal ulcers associated with disposable hydrogel contact lenses. *Am J Ophthalmol* 1989;108:113–117.

155. Dumbleton K. Noninflammatory silicone hydrogel contact lens complications. *Eye Contact Lens* 2003;29:S186–S189.

156. Tuft SJ, Matheson M. In vitro antibiotic resistance in bacterial keratitis in London. *Br J Ophthalmol* 2000;84:687–691.

157. Goldstein MH, Kowalski RP, Gordon YJ. Emerging fluoroquinolone resistance in bacterial keratitis: a 5-year review. *Ophthalmology* 1999;106:1313–1318.

158. Alexandrakis G, Alfonso EC, Miller D. Shifting trends in bacterial keratitis in south Florida and emerging resistance to fluoroquinolones. *Ophthalmology* 2000;107:1497–1502.

159. Freitas D, Alvarenga L, et al. An outbreak of *Mycobacterium chelonae* infection after LASIK. *Ophthalmology* 2003;110:276–285.

160. Boonpasart S, Kasetsuwan N, Puangsricharern V, et al. Infectious keratitis at King Chulalongkorn Memorial Hospital: a 12-year retrospective study of 391 cases. *J Med Assoc Thai* 2002;85: S217–S230.

161. Kunimoto DY, Sharma S, et al. Corneal ulceration in the elderly in Hyderabad, south India. *Br J Ophthalmol* 2000;84:54–59.

162. Srinivasan M, Gonzales CA, et al. Epidemiology and aetiological diagnosis of corneal ulceration in Madurai, south India. *Br J Ophthalmol* 1997;81:965–971.

163. Hagan M, Wright E, Newman M, et al. Causes of suppurative keratitis in Ghana. *Br J Ophthalmol* 1995;79:1024–1028.

164. Vajpayee RB, Ray M, et al. Risk factors for pediatric presumed microbial keratitis: a case-control study. *Cornea* 1999;18:565–569.

165. Whitley RJ, Kimberlin DW, Roizman B. Herpes simplex viruses. *Clin Infect Dis* 1998;26:541–553.

166. Wishart MS, Darougar S, Viswalingam ND. Recurrent herpes simplex virus ocular infection: epidemiological and clinical features. *Br J Ophthalmol* 1987;71:669–672.

167. Wilhelmus KR, Falcon MG, Jones BR. Bilateral herpetic keratitis. *Br J Ophthalmol* 1981;65:385–387.

168. Brandt BM, Mandleblatt J, Asbell PA. Risk factors for herpes simplex-induced keratitis: a case-control study. *Ann Ophthalmol* 1994;26:12–16.

169. Pramod NP, Rajendran P, Kannan KA, et al. Herpes simplex keratitis in South India: clinico-virological correlation. *Jpn J Ophthalmol* 1999;43:303–307.

170. Hodge WG, Margolis TP. Herpes simplex virus keratitis among patients who are positive or negative for human immunodeficiency virus: an epidemiologic study. *Ophthalmology* 1997;104: 120–124.

171. Herpetic Eye Disease Study Group. Acyclovir for the prevention of recurrent herpes simplex virus eye disease. Herpetic Eye Disease Study Group. *N Engl J Med* 1998;339:300–306.

172. Wilhelmus KR, Gee L, et al. Herpetic Eye Disease Study: a controlled trial of topical corticosteroids for herpes simplex stromal keratitis. *Ophthalmology* 1994;101:1883–1895.

173. Barron BA, Gee L, et al. Herpetic Eye Disease Study: a controlled trial of oral acyclovir for herpes simplex stromal keratitis. *Ophthalmology* 1994;101:1871–1882.

174. Kilgore PE, Kruszon-Moran D, Seward JF, et al. Varicella in Americans from NHANES III: implications for control through routine immunization. *J Med Virol.* 2003;70 Suppl 1:S111–S1118.

175. Starr CE, Pavan-Langston D. Varicella-zoster virus: mechanisms of pathogenicity and corneal disease. *Ophthalmol Clin North Am* 2002;15:7–15.

176. Pavan-Langston D. Ophthalmic zoster. In: Arvin AM, Gershon AA, eds. *Varicella zoster virus: virology and clinical management.* Cambridge, United Kingdom: Cambridge University Press, 2000: 276–298.

177. Womack LW, Liesegang TJ. Complications of herpes zoster ophthalmicus. *Arch Ophthalmol* 1983;101:42–45.

178. Hodge WG, Seiff SR, Margolis TP. Ocular opportunistic infection incidences among patients who are HIV positive compared to patients who are HIV negative. *Ophthalmology* 1998; 105:895–900.

179. Severson EA, Baratz KH, Hodge DO, et al. Herpes zoster ophthalmicus in Olmsted county, Minnesota: have systemic antivirals made a difference? *Arch Ophthalmol* 2003;121:386–390.

180. Radford CF, Lehmann OJ, Dart JK. *Acanthamoeba* keratitis: multicentre survey in England 1992–6. National *Acanthamoeba* Keratitis Study Group. *Br J Ophthalmol* 1998;82: 1387–1392.

181. Radford CF, Bacon AS, Dart JK, et al. Risk factors for *Acanthamoeba* keratitis in contact lens users: a case-control study. *BMJ* 1995;310:1567–1570.

182. Mathers WD, Sutphin JE, Lane JA, et al. Correlation between surface water contamination with amoeba and the onset of symptoms and diagnosis of amoeba-like keratitis. *Br J Ophthalmol* 1998;82:1143–1146.

183. Meier PA, Mathers WD, et al. An epidemic of presumed *Acanthamoeba* keratitis that followed regional flooding: results of a case-control investigation. *Arch Ophthalmol* 1998;116:1090–1094.

184. Stehr-Green JK, Bailey TM, et al. *Acanthamoeba* keratitis in soft contact lens wearers: a case-control study. *JAMA* 1987; 258:57–60.

185. Donzis PB, Mondino BJ, Weissman BA, et al. Microbial contamination of contact lens care systems. *Am J Ophthalmol* 1987;104:325–333.

186. Kilvington S, Larkin DF, White DG, et al. Laboratory investigation of *Acanthamoeba* keratitis. J Clin Microbiol 1990;28: 2722–2725.

187. Tanure MA, Cohen EJ, Sudesh S, et al. Spectrum of fungal keratitis at Wills Eye Hospital, Philadelphia, Pennsylvania. *Cornea* 2000;19:307–312.

188. Gopinathan U, Garg P, et al. The epidemiological features and laboratory results of fungal keratitis: a 10-year review at a referral eye care center in south India. *Cornea* 2002;21:555–559.

189. Wong TY, Fong KS, Tan DT. Clinical and microbial spectrum of fungal keratitis in Singapore: a 5-year retrospective study. *Int Ophthalmol* 1997;21:127–130.

190. Panda A, Sharma N, Das G, et al. Mycotic keratitis in children: epidemiologic and microbiologic evaluation. *Cornea* 1997;16: 295–299.

191. Dunlop AA, Wright ED, et al. Suppurative corneal ulceration in Bangladesh: a study of 142 cases examining the microbiological diagnosis, clinical and epidemiological features of bacterial and fungal keratitis. *Aust N Z J Ophthalmol* 1994;22:105–110.

192. Mselle J. Fungal keratitis as an indicator of HIV infection in Africa. *Trop Doct* 1999;29:133–135.

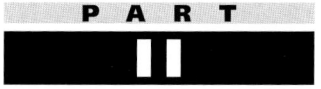

PART

II

CLINICAL TOPICS

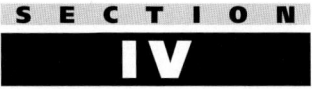

INFECTIOUS DISEASE

BACTERIAL KERATINS AND CONJUNCTIVITIS

12

BACTERIOLOGY

REGIS P. KOWALSKI AND JULES L. BAUM

Bacteria are single-celled prokaryotes and one of the earliest life forms. Although bacteria naturally inhabit many exterior and interior areas of the human body, the normal human cornea harbors no colonizing bacteria, but bacteria from the eyelids constantly contaminate the ocular surface. Host defense mechanisms of the eye and adnexa provide excellent corneal protection for the elimination of microbes through (a) mechanical, (b) immunologic, (c) chemical, and (d) innate mechanisms (1).

Bacteria colonize the cornea in infection, or some other pathologic process that compromises basic defense mechanisms, thus allowing growth. Bacteria that cause disease are labeled as pathogens because they possess virulence factors that enable the survival of these organisms in the cornea. These virulence factors include specific antigens, proteolytic enzymes, hemolysins, and toxins (2). In general, nonpathogens do not possess significant virulence factors, but under compromised conditions, may gain access to the cornea. Bacteria become established in the cornea after a breakdown of the corneal epithelium due to mechanical or nutritional stress, and proliferate under continued favorable conditions for bacterial growth (3).

The cornea may become infected from a pathogen in a wide range of bacteria, classified in part by the staining characteristics of the cell wall. The classic differential staining system is based on the Gram stain, which separates bacteria into gram-positive and gram-negative bacteria (Fig. 12-1). The staining procedure starts with placement of a corneal tissue specimen or a suspension of bacteria isolated from culture media on a glass microscope slide. The specimen is air-dried and fixed with methanol or a comparable fixative. In consecutive steps, it is stained with crystal violet, rinsed with tap water, stained with iodine, decolorized with alcohol (alcohol/acetone mixture), and counterstained with safranin. Gram-positive bacteria have a high content of peptidoglycan and a low content of lipid compared with gram-negative bacteria. When the lipid layer is dissolved, crystal violet and iodine form a complex in the cell wall that appears blue under microscopic examination, denoting gram-positive bacteria. Gram-negative bacteria

appear red because the lipid layer is not removed by the decolorizing step. A blue crystal violet complex can not form in the cell wall and safranin counterstains the bacteria. Other stains, such as an acid-fast stain, are also used to differentiate *Mycobacterium* species from other bacteria (4). Gram-positive bacteria are more frequently isolated from patients with keratitis than are gram-negative bacteria. In our laboratory (The Charles T. Campbell Ophthalmic Microbiology Laboratory, Pittsburgh, PA, 1993 to 2002), 56% of the bacterial keratitis isolates were gram-positive and 44% were gram-negative (Fig. 12-2). This ratio is consistent with other reports from China (60.2% vs. 39.6%) (5), England (54.7% vs. 45.3%) (6), and Boston (60% vs. 40%) (7).

BACTERIAL IDENTIFICATION METHODS

The vast majority of bacteria are easily cultivated in the basic microbiology laboratory using culture media. A broth-based agar medium supplemented with 5% to 10% sheep blood (blood agar), a chocolate agar (red cells partially lysed by heat) plate, and an optional mannitol salt agar plate will isolate almost all corneal bacterial pathogens. Anaerobic media such as enriched thioglycollate broth medium and broth-based agar media incubated under anaerobic conditions suffice for anaerobic bacterial isolation. Most bacteria appear on culture media with distinct characteristics that allow for immediate identification. Colony shape, size, color, and edge appearance, medium color changes due to production of end products (e.g., mannitol salt agar), and hemolysis of blood in supplemented media (i.e., beta-, alpha-*Streptococci*) due to production of lysins are examples of identification characteristics. As a rule, most bacteria can be identified to a bacterial genus or as gram-positive or gram-negative by appearance, but further identification to species requires the use of biochemicals (e.g., indole, glucose fermentation), antisera (e.g., coagulase), and changing growth conditions (e.g., *Haemophilus* growth factors). Bacteria are also characterized by specific oxygen requirements. Strict aerobic

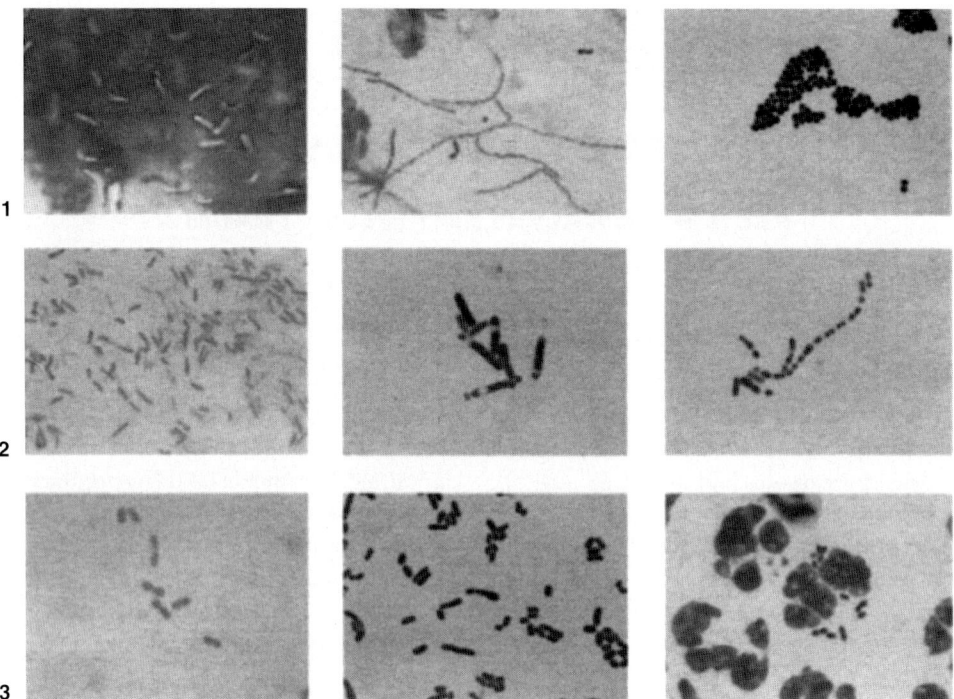

FIGURE 12-1. Microphotographs of gram-positive (blue) and gram-negative (red) bacteria that infect the cornea. (Original magnification × 100, oil immersion; photographed by Lisa M. Karenchak.) *Row 1, left*: diplococci (*Streptococcus pneumoniae*); *row 1, middle*: pleomorphic rods (diphtheroids); *row 1, right*: diplobacilli (*Moraxella*). *Row 2, left*: chain of cocci (*Streptococcus*); *row 2, middle*: rods with endospores (*Bacillus*); *row 2, right*: rods (*Pseudomonas aeruginosa*). *Row 3, left*: grapelike clusters of cocci (*Staphylococcus aureus*); *row 3, middle*: thin filaments (*Actinomyces*); *row 3, right*: nonstaining ghost rods (*Mycobacterium chelonae*). (See color figure.)

bacteria (aerobes) require oxygen for growth, whereas oxygen is toxic to other bacteria. These bacteria are classified as anaerobes. Many bacteria are facultative anaerobes in that growth occurs under either aerobic or anaerobic conditions. Bacteria also grow better at certain temperature and atmospheric conditions. In general, bacteria are incubated for isolation at body temperature (37°C or 98.6°F) and under

a 6% CO_2 atmospheric condition. *Mycobacteria* require different incubating temperatures, different light conditions, and extended incubation periods for isolation and identification.

Antibiotic susceptibility patterns are often used to identify and characterize bacteria. Susceptibility to vancomycin usually denotes a gram-positive bacteria, whereas bacitracin resistance is a characteristic of *Haemophilus* species. *Staphylococcus aureus* that are resistant to oxacillin are designated as methicillin resistant. Tables 12-1 and 12-2 include the susceptibility patterns of bacterial keratitis pathogens isolated from the Charles T. Campbell Ophthalmic Microbiology Laboratory 1993 to 2002. Although this chapter does not deal with keratitis therapy, susceptibility patterns are important in epidemiology and strain characterization. Minimum inhibitory concentrations or disk diffusion patterns using standard methods are determined and compared with established standards that interpret susceptibility (8,9). In the United States, bacterial susceptibility is determined using the serum standards established by the National Committee of Clinical Laboratory Standards (NCCLS). Most general laboratories do not test all the antibiotics presented in Tables 12-1 and 12-2 because some of these antibiotics are not used for treatment of systemic disease. There are no standards for inter-

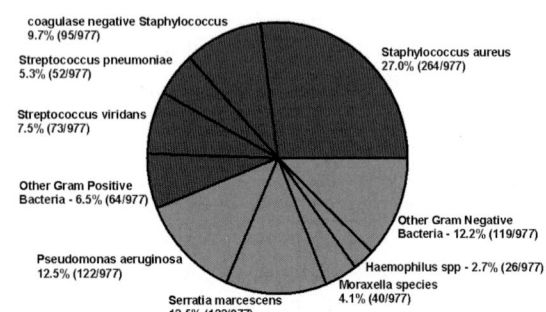

FIGURE 12-2. Distribution of bacteria isolated from cases of keratitis (1993 to 2002). Gram-positive bacteria comprised 56% of isolates, and gram-negative bacteria 44%. (Courtesy of the Charles T. Campbell Ophthalmic Microbiology Laboratory, The University of Pittsburgh Medical Center, Pittsburgh, PA.)

TABLE 12-1. SUSCEPTIBILITY OF GRAM-POSITIVE BACTERIAL ISOLATES FROM KERATITIS TO COMMON ANTIBIOTICS (PERCENTAGE SUSCEPTIBLE, 1993–2002)

Bacteria	No.	BAC	CHL	VAN	GEN	CIP	OFX	TRI	PB	CEF	TOB	SULF	OXA
Staphylococcus aureus	264	97	98	100	89	71	74	89	1	92	72	95	63
Coagulase-negative staphylococci	95	94	90	100	66	45	45	55	25	88	64	78	26
Streptococcus pneumoniae	52	100	94	100	4	54	79	22	2	100	0	94	
Streptococcus viridans	73	100	97	100	42	33	75	43	4	99	22	100	
Beta-hemolytic streptococci	8	100	100	100	25	63	88	25	0	100	0	38	
Nutritionally variant streptococci	6	50	100	100	17	33	100	25	0	83	0	17	
Enterococcus species	10	80	40	90	10	40	50	60	0	20	10	30	
Nonhemolytic streptococci	2	100	100	100	0	0	0	0	0	50	0	0	
Diphtheroids	32	91	84	100	81	58	65	6	91	91	78	75	
Bacillus species	5	40	80	100	100	100	100	100	60	80	100	100	

BAC, bacitracin; CHL, chloramphenicol; VAN, vancomycin; GEN, gentamicin; CIP, ciprofloxacin; OFX, ofloxacin; TRI, trimethoprim; PB, polymyxin B; CEF, cefazolin; TOB, tobramycin; SULF, sulfasoxazole; OXA, oxacillin.
(Data courtesy of the Charles T. Campbell Ophthalmic Microbiology Laboratory, The University of Pittsburgh Medical Center, Pittsburgh, Pennsylvania.)

pretation of antibacterial susceptibility for bacterial keratitis isolates because therapy is topical instead of systemic. NCCLS susceptibility interpretations can be used for ocular isolates if the assumption is made that the antibiotic concentration in the ocular tissue is at least as great as the antibiotic concentrations achieved in the blood serum.

Some bacteria that are implicated in corneal infection cannot be easily isolated on routine media because of their nutritional requirements and fastidious nature, as well as

TABLE 12-2. SUSCEPTIBILITY OF GRAM-NEGATIVE BACTERIAL ISOLATES FROM KERATITIS TO COMMON ANTIBIOTICS (PERCENTAGE SUSCEPTIBLE; 1993-2002)

Bacteria	No.	BAC	CHL	VAN	GEN	CIP	OFX	TRI	PB	CEF	TOB	SULF
Pseudomonas aeruginosa	122	0	0	0	96	97	92	0	100	0	98	2
Serratia marcescens	122	0	89	0	99	100	100	84	3	0	88	84
Serratia liquefaciens	4	0	100	0	100	100	100	100	100	0	100	100
Serratia species	7	0	100	0	100	100	100	83	43	0	100	67
Moraxella species	40	100	100	98	100	100	100	5	100	98	100	100
Haemophilus species	26	4	100	4	77	100	100	85	96	56	81	65
Acinetobacter species	20	10	25	15	100	95	95	0	95	10	95	100
Enterobacter species	18	0	94	6	100	100	100	86	100	50	100	100
Hafnia alvei	1	0	100	0	100	100	100	—	0	0	100	100
Klebsiella species	5	0	80	0	100	100	100	50	100	100	100	80
Escherichia coli	10	10	90	0	100	100	100	100	100	90	100	90
Citrobacter species	2	0	100	0	100	100	100	100	100	50	100	100
Shigella sonnei	1	0	100	0	100	100	100	100	100	100	100	100
Proteus mirabilis	14	0	92	0	100	100	100	57	0	86	100	100
Proteus vulgaris	2	0	50	0	100	100	100	—	0	50	100	100
Morganella morganii	4	0	100	0	100	100	100	50	0	0	100	100
Providencia stuartii	1	0	0	0	0	0	0	0	0	0	0	—
Branhamella catarrhalis	8	100	100	13	100	100	88	0	100	75	100	88
Neisseria subflava	1	100	100	100	100	100	100	—	100	100	100	100
Pasteurella haemolytica	1	0	0	100	100	100	100	—	100	100	100	100
Capnocytophaga species	1	100	100	50	100	100	100	100	100	50	100	100
Alcaligenes species	7	0	43	0	29	71	86	0	100	0	29	100
Flavobacterium species	3	66	66	100	33	100	100	—	33	33	0	100
Stenotrophomonas maltophilia	4	0	67	25	25	75	75	0	75	0	25	100
Burkholderia cepacia	1	0	0	0	0	100	100	0	100	0	0	100
Brevundimonas vesicularis	1	0	—	100	0	0	100	—	100	0	0	100
Pseudomonas stutzeri	1	0	—	0	100	100	100	—	100	0	100	0
Pseudomonas species	1	0	0	0	100	0	0	0	0	0	100	100

BAC, bacitracin; CHL, chloramphenicol; VAN, vancomycin; GEN, gentamicin; CIP, ciprofloxacin; OFX, ofloxacin; TRI, trimethoprim; PB, polymyxin B; CEF, cefazolin; TOB, tobramycin; SULF, sulfasoxazole.
(Data courtesy of the Charles T. Campbell Ophthalmic Microbiology Laboratory, The University of Pittsburgh Medical Center, Pittsburgh, Pennsylvania.)

antibiotic pretreatment. Serologic testing for the presence of antibody and molecular techniques to detect specific DNA sequences may be helpful to support the presence of these bacteria as etiologic agents.

GRAM-POSITIVE BACTERIA

The predominant gram-positive bacteria that infect the eye are *S. aureus*, coagulase-negative staphylococci, *Streptococcus pneumoniae*, *Streptococcus viridans*, and less frequent isolates that include *Bacillus* species, beta-, alpha-, and gamma-hemolytic *Streptococcus*, *Enterococcus* species, and diphtheroids. Normal bacterial eyelid flora such as coagulase-negative staphylococci, diphtheroids, and *Micrococcus* species may also contaminate the cornea (1). For ocular isolates, these genera can be separated using the Gram stain, colony morphology, coagulase test, catalase test, optochin test, and PYR (pyrrolidonyl aminopeptidase) test.

Staphylococcus aureus

S. aureus is a normal inhabitant of the skin, throat, and other parts of the human body. Spread to the cornea is probably from the eyelid margin or fingers that have been contaminated from the adjacent body flora or the environment. In general, *S. aureus* infects the cornea and causes a suppurative ulcer that could lead to permanent loss of vision and perforation. Presence of *S. aureus* on the eyelid margin can also lead to antigen–antibody hypersensitivity that produces catarrhal infiltrates in the peripheral cornea near the limbus (10,11).

S. aureus (12) are gram-positive cocci (0.5 to 1.5 μm) that appear microscopically in pairs or grapelike clusters, and grow on routine culture media within 18 to 24 hours. On broth-based agar media supplemented with blood, 6- to 8-mm, golden-pigmented colonies appear that are surrounded by beta (clear) hemolysis. *S. aureus* are nonmotile, non–spore forming, facultative anaerobes, and are usually encapsulated. Biochemically, *S. aureus* are catalase positive and coagulase positive. The latter test distinguishes *S. aureus* from the other *Staphylococcus* species and *Micrococcus*, although two other *Staphylococcus* species (*Staphylococcus intermedius* and *Staphylococcus hyicus*) that are animal pathogens are also coagulase positive.

"Wild-type" *S. aureus* is usually susceptible to all the antibiotics in Table 12-1 except polymyxin B. The widespread use of aminoglycosides in the 1970s, the use of systemic penicillins and cephalosporins, and the introduction of the fluoroquinolones in the 1990s have produced increased resistance and multiresistant isolates of *S. aureus*. In fact, fluoroquinolone resistance closely correlates with methicillin resistance in *S. aureus* (13). *S. aureus* are highly susceptible to vancomycin, bacitracin, chloramphenicol, cefazolin, and sulfasoxazole.

Coagulase-Negative Staphylococci

The genus *Staphylococcus* consists of 32 species and 15 subspecies, of which three species are coagulase positive and 29 species comprise the group coagulase-negative staphylococci (12). Coagulase-negative staphylococci are normal inhabitants of the human body, especially the skin, mucous membranes, and the eyelid margin. Microscopically, coagulase-negative staphylococci appear, similar to *S. aureus*, as gram-positive cocci in pairs and grapelike clusters, but appear on blood agar isolation medium as white to grayish colonies within 24 to 48 hours of incubation. These bacteria are also nonmotile and non–spore-forming, facultative anaerobes, usually unencapsulated, catalase positive, and, of course, coagulase negative. Coagulase-negative staphylococci are not easily speciated and multiple biochemical tests are required. The most common coagulase-negative staphylococci implicated in corneal disease are *Staphylococcus epidermidis*, *Staphylococcus warneri*, *Staphylococcus capitis*, *Staphylococcus hominis*, *Staphylococcus xylosus*, *Staphylococcus simulans*, *Staphylococcus equorum*, and *Staphylococcus lugdunensis* (14).

As in the case of *S. aureus*, coagulase-negative staphylococci have acquired antibiotic resistance to a few antibiotics that are frequently used for treating ocular infections. Table 12-1 depicts a 55% resistant rate for coagulase-negative staphylococci to fluoroquinolone antibiotics, and decreased resistance to many other frequently used ophthalmic antibiotics. Coagulase-negative staphylococci display high susceptibility to vancomycin, bacitracin, and chloramphenicol.

Although not members of the coagulase-negative staphylococci, *Micrococcus* species (*Micrococcus luteus*, *Micrococcus lylae*) are also gram-positive cocci that can be isolated from a compromised human cornea, but their presence may be as saprophytes or contaminants from the eyelid margin. *Micrococcus* species appear microscopically as gram-positive cocci in groups of four (tetrads), and appear distinctively on agar media as yellow colonies. *Micrococcus* is differentiated from *Staphylococcus* by testing for susceptibility to 0.04 units of bacitracin and resistance to 200 μg/mL of lysostaphin.

Streptococcus and Related Bacteria

Streptococcus species are normal inhabitants of the human alimentary, respiratory, and genital tracts in addition to transient isolates from the skin and other mucous membranes. Streptococci can be normal isolates of the eyelids and conjunctiva especially in children. *Streptococcus* species are first characterized by their hemolysis patterns on blood-supplemented agar media. Beta-hemolytic streptococci lyse red blood cells completely and a clear halo appears around a colony. Alpha-hemolytic streptococci partially lyse the red blood cells and a greenish halo appears around a colony. Gamma-hemolytic or nonhemolytic streptococci have no hemolysis pattern around a colony. All beta-hemolytic streptococci, if isolated from the cornea, should be treated as pathogens regardless of their species or Lancefield antigen type. *Streptococcus pyogenes*, which is Lancefield type A, can be identified by a positive PYR test. Antisera and other biochemical tests can be used to identify other species, but this is usually not necessary for ocular isolates. Alpha-hemolytic streptococci are difficult to identify as species and are usually grouped as *Streptococcus pneumoniae* and *Streptococcus viridans*. *S. pneumoniae* is differentiated from other alpha-hemolytic streptococci with a positive optochin and bile esculin hydrolysis test, a depressed colony center on blood agar medium, and a sometimes gelatinous appearance on culture media. The *S. viridans* group is divided into five subgroups: *Streptococcus mitis, Streptococcus anginosus, Streptococcus mutans, Streptococcus salvarius*, and *Streptococcus bovis* (15). Gamma-hemolytic or nonhemolytic streptococci are identified as group B streptococci and must be separated from *Enterococcus* species using the PYR test, which is positive for the latter.

Streptococci appear microscopically as gram-positive cocci, usually coccoid or coccobacilli shaped, and can appear as chains of cocci in broth medium. Streptococci are distinguished from *Staphylococcus* and *Micrococcus* species by a negative catalase reaction, are facultative anaerobes, and grow much better in a 5% CO_2 atmosphere at 37°C.

Streptococcus species are frequent bacterial agents of infectious keratitis (Fig. 12-2), which can present with ulcers, recalcitrant graft infections, and crystalline keratopathy (16). *S. pneumoniae* is another frequent bacterial pathogen of ulcerative keratitis, whereas *S. viridans* is usually a less virulent pathogen. Beta-hemolytic streptococci and nonhemolytic (group B) streptococci have also been isolated from cases of infectious keratitis.

In general, streptococci demonstrate excellent *in vitro* susceptibility to vancomycin, cefazolin, bacitracin, chloramphenicol, and sulfacetamide. Susceptibility to aminoglycoside antibiotics is generally low. Although *in vitro* susceptibility to fluoroquinolones is intrinsically low according to systemic parameters (17), it may not correlate to *in vivo* ocular success. High resistance to polymyxin B is consistent with all streptococci and related species.

Enterococcus species are normal inhabitants of the gastrointestinal tract and the female genital tract, and were once included in the genus *Streptococcus*. *Enterococcus* species are gram-positive, ovoid cocci, or coccobacilli, and can be isolated readily on broth medium with or without red blood cell supplementation. These bacteria are facultative anaerobes, PYR positive, and slightly catalase positive, and are considered to be nonhemolytic on blood-supplemented media (but alpha-hemolysis can be present). *Enterococcus faecalis* is the most common species isolated from the eye,

either as a conjunctiva contaminant or a corneal pathogen. *Enterococcus faecium* and other species have not been reported as major ocular pathogens. Antibiotic susceptibility profiles demonstrate varying levels of reduced susceptibility, with the highest susceptibility to vancomycin.

A little-known bacterial genus that represents an important corneal pathogen is *Abiotrophia*. This genus is commonly known as nutritionally variant streptococci. Nutritionally variant streptococci have been implicated in crystalline keratopathy and low-grade recalcitrant corneal infections. Nutritionally variant streptococci appear on Gram stain as a mixture of gram-variable cocci and pleomorphic rods that resemble diphtheroids. These bacteria can be very fastidious in their growth and require chocolate agar and a CO_2 atmosphere. The *in vitro* susceptibility profiles demonstrate high susceptibility to vancomycin, chloramphenicol, and ofloxacin, and slightly reduced susceptibility to cefazolin.

Diphtheroids

The term *diphtheroids* is used as a general classification for bacteria that appear microscopically as gram-positive pleomorphic rods (1). The diphtheroids include at least 32 genera of bacteria that are generally aerobic non–spore formers. *Corynebacterium* and *Propionibacterium* are the most common diphtheroids isolated from the conjunctiva, eyelid, and compromised cornea. The most common ocular *Corynebacterium* species are *hofmani, xerosis, renale*, and *mycetoides* (18). Diphtheroids grow well on blood-supplemented media, under a CO_2 atmosphere, but may require an additional day or two to appear as colonies. *Propionibacterium* species such as *Propionibacterium acnes* prefer anaerobic conditions for growth but will appear aerobically at approximately 5 to 7 days on chocolate agar. Enriched thioglycollate, a liquid broth medium, is an excellent growth broth for the isolation of anaerobic bacteria such as *Propionibacterium*.

Diphtheroids have been reported as causative agents in infectious keratitis, but their role as corneal pathogens is uncertain and their presence on a diseased cornea may be as a saprophyte (19,20). *Corynebacterium diphtheriae* and *Listeria monocytogenes* are corneal pathogens that can penetrate the corneal epithelium without prior trauma (3). *C. diphtheriae* can be isolated on routine culture media but, when suspected, cystine-tellurite blood agar or Tinesdale medium should be used for easier identification. *L. monocytogenes* can be easily misidentified as nonhemolytic streptococci. On closer inspection, a thin zone of hemolysis surrounds the colony on blood agar, and the identification can be confirmed with tumbling motility and a positive CAMP test (named for the initials of its four discoverers), observing for enhanced beta-hemolysis. In general, diphtheroids demonstrate good *in vitro* susceptibility to most antibiotics, with the exception of trimethoprim.

Bacillus

Bacillus species are ubiquitous in nature and are commonly isolated from the eyelid margin. *Bacillus* species are observed microscopically as large, gram-positive rods, but sometimes as gram-variable or gram-negative rods in older cultures. On blood agar medium, colonies can be small but are often large, dry but sometimes gelatinous, spreading across the medium, and beta-hemolysis surrounding the colonies can be present. These bacteria are spore formers, catalase positive, and motile, grow aerobically or as facultative anaerobes, and can survive under a wide range of temperatures. Although easy to identify to the genus level, identification to the species level is more complex and unnecessary in most cases. Laboratory certifying agencies would prefer, unless appropriate biochemical testing is undertaken to identify species, that the term "*Bacillus* species" be reported in order not to misidentify isolates that could be highly contagious "terrorism" isolates. Most species are opportunistic pathogens, but *Bacillus anthracis*, a "terrorism" pathogen, can infect the cornea. *Bacillus cereus* is the most important corneal pathogen (21). It appears as large, grainy, dry, beta-hemolytic colonies on agar medium supplemented with 5% sheep blood. *Bacillus* species demonstrate high *in vitro* susceptibility to vancomycin, the aminoglycosides, the fluoroquinolones, and sulfacetamide antibiotics.

Nocardia

Nocardia are members of the medically important actinomycetes, which are ubiquitous in the environment throughout the world in soil, water, and organic matter. *Nocardia* species appear microscopically as gram-positive, branching, filamentous bacteria, are aerobic, nonmotile, and partially acid-fast, and appear on routine isolation media as white, tiny, dry colonies (22). The cocultivation of other bacteria (mixed infection) can delay the appearance of *Nocardia* and subculture is usually required to confirm identification and to distinguish them from other actinomycetes, which is very cumbersome for most laboratories. Although rare pathogens, *Nocardia* have been implicated in corneal infections associated with trauma, contact lens wear, and laser *in situ* keratomileusis surgery (23). The reported pathogenic species are *Nocardia asteroides* and *Nocardia brasiliensis* (24,25). Antibiotic susceptibility testing indicates excellent susceptibility to sulfacetamides, trimethoprim-sulfamethoxazole, and amikacin, but susceptibility testing may vary with different species and isolates. A case of keratitis due to a highly resistant isolate of *Nocardia farcinica* has been reported (26).

Mycobacterium

The genus *Mycobacterium* includes bacteria that are free living in soil and water but also species that are obligate parasites and opportunistic pathogens. Although the high lipid content of the cell wall resists staining, *Mycobacterium* species are considered gram-positive bacteria that are slightly curved or straight bacilli. On Gram stain, *Mycobacterium* species may appear as "ghosts" or beaded gram-positive rods (Fig. 12-1). When *Mycobacterium* species are suspected, special acid-fast stains of specimens or culture growth should be used to confirm the suspicion and provide preliminary laboratory identification. The isolation of mycobacteria is a specialization in the large general laboratory. Many small laboratories refer mycobacteria specimens to a large central laboratory for processing. Isolation of different *Mycobacterium* species is a function of different incubation periods (2 days to 8 weeks), incubating temperatures (28°C, 30°C, 37°C, 42°C), special lighting conditions (light, darkness), and isolation medium. The screening for all species of mycobacteria is complex and probably unnecessary for ocular specimens because only a few fast-growing species of mycobacteria (*Mycobacterium chelonae* and *Mycobacterium fortuitum*) have been implicated in keratitis and refractive surgery (27–29). These species can usually be isolated on routine broth-based agar supplemented with 5% to 10% sheep blood and chocolate agar, but may still require a week to appear as colonies (30). Routine mycobacterial isolation media [i.e., Lowenstein-Jensen, Middlebrook 7H9 (liquid medium)] may also be appropriate for culture isolation. The optimal growing temperature for the fast-growing *Mycobacterium* species is 28°C. Colony morphology varies from rough to smooth, nonpigmented colonies. Other *Mycobacterium* species (*Mycobacterium avium-intracellulare*, *Mycobacterium nonchromogenicum*, *Mycobacterium triviale*, *Mycobacterium smegmatis*, and *Mycobacterium asiaticum*) have been isolated from cases of keratitis (31). *Mycobacterium tuberculosis* infections, in patients with ocular manifestations, are not sequestered to the eye but extend from previous pulmonary infection (32). Laboratories should be notified of prior *M. tuberculosis* infection when specimens for mycobacterial cultures are submitted. *Mycobacterium* species can be multiresistant, but *in vitro* susceptibility to amikacin and clarithromycin is common (31).

GRAM-NEGATIVE BACTERIA

The predominant gram-negative bacteria that infect the cornea are *Pseudomonas aeruginosa*, *Serratia marcescens*, *Moraxella* species, and *Haemophilus* species. A varied assortment of other gram-negative bacteria are also corneal pathogens, but at a lesser frequency. These less frequent pathogens spread to the cornea from the adnexa, skin flora, and contact lenses, as well as with poor hygiene and inoculation from the fingers. Most bacteria can be initially identified as gram-negative from the observation of colony morphology on culture. Often the genus of the isolate can also be determined (e.g., *Pseudomonas*, *Proteus*, *Haemophilus*), but in many cases the genus and species must be determined using biochemicals. Most gram-negative bacteria causing corneal infections appear microscopically as rods, with a rare infection stemming from cocci (e.g., *Neisseria gonorrhoeae*, *Neisseria meningitidis*, *Branhamella catarrhalis*). Once gram-negative rods are identified, colonies from culture are tested for cytochrome oxidase using the oxidase test. In general, oxidase-positive gram-negative organisms are glucose nonfermenters (e.g., *Pseudomonas*, *Moraxella*) and oxidase-negative bacteria are glucose fermenters (e.g., *Serratia*, *Escherichia coli*), but this rule does not hold for all gram-negative pathogens. Glucose nonfermenters are further identified using batteries of enzymatic tests and biochemical reactions (reduction of nitrates, indole production, acidification of glucose, arginine dihydrolase, urease, esculin hydrolysis, gelatin hydrolysis, and β-galactosidase), and sugar assimilations. Glucose fermenters are also identified with batteries of enzymatic tests and biochemical reactions (β-galactosidase, arginine dihydrolase, lysine decarboxylase, ornithine decarboxylase, citrate utilization, hydrogen sulfide production, urease, tryptophan deaminase, indole production, acetoin production, and gelatin hydrolysis), as well as the fermentation/oxidation reaction of sugars.

Pseudomonas aeruginosa

P. aeruginosa is a medically important gram-negative rod that is ubiquitous in water, soil, and plants. It is rarely part of the normal flora of healthy humans but is commonly found in domestic and hospital environments. *P. aeruginosa* are aerobic, oxygen-loving bacteria that appear microscopically as gram-negative, slender rods. It is a hardy bacterium that easily grows on routine culture media and prefers incubation temperatures of 30°C to 37°C, but will grow at 42°C. On trypticase broth supplemented with 5% sheep blood, *P. aeruginosa* presents as grayish or greenish, metallic-appearing to very gelatinous colonies and spread across the agar plate over several days of incubation. Culture plates with *P. aeruginosa* growth exude a sweet, grape-like odor, and growth on media unsupplemented with blood cells (i.e., Mueller-Hinton) displays a characteristic blue-green pigment. From corneal specimens, *P. aeruginosa* can be identified presumptively by Gram stain, colony morphology, and the oxidase test.

Although *P. aeruginosa* is considered an opportunistic pathogen, it possesses virulence factors (exotoxin A, proteolytic enzymes) and pili to attach to cells, and it produces alginate, a polysaccharide polymer that inhibits phagocytosis. These characteristics make *P. aeruginosa* a formidable pathogen to combat in systemic infections (e.g., pneumonia in patients with cystic fibrosis, wound infections, burn patients) and keratitis. Wearers of contaminated contact lenses, debilitated patients with frequent corneal epithelial

breakdown, intensive care unit patients with systemic infections and corneal exposure are all at risk for *P. aeruginosa* corneal ulcers.

In general, wild-type isolates of *P. aeruginosa* have demonstrated excellent *in vitro* susceptibility to the fluoroquinolones, aminoglycosides, polymyxin B, ceftazidime, and piperacillin. *P. aeruginosa* is resistant to vancomycin, cefazolin, and other narrow-spectrum antibiotics against gram-positive organisms. Isolates from systemic infections and reports of keratitis isolates from India (33) and Miami, Florida (34) have demonstrated increased antibiotic resistance to the fluoroquinolones and other antibiotics.

Serratia marcescens

S. marcescens is part of the normal gastrointestinal flora and is a frequent contaminant of contact lens cases and solutions. As a skin contaminant, it can spread from person to person in a hospital setting, and it is probably introduced to the cornea from contact lenses, the eyelid margins, and fingers. It is an opportunistic pathogen that produces several virulence factors (endotoxin, capsules, and adherence proteins), which, along with corneal epithelial breakdown due to contact lenses or trauma, can lead to corneal ulceration. *S. marcescens* appear microscopically as gram-variable, short, thin, rods, and sometimes as coccobacilli, and can be isolated readily on routine culture media. On broth-based agar medium supplemented with 5% sheep blood, *S. marcescens* colonies appear as large, shiny, grayish or sometimes reddish colonies. It can be suspected based on Gram stain, a negative oxidase test, a reddish colony, and *in vitro* resistance to polymyxin B. Definitive identification requires a battery of biochemical and sugar fermentation/oxidation tests to differentiate it from other glucose-fermenting bacteria. *S. marcescens* demonstrates high *in vitro* susceptibility to the fluoroquinolones and aminoglycosides (gentamicin susceptibility is greater than tobramycin susceptibility), and intermediate susceptibility (>80%) to chloramphenicol, trimethoprim, and sulfasoxazole. Unlike many other gram-negative bacteria, *S. marcescens* is resistant to polymyxin B.

Moraxella

Moraxella species are opportunistic bacteria that do not produce high morbidity systemically but can be etiologic agents in chronic conjunctivitis and acute keratitis (35,36). Microscopically, *Moraxella* are distinctive as a gram-negative, brick-shaped diplobacilli, and may appear gram-positive. They can be isolated on broth-based agar medium supplemented with 5% sheep blood, but growth generally requires a CO_2 atmosphere and several days of incubation. Frequently, *Moraxella* can be observed on Gram- and Giemsa-stained corneal tissue with the absence of a positive culture. Colonies on blood agar appear grayish, sometimes pitted, and a hazy "beach" can surround the colony. *Moraxella* species are oxidase-positive glucose nonfermenters, reduce nitrate to nitrite, and generally are negative to many biochemical and sugar assimilation tests. Although usually not identified to the species, it is believed that *Moraxella lacunata* is the primary ocular pathogen. *Moraxella catarrhalis* is another ocular pathogen, but is described along with the genus *Branhamella*. *Moraxella* demonstrate high *in vitro* susceptibility to most ocular antibiotics except trimethoprim.

Haemophilus

Haemophilus species are normal flora of the upper respiratory tract and are key pathogens implicated in pneumonia, meningitis, cellulitis, bacteremia, and venereal infections (37). In the eye, *Haemophilus* species are a frequent cause of conjunctivitis (especially in children, but all age groups are affected), orbital cellulitis, bleb infections that sometimes lead to endophthalmitis, and keratitis. *Haemophilus infuenzae* is the most common species isolated from ocular infections, but other species (*Haemophilus parainfluenzae*, *Haemophilus parahaemolyticus*, *Haemophilus paraphrophilus*) can be infectious (38,39). *Haemophilus ducreyi* is an invasive pathogen that does not require corneal epithelial trauma to induce keratitis and ulceration (3). *Haemophilus* species often appear in ocular scrapings and culture medium as pale-staining, gram-negative, tiny coccobacilli. These bacteria require hemin (X factor) and nicotine adenine dinucleotide (NAD, V factor) for growth. *Haemophilus* species do not grow routinely on blood-supplemented media unless X and V factors are provided by other bacteria (e.g., *S. aureus*) as metabolic byproducts. Their growth around other bacteria on blood-supplemented media is known as the "satellite phenomenon." Chocolate agar contains X and V factors and is the choice medium for isolating *Haemophilus* species, which appear as small, gray colonies with a pungent musty odor. The key characteristics for *Haemophilus* species identification are growth on chocolate agar, no growth on blood (except for satellite colonies), and bacitracin resistance. A special medium (*Haemophilus* test medium) is required to test for *in vitro* antibiotic susceptibility. *Haemophilus* species demonstrate excellent susceptibility to chloramphenicol, fluoroquinolones, and polymyxin B; intermediate susceptibility (>77%) to aminoglycosides and trimethoprim; and general resistance to bacitracin and vancomycin.

GRAM-NEGATIVE GLUCOSE NONFERMENTERS

Gram-negative glucose nonfermenters are an important group of opportunistic bacteria that are frequent pathogens involved in pneumonia, wound, and other systemic infec-

tions. These water and soil inhabitants are frequent contaminants of contact lens cases and can cause infectious keratitis (i.e., contact lens induced, graft infections, and crystalline keratopathy) (40–44). Gram-negative glucose nonfermenters can be readily isolated on routine culture media but do not grow well under anaerobic or reduced oxygen conditions. After isolation, these bacteria are grouped as either oxidase positive or oxidase negative. An experienced clinical microbiologist can distinguish whether the oxidase-negative bacteria should be further identified as glucose nonfermenters or fermenters based on colony pigment, colony morphology, and susceptibility patterns. This group of bacteria can be difficult to identify as to genus and species because of inconsistent biochemical and enzyme reactions. These bacteria are often reidentified and placed into new genera. For instance, *Stenotrophomonas maltophilia* was previously designated as *Pseudomonas maltophilia* and *Xanthomonas maltophilia*; *Burkholderia cepacia* was once *Pseudomonas cepacia*; and some *Alcaligenes* species have been renamed *Achromobacter*. Although the list may be incomplete (3), the important oxidase-positive glucose nonfermenters implicated in keratitis include the genera *Alcaligenes*, *Pseudomonas*, *Achromobacter*, *Flavobacterium*, *Comamonas*, and *Burkholderia*. The important oxidase-negative glucose nonfermenters are *Acinetobacter* and *Stenotrophomonas*. The antibiotic *in vitro* susceptibility patterns vary from species to species, but many of these bacteria are highly susceptible to sulfasoxazole (Table 12-2).

GRAM-NEGATIVE GLUCOSE FERMENTERS

Gram-negative glucose fermenters are ubiquitous bacteria that are found in the environment (water and soil) and are part of the normal gastrointestinal flora of humans and animals. These bacteria are responsible for high morbidity and mortality in the hospital setting (i.e., surgical infections, bacteremia, pneumonia) and food industry (i.e., gastrointestinal infections, food poisoning). As opportunistic pathogens, gram-negative glucose fermenters can be involved in infectious keratitis in infirm, contact lens–wearing patients, and in patients with poor hygenic habits. In general, gram-negative glucose fermenters are oxidase negative and easily isolated on routine culture media. The colonies are usually large with a glassy (mucoid) appearance. These bacteria are usually easy to identify to the genus and species levels with biochemical, fermentative/oxidative, and enzymatic reactions. Some bacteria such as *Proteus* are very motile and cover the culture medium with a swarm layer of bacteria. *E. coli* and *Proteus* have distinctive pungent odors that also provide rapid identification. The most common gram-negative glucose fermenters implicated in keratitis infections are *Enterobacter* species (*Enterobacter cloacae*, *Enterobacter agglomerans*, *Enterobacter aerogenes*), *Klebsiella species* (*Klebsiella pneumoniae*, *Kleb-*

siella oxytoca), Serratia liquefaciens, Citrobacter (Citrobacter freundii, Citrobacter diversus), Proteus species (Proteus mirabilis, Proteus vulgaris), E. coli, Hafnia alvei, Shigella species, Morganella morganii, and Providencia stuartii. As with the glucose nonfermenters, this list is not complete, and under certain circumstances this group of bacteria contains many bacteria that have a potential for infecting the cornea. Gram-negative glucose fermenters (Table 12-2) demonstrate high *in vitro* susceptibility to the aminoglycosides, fluoroquinolones, and sulfasoxazole, very poor susceptibility to bacitracin and vancomycin, but varied susceptibility to cefazolin. Serratia species, H. alvei, Proteus species, M. morganii, and P. stuartii are resistant to polymyxin B.

GRAM-NEGATIVE COCCI

Although gram-negative cocci are infrequent corneal pathogens, infections from N. gonorrhoeae and N. meningitidis can produce a severe keratitis. N. gonorrhoeae is not part of the normal flora of humans and is usually transmitted from person to person through intimate sexual contact. N. meningitidis is part of the normal human nasopharynx, and person-to-person spread is believed to have clinical significance. Both organisms appear microscopically on Gram stain as kidney bean–shaped, gram-negative diplococci, and grow optimally on chocolate agar or special Thayer-Martin agar medium at 35°C to 37°C under a 5% to 10% CO_2 humidified atmosphere. The colonies are usually grayish and nonpigmented, and react positively to the oxidase test. Although the genus level is rapidly determined, species identification requires additional tests for differentiation. In general, the acidification results of sugars (glucose, fructose, maltose, lactose, and sucrose) and growth on nutrient agar at 35°C distinguish between N. gonorrhoeae and N. meningitidis. Other Neisseria species (Neisseria flavescens, Neisseria sicca, Neisseria subflava) that are part of the normal nasopharyngeal flora can be cultured from the cornea as mixed flora with S. viridans, Staphylococcus species, Micrococcus, and diphtheroids. These bacteria usually grow on routine culture media, are oxidase positive, and are pigmented.

Another, less frequent corneal pathogen is Branhamella catarrhalis, which is a normal commensal bacteria of the upper respiratory tract but is the causative agent in systemic, respiratory, and ocular disease (conjunctivitis, keratitis) (45,46). B. catarrhalis, which was formerly a member of the Neisseria genus, is now part of the genus Moraxella but is distinctively different from Moraxella lacunata in its Gram stain appearance (B. catarrhalis are truer cocci), colony presentation, and biochemical utilization. B. catarrhalis isolates readily on routine culture media (blood and chocolate agar) and presents with a dry, slightly yellowish colony that is oxidase positive. Biochemically, B. catarrhalis does not produce acid from sugars,

but produces DNAase and lipase. B. catarrhalis demonstrates excellent *in vitro* susceptibility to bacitracin, chloramphenicol, aminoglycosides, fluoroquinolones, and polymyxin B, but poor susceptibility to vancomycin and trimethoprim.

SPIROCHETES

Treponema pallidum and Borrelia burgdorferi are two spirochetes that have been implicated in corneal disease (47–49). Spirochetes appear microscopically as long, slender, gram-negative rods and require a living host to multiply because no natural reservoir is available in the environment (50). T. pallidum infections result in syphilis, a venereal disease that, left untreated, can spread to other parts of the body, including the cornea. Corneal infection leads to an immunologic interstitial keratitis. There are no routine culture isolation techniques, but patients with a past history of syphilis infection and unexplained ocular inflammation should be screened serologically with the fluorescent treponemal antibody absorption (FTA-ABS) and Venereal Disease Research Laboratory (VDRL) tests. Borrelia burgdorferi is the causative agent of Lyme disease and requires a tick (Ixodes) as the host to spread. The tick is commonly found on deer and rodents and infects unsuspecting humans through bites that inject the spirochete. If left untreated, infection spreads systemically throughout the body, sometimes involving the cornea. Corneal inflammation is immunologic and must be detected with serologic tests to detect elevations in antibody because there are no routine methods for isolation. Polymerase chain reaction and staining of tissues with special stains (Warthin-Starry silver stain) may be helpful in obtaining a laboratory diagnosis.

ANAEROBIC AND MICROAEROPHILIC BACTERIA

The role of anaerobic bacteria as corneal pathogens may be underdiagnosed because of the special conditions required for isolation and detection (51). Anaerobic bacteria (e.g., Clostridium perfringens) can be found in the environment as spores, waiting for the right conditions (i.e., decrease in oxygen, adequate nutrients) to multiply. Some anaerobic bacteria can be found in body areas where the oxygen concentration is decreased (e.g., lacrimal glands, oral cavity). A diseased cornea with a low oxygen tension and infected with other bacteria that further reduce the oxygen concentration may be susceptible to a coanaerobic infection. In general, corneal specimens should be plated on chocolate agar or special anaerobic blood agar and incubated under anaerobic conditions. Anaerobic conditions can be maintained with an anaerobic bag or a jar. Enriched thioglycollate broth supplemented with vitamin K and hemin should also be inoculated. Corneal specimens planted on media should be placed under anaerobic conditions within 30 minutes and the media should be monitored every 72 hours for growth for 2 weeks before cultures are deemed negative for anaerobes. Keratitides due to gram-positive infection (*Propionibacterium, Peptostreptococcus, Actinomyces,* and *Clostridium)* are more common than those due to gram-negative organisms (*Bacteroides*) (51–53).

Capnocytophaga species are corneal pathogens that grow best at reduced oxygen conditions and prefer a CO_2 environment for isolation on routine culture media (54). These bacteria can be found in the subgingival surfaces and oral cavities of humans and other animals, and are generally opportunistic in debilitated patients in whom infection is usually due to endogenous spread (55,56). Microscopically, *Capnocytophaga* species appear as gram-negative, fusiform rods with one end rounded and the other end tapered. On culture media, growth may require 2 to 7 days and appears as beige to yellowish colonies with outgrowths indicative of gliding motility. *Capnocytophaga* species are oxidase negative, catalase negative, indole negative, and susceptible to the aminoglycosides, fluoroquinolones, and other broad-spectrum antibiotics.

REFERENCES

1. Kowalski RP, Roat MI. Normal flora of the human conjunctiva and eyelid. In: Tasman W, Jaeger EA, eds. *Duane's foundations of clinical ophthalmology*. Philadelphia: Lippincott Williams & Wilkins, 1998:1–11.
2. Burd EM. Bacterial keratitis and conjunctivitis—bacteriology: scientific foundations and clinical practice. In: Smolin G, Thoft RA, eds. *The cornea*, 3rd ed. Boston, Little, Brown, 1994:115–124.
3. Foulks GN, Gordon JS, Kowalski RP. Bacterial infections of the conjunctiva and cornea. In: Albert DM, Jakobiec FA, eds. *Principles and practices of ophthalmology*. Philadelphia: WB Saunders, 2000:893–905.
4. Forbes BA, Sahm DF, Weissfeld AS, eds. Role of microscopy in the diagnosis of infectious diseases. In: *Bailey & Scott's diagnostic microbiology*, 11th ed. St. Louis: Mosby, 1998:125.
5. Sun X, Wang Z, Luo S, et al. Distribution and shifting trends of the pathogens for bacterial keratitis. *Chin J Ophthalmol* 2002;38:292–294.
6. Tuft SJ, Matheson M. In vitro antibiotic resistance in bacterial keratitis in London. Br J Ophthalmol 2000;84:687–691.
7. Gudmundsson OG, Ormerod LD, Kenyon KR, et al. Factors influencing predilection and outcome in bacterial keratitis. *Cornea* 1989;8:115–121.
8. National Committee for Clinical Laboratory Standards. *Methods for dilution antimicrobials susceptibility tests for bacteria that grow aerobically*, 4th ed. Approved standard. NCCLS document M7-A5, vol 20, no 2. Villanova, PA: National Committee for Clinical Laboratory Standards, 2000.
9. National Committee for Clinical Laboratory Standards. *Performance standards for antimicrobial disk susceptibility tests*, 7th ed. Approved standard. NCCLS document M2-A7, vol 17, no 1. Villanova, PA: National Committee for Clinical Laboratory Standards, 2000.
10. Mondino B, Kowalski RP. Phlyctenulae and catarrhal infiltrates. *Arch Ophthalmol* 1982;99:1968–1971.
11. Mondino B, Cruz TA, Kowalski RP. Immune responses in rabbits with phlyctenulae and catarrhal infiltrates. *Arch Ophthalmol* 1983; 101:1275–1277.
12. Kloos WE, Bannerman TL. *Staphylococcus* and *Micrococcus*. In: Murray PR, Baron EJ, Pfaller MA, et al., eds. *Manual of clinical microbiology*, 7th ed. Washington, DC: American Society for Microbiology, 1999:264–282.
13. Wilkinson PS, Kowalski RP, Gordon JS. Are there other antibiotics besides vancomycin for treating MRSA (methicillin-resistant *Staphylococcus aureus*) keratitis? *Invest Ophthalmol* 2001;42(4, suppl):1374.
14. Pinna A, Zanetti S, Sotgiu M, et al. Identification and antibiotic susceptibility of coagulase negative staphylococci isolated in corneal/external infections. *Br J Ophthalmol* 1999;83:771–773.
15. Ruoff KL, Whiley RA, Beighton D. *Streptococcus*. In: Murray PR, Baron EJ, Pfaller MA, et al., eds. *Manual of clinical microbiology*, 7th ed. Washington, DC: American Society for Microbiology, 1999:283–296.
16. Ormerod LD, Ruoff KL, Meisler DM, et al. Infectious crystalline keratopathy: role of nutritionally variant streptococci and other bacterial factors. *Ophthalmology* 1991;98:159–169.
17. Kowalski RP, Karenchak LM, Romanowski EG. Infectious disease: changing antibiotic susceptibility. *Ophthalmol Clin North Am* 2003;16:1–9.
18. Linnoli O, Marconi S. Studies in the conjunctival bacterial flora. *Ann Sclavo* 1976;18:733–742.
19. Heidemann DG, Dunn SP, Diskin JA, et al. *Corynebacterium striatum* keratitis. *Cornea* 1991;10:81–82.
20. Rubenfeld RS, Cohen EJ, Arentsen JJ, et al. Diphtheroids as ocular pathogens. *Am J Ophthalmol* 1989;108:251–254.
21. Donzis PB, Mondino BJ, Weissman BA. *Bacillus* keratitis associated with contaminated contact lens care systems. *Am J Ophthalmol* 1988;105:195–197.
22. Sridhar MS, Gopinathan U, Garg P, et al. Ocular *Nocardia* infections with special emphasis on the cornea. *Surv Ophthalmol* 2001;45:361–378.
23. Sridhar MS, Sharma S, Garg P, et al. Treatment and outcome of *Nocardia* keratitis. *Cornea* 2001;20:458–462.
24. Tseng SH, Chen JJ, Hu FR. *Nocardia brasiliensis* keratitis successfully treated with therapeutic lamellar keratectomy. *Cornea* 1996;15:165–167.
25. Newmark E, Polack FM, Ellison AC. Report of a case of *Nocardia asteroides* keratitis. *Am J Ophthalmol* 1971;72: 813–815.
26. Eggink CA, Wesseling P, Boirin P, et al. Severe keratitis due to *Nocardia farcinica*. *J Clin Microbiol* 1997;35:999–1001.
27. Gottsch JD, Gilbert ML, Goodman DF, et al. Excimer laser ablative treatment of microbial keratitis. *Ophthalmology* 1991; 98:146–149.
28. Richardson P, Crawford GJ, Smith DW, et al. *Mycobacterium chelonae* keratitis. *Aust N Z J Ophthalmol* 1989;17: 195–196.
29. Freitis D, Alvarenga L, Sampaio J, et al. An outbreak of *Mycobacterium chelonae* infection after LASIK. *Ophthalmology* 2003;110:276–285.
30. Forbes BA, Sahm DF, Weissfeld AS, eds. *Mycobacteria*. In: *Bailey and Scott's diagnostic microbiology*, 11th ed. St. Louis: Mosby, 2002:240–271.
31. Ford, JG, Huang AJW, Plugfelder SC, et al. Nontuberculous mycobacterial keratitis in south Florida. *Ophthalmology* 1998; 105:1652–1658.
32. Sheu SJ, Shyu JS, Chen LM, et al. Ocular manifestations of tuberculosis. *Ophthalmology* 2001;108:1580–1585.
33. Garg P, Sharma S, Rao GN. Ciprofloxacin-resistant *Pseudomonas* keratitis. *Ophthalmology* 1999;106:1319–1323.

34. Chaudhry NA, Flynn HW, Murray TG, et al. Emerging ciprofloxacin-resistant *Pseudomonas aeruginosa*. *Am J Ophthalmol* 1999;128:509–510.
35. Kowalski RP, Harwick JC. Incidence of *Moraxella* conjunctival infection. *Am J Ophthalmol* 1986;101:437–440.
36. Cobo LM, Coster DJ, Peacock J. *Moraxella* keratitis in a nonalcoholic population. *Br J Ophthalmol* 1981;65:683–686.
37. Foweraker JE, Cooke NJ, Hawkey PM. Ecology of *Haemophilus influenzae* and *Haemophilus parainfluenzae* in sputum and saliva and effects of antibiotics on their distribution in patients with lower respiratory tract infections. *Antimicrob Agents Chemother* 1993;37:804.
38. Forbes BA, Sahm DF, Weissfeld AS, eds. *Haemophilus*. In: *Bailey & Scott's diagnostic microbiology*, 11th ed. St. Louis: Mosby, 1998:462–468.
39. Balouris CA, Kowalski RP, Karenchak LM. Susceptibility testing of ocular *Haemophilus*. ARVO Abstracts. *Invest Ophthalmol Vis Sci* 1991;32[4 Suppl]:1172(abstr).
40. Siganos DS, Tselentis IG, Papatzanaki ME, et al. *Achromobacter xylosoxidans* keratitis following penetrating keratoplasty. *Refract Corneal Surg* 1993;9:71–73.
41. Penland RL, Wilhelmus KR. *Stenotrophomonas maltophilia* ocular infections. *Arch Ophthalmol* 1996;114:433–436.
42. Doiz O, Liorente MT, Mateo A, et al. Corneal abscess by *Flavobacterium indologenes*: a case report. *Enferm Infecc Microbiol Clin* 1999;17:149–150.
43. Lema I, Gomez-Torreiro M, Rodriguez-Ares MT. *Comamonas acidovorans* keratitis in a hydrogel contact lens wearer. *CLAO J* 2001;27:55–56.
44. Khater TT, Jones DB, Wilhelmus KR. Infectious crystalline keratopathy caused by gram-negative bacteria. *Am J Ophthalmol* 1997;124:19–23.
45. Wilhelmus KR, Peacock J, Coster DJ. *Branhamella* keratitis. *Br J Ophthalmol* 1980;64:892–895.
46. Heidemann DG, Alfonso E, Forster RK, et al. *Branhamella catarrhalis* keratitis. *Am J Ophthalmol* 1987;103:576–581.
47. Tamesis RR, Foster CS. Ocular syphilis. *Ophthalmology* 1990; 97:1281–1287.
48. Baum J, Barza M, Weinstein P, et al. Bilateral keratitis as a manifestation of Lyme disease. *Am J Ophthalmol* 1988;105:75–77.
49. Orlin SE, Lauffer JL. Lyme disease keratitis. *Am J Ophthalmol* 1989;107:678–680.
50. Baron EJ, Peterson LR, Finegold SM, eds. Spirochetes and other spiral-shaped organisms. In: *Bailey & Scott's diagnostic microbiology*, 9th ed. St. Louis: Mosby, 1994:445–450.
51. Perry LD, Brinser JH, Kolodner H. Anaerobic corneal ulcers. *Ophthalmology* 1982;89:636–642.
52. Eiferman RA, Ogden LL, Snyder J. Anaerobic peptostreptococcal keratitis. *Am J Ophthalmol* 1985;100:335–336.
53. Volkov VV, Gatsu AF, Kocherovets VI. Non-clostridial anaerobes as a cause of post-traumatic keratitis. *Vestn Oftalmol* 1990; 106:61–63.
54. Alexandrakis G, Palma LA, Miller D, et al. *Capnocytophaga* keratitis. *Ophthalmology* 2000;107:1503–1506.
55. Chodosh J. Cat's tooth keratitis: human corneal infection with *Capnocytophaga canimorsus*. *Cornea* 2001;20:661–663.
56. Ormerod LD, Foster CS, Paton BG, et al. Ocular *Capnocytophaga* infection in an edentulous, immunocompetent host. *Cornea* 1988;7:218–222.

13.1

BACTERIAL KERATITIS

TERRENCE P. O'BRIEN

Keratitis may result from noninfectious stimuli or through exposure to or invasion by infectious organisms. Microbial keratitis is a common, potentially sight-threatening ocular infection caused by bacteria, viruses, fungi, or parasites (1). Sequelae from microbial keratitis constitute a leading cause of corneal blindness worldwide. The clinical challenge is to distinguish microbial keratitis from other noninfectious inflammatory conditions of the cornea resulting from trauma, hypersensitivity, and other immune-mediated reactions. Recognition of clinical signs raising suspicion for a bacterial cause as opposed to the other potential infectious organisms provides a further challenge.

Although there are no unanimously specific clinical signs that confirm infection or suggest definite bacterial cause, the clinician should assess and define the distinctive corneal signs based on the status of the epithelium (intact or ulcerated), type of stromal inflammation (suppurative or nonsuppurative), and the site of the stromal inflammation (focal, diffuse, multifocal, or marginal). When there is sufficient evidence based on clinical examination to raise the suspicion for a possible infectious etiology, laboratory studies are required to establish identity of the specific causative organism(s) and for determination of antimicrobial susceptibility. Based on the clinical setting and risk factors, features of clinical examination, results from laboratory investigation, and knowledge of the potential corneal pathogens, a therapeutic plan is initiated (2). Modification of the therapeutic plan is subsequently based on clinical response, results of *in vitro* susceptibility determination, and tolerance of the antimicrobial agents. With careful clinical monitoring, adjunctive anti-inflammatory therapy is considered; antimicrobial therapy is then terminated and any residual structural alterations corrected.

This chapter describes the principal bacterial causative organisms, risk factors, pathogenetic mechanisms, histopathology, clinical features, laboratory diagnostic techniques, and the medical and surgical therapies for bacterial keratitis.

PRINCIPAL CAUSES

There are four principal groups of bacteria that are most frequently responsible (3): Micrococcaceae (*Staphylococcus*,

Micrococcus), the *Streptococcus* species, the *Pseudomonas* species, and the Enterobacteriaceae (*Citrobacter*, *Klebsiella*, *Enterobacter*, *Serratia*, *Proteus*). However, virtually any bacteria can potentially cause keratitis under certain favorable conditions. A classification of the medically important bacteria based on type, Gram stain, and oxygen requirements for growth is provided in Table 13.1-1. The flora of the ocular surface and the environment in which the person lives influence the type of infection that develops. Ambient temperature and humidity have a major role in determining the microorganisms found in the environment. Pathogens isolated from cases of microbial keratitis vary among geographic locations according to the local climate and occupational risk factors. Differences were reported in isolates from patients with suppurative keratitis from Ghana and southern India, both of which are at similar tropical latitudes (4). There were differences found in the bacterial isolates, with *Pseudomonas* species the most frequent isolate from Ghana and *Streptococcus* species the most common isolate from southern India. Geographic variations also exist in the relative frequency of different bacterial organisms as causative agents in keratitis in the United States. Pneumococcus (*Streptococcus pneumoniae*) was a frequently encountered causative organism of bacterial keratitis in previous clinical reports because of its association with chronic dacryocystitis (5). Pneumococcus has decreased in frequency as a causative organism in developed countries with available effective antibiotics and with refinements in techniques for dacryocystorhinostomy. In developing countries, the pneumococcus may remain an important cause of infectious corneal ulceration (6–8). Other gram-positive organisms, especially among the *Staphylococcus* species, continue to be the most commonly isolated causes of bacterial keratitis. *Staphylococcus aureus* is among the most frequent causative organisms in bacterial keratitis in the Northern and North Eastern United States and Canada, both in normal hosts and in compromised corneas (9). In Great Britain, the most common organisms isolated in bacterial keratitis are *S. aureus*, *S. pneumoniae*, *Pseudomonas*, and *Moraxella* (10).

Once an infrequent isolate, *Pseudomonas* species became increasingly isolated as causative organisms in keratitis. *Pseudomonas* has been reported as the most commonly

TABLE 13-1. CLASSIFICATION OF IMPORTANT BACTERIA IN MICROBIAL KERATITIS

Gram-negative rods
  Pseudomonadaceae
    Pseudomonas
	Gram-negative cocci and coccobacilli (aerobes)
	  Neisseriaceae
	    Neisseria
	    Moraxella
	    Acinetobacter
		Bacillus
		Clostridium

Azotobacteraceae
  Azotobacter
		Actinomycetes and related organisms
		  Coryneform group of bacteria
		    Corynebacterium

Gram-negative facultatively anaerobic rods
  Enterobacteriaceae
    Escherichia
    Citrobacter
    Klebsiella
    Serratia
    Proteus
	Gram-positive aerobic and/or facultatively
	  anaerobic cocci
	  Micrococcaceae
	    Micrococcus
	    Staphylococcus
		Propionibacteriaceae
		    Propionibacterium
		    Eubacterium
		Actinomycetaceae
		    Actinomyces
		    Arachnia

	Streptococcaceae
	    Streptococcus
	    Pediococcus
	    Aerococcus
		Bifidobacterium
		    Bacterionema

Genera of uncertain affiliation
  Actinobacillus
  Flavobacterium
  Haemophilus
		Mycobacteriaceae
		    Mycobacterium

Gram-negative anaerobic rods
Bacteroidaceae
  Bacteroides
  Fusobacterium
	Gram-positive anaerobic cocci
	  Peptococcaceae
	    Peptococcus
	    Peptostreptococcus
	
	Endospore-forming rods and cocci
	  Bacillaceae
		Nocardiaceae
		    Nocardia
		
		Streptomycetaceae
		    Streptomyces

isolated organism in the southern regions of the United States (11,12). The increasing prevalence of *Pseudomonas* in otherwise healthy individuals was found largely in association with daily- or extended-wear soft contact lenses (13–19). *Pseudomonas* is widely distributed in nature and is capable of being a contaminant in the hospital environment, in fluorescein sodium solutions, in cosmetics, and organic carbon substances (20). *Pseudomonas* has long been recognized as a potential opportunistic pathogen in burn patients, patients with altered consciousness, patients with exposure, and in individuals maintained on mechanical ventilatory assistance.

Shifting trends in bacterial keratitis in south Florida were observed and reported during the 1990s (21). *S. aureus* and *Pseudomonas aeruginosa* represented 19.4% and 25.7%, respectively, of the total bacterial isolates during this period. However, a gradual increase was documented in the number of *S. aureus* keratitis isolates (29% of gram-positive organisms in 1990 versus 48% in 1998, *p* = .01) coupled with a decrease in the number of *P. aeruginosa* isolates (54% of gram-negative organisms in 1990 vs. 46% in 1998). A decrease in the incidence of contact lens–associated keratitis and *P. aeruginosa* isolates in this group of patients was documented. *Serratia marcescens* and *P. aeruginosa* were most commonly isolated in contact lens–associated keratitis (18% each).

Distribution and shifting trends of bacterial keratitis in north China were reported over the period of 1989 to 1998 (22). The data of 2220 corneal isolates were reviewed retrospectively. Positive culture was recovered in 490 isolates. Gram-positive cocci and gram-negative bacilli represented 51% and 39.4%, respectively. *P. aeruginosa* was

the most common pathogen (32.2%). A gradual increase in the percentage of gram-positive cocci was coupled with a decrease of gram-negative bacilli. *P. aeruginosa* and coagulase-negative *Staphylococcus* were the most common pathogens in bacterial keratitis in north China.

Moraxella, a gram-negative aerobic bacterium, may be a causative agent of keratitis in malnourished individuals and patients with alcoholism, diabetes, and other debilitating conditions (5,9,20). *Moraxella* may also cause bacterial keratitis in healthy patients. *Moraxella* is present in 0.3% of normal eyelids and in up to 0.8% of inflamed eyelids (23).

The indigenous bacteria, including coagulase-negative *Staphylococcus*, *Corynebacterium*, and *Propionibacterium* species, are increasing in frequency of isolation from bacterial keratitis cases because of their proximity to the cornea and the potential for direct inoculation (24). There are a number of species of coagulase-negative *Staphylococcus*. Although *Staphylococcus epidermidis* has been reported as the most frequently isolated from ocular sources, with newer, highly specific laboratory identification systems, it is possible that other coagulase-negative staphylococci may be increasingly implicated as causative organisms. In a multicenter, prospective, randomized comparative study of therapy for bacterial keratitis, coagulase-negative *Staphylococcus* species were among the most frequently encountered causative organisms (25).

Since the development of a vaccine against *Corynebacterium diphtheriae*, isolation of the organism from the eye is rare. Corneal involvement with *C. diphtheriae* is infrequent and typically observed after a reaction to diphtheria toxin (26). By virtue of the activity of its toxin, *C. diphtheriae* may penetrate intact corneal epithelium to produce keratitis.

Other *Corynebacterium* species have been recovered from infectious corneal ulcerations. The precise causative role of these *Corynebacterium* species has occasionally been uncertain. Cases in which *Corynebacterium* species have been the sole organisms isolated have increased the awareness of their potential as important causative organisms of keratitis (27,28). *Corynebacterium xerosis* and *Corynebacterium striatus* are the species that have been most commonly recovered. *C. xerosis* may be a coinfectious agent frequently associated with *Moraxella* infections.

Propionibacterium species are non–spore-forming anaerobic bacteria that have been implicated after sequestration in the capsular bag as a specific cause of chronic pseudophakic endophthalmitis (29). *Propionibacterium* species are also capable of causing keratitis in healthy and compromised corneas.

Gram-positive aerobic bacilli are widespread in nature and are usually of low virulence. They may produce infections of the cornea when host resistance is lowered (30). *Bacillus cereus* has been associated with severe posttraumatic endophthalmitis after penetrating injury with vegetable or metallic matter. Specific enzymes and toxins, including hemolysins, enterotoxins, and emetic toxin, are produced by this organism. These virulence factors may be particularly destructive to the retina and responsible for fulminant destruction (31,32). *B. cereus* keratitis may follow foreign body injury (33). Other *Bacillus* species that have been implicated as causative agents of bacterial keratitis include *Bacillus brevis*, *Bacillus coagulans*, *Bacillus laterosporus*, *Bacillus licheniformis*, and *Bacillus thuringiensis* (30,34–35).

Organisms less frequently associated with keratitis include *Serratia* (36), *Proteus*, and *Azotobacter* (37). *S. marcescens* corneal ulcerations have been associated with contact lens wear (36) and contaminated eyedrops (38).

Other aerobic gram-negative organisms capable of causing keratitis include *Neisseria gonorrhoeae* and *Neisseria meningitidis*. *N. gonorrhoeae* may produce consecutive keratitis during an episode of untreated or inadequately treated purulent conjunctivitis. *Neisseria* species can cause marked conjunctival chemosis and infiltration with polymorphonuclear neutrophils. The edematous infiltrated conjunctiva may then drape over the peripheral cornea, resulting in exposure to neutrophilic lytic enzymes capable of producing epithelial ulceration. The pace of inflammation may result in rapid stromal thinning and perforation. It is imperative to verify the presence of the gonococcus by culture because *Acinetobacter*, which is morphologically identical on smears to the gonococcus, can also cause corneal perforation.

Non–spore-forming anaerobic bacteria are principal flora of the skin, oral cavity, gastrointestinal tract, and other mucous membranes. These anaerobic bacteria are capable of causing keratitis and other ocular infections (39). The most frequently isolated organisms are *Peptostreptococcus*, *Peptococcus*, and *Propionibacterium* (40,41). Spore-forming anaerobic bacteria such as *Clostridium* species may be rarely encountered as causes of infectious corneal ulceration, especially after contamination with soil (42). The presence of *Clostridium* infection may be suggested by gas bubbles observed in the corneal tissue or anterior chamber (43). *Listeria monocytogenes* is a facultatively anaerobic, gram-positive rod that is infrequently isolated as a cause of severe, suppurative keratitis, especially among animal caretakers (44). The organism is an intracellular pathogen which may also cause endophthalmitis with pigment dispersion, dark hypopyon, and elevated intraocular pressure (45).

In studies that used adequate methods for recovery of anaerobes, these bacteria were isolated from approximately a third of patients with conjunctivitis, half of the time in pure culture (46). The predominant recovered anaerobes were *Clostridium* species, gram-negative anaerobic bacilli, and *Peptostreptococcus* species. Anaerobic bacteria were also recovered from patients who wore contact lenses and had conjunctivitis. Anaerobic bacteria were also reported in cases of keratitis (46). The most frequently recovered anaerobes were *Propionibacterium*, *Peptostreptococcus*, *Clostridium*, *Prevotella*, and *Fusobacterium* species. The most frequently recovered anaerobes from dacryocystitis were *Peptostreptococcus*, *Propionibacterium*, *Prevotella*, and *Fusobacterium* species.

Members of the actinomycetes and related organisms, including *Nocardia*, are known to resemble bacteria more than fungi. These gram-positive, branching filamentous organisms have been causally linked with infections of the lacrimal system, yet are rarely encountered as isolates from bacterial keratitis (47). *Nocardia* organisms are ubiquitously present in soil and may cause infectious corneal ulceration after trauma (48).

Primary tuberculous keratitis is now extremely rare. Nontuberculous mycobacteria, including *Mycobacterium fortuitum* (49,50), *Mycobacterium chelonae* (51,52), *Mycobacterium gordonae* (53), and *Mycobacterium avium-intracellulare* (54), are all capable of causing an indolent, intractable keratitis, especially after injury with a foreign body or after office surgical procedures (55). A case of keratitis with extension into the sclera has been reported due to *Mycobacterium marinum* (56).

Acute and delayed-onset mycobacterial keratitis after laser *in situ* keratomileusis (LASIK) has been reported with increasing frequency and in clusters or outbreaks at some outpatient laser vision correction centers around the world (57). Infectious keratitis after LASIK is a potentially vision-threatening complication (58). Onset of symptoms varies depending on causative agents. Furthermore, atypical organisms in the interface or beneath the flap can pose both diagnostic and therapeutic dilemmas. Location in the interface can make it more difficult to culture the organisms and prevent adequate penetration of topical antibiotics. In seven patients, *Mycobacterium szulgai* keratitis developed from 7 to 24 weeks after LASIK (59). Nontuberculous mycobacteria were identified 1 month after the flaps were cultured. Pulsed-field gel electrophoresis (PFGE) was used to type the isolates, and treatment was modified based on susceptibilities. *M. szulgai* was identified in five patients for whom cultures were performed, but response to empirical therapy based on cultures proved unsatisfactory. The keratitis resolved in all patients with treatment including clarithromycin based on susceptibilities. Medical therapy was sufficient, although one patient required flap amputation. Six of seven patients recovered best corrected visual acuity (BCVA), whereas one patient lost one line of BCVA. Two patients lost one line of postoperative uncorrected visual acuity (UCVA), two patients gained one line of UCVA, and three patients recovered postoperative UCVA. PFGE analysis revealed that the *M. szulgai* strains were identical, and the infection source was contaminated ice used to chill syringes for saline lavage. Nontuberculous mycobacterial keratitis after LASIK is a diagnostic and management challenge. This cluster and other outbreaks underscore the importance of adherence to sterile protocol during LASIK.

The incidence of ocular lesions of leprosy varies from approximately 15% of patients with tuberculoid leprosy to approximately 100% of the patients with long-standing lepromatous leprosy (60). *Mycobacterium leprae* is the causative agent of keratitis and may invade along peripheral corneal nerves (61,62).

Spirochetal infection with *Treponema pallidum* may result in a nonsuppurative stromal keratitis as a rare complication of acquired primary or secondary syphilis (63). Nonsyphilitic spirochetal infection of the cornea may occur in Lyme disease. A nonsuppurative, deep stromal keratitis similar to that observed in syphilis may be caused by the spirochete *Borrelia burgdorferi* (64). Organisms less frequently causing bacterial keratitis include *Aeromonas hydrophilia* (65), *Moraxella catarrhalis* (66), *Pasteurella multocida* (67), and complex, gram-negative bacilli, including *Methylobacterium* (*Pseudomonas*) *mesophilica*, *Capnocytophaga* species, and *Alcaligenes xylosoxidans* subsp. *denitrificans*.

RISK FACTORS

Bacterial keratitis typically occurs in eyes having one or more predisposing risk factors (68). Although the eye is constantly exposed to a large number of bacteria, it is a tribute to the natural host defense mechanisms that only a small portion of these microorganisms result in corneal infection. The microflora of the eye is diverse and continuously changing (69). To maintain ocular health, the various pathogenic bacteria on the ocular surface must be eliminated before proliferation and infection. There are several mechanisms to protect the surface of the eye from infectious agents. The eyelids provide a physical barrier to protect against organisms gaining direct access to the eye. The preocular tear film provides natural irrigation to remove organisms (70). The tear film contains secretory immunoglobulins, complement components, and various enzymes, including

lysozyme, lactoferrin (71), betalysins, orosomucoid, and ceruloplasmin (72). The mucin layer of the tear film produced by goblet cells acts as a mechanical protective barrier that can trap and remove potentially pathogenic organisms. The normal ocular flora provide a balance to help prevent overgrowth of exogenous organisms. The conjunctiva contains subepithelial mucosal-associated lymphoid tissue with a collection of lymphoid cells having specific defensive functions (73). T-cell lymphocytes are present in the conjunctiva in a ratio to B lymphocytes of approximately 20:1 in the substantia propria (74). Polymorphonuclear neutrophils (PMN) may be attracted to the cornea by chemotactic factors. Immunoglobulin G (IgG) in tears may assist by binding to bacteria, fixing complement, or enhancing phagocytosis. Cell-mediated immunity has an important role in the ocular defense against certain bacteria, especially intracellular pathogens. The cellular immune response may be initiated on the ocular surface by a specialized type of dendritic cell known as a *Langerhans cell*. The Langerhans cells are found in high density at the sclerocorneal limbus and diffusely throughout the bulbar conjunctiva (75). There are normally few Langerhans cells present in the central cornea (76). Langerhans cell surface expresses human leukocyte antigen DR (class II histocompatibility antigen), Ia antigen, and receptors for complement and the Fc portion of immunoglobulin (75). The Langerhans cells have an important role in the processing of bacterial antigens and their presentation to T cells.

Perhaps the most important defense barrier for the cornea is an intact epithelial layer. Most corneal infections result from trauma to the corneal epithelium. Alteration of any of the local or systemic defense mechanisms may also predispose the host to corneal infection. Eyelid abnormalities, including ectropion with exposure, entropion with trichiasis, or lagophthalmos, may be local factors contributing to corneal infection. Abnormalities of the preocular tear film, including aqueous tear layer insufficiency, mucin layer deficiencies from goblet cell loss or dysfunction, and lipid layer instability, may predispose to bacterial keratitis. Lacrimal drainage obstruction may interfere with the lubricating mechanical defense function. The inappropriate use of topical antibiotics could eliminate the natural protection provided by normal ocular flora and predispose to development of opportunistic infections of the cornea.

The use of topical corticosteroids can create a localized immunosuppression and present a major risk factor for bacterial keratitis. Corticosteroids prevent neutrophil migration in response to chemotactic factors released during microbial infection (77). Impairment in opsonization is a well-known predisposing factor to infection with encapsulated bacteria, including *S. pneumoniae*, *Streptococcus pyogenes*, *Haemophilus influenzae*, and certain strains of *P. aeruginosa*. Premature infants, patients with immunoglobulin deficiencies, asplenic individuals, and patients with sickle cell disease (78) or systemic lupus erythematosus all may have impaired opsonization.

Passive acquired maternal immunity begins to decline around 3 to 6 months of age before development of actively acquired immunity. This is a relative period of vulnerability for young children to infection with encapsulated bacteria, particularly *H. influenzae* (79). This provides the rationale for immunization with the type B conjugated vaccine against *H. influenzae*.

Individuals with functionally abnormal leukocytes may be more susceptible to development of marginal keratitis and blepharoconjunctivitis in part because of a loss of control over normal eyelid flora (80). A variety of systemic conditions can result in compromise, including use of immunosuppressive drugs, extensive body burns, pregnancy, chronic alcoholism, severe malnutrition, immunodeficiency syndromes, including acquired immunodeficiency syndrome (AIDS), drug addiction, malignancy, infancy, and old age (81). Corneal infection may be facilitated in the systemically compromised host. Patients with AIDS do not appear to have an increased risk for bacterial keratitis, yet may have a more fulminant clinical course (82,83). Severe *Pseudomonas* keratitis may develop in patients with AIDS, especially in association with contact lens wear (82).

Because the intact corneal epithelial barrier is such an important first line of defense, development of an epithelial defect represents a major risk factor for infection. Corneal abrasion, foreign body, or erosion may precipitate development of bacterial keratitis. Conditions that result in reduction of the integrity and adherence of the corneal epithelium, including bullous keratopathy, chemical injury, contact lens wear, prior viral infection, especially with herpes simplex virus, and corneal anesthesia (neurotrophic keratopathy), may predispose to development of corneal infection. Toxic epithelial changes from topical medications, including antiviral drugs, antibiotics, or anesthetics, may compromise the host for development of bacterial keratitis. The inhalational use of cocaine may lead to a relative systemic anesthetic state along with hallucinogenic stupor, loss of blink reflex, and development of infectious keratitis (84). Prescribed topical ocular medications may become contaminated and result in bacterial keratitis, including severe gram-negative infection with *Pseudomonas*, *Serratia*, and *Proteus* (85,86). Even microtrauma to the corneal epithelium may predispose to subsequent adherence and invasion of microorganisms. Seemingly trivial trauma with contaminated matter, foreign bodies, makeup, or contact lenses, including cosmetic costume plano lenses, can result in organism inoculation (87).

Contact lens wear of any type has been increasingly recognized as a major principal risk factor for microbial keratitis (13–19,88). Several investigations of contact lens–associated corneal infection have determined a greater risk with extended-wear soft contact lenses and overnight wear compared with daily-wear hard or soft lenses (89–91). The risk of ulcerative keratitis was found to be 10 to 15 times greater with extended-wear soft contact lens use than with those lenses worn on a daily basis (91). Continuous wear may result in cumulative risk because the longer lens wear was extended on a continuous basis, the greater the overall risk. From these early studies, it was estimated that the number of individuals contracting microbial keratitis in the United States because of extended-wear contact lenses is approximately 8000 per year (90). Smoking may be an additional risk factor for development of ulcerative keratitis among users of soft contact lenses (91). Extended wear with continuous overnight use promotes tissue hypoxia, as well as decreased tear flow beneath the contact lens, hampering the defensive cleansing function of the preocular tear film and the eyelids. Smoking may also contribute to relative corneal hypoxia, as in other body sites.

The introduction of disposable contact lenses was embraced with considerable enthusiasm in ophthalmology because it was postulated that by eliminating the frequent handling related to daily insertion, removal, and cleaning, these disposable lenses would have a reduced chance of contamination, possibly reducing the frequency of contact lens–associated infection (92). Use of disposable extended-wear contact lenses, however, does not appear to have significantly decreased the risk (93–96). Using contact lenses on a daily-wear basis is relatively safer, but still may result in ulcerative keratitis, with an estimated annual incidence of 3 per 10,000 contact lens wearers (90). Aphakic contact lens wearers have an estimated six to nine times greater rate of infectious corneal ulceration compared with cosmetic contact lens wearers (97). Individuals using aphakic contact lenses may be either young or elderly with relative systemic immunosuppression. In addition, the increased risk among aphakic contact lens wearers may be due to prolonged continuous wear with increased corneal hypoxia and epithelial trauma from thick aphakic contact lenses, or to reduced localized defense mechanisms after ocular surgery.

Gram-negative organisms, especially *Pseudomonas*, are the most common organisms associated with contact lens–related bacterial keratitis (19,88,98,99) (Fig. 13.1-1). With approximately 25 million individuals using contact lenses in the United States, corneal infection is a relatively rare occurrence. Poor contact lens hygiene practices increase the likelihood for development of corneal infection, yet microbial infection may also occur in individuals after proper lens hygiene techniques (100).

Keratorefractive surgery may introduce potential pathogens deep into the stroma after radial keratotomy (Fig. 13.1-2) and can result in bilateral, simultaneous keratitis after bilateral surgery (101–103). Disruption of the corneal epithelial layer after excimer laser photorefractive keratectomy with or without placement of a therapeutic soft contact lens may be an additional risk factor for the development of bacterial keratitis (104,105).

Patients who have undergone penetrating keratoplasty are at increased risk for bacterial keratitis because of adjunctive

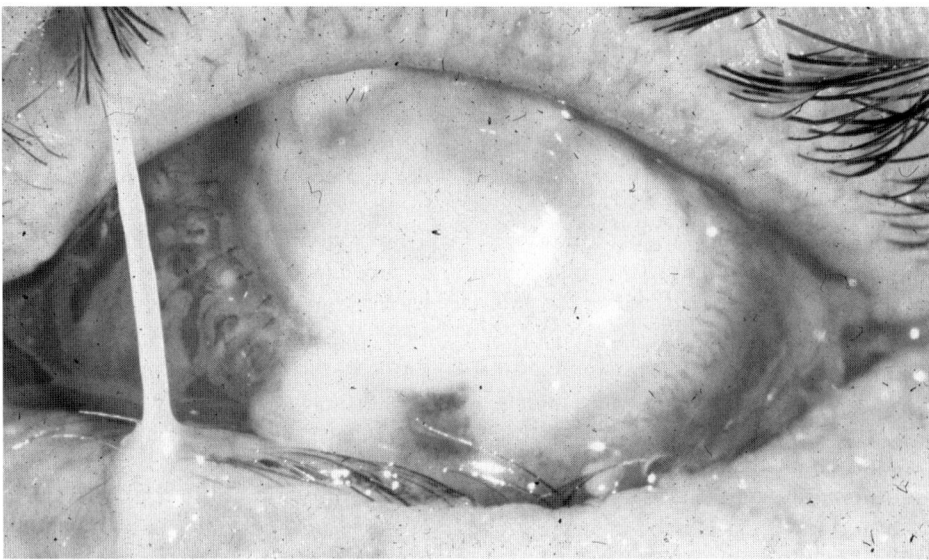

FIGURE 13.1-1. Suppurative keratitis in a patient who had been wearing extended-wear soft contact lenses around the clock, and now has *Pseudomonas* keratitis with hypopyon.

chronic topical corticosteroid use, therapeutic soft contact lens placement, and loose sutures (106–108) (Fig. 13.1-3).

Traumatic and systemic disease may be frequently associated and increase the risk for development of bacterial keratitis in children (109–111). Before 3 years of age, *Pseudomonas* was the most common organism recovered, whereas in older children, *S. aureus, S. pneumoniae,* and *P. aeruginosa* were the most common causative organisms in a series of children with bacterial keratitis (110). Because of potential delay in diagnosis and difficulty in

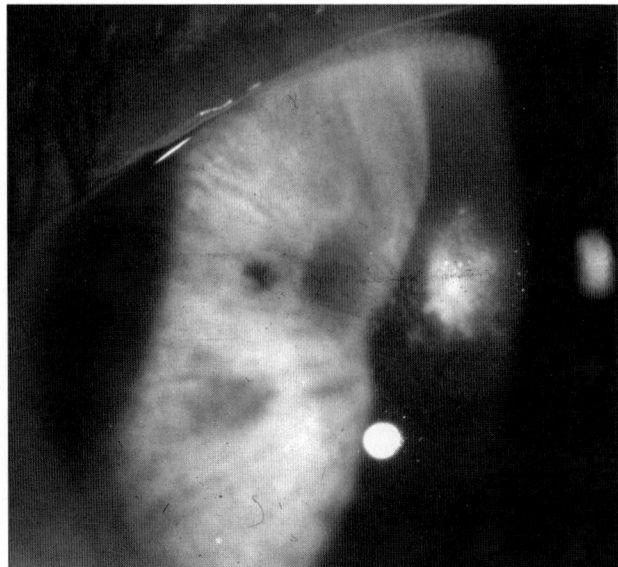

FIGURE 13.1-2. Infection at the interface in a patient who previously had undergone laser *in situ* keratomileusis keratorefractive surgery.

the delivery of therapy, surgical intervention may be required (110,111).

A retrospective analysis of hospital records of patients with bacterial keratitis in Paris, France was conducted to identify predisposing factors and to define clinical and microbiologic characteristics of bacterial keratitis in current practice (112). The study included 300 cases (291 patients) of presumed bacterial keratitis. Potential predisposing factors, usually multiple, were identified in 90.6% of cases. Contact lens wear was the main risk factor (50.3%), whereas trauma or a history of keratopathy was found in 15% and 21% of cases, respectively. An organism was identified in 201 eyes (68%). Eighty-three percent of the infections involved gram-positive bacteria, 17% involved gram-negative bacteria, and 2% were polymicrobial. Gram-negative bacteria were associated with severe anterior chamber inflammation, as well as greater surface of infiltrates. Ninety-nine percent of ulcers resolved with treatment. However, only 60% of patients had visual acuity better than the level at admission, and 5% had a very poor visual outcome (112).

Orthokeratology is a process by which the corneal curvature is flattened by sequentially fitting rigid, gas-permeable contact lenses of decreasing central curvature. There has been a resurgence of interest in the procedure with the recent introduction of reverse-geometry lenses. Although promising results have been described in reducing the myopic refractive error, the use of these lenses can be associated with corneal problems, as reported in an observational case series that identified six children with orthokeratology-related corneal ulcers (113).

Consecutive cases of orthokeratology lens (OKL)–related corneal ulcers in children presenting to a tertiary

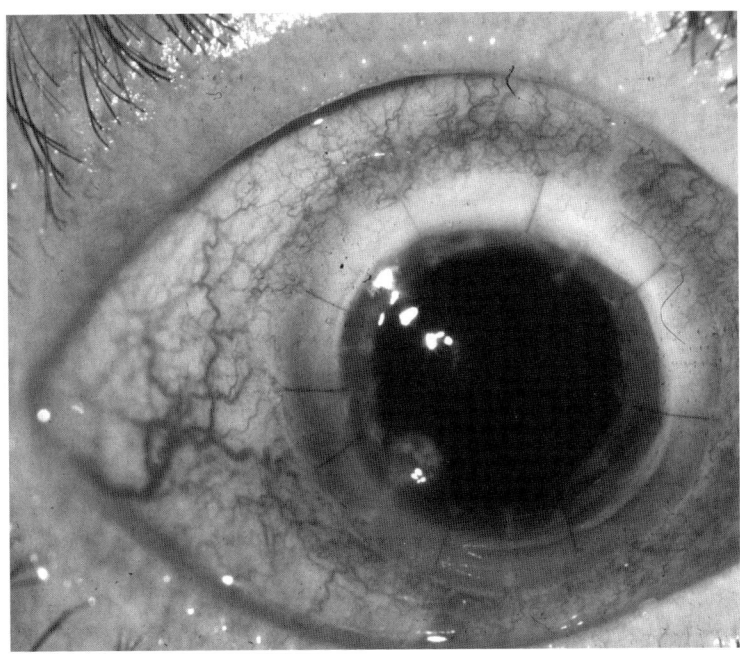

FIGURE 13.1-3. Suture abscess in a patient with corneal transplantation, in whom suture loosening was associated with microbial infestation along the suture tract. The suture has now been removed and the patient is on topical antibiotics.

referral center (March 1999 to June 2001) were reviewed for preinfection and postinfection visual acuity, refraction, and any organisms identified. Six children between the ages of 9 and 14 years (mean, 12.1 years) were treated. The male–female ratio was 1:5. All cases were unilateral, with equal numbers of left and right eyes. All children wore the OKL at night for 8 to 12 hours, with the onset of infection between 3 and 36 months (mean, 16.6 months) of OKL wear. All of the patients suffered a resultant BCVA loss. Five of the six cases were culture positive for *P. aeruginosa* (113). In view of the temporary benefits of orthokeratology, together with a known increased risk of infection associated with overnight lens wear, parents of children considering orthokeratology must be informed and warned of the potential for permanent loss of vision. The ophthalmic community should have a heightened awareness of the associated complications.

PATHOGENESIS

The pathogenesis of ocular infectious disease is determined by the intrinsic virulence of the microorganism, the nature of the host response, and the anatomic features of the site of the infection (114). The avascular, clear anatomic structure of the cornea with its specialized microenvironment predisposes to potential alteration and destruction by invading microorganisms, virulence factors, and host response factors. The intrinsic virulence of an organism relates to its ability to invade tissue, resist host defense mechanisms, and produce tissue damage (115). Penetration of exogenous bacteria into the corneal epithelium typically requires a defect in the surface of the squamous epithelial layer. By virtue of specialized enzymes and virulence factors, a few bacteria, such as *N. gonorrhoeae*, *N. meningitidis*, *C. diphtheriae*, *Shigella*, and *Listeria*, may directly penetrate corneal epithelium to initiate stromal suppuration.

Bacteria colonize host cells by engaging adhesins at their surface with receptors on the host cell surface. Specific receptors are often required by many adhesins to achieve binding. Besides adherence, microbial adhesins also contribute to subsequent interactions. Virulence factors may initiate microbial invasion or secondary effector molecules may assist the infective process. Upregulation or downregulation of host defense mechanisms may be involved. Adhesins may also be toxins (116). Therefore, receptor recognition is only the first step in the pathogenesis of infection directed by microbial adhesin molecules (117).

Many bacteria display several adhesins on fimbriae (pili) and nonfimbriae structures. Such adhesive proteins may recognize carbohydrates on host cells; alternatively, protein–protein interactions can also occur.

Certain bacteria exhibit differential adherence to corneal epithelium. The adherence of *S. aureus*, *S. pneumoniae*, and *P. aeruginosa* to ulcerated corneal epithelium is significantly higher than that of other bacteria and may account in part for their frequent isolation (118).

P. aeruginosa has many virulence factors that contribute to pathogenesis. Cell-associated structures such as pili (119) and flagella (120), and extracellular products, such as alkaline protease (121), elastase (121), exoenzyme S (116), exotoxin A (122), endotoxin (123), slime polysaccharide (124), phospholipase C (121), and leukocidin (121), are associated with virulence, invasiveness, and colonization. Whereas gram-positive bacteria, including *S. aureus*, adhere to host tissues through fibronectin and collagen (125),

P. aeruginosa attaches to cell surfaces that lack fibronectin (126). Bacteria adhere to injured cornea (127), to exposed corneal stroma (128), or to immature nonwounded cornea (129). The corneal epithelial receptors for *Pseudomonas* species are glycoproteins (130,131).

Pili (fimbriae) are thin (4 to 10 nm in diameter) protein filaments that are located on the surfaces of many bacteria. *In vitro* studies indicate purified pili successfully compete for binding with cold bacteria by saturating available binding sites on the ocular surface (132). Monoclonal antibodies specific for *Pseudomonas* pili and a peptide-conjugated alkaline phosphatase allowed identification of host corneal receptor molecules (133). Characterization of these receptor proteins indicates that carbohydrates are necessary for receptor activity (131). In competitive inhibition experiments, sialic acid was the only aminosugar able completely to inhibit pilus binding to mouse corneal epithelial proteins. Pili have been used to protect against *P. aeruginosa* keratitis (132). Pili, however, have considerable antigenic variation between strains (134). Bacteria also possess an array of other virulence factors, including non-pilus adhesins (135). Some clinical isolates of *P. aeruginosa* from keratitis are reportedly nonpiliated (136).

Flagella are subcellular filamentous organelles (16 to 18 nm in diameter) originating in the cell membrane and extending to 15 to 20 μm from its surface. These organelles are responsible for bacterial motility, which is important for dissemination of infection (137). The flagellum has a helicofilament composed of cell-assembling subunits of the protein flagellin. More than 95% of *P. aeruginosa* clinical isolates are flagellated (138). Because flagella contain aminospecific proteins and have a large surface exposure available for antibody binding, they have been considered as the basis for vaccine development. Much research examining the flagellum as a virulence factor in *P. aeruginosa* infection or as a vaccine candidate has focused on the burned-mouse model (139). A loss of virulence was observed in flagella-deficient mutants active or passive systemic, as well as topical immunization with flagella or topical antiflagellar antibody homologous to the infecting strain of bacteria, protects mice against *P. aeruginosa* corneal infection (140).

In addition to adhesins, the adherence of *P. aeruginosa* and *N. gonorrhoeae* is guided by glycocalyx, a biologic slime that enables them to adhere to susceptible cells, producing slime aggregates that are resistant to phagocytosis (141). Similar coatings may form on contact lenses to facilitate the adherence of bacteria to the lens material (142).

After adherence of microorganism to the cornea and initiation of infection, the complex tissue reactions of the host response occur, including inflammation, neovascularization, cellular and humoral immune responses, and stromal degradative processes.

A variety of cytokines may be released in response to corneal infection. During inflammation, leukocyte adhesion to the vascular endothelium is enhanced by interleukin-1 (IL-1) and tumor necrosis factor (TNF), products of macrophages and T lymphocytes (143). IL-1 is a known potent intracellular mediator of inflammation and chemotaxis for neutrophils. TNF stimulates immunocompetent cells and induces release of IL-1 and IL-6 from macrophages and other cells (144). Bacterial exotoxin-A downregulates TNF, IL-1, and lymphotoxin by inhibiting the cells' ability to produce these cytokines (145).

Neutrophil infiltration after corneal infection is a principal host defense mechanism. The host inflammatory response to *Pseudomonas* species has been studied in mice designated as susceptible or resistant. Susceptible mice are unable to clear the cornea, whereas resistant mice may restore corneal clarity within 1 month after ocular challenge (146). Resistant mice appear to have a larger number of corneal leukocytes present initially. The resistant mice also have a shorter duration of inflammatory cell and bacterial residence in the cornea compared with susceptible mice.

If neutrophils are experimentally depleted, many resistant animals succumb to lethal *Pseudomonas* sepsis within 48 hours (147). In aged mice, deficiencies of neutrophilic phagocytosis have been observed. These observations may partially explain the clinically apparent age-related susceptibility of individuals to corneal infection.

Preimmunization of rats with phenol-killed *Pseudomonas* organisms still results in massive corneal stromal degradation caused by neutrophil migration in the absence of viable bacteria. Naive, unimmunized mice show little stromal destruction during early infection, despite the presence of numerous bacteria in the cornea. Thus, immune recognition is involved in the host response to *Pseudomonas* corneal infection and is apparently required for phagocytosis, but not for neutrophil recruitment (148).

Models of experimental *P. aeruginosa* ocular disease also indicate the importance of the third component of complement (C3) in host resistance to corneal infection. Resistant mice experimentally depleted of C3 by cobra venom and then inoculated with *Pseudomonas* organisms to the cornea respond with delayed leukocyte mobility, bacterial persistence in the cornea, and subsequent scarring and opacification (149).

In addition to organism factors, host lysosomal enzymes and oxidative substances produced by neutrophils, keratocytes, and epithelial cells may significantly contribute to the destruction caused by *Pseudomonas* keratitis (150). Two eukaryotic gelatinase species have been characterized, including a type IV collagenase (72 kD) and a type V collagenase (90 to 100 kD) (151). Corneal epithelial cells produce predominantly the 92-kD form of progelatinase, whereas stromal fibroblasts synthesize predominantly the 72-kD progelatinase (152). The progelatinase is cleaved by *Pseudomonas* elastase to produce the active form (153).

A variety of bacterial toxins and enzymes may be produced during corneal infection to contribute to destruction of the corneal substance. *P. aeruginosa* produce many toxic substances capable of causing necrotic central corneal ulceration. Toxin-A inhibits protein synthesis much as diphtheria toxin by catalyzing the transfer of the adenosine 5'-diphosphate ribose (ADPR) portion of nicotinamide adenine dinucleotide to mammalian elongation factor II. With staphylococcal keratitis, alpha-toxin, but not protein A, is a major virulence factor mediating corneal destruction (154). Advances in our understanding of host innate and adaptive immune responses to experimental infection with *P. aeruginosa* have been made using a variety of animal models, including inbred murine models that are classed as resistant (cornea heals) versus susceptible (cornea perforates) (155). Evidence has been provided that sustained IL-12–driven interferon (IFN)-γ production in dominant T-helper-1 responder strains such as C57BL/6 (B6) contributes to corneal destruction and perforation, whereas IL-18–driven production of IFN-γ in the absence of IL-12 is associated with bacterial killing and less corneal destruction in dominant T-helper-2 responder strains such as BALB/c. The critical role of IL-1 and chemotactic cytokines such as macrophage inflammatory protein-2 in PMN recruitment and the critical role of this cell in the innate immune response to bacterial infection is reviewed (155). Regulation of PMN persistence is also discussed, and evidence provided that persistence of PMN in B6 cornea is regulated by CD4$^+$ T cells, whereas macrophages regulate PMN number in the cornea of BALB/c mice (155). The studies provide a better understanding of the inflammatory mechanisms that are operative in the cornea after *P. aeruginosa* challenge and are consistent with long-term goals of providing targets for alternative or adjunctive treatment for this disease. Future studies will be aimed at better defining the role of Toll receptors, neuropeptides (as unconventional modulators of the immune response), and exploitation of disease control by new techniques, such as RNA silencing (155).

In summary, the pathogenesis of bacterial keratitis initially requires the adherence of bacteria to disrupted or normal corneal epithelium. Adhesins are microbial proteins that direct the high-affinity binding to specific cell surface components. These adhesins are able to promote bacterial entry into the host cell, derange leukocyte migration, activate plasmin, and induce cytokine production. In addition, they may act as toxins directly. Adhesins recognize carbohydrate and protein moieties on the host cell surface. Most bacteria can display a number of adhesins. Although the cognate oligosaccharides for bacterial adhesins are known, the molecules bearing these determinants are not well characterized. Integrins are a family of glycoproteins mediating cell–cell and cell–extracellular matrix recognition. Many bacterial pathogens have coopted the existing integrin-based system, masking ancillary ligand recognition in a form of mimicry. Once the bacterial pathogen has adhered to the corneal epithelial surface, the next step in establishing infection is invasion into the corneal stroma. Bacterial invasion is facilitated by proteinases that degrade basement membrane and extracellular matrix and cause cell lysis. Proteinases may be derived from bacteria, corneal cells, and migrating leukocytes. Corneal matrix metalloproteinases (MMPs) are excreted in an inactive form, but are activated during infection by bacterial proteinase. Corneal proteinase production may also be induced during the course of infection. The invasion of bacteria into the cornea is facilitated by a number of exotoxins, including *P. aeruginosa* phospholipase, heat-stable hemolysin, and exotoxin-A, which leads to stromal necrosis. Once bacterial invasion into the cornea has ensued, infection is further facilitated by a complex sequence leading to interruption of the host immune response. Exopolysaccharide formation by both gram-positive and gram-negative bacteria results in local immunosuppressive effects. Certain bacteria with capsular polysaccharide also have immunosuppressive properties, including interference with phagocytosis. Proteases degrade complement components, immunoglobulins, and cytokines and may inhibit leukocyte chemotaxis and lymphocyte function. Toxin-A inhibits protein synthesis much as diphtheria toxin by catalyzing the transfer of the ADPR portion of nicotinamide adenine dinucleotide to mammalian elongation factor-II. Exoenzyme-S is another ADP-ribosyl transferase that may act as an adhesin and also contribute to dissemination of the organism.

Two specific bacterial proteases, elastase and alkaline protease, cause marked destruction of the cornea when injected intrastromally (156,157). Intrastromal injection of purified elastase alone also results in severe corneal damage. Inhibition of elastase activity with 2-mercaptoacetyl-L-phenylalanine-L-leucine (158) prevents keratolysis. The proteases contribute to the pathogenesis of keratitis by degrading basement membrane (159), laminin, proteoglycans, extracellular matrix (160), and collagen (161). In addition, the bacterial proteases inhibit host defense systems by degrading immunoglobulins, IFN, complement, IL-1, IL-2, and TNF (156). Such interference results in decreased neutrophil chemotaxis, T-lymphocyte function, and natural killer cell function. Mutants deficient for alkaline protease do not establish corneal infection, suggesting that this protease is an important initiating factor (162). A bacterial heat-labile phospholipase C has been shown in antibody/substrate specificity studies to be produced in mouse ocular infections, suggesting its role as a potential virulence factor (163). Bacterial lipopolysaccharide stimulates neutrophil migration and infiltration into the cornea with subsequent corneal scarring and opacification (164).

Bacterial exotoxins are released by actively replicating organisms, and some endotoxins are released only after the death of the organism. These enzymes and toxins have been shown to persist in the cornea for a protracted period and continue to cause stromal destruction after the death of the

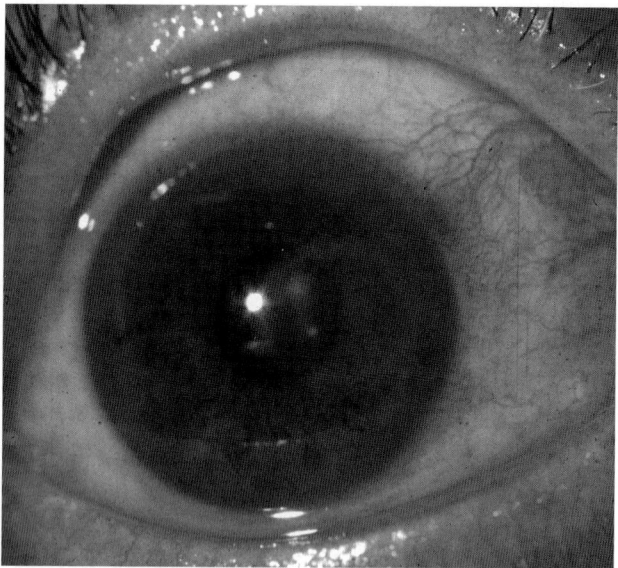

FIGURE 13.1-4. Wessely ring, much as might be seen in an antigen–antibody reaction on an Ouchterlony plate (or "immune ring").

pathogen. Most of the bacterial exotoxins are thermal labile and have antigenic properties. Gram-positive bacteria elaborate a variety of biologically active and immunologically distinct toxins. Coagulase-positive strains of staphylococci are the most pathogenic, and elaborate other extracellular enzymes, such as staphylokinase, lipase, hyaluronidase, DNase, coagulase, and lysozyme. Coagulase-negative staphylococci, including *S. epidermidis*, also produce potentially destructive toxin (165). Streptococcal toxins include streptolysin O and S, erythrogenic toxin, and the enzymes hyaluronidase, streptodornase, and streptokinase. The invasiveness of *S. pneumoniae* is aided by collagenase activity (166), although the organism may be inherently invasive without toxin production.

The lipopolysaccharides composing the endotoxins in the cell wall of gram-negative bacteria may be released on the death of the organism. These lipopolysaccharides may result in the production of stromal rings (Fig. 13.1-4). These rings have been shown to consist of polymorphonuclear leukocytes in the corneal stroma, which have been chemoattracted by the alternative complement pathway (167,168). In addition to gram-negative bacterial keratitis, such ring infiltrates have been described in fungal, viral, and *Acanthamoeba* keratitis. In nonbacterial corneal infection, these stromal rings are thought to result from antigen–antibody precipitants (immune rings).

CLINICAL FEATURES

Once corneal infection is established, there are no absolutely specific clinical symptoms to confirm infection or exclusively distinctive biomicroscopic signs to distinguish

the responsible organism(s). The determinants of clinical presentation include the strain (virulence) of the responsible organism(s), the method of inoculation or introduction, the time interval from inoculation, the antecedent status of the cornea, prior or concomitant antimicrobial corticosteroid therapy, and other host factors (115).

Because of the rich innervation of the cornea, the most common symptom of inflammatory lesions of the cornea is pain. Movement of the eyelids over ulcerated corneal epithelium intensifies the pain. Therefore, examination of patients with suspected microbial keratitis is greatly facilitated by instillation of topical anesthetic. Keratitis is usually accompanied by a variable decrease in vision. Reflex tearing, photophobia, and blepharospasm are common. A discharge, which is a distinctive feature of conjunctivitis, is usually absent in patients with keratitis, unless an associated purulent conjunctivitis is present, such as with gonococcal, pneumococcal, and *Haemophilus* infections. The conjunctiva may be variably hyperemic and a nonspecific papillary reaction may vary in intensity, depending on the severity of the keratitis. The preocular tear film in bacterial keratitis can be observed by slit-lamp microscopy to contain inflammatory cells and debris. Ipsilateral lid edema may be variably observed with bacterial keratitis. In addition to conjunctival hyperemia, chemosis may develop, especially with highly virulent causative organisms.

The hallmark clinical signs that are distinctive for suspected infectious keratitis include an ulceration of the epithelium with suppurative stromal inflammation that is either focal or diffuse (Fig. 13.1-5). Multifocal suppurative inflammation in the cornea is suggestive of mixed infection (polymicrobial keratitis) (169). Polymicrobial keratitis has

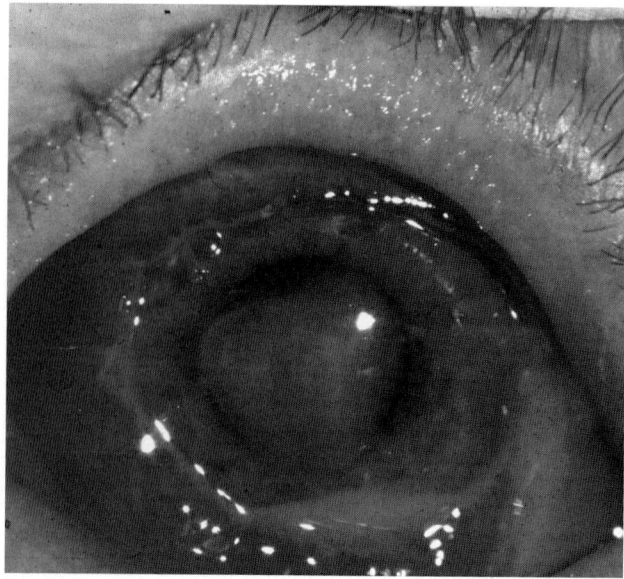

FIGURE 13.1-5. Microbial keratitis with stromal infiltration with inflammatory cells, and associated reactive hypopyon.

been observed in from 6% to 56% of overall cases (170,171). Microbial keratitis may occasionally present with an intact epithelium and nonsuppurative multifocal stromal inflammation. The presence of diffuse cellular infiltration in the adjacent stroma and an anterior chamber cellular reaction is highly suggestive for infectious keratitis. The anterior chamber reaction may range from mild flare and cells to severe layered hypopyon formation.

The hypopyon in bacterial keratitis is usually sterile when Descemet's membrane is intact. Hypopyon may also be present with mycotic keratitis and severe necrotizing viral stromal keratitis. Certain noninfectious conditions may be accompanied by hypopyon formation, including Behçet's syndrome, severe alkali injury, therapeutic soft contact lens use, and abuse of topical anesthetic agents.

If the antecedent status of the cornea is abnormal, the clinical signs and symptoms may be nondistinctive. Interpretation of the clinical signs may be difficult if there has been prior corneal inflammation, uveitis, and structural abnormalities. Careful monitoring of symptoms of pain and redness, as well as increasing epithelial or stromal ulceration, increasing anterior chamber inflammatory reaction, or an overall acute deterioration in the clinical status, should elevate the index of suspicion for infection (172). Prior treatment with antibiotic therapy can blunt the clinical symptoms and signs of corneal infection. Prior treatment with corticosteroids may enhance the likelihood of invasion by opportunistic organisms and dampen the clinical signs of inflammation associated with bacterial keratitis. Corticosteroids and other immunosuppressive agents may retard host defense mechanisms and inhibit chemotaxis, neutrophil migration, phagocytosis, degranulation, and lysosomal enzyme release. The use of corticosteroids before infection may also result in severe rebound inflammation in the stroma on abrupt cessation of corticosteroid therapy during the course of infection. Such a rebound inflammation may confound the clinician's ability to monitor the initial response to therapy. Surreptitious use of over-the-counter vasoconstrictor medicines may mask conjunctival hyperemia. The marked corneal toxicity of particular agents, including aminoglycosides, topical anesthetics, topical antivirals, and topical amphotericin B, can mimic bacterial keratitis by causing epithelial and stromal ulceration, stromal infiltration, and anterior chamber inflammatory reaction. Prior contact lens wear can also alter the clinical presentation of bacterial keratitis. Infection associated with contact lenses may be multifocal with diffuse epithelial and stromal infiltration. Given the ability of bacteria to bind to contact lenses, individuals presenting with corneal abrasions in association with contact lens wear should be suspected of having possible early bacterial keratitis. Placing a patch over a corneal epithelial abrasion associated with contact lens wear may create conditions favorable for the development of infectious keratitis (173).

Prompt clinical recognition of bacterial corneal infection is essential to successful management. The patient's symptoms and clinical biomicroscopic signs alone may be insufficient reliably to diagnose bacterial keratitis. In a study of patients hospitalized for ulcerative keratitis, diagnostic evaluations disclosed that 65% of the patients had nonbacterial keratitis (14). The differential diagnosis of bacterial keratitis may be particularly difficult in cases of herpes simplex viral keratitis, neurotrophic ulceration, marginal ulcerative and infiltrative keratitis from multiple causes, toxic keratopathy, and those diseases characterized by persistent epithelial or anterior stromal ulceration. With herpes, a prior history of herpetic infection and a relative asymmetrically diminished corneal sensation may be helpful to distinguish herpes simplex viral from bacterial keratitis. Patients with keratoconjunctivitis sicca may be especially sensitive to the toxic effects of topical medication, which can result in keratolysis and perforation in the absence of stromal cellular infiltration.

A clinical assessment of the severity of the bacterial keratitis should be made at the initial presentation. Careful measurement and documentation of objective parameters for comparative analysis with subsequent remeasurements are important to monitor the clinical course. Using the adjusting slit beam on the biomicroscope, the overall size of the epithelial involvement can be measured by recording the diameter in two dimensions. Similarly, the area of stromal ulceration can be measured in two meridians. An estimate of the depth of stromal ulceration should be determined by comparing adjacent uninvolved corneal thickness. Slit-lamp photographs are helpful for documentation and monitoring of the clinical course. Initial corneal topographic analysis may be helpful in select cases. Detailed clinical drawings with measurements of the size and depth of infiltration should be recorded at each visit. Additional features to assess include the intensity of suppuration and edema, thickness of the stroma, accompanying scleral suppuration, the degree of anterior chamber and iris inflammation, secondary glaucoma, and the rate of progression or pace of inflammation. A grading system based on the characteristics, including the size of the ulceration in millimeters, percentage depth of ulceration, intensity or density of infiltration, and scleral involvement may provide a guide to the aggressiveness of therapy. More detailed grading systems have been described (174).

Certain characteristic clinical features may be suggestive of specific corneal pathogens, although clinical observation alone should not replace laboratory investigation with corneal scrapings for smears and culture (172,175,176). Gram-positive cocci typically cause localized, round or oval ulcerations with grayish-white stromal infiltrates having distinct borders and minimal surrounding epithelial edema (Fig. 13.1-6). Staphylococcal keratitis is more frequently encountered in compromised corneas, such as with bullous keratopathy, chronic herpetic keratitis, keratoconjunctivitis sicca, ocular rosacea, or atopic keratoconjunctivitis. With

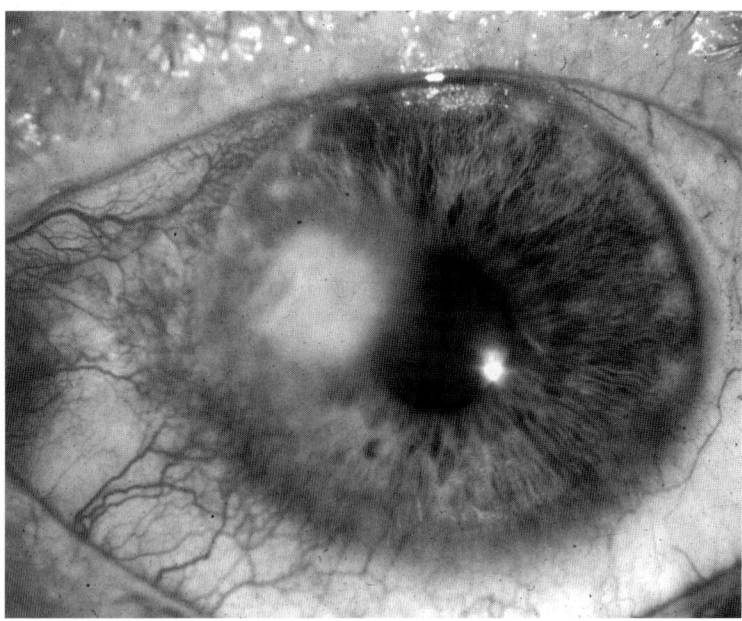

FIGURE 13.1-6. Corneal ulcer with a relatively well circumscribed stromal infiltrative inflammatory cells, in a patient whose cultures of scrapings taken at the time of the initial visit disclosed *Staphylococcus aureus*.

delay in presentation and long-standing infection, both coagulase-positive and coagulase-negative staphylococcal keratitis may cause severe intrastromal abscess and corneal perforation.

Staphylococcus is a common inhabitant of the normal ocular flora. Coagulase-negative staphylococci may be recovered from eyelid cultures in over 85% of healthy subjects, whereas *S. aureus* has been documented in 15% of eyelid cultures (177). Excessive colonization of the anterior lid margin with staphylococci may be associated with hypersensitivity (type III), marginal infiltrative keratitis, or peripheral ulceration. In compromised corneas, superinfections with *S. aureus* may present with an atypical appearance. In these abnormal corneas, *S. aureus* infection may result in marked suppuration with a deep stromal abscess. An accompanying large hypopyon or endothelial fibrin plaque is usually present and larger than anticipated, based on the area of ulceration. *S. epidermidis* typically has a more indolent clinical course, yet may also lead to deep stromal abscess and the potential for corneal perforation.

After trauma, *S. pneumoniae* keratitis may present with a deep, oval, central stromal ulceration having serpiginous edges (Fig. 13.1-7). There is typically dense stromal abscess formation with radiating folds in Descemet's membrane and moderate accompanying stromal edema. Hypopyon with retrocorneal fibrin deposition is a common clinical feature. Progression to corneal perforation is possible. Some strains of *S. pneumoniae* (designated S strains) are encapsulated, whereas others (the R strains) are not. Virulence for corneal infection is not totally dependent on encapsulation because R strains have been recovered from clinical keratitis (178). An abnormal antecedent cornea may modify the classic serpiginous, hypopyon ulcer described after trauma with *S. pneumoniae* infection. Beta-hemolytic streptococci

may cause severe corneal infection with dense suppuration, which may progress to perforation. A distinct, indolent, pauciinflammatory-appearing crystalline keratopathy has been observed in association with streptococcal corneal infection (179–183).

Gram-negative corneal infection typically follows a rapid-paced inflammatory destructive course or, alternatively, a less commonly encountered, slowly progressive

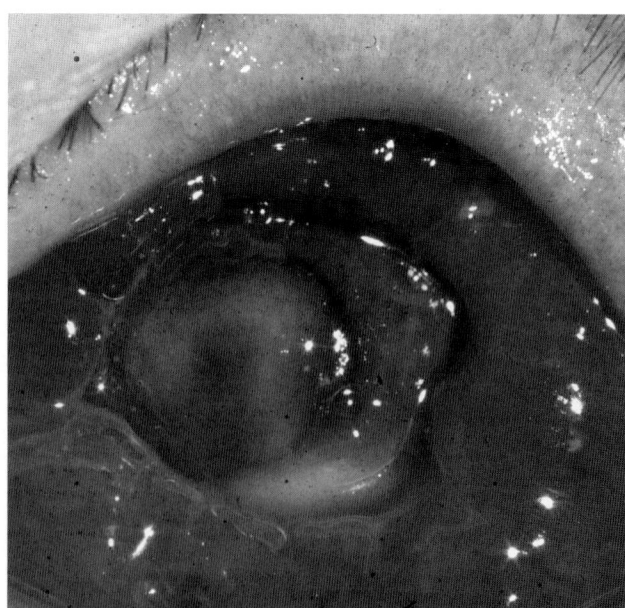

FIGURE 13.1-7. Microbial keratitis with associated hypopyon, stromal inflammatory cell infiltration, and minimal loss of stroma up to this point. Note the extensive nature of the infiltrate, however, and the undulating, "serpiginous" nature of the edges of the infiltrate in this patient whose cultures grew *Streptococcus pneumoniae*.

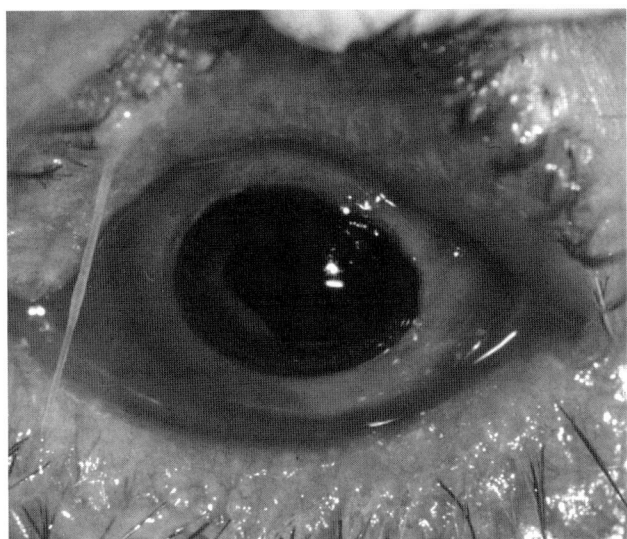

FIGURE 13.1-8. Complete dissolution of the corneal stroma in a patient with *Pseudomonas* keratitis. The glistening light reflex is from Descemet's membrane.

indolent ulceration. *P. aeruginosa* has the most distinctive clinical course after corneal infection. There is a loss of corneal transparency with adjacent peripheral inflammatory epithelial edema and a "ground-glass" stromal appearance. The keratitis may progress rapidly, even with appropriate treatment, into a deep stromal abscess (Fig. 13.1-8) spreading concentrically to form a ring ulcer with large hypopyon (Fig. 13.1-9). Complete stromal keratolysis with perforation may occur, even after apparent clinical improvement.

A less common clinical presentation of *Pseudomonas* keratitis behaves in a more indolent fashion and the organism may not possess similar virulence factors, including proteoglycanolytic enzymes, as discussed in the pathogenesis section. Other gram-negative rods may cause slower-paced ulcerative keratitis in previously compromised corneas with less intense anterior chamber inflammatory reaction and less specific distinguishing features. *Proteus* may have a fulminant course similar to *Pseudomonas* without trauma. *Klebsiella* is more often associated with infection as a consequence of chronic epithelial disease. *S. marcescens* may be an opportunistic pathogen causing contact lens–associated keratitis (36). *Moraxella* was originally discovered as an ocular pathogen. *Moraxella* may colonize the nasopharynx and produce keratitis after trauma in debilitated, alcoholic, malnourished, or diabetic patients. The large, boxlike diplobacilli and pleomorphic gram-negative rods of non-*liquefaciens Moraxella* may be observed in corneal scrapings from nonalcoholic patients in the presence of a preexisting epithelial defect (23). The typical clinical features of *Moraxella* keratitis include an indolent corneal ulceration with mild to moderate anterior chamber reaction. The ulceration is usually oval with a predilection for the inferior portion of the cornea (Fig. 13.1-10). In some cases of *Moraxella* keratitis, moderately severe stromal and anterior chamber reactions may develop, with endothelial decompensation and possible perforation (184).

A rapidly paced, hyperpurulent conjunctivitis with marked hyperemia, chemosis, and corneal epithelial ulceration with

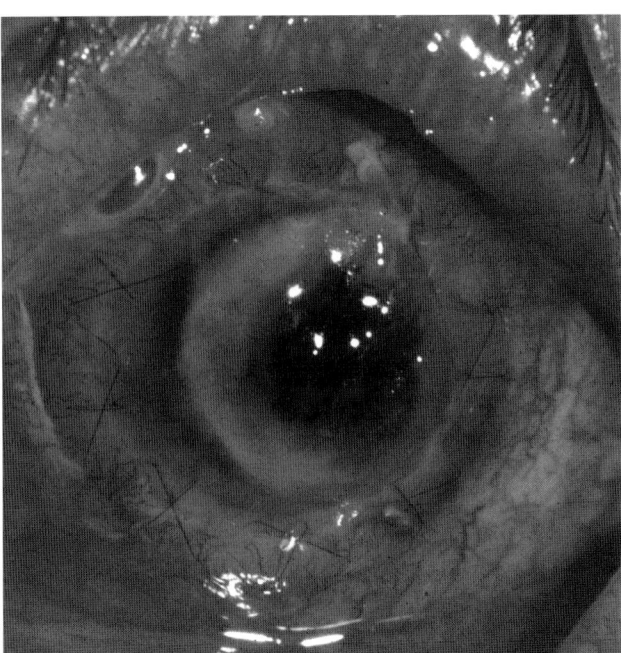

FIGURE 13.1-9. Ring infiltrate in a corneal graft of a patient on chronic topical steroids. Treatment of the infection necessitated significant reduction in topical steroid administration, resulting in corneal graft rejection.

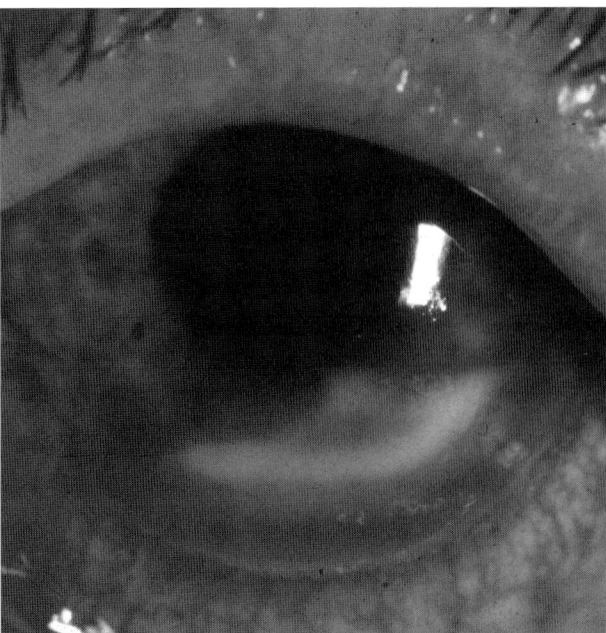

FIGURE 13.1-10. *Moraxella* corneal ulcer, with an inflammatory infiltrate in an arcuate, scimitar pattern in the inferior aspect of the cornea.

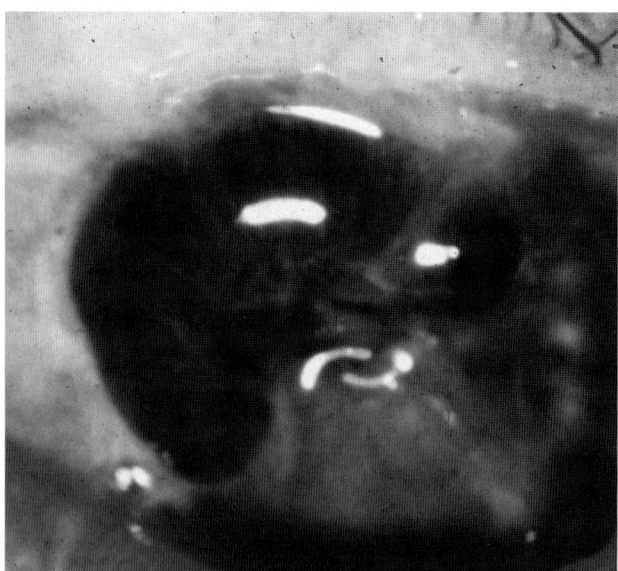

FIGURE 13.1-11. Corneal ulcer with perforation in a patient with *Neisseria* gonococcus infection. The process began just 5 days earlier, illustrating the rapidity with which the process can progress, with dissolution of the corneal stroma.

stromal infiltration should suggest infection with *N. gonorrhoeae*, or *N. meningitidis* (Fig. 13.1-11). A rapid and devastating keratitis may also follow trauma and contamination with *B. cereus*. *B. cereus* keratitis corneal infection is characterized by a distinctive stromal ring infiltrate remote from the site of injury with rapid progression to stromal abscess, corneal perforation, and intraocular extension with destruction mediated by specific exotoxins (32). The presence of a distinctive air bubble in the anterior chamber or in the corneal stromal beneath the epithelium, especially after trauma with contaminated soil, should suggest possible infection with spore-forming *Clostridium* species (42).

Corneal infections with *Nocardia*, *Actinomyces*, and *Streptomyces* typically follow an indolent clinical course, which may simulate mycotic keratitis with hyphal edges, satellite lesions, and elevated epithelial lesions. A chronic epithelial defect with "calcareous" bodies at the edges of epithelial ulceration was caused by *Nocardia asteroides* (185).

The vast majority of ocular infections by nontuberculous mycobacterial species involve the cornea and are principally due to the rapid growers, *M. fortuitum* and *M. chelonae* (186). *M. fortuitum* has been recognized as an opportunistic pathogen capable of causing intractable keratitis frequently resistant to multiple antibiotics (49). Between 1965 and 1974, virtually all of the reported cases of keratitis secondary to nontuberculous mycobacteria were attributed to *M. fortuitum*. In more recent years (1978–1995), there has been a preponderance of *M. chelonae* isolates accounting for the majority of reported corneal infections (187–191). Clinically, the nontuberculous mycobacteria produce relatively slowly progressive keratitis, which may mimic the course of disease due to other indolent organisms,

such as fungi or anaerobic bacteria. Environmental exposure is the most common route of inoculation and many patients have a history of antecedent trauma or prior surgery, such as penetrating keratoplasty or radial keratotomy. Clinical infection usually develops 2 to 8 weeks after the corneal trauma; however, delayed-onset keratitis occurring 2 years after radial keratotomy has been reported (191). Treatment with topical corticosteroids before the identification of the infection frequently occurs. Experimental studies have suggested that *M. fortuitum* keratitis in rabbits is made worse by corticosteroid use (192). The typical clinical features of nontuberculous mycobacterial keratitis include a relative paucity of suppuration, although dense stromal abscesses may form and rarely corneal perforation may occur. Multifocal lesions may be observed at the time of presentation and satellite lesions may also develop as the infection worsens. The presenting corneal lesion has occasionally been linear and pseudodendritiform, with accompanying epithelial ulceration. In partially treated cases, the lack of response to conventional antibiotic therapy is frequently a clue to the diagnosis. In addition to the more typical clinical features, a broad spectrum of unusual presentations has been reported, including ring stromal infiltrate (193) and crystalline keratopathy (194).

HISTOPATHOLOGY

Histopathologic analysis of bacterial keratitis discloses distinct stages of progressive infiltration, active ulceration, regression, and healing (175). The progressive stage includes adherence and entry of the organism, diffusion of toxins and enzymes, and resultant tissue destruction. Shortly after adherence, polymorphonuclear leukocytes arrive at the corneal wound site (141). Stromal damage from bacterial and neutrophil enzymes facilitates progressive bacterial invasion of the cornea. Penetration into the corneal stroma is accompanied by loss of the bacterial glycocalyx envelope. Initially, the neutrophils arrive in the tear film and enter the cornea through the wound, followed by radial spread through the stroma to the limbus. As infection progresses, limbal vessel ingrowth may deliver neutrophils to the site. In the second stage, active ulceration, the clinical severity varies with the virulence of the organism and toxin production. There may be progressive tissue necrosis with subsequent sloughing of the epithelium and stroma, resulting in a sharply demarcated ulcer with a surrounding infiltration of neutrophils. The necrotic base of the ulcer is surrounded by heaped-up tissue. If organisms penetrate deeper into posterior stroma, progressive keratolysis with stromal thinning may result in descemetocele formation. Corneal perforation may ensue as the next stage.

The third or regressive stage is characterized by an improvement in the clinical signs and symptoms. The natural host defense mechanisms predominate and humoral and cellular immune defenses combine with antibacterial therapy to retard bacterial replication, promote phagocytosis of the organism and cellular debris, and halt destruction of stromal collagen.

In the regression phase, a distinct demarcation line may appear as the epithelial ulceration and stromal infiltration consolidate and the edges become rounded. In ulcerative keratitis of long duration, vascularization of the cornea may ensue.

In the final phase or healing stage, the epithelium resurfaces the central area of ulceration and the necrotic stroma is replaced by scar tissue produced by fibroblasts. The reparative fibroblasts are derived from histiocytes and keratocytes that have undergone transformation. Areas of stromal thinning may be partially replaced by fibrous tissue. New blood vessel growth directed toward the area of ulceration occurs with delivery of humoral and cellular components to promote further healing. Bowman's layer does not regenerate, but is replaced with fibrous tissue. New epithelium slowly resurfaces the irregular base. Vascularization gradually disappears, but sometimes a residue of "ghost vessels" remain. The fibrous scar tissue variably produces corneal opacity, although there may be fading of the scar over time with return of relative translucency.

With severe bacterial keratitis, the progressive stage may advance beyond the point where the regressive stage can lead to the healing stage. In such severe ulcerations, stromal keratolysis may progress to corneal perforation with iris prolapse to plug the defect in Descemet's membrane (Fig. 13.1-12). Uveal blood vessels may the participate in sealing the perforation, resulting in an adherent vascularized leukoma.

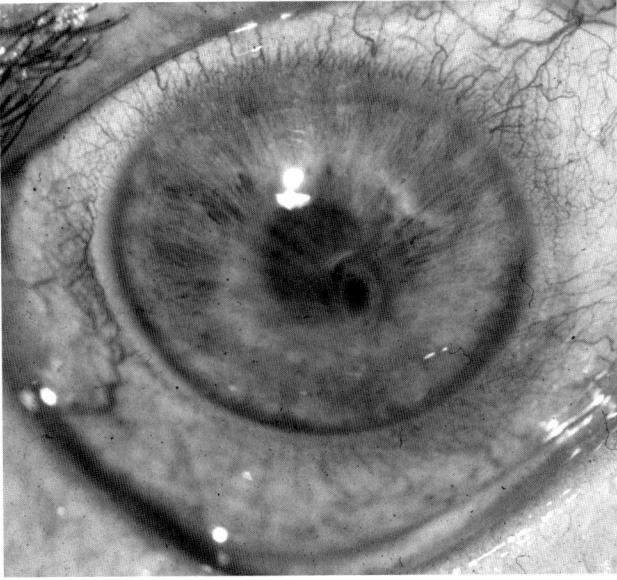

FIGURE 13.1-12. Bacterial corneal ulcer with progression to perforation, with the perforation now plugged with iris.

DIAGNOSIS

Based on the presenting clinical history, antecedent risk factors, predisposing ocular and systemic diseases, and distinctive clinical signs, an index of clinical suspicion for infectious keratitis versus a nonmicrobial process is formulated. As discussed earlier, multiple factors may alter the typical clinical features of infectious keratitis. Antecedent partial antibiotic therapy or combination antibiotic–corticosteroid therapy may mask or blunt the distinctive clinical features. The timing of clinical presentation may confound the clinician because early in the course it may be difficult to distinguish features of infectious versus noninfectious corneal processes. Noninfectious ulcerative keratitis may present a clinical dilemma if accompanied by significant corneal inflammation. In patients with longstanding persistent epithelial defects, especially postkeratoplasty, stromal infiltration may develop that mimics infectious keratitis. Similarly, individuals with neurotrophic or exposure keratopathy may have ulcerations accompanied by stromal inflammation, which may be indistinguishable from bacterial keratitis. Indolent corneal ulcerations after herpetic keratitis may also resemble the clinical features of infectious corneal ulceration. Particularly difficult to differentiate from early infectious keratitis are the noninfectious immune infiltrates associated with anterior blepharitis or contact lens wear (195).

The reality is that the suggestive biomicroscopic appearance and clinical course alone are insufficient for definitive diagnosis. The preponderance of clinical evidence raises the index of clinical suspicion, but laboratory diagnosis is required for confirmation of corneal infection.

Laboratory Investigation

Clearly, laboratory diagnosis of ocular infection by definitive culturing is the gold standard of clinical management (196). Although it is the preferred approach, microbial culture is often not a practical or a prevailing one for many ophthalmologists (92). Bypassing the step of culturing by opting directly for empirical therapy is a standard office-based approach for some ophthalmologists (197). In a survey of U.S. ophthalmologists on the West Coast who managed an average of approximately 10 cases of ulcerative keratitis annually, only 23% stated that corneal scrapings for microscopic analysis of stained smears and cultures were always necessary. Another 57.3% indicated that scraping for smears and cultures were necessary only in the presence of large or clinically severe ulcers. Only 3.3% stated that cultures were always unnecessary in the management of ulcerative keratitis. Finally, 16.4% of the survey respondents used various other criteria to selectively decide on the need for laboratory investigation in management of ulcerative keratitis (197). Such discrepancies between preferred laboratory investigation and prevailing clinical practice may be due in part to previously observed low diagnostic yields with smears and culture, increasing health care costs required to maintain the equipment necessary for proper laboratory investigation, and the belief that empirical antibiotic therapy may be associated with a high success rate (198).

Given a high index of clinical suspicion for infectious keratitis, cost-effective laboratory investigation having a high diagnostic yield remains desirable for guiding antibiotic therapy and optimal management of bacterial keratitis. Obtaining clinical material for laboratory analysis and microbial culture is an important step in the management of suspected infectious keratitis. A standard, thorough methodology should be adopted in all such cases, designed to maximize the yield of recovery of potential corneal pathogens. Knowledge of the likely responsible organisms, including aerobic and anaerobic non–spore-forming bacteria and the possibility of filamentous fungi and yeast, viruses, and protozoa, is important to select the proper laboratory methodology. Standard laboratory procedures can usually recover most organisms by stain or culture (196). In a study assessing the value of Gram stain in management of suppurative keratitis in a developing country, 127 cases of microbial keratitis were examined to determine the relative contributions of Gram stain and culture to diagnosis of the causative organism (199). There were 107 culture-proven cases of microbial keratitis among the 127 patients. Gram stain was positive in 89 cases, which represents 70% of the total and 83% of all culture-proven cases. In 20 cases (16%), no organism was isolated on Gram stain or culture. The results of this study supported the use of both Gram stain and culture in isolation of the causative organisms of suppurative keratitis. With special clinical circumstances, more selective diagnostic techniques and culture media may be indicated.

A retrospective analysis of comparative data from a prospectively collected database was conducted to determine the sensitivity, specificity, and predictive values of Gram and potassium hydroxide with calcofluor white (KOH+CFW) stains in the diagnosis of early and advanced microbial keratitis (200). Patients with nonviral microbial keratitis seen between February 1991 and December 1998 were included in the study. The type of bacteria seen on Gram stain was determined from 251 corneal scrapings from patients with early keratitis and 841 corneal scrapings from patients with advanced keratitis. The presence of fungi in corneal scrapings was determined by KOH+CFW stain of 114 and 363 scrapings from patients with early and advanced keratitis, respectively. The smear findings were compared with culture results to analyze specificity, sensitivity, and predictive values of the staining techniques. The sensitivity of Gram stain in the detection of bacteria was 36.0% in early and 40.9% in advanced keratitis cases; however, the specificity was higher in both groups (84.9% and 87.1%, respectively). Comparatively, the sensitivity and specificity of

fungal detection were higher using KOH+CFW in early (61.1% and 99.0%, respectively) as well as advanced keratitis (87.7% and 83.7%, respectively). Predictive values were high for KOH+CFW in fungus detection, whereas they were poor for Gram stain in bacteria detection. In advanced keratitis cases, the false-positive rate was higher in fungal detection (16.3%) than in bacterial detection (10.3%), whereas the false-negative rate was significantly higher in bacterial detection compared with fungal detection (59.1% vs. 12.3%, $p <$ .0001). In early keratitis, on the other hand, both false-positive and false-negative results for bacterial detection were significantly higher than for fungal detection. Decisions can reliably be based on KOH+CFW staining of corneal scrapings for initiation of antifungal therapy in mycotic keratitis. The results of Gram staining, on the other hand, have limited value in therapeutic decisions for bacterial keratitis (200).

A routine method for obtaining and maintaining standard materials and media for the collection, transport, and culture of the material from corneal scrapings should be established (196–201). If space allows, a special room devoted to maintaining the required supplies is optimal. Alternatively, assembling a special kit or tray in the office with the required materials facilitates performing laboratory investigation without delay. Specimens should be obtained for laboratory microbiologic investigation at the time of presentation immediately after documenting the clinical findings with careful slit-lamp drawings or photography. Clinical material should always be obtained before the initiation of antibiotic treatment. If the patient has been partially treated and the keratitis is mild or moderately severe, consideration should be given to suspending antibiotic therapy for a period of 12 hours before return for laboratory investigation. If the keratitis is judged to be severe with a rapid pace of inflammation, specimens should be obtained without delay and antibiotic therapy commenced immediately.

A specified sequence for obtaining clinical material for laboratory investigation should be followed for each patient with suspected infectious keratitis. Eyelid and conjunctival specimens may be collected for culture and compared with results from corneal culture. The clinical value of eyelid and conjunctival cultures may be limited, however, and even misleading in management of infectious keratitis (196). The primary site of infection yields the most valuable microbiologic information. If external ocular cultures are desired, the isolation of microorganisms from the eyelid and conjunctiva is enhanced by the use of moistened calcium alginate swabs. Cotton swabs should be avoided because they contain fatty acids, which have an inhibitory effect on bacterial growth. Conjunctival cultures should be taken first to prevent possible contamination by lid flora escaping into the preocular tear film. Topical anesthetics are not required for patient comfort and should be avoided for conjunctival cultures because the preservatives may have bacteriostatic properties. Several schemes have been described for the proper technique in obtaining and processing material for culture (196,201,202). The lower eyelids should be depressed while the patient looks up to expose the lower conjunctival cul de sac. Using the moistened calcium alginate swab, the lower conjunctival cul de sac should be wiped twice from temporal to nasal to avoid contamination from touching the eyelid margin. The right conjunctival culture may be inoculated in the upper right quadrant of each plate with a horizontal streak. In a similar manner, the left conjunctival culture should be inoculated in the lower right quadrant of each plate using a horizontal streak. Eyelid cultures are obtained using a moistened calcium alginate–tipped swab and carefully wiping along the lower eyelashes from the temporal to the nasal margin. The right eyelid culture may then be inoculated in the upper left quadrant of each plate using the letter "R." The left lid culture should be inoculated in the lower left quadrant of each plate using the "L." Care should be taken to communicate with the microbiology laboratory to avoid potential confusion in processing and interpretation.

The most valuable information comes from direct culture of the involved site. Because the cornea may have relatively few infectious organisms compared with other body sites, material from corneal scrapings should be inoculated directly onto the culture media rather than placed into carrier or transport media. Direct plating onto selective media improves the likelihood of recovery, especially with a small number of organisms and potentially fastidious organisms (196). To obtain corneal scrapings comfortably, topical anesthetic is first instilled. Proparacaine hydrochloride 0.5% has the fewest inhibitory effects on organism recovery. Use of tetracaine, cocaine, and other topical anesthetics may significantly reduce organism recovery owing to bacteriostatic effects. A platinum spatula with a rounded flexible tip may be modified with a honing stone to create a narrow-tapered, roughened edge to facilitate removal of corneal material (202). The platinum spatula should be heat sterilized in an alcohol lamp flame and allowed to cool before scraping the cornea. Having several spatulas available may expedite specimen collection. An alternative to the platinum spatula that does not require heat sterilization is the number 15 Bard-Parker (Becton-Dickinson, Franklin Lakes, NJ) surgical blade. The blade is sterile in a single-use package. The rounded tip facilitates obtaining corneal specimens.

Corneal scrapings should be performed along the edge and the base of the ulcerative keratitis lesion. Multiple samples from all areas of the ulceration should be obtained for maximum yield. Certain organisms, such as *S. pneumoniae*, are recovered more readily from the active edge of the corneal ulceration, whereas other organisms, including *Moraxella*, are more likely to be present at the base of the ulceration. The overall yield in recovery is enhanced with multiple corneal scrapings. In some small, mildly severe and nonsuppurative cases of ulcerative keratitis, there may be insufficient material to inoculate all media. In advanced, severe keratitis with marked stromal keratolysis and descemetocele

formation, the number of scrapings may be limited by necessity. Care should be taken to avoid the cilia and eyelids to reduce growth of nonpathogenic contaminants. The selective media agar plates are inoculated by streaking the platinum spatulas lightly over the surface to produce a row of separate inoculation marks in a "C" configuration (C-streaks). New materials should be obtained for each row of C-streaks. Calcium alginate swabs moistened with trypticase soy broth provide another method for collecting corneal specimens (81). A comparative study found a statistically significant higher retrieval rate of bacteria from cases of bacterial keratitis using a moistened calcium alginate swab versus the platinum spatula (171). A prospective comparative evaluation of a Bard-Parker number 15 blade and a moistened calcium alginate swab in the collection of corneal material was conducted on 30 consecutive cases of bacterial (n = 17), fungal (n = 11), and mixed (n = 2) cases of microbial keratitis (203). The calcium alginate swab yielded significantly greater growth than the blade in mycotic ulcers. However, the difference between the two methods was not significant for bacterial and mixed ulcers. Based on these investigations, a modified approach using both a platinum spatula or Bard-Parker blade and a moistened calcium alginate swab to create separate C-streaks may provide the highest yield. Using the C-streak method of inoculation provides the means of distinguishing valid growth from plate contamination. Growth on the C-streak is considered to be significant, whereas growth close to the edge of the plate outside of the C-streaks likely represents contamination. In some cases, the corneal epithelium may be intact or minimally disrupted and it is necessary to break the corneal epithelium, using the blade to gain access to the site of suspected infectious keratitis. In cases of deep stromal keratitis, microsurgical scissors, a number 11 Bard-Parker blade (Becton-Dickinson), or a small trephine may be required to sample the cornea adequately. The accompanying intraocular inflammation or layered hypopyon is most often sterile in microbial keratitis, wherein Descemet's membrane remains intact. Obtaining aqueous humor by anterior chamber paracentesis for smear or culture is contraindicated in most circumstances to avoid the potential risks of inadvertent intraocular inoculation of organisms.

After directly inoculating the choice specimen onto the selective media plates, microscopic slides of corneal scrapings are then made using precleaned glass. The specimens should be placed in the center of the slide over an area of approximately 1 cm in diameter. Pre-etched circles on the slide allow easy placement of material in a central location for later localization. The microscopic slides should be fixed immediately by immersion in 95% methanol for approximately 5 minutes. Heat fixation should be avoided to reduce the likelihood of disrupting the morphology or staining characteristics of the organisms. At least two microscopic slides should be obtained for routine staining and a third should be held for possible special stains.

Impression cytology has been used previously as a diagnostic technique for a variety of ocular conditions. A simple conjunctival biopsy technique has been reported using impression cytology (204). A millipore filter paper was pressed on the bulbar conjunctiva to remove cells from the surface of the epithelium. Other investigators have used the impression technique to acquire cells for cytologic analysis in dry eye (205–207). The technique has been extensively studied for its utility in early detection of vitamin A deficiency in xerophthalmia (208). Impression techniques have also been applied successfully in debridement of herpes simplex dendritic epithelial keratitis (209,210). Ocular impression debridement was successful in isolation of *Acanthamoeba* from the elevated epithelial lines in two cases of superficial *Acanthamoeba* keratitis (211). Impression debridement has also been investigated for its potential in the diagnosis of suspected infectious keratitis. The technique of impression debridement may provide a safe, effective adjunctive method for conventional diagnosis of infectious keratitis in superficial cases and for collection of microbial nucleic acids for molecular microbiologic organism identification.

Stains

The Gram stain is the most widely used standard microbiologic stain and its results have been advocated as a guide to the initiation of treatment of bacterial keratitis. Acridine orange is a fluorochromatic dye stain that requires a fluorescent microscope. RNA and single-stranded prokaryotic DNA stain a brilliant orange-red, whereas double-stranded eukaryotic DNA stains light green. When buffered at acidic pH 3.5 to 4.0, acridine orange stains bacteria, yeast cells, and chlamydial inclusion bodies orange-red. Filamentous fungi usually stain bright green. Acridine orange is commercially available (Difco, Detroit, MI) and the procedure can be performed in a few minutes. A stained acridine orange slide positive for bacteria can be restained with Gram stain or other vital stains for further reaction identification. The acridine orange stain has been shown to be a sensitive screening test of value in microbial keratitis in both animal and human keratitis (212,213).

Although acridine orange is a highly sensitive screening method for analyzing smears from corneal scrapings, the more traditional Gram and Giemsa stains are of specific value in the initial management of bacterial keratitis. Gram and Giemsa staining of corneal smears confirm the presence of a microorganism and distinguish the type (bacteria vs. fungus) while providing clues to suggest the specific subgroup of organisms. Gram staining may be simply performed in 5 minutes. After fixation of the slide in methyl alcohol, the slide is flooded with crystal gentian violet for 1 minute. The slide is then rinsed with water and flooded with Gram's iodine for 1 minute. The slide is again rinsed with water, then decolorized with acid alcohol for 20 seconds. After rinsing with water, the slide is counterstained by flooding with safranin for 1 minute. The slide is rinsed with water for a final time and then allowed to air or blot dry. Gram stain classifies bacteria into two major groups based on distinct differences in the cell wall. Gram-positive bacteria retain the gentian violet–iodine complex and appear blue-purple (Fig. 13.1-13).

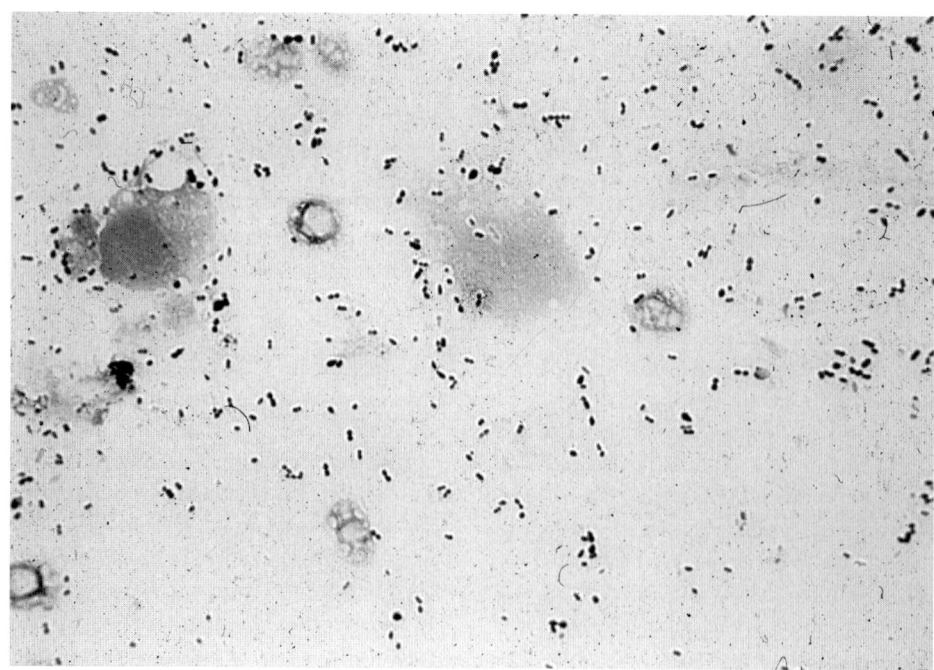

FIGURE 13.1-13. Smear from corneal scraping taken from a patient with suppurative keratitis. Note the lancet-shaped diplococci, almost diagnostic of *Streptococcus pneumoniae*.

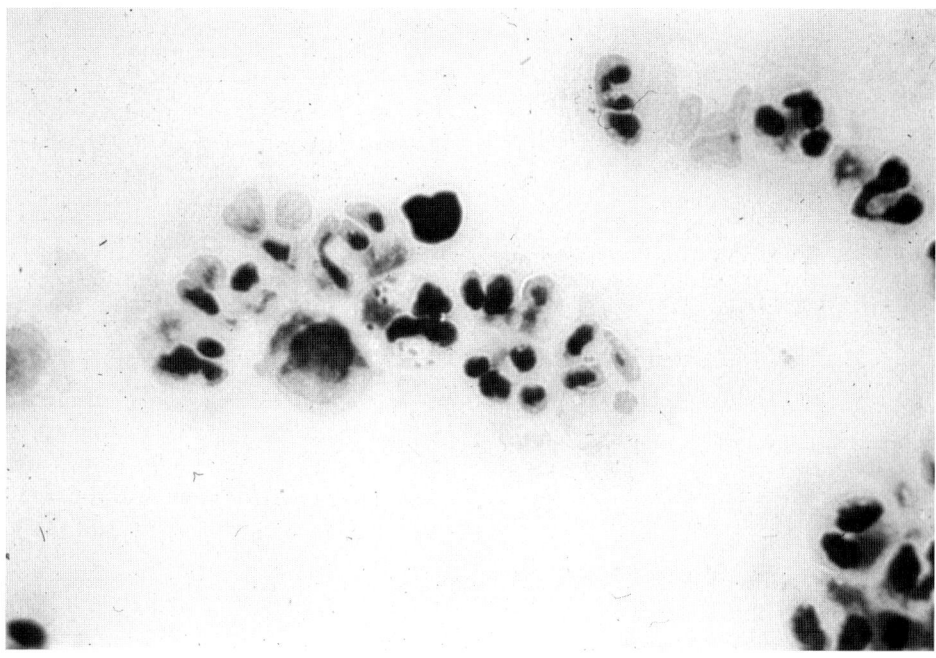

FIGURE 13.1-14. A Gram-stained specimen similar to that shown in Fig. 48–14, although from a different patient, illustrating (with some difficulty) intracellular gram-negative diplococci, almost pathognomonic for *Neisseria* species.

Gram-negative bacteria lose the gentian violet–iodine complex with the decolorization step and appear pink when counterstained with safranin (Fig. 13.1-14). The 5-minute Gram stain is preferred over the 15-second modified stain. If done properly, Gram staining may correctly identify the pathogen in up to 75% of cases caused by a single organism and in 37% of polymicrobial cases (169). The Gram stain was accurate in 61% of cases of bacterial keratitis overall. Slides must be carefully and thoroughly analyzed for correct interpretation. Gram-negative organisms may be more difficult to visualize in corneal scraping specimens than gram-positive organisms (Fig. 13.1-14). Caution must be exercised with artifacts that may accompany Gram staining, including stained deposits, carbon particles, talcum powder, sodium chloride crystals, and melanin and granules. Precipitated gentian violet may mimic the appearance of gram-positive cocci. If the Gram staining reagents are not used frequently, yeast may grow in the solutions. Periodic filtering may help remove confusing particles.

The two stains most frequently used to determine the types of inflammatory reaction present are the Giemsa stain and the Wright-Giemsa stain. The Giemsa stain may be useful in distinguishing bacteria from fungi. It uses eosin, methylene blue, and azure dyes. With the Giemsa technique, bacteria appear dark blue. Fungal hyphae absorb the stain and generally appear purple or blue. The traditional Giemsa stain takes up to 60 minutes to perform. A rapid 15-minute modification of the stain is also available. The Giemsa stain identifies normal and inflammatory cells. In addition to bacteria and fungi, identification of chlamydial inclusion bodies and the cysts and trophozoites of *Acanthamoeba* species may be facilitated with Giemsa stain.

Special stains include the use of carbolfuchsin or Ziehl-Neelsen acid-fast stain for identification of suspected *Mycobacterium*, *Actinomyces*, or *Nocardia*. Some of these organisms contain a specific lipid wax fraction that is resistant to decolorization by strong mineral acids after staining with basic carbolfuchsin. *Mycobacterium* organisms are acid fast, *Nocardia* stain variably, and *Actinomyces* is non–acid fast. Fluorochrome stain may also be used for identifying *Mycobacterium*.

Fluorescent stains like acridine orange have a major advantage of being highly sensitive in their ability to detect small numbers of microorganisms. This extraordinary sensitivity is a favorable characteristic for detection of organisms in bacterial keratitis, where the numbers may be small (Fig. 13.1-15). In addition to the acridine orange stain, the calcofluor-white stain is commercially available (Fungi-Fluor; Polysciences, Warrington, PA) and has been used to screen smears obtained from corneal scrapings. Calcofluor-white binds to chitin and cellulose. It has been used in the laundry industry as a whitening agent. Because the cell walls of yeast and filamentous fungi contain chitin and cellulose, these organisms stain bright green with calcofluor-white under epifluorescent microscopy (214,215). The cysts of *Acanthamoeba* species have a high content of chitin and cellulose and also stain bright green with calcofluor white (216,217). The trophozoites of *Acanthamoeba* stain reddish-orange.

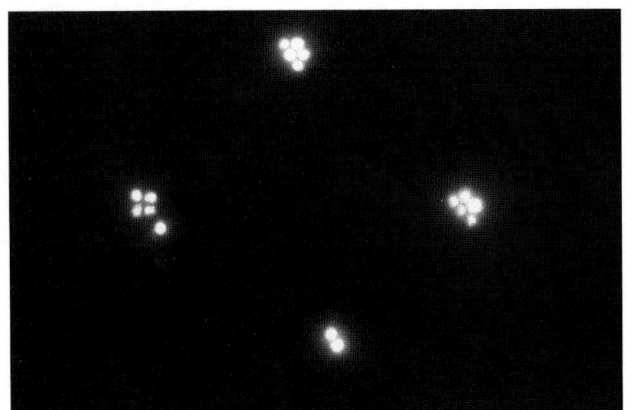

FIGURE 13.1-15. Acridine specimen for fluorescence microscopy. Note the cocci on this smear.

A fluorescent Gram stain has been commercially developed (Baclight; Molecular Probes, Inc., Eugene, OR), which differentially stains live gram-positive bacteria a reddish-orange and gram-negative bacteria bright green using fluorescent microscopy without the need for fixative. This commercially available fluorescent Gram stain has some utility in screening material from ocular infections (218).

Culture Media

Enriched media and differential selective media are the two principal forms of culture media used in clinical microbiology. For the isolation of fastidious microorganisms, enriched media such as blood and chocolate agar are preferred. Differential selective media contain an agent used to inhibit the growth of certain organisms while promoting growth of other, slower-growing organisms, or a carbohydrate having an acid–base indicator. Examples of differential selective media include mannitol salts agar, and all other media used to isolate gram-negative enteric bacilli. The culture media recommended for evaluation of suspected microbial keratitis have the potential to support the growth of the principal bacteria and fungi responsible for keratitis (196) (Table 13.1-2). Isolation and identification of other microorganisms may require selection of special media.

Media should be stored in a special devoted refrigerator and restocked frequently to avoid contamination. The recovery of bacterial organisms from ocular cultures may be increased by warming all refrigerated media to room temperature before direct inoculation.

Blood agar is the standard medium for the isolation of aerobic bacteria at 35°C. Blood agar also supports the growth of most saprophytic fungi at room temperature. The agar is derived from seaweed and produces optimal surface moisture, whereas the addition of 5% to 10% red blood cells provides nutrients and an index of hemolysis (196). Rabbit and horse serum are preferred for supporting growth of *Haemophilus*, but are more expensive than sheep blood, which is usually used.

Chocolate agar is prepared by the heat denaturation of blood and provides hemin (X factor) and diphosphopyridine nucleotide (V factor) essential for the growth of *Haemophilus*. Chocolate agar is also ideal for isolation of *Neisseria* and *Moraxella*. Chocolate agar should be incubated at 35°C with 10% carbon dioxide.

Thioglycolate broth supports growth of a number of aerobic and anaerobic bacteria at 35°C. Thioglycolate broth contains the basic nutrients for supporting growth of aerobic bacteria and also contains a sulfhydryl compound that acts as an oxygen-reducing agent to facilitate recovery of anaerobic bacteria. Thiol broth has 0.1% semisolid agar to prevent convection currents and special complexes to promote the growth of aerobic bacteria, as well as obligate and facultatively anaerobic organisms. It may also support a number of saprophytic fungi. The tubes should be carefully

TABLE 13-2.

Medium	Purpose	Incubation temperature
Routine		
Soybean casein digest broth (tryptic or trypticase soy broth)	Saturation of swabs	
Blood agar plate	Aerobic and facultatively anaerobic bacteria, fungi	35°C
Chocolate agar plate	Aerobic and facultatively anaerobic, *Neisseria Haemophilus*	35°C
Thioglycolate broth	Aerobic and anaerobic bacteria	35°C
Sabouraud's dextrose agar plate and antibiotic	Fungi	Room temperature
Brain-heart infusion (BHI) broth with antibiotic	Fungi	Room temperature
Special		
Brucella blood agar plate	*Anaerobic* bacteria	35°C (anaerobic system)
Thayer-Martin agar plate	*Neisseria*	35°C
Middlebrook-Cohn agar start	*Mycobacterium, Nocardia*	35°C

Modified from Wilhelmus KR, Liesegang TG, Osato MS, and Jones DB: Cumitech 13A: Laboratory Diagnosis of Ocular Infections. Coordinating Ed., S.C. Specter, American Society of Microbiology, Washington, D.C., 1994.

stored and transported in an upright position to allow gravitational settling of the semisolid agar. Thioglycolate may be modified through the addition of polysorbate (Tween 80), vitamin K, and hemin to facilitate recovery of certain bacteria and to inactive antimicrobial agents transferred in the inocula (39). A disadvantage of thioglycolate and thiol for isolation of anaerobic bacteria is an inability to restrict overgrowth of aerobic organisms. The ideal media to use for isolation of anaerobic bacteria are prereduced anaerobically sterilized (PRAS) media. A PRAS *Brucella* blood agar plate enriched with vitamin K and hemin allows the majority of anaerobes to grow within 4 to 7 days. The anaerobic media should not be exposed to air any longer than necessary and should be incubated in an anaerobic system, such as an anaerobic jar, anaerobic bag system, or anaerobic chamber (196). In the GasPak Pouch system (Becton-Dickinson, Cockeysville, MD), a packet containing sodium borohydride, sodium bicarbonate, and citric acid generates hydrogen and CO_2 after the addition of water to create an anaerobic environment.

If fungal keratitis is suspected, Sabouraud glucose and peptone agar is readily available as a universal nonselective medium. The Sabouraud agar should not contain cycloheximide, which may inhibit the saprophytic fungi commonly responsible for ocular infections (196,219). Specimens in Sabouraud agar are incubated at room temperature. After primary growth, the fungi isolated are transferred to sporulating medium. Brain–heart infusion broth with neopeptone incubated in a platform shaker at room temperature enhances the recovery of filamentous fungi and yeasts. It provides the fungal elements with a more even exposure to the essential nutrients, resulting in faster growth with the smaller inoculum typically found in ocular infection (196).

Thayer-Martin medium is a chemically enriched chocolate agar that suppresses the growth of inhibitory contaminants and selectively allows the isolation of *N. gonorrhoeae*.

For isolation of nontuberculous *Mycobacterium* species, Middlebrook 7H11 agar or Lowenstein-Jensen medium can be used. Direct inoculation of the media without treatment with decontaminating agents can be performed. *Nocardia* species can be isolated using either blood agar, Sabouraud dextrose agar, or brain–heart infusion broth. *Actinomyces* species are best isolated using an anaerobic blood agar plate incubated under anaerobic conditions.

As a clinical routine for microbiologic evaluation of the patient with suspected microbial keratitis, direct inoculation of material from corneal scrapings onto blood, chocolate, and Sabouraud agar plates with C-streaks provides the support for growth of most bacterial and fungal pathogens. Liquid thioglycolate or thiol broth is then inoculated by transferring the material from corneal scrapings from the spatula or surgical blade to a cotton-tipped applicator or calcium alginate swab. The swab is then inserted into the bottom of the tube to enhance growth of possible anaerobic pathogens.

Aerobic cultures of the cornea should be held for 7 days before being reported as no growth. Anaerobic cultures of ocular specimens should be incubated for a minimum of 7 days and a maximum of 14 days before being reported as no growth. Mycobacterial and fungal cultures should be held for 4 to 6 weeks before being reported as no growth.

The results of corneal cultures should be interpreted with regard to the clinical situation, the adequacy of sampling, and the possibility of contamination by organisms present on the skin, eyelids, and conjunctiva. Supportive evidence for a pathogenic role of a species is growth on two or more media, heavy growth of the organism (interpretable only on solid media), and a Gram stain directly smeared from the lesion containing organisms compatible with those isolated from culture. Although liquid media provide a highly sensitive method for demonstrating a pathogen, a positive culture from broth is less specific than is a positive culture from solid media because quantification is lacking from broth cultures. The clinician must be careful in interpretation of cultures negative for growth. Some negative cultures represent true noninfectious keratitis (sterile infiltrates), whereas others may be a consequence of partial prior antibiotic treatment, inadequate sampling methods, improper selection of media and incubation conditions, and false interpretation of data (172).

Although culture on standard bacteriologic media remains the gold standard for diagnosis of suspected bacterial keratitis (196), ancillary laboratory techniques, including refinements in agglutination, labeled antibody, enzyme immunoassay, gas and high-performance liquid chromatography, molecular methods, and animal cell culture, may also be valuable aids for pathogen identification. There has been increasing enthusiasm in clinical microbiology for rapid, highly specific, and sensitive molecular methods for organism detection. The acceptance of nucleic acid hybridization–based assays by microbiologists has steadily increased. A variety of DNA probe assays are now used routinely in many diagnostic laboratories, both for culture confirmation and for the direct detection of pathogens from clinical samples. At present, however, DNA probes and nucleic acid amplification techniques are most useful for the characterization of microorganisms for which standard culture methods are difficult, extremely expensive, or not readily available. DNA amplification techniques have a high level of sensitivity in the direct detection of microbial DNA in clinical specimens. Nucleic acid amplification methods are diverse and constantly changing. Such techniques may be assigned to one of three general categories: (a) target amplification systems, such as polymerase chain reaction, cell-sustaining sequence replication, or strand displacement amplification; (b) probe amplification systems, which include Qb replicase or the ligase chain reaction; and (c) signal amplification, in which the signal generated from each probe molecule is increased by using compound probes or branched-probe technology. Commercialization of these techniques is bringing molecular microbiology into the clinical microbiology laboratory. As the techniques become refined, simplified, and commercialized, it is likely that they will be used more frequently in the molecular detection and identification of microorganisms, including those causing ocular infectious diseases. However, expensive molecular diagnostic procedures should not be used to replace procedures currently in place, which have a proven track record of cost-effectiveness, rapidity, sensitivity, and reliability. Of note, despite their high sensitivity and rapidity, nucleic acid amplification procedures are unlikely to replace conventional culture methods. The results of nucleic acid amplification procedures and the results of culture may represent different situations. The nucleic acid amplification procedure determines whether DNA or RNA from a particular organism is present in the ocular tissue. These methods disclose no information concerning the viability of the organism (i.e., methods can detect DNA from dead organisms) or whether the organism is directly involved in the ocular infectious process. Culture unequivocally demonstrates the viability of the organism and strongly suggests involvement in infection. DNA and RNA probes have been used to analyze vitreous specimens to assist in identification of agents of infectious retinitis (220–222). Nucleic acid probes have also been applied to conjunctival specimens for identification of chlamydial and viral ocular pathogens (223). Analysis of debrided corneal epithelium with DNA probes has confirmed herpes simplex virus keratitis (224). The polymerase chain reaction has also been used to detect varicella zoster virus DNA in disciform keratitis (225).

Antimicrobial Susceptibility Testing

Effective antimicrobial therapy embodies the idea of selective toxicity and requires that the antimicrobial agent reach the site of corneal infection in sufficient concentration to inhibit and preferably kill the causative microorganism, while causing minimal to no toxicity to the host (226). Several factors modulate the interaction between drug, microorganism, and host. Only the clinical ophthalmologist, having knowledge of the necessary laboratory data, can evaluate the precise interactions and integrate the entire complex in order to initiate a rational therapeutic decision.

Standard disk diffusion or microdilution techniques are the preferred laboratory methods for antimicrobial susceptibility testing of bacterial ocular isolates (227–231). One of the limitations of ocular antimicrobial susceptibility testing is that the results of agar disk diffusion tests relate to levels of drug in serum rather than to concentrations of antibiotics achievable in ocular tissues. Minimum inhibitory concentration (MIC) determinations by broth microdilution methods provide more useful information with ocular infections than simply designating an isolate as sensitive or resistant. The quantitative MIC can be compared with the antimicrobial concentration expected at the site of infection.

For microbial keratitis, approximate drug levels are based on experimental data after treatment by topical and intravitreal routes, respectively (196). It is not practical to measure antimicrobial drug levels in ocular tissue because of the difficulty in safely obtaining ocular fluids or tissue for analysis. The precise resistance breakpoints for ocular isolates have not been determined because of the lack of data on actual drug concentrations in ocular tissues with bacterial keratitis. Extrapolating from experimental data, an ocular isolate may be designated susceptible if its MIC is less than the expected sustained antibiotic concentration in the infected ocular tissue compartment. Although the MIC by definition implies a static effect, bactericidal effect can be estimated by subculturing the clear broth onto antibiotic-free solid media. The result—for example, a reduction of growth by 99.9% below that of the control—is called the *minimum bactericidal concentration* (MBC). In addition to the MIC and MBC, two other outcomes worth noting are the minimum antibacterial concentration (MAC) (232) and the postantibiotic effect (PAE) (233). The MAC is the inhibitory effect that is observed in 5.5 hours in which 90% of the bacterial population is inhibited and that causes an ultrastructural morphologic defect in the organism. The PAE is the result observed after a bacterial population is exposed to antibiotics for approximately 1 hour, followed by removal of the antibiotic by either dilution or enzymatic treatment and then subculturing the surviving population at timely intervals to determine the numbers that remain. Both the MAC and the PAE are most relevant to the activity of antimicrobial agents against bacteria over time and thereby represent a truer paradigm of microorganism–drug interaction.

Another concept useful for evaluating certain pathogens and antibiotic agents is the mutant prevention concentration (MPC). A window can be defined in which mutants may be selected, and the MPC represents that concentration which kills the bacteria completely, thus preventing selection of mutants (231).

Controversy has arisen as to the precise role and value that microbial culture results exert in the management of suspected acute bacterial keratitis (234). To examine how the corneal culture result is associated with the antibacterial treatment response rate of ulcerative keratitis, a prospective cohort study was conducted to determine whether culture confirmation affects the relative treatment effect in randomized clinical trials of bacterial keratitis. The influence of a positive bacterial culture on the rates of antibacterial improvement and cure was estimated by proportional hazards regression among 608 patients with ulcerative keratitis treated with topical ciprofloxacin monotherapy. The interaction of culture confirmation on the relative cure rates of 735 patients enrolled in 4 clinical trials comparing fluoroquinolone monotherapy with combined cephalosporin and aminoglycoside therapy was evaluated by metaregression. Bacterial keratitis that was culture positive and larger than 4 mm had a 37% [95% confidence interval (CI), 20%–51%] slower improvement rate and a 56% (95% CI, 41%–67%) slower cure rate during ciprofloxacin therapy. Among randomized clinical trials, the culture result did not modify the relative effect of treatments having similar 1-week cure rates. Culture confirmation affects the antibacterial therapeutic response rate of ulcerative keratitis and, although not modifying the comparative effect of equivalent antibacterial treatments, facilitates generalizability of clinical trials of bacterial keratitis (235).

Corneal Biopsy

Corneal trauma may result in inoculation of organisms deep into the stroma. With deep suppurative stromal keratitis, a vertical or oblique incision can allow sampling using a sterile needle or minispatula (196). A sterile 7-0 silk suture may be passed through a deep stromal focus of infection and then cut into separate sections for inoculation onto specific culture media. Alternatively, a deep lamellar excision can be performed to reach a focal corneal abscess (236,237). If there is no access to a sequestered site of deep stromal suppuration, a corneal biopsy may be performed using a disposable skin punch or a small corneal trephine (238–241) (Fig. 13.1-16). The superficial cornea is incised and deepened with a surgical blade (# 11 Bard-Parker) to approximately 0.2 mm. Lamellar dissection is then performed using a sharp blade or microsurgical scissors. The biopsy specimen is carefully excised with fine-tooth forceps, with

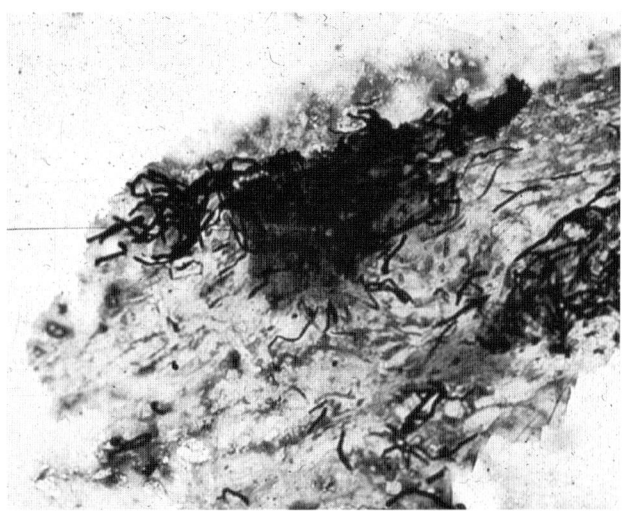

FIGURE 13.1-17. The corneal biopsy described in Fig. 13.1-16 has been fixed and stained with, among others, Gomori methenamine silver, which shows the hyphal forms in the tissue, establishing the diagnosis of filamentous fungal keratomycosis.

care taken to avoid crushing the specimen. The specimen may be placed in a sterile Petri dish for sectioning. The exposed base of the deep bed of the biopsy site may be scraped for additional culture. Corneal tissue specimens are transported to the microbiology laboratory in a sterile liquid medium, such as trypticase soy broth or sterile saline without preservatives. Tissue grinding can then be performed and the tissue homogenate plated on multiple selective media. A portion of the tissue is then processed for histopathologic analysis using special stains as indicated (241) (Fig. 13.1-17).

The *Limulus* lysate assay has been used in the diagnosis of infective keratitis when gram-negative organisms are suspected (242). Circulating cells (amebocytes) in the coelomic fluid of the horseshoe crab, *Limulus polyphemus*, gel in the presence of lipopolysaccharide located in the cell wall of gram-negative organisms. Corneal scrapings should be emulsified in rehydrated amebocyte lysate reagent in a test tube, which is incubated along with a control tube. Possible slight contamination of the glass with lipopolysaccharide can reduce the clinical usefulness of the *Limulus* lysate test. Contact lens cases and solutions can be tested for gram-negative endotoxin by the *Limulus* lysate assay, but must be diluted because of the presence of inhibitory substances (243).

Direct fluorescent monoclonal antibodies directed against specific corneal pathogens may assist in specific diagnosis. Lectins have also been suggested for use in diagnosis of specific corneal pathogens (244).

Noninvasive *in vivo* confocal microscopy offers another potential source of clinical information to assist diagnosis in suspected infectious keratitis (245). The tandem-scanning confocal microscope has received approval by the

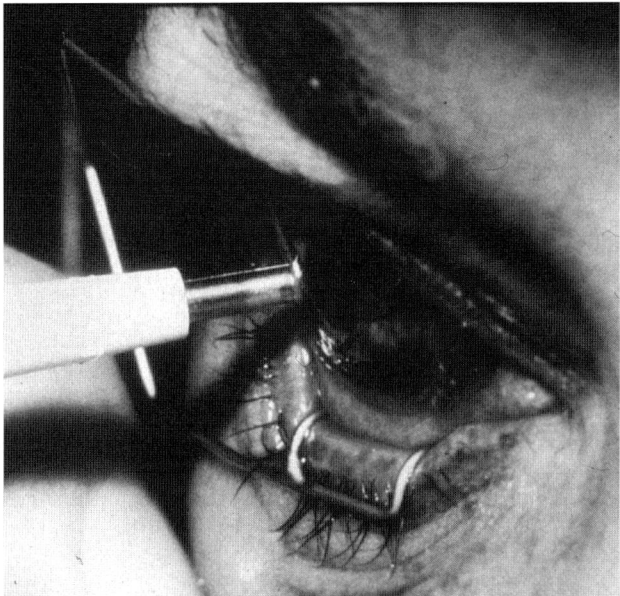

FIGURE 13.1-16. A sterile, 4-mm skin biopsy trephine being used for partial-thickness trephination of a patient with a corneal ulcer, suspected to be microbial but not responding to aggressive fortified antibiotic therapy and with negative cultures. The resulting tissue plug was subjected to histopathologic analysis, the results of which were shown in Fig. 13.1-17.

U.S. Food and Drug Administration (FDA) for general clinical use. The tandem-scanning slit-lamp confocal microscope allows real-time viewing of structures in the living cornea at the cellular level in four dimensions (*x*, *y*, *z*, and time). Using tandem-scanning confocal microscopy, distinct morphologic characteristics of filamentous and yeast fungal keratitis, *Acanthamoeba* keratitis, and infectious crystalline keratopathy due to streptococcal species were readily discernible *in vivo* (246). The current resolution of commercially available tandem-scanning slit-lamp confocal microscopes limits the usefulness of the instrument as a diagnostic tool for microbial keratitis (247). These limitations relate to instrument configuration, movement of either the tissue or the microscope, difficulty in returning to the area of interest for serial examination, the lack of distinctive morphology of some pathogens, and overall limited resolution of the microscope.

TREATMENT

In general, because of the potential rapid destruction of corneal tissue that may accompany bacterial keratitis, if there is a clinical suspicion suggestive of a bacterial pathogen, the patient should be treated appropriately for bacterial keratitis until a definitive diagnosis is established. The objective of therapy in bacterial keratitis is rapidly to eliminate the infective organism, reduce the inflammatory response, prevent structural damage to the cornea, and promote healing of the epithelial surface (3).

With suspected infectious keratitis, the clinician has the option based on the clinical impression and severity of the keratitis of initiating specific directed or broad-spectrum antimicrobial therapy, or deferring treatment pending the results of laboratory investigation, or monitoring clinical signs. The initial therapy selection is based on the clinical features, antecedent risk factors, and familiarity with the most likely responsible corneal pathogen(s) and their respective antimicrobial susceptibility patterns (248).

A basic plan for therapy of severe suppurative keratitis depends on the results of Gram stains on smears from diagnostic corneal scrapings (2). Inherent in such a therapeutic plan is confidence in the quality of specimen obtained and the technical proficiency of the microbiology laboratory in the processing and interpretation of the clinical material. Evaluation of diagnostic smears with Gram stain is a relatively insensitive method for diagnosis of bacterial keratitis. With optimal conditions, pathogens can be identified with microscopic analysis of Gram-stained smears in approximately 75% of monobacterial keratitis and 37% of polybacterial keratitis cases (3). Screening of smears from corneal scrapings with acridine orange and fluorescent microscopy is more sensitive than Gram staining (212,213), raising the sensitivity to approximately 80%. Given the 20% to 30% possibility of a false-negative interpretation of

smears from corneal scrapings, the ophthalmologist must base initial therapy on the clinical assessment of severity. If the Gram stain is equivocal or there is uncertainty in interpretation of diagnostic smears, broad-spectrum antibiotic coverage should be initiated in the initial treatment of all cases of severe suppurative microbial keratitis because the consequences of inappropriate or inadequate therapy can be devastating (170).

The design for drug administration in severe suppurative keratitis includes antibiotics administered frequently. Because of the rapid evolution to perforation in keratitis due to virulent pathogens and visual loss secondary to central corneal scarring, many patients with bacterial keratitis having significant ulceration may require hospitalization in the absence of adequate support and assistance. The high frequency and intense dosage scheduling of antimicrobial therapy often requires assistance of trained nursing personnel. Frequent antibiotic administration required for therapy of severe bacterial keratitis can often fatigue even highly motivated patients and family members, resulting in decreased compliance. In the absence of severe fulminant keratitis with impending perforation, patients with mild to moderate keratitis may be managed as outpatients with close monitoring (249). Indeed, the availability of highly potent topical antibacterial solutions has permitted outpatient management of bacterial keratitis in all but the most severe cases.

With the goal of rapid cessation of replication and elimination of the bacterial pathogen, selection of appropriate therapy requires an effective drug with minimal toxicity. The results of laboratory investigations assist the clinician in selecting the most specific and efficacious treatment based on results from microbial culture and antimicrobial susceptibility data.

Antibiotic Therapy

The large number of active antimicrobial drugs available to the treating clinician offers the patient with bacterial keratitis a greater chance for cure with less drug-related toxicity while providing alternative choices despite the continuing emergence of drug-resistant pathogenic organisms. In addition to considering the possible organisms involved, the most effective classes of antibacterial agents, and the possibility of organism resistance, variation in patient response, that is, predicting the response of an individual patient to both the organism and the proposed therapy, aids the ophthalmologist in determining the most effective, least toxic agent or agents for treatment. Additional criteria required to identify the actual drug(s) of choice for a particular patient include outpatient versus inpatient management and cost.

Although some organisms continue to be predictably susceptible to selected antimicrobial agents, the development of clinically important resistant isolates is common because of the high selective pressures applied by intense antibiotic use. Mechanisms of organism resistance include plasmid transfer, either by conjugation or transduction, alteration of permeation, chromosomal mutations, and active efflux. The rate of the emergence of mutation and the extent of resistance may vary between organisms and from drug to drug. Depending on the mechanism and degree of resistance, the administration of larger dosages of drug that do not cause serious adverse effects may be adequate for clinical cure. With corneal infection, an advantage is direct accessibility through the topical route of administration to achieve high tissue concentrations without significant systemic or local side effects. In contrast, effective treatment of certain infections, such as nontuberculous mycobacterial keratitis, often requires combinations of antimicrobial drugs to avoid the rapid development of highly resistant strains that appear when single-agent therapy is used. Antimicrobial susceptibility testing is recommended whenever there is doubt about the potential susceptibility of a given pathogen. Patterns of antimicrobial susceptibility may vary from one geographic area to another, among different hospitals in a given area, between clinics in a single building, and between community-acquired and hospital-acquired infections. With community-acquired bacterial keratitis, antibiotic resistance is infrequently encountered and usually surmounted with intensive topical dosing. Nosocomial corneal infections, such as those sustained in patients with exposure keratopathy maintained on chronic mechanically assisted ventilation in intensive care or burn units, should be monitored closely for high-level organism resistance.

Apart from the virulence of the organism, severity of corneal infection is determined in part by the age, genetic makeup, and general health of the patient. Deficiencies of humoral and cellular defense mechanisms negatively affect patient response to therapy. Factors that may limit the use of a particular agent in an individual include a reliable history of an allergic reaction to the antibiotic (rash, urticaria, angioedema, wheezing, or anaphylaxis), potential adverse interactions, and predictable adverse effects in certain clinical situations (e.g., use of tetracyclines in young children or pregnant women).

Outpatient versus inpatient drug therapy modes are distinguished primarily by the severity of the keratitis and the anticipated compliance with treatment. Among possible efficacious alternatives, low toxicity and ease of administration are the most important factors in selection of drug therapy for outpatients. Potency of the antiinfective agent with requirement for less frequent administration may improve compliance. With severe keratitis and the potential for permanent structural alteration, the rapid attainment of inhibitory, preferably bactericidal concentration within corneal tissues is the primary consideration, often overriding factors such as convenience and localized toxicity.

The impact of drug cost is an increasingly important variable in therapeutic choices. Because of the potential devastating affects of severe keratitis, the ophthalmologist's primary responsibility is selection of the antimicrobial agent that is most likely to effect a complete cure in the shortest time. In some instances, selection of an appropriate, equally effective, but less expensive preparation may ensure compliance in patients with mild to moderate keratitis. The ophthalmologist should make therapeutic comparisons based on unbiased sources of information assessing the cost of equally effective preparations.

Specific Agents

Penicillins

After Fleming's announcement of his discovery of penicillin (250), 10 years elapsed before it was established as a major chemotherapeutic agent (251,252). Interestingly, ophthalmologists performed the first encouraging experiments demonstrating the usefulness of penicillin, even impure and weak penicillin, in the treatment of pneumococcal conjunctivitis in 1932 (253,254). The case notes in 1930 and 1931 of the late Mr. A. B. Nutt, an assistant ophthalmic surgeon at Sheffield Royal Infirmary, show that three patients with gonococcal neonatal ophthalmia, one with a staphylococcal eye infection, and one with a pneumococcal eye infection were all treated successfully (255). Thus, ophthalmology played an important role between 1929 and 1940 in introducing the antibiotic era. All penicillins contain a common nucleus (6-aminopenicillanic acid) composed of a thiazolidine ring and a beta-lactam ring connected to a side chain. The intact beta-lactam ring is necessary for biologic activity, but the side chain primarily determines the spectrum of antibacterial activity, relative susceptibility to the action of beta-lactamases and acids, and the pharmacokinetic properties. Natural penicillin G is extracted from cultures of *Penicillium chrysogenum*. Semisynthetic penicillins usually are prepared by adding side chains to the basic nucleus.

The mechanism of action of penicillins is through interference with cell wall synthesis to exert a bactericidal effect on actively dividing cells. Bacterial cell wall synthesis is a complex process involving numerous enzymes. The third stage of bacterial cell wall synthesis occurs outside the cell membrane and involves cross-linking of linear peptidoglycan polymers by peptide bonds, thus completing the formation of the tough outer envelope of the bacterial cell. Penicillins are inhibitors of transpeptidation (256). In gram-positive species, cell wall lysis also seems to depend on the ability of penicillin to decrease the availability of an inhibitor of bacterial murein hydrolase, a cell wall autolytic enzyme whose normal function is unclear. Thus, the penicillins may increase breakdown of the cell wall, as well as inhibit synthesis.

A number of penicillin-binding proteins (PBPs) have been identified in association with bacterial cell membranes from both gram-positive and gram-negative bacteria

(257). These proteins form covalent complexes with penicillin and have been shown to be enzymes, such as transpeptidases, transglycosylases, and carboxypeptidases, that are involved in bacterial cell wall division, cell wall elongation, septum formation, and the maintenance of cell shape. The PBPs of gram-negative and gram-positive bacteria differ extensively. The selective affinity patterns of beta-lactam antibiotics for PBPs of different bacterial species vary with the agent and provide the basis for distinctive structural or physiologic effects caused by the antimicrobial agent (258).

The antimicrobial spectrum of penicillin G for susceptible gram-positive cocci includes *S. pyogenes* (group A), *Streptococcus agalactiae* (group B), nonenterococcal group D streptococci (e.g., *Streptococcus bovis*), *viridans* streptococci, *S. pneumoniae* (relatively resistant or absolutely resistant strains to penicillins now exist), anaerobic streptococci (*Peptostreptococcus*), *Peptococcus*, and microaerophilic streptococci. Enterococci (e.g., *Enterococcus faecalis* and *Enterococcus faecium*) are less susceptible than other streptococci, but penicillin G is also recommended in enterococcal infections. Most strains of *S. aureus* produce beta-lactamase and are resistant.

Susceptible gram-positive bacilli include *Bacillus anthracis*, most strains of *C. diphtheriae*, *L. monocytogenes*, *Erysipelothrix rhusiopathiae*, most clostridia (e.g., *Clostridium perfringens*, *Clostridium tetani*), and *Eubacterium*. Penicillin G may be effective for susceptible gram-negative cocci, including *N. gonorrhoeae* and *N. meningitidis*. With the Southeast Asia conflict, penicillin-resistant *Neisseria* strains, especially penicillinase-producing *N. gonorrhoeae*, were introduced and have become widespread in the United States. Thus, penicillin is no longer recommended for empirical therapy of presumptive *N. gonorrhoeae* infections.

Susceptible gram-negative bacilli include *P. multocida* (259), *Streptobacillus moniliformis*, and *Spirillum minor*. Although many strains of *H. influenzae* are susceptible *in vitro*, an amino-penicillin (e.g., ampicillin or amoxicillin) is usually preferred over penicillin G. Beta-lactamase–producing *H. influenzae* are resistant.

Among gram-negative anaerobic bacilli, most *Fusobacterium* and oropharyngeal strains of *Bacteroides* are susceptible. However, some strains may be resistant, and the *Bacteroides fragilis* group are usually resistant. Most other gram-negative bacilli are resistant to penicillin G, including important pathogens, such as *P. aeruginosa* and other Enterobacteriaceae.

Actinomyces strains are usually susceptible to penicillin G, but *Nocardia* are resistant. Spirochetes such as *Treponema pallidum*, *Leptospira*, and *Borrelia burgdorferi*, the causative agent of Lyme disease, are susceptible. Mycobacteria, mycoplasmas, chlamydiae, fungi, amoebae, and viruses are all resistant to penicillin.

Mechanisms of resistance to penicillin antibiotics include inactivation by bacterial beta-lactamases, decreased permeability of the bacterial cell wall to the penicillin, prohibiting the antibiotic from reaching the appropriate binding proteins, alterations in PBPs, and tolerance. In therapy of ocular infections, the most important consideration is acquired resistance due to the production of inactivating enzymes (beta-lactamases) by staphylococci and gram-negative bacteria. The beta-lactam ring of the penicillin nucleus is cleaved by the action of beta-lactamase, resulting in the formation of inactive penicilloic acid derivatives. Staphylococcal beta-lactamases are encoded by plasmids that can be transferred from one bacterium to another by transduction. A high percentage (70% to 90%) of clinical ocular isolates of staphylococci produce beta-lactamase, limiting the utility of penicillin as an empirical initial therapeutic agent.

Tolerance to penicillin has been reported primarily in gram-positive bacteria, such as *viridans* streptococci, *S. pneumoniae*, *E. faecalis*, and *S. aureus* (260). Tolerance may be suggested *in vitro* by large differences observed between the measured MIC and the MBC, which is typically much higher. Another limiting clinical use factor is the incidence of hypersensitivity, estimated at between 1% and 10%. Among antiinfectives, penicillins cause the largest number of allergic reactions and are the most common cause of anaphylaxis in the United States. Most allergic hypersensitivity reactions are limited to skin rash, contact dermatitis, low-grade fever, and eosinophilia. Both the major and minor antigenic determinants of penicillins can cause IgE-mediated hypersensitivity reactions. However, minor determinants are the major cause of systemic anaphylactic reactions. Skin testing with penicilloyl-polylysine (Pre-Pen), penicillin G, and a minor determinant mixture of penicilloic and penilloic acids is a highly efficient procedure for detecting individuals with circulating IgE antipenicillin antibodies who are at risk for severe allergic reactions. In individuals with serious infections who cannot receive alternate non–cross-reacting antiinfectives, acute desensitization may be considered.

To expand the serum half-life and serum concentration of penicillin administered systemically, ciliary body and renal excretion of penicillin can be partially blocked with administration of adjunctive 0.5 g of probenecid given orally every 6 hours. Probenecid should not be administered to children younger than the age of 2 years. Caution must be exercised with high-dose parenteral administration of penicillins to individuals having renal or cardiac disease because of the potential danger of potassium overload. Every 1 million units of penicillin supplies 1.7 mEq of potassium.

In general, penicillins have proven to be the safest antibiotics for use during pregnancy. There is no evidence that penicillins are teratogenic (261).

Semisynthetic Penicillin. Penicillinase-resistant (antistaphylococcal) penicillins include methicillin sodium, oxacillin, cloxacillin, dicloxacillin sodium, and nafcillin. These agents are indicated principally for therapy of infection due to penicillinase-producing staphylococci. Increasing resistance of strains of *S. aureus* and, to a greater extent, *S. epidermidis* to the penicillinase-resistant penicillins has been observed, especially with nosocomial infections. Such strains are also resistant to the cephalosporins.

Although some gram-positive bacilli (e.g., *C. perfringens*, *C. diphtheriae*, *L. monocytogenes*) are susceptible *in vitro*, the semisynthetic antistaphylococcal penicillins are not recommended for therapy of infections caused by these organisms. Caution must be exercised in individuals with a history of allergy to penicillin G before consideration of administration of semisynthetic penicillins. Untoward effects of semisynthetic penicillins are usually mild and most commonly consist of allergic reactions similar to those elicited by penicillin G. Neutropenia has been reported in 10% to 20% of patients receiving nafcillin (262). The neutropenia is reversible on discontinuation of the drug. Interstitial nephritis has been associated with the use of methicillin more frequently than with other antistaphylococcal penicillins. Men are more frequently affected than women. The nephrotoxicity does not appear to be dose related. Methicillin-induced nephrotoxicity may begin 1 to 2 weeks after initiation of therapy and is characterized by fever, rash, eosinophilia, hematuria, proteinuria, and leukocyturia (263).

Amino-Penicillins. Another group of semisynthetic penicillins includes the amino-penicillins, such as ampicillin, amoxicillin, bacampicillin, and cyclacillin. The antibacterial spectrum of activity for amino-penicillins is comparable with that of penicillin G and the antistaphylococcal penicillins (264). The amino-penicillins are slightly more active against *E. faecalis* and *L. monocytogenes*. The amino-penicillins are also susceptible to beta-lactamases, thereby making them ineffective against most staphylococci which are resistant. Many strains of *H. influenzae* are susceptible, but beta-lactamase–producing strains are continually emerging. Ampicillin and other amino-penicillins are usually well tolerated. Adverse reactions are typically mild, consisting most often of skin rashes or diarrhea. The incidence of diarrhea is approximately 10% in adults and 20% in children. Amoxicillin has a slightly lower tendency to cause diarrhea (265).

Antipseudomonal Penicillins. The antipseudomonal penicillins are semisynthetic derivatives that include the carboxypenicillins, carbenicillin and ticarcillin; the acylureidopenicillins, azlocillin and mezlocillin; and the piperazine penicillin, piperacillin (266). These agents have an extended spectrum of activity to include *Pseudomonas* species. Like the other semisynthetic penicillins, these agents are also susceptible to various beta-lactamases elaborated by gram-positive and gram-negative bacteria. Piperacillin appears to have the greatest *in vitro* antipseudomonal activity, followed by azlocillin, mezlocillin, ticarcillin, and carbenicillin (267). Whether the observed *in vitro* differences are of clinical relevance, especially with topical ocular dosing, is unresolved (268). The antipseudomonal penicillins appear to have activity against many strains of *Acinetobacter*. Other gram-negative anaerobic bacteria, including *Fusobacterium* and *Bacteroides*, also appear susceptible. There has been increasing resistance among strains of gram-negative bacilli to the antipseudomonal penicillins. Thus, susceptibility testing before instituting therapy is recommended, especially if the agents are to be used alone. The antipseudomonal penicillins are relatively well tolerated, but any of the adverse reactions associated with the use of penicillins may also occur with these derivatives. Neutropenia, eosinophilia, and abnormal blood clotting, especially with carbenicillin, have been reported. In high concentrations, carbenicillin combined with adenosine phosphate receptors in platelets and prevented normal platelet aggregation, thereby leading to a dose-related prolongation of bleeding time. Antipseudomonal penicillins may also activate aminoglycosides, particularly gentamicin and tobramycin. Therefore, these antibiotics should not be mixed together before administration. *In vivo* antagonism may also occur (269).

Cephalosporins

Like the penicillins, cephalosporins contain a beta-lactam ring that is necessary for antibacterial activity. The apparent nucleus of cephalosporins is 7-aminocephalosporanic acid (7-ACA). This compound is a fermentation product of *Cephalosporium acremonium*, cephalosporin C. 7-ACA is composed of a dyhydrothiazine ring and a beta-lactam ring. This structure is resistant to the action of penicillinases produced by staphylococci. The basic cephalosporin nucleus may be modified with various side chains to change antibacterial activity, stability to beta-lactamases, metabolism, and pharmacokinetic properties. The cephalosporins have historically been classified as first-, second-, or third-generation compounds based on their activity against gram-negative bacteria. First-generation cephalosporins were the initial agents developed, having generally excellent gram-positive activity but a narrower gram-negative antibacterial spectrum. Second-generation cephalosporins in general are more active against gram-negative bacteria than first-generation analogs. These compounds may have slightly less activity against gram-positive pathogens than first-generation analogs. The third-generation cephalosporins are even more active and have a still broader *in vitro* and *in vivo* spectrum of activity against gram-negative bacteria. They have increased stability to beta-lactamases produced by many gram-negative bacteria. In general, third-generation cephalosporins are less active against -gram-positive bacteria than first-generation cephalosporins (270).

Cephalosporins inhibit the third and final stage of bacterial cell wall formation by preferentially binding to one or more PBPs that are in the cytoplasmic membrane beneath the cell walls of susceptible bacteria. Cephalosporins are primarily bactericidal antibiotics, and the intrinsic activity of the cephalosporin depends in part on its binding affinity to the PBPs. Mechanisms of resistance to cephalosporins include (a) inactivation by bacterial beta-lactamases, (b) decreased permeability of the bacterial cell, and (c) alterations in PBPs. Beta-lactamase inactivation and altered permeability are the most important resistance mechanisms clinically observed in gram-negative bacteria. Decreased affinity for PBPs occurs with some gram-positive bacteria.

Cephalosporins are generally well tolerated, with hypersensitivity reactions being the most common systemic adverse effects. They are particularly well tolerated with topical ocular application. The principal systemic adverse reactions include rashes accompanied by fever and eosinophilia. Immediate-type IgE-mediated reactions are less common with cephalosporins than with penicillins. Although the chemical structures of cephalosporins and penicillins are similar, cross-hypersensitivity reaction between the two groups of antibiotics is quite low. Perhaps fewer than 5% of individuals with a history of penicillin allergy, including anaphylactic reaction, also display allergy to cephalosporins (271). Despite this low incidence, it is recommended to avoid use of cephalosporins in individuals who experience immediate hypersensitivity reactions to penicillins because of the potential severity of these reactions.

Hematologic reactions, including bleeding, have been reported with cephalosporins containing a methylthiotetrazole side chain. The methylthiotetrazole side chain appears to interfere with hepatic vitamin K metabolism, resulting in hypoprothrombinemia and prolongation of prothrombin time. A second important mechanism might be the eradication of vitamin K–producing intestinal microorganisms (272). Administration of vitamin K reverses the hypoprothrombinemia, and in some patients prophylactic vitamin K administration should be considered. Moxalactam, a third-generation cephalosporin, has caused prolonged bleeding times owing to a dose-dependent inhibition of platelet function (273). Gastrointestinal disturbances may occur after cephalosporin use, including anorexia, nausea, vomiting, and diarrhea. The risk of cephalosporin administration during pregnancy to the fetus has not been fully established, yet, as with the penicillins, there is little evidence of teratogenicity.

First-generation cephalosporins have been used frequently as prophylactic agents for surgical procedures. Cefazolin is usually preferred to other first-generation cephalosporins because of its superior pharmacokinetic properties, including higher plasma protein binding, lower volume of distribution, and slower rate of elimination, which result in higher and more sustained serum concentrations.

Because of its excellent activity against gram-positive pathogens and relatively low toxicity after topical administration, cefazolin has been the most commonly used first-generation cephalosporin for therapy of bacterial keratitis. It is most frequently used in combination with an agent effective against gram-negative organisms if there is polybacterial keratitis or if the causative organisms are unknown.

Cephalosporins are relatively lipid soluble and do not penetrate well into ocular tissues. Second-generation cephalosporins may be slightly less lipid soluble and penetrate better into ocular tissues. Ceftazidime, a third-generation cephalosporin having antipseudomonal activity, has been shown effective in experimental models of *Pseudomonas* keratitis in rabbits (274,275). Ceftazidime has been used clinically for topical therapy of bacterial keratitis in humans. Like other third-generation cephalosporins, ceftazidime has some activity against gram-positive organisms, slightly less than cefazolin, yet has antipseudomonal activity, unlike first-generation cephalosporins. All beta-lactam antibiotics are somewhat unstable in solution, which may limit their activity with topical application for bacterial keratitis (276).

Other Beta-Lactam Antibiotics

Imipenem is the first of a new class of beta-lactam antibiotics called the *carbapenems* (277). Imipenem is the *N*-formimidoyl derivative of thienamycin, an antibiotic isolated from *Streptomyces cattleya*. It has the fused ring lactam of the penicillins with a substitution of carbon for sulfur and an unsaturated five-member ring (278).

To prevent active renal metabolism, imipenem is administered in a 1:1 fixed-ratio combination with cilastatin, a specific inhibitor of dipeptidase metabolism. Imipenem has potent activity against most clinically important species of bacteria, including isolates that are resistant to other antibiotics. It is rapidly bactericidal against most bacteria that it inhibits. The antibacterial effect of imipenem is achieved by binding to critical PBPs of susceptible gram-positive and gram-negative bacteria. Imipenem has marked stability to attack by both plasmid-and chromosome-mediated beta-lactamases of most bacterial species. Imipenem also penetrates well through the outer membrane of gram-negative bacteria.

Imipenem has excellent activity against most gram-positive bacteria, including penicillinase-producing strains of *S. aureus* and coagulase-negative staphylococci. Variable activity is demonstrated against methicillin-resistant staphylococci. Imipenem has excellent activity against *Streptococcus* species, including some activity against penicillin-resistant pneumococci. Imipenem is also extremely active against most species of gram-negative aerobic bacteria. Imipenem has potency similar to that of ceftazidime against *P. aeruginosa*, and is very active against *Acinetobacter. Stenotrophomonas maltophilia* (formerly *Xanthomonas maltophilia* and *Pseudomonas maltophilia*) and *Burkholderia cepacia* (formerly *Pseudomonas cepacia*) are resistant.

Imipenem is reasonably well tolerated and has an adverse reaction profile similar to most other beta-lactam antibiotics. The most common clinical adverse reactions to imipenem/cilastatin were those involving the gastrointestinal tract after systemic administration. The drug is well tolerated after topical ocular administration. Topical imipenem therapy of aminoglycoside-resistant *Pseudomonas* keratitis has been successful in an experimental model in rabbits (279).

Aztreonam is the first of a new class of beta-lactam antimicrobial agents called *monobactams* (280). The monobactams are unique compared with the penicillins, cephalosporins, and carbapenems, which have fused double-ring nuclei, in that they are monocyclic beta-lactam agents containing 3-aminomonobactamic acid as the basic nucleus.

Monobactams were isolated from naturally occurring bacteria, but exhibited poor antibacterial properties. Aztreonam is a totally synthetic monobactam that has potent activity against aerobic gram-negative bacteria, including *P. aeruginosa*, and excellent stability to beta-lactamases. *N. gonorrhoeae*, *N. meningitidis*, and *H. influenzae*, including beta-lactamase–producing strains of these species, are highly susceptible. Aztreonam has potency comparable with third-generation cephalosporins against most Enterobacteriaceae. It is active against most strains of *P. aeruginosa*, including strains that are resistant to other antipseudomonal antibiotics. It is slightly less potent than ceftazidime against *P. aeruginosa*. Aztreonam has minimal activity against other *Pseudomonas* species and is not active against *Acinetobacter*. Aztreonam interacts poorly with the PBPs of gram-positive bacteria and anaerobes and therefore is inactive against most of these organisms.

Aztreonam is usually well tolerated after systemic administration, with an adverse reaction profile resembling that of most other beta-lactam antibiotics (281). Aztreonam has been associated with nephrotoxicity, neurotoxicity, and coagulopathies (282).

Although the retinal toxicity of aztreonam has been investigated in albino and pigmented rabbits after intravitreal administration (283), there is little clinical experience with the use of topical aztreonam for therapy of severe gram-negative bacterial keratitis.

Glycopeptides

Vancomycin is a glycopeptide antibiotic with activity against penicillin-resistant staphylococci. Vancomycin is derived from *Streptomyces orientalis*. Vancomycin inhibits the biosynthesis of peptidoglycan polymers during the second stage of bacterial cell wall formation. The primary site of action is distinct from that of the beta-lactam antibiotics. Vancomycin is usually bactericidal for replicating microorganisms. It is primarily active against gram-positive bacteria and remains one of the most potent antibiotics

against *S. aureus* and coagulase-negative staphylococci, including methicillin-resistant strains. streptococci (including penicillin G–resistant strains) are highly susceptible to vancomycin. Vancomycin also has excellent activity against a variety of gram-positive bacilli, including clostridia, corynebacteria, *Bacillus* species, *L. monocytogenes*, *Actinomyces* species, and lactobacilli. Other gram-negative bacilli, mycobacteria, *Bacteroides*, and fungi are resistant (284). Bacterial resistance rarely develops during therapy with vancomycin. Of increasing concern is the development of plasmid-mediated vancomycin-resistant enterococcal strains (285).

A nonimmunologic, dose-dependent, histamine-mediated reaction can occur with rapid intravenous administration of vancomycin, causing the "red man's syndrome." This reaction is characterized by flushing, tingling, pruritus, tachycardia, an erythematous macular rash, and systemic arterial hypotension (286). Ototoxicity is the most serious adverse effect of vancomycin, manifested by auditory nerve damage and hearing loss that may be irreversible (287). Dose-dependent nephrotoxicity may occur with vancomycin administration, especially with concomitant aminoglycoside therapy (288). Vancomycin has a high molecular weight and the osmolarity of formulations for ocular administration must be considered. Lower concentrations are reasonably well tolerated after topical administration. Subconjunctival injection may cause sloughing. Vancomycin is considered the topical therapeutic agent of choice for staphylococcal infections when penicillin or cephalosporins cannot be administered, or if the organism is resistant to these antibiotics (289).

Teicoplanin is a glycopeptide antibiotic obtained by the fermentation of *Actinoplanes teichomyceticus* and is chemically related to vancomycin. The *in vitro* and *in vivo* antimicrobial properties of teicoplanin are similar to those of vancomycin. Teicoplanin blocks bacterial cell wall synthesis by inhibiting peptidoglycan polymerization (290). Teicoplanin is active only against gram-positive bacteria and is usually bactericidal, except against enterococci and *Listeria*. As with vancomycin, development of resistance to teicoplanin is uncommon. Teicoplanin may cause some nephrotoxicity, but ototoxicity is not a worrisome adverse effect as with vancomycin. There is little investigational or clinical information regarding the use of topical teicoplanin for therapy of resistant gram-positive keratitis.

Aminoglycosides

Aminoglycosides were discovered as a result of systematic screening of soil actinomycetes for the elaboration of antimicrobial substances. Streptomycin, the first clinically useful aminoglycoside, was isolated in 1944.

Aminoglycosides contain a six-member aminocyclitol ring (aglycone) with a variety of amino and nonamino sugars attached by glycosidic linkages. Variations within families of aminoglycosides result from differences in the side chains on the amino sugars or on the aglycone. Under aerobic conditions, the aminoglycosides are bactericidal for susceptible bacteria. Aminoglycosides must be actively transported across the cytoplasmic membrane into a bacterium (291). Aminoglycoside antibiotics have a selective affinity to the bacterial 30S and 50S ribosomal subunits to produce a nonfunctional 70S initiation complex that in turn results in the inhibition of bacterial cell protein synthesis (292). Other antibiotics that impair protein synthesis (e.g., chloramphenicol, tetracycline) are usually only bacteriostatic, whereas the aminoglycosides are usually bactericidal. The binding of aminoglycoside to ribosomes may accelerate subsequent transport of antibiotic with progressive disruption of the cytoplasmic membrane, loss of permeability control, and cell death (291). The active transport of aminoglycosides across bacterial cell membranes is inhibited by divalent cations, hyperosmolarity, reduced pH, and anaerobic conditions. Thus, the clinical activity of aminoglycosides is markedly reduced in the anaerobic environment of a tissue abscess. Aminoglycosides induced prolonged postantibiotic effects lasting from 2 to 7 hours against aerobic gram-negative bacilli, both *in vitro* and in experimental models (293).

Aminoglycosides are principally active against aerobic and facultative gram-negative bacilli. Enterobacteriaceae are usually susceptible, although *Salmonella* and *Shigella* species are less susceptible *in vivo*. Widespread use of aminoglycosides has resulted in the emergence of resistant strains achieved by alteration of the bacterial ribosome, decreased antibiotic uptake, and enzymatic inactivation of the drugs. In clinical practice, enzymatic inactivation of the aminoglycoside is the most important type of resistance encountered. Bacterial conjugation transmits extrachromosomal genes (plasmids) that cause the production of enzymes that modify the aminoglycosides by acetylation of specific amino groups or phosphorylation of specific hydroxyl groups (294).

Certain aminoglycosides remain active against *P. aeruginosa*, including tobramycin, gentamicin, amikacin, and netilmicin. For severe keratitis, aminoglycosides may be combined with an antipseudomonal penicillin or antipseudomonal cephalosporin.

Aminoglycosides are also active against aerobic gram-negative bacilli, including *Acinetobacter* and *Haemophilus* species. Because of the accompanying toxicity of aminoglycoside therapy, *Haemophilus* infections are usually treated with more effective, less toxic antibiotics. Among gram-positive cocci, only staphylococci (e.g., *S. aureus*) are inhibited by the aminoglycosides. Aminoglycosides, however, are seldom used as the sole agents in serious staphylococcal keratitis because less toxic, more effective agents are available. Although the gram-positive rods of *Bacillus*, *Listeria*, and *Corynebacterium* are susceptible to gentamicin, tobramycin, and amikacin, aminoglycosides are rarely used for therapy of infections caused by these organisms. With

L. monocytogenes, ampicillin plus aminoglycoside therapy provides synergy. Aminoglycosides generally are inactive against anaerobic bacteria, including clostridia and *Bacteroides*.

Aminoglycosides have a low therapeutic–toxic ratio compared with most other antibiotics. The most severe adverse reactions include irreversible ototoxicity, nephrotoxicity, and neurotoxicity. Topical ocular use frequently results in conjunctival hyperemia, punctate keratopathy, and occasionally pseudomembranous conjunctivitis.

Tobramycin usually has slightly better *in vitro* antibacterial activity against *Pseudomonas* isolates compared with gentamicin. No difference in efficacy of tobramycin versus gentamicin in gentamicin-resistant strains in *Pseudomonas* keratitis was observed in one study (295). Occasionally, an aminoglycoside-resistant strain of *Pseudomonas* lacking susceptibility to tobramycin and gentamicin may be susceptible to amikacin sulfate (296). Amikacin is susceptible to only two of the known aminoglycoside-inactivating enzymes. Therefore, it is active against many gentamicin- and tobramycin-resistant strains of aerobic gram-negative bacilli. Bacterial strains that are resistant to amikacin usually have a defective aminoglycoside transport mechanism. Thus, these mutants typically exhibit cross-resistance to all other aminoglycosides.

Although fortified aminoglycoside topical therapy for bacterial keratitis may be associated with significant toxicity to the ocular surface, no serious effects have been observed with standard 0.3% concentration aminoglycoside therapy with moderate topical administration (297–300). Neomycin is an aminoglycoside antibiotic that is sometimes formulated in combination with other antibiotics (e.g., polymyxin-B, bacitracin, or gramicidin) for topical administration. Neomycin has relatively poor activity against *Pseudomonas* species. It is effective against many strains of *H. influenzae*, *Escherichia coli*, and *Proteus*. Topical administration of neomycin solution is associated with conjunctival and skin hypersensitivity reactions in 15% to 20% of individuals.

Fluoroquinolones

The most recent class of antibacterial agents to receive FDA approval for the indication of therapy of bacterial keratitis are the fluoroquinolone compounds. The fluoroquinolones were serendipitously discovered in 1962, during the purification of chloroquine. Nalidixic acid, the first member of the quinolone class, was principally used for therapy of gram-negative infections. The addition of a fluorine to the 6-position of the basic quinolone nucleus expanded the antibacterial spectrum greatly, and compounds having 1000 times the activity of nalidixic acid were soon synthesized. The fluoroquinolones are rapidly bactericidal in action and exert their effects by variably inhibiting the action of bacterial DNA gyrase, an enzyme essential for bacterial DNA synthesis (301–303). The commercially available fluoroquinolones (ciprofloxacin, norfloxacin, ofloxacin, gatifloxacin, and moxifloxacin) for topical ophthalmic use have similar antimicrobial spectra that include most aerobic gram-negative and some gram-positive bacteria. Fluoroquinolones are highly active against most Enterobacteriaceae. In particular, fluoroquinolones are highly active against *P. aeruginosa*, including strains that are resistant to other bacterial agents (304). Ciprofloxacin has the most potent *in vitro* activity of the ophthalmic fluoroquinolones currently commercially available against *P. aeruginosa*. The significance of *in vitro* differences between the fluoroquinolones for clinical usefulness depends on other factors, such as pharmacokinetic properties and relative toxicities. For topical ocular application, comparative *in vivo* human clinical trials between fluoroquinolones have not been conducted.

Although fluoroquinolones are active against *P. aeruginosa*, they are less active against non-*aeruginosa* pseudomonads, including *S. maltophilia* and *B. cepacia*. Most strains of *Acinetobacter* are susceptible to ciprofloxacin or ofloxacin. Norfloxacin and enoxacin are considerably less active. Ciprofloxacin and ofloxacin are the most active of the commercially available ophthalmic agents against gram-positive bacteria, including coagulase-negative and coagulase-positive, as well as methicillin-resistant staphylococcal strains (305). Streptococci, including *S. pyogenes* (group A, *S. agalactiae*), group B, *S. pneumoniae*, and *viridans* streptococci, and *E. faecalis* (enterococci) are only moderately susceptible to ciprofloxacin and ofloxacin. Norfloxacin and enoxacin are even less active (306,307).

The gram-negative coccobacilli, *H. influenzae* and *Haemophilus ducreyi* (308), and the gram-negative cocci *N. gonorrhoeae*, *N. meningitidis*, and *M. catarrhalis* are all highly susceptible to the fluoroquinolones, including beta-lactamase–producing strains of these organisms.

The fluoroquinolones are active *in vitro* against some intracellular pathogens. Ciprofloxacin and ofloxacin have some activity against *Mycobacterium tuberculosis* and certain nontuberculous mycobacteria (309). Ciprofloxacin and ofloxacin also have activity *in vitro* against *Chlamydia trachomatis* (310–312).

In general, anaerobic bacteria have shown limited susceptibility to the fluoroquinolones, although ciprofloxacin and ofloxacin demonstrate partial activity against some species (313,314).

Resistance to the fluoroquinolones is principally due to chromosomal mutations. Mutations involving Gy^r, the A subunit of DNA gyrase, usually produce high-level resistance to nalidixic acid and a lower level of resistance to fluoroquinolones. Mutations in the Gy^r B subunit of DNA gyrase produce variable effects (315,316). Mutations unrelated to DNA gyrase also produce resistance to the quinolones. Many of these mutations appear to involve the permeation of the quinolones into the gram-negative cell (317–319). Fluoroquinolones penetrate into

the gram-negative cell by passive diffusion through porins (outer membrane proteins) and exposed lipid domains on the outer membrane of bacteria (320). The hydrophobicity of a given quinolone agent alters the relative importance of each pathway. Alterations in outer membrane proteins or lipopolysaccharides of gram-negative cells may influence the susceptibility to fluoroquinolones (321). When mutations affecting permeation are involved, cross-resistance between fluoroquinolones is often encountered (322). Considerable concern has been generated regarding the emerging resistance to fluoroquinolones among staphylococci (323).

Although there has been evidence for development of resistance to fluoroquinolones based on *in vitro* susceptibility testing among ocular isolates, until recently there have been no clinically significant observations of fluoroquinolone resistance with topical therapy for keratitis. However, clinical cases of bacterial keratitis exhibiting resistance to ciprofloxacin treatment have been reported (324,325). The clinician selecting single-agent fluoroquinolone therapy should be aware of the potential gaps in the spectra of activity, especially against streptococci, enterococci, non-*aeruginosa* pseudomonads, and anaerobes, and be prepared to modify treatment accordingly (326). Although the fluoroquinolones have only relatively recently received FDA approval for treatment of ocular infections, there is already considerable clinical experience with treatment of bacterial keratitis. Fluoroquinolones were tested early on for their potential in the topical therapy of experimental bacterial keratitis (327,328). Topical ciprofloxacin (3 mg/mL) and ofloxacin (3 mg/mL) were found to penetrate well into stromal tissue and to be effective in eradicating *Pseudomonas* organisms compared with controls (327,329). Topical enoxacin was also found to be effective against *Pseudomonas* organisms in an experimental model of keratitis (328). Based on its excellent activity in experimental bacterial keratitis, topical ciprofloxacin therapy for bacterial keratitis in humans was assessed in an open-label, nonrandomized clinical trial initially (330). In this noncomparative treatment trial, ciprofloxacin 0.3% topical solution was found to be highly effective in therapy of acute bacterial keratitis and reasonably well tolerated by the ocular surface. Crystalline white ciprofloxacin precipitates were observed in the area of epithelial ulceration in 16% of patients (330). Such crystalline drug precipitation occurs with higher frequency in eyes treated with ciprofloxacin than in those treated with norfloxacin or ofloxacin, consistent with differences in fluoroquinolone compound pH solubility profiles (331). Comparative pharmacokinetic data suggest that this precipitation may reduce the active concentration of drug in the stroma at the site of infection (332).

Such crystalline deposition has the potential disadvantage of decreasing visualization of the stromal infiltrate immediately deep to the precipitate for clinical monitoring of therapeutic progress. There is evidence that ciprofloxacin precipitation may also prevent or delay reepithelialization of a corneal defect (333). The crystalline corneal precipitates of ciprofloxacin usually spontaneously resolve with cessation of therapy.

An ophthalmic ointment preparation of ciprofloxacin 0.3% has been shown to be effective in the therapy of experimental *Pseudomonas* keratitis in rabbits (334). A multicenter, nonrandomized, noncomparative clinical trial has shown favorable efficacy of 0.3% ciprofloxacin ophthalmic ointment in the treatment of bacterial keratitis (335).

The first, multicenter, randomized, comparative clinical trial assessing the efficacy of ofloxacin 0.3% solution versus fortified cefazolin and tobramycin has shown favorable, comparable efficacy of single-agent fluoroquinolone therapy versus fortified antibiotics (25). A similarly designed, randomized, double-masked, comparative trial evaluating the efficacy of ciprofloxacin 0.3% solution versus fortified cephalosporin and aminoglycoside has shown comparable results for single-agent fluoroquinolone therapy (336). In a comparative, double-masked trial of ofloxacin versus fortified cephalosporin and aminoglycoside, there was no significant difference observed in efficacy, yet the fortified antibiotics did exhibit significantly enhanced toxicity compared with single-agent ofloxacin treatment (25).

Norfloxacin is also available as a topical ophthalmic solution. Norfloxacin is generally less active *in vitro* and *in vivo* against gram-positive organisms and most gram-negative organisms compared with ciprofloxacin and ofloxacin. Topical norfloxacin ophthalmic solution has FDA approval for the treatment of bacterial conjunctivitis, but not for keratitis. Topical norfloxacin exhibits greater corneal epithelial toxicity than topical ciprofloxacin or ofloxacin, similar to the toxicity profile observed with the combination of a cephalosporin and an aminoglycoside (337).

Expanded-spectrum fluoroquinolones have a greater activity, especially against gram-positive pathogens (338–340). Temafloxacin, an aqueous-soluble fluoroquinolone, exhibited excellent activity against gram-positive bacteria, including streptococci and gram-negative bacteria, including *Pseudomonas*. Although temafloxacin was tolerated in several animal models of ocular infection, it exhibited a significant incidence of serious adverse reactions with systemic use, prompting its worldwide voluntary withdrawal (341). Several trifluoronated fluoroquinolones with an extended spectrum of activity against gram-positive and gram-negative aerobic and anaerobic bacteria have shown promise in experimental models of bacterial keratitis (328).

Studies investigating the therapeutic role of trovafloxacin mesylate, a newer-generation fluoroquinolone with an expanded spectrum of activity, in the treatment of experimental bacterial keratitis were reported (342). Susceptibility studies were performed on various strains of ocular isolates to determine the MIC of trovafloxacin compared with ciprofloxacin and ofloxacin, using the E-test method. Pharmacokinetic studies were performed by a single topical administration of trovafloxacin to rabbit eyes with either an intact or denuded corneal epithelium. Aqueous humor, vitreous, and corneal concentrations of trovafloxacin were determined at different time points. Experimental bacterial keratitis studies were performed in rabbit eyes. Three identical studies were conducted using *S. aureus*, *S. pneumoniae*, or *P. aeruginosa*. Therapy groups included 0.5% trovafloxacin, 0.3% ciprofloxacin, 0.3% ofloxacin, and isotonic sodium chloride solution. After 12 hours of eyedrops administration, corneas were excised, homogenized, and serially plated. *In vitro* susceptibility study findings indicated that the MIC of trovafloxacin was significantly lower than the MIC of ciprofloxacin and ofloxacin for *S. aureus*, *S. pneumoniae*, and *H. influenzae*, lower than the MIC of ciprofloxacin and ofloxacin for *S. epidermidis*, and intermediate between ciprofloxacin and ofloxacin for *P. aeruginosa*. Pharmacokinetic studies showed a significant concentration of trovafloxacin in the treated corneas, especially in eyes with a denuded epithelium. All serum samples had undetectable trovafloxacin concentrations. Experimental keratitis studies showed a statistically significant decrease of colony-forming units in trovafloxacin-treated eyes in the *S. aureus* model and a similar decrease in the *S. pneumoniae* and *P. aeruginosa* models. Topical 0.5% trovafloxacin proved to be an effective ocular medication for the therapy of gram-positive and gram-negative keratitis. Trovafloxacin may provide an excellent therapeutic alternative in bacterial keratitis (342).

Lomefloxacin 0.3% solution has shown long-lasting tear levels and good corneal penetration in human and animal studies (343,344). Preclinical studies also demonstrated adequate efficacy for therapy of ocular infection, including endophthalmitis (345). Clinical studies in humans have shown adequate efficacy of lomefloxacin 0.3% solution in therapy of external infections of the eye (346,347). The *in vitro* spectrum of activity is comparable with that of norfloxacin. Its potency is less than that of ciprofloxacin, ofloxacin, levofloxacin, gatifloxacin, or moxifloxacin.

A study in Thailand compared the efficacy and safety of topical lomefloxacin 0.3% with topical ciprofloxacin 0.3% for treating mildly severe suspected bacterial corneal ulcers (348). This prospective, randomized, double-masked, controlled clinical trial was conducted on 41 patients (41 eyes) with suspected bacterial corneal ulcers who were randomized into 2 groups: 23 patients were in the lomefloxacin group and 18 patients in the ciprofloxacin group. All of these corneal ulcers were scraped for Gram stain, KOH preparation, and microbiologic cultures before starting treatment. Topical lomefloxacin was found to be equivalent clinically and statistically with topical ciprofloxacin. No statistically significant treatment differences were found between lomefloxacin (100%) and ciprofloxacin (100%) in terms of success rate. Similarly, no differences were noted in the time to cure (*p* > .05), treatment failure, or the resolution of the clinical signs and symptoms (*p* > .05). The adverse effects of lomefloxacin were superficial punctate keratitis (26.1%) and irritation (8.7%), whereas those of ciprofloxacin were superficial punctate keratitis (22.2%), white precipitate (11.1%), and irritation (11.1%). However, no statistically significant differences in these adverse effects were found between the two groups (*p* > .05). The investigators concluded that lomefloxacin ophthalmic solution (0.3%) is equivalent clinically and statistically to ciprofloxacin ophthalmic solution (0.3%) for the treatment of mildly severe presumed bacterial corneal ulcers, without statistically significant differences in adverse effects and discomfort (348).

A "fortified" preparation of levofloxacin, the L-isomer of ofloxacin, at a concentration of 1.5% (15 mg/mL) has received FDA approval for the indication of acute bacterial keratitis. Further postmarketing surveillance is required to monitor carefully for cytotoxicity and to balance safety with efficacy.

To estimate how a corneal isolate's MIC for a fluoroquinolone agent affects the rate of clinical response of bacterial keratitis to fluoroquinolone therapy, a prospective cohort study was conducted (349). Six hundred sixty-three individuals with suspected bacterial keratitis underwent diagnostic corneal scraping and were treated with topical 0.3% ciprofloxacin solution or ointment. Of 407 patients with culture-confirmed bacterial keratitis, improvement and cure rates with ciprofloxacin monotherapy were estimated for 391 who had *in vitro* ciprofloxacin susceptibility of the principal corneal isolate. Slit-lamp biomicroscopic assessment was used to determine clinical improvement of corneal inflammation and clinical cure with complete reepithelialization. Adjusted rates of improvement and of cure were reduced, respectively, by 43% (95% CI, 8%–64%) and by 29% (95% CI, 0%–49%) among corneal infections having a ciprofloxacin MIC above 1 µg/mL compared with those with more sensitive isolates. Corneal infections by relatively ciprofloxacin-resistant bacteria responded more slowly to ciprofloxacin therapy. Antibacterial susceptibility testing of corneal cultures may predict the fluoroquinolone therapeutic response rate of bacterial keratitis (349).

A comparison of the *in vitro* susceptibility patterns and the MICs of gatifloxacin and moxifloxacin (fourth-generation fluoroquinolones) with ciprofloxacin and ofloxacin (second-generation fluoroquinolones) and levofloxacin (third-generation fluoroquinolone) using bacterial keratitis isolates was conducted. The goal was to determine whether the 8-methoxy fluoroquinolones offer any advantages over the second- and third-generation fluoroquinolones. In contrast to an epidemiologic prevalence study, this study was designed to compare the relative susceptibility of each bacterial group to different fluoroquinolones by deliberate selection of representative isolates that were both susceptible and resistant to second-generation fluoroquinolones. In retrospect,

the MICs of 177 bacterial keratitis isolates were determined to ciprofloxacin, ofloxacin, levofloxacin, gatifloxacin, and moxifloxacin using E-tests. A relative susceptibility analysis was performed for each bacterial group that included separate bacterial groups that were resistant to second-generation fluoroquinolones. For most keratitis isolates, there were no susceptibility differences among the five fluoroquinolones. The fourth-generation fluoroquinolones did, however, demonstrate increased susceptibility for *S. aureus* isolates that were resistant to ciprofloxacin, levofloxacin, and ofloxacin. In general, ciprofloxacin demonstrated the lowest MICs for gram-negative bacteria. The MICs of 8-methoxy fluoroquinolones were statistically lower than the MICs of second-generation fluoroquinolones for all gram-positive bacteria tested. Comparing the two fourth-generation fluoroquinolones, moxifloxacin demonstrated lower MICs for most gram-positive bacteria, whereas gatifloxacin demonstrated lower MICs for most gram-negative bacteria. The authors concluded that based on *in vitro* testing, the fourth-generation fluoroquinolones may offer some advantages over those currently available for the treatment of bacterial keratitis (350).

To assess the value of a therapeutic index for corneal infections, investigators explored the prognostic importance of a ratio of the achievable corneal level for a fluoroquinolone to the fluoroquinolone's MIC for corneal isolates of 391 patients with bacterial keratitis (351). The peak concentration and the area under the concentration curve (AUC) in the cornea were estimated from reported values achieved with topical ciprofloxacin. The inhibitory quotient was calculated as the ratio of the estimated peak achievable corneal ciprofloxacin concentration to the ciprofloxacin MIC of keratitis isolates, and the area under the inhibitory curve (AUIC) was defined as the expected 24-hour AUC divided by the MIC. The probability of clinical improvement of ciprofloxacin-treated bacterial keratitis was 90% or more if ciprofloxacin's inhibitory quotient was above 8 or the AUIC was greater than 151. The author concluded that a pharmacodynamic index relating corneal pharmacokinetic and susceptibility concentrations may correlate with the clinical response of bacterial keratitis to fluoroquinolone therapy (351).

A study to assess the effectiveness of a fourth-generation fluoroquinolone for prophylaxis against multiple drug–resistant staphylococcal keratitis after lamellar keratectomy in a rabbit model was conducted (352). Rabbits underwent unilateral lamellar keratectomy using a manual microkeratome followed by the placement of 1000 colony-forming units of log-phase *S. aureus* bacteria under each flap. Eyes (seven in each group) were randomized and treated with one of the following agents: sterile balanced salt solution, gatifloxacin (0.3%), ciprofloxacin (0.3%), or levofloxacin (0.5%) immediately and 6, 12, and 18 hours after surgery. Infectious infiltrates developed in five of seven eyes in each group treated with ciprofloxacin, levofloxacin, and balanced salt solution. Gatifloxacin-treated eyes did not develop clinical infection and exhibited lower mean inflammation scores ($p < .01$ compared with the other groups). The fourth-generation fluoroquinolone, gatifloxacin, is an effective prophylaxis against the development of keratitis after lamellar keratectomy in rabbits with an organism resistant to methicillin, levofloxacin, and ciprofloxacin (352).

In summary, there is considerable experimental and clinical experience with the use of fluoroquinolone solutions for therapy of ocular infections (353). Their high potency and generally excellent activity against the most frequent gram-positive and gram-negative ocular pathogens, bactericidal mode of action, bioavailability, and biocompatibility make fluoroquinolones an excellent initial choice for the topical therapy of bacterial keratitis.

For severe cases however, a combination of a cephalosporin and a fluoroquinolone should be considered.

The fluoroquinolone solutions are reasonably well tolerated with topical application. With frequent topical dosing, precipitation of certain fluoroquinolones (e.g., ciprofloxacin) may delay reepithelialization. Some additional concerns have been raised about corneal toxicity of certain fluoroquinolones with topical administration.

The use of topical fluoroquinolones to treat microbial keratitis is associated with an increased incidence of corneal perforation compared with other standard treatments (354). This study examined the effects of topical fluoroquinolones on corneal collagen and keratocytes in intact rabbit corneas and corneas with an epithelial defect.

Studies consisted of one group of intact corneas and one group of corneas where a 6-mm epithelial defect was created with a surgical scrape. In each group, eyes were randomly assigned to one of four topical medications [0.3% ciprofloxacin, 0.3% ofloxacin, fortified antibiotics (1.36% tobramycin, 5% cefazolin), or Tears Naturale (Alcon Laboratories, French's Forest, New South Wales, Australia)]. Two drops were instilled hourly for 48 hours and then every 2 hours for an additional 48 hours. At 96 hours, the corneas were removed and processed for light microscopy, immunohistology for collagen IV, V, and VI, and apoptosis staining.

In intact rabbit corneas, there was no demonstrable difference between treatment groups. In corneas with an epithelial defect, both fluoroquinolones delayed epithelial healing compared with fortified antibiotics or tears. Keratocyte loss was seen in all groups and was greatest in the ofloxacin group. Median stromal thicknesses with keratocyte loss were ofloxacin 30%; ciprofloxacin 10%; fortified antibiotics 7.5%; and tears 15% (ofloxacin vs. tears, Mann-Whitney U-test = 16.0; $p = .09$). Keratocyte loss did not correlate with the amount of demonstrable apoptosis. Collagens IV, V, and VI showed no differences between treatments.

These results suggest that ofloxacin is potentially cytotoxic to corneal keratocytes. Such an effect could lead to the observed increased incidence of corneal perforation in

microbial keratitis (354). MMPs play an important role in extracellular matrix deposition and degradation. Based on previous clinical observations of corneal perforations during topical fluoroquinolone treatment, an evaluation of the comparative effects of various fluoroquinolone eye drops on the expression of MMPs in cornea was conducted (355). Rats were divided into two experimental groups: intact and wounded corneal epithelium. Uniform corneal epithelial defects were created in the right eye with application of 75% alcohol in the center of the tissue for 6 seconds. The treatment groups were tested as follows: (a) tear drops: carboxymethylcellulose sodium 0.5 % (Refresh; Allergan); (b) ciprofloxacin 0.3% (Ciloxan; Alcon); (c) ofloxacin 0.3% (Ocuflox; Allergan); and (d) levofloxacin 0.5% (Quixin; Santen). Eyedrops were administered six times a day for 48 hours. Rats were sacrificed at 48 hours. Immunohistochemical analysis and zymography were conducted using antibodies specific to MMP-1, MMP-2, MMP-8, and MMP-9.

MMP-1, MMP-2, MMP-8, and MMP-9 expression was detected at 48 hours in undebrided corneal epithelium groups treated with the topical fluoroquinolones. No statistical difference was observed in quantitative expression of MMPs among ciprofloxacin 0.3%, ofloxacin 0.3%, and levofloxacin 0.5%. When the artificial tear group and the fluoroquinolone groups with corneal epithelial defects were compared, increased expression of MMPs was observed as a result of the wound healing process. However, the fluoroquinolone-treated group exhibited statistically significantly higher levels of MMPs expression.

This study provides preliminary evidence that topical application of fluoroquinolone drugs can induce the expression of MMP-1, MMP-2, MMP-8, and MMP-9 in the undebrided corneal epithelium compared with artificial tear eyedrops (355).

Potential increasing resistance among ocular isolates is also of theoretical concern, including a rise in resistance to fluoroquinolones among isolates from human keratitis (356). The ophthalmologist should be wary of the potential gaps in the spectrum of antibacterial coverage, including streptococci, enterococci, non- *aeruginosa* pseudomonads, and anaerobes, even with newer 8-methoxy fluoroquinolones. Trials assessing the efficacy and safety of newer fluoroquinolone solutions with an expanded spectrum of activity against gram-positive pathogens and anaerobes in therapy of acute bacterial keratitis seem warranted.

Macrolides and Lincosamides

Erythromycin was the first member of the macrolide family, discovered in soil extracts containing *Streptomyces erythreus* in the Philippines in 1954. Macrolides contain a macrocyclic lactone ring to which sugars are attached. Erythromycin inhibits bacterial protein synthesis by reversibly binding to the 50S ribosomal unit, thereby preventing elongation of the peptide chain, most likely through interference with the translocation step. Erythromycin does not bind to mammalian 80S ribosomes, accounting in part for its selective toxicity (357). Because chloramphenicol and the lincosamides have binding sites that overlap with the macrolides, the binding of one of these antibiotics to the ribosome may inhibit the reaction of the other (257). Thus, there are no clinical indications for the concurrent use of these antibiotics. Erythromycin may be either bacteriostatic or bactericidal depending on the concentration of drug, organism susceptibility, the growth rate the size of the inoculum. Erythromycin is inactivated in an acid medium, such as with an abscess cavity.

Erythromycin has a relatively broad spectrum of activity, especially against most gram-positive and some gram-negative bacteria. Variable activity against actinomycetes, spirochetes, chlamydiae, and certain nontuberculous mycobacteria has been shown (358). *S. pneumoniae* and *S. pyogenes* (group A, beta-hemolytic streptococci) are both highly susceptible to erythromycin, although occasional strains may be resistant. Erythromycin also has generally good activity against most *viridans* and anaerobic streptococci. It has variable activity against enterococci. Many *S. aureus* and coagulase-negative staphylococci are susceptible, although there may be increasing resistance, especially among hospital-acquired isolates or those resistant to methicillin (358).

Susceptible gram-positive bacilli include *B. anthracis*, *Clostridium*, *C. diphtheriae*, and *L. monocytogenes*. Many strains of *C. perfringens* are only moderately susceptible. Erythromycin is active against some actinomycetes, although *N. asteroides* has variable susceptibility.

Most strains of *N. gonorrhoeae* and *N. meningitidis* are susceptible to erythromycin. *M. catarrhalis* also are generally susceptible to erythromycin. Among gram-negative bacilli, *Eikenella corrodens* and *H. ducreyi* are susceptible. Many strains of *H. influenzae* are only moderately susceptible. Oropharyngeal species of *Bacteroides* are usually susceptible, but *B. fragilis* strains are resistant to erythromycin. Many *Fusobacterium* strains also are resistant.

Most aerobic gram-negative bacilli are resistant to erythromycin. The cell envelopes of most gram-negative bacilli prevent the passive diffusion of erythromycin into the cell. The susceptibility of gram-negative bacteria is increased in an alkaline medium because the ionization of erythromycin, a weak base, is reduced, making relatively more drug available in a form that can readily enter the cell. Erythromycin is rarely, if ever, indicated in infection caused by gram-negative bacteria.

Various mechanisms of resistance to erythromycin have been observed, including an alteration in a protein component of the bacterial 50S ribosomal subunit resulting in decreased binding affinity for erythromycin. This one-step, high-level resistance has been shown to be due to a chromosomal mutation. Erythromycin has enjoyed wide use as

an effective, nontoxic alternative to penicillin G for penicillin-allergic individuals. The large macrocyclic lactone ring with attached sugars results in a highly insoluble molecule, and thus erythromycin is available as an ophthalmic agent only in ointment form. The ointment form is one of the best tolerated, least toxic topical ophthalmic antibiotics. Because of its relative lack of solubility and availability in the ointment preparation, penetration into the cornea is suboptimal. With systemic use, erythromycin rarely causes adverse reactions. Gastrointestinal irritation with nausea, vomiting, and diarrhea are the most common adverse effects reported. Hypersensitivity reactions, such as skin rashes, drug, fever, and eosinophilia, rarely occur. One of the more serious adverse affects from systemic erythromycin use is cholestatic hepatitis. This has been especially seen with erythromycin estolate. Although safety during pregnancy has not been well established, congenital defects have not been reported despite widespread use.

Newer 14- and 16-member macrolides, including azithromycin, clarithromycin, and roxithromycin, have expanded serum half-lives and higher tissue levels. These favorable pharmacokinetic properties make the newer macrolides potentially exciting for therapy of intracellular pathogens, including *C. trachomatis*, nontuberculous mycobacteria, and others. Topical suspensions of clarithromycin (359,360) and azithromycin (360) have been assessed for their potential in treatment of nontuberculous mycobacterial infections. Because of their poor solubility and limited penetration into the cornea, the newer macrolides may have a limited role in therapy for bacterial keratitis.

The lincosamides include lincomycin, an antibacterial agent produced by *Streptomyces lincolnensis*, and its semisynthetic derivative, clindamycin. These drugs contain an amino acid link to an amino sugar. Clindamycin (7-chloro-7-deoxylincomycin) differs structurally from lincomycin by the substitution of a chlorine atom for a hydroxyl group on the parent molecule. This slight chemical modification increases the antibacterial potency of clindamycin over lincomycin. Clindamycin inhibits bacterial protein synthesis by binding to the 50S ribosomal subunit and preventing elongation of the peptide chain by interfering with peptidyl transfer (361). Clindamycin is primarily bacteriostatic. However, like erythromycin under certain conditions, clindamycin may demonstrate bactericidal activity against some organisms.

The lincosamides are active against most gram-positive and anaerobic gram-negative bacteria (362). Clindamycin resembles erythromycin in its *in vitro* activity against streptococci, *S. pneumoniae*, and *viridans* streptococci. Enterococci are generally resistant to clindamycin. Clindamycin also has generally excellent activity against both penicillinase- and non–penicillinase-producing *S. aureus*. Occasional resistance may be observed. *C. diphtheriae* are susceptible. One of the principal advantages of clindamycin is its generally excellent activity against anaerobic organisms, including *Propionibacterium, Eubacterium, Peptococcus, Peptostreptococcus, Veillonella* species, clostridia, *Bacteroides*, and several *Actinomyces* species. Most aerobic gram-negative bacteria are resistant to the lincosamides. Most *Nocardia* are also resistant. Mechanisms of resistance include alterations in the 50S ribosomal binding site or in the 23S RNA component of the 50S subunit (363). High-level plasmid-mediated, transferable clindamycin resistance has also demonstrated, with resistance to erythromycin also carried on these genes (363).

Clindamycin may be indicated as an alternative antibiotic for infections caused by susceptible gram-positive cocci, including staphylococci and streptococci, in patients who are allergic to both penicillins and cephalosporins.

Clindamycin in combination with pyrimethamine is a useful treatment for ocular and central nervous system toxoplasmosis, particularly in patients with AIDS who are unable to tolerate sulfonamides (364). Topical clindamycin solutions have also been effective in the management of acne.

Lincosamides are usually well tolerated. A common adverse effect of clindamycin administration is diarrhea. The lincosamides are capable of causing antibiotic-associated pseudomembranous colitis, which can be fatal. Antibiotic-associated pseudomembranous colitis has been estimated to occur in less than 0.01% to more than 10% of patients (365). Oral vancomycin therapy may be effective in the treatment of antibiotic-associated *Clostridium difficile* colitis (366).

Tetracyclines and Chloramphenicol

Tetracyclines. Tetracycline antibiotics were discovered after systematic screening of soil samples from many parts of the world for antibiotic-producing microorganisms. Tetracyclines are naturally derived compounds from various species of *Streptomyces*. Doxycycline is derived semisynthetically from oxytetracycline, and minocycline is prepared by chemical modification of tetracycline. All tetracyclines contain a hydronaphthacene nucleus consisting of four fused rings (367). Various substitutions on the basic structure may result in different properties among the tetracycline analogs. The tetracyclines are broad-spectrum antibacterial agents. Doxycycline and minocycline have increased lipophilicity compared with the parent tetracycline compound, and therefore penetrate better into adnexal and ocular tissues after oral administration. Tetracyclines interfere with protein synthesis by blocking the attachment of aminoacyl transfer RNA to the acceptor site on the messenger RNA–ribosome complex. The antibiotic binds primarily at the bacterial 30S ribosomal subunit. Tetracyclines are usually bacteriostatic at clinically achievable serum levels. Tetracyclines are effective *in vitro* against a great variety of bacteria, including gram-positive, gram-negative, aerobic, and anaerobic organisms. In addition, they show activity against many intracellular pathogens, including *Chlamydia*, and even some spirochetes (367).

Many strains of staphylococci are resistant to tetracyclines, although minocycline has greater antistaphylococcal activity than other analogs. Although tetracyclines show generally good activity against streptococci, they are usually not used to treat streptococcal infections because many strains are resistant and more effective drugs, such as penicillin G, erythromycin, and cephalosporins, are available. Tetracyclines are active against a number of gram-positive bacilli, including *B. anthracis, Clostridium,* and *L. monocytogenes*. Tetracyclines represent alternatives to penicillin G for infections caused by certain *Actinomyces*, and minocycline has activity against *N. asteroides*. Although many *N. gonorrhoeae* isolates are susceptible to tetracyclines, there has been an increasing emergence of tetracycline-resistant strains, and thus tetracyclines no longer are recommended as first-line drugs for gonococcal infections (368). *M. catarrhalis* are susceptible to the tetracyclines, especially doxycycline (369). Tetracyclines are active against a number of gram-negative bacilli, including *P. multocida, E. corrodens,* and *Francisella tularensis*. Many strains of *H. influenzae* are also susceptible. Most strains of Enterobacteriaceae and *P. aeruginosa* are resistant. Tetracyclines are the agents of choice for therapy of *C. trachomatis* and other chlamydial infections. Tetracyclines are also active against *B. burgdorferi*, the agent of Lyme disease. The nontuberculous mycobacteria *M. fortuitum* and *M. marinum* are susceptible to doxycycline and minocycline, respectively.

The primary mechanism of resistance to tetracyclines is decreased accumulation by the bacterial cell due to alterations in the energy-dependent transport process. Tetracycline resistance can be passed from one organism to another by transfer of small plasmids. Resistance to one tetracycline usually implies resistance to all. Tetracyclines are usually well tolerated, although there may be a high incidence of variable gastrointestinal intolerance. High-dose parenteral administration may result in liver damage, sometimes associated with pancreatitis. Tetracyclines are deposited in developing bones and teeth, where they can chelate with calcium to form a tetracycline–calcium orthophosphate complex. This danger is greatest from mid-pregnancy to approximately 3 years of age, but it may continue to 7 years of age and perhaps longer. Because of these adverse effects, tetracyclines should not be used during the last half of pregnancy or in children younger than 8 years of age.

Therapy with tetracyclines may result in reactions on exposure to the sun or other sources of ultraviolet light. Exaggerated sunburn reaction may occur with tetracyclines, especially with doxycyclines, because of accumulation of the drugs in the skin.

Tetracyclines may also cause pseudotumor cerebri, with increased intracranial pressure, meningeal irritation, and papilledema.

Extended dosing may result in reduction of normal bacterial flora and oral and anogenital superinfection with *Candida*.

Tetracycline is relatively insoluble and is available commercially only as a topical suspension with oil or as an ointment. It has relatively good ocular penetration with these forms. It has been used principally for therapy of external ocular infections.

Chloramphenicol. Chloramphenicol is a broad-spectrum antibiotic originally derived from *Streptomyces venezuelae*, but now prepared synthetically. Chloramphenicol also acts by inhibiting bacterial protein synthesis. It binds reversibly to the 50S subunit of the bacterial 70S ribosome and prevents the attachment of the amino acid–containing end of the aminoacyl-tran to the acceptor site on the ribosome. Chloramphenicol usually is bacteriostatic and can show bactericidal activity against certain common meningeal pathogens at therapeutic concentrations. The use of chloramphenicol has been limited by its toxicity, including a dose-dependent bone marrow depression. Mammalian mitochondria contain 70S ribosomes with physical characteristics similar to those found in bacterial cells. Many adverse affects appear to result from inhibition of protein synthesis in host mitochondria.

Chloramphenicol has been used widely worldwide for therapy of ocular infections. It is active *in vitro* against a wide variety of bacteria, including gram-positive, gram-negative, aerobic, and anaerobic organisms. In addition, chloramphenicol displays activity against chlamydiae and spirochetes. Chloramphenicol has good activity against streptococci, with variable susceptibility among enterococci. Many strains of *S. aureus* are susceptible, but resistant strains may be encountered, especially in areas with heavy use. Anaerobic gram-positive cocci, such as *Peptococcus* and *Peptostreptococcus*, are susceptible. Gram-positive bacilli, including *Bacillus* species, *L. monocytogenes*, *C. diphtheriae*, clostridia, and *Eubacterium*, are susceptible to chloramphenicol. Most strains of *N. gonorrhoeae* and *N. meningitidis* are susceptible. Chloramphenicol has been used in certain clinical situations because of its generally excellent activity against *H. influenzae* where resistance to other agents is suspected. Response of Enterobacteriaceae to chloramphenicol is variable. *P. aeruginosa* organisms are uniformly resistant to chloramphenicol.

Chloramphenicol resistance among gram-negative bacteria appears to be due to drug inactivation by an acetyl transferase that is plasmid mediated. Resistance to chloramphenicol in gram-positive bacteria also appears to develop by a similar mechanism.

Chloramphenicol has a relatively low therapeutic–toxic ratio and has been implicated in fatal aplastic anemia. Bone marrow hypoplasia occurs in two forms. One is a dose-related bone marrow suppression resulting in pancytopenia, which is usually reversible after discontinuation of the drug (370,371). A more serious sequela of chloramphenicol administration is a fatal idiosyncratic aplastic anemia, which has been estimated to occur after topical ocular administration at a frequency of 1:50,000 (372). Because the dose-related bone marrow depression can occur in any patient and is reversible, serial blood monitoring should be conducted in all patients receiving chloramphenicol. The drug should be discontinued, or at least the dosage should be reduced, when there is evidence of bone marrow depression, such as white blood cell count less than 3000/mm³ (373).

Although chloramphenicol has enjoyed considerable worldwide use given its broad spectrum of antibacterial activity, selection of an alternative agent should be considered wherever possible because of the potential serious adverse reactions.

Sulfonamides and Trimethoprim

Sulfonamides ushered in the modern antimicrobial chemotherapeutic era in the early 1930s. Sulfonamides have a structure similar to para-aminobenzoic acid (PABA), a precursor required by bacteria for folic acid synthesis. Various sulfonamides have different heterocyclic aromatic substitutions on the sulfonamide group. These chemical modifications result in differing antibacterial activities, as well as variations in drug absorption, solubility, and tolerance (374).

As structural analogs of PABA, the sulfonamides competitively inhibit the synthesis of dihydropteroic acid, the immediate precursor of dihydrofolic acid from PABA pteridine. This inhibition does not affect mammalian cells because they lack the ability to synthesize folic acid and thus require preformed folic acid. The sulfonamides are primarily bacteriostatic at therapeutic concentrations. Under certain conditions of low thymine concentrations, exposure to sulfonamides can be bactericidal because of a "thymineless death." The inhibition of bacterial growth induced by sulfonamides may be reversed with the addition of certain agents, such as thymidine, purines, methionine, and serine, to the growth medium. Such reversal of inhibition may have clinical importance in necrotic tissue, where breakdown of cells may result in the release of these substances. The sulfonamides are active against gram-positive and gram-negative bacteria, although susceptibilities often are variable, even among susceptible pathogens. In addition to antibacterial activity, sulfonamides have an antiprotozoal activity and are used in combination with pyrimethamine against ocular toxoplasmosis. Sulfonamides may be useful for therapy of conjunctivitis due to *H. influenzae* or other gram-positive organisms (375). Sulfonamides have been the preferred drugs for nocardiosis and have been active against *Nocardia* keratitis (376). Sulfonamides have some activity against chlamydiae (374).

Many bacteria become highly resistant to sulfonamides during therapy owing to chromosomally or plasmid-mediated transference. Acquired resistance to the sulfonamides is widespread and severely limits their clinical usefulness. Significant resistance among staphylococci and streptococci may be encountered. An *in vitro* comparison of the susceptibility of ocular isolates from conjunctivitis and blepharitis determined that 87% of the ocular isolates were susceptible to sulfa drugs (375). The sulfonamides are capable of producing a wide variety of adverse reactions that may affect a number of organ systems, including the blood and bone marrow, skin, kidney, liver, and nervous system. Hypersensitivity reactions affecting the skin and mucous membranes may occur, including severe toxic epidermal necrolysis and erythema nodosum. The sulfonamides may also provoke erythema multiforme in its severe form, Stevens-Johnson syndrome, especially in children. This syndrome involving both the skin and mucous membranes may be fatal in 5% to 25% of patients (377). Hematologic adverse effects may occur, including agranulocytosis, hemolytic or aplastic anemia, leukopenia, thrombocytopenia, and methemoglobinemia. Hemolytic anemia has been observed in patients both with and without glucose-6-phosphate dehydrogenase deficiency. With prolonged therapy with any sulfonamide, monitoring of blood parameters should be carried out.

Trimethoprim. Trimethoprim is a 2,4-diaminopyrimidine that inhibits bacterial hydrofolate reductases, but not mammalian enzymes. This bacterial enzymatic inhibition prevents the formation of tetrahydrofolic acid, which is essential for growth of certain bacteria. Trimethoprim is often combined with a sulfonamide to result in a synergistic antibacterial effect due to the sequential blockade of two steps in the same biosynthetic pathway. The lack of tetrahydrofolic acid ultimately prevents DNA replication. Trimethoprim may be bacteriostatic or bactericidal, depending on the clinical conditions. With severe necrotic infections, there may be cellular breakdown and release of thymine and thymidine. Under these circumstances, possibly encountered with suppurative keratitis, the action of trimethoprim may be inhibited. Trimethoprim is active *in vitro* against many gram-positive cocci, although there is increasing resistance observed among certain staphylococci. Trimethoprim has minimal activity against enterococci. Some gram-positive bacilli, such as *C. diphtheriae* and *L. monocytogenes*, are also susceptible. Most anaerobes are resistant. *P. aeruginosa* is resistant to trimethoprim.

Several mechanisms may confirm resistance to trimethoprim. Thymine- or thymidine-dependent bacterial mutants are intrinsically resistant. Organisms may develop resistance to trimethoprim through alteration of dihydrofolic reductase or by decreasing permeability of bacteria to the drug (378). Acquired resistance to trimethoprim can be mediated by both chromosomal and plasmid mechanisms. Trimethoprim generally is well tolerated, although there may be hypersensitivity reactions, including pruritus and skin rash. Cautions should be used with trimethoprim dosing in patients with possible folate deficiency (malnourished or debilitated patients, alcoholic patients, pregnant women, patients with seizures receiving phenytoin, or patients with malabsorption syndrome). Folinic acid can be administered concomitantly to prevent the antifolic effects of trimethoprim without

reducing its antibacterial efficacy. Trimethoprim is usually contraindicated in pregnant women.

Trimethoprim is usually used in ophthalmology as a combination preparation with polymyxin-B for the treatment of external ocular infections (379). Caution should be exercised with topical therapy using trimethoprim—polymyxin-B in therapy of *Neisseria* conjunctivitis because neither agent has reasonable activity against this potentially blinding ocular pathogen (380).

Rifampin

Rifampin is a semisynthetic derivative of rifamycin-B and has been used primarily in the treatment of tuberculosis. Rifampin binds to the beta subunit of bacterial DNA–dependent RNA polymerase, thus blocking initiation of RNA synthesis in susceptible bacteria. By virtue of its mechanism of action, rifampin is bactericidal. Rifampin has extremely potent antistaphylococcal activity, including methicillin-resistant strains (381). Most streptococci are also susceptible to rifampin, including *viridans* streptococci. Rifampin is less active against enterococci. Rifampin is active against *M. tuberculosis*, as well as nontuberculous mycobacteria. Gram-negative bacilli are usually resistant to rifampin. A prominent problem limiting usefulness of rifampin therapy is the rapid development of high-level resistance due to mutations altering the beta subunit of RNA polymerase. Rifampin has been principally used in ophthalmology for therapy of nontuberculous mycobacterial keratitis. Rifampin is generally well tolerated with systemic use. Red discoloration of the urine and other secretions, including tears, is a common result of rifampin therapy. Permanent staining of soft contact lenses may result from rifampin treatment.

Spectinomycin

Spectinomycin hydrochloride is an aminocyclitol antibiotic that is produced by a strain of *Streptomyces spectabilis*. It has different physical and biologic properties from the aminoglycosides. Spectinomycin inhibits protein synthesis by interacting with the 30S bacterial ribosomal unit. It is most often bacteriostatic, but may be bactericidal for some pathogens, especially *N. gonorrhoeae*. Because of its activity against most strains of *N. gonorrhoeae*, including penicillinase-producing strains, chromosomally mediated resistant *N. gonorrhoeae*, and high-level tetracycline-resistant *N. gonorrhoeae*, it has been used as an alternative to penicillins and tetracyclines. *C. trachomatis* and *T. pallidum* are resistant to the action of spectinomycin. Spectinomycin may be considered for ophthalmic use in treatment of severe gonococcal keratoconjunctivitis in penicillin- and cephalosporin-allergic patients (382). Spectinomycin-resistant clinical isolates have been reported, including a few strains that produced penicillinase (383). A high prevalence of spectinomycin-resistant *N. gonorrhoeae* was associated with treatment failures (8.2%) in U.S. military personnel stationed in the Republic of Korea, where spectinomycin had become the primary treatment for gonococcal infections (384). Adverse effects of spectinomycin occur infrequently, but include pain at the site of injection, nausea, vomiting, and abdominal cramping. Spectinomycin does not appear to be teratogenic, although its safety during pregnancy has not been established. Spectinomycin has been used effectively to treat gonorrheal infection in prepubertal children.

Peptide Antibiotics

Peptide antibiotics, including bacitracin, gramicidin, and polymyxin, share a common structure, consisting of peptide-linked amino acids. Bacitracin is a mixture of polypeptide antibiotics produced by a strain of *Bacillus subtilis*. These compounds are bactericidal and inhibit the formation of linear peptidoglycans that are major components of the bacterial cell wall. Most gram-positive bacteria, including staphylococci, streptococci, and *C. difficile*, are susceptible to bacitracin. Although bacitracin is active against *Neisseria* and *H. influenzae*, most other gram-negative bacteria are resistant. The peptide antibiotics have severe nephrotoxicity, limiting their systemic use. Bacitracin is most commonly used topically and is frequently combined with other antibiotics, such as neomycin or polymyxin-B, to increase the antibacterial spectrum. Polymyxin-B and polymyxin-E are bactericidal and alter cell membrane permeability. They are active against gram-negative organisms, including *Pseudomonas*. They are frequently combined with bacitracin or trimethoprim to expand their spectrum of antibacterial activity. The peptide antibiotics are insoluble and are available for ophthalmic use in ointment form.

Fusidic acid is a bactericidal agent having good antistaphylococcal activity. It had been used in the past to treat severe systemic staphylococcal infections, but is now commercially available in Europe (Fucithalmic) as a topical ophthalmic preparation. Pharmacokinetic studies indicate good corneal penetration, even with intact epithelium. Fusidic acid is effective against beta-lactamase–producing and methicillin-resistant staphylococci. Fusidic acid has been shown to be safe and effective in the therapy of staphylococcal keratitis (385).

Antimicrobial peptides isolated from natural sources have promising *in vitro* activity against a variety of corneal pathogens. Cecropins are antimicrobial peptides (30 to 35 amino acids) isolated from the hemolymph of the *Cecropia* moth. Previous studies have demonstrated their antimicrobial efficacy against a variety of pathogens, including both gram-positive and gram-negative bacteria, fungi, protozoa, and envelope viruses. *In vitro* antimicrobial susceptibility determinations against human clinical ocular isolates show promising activity (386).

Routes of Administration

One of the fundamental principles of pharmacotherapy is to maximize the amount of drug that reaches the site of action so that sufficient concentrations are achieved to

cause a beneficial therapeutic effect (387). Topical application is the mainstay of ocular drug delivery systems and the topical route is the preferred method of application of antibiotics in therapy for bacterial keratitis (388–390). Eyedrops are the most common route of antibiotic delivery to the eye. Other topical preparations, including ointments, gels, and sustained-release vehicles, are used to achieve higher concentrations of antibiotics in the corneal stroma. Drug penetration into the cornea may be increased with higher concentrations, greater lipophilicity, more frequent applications, and enhanced contact time using certain vehicles (391,392). The corneal epithelium represents a potential barrier to antibiotic penetration, and absence of the epithelium, as with ulcerative keratitis, often enhances drug penetration. Fortified concentrations of antibiotics are more effective and preferred to the commercial strength of many antibiotics (388). Fluoroquinolone antibiotics may be effective at their commercial concentrations in therapy for bacterial keratitis given their relatively high potency (25,330,336). Fortified topical antibiotics applied every 30 minutes are equally effective as administration every 15 minutes (393). To achieve peak corneal concentrations rapidly, a loading dose of antibiotic is initiated, followed by frequent, repetitive administration (394). Antibiotic solutions are preferred to ointment formulations because of the ease of altering the concentration of the solution as opposed to the ointment form. Ointments have the theoretical advantages of prolonged contact time, lubricating properties for the ocular surface, high viscosity to resist dilution with reflex tearing, and ease of administration. Peak corneal drug concentrations may be limited compared with achievable levels with antibiotic solutions because the ointment must dissolve in the preocular tear film before it can penetrate into the cornea (395). Antibiotic ointment preparations do not appear to deter wound healing (396). Fortified antibiotics are prepared by diluting the desired amount of parenteral compound with an appropriate vehicle, such as artificial tear solution or balanced salt solution (Table 13.1-3). Caution should be exercised to avoid mixing two antibiotics together. Different antibiotic chemical structures may result in varying stabilities in aqueous solution. Fortified cephalosporins and aminoglycosides remain stable and maintain potency in aqueous solution for at least 1 week without significant loss of antibiotic activity (397).

The initial loading dose of antibiotic is achieved with topical administration of one drop every 2 minutes for five applications. Antibiotics are then administered every 30 minutes (alternating drugs when multiple antibiotics are used for the first 24 to 36 hours, depending on initial clinical judgment of severity). If there is difficulty obtaining fortified antibiotic formulations, therapy should be initiated with very frequent commercial-strength antibiotic applications without delay. An advantage of the available fluoroquinolone ophthalmic solutions is their high potency, stability at room temperature, and broad spectrum of

TABLE 13-3.

Antibiotic	Method	Final concentration
Bacitracin	Remove 9 mL of solution from a 15 mL tear substitute bottle. Add 3 mL of solution to each of 3 commercial vials of bacitracin (50,000 U each).	9,600 U/mL
Carbenicillin	Reconstitute 1 vial of carenicillin (1 g) with 9.5 mL of sterile water. Add 1.0 mL of reconstituted carbenicillin into 15 mL tear substitute bottle (15 mL + 1 mL = 16 mL).	6.2 mg/mL
Cefazolin	Add 10 mL artificial tears to 500 mg vial of cefazolin powder; mix, remove, and place into empty artificial tear drop bottle.	50 mg/mL
Cephaloridine	Remove 2 mL of solution from a 15 mL tear substitute bottle and discard. Add 2 mL of sterile saline to 1 ampule of chephaloridine (500 mg). Replace 2.4 mL of reconstituted cephaloridine into tear bottle (13 mL + 2.4 mL = 15.4 mL).	32 mg/mL
Cephalothin	Remove 6 mL of solution from a 15 mL tear substitute bottle. Add 6 mL of solution to 1 ampule of cephalothin (1 g). Replace 6.4 mL of reconstituted cephalothin into tear bottle (9 mL + 6.4 mL = 15.4 mL).	65 mg/mL
Gentamicin	Add 2 mL parenteral gentamicin (40 mg/mL) to 5 mL bottle of commercial ophthalmic gentamicin (3 mg/mL).	14 mg/mL
Neomycin	Remove 2 mL of solution from a 15 mL tear substitute bottle. Add 2 mL of solution to 1 vial of neomycin (500 mg). Replace 2 mL of reconstituted Neomycin into tear bottle (13 mL + 2 mL = 15 mL).	33 mg/mL
Oxacillin	Remove 7 mL of solution from a 15 mL tear substitute bottle. Add 7 mL of Solution to 1 ampule of oxacillin (1 g). Replace 7.2 mL of reconstituted Oxacillin into tear bottle (8 mL + 7.2 mL = 15.2 mL).	66 mg/mL
Penicillin G	Remove 5 mL of solution from a 15 mL tear substitute bottle. Add 5 mL of solution to 1 vial of penicillin G (5 million units). Replace 5 mL of reconstituted penicillin into tear substitute bottle (10 mL + 5 mL = 15 mL).	333,000 U/mL
Tobramycin	Add 2 mL parenteral tobramycin (40 mg/mL) to 5 mL bottle of commercial Opthalmic tobramycin (3 mg/mL).	14 mg/mL
Vancomycin	Remove 9 mL of solution from a 15 mL tear sbstitute bottle and discard. Add 10 mL of sterile water to 1 vial of vancomycin (500 mg). Replace 10.2 mL of reconstituted vancomycin into tear bottle (6 mL + 10.2 mL = 16.2 mL).	31 mg/mL

* All fortified antibiotic preparations should be conducted under sterile conditions by individuals with proper expertise and training.

antibacterial activity at commercial strengths. Subconjunctival injection of antibiotics can result in high corneal drug concentrations by diffusion and by leakage through the injection site (398). Topical fortified tobramycin therapy resulted in a greater reduction of *Pseudomonas* organisms than did subconjunctival injection of tobramycin in experimental keratitis (141). Topical administration of fortified antibiotics appears just as effective as subconjunctival antibiotic injection for therapeutic effect (399,400). Subconjunctival administration of antibiotics may provoke patient anxiety, pain, subconjunctival hemorrhage, and conjunctival scarring. Depending on the pH and osmolarity of the agent administered, injection may result in significant toxicity to the conjunctiva. Toxicity may lead to conjunctival scarring, which may make any subsequent conjunctival surgery more difficult. With conjunctival chemosis and inflammation, the potential for inadvertent penetration and intraocular administration is an additional concern. Based on the clinical evidence, there appears to be no therapeutic advantage of subconjunctival antibiotic administration versus topical fortified application (401–403).

Subconjunctival antibiotic injections may be indicated in certain clinical situations, such as impending corneal perforation, where fortified topical antibiotics cannot be reliably delivered because of patient compliance. The pain from subconjunctival injections may be reduced by adjusting the pH of the antibiotic solution where possible. The conjunctiva may be anesthetized with topical proparacaine and injection of subconjunctival lidocaine 1% solution (0.25 mL delivered through a 30-gauge needle) before antibiotic administration in the same area. Subconjunctival injections may be repeated every 12 to 24 hours at separate sites during the initial 24 to 48 hours. Continuous lavage of antibiotic may deliver a high concentration and mechanical irrigation to remove potential virulence factors (404,405). Continuous lavage or infusion through a scleral contact lens (Mediflow) is costly and impractical owing to the requirement of patient immobilization. In addition, such therapy may result in epithelial trauma, cumulative toxicity of the ocular surface, or systemic toxicity. Hydrophilic soft contact lenses may act as a tear film antibiotic retention device and enhance penetration by prolonging the relative contact time (406,407). If corneal ulceration is marked, the temporary use of a therapeutic soft contact lens may facilitate stromal repair and promote reepithelialization by protecting the corneal surface from mechanical trauma of lid movement. Collagen corneal shields soaked in antibiotic solutions have also been shown to increase antibiotic penetration compared with therapeutic soft contact lenses (408,409). Collagen corneal shields have been effective adjuncts in the therapy of experimental bacterial keratitis (410). Polymer inserts have also been designed to prolong the presence of drug in the preocular tear film (411). Temporary intracanalicular collagen implants may also prolong the retention of antibiotics in tears and increase stromal concentrations to enhance bacterial killing in experimental keratitis (412). Liposomal systems have been designed to improve the interaction of drugs with the corneal surface, potentially enhancing the safe delivery of antibiotics (413). Transcorneal iontophoresis of antibiotics has also been used to increase attainable drug concentrations and efficacy of antibacterial therapy (414,415).

Antibiotics administered by the parenteral route are relatively poorly absorbed into the noninflamed eye. Bactericidal corneal tissue levels can be achieved only at the risk of systemic toxicity. Bacterial keratitis with accompanying ocular inflammation may enhance the ocular penetration of systemic antibiotics (416). Severe gonococcal keratoconjunctivitis should be treated with systemic antibiotics in addition to topical antibiotics to prevent possible ulcerative keratolysis and perforation. Severe keratitis due to *H. influenzae* or *P. aeruginosa* in young children should be treated with parenteral as well as local antibiotics to reduce the risk of systemic spread (417). Parenteral antibiotics are indicated in severe keratitis with impending perforation, perforated infections with potential for intraocular spread, after perforating injuries to the corneosclera, or with contiguous scleral involvement.

Selection of Antibiotic Therapy

The objective for initial antibiotic selection in therapy for bacterial keratitis is rapid elimination of the corneal pathogen(s). No single topical antibiotic is effective against all potential organisms causing bacterial keratitis. Thus, selection of an antimicrobial agent or agents with a broad spectrum of activity, including the most likely gram-positive and gram-negative corneal pathogens, is desirable. Historically, a combination of two compounds, with one directed against the gram-positive pathogens and the other against the gram-negative organisms, was considered a rational initial treatment choice (3). Although penicillin G is superior in activity against *S. pneumoniae* and other streptococci, the frequency of penicillinase-producing staphylococci and other organisms requires a penicillinase-resistant agent. Cephalosporins evolved as the drug of choice against unidentified gram-positive cocci. Cefazolin (50 mg/mL) is well tolerated by the ocular surface with topical and subconjunctival routes of administration. In addition, it can be used in therapy of selected patients with a prior history of allergy to penicillin.

Aminoglycosides were the preferred initial antibiotic choice for therapy of suspected gram-negative keratitis.

Gentamicin evolved as the initial aminoglycoside agent of choice because of its favorable pharmacokinetics and excellent activity against *Pseudomonas*, *Klebsiella*, *Enterobacter*, and other gram-negative species. With the emergence of gentamicin-resistant strains of *P. aeruginosa* (296), tobramycin has become an alternate initial choice. Approximately 10% of corneal isolates of *Pseudomonas* may be resistant to aminoglycosides, with some strains being resistant to gentamicin but sensitive to tobramycin (418).

In addition to coverage of gram-positive cocci, the cephalosporins may provide some activity against gram-negative rods. The third-generation cephalosporins provide greater gram-negative coverage, yet have less gram-positive activity than first-generation cephalosporins. Combined therapy with topical fortified cefazolin (or another cephalosporin) and tobramycin (or gentamicin) became the rational initial therapeutic recommendation for polybacterial keratitis or when results of Gram staining were equivocal (3). Aminoglycosides, especially tobramycin, have considerable toxicity when administered topically at frequent intervals for a prolonged period (300).

The fluoroquinolone class of antibiotics possesses potent bactericidal activity against the broad spectrum of gram-negative aerobic bacteria and many gram-positive bacteria, including penicillinase-producing and methicillin-resistant staphylococci. The fluoroquinolones have been shown in several independent clinical trials to provide as safe and effective therapy for acute bacterial keratitis as combination fortified antibiotic treatment (25,336).

The potential role of three topical fluoroquinolones was also evaluated in the treatment of bacterial keratitis by means of a laboratory database (353). Antibiotic susceptibilities were determined for 153 isolates from patients with bacterial keratitis. Results were analyzed for each fluoroquinolone individually and in combination with cefazolin. Predicted susceptibility to each cefazolin–fluoroquinolone combination (98.7%) was superior to that for single-agent therapy with ofloxacin (88.2%), ciprofloxacin (82.3%), or norfloxacin (80.4%; $p = .0002$). A cefazolin–fluoroquinolone combination (98.7%) was comparable with a cefazolin–gentamicin combination (97.4%). The investigators concluded that combination therapy with cefazolin and a fluoroquinolone offers a reasonable alternative for the treatment of bacterial keratitis (353). Single-agent therapy with fluoroquinolones for vision-threatening bacterial keratitis is not advised.

8-Methoxy fluoroquinolones are designed to provide an expanded spectrum of activity against gram-positive ocular pathogens. In a laboratory study, MICs for gatifloxacin and moxifloxacin were determined *in vitro* against bacterial strains that were isolated from suspected cases of bacterial keratitis and endophthalmitis (419). The ocular isolates included seven gram-positive, four gram-negative, and three atypical bacterial species. Gatifloxacin and moxifloxacin exhibited similar activity against six gram-positive organisms: *S. epidermidis, S. aureus, S. pneumoniae, S. pyogenes, B. cereus,* and *E. faecalis.* The MIC values for the drugs at which 90% of the isolates were inhibited (MIC_{90}) ranged from 0.08 to 0.57 mg/mL and were comparable with previously published values against isolates from patients with systemic infections. The MIC_{90} for gatifloxacin against *Streptococcus viridans* was 0.22 mg/mL, compared with 0.73 mg/mL for moxifloxacin ($p = .011$). Among the gram-negative isolates, the mean MIC_{90} for gatifloxacin against *P. aeruginosa* was 1.28 mg/mL, compared with 2.60 mg/mL for moxifloxacin ($p = .023$). MIC_{90} values for gatifloxacin against *Klebsiella pneumoniae* and *Enterobacter aerogenes* were one-fourth to one-fifth the values for moxifloxacin. For the atypicals, the MIC_{90} values for gatifloxacin against *N. asteroides* and *M. chelonae* were one-fourth the corresponding values for moxifloxacin. Gatifloxacin demonstrated a broad spectrum of activity against several key ocular pathogens tested in this study, and was at least as effective as moxifloxacin against these pathogens.

Penicillin G at a concentration of 100,000 U/mL remains the initial drug of choice for keratitis caused by streptococcal species, including *S. pneumoniae.* Some penicillin-resistant pneumococcal strains have recently been identified. Penicillinase-producing strains of *N. gonorrhoeae* have been introduced and observed in ocular infections. Because of a relatively high prevalence of *N. gonorrhoeae* resistant to penicillin, alternate drug choices, such as ceftriaxone, should be selected. If gram-positive branching filaments are observed on microscopic examination of smears from corneal scrapings, penicillin may be an appropriate choice for the possible Actinomycetales organism pending final identification.

In South America, the *in vitro* susceptibility of the most common ocular bacterial isolates to several antibiotics was assessed to verify changing trends in antibiotic susceptibility over a 15-year period (356). All cultures positive for *S. aureus,* coagulase-negative staphylococci, *Streptococcus* species, and *Pseudomonas* species in conjunctival ($n = 4585$) and corneal ($n = 3779$) specimens from 1985 to 2000 were evaluated. Susceptibility tests were performed against amikacin, gentamicin, neomycin, tobramycin, ciprofloxacin, norfloxacin, ofloxacin, cephalothin, and chloramphenicol. Amikacin and neomycin showed an improvement of their sensitivity during the study period (88% to 95% and 50% to 85%, respectively) for corneal and conjunctival samples. Gentamicin and tobramycin revealed a decrease in sensitivity over time, from 95% to less than 80% in corneal and conjunctival samples. Ciprofloxacin, norfloxacin, and ofloxacin demonstrated generally good sensitivity to all evaluated bacteria [better in conjunctiva (95%) than in cornea (90%)]. Sensitivity of *S. aureus* to cephalothin decreased during the study, but was still 98% for coagulase-negative staphylococci.

Chloramphenicol displayed reasonable sensitivity against *S. aureus* (85% in corneal and 92% in conjunctival samples), coagulase-negative staphylococci (87% and 88.5%, respectively), and *Streptococcus* species (95% and 96%, respectively). Gentamicin, tobramycin, and cephalothin demonstrated a decrease in *in vitro* susceptibility to all tested pathogens. The fluoroquinolones remained a good choice in the treatment of ocular infections, with high susceptibility in all pathogens tested. Chloramphenicol also revealed an increase in its effectiveness to all bacteria evaluated (356).

Modification of Therapy

The results of microbial culture and antimicrobial susceptibility testing data may suggest a modification from the initial therapeutic plan. If the identified organism is likely to be significantly more susceptible to an antibiotic other than the one originally selected, or if antibacterial susceptibility testing confirms resistance, the more effective drug may be substituted. If combination broad-spectrum therapy was initially selected and a single organism is isolated, the less effective agent may be discontinued. If microbial culture fails to grow a causative organism, clinical judgment must be exercised to guide further antimicrobial therapy.

Any modification of therapy should be based on the clinical response and patient tolerance to initial therapy, as well as the laboratory data. The initial judgment of clinical severity also affects decisions to modify therapy. If there is substantial clinical improvement on the initial antibiotic course, there may be no advantage to selection of an alternative agent.

For anaerobic organisms, including gram-positive cocci or gram-negative rods, penicillin remains the preferred agent. Aerobic and anaerobic gram-positive rods may also respond to penicillin therapy. Combination trimethoprim (16 mg/mL) and sulfamethoxazole (80 mg/mL) eyedrops is effective treatment for *Nocardia* keratitis (376). Sulfonamides, tetracyclines, erythromycin, or amikacin may be alternative agents.

Previously recommended initial therapy of acid-fast–stained positive corneal scrapings in suspected microbial keratitis was topical amikacin 10 to 20 mg/mL, one drop every half hour as indicated (420). Subconjunctival amikacin 20 mg in 0.5 mL may be adjunctively administered. Systemic amikacin is not routinely used, but may be added in selected cases with corneal perforation or extension of infection to involve the sclera. Other antibiotics reported to be effective against a significant number of isolates of *M. fortuitum* and *M. chelonae* include cefoxitin, ciprofloxacin, clarithromycin, doxycycline, erythromycin, gatifloxacin, imipenem, kanamycin, moxifloxacin, netilmicin, ofloxacin, and tobramycin. Sulfamethoxazole may sometimes have significant activity.

The fluoroquinolones have been shown to be active against the most important nontuberculous mycobacteria causing keratitis, including some species that are highly resistant to standard antituberculous drugs. *M. fortuitum* is highly susceptible to ciprofloxacin, levofloxacin, ofloxacin, gatifloxacin, and moxifloxacin (421,422). The MICs of ciprofloxacin have varied from 0.01 to 12.5 μg/mL. The MICs of ofloxacin have ranged from 0.03 to 1.2 μg/mL, and no resistant strains have been identified. Experimental animal models and isolated clinical reports (423) have suggested that topical ciprofloxacin alone or in combination with topical amikacin may be useful in the treatment of *M. fortuitum* keratitis. Experimental studies assessing the *in vivo* efficacy of newer macrolides, including clarithromycin and azithromycin (359,360), suggest a potential role in the therapy of *M. fortuitum* keratitis. The - 8-methoxy fluoroquinolone agents gatifloxacin and moxifloxacin may have greater activity compared with earlier fluoroquinolones against the most common species of nontuberculous mycobacteria causing keratitis after LASIK.

The therapy of nontuberculous mycobacterial keratitis is complicated by the relatively poor correlation between *in vitro* susceptibility profiles and clinical behavior. After initial response, the infection may worsen, even if the pathogen remains "sensitive" by *in vitro* susceptibility testing. Multiple agents may be required in combination for an extended duration. Adjunctive surgical debridement may be required in select cases to debulk organisms and improve access of the antibiotic agents to the interlamellar space. With post-LASIK nontuberculous infections, surgical amputation of the flap may rarely be required to bring the infection under control.

The response of bacterial keratitis to antibiotic therapy must be monitored with frequent clinical observation. Slit-lamp biomicroscopic examination twice daily on hospitalized patients should be performed. The response to therapy may be difficult to appreciate with assessment in the first few days because of organism and host factors increasing inflammation, and the reaction to corneal scrapings, as well as frequent local antibiotics. Within 48 to 72 hours of effective bactericidal therapy, the progression of keratitis is halted. The stromal infiltrate consolidates, the anterior chamber inflammation subsides, and the epithelial and stromal healing begins. Clinical response varies depending on the responsible pathogen, duration of infection, antecedent factors, and host response. After 36 to 48 hours, the frequency of antibiotic administration can be tapered. Caution with cessation of therapy is recommended for organisms that may persist in corneal tissue, such as *P. aeruginosa*, and prolonged therapy may be required. The principal end points of treatment are reepithelialization and nonprogression of stromal infiltrates. The patient should be monitored for tolerance of antimicrobial agents because toxicity may retard epithelial and stromal healing. In addition,

resistant organisms may fail to respond appropriately to topical therapy.

Adjunctive Therapy

Because of the rich innervation of the cornea, ulcerative keratitis is frequently accompanied by significant pain. Pain control with acetaminophen or other analgesics may result in improved patient comfort and more effective delivery of the treatment regimen. Topical cycloplegic agents should be administered to relieve ciliary spasm, alleviate pain, and prevent the formation of synechiae. Topical 0.25% scopolamine or homatropine 5% used three to four times daily is usually adequate. Significant intraocular inflammation may result in a secondary glaucoma. Elevated intraocular pressure should be monitored and treated with a topical β-adrenergic blocker or topical or oral carbonic anhydrase inhibitors as required for control. Most patients can be effectively managed as outpatients if there is an adequate support system to allow compliance with the treatment plan.

Patching should be avoided in the initial therapy of bacterial keratitis because this may result in a microenvironment favorable to accelerated organism replication. After eradication of the causative bacteria, patching may be applied to assist reepithelialization. Therapeutic soft contact lenses may be a useful adjunct to assist epithelial healing. Antibiotic administration should continue over the therapeutic soft contact lens. Caution should be exercised because infection may occasionally complicate therapeutic soft contact lens use (424). The therapeutic lens may provide some tectonic support with impending or microscopic corneal perforation.

One of the principal objectives of therapy for bacterial keratitis is to prevent tissue destruction and irreversible structural alterations. A number of adjunctive modalities have been suggested to reduce the destructive effects of various enzymes released with progressive bacterial keratitis. Injured corneal epithelium, infiltrating neutrophils, and some bacterial organisms elaborate various enzymes that contribute to stromal keratolysis. Collagenase is also produced by host corneal tissue. Enzyme inhibitors, including disodium edetate (EDTA, 0.05 M), acetylcysteine (Mucomyst, 20%), or heparin 2%, have been shown effective experimentally (425–427).

MMPs play an important role in corneal wound healing and in pathologic conditions. The activity of these proteases is regulated by the presence of tissue inhibitors of metalloproteinases. Infectious ulcerative keratitis may be modified by controlling the MMP activity in the tissue. MMP-2 is a normal constituent of the corneal stroma, but MMP-9 is found under pathologic conditions and after corneal wounding. Both MMP-2 and MMP-9 have the capacity to degrade basement membrane collagens (types IV and VII). Transforming growth factor-β augments the expression of MMP-9 in corneal tissue. Synthetic inhibitors of MMP have been shown to inhibit proteases from *P. aeruginosa in vitro* and to prevent experimental *Pseudomonas* keratitis (423). In addition, synthetic MMP inhibition may potentiate the antiangiogenic effect of high-dose prednisolone for inhibition of endotoxin-induced corneal neovascularization in rabbits (429). Clinical trials assessing the potential adjunctive role of synthetic MMP inhibitors are nearing completion.

The precise role and the timing of adjunctive topical corticosteroid use in the therapy of bacterial keratitis are controversial. Reduction in the host inflammatory response, which may contribute to corneal destruction, provides the rationale for corticosteroid use. Corticosteroids effectively decrease the host inflammatory response initiated by bacterial exotoxins or endotoxins and lytic enzymes released from PMNs. Several experimental studies have failed to demonstrate any deleterious effect from the addition of topical corticosteroids to concomitant bactericidal therapy for bacterial keratitis (430–432). Microbial cultures from patients with keratitis after 3 days of gentamicin therapy grew more bacteria in individuals receiving topical corticosteroids, with a longer treatment course required to eradicate the infection using this combined treatment (433). Combined antibiotic therapy with adjunctive corticosteroids did not improve the clinical course of experimental *Pseudomonas* keratitis compared with treatment with antibiotic alone, regardless of the timing or strength of corticosteroid therapy (434). Enhancement or recurrence of *Pseudomonas* keratitis has been observed with concomitant corticosteroid and antibiotic treatment (435,436).

Prior use of corticosteroids may mask the clinical signs of stromal and intraocular inflammation, such that bacterial invasion may not be detected. Antecedent use establishes the potential for severe rebound stromal inflammation with keratolysis after withdrawal of corticosteroids during the initial management of infection. Severe keratitis with marked stromal thinning may accelerate to corneal perforation with corticosteroid use.

Corticosteroids may have a limited role in the therapy of bacterial keratitis to suppress the deleterious effects of inflammation once effective bactericidal therapy has eliminated or reduced the pathogen(s). With gram-positive keratitis, judicious topical application of corticosteroid may be initiated after several days of intensive, specific antimicrobial therapy. In confirmed gram-negative infection, or if there is doubt regarding a possible gram-negative coinfection, corticosteroid therapy should be deferred for a longer period of aggressive, specific topical antibiotic therapy. Some clinicians recommend withholding steroids if clinical improvement is progressing without steroids, using steroids only after several days of antibiotics if there is persistent inflammation that does not seem to improve, administering concomitant antibiotic coverage when steroids are used, avoiding steroids in thin corneas with threatening perforation, and using steroids for 24 hours before a therapeutic penetrating keratoplasty for active bacterial keratitis (437). Topical corticosteroids may be administered in low concentrations and infrequent dosing for 1 to 2 days on a trial basis to monitor for adverse effects, and increased as indicated. Long-acting periocular corticosteroids and oral corticosteroids should be avoided in bacterial keratitis.

An evidence-based update on the decision to use adjunctive corticosteroids searched publications from 1950 to 2000 that evaluated the effect of corticosteroids on bacterial keratitis in animal experiments, case reports and series, case-comparison and cohort studies, and clinical trials, systematically identified by electronic and manual search strategies (438). The use of a topical corticosteroid before the diagnosis of bacterial keratitis significantly predisposed to ulcerative keratitis in eyes with preexisting corneal disease [odds ratio (OR), 2.63; 95% CI, 1.41–4.91]. Once microbial keratitis occurred, prior corticosteroid use significantly increased the odds of antibiotic treatment failure or other infectious complications (OR, 3.75; 95% CI, 2.52–5.58). However, the effect of a topical corticosteroid with antibiotics after the onset of bacterial keratitis was unclear. Experimental models suggested likely advantages, but clinical studies did not show a significant impact of topical corticosteroid therapy on the outcome of bacterial keratitis (OR, 0.62; 95% CL, 0.25–1.54). Topical corticosteroids increase the risk of infectious complications affecting the cornea but may or may not have an effect during antibacterial therapy. Given the unproven role of corticosteroids in the adjunctive treatment of bacterial keratitis, a prospective, randomized trial to gather information to provide guidance for this common condition seems justified (438).

Cryotherapy has been applied in experimental animal models with demonstration of bactericidal effects (439). Cryotherapy may be useful in select cases of focal peripheral corneal ulcerations or in *Pseudomonas* sclerokeratitis (440,441). Caution should be exercised with the administration of cryotherapy because severe toxic effects may be additive to the keratitis process.

The precise role for adjunctive topical nonsteroidal therapy for bacterial keratitis is not determined. Diclofenac sodium 0.1% therapy did not adversely affect the results of antibiotic therapy with gentamicin 0.3% in the treatment of experimental *Pseudomonas* keratitis (442). In an experimental model of *Pseudomonas* keratitis in rabbits, recurrence was observed in 85% of steroid-treated rabbits versus 12.5% of flurbiprofen-treated rabbits (443). Conversely, in a *S. pneumoniae* model, there were no recurrences experienced, either with steroids or nonsteroidal topical treatment (443).

The application of tissue adhesive (isobutyl cyanoacrylate or other analogs) has been recommended in progressive stromal keratolysis, thinned descemetoceles, or small, perforated infectious ulcerations. The tissue adhesive may have some inherent antibacterial activity (444). It is toxic to corneal endothelium and thus should be applied only for small perforations. Tissue glue is useful to restore the integrity of the anterior segment and to postpone the need for surgery until antibiotic and antiinflammatory therapy have reduced the ocular inflammation. The edges and bed of the ulceration should be debrided and dried with methylcellulose sponges before the application of tissue adhesive. A therapeutic soft contact lens should be placed over the tissue adhesive to prevent irritation and to protect the glue from mechanical effects of the eyelids. Tissue toxicity, microbial colonization, use of therapeutic soft contact lenses, and long-term broad-spectrum antibiotics may precipitate tissue adhesive–related microbial keratitis (445). Masking of the underlying infection and the development of resistant organisms should be considered when using tissue adhesive.

Excimer laser photoablative treatment of microbial keratitis has been investigated in experimental animal models (446,447). Results of these investigations indicate that advanced stromal keratitis with deep suppuration cannot be eradicated using the excimer laser. Because corneas may be perforated inadvertently during treatment, excimer laser therapy of infectious keratitis should be approached with caution and used only for very select superficial and well-circumscribed lesions. Carbon dioxide laser therapy has also been investigated in experimental *P. aeruginosa* keratitis (448).

Corneal patch grafting may be an alternative to the application of tissue adhesives for small corneal perforations resulting from bacterial keratitis. Small partial conjunctival flaps may be used in peripheral ulcerations to assist with healing, but are not recommended for use in impending or perforated central bacterial keratitis. If there is a large perforation or a residual necrotic cornea, a therapeutic penetrating keratoplasty may be indicated (449). Maximal antibiotic therapy to eradicate the corneal pathogen(s) and to reduce inflammation is recommended before surgery. In addition to topical intensive antibiotic treatment, parenteral antibiotic therapy should be instituted in the perioperative period. The surgeon must select a large trephine to excise completely the area of infection. A free-hand dissection may be required in limbal-to-limbal suppurative keratitis. Sclerocorneal grafting may be performed, although with a limited postoperative success owing to glaucoma, rejection, and other problems. An oversized graft (0.50 to 0.75 mm) is recommended. A portion of the corneal button should be excised and placed in tissue media for grinding and culture of the tissue homogenate. The remainder of the specimen should be submitted for histopathologic study, including special stains for light microscopy and electron microscopy where indicated. Placement of interrupted sutures is recommended over continuous running sutures, given the intense inflammatory reaction. Aggressive topical corticosteroids should be

applied in the postoperative period along with concomitant antibiotic therapy as indicated. Parenteral therapy should be continued if there is suspicion of intraocular dissemination. Therapeutic penetrating keratoplasty was successful in restoring anatomic and visual results in 75% of grafts performed for bacterial keratitis in one study (450).

Complicated cataract may result from severe bacterial keratitis (451). Cataract may result from bacterial toxins, iridocyclitis, and treatment toxicity. Cataract formation may result from severe bacterial keratitis alone, but is probably enhanced by concurrent treatment with high-dose topical corticosteroids. Surgical rehabilitation may require combined cataract extraction with penetrating keratoplasty, depending on the degree of corneal scarring and opacification with cataract formation.

REFERENCES

1. O'Brien TP, Green WR. Keratitis. In: Mandell GL, et al., eds. *Principles and practice of infectious diseases*, 4th ed. New York: Churchill Livingstone, 1995:1110.
2. Jones DB. A plan for antimicrobial therapy in bacterial keratitis. *Trans Am Acad Ophthalmol Otolaryngol* 1975;79:95.
3. Jones DB. Initial therapy of suspected microbial corneal ulcers: II. Specific antibiotic therapy based on corneal smears. *Surv Ophthalmol* 1979;24:97.
4. Leck AK, Thomas PA, Hagan M, et al. Aetiology of suppurative corneal ulcers in Ghana and south India, and epidemiology of fungal keratitis. *Br J Ophthalmol* 2002;86:1211.
5. Thygeson P: Acute central (hypopyon) ulcers of the cornea. *Calif Med* 1948;69:18.
6. Carmichael TR, Wolpert M, Koornhof WJ. Corneal ulceration at an urban African hospital. *Br J Ophthalmol* 1985;69:920.
7. Upadhyay MP, et al. Epidemiologic characteristics, predisposing factors and etiologic diagnosis of corneal ulceration in Nepal. *Am J Ophthalmol* 1991;111:92.
8. Srinivasan M, Gonzales CA, George C, et al. Epidemiology and aetiological diagnosis of corneal ulceration in Madurai, south India. *Br J Ophthalmol* 1997;81:965.
9. Asbell P, Stenson LS. Ulcerative keratitis: Survey of thirty years' laboratory experience. *Arch Ophthalmol* 1982;100:77.
10. Coster DJ, Wilhelmus K, Peacock J, et al. Suppurative keratitis in London. In: Trevor-Roper T, ed. *The cornea in health and disease*. London: Academic Press, 1981:395.
11. Liesegang TJ, Forster RK. Spectrum of microbial keratitis in south Florida. *Am J Ophthalmol* 1980;90:38.
12. Ostler HB, Okumoto M, Wilkey C. The changing pattern of the etiology of central bacterial corneal (hypopyon) ulcers. *Trans Pacif Coast Otol Ophthalmol Soc* 1976;57:235.
13. Adams CP, Cohen EJ, Laibson PR, et al. Corneal ulcers in patients with cosmetic extended wear contact lenses. *Am J Ophthalmol* 1983;96:705.
14. Musch DC, Sugar A, Meyer RF. Demographic and predisposing factors in corneal ulceration. *Arch Ophthalmol* 1983;101:1545.
15. Hassman G, Sugar J. *Pseudomonas* corneal ulcer with extended-wear soft contact lens for myopia. *Arch Ophthalmol* 1983;101:1549.
16. Weissman BA, Mondino BJ, Pettit TH, et al. Corneal ulcers associated with extended wear soft contact lenses. *Am J Ophthalmol* 1984;97:476.

17. Galentine PJ, Cohen EJ, Laibson PR, et al. Corneal ulcers associated with contact lens wear. *Arch Ophthalmol* 1984;102:891.
18. Lemp MA, Blackman HJ, Wilson LA, et al. Gram-negative corneal ulcers in elderly aphakic eyes with extended-wear lenses. *Ophthalmology* 1984;90:60.
19. Driebe WT Jr. Present status of contact lens-induced corneal infections. *Ophthalmol Clin North Am* 2003;16:485.
20. Vastine D. Infections of the ocular adnexa and cornea. In: Peyman GA, Sanders DR, Kohlbert MF, eds. *Principles and practice of ophthalmology*, vol 1. Philadelphia: WB Saunders, 1980:281.
21. Alexandrakis G, Alfonso E, Miller D. Shifting trends in bacterial keratitis in south Florida. *Ophthalmology* 2000;107:1497.
22. Sun X, Deng S, Li R, et al. Distribution and shifting trends of bacterial keratitis in north China (1989–98). *Br J Ophthalmol* 2004;88:165.
23. Cobo LM, Coster DJ, Peacock J. *Moraxella* keratitis. In: Trevor-Roper T, ed. *The cornea in health and disease.* London: Academic Press, 1981:409.
24. Smolin G, Tabbara K, Whitcher J. Lids. In: *Infectious diseases of the eye.* Baltimore: Williams & Wilkins, 1984:24.
25. O'Brien TP, Maguire M, Fink N, et al. Efficacy of ofloxacin vs cefazolin and tobramycin in the therapy for bacterial keratitis: report from the Bacterial Keratitis Study Research Group. *Arch Ophthalmol* 1995;113:1257.
26. Chandler JW, Milan DF. Diphtheria corneal ulcers. *Arch Ophthalmol* 1978;96:53.
27. Rubinfeld RS, et al. Diphtheroids as ocular pathogens. *Am J Ophthalmol* 1989;108:251.
28. Heideman DG, et al. *Corynebacterium striatum* keratitis. *Cornea* 1991;10:81.
29. Meisler DM, Palestine AG, Vastine DW, et al. Chronic *Propionibacterium* endophthalmitis after extracapsular cataract extraction and intraocular lens implantation. *Am J Ophthalmol* 1986;102:733.
30. VanBusterveld OP, Richards RD. *Bacillus* infections of the cornea. *Arch Ophthalmol* 1965;74:91.
31. Young EJ, et al. Panophthalmitis due to *Bacillus cereus*. *Arch Intern Med* 1980;140:559.
32. O'Day DM, Smith RS, Gregg CR, et al. The problem of *Bacillus* species infection, with special emphasis on the virulence of *Bacillus cereus*. *Ophthalmology* 1981;88:833.
33. O'Day DM, Ho PC, Andrews JS, et al. Mechanism of tissue destruction in ocular *Bacillus cereus* infections. In: Trevor-Roper T, ed. *The cornea in health and disease.* London: Academic Press, 1981:403.
34. Samples JR, Buettner H. Ocular infections caused by a biological insecticide. *J Infect Dis* 1983;148:614.
35. Tabbara KF, Tarabay N. *Bacillus licheniformis* corneal ulcer. *Am J Ophthalmol* 1979;87:717.
36. Lass JF, Haaf J, Forster CS, et al. Visual outcome in eight cases of *Serratia marcescens* keratitis. *Am J Ophthalmol* 1981;92:384.
37. Liesegang TJ, Jones DB, Robinson NM. *Azotobacter* keratitis. *Arch Ophthalmol* 1981;99:1578.
38. Templeton WC, Eiferman RA, Snyder JW, et al. *Serratia* keratitis transmitted by contaminated eye droppers. *Am J Ophthalmol* 1982;93:723.
39. Jones DB, Robinson NM. Anaerobic ocular infections. *Trans Am Acad Ophthalmol Otol* 1977;83:390.
40. Perry LD, Brinser JF, Kolodner H. Anaerobic corneal ulcers. *Ophthalmology* 1982;89:636.
41. Liesegang TJ. Anaerobic corneal ulcers [discussion]. *Ophthalmology* 1982;89:641.
42. Stern GA, Hodes BL, Stock EL. *Clostridium perfringens* corneal ulcer. *Arch Ophthalmol* 1979;97:661.
43. Ostler HB, Thygeson P, Okumoto M. Infectious diseases of the eye: III. Infections of the cornea. *J Cont Ed Ophthalmol* 1978;40:11.
44. Zaidman GW, Coudron P, Piros J. *Listeria monocytogenes* keratitis. *Am J Ophthalmol* 1990;109:334.
45. Eliott D, O'Brien TP, Green WR, et al. Elevated intraocular pressure, pigment dispersion, and dark hypopyon in endogenous endophthalmitis from *Listeria monocytogenes*. *Surv Ophthalmol* 1992;37:117.
46. Brook I. Ocular infections due to anaerobic bacteria. *Int Ophthalmol* 2001;24:269.
47. Duke-Elder S, Leigh AG. Inflammations of the cornea. In: *Systems of ophthalmology series*, vol 8, part II: *Diseases of the outer eye.* St. Louis: Mosby, 1965:789.
48. Hirst LW, Harrison GK, Merz EJ, et al. *Nocardia asteroides* keratitis. *Br J Ophthalmol* 1979;63:449.
49. Turner L, Stinson I. *Mycobacterium fortuitum* as a cause of corneal ulcers. *Am J Ophthalmol* 1965;60:329.
50. Lazar M, Nemet P, Bracha R, et al. *Mycobacterium fortuitum* keratitis. *Am J Ophthalmol* 1974;78:530.
51. Meisler DM, Friedlaender MH, Okumoto M. *Mycobacterium chelonei* keratitis. *Am J Ophthalmol* 1982;94:398.
52. Gangadharan PRJ, Lanier JD, Jones DB. Keratitis due to *Mycobacterium chelonei*. *Tubercle* 1978;59:55.
53. Moore MB, Newton C, Kaufman HE. Chronic keratitis caused by *Mycobacterium gordonae*. *Am J Ophthalmol* 1986;102:516.
54. Knapp A, Stern GA, Hood CI. *Mycobacterium avium-intracellulare* corneal ulcer. *Cornea* 1987;6:175.
55. Newman PE, Goodman RA, Waring GA, et al. A cluster of cases of *Mycobacterium chelonei* keratitis associated with out-patient office procedures. *Am J Ophthalmol* 1984;97:344.
56. Schonherr U, Naumann GOH, Lang GK, et al. Sclerokeratitis caused by *Mycobacterium marinum*. *Am J Ophthalmol* 1989;108:607.
57. Solomon R, Donnenfeld ED, Azar DT, et al. Infectious keratitis after laser in situ keratomileusis: results of an ASCRS survey. *J Cataract Refract Surg* 2003;29:2001.
58. Karp CL, Tuli SS, Yoo SH, et al. Infectious keratitis after LASIK. *Ophthalmology* 2003;110:503.
59. Fulcher SF, Fader RC, Rosa RH Jr, et al. Delayed-onset mycobacterial keratitis after LASIK. *Cornea* 2002;21:546.
60. Allen JH, Byers JL. The pathology of ocular leprosy: I. Cornea. *Arch Ophthalmol* 1960;64:216.
61. Elliott DC. An interpretation of the ocular manifestations of leprosy. *Ann NY Acad Sci* 1951;54:84.
62. Pillat A. Leprosy bacilli in the scraping from the diseased cornea in a leper and comments on keratitis punctata superficialis laprosa. *Arch Ophthalmol* 1930;3:306.
63. Woods AC. Syphilis of the eye. *Am J Syphil Gonor Vener Dis* 1943;27:133.
64. Baum J, Bavza M, Weinstein P, et al. Bilateral keratitis as a manifestation of Lyme disease. *Am J Ophthalmol* 1988;105:75.
65. Feaster FT, Nisbet RN, Barber JC. *Aeromonas hydrophilia* corneal ulcer. *Am J Ophthalmol* 1978;85:114.
66. Wilhelmus KR, Peacock J, Coster BJ. *Branhamella* keratitis. *Br J Ophthalmol* 1980;64:892.
67. Purcell JJ, Krachmer JH. Corneal ulcer caused by *Pasteurella multocida*. *Am J Ophthalmol* 1977;83:540.
68. Gudmundsson OG, et al. Factors influencing predilection and outcome in bacterial keratitis. *Cornea* 1989;8:115.
69. Allansmith MR, Ostler HB, Butterworth M. Concomitance of bacteria in various areas of the eye. *Arch Ophthalmol* 1969;82:37.
70. Selinger DS, Seilinger RC, Reed WP. Resistance to infection of the external eye: the role of tears. *Surv Ophthalmol* 1979;24:33.
71. Broekhuyse RM. Tear lactoferrin: a bacteriostatic and complexing protein. *Invest Ophthalmol* 1974;13:550.
72. Friedland BR, Anderson DR, Forster RK. Non-lysozyme antibacterial factors in human tears. *Am J Ophthalmol* 1972;74:52.

73. Jakobiec FA, Lefkowitch J, Knowles DM. II. B- and T-lymphocytes in ocular disease. *Ophthalmology* 1984;91:635.

74. Saks EH, Rosemary W, Jakobiec FA, et al. Lymphocyte subpopulations in the normal human conjunctiva: a monoclonal antibody study. *Ophthalmology* 1986;93:1278.

75. Gillette TE, Chandler JW, Greiner JV. Langerhans cells of the ocular surface. *Ophthalmology* 1982;89:700.

76. Chandler JW, Cummings M, Gillette TE. Presence of Langerhans cells in the central corneas of normal human infants. *Invest Ophthalmol Vis Sci* 1985;26:113.

77. Fauci AS, Dale DC, Balow JE. Glucocorticoid therapy: mechanisms of action and clinical considerations. *Ann Intern Med* 1976;84:304.

78. Winkelstein JA, Drachman RH. Deficiency of pneumococcal serum opsonization activity in sickle cell disease. *N Engl J Med* 1968;279:459.

79. Londer L, Nelson DL. Orbital cellulitis due to *Hemophilus influenzae*. *Arch Ophthalmol* 1974;91:89.

80. Palestine AG, Meyers SM, Fauci AS, et al. Ocular findings in patients with neutrophil dysfunction. *Am J Ophthalmol* 1983; 95:598.

81. Allen HF. Current status of prevention, diagnosis, and management of bacterial corneal ulcers. *Ann Ophthalmol* 1971;3:235.

82. Nanda M, Pflugfelder SC, Holland S. Fulminant *Pseudomonas* keratitis and scleritis in human immunodeficiency virus infected patients. *Arch Ophthalmol* 1991;109:503.

83. Pepose JS. A patient with AIDS presents with keratoconjunctivitis [questions and answers]. *Arch Ophthalmol* 1990;108:1224.

84. Sachs R, Zagelbaum BM, Hersh PS. Corneal complications associated with the use of crack cocaine. *Ophthalmology* 1993;100:187.

85. Schein OD, et al. Microbial keratitis associated with contaminated ocular medications. *Am J Ophthalmol* 1988;105:361.

86. Schein OD, et al. Microbial contamination of in-use ocular medications. *Arch Ophthalmol* 1992;110:82.

87. Wilson SE, et al. Corneal trauma and infection caused by manipulation of the eyelashes after application of mascara. *Cornea* 1990;9:181.

88. Wilhelmus KR. Review of clinical experience with microbial keratitis associated with contact lenses. *CLAO J* 1987;13:211.

89. Koidou-Tsiligianni A, Alfonso E, Forster RK. Ulcerative keratitis associated with contact lens wear. *Am J Ophthalmol* 1989; 108:64.

90. Poggio EC, et al. The incidence of ulcerative keratitis among users of daily wear and extended wear soft contact lenses. *N Engl J Med* 1989;321:779.

91. Schein OD, et al. The Microbial Keratitis Study Group: the relative risk of ulcerative keratitis among users of daily wear and extended wear soft contact lenses: a case control study. *N Engl J Med* 1989;321:773.

92. O'Brien TP. Approach to the patient with ocular infection. In: O'Brien TP, ed. *Ocular infection: preferred vs. prevailing practices*. Deerfield, IL: Discovery International, 1994:1.

93. Matthews TD, Frazer DG, Minassian OC, et al. Risks of keratitis and patterns of use with disposable soft contact lenses. *Arch Ophthalmol* 1992;110:1559.

94. Buehler PO, Schein OD, Stamler JF, et al. Increased risk of ulcerative keratitis among disposable soft contact lens users. *Arch Ophthalmol* 1992;110:1555.

95. Cohen EJ, et al. Corneal ulcers associated with contact lenses, including experience with disposable contact lenses. *CLAO J* 1991;17:173.

96. John T. How safe are disposable soft contact lenses? *Am J Ophthalmol* 1991;111:766.

97. Glynn RJ, et al. The incidence of ulcerative keratitis among aphakic contact lens wears in New England. *Arch Ophthalmol* 1991;109:104.

98. Bowden FW, Cohen EJ. Corneal ulcerations with contact lenses. *Ophthalmol Clin North Am* 1989;2:267.

99. Wahl JC, Katz HR, Abrams DA. Infectious keratitis in Baltimore. *Ann Ophthalmol* 1991;23:234.

100. Bowden FW, et al. Patterns of lens care practices and lens product contamination in contact lens associated microbial keratitis. *CLAO J* 1989;15:49.

101. Szerenyi K, McDonnell JM, Smith RE, et al. Keratitis as a complication of bilateral, simultaneous radial keratotomy. *Am J Ophthalmol* 1994;117:462.

102. Beldavs RA, Al-Ghandi S, Wilson LA, et al. Bilateral microbial keratitis after radial keratotomy. *Arch Ophthalmol* 1993; 111:440.

103. Leidenix MJ, Lundergan MK, Pfister D, et al. Perforated bacterial corneal ulcer in a radial keratotomy incision secondary to minor trauma. *Arch Ophthalmol* 1994;112:1513.

104. Sampath R, Ridgway AE, Leatherbarrow B. Bacterial keratitis following excimer laser photorefractive keratectomy: a case report. *Eye* 1994;8:481.

105. Donnenfeld ED, O'Brien TP, Solomon R, et al. Infectious keratitis after photorefractive keratectomy. *Ophthalmology* 2003;110:743.

106. Tuberville AW, Wood TO. Corneal ulcers in corneal transplants. *Curr Eye Res* 1981;8:479.

107. Leahy AB, Avery RL, Gottsch JD, et al. Suture abscesses after penetrating keratoplasty. *Cornea* 1993;12:489.

108. Tavakkoli H, Sugar J. Microbial keratitis following penetrating keratoplasty. *Ophthalmic Surg* 1994;25:356.

109. Clinch TE, Palmon FE, Robinson MJ, et al. Microbial keratitis in children. *Am J Ophthalmol* 1994;117:65.

110. Ormerod LD, Gomez DS, Murphree AL, et al. Microbial keratitis in children. *Ophthalmology* 1986;93:449.

111. Cruz OA, Sabir SM, Capo H, et al. Microbial keratitis in childhood. *Ophthalmology* 1993;100:192.

112. Bourcier T, Thomas F, Borderie V, et al. Bacterial keratitis: predisposing factors, clinical and microbiological review of 300 cases. *Br J Ophthalmol* 2003;87:834.

113. Young AL, Leung AT, Cheng LL, et al. Orthokeratology lens-related corneal ulcers in children: a case series. *Ophthalmology* 2004;111:590.

114. O'Brien TP, Hazlett LD. Pathogenesis of ocular infection. In: Pepose JS, Holland GN, Wilhelmus KR, eds. *Ocular infection and immunity*. St. Louis: Mosby, 1996:200.

115. Jones DB. Pathogenesis of bacterial and fungal keratitis. *Trans Ophthalmol Soc UK* 1978;98:367.

116. Baker NR. *Pseudomonas aeruginosa* exoenzyme S is an adhesin. *Infect Immun* 1991;59:2859.

117. Hoepelman AIM, Tuomanen EL. Consequences of microbial attachment: directing host cell functions with adhesins. *Infect Immun* 1992;60:1729.

118. Reichert R, Stern GA. Quantitative adherence of bacteria to human corneal epithelial cells. *Arch Ophthalmol* 1984;102:1394.

119. Doig P, et al. Role of pili in the adhesion of *Pseudomonas aeruginosa* to human respiratory epithelial cells. *Infect Immun* 1988; 56:1641.

120. Holder IA, Naglich JG. Experimental studies of the pathogenesis of infection due to *Pseudomonas aeruginosa* infection. *J Trauma* 1986;26:118.

121. Nicas TI, Iglewski BH. Toxins and virulence factors of *Pseudomonas aeruginosa*. In: Sokatch JR, ed. *The bacteria*, vol X: *The biology of* Pseudomonas. New York, Academic Press, 1986.

122. Iglewski BH, Liu PV, Kabat D. Mechanism of action of *Pseudomonas aeruginosa* exotoxin A: adenosine diphosphate-ribosylation of mammalian elongation factor II in vitro and in vivo. *Infect Immun* 1977;15:138.

123. Cryz SJ, et al. Role of lipopolysaccharide and virulence of *Pseudomonas aeruginosa*. *Infect Immun* 1984;44:508.

124. Costerton JW. *Pseudomonas aeruginosa* in nature and diseases. In: Sabath LD, ed. Pseudomonas aeruginosa: *the organism, the disease it causes and their treatment*. Bern, Switzerland: Hans Huber, 1980.

125. Patti JM, Allen PL, McGavin MJ, et al. MSCRAMM-mediated adherence of microorganisms to host tissues. *Annu Rev Microbiol* 1994;48:585.

126. Woods DE, et al. Role of fibronectin in the prevention of adherence of *Pseudomonas aeruginosa* to buccal cells. *J Infect Dis* 1981; 143:784.

127. Hazlett LD, et al. Evidence for *N*-acetylmanosomine as an ocular receptor for *P. aeruginosa* adherence to scarified cornea. *Invest Ophthalmol Vis Sci* 1987;28:1978.

128. Stern GA, Weitzenkorn D, Valenti J. Adherence of *Pseudomonas aeruginosa* to the mouse cornea: epithelial v. stromal adherence. *Arch Ophthalmol* 1982;100:1956.

129. Hazlett LD, Moon MM, Berk R. In vivo identification of sialic acid as the ocular receptor for *Pseudomonas aeruginosa*. *Infect Immun* 1986;51:687.

130. Hazlett LD, et al. *Pseudomonas aeruginosa* pili mediate binding to human corneal epithelial glycoproteins. Presented at the 10th International Congress Eye Research, Stresa Italy, 1992.

131. Rudner XL, et al. Corneal epithelial glycoproteins exhibit *Pseudomonas aeruginosa* pilus binding activity. *Invest Ophthalmol Vis Sci* 1992;33:2185.

132. Liu X, Hazlett LD, Berk RS. Systemic and topical protection studies using *Pseudomonas* flagella or pili. *Invest Ophthalmol Vis Sci* 1990;31:449.

133. Rudner XL, et al. *Pseudomonas aeruginosa* pili interact differently with glycosylated proteins of immature cornea. *Invest Ophthalmol Vis Sci* 1992;33:844.

134. Lee KK, et al. Mapping the surface regions of *Pseudomonas aeruginosa* PAK pili: the importance of the C-terminal region of adherence to human buccal epithelial cells. *Mol Biol* 1989; 3:1493.

135. Saiman L, Ishimoto K, Lory S, et al. The effect of piliation and exoproduct expression on the adherence of *Pseudomonas aeruginosa* to receptor monolayers. *J Infect Dis* 1990;161:541.

136. Baum J, Panjwani NJ. Adherence of *Pseudomonas* to soft contact lenses and cornea: mechanisms and prophylaxis. In: Cavanaugh HD, ed. *The cornea: transactions of the World Congress on the Cornea III*. New York: Raven Press, 1988.

137. Drake D, Montie TC. Flagella, motility, and invasion virulence of *Pseudomonas aeruginosa*. *J Gen Microbiol* 1988;134:43.

138. Ansorg RA, et al. Differentiation of the major flagellar antigens of *Pseudomonas aeruginosa* by the slide coagulation technique. *J Clin Microbiol* 1984;20:84.

139. Montie TC, et al. Motility, virulence, and protection with the flagella vaccine against *Pseudomonas aeruginosa* infection. *Antibiot Chemother* 1987;39:233.

140. Rudner XL, Hazlett LD, Berk RS. Systemic and topical protection studies using *Pseudomonas aeruginosa* flagella in an ocular model of infection. *Curr Eye Res* 1992;11:727.

141. Hyndiuk RA. Experimental *Pseudomonas* keratitis: I. Sequential electron microscopy; II. Comparative therapy trials. *Trans Am Ophthalmol Soc* 1981;79:541.

142. Koch JM, et al. Experimental *Pseudomonas aeruginosa* keratitis from extended wear of soft contact lenses. *Arch Ophthalmol* 1990;108:1453.

143. Cotran RS. New roles for the endothelium in inflammation and immunity. *Am J Pathol* 1987;29:407.

144. Fajardo LF. The complexity of endothelial cells: a review. *Am J Clin Pathol* 1989;92:241.

145. Staugas REM, et al. Induction of tumor necrosis factor (TNF) and interleukin-I (IL-I) by *Pseudomonas aeruginosa* and exotoxin A-induced suppression of lymphoproliferation and TNF, lymphotoxin, gammainterferon, and IL-I production in human leukocytes. *Infect Immun* 1992;60:3162.

146. Berk RS, Beisel K, Hazlett LD. Genetic studies on the murine corneal response to *P. aeruginosa*. *Proc Soc Exp Biol Med* 1983;172:488.

147. Hazlett LD, Rosen D, Berk RS. Experimental *Pseudomonas* eye infection in cyclophosphamide-treated mice. *Invest Ophthalmol Vis Sci* 1977;16:649.

148. Twining S, Lohr KM, Moulder JE. The immune system in the experimental keratitis: a model and early effects. *Invest Ophthalmol Vis Sci* 1986;27:507.

149. Cleveland RP, et al. The role of complement in *Pseudomonas* ocular infections. *Invest Ophthalmol Vis Sci* 1983;24:237.

150. Steuhl KP, et al. The effect of immunization on corneal infection by *Pseudomonas aeruginosa*. *Invest Ophthalmol Vis Sci* 1987;28:1559.

151. Hibbs MS, et al. Gelatinase (type IV collagenase) immunolocalization in cells and tissues: use of an anti-serum to rabbit bone gelatinase that identifies high and low Mr forms. *J Cell Sci* 1989;92:487.

152. Fini ME, Girard MT. Expression of collagenolytic/gelatinolytic metalloproteinase by normal cornea. *Invest Ophthalmol Vis Sci* 1990;31:1779.

153. Kirschner SE, Twining SS. The effect of *Pseudomonas aeruginosa* exoproducts on corneal proteases. ARVO Abstracts. *Invest Ophthalmol Vis Sci* 1990;31[4 Suppl]:487(abstr).

154. Callegan MC, Engel LS, Hill JM, et al. Corneal virulence of *Staphylococcus aureus*: roles of alpha-toxin and protein A in pathogenesis. *Infect Immun* 1994;62:2478.

155. Hazlett LD. Corneal response to *Pseudomonas aeruginosa* infection. *Prog Retin Eye Res* 2004;23:1.

156. Howe TR, Iglewski BH. Isolation and characterization of alkaline protease-deficient mutants of *Pseudomonas aeruginosa* in vitro and in vivo. *Infect Immun* 1984;3:1058.

157. Ohman DE, Barns RP, Iglewski BH. Corneal infection in mice with toxin-A and elastase mutants of *Pseudomonas aeruginosa*. *J Infect Dis* 1980;142:547.

158. Burns FR, Gray RP, Patterson CA. Inhibition of alkali-induced corneal ulceration and perforation by A thio peptide. *Invest Ophthalmol Vis Sci* 1990;31:107.

159. Heck LW, Morihara K, Abrahamson DR. Degradation of soluble laminin and depletion of tissue-associated basement laminin by *Pseudomonas aeruginosa* elastase and alkaline protease. *Infect Immun* 1986;54:149.

160. Twining SS, Davis SD, Hyndiuk RA. Relationship between proteases and descemetocele formation in experimental *Pseudomonas* keratitis. *Curr Eye Res* 1986;5:503.

161. Bejarano PA, et al. Degradation of basement membranes by *Pseudomonas aeruginosa* elastase. *Infect Immun* 1989;57:3783.

162. Kharazami A. Mechanisms involved in the evasion of host defense by *Pseudomonas aeruginosa*. *Immunol Lett* 1991;30:201.

163. Preston M, et al. Kinetics of serum, tear, and corneal antibody responses in resistant and susceptible mice intracorneally infected with *Pseudomonas aeruginosa*. *Infect Immun* 1992;60: 885.

164. Kreger AS, et al. Immunization against experimental *Pseudomonas aeruginosa* and *Serratia marcescens* keratitis vaccination with lipopolysaccharide endotoxin and proteases. *Invest Ophthalmol Vis Sci* 1986;27:932.

165. Valenton MJ, Okumoto M. Toxin producing strains of *Staphylococcus epidermidis*. *Arch Ophthalmol* 1973;89:187.

166. Jelyaszewicz J, Wadstrom T, eds. *Bacterial toxins in cell membranes*. London: Academic Press, 1978.

167. Mondino BJ, Rabin BS, Kessler E, et al. Corneal rings with gram negative bacteria. *Arch Ophthalmol* 1977;95:2222.

168. Belmont JB, Ostler HB, Chandler RD, et al. Non-infectious ring-shaped keratitis associated with *Pseudomonas aeruginosa*. *Am J Ophthalmol* 1982;93:338.

169. Jones DB. Polymicrobial keratitis. *Trans Am Ophthalmol Soc* 1981;79:153.

170. Baum JL, Jones DB. Initial therapy of suspected microbial corneal ulcers. *Surv Ophthalmol* 1979;24:97.

171. Benson WH, Lanier JD. Comparison of techniques for culturing corneal ulcers. *Ophthalmology* 1992;99:800.

172. Liesegang TJ. Bacterial and fungal keratitis. In: Kaufman HE, Barron BA, McDonald MB, et al., eds. *The cornea*. New York: Churchill Livingstone, 1988:217.

173. Clemons CS, et al. *Pseudomonas* ulcers following patching of corneal abrasions associated with contact lens wear. *CLAO J* 1987;13:161.

174. Harrison SM. Grading corneal ulcers. *Ann Ophthalmol* 1975; 7:537.

175. Ogawa GSH, Hyndiuk RA. Clinical disease: bacterial keratitis and conjunctivitis. In: Smolin G, Thoft RA, eds. *The cornea*, 3rd ed. Boston: Little, Brown, 1994:125.

176. Arffa RC. Infectious ulcerative keratitis: bacteria. In: *Grayson's diseases of the cornea*. St. Louis: Mosby, 163.

177. McCulley JP, Dougherty JM. Blepharitis associated with acne rosacea and seborrheic dermatitis. *Int Ophthalmol Clin* 1985;25:159.

178. Okumoto M, Smolin G. Pneumococcal infections of the eye. *Am J Ophthalmol* 1974;77:346.

179. Gorovoy MS, Stern GA, Hood I, et al. Intrastromal non-inflammatory bacterial colonization of a corneal graft. *Arch Ophthalmol* 1983;101:1749.

180. Meisler DM, Langston RHS, Naab TJ, et al. Infectious crystalline keratopathy. *Am J Ophthalmol* 1984;97:337.

181. Samples JR, Baumgartner SD, Binder PS. Infectious crystalline keratopathy: an electron microscopic analysis. *Cornea* 1985;4:118.

182. Reiss GR, Campbell RJ, Bourne WM. Infectious crystalline keratopathy. *Surv Ophthalmol* 1986;31:69.

183. Matoba AY, O'Brien TP, Wilhelmus KR, et al. Infectious crystalline keratopathy due to *Streptococcus pneumoniae*. *Ophthalmology* 1994;101:1000.

184. Stern GA. *Moraxella* corneal ulcers: poor response to medical treatment. *Ann Ophthalmol* 1982;14:295.

185. Perry HD, Nauheim JS, Donnefeld ED. *Nocardia asteroides* keratitis presenting as a persistent epithelial defect. *Cornea* 1989;8:41.

186. O'Brien TP, Matoba AY. Non-tuberculous mycobacterial ocular infections. In: Pepose JS, Holland GN, Wilhelmus KR, eds. *Ocular immunity and infection*. St. Louis: Mosby, 1995.

187. Robin JB, Beatty RF, Dunn S, et al. *Mycobacterium chelonei* keratitis after radial keratotomy. *Am J Ophthalmol* 1986; 102:72.

188. Mirate DJ, Hull DS, Steel JH Jr, et al. *Mycobacterium chelonei* keratitis: a case report. *Br J Ophthalmol* 1983;67:324.

189. Matoba AY. *Mycobacterium chelonei* keratitis. *Am J Ophthalmol* 1987;103:595.

190. Dugel PU, Holland GN, Brown HH, et al. *Mycobacterium chelonei* keratitis. *Am J Ophthalmol* 1988;105:661.

191. Matoba AY, Torres J, Wilhelmus KR, et al. Bacterial keratitis after radial keratotomy. *Ophthalmology* 1989;96:1171.

192. Paschal JF, Holland GN, Sison RF, et al. *Mycobacterium fortuitum* keratitis: clinical pathologic correlates and corticosteroid effects in an animal model. *Cornea* 1992;11:493.

193. Richardson P, Crawford GJ, Smith DW, et al. *Mycobacterium chelonae* keratitis. *Aust N Z J Ophthalmol* 1989;17:195.

194. Hu FR. Infectious crystalline keratopathy caused by *Mycobacterium fortuitum* and *Pseudomonas aeruginosa*. *Am J Ophthalmol* 1990;109:738.

195. Stein RM, et al. Infected vs. sterile corneal infiltrates in contact lens wearers. *Am J Ophthalmol* 1988;105:632.

196. Wilhelmus KR, Liesegang TG, Osato MS, et al. *Laboratory diagnosis of ocular infections*. Cumitech 13A. Washington, DC: American Society of Microbiology, 1994.

197. McDonnell PJ, Nobe J, Gauderman WJ, et al. Community care of corneal ulcers. *Am J Ophthalmol* 1992;114:531.

198. Kowal VO, Mead MD. Community acquired corneal ulcers: the impact of cultures on management. *Invest Ophthalmol Vis Sci* 1992;33:1210.

199. Williams G, McClellan K, Billson F. Suppurative keratitis in rural Bangladesh: the value of Gram stain in planning management. *Int Ophthalmol* 1991;15:131.

200. Sharma S, Kunimoto DY, Gopinathan U, et al. Evaluation of corneal scraping smear examination methods in the diagnosis of bacterial and fungal keratitis: a survey of eight years of laboratory experience. *Cornea* 2002;21:643.

201. Brinser JH, Weiss A. Laboratory diagnosis in ocular disease. In: Tazman W, Jaeger EA, eds. *Duane's clinical ophthalmology*, vol 4. Philadelphia: JB Lippincott, 1990:1.

202. Hyndiuk RA, Seideman S. Clinical and laboratory techniques in external ocular disease and endophthalmitis. In: Fedukowicz H, ed. *External infections of the eye: bacterial, viral, and mycotic*, 2nd ed. New York: Appleton-Century-Crofts, 1978:258.

203. Jakob P, Gopinathan U, Sharma S, et al. Calcium alginate swab versus Bard Parker blade in the diagnosis of microbial keratitis. *Cornea* 1995;14:360.

204. Egbert PR, Lauber S, Maurice DM. A simple conjunctival biopsy. *Am J Ophthalmol* 1977;84:798.

205. Nelson JD. Ocular surface impressions using cellulose acetate filter material: ocular pemphigoid. *Surv Ophthalmol* 1982;27:67.

206. Nelson JD, Havener VR, Cameron JD. Cellulose acetate impressions of ocular surface: dry eye states. *Arch Ophthalmol* 1983;101:1869.

207. Wittpenn JR, Tseng SCG, Sommer A. Detection of early xerophthalmia by impression cytology. *Arch Ophthalmol* 1986; 104:237

208. Natadisastra G, Wittpenn JR, West KP Jr, et al. Impression cytology for detection of vitamin-A deficiency. *Arch Ophthalmol* 1987;105:1224.

209. Wittpenn JR, Pepose JS. Impression debridement of herpes simplex dendritic keratitis. *Cornea* 1986;5:245.

210. Nakagawa H, Uchida Y, Takamura E, et al. Diagnostic impression cytology for herpes simplex keratitis. *Jpn J Ophthalmol* 1993; 37:505.

211. Florakis GJ, Folberg R, Krachmer JH, et al. Elevated corneal epithelial lines in *Acanthamoeba* keratitis. *Arch Ophthalmol* 1988;106:1202.

212. Gomez JT, Robinson NN, Osato MS, et al. Comparison of acridine orange and Gram stains in bacterial keratitis. *Am J Ophthalmol* 1988;106:735.

213. Groden LR, Rodnite J, Brinser JH, et al. Acridine orange and Gram stains in infectious keratitis. *Cornea* 1990;9:122.

214. Sutphin JE, et al. Improved detection of oculomycoses using induced fluorescence with cellufluor. *Ophthalmology* 1986;93:416.

215. Arffa RC, et al. Calcofluor-white and ink-potassium hydroxide preparations for identifying fungi. *Am J Ophthalmol* 1985; 100:719.

216. Wilhelmus KR, et al. Rapid diagnosis of *Acanthamoeba* keratitis using calcofluor-white. *Arch Ophthalmol* 1986;104:1309.

217. Marines HM, Osato MS, Font RL. The Value of calcofluor-white in the diagnosis of mycotic and *Acanthamoeba* infections of the eye and adnexa. *Ophthalmology* 1987;94:23.

218. Hahn TW, Osterhout GJ, O'Brien TP, et al. Utility of a rapid fluorescent Gram stain for recognition of live bacteria in ocular infection. *Invest Ophthalmol Vis Sci* 1995;36:3686.

219. O'Brien TP, Green WR. Fungus infections of the eye in periocular tissues. In: Garner A, Klintworth GK, eds. *Pathobiology of ocular disease: a dynamic approach.* New York: Marcel Dekker, 1994:299.

220. Aouizerte FJ, Cazenave L, Poirier P, et al. Detection of *Toxoplasma gondii* in aqueous humor by the polymerase chain reaction. *Br J Ophthalmol* 1993;77:107.

221. Delapaz MA, Young LHY. Acute retinal necrosis syndrome. *Semin Ophthalmol* 1993;8:61.

222. Fox GM, Crouse CA, Chuang EL, et al. Detection of herpes virus DNA in vitreous and aqueous specimens by the polymerase chain reaction. *Arch Ophthalmol* 1991;109:266.

223. Talley AR, Garcia-Ferrer KA, Laycock LR, et al. Comparative diagnosis of neonatal chlamydial conjunctivitis by polymerase chain reaction and McCoy cell culture. *Am J Ophthalmol* 1994;117:50.

224. Kowalski RP, Gordon YJ, Romanowski T, et al. A comparison of enzyme immunoassay and polymerase chain reaction with the clinical examination for diagnosing ocular herpetic disease. *Ophthalmology* 1993;100:530.

225. Yu DD, Lemp MA, Mathers WD, et al. Detection of varicella-zoster virus DNA and disciform keratitis using polymerase chain reaction. *Arch Ophthalmol* 1993;111:167.

226. Amsterdam D. The MIC: myth and reality. *Antimicrobic News Lett* 1992;8(2):9.

227. National Committee for Clinical Laboratory Standards. *Performance standards for antimicrobial susceptibility test,* 5th ed. Approved standard M2-A5. Villanova, PA: National Committee for Clinical Laboratory Standards, 1993.

228. National Committee for Clinical Laboratory Standards. *Methods for dilution antimicrobial susceptibility test for bacteria that grow aerobically,* 3rd ed. Approved standard M7-A3. Villanova, PA: National Committee for Clinical Laboratory Standards, 1993.

229. National Committee for Laboratory Clinical Standards. *Methods for antimicrobial susceptibility testing of anaerobic bacteria,* 3rd ed. Approved standard M11-A3. Villanova, PA: National Committee for Clinical Laboratory Standards, 1993.

230. Neuman MA, Sahm DF, Thornsberry C, et al. *New developments in antimicrobial agent susceptibility testing: a practical guide.* Cumitech 6A. Washington, DC: American Society for Microbiology, 1991.

231. Sahm DF, Neuman MA, Thornsberry C, et al. *Current concepts and approaches to antimicrobial susceptibility testing.* Cumitech 25. Washington, DC: American Society for Microbiology, 1988.

232. Lorian V. Effect of low antibiotic concentrations on bacteria. In: Lorian V, ed. *Antibiotics and laboratory medicine,* 2nd ed. Baltimore: Williams & Wilkins, 1985:596.

233. Craig WA, Gudmundsson S. The post-antibiotic effect. In: Lorian V, ed. *Antibiotics and laboratory medicine,* 2nd ed. Baltimore: Williams & Wilkins, 1985:515.

234. Drlica K. The mutant selection window and antimicrobial resistance. *J Antimicrob Chemother* 2003;52:11.

235. Wilhelmus KR, Schlech BA. Clinical and epidemiological advantages of culturing bacterial keratitis. *Cornea* 2004;23:38.

236. Hwang DG. Lamellar flap corneal biopsy. *Ophthalmic Surg* 1993;24:512.

237. Brooks JG, Coster DJ. Non-ulcerative fungal keratitis diagnosed by posterior lamellar biopsy. *Aust N Z J Ophthalmol* 1993;21:115.

238. Friedlaender MH. Corneal biopsy. *Int Ophthalmol Clin* 1988;28:101.

239. Newton C, Moore MB, Kaufman HE. Corneal biopsy in chronic keratitis. *Arch Ophthalmol* 1987;105:577.

240. Whitehouse G, Reid K, Hudson B, et al. Corneal biopsy in microbial keratitis. *Aust N Z J Ophthalmol* 1991;19:193.

241. Lee P, Green WR. Corneal biopsy: indications, techniques, and a report of 87 cases. *Ophthalmology* 1981;97:718.

242. Walters RW, Jorgensen JH, Calzada D, et al. Limulus lysate assay for early detection of certain gram-negative corneal infections. *Arch Ophthalmol* 1979;97:875.

243. Alfonso EC, Miller D. Rapid detection of gram-negative endotoxin contamination of contact lens saline solutions. *Arch Ophthalmol* 1992;110:1763.

244. Robin JB, Chan R, Andersen BR. Rapid visualization of *Acanthamoeba* using fluorescein-conjugated lectins. *Arch Ophthalmol* 1988;106:1273.

245. Cavanagh HD, Petroll WM, Alizadeh H, et al. Clinical and diagnostic use of in vivo confocal microscopy in patients with corneal disease. *Ophthalmology* 1993;100:1444.

246. Essepian GP, Rhapal RK, O'Brien TP. Non-invasive diagnosis of infectious keratitis using confocal microscopy. *Invest Ophthalmol Vis Sci* 1994;35:1936.

247. Irvine JA, Ariyasu R. Limitations in tandem scanning confocal microscopy as a diagnostic tool for microbial keratitis. *Scanning* 1994;16:307.

248. Wilhelmus KR. Bacterial corneal ulcer. *Int Ophthalmol Clin* 1984;24:1.

249. Groden LR, Brinser JH. Out-patient treatment of microbial corneal ulcers. *Arch Ophthalmol* 1986;104:84.

250. Fleming A. On the anti-bacterial action of cultures of a *Penicillium* etc. *Br J Exp Pathol* 1929;10:226.

251. Chain E, Florey HW, Gardner AD, et al. Penicillin as a chemotherapeutic agent. *Lancet* 1940;2:226.

252. Abraham EP, Chain E, Fletcher CM, et al. Further observations on penicillin. *Lancet* 1941;2:177.

253. Hare R. *The birth of penicillin.* London: George Allen and Unwin, 1970.

254. Hare R. New light on the history of penicillin. *Med Hist* 1982;26:1.

255. Howie J. Penicillin: 1929–40. *BMJ* 1986;293:158.

256. Tomasz A. Mechanism of irreversible antimicrobial effects of penicillins, how beta-lactam antibiotics kill and lyse bacteria. *Annu Rev Microbiol* 1979;33:113.

257. Pratt WB, Fekety R. *The antimicrobial drugs.* New York: Oxford University Press, 1986:85–152.

258. Tomasz A. Penicillin-binding proteins and antibacterial effectiveness of beta-lactam antibiotics. *Rev Infect Dis* 1986;8[Suppl 3]:S260.

259. Ho AC, Rapuano CJ. *Pasteurella multocida* keratitis and corneal laceration from a cat scratch. *Ophthalmic Surg* 1993;24:345.

260. Handwerger S, Tomasz A. Antibiotic tolerance among clinical isolates of bacteria. *Rev Infect Dis* 1985;7:368.

261. Chow AW, Jewesson PJ. Pharmacokinetics and safety of antimicrobial agents during pregnancy. *Rev Infect Dis* 1985;7:287.

262. Conte JE, Barriere SL. *Manual of antibiotics and infectious diseases,* 5th ed. Philadelphia: Lea & Febiger, 1984:63–64.

263. Ditlove J, et al. Methicillin nephritis. *Medicine (Baltimore)* 1977;56:438.

264. Wright AJ, Wilkowske CJ. Penicillins. *Mayo Clin Proc* 1987;62:806.

265. Neu HC. Amoxicillin. *Ann Intern Med* 1979;90:356.

266. Eliopoulos GM, Moellering RC Jr. Azlocillin, mezlocillin, and piperacillin: new broad-spectrum penicillins. *Ann Intern Med* 1982;97:755.

267. Norris SM. Penicillins with anti-pseudomonal activity. *Infect Control* 1985;6:165.

268. Neu HC. Carbenicillin and ticarcillin. *Med Clin North Am* 1982;66:61.

269. Mangini RJ, ed. *Drug interaction facts.* St. Louis: JB Lippincott, 1984:14.

270. Donowitz GR, Mandell GL. Cephalosporins. In: Mandell GL, et al., eds. *Principles and practices of infectious diseases*, 3rd ed. New York: Churchill Livingstone, 1990:246.

271. Anderson JA. Cross-sensitivity to cephalosporins in patients allergic to penicillin. *Pediatr Infect Dis J* 1986;5:557.

272. Bang NU, Kammer RB. Hematologic complications associated with beta-lactam antibiotics. *Rev Infect Dis* 1983;5[Suppl 2]: S380.

273. Weitekamp MR, Abber RC. Prolonged bleeding times and bleeding diathesis associated with moxalactam administration. *JAMA* 1983;249:69.

274. O'Brien TP, Sawusch MR, Dick JD, et al. Comparative topical ceftazidime versus aminoglycoside therapy of experimental *Pseudomonas* keratitis. Presented at the 47th Wilmer Residents Association Meeting, The Wilmer Eye Institute, Johns Hopkins University School of Medicine, Baltimore, April, 1987.

275. Kremer I, Robinson A, Braffman M, et al. The effect of topical ceftazidime on *Pseudomonas* keratitis in rabbits. *Cornea* 1994; 13:360.

276. Lambert HP, et al., eds. Ceftazidime in clinical practice. *J Antimicrob Chemother* 1983;12[Suppl A].

277. Neu HC. Other beta-lactam antibiotics. In: Mandell GL, et al., eds. *Principles and practices of infectious diseases*, 3rd ed. New York: Churchill Livingstone, 1990:257.

278. Birnbaum J, et al. Carbapenems, new class of beta-lactam antibiotics: discovery and development of imipenem/cilastatin. *Am J Med* 1985;78[Suppl 6A]:3.

279. Sawusch MR, O'Brien TP, Gottsch JD, et al. Topical imipenem therapy of aminoglycoside-resistant *Pseudomonas* keratitis in rabbits. *Am J Ophthalmol* 1988;106:77.

280. Sykes RB, Bonner DP. Aztreonam: first monobactam. *Am J Med* 1985;78[Suppl 2A]:2.

281. Henry SA, Bendush CP. Aztreonam: worldwide overview of treatment of patients with gram-negative infections. *Am J Med* 1985;78[Suppl 2A]:57.

282. Tartaglione TA, et al. In vitro and in vivo studies of effect of aztreonam on platelet function and coagulation in normal volunteers. *Antimicrob Agents Chemother* 1986;30:73.

283. Lowenstein A, Zemel E, Lazar M, et al. Retinal toxicity of two antibiotic drugs: aztreonam and imipenem. *Invest Ophthalmol Vis Sci* 1993;34:3570.

284. Cheung RPF, Dipiro JT. Vancomycin: update. *Pharmacotherapy* 1986;6:153.

285. Leclercq R, et al. Plasmid-mediated resistant to vancomycin and teicoplanin in *Enterococcus faecium*. *N Engl J Med* 1988;319:157.

286. Garrelts JC, Peterie JD. Vancomycin and the "red man's syndrome." *N Engl J Med* 1985;12:235.

287. Bailie GR, Neal D. Vancomycin ototoxicity and nephrotoxicity. *Rev Med Toxicol* 1988;3:376.

288. Farber BF, Moellering RC Jr. Retrospective study of toxicity of preparations of vancomycin from 1974 to 1981. *Antimicrob Agents Chemother* 1983;23:138.

289. Wilhelmus KR. Vancomycin revisited [editorial]. *Cornea* 1982; 1:103.

290. Somma S, et al. Teicoplanin, a new antibiotic from *Actinoplanes teichomyceticus*. *Antimicrob Agents Chemother* 1984;26:917.

291. Bryan LE. Mechanisms of action of aminoglycoside antibiotics. In: Root RK, Sande MA, eds. *Contemporary issues in infectious diseases*, vol 1: *New dimensions in antimicrobial therapy*. New York: Churchill Livingstone, 1984:17.

292. Tanaka N. Mechanism of action of aminoglycoside antibiotics. In: Umezawa H, Hooper IR, eds. *Handbook of experimental pharmacology*, vol 62. New York: Springer-Verlag, 1982:221.

293. Craig WA, Vogelman B. Post-antibiotic infection [editorial]. *Ann Intern Med* 1987;106:900.

294. Hare RS, Miller GH. Mechanisms of aminoglycoside resistance. *Antimicrobic News Lett* 1984;1:77.

295. Smolin G, Okumoto M, Wilson FM. The effect of tobramycin on gentamicin-resistant strains in *Pseudomonas* keratitis. *Am J Ophthalmol* 1974;77:583.

296. Roussel TJ, et al. Resistant *Pseudomonas* keratitis. *J Ocul Ther Surg* 1984;3:136.

297. Petroutsos G, et al. Antibiotics in corneal epithelial wound healing. *Arch Ophthalmol* 1983;101:1775.

298. Petroutsos G, Guimaraes R, Pouliquen Y. The effect of concentrated antibiotics on the rabbit corneal epithelium. *Int Ophthalmol* 1984;7:65.

299. Stern GA, et al. Effect of topical antibiotic solutions on corneal epithelial wound healing. *Arch Ophthalmol* 1983;101:644.

300. Wilhelmus KR, Gilbert ML, Osato MS. Tobramycin in ophthalmology. *Surv Ophthalmol* 1987;32:111.

301. Smith JT. The mode of action of 4-quinolones and possible mechanisms of resistance. *J Antimicrob Chemother* 1986; 18[Suppl D]:21.

302. Courtright JB, Turowski DA, Sonstein SA. Alteration of bacterial DNA structure, gene expression, and plasmid encoated antibiotic resistance following exposure to enoxacin. *J Antimicrob Chemother* 1988;21[Suppl B]:1.

303. Hooper DC, Wolfson JS. Mode of action of the quinolone antimicrobial agents. *Rev Infect Dis* 1988;10[Suppl 1]:S14.

304. Forward KR, et al. Comparative activities of norfloxacin and fifteen other antipseudomonal agents against gentamicin-susceptible and resistant *Pseudomonas aeruginosa* strains. *Antimicrob Agents Chemother* 1983;24:602.

305. Smith SM. In vitro comparison of A-56619, A-56620, amifloxacin, ciprofloxacin, enoxacin, norfloxacin, and ofloxacin against methicillin-resistant *Staphylococcus aureus*. *Antimicrob Agents Chemother* 1986;29:325.

306. King A, Phillips I. The comparative in vitro activity of eight newer quinolones and nalidixic acid. *J Antimicrob Chemother* 1986;18[Suppl D]:1.

307. Neu HC. Microbiologic aspects of fluoroquinolones. *Am J Ophthalmol* 1991;112[Suppl]:15S.

308. Wall RA, et al. Comparative in vitro activity of twelve -four quinolone antimicrobials against *Haemophilus ducreyi*. *J Antimicrob Chemother* 1985;16:165.

309. Fenlon CH, Cynamon MH. Comparative in vitro activities of ciprofloxacin and other four-quinolones against *Mycobacterium tuberculosis* and *Mycobacterium avium-intracellulare*. *Antimicrob Agents Chemother* 1986;29:386.

310. Heessen FWA, Muytjens HL. In vitro activities of ciprofloxacin, norfloxacin, pipemidic acid, cinoxacin, and nalidixic acid against *Chlamydia trachomatis*. *Antimicrob Agents Chemother* 1984;25:123.

311. Aznar J, et al. Activities of new quinolone derivatives against genital pathogens. *Antimicrob Agents Chemother* 1985;27:76.

312. How SJ, Hobson D, Hart CA, et al. A comparison of the in vitro activity of antimicrobials against *Chlamydia trachomatis* examined by Giemsa and a fluorescent antibody stain. *J Antimicrob Chemother* 1985;15:399.

313. Sutter VL, et al. Comparative activity of ciprofloxacin against anaerobic bacteria. *Antimicrob Agents Chemother* 1985;27:427.

314. Goldstein EJC, Citron DM. Comparative activity of quinolones against anaerobic bacteria isolated at community hospitals. *Antimicrob Agents Chemother* 1985;27:657.

315. Yamagishi JI, Yoshida H, Yamayoshi M, et al. Nalidixic acid-resistant mutations of the gyr B gene of *Escherichia coli*. *Mol Genet* 1986;204:367.

316. Yamagishi JI, Furutani Y, Inoue S, et al. Nalidixic acid resistant mutations related to DNA gyrase activity. *J Bacteriol* 1981; 148:50.

317. Robillard NJ, Scarpa AL. Genetic and physiologic characterization of ciprofloxacin resistance and *Pseudomonas aeruginosa* PAO. *Antimicrob Agents Chemother* 1988;32:535.

318. Hirai K, Suzue S, Iriqura T, et al. Mutations producing resistance to norfloxacin and *Pseudomonas aeruginosa*. *Antimicrob Agents Chemother* 1987;31:582.

319. Daikos GL, Lolans VT, Jackson GG. Alterations in outer membrane proteins of *Pseudomonas aeruginosa* associated with selective resistance to quinolones. *Antimicrob Agents Chemother* 1988;32:785.

320. Chapman JS, Georgopapadoakou NH. Routes of quinolone permeation in *Escherichia coli*. *Antimicrob Agents Chemother* 1988;32:438.

321. Hirai K, Aoyama H, Iriqura T, et al. Differences in susceptibility to quinolones of outer membrane mutants of *Salmonella* type *typhimurium* and *Escherichia coli*. *Antimicrob Agents Chemother* 1986;29:535.

322. Sanders CC, Sanders WE Jr, Georing RV, et al. Selection of multiple antibiotic resistance by quinolone, beta-lactams, and aminoglycoside with special reference to cross-resistance between unrelated drug classes. *Antimicrob Agents Chemother* 1984;26:79.

323. Trucksis M, Hooper DC, Wolfson JS. Emerging resistance to fluoroquinolones in staphylococci: an alert [editorial]. *Ann Intern Med* 1991;114:424.

324. Snyder ME, Katz HR. Ciprofloxacin-resistant bacterial keratitis. *Am J Ophthalmol* 1992;114:336.

325. Maffett M, O'Day DM. Ciprofloxacin-resistant bacterial keratitis. *Am J Ophthalmol* 1993;115:545.

326. Newman M, Esanu A. Gaps and prospective of new fluoroquinolones. *Drugs Exp Clin Res* 1988;14:385.

327. O'Brien TP, Sawusch MR, Dick JD, et al. Topical ciprofloxacin treatment of *Pseudomonas* keratitis in rabbits. *Arch Ophthalmol* 1988;106:1444.

328. Sugar A, Cohen MA, Bien PA, et al. Treatment of experimental *Pseudomonas* corneal ulcers with enoxacin, a quinolone antibiotic. *Arch Ophthalmol* 1986;104:1230.

329. Gritz DC, McDonnell PJ, Lee TY, et al. Topical ofloxacin in the treatment of *Pseudomonas* keratitis in a rabbit model. *Cornea* 1992;11:143.

330. Leibowitz HM, et al. Clinical evaluation of ciprofloxacin 0.3% ophthalmic solution in treatment of bacterial keratitis. *Am J Ophthalmol* 1991;112[Suppl]:34S.

331. Essepian JP, Rajpal R, O'Brien TP. Tandem scanning confocal microscopic analysis of ciprofloxacin corneal deposits in vivo. *Cornea* 1995;14:402.

332. O'Brien TP, Osterhout G, Dick JD. Comparative ocular penetration of topical ofloxacin and ciprofloxacin in rabbits. ARVO Abstracts. *Invest Ophthalmol Vis Sci* 1993;34[4 Suppl]:859.

333. Kanellopoulos AJ, Miller F, Wittpenn JR. Deposition of ciprofloxacin to prevent re-epithelialization of a corneal defect. *Am J Ophthalmol* 1994;117:258.

334. Hobden JA, O'Callaghan RJ, Insler MS, et al. Ciprofloxacin ointment versus ciprofloxacin drops for therapy of experimental *Pseudomonas* keratitis. *Cornea* 1993;12:138.

335. Wilhelmus KR, Hyndiuk RL, Caldwell DR, et al. 0.3% Ciprofloxacin ophthalmic ointment in the treatment of bacterial keratitis: the Ciprofloxacin Ointment/Bacterial Keratitis Study Group. *Arch Ophthalmol* 1993;111:1210.

336. Hyndiuk RA, Eiferman RA, Caldwell DL, et al. Comparison of ciprofloxacin 0.3% (Ciloxan) solution to fortified tobramycin/cefazolin in treatment of bacterial corneal ulcers. *Ophthalmology* 1996;103:1854.

337. Cutarelli PE, et al. Topical fluoroquinolones: antimicrobial activity and in vitro corneal epithelial toxicity. *Curr Eye Res* 1991;10:557.

338. Fugimaki K, Noumi T, Saikawa I, et al. In vitro and in vivo antibacterial activities of T-3262, a new fluoroquinolone. *Antimicrob Agents Chemother* 1988;32:827.

339. Fernandes PB, Chu DTW, Swanson RN, et al. A-61287 (A-60969): a new fluoronapthirodine with activity against both aerobic and anaerobic bacteria. *Antimicrob Agents Chemother* 1988;32:27.

340. Gargallo D, Morris M, Coll R, et al. Activity of E-3846, a new fluoroquinolone, in vitro and in experimental cystitis and pyelonephritis in rats. *Antimicrob Agents Chemother* 1988;32:636.

341. Abbott Laboratories. Temafloxacin (Omniflox): worldwide withdrawal. Drug recall notice. Chicago: Abbott Laboratories, June 6, 1992.

342. Barequet IS, Denton P, Osterhout GJ, et al. Treatment of experimental bacterial keratitis with topical trovafloxacin. *Arch Ophthalmol* 2004;122:65.

343. Ooishi M, Oomomo A, Sakaue F, et al. Studies on intraocular penetration of MY-198 (lomefloxacin) eyedrops. *Acta Soc Ophthalmol Jpn* 1988;92:1825.

344. Kodama T. Penetration of lomefloxacin ophthalmic solution into the human aqueous humor. *Jpn Rev Ophthalmol* 1991;85:492.

345. Hatano H, Inoue K, Shia S, et al. Application of topical lomefloxacin against experimental *Pseudomonas* endophthalmitis in rabbits. *Acta Ophthalmol* 1993;71:666.

346. Uchida Y, et al. Evaluation of lomefloxacin ophthalmic solution: a multi-center phase-two double-blind clinical trial. *Jpn Rev Ophthalmol* 1990;84:51.

347. Uchida Y, et al. Clinical efficacy of topical lomefloxacin in bacterial infections of the external eye: a multi-center-double-blind phase III study. *Folia Ophthalmol Jpn* 1991;42:59.

348. Booranapong W, Kosrirukvongs P, Prabhasawat P, et al. Comparison of topical lomefloxacin 0.3 per cent versus topical ciprofloxacin 0.3 per cent for the treatment of presumed bacterial corneal ulcers. *J Med Assoc Thai* 2004;87:246.

349. Wilhelmus KR, Abshire RL, Schlech BA. Influence of fluoroquinolone susceptibility on the therapeutic response of fluoroquinolone-treated bacterial keratitis. *Arch Ophthalmol* 2003;121:1229.

350. Kowalski RP, Dhaliwal DK, Karenchak LM, et al. Gatifloxacin and moxifloxacin: an in vitro susceptibility comparison to levofloxacin, ciprofloxacin, and ofloxacin using bacterial keratitis isolates. *Am J Ophthalmol* 2003;136:500.

351. Wilhelmus KR. Evaluation and prediction of fluoroquinolone pharmacodynamics in bacterial keratitis. *J Ocul Pharmacol Ther* 2003;19:493.

352. Tungsiripat T, Sarayba MA, Kaufman MB, et al. Fluoroquinolone therapy in multiple-drug resistant staphylococcal keratitis after lamellar keratectomy in a rabbit model. *Am J Ophthalmol* 2003;136:76.

353. Bower KS, Kowalski RP, Gordon YJ. Fluoroquinolones in the treatment of bacterial keratitis. *Am J Ophthalmol* 1996;121:712.

354. Pollock GA, McKelvie PA, McCarty DJ, et al. In vivo effects of fluoroquinolones on rabbit corneas. *Clin Exp Ophthalmol* 2003;31:517.

355. Reviglio VE, Hakim MA, Song JK, et al. Effect of topical fluoroquinolones on the expression of matrix metalloproteinases in the cornea. *BMC Ophthalmol* 2003;3:10.

356. Chalita MR, Hofling-Lima AL, Paranhos A Jr, et al. Shifting trends in in vitro antibiotic susceptibilities for common ocular isolates during a period of 15 years. *Am J Ophthalmol* 2004;137:43.

357. Mao JCH, et al. Biochemical basis for selective toxicity of erythromycin. *Biochem Pharmacol* 1970;19:391.

358. Washington JA II, Wilson WR. Erythromycin: microbial and clinical prospective after thirty years of clinical use. Parts I and II. *Mayo Clin Proc* 1985;60:189.

359. Field AJ, Backhoff IK, Dick JD, et al. Comparative topical treatment of *Mycobacterium fortuitum* keratitis in rabbits. *Invest Ophthalmol Vis Sci* 1993;34:737.

360. Husain SE, Matoba AY, Husain N, et al. Antimicrobial efficacy of clarithromycin and azithromycin against *Mycobacterium chelonae* and *Mycobacterium abscessus*. *Invest Ophthalmol Vis Sci* 1993;34:729.

361. Davis BD. Protein synthesis. In: Davis BD, et al., eds. *Microbiology*, 3rd ed. Hagerstown, MD: Harper & Row, 1980:229.

362. Steigbigel NH. Erythromycin, lincomycin, and clindamycin. In: Mandell GL, et al., eds. *Principles and practices of infectious diseases*, 2nd ed. New York: John Wiley and Sons, 1984:224.

363. Tally FP, et al. Susceptibility of the *Bacteroides fragilis* group in the United States in 1981. *Antimicrob Agents Chemother* 1983; 23:536.

364. Danneman BR, et al. Treatment of toxoplasmic encephalitis with intravenous clindamycin. *Arch Intern Med* 1988;148: 2477.

365. Fekety R. Antibiotic-associated pseudomembranous colitis. *Clin Microbiol Newslett* (Preview Issue), October, 1978.

366. Fekety R, et al. Treatment of antibiotic-associated *Clostridium difficile* colitis with oral vancomycin: comparison of two dosage regimens. *Am J Med* 1989;86:15.

367. Williams DN. Tetracycline. In: Peterson PK, Verhoef J, eds. *The antimicrobial agents annual/3*. New York: Elsevier, 1988:218.

368. Hook EW III, Holmes KK. Gonococcal infections. *Ann Intern Med* 1985;102:229.

369. Kallings I. Sensitivity of *Branhamella catarrhalis* to oral antibiotics. *Drugs* 1986;31[Suppl 3]:17.

370. Carpenter G. Chloramphenicol eye-drops in marrow aplasia. *Lancet* 1975;2:326.

371. Rosenthal RL, Blackman A. Bone marrow hypoplasia following use of chloramphenicol eyedrops. *JAMA* 1965;191:136.

372. Abramowicz M. Chloramphenicol ophthalmic formulation. *Med Lett Drugs Ther* 1980;22:96.

373. Bartlett JG. Chloramphenicol. *Med Clin North Am* 1982; 66:91.

374. Mandell GL, Sande MA. Antimicrobial agents: sulfonamides, trimethoprim-sulfamethoxazole, a urinary tract antiseptics. In: Gilman AG, et al., eds. *The pharmacological basis of therapeutics*, 6th ed. New York: Macmillan, 1980:1106.

375. Everett SL, Kowalski RP, Karenchak LM, et al. An in vitro comparison of the susceptibilities of bacterial isolates from patients with conjunctivitis and blepharitis to newer and established antibiotics. *Cornea* 1995;14:382.

376. Donnenfeld ED, Cohen EJ, Barza M, et al. Treatment of *Nocardia* keratitis with topical trimethoprim-sulfamethoxazole. *Am J Ophthalmol* 1985;99:601.

377. Araujo OE, Flowers FP. Stevens-Johnson syndrome. *J Emerg Med* 1984;2:129.

378. Huovinen P, et al. Trimethoprim resistance of *Escherichia coli* in out-patients in Finland after ten years use of plain trimethoprim. *J Antimicrob Chemother* 1985;16:435.

379. Van Rensburg SFJ, Gibson JR, Harvey SG, et al. Trimethoprim-polymyxin ophthalmic solution in the treatment of bacterial conjunctivitis. *Pharma Therapeutica* 1982;3:274.

380. Abramowicz M. Trimethoprim-polymyxin-B for bacterial conjunctivitis. *Med Lett Drugs Ther* 1990;32:71.

381. Thornsberry C, et al. Rifampin: spectrum of antibacterial activity. *Rev Infect Dis* 1983;5[Suppl 3]:S412.

382. U.S. Department of Health and Human Services, Division of Sexually Transmitted Diseases. Sexually transmitted diseases treatment guidelines. *MMWR Morb Mortal Wkly Rep* 1989;38(S8):5.

383. Ashford WA, et al. Spectinomycin-resistant penicillinase-producing *Neisseria gonorrhoeae*. *Lancet* 1981;2:1035.

384. Boslego JW, et al. Effect of spectinomycin use on prevalence of spectinomycin-resistant in a penicillinase-producing *Neisseria gonorrhoeae*. *N Engl J Med* 1987;317:272.

385. Tabbara K, Antonios S, Alvarez H. Effects of fusidic acid on staphylococcal keratitis. *Br J Ophthalmol* 1989;73:136.

386. Gunshefski L, Mannis MJ, Culler JS, et al. In vitro antimicrobial activity of shiva-11 against ocular pathogens. *Cornea* 1994; 13:237.

387. O'Brien TP, Reynolds IA. Basic ocular pharmacotherapy. *J Ophthalmol Nurs Tech* 1995;14:160.

388. Shell JW. Pharmacokinetics of topically applied ophthalmic drugs. *Surv Ophthalmol* 1982;26:207.

389. Lesar TS, Fiscella RG. Antimicrobial drug delivery to the eye. *Drug Intell Clin Pharm* 1985;19:642.

390. Barza M. Antibacterial agents in the treatment of ocular infections. *Infect Dis Clin North Am* 1989;3:533.

391. Davis SD, Sarff LD, Hyndiuk RA. Topical tobramycin therapy of experimental *Pseudomonas* keratitis: an evaluation of some factors that potentially enhance efficacy. *Arch Ophthalmol* 1978;96:123.

392. Kupferman A, Leibowitz HM. Topical antibiotic therapy of *Pseudomonas aeruginosa* keratitis in guinea pigs. *Arch Ophthalmol* 1979;97:1699.

393. Davis SD, Sarff LD, Hyndiuk RA. Antibiotic therapy of experimental *Pseudomonas* keratitis in guinea pigs. *Arch Ophthalmol* 1977;95:1638.

394. Glasser DB, Gardner S, Ellis JG, et al. Loading doses and extended dosing intervals in topical gentamicin therapy. *Am J Ophthalmol* 1985;99:329.

395. Robin JS, Ellis PP. Ophthalmic ointments. *Surv Ophthalmol* 1978;22:335.

396. Hanna C, Hof HC, Smith WG. Influence of drug vehicle on ocular contact time of sulfacetamide sodium. *Ann Ophthalmol* 1985;17:560.

397. Osborn E, Baum JL, Ernst C, et al. The stability of ten antibiotics in artificial tears. *Am J Ophthalmol* 1976;82:775.

398. Baum J, Barza M, Hsushan D, et al. Concentration of gentamicin in experimental corneal ulcers. *Arch Ophthalmol* 1974;92:315.

399. Kupferman A, Leibowitz HM. Antibiotic therapy of bacterial keratitis: topical application or a periocular injection? *Invest Ophthalmol Vis Sci* 1980;19:112.

400. Baum JL, Barza M. Topical versus subconjunctival treatment of bacterial corneal ulcers. *Ophthalmology* 1983;90:162.

401. Stern GA, Driebe WT. The effect of fortified antibiotic therapy on the visual outcome of severe bacterial corneal ulcers. *Cornea* 1982;1:341.

402. Liebowitz HM, Ryan WJ, Kupferman A. Route of antibiotic administration in bacterial keratitis. *Arch Ophthalmol* 1981;99:1420.

403. Baum J. Treatment of bacterial ulcers of the cornea in the rabbit: a comparison of administration by eyedrops and subconjunctival injections. *Trans Am Ophthalmol Soc* 1982;80:369.

404. Hessburg PC. Treatment of *Pseudomonas* keratitis in humans. *Am J Ophthalmol* 1966;61:896.

405. Burris TE, Newsom DI, Rowsey JJ. Hessburg subpalpebral antibiotic lavage of *Pseudomonas* corneal and corneoscleral ulcers. *Cornea* 1982;1:347.

406. Matoba AY, McCulley JP. The effect of therapeutic soft contact lenses on antibiotic delivery to the cornea. *Ophthalmology* 1985;92:97.

407. Busin M, Goebbels M, Spitznas M. Medicated bandage lenses for sustained gentamicin release. *Ophthalmology* 1987;94[Suppl]: 124.

408. O'Brien TP, Sawusch MR, Dick JD, et al. Use of collagen corneal shields versus soft contact lenses to enhance penetration of topical tobramycin. *J Cataract Refract Surg* 1988; 14:505.

409. Unterman SR, Rootman DS, Hill JM, et al. Collagen shield drug delivery: therapeutic concentrations of tobramycin in the rabbit cornea and aqueous humor. *J Cataract Refract Surg* 1988;14:500.

410. Sawusch MR, O'Brien TP, Dick JD, et al. Use of collagen corneal shields in the treatment of bacterial keratitis. *Am J Ophthalmol* 1988;106:279.

411. Baum JL, Barza M, Weinstein L. Preferred routes of antibiotic administration in treatment of bacterial ulcers of the cornea. *Int Ophthalmol Clin* 1973;13:31.

412. Gilbert ML, Wilhelmus KR, Osato MS. Intracanalicular collagen implants enhance topical antibiotic bioavailability. *Cornea* 1986;5:167.

413. Schaeffer HE, Krohn DL. Liposomes and topical drug delivery. *Invest Ophthalmol Vis Sci* 1982;22:220.

414. Rootman DS, Hobden JA, Jantzen JA, et al. Iontophoresis of tobramycin for treatment of experimental *Pseudomonas* keratitis in rabbits. *Arch Ophthalmol* 1988;106:262.

415. Callegan MC, O'Callaghan RJ, Hill JM. Pharmacokinetic considerations in the treatment of bacterial keratitis. *Clin Pharmacokinet* 1994;27:129.

416. Cunha-Vaz J. The blood-ocular barriers. *Surv Ophthalmol* 1979;23:279.

417. Burns RP, Rhodes DM. *Pseudomonas* eye infection as a cause of death in premature infants. *Arch Ophthalmol* 1961;65:517.

418. Gelender H, Rettich C. Gentamicin-resistant *Pseudomonas aeruginosa* corneal ulcers. *Cornea* 1984;3:21.

419. Callegan MC, Ramirez R, Kane ST, et al. Antibacterial activity of the fourth-generation fluoroquinolones gatifloxacin and moxifloxacin against ocular pathogens. *Adv Ther* 2003; 20:246.

420. Swenson JM, Wallace RJ Jr, Silcox VA, et al. Antimicrobial sensitivity of five subgroups of *Mycobacterium fortuitum* and *Mycobacterium chelonae*. *Antimicrob Agents Chemother* 1985; 28:807.

421. Gay JD, Deyoung DR, Roberts GD. In vitro activity of norfloxacin and ciprofloxacin against *Mycobacterium tuberculosis*, *M. avium* complex, *M. chelonei*, *M. fortuitum*, and *M. kansasii*. *Antimicrob Agents Chemother* 1984;26:94.

422. Wallace RJ, Bedsole G, Sumter G, et al. Activities of ciprofloxacin and ofloxacin against rapidly growing mycobacteria with demonstration of acquired resistance following single-drug therapy. *Antimicrob Agents Chemother* 1990;34:65.

423. Hwang DG, Biswell R. Ciprofloxacin therapy of *Mycobacterium chelonae* keratitis. *Am J Ophthalmol* 1993;115:114.

424. Brown SI, Bloomfield S, Pearce DB, et al. Infections with a therapeutic soft lens. *Arch Ophthalmol* 1974;91:275.

425. Slansky HH, Dohlman CH, Berman MB. Prevention of corneal ulcers. *Trans Am Acad Ophthalmol Otolaryngol* 1971; 75:1208.

426. Ellison A, Poirier R. Therapeutic effects of heparin on *Pseudomonas*-induced corneal ulceration. *Am J Ophthalmol* 1976;82:619.

427. Mehra KS, Singh R, Bhatia RPS. Lysozyme in corneal ulcer. *Ann Ophthalmol* 1975;7:1470.

428. Barletta JP, Balch KC, Dimova HG, et al. Inhibition of *Pseudomonas* corneal ulcers by a synthetic matrix metalloproteinase inhibitor (Galardin). *Invest Ophthalmol Vis Sci* 1993; 34:1749.

429. Brown M, Li WW, Dutt S, et al. A synthetic metalloproteinase inhibitor potentiates the anti-angiogenic effect of prednisolone in the cornea. *Invest Ophthalmol Vis Sci*

430. Davis SD, Sarff LD, Hyndiuk RA. Corticosteroid in experimentally induced *Pseudomonas* keratitis. *Arch Ophthalmol* 1978; 96:126.

431. Smolin G, Okumoto M, Leong-Sit L. Combined gentamicin-tobramycin-corticosteroid treatment: II. Effect on gentamicin-resistant *Pseudomonas* keratitis. *Arch Ophthalmol* 1980;98:473.

432. Badenoch PR, Hay GJ, McDonnell PJ, et al. A rat model of bacterial keratitis: effect of antibiotics and corticosteroids. *Arch Ophthalmol* 1985;103:718.

433. Leibowitz HM, Kupferman A. Topically administered corticosteroids: effect on antibiotic treated bacterial keratitis. *Arch Ophthalmol* 1980;98:1237.

434. Bohigian GM, Foster CS. Treatment of *Pseudomonas* keratitis in a rabbit with antibiotic steroid combination. *Invest Ophthalmol Vis Sci* 1977;16:553.

435. Harbin T. Recurrence of corneal *Pseudomonas* infection after topical steroid therapy. *Am J Ophthalmol* 1964;58:670.

436. Burns RP. *Pseudomonas aeruginosa* keratitis: mixed infections of the eye. *Am J Ophthalmol* 1969;67:257.

437. Stern GA, Buttross M. Use of corticosteroids in combination with antimicrobial drugs in the treatment of infectious corneal disease. *Ophthalmology* 1991;98:847.

438. Wilhelmus KR. Indecision about corticosteroids for bacterial keratitis: an evidence-based update. *Ophthalmology* 2002; 109:835.

439. Alpren TVP, Hyndiuk RA, Davis SD, et al. Cryotherapy for experimental *Pseudomonas* keratitis. *Arch Ophthalmol* 1979; 97:711.

440. Codere F, Brownstein S, Jackson B. *Pseudomonas aeruginosa* scleritis. *Am J Ophthalmol* 1981;91:706.

441. Eiferman RA. Cryotherapy of *Pseudomonas* keratitis and scleritis. *Arch Ophthalmol* 1979;97:1637.

442. Nassaralla BA, Wang XW, Wee WR, et al. Effect of diclofenac sodium on antibiotic treatment of experimental *Pseudomonas* keratitis. *Invest Ophthalmol Vis Sci* 1994;36:4721.

443. Gritz DZ, Kwitko S, Trousdale MD, et al. Recurrence of microbial keratitis concomitant with anti-inflammatory treatment in an animal model. *Cornea* 1992;11:404.

444. Eiferman RA, Snyder JW. Antibacterial effect of cyanoacrylate glue. *Arch Ophthalmol* 1983;101:958.

445. Cavanaugh TB, Gottsch JD. Infectious keratitis in cyanoacrylate adhesive. *Am J Ophthalmol* 1991;111:466.

446. Gottsch JD, Gilbert ML, Goodman DF, et al. Excimer laser ablative treatment of microbial keratitis. *Ophthalmology* 1991;98:146.

447. Serdarevic O, et al. Excimer laser therapy for experimental candida keratitis. *Am J Ophthalmol* 1985;99:534.

448. Sarno EM, et al. Carbon dioxide laser therapy of *Pseudomonas aeruginosa* keratitis. *Am J Ophthalmol* 1984;97:791.

449. Kirkness CM, Ficker LA, Steele AD, et al. The role of penetrating keratoplasty in the management of microbial keratitis. *Eye* 1991;5:425.

450. Killingsworth DW, Stern GA, Driebe WT, et al. Results of therapeutic penetrating keratoplasty. *Ophthalmology* 1993;100:534.

451. Lotti R, Dart JK. Cataract as a complication of severe microbial keratitis. *Eye* 1992;6:400.

BACTERIAL CONJUNCTIVITIS

SCOTT D. BARNES AND C. STEPHEN FOSTER

Bacterial conjunctivitis affects all ages and is seen in all geographic locations, and it is the most common bacterial infection of the eye (1). Conjunctivitis may occur as a consequence of infection by viruses, bacteria, parasites, or fungi, and it may also occur as a consequence of trauma, malignancy, autoimmunity, allergy, and nonimmunologic skin conditions, such as acne rosacea. But the clinical characteristics of bacterial conjunctivitis are so typical of bacterial infections that one is rarely faced with some puzzling diagnostic dilemma when confronted by a patient with bacterial conjunctivitis. The one exception to this generalization occurs when the patient has chlamydial conjunctivitis, which is often chronic and which usually lacks the most tell-tale characteristic of most other bacterial infections of the outer eye, purulent discharge.

HISTORY

Purulent or catarrhal conjunctivitis has been recognized and written about by all developed societies, with clear descriptions in Chinese, Indian, Greek, and Egyptian writings extending back over the past 3500 years. The first written documentation of the recognition that it could be contagious probably dates from the early 18th century, and in the latter part of that century, Neisser, Koch, and Weekes identified the causative bacterial agents in patients with ophthalmia neonatorum and in patients with Egyptian ophthalmia.

EPIDEMIOLOGY

Precise data on the prevalence of bacterial conjunctivitis are difficult to obtain, but it is clear that it is more frequent in the young than in the elderly, and that it has seasonal peaks, with the winter and spring being the times of the year of highest reporting. The annual incidence among naval recruits in the 1980s was reported as 0.0025% of the population (2).

RISKS AND TRANSMISSION

As might be expected, the predominant risk for increased susceptibility to bacterial conjunctivitis includes systemic immunocompromise, local (ocular) immunocompromise (e.g., chronic use of topical steroid), and general debilitation (malnutrition, alcoholism). Transmission is most commonly from hand to eye, but can be from genitals to eye or from contiguous spread from nasolacrimal system or eyelid infection. Probably an underappreciated source of infestation is through the use of eye makeup harboring steadily increasing numbers of bacteria. And, finally, transfer of secretions from one person to another by flies or other insects, as in the case of transmission of trachoma in endemic areas, is a clear source of microbial transmission.

It is for this reason that this entity is the first to be addressed in this chapter, before moving on to the more "classic" bacterial infections that can produce bacterial conjunctivitis.

CHLAMYDIAL CONJUNCTIVITIS

Chronic follicular conjunctivitis (inclusion conjunctivitis) can be caused by chlamydia. The same serotypes (there are several, identifiable by monoclonal antibodies) that cause conjunctivitis in the adult can lead to neonatal conjunctivitis if an infected mother transmits the pathogen to the newborn during vaginal delivery. Repeated infections with *Chlamydia trachomatis* serotypes A, B, Ba, and C can cause trachoma, a chronic follicular keratoconjunctivitis that remains the most common cause of preventable blindness in the world. In addition, several cases of Parinaud's oculoglandular syndrome have been reported with lymphogranuloma venereum, a sexually transmitted disease characterized by painful inguinal lymphadenopathy and caused by *C. trachomatis* serotypes L1 through L3.

Adult Inclusion Conjunctivitis

C. trachomatis can cause a chronic follicular conjunctivitis in adults and neonates. The adult form is usually sexually transmitted, with conjunctivitis developing in an estimated 1 in 300 patients with genital chlamydia (1), but it can occur with orogenital or hand-to-eye transmission of secretions (3). The

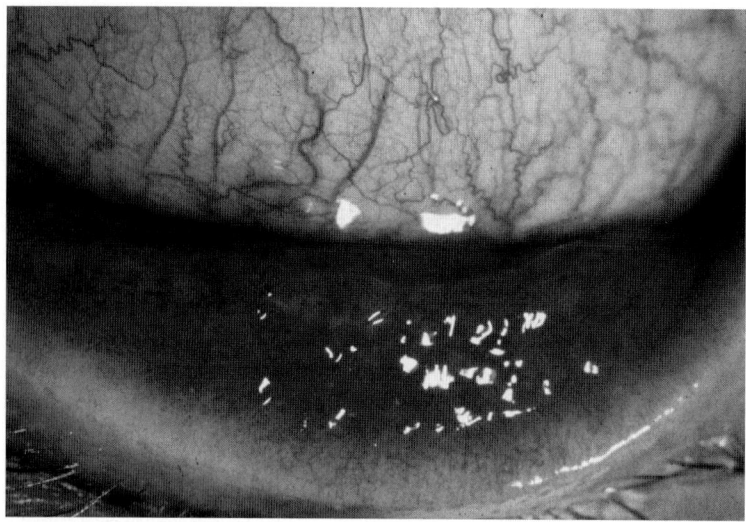

FIGURE 13.2-1. Clearly obvious follicular conjunctivitis with inflammation of the tarsal conjunctiva and formation of follicles. A slight watery discharge is also present. Conjunctival scrapings disclosed inclusion bodies, and the fluorescent antibody test disclosed unequivocal evidence of infection with the inclusion conjunctivitis agent.

most common presentation is that of unilateral red eye (although it can be bilateral), preauricular adenopathy, papillary hypertrophy, marked hyperemia, mucopurulent discharge, and a follicular reaction (Fig. 13.2-1). Men often have a concomitant urethritis; women may have asymptomatic chronic cervicitis. Corneal involvement may quickly follow the conjunctivitis, resulting in punctate keratitis, epidemic keratoconjunctivitis–like infiltrates, and superior limbal pannus (neovascularization). Corneal scarring and neovascularization are less common with inclusion conjunctivitis than with trachoma, and the upper and lower palpebral conjunctiva are often equally involved as opposed to the preferentially affected upper conjunctiva in trachoma. However, severe inclusion conjunctivitis may be associated with a chronic, relapsing course leading to characteristics usually seen in trachoma.

Treatment of Adult Inclusion Conjunctivitis

Because of the prominent mode of sexual transmission of this form of conjunctivitis, it is important simultaneously to treat all known partners. Failure to do so often results in more serious sequelae associated with reinfections. Topical antibiotics are relatively ineffective; systemic therapy is the mainstay of treatment. Tetracycline, doxycycline, azithromycin, ofloxacin or erythromycin are given for 3 weeks, with caution to avoid tetracycline in young children and pregnant or lactating women.

Trachoma

C. trachomatis serotypes A through C are responsible for trachoma. The severely blinding condition is endemic in many developing countries, especially in areas of close overcrowding and poor sanitation. Trachoma is usually the result of multiple untreated infections rather than a one-time event.

The initial follicular conjunctivitis begins in the upper palpebral conjunctiva, followed by limbal follicles. Papillary hypertrophy, mucopurulent discharge, superior corneal pannus (neovascularization), and epithelial keratitis are early features of the disease. Later stages are marked by cicatrization of the conjunctiva, cornea, and eyelids.

Sequelae of Trachoma

The blinding complications of trachoma are the result of the corneal exposure and ulceration due to the conjunctival scarring and lid deformities (4) (Fig. 13.2-2). Two classic findings are Arlt's line and Hebert's pits. Arlt's line is the horizontal line of conjunctival scarring found along the superior palpebral conjunctiva (Fig. 13.2-3). Hebert's pits are the sharply demarcated erosions near the limbus now filled with epithelium after the cicatrization of the limbal

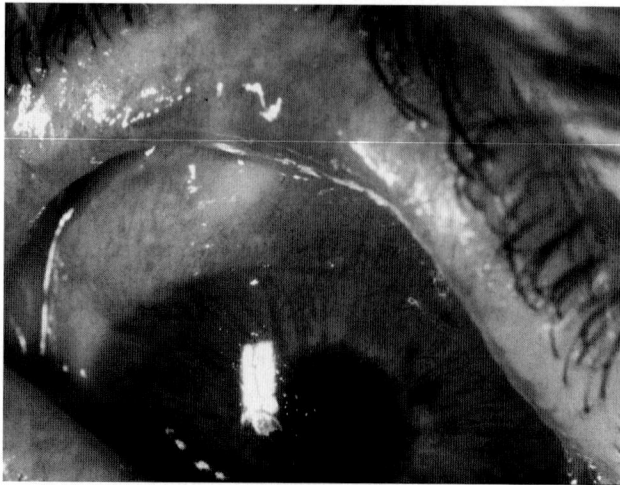

FIGURE 13.2-2. Cicatrizing conjunctivitis involving especially the tarsal conjunctiva in a patient with trachoma.

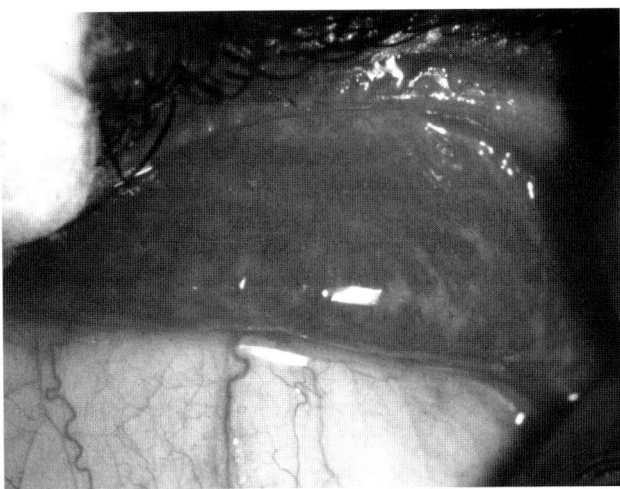

FIGURE 13.2-3. Flipped upper lid, showing the linear subepithelial fibrosis in the tarsal conjunctiva of a patient who previously had trachoma, now on treatment and resolving. Note, in particular, the horizontal linear line going across the entire horizontal extent of the lid, approximately 2 to 3 mm posterior to the lid margin: Arlt's line.

follicles (Fig. 13.2-4). Once the regression of the superior pannus occurs, a diffuse corneal haze may be seen. Eyelid deformities are the result of the conjunctival scarring. Lids can be turned inward (entropion) or outward (ectropion) and lashes can be directed against the cornea (trichiasis), all of which contribute to an irregular ocular surface. Such irregularities can cause corneal scars, ulcers, neovascularization, and even perforation.

Treatment of Trachoma

Systemic tetracycline or erythromycin is given for 3 weeks. The clinical response can often take several months; topical tetracycline or erythromycin is often used in endemic areas twice daily for 5 days each month for 6 months (5). This

repeated topical treatment is especially useful in situations where repeat infection is likely. Loosely based on the smallpox eradication efforts, widespread prophylactic systemic antibiotics have been tried in endemic areas in an attempt to eliminate the disease. A single dose of azithromycin was proposed as a good choice for the eradication theory (6).

Lymphogranuloma Venereum

Certain serotypes of *C. trachomatis* (L1, L2, L3) have been associated with systemic lymphogranuloma venereum. The associated conjunctivitis is often mild and unilateral, producing a scant watery discharge. Although the conjunctivitis appears mild, there is rather impressive edema in the upper and lower eyelids. In addition to the usual preauricular lymphadenopathy, the nodes in the parotid and submaxillary region are also involved. There is a report of lymphogranuloma venereum conjunctivitis causing a keratitis leading to a corneal perforation in a patient with acquired immunodeficiency syndrome (7). Treatment is similar to that for inclusion conjunctivitis.

THE MORE CLASSIC CAUSES OF BACTERIAL CONJUNCTIVITIS

Patients with bacterial conjunctivitis usually present with a history of a rapid onset of unilateral lid edema, conjunctival hyperemia, and mucopurulent discharge. The opposite eye very often becomes involved with the same problem within 48 hours of the onset of the disorder. *Staphylococcus* and *Corynebacterium* species are the most common organisms to colonize the lids and conjunctiva and consequently are the most common causes of infectious conjunctivitis (8). Although almost any bacterial organism can cause conjunctivitis, the most common etiologies are *Staphylococcus* species, *Streptococcus pneumoniae*, *Haemophilus* species,

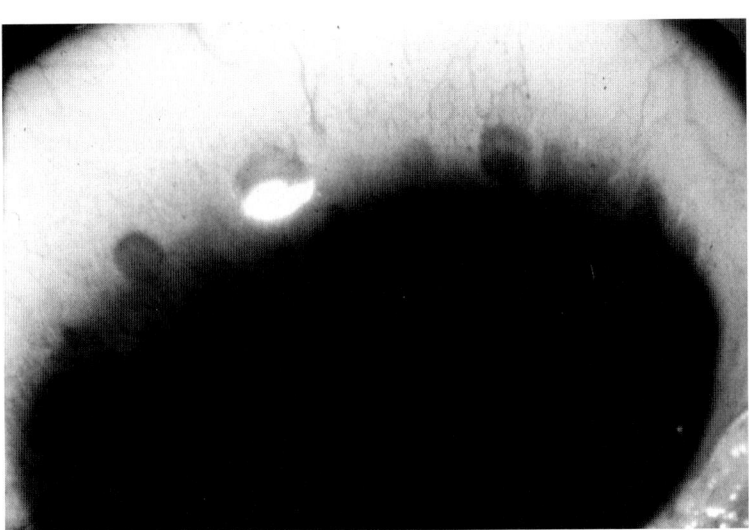

FIGURE 13.2-4. Depressions at the corneoscleral limbus in a patient who had trachoma many years before this photograph was taken. These are the so-called Herbert's pits.

Moraxella, Corynebacterium diphtheriae, Neisseria species, and enteric gram-negative rods (9).

Pathogenesis

The pathogenesis of bacterial conjunctivitis often involves a compromised epithelial surface because an intact epithelium is an effective barrier to most organisms. But *Neisseria gonorrhoeae, C. diphtheriae, Haemophilus aegyptius,* and *Listeria monocytogenes* can penetrate the intact, healthy conjunctival epithelium through specialized attachments or toxins (5). Injured epithelium or specialized attachments allow adhesion, which then results in the entry of bacteria. Proteases, coagulases, collagenases, and fibrinolysins, combined with toxins, such as those seen in *Staphylococcus* and *Pseudomonas* species, disrupt tissue, allowing further bacterial entry (10). Bacterial conjunctivitis can be clinically categorized as acute, hyperacute, and chronic, based on various features.

Acute Bacterial Conjunctivitis (Mucopurulent)

S. aureus, S. pneumoniae, and *Haemophilus influenzae* are the most common organisms that cause acute bacterial conjunctivitis. The acute conjunctivitis is marked by unilateral hyperemia, tearing, mucopurulent discharge, and matting of the eyelids (Fig. 13.2-5). *S. aureus* is the most common causative agent in adults and children; *S. pneumoniae* and *H. influenzae* occur more commonly in children than in adults (11). *H. influenzae* is often associated with systemic infections, such as upper respiratory disease, and usually requires systemic antibiotics, a fact that is well to emphasize to ophthalmologists, lest preoccupation with the eyes distract the ophthalmologist from the important systemic component of the problem, with potentially fatal

consequences if appropriate systemic therapy is not administered. *Viridans* streptococci and *Streptococcus pyogenes* can also produce an acute conjunctivitis, often with an associated membranous reaction. Gram-negative rods, other than *Haemophilus* species, rarely cause acute conjunctivitis in the immunocompetent patient, but certainly can do so in the immunocompromised individual.

Treatment of Acute Bacterial Conjunctivitis

Appropriate laboratory confirmation of the clinical diagnosis of bacterial conjunctivitis through cultures and isolation of the causative microbe is important, especially to guide treatment in the event that the first antibiotic chosen by the ophthalmologist is not curative. Although many mild conjunctival infections may resolve on their own, topical antibiotic treatment speeds resolution and reduces severity and morbidity (12). Treatment with a broad-spectrum bactericidal agent such as fluoroquinolone for 7 days is our preferred therapy for acute bacterial conjunctivitis. Appropriate alternative antimicrobial agents may be selected based on the culture results.

Hyperacute Bacterial Conjunctivitis (Purulent)

The most common cause of hyperacute conjunctivitis is *N. gonorrhoeae*; a less severe form can be seen with *Neisseria meningitidis* (13). This severe disease is most common in neonates, sexually active adolescents, and young adults. The most impressive characteristic is the copious, thick, yellowish-green purulent discharge (Fig. 13.2-6). Marked chemosis, painful hyperemia, and eyelid edema are seen. In contrast to most cases of bacterial conjunctivitis, there is often also tender preauricular adenopathy. There may be conjunctival membrane formation, and the condition may

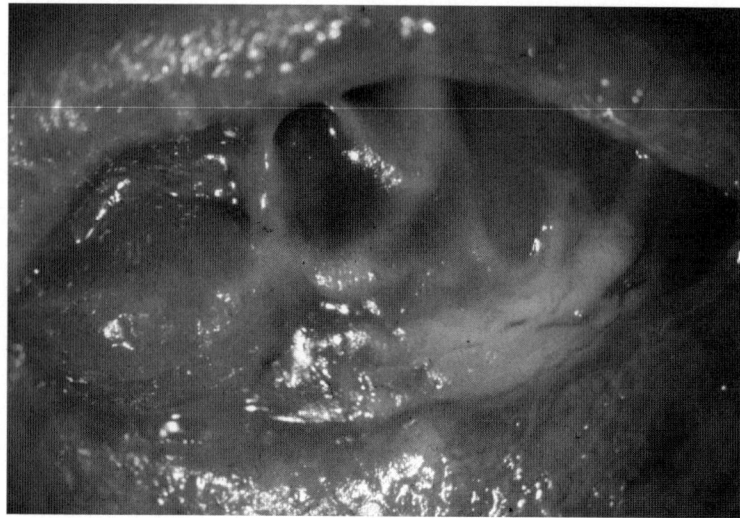

FIGURE 13.2-5. Purulent conjunctivitis, with obvious, intense conjunctival inflammation and a mucopurulent discharge, staining of smears from which gram-positive cocci were noted, and cultures of which grew abundant numbers of *Streptococcus pneumoniae*.

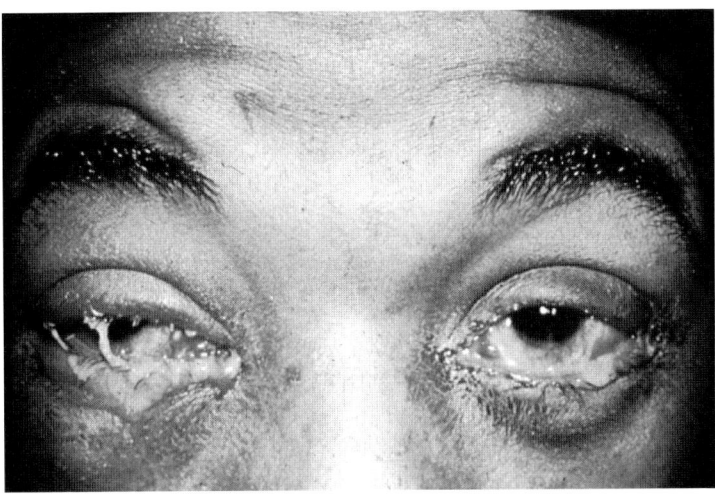

FIGURE 13.2-6. Bilateral purulent conjunctivitis in a patient who also had a urethral discharge. The conjunctival secretions and the urethral discharge all showed the same features: Gram-negative intracellular diplococci, which grew out as *Neisseria gonorrhoeae* in culture in chocolate agar plates.

rapidly progress to corneal infection, ulceration, and perforation; *Neisseria* species can penetrate an intact corneal epithelium in as little as 24 hours.

Treatment of Hyperacute Bacterial Conjunctivitis

Laboratory evaluation (Gram stain and culture) is critically important for patients with hyperacute conjunctivitis; the treatment for *Neisseria* conjunctivitis is different from that for almost every other bacterial entity: Systemic therapy is essential. Topical antibiotics can augment treatment, but systemic therapy is the mainstay of therapy for patients with *Neisseria* infections. The prevalence of penicillin-resistant organisms has made ceftriaxone the treatment of choice. Gonococcal conjunctivitis without corneal involvement may be treated with one intramuscular injection of ceftriaxone; corneal involvement usually requires hospitalization for a 3-day course of intravenous treatment. Patients with penicillin allergies may be treated with intramuscular spectinomycin or oral fluoroquinolones. Topical antibiotic ointments/solutions are also used, but the most important topical therapy is the frequent (every 30 to 60 minutes) irrigation (with saline) of the conjunctival surface and fornices to remove the inflammatory cells, proteolytic enzymes, and debris, which may be toxic to the ocular surfaces. And because up to one third of patients with gonococcal conjunctivitis also have chlamydia, concurrent treatment with tetracycline, doxycycline, or azithromycin may be indicated.

Chronic Bacterial Conjunctivitis

The most common causes of chronic bacterial conjunctivitis are the *Staphylococcus* species (14). Staphylococcal infections can be difficult to eradicate because the eyelid margins and surrounding skin are heavily populated with staphylococci. Associated exotoxins are thought to be responsible for the effect on the conjunctiva, lids, and cornea.

A diffuse hyperemia, minimal mucopurulent discharge, and conjunctival thickening with either a follicular or papillary reaction are common (Fig. 13.2-7). Eyelid involvement may be manifest as redness, telangiectasia, loss of lashes, thickening, and recurrent hordeola ("stye"), and ulceration at the base of the eyelashes may be seen. Maceration and ulceration of the inner and outer canthal angles may be seen in chronic blepharoconjunctivitis caused by *Moraxella* species. Chronic staphylococcal blepharoconjunctivitis may lead to marginal corneal ulceration likely due to an immune-mediated hypersensitivity reaction. Gram-negative bacteria are more common in cases of chronic conjunctivitis than they are in cases of acute conjunctivitis (15), and intestinal flora organisms can be associated with chronic conjunctivitis: *Proteus mirabilis* is the

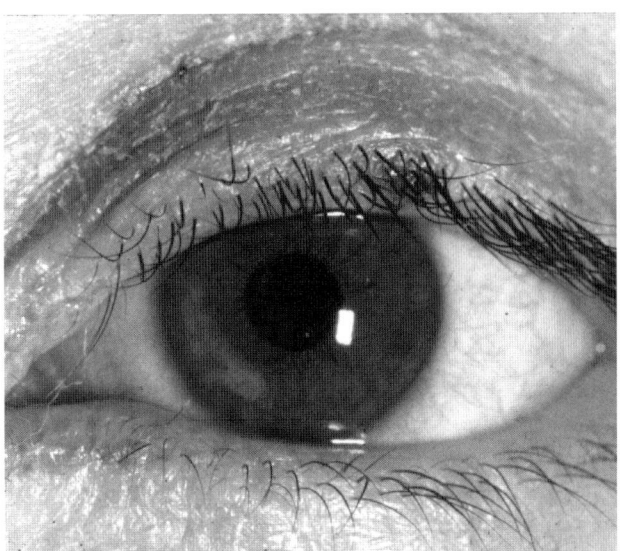

FIGURE 13.2-7. Chronic conjunctivitis with minimal discharge but with significant chronic ocular irritation. Note the characteristics of the lid skin superior to the superior lash line, with the scaly deposits in this patient with seborrheic blepharitis and chronic conjunctivitis.

most common, but *Klebsiella pneumoniae, Escherichia coli,* and *Serratia marcescens* have also been reported.

Treatment of Chronic Bacterial Conjunctivitis

Treatment of this type of bacterial conjunctivitis demands appropriate antibiotic therapy combined with aggressive lid hygiene and possible evaluation of the lacrimal system. Laboratory evaluation may guide appropriate antibiotic treatment. Lid hygiene, with warm compresses, eyelid scrubs using nontearing shampoo, and lid massage to "milk" the meibum daily from the meibomian glands and ductules (the meibomian orifices may harbor the bacteria) is an essential part of the appropriate care program. The lacrimal canaliculi/sac may also serve as a bacterial reservoir, and this possibility should be investigated, with irrigation and culture of material massaged from or refluxing from the lacrimal system. Antibiotic irrigation and oral antibiotic administration are required if lacrimal system participation in the harboring of the microbes is proven or even highly suspected. The staphylococcal hypersensitivity reaction in the cornea may require mild topical corticosteroid treatment to reduce the associated inflammation. Oral tetracycline or doxycycline may be beneficial in more severe infections.

NEONATAL CONJUNCTIVITIS (OPHTHALMIA NEONATORUM)

Any conjunctivitis occurring within the first 4 weeks of life is classified as ophthalmia neonatorum (16). Conjunctivitis in the newborn can be bacterial, viral, chlamydial, or a toxic reaction to chemicals. Specific identification of the cause is particularly important because there is often a potentially serious systemic infection associated with the localized ocular condition.

Chemical Conjunctivitis

In 1881, Credé introduced the use of topical silver nitrate as a prophylaxis against neonatal gonococcal infection (17). The self-limited conjunctivitis, present in approximately 90% of treated newborns, usually begins a few hours after delivery and resolves in 24 to 36 hours (18). The severity of the symptoms has been reduced with the advent of the single-use, buffered ampules; before availability of the ampules, the solution was kept in large, multidose bottles that allowed for a more concentrated dose when samples were taken from the bottom of the bottle. Although quite effective against *N. gonorrhoeae*, silver nitrate has little effect on bacteria and essentially no effect on chlamydia or viruses (19). Silver nitrate may injure epithelial cells to such a degree that they are more susceptible to the entry of other microbial agents. Silver nitrate may still be used in some areas, but many hospitals have changed their protocols to

erythromycin or tetracycline ointment. Povidone-iodine (Betadine) is inexpensive and quite effective against many microbial agents; it is becoming more widely used as a prophylaxis agent for newborns, especially in developing countries. The associated chemical conjunctivitis is similar in nature and course to that seen with silver nitrate.

Neonatal Chlamydial Conjunctivitis

The most frequent cause of neonatal conjunctivitis in the United States is *C. trachomatis* (20). Up to 3 million new cases of chlamydial infection occur annually (21), with 4% to 10% of all pregnant women in the United States diagnosed with chlamydia (22). Untreated mothers have infants with a 30% to 40% chance of conjunctivitis and a 10% to 20% chance for development of pneumonia (23). A unilateral or bilateral discharge begins 5 to 14 days after delivery. Chlamydial conjunctivitis in the neonate differs from that in the adult in a number of ways. No follicular response is seen in the neonate because of the immature immune system's inability to form such a reaction. The amount of mucopurulent discharge is greater in the neonate, as is the propensity to form membranes on the palpebral conjunctiva. The infection in neonates is more responsive to topical medications. Although the typical conjunctivitis is mild and self-limiting, severe cases may result in conjunctival scarring, with corneal pannus and scarring. If erythromycin or tetracycline ointment is applied to the conjunctival surface within an hour of delivery, the chance for development of chlamydial conjunctivitis is reportedly almost zero (23). However, topical medications cannot treat the pneumonitis and otitis media that can accompany the conjunctivitis. Two weeks of oral erythromycin is given to the newborn with laboratory-proven chlamydial conjunctivitis; a second course may be given if adequate resolution is not achieved with the initial treatment. The mother and her sexual partners must also be treated with oral erythromycin or tetracycline (caution in breast-feeding) for 1 week.

Gonococcal Conjunctivitis

The incidence of neonatal gonococcal conjunctivitis has dropped dramatically with effective prenatal screening and prophylactic antimicrobials in newborns. The clinical presentation begins with a hyperacute, bilateral conjunctival discharge appearing within the first 24 to 48 hours after delivery. The associated purulent exudate is often so profuse that it reappears immediately on cleaning of the eye. Conjunctival membrane formation is not uncommon. *N. gonorrhoeae* can penetrate an intact epithelial surface and quickly invade the cornea, causing ulceration, perforation, and even endophthalmitis if the infection is not promptly treated. Other localized gonococcal infections such as rhinitis and proctitis may be present, as well as the rare but more severe disseminated infection with arthritis, meningitis, pneumonia, and septicemia, which could lead to infant death. With resistance emerging against penicillin, tetracycline, and even the fluoroquinolones, a single dose of intramuscular or intravenous ceftriaxone 25 to 50 mg/kg (maximum 125 mg) is the preferred treatment (24). Hospitalization and hourly saline irrigation of the conjunctival fornices is recommended and if corneal involvement cannot be excluded owing to the copious exudation. Topical antibiotics are applied after each irrigation (25).

Nongonococcal Bacterial Conjunctivitis

Numerous organisms may cause bacterial conjunctivitis in the newborn. Most infections are associated with gram-positive organisms such as the *Staphylococcus* and *Streptococcus* species. Gram-negative organisms such as the *Haemophilus* and *Enterobacter* species, *E. coli*, *Proteus mirabilis*, *K. pneumoniae*, and *S. marcescens* have been less commonly implicated (26). Although *Pseudomonas aeruginosa* is a very rare cause of neonatal conjunctivitis, it deserves special consideration because of its ability rapidly to cause corneal ulceration and possible perforation (27).

Although symptoms can present any time within the first month of life, nongonococcal bacterial conjunctivitis usually presents 2 to 5 days after delivery. The clinical presentation consists of periorbital edema, chemosis, and conjunctival hyperemia and discharge. There is a higher incidence when obstruction of the nasolacrimal system is present. Conjunctival scrapings for Gram stain and cultures allow for appropriate treatment—usually erythromycin ointment for gram-positive organisms, and either gentamicin or tobramycin ointment for gram-negative organisms.

Viral (Herpetic) Conjunctivitis

Herpetic conjunctivitis in the neonate is rare but can be associated with significant morbidity and mortality. Herpes simplex virus (HSV) types 1 and 2 can be associated with conjunctivitis. In theory, HSV-1 can be transmitted to the infant through oral secretions from an adult or sibling with an active "cold sore," but the more common etiology is through contact with HSV-2 while passing through an infected birth canal. The edema, conjunctival injection, and tearing usually begin within the first 2 weeks of life and may be followed by keratitis or keratouveitis.

Diagnosis may be confirmed by Gram and Giemsa stains or viral cultures/immunoassays. Localized cases are treated with frequent trifluorothymidine drops for 1 week. Systemic cases, often marked by pneumonitis, meningitis, and septicemia, usually require systemic acyclovir. As with most causes of ophthalmia neonatorum, good prenatal care with frequent culture and treatment of infected mothers can significantly reduce the incidence of herpetic conjunctivitis of the newborn.

PARINAUD'S OCULOGLANDULAR CONJUNCTIVITIS

This classification describes a type of conjunctivitis that has numerous associated etiologies, including bacterial, viral, parasitic, mycobacterial, syphilitic, leukemic, and fungal agents. The red eye, mucopurulent discharge, and foreign-body sensation are accompanied by one or more granulomatous nodules on the palpebral conjunctiva. There is usually a visibly enlarged preauricular or submandibular lymph node on the involved side. This follicular conjunctivitis is associated with a fever and possible rash. Infection with *Bartonella henselae*, or cat-scratch disease, is the most common cause, but tularemia, tuberculosis, syphilis, lymphoma, mumps, Epstein-Barr virus, sporotrichosis, and sarcoidosis have all been implicated as potential causes.

Cat-scratch disease often resolves spontaneously, but 1 month of topical and systemic antibiotic therapy has been described. Because of the host of causative etiologies, an extensive workup may be warranted and the identified cause given the appropriate systemic treatment.

REFERENCES

1. Tullo AB, Richmond SJ, Easty PL. The presentation and incidence of paratrachoma in adults. *J Hyg (Lond)* 1981;87:63–69.
2. Heggie AD. Incidence and etiology of conjunctivitis in Navy recruits. *Mil Med* 1990;1:155.
3. Dawson CR, Schachter J. TRIC agent infections of the eye and genital tract. *Am J Ophthalmol* 1967;63:1288–1298.
4. Dawson CR, Jones BR, Tarizzo M. *Guide to trachoma control.* Geneva: World Health Organization, 1981:56.
5. Buchanan TM. Surface antigens pili. In: Roberts RB, ed. *The gonococcus.* New York: John Wiley, 1981:256–272.
6. Tabbara KF, AbuEl-Asrar AM, Al-Omar O, et al. Single-dose azithromycin in the treatment of trachoma: a randomized, controlled study. *Ophthalmology* 1996;103:842–846.
7. Buus DR, Pflugfelder SC, Schachter J, et al. Lymphogranuloma venereum conjunctivitis with a marginal corneal perforation. *Ophthalmology* 1988;95;799–802.
8. Perkins RE, Kundsin RB, Pratt MV. Bacteriology of normal and infected conjunctiva. *J Clin Microbiol* 1975;1:147–149.
9. Mannis MJ, Plotnick RD. Bacterial conjunctivitis. In: Tasman W, Jaeger EA, eds. *Duane's clinical ophthalmology*, vol 4. Philadelphia: Lippincott Williams & Wilkins, 1998:5.1–5.7.
10. Hyndiuk RA. Experimental *Pseudomonas* keratitis. *Trans Am Ophthalmol Soc* 1981;79:541–624.
11. Foulks GN, Austin R, Knowlton G. Clinical comparison of topical solutions containing trimethoprim in treating ocular surface bacterial infections. *J Ocul Pharmacol* 1988;4:111–115.
12. Leibowitz HM. Antibacterial effectiveness of ciprofloxacin 0.3% ophthalmic solution in the treatment of bacterial conjunctivitis. *Am J Ophthalmol* 1991;112:29S.
13. Brooke I, Bateman JB, Pettit TH. Meningococcal conjunctivitis. *Arch Ophthalmol* 1979;97:890–891.
14. Thygeson P, Kimura SJ. Chronic conjunctivitis. *Trans Am Acad Ophthalmol Otolaryngol* 1963;67:494–517.
15. Gutierrez EH. Bacterial infections of the eye. In: Locatcher-Khorazo D, ed. *Microbiology of the eye.* St. Louis: CV Mosby, 1972:5.

16. Chandler JW. Neonatal conjunctivitis. In: Tasman W, Jaeger EA, eds. Duane's clinical ophthalmology, vol 4. Philadelphia: Lippincott-Raven, 1995;6.1–6.7.

17. Cred<aae> CSF. Die Verhutung der Augenentzundung der Neugenborenen. *Arch Gynakkol* 1881;17:50–55.

18. Nishida H, Risemberg HM. Silver nitrate ophthalmic solution and chemical conjunctivitis. *Pediatrics* 1975;56:368–373.

19. Laga M, Plummer FA, Piot P, et al. Prophylaxis of gonococcal and chlamydial ophthalmia neonatorum: a comparison of silver nitrate and tetracycline. *N Engl J Med* 1988;318:653–657.

20. Sutphin JE Jr, Chodosh J, Dana MR, et al. Section 8: External disease and cornea. In: Liesegang TJ, Deutsch TA, Grand MG, eds. *Basic and clinical science course*. San Francisco: American Academy of Ophthalmology, 2002:161.

21. Centers for Disease Control. *Chlamydia trachomatis* infections: policy guidelines for prevention and control. *MMWR Morb Mortal Wkly Rep* 1985;34:53S–74S.

22. Holmes KK. The *Chlamydia* epidemic. *JAMA* 1981;245:1718–1723.

23. Harrison HR, English MG, Lee CK, et al. *Chlamydia trachomatis* infant pneumonitis: comparison with matched controls and other infant pneumonitis. *N Engl J Med* 1978;298:702–708.

24. Centers for Disease Control and Prevention. Sexually transmitted diseases treatment guidelines 2002. *MMWR Morb Mortal Wkly Rep* 2002;51:36–42.

25. Committee on Infectious Diseases, American Academy of Pediatrics. Gonococcal infections. In: Pickering LK, ed. *2000 Red Book: Report of the Committee on Infectious Diseases*, 25th ed. Elk Grove Village, IL: American Academy of Pediatrics, 2000:256.

26. Prentice MJ, Hutchinson GR, Taylor-Robinson D. A microbiological study of neonatal conjunctivae and conjunctivitis. *Br J Ophthalmol* 1977;61:601–607.

27. Burns RP, Rhodes DH Jr. *Pseudomonas* eye infection as a cause of death in premature infants. *Arch Ophthalmol* 1961;65:517–525.

14

VIRAL DISEASE OF THE OCULAR ANTERIOR SEGMENT: BASIC SCIENCE AND CLINICAL DISEASE

DEBORAH PAVAN-LANGSTON

VIRUSES

General Characteristics

Unlike bacteria, fungi, and protozoa, viruses are obligate intracellular parasites dependent on the biosynthetic pathways of the host cell for replication. They may infect bacteria, certain other viruses, plants, and animals. This chapter focuses on animal viruses that infect the eye directly or through systemic viral illness.

Classification and Structure

The parasitic nature of viruses is a result of their simple construction: a nucleic acid core of single- or double-stranded RNA or DNA within a protein coat (the capsid). Some viruses, such as the herpesviruses, have their nucleocapsid (core plus capsid) surrounded by a lipoprotein coat, the envelope. This envelope contains components of both host cell membrane and virus-specific protein subunits (Fig. 14-1). This combination confers immunologic immunity and is critical to early infection events. The most commonly used criteria of classification include both physical and biochemical characteristics, such as type of nucleic acid and capsid, size and morphology (e.g., presence or absence of an envelope), as well as tissue and host tropism and means of replication (1–4).

Virion size is measured in nanometers (nm), with the clinically important viruses ranging from 18 nm (parvoviruses, associated with adenovirus) to 300 nm (poxvirus). The repetitive structural protein pattern of the capsid reduces the amount of viral genome that must be used for encoding the capsid components. Animal viruses have three types of symmetry: icosahedral, helical , and complex symmetry, with the first two being the simplest in structure. The helical viruses have repeating subunits of capsids bound along the helical spiral of the viral nucleic acid core. The icosahedral symmetry is nearly spherical, with multiple axes of rotational symmetry around the core.

Replication

RNA viruses usually synthesize all viral products simultaneously, whereas DNA virus replication is divided into four multistep phases or periods (2–5). The *early phase* involves viral recognition of an appropriate target cell, attachment to and penetration of the cell plasma membrane, intracytoplasmic uncoating of the viral nucleic acid, and, with some viruses, delivery of the genome to the nucleus. Once the genome is uncoated in the early phase, infectivity and identifiable structure are lost, thus beginning the *eclipse period*. This period ends with appearance of new virions after virus assembly. The *late phase* includes synthesis of early messenger RNA (mRNA) and nonstructural proteins, replication of the genome, late mRNA and structural protein synthesis, posttranslational modification of protein such as phosphorylation, and assembly of new virions (ending the eclipse phase). The *latent period* includes the eclipse phase and ends with release of virus. One cell may produce 100,000 particles (virions), but only 1% to 10% may be infectious. The noninfectious defective virions result from mutations and errors in manufacture.

Viral recognition of and binding to a host cell is a function of the types of receptors on the cell species (host range), the cell type (tissue tropism), or both. For example, the herpesvirus Epstein-Barr virus (EBV), which causes mononucleosis, has a very limited host range and tissue tropism because it binds to the C3d receptor on human B lymphocytes. The attachment structure for a capsid virus (no envelope) may be part of the capsid or a protein extending from it. The receptors on the cell may be proteins or carbohydrates on glycoproteins or glycolipids. Enveloped viruses have specific glycoproteins as attachment structures.

Most viruses enter the cell by receptor-mediated endocytosis through cell endosomes or by direct injection into the cell through viropexis. After uncoating, the genome of DNA viruses (with the exception of poxviruses) is delivered to the cell nucleus, whereas most RNA viruses remain in the cytoplasm for the entire replicative cycle. Regardless of

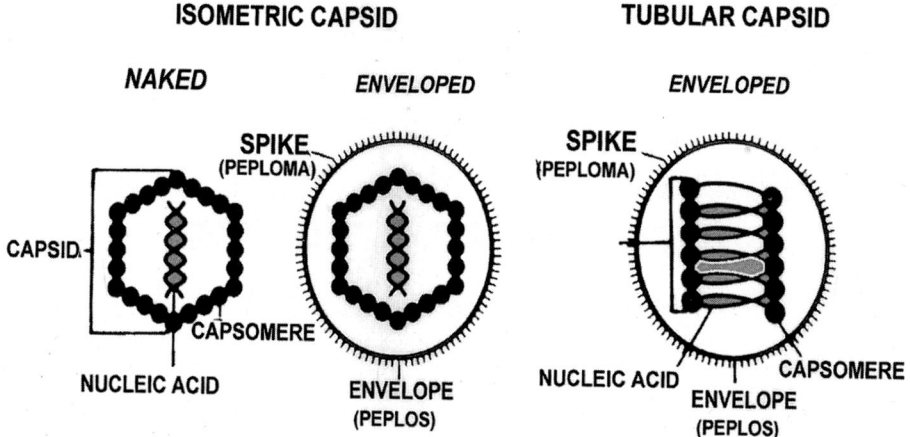

FIGURE 14-1. Diagrams of viral taxonomic groups discussed in this chapter, showing relative size and structure. (Adapted in part from Kinchington P. Virology. In: Smolin G, Thoft R, eds. *The cornea*, 3rd ed. Boston: Little, Brown 1994:169–183.)

whether the infecting nucleic acid is DNA or RNA, the critical step of translation depends on the production of mRNA using the viral genome as the template. The host cell enzymes for making mRNA from a DNA template are all intranuclear and therefore inaccessible to RNA viruses, which are all cytoplasmic. Host cells lack the enzymes to make mRNA from an RNA template. As a result, positive-stranded RNA viruses serve as their own mRNA templates. With negative-stranded RNA viruses, such as human immunodeficiency virus (HIV), the RNA polymerase, reverse transcriptase, facilitates the making of positive-stranded mRNA, leading to viral RNA production (2).

Virion assembly depends on where the genome replication occurred and whether the final product is a naked capsid or an enveloped virus. Capsid viruses may be assembled around the new genomes or built as empty structures to be filled with the genome later in the cycle. With enveloped viruses, after the nucleocapsid is formed, new viral glycoproteins are sent to cellular membranes by vesicular transport. The envelope is acquired after the nucleocapsid associates with the viral glycoprotein–containing regions of host cell membranes in the budding process. This process may occur at the plasma membrane with release (RNA viruses), in the endoplasmic reticulum en route to the surface (flaviviruses), or at the nuclear membrane with release into the endoplasmic reticulum and transport to the surface. In all cases the virion is released by exocytosis, cell lysis, or by cell-to-cell bridges (herpesviruses) (1–4).

IMMUNE RESPONSE TO VIRAL INFECTION

Host immune response to viral invasion involves both nonspecific (natural) and specific (acquired) defenses (4,6–8). The nonspecific category includes the complement system, primitive cellular immunity (macrophages and natural killer cells), and interferon, none of which requires previous exposure to the viral antigens. The interferons, in particular, inhibit virtually all phases of viral infection from penetration to assembly, but interferons may also cause a damaging inflammatory response.

Specific immune responses take a few days to begin and are stimulated by viral proteins that are part of the virus particle or on the surface of infected cells, resulting in B- and T-lymphocyte activation. The viral antigens react with macrophages with type II histocompatibility antigens on the surface, thus precipitating both humoral (B cells) and cellular (T cells) immunity. Neutralizing antibodies bind virus, making it noninfectious. Other antibodies do not affect infectivity but bind the virus and stimulate phagocytosis or the complement system, which result in viral death. Complement may lyse free virus and virus-infected cells in the presence of antibody (4,6–8).

Specific cell-mediated immunity (CMI) includes activation of cytotoxic T-lymphocytes and delayed-type hypersensitivity T cells by viral proteins on the host cell membrane, not by soluble antigen (6–8). The cytotoxic T lymphocytes destroy cells and present viral antigen on their cell membrane surfaces. Delayed-type T cells secrete lymphokines chemotactic for macrophages and neutrophils. Helper T cells facilitate both B- and T-cell activity, and suppressor T cells downregulate the antiviral immune response. As is noted later in the discussion of herpetic disease, the immune response may, on occasion, be more destructive than the infectious disease itself.

LABORATORY DIAGNOSTIC TECHNIQUES

The general laboratory methods used to confirm clinical diagnosis include (a) direct-view morphology, (b) immunomorphology, (c) immunologic virology, (d) viral culture, (e) serology, and (f) molecular virology (1–3, 9,10).

Direct-view morphology includes cytologic testing and electron microscopy. Scrapings are taken directly from the lesions for cytology and smeared on a glass slide, fixed in Bouin's solution for 1 hour, and stained with Giemsa, Tzanck, hematoxylin and eosin, or Papanicolaou stain before light microscopy examination. This technique is useful for rapid diagnosis of the herpesviruses, herpes simplex virus (HSV), varicella zoster virus (VZV), and cytomegalovirus (CMV), as well as measles and rabies infection; it is not as specific or sensitive as viral isolation or immunotesting. Typical changes include change in cell morphology, cell lysis, vacuoles, syncytia, and inclusion bodies. Syncytia are multinucleated giant cells formed by viral fusion of adjacent cells. The herpesviruses, HIV, and paramyxoviruses induce this fusion. Inclusion bodies are either histologic changes in the cells due to viral components or virus-induced changes in cell structure. Cowdry type A inclusions, seen in HSV and VZV infections, are brilliant, large intranuclear inclusions surrounded by a halo separating them from the nuclear membrane. CMV may induce nuclear owl's eye inclusions, and adenovirus produces smudgy eosinophilic nuclear inclusions. Molluscum contagiosum virus and poxvirus may cause eosinophilic cytoplasmic inclusions, and rabies may cause Negri bodies, rabies virus inclusions in brain tissue (1–3,10).

Electron microscopy is not a standard laboratory test but can be very useful if sufficient viral particles (10^6 to 10^7) are present, and particularly if virus-specific antibody has been added to the sample to cause viral clumping, thus facilitating detection and identification of the virus (immunoelectron microscopy). Definitive diagnosis often cannot be made, however, because many viruses such as the herpesviruses are indistinguishable by electron microscopy.

Immunomorphology includes the immunofluorescence and immunoperoxidase techniques. Direct, indirect, and anti-complement immunofluorescent staining are used for detection of viral antigens in infected cells. Scrapings are taken from the lesion and smeared on a glass slide. In the direct method, the slide is treated with fluorescein-conjugated virus-specific antibody, and incubated for 30 to 60 minutes before buffered saline washing. Reading is under fluorescent microscopy. This is an easier and faster technique than the indirect, but it is less sensitive. In the indirect method, step one is covering the slide with unlabeled virus-specific antibody, step two washing and applying normal serum to decrease nonspecific antibody binding, and step 3 coating the slide with a fluorescein-labeled, anti-immunoglobulin conjugate. This is more sensitive because more label can be bound to the antigen. Immunofluorescence is routinely used to detect herpesvirus, adenovirus, CMV, mumps, measles, respiratory syncytial virus, and rabies (1,2,10,11).

Immunoperoxidase is a commonly used staining technique that uses antibody conjugated with enzymes such as horseradish peroxidase rather than fluorescein as an indicator. The technique is similar to direct immunofluorescence after normal serum overlay to decrease nonspecific staining. The peroxidase enzyme produces an orange-brown precipitate localized at the binding sites in the specimen. This technique has the advantage of being more permanent and being read under light rather than fluorescent microscopy, thus allowing viewing of adjacent tissues for histopathologic analysis (1,3,10–12).

Immunologic virology involves enzyme immunoassay (EIA) for the detection of viral antigen on the cell surface or within the cell. The enzyme-linked immunosorbent assay (ELISA), radioimmunoassay, and latex agglutination are used to detect virus or antigen released from infected cells (1,2,10). ELISA tests come in a variety of commercially available formats for detection of several viruses by solid-phase or membrane-phase technique. In the solid-phase test, virus-specific antibody is bound to a solid surface such as a plastic microtiter well or tube. In membrane tests, the solid surface is replaced by a membrane. The specimen is put in and captured by the antibody. It is then detected by binding of an enzyme-linked antibody to the antigen, washing, and adding a colorimetric substrate of the enzyme. Solid-phase tests are best suited for batch testing, whereas membrane tests may be used in single tests with little equipment in the physician's office to detect HSV types 1 and 2 (differentiating from VZV), CMV, adenovirus, and rubella (13,14). Advances in ELISA methodology include fluorescent and enzymatic labels, antibody-capture formats, and monoclonal antibodies, thus making ELISA a frontrunner in routine serologic assay techniques.

Viral culture and isolation is still the gold standard of diagnostic virology. Tissue culture cells are used to grow viruses. Primary cell cultures are cells trypsinized free from animal tissue and grown in monolayers in tubes or flasks. Diploid cell lines are a single cell type that may be passed in sequential generations several but a finite number of times before dying out. Tumor cell lines originate from patient cancers and are immortalized, being passed indefinitely without senescing. Human fetal diploid cells are fibroblastic and support the culture of a wide variety of viruses, including HSV, VZV, CMV, adenovirus, picornavirus. Hep-2, a continuous cell line from a human cancer, also supports many viruses such as adenovirus, HSV, and respiratory syncytial virus. Primary monkey kidney cells are excellent for growth of myxoviruses, some adenoviruses, and enterovirus (3,10).

After tissue culture inoculation of the clinical specimen, the virus may first be detected with light microscopy by changes in the cell monolayer, called *cytopathic effect*. This is usually a rounding up and ballooning of infected cells that may pull away from the monolayer to leave open "plaques." HSV can produce cytopathic effect within 1 to 2 days, whereas CMV, adenovirus, and rubella may take up to 1 month. The virus is identified by virus-specific antibody tests such as immunofluorescence, immunoperoxidase, EIA, or ELISA tests. These techniques may even be used in the pre–cytopathic effect stage to speed up diagnosis (1,13).

Serologic test methods involve both quantitative and qualitative evaluation of humoral immunity and antibody production. This may be done by using specific viral antibodies to identify unknown viral isolates or antigens, as noted in the discussion of viral tissue culture, or antibody may be identified using panels of known antigens or for the quantitation of antibody in the sera of infected patients. Methods used for antibody quantitation, discussed previously or elsewhere in this chapter, include viral neutralization, complement fixation, hemagglutination inhibition, ELISA, Western immunoblotting, immunofluorescence, latex particle agglutination, and gel immunodiffusion. Complement-fixing antibodies are quite transient, whereas neutralizing antibodies are often present for years after infection.

ELISA tests are used for viral antigen detection, but are particularly useful for detection of immunoglobulin M (IgM) in the presence of IgG. Only IgM antibodies, if present in the serum, are bound to the solid phase and therefore easily detectable. This is important diagnostically because IgM antibodies appear early during infection and last only a few weeks, whereas IgG appears after 1 or 2 weeks but lasts for years. Quantitative documentation of a fourfold rise in either IgM or IgG strongly supports the diagnosis. Serum should be drawn as soon as possible in the acute illness and again 2 to 3 weeks later for comparative titers. Finding a positive IgM in a single specimen may also be diagnostic in a very ill patient (e.g. Ebola virus) or a patient with ongoing infection (e.g., HIV). Elevation of IgM may also indicate reactivation of a latent infection. IgM detection is most useful in diagnosis of VZV, EBV, CMV, measles, rubella, coxsackieviruses, and hepatitis. Finding IgM in a newborn is diagnostic of intrauterine infection because IgM does not cross the placental barrier (2,4,10,15).

Viral neutralization testing is of value only if a change in titer can be demonstrated in two samples, acutely and at 3 to 4 weeks, because these antibodies last for years after an infection. Change in titer is shown by adding sequential dilutions of serum to tissue culture growing the virus. The titer is the reciprocal of the highest dilution at which the viral cytopathic effect in inhibited.

Complement fixation testing is based on the fact that complement, a complex of multiple plasma proteins that act sequentially to lyse infected cells, combines with viral antigen only in the presence of virus-specific antibody. Antigen and complement are mixed with the patient's serum. If complement is bound by the effective complex, there will be no hemolysis when this is mixed with hemolysin-sensitized sheep red cells. If complement is free because the antigen and antiserum did not match, there will be hemolysis. The test can be arduous and yield nonspecific results.

Agglutination tests detect viral antigens based on the visible clumping of particles, such as latex, red blood cells, or polystyrene, to which virus-specific antibody has been absorbed. This is not commonly used in ocular disease diagnosis. Agglutination of red blood cells occurs in the presence of vaccinia, adenovirus, rubella, mumps, measles, and Newcastle disease. Acute and convalescent host serum is added to a known viral antigen concentration. If the serum inactivates the virus antigen, there will be no agglutination and diagnosis is made. A diagnosis of primary infection, however, requires a fourfold rise in serum antibody titer between acute and convalescent sera. This test is usually done at reference laboratories.

Molecular virology uses recombinant DNA or RNA technology in highly specific tests to detect viral nucleic acids rather than viral protein antigen. Genetic structure and sequence are the distinguishing factors of the family, type, and strain of virus. The unique electrophoretic patterns of RNA viruses or the DNA fragment lengths obtained through restriction endonuclease treatment of nucleic acid samples yield highly specific and sensitive diagnostic data. DNA probes can be made with sequences complementary to specific regions of a known viral genome. These probes are labeled radioactively or with fluorescein or peroxidase, bind the complementary sites in the viral DNA under investigation, and are then read against known probes and viral nucleic acid by autoradiography or under fluorescent or light microscopy. Genetic sequences can also be detected in fixed tissue by *in situ* hybridization, thus revealing cellular location of the nucleic acid. Other detection techniques include Southern blot (DNA virus) and Northern blot (RNA virus), in which patient viral genome fragments are blotted onto nitrocellulose filters and then detected on the filter by their hybridization to DNA or RNA/DNA probes with autoradiography or EIA-like methods (1–3).

Amplification techniques have been developed to further the application and usefulness of this technique. The best known is the *polymerase chain reaction* (PCR). This technique allows a single copy of a genome to be amplified *in vitro* more than a millionfold in just a few hours (16). This amplification allows the detection and identification of very small amounts of viral nucleic acids using labeled probes in a hybridization assay. PCR can also be modified to detect viral RNA by use of reverse transcriptase to convert RNA to DNA before running the sample. A new version of this test, the real-time quantitative PCR, is an amplification reaction performed using fluorescent probes or DNA intercalating dyes that increase in fluorescence as it quantifies the pathogen load (17). It has a sensitivity of fewer than 10 organisms for all pathogens. Nucleic acid hybridization is quickly becoming the procedure of choice for diagnostic testing in many laboratories.

CHARACTERISTICS OF THE MAJOR OCULAR VIRAL PATHOGEN FAMILIES

Herpesviruses

Family: Herpesviridae
Subfamilies:

Alphaherpesvirinae
Genus: Simplexvirus (HSV types 1 and 2)
Genus: Varicellovirus (VZV)
Betaherpesvirinae
Genus: Cytomegalovirus
Genus: Roseolovirus
Genus: Human herpesvirus 7
Gammaherpesvirinae (lymphoproliferative)
Genus: Lymphocryptovirus (EBV)
Genus: Human herpesvirus 8 (Kaposi's sarcoma)

The members of this family include HSV types 1 and 2, VZV, CMV, EBV, human herpesviruses 6 (HHV6, roseola), 7 (HHV7, lymphoproliferative) and 8 (HHV8, Kaposi's sarcoma). These DNA viruses have several characteristics in common, including morphology, mode of replication, ability to cause lytic disease or establish recurrent and latent infections, ability to encode proteins and enzymes in interaction with the host cell, and CMI as the key to control infection but, in some cases, worsen disease (2–4).

These large (150 to 200 nm), enveloped viruses contain a linear, double-stranded DNA within an icosadeltahedral capsid that is surrounded by a glycoprotein-containing envelope derived from the host cell membrane (Fig. 14-2). The HSV

DNA VIRUSES

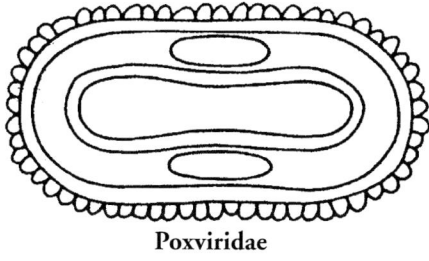

Poxviridae

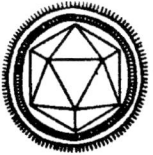 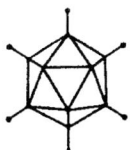 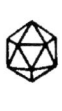

Herpesviridae   Adenoviridae   Papovaviridae

RNA VIRUSES

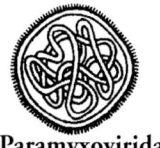 

Paramyxoviridae   Retroviridae   Picoma-viridae   Togaviridae

FIGURE 14-2. Diagram showing structural components of naked and enveloped viruses. (Adapted in part from Kinchington P. Virology. In: Smolin G, Thoft R, eds. *The cornea*, 3rd ed. Boston: Little, Brown 1994:169–183.)

genome encodes approximately 80 proteins, half of which are needed for viral replication and the others for the virus' interaction with host cells and an immune response. The glycoproteins are encoded by the virus for purposes of attachment, fusion, replication, and avoiding immune control. The last works by IgG binding to viral gE/gI glycoproteins, thereby camouflaging virus and virus-infected cells and reducing antibody effectiveness.

HSV-1 and HSV-2 are spread by vesicle fluid, saliva, and vaginal secretions. They may infect most types of human and nonhuman cell types, causing lytic infection of epithelial cells and fibroblasts and latent infection in neurons. Cells that support latent infection transcribe only certain genes without genome replication. With reactivation there is progression to early and late gene expression, leading to lytic infection and cell death (3). Triggers of reactivation are not completely understood. In animal models of latency, corneal intrastromal injection, neurosurgical disturbance of the fifth cranial nerve, iontophoresis, and corneal trauma may all induce reactivation, but the final common pathway for this reactivation is unknown. The resulting clinical disease may vary in severity depending on neurovirulence and pathogenicity, and variations in host system response (4,18,19).

Transcription of the viral genome and protein synthesis proceeds in three phases: (a) immediate early protein (alpha) gene transcription through DNA-binding proteins; (b) early proteins (beta) producing more transcription factors and enzymes such as DNA polymerase and thymidine kinase (TK); and (c) late proteins (gamma) with production of structural proteins triggered by genome replication. The remainder of reproduction proceeds as described previously in the section on Replication. HSV production of TK in the beta phase is a critical factor that makes it susceptible to several antiviral agents. If the infection is to be a latent one (i.e., neuronal), the only region of the genome transcribed generates the latency-associated transcripts. These RNAs are not translated into protein and replication does not proceed until there is viral reactivation (3,19).

VZV primary infection manifests as chickenpox, which is acquired through the respiratory tract and disseminated by viremia, ultimately becoming latent in the sensory ganglia. As reactivated disease, it is zoster or shingles. The virus is morphologically identical to HSV but, unlike the latter, there is no reported antigenic variation among VZV strains (20,21). VZV and HSV share several minor antigens, at least six glycoproteins, replicative pathways, the ability to establish latent neuronal infection and recurrent disease, characteristic blister-like skin and mucous membrane lesions, the encoding of TK that makes it susceptible to several antiviral drugs, and control of infection by CMI (2,3,5). The glycoproteins are potent inducers of antibody and may be an integral part of HSV and VZV vaccines in the future (22). These herpesviruses also share a role as the most common infectious causes of anterior segment visual loss in the developed world (23). VZV is fastidious and hard to recover from clinical samples. Human fibroblast lines are best for tissue culture recovery, and likelihood of recovery is increased by culturing vesicular fluid located around the eye or on the V-1 dermatome. Cytopathic effect appears between 5 and 28 days in culture. Because of this difficulty, VZV is usually identified by immunofluorescence, viral neutralization, or PCR (1,10,13,24–27). The FAMA test (fluorescent antibody to membrane antigen) is useful for diagnosis of skin scrapings or biopsies. Cytopathologic results are similar to those of HSV, with Cowdry-type intranuclear inclusions and syncytia.

CMV is a lymphotrophic herpesvirus and contains the largest genome in this family. It infects up to 2.5% of all newborns and 50% of the world's adult population and is a frequent cause of congenital defects and an opportunistic virus in immunocompromised patients (2,10,28). Although CMV rarely causes problems in the immunocompetent host (other than CMV mononucleosis), with the dramatic rise in the number of immunosuppressed patients due to HIV infection and iatrogenic immunosuppression in the past two decades, CMV retinitis has become a major cause of visual morbidity and vision loss (29–31). All layers of the retina are damaged, and both intranuclear and intracytoplasmic inclusions are present.

Unlike other viruses, where either DNA or RNA are carried into the host cell, research indicates that CMV carries mRNA in the virion and that this is the source of infection. The virus replicates only in human cells, but these include a wide variety such as epithelial cells, fibroblasts, and macrophages. It establishes both persistent and latent infection, often asymptomatic, in mononuclear leukocytes, bone marrow, kidney, and heart. The virus has been isolated from virtually all forms of body fluid, from tears to blood or breast milk. Transmission is by the congenital, oral, and sexual routes, blood transfusion, and tissue transplantation. Diagnosis is made by a wide variety of tests such as isolation, immunoassays, and PCR testing, as discussed earlier. Serology is useful only for primary infection because of the persistence of the infection. Histopathology or cytology may show the diagnostic "owl's eye" inclusion body (32,33).

EBV is the epitome of a lymphotrophic virus. It infects the B lymphocyte (B cell) and some epithelial cells of the nasopharynx, and causes or is causally associated with a variety of diseases such as infectious mononucleosis, endemic Burkitt's lymphoma, Hodgkin's disease, and nasopharyngeal carcinoma. This limited tissue tropism is a result of the limited cellular expression of its receptor. By the third decade of life, 90% of adults are positive for EBV antibody (2). Contagion rate is low, with most cases of mononucleosis contracted by intimate contact with an asymptomatic person shedding EBV from the oropharyngeal epithelium. Active infection may persist for years in mucosa-associated lymphoid tissue (34,35). The virus has never been isolated from tear film.

EBV encodes more than 70 proteins, various groups of which are expressed depending on type of infection: replicative, latent, or immortalization. During replicative infection, transcription and translation of the ZEBRA transcriptional activator protein activates the early viral genes, leading ultimately to synthesis of viral DNA, capsid, and glycoproteins. The viral proteins produced during the replicative infection are serologically defined as early antigen, viral capsid antigen, and membrane antigen, all of which are diagnostically useful in serologic testing (3,4). If the infection is a nonpermissive B-cell disease (latent), the cells contain only a few circular, plasmid-like EBV genomes that replicate only when the cell replicates. Immediate early genes are expressed along with Epstein-Barr nuclear antigens, which are also diagnostically useful. EBV is unique among herpesviruses in its ability to immortalize B cells.

The Epstein-Barr nuclear antigens and certain membrane proteins are DNA-binding proteins essential for establishing and maintaining infection and immortalization. They activate cell growth and prevent cell apoptosis (programmed cell death). The EBV genome is an episome in latent state and continuously expresses EBV nuclear antigen. B-cell production results in an IgM antibody to the Paul-Bunnell antigen, the heterophile antibody, another protein of diagnostic use. T cells usually control B-cell proliferation but, if control is lost, lymphoma will develop (2,3).

HHV8 DNA is most likely transmitted sexually. It has been detected in 95% of biopsy specimens from Kaposi's sarcoma, primary effusion lymphoma, and multicentric Castleman's disease through PCR testing and Southern blot analysis (36). It has also been found in the peripheral monocytes of HIV-positive patients. The virus may infect B cells, null cells, vascular endothelial cells, and perivascular spindle cells (37). HHV8 encodes proteins homologous to human proteins that enhance the growth and prevent apoptosis of infected and surrounding cells. This in turn promotes growth of polyclonal Kaposi's sarcoma cells in immunosuppressed patients. It is also found in the B cells of approximately 10% of immunocompetent people.

Adenoviruses

Family: Adenoviridae
Genus: Mastadenovirus (mammals), human adenovirus

There are approximately 100 serotypes of adenovirus, of which at least 47 infect humans. They are subtyped on the basis of DNA homology and hemagglutination patterns into six subgroups, A through F. There is 90% genomic homology within an adenoviral type and 20% homology between adenoviral types. Adenoviruses are nonenveloped, icosadeltahedron viruses (70 to 90 nm in diameter) with linear double-stranded DNA at the core. The capsid is made of 240 capsomeres that consist of hexons and 12 pentons. Each penton has a fiber that contains the viral attachment proteins, which have viral specific antigens and can also act as hemagglutinins (38,39) (Fig. 14-2).

The viruses are highly epitheliotropic with a small host range. The diseases caused include respiratory and gastrointestinal infections, hepatitis, cystitis, and keratoconjunctivitis. These viruses are endemic and cause illness year round. Ocular disease is transmitted primarily through direct contact with infected material such as saliva fomites or contaminated towels, or through bathing in a contaminated swimming pool. Immunity is lifelong but type specific (4,38,39). Replication of a single virus takes approximately 36 hours and produces 10,000 progeny. The virus binds to the host cell surface first by the penton fiber attaching to a glycoprotein, and then enters the cell by receptor-mediated endocytosis in a coated vesicle. The virus lyses the endosome and the DNA is delivered to the cell nucleus. Genomic transcription occurs on both viral DNA strands and in both directions at different times in the cycle. Early transcription produces 20 nonstructural proteins that stimulate cell growth and viral DNA replication. After early replication ends there is concurrent production of viral DNA in the nucleus mediated by DNA polymerase, and late transcription of structural proteins. Capsid proteins are produced in the cytoplasm and the capsids are then transported to the nucleus for DNA insertion. The process is inefficient, with only 1 infectious unit produced per 11 to 2300. The virus is released on cell lysis (4,38,39).

Diagnosis may be made in the office or in the laboratory. Adenoclone (Cambridge Bioscience, Worcester, MA) is an EIA that detects adenoviral antigen on conjunctival swabs (40). It is simple, rapid (1 hour), and inexpensive, and is 81% sensitive and 100% specific if taken within 1 week of disease onset. Laboratory diagnosis can be made by direct detection in clinical specimens or by viral isolation on human embryonic kidney or human HeLa or HEp-2 cell lines, with subsequent identification using fluorescent antibody or ELISA tests. Serotyping may be done after isolation from tissue culture. Other tests include serology of acute and convalescent sera, especially hemagglutination inhibition. A fourfold rise in antibody titer is diagnostic of adenoviral infection (4,10).

Poxviruses

Family: Poxviridae
Subfamily: Chordopoxvirinae
Genus: Orthopoxvirus: vaccinia, smallpox (variola)
Genus: Molluscipoxvirus: molluscum contagiosum virus, orf

The members of this virus family are the largest and most complex of all animal viruses, being almost visible on light microscopy and measuring 230 × 300 nm in a morphologically complex, bricklike shape with (3,41). The natural hosts for poxvirus that can infect humans are vertebrates in the bovine family. With the exception of smallpox and molluscum contagiosum, human infection occurs through accidental or occupational exposure. Smallpox and molluscum are spread from human to human. Smallpox is very contagious and spread primarily by the respiratory route and to some extent by contact with dried, but living virus, on cloth or other materials. Dissemination in the host then occurs by lymphatic and cell-associated viremia. Molluscum is spread by direct physical contact or by contact with infected material such as a towel. The lesions do not spread extensively.

Poxvirus replication is unique among the DNA agents in that the entire cycle occurs in the host cell cytoplasm. The virion therefore carries several enzymes, including DNA-dependent RNA polymerase, to allow this cytoplasmic replication. After fusion into the cytoplasm through host phagocytic vacuoles, viral RNA polymerase transcribes approximately half of the viral genome into early mRNA. The subsequent protein products include an enzyme that completes uncoating, plus TK and other enzymes (42,43). After uncoating, DNA synthesis begins and host macromolecular synthesis is stopped during this 1.5- to 6-hour period. The areas of DNA construction are seen as inclusion bodies in the cytoplasm. The viral DNA genome is then transcribed, but only late mRNAs are translated to structural proteins. Assembly of DNA and capsid then occurs and is completed by *de novo* synthesis of viral membrane by the poxviruses themselves. This viral membrane confers infectivity. Nucleocapsids that bud through taking just the host membrane are not infectious (43) (Fig. 14-2).

Smallpox and vaccinia have only recently become infectious agents of concern again, the former having been eliminated from the world by 1980. Now, however, it is a potential bioterrorism agent. Along with its preventative, vaccinia vaccination, both of these agents are of importance in ocular disease such as cellulitis, conjunctivitis, and acute or chronic keratitis or iritis. Useful diagnostic tests are not routine serologic tests but ELISA, radioimmunoassay, or monoclonal antibody assays (2,10,41).

Human Immunodeficiency Virus

Family: Retroviridae
Subfamily: Lentivirinae
Genus: Lentivirus (HIV types 1 and 2)
Genus: HTLV-BLV (human T-lymphotropic virus types 1 and 2–bovine leukemia virus)

The Lentivirinae, as the name implies, are characterized by very long incubation and latency periods (2,44). These medium-sized viruses (80 to 130 nm) have a positive-sense, single-stranded RNA genome, the viral enzymes protease, reverse transcriptase, and integrase, and a viral capsid.

There is broad genetic variability because of a very high level of virus turnover and low fidelity of reverse transcripts (2,10,45). These viruses share tissue tropism for the hematopoietic and neurologic systems and the ability to cause immunosuppression: acquired immunodeficiency syndrome (AIDS) in the case of HIV. More than 30 million adults and 10 million children are infected worldwide. In the United States and Europe, HIV-1 is the most common etiologic agent of this severe and often fatal illness. HIV-2 is more common in western Africa. It has a 55% homology with HIV-1 but causes a more benign clinical course with a much lower viral load in infected persons compared with HIV-1. Furthermore, HIV-2 is less frequently transmitted either sexually or vertically through a family.

Both HIV type 1 and 2 genomes have three genes common to all retroviruses: *gag*, *pol*, and *env*. The cell-derived viral membrane contains transmembrane glycoproteins gp41 and gp120, crucial to viral adherence. Gp120 binds to CD4 receptors on human T lymphocytes, and gp41 is necessary for fusion. After penetration, the virus uncoats and transcription of viral RNA proceeds through reverse transcriptase. HIV DNA then inserts itself into the host cell genome. The virus may remain latent, producing little or no mRNA, or be active, with virus-encoded RNA and proteins produced. Viral assembly takes place in the cytoplasm and viral exit is by budding through the host membrane (2,4,45,46) (Fig. 14-2).

Transmission is largely through unprotected sex and intravenous (IV) drug use with contaminated needles. Others at risk are recipients of blood transfusions and newborns of infected mothers. There is currently no preventive vaccine. The virus infects a variety of tissues, including blood, brain, lymph nodes, marrow, skin, and bowel (47). In the eye, it is permissive for anterior and posterior segment opportunistic infections and may itself cause disease of various structures of the anterior segment.

Diagnosis may be made by viral isolation (which takes up to 5 weeks), or the much faster techniques of serology or nucleic acid detection (2,10,48). The reliability of diagnosis is affected by the length of time between transmission and the time of testing. Serology, such as the enzyme immunoassay for IgG antibodies to HIV using viral lysate or recombinant proteins and the antigen, is of great value as a rapid and sensitive screening test. ELISA is also very sensitive for HIV-1, HIV-2, and HTLV, and is used for blood donation screening. Because of its lower specificity, however, the results are always confirmed by Western blot, immunoprecipitation, or indirect immunofluorescence. Western blot detects antibody to the specific HIV antigens p24, gp41, or gp 120. Antibody may be detected within 2 to 6 weeks of transmission but may take longer. If results are still equivocal, as in an early infection, detection of viral RNA by PCR is a reliable method of diagnosis (1,10,49). These immunologic/molecular virologic tests produce results in hours to a day or two.

The risk for development of AIDS in asymptomatic HIV-positive patients may be predicted with reasonable reliability by determining the number CD4$^+$ helper T lymphocytes and viral load in the peripheral blood (CD4$^+$ helper lymphocytes <200 cells/mL, viral burden >10^7 plasma HIV RNA copies/mL). This test, coupled with testing plasma HIV RNA levels, is a useful guideline for eligibility for antiretroviral or other antiviral therapy (e.g., for CMV retinitis), predicting disease progression, and monitoring disease control.

Human Papillomaviruses

Family: Papovaviridae
Genus: Papillomavirus: human papillomavirus (HPV)

The papillomaviruses are common throughout nature, highly epitheliotropic, genus-specific, and found most often among higher vertebrates (2,4,50). In humans, the viruses have been associated with warts, dysplasias, and carcinomas of the genital tract and conjunctiva (51,52). Mucosal areas are infected by HPVs 6, 11, 16, and 18, whereas skin sites are infected by HPVs 1 through 4. The viruses cannot be grown in tissue culture. Differentiation of the 70 different HPV types and understanding the reproductive cycle has been aided by molecular and immunologic virologic technology (1,3,10).

HPV is a nonenveloped, relatively small, 45- to 55-nm icosahedral structure containing linear double-stranded DNA complexed with histones of cellular origin (4,50,52). Genomic structure among the various papilloma viruses is similar and the major capsid protein represents 80% of the total viral protein (Fig. 14-2). The viral genome is divided into three areas: early, late, and regulatory. In replication, the early regions are necessary for transformation and the late region controls transcription and replication (51).

Diagnosis is based on morphology under electron microscopy and viral nucleic acid detection. Immunoperoxidase testing may be performed but is unreliable in intraepithelial neoplasia and invasive carcinoma because of absence of HPV antigens. Southern blot technique and *in situ* hybridization are useful, but limitations in our knowledge of the role of HPV in malignancy make the significance of detecting HPV DNA in lesions unclear (10,50,52).

Paramyxoviruses

Family: Paramyxoviridae
Genus: Paramyxovirus (mumps, parainfluenza, Newcastle disease)
Genus: Morbillivirus (measles virus)
Genus: Pneumovirus (respiratory syncytial virus)

The paramyxoviruses have similar morphology and protein components and a common capacity to induce syncytia and multinucleated giant cells (cell–cell fusion).

The major diseases caused by these agents are often common childhood infections that are now largely prevented through vaccination in the United States but remain a problem in underdeveloped nations (2,3). The viruses are large (156 to 300 nm) with a negative-sense, single-stranded RNA in a helical nucleocapsid surrounded by an environmentally labile membrane. Replication begins by viral hemagglutination protein attachment to the cell surface. A viral F transenvelope protein allows penetration by membrane fusion. Cells lacking the enzyme necessary to cleave the F protein are not permissive for viral infection. After penetration, viral RNA polymerase transcribes the negative-stranded RNA viral genome. Viral gene transcription and translation occur in the cytoplasm. The nucleocapsids assemble here as well and align along sites of membrane hemagglutination protein and F viral protein insertion. Exit is by budding with the acquisition of a host cell lipid envelope (2–4,10) (Fig. 14-2).

Both measles and mumps are highly contagious and transmitted by respiratory droplets (2,53–55). Measles has only one antigenic type. The incubation period after exposure is 9 to 11 days, with local replication in the respiratory tract preceding viremia, with seeding of leukocytes and the reticuloendothelial system. This is followed by a secondary viremia that seeds the skin (maculopapular rash), cornea, and conjunctiva. One third of infected patients do not manifest clinical disease but may transmit it. Diagnosis is based on clinical findings, but the virus may be grown in simian or human tissue culture, and shell-vial immunoassay and reverse transcription PCR are used for definitive tissue diagnosis such as in the late measles complication, subacute sclerosing panencephalitis (10). Acute and convalescent antibody titers are diagnostic if there is a fourfold rise.

Mumps has an incubation period of 7 to 25 days, averaging 8 days (2,53). Acquired by respiratory inhalation of virions, replication occurs in the upper respiratory tract, followed by a viremia and viral spread to other organ systems such as the parotid gland, testicles, ovaries, and brain (4,56). Ocular involvement may be widespread in both anterior and posterior segments. Diagnosis is usually clinical but fluorescent antibody stainings of conjunctival scrapings are also reliable. Other diagnostically useful tests include acute and convalescent sera, neutralization complement fixation and hemagglutination, and ELISA testing.

Newcastle disease virus is a helically symmetric, pleomorphic virus with a negative-stranded RNA at the core surrounded by a lipoprotein envelope containing hemagglutination and fusion glycoprotein fibers (2,10,53). Human infection is usually accidental from exposure to infected chickens. The incubation period is 1 to 2 days, followed by a conjunctivitis (57). Virus culture is possible but rarely used.

Togaviruses

Family: Togaviridae
Genus: Rubivirus: rubella virus (German measles)

Rubella virus is an enveloped, relatively small (50 to70 nm) icosahedral agent. Like measles, there is only one serotype (Fig. 14-2). Transmission is by inhalation of droplets from an infected patient. The illness is subclinical or mild, causing rash, fever, and lymphadenopathy, but its consequences for the unborn child of an infected woman can be devastating both systemically and ophthalmologically (2,58–60).

Diagnosis is based on serologic detection of anti-rubella antibodies or viral isolation (10). Viral shedding may remain positive up to 18 months after the acute illness. Because no cytopathic effect is produced in tissue culture such as simian or human kidney cells supporting viral replication, fluorescent antibody staining is used to shorten detection time to 48 to 96 hours rather than waiting for enterovirus interference testing. Detection of rubella IgM in infants is also diagnostic, whereas IgG is not because it crosses the placental barrier.

Coxsackieviruses

Family: Picornaviridae
Genus: Enterovirus: coxsackieviruses, human enteroviruses

The enteroviruses are in the same genus as the polioviruses. There are 67 serotypes in the enterovirus group. These are all very small viruses (30 nm) with a single strand of positive-sense RNA at the core and surrounded by a nonenveloped viral capsid (Fig. 14-2). These viruses may cause a wide variety of illnesses involving a wide variety of organ systems, including encephalitis, myocarditis, pleurodynia, neonatal sepsis, polio, peripheral neuritis, and acute hemorrhagic conjunctivitis (2,61). No serotype is associated with any one illness.

OCULAR ANTIVIRAL AGENTS: LABORATORY AND CLINICAL STUDIES*

Of the 10 ocular antiviral agents discussed in the following sections, the last 4 are essentially used only for CMV retinitis despite activity against herpetic, adenoviral, or vaccinia viral infection (23,62–65). They are, however, occasionally used for the latter infections because of resistance to the first six drugs or because of ongoing studies into their potential use in ocular viral disease. Their review is brief and oriented to treatment of anterior segment disease.

---

* Adapted in part from Pavan-Langston D. Ocular pharmacology of antiviral drugs. In: Tasman W, Jaeger E, Wilhelmus K, eds. *Duane's foundations of clinical ophthalmology.* Philadelphia: Lippincott Williams & Wilkins 2004, vol 2, ch 100, 1–24.

Idoxuridine

Structure

Idoxuridine (5-iodo-2′-deoxyuridine; IDU; Herplex), a pyrimidine antimetabolite introduced commercially in 1962, was the first drug used to control human viral disease (66,67). Structurally, idoxuridine is a thymidine analog with the 5′-methyl group replaced by iodine. Because of the development of better and more convenient drugs, idoxuridine's use and marketing have dropped dramatically in recent years.

Mechanism of Action

Idoxuridine is incorporated as a thymidine analog preferentially into viral DNA over cellular DNA because the former replicates more rapidly in infected cells (68,69). The drug is not selectively activated but is phosphorylated by both viral and cellular kinases. The idoxuridine triphosphate (IDU-TP) also inhibits the virus-specific DNA polymerase more than the host cell polymerases. Idoxuridine may interact specifically with deoxythymidine monophosphate synthetase, or it may be incorporated directly into DNA as idoxuridine monophosphate (70). Substitution of idoxuridine for thymidine in the DNA chain leads to abnormal transcription and translation, thus producing defective viral progeny. Its incorporation into some host DNA adds to the toxicity of the agent.

Although idoxuridine and its phosphorylated metabolites inhibit a variety of cellular enzymes, idoxuridine action as an antiherpetic agent may also be at a viral biosynthetic level before incorporation into the viral genome. Phosphorylation of idoxuridine to IDU-TP allows this compound to mimic deoxythymidine triphosphate, and subsequently IDU-TP may exert either an allosteric or a feedback inhibitory effect at the level of deoxythymidine kinase, deoxycytidine monophosphate deaminase, or cytidine diphosphate reductase, ultimately terminating viral replication (66,70).

The toxic effects of idoxuridine are magnified in tissues undergoing rapid cellular DNA synthesis (71). Clinical trials using the drug systemically for HSV encephalitis revealed that the drug was minimally effective and highly toxic (72). The drug is teratogenic and mutagenic, and potentially carcinogenic. For these reasons it is not used as a systemic agent.

In the eye, adverse reactions to topical idoxuridine include contact dermatitis, punctate epithelial keratopathy, follicular conjunctivitis, lacrimal punctal occlusion, and lid margin keratinization (73). Controlled studies on the effects of antivirals on corneal epithelial and stromal wounds indicate that idoxuridine is the most toxic of the commonly used topical antiviral drugs, interfering primarily with stromal healing and causing toxic epithelial changes (74).

Penetration and Pharmacokinetics

Pavan-Langston and coworkers demonstrated that in rabbits treated with 0.5% idoxuridine ointment, the drug did not penetrate the intact cornea (75). In human ocular penetration studies, idoxuridine, as the parent nucleoside, did not enter the aqueous humor. Instead, a metabolic breakdown product of idoxuridine, uracil, was detected in the aqueous. Only in patients in whom the corneal epithelium was damaged did idoxuridine penetrate the corneal barrier. When administered systemically (IV, intramuscularly, or subcutaneously), the drug is dehalogenated and rapidly metabolized; 50% to 75% is excreted within 4 to 5 hours after systemic administration in animals (76,77).

Efficacy

Idoxuridine is used topically for HSV keratoconjunctivitis. It is, however, effective in vaccinia keratitis (78–80). *In vitro* studies demonstrated that idoxuridine did not affect the adsorption of HSV in tissue culture cell monolayers, nor did it alter the infectivity of extracellular herpesvirus. idoxuridine did stop viral replication after it had begun and resulted in at least a 2–log-unit diminution in viral titer 24 hours posttreatment (81). The antiviral efficacy of idoxuridine was substantiated by numerous controlled clinical trials (82,83). Healing rates vary from approximately 75% in complicated cases to 90% in straightforward dendritic or geographic keratitis. When 0.1% idoxuridine was instilled into the eyes of patients with dendritic lesions, relief was noted within 12 to 24 hours after initiation of therapy. By 72 hours, notable healing of the epithelium occurred. Idoxuridine is highly effective in treating infectious corneal epithelial herpetic disease but is ineffective in HSV-induced iritis, stromal keratitis, and other forms of HSV intraocular infection (82,84). It is also less effective than trifluridine and vidarabine if topical steroids are being used concomitantly (85,86).

Idoxuridine use essentially stopped with the advent of newer, more convenient drugs; recommended therapy when used is 0.1% every 1 to 2 hours by day and 0.5% idoxuridine ointment at bedtime for 14 days.

Resistance

HSV resistance to idoxuridine is through modification of the TK gene. Clinically resistant virus strains isolated from patients or created by serial passage through idoxuridine-containing medium all had the common finding of reduced TK activity, sometimes to as low as 5.6% of that of the wild type or the parental strain (87,88). This has significance in this time of the increasing emergence of resistant viral strains during treatment of immunosuppressed patients. Idoxuridine-resistant HSV showed cross-resistance to bromovinyldeoxyuridine and to acyclovir, intermediate resistance to trifluridine, and full sensitivity to vidarabine and ganciclovir (88).

Trifluridine (Trifluorothymidine)

Structure

Trifluridine or trifluorothymidine [5-trifluoromethyl-2′-deoxyuridine, 2′-deoxy-5-(trifluoromethyl) uridine; TFT; F_3T; Viroptic] is a fluorinated pyrimidine nucleoside. Structurally, it is an analog of the deoxyribonucleoside thymidine and is virtually identical to idoxuridine with the exception of three fluorine atoms attached to a methyl radical replacing the iodine (89). As a pyrimidine nucleoside analog, trifluridine inhibits DNA viruses, and because of its structure, it is incorporated rapidly into growing host cell types (e.g., bone marrow.)

Mechanism of Action

Although the specific mechanism of trifluridine inhibition of active herpesvirus production is not entirely certain, its antiviral activity appears similar to that of idoxuridine and results from the effect of the drug on viral DNA synthesis (89). Trifluridine can exert its inhibition at several stages in the viral biosynthetic pathway, starting from 2-deoxyuridine-5′-monophosphate to DNA synthesis. Trifluridine acts as a competitive inhibitor of thymidine (90). The drug is initially phosphorylated to trifluridine monophosphate, which is a potent inhibitor of thymidylate synthetase (91). After phosphorylation to the triphosphate form, the compound competitively inhibits incorporation of thymidine triphosphate into viral DNA.

Toxicity

The drug is cytotoxic, teratogenic, mutagenic, and potentially carcinogenic, and is sufficiently toxic that it is not used systemically (92,93). *In vivo* treatment of normal rabbit corneas with trifluridine caused no adverse effects or evidence of corneal toxicity (94). However, when rabbit corneas with standardized epithelial defects were treated with either 1% or 0.1% trifluridine drops eight times a day for 8 days, pathologic changes in the regenerating epithelium were observed. Stromal wound healing appears to be affected by trifluridine therapy (tensile strength was significantly reduced 12 days after wounding and treatment with 1% trifluridine) (95).

Penetration Studies and Pharmacokinetics

The biphasic solubility profile of trifluridine enhances the transport of the intact, active drug across the cornea. The mechanism of penetration (as for idoxuridine and vidarabine) appears to be by nonfacilitated diffusion as demonstrated by linear penetration kinetics through excised, perfused rabbit corneas and the lack of demonstrable saturation kinetics (96). In a controlled study, trifluridine penetrated the corneal epithelium faster than idoxuridine and vidarabine. The presence or absence of an intact epithelial cell layer did not significantly alter trifluridine distribution. However, the concentration of trifluridine in the aqueous was increased in debrided or damaged corneas, and the rate of penetration was doubled (97). Trifluridine (1%, four times a day) administered to both infected rabbit eyes and patients with a history of recurrent herpetic keratitis penetrated the corneal stroma and achieved therapeutic levels (5.3 to 18 μg/mL) (96–98).

The parent compound is hydrolyzed to 5-carboxy-2′-deoxyuridine within 3 to 5 hours at 37°C and pH 7.2 (97,99,100). This metabolite has little or no antiviral activity. *In vivo*, trifluridine is hydrolyzed to 5-carboxyuracil or 5-carboxyuridine with the loss of the inorganic fluoride. The rate of elimination of trifluridine correlates with the rate of trifluridine metabolism. Monophosphate, diphosphate, and triphosphate trifluridine metabolites are found in body tissues The short serum half-life (12 to 30 minutes) and toxicity of trifluridine prevent the use of this drug in systemic herpetic infections.

Efficacy

Trifluridine interferes not only with the replication of HSV-1 and HSV-2 but has an effect on vaccinia and certain adenoviruses (101). Trifluridine (0.2 to 1.7 μg/mL) inhibits the cytopathic effects of HSV-1 by 50% in plaque reduction assay (102). Plaque formation was reduced by over 98% when HSV-1 grown into Vero cells was treated with 17 μg/mL trifluridine (103). Trifluridine activity *in vitro* is comparable to that of idoxuridine, and trifluridine is considerably more active on a weight-for-weight basis than is vidarabine. As observed for both idoxuridine and vidarabine, the strain of HSV-1 appears to be of major importance in determining the relative antiviral efficacy. Trifluridine was shown to inhibit five strains of HSV-1 within a narrow range; however, the susceptibility of five HSV-2 strains was variable, with two strains being insensitive at the maximum nontoxic concentration (104).

Trifluridine was more potent on a weight-for-weight basis than idoxuridine in the treatment of HSV-1 herpetic keratitis in rabbits. When trifluridine and idoxuridine were compared with respect to their ability to eradicate virus from the preocular tear film, no virus was recovered on days 2 and 4 of the 7-day treatment with trifluridine. However, HSV-1 was present in idoxuridine treated eyes throughout the treatment regimen (82,105). Two days after discontinuation of therapy, rebound virus shedding had occurred in both the trifluridine and idoxuridine groups, with virus titers higher than those observed in control, placebo-treated animals. These results indicate that a critical time period exists in an acute herpetic infection during which continued presence of the antiviral is necessary to control rebound virus shedding, even though infectious virus cannot be detected in the tear film. Clinical studies comparing topical 1% trifluridine with 0.1% idoxuridine drops, 3.0% vidarabine, or acyclovir ointments have shown that, overall, the latter two drugs and trifluridine have efficacy rates of 90% to 95% regardless of whether steroids are in use (85,106–110). The idoxuridine overall efficacy rate was approximately 76%, dragged down by apparent decreased efficacy in the face of steroid use in some patients, or perhaps by its having been in clinical use so long that certain organisms had become resistant or patients had become allergic to the agent. Although trifluridine had a slight edge over all other drugs in the face of concomitant steroid therapy, no statistical difference could be shown.

Resistance

Resistance to trifluridine is rare and is discussed in the section on idoxuridine (88,111).

Vidarabine

Because of the availability of trifluridine and oral antivirals, vidarabine (9-B-D-arabinofuranosyladenine, vidarabine, ara-A, Vira-A) is no longer commercially available in the United States. For special conditions such as ocular vaccinia, however, it is available through compounding pharmacists.

Structure

9-B-D-Arabinofuranosyladenine is a purine arabinosyl nucleoside structurally similar to deoxyguanosine (112).

Mechanism of Action

Like all current antivirals, vidarabine is virostatic. Its biologic activity is due in part to intracellular phosphorylation, first to the monophosphate form (ara-A-MP) and subsequently to diphosphate and triphosphate forms (ara-A-DP, ara-A-TP) by cellular enzymes. Vidarabine inhibits viral DNA synthesis by several mechanisms. Direct incorporation into DNA as ara-A-MP results in DNA chain termination. The triphosphorylated form, ara-A-TP, inhibits terminal deoxynucleotidyl transferase and DNA polymerase (δ and β). Ara-A-DP and ara-A-TP also inhibit the activity of ribonucleotide reductase enzymes (113–115).

Toxicity

After systemic or topical administration, vidarabine is converted to a hypoxanthine arabinoside derivative (ara-HX); this metabolite has only 20% of the antiviral potency of the parent compound (116). The toxicity of vidarabine, administered systemically or topically, is negligible over a wide range of pharmacologic dosages. A major problem in systemic administration of vidarabine is that the compound's relative insolubility requires the use of large volumes of fluid, which can tax cardiovascular and renal homeostatic mechanisms. The drug is also teratogenic and mutagenic, and has carcinogenic potential (117). As a result, vidarabine is used systemically only as an alternative to acyclovir or ganciclovir in drug-resistant, life-threatening HSV or VZV infections.

Vidarabine administered topically to rabbits did not impair wound healing as measured by planimetry and histopathologic examination. However, stromal wound strength of corneas treated topically with vidarabine or idoxuridine was less than that of wounds treated with placebo ointment (74).

Penetration and Pharmacokinetics

Ocular penetration studies have shown that topically applied vidarabine crosses the corneal barrier in minor amounts in corneas with intact epithelium. The deaminated semiactive metabolite ara-HX was found in the aqueous in significant amounts after topical vidarabine treatment (75,97). Application of 3% vidarabine in a water-miscible cream produced corneal levels of 20 μg/mL, whereas the same concentration in petrolatum ointment produced levels of only 4.5 μg/mL.

After IV administration, vidarabine is rapidly deaminated by adenosine deaminase to the less effective ara-HX form or other noneffective metabolites. Plasma levels of ara-HX are directly related to the rate of vidarabine infusion. Vidarabine's plasma half-life is approximately 3.5 hours, and the metabolite ara-HX is well distributed in tissues. Ara-HX readily crosses the blood–brain barrier and attains concentrations within 35% of plasma levels in the cerebrospinal fluid (CSF) (116,118). To enhance the antiviral efficacy of vidarabine therapy, potent inhibitors of adenosine deaminase, which stop the conversion of vidarabine to ara-HX, have been used. These inhibitors have enhanced the virucidal activity (by 20-fold) and the cytotoxic activity of vidarabine *in vitro* and *in vivo* (119,120).

Efficacy

Vidarabine has a broad antiviral spectrum that includes many DNA viruses (HSV-1, HSV-2, vaccinia, VZV, CMV, and pseudorabies virus); it has little or no effect against RNA viruses (80,84,121–123). Plaque reduction assays using several different herpesvirus strains indicated a high degree of strain variability. As is the case with idoxuridine, the cell type, virus passage, and virus strain all significantly affect the antiviral activity of vidarabine. Vidarabine is highly effective against idoxuridine-resistant HSV-1 and HSV-2 *in vitro* (80).

In the eye, topical vidarabine 3% ointment has been found effective in herpetic keratitis and keratouveitis in both animal models and in humans (86,107,124). In one study of 69 patients with external ocular herpetic keratitis, vidarabine proved to be equal to idoxuridine in reducing tear film viral titers and in promoting corneal reepithelialization (125). Vidarabine was significantly less toxic than idoxuridine and caused healing of herpetic lesions clinically resistant to idoxuridine. Other studies in patients with extensive dendrogeographic ulcerations substantiate these findings (124). Fewer treatment failures occurred with vidarabine (9.5%) compared with idoxuridine (18.8%) in a study of more than 300 patients with ocular herpes (86). Several studies referenced in this section and the section on trifluridine indicate that there is no statistically significant difference between topical vidarabine, trifluridine, and acyclovir therapy of HSV keratitis (HSK) (107,109,124).

Systemic vidarabine has also been effective in therapy of varicella and in herpes zoster ophthalmicus (HZO), although it is now in distant fourth place behind valacyclovir, famciclovir, and acyclovir in this regard. Whitley et al. reported that vidarabine therapy (10 mg/kg/day for 5 days) of varicella in immunocompromised patients reduced fever duration, lesion count, and systemic morbidity significantly compared with placebo (122). A Collaborative Antiviral Study Group report on vidarabine therapy of zoster infection (including HZO) in immunocompromised patients noted that the same therapy used for varicella, mentioned previously, resulted in more rapid cessation of viral shedding and increased healing rate of lesions (126). Postherpetic neuralgia (PHN) could not be evaluated. Its role in TK-negative, acyclovir-resistant HSV mutants continues to make this drug of interest (127–129).

Resistance

Resistance to vidarabine appears related to viral DNA polymerase rather than to TK. Mutant, vidarabine-resistant viruses with changes in the DNA polymerase gene have been isolated (130,131). This resistance was mapped to a 0.8-kb region in the *pol* gene and makes viral DNA polymerase less susceptible to ara-A-TP (130,132). Although other gene products may be affected, most HSV mutations have been found to code for the carboxyl-terminal portion of the viral DNA polymerase (133). Such DNA polymerase mutation is of clinical significance because mutant HSV is resistant not only to vidarabine but to the other common agents that use this antiviral mechanism. Resistance to

vidarabine is uncommon and is discussed with reference to its use in HSV and VZV infections resistant to other antivirals (idoxuridine, acyclovir).

Acyclovir

Structure

Acyclovir [9-(2-hydroxyethoxymethyl)guanine; acyclovir, acycloguanosine (Zovirax)] is a synthetic compound that was designed to mimic substrates for model enzyme systems. Acyclovir is an analog of guanosine or deoxyguanosine in which the 2′- and 3′-carbon atoms are missing. Acyclovir was the first compound engineered to have selective *in vitro* and *in vivo* antiviral activity (102,134,135).

Mechanism of Action

The major modes of action of acyclovir are viral DNA chain termination and rapid inactivation of viral DNA polymerase. Acyclovir is phosphorylated (activated) to acyclovir monophosphate (ACV-MP) specifically by herpesvirus-encoded TK, thereby largely bypassing activation in any but infected cells (102,134). This markedly reduces toxicity and increases specificity. ACV-MP is further phosphorylated to ACV diphosphate (ACV-DP) and ACV triphosphate (ACV-TP) by viral and cellular enzymes. ACV-TP competes for deoxyguanosine triphosphate, the natural substrate for virus-specific DNA polymerase, and is incorporated irreversibly as ACV-MP onto the growing viral DNA chains, thus causing chain termination (136,137). Termination occurs because acyclovir lacks the 3′ hydroxyl group needed to react with incoming nucleotides. DNA polymerase then binds irreversibly to the acyclovir-terminated chain and the entire enzyme complex is metabolically inactive. Little to no inactivation of cellular polymerase occurs (102,136–138). Elion and coworkers have determined that ACV-TP inhibits HSV DNA polymerase (DNA nucleotidyl transferase) 10 to 30 times more efficiently than cellular DNA polymerase, another factor in reducing toxicity (133,134). Approximately a 3000-fold concentration increase in acyclovir (above that which is virucidal) is needed to inhibit host cell growth.

Toxicity

Because acyclovir is activated specifically by herpesvirus-coded TK, it was anticipated that the drug would be relatively nontoxic. After corneal application of 3% acyclovir ointment, no toxic corneal effects were noted, and the quality and rate of reepithelialization and stromal wound strength of the cornea were not impaired (74). Clinical study did note rare diffuse punctate keratitis that cleared after discontinuation of acyclovir therapy, but this apparent toxicity was thought to be a function of the drug vehicle (139).

The only important metabolite of acyclovir is 9-carboxymethoxy-methyl guanine, an inactive compound that accounts for up to 14% of acyclovir dosage administered to humans (140). Renal clearance of acyclovir ranges from 75% to 80% of the total body clearance and is substantially greater than the clearance of creatinine, indicating that glomerular filtration and tubular secretion mechanisms (possibly the organic acid secretory system) are involved (141). The drug may rarely cause renal failure when given in high doses (>5 mg/kg) IV if there is renal insufficiency or dehydration. Hydration of all patients should be monitored and patients with renal insufficiency should have reduced doses and prolongation of the intervals between dosing to minimize this risk. Rare central nervous system (CNS) toxicity, delirium tremens, and coma have been reported (142). Other common side effects are gastrointestinal distress and headache. There is no evidence that acyclovir is a carcinogen or teratogen, and, at therapeutic doses, there is no effect on the hematopoietic or immune systems (143).

Penetration and Pharmacokinetics

Acyclovir can be administered safely and effectively by IV or subconjunctival injection, orally, or topically. Its adsorption after oral administration is variable and appears to be species dependent (140,143–145). Animal studies have indicated that after oral administration in mice, 50% of the acyclovir is adsorbed and peak plasma concentrations occur 2 to 4 hours after ingestion (141).

In humans, oral adsorption of acyclovir is incomplete, with bioavailability of the drug ranging between 15% and 30% of the dosage (146). Peak plasma concentrations occur 1.5 to 2.5 hours after administration, and steady-state plasma concentrations after multiple oral doses of 2.5, 5, 10 and 15 mg/kg administered every 8 hours were 6.7, 9.7, 20, and 20.6 μg/mL, respectively. These values are similar to the peak plasma concentrations observed after equivalent single oral doses, and it was concluded that acyclovir does not accumulate in plasma after repetitive dosing. Oral dosing of 200 mg every 4 hours reaches steady-state levels ranging from 1.4 to 4.0 μM, which is inhibitory for HSV-1 and HSV-2, but doses of 800 mg orally (PO) five times daily are needed to yield peak and trough serum levels, respectively, of 6.9 μM and 3.5 μM to inhibit most strains of VZV (147–149).

Studies by Hung et al. and Collum et al. on the concentrations of acyclovir in the tear film and aqueous in patients on 400 mg PO five times daily showed levels of 3.28 μM (0.96 to 8.79 μM) and 3.26 μM (1.10 to 5.39 μM), respectively, 4 hours after the last oral dose (147,150). The mean ED$_{50}$ (effective dose reducing viral plaque count in tissue culture by 50%) for HSV-1 ranges from 0.15 to 0.18 μM to 0.1 to 1.6 μM, which indicated that the tear and aqueous levels achieved were well in excess of that

which should be needed to eliminate the virus (68,148,150–152). This is not always the case. Stromal HSV particles may persist in the face of prolonged, therapeutic doses of oral acyclovir (153). Drug resistance may have played a role in this finding. Compared with HSV, the inhibitory doses for VZV are much higher, at 3 to 4 μM, resulting in the need for fourfold higher drug dosing, as noted earlier, and less leeway in terms of resistance (152).

After topical instillation of 3% acyclovir ointment in the inferior cul de sac of 25 eyes (every 5 hours for four to six doses before cataract extraction), the mean acyclovir concentration in the aqueous humor was 1.7 μg/mL, which falls within the therapeutic range (152,154). Cutaneous adsorption of acyclovir may occur through damaged skin, but systemic adsorption is limited.

Total-body distribution of IV ^{14}C-acyclovir has been studied in several animal species (144). Acyclovir rapidly entered all tissues after administration in both mice and rats. In humans with normal kidney function the serum half-life is approximately 3 hours. IV dosing of 5 mg/kg three times daily resulted in serum ID$_{50}$ levels (inhibitory dose reducing viral plaque count in tissue culture by 50%) well above those needed for HSV-1 and HSV-2 at all times, but a dosage of 10 mg/kg three times daily was necessary to avoid trough levels that fell below the ID$_{50}$ of several VZV strains (144,148,154,155). Multidose IV therapy with 400 to 1200 mg/m^2 every 8 hours resulted in acyclovir concentrations in kidney, lung, and brain that were 1000%, 131%, and 25% to 70% of plasma levels, respectively (156). CSF acyclovir levels were approximately 50% of corresponding plasma levels. The rapid penetration of acyclovir into the CSF has made this drug an important compound for treating focal and disseminated CNS herpetic infections. Further information is given in the section on valacyclovir, later.

Intravitreal levels in humans 2 hours after 13 mg/kg IV acyclovir were at inhibitory levels for HSV-1 and HSV-2, VZV, and EBV (147). Regular acyclovir dosing of 5 mg/kg three times daily yielded concentrations of 8.8 to 11.0 μM, well in excess of the inhibitory dose for HSV-1 and HSV-2, VZV, and EBV, as did 25 mg of subconjunctival acyclovir (157).

Clinical Efficacy

In vitro studies with acyclovir have demonstrated that this compound has a broad antiviral spectrum, including HSV-1, HSV-2, VZV, EBV, and, to a much lesser extent, CMV (135). It is not effective against vaccinia. Acyclovir is 160 times more potent than vidarabine and 10 times more potent than idoxuridine (158,159). Inhibitory doses for various viruses were noted previously.

Herpes Simplex Virus

Acyclovir (100 μg/mL) has been used in a drug-induced suppression model of HSV-1 infection in trigeminal ganglion cells. In this system, it produces a suppressed HSV-1 infection that is functionally identical to HSV-1 latency *in vivo*. Acyclovir has also been shown to suppress the reactivation of latent virus in explanted trigeminal ganglia (160). Latency was not eradicated, however, as demonstrated by an increase in viral titer after acyclovir removal. The rabbit eye model of HSV-1 infection has been used extensively to assess the *in vivo* efficacy of acyclovir (161,162).

It is not within the purview of this chapter to cover in fine detail the multiple clinical uses of acyclovir, except to note that this important drug is indicated or has been effective in the following conditions: (a) primary genital HSV (PO or IV), (b) recurrent genital HSV in immunocompetent patients (PO), (c) mucocutaneous HSV in immunocompromised patients (PO or IV), (d) HSV encephalitis (IV), (e) neonatal HSV (IV), (f) varicella in immunocompetent (PO) or immunocompromised patients (IV then PO), (g) herpes zoster in immunocompetent (PO) or immunocompromised patients (IV the PO), and (h) possibly EBV infections (PO) (107,127, 163–165).

Multiple clinical studies on infectious HSV epithelial keratitis comparing topical 3% acyclovir with 3% vidarabine ointment, 0.1% idoxuridine drops, or 1.0% trifluridine drops in recommended doses revealed no statistically significant difference among the four drugs, although there was a trend suggesting that trifluridine, acyclovir, and possibly vidarabine were superior to idoxuridine if concomitant steroids were given (23,109,124,139,149, 164,166–169). Acyclovir ophthalmic ointment is not commercially available in the United States although it is marketed in other countries.

Oral acyclovir 400 mg five times daily is equivalent to topical acyclovir in treating epithelial keratitis, with 90% of patients healing their ulcers in a mean of 5 days (147,170–172). Two hundred milligrams PO five times daily healed 18 of 19 patients with combined HSV epithelial and stromal keratitis in 5 to 21 days (171). The therapeutic pediatric dosage is 20 to 40 mg/kg/day for 7 to 14 days as a pediatric elixir (200 mg/tsp) (170).

Between 1994 and 2001, eight multicenter studies on the efficacy of oral acyclovir or topical steroids, or both, on various forms of ocular HSV were reported from the Herpetic Eye Disease Study (HEDS) (173–180). The results may be briefly summarized as follows:

1. After resolution of any form of ocular HSV, 1 year of acyclovir 400 mg twice daily significantly reduced recurrence of herpetic disease during that time and without rebound up to 6 months after acyclovir was stopped.
2. There was no statistically significant benefit of acyclovir 400 mg five times daily for 10 weeks in treating active HSV stromal keratitis already being treated with steroids and trifluridine.
3. Steroids were significantly better than placebo in resolving active stromal keratitis, and postponing

steroids slowed resolution but showed no difference in outcome by 6 months.
4. Treatment of iritis with acyclovir 400 mg five times daily for 10 weeks in patients already on steroids and trifluridine may possibly have some beneficial effect.
5. A 3-week course of acyclovir 400 mg five times daily for patients with epithelial keratitis already on trifluridine did not alter the subsequent incidence of stromal keratitis or iritis.
6. Acyclovir 400 mg twice daily for 1 year significantly reduced the recurrence of HSV stromal or epithelial keratitis, with greatest benefit in the stromal group.
7. Previous stromal, but not epithelial, keratitis markedly increased the risk of recurrent similar disease in the future.
8. Psychological stress, sun exposure, contact lens wear, or systemic illness could not be shown to be triggers for HSV reactivation.
9. The number of past episodes of either epithelial or stromal keratitis was strongly associated with the likelihood of a recurrence.
10. Long-term oral acyclovir significantly lowers recurrence of either form of HSK, but is more effective in preventing recurrence in stromal than in epithelial disease.

It should be noted that prophylactic use of oral antivirals is legitimate but defined as "off label" use.

In a study of 105 patients with HSK, Wu and Chen reported an even more positive prophylactic effect in preventing recurrent epithelial HSV in patients who had not undergone keratoplasty than did the HEDS (174,181). Using low-dose acyclovir at 300 mg/day for 1 year, they found statistically significant differences between treated and control groups: 5 recurrences of epithelial and 1 case of stromal keratitis in the acyclovir group, and 14 cases of epithelial and 4 cases of stromal keratitis in the untreated control group. The epithelial data conform with those reported by Simon and Pavan-Langston (182).

There are additional indications for oral acyclovir in patients with herpetic keratitis. These include use as an adjunct to topical antivirals in patients with atopic disease or in immunosuppressed patients, especially in patients with AIDS (23,127,183–186). Oral or IV therapy is determined on the basis of severity of immunosuppression in AIDS (CD4$^+$ T-helper lymphocytes <200 cells/mL, viral burden >10^5 to 10^7 plasma HIV RNA copies/mL) and degree of illness (187). Dosage in atopy of 400 mg PO three times to four daily for 2 to 3 weeks is usually quite effective. Another indication is use in those patients who are unable or unwilling to take topical antiviral agents for epithelial keratitis, such as those with crippling arthritis, children or uncooperative adults, those whose occupation makes topical agents difficult to use, and those with ocular toxic medicamentosa from local antivirals. Adult dosage is 400 mg PO three to five times daily, and for children, 20 to 40 mg/kg in divided doses for 7 to 10 days. Prophylaxis of HSV epithelial recurrences with oral acyclovir in patients post–HSV keratoplasty is effective and indicated. It is discussed in further detail later in the section on Surgical Factors and Management (182,188–190).

Varicella Zoster Virus/Herpes Zoster Ophthalmicus

The role of acyclovir in HZO is now well established (23,149,151,164,184,191–197). In studies of topical acyclovir, McGill and coworkers reported that 5% acyclovir ointment five times daily was highly effective in resolving zoster epithelial keratitis and in significantly reducing the incidence of recurrent disease compared with topical steroids (198,199). In addition, the combination of topical steroid and acyclovir was found to be less effective than acyclovir alone, and there was no difference among groups in resolution of stromal keratitis, iritis, scleritis, or secondary glaucoma. In contrast, Marsh and Cooper reported an overall trend for more rapid resolution of inflammation in patients with HZO treated with the acyclovir–steroid combination, compared with the progressive ocular inflammation noted in patients treated with topical acyclovir alone (200). No patient received systemic acyclovir or corticosteroids. The study concluded that topical steroids were useful in the management of the inflammatory aspects of HZO and that there was no clear benefit of topical acyclovir ophthalmic ointment when used alone.

Conversely, Zaal et al. have reported that at 3 months after onset of HZO, patients who received 3% topical acyclovir had longer durations of periocular lesions and significantly more visual loss compared with the group receiving oral acyclovir, and that chronic disease developed in all patients put on combined topical acyclovir and dexamethasone drops (201). Acyclovir ointment is not available in the United States, but is in use in Europe and South America. The aforementioned studies and the data on systemic acyclovir all suggest that the systemic route is the one to use in treating VZV.

In immunocompetent patients, acyclovir 800 mg PO five times daily for 7 to 14 days (average, 10 days) results in more rapid resolution of viral shedding, acute neuralgia, and new skin lesions, and a reduced incidence of pseudodendritiform keratopathy, stromal keratitis, and iritis. There was variable effect on PHN, depending on the study, and no effect on corneal hypesthesia or neurotrophic ulceration. With the exception of PHN, acyclovir compares favorably with famciclovir and valacyclovir (see later). In the presence of immunosuppression, where HZO tends to be more severe and slow to respond to therapy, initial treatment with IV acyclovir is indicated (1500 mg/m²/d in three divided doses = 10 to 15 mg/kg every 8 hours) for 7 to 10 days, followed by acyclovir 800 mg PO five times

daily for 6 to 14 weeks. This dosage is similar to that used in acute retinal necrosis (202,203). Because patients with HZO are at increased risk for complications, several studies have been conducted demonstrating that use of oral acyclovir in ophthalmic zoster has a high therapeutic efficacy. Compared with placebo, acyclovir therapy, 800 mg PO five times daily for 7 to 10 days, induces a prompt resolution of skin rash, cessation of pain, more rapid healing, reduced duration of viral shedding, and reduced duration of new lesion formation. There is also a significant reduction in the incidence and severity of acute dendritiform keratopathy, scleritis, episcleritis, iritis, the incidence (but not the severity if it occurred) of corneal stromal immune keratitis, and the incidence of late-onset ocular inflammatory disease (e.g., episcleritis, scleritis, iritis) (197,204–207). Effect on PHN was variable, with some reports showing no efficacy, and others notable decrease in severity and incidence (197,202,206–209). Two studies noted that higher dosages of oral acyclovir, 800 mg given orally five times daily, for 7 to 10 days had beneficial effects similar to those noted by others, but also reduced the prevalence of localized zoster-associated neurologic symptoms such as paresthesia, dysesthesia, and hyperesthesia. With the exception of PHN, acyclovir compares favorably with famciclovir and valacyclovir (see later) (207,210). The current U.S. Food and Drug Administration (FDA)–approved adult dose for HZO is 800 mg PO five times daily for 7 days.

The FDA-approved dosing recommendations for acyclovir are as follows: (a) genital HSV, 200 mg PO five times daily for 10 days (first episode) or for 5 days (recurrence); (b) HSV prophylaxis, 400 mg PO twice daily; (c) acute zoster, 800 mg PO five times daily for 7 to 10 days; (d) IV, 5 to 10 mg/kg every 8 hours, each dose over 1 hour; (e) safety and efficacy of acyclovir not established in children younger than 2 years of age; (f) varicella, 20 mg/kg PO four times daily for 5 days; and (g) use adult dose if patient weighs 40 kg. The American Association of Pediatrics does not recommend routine use of acyclovir for varicella, but consider use if patient is older than 12 years of age, has chronic cutaneous or pulmonary disease, or is on long-term steroid or salicylate treatment. Off-label use of acyclovir in HIV-positive adults is as follows: (a) genital HSV, 400 mg PO three time daily for 7 to 10 days, and for 5 to 10 days for recurrence; and (b) genital HSV prophylaxis, 400 to 800 mg PO two to three times daily (211,212). Ocular doses are usually adapted from genital HSV study doses if there has been no specific ocular study done.

Resistance

An important consideration in the use of TK-activated antivirals is the development of resistant HSV strains. *In vitro* studies have shown that acyclovir resistance can be manifested by (a) a lack of viral TK (TK⁻), (b) altered substrate specificity of viral TK such that it phosphorylates thymidine but not acyclovir, and (c) a viral DNA polymerase gene mutation to alter the enzyme such that it is not inhibited by ACV-TP. By far the most common mechanism of resistance is TK⁻ mutation (213,214).

Acyclovir-resistant HSV and VZV mutants are rarely seen in immunocompetent patients, but resistant strains are being encountered ever more frequently in immunodeficient patients (215–217). The AIDS epidemic has accelerated this because of large numbers of patients on long-term acyclovir therapy. Despite the TK⁻ status of most mutants, severe mucocutaneous disease may result. Vidarabine and foscarnet are reasonable alternative drugs because they do not require TK for activation (131,218,219). Sonkin et al. have reported isolation of an acyclovir-sensitive HSV with normal TK activity from a patient who had undergone keratoplasty on postoperative day 22 (220). Five and 7 days later, as the clinical course deteriorated, acyclovir-resistant HSV with deficient TK activity was isolated. Despite sensitivity to foscarnet, the graft eventually failed.

Valacyclovir

Structure

Valacyclovir (VCV; Valtrex) is the L-valine ester of acyclovir. This prodrug was synthesized to enhance greatly the oral absorption of acyclovir from the gastrointestinal tract. It undergoes an almost complete first-pass conversion to acyclovir and L-valine through enzymatic hydrolysis. The bioavailability of acyclovir is enhanced three to five times by this prodrug and is not altered by the simultaneous administration of food.

After enzymatic conversion to acyclovir, a 1-g dose of valacyclovir gives peak plasma concentrations of 5 to 6 μg/mL of acyclovir, a therapeutic dose for both HSV and VZV (221–224). One gram of valacyclovir orally four times daily gives a concentration–time curve of acyclovir similar to that with the IV administration of 5 mg/kg of body weight of acyclovir every 8 hours (222).

Mechanism of Action

After enzymatic conversion to acyclovir, the mechanism of action of valacyclovir is identical to that discussed previously for acyclovir.

Toxicity

In general, toxicity is negligible and patient tolerance is excellent (225). Carcinogenicity, tumorigenicity, fertility, and mutagenicity studies on valacyclovir were negative (222). Although acyclovir does cross the placenta, it was found

that the rate of birth defects in infants of women on acyclovir during pregnancy was the same as the general population. The registry of patients studied was too small to make definitive conclusions about the safety of the drug in the fetus.

Valacyclovir does, however, have a *potential significant toxicity in immunosuppressed patients*. Thrombotic thrombocytopenic purpura/hemolytic-uremic syndrome has been reported in bone marrow or renal transplant recipients or HIV-positive patients who were taking high doses of valacyclovir for prolonged periods. This drug therefore is not indicated in immunocompromised patients. There have been no such adverse reports in immunocompetent patients (183,222).

Penetration and Pharmacokinetics

The pharmacodynamics of valacyclovir are similar to those of acyclovir (221,222,224,226). Acyclovir is widely distributed through all body organs and fluids, including the brain, CSF, vaginal mucosa, uterus, seminal and herpetic vesicular fluids, liver, and kidneys. Although there are no studies on the intraocular penetration of valacyclovir, it seems safe to assume that drug titers are similar to or higher than those discussed previously for acyclovir. Acyclovir concentrations after oral valacyclovir are approximately 50% of plasma levels. After multiple doses of 1 g of valacyclovir, these levels are 5 to 5.5 g/mL. Eighty to 89% of drug is eliminated by the kidneys as acyclovir. Mean renal clearance of acyclovir exceeds creatinine clearance, indicating that renal tubular secretion is actively involved in elimination of drug, which is 99% acyclovir.

Clinical Efficacy

Valacyclovir's antiviral activity, in descending order of *in vitro* susceptibility, is HSV-2, HSV-1, VZV, EBV, HHV6, HHV8, HHV7, and CMV (224,227–230). It is not effective against vaccinia. The primary FDA-approved clinical uses of valacyclovir are for treatment of herpes zoster and herpes simplex (222,224,231,232).

Clinical studies comparing valacyclovir 1 g PO three times daily with acyclovir 800 mg PO five times daily in 1141 immunocompetent patients with herpes zoster (35 with HZO) indicated that the drugs were equivalent in ability to accelerate dermal healing and reduce the duration of virus shedding, but that valacyclovir was significantly better in acute pain resolution and reduced duration of PHN up to 1 year of follow-up (196,224). There was no difference if drugs were given 7 or 14 days. Further, studies on PHN revealed that the medium time to pain resolution was 38 days with valacyclovir and 51 days with acyclovir (*p* < .03). Other studies support the good efficacy of valacyclovir in herpes zoster, particularly if started within 72 hours of rash onset (22,233–236).

The only ocular study compared acyclovir with valacyclovir in 121 immunocompetent patients with acute HZO, and reported an incidence of keratitis, uveitis, and episcleritis that was similar in both groups (237). Neither group had any incidence of neurotrophic keratitis or scleritis, and acute pain was noted in approximately two thirds of each group. It was concluded that valacyclovir was a valid alternative to acyclovir in treatment of HZO, but, like famciclovir (see later), was superior in acute and long-term pain inhibition and in patient compliance, with only three-times-daily dosing.

Clinical studies in immunocompetent patients using the well-tolerated valacyclovir 1000 mg PO three times daily indicate equivalent efficacy with acyclovir 400 mg PO five times daily in acute zoster.

Currently used dosages have been adopted from genital HSV studies (231,232). These reports indicate that for acute HSV infection, valacyclovir 1000 mg PO every day for 10 days is as effective as acyclovir at 200 mg PO five times daily for the same time period. For recurrent genital HSV, valacyclovir therapy is 500 mg PO two times daily for 3 days, and for suppression of recurrent episodes of HSV, 1 g PO every day (226,231, 232,238). The same valacyclovir dose has been used for long-term prophylaxis up to one year with no adverse side effects in immunocompetent patients.

The FDA approved dosages of valacyclovir are (a) for primary genital HSV, 1 g PO two times daily for 10 days; (b) for genital HSV prophylaxis in HIV-positive patients, 500 mg PO twice daily; (c) for varicella in young adults, 500 mg PO three times daily for 5 days; (d) and for orolabial HSV in immunocompetent patients, 2 g PO q12h × 2 treated as soon as possible (controversial use). Off-label use is for varicella in adolescents at 500 mg PO three times daily for 5 days (212,239). Ocular use is also off label, with doses as used in the above clinical studies. However, in some severely immunocompromised HIV-positive patients, thrombocytopenic purpura/hemolytic uremic-syndrome developed, with a few deaths (22). As a result, this drug is not FDA approved for use in immunocompromised patients.

A more recent application for valacyclovir is the inhibition of ocular HSV reactivation after excimer laser keratectomy or laser *in situ* keratomileusis (240,241). The effective dose in the experimental model was 150 mg/kg/day for 2 weeks. Human trials are now underway.

Resistance

The mechanism of resistance of herpesviruses, most commonly VZV, to valacyclovir is similar to that for acyclovir—that is, the vast majority are TK deficient (226). Although VZV resistance emerging from valacyclovir treatment of immunocompetent patients is very rare, the incidence of acyclovir-resistant VZV in immunosuppressed patients is increasing. It is most common in HIV-positive individuals, but occasionally is seen in organ transplant recipients (213–215). Alternative therapy in these cases would be IV foscarnet (202,242).

Famciclovir

Structure

Famciclovir (Famvir) is the orally bioavailable diacetyl ester of 6-deoxy-penciclovir. Penciclovir itself is an acyclic guanine derivative similar to acyclovir in structure, mechanism of action, and antiviral activity.

Mechanism of Action

Penciclovir and acyclovir differ qualitatively in rates of phosphorylation, concentration of triphosphate derivatives, stability, and affinity for viral DNA polymerase (243–245). The intracellular activity of penciclovir is very long even when extracellular titers are low—for example, 10 to 20 hours and 9 hours in HSV- and VZV-infected cells, respectively, compared with less than 1 hour for acyclovir (ACV-TP) in similarly infected cells (246). Further, penciclovir triphosphate (PCV-TP), a nonobligate DNA chain terminator, is more effective than ACV-TP, an obligate chain terminator, in inhibiting HSV DNA polymerase–mediated DNA chain elongation (243,247).

Toxicity

Penciclovir's preferential phosphorylation in herpesvirus-infected cells far exceeds that of acyclovir, but the minimal phosphorylation of penciclovir in uninfected cells and the low activity of PCV-TP against cellular DNA polymerases explains penciclovir's and its derivative, famciclovir's, lack of toxicity in cell culture and in clinical studies (244,245). There was no significant difference in adverse experiences such as headaches, nausea, and diarrhea between patients with zoster and genital herpes infections receiving oral famciclovir or placebo up to 18 weeks in masked studies. Laboratory abnormalities and results of hematologic analyses, clinical chemistries, semen analyses, and urinalyses were similar in both famciclovir and placebo groups (248,249).

Penetration and Pharmacokinetics

Although penciclovir is very poorly absorbed from the gastrointestinal tract, famciclovir has an absorption rate of 77% after oral administration. The metabolite, penciclovir, is not further broken down but is eliminated unchanged in the urine, with a half-life of approximately 2 hours after IV administration (244,245,250). As noted in the section on Mechanism of Action, intracellular PCV-TP activity persists despite low extracellular titers.

Efficacy

Famciclovir's efficacy is similar to that of acyclovir. *In vitro* activity includes HSV-1, HSV-2, VZV, and EBV. It is not effective against vaccinia. Penciclovir's *in vitro* activity against VZV equals that of acyclovir, with a mean EC_{50} in tissue culture of 3 to 4 μg/mL (244,245,250). In experimental HSK in rabbits, oral famciclovir twice daily at doses of 60 to 500 mg/kg body weight, regardless of dose, resulted in significant reduction in keratitis and HSV-1 genomes in the trigeminal ganglion, as well as improved survival. These data suggest that oral famciclovir may reduce the morbidity of HSV in clinical situations (231,251–255).

Clinical studies in several hundred immunocompetent patients with nonophthalmic zoster infection have been quite successful. Famciclovir, 500 mg PO three times daily, was compared with placebo or with acyclovir 800 mg five times daily for 7 days. Results were clearly superior to placebo and similar to acyclovir both in stopping viral shedding and accelerating dermal healing. Perhaps more important, famciclovir had a significantly greater effect on reduction of PHN compared with placebo or acyclovir. With an incidence of just over 50% in all groups, the median time to resolution of the neuralgia was 55 and 62 days in the famciclovir groups, compared with 128 days in the placebo group. These are also more favorable data on PHN than those seen in acyclovir-treated patients (253,256). A study comparing valacyclovir with famciclovir showed the drugs to be comparable in nonocular VZV infection in terms of cutaneous healing and pain resolution (235). This further affirms the superiority of both famciclovir and valacyclovir over acyclovir in acute zoster and, more important, PHN.

In HZO, a randomized, double-masked study on 454 patients comparing famciclovir 500 mg PO three times daily with acyclovir 800 mg PO five times daily revealed that both drugs were equally effective in all parameters of ocular disease (252). The effects on neuralgia were not reported.

The drug is FDA-approved for treatment of herpes zoster infection at dosages of 500 mg TID/day PO for 7 days. Dosage for recurrent genital herpes simplex is 125 mg PO twice daily for 5 days, and for herpes prophylaxis, 250 mg PO twice daily for a year or more. For acute orolabial HSV infection, the dose is 500 mg PO twice daily for 7 days (212,239). Ocular use is also off label, with doses as used in the aforementioned clinical studies.

Resistance

There have not yet been cases of reported resistance.

Ganciclovir

Structure

Ganciclovir [9-(1,3-dihydroxy-2-propoxy)methylguanine; DHPG; GCV; Cytovene, Cymevene] was the first of the five currently FDA-approved agents for treatment of CMV retinitis in immunosuppressed patients. It is also active, however, against HSV, VZV, and EBV. This nucleoside analog of deoxyguanosine is similar in structure to acyclovir, with the addition of a terminal hydroxymethyl group in the acyclic sugar (257). The active form is ganciclovir-5'-triphosphate.

Mechanism of Action

Like acyclovir, ganciclovir activation in HSV and VZV infection begins with its monophosphorylation by virus-specific TK. Because ganciclovir is a far better substrate for viral TK, nearly 10-fold more ganciclovir triphosphate than ACV-TP is formed in HSV-1–infected cells (68,257,258). The triphosphate, in turn, selectively inhibits viral DNA polymerase.

Toxicity

Ganciclovir is effectively not metabolized by the body and its clearance depends on the kidneys. Although plasma levels and half-life increase with reduced renal function, the drug is not nephrotoxic. Toxicity is primarily hematopoietic, with neutropenia and thrombocytopenia, usually reversible, occurring in approximately 40% and 20% of patients, respectively, and often obviating use or limiting dosage of other myelosuppressive agents such as trimethoprim-sulfamethoxazole, amphotericin B, and zidovudine, but it may be used with other anti-HIV dideoxynucleotides (259–261). Half of each group sustains dose-limiting hematologic suppression; neutropenia is seen more frequently in patients with AIDS and thrombocytopenia in patients immunosuppressed due to other causes. Other, less frequent side effects include nausea, neurotoxicity, hepatic dysfunction, fever, and local rash or phlebitis (ganciclovir = pH 11). Ganciclovir is also carcinogenic and teratogenic, and induces azoospermia (127).

Penetration and Pharmacokinetics

Ganciclovir's oral bioavailability is quite poor, less than 3%, necessitating IV or, as noted later, topical administration (261,262). Oral ganciclovir is available for clinical use, but its poor bioavailability (6% to 9%) and the development of valganciclovir have greatly curtailed its use (263).

Efficacy

Although ganciclovir is as active as acyclovir against HSV-1, HSV-2, VZV, and EBV, given its toxic nature, it is used only in life- or vision-threatening CMV infections. In addition to its FDA-approved uses, ganciclovir has notable potential as a topical anti-HSV agent. Clinical trials have shown that 0.15% ganciclovir gel or 3% acyclovir ointment three to five times per day over 1 week was therapeutically equivalent, but that ganciclovir had superior local tolerance (264).

Resistance

Ganciclovir-resistant CMV strains have been isolated in up to 27% of patients with retinitis receiving treatment for 9 months or longer (265). The mutation giving resistance to ganciclovir is in either the UL97 or UL54 gene. Genotypically resistant virus developed increasing phenotypic resistance with time and continued ganciclovir therapy. Change in therapy may allow a shift in virus population and the CMV genotype identified. Cidofovir, foscarnet, and vidarabine are alternatives in the face of ganciclovir resistance.

Cidofovir

Structure

Cidofovir [(S)-9-(3-hydroxy-2-phosphonylmethoxypropyl) cytosine; HPMPC; CDV; Vistide; Forvade] is an acyclic nucleotide analog derived from phosphonoformic acid. It is currently FDA approved in combination with probenecid for treatment of CMV retinitis in HIV-positive patients (266,267). Of equal interest, however, is the finding that this drug may be effective against several viruses of ocular importance, including HSV, vaccinia, and smallpox (268–272).

Mechanism of Action

The drug does not require activation by viral-encoded TK, and phosphorylation of cidofovir is independent of virus infection. The mechanism of action is through cidofovir diphosphate, which inhibits viral DNA polymerase at concentrations 50-fold lower than the level that inhibits cellular polymerases (268). The decreased rate of viral DNA synthesis is due to incorporation of cidofovir into the growing viral DNA chain (273,274). The drugs resist degradation by esterases and persist intracellularly up to 65 hours. This may allow drug-carrying cells to resist replication for several days when challenged by virus after therapy has been discontinued.

Toxicity

Cidofovir is carcinogenic in rats and potentially so in humans. At 65 times the recommended dose, it causes chromosomal alterations in red blood cells *in vitro*. It inhibits spermatogenesis and is embryotoxic in laboratory animals (273–275). Pediatric use should be with caution because of the carcinogenic potential and reproductive toxicity.

The major dose-limiting toxicity of cidofovir is nephrotoxicity in 50% of patients on the maintenance dose of 5 mg/kg body weight every other week. There is an early increase in serum creatinine and proteinuria, and later glucosuria when proximal tubular damage occurs. Neutropenia occurs in 20% of patients on maintenance. Interestingly, ocular hypotony was noted in several patients on maintenance (273).

Penetration and Pharmacokinetics

Pharmacokinetic studies *in vitro* show slow elimination, with a half-life of 22 hours, which supports use of intermittent dosing to achieve efficacy while minimizing toxicity (273,274). Protein binding is minimal (<6%) and the time to peak serum concentration is at the end of the infusion. Peak serum concentration with a 1-hour infusion of cidofovir 5 mg/kg body weight with probenecid is approximately 19 μg/mL. Approximately 70% of cidofovir is recovered unchanged in human urine within 24 hours.

Efficacy

Cidofovir is effective against many herpesviruses, including HSV-1, HSV-2, VZV, EBV, and ganciclovir-resistant and-sensitive CMV, as well as against vaccinia virus and several adenoviruses (266,267,273,275–277). Comparison of topical 1% and 0.5% cidofovir with trifluridine and acyclovir in the rabbit HSV-1 keratitis model showed that both concentrations of cidofovir were significantly better than either of the other two drugs. (232, 233) Snoeck et al. have reported *in vitro* studies on vaccinia that of both phosphonate derivatives, cidofovir (HPMPC) proved to be the most therapeutically effective and most promising agent for both vaccinia and smallpox (271).

Cidofovir is of interest as a potential treatment for adenovirus. Romanowski et al. have reported *in vitro* efficacy against adenovirus types 1, 5, 8, and 19. In the rabbit model, 0.5% cidofovir twice daily for 7 days showed significant efficacy against adenovirus types 1, 5, and 6, all important strains in epidemic forms of the ocular disease (278,279). Antiviral prophylaxis against adenovirus-5 infection with twice-daily dosing of 0.5% or 1% drops was also highly effective at blocking viral replication (280).

Resistance

In experimental adenoviral ocular infection, treatment with 0.5% cidofovir twice daily for 7 days of known cidofovir-resistant strains showed no therapeutic effect compared with the parental adenovirus-5 strain in the rabbit model (276). In CMV retinitis, clinical resistance to intravitreal cidofovir was found in 5% of patients and was associated with prior oral ganciclovir or IV cidofovir. Resistance-associated mutations were found in the UL97 and polymerase genes. Resistant CMV disease can result from a local infection independent of a systemic site of CMV infection (281).

Foscarnet

Structure

Foscarnet (phosphonoformic acid; PFA; Foscavir) is a pyrophosphate derivative of phosphonoacetic acid. It differs from all previously discussed antivirals in that it is not a nucleoside analog (282,283). It is FDA approved for treatment of CMV retinitis in immunosuppressed patients, but is also of use in certain drug-resistant ocular viral infections, such as HSV and VZV.

Mechanism of Action

Antiviral action is through a selective and noncompetitive inhibition of viral-specific DNA polymerases and RNA polymerases (reverse transcriptases) at concentrations not affecting cellular polymerases (284). Because the reaction is reversible, the drug is virostatic, with viral replication restarting on removal of the agent. Because foscarnet does not require phosphorylation and directly affects the pyrophosphate binding site on viral polymerases, it is a therapeutically useful agent against resistant TK^- herpesviruses. Because of its anti–viral reverse transcriptase effect, it has efficacy against HIV (68,128, 218,219,242,284,285).

Toxicity

Renal toxicity may occur in up to 45% of patients with AIDS with resulting azotemia and the need for constant monitoring of creatinine levels in all patients on the drug (282,286). The drug is excreted unmetabolized by renal tubular secretion and glomerular filtration. Toxicity may be due, in part, to foscarnet interference with renal phosphate secretion (287,288). This nephrotoxicity may be avoided or minimized in a number of cases by using intermittent foscarnet dosing rather than constant infusion and by maintaining excellent patient hydration. Elevated creatinine levels almost invariably return to normal (if due to drug) within 2 to 4 weeks of reducing or ceasing foscarnet administration. Electrolyte changes must also be monitored because the serum calcium may become quite high or low, a problem in itself, and one that makes concomitant use of other drugs that affect calcium balance, such as pentamidine, more precarious (289). Similarly, serum phosphorus and magnesium levels should be monitored.

Other toxic side effects include anemia in up to 50% of patients, hepatic enzyme elevation, CNS dysfunction, headaches, nausea and other gastrointestinal disturbance, mucous membrane erosions, and nephrogenic diabetes insipidus (282,288). Neutropenia and thrombocytopenia are not seen with foscarnet therapy.

Penetration and Pharmacokinetics

Oral absorption of foscarnet is very poor, resulting serum levels negligible, and gastrointestinal irritation common (282,288). The IV induction dose at the recommended regimen of 60 mg/kg over 1 to 2 hours three times daily results in peak plasma levels above the ID_{50} for most CMV (100 to 300 μM), HIV (132 μM), and HSV (100 μM) strains (128,282,288). CSF levels are approximately 43% of plasma levels (282). The half-life is 4 hours, and no drug is detectable in the serum by 24 hours, having been cleared by the kidneys unmetabolized. Unlike other antivirals, part of the foscarnet dose sequesters in the bone marrow for as long as several months (275). Over a 7-day period, up to 20% of the administered dose may be deposited in the marrow of patients with AIDS. This may be related to the calcium fluctuations seen in some patients.

Efficacy

Foscarnet is effective against all known human herpesviruses—CMV, HSV-1 and HSV-2, VZV, and EBV— and against the retrovirus, HIV. The primary therapeutic indication is the treatment of CMV retinitis in immunosuppressed patients. Other indications include any systemic form of life-threatening CMV infection, as well as acyclovir-resistant mucocutaneous HSV or VZV infection in immunocompromised patients (282). Doses of 60 mg/kg IV three times daily for 2 to 3 weeks and 90 to 120 mg/kg/day as maintenance are as effective as ganciclovir in CMV retinitis (282,290). Clinical response takes approximately 1 week. Because it does not need viral TK or other enzyme-dependent phosphorylation to be activated, the drug is also of use, and superior to vidarabine, in treatment of the acyclovir-resistant HSV and VZV infections most commonly seen in patients with AIDS (218,219,282).

Resistance

Recent reports of foscarnet-resistant HSV involved virus that was also acyclovir resistant (291). There was no relationship to the TK gene found to explain the acyclovir resistance. Four patients had undergone allogeneic stem cell transplantation. One was cured with valacyclovir and two with cidofovir, but the fourth patient died despite cidofovir treatment. A leukemic child with foscarnet-resistant HSV stomatitis responded well to a course of cidofovir (292).

HERPES SIMPLEX OCULAR DISEASE

HSV, the most ubiquitous communicable infectious virus in humans, is the causal agent of a wide variety of chronically recurring diseases. Ocular herpes simplex, caused primarily by type 1 (oral) but occasionally by type 2 (genital) HSV, is the leading infectious cause of corneal blindness in the United States, with approximately 500,000 cases reported annually (4,184,293,294). Recurrent herpes labialis and dermatitis, also usually caused by HSV-1, afflicts approximately one third of the world population; one half of these people experience more than one attack annually. Herpes genitalis, caused primarily by HSV-2, is the second most common venereal disease in this country, with approximately 100,000 cases reported annually (2,295). In neonates and children, the primary attack of HSV can be devastating. It may be associated with herpetic encephalitis and dissemination of infection, which have very high degrees of morbidity and mortality. Immunologically compromised patients, such as those with atopy, patients with leukemia, and organ transplant recipients, are also at high risk of severe systemic and ocular herpetic infections (2,184,185,294,296–302).

Incidence and Epidemiology

In contrast to the extensive data available on the epidemiology of extraocular HSV infection, little is known about the epidemiology of ocular infections. Nonetheless, information derived from nonocular herpetic studies is of use in understanding many aspects of the often visually debilitating ocular involvement.

The only natural reservoir of HSV is humans, with sources of infection being children with primary disease, adults with recurrent disease, and children and adults as healthy asymptomatic carriers. There is a very high incidence of herpetic neutralizing antibodies in children younger than 6 months of age, presumably from passive transfer through the placenta. This incidence then falls to approximately 20% in children from 6 months to 1 year of age, and then rises slowly to approximately 60% by age 15 to 25 years (2,294,303,304). In a sociologic study, Smith et al. demonstrated a decrease in the incidence of herpetic antibodies in a large population in England. They attributed this to a general improvement in the social environment, improved housing conditions, and better general hygiene (305).

Transmission of the virus appears to be primarily by direct contact. In the head area, this would be salivary droplets or direct oral contact leading to a primary infection, usually around the mouth. Occasionally, silent shedding with no apparent lesions may be the cause of viral spread to other patients (301). Although the primary illness is manifested clinically in only approximately 1% to 6% of patients infected with virus, the virus still has access

by the oral route to the trigeminal ganglion, the ganglion that innervates the eye (305–307). The incubation period between contact and disease is from 3 to 9 days.

In an epidemiologic study on 141 patients with documented infectious epithelial HSK, Bell et al. found an overall predominance of male patients in the 80 patients older than 40 years of age (1.67:1.0; $p < .03$) (295). Of the 65 patients with more than one episode, 34% had a mean recurrence rate of one or more episodes annually and 68% had one or more recurrences every 2 years. The median interval between episodes was 1.5 years (range, 1.7 months to 20.8 years). No patient risk factors for frequent recurrence or for severity of disease (age of entering into study, age of first ocular episode, sex, or source of primary eye care) were noted. However, 46% of 57 recurrences in 27 patients occurred during the winter months of November through February, suggesting a possible role for upper respiratory tract infections in the pathogenesis of infectious ocular herpes.

Liesegang et al. found no seasonal trends in incidence, although rates increased with time (293). The overall prevalence of a history of ocular herpes was 149 cases per 100,000 population, and initial ocular episodes included incidences of 54% for blepharitis and conjunctivitis, 63% for epithelial keratitis, 6% for stromal keratitis, and 4% for uveitis. In a similar but prospective study by Shuster and coworkers of 119 percent with ocular herpes, the recurrence rates were somewhat lower, with 24% of patients having recurrences within 1 year and 33% within 2 years. This may reflect a difference in recurrence rates in the northeastern United States as opposed to the South and West. Shuster and colleagues also found no correlation between the rate of recurrence and either sex or age of the patient, but did note a general correlation between short intervals between past attacks and short intervals between future recurrences. This conforms with the HEDS data (177,308).

There is currently no vaccine for HSV, although killed, subunit, vaccinia hybrid, and DNA vaccines are under development to prevent spread of the virus and to treat infected patients. Glycoprotein D is used in several subunit vaccines, and live, defective mutant viruses lacking critical genes are being used in disabled infectious single-cycle vaccines. This latter vaccine produces noninfectious virions in the inoculated host (3).

Clinical Features

Ocular herpes may be classified into three general groups: congenital and neonatal, primary, and recurrent.

Congenital and Neonatal Ocular Herpes

HSV infection in the newborn may be acquired at one of three periods: intrauterine (5%), peripartum (10%), and postpartum (85%). The first category occurs in 1/300,000 births, with ophthalmic of microphthalmia, retinal dysplasia, optic atrophy, and chorioretinitis (309). There are also often marked skin, vital organ, and neurologic lesions.

HSV infections in the latter two periods are further classified as skin, eyes, or mouth (SEM), with or without the other involvement seen in intrauterine infections. SEM presents at 10 to 12 days of age, whereas CNS disease usually appears at 16 to 19 days of age (309). Ocular herpes may include one or all of the following: conjunctivitis, epithelial keratitis, stromal immune reaction, cataracts, and necrotizing chorioretinitis (310,311). One third of neonates with HSV have CNS disease with or without SEM. In the era before the availability of IV vidarabine and acyclovir, only 18% of neonates had HSV disease limited to SEM. With the advent of acyclovir, this number has risen to 43% (166,309). Similarly, in the pre–systemic antiviral era, 38% of SEM neonates had developmental problems by 1 year of age. With vidarabine and acyclovir, these numbers dropped to 12% and 2%, respectively.

Hutchison et al. recovered HSV-1 from the eye of an infant, a dizygotic twin, born with active herpetic keratitis (312). The mother had no evidence of cervical herpes by culture or serial immune titers, delivery was by cesarean section, and there had been no premature rupture of the membranes. It was hypothesized (but it could not be proved) that the infection was acquired *in utero* by the transplacental, not the ascending, route. Periocular HSV infection also developed in the second twin a few days after birth. Both infants were treated with topical idoxuridine and, because of the chance of disseminated disease, systemic vidarabine, and both made a full recovery.

Although the vast majority of all ocular herpes infections are caused by HSV-1, because of the usual nature of acquisition, 80% of neonatal cases are caused by HSV-2 (298). Despite the unusual case reported by Hutchinson et al., neonatal disease is almost invariably secondary to direct exposure to an HSV-2–infected birth canal during the late prenatal period or during passage through an infected canal at birth itself (312). Inoda and colleagues reported a 3-year-old boy with stromal keratitis and iritis of unknown etiology. PCR testing of the aqueous fluid revealed HSV-2 as the causative pathogen. The patient recovered on acyclovir and steroid therapy (313). Multiple recurrences are far more common with genital and oral herpes than with ocular disease. Studies have shown an 89% recurrence rate for genital and a 42% recurrence rate for oral HSV infection over a 1-year period. In contrast, the ocular herpes recurrence rate was 40% over a 5-year period, which is fortunate, considering the visual consequences (184,314).

Infants' "protective" transplacental antibodies are not sufficient to protect them completely from ocular disease, although they may escape life-threatening visceral involvement. In almost all reported cases, there has been an associated vesicular eruption of the skin, which is a most useful finding when the physician is faced with the need for a very rapid diagnosis. The clinical course of the ocular disease is similar to that encountered with primary or recurrent infections, depending on whether the infant has passively acquired transplacental antibody from the mother. Epithelial ulcers ultimately respond to antiviral therapy, but stromal involvement may clear or leave a nebulous scar. In the absence of superinfection, the skin lesions heal without scarring. An *emergency* pediatric or infectious disease consult is essential because IV acyclovir should be started urgently to minimize serious systemic complications of infection (315).

Primary Ocular Herpes

As noted earlier, most newborns are protected, in part, by maternal anti-herpetic antibodies transferred passively across the placenta *in utero*. This partial protection lasts for approximately 6 months, at which time the passively received antibodies have dwindled to negligible titers and the child becomes nonimmune and susceptible to a primary attack of HSV Fortunately, more than 94% of children do not suffer overt disease when they finally do contract the virus; those who do have overt disease usually manifest it about the mouth and not the eye. All those who are infected (60% by the age of 5 years) then become viral carriers, with the agent resting in latent state in the sensory (trigeminal ganglion) and autonomic nervous systems (304,316–322).

Although HSV has been isolated from the tear film of patients with no history of ocular herpes, studies on patients with a known history of herpetic keratitis show them to have no greater risk of asymptomatic shedding than does the normal population (323). In addition, tear antibodies to HSV-1 may be detected in the absence of detectable parotid saliva or serum antibodies. This suggests that the ocular surface may be an initial infection site for HSV in some healthy, clinically normal subjects and that there may be a preferential homing of committed B lymphocytes to the ocular mucosal surface (324). It is not yet determined what role, if any, these findings have in terms of latency and recurrent disease.

Primary ocular involvement may present as an acute follicular conjunctivitis or keratoconjunctivitis with nonsuppurative preauricular adenopathy and often with notable vesiculating periocular skin involvement (Fig. 14-3A). Pseudomembranes may be present in the fornices. In the absence of skin vesiculation, differentiation from adenoviral infection is aided by a careful search of the lid margins for signs of herpetic blistering.

Primary HSK is often atypical. Initially, there may be just a nonspecific, diffuse punctate keratitis that evolves into multiple scattered microdendritic figures. There may be wandering linear serpiginous ulcers across the entire corneal surface (184). The diffuse nature of this primary epithelial involvement is probably a function of the host's nonimmune state, which allows more widespread ulceration. Primary

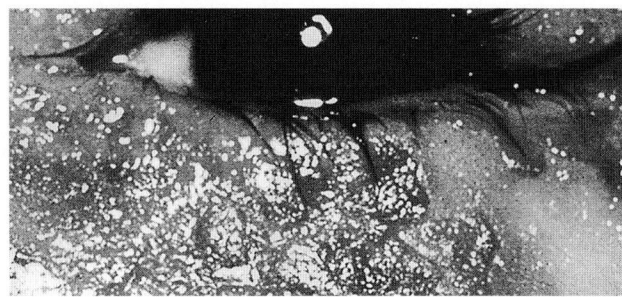
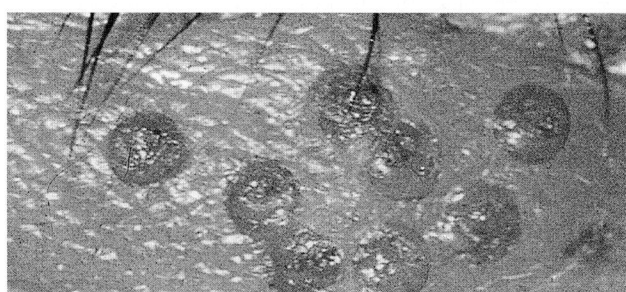

FIGURE 14-3. A: Acute primary herpes simplex virus (HSV) blepharitis with confluent vesicles on hyperemic base. **B:** Recurrent HSV vesicles on lower lid showing much more localized lesions than in primary disease.

disease is, as a rule, confined to the epithelium in terms of clinical findings. Stromal involvement is not usually seen in this phase of the disease, presumably because the host is not immunologically programmed against the virus.

Primary ocular herpes should not be confused with "first ocular occurrence." The former is a first encounter with the virus, whereas the latter is the first eye involvement with HSV in a patient who has had a subclinical oral or nasal infection and is immune. First ocular occurrence is, therefore, similar to recurrent ocular herpes as described later.

Recurrent Ocular Herpes

Patients with recurrent herpes have both cellular and humoral immunity against the virus. The disease may present as any one or a combination of the following:

Blepharoconjunctivitis
Episcleritis, scleritis
Corneal:
Epithelial disease
Infectious ulceration
Trophic (metaherpetic) ulceration
Stromal disease
Viral necrotizing keratitis
Interstitial keratitis, immune rings, and limbal vasculitis
Disciform keratitis

Endotheliitis
Iridocyclitis and trabeculitis

Blepharoconjunctivitis, Episcleritis, and Scleritis

Blepharoconjunctivitis is a much more localized infection than that seen in primary disease. Vesicles are localized rather than diffuse, starting as red papules that form clear vesicles, break, and scab over to heal without scarring (Fig. 14-3B). Virus is present for approximately 3 days in the lesions, although the lesions themselves take approximately 1 week to heal. Conjunctivitis is usually diffuse and watery. Occasionally, rose bengal or fluorescein staining reveals a conjunctival dendritic ulcer. Episcleritis and scleritis may occasionally occur and are slowly responsive to topical or oral nonsteroidal antiinflammatory agents (NSAIDs) such as ketorolac drops four times daily and ibuprofen. Topical steroids are effective in NSAID-unresponsive cases.

Epithelial Disease

Infectious Ulceration. HSV-induced eruptions of the corneal epithelium are characteristically thin, branching dendritic ulcers; wider, branching dendrogeographic ulcers; or map-shaped geographic lesions (Fig. 14-4). All are caused by live virus. Little inflammatory cell reaction-neutrophils but no lymphocytes-is seen in this form of ocular herpes, but many free viruses lie in intracellular and extracellular locations, particularly in the basal epithelium (325).

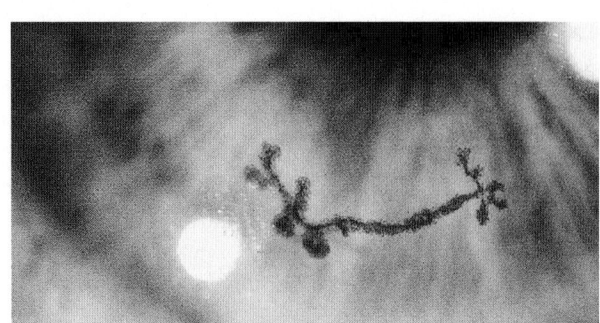
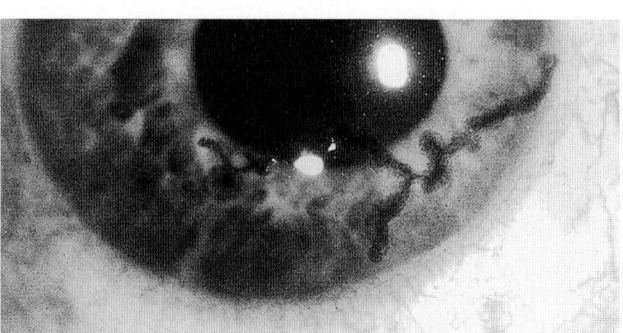

FIGURE 14-4. A, B: Two examples of herpes simplex virus corneal dendritic ulcers with terminal bulbs at the end of each branch.

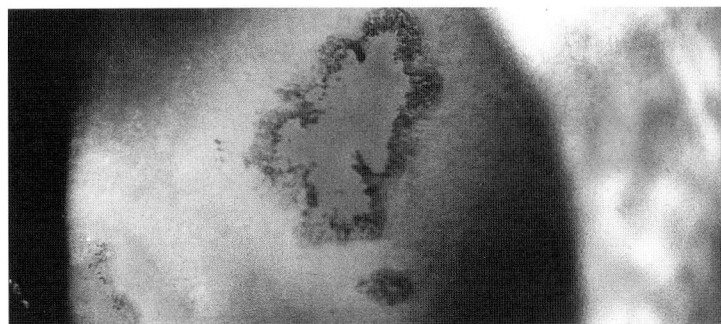

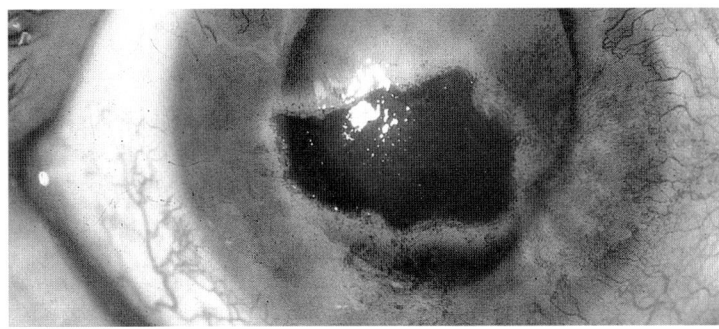

FIGURE 14-5. A, B: Two examples of scallop-edged infectious herpes simplex virus geographic corneal ulcers. These may be differentiated from trophic mechanical ulcers in that the latter have smoother, thicker edges.

Signs and symptoms include tearing, irritation, photophobia, and often blurring of vision. Because the only presenting clinical finding may be a watery conjunctivitis, the patient should be asked about any trauma, previous corneal ulcers, inflammation inside the eye (iritis), nasal or oral cold sore, genital sores, recent use of topical or systemic steroid or immunosuppressive drugs, and immunologic deficiency states such as HIV positivity, malignancy, organ transplantation, or chronic eczema.

If corneal examination reveals dendritic or even geographic ulceration, the infectious agent is HSV until proved otherwise. In herpes, corneal sensation is reduced in approximately 70% of patients (326). It is almost never totally absent, as often seen in zoster keratitis. Marked stromal scarring as seen in more chronic forms of herpes results in a more marked decrease in sensitivity. Initially, the corneal lesions begin as a fine, transient, punctate keratitis that coalesces to form dendritic, dendrogeographic, or geographic ulcers (Fig. 14-5). In an eye that has had many recurrences or is receiving steroids without antiviral prophylaxis, the more subtle stages may be bypassed and the cornea may simply break down in rapidly forming geographic ulceration.

The actual incidence of infectious epithelial HSK in immunocompetent patients may be much higher than suspected clinically. Kodama et al., using immunofluorescent staining and corneal sensitivity testing, reported that of 48 eyes with diagnoses of nonherpetic conditions, 11 had positive reactions on immunofluorescent staining and 8 (73%) had decreased corneal sensitivity (326). The diagnosis in nine of these patients was recurrent erosion and in two, nonherpetic superficial punctate keratitis. Conversely, only 30% of eyes not suspected of having

herpes keratitis and having negative findings on immunofluorescent staining still had decreased corneal sensitivity. Clinically, the nine "recurrent erosion" eyes that were not correctly diagnosed clinically as herpetic were described as having epithelial defects that were oval and central with hazy surrounding edges. Superficial stromal opacities were occasionally observed. It is likely, then, that had these eyes been correctly diagnosed as herpetic, they would not have been placed into the category of sterile trophic mechanical ulceration and therapy incorrectly directed toward lubrication and therapeutic lenses.

Contrary to common opinion, recurrent epithelial infections are not always due to the patient's original HSV strain. Remeijer et al. have reported a study on 30 patients in whom sequential corneal HSV-1 isolates revealed that 63% were genotypically the same from recurrence to recurrence, whereas 37% were actually genetically different (327). Four of 11 patients in the latter group had undergone keratoplasty between recurrences, but otherwise no other risk factor could be identified for infection with exogenous strains.

Infectious HSK in patients with AIDS is not entirely identical to that encountered in the immunocompetent patient. It has been reported that the incidence of HSV infection was no greater than in the general population, but recurrences of herpetic disease were more frequent in the HIV-positive population, with some patients having two to three recurrences over an average period of 17 months (183,299,328). These recurrences also tended to be lengthier than the initial episodes, with a clinical course requiring 2 to 4 weeks of topical therapy and a mean healing time of 3 weeks. There is little to no stromal infiltration under these ulcers, presumably as a result of the immunosuppressed state of the patients. Immunocompetent patients usually had a recurrence-free interval of at least 18 months (295,308,314). Other reports on HIV-positive patients and patients with eczema noted that they benefitted from the use of oral acyclovir in more rapid resolution of their recurrent episodes of infectious disease (299,329).

Hodge and Margolis have reported a large, controlled study on ocular HSV in HIV-positive patients (330). There were 1800 HIV-positive patient visits and 48,200 HIV-negative patient control visits. Although they also found no increased incidence of HSK, unlike earlier reports, there was no significant difference between HIV-positive and control patients in lesion type (epithelial and stromal), lesion location (peripheral vs. central), response time to topical trifluridine or oral acyclovir therapy (HIV-positive = 17 days; HIV-negative = 18 days), ultimate visual outcome, and time to first recurrence (347 days for HIV-positive vs. 321 days for HIV-negative). Only the recurrence rate was significantly higher in HIV-positive patients, being on average 1/587 days for HIV-positive patients and 1/1455 days for HIV-negative patients.

The pathogenesis of the branching ulceration typical of herpes epithelial keratitis has never been elucidated. The popular concept that it is related to neuronal distribution has been disproved (331). The pattern may simply be a function of viral linear spread by contiguous cell-to-cell movement. In HSV keratoplasties, the epithelium may occasionally heal in a superficial hypertrophic dendriform epitheliopathy pattern that may be confused with infectious dendritic ulcers. These lesions are sterile, however, and refractory to all treatment except therapeutic soft contact lenses (332).

Ulcerations occasionally occur within 2 mm of the limbus. These tend to be much more resistant to antiviral therapy than are central herpetic infections. Corneal sensation may remain normal in these marginal ulcers. These lesions must be differentiated from staphylococcal immune marginal ulcerations because the latter respond to steroid therapy and the former may worsen with such therapy.

Stromal reaction is usually absent or mild and confined to the anterior layers in milder epithelial infections. On occasion, however, even mild epithelial infection may be associated with notable stromal edema and iritis. These eyes are more likely to go on to chronic recurrent immune disease and scarring, resulting in visual loss. Concurrent or future stromal disease may be minimized, as well as the healing rate enhanced, by gentle debridement of the infected epithelium with a sterile cotton-tipped applicator before instituting antiviral chemotherapy (110,333). Such debridement is thought to remove much of the immune-inciting antigen that could penetrate to deep stromal layers.

Trophic (Metaherpetic) Ulceration. Occasionally, despite adequate antiviral therapy, epithelial ulcers do not completely heal or, having healed, break down again in an ovoid or dendritiform pattern. This is called trophic, or "metaherpetic," keratopathy. This chronic sterile ulceration is secondary to interacting adverse factors, including impaired corneal innervation, abnormal tear film stability, and damaged basement membrane (125,334). Corneal epithelial cells normally lie on top of their basement membrane attached by hemidesmosomes, rather than interdigitating with the membrane. If the basement membrane is damaged during the infection or if the tear film lubricates poorly, the basement membrane takes at least 12 to 15 weeks to repair itself and thus slows adequate healing of the overlying epithelium (334). Gundersen's classic study on the occurrence of trophic ulcers in several hundred patients with herpes revealed that trophic ulcers developed in 17% of patients receiving no therapy at all (335). Twenty-six percent treated with partial 10% iodine scrubs of the affected epithelium and 38% of those undergoing total epithelial removal with iodine scrubs acquired this condition.

Clinically, a trophic ulcer may be distinguished from an actively infected viral ulcer by the appearance of its edge. Trophic ulcers have gray, thickened borders formed by heaped-up epithelium unable to move across or adhere to the damaged ulcer base (Fig. 14-6A). In contrast, actively infected ulcers have discrete, flat edges that may change

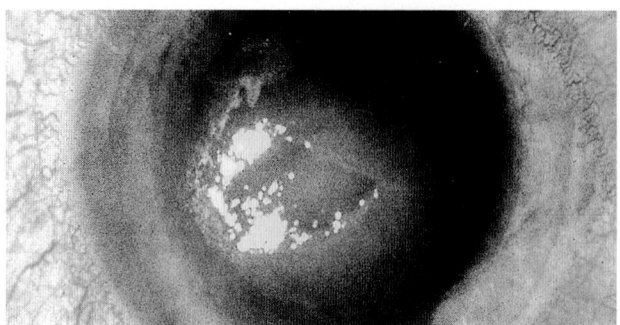
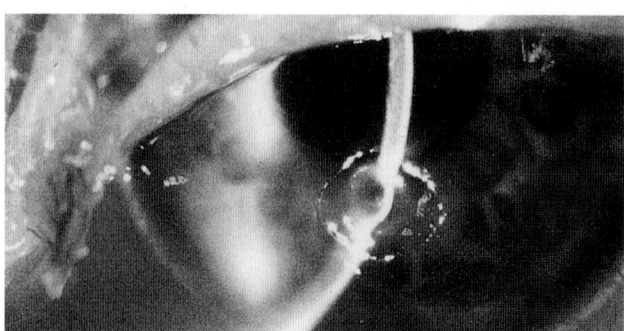

A   B

FIGURE 14-6. A: Thick-edged, sterile herpes simplex virus (HSV) trophic mechanical ulcer over active immune disciform keratitis. **B:** HSV trophic ulcer persisting over several months with subsequent melting (thinning) down to Descemet's membrane (descemetocele) and impending perforation.

their configuration as the ulcer erodes newly infected epithelium. Persistence of trophic ulceration over several weeks or months poses a threat to the integrity of the globe. The longer the ulcer is present, the greater the chance of collagenolytic activity with subsequent stromal melting (thinning) down to Descemet's membrane, and perforation (Fig. 14-6B). This is particularly true in male patients and if the ulcer is located in the central cornea away from peripheral vascularization, which scars but heals (336,337).

Stromal Disease

Stromal disease may be divided into four to five categories according to currently accepted pathogenetic mechanisms: antigen-antibody-complement (AAC)–mediated immune disease characterized by viral interstitial keratitis, immune rings, and limbal vasculitis; and delayed hypersensitivity immune disease characterized by disciform edema/endotheliitis. The latter two are considered two separate categories by some authorities (i.e., disciform keratitis and endotheliitis). Endotheliitis is often associated with elevated intraocular pressure (23,297,338–340).

Interstitial Keratitis, Immune Rings, and Limbal Vasculitis. All three forms of herpetic AAC-mediated disease are thought to be due to immune complex hypersensitivity (125,184,341,342). The interstitial keratitis is a necrotizing keratitis (unlike disciform disease, which is nonnecrotizing). Interstitial keratitis presents clinically as single or multiple areas of dense, white infiltrates (Fig. 14-7). After several weeks of smoldering, deep leashes of vessels often move in as if in pursuit of the infiltrate(s). These lesions may remain small

and focal or become so severe as to give the cornea a red (vessels) and white (interstitial keratitis) mottled pattern on unaided view. They resemble bacterial or fungal infiltrates, but are far more indolent and usually run a course of many months.

A number of studies have reported presence of viral particles in HSK. We have reported two patients with ulcerative necrotizing HSK who despite months of topical and systemic antiviral therapy had numerous intact virions noted in the stromal keratocytes and extracellular lamellae on electron microscopic examination of the keratoplasty buttons (153). Using immunohistochemical stainings for HSV-1 antigens, Holbach et al. reported that 91% of 22 keratectomy specimens from patients with ulcerative necrotizing keratitis displayed HSV antigens (343). These antigens were located primarily in stromal keratocytes and the extracellular stroma, and less commonly in the endothelial and epithelial cells. Conversely, only 11% of 36 keratectomy specimens from patients with nonulcerative, nonnecrotizing keratitis or disciform stromal scarring had similar viral antigen staining. Histopathologic studies on a perforated graft with necrotizing stromal keratitis revealed that the endothelium and keratocytes contained viral inclusion bodies and antigens, indicating that a productive endothelial and stromal herpes infection can lead to graft failure and necrotizing stromal disease (344). Interstitial HSK is the most likely form of ocular herpes to recur in a new graft (153,345,346).

Indeed, molecular biologic studies on both animal models and human keratoplasty buttons have also provided evidence of a persistent or latent infection in peripheral

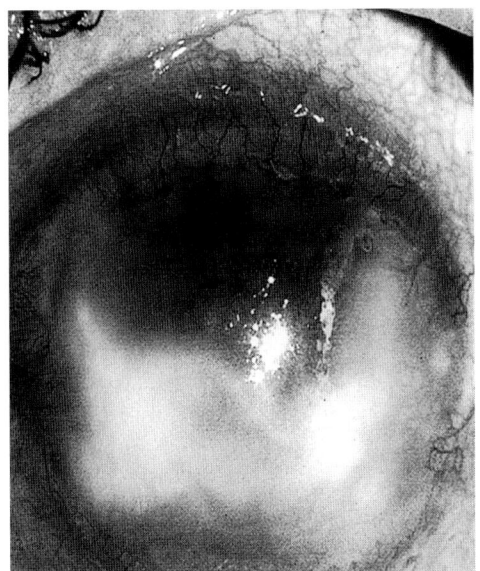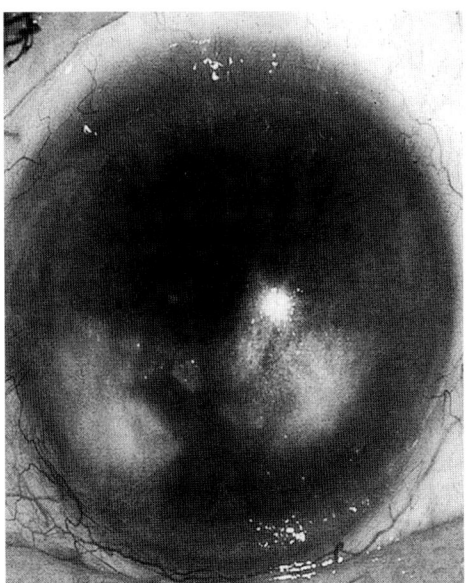

A   B

FIGURE 14-7. A: Dense, white, necrotic herpes simplex virus interstitial keratitis with 360 degrees of neovascularization. **B:** Same eye 1 year later after slowly tapered topical steroid therapy.

nonneural tissues, including the cornea (347–349). The discovery of live virus or viral antigen throughout all corneal layers in up to 25% of patients with herpetic keratitis substantiates the view that some stromal disease is due to active infection or a combination of infection and the immune processes discussed later (153,344,346,350).

Immune (Wessely) rings in the anterior stroma and limbal vasculitis are thought to be two other clinical manifestations of AAC-mediated disease (351–356). Limbal vasculitis is usually focal, although one or more quadrants may be involved in an edematous, hyperemic reaction sufficiently severe to cause dellen formation. There is little to no tendency for these vessels to invade the cornea in the absence of associated interstitial keratitis (Fig. 14-8A). The immune ring does not seem to incite major neovascularization but, not uncommonly, patches of interstitial keratitis may be associated with the ring and stimulate the growth of vessels (Fig. 14-8B and C).

Disciform Keratitis. Disciform edema of the cornea is a well-known adverse consequence of ocular herpes.

It is categorized by some authorities as an entity separate from endotheliitis and by others as disciform keratitis/endotheliitis. It is currently believed that the pathogenesis of this lesion is a delayed hypersensitivity reaction to HSV-antigenic changes of the surface membranes of stromal cells and to the antigenically provocative residue of the viral invasion. The reaction itself is characterized histopathologically by a mixture of sensitized lymphocytes, plasma cells, macrophages, and neutrophils, as described later in the section on Immune Defense Mechanisms, under Pathogenesis (346,351,357).

Clinically, the milder to moderate forms of disciform disease present as focal, often disc-shaped stromal edema (Fig. 14-9). There is no necrosis or neovascularization, but there may be fine keratic precipitates attacking the endothelium just in the involved area, and there may be iritis. In some cases there is no anterior chamber reaction, yet keratic precipitates are present, which suggests that these programmed lymphocytes are particularly attracted to the focal corneal antigen in the endothelium or deep stroma. In

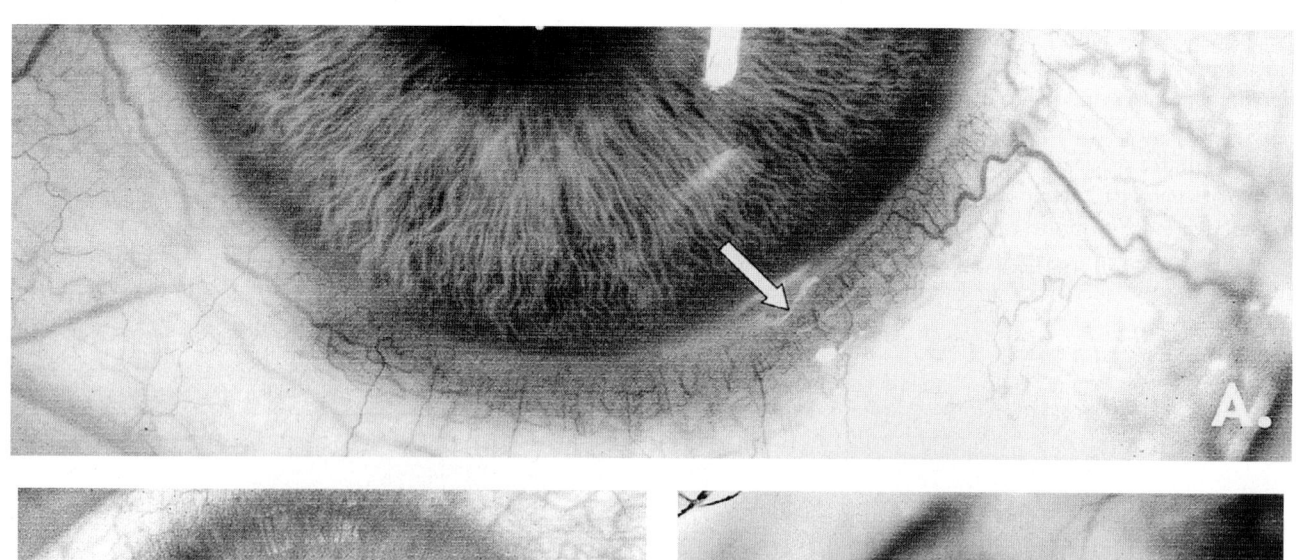

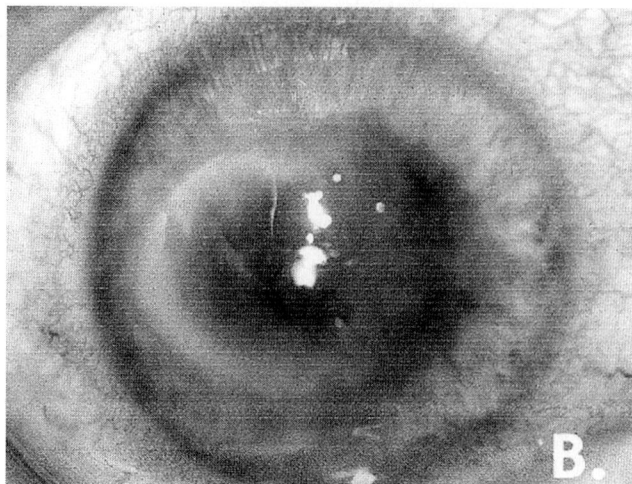

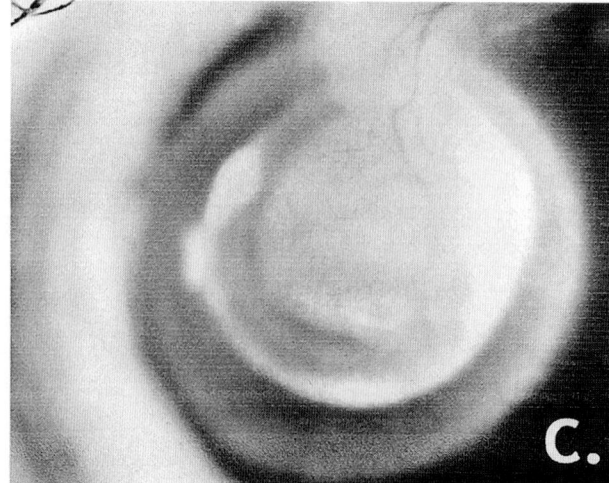

FIGURE 14-8. A: Herpes simplex virus (HSV) limbitis (*arrow*) with local edema and hyperemia due to local Arthus reaction. **B, C:** Single and double HSV immune rings in stroma. Double ring has a deep leash of vessels feeding to central cornea.

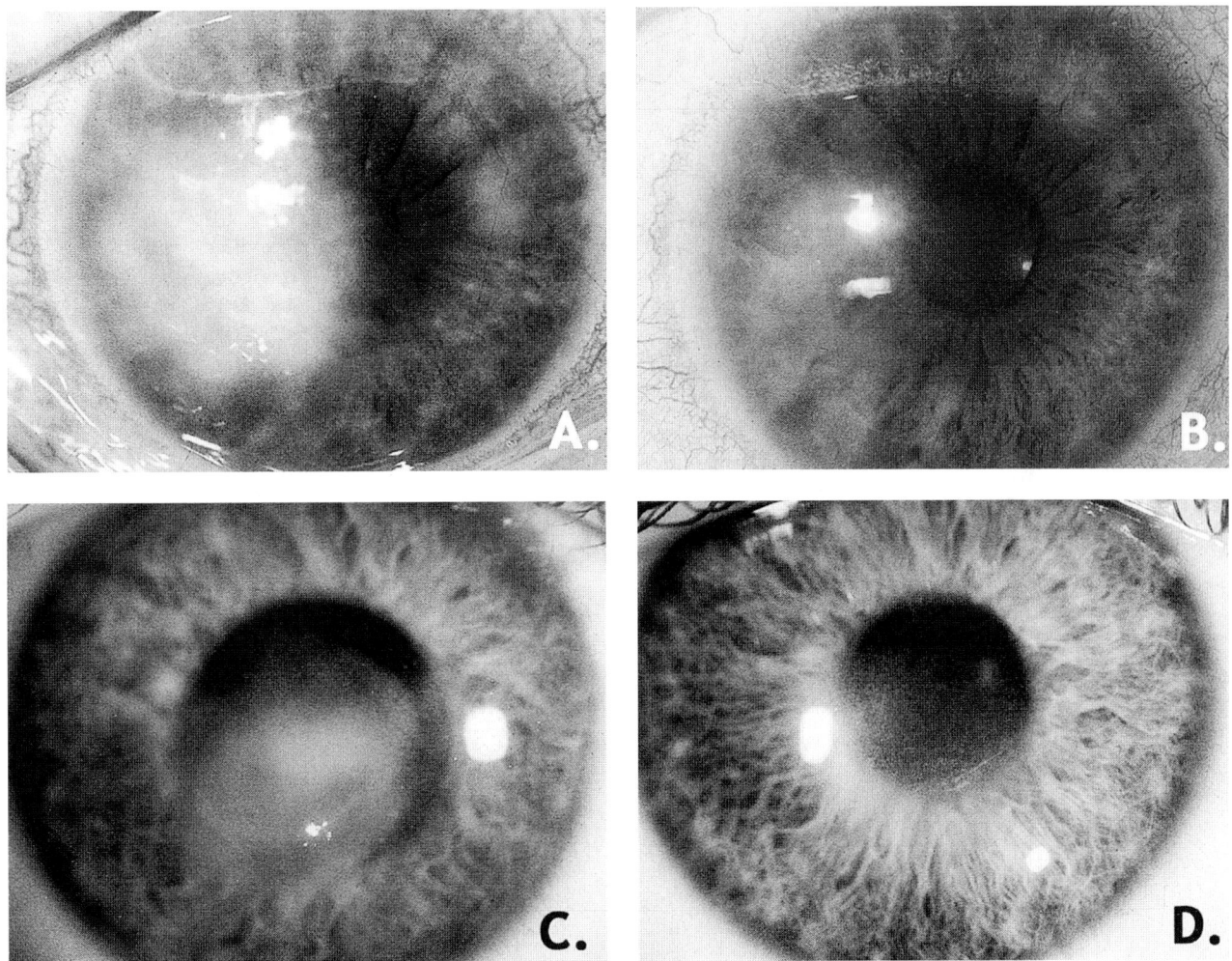

FIGURE 14-9. A: Active herpes simplex virus disciform edema without necrosis, seen with interstitial keratitis. **B:** Same eye as in **A** 2 weeks after starting topical steroids therapy. **C:** Active disciform edema in 5-year-old boy with history of recent eye trauma. There were no previous dendrites or facial cold sores. **D:** Same eye as **C** 6 months later, after topical steroids were discontinued.

the more severe cases of disciform disease, the stromal edema is more diffuse, Descemet's folds are present, and deep and superficial neovascularization may occur. Focal bullous keratopathy may develop, which indicates both that the endothelium is severely compromised by the inflammatory attack and that an abnormal amount of fluid is being driven into the cornea by hydrostatic pressure. In the most severe cases, the bullae rupture, and the cornea may become ulcerated with subsequent necrosis and melting. In moderate to severe cases of disciform disease, iritis is almost invariably present.

Patches of viral interstitial keratitis, immune rings, or limbal vasculitis may be found in eyes with active disciform edema. This combined AAC-mediated disease and delayed hypersensitivity reaction may be mild and readily amenable to therapy, or more severe and stubbornly unresponsive to the most assiduous treatment.

Endotheliitis, Trabeculitis, and Secondary Glaucoma. Progressive endotheliitis with or without uveitis may be

associated with dendritic ulceration, disciform edema, or marked elevation in intraocular pressure (340). Pure HSV endotheliitis may be characterized by a line of keratic precipitates demarcating edematous and nonedematous corneal zones (340). One HSV patient who had not undergone keratoplasty had progression of a "rejection line" across the endothelium with overlying stromal edema and a sudden rise in intraocular pressure to 60 mm Hg just 2 weeks after a dendritic ulcer had been treated (D. Pavan-Langston, unpublished data). There was no associated iritis, and the pressure rise was attributed to an inflammatory trabeculitis. The glaucoma responded to intensive topical and subconjunctival steroid therapy and short-term antiglaucoma measures, but the corneal edema was irreversible.

Sundmacher and Neumann-Haefelin have reported that elevated intraocular pressure was strongly predictive of the presence of intact viral particles in the aqueous humor of

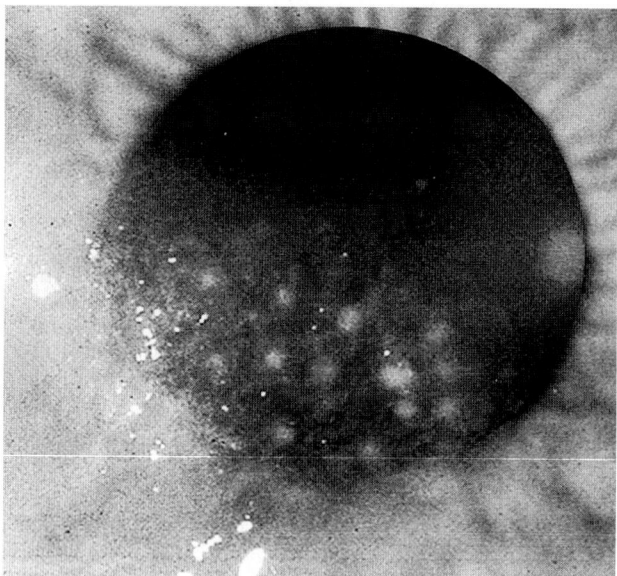

FIGURE 14-10. Herpes simplex virus endotheliitis with disciform edema. Lymphocytic keratic precipitates cling to endothelium. The anterior chamber is entirely clear, with no evidence of iritis.

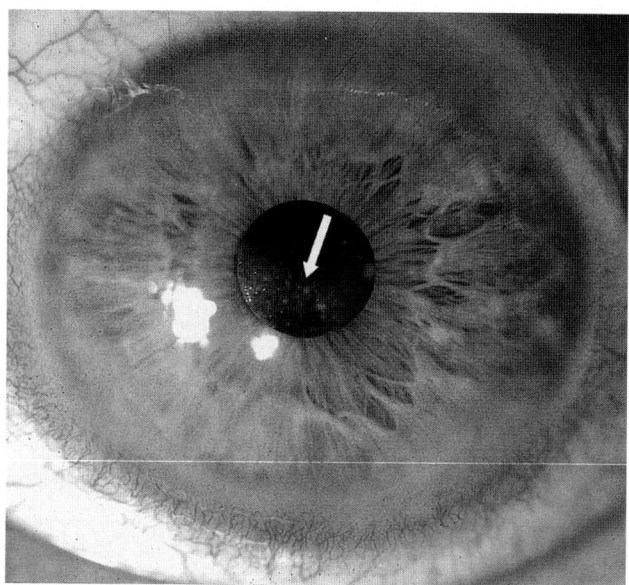

FIGURE 14-11. Acute herpes simplex virus iritis with 360 degrees of limbal ciliary flush, keratic precipitates, and cells and flare in the anterior chamber.

such patients (338,358,359). Despite this finding, topical antiviral therapy had no effect. Systemic acyclovir also has little efficacy in this condition. Topical steroids and antiglaucoma medications are the mainstay of therapy.

Vogel et al. have reported a case of HSV endotheliitis in which the inflammatory infiltrate along Descemet's membrane and the endothelium consisted mostly of CD4+ T lymphocytes with only a few neutrophils, macrophages, and CD20+ B lymphocytes (Fig. 14-10). No viral particles or antigen could be demonstrated, indicating that herpetic endotheliitis and graft rejection endotheliitis may be histologically similar, and that viral particles are not necessarily required (360). Several other patients with documented HSK have been shown to have unilateral stromal edema, aqueous flare and cells, and endothelial cell swelling or guttata-like defects in the endothelial mosaic (340,361–363). This all indicates that viral cytolysis or attack by immunocompetent cells may result in the endothelial cell damage. Extension of this process into the trabecular meshwork appears to be the etiology of the secondary glaucoma, which is highly responsive to steroid therapy.

Iridocyclitis

Recurrent nongranulomatous HSV iridocyclitis may occur without known prior keratitis or without concomitant keratitis. In the presence of active keratitis, however, there is almost invariably some uveal inflammation caused either by reaction to viral antigen in the iris or by the irritative effects of the keratitis. Clinically, there is often circumlimbal ciliary flush, keratic precipitates on the corneal endothelium, and, of course, cells and flare in the aqueous (Fig. 14-11).

Multiple recurrences may lead to diffuse iris atrophy and posterior synechia formation to the lens (Fig. 14-12). If trabeculitis is present, there is usually a secondary glaucoma unless aqueous production has been markedly reduced by inflammation in the ciliary body.

The pathogenesis of this uveitis is not well understood. Complete viral organisms have been found in the aqueous in several cases and, in one instance, in a retrocorneal membrane (338,364,365). The immune inflammatory component is characterized by diffuse lymphocytic infiltration of the iris stroma, and, on retroillumination, diffuse pigment epithelial defects may be noted. In severe cases there may be anterior chamber fibrin exudate, hypopyon, iris edema, and posterior synechia formation.

In studies on the clinical nature and visual outcome in patients with HSV or VZV iritis, the disease was remitting and recurrent in HSV and chronic in VZV cases (366). Secondary glaucoma was the most common complication in both groups (54% HSV, 38% VZV). Posterior pole complications included cystoid macular edema, epiretinal membrane, papillitis, retinal fibrosis, and detachment (8% HSV, 25% VZV). Treatment modalities were similar for both groups, but periocular and systemic steroids were used more frequently in HSV than in VZV (60% vs. 25%). Legal blindness was also similar for both groups at 20%.

Pathogenesis

Latency and Reactivation

Much of the scarring caused by herpesvirus infection is the result of its pattern of recurrence. With each new attack, more permanent damage may be left.

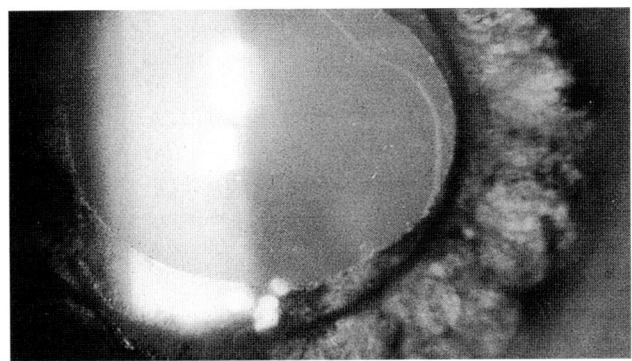
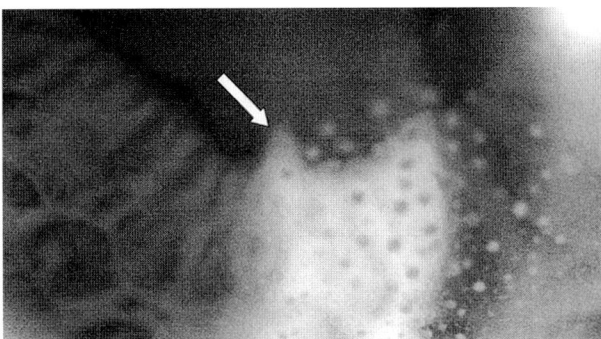

FIGURE 14-12. A: Chronic recurrent herpes simplex virus (HSV) iridocyclitis has resulted in diffuse iris atrophy of the stroma, sphincter, and pigment epithelium. **B:** Acute recurrent HSV iritis with keratic precipitates and posterior iris synechiae (*arrow*).

Latency with the ability for subsequent reactivation to the infectious state characterizes all members of the herpesvirus family. Whether viral latency is a static or smoldering but dynamic state is as yet undetermined. Viral DNA has been found in latently infected human ganglia and corneas by molecular biologic techniques, including *in situ* hybridization, slot blot analysis, and PCR (318,348,349,367–369). The ICPO (infected-cell protein number zero) or junctional region of the viral genome is retained in the host cell nucleus during the latent viral state, and viral RNA transcribed from the opposite region on the DNA strand may be involved in, but not required to maintain latency or prevent reactivation. Reactivation from latency results in the production of large amounts of this RNA, referred to as *antisense RNA*, and results in a cascade of events leading to production of viral polypeptides and ultimately intact infectious virions (368, 370,371).

In a study of 110 patients by Kaye et al., HSV-1 DNA and antigen were found in 82% and 74%, respectively, of 52 corneas with documented history of HSK and in 22% and 15%, respectively, of corneas from patients with no history of HSK (372). Furthermore, VZV DNA or antigen, but not CMV or EBV, were found significantly more frequently in specimens where there was a history of HSK (*p* < .001). All of this has a bearing on herpes "recurring" in herpetic and nonherpetic keratoplasties, as discussed later in the section on Surgical Factors and Management.

Within 1 to 2 days of the primary infection about the face or eyes, the virus has traveled by retrograde axoplasmic flow to the trigeminal ganglia, ciliary ganglia, mesocephalic nucleus of the brainstem, and the sympathetic ganglia, where it enters a latent or dormant state over the ensuing 2 to 3 weeks (320–322,369,373,374). Although any of the sites, or even the cornea itself, may be a source of virus in recurrent disease, the trigeminal ganglion appears to be the main source of reactivated HSV. As discussed earlier in the section on Primary Ocular Herpes, an initial oral facial infection may establish latent virus in the ganglion and subsequent reactivation may result in viral migration

peripherally through the ophthalmic division of the fifth nerve, causing a first ocular infection rather than recurring sores about the nose or mouth (341,375,376). Because of the presence of CMI and humoral antibody resulting from the primary infection, these first ocular recurrences resemble any other recurrent ocular herpetic disease.

Bilateral infection is uncommon and occurs in less than 2% of immunocompetent patients, most of whom are younger than 10 years of age (377). Atopic or other immunoincompetent patients have a notably higher incidence of bilateral disease (185,378). Souza et al., in their study of 544 patients with ocular HSV, found that in contrast to unilateral HSK, patients with bilateral disease had underlying atopy or immune deviations and followed more protracted clinical courses (379). Long-term acyclovir, 400 mg PO twice daily, significantly reduced the incidence of recurrence of all forms of HSV in the bilateral disease group.

Although local ocular cellular and humoral immune mechanisms (secretory IgA) may determine whether an active infection will be established or reactivated virus simply neutralized on the ocular surface, circulating antibodies have little to no influence on the development of recurrent disease. Systemic antibody titers remain unchanged during and between recurrences, or may rise to high levels in the absence of an overt episode of infectious disease (304,351,380,381).

Data on the character of different viral strains have also indicated that some herpes strains are more likely to cause repeated and severe disease, whereas other strains rarely, if ever, cause recurrences and consequently cause little disease after the primary infection (382,383). In one study, recombinant HSV DNA analysis revealed that the differences in ocular disease patterns may be genetically determined by specific sites on the chromosomes of various substrains of virus (384). A human clinical isolate may, in fact, be composed of more than one substrain, each of which may cause a different form of ocular disease, epithelial or stromal (385). In another study, an isolate initially caused just mild epithelial disease, but with repeated passage (analogous to recurrences) there was a spontaneous selection for a more virulent neurotrophic substrain that caused severe epithelial ulceration and death from encephalitis in inoculated animals. This suggests that one factor in worsening clinical disease with multiple recurrences is the possible natural selection of more virulent substrains already colonizing a patient's ganglia.

The question of whether the first HSV infection and latency in the ganglia can prevent subsequent latent infection by different strains has yet to be resolved. It was initially reported that the first virus strain would block a later infecting strain from establishing latency (386). This raised hopes that early vaccination with benign, nonrecurring strains of HSV might prevent establishment of chronic latent infection by a more virulent recurring strain and thus prevent debilitating ocular or other herpetic disease. It was subsequently reported, however, that although previous inoculation with a benign strain of virus can reduce the severity of keratitis, increase survival rates, and decrease the frequency of recovery of latent virus when a more virulent HSV superinfection occurs, this protection is incomplete (387). More than one strain of virus was, in fact, isolated from the same trigeminal ganglion in several animals. In addition, the previously mentioned recovery of more than one substrain of virus from a human isolate indicates that there is a direct correlation between the experimental data and what occurs clinically (385). This ability of HSV substrains to coexist in the ganglia would suggest only limited potential success of live attenuated vaccination as an approach to preventing recurrent herpetic disease. In human studies, Remeijer et al. have reported that 37% of recurrent HSK is due to a strain different from the strain of the previous attack (discussed previously in the section on Infectious Ulceration, under Recurrent Ocular Herpes) (327).

In studies on the effect of oral famciclovir or topical trifluridine on corneal disease and latency, Loutch et al. found that starting famciclovir or trifluridine the day of ocular inoculation with HSV resulted in a significant reduction in the severity of keratitis and viral copy numbers in the trigeminal ganglion in the famciclovir group compared with the control and trifluridine groups (251). It remains to be seen if long-term famciclovir therapy in animals or humans will reduce recurrence rates by reducing virus in the ganglion and whether that effect will persist even after famciclovir is stopped.

The wide variety of factors able to induce herpetic eruptions in humans (sunlight, local trauma, heat, fever, menstruation, immunologic manipulation, infectious disease, surgery, and emotional stress) have been reviewed in the last two decades (184,318,374,376). Spontaneous reactivation of virus is not common in laboratory animals but can be provoked by stimuli such as anaphylactic shock, epinephrine, iontophoresis with epinephrine and 6-hydroxydopamine, prostaglandins, ultraviolet light, electrical stimulation of

the trigeminal ganglion, and epilation (319,388–391). Attempts to reactivate HSV by immunosuppressive agents alone have been generally unsuccessful. However, Openshaw et al. demonstrated reactivation of latent HSV in up to 70% of the animals treated with the immunosuppressive drug cyclophosphamide, x-rays, or both (370).

A number of human studies have confirmed that both prostamide analogs used in therapy of glaucoma (e.g., bimatoprost, latanoprost) and various forms of anterior segment laser surgery notably increase the incidence of recurrent ocular herpes, whether epithelial or stromal (240,241,392–394). Laser-induced reactivations may be prevented with prophylactic use of oral antivirals in animal studies. Valacyclovir 500 mg three times daily, famciclovir 250 twice daily, or acyclovir 400 mg three times daily starting 1 day before surgery and continuing for approximately 2 weeks after surgery have been effective in blocking recurrence (author's personal experience).

The HEDS study on risk factors for recurrence did not confirm psychological stress, sun exposure, or systemic illness as related to recurrence (177). Because the weekly log used in the study did not record events within 72 hours (or longer), triggering factors such as the latter two would have been missed in data analysis. The wide variety of factors that appear capable of affecting recurrence rates in humans and animals are primarily forms of physical stress or alterations in the immune status of the host. Questioning patients carefully often reveals such factors occurred within a few days before onset of disease. Such factors should be taken into account and, if possible, ameliorated when evaluating the best overall management of patients with ocular herpes.

Immune Defense Mechanisms

The byproducts of viral replication and immune alteration of the cornea and iris play an important role in many destructive corneal conditions, including necrotizing keratitis, immune rings, limbal vasculitis, disciform edema, and uveitis (79,101,141,153,343,344,346,350). The pathogenesis of these manifestations of herpetic disease has yet to be fully elucidated, but much has been established recently through animal models and histopathologic study of human corneal transplants (327,346,372,395). Intact HSV is found in some transplant specimens; therefore, as noted earlier in the section on Interstitial Keratitis, Immune Rings, and Limbal Vasculitis, it seems likely that in many cases the persistence of incomplete viral antigens and the viral immune alteration of cell membranes in the corneal stroma incite inflammatory reactions that involve programmed host lymphocytes, antiviral antibodies, serum complement, neutrophils, and macrophages (343,344,376). In other cases, viral byproducts are not found (360).

Another factor is the finding that HSV strains that cause stromal disease secrete greater amounts of glycoproteins than do strains that produce primarily epithelial disease (382). This suggests that some stromal disease is a host immune response to the antigenic glycoproteins produced in the ocular tissues by the infecting HSV strain. The clinical response to steroid therapy may also be determined by the viral genome (383). Consequently, one may conclude that both host immune factors and viral characteristics play key roles in determining the ultimate expression of clinical disease in ocular herpes. Further study of the role of hypersensitivity and virus replication is still in progress.

It has been shown that herpetic stromal keratitis may develop in the absence of viral antigen recognition through the activation of bystander T lymphocytes in nonimmune animals, and that $CD4^+$ and $CD8^+$ T lymphocytes participate in HSK (396). Similarly, interleukin (IL)-12 and IL-17 have been shown to play a key role in inflammatory diseases characterized by massive infiltration of neutrophils. Human studies indicate that IL-17 plays an important role in the initiation or perpetuation of the immune disease in HSK by modulating the secretion of proinflammatory and neutrophil chemotactic factors by corneal resident fibroblasts (397,398). The extent to which the host inflammatory response may be beneficial to the eye in terms of ridding the cornea of viral antigens, as opposed to being detrimental in causing matrix destruction, is not yet clear. It is likely that inflammation may be involved in both roles simultaneously. It would be highly useful to be able to separate these two functions and to know when and if there is an appropriate time to use antiinflammatory agents before irreversible damage to the cornea ensues.

Host factors, including hereditary characteristics (human leukocyte antigen [HLA] type), systemic immune diseases (atopy), and other forms of immune incompetence and hyperimmunity, have long been thought to play a role in the nature and severity of the reaction to herpetic antigen. Studies of HLA type, particularly HLA-DR, HLA-A2, and HLA-A3, have been of interest, but the results are at variance with one another, with some investigators reporting a positive correlation and others a negative one (355,399). The ability to identify the high-risk patient and predict the prognosis would greatly enhance our management not only of ocular disease but of herpetic infections elsewhere in the body. It is established, however, that atopic or otherwise immune-altered patients are at greater risk for bilateral and prolonged disease compared with immunocompetent patients (379).

Vaccination to prevent HSK is still in the investigational stage. Inoue et al. have reported that DNA immunization using HSV-1 gD (glycoprotein D) or gD-IL-2 (chimeric gene of gD and human IL-2) was significantly better at suppressing stromal, but not epithelial, keratitis, in mice compared with mock-vaccinated controls (400). Similarly, vaccination of mice with virion host shutoff–deficient (vhs−) HSV resulted in significant reduction in corneal disease compared with controls (401). There are no human ocular studies done in this area, but HSV-2 gD vaccine has been reported as effective against contracting genital HSV in women negative for both HSV-1 and HSV-2 at entry into the study. Men did not benefit regardless of HSV immunity status (402).

Diagnosis

See the section on Laboratory Diagnostic Techniques, previously, for greater detail (1,2,10).

Diagnosis of either primary or recurrent ocular HSV infection may be assisted by the Tzanck technique, staining epithelial scrapings taken from the skin or corneal ulcers. Microscopic examination of the Giemsa-stained smear may, but does not invariably, reveal typical eosinophilic viral inclusion bodies of Lipschütz in the nuclei. Other stains used are Wright, hematoxylin-eosin, Papanicolaou methylene blue, and Paragon multiple. The epithelial cells themselves show ballooning degeneration, and a monocytic white cell infiltrate characteristic of viral infection is always present. A more definitive diagnosis can be made if a viral culture can be performed within several days of the onset of disease. Swabbing the ulcerated areas and immediately inoculating into tissue culture results in a viral isolation rate of approximately 70% if antiviral agents have not been used recently. The virus isolate may then be typed as HSV-1 or HSV-2 (2,10,184).

Primary herpes can be differentiated from first ocular occurrence of recurrent disease by drawing paired sera. The initial clotted blood sample should be drawn when the patient is first seen during the acute phase, and the second sample 4 to 6 weeks later. These may be sent to the state laboratory for titers against both HSV-1 and HSV-2. Negligible titers in the first blood sample but appreciable titers in the second indicate a primary infection in a previously nonimmune patient with subsequent appearance of anti-HSV antibodies. As noted earlier, fluctuations in titers occur independently of the presence or absence of clinical recurrence and are therefore meaningless in all but primary infections (304).

Additional, more sophisticated, sensitive, and selective tests require more complicated technology and equipment. These tests are worthwhile, however, in cases where the diagnosis remains in doubt. They include immunomorphologic evaluation of scrapings from vesicles, for example, immunofluorescent electron microscopy, immunoperoxidase staining, radioimmunoassay, agar gel immunodiffusion, and DNA probes. Serologic evaluation tests include fluorescent antibody staining of membrane antigen, immune adherence hemagglutination assay, ELISA, complement fixation, and neutralization tests. Of these, the most readily available and extremely sensitive test is the commercially marketed HerpChek (DuPont, Wilmington, DE), which is available in a simple kit form and is based on the ELISA system (1,2,10,403–405).

Treatment of Ocular Herpes Simplex

Antiviral Drugs

The pharmacology and clinical efficacy of these agents are discussed in detail in the section on Ocular Antiviral Agents: Laboratory and Clinical Studies, earlier.

Of the 10 antiviral agents with proven efficacy against ocular HSV, only four are in active clinical use: trifluridine (Viroptic) drops, acyclovir (oral; Zovirax; or 3% ointment outside the United States), famciclovir (oral; Famvir), and valacyclovir (oral; Valtrex). Idoxuridine (Stoxil, Dendrid, Herplex) and vidarabine (Vira-A) were recently discontinued from manufacture, although the latter may be obtained as a 3% ointment for five times daily application from compounding pharmacists if needed in resistant cases or for vaccinia.

Those patients in whom short-term oral acyclovir, famciclovir, or valacyclovir, with or without topical antiviral therapy, may be indicated include (a) patients with primary HSK or recurrent epithelial dendritic or geographic keratitis; (b) patients with infectious epithelial keratitis and atopic disease such as eczema; (c) immunosuppressed patients such as those with AIDS or blood dyscrasias, and organ transplant recipients; (d) patients who for physical or emotional reasons are unable to instill topical medication (e.g., those with rheumatoid arthritis, or children); and (e) those whose occupation prevents them from being able to instill medication as directed. In moderately to severely immunosuppressed patients, IV acyclovir may be required in place of oral dosing because of the superior serum levels that are more rapidly and more reliably achieved using this route. IV dosage of acyclovir is 5 mg/kg of body weight every 8 hours for at least 3 to 6 days before switching to oral acyclovir. In some patients, a full 10 days of IV acyclovir therapy may be required. Patients in whom long-term (more than 6 months to 1 year) oral acyclovir, famciclovir, or valacyclovir prophylactic therapy is indicated include those with HSV stromal keratitis and patients with HSV infection who have undergone keratoplasty (23,182,188,190,202,406).

In an extensive literature review to determine the efficacy of various antiviral drugs in ocular epithelial herpes, Wilhelmus reported data on 4251 patients (110). He found the following:

1. Acyclovir or trifluridine were better than idoxuridine at 1 week and, at 2 weeks, trifluridine, vidarabine, and acyclovir were all better than idoxuridine for both dendritic and geographic keratitis.
2. Other agents such as bromovinyldeoxyuridine, ganciclovir, and foscarnet were equivalent to trifluridine or acyclovir.
3. Oral acyclovir was equivalent to topical acyclovir ointment and use of the oral form did not hasten healing when used in combination treatment with a topical antiviral.
4. Antiviral agents did not increase the speed of healing compared with debridement, but reduced the risk of recurrent epithelial keratitis.
5. The combination of debridement with topical antiviral seemed to be better than either treatment alone.
6. Combined topical antiviral therapy and interferon was better than an antiviral alone at 7 days, but not at 14 days.

In studies on the cost-effectiveness of using a prophylactic oral antiviral (acyclovir) to prevent recurrent HSV infection, Lairson et al. found that treatment cost $8532.00 per HSV episode averted (407). Because of the importance, however, of preventing vision loss and time away from work, it was concluded that the decision to use prophylaxis had to be made on a case-by-case basis. This would be particularly important in view of the HEDS data on stromal keratitis (178).

Corticosteroid Therapy

Corticosteroids are excellent antiinflammatory agents that interfere with the function and distribution of immunologically competent lymphocytes, ameboid white cell migration, and the release of cellular digestive enzymes through physiologic stabilization of lysosomal membranes (408–411). Ocular studies on the effect of topical steroids in herpes indicate that there is local inhibition of antibody-forming cells (B lymphocytes) in the cornea and uveal tract. Because there is only a transient effect on the number of B lymphocytes in the draining lymph nodes and none on circulating antibody response, the host is still capable of mounting an immune reaction once the inflammation-inhibiting steroids are removed (352). Although it is known that both topical and systemic corticosteroids worsen herpetic infection in the absence of antiviral prophylaxis, it has been reported that these drugs do not increase the incidence of recurrence but only its severity, if infectious disease does recur spontaneously (412).

Steroids have also been found to inhibit the formation of both mucopolysaccharides and collagen, two substances critical to the integrity of the corneal matrix and structure. The role of steroids in enhancing the release of collagenolytic enzymes is also of concern in cases of corneal thinning and melting. It was reported, however, that 1% medroxyprogesterone acetate (Provera) treatment of herpetic keratitis in animals resulted in the suppression of both latent and active collagenase, thus inhibiting melting (thinning) phenomena (357). This was correlated clinically and histologically with a marked reduction in the neutrophil infiltrate and stromal neovascularization, compared with results in control animals. Epithelial infectious disease was enhanced but could be eliminated by concomitant antiviral therapy. It was believed that medroxyprogesterone acetate, which has an antiinflammatory efficacy roughly equivalent to that of 0.2% prednisolone, was a safer steroid to use in herpetic cases threatened by corneal melting. Clinical use in patients with inflamed but melting corneas appears to bear this out.

Factors arguing for the use of steroids in ocular herpes, then, are significant inhibition of (a) cellular infiltration, (b) toxic hydrolytic enzyme release, (c) scar tissue formation, and (d) neovascularization. On the negative side, steroids (a) suppress the normal inflammatory responses, which may allow deeper spread of a potentially superficial viral infection; (b) cause possible "corneal addiction" to steroids by allowing buildup of leukocyte-attracting antigen, the reaction to which must be constantly suppressed; (c) open the cornea to opportunistic bacterial or fungal infection through suppression of the immune defense system; (d) enhance collagenolytic enzyme production (most steroids); and (e) cause the well-known side effects of steroid glaucoma and cataract.

Having once committed a patient to topical steroid therapy, it is sometimes difficult to withdraw treatment. If the steroids are stopped too abruptly, recrudescence of the immune disease may occur and the drugs will have to be reinstituted. Some patients are unable to stop taking these drugs without an inflammatory flare-up, and may have to continue using "homeopathic" steroid drops once or twice weekly.

A useful rule of thumb to follow in tapering steroids is the *50% reduction technique*—that is, each dosage reduction is never more than half of the current level of therapy. An example of this would be to have a patient take 1% prednisolone every 2 hours while awake for 2 to 3 days, then every four times a day for a week, followed by 1 to 3 weeks at levels of three times a day, with succeeding 1- to 3-week periods of twice daily, then once daily. At this point, the patient would be switched to 0.125% prednisolone four times a day and a similar taper carried out over a several-week period. If a patient is unable to go below 1% prednisolone two or three times daily, the patient should be carried at these levels to control inflammatory damage, but regular, periodic attempts at tapering should be made. Less severe disease would warrant starting steroid therapy at levels well below 1% every 3 hours: for example, prednisolone 0.125%, rimexolone, or loteprednol two or three times daily.

Cyclosporine in Herpetic Keratitis

With the recent FDA approval of topical cyclosporine for treatment of the inflammatory component of dry eyes, the potential role of this agent in ocular herpes is being explored. It would appear to be of particular use in cases involving steroid glaucoma.

An early report that herpetic epithelial keratitis persisted in a corneal graft until cyclosporine was discontinued indicated that the drug has the same potential to enhance the infectious component of this illness as steroids (413).

Cyclosporine use should, therefore, be covered with an antiviral agent prophylactically. Gunduz and Ozdemir treated 10 patients with HSK using 2% cyclosporine drops four times daily and acyclovir 3% ointment five times daily for 2 months. In all patients the stromal disease completely resolved, and visual acuity increased by at least two Snellen lines in 8 of the 10 patients. There were no episodes of epithelial infections (414). A similar study in 18 patients reported that HSK resolved in 14 patients with nonnecrotizing keratitis, and in 2 of 4 eyes with necrotizing keratitis (415).

Patients who have undergone keratoplasty would also appear to benefit from use of cyclosporine drops. Perry et al. reported the successful use of cyclosporine in three cases of therapeutic keratoplasty for mycotic keratitis (416). All were treated with cyclosporine 0.5% drops twice daily from 15 to 42 months. Two grafts remained clear, although the third failed because of preexisting epithelial disease. There was no recurrence of mycosis. Another report on the use of 2% cyclosporine started 48 hours before surgery in four patients with melting metaherpetic keratitis showed notable quieting of the inflammation without further thinning. This was presumably due to inhibition of T-lymphocyte activity (417). Systemic cyclosporine does not appear to be as successful. Inoue et al. were unable to find a difference in incidence of rejection or improvement in the rate of graft clarity in graft recipients receiving topical steroid and oral cyclosporine or control (418). Average follow-up was 5.4 months.

Medical Treatment

Antiviral agents for treatment of HSV are discussed in detail in the section on Ocular Antiviral Agents: Laboratory and Clinical Studies, earlier (Table 14-1).

Primary Ocular and Periocular Herpes Simplex Virus Infections

In the immunologically competent host, herpetic skin lesions remain fairly localized and are a self-limited disease that resolves without scarring without specific therapy. Specific antiviral therapy is recommended, however, and may be outlined as follows:

1. In the absence of corneal ulceration, administer a prophylactic topical or oral antiviral until the skin lesions are resolving (approximately 7 to 10 days). Oral antivirals are used in patients unable or unwilling to use topical medication (e.g., children, adults with disabling arthritis).
   a. Acyclovir 400 mg PO three to five times daily for 14 days *or*
   b. Famciclovir 125 to 250 mg PO twice daily for 14 days *or*
   c. Valacyclovir 500 mg PO twice daily for 14 days *or*
   d. Trifluridine 1% drops nine times daily for 5 days, then five times daily for 9 days

TABLE 14-1. ANTIVIRAL MEDICATIONS USED IN HERPES SIMPLEX KERATITIS[a]

Drug	Dosage
Acute infection	
Trifluridine (Viroptic) 1% drops	9 times daily for 7 days; may decrease dose to 5 times daily after 7 days if ulcer healed
Acyclovir (Zovirax) 400-mg pill[b]	tid to bid for 14–21 days.
Famciclovir (Famvir) 500-mg pill[c]	bid for 14–21 days.
Valacyclovir (Valtrex) 1-g pill[c] (immunocompetent patients)	bid for 14–21 days.
Prophylaxis[d]	
Acyclovir (Zovirax) 400-mg pill[b,c]	bid for 12–18 mo
Famciclovir (Famvir) 250-mg pill[c]	bid for 12–18 mo
Valacyclovir (Valtrex) 500-mg pill[c] (immunocompetent patients)	bid for 12–18 mo

[a]Topical or systemic medication. In immunocompromised patients, a topical may be combined with a systemic agent and continued longer than the indicated period.
[b]Pediatric syrup, 200 mg/tsp.
[c]Not approved by the U.S. Food and Drug Administration for this specific purpose.
[d]Against recurrent stromal keratitis, with high steroid use, in graft rejection, or in postoperative grafts.

2. In the presence of corneal ulceration, gently debride the ulcers with a sterile cotton-tipped applicator after application of topical anesthetic drops, followed by topical or oral antivirals as previously for 14 to 21 days.
3. Apply topical antibiotics twice daily if the cornea is ulcerated.
4. Apply topical antibiotic ointment twice daily to ulcerated skin. Keep area clean with gentle lukewarm or cool soaks (soft facecloth, cotton balls) for 5 minutes twice daily until skin lesions are resolving.
5. Administer cycloplegics if iritis is present (rare).
6. Use eye shields or hand restraints with young children if there is eye rubbing.

Primary corneal disease responds slowly but well to therapy, and the eye, like the skin, usually heals without scarring because of the absence of immune reaction.

Recurrent Infectious Epithelial Herpes (Dendritic, Geographic Ulcers)

Therapy for recurrent infectious herpes is in many ways similar to that for primary disease, and may be outlined as follows:

1. Gently debride involved epithelium with a sterile cotton-tipped applicator.
2. Use topical or oral antivirals for 14 to 21 days as described in the previous section. If ulceration persists after this period, consider therapy for sterile trophic ulceration. In an immunosuppressed patient, lack of healing or spread may be due to viral resistance. Change therapy to alternative drug class (see section on Resistance, under Antiviral Drugs, earlier).
3. Apply topical antibiotics while the corneal is ulcerated.
4. Administer cycloplegics, if needed, for mild iritis. See section on Iridocyclitis and Trabeculitis, later, for steroid indications and use.

With antiviral chemotherapy arresting virus replication until the infected cells slough from the eye, or with debridement, the infectious epithelial disease heals 90% of the time without complication and usually without the need for an antiinflammatory drug. Limbal ulcers are more resistant to healing but eventually close over, usually with little scarring. There is no place for the use of steroids in infectious epithelial disease uncomplicated by stromal immune reaction.

Trophic Postinfectious Ulcers

Therapy for trophic ulcers (metaherpetic herpes) is aimed at protecting the damaged basement membrane by lubrication and soft contact lens therapy. Rarely is a conjunctival flap used today, and stem cell transplantation is in the earliest stages of study for this condition. In the presence of underlying stromal inflammatory disease that may interfere with basement membrane healing, gentle topical steroids may also be indicated.

Multiplying virus does not cause the trophic form of disease. Therefore, the only indication for antiviral therapy would be as prophylaxis against recurrent HSK. Oral antivirals are best because topical agents may interfere with healing owing to toxic medicamentosa. Gently removing all corneal epithelium results in regrowth of the epithelium up to the borders of the ulcer and possibly across it, but often the cells are still unable to adhere to the damaged ulcer base and the surface breaks down again.

Therapeutic wear of thin soft contact lenses has greatly increased the frequency and rapidity of healing of trophic ulcers. The soft lenses work by splinting and protecting the cornea from abrasive lid action and by keeping the ulcer well lubricated by reducing tear film evaporation. They may be worn for just a few weeks if healing is rapid, or for many months if it is slow. Lenses should be replaced if notable deposits build up.

If a mild steroid is needed for inflammation control, 1% medroxyprogesterone acetate drops two to four times daily are safer than prednisolone. Medroxyprogesterone downregulates conversion of latent to active collagenase without major interference with collagen matrix formation (357).

Once healing is achieved, lubrication with bland ointment or artificial tears should be continued for 2 to 3 months to prevent lid action from abrading the newly healed epithelium from the still-fragile ulcer base. If stromal melting does begin, it may be slowed, or even stopped, with the addition of collagenase inhibitors such as tetracycline, 250 mg PO twice daily, or doxycycline, 100 mg PO once daily, which apparently work through chelation of essential zinc in collagenase (419). Doxycycline is the most effective and may be given once daily (*not* with milk products or vitamins with minerals).

The use of cyanoacrylate glue has helped greatly in forestalling emergency surgery, but is not yet approved by the FDA for use in the eye; informed consent should be obtained (420). If corneal melting and thinning progress, the epithelium should be gently debrided away from the ulcer edge and the polyethylene applicator tube containing tissue adhesive gently touched to the ulcer base several times until the area is well covered. Cyanoacrylate adhesive can also be applied with a 25-gauge needle (Fig. 14-13). Sterile saline solution may be dripped on at the end of the procedure to hasten polymerization. A soft contact lens is then applied for continuous wear to protect the lids from irritation by the rough surface of the glue. Antibiotic drops are instilled twice daily. The glue usually detaches after a

couple of weeks. Unfortunately, some mechanical healing defects persist in some patients and melting progresses despite all efforts, ultimately requiring surgical intervention.

Treatment of trophic ulcers may be outlined as follows:

1. For small ulcers (<2 mm) or rough epithelium that threatens to break down, initiate a trial of copious lubrication with antibiotic ointment three times daily and at bedtime, with artificial tears in between ointment doses.
2. For larger ulcers or failure of step #1, therapeutic contact lenses (Permalens, Kontur) should be worn continuously, around the clock, with twice-daily administration of antibiotic drops. No ointments should be used because they dislodge the lenses.
3. Administer artificial tears four to five times per day while the lens is in and for 3 or more months after removal.
4. A mild steroid is warranted if active stromal keratitis is present (e.g., prednisolone 1/8% twice daily, or one of the newer topical steroids, rimexolone or loteprednol).
5. Administer doxycycline, 100 mg PO once daily or tetracycline, 250 mg PO twice daily to inhibit collagenase.
6. Administer cycloplegics if iritis is present or if the patient is not tolerating the thin soft contact lenses well.
7. Consider cyanoacrylate tissue glue (Dermabond, EpiDermGlu) in ulcer bed if there is active melting

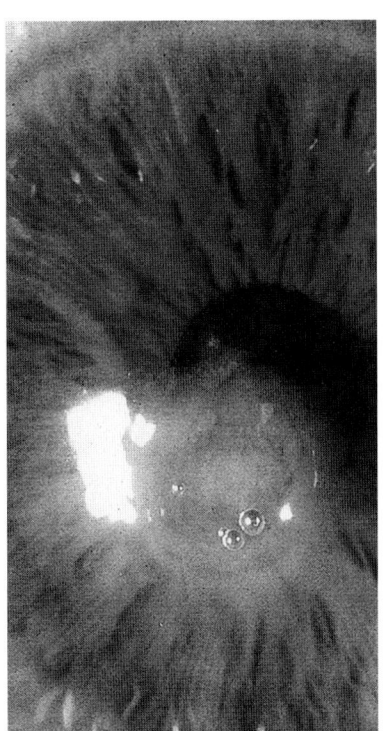 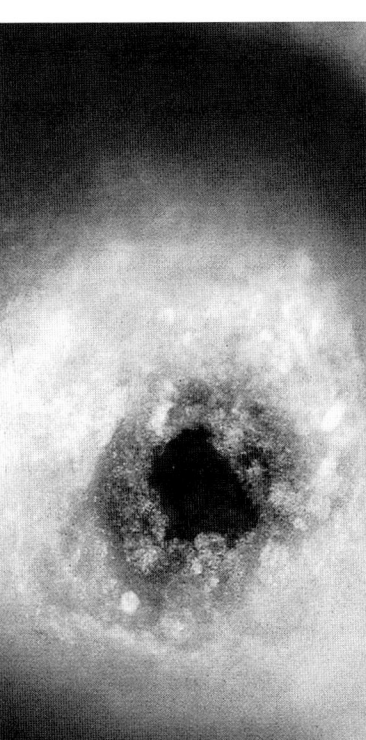 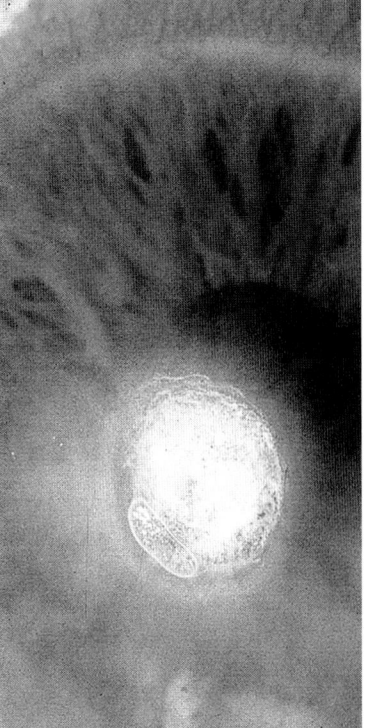

A B,C

FIGURE 14-13. A: Melting herpes simplex virus trophic ulcer neglected by patient. **B:** Ulcer ultimately perforated in the absence of treatment. Anterior chamber is flat. **C:** Perforation was sealed with cyanoacrylate tissue adhesive to reform the chamber. Unfortunately, the ulcer continued to melt, the glue dislodged, and emergency penetrating keratoplasty was performed.

(thinning). Cover glue with medium-thickness soft contact lens (Plano T) (23,420). Reduce topical steroid if possible, although tissue adhesive sealing of the ulcer provides protection from the melting influence of the steroid.

8. Use a patch graft or conjunctival flap if all else fails. Corneal transplantation should be done in an inflamed eye only if corneal perforation threatens and gluing or patch graft is not possible or successful.

Herpetic Interstitial Keratitis, Immune Rings, Limbal Vasculitis, and Disciform Keratitis/Endotheliitis

Although all three forms of AAC-mediated disease are thought to be generally responsive to steroids, there is often residual lipid-like deposition in interstitial keratitis and fibrotic scarring in immune rings. Vision may, therefore, be compromised despite treatment if the central visual axis is involved. Interstitial keratitis, immune rings, and limbal vasculitis all tend to resolve spontaneously in several weeks to months, but with scarring—especially with interstitial keratitis. Neovascularization should regress to fine or ghost vessels. An overlying irregular astigmatism often smooths out with time if there is no recurrence of disease. Stromal disciform disease, largely a lymphocyte-mediated inflammatory reaction, is highly steroid sensitive and may clear with little scarring or leave a notable gray haze primarily in the anterior stroma. If a major attack on the endothelium is allowed to continue unmitigated by therapy, a potentially reversible bullous keratopathy may be converted to a permanent state owing to irreversible damage to the endothelium.

Intact virus particles and HSV antigens have been demonstrated in some of the corneas of patients with interstitial keratitis or disciform keratitis/endotheliitis (153,343, 344,346,350). This suggests that antiviral agents might play a role in at least these forms of stromal HSV infection. It was noted, however, that these particles were present in some cases despite weeks of therapy with topical trifluridine or vidarabine and systemic acyclovir. Further, the HEDS studies indicated that although oral acyclovir was effective in preventing recurrence of stromal keratitis, it had no statistically beneficial effect if combined with topical trifluridine and steroid therapy compared with trifluridine and steroids alone (175,178). In general, steroids remain the prime therapeutic mode for *active* stromal disease, with antiviral drugs used primarily as prophylaxis against recurrent infectious disease.

Therapeutically, a general guideline for treating interstitial keratitis, immune rings, limbal vasculitis, and disciform keratitis/endotheliitis is that if steroids have never been used in a particular eye, the physician should try not to use them. In addition to the usual risks, once steroids have been used, their use will usually be necessary again to resolve any future recurrences. Treatment is started at the dosage the physician believes is warranted to bring the process under control, and

then tapered slowly. Should the inflammatory process recur during steroid dosage reduction, the drug should be increased to higher dosages for a few weeks and tapering attempted again as the process quiets down. This process may go on for months and be frustrating to physician and patient alike. Good, supportive communication with the patient helps to alleviate this situation.

Therapy is outlined as follows:

1. In mild, off-visual-axis cases, no treatment is necessary, but use artificial tears for lubrication of potentially unhealthy epithelium.
2. In moderate to severe cases, especially with neovascularization, start with the lowest dose of steroids needed to bring process under control (e.g., 1% prednisolone or one of the newer steroids, loteprednol or rimexolone, four times daily). Begin to taper slowly as disease comes under control. Progress downward with stronger steroid to weaker steroid. The lower the dose of steroid, the longer it is used. Below once daily, go to once every other day, then to three times per week, and so forth, over several months as needed. Some patients will never be able to go below once-daily dosing to keep their disease under control, and some may need to be at four times daily levels for many weeks before tapering may be done without rebound inflammation. Monitor for side effects and treat steroid-induced glaucoma if it occurs.
3. Secondary glaucoma may be due to trabeculitis, in which case therapy is a topical steroid such as 1% prednisolone four times daily and, if warranted, a nonprostamide analog antiglaucoma drop such as brimonidine (Alphagan) or a beta-blocker. If the pressure does not respond to steroid therapy within 1 week, or if the patient was already on a steroid and the pressure goes up because the rise was (unknowingly) due to steroid-induced glaucoma in the first place, reduce or stop the steroids and continue glaucoma treatment. It is often difficult to know which way to go with the steroid if the patient is already on it, even in low dose. It is advisable to tell the patient at the beginning that treatment may have to be reversed if the response is not satisfactory.
4. Administer cycloplegics as needed for mild iridocyclitis.
5. If iridocyclitis is moderate to severe, use steroids as described in #2.
6. Administer acyclovir 400 mg PO twice daily (or famciclovir or valacyclovir; Table 14-1) or trifluridine drops five times daily as prophylaxis if steroids are used more than twice daily.
7. Apply topical antibiotic ointment at bedtime as prophylaxis if topical steroids are used.
8. Apply artificial tears four to six times per day to lubricate roughened epithelium.
9. If the epithelium is ulcerated and melting, reduce or stop topical steroids. If iritis or trabeculitis must be treated urgently, use systemic prednisone (20 to 30 mg

PO twice daily for 7 to 10 days), then taper over 7 days to control intraocular inflammation until the epithelium is healed, glued, or otherwise under control and topical steroids may be started.

10. If, with treatment, the eye remains uninflamed with little or no steroid for several months but vision is poor due to HSK scarring, keratoplasty may reasonably be performed.

11. The following may be used as prophylaxis against recurrent stromal keratitis (no effect on active disease): acyclovir 400 mg PO twice daily, or famciclovir 125 to 250 mg twice daily, or valacyclovir (immunocompetent patients only) 500 mg PO twice daily for 1 year or more.

Combined Epithelial and Stromal Disease

When a patient has epithelial ulceration and active stromal disease, the physician may be placed squarely between Scylla and Charybdis in making therapeutic decisions. If steroids are chosen to control the stromal inflammation, the surface process may worsen if it is infectious. If the surface disease is thought to be infectious, full antiviral therapy must precede any use of steroids. This contains the infectious process before any aggravating effects of steroids can occur. Should the ulcers worsen because of the steroids, the frequency or concentration of the steroids should be reduced until the ulcers are under control and healing.

If the surface process is an indolent trophic ulcer, the usual ophthalmic steroid drops may enhance the chances of stromal melting. As discussed previously, milder steroids such as loteprednol or rimexolone or use of 1% medroxyprogesterone acetate drops may be advisable in a situation in which the stromal reaction must be controlled or is interfering with healing of the trophic ulcer. In addition, the usual soft contact lens, prophylactic antibiotics and antivirals, and lubricants should be used to treat the trophic ulcer. If melting does progress, cyanoacrylate tissue adhesive, as discussed previously in the section on Trophic Postinfectious Ulcers, should be considered.

Iridocyclitis and Trabeculitis

Because iridocyclitis and trabeculitis are basically immune reactions to viral antigen and, in some cases, intact virus, therapy is primarily topical or systemic steroids. Topical steroids are used if epithelium is intact. In the presence of ulcerative keratitis, and particularly if there is corneal melting or thinning, tissue glue should be applied to seal the ulcer and topical steroid should be minimized to the level needed to control the inflammatory reaction. Systemic steroids do reach the uveal tract and trabecular meshwork in therapeutic levels, but are negligible in the corneal stroma. Preferred therapy for iritis and trabeculitis, then, is a topical steroid in the absence of ulceration and a systemic steroid in the presence of ulceration. Concomitant topical medication should be continued as indicated in the following.

The treatment of herpetic iritis may be summarized as follows:

1. Administer cycloplegics only for mild iritis, coupled with following treatment steps for more severe disease.
2. Topical steroid therapy may range from every 2 to 3 hours for severe iritis to once daily for mild disease. Once the inflammation is under control, gradual tapering should begin. Total cessation may be attempted when the treatment is every 3 days.
3. If the cornea has ulcerated or is melting, topical steroids should be reduced or stopped, and prednisolone (20 to 30 mg PO) may be given twice daily for 7 to 14 days, then tapered over 10 days. Appropriate treatment for the corneal condition is given during this period.
4. Oral antiviral agents twice daily (acyclovir, famciclovir, valacyclovir, or antiviral trifluridine drops five times daily) plus antibiotic once daily are advisable if strong topical steroids are used more often than two to three times per day.
5. Nonprostamide agonists such as brimonidine or beta-blockers should be given if secondary glaucoma is present.

Surgical Factors and Management

Keratoplasty

In the face of a significantly scarred or chronically diseased eye, penetrating keratoplasty is the procedure of choice in many herpetic patients (12,54). Improved surgical techniques and medical management now justify penetrating keratoplasty not just to restore vision in a relatively quiet eye but in an eye with significant ulceration or perforation, or to remove the viral antigenic material lodged in the cornea and inciting repeated immune inflammatory episodes (421).

Herpes simplex–scarred corneas, unlike those scarred by herpes zoster, may undergo transplantation with reasonable surety of success in large part because of less corneal anesthesia from ganglionic damage. In a study evaluating factors bearing on success or failure in herpetic keratoplasty, Langston et al. found that factors leading to a success rate greater than 80% included (a) operation on an uninflamed eye; (b) no deep neovascularization, or, if present, neovascularization involving less than one quadrant; (b) use of fine (no. 10-0 nylon) sutures; and, most important of all, (d) use of very high doses of topical steroids in the immediate postoperative period and tapered use of steroids over the ensuing 3 or more months (422). Recurrence of dendritic disease in the graft was the same (15% within 2 years) regardless of the level of steroid used. Antiviral prophylaxis was commonly in use when steroids were used. Postoperative complications such as wound synechiae, graft rejection, and secondary glaucoma were more frequent in low-dosage steroid groups, and the incidence of wound dehiscence in the high-dosage steroid group was negligible (Fig. 14-14).

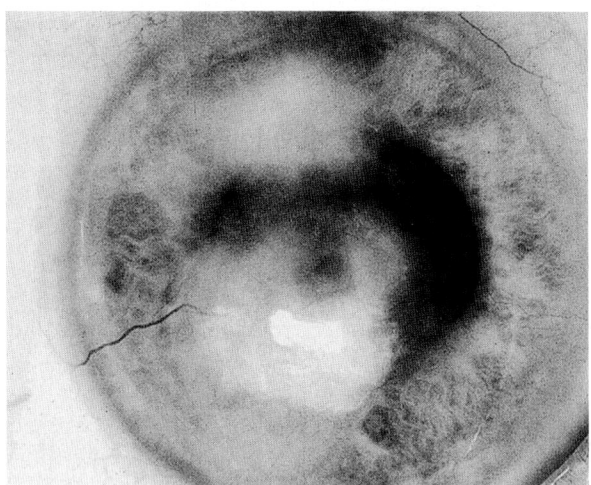
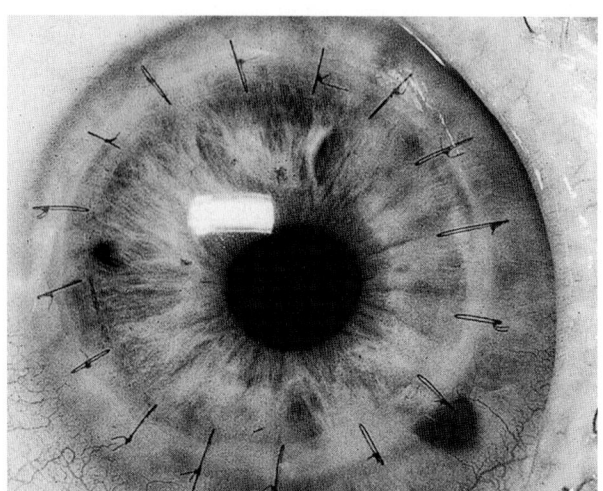

FIGURE 14-14. A: Old, quiescent scarring from herpes simplex virus interstitial keratitis. **B:** Same eye 1 year after penetrating keratoplasty. Uncorrected vision is 20/30.

Cohen et al. also reported a high overall success rate (80%) in 107 patients with HSV infection who underwent grafting, although the 7 patients with active disease at the time of surgery had a lower overall success rate when analyzed separately (423). Unlike previous studies, however, there was no statistically significant correlation between preoperative vascularization and rejection, clarity, or final visual acuity. There was also no greater incidence of recurrent dendritic keratitis in the grafts (19%) when steroids were used without prophylactic antivirals. Langston et al. reported a 15% recurrence rate in the presence of antiviral therapy, and Fine and Cignetti reported a 12% recurrence rate with no antivirals given (422,424). One additional finding by Cobo et al. was that epithelial herpetic recurrences occurred in 32% of eyes undergoing treatment for allograft rejection (425). No antiviral prophylaxis was used in these eyes or eyes with uncomplicated keratoplasties still receiving high-dose postoperative steroids; yet in the latter group, the epithelial recurrence rate was only 6%. This suggests that antiviral prophylaxis may not be necessary except in those cases in which allograft rejection is occurring.

A study by Ficker et al. on the effects of changing management in improving the prognosis for herpetic keratoplasty revealed that the improved use of prophylactic antivirals and corticosteroids increased the success rate in grafting inflamed eyes to a rate comparable with that in quiescent eyes (426). Their expected long-term survival rate for first grafts in quiet eyes was 70% using survival curves not used in previous studies. They also noted that success rate increased with the use of interrupted sutures (no. 10-0 nylon), extracapsular cataract techniques where extraction was indicated, prompt removal of loose sutures (a trigger factor for both rejection and herpetic recurrence), adequate topical steroid treatment to ensure a quiescent eye, and topical antiviral prophylaxis during intensive steroid treatment for rejection (but no antiviral therapy was used as routine postoperative management). Because the survival rate for secondary grafts was significantly worse than that for primary grafts, it was emphasized that immediate and intensive treatment of complications of first grafts was essential. The incidence of herpes simplex recurrence was 15%, similar to that in previously reported studies, with 89% of these being epithelial and 11% stromal. In addition, Mannis et al. have reported the occurrence of herpes between 3 and 11 months after surgery in grafts in eyes with no history of HSV infection, thus raising the index of suspicion for this infection in cases of late-onset epithelial defects in any graft (427). The detection of HSV DNA in two corneal donor buttons that had degenerated during preoperative storage and in the failed graft of one of the donor pairs used, and the finding of HSV in corneal donor rims, require that surgeons be ever-vigilant for this organism (395,428).

HSV trigeminal ganglion latency as a source of recurrent infection was already well documented when reports of HSV corneal latency and persistence of HSV in ocular tissues began to appear in the late 1980s (307,316,317, 348,349,368,376). More recent studies on the relationship between HSV and graft success or failure have shed considerable light on the cause of some failures and the need for certain forms of postoperative management. Liekfeld et al. performed micro-ELISA assays for HSV, VZV, and CMV on aqueous taken from 24 herpetic eyes and found antibodies against HSV in 50%, against HSV and VZV in 25%, and against VZV alone in 3.6%, and no antibodies in 22%. They suggested the use of perioperative and postoperative antivirals as advisable, but also pointed out that approximately one fourth of patients may not need this prophylaxis (429). PCR studies for viral DNA on 31 herpetic corneal buttons taken at keratoplasty and 78 nonherpetic eyes revealed that in the HSK specimens, one third were positive for HSV-1, 3% for HSV-2, and 19% for VZV (430). In nonherpetic specimens, HSV-1 DNA was detected in 17%, including eight grafts that failed without clinically obvious HSV disease or a history thereof. In a similar report, four nonherpetic patients with unexplained primary graft failure were found to be culture positive for external HSV, and PCR positive in aqueous, corneal graft, and iris tissue testing (431).

The origin of HSV recurrence in recurrent disease has until recently been assumed to be the patient's own re-activated latent HSV. As noted earlier, Remeijer and colleagues' study of 30 patients revealed that 63% were genotypically the same from recurrence to recurrence, whereas 37% were actually genetically different, suggesting a significant number of recurrent HSK cases may be exogenously acquired (327). Animal studies by Zheng et al. on the phenomenon of transmission of HSV by keratoplasty revealed that corneas from latently infected rabbits contain HSV-1 DNA that can replicate after induced reactivation, and that viral migration may be both anterograde or retrograde between donor cornea and recipient rim and trigeminal ganglion (432,433). Further, lamellar keratoplasty induces HSV-1 shedding and recurrent epithelial lesions in rabbits latently infected with HSV-1 before surgery, but not in uninfected control animals (434).

All of these human and animal studies again indicate that HSV is an important cause of recurrent disease and graft failure even in "nonherpetic" eyes, and that prophylactic antivirals should be an integral part of therapy (Fig. 14-15). Prophylaxis of HSV epithelial recurrences in patients post-HSV keratoplasty with oral acyclovir is effective and indicated. A number of studies report significant efficacy in protecting grafts from recurrent HSV disease, the direct cause of failure in approximately 15% of cases (182,188–190). The

generally recommended dosage is 400 mg acyclovir PO twice daily for 12 to 18 months postkeratoplasty. Akova et al. reported successful use of lower-dose acyclovir postkeratoplasty, using 400 mg acyclovir PO once daily for 1 year after surgery in treated groups and no acyclovir in the control groups in a study on 35 patients with HSK (435). After 25 to 30 months of follow-up, the acyclovir group had statistically fewer recurrences compared with the control patients. Two recurrences occurred after acyclovir was stopped. The worst prognosis in both groups was in those eyes with necrotizing keratitis, but it was still statistically better in the acyclovir group. These findings are in agreement with those noted in long-term oral acyclovir or valacyclovir prophylaxis of recurrent genital HSV, including return to pretreatment recurrence pattern with cessation of therapy (436–438).

Given our evolving understanding of the factors involved in HSV keratoplasty, it is important to know how they are effecting clinical outcomes. In Jonas and coworkers' study of 245 patients, there were 29 cases of HSK, 77 cases of keratoconus, 46 with nonherpetic scars, 24 cases of Fuchs' dystrophy, and 69 cases of pseudophakic/aphakic bullous keratopathy (439). Follow-up was at 1 year. Interestingly, the visual acuity was significantly higher in the keratoconus group, followed very closely by the patients with HSK. The worst group was the bullous keratopathy group. The main predictive factors for visual outcome were reason for keratoplasty and graft size.

Another report on prognostic factors, rejection, and recurrence of HSK in keratoplasty for HSV leukoma revealed a significant difference in rejection rate between herpetic eyes (45%) and nonherpetic control eyes (5%), mostly within the first year (440). Recurrent HSV disease

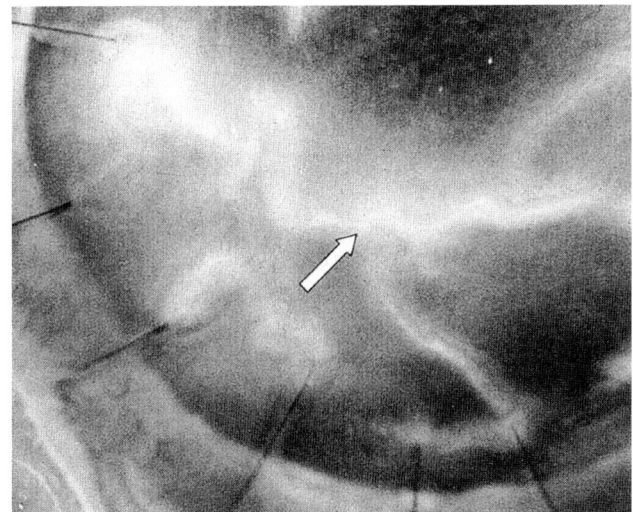 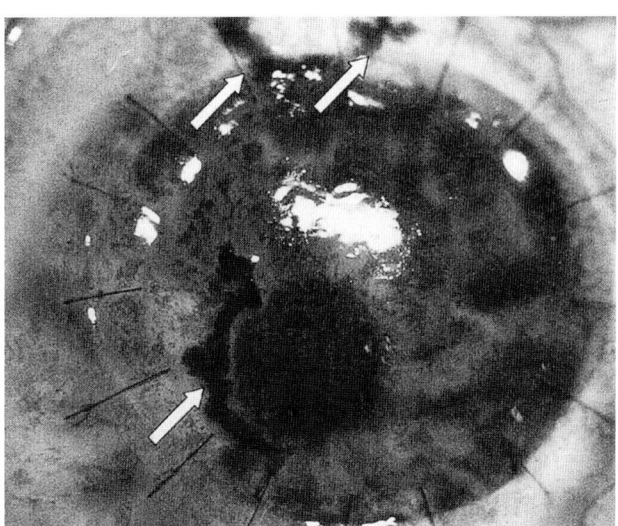

FIGURE 14-15. A: Giant herpes simplex virus (HSV) dendritic ulcer in penetrating keratoplasty (*arrow*). Graft ultimately failed despite steroids and antiviral therapy. **B:** Scattered HSV dendrites in keratoplasty and on host rim (*arrows*). Oral antivirals were initiated along with continued steroid and antibiotic coverage, with resultant clearing of graft. Antivirals were given for a total of 18 months after this episode, and steroids slowly tapered.

occurred within 3 years, and earlier than graft rejections. These authors did not mention use of antiviral prophylaxis, which may account for their poor HSK outcome. They did conclude that in HSV leukoma grafts, steroid therapy is important in the first year to suppress graft rejection but then should be reduced because of the greater increase in the chance for recurrent HSV infection.

Conversely, Halberstadt et al. reported a 5-year follow-up study on 384 patients who had undergone keratoplasty, 186 with HSK and 198 with nonherpetic disease (441). Using both systemic antiviral prophylaxis and local steroid therapy, they found that although the HSV group had significantly more corneal vascularization, more epithelial defects, lower corneal sensitivity, and more graft rejection episodes, and required larger grafts, the postoperative course of visual acuity, endothelial cell count, and rate of graft failures were similar in both groups. After 5 years, the cumulative probability of graft survival in HSK was 41%, and 50% in non-HSV eyes (*p* not significant). The combined use of systemic antiviral prophylaxis and judicious steroid therapy was credited for this good outcome.

Glaucoma is one other factor of significance in determining success or failure of graft outcome in HSK. A study of 122 repeat keratoplasties with a mean duration of 89 months after the primary graft had a minimum follow-up of 6 months (442). Significant risk factors for development of postoperative glaucoma were HSK and previous graft rejection compared with all other groups. The incidence of glaucoma increased with an increased number of keratoplasties in an eye, and included, in decreasing order of frequency: closed-angle (59%), steroid-induced (21%), open-angle (11%), angle recession (3%), and miscellaneous (6%). In all keratoplasties, but particularly in those performed for HSK, close monitoring and early therapy are warranted to increase survival rate of transplants in eyes affected by glaucoma. HSK is a notable risk factor in this.

In brief, it would appear that five major factors emerge as crucial to long-term survival of keratoplasty in herpetic eyes: (a) use of fine, interrupted sutures (less trauma on removal); (b) intensive postoperative topical steroids to suppress inflammation, with taper over 1 year; (c) acyclovir 400 mg PO twice daily for 12 to 18 months [or famciclovir, or valacyclovir prophylaxis (Table 14-1) against recurrence of HSV infection in graft]; (d) monitoring and early management of glaucoma; and (e) full antiviral prophylaxis (oral or topical) during intensive topical steroid therapy for rejection. Because of the significantly worse survival rate in regrafts, the importance of immediate and intensive treatment of complications of first grafts is emphasized.

Conjunctival Flap, Tarsorrhaphy, and Lamellar Keratoplasty

As judiciously administered steroids, antiviral drugs, and adjunctive therapy have come into greater use, there is less indication for the conjunctival flap. In previous years the

flap was used to quiet down an inflamed, ulcerated, melting eye that could not be controlled with the then-available therapy (443). A graft placed in an inflamed eye would almost certainly have a difficult postoperative course. Nonetheless, this technique, as well as that of conjunctival transplant or patch grafting, has been used with considerable success in situations where a transplant might be at high risk (444). This may occur in particular with an unreliable or severely ill patient or in cases where a holding action is desired if an ulcer is too large for gluing or the eye is considered too inflamed for keratoplasty in an acute situation. A penetrating keratoplasty may be placed through the flap at a later time when the eye in no longer inflamed. Similarly, partial tarsorrhaphy may be used as adjunctive therapy to a therapeutic contact lens where protection and healing of the recalcitrant ulcerated surface are the immediate aims. Lamellar keratoplasty has been used in the past for this same purpose or in the presence of very superficial scarring in the hopes of restoring vision without the risk of rejection of a full-thickness transplant. This technique has largely fallen into disfavor because of its low success rate in achieving satisfactory visual results, and because of the recent studies cited in the section on viral stromal keratitis indicating that virus or viral antigens may be present in corneal tissue deep to the lamellar keratoplasty and thus be a threat to its ultimate integrity (153,346,395,445,446).

VARICELLA ZOSTER VIRUS (VZV) OCULAR DISEASE

The varicella or chickenpox virus and herpes zoster virus are the same organism: the varicella zoster virus (VZV).

Incidence and Epidemiology

Contact with VZV in this country is almost universal, with seropositive reactions in 80% to 90% by adolescence and approaching 100% by middle age (22,447). Approximately 2.8 million cases occur annually, with the vast majority occurring in children younger than 9 years of age. Spread of the disease is largely by saliva droplets or direct contact with an infected rash [chickenpox (varicella) or zoster] or recently contaminated material. The incubation period is 12 to 17 days after contact. Local infection of the nasopharynx, or rarely through the skin, is followed by waves of viremia and seeding of the reticuloendothelial cells, skin, viscera, and ganglia. The maculopapulovesicular rash appears in successive crops; lesions in various stages are present simultaneously. The contagious period starts approximately 1 day before rash and continues approximately 1 week after the appearance of each crop of lesions or until the cutaneous sores crust over (21,22,184,192, 195,448–451).

Despite this long incubation period, antibody production is fairly slow and sequential, with the first formed being against structural glycoproteins and nucleocapsid protein in several days to 2 weeks. Two months later, antibodies to a wider variety of viral proteins appear, and most disappear within 3 to 4 months. Antibodies to the immunodominant gp66, gp118, gp98, and gp62 last for years, however, and are very good markers for previous varicella infection. If there is a subclinical reinfection after exogenous exposure there is a general rise in anti-glycoprotein antibody levels, especially to gp98 and gp62, but not of the magnitude seen with endogenous reactivation of VZV (452).

Clinical Disease

Eye findings in varicella may be those of congenital varicella syndrome or those of the more common, generalized varicella most commonly seen in young children (22,184, 447–450,453).

Congenital Varicella Syndrome

If the mother contracts varicella during the first or second trimester of pregnancy, the fetus may become infected and significantly deformed (256,454). Systemic findings may include hemiparesis, bulbar palsies, cicatricial skin lesions in a dermatomal distribution, developmental delay, and learning difficulties. Ocular findings may include chorioretinitis, optic nerve atrophy or hypoplasia, congenital cataract, and Horner's syndrome. There is no definitive therapy for congenital varicella syndrome, which strengthens the argument for vaccination of all women with no history of previous varicella (454–456). Five to 15% of women of childbearing age are susceptible to this virus.

Classic Varicella Ocular Findings

This infection may involve any structure in the anterior segment. Lesions may occur on the lids, or on the conjunctiva in the form of small vesicular or papular eruptions at the limbus. These usually resolve without difficulty, but rarely may turn to very red, painful, punched-out ulcers with secondary reaction in the eye. Small phlyctenule-like lesions may erupt, most commonly at the corneal limbus (22,184,450). It is unclear whether these are due to live virus or an immune phlyctenule-like reaction, or both. The cornea may develop superficial punctate keratitis or wispy, branching dendritic ulcers without terminal knobs (herpes simplex ulcers have knob-shaped endings on their branches) (453,457–460). These lesions are thought to be infectious. Similar lesions in HZO are PCR positive for VZV DNA (25). Months after the acute disease, disciform keratitis similar to that seen in HSV disease may develop (461). This disciform reaction is steroid responsive but

may recur and cause scarring similar to HSK. A report of perforation of an ulcer of unknown etiology 7 months after uncomplicated varicella proved, on PCR and electron microscopic study, to be due to delayed primary varicella keratitis (462).

Less frequently reported varicella findings in the eye include iritis (occasionally fibrinous), lid necrosis, interstitial keratitis with neovascularization, dendritic keratitis, neurotrophic ulceration with corneal melting, extraocular muscle palsies, internal ophthalmoplegia, cataract, chorioretinitis, and optic neuritis (23,450,453,457,459,463–465).

Diagnosis and Treatment

Ocular chickenpox is diagnosed on the basis of an acute or recent history of the systemic disease with ocular or periocular involvement with the vesicles–pustules. FDA-approved treatment of acute disease is acyclovir 20 mg/kg PO four times daily for 5 days, or the adult dose of 800 mg PO four times daily for 5 days if the patient weighs more than 40 kg. The American Association of Pediatrics does not recommend routine use of acyclovir (212). Consider its use if the patient is older than 12 years, has chronic cutaneous or pulmonary disease, or has a history of long-term steroid or salicylate use.

Infectious chickenpox of the lid, conjunctiva, or cornea (dendritic or rarely geographic keratitis) may be ameliorated by trifluridine applied nine times daily over a 7- to 10-day period plus a topical antibiotic. Good hygiene to keep the skin area clean (tepid soaks and patting dry) is important. Late-onset immune stromal disease would be treated in a manner similar to stromal herpes simplex or zoster infection with gradual tapering of the steroids. Antivirals are not indicated in this stage of disease, although antibiotic ointment at bedtime is recommended when higher doses of topical steroid (more than 1% prednisolone twice daily) are in use. Steroids should probably not be used during the acute infectious disease because this may enhance the viral process. IV acyclovir may be used in severe cases.

Varicella Vaccine

The 1995 FDA approval of a live, attenuated VZV vaccine, the Oka strain, for the immunization of healthy people of all ages (infancy to adulthood) who have not had previous varicella, thereby reducing the incidence of varicella and its complications, was hailed, rightly so, as a major step forward in controlling this disease and a potential key to reducing the incidence of zoster (202,466). How long the vaccine was effective was not yet established. It was known, however, that although the postvaccination antibodies decline over the years in adults and leukemic children, this does not happen in healthy children studied for 10 to 20 years (456,467–469). CMI may continue to protect vaccinees long after antibody levels are low, but periodic booster shots of the vaccine may also be necessary to maintain protection, much as we repeat booster tetanus and other vaccines. The recent observation that acute varicella may, in fact, develop in vaccinated children showed that the children immunized 3 years before exposure were at greatest risk for development of disease, but also that vaccinated children were much less likely to have moderate or severe disease (470).

Given the increasing average age of our population, the effect of vaccination on preventing zoster is still not completely elucidated, but data are promising. Studies on the effect of giving live, attenuated VZV vaccine (Oka strain) showed a significant increase in VZV CMI in a healthy, elderly (55 to 75 years of age) population (471). No relationship between vaccine dose and the intensity of the specific response was noted. In leukemic children, the incidence of zoster was 15% in unvaccinated control patients, compared with just 3% in vaccinated patients, possibly reflecting a lower rate of latency after vaccination compared with that seen in natural disease, because there is no skin infection (472,473). Data in the normal population indicate that the incidence of zoster is much lower in vaccinated healthy children and adults compared with those who suffered a natural infection (474). There has, however, been one case of zoster ophthalmicus occurring in a child 5 years after vaccination at 3 years of age, but it could not be proven whether this was due to the vaccine strain or to a natural strain of VZV (475). In another report, however, a child in whom zoster sclerokeratitis and uveitis developed 3 years after vaccination proved to have wild-type virus, not reactivation of the vaccine's Oka strain (476).

HERPES ZOSTER OPHTHALMICUS

Incidence and Epidemiology

Herpes zoster is a recurrent infection with varicella virus, endogenous (reactivated latent virus) or exogenous, that accounts for an estimated 500,000 cases of infectious dermatitis annually in this country (236). Up to 20% of the population will have zoster at some time in life (477). The chance of members of this group having a second attack of zoster is also 20% (478). Of every 1000 people living to age 85 years, 500 will have had one attack of dermatomal zoster and 10 will have had two attacks. The aging process and depressed CMI response greatly enhance the risk for development of zoster (477,479–482). Hope-Simpson reported that the incidence of zoster rises steadily until the age of 20 years, and plateaus at three cases per 1000 people per year for ages 20 to 49 years (483). The incidence then rises sharply to peak at 10 cases per 1000 people aged 80 to 89 years. This may be correlated directly with a decline in the CMI response with age (192,479,484). Elderly patients, healthy except for the development of zoster, show

little CMI response during the first 5 days after the eruption of the skin rash. The usual anamnestic CMI response time to recurrent VZV is less than 3 days, if not immediate (485). Immunosuppressed patients (e.g., those with AIDS or blood dyscrasias, organ transplant recipients) as well as patients with cancer, especially lymphoproliferative disorders, are at greater risk for reactivation of latent VZV and for more severe disease when it occurs because of their inability to mount an anamnestic T-cell response (477,480, 482,486,487).

Early studies indicated that occult or overt malignant disease is present with significantly greater frequency in patients with zoster than in the normal population and should be counted as an adverse factor in the pathogenesis of the disease (488–490). More recent studies contradicted these findings, however, with one noting that only 15% of the patients with HZO had the malignant disease several years before the onset of the ocular infection (22,192,204,477,490–492). This figure does not differ from the incidence in the nonzoster population. A search for occult malignancy is not warranted in otherwise healthy patients with VZV disease. Herpes zoster may develop, however, in HIV-positive patients who are asymptomatic and undiagnosed as positive. It is now believed that, in the absence of other extenuating factors, HIV serologic testing would be appropriate in any patient younger than 50 years of age in whom zoster develops (236,477,478,493–495) (Fig. 14-16).

HZO is second only to thoracic zoster in frequency (26). Two Mayo Clinic reviews of all zoster cases occurring between 1935 and 1949 and between 1949 and 1959 reported a frequency of 9% to 16% for trigeminal zoster (481,496). This is at the low end of the scale for involvement of the ocular branch of the cranial nerve, which varies in frequency from 8% to 56% in other studies (22,192,204, 490–492). Approximately 50% to 72% of patients with periocular zoster will have involvement of the ocular structures, develop chronic disease, and possibly sustain a moderate to severe degree of visual loss (366).

Relationship between Neuronal Patterns and Disease

The cranial nerves are second to the thoracic nerves as the most common area where herpes zoster may develop (497). Of the three divisions of the fifth (trigeminal) cranial nerve, the first is by far the one most frequently affected. VZV occasionally affects the maxillary division, but rarely affects the mandibular division (498).

Within the first division of the fifth nerve, the frontal branch stands out as most often involved, through its supraorbital and supratrochlear branches. These branches go to the upper lid, forehead, and superior conjunctiva. The nasociliary branch is the primary sensory nerve to the eyeball. Through its infratrochlear division, it supplies the lacrimal sac, conjunctiva, skin of both lids, and root of the

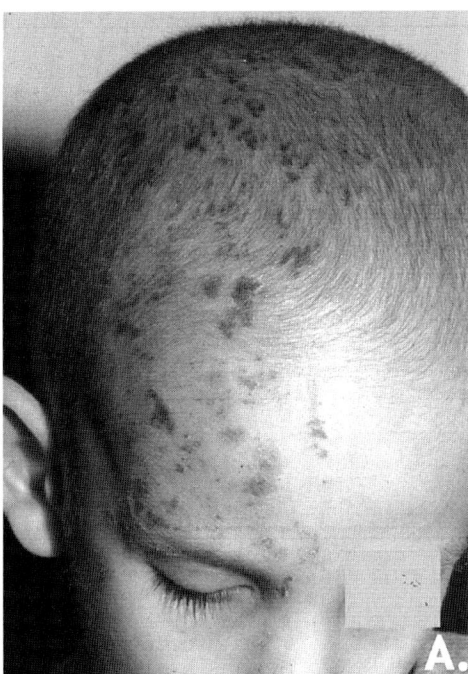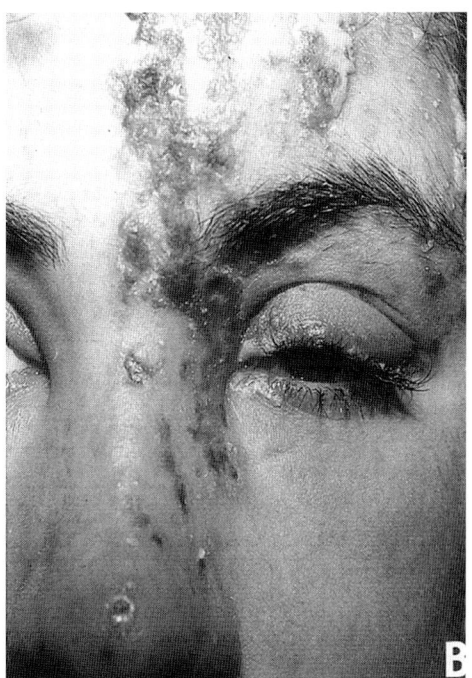

FIGURE 14-16. A: A 7-year-old girl under treatment for leukemia developed herpes zoster ophthalmicus (HZO) responsive to oral famciclovir. **B:** Eighteen-year-old immunocompetent woman with acute HZO. Results of immune workup were completely normal. Oral valacyclovir was given within 48 hours of rash onset and patient recovered without sequelae.

nose. The most critical division of this nerve, however, is the nasal branch. With sympathetic branches from the ciliary ganglion, the nasal branch of the nasociliary nerve innervates the sclera, cornea, iris, ciliary body, and choroid through the long and short ciliary nerves, as well as the tip of the nose through the nasal nerve proper. This direct neural connection to so many critical structures in the eye allows herpes zoster reactivated from latency to cause devastating and chronic disease in a previously healthy eye. This direct connection, along with diffuse spread of the virus through the orbital tissues to other cranial and autonomic nerves and the CNS, allows herpes zoster to cause a variety of reactions mimicked by no other infectious entity (497–499).

The list of complications is protean: scarred lid retraction; paralytic ptosis; conjunctivitis; scleritis; keratitis; iridocyclitis; hemorrhagic retinitis; acute retinal necrosis; choroiditis; papillitis; retrobulbar neuritis; optic atrophy, Argyll Robertson pupil; partial or complete third, fourth, or sixth nerve palsy; isolated pupillary paralysis; internuclear ophthalmoplegia, acute and chronic glaucoma; orbital apex syndrome; PHN; inflammatory syndromes; and sympathetic ophthalmia (22,23,194,406,491,500).

Clinical Features

In HZO, virtually any ocular structure may be involved (22,184,194,195,478,488,492,501–503).

Dermal, Extraocular Muscle, and Orbital Involvement

The illness is heralded by headache, malaise, and dysesthesia, but rarely fever, followed 24 to 48 hours later by neuralgia and dysesthesia, and 2 to 3 days after that by hyperemic, hyperesthetic edema of the involved dermatome, which erupts with multiple crops of watery blisters that continue to form over 3 to 5 days (Fig. 14-17A). The blisters become turbid and crust over, often with hemorrhagic scabs, over 7 to 10 days. Virus may be cultured from the vesicles for up to a week in uncomplicated zoster, but for much longer in immunosuppressed patients. Two to 20% of patients have several vesicles scattered elsewhere on the body, indicating viremia (480,481). Unlike herpes simplex skin infections, herpes zoster involves epidermis down to the corium and forms deep eschars that may leave permanent pitted scars that may perfectly map out the dermatome. The skin and any ocular ulceration may take weeks to heal, with subsequent ptosis, lid retraction, or sloughing of lashes and lid tissues (22,184,450,488,504). It is also of note that HSV disease may closely mimic VZV dermatitis. In one case report, PCR was used to prove that the "zoster dermatitis" was, in fact due to HSV (505).

The severity of the skin and periocular involvement may be so great as to resemble a bacterial orbital cellulitis, with a notable contralateral sterile cellulitis in the adnexa of the uninvolved eye as well (Fig. 14-17B). Palsies of cranial

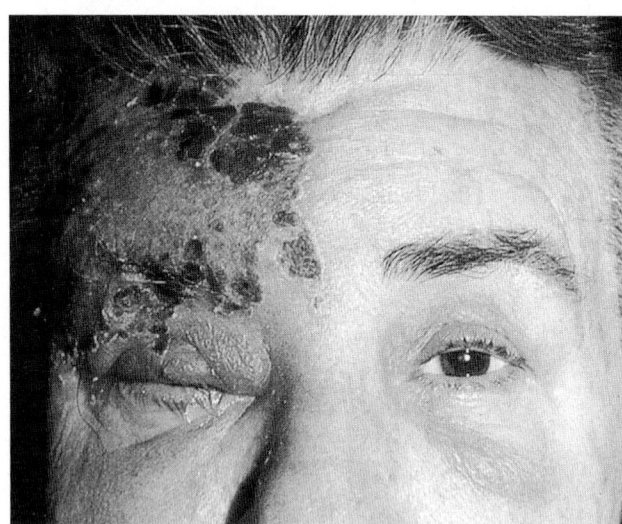
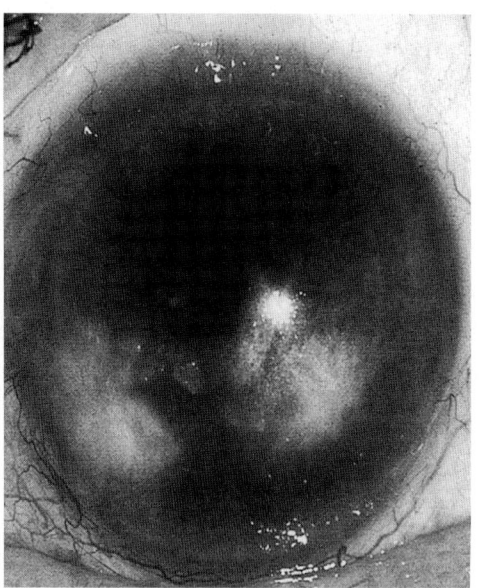

FIGURE 14-17. A. Sixty-six-year-old woman with resolving acute herpes zoster ophthalmicus that had taken the form of an acute cellulitis. Note sympathetic edema and hyperemia of contralateral lids. **B.** Same patient 4 months later with residual corneal scarring.

nerves III, IV, and VI are not uncommon, and with the exception of an almost invariable residual partial ptosis, these clear completely, independent of initial severity (Fig. 14-18). Other palsies include internuclear ophthalmoplegia, isolated iris sphincter paralysis, and Horner's syndrome (506–509). It is thought that the extraocular muscle palsies and orbital edema seen in HZO may be the result of perineuritis and perivasculitis associated with the generalized orbit inflammation (508,510,511). Fortunately, the vast

majority of muscle palsies resolve spontaneously. Acute dacryoadenitis may also occur and present only as severe ocular pain and red eye (512). Magnetic resonance imaging showed enlargement of the lacrimal gland. Two days later, iridocyclitis and V-1 dermatomal skin lesions developed. Oral acyclovir quickly resolved the entire clinical situation. Superior orbital syndrome is not infrequent in the elderly and immunocompromised patient with VZV infection (503). It may be associated with meningoencephalitis. Because of the risk of irreversible damage to the cranial nerves passing through the superior orbital fissure, systemic steroids should seriously be considered to reduce orbital tissue swelling. The patient's immune status should be figured into this equation, however.

Conjunctivitis, Episcleritis, and Scleritis

Conjunctivitis is second only to lid involvement in frequency of occurrence and is rarely seen without eruption of the periocular skin. Conjunctival herpes zoster may present as a watery follicular reaction with or without petechial reaction and regional adenopathy, or as a necrotizing membranous inflammation. Episcleritis or a scleritis that may be flat and diffuse or focal with nodular elevations is fairly common (Fig. 14-19). Inflammation may occur acutely or months after the original skin disease, and become recurring. The lesions are believed to have an immune etiology to residual antigen or possibly "subclinical" reactivation of VZV. Resolution of diffuse, flat scleritis is usually uneventful; the nodular form may lead to scleral thinning and staphyloma formation. Rarely, a 360-degree limbal scleritis

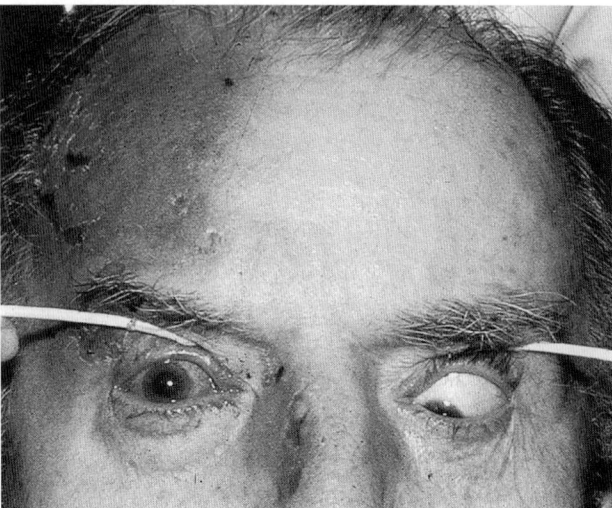

FIGURE 14-18. Seventy-two-year-old man 2 months after acute herpes zoster ophthalmicus with residual complete third, fourth, and sixth nerve palsies, with onset during first week of acute illness. By 12 months, all paresis had resolved.

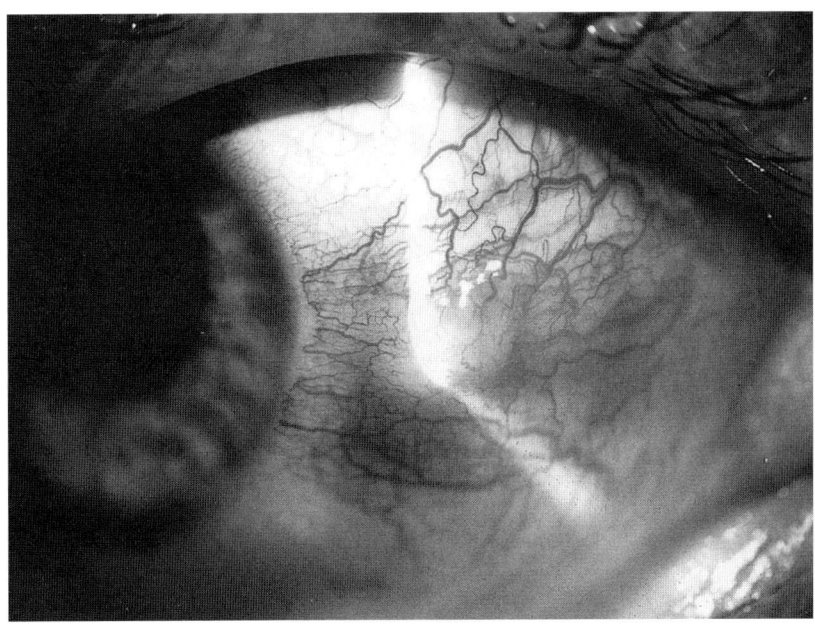

FIGURE 14-19. Herpes zoster ophthalmicus (HZO) nodular episcleritis, onset 1 year after acute HZO. The HZO was moderately responsive to topical steroids and cleared over 4 months with added oral ibuprofen.

or vasculitis may develop, resulting in anterior segment ischemia (500). VZV infection should be considered in any patient presenting with episcleritis, scleritis, or iritis. A 9-year-old child presented with scleritis, marginal keratitis, mild glaucoma, marked iritis, and rare skin vesicles 3 years after varicella vaccination (476). Amplified DNA taken from the skin revealed wild-type VZV, not the Oka strain of the vaccine, indicating an exogenous infection despite previous vaccination. All of these conditions are variably responsive to topical steroids and, in some cases, to NSAIDs such as ibuprofen 400 mg PO three times daily.

Keratitis

Liesegang's study of 94 patients with HZO reveals that two thirds had corneal involvement (500). This took the form of punctate keratitis (51%), pseudodendrites (51%), anterior stromal infiltrates (41%), sclerokeratitis (1%), keratouveitis-endotheliitis (34%), peripheral ulcerative keratitis (7%), delayed mucous plaques (13%), disciform keratitis (10%), neurotrophic keratitis (25%), and exposure keratitis (11%). A delayed limbal vasculitis with or without anterior ischemic necrosis was also noted on rare occasions.

Corneal disease may precede, accompany, or follow the acute disease by months to years and may recur in any of its many forms. The acute epithelial disease is considered infectious and may present as a diffuse superficial punctate keratitis or, more commonly, as migratory dendritic lesions that at first could be confused with herpes simplex. Pavan-Langston and McCulley isolated VZV from these dendrites (513). They reported branching, superficial, grayish linear lesions, appearing to be painted on the corneal surface. VZV may be isolated from the ulcers of acute HZO, but

not from late-onset dendrites. PCR studies, however, reported detection of VZV DNA in several late-onset pseudodendrites in immunocompetent and immunocompromised patients (25) (Fig. 14-20). In this study, electron microscopy of a corneal button taken from a patient with lymphoma with pseudodendrites revealed numerous mature and immature viral particles in the epithelial basal cells and myeloid bodies in the keratocytes. Piebenga and Laibson also described herpes zoster dendrites (the delayed mucous plaques described by Liesegang) that were culture negative but appeared as heaped-up, superficial, plaquelike lesions, coarser than herpes simplex dendrites but lacking terminal bulbs (an important differentiating point) and staining poorly with fluorescein (514). Liesegang's "delayed corneal mucous plaques" appear in approximately 13% of patients, up to 2 years after acute VZV disease (500,515). They cause a foreign body sensation and are elevated, coarse, gray-white, swollen epithelial cells piled in plaques or a dendritiform shape on the surface of the cornea. They are both migratory and transitory and are usually associated with a neurotrophic keratitis (75%) or previous corneal inflammation (100%).

Zaal et al. reported a longitudinal study on VZV DNA on the conjunctival and corneal surfaces associated with acute HZO of less than 7 days' duration (516). At entrance into the study, 19 of the 21 patients were PCR positive for VZV DNA; 6 had no ocular inflammation. All were treated with 1 g valacyclovir three times daily for 10 days. Continued weekly testing revealed that DNA could be detected from 2 to 34 days after rash onset in different study patients, with longer duration of DNA presence in patients older than 66 years of age. The authors concluded that VZV DNA shedding is highly variable, age dependent, and probably related to host immune status.

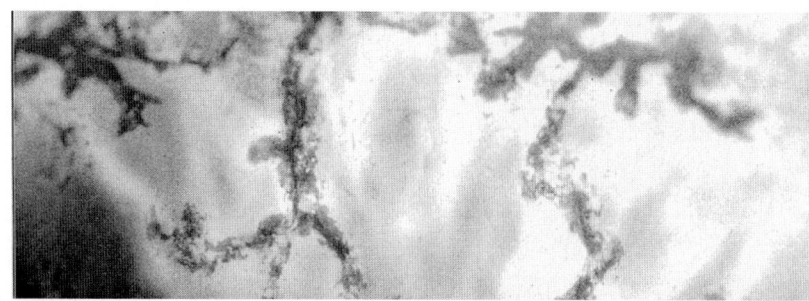

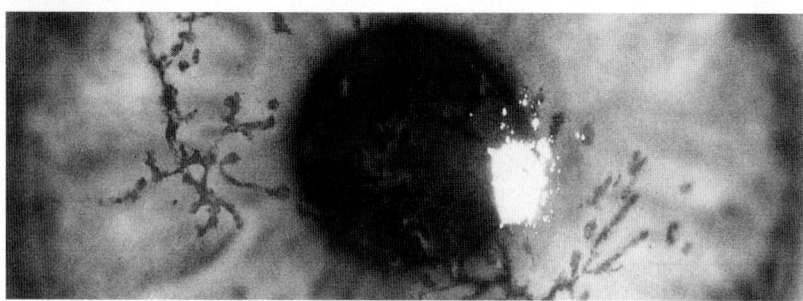

FIGURE 14-20. A: Late-onset limbal dendrites 8 months post acute herpes zoster ophthalmicus (HZO). The lesions resolved without treatment. **B:** Acute HZO dendrites that cleared during oral antiviral treatment for acute disease. Note wispy nature of dendrites in **A** and **B**, and lack of terminal bulbs seen in herpes simplex virus dendrites. Lesions in **A** and **B** were positive for zoster DNA by polymerase chain reaction.

Stromal Immune Disease

Immune keratitis similar in appearance to HSV stromal disciform edema/endotheliitis may occur any time after the acute illness, most commonly first appearing within 3 to 4 months. As with HSK, there may be focal or local stromal edema and associated keratic precipitates. Other immune reactions include necrotizing interstitial keratitis with neovascularization, Wessely rings, or limbal vasculitis (Fig. 14-21). If there is an associated interstitial keratitis, there is increased chance of deep neovascularization with lipid deposition and fibrovascular scarring. The response of this lymphocytic/plasma cell/macrophage immune reaction to steroids is rapid to moderate initially, but tapering of steroids is frequently slow, with many patients requiring minimal daily doses to prevent rebound immune disease (23,478,511,517). Assay for VZV DNA has been positive in some reported cases (518–521). Stromal forms of VZV disease are clinically difficult, if not impossible to differentiate from stromal herpes simplex disease, and may represent the same immune pathogenetic mechanisms (369).

Neuroparalytic Keratopathy (Neurotrophic Ulcers)

Corneal sensation may be markedly diminished in even the mildest cases of clinically manifest herpes zoster keratitis. Sixty percent of patients have moderate to complete corneal anesthesia (neuroparalysis) secondary to the destructive VZV ganglionitis and to aqueous tear deficiency due to loss of the nasolacrimal reflex (369,492,500,522,523). The anesthesia may be evident at the time of onset of HZO or may develop over the next 2 to 3 weeks (524,525). It is almost invariably greater than that seen with HSK of comparable severity because the anesthesia is related more to the ganglionic damage than to corneal changes.

In general, the more intact the corneal sensation, the better the prognosis for the cornea. This should be tested in comparison with the normal contralateral eye at each examination during the first several weeks after onset.

Anesthetic epithelial breakdown similar to that seen after trigeminal ganglion ablation comprises one of the most dangerous forms of herpes zoster keratitis. One fourth of all patients with HZO develop clinical signs of neurotrophic keratitis due to permanent corneal anesthesia. Early clinical findings include a dull or irregular

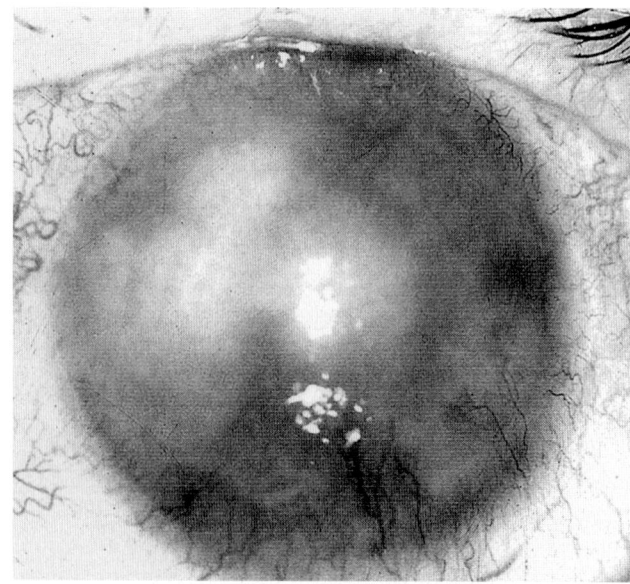

FIGURE 14-21. Active, necrotic herpes zoster ophthalmicus interstitial keratitis (IK) with 260 degrees of deep neovascularization. Corneal sensation was zero. IK resolved and vessels regressed over 2 years with gentle topical steroid therapy. No antivirals were indicated.

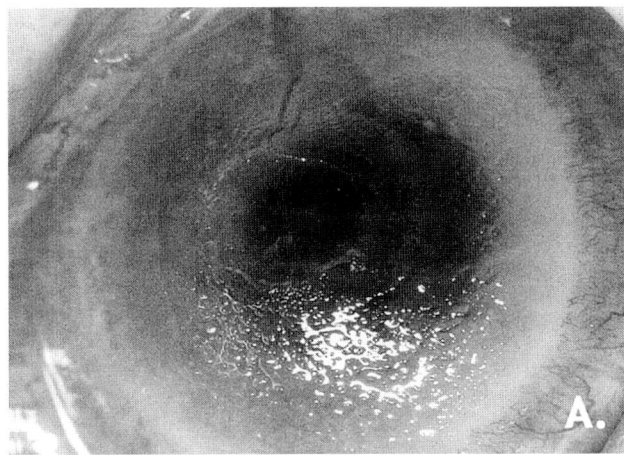 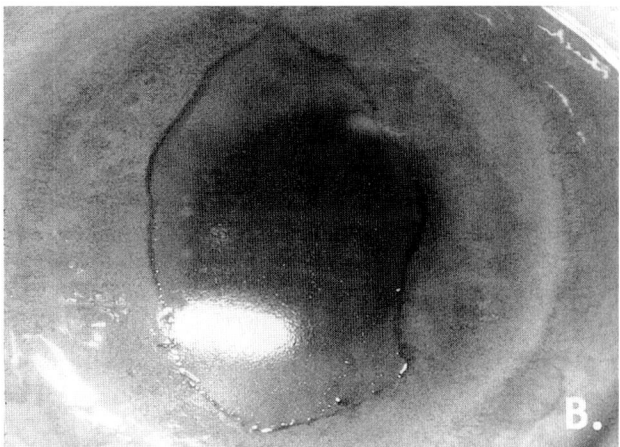

FIGURE 14-22. A: Unhealthy, irregular epithelium in herpes zoster ophthalmicus cornea with zero sensation because of ganglionic damage. Patient refused therapeutic contact lens and continued lubrication. **B:** Same eye 1 week later with large trophic ulcer that might have been prevented had a thin soft contact lens been applied earlier.

corneal surface with a mild, coarse, punctate epithelial keratitis (Fig. 14-22A). Subsequently, a diffuse epithelial haze or edema with fine intraepithelial vesicles may develop. As noted, the tear film is highly unstable and blink frequency is reduced in these anesthetic eyes, thus further aggravating the condition. There is an exposure pattern in 40% of patients so affected. As the corneal epithelium becomes progressively more unhealthy, oval epithelial defects may develop in the palpebral fissure or lower corneal area with subsequent melting and corneal thinning (Fig. 14-22B). Melting is most commonly seen in patients with previous keratouveitis (80%) (478,500,523).

Incipient ulcers may often be aborted by copious artificial tear lubrication (plus antibiotic prophylaxis) and lateral tarsorrhaphy. A lower punctal plug is also advisable to increase natural lubrication. If all fails and the epithelium is about to break or an ulcer develops but does not melt, soft contact lens wear with continued tear lubrication and antibiotic drop prophylaxis should be started (Fig. 14-23). Ointments will dislodge the lens. If the ulcer begins to melt, cyanoacrylate gluing is in order (see previous section on therapy of HSV trophic ulcers; Fig. 14-24). Neovascularization in these cases is a good sign and should be allowed to take place because healing often accompanies

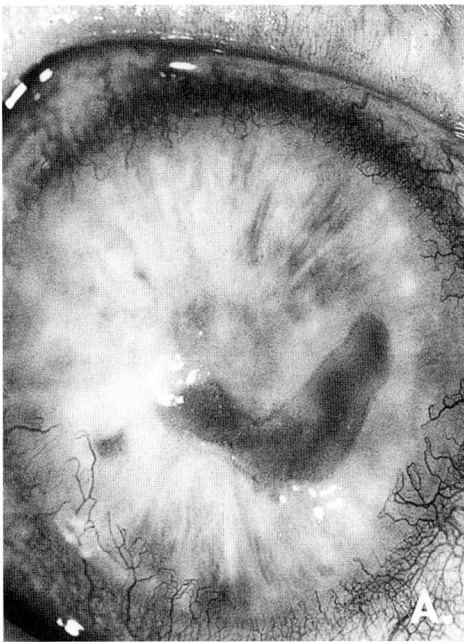 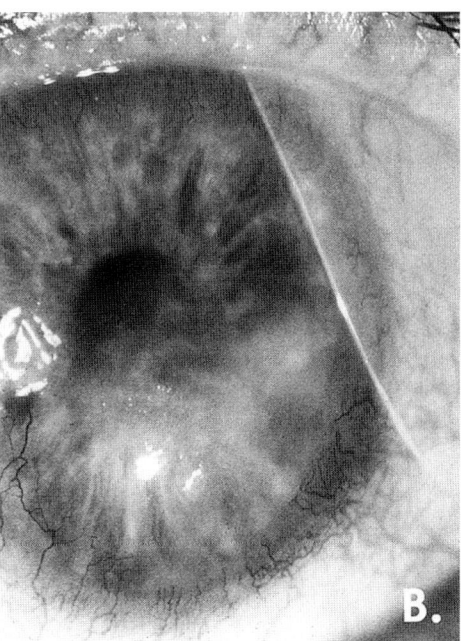

FIGURE 14-23. A: Herpes zoster ophthalmicus trophic ulcer with early melt. **B:** Treatment with thin soft contact lens (seen to right), topical antibiotic, and tear lubrication resulted in healing within 6 weeks.

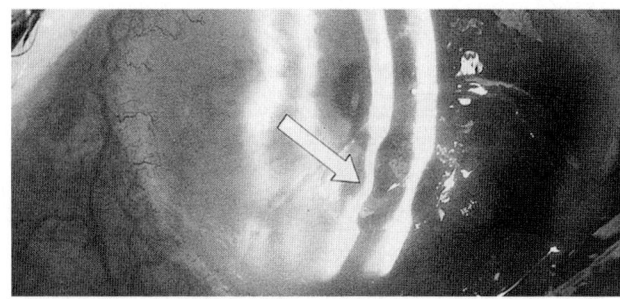 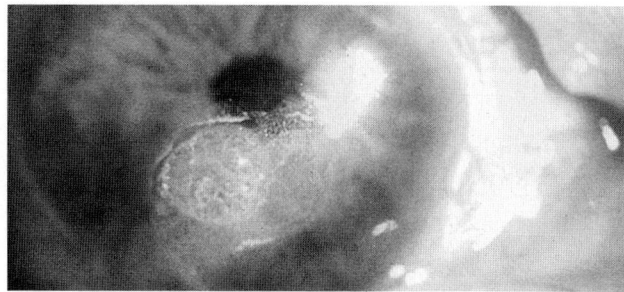

A

B

FIGURE 14-24. A: Herpes zoster ophthalmicus trophic ulcer in anesthetic cornea with melting down to descemetocele. **B:** Same eye with descemetocele just sealed with cyanoacrylate tissue adhesive. Plano T lens has not yet been put in to protect lids from roughness of adhesive. Over 6 months, stroma healed in under glue to 20% of normal thickness; epithelium healed in under glue and dislodged it. Eye subsequently did well with copious lubrication.

the process. Because many of these eyes are poor surgical risks, it is unlikely that a keratoplasty graft would ultimately be placed in the cornea (Fig. 14-25). Complete loss of sensation is not invariably associated with neurotrophic disease, however, and patients with totally anesthetic eyes may maintain clear corneas for years, but should still be protected with lubrication.

Iridocyclitis

The anterior uveal tract is involved in HZO second only to the cornea in frequency. Like corneal disease, this involvement may occur during the acute illness, months later, or

both. Clinically, the inflammation is characterized by the symptoms of pain, decreased vision, and photophobia, and the signs of ciliary hyperemia, keratic precipitates, and iris edema. In the more severe cases, there may be anterior peripheral and posterior synechia formation with a fibrinous exudate (Fig. 14-26A). Womack and Liesegang reported anterior uveitis in 43% of their patients. This is in agreement with other studies, as were the characteristic findings of striate keratopathy, vascular dilatation, posterior synechiae, sectoral pigment iris atrophy, and sphincter damage (492). Herpes zoster iritis differs from herpes simplex iritis in that the former is a lymphocytic/plasma cell vasculitis, whereas the latter is a diffuse lymphocytic infiltrate of the iris

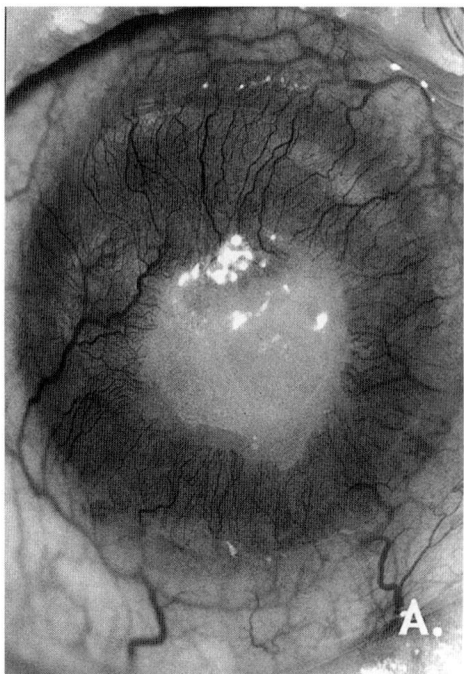 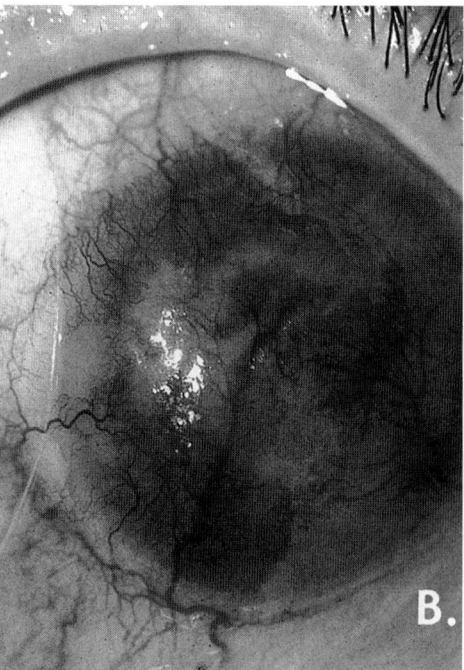

FIGURE 14-25. A: Herpes zoster ophthalmicus soft trophic ulcer in anesthetic cornea gradually being healed by vascular pannus. **B:** Same eye 6 months after thin soft contact lens application, with pannus complete and inflammation resolving.

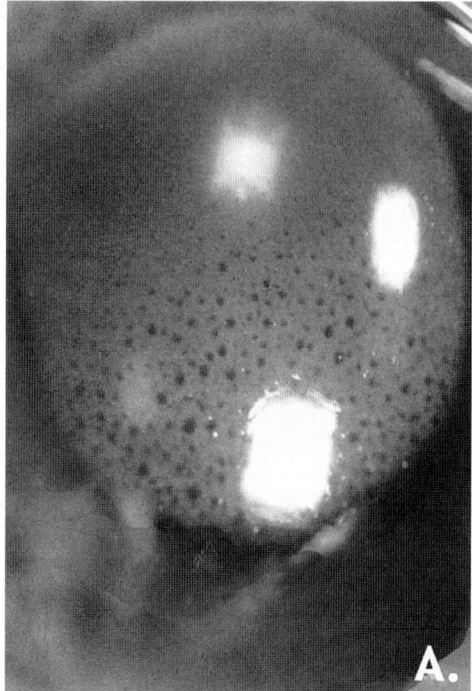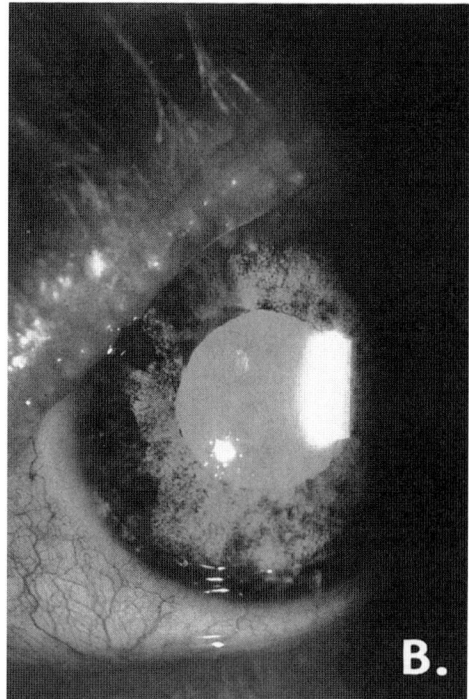

FIGURE 14-26. A: Herpes zoster ophthalmicus (HZO) iritis with keratic precipitates, pupil distortion, and early posterior synechiae forming inferiorly. **B:** Chronic recurrent HZO iridocyclitis with massive confluent iris stromal and epithelial atrophy, with the usual sector appearance of zoster iris atrophy.

stroma (there may be an associated ischemic limbal vasculitis). Fluorescein angiography reveals occlusion of iris vessels at the sites of atrophy. This differs from the iris atrophy seen with HSV disease, which causes sharply defined borders and scalloped margins with the iris arterioles patent in the involved areas. Because of the vasculitis mode of disease, HZO characteristically causes sectoral (rather than diffuse, as seen with HSV) iris atrophy in 17% to 25% of patients (491,492,526) (Fig. 14-26B). Acute or late-onset uveitis may be due to immune reaction to the antigenic residua of this virus or to new virus production (201). VZV DNA has been detected in the aqueous and iris stroma in cases of zoster sine herpete (ZSH; see later) (527,528). Additional studies indicated that an absent or poor VZV delayed hypersensitivity response correlates with increased severity of VZV uveitis and may also prove to be a useful diagnostic test in ZSH (529). As a result of the vasculitis and ischemia, zoster iritis may also cause hypopyon, hyphema, heterochromia iridis, sympathetic ophthalmia, hypotony, and phthisis (376,490,511).

In studies comparing the morbidity and visual outcome of HSV and VZV uveitis, 25% of patients with VZV disease had posterior pole complications such as cystoid macular edema, epiretinal membranes, papillitis, and retinal fibrosis and detachment, whereas only 8% of patients with HSV infection had such adverse effects (366). The most frequent ocular complication in both groups was glaucoma,

with 54% for HSV and 38% for VZV. Periocular and systemic steroids were required in more patients with HSV disease (60%) compared with VZV disease (25%). Despite these differences, in the end the visual outcomes were similar in the two groups, with 20% of patients with HSV and 21% of patients with VZV disease being legally blind in the involved eye. In a similar study on 34 patients with HZO, 68% had a single episode of iritis, whereas 32% had chronic relapsing uveitic disease (530). Nine percent had bilateral iritis and 15% had visual loss of greater than two lines (Snellen). This loss was related to other HZO complications, however, not to the iritis.

Glaucoma

The potential reduction in intraocular pressure resulting from herpes zoster inflammatory necrosis of the ciliary body and pars plicata may be more than counterbalanced by impairment of outflow facility by pigment and cellular debris clogging the trabecular network, acute trabeculitis, or secondary angle closure caused by anterior synechia formation (201,478,488,511) (Fig. 14-27). Depending on the resulting imbalance between decreased aqueous production and outflow blockage, intraocular pressure may range from abnormally low to marked secondary glaucoma. This elevated pressure may be acute or transient, or turn into a chronic problem that far outlasts the initial

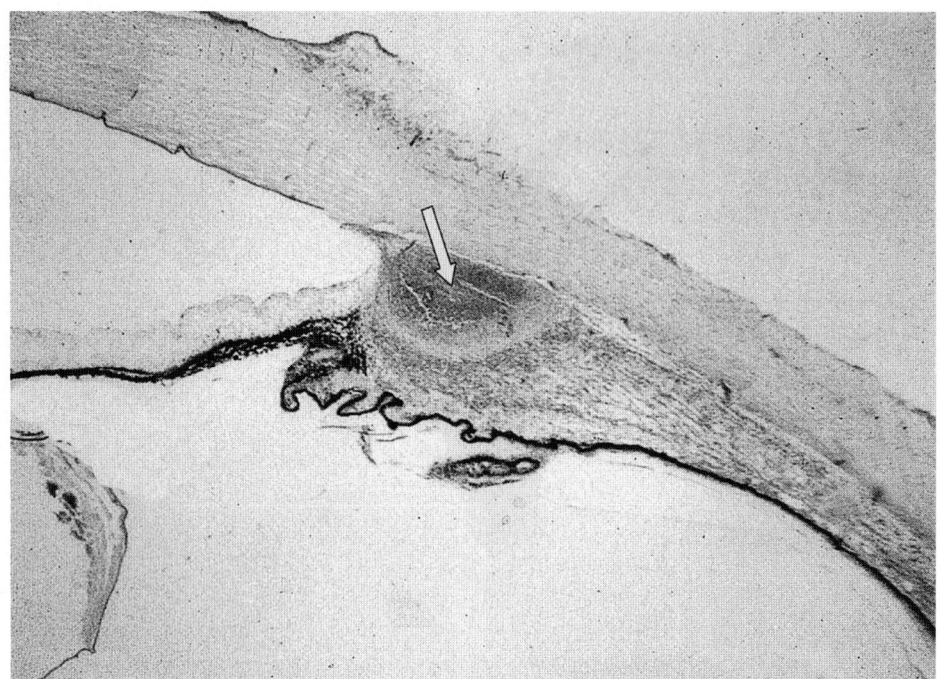

FIGURE 14-27. Histopathology of acute trabeculitis (*arrow*) showing meshwork clogged with lymphocytic infiltrate. Ciliary body is also infiltrated with monocytes.

disease. It is the most common secondary complication of VZV uveitis, occasionally requiring surgical intervention (366). Topical beta-blockers, prostamide analogs, and systemic or topical carbonic anhydrase inhibitors may all be used effectively to treat both the acute and the chronic aspects of this secondary glaucoma.

Acute and Postherpetic Neuralgia and Postherpetic Itch

There are four types of pain or discomfort: PHN is a constant aching or burning, a sudden lancinating pain, or allodynia (nonpainful stimuli perceived as painful), and postherpetic itch (PHI) is constant or intermittent itching in the involved area. Change in behavior is not uncommon in patients with PHN/PHI. It may be manifested by sleep disturbance, lassitude, anorexia, weight loss, constipation, and depression. In a study of 916 patients with zoster by deMoragas and Kierland, acute neuralgia occurred in 12% of patients younger than 20 years of age, in 40% of those in the third and fourth decade, and in only 20% of those patients 60 years of age and older (531). In contrast, in this same study population, chronic PHN pain lasting more than 1 year occurred in less than 4% of patients 20 years of age or younger and in 10% of patients in the third and fourth decades of life, but the incidence rose to nearly 50% for those patients in the sixth and seventh decades of life. Similarly, Womack and Liesegang noted PHN persisting in 17% of their patients with the most severe cases who were

60 through 80 years of age (492). Maximum recovery is usually achieved by 2 years, with little change in status after that time.

The pain of acute neuralgia experienced by almost all patients during the early phases of illness is attributed to an acute swelling of the trigeminal ganglion associated with a marked neural vasculitis with lymphocytic/plasma cell/macrophage infiltrate, necrosis of nerve cells and axons, focal hemorrhage, and a similar inflammatory reaction in the periocular tissues. Viral inclusion bodies are noted in the neuronal and satellite cell nuclei of the trigeminal ganglion and in areas of vasculitis (22,517,518). The pain may be so severe as to be accompanied by sympathetic hyperactivity such as tachypnea, tachycardia, diaphoresis, mydriasis, and severe anxiety.

The risk and prognostic factors for PHN/PHI and focal sensory denervation include (a) patient age, (b) severity of acute neuralgia, (c) ocular inflammation, (d) extent of acute skin rash, and (e) nontrigeminal cranial nerve involvement (522,532). In HIV-positive patients, an additional study found that PHN was correlated with baseline acute pain, pain at 1 month, and duration of skin lesions (533). These findings suggest that the ability of the immune system to control the acute disease is directly related to the development and severity of chronic VZV neuropathy. The cause of PHN/PHI appears to be multifactorial. Some investigators have produced evidence indicating the neuropathy to be predominantly a deafferentation-type central pain syndrome, whereas others have produced data indicating that activity of remaining peripheral nociceptors (skin pain transmitters) plays a critical role.

The deafferentation studies indicate that both PHN and PHI appear related to loss of peripheral sensory neurons (534–536). In Oaklander's studies, skin biopsies were obtained from 38 adults with or without PHN at least 3 months after healing of shingles (zoster lesions) on the torso. The density of remaining nerve endings in skin previously affected by shingles was determined. The overlap between subjects with and without PHN was small. Of 19 subjects without PHN, 17 had more than 670 neurites/mm² skin surface area, and 18 of 19 subjects with PHN had 640 or fewer neurites/mm². It was thought that this indicated that PHN may be a "phantom-skin" pain associated with loss of nociceptors. This threshold of approximately 650 neurites/mm² skin surface had not been previously reported. It suggested that the absence of pain after shingles may require the preservation of a minimum density of primary nociceptive neurons, and that the density of epidermal innervation may provide an objective correlate for the presence or absence of PHN pain (536). Other proposed mechanisms for PHN/PHI are that both may result from hyperactivity of hypoafferented central itch- and pain-specific neurons, selective preservation of peripheral pain and itch fibers from unaffected adjacent dermatomes, or an imbalance between inhibition and excitation of second-order sensory neurons (534,537). These authors further demonstrated that the relative contributions of peripheral and central mechanisms to the pathophysiology of PHN/PHI may vary with time (535) (Fig. 14-28).

The proposed mechanism for nociceptor hyperactivity is that the period of acute disease initiates peripheral nociceptor-evoked CNS hyperexcitability and axonal lesions that may induce the growth of ectopically discharging nociceptor nerve endings (22). At autopsy, patients with PHN have histopathologic lesions both in the peripheral nerves and in the dorsal horn and spinal cord, changes not seen in patients with VZV disease who recover without PHN (538). A further difference is that VZV-specific proteins have been found in the monocytes of patients with PHN months or years after the acute disease, indicating persistence, reactivation, and expression of VZV in patients with chronic pain (539).

Zoster Sine Herpete (ZSH)

Iritis, disciform keratitis, and facial palsy (Bell's palsy) may all be due to ZSH. ZSH is defined as reactivated VZV that causes only neurologic symptoms such as dermatomal

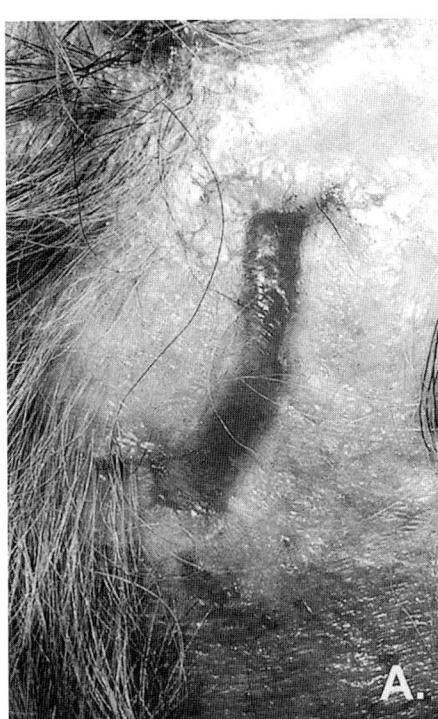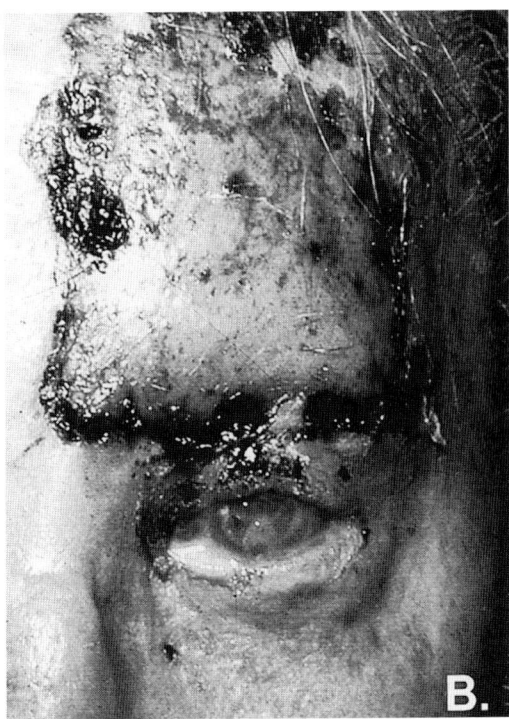

FIGURE 14-28. A: Deep gouge in scalp down to bone at lower end due to persistent scratching of postherpetic itch (PHI) in anesthetic V-1 tissues. **B:** Failure to heal 8 months after acute herpes zoster ophthalmicus because of scratching in V-1 area afflicted with severe itch, but without other sensation to curb patient's action. Anesthetic cornea is also ulcerated and melting. Treatment with lateral tarsorrhaphy, thin soft contact lens, antibiotics, and lubrication ultimately healed cornea. Diphenhydramine (Benadryl), lidocaine ointment, and gabapentin (Neurontin) partially alleviated the PHI.

neuralgia or neuropathy, and, on occasion, ocular inflammation. There is, by definition, no rash (540).

Any unexplained acute granulomatous iritis, with or without elevated intraocular pressure, should be suspect for HZO. In studies on nine patients with suspected ZSH with iritis and secondary glaucoma, the aqueous humor was positive for VZV DNA in the early stages of disease, and pigmented keratic precipitates and typical sectoral iris atrophy were residua (541). The aqueous was also positive for VZV DNA in a 65-year-old man with bilateral granulomatous iritis, secondary glaucoma unresponsive to steroid therapy, and no rash (542). The inflammatory disease responded promptly to oral acyclovir, but there was residual iris sector atrophy. Facial palsy (Bell's palsy) may also be due to ZSH (543). Thirteen patients with acute facial palsy who were PCR positive for VZV DNA were treated within 7 days of onset using acyclovir–prednisone therapy, and all recovered completely.

Noncontact *in vivo* photomicrography on seven patients with ZSH revealed that all patients had corneal epithelial changes at presentation and that new changes developed over 2 weeks. The smallest lesions noted were 10 to 25 μm in diameter and large foci were 100 to 200 μm. Three of three corneas tested were PCR positive for VZV DNA (544). This was also noted in a similar study on patients with overt HZO (545). In the latter study, pseudodendrites developed in two patients and white plaques developed in some, but there were no ulcers. Disciform keratitis may also occur as a manifestation of ZSH. VZV DNA had been detected in the aqueous of such a patient, whereas HSV and CMV assays were negative (546). Treatment for ZSH is similar to that for the other complications of HZO, including oral antivirals, steroids, and PHN inhibitors.

Pathogenesis and Histopathology

There are two chief mechanisms for development of herpes zoster: (a) reactivation of latent virus in the sensory ganglion, virus left there during the primary illness of chickenpox; and (b) contact with exogenous virus through direct or indirect contact with a patient with active chickenpox or zoster (192,547,548). Both result from decreased and, therefore, permissive VZV CMI immunocompetence. The incubation period after known exposure to the virus is a few days to 2 weeks (488,490,547). This period is not known in cases of endogenous zoster, but endogenous disease is by far the most common form.

During acute chickenpox, the virus travels by viremia and retrograde neuronal spread from infected skin cells such that the virus infects and becomes latent in multiple ganglia along the entire neural axis. The complete viral genome becomes latent in most dorsal root and cranial ganglia: 65% to 90% of trigeminal, 50% to 80% of thoracic, and 70% of geniculate ganglia (22,26,27,549).

Attempts to recover VZV from ganglia at autopsy have been unsuccessful, although the virus has been recovered if active VZV existed in the corresponding dermatome at the time of death (498,550). Because the total amount of latent VZV (0.01% to 0.15% of ganglionic cells) is low, most methods to detect it have failed (317). During active infection it is known that virus replicates both in neural and nonneuronal satellite cells. By using a combination of *in situ* PCR and *in situ* hybridization, VZV DNA has been found to exist only in the neuronal nuclei during latent infection (551).

Although it is clear that competent CMI is essential to prevent clinical VZV disease, the immune response does not completely prevent reactivation. It appears that subclinical infections occur in both immunocompetent and immunocompromised patients several times during life (552,553). This appears to "reboot" the VZV CMI system such that the CMI acts to inhibit spread of VZV in the ganglion and subsequent spread to the skin or eye. During these subclinical reactivations, there is also a rapid rise in the VZV glycoprotein antibody level, with the greatest increase in antibodies to gp98 and gp62, which persist for at least 2 years (452). Occasionally there may be partial breakthrough in the form of recurrent dermatomal pain, corneal pseudodendrites, or even a marked uveitis. With or without a previous history of overt herpes zoster, these VZV reactivations without dermal eruption are classified as ZSH (discussed later). During these contained recurrences, there is a marked boost in T-cell response, and incomplete VZV DNA is present in peripheral mononuclear cells (540,554). The ability of CMI to contain these recurrences determines whether a patient will one day have a full-blown attack of herpes zoster.

Reactivating VZV causes inflammation and hemorrhagic necrosis often associated with neuritis, leptomeningitis, segmental myelitis, and related motor and sensory root degeneration (525). There may be retrograde viral spread to the brainstem and spinal cord to damage the corresponding sensory nuclei, as well as to regional arteries and the CNS. Postmortem examination of those who die of VZV disease shows satellitosis, lymphocytic infiltration and necrosis of the ganglia, and viral particles in granulomatous arteritis (555). Cerebrovascular accident is not infrequent (556). Virus particles have also been found in acute VZV disease in the trigeminal ganglion and its axons, in CNS tissues, and in the arterial walls of ocular and CNS tissues by electron microscopy and immunofluorescence (524). There is VZV DNA in peripheral mononuclear cells (557).

Reports on the histopathology of acute and chronic HZO revealed, in the acute cases, normal cornea or episcleral and corneal inflammation with macrophages in the endothelium, nongranulomatous inflammation (lymphocytes, plasma cells) of the iris and ciliary body with extension into the choroid, and macrophage and other inflammatory cell infiltration of the trabecular meshwork (511,517,518). All of these abnormalities appeared to be reversible. In other patients, a severe retinitis was noted over areas of intense granulomatous choroiditis containing epithelioid and giant cells with areas of hemorrhage. Similarly, the optic nerve, meninges, and central retinal vessels could be involved in a granulomatous inflammation, with the primary site of involvement being the optic nerve itself and secondarily the posterior ciliary nerves. Late findings included lymphocytic infiltration of the posterior ciliary nerves and vessels, a pathognomonic sign of VZV disease, chronic inflammation of the iris and ciliary body with necrosis, granulomatous choroiditis or giant cell arteritis, and perivasculitis. The mechanism for chronic smoldering VZV inflammatory damage to the eye is not fully known, but immune reaction against recurring viral reactivation or persistent viral antigen is suspect (201,518).

In anterograde spread, the virus travels down the fifth cranial nerve axons to the skin, resulting in a demyelination, granulomatous, mononuclear cellular infiltration, and consequent fibrotic scarring of peripheral nerves and end organs (skin and eye) affected. Acute skin and conjunctival vesicles and dendritic ulcers are infectious in etiology. The skin eruption is simultaneous, with a strong VZV-specific T-cell proliferation. Current evidence as to the pathogenesis of stromal disease indicates that, as in herpes simplex, an AAC-mediated reaction is responsible for the Wessely immune rings, necrotizing interstitial keratitis, and limbal vasculitis (local Arthus reaction) (22,184,195,500). The diffuse or local gray stromal edema of disciform disease and iritis is thought to be primarily a lymphocyte-mediated delayed hypersensitivity reaction to virus or viral antigen. The chronic HZO keratitis may be noted to have a giant cell reaction at the level of Descemet's membrane, and VZV DNA may be detected in human corneas at least 8 years after the acute event (517,519). In addition, mechanical healing problems (trophic ulcers) may result from the abnormal precorneal tear film encountered with neurotrophic changes, exposure, and scarred meibomian gland orifices. The neurotrophic changes and density of corneal anesthesia are a function of the ganglionic damage (524,525).

Diagnosis

See the section on Laboratory Diagnostic Techniques, previously, for greater detail (1,2,10).

Diagnosis of HZO is usually by clinical impression. The direct immunofluorescence assay is more specific and sensitive than any of the other tests mentioned here, and has the advantage of lower cost and more rapid time to execute (10). However, as noted earlier in the section on Laboratory Diagnostic Techniques, virus may be cultured (with some difficulty because of its fastidious nature) from the skin vesicles and ocular lesions for up to 7 days after their appearance, or longer in the immunosuppressed patient.

Giemsa staining of scrapings taken from the lesions often reveals eosinophilic intranuclear inclusion bodies in the epithelium indicative of herpesvirus, but not distinguishing between zoster or simplex. There are also a ballooning degeneration of the epithelial cells, multinucleated giant cells, and a monocytic infiltrate compatible with some sort of herpetic viral infection.

Other diagnostic tests of greater complexity and specificity include PCR, immunomorphologic evaluations such as immunofluorescence electron microscopy, immunoperoxidase, radioimmunoassay, ELISA, and agar gel immunodiffusion. Serologic evaluations include fluorescent antibody staining for membrane antigen, immune adherence hemagglutination assay, neutralization, complement fixation, radioimmunoassay, and agar gel protein fractionation (10,22,478).

Medical Treatment

Antiviral Drugs

Antiviral agents for HZO are discussed in detail in the section on Ocular Antiviral Agents: Laboratory and Clinical Studies, earlier.

One question that continues to be raised is, "Should every patient with herpes zoster receive antiviral treatment?" Gnann has recommended that treatment be given to those at high risk for complications: age older than 50 years, immunocompromise, moderately severe to severe pain at presentation, greater degree of skin surface involvement, and those with HZO (236). In a study on the effect of antiviral therapy on complications of HZO from 1976 through 1998, comparing treated with untreated patients ($N = 324$ total), the probability of adverse outcome was 9% in untreated patients and 2% in treated patients (558). The mean time to initiation of treatment in those in whom stromal keratitis, corneal edema, scleritis, uveitis, or glaucoma developed was 4.8 days, compared with 3.8 days ($p = .006$) for those in whom such complications did not develop. Neurotrophic disease was significantly less frequent in treated patients, probably because of drug inhibition of ganglionic damage. Differences between different drugs used and PHN were not addressed. The study, however, strongly supports the early and routine use of systemic antivirals for HZO.

As noted earlier in the section on Ocular Antiviral Agents: Laboratory and Clinical Studies, famciclovir and valacyclovir both have better bioavailability, require less frequent dosing, and are statistically better than acyclovir in inhibiting PHN (559,560).

Corticosteroids

Topical steroids are therapeutically useful in the management of manifestations of zoster vasculitis such as scleritis, stromal keratitis, interstitial keratitis, and uveitis. In addition, they suppress nonspecific inflammation and immune-mediated diseases, including anterior stromal infiltrates, stromal disciform reaction, corneal mucous plaques, sclerokeratitis, serpiginous ulceration, and keratouveitis (22,184,195,376,478).

The role of systemic corticosteroids in acute HZO and in the prevention of PHN is now controversial. A series of open and controlled studies indicated that systemic steroids had a significant beneficial effect on the control of keratitis, uveitis, secondary glaucoma, and PHN (488,561–563). One of the strongest studies favoring systemic steroid treatment for the prevention of long-term neuralgia was reported by Keczkes and Basheer (564). Forty otherwise healthy patients with HZO were treated with either 40 mg of prednisone given orally daily tapered over 4 weeks (20 patients) or carbamazepine, a drug used for trigeminal neuralgia, 100 mg given orally four times daily for 4 weeks (20 patients). Sixty-five in the carbamazepine group had PHN lasting up to 2 years, whereas only 15% of the prednisone group had long-term neuralgia that lasted only 6 months. There was no dissemination of infection in either group.

Esmann and coworkers, however, contradicted these findings in a masked, controlled study (565). These workers reported that high-dose oral prednisolone even in combination with oral acyclovir did not prevent PHN. This suggested that the carbamazepine may have been the effective agent in Keczkes and Bashheer's study (564). Seventy-eight patients older than the age of 60 years and with acute VZV infections of less than 4 days' duration were treated prospectively in a double-masked study. Therapy was either 225 mg of prednisolone or calcium lactate over a 10-day period plus acyclovir, 300 mg given orally five times daily for 7 days. Twelve of these patients had HZO. Although the acute pain was relieved more rapidly in the steroid-treated group, the long-term results were not significantly different. Twenty-three percent of both the placebo- and the steroid/acyclovir-treated patients had persistent neuralgia at 6 months after the onset of illness. A greater percentage (29%) of patients with HZO had long-term neuralgia compared with patients with nontrigeminal forms of the disease (22%).

The most definitive studies on the role of steroids in this illness were two large, controlled clinical trials combining acyclovir with corticosteroids. Two hundred eight immunocompetent patients older than 50 years of age with localized herpes zoster of less than 72 hours' duration were enrolled in one study by Whitley et al. (566). Acyclovir or a matched placebo was given orally, 800 mg five times daily, for 21 days. Prednisone or a matched placebo was given orally at 60 mg/day for the first 7 days, 30 mg/day for days 8 to 14, and 15 mg/day for days 15 to 21. Patients receiving both had a moderate but statistically significant acceleration in the rate of cutaneous healing and relief of acute pain. There was also improved quality of life: less need for analgesics, more uninterrupted sleep, and shorter time to resumption of usual activities. The study by Wood et al. produced similar results. Neither study demonstrated any effect on PHN (566,567).

Because of the lack of a clearly beneficial effect of systemic steroids in acute zoster, the well-known adverse side effects of these drugs, and the risk of disseminated infectious disease, the use of systemic steroids to prevent acute and long-term pain must be carefully assessed. It would appear advisable to limit the use of systemic corticosteroids to those immunocompetent, nondiabetic patients experiencing the vasculitic complications of HZO such as severe scleritis, uveitis, and orbital apex syndrome, and those at minimal risk for adverse steroid reaction to achieve faster improvement in quality of life (478,566–568).

Pharmacologic Agents for Postherpetic Neuralgia/Postherpetic Itch

Tricyclic Antidepressants

Evidence is strong that *PHN/PHI may be prevented or greatly inhibited* by combining antiviral famciclovir or valacyclovir with tricyclic antidepressants or anticonvulsants, as well as strong analgesics *at the onset of acute VZV illness* (236,533,569).

In recent years, the use of psychotropic medication for the treatment of chronic pain, particularly the tricyclic antidepressants, has become an important therapeutic modality in managing neuralgia of any etiology (570,571). The proposed mechanisms of action of the tricyclic antidepressants include alteration of transport or activity of substances involved in inflammation at the tissue level, such as serotonin, and inhibition of prostaglandin synthetase, an enzyme crucial to inflammation; and modification of blood protein-binding capacity, a characteristic noted with conventional antiinflammatory drugs (570).

In a placebo-controlled study, Watson and coworkers noted a significant clinical value in the use of the tricyclic antidepressant amitriptyline (25 to 150 mg PO every day) in older patients with PHN (572). The positive response rate was 60%, with very severe pain becoming milder but not entirely alleviated. Therapeutic response was noted within 3 weeks, yet serum drug levels were consistently below those associated with antidepressant activity. Increasing dosage resulted in increased pain in some patients, suggesting a therapeutic window for the analgesic dose of the tricyclic antidepressants. Similarly, Kvinesdal and coworkers used imipramine (100 mg PO daily) in nondepressed patients with severe diabetic neuropathy (571). Analgesia was successfully achieved at serum levels half that required for antidepressant effect and occurred within 2 weeks of initiating therapy.

As work in this area continued, different tricyclic antidepressants were tried and some compared with each other.

Watson et al. believed that nortriptyline, a noradrenergic metabolite of amitriptyline, might be more effective. In a study of 33 patients with VZV PHN, 68% had at least a good response to either amitriptyline or nortriptyline, with no difference between the two drugs regarding the pain parameters studied (573). There was also no change in the rating scales for depression in either group despite the relief of pain. Intolerable side effects, however, were more common with amitriptyline, making nortriptyline the drug of choice between these two.

There are no data to suggest superiority of one tricyclic antidepressant over another in analgesic efficacy, but side effects are a differentiating matter. Selection of one of these drugs for therapy of PHN, then, depends on potential side effects. Amitriptyline, imipramine, and doxepin have greater anticholinergic, cardiac, and CNS side effects than do nortriptyline and desipramine. In addition, desipramine may be less sedating to a more quiescent patient, whereas amitriptyline or doxepin may be of greater benefit in the agitated or anxious patient. The presence of bradycardia or heart block is an indication for using nortriptyline. The common dosage for amitriptyline, doxepin, and desipramine is 25 to 50 mg PO at bedtime, with increasing dosage every 7 to 14 days if necessary and if tolerated, until a dosage of 75 to 100 mg/day is achieved. Because of their sedating effect, these drugs are usually given in a single dose at bedtime.

Alternative therapy to the tricyclic antidepressants includes the combination of neuroleptic agents such as the tranquilizer perphenazine and amitriptyline (Triavil, 2 to 10 tablets, or Etrafon, 2 to 10 tablets) three to four times daily for patients with PHN and mixed anxiety and agitation with symptoms of depression. This is a particularly effective combination in patients younger than the age of 50 years. In older patients, however, there is increased risk of tardive dyskinesia and other extrapyramidal reactions such as motor restlessness and oculogyric crisis (570,574,575). Should any of these side effects present themselves, the medication should be stopped immediately. On resolution of the side effects, tricyclic antidepressant therapy alone may be undertaken to control the PHN.

Anticonvulsants, Narcotic Analgesics, and Intrathecal Steroids

The anticonvulsant gabapentin (Neurontin) 600 mg PO two to six times daily is frequently very effective at controlling PHN as a single agent, and may be given intermittently or continuously for months to years as tolerated or needed (569,576,577). Tapering may be attempted periodically. Another anticonvulsant in this same family has also been reported to have very good effects in PHN. Pregabalin 600 mg/day versus no treatment in control patients with VZV disease showed significantly decreased mean pain scores, improved sleep, and general global improvement

(578). Zonisamide (Zonegran) 200 to 600 mg/day is a third anticonvulsant useful in management of PHN. All three drugs are reported as safe, well tolerated, and efficacious. Their use for VZV neuropathic pain is off-label.

For patients not responding satisfactorily to single-agent therapy, gabapentin and a tricyclic antidepressant such as nortriptyline or desipramine may be combined for additive effect. If the combination is still not totally effective or if one or both drugs are not tolerated in treatment of PHN, slow-release opioids such as oxycodone-SR (OxyContin-SR) 10 to 20 mg PO every 12 hours may be added or given as a single agent to provide relief (579,580). Because of the slow release, there is no "high," and therefore little chance of addiction when taken by the appropriate oral route. The combination of either doxepin or amitriptyline with a narcotic analgesic reduced pain intensity more than either an antidepressant or a narcotic drug alone in patients with chronic neuralgia (581). Because of amitriptyline's less desirable side effect profile, combination of desipramine or nortriptyline with an opioid analgesic for recalcitrant cases seems more desirable (e.g., nortriptyline 50 mg at bedtime and oxycodone slow-release 10 to 40 mg PO every 12 hours). Again, periodic tapering should be attempted because PHN may decrease spontaneously over time.

Use of intrathecal methylprednisolone for intractable PHN is still under study. Initial results have been quite favorable, but because of the nature of the treatment larger series of patients are being evaluated (582). Surgical ablation of the trigeminal ganglion is now contraindicated because of poor postoperative results coupled with significant potential complications due to the induced sensory paralysis.

Topical Agents: Capsaicin, Lidocaine Patches, Diphenhydramine Cream, and Oral Diphenhydramine

Substance P is a tachykinin peptide that acts as a neurotransmitter in peripheral pain impulses. Capsaicin (Zostrix) depletes substance P from the small sensory peripheral and central neurons and prevents reaccumulation at these sites. Watson's study using open-label capsaicin 0.025% four times daily on 31 men and women with median age of 71 years and median duration of severe PHN of 2 years noted a positive therapeutic response rate in 76% of patients within 4 weeks (583). In subsequent studies, he came to believe that much of the "success" was due to placebo effect and that his clinical experience indicated only a modest effect in many patients. He noted that most failed to find relief, found the relief unsatisfactory, or were unable to tolerate the burning sensation. Occasional patients appeared to have a very good result, and those unusual cases may not have been reflected by clinical trials (584). In general, topical capsaicin is *not* satisfactory as a sole therapy for chronic painful conditions, although it may serve as an adjuvant to other approaches.

Lidocaine (Lidoderm) skin patches are also effective for both PHN and PHI in application over the forehead and scalp as needed (534). Diphenhydramine (Benadryl) cream to the affected area or oral diphenhydramine 25 to 50 mg at bedtime and as tolerated by day also reduces PHI in a number of patients.

Injected Anesthetics

For severe pain in acute HZO, frontal and nasal nerve blocks are effective in controlling pain not controlled by drugs, particularly in the elderly (585,586). Bupivacaine, epinephrine, and clonidine are injected at the frontal and nasal branch levels of the ophthalmic nerve. The effect lasts approximately 5 days and this simple injection can be repeated if necessary. Stellate ganglion block may also be effective if given within 14 days of onset of the rash. (587). A 10-mL mixture of plain 1% lidocaine and 0.5% bupivacaine is injected at the level of the C5-6 vertebrae with the head extended. This should be done by an anesthesiologist or neurosurgeon experienced in the technique.

Surgical Procedures

The most common indications for a surgical procedure in HZO are exposure keratopathy and anesthetic cornea. If lid closure is good but the tear meniscus low or unstable, punctal plugs may suffice. In the more severe forms of the illness, significant scarring or partial destruction of lid tissue interferes with blinking and normal lid closure during sleep. If lid structures are basically intact but closure is incomplete because of scarring, a lateral or lateral and medial tarsorrhaphy with ointment at bedtime should suffice to protect the globe. If lid tissue has actually been lost, plastic reconstruction involving the swinging of flaps may be necessary. This should be done by a surgeon experienced with such procedures because the remaining lid tissues are often friable and hold sutures poorly.

In the partially or totally anesthetic cornea where the epithelium is gray, unhealthy, or prone to recurrent breakdown, partial tarsorrhaphy is also indicated. It is may also be advisable to use a therapeutic contact lens in these cases. Wherever medial and lateral tarsorrhaphy is used, an open area must be left between the lids to allow the physician an adequate view of the underlying globe (Fig. 14-29).

If corneal melting occurs, sealing the area with the sterile cyanoacrylate glue (see section on therapy of HSV trophic ulcers, earlier) and inserting a Plano T therapeutic lens to cover the rough surface of the glue are indicated. The patient should be informed that this gluing procedure is not FDA approved for the eye, however. With time, the cornea almost invariably heals under the glue and the glue dislodges spontaneously or a corneal pannus grows in and

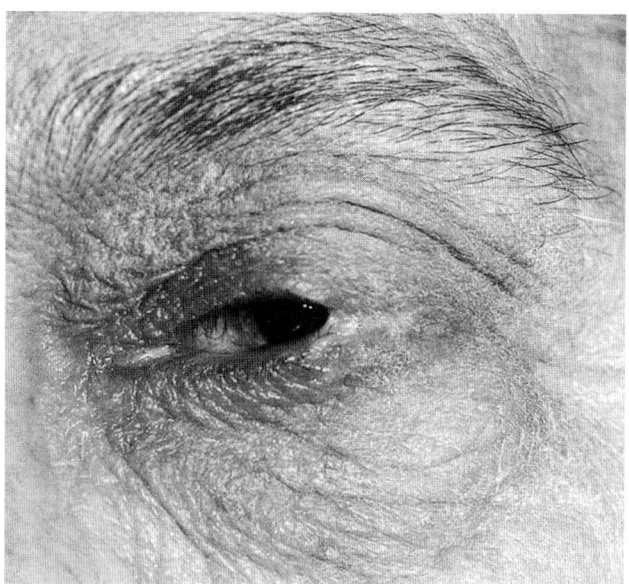

FIGURE 14-29. Lateral tarsorrhaphy with 50% closure of palpebral fissure to protect totally anesthetic cornea, which had begun to ulcerate. Thirty percent closures are often more cosmetically acceptable to patients and also protect the cornea.

heals the surface under the glue. Good alternative but more extensive surgical procedures include the pulling down of a conjunctival flap if the tissue has not been too severely scarred by the disease or the placing of conjunctival transplants from the contralateral eye. Stem cell transplantation from the contralateral eye is still under study.

Keratoplasty is potentially complicated in HZO. Anesthetic corneas heal poorly, and the transplanted eye is prone to melting and superinfection. A cornea that has scarred but retained a reasonable amount of sensation is perhaps the best situation in which keratoplasty might succeed. Any major surgical procedure, such as transplantation or cataract extraction, should be deferred, if possible, until the eye is uninflamed. The longer it is deferred beyond this point, the better (588). Cataract extractions that must be performed for mature lenses are best done with care taken to avoid incisions in an anesthetic cornea. The visual acuity can be diminished by the lipid keratopathy that persists after the HZO has subsided. Argon laser has been used to diminish the deposition of lipid (589).

If keratoplasty is performed, however, a lateral tarsorrhaphy should be done at the same time to protect the graft. Reed et al. performed penetrating keratoplasty on 12 patients with HZO, 5 of whom had neurotrophic ulceration (590). Lateral tarsorrhaphy was performed in 10 patients to prevent postoperative breakdown of the corneal epithelium. At average follow-up of 3 years, 83% of the grafts were clear and 75% of the eyes had vision at 20/80 or greater. Similarly, Marsh and Cooper reported that tarsorrhaphy led to rapid epithelial healing in grafted zoster eyes, vision of 6/12 or better in six of seven eyes undergoing keratoplasty, and clear grafts for 2 to 9 years of follow-up (591). Neovascularization was closed with the argon laser before surgery. Eighteen additional patients with HZO underwent successful cataract extraction, 12 receiving posterior chamber implants. Trabeculectomies were successful in seven patients with zoster glaucoma, although cataracts subsequently developed in five. In a review of 15 patients (12 VZV, 3 varicella keratopathy), Tanure et al. reported placing lateral tarsorrhaphies at the time of four of the grafts (592). Three patients had steroid-responsive rejections, and two failed (one primary and one neurotrophic). At an average follow-up of 50 months, 87% of the grafts remained clear and the best-corrected visual acuity was 20/100 or better in 53% of eyes. The authors thought that useful visual rehabilitation could be achieved in VZV-infected eyes but that careful postoperative follow-up, frequent lubrication, and lateral tarsorrhaphies to protect the surface were major factors in enhancing chances of a successful outcome. A newer procedure, the keratoprosthesis, holds great promise for success in many of the most severe cases, however (593).

Summary of Therapeutic Approaches

Because HZO can cause such devastating damage, a fairly vigorous therapeutic approach should be taken in an attempt to prevent severe complications. Therapeutic guidelines are given in the following sections (Table 14-2).

Prevention

VZV vaccination boosters to prevent zoster are under study (471,594). Recent studies have shown that the VZV vaccine in children begins to lose efficacy after a few years and should probably be repeated (595).

Acute Disease

1. Antivirals: Administer famciclovir 500 mg PO three times daily or valacyclovir 1 g PO three times daily for 7 days, preferably starting within 72 hours of rash onset. As a second-line antiviral if the first two are not available, give acyclovir 800 mg PO five times daily for 7 to 10 days. Acyclovir affords dubious protection against PHN compared with famciclovir or valacyclovir. For immunocompromised patients, acyclovir can be given at dosages of 10 mg/kg IV every 8 hours for 7 days in adults and 500 mg/m^2 every 8 hours for children younger than 12 years of age (FDA-approved dosages). Famciclovir but not valacyclovir may be used in immunocompromised patients.
2. Simultaneously with antivirals, start nortriptyline or desipramine 25 to 50 mg PO at bedtime to inhibit acute pain and minimize or prevent PHN, particularly in patients older than 50 years. Add gabapentin 300 mg four times daily to 600 mg six times daily, or zonisamide 100 to 600 mg/day if needed.
3. For superficial punctate keratitis or dendritic keratitis, apply topical antibiotic. Oral antivirals may heal the lesions. Topical antivirals are often ineffective.
4. For moderate to severe corneal or scleral inflammatory disease, apply topical steroids ranging from 0.125% prednisolone two to four times daily, up to 0.1% dexamethasone in a frequency as disease warrants. Taper over a several-week period.
5. If disease is mild or there is no pain or ocular involvement, apply warm compresses or Burrow's solution compresses for 15 minutes, four times daily until scabbing has cleared.
6. For iritis, administer cycloplegics (homatropine, atropine) and topical steroids as needed.
7. Administer nonnarcotic or narcotic analgesics for acute neuralgia on days 1 through 3. If there is no resolution of pain or an increase in neuralgia, consider systemic prednisone in the immunocompetent patient at a dosage of 20 mg PO three times a day for 3 days, 15 mg PO twice daily for 3 days, and 15 mg PO once daily for 3 days. Continue oral antiviral. Systemic steroids may also be useful for severe orbital edema with superior orbital fissure syndrome and to hasten the patient's return to a more comfortable, functional life.
8. Frontal and nasal nerve or stellate ganglion block may be used for severe pain uncontrolled by medical means. It is best if it is administered by an anesthesiologist experienced in this area.
9. Use artificial tears and ointments for exposure keratitis or unstable tear film.

Long-Term or Chronic Problems

1. For exposure or corneal ulceration use a high-water-content therapeutic soft contact lens (Permalens, Kontur), with or without cyanoacrylate tissue adhesive, punctal plugs, lateral tarsorrhaphy, conjunctival flap, or transplantation, as described in text.
2. For late pseudodendritic keratitis, use antibiotic lubrication only, or, for persistent lesions, there is a variable response to topical or systemic antivirals. Trial and error must be used.
3. For immune stromal disciform, interstitial keratitis, limbal vasculitis, episcleritis, or scleritis: Depending on the severity of the inflammation, starting therapy may range from 1% prednisolone or 0.1% dexamethasone every 2 hours while awake to just two or three times daily. Tapering the dose in 50% reduction steps begins as the immune disease lessens and is continued over several weeks to months by switching to weaker dilutions of prednisolone (e.g., 0.125%), or to intermediate-strength rimexolone, or from once-daily to every-other-day dosing.

TABLE 14-2. THERAPY OF HERPES ZOSTER OPHTHALMICUS

Acute disease

Antivirals (treat for 7 days, preferably starting within 72 h of onset of rash)
  a. Famciclovir (Famvir) 500 mg PO tid (immunocompetent or compromised) *or*
  b. Valacyclovir (Valtrex) 1 g PO tid (immunocompetent), *or*
  c. Acyclovir (Zovirax) 800 mg PO five times daily
  d. Immunocompromised patients: intravenous acyclovir for 10 days, 10 mg/kg q8h in adults and 500 mg/m² q8h for children younger than 12 y of age

Pain prevention/management
  a. TCAs (e.g., nortriptyline, desipramine) 25–75 mg PO qhs or divided dose × 3 mo (or longer PRN), starting lowest dose with antivirals or as early as possible after acute disease onset, increasing over 2–3 wk PRN. Caution in patients with cardiac disease.
  b. Nonnarcotic or short-term narcotic analgesics (e.g., oxycodone, codeine, propoxyphene)

Dermatitis therapy
  a. Cool to tepid wet compresses (if tolerated) to keep dermatitis clean

Ocular anterior segment
  a. Exposure keratopathy (poor lid closure): topical antibiotic ophthalmic ointment tid
  b. Dendriform keratopathy: therapy × 2–3 wk (variably effective):
     1. 3% vidarabine ointment, *or*
     2. 1% trifluridine five times daily, *or*
     3. Oral antivirals (see above)
  c. Immune keratopathy, episcleritis, scleritis, or iritis:
     1. Topical steroids (1%–0.125% prednisolone, 0.1% dexamethasone, 1% rimexolone, 0.2%–0.5% loteprednol) q3–4h to qid PRN based on disease severity. Slow taper. Antibiotic drops/ointment prophylaxis.
     2. Oral nonsteroidal antiinflammatory drugs (e.g., ibuprofen 400 mg PO bid—tid)
     3. Topical antivirals unnecessary
     4. Cycloplegia PRN for iritis (scopolamine qd)

Glaucoma
     1. Topical beta blockers (e.g., timolol or carteolol bid)
     2. Add PRN latanoprost qd, brimonidine, unoprostone, or dorzolamide bid
     3. *No* miotics (e.g., pilocarpine)
     4. Topical steroids if glaucoma due to inflammatory trabeculitis

Chronic/recurrent disease

Dendriform or immune keratopathy, episcleritis, scleritis, iritis
     1. See acute HZO, above

Tenuous, hazy epithelium in anesthetic cornea
     1. Early lateral tarsorrhaphy and lubrication with artificial tears and tear ointments
     2. Allow vascularization to progress to aid in healing any ulcer
     3. Topical steroids with caution and only at low doses to minimize any inflammation

Exposure keratopathy (poor lid closure) or corneal ulceration or thinning
     1. Lateral tarsorrhaphy
     2. Therapeutic soft contact lens (e.g., Permalens or Kontur) lenses.
     3. Tissue adhesive (e.g., Dermabond, EpiDermGlu) for progressive thinning
     4. Conjunctival flap, transplant or keratoprosthesis (see Surgical Factors and Management)

Glaucoma
     See acute HZO, above

Postherpetic neuralgia (drugs below may be used additively)
     1. TCAs (e.g., nortriptyline, desipramine): 25 mg titrated up to 75 mg qhs PRN or divided dose. Caution if patient has cardiac disease.
     2. Gabapentin (Neurontin): 300 mg PO bid starting dose. Efficacy may not be reached until 600 mg bid six times daily. Some may not respond at all.
     3. Slow-release opioids added if TCAs ± gabapentin not sufficiently effective: oxycodone (OxyContin-SR) 10–40 mg PO q12h
     4. Capsaicin cream qd—tid to skin as tolerated
     5. Lidocaine skin patches or cream, 12 h on, 12 h off painful skin area
     6. Frontal or nasal nerve block
     7. Trigeminal ganglion ablation contraindicated

HZO, herpes zoster ophthalmicus; PO, orally; PRN, as needed; TCA, tricyclic antidepressant.
(Adapted from Pavan-Langston D. Ophthalmic zoster. In: Watson CPN, Gershon A, eds. *Herpes zoster and postherpetic neuralgia*. Amsterdam: Elsevier Science, 2001:119–129.)

The latter two steroids or reduced dosing schedule have less propensity to elevate the intraocular pressure.

4. Iritis therapy is similar to that of stromal immune keratitis. Treat any secondary glaucoma: (a) trabeculitis therapy is strong topical steroids with glaucoma drops. Pressure should drop quickly (days) if inflammatory trabeculitis is the cause and is responding to steroids. (b) Glaucoma due to debris or partial synechial angle closure is treated with drops: Beta-blockers (e.g., timolol, betaxolol, levobunolol), alpha-adrenergic agents (e.g., brimonidine), carbonic anhydrase inhibitors (e.g., brinzolamide, dorzolamide), or prostaglandin inhibitors (e.g., latanoprost, bimatoprost) may be used once or twice daily alone or in combination with the other drug groups just named. Prostaglandin inhibitors may, however, increase inflammation.

5. For chronic PHN, use tricyclic antidepressants (nortriptyline or desipramine) alone or in combination with gabapentin or zonisamide, as in step #1 under Acute Disease, or narcotic analgesics as described previously.

6. For PHN and/PHI (itch), apply capsaicin cream once to twice daily, or lidocaine patches. Apply diphenhydramine cream to involved skin. Oral diphenhydramine 25 to 50 mg may also help PHI. The duration of treatment is several months to several years.

EPSTEIN-BARR VIRUS

EBV, like all members of the family Herpesviridae, is a common cause of lifelong infection in humans. This DNA virus is encountered worldwide. EBV-specific antibodies are present in up to 50% to 85% of children younger than 4 years of age living in socioeconomically underdeveloped countries, and in 26% to 82% of college students (2,596–599). EBV infection in young children produces little to no overt clinical disease. By the teenage years or adulthood, however, the classic picture of infectious mononucleosis (IM) is seen, with fever, extensive lymphadenopathy, pharyngitis, hepatitis, lymphocytosis, myositis, polyarthritis, pericarditis, and follicular conjunctivitis (599–601). The disease is transmitted by upper respiratory fomites.

Epstein-Barr Virus Ocular Disease

The ocular manifestations of EBV infection, particularly those associated with or after IM, include a wide range of neuroophthalmic, posterior segment, and anterior segment findings. Neuroophthalmic and posterior manifestations include papilledema, optic neuritis, and cranial nerve palsies. Anterior segment findings include follicular conjunctivitis, flat or nodular episcleritis, subconjunctival hemorrhaging, iritis or panuveitis, oculoglandular syndrome, infectious dendritiform epithelial keratitis, stromal keratitis,

and occasionally a membranous follicular conjunctivitis. In one 14-year-old girl, EBV infection presented as exophthalmos and ocular muscle swelling (602). EBV genome was detected in activated T lymphocytes and local muscle biopsies. The patient responded to immunosuppressive treatment with steroids and cyclophosphamide. Meisler et al. have reported EBV Parinaud's oculoglandular syndrome (603). In another orbital case, EBV dacryoadenitis resulted in severe keratoconjunctivitis sicca in a 10-year-old boy (604). Serologic and immunohistologic data confirmed the diagnosis and the histopathology of the lacrimal gland was similar to that of primary Sjögren's syndrome. Treatment with acyclovir and cyclosporine was highly successful.

HIV-positive patients are reported to have a higher incidence of Sjögren's syndrome than the average population. EBV has been found in the tear film of 12 HIV-positive patients with marked keratoconjunctivitis sicca (605). EBV was not found in the tear film of 20 normal control subjects, and was found in 4 of 15 HIV-negative patients with Sjögren's syndrome (not significantly different from control subjects), and in 12 of 19 HIV-positive patients with Sjögren's syndrome ($p < .01$). Pflugfelder has also noted EBV in HIV-negative patients with dry eye (35). Further molecular evidence for the probable role of EBV in ocular inflammation is reported in two patients with acute conjunctivitis as the presenting signs of systemic EBV disease (606). *In situ* hybridization studies on conjunctival biopsies were positive for EBV genome.

The keratitis of EBV may be unilateral or bilateral, with onset 1 to 4 weeks after the acute IM or a flulike illness compatible with IM (607–610). Patients complain of symptoms of irritation, watering, photophobia, and blurred vision. There is a characteristic conjunctival hyperemia during the acute phase. Rarely, patients experience recurrent bouts of EBV keratitis in both eyes without the associated red eye. There is one report of development of nodular scleritis in a patient 4 years after occurrence of an acute EBV keratitis (607,608,611,612). In another report on screening 12 cadaveric normal eyes for EBV DNA, 70% of the eyes were positive in at least one sample taken from the eyes (613). Only the optic nerves were consistently negative for EBV DNA. This suggests that EBV may be involved in ocular disease more than is recognized, but also that we need specific criteria to implicate this virus in ocular disease.

Because of the apparent immune basis to EBV keratitis and iritis, both forms of this anterior segment disease are commonly responsive to topical steroid therapy. Wong and coworkers reported three cases of chronic EBV systemic infection associated with keratitis and iritis responsive to 1% prednisolone drops given four times a day over a 3-week period (614). There are no reports concerning management of the infectious microdendritic epithelial keratitis with antivirals and no reason to believe that any of the commercially available antiviral agents would be therapeutically useful. The epithelial phase of EBV infection is apparently self-limited without therapeutic intervention. The epithelial keratitis may mimic HSV disease with superficial punctate keratitis or multiple microdendritic lesions. EBV has been cultured from these lesions or detected by ELISA testing of corneal, conjunctival, and tear film samples taken from patients demonstrating these changes (597,606,608–611,614).

Rarely, stromal keratitis may develop. The stromal disease is thought to be due to an immune reaction to EBV or EBV antigen–bearing cells in the cornea. EBV persists in the host as a chronic low-grade infection, particularly of the B lymphocyte. Because of this chronicity of virus shedding, there is persistent stimulation of the immune system, and the cornea occasionally responds to this. Clinically, there are two recognized forms of EBV stromal keratitis, using the classification of Matoba and coworkers (597,608–610,614). The anterior stromal form has clearly demarcated areas of granular, circular, or ring-shaped opacities ranging in size from 0.1 to 2 mm (Fig. 14-30). These are distributed across the cornea and associated with variable degrees of superficial and deep neovascularization. Stroma between lesions is spared, with consequent preservation of good to normal vision. The overlying epithelium is intact, but may occasionally display a mild punctate stain. EBV anterior stromal disease may be differentiated from adenovirus infection in that the latter produces softer infiltrates sequential to an acute red eye and punctate epithelial keratitis. In addition, adenoviral infiltrates tend to be confined to the subepithelial and anterior stromal area, whereas EBV infiltrates are more pleomorphic and may penetrate to the mid-stroma. They frequently develop in the absence of epithelial keratitis or red eye. The second form of EBV keratitis resembles syphilitic interstitial keratitis or HSV stromal keratitis. It is characterized by a blotchy, peripheral, full-thickness or deep stromal infiltrate that may or may not attract neovascularization. As noted previously, the probable immune nature of the keratitis makes it amenable to topical steroid therapy.

An acute or chronic, smoldering iritis with or without development or secondary cataract and macular edema may be seen in EBV ocular inflammatory disease. This uveal involvement characteristically develops several months after the onset of acute IM. Morishima et al. have reported a case if uveitis associated with chronic active EBV infection in a 7-year-old girl (615). The patient had fever and hepatosplenomegaly followed by left facial nerve palsy. Eye examination showed right iridocyclitis and bilateral optic disc edema. EBV antibody titers were highly elevated. The patient responded dramatically well in all parameters to treatment with topical and systemic steroids, IL-2, and splenectomy.

Diagnosis

The diagnosis of IM has classically been by detection of heterophil antibodies, which are IgM type and indicative of an acute infection. IgM antibodies are found in 85% of patients. In heterophil-negative patients, diagnosis may be made by detection of antibodies to EBV capsid antigen or Epstein-Barr nuclear antigen. Patients with acute disease have elevated titers of viral capsid antigen antibodies, but Epstein-Barr nuclear antigen antibodies do not appear for several weeks or months after the acute infection. Both antibodies persist throughout life (596,597,609,616). A fourth test, the Monospot, is also highly reliable and readily available to clinicians through commercial and

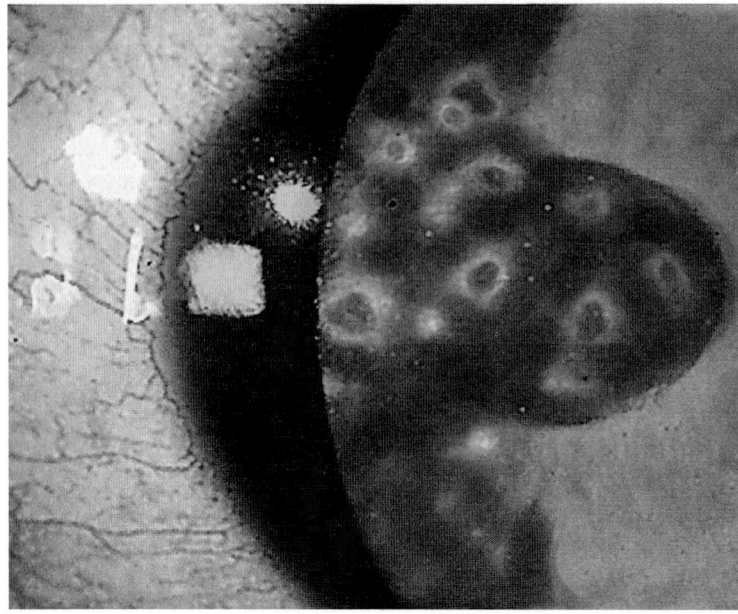

FIGURE 14-30. Epstein-Barr virus (EBV) keratitis with subepithelial infiltrates and circular or ring-shaped opacities. Stroma between lesions is spared, with preservation of good vision. The EBV anterior stromal disease may be differentiated from adenoviral disease because the latter produces softer infiltrates sequential to an acute red eye and punctate epithelial keratitis.

hospital laboratories. See the section on Laboratory Diagnostic Techniques, earlier, for greater detail (2,10).

Treatment

Treatment for ocular EBV disease is a two-pronged approach. Topical steroids for keratitis, iritis, scleritis, and other anterior segment disease are often coupled with systemic treatment of the systemic disease with immunosuppressants and, in some cases, splenectomy.

ADENOVIRAL KERATOCONJUNCTIVITIS

The Adenoviridae family of viruses shares a common group complement-fixing antigens and has 47 known serotypes that are classified into six subgroups (A through F) according to hemagglutination reactions (2,10,617). These very stable, ether-resistant organisms, found worldwide, cause infections of the upper respiratory tract and the eye (23,39,618). These are reviewed in detail in the section on Classification and Structure of viruses, earlier.

Epidemiology

In 1889, the first description of an adenoviral ocular epidemic was given by Fuchs in Austria (619). He described 36 cases as an acute catarrhal conjunctivitis followed by multiple, discrete, round corneal subepithelial lesions lasting for up to 2 years (620,621). Over the next half century, several other epidemics were reported from East Asia to the United Sates to Europe. Perhaps the most important of these occurred in Hawaii and on the West Coast of the United States during World War II (622–624). It was dubbed "shipyard eye" and subsequently *epidemic keratoconjunctivitis* (EKC) because the severity of the epidemic was such that many of the military shipyards had to be closed for weeks, notably damaging the war effort in the Pacific Rim. The identified strain of virus was Ad 8 (625). Other major EKC epidemics were later caused by type 19 (1959) and type 37 (1981) (626,627).

At least 19 different serotypes have been reported as the cause of epidemic or sporadic cases of conjunctivitis or keratoconjunctivitis (628). The serotypes commonly associated with EKC are Ad 8, 19, and 37, with pharyngeal conjunctival fever (PCF) Ad 3 and 7, and with nonspecific follicular conjunctivitis (NFC) Ad 1, 2, 4, 5, and 6 (619). The most severe ocular disease is usually noted in patients with Ad 8 adenoviral infection. An intermediate-type adenovirus has been isolated from both the eyes and cervix in women with active EKC and PCF syndromes, and Ad 19 has also been isolated from the genital tracts of both men and women with adenoconjunctivitis (629,630). The likely existence of an endemic infection in any community is the probable source of intermittent spread to hospitals,

industrial areas, and other large institutions, which may also serve as the sites of epidemics (631). PCF and NFC are also most commonly associated with respiratory and gastrointestinal illness, particularly in children.

Despite documentation of numerous adenoviral infections worldwide, specific data on the exact incidence of adenoviral ocular disease are not available. Nonetheless, although much adenoviral conjunctivitis goes undiagnosed or unseen by a physician, this virus family is very likely the most common cause of external ocular viral infection in the world. EKC occurs mainly in adults between the ages of 20 and 40 years, with men and women equally affected, whereas PCF and is seen more commonly in children. Approximately 10% of all children younger than 5 years of age are seropositive; Ad 1, 2, 3, 5, and 6 are thought to be endemic and a major cause of respiratory infections in children. Race, social status, and nutritional status are not considered risk factors (39,619,628).

Because there is no known animal carrier of this virus, humans are the only reservoir. Serologic studies have shown that there is a low level of natural immunity in the general population of the United States and European countries to offer protection against EKC. This lack of immune protection would appear to account for ocular adenovirus infections occurring primarily in epidemic form (e.g., there is less than 10% immunity for Ad 8). The pattern of adenoviral disease in Asia and Africa is that of an endemic disease, with 25% to 85% of the general population having positive serology to Ad 8. Clinical cases of ocular adenoviral infection tend to be sporadic (100,632). The incidence of acute disease in the general population is generally low (0.03% to 1.10%). In situations where there is close contact, however, the attack rate is high (10% to 32%), such as in camps, homes, and prisons. The primary mode of spread appears to be direct contact with contaminated secretions on such surfaces as towels, bed linens, clothing, and soap, in swimming pools, and by physical intimacy, and probably by salivary and nasal airborne droplet (39,619,621). It would also appear that there are continual changes in the genome of adenoviruses, but that these are usually contained within the population at a subclinical level. On occasion, however, a genotypic change may enhance pathogenicity such that clinical disease in sporadic or epidemic form ensues (39).

The ophthalmologist's office or hospital setting also presents a unique opportunity for the start of an epidemic through use of a tonometer on sequential patients without adequate sterilization after use on one patient infected with adenovirus. Another excellent mode of spread is the contaminated hands of the doctor or staff; a single handshake with an infected patient will spread the organism. Further risk is in the waiting room. This hardy virus may survive for hours in a desiccated but viable form on the furniture and magazines patients share (39,619,633–635). Disease transmission may be prevented by physicians and paramedical personnel by frequent and adequate handwashing and by the cleansing of ophthalmic instruments, especially tonometers, between patient examinations (alcohol swabs or Dakin's solution followed by careful rinse). This is particularly important when examining any patient with a red eye or during times of adenovirus epidemic in the community. Patients should be advised, whether in the home or institutional setting, to avoid close personal contact for at least 2 weeks and to use their own towels and facecloths, avoiding sharing with those who are not infected (631,636). Hard and soft contact lens sterilization studies using Ad 8 and 19 have shown that both viruses survive hydrogen peroxide and heat sterilization systems. This strongly suggests that contact lens wearers who contract acute adenoviral ocular infection should simply dispose of their contacts and buy new ones after the illness has resolved (637).

Clinical Syndromes

Epidemic Keratoconjunctivitis

The more serious of the adenoviral ocular illnesses is EKC (23,39,618,638–640). This entity is usually associated with Ad 8 and 19, but has also been reported with multiple serotypes, including Ad 2 to 4, 7 to 11, 14, 16, and 29 (631,641). Serotypes other than Ad 8 and 19 may produce a similar clinical picture to the latter but do not have the tendency to cause widespread epidemic disease.

The acute ocular disease usually attacks young adults during the fall and winter months and is unilateral in two thirds of patients. Systemic symptoms with EKC are uncommon, but it may occasionally present as a flulike illness with fever, respiratory symptoms, myalgias, diarrhea, nausea, and vomiting. EKC differs from PCF in that the latter is far more commonly associated with systemic illness and bilateral ocular involvement. The incubation period after exposure is approximately 8 days, at which time there may be the onset of acute tearing, foreign body sensation, and photophobia, followed by lid and conjunctival edema and hyperemia, follicular and papillary conjunctival response with or without hemorrhage or membrane formation, and tender preauricular nodes (Figs. 14-31 and 14-32A). Tear film viral titer increases steadily during the first week of illness, although there are reports that viral titers during acute disease may vary with serotype (e.g., Ad 3 and 4 are highest during the first week, whereas Ad 8 is highest during the second week) (39,621,642). Lid edema may become so severe as to resemble a cellulitis. In some patients a serous/hemorrhagic exudate forms on the conjunctiva, forming true membranes (which bleed when removed) or pseudomembranes. These membranes may rub mechanical ulcers in the corneal epithelium. The predominant cell type in these membranes is the neutrophil. Dry eye or symblepharon formation may be a long-term sequela of this conjunctival damage (Fig. 14-32B). Conversely, the lacrimal punctum may scar, resulting in chronic epiphora. In those patients in whom the disease goes on to bilaterality, the second eye becomes involved within 4 to 5 days but usually much less severely than the first eye, probably because of partial immune protection of the host (23,39,618,639,640).

The patients are moderately uncomfortable during the conjunctivitis stage, but more severe pain comes with the

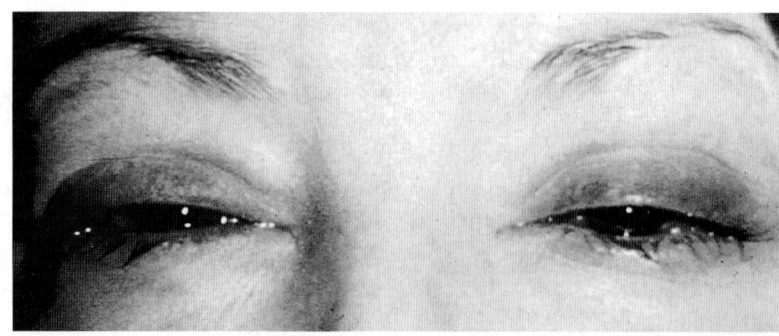
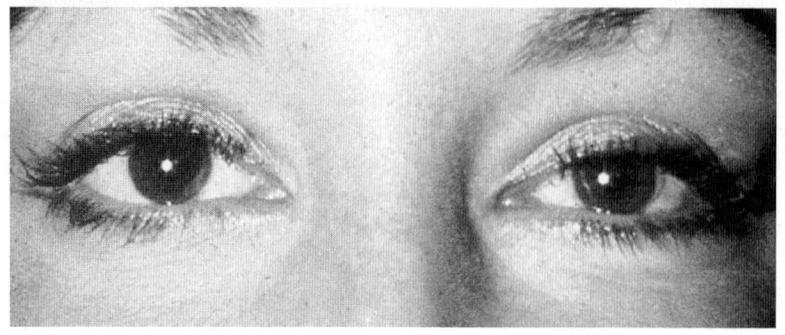

FIGURE 14-31. A: Acute adenoviral blepharoconjunctivitis with lid and conjunctival edema and erythema with watery discharge. **B:** Same patient 6 weeks later with total resolution of disease and no sequelae.

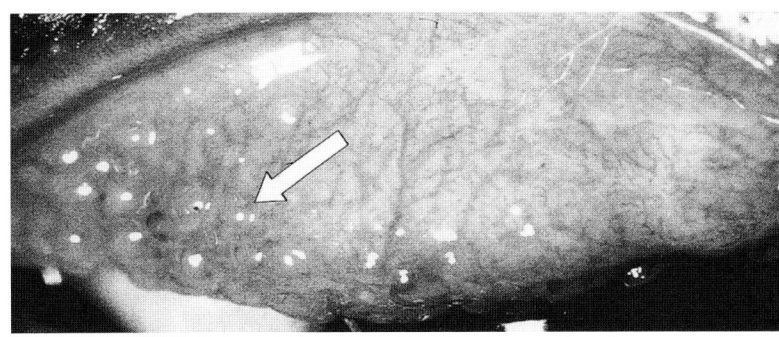

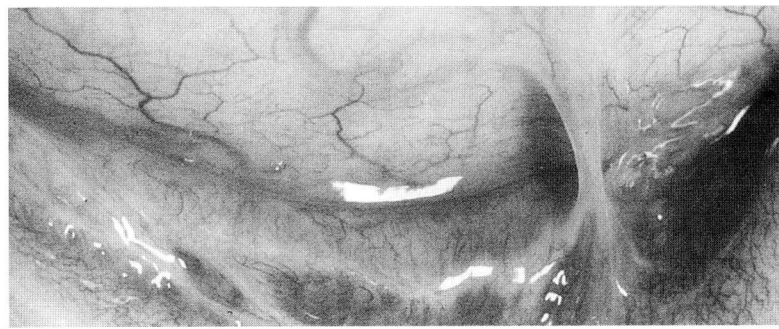

FIGURE 14-32. A: Acute follicular conjunctivitis of adenoviral infection. **B:** Symblepharon formation and dry eye after severe adenoviral blepharoconjunctivitis.

development of keratitis, which occurs in approximately 80% of patients and begins around the eighth day after onset of the acute disease, during which period the corneal epithelial cells have been infected. This adenoviral keratitis is heralded by marked discomfort or pain, photophobia, lacrimation, and blepharospasm. These symptoms persist until the acute epithelial phase subsides, usually within a week or two, by which time the conjunctivitis has also begun to resolve.

The keratitis evolves through four stages (39,184,639, 643–645). Stage 1 is a diffuse, fine, superficial epithelial punctate keratitis caused by live virus. At approximately 1 week this progresses to stage 2, which is a coalescence of these lesions to focal, punctate, slightly raised, whitish epithelial lesions that stain with fluorescein. These lesions last for approximately 10 days. Electron microscopic studies of the acute epithelial stage show viral replication in these surface cells (639). The punctate epithelial lesions are made up of groups of epithelial cells swollen from the viral infection (646). Fusion of the cells leads to syncytia formation and loss of cell contents results in plica formation of many cell surfaces. Two types of inclusion bodies have been detected: intranuclear vacuole inclusions containing homogeneous material, and intranuclear vacuolar inclusions that were round, dense bodies developing in the homogeneous material. The dense bodies contained the replicating and maturing virus particles. With cell rupture, these viral bodies become extracellular and free to spread elsewhere.

In the presence of a lid membrane, a mechanical geographic ulcer mimicking HSK may develop (620,639,640) (Fig. 14-33). Chodosh et al. reported six cases of adenovirus-positive, HSV-negative dendritic, geographic, or dendrogeographic ulcerative keratoconjunctivitis (645). The serotypes isolated were Ad 3, 8, and 19. Another atypical adenoviral course is an association of adenovirus with acute posterior multifocal placoid pigment epitheliopathy. This has been described with Ad 5 infection (647).

The replicating viruses are believed to establish the antigen for the delayed hypersensitivity reaction that produces the subepithelial infiltrates of the later and more chronic stages. By 2 weeks, all replicating virus has been terminated by the host immune response, and within a few days the

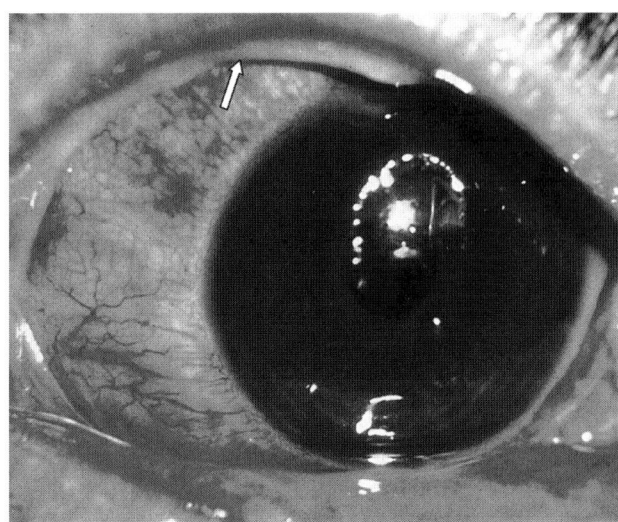

FIGURE 14-33. Acute adenoviral blepharoconjunctivitis with diphtheric-like true membrane formation under the upper lid. Membrane is rubbing a mechanical epithelial defect into the corneal epithelium. A thin soft contact lens was placed to protect and heal the cornea until the membrane resolved.

epithelial lesions become combined epithelial and subepithelial areas as stage 3. Over the next few days the disease enters stage 4, which is characterized by subepithelial, whitish macular lesions or nebulae that no longer stain with fluorescein (Fig. 14-34). The keratitis typically involves the central cornea in clumps or rows of macular opacities, but may reach the periphery and reach maximum density by the third or fourth week of the illness. If the second eye is involved the number of infiltrates is usually less, presumably because of a less severe corneal infection and less antigen deposition. Occasionally, lesions coalesce to form scallop-edged nummular opacities 1 to 2 mm in diameter that in severe cases may mimic HSK. These subepithelial nebulae may last several months, causing glare and diminished vision before gradually self-resolving.

Histopathologic studies of chronic adenoviral keratitis are rare owing to lack of tissue samples in this self-limited disease. Studies on corneal specimens taken from two patients who underwent lamellar keratoplasty for permanent visual loss after documented adenoviral keratitis 2 years earlier revealed lymphocytes, histiocytes, and fibroblasts in the deep layers of the epithelium and in the anterior stroma. These were associated with breaks in Bowman's membrane (39,632,648). The virus could not be recovered by culture, nor was it visualized by electron microscopy or indirect immunofluorescence. These studies lend support to the belief that the infiltrates seen in adenoviral keratitis are the result of host immune and inflammatory response to residual viral antigen resulting from the acute infection. These data have been further supported in the rabbit model of Ad 5 keratitis.

Pharyngoconjunctival Fever

The ocular disease of PCF is similar to EKC except that the keratitis is usually mild and bilateral, and subepithelial infiltrates are less frequent and more transient. PCF is commonly caused by Ad 3, 4, and 7, but it has been associated with Ad 1, 5, 6, and 14. It has been isolated from conjunctiva, nasopharynx, and feces (23,618,649). PCF is an acute and highly infectious illness characterized by fever, pharyngitis, acute follicular conjunctivitis, which may be hemorrhagic, and regional lymphoid hyperplasia with tender, enlarged preauricular adenopathy. It is seen predominantly in the young and institutionalized people, with epidemics occurring within families, schools, and military organizations.

As with EKC, transmission is by contact with infected upper respiratory droplets or fomites, or in swimming pools. Communicability is 100% during the first few days to 0% by 10 to 15 days after the onset of symptoms. After exposure, the incubation period is 5 to 12 days (most commonly 8 days) before onset of illness. The patient experiences a sudden or gradual onset of fever that may range from 100°F to 104°F, lasting up to 10 days (23,39, 618). Other systemic symptoms associated with fever are myalgia, malaise, and, often, gastrointestinal disturbances.

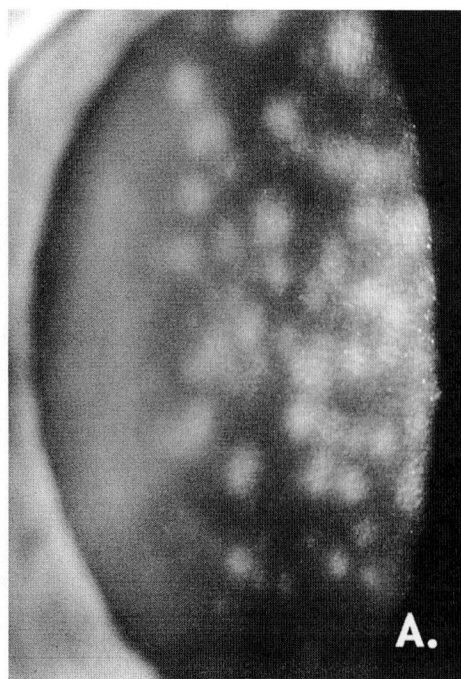 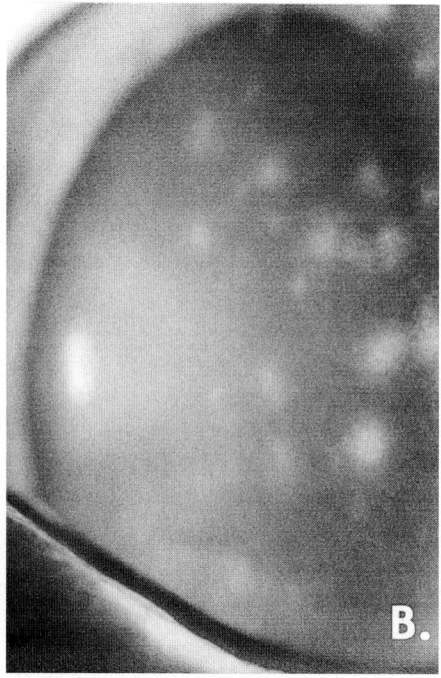

FIGURE 14-34. A: Adenoviral subepithelial infiltrates causing severe photophobia 1 month after acute disease. Polarized clip-ons were given and low-dose steroid drops were tapered over 2 months to relieve symptoms. **B:** Same eye 5 months after acute disease and 2 months after steroids were stopped.

The pharyngitis may be mild or quite painful. There is typically a reddened posterior oropharynx covered with glassy follicles and nontender cervical lymphadenopathy.

Ocular disease initial symptoms range from slight itching and burning to marked irritation and tearing and some photophobia. The lids are swollen within 48 hours. The conjunctivitis presents initially as a diffuse hyperemia that is maximal in the lower fornix but extends throughout the palpebral mucosa and onto the bulbar conjunctiva. Chemosis may give a slightly gelatinous appearance to this tissue, and follicle formation, although not invariable, is always more severe in the lower lid than in the upper. The discharge is serous, and there may be slight crusting on the lids. If there is no pseudomembrane, mucopurulence is scant. Scrapings reveal a predominantly mononuclear exudate without characteristic features. If a membrane is present, the predominant inflammatory cell type is the neutrophil. The lower lid is somewhat tender to palpation and occasionally ecchymotic, giving the patient the appearance of recent orbital trauma. PCF may be unilateral or bilateral, with the second eye having onset 1 to 3 days after the first. In this event, the second eye has less severe disease than the first and resolves more quickly.

A punctate keratitis may appear a few days to a week after the onset of symptoms. This begins as small epithelial dots that stain with fluorescein and progresses to combined epithelial and subepithelial, focal, whitish lesions that may or may not stain, and finally to nonstaining subepithelial infiltrates. It is similar to that of EKC but not as severe or prolonged. Virus may be cultured during the acute epithelial stage, but the stromal infiltrates are thought to be immune complexes against residual viral antigen (620,639,640,646). These infiltrates are usually scattered primarily in the central corneal area. The entire illness is usually acute and transient, resolving over a few days to 3 weeks. The subepithelial infiltrates are usually mild, but fade over a few months. Their histopathologic features and immune origin are believed to be similar to those described for EKC (39,632,648). If in the visual axis, they may cause some visual disturbance.

Nonspecific Follicular Conjunctivitis

NFC may be caused by any of the ocular adenoviruses, but is usually sufficiently mild not to be seen in the physician's office. It may occur in children or adults and may be caused by any of the serotypes that also cause EKC or PCF. Because keratitis does not develop and the conjunctivitis remains mild, these patients are usually treated by pediatricians or family physicians. The clinical disease resolves without residua over a 7- to 10-day period. Its importance stems from its serving as the reservoir of the adenovirus serotypes that may ultimately spark a more severe, widespread epidemic in the community (23,39,618).

Chronic Adenoviral Keratoconjunctivitis

Chronic adenoviral keratoconjunctivitis is an uncommon and often unrecognized cause of disturbing anterior segment inflammatory and scarring disease. It is caused by a variety of adenovirus serotypes (643,650,651). The syndrome is characterized by a prolonged course of intermittent exacerbation of tearing, redness, and photophobia. The clinical history commonly reveals an episode of acute conjunctivitis several months in the past. In the chronic state, the cornea may or may not have subepithelial opacities or active focal superficial keratitis. Ad 2, 3, 4, and 19 have been isolated as late as 12 months after the onset of chronic keratoconjunctivitis. These cases had either active epithelial keratitis, recurrent conjunctivitis with subepithelial opacities, or chronic recurrent papillary conjunctivitis. The total duration of disease may well exceed 1 1/2 years (643,650,651). Because the conjunctival reaction is primarily papillary, the clinician may be confused by the absence of follicles in what is, in fact, a viral disease. The diagnosis in suspected cases may be made by virus isolation from cornea or conjunctiva, by PCR assay for adenoviral DNA, or by testing for serotype-specific neutralizing and hemagglutination-inhibiting antibody in the absence of other bacterial, viral, or toxic systemic illness that might mimic chronic adenoviral keratoconjunctivitis. Early topical steroid use appears to be unrelated to the development of this chronic disease.

Diagnosis

Diagnostic techniques for adenovirus are discussed in detail earlier in this chapter (see sections on Laboratory Diagnostic Techniques, and Characteristics of the Major Ocular Viral Pathogen Families). These include cytologic scrapings that reveal a mixed lymphocytic and neutrophil infiltrate and degenerated epithelial cells. Giemsa staining for inclusions may reveal early eosinophilic intranuclear bodies and late basophilic intranuclear bodies (619). These are both homogeneous and small, dense bodies containing virus (646). Viral cultures are positive 82% of the time if taken during the first week of the disease, but by the end of the third week less than 25% of the patients continue to spill virus (652). Alternative diagnostic techniques include paired blood specimens, with the first drawn within 7 days of the onset of symptoms and the second 2 to 3 weeks later. A fourfold or greater increase in humoral antibody to adenovirus is indicative of recent infection. Other rapid laboratory diagnostic tests include immunofluorescence, EIA (Andenoclone, Cambridge Bioscience, Worcester, MA), ELISA, and electron microscopy (10,618,621).

Treatment

Specific therapy of ocular adenoviral infection is still under development. Antibiotics and commercially available antivirals are ineffective, although the virus is sensitive *in vitro* to trifluridine (80,638,653,654). Cidofovir is discussed in detail in the section on Antiviral Drugs, earlier. This antimetabolite, which is FDA approved for therapy of CMV infection, also holds considerable hope as the first effective antiviral agent in ocular adenoviral disease (269,279). In the adenoviral rabbit model, topical 0.5% cidofovir twice daily for 7 days showed significant antiviral activity against Ad 1, 5, and 6 (655). Antiviral prophylaxis studies against Ad 5 infection using 0.5% and 1% twice-daily dosing conferred effective prophylaxis against viral infection, with the 1% formulation eliminating all replication after day zero (280). Although the results of clinical studies have yet to be reported, because of its FDA approval for CMV retinitis, cidofovir has the potential for off-label use, or for FDA approval as a topical agent for adenoviral infection if future clinical data are positive. Because the subepithelial corneal opacities seen in postacute disease are immunologic in origin and the conjunctival disease is self-limited, cidofovir therapy does not appear to have a role in adenoviral ocular sequelae. A possible exception to this is proven chronic adenoviral conjunctivitis (643,650,651).

Topical steroid therapy is controversial in acute adenoviral ocular disease. Steroids have been used to provide notable symptomatic and inflammatory relief in those patients with severe conjunctival reactions such as marked inflammation, edema, pseudomembrane, or early symblepharon formation. Against steroid use during the acute infectious disease, however, are two Ad 5 rabbit studies that have shown that use of 1% prednisolone four times daily for as little as 3 days significantly enhanced the replication of virus in the treated eyes compared with controls (656). Further, use of limited-potency steroids such as 0.12% prednisolone, 0.1% fluorometholone, or 1% rimexolone four times daily for 3 days also significantly enhanced Ad 5 replication. The authors concluded that although these drugs may offer symptomatic relief, they may also delay viral clearance and increase the spread of epidemics (657). In an Ad 5 rabbit study on use of topical NSAIDs (ketorolac and diclofenac) concurrent with cidofovir, it was found that neither drug diminished that antiviral agent's efficacy, nor did it prevent formation of corneal subepithelial infiltrates (658). Nonetheless, the topical NSAIDs may have a role in enhancing patient comfort during the acute inflammatory illness, and are safer than steroids. Further comfort is given by use of polarized clip-on lenses to cut glare.

Use of topical steroids for the subepithelial infiltrates that appear at 10 to 14 days after disease onset is also controversial. These drugs unquestionably provide relief for many patients with discomfort, photophobia, glare, and visual loss due to the infiltrates. After steroid-induced resolution of the corneal nebulae, the drugs may be slowly tapered over several weeks, usually without difficulty. There are some patients, however, for whom steroids have no beneficial therapeutic effect on the ultimate clinical outcome. Laibson and associates have shown that the subepithelial infiltrates often recur when steroids are discontinued and that only time will ultimately resolve their presence (620). The return of visual disability with steroid discontinuation often necessitates resuming the steroids, and a self-limiting disease may be prolonged for months to years as steroid tapering is prolonged. This adds the further risk of long-term steroid use to an already disabling illness.

Without steroid treatment, the corneal infiltrates ill almost invariably recede spontaneously over a period of weeks, months, or rarely, years, and vision improves. As noted in the discussion of the histopathology of EKC, infiltrates appear to be the result of immune inflammatory cells attracted to viral antigen in the anterior cornea (632,648). They may usually be suppressed by topical steroids, but until the inciting antigen washes out over a several-month period, the infiltrates will simply reappear when immune suppression is released on discontinuation of steroids. The author has, however, seen one patient who had vision-debilitating (20/80 OU) subepithelial infiltrates 3 years after the acute disease; the infiltrates were unresponsive to steroids and NSAIDs. In such cases, lamellar keratoplasty or possibly excimer laser treatment may provide visual relief (39,648).

The therapy of adenoviral keratoconjunctivitis may be summarized as follows and is in general palliative:

1. Antivirals are ineffective, with the possible exception of cidofovir.
2. Consider topical NSAIDs (ketorolac, diclofenac) four times daily and oral NSAIDs (ibuprofen 400 mg PO two to three times daily) for relief of inflammatory ocular disease. There is no effect on viral replication or appearance of corneal infiltrates.
3. Administer cycloplegia as needed for iritis (rare).
4. Apply topical antibiotic ointment to lubricate and protect the cornea in presence of membranes.
5. Use ice packs, antipyretics, and dark glasses as needed.
6. Practice prophylaxis against disease spread by careful washing of hands and instruments by medical personnel working on the eye.
7. Infected medical personnel should terminate their duties immediately for 2 weeks after onset of disease when virus transmission becomes unlikely.
8. Infected patients should avoid oral or close contact with family members or associates, not attend work or school for the first 2 weeks of illness, and use separate linens. Wash hands frequently with antiseptic soap.
9. For chronic protracted cases use topical NSAID (e.g., diclofenac or ketorolac) four times daily. Consider conjunctival biopsy for testing for persistent adenoviral replication.
10. Use polarized clip-ons to cut photophobic glare.
11. For truly debilitating visual disturbance or loss, use mild topical steroids to relieve symptoms and infiltrates temporarily. These should be reserved for

severe cases only (i.e., photophobia, membrane or pseudomembrane formation, or visual loss). Inform the patient before starting therapy that steroids will ultimately have to be tapered and symptoms may recur.

ACQUIRED IMMUNODEFICIENCY SYNDROME

The retrovirus HIV-1 is the etiologic agent of AIDS. Because the virus replicates in CD4$^+$ T lymphocytes, the agent is transmitted by blood, blood products, and other body fluids such as semen, breast milk, saliva, and tears. Recent estimates from the World Health Organization and Joint United Nations Program on HIV/AIDS indicate that in the past 20 years more than 50 million people have been infected worldwide, and 22 million have died of this disease (302,659). It is estimated that 15,000 to 20,000 new infections occur daily. The Centers for Disease Control and Prevention (CDC) estimates that 300,000 individuals in the Unites States are unaware that they are currently infected with HIV and that over 23,000 health care workers have AIDS (660–662).

The transmission of the viral infection is primarily through the cellular immune system aided by striking virus-induced immunologic abnormalities in the infected T-helper lymphocyte population. With disease progression there is reversal of the T-lymphocyte helper/suppressor (T4/T8) ratio from a normal of 1.1 to 3.5 to levels far below 1. Reduced lymphokine production, inhibition of mitogen and antigen response, depressed clonal expansion, and decreased ability to assist B lymphocytes in immunoglobulin production are other debilitating immune changes. The ocular disease seen in AIDS is in part related to the finding that B lymphocytes in patients with AIDS are polyclonally activated and spontaneously secrete antibody. This results in elevated total serum immunoglobulin levels, primarily IgG and IgA, resulting in circulating immune complexes that ultimately infarct small blood vessels. Unfortunately, these B lymphocytes do not, however, respond to the normal signals for proliferation and differentiation and do not usually respond to common immunizations or new antigens. Monocytes lose their ability to kill certain target cells, secrete IL-1, and migrate chemotactically. There is also impairment of natural killer cell immune surveillance and virus-specific T-cytotoxic lymphocyte function. HIV infection results in progressive decline in the immune system, with the result that the eye, among other organs of the body, suffers an increased incidence of multiple opportunistic infections and malignant diseases, conditions rarely seen before the AIDS epidemic and normally held in check by an intact immune surveillance system (2,23,187, 302,663,664)

HIV-related ocular disease is not a good sign prognostically because those patients with anterior or posterior segment disease are significantly more immunosuppressed than HIV-positive patients without eye findings (187, 665–668). The most common findings are in the posterior segment and include Roth's spots, microaneurysms, cotton-wool spots (immune complex infarctions), retinal hemorrhages, ischemic maculopathy, retinal periphlebitis, and papilledema. Opportunistic infectious retinitis can be caused by HSV, VZV, CMV, *Cryptococcus*, *Toxoplasma*, *Candida*, *Mycobacterium avium-intracellulare*, microsporidia, and potentially any other known infectious agent (Fig. 14-35).

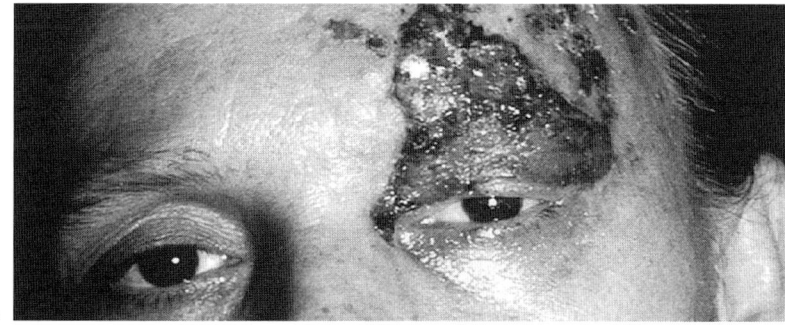

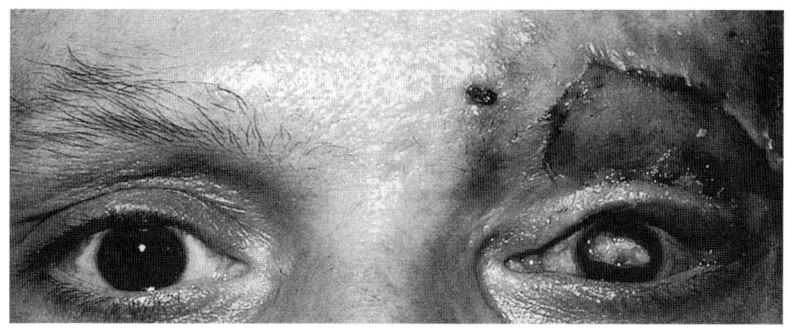

FIGURE 14-35. A: Thirty-four-year-old human immunodeficiency virus–positive woman with slowly resolving herpes zoster ophthalmicus. **B:** Same patient 1 year later with persistent nonhealing of skin and melting trophic ulcer, recovering from *Staphylococcus aureus* superinfection.

Anterior segment findings include conjunctival microvascular disease, dry eye, allergic or infectious conjunctivitis, microsporidial keratoconjunctivitis, HZO, HSK, molluscum contagiosum, fungal keratitis, bacterial keratoconjunctivitis, and Kaposi's sarcoma (23,663,669). AIDS conjunctivitis is infectious (HIV-positive) but nonspecific, with diffuse hyperemia, irritation, and tearing. This is transient and requires no specific therapy other than ocular decongestants. Dry eye syndrome develops in approximately 20% of patients with AIDS. This is thought to be the result of HIV-mediated inflammatory destruction of accessory and primary lacrimal glands, much as occurs in Sjögren's syndrome (670).

The cornea may be affected by an HIV-induced diffuse superficial keratitis with iritis, herpes-like dendritic ulcerations (HSV culture negative), or a stromal interstitial keratitis. Opportunistic infections include Kaposi's sarcoma (HHV8), HSV, VZV, and a variety of bacterial and fungal organisms. The most common bacteria are *Staphylococcus aureus*, *Staphylococcus epidermidis*, and *Pseudomonas aeruginosa*. Microsporidia are common intracellular protozoans that can cause a punctate epithelial keratopathy that is treated with oral antifungals (itraconazole, albendazole) (184,302,663,668). Bilateral ulcerative keratitis similar to herpetic geographic ulceration has been reported in patients with AIDS. Immunofluorescence studies on these corneas taken at autopsy, however, failed to reveal any HSV antigen, thus raising the question whether this was truly HSV disease or secondary to invasion by HIV. HZO is a well-known presenting symptom in previously undiagnosed HIV-positive patients (486,493,495). The course and management of HSV infection and HZO are discussed in earlier sections of this chapter.

Peripheral ulcerative keratitis, similar to that seen in other immunologic disorders in which circulating immune complexes are found, has now been reported in a patient with AIDS-related complex. The disorder was thought to be due to high levels of circulating immune complexes that created anterior segment microinfarctions affecting the integrity of the peripheral cornea. This mechanism is similar to that believed to be operative in AIDS/CMV retinitis (665,671). AIDS peripheral ulcerative keratitis may be treated by sealing with cyanoacrylate tissue adhesive and covering with Plane T therapeutic soft contact lenses, with prophylactic antibiotic drops and cycloplegia. With neovascularization of the stroma over several weeks, the ulcer generally heals, dislodges the glue, and leaves a scarred but intact cornea (see the section on treatment of HSV trophic ulcers, earlier).

Kaposi's sarcoma occurs in approximately 20% of patients with AIDS (672). It is believed to be caused by HHV8 because this virus is found in 90% of tissue samples taken from AIDS-associated Kaposi's sarcoma. The disease may occur anywhere on the body, including the face (Fig. 14-36A). The lids and conjunctiva may appear to have lymphomatous-like tumors (36,673). Conjunctival involvement occurs in 10% of patients with AIDS and is more frequently found in the inferior cul de sac. It may be missed without retraction of the lower lid on examination. Sarcoma of the lid presents as a deep red subconjunctival

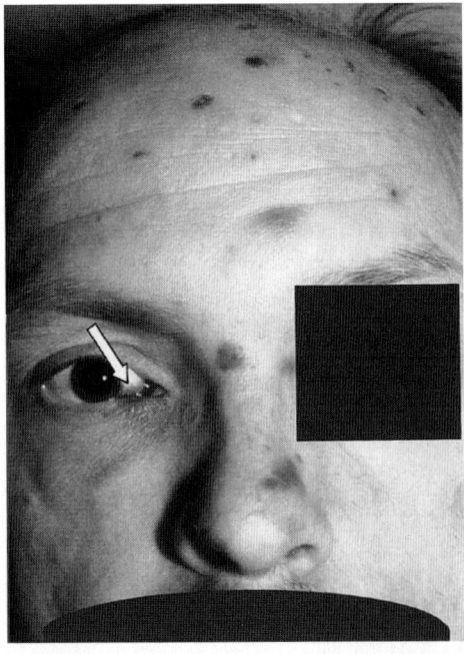
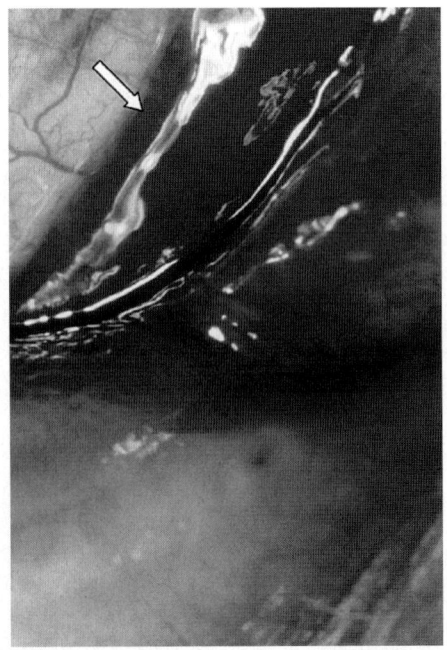

FIGURE 14-36. A: Thirty-year-old human immunodeficiency virus–positive man with multiple Kaposi's sarcoma lesions scattered over his face and scalp. Medial canthal sarcoma (*arrow*) can be seen in the right eye. **B:** Close-up of medial canthal sarcoma in **A** showing lesion that resembles conjunctival lymphoma.

mass that may appear to be a hemorrhage (Fig. 14-36B). The masses may be focal nodules or diffuse infiltrative lesions.

The causal relationship between HHV8 and Kaposi's sarcoma has not been proven conclusively. Dugel and colleagues reported finding multiple immature retrovirus particles in conjunctival nodules in eyes with conjunctival Kaposi's sarcoma, but no particles in the sarcoma tissue itself (674). Nakamura and coworkers showed that HIV-infected cells release a factor that greatly enhances the growth of Kaposi's sarcoma cells in culture (675). Elucidating the possible role of retroviruses in the growth of Kaposi's sarcoma may give key information about the pathogenesis of this increasingly more common ocular malignancy. The most effective therapy for the sarcoma is treatment of the underlying HIV disease itself. Local cryotherapy, radiation therapy, and local excision have only transient efficacy.

Iritis occurs in approximately 50% of patients, particularly with HIV, HSV, or VZV keratitis. It is usually responsive to topical steroids, dilation, and appropriate antiviral (antiherpes, anti-HIV) therapy. VZV disease has a far greater increase in incidence than HSV disease in HIV-positive patients compared with the HIV-negative population (668,676).

The AIDS epidemic has posed new problems in ocular surgery. HIV-1 has been isolated from multiple ocular tissues, including the tears, conjunctiva, cornea, iris, vitreous, and retina (666,677–680). This poses an epidemiologic concern not only in that the eye may be an as-yet-unproven source of spread of disease but in the implications for corneal transplantation. Eye banks now screen all potential donors for HIV. The ELISA test is very good for widespread epidemiologic screening, and Western blot analysis is a more specific test capable of detecting HIV at earlier stages of infection. Unfortunately, its results may be falsely negative even when results of an ELISA test are repeatedly positive (681).

With 25,000 corneal transplants being performed annually in the United States, the risk of transmitting HIV through donor corneal tissue despite negative serologic testing is a valid concern to physicians and patients alike. In a mathematical model, Goode and associates calculated that the risk of a patient undergoing corneal transplantation receiving a transplant from an HIV-infected donor with negative serology is only 0.03% (681). This increases by a factor of 10, however, when tissue from donors at high risk for AIDS is used (e.g., homosexuals, drug addicts, transfusion patients). Nonetheless, it was felt that the current screening procedures are probably adequate to prevent transmission of HIV by corneal transplantation, but increased vigilance for high-risk donor populations is appropriate. Thus far there has been no report of HIV transmission through penetrating keratoplasty.

Diagnosis

Diagnostic techniques are discussed in detail in the section on Characteristics of Major Ocular Viral Pathogen Families,

earlier. Serologic tests such as the enzyme immunoassay for IgG antibodies to HIV using viral lysate or recombinant proteins and the antigen are of great value as rapid and sensitive screening tests. ELISA is also very sensitive for HIV-1, HIV-2, and human T-cell lymphotrophic virus and is used for blood donation screening. Because of its lower specificity, however, the results are always confirmed by Western blot, immunoprecipitation, or indirect immunofluorescence (2,10).

Therapy

It is beyond the purview of this chapter to cover in detail the newest and ever-changing therapeutic modalities for HIV infection. With the advent of highly active antiretroviral therapy (HAART), a combination of three or more anti-HIV agents, the natural history of the disease has changed and the long-term survival rate greatly increased (682). Patients live longer with higher $CD4^+$ cell counts and little to no detectable virus load, thus vastly improving the quality of life for these patients. Some have been able partially to reconstitute their $CD4^+$ T-lymphocyte immune system to help further prevent opportunistic infection or malignancy.

POXVIRUSES

The poxviruses include the viruses responsible for variola (smallpox), its bovine derivative, vaccinia, orf, and molluscum contagiosum. These large DNA viruses share a common group antigen, and have a primary affinity for the skin and mucous membranes (683,684).

Molluscum Contagiosum

This cutaneous disease is caused by a virus of Molluscipoxvirus genus and usually results in a benign, self-limited papular eruption of multiple, small, pink, umbilicated tumors on the skin and mucous membranes (Fig. 14-37). It is usually limited exclusively to humans, although there are a few isolated reports of molluscum contagiosum occurring in birds, chimpanzees, dogs, and horses. Transmission requires direct contact with infected hosts or contaminated fomites. The virus is found worldwide but has a higher incidence in children, sexually active adults, and those who are immunodeficient, whether by AIDS or atopy (618,685,686).

Molluscum contagiosum lesions of the lid margin may cause an irritating chronic follicular conjunctivitis with punctate keratitis, superior corneal vascular pannus, and cicatricial punctal occlusion. Lesions may also occur several millimeters away from the lid margins yet still cause a follicular conjunctivitis that is culture positive for virus (2,618,619,687). Molluscum contagiosum lesions confined to cornea or

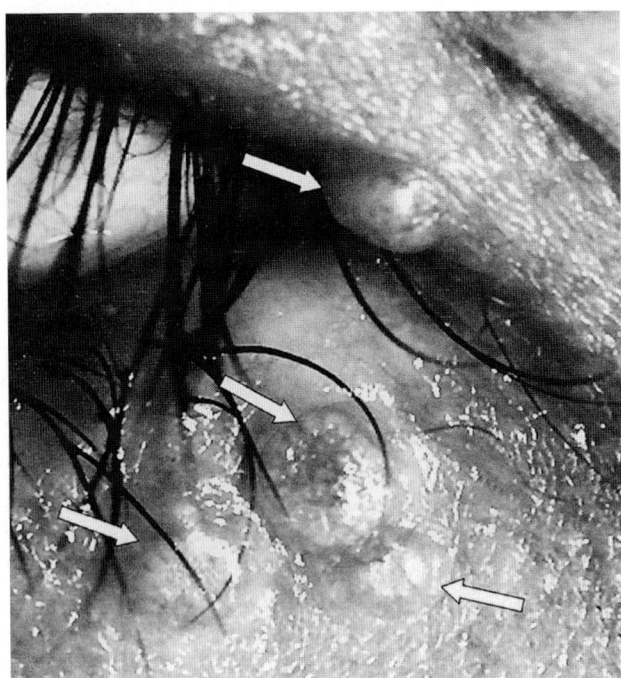

FIGURE 14-37. Multiple molluscum contagiosum lesions at lateral canthus region of human immunodeficiency virus (HIV)–positive patient (*arrows*). Lesions were associated with chronic conjunctivitis due to seeding of virus into the area. Repeated excisions of lesions were followed by repeated recurrences of disease because of HIV-positive status.

conjunctiva alone are rare but not unheard of. They are usually seen in patients with immune dysfunction (686).

Immunohistochemical analysis of biopsy specimens show T lymphocytes and a few macrophages consistently present in the adjacent dermis and epidermis but not infiltrating the molluscum contagiosum lesions themselves (688). The lesions themselves consist of acanthotic epidermis with central craters filled with epithelial cells containing intracytoplasmic inclusion bodies. There is cross-reactivity of T-cell antibody to the molluscum contagiosum bodies. Giemsa stain reveals the viral particle inclusions 12 to 24 hours after infection. Unlike many other poxviruses, molluscum contagiosum virus cannot be grown productively in tissue culture and does not produce long-term cytopathic effects that can be passaged to fresh tissue cultures (2,10).

Treatment in the immunologically normal host may range from simple observation as the lesions resolve spontaneously to simple excision, laser therapy, or possibly antiviral therapy. The keratoconjunctivitis resolves with removal of the molluscum contagiosum lesions. Successful treatment of molluscum contagiosum with pulsed dye laser over a 28-month period in 43 patients has been reported (689). All of the 1250 lesions treated resolved and 35% of patients had no new lesions after two treatments. There were no complications noted.

In HIV-positive patients, the lesions may be particularly stubborn and recur within 6 to 8 weeks of repeated excisional treatments. As with all HIV disease, the most effective treatment is treating the systemic disease itself with HAART (682). Chemotherapy is just coming of age in terms of treating poxvirus infections. Cidofovir, the broad-spectrum antiviral agent effective against herpesviruses, is also effective against poxviruses such as vaccinia, cowpox, and monkey pox in animal models, against variola *in vitro*, and, in human studies, against molluscum contagiosum. It is currently formulated in gel or cream form or as intranasal aerosol or peroral as a lipid prodrug as indicated against these latter infections (690,691).

Variola (Smallpox)

Variola, until recently considered an extinct threat to humankind, has again come into prominence as a very real threat in the form of a bioterrorist weapon (692,693). As a result, we are now dealing with reeducating ourselves about the potential complications of both variola and the vaccine against it, vaccinia. After an 8- to 12-day incubation period, systemic smallpox has a 2- to 3-day prodrome of flulike illness followed by abrupt onset of severe illness with high fever, myalgia, headache, prostration, and often severe abdominal pain. A maculopapular rash appears in 1 to 2 days in the oropharynx, face, and arms and spreads centrally, rapidly becoming vesicular and then pustular, sometimes associated with hemorrhage. The lesions are countless, firm, and elevated and involve the palms and soles. Most deaths occur during the second week of illness (693,694). Over the next 3 weeks, the lesions scab and fall off, leaving deep, depigmented, pitted scars.

Ten to 20% of patients have severe ocular complications (684,695). Approximately 5 days after the onset of clinical disease, an exanthematous, watery conjunctivitis may develop and frequently clear without complication. In a few patients, however, pustules appeared on the bulbar conjunctiva. These are painful with great inflammatory reaction and purulent discharge, often extending to the cornea, causing inflammation, scarring, and even perforation with loss of the eye. Bacterial infection is not infrequent in these corneal ulcers and contributes to the ocular damage if untreated.

Diagnosis

This is discussed in detail in the section on Characteristics of the Major Ocular Viral Pathogens, earlier. Clinical impression with history of exposure, viral culture, and immunohistochemistry are the primary techniques.

Treatment

Specific treatment is currently not established. Suspect cases should be placed in a negative-pressure room, if available, and vaccinated, especially if the illness is in early stage. A promising but unproven treatment, however, is systemic and topical cidofovir. As noted previously in the discussion of molluscum contagiosum, this broad-spectrum antiherpes agent is also effective against poxviruses such as vaccinia, cowpox, and monkey pox in animal models, and against variola *in vitro* (690,691). Isothiazole thiosemicarbazone given soon after documented exposure may prevent death but not disfigurement (696). Penicillinase-resistant antimicrobial agents should be used if the skin lesions are secondarily infected or if infection is near or involves the eyes. Daily rinsing of the eyes is important in severe cases. Adequate hydration and nutrition are important because much fluid is lost through fever and weeping lesions. There are no data showing that prophylaxis or treatment of active disease with vaccinia immune globulin (VIG) has any effect.

Ocular Vaccinia

Epidemiology and Historical and Present Status

Bioterrorism has put vaccinia and its potential ocular and other complications back on the list of infections "to know about" (694,697). Because the disease against which it was used, variola, was considered extinct and the risk of vaccination outweighed the benefits, especially in children and the immunocompromised, compulsory childhood smallpox vaccination in the United States was stopped in 1972, vaccination of health care workers in 1976, and vaccination of the military in the early 1990s (698). However, because of growing concerns about the potential use of smallpox as an agent of bioterrorism, the U.S. Department of Health and Human Services has recommended that smallpox vaccination be reinstated for U.S. military personnel and bioterrorism first-responder units, followed by primary and ancillary health care personnel (697–700).

Mack has reported that "current policy is to promote vaccination, initially 500,000 hospital-selected health care providers and subsequently to as many as 10 million others" (701). Because of the large number of immunosuppressed people in the population [organ transplants, cancer, use of immunosuppressive drugs, HIV infection (known and unknown), and the expansion of intensive care units and neonatal nurseries], it is anticipated that the complication rate will be several times that of the previous vaccination era (702). With a death rate of 3 per million, vaccinating 250,000 people will result in 1 to 2 deaths. The number of deaths in the event of a smallpox terrorist attack in 250,000 unvaccinated people, however, would be 75,000 people. The risk of such an attack must be weighed against the risk of vaccinia complications based on the evolving geopolitical situation. The nonfatal complication rate is undetermined but expected to be notably higher than previously.

With an overall complication rate of 0.004% and one death per million vaccinations, vaccination with vaccinia is considered a relatively safe and effective preventative against smallpox. The complication rate is higher, however, than with other vaccines, and the complications can be quite severe (693,701,703,704). Most complications occur in the person who has been vaccinated. Because it is a live virus vaccine, however, the virus can be inadvertently transmitted from the vaccinee to other sites in his or her own body or to other people in contact. The inoculation site can shed infectious virus for up to 21 days, until the dried scab detaches. The more serious complications that can follow infection with the vaccinia virus include the following:

1. Accidental infection from unintentional inoculation of vaccinia virus on the face or elsewhere in immunocompetent individuals.
2. Eczema vaccinatum, which usually occurs in individuals with eczema (or other atopic dermatitis) or a history of eczema, producing fever, lymphadenopathy, and widespread, often confluent lesions, especially on the face and limbs (Fig. 14-38).
3. Vaccinia necrosum (progressive vaccinia), which occurs primarily in immunocompromised individuals with T-cell deficiency. The vaccination site does not heal and infection spreads locally and may result in death.
4. Postvaccinial encephalitis, which is seen in otherwise healthy primary vaccinees younger than 1 year of age up to adults receiving primary vaccination. It has not been reported in secondary acquired vaccinia. Up to 25% of primary vaccinees with encephalitis die, and 25% have permanent neurologic sequelae (703–705).

As a rule, then, vaccination with the current live virus vaccine (Dryvax) should not be given to patients who have immunologic disorders, severe eczema, or pregnancy, nor should such individuals be exposed to recent vaccinees (692,693,704).

Clinical Disease

The most common route of spread to the eye is by autoinoculation from the patient's vaccination site through contaminated fingers to his or her own face or to that of another person in close contact (692,704,706) (Fig. 14-39). The incidence is low, at 1 case of ocular vaccinia per 40,000 vaccinations. Other proposed routes of transmission include health care workers carrying virus on their clothes, or fomites from the nasopharynx of vaccinees. Secondary cases manifest between 8 and 18 days after exposure. A primary accidental self-inoculation may appear between 5 and 11 days. Dissemination of vaccinial disease is expected to be minimized by techniques not used in the previous vaccination era, including use of an occlusive dressing at the vaccination site, as well as infection control

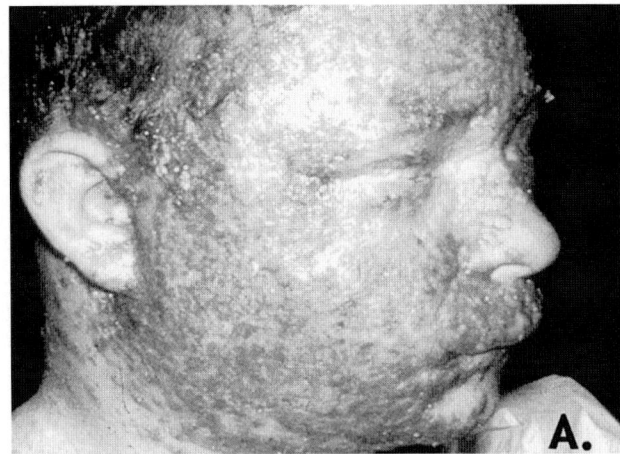
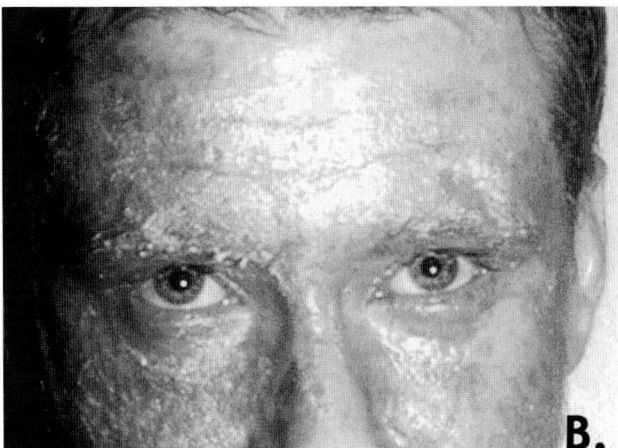

FIGURE 14-38. A: Acute eczema vaccinatum in 20-year-old military recruit with history of eczema. There is diffuse dissemination of confluent lesions about the face associated with significant edema, and multiple, nonconfluent lesions over the trunk. **B:** Same patient 1 month later with almost complete resolution of disease and very minimal scarring.

procedures, including hand and equipment hygiene and sterilization procedures (702).

A study by Ruben and Lane indicated that not only were the ocular complications of vaccination infrequent, they were not notably vision-threatening (706). The incidence of keratitis was 1.2 cases per million primary vaccinations. Of 328 cases of ocular vaccinia, 70% were in primary vaccinees, 58% of whom were younger than 4 years of age. The time of onset ranged from 1 to 15 days postexposure, with most occurring between 3 and 11 days. Only 22 cases involved the cornea and only 2% of noncorneal cases had residual ocular damage, none severe. Eighteen percent (4 of 22) of the patients with keratitis had

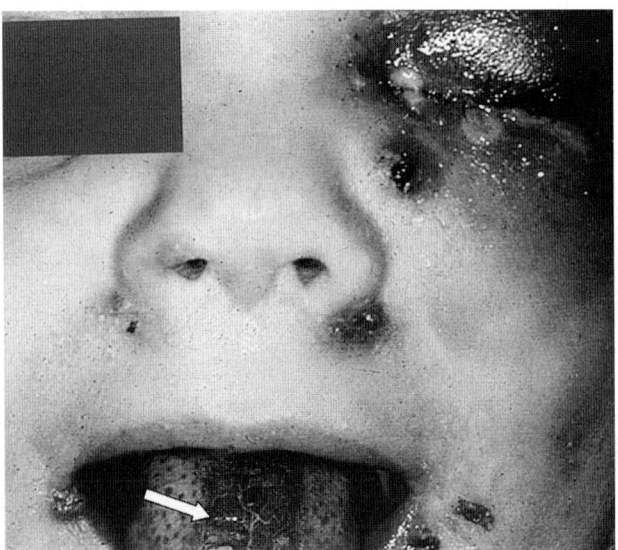

FIGURE 14-39. Three-year-old thumb-sucking boy with dissemination of his vaccination to lids and conjunctiva, face, and tongue (*arrow*). Ocular treatment with vidarabine ointment resulted in resolution of eye disease within 6 days. Other lesions resolved over 2 weeks.

residual minor scarring. Treatment involved 336 of 348 patients receiving VIG and 28 patients receiving idoxuridine. It was not stated whether VIG was also given to these patients or whether they had corneal involvement. The authors concluded that ocular involvement was more severe in primary vaccinees than in revaccinated patients, that the residua in noncorneal cases were strikingly low, and that reexamination of the corneal cases 5 years later revealed either no residua, minor corneal scarring, and one case with a few ghost vessels at the limbus and one with minor subepithelial opacity that responded to steroid drops three times weekly.

Lid and conjunctival involvement is the most common form of ocular vaccinia and is similar to that seen on the arm at the site of the intentional vaccination: formation of vesicles that progress to indurated pustules that umbilicate to open sores, scab, and may occasionally scar, leaving depigmented marks in the skin (Fig. 14-40). Vaccinia lesions may be differentiated from those of herpes simplex or zoster in that the latter two have a clear vesicle stage that then scabs without going through a pustular stage and, in the case of zoster, respect a dermatomal distribution. Vaccinia lesions can produce severe lid swelling and periorbital erythema in a true orbital cellulitis (Fig. 14-41). There is often preauricular or submandibular lymphadenopathy. Eyelid lesions can progress to scarring and madarosis, and be accompanied by symblepharon formation (79,692, 706–708). The differential diagnosis of vaccinia lesions of the eyelid or ocular adnexa includes molluscum contagiosum, keratoacanthoma, bacterial blepharitis, and HSV or VZV infection (692).

Vaccinial keratitis after autoinoculation is uncommon, as noted in Ruben and Lane's reports of 1.2 cases per million primary vaccinations (704,706). Other studies have reported a somewhat higher incidence of postvaccinial keratitis in 6% to 37% of vaccinia cases with ocular involvement (707,709).

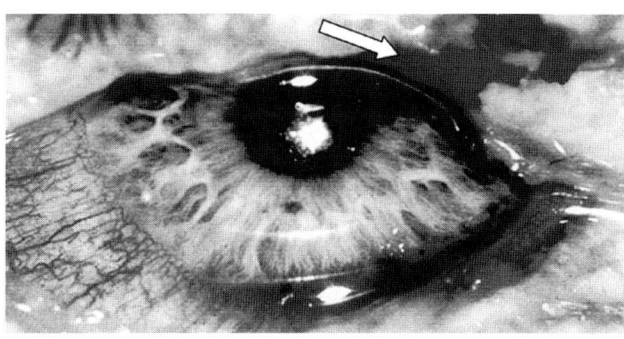
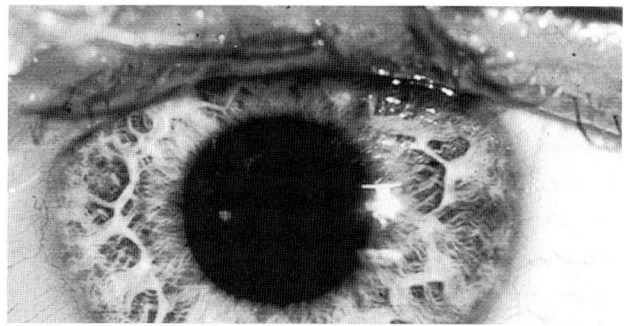

A   B

FIGURE 14-40. A: Acute vaccinial blepharoconjunctivitis with active bleeding (*arrow*) from the lid lesions. **B:** Same eye 14 days later with almost complete healing and no significant sequelae. Treatment was idoxuridine drops.

The lower incidence of keratitis in revaccinees would appear to be a reflection of the partially protected immune status of the previously vaccinated patient.

The vaccinial keratitis itself ranges from mild superficial punctate keratitis to necrotic interstitial or disciform stromal keratitis with keratic precipitates. There may be melting with or without bacterial superinfection and ultimately perforation (Fig. 14-42A). Epithelial punctate lesions stain with rose bengal early in the course of the disease, and may later coalesce to form a geographic pattern that may resemble that seen with herpetic disease. Stromal disease may present as punctate epithelial keratitis and evolve to scattered subepithelial opacities or an immune edema and haze similar to that seen with herpetic keratitis, and usually is responsive to topical steroid therapy (692,710) (Fig. 14-42B).

Diagnosis

Laboratory diagnostic techniques are discussed in greater detail in the earlier sections on Laboratory Diagnostic Techniques, and Poxviruses (under Characteristics of the Major Ocular Viral Pathogen Families). In making a diagnosis of ocular or other vaccinia, a history of recent smallpox vaccination or exposure to a recent vaccinee is critical and highly suggestive information. If the ophthalmologist finds that he or she is dealing with a patient manifesting suspect ocular or facial lesions and recently exposed to vaccinia, the entire office staff should follow infection control procedures, including hand and equipment hygiene and sterilization procedures. The examination room should be closed after the patient leaves, and antisepsis sprays similar to those used after examination of acute adenovirus cases used for cleaning. Pregnant, atopic, or immunosuppressed office workers should not be involved in patient care (692).

Smears taken from discharge and lesions reveal polymorphonuclear cells in the purulent material and eosinophilic cytoplasmic inclusion bodies (Guarnieri bodies) in the epithelial cells. The virus may be cultured in a variety of tissue cultures, including HeLa cells, rabbit or monkey kidney cells, MRC-5 human embryonic lung

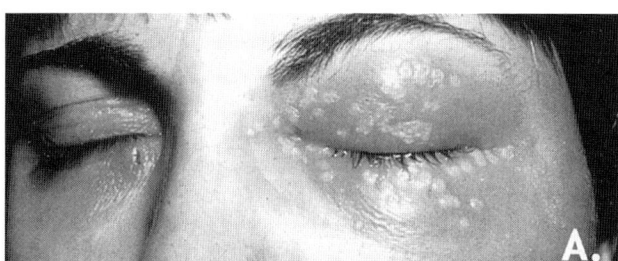
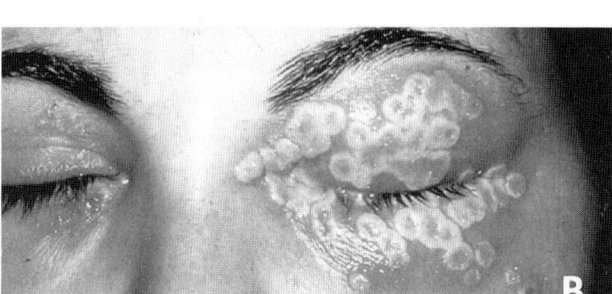
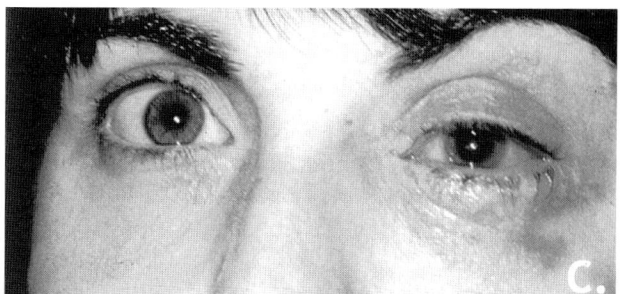

FIGURE 14-41. A: Mother exposed to child's vaccination 1 week before these early vesiculopustular lesions appeared (day 2 of lesions). **B:** Same patient on day 5, with progression and confluence of pustules and lid edema. **C:** Same patient on day 21, showing marked resolution of disease and no notable scarring. Treatment was vidarabine ointment. (Adapted in part from Pavan-Langston D. Viral disease of the cornea and external eye. In: Albert D, Jakobiec F, eds. *Principles and practice of ophthalmology*, 2nd ed. Philadelphia: WB Saunders 2000:846–893; and Pepose JS, Margolis TP, LaRussa P, et al. Ocular complications of smallpox vaccination. *Am J Ophthalmol* 2003;136:343–352.)

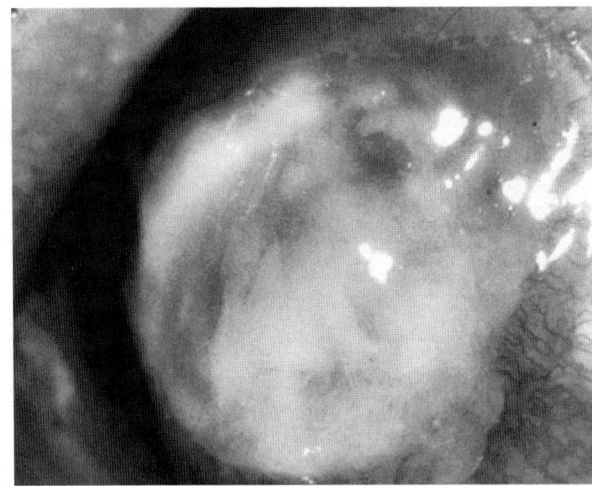
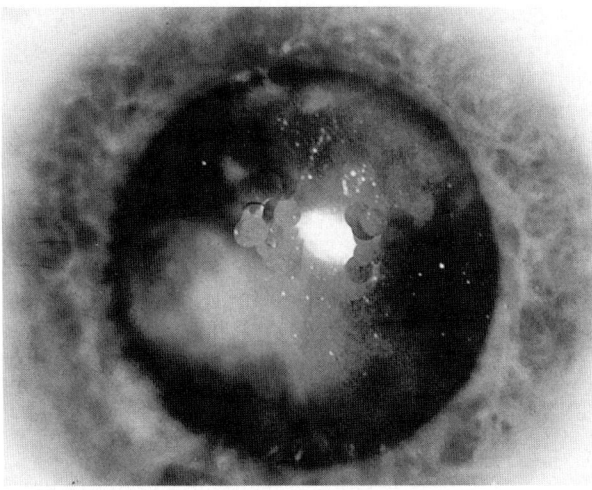

A

B

FIGURE 14-42. A: Severe vaccinial pock of cornea with necrosis and melting. Repeated cultures for superinfection were negative. Culture for vaccinia was positive. **B:** Vaccinial immune keratitis that developed 3 weeks after vaccinial blepharoconjunctivitis with diffuse punctate corneal lesions. Chronic keratitis responded to low-dose steroids, but residual scarring persisted. No vaccinia immune globulin was given during illness. (Adapted in part from Pavan-Langston D. Viral disease of the cornea and external eye. In: Albert D, Jakobiec F, eds. *Principles and practice of ophthalmology*, 2nd ed. Philadelphia: WB Saunders 2000:846–893; and Pepose JS, Margolis TP, LaRussa P, et al. Ocular complications of smallpox vaccination. *Am J Ophthalmol* 2003; 136:343–352.)

fibroblasts, and human embryonic kidney cells (2,10). Electron microscopic studies of thin sections of infected cells reveal the 300 × 200 nm, brick-shaped vaccinia virus particles, usually located in the cell cytoplasm. Rapid laboratory diagnosis of vaccinia infection using real-time PCR may allow rapid analysis of autoclaved suspensions, thereby limiting contact with infectious samples (711). Specific diagnosis can also be confirmed by restriction endonuclease analysis of infected cell DNA extracts and by other tests discussed previously (Fig. 14-43).

Treatment

There are no reported masked, controlled human studies on the efficacy of antivirals or VIG on ocular vaccinia (692). Only VIG is licensed for the treatment of complications of vaccinia vaccination. This immunoglobulin fraction of plasma from persons recently vaccinated with the smallpox vaccine is currently administered intramuscularly, but a new formulation will allow IV administration. It is available only through an Investigational New Drug protocol from the CDC in Atlanta (699,712). It has been effective for the treatment of eczema vaccinatum, and some cases of progressive vaccinia.

VIG's use in ocular vaccinia is best demonstrated in treatment of lid and conjunctival lesions as an intramuscular but not as a topical medication. Jones et al. reported four cases of severe orbital cellulitis responding within 1 day to intramuscular VIG. Topical VIG was found to be only possibly useful as prophylaxis against corneal

infection (79). Ellis et al. reported six cases, three with keratitis, all treated successfully with intramuscular VIG, two receiving three doses and one receiving seven doses over a several-day period (713). There were no residua except steroid-responsive, minimal stromal edema and 20/40 vision in the one patient with keratitis who received topical as well as intramuscular VIG. As noted previously, Ruben and Lane reported their accumulated experience of 348 patients with of ocular vaccinia, 22 with keratitis, of whom 336 were treated with intramuscular VIG and 28 with idoxuridine with or without VIG (706). Only 2% of noncorneal cases had residua, none severe (lid scarring, madarosis, or punctual stenosis with epiphora). Of the 22 patients with keratitis, only 4 (18%) at 5-year follow-up had any findings (i.e., 1 case each of mild focal corneal thickening not involving the visual axis, peripheral ghost vessels, epithelial and subepithelial opacities, and scattered subepithelial infiltrates). Further supportive anecdotal evidence for intramuscular VIG was reported by Kempe, who treated two brothers with identical cases of vaccinia keratitis (714). The brother treated with intramuscular VIG improved in 24 hours and healed with no scar. The untreated brother took 4 weeks to heal and was left with corneal scarring.

It is unclear whether VIG contributes to corneal scarring. In an unmasked, controlled rabbit study, animals receiving intramuscular VIG daily for 5 days had some corneal scarring, whereas animals receiving intramuscular VIG once with or without daily topical idoxuridine or topical VIG, or no treatment at all, had no scarring and did

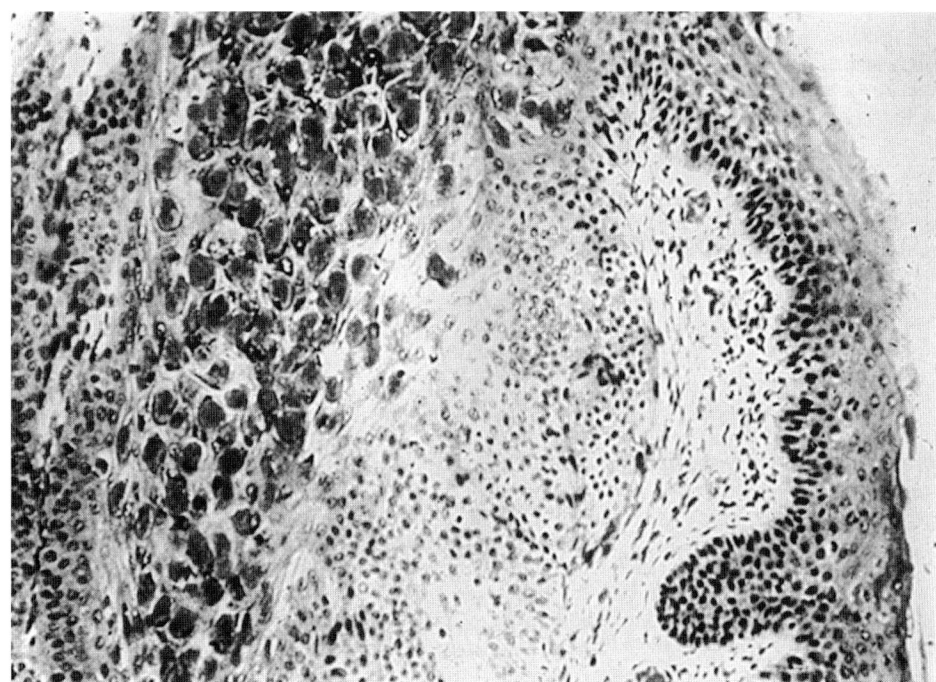

FIGURE 14-43. Histopathologic appearance of early vaccinial vesiculopustular skin lesion showing mixed neutrophil and monocytic cells in the center of the vesicle and giant cells at the base of the lesion (left side). Eosinophilic cytoplasmic inclusion bodies were seen in some cells in this area. (Original magnification: 40 ×, H&E stain)

not demonstrate any difference in clinical course or viral shedding period (715). It seems unlikely, given the cases cited previously where patients received single or multiple doses of intramuscular VIG and had no corneal scarring, and the evidence in the literature that vaccinial keratitis may be a scarring disease in the absence of VIG, that VIG be contraindicated in the presence of keratitis if there are other indications for its use in vaccinial disease (706,713,714,717–719). Use of VIG is recommended in moderate to severe blepharitis or blepharoconjunctivitis when keratitis is not present. If keratitis accompanies these conditions, intramuscular VIG need not be withheld, but should be used judiciously, usually in a single dose or two doses 48 hours apart. There is possible, but unproven, risk of corneal scar formation if large doses are given over several days. If VIG is indicated based on such serious disease as eczema vaccinatum, progressive vaccinia, or encephalitis, its use or dosing should not be withheld even if keratitis is present.

Although no topical antiviral is FDA approved for the treatment of ocular vaccinia, idoxuridine, trifluridine, or cidofovir drops or vidarabine ointment have been shown to be effective in animal and uncontrolled human reports. Acyclovir is not effective against vaccinia by *in vitro* antiviral screening (78,80,101,123,271,690,691,719). The effective antivirals may, therefore, be used off-label for this purpose. In teenagers and adults, trifluridine drops nine times daily for 14 days are recommended and are readily available.

Topical 3% vidarabine ointment may be preferable for use in children because the ointment preparation allows less frequent dosing and is less stinging than trifluridine. Vidarabine ointment is no longer commercially available, but may be obtained through compounding pharmacists. If, however, vidarabine cannot be obtained or the patient would tolerate drops, *trifluridine may be used in children just as it is in ocular herpes simplex in the doses indicated for adults* (i.e., nine times daily for 14 days). Topical antiviral drugs should be used as prophylaxis to protect the conjunctiva and cornea if vaccinia lesions are present on the eyelid. If, despite all efforts, there is a permanently visually disabling scar or leukoma, lamellar or penetrating keratoplasty has a generally favorable prognosis in the absence of corneal neovascularization or active inflammation (720).

Treatment of vaccinial ocular disease is summarized in the following. If vidarabine is not available for children, use trifluridine in the doses recommended for adults (692). It is the author's recent personal experience treating military recruits with ocular vaccinia that a full dose of Viroptic nine times daily is needed to treat infection effectively.

1. Blepharitis
   Mild to moderate (some pustules, mild edema, no fever)
   Prophylaxis of the conjunctiva and cornea: Adults: trifluridine (Viroptic) drops nine times daily for 2 weeks; children: vidarabine 3% ointment (Vira-A)

two to five times daily for 2 weeks; topical antibiotic to the conjunctiva

Moderately severe to severe (pustules, notable edema, hyperemia, lymphadenopathy, cellulitis, fever)

VIG 100 mg/kg intramuscularly; repeat in 48 hours if not improved

Adults: trifluridine drops nine times daily for 2 weeks; children: vidarabine 3% ointment two to five times daily for 2 weeks

2. Conjunctivitis with or without blepharitis but without keratitis

Mild to moderate (mild hyperemia and edema, no membranes or focal lesions)

Adults: trifluridine drops nine times daily for 2 weeks; children: vidarabine 3% ointment two to five times daily for 2 weeks

The majority of ophthalmic consultants at the CDC consultants meeting in October, 2002 recommended intramuscular VIG 100 mg/kg, one dose, for moderate disease (699).

Severe: (marked hyperemia, edema, membranes, focal lesions, lymphadenopathy, fever)

VIG 100 mg/kg; repeat in 48 hours if not improved. Adults: trifluridine drops nine times daily for 2 weeks; children: vidarabine 3% ointment two to five times daily for 2 weeks. Topical antibiotic to the conjunctiva.

3. Keratitis with mild or moderate blepharitis

Mild (gray epitheliitis, no ulcer, no stromal haze or infiltrate)

Adults: Trifluridine drops nine times daily for 2 weeks; children: vidarabine 3% ointment two to five times daily for 2 weeks

Topical antibiotic ointment once daily for 10 days

Moderate (ulcer, but no stromal haze or infiltrate)

Same treatment as for mild disease, but use topical antibiotic four times daily for 10 days or until ulcer healed

Severe (ulcer, stromal haze or infiltrate)

Same treatment as for moderate disease, but after epithelium is healed (at approximately 7 to 10 days), add moderate- to low-dose steroid to decrease immune reaction (e.g., prednisone 0.125%, loteprednol 0.5% to 0.2%, rimexolone 1%, and taper slowly). Topical antiviral prophylaxis is advisable to cover corticosteroid use for 2 to 3 weeks after acute disease.

4. Keratitis with severe blepharitis or conjunctivitis

Trifluridine drops nine times daily for 2 weeks; children: vidarabine 3% ointment two to five times daily for 2 weeks

Topical antibiotic four times daily for 10 days

Consider VIG intramuscularly 100 mg/kg, one dose; consider repeat in 48 hours if no improvement. After epithelium is healed (at approximately 7 days), add moderate- to low-dose steroid to decrease immune

reaction, if present (e.g., prednisone 0.125%, loteprednol 0.5% to 0.2%, or rimexolone 1%, and taper slowly). Topical antiviral prophylaxis is advisable to cover corticosteroid use for 2 to 3 weeks after acute disease.

5. Iritis

Treat as for other eye conditions noted previously.

After corneal epithelium is healed, add moderate- to low-dose steroid to decrease inflammatory reaction (e.g., prednisone 0.125%, loteprednol 0.5% to 0.2%, or rimexolone 1%, and taper slowly).

PAPILLOMAVIRUSES (HUMAN PAPILLOMAVIRUS)

Neoplastic and Nonneoplastic Relationships

Of the 70 different strains of HPV, the ones most associated with ocular disease are HPVs 6, 11, 16, and 18, which infect mucosal areas, and HPVs 1 through 4, which infect skin sites. This DNA virus is ubiquitous and spread by contact. After initial inoculation, the virus grows to create a lesion that may lead to further autoinoculation, causing a multicentric infection. Conjunctival intraepithelial neoplasia (CIN) is of particular interest. In studies on 10 consecutive patients who underwent excision of CIN and five non-CIN control patients, reverse transcriptase *in situ* PCR technique was used to search for the presence of HPV mRNA (721). HPV-16 DNA and mRNA were found in five CIN specimens, and HPV-18 DNA and mRNA were present in the remaining five CIN specimens. Further, in each of the CIN specimens, 20% to 40% of the dysplastic cells expressed the HPV E6 region. No HPV DNA or mRNA was detected in any of the control specimens or in any of the clinically uninvolved conjunctival specimens ($p < .001$).

Other studies indicate that HPV may be associated with a variety of conjunctival conditions. In a PCR study of 96 neoplastic and nonneoplastic lesions and 19 conjunctival samples free from overt disease, HPV types 16 and 18 DNA was identified in 57% of *in situ* squamous cell carcinoma specimens, in 55% of invasive squamous cell carcinoma specimens, in 20% of climatic droplet keratopathy specimens, in 35% of scarred corneas, and in 32% of normal conjunctival tissue obtained during routine cataract extractions (722). It is this type of data that makes the exact relationship between viral papillomas and neoplastic transformation unclear.

Clinical Disease

The papillomas are fleshy, pinkish-red, shiny, and elevated with prominent internal blood vessels present as multiple vascular loops in a fibrovascular core (52). The lesions may be broad and low (sessile) or pedunculated on a stalk, and located on the palpebral, fornical, or bulbar conjunctiva, on the lacrimal puncta or caruncle, or in the canaliculus. Limbal or corneal involvement is unusual and may be associated with fibrovascular pannus or punctate keratitis. In HIV-positive or other immunocompromised patients, lesions may be bilateral, multiple, and large. Symptoms may vary from none to irritation, foreign-body sensation, tearing, itching, mucoid discharge, photophobia, and blurred vision.

Diagnosis

Diagnosis is made by clinical observation and histopathologic study of excised specimens.

Treatment

Many viral papillomas regress spontaneously over 1 to 2 years, making observation of asymptomatic or mildly symptomatic patients a good option. Common therapy, however, for those who need treatment of conjunctival lesions is surgical excision, cryotherapy, or both. Unfortunately, with either of these techniques alone, seeding may take place during the procedure(s), resulting in recurrence of infection. The most effective method to prevent this is a combination of techniques by freezing the entire lesion and gently lifting it slightly from the surface to permit excision of the papilloma, stalk, and base plus some surrounding normal tissue. Then, freeze-thaw is applied twice to the base of the area excised using a cryoprobe. Electrodesiccation or heat cautery is useful for lid papillomas. In the former, an electric needle is inserted in the lesion and heat applied until the tissue begins to bubble. The lesion is then curetted. With heat cautery, the lesion is excised and cautery applied to the base.

Because of the less than stellar success in treating ocular papillomatosis, chemotherapy is now of interest. Initial clinical trials point to the efficacy of topical cidofovir (1% ointment) in the treatment of pharyngeal, laryngeal, and anogenital HPV infections (723,724). Cidofovir is now being pursued in the topical treatment of the papillomaviruses.

PARAMYXOVIRUS OCULAR DISEASE

The paramyxoviruses include the RNA viruses of measles (rubeola), mumps, and Newcastle disease.

Measles

Measles has an incubation period of approximately 2 weeks after exposure and begins with fever and follicular conjunctivitis, followed a few days later by a maculopapular skin rash (2). In addition to the acute watery conjunctivitis, measles infection of the eye produces a punctate keratitis, and, infrequently, Koplik's spots on the conjunctiva or semilunar fold. Photophobia may be severe but is self-limited and leaves no visual deficit. Rarely, an immune interstitial keratitis may occur (55,725).

In a report by Kayikcioglu et al. on the ocular findings in a measles epidemic among healthy young adults treated in the right eye with diclofenac four times daily and nothing in the left eye, the following study results were noted (726). Forty patients (65.6%) had measles conjunctivitis with bulbar and tarsal conjunctival hyperemia, of whom five had increased mucus secretion. Thirty-five (57.4%) had superficial punctate corneal epithelial lesions that stained with fluorescein, and some subepithelial nebulae. Ten patients had corneal lesions without obvious conjunctival disease. Twelve of the 14 patients who had subconjunctival hemorrhages had bilateral lesions, mostly in the superonasal quadrant. The time to disappearance of corneal lesions was 4.5 ± 3.2 days in the diclofenac-treated right eyes, and 4.1 ± 3.8 days in the left eyes. There was no significant difference in the healing time between the two eyes ($p = .75$). The authors concluded that although measles did not cause serious ocular complications in healthy patients, the often painful keratitis was unresponsive to diclofenac sodium eyedrops with respect to both healing time and end result.

In immunocompromised patients or in patients living in developing nations where there are nutritional deficiencies, particularly vitamin A deficiency, measles keratitis may be a perforating, blinding disease (727). Generalized measles infection may result in severe keratitis, keratomalacia, pneumonia, myocarditis, encephalitis, and death. Tuberculosis has been known to reactivate after measles infection in developing nations (728).

Mumps

Mumps infection follows an incubation period of 7 to 10 days and is usually associated with the systemic findings of fever, malaise, parotitis (90%), orchitis in male patients (25%), and mastitis in female patients (15%), with rare meningoencephalitis (729). The virus may also involve the ocular adnexa, causing a severe dacryoadenitis, sudden orbital pain, and swelling that produces a tender lacrimal fossa mass. A catarrhal conjunctivitis is common, and a punctate epithelial keratitis or severe stromal keratitis with decrease in vision may develop along with severe photophobia and lacrimation, but often little discomfort (730). The stromal disciform keratitis is often unilateral and may begin within a week of onset of the epithelial disease. Despite marked stromal edema, the disease ultimately resolves spontaneously (731,732). Mumps may also induce episcleritis, scleritis, uveitis, and a variety of posterior segment inflammatory lesions and extraocular muscle palsies. Severe intraocular inflammatory disease is usually seen only in immunosuppressed patients.

Newcastle Disease

Newcastle disease virus causes a limited infection seen primarily in poultry workers and laboratory technicians. It has a short incubation period of 18 to 48 hours after exposure, which is usually to infected poultry. Systemic disease is mild with fever, headache, and malaise lasting approximately 48 hours. Ocular clinical findings are usually a unilateral follicular and papillary conjunctivitis with hyperemia, edema, and chemosis usually in the lower fornix, mild tearing, and preauricular adenopathy (57,733). There may be a fine punctate epithelial keratitis with infrequent subepithelial infiltrates. The keratitis resolves in approximately 4 days. The illness is self-limiting with no sequelae and does not require therapy.

Diagnosis

Diagnosis is made by clinical impression and confirmed by isolation of virus from the throat, blood, or mucous membranes or by determination of humoral antibody response. The paramyxoviruses may be cultured for complement fixation and hemagglutination inhibition serologic identification or ELISA assay. Histopathologic findings in scrapings are typical of the paramyxoviruses, with intranuclear and intracytoplasmic eosinophilic inclusion bodies and multinucleated giant cells (10).

Treatment

There is no specific treatment for paramyxovirus infection. Supportive aids such as ibuprofen, cold compresses, oral fluids, and darkening the room (if there is photophobia) alleviate symptoms. Topical NSAIDs (diclofenac, ketorolac), steroids, and cycloplegia may be useful if inflammation is moderate to moderately severe. Systemic steroids may serve only to disseminate disease. Immunosuppressed patients should be put on antibacterial drops or ointment to protect the cornea from secondary bacterial infection (60,727). Most important is prevention in the form of routine rubeola and mumps vaccination in children older than 1 year. This not only prevents rubeola but has greatly reduced the incidence of neurologic complications, including acute sclerosing panencephalitis. There is no vaccine for Newcastle disease.

PICORNAVIRUSES

Acute Hemorrhagic Conjunctivitis

Acute hemorrhagic conjunctivitis (AHC), also known as Apollo 11 disease, is a highly contagious ocular infection caused by the enteroviruses (EVs), members of the picornavirus family. The EVs include several renowned and

dangerous RNA organisms: poliovirus, coxsackievirus A and B, and the echoviruses (2). The specific viruses most commonly associated with AHC are EV70 and coxsackievirus A24, but reports from East Asia indicate that other picornaviruses not cross-reacting with known EVs may also induce the disease (618,734–736). For years, only EV70 was thought to cause the disease, but serologic characterization and nucleotide sequencing revealed that EV70 and coxsackievirus A24 were separate viruses that caused identical clinical presentations (737). Because the viruses are difficult to isolate, reverse transcription PCR has been used successfully to detect EV70 specifically in patients with AHC who were culture negative (738).

With the exceptions of adenovirus infection and perhaps Newcastle disease, AHC differs from other external ocular infections by its proclivity to assume epidemic proportions and its clinical presentation. It may, during times of epidemic, afflict from tens of millions of people in densely populated, humid areas of East Asia to several hundred people in Western countries (734,739).

Disease is spread by fomites and direct inoculation of the conjunctiva from contaminated fingers (740). The conjunctiva is thought to be the primary site of replication of both EV70 and coxsackievirus A24. The incubation period after exposure is 1 to 2 days, followed by the sudden onset of acute orbital pain or foreign-body sensation, photophobia, profuse tearing, and lid edema. Diagnostic neutralizing antibodies against both viruses are present in the tear film within 24 hours and may contribute to the short duration of the disease (741). Progression of disease is rapid over the ensuing 24 hours, with development of hyperemic conjunctival chemosis and characteristic subconjunctival petechial or sheetlike hemorrhages that appear as concentric ridges encircling the corneal limbus, fine superficial punctate erosions of the cornea, and preauricular adenopathy. Symptoms resolve within 3 to 5 days without notable ocular damage. There are no subepithelial infiltrates, which helps to differentiate this from other viral infections, particularly adenovirus. There is frequently an associated superficial punctate keratitis and preauricular adenopathy, and the entire clinical picture may initially resemble acute adenoviral keratoconjunctivitis. Systemic symptoms may or may not be present and include malaise, myalgia, and upper respiratory tract symptoms similar to influenza (734,735,739). Rarely, there may be a radiculomyelitis.

Diagnosis

Diagnosis is by clinical observation and awareness of other contact cases or presence of ongoing epidemic.

Treatment

Therapy is essentially supportive, with bed rest, analgesics, and cool compresses. Antibiotics and steroids have no established role. The subconjunctival hemorrhage clears over 1 to 2 weeks.

TOGAVIRUSES

The togaviruses include the agents of rubella (German measles) and the arbovirus group B agents of yellow fever, dengue, and sandfly fever. Every togavirus may cause conjunctival hyperemia, lid edema, photophobia, and lacrimation. Clinical disease resolves spontaneously and does not require therapy. Only congenital rubella presents a significant threat to vision, if not to life.

Congenital Rubella Syndrome

Congenital rubella syndrome (CRS) results from maternal infection with this virus during the first or second trimester of pregnancy. The numerous ocular findings include microphthalmia, corneal opacity, microcornea, keratoconus, iris hypoplasia, cataracts, glaucoma, retinopathy, and subretinal neovascularization. The incidence of keratoconus in these patients is much higher than in the general population, and patients may have full-blown hydrops (58,60,742,743). Surgical procedures on these affected eyes are risky because of the postoperative inflammation and occasional persistence of live virus in the crystalline lenses.

In a study from India, in 40 eyes in 22 children with CRS (median age, 6 months), visual acuity at 5-year follow-up was 6/24 or better in only 6 eyes (15.0%). Twenty-two eyes (55.0%) had visual acuity of less than 3/60. Postoperative complications included transient corneal edema in 18 (45.0%) eyes, glaucoma in 5 (12.5%) eyes, after-cataract in 1 (2.5%) eye, and hyphema in 1 (2.5%) eye. Visual outcome disorders included deprivation amblyopia, glaucoma, optic atrophy, corneal opacity, and after-cataract. Associated systemic disorders included neurologic problems in 15 (68.2%), hearing loss in 12 (54.6%), cardiovascular problems in 9 (40.9%), and speech abnormalities in 7 (31.8%) children (744). The authors concluded that their rather discouraging results vastly increased the need for prevention of CRS with rubella vaccination of all unvaccinated women of childbearing age and early vaccination of female children.

In O'Neill's study on a cohort of 34 cases with CRS demonstrated by virus isolation, the early and long-term outcomes of CRS in an industrialized society (United States) were different with respect to lack of corneal findings (no surgery was done on these eyes), but not more encouraging (745). He reported that both persistent and delayed-onset effects may continue or occur as late as 30 years after original infection, in all likelihood owing to persistence of virus in the affected organs. The two most important factors contributing to the varied outcomes of prenatal infection were the presence of maternal immunity during early gestation and the stage of gestation during which fetal exposure occurs in a nonimmune mother.

Data review revealed little corneal disease. Cataracts were present in 29 (85%), 21 (63%) of which were bilateral. Microphthalmia was present in 28 (82%) of the 34 infants and was bilateral in 22 (65%). Glaucoma was found in 11 cases (29%) and presented either as a transient occurrence with early cloudy cornea in microphthalmic eyes (4 patients), as the infantile type with progressive buphthalmos (1 patient), or as a later-onset, aphakic glaucoma many months or years after cataract aspiration in 11 eyes of 6 patients. Rubella retinopathy was present in most patients, although an accurate estimate of its incidence or laterality was not possible because of the frequency of cataracts and nystagmus and the difficulty in obtaining adequate fundus examinations (745).

Acquired German Measles

Acquired German measles produces a less worrisome ocular disease in 70% of children and adults with this viral exanthem. The incubation period after exposure is 5 to 7 days, at which time a mild catarrhal or follicular conjunctivitis frequently occurs. In 2% of patients, a fine punctate epithelial keratitis associated with photophobia and tearing may develop. The corneal lesions are central and have their onset approximately 1 week after appearance of the rash (60,746,747). Late ocular disease has not been reported, and the acute disease is self-limited, requiring no therapy.

ACKNOWLEDGMENTS

The author has been supported by the Georgianna Stevens Fund, Boston and San Francisco, and the Nancy and Vanderburgh Johnstone Fund, Chicago.

REFERENCES

1. Laboratory methods in basic virology. In: Baron E, Peterson L, Finegold S, eds. *Bailey and Scott's diagnostic microbiology*, 9th ed. St. Louis, Mosby-Year Book, 1994:634–688.
2. Fields B, Knipe D, Howley P, eds. *Virology*, 3rd ed, vols 1 and 2. Philadelphia: Lippincott-Raven, 1996.
3. Murray P, Rosenthal K, Kobayashi G, et al. Viral classification, structure and replication; Laboratory diagnosis of viral disease; Adenoviruses; Human herpesviruses; Poxviruses; Paramyxoviruses. In: *Medical microbiology*. St. Louis: Mosby, 2002:48–65, 449–457, 467–473, 475–498, 499–504, 523–524.
4. Liesegang T. Ocular virology. In: Albert D, Jakobiec F, eds. *Principles and practice of ophthalmology*, 2nd ed. Philadelphia: WB Saunders, 2000:171–198.
5. Alcamo I. *Fundamentals of microbiology*. Boston: Jones and Bartlett, 2001:343–395.
6. Newell C, Martin S, Sendele D, et al. Herpes simplex virus-induced stromal keratitis: role of T-lymphocyte subsets in immunopathology. *J Virol* 1989;63:769–775.

7. Streilein J. Regional immunology of the eye. In: Pepose J, Holland G, Wilhelmus K, eds. *Ocular infection and immunity.* St. Louis: Mosby, 1996:19–33.

8. Hendricks R, Tang Q. Cellular immunity and the eye. In: Pepose J, Holland G, Wilhelmus K, eds. *Ocular infection and immunity.* St. Louis: Mosby, 1996:71–96.

9. Ahonen R, Vannas A. Clinical comparison between herpes simplex and herpes zoster ocular infections. In: Maudgal P, Missotten L, eds. *Herpetic eye diseases.* Dordrecht, the Netherlands: W. Junk, 1985:389.

10. Laboratory diagnosis of viral disease. In: White D, Fenner F, eds. *Medical virology,* 4th ed. San Diego: Academic Press, 1994:191–218.

11. Walpita P, Darougar S. Double-label immunofluorescence method for simultaneous detection of adenovirus and herpes simplex virus from the eye. *J Clin Microbiol* 1989;27:1623–1625.

12. Walpita P, Darouger S, Marsh RJ, et al. Development of an immunofluorescence test for the serodiagnosis of herpes zoster ophthalmicus. *Br J Ophthalmol* 1986;70:431–434.

13. Mann L, Woods G. Rapid diagnosis of viral pathogens. *Clin Lab Med* 1995;15:389–405.

14. Dunkel E, Pavan-Langston D, Fitzpatrick K, et al. Rapid detection of herpes simplex virus antigen in human ocular infections. *Curr Eye Res* 1988;7:661.

15. Gleaves C, Hondinka R, Johnston S, et al. Cumtech 15A. In: Baron E, ed. *Laboratory diagnosis of viral infections.* Washington, DC: American Public Health Association, 1994:38–56.

16. Forghani B, Hagens S. Diagnosis of viral infections by antigen detection. In: Lennette E, Lennette D, Lennette E, eds. *Diagnostic procedures for viral, rickettsial, and chlamydial infections.* Washington, DC: American Public Health Association, 1995:79–96.

17. Dworkin L, Gibler T, Van Gelder R. Real-time quantitative polymerase chain reaction diagnosis of infectious posterior uveitis. *Arch Ophthalmol* 2002;120:1534–1539.

18. Dunkel E, Pavan-Langston D. HSV-induced reactivation: contribution of epinephrine after corneal iontophoresis. *Curr Eye Res* 1987;6:75–84.

19. Fraser N, Valyi-Nagy T. Viral, neuronal, and immune factors which may influence herpes simplex virus (HSV) latency and reactivation. *Microb Pathog* 1993;15:83–91.

20. Liesegang T. Varicella zoster viral disease. In: Tasman W, Haeger E, eds. *Duane's foundations of clinical ophthalmology.* Philadelphia: JB Lippincott, 1991;v1,ch1:1–10.

21. Gershon A, Forghani B. Varicella-zoster virus. In: Lennette E, Lennette D, Lennette E, eds. *Diagnostic procedures for viral, rickettsial, and chlamydial infections.* Washington, DC: American Public Health Association, 1995:601–613.

22. Liesegang T. Varicella-zoster virus eye disease: review. *Cornea* 1999;18:511–531.

23. Pavan-Langston D. Viral disease of the cornea and external eye. In: Albert D, Jakobiec F, eds. *Principles and practice of ophthalmology,* 2nd ed. Philadelphia: WB Saunders, 2000: 846–893.

24. Cohen P. Tests for detecting herpes simplex virus and varicella zoster infections. *Dermatol Clin* 1994;12:51–68.

25. Pavan-Langston D, Yamamoto S, Dunkel E. Delayed herpes zoster pseudodendrites. *Arch Ophthalmol* 1995;113: 1381–1385.

26. Mahalingam R, Wellish M, Wolfe W, et al. Latent varicella-zoster viral DNA in human trigeminal and thoracic ganglia. *N Engl J Med* 1990;323:627–631.

27. Mahalingam R, Wellish M, Lederer D, et al. Quantitation of latent varicella-zoster virus DNA in human trigeminal ganglia by polymerase chain reaction. *J Virol* 1993;67: 2381–2384.

28. Landini M. New approaches and perspectives in cytomegalovirus diagnosis. *Prog Med Virol* 1993;40:157–177.

29. Pavan-Langston D, Dunkel E. Ocular pharmacology of antiviral drugs. In: Tasman W, Jaeger E, eds. *Duane's foundations of clinical opthalmology.* Philadelphia: Lippincott-Raven, 1995, vol 2, ch 100:1–24.

30. Palestine A, Rodriques M, Macher A, et al. Ophthalmic involvement in acquired immune deficiency syndrome. *Ophthalmology* 1984;91:1092–1099.

31. Palestine AG, Stevens G Jr, Lane HC, et al. Treatment of cytomegalovirus retinitis with dihydroxy propoxymethyl guanine. *Am J Ophthalmol* 1986; 101:95–101.

32. Adler SP. Cytomegalovirus and child day care. *N Engl J Med* 1989;321:1290–1296.

33. Borisch B, Gerhard J, Scholl B, et al. Detection of human cytomegalovirus DNA and viral antigens in tissues of different manifestations of CMV infection. *Virchows Arch B Cell Pathol* 1988;55:93–99.

34. Pflugfelder S, Crouse C, Atherton S. Ophthalmic manifestations of Epstein-Barr virus infection. *Int Ophthalmol Clin* 1993;33:95–101.

35. Pflugfelder S, Tseng S, Pepose J, et al. Epstein-Barr virus infection and immunologic dysfunction in patients with aqueous tear deficiency. *Ophthalmology* 1990;97:313.

36. Moore P, Chang Y. Detection of herpes-like DNA sequences in Kaposi's sarcoma in patients with and without HIV infection. *N Engl J Med* 1995;332:1181–1185.

37. Humphrey R, O'Brien T, Newcomb F, et al. Kaposi's sarcoma-associated herpesvirus in a new transmissible virus that infects B cells. Blood 1996;88:297–301.

38. Hierholzer J. Adenoviruses. In: Murray P, Baron E, Pfaler M, eds. *Manual of clinical microbiology.* Washington, DC: ASM Press, 1995:947–955.

39. Gordon Y, Aoki K, Kinchington P. Adenovirus keratoconjunctivitis. In: Pepose J, Holland G, Wilhelmus K, eds. *Ocular infection and immunity,* St. Louis: Mosby, 1996:877–894.

40. Kowalski R, Gordon Y. Comparison of direct rapid tests for the detection of adenovirus antigen in routine conjunctival specimens. *Ophthalmology* 1989;96:1106–1109.

41. Behbehani A. Poxviruses. In: Lennette E, Lennette D, Lennette E, eds. *Diagnostic procedures for viral, rickettsial, and chlamydial infections.* Washington, DC: American Public Health Association, 1995:511–520.

42. Baxby D. Identification and interrelationships of the variola/vaccinia virus genomes. *Prog Med Virol* 1975;19: 215–246.

43. Stern W, Dales S. Biogenesis of vaccinia: relationship of the envelope to virus assembly. *Virology* 1976;75:242–255.

44. McCune J. Viral latency in HIV disease. *Cell* 1995;82: 183–188.

45. Fauci A. AIDS: newer concepts in the immunopathogenic mechanisms of human immunodeficiency virus disease. *Proc Assoc Am Physicians* 1995;107:1–7.

46. Haseltine W, Wong-Staal F. The molecular biology of the AIDS virus. *Sci Am* 1988;259(40):52–62.

47. Kaplan M. Pathogenesis of HIV. *Infect Dis Clin North Am* 1994;8:279–288.

48. Proffitt M, Yen-Lieberman B. Laboratory diagnosis of human immunodeficiency virus infection. *Infect Dis Clin North Am* 1993;7:203–219.

49. Ou C, Kwok S, Mitchell S, et al. DNA amplification for direct detection of HIV-1 in DNA of peripheral blood mononuclear cells. *Science* 1988;239:295–297.

50. Lorincz A. Human papilloma viruses. In: Lennette E, Lennette D, Lennette E, eds. *Diagnostic procedures for viral, rickettsial, and chlamydial infections.* Washington, DC: American Public Health Association, 1995:465–480.

51. Bardenstein D, Lass J. Periocular involvement of papillomavirus and molluscum contagiosum virus. In: Tasman W, Jaeger E, eds. *Duane's foundations of clinical ophthalmology.* Philadelphia: Lippincott-Raven, 1996:1–17.

52. Prasad C. Pathobiology of human papilloma viruses. *Clin Lab Med* 1995;15:685–704.

53. Kleiman M, Leland D. Mumps virus and Newcastle disease virus. In: Lennette E, Lennette D, Lennette E, eds. *Diagnostic procedures for viral, rickettsial, and chlamydial infections.* Washington, DC: American Public Health Association, 1995:455–463.

54. Atkinson W. Epidemiology and prevention of measles. *Dermatol Clin* 1995;13:553–559.

55. Boniuk V. Rubeola (measle, morbilli). In: Pavan-Langston D, ed. *Ocular viral disease.* Boston: Little, Brown, 1975:243–256.

56. Librach I. Ocular symptoms in glandular fever. *Br J Ophthalmol* 1956;40:619–624.

57. Wood T. Newcastle disease. In: Pepose J, Holland G, Wilhelmus K, eds. *Ocular infection and immunity.* St. Louis: Mosby, 1996: 873–876.

58. Chernsky M, Mahoney J. Rubella virus. In: Murray P, Baron E, Pfaler M, eds. *Manual of clinical microbiology.* Washington, DC: ASM Press, 1995:968–973.

59. Best J, O'Shea S. Rubella virus. In: Lennette E, Lennette D, Lennette E, eds. *Diagnostic procedures for viral, rickettsial, and chlamydial infections.* Washington, DC: American Public Health Association, 1995:583–600.

60. Boniuk V. Rubella and congenital rubella syndrome. In: Pavan-Langston D, ed. *Ocular viral disease.* Boston: Little, Brown, 1975:229–242.

61. Rotbart H. Enteroviruses. In: Murray P, Baron E, Pfaler M, eds. *Manual of clinical microbiology.* Washington, DC: ASM Press, 1995:1004–1011.

62. Balfour H. Antiviral drugs. *N Engl J Med* 1999;340:1255–1268.

63. Pavan-Langston D. Ocular pharmacology of antiviral drugs. In: Jaeger E, Tasman W, Wilhelmus K, eds. *Duane's foundations of clinical ophthalmology.* Philadelphia: Lippincott Williams & Wilkins, 2004, v2, ch 100:1–24.

64. O'Brien W. Antiviral agents. In: Tabbara K, Hyndiuk R, eds. *Infections of the eye,* 2nd ed. Boston: Little, Brown, 1996: 269–280.

65. Chau Tran TH, Cassoux N, Bodaghi B, Lehoang P. Successful treatment with combination of systemic antiviral drugs and intravitreal ganciclovir injections in the management of severe necrotizing herpetic retinitis. *Ocul Immunol Inflamm* 2003 Jun;11(2):141–144.

66. Prusoff W. Synthesis and biological activities of iododeoxyuridine, an analog of thymidine. *Biochim Biophys Acta* 1959;32:295.

67. Kaufman H, Martola E, Dohlman C. Use of idoxuridine in treatment of herpes simplex keratitis. *Arch Ophthalmol* 1962; 68:235.

68. Hirsch M, Kaplan J. Antiviral agents. In: Fields D, Knipe D, eds. *Virology.* New York: Raven Press, 1990:441.

69. Prusoff W, Ward D. Nucleoside analogues with antiviral activity. *Biochem Pharmacol* 1976;25:1233.

70. Kaplan A, Ben-Porat T. Mode of antiviral action of 5 iodouracil deoxyriboside. *J Mol Biol* 1966;19:320.

71. Tamm I. Symposium of the experimental pharmacology and clinical use of antimetabolites: III. Metabolic antagonists and selective virus inhibition. *Clin Pharmacol Ther* 1960;1:777.

72. Boston Interhospital Viral Study Group and the NIAID-Sponsored Cooperative Antiviral Clinical Study. Failure of high dose 5-iodo-2′-deoxyuridine in the therapy of herpes simplex encephalitis. *N Engl J Med* 1975;292:599–603.

73. Aronson S, Moore T. Antiviral properties of idoxuridine during steroid treatment of herpes stromal keratitis. *Ann NY Acad Sci* 1970;173:96.

74. Lass J, Langston R, Foster C, et al. Antiviral medications and corneal wound healing. *Antiviral Res* 1984;4:143.

75. Pavan-Langston D, et al. Intraocular penetration of Ara A and IDU-therapeutic implications in clinical herpetic uveitis. *Trans Am Acad Ophthalmol Otolaryngol* 1973;77:455.

76. Smith K. Some biologic aspects of herpesvirus-cell interactions in the presence of 5-iodo-2′-deoxyuridine: cytotoxicity. *J Immunol* 1963;91:582.

77. Smith K, Dukes C. Effects of 5′-iodo 2′-deoxyuridine on herpesvirus synthesis and survival in infected cells. *J Immunol* 1964;92:550.

78. Jack M, Sorenson R. Vaccinial keratitis treated with IDU. *Arch Ophthalmol* 1963;69:730–732.

79. Jones B, Al-Hussaini M. Therapeutic considerations in ocular vaccinia. *Trans Ophthalmol Soc UK* 1964;83:613–631.

80. Pavan-Langston D, Dohlman C. A double blind clinical study of adenine arabinoside therapy of viral keratoconjunctivitis. *Am J Ophthalmol* 1972;74:81.

81. Delamore I, Prusoff W. Effect of 5′-iodo-2′-deoxyuridine on the biosynthesis of phosphorylated derivatives of thymidine. *Biochem Pharmacol* 1962;11:101.

82. Dohlman C, Zucker B. Long-term treatment with IDU and steroids. *Arch Ophthalmol* 1965;74:172.

83. Patterson A, Fox A, Davies G, et al. Controlled studies of IDU in the treatment of herpetic keratitis. *Trans Ophthalmol Soc UK* 1963;83:583.

84. Pavan-Langston D, Buchanan R. Vidarabine therapy of simple and IDU-complicated herpetic keratitis. *Trans Am Acad Ophthalmol Otolaryngol* 1976;81:813.

85. Fardeau C, Langlois M, Nugier F, et al. Cross-resistances to antiviral drugs of IUdR-resistant HSV-1 in rabbit keratitis and in vitro. *Cornea* 1993;12:19–24.

86. Pavan-Langston D, Foster C. Trifluorothymidine and idoxuridine therapy of ocular herpes. *Am J Ophthalmol* 1977; 84:818.

87. Heidelberger C, King D. Trifluorothymidine. *Pharmacol Ther* 1979;6:427–442.

88. Funderburgh M, Funderburgh J, Chandler J. Thymidine kinase activity of ocular herpes simplex isolates resistant to IUDR therapy. *Invest Ophthalmol Vis Sci* 1986;27:1546–1548.

89. Wigdahl B, Parkhurst J. HEp-2 cell and herpes simplex virus type 1-induced deoxythymidine kinases: inhibition by derivatives of 5-trifluoromethyl-2′-deoxyuridine. *Antimicrob Agents Chemother* 1978;14:470.

90. De Clercq E, Descamps J, Huang G, et al. 5-Nitro-2′-deoxyuridine and 5-nitrodeoxyuridine 5′-monophosphate antiviral activity and inhibition of thymidylate synthetase in vivo. *Mol Pharmacol* 1978;14:422.

91. U.S. Pharmacopeia: trifluridine. In: *United States Pharmacopeia drug information.* Englewood, CO: Micromedics, 2000: 3054–3057.

92. De Clercq E. 5′-Substituted 2′-deoxyuridines which inhibit herpes simplex virus replication. *Adv Ophthalmol* 1979;38:204.

93. Kaufman H, Heidelberger C. Therapeutic antiviral action of 5-trifluoromethyl-2′-deoxyuridine in herpes simplex keratitis. *Science* 1964;145:585.

94. Foster C, Pavan-Langston D. Corneal wound healing and antiviral medication. *Arch Ophthalmol* 1977;95:2062.

95. Sugar J, Varnell E, Centifanto Y, et al. Trifluorothymidine treatment of herpetic iritis in rabbits and ocular penetration. *Invest Ophthalmol Vis Sci* 1973;12:532.

96. O'Brien W, Edelhauser H. The corneal penetration of trifluorothymidine, adenine arabinoside, and idoxuridine. *Invest Ophthalmol Vis Sci* 1977;16:1093.

97. Pavan-Langston D, Nelson D. Intraocular penetration of trifluorothymidine. *Am J Ophthalmol* 1979;87:814.

98. O'Brien W. Antiviral agents. In: Tabbara K, Hyndiuk R, eds. *Infections of the eye*. Boston: Little, Brown, 1986:257.

99. Clough D, Wigdahl B, Parkhurst J. Biological effects of 5-carboxy-2'-deoxyuridine: hydrolysis product of 5-trifluoromethyl-2'-deoxyuridine. *Antimicrob Agents Chemother* 1978; 14:126.

100. Guyer B, O'Day D, Hierholzer J, et al. Epidemic keratoconjunctivitis: types 8 and 19. *J Infect Dis* 1975;132:142.

101. Hyndiuk R, Seideman S, Leibsohn J. Treatment of vaccinial keratitis with trifluorothymidine. *Arch Ophthalmol* 1976;94: 1976.

102. Lin T, Chai C, Prusoff W. Synthesis and biological activities of 5-trifluoromethyl-5'-azido-2,5' dideoxyuridine and 5-trifluoromethyl-5'-amino-2',5'-dideoxyuridine. *J Med Chem* 1976; 19:915.

103. Collins P, Bauer D. Comparison of activity of herpes virus inhibitors. *J Antimicrob Chemother* 1977;3[Suppl A]:73.

104. Reyes P, Heidelberger C. Fluorinated pyrimidines: XXVI. mammalian thymidylate synthetase. *Mol Pharmacol* 1965; 1:14.

105. Coster D, McKinnon JR, McGill JI, et al. Clinical evaluation of adenine arabinoside and trifluorothymidine in the treatment of corneal ulcers caused by herpes simplex virus. *J Infect Dis* 1976;133[Suppl A]:173.

106. Liesegang T. Ocular virology. In: Albert D, Jakobiec F, eds. *Principals and practice of opthalmology*. Philadelphia: WB Saunders. 1:171–198.

107. La Lau C, Oosterhuis J, Versteeg J, et al. Acyclovir and trifluorothymidine in herpetic keratitis: a multicenter trial. *Br J Ophthalmol* 1982;66:506–508.

108. Kaufman H. In vivo studies with antiviral agents. *Ann NY Acad Sci* 1965;130:168.

109. Hyndiuk R, Raimundo E, Charlin T, et al. Trifluridine in resistant human herpetic keratitis. *Arch Ophthalmol* 1978; 96:1839.

110. Wilhelmus K. The treatment of herpes simplex virus epithelial keratitis. *Trans Am Ophthalmol Soc* 2000;98:505–532.

111. Lee W, Benitez G, Goodman L, et al. Potential anticancer agents: XI. synthesis of the B-anomer of 9-(D-arabinofuransyl)-adenine. *J Am Chem Soc* 1960;82:2648.

112. Muller W, Maidhof A, Zahn RK, et al. Effect of 9-B-D-arabinofuranosyladenine on DNA synthesis in vivo. *Cancer Res* 1977;37:2282–2290.

113. Moore E, Cohen C. Effect of arabinomononucleotides con ribonucleotides reduction by an enzyme system from rat tumor. *J Biol Chem* 1976;242:2116.

114. Wagar M, Burgoyne L, Athinson M. Deoxyribonucleic acid synthesis in mammalian nuclei: incorporation of deoxyribonucleotides and chain-terminating nucleotide analogues. *Biochem J* 1971;121:803.

115. Brink J, LePage G. Metabolism and distribution of 9-B-D-arabinofuransyladenine in mouse tissue. *Cancer Res* 1964; 24:1042.

116. Kurtz S, Fitzgerald J, Schardein J. Comparative animal toxicology of vidarabine and its 5'-monophosphate. *Ann NY Acad Sci* 1977;284:6.

117. Sidwell R, Dixon G, Sellers S, et al. In vivo antiviral properties of biologically active compounds: II. studies with influenza and vaccinia viruses. *Appl Microbiol* 1968;16:370.

118. Sawa T, Fukagawa Y, Homma I, et al. Mode of inhibition of coformycin on adenosine deaminase. *J Antibiot* 1967; 20A:227.

119. Woo P, Dion H, Lange S. A novel adenosine and Ara-A deaminase inhibitor. *J Heterocycl Chem* 1974;11:641.

120. Shannon W. Adenine arabinoside: antiviral action in vitro. In: Pavan-Langston D, Buchanan R, Alford C, eds. *Adenine arabinoside: an antiviral agent*. New York: Raven Press, 1975:1–43.

121. Nesburn A, Robinson C, Dickenson R. Adenine arabinoside effect on experimental idoxuridine-resistant herpes simplex infection. *Invest Ophthalmol Vis Sci* 1974;13:302.

122. Whitley R, Hilty M, Haynes R, et al. Adenine arabinoside therapy of herpes zoster in the immunosuppressed. *N Engl J Med* 1976;294:1193–1199.

123. Hyndiuk R, Seideman S, Leibsohn J. Treatment of vaccinial keratitis with vidarabine. *Arch Ophthalmol* 1976;94:1363.

124. Coster D, Wilhelmus K, Michaud R, et al. A comparison of acyclovir and idoxuridine as treatment for ulcerative herpetic keratitis. *Br J Ophthalmol* 1980;64:763.

125. Falcon M, Jones B, Williams HP, et al. Management of herpetic eye disease. *Trans Ophthalmol Soc UK* 1977;97:345.

126. Hirsch MS, Schooley RT. Resistance to antiviral drugs: the end of innocence. *N Engl J Med* 1989;320:313–314.

127. Teich SA, Cheung TW, Friedman AH. Systemic antiviral drugs used in ophthalmology. *Surv Ophthalmol* 1992;37:19–53.

128. Larder B, Darby G. Susceptibility to other antiherpes drugs of pathogenic variants of herpes simplex virus selected for resistance ot acyclovir. *Antimicrob Agents Chemother* 1986;29: 894–898.

129. Coen D, Aschman D, Gelep P, et al. Fine mapping and molecular cloning of mutations in the herpes simplex virus DNA polymerase locus. *J Virol* 1984;49:236–247.

130. Coen D. General aspects of drug resistance with special reference to herpes simplex virus. *J Antimicrob Chemother* 1986; 18[Suppl B]:1–10.

131. Fleming HJ, Coen D. Herpes simplex virus mutants resistant to arabinosyladenine in the presence of deoxycoformycin. *Antimicrob Agents Chemother* 1984;26:382–387.

132. Gibbs J, Chiou H, Hall J, et al. Sequence and mapping analyses of the herpes simplex virus DNA polymerase gene predict a C-terminal substrate binding domain. *Proc Natl Acad Sci U S A* 1985;82:7969–7973.

133. Elion G, Furman P, Fyfe J, et al. Selectivity of action of an antiherpetic agent 9-(1-hydroxyethoxymethyl) guanine. *Proc Natl Acad Sci U S A* 1977;74:5716.

134. Furman P, St. Clair M, Spector T. Acyclovir triphosphate is a suicide inactivator of the herpes simplex virus DNA polymerase. *J Biol Chem* 1984;259:9575–9579.

135. Wagstaff A, Faulds D, Goa KA. Acyclovir, a reappraisal of its antiviral activity, pharmacokinetic properties and therapeutic efficacy. *Drugs* 1994;47:153–205.

136. Davidson R, Kaufman E, Crumpacker C, et al. Inhibition of herpes simplex virus transformed and nontransformed cells by acycloguanosine: mechanisms of uptake and toxicity. *Virology* 1981;113:9.

137. Mertz G, Eron L, Kaufman R, et al. Prolonged continuous versus intermittent oral acyclovir treatment in normal adults with frequently recurring genital herpes simplex virus infection. *Am J Med* 1988;85(2A):14–19.

138. DeMiranda P, Good S, Krasny H, et al. Metabolic fate of radioactive acyclovir in humans. *Am J Med* 1982;73:215.

139. Markham R, Carter C, Scobie M, et al. Double-blind clinical trial of adenine arabinoside and idoxuridine in herpetic corneal ulcers. *Trans Ophthalmol Soc UK* 1977;97:333.

140. Laskin O. Clinical pharmacokinetics of acyclovir. *Clin Pharmacokinet* 1983;8:187.

141. Feldman S, Rodman J, Gregory B. Excessive serum concentrations of acyclovir and neurotoxicity. *J Infect Dis* 1988;157: 385–388.

142. Moore HJ Jr, Szczech GM, Rodwell DE, et al. Preclinical toxicology studies with acyclovir: teratologic, reproductive, and neonatal tests. *Fundam Appl Toxicol* 1983;3:560–568.

143. Steele R, Marmer D, Keeney R. Comparative in vitro immuno-toxicology of acyclovir and other antiviral agents. *Infect Immun* 1980;28:957–962.

144. Strauss S, Smith H, Brickman C, et al. Acyclovir for chronic mucocutaneous herpes simplex virus infection in immunosuppressed patients. *Ann Intern Med* 1982;96:270.

145. DeMiranda P, Blum M. Pharmacokinetics of acyclovir after intravenous and oral administration. *J Antimicrob Chemother* 1983;12[Suppl B]:29–37.

146. Dorsky D, Crumpacker C. Drugs five years later: acyclovir. *Ann Intern Med* 1987;107:859–874.

147. Collum L, Akhtar J, McGettrick P. Oral acyclovir in herpetic keratitis. *Trans Ophthalmol Soc UK* 1985;104:629.

148. McKendrick M, Case C, Burke C, et al. Oral acyclovir in herpes zoster. *Antimicrob Agents Chemother* 1984;14:661–665.

149. McKendrick M, McGill J, White J, et al. Oral acyclovir in acute herpes zoster. *BMJ* 1986;293:1529–1532.

150. Hung S, Patterson A, Rees P. Pharmacokinetics of oral acyclovir (Zovirax) in the eye. *Br J Ophthalmol* 1984;68:192–195.

151. Biron K, Elion GB. In vitro susceptibility of varicella zoster virus to acyclovir. *Antimicrob Agents Chemother* 1980;18:443–447.

152. Poirier R, Kinham J, Hutcherson J. Human aqueous penetration of topically applied acyclovir ophthalmic ointment 3%. *Am J Med* 1982;73:393.

153. Brik D, Dunkel E, Pavan-Langston D. Persistent herpes simplex virus in the corneal stroma despite topical and systemic antiviral therapy. *Arch Ophthalmol* 1994;111:522–527.

154. DeMiranda P, Krasny H, Page D, et al. Species differences in the disposition of acyclovir. *Am J Med* 1982;73:31.

155. Balfour HJ. Acyclovir. In: Peterson P, Verhoeft J, eds. *Antimicrobial agents annual 3*. Amsterdam: Elsevier, 1988:345–360.

156. Schulman J, Peyman GA, Hortom MB, et al. Intraocular 9-[(2-hydroxy-l-(hydroxymethyl) ethoxy] methyl) guanine levels after intravitreal and subconjunctival administration. *Ophthalmic Surg* 1986;17:429–432.

157. Centifanto Y, Kaufman H. 9-(2-Hydroxyethoxymethyl) guanine as an inhibitor of herpes simple virus replication. *Chemotherapy* 1979;25:279.

158. Pagano J, Sixbey J, Lin J. Acyclovir and Epstein-Barr virus infection. *J Antimicrob Chemother* 1983;12:113.

159. Dunkel EC, Green MT, Rosborough JP. Suppression of HSV-1 infection in trigeminal ganglion cells: an in vitro model of latency. *Invest Ophthalmol Vis Sci* 1984;25:525–533.

160. Pavan-Langston D, Campbell R, Lass J. Acyclic antimetabolite therapy of experimental herpes simplex keratitis. *Am J Ophthalmol* 1978;86:618.

161. Goldberg LH, Kaufman RH, Kurtz TO, et al. Continuous five-year treatment of patients with frequently recurring genital herpes simplex virus infection with acyclovir. *J Med Virol* 1993;1:45–50.

162. Trousdale M, Dunkel E, Nesburn A. Effect of acyclovir on acute and latent herpes simplex virus infections in the rabbit. *Invest Ophthalmol Vis Sci* 1980;19:1336.

163. Wade J, Hintz M, McGuffin R, et al. Treatment of cytomegalovirus pneumonia with high-dose acyclovir. *Am J Med* 1982;73:249.

164. Whitley RJ, Gnann JJ Jr. Acyclovir: a decade later. *N Engl J Med* 1992;327:782–789.

165. Kinghorn G. Long-term suppression with oral acyclovir of recurrent herpes simplex virus infections in otherwise healthy patients. *Am J Med* 1988;85(2A):26–29.

166. Pavan-Langston D, Buchanan R, Alford C. *Adenine arabinoside: a new antiviral*. New York: Raven Press, 1975.

167. Pavan-Langston D, et al. Acyclovir and vidarabine in the treatment of ulcerative herpes simplex keratitis. *Am J Ophthalmol* 1981;92:829.

168. McCulley J, Binder PS, Kaufman HE, et al. A double-blind, multicenter clinical trial of acyclovir vs idoxuridine for treatment of epithelial herpes simplex keratitis. *Ophthalmology* 1982;89:1195–1200.

169. Laibson P, Pavan-Langston D, Yeakley WR, et al. Acyclovir and vidarabine for the treatment of herpes simplex keratitis. *Am J Med* 1982;73(1A):281.

170. Schwartz G, Holland G. Oral acyclovir for the management of herpes simplex keratitis in children. *Ophthalmology* 2000;107:278–282.

171. Schwab I. Oral acyclovir in the management of herpes simplex ocular infections. *Ophthalmology* 1988;95:423.

172. Collum L, McGettrick P, Akhtar J, et al. Oral acyclovir (Zovirax) in herpes simplex dendritic corneal ulceration. *Br J Ophthalmol* 1986;70:435–438.

173. Herpetic Eye Disease Study Group. A controlled trial of oral acyclovir for the prevention of stromal keratitis or iritis in patients with herpes simplex virus epithelial keratitis. *Arch Ophthalmol* 1997;115:703–712.

174. Wilhelmus KR, Beck RW, Moke PS, et al, for the Herpetic Eye Disease Study Group. Acyclovir for the prevention of recurrent herpes simplex virus eye disease. *N Engl J Med* 1998;339:300–306.

175. Barron B, Gee L, Hauck WW, et al, for the Herpetic Eye Disease Study Group. A controlled trial of acyclovir for herpes simplex stromal keratitis. *Ophthalmology* 1994;101:1871–1882.

176. Wilhelmus K, Gee L, Hauck WW, et al, for the Herpetic Eye Disease Study Group. A controlled trial of topical corticosteroids for herpes simplex stromal keratitis. *Ophthalmology* 1994;101:1883–1896.

177. Herpetic Eye Disease Study Group. Predictors of recurrent herpes simplex virus keratitis. *Cornea* 2001;20:123–128.

178. Herpetic Eye Disease Study Group. Oral acyclovir for herpes simplex virus eye disease: effect on prevention of epithelial keratitis and stromal keratitis. *Arch Ophthalmol* 2000;118:1030–1036.

179. Herpetic Eye Disease Study Group. A controlled trial of oral acyclovir for iridocyclitis caused by herpes simplex virus. *Arch Ophthalmol* 1996;114:1065–1072.

180. Herpetic Eye Disease Study Group. Psychological stress and other potential triggers for recurrences of herpes simplex virus eye infections. *Arch Ophthalmol* 2000;118:1617–1625.

181. Wu X, Chen X. Acyclovir for the treatment and prevention of recurrent infectious herpes simplex keratitis. *Chin Med J (Engl)* 2002;115:1569–1572.

182. Simon A, Pavan-Langston D. Long-term oral acyclovir therapy: effect on recurrent infectious herpes simplex keratitis in patients with and without grafts. *Ophthalmology* 1996;103:1399–1405.

183. Pepose JS. External ocular herpesvirus infections in immunodeficiency. *Curr Eye Res* 1991;10[Suppl]:87–95.

184. Pavan-Langston D. Cornea and external disease. In: Pavan-Langston D, ed. *Manual of ocular diagnosis and therapy*. Philadelphia: Lippincott Williams & Wilkins, 2002:67–129.

185. Margolis T, Ostler B. Treatment of ocular disease in eczema herpeticum. *Am J Ophthalmol* 1990;110:274.

186. Pavan-Langston D. Herpes keratitis: clinical features, diagnosis, treatment and prophylaxis. In: Remington J, ed. *Current clinical topics in infectious disease*. Boston: Blackwell Science, 2000:298–324.

187. Dunn J, Holland G. Human immunodeficiency virus infection and AIDS. In: Tabbara K, Hyndiuk R, eds. *Infections of the eye*, 2nd ed. Boston: Little, Brown, 1996:625–644.

188. Tambasco F, Cohen EJ, Nguyen LH, et al. Oral acyclovir after penetrating keratoplasty for herpes simplex keratitis. *Arch Ophthalmol* 1999;117: 445–449.

189. Colin J, Robinet A, Malet F. Traitement preventif des keratites herpetiques par l'acyclovir en comprimes. *J Fr Ophthalmol* 1993;16:6–9.

190. Barney N, Foster C. A prospective randomized trial of oral acyclovir following penetrating keratoplasty for herpes. *Cornea* 1994;13:232–236.

191. Margolis T, Milner MS, Shama A, et al. Herpes zoster ophthalmicus in patients with human immunodeficiency virus infection. *Am J Ophthalmol* 1998;125:285–291.

192. Weller T. Varicella-zoster virus: history, perspective, and evolving concerns. *Neurology* 1995;45[Suppl 8]:S9–S10.

193. Wood M, Shukla S, Fiddian AP, et al. Treatment of acute herpes zoster: effect of early versus late therapy with acyclovir and valaciclovir on prolonged pain. *J Infect Dis* 1998;178[Suppl]:S81–S84.

194. Pavan-Langston D. Ophthalmic zoster. In: Watson CPN, Gershon A, eds. *Herpes zoster and postherpetic neuralgia.* Amsterdam: Elsevier Science, 2001:119–129.

195. Pavan-Langston D. Clinical manifestations and therapy of herpes zoster ophthalmicus. *Compr Ophthalmol Update* 2002;3: 217–225.

196. Colin J, Prisant O, Cochener B, et al. A double blind randomized trial to compare the efficacy and safety of valaciclovir and acyclovir for treatment of herpes zoster ophthalmicus. *Ophthalmology* 2000;107:1507–1511.

197. Cobo L, Gomez-Carpio M, Ramirez J, et al. Oral acyclovir in the treatment of acute herpes zoster ophthalmicus. *Ophthalmology* 1986;93:763.

198. McGill J, Chapman C. Comparison of topical acyclovir with steroids in the treatment of herpes zoster keratouveitis. *Br J Ophthalmol* 1983;67:746.

199. McGill J, Chapman C, Copplestone A, et al. Review of acyclovir treatment of ocular herpes zoster and skin infections. *J Antimicrob Chemother* 1983; 12[Suppl B]:45.

200. Marsh R, Cooper M. Double masked trial of topical acyclovir and steroids in the treatment of herpes zoster ocular inflammation. *Br J Ophthalmol* 1991;75:542.

201. Zaal M, Maudgal PC, Rietveld E, et al. Chronic ocular zoster. *Curr Eye Res* 1991;10: 125–130.

202. Pepose J. The potential impact of varicella vaccine and new antivirals on ocular disease related to varicella-zoster virus. *Am J Ophthalmol* 1997;123:243–249.

203. Duker J, Blumenkranz M. Diagnosis and management of the acute retinal necrosis (ARN) syndrome. *Surv Ophthalmol* 1991;35:327–343.

204. Cobo L, Foulks GN, Liesegang T, et al. Oral acyclovir in the therapy of acute Herpes zoster ophthalmicus: an interim report. *Ophthalmology* 1985;92:1574–1583.

205. Borruat F, Buechi ER, Piguent B, et al. Prevention of ocular complications of herpes zoster ophthalmicus by adequate treatment with acyclovir. *Klin Monatsbl Augenheilkd* 1991;198: 358–360.

206. Harding S, Porter S. Oral acyclovir in herpes zoster ophthalmicus. *Curr Eye Res* 1991;10[Suppl]:177–182.

207. Hoang-Xuan T, Buechi ER, Herbort CP, et al. Oral acyclovir for herpes zoster ophthalmicus. *Ophthalmology* 1992;99: 1062–1071.

208. Aylward G, Claoue CM, Marsh RJ, et al. Influence of oral acyclovir on ocular complications of herpes zoster ophthalmicus. *Eye* 1994;8:70–74.

209. McGill J, White J. Acyclovir and post-herpetic neuralgia and ocular involvement. *BMJ* 1994;309:1124–1128.

210. Herbort CP, Buechi ER, Piguet B, et al. High-dose oral acyclovir in acute herpes zoster ophthalmicus: the end of the corticosteroid era. *Curr Eye Res* 1991;10[Suppl]:171–175.

211. U.S. Pharmacopeia: acyclovir. In: *United States Pharmacopeia drug information.* Englewood, CO: Micromedics, 2000:25–33.

212. Antimicrobials–antivirals: antiherpes. In: *Tarascon pocket pharmacopoeia.* Loma Linda, CA: Tarascon, 2003:40–41.

213. Morfin F, Thouvenot D, De Turenne-Tessier M, et al. Phenotypic and genetic characteristics of thymidine kinase from classical strains of varicella zoster virus resistant to acyclovir. *Antimicrob Agents Chemother* 1999;43:2412–2416.

214. Boivin G, Edelman CK, Pedneault L, et al. Phenotypic and genotypic characterization of acyclovir-resistant varicella zoster virus isolates from persons with AIDS. *J Infect Dis* 1994;170: 68–75.

215. Ida M, Kageyama S, Sato H, et al. Emergence of resistance in acyclovir and penciclovir in varicella zoster virus and genetic analysis of acyclovir-resistant variants. *Antiviral Res* 1999;40: 155–166.

216. Jacobson MA, Berger TG, Fikrig S, et al. Acyclovir-resistant varicella zoster virus infection after chronic oral acyclovir therapy in patients with the acquired immunodeficiency syndrome (AIDS). *Ann Intern Med* 1990;112:187–191.

217. Bodaghi B, Mougin C, Michelson S, et al. Acyclovir-resistant bilateral keratitis associated with mutations in the HSV-1 thymidine kinase gene. *Exp Eye Res* 2000;71:353–359.

218. Safrin S, Assaykeen T, Follensbee S, et al. Foscarnet therapy for acyclovir-resistant mucocutaneous herpes simplex virus infection in 26 AIDS patients. *J Infect Dis* 1990;161:1078–1084.

219. Chatis P, Miller CH, Schrager LE, et al. Successful treatment with foscarnet of an acyclovir-resistant mucocutaneous infection with herpes simplex virus in a patient with acquired immunodeficiency syndrome. *N Engl J Med* 1989;320:297–300.

220. Sonkin P, Baratz KH, Frothingham R, et al. Acyclovir-resistant herpes simplex virus keratouveitis after penetrating keratoplasty. *Ophthalmology* 1992; 99:1805–1808.

221. Soul-Lawton J, Seaber I, On N, et al. Absolute bioavailability and metabolic disposition of valaciclovir L-valyl ester of acyclovir following oral administration to humans. *Antimicrob Agents Chemother* 1995;39:2759–2764.

222. Ormrod D, Goa K. Valaciclovir: a review of its use in the management of herpes zoster. *Drugs* 2000;59:1317–1340.

223. Burnette T, deMiranda P. Purification and characterization of an enzyme from rat live that hydrolyzes 256487, the L-valyl ester prodrug of acyclovir (Zovirax). *Antiviral Res* 1993; 20[Suppl 1]:115.

224. Beutner K, Friedman DJ, Forszpaniak C, et al. Valaciclovir compared with acyclovir for improved therapy for herpes zoster in immunocompetent adults. *Antimicrob Agents Chemother* 1995;39:1546–1553.

225. Weller S, Blum M, Smiley M. Phase I pharmacokinetics of the acyclovir prodrug, valacyclovir. *Antiviral Res* 1993;20[Suppl 1]:144.

226. Perry C, Faulds D. Valaciclovir: a review of its antiviral activity, pharmacokinetic properties, and therapeutic efficacy in herpesvirus infections. *Drugs* 1996;52:754–772.

227. Takahashi K, Suzuki M, Iwata Y, et al. Selective activity of various nucleoside and nucleotide analogues against human herpesvirus 6 & 7. *Antivir Chem Chemother* 1997;81:24–31.

228. Kedes D, Ganem D. Sensitivity of Kaposi's sarcoma-associated herpes virus replication to antiviral drugs. *J Clin Invest* 1997;99:2082–2086.

229. Medveczky M, Horvath E, Lund T, et al. In vitro antiviral drug sensitivity of the Kaposi's sarcoma associated herpes virus. *AIDS* 1997;11:1327–1332.

230. Neyts J, De Clercq E. Antiviral drugs susceptibility of human herpes virus 8. *Antimicrob Agents Chemother* 1997;41:2754–2756.

231. Tyring S, Douglas JM Jr, Corey L, et al. A randomized, placebo-controlled comparison of oral valacyclovir and acyclovir in immunocompetent patients with recurrent genital herpes infections. *Arch Dermatol* 1998;134:185–191.

232. Fife K, Barbarash RA, Rudolph T, et al. Valaciclovir versus acyclovir in the treatment of first-episode genital herpes infection: results of an international, multicenter, double blind, randomized clinical trial. *Sex Transm Dis* 1995;24:481–486.

233. Fiddian A. Antiviral drugs in development for herpes zoster. *Scand J Infect Dis Suppl* 1996;100:51–54.

234. Herne K, Cirelli R, Lee P, et al. Antiviral therapy of acute herpes zoster in older patients. *Drugs Aging* 1996;8:97–112.

235. Tyring S, Beutner KR, Tucker BA, et al. Antiviral therapy for herpes zoster: randomized controlled clinical trial of valacyclovir and famciclovir therapy in immunocompetent patients 50 years and older. *Arch Fam Med* 2000;9:863–869.

236. Gnann JJ, Whitley R. Clinical practice: herpes zoster [review]. *N Engl J Med* 2002;347:340–346.

237. Colin J, Prisant O, Cochener B, et al. Comparison of the efficacy and safety of valaciclovir and acyclovir for the treatment of herpes zoster ophthalmicus: a double-blind trial to compare valaciclovir and aciclovir. *Ophthalmology* 2000;107:1507–1512.

238. Bodsworth N, Crooks RJ, Borelli S, et al. Valaciclovir versus aciclovir in patient initiated treatment of recurrent genital herpes. *Genitourin Med* 1997;73:110–116.

239. U.S. Pharmacopeia—Famvir. In: *United States Pharmacopeia drug information*. Englewood, CO: Micromedics, 2000:1501–1503.

240. Dhaliwal D, Romanowski EG, Yates KA, et al. Valaciclovir inhibition of recovery of ocular herpes simplex virus type 1 after experimental reactivation by laser in situ keratomileusis. *J Cataract Refract Surg* 2001;27:1288–1293.

241. Asbell P. Valaciclovir for prevention of recurrent herpes simplex virus eye disease after excimer laser photokeratectomy. *Trans Am Ophthalmol Soc* 2000;98:285–303.

242. Safrin S, Berger TG, Gilson I, et al. Foscarnet therapy in five patients with AIDS and acyclovir-resistant varicella-zoster virus infection. *Ann Intern Med* 1991;115:19–21.

243. Earnshaw D, Bacon TH, Darlison SJ, et al. Mode of antiviral action of penciclovir in MRC-5 cells infected with herpes simplex virus type 1 (HSV-1), HSV-α, and varicella-zoster virus. *Antimicrob Agents Chemother* 1992;36:2747–2757.

244. Vere Hodge R, Cheng Y-C. The mode of action of penciclovir. *Antivir Chem Chemother* 1993;4[Suppl 1]:13–24.

245. Boyd M, Safrin S, Kern E. Penciclovir: a review of spectrum of activity, selectivity, and cross-resistance pattern. *Antivir Chem Chemother* 1993;4[Suppl 1]:25–36.

246. deGreef H. Famciclovir, a new oral antiherpes drug: results of the first controlled clinical study demonstrating its efficacy and safety in the treatment of uncomplicated herpes zoster in immunocompetent patients. *Int J Antimicrob Agents* 1994;4:241–246.

247. Weinberg A, Bates BJ, Masters HB, et al. In vitro activities of penciclovir and acyclovir against herpes simplex virus types 1 and 2. *Antimicrob Agents Chemother* 1992;36:2037–2038.

248. Sacks S, Aoki FY, Diaz-Mitoma F, et al. Patient-initiated twice-daily oral famciclovir for early recurrent genital herpes. *JAMA* 1996;276:44–49.

249. Sacks S, Portnoy J, Tyrell LD, et al. Topical Edoxudine 3% cream: a double-blind, placebo controlled trial of the effect of chronically administered oral famciclovir on sperm production in men with recurrent genital herpes infection. *Antiviral Res* 1994;23[Suppl 1]:72.

250. Pue M, Benet L. Pharmacokinetics of famciclovir in man. *Antivir Chem Chemother* 1993;4(Suppl 1):47–55.

251. Loutsch J, Sainz B Jr, Marquart ME, et al. Effect of famciclovir on herpes simplex virus type 1 corneal disease and establishment of latency in rabbits. *Antimicrob Agents Chemother* 2001;45:2044–2053.

252. Tyring S, Engst R, Corriveau C, et al. Famciclovir for ophthalmic zoster: a randomised aciclovir controlled study. *Br J Ophthalmol* 2001;85:576–581.

253. Tyring S, Barbarash RA, Nahlik JE, et al. Famciclovir for the treatment of acute herpes zoster: effects on acute disease and post-herpetic neuralgia. *Ann Intern Med* 1995;123:89–96.

254. Tyring S. Efficacy of famciclovir in the treatment of herpes zoster. *Semin Dermatol* 1996;15[2 Suppl 1]:27–31.

255. deGreef H. Famciclovir, a new oral antiviral drug: its efficacy and safety in the treatment of uncomplicated herpes zoster in immunocompetent patients. *Int J Antimicrob Agents* 1995;4:241–246.

256. Huse D, Schainbaum S, Kirsch AJ, et al. Economic evaluation of famciclovir in reducing the duration of post herpetic neuralgia. *Am J Health Syst Pharm* 1997;54:1180–1184.

257. Ashton W, Karkas JD, Field AK, et al. Activation by thymidine kinase and potent antiherpetic activity of 2′-nor-2′-deoxyguanidine (2′NDG). *Biochem Biophys Res Commun* 1982;108:1716–1721.

258. Biron K, Stanat SC, Sorrell JB, et al. Metabolic activation of the nucleoside analog 9-[2-hydroxy-1-(hydroxymethyl) ethoxy] methylguanine in human diploid fibroblasts infected with human cytomegalovirus. *Proc Natl Acad Sci USA* 1985;82:2473–2477.

259. Buhles WC Jr, Mastre BJ, Tinker AJ, et al. Ganciclovir treatment of life or sight-threatening cytomegalovirus infection: experience in 314 immunocompromised patients. *Rev Infect Dis* 1988;10[Suppl]:S495–S506.

260. Causey D. Concomitant ganciclovir and zidovudine treatment for cytomegalovirus retinitis in patients with HIV infection: an approach to treatment. *J Acquir Immune Defic Syndr* 1991;4[Suppl 1]:S16–S21.

261. Jacobson M, de Miranda P, Cederberg DM, et al. Human pharmacokinetics and tolerance of oral ganciclovir. *Antimicrob Agents Chemother* 1987;31:1251–1254.

262. Matthews T, Boehme R. Antiviral activity and mechanism of action of ganciclovir. *Rev Infect Dis* 1988;10[Suppl 3]:S490–S494.

263. Anderson R, Griffy KG, Jung D, et al. Ganciclovir absolute bioavailability and steady state pharmacokinetics after oral administration of two 3000-mg/d dosing regimens in human immunodeficiency virus and cytomegalovirus-seropositive patients. *Clin Ther* 1995;17:425–432.

264. Colin J, Hoh HB, Easty DL, et al. Ganciclovir ophthalmic gel (Virgan; 0.15%) in the treatment of herpes simplex keratitis. *Cornea* 1997;16:393–399.

265. Jabs D, Martin BK, Forman MS, et al. Longitudinal observations on mutations conferring ganciclovir resistance in patients with acquired immunodeficiency syndrome in cytomegalovirus retinitis: the Cytomegalovirus and Viral Resistance Study Group report #8. *Am J Ophthalmol* 2001;132:700–710.

266. Bronson J, Ghazzouli I, Hitchcock MJ, et al. Synthesis and antiviral activity of the nucleoside analogue (S)-1-(3-hydroxy-2-phosphoylmethoxypropyl) cytosine. *J Med Chem* 1989;32:1457–1463.

267. Martin J, Hitchcock M. Phosphonomethyl ether compounds as antiviral agents. *Transplant Proc* 1991;23:156–158.

268. De Clercq E. Therapeutic potential of HPMPC as an antiviral drug. *Rev Med Virol* 1993;3:85–96.

269. Gordon Y, Romanowski E, Araullo-Cruz T. Topical HPMPC is the first effective broad spectrum antiviral to inhibit both HSV-1 and adenovirus in the NZ rabbit eye models. *Invest Ophthalmol Vis Sci* 1993;34[Suppl]:1396.

270. Gordon Y, Romanowski E, Araullo-Cruz T. HPMPC, a broad-spectrum topical antiviral agent, inhibits herpes simplex virus type 1 replication and promotes healing of dendritic keratitis in the rabbit ocular model. *Cornea* 1994;13:516–520.

271. Snoeck R, Holly A, Dewolf-Peeters C, et al. Antivaccinia activities of acyclic nucleoside phosphonate derivatives in epithelial

cells and organotypic cultures. *Antimicrob Agents Chemother* 2002;46:3356–3361.

272. Snoeck R, De Clercq E. Treatment of herpes simplex virus infections. *Infect Med* 1999;16:249–265.

273. U.S. Pharmacopeia—cidofovir. In: *United States Pharmacopeia drug information.* Englewood, CO: Micromedics, 2000: 895–896.

274. Ho HT, Woods KL, Bronson JJ, et al. Intracellular metabolism of the anti-herpes agent, (S)-1-[3-hydroxy-2-(phosphonyl-methoxy) propyl] cytosine. *Mol Pharmacol* 1992;41:197–202.

275. Snoeck R, Sakuma T, De Clercq E, et al. (S)-1-(3-hydroxy-2-phosphonylmethoxy-propyl) cytosine, a potent and selective inhibitor of human cytomegalovirus replication. *Antimicrob Agents Chemother* 1988;32:1839–1844.

276. Romanowski E, Gordon YJ, Araullo-Cruz T, et al. The antiviral resistance and replication of cidofovir-resistant adenovirus variants in the New Zealand white rabbit ocular model. *Invest Ophthalmol Vis Sci* 2001;42:1812–1815.

277. DeClerq E. Vaccinia and cidofovir. *Antimicrob Agents Chemother* 2002;46:3356– 3361.

278. Romanowski E, Bartels S, Gordon Y. Comparative antiviral efficacies of cidofovir, trifluridine and acyclovir in the HSV-1 rabbit keratitis model. *Invest Ophthalmol Vis Sci* 1999; 40:378–384.

279. Romanowski E, Gordon Y. Efficacy of topical cidofovir on multiple and adenoviral serotypes in the New Zealand ocular model. *Invest Ophthalmol Vis Sci* 2000;41:460–463.

280. Romanowski E, Yates K. Antiviral prophylaxis with twice daily topical cidofovir protects against challenge in the adenovirus type 5/New Zealand rabbit ocular model. *Antiviral Res* 2001; 52:275–280.

281. Smith I, Tashintuna I, Rahhal FM, et al. Clinical failure of CMV retinitis with intravitreal cidofovir is associated with antiviral resistance. *Arch Ophthalmol* 1998;116:178–185.

282. U.S. Pharmacopeia—foscarnet. In: *United States Pharmacopeia drug information.* Englewood, CO: Micromedics, 2000: 1601–1604.

283. Oberg B. Antiviral effects of phosphonoformate (PFA foscarnet sodium). *Pharmacol Ther* 1983;19:387–415.

284. Cheng YC, Grill S, Derse D, et al. Mode of action of PFA as an antiherpes simplex agent. *Biochim Biophys Acta* 1981;652: 90–98.

285. Erlich K, Mills J, Chatis P, et al. Acyclovir-resistant herpes simplex virus infections in patients with the acquired immunodeficiency syndrome. *N Engl J Med* 1989;320:293–296.

286. Fanning M, Read SE, Benson M, et al. Foscarnet therapy of cytomegalovirus retinitis in AIDS. *J Acquir Immune Defic Syndr* 1990;3:472–479.

287. Sjovall J, Bergdahl S, Movin G, et al. Pharmacokinetics of foscarnet and distribution to cerebrospinal fluid after intravenous infusion in patients with human immunodeficiency virus infection. *Antimicrob Agents Chemother* 1989;33:1023–1031.

288. Sjovall J, Karlsson A, Ogenstad S, et al. Pharmacokinetics and absorption of foscarnet after intravenous and oral administration to patients with human immunodeficiency virus. *Clin Pharmacol Ther* 1988;44:65–73.

289. Youle M, Clarbour J, Gazzard B, et al. Severe hypocalcemia in AIDS patients treated with foscarnet and pentamidine. *Lancet* 1988;1:1455–1456.

290. Palestine AG, Polis MA, De Smet MD, et al. A randomized controlled trial of foscarnet in the treatment of cytomegalovirus retinitis in patients with AIDS. *Ann Intern Med* 1991;115: 665–673.

291. Venard V, Dauendorffer JN, Carret AS, et al. Infection due to acyclovir resistant herpes simplex virus in patients undergoing allogeneic hematopoietic stem cell transplantation. *Pathol Biol (Paris)* 2001;49:553–558.

292. Bryant P, Sasadeusz J, Carapetis J, et al. Successful treatment of foscarnet-resistant herpes simplex stomatitis with intravenous cidofovir in a child. *Pediatr Infect Dis J* 2001;20:1083–1086.

293. Liesegang T, Melton LJ 3rd, Daly PJ, et al. Epidemiology of ocular herpes simplex: incidence in Rochester, MN, 1950–1982. *Arch Ophthalmol* 1989;107:1160–1166.

294. Pepose J, Leib DA, Stuart PM, et al. Herpes simplex virus diseases: anterior segment of the eye. In: Pepose J, Holland G, Wilhelmus K, eds. *Ocular infection and immunity.* St. Louis: Mosby, 1996:905–932.

295. Bell D, Holman R, Pavan-Langston D. Epidemiologic aspect of herpes simplex keratitis. *Ann Ophthalmol* 1982;14:421.

296. Hooks J. Ocular virology. In: Tabbara K, Hyndiuk R, eds. *Infections of the eye,* 2nd ed. Boston: Little, Brown, 1996:99–114.

297. Hyndiuk R, Glasser D. Herpes simplex keratitis. In: Tabbara K, Hyndiuk R, eds. *Infections of the eye,* 2nd ed. Boston: Little, Brown, 1996:361–386.

298. Nahmias A, Alford C, Korones S. Infection of the newborn with herpesvirus hominis. *Adv Pediatr* 1970;17:185.

299. Young T, Robin JB, Holland GN, et al. Herpes simplex keratitis in patients with acquired immune deficiency syndrome. *Ophthalmology* 1989;96:1476.

300. Schuman J, et al. Acquired immune deficiency syndrome. *Surv Ophthalmol* 1987;31:384–395.

301. Pavan-Langston D. *Living with herpes.* New York: Doubleday, 1983.

302. Moraes JH. Ocular manifestations of HIV/AIDS. *Curr Opin Ophthalmol* 2002;13:397–403.

303. Scott T. Epidemiology of herpetic infections. *Am J Ophthalmol* 1957;43:134.

304. Buddingh G, Schrum DI, Lanier JC, et al. Studies on the natural history of herpes simplex infections. *Pediatrics* 1953;11: 595–610.

305. Smith I, Peutherer J, MacCallum F. The incidence of herpesvirus hominis antibody in the population. *J Hyg (Camb)* 1967;65:395.

306. Lehner T, Wilton J, Shilltoe E. Immunological basis for latency, recurrences and putative oncogenicity of herpes simplex virus. *Lancet* 1975;2:60.

307. Stevens J, Wagner EK, Devi-Rao GB, et al. RNA complimentary to a herpes virus alpha gene mRNA is prominent in latently infected neurones. *Science* 1987;235:1056.

308. Shuster J, Kaufman H, Nesburn A. Statistical analysis of the rate of recurrence of herpes virus ocular epithelial disease. *Am J Ophthalmol* 1981;91:328.

309. Kimberlin D. Herpes simplex virus infections in the neonatal period. *Infect Med* 2002;19:462–474.

310. Cibis A, Bunde R. Herpes simplex virus induced congenital cataracts. *Arch Ophthalmol* 1971;85:220.

311. Hagler W, Walters P, Nahmias A. Ocular involvement in neonatal herpes simplex virus infection. *Arch Ophthalmol* 1969;82:169.

312. Hutchison D, Smith R, Haughton D. Congenital herpetic keratitis. *Arch Ophthalmol* 1975;93:70.

313. Inoda S, Wakakura M, Hirata J, et al. Stromal keratitis and anterior uveitis due to herpes simplex virus-2 in a young child. *Jpn J Ophthalmol* 2001;45:618–621.

314. Wilhelmus K, Coster DJ, Donovan HC, et al. Prognostic indicators of herpetic keratitis: analysis of a five year observation period after corneal ulceration. *Arch Ophthalmol* 1981;91:1578.

315. Azazi M, Gunilla M, Forsgren M. Late ophthalmologic manifestations of neonatal herpes simplex virus infection. *Am J Ophthalmol* 1990;109:1–7.

316. Croen K, Ostrove JM, Dragovic LJ, et al. Latent herpes simplex virus in human trigeminal ganglia: detection of an immediate early gene "anti-sense" transcript by in situ hybridization. *N Engl J Med* 1987;317:1427.

317. Croen K, Ostrove JM, Dragovic LJ, et al. Patterns of gene expression and sites of latency in human ganglia are different for varicella-zoster and herpes simplex viruses. *Proc Natl Acad Sci U S A* 1988;85:9773–9777.

318. Liesegang T. The biology and molecular aspects of herpes simplex and varicella zoster virus infections. *Ophthalmology* 1992;99:781–799.

319. Nesburn AB, Green MT, Radnoti M, et al. Reliable in vitro model for latent herpes simplex virus reactivation with peripheral virus shedding. *Infect Immun* 1977;15:772.

320. Baringer J. The virology of herpes simplex virus infection in humans. *Surv Ophthalmol* 1976;21:171.

321. Baringer J, Swoveland P. Recovery of herpes simplex virus from human trigeminal ganglions. *N Engl J Med* 1973;288:648.

322. Bastian F, Rabson AS, Yee CL, et al. Herpesvirus hominis: isolation from human trigeminal ganglion. *Science* 1972;178:306.

323. Kaye S, Madan N, Dowd TC, et al. Ocular shedding of herpes simplex virus. *Br J Ophthalmol* 1990;74:114.

324. Coyle P, Sibony P. Viral antibodies in normal tears. *Invest Ophthalmol Vis Sci* 1988;29:1552.

325. VanHorn D, Edelhauser H, Schultz R. Experimental herpes simplex keratitis: early alterations of corneal epithelium and stroma. *Arch Ophthalmol* 1970;84:67.

326. Kodama T, Hayasaka S, Setogawa T. Immunofluorescent staining and corneal sensitivity in patients suspected of having herpes simplex keratitis. *Am J Ophthalmol* 1992;113:187.

327. Remeijer L, Maertzdorf J, Buitenwerf J, et al. Corneal herpes simplex virus type 1 superinfection in patients with recrudescent herpetic keratitis. *Invest Ophthalmol Vis Sci* 2002;43:358–363.

328. Binder P. Review of treatment of ocular herpes simplex infections in the neonate and immunocompromised host. *Cornea* 1985;3:178.

329. Nimura M, Nishikawa T. Treatment of eczema herpeticum with oral acyclovir. *Am J Med* 1988;85:49–54.

330. Hodge W, Margolis T. Herpes simplex virus keratitis among patients who are positive or negative for human immunodeficiency virus. *Ophthalmology* 1997;104:120–124.

331. Baum J. Morphogenesis of the dendritic figure in herpes simplex keratitis: a negative study. *Am J Ophthalmol* 1970;70:722.

332. Mannis M, Garcia-Ferrer FJ, Davitt S. Superficial hypertrophic dendriform epitheliopathy post-keratoplasty. *Cornea* 1998;17:257–261.

333. Wilhelmus K. Interventions for herpes simplex virus epithelial keratitis [review]. *Cochrane Database Syst Rev* 2001;(1):CD002898.

334. Kaufman H. Epithelial erosion syndrome: metaherpetic keratitis. *Am J Ophthalmol* 1964;57:983.

335. Gundersen T. Herpes corneas: treatment with strong solution of iodine. *Arch Ophthalmol* 1936;12:225.

336. Cavanagh C, Colley A, Pihlaja D. Persistent corneal epithelial defects. *Int Ophthalmol Clin* 1979;19:197.

337. Cavanagh H. Herpetic ocular disease: therapy of persistent epithelial defects. *Int Ophthalmol Clin* 1975;15:67.

338. Sundmacher R, Neumann-Haefelin D. Herpes simplex virus isolations from the aqueous of patients suffering from focal iritis, endotheliitis, and prolonged disciform keratitis with glaucoma. *Surv Ophthalmol* 1981;27:342.

339. Kaufman H, Rayfield M. Viral conjunctivitis and keratitis. In: Kaufman H, et al., eds. *The cornea.* New York: Churchill Livingstone, 1988:299–332.

340. Robin J, Stergner J, Kaufman H. Progressive herpetic corneal endotheliitis. *Am J Ophthalmol* 1985;100:336.

341. Jones B, Falcon MG, Cantell K, et al. Symposium on herpes simplex eye disease: objectives in therapy. *Trans Ophthalmol Soc UK* 1977;97:305.

342. Pepose J. Herpes simplex keratitis: role of viral infection versus immune response. *Surv Ophthalmol* 1991;35:345–352.

343. Holbach L, Font R, Naumann G. Herpes simplex stromal and endothelial keratitis. *Ophthalmology* 1990;97:722.

344. Holbach L, Asano N, Naumann G. Infection of the corneal endothelium in herpes simplex keratitis. *Am J Ophthalmol* 1998;126:592–594.

345. Weiss N, Jones B. Problems of corneal grafting in herpetic keratitis. *Ciba Found Symp* 1973;15:220.

346. Dawson C, Togni B, Moore T Jr. Structural changes in chronic herpetic keratitis: studied by light and electron microscopy. *Arch Ophthalmol* 1968;79:740.

347. O'Brien W, Taylor J. The isolation of herpes simplex virus from rabbit corneas during latency. *Invest Ophthalmol Vis Sci* 1989;30:357.

348. Sabbaga E, Pavan-Langston D, Bean KM, et al. Detection of HSV nucleic acid sequences in the cornea during acute and latent ocular disease. *Exp Eye Res* 1988;47:545.

349. Rong B, Pavan-Langston D, Weng QP, et al. Detection of HSV thymidine kinase and latency-associated transcript gene expression in human herpetic corneas by polymerase chain reaction. *Invest Ophthalmol Vis Sci* 1991;32:1808.

350. Tullo A, Easty DL, Shimeld C, et al. Isolation of herpes simplex virus from corneal discs of patients with chronic stromal keratitis. *Trans Ophthalmol Soc UK* 1985;104:159.

351. Meyers R. Immunology of herpes simplex virus infection. *Int Ophthalmol Clin* 1975;15:37.

352. Meyers R, Smolin G, Hall JM, et al. Effect of local corticosteroids on antibody-forming cells in the eye and draining lymph nodes. *Invest Ophthalmol Vis Sci* 1975;14:138.

353. Meyers R, Chitjian P. Immunology of herpesvirus infection: immunity to herpes simplex virus in eye infections. *Surv Ophthalmol* 1976;21:194.

354. Meyers-Elliott R, Pettit T, Maxwell W. Viral antigens in the immune ring of herpes simplex stromal keratitis. *Arch Ophthalmol* 1980;98:897.

355. Meyers-Elliott R, Elliott JH, Maxwell WA, et al. HLA antigens in herpes stromal keratitis. *Am J Ophthalmol* 1980;89:54.

356. Meyers R, Pettit T. Corneal immune response to herpes simplex virus antigens. *J Immunol* 1973;110:575.

357. Lass J, Berman MB, Campbell RC, et al. Treatment of experimental herpetic interstitial keratitis with medroxyprogesterone. *Arch Ophthalmol* 1980;98:520.

358. Sundmacher R, Neumann-Haefelin D. Herpes simplex virus isolation from the aqueous of patients suffering from focal iritis, endotheliitis and prolonged disciform keratitis with glaucoma. *Klin Monatsbl Augenheilkd* 1979;175:488.

359. Sundmacher R. A clinico-virologic classification of herpetic anterior segment disease with special reference to intraocular herpes. In: Sundmacher R, ed. *Herpetic eye disease.* Munich: JF Bergmann Verlag, 1981:203.

360. Vogel A, Schneide RH, Loffler K. Histopathology of herpetic corneal endotheliitis: a case report [in German]. *Klin Monatsbl Augenheilkd* 2002;219:449–453.

361. Vannas A, Ahonen R. Herpetic endothelial keratitis. *Acta Ophthalmol* 1981;59:296.

362. Vannas A, Ahonen R, Makitie J. Corneal endothelium in herpetic keratouveitis. *Arch Ophthalmol* 1983;101:913.

363. Sutcliffe E, Baum J. Acute idiopathic corneal endotheliitis. *Ophthalmology* 1984;91:1161.

364. Pavan-Langston D, Brockhurst R. Herpes simplex panuveitis: a clinical report. *Arch Ophthalmol* 1969;81:783.

365. Collin H, Abelson M. Herpes simplex virus in human cornea, retrocorneal fibrous membrane and vitreous. *Arch Ophthalmol* 1976;94:1726.

366. Miserocchi, E, Waheed NK, Dios E, et al. Visual outcome in herpes simplex virus and varicella zoster virus uveitis. *Ophthalmology* 2002;109:1532–1537.

367. Pavan-Langston D, Rong B, Dunkel E. Extraneuronal herpetic latency: animal and human corneal studies. *Acta Ophthalmol* 1989;67[Suppl 192]:135.

368. Openshaw H, Asher LV, Wohlenberg C, et al. Acute and latent infection of sensory ganglia with herpes simplex virus: immune control and virus reactivation. *J Gen Virol* 1979;44:205.

369. Straus S. Clinical and biological differences between recurrent herpes simplex virus and varicella-zoster virus infections. *JAMA* 1989;262:3455–3458.

370. Openshaw H, Puga A, Notkins A. Herpes simplex virus infection in sensory ganglia: immune control, latency, and reactivation. *Fed Proc* 1979;38:2660–2664.

371. Puga A, Rosenthal JD, Openshaw H, et al. Herpes simplex virus DNA and mRNA sequences in acutely and chronically infected trigeminal ganglia of mice. *Virology* 1978;89:102–111.

372. Kaye S, Baker K, Bonshek R, et al. Human herpesviruses in the cornea. *Br J Ophthalmol* 2000;84:563–571.

373. Klein R. The pathogenesis of acute, latent, and recurrent herpes simplex infections. *Arch Virol* 1982;72:143–168.

374. Klein R. Pathogenic mechanisms of recurrent herpes simplex virus infections. *Arch Virol* 1976;51:1.

375. Claoue C, Hill T, Blyth W, et al. Clinical findings after zosteriform spread of herpes simplex virus to the eye of the mouse. *Curr Eye Res* 1987;6:281.

376. Liesegang T. Ocular herpes simplex infection: pathogenesis and current therapy. *Mayo Clin Proc* 1988;63:1092.

377. Wilhelmus K, Falcon M, Jones B. Bilateral herpetic keratitis. *Br J Ophthalmol* 1981;65:385.

378. Garrity J, Liesegang T. Ocular complications of atopic dermatitis. *Can J Ophthalmol* 1984;19:21.

379. Souza P, Holland E, Huang A. Bilateral herpetic keratoconjunctivitis. *Ophthalmology* 2003;110:493–496.

380. Centifanto Y, Little J, Kaufman H. Relationship between virus chemotherapy, secretory antibody formation and recurrent herpetic disease. *Ann NY Acad Sci* 1973;173:649.

381. Hammer H, Dobozy A. Cell mediated immunity to herpes virus type I in patients with recurrent corneal herpes simplex. *Acta Ophthalmol* 1980;58:161.

382. Spear P. Glycoproteins specified by herpes simplex viruses. In: Roizman B, ed. *The herpesviruses*. New York: Plenum Press, 1985:315.

383. Kaufman H, Varnell ED, Centifanto YM, et al. Effect of the herpes simplex virus genome on the response of infection to corticosteroids. *Am J Ophthalmol* 1985;100:114.

384. Centifanto-Fitzgerald Y, Yamaguchi T, Kaufman HE, et al. Ocular disease pattern induced by HSV is genetically determined by specific region of viral DNA. *J Exp Med* 1982;155:475.

385. Centifanto-Fitzgerald Y, Caldwell DR, Yates F. Herpes simplex virus: recurrent and nonrecurrent strains. *Proc Soc Exp Biol Med* 1987 Sep;185(4):484–492.

386. Centifanto-Fitzgerald Y, Varnell E, Kaufman H. Initial HSV-1 injection prevents ganglionic superinfection by other strains. *Infect Immun* 1982;35:1125.

387. Gordon Y, Araullo-Cruz T. Herpesvirus inoculation of cornea. *Am J Ophthalmol* 1984;97:482.

388. Blyth W, Hill TJ, Field HJ, et al. Reactivation of herpes simplex virus infection by ultraviolet light and possible involvement of prostaglandins. *J Gen Virol* 1976;33:547.

389. Laibson P, Kilbrick S. Reactivation of herpetic keratitis by epinephrine in rabbit. *Arch Ophthalmol* 1966;75:254.

390. Shimomura Y, et al. HSV-1 shedding by iontophoresis of 6-hydroxydopamine followed by topical epinephrine. *Invest Ophthalmol Vis Sci* 1983;24:1588.

391. Willey DE, Trousdale MD, Nesburn AB. Reaction of murine latent HSV infection by epinephrine iontophoreses. *Invest Ophthalmol Vis Sci* 1984;25:945.

392. Wand M, Gilbert C, Liesegang T. Latanoprost and herpes simplex keratitis. *Am J Ophthalmol* 1999;127:602–604.

393. Kroll D, Schuman J. Reactivation of herpes simplex virus keratitis after initiating bimatoprost treatment for glaucoma. *Am J Ophthalmol* 2002;133:401–403.

394. Perry H, Doshi SJ, Donnenfeld ED, et al. Herpes simplex reactivation following laser in situ keratomileusis and subsequent corneal perforation. *CLAO J* 2002;28:69–71.

395. Remeijer L, Maertzdorf J, Doornenbal P, et al. Herpes simplex virus 1 transmission through corneal transplantation. *Lancet* 2001;357:442–448.

396. Banerjee K, Deshpande S, Zheng M, et al. Herpetic stromal keratitis in the absence of viral antigen recognition. *Cell Immunol* 2002;219:108–118.

397. Maertzdorf J, Osterhaus A, Verjans G. IL-17 expression in human herpetic stromal keratitis: modulatory effects on chemokine production by corneal fibroblasts. *Immunology* 2002;169:5897–5903.

398. Osorio Y, Wechsler SL, Nesburn AB, et al. Reduced severity of HSV-1-induced corneal scarring in IL-12-deficient mice. *Virus Res* 2002;90:317–326.

399. Foster CS, Dubey DP, Stux S, et al. HLA phenotypic expression in patients with recurrent and non-recurrent herpes simplex keratitis. In: Sundmacher R, ed. *Herpetic eye diseases*. Munich: JF Bergmann Verlag, 1981:85.

400. Inoue T, Inoue Y, Hayashi K, et al. Effect of herpes simplex virus-1 gD or gD-IL-2 DNA vaccine on herpetic keratitis. *Cornea* 2002;21[7 Suppl]:S79–S85.

401. Keadle T, Laycock KA, Morris JL, et al. Therapeutic vaccination with vhs(−) herpes simplex virus reduces the severity of recurrent herpetic stromal keratitis in mice. *J Gen Virol* 2002; 83:2361–2365.

402. Stanberry L, Spruance SL, Cunningham AL, et al. Glycoprotein-D-adjuvant vaccine to prevent genital herpes. *N Engl J Med* 2002;347:1652–1661.

403. Koneman E, Allen S, Dowell VJ. *Color atlas and textbook of diagnostic microbiology*. Philadelphia: JB Lippincott, 1988: 691–764.

404. Pavan-Langston D, Dunkel E. A rapid clinical diagnostic test for herpes simplex infectious keratitis. *Am J Ophthalmol* 1988;107:675.

405. Solomon A. New diagnostic tests for herpes simplex and varicella zoster infections. *J Am Acad Dermatol* 1988;18:218–221.

406. Pavan-Langston D. Herpes keratitis: clinical features, diagnosis, treatment and prophylaxis. In: Remington J, ed. *Current clinical topics in infectious disease*. Boston: Blackwell Science, 2000:298–324.

407. Lairson D, Begley CE, Reynolds TF, et al. Prevention of herpes simplex virus eye disease: a cost-effectiveness analysis. *Arch Ophthalmol* 2003;121:108–112.

408. Foster CS. Nonsteroidal anti-inflammatory and immunosuppressive agents. In: Lamberts D, Potter D, eds. *Clinical ophthalmologic pharmacology*. Boston: Little, Brown, 1987:173.

409. Kleinert R. Corticosteroid use in ocular infectious disease. In: Tabbara K, Hyndiuk R, eds. *Infections of the eye*. Boston: Little, Brown, 1986:293.

410. Kleinert R, Palmer M. Antiinflammatory agents. In: Tabbara K, Hyndiuk R, eds. *Infections of the eye*, 2nd ed. Boston: Little, Brown, 1996:301–322.

411. Pavan-Langston D, Dunkel E. Corticosteroids, immunosuppressive agents, and non-steroidal anti-inflammatory drugs. In: *Handbook of ocular drug therapy and ocular side effects of systemic drugs*. Boston: Little, Brown, 1991:182.

412. Kibrick S, Takahashi GH, Leibowitz HM, et al. Local corticosteroid therapy and reactivation of herpetic keratitis. *Arch Ophthalmol* 1971;86:694.

413. Field A, Gottsch J. Persisting epithelial herpes simplex keratitis while on cyclosporin-A ointment. *Aust N Z J Ophthalmol* 1995;23:333–334.

414. Gunduz K, Ozdemir O. Topical cyclosporin as an adjunct to topical acyclovir treatment in herpetic stromal keratitis. *Ophthalmic Res* 1997;29:405–408.

415. Heiligenhaus A, Steuhl K. Treatment of HSV-1 stromal keratitis with topical cyclosporin A: a pilot study. *Graefes Arch Clin Exp Ophthalmol* 1999;237:435–438.

416. Perry H, Donnenfeld ED, Kanellopoulos AJ, et al. Topical cyclosporin A in the management of therapeutic keratoplasty for mycotic keratitis. *Cornea* 1997;16:284–288.

417. Goichot-Bonnat L, Chemla P, Pouliquen Y. Use of cyclosporin A eyedrops in the prevention of corneal graft rejection in man: I. preoperative development of 4 eyes with metaherpetic keratitis). *J Fr Ophtalmol* 1987;10:207–211.

418. Inoue K, Kimura C, Amano S, et al. Long-term outcome of systemic cyclosporine treatment following penetrating keratoplasty. *Jpn J Ophthalmol* 2001;45:378–382.

419. Burns F, Stack MS, Gray RD, et al. Inhibition of purified collagenase from alkali-burned rabbit corneas. *Invest Ophthalmol Vis Sci* 1989;30:1569.

420. Refojo M, Dohlman C, Koliopoulos J. Adhesives in ophthalmology: a review. *Surv Ophthalmol* 1971;15:217.

421. Foster C, Dunkin J. Penetrating keratoplasty for herpes simplex keratitis. *Am J Ophthalmol* 1981;92:336.

422. Langston R, Pavan-Langston D, Dohlman C. Penetrating keratoplasty for herpetic keratitis: prognostic and therapeutic determinants. *Trans Am Acad Ophthalmol Otolaryngol* 1975; 79:577.

423. Cohen E, Laibson P, Arentsen J. Corneal transplantation for herpes simplex keratitis. *Am J Ophthalmol* 1983;95:645.

424. Fine M, Cignetti F. Penetrating keratoplasty in herpes simplex keratitis. *Arch Ophthalmol* 1977;95:1755.

425. Cobo L, Coster D, Rice N, et al. Prognosis and management of corneal transplantation for herpetic keratitis. *Arch Ophthalmol* 1980;98:1755.

426. Ficker L, Kirkness C, Rice N, et al. Changing management and improved prognosis for corneal grafting and herpes simplex keratitis. *Ophthalmology* 1989;96:1587.

427. Mannis M, Plotnik R, Schwab I, et al. Herpes simplex dendritic keratitis after keratoplasty. *Am J Ophthalmol* 1991;111: 480–484.

428. Cleator G, Klapper P, Dennett C, et al. Corneal donor infection by herpes simplex virus: herpes simplex virus DNA in donor corneas. *Cornea* 1994;13:294–304.

429. Liekfeld A, Jaeckel C, Pleyer U, et al. Analysis of the aqueous humor in keratoplasty patients with keratitis: initial results [in German]. *Ophthalmologie* 2001;98:456–459.

430. van Gelderen B, Van der Lelij A, Treffers WF, et al. Detection of herpes simplex virus type 1, 2 and varicella zoster virus DNA in recipient corneal buttons. *Br J Ophthalmol* 2000;84: 1238–1243.

431. De Kesel R, Koppen C, Ieven M, et al. Primary graft failure caused by herpes simplex virus type 1. *Cornea* 2001;20: 187–190.

432. Zheng X. Reactivation and donor-host transmission of herpes simplex virus after corneal transplantation. *Cornea* 2002;21 [7 Suppl]:S90–S93.

433. Zheng X, Marquart ME, Loustch JM, et al. HSV-1 migration in latently infected and naive rabbits after penetrating keratoplasty. *Invest Ophthalmol Vis Sci* 1999;40:2490–2497.

434. Zheng X. Reactivation of herpes virus after lamellar keratoplasty. *Jpn J Ophthalmol* 1999;43:257–261.

435. Akova Y, Onat M, Duman S. Efficacy of low-dose and long-term oral acyclovir therapy after penetrating keratoplasty for herpes simplex keratitis. *Ocul Immunol Inflamm* 1999;7: 51–60.

436. Kaplowitz L, Baker D, Gelb L, et al. Prolonged continuous acyclovir treatment of normal adults with frequently recurring genital herpes simplex virus infection. *JAMA* 1991;265:747.

437. Mindel A, Long-term clinical and psychological management of genital herpes. *J Med Virol* 1993;1:39–44.

438. Corey L. Once daily antiherpetic agent for suppression of genital herpes. *Pharmacol Ther* 2002;27:546–547.

439. Jonas J, Rank R, Budde W. Visual outcome after allogenic penetrating keratoplasty. *Graefes Arch Clin Exp Ophthalmol* 2002;240:302–307.

440. Tabuchi K, Iwasaki Y, Shoji J, et al. Clinical study on surgical outcome of penetrating keratoplasty for herpetic leukoma [in Japanese]. *Nippon Ganka Gakkai Zasshim* 2002;106:293–296.

441. Halberstadt M, Machens M, Gahlenbek KA, et al. The outcome of corneal grafting in patients with stromal keratitis of herpetic and non-herpetic origin. *Br J Ophthalmol* 2002;86:646–652.

442. Rumelt S, Bersudsky V, Blum-Hareuveni T, et al. Preexisting and postoperative glaucoma in repeated corneal transplantation. *Cornea* 2002;21:759–765.

443. Gundersen T. Conjunctival flaps in treatment of corneal disease. *Arch Ophthalmol* 1958;6:880.

444. Thoft RA. Conjunctival transplantation. *Arch Ophthalmol* 1977;95:1425.

445. Rosenfeld S, Alfonso E, Gollamudi S. Recurrent herpes simplex infection in a conjunctival flap. *Am J Ophthalmol* 1993; 116:242–243.

446. Sharma N, Gupta V, Vanathi M, Agarwal T, Vajpayee RB, Satpathy G. Microbial keratitis following lamellar keratoplasy. *Cornea* 2004 Jul;23(5):472–478.

447. Preblud S, et al. Chicken pox in the United States 1972–1977. *J Infect Dis* 1979;140:257–263.

448. Preblud S. Age specific risks of varicella complication. *Pediatrics* 1981;68:14.

449. Cherry J. Chicken pox transmission. *JAMA* 1983;250:2060.

450. Wilson FI. Varicella and herpes zoster ophthalmicus. In: Tabbara K, Hyndiuk R, eds. *Infections of the eye*, 2nd ed. Boston: Little, Brown, 1996:387–400.

451. Gershon A, Steinberg S. Antibody responses to varicella-zoster virus and the role of antibody in host defense. *Am J Med* Sci 1981;282:12–17.

452. Weigle KA, Grose C. Molecular dissection of the humoral immune response to individual varicella-zoster viral proteins during chickenpox, quiescence, reinfection, and reactivation. *J Infect Dis* 1984;149:741–749.

453. Edwards T. Ophthalmic complications of varicella. *J Pediatr Ophthalmol* 1965;2:37.

454. Lambert SR, Taylor D, Kriss A, et al. Ocular manifestations of the congenital varicella syndrome. *Arch Ophthalmol* 1989; 107:52.

455. Gershon A. Varicella in mother and infant. In: Krugman S, Gershon A, eds. *Infections of the fetus and the newborn infant*. New York: Alan R. Liss, 1975.

456. Gershon A. Varicella-zoster virus: prospects for control. *Adv Pediatr Infect Dis* 1995;10:93–124.

457. deFreitas D, Sato E, Pavan-Langston D, et al. Delayed onset varicella keratitis. *Cornea* 1992;11:471–474.

458. Nesburn A, Borit A, Pentelei-Molnar J, et al. Varicella dendritic keratitis. *Invest Ophthalmol* 1974;13:764.

459. Strachman J. Uveitis associated with chicken pox. *J Pediatr* 1955;46:327.

460. Uchida Y, Kaneko M, Hayashi K. Varicella dendritic keratitis. *Am J Ophthalmol* 1980;89:259.

461. Wilhelmus K, Hamill M, Jones D. Varicella disciform stromal keratitis. *Am J Ophthalmol* 1991;111:575–580.

462. Power W, Hogan N, Hu S, et al. Primary varicella-zoster keratitis diagnosis by polymerase chain reaction. *Am J Ophthalmol* 1997;123:252–254.

463. Knoll L, Watson A. Internal ophthalmoplegia following chicken pox. *Can J Ophthalmol* 1976;11:267.

464. Robb R. Cataracts acquired following varicella infection. *Arch Ophthalmol* 1972;87:352.

465. Taylor D, Ffytche T. Optic disc pigmentation associated with a field defect following chicken pox. *J Pediatr Ophthalmol* 1976;13:80.

466. Centers for Disease Control and Prevention. Licensure of varicella virus vaccine, live. *MMWR Morb Mortal Wkly Rep* 1995;44:264.

467. Asano Y, Suga S, Yoshikawa T, et al. Experience and reason: twenty-year follow-up of protective immunity of the Oka strain live varicella vaccine. *Pediatrics* 1994;94:524–526.

468. Gershon AA, Steinberg SP, Gelb L, et al. Live attenuated varicella vaccine use in immunocompromised children and adults. *Pediatrics* 1986;78[Suppl]:757–762.

469. Kuter B, Weibel RE, Guess HA, et al. Oka/Merck varicella vaccine in healthy children: final report of a 2-year efficacy study and 7-year follow-up studies. *Vaccine* 1991;9:643–647.

470. Galil K, Lee B, Strome T, et al. Outbreak of varicella at a day-care center despite vaccination. *N Engl J Med* 2002;347:1909–1915.

471. Trannoy E, Berger R, Hollander G, et al. Vaccination of immunocompetent elderly subjects with a live attenuated Oka strain of varicella zoster virus: a randomized, controlled, dose-response trial. *Vaccine* 2000;18:1700–1706.

472. Hardy I, Gershon A, Sterinberg S, et al. The incidence of zoster after immunization with live attenuated varicella vaccine: a study in children with leukemia. *N Engl J Med* 1991;325:1545–1550.

473. Brunell P, Taylor-Wiedeman J, Geiser C, et al. Risk of herpes zoster in children with leukemia: varicella vaccine compared with history of chickenpox. *Pediatrics* 1986;77:53–56.

474. White C. Letter to the editor. *Pediatrics* 1992;89:354.

475. Matsubara K, et al. Herpes zoster in a normal child after varicella vaccination. *Acta Paediatr Jpn* 1995;37:648–650.

476. Naseri A, Good W, Cunningham EJ. Herpes zoster virus sclerokeratitis and anterior uveitis in a child following varicella vaccination. *Am J Ophthalmol* 2003;135:415–417.

477. Ragozzino M, et al. Risk of cancer after herpes zoster: a population based study. *N Engl J Med* 1982;307:393.

478. Liesegang T. Diagnosis and therapy of herpes zoster ophthalmicus. *Ophthalmology* 1991;98:1216–1229.

479. Miller A. Selective decline in cellular immune response to varicella-zoster in the elderly. *Neurology* 1980;30:582.

480. Dolin R, Reichman RC, Mazur MH, et al. Herpes zoster varicella infections in immunosuppressed patients. *Ann Intern Med* 1978;89:375.

481. Ragozzino M, Melton LJ 3rd, Kurland LT, et al. Population based study of Herpes zoster and its sequellae. *Medicine (Baltimore)* 1982;61:310.

482. Rand K, Rasmussen LE, Pollard RB, et al. Cellular immunity and herpes virus infections in cardiac transplant patients. *N Engl J Med* 1977;296:1372.

483. Hope-Simpson R. The nature of herpes zoster: a long term study and a new hypothesis. *Proc Soc Med* 1965;58:9.

484. Berger R, Florent G, Just M. Decrease of the lymphoproliferative response to varicella zoster antigen in the aged. *Infect Immun* 1981;32:24.

485. Kumagai T, Chiba Y, Wataya Y, et al. Development and characteristic of the cellular immune response to infection with varicella-zoster virus. *J Infect Dis* 1980;141:7.

486. Cole E, Meisler DM, Calabrese LH, et al. Herpes zoster ophthalmicus and acquired immune deficiency syndrome. *Arch Ophthalmol* 1984;102:1027.

487. Whitley R, Soorg SJ, Dolin R, et al. Early vidarabine therapy to control the complications of herpes zoster in immunosuppressed patients. *N Engl J Med* 1982;307:971.

488. Scheie H. Herpes zoster ophthalmicus. *Trans Ophthalmol Soc UK* 1970;90:899.

489. Goodman R, Jaffe E, Filler R, et al. Herpes zoster in children with stage I–III Hodgkin's disease. *Radiology* 1976;118:429.

490. Edgerton A. Herpes zoster ophthalmicus: report of cases and review of literature. *Arch Ophthalmol* 1945;34:40–62.

491. Liesegang T. Varicella-zoster virus: systemic and ocular features. *J Am Acad Dermatol* 1984;11:165.

492. Womack L, Liesegang T. Complications of herpes zoster ophthalmicus. *Arch Ophthalmol* 1983;101:42.

493. Freidman-Kein A. Herpes zoster: a possible clinical sign for development of acquired immune deficiency syndrome in high risk individuals. *J Am Acad Dermatol* 1986;14:1023–1028.

494. Pavan-Langston D. Major ocular viral infections. In: Galasso G, Whitley R, Merrigan T, eds. *Antiviral agents and viral diseases of man.* New York: Raven Press, 1990:183.

495. Sandor E, Millman A, Croxson TS, et al. Herpes zoster ophthalmicus in patients at risk for the acquired immune deficiency syndrome (AIDS). *Am J Ophthalmol* 1986;101:153.

496. Kurland L. Descriptive epidemiology of selected neurological and myopathic disorders with particular reference to a survey in Rochester, Minnesota. *J Chronic Dis* 1958;8:378.

497. Ruppenthal M. Changes of the central nervous system in herpes zoster. *Acta Neuropathol (Berl)* 1980;52:59.

498. Esiri M, Tomlinson A. Herpes zoster: demonstration of virus in trigeminal nerve and ganglion by immunofluorescence and electron microscopy. *J Neurol Sci* 1972;15:35–38.

499. Pratesi R, Freemon F, Lowry J. Herpes zoster ophthalmicus with contralateral hemiplegia. *Arch Neurol* 1977;34:640.

500. Liesegang T. Corneal complications from herpes zoster ophthalmicus. *Ophthalmology* 1985;92:316.

501. Marsh R. Ophthalmic herpes zoster. *Br J Hosp Med* 1976;15:609–618.

502. Sauer G. Herpes zoster. *Arch Dermatol* 1955;71:488–491.

503. Yong V, Yip C, Yong V. Herpes zoster ophthalmicus and the superior orbital fissure syndrome. *Singapore Med J* 2001;42:485–486.

504. Uchida Y, Kaneko M, Onishi Y. Ophthalmic herpes zoster without eruption. In: Henkind P, ed. *Acta: XXIV International Congress of Ophthalmology.* Philadelphia: JB Lippincott, 1983:876.

505. Yamamoto S, Shimomura Y, Kinoshita S, et al. Differentiating zosteriform herpes simplex from ophthalmic zoster. *Arch Ophthalmol* 1994;112:1515–1516.

506. Al-Abdulla N, Rismondo V, Minkowski JS, et al. Herpes zoster vasculitis presenting as giant cell arteritis with bilateral internuclear ophthalmoplegia. *Am J Ophthalmol* 2002;134:912–914.

507. Sodhi P, Goel J. Presentations of cranial nerve involvement in two patients with herpes zoster ophthalmicus. *J Commun Dis* 2001;33:130–135.

508. Pandey P, Chaudhuri Z, Sharma P. Extraocular muscle and facial paresis in herpes zoster ophthalmicus. *J Pediatr Ophthalmol Strabismus* 2001;38:363–366.

509. Hallas P. Pupillary paresis: a rare complication of varicella zoster eye infection [in Danish]. *Ugeskr Laeger* 2001;163:5835–5836.

510. Archambault P, Wise JS, Rosen J, et al. Herpes zoster ophthalmoplegia: report of six cases. *J Clin Neuroophthalmol* 1988;8:185–193.

511. Naumann G, Gass J, Font R. Histopathology of herpes zoster ophthalmicus. *Am J Ophthalmol* 1968;65:533.

512. Obata H, Yamagami S, Saito S, et al. A case of acute dacryoadenitis associated with herpes zoster ophthalmicus. *Jpn J Ophthalmol* 2003;47:107–109.

513. Pavan-Langston D, McCulley J. Herpes zoster dendritic keratitis. *Arch Ophthalmol* 1973;89:25.

514. Piebenga L, Laibson P. Dendritic lesions in herpes zoster ophthalmicus. *Arch Ophthalmol* 1973;90:268.

515. Marsh R, Cooper M. Ophthalmic zoster: mucous plaque keratitis. *Br J Ophthalmol* 1987;71:725–728.

516. Zaal M, Volker-Dieben HJ, Weinesen M, et al. Longitudinal analysis of varicella-zoster virus DNA on the ocular surface associated with herpes zoster ophthalmicus. *Am J Ophthalmol* 2001;131:25–29.

517. Hedges T III, Albert D. The progression of the ocular abnormalities of herpes zoster: histopathologic observations of nine cases. *Ophthalmology* 1982;89:169–177.

518. Wenkel H, Rummelt V, Fleckenstein B, et al. Detection of varicella zoster virus DNA and viral antigen in human eyes after herpes zoster ophthalmicus. *Ophthalmology* 1998;105:1323–1330.

519. Wenkel H, Rummelt C, Rummelt V, et al. Detection of varicella zoster virus DNA and viral antigen in human cornea after herpes zoster ophthalmicus. *Cornea* 1993;12:131–137.

520. Yu D, Lemp MA, Mathers WD, et al. Detection of varicella-zoster virus DNA in disciform keratitis using polymerase chain reaction. *Arch Ophthalmol* 1993;111:167–168.

521. Green W, Zimmerman L. Granulomatous reaction of Descemet's membrane. *Am J Ophthalmol* 1967;64:555.

522. Zaal M, Volker-Dieben H, D'Amaro J. Risk and prognostic factors of postherpetic neuralgia and focal sensory denervation: a prospective evaluation in acute herpes zoster ophthalmicus. *Clin J Pain* 2000;16:345–351.

523. Heigle T, Pflugfelder S. Aqueous tear production in patients with neurotrophic keratitis. *Cornea* 1996;15:135–138.

524. Nagashima K, Nakazawa M, Endo H. Pathology of the human spinal ganglia in varicella-zoster virus infection. *Acta Neuropathol (Berl)* 1975;33:105–117.

525. Ghatak N, Zimmerman H. Spinal ganglion in herpes zoster. *Arch Pathol* 1973;95:411–415.

526. Marsh R, Easty D, Jones B. Iritis and iris atrophy in herpes zoster ophthalmicus. *Am J Ophthalmol* 1974;78:255.

527. Yamamoto S, Tada R, Shimomura Y, et al. Detecting varicella-zoster virus DNA in iridocyclitis using polymerase chain reaction: a case of zoster sine herpete. *Arch Ophthalmol* 1995;113:1358–1359.

528. Nakashizuka H, Yamazaki Y, Tokumaru M, et al. Varicella-zoster viral antigen identified in iridocyclitis patient. *Jpn J Ophthalmol* 2002;46:70–73.

529. Kezuka T, Sakai J, Minoda H, et al. A relationship between varicella-zoster virus-specific delayed hypersensitivity and varicella-zoster virus-induced anterior uveitis. *Arch Ophthalmol* 2002;120:1183–1188.

530. Thean J, Hall A, Stawell R. Uveitis in herpes zoster ophthalmicus. *Clin Exp Ophthalmol* 2001;29:406–410.

531. deMoragas J, Kierland R. The outcome of patients with herpes zoster. *Arch Dermatol* 1957;75:193.

532. Opstelten W, Mauritz JW, de Wit NJ, et al. Herpes zoster and postherpetic neuralgia: incidence and risk indicators using a general practice research database. *Fam Pract* 2002;19:471–475.

533. Harrison R, Soong S, Weiss HL, et al. A mixed model for factors predictive of pain in AIDS patients with herpes zoster. *J Pain Symptom Manage* 1999;17:410–417.

534. Oaklander A, Cohen S, Raju S. Intractable postherpetic itch and cutaneous deafferentation after facial shingles. *Pain* 2002;96:9–12.

535. Pappagallo M, Oaklander AL, Quatrono-Piacentini AL, et al. Heterogenous patterns of sensory dysfunction in postherpetic neuralgia suggest multiple pathophysiologic mechanisms. *Anesthesiology* 2000;92:691–698.

536. Oaklander A. The density of remaining nerve endings in human skin with and without postherpetic neuralgia after shingles. *Pain* 2001;92:139–145.

537. Oaklander A, Rissmiller J. Postherpetic neuralgia after shingles: an under-recognized cause of chronic vulvar pain. *Obstet Gynecol* 2002;99:625–628.

538. Watson C, Deck JH, Morshead C, et al. Post-herpetic neuralgia: further post-mortem studies of cases with and without pain. *Pain* 1991;44:105–117.

539. Vafai A, Murray RS, Wellish M, et al. Expression of varicella-zoster virus and herpes simplex virus in normal human trigeminal ganglia. *Proc Natl Acad Sci USA* 1988;85:2362–2366.

540. Gilden D, Wright RR, Schneck SA, et al. Zoster sine herpete: a clinical variant. *Ann Neurol* 1994;35:530–533.

541. Kashiwase M, Sakai J, Usui M. Uveitis associated with zoster sine herpete: diagnosis and clinical findings [in Japanese]. *Nippon Ganka Gakkai Zasshim* 2000;104:97–102.

542. Nakamura M, Tanabe M, Yamada Y, et al. Zoster sine herpete with bilateral ocular involvement. *Am J Ophthalmol* 2000;129:809–810.

543. Furuta Y, Ohtani F, Mesuda Y, et al. Early diagnosis of zoster sine herpete and antiviral therapy for the treatment of facial palsy. *Neurology* 2000;55:708–710.

544. Tabery H. Corneal epithelial keratitis in herpes zoster ophthalmicus: "delayed" and "sine herpete." A non-contact photomicrographic in vivo study in the human cornea. *Eur J Ophthalmol* 2002;12:267–275.

545. Tabery H. Morphology of epithelial keratitis in herpes zoster ophthalmicus: a non-contact photomicrographic in vivo study in the human cornea. *Acta Ophthalmol Scand* 2000;78:651–655.

546. Silverstein B, Chandler D, Neger R, et al. Disciform keratitis: a case of herpes zoster sine herpete. *Am J Ophthalmol* 1997;123:254–255.

547. Thomas M, Robertson W. Dermal transmission of a virus as a cause of shingles. *Lancet* 1968;2:1349.

548. Weller T. Varicella and herpes zoster: changing concepts of the natural history, control, and importance of a not so benign virus. Parts 1 and 2. *N Engl J Med* 1983;309:1362–1368, 1434–1440.

549. Gilden D, Vafai A, Shtram Y, et al. Varicella-zoster virus DNA in human sensory ganglia. *Nature* 1983;306:478–480.

550. Bastian F, Rabson FO, Yee CL, et al. Herpes virus varicella isolated from human dorsal root ganglia. *Arch Pathol* 1974;97:331–336.

551. Dueland A. Latency and reactivation of varicella zoster virus infections. *Scand J Infect Dis Suppl* 1996;100:46–50.

552. Wilson A, Sharp M, Koropchak CM, et al. Subclinical varicella-zoster virus viremia, herpes zoster, and T-lymphocyte immunity to varicella-zoster viral antigens after bone marrow transplantation. *J Infect Dis* 1992;165:119–126.

553. Gilden D, Dueland AN, Devlin ME, et al. Varicella-zoster virus reactivation without rash. *J Infect Dis* 1992;166[Suppl 1]:S30–S34.

554. Lewis G. Zoster sine herpete. *BMJ* 1958;2:418.

555. Doyle P, Gibson G, Dohlman C. Herpes zoster ophthalmicus with contralateral hemiplegia: identification of cause. *Ann Neurol* 1983;14:84–85.

556. Bhat G, Mathur DS, Saxena GN, et al. Granulomatous angiitis of the central nervous system associated with herpes zoster. *J Assoc Physicians India* 2002;50:977–978.

557. Gilden D, Devlin DH, Wellish M, et al. Persistence of varicella-zoster virus DNA in blood mononuclear cells of patients with varicella or zoster. *Virus Genes* 1989;2:299–305.

558. Severson E, Baratz EA, Hodge DO, et al. Herpes zoster ophthalmicus in Olmsted County, Minn: have systemic antivirals made a difference? *Arch Ophthalmol* 2003;121:386–390.

559. Nikkels A, Pierard G. Oral antivirals revisited in the treatment of herpes zoster: what do they accomplish? *Am J Clin Dermatol* 2002;3:591–598.

560. Wood M, Shukla S, Fiddian AP, et al. Treatment of acute herpes zoster: effects of early (<48h) versus late (>48–72 h) therapy with acyclovir or valacyclovir on prolonged pain. *J Infect Dis* 1998;178: S81–S84.

561. Bergaust B, Westby R. Zoster ophthalmicus: local treatment with cortisone. *Acta Ophthalmol* 1967;45:787.

562. Carter A, Royds J. Systemic steroids in herpes zoster. *BMJ* 1957;2:746.

563. Elliott R. Treatment of herpes zoster with high doses of prednisone. *Lancet* 1964;2:610.

564. Keczkes K, Basheer A. Do corticosteroids prevent post-herpetic neuralgia? *Br J Dermatol* 1980;101:551.

565. Esmann V, Geil JP, Kroon S, et al. Prednisolone does not prevent post-herpetic neuralgia. *Lancet* 1987;2:126.

566. Whitley R, Weiss H, Gnann JW Jr, et al. Acyclovir with and without prednisone for the treatment of herpes zoster: a randomized, placebo-controlled trial. The National Institute of Allergy and Infectious Diseases Collaborative Antiviral Study Group. *Ann Intern Med* 1996;125:376–383.

567. Wood M, Johnson RW, McKendrick MW, et al. A randomized trial of acyclovir for 7 days and 21 days with and without prednisolone for treatment of acute herpes zoster. *N Engl J Med* 1994;330:896–900.

568. Merselis J, Kaye D, Hook E. Disseminated herpes zoster. *Arch Intern Med* 1961;113:679.

569. Bowsher D. The effects of preemptive treatment of postherpetic neuralgia with amitriptyline: a randomized, double-blind, placebo-controlled trial. *J Pain Symptom Manage* 1997;13: 327–331.

570. Satterthwaite J, Tollison C, Kriegel M. Use of tricyclic antidepressants for the treatment of intractable pain. *Compr Ther* 1990;16:10.

571. Kvinesdal B, Molin J, Froland A, et al. Imipramine treatment of painful diabetic neuropathy. *JAMA* 1984;251:1727.

572. Watson C, Evans R, Reed K. Amitriptyline vs placebo in postherpetic neuralgia. *Neurology* 1982;32:671.

573. Watson C, Vernich L, Chipman M, et al. Nortriptyline versus amitriptyline in postherpetic neuralgia: a randomized trial. *Neurology* 1998;51:1166–1171.

574. Hurtig H. Fluphenazine and post-herpetic neuralgia. *JAMA* 1990;263:2750.

575. Murphy T. Post-herpetic neuralgia. *JAMA* 1989;262:3478.

576. Galen B. Neuropathic pain of peripheral origin: advances in pharmacologic treatment. *Neurology* 1995;45[Suppl 9]: S17–S25.

577. Dworkin R, Schmader K. Treatment and prevention of postherpetic neuralgia [review]. *Clin Infect Dis* 2003;36:877–882.

578. Dworkin R, Corbin AE, Young JP Jr, et al. Pregabalin for the treatment of postherpetic neuralgia: a randomized, placebo-controlled trial. *Neurology* 2003;60:1274–1283.

579. Watson C. The treatment of neuropathic pain: antidepressants and opioids [review]. *Clin J Pain* 2000;16[2 Suppl]:S49–S55.

580. Watson C, Babul N. Efficacy of oxycodone in neuropathic pain: a randomized trial in postherpetic neuralgia. *Neurology* 1998;50:1837–1841.

581. Levine J, Gordon NC, Smith R, et al. Desipramine enhances opiate postoperative analgesia. *Pain* 1986;27:45.

582. Kotani N, Kushikata T, Hashimoto H, et al. Intrathecal methylprednisolone for intractable postherpetic neuralgia. *N Engl J Med* 2000;343:1514–1519.

583. Watson P. Therapeutic advances in the management of postherpetic neuralgia. *Geriatr Med Today* 1988;70:20.

584. Watson C. Topical capsaicin as an adjuvant analgesic [review]. *J Pain Symptom Manage* 1994;9:425–433.

585. Gain P, Thuret G, Chiquet C, et al. Facial anesthetic blocks in the treatment of acute pain during ophthalmic zoster [in French]. *J Fr Ophtalmol* 2003;26:7–14.

586. Gain P, Thuret G, Chiquet C, et al. Frontal and nasal nerve blocks in the treatment of severe pain in acute ophthalmic zoster. *Anesth Analg* 2002;95:503.

587. Harding S, Lipton JR, Wells JC, et al. Relief of acute pain in herpes zoster ophthalmicus by stellate ganglion block. *Br Med J* 1986;292:1428.

588. Makensen G, Sundmacher R, Witschel D. Late wound complications after circular keratotomy for zoster keratitis. *Cornea* 1984;3:95.

589. Marsh RJ, Marshall J. Treatment of lipid keratopathy with the argon laser. *Br J Ophthalmol* 1982;66:127–135.

590. Reed J, Joyner S, Knauer W III. Penetrating keratoplasty for herpes zoster keratopathy. *Am J Ophthalmol* 1989;107:257.

591. Marsh R, Cooper M. Ocular surgery in ophthalmic zoster. *Eye* 1989;3:313–317.

592. Tanure M, Cohen EJ, Grewel S, et al. Penetrating keratoplasty for varicella-zoster virus keratopathy. *Cornea* 2000;19:135–139.

593. Yaghouti F, Dohlman C. Innovations in keratoprosthesis: proved and unproved. In: Jakobiec F, Krystolik M, eds. *Surgical advances in ophthalmology*. Philadelphia: Lippincott Williams & Wilkins, 1999:27–36.

594. Chapman R, Cross K, Fleming D. The incidence of shingles and its implications for vaccination policy. *Vaccine* 2003;21: 2541–2547.

595. Wack R. An outbreak of varicella despite vaccination. *N Engl J Med* 2003;348:1405–1407.

596. Henle W, Henle G. Serodiagnosis of infectious mononucleosis. *Resident Staff Phys* 1981;27:37.

597. Matoba A. Epstein-Barr virus diseases. In: Pepose J, Holland G, Wilhelmus K, eds. *Ocular infection and immunity*. St. Louis: Mosby, 1996:958–969.

598. Niederman J, Evans AS, Subrahmanyan L, et al. Prevalence, incidence and persistence of EB virus antibody in young adults. *N Engl J Med* 1970;272:361.

599. Straus S. Epstein-Barr virus and human herpesvirus type VI. In: Galasso GJ, Whitley R, Merigan TC, eds. *Antiviral agents and viral diseases of man*. New York: Raven Press, 1990:647.

600. Stagno S, Whitley R. Herpes virus infections of pregnancy. Parts I and II: cytomegalovirus and Epstein-Barr virus infections. *N Engl J Med* 1985;313:1270–1275, 1327–1332.

601. McCallum R. Infectious mononucleosis and the Epstein-Barr virus. *J Infect Dis* 1970;121:347.

602. Sugiyama K, Ito M, Ichimi R, et al. A case of Epstein-Barr virus infection with exophthalmos and ocular muscle swelling. *Acta Paediatr Jpn* 1997;39:694–697.

603. Meisler D, Bosworth D, Krachmer J. Ocular infectious mononucleosis manifested as Parinaud's oculoglandular syndrome. *Am J Ophthalmol* 1981;92:722.

604. Merayo-Lloves J, Baltatzis S, Foster CS. Epstein-Barr virus dacryoadenitis resulting in keratoconjunctivitis sicca in a child. *Am J Ophthalmol* 2001;132:922–923.

605. Willoughby C, Baker K, Kaye SB, et al. Epstein-Barr virus (types 1 and 2) in the tear film in Sjögren's syndrome and HIV infection. *J Med Virol* 2002;68:378–383.

606. Slobod K, Sandlund JT, Spiegel PH, et al. Molecular evidence of ocular Epstein-Barr virus infection. *Clin Infect Dis* 2000;31: 184–188.

607. Aaberg T, O'Brien W. Expanding ophthalmologic recognition of Epstein-Barr virus infections. *Am J Ophthalmol* 1987;104:420.

608. Matoba A, McCulley J. Epstein-Barr virus and its ocular manifestations. In: Darrell RW, ed. *Viral diseases of the eye*. Philadelphia: Lea & Febiger, 1985.

609. Matoba A, Wilhelmus K, Jones D. Epstein-Barr viral stromal keratitis. *Ophthalmology* 1986;93:1986.

610. Wilhelmus K. Ocular involvement in infectious mononucleosis. *Am J Ophthalmol* 1981;91:117.
611. Pflugfelder S, Huang C, Crouse C. Epstein-Barr virus keratitis after a facial chemical peel. *Am J Ophthalmol* 1990;110:571.
612. Pinnolis M, McCulley J. Nummular keratitis associated with infectious mononucleosis. *Am J Ophthalmol* 1980;89:791.
613. Chodosh J, Gan Y, Sixbey J. Detection of Epstein-Barr virus genome in ocular tissues. *Ophthalmology* 1996;103:687–690.
614. Wong K, D'Amico DJ, Hedges TR 3rd, et al. Ocular involvement associated with chronic Epstein-Barr virus disease. *Arch Ophthalmol* 1987;105:788–792.
615. Morishima N, et al. A case of uveitis associated with chronic active Epstein-Barr virus infection. *Ophthalmologica* 1996;210:186–188.
616. Henle G, Henle W. Immunofluorescence, interference and complement fixation techniques in detection of the herpes-type virus in Burkitt tumor cell lines. *Cancer Res* 1967;27:2442.
617. Fife K, Crumpacker CS, Mertz GJ, et al. Recurrence and resistance patterns of herpes simplex virus following cessation of > 6 years of chronic suppression with acyclovir. *J Infect Dis* 1994;169:1338–1341.
618. Ogawa G, Vastine D. Nonherpetic viral keratitis. In: Tabbara K, Hyndiuk R, eds. *Infections of the eye*, 2nd ed. Boston: Little, Brown, 1996:401–422.
619. Asbell P. Viral conjunctivitis. In: Tabbara K, Hyndiuk R, eds. *Infections of the eye*, 2nd ed. Boston: Little, Brown, 1996:453–470.
620. Laibson P, et al. Corneal infiltrates in epidemic keratoconjunctivitis: response to double blind corticosteroid therapy. *Arch Ophthalmol* 1970;84:36.
621. Gordon Y. Adenovirus and other nonherpetic viral diseases. In: Smolin G, Thoft R, eds. *The cornea*, 3rd ed. Boston: Little, Brown, 1994:215–228.
622. Holmes WJ. Epidemic infectious conjunctivitis. *Hawaii Med J* 1941;1:11.
623. Rieke FE. Epidemic conjunctivitis of presumed virus causation: report of an estimated six hundred cases in one shipyard. *JAMA* 1942;119:942.
624. Hogan M, et al. Adenoviral keratitis. *Am J Ophthalmol* 1942;25:1059–1063.
625. Jawetz E, Kimura S, Nicholas AN. New type of APC virus from epidemic keratoconjunctivitis. *Science* 1955;122:1190–1196.
626. de Jong JC, Wigand R, Wadell G, et al. Adenovirus 37: Identification and characterization of a medically important new adenovirus type of subgroup D. *J Med Virol* 1981;7:105–109.
627. Bell SD, McComb DE, Murray ES, et al. Adenoviruses isolated from Saudi Arabia. *Am J Trop Med Hyg* 1959;8:492–496.
628. Ford E, Nelson KE, Warren D. Epidemiology of epidemic keratoconjunctivitis. *Epidemiol Rev* 1987;9:244–249.
629. Harnett G, Newnham W. Isolation of adenovirus type 19 from the male and female genital tracts. *Br J Vener Dis* 1981;57:55.
630. Schaap G, de Jong JC, van Bijsterveld OP, et al. A new intermediate adenovirus type causing conjunctivitis. *Arch Ophthalmol* 1979;97:2336–2338.
631. Laibson P, Ortolan G, Dupre-Strachan S. Community and hospital outbreak of epidemic keratoconjunctivitis. *Arch Ophthalmol* 1968;80:467.
632. Tullo A. The adenoviruses. In: Easty DL, ed. *Virus disease of the eye*. Chicago: Year Book Medical, 1985:257–270.
633. Gordon Y, Gordon RY, Romanowski E, et al. Prolonged recovery of desiccated adenoviral serotypes 5, 8, and 19 from plastic and metal surfaces in vitro. *Ophthalmology* 1993;100:1835–1839.
634. Azar M, Dhaliwal DK, Bower KS, et al. Possible consequences of shaking hands with your patients with epidemic keratoconjunctivitis. *Am J Ophthalmol* 1996;121:711–712.
635. Sprague JB, Hierholzer JC, Currier RW 2nd, et al. Epidemic keratoconjunctivitis: a severe industrial outbreak due to adenovirus type 8. *N Engl J Med* 1973;289:1341–1346.
636. O'Day D, Guyer B, Hierholzer JC. Clinical and laboratory evaluation of epidemic keratoconjunctivitis due to adenoviruses type 8 and 19. *Am J Ophthalmol* 1976;81:207.
637. Kowalski R, Sundar-Raj CV, Romanowski EG, et al. The disinfection of contact lenses contaminated with adenovirus. *Am J Ophthalmol* 2001;132:777–779.
638. Waring GO, Laibson PR, Satz JE, et al. Use of vidarabine in epidemic keratoconjunctivitis due to adenovirus types 3, 7, 8 and 19. *Am J Ophthalmol* 1976;82:71.
639. Dawson C, Hanna L, Togni B. Adenovirus type 8 infections in the United States: IV. observations on the pathogenesis of lesions in severe eye disease. *Arch Ophthalmol* 1972;87:258.
640. Dawson C, Hanna L, Wood TR, et al. Adenovirus type 8 keratoconjunctivitis in the United States: III. epidemiologic, clinical and microbiologic features. *Am J Ophthalmol* 1970;69:473–480.
641. D'Angelo L, Hierholzer JC, Keenlyside RA, et al. Pharyngoconjunctival fever caused by adenovirus type 4: report of a swimming pool related outbreak. *J Infect Dis* 1979;140:42.
642. Roba L, Kawalski RP, Gordon AT, et al. Adenoviral ocular isolates demonstrate serotype-dependent differences in in vitro infectivity titers and clinical course. *Cornea* 1995;14:388–393.
643. Darougar S, Viswalingam M, Treharne JD, et al. Epidemic keratoconjunctivitis and chronic papillary conjunctivitis in London due to adenovirus type 19. *Br J Ophthalmol* 1977;61:76.
644. Pavan-Langston D. Major ocular viral infections: herpes simplex, adenovirus, Epstein Barr virus, pox. In: Galasso G, Merrigan T, Whitley R, eds. *Antiviral agents and viral diseases of man*, 4th ed. New York: Lippincott-Raven, 1997:187–229.
645. Chodosh J, et al. Adenoviral epithelial keratitis. *Cornea* 1995;14:167–174.
646. Maudgal P. Cytopathology of adenovirus keratitis by replica technique. *Br J Ophthalmol* 1990;74:670–675.
647. Azar P Jr, Gohd RS, Waltman D, et al. Acute posterior multifocal placoid pigment epitheliopathy associated with an adenovirus type V infection. *Am J Ophthalmol* 1975;80:1003.
648. Lund O, Stefani F. Corneal histology after epidemic keratoconjunctivitis. *Arch Ophthalmol* 1978;96:2085–2088.
649. Pavan-Langston D. Herpetic infections. In: Smolin G, Thoft R, eds. *The cornea*, 3rd ed. Boston: Little, Brown, 1994:183–214.
650. Boniuk M, Phillips CA, Friedman JB. Chronic adenovirus type 2 keratitis in man. *N Engl J Med* 1965;273:924.
651. Pettit T, Holland G. Chronic keratoconjunctivitis associated with ocular adenovirus infection. *Am J Ophthalmol* 1979;88:748.
652. Gibson J, Doraugar S, McSwiggan DA, et al. Comparative sensitivity of a cultural test and the complement fixation test in the diagnosis of adenovirus ocular infection. *Br J Ophthalmol* 1979;63:617.
653. Ward J, Siojo L, Waller S. A prospective, masked clinical trial of trifluridine, dexamethasone, and artificial tears in the treatment of epidemic keratoconjunctivitis. *Cornea* 1993;12:216–221.
654. Dudgeon J, Bhargava S, Ross C. Treatment of adenovirus infection of the eye with 5-iodo-2-deoxyuridine: a double blind trial. *Br J Ophthalmol* 1969;53:530.
655. Romanowski E, Gordon Y. Efficacy of topical cidofovir on multiple adenoviral serotypes in the New Zealand rabbit ocular model. *Invest Ophthalmol Vis Sci* 2000;41:460–463.
656. Romanowski E, Yates K, Gordon Y. Short-term treatment With a potent topical corticosteroid of an acute ocular adenoviral infection in the New Zealand white rabbit. *Cornea* 2001;20:657–660.

657. Romanowski E, Yates K, Gordon Y. Topical corticosteroids of limited potency promote adenovirus replication in the Ad5/NZW rabbit ocular model. *Cornea* 2002;21:289–291.

658. Romanowski E, Gordon Y. Effects of diclofenac or ketorolac on the inhibitory activity of cidofovir in the Ad5/NZW rabbit model. *Invest Ophthalmol Vis Sci* 2001;42:158–162.

659. Centers for Disease Control and Prevention. The global HIV and AIDS epidemic. *MMWR Morb Mortal Wkly Rep* 2001;50:434–439.

660. Centers for Disease Control and Prevention. Surveillance of health care workers with HIV/AIDS. Available at: http://www.cdc.gov/hiv/pubs/facts/hchsurv.htm. Accessed September 13, 2002.

661. Walensky R, Losina E, Steger-Craven KA, et al. Identifying undiagnosed human immunodeficiency virus. *Arch Intern Med* 2002;162:887–892.

662. Hazeltine W. Silent HIV infections. *N Engl J Med* 1989; 320:1487.

663. Ryan M, Pavan-Langston D, Durand M. AIDS and the anterior segment. *Int Ophthalmol Clin* 1997;38:241–264.

664. Jabs D. Ocular manifestations of HIV infection. *Trans Am Ophthalmol Soc* 1995;93:623–683.

665. Pepose J, Holland GN, Nestor MS, et al. Acquired immune deficiency syndrome: pathogenic mechanisms of ocular disease. *Ophthalmology* 1985;92:472–484.

666. Pepose J, et al. Cellulogic markers after the transplantation of corneas from donors infected with human immunodeficiency virus. *Am J Ophthalmol* 1987;103:798.

667. Grossniklaus H, Frank K, Tomsak R. Cytomegalovirus retinitis and optic neuritis in acquired immune deficiency syndrome. *Ophthalmology* 1987;94:1601.

668. Cunningham EJ, Margolis T. Ocular manifestations of HIV infection. *N Engl J Med* 2000;339:236–244.

669. Chronister C. Review of external ocular disease associated with aids and HIV infection [review]. *Optom Vis Sci* 1996;73: 225–230.

670. Lucca J, Farris RL, Bielory L, et al. Keratoconjunctivitis sicca in male patients infected with human immunodeficiency virus type 1. *Ophthalmology* 1990;97:1008–1010.

671. Pflugfelder S, Saulson R, Ullman S. Peripheral corneal ulceration in a patient with AIDS-related complex. *Am J Ophthalmol* 1987;104:542.

672. Zuccati G, Tiradritti L, Mastrolorenzo A, et al. AIDS-related Kaposi's sarcoma of the eye. *Int J STD AIDS* 1991;2:136–137.

673. Foreman K, Friborg J Jr, Kong WP, et al. Propagation of human herpesvirus from AIDS-associated Kaposi's sarcoma. *N Engl J Med* 1997;336:163–171.

674. Dugel, P, Gill PS, Frangieh GT, et al. Ocular adnexal Kaposi's sarcoma in acquired immunodeficiency syndrome. *Am J Ophthalmol* 1990;110:500–503.

675. Nakamura S, Salahuddin SZ, Biberfeld P, et al. Kaposi's sarcoma cells: long term culture with growth factor from retrovirus-infected CD4+ T cells. *Science* 1988;242:426–430.

676. Cunningham EJ. Uveitis in HIV positive patients. *Br J Ophthalmol* 2000;84:233–235.

677. Conway M, Insler M. Identification and incidence of human immunodeficiency virus antibodies and hepatitis B virus antigens in corneal donors. *Ophthalmology* 1988;95:1463.

678. Doro S, Navia BA, Kahn A, et al. Confirmation of HTLV-III virus in cornea. *Am J Ophthalmol* 1986;102:390–391.

679. Cantrill H, Henry K, Jackson B, et al. Recovery of human immunodeficiency virus from ocular tissues in patients with acquired immune deficiency syndrome. *Ophthalmology* 1988;95: 1458–1462.

680. Fujikawa L, Salahuddin SZ, Ablashi D, et al. HTLV-III in the tears of AIDS patients. *Ophthalmology* 1986;93:1479.

681. Goode S, Hertzmark E, Steinert RF. Adequacy of the ELISA test for screening corneal transplant donors. *Am J Ophthalmol* 1988;106:463.

682. Kilby J, Eron J. Novel therapies based on mechanisms of HIV-1 cell entry. *N Engl J Med* 2003;348:2228–2238.

683. Pepose J, Esposito J. Molluscum contagiosum, orf, and vaccinia. In: Pepose J, Holland G, Wilhelmus K, eds. *Ocular infection and immunity*. St. Louis: Mosby, 1996:846–856.

684. Koplan J, Hicks J. Smallpox and vaccinia in the United States—1972. *J Infect Dis* 1974;129:224.

685. Bikowski JB Jr. Molluscum contagiosum: the need for physician intervention and new treatment options. *Review Cutis* 2004 Mar;73(3):202–206.

686. Ingraham H, Schoenleber D. Epibulbar molluscum contagiosum. *Am J Ophthalmol* 1998;125:394–396.

687. Gonnering R, Kronish J. Treatment of periorbital molluscum contagiosum by incision and curettage. *Ophthalmic Surg* 1988; 19:325–329.

688. Charteris D, Bonshek R, Tullo A. Ophthalmic molluscum contagiosum: clinical and immunopathological features. *Br J Ophthalmol* 1995;79:476–481.

689. Hancox J, Jackson J, McCagh S. Treatment of molluscum contagiosum with the pulsed dye laser over a 28-month period. *Cutis* 2003;71:414–416.

690. De Clercq E. Cidofovir in the therapy and short-term prophylaxis of poxvirus infections [review]. *Trends Pharmacol Sci* 2002;23:456–458.

691. Neyts J, De Clercq E. Therapy and short-term prophylaxis of poxvirus infections: historical background and perspectives. *Antiviral Res* 2003;57:25–33.

692. Pepose JS, Margolis TP, LaRussa P, et al. Ocular complications of smallpox vaccination. *Am J Ophthalmol* 2003;136:343–352.

693. Breman J, Henderson D. Diagnosis and management of smallpox. *N Engl J Med* 2002;346:1300–1308.

694. Maki D. National preparedness for biological warfare and bioterrorism: smallpox and the ophthalmologist. *Arch Ophthalmol* 2003;121:710–711.

695. Chirambo M, Benezra D. Causes of blindness among students in blind school institutions in a developing country. *Br J Ophthalmol* 1976;60:665–668.

696. Sharma R. Clinical assessment of an isothiazole thiosemicarbazone against smallpox. *J Indian Med Assoc* 1968;51:610–615.

697. Henderson D, Inglesby TV, Bartlett JG, et al. Smallpox as a biological weapon: medical and public health management (consensus statement). *JAMA* 1999;281:2127–2137.

698. Cono J, Casey CG, Bell DM, Centers for Disease Control and Prevention. Smallpox vaccination and adverse reactions: guidance for clinicians. *MMWR Morb Mortal Wkly Rep* 2003; 52(RR-4):1–28.

699. Centers for Disease Control and Prevention. *Summary of October 2002 ACIP smallpox vaccination recommendations*. Atlanta: Centers for Disease Control and Prevention. (Also available at: http://www.bt.cdc.gov/agent/smallpox/vaccination/acip-recs-oct2002.asp.)

700. Bozzette S, et al. A model for a smallpox-vaccination policy. *N Engl J Med* 2003;348:416–425.

701. Mack T. A different view of smallpox and vaccination. *N Engl J Med* 2003;348:460–463.

702. Sepkowitz K. How contagious is vaccinia? *N Engl J Med* 2003;348:439–446.

703. Neff J, Lane JM, Fulginiti VA, et al. Contact vaccinia: transmission of vaccinia from smallpox vaccination. *JAMA* 2002; 288:1901–1905.

704. Lane J, Ruben FL, Neff JM, et al. Complications of smallpox vaccination 1968: national survey in the United States. *N Engl J Med* 1969;281:1201–1208.

705. Goldstein J, Neff JM, Lane JM, et al. Smallpox vaccination reactions, prophylaxis and therapy of complications. *Pediatrics* 1975;55:342–347.

706. Ruben F, Lane J. Ocular vaccinia: epidemiologic analysis of 348 cases. *Arch Ophthalmol* 1970;84:45–51.

707. Ellis P, Winograd L. Current concepts of ocular vaccinia. *Trans Proc Coast Otoophthalmol Soc* 1963;44:141–148.

708. Semba R. The ocular complications of smallpox and smallpox immunization. *Arch Ophthalmol* 2003;121:715–719.

709. Sedan J, Ourgaud A, Guillot P. Les accidents oculaires d'origine vaccinale observes dans le Department des Bouches-du-Rhone au cours de l'epidemie variolique de l'hiver 1952. *Ann Oculist* 1953;186:34–61.

710. Perera C. Vaccinial disciform keratitis. *Arch Ophthalmol* 1940;24:352–356.

711. Espy M, Uhl JR, Sloan LM, et al. Detection of vaccinia virus, herpes simplex virus, varicella-zoster virus, and *Bacillus anthracis* DNA by LightCycler polymerase chain reaction after autoclaving: implications for biosafety of bioterrorism agents. *Mayo Clin Proc* 2002;77:624–628.

712. Centers for Disease Control and Prevention. Smallpox fact sheet: smallpox overview 2002. Available at: http://www.cdc.gov/smallpox.

713. Ellis P, Winograd L. Ocular vaccinia a specific treatment. *Arch Ophthalmol* 1962;68:600.

714. Kempe C. Studies on smallpox and complications of smallpox vaccination. *Pediatrics* 1960;26:76–89.

715. Fulginiti V, et al. Therapy of experimental vaccinial keratitis. *Arch Ophthalmol* 1965;74:539–544.

716. Rennie A, Cant JS, Foulds WS, et al. Ocular vaccinia. *Lancet* 1974;7909:273–275.

717. Jones BR, Al-Hussaini MK. Therapeutic considerations in ocular vaccinia. *Trans Ophthalmol Soc UK* 1964;83:613–631.

718. Perera C. Vaccinial disciform keratitis. *Arch Ophthalmol* 1940;24:352–356.

719. Elion G, Rideout JL, de Miranda P, et al. Biological activities of some purine arabinosides. *Ann NY Acad Sci* 1975;255:468–480.

720. Sugar A, Meyer R. Smallpox and vaccinia. In: Darrell RW, ed. *Viral diseases of the eye*. Philadelphia: Lea & Febiger, 1985: 121–127.

721. Scott I, Karp C, Nuovo G. Human papillomavirus 16 and 18 expression in conjunctival intraepithelial neoplasia. *Ophthalmology* 2002;109:542–547.

722. Karcioglu Z, Issa T. Human papilloma virus in neoplastic and non-neoplastic conditions of the external eye. *Br J Ophthalmol* 1997;81:595–598.

723. De Clercq E. Highlights in the development of new antiviral agents [review]. *Mini Rev Med Chem* 2002;2:163–175.

724. De Clercq E. Therapeutic potential of Cidofovir (HPMPC, Vistide) for the treatment of DNA virus (i.e. herpes-, papova-, pox- and adenovirus) infections. *Verh K Acad Geneeskd Belg* 1996;58:19–47.

725. Haltia M, Tarkkanen A, Veheri A, et al. Measles retinopathy during immunosuppression. *Br J Ophthalmol* 1978;62:356.

726. Kayikcioglu O, Kir E, Soyler M, et al. Ocular findings in a measles epidemic among young adults. *Ocul Immunol Inflamm* 2000;8:59–62.

727. Sommer A. *Vitamin A deficiency and its consequences: a field guide to detection and control*, 3rd ed. Geneva: World Health Organization, 1994.

728. Sandford-Smith J. *Eye diseases in hot climates*, 3rd ed. Oxford: Butterworth Heinemann, 1997:352.

729. Wolinsky J, Server A. Mumps virus. In: Fields B, Knipe D, Melnick J, eds. *Virology*. New York: Raven Press, 1985: 1255–1284.

730. Mickatavatge R, Amadur J. A case report of mumps keratitis. *Arch Ophthalmol* 1963;69:758.

731. Meyer R, Sullivan J, Oh J. Mumps conjunctivitis. *Am J Ophthalmol* 1974;78:1022.

732. Riffenburgh R. Ocular manifestations of mumps. *Arch Ophthalmol* 1961;66:739.

733. Keeney A, Hunter M. Human infection with the Newcastle virus of fowls. *Arch Ophthalmol* 1950;44:573–580.

734. Rosa R, Alfonso E. Enterovirus keratoconjunctivitis. In: Pepose J, Holland G, Wilhelmus K, eds. *Ocular infection and immunity*. St. Louis: Mosby, 1996:895–904.

735. Mitsui Y, Kajima M, Matsumara K, et al. Hemorrhagic conjunctivitis: a new type of epidemic viral keratoconjunctivitis. *Rev Int Trach* 1972;49:63–79.

736. Baum J. Hemorrhagic conjunctivitis: a new type of epidemic viral keratoconjunctivitis. *Surv Ophthalmol* 1973;17:489.

737. Natori K, Yamazaki S, Miyamura K, et al. Genetic relationship between two enteroviruses causing the acute hemorrhagic conjunctivitis syndrome. *Intervirology* 1984;22:97–103.

738. Uchio E, Yamazaki K, Aoki K, et al. Detection of enterovirus 70 by polymerase chain reaction in acute hemorrhagic conjunctivitis. *Am J Ophthalmol* 1996;122:273–275.

739. Whitcher J, Schmidt NJ, Mabrouk R, et al. Acute hemorrhagic conjunctivitis in Tunisia. *Arch Ophthalmol* 1975;94:51.

740. Wright P, Strauss G, Langford M. Acute hemorrhagic conjunctivitis [review]. *Am Fam Physician* 1992;45:173–178.

741. Langford M, Barber JC, Sklar VE, et al. Virus-specific, early appearing neutralizing activity and interferon in tears of patients with acute hemorrhagic conjunctivitis. *Curr Eye Res* 1985;4:233–239.

742. Vijayalakshmi P, Kakkar G, Samprathi A, et al. Ocular manifestations of congenital rubella syndrome in a developing country. *Indian J Ophthalmol* 2002;50:307–311.

743. Boger W III, Peterson R, Robb R. Keratoconus and acute hydrops with congenital rubella syndrome. *Am J Ophthalmol* 1981;91:231.

744. Vijayalakshmi P, Srivastava KK, Poornima B, et al. Visual outcome of cataract surgery in children with congenital rubella syndrome. *J AAPOS* 2003; 7:91–95.

745. O'Neill J. The ocular manifestations of congenital infection: a study of the early effect and long-term outcome of maternally transmitted rubella and toxoplasmosis. *Trans Am Ophthalmol Soc* 1998;96:813–879.

746. Smolin G. Report of a case of rubella keratitis. *Am J Ophthalmol* 1972;74:436.

747. Hara J, Fujimoto F, Ishibashi T, et al. Ocular manifestations of the 1976 rubella epidemic in Japan. *Am J Ophthalmol* 1979; 87:642–645.

FUNGAL KERATITIS, CONJUNCTIVITIS, AND CANALICULITIS

FUNGAL KERATITIS, CONJUNCTIVITIS, AND CANALICULITIS: MYCOLOGY

MARLENE L. DURAND

INTRODUCTION TO FUNGI

On the phylogenetic tree, fungi are closer to animals and plants than they are to bacteria. Like plants and animals, fungi are eukaryotes, have a separate membrane-bound nucleus, many membrane-bound organelles such as mitochondria, sterols in their cell membranes, DNA that contains noncoding regions, and 80S ribosomes (bacteria have 70S) (1). Fungi, like animals, need preformed organic compounds as energy sources. The ancestor of fungi may be a protozoan (1).

Fungi are helpful and harmful to humans. Fungi cause 70% of all major crop diseases. They were responsible for the Irish potato famine of the 1840s, which led to the starvation of 1 million people, and for Dutch elm disease and the American chestnut blight, which permanently altered U.S. hardwood forests. On the other hand, fungi have provided leavening for bread, fermentation of alcohol, and important therapeutic agents (penicillins, cephalosporins, aminoglycosides, amphotericin, cyclosporine).

EPIDEMIOLOGY

Fungi are ubiquitous in the environment. Their spores can survive extremes of heat, cold, and desiccation, and are present in high concentration in the air. Outdoor and indoor air concentrations in temperate climates are typically 1500 and 1000 spores per cubic meter, respectively, although they may reach as high as 50,000 spores per cubic meter (2). Humans constantly breathe in fungal spores, and molds may be isolated from nasal mucus in 100% of randomly sampled individuals (3). Despite this, invasive fungal infections rarely develop in immunocompetent people.

The ocular surface is also exposed to fungi, but keratomycosis is rare. Fungi, particularly *Candida* species, are often part of the normal conjunctival flora (4). Fungi have been cultured from 24% of contact lens cases from asymptomatic cosmetic lens wearers, yet keratomycosis in a contact lens wearer is so rare as to be worthy of a case report (5,6). As in systemic fungal infections, fungi invade the ocular surface only when it is compromised, either from surface disease, topical steroid use, or trauma. Ocular trauma, especially involving vegetable matter, is the most common risk factor for keratomycosis and accounts for 50% of cases in most series. Trauma may be minor, and farmers who live in tropical climates are at particular risk.

Worldwide, fungal keratitis due to molds is one of the most common causes of infectious keratitis. Most cases occur in hot, humid climates. In India, Nepal, Bangladesh, Ghana, and Paraguay, fungi cause 20% to 60% of all infectious keratitis cases (Table 15-1). Keratomycosis is uncommon in temperate regions such as the northern United States and western Europe, where it accounts for at most 3% of keratitis cases (7,8). It is more common in the southern United States, and fungi cause 16% of microbial keratitis cases in Florida (9).

FUNGAL STRUCTURE

Fungi have a nucleus, membrane-bound organelles, a cell wall that contains chitin, and a cell membrane that contains ergosterol (mammalian cell membranes contain cholesterol). Fungal cells are larger than bacteria. *Staphylococcus aureus* is 1 μm in diameter, for example, whereas *Candida* is 4 to 6 μm.

Fungi take the form of either yeasts or molds. Yeasts are usually unicellular and grow by budding. In budding, the nucleus undergoes mitosis and a daughter cell pinches off to form a new cell containing the new nucleus. Molds, also called *filamentous fungi*, are composed of hyphae and are multicellular. Molds grow by extension and branching of hyphae. A hypha is a rigid tube that grows only at the tip. It contains cytoplasm that continuously moves toward the growing tip to supply it with materials for growth, leaving behind a vacuolated base that may undergo autolysis (Fig. 15-1). There is little difference between septate and aseptate hyphae because septa have pores through which cytoplasm and nuclei pass to reach the growing tip.

Although most fungi are always yeasts or always molds, some take either form depending on temperature. These

TABLE 15-1. KERATOMYCOSES AS A PERCENTAGE OF TOTAL CULTURE-POSITIVE KERATITIS CASES

Author	Country	No. Culture-Positive Keratitis Cases	Fungal
Upadhyay (24)	Nepal	324	21%
Sundaram (25)	India (Madras)	150	45%
Kotigadde (26)	India (Karnataka)	295	23%
Srinivasan (27)	India (Madurai)	297	52%
Dunlop (28)	Bangladesh	142	36%
Mino De Kaspar (29)	Paraguay	45	58%
Leck et al. (17)	Ghana/India	1090	42%

fungi are called *dimorphic*, and are yeasts *in vivo* and at 37°C but molds in the environment and at 25°C. They include the *endemic mycoses* (those that are geographically restricted): *Histoplasma*, *Blastomyces*, *Coccidioides*, and *Paracoccidioides*. None of them is an important cause of keratomycosis.

Fungi reproduce by spores. Spores may be sexual as a result of fusion of two cells followed by meiosis, or asexual (mitosis only). The asexual spores of medically important fungi are called *conidia*.

CLASSIFICATION

There are 250,000 species of fungi, although few are human pathogens (10). Until recently, the only effective antifungal for treating systemic fungal infections was amphotericin B, and the identity of the species of *Candida* or genus of mold seemed unimportant from a therapeutic standpoint. Now, with the advent of many new antifungal agents whose activity varies with fungal species, fungal identification has taken on new importance.

Although terminology is in flux, all fungi may be placed in seven phyla or groups: Oomycota, Chytridiomycota, Zygomycota, Ascomycota, Basidiomycota, and Deuteromycota. These groups are based on septation, growth, and reproductive characteristics. Deuteromycota, also called Fungi Imperfecta, include all fungi that reproduce only asexually. Most human pathogens, including the major agents of keratomycosis, are in this group (Table 15-2). Deuteromycetes include the yeasts *Candida* and *Cryptococcus* and the molds *Aspergillus*, *Fusarium*, *Curvularia*, *Alternaria*, and others. Deuteromycete molds are divided into the families Moniliaceae and Dematiaceae, based on the color of the unstained hyphae when viewed through a light microscope. Molds whose hyphae have white or light-colored walls are called *hyaline fungi* and are classified in the family Moniliaceae. Molds with brown or black-pigmented walls are *dematiaceous fungi* (family Dematiaceae). The pigment is due to melanin in the hyphal walls. Note that color does not refer to the color of the mycelial colonies growing on agar and visible to the unaided eye. Many hyaline molds form pigmented colonies, usually due to pigmented conidia.

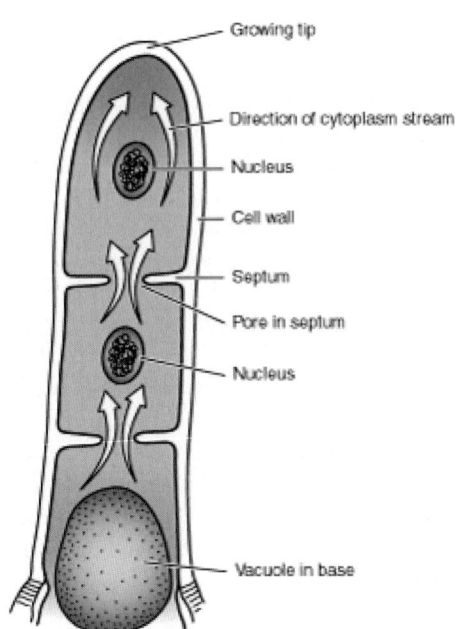

FIG. 15-1. Diagram of a mold hypha.

TABLE 15-2. CLASSIFICATION OF THE MOST IMPORTANT PATHOGENS OF KERATOMYCOSES (ALL ARE IN THE GROUP DEUTEROMYCOTA)

Fungi	
Yeast (*Candida*)	Molds
Candida	Moniliaceae (light-colored)
	Fusarium
C. albicans	Aspergillus
C. tropicalis	Penicillium
C. parapsilosis	
C. glabrata	Dematiaceae (brown)
C. krusei	Curvularia
	Exserohilum, Bipolaris,
	Alternaria

MOLDS VERSUS YEASTS

In general, infections due to molds are much more difficult to diagnose and treat than are those due to yeasts. *Candida*, the major pathogenic yeasts, are as easy to Gram stain and culture as common bacteria and have similar media requirements. Molds require special media and incubation temperature, and may take days to grow. Even with optimal culture techniques, cultures from specimens infected with molds are often falsely negative, whereas this is rare in *Candida* infections. Ocular and systemic infections due to molds are also much more difficult to treat than are those due to *Candida*. A recent report noted that only 8% of 84 patients with endogenous *Aspergillus* endophthalmitis recovered useful vision, in contrast to the 76% to 100% vision recovery rates reported for patients with intraocular candidiasis (11). Similarly, attributable mortality from systemic *Aspergillus* infection (invasive pulmonary aspergillosis in bone marrow transplant recipients) is much higher than from candidemia (85% vs. 38%) (12).

STAINS AND CULTURE TECHNIQUES

Stains

In the microbiology laboratory, Gram stain readily shows the budding yeasts of *Candida* species, which stain grampositive, but may fail to stain the hyphae of molds. The best stain for fungi is Calcofluor white. This fluorescent reagent stains chitin in fungal cell walls and is used in combination with potassium hydroxide, which removes nonfungal elements (e.g., tissue cells) from the specimen. The fungi fluoresce when viewed with a fluorescent microscope.

In histopathology sections, hematoxylin and eosin (H&E) and periodic acid-Schiff stain fungi, but Gomori methenamine silver (GMS) stain is considered the best fungal stain. Fungi appear black with this stain. The advantage of tissue biopsy and histopathologic staining is that this can distinguish fungal infection (tissue invasion) from surface colonization, whereas culture cannot.

Culture

The likelihood of culturing mold from infected tissue is higher if a tissue biopsy, rather than swabs, is submitted for culture. However, a portion of this biopsy specimen should be plated directly on fungal culture media, and not ground up in the microbiology laboratory. Laboratories routinely grind up tissue samples with a mortar and pestle before plating to allow even distribution of the specimen on various media, and this grinding disrupts fungal hyphae and reduces the chance of a positive culture.

Specimens should be planted on routine and fungal culture media. *Candida* species grow rapidly (2 days) on standard bacterial culture media such as blood agar, but molds grow more slowly, especially because bacterial culture plates are incubated at 37°C, which is too hot for some molds. Molds are best grown on nonselective media such as Sabouraud dextrose and brain heart infusion (SABHI) agar, and should be incubated at 25°C to 30°C. Most fungi that cause keratomycosis grow within 5 days.

Candida colonies resemble bacterial colonies and are smooth, white to tan mounds. *Candida albicans* can be distinguished from other *Candida* species by the germ-tube test, in which an inoculum of the colony is placed in broth and incubated at 37°C (less than 4 hours is needed). Only *C. albicans* forms elongated hyphae (germ tubes). *C. albicans* can also be identified by growing the organism on special agar containing chromogenic substrates (e.g., Chromagar; Hardy Diagnostics, Santa Maria, CA). *C. albicans* forms green colonies on Chromagar, whereas *Candida tropicalis* colonies are blue-gray.

Molds form a fuzzy mass on culture plates. Pigmentation of mold colonies depends on the culture media used as well as the type of mold and age of the culture. Hyaline mold colonies may be white initially but pigmented with sporulation. On Sabouraud dextrose agar, mature colonies of *Aspergillus fumigatus* are blue-green, *Aspergillus flavus* yellow-green, and *Aspergillus niger* black.

Laboratory Contaminants

Distinguishing *Aspergillus* laboratory contaminants from true infection can be difficult. Because *Aspergillus* spores are ubiquitous in the air, they may contaminate the culture plate while it is being planted with the clinical sample, leading to false-positive cultures. *A. niger* is the most common fungal cause of laboratory contamination. To distinguish a contaminant from a true-positive culture requires clinical suspicion and examination of the culture plates. When a specimen is planted, either a visible fragment of tissue is placed on the agar, or the sample is inoculated using a metal loop that leaves visible wavelike streaks in the agar surface. If the fungus is not growing on either the tissue fragment or on the streaks, one should suspect it is a laboratory contaminant, especially if the fungus is *A. niger*.

YEASTS

Nearly all systemic yeast infections are due to *Candida* and *Cryptococcus*. Other yeasts (e.g., *Malassezia*, *Trichosporon*, *Saccharomyces*, *Rhodotorula*) are unusual causes of invasive disease. With rare exceptions, all keratomycoses due to yeasts are caused by members of the genus *Candida*.

Candida

Candida species are part of the normal oral and gastrointestinal flora, and are normal skin and ocular surface colonizers.

TABLE 15-3. SYSTEMIC *CANDIDA* INFECTIONS BY SPECIES

Species	Percentage of Candidemias[a]	Susceptibility to Fluconazole[b]
Candida albicans	54%	S
Candida glabrata	16%	S-DD to R
Candida parapsilosis	15%	S
Candida tropicalis	8%	S (some strains R)
Candida krusei	2%	R
Other species	5%	

S, susceptible; S-DD, susceptible, dose-dependent; R, resistant.
[a]Pfaller MA, Jones RN, Doern GV, et al. Bloodstream infections due to Candida species: SENTRY antimicrobial surveillance program in North America and Latin America, 1997–1998. *Antimicrob Agents Chemother* 2000;44:747–751.
[b]Perea S, Patterson TF. Antifungal resistance in pathogenic fungi. *Clin Infect Dis* 2002;35:1073–1080.

They typically cause invasive disease only when there is a breach in host defense (e.g., indwelling intravenous catheter, ocular surface disease). They are the most important cause of systemic nosocomial fungal infections, and were the fourth most common cause of nosocomial bloodstream infections in a 1996 surveillance of 4700 nosocomial bacteremias and fungemias (13). Although there are more than 100 species of *Candida*, *C. albicans* is the most important, accounting for 50% to 60% of *Candida* infections (Table 15-3). Most cases of *Candida* keratitis are also due to *C. albicans*, although a 10-year review (1982–1992) of keratomycosis cases in Florida found more cases of *Candida parapsilosis* than *C. albicans* (11 versus 4) (14).

It is important to distinguish *C. albicans* from other *Candida* species in systemic infections because fluconazole can reliably be used only for *C. albicans*. *C. albicans* can be readily distinguished from other species by the germ-tube test (see earlier). Nearly all *C. albicans* strains are susceptible to fluconazole. Non-*albicans* species of *Candida* may be resistant, and the frequency of resistance varies with the species. Assuming that the new *in vitro* susceptibility testing for *Candida* species correlates with clinical outcome (and this is not always true) (15), nearly all *C. tropicalis* strains are fluconazole susceptible. Most *C. parapsilosis* strains are susceptible, but some are azole resistant. *Candida glabrata*

(formerly called *Torulopsis glabrata*) strains usually show bimodal susceptibility, with some very resistant [minimum inhibitory concentration (MIC) >64 μg/mL] and others showing dose-dependent susceptibility (MIC >8 and $\leq$32 μg/mL). *Candida krusei* is intrinsically resistant to fluconazole and itraconazole. All *Candida* species are susceptible to amphotericin with one exception, *Candida lusitaniae*, which has intrinsic and acquired resistance (16).

MOLDS

The most important causes of keratomycoses worldwide are molds. *Fusarium* and *Aspergillus* account for nearly two thirds of published cases (17). Dematiaceous fungi, such as *Curvularia* and *Alternaria*, are the third most common (Table 15-4)

Aspergillus

Aspergillus is a major pathogen of humans and causes three syndromes: invasive disease, noninvasive disease (aspergilloma), and allergic disease (e.g., allergic bronchopulmonary aspergillosis). Systemic invasive disease occurs almost exclusively in immunocompromised hosts, particularly bone marrow transplant recipients. Aspergilloma occurs in otherwise healthy hosts in either a sinus or lung cavity and is noninvasive. Allergic sinus aspergillosis and allergic bronchopulmonary aspergillosis occur in otherwise healthy hosts and represent allergies to the inhaled and mucustrapped hyphae rather than infection. *Aspergillus* keratitis represents a form of superficially invasive disease.

Although there are over 200 species, 95% of all *Aspergillus* infections are caused by *A. fumigatus*, *A. flavus*, and *A. niger* (18). *A. fumigatus* is the most common of these. Pathogenic *Aspergillus* species produce proteolytic enzymes such as elastase, and these may be virulence factors. All species are common in soil, dust, vegetable matter, and air. Conidia (spores) are often prevalent in fireproof ceiling tiles and insulation, and hospital construction projects have been associated with nosocomial outbreaks of invasive *Aspergillus* infection in immunocompromised patients.

TABLE 15-4. FREQUENCY OF VARIOUS FUNGI RESPONSIBLE FOR KERATOMYCOSES WORLDWIDE

Fungus	Hyderabad (30)	New Delhi (31)	Singapore (32)	Ghana (17)	Florida (33)
Fusarium	38%	11%	52%	42%	52%
Aspergillus	30%	40%	17%	17%	4%
Penicillium		7%	3%	0	2%
Curvularia	4%	7%	3%	1%	9%
Other Dematiaceae[a]	16%	17%		6%	10%
Candida		1%	10%	1%	8%
Total no. of cases	557	211	29	109	240

[a]Other Dematiaceae include *Exserohilum*, *Bipolaris*, *Alternaria*, *Cladosporium*, and others.

A. fumigatus tolerates a temperature range from 20°C to 50°C, so grows readily at body temperature. *Aspergillus* grows quickly on most culture media and grows at room temperature or at the usual bacterial incubation temperature (37°C). Growth is usually apparent in 2 to 3 days. All species have septate hyphae that branch at acute angles. Diagnosis of *Aspergillus* infection, as with all molds, requires growth of the organism into a mycelial mass on culture media, then examination of the hyphae and conidial heads (sporulating tips) under the microscope. The morphology of conidial heads varies by fungal genus. *Aspergillus* hyphal walls are hyaline, but colonies growing on culture plates may be pigmented, mostly because of pigmented conidia.

Fusarium

Fusarium is common in the soil and is an important plant pathogen. It may cause localized infection after trauma in otherwise healthy patients. Invasive systemic disease occurs only in immunocompromised patients and has a high mortality rate. *Fusarium* may be a nosocomial pathogen, and at one cancer institute the hospital water system was found to be a reservoir (19). Patients were most likely exposed from aerosolization of the organism that occurred during showering. *Fusarium solani* is the most common species, but *Fusarium oxysporum*, *Fusarium moniliforme*, and *Fusarium proliferatum* are also pathogens. In keratomycoses, *F. oxysporum* and *F. solani* are the most common species (14). *Fusarium*, like *Aspergillus*, has hyaline, septate, branching hyphae with diameters of 3 to 8 μm. *Fusarium* grows rapidly on many types of media, and mycelial colonies are various colors. *Fusarium* is identified microscopically by its sickle- or banana-shaped macroconidia and clusters of fusiform microconidia.

Dematiaceous Fungi

Dematiaceous fungi have melanin in their hyphal walls, so are dark pigmented (olive, brown, black) when viewed with a light microscope. Colonies assume their characteristic dark color only on certain media such as potato dextrose agar. On Sabouraud plates, they are often salmon-colored.

In a series by Garg and colleagues of 88 cases of keratomycosis due to dematiaceous fungi in India, half of the fungi did not sporulate so could not be further identified (20). Of the remaining half, *Curvularia* was most common (23% of all cases), followed by *Exserohilum* and *Bipolaris* (15% combined). *Curvularia* was also the most common dematiaceous fungus in the Florida series (14). *Curvularia* and *Exserohilum* grow rapidly, whereas *Bipolaris* grows more slowly, with mature colonies formed within a week. All three have septate hyphae.

Dematiaceous fungi may appear dark in tissues as well, although not always. In Garg and colleagues' study, only

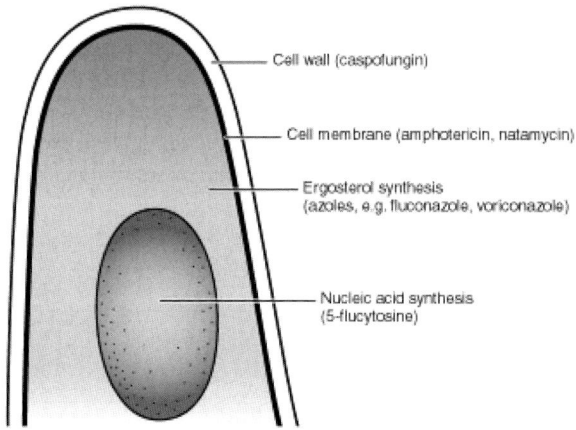

FIG. 15-2. Diagram showing site of action of antifungal agents in the fungal cell.

27% of corneal ulcers caused by dematiaceous fungi appeared to be darkly pigmented macroscopically. There may be two explanations for this. First, tissue inflammation may mask fungal color. Second, two of the common causes of dematiaceous keratomycosis, *Curvularia* and *Bipolaris*, often appear hyaline in tissue because of minimal formation of melanin (21). In pathologic sections, pigmentation may be difficult to see with H&E stain, and would not be seen with GMS stain. The Masson-Fontana stain stains melanin and is often helpful in identifying dematiaceous fungi.

ANTIFUNGAL AGENTS

Amphotericin was introduced 50 years ago and, until the 1980s, was the only systemic antifungal agent available. In the past 20 years, there has been a dramatic increase in systemic and mucosal fungal infections that has paralleled the acquired immunodeficiency syndrome epidemic and the increase in patients undergoing bone marrow or solid organ transplantation. As a consequence, there has been a resurgence in antifungal drug development. This has resulted in new agents with promising activity not only against *Candida* species, but against the more difficult-to-treat molds. The site of action of the current and experimental antifungal agents is illustrated in Fig. 15-2.

Polyenes

The polyenes (amphotericin, nystatin, natamycin) bind to ergosterol in the fungal cell membrane, leading to osmotic disruption and leakage of potassium. Amphotericin B inserts itself into the membrane, creating membrane pores. The ability of polyenes to bind weakly to cholesterol, the sterol in mammalian cell membranes, contributes to their toxicity. Only amphotericin can be given systemically, and it has significant renal toxicity. This toxicity is greatly reduced if the amphotericin is complexed with lipid, such as the spherical liposomes in AmBisome (Fujisawa). AmBisome appears to be as effective in treating systemic fungal infections as amphotericin B, but costs 10 times as much. Amphotericin is active against nearly all yeasts and molds, although clinical success is much higher against yeast than mold infections. Fungi resistant to amphotericin include *Candida lusitaniae*, *Trichosporon beigelii*, *Aspergillus terreus*, and *Scedosporium apiospermum* (the asexual counterpart of *Pseudallescheria boydii*).

Azoles

The azoles include topical (clotrimazole, miconazole, econazole) and systemic agents (the imidazole ketoconazole, and the triazoles fluconazole, itraconazole, and voriconazole). They act by inhibiting ergosterol synthesis, thereby disrupting the fungal cell membrane. Because amphotericin requires the presence of ergosterol in the cell membrane to be effective, there has been concern that azoles and amphotericin may be antagonistic. Whether this is true clinically is controversial.

Ketoconazole was the first useful systemic azole, but its activity is limited to yeasts and dimorphic fungi (e.g., *Histoplasma*). It has been replaced in clinical practice by fluconazole, which is much more active and better tolerated.

Fluconazole is very effective against most yeasts, though *C. krusei* and some *C. glabrata* are resistant. It is as effective as amphotericin against candidemia due to sensitive strains. It has no significant activity against molds, such as *Aspergillus* and *Fusarium*. Unlike the other azoles, fluconazole is water soluble. The major toxicity is hepatic.

Itraconazole was the first azole with activity against molds in addition to yeasts, but because of poor absorption of the capsules, it has proved disappointing. Recently, an oral solution has become available that allows nearly complete absorption and much better potency against *Aspergillus*. An intravenous formulation is also now available. Itraconazole may have significant drug–drug interactions (e.g., cyclosporine, phenytoin, rifabutin) that must be monitored.

Voriconazole was approved in 2002 as a new triazole with excellent oral absorption and broad-spectrum efficacy against both yeasts and molds. A recent study of invasive aspergillosis found voriconazole to be superior to amphotericin, producing complete or partial responses in 53% of patients, versus 32% in the amphotericin group (22). In addition to activity against *Aspergillus*, voriconazole appears to have activity against *Fusarium* and dematiaceous fungi. Visual scotomas occur in 30% of patients while on voriconazole, but these are transient and reversible.

Posaconazole is an experimental triazole that appears to have very good activity against molds, including *Aspergillus*, *Fusarium*, dematiaceous fungi, and Zygomycetes (e.g. mucormycosis). Clinical experience is limited at this point.

Echinocandins

Echinocandins are a new class of antifungals that, unlike the polyenes and azoles, do not target ergosterol but rather the fungal cell wall. Caspofungin is the only approved echinocandin at present. Echinocandins inhibit fungal cell wall formation by binding to the enzyme β-1,3 glucan synthase. Because mammalian cells lack cell walls, echinocandins are expected to have few side effects. Caspofungin is increasingly used to treat fluconazole-resistant *Candida* infections, and in combination with voriconazole to treat invasive aspergillosis.

Flucytosine

Flucytosine acts as a false nucleoside when taken up by the fungal cell, inhibiting nucleic acid synthesis. It is used for synergistic activity with amphotericin against some infections due to *Cryptococcus*, *Candida*, and *Aspergillus*. It has myelosuppressive and hepatic toxicities.

SUSCEPTIBILITY TESTING

In 1997 and 1998, the National Committee for Clinical Laboratory Standards established standards for MIC breakpoints for yeast and molds. These were intended to be the basis for *in vitro* antifungal susceptibility testing. However, the correlation between susceptibility testing for fungi and clinical outcome is still poor. There is some correlation for fluconazole susceptibility in *Candida*, although not as good as the correlation for susceptibility testing in bacteria. In bacterial infections, clinical success rates of over 80% are achieved when the patients are treated with antibiotics to which the organism is sensitive, whereas only 4% of patients are effectively treated when the organism is resistant to the antibiotic used (23). With fluconazole testing in *Candida* species, these rates are closer to 90% and 60%, respectively (23), so that resistance does not reliably predict clinical failure. There is no correlation between *in vitro* susceptibility results for molds and clinical outcome, and susceptibility testing is not recommended (15).

REFERENCES

1. Deacon JW. *Modern mycology*, 3rd ed. London, Blackwell Science, 1997:3.
2. Santilli J, Rockwell W. Fungal contamination of elementary schools: a new environmental hazard. *Ann Allergy Asthma Immunol* 2003;90:175.
3. Ponikau JU, Sherris DA, Kern EB, et al. The diagnosis and incidence of allergic fungal sinusitis. *Mayo Clinic Proc* 1999;74: 877–884.
4. Ando N, Takatori K. Fungal flora of the conjunctival sac. *Am J Ophthalmol* 1982;94:67–74.

5. Choi DM, Goldstein MH, Salierno A, et al. Fungal keratitis in the daily disposable soft contact lens wearer. *CLAO J* 2001;27: 111–112.

6. Foroozan R, Eagle RC Jr, Cohen EJ. Fungal keratitis in a soft contact lens wearer. *CLAO J* 2000;26:166–168.

7. Coster DJ, Wilhelmus J, Peacock J, et al. Suppurative keratitis in London. In: Trevor-Roper PD, ed. *VIth Congress of The European Society of Ophthalmology: The cornea in health and disease.* International Congress and Symposium Series No. 40. London: Academic Press, 1981:395–398.

8. Neumann M, Sjostrand J. Central microbial keratitis in a Swedish City population: a three-year prospective study in Gothenburg. *Acta Ophthalmol (Copenh)* 1993;71:160–164.

9. Forster RK. Conrad Berens Lecture: the management of infectious keratitis as we approach the 21st century. *CLAO J* 1998;24:175–180.

10. Dixon DM, Rhodes JC, Fromtling RA. Taxonomy, classification, and morphology of the fungi. In: Murray PR, ed. *Manual of clinical microbiology*, 7th ed. Washington, DC: American Society of Microbiology Press, 1999:1161.

11. Riddell J IV, McNeil SA, Johnson TM, et al. Endogenous *Aspergillus* endophthalmitis: report of 3 cases and review of the literature. *Medicine (Baltimore)* 2002;81: 311–320.

12. Pfaller MA, Wenzel RP. The epidemiology of fungal infections. In: Anaissie EJ, McGinnis MR, Pfaller MA, eds. *Clinical mycology.* New York: Churchill Livingstone, 2003:5.

13. Pfaller MA, Jones RN, Messer SA, et al., and the SCOPE Participant Group. National surveillance of nosocomial bloodstream infections due to species of *Candida* other than *Candida albicans*: frequency of occurrence and antifungal susceptibility in the SCOPE Program. *Diagn Microbiol Infect Dis* 1998; 30:121.

14. Rosa RH Jr, Miller D, Alfonso EC. The changing spectrum of fungal keratitis in south Florida. *Ophthalmology* 1994;101: 1005–1013.

15. Rex JH, Pfaller MA. Has antifungal susceptibility testing come of age? *Clin Infect Dis* 2002;35:982–989.

16. Perea S, Patterson TF. Antifungal resistance in pathogenic fungi. *Clin Infect Dis* 2002;35:1073–1080.

17. Leck AK, Thomas PA, Hagan M, et al. Aetiology of suppurative corneal ulcers in Ghana and south India, and epidemiology of fungal keratitis. *Br J Ophthalmol* 2002;86: 1211–1215.

18. Richardson MD, Kokki M. *Aspergillus*. In: Annaissie EJ, McGinnis MR, Pfaller MA, eds. *Clinical mycology*. New York: Churchill Livingstone, 2003:273.

19. Anaissie EJ, Stratton SL, Dignani MC, et al. Pathogenic *Aspergillus* species recovered from a hospital water system: a three-year prospective study. *Clin Infect Dis* 2002;34:780.

20. Garg P, Gopinathan U, Choudhary K, et al. Keratomycosis: clinical and microbiologic experience with dematiaceous fungi. *Ophthalmology* 2000;107:574–580.

21. Schell WA, Salkin IF, Pasarell L, et al. *Bipolaris, Exophiala, Scedosporium, Sporothrix*, and other dematiaceous fungi. In: Murray PR, ed. *Manual of clinical microbiology*, 7th ed. Washington, DC: American Society of Microbiology Press, 1999: 1295.

22. Herbrecht R, Denning DW, Patterson TF, et al. Voriconazole versus amphotericin B for primary therapy of invasive aspergillosis. *N Engl J Med* 2002;347:408–415.

23. Lorian V, Burns L. Predictive value of susceptibility tests for the outcome of antibacterial therapy. *J Antimicrob Chemother* 1990; 25:175–181.

24. Maeda N, Klyce SD, Hamano H. Alteration of corneal asphericity in rigid gas permeable contact lens induced warpage. *CLAO J* 1994;20:27–31.

25. Maeda N, Klyce SD, Smolek MK, et al. Disparity of keratometry-style readings and corneal power within the pupil after refractive surgery for myopia. *Cornea* 1997;16:517–524.

26. Wilson SE, Klyce SD. Quantitative descriptors of corneal topography: a clinical study. *Arch Ophthalmol* 1991;109:349–353.

27. Maloney RK, Bogan SJ, Waring GO. Determination of corneal image-forming properties from corneal topography. *Am J Ophthalmol* 1993;115:31–41.

28. Holladay JT. Corneal topography using the Holladay Diagnostic Summary. *J Cataract Refract Surg* 197;23:209–221.

29. Hjortdal JO, Erdmann L, Bek T. Fourier analysis of videokeratographic data: a tool for separation of spherical, regular astigmatic and irregular astigmatic corneal power components. *Ophthalmic Physiol Opt* 1995;15:171–185.

30. Olsen T, Dam-Johansen M, Bek T. Evaluating surgically induced astigmatism by Fourier analysis of corneal topography data. *J Cataract Refract Surg* 1996;22:318–323.

31. Oshika T, Tomidokoro A, Maruo K, et al. Quantitative evaluation of irregular astigmatism by Fourier series harmonic analysis of videokeratography data. *Invest Ophthalmol Vis Sci* 1998;39: 705–709.

32. Seiler T, Reckmann W, Maloney RK. Effective spherical aberration of the cornea as a quantitative descriptor in corneal topography. *J Cataract Refract Surg* 1993;19[Suppl]:155–165.

33. Camp JJ, Maguire LJ, Cameron BM, et al. A computer model for the evaluation of the effect of corneal topography on optical performance. *Am J Ophthalmol* 1990;109:379–386.

16

FUNGAL INFECTIONS

**EDUARDO C. ALFONSO, RICHARD K. FORSTER,
PRASHANT GARG, AND SAVITRI SHARMA**

FUNGAL KERATITIS

Fungal keratitis is one of the most challenging types of microbial keratitis for the ophthalmologist to diagnose and treat. There has been an increase in the awareness and recognition of the clinical signs of fungal keratitis, particularly in geographic areas where these infections tend to be more commonly seen (e.g., rural areas and areas of warm climates). This has led to better and more frequent diagnosis and to improved management. Fungal keratitis remains a therapeutic challenge because its management is restricted by the paucity of effective antifungal agents and by the extent to which they can penetrate into corneal tissue. It is important, therefore, to understand the clinical picture presented by mycotic keratitis, and, as an aid in interpreting culture results, to know the fungi that most commonly cause it. Above all, it is important to have a rational and informed approach to the use of both diagnostic laboratory techniques and antifungal compounds and therapeutic alternatives. Here we review the current status of mycotic keratitis.

Incidence

The incidence of fungal keratitis is low (6% to 20%) when compared to bacterial keratitis in various series of microbial corneal ulcers, with more numerous reports of fungal keratitis from the southern United States (1–3). It continues to be a disease most commonly encountered in patients who come from a rural setting. *Aspergillus* sp. may be the most common organism responsible for fungal keratitis worldwide (4). *Candida* sp. and *Aspergillus* sp. are most frequently isolated in fungal keratitis in the northern United States, whereas *Fusarium* sp. predominates in the southern United States (5–7). *Fusarium solani* was the most commonly isolated organism in two series of fungal keratitis from South Florida (1,8). In a more recent study *Fusarium oxysporum* was the most common species (37%), followed by *Fusarium solani* (24%) (9). *Candida* sp., *Curvularia* sp., and *Aspergillus* sp. were the next most common fungal

isolates in order of decreasing frequency. *Fusarium* sp. has been reported as an isolate in fungal keratitis in many regions of the world. The largest series of fungal keratitis are reported from India, with the most common fungal isolates being *Aspergillus* sp. (27% to 64%), followed by *Fusarium* sp. (6% to 32%), *Penicillium* sp. (2% to 29%), and a number of other rare organisms (10–12). Increased awareness of the occurrence and frequency of fungal keratitis, better recognition of the clinical features of these infections, and improved laboratory diagnostic techniques of direct examination of stained smears and culture of the causative fungi have all led to an increase in the frequency of correct diagnosis. The growing population in southern climates has probably also contributed to greater interest in diagnosing mycotic infections (13). Numerous case reports of less usual organisms have been reported as a cause of keratomycosis. Proper identification is important for future exposure prevention and for determining the best treatment modalities (14–20).

Etiology

Although there have been many different fungi associated with corneal infections, certain genera and species seem to predominate. Infections caused by the same or related species may present a generally similar picture and respond similarly to antifungal agents *in vitro* and clinically. Fungi gain access into the corneal stroma through a defect in the epithelial barrier. This defect is most often due to external trauma, including contact lenses, a compromised ocular surface, or previous surgery. Once in the stroma, fungi multiply and can cause tissue necrosis and a host inflammatory reaction. They can even penetrate deep into the stroma and through an intact Descemet's membrane. It is thought that once fungi gain access into the anterior chamber or to the iris and lens, eradication of the organism becomes extremely difficult. Likewise, organisms that extend from the cornea into the sclera become difficult to control. Blood-borne growth inhibiting factors may not reach the avascular tissues of the eye, such as the cornea, anterior chamber, and sclera, which may explain why fungi continue

TABLE 16-1. FUNGAL ISOLATES FROM KERATITIS, BASCOM PALMER EYE INSTITUTE, MIAMI. 1982-2003

Hyaline (molds)	N	% culture positive isolates
Aspergillus species		
A. terreus	3	
A. fumigatus	6	
A. flavus	3	
A. glaucus	8	
A. niger	1	
Aspergillus species, NOS	3	
Total	24	6%
Fusarium Species		
F. oxysporum	151	
F. solani	46	
F. moniliforme	1	
Fusarium species, NOS	6	
	204	51%
Acremonium species	8	2%
Cylindrocarpon species	3	<1%
Mucor species	1	<1%
Rhizopus species	1	<1%
Paecilomyces species	12	3%
Scedosporium apiosperum (Pseudallescheria boydii)	2	<1%
Dematiaceous (mold)		
Curvularia species		
C. senegalensis	5	1%
C. verruculosa	1	<1%
Curvularia species, NOS	31	8%
	37	9%
Colleotricum species		
C. dematium	3	
C. gloeosporoides	3	
Colleotricum species, NOS	8	
	14	3%
Alternaria species, NOS	2	<1%
Lasiodiplodia theobromae	3	<1%

to grow and persist in these areas despite treatment. It also may be the reason why a conjunctival flap sometimes can help limit fungal growth (i.e., by bringing to avascular tissue blood-borne growth-inhibiting factors (21).

Over the last several years we have been able to recognize and catalog certain fungi as frequent or repeated causes of mycotic keratitis. In Miami, *Fusarium* sp. are the most commonly isolated filamentousous fungi and *Candida* sp. the most common yeast (Table 16-1). A list of the more frequent causes of fungal keratitis include, in addition to *Fusarium* sp., *Aspergillus fumigatus* and *Aspergillus flavus*, *Paecilomyces lilacinus*, and *Petriellidium boydii*; the pigmented fungi (22), species of *Curvularia*, *Drechslera*, *Alternaria*, and *Phialophora*; as well as tropical fungi such as *Lasiodiplodia* and *Colletotrichum*, which are associated with lesions in plants. Any of these species

isolated from corneal ulcerative stromal inflammation would be highly suspect as being the causative agent, as are other fungi when they are isolated from carefully made cultures (see Laboratory Diagnosis, below). Although *Fusarium* sp. may be especially common as a cause of keratitis in southern Florida, it is also by far the most common isolate in other parts of the United States, other Western Hemisphere nations, and in fact all parts of the world. Before 1974, nearly 50% of reported cases of keratomycosis were attributed to *Aspergillus*; nearly 25% to *C. Albicans*; and the remaining 25% to diverse fungi among which *F. solani* was increasingly commonly identified after 1970 (23). This change in isolated organisms prevalence probably resulted from improved mycologic identification rather than from a real change in prevalence. Most of the fungi causing keratitis are opportunistic organisms and are ubiquitous as plant pathogens or in the soil. How they become established in the corneal stroma after minor trauma, presumably involving implantation of the organism from some outdoor plant material, is not completely understood. But there are many cases in which the association between infection (after trauma or injury to the cornea) and plant material is well documented.

An early report of fungal ulcers from southern Florida showed an absence of keratitis during the hot, humid, rainy months of June to September (24). In recent years, however, fungal keratitis, most frequently caused by filamentous fungi other than *F. solani* and yeasts, has also been seen during the summer months. November and March, usually dry, cool, and windy months in southern Florida, remain the peak months for the occurrence of fungal keratitis (1). There is possibly an association of keratitis with dry, windy weather following a wet period suitable for fungus growth.

Zygomycetes (Phycomycetes) and dermatophytes (ringworm fungi) are rarely reported as causes of fungal keratitis. But many, or perhaps most, fungi may have the potential to cause keratitis, given the right combination of organism, trauma leading to implantation, and host factors. However, the most common causes are those most frequently encountered after apparently negligible trauma.

Clinical Features

Risk Factors

Trauma is the most frequent risk factor for the onset of fungal keratitis; it was the major risk factor in 44% of patients in a recent study (9). Trauma most often occurs outdoors and involves plant matter. Gardeners using motorized lawn mowers and trimmers are specially predisposed (9,25,26).

Fungal keratitis can also be associated with contact lens wear, and fungi have been recovered from contact lenses (27–31). The incidence of fungal keratitis in contact lens wearers has been reported as 4% for cosmetic (phakic and aphakic) contact lens wearers and in 27% in therapeutic lens users (32,33). Filamentous fungi are more commonly associated with cosmetic lens wear, and yeasts with therapeutic lens use (34). In large series of contact lens–related microbial keratitis, few cases of fungal keratitis were associated with contact lens wear. The decreased number of fungal infections in contact lens wearers compared to noncontact lens wearers is statistically significant (35). Similar findings have been reported from India (36) and Singapore (37). It has been theorized that this difference could be due to a lower association between contact lens wear and other risk factors for fungal keratitis or a protective mechanism against fungal invasion into the cornea by the presence of the contact lens.

The use of topical and systemic corticosteroids has been associated with the development of and worsening of fungal keratitis. Steroids impair the host immunologic response to the microbial invader (38,39). Topical anesthetic abuse has also been associated as a risk factor for *Candida* keratitis (40).

Patients with vernal or allergic conjunctivitis may also be predisposed to fungal keratitis (41). It has also been reported in atopic patients (42).

Corneal transplant and refractive surgery have also been associated with fungal keratitis (43,44). Predisposing factors for the development of fungal keratitis in patients after keratoplasty include loose sutures, chronic topical steroid use, chronic antibiotic use, contact lens wear, graft failure, and persistent epithelial defects (44–46). The contamination of donor corneas is of special concern because no antifungal is routinely used in the preparation of the donor globe or in the solution used to preserve the tissue before transplantation (47). Routine culture of donor rims and media may aid in the identification of the organism and prompt initiation of antifungal treatment (48).

Fungal keratitis has been reported to be associated with refractive surgery (43,53). It can occur in the immediate postoperative period or later. The early form may be associated with the direct surgical contamination of the cornea. The late form is usually associated with trauma (54). It was associated with contamination from a pet in one case report (55). Mild trauma allows the organisms to penetrate through the diseased epithelium directly into the stroma, avoiding Bowman's layer (56,57). Delayed diagnosis may worsen the outcome of fungal keratitis after refractive surgery (58–60). It can also occur after enhancement procedures (61).

Systemic diseases associated with inmunosuppression may increase the risk for the development of fungal keratitis. One series reported a 12% incidence of diabetes mellitus in a group of patients with fungal keratitis; the incidence of diabetes mellitus in the United States is estimated to be only 1% of the population (9). Patients chronically ill and hospitalized in intensive care units also may be predisposed to the development of fungal keratitis, usually with *Candida* sp. In a series from Africa, HIV-positive patients were more likely to develop fungal keratitis compared to non-HIV patients (49). In patients with leprosy, fungal ulcers may be more common (50).

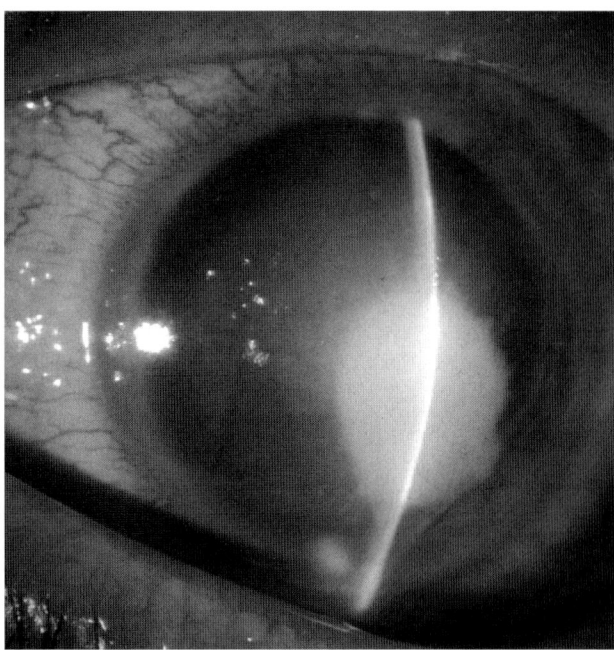

FIGURE 16-1. Slit lamp biomicroscopic view of fungal keratitis (*Fusarium solani*) with dry infiltrate elevated above the level of the corneal surface.

Keratomycosis in children is usually associated with trauma with organic matter. In one series fungal keratitis comprised 18% of all cases of keratitis cultured in children (51). It may be difficult to establish a history of trauma with organic matter in pediatric patients, and so all children with keratitis should be cultured for fungi (52).

The salient features of fungal keratitis have been described, and although satellite lesions, presumed immune rings, and endothelial plaques may not be unique to fungal keratitis, these features and the following ones should elevate one's suspicion of a fungal infection: stromal infiltrates with feathery, hyphate edges; and infiltrates that tend to be dry, gray, and somewhat elevated above the level of the corneal surface (Figs. 16-1 and 16-2) (62). Keratitis caused by yeasts may be more localized and have a "collar button" configuration, often with a small ulceration and an expanding although discrete stromal infiltrate (Fig. 16-3). But whether or not these suggestive slit-lamp features exist, any corneal stromal infiltrate with ulceration, or even with an intact epithelium, should be considered a microbial infection, and fungus can be the microbe (63). A complete microbiologic diagnostic workup, including harvesting of material for the isolation of bacteria, fungi, and *Acanthamoeba*, should be performed in all patients with such infiltrates (64). Unrecognized and undiagnosed fungal keratitis inadvertently treated with corticosteroids will worsen. Herpes keratitis may be the condition most commonly confused with keratomycosis (65).

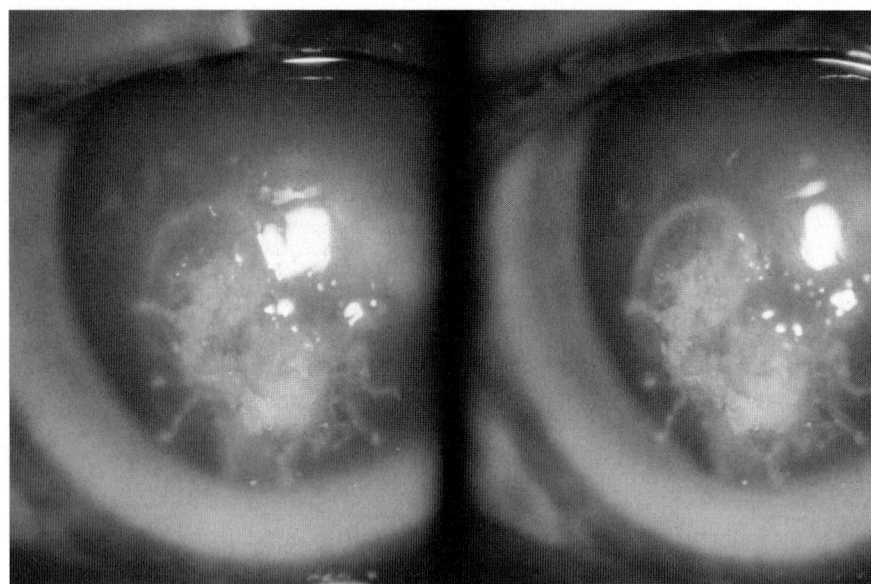

FIGURE 16-2. Stromal infiltrate with pseudopods, satellites, and hypopyon. *Fusarium solani.*

The confocal microscope now affords a unique way of clinically investigating cases of microbial keratitis, and specifically finding fungal organisms in the stroma (66,67).

Laboratory Diagnosis

After a careful clinical history is obtained and the clinical features of the stromal keratitis are documented, the next essential step is to promptly perform laboratory studies (68,69). Corneal scrapings are best obtained with a sharpened spatula or a surgical blade. This method is preferred to the use a calcium alginate, Dacron/rayon swab, or a sponge-type material. The organisms may be deep in the tissue and not accessible to swabbing. Scraping also provides for initial debridement of organisms and of epithelium, which may provide a barrier to antifungal drug penetration. A diamond-tipped motorized burr may also be useful to obtain the scrapings. When corneal scrapings are negative, a diagnostic superficial keratectomy or corneal biopsy may be performed. A 2- to 3-mm sterile disposable dermatologic trephine is advanced into the anterior corneal stroma to incorporate both infected and adjacent clear cornea. The visual axis should be avoided if possible. But we would emphasize that the primary goal must not be a compromised biopsy of the infiltrate, even if it is in the visual axis and even if it is deep. The base is then undermined with a surgical blade to complete the lamellar keratectomy (70,71). The corneal biopsy specimen should be submitted for smears, cultures, and histopathologic examination. In some cases of deep keratitis with an intact overlying epithelium and stroma, a 27-gauge hypodermic needle or a 6–0 silk suture can be introduced into the infiltrate to obtain a specimen for culture.

A corneal biopsy has been shown to have better yield than scrapings for recovering fungi. In animal experiments, corneal scrapings found three of 10 specimens positive for *C. albicans*, five of 10 for *F. solari*, and six of 10 for *A. fumigatus* corneal biopsy specimens demonstrated fungal elements in all inoculated eyes (72). Furthermore, comparing the value of direct examination and culture of biopsy specimens, cultures found seven of 10 specimens positive for *C. albicans*, and eight of 10 for *F. solani* and *A. fumigatus*; direct examination demonstrated positive-positive fungal elements in all specimens (73). Alexandrakis et al. (70) also demonstrated an increased recovery rate of organisms from corneal biopsy specimens from recalcitrant, culture-negative cases. In initial cases of keratitis the corneal biopsy has also been shown to have an increased recovery rate of organisms (9). An anterior chamber tap can be performed to isolate fungal

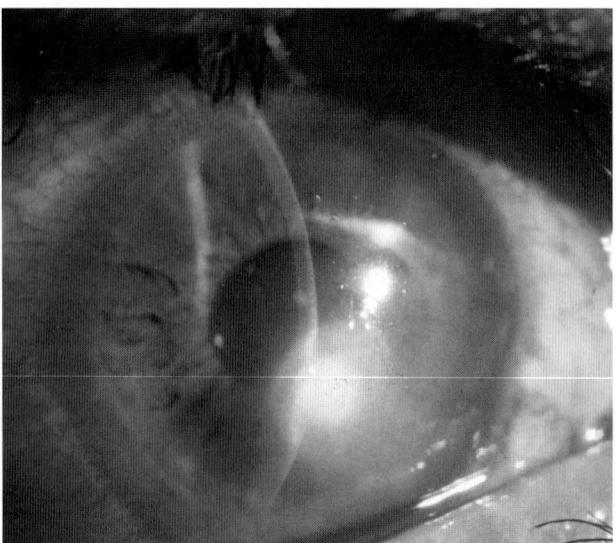

FIGURE 16-3. Stromal keratitis caused by mixed infection with *Candida* parapsilosis and *Fusarium oxysporum.* Note the more localized, discrete infiltrate underlying the small ulceration.

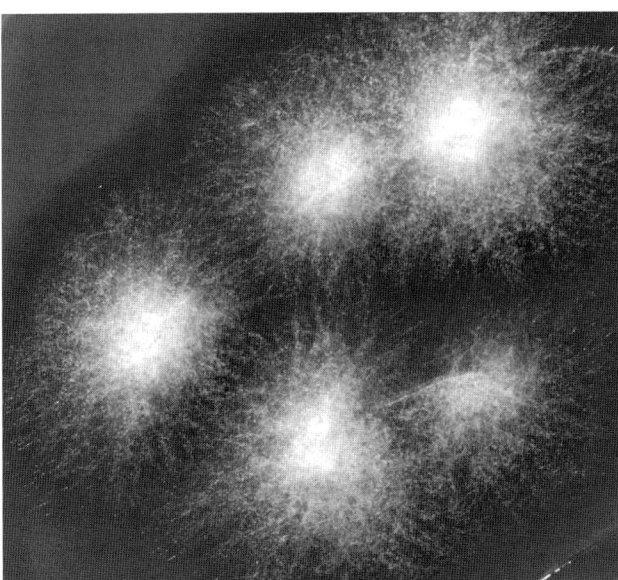

FIGURE 16-4. C streaks with early growth *of Fusarium solani* 48 hours after inoculation.

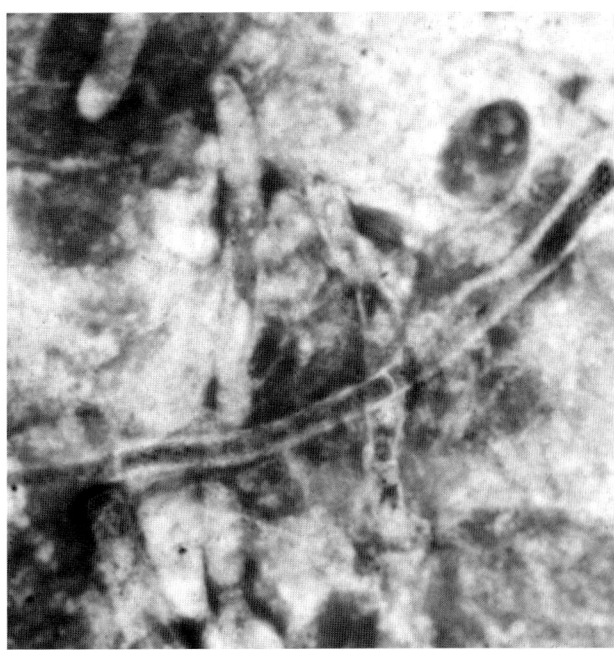

FIGURE 16-5. Giemsa-stained corneal scraping. Note that fungal cell walls and septa do not stain.

organisms that may have penetrated through an intact Descemet's membrane. Under aseptic conditions, the hypopyon and or endothelial plaque can be aspirated and submitted for laboratory examination (74).

We routinely inoculate two blood agar plates: one to be maintained at room temperature for fungus growth, and the other at body temperature (35–37°C) for bacterial growth. A Sabouraud agar plate containing gentamicin (50 μ/mL) but without cycloheximide (which inhibits saprophytic fungi) should also be inoculated and incubated at room temperature. A chocolate agar plate is incubated at 37°C in a candle jar. Thioglycolate broth is also routinely inoculated and incubated for possible anaerobic growth at 35° to 37°C. By convention, to indicate the site of inoculation on solid medium, harvested material is inoculated in the form of a "C" streak, with each row of "C" streaks on each medium being made from a separate scraping (Fig. 16-4). Therefore, it is apparent that in order to produce two or three rows of "C" streaks, 10 to 15 individual scrapings of the corneal inflammatory material are required. In addition to the cultures, scraped material is placed on three or four slides for Gram's and Giemsa stains as well as on a gelatin- or albumin-coated slide to be used for Gomori methenamine-silver stain. If adequate corneal material is available, it is appropriate to smear an additional slide that can be held in reserve for special or repeat stains.

Review of laboratory results in cases of culture-proved keratitis indicates that Gram's stains of corneal scrapings were positive for hyphal elements in 55% of the cases, and Giemsa stains in 66% (Fig. 16-5) (1). A shortened technique for the preparation of the Gomori methenamine-silver stain for fungi has proved highly reliable in confirming the diagnosis of fungal keratitis from scrapings (Fig. 16-6) (75). The stain can also be used for restaining

Gram- and Giemsa-stained slides and will often reveal hyphae not clearly shown by the other staining procedures. In a series of 133 culture-proved cases of fungal keratitis Gram's and Giemsa stains were performed in 94 cases (1). Fungal hyphae were present on two or more slides in 60% of these and on only one slide in 21%. No hyphae were seen in 19%. Other methods of examining smears in patients with suspected fungal keratitis are potassium hydroxide (10% to 20%) wet preps (76), acridine orange staining, Grocott's methenamine silver technique (77), lectins (78), and calcofluor white preparations (69,75,79–81).

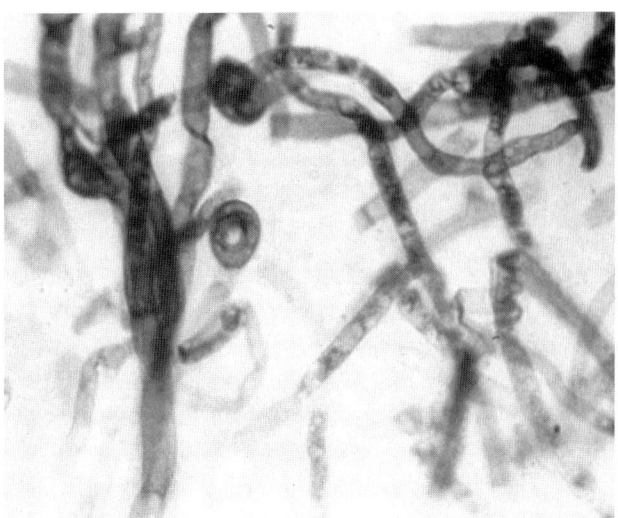

FIGURE 16-6. Gomori's methenamine-silver stain of corneal scraping. Note the staining of cell walls and septa.

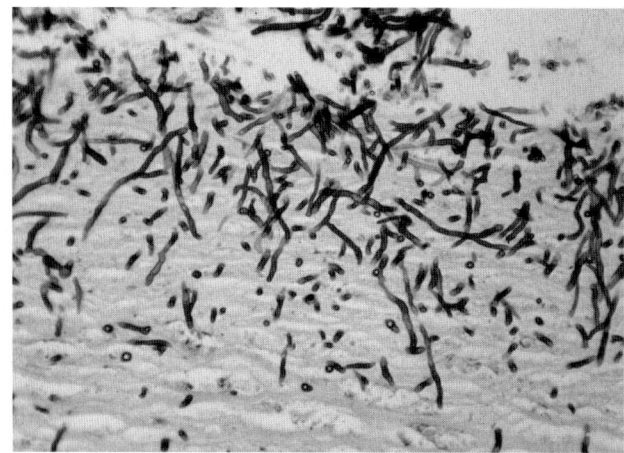
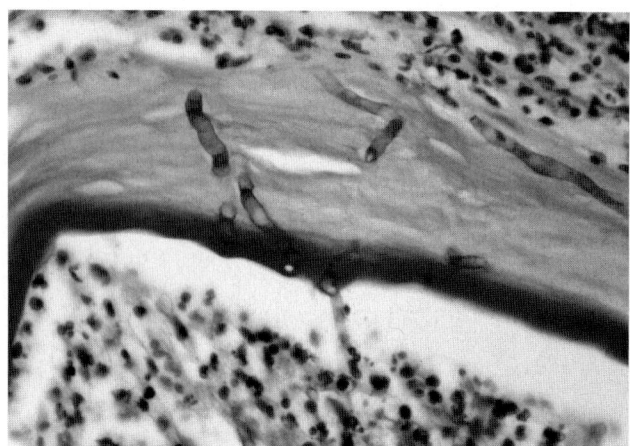

A   B

FIGURE 16-7. A: Gomori methenamine-silver stain of keratoplasty specimen showing fungal organisms. **B:** Penetrating keratoplasty specimen showing abscess formation and arrangement of the hyphal elements perpendicular to the corneal lamellae.

Although Sabouraud agar with gentamicin and without cycloheximide incubated at room temperature is still the most sensitive medium for isolating fungi, sheep or rabbit blood agar incubated at room temperature is nearly as successful. Blood agar at 37°C was positive for fungi in about 35% of the cases, and liquid brain-heart infusion (BHI) medium maintained on a rotary shaker at room temperature was positive for fungi in about 50% of cases. Fungal isolates were detected on one or more media in 84 of 105 consecutive cases and on only one medium in 21 cases. In each instance of growth limited to a single medium, the presence of fungus was confirmed by microscopic examination of the scraping. Increasing the humidity of the medium by placing the inoculated agar plates in plastic bags has also been recommended for enhancement of fungal growth (82).

Almost all ocular fungal isolates grow and become evident in 48 to 72 hours. Most, in fact, are visible with the dissecting microscope or naked eye within less than 36 hours. But one should wait a week before declaring a culture negative for fungi. One report indicated slower growth of fungi from eye cultures and a lower incidence of detection by solid media or stained scrapings (83). However, this is in sharp contrast to the results obtained in a series of 134 isolations from 133 ocular fungus infections (1).

Newer methods for the identification of fungi, although still not widely available, include immunofluorescence staining, electron microscopy, and polymerase chain reaction (84–87). Fungi have been recovered from topically applied medications, cosmetics, contact lenses, and their storage and cleaning solutions in patients with fungal keratitis. These items, therefore, should be obtained from the patient at the initial visit. Cultures and smears should be obtained to increase the chances of identifying the causative organism (88–90).

There is little evidence that topical antibiotics aggravate fungal keratitis. Likewise, fungi do not seem to alter or

contribute to the normal ocular flora of the conjunctival surface and the cul-de-sac. (See the first section of this chapter for the culture characteristics of the fungi.)

Histopathology

The classic histopathologic findings in fungal keratitis include two features that are considered to be suggestive of progressive pathogenicity: fungal hyphal elements oriented perpendicular to the normal corneal lamellae, and a tendency for hyphal elements to penetrate intact Descemet's membrane (91). We examined over 30 ocular specimens histopathologically (Fig. 16-7); some were whole eyes, but 29 were therapeutic penetrating keratoplasty specimens after medical treatment failures in which the infection had progressed to frank or impending perforation (92). We noted the presence of limbal infiltrates (Fig. 16-8) and a tendency toward progressive keratitis in cases of impending

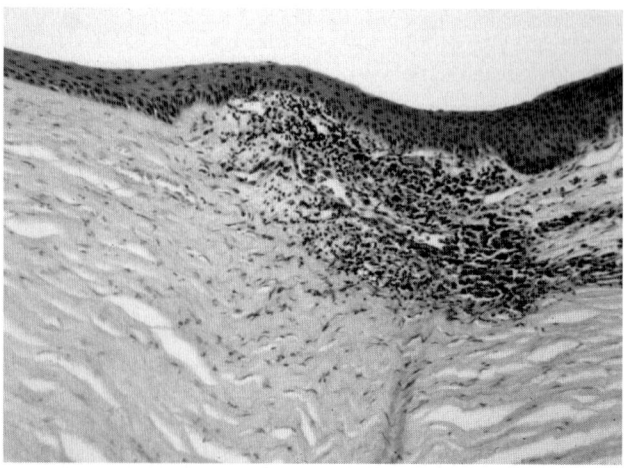

FIGURE 16-8. Limbal infiltrate with round cells and plasma cells associated with progressive stromal ulceration.

perforation and abscess formation. We also recognized the following syndrome: After initial laboratory proof of fungal keratitis and treatment with topical antifungal agents, there was initial improvement, followed, after approximately 2 weeks of therapy, by progressive ulceration that necessitated penetrating keratoplasty or keratectomy with a conjunctival flap. In these cases, abnormal degenerated hyphal forms were seen histopathologically, sometimes associated with negative cultures obtained at the time of surgery (92,93). This finding suggests the need to evaluate factors that contribute to progressive keratitis even in the presence of antifungal treatment that leaves nonviable fungal elements in the corneal stroma. A localized inflammatory reaction at the limbus characterized by a collection of round cells and plasma cells was also observed in some of these histopathologic specimens. This suggests that immune mechanisms contribute in some instances to progressive ulceration.

Progressive keratitis in laboratory animals is difficult to establish without corticosteroids, and fungal keratitis has to date been reported infrequently in animals such as the dog and horse (see the first section of this chapter).

Antifungal Agents

Although less frequently encountered than bacterial keratitis, fungal infections of the cornea remain difficult to treat, and most ophthalmologists are understandably uncertain in managing cases of presumed or culture-positive fungal keratitis.

The major problems in management are (a) choice of antifungal agents, (b) management of deep keratitis, and (c) delivery of antifungal therapy. The major limiting factors to successful management include (a) the sensitivity of the fungal infection to antimicrobial therapy, (b) the penetration of the antifungal agents into and through the cornea, (c) bioavailability and delivery of the drug, and (d) toxicity of the antifungal agents.

In the case of bacterial keratitis, the available agents penetrate the cornea well, there is a choice of nontoxic available agents, sensitivity patterns are reproducible and rapid, and there is a high correlation between *in vitro* and *in vivo* effects. In contrast, antifungal agents in general are of low solubility and penetrate nonlipid layers poorly, they tend to be toxic at adequate therapeutic concentrations, and there is marked and noticeable variability between the *in vitro* sensitivity patterns compared to *in vivo* efficacy. The pharmacokinetics, the effect of the immune response, and other unknown drug-microbe interactions are not well understood.

The major groups of antifungal agents are the polyenes, including amphotericin B, natamycin, and nystatin; the azoles, including clotrimazole, miconazole, ketoconazole, and fluconazole; and flucytosine. Before 1969, most cases of fungal keratitis were treated with topical amphotericin B (24). Successful treatment was variable and toxicity was (is) a problem. Subsequently, during the 1970s, the related polyene antifungal agent natamycin was used investigationally

and became another treatment choice (94). In 1979 the Food and Drug Administration approved natamycin (Natacyn) for topical ocular use and Alcon Laboratories (Ft. Worth, Texas) made a 5% suspension commercially available on a case-by-case basis. Failure of infections to heal when treated with natamycin has been due to microbial resistance, to poor tissue penetration, and to as yet unidentified factors contributing to progressive keratitis (94,95).

O'Day and associates (96), in a series of experiments using an animal model of *Candida* keratitis, compared polyenes (amphotericin B and natamycin) with azoles, (miconazole and ketozonazole), and new triazole agents (fluconazole and saperconazole). They reported that amphotericin penetrated the cornea better than the polyene natamycin, and that the imidazoles penetrated poorly. In contrast, in a comparative study of corneal penetration of topical amphotericin B and natamycin, O'Day and associates (97) in 1986 reported the corneal uptake and penetration of C-labeled 0.15% amphotericin B and 5% natamycin in rabbits. Corneal levels of natamycin were substantially higher than those of amphotericin B. In corneas debrided of epithelium, both entered the stroma and aqueous, whereas in corneas with intact epithelium natamycin entered in greater amounts than amphotericin B. Further investigation of the influence of the corneal epithelium on the efficacy of topical antifungal agents reported by O'Day and associates (98) in 1984, employing a model of deep stromal *C. albicans* infection in rabbits, and comparing the efficacy of six topical antifungal agents in the presence of intact and debrided epithelium. In corneas debrided daily, the polyenes (amphotericin B and natamycin) exhibited significant antifungal effect. Removal of the epithelium adversely affected the efficacy of flucytosine; the imidazoles were not efficacious in this model. However, in 1992 O'Day and coworkers (99) demonstrated that the triazole saperconazole was effective in the management of *Aspergillus* species and *C. albicans* infections, and penetrates the cornea when applied topically to potential therapeutic levels. These animal penetration and efficacy studies suggest that the epithelium is an important barrier to penetration.

With the exception of penicillin, the mechanism of action of few antibiotics has been studied as extensively as that of the antifungal polyenes. These agents exert their effect by binding to sterols present in the cell membrane (100). They have no effect on cell membranes in which sterols are absent. They also have a greater affinity for ergosterol present in the fungus membrane, than for cholesterol in the animal membrane. This probably accounts for their *in vivo* selective antifungal effect in the treatment of mycotic disease in animals. However, their affinity for cholesterol is considerable, which makes them relatively toxic. Of the three principal polyene antimycotics used in medicine, amphotericin B, nystatin, and natamycin, only amphotericin B can be administered systemically, although its use and effectiveness are compromised by its toxicity. Functionally, the polyene antibiotics are divided into two

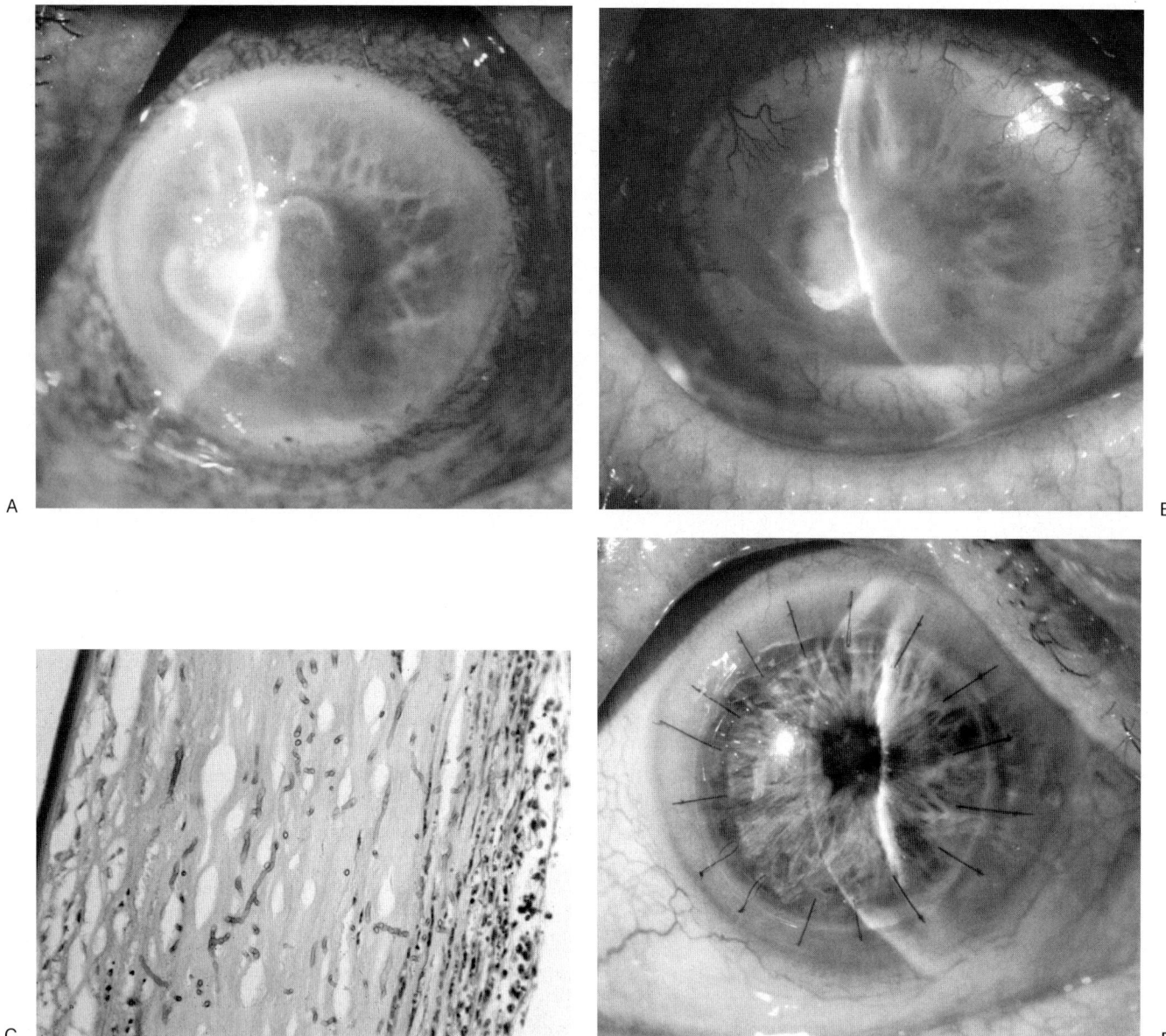

FIGURE 16-9. A: Indolent paracentral ulceration with necrotic borders initially seen 2 months after the onset of symptoms. Initial management was with bandage contact lens, topical cortico-steroids, and antibiotics. Gram's and Giemsa stains demonstrate hyphal elements. *Curvularia senegalensis.* **B:** Six weeks following natamycin therapy with progressive thinning and impend-ing perforation. **C:** Histopathology from therapeutic penetrating keratoplasty. Note the superfi-cial polymorphonuclear leukocyte response with hyphal elements throughout the depth of the cornea. **D:** Seven weeks postoperatively, preceding removal of interrupted sutures used in thera-peutic keratoplasty.

classes: large polyenes such as amphotericin B, and smaller polyenes such as natamycin. Although both bind to sterols, they differ in their subsequent effect on the cell membranes as a consequence of their relative size. The larger polyenes approximate the length of the cell membrane phospholipid and form narrow circular channels for the passage of potassium chloride and other ions. This free passage leads to electrolyte imbalance and subsequent death of the cell. However, the lethal effect of the large polyenes may be blocked or reversed by osmotic and electrolyte control of the surrounding medium. In contrast, the molecular length of the small polyenes such as natamycin, instead of forming channels, accumulate on the membrane, forming "blisters" that disrupt and cause the sterol phospholipid film to break down. This phenomenon is not reversible by osmotic or elec-trolyte control, and therefore the fungicidal end point of natamycin as observed *in vitro* tends to be more absolute. Whether or not these differences between the small and large

TABLE 16-2 SUSCEPTIBILITY DATA FOR KERATITIS FUNGAL ISOLATES. BASCOM PALMER EYE INSTITUTE

Susceptibility Data for Frequent Ocular Fungal Pathogens	Amphotericin B	Natamycin	Miconazole	ketoconazole	Fluconazole	Itraconazole	Voriconazole	Posconazole	5-Flucytocine
Fusarium solani	MS❷	MS❶	R	R	R	R	MS	MS	R
Fusarium oxysporum	MS❷	MS❶	R	R	R	R	MS	MS	R
Fusarium species									
Curvularia species	S❷	S❶	S❷	S❷	MS	MS	S	NA	R
Colleotrichum species	S❶	S❶	S	S❷	R	MS	S	NA	R
Aspergillus fumigatus	S❶	S❶	MS	S	R	MS❷	S	S	R
Aspergillus species	S❶	S❶	MS	S	R	MS❷	S	S	R
Paecilomyces lilacinus	R	R	S❶	S❷	R	R	S❷	NA	R
Paecilomyces varioti	S❶	S	S❶	S❷	R	MS	S❷	NA	R
Candida albicans	S❶	S❶	MS	S❷	MS	MS	S	S	S
Candida parapsilosis	S❶	S❶	S	S❷	S	S	S	S	S
Candida tropicalis	S❶	S❶	S	S❷	MS	MS	S	S	S

S = >90% susceptible in vitro (usually clinically effective)
MS = 60–89% susceptible in vitro (variably clinically efective)
R = <60% susceptible in vitro (usually not clinically effective)
❶ = First drug of coice
❷ = Second drug of choice

Note: In vitro results do not always correlate with clinical response. Factors that may impact interaction include host's immune status, drug bioviability and stage of infection.

References

1. Susceptibility Data-Bascom Palmer Eye Institute 1982–2002.
2. Sutton DA, Fothergill AW, Rinaldi, MG. Guide to Clinically Significant Fungi, Willians & Wilkins, Baltimore, 1998.
3. Seal DV, Bron AJ, Hay J. Ocular Infections. Investigation and Treatment in Practice. Mosby, St. Louis, 1998.
4. Hoog GS, Guarro J, Gene J, Figueras MJ. Atlas of Clinical Fungai, 2nd ed. Universitat Rovira I Virgili, Reus, Spain 2000.
5. Anaissie EJ, McGinnis MR, Pfaller MA. Clinical Mycology. Churchhill & Livingstone, New York, 2003.

polyenes is of clinical importance is unknown, and in general the polyene antibiotics can be relied on to be effective *in vitro* against almost all fungi.

The azole compounds such as miconazole, ketoconazole, clotrimazole and fluconazole owe their antifungal effect to two mechanisms (101): interference with the synthesis of ergosterol in the fungus membrane, and a direct action causing the membranes to become leaky. Clotrimazole has a greater tendency to bind to fatty acids than do miconazole or ketoconazole, but it is also more toxic and cannot be administered systemically. Unlike the polyenes and the azoles, which act on the cell membrane, flucytosine is incorporated into the fungal RNA and interferes with protein synthesis (102).

In Vitro Antifungal Sensitivities

It is not practical for the clinical ophthalmologist to send a corneal isolate to a microbiology laboratory and ask for identification and sensitivity studies in order to initiate and plan therapeutic management (103). Many laboratories are not equipped or experienced to perform sensitivity studies on fungi. Such laboratories, even if regional, with the necessary expertise, may exhibit variability within their own results with the same or different fungi and may take days to weeks to perform the tests. Once obtained, the *in vitro* data and the clinical sensitivity response may not correlate. It is most practical to consult published tables of sensitivities for general groups of identified fungi against common available antifungal agents (Table 16-2). Recent studies suggest that careful clinical monitoring of the infiltrate and antifungal testing may play a role in the outcome of the treatment (104).

The Role of Steroids

O'Day and associates (105) also examined the influence of topical corticosteroids on the efficacy of antifungal agents. They observed that corticosteroids adversely influence the efficacy of natamycin, flucytosine, and miconazole. Amphotericin B appeared unaffected in concentrations of 0.50% to 0.15%, an accepted therapeutic dosage.

In an attempt to take advantage of the *in vitro* sensitivity patterns exhibited by amphotericin B, Wood and Williford

(106) demonstrated that amphotericin B at a concentration of 0.15% is clinically effective and relatively nontoxic. O'Day and associates (107) also examined the efficacy of topical amphotericin B methyl ester in two models of yeast infection in rabbit eyes, and demonstrated that efficacy was dose related in the superficial model and that the antifungal activity did not deteriorate in the presence of 1% prednisolone acetate using 1% amphotericin B methyl ester. In a model of deep stromal infection, 1% amphotericin B methyl ester was highly efficacious when corneal epithelium was absent, and with intact epithelium a reduced but significant effect was noted.

Robinson and associates (108) examined the comparative efficacy of newer azole antifungal agents against human ocular isolates. *In vitro* minimum inhibitory concentration demonstrated that the polyenes remain the agents of choice for the treatment of yeast and filamentous fungal infections of the eye. However, encouraging results with the use of fluconazole following oral administration were reported by O'Day (109) in 1990, who demonstrated ocular penetration and distribution of oral fluconazole in rabbits. Brooks and associates (110), using an experimental *C. albicans* keratitis model in the rabbit, found that the triazole antifungal agents such as fluconazole, saperconazole, and itraconazole are effective in the treatment of experimental *C. albicans* keratitis and appear to be equivalent to and potentially less toxic than amphotericin B. A case series of 15 patients treated with topical dermatologic diluted clotrimazole (0.5%) and a polyene showed adequate response to treatment (111).

In general, antiseptics have received a mixed review in the literature as to their effectiveness in the treatment of fungal keratitis. Povidone iodine, polyhexamethylene biguanide, and others have been used in animal models (112,113). Chlorhexidine has been suggested as a potential treatment for fungal keratitis (114). Some of the newer antifungal available for systemic use have been tried topically. Voriconazole is one such medication that may be promising for the treatment of keratitis (115).

Modifications in the topical delivery of antimicrobial agents by iontophoresis and more recently by collagen shields may permit the enhancement of antifungal delivery. Schwartz and associates (116) reported the collagen shield delivery of amphotericin B. They investigated the ability of collagen shield therapeutic contact lenses to release amphotericin B levels compared to frequent-drop therapy over 6 hours. They observed that presoaked collagen shields release most amphotericin B within the first hour of elution and that amphotericin B delivery by collagen shields is comparable to that by frequent-drop therapy. This suggests the potential benefit of added convenience and compliance (116).

Medical Management

Prompt, appropriate, rational therapy for fungal keratitis rests on clinical evaluation and laboratory investigation.

TABLE 16-3. RECOMMENDED DOSES OF AVAILABLE TOPICAL AND SUBCONJUNCTIVAL ANTIMYCOTICS

Antimycotic	Topical	Subconjunctival
Amphotericin B	1.0–2.5 mg/ml	0.5–1.0 mg
Natamycin	50 mg/ml	
Nystatin	50,000 units/ml	
Miconazole	10 mg/ml	5–10 mg
Ketoconazole	10–20 mg/ml	
Fluconazole	2 mg/ml	
Voriconazole	10 mg/ml	
Flucytosine	10 mg/ml	

Since about 75% to 80% of cases of stromal keratitis confirmed by culture to have a fungal cause can be detected by microscopic examination of the scraped material after appropriate staining, it is reasonable to restrict initial antifungal therapy to those cases with a fungus-positive scraping. If by 24 hours after scraping the culture growth is consistent with a bacterial infection, then in spite of the clinical history and appearance, therapy should not include an antifungal agent. On the other hand, a scraping positive for fungal elements or the appearance of fungal growth by 36 to 48 hours after culture should prompt the initiation of antifungal therapy (Table 16-3).

At this time therapy should be started with 5% natamycin suspension (50 mg/mL), usually hourly during the day and every 2 hours at night. The therapy should also include cycloplegic agents and careful monitoring of the intraocular pressure with use of appropriate antiglaucoma medications when indicated. As with other forms of keratitis, in fungal corneal infections immediate or prompt improvement in the clinical picture is unusual; one must be patient and allow time for stabilization, lack of progression, and finally improvement in the corneal stromal infiltrate and ulceration.

If the infection appears to be progressing in the presence of a confirmed fungal cause, particularly when there is a deep stromal infiltrate or prior use of corticosteroids, then consideration should be given to adding or substituting another antifungal agent such as miconazole (117) or amphotericin B (96). In the case of fungal keratitis due to *Aspergillus* that is not responding satisfactorily to topical natamycin, itraconazole or miconazole are good second choices. Since *Paecilomyces* species tend to be relatively resistant to the polyene antimycotics, 1% miconazole or 1% to 2% ketoconazole (118) should be used. In the case of infections due to *Fusarium* species that do not respond clinically to natamycin, 0.10% to 0.25% amphotericin B should be alternated hourly with natamycin.

Miconazole, available as a 1% solution (10 mg/ml) (Monistat), can be used hourly or more frequently topically and can be injected periocularly or subconjunctivally in a dosage of 10 mg. In our experience, injectable miconazole appears much less locally toxic than amphotericin B. It must be emphasized, however, that a body of data similar to that for natamycin testifying to the efficacy of imidazole compounds does not exist, and the presumption of better penetration into the corneal stroma is also not fully proved.

The management of yeast keratitis (*C. albicans*) can be more difficult than that of infections with filamentous fungi because in cases of yeast infection there are often underlying local ocular abnormalities and sometimes general defects in host resistance. Since yeast infections tend to occur in either immunosuppressed or locally compromised eyes, there appears to be a greater disparity in antifungal sensitivities among cases of *Candida* infection than among infections with filamentous fungi. Therefore, one must attempt to stabilize the ocular surface and consider using antifungal agents more specifically directed against yeast infections such as flucytosine. Yeasts grow quickly and usually become evident on culture by 24 to 36 hours, and they can perhaps be best treated by combined therapy using natamycin, nystatin, miconazole, ketoconazole, fluconazole, voriconazole, and flucytosine. Sensitivity studies should be performed with the particular yeast since there is a high incidence of both acquired resistance and de novo resistance to flucytosine. Clinically, nystatin was the first antifungal polyene to be used. Although not commercially available as an ocular medication, it can be prepared as an eye drop in a concentration of 50,000 units/mL. The dermatologic cream preparation can also be utilized for ocular infections. Its use in yeast infections is traditional, although it does not appear to be as effective against yeast infections as natamycin is against filamentous fungi.

Usually stabilization or improvement in the ulceration and stromal infiltrate is evident within 48 to 72 hours, at which time the frequency of topical application of antimycotics can be reduced during the nighttime hours, and then subsequently the daytime application can be tapered to every 2 hours, with further reduction in the frequency as clinical improvement continues. The length of time required for topical treatment has not been firmly established clinically or experimentally. Guidelines have been derived from retrospective clinical reviews. Jones et al. (95) reported an average of 30 days of treatment for *Fusarium* keratitis with natamycin. In one review, the average length of treatment with topical treatment was 39 days (9).

In general, the length of treatment is longer than that for cases of bacterial keratitis. The clinician must determine the length of treatment for each individual based on clinical response. Problems that can arise from prolonged treatment are due to toxicity. The inflammatory response from this toxicity can be confused with persistent infection. If toxicity is suspected and if adequate treatment has been given for at least 4 to 6 weeks, treatment should be discontinued and the patient carefully observed for evidence of recurrence.

Subconjunctival injections of antifungals can cause local toxicity and pain, and are therefore not commonly used. Miconazole is the best tolerated subconjunctival antifungal agent (5 to 10 mg of a 10 mg/mL suspension). It is reserved for severe cases of keratitis, scleritis, and endophthalmitis (119).

The use of systemic antifungal agents is generally not indicated in the management of fungal keratitis. The most frequently used oral antifungal has been ketoconazole. Reports suggest that fluconazole may penetrate better into the cornea after systemic administration than some of the other azoles and may be associated with fewer systemic side effects (109). Systemic antifungal agents are recommended in cases of severe deep keratitis, scleritis, endophthalmitis, and after penetrating keratoplasty for a fungal infection.

The use of topical corticosteroids in the treatment of fungal infections can be problematic (120). In an experimental model, topical corticosteroid worsened the disease when given alone and adversely influenced the efficacy of natamycin, flucytosine, and miconazole when given in combination (105). Similar results have been reported in clinical series of patients (9). A recent animal model of *Candida* keratitis suggests that topical steroids started after the infectious keratitis has been controlled may be beneficial (121). Our current regimen is to not consider topical steroids until after at least 2 weeks of antifungal treatment and clear clinical evidence of control of the infection. Careful follow-up is required to ensure that improvement is taking place. The steroid drop is used in conjunction with the topical antifungal and never without. Usually steroid treatment is carried on for 2 to 3 weeks.

Collagen shields soaked in amphotericin increase the concentration of the drug in the initial treatment periods (116). The excimer laser has been used in rabbits to ablate surface infection of fungal organisms (122). Rao et al. (123) showed the potential fungistatic capabilities of tissue glue. Preliminary experience suggests that intracameral injections of amphotericin B may have a role in the management of deep keratomycoses (124). It is hoped that future treatment modalities will be based on better understanding of the pathophysiology of fungal keratitis. As we gain more knowledge at the molecular level, better medical treatments will be available (125).

In about one third of fungal infections, especially in those patients who may have inadvertently received corticosteroids topically, periocularly, or systemically (105), medical therapy is not successful and the inflammatory process may progress, leading to either impending perforation with descemetocele formation or a frank perforation. In those cases surgical intervention is indicated.

Surgical Management

Fungal keratitis can easily become a surgical disease because of the delay in initiating medical treatment or the inability to obtain antifungal medications. Debridement with a spatula or blade is the simplest form of surgical intervention and is usually performed at the slit lamp under topical anesthesia. Debridement is performed every 24 to 48 hours and works by debulking organisms and necrotic material and by enhancing the penetration of the topical antifungal. A biopsy may be used not only for a diagnosis but also as a therapeutic intervention (126). One third of fungal infections result in surgical intervention because of medical treatment failures or corneal perforations (92). The most often performed surgery in these cases are therapeutic penetrating keratoplasty, and a small percentage has been treated with a conjunctival flap. A recent report looked at the benefits of lamellar keratoplasty (127). The main goal of surgical intervention is to control the infection and maintain the integrity of the globe (Fig. 16-9). An optical keratoplasty can then be performed at a later time (94). Keratoplasty may be needed early with a reported average of within 4 weeks of presentation, primarily because of medical treatment failures; in some cases it may be required because of recurrence of infection (9). If the infection progresses until it involves the limbus or sclera, unfavorable outcomes secondary to scleritis, endophthalmitis, and recurrences are more common (128–130).

In cases of fungal scleritis and keratoscleritis cryotherapy has been used with topical antifungal agents (131). It is applied using a retinal cryoprobe; two freeze-thaw cycles of several seconds are applied primarily to the borders of the infection where the organisms are presumably replicating and invading subconjunctival antifungals injected, and the area is left exposed. These patients are usually continued on both topical and systemic antifungal agents (132). (See further details in the section on fungal scleritis.) The keratoplasty technique is similar to that performed for other forms of microbial keratitis (133). The size of the trephination should have a diameter that leaves a 1- to 1.5-mm area of apparent noninfected cornea. This may decrease the chances of recurrence or persistence of the infection adjacent to the trephination. Interrupted sutures with slightly longer bites should be used to avoid cheese wiring of the suture if the edge of the recipient becomes infected or necrotic (92). Irrigation of the anterior segment with an antifungal can be performed to eliminate any organisms using the concentration for the treatment of endophthalmitis. Affected intraocular structures including the iris, lens, and vitreous should be excised. The specimens removed should be submitted to both the microbiology and pathology laboratories for culture and fixed section examination. If involvement of intraocular structures or endophthalmitis is suspected, an antifungal agent should be injected intraocularly at the time of keratoplasty. Recommended intraocular antifungal agents that can be used for injection and irrigation include amphotericin B (5 μg/0.1 mL) or miconazole (25 μg/0.1 mL).

Following penetrating keratoplasty, topical antifungal agents should be continued to prevent recurrence of infection. In addition, systemic ketoconazole, fluconazole, or

voriconazole may be used (134). If the pathology laboratory reports that no organisms were seen at the edge of the corneal specimen, antifungals could be stopped after 2 weeks and the patient followed carefully for recurrences. A report from the microbiology laboratory regarding growth of organisms from the corneal or intraocular tissues should indicate the need for more prolonged topical and systemic antifungal therapy, possibly for 6 to 8 weeks.

The use of topical corticosteroids should be avoided in the immediate postoperative period. Corticosteroids may be used once the infection is under control for several weeks. Although the main goal of penetrating keratoplasty in fungal keratitis is to eliminate the infecting organism, a secondary goal is the maintenance of a clear corneal transplant for optical reasons. Even if graft failure or rejection occurs, the patient can undergo a second optical keratoplasty once the rejection is controlled (135). The effects of cyclosporin A has been investigated in the laboratory and clinically and seems to be of help in postkeratoplasty patients. Cyclosporin A is an antifungal that can also help prevent the inmune response. This dual action makes it ideal for use in this clinical condition (136,137).

Therapeutic penetrating keratoplasty has been reported as having better results than medical therapy (138). Other surgical procedures that have been used include conjunctival flap, keratectomy, and lamellar or penetrating graft followed by flap (139). Several authors have recommended excisional keratectomy and inlay conjunctival flap as the procedure of choice in fungal keratitis, especially in peripheral ulcers refractory to medical therapy. A consideration when a flap and lamellar keratoplasty are used is that the fungal organisms can be trapped in the intralamellar space, keeping them isolated from the antifungal therapy and the host immune response, thereby leading to the potential for persistence or recurrence of the infection.

FUNGAL CONJUNCTIVITIS

Although the normal flora of the conjunctiva principally consists of aerobic bacteria, the transient flora in the conjunctival sac may include fungi (140,141). The reported incidence of normal fungal flora in the eye varies from 2.9% to 37.1% (141,142). These figures basically seem to reflect the natural environment of the place of study. Seasonal fluctuations have been reported in the incidence and type of fungi in the conjunctival sac of healthy subjects (140). Although some studies have reported a higher incidence in diseased eyes compared to normal eyes (143), others have shown no difference (140). Corticosteroid administration has been shown to increase fungal colonization of the conjunctiva (140,144). Filamentous fungi such as *Cladosporium* spp., *Fusarium* spp., *Alternaria* spp., *Aspergillus* spp., and yeast-like fungi such as *Candida* spp. are some of the fungal species recovered from conjunctival sacs of healthy individuals (140). When appropriate culture conditions and media are used, indigenous ocular flora of *Malassezia furfur* (*Pityrosporum ovale*) can be recovered (145). A majority of these species remain benign passersby in the conjunctiva and do not cause infection (146). Thus, fungal conjunctivitis is a rare condition. In a period of over 2 years, a high-volume tertiary eye care center in south India saw two patients with fungal conjunctivitis associated with chronic dacryocystitis caused by *Candida* spp. and one patient with *Aspergillus flavus* infection of the conjunctiva secondary to scleral buckle exposure (unpublished data).

Predisposing Factors

Apart from causing an increase in colonization of conjunctiva with fungi, prolonged use of topical antibacterial antibiotics and corticosteriods may predispose to fungal infection of the conjunctiva. The principal routes of inoculation with fungi are air, fomites, hand-to-eye contact, contaminated eye drops, and migration from surrounding ocular adnexa including chronic dacryocystitis. Endogenous conjunctivitis is extremely rare. Although keratoconjunctivitis sicca is common in HIV-infected patients, the inflammation is usually noninfectious and self-limited (147).

Clinical Features

Conjunctival fungal infections may be pleomorphic. The infection may be superficical, deep, or proliferative (148). Superficial lesions are nongranulomatous and are confined to the epithelium and its appendages. They may be caused by *Candida albicans, Microsporum* spp., *Trichophyton* spp., *Cephalosporium* spp., *Pityrosporum ovale*, etc. The last is generally associated with seborrheic conjunctivitis secondary to blepharitis and may be associated with superficial punctate keratitis (149). Deep conjunctivitis may present as a granulomatous nodular conjunctivitis, most often caused by *Sporothrix schenkii*. Like most fungi it is a saprophyte and most likely gets implanted in the conjunctiva upon abrasion or injury. The lesions may become purulent and present concomitantly with local adenopathy. Intraocular complications are rare, but perforation of the sclera has been reported. Proliferative conjunctivitis may be granulomatous and is caused by a variety of fungi such as *Aspergillus* spp., *Rhinosporidium seeberi, Blastomyces* spp., *Coccidioides immitis, Paracoccidioides brasiliensis*, etc. Reports of conjunctivitis caused by these fungi are exceedingly rare and most have appeared in the literature prior to the 1960s with the exception of rhinosporidial infection. *R. seeberi* defies Koch's postulates in being as yet uncultivable. Nevertheless, it is accepted as a fungus and is associated with chronic infection of mucous membranes at various sites including the conjunctiva (150). The eye is involved in ~15% of patients with rhinosporidiosis. First described in India in 1912, the infection is common in Southeast Asia, especially

Sri Lanka. The conjunctival lesions are characterized by polypoid growth situated in upper or lower palpebral or bulbar conjunctiva. The lesion may resemble a ruptured chalazion and a creamy exudate may be expressed. The surrounding conjunctiva may appear normal.

In addition to direct inoculation and infection, fungi may cause immune-mediated conjunctivitis. Immediate type of hypersensitivity (type 1)-based hay fever conjunctivitis may be caused in some individuals by fungal spores present in the environment. *Tinea capitis* infection of the scalp may be associated with inflammatory conjunctivitis, which is most likely a manifestation of type IV hypersensitivity (delayed hypersensitivity reaction).

Diagnosis

The choice of sampling technique depends on the type of lesion. Sterile calcium alginate or cotton-tipped swabs moistened with sterile saline, may be used for collection of conjunctival discharge. The swabs are gently rolled over the inferior tarsal conjunctiva and fornix while the patient looks up and the physician pulls down the lower lid. No anesthetic is required. For dry lesions it may be necessary to use a spatula or surgical blade No. 15 on a Bard Parker handle to obtain conjunctival scraping under topical anesthesia. Conjunctival biopsy may be required for deep lesions or polypoidal lesions.

The swabs and scrapings may be processed in a similar manner, by making smears for Gram and Giemsa stain and culture on Sabouraud dextrose agar, brain-heart infusion broth, blood agar, and thioglycollate broth. Special stains for fungus such as periodic acid-Schiff (PAS) and Gomori methenamine silver (GMS) stain may also be done on smears from conjunctival scrapings. Paraffin sections of biopsy tissue are subjected to these special stains apart from the routine hematoxylin and eosin (H&E) stain for the detection of fungal elements. A portion of the biopsy sample may also be sent for culture without fixation in formaldehyde. The results of all diagnostic tests must always be correlated with each other and with the clinical features. The microscopic and culture characteristics of various fungi have been dealt with elsewhere in this chapter. Infection with Actinomycetes (higher bacteria) such as *Actinomyces* spp., *Nocardia* spp. need to be differentiated from fungal infections as the treatment strategy is entirely based on it.

Treatment

Although *Actinomyces* spp. and *Nocardia* spp. respond to penicillin, sulfonamides or broad-spectrum antibiotics, fungi do not. For superficial conjunctivitis, 2% topical miconazole, 5% natamycin, or 2% clotrimazole may be effective. Systemic therapy in the form of oral ketoconazole and fluconazole have been found effective for deep or proliferative conjunctivitis. Oral iodides, used earlier, are currently not preferred because of toxicity. *Candida* spp. are especially susceptible to nystatin and amphotericin B topical drops (149). Surgical excision is the treatment of choice for growth like lesions, especially rhinosporidiosis.

FUNGAL SCLERITIS

Inflammatory scleral disease is frequently associated with autoimmune disorders and is occasionally caused directly by an infective agent (151). Fungal infections primarily involving the sclera are extremely rare, but have been reported after trauma (152–154), retinal detachment surgery (155–158), treatment of pterygium (159–166), cataract surgery (167–171), and in association with systemic fungal infection (172,173). Diagnosis of the condition is often difficult because the clinical picture may appear identical to that caused by immune-mediated disease. Lack of suspicion is one of the causes of delayed diagnosis. In addition, because organisms lie deep in the stroma, negative microbiology is a frequent finding in these cases. Because of a mistaken diagnosis of noninfectious scleritis, many of these cases are initially treated with corticosteroids or other immunosuppressive agents that lead to diffuse spread of infection. The outcome of fungal scleritis is usually disappointing due to delayed diagnosis, prior corticosteroid or immunosuppressive therapy, and poor penetration of the available antifungal agents through sclera.

Pathogenesis

Fungal infection of the sclera usually occurs following (a) an accidental or surgical trauma, (b) as an extension from adjacent focus such as keratitis, and (c) rarely as endogenous infection.

Exogenous Infection

The most common mode of infection in fungal scleritis is exogenous infection via an accidental or surgical trauma. Fungal scleritis usually occurs after trauma with vegetable matters. The interval between trauma and the onset of the clinical manifestations is usually long in these cases (152–154).

Ocular surgery is a significant predisposing cause of microbial scleritis. Fungal scleritis has been reported following cataract surgery including surgery with self-sealing scleral tunnel incision (167–171). Scleritis can occur in association with postcataract endophthalmitis also. Pterygium excision is another important predisposing factor for fungal scleritis. The complication has been reported after bare sclera technique but more often after beta irradiation therapy and use of antimetabolites (159–166). Avascular scleral necrosis and an overlying epithelial defect predispose these patients to infectious scleritis.

Infection after retinal detachment surgery with scleral buckling is a potential long-term complication with incidence varying from less than 1% to over 3% (174). Infection and extrusion are most likely to occur after reoperations and with the use of multiple sponges and encircling elements. The organisms are usually introduced into the surgical field at the time of surgery, but inoculation may occur later if the ocular surface is abnormal. Although scleritis is most frequently an aseptic, immune-mediated inflammation that can occasionally be initiated by surgical (surgically induced necrotizing scleritis) trauma, the possibility of infectious scleritis after surgery must be considered when there is no history of immune disease and when the disease characteristics are atypical of immune-mediated scleral inflammation.

Another mode of scleral involvement is the spread of infection from contiguous structures such as cornea or choroid. Fungal infection of cornea may extend to involve the limbus and adjacent sclera (175). Various underlying ocular or systemic conditions such as use of topical corticosteroids, disciform keratitis, penetrating keratoplasty, renal failure, diabetes mellitus, HIV infection, and advanced age increase susceptibility to such an extension.

Endogenous Infection

Fungal infection of sclera may result from septic emboli released from systemic infection or an infecting focus elsewhere in the body. The emboli may localize in the sclera inducing nodular scleritis, which may progress to abscess formation with slow suppuration. Such patients are usually quite ill with a systemic infection. At times, the scleritis may also result from hypersensitivity reaction induced by infectious agents.

Organisms

Although yeasts has been isolated (156,164), the most common fungi that cause scleritis are the filamentous fungi. Various fungi isolated from cases of scleritis are *Aspergillus* (153,154,159,164,168,170,171), *Acremonium* (176), *Lasiodiplodia* (177), *Paecilomyces* (167), *Sporotrichum, Blastomyces, Coccidiomycosis, Mucormycosis* (155), *Fusarium* (160,161), *Scedosporium* (157,160–163), *Aureobasidium pullulans* (175), *Rhizopus* (169), *Petriellidium boydii* (160,161), dimorphic fungi such as *Sporothrix schenckii* (152), and *Rhinosporidium seeberi* (177–179), an organism of uncertain taxonomic position.

Clinical Presentation

Fungal scleritis usually presents as slowly progressive scleral necrosis with suppuration. Initially the lesion appears as localized, firm, tender scleral nodule indistinguishable from immune-mediated scleritis. Soon this scleral nodule assumes the appearance of an abscess with ulceration of overlying

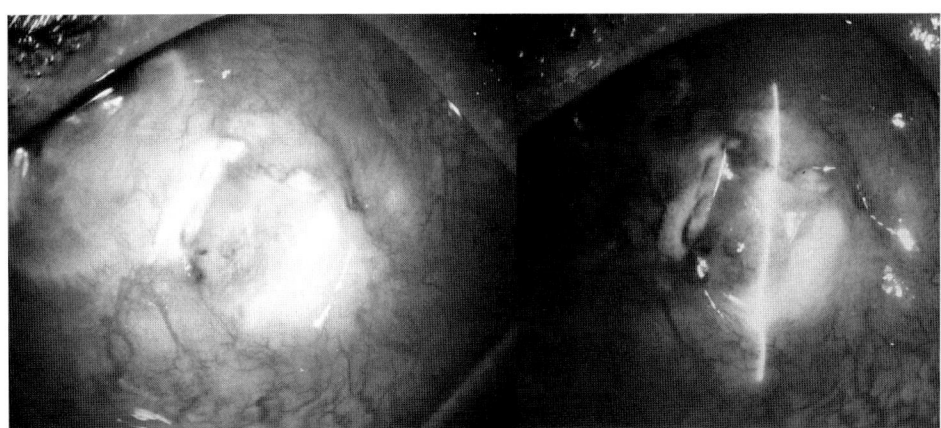

FIGURE 16-10. Fungal scleritis caused by *Aspergillus flavus*. Note scleral necrosis with suppuration.

conjunctiva and suppuration (Fig. 16-10). At this stage, scleral lesion is associated with intense conjunctival reaction, purulent discharge, and variable intraocular inflammation. Some cases may show development of multifocal infectious nodules (Fig. 16-11). The condition occasionally mimics pseudotumor or orbital cellulitis producing painful proptosis. These cases of posterior scleritis have associated serous retinal detachment (161). Unless diagnosed in time and managed appropriately, perforation and intraocular spread of infection occurs with subsequent loss of the eye.

Patients with fungal infection of scleral buckle present with variable lid edema, localized or generalized conjunctival injection, and purulent discharge. Examination shows extrusion of the buckle with tenderness at the site of extrusion. This may be associated with abscess formation. In cases with delayed presentation, the retina over the buckle becomes white with the development of localized vitreous reaction or endophthalmitis. On removing the explant, multiple discrete white lesions are noted on the scleral surface underneath and around the explant site. These are

presumed to represent fungal colonies. The explant itself may be blackened and frayed, containing fungal colonies on its surface.

Patients who develop this complication after pterygium surgery show an avascular and necrotic sclera with an overlying calcific plaque. Patients developing infection of the cataract surgery wound show suppurative necrosis of the sclera at the site of the incision associated with infiltration of the adjoining cornea and variable anterior chamber reaction (Fig. 16-12).

Diagnosis

Although the systemic immune-mediated diseases are the main possibilities in the differential diagnosis of scleritis, it is important to rule out infectious etiology in suppurative lesions. This differentiation is important because corticosteroid therapy or immunosuppressive therapy, often used in immune-mediated scleritis is contraindicated in infectious scleritis. A thorough history, detailed ocular examination, and a complete general physical examination, looking especially for signs of infection or evidence of a collagen vascular disease, is essential. Fungal scleritis should be suspected in cases of slow but progressive scleral necrosis with suppuration, especially if there is a history of accidental or surgical trauma, and debilitating ocular or systemic disease. If the lesion is adjacent to keratitis, a characteristically dry, raised infiltrate with feathery edge, satellite lesion, and endothelial plaque helps in diagnosis. In other cases, laboratory workup is necessary to rule out active infection.

Laboratory Workup

In patients with suppurative scleral lesion, laboratory workup helps establish diagnosis and identification of the causative organisms. In ulcerative lesions, scraping should be done using a sterile surgical blade or Kimura's spatula. The material so obtained should be smeared on glass slides for microscopic examination and onto agar plates and broth for culture. The

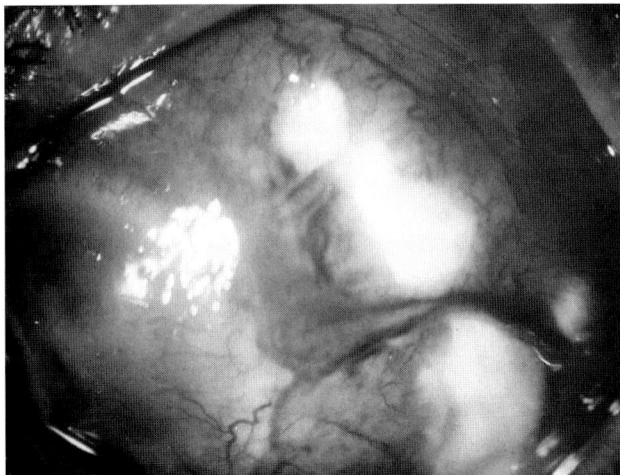

FIGURE 16-11. Multifocal infiltrate in fungal scleritis.

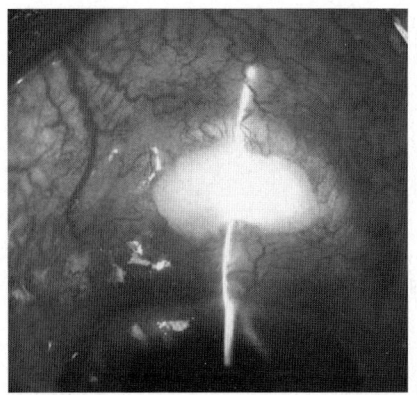
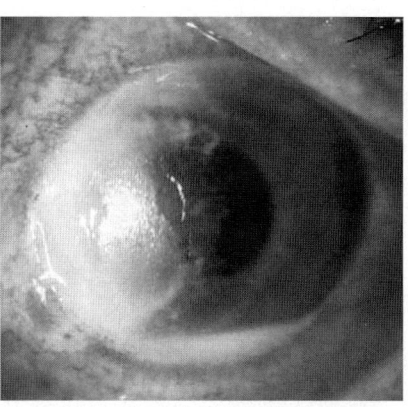

A   B

FIGURE 16-12. Fungal infection of self-sealing wound of cataract surgery. **A:** Infection of scleral tunnel incision. **B:** Infection of temporal corneal incision.

media usually inoculated include blood agar, chocolate agar, Sabouraud dextrose agar (SDA), potato dextrose agar (PDA), nonnutrient agar (NNA), thioglycollate broth, and brain-heart infusion broth. However, one must remember that negative microbiology from scrapings is a frequent finding and does not exclude an infection, because organisms may be present only in the deep stroma (170).

If fungal infection is the primary clinical suspicion, but the initial microbiology workup is negative and the patient is not improving on initial broad-spectrum antibacterial therapy, scleral or corneoscleral biopsy is recommended. The procedure involves dissection of the conjunctiva, Tenon's capsule, and episclera to expose the scleral lesion. Lamellar dissection of the sclera is then performed from the edge of the lesion. The biopsy specimen is divided into two halves; one half is sent in saline for microbiology evaluation and the other half is sent in formaline for histopathology evaluation. The sections are examined using routine (H&E) and special stains including PAS and GMS stain for fungal identification.

Anterior chamber paracentesis is indicated in cases of corneoscleral involvement with endothelial exudates. The procedure is performed using an adequate-sized needle (22 gauge). The harvested material is either directly inoculated on culture media or immediately transported to the microbiology laboratory.

Treatment

Medical treatment of fungal scleritis is limited by the paucity of approved antifungal drugs, poor penetration of available agents, and their fungistatic rather than fungicidal property. Therefore, although therapy for confirmed fungal scleritis is initially medical, surgery may be required in a significant proportion of cases. The therapy is started with local and systemic administration of the following antifungal agents: amphotericin B, flucytosine, topical miconazole (2%), topical econazole, topical natamycin (5%), fluconazole, or itraconazole. Amphotericin B and fluconazole have an excellent activity against yeast but relatively poor activity against filamentous fungi. In addition, amphotericin B is irritant to

ocular tissues, and penetrates the anterior chamber and vitreous poorly, achieving levels below minimum inhibitory concentrations when administered via subconjunctival or intravenous route. Nevertheless, when used with other azole antifungals, amphotericin B can have an additive effect against certain isolates. Natamycin is effective against many filamentous fungi. It is available as a 5% suspension. Miconazole and econazole have also been found to be effective against filamentous fungi. They show a good penetration of ocular tissue (157). Carlson and associates (168) reported successful outcome using itraconazole 200 mg/day in a patient with *A. flavus* scleritis after cataract surgery (168). In a recent publication Kim and associates (158) reported successful management of fungal scleritis using voriconazole. A saturated solution of potassium iodide (50 mg/mL) 10 drops orally three times daily increasing to 24 drops three times daily was successful in treating *S. schenckii* scleritis (152). It has to be borne in mind, however, that massive inflammatory reaction may occur after initiation of medical therapy. These may represent an immunologic response to fungal cell death rather than actual disease progression. Corticosteroids and immunosuppressive agents should be avoided to prevent acceleration of fungal infection.

Although there are reports of successful management, the outcome of fungal scleritis with medical therapy alone has been uniformly poor. This poor prognosis is attributed mainly to the poor penetration of topical or systemic antifungal agents into avascular sclera and the ability of microbial organisms to reside in deep intrascleral lamellae. Patients with scleritis refractory to medical treatment or complicated by scleral abscess should have surgical intervention.

The surgical intervention involves scleral excision and debridement of the ulcer base coupled with cryotherapy of the ulcer margin. This procedure helps by debulking the infection and facilitating topical antifungal penetration (154,160,162,164,170,175,176). In cases with diffuse scleral involvement or intrascleral dissemination, repeated debridement may be required. Antifungal treatment needs to be continued for a long period after the infection has clinically resolved, as viable fungi can still be found in tissues even after debridement and topical and systemic antifungal therapy (157,160).

Patients with scleral buckle infection require immediate removal of the buckling elements and sutures (157). It is better to accept the risk of detachment to achieve resolution of the infection rather than run the risk of loss of the eye. At the time of surgery, the scleral surface underneath and around the buckle must be examined carefully. All discrete white lesions, which represent fungal colonies, must be cleared, taking care not to further disseminate the infection, and the area washed with 5% povidone iodine (157).

Occasionally, an emergency graft may be necessary if there is impending perforation. In such cases excision of as much necrotic tissue as possible is necessary. In other situations early grafts should be avoided as the grafts performed prior to adequate debridement and antifungal therapy have a high risk of necrosis and sloughing.

CANALICULITIS

Fungal infection of the lacrimal canaliculus is an uncommon condition. Of the various organisms responsible, by far the most commonly described has been *Actinomyces* species (an anaerobic, nonsporulating, filamentous bacterium); true fungi such as *Candida albicans* and *Aspergillus niger* are less common causes of canaliculitis (180).

Clinical Features

Patients with canaliculitis present with chronic, unilateral, mucoid, or mucopurulent conjunctivitis associated with epiphora. Examination reveals swelling of the medial half of the lid margin along with erythema of the overlying skin and hyperemia of the medial palpebral and bulbar conjunctiva. The punctum of the involved canaliculus becomes prominent and inflamed. A posteriorly directed pressure on the medial eyelid produces a milky, yellow, or blood-tinged discharge from the punctum. In cases of *Aspergillus niger* infection, the infected punctum and canaliculus show characteristic black pigmentation. Probing of the involved canaliculus demonstrates obstruction with a grating sensation, and irrigation offers resistance to flow, but the distal lacrimal drainage system may be patent.

Diagnosis

Canaliculitis must be considered in the differential diagnosis of all cases of unexplained epiphora associated with segmental lid and conjunctival inflammation. Pressure over the inflamed eyelid segment will express creamy-white pus from the involved punctum. The expressed material may contain characteristic granular concretions (dacryoliths) (180,181). Absence of reflux on pressure over the lacrimal sac area will help differentiate canaliculitis from chronic dacryocystitis.

To identify causative organisms the expressed material should be examined microscopically as well as cultured using both anaerobic and aerobic techniques. Because *Actinomyces* species and other filamentous bacteria are the most common causes of canaliculitis, care must be taken to differentiate filamentous bacteria from true fungi on smear examination.

Treatment

The most effective treatment of fungal canaliculitis is thorough curettage of infected material followed by a course of topical antifungal agents (182). It is important to understand that the responsible organisms usually reside in diverticula of canaliculus; therefore, repeat curettage and even canaliculotomy may be necessary to eliminate the infection. Amphotericin B (1–5 mg/mL) is used as irrigating fluid at the time of curettage. After surgical drainage, natamycin (5%) or Amphotericin B 5 mg/mL eyedrops are used as adjunctive to surgical approach.

REFERENCES

1. Liesegang TJ, Forster RK. Spectrum of microbial keratitis in South Florida. *Am J Ophthalmol* 1980;90:38–47.
2. Alfonso E, Mandelbaum S, Fox MJ, et al. Ulcerative keratitis associated with contact lens wear *Am J Ophthalmol* 1986;101:429–433.
3. Koidou-Tsiligianni A, Alfonso EC, Forster RK. Ulcerative keratitis associated with contact lens wear. *Am J Ophthalmol* 1989;108:64–67.
4. Foster CS. Fungal keratitis. *Infect Dis Clin North Am* 1992;6:851–857.
5. Jones DB. Diagnosis and management of fungal keratitis. In: Tasman W, Jaeger EA, eds. *Duane's clinical ophthalmology*, rev ed, vol 4. Philadelphia:, JB Lippincott, 1993.
6. Chin GN, Hyndiuk RA, Kwasny GP, et al. Keratomycosis in Wisconsin. *Am J Ophthalmol* 1975;79:121–125.
7. Doughman DJ, Leavenworth NM, Campbell RC, et al. Fungal keratitis at the University of Minnesota: 1971–1981. *Trans Am Ophthalmol Soc* 1982;80:235–247.
8. Jones DB, Sexton RR, Rebell G. Mycotic keratitis in South Florida: a review of thirty-nine cases. *Trans Ophthalmol Soc UK* 1970;89:781–797.
9. Rosa RH, Miller D, Alfonso EC. The changing spectrum of fungal keratitis in South Florida. *Ophthalmology* 1992;4101:1005–1113.
10. Srinivasan R, Kanungo R, Goyal JL. Spectrum of oculomycosis in South India. *Acta Ophthalmol* (Copenh) 1991;69:744–749.
11. Gopinathan U, Garg P, Fernandes M, et al. The epidemiological features and laboratory results of fungal keratitis: a 10-year review at a referral eye care center in South India. *Cornea* 2002;21(6):555–559.
12. Leck AK, Thomas PA, Hagan M, et al. Aetiology of suppurative corneal ulcers in Ghana and south India, and epidemiology of fungal keratitis. *Br J Ophthalmol* 2002;86(11):1211–1215.
13. Jones DB. Diagnosis and Management of Fungal Keratitis. In: Tasman W, Jaeger E, eds. *Duane's clinical ophthalmology*, vol 4. Philadelphia: Lippincott, 1986:1–22.
14. Wilhelmus KR, Jones DB. Curvularia keratitis, discussion 130–132. *Trans Am Ophthalmol Soc* 2001;99:111–130.

15. Rishi K, Font RL. Keratitis caused by an unusual fungus, Phoma species. *Cornea* 2003;22(2):166–168.

16. Guarro J, Hofling-Lima AL, Gene J, et al. Corneal ulcer caused by the new fungal species Sarcopodium oculorum. *J Clin Microbiol* 2002;40(8):3071–3075.

17. Wu Z, Ying H, Yiu S, et al. Fungal keratitis caused by Scedosporium apiospermum: report of two cases and review of treatment, *Cornea* 2002;21(5):519–523; Comment in *Cornea* 2003;22(1):92.

18. Shin JY, Kim HM, Hong JW.Keratitis caused by Verticillium species. *Cornea* 2002;21(2):240–242.

19. Yamamoto N, Matsumoto T, Ishibashi Y. Fungal keratitis caused by Colletotrichum gloeosporioides. *Cornea* 2001;20(8): 902–903.

20. Jani BR, Rinaldi MG, Reinhart WJ. An unusual case of fungal keratitis: Metarrhizium anisopliae. *Cornea* 2001;20(7):765–768.

21. Atlas RM. *Basic and practical microbiology.* New York: Macmillan, 1986.

22. Forster RK, Rebell G, Wilson LA. Dematiaceous fungal keratitis: clinical isolates and management. *Br J Ophthalmol* 1975; 59:372.

23. Jones BR. Principles in the management of oculomycosis. *Trans Am Acad Ophthalmol Otolaryngol* 1975;79:15.

24. Jones DB, Sexton RR, Rebell G. Mycotic keratitis in South Florida: a review of 39 cases. *Pans Ophthalmol Soc U.K* 1969; 89:781.

25. Clinch TE, et al. Fungal keratitis from nylon line lawn trimmers. *Am J Ophthalmol* 1992;114:437–440.

26. Srinivasan M, Gonzales CA, George C, et al. Epidemiology and aetiological diagnosis of corneal ulceration in Madurai, south India. *Br J Ophthalmol* 1997;81(11):965–971.

27. Kremer I, Goldenfeld M, Shmueli D. Fungal keratitis associated with contact lens wear after penetrating keratoplasty. *Ann Ophthalmol* 1991;23:342–345.

28. Strelow SA, Kent HD, Eagle RC Jr, et al. A case of contact lens related *Fusarium solani* keratitis. *CLAO J* 1992;18:125–127.

29. Yamamoto GK, Pavan-Langston D, Stowe GC III, et al. Fungal invasion of therapeutic soft contact lens and cornea. *Ann Ophthalmol* 1979;1731–1735.

30. Berger RO, Streeten BW. Fungal growth in aphakic soft contact lenses. *Am J Ophthalmol* 1981;91:630–633.

31. Churner R, Cunningham RD. Fungal-contaminated soft contact lenses. *Ann Ophthalmol* 1983;15:724–727.

32. Wilhelmus KR, et al. Fungal keratitis in contact lens wearers. *Am J Ophthalmol* 1988;106:708–714.

33. Wilhelmus KR. Review of clinical experience with microbial keratitis associated with contact lenses. *CLAO J* 1987;13:211–214.

34. Hofling-Lima AL, Roizenblatt R. Therapeutic contact lens-related bilateral fungal keratitis. *CLAO J* 2002;28(3):149–150.

35. Alfonso E, Mandelbaum S, Fox MJ, et al. Ulcerative keratitis associated with contact lens wear. *Am J Ophthalmol* 1986;101: 429–433.

36. Sharma S, Gopalakrishnan S, Aasuri MK, et al. Trends in contact lens-associated microbial keratitis in Southern India. *Ophthalmology* 2003;110(1):138–143.

37. Wong TY, Ng TP, Fong KS, et al. Risk factors and clinical outcomes between fungal and bacterial keratitis: a comparative study. *CLAO J* 1997;23(4):275–281.

38. Mitsui Y, Hanabusa J. Corneal infections after cortisone therapy. *Br J Ophthalmol* 1955;39:244–250.

39. Forster RK, Rebell G. Animal model of *Fusarium solani* keratitis. *Am J Ophthalmol* 1975;79:510–515.

40. Chern KC, Meisler DM, Wilhelmus KR, et al. Corneal anesthetic abuse and Candida keratitis. *Ophthalmology* 1996;103(1):37–40.

41. Sridhar MS, Gopinathan U, Rao GN. Fungal keratitis associated with vernal keratoconjunctivitis. *Cornea* 2003;22(1):80–81.

42. Vajpayee RB, Gupta SK, Bareja U, et al. Ocular atopy and mycotic keratitis. *Ann Ophthalmol* 1990;22:369–372.

43. Verma S, Tuft SJ. Fusarium solani keratitis following LASIK for myopia. *Br J Ophthalmol* 2002;86(10):1190–1191.

44. Fong LP, Ormerod LD, Kenyon KR, et al. Microbial keratitis complicating penetrating keratoplasty. *Ophthalmology* 1988;94: 1269–1275.

45. Driebe WT, Stern GA. Microbial keratitis following corneal transplantation. *Cornea* 1983;2:41–45.

46. Tseng SH, Ling KC. Late microbial keratitis after corneal transplantation. *Cornea* 1995;14(6):591–594.

47. Kloess PM, Stulting RD, Waring GO III, et al. Bacterial and fungal endophthalmitis after penetrating keratoplasty. *Am J Ophthalmol* 1993;115:309–316.

48. Sutphin JE, Pfaller MA, Hollis RJ, et al. Donor-to-host transmission of Candida albicans after corneal transplantation *Am J Ophthalmol* 2002;134(1):120–121.

49. Mselle J. Fungal keratitis as an indicator of HIV infection in Africa. *Trop Doct* 1999;29(3):133–135.

50. John D, Daniel E. Infectious keratitis in leprosy. *Br J Ophthalmol* 1999;83(2):173–176.

51. Cruz OA, Sabir SM, Capo H, et al. Microbial keratitis in childhood. *Ophthalmology* 1993;100:192–196.

52. Panda A, Sharma N, Das G, et al. Mycotic keratitis in children: epidemiologic and microbiologic evaluation. *Cornea* 1997;16(3): 295–299.

53. Panda A, Das GK, Vanathi M, et al. Corneal infection after radial keratotomy. *J Cataract Refract Surg* 1998;24(3):331–334.

54. Karp CL, Tuli SS, Yoo SH, et al. Infectious keratitis after LASIK. *Ophthalmology* 2003;110(3):503–510.

55. Tuli SS, Yoo SH. Curvularia keratitis after laser in situ keratomileusis from a feline source. *J Cataract Refract Surg* 2003; 29(5):1019–1021.

56. Maskin SL, Alfonso E. Fungal keratitis after radial keratotomy. *Am J Ophthalmol* 1992;114:369–370.

57. Gussler JR, Miller D, Jaffee M, et al. Infection after radial keratotomy. *Am J Ophthalmol* 1995;119:798–799.

58. Periman LM, Harrison DA, Kim J. Fungal keratitis after photorefractive keratectomy: delayed diagnosis and treatment in a co-managed setting. *J Refract Surg* 2003;19(3):364–366.

59. Pushker N, Dada T, Sony P, et al. Microbial keratitis after laser in situ keratomileusis. *J Refract Surg* 2002;18(3):280–286.

60. Kouyoumdjian GA, Forstot SL, Durairaj VD, et al. Infectious keratitis after laser refractive surgery. *Ophthalmology* 2001;108(7): 1266–1268.

61. Kuo IC, Margolis TP, Cevallos V, et al. Aspergillus fumigatus keratitis after laser in situ keratomileusis. *Cornea* 2001;20(3): 342–344.

62. Kaufman HE, Wood RM. Mycotic keratitis. *Am J Ophthalmol* 1965;59:993.

63. Sevel D, Kassar B. Suppurative keratitis and fungal keratitis. *Trans Ophthalmol Soc N Z* 1973;25:228–232.

64. Jones DB. Decision-making in the management of microbial keratitis. *Ophthalmology* 1981;88:814.

65. Forster RK, Rebell G. The diagnosis and management of keratomycoses. I. Cause and diagnosis. *Arch Ophthalmol* 1975; 93:975.

66. Avunduk AM, Beuerman RW, Varnell ED, et al. Confocal microscopy of Aspergillus fumigatus keratitis. *Br J Ophthalmol* 2003;87(4):409–410.

67. Winchester K, Mathers WD, Sutphin JE. Diagnosis of Aspergillus keratitis in vivo with confocal microscopy. *Cornea* 1997;16(1):27–31.

68. Rebell G, Forster RK. Fungi of keratomycosis. In: Lennette EH, ed. *Manual of clinical microbiology*, 3rd ed. Washington, DC: American Society for Microbiology, 1980:553–561.

69. Wilson LA, Sexton RR. Laboratory diagnosis in fungal keratitis. *Am J Ophthalmol* 1968;66:646.
70. Alexandrakis G, Haimovici R, Miller D, et al. Efficacy of diagnostic corneal biopsy in refractory and nonulcerative microbial keratitis. *Ophthalmology* 2000;129(5):571–576.
71. Rosa RH, Alfonso EC. Infectious keratitis: fungal keratitis. In: Stenson SM, ed. *Surgical management in external diseases of the eye.* New York: Igaku-Shoin, 1995.
72. Ishibashi Y, Kaufman HE. Corneal biopsy in the diagnosis of keratomycosis. *Am J Ophthalmol* 1986;101:288–293.
73. Ishibashi Y, Hommura S, Matsumoto Y. Direct examination vs culture of biopsy specimens for the diagnosis of keratomycosis. *Am J Ophthalmol* 1987;103:636–640.
74. Sridhar MS, Sharma S, Gopinathan U, et al. Anterior chamber tap: diagnostic and therapeutic indications in the management of ocular infections. *Cornea* 2002;21(7):718–722.
75. Forster RK, Wirta MG, Solis M, et al. Methenamine-silver-stained corneal scrapings in keratomycoses. *Am J Ophthalmol* 1976;82:261.
76. Sharma S, Silverberg M, Mehta P, et al. Early diagnosis of mycotic keratitis: predictive value of potassium hydroxide preparation. *Indian J Ophthalmol* 1998; 46(1):31–35.
77. Vemuganti GK, Naidu C, Gopinathan U. Rapid detection of fungal filaments in corneal scrapings by microwave heating-assisted Grocott's methenamine silver staining. *Indian J Ophthalmol* 2002;50(4):326–328.
78. Garcia ML, Herreras JM, Dios E, et al. Evaluation of lectin staining in the diagnosis of fungal keratitis in an experimental rabbit model. *Mol Vis* 2002;8:10–16.
79. Kanungo R, Srinivasan R, Rao RS. Acridine orange staining in early diagnosis of mycotic keratitis. *Acta Ophthalmol (Copenh)* 1991;69:750–753.
80. Thomas PA. Mycotic keratitis—an underestimated mycosis. *J Med Vet Mycol* 1994;32:235–256.
81. Sharma S, Kunimoto DY, Gopinathan U, et al. Evaluation of corneal scraping smear examination methods in the diagnosis of bacterial and fungal keratitis: a survey of eight years of laboratory experience. *Cornea* 2002 Oct;21(7):643–647.
82. O'Day DM. Selection of appropriate antifungal therapy. *Cornea* 1987;6:238–245.
83. O'Day DM, et al. Laboratory isolation techniques in human experimental fungal infections. *Am J Ophthalmol* 1979;87:688.
84. Bock M, et al. Polymerase chain reaction-based detection of dermatophyte DNA with a fungus-specific primer system. *Mycoses* 1994;37:79–84.
85. Makimura K, Murayama SY, Yamaguchi H. Specific detection of *Aspergillus* and *Penicillium* species from respiratory specimens by polymerase chain reaction. *Jpn J Med Sci Bio* 1994;47:141–156.
86. Gaudio PA, Gopinathan U, Sangwan V, et al. Polymerase chain reaction based detection of fungi in infected corneas. *Br J Ophthalmol* 2002;86(7):755–760.
87. Ferrer C, Colom F, Frases S, et al. Detection and identification of fungal pathogens by PCR and by ITS2 and 5.8S ribosomal DNA typing in ocular infections. *J Clin Microbiol* 2001;39(8):2873–2879.
88. Pereira IC, Alfonso EC. Evaluation of contamination of in use ophthalmic medications. *Arq Bras Oftalmol* 1992;55:15–18.
89. Schein OD, et al. Microbial contamination of in-use ocular medications. *Arch Ophthalmol* 1992;110:82–85.
90. Martins EN, Farah ME, Alvarenga LS, et al. Infectious keratitis: correlation between corneal and contact lens cultures. *CLAO J* 2002;28(3):146–148.
91. Naumann G, Green WR, Zimmerman LE. Mycotic keratitis. A histopathologic study of 73 cases. *Am J Ophthalmol* 1967;64:668.
92. Forster RK. The role of excisional keratoplasty in microbial keratitis. In: Cavanagh HD, ed. *The cornea: transactions of the World Congress on the Cornea 111.* New York: Raven, 1988:529–533.
93. Forster RK, Rebell G. Therapeutic surgery in failures of medical treatment for fungal keratitis. *Br J Ophthalmol* 1975;59:366.
94. Forster RK, Rebell G. The diagnosis and management of keratomycoses. II. Medical and surgical management. *Arch Ophthalmol* 1975;93:1134.
95. Jones DB, Forster RK, Rebell G. *Fusarium solanae* keratitis treated with natamycin (pimaricin). *Arch Ophthalmol* 1972;88:147.
96. O'Day DM, Robinson R, Head WS. Efficacy of antifungal agents in the cornea. I. A comparative study. *Invest Ophthalmol Vis Sci* 1983;24:1098.
97. O'Day DM, et al. Corneal penetration of topical amphotericin B and natamycin. *Curr Eye Res* 1986;5:877.
98. O'Day DM, et al. Influence of the corneal epithelium on the efficacy of topical antifungal agents. *Invest Ophthalmol Vis Sci* 1984;25:855.
99. O'Day DM, et al. Ocular pharmacokinetics of saperconazole in rabbits. A potential agent against keratomycoses *Arch. Ophthalmol* 1992;110:550.
100. Kotler-Brajtburg J, et al. Classification of polyene antibiotics according to chemical structure and biological effects. *Antimicrob Agents Chemother* 1979;15:716.
101. Sud IJ, Feingold DS. Heterogeneity of action mechanisms among antimycotic imidazoles. *Antimicrob Agents Chemother* 1981;20:71.
102. Wagner GE, Shadomy S. Studies on the mode of action of 5-fluorocytosine in *Aspergillus* species. *Chemotherapy* 1979;25:61.
103. Shadomy S. Susceptibility Testing with Antifungal Drugs. In: Lennette EH, ed. *Manual of clinical microbiology,* 4th ed. Washington, DC: American Society for Microbiology, 1985:991–999.
104. Vemuganti GK, Garg P, Gopinathan U, et al. Evaluation of agent and host factors in progression of mycotic keratitis: a histologic and microbiologic study of 167 corneal buttons. *Ophthalmology* 2002;109(8):1538–1546.
105. O'Day DM, et al. Efficacy of antifungal agents in the cornea. II. Influence of corticosteroids. *Invest Ophthalmol Vis Sci* 1984; 25:331.
106. Wood TO, Williford W. Treatment of keratomycosis with amphotericin B 0.15%. *Am J Ophthalmol* 1976;81:847.
107. O'Day DM, et al. Efficacy of antifungal agents in the cornea. IV Amphotericin B methyl ester. *Invest Ophthalmol Vis Sci* 1984;25:851.
108. Robinson N, Penland R, Osato M. Comparative efficacy of new azole antifungal agents against human ocular isolates. *Invest Ophthalmol Vis Sci* 1990;31(suppl):451.
109. O'Day DM. Orally administered antifungal therapy for experimental keratomycosis. *Trans Am Ophthalmol Soc* 1990;88:685.
110. Brooks JG, et al. Comparative topical triazole therapy of experimental *Candida albicans* keratitis. *Invest Ophthalmol Vis Sci* 1990;31(suppl):570.
111. Mselle J. Use of topical clotrimazole in human keratomycosis. *Ophthalmologica* 2001;5(5):357–360.
112. Panda A, Ahuja R, Biswas NR, et al. Role of 0.02% polyhexamethylene biguanide and 1% povidone iodine in experimental Aspergillus keratitis. *Cornea* 2003;22(2):138–141.
113. Fiscella RG, Moshifar M, Messick CR, et al. Polyhexamethylene biguanide (PHMB) in the treatment of experimental Fusarium keratomycosis. *Cornea* 1997;16(4):447–449.
114. Rahman MR, Johnson GJ, Husain R, et al. Randomised trial of 0.2% chlorhexidine gluconate and 2.5% natamycin for fungal keratitis in Bangladesh. *Br J Ophthalmol.* 1998;82(8):919–925.
115. Shah KB, Wu TG, Wilhelmus KR, et al. Activity of voriconazole against corneal isolates of Scedosporium apiospermum. *Cornea* 2003;22(1):33–36.

116. Schwartz SD, et al. Collagen shield delivery of amphotericin B. *Am J Ophthalmol* 1990;109:701.
117. Foster CS. Miconazole therapy for keratomycosis. *Am J Ophthalmol* 1981;91:622.
118. Sud IJ, Feingold DS. Heterogeneity of action mechanisms among antimycotic imidazoles. *Antimicrob Agents Chemother* 1981;20:71.
119. Scott IU, Flynn HW Jr, Feuer W, et al. Endophthalmitis associated with microbial keratitis. *Ophthalmology* 1996;103(11):1864–1870.
120. Stern GA, Buttross M. Use of corticosteroids in combination with antimicrobial drugs in the treatment of infectious corneal disease. *Ophthalmology* 1991;98:847–853.
121. Schreiber W, Olbrisch A, Vorwerk CK, et al. Combined topical fluconazole and corticosteroid treatment for experimental Candida albicans keratomycosis. *Invest Ophthalmol Vis Sci.* 2003; 44(6):2634–2643.
122. Frucht-Pery J, et al. The effect of the ArF excimer laser on *Candida albicans* in vitro. *Graefes Arch Clin Exp Ophthalmol* 1993; 231:413–415.
123. Rao GN, Reddy MK, Vagh MM. Results of cyanoacrylate tissue adhesive application in active filamentous fungal keratitis. Presentation at the Castroviejo Cornea Society, San Francisco, October 29, 1994.
124. Kuriakose T, Kothari M, Paul P, et al. Intracameral amphotericin B injection in the management of deep keratomycosis. *Cornea* 2002;21(7):653–656.
125. Gopinathan U, Ramakrishna T, Willcox M, et al. Enzymatic, clinical and histologic evaluation of corneal tissues in experimental fungal keratitis in rabbits. *Exp Eye Res* 2001;72(4):433–442.
126. Kompa S, Langefeld S, Kirchhof B, et al. Corneal biopsy in keratitis performed with the microtrephine. *Graefes Arch Clin Exp Ophthalmol* 1999;237(11):915–919.
127. Xie L, Shi W, Liu Z, et al. Lamellar keratoplasty for the treatment of fungal keratitis. *Cornea* 2002;21(1):33–37.
128. Xie L, Dong X, Shi W. Treatment of fungal keratitis by penetrating keratoplasty. *Br J Ophthalmol* 2001;85(9):1070–1074.
129. Dursun D, Fernandez V, Miller D, et al. Advanced fusarium keratitis progressing to endophthalmitis. *Cornea* 2003;22(4): 300–303.
130. Wang MX, Shen DJ, Liu JC, et al. Recurrent fungal keratitis and endophthalmitis. *Cornea* 2000;19(4):558–560.
131. Reynolds MG, Alfonso E. Treatment of infectious scleritis and keratoscleritis. *Am J Ophthalmol* 1991;112:543–547.
132. Alfonso EC. Surgical management of ocular infections. In: Infectious diseases of the eye. Bialasiewicz AA, Schaal KD (eds.) Buren, The Netherlands, Aeolus Press 1994;7:255–258.
133. Sony P, Sharma N, Vajpayee RB, et al. Therapeutic keratoplasty for infectious keratitis: a review of the literature. *CLAO J* 2002;28(3):111–118.
134. Comparison of efficacy of topical and oral fluconazole treatment in experimental Aspergillus keratitis. *Curr Eye Res* 2003;26(2):113–117.
135. Cristol SM, Alfonso EC, Guildford JH, et al. Results of large penetrating keratoplasty in microbial keratitis. *Cornea* 1996; 15(6):571–576.
136. Bell NP, Karp CL, Alfonso EC, et al. Effects of methylprednisolone and cyclosporine A on fungal growth in vitro. *Cornea* 1999;18(3):306–313.
137. Perry HD, Doshi SJ, Donnenfeld ED, et al. Topical cyclosporin A in the management of therapeutic keratoplasty for mycotic keratitis. *Cornea* 2002;21(2):161–163. Comment in *Cornea* 2003;22(1):92–93.
138. Killingsworth DW, et al. Results of therapeutic penetrating keratoplasty. *Ophthalmology* 1993;100:534–541.
139. Polack FM, Kaufman HE, Newmark E. Keratomycosis: medical and surgical treatment. *Arch Ophthalmol* 1971;85:410–416.
140. Ando N, Takatori K. Fungal flora of conjunctival sac. *Am J Ophthalmol* 1982;94:67–74.
141. Williamson J, Gordon AM, Wood R, et al. Fungal flora of the conjunctival sac in health and disease. *Br J Ophthalmol* 1968;52:127.
142. Gopinathan U, Stapleton F, Sharma S, et al. Microbial contamination of hydrogel contact lenses. *J Appl Microbiol* 1997;89: 389–398.
143. Sinha BN, Das MS. Bacterial and fungal flora of the conjunctival sacs in healthy and diseased eyes. *J Indian Med Assoc* 1968;51:217.
144. Mitsui Y, Hanabusa J. Corneal infection after cortisone therapy. *Br J Ophthalmol* 1955;39:244.
145. Aintey R, Smith B. Fungal flora of the conjunctival sac in healthy and diseased eyes. *Br J Ophthalmol* 1965;49:505–515.
146. Burns RP. Indigenous flora of the lids and conjunctiva. In: Tasman W, Jaeger EA, eds. *Duan's foundations of clinical ophthalmology,* vol 2. Philadelphia: JB Lippincott, 1994.
147. Holland GN, Pepose JS, Pettit TH, et al. Acquired immunodeficiency syndrome: ocular manifestations. *Ophthalmology* 1983; 90:859–878.
148. Duke-Elder S. Inflammations of the conjunctiva. In: *Diseases of the outer eye, vol 8, System of Ophthalmology.* St. Louis: CV Mosby, 1965:385.
149. Thomas PA. Tropical ophthalmomycoses. In: Seal DV, Bron AJ, Hay J, eds. *Ocular infection investigation and treatment in practice.* London: Martin Dunitz, 1998:128.
150. Arsecularatne SN. Recent advances in rhinosporidiosis and *Rhinosporidium seeberi. Indian J Med Microbiol* 2002;20: 119–131.
151. Watson PG. Diseases of the sclera and episclera. In: Duane TD, Jaeger EA, eds. *Clinical ophthalmology,* vol 4. Philadelphia: JB Lippencott, 1995:1–45.
152. Brunette I, Stulting RD. Sporothrix schenckii scleritis. *Am J Ophthalmol* 1992;114:370–371.
153. Rodriguez-Ares MT, De Rojas Silva MV, Pereiro M, et al. Aspergillus fumigatus scleritis. *Acta Ophthalmol Scand.* 1995;73: 467–469.
154. Jager MJ, Chodosh J, Huang AJW, et al. Aspergillus niger as an unusual cause of scleritis and endophthalmitis. *Br J Ophthalmol* 1994;78:584–586.
155. Lincoff HA, McLean JM, Nano H. Scleral abscess. I. A complication of retinal detachment buckling procedures. *Arch Ophthalmol* 1965;74:641–648.
156. Milauskas AT, Duke JR. Mycotic scleral abscess: report of a case following a scleral buckling operation for retinal detachment. *Am J Ophthalmol* 1967;63:951–954.
157. Bhermi G, Gillespie I, Mathalone B. Scedosporium fungal infection of a sponge explant. *Eye* 2000;14:247–249.
158. Kim JF, Perkins SL, Harris GJ. Voriconzole treatment of fungal scleritis and epibulbar abscess resulting from scleral buckle infection. *Arch Ophthalmol* 2003;121:735–737.
159. Margo CE, Polack FM, Mood CI. Aspergillus panophthalmitis complicating treatment of pterygium. *Cornea* 1988;7:285–289.
160. Moriarty AP, Crawford GJ, McAllister IL, et al. Fungal corneoscleritis complicating beta-irradiation-induced scleral necrosis following pterygium excision. *Eye* 1993;7:525–528.
161. Moriarty AP, Crawford GJ, McAllister IL, et al. Severe corneoscleral infection. A complication of beta irradiation scleral necrosis following pterygium excision. *Arch Ophthalmol* 1993; 111:947–951.
162. Sullivan LJ, Snibson G, Joseph C, et al. Scedosporium prolificans sclerokeratitis. *Aust N Z J Ophthalmol* 1994;22:207–209.
163. Kumar B Crawford GJ, Morlet GC. Scedosporium prolificans corneoscleritis: a successful outcome. *Aust N Z J Ophthalmol* 1997;25:169–171.

164. Huang FC, Huang SP, Tseng SH. Management of infectious scleritis after pterygium excision. *Cornea* 2000;19:34–39.

165. Lin CP, Shih MH, Tsai MC. Clinical experience of infectious scleral ulceration: a complication of pterygium operation. *Br J Ophthalmol* 1997;81:980–983.

166. Hsiao CH, Chen JJ, Huang SC, et al. Intrascleral dissemination of infectious scleritis following pterygium excision. *Br J Ophthalmol* 1998;82:29–32.

167. Podedworny W, Suie T. Mycotic infection of the sclera. *Am J Ophthalmol* 1964;57:494.

168. Carlson AN, Foulks GN, Perfect JR, et al. Fungal scleritis after cataract surgery. Successful outcome using itraconzole. *Cornea* 1992;11:151–154.

169. Locher DH, Adesina A, Wolf TC, et al. Postoperative Rhizopus scleritis in a diabetic man. *J Cataract Refract Surg.* 1998;24:562–565.

170. Bernauer W, Allan BD, Dart JK. Successful management of Aspergillus scleritis by medical and surgical treatment. *Eye* 1998;12:311–316.

171. Mendicute J, Orbegozo J, Ruiz M, et al. Keratomycosis after cataract surgery. *J Cataract Refract Surg* 2000;26:1660–1666.

172. Stenson S, Brookner A, Rosenthal S. Bilateral endogenous necrotizing scleritis due to Aspergillus oryzae. *Ann Ophthalmol* 1982;14:67.

173. Hemady R, Sainz de la Maza M, Raizman MB, et al. Six cases of scleritis associated with systemic infection. *Am J Ophthalmol* 1992;114:55.

174. Hahn YS, Lincoff A, Lincoff H, et al. Infection after sponge implantation for scleral buckling. *Am J Ophthalmol* 1979;87:180.

175. Gupta V, Chawla R, Sen S. Aureobasidium pullulans scleritis following keratoplasty: a case report. *Ophthalmic Surg Laser* 2001;32:481–482.

176. Reynolds MG, Alfonso E. Infectious scleritis and keratoscleritis: management and outcome. *Am J Ophthalmol* 1991;112:543–547.

177. Slomovic AR, Forster RK, Gelender H. Hasiodiplodia theobrome panophthalmitis. *Can J Ophthalmol* 1985;20:225.

178. Kuriakose ET. Oculosporidiosis. Rhinosporidiosis of the eye. *Br J Ophthalmol* 1963;47:346.

179. Lamba PA, Shucka KN, Ganapathy M. Rhinosporidium granuloma of the conjunctiva with scleral ectasia. *Br J Ophthalmol* 1970;54:565.

180. Demant E, Hurwitz JJ. Canaliculitis: Review of 12 cases. *Can J Ophthalmol* 1980;15:73.

181. Wolter JR. *Pitryosporum* species associated with dacryoliths in obstructive dacryocystitis. *Am J Ophthalmol* 1977;806:84.

182. Pavklack MA, Frueh BR. Through curettage in the treatment of chronic canaliculitis. *Arch Ophthalmol* 1992;110:202.

PARASITIC KERATITIS AND CONJUNCTIVITIS

JOSEPH TAUBER AND FAISAL JEHAN

Parasitic ocular infections are a common cause of worldwide ocular morbidity and vision loss. The incidence of parasitic ocular infections is increasing, due in part to the worldwide epidemic of AIDS, the increase in airline travel across the world, increased contact lens wear, and the increase in movement of refugee populations across traditional national boundaries. This chapter is not intended as an encyclopedic review of every known parasite, but instead aims to present and review the major classes of parasitic infections affecting the cornea. Some of the most common parasitic ocular infections, such as toxoplasmosis and toxocariasis, are discussed in separate chapters. Millions of persons worldwide suffer from onchocerciasis, although far fewer are infected with dracunculiasis. The reader interested in rarer entities is referred to textbooks of parasitology (1,2). Parasitic ocular infections are discussed in groups according to the class of infecting organism.

INFECTIONS CAUSED BY PROTOZOA

The most frequently encountered parasitic ocular infections are caused by Protozoan species, including *Acanthamoeba, Entamoeba, Microsporidia*, the hemoflagellates *Trypanosoma* and *Leishmania, Toxoplasma* and *Giardia*.

Acanthamoeba

Acanthamoeba are small, free-living ubiquitous protozoans that have been isolated from fresh water, sea water, ocean sediment, arctic ice, swimming pool water (even frozen), bottled water, soil, vegetable matter, dialysis treatment units, contact lens cases, and even air (3). One study based on air sampling estimated that a human inhales, on average, two *Acanthamoeba* organisms per day (4). In contrast to many other protozoans, *Acanthamoeba* is not naturally parasitic and does not require a host. It feeds on bacteria, fungi, and other organisms and thrives where these microorganisms exist in large numbers, such as in biofilms on the walls of hot tubs. Contact with humans is largely accidental and infection is rare and opportunistic (5). Up to 100% of normal persons demonstrate serum immunoglobulin G (IgG) antibodies against *Acanthamoeba* species (6). *Acanthamoeba* has been recovered from human nasal cavities, throats, intestines, lung tissue, and cornea (3,7). Classification of the more than 50 known strains of *Acanthamoeba* species has been a subject of debate (8,9), but reports classify 22 species into three groups that differ in morphologic characteristics. Because these morphologic characteristics can vary with local environmental conditions, immunofluorescence, isoenzyme profiles, and restriction fragment length polymorphism (RFLP) patterns of whole-cell or ribosomal DNAs have been used in species identification (10–13).

Acanthamoeba exist in two life forms, an active trophozoite and a dormant cyst. Trophozoites are the infectious form and measure from 15 to 45 μm in diameter. Encystment of trophozoites is the major factor accounting for the severity of *Acanthamoeba* infections. Encystment occurs as a result of pH changes or adverse changes in oxygen or food supply, but the exact stimulus that directs conversion between life forms in corneal tissue remains unknown (14). The cyst form is slightly smaller than the trophozoite (15 to 28 μm length), double walled, and can remain dormant but viable for years before resuming the trophozoite form (4). Cysts are resistant to wide extremes of temperature, desiccation, and many antimicrobial and disinfectant chemicals that have been shown effective against the trophozoites (15–17). Cysts may be impervious to inorganic chlorine up to 50 parts per million (ppm), whereas trophozoites are sensitive at 2 ppm, which is still in excess of levels found in public water supplies (<1 ppm) (18). Only some of the known strains of *Acanthamoeba* are pathologic in humans (*A. castellanii, A. culbertsoni, A. hatchetti, A. lugdunensis, A. polyphaga, A. quina, A. rhysodes, A. griffini*), possibly due to species differences in tissue adhesion or protease production (18–22). The earliest reported infections in humans involved the central nervous system (CNS) in immunocompromised patients (3,9), but keratitis due to *Acanthamoeba* was reported in immunocompetent patients in the early

1970s (23). Cutaneous infections may occur with or without CNS involvement (9).

The first published report of *Acanthamoeba* keratitis was in 1974 (24). Uncertainty remains about whether earlier cases had gone unrecognized or unreported, or whether this was a new disease. Five retrospective studies of histopathologic specimens identified evidence of only four cases of amebic infection (25–29). Isolated case reports followed until a relative "epidemic" of cases appeared worldwide, but especially in the United States and Great Britain in the early 1980s, with many of these cases occurring in contact lens-wearing patients (30). Hard, rigid gas-permeable, daily-wear soft, extended-wear soft, and disposable contact lenses have all been associated with *Acanthamoeba* keratitis, but most cases have involved daily-wear soft contact lenses (31). Often, patients had mixed their own saline solution using large jugs of water and salt tablets or had other nonhygienic lens care habits. *Acanthamoeba* adherence to contact lens surfaces and contact lens cases is a significant factor in pathogenicity (32). Most commercially available contact lens disinfectants are ineffective at killing *Acanthamoeba*, although thermal disinfection is reliable (33). As many as 85% of *Acanthamoeba* keratitis cases occur in contact lens-wearing patients (30), but other risk factors have been defined, including trauma, corneal transplantation, and exposure to infected lake water, sea water, or hot tubs (34–36). Cases in non-contact lens-wearing patients are most often associated with trauma, exposure to contaminated water or penetrating keratoplasty (37–40). Many idiopathic cases have also been reported. The incidence of *Acanthamoeba* keratitis has been estimated between 1.2 and 3.0 cases per million (41).

Variability in presentation is one of the hallmarks of *Acanthamoeba* keratitis. Severe pain, frequently in excess of objective findings, is a common feature (42), as are symptoms of foreign-body sensation, photophobia, and tearing (42). The majority of cases are unilateral, but bilateral cases have been reported in 7.5% of cases (41).

Clinical signs vary with the stage of presentation, and disease progression is often slow. In very early corneal infection, only conjunctival hyperemia with superficial epithelial irregularities (microerosions, pseudodendrites, opacification, microcystic edema, or a diffuse granularity) may be seen (4,43). Despite corneal hypesthesia, severe pain thought to be secondary to keratoneuritis is common. In later stages, multifocal, nummular anterior stromal infiltrates develop, and may coalesce into annular or crescentic opacities (Fig. 17-1). Disciform keratitis may occur. A ring infiltrate, initially vague, with intact central epithelium, has been described by some as pathognomonic of *Acanthamoeba* keratitis (44). In later stages, the ring often appears more dense and discrete, and the central epithelium sloughs, facilitating stromal necrosis. Anterior chamber reaction is rare. The pathogenesis of the ring infiltrate is uncertain. Residual antigen may cause inflammation in the absence of active trophozoite infection. Cysts have been shown to induce corneal stromal inflammation as long as 31 months following antiamebic therapy (45). Focal stromal edema with intrastromal inflammatory infiltration is common and radially oriented perineural infiltration (keratoneuritis) has been described (43) (Fig. 17-2).

Later, continued inflammation and presumed release of proteases and collagenases lead to stromal lysis and sometimes to descemetocele formation or perforation. Less common sequelae may include secondary immune-mediated scleritis (46), iritis (47), and corneal neovascularization.

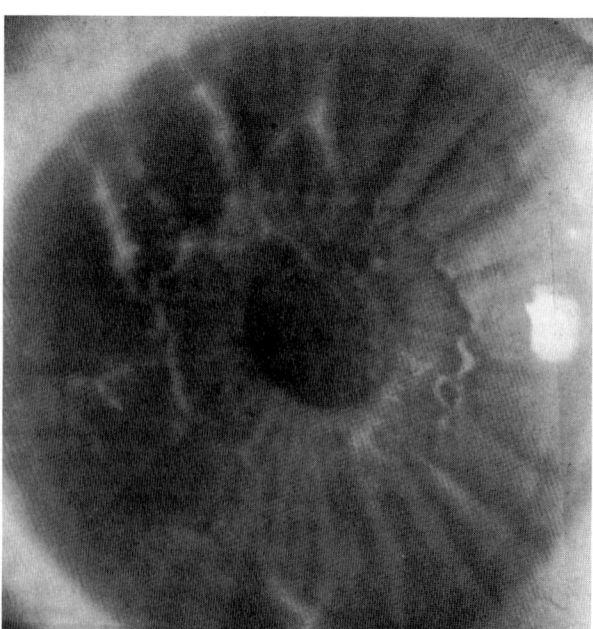

FIGURE 17-2. Perineural infiltrates during early stage of *Acanthamoeba* keratitis.

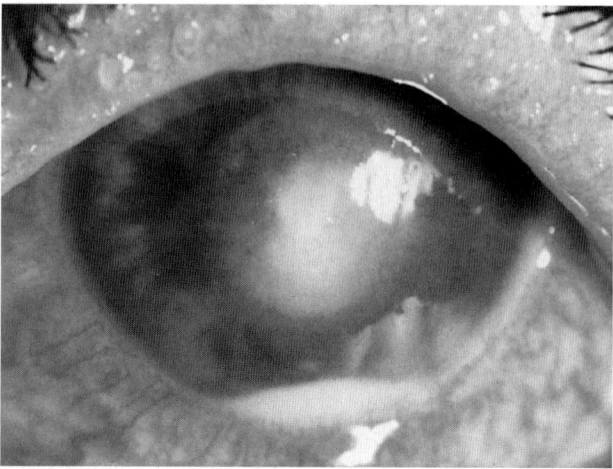

FIGURE 17-1. Acanthamoeba keratitis with hypopyon.

TABLE 17-1. REPORTED FREQUENCIES OF CLINICAL SIGNS IN ACANTHAMOEBA KERATITIS

Pain	50–100%
Reduced corneal sensation	29%
Epithelial defects, erosions	60%
Stromal ring infiltrate	6–29%
Other stromal infiltrate	33%
Radial keratoneuritis	2–57%
Limbitis	84–94%
Hypopyon	39%
Cataract	20%

Chorioretinitis following keratitis (48) and a culture-positive anterior chamber paracentesis (49) have been reported. Herpetic keratitis is often the most commonly considered differential diagnosis, and may delay the diagnosis of *Acanthamoeba* infection (50). The appearance of satellite lesions in later stages can mimic fungal keratitis. In some studies, the mean delay to diagnosis was 42 to 48 days (51,52) and may be longer in non-contact lens-wearing patients (53). Clinical signs in *Acanthamoeba* keratitis are listed in Table 17-1.

Diagnosis

Accurate diagnosis of *Acanthamoeba* infection requires microbiologic confirmation and should not be made wholly on clinical grounds. All available sources for culture should be exploited, including contact lens solutions and cases, well water, or hot tub water samples. Diagnosis is most often confirmed by direct inoculation of corneal scrapings onto appropriate culture media or submission of scrapings from the base of ulcers for histopathologic examination. Sometimes, direct incision into the stroma to reach deeper infiltrates or excisional corneal biopsy is necessary to obtain adequate tissue samples. Corneal buttons obtained at the time of keratoplasty should always be submitted for both histopathologic examination and culture. Recently, confocal microscopy has been reported as a tool to identify cysts or trophozoites *in vivo* (54,55), but debate about the validity of these findings has tempered early enthusiasm about this technology as a noninvasive diagnostic tool.

Culture specimens should be directly inoculated onto culture media at the slit lamp or in the operating room. *Acanthamoeba* organisms grow poorly on media typically used for bacterial keratitis sampling (blood agar, chocolate agar, Sabouraud agar). Early reports recommended culture on nonnutrient agar seeded with an overlay of bacteria, usually gram-negative rods (e.g., *Escherichia coli, Enterobacter aerogenes, Klebsiella pneumoniae,* or *Xanthomonas maltophilia*). Examination of culture plates reveals "trails" that motile trophozoites leave on the agar surface as they ingest bacteria (Fig. 17-3). *Acanthamoeba* will grow on commercially available buffered charcoal yeast extract (BCYE) (56) and tryptic soy agar with horse or rabbit blood (57). In one review of 106 cases, 43.4% of cases were culture positive (52).

Histopathologic studies have demonstrated both trophozoites and cysts using methenamine-silver, periodic acid-Schiff (PAS), Masson trichrome, and iron-hematoxylin-and-eosin stains (58,59). Fluorescent microscopy can be done using calcofluor white, fluorescein-conjugated lectins such as

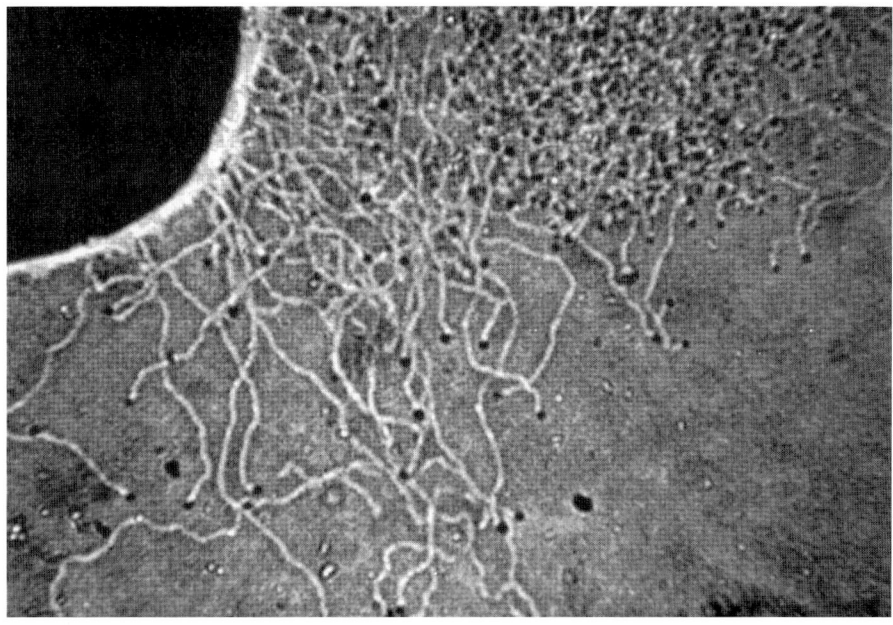

FIGURE 17-3. Migration of *Acanthamoeba* organisms on a culture plate.

concanavalin A and wheat-germ agglutinin, and immunofluorescent stains, and immunoperoxidase staining is available (3,60–62). A reculture technique has been proposed as a laboratory standard for *in vitro* sensitivity testing (63), but is not widely performed (64). Both trophozoiticidal and cysticidal concentrations can be measured, but correlation with clinical efficacy has not been demonstrated.

Treatment

Early reports of *Acanthamoeba* keratitis treatment were characterized by failures of medical treatment, recurrence following surgical intervention, and frequent loss of vision. Some medical cures were reported with combinations of amebicidal drugs (65–69), but treatment failures were common and prolonged duration of therapy was required (50,70,71). Better results were achieved when treatment was begun early in the course of disease (70,72).

Medical therapy has employed aminoglycosides, polymeric biguanides, diamidines, and imidazoles, usually in combinations (43,69). Most of these medications are prescribed to be instilled initially every hour and then slowly tapered. To date, no report has recommended standardization of the therapeutic regimen (73). Among the aminoglycosides, neomycin, commercially available as an 8-mg/mL solution or fortified to 20 mg/mL, has been demonstrated to have antiamebic efficacy. Paromycin 10 mg/mL has also been used. Polymeric biguanides, commercially available as environmental biocides (Baquacil, a swimming pool disinfectant), have been used with success in the treatment of *Acanthamoeba* keratitis (43,69). Diluted to a 0.02% concentration, progressive ocular surface toxicity often forces discontinuation of therapy. The mechanism of action of this agent is believed to be interference with cytoplasmic membrane integrity and inhibition of essential respiratory enzymes (69). Chlorhexidine 0.02% to 0.1% is another cationic antiseptic agent that has shown good efficacy at eradicating *Acanthamoeba*, and it also acts by disrupting membrane function (63,74). Because of the lower surface toxicity as compared with polyhexylmethylbiguanide (PHMB), chlorhexidine has emerged as a favored treatment, whether alone or in combination with other agents (43). Aromatic diamidines such as Brolene (propamidine isethionate 0.1% solution), pentamidine isethionate, and dibromopropamidine ointment are available in eyedrop or ointment preparations. These agents act by inhibition of S-adenosylmethionine decarboxylase or by direct interaction with amebic nucleic acids (63). Limited bioavailability, induction of encystment, and acquired resistance have all been suggested as causes of treatment failures with Brolene. Imidazoles, which also act by affecting membrane permeability, have been used both as topical preparations and systemically administered (75). Oral therapy with itraconazole or ketoconazole may have an important role in adjunctive therapy. Miconazole 1% to 2% and clotrimazole 1% to 2%

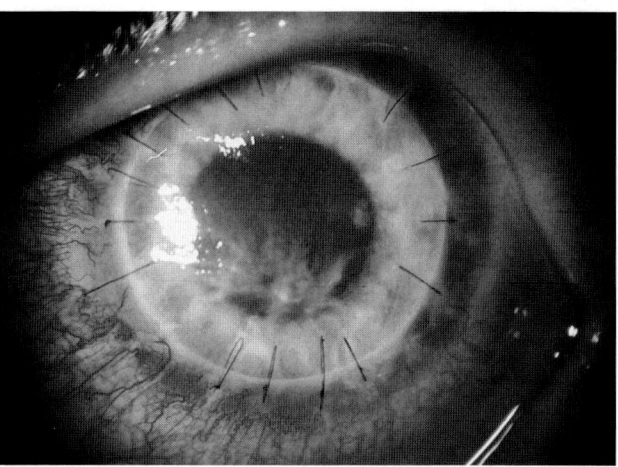

FIGURE 17-4. Recurrent *Acanthamoeba* keratitis following second keratoplasty in a 29-year-old contact lens wearer.

have been used in therapy with success, but ocular surface toxicity is common and these drugs are amebistatic rather than amebicidal (76).

As is true in other infectious scenarios, the role of topical corticosteroids is controversial. Controlling the severe stromal and scleral inflammatory process is important, but inhibition of host defense mechanisms may prolong the course of disease or even significantly worsen outcomes (77,78). Some reports have indicated worse outcomes in cases of early steroid use, and have recommended delaying steroids until after effective antiamebic therapy is confirmed. Steroids have been shown to promote conversion of cysts to trophozoites (79).

Surgical intervention should be delayed until there is clear evidence of control of amebic replication, and should not be employed as a strategy to debulk the cornea of amebic load (80). Penetrating keratoplasty is occasionally required to maintain the structural integrity of the globe (81), but vigorous attempts should be made to forestall surgical intervention as long as possible (9,82). Recurrence of disease following penetrating keratoplasty has been frequently reported (43,82), often as a crescentic infiltrate near the graft–host junction, and results in reduced likelihood of vision preservation (Fig. 17-4). As in cases of fungal keratitis, postoperative treatment with topical cyclosporine is recommended for prophylaxis against rejection rather than topical steroids. Penetrating keratoplasty is best reserved for optical rehabilitation in quiescent, medically cured eyes (82).

Entamoeba histolytica Infections

Entamoeba species are endemic worldwide, but thrive in contaminated water supplies in areas of poor sanitation. Entamoeba species exist in three life forms: a trophozoite (12–60 μm), precyst, and cyst (10–20 μm). The most common route of infection is fecal to oral transmission.

Infection follows ingestion of even small numbers of cysts. Excystment occurs in the small intestine, but trophozoite maturation and encystment occur in the large intestine. Gastrointestinal infection is the most common clinical presentation of infection, but extragastrointestinal spread occurs. *Entamoeba histolytica* has been reported to infect the external tissues of the eye, presumably following fecal-ocular transmission (83).

Diagnosis is made on the basis of direct visualization of trophozoites in infected material, usually stool specimens. Trichrome, iron-hematoxylin, PAS, and immunofluorescence techniques have all been used to enhance detection of entamoebic trophozoites. Serologic tests are available, but their usefulness in the diagnosis of ocular entamoebiasis is unknown.

Microsporidiosis

Microsporidia are ubiquitous, obligate intracellular spore-forming protozoan parasites, prevalent in numerous wild and domesticated animal hosts (84). *Microsporidia* organisms exist in three developmental stages within infected cells: infective, proliferative (binary or multiple fission), and sporogony. Sporogony results in spore production, ranging from 1 to 20 μm, with the coiled polar filament or tubule characteristic of *Microsporidia*. Classification of over 100 species into 144 genera is made by morphologic features such as the number of coils, number of nuclei, or presence of vacuoles (85,86).

Only five genera of *Microsporidia* are known to cause human disease (*Nosema, Encephalitozoon, Enterocytozoon, Pleistophora,* and *Septada*) (87). Most cases have involved immunocompromised hosts, especially AIDS patients (88–90), though sporadic cases have occurred in immunocompetent patients (91). *Microsporidia* infections are usually transmitted by fecal-oral, transplacental, or transovarial routes; ocular infection more often occurs by direct inoculation. Enteritis is the most common manifestation of human *Microsporidia* infection, occurring in as many as 30% of AIDS patients (86), but disseminated infections may produce peritonitis, sinusitis, pulmonary, renal, cardiac, hepatic, or CNS disease (86,90,92).

Microsporidia keratitis was first reported in 1990, although there were prior case reports of ocular infection (93). Ocular disease is most common in AIDS patients or following trauma (94–98). Ocular findings of microsporidial infection include conjunctival injection, mixed follicular-papillary tarsal conjunctival reaction, and punctate epithelial keratopathy. Most cases present as a coarse, granular epithelial keratitis with small foci of anterior stromal infiltration (Fig. 17-5). Hyphema and necrotizing keratitis have been reported (85).

Two clinical presentations of *Microsporidia* keratitis have been described. Immunocompromised or AIDS patients usually present with bilateral conjunctival inflammation

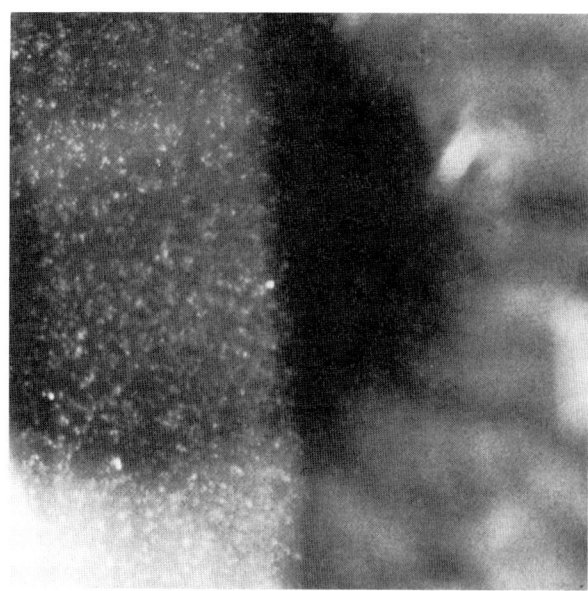

FIGURE 17-5. Microsporidial keratoconjunctivitis presenting as punctate epithelial keratopathy. (From Lowder CY, et al. Microsporidia infection of the cornea in a man seropositive for human immunodeficiency virus. *Am J Ophthalmol* 1990;109:242. Published with permission from the *American Journal of Ophthalmology.* Copyright by the Ophthalmic Publishing Company.)

and coarse epitheliopathy usually related to *Encephalitozoon* spp. (96,99,100), thought to reach the cornea through systemic dissemination. The characteristic coarse or punctuate epitheliopathy may extend to the limbus, but significant stromal involvement, bacterial superinfection, or iritis is rare. Healthy immunocompetent patients may present with unilateral conjunctival inflammation with focal stromal keratitis, usually related to exogenous infection with *Nosema* spp. (94,95). Stromal involvement may extend to deeper layers, taking on a disciform appearance similar to herpetic keratitis.

Diagnosis requires demonstration of oval *Microsporidia* spores in specimens obtained during superficial corneal scraping, or more rarely from biopsy. Spores stain gram positive and may show a PAS-positive body at one end of the oval spore, but staining is variable with routine methods such as Giemsa, Gomori silver, or acid-fast staining. Calcofluor white staining is better for light microscopic diagnosis, but electron microscopy is preferred for revealing the characteristic coiled tubules within the spore coat of *Microsporidia.* Without electron microscopy, spores may be confused with *Toxoplasma gondii, Histoplasma capsulatum,* or *Leishmania* (101). Polymerase chain reaction (PCR) is available as a diagnostic research tool only. Serologic testing and culture are unreliable (86,94,102,103).

Reports of medical treatment of *Microsporidia* keratitis have demonstrated poor results with topical antibiotics, metronidazole, or thiabendazole, but better results with topical propamidine isethionate 0.1% (Brolene) (99) or topical fumagillin (91,101,104,105). Benzimidazoles such as albendazole have a long history of use against numerous helminthic infections, but have resulted in inconsistent clearing of *Microsporidia* infections (86). Fumagillin is an antiamebic compound isolated from *Aspergillus fumigatus* in 1949. The mechanism of action of fumagillin is not well understood (86). In AIDS patients, best results have been reported with topical fumagillin or systemic albendazole (106), but successful reports of treatment with metronidazole and oral itraconazole have been published (86,100). There is no validated model for *in vitro* sensitivity testing. Surgical treatment for significant stromal involvement involving penetrating keratoplasty with cryotherapy has been reported (90,107,108).

Hemoflagellate Infections

The hemoflagellates include the *Trypanosoma* and *Leishmania* species as well as *Toxoplasma* and *Giardia*. Different life forms present within each species.

Trypanosomes

Two distinctive diseases caused by *Trypanosoma* species have been well described. Over 10 million people in Latin America are thought to be infected with Chagas' disease or trypanosomiasis, caused by *Trypanosoma cruzi*. The organism lives within the gastrointestinal system of the reduvid bug and is passed into the feces. During feeding, the bug defecates and organisms gain entry into fresh bite wounds. Transmission of infection has also been reported transplacentally, via consumption of contaminated foods, blood transfusions, breast-feeding, and laboratory accidents. Clinical disease is usually cutaneous, characterized by the chagoma or hard cutaneous nodule. Once the parasite enters the bloodstream, generalized lymphadenopathy, splenomegaly, hepatomegaly, myocarditis, or meningoencephalitis may result. Most patients recover within months, but fatal cases have been reported. Ocular involvement is usually eyelid swelling or chagoma of the lid or lacrimal gland (109). Conjunctival edema and erythema or dacryoadenitis may be associated with generalized lymphadenopathy.

African trypanosomiasis, or African sleeping sickness, is caused by *Trypanosoma brucei gambiense* and *Trypanosoma brucei rhodesiense*. Transmission is via the bite of the tsetse fly in sub-Saharan Africa. Systemic disease may present in various ways, including meningoencephalitis, myocarditis, hepatosplenomegaly or cutaneous nodules. Central nervous system involvement may follow lymphatic spread of trypanosomes. Ocular involvement is usually eyelid edema (110). Interstitial keratitis and anterior uveitis have been described (110,111).

Laboratory diagnostic methods include examination of wet mounts of whole blood or Giemsa staining of blood smears, buffy coat, or cerebrospinal fluid samples to identify extracellular trypanosomes. If involved, lymph node aspirates or biopsies, bone marrow biopsies, or biopsy of cutaneous lesions may yield organisms. Trypanosomes can be cultured on Novy-MacNeal-Nicolle agar or in tissue culture (112), but standardized techniques remain in development. Serologic testing is available but infrequently used. Enzyme-linked immunosorbent assay (ELISA), indirect immunofluorescence, radial immunodiffusion, immunoprecipitation, and indirect agglutination are useful epidemiologic tools, although they are not presently standardized (113).

Systemic treatment with oral nifurtimox or benzimidazole is effective in early stages of American trypanosomiasis. For African trypanosomiasis, early-stage parenteral therapy includes suramin or pentamidine. Systemic treatment can limit corneal scarring and neovascularization if stromal keratitis is present. Intravenous medication is used for central nervous system involvement.

Leishmaniasis

Leishmaniasis is considered by the World Health Organization (WHO) as one of the six major tropical diseases. There are estimated to be 10 million to 12 million infected persons worldwide, with about 2 million new cases recognized annually and nearly 400 million people at risk for infection (114). Leishmaniasis is classified into Old and New World cutaneous leishmaniasis, mucocutaneous, and visceral leishmaniasis (kala-azar), each caused by various *Leishmania* species with unique animal reservoirs and insect vectors. Despite attempts at controlling the disease, new endemic areas have developed due to immigration (115) between developing countries. There are endemic areas on every continent except Australia (116), but especially in India and Afghanistan, the rural Middle East, Northern and Eastern Africa, and South America. Cases of a variant of visceral leishmaniasis were reported among American military personnel after Operation Desert Storm (117). Leishmaniasis is transmitted through the bite of *Phlebotomus* or *Lutzomyia* species sandflies.

Leishmania spp. exist in two forms, the promastigote or infective stage, and the amastigote stage, which undergoes intracellular binary fission after phagocytosis by circulating macrophages. Local replication of organisms results in papular lesions that may granulate or ulcerate. Transport of infected macrophages via the lymphatic system may lead to distant subcutaneous nodules or lymphangiitis. Systemic dissemination (visceral leishmaniasis) via the reticuloendothelial system leads to hepatosplenomegaly, hypersplenism, and secondary pancytopenia.

Leishmaniasis of the eye is extremely rare (118–123). Visceral leishmaniasis has been associated with retinal hemorrhages and anterior uveitis, whereas cutaneous and mucocutaneous infections have been mostly associated with eyelid manifestations (116). Cutaneous leishmaniasis may involve any area of exposed skin, but involves the eyelid only rarely, thought likely due to lid movement during blinking (120,124,125). Solitary or multiple lesions on the face or extremities are typical (120,121,126). Cicatricial entropion or ectropion may result from prolonged lid inflammation. Eyelid lesions may progress to conjunctival involvement, with granuloma formation or chronic conjunctivitis with scarring (109,120,127,128). Progressive disease can involve the lacrimal drainage structures and can produce cicatricial entropion or ectropion. The cornea may be involved via hematogenous spread of organisms or via contiguous spread of disease from the eyelids, beginning with punctate epithelial keratitis and progressing to limbal keratitis or generalized stromal keratitis with neovascularization and scarring (128,129). Necrosis may develop leading to ulceration and perforation, necessitating enucleation (130). Three additional cases have been reported leading to blindness (131).

Leishmania infection in canines has been reported to include ocular manifestations in 24% and exclusive ocular or periocular involvement in 15% of dogs (132). Anterior uveitis is common in canine infection, with elevated immune complexes and elevated antinuclear antibody titers (132).

Definitive diagnosis requires direct demonstration of amastigotes within infected tissues. Scraping, biopsy, or needle aspiration of the leading edge of cutaneous or eyelid lesions or conjunctival granulomas can provide a diagnostic specimen for laboratory evaluation. Staining with hematoxylin and eosin (H&E), Giemsa, or the Wilder reticulum stain demonstrates amastigotes (133). DNA hybridization, indirect immunofluorescence, and isoenzyme analysis have also been used to identify leishmania infection. Culture of *Leishmania* organisms is unreliable, although positive cultures have been obtained using blood agar plates, Schneider's insect medium, and Novy-MacNeal-Nicolle (NNN) medium as well as tissue culture procedures. Serologic testing is useful only for visceral leishmaniasis.

Treatment of leishmaniasis varies with the form of clinical disease. Cutaneous leishmaniasis tends to heal spontaneously or responds to cryotherapy or local curettage. Systemic treatment with oral allopurinol or pentavalent antimony compounds, such as Glucantime and Pentosam, is the most successful for visceral disease. Pentamidine and antifungal agents such as amphotericin-B, itraconazole, and ketoconazole have been used with success (116).

Giardiasis

Giardiasis is one of the most common parasitic diarrheal diseases in the world today, with highest prevalence rates in developing countries (134,135). In the United States, outbreaks and high prevalence rates have been reported in daycare centers and on Native-American reservations. *Giardia lamblia* is a flagellated protozoan of the Mastigophora subphylum. The cyst form infects humans following ingestion

of contaminated water or via fecal-oral transmission. Colonization of the upper gastrointestinal tract leads to enteritis and moderate diarrhea and dehydration. Infection may be relatively asymptomatic in adults, but is much more symptomatic in children (136). In infants, severe dehydration is associated with death. In several reports, 10% to 20% of symptomatic children had ocular changes caused by the parasite (136,137). Ocular findings associated with *Giardia* infection were first reported in 1938 (138) and have been described many times since, most often a "salt and pepper" fundus appearance, thought to be immune-mediated (136). Anterior and posterior uveitis have been reported, as has chorioretinitis and optic disc pallor (139–143).

Diagnosis is usually made by laboratory analysis of stool samples, but both immunofluorescence and ELISA testing for *Giardia* antigen are available. Treatment options include a 7- to 10-day course of oral metronidazole or Furoxone, or nitazoxanide for 3 days. Outside of the U.S., single-dose treatment with tinidazole is another option.

INFECTIONS CAUSED BY NEMATODES

Classification of nematodes into subclasses and orders is complex and is being revised by findings in DNA sequencing (144,145). Of the two classes of nematodes, the Enoplea, which includes the orders Trichurida and Mermithida, is considered the more primitive. Trichurida (which includes *Trichinella*) are parasites of vertebrates and (rarely humans), while Mermithida parasitizes insects. The second class, Rhabditea, includes the orders Rhabditita (including *Strongyloides*), Strongylida (hookworms), Ascaridida including *Ascaris*, the common earthworm), and Spirurida (filariae). The life cycle of nematodes is complex, consisting of an egg, four larval stages, and an adult stage. For most nematodes, it is the third larval stage that is infectious.

Of the thousands of species of nematodes, generally called roundworms, relatively few cause recognized clinical human infection. Only several species of filariae are considered pathogenic for humans and even fewer have been reported to produce ocular manifestations. The filariae have similar life cycles and are transmitted by blood-sucking mosquitos or flies. Unlike infections caused by other blood parasites, filarial infections cannot be transferred by microfilariae in infected blood samples; filariasis can be acquired only from the vector that harbors the infective third larval stage. Recovery of a live intraocular nematode is rare, but has been reported with *Gnathostoma, Parastrongylus*, and several microfilariae, mostly in Southeast Asian countries (146).

Wuchereria bancrofti and *Brugia malayi* Infections

Filariasis may produce primarily cutaneous disease, lymphatic disease, or body cavity disease, according to the primary habitat of the adult worm in the vertebrate host. Bancroftian filariasis is characterized as a lymphatic filariasis, with a worldwide prevalence of over 90 million, highest in the tropics. Mortality is rare but morbidity is common, due to the presence of adult worms in the body or due to immunologic reaction within the host. The insect vectors of Bancroftian filariasis are mosquitoes of the genera *Aedes, Anopheles, Culex,* and *Mansonia.* Symptoms of systemic infection may include fever, inguinal or axillary adenopathy, testicular pain or swelling, or cough and dyspnea (147,148).

Subconjunctival infection with demonstration of a live worm can occur through direct migration of the adult worm or via vascular or lymphatic deposition of microfilariae with subsequent maturation into an adult worm. Massive swelling of the eyelid has been described related to obstruction of the lymphatic system (149–151) and retinal involvement has been reported (152). Laboratory diagnosis is traditionally based on demonstration of microfilariae in peripheral blood. Multiple blood samples may be necessary to detect low-level infection due to the periodicity of microfilarial shedding. Provocation of normally nocturnal shedding may be accomplished with systemic diethylcarbamazine therapy. Eosinophilia is commonly observed.

Treatment options include systemic ivermectin, diethylcarbamazine, or albendazole (153).

Onchocerciasis

Onchocerciasis, commonly called "river blindness," is caused by the filarial nematode *Onchocerca volvulus.* Onchocerciasis causes eye and skin disease in endemic areas along rivers and streams where its insect vector breeds, and has been reported to occur in 37 countries in Central Africa, northern portions of South America, and the Arabian peninsula. Of the estimated 17.7 million people who are infected, 270,000 are blind and 500,000 have severe visual impairment (154). In hyperendemic areas almost every person is infected and about half of the population is eventually blinded by the disease (155).

Onchocerca volvulus is transmitted by black flies of the genus *Simulium.* When an infected human is bitten by a female black fly obtaining a blood meal, anticoagulants in the saliva allow the fly to ingest *O. volvulus* microfilaria. After 6 to 12 days, the microfilariae become infective larvae that enter the subcutaneous tissues of a new host during the fly's next blood meal (156). Once in the human host, larvae become adult worms in approximately 12 months, occasionally living free within tissues but more often becoming encapsulated in fibrous nodules derived from the host. The adult female worm is long and thin, measuring up to 50 cm in length, whereas males vary from 2.5 to 5 cm in length. Gravid females produce thousands of microfilariae daily for 12 to 15 months following infection and may live up to 15 years. Microfilariae move freely within tissues and

lymphatic vessels, measure 250 to 300 μm in length, and live up to 2 years (157).

The severity of systemic disease varies widely from asymptomatic infection to disfiguring skin changes. Tissue pathology and clinical symptoms are due to host inflammatory response to dead or dying microfilariae; live microfilariae elicit little inflammation.

Onchocercomas are subcutaneous nodules that develop when adult worms become encapsulated in thick fibrous capsules in host tissue. Onchocercomas may contain several worms and are usually nontender when found on the trunk, limbs, or scalp, but may cause pain or discomfort when periosteum of bone is involved.

In the skin, degenerating microfilariae induce an inflammatory reaction that manifests as a maculopapular rash, pruritus, edema, or draining pustules containing microfilariae. Chronic skin changes include depigmentation, lichenification and thickening, or atrophy with loss of elasticity and early wrinkling (158,159). In areas of dermatitis, lymphadenopathy may also be present.

Similar to cutaneous pathology, ocular lesions are caused by the host immune response to dead microfilariae. All ocular structures may be affected, including the conjunctiva and cornea, anterior segment structures, and the posterior segment. In affected eyes conjunctival hyperemia and chemosis are often present. Other findings include ciliary injection, photophobia, or epiphora. Conjunctival nodules containing microfilariae have also been reported (160). The spectrum of corneal involvement ranges from a less severe and reversible punctate keratitis to sclerosing keratitis and iridocyclitis that cause permanent visual loss.

Microfilariae may migrate from the skin and conjunctiva through the limbus into anterior corneal stroma (161). Microfilariae within the cornea can be visualized at the slit lamp, with live microfilariae appearing coiled and producing little inflammatory response, and dead microfilariae appearing straight and immobile (162). As microfilariae die, either naturally or by chemotherapy, a localized inflammatory response ensues, causing a punctate keratitis and hazy, fluffy, or snowflake corneal opacities located in the anterior stroma measuring 0.3 to 0.7 mm in diameter (163–165). Punctate keratitis usually heals without scarring in several days to weeks. Other reported corneal findings may include flaky crystalline deposits or lattice-type changes in the peripheral cornea (166).

With prolonged exposure to massive invasion of the cornea by microfilariae, an irreversible sclerosing keratitis develops. The first sign of sclerosing keratitis is haze in the peripheral cornea adjacent to the limbus at the 3 o'clock and 9 o'clock positions. As disease progresses, the peripheral haze opacifies and spreads like two tongues around the inferior peripheral cornea, becoming a confluent zone involving the entire lower limbus. Once haze reaches the visual axis, vision loss and ultimately blindness ensues. Progressive vessel ingrowth may occur until the entire cornea is vascularized and opaque (161,163–165,167).

Anterior chamber and ciliary body microfilariae lead to iridocyclitis, more often chronic than acute, with posterior synechiae, pupillary block, secondary cataract, or secondary glaucoma (168). Iris involvement may lead to an inferiorly distorted, pear-shaped pupil or atrophy (163,164). Pigment may be seen on the posterior corneal surface and anterior lens capsule. Complications of iridocyclitis are probably the main cause of visual loss in Central America (169).

Microfilariae may enter the posterior segment along the posterior ciliary vessels and lead to slowly progressive retinal pigment epithelium (RPE) atrophy and chorioretinal scarring. Active inflammation is rarely seen and subretinal fibrosis may be present. Microfilariae involving the optic nerve may lead to acute optic neuritis and eventual optic atrophy (170,171).

Diagnosis is suspected with typical skin and ocular findings in patients living in or traveling from endemic areas. Diagnosis in heavily infected persons is made by microscopically counting microfilariae emerging from small skin snips immersed in saline. With low infection levels, the Mazzotti test is diagnostic when oral diethylcarbamazine (DEC) kills skin microfilariae, eliciting an intense pruritus. Alternatively, the patch test may diagnose infection by noting an inflammatory reaction of the skin after the application of topical DEC (172). Highly sensitive and specific PCR tests and enzyme-linked immunosorbent assay tests are also available (173).

Since its introduction in the 1980s, oral ivermectin has replaced oral DEC as the treatment of choice for onchocerciasis. DEC is no longer used because it rapidly kills microfilariae, causing anterior uveitis, acute stromal keratitis, and an adverse Mazzotti reaction characterized by severe pruritus, rash, fever, facial edema, arthralgias, hypotension, and even (rarely) death. Intravenous sumarin, also associated with severe adverse reactions, has a limited role in patients unresponsive to ivermectin treatment. Nodulectomy with surgical removal of adult worms, particularly when involving head nodules in children, can be performed to reduce microfilarial counts and reduce ocular complications (174).

Ivermectin in a single dose of 150 µg/kg is well tolerated and is effective in reducing microfilarial burdens and symptoms when used semiannually, and it improves or cures onchocercal punctate keratitis, sclerosing keratitis, anterior uveitis, and optic nerve disease. It rapidly reduces microfilarial counts within 48 hours and blocks the release of microfilariae from the adult female uterus for up to 6 months (175,176). Mass distribution of ivermectin combined with vector control programs have been successful in reducing disease in endemic countries, and continue to show promise in ongoing efforts to eliminate onchocerciasis worldwide (177).

Newer treatment strategies directed against endosymbiotic *Wolbachia* bacteria in adult worms have also shown promise. Experimental evidence indicates that *Wolbachia* endotoxins have a role in the development of both keratitis and the adverse effects of microfilaricidal drugs. Additionally, fertility of the adult female worm is dependent on *Wolbachia*. When combined with ivermectin, anti-*Wolbachia* therapy with oral doxycycline significantly reduces long-term microfilarial counts compared to ivermectin alone (178).

Loiasis

Loiasis results from subcutaneous infection by the filarial nematode *Loa loa*. The parasite is endemic in the rain forests of central and western Africa where its vectors, flies of the *Chrysops* species, known in Africa as red flies, breed (179). It is estimated that up to 20 million people and 40% of the population in endemic regions may be infected. (180).

The life cycle begins when a biting female fly ingests microfilaria during a daytime blood meal from an infected human. The microfilaria then penetrates the gut wall, molt, and become infective larvae in the mouthparts of the fly after 10 to 12 days. When the infected fly bites a new human host, larvae are deposited under the skin, where they take 6 to 12 months to mature into adult worms (181).

Adult *Loa loa* are thin transparent worms that continually migrate through human subcutaneous tissues at a rate of 1 cm per minute. Males measure 3 to 4 cm and females 5 to 7 cm in length. After adult male and female worms mate, females excrete microfilaria that enter the bloodstream with diurnal periodicity, with a peak concentration of microfilaria between 10 AM and 2 PM. Adults may survive in humans for up to 15 years (182).

Systemic disease manifestations result from migration of the worm under the skin and subcutaneous tissues and include recurrent, nonpainful, localized areas of edema called Calabar swellings (183). Resulting from a localized inflammatory reaction to *Loa loa* antigens, Calabar swellings vary in size, last 1 to 3 days, and are most commonly seen on the extremities.

Systemic symptoms of loiasis include pruritus, fever, myalgias, arthralgias, and malaise. Peripheral eosinophilia and systemic symptoms are usually more pronounced in individuals from nonendemic areas who become infected, whereas filaremia is more common in the endemic population (184). Severe but less common complications of loiasis include encephalitis in patients who have undergone treatment with diethylcarbamazine, endomyocardial fibrosis, and glomerulonephritis.

Migration of the adult worm underneath the conjunctiva may be the presenting symptom in loiasis, causing an intense conjunctivitis, itching, pain, and transient eyelid edema. The adult worm may be seen or felt by the patient migrating from the conjunctiva to the eyelid or across the bridge of the nose (185). The overlying conjunctiva may be quiet, injected, edematous, or may demonstrate subconjunctival hemorrhages. Small adult worms may cause atypical findings, including yellow nodules in the bulbar conjunctiva or edema of the eyelids and face known as bung-eye or bug-eye (186–188).

Patients treated systemically may develop an intense inflammatory reaction of the conjunctiva surrounding the dead worm, causing an intense conjunctivitis, keratitis, or iridocyclitis (189). Hemorrhages of the palpebral conjunctiva and retinal lesions observed in patients treated with systemic ivermectin are uncommon and may be related to the same vascular pathological process that occurs in patients who develop *Loa-loa*—related encephalopathies (190). Rare cases of anterior chamber, vitreous, and retinal worms causing retinal artery occlusion have been reported (191–193).

Diagnosis is made clinically based on travel history or residence in an area of endemicity, Calabar swellings, unexplained eosinophilia, or visualization of a subconjunctival worm. Because microfilaremia exhibits diurnal periodicity, blood samples should be collected during daytime hours to assist in diagnosis. Demonstration of sheathed microfilaria measuring approximately 250 nm in length containing nuclei extending to the tip of the tail, or identification of the adult worm removed from subcutaneous or subconjunctival tissue is diagnostic. Serologic testing may be useful, but generally has low specificity due to cross-reactions with other filariases (194).

Although systemic diethylcarbamazine is effective in treating microfilaremia, patients with high microfilarial burdens are at risk of meningoencephalitis and renal failure due to massive release of antigens from dying microfilaria. In such cases concomitant use of corticosteroids should be administered. Ivermectin also has been shown to effectively reduce microfilaremia in a single dose in low-to-moderate parasitemia (195,196). Patients unable to tolerate systemic treatment with diethylcarbamazine may benefit from apheresis or systemic albendazole treatment (197–199).

Treatment of ocular loiasis consists of surgically extracting the adult worm (Fig. 17-6). Topical anesthesia, bright light from the slit lamp, or manipulation of the worm with forceps may irritate the worm and cause it to migrate and disappear into deeper subconjunctival or subcutaneous tissues. For surgical removal, a single conjunctival incision is made adjacent to the worm. The worm may then be removed by grasping it with forceps. If motile, the worm may be immobilized by passing a suture under the worm and then tying a knot around it, grasping it with a second pair of forceps, or applying a cryoprobe to the worm (199,200). Pathologic examination of excised worms is important for differentiation from other filarial nematodes.

Dirofilariasis

Dirofilarial infection is rare, with approximately 800 total reported cases (201). Two clinical variants occur throughout areas of Africa, Europe, Asia, South America, and the United States, with the highest incidence of disease in Italy. Subcutaneous dirofilariasis is caused by *Dirofilaria repens (D. conjunctivae), D. tenuis, D. striata*, and *D. ursi*—like worms. The dog heartworm, *D. immitis*, causes pulmonary dirofilariasis, and rare cases of ocular infection with *D. immitis* have been reported (202–204).

Little is known about the transmission of this zoonotic infection. Mosquitoes are thought to transmit the subcutaneous parasite to humans from infected raccoons, cats, or

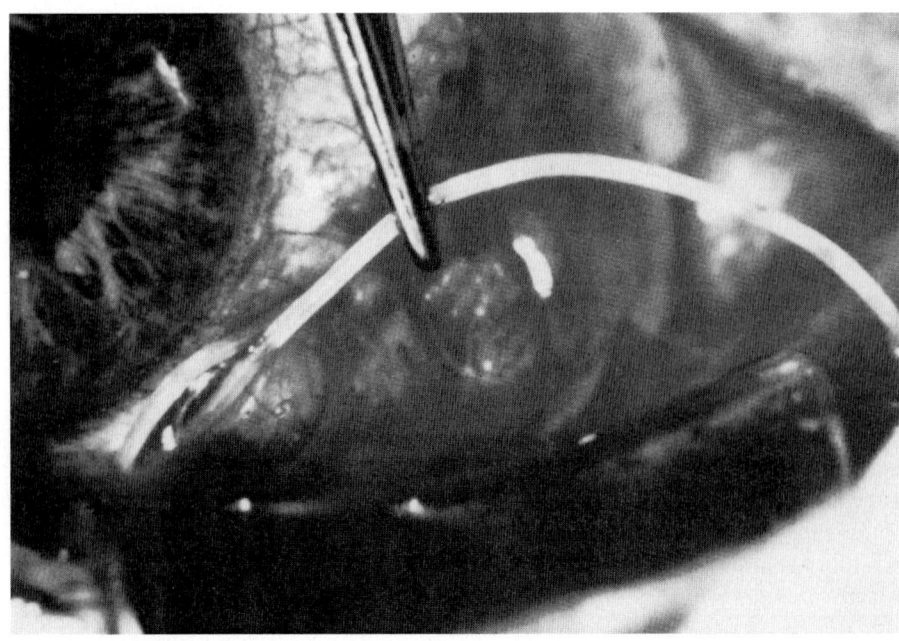

FIGURE 17-6. Adult worm being removed from the conjunctiva of a patient with loiasis.

dogs. Humans are accidental dead-end hosts. In humans, the parasites may reach maturity, but no microfilariae are seen in tissues surrounding the worm or in the circulation. Mature worms may measure up to 9.5 cm in length (205,206).

Subcutaneous dirofilariasis occurs anywhere in the body, most commonly in the scrotum, breast, arm, and leg. It presents as a painless subcutaneous nodule, occasionally becoming tender, painful, erythematous, or migratory (207).

Ophthalmic involvement includes infection of orbital, periorbital, subconjunctival, or intraocular tissues (208,209). Subcutaneous lesions in the periocular region may be described as a mass, cyst, abscess, or nodule, causing itching, swelling, or pain. Orbital involvement can present with diplopia, ptosis, and other symptoms suggestive of an orbital mass (208,210). Subconjunctival infections most commonly present as tearing and a foreign-body sensation, and may be mistaken for a nonspecific allergic conjunctivitis. Ocular signs include conjunctival chemosis and inflammation overlying a visible coiled or motile worm, but the conjunctiva overlying the worm may be uninflamed.

Diagnosis is made by histopathologic identification of the worm from a biopsy specimen. In early lesions, histologic specimens show a coiled, degenerating worm in abscess tissue. Chronic lesions show necrotizing granulomatous inflammation, containing epithelioid cells, foreign-body giant cell, histiocytes, and eosinophils (205). Important morphologic features seen microscopically include a thick, multilayered cuticle with longitudinal ridges. Serologic tests have low specificity and thus are of little value, though serum antibodies against *D. repens* have been monitored after surgery using immunoenzymatic assays to confirm cure of infection (211). No chemotherapeutic agents are effective for dirofilariasis. The only known treatment is surgical extraction of the worm.

Dracunculus medinensis Infections

Dracunculus medinensis, commonly known as guinea worm or "fiery serpent," is a parasite of the dog, horse, cow, wolf, leopard, monkey, and baboon that also commonly infects humans. The majority of human infections occur in parts of West Africa, East Africa, and India.

The WHO, in a worldwide effort to eradicate this parasite, has reported a reduction in prevalence of cases from 3.5 million in 1986 to only 130,000 in 1995. Dracunculiasis is currently estimated to have a prevalence of 100,000 cases worldwide. *Dracunculus* depends on water for transfer, and is endemic in areas where drinking water sources are limited, with many people using a common source. In a testimony to the antiquity of this infectious disease, it has been speculated that the serpent depicted in the medical caduceus represents the guinea worm.

Female worms are found in or just beneath the skin in infected persons, often in the feet, ankles, or legs. The adult worms can be up to 1 m in length, making this one of the longest known nematodes. Release of juvenile worms into the skin produces an intense allergic reaction, extreme pain, and a papular skin eruption. Ulceration allows the juvenile worms to be released, often into water used to soothe the irritated skin. Humans are infected when they drink water containing infected intermediate hosts, such as copepods or crustaceans. Once in the human, the juvenile worms migrate from the intestinal tract, through the abdominal cavity, and into the subcutaneous connective tissues. Fertilization of female worms produces new juveniles, with complete development of the parasite requiring about 1 year. Bacterial superinfection of cutaneous sores may occur.

Ocular involvement is rare. However, in one well-documented case report, a bulbar conjunctival swelling revealed a dead adult female guinea worm (212).

Isolation of the female worm from the skin ulcer is diagnostic for dracunculiasis. Serologic tests are of limited value because they are nonspecific. The most commonly employed treatment is "stick therapy," in which the female worm is attached to a small stick and removed by slowly winding the worm on to the stick. Complete removal may require months (212,213).

Thelaziasis

Thelaziasis, also known as circumocular filariasis, is caused by a spiruroid nematode that resides in the conjunctival fornices of mammals. Two species are known to infect humans. *Thelazia callipaeda*, also known as the oriental eyeworm, is found in China, India, Thailand, Korea, and Japan, and *Thelazia californiensis* is found in the western United States (214). Definitive hosts include the dog, cat, horse, fox, coyote, sheep, bear, and deer. Flies, including those of the *Drosophila* family, are thought to be the intermediate host. Thelaziasis results when eggs in the ocular secretions of an infected host are ingested by flies, develop into larvae, and are deposited onto the conjunctiva of humans where they develop into adult worms that are creamy white, 1 to 1.5 cm long, and thread-like. Although *Thelazia* species lack the rows of hooks and spines that enable its close relative *Gnathostoma spinigerum* to invade and destroy intraocular tissues, one case of vitreous thelaziasis has been reported (215).

Ocular disease manifestations result from the worm residing in the conjunctival fornices. Symptoms include excessive tearing, pain, irritation, redness, itching, or foreign-body sensation. Slit-lamp examination may reveal a nonspecific papillary or follicular conjunctivitis, chemosis, or corneal scarring. The worm may be found in either the superior or inferior conjunctival fornix, and may be seen moving across the cornea. Repeated movement of the parasite across the cornea may cause corneal opacification and scarring (216–219). The number of worms present usually varies from one to five, and small worms may be missed on initial examination and cause persistent symptoms as they grow (220,221).

Treatment of thelaziasis involves removal of the organism from the ocular surface with forceps after instillation of topical anesthetic. Diagnosis is established by microscopic identification of the parasite.

Gnathostomiasis

Gnathostoma species are nematodes that cause enteritis in tigers, leopards, mink, otters, cats, and dogs (222). Infection localizes in the gastric wall, leading to shedding of eggs into the feces. After infection and transmission through two intermediate hosts, it is the third-stage larva, encysted in muscle tissue of chickens, pigs, ducks, frogs, or snakes, that is infective for humans. Infection occurs after ingestion of infected undercooked meat or fish. Humans are nondefinitive hosts, in whom larvae never mature.

Gnathostomiasis is a rare infection, with most cases reported from the Southeast Asia and Latin America (223,224). In Thailand, 6% of subarachnoid hemorrhages and 18% of those in infants and children are due to gnathostomiasis. Infection is thought to be caused by ingestion of infectious third-stage larvae from raw or undercooked meat. The most commonly reported clinical manifestation is subcutaneous swelling, which may be migratory, but eosinophilic meningitis, pulmonary infection, and gastrointestinal tract inflammation have all been reported. *Gnathostoma* species have been reported to cause ocular infection in 12 individuals (146). Ocular disease is a result of movement of larva through ocular tissues and also to immunologic and inflammatory reaction. Reported ocular findings include orbital cellulites, conjunctivitis, corneal ulceration, uveitis, cataract, vitreitis, vitreous hemorrhage, retinal detachment, and retinal artery occlusion (225–227).

Diagnosis is typically made by examination of extracted worms by reference laboratories. Treatment is limited to surgical removal of the parasite, which is *Gnathostoma spinigerum* in most reports of human ocular infection.

Angiostrongyliasis

Parastrongylus cantonensis is a rodent lungworm commonly encountered in Southeast Asian countries. It is a well-recognized cause of eosinophilic meningitis or meningoencephalitis in many Pacific islands and Southeast Asia, with over 50 reported cases (228). The parasite normally cycles between rodents and several land mollusks. It is thought that human infection occurs following ingestion of infected snails or slugs or possibly raw vegetables contaminated by larvae from infected mollusks. Ocular angiostrongyliasis has been reported in approximately 18 human cases (229), including one case in Japan (228). Ocular findings have included uveitis and retinal detachment. Though live parasites are recoverable in only 20% of cases, recovery of live worms has been

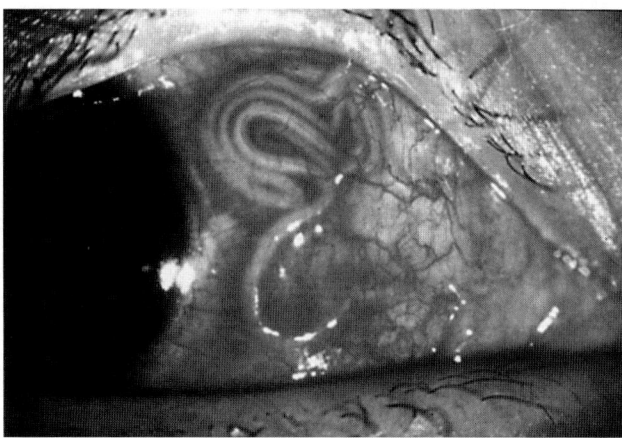

FIGURE 17-7. Subconjunctival *Macacanema formosana* worm at slit-lamp examination. (From Lau LI, Lee FL, Hsu WM, et al. Human subconjunctival infection of Macacanema formosana: the first case of human infection reported worldwide. *Arch Ophthalmol* 2002;120:643–644, with permission.)

reported from both the anterior chamber and the subretinal space (228,229).

Macacanema formosana Infection

Macacanema formosana is a nematode first identified and described in 1963. It has only has recently been reported to cause ocular infection in humans (230,231). This filarial worm has been identified in as many as 42% of Taiwanese monkeys, but without clinical evidence of ocular infection. In the first reported human case, a 7.5-cm-long worm was extracted from the subconjunctival space (Fig. 17-7). No definitive information is known about transmission of infection.

INFECTIONS CAUSED BY CESTODES

Cestodes or tapeworms are ribbon-shaped hermaphroditic flatworms. Cestodes have a scolex or "holdfast segment" with barbs used for anchoring in the intestinal tract of hosts. The life cycle involves a definitive and one or more intermediate hosts, in which infective larva develop.

Cysticercosis

Cysticercosis has been estimated to affect 50 million people worldwide, and is the most commonly diagnosed parasitic infection of the CNS (232,233). Endemic areas include Mexico, East Asia, sub-Saharan Africa, India, and Latin America. One thousand new cases are diagnosed in the U.S. annually. Hispanic and Asian populations in the U.S. are affected more frequently, due to immigration from endemic areas. Infection is caused by the larval form of

Taenia solium, known as the pork tapeworm. Disease follows ingestion of *T. solium* eggs from undercooked pork or via fecal-oral transmission from an infected intermediate host (e.g., pigs). Cysticerci, or larval cysts, may develop in skin, skeletal muscle, cardiac, ocular, and neuronal tissues. Inflammation caused by degenerating cysts leads to granuloma formation and calcification. Clinical signs vary according to the number of cysts and the infected organ, and may include seizures, meningoencephalitis, cerebrovascular occlusions, cardiac arrhythmias, and systemic vasculitis (234).

Ocular manifestations, usually unilateral (235), have been reported in 13% to 46% of patients (236). In early series, 67% of cases presented as subconjunctival granulomas (237). Both extraocular (orbit or extraocular muscles) and intraocular disease has been reported, including nystagmus, papilledema, and intravitreal and subretinal cysts (236). Extraocular involvement presents as proptosis or restriction of movement, which may also be due to cranial nerve palsy. Intraocular disease presents as exudative retinal detachment or chorioretinitis (Fig. 17-8). Intraocular larval death may lead to endophthalmitis.

Diagnosis is usually made using a combination of imaging studies (which typically show calcified granulomas) and serologic testing. ELISA testing and the newer ELISA are reported as 80% to 100% sensitive (238). Stool testing is insensitive and nonspecific.

Treatment options include praziquantel and albendazole, but corticosteroids are often required to limit host inflammatory responses. Early reports indicated that medical therapy was not useful in cases of ocular involvement (236). More recent reports have shown excellent preservation of vision with modern vitreoretinal surgical

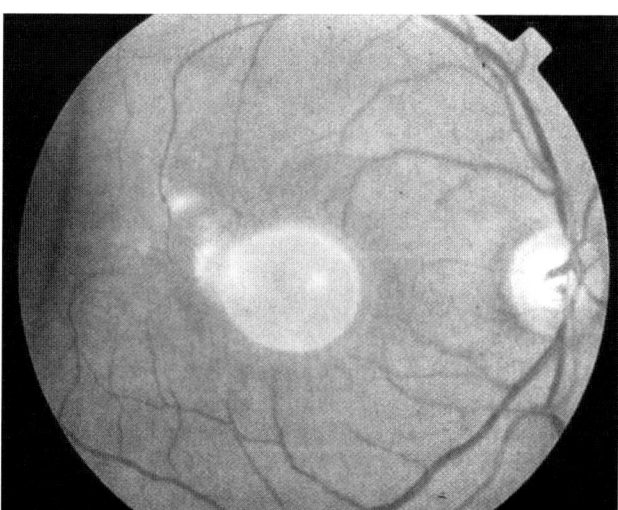

FIGURE 17-8. Subretinal cyst in cysticercosis. (From Sharma T, Sinha S, Shah N, et al. Intraocular cysticercosis: clinical characteristics and visual outcome after vitreoretinal surgery. *Ophthalmology* 2003;110:996–1004, with permission.)

techniques (235). Early removal of cysts is the treatment of choice.

INFECTIONS CAUSED BY TREMATODES

Schistosomiasis

Schistosomiasis is estimated to currently have infected over 200 million people in over 70 countries worldwide, but especially in endemic areas of Africa, the Caribbean, Central and South America, Asia, and the Middle East. Human schistosomiasis is caused by *Schistosoma japonicum, Schistosoma mansoni,* and *Schistosoma haematobium.* Human infection follows prolonged freshwater contact with contaminated water containing the schistosomal cercariae.

Organisms enter the body and migrate to blood vessels and then to lungs and liver, where maturation into adult worms occurs. Adult worms then migrate to venous plexuses, where they may live for 5 to 10 years, producing hundreds or thousands of eggs daily. Human disease is a result of an inflammatory or fibro-occlusive reaction to the eggs. A discussion of the clinical features of systemic infection is beyond the scope of this chapter (239,240). Reports of ocular involvement have included subconjunctival granulomas (241,242), APMPPE-like retinal pigment epithelial inflammation (243,244), retinitis, and uveitis (245).

The definitive laboratory diagnostic procedure is the demonstration of specific schistosome eggs in stool or urine specimens. Thick smears or concentration techniques are often required.

Serologic testing, including detection of schistosome antigens and antibodies directed against these antigens, is useful. Treatment options include praziquantel, oxamniquine, and metrifonate.

Ophthalmia Nodosa and Insect Stings

Barbed hairs from vegetation or insects are capable of penetrating the corneal stroma and migrating into the anterior chamber, causing a range of ocular findings, broadly known as ophthalmia nodosa. Findings include an acute allergic reaction, chronic mechanical keratoconjunctivitis from retained hairs and eye rubbing, conjunctival granulomas, intracorneal hairs, stromal keratitis, and iritis. The anterior chamber may be penetrated and vitreoretinal involvement may lead to vitreitis, macular edema, papillitis, or endophthalmitis (246–248).

Insect stings of the cornea may also lead to severe stromal inflammation and iritis. Inflammation and toxic reactions are due to various components of bee or wasp venom, including phospholipase and hyaluronidase (249,250). Additionally, beetles and other insects can fly into the conjunctival fornices and release cantharidin and other toxic substances when squashed, leading to a keratoconjunctivitis (251).

Treatment of ophthalmia nodosa and insect stings includes prompt identification and removal of any insect material. The conjunctival fornices should be irrigated and any accessible hairs mechanically removed immediately. Because the hair is barbed, excision of a small area of surrounding corneal tissue may be required. Inflammation is treated with topical application or peribulbar injection of corticosteroids (252,253).

INFECTIONS ASSOCIATED WITH ARTHROPODS

Although not parasites in the traditional sense, external or ectoparasites can cause ocular and periocular inflammation. This category of infection includes ticks, mites, and other insect bites.

Phthiriasis

Phthiriasis palpebrarum is an uncommon cause of blepharitis and conjunctivitis that occurs when the pubic louse *Phthirus pubis* infests the eyelashes. Adult lice and nits (louse eggs) cling to the eyelashes, leaving blood-tinged deposits of excreta on the lashes and eyelid margin and blue spots at the site of bites. A rare case of marginal keratitis has been reported (254). The adult's predilection for causing phthiriasis is due to the grasping span of its hindlegs, which corresponds to the space between adjacent cilia and pubic hairs (Fig. 17-9) (255).

Mechanical removal of lice at the slit lamp is accomplished by plucking or maximally trimming the lashes. Other treatment modalities include benzene hexachloride cream, mercuric oxide ointment, malathion drops or shampoo, cryotherapy, or argon laser photocoagulation (256–258). Nits hatch every 7 to 10 days, so follow-up during this interval is recommended. Lice on other body sites are treated with lindane or pyrethrin shampoo. Clothing, linens, and grooming instruments should be laundered in hot water.

External Ophthalmomyiasis

Ophthalmomyiasis results from infestation of the ocular structures by fly larvae, and is classified as external, internal, or orbital. External ophthalmomyiasis, most commonly caused by the sheep botfly *Oestrus ovis*, results from the deposition of larvae on the conjunctiva or eyelids (259). *O. ovis* larvae are normally deposited in the nostrils of sheep or goats then mature in the nasal or frontal sinuses. Mature larvae then wiggle out of the nostrils or are sneezed out by the host and fall to the ground to pupate. In humans, deposited larvae cause inflammation but do not mature. Other reported species causing ophthalmomyiasis include *Dermatobia hominis*, *Rhinoestrus purpureus*, *Gasterophilus* species, *Cuterebra* species, and various species of calliphorid flies such as *Chrysomyia bezziana* and *Cochliomyia* species (260,261).

Symptoms consist of an acute foreign-body sensation, burning, itching, redness, photophobia, or epiphora. Findings include eyelid edema, follicular conjunctivitis, small conjunctival hemorrhages, and superficial punctate keratitis resulting from movement of the larvae across the cornea (262). Motile

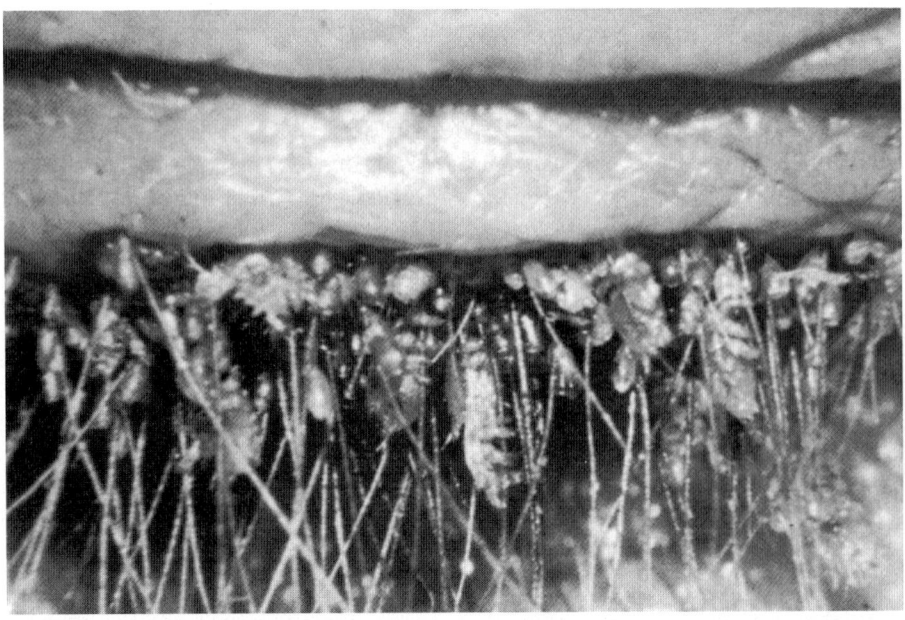

FIGURE 17-9. Lice adhering to lashes.

larvae crawling along the conjunctiva tend to avoid light from the slit-lamp beam. Some species of botfly larvae are able to burrow into tissues and cause internal or orbital ophthalmomyiasis, resulting in subretinal tracks in the posterior segment, infestation and inflammation of the orbit, or intracorneal involvement (263–265).

Treatment consists of topical anesthetic agents to slow the maggots, followed by forceps removal. Species identification is made by microscopic examination of larva morphology (266).

REFERENCES

1. Tsieh S, ed. *Parasitic disorders: pathology, diagnosis and management.* Baltimore: William & Wilkins, 1999.
2. Cox FEG, ed. *Modern parasitology: a textbook of parasitology.* Oxford; Boston: Blackwell Scientific Publications, 1993.
3. De Jonckheere JF. Ecology of Acanthamoeba. *Rev Infect Dis* 1991;13(suppl 5):S385–387.
4. De Jonckheere JF. Epidemiology. In: Rondanelli EG, ed. *Amphizoic amoeba. Human Pathology.* Padua, Italy: Piccin Nuova Libraria, 1987:127–147.
5. Illingworth CD, Cook SD. Acanthamoeba keratitis. *Surv Ophthalmol* 1998;42:493–508.
6. Fritsche TR, Gautom RK, Seyedirashti S, et al. Occurrence of bacterial symbionts in Acanthamoeba spp. isolated from corneal and environmental specimens and contact lenses. *J Clin Microbiol* 1993;31:1122–1126.
7. Byers TJ, Hugo ER, Stewart VJ. Genes of Acanthamoeba: DNA, RNA and protein sequences (a review). *J Protozool* 1990; 37:17S–25S.
8. Kilvington S, Beeching JR, White DG. Differentiation of Acanthamoeba strains from infected corneas and the environment by using restriction endonuclease digestion of whole-cell DNA. *J Clin Microbiol* 1991;29:310–314.
9. Marciano-Cabral F, Cabral G. Acanthamoeba spp. as agents of disease in humans. *Clin Microbiol Rev* 2003;16:273–309.
10. Visvesvara, GS, Mirra SS, Brandt FH, et al. Isolation of two strains of *Acanthamoeba castellanii* from human tissue and their pathogenicity and isoenzyme profiles. *J Clin Microbiol* 1983; 18:1405–1412.
11. Yagita K, Endo T. Restriction enzyme analysis of mitochondrial DNA of Acanthamoeba strains in Japan. *J Protozool* 1990;37: 570–575.
12. Byers TJ, Kim BG, King LE. Molecular aspects of the cell cycle and encystment of Acanthamoeba. *Rev Infect Dis* 1991;13 (suppl 5):S373–S384.
13. De Jonckheere JF, van de Voorde H. Differences in destruction of cysts of pathogenic and nonpathogenic Naegleria and Acanthamoeba by chlorine. *Appl Environ Microbiol* 1976;31: 294–297.
14. Chang JCH, Ossoff SF, Lobe DC, et al. UV inactivation of pathogenic and indicator microorganisms. *Appl Environ Microbiol* 1985;49:1361–1365.
15. Khan NA, Jarroll EA, Panjwani N, et al. Proteases as markers for differentiation of pathogenic and nonpathogenic species of Acanthamoeba. *J Clin Microbiol* 2000;38:2858–2861.
16. Aksozek A, McClellan K, Howard K, et al., Resistance of Acanthamoeba castellianii cysts to physical, chemical, and radiological conditions. *J Parasitol* 2002;88:621–623.
17. Kilvington S, Hughes R, Byas J, et al. Activities of therapeutic agents and myristamidopropyl dimethylamine against

18. Leher HF, Silvany R, Alizadeh H, et al. Mannose induces the release of cytopathic factors from Acanthamoeba castellanii. *Infect Immun* 1998;66:5–10.
19. Yang ZT, Cao ZY, Panjwani N. Pathogenesis of Acanthamoeba keratitis carbohydrate mediated host-parasite interactions. *Infect Immun* 1997;65:439–445.
20. He YG, Niederkorn JY, McCulley JP, et al. In vitro and in vivo collagenolytic activity of Acanthamoeba castellanii. *Invest Ophthalmol Vis Sci* 1990;31:2235–2240.
21. Ma P, Visvesvara AJ, Martinez FH, et al. Naegleria and Acanthamoeba infections: review. *Rev Infect Dis* 1990;143:662–667.
22. Nagington J, Watson PG, Playfair TJ, et al. Amoebic infection of the eye. *Lancet* 1974;2:1537–1540.
23. Ashton N, Stamm W. Amoebic infection to the eye. *Trans Ophthalmol Soc UK* 1975;95:214–220.
24. Lund OE, Stephani FJ, Dechant W. Amoebic keratitis: a clinicopathologic case report. *Br J Ophthalmol* 1978;62:373–375.
25. Kelly LD. Reevaluation of host corneal tissue 1955 to 1970: calcofluor white staining for occult Acanthamoeba infection. *Ann Ophthalmol* 1992;24:345–346.
26. Cohen EJ, Fulton JC, Hoffman CJ, et al. Trends in contact lens-associated corneal ulcers. *Cornea* 1996;15:566–570.
27. Stehr-Green JK, Bailey TM, Visvesvara GS. The epidemiology of Acanthamoeba keratitis in the United States. *Am J Ophthalmol* 1989;107:331–336.
28. Radford CF, Bacon AS, Dart JK, et al. Risk factors for Acanthamoeba keratitis in contact lens users: a case control study. *Br Med J* 1995;310:1567–1570.
29. Leger F, Vital C, Negrier ML, et al. Histologic findings in a series of 1540 corneal allografts. *Ann Pathol* 2001;21:6–14.
30. Ludwig IH, Meisler DM, Rutherford I, et al. Susceptibility of Acanthamoeba to soft contact lens disinfection systems. *Invest Ophthalmol Vis Sci* 1986;27:626–628.
31. Centers for Disease Control. Acanthamoeba keratitis associated with contact lenses-United States. *MMWR* 1986;35:405–408.
32. Khan NA. Pathogenicity, morphology and differentiation of Acanthamoeba. *Curr Microbiol* 2001;43:391–395.
33. Centers for Disease Control. Acanthamoeba keratitis in soft contact lens wearers. *MMWR* 1987;36:397–398,403–404.
34. Stehr-Green, JK, Bailey TM, Brandt FH, et al. Acanthamoeba keratitis in soft contact lens wearers. A case-control study *JAMA* 1987;285:57–60.
35. Chang PCT, Soong HK. Acanthamoeba keratitis in non-contact lens wearers. *Arch Ophthalmol* 1991;109:463–464.
36. Parrish CM, Head WS, O'Day DM, et al. Acanthamoeba keratitis following keratoplasty without other identifiable risk factors. *Arch Ophthalmol* 1991;109:471.
37. Sharma S, Srinivasan M, George C. Acanthamoeba keratitis in non-contact lens wearers. *Arch Ophthalmol* 1990;108: 676–678.
38. Zanetti S, Fiori PL, Pinna A, et al. Susceptibility of Acanthamoeba castellanii to contact lens disinfecting solutions. *Antimicrob Agents Chemother* 1995;39:1596–1598.
39. McCulley JP, Alizadeh H, Niederkorn JY. The diagnosis and management of Acanthamoeba keratitis. *CLAO J* 2000;26: 47–51.
40. Lindquist TD. Treatment of Acanthamoeba keratitis. *Cornea* 1998;17:11–16.
41. Radford CF, Lehmann OJ, Dart JK. Acanthamoeba keratitis: multicentre survey in England 1992-1996. National Acanthamoeba Keratitis Study Group. *Br J Ophthalmol* 1998;82:1387–1392.
42. Theodore FH, Jakobiec FA, Juechter KB, et al. The diagnostic value of a ring infiltrate in Acanthamoebic keratitis. *Ophthalmology* 1985;92:1471–1479.

Acanthamoeba isolates. *Antimicrob Agents Chemother* 2002;46: 2007–2009.

43. Mannis MJ, Tamaru R, Roth AM, et al. Acanthamoeba sclerokeratitis: determining diagnostic criteria. *Arch Ophthalmol* 1986; 104:1313–1317.

44. Mietz H, Font RL. Acanthamoeba keratitis with granulomatous reaction involving the stroma and anterior chamber. *Arch Ophthalmol* 1997;115:259–263.

45. Yang YF, Matheson M, Dart JK, et al. Persistence of Acanthamoeba antigen following Acanthamoeba keratitis. *Br J Ophthalmol* 2001;85:277–280.

46. Berger ST, Mondino BJ, Hoft RH, et al. Successful medical management of Acanthamoeba keratitis. *Am J Ophthalmol* 1990; 110:395–403.

47. Alizadeh H, Niederkorn JY, McCulley JP. Acanthamoeba keratitis. In: Krachmer JH, Mannis MJ, Holland EJ, eds. *Cornea.* St. Louis: Mosby, 1997:1267–1273.

48. Moshari A, McLean IW, Dodds MT, et al. Chorioretinitis after keratitis caused by Acanthamoeba. Case report and review of the literature. *Ophthalmology* 2001;108:2232–2236.

49. McClellan K, Coster DJ. Acanthamoeba keratitis diagnosed by paracentesis and biopsy and treated with propamidine. *Br J Ophthalmol* 1987;71:734–736.

50. Bernauer W, Duguid GI, Dart JK. Early clinical diagnosis of Acanthamoeba keratitis. A study of 70 eyes. *Klin Monatsbl Augenheilkd* 1996;208:282–284.

51. Tabin G, Taylor H, Snibson G, et al. Atypical presentation of Acanthamoeba keratitis. *Cornea* 2001;20:757–759.

52. Penland RL, Wilhelmus KR. Laboratory diagnosis of Acanthamoeba keratitis using buffered charcoal-yeast extract agar. *Am J Ophthalmol* 1998;126:590–592.

53. Penland, RL, Wilhelmus KR. Comparison of axenic and monoxenic media for isolation of Acanthamoeba. *J Clin Microbiol* 1997;35(4):915–922.

54. Kaldawy RM, Sutphin JE, Wagoner MD. Acanthamoeba keratitis after photorefractive keratectomy. *J Cataract Refract Surg* 2002;28:364–368.

55. Mathers WD, Nelson SE, Lane JL, et al. Confirmation of confocal microscopy diagnosis of acanthamoeba keratitis using polymerase chain reaction analysis. *Arch Ophthalmol* 2000;118:178–183.

56. Cohen EJ, Buchanan HW, Laughrea JPA, et al. Diagnosis and management of Acanthamoeba keratitis. *Am J Ophthalmol* 1985; 100:389–395.

57. Epstein, RLJ, Wilson LA, Visvesvara GS, et al. Rapid diagnosis of Acanthamoeba keratitis from corneal scrapings using indirect fluorescent antibody staining. *Arch Ophthalmol* 1986;104:1318–1321.

58. Marines HM, Osato MS, Font RL. The value of calcofluor white in the diagnosis of mycotic and Acanthamoeba infections of the eye and ocular adnexa. *Ophthalmology* 1987;94:23–26.

59. Silvany RE, Luckenbach MW, Moore MB. The rapid detection of Acanthamoeba in paraffin-embedded sections of corneal tissue with calcofluor white. *Arch Ophthalmol* 1987;105:1366–1367.

60. Wilhelmus KR, Osato MS, Font RL, et al. Rapid diagnosis of Acanthamoeba keratitis using calcofluor white. *Arch Ophthalmol* 1986;104:1309–1312.

61. Wysenbeek, YS, Blank-Porat D, Harizman N, et al., The reculture technique. Individualizing the treatment of Acanthamoeba keratitis. *Cornea* 2000;19(4):464–467.

62. Osato MS, Robinson NM, Wilhelmus KR, et al. In vitro evaluation of antimicrobial compounds for cysticidal activity against Acanthamoeba. *Rev Infect Dis* 1991;13(suppl 5):S431–S435.

63. Wright P, Warhurst D, Jones BR. Acanthamoeba keratitis successfully treated medically. *Br J Ophthalmol* 1985;69:778–782.

64. Auran JD, Starr MB, Jakobiec FA. Acanthamoeba keratitis. A review of the literature. *Cornea* 1987;6:2–26.

65. Gibson DW, Duke BO, Connor DH. Onchocerciasis: a review of clinical, pathologic and chemotherapeutic aspects, and vector control program. *Prog Clin Parasitol* 1989;1:57–103.

66. Laborde RP, Kaufman HE, Beyer WB. Intracorneal ophthalmomyiasis. *Arch Ophthalmol* 1988;106:880–881.

67. Varga JH, Wolf TC, Jensen HG, et al. Combined treatment of Acanthamoeba keratitis with propamidine, neomycin, and polyhexamethylene biguanide. *Am J Ophthalmol* 1993;115: 466–470.

68. Larkin DFP, Kilvington S, Dart JKG. Treatment of Acanthamoeba keratitis with polyhexamethylene biguanide. *Ophthalmology* 1992;99:185–191.

69. Alizadeh H, Niederkorn J, McCulley JP. Amoebic diseases of the eye. In: Zimmerman TJ, Kooner KS, Sharir M, et al., eds. *Textbook of ocular pharmacology.* Philadelphia: Lippincott-Raven, 1997:565–573.

70. Bacon AS, Dart JKG, Ficker LA, et al. Acanthamoeba keratitis: the value of early diagnosis. *Ophthalmology* 1993;100:1238–1243.

71. Seal D, Hay J, Kirkness C, et al. Successful medical therapy of Acanthamoeba keratitis with topical chlorhexidine and propamidine. *Eye* 1996;10:413–421.

72. Ishibashi Y, Matsumoto Y, Kabala T, et al. Oral itraconazole and topical miconazole with débridement for Acanthamoeba keratitis. *Am J Ophthalmol* 1990;109:121–126.

73. Kumar R, Lloyd D. Recent advances in the treatment of Acanthamoeba keratitis. *CID* 2002;35:4343–4441.

74. Schuster FL, Jacob LS. Effects of magainins on ameba and cyst stages of Acanthamoeba polyphaga. *Antimicrob Agents Chemother* 1992;36:1263–1271.

75. Park DH, Palay DA, Daya SM, et al. The role of topical corticosteroids in the management of Acanthamoeba keratitis. *Cornea* 1997;16:277–283.

76. Rabinovitch T, Weissman SS, Ostler B, et al. Acanthamoeba keratitis: clinical signs and analysis of outcome. *Rev Infect Dis* 1991;13(suppl 5):S427.

77. Osato M, Robinson N, Wilhelmus KR, et al. Morphogenesis of Acanthamoeba castellanii: titration of the steroid effect. *Invest Ophthalmol Vis Sci* 1986;27(suppl):37.

78. Hargrave SL, McCulley JP, Husseini Z, the Brolene Study Group. Results of a combined propamidine isethionate and neomycin therapy for Acanthamoeba keratitis. *Ophthalmology* 1999;106:952–957.

79. McClellan K, Howard K, Niederkorn JY, et al. Effect of steroids on Acanthamoeba cysts and trophozoites. *Invest Ophthalmol Vis Sci* 2001;42:2885–2893.

80. O'Day DM, Head WS. Advances in the management of keratomycosis and Acanthamoeba keratitis. *Cornea* 2000;19: 681–687.

81. Sony P, Sharma N, Vajpayee RB, et al. Therapeutic keratoplasty for infectious keratitis: a review of the literature. *CLAO J* 2002; 28:111–118.

82. Ficker LA, Kirkness C, Wright P. Prognosis for penetrating keratoplasty in Acanthamoeba keratitis. *Ophthalmology* 1993;100: 105–110.

83. Beaver PC, Villegas AL, Cuello C, et al. Cutaneous amebiasis of the eyelid with extension into the orbit. *Am J Trop Med Hyg* 1978;27:1133–1136.

84. Canning EU, Lom J. *The microsporidia of vertebrates.* New York: Academic Press, 1986.

85. Klotz SA, Penn CC, Negveskey GJ, et al. Fungal and parasitic infections of the eye. *Clin Microbiol Rev* 2000;13:662–685.

86. Costa SF, Weiss LM. Drug treatment of microsporidiosis. *Drug Ref Updates* 2000;3:384–399.

87. Lowder CY, McMahon JT, Meisler DM, et al. Microsporidial keratoconjunctivitis caused by Septata intestinalis in a patient with acquired immunodeficiency syndrome. *Am J Ophthalmol* 1996;121:715–717.

88. Canning EU, Hollister WS. Human infections with microsporidia. *Rev Med Microbiol* 1992;3:35–42.

89. Orenstein JM. Microsporidiosis in the acquired immunodeficiency syndrome. *J Parasitol* 1991;77:843–864.

90. Weber RR, Bryan DA, Schwartz A, et al. Human microsporidial infections. *Clin Microbiol Rev* 1994;7:426–461.

91. Theng J, Chan C, Ling ML, et al. Microsporidial keratoconjunctivitis in a healthy contact lens wearer without human immunodeficiency virus infection. *Ophthalmology* 2001;108:976–978.

92. Rossi P, Urbani C, Donelli G, et al. Resolution of microsporidial sinusitis and keratoconjunctivitis by itraconazole treatment. *Am J Ophthalmol* 1999;127:210–212.

93. Lowder CY, Wilson LA. Microsporidiosis. In: Pepose JS, Holland EJ, Wilhelmus KR, eds. *Ocular infection and immunity*. St. Louis: Mosby, 1996:1072–1079.

94. Ashton N, Wirasinha PA. Encephalitozoonosis (nosematosis) of the cornea. *Br J Ophthalmol* 1973;57:669–674.

95. Pinnolis M, Egbert PR, Font RL, et al. Nosematosis of the cornea: case report, including electron microscopic studies. *Arch Ophthalmol* 1981;99:1044–1047.

96. Friedberg DN, Stenson SM, Orenstein JM, et al. Microsporidial keratoconjunctivitis in acquired immunodeficiency syndrome. *Arch Ophthalmol* 1990;108:504–508.

97. Lowder CY, Meisler DM, McMahon JT, et al. Microsporidia infection of the cornea in a man seropositive for human immunodeficiency virus. *Am J Ophthalmol* 1990;109:242–244.

98. Shadduck JA. Human microsporidiosis and AIDS. *Rev Infect Dis* 1990;162:773–776.

99. Metcalfe TW, Doran RM, Rowlands PL, et al. Microsporidial keratoconjunctivitis in a patient with AIDS. *Br J Ophthalmol* 1992;76:177–178.

100. Yee RW, Fermin TO, Martinez JA, et al. Resolution of microsporidial epithelial keratopathy in a patient with AIDS. *Ophthalmology* 1991;98:196–201.

101. Garvey MJ, Ambrose PG, Ulmer JL. Topical fumagillin in the treatment of microsporidial keratoconjunctivitis in AIDS. *Ann Pharmacother* 1995;29:872–874.

102. Didier ES, Shadduck J, Didier P, et al. Studies on ocular microsporidia. *J Protozool* 1991;38:635–638.

103. Didier ES, Didier PJ, Friedberg DN, et al. Isolation and characterization of a new human microsporidian, *Encephalitozoon hellem* (n., sp.), from three AIDS patients with keratoconjunctivitis. *J Infect Dis* 1991;163:617–621.

104. Diesenhouse MC, Wilson LA, Corrent GF, et al. Treatment of microsporidial keratoconjunctivitis with topical fumagillin. *Am J Ophthalmol* 1993;115:293–298.

105. Shadduck JA. Effect of fumagillin on in vitro multiplication of *Encephalitozoon cuniculi*. *J Protozool* 1980;27:202–208.

106. Didier ES. Effects of albendazole, fumagillin and TNP-470 on microsporidial replication in vitro. *Antimicrob Agents Chemother* 1997;41:1541–1546.

107. Rosberger DF, Serdarevic ON, Erlandson RA, et al. Successful treatment of microsporidial keratoconjunctivitis with topical fumagillin in a patient with AIDS. *Cornea* 1993;12:261–265.

108. Gritz DC, Holsclaw DS, Neger RE, et al. Ocular and sinus microsporidial infection cured with systemic albendazole. *Am J Ophthalmol* 1997;124:241–243.

109. Kean BH. Cutaneous leishmaniasis on the Isthmus of Panama. *Arch Dermatol Syph* 1944;50:237.

110. Rodger FC. *Eye disease in the tropics*. Edinburgh: Churchill Livingstone, 1981:83–84.

111. Daniels CW. Trypanosome keratitis. *Br J Ophthalmol* 1918;2:83.

112. Brun R, Jenni I. Cultivation of African and South American trypanosomes of medical or veterinary importance. *Br Med Bull* 1985;41:122–129.

113. Voller A, Bidwell DE, Bartlett, A, et al. A comparison of isotopic and enzyme-immunoassays for tropical parasitic diseases. *Trans R Soc Med Hyg* 1977;71:431–437.

114. The Expert Committee. Control of the leishmaniases: report of a WHO Expert Committee. *WHO Tech Rep Ser* 1990;793:1–158.

115. Abrishami M, Soheilian M, Farahi A, et al. Successful treatment of ocular leishmaniasis. *Eur J Dermatol* 2002;12:88–89.

116. Wunderle IIH, de Kaspar HM, Cabrera E, et al. Ocular alterations in patients with cutaneous and mucocutaneous leishmaniasis. *Trop Doc* 2003;33:112–115.

117. Magill AJ, Grogl M, Gasser RA, et al. Visceral infection caused by Leishmania tropica in veterans of Operation Desert Storm. *N Engl J Med* 1993;328:1383–1387.

118. Rodriguez N, Guzman B, Rodas A, et al. Diagnosis of cutaneous leishmaniasis and species discrimination of parasites by PCR and hybridization. *J Clin Microbiol* 1994;32:2246–2252.

119. Pearson RD, de Queiroz Sousa A. Clinical spectrum of leishmaniasis. *Clin Infect Dis* 1996;22:1–13.

120. O'Neill DP, Deutsch J, Carmichael AJ, et al. Eyelid leishmaniasis in a patient with neurogenic ptosis. *Br J Ophthalmol* 1991;75:506–507.

121. Nandy A, Addy M, Chowdhury AB. Leishmanial blepharoconjunctivitis. *Trop Geogr Med* 1991;43:303–306.

122. El Hassan AM, El-Sheikh EA, Eltoum IA, et al. Past kala-azar anterior uveitis: demonstration of leishmania parasites in the lesion. Trans R Soc Trop Med Hyg 1991;85:471–473.

123. Ferrari TC de Abreu, Guedes ACM, et al. Isolation of leishmania sp from aqueous humor of a patient with cutaneous disseminated leishmaniasis and bilateral iridocyclitis (preliminary report). *Rev Inst Med Trop Sao Paolo* 1990;32:296–298.

124. Ozdemir Y, Kulacoglu S, Cosar CB, et al. Ocular leishmaniasis. *Eye* 1999;13:666–667.

125. Aouchiche M, Hartani D. Manifestations ophtalmologiques des leishmanioses cutanees. *Med Trop* 1981;41:519–522.

126. Satici A, Gurler B, Gurel MS, et al. Mechanical ptosis and lagophthalmos in cutaneous leishmaniasis. *Br J Ophthalmol* 1998;82:975.

127. Sodaify M, Aminiari A, Resaei H. Ophthalmic leishmaniasis. *Clin Exp Dermatol* 1981;6:485–488.

128. Roizenblatt J. Interstitial keratitis caused by American (mucocutaneous) leishmaniasis. *Am J Ophthalmol* 1979;87:175.

129. Cairns JE. Cutaneous leishmaniasis (Oriental sore). A case with corneal involvement. *Br J Ophthalmol* 1968;52:481–483.

130. Reinecke P, Gabbart HE, Strunk W, et al. Ocular scleromalacia caused by leishmaniasis: a rare cause of scleral perforation. *Br J Ophthalmol* 2001;85:240–241.

131. Kumar PV, Roozitalab MH, Lak P, et al. Ocular leishmaniasis, a case of blindness. *Im J Med Sci* 1993;18:106–111.

132. Pena MT, Roura X, Davidson MG. Ocular and periocular manifestations of leishmaniasis in dogs: 105 cases (1993-1998). *Vet Ophthalmol* 2000;3:35–41.

133. Chu FC, Rodriguez MM, Cogan GG, et al. Leishmaniasis affecting the eyelids. *Arch Ophthalmol* 1983;101:84–91.

134. Pickering LK, Engelkirk PG. *Giardiasis lamblia*. Pediatr Clin North Am 1988;35:565–572.

135. Larson SC. Traveler's diarrhea. *Emerg Med Clin North Am* 1997;15:179–189.

136. Corsi A, Nucci C, Knafelz D, et al. Ocular changes associated with Giardia lamblia infection in children. *Br J Ophthalmol* 1998;82:59–62.

137. Pettoello Mantovani M, Giardino I, Magli A, et al. Intestinal giardiasis associated with ophthalmologic changes. *J Pediatr Gastroenterol Nutr* 1990;11:196–200.

138. Barraquer I. Sur la coincidence de la lambiase et de certains lesions du fond de l'oeill. *Bull Soc Pathol Exot* 1938;31:55–58.

139. Carroll ME, Anast BP, Birch CL. Giardiasis and uveitis. *Arch Ophthalmol* 1961;65:775–778.

140. Djabri SE, Diallinas N. L'importance de la lambliase comme facteur etiologique dans le chorioretinite centrale sereuse. *Ophthalmologica* 1964;147:264–272.

141. Knox DL, King J. Retinal arteritis, iridocyclitis and giardiasis. *Ophthalmology* 1982;89:1303–1308.

142. Druault Toufesco N. Les lesions maculaires en rapport avec le parasite intestinaux. *Bull Soc Fr Ophtal* 1960;73:145–151.

143. Collier M, Adias L. Lambliase et emorragie du vitre. *Bull Soc Med Pau* 1961;43:133–139.

144. Blaxter ML, De Ley P, Garey JR, et al. A molecular evolutionary framework for the phylum Nematoda. *Nature* 1998;392:71–75.

145. De Ley P, Blaxter ML. Systematic position and phylogeny. In: Lee DL, ed. *The biology of nematodes.* London: Taylor and Francis, 2002:1–30.

146. Biswas J, Gopal L, Sharma T, et al. Intraocular *Gnathostoma spinigerum.* Clinicopathologic study of two cases with review of literature. *Retina* 1994;14:438–444.

147. Dreyer G, Noroes J, Figueredo-Silva J. Pathogenesis of lymphatic disease in bancroftian filariasis: a clinical perspective. *Parasitol Today* 2000;16:544–548.

148. Nanduri J, Kazura JW. Clinical and laboratory aspects of filariasis. *Clin Microbiol Rev* 1989;2:39–50.

149. Dissanaike AS, Hock AC, Min TS. Mature female filaria probably *Brugia spp.* from the conjunctiva of man in West Malaysia. *Am J Trop Med Hyg* 1974;23:1023–1026.

150. Joon-Wah, M, Singh D, Sukoaryono J, et al. *Brugia malayi* infection of the human eye: a case report. *Southeast Asian J Trop Med Pub Health* 1974;5:226–229.

151. Anandakannan K, Gupta CP. Microfilaria malayi in uveitis: case report. *Br J Ophthalmol.* 1977;61:263–264.

152. Gupta A, Agarwal A, Dogra MR. Retinal involvement in *Wucheria bancrofti* filariasis. *Acta Ophthalmol* 1992;70:832–835.

153. Dunyo SK, Nkrumah FK, Simonsen PE. Single-dose treatment of *Wucheria bancrofti* with ivermectin and albendazole alone or in combination: evaluation of the potential for control at 12 months after treatment. *Trans R Soc Trop Med Hyg* 2000;94: 437–443.

154. World Health Organization. Onchocerciasis and its control. *World Health Organ Tech Rep Ser* 1995;852:1–103.

155. Sabrosa NA, Zajdenweber M. Nematode infections of the eye: toxocariasis, onchocerciasis, diffuse unilateral subacute neuroretinitis, and cysticercosis. *Ophthalmol Clin North Am* 2002;15: 351–356.

156. Strickland GT. *Hunter's tropical medicine and emerging infectious diseases,* 8th ed. Philadelphia: WB Saunders, 2000:756–758.

157. Burnham G. Onchocerciasis. *Lancet* 1998;35:1341–1346.

158. Hagan M. Onchocercal dermatitis: clinical impact. *Ann Trop Med Parasitol* 1998;92(suppl 1):S85–96.

159. Elgart ML. Onchocerciasis and dracunculosis. *Dermatol Clin* 1989;7:323–330.

160. Semba RD, Day SH, Spencer WH. Conjunctival nodules associated with onchocerciasis. *Arch Ophthalmol* 1985;103:823–824.

161. Tonjum AM, Thylefors B. Aspects of corneal changes in onchocerciasis. *Br J Ophthalmol* 1978;62:458–461.

162. Anderson J, Fuglsang H. Living microfilariae of *Onchocerca volvulus* in the cornea. *Br J Ophthalmol* 1973;57:712.

163. Von Noorden GK, Buck AA. Ocular onchocerciasis. An ophthalmological and epidemiological study in an African village. *Arch Ophthalmol* 1968;80:26–34.

164. Budden FJ. Natural history of onchocerciasis. *Br J Ophthalmol* 1957;41:214–227.

165. Rodger FC, Chir M. The pathogenesis and pathology of ocular onchocerciasis. *Am J Ophthalmol* 1960;49:104–135.

166. Babalola OE, Murdoch IE. Corneal changes of uncertain etiology in mesoendemic onchocercal communities of Northern Nigeria. *Cornea* 2001;20:183–186.

167. Ridley H. Ocular onchocerciasis, including an investigation in the Gold Coast. *Br J Ophthalmol* 1945;10(suppl);5–58.

168. Schlaegel TF Jr. Uveitis and miscellaneous parasites. *Int Ophthalmol Clin* 1977;17:177–194.

169. Cooper PJ, Proano R, Beltran C, et al. Onchocerciasis in Ecuador: ocular findings in Onchocerca volvulus infected individuals. *Br J Ophthalmol* 1995;79:157–162.

170. Bird AC, Anderson J, Fuglsang H. Morphology of posterior segment lesions of the eye in patients with onchocerciasis. *Br J Ophthalmol* 1976;60:2–20.

171. Semba RD, Murphy RP, Newland HS, et al. Longitudinal study of lesions of the posterior segment in onchocerciasis. *Ophthalmology* 1990;97:1334.

172. Boatin BA, Toe L, Alley ES, et al. Detection of *Onchocerca volvulus* infection in low prevalence areas: a comparison of three diagnostic methods. *Parasitology* 2002;125:545–552.

173. Bradley JE, Unnasch TR. Molecular approaches to the diagnosis of onchocerciasis. *Adv Parasitol* 1996;37:57–106.

174. Fuglsang H, Anderson, J. Further observations on the relationship between ocular onchocerciasis and the head nodule, and on the possible benefit of nodulectomy. *Br J Ophthalmol* 1987;62:445.

175. Taylor HR. Ivermectin treatment of ocular onchocerciasis. Acta Leiden 1990;59:201.

176. Abiose A, Jones BR, Cousens SN, et al. Reduction in incidence of optic nerve disease with annual ivermectin to control onchocerciasis. *Lancet* 1993;341:130–134.

177. Dadzie Y, Neira M, Hopkins D. Final report of the Conference on the eradicability of Onchocerciasis. *Filaria J* 2003;2:1–141.

178. Hoerauf A, Buttner DW, Adjei O, et al. Onchocerciasis. *BMJ* 2003;326:207–210.

179. Nelson GS. Filarial infections as zoonosis. *J Helminthol* 1965; 39:229–250.

180. Wahl G, Georges AJ. Current knowledge on the epidemiology, diagnosis, immunology, and treatment of loiasis. *Trop Med Parasitol* 1995;46:287–291.

181. Garcia, LS. *Diagnostic medical parasitology,* 4th ed. Washington, DC: ASM Press, 2001.

182. Oberg MS, McGown BA, Kleiman DA. Loiasis 15 years after exposure. *Tex Med* 1987;83:36–37.

183. Argyll-Robertson D. Case of Filaria loa in which the parasite was removed from under the conjunctiva. *Trans Ophthalmol Soc UK* 1895;15:137–167.

184. Klion AD, Massougbodji A, Sadeler BC, et al. Loiasis in endemic and nonendemic populations: immunologically mediated differences in clinical presentation. *J Infect Dis* 1991;163: 1318–1325.

185. Duke-Elder S, ed. *System of ophthalmology. Volume XIII Part 1: Diseases of the eyelids: filariasis.* St. Louis: CV Mosby, 1974:188–193.

186. Nnochiri E. The causal agent of the ocular syndrome of the Kampala eye worm. *E Afr Med J* 1972;49:198.

187. Poltera AA. The histopathology of ocular loiasis in Uganda. *Trans R Soc Trop Med Hyg* 1973;67:819–829.

188. Reisman J, Krolman GM, Hogg GR. Conjunctival *Loa loa. Can J Ophthalmol* 1974;9:379–381.

189. Geldelman D, Blumberg R, Sadun A. Ocular Loa Loa with cryoprobe extraction of subconjunctival worm. *Ophthalmology* 1984; 91:300–303.

190. Fobi G, Gardon J, Santiago M, et al. Ocular findings after ivermectin treatment of patients with high Loa loa microfilaremia. *Ophthalmol Epidemiol* 2000;7:27–39.

191. Satyavani M, Rao KN. Live male adult *Loa loa* in the anterior chamber of the eye a case report. *Indian J Pathol Microbiol* 1993; 36:154–157.

192. Corrigan MJ, Hill DW. Retinal artery occlusion in loiasis. *Br J Ophthalmol* 1968;52:477–480.

193. Osuntokun O. Filarial worm *Loa loa* in the anterior chamber. *Br J Ophthalmol* 1975;59:166–167.

194. Jaoko WG. *Loa loa* antigen detection by ELISA: a new approach to diagnosis. *East Afr Med J* 1995;72:176–179.

195. Martin-Prevel Y, Cosnefroy JY, Tshipamba P, et al. Tolerance and efficacy of single high-dose ivermectin for the treatment of loiasis. *Am J Trop Med Hyg* 1993;48:186–192.

196. Duong TH, Kombila M, Ferrer A, et al. Reduced *Loa loa* microfilaria count ten to twelve months after a single dose of ivermectin. *Trans R Soc Trop Med Hyg* 1997;5:592–593.

197. Muylle L, Taelman H, Moldenhauer R, et al. Usefulness of apheresis to extract microfilarias in management of loiasis. *Br Med J (Clin Res Ed)* 1983;287:519–520.

198. Klion AD, Horton J, Nutman TB. Albendazole therapy for loiasis refractory to diethylcarbamazine treatment. *Clin Infect Dis* 1999;3:680–682.

199. Kamgno J, Boussinesq M. Effect of a single dose (600 mg) of albendazole on *Loa loa* microfilaraemia. *Parasite* 2002;91:59–63.

200. Johnson GJ, Axmith K, Desser SS. The elusive *Loa Loa*. *Can J Ophthalmol* 1973;8:492–496.

201. Pampglione S, Rivasi F. Human dirofilariasis due to *Dirofilaria (Nochtiella) repens*: an update of world literature from 1995 to 2000. *Parassitologia* 2000;42(3-4):231–254.

202. Boreham RE, Cooney PT, Stewart PA. Dirofilariasis with conjunctival inflammation. *Med J Aust* 1997;167:51.

203. Moorehouse DE. *Dirofilaria immitis*: a cause of human intraocular infection. *Infection* 1978;6:192–193.

204. Kerkenezov N. Intra-ocular filariasis in Australia. *Br J Ophthalmol* 1962;46:607–615.

205. Font RL, Neafie RC, Perry HD. Subcutaneous dirofilariasis of the eyelid and ocular adnexa: report of six cases. *Arch Ophthalmol* 1980;98(6):1079–1082.

206. Arvantis PG, Vakalis NC, Damanakis AG, et al. Ophthalmic Dirofilariasis. *Am J Ophthalmol* 1997;123:689–691.

207. Strickland GT. *Hunter's tropical medicine and emerging infectious diseases*, 8th ed. Philadelphia: 2000.

208. Stringfellow GJ, Francis IC, Coroneo MT, et al. Orbital dirofilariasis. *Clin Exp Ophthalmol* 2002;30(5):378–380.

209. Afendulova IS. A case of an ocular form of dirofilariasis. *Vestn Oftalmol* 2000;116(2):40.

210. Strianese D, Martini A, Molfino G, et al. Orbital dirofilariasis. *Eur J Ophthalmol* 1998;8(4):258–262.

211. Ruiz-Moreno JM, Bornay-Llinares FJ, Prieto Maza G, et al. Subconjunctival infection with *Dirofilaria repens*: serological confirmation of cure following surgery. *Arch Ophthalmol* 1998;116 (10):1370–1372.

212. Verma AK. Ocular dracontiasis. *Int Surg* 1968;50:508–509.

213. Muller R. Dracunculus and Dracunculiasis. *Adv Parasitol* (Elsevier) 1971;9:73–152.

214. Knierim R, Jack MK. Conjunctivitis due to *Thelazia californiensis*. *Arch Ophthalmol* 1975;93:522–523.

215. Zakir R, Zhong-Xia Z, Chioddini P, et al. Intraocular infestation with the worm, *Thelazia callipaeda*. *Br J Ophthalmol* 1999; 83:1194–1195.

216. Singh TS, Singh KN. Thelaziasis: report of two cases. *Br J Ophthalmol* 1993;77:528–529.

217. Choudhury AR. Thelaziasis. *Am J Ophthalmol* 1969;67:773–774.

218. Chaiyaporn V, Phanich V. Thelaziasis in man in Thailand. *J Parasitol* 1969;55:941.

219. Cheung WK, Lu HJ, Liang CH, et al. Conjunctivitis caused by *Thelazia callipaeda* infestation in a woman. *J Formos Med Assoc* 1998;6:425–427.

220. Koyama Y, Ohira A, Kono T, et al. Five cases of thelaziasis. *Br J Ophthalmol* 2000;84:441.

221. Kirschner BI, Dunn JP, Ostler HB. Conjunctivitis caused by *Thelazia californiensis*. *Am J Ophthalmol* 1990;110:573–574.

222. Bunnag T. Gnathostomiasis. In: Strickland GT, ed. *Hunter's tropical medicine*. Philadelphia: WB Saunders 1991:764–767.

223. Despommier DD. Tissue nematodes. In: Long SS, Pickering LK, Prober CG, eds. *Principles and practice of pediatric infectious diseases*. New York: Churchill Livingstone. 1997:1469–1476.

224. Rojas-Molina N, Pedraza-Sanchez S, Torres-Bibiano B, et al. Gnathostomosis, an emerging foodborne zoonotic disease in Acapulco, Mexico. *Emerg Infect Dis* 1999;5:264–266.

225. Choudhury AR. Ocular gnathostomiasis. *Am J Ophthalmol* 1970; 70:276–278.

226. Teekhasaenee C, Ritch R, Kanchanaranya C. Ocular parasitic infection in Thailand. *Rev Infect Dis* 1986;8:350–356.

227. Kittiponghansa S, Prabriputaloong A, Pariyanonda S, et al. Intracameral gnathostomiasis: a cause of anterior uveitis and secondary glaucoma. *Br J Ophthalmol* 1987;71:618–622.

228. Toma H, Matsumura S, Oshiro C, et al. Ocular angiostrongyliasis without meningitis symptoms in Okinawa, Japan. *J Parasitol* 2002;88:211–213.

229. Dissanaike AS, Ihalamulla RL, de S Naotunne T, et al. Third report of ocular parastrongyliasis (angiostrongyliasis) from Sri Lanka. *Parassitologia* 2001;43:95–97.

230. Lau LI, Lee FL, Hsu WM, et al. Human subconjunctival infection of *Macacanema formosana*: the first case of human infection reported worldwide. *Arch Ophthalmol* 2002;120:643–644.

231. Natarajan R. Another case of human subconjunctival infection by Macacanema formosana. *Arch Ophthalmol* 2003;121: 584–585.

232. Botero D, Tanowitz HB, Weiss LM, et al. Taeniasis and cysticercosis. *Infect Dis Clin North Am* 1993;7:683–697.

233. Pushker N, Bajaj MS, Chandra M. Ocular and orbital cysticercosis. *Acta Ophthalmol Scand* 2001;79:408–413.

234. Del Brutto OH. Cysticercosis and cerebrovascular disease: a review. *J Neurol Neurosurg Psychiatry* 1992;55:252–254.

235. Sharma T, Sinha S, Shah N, et al. Intraocular cysticercosis: clinical characteristics and visual outcome after vitreoretinal surgery. *Ophthalmology* 2003;110:996–1004.

236. Lombardo J. Subretinal cysticercosis. *Optom Vis Sci* 2001;78: 188–194.

237. Kapoor S. Ocular cysticercosis in India. *Trop Geog Med* 1978;30: 253–256.

238. White AC. Neurocysticercosis: updates on epidemiology, pathogenesis, diagnosis and management. *Annu Rev Med* 2000;51: 187–206.

239. Bergquist NR. Schistosomiasis: from risk assessment to control. *Trends Parasitol* 2002;18:309–314.

240. Cox FE. History of human parasitology. *Clin Microbiol Rev* 2002;15:595–612.

241. Newton JC, Kanchanaranya C, Previte LR Jr. Intraocular *Schistosoma mansoni*. *Am J Ophthalmol* 1968;65:774–778.

242. Welsh NH. Bilharzial conjunctivitis. *Am J Ophthalmol* 1968; 66:933–938.

243. Dickinson AJ, Rosenthal AR, Nicholson KG. Inflammation of the retinal pigment epithelium: a unique presentation of ocular schistosomiasis. *Br J Ophthalmol* 1990;74:440–442.

244. Milligan A, Burns DA. Ectopic cutaneous schistosomiasis and schistosomal ocular inflammatory disease. *Br J Ophthalmol* 1988; 119:793–798.

245. Bialasiewicz AA, Hassenstein A, Schaudig U. Subretinal granuloma, retinal vasculitis and keratouveitis with secondary open-angle glaucoma in schistosomiasis. *Ophthalmologe* 2001;98: 972–975.

246. Cadera W, Pachtman MA, Fountain JA, et al. Ocular lesions caused by caterpillar hairs (ophthalmia nodosa). *Can J Ophthalmol* 1984;19:40–44.

247. Hered RW, Spaulding AG, Sanitato JJ, et al. Ophthalmia nodosa caused by tarantula hairs. *Ophthalmology* 1988;95:166–169.

248. Teske SAH, et al. Caterpillar-induced keratitis. *Cornea* 1991; 10:317.

249. Grub M, Mielke J, Schlote T. Bee sting of the corneaæa case report. *Klin Monatsbl Augenheilkd* 2001;218:747–750.

250. Miyashita K. Wasp sting-induced linear keratitis. *Ann Ophthalmol* 1992;24:143–145.

251. Poole TR. Blister beetle periorbital dermatitis and keratoconjunctivitis in Tanzania. *Eye* 1998;12:883–885.

252. Lasudry JG, Brightbill FS. Ophthalmia nodosa caused by tarantula hairs. *J Pediatr Ophthalmol Strabismus* 1997;34:197–198.

253. Fraser SG, Dowd TC, Bosanquet RC. Intraocular caterpillar hairs (setae): clinical course and management. *Eye* 1994;8:596–598.

254. Ittyerah TP, Fernandez ST, Kutty KN. Marginal keratitis produced by phthirus pubes. *Indian J Ophthalmol* 1976;24:21–22.

255. Couch JM, Green WR, Hirst LW, et al. Diagnosing and treating Phthirus pubis palpebrarum. *Surv Ophthalmol* 1982;26:219–225.

256. Ashkenazi I, Desatnik HR, Abraham FA. Yellow mercuric oxide: a treatment of choice for phthiriasis palpebrarum. *Br J Ophthalmol* 1991;75:356–358.

257. Awan KJ. Argon laser phototherapy of phthiriasis palpebrarum. *Ophthalmic Surg* 1986;17:813–814.

258. Mansour AM. Photo essay: phthiriasis palpebrarum. *Arch Ophthalmol* 2000;118:1458–1459.

259. Reingold WJ, Robin JB, Leipa D, et al. Oestrus ovis ophthalmomyiasis externa. *Am J Ophthalmol* 1984;97:7–10.

260. Wilhelmus KR. Myiasis palpebrarum. *Am J Ophthalmol* 1986; 101(4):496–498.

261. Chodosh J, Clarridge JE, Matoba A. Nosocomial conjunctival ophthalmomyiasis with cochliomyia macellaria. *Am J Ophthalmol* 1991;111(4):520–521.

262. Cameron JA, Shoukrey NM, Al-Garni AA. Conjunctival ophthalmomyiasis caused by the sheep nasal botfly (*Oestrus ovis*). *Am J Ophthalmol* 1991;112:331–333.

263. Ziemianski MC, Lee K, Sabates FN. Ophthalmomyiasis interna. *Arch Ophthalmol* 1980;98:1588–1589.

264. Kersten RC, Shoukrey NM, Tabbara KF. Orbital myiasis. *Ophthalmology* 1986;93:1228–1232.

265. Perry DP, Donnenfeld ED, Font RL. Intracorneal ophthalmomyiasis. *Am J Ophthalmol* 1990;109:741–742.

266. Gutierrez Y. *Diagnostic pathology of parasitic infections with clinical correlations,* 2nd ed. New York: Oxford University Press, 2000:728.

CHLAMYDIAL KERATITIS AND CONJUNCTIVITIS

ELISABETH M. MESSMER

PREVALENCE

Chlamydiae have long been important causes of ocular infections and are still the second leading cause of blindness in Africa (1,2). Trachoma is one of the oldest recorded diseases of mankind, documented in the Egyptian Eber's papyrus in 1900 BC (2,3). It is still endemic in sub-Saharan Africa, including Ghana, Mali, and Tanzania, as well as eastern Mediterranean countries such as Iraq, Saudi Arabia, United Arab Emirates, Qatar, and Oman (1,2,4,5). According to the World Health Organization (WHO) there are 146 million people worldwide with active trachoma (2). It is one of the greatest single causes of preventable blindness and impaired vision in the world today (6). Western Europe and the United States have been trachoma free in the last century, correlating with economic development, and in Southeast Asia progress is being made for the same reason (4). Transmission of the chlamydial agent causing trachoma is by eye-to-eye or hand-to-eye contact. The disease is usually acquired in early childhood. Chronic inflammation from recurrent infections leads to conjunctival scarring and blinding complications in adults. A number of environmental factors such as low living standard and poor hygiene, influence prevalence and severity of trachoma.

The second ocular disease caused by *Chlamydia trachomatis* is adult inclusion conjunctivitis, also called paratrachoma. Reported prevalences range from zero to 28% (7–10), but population selection biases, the absence of controls, and differing diagnostic assays used in these studies explain the wide range of results. Adult inclusion conjunctivitis typically occurs in sexually active young adults following transfer of bacteria from the genitalia to the eye. There is a high incidence of cervical or urethral chlamydia in these individuals (9–11).

With the advent of widespread neonatal ocular prophylaxis, gonococcal infections have decreased and *C. trachomatis* is now the most common cause of ophthalmia neonatorum in industrialized countries as well as in several developing countries (12–15). It may be responsible for 20% to 73% of all cases of neonatal conjunctivitis (16–18). In developing countries the prevalence of genital chlamydial infection in pregnant women ranges from 7% to 29%. One third of infants exposed at birth will develop chlamydial disease (2,14). In North America and Europe, 2% to 6% of all newborns are infected with neonatal chlamydiae (19). However, the incidence of *C. trachomatis* conjunctivitis is declining, as shown in Argentina with 4.39/1,000 live births in 1995 down to 0.78/1000 live births in 1998 (2).

EPIDEMIOLOGY

Trachoma

Although trachoma has been declining in many areas of the world, estimates suggest that approximately 2.2 million people are blind from trachoma in Africa (1) and trachoma is responsible for 6 million blinded people or 15% of world's blindness. In some areas trachoma is holoendemic—every child acquires active trachoma and every adult shows evidence of conjunctival scarring. Corneal opacification from trachoma was found to be responsible for 20.6% of all blindness in Jimma zone, Ethiopia (22) and for 4.5% of blind individuals in the Central African Republic (23). Investigations in highly endemic sub-Saharan Africa have shown that women account for about 75% of all trachomatous trichiasis and subsequent blindness due to corneal scarring (1). A survey in Saudi Arabia revealed that over 3.5% of the population showed corneal scars, about half of them due to trachoma (5). However, trachoma is extremely variable, and a high incidence of trachoma in an area may not necessarily be correlated with a high degree of visual impairment (2). The duration of disease and infection is markedly age-dependent. The estimated median duration of disease was 13.2 weeks in 0- to 4-year-old subjects and 1.7 weeks in those age 15 and over in a study by Bailey et al. (24). The cumulative incidence rate of disease was reduced threefold, with age mostly attributable to a more rapid disease resolution.

The risk of acquiring *C. trachomatis* is strongly linked with environmental and behavioral characteristics. Numerous studies have demonstrated that limited access to water supplies, low water consumption by the household, the presence of flies, and poor hygiene are all risk factors for becoming infected with *C. trachomatis* (25). The infection is usually transmitted by ocular secretions from contaminated fingers, clothes, and aerosolized nasopharyngeal secretions (26). The basic pattern is mother-to-child transfer. The higher incidence of acute disease and blindness in women may be explained by their lower status in society, their permanent close contact with children and common applicators used to apply eye makeup (1,2). Face flies are found commonly in seasons with the highest prevalence of active trachoma and are believed to feed on ocular discharges, but it has been difficult to quantify the role of flies in transmission. Reducing fly densities in rural African villages, however, has been demonstrated to reduce active disease (27) as has the introduction of face washing (28). Although malnutrition is common in hyperendemic areas, no relationship was found between nutritional status and trachoma in preschool children (29).

Coinfection with other bacteria occurs often and may facilitate transmission and proliferation of chlamydia. Moreover, bacterial conjunctivitis may cause disastrous sequelae in eyes already infected with trachoma, and bacterial infection may play a greater role than trachoma in producing blinding complications (30).

Adult Inclusion Conjunctivitis

Chlamydia was the causative organism in 2% of patients with acute conjunctivitis in a study performed in Australia (9). A distinctive feature was the long delay before a definitive diagnosis of ocular chlamydial infection was made.

Inclusion conjunctivitis is an oculogenital disease and as such, its epidemiology differs dramatically from that of trachoma. It was originally described in Europe as "swimming pool conjunctivitis," contracted from swimming in contaminated pools (31). Today proper chlorination has eliminated chlamydiae from this source, but nongenital infection may occur with bathing in unchlorinated water (9). Adult inclusion conjunctivitis is usually transmitted by autoinoculation from genital secretions or by genital-to-eye-inoculation by an infected sexual partner. At present, a minimum of 70% of women (and possibly all) with chlamydial conjunctivitis are estimated to have genital *C. trachomatis* infection, which is mostly asymptomatic. Chronic disease of the female genital tract may produce pelvic inflammatory disease, tubal blockage, ectopic pregnancy, and infertility (9,32,33). Also 54% of men with chlamydial conjunctivitis had a positive chlamydial urethral culture, and 70% of these patients had no genital symptoms (34). Up to 32% of men and 63% of women with genital *Neisseria gonorrhoeae* have coexistent chlamydial infections, and it has been suggested

that *N. gonorrhoeae* can activate latent Chlamydia (35). Eye-to-eye transmission is possible, but extremely rare (9).

Neonatal Inclusion Blennorrhea

Intrapartum transmission of neonatal chlamydial ocular infection from the mother's genital tract was first described by Halberstaedter and von Prowazek (36) in 1909. Characteristic inclusion bodies were found in specimens from eyes of infected newborns as well as from the cervices of their mothers. Subsequently, Lindner (37) demonstrated infectious agents in urethral swabs from fathers of infants with neonatal inclusion conjunctivitis. Without prophylaxis, the transmission rate from an infected mother to her infant is approximately 50%, with the risk of development of conjunctivitis being 30% to 40% for infected babies (38). Although infection is thought to typically occur as the fetus passes through an infected birth canal, a study suggests bacterial transmission to infants' eyes from their nasopharyngeal passages or those of their caregivers after birth (39). Moreover, a transmembrane or transplacental route of infection may be involved in early chlamydial infections in infants delivered by cesarean section (40).

CLINICAL FEATURES

Trachoma

The initial infection of trachoma is characterized by an abrupt nonspecific conjunctivitis, followed by follicle formation at about the third week (Fig. 18-1). The symptoms appear within 5 to 7 days postinoculation. A purulent discharge consisting of mixed inflammatory cells may develop, along with a tender preauricular lymph node. Conjunctival follicles grow, and peripheral corneal follicles as well as a marked trachomatous pannus develop. Later, large papillae may mask the typical gelatinous follicles. Resolving limbal follicles leave

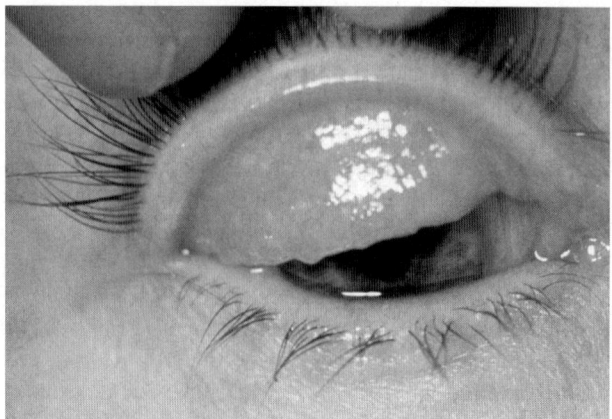

FIGURE 18-1. Follicular conjunctivitis in trachoma.

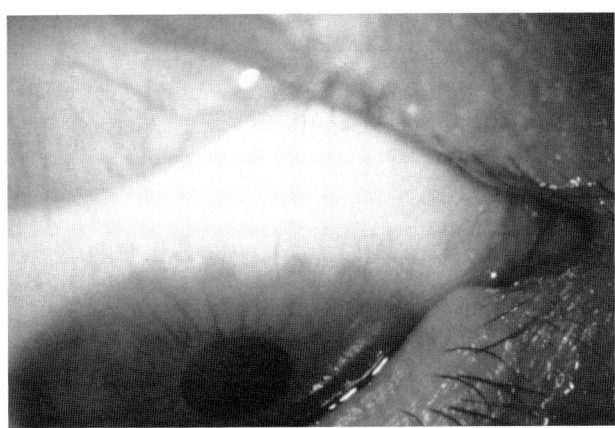

FIGURE 18-2. Peripheral Herbert pits after resolution of limbal follicles in trachoma.

TABLE 18-1. STAGES OF TRACHOMA, ACCORDING TO MACCALLAN, 1931

Stage I	Early stage of follicles
Stage IIa	Large and gelatinous follicles
Stage IIb'	Papillary enlargement as well as follicles
Stage IIb''	Follicles with the added complication of spring catarrh
Stage IIc	Trachoma complicated by gonococcal conjunctivitis
Stage III	Cicatrization has commenced
Stage IV	Cicatrization is complete

of ocular trachoma (Table 18-2) (45). Trachoma is divided into two inflammatory stages (follicular inflammation, TF; trachomatous inflammation intense, TI) and three stages associated with scarring (trachomatous scarring, TS; trachomatous trichiasis, TT; corneal opacity, CO). This classification system demonstrated high interobserver reliability in trachoma studies.

Adult Inclusion Conjunctivitis

Symptoms of adult inclusion conjunctivitis, such as redness, foreign-body sensation, photophobia, and mucopurulent discharge, typically begin 2 days to 3 weeks after inoculation (19). Examination reveals a follicular conjunctivitis, mainly localized to the inferior tarsal conjunctiva, associated with papillary hypertrophy (Figs. 18-4 and 18-5). Usually, the infection is bilateral, but Garland et al. (9) reported monocular inclusion conjunctivitis in the majority of their patients. Nontender lymphadenopathy of the ipsilateral preauricular nodes may also be present. Corneal complications include a superficial punctate keratitis as well as pannus formation. This superficial micropannus, however, is distinct from the severe macropannus developing in trachoma. Marginal and central subepithelial infiltrates as well as epidemic keratoconjunctivitis-like subepithelial lesions may occur (19,46,47). If adult inclusion conjunctivitis is left untreated, it usually heals spontaneously but may persist for longer than a year. Few cases will lead to conjunctival or corneal scarring. Coinfection with adenovirus is rare but must be suspected in prolonged follicular keratoconjunctivitis (48). Anterior uveitis may complicate inclusion conjunctivitis. Moreover, antibodies to *C. trachomatis* are significantly increased in acute anterior uveitis compared to healthy controls or other forms of uveitis (49). A common genetic predisposition to *Chlamydia* infection and acute anterior uveitis in the context of human leukocyte antigen (HLA)-B27-positivity may be responsible for this phenomenon. Reactive arthritis occurs in approximately 2% to 4% of patients after previous infections mainly of the urogenital tract with *C. trachomatis* or of the gut with enterobacteriae (50). Although HLA-B27 is found in only approximately 50% of patients with acute reactive arthritis, HLA-B27 seems

typical Herbert's peripheral pits (Fig. 18-2). Cicatricial changes of the conjunctiva and the underlying tarsus lead to entropion formation and trichiasis. Often a heavy linear scar parallel with and 1 to 2 mm from the lid margin extends across the entire lid (Arlt's line, Fig. 18-3) (41). Untreated lid deformities and added superinfection may progress to corneal complications and severe visual loss. Whereas in early disease epiphora dominates, advanced disease may cause severe keratoconjunctivitis sicca due to atrophy of meibomian glands, loss of mucus-secreting cells, and occlusion of the tear lacrimal ducts (42,43). Lacrimal system complications observed in severe, inactive disease include dacryocystitis, dacryocystocele, and dacryocutaneous fistula (43).

Two classification schemes are used to categorize the stages of trachoma, the MacCallan system dating back to 1908, and that of the WHO (44,45). MacCallan (44) divided the course of trachoma into four stages, based on developmental changes in the follicles, papillary hypertrophy, and scar formation (Table 18-1). His classification is useful for epidemiologic studies, but it neglects the intensity of the inflammatory reaction in chlamydial disease. The WHO uses a simple grading scheme for clinical assessment

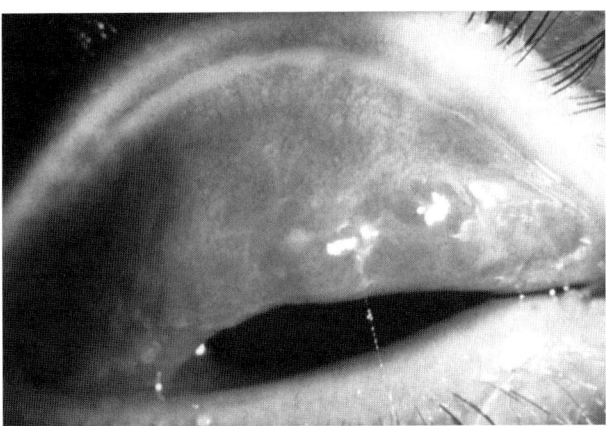

FIGURE 18-3. Trachoma. Cicatrizing conjunctivitis.

TABLE 18-2. STAGES OF TRACHOMA ACCORDING TO THE WHO, 1987

Clinical Findings	WHO Grade	Code
≥5 follicles in the upper tarsal conjunctiva; Follicles must be ≥0.05 mm in diameter	trachomatous inflammation follicular	TF
Pronounced inflammatory thickening of the tarsal conjunctiva which obscures half of the normal deep tarsal vessels	trachomatous inflammation intense	TI
Presence of easily visible scars in the tarsal Conjunctiva	trachomatous Conjunctival scarring	TS
At least one eyelash rubs against the eyeball; also includes evidence of recent removal of an in-turned lash	trachomatous trichiasis	TT
Easily visible corneal opacity present over the Pupil that is so dense that at least part of the pupil margin is blurred when seen through the opacity	corneal opacity	CO

to be crucials for the development of sacroiliitis and chronic spondyloarthropathy (50).

Twelve of 84 infected volunteers (14%) developed symptoms of otitis media in experimental inclusion conjunctivitis (47). *C. trachomatis* was cultured from the middle ear aspirates of patients with acute otitis media with and without effusion and chronic otitis media (51). In animal experiments otitis could be induced by direct inoculation into the middle ear as well as indirectly by infection of the nasopharynx and the conjunctiva (51,52).

Neonatal Inclusion Blennorrhea

Symptoms of neonatal inclusion conjunctivitis appear 5 to 12 days postpartum (earlier with premature rupture of amniotic membranes). Acute infection typically presents with binocular lid edema, conjunctival hyperemia, papillary hypertrophy, and copious mucopurulent discharge (Fig. 18-6). A follicular reaction, indicating the formation of secondary germinal centers, cannot be established in newborns before 6 to 8 weeks, but may develop in chronic disease. It may be extremely difficult to differentiate between chlamydial and other bacterial causes of conjunctivitis on the basis of physical examination. Moreover, more than one organism was isolated from the conjunctiva in 50% of

cases with chlamydial conjunctivitis (17). Age of presentation, however, is about 1 week later in infants with other bacterial infections compared to *Chlamydia* (17).

Corneal manifestations similar to those of adult inclusion conjunctivitis such as superficial punctate keratopathy, fine micropannus, and peripheral subepithelial infiltrates have been described in newborns. Conjunctival and corneal scarring are possible sequelae (53). Untreated, neonatal inclusion blennorrhea may pursue a prolonged course with systemic involvement. A high incidence of pharyngeal infection is found in babies with isolation-positive chlamydial conjunctivitis. Lower respiratory tract infections, including pneumonitis, otitis media, proctitis, and vulvovaginitis, may complicate neonatal ocular disease (38,54).

PATHOGENESIS, PATHOLOGY, AND IMMUNOLOGY

Chlamydia are unique among bacteria in that they are obligate intracellular gram-negative organisms with a complex intracellular development cycle that consists of an infectious metabolically inactive elementary body and a noninfectious, metabolically active reticulate body. They are unable to produce adenosine triphosphate and thus are energy para-

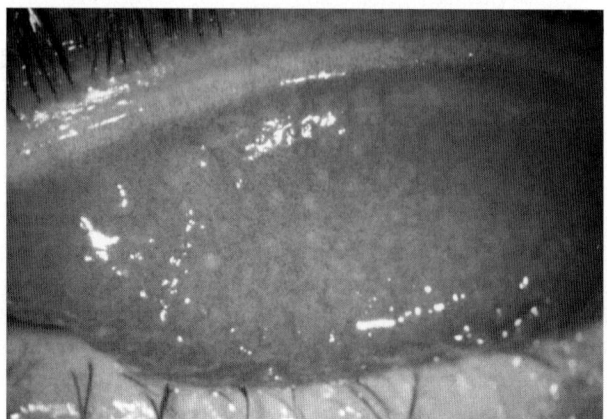

FIGURE 18-4. Adult inclusion conjunctivitis. Follicular conjunctivitis localized to the inferior tarsal conjunctiva

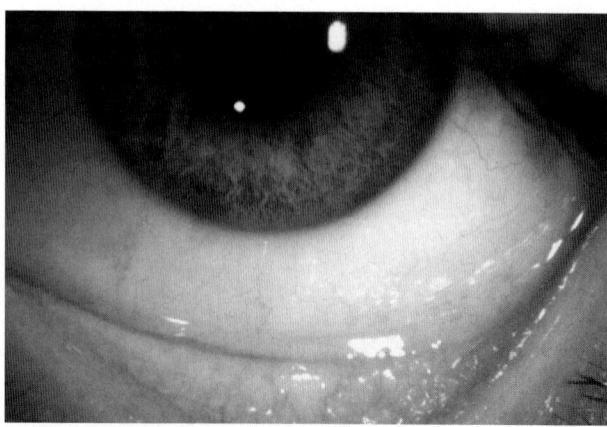

FIGURE 18-5. Adult inclusion conjunctivitis. Follicular conjunctivitis of the upper tarsal conjunctiva.

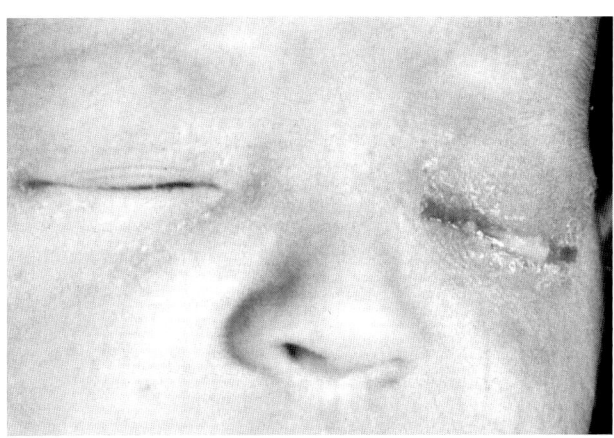

FIGURE 18-6. Neonatal inclusion conjunctivitis with lid edema and copious mucopurulent discharge.

sites (55). Because of their singular biologic character, the chlamydiae are assigned their own order, the Chlamydiales, consisting in turn of one family, the Chlamydiaceae, two genera, the *Chlamydia* and the *Chlamydophila,* and nine species. Human chlamydial infection is often caused by *Chlamydia trachomatis*, less frequently by *Chlamydophila pneumoniae*, and rarely by *Chlamydophila psittaci, Chlamydophila abortus,* or *Chlamydophila felis* (56). *C. trachomatis* isolates are commonly classified into 15 distinct serovars, designated A-K, L1–L3, and MoPn, which is a mouse adapted strain. Serovars A-C cause trachoma, serovars D-K (and occasionally, variants of B or Ba) are primarily associated with sexually transmitted infections, and serovars L1-L3 cause lymphogranuloma venereum (57,58). *C. trachomatis* is essentially a pathogen of mucosal surfaces, infecting and replicating within epithelial cells. The infected cell ruptures, releasing thousands of elementary bodies.

The pathophysiology of chronic chlamydial disease is still unknown in detail, but most likely depends on both parasite and host factors. Recent data provide compelling evidence for a chlamydial cytotoxin for epithelial cells present in the elementary body and delivered to host cells very early during infection. This cytotoxin may also provide a mechanism for immune evasion compatible with the clinical characteristics of persistent oculogenital infections (57). Infection with *C. trachomatis* leads to the upregulation of several functionally important genes in the host cell such as *IL-11, LIF,* chemokine gene *MIP2a,* transcription factor genes, apoptosis-related genes, and adhesion molecule genes such as *ICAM-1* (59). Chlamydia seems to reprogram the host cells at various key positions that act as intra- or intercellular switches (59).

Ocular infections are characterized by distinct immunologic and pathologic responses to the different chlamydial strains causing either trachoma or inclusion conjunctivitis. The immune response seems to confer partial protection against subsequent infection, yet appears also to be responsible for much of the observed pathology and tissue de-

struction seen in trachoma. In trachoma, repeated infection with the causative organism, perhaps exacerbated by superinfection with other organisms, is necessary to cause severe conjunctival scarring and blinding complications. The stimulus for continual inflammation may not be from repeated exposure to chlamydial surface antigens but may rather be due to a labile product released by the living organisms (60). Cellular responses elicited in nonimmune cells (i.e., mucosal epithelial cells) infected by chlamydiae may be necessary and sufficient to account for chronic and intense inflammation and the promotion of cellular proliferation, tissue remodeling, and scarring (61). Inflammatory cells become activated in both an antigen-nonspecific and, for reinfection, an antigen-specific manner to produce their own repertoire of cytokines and growth factors (61).

Both humoral and cell-mediated immune responses are involved. Target antigens are the major outer membrane protein (MOMP) and heat shock proteins (HSP60) (62,63). Antichlamydial antibodies can neutralize chlamydiae and block attachment and internalization of the organism (62). Experimental studies in monkeys and human indicate that tear immunoglobulins, especially immunoglobulin A (IgA), may play a vital role in mediating protective immunity (64,65). But antibodies may limit the extent of chlamydial multiplication and prevent more invasive disease rather than to effect a cure (66). Moreover, antichlamydial antibodies do not protect against reinfection (67,68). Serum IgG antichlamydia antibody was detected in 42% of patients with trachoma and in 37% of patients with acute inclusion conjunctivitis by Numazaki et al. (69). Antichlamydial IgM was present in 13% of patients with trachoma and in 33% of patients with acute inclusion conjunctivitis. Forty percent of the trachoma patients and 34% of patients with inclusion conjunctivitis were IgA-positive. However, antichlamydial IgG and IgA was also present in 25% and 22% of healthy controls, respectively, compared to IgM, which was positive in only 2% of the healthy population (69). IgA antibodies in tears were detected as early as 5 days after onset of clinical symptoms in patients with inclusion conjunctivitis. The IgA response in tears was not significantly correlated with the severity of the ocular infection, whereas serum IgA titers increased with the severity of clinical findings (70–72). In neonatal inclusion blennorrhea, passively transferred maternal antibodies supposedly do not confer any protection against the transmitted chlamydiae. The detection of IgA antibodies in tears and serum among chlamydia-positive neonates without corresponding maternal antibodies may suggest a production of antichlamydial IgA antibodies in the newborn. The antibody response in serum of newborns with chlamydial conjunctivitis is poor, as would be expected (70–72).

Stimulating a strong humoral immune response by immunization with whole bacteria or detergent extracts was evaluated for trachoma control. The results were disappointing; the protection observed was either short lived (73) or the duration and intensity of disease was actually exacerbated by vaccination (74,75).

Cell-mediated immune mechanisms are important components in the response to trachoma. Courtright et al. (71) demonstrated that factors related to an individual's cellular response are essential to the development of conjunctival scarring. Trachomatous scarring was less pronounced in multibacillary leprosy patients (with suppressed cell-mediated immunity) and was more severe in paucibacillary leprosy patients (with enhanced cell-mediated immunity) compared to their healthy siblings (70,71). A vigorous T- and B-lymphocyte response with a surprising preponderance of T cells is evident in the conjunctiva during acute chlamydial infection in monkeys (76). Eyelid specimens from trachomatous entropion also exhibited a vast amount of T cells (77). In conjunctival biopsies of trachoma patients with extensive fibrosis, T-helper cells predominated over B lymphocytes (78). Strong T-helper-1 (Th1)-type responses are thought to play a role in resolution of infection, whereas Th2-type responses seem to be involved in scarring (79,80). HLA-A28 (A*6802) haplotype was significantly associated with advanced trachoma in an endemic population in Gambia. This may be due to an immunopathologic HLA-A*6802-restricted cytotoxic T-lymphocyte response (70).

C. trachomatis infection stimulates a number of local cytokines such as interleukin (IL)-1β, IL-12, transforming growth factor-β1 (TGF-β1), tumor necrosis factor-α (TNF-α), and interferon-γ (IFN-γ), which favor a strong cell-mediated and proinflammatory response in both the early and later manifestations of trachoma (81,82). IL-1 and TNF-α are potent stimulators of tissue remodeling, inducing collagenase production from fibroblasts, whereas TGF-β plays an important role in progressive scarring in chronic infection (81). IFN-γ facilitates control of the replicative form of the bacterium by limiting intracellular pools of tryptophan and by inducing nitric oxide synthase (iNOS) activity. Chlamydia exposed to IFN-γ differentiate into large, morphologically aberrant persistent bodies (PBs) and may express decreased levels of surface structural proteins while expressing baseline or increased levels of inflammatory proteins. A decrease of IFN-γ in the microenvironment leads to reentry of PBs into the productive life cycle, systemic dissemination, or chronic chlamydial persistence (82,83).

The histopathology of trachoma shows chronic inflammation with papillary hypertrophy of the epithelium, lymphoid infiltration of the subepithelial tissue with the formation of follicles, and subsequent reactive proliferation of connective tissue (41). Alterations of extracellular matrix components and collagen metabolism with formation of new collagen type I, III, IV, and V was noted in the conjunctiva of patients with active trachoma. Scarred trachoma conjunctiva is characterized by a marked increase in basement membrane collagen types IV and V and a decrease in colla-

gen types I and III (78). Biopsies of tarsal plates and palpebral conjunctiva in patients with inactive trachoma revealed a subepithelial, thick, fibrous membrane adherent to the tarsus, hyaline degeneration of the tarsal plate with focal replacement by adipose tissue, atrophy of the meibomian glands with thickening of the acinar basement membrane, loss of goblet cells, and presence of retention cysts (42). Primary and secondary orbicularis oculi muscle changes, such as degenerated fibers, increased connective tissue, and edema, may contribute to the development of trachomatous entropion and trichiasis (84). Lacrimal sac biopsies showed the same cicatrizing changes seen in conjunctival biopsies (43).

DIAGNOSIS

Clinically active-appearing trachoma is not always a reliable marker of active infection, particularly in teenagers and after treatment. Of clinically active-appearing children aged 1 to 5 years, 78% were actively infected, as determined by ligase chain reaction analysis to detect chlamydial DNA, versus only 17% of those aged 11 to 15 years (85).

The conventional techniques for diagnosing chlamydial keratoconjunctivitis include conjunctival cytologic investigation, inoculation of susceptible cell lines followed by observation for cytopathic effect or visualization using various chemical or immunologic staining techniques, examination of blood or tears for various classes of antibodies, and detection of chlamydial antigens in conjunctival and corneal specimens (86). However, the pitfalls of these conventional techniques are numerous (see below). Diagnostic tests based on nucleic acid amplification techniques are likely to play an increasingly important role in the diagnosis of ocular *C. trachomatis* infection (87). Based on the literature documenting coinfection of chlamydia in patients with gonococcus, testing for both gonococci and chlamydia of the genital tract in patients with chlamydial conjunctivitis is recommended (11). Serologic testing for syphilis should also be performed (11).

Cytology

In 1909 Halberstaedter and von Prowazek identified inclusions in conjunctival scrapings by means of Giemsa staining (36). Electron microscopically, these inclusions are detected in the host perikarya and contain highly infectious elementary bodies (88). Giemsa stained conjunctival scrapings are still used to confirm chlamydial disease, but the sensitivity of this method is variable and is lower than most of the other tests (89). Both neutrophils and lymphocytes are common, and the predominate cell type in the inflammatory infiltrates does not allow one to differentiate between chlamydial and viral infections. More sensitive cytologic features include the presence of plasma cells, Leber cells, blastoid cells, and multinucleated giant cells (90).

Culture

Culture of eye swabs on cycloheximide-treated McCoy cells (mouse fibroblasts) remains the "gold standard" for chlamydial diagnosis in ocular and genitourinary disease, with a specificity of 100%, but a sensitivity that varies from 65% to 85% (91,92). HeLa229 cells (derived from human cervical carcinoma cells) and BHK-21 cells (baby hamster kidney cells) may also be used for culture (93). After 48 to 72 hours of growth, infected cells develop characteristic intracytoplasmic inclusions, which are detected by staining with a fluorescein-conjugated monoclonal antibody specific for the MOMP of *C. trachomatis*. Efficient isolation in cell culture requires that the sample be plated as quickly as possible after collection or stored under optimal conditions to maintain the infectious elementary bodies. The main disadvantages of the culture technique are its time delay to final report, complexity, and susceptibility to microbial overgrowth and cell toxicity (87,94). Cell culture, however, is still the first choice when results will be used as evidence in legal investigations (95). In addition, cell culture is the only method by which a clinical isolate can be obtained for antimicrobial susceptibility testing (95).

Antigen Tests

Direct Fluorescein Antibody Test

The direct fluorescein antibody (DFA) test uses fluorescein-conjugated antibodies that bind specifically to bacterial antigen (MOMP or lipopolysaccharide, LPS) in smears. It shows a sensitivity of up to 100% in comparison with culture in neonatal eye infections (96). Commercially available DFA assays (Syva MicroTrak) show sensitivities of 60% to 93% in cervical specimens, with excellent specificities (97,98). However, laborious microscopic examinations of each specimen by highly skilled and experienced personnel is necessary. Moreover, the assay is suitable only for the examination of a small sample size.

Immunoassays

Enzyme immunoassays (EIAs) are able to detect chlamydial LPS with a monoclonal or polyclonal antibody that has been linked to an enzyme. The enzyme converts a colorless substrate into a colored product, which is detected by a spectrophotometer. EIAs have the advantage of low cost and suitability for testing large numbers of specimens. They typically require specialized equipment and trained personnel to perform the tests and interpret the results. Cross-reaction with LPS of other microorganisms may cause false-positive results (99). Commercially available tests such as MicroTrak EIA (Syva), Pathfinder EIA (Sanofi, Kallestad), and Abbott's Chlamydiazyme EIA are screening devices with sensitivities ranging from 50% to 85% (98,100,101).

The BioStar optical immunoassay is a rapid, self-contained chlamydial test based on changes in the reflection of light. It revealed a high sensitivity (100%) and specificity (93%) in the diagnosis of neonatal chlamydial conjunctivitis (102). In endocervical swab specimens sensitivity was 74% compared to polymerase chain reaction (PCR) and cell culture (97).

Nucleic Acid Probe (NAP) Test

Two nucleic acid hybridization assays are Food and Drug Administration (FDA)-approved to detect chlamydia, the Gen-Probe PACE and the Digene Hybrid Capture. Both tests can detect *C. trachomatis* and *N. gonorrhoeae* in a single specimen. The Gen-Probe PACE system uses a chemiluminescent labeled, single-stranded DNA probe that is complementary to the ribosomal RNA of the target organism "chlamydia." After the ribosomal RNA is released from the organism by heating, the labeled DNA probe combines with the chlamydia ribosomal RNA to form a stable DNA:RNA hybrid that can be measured in the Gen-Probe luminometer. NAP tests are effective for large-scale screening, and viable organisms are not required. These tests provide a rapid result (3 to 5 hours), are relatively inexpensive and require only moderate technical skill. Specimen may be stored or transported for ≤7 days without refrigeration before receipt and testing by the laboratory (95). NAP tests, however, are less sensitive (60–79%) compared to the nucleic acid amplified tests (101,103,104). In addition, their specificity is less than that of cell culture.

Nucleic Acid Amplification Tests (NAATs)

The common characteristic among NAATs is that they are designed to amplify nucleic acid sequences that are specific for the organism being detected. Similar to other nonculture tests, NAATs do not require viable organisms. NAATs are technically demanding, and special areas within laboratories must be utilized in order to run these tests due to the increased potential for cross-contamination of the specimens. Specimen transport and storage times are critical. The NAATs are not FDA-approved for conjunctival specimens. The tests are expensive, with a turnaround time of 1 to 3 days (95). PCR appears to be equally specific and at least equally sensitive compared to McCoy cell culture, and superior to direct immunofluorescence in the diagnosis of chlamydial infections (86,87,105).

Bobo et al. (106) investigated the use of PCR in 234 Tanzanian children with no signs of trachoma, follicular trachoma, or intense inflammatory trachoma. PCR detected *C. trachomatis* in 24%, 54%, and 95% of the individuals, whereas direct immunofluorescence against chlamydial antigen was positive in 1%, 28%, and 60%, respectively. In addition, this study demonstrated the suitability of PCR for field work, owing to ease of specimen collection and transport.

A commercially available PCR assay, Roche Amplicor, was found to be equivalent to culture concerning sensitivity, specificity, as well as positive and negative predictive values in neonatal conjunctivitis (107). Other commercially available nucleic acid amplification systems for the detection of *C. trachomatis* use ligase chain reaction (Abbott LCx), strand displacement amplification to amplify *C. trachomatis* DNA sequences in the cryptic plasmid (BDProbeTec), or transcription-mediated amplification (Gen-Probe APTIMA) to detect a specific 23S ribosomal RNA target (95). The performance of these tests has been demonstrated to be comparable (100,103,108,109).

In addition to being a diagnostic method, PCR is a valuable epidemiologic tool for detecting and genotyping ocular strains of *C. trachomatis* (110). Although PCR achieves the accuracy needed for diagnosis of ocular chlamydial infections, it still lacks the speed and simplicity required for an office-based test. Future developments will allow the simultaneous investigation of several pathogens (multiplex PCR) (111). Pooling specimens before testing for *C. trachomatis* and *N. gonorrhoeae* with NAATs has been proposed as a method of reducing costs (112).

Antichlamydial Antibodies

Serum

Antichlamydial antibodies in serum samples help support a chlamydial diagnosis in cases of chronic disease when results of culture and nonculture tests prove negative. Serotests, however, cannot compete in sensitivity and specificity with antigen detection. Antichlamydial IgA occurs 10 days after infection and has a half-life of 5 to 6 days. It is, therefore, a good marker for persistent or recurrent infections or for an active carrier state (105). IgG appears approximately 2 weeks after infection and may persist for years in detectable concentrations, indicating a previous infection or an inactive disease state (105).

Serotests differ in sensitivity and specificity, depending on the antigen employed. Most of the tests are based on two different surface antigens of the outer cell wall, MOMP and a LPS. MOMP has species-, subspecies- and serotype-specific epitopes, whereas LPS is genus-specific. The first immune response to infections with *C. trachomatis* is anti-LPS, followed by anti-MOMP. Therefore, tests that use LPS as an antigen are not species-specific, but are sensitive and detect the early immune response. In patients with chronic chlamydial infections, this response is likely to be missed, resulting in a false-negative result. Tests that employ MOMP as the antigen are species-specific, but less sensitive, and detect the late immune response (105). Screening for antichlamydial antibodies may be performed with an indirect immunoperoxidase assay or with enzyme-linked immunosorbent assay (ELISA).

The value of a positive antibody test is debated, and many agree that a positive antibody response alone cannot

justify antibiotic treatment. Conversely, patients with positive conjunctival specimens and negative serology could have early disease with the potential for a better response to antichlamydial therapy (113).

Tears

Detection of antichlamydial antibodies in tears may offer further diagnostic help. Antichlamydial antibodies were found in tears of 88% of patients with antigen-proven chlamydial conjunctivitis. However, 40% of patients with antigen-negative conjunctival specimen also had tear antibodies against chlamydia. Antichlamydial antibodies were also found in tears of eight patients (32%) with urethritis (114).

Differential Diagnosis

Adult inclusion conjunctivitis and trachoma must be differentiated from other forms of follicular conjunctivitis, such as viral diseases, including adenoviral infections, herpes simplex blepharoconjunctivitis, and *Molluscum contagiosum*, drug toxicity (dipivefrin, antivirals, etc.), and acute hemorrhagic conjunctivitis (e.g., enteroviral). Allergic keratoconjunctivitis, though typically associated with a prominent papillary reaction, may be confused with chronic chlamydial disease. Moreover, the presence of eosinophils in conjunctival swabs of patients with adult inclusion conjunctivitis reflects the problem of some degree of allergic sensitizing capacity of chlamydia, and, conversely, the possibility that chlamydia may easily develop in subjects with preexisting allergic conjunctivitis (115).

End-stage trachoma must be distinguished from other causes of conjunctival cicatrization, such as ocular cicatricial pemphigoid, thermal and chemical burns, Stevens-Johnson syndrome, ocular rosacea, and atopic keratoconjunctivitis (116).

The differential diagnosis of neonatal inclusion conjunctivitis is complicated by the fact that the newborn's immune system is not capable of mounting a follicular reaction in the conjunctiva. Hyperemia, papillary hypertrophy and mucopurulent discharge are the ocular clinical signs, regardless of the pathogen involved. Conjunctival scrapings and cultures must rule out a bacterial infection, especially gonococcus. Laboratory testing for *Chlamydia* can readily establish the correct diagnosis. Other bacteria implicated in neonatal conjunctivitis include *Staphylococcus aureus*, *Haemophilus influenzae*, *Streptococcus pneumoniae*, *Branhamella catarrhalis*, *Haemophilus parainfluenzae*, streptococcus group D, *Pseudomonas aeruginosa*, *Proteus mirabilis*, and *Klebsiella pneumoniae* (38).

Chemical conjunctivitis caused by the instillation of silver nitrate into the newborn's eyes after birth produces a mild transient conjunctival injection and tearing with variable purulence, which normally subside within 24 to 48 hours (117). Viral conjunctivitis is uncommon in the newborn, and 70% are caused by Herpes simplex virus type 2. The onset of clinical disease is usually within the first 2 weeks of life, with signs of skin lesions and conjunctivitis with little purulence preceding corneal involvement (38).

TREATMENT

Trachoma

Vaccine Trials

Following limited success in preventing trachoma in primates using killed whole organisms given parenterally, several large field trials were undertaken in humans in the 1960s in Taiwan, Saudi Arabia, Italy, and Gambia (118). The vaccines were ultimately unsuccessful. In some cases, vaccination led to exacerbation of trachoma on rechallenge, highlighting the importance of immune responses in causing pathosis in chlamydial infection (74,119).

Therapy

Studies from Gambia, Saudi Arabia, and Egypt have demonstrated that a single dose of azithromycin (20 mg/kg), a long-acting azalide antibiotic, is effective in eradicating *C. trachomatis* from more than 70% of an infected population (120–122). The fact that more than 20% of subjects failed to resolve clinical signs of disease was due to the high rate of reinfection rather than treatment failure (2). Antibiotic levels above the 90% minimal inhibitory concentration for *C. trachomatis* were detected after 4 days in all tear samples and after 14 days in all conjunctival tissue specimen following a single 1-g oral dose of azithromycin (123). Single-dose oral azithromycin was superior to a 6-week course of tetracycline eye ointment twice daily applied by caregivers (124). Multiple doses of oral azithromycin (once a week for 3 weeks) may be even more effective for treating communities (125). Dose reduction according to weight (15 to 30 mg/kg) or height is necessary in the treatment of children with trachoma (126). Lietman et al. (127) used a mathematical model on available epidemiologic data to predict the frequency of treatment necessary to eradicate trachoma. They recommend up to biannual treatment in hyperendemic communities and suggest that even a few chlamydial infections within such communities may eventually lead to pretreatment levels of infection (127). Administration of a single antibiotic en masse to large communities does pose a risk for development of resistance (128,129), but macrolide-resistant streptococcus pneumoniae did not persist until the next scheduled annual treatment (130).

The second major treatment goal in trachoma is the avoidance of ocular complications associated with trachomatous trichiasis of the upper lid. Tarsal rotation was the most effective procedure in a clinical trial in Oman including 384 lid surgeries for trachoma. It was successful in 80% of cases with minor trichiasis, compared with success rates of 29% for electrolysis and 18% for cryoablation. Tarsal rotation was also successful in 77% of cases of major trichiasis compared to a 41% success rate for tarsal advance and rotation (131). Poor attendance for lid surgery remains a problem in the developing world, due to ignorance and lack of time and money (132).

The outcome of penetrating keratoplasty in trachoma patients is usually poor because of extensive pannus formation and adnexal and ocular surface problems, but limited visual rehabilitation may be achievable (133).

Prevention Programs

Because of the difficulty of treating visual loss in trachoma once it has occurred, public health prevention programs are the most cost-effective means of decreasing this problem. Trachoma prevention strategies target defined risk factors such as poverty, crowding, and lack of safe water. Emerging treatment strategies are based on the "SAFE" protocol, adopted by the WHO to eradicate trachoma by 2020. "SAFE" includes *s*urgery for trichiasis, *a*ntibiotic treatment of clinically active chlamydial infection, the promotion of *f*acial cleanliness, and the improvement of *e*nvironmental conditions such as providing safe water and adequate disposal of feces (134). Face washing significantly decreased the prevalence of severe inflammatory trachoma in villages with intensive educational intervention (135). The reduction of fly populations in intervention villages decreased the prevalence of active trachoma by 61% after 3 months (136).

Adult Inclusion Conjunctivitis

Adult inclusion conjunctivitis in theory could be treated with topical tetracycline or erythromycin, but due to the high prevalence and association with genitourinary and epipharyngeal infection, systemic antibiotics are the treatment of choice (137). Sexual partners should be treated as well to decrease the rate of reinfection. Effective antichlamydial agents include tetracyclines, macrolides, and some of the quinolones (137). A single 1-g dose of azithromycin is established as the first line treatment of chlamydial urethritis/cervicitis (138). A single 1-g azithromycin therapy was as effective as standard 10-day treatment with doxycycline (100 mg twice daily) to eradicate chlamydia in the treatment of adult inclusion conjunctivitis. Clinical cure was observed in 60% and 69% of patients treated with azithromycin and doxycycline, respectively (139). Incomplete disappearance of signs and symptoms was related to slow regression of the follicular reaction, which may need several weeks to subside (122,137,139). All patients with adult inclusion conjunctivitis should undergo further conjunctival scrapings for detection of *C. trachomatis* at least 3 weeks after completing the course of antibiotics (113). Topical steroids are indicated in associated anterior uveitis (47). Although anecdotal reports have suggested that topical corticosteroids may reactivate chlamydial infection (140), an animal model of trachoma failed to support this finding (141).

Neonatal Inclusion Blennorrhea

Inclusion conjunctivitis is often complicated by respiratory tract infections such as epipharyngitis and pneumonia. Therefore, treatment must include systemic antibiotics. Treatment with erythromycin (200 mg/d) or roxithromycin (50 mg/d) divided into two doses were similarly successful in the clinical cure. One month after commencing therapy, however, several newborns were culture-positive for *C. trachomatis* in samples from eye or nasopharynx (142). No reports have been published on the experience with azithromycin in neonatal inclusion blennorrhea, but it is used in the treatment of trachoma in children <1 year in a recommended dosage of 15 to 30 mg/kg (126).

The prophylaxis of ophthalmia neonatorum shortly after birth has been a matter of debate. Prophylaxis is performed with silver nitrate 1% (Crede's prophylaxis), tetracycline ophthalmic ointment (1%), 0.5% erythromycin, gentamicin, neomycin, or chloramphenicol (143). Some studies refute the usefulness of ocular prophylaxis at all (144), and prophylaxis has been discontinued in a number of facilities. Other institutions still perform ocular prophylaxis, but the agent chosen is mainly determined by pediatricians, governmental regularities, and hospital policy (144). Povidone-iodine (PVP-I) has excellent chlamydicidal activity, is well tolerated, and may substitute other substances in the future (145). In a controlled trial of 2.5% PVP-I as prophylaxis against ophthalmia neonatorum involving 3,117 newborns in Kenya, PVP-I proved to be more effective against *C. trachomatis* than silver nitrate or erythromycin (146).

Other Ocular Chlamydial Infections

Human infections may be caused by chlamydiaceae other than *C. trachomatis*, including *Chlamydophila pneumoniae, Chlamydophila psittaci, Chlamydophila abortus*, and *Chlamydophila felis*. A survey of 41 selected patients with conjunctivitis revealed infection with nontrachomatis chlamydiae in four patients (147), indicating that these infections may be more frequent than presumed but remain undetected unless specifically looked for.

C. pneumoniae

C. pneumoniae infections and reinfections are common in the adult population, the seroprevalence being over 50% in many countries (148). *C. pneumoniae* (Taiwan acute respiratory agent, TWAR) was first isolated from the conjunctiva of a pa-

tient with trachoma in 1965 (149). It has since been reported as an ocular pathogen only from a laboratory accident. Clinically, a papillary conjunctivitis was found with no significant preauricular lymphadenopathy (147).

C. pneumoniae has the capacity to establish persistent infections that comply with theories to link infection and autoimmunity. *C. pneumoniae* has been associated with atherosclerosis (150) and reactive arthritis (151). In ocular disease, elevated IgG antibodies to *C. pneumoniae* are associated with nonarteritic ischemic optic neuropathy (152). Moreover, IgA antibodies to *C. pneumoniae* heat shock protein (Cpn Hsp60) were significantly elevated in patients with acute anterior uveitis, and complications such as cataract and cystoid macular edema were increased in uveitis patients with positive IgA titers to Cpn Hsp60 (153).

C. psittaci

C. psittaci is the causative agent of human psittacosis and guinea pig inclusion conjunctivitis. Few cases of follicular conjunctivitis in humans have been attributed to *C. psittaci* (147,154–158). Most of the patients had contact with animal or laboratory *C. psittaci* strains. The follicular reaction was not limited to the upper and lower tarsal conjunctiva but also involved the bulbar conjunctiva in some patients. A superficial punctate keratitis was common, whereas corneal pannus formation was rarely observed in patients with *C. psittaci* associated conjunctivitis.

C. felis

C. felis is a frequent cause of infectious conjunctivitis in kittens (109). Follicular conjunctivitis in humans due to *C. felis* is rare and typically acquired from cats (109,154,158). Clinical suspicion and detection of nontrachomatis chlamydial inclusions in the cell culture by immunofluorescence with the family-specific anti-LPS antibody are important for prompt diagnosis. Prolonged antibiotic treatment is necessary to treat human *C. felis* conjunctivitis (109). PCR testing for *C. felis* and all other chlamydia known to infect humans may be available in the future (109).

REFERENCES

1. Lewallen S, Courtright P. Blindness in Africa: present situation and future needs. *Br J Ophthalmol* 2001;85:897–903.
2. Whitcher JP, Srinivasan M, Upadhyay MP. Corneal blindness: a global perspective. *Bull WHO* 2001;79:214–221.
3. Estes JW. *The medical skills of ancient Egypt.* Canton, MA: Science History Watson Publishing International, 1989.
4. Lietman TM. Trachoma control: the end of the beginning? *Ophthalmology* 2001;108:2163–2164.
5. Tabbara KF. Blindness in the eastern Mediterranean countries. *Br J Ophthalmol* 2001;85:771–775.
6. Executive Board of the WHO. *Global elimination of blinding trachoma.* Geneva: WHO,1998.

7. Coppens I, Abu el-Asrar AM, Maudgal PC, et al. Incidence and clinical presentation of chlamydial keratoconjunctivitis: a preliminary study. *Int Ophthalmol* 1988;12:201–205.
8. Fitch CP, Rapoza PA, Owens S, et al. Epidemiology and diagnosis of acute conjunctivitis at an inner-city hospital. *Ophthalmology* 1989;96:1215–1220.
9. Garland SM, Malatt A, Tabrizi S, et al. Chlamydia trachomatis conjunctivitis. Prevalence and association with genital tract infection. *Med J Aust* 1995;162:363–366.
10. Olafsen LD, Storvold G, Melby K. A microbiological study of conjunctivitis with emphasis on Chlamydia trachomatis, in northern Norway. *Acta Ophthalmol (Copenh)* 1986;64:463–470.
11. Pamel GJ, Feldman ST. Chlamydial conjunctivitis and genital gonorrhea in pregnancy. *Arch Ophthalmol* 1990;108:327.
12. Ophthalmia neonatorum. *Afr Health* 1995;17:30.
13. Dannevig L, Straume B, Melby K. Ophthalmia neonatorum in northern Norway. I: Epidemiology and risk factors. *Acta Ophthalmol (Copenh)* 1992;70:14–18.
14. Laga M, Plummer FA, Nzanze H, et al. Epidemiology of ophthalmia neonatorum in Kenya. *Lancet* 1986;2:1145–1149.
15. Schachter J, Grossman M, Holt J, et al. Prospective study of chlamydial infection in neonates. *Lancet* 1979;2:377–380.
16. Heggie AD, Jaffe AC, Stuart LA, et al. Topical sulfacetamide vs oral erythromycin for neonatal chlamydial conjunctivitis. *Am J Dis Child* 1985;139:564–566.
17. Rapoza PA, Quinn TC, Kiessling LA, et al. Epidemiology of neonatal conjunctivitis. *Ophthalmology* 1986;93:456–461.
18. Schaller U, Klauss V. Is Credé's prophylaxis for ophthalmia neonatorum still valid? *Bull WHO* 2001;79:262–266.
19. An BB, Adamis AP. Chlamydial ocular diseases. *Int Ophthalmol Clin* 1998;38:221–230.
20. Di Bartolomeo S, Mirta DH, Janer M, et al. Incidence of Chlamydia trachomatis and other potential pathogens in neonatal conjunctivitis. *Int J Infect Dis* 2001;5:139–143.
21. Roodhooft JM. Leading causes of blindness worldwide. *Bull Soc Belge Ophtalmol* 2002;283:19–25.
22. Zerihun N, Mabey D. Blindness and low vision in Jimma Zone, Ethopia: results of a population-based survey. *Ophthalmic Epidemiol* 1997;4:19–26.
23. Schwartz EC, Huss R, Hopkins A, et al. Blindness and visual impairment in a region endemic for onchocerciasis in the Central African Republic. *Br J Ophthalmol* 1997;81:443–447.
24. Bailey R, Duong T, Carpenter R, et al. The duration of human ocular Chlamydia trachomatis infection is age dependent. *Epidemiol Infect* 1999;123:479–486.
25. Marx R. Social factors and trachoma: a review of the literature. *Soc Sci Med* 1989;29:23–34.
26. Mabey D, Bailey R. Eradication of trachoma worldwide. *Br J Ophthalmol* 1999;83:1261–1263.
27. Emerson PM, Lindsay SW, Walraven GE, et al. Effect of fly control on trachoma and diarrhoea. *Lancet* 1999;353:1401–1403.
28. West SK, Congdon N, Katala S, et al. Facial cleanliness and risk of trachoma in families. *Arch Ophthalmol* 1991;109:855–857.
29. Fine D, West S. Absence of a relationship between malnutrition and trachoma in preschool children. *Ophthalmic Epidemiol* 1997;4:83–88.
30. Brilliant LB, Pokhrel RP, Grasset NC, et al. Epidemiology of blindness in Nepal. *Bull WHO* 1985;63:375–386.
31. Huntemüller, Paderstein. Clamydozoen-Befunde bei Schwimmbad-Conjunktivitis I: Klinischer Teil. *Dtsch Med Wochenschrift* 1913;39:66.
32. Brunham RC, Binns B, Guijon F, et al. Etiology and outcome of acute pelvic inflammatory disease. *J Infect Dis* 1988;158:510–517.
33. Brunham RC, Peeling R, Maclean I, et al. Chlamydia trachomatis-associated ectopic pregnancy: serologic and histologic correlates. *J Infect Dis* 1992;165:1076–1081.
34. Postema EJ, Remeijer L, van der Meijden WI. Epidemiology of genital chlamydial infections in patients with chlamydial conjunctivitis; a retrospective study. *Genitourin Med* 1996;72:203–205.
35. Batteiger BE, Fraiz J, Newhall WJ, et al. Association of recurrent chlamydial infection with gonorrhea. *J Infect Dis* 1989;159:661–669.
36. Halberstaedter L, von Prowazek S. Über Chlamydienbefunde bei Blenorrhoea neonatorum non gonorrhoica. *Berl Klin Wochenschrift* 1909;46:1839–1840.
37. Lindner K. Zur Ätiologie der gonokokkenfreien Urethritis. *Wien Klin Wochenschr* 1910;23:283–284.
38. de Toledo AR, Chandler JW. Conjunctivitis of the newborn. *Infect Dis Clin North Am* 1992;6:807–813.
39. Krohn MA, Hillier SL, Bell TA, et al. The bacterial etiology of conjunctivitis in early infancy. Eye Prophylaxis Study Group. *Am J Epidemiol* 1993;138:326–332.
40. Shariat H, Young M, Abedin M. An interesting case presentation: a possible new route for perinatal acquisition of Chlamydia. *J Perinatol* 1992;12:300–302.
41. Spencer WH, Zimmerman LE. *Ophthalmic pathology,* 3rd ed. Philadelphia: WB Saunders, 1985.
42. al Rajhi AA, Hidayat A, Nasr A, et al. The histopathology and the mechanism of entropion in patients with trachoma. *Ophthalmology* 1993;100:1293–1296.
43. Tabbara KF, Bobb AA. Lacrimal system complications in trachoma. *Ophthalmology* 1980;87:298–301.
44. MacCallan AF. The epidemiology of trachoma. *Br J Ophthalmol* 1931;369–412.
45. Thylefors B, Dawson CR, Jones BR, et al. A simple system for the assessment of trachoma and its complications. *Bull WHO* 1987;65:477–483.
46. Darougar S, Viswalingam ND. Marginal corneal abscess associated with adult chlamydial ophthalmia. *Br J Ophthalmol* 1988;72:774–777.
47. Dawson, C, Wood TR, Rose L, et al. Experimental inclusion conjunctivitis in man. 3. Keratitis and other complications. *Arch Ophthalmol* 1967;78:341–349.
48. Mellman-Rubin TL, Kowalski RP, Uhrin M, et al. Incidence of adenoviral and chlamydial coinfection in acute follicular conjunctivitis. *Am J Ophthalmol* 1995;119:652–654.
49. Aguettaz JM, Vadot E, Mouillon M, et al. [Epidemiological approach of the role of Chlamydiae in uveitis]. *J Fr Ophtalmol* 1987;10:679–682.
50. Sieper J. Pathogenesis of reactive arthritis. *Curr Rheumatol Rep* 2001;3:412–418.
51. Ogawa H, Hashiguchi K, Kazuyama Y. Isolation of Chlamydia trachomatis from the middle ear aspirates of otitis media. *Acta Otolaryngol* 1990;110:105–109.
52. Weber PC, Koltai PJ. Chlamydia trachomatis in the etiology of acute otitis media. *Ann Otol Rhinol Laryngol* 1991;100:616–619.
53. Mordhorst CH, Dawson C. Sequelae of neonatal inclusion conjunctivitis and associated disease in parents. *Am J Ophthalmol* 1971;71:861–867.
54. Rees E, Tait IA, Hobson D, et al. Persistence of chlamydial infection after treatment for neonatal conjunctivitis. *Arch Dis Child* 1981;56:193–198.
55. Peeling RW, Brunham RC. Chlamydiae as pathogens: new species and new issues. *Emerg Infect Dis* 1996;2:307–319.
56. Hartley JC, Kaye S, Stevenson S, et al. PCR detection and molecular identification of Chlamydiaceae species. *J Clin Microbiol* 2001;39:3072–3079.
57. Belland RJ, Scidmore MA, Crane DD, et al. Chlamydia trachomatis cytotoxicity associated with complete and partial cytotoxin genes. *Proc Natl Acad Sci U S A* 2001;98:13984–13989.
58. Riordan-Eva P. Nomenclature of chlamydia. *Int Ophthalmol* 1988;12:15–17.

59. Hess S, Rheinheimer C, Tidow F, et al. The reprogrammed host: Chlamydia trachomatis-induced up-regulation of glycoprotein 130 cytokines, transcription factors, and antiapoptotic genes. *Arthritis Rheum* 2001;44:2392–2401.

60. Taylor HR, Johnson SL, Schachter J, et al. Pathogenesis of trachoma: the stimulus for inflammation. *J Immunol* 1987;138:3023–3027.

61. Stephens RS. The cellular paradigm of chlamydial pathogenesis. *Trends Microbiol* 2003;11:44–51.

62. Brunham RC, Peeling RW. Chlamydia trachomatis antigens: role in immunity and pathogenesis. *Infect Agents Dis* 1994;3:218–233.

63. Morrison RP, Belland RJ, Lyng K, et al. Chlamydial disease pathogenesis. The 57-kD chlamydial hypersensitivity antigen is a stress response protein. *J Exp Med* 1989;170:1271–1283.

64. Bailey RL, Kajbaf M, Whittle HC, et al. The influence of local antichlamydial antibody on the acquisition and persistence of human ocular chlamydial infection: IgG antibodies are not protective. *Epidemiol Infect* 1993;111:315–324.

65. Caldwell HD, Stewart S, Johnson S, et al. Tear and serum antibody response to Chlamydia trachomatis antigens during acute chlamydial conjunctivitis in monkeys as determined by immunoblotting. *Infect Immun* 1987;55:93–98.

66. Kunimoto D, Brunham RC. Human immune response and Chlamydia trachomatis infection. *Rev Infect Dis* 1985;7:665–673.

67. Orenstein NS, Mull JD, Thompson SE III. Immunity to chlamydial infections of the eye. V. Passive transfer of antitrachoma antibodies to owl monkeys. *Infect Immun* 1973;7:600–603.

68. Watson RR, Mull JD, MacDonald AB, et al. Immunity to chlamydial infections of the eye. II. Studies of passively transferred serum antibody in resistance to infection with guinea pig inclusion conjunctivitis. *Infect Immun* 1973;7:597–599.

69. Numazaki K, Chiba S, Aoki K, et al. Detection of serum antibodies to Chlamydia pneumoniae in patients with endogenous uveitis and acute conjunctivitis. *Clin Infect Dis* 1997;25:928–929.

70. Conway DJ, Holland MJ, Campbell AE, et al. HLA class I and II polymorphisms and trachomatous scarring in a Chlamydia trachomatis-endemic population. *J Infect Dis* 1996;174:643–646.

71. Courtright P, Lewallen S, Howe R. Cell-mediated immunity in trachomatous scarring. Evidence from a leprosy population. *Ophthalmology* 1993;100:98–104.

72. Herrmann B, Stenberg K, Mardh PA. Immune response in chlamydial conjunctivitis among neonates and adults with special reference to tear IgA. *APMIS* 1991;99:69–74.

73. Ward ME. Chlamydial vaccines—future trends. J Infect 1992;25(suppl 1):11–26.

74. Grayston JT, Wang SP, Lin HM, et al. Trachoma vaccine studies in volunteer students of the National Defense Medical Center. II. Response to challenge eye inoculation of egg grown trachoma virus. *Chin Med J* 1961;8:312.

75. MacDonald AB, McComb D, Howard L. Immune response of owl monkeys to topical vaccination with irradiated Chlamydia trachomatis. *J Infect Dis* 1984;149:439–442.

76. Whittum-Hudson JA, Taylor HR, Farazdaghi M, et al. Immunohistochemical study of the local inflammatory response to chlamydial ocular infection. *Invest Ophthalmol Vis Sci* 1986;27:64–69.

77. Guzey M, Ozardali I, Basar E, et al. A survey of trachoma: the histopathology and the mechanism of progressive cicatrization of eyelid tissues. *Ophthalmologica* 2000;214:277–284.

78. Abu el-Asrar AM, Geboes K, Missotten L. Immunology of trachomatous conjunctivitis. *Bull Soc Belge Ophtalmol* 2001;280:73–96.

79. Darville T, Andrews CW Jr, Sikes JD, et al. Mouse strain-dependent chemokine regulation of the genital tract T helper cell type 1 immune response. *Infect Immun* 2001;69:7419–7424.

80. Igietseme JU, Ramsey KH, Magee DM, et al. Resolution of murine chlamydial genital infection by the adoptive transfer of a biovar-specific, Th1 lymphocyte clone. *Reg Immunol* 1993;5:317–324.

81. Bobo L, Novak N, Mkocha H, et al. Evidence for a predominant proinflammatory conjunctival cytokine response in individuals with trachoma. *Infect Immun* 1996;64:3273–3279.

82. Perry LL, Feilzer K, Caldwell HD. Immunity to Chlamydia trachomatis is mediated by T helper 1 cells through IFN-gamma-dependent and -independent pathways. *J Immunol* 1997;158:3344–3352.

83. Beatty WL, Morrison RP, Byrne GI. Reactivation of persistent Chlamydia trachomatis infection in cell culture. *Infect Immun* 1995;63:199–205.

84. Guzey M, Basar E, Ermis SS, et al. Pretarsal and marginal orbicularis oculi muscle fiber changes in trachomatous cicatricial entropion: histopathological evaluation. *Eur J Ophthalmol* 1999;9:89–92.

85. Bird M, Dawson CR, Schachter JS, et al. Does the diagnosis of trachoma adequately identify ocular chlamydial infection in trachoma-endemic areas? *J Infect Dis* 2003;187:1669–1673.

86. Elnifro EM, Cooper RJ, Klapper PE, et al. Diagnosis of viral and chlamydial keratoconjunctivitis: which laboratory test? *Br J Ophthalmol* 1999;83:622–627.

87. Elnifro EM, Storey CC, Morris DJ, et al. Polymerase chain reaction for detection of Chlamydia trachomatis in conjunctival swabs. *Br J Ophthalmol* 1997;81:497–500.

88. Patton DL, Chan KY, Kuo CC, et al. In vitro growth of Chlamydia trachomatis in conjunctival and corneal epithelium. *Invest Ophthalmol Vis Sci* 1988;29:1087–1095.

89. Schachter J, Moncada J, Dawson CR, et al. Nonculture methods for diagnosing chlamydial infection in patients with trachoma: a clue to the pathogenesis of the disease? *J Infect Dis* 1988;158:1347–1352.

90. Wilhelmus KR, Robinson NM, Tredici LL, et al. Conjunctival cytology of adult chlamydial conjunctivitis. *Arch Ophthalmol* 1986;104:691–693.

91. LeBar W, Herschman B, Jemal C, et al. Comparison of DNA probe, monoclonal antibody enzyme immunoassay, and cell culture for the detection of Chlamydia trachomatis. *J Clin Microbiol* 1989;27:826–828.

92. Peterson EM, Oda R, Alexander R, et al. Molecular techniques for the detection of Chlamydia trachomatis. *J Clin Microbiol* 1989;27:2359–2363.

93. Ripa KT. Microbiology diagnosis of chlamydia trachomatis infection. *Infection* 1982;10 (suppl 1):S19–24.

94. Talley AR, Garcia-Ferrer F, Laycock KA, et al. Comparative diagnosis of neonatal chlamydial conjunctivitis by polymerase chain reaction and McCoy cell culture. *Am J Ophthalmol* 1994;117:50–57.

95. Johnson RE, Newhall WJ, Papp JR, et al. Screening tests to detect Chlamydia trachomatis and Neisseria gonorrhoeae infections—2002. *MMWR Recomm Rep* 2002;51:1–38.

96. Stamm WE. Laboratory diagnosis of chamydial infection. In: Bowie WR, Caldwell HD, Jones RP, et al., eds. *Chlamydial infections.* Cambridge: Cambridge University Press, 1990:459–470.

97. Pate MS, Dixon PB, Hardy K, et al. Evaluation of the Biostar Chlamydia OIA assay with specimens from women attending a sexually transmitted disease clinic. *J Clin Microbiol* 1998;36:2183–2186.

98. LeBar W, Schubiner H, Jemal C, et al. Comparison of the Kallested Pathfinder EIA, cytocentrifuged direct fluorescent antibody, and cell culture for the detection of Chlamydia trachomatis. *Diagn Microbiol Infect Dis* 1991;14:17–20.

99. Kellogg JA, Seiple JW, Hick ME. Cross-reaction of clinical isolates of bacteria and yeasts with the chlamydiazyme test for

chlamydial antigen, before and after use of a blocking reagent. *Am J Clin Pathol* 1992;97:309–312.

100. Lauderdale TL, Landers L, Thorneycroft I, et al. Comparison of the PACE 2 assay, two amplification assays, and Clearview EIA for detection of Chlamydia trachomatis in female endocervical and urine specimens. *J Clin Microbiol* 1999;37:2223–2229.

101. Newhall WJ, Johnson RE, DeLisle S, et al. Head-to-head evaluation of five chlamydia tests relative to a quality-assured culture standard. *J Clin Microbiol* 1999;37:681–685.

102. Roblin PM, Gelling M, Kutlin A, et al. Evaluation of a new optical immunoassay for diagnosis of neonatal chlamydial conjunctivitis. *J Clin Microbiol* 1997;35:515–516.

103. Black CM, Marrazzo J, Johnson RE, et al. Head-to-head multicenter comparison of DNA probe and nucleic acid amplification tests for Chlamydia trachomatis infection in women performed with an improved reference standard. *J Clin Microbiol* 2002;40:3757–3763.

104. Wylie JL, Moses S, Babcock R, et al. Comparative evaluation of chlamydiazyme, PACE 2, and AMP-CT assays for detection of Chlamydia trachomatis in endocervical specimens. *J Clin Microbiol* 1998;36:3488–3491.

105. Haller EM, Auer-Grumbach P, Stuenzner D, et al. Evaluation of two nonculture antigen tests and three serotests for detection of anti-chlamydial antibodies in the diagnosis of ocular chlamydial infections. *Graefes Arch Clin Exp Ophthalmol* 1996;234:510–514.

106. Bobo L, Munoz B, Viscidi R, et al. Diagnosis of Chlamydia trachomatis eye infection in Tanzania by polymerase chain reaction/enzyme immunoassay. *Lancet* 1991;338:847–850.

107. Hammerschlag MR, Roblin PM, Gelling M, et al. Use of polymerase chain reaction for the detection of Chlamydia trachomatis in ocular and nasopharyngeal specimens from infants with conjunctivitis. *Pediatr Infect Dis J* 1997;16:293–297.

108. Goessens WH, Mouton JW, van der Meijden WI, et al. Comparison of three commercially available amplification assays, AMP CT, LCx, and COBAS AMPLICOR, for detection of Chlamydia trachomatis in first-void urine. *J Clin Microbiol* 1997;35:2628–2633.

109. Hartley JC, Stevenson S, Robinson AJ, et al. Conjunctivitis due to Chlamydophila felis (Chlamydia psittaci feline pneumonitis agent) acquired from a cat: case report with molecular characterization of isolates from the patient and cat. *J Infect* 2001;43:7–11.

110. Isobe K, Aoki K, Itoh N, et al. Serotyping of Chlamydia trachomatis from inclusion conjunctivitis by polymerase chain reaction and restriction fragment length polymorphism analysis. *Jpn J Ophthalmol* 1996;40:279–285.

111. Elnifro EM, Cooper RJ, Klapper PE, et al. Multiplex polymerase chain reaction for diagnosis of viral and chlamydial keratoconjunctivitis. *Invest Ophthalmol Vis Sci* 2000;41:1818–1822.

112. Kapala J, Copes D, Sproston A, et al. Pooling cervical swabs and testing by ligase chain reaction are accurate and cost-saving strategies for diagnosis of Chlamydia trachomatis. *J Clin Microbiol* 2000;38:2480–2483.

113. Carta F, Zanetti S, Pinna A, et al. The treatment and follow up of adult chlamydial ophthalmia. *Br J Ophthalmol* 1994;78:206–208.

114. Haller EM, Auer-Grumbach P, Stuenzner D, et al. Detection of antichlamydial antibodies in tears: a diagnostic aid? *Ophthalmology* 1997;104:125–130.

115. Reccia R, Del Prete A, Scala A, et al. Direct immunofluorescence and scraping conjunctival cytology in the study of 912 patients affected by microfollicular conjunctivitis. *Ophthalmologica* 1994;208:295–297.

116. Faraj HG, Hoang-Xuan T. Chronic cicatrizing conjunctivitis. *Curr Opin Ophthalmol* 2001;12(4):250–257.

117. Nishida H, Risemberg HM. Silver nitrate ophthalmic solution and chemical conjunctivities. *Pediatrics* 1975;56:368–373.

118. Sowa S, Sowa J, Collier LH, et al. Trachoma vaccine field trials in the Gambia. *J Hyg (Lond)* 1969;67:699–717.

119. Grayston JT, Wang SP, Yeh LJ, et al. Importance of reinfection in the pathogenesis of trachoma. *Rev Infect Dis* 1985;7:717–725.

120. Tabbara KF, Abu-el-Asrar A, al Omar O, et al. Single-dose azithromycin in the treatment of trachoma. A randomized, controlled study. *Ophthalmology* 1996;103:842–846.

121. Dawson CR, Schachter J, Sallam S, et al. A comparison of oral azithromycin with topical oxytetracycline/polymyxin for the treatment of trachoma in children. *Clin Infect Dis* 1997;24:363–368.

122. Bailey RL, Arullendran P, Whittle HC, et al. Randomised controlled trial of single-dose azithromycin in treatment of trachoma. *Lancet* 1993;342(8869):453–456.

123. Tabbara KF, al Kharashi SA, al Mansouri SM, et al. Ocular levels of azithromycin. *Arch Ophthalmol* 1998;116:1625–1628.

124. Bowman RJ, Sillah A, Van Dehn C, et al. Operational comparison of single-dose azithromycin and topical tetracycline for trachoma. *Invest Ophthalmol Vis Sci* 2000;41:4074–4079.

125. Schachter J, West SK, Mabey D, et al. Azithromycin in control of trachoma. *Lancet* 1999;354:630–635.

126. Munoz B, Solomon AW, Zingeser J, et al. Antibiotic dosage in trachoma control programs: height as a surrogate for weight in children. *Invest Ophthalmol Vis Sci* 2003;44:1464–1469.

127. Lietman T, Porco T, Dawson C, et al. Global elimination of trachoma: how frequently should we administer mass chemotherapy? *Nat Med* 1999;5:572–576.

128. Kalayoglu MV. Ocular chlamydial infections: pathogenesis and emerging treatment strategies. *Curr Drug Targets Infect* Disord 2002;2:85–91.

129. Chern KC, Shrestha SK, Cevallos V, et al. Alterations in the conjunctival bacterial flora following a single dose of azithromycin in a trachoma endemic area. *Br J Ophthalmol* 1999;83:1332–1335.

130. Gaynor BD, Holbrook KA, Whitcher JP, et al. Community treatment with azithromycin for trachoma is not associated with antibiotic resistance in Streptococcus pneumoniae at 1 year. *Br J Ophthalmol* 2003;87:147–148.

131. Reacher MH, Munoz B, Alghassany A, et al. A controlled trial of surgery for trachomatous trichiasis of the upper lid. *Arch Ophthalmol* 1992;110:667–664.

132. Bowman RJ, Faal H, Jatta B, et al. Longitudinal study of trachomatous trichiasis in The Gambia: barriers to acceptance of surgery. *Invest Ophthalmol Vis Sci* 2002;43:936–940.

133. Kocak-Midillioglu I, Akova YA, Kocak-Altintas AG, et al. Penetrating keratoplasty in patients with corneal scarring due to trachoma. *Ophthalmic Surg Lasers* 1999;30:734–741.

134. Bailey R, Lietman T. The SAFE strategy for the elimination of trachoma by 2020: will it work? *Bull WHO* 2001;79:233–236.

135. Dolin PJ, Faal H, Johnson GJ, et al. Trachoma in The Gambia. *Br J Ophthalmol* 1998;82:930–933.

136. Baral K, Osaki S, Shreshta B, et al. Reliability of clinical diagnosis in identifying infectious trachoma in a low-prevalence area of Nepal. *Bull WHO* 1999;77:461–466.

137. Nakagawa H. Treatment of chlamydial conjunctivitis. *Ophthalmologica* 1997;211(suppl 1):25–28.

138. CDC. Guidelines for the treatment of sexually transmitted diseases. *MMWR* 1998;47:1–111.

139. Katusic D, Petricek I, Mandic Z, et al. Azithromycin vs doxycycline in the treatment of inclusion conjunctivitis. *Am J Ophthalmol* 2003;135:447–451.

140. Ormsby HL, Thompson GA, Cousineau GG, et al. Topical therapy in inclusion conjunctivitis. *Am J Ophthalmol* 1952;35:1811.

141. Taylor HR, Johnson SL, Schachter J, et al. An animal model of trachoma: IV. The failure of local immunosuppression to reveal inapparent infection. *Invest Ophthalmol Vis Sci* 1983;24:647–650.

142. Stenberg K, Mardh PA. Treatment of chlamydial conjunctivitis in newborns and adults with erythromycin and roxithromycin. *J Antimicrob Chemother* 1991;28:301–307.

143. Assadian O, Assadian A, Aspock C, et al. Prophylaxis of ophthalmia neonatorum—a nationwide survey of the current practice in Austria. *Wien Klin Wochenschr* 2002;114:194–199.

144. Chen JY. Prophylaxis of ophthalmia neonatorum: comparison of silver nitrate, tetracycline, erythromycin and no prophylaxis. *Pediatr Infect Dis J* 1992;11:1026–1030.

145. Wutzler P, Sauerbrei A, Klocking R, et al. Virucidal and chlamydicidal activities of eye drops with povidone-iodine liposome complex. *Ophthalmic Res* 2000;32:118–125.

146. Isenberg SJ, Apt L, Wood M. A controlled trial of povidone-iodine as prophylaxis against ophthalmia neonatorum. *N Engl J Med* 1995;332:562–566.

147. Lietman T, Brooks D, Moncada J, et al. Chronic follicular conjunctivitis associated with Chlamydia psittaci or Chlamydia pneumoniae. *Clin Infect Dis* 1998;26:1335–1340.

148. Kuo CC, Jackson LA, Campbell LA, et al. Chlamydia pneumoniae (TWAR). *Clin Microbiol Rev* 1995;8:451–461.

149. Grayston JT, Kuo CC, Wang SP, et al. A new Chlamydia psittaci strain, TWAR, isolated in acute respiratory tract infections. *N Engl J Med* 1986;315:161–168.

150. Saikku P, Leinonen M, Mattila K, et al. Serological evidence of an association of a novel Chlamydia, TWAR, with chronic coronary heart disease and acute myocardial infarction. *Lancet* 1988;2:983–986.

151. Hannu T, Puolakkainen M, Leirisalo-Repo M. Chlamydia pneumoniae as a triggering infection in reactive arthritis. *Rheumatology (Oxford)* 1999;38:411–414.

152. Weger M, Haas A, Stanger O, et al. Chlamydia pneumoniae seropositivity and the risk of nonarteritic ischemic optic neuropathy. *Ophthalmology* 2002;109:749–752.

153. Huhtinen M, Puolakkainen M, Laasila K, et al. Chlamydial antibodies in patients with previous acute anterior uveitis. *Invest Ophthalmol Vis Sci* 2001;42:1816–1819.

154. Dawson CR. Lids, conjunctiva, and lacrimal apparatus. Eye infections with chlamydia. *Arch Ophthalmol* 1975;93:854–862.

155. Dean D, Shama A, Schachter J, et al. Molecular identification of an avian strain of Chlamydia psittaci causing severe keratoconjunctivitis in a bird fancier. *Clin Infect Dis* 1995;20:1179–1185.

156. Ostler HB, Schachter J, Dawson CR. Acute follicular conjunctivitis of epizootic origin. Feline pneumonitis. *Arch Ophthalmol* 1969;82:587–591.

157. Schachter J, Arnstein P, Dawson CR, et al. Human follicular conjunctivitis caused by infection with a psittacosis agent. *Proc Soc Exp Biol Med* 1968;127:292–295.

158. Schachter J, Ostler HB, Meyer KF. Human infection with the agent of feline pneumonitis. *Lancet* 1969;1:1063–1065.

IMMUNOLOGIC DISEASE

CONJUNCTIVITIS

ATOPIC CONJUNCTIVITIS

NEAL P. BARNEY

Atopy refers to hypersensitivities in persons with a hereditary background of allergic diseases as first described by Cocoa and Cooke (1). The major, most commonly recognized atopic conditions include eczema (atopic dermatitis), asthma, hay fever, and allergic rhinitis. Atopic conditions affect 10% to 20% of the population. Atopic ocular disease includes seasonal allergic conjunctivitis (SAC), perennial allergic conjunctivitis (PAC), vernal keratoconjunctivitis (VKC), atopic keratoconjunctivitis (AKC), and giant papillary conjunctivitis (GPC). VKC and AKC may cause significant complications and lead to loss of vision. Type I hypersensitivity reaction of the ocular surface is the putative mechanism in SAC and PAC but is not the only pathophysiologic mechanism in VKC and AKC.

ALLERGIC CONJUNCTIVITIS: SEASONAL/PERENNIAL

Allergic conjunctivitis (AC) is a bilateral, self-limiting, allergic conjunctival inflammation. It occurs in sensitized individuals (no gender difference) and is initiated by allergen binding to immunoglobulin E (IgE) antibody on resident mucosal mast cells. Its importance is related more to its frequency than to its severity. The two forms of AC are defined by whether the inflammation occurs seasonally (spring, fall, SAC) or perennially (year-round, PAC). The inflammatory symptoms are similar for both entities; seasonal allergic conjunctivitis ("hay fever conjunctivitis") is more common. SAC accounts for the majority of cases of AC and is related to atmospheric pollens (e.g., grass, trees, ragweed) that appear during specific seasons. Perennial allergic conjunctivitis is often related to animal dander, dust mites, or other allergens that are present in the environment year-round. Both SAC and PAC must be differentiated from the sight-threatening allergic diseases of the eye, AKC and VKC.

Demographics

Prevalence estimates for allergic conjunctivitis are difficult because allergies in general tend to be considerably underreported. A survey conducted by the American College of

Allergy, Asthma, and Immunology (ACAAI) found that 35% of families interviewed experience allergies. Of these, at least 50% report associated eye symptoms. Most reports agree that allergic conjunctivitis affects up to 20% of the population, i.e., 60 million individuals in the United States (2). Importantly, 60% of all allergic rhinitis sufferers have associated allergic conjunctivitis. The distribution of SAC depends largely on the climate. For example, in the United States grass pollen—induced SAC generally occurs in the Gulf Coast and southwestern areas of the country from March to October, and from May to August in most of the rest of the country. Conversely, ragweed pollen—induced SAC occurs in most of the country during August through October, but in the southernmost states it can begin as early as July and stretch out through November. Tree pollens can become a problem as early as January in the south, and March in the north.

Symptoms

The dominant symptom reported in allergic conjunctivitis is ocular itching. Itching can range from mild to severe. Other symptoms include tearing (watery discharge), redness, swelling, burning, a sensation of fullness in the eyes or eyelids, an urge to rub the eyes, sensitivity to light, and occasionally blurred vision. As stated previously, allergic conjunctivitis is often associated with symptoms of allergic rhinitis.

Signs

Mild conjunctival hyperemia and chemosis are typical signs seen in patients with SAC. Hyperemia is the result of vascular dilatation; chemosis occurs because of altered permeability of postcapillary venules (Fig. 19-1). "Allergic shiners" (periorbital darkening), due to a transient increase of periorbital pigmentation resulting from the decreased venous return in the skin and subcutaneous tissue, are also common.

Pathophysiology

It has been understood for some time that antigen cross-linking of IgE antibody bound to the high-affinity IgE

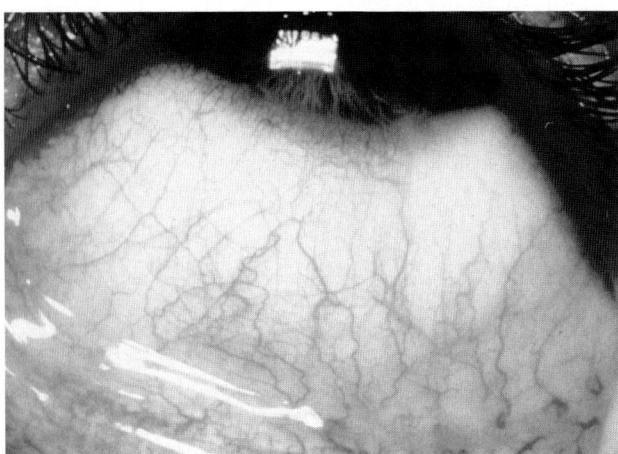

FIGURE 19-1. Seasonal allergic conjunctivitis showing chemosis and hyperemia.

receptor (FcεRI) on mast cells induces release of both preformed (granule associated, e.g., histamine and tryptase) and newly synthesized mediators (e.g., arachidonic acid metabolites), which have diverse and overlapping biologic effects. Both tissue staining and tear film data have implicated the mast cell and IgE-mediated release of its mediators in the pathophysiology of the ocular allergic inflammatory response. Additionally, a number of clinical studies examining topical antihistamine, mast cell stabilizing, and dual-acting drugs have demonstrated relief of allergic conjunctivitis symptoms (see Treatment, below).

Synthesis of inflammatory mediators varies according to the phenotype and tissue location of the mast cell. Granule-associated neutral proteases (tryptase and chymase) unique to mast cells are generally accepted as the most appropriate phenotypic markers to categorize human mast cells into subsets. Mast cells on this basis have been divided into MC_T (tryptase) and MC_{TC} (tryptase/chymase) phenotypes. The phenotype of normal human conjunctival mast cells has been well-documented using immunostaining of conjunctival biopsy specimens. Mast cells are rarely present in the normal human conjunctival epithelium, but when they are found, they appear to be limited to the MC_T phenotype. Mast cells (MC_T phenotype) and eosinophils are found to be increased in the conjunctival epithelium of individuals with SAC and PAC. In the substantia propria of the normal human conjunctiva, 95% are of the MC_{TC} phenotype (3–5). The total number of mast cells (MC_{TC} phenotype) is also increased in the substantia propria of individuals with AC (3).

Clinical evidence for mast cell activation is found in SAC and PAC. Tear film analysis of patients consistently reveals the presence of IgE antibody, histamine (6), and tryptase (7). There are granule associated, preformed (histamine, tryptase, bradykinin) and arachidonic acid derived, newly formed (leukotrienes, prostaglandins) mediators present in patients with ocular allergy. Preformed mediators are released immediately upon allergen exposure, whereas roughly 8 to 24 hours are required for release of newly formed mediators. These mediators are known to have overlapping biologic effects that contribute to the characteristic ocular itching, redness, and watery discharge associated with allergic eye disease. Histamine is involved in the regulation of vascular permeability, smooth muscle contraction, mucus secretion, inflammatory cell migration, cellular activation, and modulation of T-cell function (8). Arachidonic acid metabolites and tryptase originating from mast cells also have been shown to be specifically involved in the regulation of many of these same processes. Mast cells also synthesize cytokines and chemokines. Less well documented and defined are the effects of these mediators in the ocular allergic inflammatory process. Cytokines stored in mast cells are likely the first signals initiating infiltration of inflammatory white blood cells, such as eosinophils. Once these cells arrive, they gain access to the conjunctival surface by moving through the already dilated capillaries.

Immunohistochemical staining of human conjunctival tissue biopsies shows that inflammatory cytokines interleukin-4 (IL-4), IL-5, IL-6, and tumor necrosis factor-α (TNF-α) are localized to mast cells in normal and allergic conjunctivitis (9). These cytokines are consistent with a T-helper-2 (Th2) cytokine profile. Inflammatory cytokines (e.g., TNF-α) have also been measured in human tears (10–13). Although it is difficult *in vivo* to determine the cellular source of cytokines in tears, recent studies comparing allergic to nonallergic subjects indicate that cytokine levels may be important indicators of ocular allergy (14). It has been demonstrated that tears from allergic donors (when compared to nonallergic donors) contained significantly less of the antiinflammatory cytokine, IL-10, and a trend toward decreased levels of the Th1 cytokine, interferon-γ (IFN-γ)–(14). Finally, IgE-mediated release of histamine and cytokines from mast cells can also initiate secondary effects on conjunctival epithelial cells. The activation and participation of epithelial cells in allergic inflammation is an active field of research. Human conjunctival epithelial cells express H_1 receptors coupled to phosphatidylinositol turnover and calcium mobilization (15). Cytokines released from mast cells upregulate intercellular adhesion molecule 1 (ICAM-1) expression on conjunctival epithelial cells (16). This has become a hallmark of allergic inflammation. ICAM-1 appears to play a critical role in the migration of inflammatory cells, and is rapidly expressed following ocular allergen provocation.

Diagnosis

An individual suspected of having allergic conjunctivitis should have a thorough ocular, medical, and medication history. This will help greatly in differentiating AC from other ocular processes. This history should establish whether the process is acute, subacute, chronic, or recurrent. It should further delineate whether the symptoms and signs are unilateral or bilateral, and whether they are associated with any specific environmental or work-related exposure. Ocular symptoms such as tearing, irritation, stinging, and burning are nonspecific. A history of significant ocular itching and a personal or family history of hay fever, allergic rhinitis, asthma, or atopic dermatitis are suggestive of ocular allergy. Viral and bacterial infections of the eye may mimic allergic conjunctivitis. Because AC is secondary to environmental allergens as opposed to transmission by eye-hand contact (infectious etiology), SAC and PAC usually present with bilateral symptoms. Patients complain of watery discharge or increased tearing. Redness is mild and chemosis may be present. Symptoms are often greater than signs. Vision, pupil shape, ocular movement, light reactivity, and the red retinal reflex remain normal in allergic conjunctivitis. Dry eye (secondary to a decrease of the aqueous portion of the tear film) gives symptoms suggestive of foreign body in the eye and may result in conjunctival redness. Similar symptoms are possible from anticholinergic side effects of systemic medications. Typically, itch is not reported with dry eye. Medication history should include questions concerning the patient's use of over-the-counter topical ocular medications, cosmetics, contact lenses, and systemic medications. Any of these can produce acute or chronic conjunctivitis. This inquiry should include direct questions and should not rely on the patient to volunteer information. Many individuals do not appreciate the potential for nonprescription topical ocular medications to cause eye symptoms or partially treat AC.

Treatment

Allergic conjunctivitis can be debilitating to some degree and may cause some individuals affected to seek any type of help for relief of symptoms. The itching and tearing may be unbearable and sleepless nights frequent. Ocular allergic conjunctivitis symptoms may be worse than the nasal symptoms in those suffering from rhinoconjunctivitis. Furthermore, treatment of the nasal symptoms with topical nasal steroids may help the rhinitis, but not be effective for relieving ocular symptoms.

Management of allergic conjunctivitis, therefore, is primarily aimed at alleviating symptoms. Establishing the cause is the first step in treating allergic conjunctivitis. The best treatment is avoidance of the specific allergen, which, unfortunately, is sometimes not possible. But evaluation by an allergist, determination of sensitivities, and education about allergen avoidance through the use of filtering systems, barriers (bedding), special cleaning products, and vacuum sweepers can be of enormous help to the allergic patient. Avoidance of scratching or rubbing, application of cool compresses, artificial tears, and refrigeration of topical ocular medications are practical interventions to alleviate discomfort. Although oral antihistamines may help to relieve eye

discomfort, this may also decrease tear production, causing more ocular symptoms.

The treatment of choice for mild to moderate AC is a dual-acting topical ocular medication (mast cell stabilizer and antihistamine effect: azelastine, ketotifen, or olopatadine). The mast cell stabilizing component of these drugs benefits patients most if treatment is started before the height of symptom onset. Patients usually note rapid onset of relief of itch upon drop instillation, as most dual-action medications have high H_1 receptor affinity. Drug dosing varies from two to four times per day and efficacy is judged best by symptom relief.

In severe disease, combination therapy may be recommended. This therapy may include topical medications [antihistamines, mast cell stabilizers, nonsteroidal antiinflammatory drug (NSAIDs), or combinations], and oral antihistamines. NSAIDs inhibit cyclooxygenase, resulting in decreased formation of prostaglandins and thromboxanes, but not leukotrienes. Therefore, these compounds are useful in controlling itching and some inflammation, but not the infiltration of inflammatory cells. In extreme cases, use of a topical steroid four times a day should be considered. All patients receiving topical steroids should have their intraocular pressure measured frequently. Immunotherapy performed by an allergist may be beneficial in decreasing the severity of future ocular allergy symptoms.

VERNAL KERATOCONJUNCTIVITIS
Definition

VKC is a chronic, bilateral conjunctival inflammatory condition found in individuals predisposed by their atopic background. An excellent review of the history and description of this disease was published by Buckley (17) in 1988. Beigelman's (18) 1950 monograph, *Vernal Conjunctivitis,* continues to be the most exhaustive compilation of information on this disease and is unmatched in current times. The list of easily recognized names in ophthalmology to have published on this entity is formidable: Arlt (19), Desmarres (20), von Graefe (21), Axenfeld (22), Trantas (23), and Herbert (24).

Demographics

In 2000, Bonini et al. (25) reviewed a series of 195 patients with VKC as the only allergic manifestation in 58.5% of patients. The onset of VKC generally occurs before age 10, it lasts 2 to 10 years, and it usually resolves during late puberty. Only 11% of patients were older than 20 years of age in the Bonini series (25). Males predominate in the younger ages, but the male-female distribution is nearly equal in the older patients. Young males in dry, hot climates are those primarily affected. The Mediterranean area and West Africa are areas of the greatest numbers of patients. It is relatively unusual in most of North America and Western Europe. There is a significant history of other atopic manifestations such as eczema or asthma in 40% to 75% of patients with VKC (25). A family history of atopy is found in 40% to 60% of patients (25). Seasonal exacerbation, as the name implies, is common, but patients may have symptoms year-round.

Symptoms

Severe itching and photophobia are the main symptoms. Associated foreign-body sensation, ptosis, thick mucous discharge, and blepharospasm also occur.

Signs

The signs are confined mostly to the conjunctiva and cornea; the skin of the lids and lid margin are relatively uninvolved compared to AKC. The conjunctiva develops a papillary response, principally of the limbus or upper tarsus. The tarsal papillae are discrete, greater than 1 mm in diameter, have flattened tops that may stain with fluorescein, and occur more frequently in European and North American patients (17). Thick, ropy mucus tends to be associated with the tarsal papilla (Fig. 19-2). These are the classic "cobblestone papillae."

Limbal papillae tend to be gelatinous and confluent, and they occur more commonly in African and West Indian patients (17) (Fig. 19-3). Horner-Trantas dots, which are collections of epithelial cells and eosinophils, may be found at any meridian around the limbus (22). These changes may lead to superficial corneal neovascularization. The forniceal conjunctiva usually does not show foreshortening or symblepharon formation.

The corneal findings may be sight threatening. Buckley (17) describes in detail the sequence of occurrence of corneal pathogenesis. Mediators from the inflamed tarsal conjunctiva cause a punctate epithelial keratitis. Coalescence of these areas leads to frank epithelial erosion, leaving Bowman's membrane intact. If, at this point, inadequate or no treatment is rendered, a plaque containing fibrin and mucus deposits over the epithelial defect (26). Epithelial healing is then impaired, and new vessel growth is encouraged. This so-called shield ulcer (Fig. 19-4) usually has

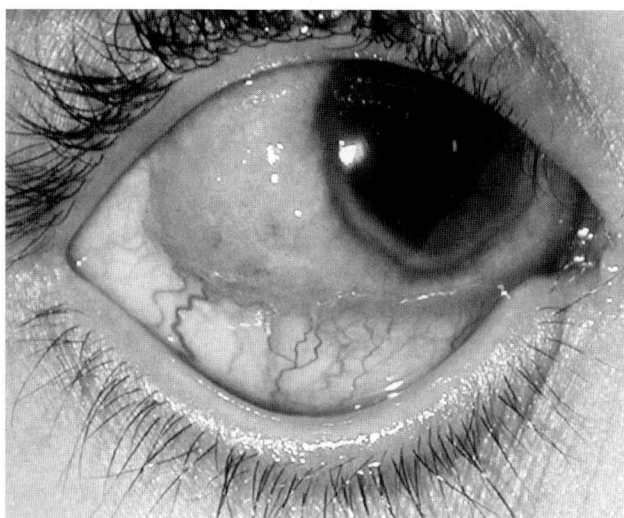

FIGURE 19-3. Limbal vernal lesion.

its lower border in the upper half of the visual axis. With resolution, the ulcerated area leaves a subepithelial ringlike scar. The peripheral cornea may show a waxing and waning, superficial stromal, and gray-white deposition termed pseudogerontoxon. Iritis is not reported to occur in VKC.

Pathophysiology

Biopsy of a tarsal conjunctival papilla in VKC reveals distinct findings. The epithelium contains large numbers of mast cells and eosinophils, neither of which are found in normal individuals (27,28). Human mast cells may be categorized based on the presence of neutral proteases (29). The epithelium of VKC patients contains mast cells predominantly of the type containing the neutral proteases tryptase and chymase (2). Basophils are found in the epithelium, which may indicate one form of a delayed type hypersensitivity reaction is occurring. Leonardi et al. (28) demonstrated eosinophils,

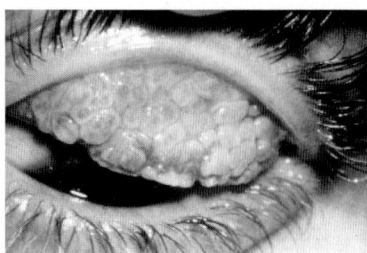

FIGURE 19-2. Flat-topped giant papillae of vernal keratoconjunctivitis (VKC).

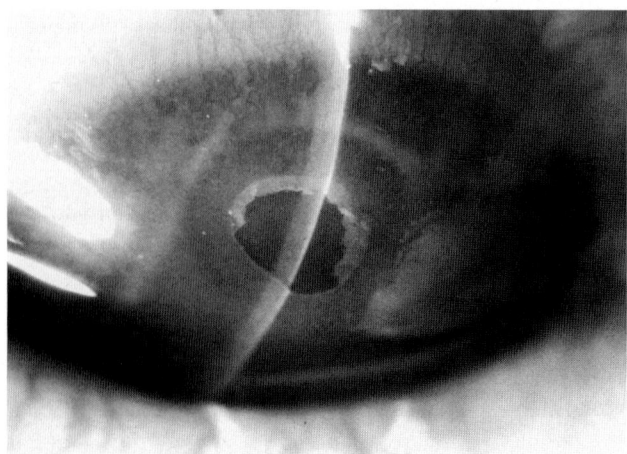

FIGURE 19-4. Shield ulcer in VKC. (Courtesy of Devon Harrison, M.D.)

TABLE 19-1. COMPARISON OF VERNAL KERATOCONJUNCTIVITIS (VKC) AND ATOPIC KERATOCONJUNCTIVITIS (AKC)

	VKC	AKC
Age	Younger	Older
Sex	Males > females	No predilection
Duration of disease	Limited; resolves at puberty	Chronic
Time of year	Spring	Perennial
Conjunctival involvement	Upper tarsus	Lower tarsus
Conjunctival cicatrization	Rare	Common
Cornea	Shield ulcer	Persistent epithelial defects
Corneal scar	Common; not vision threatening	Common; vision threatening
Corneal vascularization	Rare	Common

neutrophils, and mononuclear cells in the hyperplastic epithelium. Brush cytology of the conjunctival epithelium from patients with VKC showed more eosinophils and neutrophils in patients with corneal erosion or ulcer than in those without (30). Goblet cell density is not found to be elevated in the conjunctival epithelium of VKC (31). Eosinophil major basic protein is deposited diffusely throughout the conjunctiva of VKC patients, including the epithelium (32).

The substantia propria contains elevated numbers of mast cells compared to normal individuals (27,28). The predominant mast cell subtype found contains tryptase and chymase (2). Forty-six percent of the mast cells in the substantia propria contain basic fibroblast growth factor (bFGF) (33). This may serve as a source of fibroblast growth and production of collagens. Eosinophil major basic protein granules are found close to mast cells in VKC (32). As in the epithelium, the substantia propria contains increased numbers of eosinophils and basophils compared to normal tissue (27). A unique profile of lymphocytes is found. T-cell clones can be isolated from biopsy specimens of VKC tarsal conjunctiva. These CD4 T-cell clones show helper function for IgE synthesis *in vitro* and produce IL-4 (34). Calder et al. (35), in separate work, found IL-5 expressed in T-cell lines from vernal biopsy specimen. Cognate interaction with T cells and the presence of IL-4 are needed for B-cell production of IgE (34). This would support the suggestion that IgE is produced locally. The substantia propria also has an increased amount of collagen. Fibroblasts from the tarsal conjunctival biopsy of VKC patients can be induced to proliferate by histamine and epithelium-derived growth factor (28). Cyclosporin A, which can be used effectively in VKC, has been shown *in vitro* to reduce collagen production and induce apoptosis of conjunctival fibroblasts from VKC patients (36).

The corneal epithelium of VKC patients expresses ICAM-1, an important cell adhesion molecule (37). Eosinophil peroxidase in contact with human corneal epithelial cells causes disruption of cell adhesion (38). Eosinophil major basic protein (EMBP) and cationic protein (ECP) are proinflammatory, and EMBP has been shown to be cytotoxic to corneal epithelium. *In vitro*, both of these damage the monolayers of human corneal epithelial cells but not the stratified corneal epithelial cells in culture (39).

Specific IgE and IgG have been isolated from the tears of VKC patients (40,41). Histamine (6) and tryptase (7) are elevated in the tears of VKC patients. The serum of VKC patients has been found to contain decreased levels of histaminase and increased levels of nerve growth factor (42,43). Finally, VKC is reported to occur in patients with the hyperimmunoglobulin E syndrome (44).

Diagnosis

The diagnosis is relatively straightforward, based on the history and presentation of findings. As indicated previously, VKC occurs predominantly in young boys living in warm climates. These patients have intense photophobia, ptosis, and the characteristic finding of giant papillae. The principal differential diagnostic entity is AKC. The two are compared and contrasted in Table 19-1. Tear fluid analysis and cytology, conjunctival scraping for cytology and biopsy are rarely needed to assist in establishing the diagnosis.

Treatment

As with any atopic condition, avoidance of allergens is important. This is often difficult for VKC patients because of the possible large number of antigens to which they react. Seasonal removal of affected children from their home to a reduced allergen climate is usually not practical for most families. What is practical and should not be overlooked is alternate occlusive therapy, as an allergen avoidance strategy. Hyposensitization in VKC has limitations. It is not feasible to desensitize children with VKC to all of the allergens to which they are responsive. Moreover, some suggest that although skin and lung respond to hyposensitization, the conjunctiva often does not (2).

For the patient with a significant seasonal exacerbation, a short-term, high-dose pulse regimen of topical steroids is commonly necessary. Usually, dexamethasone 0.1% or prednisolone phosphate 1% eight times daily for 1 week brings excellent relief of symptoms. This should be tapered rapidly to as little as is needed to maintain patient comfort. As in any chronic ocular inflammatory disease, the risks of prolonged use of corticosteroids are cataract and glaucoma. Thus any limited use of steroids should include additional measures to sustain decreased inflammation. Cromolyn sodium, a mast cell stabilizer, has repeatedly been shown to be effective in patients with VKC (45–47). At the time of an exacerbation, the patient should be given a steroid pulse dose as outlined earlier and begin taking cromolyn or dual-acting drug such as olopatadine, ketotifen, or azelastine, concurrently to begin mast cell stabilization and antihistamine treatment. Other drugs that have undergone clinical trials for VKC are available and are listed in Table 19-2.

Oral medications that have a role in VKC treatment include steroids, antihistamines, and NSAIDs. For the care of severe bilateral vision-threatening disease, oral steroids may be used, but using this treatment for VKC alone is unusual. Maximizing the use of nonsedating antihistamines is often helpful. Oral aspirin has been effective, often requiring a dose as high as 2,400 mg daily (48,49).

Topical cyclosporin A (CsA) shows promise in the treatment of VKC. The release of IL-2 is diminished with cyclosporin A, thus reducing the expansion of certain T-cell clones. Several studies have demonstrated the effectiveness of CsA in VKC therapy (50–57).

The corneal shield ulcer is a vision-threatening complication of VKC. Treatment may include antibiotic-steroid ointment and occlusive therapy. If a plaque forms in the ulcer bed, a superficial keratectomy is sometimes beneficial in promoting epithelial healing (58). Recently, phototherapeutic keratectomy (59) and keratectomy with amniotic membrane graft placement have been shown effective (60).

Climatotherapy may be beneficial. This may involve simple measures, such as cool compresses over the closed lids. Maintenance of an air-conditioned environment or relocation to a cool, dry climate are most helpful during seasonal exacerbations. The economic and geographic restrictions of these measures are obvious.

Surgical procedures are primarily of historic significance. Cryoablation of upper tarsal cobblestones is reported to render short-term improvement. However, scar formation from this may lead to lid and tear film abnormalities. The risk of these adverse permanent changes is probably not warranted in this usually self-limited disease. Surgical removal of the upper tarsal papilla in combination with forniceal conjunctival advancement or buccal mucosal grafting may result in obliteration of the fornix (61). Injection of short- or long-acting steroids into the tarsal papilla has been shown effective at reducing their size (62–64).

The therapy of the future will be directed toward diminishing mast cell number or function and immunomodulation of the cell-mediated response.

ATOPIC KERATOCONJUNCTIVITIS

Definition

AKC is a bilateral, chronic inflammation of the conjunctiva and lids associated with atopic dermatitis. Hogan (65), in 1953, was the first to describe the findings of chronic conjunctivitis and keratitis in patients with atopic dermatitis. Three percent of the population has atopic dermatitis (66,67). From 15% to 67.5% of patients with atopic dermatitis have ocular involvement, usually AKC (66–68).

Demographics

The onset of AKC is usually in the second through fifth decade. Recent series of patients report the onset of symptoms between the ages of 7 and 76 (69–71). The male-female ratio is reported as 2.4:1 (69) to slightly fewer males than females (70). No racial or geographic predilection is reported.

Symptoms

Itching is the major symptom of AKC. This may be more pronounced in certain seasons or it may be perennial. Other symptoms, in decreasing order of frequency, include watering, mucous discharge, redness, blurring of vision, photophobia, and pain (69). Exacerbation of symptoms most frequently occurs in the presence of animals (69).

Signs

Signs of AKC include skin, lid margin, conjunctival, corneal, and lens changes (Table 19-3). The periocular skin often shows a scaling, flaking dermatitis with a reddened base (Fig. 19-5). The lids may become lichenified and woody, developing cicatricial ectropion and lagophthalmos. Lateral canthal ulceration, cracking, and madarosis

TABLE 19-2. DRUGS USED IN CLINICAL TRIALS FOR THE TREATMENT OF VERNAL KERATOCONJUNCTIVITIS SINCE 1992

Antihistamine	
Levocabastine	0.05%
Nonsteroidals	
Flurbiprofen	0.03%
Ketoralac	0.5%
Indomethacin	1.0%
Mast cell stabilizers	
Nedocromil sodium	2%
Sodium cromoglycate	2% or 4%
Lodoxamide	0.1%
Steroids (Topical)	
Fluorometholone	0.1%
Mepragoside gel	0.5%
Antibiotics	
Mitomycin C	0.01%

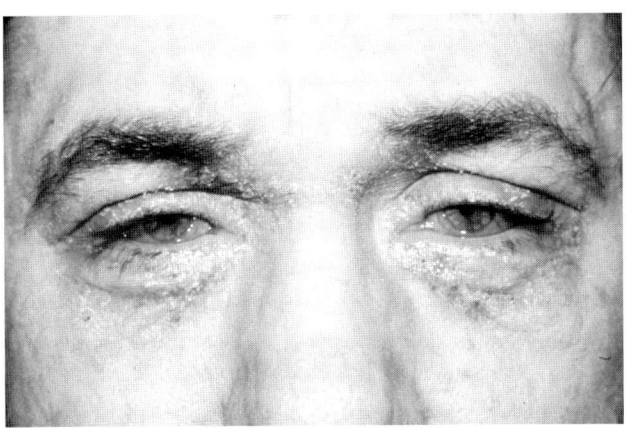

FIGURE 19-5. Severe periocular and lid involvement of atopic keratoconjunctivitis (AKC).

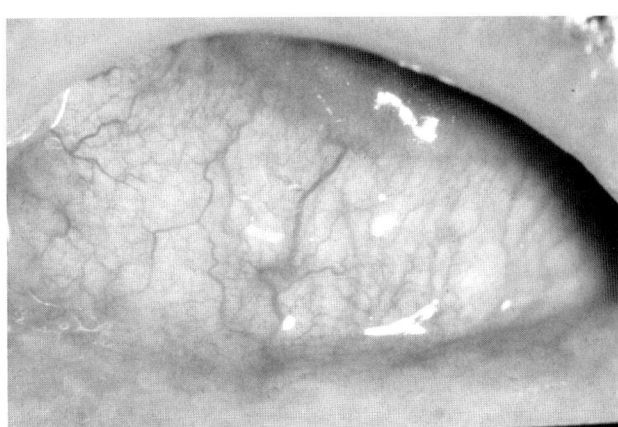

FIGURE 19-6. Lower tarsal conjunctiva in AKC. Note the fornix foreshortening and pale edema.

are common. This may even be the principal manifestation in a minority of cases. The lid margins may show loss of cilia, meibomianitis, keratinization, and punctal ectropion. The conjunctiva of the tarsal surfaces has a papillary reaction, follicles, and possibly a pale white edema (Fig. 19-6). In contrast to VKC, the papillary hypertrophy of AKC is more prominent in the inferior conjunctival fornix. Subepithelial fibrosis is present in many, fornix foreshortening in some, and symblepharon in a few. The bulbar conjunctiva may have few findings besides erythema and chemosis. A perilimbal, gelatinous hyperplasia may occur. Horner-Trantas dots have been reported to occur in patients with AKC (72).

Significant vision loss in patients with AKC usually results from corneal pathology. Punctate epithelial keratopathy is the most common corneal problem. Persistent epithelial defects, scarring, microbial ulceration, and neovascularization are the main corneal causes for decreased vision (Table 19-3). Penetrating keratoplasty typically results in similar surface problems but has been shown to improve vision in some (73). Herpetic keratitis is reported to occur in 14% to 17.8% of AKC patients, and keratoconus occurs in 6.7% to 16.2% (69,70).

Anterior uveitis and iris abnormalities are not reported. The prevalence of cataract associated with AKC is difficult to determine, because steroids are so frequently used in the

TABLE 19-3. CLINICAL SIGNS IN PATIENTS WITH ATOPIC KERATOCONJUNCTIVITIS

Condition	Foster and Calogne (N = 45)	Tuft et al (N = 37)	No. of patients %	No. of patients %
Lids				
Eczema	28	62.2	30	81
Blepharitis	25	55.6	33	89
Meibomianitis	25	55.6	–	–
Tarsal margin keratinization	13	28.9	–	–
Trichiasis	8	17.8	6	16.2
Madarosis	6	13.8	–	–
Punctal ectropion	–	–	18	48.6
Ectropion	5	11.1	–	–
Entropion	2	4.4	–	–
Conjunctiva				
Subepithelial fibrosis	26	57.8	26	70.2
Fornix foreshortening	13	28.9	–	–
Symblepharon	12	26.7	10	27
Giant papillae	11	24.4	11	29.7
Follicles	6	13.3	5	13.5
Cornea				
Superficial punctate keratitis	24	53.3	37	100
Neovascularization	17	37.8	24	64.8
Persistent epithelial defects	17	37.8	4	10.8
Filamentary keratitis	2	4.4	1	2.7

treatment of the disease. The lens opacity typically associated with AKC, however, is an anterior or posterior subcapsular cataract. This cataract often has the configuration of a Maltese cross. Retinal detachment with or without previous cataract surgery is the principal reported posterior manifestation of AKC (74–76).

Pathophysiology

AKC is driven by both type I and type IV hypersensitivity mechanisms. Evidence of the pathologic process comes from histologic and immunohistochemical analysis of conjunctival biopsy specimens and from tear fluid analysis for mediators and cells.

Mast cells and eosinophils are found in the conjunctival epithelium of AKC patients but not in normal individuals. Mast cells in the epithelium of AKC patients contain predominantly tryptase as the neutral protease (5). Goblet cell density and squamous metaplasia are then examined by impression cytology (77). The epithelium may become involuted, allowing pseudotubule structures to form (70). Antibodies to human leukocyte antigen (HLA)-DR stain diffusely throughout the epithelium (78). This suggests an upregulation of antigen presentation. There is an increase in the CD4/CD8 ratio in AKC over normal conjunctival epithelium (78). This increase of CD4 or helper T cells probably serves to amplify the immune response that is occurring.

The substantia propria in AKC has an increased number of mast cells compared to normal. Eosinophils, never found in normal structures, are present in the substantia propria in AKC. These eosinophils are found to have increased numbers of activation markers on their surface (79). A large number of mononuclear cells are present in the substantia propria. Fibroblast numbers are increased, and there is an increased amount of collagen compared to that in the conjunctiva of normal individuals. In addition, the substantia propria demonstrates increased CD4/CD8, B cells, HLA-DR staining, and Langerhans' cells (78). The T-cell receptor on lymphocytes in the substantia propria is predominantly of the α or β subtype (78). The T-cell population of the substantia propria includes CD4 and memory cells (80). Th2 cytokines predominate in allergic disease, yet lymphocytes with Th1 cytokines have been found in the substantia propria of AKC patients (81).

Tears of AKC patients contain increased levels of IgE, eosinophil cationic protein, T-helper cells, activated B cells, decreased eotaxin, eosinophil neurotoxin, soluble IL-2 receptor, IL-4, IL-5, and osteopontin (9,68,70,82–87). Schirmer values are depressed (56% of patients less than 5 mm). Dysfunctional cellular immune response in AKC patients is demonstrated by reduction or abrogation of the cell-mediated response to *Candida* and the inability of some patients to become sensitized to dinitrochlorobenzene. Serum of AKC patients has been found to contain increased levels of IgE, eosinophil cationic protein, eosinophil neurotoxin, and IL-2 receptor (69,85,88,89). A recent study

shows eosinophils and their products deposited in the ulcers and stroma of corneas from AKC patients (90).

In summary, AKC patients demonstrate an increased number of conjunctival mast cells and evidence of mast cell activation. Furthermore, a complex immune cell profile implicates more than the mast cell alone, but the details of these cellular interactions remain speculative.

Diagnosis

A careful history is paramount for both diagnosis and treatment in AKC. The patient typically describes severe, persistent, periocular itching associated with dermatitis. There is usually a family history of atopy in one or both parents and commonly other atopic manifestations in the patient, such as asthma (65%) or allergic rhinitis (65%) (71). A history of seasonal or exposure-related exacerbations is usually present. History and examination reveal features to help differentiate AKC from other atopic ocular conditions. The lack of contact lens wear aids in differentiating AKC from GPC. AKC patients are usually older and have major lid involvement compared to patients with VKC. SAC patients have no or markedly diminished symptoms out of their season and show no evidence of chronic inflammation in the conjunctiva. The significant past history or concurrent presence of eczema cannot be emphasized enough as a finding in patients with AKC. The serum level of IgE is often elevated in patients with AKC. A Giemsa stain of a scraping of the upper tarsal conjunctiva may reveal eosinophils.

Treatment

The approach to treatment is multifaceted and includes environmental controls as well as topical and systemic medications. It is unlikely that the AKC patient will see the ophthalmologist without also being under the care of a medical physician. However, the patient must remove environmental irritants in both the home and the employment or school setting. The nature of the irritants may be better defined through skin testing.

The topical ocular application of a vasoconstrictor-antihistamine combination may bring transient relief of symptoms but is unlikely to intervene in the immunopathologic process or its sequelae. There is potential for overuse of vasoconstrictors due to the chronic nature of the disease. Currently available drops include naphazoline hydrochloride and pheniramine maleate or naphazoline hydrochloride and antazoline phosphate. The potent antihistamine levocabastine and emedastine offer much greater H_1 receptor antagonism than the other two over-the-counter antihistamines. The topical administration of steroids such as prednisolone acetate eight times per day for 7 to 10 days is clearly beneficial in controlling symptoms and signs. These agents must be used judiciously, because the chronic nature of the disease may encourage overuse. Patients must be instructed that steroid use must be transient only and must be carefully monitored for efficacy; they must also be warned of the potential for causing cataract and glaucoma. Prescriptions for the steroid should not be refillable, and frequent monitoring of intraocular pressure is crucial. Steroid-sparing medications, including the mast cell stabilizer sodium cromolyn 4%, have been shown to be effective in reducing itching, tearing, and photophobia and need for steroid (91,92). Disodium cromoglycate 4%, four times daily is recommended year-round in patients with perennial symptoms. If an exacerbation occurs and the patient is not taking cromolyn sodium, its use should be initiated four times daily concurrent with a short burst of topical steroids (for 7 to 10 days). From 2 to 4 weeks of dosing may be needed before cromolyn sodium becomes effective. Other mast cell stabilizers or combination mast cell stabilizers—antihistamines such as nedocromil, lodoxamide, olopatadine, azelastine, or ketotifen, may be helpful. Cyclosporine both orally and topically has been shown effective in treating AKC as well as in reducing the amount of topical steroid use (93,94).

Foster and Calonge (70) recommend maximizing the use of systemic antihistamines. H_1 receptors seem most responsible for the symptoms of AKC, and newer antagonists are fairly specific for the H_1 receptor. Only in rare cases of uncontrolled dermatitis with vision-threatening complications are oral steroids indicated. The role of systemic desensitization is similar to that in VKC. Plasmapheresis has been shown effective in the treatment of fulminant AKC (95,96).

Lid and ocular surface abnormalities may require treatment other than that directed toward the underlying pathologic condition of AKC. Trichiasis or lid position abnormalities, if contributing in any way to corneal compromise, must be corrected. Any staphylococcal blepharitis should receive adequate antibiotic treatment. If, despite adequate control of signs and symptoms of AKC, corneal punctate staining persists, artificial tears should be used to avoid the development of corneal epithelial defects. It may be extremely difficult to achieve reepithelialization of these defects, and surgical approaches have been attempted (97). Lid or ocular surface herpes simplex virus (HSV) infection should be treated with topical antiviral agents. Care should be taken in using these to achieve viral eradication without sustained use and subsequent epithelial toxicity. If frequent recurrent episodes of epithelial HSV keratitis occur, one may consider chronic oral acyclovir (400 mg orally twice daily) as prophylaxis against frequent recurrences.

Interleukin-2 (IL-2) has been used successfully to treat atopic dermatitis but has not been used specifically for AKC. After treatment with IL-2, the skin biopsy of atopic dermatitis patients shows depletion of the abnormally high number of CD4 cells but no change in the number of Langerhans' cells. The decreased CD4 count may result in the abrogation of the exaggerated antigen processing and cellular activation. The effect of IL-2 is short lived, with a return of symptoms 2 to 6 weeks after therapy ceases.

In summary, topical steroids control most patients with AKC. The chronic use of steroids must be avoided, and early in treatment, steroid sparing strategies must be considered.

GIANT PAPILLARY CONJUNCTIVITIS

Definition

Giant papillary conjunctivitis (GPC) is a chronic inflammatory process leading to the production of giant papillae on the tarsal conjunctiva lining of the upper eyelids (Fig. 19-7). Most often associated with soft contact lens wear, GPC has been reported in patients wearing soft, hard, and rigid gas-permeable contact lenses, as well as in patients with ocular prostheses and exposed sutures in contact with the conjunctiva.

Demographics

GPC may affect as many as 20% of soft contact lens wearers (98). People wearing regular (as opposed to disposable) soft contact lenses are at least ten times more susceptible to GPC than rigid (gas-permeable) contact lens wearers. Patients wearing daily-wear disposable contact lenses and those wearing rigid contact lenses are about equally affected. Patients who wear disposable contact lenses during sleep are probably three times more likely to have GPC symptoms than if the lenses are removed daily. Patients with asthma, hay fever or animal allergies may be at greater risk for GPC (99).

Symptoms

Symptoms of GPC include ocular itching after lens removal, redness, burning, increased mucus discharge in the morning, photophobia, and decreased contact lens tolerance. Blurred vision can result from deposits on the contact

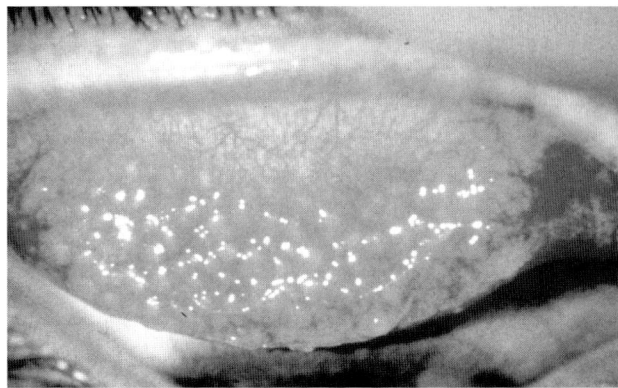

FIGURE 19-7. Greater than 1.0-mm-diameter papilla of giant papillary conjunctivitis (GPC).

lens, or from displacement of the contact lens secondary to the superior eyelid papillary hypertrophy.

Signs

Hyperemia of the conjunctiva and the characteristic giant papillae on the underside of the upper lid are often the only findings.

Pathophysiology

The onset of GPC may be the result of mechanical trauma secondary to contact lens fit or a lens edge causing chronic irritation of the upper eyelid with each blink. It is more likely, however, that a buildup of "protein" on the surface of the contact lens causes an allergic reaction in the eyelid tissue. As with AKC and VKC, tissue biopsies are the primary source of data on the pathophysiology of this GPC. Many of the published studies concerning mast cell involvement in GPC contrast the disease with VKC. Like VKC, conjunctival biopsies in GPC show mast cells of the MC_T type in the conjunctival epithelium. However, there is no significant increase in mast cells in the substantia propria, and thus no overall increase in number of mast cells present in the conjunctival tissue (2). Interestingly, whereas increased histamine is measured in tears in patients with VKC, patients with GPC have normal tear histamine levels (6,98). This can be partially explained from electron microscopy data on biopsies from patients with GPC, which has revealed less mast cell degranulation (30%) than is observed in patients with VKC (80%) (100). Tryptase has also been found in the tears from patients with GPC (101). This is not surprising, considering the fact that rubbing, alone, can result in significant increases of tryptase in tears (7). As in SAC and PAC, release of mediators from mast cells results in increased capillary permeability and inflammatory cell infiltration of eyelid tissue. Cytologic scrapings from the conjunctiva of patients with GPC exhibit an infiltrate containing lymphocytes, plasma cells, mast cells, eosinophils, and basophils. All of these factors contribute to discomfort and formation of the papillae. The differentiating pathophysiologic characteristics between GPC and VKC are important because they could be considered as possible clues to the differences in pathogenesis between these two ocular diseases.

Diagnosis

Examination of the underside of the upper eyelid will, in severe cases, reveal large papillae with red, inflamed tissue (Fig. 19-5). In milder cases of GPC, smaller papillae occur. These papillae are thought to be caused by the contact lens riding high on the surface of the eye with each blink. In very mild cases this tendency of the contact lens to ride up on the eye may contribute to the diagnosis in the absence of visible papillae. In cases of chronic GPC, tear deficiency may be a contributing factor. Redness of the upper eyelid on ocular examination is one of the earliest signs of GPC, and this observation can facilitate early diagnosis. Abnormal thickening of the conjunctiva may progress to opacification as inflammatory cells enter the tissue.

Treatment

Reducing symptoms is the primary aim in managing GPC. A reduction in the wearing time of contacts from a few hours a day to total abstinence may be required. Daily disposable contact lenses may be a consideration for persistent cases of GPC. However, in more serious cases, a more aggressive approach may be required to prevent ocular tissue damage. Over-the-counter "artificial" tears help to wash away environmental allergens and lens debris.

Topical mast cell stabilizers have proven effectiveness in the treatment of GPC (102–105). Dual acting drugs may be the best therapy for chronic GPC. A patient with GPC may require continued use of these drugs once they return to contact lens wear. Steroids have also been approved for the treatment of GPC (106). Topical steroids may be used four times per day for 2 to 4 days (107). A return to contact lens wear can usually be accomplished but may require a change in contact lens style or lens material.

REFERENCES

1. Cocoa AF, Cooke RA. On the classification of the phenomena of hypersensitiveness. *J Immunol* 1923;8:163–182.
2. Bielory L. Allergic and immunologic disorders of the eye. Part II: ocular allergy. *J Allergy Clin Immunol* 2000;106:1019–1032.
3. Irani AM, Butrus SI, Tabbara KF, et al. Human conjunctival mast cells: distribution of MCT and MCTC in vernal conjunctivitis and giant papillary conjunctivitis. *J Allergy Clin Immunol* 1990;86:34–40.
4. Morgan SJ, Williams JH, Walls AF, et al. Mast cell hyperplasia in atopic keratoconjunctivitis. An immunohistochemical study. *Eye* 1991;5:729–735.
5. Baddeley SM, Bacon AS, McGill JI, et al. Mast cell distribution and neutral protease expression in acute and chronic allergic conjunctivitis. *Clin Exp Allergy* 1995;25:41–50.
6. Abelson MB, Baird RS, Allansmith MR. Tear histamine levels in vernal conjunctivitis and other ocular inflammations. *Ophthalmology* 1980;87:812–814.
7. Butrus SI, Ochsner KI, Abelson MB, et al. The level of tryptase in human tears. An indicator of activation of conjunctival mast cells. *Ophthalmology* 1990;97:1678–1683.
8. Akdis CA, Blaser K. Histamine in the immune regulation of allergic inflammation. *J Allergy Clin Immunol* 2003;112:15–22.
9. Macleod JD, Anderson DF, Baddeley SM, et al. Immunolocalization of cytokines to mast cells in normal and allergic conjunctiva. *Clin Exp Allergy* 1997;27:1328–1334.
10. Uchio E, Ono SY, Ikezawa Z, et al. Tear levels of interferon-gamma, interleukin (IL) -2, IL-4 and IL-5 in patients with vernal keratoconjunctivitis, atopic keratoconjunctivitis and allergic conjunctivitis. *Clin Exp Allergy* 2000;30:103–109.

11. Vesaluoma M, Rosenberg ME, Teppo A, et al. Tumour necrosis factor alpha (TNFalpha) in tears of atopic patients after conjunctival allergen challenge. *Clin Exp Allergy* 1999;29:537–5142.

12. Nakamura Y, Sotozono C, Kinoshita S. Inflammatory cytokines in normal human tears. *Curr Eye Res* 1998;17:673–676.

13. Fujishima H, Takeuchi T, Shinozaki N, et al. Measurement of IL-4 in tears of patients with seasonal allergic conjunctivitis and vernal keratoconjunctivitis. *Clin Exp Immunol* 1995;102:395–398.

14. Cook EB, Stahl JL, Lowe L, et al. Simultaneous measurement of six cytokines in a single sample of human tears using microparticle-based flow cytometry: allergics vs. non-allergics. *J Immunol Methods* 2001;254:109–118.

15. Sharif NA, Xu SX, Magnino PE, et al. Human conjunctival epithelial cells express histamine-1 receptors coupled to phosphoinositide turnover and intracellular calcium mobilization: role in ocular allergic and inflammatory diseases. *Exp Eye Res* 1996;63:169–178.

16. Cook EB, Stahl JL, Miller ST, et al. Isolation of human conjunctival mast cells and epithelial cells: tumor necrosis factor-α from mast cells affects intracellular adhesion cell molecule 1 expression on epithelial cells. *Invest Ophthalmol Vis Sci* 1998;39:336–343.

17. Buckley RJ. Vernal keratoconjunctivitis. *Int Ophthalmol Clin* 1988;28:303–308.

18. Biegelman MN. *Vernal conjunctivitis.* Los Angeles: University of Southern California Press, 1950.

19. Arlt F. Physiologisch and pathologisch anatomische Bemerkungen uber die bindehaut des Auges. *Prager Vierteljahrschrift* 1846;4:73.

20. Desmarres LA. *Hypertrophie perikeratique de la conjonctive. Traite theorie et pratique des maladies des yeus,* 2nd ed. Paris: Germer Baillere, 1855.

21. von Graefe A. *Klinische Vortrage uber Augenheilkunde.* Journal Hirshberg 1871;21.

22. Axenfeld T. Rapport sur le catarrhe printanier. *Bull Mem Soc Fr Ophthalmol* 1907;24:1.

23. Trantas A. Sur le catarrhe prntanier. *Arch Ophthalmol (Paris)* 30:593–621.

24. Herbert H. Preliminary note on the pathology and diagnosis of spring catarrh. *Br Med J* 1903;735.

25. Bonini S, Lambiase A, Marchi S, et al. Vernal keratoconjunctivitis revisited: a case series of 195 patients with long-term followup. *Ophthalmology* 2000;107:1157–1163.

26. Rahi AHS. Pathology of Corneal plaque in vernal keratoconjunctivitis. In: O'Connor GR, Chandler JW, eds. *Advances in immunology and immunopathology of the eye.* New York: Masson, 1985.

27. Allansmith MR, Baird RS, Greiner JV. Vernal conjunctivitis and contact lens-associated giant papillary conjunctivitis compared and contrasted. *Am J Ophthalmol* 1979;87:544–555.

28. Leonardi A, Abatangelo G, Cortivo R, et al. Collagen types I and III in giant papillae of vernal keratoconjunctivitis. *Br J Ophthalmol* 1995;79:482–485.

29. Irani AA, Schechter NM, Craig SS, et al. Two types of human mast cells that have distinct neutral protease compositions. *Proc Natl Acad Sci U S A* 1986;83:4464–4468.

30. Miyoshi T, Fukagawa K, Shimmura S, et al. Interleukin-8 concentrations in conjunctival epithelium brush cytology samples correlate with neutrophil, eosinophil infiltration, and corneal damage. *Cornea* 2001;20:743–747.

31. Allansmith MR, Baird RS, Greiner JV. Density of goblet cells in vernal conjunctivitis and contact lens-associated giant papillary conjunctivitis. *Arch Ophthalmol* 1981;99:884–885.

32. Trocme SD, Kephart GM, Allansmith MR, et al. Conjunctival deposition of eosinophil granule major basic protein in vernal keratoconjunctivitis and contact lens-associated giant papillary conjunctivitis. *Am J Ophthalmol* 1989;108:57–63.

33. Leonardi A, Brun P, Tavolato M, et al. Growth factors and collagen distribution in vernal keratoconjunctivitis. *Invest Ophthalmol Vis Sci* 2000;41:4175–4181.

34. Romagnani S. Regulation and deregulation of human IgE synthesis. *Immunol Today* 1990;11:316–321.

35. Calder VL, Jolly G, Hingorani M, et al. Cytokine production and mRNA expression by conjunctival T-cell lines in chronic allergic eye disease. *Clin Exp Allergy* 1999;29:1214–1222.

36. Leonardi A, DeFranchis G, Fregona IA, et al. Effects of cyclosporin A on human conjunctival fibroblasts. *Arch Ophthalmol* 2001;119:1512–1517.

37. Temprano J. Corneal epithelial expression of ICAM-1 in vernal keratoconjunctivitis. *Invest Ophthalmol Vis Sci* 1995;36:1024.

38. Hallberg CK. Eosinophil peroxidase and eosinophil-derived neurotoxin toxicity on cultured human corneal epithelium. *Invest Ophthalmol Vis Sci* 1995;36:698.

39. Ward SL. The barrier properties of an in vitro human corneal epithelial model are not altered by eosinophil major basic protein or eosinophil cationic protein. *Invest Ophthalmol Vis Sci* 1995;36:699.

40. Sompolinsky D. A contribution to the immunopathology of vernal keratoconjunctivitis. *Documenta Ophthalmologica* 1982;53:61–92.

41. Ballow M, Mendelson L. Specific immunoglobulin E antibodies in tear secretions of patients with vernal conjunctivitis. *J Allergy Clin Immunol* 1980;66:112–118.

42. Mukhopadhyay K, Pradhan SC, Mathur JS, et al. Studies on histamine and histaminase in spring catarrh (vernal conjunctivitis). *Int Arch Allergy Appl Immunol* 1981;64:464–468.

43. Bonini S, Lambiase A, Levi-Schaffer F, et al. Nerve growth factor: an important molecule in allergic inflammation and tissue remodelling. *Int Arch Allergy Immunol* 1999;118:159–162.

44. Butrus SI, Leung DY, Gellis S, et al. Vernal conjunctivitis in the hyperimmunoglobulinemia E syndrome. *Ophthalmology* 1984;91:1213–1216.

45. El Hennawi M. Clinical trial with 2% sodium cromoglycate (Opticrom) in vernal keratoconjunctivitis. *Br J Ophthalmol* 1980;64:483–486.

46. Foster CS, Duncan J. Randomized clinical trial of topically administered cromolyn sodium for vernal keratoconjunctivitis. *Am J Ophthalmol* 1980;90:175–181.

47. Tabbara KF, Arafat NT. Cromolyn effects on vernal keratoconjunctivitis in children. *Arch Ophthalmol* 1977;95:2184–2186.

48. Abelson MB, Butrus SI, Weston JH. Aspirin therapy in vernal conjunctivitis. *Am J Ophthalmol* 1983;95:502–505.

49. Chaudhary KP. Evaluation of combined systemic aspirin and cromolyn sodium in intractable vernal catarrh. *Ann Ophthalmol* 1990;22:314–318.

50. Tomida I, Schlote T, Brauning J, et al. [Cyclosporin a]. *Ophthalmologe* 2002;99:761–767.

51. Pucci N, Novembre E, Cianferoni A, et al. Efficacy and safety of cyclosporine eyedrops in vernal keratoconjunctivitis. *Ann Allergy Asthma Immunol* 2002;89:298–303.

52. Gupta V, Sahu PK. Topical cyclosporin A in the management of vernal keratoconjunctivitis. *Eye* 2001;15:39–41.

53. Avunduk AM, Avunduk MC, Erdol H, et al. Cyclosporine effects on clinical findings and impression cytology specimens in severe vernal keratoconjunctivitis. *Ophthalmologica* 2001;215:290–293.

54. Mendicute J, Aranzasti C, Eder F, et al. Topical cyclosporin A 2% in the treatment of vernal keratoconjunctivitis. *Eye* 1997;11:75–78.

55. Secchi AG, Tognon MS, Leonardi A. Topical use of cyclosporine in the treatment of vernal keratoconjunctivitis. *Am J Ophthalmol* 1990;110:641–645.

56. Holland EJ, Olsen TW, Ketcham JM, et al. Topical cyclosporin A in the treatment of anterior segment inflammatory disease. *Cornea* 1993;12:413–419.

57. BenEzra D, Pe'er J, Brodsky M, et al. Cyclosporine eyedrops for the treatment of severe vernal keratoconjunctivitis. *Am J Ophthalmol* 1986;101:278–282.

58. Jones BR. Vernal keratitis. *Trans Ophthalmol Soc UK* 1961;81: 215–228.

59. Autrata R, Rehurek J, Holousova M. [Phototherapeutic keratectomy in the treatment of corneal surface disorders in children]. *Cesk Slov Oftalmol* 2002;58:105–111.

60. Sridhar MS, Sangwan VS, Bansal AK, et al. Amniotic membrane transplantation in the management of shield ulcers of vernal keratoconjunctivitis. *Ophthalmology* 2001;108:1218–1222.

61. Nishiwaki-Dantas MC, Dantas PE, Pezzutti S, et al. Surgical resection of giant papillae and autologous conjunctival graft in patients with severe vernal keratoconjunctivitis and giant papillae. *Ophthal Plast Reconstr Surg* 2000;16:438–442.

62. Saini JS, Gupta A, Pandey SK, et al. Efficacy of supratarsal dexamethasone versus triamcinolone injection in recalcitrant vernal keratoconjunctivitis. *Acta Ophthalmol Scand* 1999;77: 515–518.

63. Sethi HS, Wangh VB, Rai HK. Supratarsal injection of corticosteroids in the treatment of refractory vernal keratoconjunctivitis. *Indian J Ophthalmol* 2002;50:160–161.

64. Holsclaw DS, Whitcher JP, Wong IG, et al. Supratarsal injection of corticosteroid in the treatment of refractory vernal keratoconjunctivitis. *Am J Ophthalmol* 1996;121:243–249.

65. Hogan MJ. Atopic keratoconjunctivitis. *Am J Ophthalmol* 1953; 36:937–947.

66. Garrity JA, Liesegang TJ. Ocular complications of atopic dermatitis. *Can J Ophthalmol* 1984;19:21–24.

67. Rich LF, Hanifin JM: Ocular complications of atopic dermatitis and other eczemas. *Int Ophthalmol Clin* 1985;25:61–76.

68. Dogru M, Nakagawa N, Tetsumoto K, et al. Ocular surface disease in atopic dermatitis. *Jpn J Ophthalmol* 1999;43:53–57.

69. Tuft SJ, Kemeny DM, Dart JK, et al. Clinical features of atopic keratoconjunctivitis. *Ophthalmology* 1991;98:150–158.

70. Foster CS, Calonge M. Atopic keratoconjunctivitis. *Ophthalmology* 1990;97:992–1000.

71. Power WJ, Tugal-Tutkun I, Foster CS. Long-term follow-up of patients with atopic keratoconjunctivitis. *Ophthalmology* 1998;105: 637–642.

72. Friedlaender MH. Diseases affecting the eye and skin. In: Friedlaender MH, ed. *Allergy and immunology of the eye.* Hagerstown, PA: Harper and Row, 1979.

73. Ghoraishi M, Akova YA, Tugal-Tutkun I, et al. Penetrating keratoplasty in atopic keratoconjunctivitis. *Cornea* 1995;14:610–613.

74. Hurlbut WB, Damonkos AN. Cataract and retinal detachment associated with atopic dermatitis. *Arch Ophthalmol* 1961;52: 852–857.

75. Klemens F. Dermatose, Kataradt und ablatio retinae. *Klin Monatsbl Augenheilkd* 1966;152:921–927.

76. Yoneda K, Okamoto H, Wada Y, et al. Atopic retinal detachment. Report of four cases, a review of the literature. *Br J Dermatol* 1995;133:586–591.

77. Dogru M, Katakami C, Nakagawa N, et al. Impression cytology in atopic dermatitis. *Ophthalmology* 1998;105:1478–1484.

78. Foster CS, Rice BA, Dutt JE. Immunopathology of atopic keratoconjunctivitis. *Ophthalmology* 1991;98:1190–1196.

79. Hingorani M, Calder V, Jolly G, et al. Eosinophil surface antigen expression and cytokine production vary in different ocular allergic diseases. *J Allergy Clin Immunol* 1998;102:821–830.

80. Metz DP, Bacon AS, Holgate S, et al. Phenotypic characterization of T cells infiltrating the conjunctiva in chronic allergic eye disease. *J Allergy Clin Immunol* 1996;98:686–696.

81. Metz DP, Hingorani M, Calder VL, et al. T-cell cytokines in chronic allergic eye disease. *J Allergy Clin Immunol* 1997;100: 817–824.

82. Montan PG, van Hage-Hamsten M. Eosinophil cationic protein in tears in allergic conjunctivitis. *Br J Ophthalmol* 1996;80: 556–560.

83. Avunduk AM, Avunduk MC, Dayioglu YS, et al. Flow cytometry tear analysis in patients with chronic allergic conjunctivitis. *Jpn J Ophthalmol* 1997;41:67–70.

84. Avunduk AM, Avunduk MC, Tekelioglu Y. Analysis of tears in patients with atopic keratoconjunctivitis, using flow cytometry. *Ophthalmic Res* 1998;30:44–48.

85. Leonardi A, Borghesan F, Faggian D, et al. Tear and serum soluble leukocyte activation markers in conjunctival allergic diseases. *Am J Ophthalmol* 2000;129:151–158.

86. Fukagawa K, Nakajima T, Tsubota K, et al. Presence of eotaxin in tears of patients with atopic keratoconjunctivitis with severe corneal damage. *J Allergy Clin Immunol* 1999;103:1220–1221.

87. Uchio E, Matsuura N, Kadonosono K, et al. Tear osteopontin levels in patients with allergic conjunctival diseases. *Graefes Arch Clin Exp Ophthalmol* 2002;240:924–928.

88. Geggel HS. Successful penetrating keratoplasty in a patient with severe atopic keratoconjunctivitis and elevated serum IgE level treated with long-term topical cyclosporin A. *Cornea* 1994;13: 543–545.

89. Akova YA, Jabbur NS, Neumann R, et al. Atypical ocular atopy. *Ophthalmology* 1993;100:1367–1371.

90. Messmer EM, May CA, Stefani FH, et al. Toxic eosinophil granule protein deposition in corneal ulcerations and scars associated with atopic keratoconjunctivitis. *Am J Ophthalmol* 2002;134: 816–821.

91. Ostler HB, Martin RG, Dawson CR, The use of disodium cromoglycate in the treatment of atopic ocular disease. In: Leopold JG, Burns RD, eds. *Symposium on ocular therapy.* New York: John Wiley, 1977:99–108.

92. Jay JL. Clinical features and diagnosis of adult atopic keratoconjunctivitis and the effect of treatment with sodium cromoglycate. *Br J Ophthalmol* 1981;65:335–340.

93. Hoang-Xuan T, Prisant O, Hannouche D, et al. Systemic cyclosporine A in severe atopic keratoconjunctivitis. *Ophthalmology* 1997;104:1300–1305.

94. Hingorani M, Moodaley L, Calder VL, et al. A randomized, placebo-controlled trial of topical cyclosporin A in steroid-dependent atopic keratoconjunctivitis. *Ophthalmology* 1998;105: 1715–1720.

95. Aswad MI, Tauber J, Baum J. Plasmapheresis treatment in patients with severe atopic keratoconjunctivitis. *Ophthalmology* 1988;95:444–447.

96. Mach R, Rozsival P, Jilek D. [Steroid glaucoma in severe atopic keratoconjunctivitis. A reminder for possible therapy with plasmapheresis]. *Cesk Oftalmol* 1992;48:167–170.

97. Thoft RA. Keratoepithelioplasty. *Am J Ophthalmol* 1984; 97:1–6.

98. Allansmith MR, Korb DR, Greiner JV, et al. Giant papillary conjunctivitis in contact lens wearers. *Am J Ophthalmol* 1977; 83:697–708.

99. Begley CG, Riggle A, Tuel JA. Association of giant papillary conjunctivitis with seasonal allergies. *Optom Vis Sci* 1990;67: 192–195.

100. Henriquez AS, Kenyon KR, Allansmith MR. Mast cell ultrastructure. Comparison in contact lens-associated giant papillary conjunctivitis and vernal conjunctivitis. *Arch Ophthalmol* 1981;99:1266–1272.

101. Butrus SI, Laby DM, Zacharia JS, et al. Tryptase in tears: a marker for mast cell activation in giant papillary conjunctivitis (GPC). *Invest Ophthalmol Vis Sci* 1991;32:740.

102. Meisler DM, Berzins UJ, Krachmer JH, et al. Cromolyn treatment of giant papillary conjunctivitis. *Arch Ophthalmol* 1982; 100:1608–1610.

103. Donshik PC, Ballow M, Luistro A, et al. Treatment of contact lens-induced giant papillary conjunctivitis. *CLAO J* 1984;10: 346–350.
104. Sorkin EM, Ward A. Ocular sodium cromoglycate. An overview of its therapeutic efficacy in allergic eye disease. *Drugs* 1986; 31:131–148.
105. Allansmith MR. Pathology and treatment of giant papillary conjunctivitis. I. The U.S. perspective. *Clin Ther* 1987;9:443–450.
106. Asbell P, Howes J. A double-masked, placebo-controlled evaluation of the efficacy and safety of loteprednol etabonate in the treatment of giant papillary conjunctivitis. *CLAO J* 1997;23: 31–36.
107. Bartlett JD, Howes JF, Ghormley NR, et al. Safety and efficacy of loteprednol etabonate for treatment of papillae in contact lens-associated giant papillary conjunctivitis. *Curr Eye Res* 1993; 12:313–321.

CICATRIZING CONJUNCTIVITIS

ESEN KARAMURSEL AKPEK AND OZGE ILHAN-SARAC

Chronic cicatrizing conjunctivitis (CCC) is a broad term encompassing a spectrum of clinical disorders that result in conjunctival fibrosis and scar tissue formation. The resultant structural and functional alterations of the ocular surface can lead to loss of corneal transparency and loss of vision. Some of the conditions causing CCC are systemic diseases and thus have further potential for morbidity and even death. Therefore, it is clearly essential to identify the exact etiology of CCC early in its course, and to treat appropriately. This chapter reviews the pathogenesis, clinical and laboratory features, and management of some of the most common disorders that can cause chronic cicatricial conjunctivitis (Table 20-1).

MUCOUS MEMBRANE PEMPHIGOID

Mucous membrane pemphigoid (MMP) is a spectrum of acquired, autoimmune, subepithelial blistering diseases that primarily affect mucous membranes but may involve the skin. Morbidity is associated with scar formation and may be especially severe when mucosal surfaces such as the conjunctivae, larynx, esophagus, or urethra are involved. Bilateral, albeit frequently asymmetrical, progressive subconjunctival scar formation is the key ocular feature in ocular MMP, otherwise known as ocular cicatricial pemphigoid (OCP) (1–4). Loss of vision or even loss of the eye may result from corneal involvement.

Epidemiology

OCP is uncommon. Estimates suggest that 1 in 8,000 to 46,000 ophthalmic patients, depending on the series, have OCP (5–7). The disease may be more common than is recognized, however, given the exclusion from these numbers of patients presenting with predominantly skin or nonocular mucosal involvement. Also, the diagnosis of this disorder in its early stages is difficult, and most cases of early disease may be uncounted in the epidemiologic estimates. MMP has no geographic or racial predilection, but a genetic susceptibility has been suggested (8,9). It is a

disease of relatively older populations, with a peak of presentation between the sixth and seventh decades (range 43 to 88 years) (10). Although considered to be a disease of the elderly, in many patients, because of the subtle nature of the subepithelial fibrosis in the earliest stages of the disease, it may have begun in the fourth or fifth decade of the life. Most series report a female predilection, with a female to male ratio of approximately 2:1 (1,8).

Clinical Features

MMP is a group of chronic inflammatory, blistering diseases predominantly affecting any or all of the mucous membranes, with or without clinically apparent scar formation. OCP is one subset of this group.

Ocular Involvement

At its onset and in the early stages, OCP is usually clinically indistinguishable from any other nonspecific chronic conjunctivitis. Patients frequently complain of conjunctival irritation, burning, tearing, hyperemia, and discharge. The earliest ocular manifestation of OCP is an intermittent, unilateral chronic papillary conjunctivitis, which eventually becomes bilateral. Foreign-body sensation and photophobia can occur, as a consequence of breakdown of the corneal epithelium (11–13).

Later in the course of the disease, conjunctival bullae can form. These are rarely seen by the ophthalmologist, as they evolve quickly into ulcerous lesions, conjunctival thickening, and scarring. The earliest sign of conjunctival scarring is formation of lacy white lines of subepithelial fibrosis, commonly perivascular in localization and appearing first in the inferior fornix (1,12,14) (Fig. 20-1). Another early clinical sign is involvement of the canthal structures, leading to shallow canthal recesses (Fig. 20-2). Involvement of the medial canthus can lead to a loss of architecture, with flattening and obliteration of the normal conjunctival folds, plica, and caruncula (15). As the disease advances, progression of the subepithelial fibrosis results in "shrinkage" of the fornices and then formation of symblephara, fibrotic bands between the palpebral and bulbar conjunctiva.

TABLE 20-1. DISORDERS ASSOCIATED WITH CHRONIC CICATRIZING CONJUNCTIVITIS

Autoimmune causes
  Cicatricial pemphigoid
  Linear immunoglobulin A (IgA) disease
  Stevens-Johnson syndrome/toxic epidermal necrolysis
  Epidermolysis bullosa acquisita
  Dermatitis herpetiformis
  Bullous pemphigoid
  Paraneoplastic pemphigus
  Lichen planus
  Discoid lupus
  Lupus erythematosus
  Sjögren's syndrome
  Atopic keratoconjunctivitis
  Progressive systemic sclerosis
  Graft versus host disease

Infectious causes
  Trachoma
  Corynebacterium diphtheria
  Streptococci
  Adenovirus
  Chronic mucocutaneous candidiasis

Malignant causes
  Sebaceous cell carcinoma
  Squamous cell carcinoma
  Intraepithelial epithelioma
  Mucosa-associated lymphoid tissue lymphoma

Miscellaneous
  Ocular rosacea
  Sarcoidosis
  Conjunctival trauma (chemical or thermal)
  Ionizing radiation
  Self-induced cicatricial conjunctivitis
  Porphyria cutanea tarda
  Erythroderma ichthyosiform congenita
  Drug-induced conjunctival cicatrization

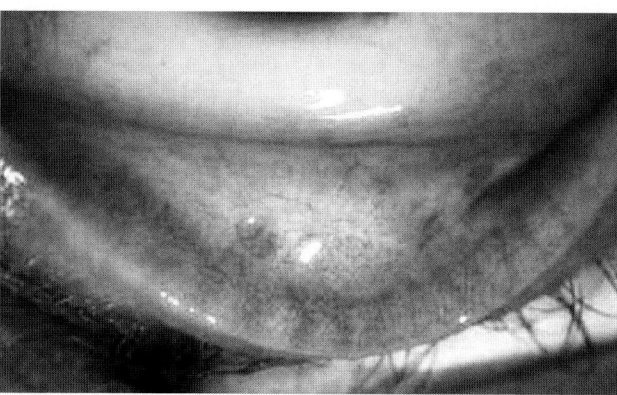

FIGURE 20-1. Lacy white lines of subepithelial fibrosis, commonly perivascular in localization in the inferior fornix and tarsal conjunctiva, representing the earliest sign of cicatrization.

with keratinization of the eyelid margins may occur. All these factors damage the corneal epithelium.

The advanced stages of the disease include blinding keratopathy, with corneal neovascularization, pseudopterygium formation, and progressive thinning and perforation. Secondary bacterial infection and ulcers may be associated with the compromised corneal epithelium. Use of topical corticosteroids, use of bandage contact lenses, chronic irritation, and epithelial defects resulting from trichiasis, meibomitis, and lagophthalmos may predispose to development of bacterial superinfections.

OCP-induced alterations in aqueous outflow may also predispose to development of glaucoma. Indeed, in a series of 111 patients, 29 (26%) had glaucoma (17). Interestingly, 27 of these patients had a history of glaucoma for a mean of 11.3 years before the diagnosis of OCP. Most had advanced glaucoma, with optic nerve damage and visual field loss.

Mucous Membrane Involvement

MMP also involves mucous membranes, other than conjunctiva. Oral lesions have been found to be the most common manifestation, occurring in 91% of patients in a series of dermatologic patients with MMP (18). In the same series, the conjunctival lesions were present in 66% of the patients.

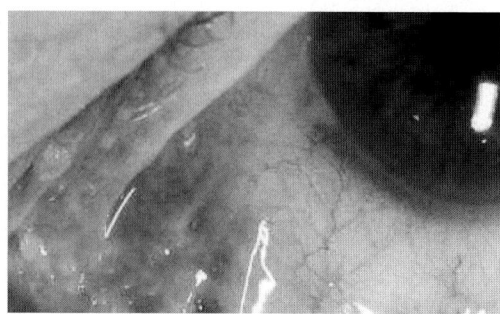

FIGURE 20-2. Involvement of the medial canthus, leading to shallow canthal recess and conjunctival subepithelial fibrosis.

Early symblephara are best demonstrated by external examination with a penlight, retracting the lower eyelid downward while the patient looks upward.

During the chronic stage, the disease manifests as a chronic conjunctivitis with cicatrix formation. Fibrosis beneath the conjunctival epithelium in the upper tarsal conjunctiva and superior fornix can cause obliteration of the ducts of the lacrimal and accessory lacrimal glands, resulting in keratoconjunctivitis sicca (13). Excessive and progressive conjunctival shrinkage later in the disease course alters the architecture of the lids and causes lagophthalmos and exposure, or entropion. Severe prolonged conjunctival cicatrization, in the absence of effective therapy, may cause ankyloblepharon, fusion of the lower eyelid to the bulbar conjunctiva, resulting in a restriction of ocular motility (1,13–16) (Fig. 20-3). Alterations in the orientation of eyelash follicles as a consequence of the scarring process can produce trichiasis and distichiasis, and squamous metaplasia

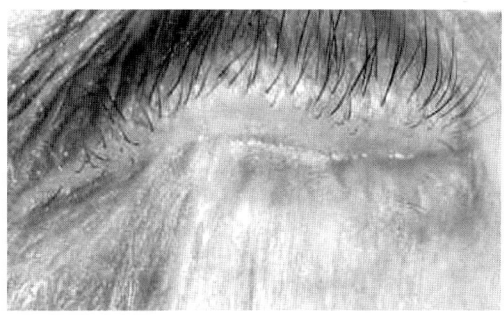

FIGURE 20-3. Ankyloblepharon, total fusion of the eyelids to the bulbar conjunctiva and cornea.

In ophthalmic series (all patients having conjunctival involvement), 15% to 50% also had oral mucosal lesions (1,10,19).

The most common finding in the mouth is desquamative gingivitis, which may be patchy or diffuse, with redness, easy bleeding, and ulcerations (14,20,21). Another form of oral mucosal involvement is vesicle and bulla formations of the oral mucosa that develop rapidly, remain intact for a few days, and then rupture (22). Involvement of the larynx, trachea, or esophagus also occurs. Esophageal involvement is not uncommon and has been reported in as many as 27% of patients (23); it may lead to heartburn, dysphagia, and fatal aspirations (24). The laryngeal and tracheal involvement with stenosis may cause difficulty in breathing, intermittent hoarseness, or dysphonia, and this requires endoscopic evaluation (25,26). Because many patients first present with ocular symptoms, ophthalmologists must inquire about signs of potential life-threatening esophageal and laryngeal involvement, such as hoarseness and difficulty in breathing or swallowing. Scarring and stenosis may lead to fatalities and thus warrant special attention and referral for evaluation.

Cutaneous Involvement

Skin lesions occur in 9% to 24% of patients with MMP, depending on the series (1,4,18). It is less frequent than mucous membrane involvement and can be of two types: (a) recurrent vesiculobullous, nonscarring eruptions that involve the extremities and inguinal area (similar to but smaller than those seen in bullous pemphigoid); or (b) localized erythematous plaques with overlying vesicles and bullae of the scalp and face that evolve into pruritic blisters that rupture and leave scars (Brusting-Perry dermatitis) (13,25).

Associated Medical Conditions

OCP can be associated with other "autoimmune" disorders. An association with rheumatoid arthritis has been noted (27) and confirmed by others (1,28). In the largest series of 130 patients with OCP, 23 patients had an associated

medical condition (1). Nineteen of the 130 (15%) had rheumatoid arthritis. Also, in the same series, three patients had systemic lupus erythematosus, and one had multiple autoimmune phenomena. Wegener's granulomatosis has also been reported to occur simultaneously with MMP (29).

Pathogenesis and Immunology

Mucous membrane pemphigoid is an autoimmune disease characterized by the presence of autoantibodies, most commonly immunoglobulin G (IgG), that bind to autoantigens located in the conjunctival epithelial basement membrane zone (BMZ), and of components of both classical and alternative complement pathways. A T-cell dysregulation, abnormal serum levels of cytokines such as interleukins (IL)-1, IL-5, IL-6, and tumor necrosis factor (TNF)-α and -β can be detected (30).

There is a genetic predisposition to OCP with an increased incidence of human leukocyte antigen (HLA)-DQB1*0301 gene (DQw7) (9). HLA-DR2 (31) and HLA-DR4 antigens (32) have also been implicated. HLA-DQ molecules on the surface of antigen-presenting cells function immunologically by presenting antigen to T cells. The DQB1*0301 gene may have a role in T-cell recognition of basement membrane antigens, resulting in production of anti-BMZ IgG autoantibodies (33).

By virtue of the genetic susceptibility, some triggering agent(s) during the patient's life can cause development of autoantibodies to the target autoantigens at the BMZ. Some identified environmental triggers include systemic practolol therapy (34) and ocular exposure to epinephrine (35), idoxuridine (36), phospholine iodide (37), and Humorsol (38). The autoantigens located in the BMZ include the β4 protein of the α6β4 integrin as a highly targeted autoantigen (39,40) and epiligrin (α3 subunit of laminin 5) (41).

Binding of the autoantibody to the target autoantigen at the epithelial BMZ is followed by activation of the complement cascade, with deposition of the complement products and inflammatory cells predominantly at the level of the basal epithelial hemidesmosome and the lamina lucida of the basement membrane (14). Lymphocytes, macrophages, dendritic cells, plasma cells, neutrophils, and mast cells are recruited to the subepithelial tissues in different compositions depending on the clinical activity of the disease. OCP is not simply an antibody-mediated disease, but rather involves T-cell dysregulation as well (42).

There is evidence that soluble factors, especially fibrogenic cytokines secreted by inflammatory cells and fibroblasts, play an important role in the immunopathogenesis of acute MMP by remodeling the matrix in the conjunctival stroma, possibly by regulating the altered metabolism of matrix proteins (43). Studies on cytokine profiles have shown an increased expression of transforming growth factor (TGF)-β (43–45) and IL-5 (30), decreased levels of serum IL-6 (45), and elevated levels of serum IL-1 and IL-1 components (46) in patients with active OCP.

The absence of fibrogenic cytokines in chronic progressive OCP provides support for the idea that fibroblasts in the conjunctiva of patients with OCP may remain functionally and morphologically abnormal after withdrawal of cytokine influences (43).

Histopathology

The characteristic conjunctival scarring in OCP is a consequence of subepithelial fibrosis. Accumulating evidence indicates that the subepithelial fibrosis is mainly caused by macrophages and by conjunctival fibroblasts (1). The number of macrophages within the conjunctival subepithelial tissue is significantly increased in OCP and reflects the activity of the disease. One study has demonstrated a relationship in OCP between local proliferation of macrophages and increased expression of macrophage–colony-stimulating factor (m-CSF), mainly by conjunctival fibroblasts and infiltrating inflammatory cells (47). Macrophages, by producing fibrogenic cytokines such as TGF-β, platelet-derived growth factor, and basic fibroblast growth factor, stimulate the proliferation and migration of the fibroblasts—the cellular elements responsible for fibrosis (12). The conjunctival fibroblasts from patients with OCP are abnormally hyperproliferative, with a decreased doubling time in tissue cultures when compared with normal cells (48). These activated fibroblasts produce an abnormal new extracellular matrix and collagen, mostly type III (49). Thus the scarring that characterizes MMP appears to be due to excessive fibroblast proliferation and abnormal collagen synthesis.

The conjunctival epithelium in OCP shows squamous metaplasia with parakeratosis and keratinization (50), associated with a decreased number or absence of mucin-producing goblet cells (51). Destruction of the goblet cells and obliteration of the lacrimal gland ductules cause severe dry eye. The inflammatory cells in the conjunctiva of OCP patients are predominantly mononuclear cells, mainly T lymphocytes. There is a threefold increase in T lymphocytes within the epithelium and a 20-fold increase within the substantia propria of bulbar conjunctival tissue of patients with OCP (42). These T cells are activated, as evidenced by the expression of IL-2 receptors on their cell surfaces. The dendritic cells are also increased, 25-fold, over normal levels. The number of macrophages and neutrophils was also found to be increased, particularly in the acute stages of the disease, and correlate with the clinical activity of the disease (44). Interestingly, the infiltrations in subacute and chronic OCP differ greatly. The number of mononuclear cells, neutrophils, CD45$^+$ cells, and CD3$^+$ cells, as well as HLA-DR expression, were significantly higher in the subacute than in the chronic disease, with some eosinophil granule proteins such as eosinophil-derived cationic protein and major basic protein in the epithelium and substantia propria of the conjunctiva in the subacute form (52). A study of the mast cell subsets in the conjunctivae in OCP revealed a predominance of connective tissue mast cells (53).

Diagnosis

Unfortunately, the diagnosis of OCP is frequently delayed because of the nonspecificity of its early symptoms and the difficulty of recognizing the early stages. Patients are usually diagnosed with MMP when they already have advanced signs of conjunctival cicatrization and ocular surface disturbances. To reduce the delay in diagnosis, a careful ocular and systemic examination must be performed for any patient with conjunctival scarring. The clinician should inquire about the presence of oral lesions, past and present oral and topical medications, any history of previous ocular infection, drug reaction, trauma, chemical burns, ionizing radiation, atopy, and conjunctival surgery. Facial skin, scalp, nasal and oral mucosa, finger and wrist joints, nail beds, and periungual folds should be closely examined for any associated systemic or iatrogenic disorders. Because MMP may lead to blindness, it is of critical importance to make the diagnosis as early as possible to allow early treatment.

Conjunctival biopsy facilitates the early diagnosis of MMP. A lower bulbar conjunctival specimen is harvested from the actively inflamed eye and divided into three equal samples for light microscopic, electron microscopic, and immunohistochemical studies. Linear immunoreactant (immunoglobulin and/or complement) deposition at the BMZ confirms the diagnosis (54,55). Other disorders such as bullous pemphigoid, epidermolysis bullosa acquisita, and paraneoplastic and drug-induced cicatrizations may produce a similar pattern. Also, absence of immunoreactant does not exclude MMP, and regrettably, false-negative biopsy occurs in a significant proportion of patients (3,12). Immunohistochemical analysis of biopsied conjunctiva by direct immunofluorescence yields a positivity rate of 50% to 60% (55,56). Routine use of the immunoperoxidase technique in immunofluorescent-negative biopsies, allied with appropriate harvesting and handling of conjunctiva, increases the diagnostic yield to more than 80% (56). Especially in cases of multiple negative biopsies, other specimens submitted for light microscopic and electron microscopic studies should be carefully examined to look for other possible causes of cicatrizing conjunctivitis.

The early diagnosis of MMP is challenging yet essential, because the ocular manifestations may be the first clinical presentation of this potentially fatal disease.

Disease Course

Mucous membrane pemphigoid runs a chronic course characterized by progressive conjunctival cicatrization and

TABLE 20-2. MONDINO'S STAGING SYSTEM

Stage	Characteristics
Fornix foreshortening (loss of inferior fornix depth)	
1	0–25%
2	25–50%
3	50–75%
4	75–100%

TABLE 20-4. MODIFICATION OF FOSTER'S STAGING SYSTEM

Stage	Characteristics
1	Subconjunctival scarring and fibrosis
2	Fornix foreshortening (loss of inferior fornix depth)
	a 0–25%
	b 25–50%
	c 50–75%
	d 75–100%
3	Presence and number of symblepharons countable (horizontal involvement by symblepharons)
	a 0–25%
	b 25–50%
	c 50–75%
	d 75–100%
4	Ankyloblepharon, frozen globe

shrinkage. Assessment of progression of conjunctival changes with some standardized assessment system is required to determine the stage and inflammatory activity of the disease. The clinician should consider drawings in conjunction with photographs of the external eye at each visit to make comparisons with the previous clinical findings.

Two established staging systems are in use for the assessment of progression in MMP. Mondino's system is based on the percentage loss of inferior fornix depth (4,21) (Table 20-2). Foster's staging system is based on the presence or absence of specific clinical signs in the lower forniceal conjunctiva (57) (Table 20-3). A modification of Foster's original classification is also in use (58) (Table 20-4).

Differential Diagnosis

MMP must be differentiated from a variety of disorders that can cause cicatrizing conjunctivitis (Table 20-1). The chronic progressive course of conjunctival cicatrization, the sine qua non of a diagnosis of MMP, can also be seen in linear IgA disease, bullous pemphigoid, epidermolysis bullosa acquisita, and drug-induced conjunctival cicatrization, in a relatively milder form. As in MMP, direct immunofluorescence shows linear immune deposits at the BMZ in linear IgA disease, epidermolysis bullosa acquisita, and bullous pemphigoid. In MMP, epidermolysis bullosa acquisita, and bullous pemphigoid, the deposits mainly consist of IgG and C3, but in linear IgA disease they are mainly IgA (59). Circulating autoantibodies may be found in all these disorders, but are observed with higher frequency and higher titers in MMP. The morphology and distribution of eruptions may help in the differential diagnosis of these conditions.

Clinically, involvement of canthal structures and upper tarsal conjunctiva is an important early clinical sign of MMP; in contrast, the conjunctival cicatrization due to

TABLE 20-3. FOSTER'S STAGING SYSTEM

Stage	Characteristics
1	Subconjunctival scarring and fibrosis
2	Fornix foreshortening, any degree
3	Presence of symblepharon, any degree
4	Ankyloblepharon, frozen globe

topical or systemic medications involves mainly the lower fornix (15,60).

Cicatrizing conjunctivitis resulting from chemical burns, radiation exposure, and membranous conjunctivitis is generally nonprogressive, unlike that in MMP (11). Stevens-Johnson syndrome should also be considered in the differential diagnosis. However, the initial acute illness, typical skin lesions, and history of exposure to a known trigger easily differentiate this condition from MMP.

Treatment

The natural history of MMP is such that, if untreated, chronic gradual progression of the inflammation leads to bilateral blindness. Early diagnosis and therapy can prevent ocular complications, but advanced stages of the disease often result in irreversible visual loss despite the institution of therapy. The objectives of management of MMP involves control of the systemic immunodysregulation, inhibition of the progressive conjunctival scarring, and maintenance of a normal relation between the eyelids and the ocular surface to prevent ocular surface disturbances. Because MMP is a systemic disease, no topical therapy is effective in controlling progression of the ocular inflammation and the scarring process. Failure of topical and subconjunctival treatment with corticosteroids, cyclosporine, mitomycin-C, and retinoids has been well demonstrated (61). Once the diagnosis is established, long-term systemic therapy must be instituted as soon as possible.

Dermatologists evaluated the efficacy of systemic corticosteroids in the early 1970s (62). Although high-dose oral prednisone was effective in preventing progression of the mucosal shrinkage, many of the patients developed unacceptable steroid-induced complications because of the high dose required. Azathioprine was then shown to be beneficial as a nonsteroidal immunomodulatory therapy (63).

Soon after came a report of the cure of a patient with systemic cyclophosphamide therapy (64). In the early 1980s the results of the first large ophthalmic case series demonstrating the efficacy of systemic immunosuppression were published, reporting cessation of the inflammation and cicatrization with azathioprine or cyclophosphamide combined with systemic steroid therapy (57). Another large study followed (21).

Formulation of a standard treatment protocol for MMP is very difficult. The therapeutic approach should take into consideration the site involved, the severity of involvement, and the rapidity of progression. The importance of considering the specific site is based on the observations that ocular involvement can lead to blindness, tracheal and laryngeal involvement can lead to airway obstruction, and genital involvement can lead to urinary and sexual dysfunction.

Diaminodiphenylsulfone (dapsone) is the usual initial chemotherapeutic agent for patients with mild to moderate inflammation and slow progression of the disease (65,66). Dapsone should not be given to patients with a history of sulfa allergy or glucose-6-phosphate dehydrogenase deficiency. It has potentially severe adverse effects such as hemolytic anemia, agranulocytosis, aplastic anemia, hepatitis, and peripheral neuropathy. A complete blood count, liver function tests, and glucose-6-phosphate dehydrogenase activity should be evaluated before initiating therapy. The usual initial therapeutic dose of dapsone is 25 mg twice daily. If the drug is tolerated well and has no side effects, the dose can be increased to 50 mg twice daily if necessary. The highest dose employed is 150 mg/day. If the patient has taken the drug for 12 weeks with no response, advancement to more conventional systemic immunosuppression with methotrexate (7.5–15 mg once weekly), or daily azathioprine (2–3 mg/kg), or daily mycophenolate mofetil (1–2 g/day) follows (49). In severe or rapidly progressive forms, the first-line treatment of choice is systemic prednisone (1 mg/kg/day) combined with cyclophosphamide (2 mg/kg/day). To avoid long-term complications, steroids should never be used as sole agents in treating MMP, and tapering of steroids should begin within 6 weeks of initiating treatment. Analyses of success rates with the recommended systemic immunosuppression approach show that approximately 6% to 10% of patients continue to experience progression of inflammation with irreversible damage to the ocular surface, despite the best treatment efforts (21,67).

In progressive cases, intravenous immunoglobulin treatment can be used as an alternative to the systemic immunosuppressive agents (68,69). Intravenous infusions of pooled human Ig, 2 to 3 g/kg/cycle divided over 3 days and repeated every 2 to 6 weeks, is the usual regimen. Intravenous Ig exhibits a number of immunomodulatory properties that are mediated by the Fc portion of IgG and by the spectrum of variable regions contained in the immunoglobulin preparations (70). Although the major component of intravenous Ig is IgG, other minor components such as solubilized lymphocyte surface molecules also exhibit immunoregulatory effects on T- and B-cell immune responses. The lack of significant side effects makes intravenous Ig a valuable therapeutic agent.

Daclizumab is a humanized IgG monoclonal antibody produced by recombinant DNA technology that specifically binds CD25 of the human IL-2 receptor expressed on activated T lymphocytes. The medication is composed of 90% human and 10% murine antibody sequences that function as an IL-2 receptor antagonist for inhibiting IL-2 binding, thus selectively inhibiting activated but not resting T cells (71). Daclizumab is administered intravenously at a dose of 1 mg/kg per treatment, with treatment every 2 weeks during the first 12 weeks of therapy, every 3 weeks until week 24 of therapy, then every 4 weeks until week 52. In total, the patient receives 18 doses of the medication during an entire year. Preliminary experience using daclizumab in the treatment of resistant cases shows promise (72).

The treatment recommendations presented here are modified from the consensus statement of the First International Consensus on Mucous Membrane Pemphigoid, published in 2002 (73).

Prolonged periods of remission without therapy can be maintained in approximately one third of patients with MMP following systemic immunosuppressive treatment. Follow-up must be continued for life, as relapses occur in 22% of those in remission off therapy (74). It is also essential to involve an expert chemotherapist for the long-term care of patients with MMP, to monitor for potential toxicity and side effects of the medications.

Rehabilitation

Management of the ocular surface problems in MMP patients is extremely important. Severe abnormalities of the tear film with dry eye can be treated with artificial tears and lubricating ointments, preferably preservative-free, or with punctal occlusion if scarring has not already occluded the puncta. In the presence of trichiasis and lid abnormalities, therapeutic contact lenses can be used in patients with sufficient forniceal depth, to prevent the cornea from epithelial breakdown. Fluid-ventilated, gas-permeable scleral lenses are a valuable tool in the management of severe ocular surface problems. In addition to enhancing vision, they have the potential to reduce greatly the disabling ocular pain and photophobia and the rate of persistent/recurrent corneal epithelial defects. The therapeutic benefits of these lenses result from the oxygenated aqueous environment created over the corneal epithelium. The oxygenated precorneal fluid compartment maintained at neutral pressure protects the epithelial surface from the desiccating effects of exposure to air and the friction generated by blinking, and avoids the shearing forces generated during the blink-induced movement of soft lenses (75).

Keratinization of the eyelids and conjunctiva stimulates the colonization of bacterial pathogens and places MMP patients at significant risk for ocular surface breakdown and bacterial blepharoconjunctivitis and keratitis. In more than 80% of patients, the eyelids or conjunctiva have colonies of potential pathogens (4), so cultures should be taken frequently and if positive, the patient should be treated with topical antibiotics.

Surgery or any mechanical manipulation of the eyelids or conjunctiva should be strictly avoided during active stages of the inflammation, because the trauma of the surgery can trigger further conjunctival inflammation with resultant additional conjunctival scarring (1,76). All surgical procedures must be delayed until the conjunctival inflammation is completely controlled. After the eye becomes quiescent, procedures involving manipulation of the eyelids and conjunctiva or cataract surgery can be performed while the patient is taking immunosuppressive therapy. Penetrating keratoplasty may be performed to restore sight in patients with corneal pathology, after controlling the primary immunologic process and aggressive treatment of the mechanical factors damaging the ocular surface, such as anatomic lid problems from scarring, conjunctival and lid margin keratinization, and trichiasis, provided that the patient does not have significant dry eye. The success of penetrating keratoplasty in these patients is generally limited because of dryness and impairment of eyelid functions (77). Limbal stem cell transplantation can be performed prior to or in combination with penetrating keratoplasty to improve outcomes, again provided that the effort is not sabotaged by a hostile environment such as dry eye, lagophthalmos, distichiasis (78). However, patients with underlying immunologically mediated diseases generally have lower success rates with these procedures than do patients with noninflammatory ocular surface diseases (79).

In patients with the final stages of MMP, keratoprosthesis is the only viable option to restore sight. Although the recent advances aimed at preventing and treating complications after keratoprosthesis surgery have improved prognosis, the potential complications are considerable: retroprosthetic membrane, glaucoma, endophthalmitis, extrusion of the prosthesis, and retinal detachment (80). Dohlman's success rate for achieving 20/200 or better vision in patients with OCP employing his keratoprosthesis is 33% after 2 years. However, at 5 years none of the seven patients retained vision better than 20/200 (80).

STEVENS-JOHNSON SYNDROME

Stevens-Johnson syndrome (SJS) is a rare, life-threatening, acute, multisystem inflammatory disorder that affects skin and mucous membranes, including the conjunctiva. A new classification, based on the pattern and distribution of cutaneous lesions, differentiates a closely related disease,

erythema multiforme major, from SJS (81). A retrospective reclassification of 76 cases (82) and a prospective international case-control study (83) supported the validity of this differentiation by demonstrating differing demographic characteristics, severity, causes, and risk factors for the two disorders.

Erythema multiforme (EM) is an acute, self-limiting disease of the skin and mucous membranes first described by von Hebra (84) in 1866. It is characterized by symmetrically distributed skin lesions, located primarily on the extremities and torso, and by a tendency for recurrences. In 1922, Stevens and Johnson (85) described two children who had fever, conjunctivitis, stomatitis, and a generalized exanthema with skin lesions distinct from EM. During the past 30 years it became widely accepted that EM and SJS, as well as toxic epidermal necrolysis (TEN), are all part of a single "EM spectrum." In both EM and SJS, pathologic changes in the earliest skin lesion consist of the accumulation of mononuclear cells around the superficial dermal blood vessels; epidermal damage is more characteristic of EM, with keratinocyte necrosis leading to multilocular intraepidermal blisters (86). However, there is little clinical resemblance between typical EM and SJS, and some researchers have proposed a reconsideration of the "spectrum" concept and a return to the original description (87–90). Some investigators suggest that the term *EM* should be restricted to acrally distributed typical targets or raised edematous papules. Depending on the presence or absence of mucous membrane erosions, the cases may be classified as EM major or EM minor (89). The term *SJS* should be used for a syndrome presenting with erythematous or purpuric macules, characterized by mucous membrane erosions and widespread blisters, often predominant on the chest (90). TEN is characterized by the most severe type of skin reaction with detachment of more than 30% of the body skin. Given the close connection between these disorders, this section necessarily discusses EM and TEN along with SJS.

Epidemiology

Both SJS and TEN are rare. The estimated incidence of SJS is approximately two to six cases per 1 million people per year, and that of TEN is 0.4 to 1.2 per million patient-years (91–93).

In a retrospective study covering a 14-year period (94), among an average of about 260,000 persons with demographic characteristics similar to those of the general population, there were about 25,000 hospital admissions per year. Of these, 61 possible cases of EM, SJS, or TEN were identified from the computerized hospital discharge files. Then, based on record review and the application of a uniform set of diagnostic criteria, 37 of the 61 patients (61%) were classified as having EM, SJS, or TEN. Of these, 16 cases (43%) were attributed to drugs administered to the patients prior to hospitalization. The overall incidence of hospitalization for EM, SJS, or TEN due to all causes was 4.2 per 10 million person-years. The incidence of TEN alone due to all causes was 0.5 per 10 million person-years. The incidence of EM, SJS, or TEN associated with drug use was 7.0, 1.8, and 9.0 per 10 million person-years for persons younger than 20 years of age, 20 to 64 years of age, and 65 years of age and older, respectively. Drug therapies with reaction rates in excess of 1 per 100,000 exposed individuals included phenobarbital (20 per 100,000); nitrofurantoin (7 per 100,000); sulfamethoxazole and trimethoprim, and ampicillin (both 3 per 100,000); and amoxicillin (2 per 100,000) (94).

SJS can produce devastating long-term ocular complications by causing conjunctival scarring. Ocular involvement occurs in 48% to 81% of patients with SJS (95–97). In a retrospective study covering a 34-year period, 366 patients admitted to hospital with EM, SJS, or TEN were identified (98). Eighty-nine patients (24%) had ocular manifestations at the time of their acute hospital stay. Ocular involvement occurred later, during the follow-up period, in 9% of patients with EM, in 69% with SJS, and in 50% with TEN. The ocular problems were more severe in patients with both SJS and TEN.

No racial or geographic predilection has been found for SJS. Although it can affect individuals of almost any age, it is most frequently seen in younger populations (86,99). There may be a slight male preponderance.

Clinical Features

All three disorders, EM, SJS, and TEN, share many clinical features. The most recent and widely accepted diagnostic criteria for these bullous skin diseases are summarized in Table 20-5 (94). SJS generally has a prodromal period of 1 to 14 days, characterized by symptoms of an upper respiratory tract infection, malaise, fever, headache, prostration, and arthralgias (86,99,100). After the prodromal period, the cutaneous and mucosal lesions begin to develop. The cutaneous lesions consist of round erythematous macules, which rapidly develop into papules, as well as vesicles, bullae, and epidermal necrosis. These lesions most often occur on the dorsal aspects of the hands and feet and the extensor surface of the extremities. The characteristic "iris" or "target" lesion is produced by hemorrhage in the vesicles and is seen as a red center surrounded by a pale zone and another red ring around the pale zone (101). Healing of the skin lesions leaves residual hyperpigmentation and scarring.

SJS may involve any mucous membrane, with a predilection for mouth, conjunctiva, and genitalia (98). The mucosal lesions are bullous, clear, or hemorrhagic, and their rupture results in membrane or pseudomembrane formation with a painful and hemorrhagic base. Epithelialization of the mucosal lesions usually occurs within a week from onset, but the acute phase of the disease usually lasts

TABLE 20-5. CLINICAL FEATURES OF BULLOUS SKIN DISEASES

Disorder	Characteristics
Erythema multiforme	Target lesions, individual lesions <3 cm in diameter, no or minimal mucous membrane involvement, <20% of body area involved
Stevens-Johnson syndrome	Less than 20% of body area involved in first 48 hours, greater than 10% body involvement, target lesions, individual lesions <3 cm in diameter, fever, mucous membrane involvement (at least two)
Toxic epidermal necrolysis	Bullae and/or erosions in >20% of body area, bullae developing on erythematous base, occurring on non-sun-exposed skin, skin peeling off in >3-cm sheets, frequent mucous membrane involvement, tender skin within 48 hours of onset of rash, fever

Adapted from Chan et al. (80)

until the end of the third week (102). The oral lesions are the most commonly seen mucosal lesions, with swollen and crusted lips.

A bilateral, symmetrical, nonspecific conjunctivitis occurs concurrently with the lesions on other mucous membranes and the skin. Sometimes, conjunctivitis may precede the skin eruption (102). In the acute phase of the disease, the severity of the conjunctival involvement varies from a mild catarrhal conjunctivitis to hemorrhagic pseudomembranous or membranous conjunctivitis with swollen, ulcerated, and crusted eyelids (103). Purulent conjunctivitis may also be seen, due to the secondary bacterial infections, most commonly gram-positive cocci (104). Anterior uveitis may also occur at the acute stages of the disease and often resolves spontaneously (95,102,105). The acute phase of the ocular involvement usually lasts 2 to 3 weeks. Devastating ocular complications such as dry eye, symblepharon and ankyloblepharon formation, conjunctival epithelial squamous metaplasia, trichiasis, distichiasis, entropion, lagophthalmos, corneal epithelial defects, corneal ulceration, neovascularization, and conjunctivalization of the cornea can occur in patients with pseudomembranous or membranous conjunctivitis (96,102,105). In these patients the conjunctiva heals with scarring. Destruction of the goblet cells and cicatrization and obstruction of the lacrimal ducts can cause severe dry eye. Obliteration of the lacrimal puncti by fibrosis may cause initial epiphora in some patients in the early stages (103). In the presence of the severe abnormalities of the tear film and eyelids, corneal complications such as epithelial erosions, ulcers, vascularization, opacification, and perforation may develop.

Pathogenesis and Immunology

The pathogenesis of SJS is poorly understood. The laboratory studies in this field are very limited, probably because of the rarity of these disorders as well as the seriousness of the patients' medical condition. Clinical and epidemiologic studies demonstrate that EM is most commonly related to herpesvirus infections or to other infections, malignancies, and is rarely related to drugs. On the other hand, SJS is nearly always related to drugs and never to herpes (90). Although drugs are the most frequent provocative factors in the pathogenesis of SJS, clinical and laboratory features fail to support a mechanism involving type I hypersensitivity reaction mediated with IgE (106).

Symptoms of drug-related SJS or TEN typically arise within 3 weeks after initiation of the therapy (94). If the patient is reexposed to the inciting drug, a reaction may begin within hours of restarting the therapy. The sulfonamides are the best-documented agents known to cause SJS in healthy patients. Anticonvulsants (phenytoin and phenylbutazone), penicillins, and salicylates are other drugs associated with SJS (107). SJS has also been observed after the use of topical medications. Ophthalmic proparacaine, sulfonamide, scopolamine, or tropicamide may be associated with SJS (108–110).

EM is mainly related to herpes simplex virus (HSV). Other less common agents in the etiology are *Mycoplasma pneumoniae, Yersinia enterocolitica*, measles, and small pox vaccination (111,112). TEN can also be associated with an infectious etiology; about one fourth of cases have been found to be associated with cutaneous staphylococcal infections in children (99).

One study suggests that immune complex formation and subsequent deposition in the cutaneous microvasculature play a role in the pathogenesis of EM (113). This study reported IgM deposition in the superficial blood vessels, along with C3, fibrin, and rarely IgA; IgG was not found. In addition, indirect immunofluorescein testing was negative for skin-reactive antibodies. In another study, serum samples from patients with EM were examined for the presence of HSV antigen in immune complexes, using the Raji cell radioimmunoassay. Immune complexes composed of antibody and HSV antigen were present in serum samples of patients with EM after HSV infection and in some cases of EM of uncertain cause (114).

A profound lymphopenia (peripheral blood lymphocyte count less than 1,000/mm³) with depletion of CD4$^+$ cells during the acute phase of the SJS has been reported (115). In contrast, CD8$^+$ cell counts were not significantly changed. Normal balance was restored after clinical recovery.

Interestingly, the T lymphocytes present in the lesions of TEN are CD8$^+$ antigen primed cytotoxic T lymphocytes, and they can exhibit, without any restimulation, a drug-specific cytotoxicity against autologous cells (116).

There may be an immunogenetic susceptibility to the development of SJS with ocular manifestations. The HLA-Bw44 antigen was found to have an increased frequency of 66.7% in white patients with SJS with ocular involvement, compared with a frequency of 20.4% in the white control population (117). Another study found that HLA-DQB1*0601 was present in 17% of patients with SJS versus 3% of control subjects, with a relative risk of 7.2 (118). None of the class II antigens tested appeared to offer a protective effect against the development of disease.

Histopathology

The clinical and histopathologic classification of EM, SJS, and TEN is difficult, given the lack of clear-cut criteria. Histopathologic specimens from patients with EM, SJS, and TEN have been reviewed based on a new clinical classification, and compared (119). No major differences could be found with respect to clinical diagnosis, gender, and age between the biopsies examined. Necrotic keratinocytes were found, ranging from individual cells to confluent epidermal necrosis. The epidermal-dermal junction showed changes ranging from vacuolar alteration to subepidermal blisters. The dermal infiltrate was superficial and mostly perivascular. It was sparse in SJS and TEN, and more pronounced in EM. Edema in the papillary dermis was evident occasionally in all clinical groups. In about half of the cases, at least one eosinophil was present in the dermis. In 10% of the sections, more than 10 eosinophils per field were visible. Eosinophils were less common in patients with the most severe forms of TEN—those with detachment of more than 30% of the skin surface area. No differences in the history of drug intake, or of infection with *Mycoplasma pneumoniae*, HSV, or other organisms, were evident between patients with or without eosinophils in their skin sections (119).

Histopathologically, skin and mucosal findings are very similar in SJS. There is a separation of epidermis and basement membrane from the dermis and areas of epithelial necrosis. Perivasculitis and edema of the superficial dermal blood vessels, which are surrounded by a small number of neutrophils and nuclear debris intermingled with mononuclear cells, characterize the histopathologic findings of the skin in acute SJS (120). Immunofluorescence reveals IgM and C3 depositions in vessel walls in more than 75% of early skin lesions (121). These immunoreactants appear as delicate granular deposits lodged in the walls of vessels of the papillary dermis. Such deposits are not present in normal, unaffected skin, although they can be induced there by injection of substances that increase vascular permeability. Factors that cause accumulation of mononuclear cells in the papillary dermis have not been fully elucidated, but receptors for the C3d fragment of C3 could be responsible (121). Factors that cause intercellular edema in the epidermis, epidermal-dermal separation, or necrotic keratinocytes are unknown. Cryoglobulins have been described, and antigens of *Herpesvirus hominus* have been measured in the cryoprecipitate of two patients who experienced EM following recurrent herpesvirus infection. EM commonly accompanies serum sickness reactions, which occur after injection of immune horse serum (von Pirquet and Schick). Such reactions are now well established as being due to circulating immune complexes in antigen excess.

Skin lesions of EM show time-dependent changes from early papular erythema to late target lesion, which consist of a peripheral elevated erythematous area and a central depressed area. In one study, circulating immune complex levels in the early papular erythema were occasionally elevated (122). Sera generated high levels of reactive oxygen species, and the nitroblue tetrazolium test revealed a positive reaction in the infiltrating cells around the blood vessels. These findings suggest that the papular erythema develops via a type III allergic reaction, followed by damage through reactive oxygen species. In the target lesion, the activity of histamine-*N*-methyltransferase, the major histamine-degrading enzyme, was markedly decreased in the peripheral elevated erythematous area, and the activity was recovering in the central clearing area. Intercellular adhesion molecule 1 (ICAM-1) and HLA-DR antigens were expressed on keratinocyte surfaces. An increased number of epidermal Langerhans' cells and CD4 cell infiltration were observed in the peripheral elevated erythematous area, and a decreased number of epidermal Langerhans' cells and CD8 cell infiltration in the central depressed area. These findings suggest that impaired histamine metabolism and cellular allergic reactions play important roles in development of the target lesion.

In skin biopsy specimens of patients with TEN, 80% of the infiltrating cells exhibited markers of macrophages, 15% were granulocytes, and only 5% were lymphocytes (almost exclusively CD8$^+$ T lymphocytes) (123). Early prenecrotic lesions showed exocytosis of mononuclear cells within the epidermis, with features of satellite cell necrosis and formation of colloid bodies. Almost all these mononuclear cells were macrophages, as evidenced by endogenous peroxidase-positive granules. These findings suggest that some kind of macrophage-mediated cytotoxicity may play a role in the necrosis of epidermal cells during TEN.

Early mucosal findings of EM and SJS demonstrate a nonspecific mononuclear perivascular inflammation and degenerative changes in the overlying epithelium, similar to skin lesions (124). In some severe cases, accumulation of the necrotic epithelial cells, neutrophils, and fibrinous exudate can produce pseudomembranes (103). True membranes can also be seen with severe necrotizing reactions.

In the late phases of TEN, conjunctival goblet cell density reveals goblet cell loss on both the interpalpebral bulbar and inferior palpebral ocular surfaces of more than 95% compared with normal eyes (125). In other ocular surface disorders, such as blepharitis and secondary keratoconjunctivitis sicca, this rate is 8%.

Various keratinization-related proteins known to play important roles in the physiologic keratinization process in human epidermis, including transglutaminase 1, involucrin, filaggrin, and the cytokeratin pair 1/10, were found to be expressed at high levels in the conjunctival tissues of patients with SJS (126,127). Hence, increased proliferation of basal epithelial cells appears to be correlated with the severity of the disease.

Diagnosis

The diagnosis of SJS is based mainly on clinical findings in both the acute and chronic phases. Laboratory investigations do not have a place in the diagnosis. New diagnostic criteria help differentiate SJS from EM and TEN (94). Skin or mucosal biopsy can be performed to confirm the diagnosis.

Disease Course

Both SJS and TEN are potentially fatal diseases. A mortality rate of 30% to 40% can be calculated for patients suffering from TEN. The prognosis for SJS patients is better, with a mortality rate of about 1% to 5% (128). Both EM and SJS can recur, sometimes requiring use of immunosuppressive agents to prevent further complications and late sequelae (129,130).

The ocular complications can be one of the lasting sequelae for survivors of these conditions. The outcome depends on the severity of the initial event, and on the initial treatment. Recurrent conjunctival inflammation unassociated with external factors such as lid margin keratinization, sicca syndrome, trichiasis, or entropion has also been reported in patients with SJS (131). The ultrastructural and immunopathologic characteristics of the conjunctiva from these patients were distinctly different from those of the conjunctiva from SJS patients without recurrent conjunctivitis, and suggested an active, immunologically mediated inflammation. Vasculitis or perivasculitis, immunoreactant deposition in vessel walls, vascular basement membrane disruption, thickening and reduplication, and a preponderance of helper T lymphocytes, macrophages, and Langerhans' cells were the notable distinguishing features in patients with recurrent conjunctival inflammation.

Sadly, SJS remains an important cause of severe, permanent, bilateral visual loss in two thirds of affected young patients, even at the best tertiary care centers, and there has been no significant improvements in prognosis within the past 40 years (98).

Differential Diagnosis

The impressive clinical picture of SJS is mimicked by few other disorders. Toxic shock syndrome, staphylococcal scalded skin syndrome, Kawasaki disease, Leiner disease, contact dermatitis, chickenpox, and burns must be considered in the differential diagnosis of the acute phase (132). It is of paramount importance to make the diagnosis at once, as the management and prognosis of these conditions are different.

The chronic ocular findings, with cicatrization, should be differentiated from ocular cicatricial pemphigoid, atopic keratoconjunctivitis, chemical burns, or ionizing radiation damage. The differential diagnosis can be made on the basis of the past history of initial acute illness and exposure to a trigger. Conjunctival biopsy can also be helpful to rule out other disorders such as cicatricial pemphigoid. Cultures can be confusing, as all the bullous skin diseases that cause detachment can secondarily cause skin colonization with various microorganisms.

Treatment

The management of cases of SJS, TEN, and EM remains difficult. In the acute phase patients are generally critically ill, and care must be provided in specialized intensive care units or in burn units (133). The main principles of symptomatic therapy are the same as for major burns: warming of the environment, correction of electrolyte disturbances, high caloric intake, and prevention of sepsis. Systemic antibiotic treatment should be considered.

The suspected immunologic origin of drug eruptions prompted the use of corticosteroids, immunosuppressive drugs, and anticytokines. The use and benefits of systemic corticosteroid therapy are controversial. Rare studies report a significantly increased rate of infections and other complications, particularly in pediatric patients with advanced TEN (134). However, several reports from one center demonstrated that high-dose (up to 4 mg/kg/day) corticosteroid therapy may be lifesaving in patients with "hypersensitivity syndrome" (visceral lesions with infiltration by activated eosinophils) (135–137). No fatalities or adverse effects due to corticosteroids were noted. The authors suggested that SJS due to a drug, a drug metabolite, or viral infection may mimic a graft-versus-host reaction in which the patient rejects skin, mucous membrane, kidney, or liver cells to which the drug, drug metabolite, or virus has bound. They proposed that corticosteroids suppress the inflammatory rejection, until the activating agent has been eliminated.

High oral doses of cyclosporine (138–140) or intravenous cyclophosphamide (141–143) have been administered to a few patients with TEN, most often following ineffective treatment with corticosteroids for 1 to 5 days. It remains doubtful that the progression of the lesions was shortened by these treatments. A few patients appeared to benefit from treatment with pentoxifylline, a drug that suppresses the production of TNF (144). But thalidomide, another suppressor of TNF production, significantly increased the death rate when tested in a double-blind placebo-controlled trial in patients with early TEN (145–147). The study was stopped because of the exceptionally high mortality rate in the treated group (10 of 12 patients died, compared with three of 10 in the placebo group). The data suggest that thalidomide is detrimental in TEN, possibly because of a paradoxical enhancement of TNF-α production.

Intravenous immunoglobulin, 1.5 to 2 g/kg, may be an effective treatment for SJS (148,149), on the basis of the ability to inhibit fas-fas ligand-mediated apoptosis. A rapid decrease in fever and shortening of the hospital stay have been reported. The potential benefit of this treatment needs confirmation by further studies.

Good hygiene of the ocular surface should be maintained during the acute stages of SJS. Patients should be seen daily. The eye surfaces should be kept moist by frequent instillation of preservative-free lubricants to maintain corneal epithelial integrity. Topical antibiotic ointments can be used to protect from superinfections, especially in patients with epithelial defect. Use of cycloplegics can be considered in patients with anterior uveitis. The role of topical steroids remains controversial; they tend to decrease the surface inflammation, but symblephara can still form (102). Topical steroids should be used judiciously, because there is a risk of superinfection particularly in patients with corneal epithelial defects. The role of topical cyclosporine for conjunctival/corneal involvement has yet to be determined, although some beneficial effect has been observed with systemic use (138–140).

Daily sweeping of fornices for lysis of symblephara is appropriate. Peeling of pseudomembranes can be attempted, but this is usually ineffective in preventing recurrence in the presence of active inflammation. Rigid symblepharon rings or large-diameter (20 or 22 mm) soft contact lenses can be used to line the palpebral surface in order to prevent symblepharon formation. Plastic wraps such as Saran Wrap can be applied to line the palpebral surface, placing one edge of the wrap in the fornix and draping it over the palpebral surface, eyelid margin, and skin, with mattress sutures to anchor it in the fornix. The wrap is left in place until the acute inflammation is over.

Patients and their first-degree relatives should be advised to avoid the responsible drug and chemically related compounds. Regulatory agencies should be notified of all cases.

Rehabilitation

The rehabilitation of patients with severe ocular surface problems resulting from SJS, EM, or TEN is challenging. Mucin-deficient keratoconjunctivitis sicca is very common. Preservative-free methylcellulose lubricants should be used frequently. Intermittent use of topical corticosteroids, and mucolytics such as 10% *N*-acetylcysteine, can control filament or abnormal mucus formation.

Trichiasis can be especially problematic. Patients with trichiasis and surface epithelial breakdown can undergo epilation, cryotherapy, argon laser treatment, electrolysis, or surgical correction (150,151). Mucous membrane grafting should be performed in an effort to protect against constant mechanical trauma to the ocular surface from epidermalization of the tarsal conjunctival surfaces, lid margin keratinization, and anatomic lid abnormalities such as entropion (152,153). Extended wear of an appropriately designed gas-permeable scleral contact lens can also be effective in promoting the healing of corneal epithelial defects in some eyes that fail to respond to therapeutic measures (154). Reepithelialization appears to be aided by a combination of oxygenation, moisture, and protection of the fragile epithelium by the scleral lens. However, microbial keratitis represents a significant risk.

Use of topical vitamin A to reverse the surface keratinization and recover the goblet cell population is controversial, although some studies report favorable results (155).

Surgical interventions should be postponed until the inflammation has completely subsided. However, amniotic membrane transplantation can be employed at early stages for patients suffering from nonhealing corneal epithelial defects (156). This procedure can serve either as a permanent therapy or as a temporizing measure until the inflammation has subsided and a definitive reconstructive procedure becomes possible. In fact, amniotic membrane was used successfully in patients with TEN who have extensive denuding of the body surface (157), long before its ocular use in SJS or TEN.

Limbal allograft transplantation with or without amniotic membrane transplantation can be attempted (79,158–160). However, long-term survival of these grafts, even in the best hands, is not good, given the extremely hostile ocular surface and the chronic-recurrent surface inflammation in this patient group. Requirement for long-term systemic immunosuppression is another factor that needs to be considered carefully for this group of patients. Cultivated corneal epithelial transplantation using denuded amniotic membrane as a carrier does not appear to have a better success rate than the conventional limbal and amniotic membrane transplantation (160).

Keratoprosthesis can be tried in patients with bilaterally very poor vision (161–163). However, among all patients requiring keratoprosthesis, those with SJS have the worst prognosis (80).

A recent report described a patient with end-stage ocular surface disease resulting from severe SJS (164). Complex surgical techniques were used, including penetrating corneal graft covered by a full-thickness lower lid skin advancement-flap to prevent impending perforation, submandibular salivary gland autotransplantation to treat the dryness, and finally osteo-odonto-keratoprosthesis to achieve visual rehabilitation. Although these procedures are complex and costly, requiring the collaborative subspecialist surgical skills of ophthalmologists and maxillofacial surgeons, gains were made well within the second year of rehabilitation, as the patient was able to take up a regular job. In view of the benefit in quality of life for the patient and the monetary savings for society, these procedures and studies for new advancements deserve support.

LINEAR IgA DISEASE

Linear IgA disease (LAD) is a chronic, acquired subepidermal blistering disease of the skin, and less frequently of the mucous membranes, characterized by homogeneous linear depositions of IgA autoantibodies along the basement membrane zone (165). Unlike skin and oral lesions, conjunctiva affected by LAD heals with scarring. The cicatrizing conjunctivitis associated with LAD is clinically indistinguishable from chronic cicatrizing conjunctivitis associated with other diseases such as cicatricial pemphigoid or SJS.

Epidemiology

Linear IgA disease is extremely rare. In a retrospective case series from Singapore, 67 patients were diagnosed with blistering skin disorders during a 2-year period (165). Bullous pemphigoid was the most common disorder, and only two patients had LAD. The incidence of LAD in Singapore was estimated as 0.26 per million population per year. The mean age of onset was 65 years, and there was no predilection for either sex. Another study found a mean annual incidence of autoimmune subepidermal bullous diseases of 10.4 per million people in France (166). The estimated overall number of new cases of these disorders was about 7 per million people per year, and the most common disorder was bullous pemphigoid. The estimated annual incidence of LAD was less than 0.5 per million people.

Clinical Features

The dermatosis in LAD is clinically similar to dermatitis herpetiformis, but unlike the latter it is not associated with gluten-sensitive enteropathy. Affected patients generally present with pruritic, urticarial plaques, papules, and blisters (167). The lesions are mainly distributed over the trunk, face, scalp, eyelids, perioral region, lower abdomen, perineum, buttock, inner thighs, and extremities. Mucous membrane involvement occurs in the majority of patients (67%), involving oral, nasal, pharyngeal, and genital mucosa and conjunctiva (168). In children, the disease often shows an annular clustering of blisters resembling a "cluster of jewels."

Ocular involvement is typically bilateral and asymmetrical. There may be blisters on the eyelid margins or on the tarsal conjunctiva. As noted above, unlike skin and oral lesions, conjunctiva affected with LAD heals with scarring. Some patients have recurrent or persistent conjunctivitis indistinguishable from that seen in ocular cicatricial pemphigoid or SJS. However, LAD conjunctivitis is usually less aggressive; only a minority of patients develop progressive conjunctival cicatrization. In these infrequent cases, patients may develop scarring of the tarsal or canthal conjunctiva, shrinkage of the conjunctival fornices, scarring of the lid margins, symblepharon formation, loss of goblet cells, corneal neovascularization, and opacification that are indistinguishable from ocular cicatricial pemphigoid (169–171).

Pathogenesis and Immunology

LAD is an autoimmune disease characterized by IgA autoantibodies directed against the epidermal BMZ. The hemidesmosome is a membrane-associated supramolecular dermal-epidermal complex that links the cytoskeleton of the basal keratinocyte to structures within the papillary dermis. Different components of this complex have been identified as autoantigens in various autoimmune bullous skin diseases. Serum from patients with LAD contains IgA autoantibodies that are directed against the hemidesmosomal transmembrane glycoprotein bullous pemphigoid antigen 180 (BP180) (172). BP180 is a member of the collagen protein family and is also referred to as type XVII collagen or BP antigen 2 (173). It is a transmembrane protein constituent of the dermal-epidermal anchoring complex. The long-held hypothesis that BP180 functions as a cell-matrix adhesion molecule has been supported by recent investigations of human disorders of the dermal-epidermal junction in which BP180 is either genetically defective or targeted by the immune system. In generalized atrophic benign epidermolysis bullosa, mutations of BP180 result in an inherited subepidermal blistering disease. Investigators have shown that various antigenic sites on the extracellular domain of this anchoring filament protein are targeted by autoantibodies in other autoimmune bullous skin diseases, including bullous pemphigoid and cicatricial pemphigoid. The strongest reactivity in LAD is observed with the C-terminal portion of BP180. Interestingly, this is also the major region recognized by autoantibodies in patients with cicatricial pemphigoid.

BP180 spans the lamina lucida of the dermal-epidermal junction (174). The BP180 ectodomain consists of 15 interrupted collagen domains. The largest noncollagenous (NC) 16A domain is located next to the cell membrane. In cicatricial pemphigoid, autoantibodies are directed to both the NC16A domain and the C-terminus of BP180 that projects into the lamina lucida/lamina densa interface of the dermal-epidermal junction. In LAD, the epidermal 97-kd and keratinocyte-derived 120-kd autoantigens (LABD97 and LAD-1, respectively) have recently been identified as the portions of the BP180 ectodomain with which the IgA autoantibodies react (175). This finding correlates with the observation that there may be significant overlap of the clinical and immunopathologic findings in LAD and cicatricial pemphigoid.

Several drugs have been implicated in the development of LAD, including vancomycin, captopril, diclofenac, cefamandole, and somatostatin (176). There is also a somewhat (about 30% to 56%) increased incidence of HLA-B8 among patients with linear IgA disease (167,168). However, the significance of this observation is uncertain, as the incidence in patients with other bullous diseases and in the general population is 20% to 30%.

Histopathology

Linear IgA disease is characterized by loss of tissue adhesion in the dermal-epidermal junction and formation of a vesicle or bulla in the lamina lucida or under the lamina densa. Cutaneous biopsy specimens from patients with LAD demonstrate subepidermal cleavage associated with a nonspecific inflammatory cell infiltrate. Multiple microabscesses, acantholysis and fibrin at the tips of papillae, and leukocytoclasis are evident (177). There may be infiltration of eosinophils in and below bullae and occasionally a linear infiltrate of eosinophils along the basement membrane. The characteristic immunofluorescence finding in LAD is a homogeneous or sometimes linear deposition of IgA, but not IgG or IgM, along the dermal-epidermal junction in uninvolved skin and along the subepithelial basement membrane of mucous membranes (167,178). Conjunctival findings are similar to those of skin. The IgA in LAD is exclusively IgA1, suggesting that mucosal IgA may not make a major contribution to the skin or mucosal deposits (179).

The lymphocytic infiltrate, consisting principally of CD4+, HLA-DR+, and CD30+ T cells, has a predominantly perivascular distribution (180). Proinflammatory cytokines, such as TNF-α and interferon-γ (IFN-γ), show a moderate focal expression on the dermal perivascular sites; IL-8 has a particularly intense staining on all the epidermal cell layers and at perivascular and vascular sites. Other cytokines, such as IL-4 and IL-5, show intracytoplasmic staining on some cells of the dermal infiltrate (probably mastocytes and lymphocytes) and at the dermal-epidermal separation sites. The specific tissue lesions of LAD seem to be the consequence of the IgA deposits at the BMZ and of the release of the cytokines, together with tissue-damage enzymes derived from neutrophils or eosinophils.

Diagnosis

The clinician should suspect LAD in any patient with a blistering skin disorder. The presence of cicatrizing conjunctivitis in preschool children, teenagers, or young adults should particularly raise the possibility of LAD (181).

The skin lesions of LAD have a heterogeneous clinical profile and may resemble those of dermatitis herpetiformis or bullous pemphigoid, with pruritic vesicles or bullae mainly distributed on the trunk and limbs. The exact diagnosis of LAD is based primarily on immunofluorescence techniques such as immune electron microscopy and Western blot analysis. The condition is distinguished from other subepithelial blistering diseases by the presence of linear IgA deposition, but not IgG or IgM, along the BMZ—a characteristic finding. Biopsy specimens from patients with dermatitis herpetiformis also demonstrate IgA deposition at the BMZ, but in a granular rather than linear form. Bullous pemphigoid specimens are characterized by primarily IgG deposition.

Specimens from the clinically uninvolved skin, blister fluid, serum, or conjunctiva may also be tested. The positivity rate for circulating IgA antibodies in serum is about 30% (182). The more sensitive indirect immunofluorescence using normal-appearing conjunctiva, instead of normal skin, gives a higher yield of positive results (183).

Disease Course

Untreated, LAD persists for life. Characteristically, the skin lesions of patients with LAD are benign and heal without scarring when treated with disease-modifying agents such as dapsone. Only a minority of patients have milia or scarring or therapy-resistant skin lesions. Dapsone treatment results in disease-free remission within about 1.9 years in the great majority of patients (184). Affected conjunctiva, however, heals with scarring. The ophthalmologic findings in these patients—subconjunctival fibrosis of the tarsal conjunctiva, shortening of fornices, and symblepharon formation—are clinically indistinguishable from the findings for other cicatrizing conjunctivitides such as cicatricial pemphigoid or SJS. Chronic ocular surface inflammation can lead to permanent vision loss due to progressive keratopathy. Treatment with systemic immunomodulating agents, therefore, is essential for patients with progressive ocular involvement.

An immune complex nephropathy can also develop in LAD, especially in younger children and adolescents, and less commonly in adults. IgA nephropathy has a variable course and is one of the most common primary types of glomerulonephritis to progress to end-stage renal disease. In fact, in about one fourth of patients IgA nephropathy progresses to terminal renal failure within 10 years of the apparent clinical onset. Its variable and often long natural history makes any prediction of outcome difficult. A retrospective multicenter study of pediatric patients examined the relationship between clinical and pathologic features and the subsequent development of end-stage renal disease. Seven variables were found to be predictive of end-stage renal disease: the presence of glomerular sclerotic changes, hypertension at biopsy, proteinuria at biopsy, old age at presentation, presence of crescents, black race, and male sex

(185). The same risk factors were documented in adult studies, especially the presence of glomerular sclerosis, proteinuria, and hypertension (186).

Differential Diagnosis

Linear IgA disease shares features of dermatitis herpetiformis, bullous pemphigoid, and cicatricial pemphigoid, all of which involve immunologically mediated pathologies at the BMZ. Clinically, the skin lesions of LAD may resemble those of dermatitis herpetiformis, with small grouped vesicles on an urticarial base. The lesions of dermatitis herpetiformis also heal without scarring. However, dermatitis herpetiformis is strongly associated with gluten-sensitive enteropathy. Also, direct immunofluorescent staining of biopsy specimens shows a granular, not linear, deposition of IgA at the dermal papillae of the dermal-epidermal junction, in patients with dermatitis herpetiformis.

Bullous pemphigoid is more common than are dermatitis herpetiformis or LAD. It is characterized by tense nongrouped bullae arising from an erythematous or urticarial base, which also resolve without scarring. Direct immunofluorescent studies show classic linear IgG deposition at the BMZ. Bullous pemphigoid and LAD also differ in the incidence of mucosal lesions. Whereas involvement of mucosal surfaces is rare in bullous pemphigoid, the prevalence of mucosal involvement is more than 60% in LAD (168). In contrast, the key similarity between LAD and cicatricial pemphigoid is the associated involvement of mucosal surfaces, most notably the conjunctiva and oral mucosa. In cicatricial pemphigoid, there is linear IgG or IgA and/or C3 deposition at the BMZ. Skin lesions are less frequent than are mucosal lesions in cicatricial pemphigoid, and when present they leave an atrophic scar after healing, i.e., the clearest distinguishing traits between cicatricial pemphigoid and LAD are the skin manifestations of the two diseases.

Treatment

The course of LAD is chronic, with rare occurrences of spontaneous remissions (187). Conventional first-line treatment for mild disease confined to skin is topical steroids. Dapsone, sulfapyridine, sulfamethoxypyridazine, corticosteroids, and immunosuppressive agents are the systemic drugs to be used in more severe cases, especially with ocular involvement (168). Generally, there is a rapid and complete clinical response, both of skin and mucosal lesions, to dapsone and sulfonamides (167,187). A decreased serum glucose-6-phosphate dehydrogenase or history of allergic reaction to sulfa antibiotic preclude the use of dapsone.

Reports of success with intravenous Ig therapy for the treatment of cutaneous involvement (188,189) and ocular involvement (190) in LAD have been published. In fact, intravenous Ig has been used successfully in many patients with various other blistering skin disorders, often after failure of conventional immunosuppressive chemotherapy. Evidence for the usefulness of intravenous Ig in the treatment of autoimmune bullous disorders is based mainly on uncontrolled trials and case reports (191). Collectively, high-dose intravenous Ig seemed effective in 81% of the patients with blistering disease, including pemphigus vulgaris, pemphigus foliaceus, bullous pemphigoid, pemphigoid gestationis, cicatricial pemphigoid, epidermolysis bullosa acquisita, and linear IgA disease. Patients were more likely to respond when intravenous Ig was used as adjunctive therapy (91% response rate) rather than as monotherapy (56% response rate). Various mechanisms of action are proposed in antibody-mediated conditions: blockade and downregulation of phagocytic function via Fc receptor, regulation of the idiotype–antiidiotype network, suppression of idiotype synthesis, T- and B-cell interference in antigen presentation, increase in suppressor lymphocytes, and intravenous Ig–cytokine interaction. Double-masked placebo-controlled trials are desirable to confirm the efficacy of intravenous Ig treatment, but the logistics of conducting such trials, given the rarity of the disorders under consideration, are imposing and formidable. A recently published consensus statement reviews the matter, and concludes that intravenous Ig therapy is an important addition to the therapeutic options available for treating autoimmune mucocutaneous blistering disease, and provides guidelines for its use (192).

Alternative, milder antiinflammatory therapies such as tetracycline and macrolide antibiotics have also been used to treat patients with LAD (193–196). Although the mode of action is speculative and the antiinflammatory mechanisms are unclear, macrolides are worth considering in children, because their use probably carries less potential risks. There are also single case reports of the use of other immunomodulatory treatments such as mycophenolate mofetil (197) and colchicine (198).

LICHEN PLANUS

Lichen planus is an autoimmune mucocutaneous condition of unknown etiology, with characteristic violaceous, polygonal, flat-topped papules and plaques commonly affecting the skin of wrists, ankles, extremities, and trunk. Mucous membranes, most typically those of the genitalia and mouth, are also involved. Conjunctival involvement is less common, but it may cause significant cicatrization indistinguishable from mucous membrane pemphigoid.

Epidemiology

Lichen planus is relatively common, with an incidence ranging from 1.4% of all patients examined at dermatology clinics to 5% of patients examined at oral medicine clinics (199). In one study, lichen planus constituted 0.38% of all dermatology outpatient diagnoses (200). The patient ages ranged from 8 to 76 years, most being in the range 20 to 49 years. Both sexes were equally affected. Mucosal involvement along with cutaneous lesions was observed in 16.8% of patients. Mucosal involvement alone is rare, occurring in only 1.1% of all cases (201).

Infrequently, lichen planus presents with ocular involvement, typically with eyelid lesions (202,203). Conjunctival involvement is even rarer, observed in 1 of 93 patients with cutaneous lichen planus in one study (204). There are only a handful of reports on the ocular involvement; most are single case reports. The largest case series includes only six patients (205).

Clinical Features

The morphologic characteristics and the site of involvement differentiate between two distinct clinical variants of lichen planus. In *cutaneous* lichen planus, the more common form, the eruptions are typically flat-topped papules, violaceous, scaly, angular, and primarily distributed on the trunk, scalp, flexor aspects of the limbs, and external genitalia. A reticulated pattern may be present atop the papule. Most lesions are slightly or profoundly pruritic. Nail involvement with dystrophy, ridging, splitting, and destruction of the matrix is often seen. In the *mucous membrane* form, the lesions involve mainly the oral mucosa and less commonly the genital mucosa. Oral lichen planus is the sole site of involvement in about 20% of patients. More commonly the oral lesions manifest as asymptomatic, subepithelial fibrosis, presenting as white to pale lilac linear reticulation or plaques on the buccal mucosal surface. The oral form may also have erosive or ulcerative lesions affecting gingiva, hard and soft palate, and esophagus. The erosive form is less common but potentially disabling (204).

The cutaneous form commonly involves the eyelids (202–204). Chronic conjunctival inflammation resulting in cicatrization can occur in the mucosal form (201,204,205). Patients present with redness, irritation, and discomfort. Subepithelial fibrosis in the upper and lower tarsal conjunctiva, foreshortening or total loss of the fornix, or symblepharon formation can occur in advanced cases. Thickening, hyperemia, and irregularity of the lid margins or trichiasis are sometimes observed. There are also reports of punctate epithelial keratitis and sicca syndrome (206–209).

Pathogenesis and Immunology

The etiopathogenesis of lichen planus is complex, with the involvement of T lymphocytes, mast cells, ICAM-1, and major histocompatibility complex class II antigens. Based on available evidence, lichen planus seems to involve a cell-mediated immunologic response to an induced antigenic change in the mucosa or skin. The immunologic process results in vacuolar degeneration, lysis, and, ultimately, liquefaction of the basal cells (210). Both antigen-specific and nonspecific mechanisms may be involved in the pathogenesis of lichen planus (211). Antigen-specific mechanisms include antigen presentation by basal keratinocytes and killing of antigen-specific keratinocytes by $CD8^+$ cytotoxic T cells. Nonspecific mechanisms include mast cell degranulation and matrix metalloproteinase activation (212). These mechanisms may combine to cause T cell accumulation in the superficial lamina propria, basement membrane disruption, intraepithelial T-cell migration, and keratinocyte apoptosis (213,214). The chronicity of lichen planus may be due in part to deficient antigen-specific TGF-β1–mediated immunosuppression (215). The initial event, however, and the factors that determine susceptibility are unknown.

Histopathology

Langerhans' cells, monocytes, and lymphocytes, infiltrating the basal layer of the epithelium and the BMZ, are the predominant cells of the inflammatory infiltrate in mucosa affected by lichen planus (216,217), suggesting a cell-mediated response. Lymphocyte-related necrosis of epithelium and nonspecific vasculitis are associated with an altered BMZ. Immunohistochemical studies of affected skin or oral mucosa demonstrate abnormal deposition in the BMZ of a fibrinogen band of variable width, with breaks and reduplications (199,217,218). Globular or cytoid body–like deposits of immunoglobulins, mainly IgM, have been detected in active lesions as well as in uninvolved skin biopsies (218). Deposition of fibrin in the papillary dermis and around follicular structures was present only in the active lichen planus papules. Although the presence of immunoglobulin cytoid bodies and fibrin was found to be highly characteristic of lichen planus, these findings were not specifically diagnostic. Morphologically identical deposits are often seen in lupus erythematosus and in chronic active eczema.

Conjunctival specimens from patients with active lichen planus have distinct characteristics (205,219). The affected epithelium is thickened, with an interface lymphocytic infiltrate along the lamina propria. Electron microscopy shows an irregular, abnormally thickened basement membrane with fragmentations and reduplications similar to the findings in oral mucosa. Direct immunofluorescence staining is remarkable for a linear and shaggy fibrinogen deposition along the BMZ. There is also positive staining for collagen IV and VII, fibrinogen, and laminin. It is of note that, unlike oral mucosa, normal conjunctiva does contain fibrinogen as a normal constituent of the basement membrane, and therefore merely finding, on direct immunofluorescence staining, fibrinogen at the basement membrane is not abnormal or

unexpected. Rather, it is the shaggy, spiked, irregular edge of the fibrinogen band that is the characteristic feature of the conjunctiva affected by lichen planus.

Diagnosis

The skin or oral lesions of lichen planus are quite typical. However, a previous diagnosis of lichen planus in a patient with cicatrizing conjunctivitis does not establish the diagnosis of conjunctival lichen planus. Lupus (discoid and systemic), bullous pemphigoid, and other autoimmune disorders are known to coexist in patients with lichen planus (220–222). Therefore, a thorough histologic analysis, including immunofluorescence staining and electron microscopic studies, is essential for a definitive diagnosis. Typical abnormal immunostaining for fibrinogen in the absence of immunoreactant deposition establishes the diagnosis.

Disease Course

In most patients the cutaneous lesions are self-limiting and follow a course of 1 to 2 years. Cutaneous lichen planus can be disabling in a small proportion of patients because of the extreme pruritus or disfigurement. Use of immunosuppressive agents may be required in these instances (223). Recurrent painful erosive lesions in patients with the mucosal form also require treatment.

There are conflicting reports on the association of lichen planus with different medical conditions such as diabetes, hepatitis C infection, and liver disease. The evidence does suggest, however, that oral cancers are more common in patients with oral lichen planus. One study reported a prevalence of 1.2% (224); another estimated a rate of developing oral carcinoma from oral lichen planus lesions as approximately 0.2% per person-year, compared with approximately 0.005% for the general adult population (225). Therefore, patients with oral lichen planus should be asked to report any changes in their lesions and/or symptoms and should be monitored at least once a year for malignant transformation.

Conjunctival involvement in patients with lichen planus can progress to irreversible damage to the ocular surface. In the largest study on the clinical characteristics of patients with conjunctival lichen planus, five of six had inferior forniceal symblepharon formation at presentation (205). In another study, both patients described had symblepharon formation along with severe corneal epitheliopathy (219). Corneal ulcers or melting and perforations have not been reported.

Differential Diagnosis

Lichen planus should be included in the differential diagnosis of any patient presenting with cicatrizing conjunctivitis. Performing appropriate investigations to distinguish conjunctival lichen planus from other autoimmune diseases, such as cicatricial pemphigoid, bullous pemphigoid, or lupus, is critical to proper management. In particular, the overlapping syndromes of lupus erythematosus and lichen planus should be considered. Electron microscopic and direct immunofluorescent studies of the affected conjunctiva aid in the definitive diagnosis of this condition.

We followed two adult patients with conjunctival lichen planus in the absence of oral or cutaneous manifestations, at the Wilmer Eye Institute, Johns Hopkins Hospital, Baltimore, Maryland. Both had advanced conjunctival involvement with symblepharon formation, keratoconjunctivitis sicca, and decreased vision due to severe corneal epitheliopathy. One of the patients (a 78-year-old white man) had been diagnosed with acne rosacea and was referred to us because of failure to respond to chronic treatment with doxycycline and topical steroids. The other patient (a 58-year-old white woman) had had rheumatoid arthritis for many years, with typical joint findings. She was being treated only with artificial tears, as her ocular symptoms were attributed to secondary Sjögren's syndrome. Both patients were diagnosed with lichen planus following a conjunctival biopsy, and were treated with topical cyclosporine. They both responded favorably within several weeks.

Treatment

Most patients with lichen planus are asymptomatic. However, some may have disfigurement or pruritus. Most cases can be treated successfully with topical corticosteroids with or without wet dressings or with occlusion. Cases of severe generalized lichen planus may require systemic corticosteroids. Chronic, aggressive lesions may need additional therapy ranging from psoralen plus ultraviolet A to retinoids or cyclosporine (226). Low-dose systemic cyclosporine may be required for patients with severe disease unresponsive to systemic steroids (227). Complications occurring during the natural course of the disease, ranging from infections to bullous disease or ulcerations, require special treatment considerations.

The most symptomatic forms of oral lichen planus are the erosive and atrophic types, with severe pain and a burning sensation in the mouth. These forms may interfere significantly with quality of life. Corticosteroids are the mainstay treatment for oral lichen planus, either systemic or high-potency corticosteroids. Most studies report favorable results with the topical steroid treatment, comparable to systemic treatment (228–230). Other forms of therapy include the use of topical cyclosporine (231–233) and retinoids (234), both systemic (etretinate) and topical (tretinoin). However, no single, standard protocol has proven effective with either systemic retinoids or topical cyclosporine. Results so far are controversial (235,236).

Topical tacrolimus appears to be a well-tolerated and effective therapy to control symptoms and clear the lesions of erosive or ulcerative oral lichen planus (237,238). However, the efficacy of this treatment needs to be evaluated in larger studies.

Reported treatments of conjunctival lichen planus have included topical and systemic cyclosporine, mycophenolate mofetil, and azathioprine (205,207,219). Topical cyclosporine should be considered alone or in combination with other medications, depending on the site and severity of involvement. It has a proven ability to accelerate apoptosis in clinically fibrotic tissues and should be considered in hyperproliferative conjunctival disorders (239). Oral cyclosporine seemed to accelerate control of the disease in four patients (205). However, toxicities were significant and dose limiting. The disease requires long-term treatment, and only one of five patients treated systemically was able to discontinue the medications while maintaining remission.

DRUG-INDUCED CONJUNCTIVAL CICATRIZATION

Chronic progressive cicatrizing conjunctivitis may arise as a rare adverse effect of certain drugs. Drug-induced conjunctival cicatrization is clinically indistinguishable from mucous membrane pemphigoid, and it has also been called pseudopemphigoid. The underlying mechanism remains unknown. The course of the disease is variable, and not always progressive after withdrawal of the causative drug. Thus the diagnosis of drug-induced conjunctival cicatrization early in the course of the process is essential in order to terminate as soon as possible potentially toxic treatment modalities.

Epidemiology

Drug-induced progressive conjunctival fibrosis and dacryostenosis was first described in 1951, caused by long-term use of topical furmethide iodide (240). Conjunctival cicatrization as an adverse effect of systemically administered drugs is exceptionally rare (241). One of the best-known systemic medications that cause conjunctival cicatrization is practolol, an early-generation beta-adrenoreceptor blocker. Patients treated with systemic practolol may suffer from not only conjunctival but also peritoneal fibrosis (242–247). In fact, for this reason, the drug was withdrawn from clinical use in 1975. Conjunctival cicatrization has also been reported in patients treated with orally administered iodides or bromides (242). However, because these patients were simultaneously treated with topically administered mercurous chloride (calomel), it is not known whether the conjunctival side effects were due to the direct toxicity of the systemic medications. Ocular side effects varying from irritation and excessive lacrimation to conjunctival fibrosis, and obstruction of the nasolacrimal canal can be observed in about 30% of patients receiving systemic 5-fluorouracil, especially for breast and gastrointestinal malignancies (248–250). This might be because the drug is excreted in significant concentrations in the tears (250).

There is a wide spectrum of conjunctival reactions to topical medications, ranging from an asymptomatic, nonspecific papillary conjunctivitis to symptomatic allergic blepharoconjunctivitis or severe cicatrizing conjunctivitis indistinguishable from mucous membrane pemphigoid. Various topical drugs have been implicated in the etiology of drug-induced cicatrizing conjunctivitis. Topical adrenaline can cause conjunctival fibrosis, secondary ocular surface alterations such as ectropion, and pigment deposits in the conjunctiva and cornea (35,251–254). The duration of exposure to the drug is an important factor in the development of sensitization to topically applied adrenaline (255). In an early study, 14 of 29 patients with "benign mucous membrane pemphigoid" had been treated with long-term topical adrenaline (256). Idoxuridine (36), guanethidine (257), dipivefrin (38,257), pilocarpine (38,257), timolol (258), echothiophate iodide (phospholine iodide) (37,257), and demecarium bromide (38) are some other drugs found to cause cicatrizing conjunctivitis. Various other medications, including prednisolone, chloramphenicol, naphthazoline, dexamethasone, betaxolol, tropicamide, tobramycin, and indomethacin, have also been implicated in the etiopathogenesis of conjunctival fibrosis and punctal stenosis, although a causal relationship could not be confirmed (259).

In a prospective study, the inferior fornix depth was measured in patients being treated with topical medications for glaucoma (60). Asymptomatic shortening of the fornices was detected in a significant proportion of the patients. Increasing age and topical medications for glaucoma (or the preservatives in the medications), used for 3 years or longer, were found to be independently associated with conjunctival shrinkage. The association of different classes of topically administered medications with conjunctival shrinkage may indicate a common pathway resulting in inflammation or toxicity.

Thimerosal (thiomersal) keratoconjunctivitis is a common problem in wearers of soft contact lenses, accounting for 32 (10%) of 312 consecutive referrals for contact lens–related problems to an ophthalmology clinic (260). The typical clinical findings consist of nonspecific conjunctival changes, limbal follicles, superficial punctate keratopathy, and superior corneal epithelial opacity. Thirteen atypical cases had superior limbitis occurring in isolation, coarse punctate keratopathy, severe keratopathy with visual loss, pseudodendritic corneal lesions, and acute conjunctival hyperemia without keratopathy. In another study, 38 patients were examined because of ocular redness, irritation, and corneal changes apparently related to soft contact lens wear. The corneal changes were transient and ranged

from faint epithelial opacities to a coarse, punctate epithelial keratopathy. Solutions containing thimerosal had been used by all of the patients for lens care, and 31 responded to an ocular challenge with a thimerosal-preserved lens lubricant. Twenty-seven of these 31 also reacted to thimerosal patch testing. Hypersensitivity to thimerosal was believed to be responsible for the clinical findings (261).

Most cases of drug-induced cicatrizing conjunctivitis arise in eyes exposed to topically used antiglaucoma medications. Despite scattered reports of scarring of the conjunctiva induced by these medications, no systematic review of the incidence of such changes has been undertaken. Most reviews focus their analyses on visual and systemic side effects.

Clinical Features

Drug-induced cicatrizing conjunctivitis presents a spectrum of clinical changes. The most common drug-related conjunctival reaction is a nonspecific papillary reaction along with conjunctival hyperemia, usually representing a nonspecific toxic reaction related to physical factors such as the pH or tonicity of the medication. Most patients with this stage remain generally symptom free over long periods of time. The symptomatic patients may have irritation, hyperemia, blepharoconjunctivitis, and corneal edema. Follicular conjunctivitis is usually of immune origin, with prominent follicle formation in the lower forniceal conjunctiva. This represents a more serious reaction and in most instances is due to the preservatives in the drug (262). In such cases, administration of preservative-free drops should be tried, and if that does not help, discontinuation of the medication is indicated; this may be curative in at least some cases (241). However, these findings are usually not striking and can easily be missed during routine ophthalmic examination. The clinician should specifically look for subtle squamous metaplasia of the conjunctival epithelium and disturbance of epithelial wetting by the tear film. Increasing keratinization may create a whitish, slightly foamy appearance, and if this remains undetected a thick white mass of keratin, or leukoplakia, can eventually form. This type of reaction has been reported with dipivefrin and metipranolol (263). Interestingly, there is a striking pharmacologic resemblance between metipranolol and practolol. Punctal stenosis, especially inferior, commonly occurs early during the disease process. Later stages can include inferior fornix foreshortening, shallowing of the canthal recesses, canthal keratinization, obliteration of the conjunctival folds, flattening of the plica and caruncula, conjunctival thickening, increased conjunctival vascularization, and subepithelial fibrosis (241,262,264).

Findings of advanced conjunctival cicatrization are sometimes evident, such as symblepharon formation, conjunctival ulceration, complete cicatrization or epidermalization, and corneal opacification with vascularization. These late findings are indistinguishable from mucous membrane pemphigoid. Progression cannot always be arrested by discontinuation of the inciting agent, at this stage.

Pathogenesis and Immunology

The exact etiopathogenesis of drug-induced cicatrizing conjunctivitis remains unknown. A chain of events starting with the induction of submucosal inflammation leads to hyperproliferation of fibroblasts and results in ocular surface cicatrix formation. The transition from inflammation to scar tissue formation in the conjunctiva seems to be mediated by the same mechanisms as those involved in wound healing and fibrosing diseases (265).

A variety of factors can activate fibroblasts and other connective tissue cells. One hypothesis suggested a direct effect of drugs in producing a toxic effect, and tissue culture studies have been performed to test this. A number of studies investigated various antiglaucoma medications and their preservatives (266–272). The results are conflicting and do not exactly support the hypothesis that antiglaucoma medications directly stimulate fibroblastic growth. Furthermore, *in vitro* studies have the inherent weakness of not truly representing the *in vivo* state. Nevertheless, the evidence suggests that, at the very least, the preservatives may have a direct cytotoxicity. The type of medication, the preservative it contains, the frequency of medication and cumulative duration of treatment, the physical properties of the preparation such as tonicity, temperature, and pH, and whether or not it is used in combination with other medications may be important factors in the process of conjunctival cicatrization.

Another possible mechanism would be an induced autoimmunity to the epithelial basement membrane, mimicking ocular involvement from mucous membrane pemphigoid. Chronic inflammation due to long-term topical medication use may be responsible for precipitating an immune phenomenon called "epitope spreading." Simply stated, epitope spreading describes an immune phenomenon whereby an autoimmune or inflammatory disease causes tissue damage in such a way that certain antigens originally "hidden" from the autoreactive T cells or B cells become "exposed" and evoke a secondary or primary immune disease. In fact, some patients with a history of long-term topical medication use, such as for glaucoma, may develop a drug-induced cicatrizing conjunctivitis, with autoantibodies to BMZ visible by direct immunofluorescein staining. Chronic low-grade conjunctival inflammation resulting from direct tissue damage from the long-term eyedrop use may possibly alter the antigenicity of the basement membrane, inducing an autoimmune reaction identical to that of mucous membrane pemphigoid. Such reaction would only occur in certain patients, perhaps those predisposed to developing pemphigoid. Indeed, some investigators have suggested that

"drug-induced cicatrization may develop in individuals who are destined to develop mucous membrane pemphigoid and who, by chance, also have an ocular disease requiring the use of a medication reported to cause cicatrisation" (257). Arguing against this theory is the fact that reported cases of drug-induced cicatrizing conjunctivitis have not been associated with extraocular mucous membrane cicatrization, although some patients with cicatricial pemphigoid never develop other mucous membrane involvement.

Histopathology

Light microscopic findings for drug-induced cicatrizing conjunctivitis appear identical to those for mucous membrane pemphigoid. Essentially one sees conjunctival subepithelial inflammation with invasion of submucosa by newly formed connective tissue, which subsequently contracts. Loss of goblet cells, epidermalization of conjunctiva with abnormally thickened epithelium, and keratinization, fibrosis, and infiltration of mononuclear cells and macrophages are typical findings (37,257,273). Scarring is uniformly present, and the subepithelial fibrosis is not associated with acantholysis (37). The localized inflammatory cell population, in particular macrophages, produces a cocktail of fibrogenic cytokines, which incites a fibroblastic reaction. The main fibrogenic cytokines thought to play a role include TGF-β, platelet-derived growth factor, basic fibroblast growth factor, and TNF-α (274).

Immunofluorescent studies of conjunctiva in patients with drug-induced conjunctival cicatrization have been inconsistent; some reported immunoreactant deposition at the basement membrane, mimicking mucous membrane pemphigoid, and some did not (36–38,257,258). One study has reported on a patient with IgA, IgD, IgE, and complement components C3 and C4 staining in plasma cells and IgG staining extracellularly in the substantia propria (37). However, there was no immunoglobulin deposition at the BMZ. One eye of the other patient in the same study had IgG deposition at the epithelial BMZ, which disappeared 3 weeks after discontinuation of the presumed inciting agent, echothiophate (37). In other studies, immunoreactant deposition either was not found or was nonspecific (36,38). Immunoperoxidase studies showed fixation of specific antibody in the corneal and conjunctival epithelium of a patient with practolol-induced cicatricial conjunctivitis (34). However, complement fixation could not be demonstrated. Thus the immune response in patients with practolol-induced ocular damage was suggested to be perhaps secondary to the epithelial disturbance rather than its cause.

Examination of conjunctival specimens by electron microscopy has revealed subepithelial inflammatory cell infiltration, advanced parakeratinization associated with flattening of superficial and intermediate epithelial cells, intracytoplasmic keratofibrils, numerous desmosomes, and reduction or complete disappearance of intercellular spaces (257). Increased numbers of desmosomes and basal lamina modifications suggested continuous damage and attempted repair.

Diagnosis

The early diagnosis of drug-induced conjunctival cicatrization is difficult. The initial symptoms are nonspecific: chronic conjunctivitis with irritation, lacrimation, and burning. Later corneal desiccation and foreign-body sensation, photophobia, and finally reduced vision due to scar formation and neovascularization can occur. Patients with end-stage disease may have complete ocular surface keratinization and ankyloblepharon formation.

The diagnosis of drug-induced conjunctival cicatrization is presumed by excluding other causes of cicatrizing conjunctivitis, in the presence of a history of topical medication use. The clinical picture of drug-induced conjunctival cicatrization and associated positive BMZ immune deposits (IgG type) fulfill the diagnostic criteria of mucous membrane pemphigoid, according to the report by the First International Consensus on Mucous Membrane Pemphigoid (73). Thus these patients should be diagnosed as having mucous membrane pemphigoid.

Disease Course

Drug-induced cicatricial conjunctivitis, in most instances, appears to behave like mucous membrane pemphigoid. Although it can occur as a nonprogressive toxic reaction that is self-limiting once the offending medication is stopped, the disease can also relentlessly progress and lead to extensive ocular surface damage with permanent loss of vision—even loss of the eye. In progressive cases, an autoimmune process is more likely to be involved rather than merely a direct toxicity from the drug (257).

Differential Diagnosis

Various disorders should be considered in the differential diagnosis of ocular cicatrix formation and conjunctival shrinkage, including chemical, thermal, or radiation trauma; infectious conjunctivitis caused by adenovirus, diphtheria, or β-hemolytic streptococci; and SJS, Sjögren's syndrome, sarcoidosis, trachoma, and mucous membrane pemphigoid (275). Obtaining a detailed history aids in the differential diagnosis.

Treatment

The first step in the treatment of drug-induced conjunctival cicatrization is to make every effort to exclude other causes of the cicatrizing conjunctivitis. Suspected medications must be withdrawn as early as possible to maximize the chance of

aborting the fibrotic process before the onset of irreversible alterations of the ocular surface. The clinician should not assume, however, that cessation of the suspect medication will result in resolution of symptoms and stabilization of the disease in all cases. Any subsequent progression of inflammation should be closely monitored. Lubrication with preservative-free artificial tears or mild steroids may give symptomatic relief if the disease is caught at an early stage. However, in a significant proportion of patients the inflammatory process progresses chronically, mimicking the course of mucous membrane pemphigoid. There is no specific treatment for these patients, and the management is identical to that for mucous membrane pemphigoid (discussed earlier in the chapter). The presence of glaucoma in the overwhelming majority of these patients requires special attention. Early surgery may be considered for those who cannot be treated with topical medications. Importantly, inflammation must be completely arrested prior to surgery; otherwise failure is inevitable because of the nature of scarring in this disorder.

SUMMARY

Cornea is a unique, highly transparent tissue, which refracts light to permit high-resolution vision. Preservation of clarity of the cornea is essential for vision, and maintenance of homeostasis of the ocular surface is essential to preserving corneal clarity. Lids, tear film, and conjunctival and corneal epithelial surfaces constantly interact to ensure an optimal environment for the cornea. Any changes in normal conjunctival morphology or function may alter the complex physicochemical system of the ocular surface and lead to loss of corneal transparency.

Cicatrizing conjunctivitis is a common denominator of a challenging group of heterogeneous conditions, with different etiologies and different treatment requirements. The severity of these conditions varies widely. The most striking feature of end-stage disease is permanent loss of vision due to loss of corneal clarity. Some of these diseases that manifest as cicatricial conjunctivitis are also associated with significant morbidity or even mortality. Attempts to reverse blindness surgically, without first addressing the underlying condition and dealing with the alterations of the ocular surface, are doomed to failure. An in-depth understanding of the nature of the conjunctival problems is fundamental to preventing blindness in these patients.

REFERENCES

1. Foster CS. Cicatricial pemphigoid. *Trans Am Ophthalmol Soc* 1986;84:527–663.
2. Mondino BJ, Brown I, Lempert S, et al. The acute manifestations of ocular cicatricial pemphigoid: diagnosis and treatment. *Ophthalmology* 1979;86:543–555.

3. Bernauer W, Broadway DC, Wright P. Chronic progressive conjunctival cicatrisation. *Eye* 1993;7:371–378.
4. Mondino BJ, Brown SI. Ocular cicatricial pemphigoid. *Ophthalmology* 1981;88:95–100.
5. Bedell AJ. Ocular pemphigus: a clinical presentation. *Trans Am Ophthalmol Soc* 1964;62:109–122.
6. Bettelheim H, Kraft D, Zehetbauer G. On the so-called ocular pemphigus (pemphigus ocularis, pemphigus conjunctivae). *Klin Monatsbl Augenheilkd* 1972;160:65–75.
7. Smith RC, Myers EA, Lamb HD. Ocular and oral pemphigus: report of case with anatomic findings in eyeball. *Arch Ophthalmol* 1934;11:635–640.
8. Drouet M, Delpuget-Bertin N, Vaillant L, et al. HLA-DRB1 and HLA-DQB1 genes in susceptibility and resistance to cicatricial pemphigoid in French Caucasians. *Eur J Dermatol* 1998;8:330–333.
9. Ahmed AR, Foster S, Zaltas M, et al. Association of DQw7 (DQB1*0301) with ocular cicatricial pemphigoid. *Proc Natl Acad Sci U S A* 1991;88:11579–11582.
10. Mondino BJ. Bullous diseases of the skin and mucous membranes. In Duane T, ed. *Clinical ophthalmology,* vol 4. Hagerstown: Harper & Row, 1991:1–19.
11. Wright P. Cicatrizing conjunctivitis. *Trans Ophthalmol Soc U K* 1986;105:1–17.
12. Faraj HG, Hoang-Xuan T. Chronic cicatrizing conjunctivitis. *Curr Opin Ophthalmol* 2001;12:250–257.
13. Mondino BJ. Cicatricial pemphigoid and erythema multiforme. *Ophthalmology* 1990;97:939–952.
14. Holsclaw DS. Ocular cicatricial pemphigoid. *Int Ophthalmol Clin* 1998;38:89–106.
15. Wright P. Enigma of ocular cicatricial pemphigoid: a comparative study of clinical and immunological findings. *Trans Ophthalmol Soc U K* 1979;99:141–145.
16. Rosser PM, Collin JR. Retractor plication for lower lid entropion in ocular cicatricial pemphigoid. *Aust N Z J Ophthalmol* 1993;21:93–97.
17. Tauber J, Melamed S, Foster CS. Glaucoma in patients with ocular cicatricial pemphigoid. *Ophthalmology* 1989;96:33–37.
18. Lever WF. Pemphigus and pemphigoid: a review of the advances made since 1964. *J Am Acad Dermatol* 1979;1:2–31.
19. Mondino BJ, Brown SI. Immunosuppressive therapy in ocular cicatricial pemphigoid. *Am J Ophthalmol* 1983;96:453–459.
20. Eversole LR. Immunopathology of oral mucosal ulcerative, desquamative, and bullous diseases: selective review of the literature. *Oral Surg Oral Med Oral Pathol* 1994;77:555–571.
21. Ahmed A, Kurgis B, Rogers R. Cicatricial pemphigoid. *J Am Acad Dermatol* 1991;24:987–1001.
22. Moschella SL, Pillsbury DM, Hurley EJ. *Dermatology.* Philadelphia: Saunders, 1975:466–468.
23. Elder MJ, Bernauer W, Leonard J, et al. Progression of disease in ocular cicatricial pemphigoid. *Br J Ophthalmol* 1996;80:292–296.
24. Hanson RD, Olsen KD, Rogers RS 3rd. Upper aerodigestive tract manifestations of cicatricial pemphigoid. *Ann Otol Rhinol Laryngol* 1988;97:493–499.
25. Nguyen QD, Foster CS. Cicatricial pemphigoid: diagnosis and treatment. *Int Ophthalmol Clin* 1996;36:41–60.
26. Ito H, Suzuki K, Hoshino T, et al. Total laryngeal stenosis in cicatricial pemphigoid. *Auris Nasus Larynx* 1991;18:163–167.
27. Spigel GT, Winkelmann RK. Cicatricial pemphigoid and rheumatoid arthritis. *Arch Dermatol* 1978;114:415–417.
28. Olsen KE, Holland EJ. The association between ocular cicatricial pemphigoid and rheumatoid arthritis. *Cornea* 1998;17:504–507.
29. Miserocchi E, Waheed NK, Baltatzis S, et al. Chronic cicatrizing conjunctivitis in a patient with ocular cicatricial pemphigoid and fatal Wegener granulomatosis. *Am J Ophthalmol* 2001;132:923–924.
30. Letko E, Bhol K, Colon J, et al. Biology of interleukin-5 in ocular cicatricial pemphigoid. *Graefes Arch Clin Exp Ophthalmol* 2002;240:565–569.
31. Yunis JJ, Mobini N, Yunis EJ, et al. Common major histocompatibility complex class II markers in clinical variants of cicatricial pemphigoid. *Proc Natl Acad Sci U S A* 1994;91:7747–7751.
32. Zaltas MM, Ahmed R, Foster CS. Association of HLA-DR4 with ocular cicatricial pemphigoid. *Curr Eye Res* 1989;8:189–193.
33. Setterfield J, Theron J, Vaughan RW, et al. Mucous membrane pemphigoid: HLA-DQB1*0301 is associated with all clinical sites of involvement and may be linked to antibasement membrane IgG production. *Br J Dermatol* 2001;145:406–414.
34. Rahi AH, Chapman CM, Garner A, et al. Pathology of practolol-induced ocular toxicity. *Br J Ophthalmol* 1976;60: 312–323.
35. Norn MS. Pemphigoid related to epinephrine treatment. *Am J Ophthalmol* 1977;83:138.
36. Lass JH, Thoft RA, Dohlman CH. Idoxuridine-induced conjunctival cicatrisation. *Arch Ophthalmol* 1983;101:747–750.
37. Patten JT, Cavanagh HD, Allansmith MR. Induced ocular pseudopemphigoid. *Am J Ophthalmol* 1976;82:272–276.
38. Hirst LW, Werblin T, Novak M, et al. Drug-induced cicatrizing conjunctivitis simulating ocular pemphigoid. *Cornea* 1982;1:121–128.
39. Chan RY, Bhol K, Tesavibul N, et al. The role of antibody to human beta4 integrin in conjunctival basement membrane separation: possible in vitro model for ocular cicatricial pemphigoid. *Invest Ophthalmol Vis Sci* 1999;40:2283–2290.
40. Kumari S, Bhol KC, Simmons RK, et al. Identification of ocular cicatricial pemphigoid antibody binding site in human beta4 integrin. *Invest Ophthalmol Vis Sci* 2001;42:379–385.
41. Hsu RC, Lazarova Z, Lee HG, et al. Antiepiligrin cicatricial pemphigoid. *J Am Acad Dermatol* 2000;42:841–844.
42. Sacks EH, Jakobiec FA, Wieczorek R, et al. Immunophenotypic analysis of the inflammatory infiltrate in ocular cicatricial pemphigoid: further evidence for a T cell-mediated disease. *Ophthalmology* 1989;96:236–243.
43. Elder MJ, Dart JK, Lightman S. Conjunctival fibrosis in ocular cicatricial pemphigoid—the role of cytokines. *Exp Eye Res* 1997;65:165–176.
44. Bernauer W, Wright P, Dart JK, et al. Cytokines in the conjunctiva of acute and chronic mucous membrane pemphigoid: an immunohistochemical analysis. *Graefes Arch Clin Exp Ophthalmol* 1993;231:563–570.
45. Lee SJ, Li Z, Sherman B, et al. Serum levels of tumor necrosis factor-alpha and interleukin-6 in ocular cicatricial pemphigoid. *Invest Ophthalmol Vis Sci* 1993;34:3522–3525.
46. Kumari S, Bhol KC, Rehman F, et al. Interleukin 1 components in cicatricial pemphigoid: role in intravenous immunoglobulin therapy. *Cytokine* 2001;14:218–224.
47. Razzaque MS, Foster CS, Ahmed A. Role of enhanced expression of m-CSF in conjunctiva affected by cicatricial pemphigoid. *Invest Ophthalmol Vis Sci* 2002;43:2977–2983.
48. Roat MI, Sossi G, Lo CY, et al. Hyperproliferation of conjunctival fibroblasts from patients with cicatricial pemphigoid. *Arch Ophthalmol* 1989;107:1064–1067.
49. Foster CS. Chronic cicatricial conjunctivitis. *CLAO* 2001;27:61–67.
50. Andersen SR, Jensen OA, Kristensen EB, et al. Benign mucous membrane pemphigoid. 3. Biopsy. *Acta Ophthalmol (Copenh)* 1974;52:455–463.
51. Kinoshita S, Kiorpes TC, Friend J, et al. Goblet cell density in ocular surface disease: a better indicator than tear mucin. *Arch Ophthalmol* 1983;101:1284–1287.

52. Heiligenhaus A, Schaller J, Mauss S, et al. Eosinophil granule proteins expressed in ocular cicatricial pemphigoid. *Br J Ophthalmol* 1998;82:312–317.

53. Hoang-Xuan T, Foster CS, Raizman MB, et al. Mast cells in conjunctiva affected by cicatricial pemphigoid. *Ophthalmology* 1989;96:1110–1114.

54. Mondino BJ, Brown SI, Rabin BS. Autoimmune phenomena of the external eye. *Ophthalmology* 1978;85:801–817.

55. Bernauer W, Elder MJ, Leonard JN, et al. The value of biopsies in the evaluation of chronic progressive conjunctival cicatrisation. *Graefes Arch Clin Exp Ophthalmol* 1994;232:533–537.

56. Power WJ, Neves RA, Rodriguez A, et al. Increasing the diagnostic yield of conjunctival biopsy in patients with suspected ocular cicatricial pemphigoid. *Ophthalmology* 1995;102:1158–1163.

57. Foster CS, Wilson LA, Ekins MB. Immunosuppressive therapy for progressive ocular cicatricial pemphigoid. *Ophthalmology* 1982;89:340–353.

58. Tauber J, Jabbur N, Foster CS. Improved detection of disease progression in ocular cicatricial pemphigoid. *Cornea* 1992;11:446–451.

59. Helm KF, Peters MS. Immunodermatology update: the immunologically mediated vesiculobullous diseases. *Mayo Clin Proc* 1991;66:187–202.

60. Schwab IR, Linberg JV, Gioia VM, et al. Foreshortening of the inferior conjunctival fornix associated with chronic glaucoma medications. *Ophthalmology* 1992;99:197–202.

61. Miserocchi E, Baltatzis S, Roque MR, et al. The effect of treatment and its related side effects in patients with severe ocular cicatricial pemphigoid. *Ophthalmology* 2002;109:111–118.

62. Hardy KM, Perry HO, Pingree GC, et al. Benign mucous membrane pemphigoid. *Arch Dermatol* 1971;104:467–475.

63. Dave VK, Vickers CF. Azathioprine in the treatment of mucocutaneous pemphigoid. *Br J Dermatol* 1974;90:183–186.

64. Brody HJ, Pirozzi DJ. Benign mucous membrane pemphigoid: response to therapy with cyclophosphamide. *Arch Dermatol* 1977;113:1598–1599.

65. Fern AI, Jay JL, Young H, et al. Dapsone therapy for the acute inflammatory phase of ocular pemphigoid. *Br J Ophthalmol* 1992;76:332–335.

66. Rogers RS 3rd, Seehafer JR, Perry HO. Treatment of cicatricial (benign mucous membrane) pemphigoid with dapsone. *J Am Acad Dermatol* 1982;6:215–223.

67. Tauber J, Sainz de la Maza M, Foster CS. Systemic chemotherapy for ocular cicatricial pemphigoid. *Cornea* 1991;10:185–195.

68. Foster CS, Ahmed AR. Intravenous immunoglobulin therapy for ocular cicatricial pemphigoid: a preliminary study. *Ophthalmology* 1999;106:2136–2143.

69. Letko E, Bhol K, Foster SC, et al. Influence of intravenous immunoglobulin therapy on serum levels of anti-beta 4 antibodies in ocular cicatricial pemphigoid: a correlation with disease activity. A preliminary study. *Curr Eye Res* 2000;21:646–654.

70. Strand V. Monoclonal antibodies and other biologic therapies. *Lupus* 2001;10:216–221.

71. Nussenblatt RB. Bench to bedside: new approaches to the immunotherapy of uveitic disease. *Int Rev Immunol* 2002;21:273–289.

72. Papaliodis GN, Chu D, Foster CS. Treatment of ocular inflammatory disorders with daclizumab. *Ophthalmology* 2003;110:786–789.

73. Chan LS, Ahmed R, Anhalt GJ, et al. The first international consensus on mucous membrane pemphigoid: definition, diagnostic criteria, pathogenic factors, medical treatment, and prognostic indicators. *Arch Dermatol.* 2002;138:370–379.

74. Neumann R, Tauber J, Foster CS. Remission and recurrence after withdrawal of therapy for ocular cicatricial pemphigoid. *Ophthalmology* 1991;98:858–862.

75. Rosenthal P, Cotter J. The Boston Scleral Lens in the management of severe ocular surface disease. *Ophthalmol Clin North Am* 2003;16:89–93.

76. Chan RY, Foster CS. A step-wise approach to ocular surface rehabilitation in patients with ocular inflammatory disease. *Int Ophthalmol Clin* 1999;39:83–108.

77. Tugal-Tutkun I, Akova YA, Foster CS. Penetrating keratoplasty in cicatrizing conjunctival diseases. *Ophthalmology* 1995;102:576–585.

78. Akpek E, Foster C. Limbal stem-cell transplantation. *Int Ophthalmol Clin* 1999;39:71–82.

79. Samson CM, Nduaguba C, Baltatzis S, et al. Limbal stem cell transplantation in chronic inflammatory eye disease. *Ophthalmology* 2002;109:862–868.

80. Yaghouti F, Nouri M, Abad JC, et al. Keratoprosthesis: preoperative prognostic categories. *Cornea* 2001;20:19–23.

81. Roujeau JC. Stevens-Johnson syndrome and toxic epidermal necrolysis are severity variants of the same disease which differs from erythema multiforme. *J Dermatol* 1997;24:726–729.

82. Leaute-Labreze C, Lamireau T, Chawki D, et al. Diagnosis, classification, and management of erythema multiforme and Stevens-Johnson syndrome. *Arch Dis Child* 2000;83:347–352.

83. Auquier-Dunant A, Mockenhaupt M, Naldi L, et al. Correlations between clinical patterns and causes of erythema multiforme majus, Stevens-Johnson syndrome, and toxic epidermal necrolysis: results of an international prospective study. *Arch Dermatol* 2002;138:1019–1024.

84. von Hebra F. *Atlas der Hautkrankheiten.* Vienna: Kaiserliche Akademie der Wissenchaften Wien, Vienna, 1866.

85. Stevens AM, Johnson FC. A new eruptive fever associated with stomatitis and ophthalmia. *Am J Dis Child* 1922;24:526–533.

86. Huff JC, Weston WL, Tonnesen MG. Erythema multiforme: a critical review of characteristics, diagnostic criteria, and causes. *J Am Acad Dermatol* 1983;8:763–775.

87. Weston WL, Morelli JG, Rogers M. Target lesions on the lips: childhood herpes simplex associated with erythema multiforme mimics Stevens-Johnson syndrome. *J Am Acad Dermatol* 1997;37:848–850.

88. Bastuji-Garin S, Rzany B, Stern RS, et al. Clinical classification of cases of toxic epidermal necrolysis, Stevens-Johnson syndrome, and erythema multiforme. *Arch Dermatol* 1993;129:92–96.

89. Roujeau JC. What is going on in erythema multiforme? *Dermatology* 1994;188:249–250.

90. Assier H, Bastuji-Garin S, Revuz J, et al. Erythema multiforme with mucous membrane involvement and Stevens-Johnson syndrome are clinically different disorders with distinct causes. *Arch Dermatol* 1995;131:539–543.

91. Mockenhaupt M, Schopf E. Epidemiology of drug-induced severe skin reactions. *Semin Cutan Med Surg* 1996;15:236–243.

92. Sane SP, Bhatt AD. Stevens-Johnson syndrome and toxic epidermal necrolysis: challenges of recognition and management. *J Assoc Physicians India* 2000;48:999–1003.

93. Rzany B, Mockenhaupt M, Baur S, et al. Epidemiology of erythema exsudativum multiforme majus, Stevens-Johnson syndrome, and toxic epidermal necrolysis in Germany (1990–1992): structure and results of a population-based registry. *J Clin Epidemiol* 1996;49:769–773.

94. Chan H, Stern R, Arndt K, et al. The incidence of erythema multiforme, Stevens-Johnson syndrome, and toxic epidermal necrolysis: a population-based study with particular reference to reactions caused by drugs among outpatients. *Arch Dermatol* 1990;126:43–47.

95. Howard GM. The Stevens-Johnson syndrome: ocular prognosis and treatment. *Am J Ophthalmol* 1963;55:893–900.

96. Arstikaitis MJ. Ocular aftermath of Stevens-Johnson syndrome. *Arch Ophthalmol* 1973;90:376–379.

97. Yetiv JZ, Bianchine JR, Owen JA Jr. Etiologic factors of the Stevens-Johnson syndrome. *South Med J* 1980;73:599–602.

98. Power WJ, Ghoraishi M, Merayo-Lloves J, et al. Analysis of the acute ophthalmic manifestations of the erythema multiforme/Stevens-Johnson syndrome/toxic epidermal necrolysis disease spectrum. *Ophthalmology* 1995;102:1669–1676.

99. Tonnesen MG, Soter NA. Erythema multiforme. *J Am Acad Dermatol* 1979;1:357–364.

100. Bianchine JR, Macaraeg PV Jr, Lasagna L, et al. Drugs as etiologic factors in the Stevens-Johnson syndrome. *Am J Med* 1968;44:390–405.

101. Courson DB. Stevens Johnson syndrome: nonspecific parasensitivity reaction? *JAMA* 1966;198:133.

102. Dohlman CH, Doughman DJ. The Stevens-Johnson syndrome. In: *Symposium on the cornea: transactions of the New Orleans Academy of Ophthalmology.* St. Louis: CV Mosby, 1972: 236–252.

103. Mondino BJ. Cicatricial pemphigoid and erythema multiforme. *Int Ophthalmol Clin* 1983;23:63–79.

104. Ormerod LD, Fong LP, Foster CS. Corneal infection in mucosal scarring disorders and Sjogren's syndrome. *Am J Ophthalmol* 1988;105:512–518.

105. Patz A. Ocular involvement in erythema multiforme. *Arch Ophthalmol* 1950; 43:244–256.

106. Merot Y, Gravallese E, Guillen FJ, et al. Lymphocyte subsets and Langerhans' cells in toxic epidermal necrolysis: report of a case. *Arch Dermatol* 1986;122:455–458.

107. Raviglione MC, Pablos-Mendez A, Battan R. Clinical features and management of severe dermatological reactions to drugs. *Drug Saf* 1990;5:39–64.

108. Ward B, McCulley JP, Segal RJ. Dermatologic reaction in Stevens-Johnson syndrome after ophthalmic anesthesia with proparacaine hydrochloride. *Am J Ophthalmol* 1978;86: 133–135.

109. Rubin Z. Ophthalmic sulfonamide-induced Stevens-Johnson syndrome. *Arch Dermatol* 1977;113:235–236.

110. Guill MA, Goette DK, Knight CG, et al. Erythema multiforme and urticaria: eruptions induced by chemically related ophthalmic anticholinergic agents. *Arch Dermatol* 1979;115: 742–743.

111. Ostler HB, Conant MA, Groundwater J. Lyell's disease, the Stevens-Johnson syndrome, and exfoliative dermatitis. *Trans Am Acad Ophthalmol Otolaryngol* 1970;74:1254–1265.

112. Lyell A. A review of toxic epidermal necrolysis in Britain. *Br J Dermatol* 1967;79:662–671.

113. Bushkell LL, Mackel SE, Jordon RE. Erythema multiforme: direct immunofluorescence studies and detection of circulating immune complexes. *J Invest Dermatol* 1980;74:372–374.

114. Kazmierowski JA, Peizner DS, Wuepper KD. Herpes simplex antigen in immune complexes of patients with erythema multiforme: presence following recurrent herpes simplex infection. *JAMA* 1982;247:2547–2550.

115. Roujeau JC, Moritz S, Guillaume JC, et al. Lymphopenia and abnormal balance of T-lymphocyte subpopulations in toxic epidermal necrolysis. *Arch Dermatol Res* 1985;277:24–27.

116. Nassif A, Bensussan A, Dorothee G, et al. Drug specific cytotoxic T-cells in the skin lesions of a patient with toxic epidermal necrolysis. *J Invest Dermatol* 2002;118:728–733.

117. Mondino BJ, Brown SI, Biglan AW. HLA antigens in Stevens-Johnson syndrome with ocular involvement. *Arch Ophthalmol* 1982;100:1453–1454.

118. Power WJ, Saidman SL, Zhang DS, et al. HLA typing in patients with ocular manifestations of Stevens-Johnson syndrome. *Ophthalmology* 1996;103:1406–1409.

119. Rzany B, Hering O, Mockenhaupt M, et al. Histopathological and epidemiological characteristics of patients with erythema exudativum multiforme major, Stevens-Johnson syndrome and toxic epidermal necrolysis. *Br J Dermatol* 1996;135:6–11.

120. Kazmierowski JA, Wuepper KD. Erythema multiforme: immune complex vasculitis of the superficial cutaneous microvasculature. *J Invest Dermatol* 1978;71:366–369.

121. Wuepper KD, Watson PA, Kazmierowski JA. Immune complexes in erythema multiforme and the Stevens-Johnson syndrome. *J Invest Dermatol* 1980;74:368–371.

122. Imamura S, Horio T, Yanase K, et al. Erythema multiforme: pathomechanism of papular erythema and target lesion. *J Dermatol* 1992;19:524–533.

123. Roujeau JC, Dubertret L, Moritz S, et al. Involvement of macrophages in the pathology of toxic epidermal necrolysis. *Br J Dermatol* 1985;113:425–430.

124. Buchner A, Lozada F, Silverman S Jr. Histopathologic spectrum of oral erythema multiforme. *Oral Surg Oral Med Oral Pathol* 1980;49:221–228.

125. Nelson JD, Wright JC. Conjunctival goblet cell densities in ocular surface disease. *Arch Ophthalmol* 1984;102:1049–1051.

126. Nakamura T, Nishida K, Dota A, et al. Elevated expression of transglutaminase 1 and keratinization-related proteins in conjunctiva in severe ocular surface disease. *Invest Ophthalmol Vis Sci* 2001;42:549–556.

127. Nishida K, Yamanishi K, Yamada K, et al. Epithelial hyperproliferation and transglutaminase 1 gene expression in Stevens-Johnson syndrome conjunctiva. *Am J Pathol* 1999;154:331–336.

128. Schopf E, Stuhmer A, Rzany B, et al. Toxic epidermal necrolysis and Stevens-Johnson syndrome: an epidemiologic study from West Germany. *Arch Dermatol* 1991;127:839–842.

129. Davis MD, Rogers RS 3rd, Pittelkow MR. Recurrent erythema multiforme/Stevens-Johnson syndrome: response to mycophenolate mofetil. *Arch Dermatol* 2002;138:1547–1550.

130. Nesbit SP, Gobetti JP. Multiple recurrence of oral erythema multiforme after secondary herpes simplex: report of case and review of literature. *J Am Dent Assoc* 1986;112:348–352.

131. Foster CS, Fong LP, Azar D, Kenyon KR. Episodic conjunctival inflammation after Stevens-Johnson syndrome. *Ophthalmology* 1988;95:453–462.

132. Coster DJ. Stevens-Johnson syndrome. In: Bernauer W, Dart JKG, Elder MJ, eds. *Cicatrising conjunctivitis (Dev Ophthalmol,* vol 28). Basel: Karger, 1997:24–31.

133. Finlay AY, Richards J, Holt PJ. Intensive therapy unit management of toxic epidermal necrolysis: practical aspects. *Clin Exp Dermatol* 1982;7:55–60.

134. Ginsburg CM. Stevens-Johnson syndrome in children. *Pediatr Infect Dis* 1982;1:155–158.

135. Cheriyan S, Patterson R, Greenberger PA, et al. The outcome of Stevens-Johnson syndrome treated with corticosteroids. *Allergy Proc* 1995;16:151–155.

136. Patterson R, Miller M, Kaplan M, et al. Effectiveness of early therapy with corticosteroids in Stevens-Johnson syndrome: experience with 41 cases and a hypothesis regarding pathogenesis. *Ann Allergy* 1994;73:27–34.

137. Tripathi A, Ditto A, Grammer L, et al. Corticosteroid therapy in an additional 13 cases of Stevens-Johnson syndrome: a total series of 67 cases. *Allergy Asthma Proc* 2000;21:101–105.

138. Hewitt J, Ormerod AD. Toxic epidermal necrolysis treated with cyclosporin. *Clin Exp Dermatol* 1992;17:264–265.

139. Renfro L, Grant-Kels JM, Daman LA. Drug-induced toxic epidermal necrolysis treated with cyclosporin. *Int J Dermatol* 1989;28:441–444.

140. Jarrett P, Rademaker M, Havill J, et al. Toxic epidermal necrolysis treated with cyclosporin and granulocyte colony stimulating factor. *Clin Exp Dermatol* 1997;22:146–147.

141. Hertl M, Bohlen H, Merk HF. Efficacy of cyclophosphamide in toxic epidermal necrolysis. *J Am Acad Dermatol* 1993;28:511.

142. Heng MC, Allen SG. Efficacy of cyclophosphamide in toxic epidermal necrolysis: clinical and pathophysiologic aspects. *J Am Acad Dermatol* 1991;25:778–786.

143. Frangogiannis NG, Boridy I, Mazhar M, et al. Cyclophosphamide in the treatment of toxic epidermal necrolysis. *South Med J* 1996;89:1001–1003.

144. Roujeau JC. Treatment of severe drug eruptions. *J Dermatol* 1999;26:718–722.

145. Wolkenstein P, Latarjet J, Roujeau JC, et al. Randomised comparison of thalidomide versus placebo in toxic epidermal necrolysis. *Lancet* 1998;352:1586–1589.

146. Klausner JD, Kaplan G, Haslett PA. Thalidomide in toxic epidermal necrolysis. *Lancet* 1999;353:324.

147. Levy R. Thalidomide in toxic epidermal necrolysis. *Lancet* 1999;353:324.

148. Brett AS, Philips D, Lynn AW. Intravenous immunoglobulin therapy for Stevens-Johnson syndrome. *South Med J* 2001;94:342–343.

149. Morici MV, Galen WK, Shetty AK, et al. Intravenous immunoglobulin therapy for children with Stevens-Johnson syndrome. *J Rheumatol* 2000;27:2494–2497.

150. Bartley G, Lowry J. Argon laser treatment of trichiasis. *Am J Ophthalmol* 1992;113:71–74.

151. Hecht SD. Cryotherapy of trichiasis with use of the retinal cryoprobe. *Ann Ophthalmol* 1977;9:1501–1503.

152. Beyer C. The management of special problems associated with Stevens-Johnson syndrome and ocular pemphigoid. *Trans Am Acad Ophthalmol Otolaryngol* 1977;83:701–707.

153. Leone CR Jr. Mucous membrane grafting for cicatricial entropion. *Ophthalmic Surg* 1974;5:24–28.

154. Rosenthal P, Cotter JM, Baum J. Treatment of persistent corneal epithelial defect with extended wear of a fluid-ventilated gas-permeable scleral contact lens. *Am J Ophthalmol* 2000;130:33–41.

155. Tseng SC, Maumenee AE, Stark WJ, et al. Topical retinoid treatment for various dry-eye disorders. *Ophthalmology* 1985; 92:717–727. [Erratum in *Ophthalmology* 1989;96:730.]

156. Solomon A, Meller D, Prabhasawat P, et al. Amniotic membrane grafts for nontraumatic corneal perforations, descemetoceles, and deep ulcers. *Ophthalmology* 2002;109:694–703.

157. Prasad JK, Feller I, Thomson PD. Use of amnion for the treatment of Stevens-Johnson syndrome. *J Trauma* 1986;26: 945–946.

158. Tsubota K, Shimazaki J. Surgical treatment of children blinded by Stevens-Johnson syndrome. *Am J Ophthalmol* 1999;128: 573–581.

159. Tseng SC, Prabhasawat P, Barton K, et al. Amniotic membrane transplantation with or without limbal allografts for corneal surface reconstruction in patients with limbal stem cell deficiency. *Arch Ophthalmol* 1998;116:431–441.

160. Shimazaki J, Aiba M, Goto E, et al. Transplantation of human limbal epithelium cultivated on amniotic membrane for the treatment of severe ocular surface disorders. *Ophthalmology* 2002;109:1285–1290.

161. Kim MK, Lee JL, Wee WR, et al. Seoul-type keratoprosthesis: preliminary results of the first 7 human cases. *Arch Ophthalmol* 2002;120:761–766.

162. Girard LJ, Hawkins RS, Nieves R, et al. Keratoprosthesis: a 12-year follow-up. *Trans Am Acad Ophthalmol Otolaryngol* 1977;83:252–267.

163. Dohlman CH, Terada H. Keratoprosthesis in pemphigoid and Stevens-Johnson syndrome. *Adv Exp Med Biol* 1998;438: 1021–1025.

164. Geerling G, Liu CS, Dart JK, et al. Sight and comfort: complex procedures in end-stage Stevens-Johnson syndrome. *Eye* 2003;17: 89–91.

165. Wong SN, Chua SH. Spectrum of subepidermal immunobullous disorders seen at the National Skin Centre, Singapore: a 2-year review. *Br J Dermatol* 2002;147:476–480.

166. Bernard P, Vaillant L, Labeille B, et al. Incidence and distribution of subepidermal autoimmune bullous skin diseases in three French regions—Bullous Diseases French Study Group. *Arch Dermatol* 1995;131:48–52.

167. Leonard JN, Haffenden GP, Ring NP, et al. Linear IgA disease in adults. *Br J Dermatol* 1982;107:301–316.

168. Wojnarowska F, Frith P. Linear IgA disease. In: Bernauer W, Dart JKG, Elder MJ, eds. *Cicatrising conjunctivitis (Dev Ophthalmol,* vol 28). Basel: Karger, 1997:64–72.

169. Leonard JN, Wright P, Williams DM, et al. The relationship between linear IgA disease and benign mucous membrane pemphigoid. *Br J Dermatol* 1984;110:307–314.

170. Aultbrinker EA, Starr MB, Donnenfeld ED. Linear IgA disease: the ocular manifestations. *Ophthalmology* 1988;95:340–343.

171. Wojnarowska F, Marsden RA, Bhogal B, et al. Childhood cicatricial pemphigoid with linear IgA deposits. *Clin Exp Dermatol* 1984;9:407–415.

172. Georgi M, Scheckenbach C, Kromminga A, et al. Mapping of epitopes on the BP180 ectodomain targeted by IgA and IgG autoantibodies in patients with the lamina lucida-type of linear IgA disease. *Arch Dermatol Res* 2001;293:109–114.

173. Zillikens D, Giudice GJ. BP180/type XVII collagen: its role in acquired and inherited disorders of the dermal-epidermal junction. *Arch Dermatol Res* 1999;291:187–194.

174. Zillikens D. BP180 as the common autoantigen in blistering diseases with different clinical phenotypes. *Keio J Med* 2002; 51:21–28.

175. Lin MS, Fu CL, Olague-Marchan M, et al. Autoimmune responses in patients with linear IgA bullous dermatosis: both autoantibodies and T lymphocytes recognize the NC16A domain of the BP180 molecule. *Clin Immunol* 2002;102:310–319.

176. Caux FA, Guidece GJ, Diaz LA, et al. Autoimmune subepithelial blistering diseases with ocular involvement. *Immunol Allergy Clin North Am* 1997;17:139–159.

177. Blenkinsopp WK, Haffenden GP, Fry L, et al. Histology of linear IgA disease, dermatitis herpetiformis, and bullous pemphigoid. *Am J Dermatopathol* 1983;5:547–554.

178. Leonard JN, Hobday CM, Haffenden GP, et al. Immunofluorescent studies in ocular cicatricial pemphigoid. *Br J Dermatol* 1988;118:209–217.

179. Wojnarowska F, Delacroix D, Gengoux P. Cutaneous IgA subclasses in dermatitis herpetiformis and linear IgA disease. *J Cutan Pathol* 1988;15:272–275.

180. Caproni M, Rolfo S, Bernacchi E, et al. The role of lymphocytes, granulocytes, mast cells and their related cytokines in lesional skin of linear IgA bullous dermatosis. *Br J Dermatol* 1999;140:1072–1078.

181. Langeland T. Childhood cicatricial pemphigoid with linear IgA deposits: a case report. *Acta Derm Venereol* 1985;65:354–355.

182. Wojnarowska F, Allen J, Collier P. Linear IgA disease. *Dermatology* 1994;189:52–56.

183. Kelly SE, Frith PA, Millard PR, et al. A clinicopathological study of mucosal involvement in linear IgA disease. *Br J Dermatol* 1988;119:161–170.

184. Kulthanan K, Akaraphanth R, Piamphongsant T, et al. Linear IgA bullous dermatosis of childhood: a long-term study. *J Med Assoc Thai* 1999;82:707–712.

185. Hogg R, Silva F, Wyatt R, et al. Prognostic indicators in children with IgA nephropathy-report of the Southwest Pediatric Nephrology Study Group. *Pediatr Nephrol* 1994;8:15–20.

186. Goumenos D, Ahuja M, Shortland JR, et al. Can immunosuppressive drugs slow the progression of IgA nephropathy? *Nephrol Dial Transplant* 1995;10:1173–1181.

187. Mobacken H, Kastrup W, Ljunghall K, et al. Linear IgA dermatosis: a study of ten adult patients. *Acta Derm Venereol* 1983;63:123–128.
188. Khan IU, Bhol KC, Ahmed AR. Linear IgA bullous dermatosis in a patient with chronic renal failure. *J Am Acad Dermatol* 1999;40:485–488.
189. Kroiss M, Vogt T, Landthaler M, et al. High-dose intravenous immune globulin is also effective in linear IgA disease. *Br J Dermatol* 2000;142:582. [Erratum 2000;142:1268.]
190. Letko E, Bhol K, Foster CS, et al. Linear IgA bullous disease limited to the eye: a diagnostic dilemma—response to intravenous immunoglobulin therapy. *Ophthalmology* 2000;107:1524–1528.
191. Jolles S. A review of high-dose intravenous immunoglobulin (hdIVIg) in the treatment of the autoimmune blistering disorders. *Clin Exp Dermatol* 2001;26:127–131.
192. Ahmed AR, Dahl MV. Consensus statement on the use of intravenous immunoglobulin therapy in the treatment of autoimmune mucocutaneous blistering diseases. *Arch Dermatol* 2003;139:1051–1059.
193. Cooper SM, Powell J, Wojnarowska F. Linear IgA disease: successful treatment with erythromycin. *Clin Exp Dermatol* 2002;27:677–679.
194. Chaffins ML, Collison D, Fivenson DP. Treatment of pemphigus and linear IgA dermatosis with nicotinamide and tetracycline: a review of 13 cases. *J Am Acad Dermatol* 1993;28:998–1000.
195. Peoples D, Fivenson DP. Linear IgA bullous dermatosis: successful treatment with tetracycline and nicotinamide. *J Am Acad Dermatol* 1992;26:498–499.
196. Yomada M, Komai A, Hashimato T. Sublamina densa-type linear IgA bullous dermatosis successfully treated with oral tetracycline and niacianamide. *Br J Dermatol* 1999;141:608–609.
197. Glaser R, Sticherlin M. Successful treatment of linear IgA bullous dermatosis with mycophenolate mofetil. *Acta Derm Venereol* 2002;82:308–309.
198. Benbenisty KM, Bowman PH, Davis LS. Localized linear IgA disease responding to colchicine. *Int J Dermatol* 2002;41:56–58.
199. Arndt KA. Lichen planus. In: Fitzpatrick TB, Arthur EZ, and Wolff K, eds. *Dermatology in general medicine,* vol 1. New York: McGraw-Hill, 1987:967–973.
200. Bhattacharya M, Kaur I, Kumar B. Lichen planus: a clinical and epidemiological study. *J Dermatol* 2000;27:576–582.
201. Handa S, Sahoo B. Childhood lichen planus: a study of 87 cases. *Int J Dermatol* 2002;41:423–427.
202. Itin PH, Buechner SA, Rufli T. Lichen planus of the eyelids. *Dermatology* 1995;191:350–351.
203. Sharma R, Singhal N. Lichen planus of the eyelids: a report of 5 cases. *Dermatol Online J* 2001;7:5.
204. Eisen D. The evaluation of cutaneous, genital, scalp, nail, esophageal, and ocular involvement in patients with oral lichen planus. *Oral Surg Oral Med Oral Pathol Oral Radiol Endod* 1999;88:431–436.
205. Thorne JE, Jabs DA, Nikolskaia OV, et al. Lichen planus and cicatrizing conjunctivitis: characterization of five cases. *Am J Ophthalmol* 2003;136:239–243.
206. Goldsmith J. Deep keratitis associated with atypical lichen planus. *Arch Ophthalmol* 1948;40:138–146.
207. Crompton DO. Immuno-suppressive drug treatment of keratitis sicca, including an example of lichen planus of the conjunctiva. *Aust N Z J Surg* 1968;38:143–146.
208. Zijdenbos L, Starink T, Spronk C. Ulcerative lichen planus with associated sicca syndrome and good therapeutic result of skin grafting. *J Am Acad Dermatol* 1985;13:667–668.
209. Hutnik CM, Probst LE, Burt WL, et al. Progressive, refractory keratoconjunctivitis associated with lichen planus. *Can J Ophthalmol* 1995;30:211–214.
210. Agarwal R, Saraswat A. Oral lichen planus: an update. *Drugs Today* 2002;38:533–547.
211. Sugerman PB, Savage NW, Walsh LJ, et al. The pathogenesis of oral lichen planus. *Crit Rev Oral Biol Med* 2002;13:350–365.
212. Zhao ZZ, Savage NW, Sugerman PB, et al. Mast cell/T cell interactions in oral lichen planus. *J Oral Pathol Med* 2002;31:189–195.
213. Khan A, Farah CS, Savage NW, et al. Th1 cytokines in oral lichen planus. *J Oral Pathol Med* 2003;32:77–83.
214. Zhou XJ, Sugerman PB, Savage NW, et al. Matrix metalloproteinases and their inhibitors in oral lichen planus. *J Cutan Pathol* 2001;28:72–82.
215. Sugermann PB, Savage NW, Seymour GJ, et al. Is there a role for tumor necrosis factor-alpha (TNF-alpha) in oral lichen planus? *J Oral Pathol Med* 1996;25:219–224.
216. Toto PD, Nadimi HT. An immunohistochemical study of oral lichen planus. *Oral Surg Oral Med Oral Pathol* 1987;63:60–67.
217. Ishii T. Immunohistochemical demonstration of T cell subsets and accessory cells in oral lichen planus. *J Oral Pathol* 1987;16:356–361.
218. Abell E, Presbury DG, Marks R, et al. The diagnostic significance of immunoglobulin and fibrin deposition in lichen planus. *Br J Dermatol* 1975;93:17–24.
219. Neumann R, Dutt CJ, Foster CS. Immunohistopathologic features and therapy of conjunctival lichen planus. *Am J Ophthalmol* 1993;115:494–500.
220. Grabbe S, Kolde G. Coexisting lichen planus and subacute cutaneous lupus erythematosus. *Clin Exp Dermatol* 1995;20:249–254.
221. De Jong EM, Van De Kerkhof PC. Coexistence of palmoplantar lichen planus and lupus erythematosus with response to treatment using acitrecin. *Br J Dermatol* 1996;134:538–541.
222. Stingl G, Holubar K. Coexistence of lichen planus and bullous pemphigoid: an immunopathological study. *Br J Dermatol* 1975;93:313–320.
223. Verma KK, Mittal R, Manchanda Y. Azathioprine for the treatment of severe erosive oral and generalized lichen planus. *Acta Derm Venereol* 2001;81:378–379.
224. Lozada-Nur F, Miranda C. Oral lichen planus: epidemiology, clinical characteristics, and associated diseases. *Semin Cutan Med Surg* 1997;16:273–277.
225. Sugerman PB, Savage NW. Oral lichen planus: causes, diagnosis and management. *Aust Dent J* 2002;47:290–297.
226. Oliver GF, Winkelmann RK. Treatment of lichen planus. *Drugs* 1993;45:56–65.
227. Levell NJ, Munro CS, Marks JM. Severe lichen planus clears with very low-dose cyclosporin. *Br J Dermatol* 1992;127:66–67.
228. Carbone M, Goss E, Carrozzo M, et al. Systemic and topical corticosteroid treatment of oral lichen planus: a comparative study with long-term follow-up. *J Oral Pathol Med* 2003;32:323–329.
229. Thongprasom K, Luengvisut P, Wongwatanakij A, et al. Clinical evaluation in treatment of oral lichen planus with topical fluocinolone acetonide: a 2-year follow-up. *J Oral Pathol Med* 2003;32:315–322.
230. Voute AB, Schulten EA, Langendijk PN, et al. Fluocinonide in an adhesive base for treatment of oral lichen planus. A double-blind, placebo-controlled clinical study. *Oral Surg Oral Med Oral Pathol* 1993;75:181–185.
231. Epstein JB, Truelove EL. Topical cyclosporine in a bioadhesive for treatment of oral lichenoid mucosal reactions: an open label clinical trial. *Oral Surg Oral Med Oral Pathol Oral Radiol Endod* 1996;82:532–536.
232. Voute A, Schulten E, Langendijk P, et al. Cyclosporin A in an adhesive base for treatment of recalcitrant oral lichen planus: an open trial. *Oral Surg Oral Med Oral Pathol* 1994;78:437–441.

233. Sieg P, Von Domarus H, Von Zitzewitz V, et al. Topical cyclosporin in oral lichen planus: a controlled, randomized, prospective trial. *Br J Dermatol* 1995;132:790–794.

234. Plewig G. Retinoids in lichen planus. *Dermatology* 1997;194: 311–312.

235. Chan ES, Thornhill M, Zakrzewska J. Interventions for treating oral lichen planus. *Cochrane Database Syst Rev* 2000;2: CD001168.

236. Cribier B, Frances C, Chosidow O. Treatment of lichen planus: an evidence-based medicine analysis of efficacy. *Arch Dermatol* 1998;134:1521–1530.

237. Kaliakatsou F, Hodgson TA, Lewsey JD, et al. Management of recalcitrant ulcerative oral lichen planus with topical tacrolimus. *J Am Acad Dermatol* 2002;46:35–41.

238. Rozycki TW, Rogers RS 3rd, Pittelkow MR, et al. Topical tacrolimus in the treatment of symptomatic oral lichen planus: a series of 13 patients. *J Am Acad Dermatol* 2002;46:27–34.

239. Leonardi A, DeFranchis G, Fregona IA, et al. Effects of cyclosporin A on human conjunctival fibroblasts. *Arch Ophthalmol* 2001;119:1512–1517.

240. Schaffer RN, Ridgway WL. Furmethide iodide in the production of dacryostenosis. *Am J Ophthalmol* 1951;34:718–720.

241. Broadway D. Drug induced conjunctival cicatrisation. In Bernauer W, Drat JKG, Elder MJ, eds. *Cicatrizing conjunctivitis (Dev Ophthalmol, vol 28).* Basel: Karger, 1997:86–101.

242. Grant WM. *Toxicology of the eye.* Springfield, IL: Charles C Thomas, 1974:653.

243. Wright P. Untoward effects associated with practolol administration: oculomucocutaneous syndrome. *Br Med J* 1975;1:595–598.

244. Wright P. Letter: Ocular reactions to beta-blocking drugs. *Br Med J* 1975;4:577.

245. Kestens PJ, Muschart JM, Koerperich G, et al. Fibrinous peritonitis and ocular reactions: a complication of practolol therapy. *Acta Gastroenterol Belg* 1977;40:175–187.

246. Cruysberg JR, Pinckers A. Ocular disorders resulting from treatment with practolol (Eraldin). *Ophthalmologica* 1977;175: 39–40.

247. Marshall AJ, Baddeley H, Barritt DW, et al. Practolol peritonitis. A study of 16 cases and a survey of small bowel function in patients taking beta adrenergic blockers. *Q J Med* 1977;46: 135–149.

248. Reeder RE, Mika RO. Ectropion secondary to bolus injection of 5-fluorouracil. *Optometry* 2001;72:112–116.

249. Loprinzi CL, Wender DB, Veeder MH, et al. Inhibition of 5-fluorouracil-induced ocular irritation by ocular ice packs. *Cancer* 1994;74:945–948.

250. Christophidis N, Vajda FJ, Lucas I, et al. Ocular side effects with 5-fluorouracil. *Aust N Z J Med* 1979;9:143–144.

251. Hoffer KJ. Pemphigoid related to epinephrine treatment. *Am J Ophthalmol* 1977;83:601.

252. Drance SM, Ross RA. The ocular effects of epinephrine. *Surv Ophthalmol* 1970;14:330–335.

253. Mooney D. Pigmentation after long-term topical use of adrenaline compounds. *Br J Ophthalmol* 1970;54:823–826.

254. D'Ostroph AO, Dailey RA. Cicatricial entropion associated with chronic dipivefrin application. *Ophthal Plast Reconstr Surg* 2001;17:328–331.

255. Theodore J, Leibowitz HM. External ocular toxicity of dipivalyl epinephrine. *Am J Ophthalmol* 1979;88:1013–1016.

256. Kristensen EB, Norn MS. Benign mucous membrane pemphigoid. 1. Secretion of mucus and tears. *Acta Ophthalmol (Copenh)* 1974;52:266–281.

257. Pouliquen Y, Patey A, Foster CS, et al. Drug-induced cicatricial pemphigoid affecting the conjunctiva: light and electron microscopic features. *Ophthalmology* 1986;93:775–783.

258. Fiore PM, Jacobs IH, Goldberg DB. Drug-induced pemphigoid: a spectrum of diseases. *Arch Ophthalmol* 1987;105: 1660–1663.

259. McNab AA. Lacrimal canalicular obstruction associated with topical ocular medication. *Aust N Z J Ophthalmol* 1998;26: 219–223.

260. Wilson-Holt N, Dart JK. Thiomersal keratoconjunctivitis: frequency, clinical spectrum and diagnosis. *Eye* 1989;3:581–587.

261. Wilson LA, McNatt J, Reitschel R. Delayed hypersensitivity to thimerosal in soft contact lens wearers. *Ophthalmology* 1981; 88:804–809.

262. Wilson FM 2nd. Adverse external ocular effects of topical ophthalmic therapy: an epidemiologic, laboratory, and clinical study. *Trans Am Ophthalmol Soc* 1983;81:854–965.

263. Derous D, de Keizer RJ, de Wolff-Rouendaal D, et al. Conjunctival keratinisation, an abnormal reaction to an ocular beta-blocker. *Acta Ophthalmol (Copenh)* 1989;67:333–338.

264. Kubo M, Sakuraba T, Arai Y, et al. A case of suspected drug-induced ocular pemphigoid. *Nippon Ganka Gakkai Zasshi* 2001;105:189–192.

265. Bernauer W, Wright P, Dart JK, et al. The conjunctiva in acute and chronic mucous membrane pemphigoid: an immunohistochemical analysis. *Ophthalmology* 1993;100:339–346.

266. Staatz WD, Radius RL, Van Horn DL, et al. Effects of timolol on bovine corneal endothelial cultures. *Arch Ophthalmol* 1981;99:660–663.

267. Takahashi N. A new method evaluating quantitative time-dependent cytotoxicity of ophthalmic solutions in cell culture: beta-adrenergic blocking agents. *Graefes Arch Clin Exp Ophthalmol* 1983;220:264–267.

268. Williams DE, Nguyen KD, Shapourifar-Tehrani S, et al. Effects of timolol, betaxolol, and levobunolol on human Tenon's fibroblasts in tissue culture. *Invest Ophthalmol Vis Sci* 1992; 33:2233–2241.

269. Wu KY, Hong SJ, Wang HZ. Effects of pilocarpine and other antiglaucoma drugs on cultured human Tenon's fibroblast cells. *J Ocul Pharmacol Ther* 1997;13:13–21.

270. Cunliffe IA, McIntyre CA, Rees RC, et al. Pilot study on the effect of topical adrenergic medications on human Tenon's capsule fibroblasts in tissue culture. *Br J Ophthalmol* 1995; 79:70–75.

271. van Beek LM, Mulder M, van Haeringen NJ, et al. Topical ophthalmic beta blockers may cause release of histamine through cytotoxic effects on inflammatory cells. *Br J Ophthalmol* 2000;84:1004–1007.

272. Simmons P, Clough S, Teagle R, et al. Toxic effects of ophthalmic preservatives on cultured rabbit corneal epithelium. *Am J Optom Physiol Opt* 1988;65:867–873.

273. Butt Z, Kaufman D, McNab A, et al. Drug-induced ocular cicatricial pemphigoid: a series of clinico-pathological reports. *Eye* 1998;12:285–290.

274. Kovacs EJ. Fibrogenic cytokines: the role of immune mediators in the development of scar tissue. *Immunol Today* 1991;12: 17–23.

275. Fiore PM. Drug-induced ocular cicatrization. *Int Ophthalmol Clin* 1989;29:147–150.

CONJUNCTIVITIS AND DRUG HYPERSENSITIVITY

HELEN K. WU

Conjunctival inflammation may result from allergic and toxic reactions to medication and is common among external eye diseases. Particularly familiar is the clinical scenario in which the treatment of an underlying infection or dry eye condition creates worsening of the red eye, due to toxicity of the medication or to its preservatives. Failure to recognize this clinical picture may lead one to assume worsening of the underlying problem and to prescribe additional medications, which can further exacerbate the ocular irritation or inflammation. Knowledge of toxic and allergic reactions to medication helps identify a rational and targeted clinical approach to patients presenting with red eye and irritation.

Both toxicity and allergy may play a role in producing ocular symptoms, and may sometimes be difficult to distinguish. In general, toxicity implies damage to the ocular surface without accompanying ocular inflammation, whereas allergy results from either the type I anaphylactoid (Prausnitz-Küstner) reaction or a type IV delayed hypersensitivity reaction. In the immediate type I hypersensitivity response, allergen combines with immunoglobulin E (IgE) attached to mast cells or basophils, which degranulate and release histamine, prostaglandins and leukotrienes, and cytokines such as tumor necrosis factor (TNF), interleukin-4 (IL-4), and IL-5. In the delayed type IV hypersensitivity reaction, the antigen is presented to naive T lymphocytes, resulting in expansion of antigen-specific activated $CD4^+$ T cells that produce a variety of cytokines. Although allergy generally requires repeated exposure to the drug and sensitization time, a toxic reaction may occur either immediately or over time.

SIGNS AND SYMPTOMS

The signs and symptoms of toxicity and allergy to medication may be similar. Symptoms of toxicity may include irritation, dryness, photophobia, pain, tearing, or blurry vision. The most common adverse reaction to topical medications is a toxic papillary keratoconjunctivitis. Although a papillary reaction is common with toxicity, follicles may also be seen. A purely follicular response of the conjunctiva

may be seen typically with certain medications, including pilocarpine, dipivefrin, carbachol, scopolamine, neomycin, ketorolac tromethamine, gentamicin, sulfacetamide, and antiviral medications, among others. With toxicity, conjunctival hyperemia and chemosis tend to be more concentrated in the inferior interpalpebral zone, with relative sparing of the superior conjunctiva. There is typically an associated punctate keratopathy but severity of corneal involvement may extend to corneal ulceration. Pseudodendrites and persistent corneal epithelial defects with a rolled edge appearance may occur. In severe cases, keratinization of the ocular surface and conjunctival scarring may also result. Predisposing factors include dry eye, a compromised ocular surface, long-term drug exposure, intensified treatment, and additive drug toxicity (1).

In allergic conjunctivitis, itching is the most common symptom. Conjunctival injection, chemosis, and eyelid and periorbital swelling may occur. A white stringy mucous discharge is common. A papillary reaction of the conjunctiva is most common in allergy, and follicles are not typically seen as an isolated response. With contact hypersensitivity, hyperemia and swelling are seen predominantly around the eyelids and periorbital area, and the inflammation may be worse inferiorly where the medication tends to drip toward the cheek.

DIAGNOSTIC TESTS

Diagnostic techniques to distinguish an allergic response from a toxic reaction include the intradermal skin test, in which a wheal and flare reaction occurs shortly after injection of the antigen within the skin, or application of the substance into the conjunctiva, with immediate conjunctival injection, chemosis, itching and lid swelling. Patch testing may be helpful in diagnosing patients with contact hypersensitivity, but a detailed clinical history is crucial in making the diagnosis. Conjunctival scrapings may show eosinophils in allergic conjunctivitis. There are no specific tests for toxicity, although toxic large basophilic granules may be seen in cells obtained from conjunctival scraping.

KERATOCONJUNCTIVITIS RELATED TO TOPICAL MEDICATIONS

Topical medications are most likely to cause keratoconjunctivitis or contact dermatitis from the medication itself, or from the preservatives or other compounds added to the preparation. The following is a discussion of medications commonly associated with toxicity and hypersensitivity reactions.

Preservatives

Although preservatives, required in multiple dose containers, are important in reducing the incidence of ocular infections associated with topical medications, they may be associated with significant toxicity to the conjunctival and corneal epithelium. Allergic reactions are also common with certain preservatives, such as thimerosal. Benzalkonium chloride, benzethonium chloride, cetylpyridinium chloride, chlorobutanol, ethylenediaminetetraacetic acid (EDTA), mercurial preservatives, paraben esters, phenylethyl alcohol, sodium benzoate, sodium propionate, and sorbic acid are preservatives that may be present in ophthalmic products. Sodium perborate is considered a less toxic preservative. Of these preservatives, benzalkonium chloride is one of the most common. This bactericidal quaternary ammonium agent may damage the corneal epithelial microvilli, with decreased adherence of the tear film to the cornea. It may increase the penetration of some medications through the corneal epithelium. In higher concentrations, it may severely damage the corneal endothelium. In addition to preservatives, a variety of chemicals may be added to ophthalmic products, including antioxidants, buffers, tonicity agents, and viscosity-increasing agents.

Contact lens wearers may be particularly at risk for allergy or toxicity from their solutions, which may include a variety of preservatives, including benzalkonium chloride, chlorhexidine, benzyl alcohol, polyaminopropyl biguanide, EDTA, and thimerosal. Because preservatives may bind to the contact lenses, toxicity may be amplified. Thimerosal, a mercury-containing preservative, is a particularly common cause of irritation, conjunctival hyperemia, and chemosis. Hypersensitivity reactions may occur in up to 10% of patients in the United States and up to 50% of patients in Japan. Clinical findings of thimerosal toxicity include redness, irritation, and epitheliopathy, which may range from faint opacities to coarser punctate lesions (2). The findings may be quite acute, mimicking adenoviral keratoconjunctivitis (3). Patients with delayed hypersensitivity to thimerosal may react to patch testing or intradermal injection (4). In patients with sensitivity to preservatives in contact lens solutions, hydrogen peroxide disinfection and preservative-free saline solution may ameliorate the symptoms. Daily disposable contact lenses are also a good alternative.

Mydriatics

In general, mydriatics are well tolerated, with transient burning and stinging upon instillation. The conjunctiva may become hyperemic, and mild punctate keratitis may be present. With prolonged use, however, atropine and homatropine may produce a contact dermatitis. An allergic response of the conjunctiva may produce papillary conjunctivitis, whereas toxicity may be associated with a follicular conjunctival response (5).

Glaucoma Medications

Glaucoma medications are widely prescribed and have virtually all been associated with local allergic or toxic reactions. They may cause ocular hyperemia and transient burning and stinging. Miotic agents, such as pilocarpine and carbachol, rarely cause allergy, although pilocarpine and carbachol may both cause conjunctival follicles. Pilocarpine may also be a cause of drug-induced ocular cicatricial pemphigoid. In patients on pilocarpine gel, a subtle diffuse superficial corneal haze may occur, persisting for several years even after cessation of the medication (6). Carbachol may result in corneal clouding and persistent bullous keratopathy. The benzalkonium chloride preservative in these medications may also be responsible for some of their side effects.

Timolol, a commonly prescribed beta-blocker, may cause a papillary or follicular conjunctival reaction, in addition to a contact dermatitis (7–9). Corneal findings may include a punctate epitheliopathy, pseudodendrites, and corneal anesthesia (10). A mild dry eye may result from decreased tear film breakup time and decreased tear secretion. Symblepharon formation and cicatrization of the conjunctiva may occur with long-term use, particularly in the inferior cul-de-sac.

Epinephrine is a topical sympathomimetic amine that is not commonly prescribed currently. It is frequently associated with reactive hyperemia. Cicatrizing conjunctival changes may occur over time, resembling ocular cicatricial pemphigoid. Blepharitis and meibomitis may occur, in addition to conjunctival epidermalization. Adrenochrome deposits in the conjunctiva, resembling dark brown or black spots, are common after prolonged use. These are the products of oxidation and polymerization of epinephrine. The cornea may appear black due to deposition of this material on a compromised corneal surface. Corneal epithelial toxicity or edema may also be observed. Use of epinephrine or any of its derivatives may induce an allergic reaction. Dipivefrin is generally much better tolerated than epinephrine, but may frequently induce a follicular conjunctivitis (11–13) as well as a contact dermatitis (13,14). Cicatrizing conjunctival changes may also occur with use of dipivefrin, but adrenochrome deposits are less frequently associated with dipivefrin compared to epinephrine (15).

Apraclonidine, an α_2-adrenergic agonist, may also cause ocular allergic conjunctivitis and contact dermatitis in 20% to 50% of patients (16). It may also be associated with a follicular conjunctivitis (17). Brimonidine, a newer α_2-adrenergic agonist, may also cause a follicular conjunctivitis. Like apraclonidine, it may cause an allergic contact dermatitis or conjunctivitis in up to 10% of patients (18). Cross-reactivity may be seen in approximately 10% to 20% of patients allergic to apraclonidine, but overall it is much better tolerated than apraclonidine (19,20).

Dorzolamide, a carbonic anhydrase inhibitor, may also cause follicular conjunctivitis, an allergic conjunctival response and contact dermatitis (21–23). Superficial punctate keratitis may occur in 10% to 15% of patients. In patients with endothelial compromise, dorzolamide may produce irreversible corneal edema (24). Brinzolamide is also a carbonic anhydrase inhibitor that may cause less stinging upon instillation (25). Because these medications are both sulfonamides, however, the same type of severe adverse reactions attributed to systemically administered sulfonamides may occur, such as Stevens-Johnson syndrome and toxic epidermal necrolysis, among others.

The prostaglandin analogs, including latanoprost, bimatoprost, travoprost, and unoprostone, may all cause ocular hyperemia initially in up to 50% of patients, but it tends to improve over time. Medications in this class may alter iris and periocular pigmentation, and cause increased length and thickness of eyelashes. Latanoprost may cause ocular allergy, with contact dermatitis (26). It is more likely to increase eosinophils in the conjunctiva than timolol and may cause ocular toxicity due to its high concentration of benzalkonium chloride and its use at bedtime, as well (27). It has been associated with reactivation of herpetic keratitis (28), as well as periocular herpetic dermatitis (29).

Antiviral Medications

Topical medications to treat herpes simplex virus include trifluorothymidine, vidarabine, and idoxuridine. Idoxuridine, in particular, may cause irritation and conjunctival inflammation, in addition to a persistent corneal epitheliopathy, which may be difficult to distinguish from the herpetic infection itself. With any of these medications, the cornea may exhibit a punctate keratopathy, corneal erosions, and pseudodendrites. With prolonged use of idoxuridine, conjunctival cicatrization may result, causing irreversible punctal occlusion and conjunctival scarring, similar to cicatricial pemphigoid (30). Vidarabine and trifluorothymidine are less likely to cause conjunctival cicatrization, but corneal epithelial dysplasia may occur with trifluorothymidine use (31). Contact dermatitis may occur more frequently with trifluorothymidine as well (32). Topical acyclovir, which is not available commercially in the United States, is a better-tolerated medication with low toxicity.

Antibiotics

Most topical antibiotics may cause some transient burning, irritation, or punctate keratitis with prolonged use. Allergic reactions in the conjunctiva and lids may occur after use of any of the medications. Neomycin is one of the most likely antibiotics to produce allergy, as well as toxicity, with up to 15% of patients experiencing sensitization of the skin and conjunctiva. Use of neomycin for longer than 7 to 10 days increases the incidence of an allergic reaction. Topical sulfonamides may also incite an allergic response, and may rarely cause Stevens-Johnson syndrome or other adverse reactions associated with systemic sulfonamide treatment. Polymixin B and topical bacitracin, on the other hand, are very well tolerated in general.

Aminoglycoside antibiotics may cause eyelid swelling, erythema, and toxicity to the corneal epithelium. Tobramycin may cause less toxicity than gentamicin, but both can adversely affect corneal epithelial wound healing. Fortified topical gentamicin may cause conjunctival necrosis, particularly in the inferior nasal bulbar conjunctiva (33,34). Several cases of pseudomembranous conjunctivitis have been reported as well (35). Penicillin and semisynthetic penicillins may result in a high incidence of allergic reactions. Cephalosporins, including commonly used cefazolin and ceftazidime, are relatively less toxic than the aminoglycosides and less likely to cause hypersensitivity reactions than the penicillins.

The fluoroquinolones are enjoying widespread use as both treatment and prophylaxis for ocular infections. This group of medications is less toxic than the aminoglycosides, and is generally well tolerated. Ciprofloxacin may produce white crystalline precipitates in the base of a corneal ulcer with frequent use. Ofloxacin may rarely cause precipitates as well (36). The newer generation fluoroquinolone moxifloxacin is currently available without preservatives; this may minimize its toxicity.

Antifungals

The three classes of antifungal medication include the polyenes, pyrimidines, and the imidazoles. Pimaricin (Natamycin) and amphotericin B are polyenes. Amphotericin B, prepared from intravenous solution, may cause corneal epithelial toxicity and wound healing defects (37). Salmon-colored nodules and yellowing of the conjunctiva may be seen after amphotericin B subconjunctival injection (38). Natamycin, which is commercially available, is well tolerated. Pyrimidines, including flucytosine, have lower toxicity. The imidazoles, such as clotrimazole, miconazole, ketoconazole, and econazole, are not commercially available for ophthalmic use, but may be adapted from other preparations. Miconazole may be to irritating to the ocular surface.

Anesthetics

The short-term use of topical anesthetics does not result in significant side effects, but prolonged use of these agents inhibits the rate of corneal epithelial wound healing by slowing epithelial cell migration and destroying corneal epithelial microvilli. The persistent epithelial defects caused by chronic use may lead to dense ring infiltrates in the corneal stroma, resembling a Wessely ring. Endothelial cell damage may also occur. Corneal perforation may result in severe cases (39).

Nonsteroidal Antiinflammatory Agents

When used in prescribed dosages, these medications have few serious side effects. Mild burning and irritation are common. Corneal sensitivity may be decreased with diclofenac, and corneal epithelial wound healing may be delayed after penetrating keratoplasty or photorefractive keratectomy. Severe punctate keratitis, ulceration, and perforation may occasionally occur when the medication is used in excess. Although allergic reactions are uncommon, these products should be avoided in patients with aspirin allergies or in those with asthma and nasal polyps.

Antineoplastic Agents

The use of topical or subconjunctival mitomycin-C and 5-fluorouracil was initially popularized as adjunctive therapy in the management of challenging trabeculectomy cases. Mitomycin-C is also currently used in the treatment of pterygium and corneal dysplasias, and to prevent corneal haze in high-risk patients undergoing photorefractive keratectomy. Both agents may be associated with conjunctival edema and delayed wound healing. Fluorouracil is particularly prone to cause superficial keratitis, and rarely corneal ulceration. Mitomycin may cause side effects similar to ionizing radiation, with potential corneal and scleral melting up to years after its administration.

DRUG-INDUCED CICATRICIAL PEMPHIGOID

The prolonged exposure of antiglaucoma or antiviral medication may lead to progressive conjunctival cicatrization, with or without obvious clinical inflammation, known as drug-induced ocular cicatricial pemphigoid. This clinical entity, previously thought to be distinct from idiopathic ocular cicatricial pemphigoid, is now felt to be a subset of genetically predisposed patients whose conjunctival changes are triggered by a medication. Light and electron microscopic findings are identical in both conditions (40). Immunofluorescent findings are also identical and circulating anti-basement membrane zone antibodies may be found in both entities (41). It is likely that these two populations share a common predispos-

ing human leukocyte antigen (HLA) haplotype (42). Treatment of this condition includes cessation of the presumed offending medication and immunosuppressive agents, such as dapsone, cyclophosphamide, and corticosteroids, if inflammation persists or the cicatrizing changes are progressive.

CONJUNCTIVAL INFLAMMATION ASSOCIATED WITH SYSTEMIC MEDICATIONS

Conjunctival inflammation secondary to systemic medications may occur infrequently due to allergic reactions or toxicity, as well. This is more commonly seen with antineoplastic agents, but may also occur with systemic nonsteroidal antiinflammatory medication, acetaminophen, diazepam, calcitonin, and phenobarbital, among others. As with many medications, antimetabolites are concentrated in the tears and may cause irritation of the conjunctiva and lid margins. Isotretinoin (Accutane) may cause blepharoconjunctivitis and dry eye syndrome (secondary to meibomitis) (43,44), in addition to subepithelial corneal opacities (45). Discoloration of the conjunctiva or sclera may be associated with chlorpromazine, tetracycline, and minocycline. Yellow-brown conjunctival pigmentation may be caused by tetracycline. Cefaclor may induce a type III hypersensitivity reaction, with mild conjunctivitis, limbal hyperemia, and peripheral corneal edema, and a serum sickness-like reaction systemically (46,47). Practolol, a beta-blocker, causes nonspecific conjunctivitis with keratoconjunctivitis sicca and conjunctival cicatrization and fornix obliteration, among multiple other serious systemic side effects, resulting in its withdrawal from clinical use. Other systemic medications, including thiabendazole and penicillamine, may also cause drug-induced pemphigoid.

Stevens-Johnson syndrome, Lyell's syndrome, and toxic epidermal necrolysis may result after ingestion of a variety of systemic medications, resulting in potentially severe conjunctival inflammation and scarring. These clinical entities are discussed at length in Chapter 20.

TREATMENT OF DRUG-INDUCED CONJUNCTIVITIS

The treatment of drug-induced toxicity or allergy involves the recognition of the problem and the cessation of the medication causing the reaction. If the problem is toxicity and further treatment is required, switching to a preservative-free or less toxic alternative may be helpful. When feasible, as many medications as possible should be stopped. Lubricating drops and ointment without preservatives may be used to ameliorate symptoms. Antihistamines or mild topical steroids also help diminish itching and other symptoms and signs of ocular allergy. If a severe corneal epitheliopathy persists, patching, bandage contact lenses, or a tarsorrhaphy should be performed. In the case of anesthetic abuse, hospitalization and observation may be warranted. Rarely, tissue adhesive, followed by penetrating or tectonic keratoplasty may be necessary for severe thinning or perforation of the cornea. In the setting of severe conjunctival inflammation secondary to drug-induced cicatricial pemphigoid or Stevens-Johnson syndrome, systemic antiinflammatory and immunosuppressive medication may be required.

SUMMARY

Drug-related conjunctivitis may result from topical or systemic medication and may be mediated by allergic or toxic mechanisms. Immediate and delayed-type hypersensitivity reactions may be responsible for allergic reactions around the conjunctiva and lids. Many commonly used topical medications and their preservatives may cause toxicity and allergy, particularly those used to treat glaucoma and infection. Contact lens wearers may be sensitive to chemicals in their solutions. Reactions to these medications or to their preservatives may result in keratoconjunctivitis or contact dermatitis, which can be misinterpreted as worsening of the underlying medical condition. Severe reactions may result in corneal epithelial wound healing problems and potential ulceration, or progressive conjunctival scarring and inflammation. Cessation of the offending agent and appropriate treatment with lubricating agents and antiinflammatory agents serve to improve patient comfort and minimize damage to the ocular surface.

REFERENCES

1. Bernauer W. Ocular surface problems following topical medication. *Klin Monatsbl Augenheilkd* 2002;219(4):240–242.
2. Wilson LA, McNatt J, Reitschel R. Delayed hypersensitivity to thimerosal in soft contact lens wearers. *Ophthalmology* 1981; 88(8):804–809.
3. Binder PS, Rasmussen DM, Gordon M. Keratoconjunctivitis and soft contact lens solutions. *Arch Ophthalmol* 1981;99(1):87–90.
4. Wilson FM 2nd. Adverse external ocular effects of topical ophthalmic therapy: an epidemiologic, laboratory, and clinical study. *Trans Am Ophthalmol Soc* 1983;81:854–965.
5. Fraunfelder FT, Fraunfelder FW, ed. *Drug-induced ocular side effects,* 5th ed. Boston: Butterworth Heinemann, 2001:263–265.
6. Johnson DH, Kenyon KR, Epstein DL, et al. Corneal changes during pilocarpine gel therapy. *Am J Ophthalmol* 1986; 101(1):13–15.
7. Baldone JA, Hankin JS, Zimmerman TJ. Allergic conjunctivitis associated with timolol therapy in an adult. *Ann Ophthalmol* 1982;14(4)364–365.
8. Fernandez-Vozmediano JM, Blasi NA, Romero-Cabrera MA, et al. Allergic contact dermatitis to timolol. *Contact Dermatitis* 1986;14(4):252.
9. Romaguera C, Grimalt F, Vilaplana J. Contact dermatitis by timolol. *Contact Dermatitis* 1986;14(4):248.
10. Van Buskirk EM. Adverse reactions from timolol administration. *Ophthalmology* 1980;87(5):447–450.
11. Coleiro JA, Sigurdsson H, Lockyer JA. Follicular conjunctivitis on dipivefrin therapy for glaucoma. *Eye* 1988;2(pt 4): 440–442.
12. Liesegang TJ. Bulbar conjunctival follicles associated with dipivefrin therapy. *Ophthalmology* 1985;92(2):228–233.
13. Gaspari AA. Contact allergy to ophthalmic dipivalyl epinephrine hydrochloride: demonstration by patch testing. *Contact Dermatitis* 1993;28(1):35–37.
14. Petersen PE, Evans RB, Johnstone MA, et al. Evaluation of ocular hypersensitivity to dipivalyl epinephrine by component eye-drop testing. *J Allergy Clin Immunol* 1990;85(5): 954–958.
15. Wandel T, Spinak M. Toxicity of dipivalyl epinephrine. *Ophthalmology* 1981;88(3):259–260.
16. Butler P, Mannschreck M, Lin S, et al. Clinical experience with the long-term use of 1% apraclonidine. Incidence of allergic reactions. *Arch Ophthalmol* 1995;113(3):293–296.
17. Wilkerson M, Lewis RA, Shields MB. Follicular conjunctivitis associated with apraclonidine. *Am J Ophthalmol* 1991;111(1):105–106.
18. Blondeau P, Rousseau JA. Allergic reactions to brimonidine in patients treated for glaucoma. *Can J Ophthalmol* 2002;37(1):21–26.
19. Williams GC, Orengo-Nania S, Gross RL. Incidence of brimonidine allergy in patients previously allergic to apraclonidine. *J Glaucoma* 2000;9(3):235–238.
20. Gordon RN, Liebmann JM, Greenfield DS, et al. Lack of cross-reactive allergic response to brimonidine in patients with known apraclonidine allergy. *Eye* 1998;12(pt 4):697–700.
21. Adamsons IA, Polis A, Ostrov CS, et al. Two-year safety study of dorzolamide as monotherapy and with timolol and pilocarpine. Dorzolamide Safety Study Group. *J Glaucoma* 1998;7(6): 395–401.
22. Mancuso G, Berdondini RM. Allergic contact blepharoconjunctivitis from dorzolamide. *Contact Dermatitis* 2001;45(4):243.
23. Shimada M, Higaki Y, Kawashima M. Allergic contact dermatitis due to dorzolamide eyedrops. *Contact Dermatitis* 2001;45 (1):52.
24. Konowal A, Morrison JC, Brown SV, et al. Irreversible corneal decompensation in patients treated with topical dorzolamide. *Am J Ophthalmol* 1999;127(4):403–406.
25. Sall K. The efficacy and safety of brinzolamide 1% ophthalmic suspension (Azopt) as a primary therapy in patients with open-angle glaucoma or ocular hypertension. Brinzolamide Primary Therapy Study Group. *Surv Ophthalmol* 2000;44(suppl 2):S155–162.
26. Jerstad KM, Warshaw E. Allergic contact dermatitis to latanoprost. *Am J Contact Dermatol* 2002;13(1):39–41.
27. Costagliola C, Prete AD, Incorvaia C, et al. Ocular surface changes induced by topical application of latanoprost and timolol: a short-term study in glaucomatous patients with and without allergic conjunctivitis. *Grafes Arch Clin Exp Ophthalmol* 2001;239(11):809–814.
28. Wand M, Gilbert CM, Liesegang TJ. Latanoprost and herpes simplex keratitis. *Am J Ophthalmol* 1999;127(5):602–604.
29. Morales J, Shihab ZM, Brown SM, et al. Herpes simplex virus dermatitis in patients using latanoprost. *Am J Ophthalmol* 2001;132(1):114–116.
30. Lass JH, Thoft RA, Dohlman CH. Idoxuridine-induced conjunctival cicatrization. *Arch Ophthalmol* 1983;101(5): 747–750.
31. Maudgal PC, Van Damme B, Missotten L. Corneal epithelial dysplasia after trifluridine use. *Graefes Arch Clin Exp Ophthalmol* 1983;220(1):6–12.
32. Pavan-Langston D, Dohlman CH. A double blind clinical study of adenine arabinoside therapy of viral keratoconjunctivitis. *Am J Ophthalmol* 1972;74(1):81–88.

33. Davison CR, Tuft SJ, Dart JK. Conjunctival necrosis after administration of topical fortified aminoglycosides. *Am J Ophthalmol* 1991; 111(6):690–693.
34. Nauheim R, Nauheim J. Bulbar conjunctival defects associated with gentamicin. *Arch Ophthalmol* 1987;105(10):1321.
35. Bullard SR, O'Day DM. Pseudomembranous conjunctivitis following topical gentamicin therapy. *Arch Ophthalmol* 1997; 115(12):1591–1592.
36. Claerhout I, Kestelyn P, Meire F, et al. Corneal deposits after the topical use of ofloxacin in two children with vernal keratoconjunctivitis. *Br J Ophthalmol* 2003;87(5):646.
37. Foster CS, Lass JH, Moran-Wallace K, et al. Ocular toxicity of topical antifungal agents. *Arch Ophthalmol* 1981;99(6):1081–1084.
38. O'Day DM, Smith R, Stevens JB, et al. Toxicity and pharmacokinetics of subconjunctival amphotericin B. An experimental study. *Cornea* 1991;10(5):411–417.
39. Rosenwasser, GO, Holland S, Pflugfelder SC, et al. Topical anesthetic abuse. *Ophthalmology* 1990;97(8):967–972.
40. Pouliquen Y, Patey A, Foster CS, et al. Drug-induced cicatricial pemphigoid affecting the conjunctiva. Light and electron microscopic features. *Ophthalmology* 1986;93(6):775–783.
41. Leonard JN, Hobday CM, Haffenden GP, et al. Immunofluorescent studies in ocular cicatricial pemphigoid. *Br J Dermatol* 1988;118(2):209–217.
42. Yunis JJ, Mobini N, Yunis EJ, et al. Common major histocompatibility complex class II markers in clinical variants of cicatricial pemphigoid. *Proc Natl Acad Sci USA* 1994; 91: 7747–7751.
43. Egger SF, Huber-Spitzy V, Bohler K, et al. Isotretinoin administration in treatment of acne vulgaris. A prospective study of the kind and extent of ocular complications. *Ophthalmologe* 1995; 92(1):17–20.
44. Bozkurt B, Irkec MT, Atakan N, et al. Lacrimal function and ocular complications in patients treated with systemic isotretinoin. *Eur J Ophthalmol* 2002;12(3):173–176.
45. Fraunfelder FT, LaBraico JM, Meyer SM. Adverse ocular reactions possibly associated with isotretinoin. *Am J Ophthalmol* 1985;100(4):534–537.
46. Murray DL, Singer DA, Singer AB, et al. Cefaclor—a cluster of adverse reactions. *N Engl J Med* 1980;303(17):1003.
47. Platt LW. Bilateral peripheral corneal edema after cefaclor therapy. *Arch Ophthalmol* 1990;108(2):175.

PHLYCTENULAR KERATOCONJUNCTIVITIS

D. REX HAMILTON AND ELIZABETH A. DAVIS

INTRODUCTION AND HISTORICAL PERSPECTIVE

Phlyctenular keratoconjunctivitis (PKC) is a localized, noninfectious inflammatory disorder of the ocular surface characterized by subepithelial nodules of the conjunctiva and/or cornea. These "phlyctenules," derived from "phlyctena," the Greek word for "blister," were first described in classical Greek and Arabic literature (1). The blister characterization, described later by Saint-Yves (2) and Wardrop (3), was likely chosen due to the tendency for the nodules to ulcerate once necrosis occurs. PKC has been reported throughout the world, most commonly as a disease of children with a higher incidence in females. The disease was initially identified in patients with positive tuberculin skin tests (4), classically in children who lived in crowded, unsanitary conditions (5). In the United States, several studies have documented PKC in Native American and Inuit patients with positive tuberculin skin tests and clinical tuberculosis (6–8). Sorsby (9) was the first to clinically implicate a hypersensitivity reaction to tuberculin protein as an etiology for PKC, finding that 85% of patients with the disorder had a positive tuberculin skin test. In recent years, as endemic tuberculosis has come under control in developed countries, other antigens have been suggested as etiologies for PKC. In 1974, Ostler and Lanier (10) published a series of five cases of PKC related to staphylococcal infection. Currently in the United States, it appears that most cases of PKC are associated with chronic staphylococcal blepharitis (11–13).

ETIOLOGY

The pathogenesis of PKC is thought to be a hypersensitivity reaction to an antigen of bacterial origin (14). Although PKC has been clinically associated with *M. tuberculosis* and other organisms (Table 22-1), the microbe that has been implicated most rigorously from an immunological standpoint in the laboratory is *Staphylococcus aureus*. Clinically,

S. aureus is the most common organism associated with PKC in the United States, via its association with chronic blepharitis. Chlamydial infection has been identified in association with PKC. Culbertson et al. (15) reported 17 cases of PKC in patients under age 18. Five of the 10 patients tested for chlamydial infection were positive. In countries where it is still highly present, however, *M. tuberculosis* remains a major cause of PKC. A study in India prospectively examined 112 patients with phlyctenular eye disease and found 77% associated with tuberculosis whereas only 6% were associated with staphylococcal blepharitis (16).

HISTOPATHOLOGY

Phlyctenules are subepithelial inflammatory nodules containing histiocytes, lymphocytes, plasma cells, and neutrophils (Fig. 22-1). Mononuclear phagocytes, dendritic Langerhans cells, and neutrophils make up the majority of the inflammatory cells in the epithelium overlying the phlyctenule with a moderate number of T lymphocytes also present. The underlying stromal inflammatory infiltrate is typically organized in perivascular cuffs with a scattered subepithelial infiltrate consisting mainly of monocyte derived cells and neutrophils. T lymphocytes are also present, whereas B lymphocytes and plasma cells are infrequent (17).

In a conjunctival lesion, mononuclear phagocytes and neutrophils infiltrate the deep tissue causing edema, which eventually resolves. In a corneal lesion, lymphocytes infiltrate under Bowman's membrane and stroma. The associated edema may lift and break down the epithelium, forming an ulcer. Bowman's membrane and anterior stroma may be destroyed and replaced with a vascularized pannus.

Animal models suggest that phlyctenular disease is a hypersensitivity reaction to an antigen, such as ribitol teichoic acid found in the cell wall of *S. aureus* (18). Mondino et al. (19–22) established the role of hypersensitivity to staphylococcal antigen in the pathogenesis of peripheral corneal infiltrates and phlyctenular disease in a rabbit model. The rabbits, previously immunized intravenously by ribitol

TABLE 22-1. ORGANISMS IMPLICATED IN THE PATHOGENESIS OF PHLYCTENULAR KERATOCONJUNCTIVITIS

Mycobacterium tuberculosis
Staphylococcus aureus
Chlamydia trachomatis[1]
Neisseria gonorrhea
Coccidioides immitis[2]
Bacillus spp.
Herpes simplex virus[3]
Leishmaniasis[4]
Ascaris lumbricoides[5,6]
Hymenolepsis nana
Candida spp.

[1] Janssen KT, Siemon P, Bialasiewicz AA. Ocular chlamydia infections in Munsterland. A clinical study of 409 patients. Ophthalmologe 1994; 91:671–675.
[2] Thygeson P. Observations on nontuberculous phlyctenular keratoconjunctivitis. Am Acad Ophth Otolaryngol Trans 1954; 58:128–132.
[3] Holland EJ, Mahanti RL, Belongia EA, et al. Ocular involvement in and outbreak of herpes gladiatorum. AJO 1992; 114:680–684.
[4] Ghosh JB. Phlyctenular conjunctivitis in kala-azar. Indian Pediatrics 1991; 28:1531.
[5] Jeffery MP. Ocular diseases caused by nematodes. AJO 1955; 40:41.
[6] Hussein AA, Nasr ME. The role of parasitic infection in the aetiology of phlyctenular eye disease. J Egypt Soc Parasitology 1991; 21:865–868.

teichoic acid (the major antigenic determinant of the *S. aureus* cell wall) developed phlyctenules after topical challenge with viable *S. aureus*. Subsequent studies have suggested that corneal antibodies to ribitol teichoic acid may be influenced not only by exposure to staphylococcal antigens in the ocular adnexa but to antigens in remote sites as well (e.g., skin) (23). These findings are consistent with the association between rosacea, a dermatologic disorder potentially related to hypersensitivity to staphylococcal antigens, and ocular external disease such as meibomian dysfunction blepharoconjunctivitis, marginal keratitis, recurrent chalazion, and phlyctenular disease (24).

CLINICAL SIGNS AND SYMPTOMS

Symptoms of PKC depend on the location of the lesion. Conjunctival lesions usually present with mild to moderate symptoms, including tearing, photophobia, burning, itching, and foreign-body sensation. The lesions may spontaneously regress as the lesion ulcerates and reepithelializes, but symptoms may persist for 2 weeks or longer. Corneal lesions typically present with more severe symptoms of the same variety and may also include blepharospasm.

Phlyctenules typically appear unilaterally, first at or near the limbus, and they may spread to the cornea or bulbar conjunctiva. Although lesions can occur anywhere on the ocular surface, they rarely occur on the palpebral conjunctiva. Conjunctival and corneal lesions may occur separately or simultaneously.

The conjunctival or limbal phlyctenule appears as a raised, pink to gray amorphous nodule, typically 1 to 2 mm in diameter with surrounding conjunctival injection (Fig. 22-2). The lesions usually soften in appearance and become less injected after 2 to 5 days. Ulceration with reepithelialization typically occurs, with the entire clinical course complete in 2 to 3 weeks.

Corneal phlyctenules usually begin at the limbus and spread centrally, perpendicular to the limbus, leaving no clear zone between the lesion and the limbus (Fig. 22-3). The vessels run in a straight course from the limbus, creating a superficial pannus. The lesions typically ulcerate, leading to moderate to severe symptoms of tearing, photophobia, burning, itching, foreign-body sensation, and blepharospasm. The peripheral area may reepithelialize, whereas the central ulcer remains active, proceeding across the cornea preceded by a gray inflammatory zone. An anterior stromal scar forms in proportion to the amount of inflammation. Occasionally, corneal phlyctenules can "wander" across the visual axis. Rarely, inflammation associated with corneal phlyctenules can lead to keratolysis and perforation (25).

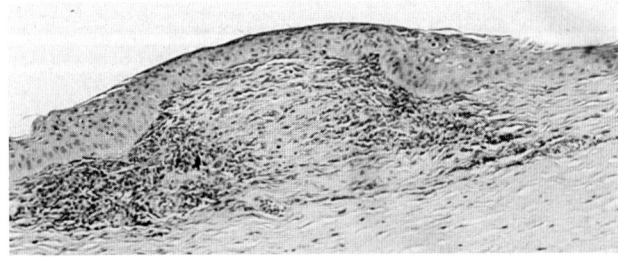

FIGURE 22-1. Histopathologic specimen of a corneal phlyctenule in a rabbit model demonstrating a subepithelial nodule consisting of a central zone of histiocytes and lymphocytes surrounded by a mantle of lymphocytes and polymorphonuclear neutrophils. (Courtesy of B. J. Mondino, M.D.)

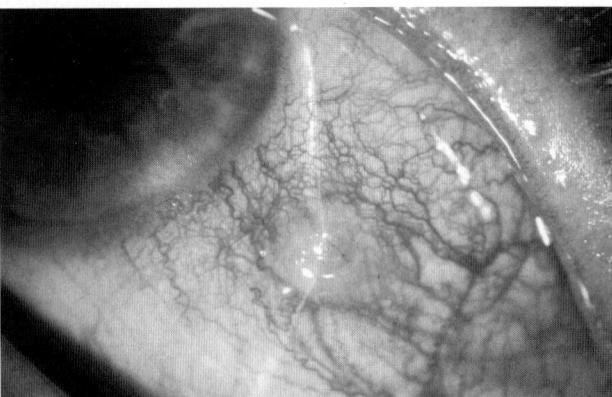

FIGURE 22-2. Conjunctival phlyctenule in a patient. This amorphous, pink to gray nodule typically appears at or near the limbus with associated conjunctival injection. The lesion commonly ulcerates, as in this example, and reepithelializes over a period of 2 weeks. Symptoms are mild to moderate and include tearing, photophobia, burning, itching, and foreign-body sensation. (Courtesy of B. J. Mondino, M.D.)

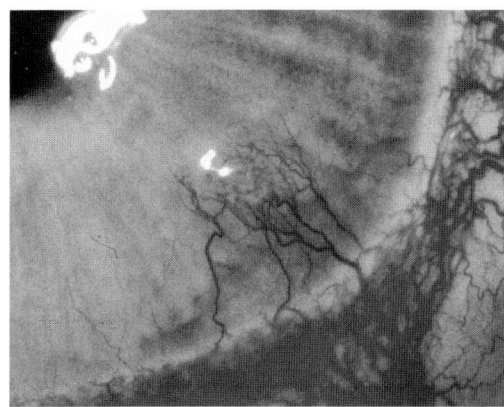

FIGURE 22-3. Corneal phlyctenule in a rabbit model. These lesions usually begin at the limbus and spread centrally, perpendicular to the limbus, leaving no clear zone between the lesion and the limbus. The vessels run in a straight course from the limbus, creating a superficial pannus. The lesions typically ulcerate, leading to moderate to severe symptoms of tearing, photophobia, burning, itching, foreign-body sensation, and blepharospasm. An anterior stromal scar forms in proportion to the amount of inflammation. (Courtesy of B. J. Mondino, M.D.)

DIFFERENTIAL DIAGNOSIS

During the nodular stage of PKC, limbal and conjunctival lesions can resemble inflamed pingueculae, nodular episcleritis, limbal papillae associated with vernal keratoconjunctivitis (VKC), or a sarcoid granuloma. Inflamed pingueculae do not ulcerate, are typically located at the 3 and 9 o'clock positions, and do not migrate onto the cornea as quickly as PKC lesions. The nodules in episcleritis are typically associated with minimal or no symptoms and do not ulcerate or migrate. Limbal papillae associated with VKC occur bilaterally and predominately in patients of African or Asian ethnicity who live in hot climates. Like PKC, VKC commonly occurs in children but, unlike PKC, occurs more often in males than females. VKC is typically a seasonal disorder, occurring most commonly in the spring in temperate zones, and this condition invariably produces significant ocular itch. The limbus has a gelatinous, hypertrophic appearance with multiple, heaped-up opalescent mounds associated with a copious, mucoid discharge. The superior palpebral conjunctiva typically has large cobblestone-like papillae. PKC lesions are typically but not always singular, unilateral, and not associated with a mucoid discharge. Sarcoid granulomas most commonly occur in the fornix or on the palpebral conjunctiva. Sarcoidosis has protean ocular manifestations, but most commonly presents with anterior granulomatous uveitis. If a conjunctival lesion is suggestive of sarcoidosis, a simple biopsy may prove diagnostic.

Prior to ulceration, corneal phlyctenules may resemble Salzmann's corneal nodules, pterygia, or staphylococcal (catarrhal) marginal infiltrates, a related entity thought to be a type III hypersensitivity reaction to antigens deposited in corneal tissue. The subepithelial fibrosis associated with Salzmann's nodular degeneration is noninflammatory and nonprogressive. Pterygia occur at the 3 and 9 o'clock positions and have a characteristic, winged appearance. Unlike PKC lesions, staphylococcal marginal infiltrates are not elevated, may ulcerate, and typically have a clear zone between the lesion and the limbus.

During the ulcerative and convalescent phase, PKC lesions can be confused with bacterial, fungal, herpes simplex virus (HSV), syphilitic, and peripheral ulcerative keratitides as well as trachoma. Bacterial or fungal keratitis is typically more centrally located, more painful, and may be associated with an anterior chamber reaction. The hallmark of HSV superficial keratitis is the dendritic epithelial lesions with corneal hypesthesia. Focal stromal edema, underlying keratic precipitates without ulceration, indicates HSV disciform keratitis.

Topical corticosteroid therapy can be quite effective in treating PKC, but may make infectious keratitis worse. Syphilitic keratitis is a late immune manifestation of congenital syphilis infection. It typically occurs in the same age group as PKC but is associated with systemic findings of congenital syphilis infection: dental deformities, bone and cartilage abnormalities, and mental retardation. The corneal disease manifests itself as a bilateral, although not necessarily simultaneous, sectoral deep keratitis with keratic precipitates. The chronic appearance is characterized by deep ghost vessels and stromal scarring. Autoimmune-related peripheral ulcerative keratitis (PUK) is a vaso-occlusive disease most often associated with systemic autoimmune disorders such as rheumatoid arthritis, Wegener's granulomatosis, systemic lupus erythematosus, polyarteritis nodosa, ulcerative colitis, relapsing polychondritis, and other inflammatory conditions such as rosacea. PUK differs from PKC in that the lesions are typically circumferential, not perpendicular to the limbus. Keratolysis is much more common in PUK than PKC, and such ulceration can happen very rapidly. In contrast to PKC, trachoma is typically characterized in the acute phase by a mucopurulent discharge and a severe follicular reaction on the superior tarsal conjunctiva. In the convalescent phase, tarsal conjunctival scarring (Arlt's line) is pathognomonic. Herbert's pits are depressions at the limbus, representing necrosis of prior limbal inflammatory follicles. Although trachoma lesions of the limbus and cornea may resemble those associated with PKC, the diagnosis typically requires the tarsal findings (see above).

TREATMENT

Although phlyctenular disease manifests itself as a hypersensitivity reaction to microbial antigens, and thus is primarily an immune-mediated disorder, the underlying organism should be treated with appropriate antibiotics. Currently, staphylococcal-related external eye diseases are the major etiologic entities associated with PKC in the United States. The persistent nature of staphylococcal/rosacea-associated blepharitis will lead to recurrences of PKC if the chronic infection is not treated. Lid hygiene together with antibiotic ointment applied to the eyelid margin may aid in reducing the bacterial colonization of the eyelids.

Phlyctenular keratoconjunctivitis is well controlled with topical corticosteroids, a feature that distinguishes the condition from other infectious etiologies in the differential diagnosis. This clinical finding of corticosteroid response further supports the laboratory evidence that PKC is primarily an immunologic disorder. If there is compelling evidence in the history or examination that a lesion might be infectious, cultures should be obtained and a broad-spectrum antibiotic should be initiated.

Oral tetracycline has been used for several decades, both as an alternative treatment for nontuberculous PKC in patients suffering from corticosteroid induced complications and to decrease the incidence of recurrent episodes. Zaidman and Brown (26) reported a series of six patients with recurrent episodes of nontuberculous PKC and progressive corneal vascularization who were treated with oral tetracycline. The treatment resulted in rapid arrest of the disease and relief of symptoms. The remission of the disease persisted in all but one patient even after cessation of the antibiotic. Culbertson et al. (15) reported a series of 17 patients under age 18 with severe, recurrent nontuberculous PKC treated with either oral tetracycline or erythromycin. The severity of the existing PKC was substantial, with significant ocular morbidity, including three perforated corneas. All patients experienced long-term remission of the PKC after completion of a course of tetracycline or erythromycin that ranged from 3 weeks to 9 months. Although the dosages and durations varied, a dose of 250 mg three times daily for 3 weeks followed by 250 mg once daily for 2 months appeared to be effective. Persistence of the remission following cessation of the antibiotic suggests that the mechanism of action is antimicrobial, reducing the bacterial burden that is the source of antigen for the hypersensitivity reaction, rather than the nonspecific antiinflammatory effect of both tetracycline and erythromycin that has been reported (27).

Tetracycline should not be used in children under age 8 because permanent tooth discoloration can occur. In addition, tetracycline is teratogenic and should be avoided in pregnant women and those attempting to become pregnant. Erythromycin appears to be an effective alternative in these patients. Other complications of tetracycline include gastrointestinal distress, photosensitivity, and benign intracranial hypertension.

Phlyctenular keratoconjunctivitis is a hypersensitivity reaction to microbial antigen, with *S. aureus* being the most common etiologic agent in the developed world. *M. tuberculosis* is still a prominent cause in the developing world and, due to its significant morbidity and mortality, should always be considered in patients with PKC. The disease, most often seen in young females, can lead to significant ocular morbidity if left untreated, and corneal involvement occurs. Fortunately, PKC responds well acutely to topical corticosteroids, and recurrences can be greatly reduced and even eliminated through the use of oral tetracycline or erythromycin.

ACKNOWLEDGMENT

The authors wish to thank Bartly J. Mondino, M.D., for his contributions to this chapter.

REFERENCES

1. Duke-Elder S, ed. *System of ophthalmology. Vol. VIII: diseases of the outer eye. Pt. 1: conjunctiva.* St. Louis: Mosby, 1965.
2. De Saint-Yves C. *Nouveau traite des maladies des yeux.* Paris: Pierre-Augustin Le Mercier, 1722:183–184.
3. Wardrop J. *Essays on the morbid anatomy of the human eye,* vol 1. Edinburgh: George Ramsay, 1808;136–137.
4. Gibson WS. The etiology of phlyctenular conjunctivitis. *Am J Dis Child* 1918;15:81–115.
5. Walkingshaw R. Phlyctenular disease and tuberculosis. *Trans Ophth Soc Aust* 1951;11:115–121.
6. Philip RN, Comstock GW, Shelton JH. Phlyctenular keratoconjunctivitis among Eskimos in southwestern Alaska. *Am Rev Respir Dis* 1965;91:171–187.
7. Thygeson P. The etiology and treatment of phlyctenular keratoconjunctivitis. *Am J Ophthalmol* 1951;34:1217–1236.
8. Fritz MN, Thygeson P, Durham DG. Phlyctenular keratoconjunctivitis among Alaska natives. *Am J Ophthalmol* 1951;34:177–184.
9. Sorsby A. The aetiology of phlyctenular ophthalmia. *Br J Ophthalmol* 1942;26:189–215.
10. Ostler HB, Lanier JD. Phlyctenular keratoconjunctivitis with special reference to the staphylococcal type. *Trans Pac Coast Oto-Ophth Soc Ann Mtg* 1974;55:237–252.
11. Thygeson P. Complications of staphylococcic blepharitis. *Am J Ophthalmol* 1969;68:446–449.
12. Thygeson P. Nontuberculous phlyctenular keratoconjunctivitis. In: Golden B, ed. *Ocular inflammatory disease.* Springfield, IL: Charles C Thomas, 1974.
13. Smolin G, Okumoto M. Staphylococcal blepharitis. *Arch Ophthalmol* 1977;95:812–816.
14. Abu El-Asrar AM, Geboes K, Maudgal PC, et al. Immunocytological study of phlyctenular eye disease. *Int Ophthalmol* 1987;10:33–39.
15. Culbertson WW, Huang AJW, Mandelbaum SH, et al. Effective treatment of phlyctenular keratoconjunctivitis with oral tetracycline. *Ophthalmology* 1993;100:1358–1366.
16. Rohatgi J, Dhaliwal U. Phlyctenular eye disease: a reappraisal. *Jpn J Ophthalmol* 2000;44:146–150.
17. Abu El-Asrar AM, Van den Oord JJ, Geboes K, et al. Phenotypic characterization of inflammatory cells in phlyctenular eye disease. *Doc Ophthalmol* 1989;70:353–362.

18. Mondino BJ. Inflammatory diseases of the peripheral cornea. *Ophthalmology* 1988;95:463–472.
19. Mondino BJ, Kowalski R, Ratajczak HV, et al. Rabbit model of phlyctenulosis and catarrhal infiltrates. *Arch Ophthalmol* 1981;92:178–182.
20. Mondino BJ, Phlyctenulae and catarrhal infiltrates: occurrence in rabbits immunized with staphylococcal cell walls. *Arch Ophthalmol* 1982;100:1968–1971.
21. Mondino BJ, Cruz TA, Kowalski RP. Immune responses in rabbits with phlyctenules and catarrhal infiltrates. *Arch Ophthalmol* 1983;101:1275–1277.
22. Mondino BJ, Occurrence of phlyctenules after immunization with ribitol teichoic acid of *Staphylococcus aureus. Arch Ophthalmol* 1984;102:461–463.
23. Mondino BJ, Brawman-Mintzer O, Adamu SA. Corneal antibodies to ribitol teichoic acid in rabbits immunized with staphylococcal antigens using various routes. *Invest Ophthalmol Vis Sci* 1987;28:1553–1558.
24. Browning DJ, Proia AD. Ocular rosacea. *Surv Ophthalmol* 1986;31:145–158.
25. Ostler HB. Corneal perforation in nontuberculous (staphylococcal) phlyctenular keratoconjunctivitis. *Am J Ophthalmol* 1975;79: 446–449.
26. Zaidman GW, Brown SI. Orally administered tetracycline for phlyctenular keratoconjunctivitis. *Am J Ophthalmol* 1981;92: 178–182.
27. Jain A, Sangal L, Basal E, et al. Anti-inflammatory effects of erythromycin and tetracycline on Propionibacterium acnes induced production of chemotactic factors and reactive oxygen species by human neutrophils. *Dermatol Online J* 2002;8:2.
28. Janssen KT, Siemon P, Bialasiewicz AA. Ocular chlamydia infections in Munsterland. A clinical study of 409 patients. *Ophthalmologe* 1994;91:671–675.
29. Thygeson P. Observations on nontuberculous phlyctenular keratoconjunctivitis. *Am Acad Ophthalmol Otolaryngol Trans* 1954; 58:128–132.
30. Holland EJ, Mahanti RL, Belongia EA, et al. Ocular involvement in and outbreak of herpes gladiatorum. *Am J Ophthalmol* 1992;114:680–684.
31. Ghosh JB. Phlyctenular conjunctivitis in kala-azar. *Indian Pediatr* 1991;28:1531.
32. Jeffery MP. Ocular diseases caused by nematodes. *Am J Ophthalmol* 1955;40:41.
33. Hussein AA, Nasr ME. The role of parasitic infection in the aetiology of phlyctenular eye disease. *J Egypt Soc Parasitology* 1991; 21:865–868.

KERATITITS

CONNECTIVE TISSUE/COLLAGEN VASCULAR DISEASES

C. STEPHEN FOSTER

The acquired connective tissue and vasculitic disorders, including rheumatoid arthritis, ankylosing spondylitis, psoriatic arthritis, reactive arthritis, systemic lupus erythematosus (SLE), polyarteritis nodosa (PAN), Wegener's granulomatosis, giant cell arteritis (GCA), relapsing polychondritis, juvenile idiopathic arthritis (JIA), scleroderma, polymyositis, and Sjögren's syndrome may all produce conjunctival, episcleral, sclera, corneal, and intraocular inflammation. Additionally, except in the case of rheumatoid arthritis, the ocular manifestations of the disease may be the feature that stimulates the patient to first seek medical care. Furthermore, for reasons that are not well understood, the eye may be one of the most exquisitely sensitive indications of very ominous, otherwise subclinical disease activity. That is, ocular inflammation may portend catastrophic extraocular vasculitis in a patient whose systemic disease appears to be in remission. Examples of this are abundant and legendary, yet few ophthalmologists and even fewer rheumatologists are aware of this phenomenon. But the evidence for this is vast (1–5). Failure to act on the occurrence of new-onset ocular inflammation in such patients with dramatically increased therapeutic vigor is generally associated with disastrous systemic outcomes. This will be addressed more fully (below) for each specific disease. But this introductory preamble is intended to indicate to the reader the primary importance of this chapter: recognition of not only the ocular manifestations of the acquired connective tissue and vasculitic disorders, but also the systemic prognostic significance of same.

RHEUMATOID ARTHRITIS

Rheumatoid arthritis (RA) is the preeminent autoimmune disease, with (especially) genetically predisposed (6–8) individuals triggered (probably) by as yet unknown microbial contact to mount inappropriate immune, inflammatory attacks on various targets, including molecules in joint synovium, with resultant chronic inflammation that produces damage to the affected joints (9–13). The arthritis is generalized and is generally symmetric, and any joint can be involved (14–16).

Systemic Manifestations

Epidemiology

The prevalence of RA is 0.5% to 1.0% in most population groups, with higher rates in some Native American groups and lower rates in Asians and Africans. Women are affected three times more frequently than men.

Pathogenesis

The evidence for a combined microbiologic, immunologic, and genetic etiology for RA is compelling (16,17). Figure 23-1 illustrates this general paradigm.

Rheumatoid factor, the classic autoantibody produced in RA, is present in the circulation and in the joint, and is present in immune complexes, which are central to the cascade of inflammatory events (18), resulting in the release of a panoply of inflammatory cytokines and destructive enzymes that result in arthritis, scleritis or tissue destruction, and scarring (9,11,13,16,19–21). The articular manifestations of RA may be ascribed to the production of a number of cytokines, including interleukin-1 (IL-1), IL-2, IL-6, and IL-8; interferon-γ; macrophage–colony-stimulating factor; tumor necrosis factor-α; and epidermal growth factor. Many of the extraarticular manifestations of RA may also be attributed to systemic effects of circulating cytokines (22).

The important role of immune complexes is suggested by findings of increased levels of immune complexes and decreased complement levels (complement consumption in the process of immune complex formation) in synovial, pericardial, and pleural fluids of RA patients (18,23–29). Cell-mediated immunity (CMI) is also important in the pathogenesis of RA. T lymphocytes predominate in the synovial infiltrate (18,23–26,28,29), with CD4$^+$/CD29$^+$ memory T cells prominent (22). Macrophages isolated from the synovium of patients with RA are capable of

RHEUMATOID ARTHRITIS: PATHOGENESIS

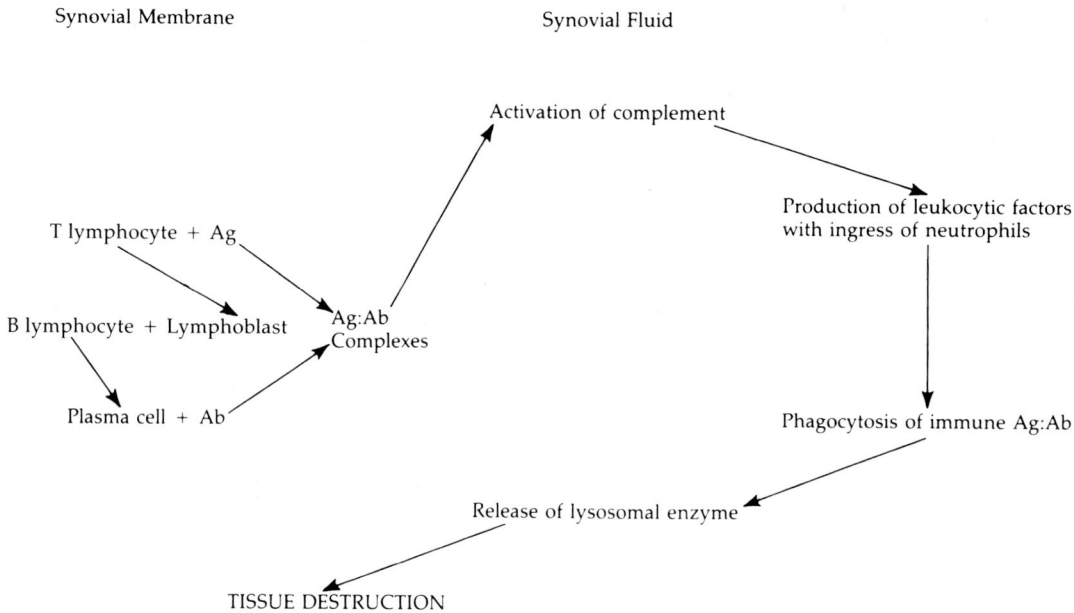

FIGURE 23-1. Proposed pathogenesis of rheumatoid arthritis. Ab, antibody; Ag, antigen. (From Zizic TM, Stevens MB. Rheumatoid arthritis and variants. In Ryan SJ Jr, Smith RE, eds. *Selected topics on the eye in systemic disease.* New York: Grune & Stratton, 1974:315–338, with permission.)

inducing neovascularization, probably via secretion of IL-1, and therefore contribute to the development of the rheumatoid synovial pannus (30).

Clinical Features

The average age of onset of RA is between 30 and 40 years. A prodrome of fatigue, malaise, loss of appetite, and weight loss may occur, with subsequent onset of morning stiffness, and then pain and swelling of the interphalangeal and metacarpophalangeal joints in the fingers and wrists. Larger joints, such as knees, ankles, shoulders, and elbows, become inflamed subsequently. The chronic progressive nature of the arthritis can lead to crippling joint damage (Fig. 23-2).

The course of RA varies from a short, mild episode of arthritis to progressive, severe, crippling disease. The longer the inflammatory activity, the less the likelihood of a remission. The sooner effective therapeutic intervention occurs, the less disability that ensues. This latter realization has prompted reevaluation of the traditional base-down pyramid model for RA therapy, with the most potent treatments (e.g., immunosuppressive medications) reserved for the apex of the pyramid, employed for only the most severe cases that had failed lesser therapy (nonsteroidal antiinflammatory agents, sulfonamides, gold). Evidence-based outcomes studies clearly indicate better outcomes, with less disability, when RA is treated more aggressively earlier in its course (31). A

reappraisal of the role of chronic daily oral corticosteroid therapy has even arisen recently for this same reason (32).

Numerous extraarticular problems are part of the RA syndrome (33). Cardiac, respiratory, central nervous system, cutaneous, eye, and reticuloendothelial system damage may occur (Table 23-1). Pulmonary complications, including pleurisy with or without effusion, rheumatoid pneumoconiosis (Caplan's syndrome), nonpneumoconiotic intrapulmonary rheumatoid nodules, and diffuse interstitial pulmonary fibrosis, are more common in men (34). Peripheral neuropathy, with a mixed sensorimotor component, occurs in less than 5% of patients with advanced RA. This neuropathy is probably caused by vasculitis of the vasa vasorum of the peripheral nerves (16,33). Cutaneous manifestations of RA include the characteristic subcutaneous nodules that occur in about 25% of patients (16). Raynaud's phenomenon, erythema nodosum, and ischemic necrosis secondary to vasculitis may also occur (35). Generalized lymphadenopathy and splenomegaly develops in some patients with RA. Felty's syndrome is characterized by rheumatoid arthritis, splenomegaly, and neutropenia.

The most obvious pathologic features of RA occur in the involved joints and surrounding tissue (9,16,33,36–38). The lesions probably begin in the synovial membrane with a proliferation of cells lining the synovium, with inflammatory cell infiltration (lymphocytes, plasma cells, and macrophages), and eventual granuloma formation, with epithelioid cells and even, in some instances, multinucleated giant cells.

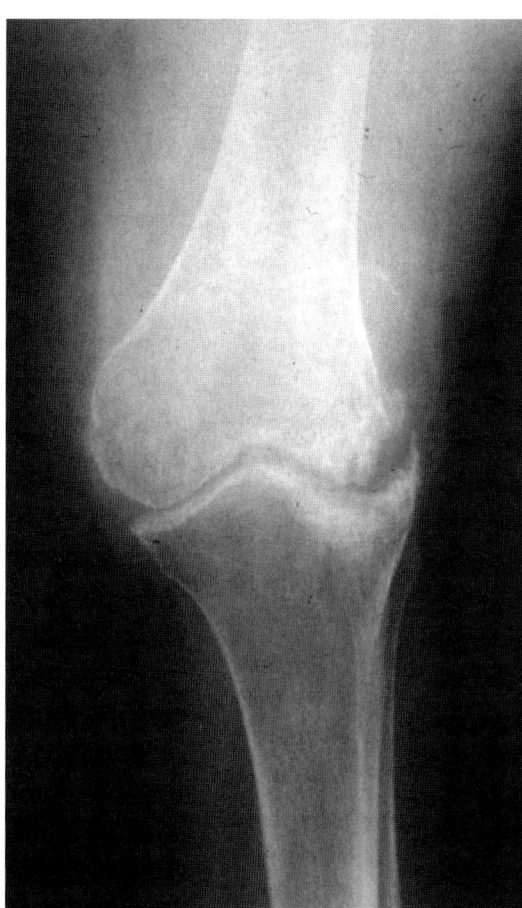

FIGURE 23-2. Typical radiographic pattern of a knee affected by rheumatoid arthritis, with narrowing of the joint space, along with new bone formation and obvious erosion on one of the tubercles.

Exudation of fluid into the synovial space occurs as a result of the inflammatory reaction, and cartilage and periosteal involvement within the joint capsule ensues, resulting in erosion of bone, formation of granulation tissue, and ultimately, destruction of the joint itself, with replacement by fibrous tissue. Loss of structure and function of the joint results in the characteristic deformities of RA (Fig. 23-3).

Rheumatoid nodules contain a central area of necrotic tissue, surrounded by palisades of lymphocytes, plasma cells, and giant cells. The nodules have a characteristic histopathologic appearance, whether they are in the joint, the eye (36,39), or other extraarticular tissue.

Ocular Manifestations

Potential ocular manifestations of RA include keratoconjunctivitis sicca (Sjögren's syndrome), scleritis, episcleritis, peripheral ulcerative keratitis (PUK), sclerosing keratitis, and keratolysis (23,40–42). Ocular complications may occur in patients with limited systemic disease but are more common in those with marked systemic complications including vasculitis, pericarditis, and rheumatoid nodules.

TABLE 23-1. EXTRAARTICULAR MANIFESTATIONS OF RHEUMATOID ARTHRITIS

Systemic Changes	Frequency
Rheumatoid nodules	Common
Systemic vasculitis	Uncommon
Ocular manifestations	
Keratoconjunctivitis sicca	Very common
Keratitis	
Marginal ulceration	Common
Marginal thinning	Common
Sclerosing keratitis	Rare
Keratolysis	Rare
Scleritis	
Diffuse anterior	Common
Nodular anterior	Uncommon
Necrotizing anterior	In severe systemic disease
Scleromalacia perforans	In long-standing disease
Posterior	Uncommon
Diffuse nodular episcleritis	Uncommon
Uveitis	Rare
Respiratory changes	Uncommon
Cardiac disease	Uncommon
Disease of lymph nodes and spleen	Uncommon
Amyloidosis	Common

Modified from Zizic TM, Stevens MB. Rheumatoid arthritis and variants. In Ryan SJ Jr, Smith RE, eds. *Selected topics on the eye in systemic disease.* New York: Grune & Stratton, 1974:315–338.

Keratoconjunctivitis Sicca

The most common ocular manifestation of RA is keratoconjunctivitis sicca (41,43). Sjögren's syndrome (dry eye and dry mouth) is present in some patients. The dry eye associated with RA is indistinguishable from dry eye in the nonrheumatoid patient. However, unexplained xerostomia and RA (or other collagen vascular diseases) with or without swelling of the salivary glands complete the syndrome described by Sjögren (23). The presence of human leukocyte antigens

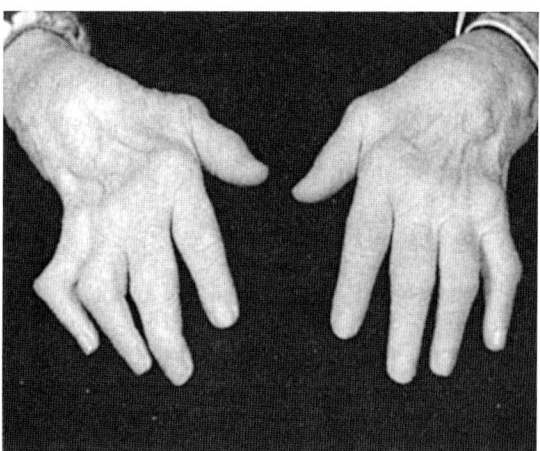

FIGURE 23-3. Characteristic joint deformities in the hands of a patient with rheumatoid arthritis.

HLA-DR3 (44), HLA-B44, and HLA-DR4 (45), hypergammaglobulinemia, and reduced T lymphocytes are frequent findings in patients with RA and Sjögren's syndrome (6,40), and the haplotypes serve to distinguish patients with these ailments from those without RA. Tear lysozyme is deficient or absent in Sjögren's syndrome (40). Increased amounts of immunoglobulin A (IgA)-, IgM-, and IgG-containing immune complexes are present in patients with primary Sjögren's syndrome and in RA patients, and IgA-containing immune complexes are more frequently found in Sjögren's patients with extraglandular manifestations (46).

Clinical manifestations of keratoconjunctivitis sicca associated with RA are those of any dry eye, including foreign-body sensation, mucous threads in the tears, and the feeling of dryness and tightness around the eyes, often worse later in the day as tears evaporate (41). Examination discloses a reduced marginal tear strip, rose Bengal staining of the conjunctiva in the interpalpebral area, corneal complications related to dry eye (superficial punctate epitheliopathy, filaments), and shortened breakup time of the tear film.

Scleritis and Episcleritis

Inflammation of the collagenous coats of the eye (sclera and cornea) is a serious complication of RA (23,39,47–51). Scleritis (Fig. 23-4) is the most common, although episcleritis and keratitis may occur. Episcleritis, nodular or diffuse, is a relatively benign problem that responds well to low-dose oral nonsteroidal antiinflammatory agents. Topical steroid therapy for episcleritis is also effective, but this treatment probably prolongs (through multiple recurrences) the total duration or "life" of the problem. Scleritis (diffuse, nodular, necrotizing (with or without {scleromalacia perforans} inflammation), and posterior) is always a serious matter, both ocularly and systemically (39,40,52–57).

Patients with scleritis characteristically have pain. Patients with episcleritis do not. Scleritis pain may be intense, and may even awaken the patient from sleep. In

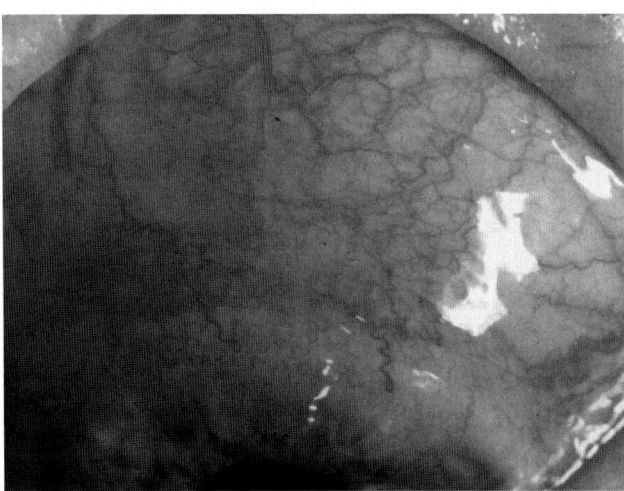

FIGURE 23-5. Scleritis, in a patient with a painful, tender eye. Note the violaceous hue to the ocular redness, as well as the loss of radiality of some of the episcleral vasculature.

nodular episcleritis, the nodule is movable over the underlying sclera. The nodule of nodular scleritis is tender to the touch and immobile. The conjunctival vascular dilation associated with episcleritis can be blanched by the use of topical phenylephrine hydrochloride (Neo-Synephrine) or epinephrine. After the overlying vessels are blanched, dilatation of the vessels in the episclera can be observed. As emphasized by Watson (56) and by Foster (58), the pattern of vessel dilatation (episcleral versus scleral) is helpful in differentiating episcleritis from scleritis.

There is a blue hue to the red eye associated with scleritis, owing to the location of the inflammation and the associated vascular dilatation of the deeper layers of sclera (Fig. 23-5). The red eye of the patient with episcleritis lacks this blue hue and hence appears bright red (Fig. 23-6).

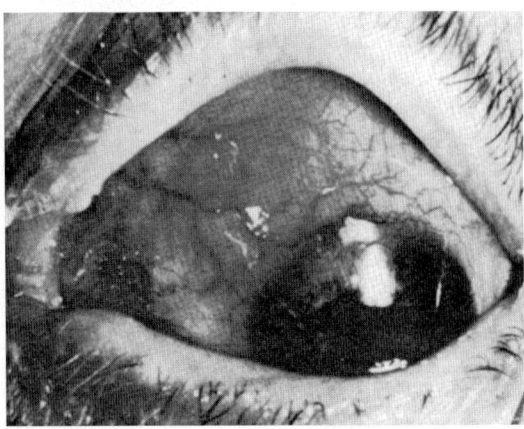

FIGURE 23-4. Localized scleritis in a patient with rheumatoid arthritis.

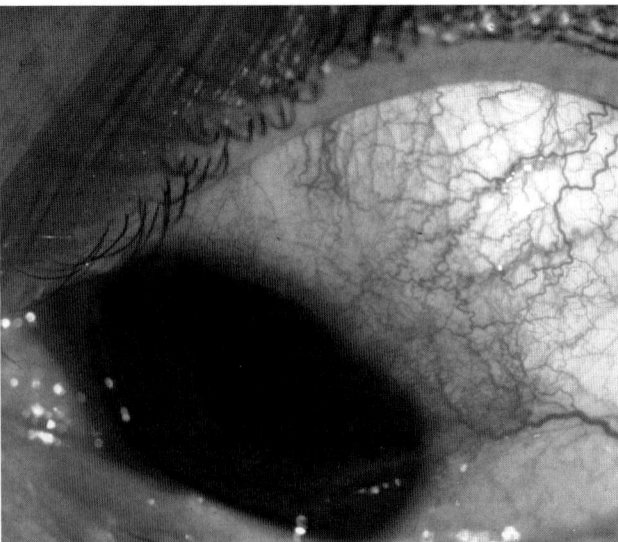

FIGURE 23-6. Episcleritis, in a patient with a red but non-painful and nontender eye. Note the bright red color of the patch of sectorial episcleritis.

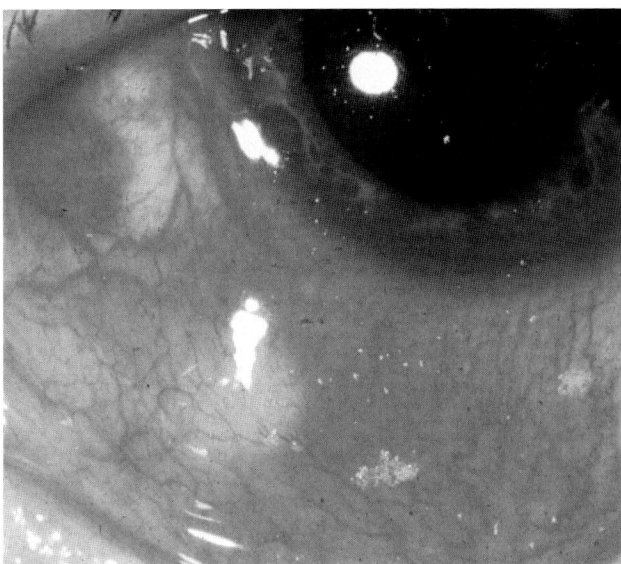

FIGURE 23-7. Nodular scleritis. Note the intensely red eye with a slight blue component to the redness. The obvious nodule is tender and immobile.

Nodular scleritis is characterized by the presence of a painful, very tender, red elevated area of sclera inflammation. The nodule is immobile (Fig. 23-7).

Necrotizing scleritis is always associated with vasculitis and ischemia, with inflammatory destruction of sclera (Fig. 23-8). Scleromalacia perforans is an equally severe necrotizing and ulcerative process, but it is relatively asymptomatic in a deceptively quiet-appearing painless eye (Fig. 23-9). There is no clinically apparent inflammation. Slow, progressive ulceration of the sclera with exposure of underlying uvea occurs, however. This form of scleritis is always associated with long-standing, severe RA (39). The inflammatory and painful variety of necrotizing scleritis may be seen in RA as well, but it is also associated with other connective tissue disorders such as Wegener's granulomatosis, polyarteritis nodosa, and relapsing polychondritis (23,39,59).

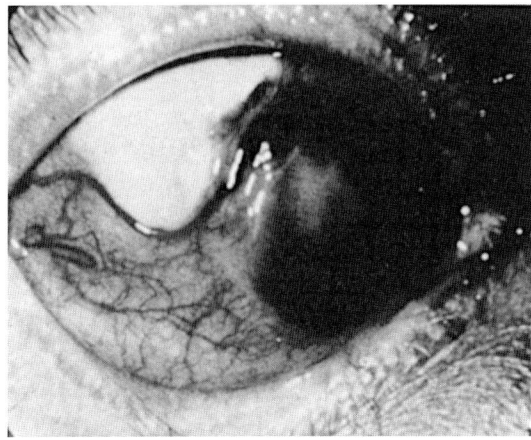

FIGURE 23-8. Active necrotizing scleritis and associated corneal marginal thinning and vascularization.

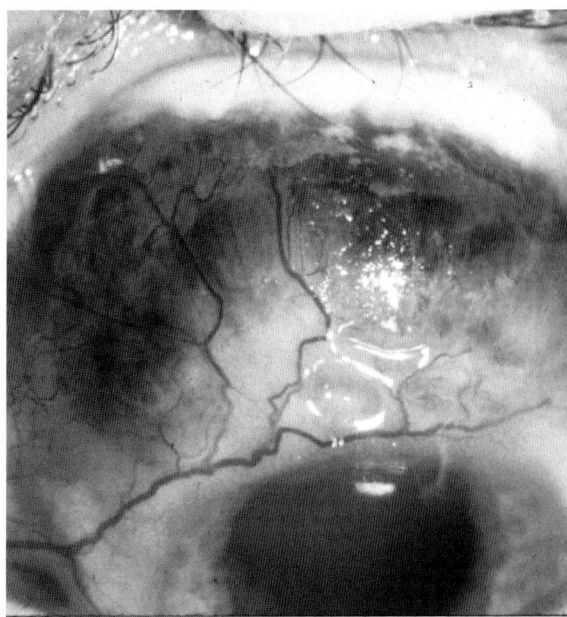

FIGURE 23-9. Scleromalacia perforans in a patient with rheumatoid arthritis. Note the lack of any clinically obvious inflammation (redness). The globe is not tender.

Anterior segment fluorescein and indocyanine green angiography reveals vaso-obliterative vasculitis in all cases of necrotizing scleritis (60,61).

Posterior scleritis in the absence of anterior scleritis may be confused with retrobulbar problems (62). Pain accentuated with eye movement is present in almost all cases. Mild proptosis, diplopia, decreased vision, and limited ductions also occur. Exudative retinal detachment, posterior choroidal folds, and vitreitis may be present (62) (Fig. 23-10). Glaucoma may also occur, as a result of associated iridocyclitis or peripheral anterior synechia, or may be steroid-induced (63).

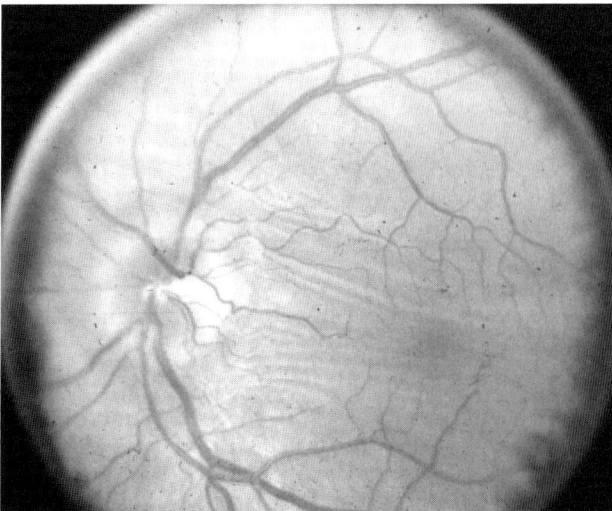

FIGURE 23-10. Fundus photograph of a patient with posterior scleritis. Note the retinochoroidal folds extending between the disk and the macula.

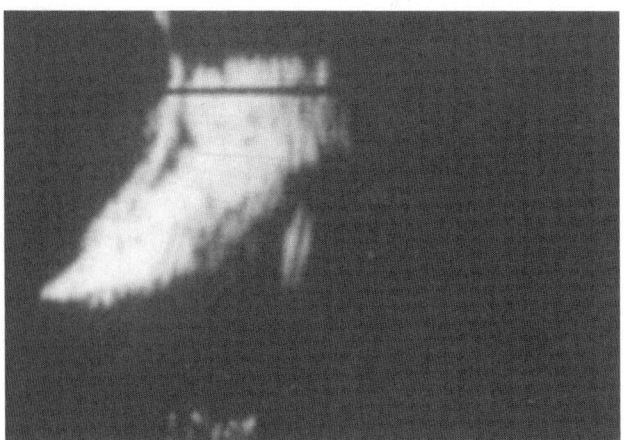

FIGURE 23-11. B-scan ultrasonography of a patient with posterior scleritis in the absence of anterior scleritis. The patient has pain, which is accentuated on binocular rotations. Note the thickening of the retinochoroid layer and the presence of edema in Tenon's space, which, at the level of the optic nerve, produces the classic so-called T sign.

Ultrasonography is especially helpful in differentiating posterior scleritis from other entities (62,64) (Fig. 23-11).

Although the exact pathogenesis of scleral and episcleral inflammation in RA has not been established, it probably has the same cause as the joint inflammation (39,56). Immune complexes are probably deposited in the sclera of patients with rheumatoid scleritis, just as they occur in the synovia of joints in RA patients (20,40). These antigen-antibody complexes, with complement, trigger the cascade of events leading to scleral (or joint) inflammation (i.e., attraction of neutrophils and release of various enzymes and other mediators followed by localized tissue destruction) (39). Intrascleral vasculitis (microangiopathy) may also occur (65,66). This may result in deep scleral intravascular coagulation, ischemic necrosis, and scleral dissolution (39,65). Both scleral inflammation and vasculitis are probably present in some patients. Histopathologic studies of patients with severe scleritis have revealed the presence of active stromal fibrocytes in the absence of inflammatory cells, suggesting that collagenous resorption may precede granuloma formation. Mast cells were also abundant (67,68).

The pathologic changes of rheumatoid scleritis include foci of fibrinoid necrosis of the sclera surrounded by palisading fibroblasts and an inflammatory component consisting largely of neutrophils, lymphocytes, and plasma cells (36,63,69,70). The amount of cellular proliferation and necrosis varies, depending on the severity and the extent of vascular involvement.

Scleritis and episcleritis occur in approximately 4% to 10% of all RA patients (39,56). However, when a patient comes to an ophthalmologist with scleritis, RA must be considered, because it is the most common cause of scleritis (and episcleritis). The frequency of RA in patients presenting with scleritis is about 30% (12). Besides history taking for RA and other collagen disorders that may also be associated with scleritis, certain laboratory tests are appropriate.

Rheumatoid factors (IgG, IgA, and IgM), uric acid, sedimentation rate, C-reactive protein, antineutrophil cytoplasmic antibody, fluorescent treponemal antibody absorption (FTA-ABS), purified protein derivative (PPD) (tuberculosis), and chest x-ray films (tuberculosis) are suggested screening tests. I also search for circulating immune complexes by the C1q binding and the Raji cell assays.

Secondary intraocular inflammation and retinal detachment frequently occurs with severe scleritis (39,47,71). Both resolve with improvement of the overlying scleritis.

Keratitis and Sclerosing Keratitis

Corneal changes may be found adjacent to areas of scleral inflammation or as the only ocular complications of RA (23,39,56). Localized inflammatory cell infiltration of the cornea, followed by development of epithelial defects and frank loss of stroma, may occur (Fig. 23-12). A relatively severe proliferation and infiltration of inflammatory cells with secondary fibrovascular invasion results in peripheral corneal scarring in some cases.

Corneal involvement in RA includes keratitis and sclerosing keratitis, peripheral corneal ulceration (furrows), and keratolysis (39,56).

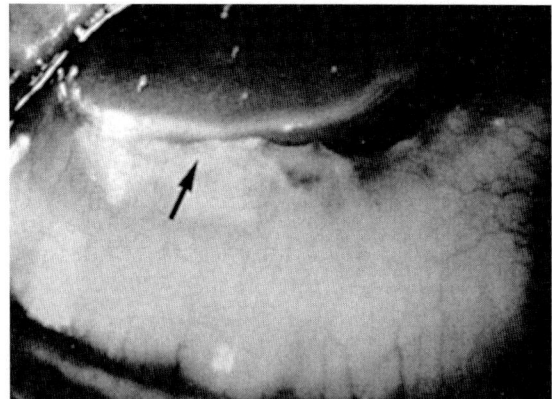

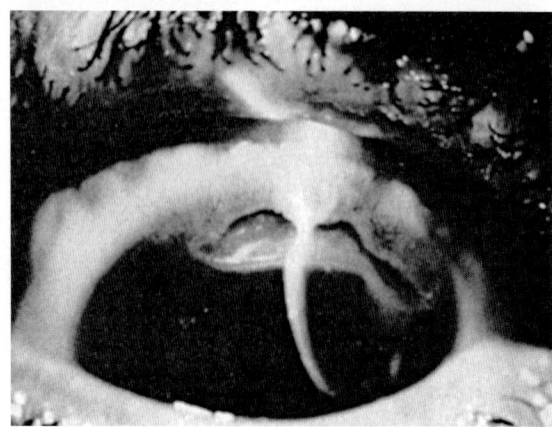

FIGURE 23-12. A: Limbal furrow in rheumatoid arthritis. There is no associated scleritis. **B:** Same patient as in **A.** Note the infiltrate *(arrow)* at the advancing edge of the furrow.

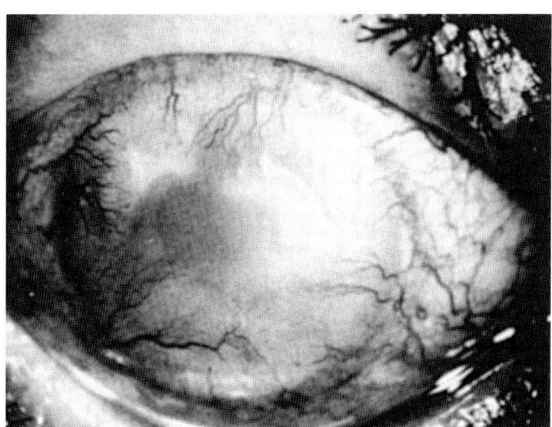

FIGURE 23-13. Sclerosing keratitis and keratolysis in a rheumatoid arthritis patient with scleritis. Note the marked vascularization of the cornea with thinning.

Sclerosing keratitis is the most common corneal complication of scleritis (39,56). The keratitis occurs in association with severe scleritis and not as an isolated corneal finding (56). This is in contradistinction to peripheral guttering of the cornea, which may occur without scleral inflammation in patients with long-standing RA.

In sclerosing keratitis, a gradual gray corneal stromal thickening progresses toward the center of the cornea, followed by vascularization (Fig. 23-13). The advancing edge may have a striate configuration with crystalline-like changes developing behind this edge. If this process extends into the visual axis, it causes a marked decrease in vision. If the associated scleritis is nodular, sclerosing keratitis is generally localized to the quadrant of the scleral nodule. However, if the scleritis is diffuse, the entire cornea may become white and vascularized. Sclerosing keratitis may lead to perforation as a result of (noninfectious) localized corneal ulceration. Lipid deposition is a late change.

Keratitis alone (sterile corneal inflammation) may also be associated with scleritis and may occur in areas adjacent to the active scleral inflammation. Such corneal inflammation has been found in 30% to 70% of patients with scleritis or episcleritis associated with RA (52,70). The corneal inflammation includes midstromal and superficial stromal infiltrates, depending on the nature of the scleritis. The infiltrates may become very diffuse and even result in corneal epithelial breakdown and ulceration. This corneal complication may take a sclerosing configuration, with ingrowth of vessels and connective tissue resulting in peripheral corneal scarring as noted above.

Peripheral Corneal Ulceration (Furrows)

Peripheral corneal ulceration occurs with or without associated scleral or episcleral inflammation (Fig. 23-14) Brown and Grayson (72) reported marginal furrows in patients with chronic RA; this is probably a more common occurrence in RA patients than has been previously reported (23,73). The thinned area, usually located inferiorly, may be very superficial at first but progresses rapidly. The peripheral corneal ulceration is often associated with a mildly inflamed conjunctiva. This mild contiguous conjunctivitis should not be confused with episcleritis.

There is usually no vascularization in the bed of the furrow, and the corneal epithelium is intact. Limbal ulceration (52,57,73,74) may also occur in association with rheumatoid scleritis, episcleritis, or sclerosing keratitis. Although the majority of such ulcers do not progress, some have resulted in marked thinning and descemetocele formation. Perforation is rare but may occur with minor trauma.

The pathogenesis of the corneal lesions is unclear. Collagenase has been found in the conjunctiva and corneal epithelium adjacent to the furrow itself (75). The pathogenesis of the scleral and corneal inflammation may be the same as that for joint disease (40); cells associated with synovial tissue (and by analogy, with scleral or corneal collagen) produce an IgG antibody in response to an unknown antigenic

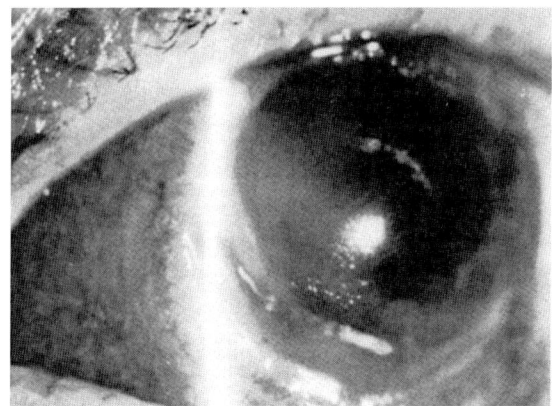
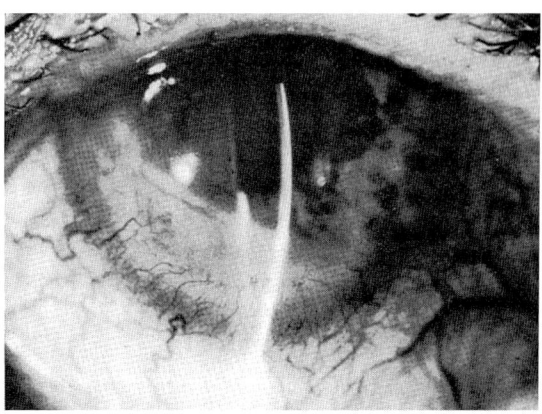

A   B

FIGURE 23-14. A: Marginal furrow with scleritis in rheumatoid arthritis. **B:** Same patient as in **A,** after local corticosteroid therapy. Note the decreased corneal edema and infiltrate and the increased neovascularization.

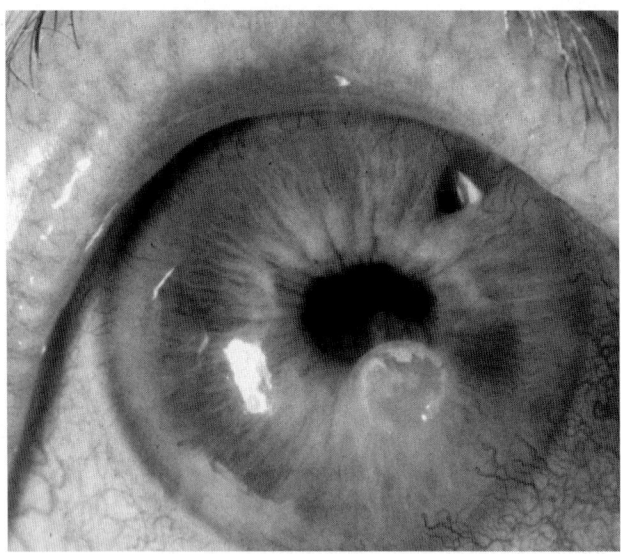

FIGURE 23-15. Paracentral keratolysis (stromal melting) with associated epithelial defect in a patient with rheumatoid arthritis.

stimulus, possibly a virus, the IgG antibody may be altered, leading to the development of autoantibodies, immune complexes are formed with the abnormal IgG, and these are deposited locally in the synovium (or sclera) (40,74); these complexes activate the complement cascade, which triggers release of mediators of inflammation, attracts neutrophils, and causes tissue destruction and tissue melting. This sequence probably occurs in the sclera and the limbus as well as in synovium. Destruction of collagen and occlusion of associated vessels results in the scleritis, ischemic necrosis, and ulceration associated with rheumatoid syndromes.

Paracentral Keratolysis

Ulceration of clear central or paracentral cornea may occur in eyes with no signs of inflammation (76) or less commonly, in cases of necrotizing scleritis (36,56,57) (Fig. 23-15). In most cases, severe aqueous tear deficiency is associated. The epithelium breaks down, superficial layers of the cornea begin to ulcerate, and a descemetocele may occur in the most severe cases. Perforation of the cornea may result rapidly, with or without minor trauma. Treatment options include the aggressive use of wetting agents, bandage contact lenses, application of tissue adhesive (prior to or after perforation), use of a protective shield, tarsorrhaphy, and tectonic keratoplasty (76–78). Patients with this problem usually respond poorly to these measures and often develop recurrent keratolysis.

Corneal Ulceration Following Cataract Surgery

A particularly devastating complication of cataract surgery in RA patients with keratoconjunctivitis sicca has been emphasized in recent years. Sterile corneal ulceration and melting have been observed days to weeks after otherwise unremarkable cataract surgery (39,79–83). Studies of penetrating keratoplasty corneal buttons has disclosed neutrophils localized near the areas of keratolysis, suggesting that collagenase derived from these neutrophils is involved in the pathogenesis of keratolysis (82). Patients who develop this problem are usually elderly women with moderate dry eyes and Sjögren's syndrome, RA, or another collagen vascular disease. Physician failure to recognize the dry eye is a major problem. Prevention of epithelial damage at the time of cataract surgery and prompt institution of therapy for dry eyes or sterile corneal ulceration are critical. Unless the underlying cause is recognized, central corneal ulceration may progress to descemetocele formation, perforation, and loss of the eye.

Diagnosis and Differential Diagnosis

The diagnosis of RA is clinical. Arthritis, rheumatoid nodules, presence of rheumatoid factor, and diagnostic radiologic findings (84,85) form the basis for the diagnosis. Guidelines for the diagnosis of RA have been established by the American Rheumatism Association (15) and more recently, by the American College of Rheumatology (86).

The most characteristic laboratory feature of RA is the presence of rheumatoid factor (16,87). There are three rheumatoid factors, antibodies to IgG; classical rheumatoid factor is IgM anti-IgG; IgG anti-IgG and IgA anti-IgG may also be produced. One or more rheumatoid factors is present in about 90% of patients with RA. Numerous rheumatoid factor tests have been developed. The most commonly used tests include the Waaler-Rose test and the latex bead agglutination test. The first employs sheep red blood cells sensitized with rabbit antibodies to sheep cells. Rheumatoid factor combines with the rabbit IgG, causing agglutination of the sheep red blood cells. Test results are positive in 60% to 70% of patients with RA (16). The latex test involves adsorbing aggregated human 7S IgG on latex particles; rheumatoid factor reacting with IgG causes flocculation of the latex particles. Results are positive in 80% to 90% of patients. An increased frequency of positive test results, and higher titers occur in patients with subcutaneous nodules, in patients with RA variants (Felty's, Sjögren's), and in patients with multiple extraarticular manifestations of RA. The development of enzyme-linked immunosorbent assays for rheumatoid factor may increase the sensitivity of rheumatoid factor measurements (88).

Rheumatoid factor is present in some patients with connective tissue diseases other than RA (16), in up to 20% of patients with scleroderma, polyarteritis nodosa, and SLE. It is usually not present in patients with ankylosing spondylitis, enteropathic arthritis, reactive arthritis, or juvenile idiopathic arthritis. Therefore, testing for rheumatoid factor is helpful in differentiating variants of rheumatoid disorders.

Anemia, leukocytosis, and elevation of the erythrocyte sedimentation rate (ESR) and of the C reactive protein (CRP) are the other typically abnormal laboratory parameters in patients with RA. Additionally, approximately 25% of patients with classic RA are antinuclear antibody positive. If neutropenia is present, Felty's syndrome should be suspected.

Treatment

Treatment of RA and its variants is very difficult and time-consuming and ideally should be orchestrated by a rheumatologist. Additionally, patients with RA have chronic problems that require not only medical treatment, but also rehabilitation services and even surgery to relieve deforming and incapacitating deformities in joints.

Almost 25% of RA patients respond initially to aspirin alone (16). Although there are potentially serious side effects associated with chronic salicylate use, salicylates remain a useful drug in the care of patients with RA. Salicylates inhibit prostaglandin synthesis. Therapeutic salicylate serum levels are 20 to 25 mg/dL. Enteric-coated aspirin may be required in patients who have gastric intolerance to the 2 to 4 g of aspirin per day generally required to achieve this serum level. If there is no clinical response despite adequate serum levels within 8 weeks, other nonsteroidal antiinflammatory drugs (NSAIDs) are generally prescribed. Naproxen, tolmetin sodium, ibuprofen, indomethacin, diclofenac, piroxicam, or one of the cyclooxygenase-2 specific (Cox-2 specific) NSAIDs may be effective. Gold salts (72,89–92) and antimalarial drugs are also employed. Antimalarials that are quinoline derivatives have a number of potential side effects, including some related to the eye. The ophthalmologist must be aware of the corneal deposits and retinal toxic changes that may occur in the retinal pigment epithelium of patients taking certain quinoline derivatives. The positive effects of these drugs can generally be achieved at a lower dosage than that which usually results in ocular toxicity (93).

Systemic corticosteroids have a very potent antiinflammatory effect, relieve pain, and maintain function of the joints in patients with RA. Steroids work rapidly and can be used initially, whereas slower-acting remittable agents take effect. Low-dose corticosteroids are often used as a substitute for NSAIDs in patients who have gastrointestinal or other intolerance to NSAIDs (94), and a recent reappraisal of the safety and efficacy of chronic low-dose systemic steroid therapy for patients with RA suggests that low doses (≤10 mg/day) of prednisone used early (within 1 year of onset of the disease) has a disease modifying effect, limiting bony progression, with limited and manageable side effects [weight gain (3 kg), ecchymoses, and osteopenia]; the drug should be stopped within 6 months. Pulsed high-dose intravenous corticosteroids (methylprednisolone) have also been used in patients with rapidly progressive RA, generally in conjunction with long-term steroid-sparing

agents such as gold, penicillamine, or other immunosuppressive disease modifying agents (52,95–97). Immunosuppressive drugs, such as azathioprine and methotrexate, have a similar favorable effect on the inflammation. These medications used to be considered if other drugs failed to induce a remission (base-down pyramid model), because of the greater potential risks associated with the chronic use of immunosuppressive medications. The risk of increased susceptibility to cancer development after the use of cytotoxic agents is an especially important consideration in the management of RA patients, with particular concern about those who harbor the Epstein-Barr virus (98). Some studies have evaluated cyclosporine as a therapeutic agent in RA (99). Although these studies have generally demonstrated a significant improvement in disease activity, problems with nephrotoxicity have limited the usefulness of cyclosporine for care of patients with RA. Immunomodulatory agents are now being employed much earlier in the course of RA, because outcomes studies have shown, quite clearly, better outcomes employing this paradigm in place of the older, more conservative base-down pyramid one.

Biologics (monoclonal antibodies directed against specific cell types and against specific cytokines) have also revolutionized the care of patients with rheumatoid arthritis. Tumor necrosis factor-α (TNF-α) is a preeminently important inflammatory cytokine found in abundance in inflamed joint effusion fluid (unlike aqueous or vitreous humor of patients with uveitis, in which TNF-α is not impressive). Anti-TNF-α therapy [etanercept (Enbrel) was the first, but infliximab (Remicade) and adelimumab (Humira) have joined in the pack], usually in combination with methotrexate but sometimes even as monotherapy, is a major advance in our care of patients with arthritis, especially those with RA. IL-1 is also a keystone in the inflammatory pathways leading to joint destruction in uveitis, and antibody therapy directed against the IL-1 receptor [kineret (Anakinra)] is another "biologic" that has been approved by the United States Food and Drug Administration (FDA), based on safety and efficacy data, for the treatment of patients with rheumatoid arthritis.

Ocular Treatment

The management of keratoconjunctivitis sicca includes replacement tear therapy, occlusion of the lacrimal drainage puncta, warm compresses and lid massage (for the invariably present meibomian gland dysfunction), and, in selected cases, therapy aimed at any active inflammatory component of the disorder (topical cyclosporine and/or steroid).

The treatment of episcleritis and scleritis is directed toward the underlying disease. Topical steroids may help while systemic medication takes effect.

Episcleritis
Although highly effective, topical steroids actually prolong the total duration of recurrences of episcleritis. Therefore,

we advocate the avoidance of steroid therapy for patients with episcleritis, and instead use only iced artificial tears topically. An oral NSAID is used for those patients who must have prompt resolution of the episcleritis. NSAID therapy is also generally our first step in treating scleritis. I prefer the Cox-2 specific NSAIDs, celecoxib (200 mg b.i.d.) and rofecoxib (25 mg/day). Diclofenac (75 mg PO b.i.d.), sustained-release indomethacin (75 mg b.i.d.), diflunisal (500 mg b.i.d.), and naproxen (500 mg b.i.d.) are nonselective NSAID alternatives. Early response to therapy includes a dramatic decrease in the deep pain of scleritis. Systemic corticosteroids are employed (1 to 1.5 mg/kg/day of prednisone) in cases of scleritis that do not adequately respond to NSAID therapy.

Immunomodulatory therapy is employed for scleritis resistant to all other forms of therapy and in cases associated with potentially lethal outcomes (necrotizing scleritis; scleromalacia perforans, cases associated with Wegener's granulomatosis, polyarteritis nodosa, relapsing polychondritis). Cyclophosphamide, methotrexate, azathioprine, mycophenolate mofetil, cyclosporine, and chlorambucil have all been used in this context (19,100–102). Cyclophosphamide is the most effective agent (19,100,102). Hemorrhagic cystitis and severe bone marrow depression are the major potential complications of its use. I prescribe 2 to 3 mg/kg/day, and in urgent care administer the drug intravenously (1 g/m²). Guidelines for managing patients on this medication for eye disease have been published (19,100). Active involvement of an experienced chemotherapist (ocular immunologist or otherwise) is mandatory in the management of such patients, especially when systemic corticosteroids or immunosuppressives are employed. Clues to improvement include rapid relief of pain, decrease in redness, and improvement of vision.

We have considerable experience in the use of the various biologics (see above) in the care of both the ocular and extraocular manifestations of RA. Remicade has been especially effective in patients with scleritis. Another biologic, not mentioned above and not FDA approved for treatment of rheumatoid arthritis or for any eye disease, is Daclizumab (Zenapax), which has also been extremely valuable to us in our care of patients with otherwise treatment-resistant ocular inflammatory disease associated with RA. This monoclonal antibody is directed against the IL-2 receptor and hence blocks the binding of IL-2 to its receptor on T lymphocytes.

Management of severe thinning associated with scleritis is difficult. Most cases do not perforate spontaneously, although such eyes are more susceptible to rupture from trauma. Homologous scleral grafts can be very difficult to accomplish but may result in salvage of the eye (23). Autologous fascia lata or periosteum has also been successfully employed to reinforce or repair areas of severe scleral thinning or perforation (23,103–106).

Therapy for sclerosing keratitis includes the use of high-dose topical corticosteroids to prevent progression of the corneal disease (56,65), and systemic therapy (corticosteroids, NSAIDs, and immunosuppressives), as outlined earlier for scleritis, is important to treat both the associated scleritis and the corneal disease.

Therapy for marginal or central thinning, ulceration, or melting associated with RA is controversial. It is important to exclude microbial infection in all cases. Keratoconjunctivitis sicca, microbial keratitis, lid margin and meibomian gland pathology, and scleritis must be identified and treated (23,107). If there is no infiltration in the corneal furrow, and a clear zone is present between the limbus and the ulcer, corticosteroids should not be used; the danger of perforation in this instance is too great (39,56,74). However, if the ulcer resembles a Mooren's ulcer, beginning at the limbus, extending centrally and circumferentially, and having a major white blood cell infiltrative component, topical steroids may be helpful (23). Frequent examinations are essential, because perforation is a distinct risk, especially with the use of topical corticosteroids. Improvement and resolution of marginal ulcers may also occur with high-dose systemic corticosteroid therapy.

Topical collagenase inhibitors such as acetylcysteine (Mucomyst 20%), 1% medroxyprogesterone, and doxycycline have all been used in the treatment of corneal melting syndromes (8 times/day) (75). I especially like systemic doxycycline, 100 mg PO b.i.d., and topical medroxyprogesterone q2h for this purpose. Hydrophilic bandage lenses may be effective in promoting healing of the ocular surface. Tissue adhesive applied to the ulcer may also be helpful, as can resection of the conjunctiva adjacent to the marginal furrow.

Immunosuppressive therapy has been employed in unusually severe cases in which topical medication did not suffice (39,56,100,101). Azathioprine, cyclophosphamide, and chlorambucil have been used to treat not only severe rheumatoid systemic disease and severe scleritis, but also the associated corneal ulceration. Cyclophosphamide is probably the most effective. Dosages must be carefully monitored as noted earlier (108).

Perforation occurs in the corneal ring ulcer or furrow. If imminent, perforation can be prevented with a ring, patch, or lamellar corneal graft or fascia lata graft (39,106). The destructive process, however, will destroy this graft too, unless the underlying immunologically driven process is modified through systemic therapy (74,107).

JUVENILE IDIOPATHIC ARTHRITIS

There are several hundred thousand patients with JIA, the most important cause of chronic and progressive crippling childhood arthritis in the United States (109–112). The prevalence of JIA is approximately 94 per 100,000 children, and the incidence is about 14 cases per 100,000 per year. The age of onset is generally between 2 and 4 years, with some cases occurring in the preteen years. JIA rarely occurs before the age of 6 months. It occurs a little more frequently in girls than in boys. The iridocyclitis and associated complications are major causes of blindness in children in this country; therefore, recognition of this syndrome and accurate classification are important. JIA-associated iritis accounted for about 80% of all cases of uveitis in children in one series from England (109). Band keratopathy is the principal corneal feature of JIA (41,85,113).

There are three relatively distinct forms of JIA, classified on the basis of disease onset: systemic onset, polyarticular onset, and oligoarticular onset (109,110,114–117).

Clinical Features

Systemic-onset JIA is a febrile, severe systemic illness with large joint involvement, splenomegaly, and lymphadenopathy (118). Iridocyclitis (or any other ocular finding) is rare in patients with systemic onset JIA (110,119). Polyarticular onset JIA accounts for about 50% of patients with JIA and is usually seen in younger children. Fever and lymphadenopathy may occur. Oligoarticular onset JIA begins with arthritis in five or fewer joints. Uveitis risk factors in JIA patients include female gender, oligoarticular onset, presence of circulating antinuclear antibodies, and the presence of HLA-DR5 or -DP2 (120). Children with oligoarticular-onset JIA are the most severely affected from the ocular standpoint (116,117). Although the arthritis may be very mild in such patients, the ocular complications are very severe and occur in up to 25% of patients (110,116,117,121). Chronic iridocyclitis is the predominant finding (122–129). The presenting symptom may be decreased vision on a routine school examination or the onset of cataract with a white pupil observed by a parent or teacher. Most of the patients have no symptoms. By the time they are examined, they may have band keratopathy, cells and flare in the anterior chamber, posterior synechiae with a bound-down pupil, secondary cataract, and secondary glaucoma. The disease is usually present bilaterally. Because of the insidious onset and chronic nature of the ocular disease, all patients with JIA should be examined by an ophthalmologist every 3 months. In patients with iridocyclitis, close follow-up is important because increased inflammation is usually not accompanied by increased symptomatology (130).

The iridocyclitis associated with JIA is frequently relentlessly progressive despite corticosteroid therapy, with eventual blindness caused by cataract and glaucoma (131,132). Vitreitis, tractional retinal detachment, macular cysts and edema, macular holes, and lesions of the choroid are not rare (133). Pathologic findings are nonspecific, with infiltrates (mononuclear cells and lymphocytes) in the ciliary body and iris (124,134–136). Plasma cells have been prominent in the iris of some patients (137).

Patients with JIA and active iridocyclitis have been found to have elevated antibody levels to human iris and retina, compared with either normal control subjects or JIA patients without active iridocyclitis (138), and antibody to retinal S antigen is found more frequently in patients with JIA and uveitis, compared with normals and with JIA patients without uveitis (134).

Although the most important ocular complication of JIA is chronic iridocyclitis, corneal complications (band keratopathy) also produce visual morbidity. Band keratopathy frequently occurs in young patients with any form of chronic inflammation but is especially prominent in patients with JIA-associated uveitis (113). The keratopathy begins in Bowman's layer, usually at the 9 and 3 o'clock position meridians, with deposition of calcium crystals. Involvement of the deep layers of the corneal epithelium progresses in a band-shape across the entire cornea. Holes in the calcium deposition may give it a Swiss-cheese appearance (Fig. 23-16). These holes may represent areas where nerves penetrate Bowman's membrane, ending in corneal epithelium.

A number of entities are associated with band keratopathy. Although it occurs as a secondary change in patients with chronic uveitis, it can also occur in individuals without other major eye problems (41,140–144). In some cases, serum calcium levels may be elevated (145).

The pathophysiology of the deposition of calcium crystals in Bowman's membrane is unclear. O'Connor (85) reviewed this problem and proposed the following mechanism: 99% of the body's calcium is in the form of bone or hydroxyapatite, a complex crystalline structure with calcium and phosphate ions. Excess calcium favors precipitation as a calcium phosphate under certain local conditions. Doughman and associates (146) believed that evaporation

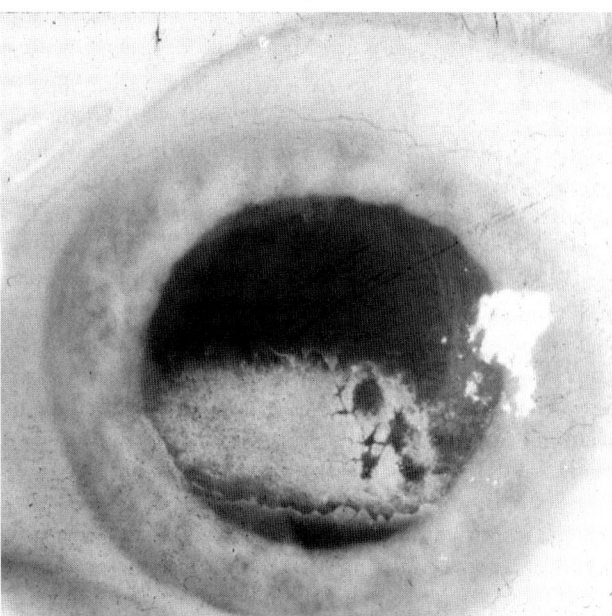

FIGURE 23-16. Band keratopathy in a patient with long-standing juvenile rheumatoid arthritis associated chronic iridocyclitis. Note the Swiss-cheese lacunae in some areas of the calcium deposition.

in the interpalpebral area resulted in deposition of calcium salts in a band configuration. In addition to the evaporation, which would favor the precipitation of calcium phosphate, O'Connor (85) implicated the diffusion of gases with a subsequent increase in local pH. Loss of carbon dioxide, which affects the ionization of carbonic acid, may result in a decrease in the availability of free hydrogen ions, and therefore increases the pH specifically in the exposed area of the cornea (interpalpebral area). Increased gaseous exchange at the surface of the exposed cornea in the interpalpebral area with a loss of carbon dioxide and an increase in pH thus would result in deposition of the calcium phosphate crystalline material composing the band. But none of this hypothetical speculation explains why chronic uveitis beginning in adulthood never results in the formation of band keratopathy, whereas chronic uveitis beginning in childhood always does.

O'Connor (85) also performed extensive histopathologic examinations on eyes with band keratopathy, including those from patients with JIA and uveitis. Calcific deposits were found in Bowman's layer, in the basement membrane of the epithelium, and in the superficial stromal lamellae. These were common changes regardless of the cause.

Serum levels of calcium are not elevated in JIA patients; however, it is postulated that in the development of bone in children, there is more circulating calcium ion available for deposition in the form of band keratopathy.

Diffuse or nodular scleritis and episcleritis can be seen in JIA patients. These patients most frequently have polyarticular arthritis and are seropositive for rheumatoid factor (147).

Diagnosis

Antinuclear antibody is present in 80% of patients with JIA who develop iridocyclitis. It is rarely present in JIA patients who do not develop iridocyclitis (148). Antibodies to a 15-kd nuclear antigen are found much more frequently in JIA patients with chronic anterior uveitis than in those without uveitis, and this may thus provide a clue to earlier diagnosis of uveitis (149). The sedimentation rate is elevated and rheumatoid factor is absent in JIA patients (41,118). The knee is the most common joint involved, and a routine knee examination and x-ray films are recommended in patients in whom JIA is suspected, even in the absence of clinically active arthritis (16,110,112). A comparison of HLAs in patients with JIA demonstrated a correlation of HLA-DR5 with the presence of eye disease and of HLA-DR1 with the absence of eye disease (150).

Uveitis in childhood results from a group of diseases that are important to differentiate. Toxocariasis, pars planitis, and toxoplasmosis are common posterior or diffuse forms of uveitis in children, and it is important to differentiate these entities because therapy and prognosis vary (109). Sarcoidosis uncommonly occurs in childhood, but it may mimic JIA (151,152). And psoriatic arthritis may

also be associated with development of uveitis. Chest x-ray films, skin testing for anergy, skin biopsy, and other tests for sarcoidosis are important in the differential diagnosis of suspicious cases of iridocyclitis in children. The presence of joint changes and the typical history help make the diagnosis of JIA.

Treatment

Steroid therapy for the chronic form of iridocyclitis in children with JIA is often ineffectual (118,126,127,131,132), but reports on more aggressive therapy have been more hopeful (109). Very early cases may present with just a few cells in the anterior chamber and no synechiae. Dilating agents alone are recommended in early cases because such patients are often subject to a long-term chronic course of corticosteroids with little hope for resolution of the process. Corticosteroids are recommended in patients in whom the anterior chamber cellular reaction increases and synechiae begin to form. At this stage, topical steroids should be titrated and every attempt made to avoid overuse of steroid. JIA patients with uveitis often have chronic flare in the anterior chamber, even in the absence of cellular reaction, because of a breakdown of the blood–aqueous barrier. Flare alone may not be an appropriate indication for corticosteroid therapy. The presence of cells in the anterior chamber, on the other hand, is an irrefutable indication for treatment. If topical corticosteroids are not effective, subtenon corticosteroid injections may be considered, and even short-term systemic corticosteroids may be appropriate. NSAIDs may be used to help control inflammation and may allow a reduction in corticosteroid dosage (153), and in some cases retention of remission of the uveitis, off all steroids, may be possible through chronic oral NSAID use. Immunomodulatory therapy must be considered for otherwise treatment-resistant cases (154,155). The presence of vitreous inflammatory cells, in particular, is an indicator for the likely need for immunosuppressive treatment in JIA patients.

Glaucoma is initially managed medically, as are all forms of secondary glaucoma (109). Miotics, however, should be avoided. The management of cataract in JIA is especially challenging. Results of standard surgery have been poor (109,131,132,156,157), and combined lensectomy and vitrectomy may be appropriate in some cases (87,109,156, 158–160). Incorporation of an intraocular lens into the surgical plan may (rarely) or may not be appropriate.

It is critically important to monitor JIA patients closely because they frequently do not complain of photophobia and redness but rather present with far-advanced uveitis, cataract, band keratopathy, and glaucoma. In general, the acute varieties of iridocyclitis associated with JIA do much better with better resolution and fewer recurrences than does the chronic variety, which has a poor prognosis (85,113).

Although formal genetic counseling is probably not warranted, there may be a genetic predisposition to develop JIA in some families (161,162). Association of JIA with various HLAs also suggests a genetic component (109,163–166).

Therapy for band keratopathy includes the use of chelating agents (85,113). A variety of techniques may be employed. In general, a topical anesthetic is applied, the epithelium is removed with a blade, and 0.37 molar (m) μg disodium ethylenediaminetetraacetic acid is applied with a well made from rubber, cardboard, plastic, or even a disposable trephine blade, for 5 minutes. Subsequent scraping of Bowman's membrane is generally sufficient to remove the calcium deposits. A cycloplegic agent and antibiotic are instilled and a semipressure patch or bandage soft contact lens applied until the epithelium heals.

RELAPSING POLYCHONDRITIS

Relapsing polychondritis (RP) is an uncommon connective tissue disease (167–170). Systemically, there is recurrent inflammation of the cartilaginous tissues throughout the body, particularly in the ears and nose. The disease occurs equally in men and women, with onset between the ages of 30 and 50 years.

The pinnae of the ears are the most commonly involved areas (171–173). The ears become red, swollen, and painful (Fig. 23-17). This gradually subsides over a period of weeks. Resorption of ear cartilage may result in flaccid,

drooping ears. Arthritis may also be seen but should not be confused with the disabling and destructive arthritis associated with RA. When nasal cartilage is involved, there is pain on movement of the nose, destruction of cartilage, and deformity of the nose (Fig. 23-18). Aortic, laryngotracheal, and costal cartilages may also be involved. The course of the systemic disease is variable, but it may be fatal if vital structures, such as the aortic ring and trachea, are involved. Cardiovascular and respiratory complications are the cause of death in such cases (59,172).

The pathogenesis of relapsing polychondritis is unknown (172). Antibodies to cartilage and to native (type 2) collagen have been found in patients with RP (59). There are no specific laboratory tests to assist in the diagnosis of RP. The sedimentation rate is usually elevated. Serum protein abnormalities and leukocytosis occur. Most patients have no rheumatoid factor, no LE cells, and negative results on serum tests for syphilis. However, there may be other associated systemic collagen disorders, (overlap syndromes), including vasculitis, Wegener's granulomatosis, Behçet's disease, or SLE. Imbalance in helper-to-suppressor T-cell ratios has been reported (174,175). Pathologic examination reveals acute inflammatory changes in the cartilage (early) or atrophy and fibrous replacement of cartilage (late) (169,170).

Therapy for the systemic disorder includes antiinflammatory agents in high doses to decrease the severe inflammatory involvement of cartilage. Prednisone, 60 to 80 mg/day or its

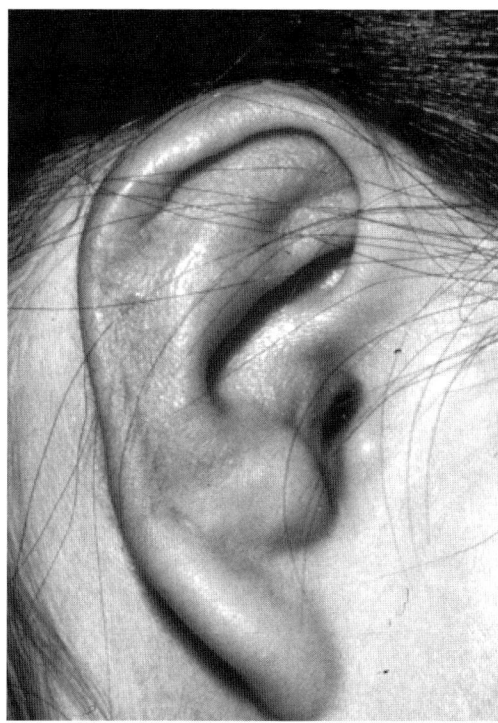

FIGURE 23-17. Ear of patient with active relapsing polychondritis. Note the erythema and swelling of the outer ear, which is quite tender to palpation. Note also the loss of supportive cartilage in the lower aspect of the outer ear as a consequence of prior attacks of inflammation.

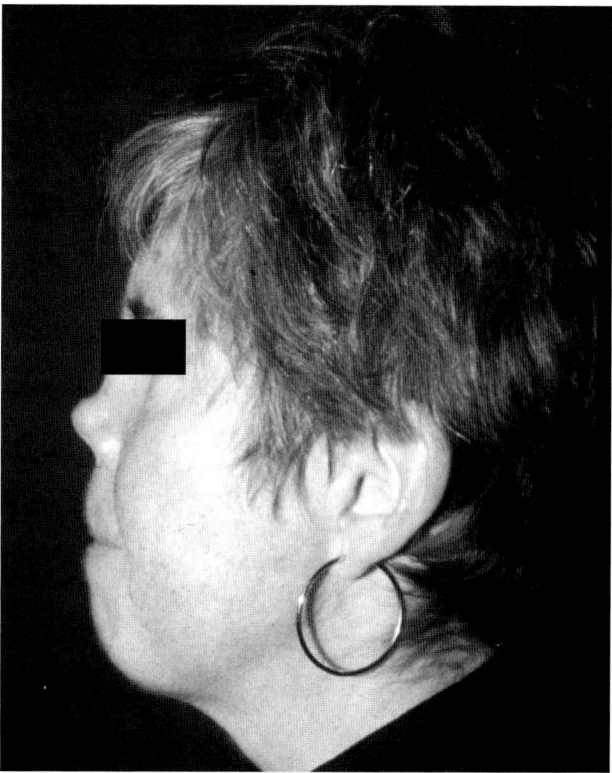

FIGURE 23-18. Relapsing polychondritis, currently inactive. Note the collapse of nasal cartilage from previous episodes of active chondritis.

equivalent, brings about a significant improvement (176). Maintenance doses of 5 to 10 mg daily may be necessary for suppression of the disease (174,177–179). Antimalarials, NSAIDs, dapsone, and immunomodulatory agents have been used with varying degrees of success (176,177,180–182).

A variety of ocular findings have been associated with relapsing polychondritis, including episcleritis (40% of cases), conjunctivitis (25% of cases), iridocyclitis, scleritis, and keratitis (179,183–190). In fact, episcleritis or conjunctivitis may be a presenting feature of relapsing polychondritis in some cases. Keratoconjunctivitis sicca, abducens nerve palsies, and exophthalmos have also been reported (159,190). Scleritis may be nodular, necrotizing, or diffuse anterior (191). Treatment with dapsone or systemic corticosteroids is usually ineffective once scleritis occurs, and immunosuppressive agents such as azathioprine and cyclophosphamide are required not only to control the scleral inflammation but also to prevent RP from evolving to tracheal, aortic, or renal involvement.

Localized peripheral corneal infiltrates with moderate progressive thinning have been reported (59). This may be associated with thinning of the sclera and staphyloma formation. Histologic and immunofluorescent studies of biopsy specimens from patients with RP scleritis have disclosed the vasculitic nature of this inflammation (191). The cause of the corneal complications is not known. The serious ocular complications of relapsing polychondritis are related to peripheral corneal ulcerations, which in rare cases may result in corneal perforation and its complications (57,176,192).

Therapy for corneal complications of relapsing polychondritis includes high-dose topical corticosteroids and management of the associated systemic disease (56,59). However, if corneal ulceration has occurred, topical steroids should be discontinued and therapy directed toward the ulceration according to the guidelines discussed earlier in this chapter for rheumatoid peripheral corneal ulcerations.

SYSTEMIC LUPUS ERYTHEMATOSUS

The modern history of systemic lupus erythematosus (SLE) began with the 1939 description by Rose and Pillsbury (192) of disseminated multiorgan involvement in this chronic, progressive disease of unknown etiology. With the publication, in 1941, of the now classic paper, "Pathology of Disseminated Lupus Erythematosus," by Klemperer, Pollack, and Baehr (193), in which the importance of vasculitis was emphasized, research interest in this disease with protean manifestations expanded greatly. SLE is a clinical syndrome of unknown etiology characterized by multisystem involvement and subject to multiple remissions and exacerbations in one or more systems. It is a chronic, often progressive, pleomorphic disease. The clinical course of

TABLE 23-2. ORGAN SYSTEM INVOLVEMENT IN SYSTEMIC LUPUS ERYTHEMATOSUS

System	Involvement
Articular	Arthralgias, arthritis, aseptic bone necrosis
Cutaneous	Rash, alopecia, photosensitivity
Renal	Glomerulonephritis
Hematologic	Anemia, leukopenia, autoantibodies
Pulmonary	Pleurisy, pleural effusion, pneumonitis
Neurologic	Behavioral disturbance, seizures, mononeuritis
Cardiovascular	Raynaud's phenomenon, vasculitis, pericarditis
Ocular	Corneal epitheliopathy, scleritis, retinopathy

SLE may be mild or severe and continuous or recurrent, with destructive inflammatory processes that can affect any organ. The organ systems are those most notably involved in SLE are shown in Table 23-2.

Epidemiology

The estimated incidence (new cases per unit of population per unit of time) of SLE has increased over the past 30 years from 0.5 in 100,000 in 1950 to between 2.7 and 7.6 in 100,000 in 1974 and 1973 (data from New York and San Francisco, respectively) (194,195). How much of this increase is a true increase in disease frequency and how much is the result of improved diagnostic capabilities is unclear, but certainly improved techniques for diagnosing SLE and increased awareness of the disease by physicians have contributed to the increase. The prevalence of SLE (the total number of cases existing at any given time) has similarly increased to between 15.5 and 50.0 cases in 100,000. This increase has resulted from the increased incidence and improved survival of patients with SLE.

Although SLE occurs in both males and females and has been reported to have its onset as early as the age of 1 year or as late as age 90, it is found primarily in women of childbearing age. Approximately 90% of patients with SLE are women, and most of them experience onset of symptoms between ages 15 and 45. Most studies show no racial predilection for this disease.

Pathogenesis

Although the fundamental cause of SLE is unknown, the best available body of scientific evidence today strongly points to a dysfunction in immunoregulation. The most reasonable hypothesis for the pathogenesis of this disease includes a genetic predisposition to the development of defective suppressor T-lymphocyte function, possibly after the perturbation of the immune system by some environmental factor. Defective T-cell function then results in inadequately controlled helper T-lymphocyte and B-lymphocyte activity, with resultant production of autoantibodies (antinuclear antibodies, antithyroid antibodies). Autoantigen-autoantibody immune complexes are formed, predominantly in the circulation, and these are then deposited in certain organs and tissues, primarily because of physical factors and molecular sieving restrictions. Activation of the complement pathway, through both classic and alternate routes, then causes, at the site of the immune complex deposition, chemotaxis of neutrophils and macrophages, release of proteolytic enzymes, and activation of the clotting cascade sequence, as well as the activation of various kinins. It appears that the bulk of the tissue damage occurring in SLE results from these latter reactions and tissue digestion by the proteolytic enzymes, particularly from neutrophils.

Patients with SLE have been shown to have decreased numbers of suppressor T lymphocytes, and those present have been shown to be functionally defective, particularly during periods of major disease activity (196–199). There is a pronounced impairment in the ability of suppressor T lymphocytes from SLE patients to control B-lymphocyte antibody synthesis. Once defective suppressor T-lymphocyte function is triggered, probably by some environmental factor in the genetically predisposed person, antilymphocyte antibodies are manufactured, along with many other autoantibodies. One of the more prominent antilymphocyte antibodies manufactured in these patients is one that is specifically reactive with suppressor T lymphocytes. The activity of this autoantibody probably further compromises suppressor T-lymphocyte function, with a resulting increase in disease activity.

In addition to the aforementioned immune alterations, a number of other abnormalities are frequently present in patients with SLE. IL-1 and IL-2 production is decreased. This might be related to prostaglandin production from monocytes of SLE patients. A soluble natural killer cell cytotoxic factor is released at significantly lower levels in SLE patients (200), mirroring or resulting in the decreased natural killer cell activity (201) that is unresponsive to exogenous beta interferon (202). Elevated levels of IgA (203), IgE (203), and anti-Ro (SSA) antibodies (205) have also been reported. An intrinsic defect in phagocytosis noted in some SLE patients may result in repeated skin infections (206).

Predisposing Factors

Family studies have provided evidence for both genetic and environmental factors in the development of SLE. Both related and unrelated household contacts of SLE patients have a higher incidence of circulating antoantibodies than does the population at large (207), and approximately 5%

of patients with SLE have family members with the disease as well. The available evidence suggests that both genetic predisposition and environmental stimuli are important in the development of serologic abnormalities and clinically apparent SLE (208).

Genetic Factors

Strong evidence for a major role of genetic susceptibility in the development of SLE has emerged from family studies, studies of monozygotic and dizygotic twins (209), genetic studies of the composition of the region on chromosome 6 where the putative immune response gene is located, and studies of the New Zealand (NZ) mouse model of SLE.

Genetic studies, primarily those involving HLA typing, have failed to show any relationship between HLA-A/B/C phenotype and SLE susceptibility. But evidence suggests that DR2 or HLA-DR3 may predispose to SLE (210,211). There is also an increased incidence of Ia-715 phenotypes in SLE patients compared to those without SLE (211). Schur (212) reported a higher incidence of SLE in patients with inherited deficiencies of complement. This is of interest, because the gene coding for synthesis of the second component of complement is believed to lie in close juxtaposition to a putative immune response gene on chromosome 6 of humans.

Environmental Factors

A great deal of evidence suggests that in the genetically susceptible person, certain environmental stimuli, such as viral infection, ultraviolet irradiation, and contact with certain drugs, induce alterations in DNA, immunoregulatory networks, or both, with resultant formation of autoantibodies, including antinuclear antibody. DeHoratius and co-workers (207) showed that unrelated persons in the same household as patients with SLE had an increased frequency of antilymphocyte antibodies, compared with the normal population. In the Nevada study of Chantler and colleagues (213), the impressive prevalence of eight cases of SLE in six different families in a community of less than 3,000 population over a 15-year period was suggestive of an environmental influence on the development of SLE.

A number of investigators have hypothesized that SLE can be caused by inappropriate immune responses to viral infection. Type C virus (oncornavirus C within the RNA Reoviridae family) endogenous xenotropic infection is commonly present in NZ mice and is transmitted vertically, during cell division, from parent to offspring. This virus has a particular tropism for thymus cells, and most investigators believe this is at least partially responsible for the thymic dysfunction and disturbed immunoregulation seen in these mice (214). Viral glycoprotein-antiviral glycoprotein immune-complex deposits are found in the nephritic kidneys of NZ black (NZB)/NZ white (NZW) mice (215). Conflicting data have been obtained in studies for type C viral antigens in humans (216–219).

Ultraviolet irradiation is another environmental factor that may trigger the development of, or aggravate, SLE in the genetically susceptible person. Twenty-five percent to 35% of SLE patients are photosensitive (compared with 1% of normal persons and 1% of patients with rheumatoid arthritis). Tan and Rodnan (220) believe that DNA damage from ultraviolet irradiation may trigger the development of SLE. About one-third of patients with SLE have antibodies against ultraviolet-damaged DNA (221).

A number of drugs are capable of altering DNA and stimulating the production of antinuclear antibodies. Fifteen percent to 70% of those patients receiving these drugs (hydralazine, procainamide, methyldopa, isoniazid, chlorpromazine, hydantoins, ethosuximide, trimethadione) over a prolonged period will develop antinuclear antibodies. Some individuals may be more genetically susceptible to development of pathologic changes from the immune complexes that result from antinuclear antibody–DNA reactions or from inappropriate immunoregulatory responses to the development of DNA alterations and the formation of antinuclear antibodies. These may be the patients who develop clinically obvious SLE after ingestion of these drugs.

Hormonal factors may influence the development or clinical expression of SLE. As has been pointed out above, for example, the disease occurs much more commonly in females than in males. And approximately 30% of female patients with SLE have a major increase in disease activity during pregnancy (222). Studies from the NZB/NZW Fl mouse model of SLE also lend support to the notion that hormonal factors may play an important role in the clinical expression of SLE (223). The evidence suggests that female sex hormones are important in triggering or permitting the immune responses that result in the development of clinically apparent SLE; it may also be that male sex hormones offer some protection against the disease.

Clinical Features

Systemic Involvement

The presenting and eventual organ systems involved in SLE are shown in Table 23-2. In its earliest phases, SLE may be relatively subtle and difficult to diagnose. Any patient exhibiting constitutional symptoms (malaise, anorexia, easy fatigability, and fever) who is found to have antinuclear antibodies in the serum should be carefully investigated for multiorgan disease typical of SLE. The benefits of making the diagnosis early stem from adequate therapy, which will decrease tissue damage over the rest of the patient's life.

Articular

Ninety-five percent of patients with SLE develop arthralgia, articular findings, or both during the course of their disease, and 55% of patients experience arthralgia as the initial manifestation of their disease. Some SLE patients (about 10%) develop deforming arthritis changes similar to those seen in rheumatoid arthritis; the most commonly affected site is the hands.

Cutaneous

Seventy percent to 80% of SLE patients develop skin lesions at some point during their lives (224), and approximately 20% have skin lesions as the initial symptom of the disease. The "butterfly rash" across the nose and cheek, occurring in about 30% of SLE patients, is one of the more notable rashes occurring in these patients. This rash is edematous and is exacerbated by ultraviolet exposure. It also commonly involves the skin of the chin and ears.

Alopecia occurs in 25% to 40% of patients with SLE; it has been emphasized that this finding commonly is associated with clinically active disease in some other organ system. The development of mucous membrane ulcers (nasal septum, larynx, pharynx, palate, vagina), petechiae or purpura, ulcerative lesions of the skin (commonly on the fingertips, around the nail folds, and on the ankles and arms), and periungual erythema and telangiectasis signifies the development of frank vasculitis.

The skin manifestations seen in discoid lupus erythematosus (DLE), the cutaneous disease that probably represents the benign end of the spectrum of lupus erythematosus, unlike the skin lesions of SLE, are destructive. Hypopigmented scars result from the cutaneous inflammation in DLE, and the alopecia that occurs is permanent. Repeated skin infections (i.e., furuncles, folliculitis) may occur.

Renal

Immune complex deposition in the kidney occurs in virtually all patients with SLE. It has been shown that even if there is no clinical evidence of renal disease in an SLE patient, kidney biopsy specimens are routinely abnormal when studied by immunofluorescence and electron microscopy. The mesangium is apparently the site of earliest involvement with immune complex deposition.

End-stage renal disease is probably the most common SLE-related cause of death in patients with SLE. Approximately 50% of SLE patients develop clinically apparent renal disease, and 10% to 20% develop renal failure. It should be emphasized, therefore, that SLE patients should be carefully and repeatedly examined for evidence of renal disease.

Neurologic

SLE-related central nervous system (CNS) changes may be the second most common SLE-related cause of death in patients with SLE. The most common neurologic manifestation is behavioral disturbance ranging from anxiety to psychosis; the second most common is grand mal seizures. Recurrent headache and organic brain syndrome can also occur. But in approximately 15% of patients with SLE, severe CNS changes occur. Multifocal disease mimicking multiple sclerosis, cranial nerve palsies, transverse myelitis, hemiparesis, and frank cerebrovascular accident with paralysis may occur. Hypothalamic, extrapyramidal, and cerebellar dysfunction may occur when the tracts or centers controlling these functions are affected.

Cardiovascular

Just as there is a high incidence of subclinical renal disease in SLE, so too, 50% of patients with SLE have pathologically demonstrable endocarditis, myocarditis, or pericarditis. The inflamed endocardium (Libman-Sacks endocarditis) can be secondarily infected.

Pulmonary

Although pulmonary disease is common in patients with SLE (occurring in 50% to 75% of SLE patients), it is usually not fatal. The most common form of pulmonary involvement is pleurisy Sixty percent to 70% of patients with lupus have abnormal results on pulmonary function tests even if they are asymptomatic from a respiratory standpoint (224). The most frequent abnormality is an impairment in the diffusion capacity. It is probably reasonable to carefully evaluate the pulmonary status of any patient with SLE periodically.

Hematologic

Nearly all patients with SLE develop normochromic anemia. This usually occurs because of impaired utilization of iron by the bone marrow, and it improves in association with improvement in the other systemic manifestations.

Ocular Involvement

Although the ophthalmologist may be the first physician to see the patient with SLE, more commonly the patient is referred to the ophthalmologist for evaluation of ocular symptoms. The most conspicuous findings are those related to the cornea and sclera, but the retinal and choroidal findings frequently serve as a better barometer of the severity and prognosis of the disease.

Corneal

The corneal manifestations of SLE are, by and large, confined to the epithelium. Although peripheral ulcerative keratitis has been reported in patients with SLE, and keratitis and neovascularization have been described in patients with discoid lupus (225–228), these lesions rarely occur in SLE. Sicca syndrome is quite common, however, in SLE patients with inadequately controlled systemic disease. Sjögren's syndrome in SLE is relatively rare and is usually mild (229).

Pillat (230) reported superficial keratitis in one of his 16 patients with SLE, and Gold and associates (231) found a 6.5% incidence of keratitis in an outpatient population of SLE patients. Spaeth (232) found, in a study of SLE patients hospitalized at the National Institutes of Health, that 88% had superficial punctate keratitis with fluorescein corneal staining. He reported that Schirmer test results were normal in these patients, and therefore the issue of whether the superficial punctate keratitis seen in patients with SLE is always truly the result of sicca syndrome or in fact is secondary to corneal epithelial damage associated with lupus disease activity is unclear. Reeves (228) described bilateral deep segmental interstitial keratitis and subsequent recurrent iritis in a patient who 1 year later developed cutaneous, articular, and hematologic manifestations of SLE. Halmay and Ludwig (226) described similar cases previously. Grayson (225) mentioned deep stromal keratitis as a rare finding in patients with SLE and Raizman and Baum (233) mentioned these changes in two patients with DLE.

Superficial punctate keratitis can also occur in patients with DLE. Doesschat (234) reported persistent superficial punctate keratitis and recurrent corneal epithelial erosion in a patient with DLE. The corneal lesions were minimal in the superior cornea, where the ocular surface was protected from the environment by the upper lid. Doesschat reported marked improvement in the keratopathy in association with systemic quinacrine hydrochloride therapy. I reported similar findings in a patient with chronic blepharoconjunctivitis and keratitis of 4 years' duration, in whom the diagnosis of DLE was made on the basis of histopathologic study of lid skin (235); systemic quinacrine hydrochloride therapy resulted in prompt resolution of the ocular lesions.

Scleral

Chemosis, recurrent episcleritis, or scleritis may occur in patients with SLE and may be the initial presenting manifestation of the disease (236,237). Scleritis is a reasonably accurate guide to the presence of major systemic activity in the SLE patient. As in the case of retinopathy, we suggest that any patient who develops scleritis be evaluated for SLE. Scleritis will resolve with adequate control of systemic disease; it will not respond to topical therapy. Uveitis is not common in patients with SLE (238). It may rarely occur in the absence of other ocular lesions but usually is seen in association with severe lupus scleritis.

Lower tarsal plaques, erosion of the lower lid margins, conjunctival scarring, and symblepharon may occur in patients with DLE (239).

Finally, iatrogenic ocular lesions occur in SLE patients treated with corticosteroids or antimalarial drugs. Cataract and (rarely) glaucoma may occur with long-term systemic corticosteroid therapy, and the retinopathy secondary to high-dose or prolonged antimalarial drug therapy is well known.

Retinal and Choroidal

A major event early in the development of lupus retinopathy is the appearance of retinal vasculitis, which is evident on

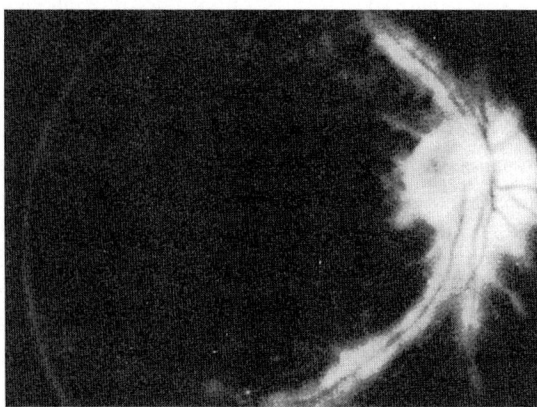

FIGURE 23-19. Fluorescein angiogram of a patient with systemic lupus erythematosus. Note the leakage of fluorescein dye from the retinal vessels, indicating retinal vasculitis.

fluorescein angiography (Fig. 23-19). Similar findings may occur in iris vessels as well (Fig. 23-20). Subtle macular or disk edema may appear next, followed by intraretinal hemorrhages and cotton-wool spots (Fig. 23-21). These latter changes may be indistinguishable from hypertensive retinopathy; it may be impossible for the clinician to decide whether the retinal lesions are secondary to hypertension or to SLE immune complex vasculitis in the SLE patient with idiopathic, renal, or iatrogenic hypertension. A combined posterior and anterior segment fluorescein angiographic search for vasculitis may be helpful in this regard.

Gold and co-workers (231) emphasized that the appearance and disappearance of retinal lesions in SLE patients parallel the systemic clinical course and that effective therapeutic control of the systemic disease is associated with a dramatic decrease in retinal lesions. Although absolute direct proof that the lesions of lupus retinopathy are caused by immune-complex vasculitis is lacking, clinical and experimental evidence to support this assumption does exist. Aronson and associates (240) found immunoglobulin and complement components in the ciliary processes and choroidal vasculature of the eyes of a patient who died of

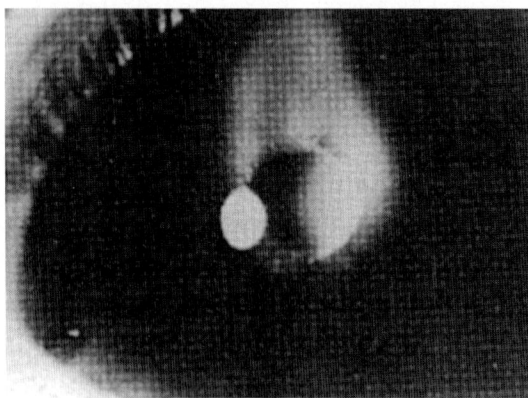

FIGURE 23-20. Fluorescein angiogram, anterior segment. Note the leak of fluorescein dye from the iris vasculature superiorly, which suggests iris vasculitis.

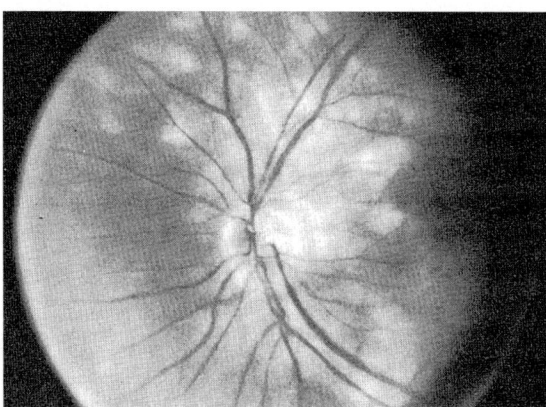

FIGURE 23-21. Elschnig spots in a patient with polyarteritis nodosa. Note the scattered light foci of various sizes, some of which have a slightly pigmented center (note in particular the small lesions at 12 o'clock and approximately 11 o'clock just distal to the venule branch). These are areas of is chemic infarct of the choriocapillaris.

SLE, and immunoglobulins and complement have been demonstrated in the ciliary body and choroidal vasculature of eyes from rabbits in an animal model of serum sickness. This suggests that whenever a patient with SLE develops retinopathy (or whenever existing retinopathy worsens), a thorough study of renal and pulmonary status should be done and the appropriate serologic studies be performed in search of systemic evidence of disease activity, with prompt, aggressive therapy and longitudinal monitoring of the ocular and systemic abnormalities. The therapeutic goal should be to suppress active disease, minimize the amount of tissue damage, and reduce the incidence of clinically important exacerbations over the lifetime of the patient.

Lupus anticoagulants and anticardiolipin antibodies are recognized markers for an increased risk of thrombosis and may also play a role in the compromise of the retinal vasculature (i.e., arterial and venous occlusions) (241).

Diagnosis and Differential Diagnosis

The diagnosis of SLE is based on a combination of clinical and laboratory criteria, which have varied over the past decade. Two of the most useful systems are those proposed by Cohen and associates (242) (and accepted by the American Rheumatism Association) and by Hahn (243) (Table 23-3).

It should be emphasized that any patient exhibiting constitutional symptoms who is found to have antinuclear antibodies in the serum should be carefully investigated for multiorgan disease typical of SLE. We have found that in addition to using both the Hahn and the American Rheumatism Association diagnostic criteria as guides, the immunofluorescent lupus band test on biopsy specimens of clinically normal skin, circulating antibodies to autologous erythrocytes, and ribonuclease-insensitive acid nuclear protein (anti-Sm) are very helpful in establishing the diagnosis of SLE. Moses and Barland (244) and others (245) emphasized

TABLE 23-3. CRITERIA FOR THE DIAGNOSIS OF SYSTEMIC LUPUS ERYTHEMATOSUS

American Rheumatism Association criteria
  Four or more of the following:
Facial rash
  Discoid lupus
  Raynaud's phenomenon
  Alopecia
  Photosensitivity
  Oral or nasopharyngeal ulcer
  Nondeforming arthritis
  ANA or LE cells
  False-positive STS results
  Proteinuria (3.5 gm/d)
  Urinary sediment cellular casts
  Pleuritis and/or pericarditis
  Psychosis and/or convulsion
  Anemia, leukopenia, and/or
    thrombocytopenia

Hahn's criteria

ANA (1 : 5) + score of 7 points

	Points
Butterfly rash	2
Rash biopsy findings compatible with SLE	2
Polyarthritis	2
Serositis	2
Glomerulonephritis biopsy findings compatible with SLE	2
LE cells	2
Rash compatible with SLE, not biopsy-proved	1
Clinical nephritis, no biopsy	1
Organic brain syndrome	1
Localizing neurologic signs	1
Alopecia	1
Raynaud's phenomenon	1
Nail-bed capillary abnormality	1
Arthralgia	1
Fever	1
Retinal cytoid bodies	1
Polymyositis	1
Myocarditis	1
Hemolytic anemia	1
Leukopenia	1
Thrombocytopenia	1
Lymphadenopathy	1
Positive results on direct Coombs' test	1
False-positive STS results	1
Antibodies to DNA	1
Hypergammaglobulinemia	1
Hypocomplementuria	1
Circulating anticoagulant	1

ANA, antinuclear antibody; LE, lupus erythematosus; SLE, systemic lupus erythematosus; STS, serologic test for syphilis.
(Data from Cohen AS, et al. Preliminary criteria for the classification of systemic lupus erythematosus. *Bull Rheum Dis* 1971;21:643, for American Rheumatism Association criteria; Hahn BH. Systemic lupus erythematosus. In: Parker CW, ed. *Clinical Immunology.* Philadelphia: Saunders, 1980:583–631.)

the usefulness of these three diagnostic laboratory tests in patients with SLE.

Frankly, we believe strongly that ocular inflammatory lesions (scleritis, uveitis, choroiditis, and retinal vasculitis)

should be added to the point score list of SLE diagnostic criteria. It is clear to us that some patients ultimately diagnosed with SLE would have been diagnosed earlier and followed more closely if their ocular inflammation had been included as a diagnostic criterion.

The other collagen vascular diseases, in their early stages, may be difficult to differentiate from SLE. Thus, the patient with RA, antinuclear antibodies, Raynaud's phenomenon, and photosensitivity may be believed to have SLE if seen before the typical radiographic joint changes of RA appear. Patients with progressive systemic sclerosis, dermatomyositis, and polymyositis may be similarly misclassified initially. A patient with prominent arthralgia, photosensitivity, antinuclear antibodies, proteinuria, Raynaud's phenomenon, digital pad infarcts, scleritis, and nasal mucosal ulceration (and possibly perforation) may be initially diagnosed as having polyarteritis nodosa. Yet all of these findings have occurred in patients with SLE, and it is only with careful longitudinal follow-up and repeated investigations that the correct diagnosis can be made. Chronic active hepatitis and mixed connective tissue disease may also mimic SLE in the early stages.

Treatment

Ocular

Therapy for the ocular surface manifestations of SLE is based on successful control of the underlying disease, as well as local therapy for the keratitis and tear deficiency. The usual therapy for sicca syndrome (tear replacement, soft contact lenses, punctal occlusion, warm compresses and lid massage, antiinflammatory medication) may produce both symptomatic and objective improvement. Topical steroid therapy may be a useful adjunct to systemic steroid and immunomodulatory therapy in the treatment of the scleritis. The retinopathy resolves only with successful control of the underlying systemic disease. This may require urgent, aggressive care, with high-dose intravenous steroid and staged sequential plasmapheresis and intravenous cyclophosphamide.

Systemic

Many patients with SLE have relatively mild disease, and they lead relatively normal lives with conservative therapy in the form of adequate rest and nutrition, use of a skin-protective sunscreen when avoidance of sun exposure is impossible, and use of salicylates and other NSAIDs for control of arthralgia, myalgia, low-grade serositis, and mild constitutional symptoms. Antimalarial therapy (e.g., hydroxychloroquine sulfate) may be the next step employed in arthralgia and arthritis control or in therapy for cutaneous lesions or mild anterior segment ocular inflammatory lesions if NSAIDs have not been effective. One must evaluate for the possibility of development of a drug-induced retinopathy (246,247).

Severe manifestations of SLE require therapy with systemic corticosteroids and immunomodulatory agents. Disabling constitutional symptoms and articular, cutaneous, and other systemic manifestations of the disease unresponsive to the aforementioned conservative therapy should be treated with the daily corticosteroid sufficient for adequate control of disease activity. Alternate-day steroid therapy is ineffective in the treatment of SLE, and most patients respond considerably better to divided daily doses (e.g., two or three times a day) than to single morning doses of corticosteroid. Severe disease affecting the central nervous, cardiovascular, pulmonary, or renal system may require initial high-dose (60 to 300 mg of prednisone/day) steroid therapy, tapered as soon as clinical improvement warrants it. In tapering daily prednisone dosage from the 60 mg/day level, a useful rule of thumb is to decrease the dosage by 10% every 3 days until 40 mg/day is reached; then the taper should be slower.

SLE renal or CNS crisis is usually treated with high-dose intravenous steroid therapy (1 to 2 g of methylprednisolone/day for 3 to 6 days) in conjunction with high-dose oral steroid (100 to 300 mg of prednisone/day). Combination corticosteroid-cytotoxic therapy is typically required in cases of severe SLE and in cases in which the systemic corticosteroids cannot be tapered below toxic levels without exacerbations of clinical disease. Cyclophosphamide may be the most effective cytotoxic agent studied for this purpose (248). Plasmapheresis for lupus crisis is also under investigation, and we have employed this treatment modality successfully on many occasions. One group of researchers found plasmapheresis especially effective in patients with high anti-DNA antibody titers (249), whereas another group reported on the lack of effect of plasmapheresis on T- and B-cell function (250).

Dapsone has been used successfully in patients with various forms of vasculitis, and it has yielded good therapeutic results in certain forms of SLE. Dapsone has been effective in patients with vasculitic urticaria, oral lesions, and the nonscarring form of chronic DLE (251,252).

POLYARTERITIS NODOSA

Kussmaul and Maier (253) described the clinical characteristics and histopathologic findings in a patient dying of multisystem involvement with the disease they called periarteritis nodosa. The name of this multisystem disease has been changed to *polyarteritis nodosa* because histopathologic study of the lesions shows that all layers of the involved vessels, rather than just the adventitial layer, have inflammatory changes. Over the century since Kussmaul and Maier's description of polyarteritis nodosa, a great many case reports, reviews, and histopathologic studies of

patients with systemic vasculitis have been published. Many of the reported cases exhibited features quite different from those in the original description of Kussmaul and Maier, and it has become clear that there is a spectrum of systemic vasculitis. Zeek (254) proposed a classification of vasculitis that has been found to be quite useful in establishing the diagnosis and formulating a plan of therapy for individual patients (Table 23-4).

Classic polyarteritis nodosa is a systemic necrotizing vasculitis that involves small and medium-size muscular arteries with segmental acute and chronic inflammatory cell infiltration of all layers of the vessel wall and infiltration of the perivascular areas. Granuloma formation with multinucleated giant cells is a histopathologic feature of classic polyarteritis nodosa. The disease is of unknown etiology. Its manifestations are protean, and it can be rapidly fatal.

There are no accurate figures on the true incidence of classic polyarteritis nodosa, but it appears to be fairly rare. It may occur in patients of any age, although is seen most

TABLE 23-4. CLASSIFICATION OF SYSTEMIC VASCULITIS

I. Polyarteritis nodosa group
  A. Classic polyarteritis nodosa of Kussmaul and Maier
  B. Allergic granulomatosis and angiitis of Churg and Strauss
  C. Overlap syndrome of systemic necrotizing vasculitis
II. Hypersensitivity vasculitis
  A. Serum sickness
  B. Schönlein-Henoch purpura
  C. Vasculitis associated with connective tissue disorders
    1. Rheumatoid arthritis
    2. Systemic lupus erythematosus
    3. Polymyositis, dermatomyositis
    4. Progressive systemic sclerosis
    5. Rheumatic fever
  D. Vasculitis associated with malignancy
  E. Vasculitis associated with mixed cryoglobulinemia
  F. Vasculitis associated with gastrointestinal disease (ulcerative colitis, Crohn's disease)
  G. Vasculitis associated with pulmonary disease (Goodpasture's syndrome)
  H. Vasculitis associated with drug or chemical hypersensitivity reactions
III. Wegener's granulomatosis
IV. Lymphomatoid granulomatosis
V. Giant cell arteritis
  A. Temporal arteritis
  B. Takayasu's arteritis
VI. Mucocutaneous lymph node syndrome
VII. Erythema nodosum
VIII. Thromboangiitis obliterans (Buerger's disease)
IX. Miscellaneous
  A. Behçet's syndrome
  B. Cogan's syndrome
  C. Stevens-Johnson syndrome
  D. Eales' disease
  E. Hypocomplementemic vasculitis
  F. Erythema elevatum diutinum
  G. Hypereosinophilic syndromes

usually in 20- to 40-year-olds. There is a 3:1 male-to-female predilection. There seems to be no racial or geographic association.

Pathogenesis

The cause of polyarteritis nodosa is unknown. It has been reported to occur in association with upper respiratory tract infections (255), drug use (particularly methamphetamine) (256), and hepatitis B antigenemia (257). Sergent and colleagues (258) reported hepatitis B antigenemia in approximately 30% of their study population with polyarteritis nodosa. Fye and associates (259) reported circulating immune complexes containing hepatitis B antigen and IgG antihepatitis B antigen in patients with polyarteritis nodosa, and Gocke and co-workers (260) demonstrated hepatitis B antigen, IgM, and complement in the vascular walls of patients with polyarteritis nodosa. These findings, coupled with the observation of decreased serum complement levels in the acute phases of the disease, plus the characteristic histopathologic findings provide strong circumstantial evidence that the disease is caused by an immune complex–mediated vasculitis. The antigen in some cases is probably microbial (261). Streptococcal infections, especially with group A, has been implicated as well as the hepatitis B virus (262,263).

Polyarteritis nodosa appears to occur as a complication in hepatitis B virus infection in approximately 1 in 500 cases (264). The finding that 30% to 50% of patients with polyarteritis nodosa are chronically infected with hepatitis B virus is especially intriguing with respect to microbe-induced immune complex vasculitis as a possible, even probable, mechanism in polyarteritis nodosa. The size and composition of the immune complexes are no doubt critical in determining clinical disease production.

Dixon and colleagues (265) provided a great deal of insight into the pathogenic mechanism of serum-sickness vasculitis, a vasculitic syndrome sharing many features with polyarteritis nodosa. They demonstrated that the vasculitis lesions were in fact induced by immune complex deposition at vascular basement membranes, with activation of complement pathways, chemotaxis of neutrophils and other inflammatory cells, and resultant tissue damage. To be pathogenic, the immune complexes had to be of a certain size, approximately 106 kd. Complexes formed in antibody excess were rapidly cleared by the phagocytic system, and complexes in great antigen excess were typically too small to be sieved and lodged at the basement membrane zone and the internal elastic lamina of arteries. The most toxic complexes were formed in slight antigen excess and were of IgG1 and IgG3 complement-fixing subtypes. These investigations also showed that increased permeability, through IgE-histamine pathways, can enhance immune complex deposition in arteriolar walls. In patients with

the serum-sickness–like prodrome of hepatitis B virus infection, the hepatitis B antigen–antihepatitis B antibody complexes contain the complement-fixing IgG1 and IgG3 subtypes (266). In contrast, circulating immune complexes in patients with hepatitis B virus infection without the prodromal vasculitic syndrome do not contain these complement-fixing antibodies. A polyarteritis-like syndrome occurs in blue foxes (*Alopex lagopus*). It has been shown that this disease is induced by a protozoon, *Encephalitozoon (Nosema) cuniculi*, and that an immune complex arteritis accounts for the pathologic lesions (267).

Platelet immune complex interactions, and antiendothelial cell antibodies may also play a role in the pathogenesis (268).

Histopathologic Findings

In contradistinction to SLE, histopathologic study of ocular tissues of patients with polyarteritis nodosa has been performed by a number of investigators. As early as 1889, Müller (269) described classic histopathologic evidence of choroidal vasculitis in a patient with polyarteritis nodosa. At least nine excellent, well-documented histopathologic reports on choroidal, retinal, and ciliary arteritis have appeared since then. There is a scattered pattern of vasculitic lesions with all stages—acute, chronic, and healing lesions—seen in the involved tissues. Acute lesions show infiltration of the vessel walls and surrounding tissues with neutrophils and eosinophils; monocytes, lymphocytes, and plasma cells surround the vessel. Endothelial swelling and proliferation, with fibrinoid necrosis of the involved vessels, occur, and this process affects all the layers of small to medium-size arteriole walls. Fibrosis and scarring mark the healed lesions.

The histopathologic features of the scleral, conjunctival, and corneal lesions of polyarteritis nodosa are strikingly nonspecific. Specimens of cornea from areas of active corneal ulceration show almost exclusively a neutrophil infiltrate; this is not surprising, because the major effector cell for collagen degradation in most forms of corneal ulceration appears to be the neutrophil (270,271). Specimens of conjunctiva that appear infiltrated adjacent to peripheral ulcerative keratitis lesions show numerous eosinophils, plasma cells, and lymphocytes in the substantia propria. Specimens of sclera from involved areas show neutrophils in areas of frank scleral destruction and necrosis, with surrounding zones of lymphocytes and plasma cells.

The exact mechanism involved, then, in production of the scleral and corneal lesions in polyarteritis nodosa is unclear. A reasonable hypothesis would be the deposition of immune complexes in sclera or corneoscleral limbus, with subsequent activation of complement pathways resulting in chemotaxis and inflammatory cell recruitment to the area of immune complex deposition.

Clinical Features

Systemic Involvement

The clinical manifestations of polyarteritis nodosa are so protean and varied that a classic characteristic description is impossible. The clinical manifestations include fever, malaise, easy fatigability, weight loss, anorexia, myalgia, muscle wasting, and arthralgia. The disease may have an abrupt or gradual onset. The initial clinical manifestations are usually related predominantly to one organ system, frequently the articular or muscular system. The clinical manifestations are usually progressive, without notable remission and exacerbation. The disease may be rapidly or slowly progressive, and as it evolves, multisystem manifestations appear. It may be rapidly fatal; renal involvement is the major cause of death.

Renal

Polyarteritis with glomerulonephritis, glomerulitis, or both may occur in patients with polyarteritis nodosa. Proteinuria, urinary sediment casts, microscopic hematuria, and progressive renal failure with renal hypertension is the usual sequence. These changes may be rapidly progressive and may be fatal, if untreated, within less than 6 months after the onset of the illness.

Cutaneous

Cutaneous lesions in polyarteritis nodosa are relatively uncommon, but the appearance of livedo reticularis, tender subcutaneous nodules, or both is an extremely helpful diagnostic sign when present.

Hematologic

Leukocytosis with neutrophilia and sometimes eosinophilia is common in polyarteritis nodosa. Because they are quite uncommon in the other connective tissue diseases with which polyarteritis nodosa may sometimes be confused, these hematologic findings may be diagnostically helpful. Results of rheumatoid factor and antinuclear antibody tests are routinely negative, and immunoglobulin levels are usually normal. Complement levels may be depressed during acute phases of the disease, and circulating immune complexes or cryoglobulins may be present in the serum.

Neurologic

Peripheral neuropathy commonly occurs in patients with polyarteritis nodosa, and the disease should always be considered in the differential diagnosis of any patient with peripheral neuritis and constitutional symptoms.

Pulmonary

Pulmonary involvement in classic polyarteritis nodosa is quite uncommon. When obvious pulmonary involvement occurs in a systemic syndrome identical to classic polyarteritis nodosa, the more likely diagnosis is either Wegener's granulomatosis or allergic granulomatosis of Churg and Strauss. Granulomatous reactions are typically present in these diseases; granulomatous reactions are not found in histopathologic specimens from patients with classic polyarteritis nodosa.

Cardiovascular

Cardiovascular disease—myocardial infarction, hypertensive cardiomyopathy, and congestive heart failure—is a major cause of death in patients with polyarteritis nodosa. Segmental coronary arteritis is a very frequent finding at autopsy.

Gastrointestinal

Gastrointestinal manifestations frequently occur in patients with polyarteritis nodosa, and the patient may present with severe abdominal pain mimicking appendicitis or cholecystitis. Superior mesenteric arteritis may produce bowel infarction with subsequent necrosis and perforation. Crohn's disease may be also associated with polyarteritis nodosa (65). More commonly, however, the gastrointestinal symptoms are less pronounced and usually consist of anorexia, nausea, vomiting, and diarrhea.

Hepatic infarction from vasculitis may occur in up to 50% of patients with polyarteritis nodosa. When cases of massive hepatic infarction secondary to surgery are excluded, nearly half of all cases of massive hepatic infarction and necrosis are found to be caused by polyarteritis nodosa.

Genital

Testicular or epididymal pain is a frequent finding in male patients with polyarteritis nodosa, and testicular biopsy is likely to reveal the characteristic histopathologic features of polyarteritis nodosa in patients with this symptom.

Ocular Involvement

Corneal

Peripheral ulcerative keratitis, morphologically similar to Mooren's ulcer (272), may occur in polyarteritis nodosa and may be the presenting manifestation of this lethal disease (236,273–275). A clinical characteristic of the keratitis in these cases is corneal ulceration at the limbus that is progressive, both centrally and circumferentially, associated with ocular pain and inflammation and with undermining of the central edge of the ulcer, resulting in an overhanging lip of cornea. Involvement of adjacent sclera has commonly been reported; this may be a distinguishing characteristic from classic Mooren's ulcer (Fig. 23-22). All forms of local therapy for these ulcers have ultimately failed. The importance of diagnosis of the underlying systemic condition and adequate systemic therapy to control it, which affords concomitant control of the destructive ocular lesions, has been emphasized (236,276,277).

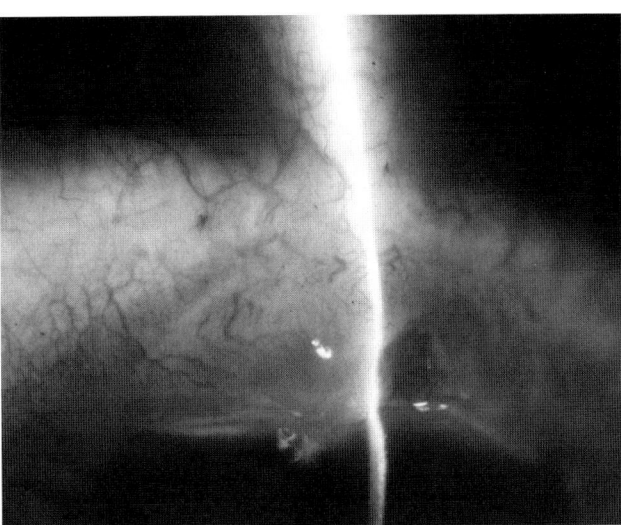

FIGURE 23-22. Scleritis with associated peripheral ulcerative keratitis. Note the clear evidence of ulceration with an overhanging lip and undermining of the edge of the overhanging lip, centrally, from the destructive process.

Conjunctival

Pale yellow, raised, and very friable conjunctival lesions have been noted in patients with PAN. The lesions had a waxy appearance and represented an area of edema and necrosis with a surrounding inflammatory reaction (278). Biopsy of the lesions was helpful in diagnosing the disease.

Scleral

The scleral lesions of polyarteritis nodosa are highly destructive and are invariably progressive unless correct diagnosis and control of the underlying systemic disease are achieved. The scleritis is always painful and may be diffuse or nodular. It may eventually progress to a necrotizing scleritis and may be associated with perforation and loss of all visual function. Our experience with similar lesions in patients with RA emphasizes the vasculitic origin of such lesions, the futility of strictly local therapy, and the ominous, lethal consequences from untreated occult systemic vasculitis (279).

Retinal and Choroidal

Choroidal vasculitis is the most common ophthalmic manifestation in polyarteritis nodosa, and it may be considerably more common than is currently recognized. Repeated longitudinal ophthalmoscopic examinations and retinal fluorescein angiograms may be especially helpful in the diagnosis of polyarteritis nodosa. Clinically symptomatic ocular involvement occurs relatively infrequently (approximately 20% of patients). Choroiditis, retinal vasculitis (with retinal edema, cotton-wool spots, hemorrhages, and irregular caliber of the retinal vessels), optic atrophy (possibly secondary to posterior ciliary vasculitis), papilledema, exudative retinal detachment, and central retinal artery occlusion are the most frequent abnormalities found. Iritis

and iridocyclitis may rarely occur (278). In addition, one may see Elschnig spots scattered throughout the posterior pole. These are isolated round, light yellow spots, one-sixth to one-third disk diameter in size, with a pigmented center. Such spots are not specific for polyarteritis nodosa, but in fact occur in a variety of systemic vasculitic syndromes. Their appearance is said to be a grave prognostic sign (280). Hypertensive retinopathy may also obviously occur with the development of renal vascular hypertension secondary to renal involvement in polyarteritis nodosa. The report by Newman and co-workers (281) of repeated monocular constriction of the visual field with sparing of central vision in a patient who was ultimately shown to have polyarteritis nodosa is of particular interest. These episodes of "peephole" vision occurring three to 12 times per day in either eye and lasting 4 to 5 minutes were shown by fluorescein angiography to be associated with incomplete choroidal filling until late in the venous phase. Autopsy findings showed impressive vasculitis of the short posterior ciliary arteries, as well as other small and medium-size orbital arteries.

CNS involvement may also result in extraocular muscle palsies, homonymous hemianopsia, amaurosis, Horner's syndrome, or nystagmus.

Diagnosis and Differential Diagnosis

The diagnosis of polyarteritis nodosa rests on histopathologic evidence of nongranulomatous vasculitis of small and medium-size arteries in a patient with multisystem clinical disease compatible with polyarteritis nodosa. There are no laboratory tests or other diagnostic data that can confirm the diagnosis.

Nodular skin lesions, symptomatic muscle, and the testes are the appropriate biopsy sites likely to reveal the characteristic histopathologic findings. Temporal artery biopsy may be useful (282). Electromyography may be helpful in selecting a suitable muscle biopsy site in the absence of muscle symptoms. Blind muscle biopsy is almost never positive. Clinically involved tissue should be biopsied as quickly as possible after the clinically apparent lesion appears. Immunoglobulin and complement components may be degraded rapidly after deposition at tissue sites. Cochrane and Koffler (283) showed that these components are undetectable 24 to 48 hours after injection into animals. This underscores the crucial importance of obtaining biopsy specimens from clinical lesions as quickly as possible after their appearance in an effort to enhance the likelihood of diagnosis.

Treatment

Ocular

Although none of the ocular lesions can be satisfactorily treated by local means, it is possible to retard progressive

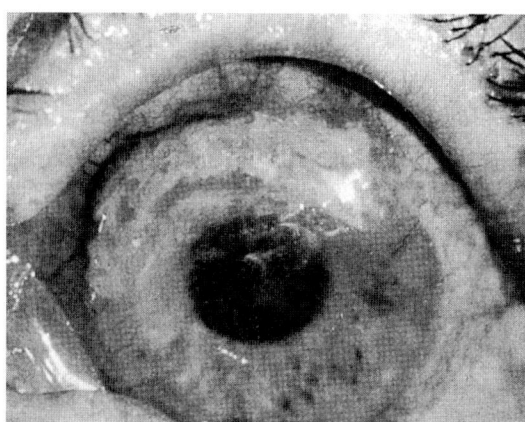

FIGURE 23-23. Anterior necrotizing scleritis and peripheral ulcerative keratitis in a patient with polyarteritis nodosa. The area of ulcerating cornea has been debrided; the necrotic, overhanging lip of cornea and the conjunctiva adjacent to the area of ulceration have been resected; and a layer of cyanoacrylate surgical adhesive has been applied in a wide area not only encompassing the area of active corneal and scleral degradation but also extending to clinically normal tissue in an effort to effect a tight bond. A soft contact lens has been applied to protect the glue from the trauma of the lid with each blink and to protect the patient against irritation of the tarsal conjunctiva by the glue.

corneal destruction in cases of peripheral ulcerative keratitis associated with polyarteritis nodosa through local means while control of the underlying systemic disease is being achieved through systemic therapy. Conjunctival resection, ulcer debridement, application of cyanoacrylate tissue adhesive to the ulcer bed and to a small rim of surrounding normal cornea and sclera, and application of a continuous-wear bandage soft contact lens may be useful while the patient is being adequately immunosuppressed (Fig. 23-23). The use of topical corticosteroids to inhibit inflammatory cell activity does not seem to be particularly effective and may in fact be harmful because of its inhibitory effect on new collagen formation. Inhibitors of collagenase synthesis, such as 1% medroxyprogesterone acetate drops, and competitive inhibitors of collagenase activity, such as acetylcysteine (20% drops), are other adjunctive forms of topical therapy that may help retard ulcer progression while the disease is being brought under control. Systemic doxycycline may also serve the same function of inhibition of matrix metalloproteinases.

Systemic

The prognosis of untreated polyarteritis nodosa is extremely grim. The disease is almost invariably relentlessly progressive, with death usually resulting from renal failure, myocardial infarction, congestive heart failure, hepatic failure, bowel perforation, cerebral infarction, or subarachnoid hemorrhage. The 5-year survival rate in untreated cases is approximately 13% (284). High-dose systemic corticosteroid therapy improves the 5-year survival rate to approximately 48% (284,285). A striking increase in 5-year

survival in patients with polyarteritis nodosa is achieved with a combination of corticosteroid and cytotoxic immunosuppressive therapy. Fauci and associates (286) documented striking complete remissions in patients with advanced polyarteritis nodosa treated with prednisone and cyclophosphamide. Lieb and colleagues (287), in a retrospective longitudinal cohort study of outcome with respect to therapy in patients with polyarteritis nodosa, found a 12% 5-year survival rate in untreated patients, a 53% 5-year survival rate in patients treated with systemic corticosteroids, and an 80% 5-year survival rate in patients treated with both corticosteroid and cytotoxic agent immunosuppression.

WEGENER'S GRANULOMATOSIS

Wegener's granulomatosis is a multisystem disease of unknown etiology, first described by Klinger (288) in 1931 and later characterized as a distinctive syndrome by Wegener (289,290). The disease is characterized by glomerulonephritis; necrotizing granulomatous vasculitis of small and medium-size pulmonary arteries and veins; necrotizing granulomatous lesions of the mucosa of sinuses, nose, and nasopharynx; and generalized necrotizing granulomatous vasculitis of other organs, including the eyes.

Epidemiology

Although not rare, Wegener's granulomatosis is uncommon. It affects males more commonly than females (3:2) and has been documented in patients of all ages from infancy to the ninth decade but has its peak incidence in the fourth and fifth decades (291). There are no obvious racial, geographic, or occupational predispositions. Bondes (292) suggested classifying an entity as purely granulomatous Wegener's granulomatosis, an early phase of the disease presenting only with extravascular granulomas primarily in the eye, nose, throat, or lung associated with an elevated antineutrophil cytoplasmic antibodies (ANCA) level. The classification may be useful in future therapeutic trials.

Pathogenesis

Although definitive proof is lacking, one of the more popular current hypotheses about the pathogenesis of the tissue destruction that occurs in Wegener's granulomatosis is that it represents immune complex-mediated vasculitis. IgG, complement component C3, and fibrin have been demonstrated in glomerular vessel walls (291,293), and immunoglobulin and complement have been found in the vascular lesions of skin (294). Circulating immune complexes have been demonstrated in the sera of patients with Wegener's granulomatosis (295). IgA levels may be elevated (296).

There may be an increased frequency of HLA-B8 or HLA-DR2 in these patients (297).

Histopathologic Findings

Lesions from the upper respiratory tract typically show extensive granulomatous inflammation with tissue necrosis and a prominent giant cell reaction. Pulmonary arteries and veins and arteries, arterioles, veins, and venules from other clinically involved organs show a necrotizing vasculitis with acute, chronic, and healing lesions all typically represented in the same organ. Neutrophils predominate in the vascular walls in the acute lesions; mononuclear cells predominate in the more chronic lesions. Fibrinoid necrosis of vascular walls is prominent, and granulomas with multinucleated giant cells may be found in and around involved vessels and scattered in isolated foci within the involved tissue. Focal and segmental necrotizing glomerulonephritis is seen in the kidney; as the disease progresses, proliferative glomerulonephritis is the predominant histopathologic feature in the kidneys. IgG and complement have been demonstrated by immunofluorescence technique in the glomeruli of renal biopsy specimens from some patients with Wegener's granulomatosis (291).

The histopathologic features of conjunctival biopsy specimens from areas adjacent to necrotizing scleritis or peripheral ulcerative keratitis are almost never diagnostic of the underlying disorder. Lymphocytes and plasma cells predominate in the substantia propria, and variable numbers of neutrophils and eosinophils may be seen. The deeper tissues (episcleral and superficial sclera), however, may show a typical granulomatous reaction with epithelioid cells and giant cells present. Specimens of ulcerating sclera commonly show neutrophils in the area of active scleral degradation, fibrinoid necrosis, and surrounding granulomatous inflammation, including, in some cases, extensive arrays of multinucleated giant cells. If intrascleral vessels have been obtained in the biopsy specimen, true necrotizing vasculitis with inflammatory cell infiltration into the vascular wall and fibrinoid necrosis of the vessel may be seen. Granulomas of the ciliary body and of the iris have been found, and necrotizing vasculitis of the anterior ciliary arteries as they lie in the rectus muscles has been demonstrated (270,298,299). Eosinophil and neutrophil degranulation has been demonstrated in orbital lesions.

Biopsy specimens of the overhanging lip of undermined cornea at the edge of a peripheral ulcerative keratitis lesion in these patients commonly show predominantly neutrophil infiltration in the area of active collagen degradation, with variable numbers of lymphocytes. The histopathologic findings abruptly change immediately adjacent to the area of active collagen degradation (limbus and sclera) to granulomatous reaction with vast numbers of plasma cells, lymphocytes, and multinucleated giant cells (300). It should be emphasized that simply obtaining

TABLE 23-5. FREQUENCY OF OCULAR LESIONS IN WEGENER'S GRANULOMATOSIS

Lesion	Frequency (%)
Scleritis and/or peripheral ulcerative keratitis	18
Proptosis or pseudotumor	18
Conjunctivitis	15
Retinal vasculitis	8
Uveitis	6
Dacryocystitis	3

biopsy specimens of conjunctiva and of ulcer margin is unlikely to yield important clues to the diagnosis.

Clinical Features

Ocular Involvement

A review of the reported cases of Wegener's granulomatosis in the world literature reveals that the eye may be involved in 50% to 60% of cases. The ocular lesion may be the first major clinical expression of the disease that stimulates the patient to seek medical attention, and hence patients with this potentially lethal disease may have their first contact with the health care system through the ophthalmologist. Table 23-5 lists the approximate frequency of ocular and orbital lesions occurring in the reported cases of Wegener's granulomatosis. External ocular complaints ranging from restricted ocular motility (297), conjunctivitis, dacryoadenitis (301), and nasolacrimal duct obstruction to proptosis, necrotizing scleritis, and peripheral ulcerative keratitis predominate (302–305). The optic nerve, retina (vasculitis or detachment), and uveal tract may be less frequently involved (277,306,307).

Corneal

Peripheral ulcerative keratitis, necrotizing scleritis, or both are reported with increasing frequency as the first major clinical manifestation of Wegener's granulomatosis. The peripheral ulcerative keratitis is frequently preceded by localized conjunctivitis or episcleritis, followed by the onset of true scleritis and the development of intrastromal peripheral corneal inflammatory infiltrates. Pain may be mild or severe. Corneal ulceration develops with breakdown of the peripheral corneal epithelium, and the crescentic peripheral corneal ulcer progresses centrally and circumferentially, producing a biomicroscopic appearance quite similar to that of Mooren's corneal ulcer, except that sclera is never involved in the latter (Fig. 23-24). Others have reported a higher frequency of corneal (28%) and scleral and episcleral involvement (38%) in Wegener's granulomatosis (308).

Scleral

Scleral involvement is invariably present in peripheral ulcerative keratitis associated with Wegener's granulomatosis, and this may be helpful in differentiating it from Mooren's ulcer.

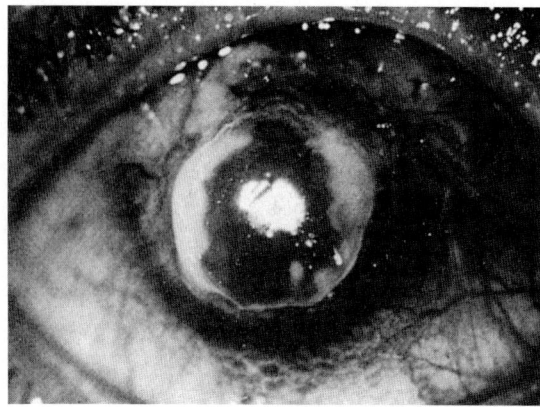

FIGURE 23-24. Peripheral ulcerative keratitis and necrotizing scleritis in a patient with undiagnosed Wegener's granulomatosis. Note the characteristic intrastromal infiltrates of inflammatory cells in advance of the underlying ulcer with an overhanging lip of ulcerating cornea. Note also the extensive involvement of the anterior sclera.

The corneal and scleral destruction progresses, often slowly but always relentlessly, in spite of all medical and surgical ocular therapy. Topical and systemic corticosteroid therapy is notably ineffective. Before the institution of immunosuppressive therapy for Wegener's granulomatosis, eyes with necrotizing scleritis, peripheral ulcerative keratitis, or both were commonly lost because of perforation and relentless tissue destruction.

Systemic Involvement

Pulmonary

Although patients with Wegener's granulomatosis may have clinical manifestations in any organ system, the most common presentation is with upper respiratory tract symptoms: recurrent epistasis; chronic rhinorrhea; painful, purulent sinusitis; chronic otitis media; hoarseness; dysphagia; cough; or pleurisy. These symptoms may have been present for weeks, months, or even years, with gradual or sudden worsening, or with the sudden onset of fever, malaise, anorexia, weight loss, and weakness. Otolaryngologic findings and pulmonary findings may be present in 98% and 52%, respectively, of the patients (306,308).

Physical examination very frequently reveals nasal, nasopharyngeal, or pharyngeal ulcerative lesions. x-ray films of the ethmoidal, frontal, or sphenoidal sinus frequently appear abnormal, and the chest x-ray film may show multiple nodular or cavitary pulmonary lesions.

Renal

Overt clinical renal symptoms are usually absent in the early phases of the disease, though microscopic hematuria and proteinuria may be found on urinalysis.

Hematologic

The erythrocyte sedimentation rate (ESR) is always elevated, and the patient usually has mild leukocytosis and mild anemia.

Mild hypergammaglobulinemia may be present, circulating autoantibodies to smooth muscle may be found, and circulating immune complexes may be detected in the serum. The test for rheumatoid factor is frequently positive. Screening for hepatitis B antigen and for antinuclear antibodies typically is negative. Delayed hypersensitivity skin test reactions may be impaired in patients with Wegener's granulomatosis.

Cutaneous

Skin lesions occur in approximately 50% of the patients; rash, petechiae, ischemic ulcers, and subcutaneous nodules may all occur.

Diagnosis

The diagnosis of Wegener's granulomatosis rests on demonstration of necrotizing granulomatous vasculitis in biopsy specimens from clinically involved upper or lower respiratory tract lesions in a patient with glomerulonephritis and a clinical history compatible with Wegener's granulomatosis.

There are few consistently abnormal immunologic laboratory test findings in study populations of patients with Wegener's granulomatosis, with the notable exception of the presence of the autoantibody ANCA (309–311). ANCAs are specific for constituents of neutrophil primary granules and monocyte lysosomes. There are different types of ANCAs. Two major categories of ANCAs can be identified by immunofluorescence microscopy with appropriate reagents, one with cytoplasmic staining (C-ANCA) and the other with perinuclear staining (P-ANCA) (312). The material identified by C-ANCA staining is proteinase 3, and that identified by P-ANCA staining is myeloperoxidase. Specific enzyme-linked immunosorbent assays (ELISAs) are now available for these separate ANCAs, and these assays are both sensitive and specific and are useful in following response to therapy (titer levels). ANCAs can be found in patients with necrotizing systemic vasculitis, such as Wegener's granulomatosis, polyarteritis nodosa, Churg-Strauss syndrome, and idiopathic crescentic glomerulonephritis (313,314).

The distribution of disease correlates to a degree with the ANCA specificity, although there is substantial overlap. Thus, patients with Wegener's granulomatosis most often have C-ANCA, and patients with renal-limited disease most often have P-ANCA (312).

Most patients also have a moderate hypergammaglobulinemia, notably IgA hypergammaglobulinemia. Mild anemia, mild leukocytosis, elevated ESR, and a weakly positive rheumatoid factor (in approximately 60% of patients) may be found. Urinalysis generally reveals proteinuria, microscopic hematuria, or granular, hyalin, or red cell casts. Chest x-ray films frequently reveal hilar enlargement and multiple nodular or cavitary pulmonary infiltrates. These infiltrates may be extremely evanescent, with changing radiographic patterns occurring rapidly. X-ray films of the paranasal sinuses are frequently abnormal. One of the earliest radiologic abnormalities is mucosal thickening of the maxillary antrum. The ethmoidal, frontal, and sphenoidal sinuses are involved in decreasing order of frequency. As sinus involvement progresses, radiographic evidence of sinus clouding, complete opacification, development of air-fluid levels, or bony destruction may appear (315).

Lethal midline granuloma has sometimes been confused with Wegener's granulomatosis. The former, however, lacks pulmonary and renal involvement and commonly has necrotizing lesions of the face as part of its features. The sinus and nasal lesions of Wegener's granulomatosis never erode the skin and face, and therefore it should not be difficult to differentiate these two diseases.

Liebow (316) described three forms of pulmonary granulomatosis that might be confused with Wegener's granulomatosis. Lymphogranulomatosis may clinically resemble Wegener's granulomatosis, but histopathologic study of clinical lesions in lymphogranulomatosis shows an active atypical lymphoreticular proliferation that is quite distinct from the necrotizing granulomatous vasculitis typical of Wegener's. Necrotizing sarcoid granulomatosis resembles Boeck's sarcoidosis histopathologically by the presence of noncaseating granulomas, but differs from sarcoidosis in that diffuse necrotizing angiitis may also be seen. Bronchocentric granulomatosis may clinically resemble Wegener's granulomatosis of the lung, but histopathologic study in the former reveals the lesions to be centered around the bronchi rather than around the vessels. Extrapulmonary lesions have not been described in this disorder. Goodpasture's syndrome, the other classic pulmonary-renal syndrome, lacks the upper respiratory manifestations of Wegener's granulomatosis and is distinguished by the presence of antiglomerular basement membrane antibody and by the positive linear immunoglobulin staining patterns of glomeruli on fluorescent antibody study of biopsy specimens.

Treatment

Ocular

Local ocular therapy will never cure the ocular lesion without successful treatment of the underlying systemic disease. However, as in the case of polyarteritis nodosa, some measures may be quite helpful in saving the eye from perforation and destruction while systemic immunosuppression is being achieved. The use of topical antibiotics, conjunctival resection, ulcer debridement, cyanoacrylate tissue adhesive, and soft contact lenses, along with anticollagenolytic agents, may be beneficial in this regard. Definitive therapy is systemic immunosuppression (236,303) (Fig. 23-25).

Systemic

Wegener's granulomatosis is a fatal disease, and the mean survival time is approximately 5 months after the onset of

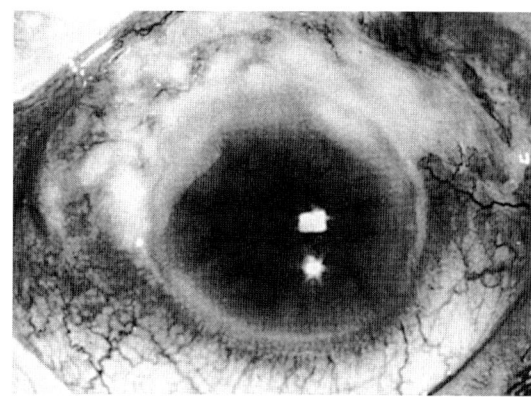

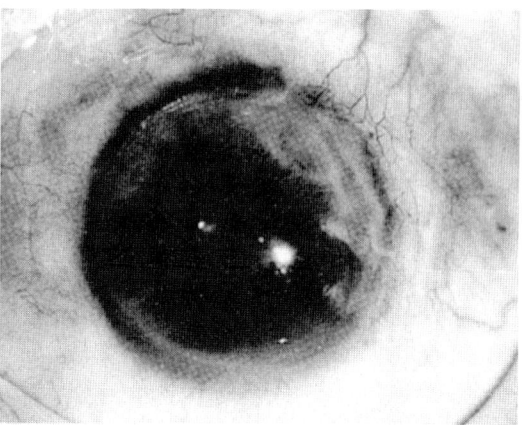

FIGURE 23-25. A: Peripheral ulcerative keratitis and necrotizing scleritis in a patient with Wegener's granulomatosis. The ulcerative process has extended counterclockwise from 8:30 o'clock to 3 o'clock. Note the intrastromal inflammatory cell infiltrates as well as the intrascleral nodules of inflammatory cells. **B:** Same eye, after conjunctival resection, ulcer debridement, cyanoacrylate tissue adhesive application, soft lens application, and systemic immunosuppression with prednisone and cyclophosphamide. Ocular inflammation and progressive corneal and scleral destruction ceased within 4 weeks of institution of systemic immunosuppression. Soft lens and surgical adhesive were removed, the patient was treated with cytotoxic therapy for 18 months, and therapy was then discontinued. He remained disease-free during a 5-year follow-up period and maintained a visual acuity of 20/20.

renal disease. Corticosteroids alone are ineffective in influencing the long-term prognosis (315). Systemic immunosuppression with cyclophosphamide and steroids, however, is extremely effective in the treatment of this disease, and long-lasting complete remissions of many years' duration have been achieved in patients with far-advanced disease in this once universally fatal illness (291,315,317). A dramatic improvement may occur after bolus corticosteroids and cyclophosphamide are given (318).

PROGRESSIVE SYSTEMIC SCLEROSIS (SCLERODERMA)

Progressive systemic sclerosis (PSS) is a multisystem disease characterized by inflammation, fibrosis, and degenerative changes of skin, vessels, synovium, and visceral organs such as the gut, kidney, heart, and lungs. The disease is of unknown etiology, and there is no known cure. The clinical course and prognosis depend on the extent of visceral involvement.

Curzio (319) may have been the first to describe the syndrome that we call scleroderma today. Gintrac (320) was the first to use the term *scleroderma* to describe the syndrome. Visceral involvement in patients with the disease was not emphasized in the medical literature until Matsui (321) did so, and in 1945 Goetz (322) proposed the name *progressive systemic sclerosis* for this multisystem disorder.

The disease appears to affect women four times more frequently than men, with an especially high degree of disparity between the two sexes during the third and fourth decades. There is no racial or geographic predilection. There is an unusually high incidence of PSS in miners (both coal and gold miners) and in other workers with major exposure to silica dust (323). HLA-A9 and HLA-DR3 are overrepresented in PSS patient cohorts (324).

Pathogenesis

Patients with PSS commonly exhibit hypergammaglobulinemia, and approximately 50% have either circulating immune complexes detectable as cryoglobulins or circulating rheumatoid factor and antinuclear antibody. A speckled pattern on the immunofluorescent test for antinuclear antibody is particularly common in patients with PSS, and an antinuclear antibody, ScL-70, now known to recognize the intranuclear enzyme topoisomerase 1, that appears to be unique to patients with PSS, has been described (220,325). Antinuclear antibodies to endothelial cells of dermal blood vessels and epithelial basal cells are also present (326). Approximately half the patients with PSS also have circulating antibodies to nuclear RNA. The relative numbers of circulating T lymphocytes in the peripheral blood may be modestly reduced, and some patients with PSS have been shown to have circulating lymphocytes that can be stimulated by skin extracts. Biopsy specimens of pathologic tissue from patients with PSS are typically negative for immunoglobulin and complement deposition, with the exception of renal vessels.

These data suggest that a reasonable working hypothesis for the pathogenesis of PSS may involve abnormalities in both the immune and the connective tissue systems, with lymphocyte sensitization to skin antigens, migration of lymphocytes into tissues, and liberation of chemotactic factors attractive to dermal fibroblasts, with resultant proliferation of the fibroblasts and overproduction of immature collagen. There may be mast cell–fibroblast interactions that contribute to the resultant pathology (325). The vascular changes seen may be secondary to these phenomena; an alternative hypothesis involves a more active role for the vascular events. It is clear that the vascular system is involved very early in the course of PSS.

Histopathologic Findings

Histopathologic study of skin biopsy specimens during the active (as opposed to the fibrotic) phase of scleromatous involvement in PSS shows almost an exclusive T-lymphocyte infiltrate (239), vascular endothelial cell proliferation with hyalinization, myxomatous degeneration of arterioles (327), perivascular mononuclear cell infiltration, and greatly increased amounts of immature collagen fibers with resultant thickening of the dermis. Increased melanin is also seen in the basal layers of the epidermis.

Clinical Features

Ocular Involvement

Corneal

The association of tear insufficiency with PSS has been well established (328,329). A high percentage (probably at least 70%) of patients with PSS have tear insufficiency, and many become symptomatic with clinical sicca syndrome (Table 23-6). Most patients with PSS also have progressive conjunctival fornix foreshortening. This should not be surprising in a disease characterized by mucosal subepithelial fibrosis. Stucchi and Geiser (330) and Horan (331) documented and emphasized the frequency of shallow fornices in patients with PSS. Extraocular muscle myositis (332) and keratitis unrelated to keratoconjunctivitis sicca may also occur (333). Transient corneal opacification has been induced by cold in a patient with Raynaud's disease (334), and telangiectasia and sludging of the conjunctival vessels have been observed (335).

Retinal

As in other collagen vascular diseases, retinopathy has, in general, been underemphasized in PSS. The incidence of choroidal vascular abnormalities in patients with PSS is probably considerably higher than that in patients with SLE. Grennan and Forrester (336) found that 53% of their study patients with PSS had patchy areas of nonperfusion of the choroidal vasculature; one patient showed abnormalities of the retinal vasculature (microaneurysmal dilatation of the terminal venules in one quadrant). The abnormalities of the choroidal vasculature were extensive and were found in patients without history of hypertension. Ophthalmoscopy had appeared normal in all the patients. The choroidal choriocapillaris and arteriolar abnormalities

TABLE 23-6. OCULAR MANIFESTATIONS IN PROGRESSIVE SYSTEMIC SCLEROSIS

Manifestation	Frequency
Sicca syndrome	70
Conjunctival shrinkage	70
Choroidal nonperfusion	50
Episcleritis	5

probably relate to the vascular endothelial basement membrane thickening, with deposition of mucopolysaccharide material in the precapillary arteriolar walls; patchy choroidal nonperfusion occurs then on the basis of vascular obliteration (337,338).

Systemic Involvement

The most common initial clinical manifestation of PSS is the appearance of Raynaud's phenomenon. Well over 95% of patients with PSS develop paroxysmal vasospasm of the fingers, ear lobes, tongue, or toes. Episodes are characterized by sudden pallor or cyanosis of the involved areas, with concomitant pain and sensations of cold and numbness. Within 10 to 15 minutes the symptoms and signs begin to resolve. Patients with these signs and symptoms have been shown to have up to a 90% decrease in nail-bed capillaries, with abnormal, dilated capillary loops.

Cutaneous
Symmetric painless finger edema generally develops at the same time as or shortly after the onset of Raynaud's phenomenon; alternatively, approximately 30% of patients may develop arthralgia along with the sausage-shaped digital edematous changes. Skin involvement of the face, forearms, and trunk may then develop, first as edematous, indurated areas of skin, followed by contraction and hardening of tissue and the development of tight, atrophic skin. Telangiectasia and dermal sclerosis of the eyelids occur.

Gastrointestinal
Esophageal dysfunction is the most common visceral abnormality in patients with PSS; it develops in over 90% of patients. The obvious clinical symptom is dysphagia, but even in those patients who do not have overt clinical symptoms of esophageal motility dysfunction, fluorometric radiographic studies have shown that nearly all have abnormal esophageal peristaltic activity, particularly in the lower third of the esophagus (339).

Articular
Articular changes are common in patients with PSS, with joint stiffness and polyarthralgia as the most frequent complaints. Fibrous deposits on tendon sheaths may produce rubs in association with movement of the affected joint, and many patients with PSS develop such creaking rubs in association with knee movement. Calcinosis—the development of subcutaneous and intracutaneous calcium deposits, particularly in the finger tips—may occur in patients with PSS; this is a prominent feature in patients with the so-called CRST (calcinosis, Raynaud's, sclerodactyly, telangiectasia) or CREST (CRST plus esophageal dysfunction) form of the disease. Such depositions produce quite characteristic radiographic changes. The explanation for the development of these depositions is unclear.

Pulmonary
Pulmonary involvement is nearly universal in patients with PSS, though many are totally asymptomatic. The most common clinical sign of pulmonary involvement is the development of exertional dyspnea. Pulmonary fibrosis has been found in up to 90% of PSS patients at autopsy (339).

Cardiac
The heart may be involved in PSS as well, with autopsy studies disclosing myocardial fibrosis. Cardiac catheterization studies have shown a high frequency of pulmonary hypertension in patients with PSS, but it is the unusual case that progresses to frank cor pulmonale.

Renal
Renal disease is the single most common cause of death in patients with PSS, and death is usually the result of severe hypertension in the patients who have had severe and rapidly progressive PSS for less than 3 years. Histopathologic study reveals extensive renal arterial and arteriolar pathologic changes as described above, with fibrinoid necrosis and deposition of immunoglobulin and complement in vessel walls.

Treatment

Therapy in PSS has been generally discouraging, although corticosteroids may relieve myositis in some patients and others may respond to cytotoxic and corticosteroid drug combinations. Plasmapheresis combined with prednisone and cyclophosphamide was successfully employed in a small group of PSS patients (340), and dimethyl sulfoxide has been employed experimentally in the treatment of PSS (341).

REFERENCES

1. Jones P, Jayson ME. Rheumatoid scleritis: a long-term follow-up. *Proc Soc Med* 1973;66:1161.
2. Erhardt CC, Mumford PA, Venables PJ, Maini RN. Factors predicting a poor life prognosis in rheumatoid arthritis: an eight year prospective study. *Ann Rheum Dis* ;48:7.
3. Foster CS, Forstot SL, Wilson LA. Mortality rate in rheumatoid arthritis patients developing necrotizing scleritis or peripheral ulcerative keratitis. Effects of immunosuppression. *Ophthalmology* 1984;91:1253.
4. Zer I, Machtey I, Kurz Os. Combined treatment of scleromalacia perforans in rheumatoid arthritis with penicillamine and plastic surgery. *Ophthalmologica* 1973;166:293.
5. Jampol LM, West C, Goldberg MF. Therapy of scleritis with cytotoxic agents. *Am J Ophthalmol* 1978;86:266.
6. Pisko EJ, et al. Ocular pathology, tear production, and tear lysozyme in rheumatoid arthritis. *J Rheumatol* 1982;9:708.
7. Svejgaard A, et al. HLA in rheumatology (editorial). *J Rheumatol* 1981;8:541.
8. Woodrow JC. Genetic aspects of the spondyloarthropathies. *Clin Rheum Dis* 1985;11:1.
9. Hollander JL, et al. Studies on the pathogenesis of rheumatoid joint inflammation: I. The "R.A. cell" and a working hypothesis. *Ann Intern Med* 196562:271.

10. Rawson AJ, Abelson NM, Hollander JL. Studies on the pathogenesis of rheumatoid joint inflammation: II. Intracytoplasmic particulate complexes in rheumatoid synovial fluids. *Ann Intern Med* 1965;62:281.

11. Ruddy S, Austen KF. The complement system in rheumatoid synovitis: I. An analysis of complement component activities in rheumatoid synovial fluids. *Arthritis Rheum* 1970;13:713.

12. Zvaifler NJ. A speculation on the pathogenesis of joint inflammation in rheumatoid arthritis. *Arthritis Rheum* 1965;8:289.

13. Zvaifler NJ. Further speculation on the pathogenesis of joint inflammation in rheumatoid arthritis. *Arthritis Rheum* 1970;13:895.

14. Nance EP, Jr, Kaye, JJ. The rheumatoid variants. *Semin Roentgenol* 1982;17:16.

15. Rodnan GP. *Primer on the rheumatic diseases,* 7th ed. New York: Arthritis Foundation, 1973:25–38.

16. Zizic TM, Stevens MB. Rheumatoid arthritis and variants. In: SJ Ryan, Jr, RE Smith, eds. *Selected topics on the eye in systemic disease.* New York: Grune & Stratton, 1974:315–338.

17. Goldstein R, Arnett FC. The genetics of rheumatic disease in man. *Rheum Dis Clin North Am* 1987;13:487.

18. Luthra HS, et al. Immune complexes in sera and synovial fluids of patients with rheumatoid arthritis: radioimmunoassay with monoclonal rheumatoid factor. *J Clin Invest* 1975;56:458.

19. Foster CS. Immunosuppressive therapy for external ocular inflammatory disease. *Ophthalmology* 1980;87:140.

20. Immune complexes in rheumatic disease (editorial). *Lancet* 1976;2:79.

21. Ishikawa H, Ziff M. Electron microscopic observations of immunoreactive cells in the rheumatoid synovial membrane. *Arthritis Rheum* 1976;19:1.

22. Cush JJ, Lipsky PE. Cellular basis for rheumatoid inflammation. *Clin Orthop* 1991;265:9.

23. Gardner KM, Rajacich GM, Mondino BJ. Ophthalmological manifestations of adult rheumatoid arthritis and cicatricial pemphigoid. *Int Ophthalmol Clin* 1985;25:1.

24. Hunder GG, et al. Pleural fluid complement, complement conversion, and immune complexes in immunologic and nonimmunologic diseases. *J Lab Clin Med* 1977;90:971.

25. Liebling MR, et al. Pulse methylprednisolone in rheumatoid arthritis: a double-blind crossover trial. *Ann Intern Med* 1981;94:71.

26. Pekin TJ Jr, Zvaifler NJ. Hemolytic complement in synovial fluid. *J Clin Invest* 1964;43:1372.

27. Van Boxel JA, Paget SA. Predominantly T-cell infiltrate in rheumatoid synovial membranes. *N Engl J Med* 1975;293:517.

28. Winchester RJ, Agnello V, Kunkel HG. Gamma globulin complexes in synovial fluids of patients with rheumatoid arthritis: partial characterization and relationship to lowered complement levels. *Clin Exp Immunol* 1970;6:689.

29. Yoshinoya S, et al. Detection and partial characterization of immune complexes in patients with rheumatoid arthritis plus Sjogren's syndrome and with Sjogren's syndrome alone. *Clin Exp Immunol* 1982;48:339.

30. Koch AE, Polverini PJ, Leibovich SJ. Stimulation of neovascularization by human rheumatoid synovial tissue macrophages. *Arthritis Rheum* 1986;29:471.

31. O'Dell JR, Haine CE, Erikson N, et al. Treatment of rheumatoid arthritis with methotrexate alone, sulfasalazine and hydroxychloroquine, or a combination of all three medications. *N Engl J Med* 1996;334:1287.

32. Conn DL, Lim SS. New role for an old friend: prednisone is a disease-modifying agent in early rheumatoid arthritis. *Curr Opin Rheumatol* 2003;15:193.

33. Gordon DA, Stein JL, Broder I. The extraarticular features of rheumatoid arthritis: A systemic analysis of 127 cases. *Am J Med* 1973;54:445.

34. Walker WC, Wright V. Pulmonary lesions and rheumatoid arthritis. *Medicine* 1968;47:501.

35. Schmid FR, et al. Arteritis in rheumatoid arthritis. *Am J Med* 1961;30:56.

36. Ferry AP. The histopathology of rheumatoid episcleral nodules: An extra-articular manifestation of rheumatoid arthritis. *Arch Ophthalmol* 1969;82:77.

37. Hollywell C, et al. Ultrastructure of synovial changes in rheumatoid disease and in seronegative inflammatory arthropathies. *Virchows Arch A Pathol Anat Histopathol* 1983;400:345.

38. Restifo RA, et al. Studies on the pathogenesis of rheumatoid joint inflammation: III. The experimental production of arthritis by the intra-articular injection of 7S gamma globulin. *Ann Intern Med* 1965;62:285.

39. Watson PG, Hazleman BL. *The sclera and systemic disorders.* London: Saunders, 1976.

40. Friedlaender MH. Ocular allergy and immunology. *J Allergy Clin Immunol* 1979;63:51.

41. Michels RG. Ocular manifestations in arthritis. In: Ryan SJ, Smith RE, eds. *Selected topics on the eye in systemic disease.* New York: Grune & Stratton, 1974:363–379.

42. Stanworth A. The association of ocular and articular disease. *Trans Ophthalmol Soc UK* 1951;71:189.

43. Thompson M, Eadie S. Keratoconjunctivitis sicca and rheumatoid arthritis. *Ann Rheum Dis* 1956;15:21.

44. Fye KH, et al. Relationship of HLA-Dw3 and HLA-B8 to Sjögren's syndrome. *Arthritis Rheum* 1978;21:337.

45. Powell TR, et al. HLA-Bw44 and HLA-DRw4 in male Sjögren's syndrome patients with associated rheumatoid arthritis. *Clin Immunol Immunopathol* 1980;17:463.

46. Bendaoud BD, et al. IgA-containing immune complexes in the circulation of patients with primary Sjögren's syndrome. *J Autoimmun* 1991;4:177.

47. Cobo M. Inflammation of the sclera. *Int Ophthalmol Clin* 1983;23:159.

48. Jayson MIV, Jones DEP. Scleritis and rheumatoid arthritis. *Ann Rheum Dis* 1971;30:343.

49. Lachmann SM, Hazleman BL, Watson PG. Scleritis and associated disease. *Br Med J* 1978;1:88.

50. Lyne AJ, Pitkeathley DA. Episcleritis and scleritis: association with connective tissue disease. *Arch Ophthalmol* 1968;80:171.

51. McGavin DDM, Williamson J, Forrester JV, et al. Episcleritis and scleritis: a study of their clinical manifestations and associations with rheumatoid arthritis. *Br J Ophthalmol* 1976;60:192.

52. Jayson MIV, Jones DEP. Rheumatoid arthritis and scleritis. *Trans Ophthalmol Soc UK* 1971;91:189.

53. Jones DB. Prospects in the management of tear deficiency states. *Trans Am Acad Ophthalmol Otolaryngol* 1977;83:693.

54. Rogers RS III, et al. Immunopathology of cicatricial pemphigoid: Studies of complement deposition. J Invest Dermatol 1977;68:39.

55. Sjögren H, Bloch KJ. Keratoconjunctivitis sicca and the Sjögren syndrome. *Surv Ophthalmol* 1971;16:145.

56. Watson PG. Disease of the sclera and episclera. In: Tasman W, Jaeger EA, eds. *Duane's clinical ophthalmology.* Philadelphia: Lippincott, 1991:1–43.

57. Watson PG, Hayreh SS. Scleritis and episcleritis. *Br J Ophthalmol* 1976;60:163.

58. Foster CS, Sainz de la Maza M. *The sclera.* New York: Springer-Verlag, 1994.

59. Gold DH. Ocular manifestations of connective tissue (collagen) disease. In: Tasman W, Jaeger EA, eds. *Duane's clinical ophthalmology.* Philadelphia: Lippincott, 1991:1–30.

60. Watson PG, Bovey E. Anterior segment fluorescein angiography in the diagnosis of scleral inflammation. *Ophthalmology* 1985;92:1.

61. Watson PG, Young RD. Changes at the periphery of a lesion in necrotising scleritis: anterior segment fluorescein angiography correlated with electron microscopy. *Br J Ophthalmol* 1985;69:656.
62. Benson WE, et al. Posterior scleritis: a cause of diagnostic confusion. *Arch Ophthalmol* 1979;97:1482.
63. Wilhelmus KR, Grierson I, Watson PG. Histopathologic and clinical associations of scleritis and glaucoma. *Am J Ophthalmol* 1981;91:697.
64. Marushak D. Uveal effusion attending scleritis posterior: a case report with A-scan and B-scan echograms. *Acta Ophthalmol* 1982;60:773.
65. Aronson SB, Elliott JH. Scleritis. In: Golden B, ed. *Ocular inflammatory disease.* Springfield, IL: Charles C Thomas, 1974:43–49.
66. Aronson SB, et al. Pathogenetic approach to therapy of peripheral corneal inflammatory disease. *Am J Ophthalmol* 1970; 70:65.
67. Young RD, Watson PG. Microscopical studies of necrotising scleritis. I. Cellular aspects. *Br J Ophthalmol* 1984;68:770.
68. Young RD, Watson PG. Microscopical studies of necrotising scleritis. II. Collagen degradation in the scleral stroma. *Br J Ophthalmol* 1984;68:781.
69. Cohen KL. Sterile corneal perforation after cataract surgery in Sjögren's syndrome. *Br J Ophthalmol* 1982;66:179.
70. Sevel D. Rheumatoid nodule of the sclera (a type of nongranulomatous scleritis). *Trans Ophthalmol Soc UK* 1965;85:357.
71. Wilhelmus KR, Watson PG, Vasavada AR. Uveitis associated with scleritis. *Trans Ophthalmol Soc UK* 1981;101:351.
72. Brown SI, Grayson M. Marginal furrows: a characteristic corneal lesion of rheumatoid arthritis. *Arch Ophthalmol* 1968;79:563.
73. Jayson MIV, Easty DL. Ulceration of the cornea in rheumatoid arthritis. *Ann Rheum Dis* 1977;36:428.
74. Bron AJ, McLendon BF, Camp AV. Epithelial deposition of gold in the cornea of patients receiving systemic therapy. *Am J Ophthalmol* 1979;88:354.
75. Eiferman RA, Carothers DJ, Yankeelov JA Jr. Peripheral rheumatoid ulceration and evidence for conjunctival collagenase production. *Am J Ophthalmol* 1979;87:703.
76. Kervick GN, et al. Paracentral rheumatoid corneal ulceration: Clinical features and cyclosporine therapy. *Ophthalmology* 1992;99:80.
77. Palay DA, et al. Penetrating keratoplasty in patients with rheumatoid arthritis. *Ophthalmology* 1992;99:622.
78. Welch C, Baum J. Tarsorrhaphy for corneal disease in patients with rheumatoid arthritis. *Ophthalmic Surg* 1988;19:31.
79. Gelender H. Descemetocele after intraocular lens implantation. *Arch Ophthalmol* 1982;100:72.
80. Insler MS, Boutros G, Boulware DW. Corneal ulceration following cataract surgery in patients with rheumatoid arthritis. *Am Intraocular Implant Soc J* 1985;11:594.
81. Maffett MJ, et al. Sterile corneal ulceration after cataract extraction in patients with collagen vascular disease. *Cornea* 1990;9:279.
82. Radtke N, Meyers S, Kaufman HE. Sterile corneal ulcers after cataract surgery in keratoconjunctivitis sicca. *Arch Ophthalmol* 1978;96:51.
83. Yang HK, Kline OR Jr. Corneal melting with intraocular lenses. *Arch Ophthalmol* 1982;100:1272.
84. Gold RH, Bassett LW, Theros EG. Radiologic comparison of erosive polyarthritides with prominent interphalangeal involvement. *Skeletal Radiol* 1982;8:89.
85. O'Connor GR. Calcific band keratopathy. *Trans Am Ophthalmol Soc* 1972;70:58.
86. Arnett FC. Revised criteria for the classification of rheumatoid arthritis. *Bull Rheum Dis* 1989;38:1.
87. Stage DE, Mannik M. Rheumatoid factors in rheumatoid arthritis. *Bull Rheum Dis* 1973;23:720.
88. Carsons S. Newer laboratory parameters for the diagnosis of rheumatic disease. *Am J Med* 1988;85:34.
89. Cooperating Clinics Committee of the American Rheumatism Association. A controlled trial of gold salt therapy in rheumatoid arthritis. *Arthritis Rheum* 1973;16:353.
90. Empire Rheumatism Council. Gold therapy in rheumatoid arthritis: final report of a multicentre controlled trial. *Ann Rheum Dis* 1961;20:315.
91. Ennis RS, Granda JL, Posner AS. Effect of gold salts and other drugs on the release and activity of lysosomal hydrolases. *Arthritis Rheum* 1968;11:756.
92. Gottlieb NL, Smith PM, Smith EM. Tissue gold concentration in a rheumatoid arthritic receiving cryotherapy. *Arthritis Rheum* 1972;15:16.
93. Morsman CDG, et al. Screening for hydroxychloroquine retinal toxicity: Is it necessary? *Eye* 1990;4:572.
94. Caldwell JR, Furst DE. The efficacy and safety of low-dose corticosteroids for rheumatoid arthritis. *Semin Arthritis Rheum* 1991;21:1.
95. Barry M. The use of high-dose pulse methylprednisolone in rheumatoid arthritis: unproved therapy. *Arch Intern Med* 1985;145:1483.
96. Williams IA, Baylis EM, English J. High dose intravenous methylprednisolone (pulse therapy) in the treatment of rheumatoid disease. *Scand J Rheumatol* 1981;10:153.
97. Williams IA, Baylis EM, Shipley ME. A double-blind placebo-controlled trial of methylprednisolone pulse therapy in active rheumatoid disease. *Lancet* 1982;2:237.
98. Dawson TM, Starkebaum G, Wood BL, et al. Epstein-Barr virus, methotrexate and lymphoma in patients with rheumatoid arthritis and primary Sjögren's syndrome: case series. *J Rheumatol* 2001;28:47.
99. Weinblatt ME, Maier AL. Disease-modifying agents and experimental treatments of rheumatoid arthritis. *Clin Orthop* 1991;265:103.
100. Foster CS, Forstot SL, Wilson LA. Mortality rate in rheumatoid arthritis patients developing necrotizing scleritis or peripheral ulcerative keratitis: effects of systemic immunosuppression. *Ophthalmology* 1984;91:1253.
101. Jampol LM, West C, Goldberg MF. Therapy of scleritis with cytotoxic agents. *Am J Ophthalmol* 1978;86:266.
102. Watson PG. The diagnosis and management of scleritis. *Ophthalmology* 1980;87:716.
103. Ghafoor SYA, Williamson J. Surgical management of scleromalacia perforans–a case report. *Scot Med J* 1983;28:357.
104. Koenig SB, Kaufman HE. The treatment of necrotizing scleritis with an autogenous periosteal graft. *Ophthalmic Surg* 1983;14:1029.
105. Koenig SB, Sanitato JJ, Kaufman HE. Long-term follow-up studies of scleroplasty using autogenous periosteum. *Cornea* 1990;9:139.
106. Torchia RT, Dunn RE, Pease PJ. Fascia lata grafting in scleromalacia perforans with lamellar corneal-scleral dissection. *Am J Ophthalmol* 1968;66:705.
107. Kenyon KR. Decision-making in the therapy of external eye disease: noninfected corneal ulcers. *Ophthalmology* 1982; 89:44.
108. Foster CS, Wilson LA, Ekins MB. Immunosuppressive therapy for progressive ocular cicatricial pemphigoid. *Ophthalmology* 1982;89:340.
109. Kanski JJ, Shun-Shin GA. Systemic uveitis syndromes in childhood: An analysis of 340 cases. *Ophthalmology* 1984;91:1247.
110. Schaller JG. Chronic arthritis in children: juvenile rheumatoid arthritis. *Clin Orthop* 1984;182:79.

111. Smith RE, Nozik R. *Uveitis: a clinical approach to diagnosis and management.* Baltimore: Williams & Wilkins, 1983:108–110,155.

112. Stoeber E. Prognosis in juvenile chronic arthritis: follow-up of 433 chronic rheumatic children. *Eur J Pediatr* 1981;135:225.

113. Edström G. Band-shaped keratitis in juvenile rheumatoid arthritis. *Acta Rheum Scand* 1961;7:169.

114. Bywaters EGL, Ansell BM. Monoarticular arthritis in children. *Ann Rheum Dis* 1965;24:116.

115. Calabro JJ, Marchesano JM. Juvenile rheumatoid arthritis. *N Engl J Med* 1967;277:696.

116. Calabro JJ, Parrino GR, Marchesano JM. Monarticular-onset juvenile rheumatoid arthritis. *Bull Rheum Dis* 1970;21:613.

117. Schaller J, Smiley WK, Ansell BM. Iridocyclitis of juvenile rheumatoid arthritis (JIA, Still's disease): a follow-up study of 76 patients. *Arthritis Rheum* 1973;16:130.

118. Smiley WK, May E, Bywaters EGL. Ocular presentations of Still's disease and their treatment. Iridocyclitis in Still's disease: its complications and treatment. *Ann Rheum Dis* 1957; 16:371.

119. Rosenbaum JT. Iridocyclitis is not characteristic of Still's disease (letter). *West J Med* 1985;143:252.

120. Kanski JJ. Juvenile arthritis and uveitis. *Surv Ophthalmol* 1990;34:253.

121. Calin A, Calin HJ. Oligoarthropathy with chronic iridocyclitis— A disease only of children? *J Rheumatol* 1982;9:105.

122. Calabro JJ, et al. Chronic iridocyclitis in juvenile rheumatoid arthritis. *Arthritis Rheum* 1970;13:406.

123. Kanski JJ. Uveitis in juvenile chronic arthritis. *Clin Exp Rheumatol* 1990;8:499.

124. Hinzpeter EN, Naumann G, Bartelheimer HK. Ocular histopathology in Still's disease. *Ophthalmic Res* 1971;2:16.

125. O'Brien JM, Albert DM. Therapeutic approaches for ophthalmic problems in juvenile rheumatoid arthritis. *Rheum Dis Clin North Am* 1989;15:413.

126. Schaller J, Kupfer C, Wedgwood RJ. Iridocyclitis in juvenile rheumatoid arthritis. *Pediatrics* 1969;44:92.

127. Smiley WK. Iridocyclitis in Still's disease: prognosis and steroid treatment. *Trans Ophthalmol Soc UK* 1965;85:351.

128. Stewart AJ, Hill RH. Ocular manifestations in juvenile rheumatoid arthritis. *Can J Ophthalmol* 1967;2:58.

129. Wolf MD, Lichter PR, Ragsdale CG. Prognostic factors in the uveitis of juvenile rheumatoid arthritis. *Ophthalmology* 1987; 94:1242.

130. Rosenbaum JT. Systemic associations of anterior uveitis. *Int Ophthalmol Clin* 1991;31:131.

131. Key SN III, Kimura SJ. Iridocyclitis associated with juvenile rheumatoid arthritis. *Am J Ophthalmol* 1975;80:425.

132. Smiley WK. The eye in juvenile rheumatoid arthritis. *Trans Ophthalmol Soc UK* 1974;94:817.

133. Okada AA, Foster CS. Posterior uveitis in the pediatric population. *Int Ophthalmol Clin* 1992;32:121.

134. Kemp AS, Searle C, Horne S. Transient Brown's syndrome in juvenile chronic arthritis. *Ann Rheum Dis* 1984;43:764.

135. Merriam JC, Chylack LT Jr, Albert DM. Early-onset pauciarticular juvenile rheumatoid arthritis: a histopathologic study. *Arch Ophthalmol* 1983;101:1085.

136. Wang FM, et al. Acquired Brown's syndrome in children with juvenile rheumatoid arthritis. *Ophthalmology* 1984;91:23.

137. Godfrey WA, Lindsley CB, Cuppage FE. Localization of IgM in plasma cells in the iris of a patient with iridocyclitis and juvenile rheumatoid arthritis. *Arthritis Rheum* 1981; 24:1195.

138. Uchiyama RC, Osborn TG, Moore TL. Antibodies to iris and retina detected in sera from patients with juvenile rheumatoid arthritis with iridocyclitis by indirect immunofluorescence studies on human eye tissues. *J Rheumatol* 1989;16:1074.

139. Petty RE, et al. Immunity to soluble retinal antigen in patients with uveitis accompanying juvenile rheumatoid arthritis. *Arthritis Rheum* 1987;30:287.

140. Cogan DG, Albright F, Bartter FC. Hypercalcemia and band keratopathy. *Arch Ophthalmol* 1948;40:624.

141. Duke-Elder S, Leigh AG. *Diseases of the outer eye. System of ophthalmology series.* St. Louis: Mosby, 1965:898.

142. Fishman RS, Sunderman FW. Band keratopathy in gout. *Arch Ophthalmol* 1966;75:367.

143. Grayson M, Keates RH. *Manual of diseases of the cornea.* Boston: Little, Brown, 1969:293.

144. Roy FH. *Ocular differential diagnosis,* 2nd ed. Philadelphia: Lea & Febiger, 1975:191–192.

145. Walsh FB, Howard JE. Conjunctival and corneal lesions in hypercalcemia. *J Clin Endocrinol* 1947;7:644.

146. Doughman DJ, et al. Experimental band keratopathy. *Arch Ophthalmol* 1969;81:264.

147. Hakin KN, Watson PG. Systemic associations of scleritis. *Int Ophthalmol Clin* 1991;31:111.

148. Schaller J, et al. Antinuclear antibodies (ANA) in patients with iridocyclitis and juvenile rheumatoid arthritis ORA, Still's disease). *Arthritis Rheum* 1973;16:130.

149. Neuteboom HG, et al. Antibodies to a 15 kD nuclear antigen in patients with juvenile chronic arthritis and uveitis. *Invest Ophthalmol Vis Sci* 1992;33:1657.

150. Malagon C, et al. The iridocyclitis of early onset pauciarticular juvenile rheumatoid arthritis: outcome in immunogenetically characterized patients. *J Rheumatol* 1992;19:160.

151. Fallahi S, et al. Coexistence of rheumatoid arthritis and sarcoidosis: difficulties encountered in the differential diagnosis of common manifestations. *J Rheumatol* 1984;11:526.

152. Sahn EE, et al. Preschool sarcoidosis masquerading as juvenile rheumatoid arthritis: two case reports and a review of the literature. *Pediatr Dermatol* 1990;7:208.

153. Olson NY, Lindsley CB, Godfrey WA. Nonsteroidal anti-inflammatory drug therapy in chronic childhood iridocyclitis. *Am J Dis Child* 1988;142:1289.

154. Hemady RK, Baer JC, Foster CS. Immunosuppressive drugs in the management of progressive corticosteroid-resistant uveitis associated with juvenile rheumatoid arthritis. *Int Ophthalmol Clin* 1992;32:241.

155. Mehra R, et al. Chlorambucil in the treatment of iridocyclitis in juvenile rheumatoid arthritis. *J Rheumatol* 1981;8:141.

156. Flynn HW Jr, Davis JL, Culbertson WW. Pars plana lensectomy and vitrectomy for complicated cataracts in juvenile rheumatoid arthritis. *Ophthalmology* 1988;95:1114.

157. Hooper PL, Rao NA, Smith RE. Cataract extraction in uveitis patients. *Surv Ophthalmol* 1990;35:120.

158. Crovato F, et al. Exophthalmos in relapsing polychondritis (letter). *Arch Dermatol* 1980;116:383.

159. Diamond JG, Kaplan HJ. Lensectomy and vitrectomy for complicated cataract secondary to uveitis. *Arch Ophthalmol* 1978;96:1798.

160. Diamond JG, Kaplan HJ. Uveitis: effect of vitrectomy combined with lensectomy. *Ophthalmology* 1979;86:1320.

161. Clemens LE, Albert E, Ansell BM. Sibling pairs affected by chronic arthritis of childhood: evidence for a genetic predisposition. *J Rheumatol* 1985;12:108.

162. Miller ML, et al. Inherited predisposition to iridocyclitis with juvenile rheumatoid arthritis: selectivity among HLA-DR5 haplotypes. *Proc Natl Acad Sci USA* 1984;81:3539.

163. Glass D, et al. Early-onset pauciarticular juvenile rheumatoid arthritis associated with human leukocyte antigen-DRw5, iritis, and antinuclear antibody. *J Clin Invest* 1980;66:426.

164. Oen K, Petty RE, Schroeder ML. An association between HLA-A2 and juvenile rheumatoid arthritis in girls. *J Rheumatol* 1982;9:916.

165. Sher MR, et al. HLA-DR and MT associations with the clinical and serologic manifestations of pauciarticular onset juvenile rheumatoid arthritis. *J Rheumatol* 1985;12:114.

166. Anderson B, Sr. Ocular lesions in relapsing polychondritis and other rheumatoid syndromes: the Edward Jackson Memorial Lecture. *Am J Ophthalmol* 1967;64:35.

167. Hilding AC. Syndrome of joint and cartilaginous pathologic changes with destructive iridocyclitis: comparison with described concurrent eye and joint diseases. *Arch Intern Med* 1952;89:445.

168. Kaye RL, Sones DA. Relapsing polychondritis: clinical and pathologic features in fourteen cases. *Ann Intern Med* 1964;60:653.

169. Verity MA, Larson WM, Madden SC. Relapsing polychondritis: report of two necropsied cases with histochemical investigation of the cartilage lesion. *Am J Pathol* 1963;42:251.

170. Campbell SM, Montanaro A, Bardana EJ. Head and neck manifestations of autoimmune disease. *Am J Otolaryngol* 1983;4:187.

171. Dolan DL, Lemmon GB Jr, Teitelbaum SL. Relapsing polychondritis: analytical literature review and studies on pathogenesis. *Am J Med* 1966;41:285.

172. Kovarsky J. Otorhinolaryngologic complications of rheumatic diseases. *Semin Arthritis Rheum* 1984;14:141.

173. Check IJ., et al. T helper-suppressor cell imbalance in pyoderma gangrenosum, with relapsing polychondritis and corneal keratolysis. *Am J Clin Pathol* 1983;80:396.

174. Meyer O, et al. Relapsing polychondritis—Pathogenic role of anti-native collagen type II antibodies: a case report with immunological and pathological studies. *J Rheumatol* 1981;8:820.

175. Michelson JB. Melting corneas with collapsing nose. *Surv Ophthalmol* 1984;29:148.

176. Calin A. The management of collagen diseases. *Ration Drug Ther* 1980;14:1.

177. McAdam LP, et al. Relapsing polychondritis: prospective study of 73 patients and a review of the literature. *Medicine* 1976;55:193.

178. McKay DAR, Watson PG, Lyne AJ. Relapsing polychondritis and eye disease. *Br J Ophthalmol* 1974;58:600.

179. Barranco VP, Minor DB, Solomon H. Treatment of relapsing polychondritis with dapsone. *Arch Dermatol* 1976;112:1286.

180. Kristensen EB, Norn MS. Benign mucous membrane pemphigoid: I. Secretion of mucus and tears. *Acta Ophthalmol* 1974; 52:266.

181. MacSween RNM, et al. Occurrence of antibody to salivary duct epithelium in Sjögren's disease, rheumatoid arthritis, and other arthritides: a clinical and laboratory study. *Ann Rheum Dis* 1967;26:402.

182. Anderson B Sr. Ocular lesions in relapsing polychondritis and other rheumatoid syndromes. *Trans Am Acad Ophthalmol Otolaryngol* 1967;71:227.

183. Barth WF, Berson EL. Relapsing polychondritis, rheumatoid arthritis and blindness. *Am J Ophthalmol* 1968;66:890.

184. Bergaust B, Abrahamsen AM. Relapsing polychondritis: report of a case presenting multiple ocular complications. *Acta Ophthalmol* 1969;47:174.

185. Hughes RAC, et al. Relapsing polychondritis: three cases with a clinico-pathological study and literature review. *Q J Med* 1972;41:363.

186. Magargal LE, et al. Ocular manifestations of relapsing polychondritis. *Retina* 1981;1:96.

187. Matas BR. Iridocyclitis associated with relapsing polychondritis. *Arch Ophthalmol* 1970;84:474.

188. Rucker CW, Ferguson RH. Ocular manifestations of relapsing polychondritis. *Trans Am Ophthalmol Soc* 1964;62:167.

189. Rucker CW, Ferguson RH. Ocular manifestations of relapsing polychondritis. *Arch Ophthalmol* 1965;73:46.

190. Hoang-Xuan T, Foster CS, Rice BA. Scleritis in relapsing polychondritis: Response to therapy. *Ophthalmology* 1990;97:892.

191. Matoba A, et al. Keratitis in relapsing polychondritis. *Ann Ophthalmol* 1984;16:367.

192. Rose E, Pillsbury DM. Acute disseminated lupus erythematosus—a systemic disease. *Ann Intern Med* 1939;12:951.

193. Klemperer P, Pollack AD, Baehr G. Pathology of disseminated lupus erythematosus. *Arch Pathol* 1941;32:569.

194. Fessel WJ. SLE in the community: incidence, prevalence, outcome and first symptoms; the high prevalence in black women. *Arch Intern Med* 1974;134:1027.

195. Siegel M, Lee SL. The epidemiology of systemic lupus erythematosus. *Semin Arthritis Rheum* 1973;3:1.

196. Abdou NI, et al. Suppressor T cell abnormality in idiopathic systemic lupus erythematosus. *Clin Immunol Immunopathol* 1976;6:192.

197. Alarcon-Segovia D, Ruiz-Arguelles A. Decreased circulating thymus-derived cells with receptors for the Fc portion of immunoglobulin G in systemic lupus erythematosus. *J Clin Invest* 1978;62:1390.

198. Fauci AS, et al. Immunoregulatory aberrations in systemic lupus erythematosus. *J Immunol* 1978;121:1473.

199. Messner RP, Lundstrom FD, Williams RC Jr. Peripheral blood lymphocyte cell surface markers during the course of SLE. *J Clin Invest* 1973;52:3046.

200. Sibbitt WL Jr, Mathews PM, Bankhurst AD. Impaired release of a soluble natural killer cytotoxic factor in systemic lupus erythematosus. *Arthritis Rheum* 1984;27:1095.

201. Kaufman DB. Natural killer augmentation in systemic lupus erythematosus. *Arthritis Rheum* 1982;25:5621.

202. Tsokos GC, et al. Natural killer cells and interferon responses in patients with systemic lupus erythematosus. *Clin Exp Immunol* 1982;50:239.

203. Hall RP, et al. IgA-containing circulating immune complexes in dermatitis herpetiformis, systemic lupus erythematosus and other diseases. *Clin Exp Immunol* 1980;40:431.

204. Rebhun J, et al. Systemic lupus erythematosus activity and IgE. *Ann Allergy* 1983;50:34.

205. Scopelitis P, Biundo JJ, Alspaugh MA. Anti SSA antibody and other antinuclear antibodies in systemic lupus erythematosus. *Arthritis Rheum* 1980;23:287.

206. Rebora A, et al. Repeated skin infections as a manifestation of lupus erythematosus. *Arch Dermatol* 1982;118:213.

207. DeHoratius RJ, Pillarsetty R, Messner RP. Antinucleic acid antibodies in systemic lupus erythematosus patients and their families: Incidence and correlation with lymphocyte antibodies. *J Clin Invest* 1975;56:1149.

208. Tan EM. Sunlight as a potential aetiological factor in systemic lupus erythematosus. In: Hughes GR, ed. *Modern topics in rheumatology*. Chicago: Year Book, 1976:99–106.

209. Block SR, et al. Studies of twins with systemic lupus erythematosus: a review of the literature and presentation of twelve additional sets. *Am J Med* 1975;59:533.

210. Gibosky A, et al. Disease associations of the Ia-like human alloantigens: contrasting patterns in rheumatoid arthritis and systemic lupus erythematosus. *J Exp Med* 1978;148:1728.

211. Reinertsen JL, et al. B-lymphocyte alloantigens associated with systemic lupus erythematosus. *N Engl J Med* 1978;299:515.

212. Schur PH. Complement in lupus. *Clin Rheum Dis* 1975;1:519.

213. Chantler S, Hanson J, Jacobson J. Incidence of nuclear antibodies in patients and in related and in unrelated groups from a community with "microepidemic" of systemic lupus erythematosus. *Clin Immunol Immunopathol* 1973;2:9.

214. Phillips PE. The role of viruses in SLE. *Clin Rheum Dis* 19751:505.

215. Yoshiki T, et al. The viral envelope glycoprotein of murine leukemia viruses and the pathogenesis of immune complex nephritis in New Zealand mice. *J Exp Med* 1974;140:1011.

216. Haase AT, et al. Role of DNA intermediates in persistent infections caused by RNA viruses. In: Schlessinger D, ed. *Microbiology.* Washington, DC: American Society of Microbiology, 1977:478–483.

217. Mellors RC, Mellors JW. Type C RNA virus expression in systemic lupus erythematosus: New Zealand mouse model and human disease. *Arthritis Rheum* 1968;21:568.

218. Panem S, et al. C-type virus expression in systemic lupus erythematosus. *N Engl J Med* 1976;295:470.

219. Phillips PE. Type-C oncornavirus studies in systemic lupus erythematosus. *Arthritis Rheum* 1978;21:576.

220. Tan EM, Rodnan GP. Profile of antinuclear antibodies in progressive systemic sclerosis (PSS). *Arthritis Rheum* 1975;18:430(abst).

221. Tan EM, et al. Deoxyribonucleic acid (DNA) and antibodies to DNA in the serum of patients with systemic lupus erythematosus. *J Clin Invest* 1976;45:1732.

222. Zurier RB. SLE in pregnancy. *Clin Rheum Dis* 1975;1:613.

223. Steinberg AD, Reinertsen JL. Lupus in New Zealand mice and in dogs. *Bull Rheum Dis* 1978;28:940.

224. Dubois EL. *Lupus erythematosus,* 2nd ed. Los Angeles: University of Southern California Press, 1974.

225. Grayson M. *Diseases of the cornea.* St. Louis: Mosby, 1979:314–333.

226. Halmay O, Ludwig K. Bilateral bandshaped deep keratitis and iridocyclitis in systemic lupus erythematosus. *Br J Ophthalmol* 1964;48:558.

227. Henkind P, Gold DH. Ocular manifestations of rheumatic disorders: natural and iatrogenic. *Rheumatology* 1973;4:13.

228. Reeves JA. Keratopathy associated with systemic lupus erythematosus. *Arch Ophthalmol* 1965;74:159.

229. Ribrioux A. Sjögrens syndrome in systemic lupus erythematosus. *J Rheumatol* 1990;17:201.

230. Pillat A. Uber das Vorkommen von Choroiditis bei Lupus erythematodes. *Graefes Arch Klin Exp Ophthalmol* 1934;133:566.

231. Gold DH, Morris DA, Henkind P. Ocular findings in SLE. *Br J Ophthalmol* 1972;56:800.

232. Spaeth GL. Corneal staining in systemic lupus erythematosus. *N Engl J Med* 1967;276:1168.

233. Raizman MB, Baum J. Discoid lupus keratitis. *Arch Ophthalmol* 1989;107:545.

234. Doesschat JT. Corneal complications in lupus erythematosus discoidus. *Ophthalmologica* 1956;132:153.

235. Foster CS. Ocular surface manifestations of neurological and systemic diseases. *Int Ophthalmol Clin* 1979;19:207.

236. Foster CS. Immunosuppressive therapy in external ocular inflammatory disease. *Ophthalmology* 1980;87:140.

237. Leahey AB, et al. Chemosis as a presenting sign of systemic lupus erythematosus. *Arch Ophthalmol* 1992;110:609.

238. Drosos AA, et al. Unusual eye manifestations in systemic lupus erythematosus patients. *Clin Rheumatol* 1989;8:49.

239. Fleischmajer R, Perlish JS, Reeves JRT. Cellular infiltrates in scleroderma skin. *Arthritis Rheum* 1977;20:975.

240. Aronson AJ, et al. Immune complex deposition in the eye in systemic lupus erythematosus. *Arch Intern Med* 1979;139:1312.

241. Fitzpatrick EP, Chesen N, Rahn EK. The lupus anticoagulant and retinal vasoocclusive disease. *Am J Ophthalmol* 1990;22:148.

242. Cohen AS, et al. Preliminary criteria for the classification of systemic lupus erythematosus. *Bull Rheum Dis* 1971;21:643.

243. Hahn BH. Systemic lupus erythematosus. In: Parker CW, ed. *Clinical immunology.* Philadelphia: Saunders, 1980:583–631.

244. Moses S, Barland P. Laboratory criteria for a diagnosis of systemic lupus erythematosus. *JAMA* 1979;242:1039.

245. Burge SM, et al. The lupus hand test in oral mucosa, conjunctiva, and skin. *Br J Dermatol* 1989;121:743.

246. Kerdel F, et al. Antimalarial agents and the eye. *Dermatol Clin* 1992;10:513.

247. Weiner A, et al. Hydroxychloroquine retinopathy. *Am J Ophthalmol* 1991;112:528.

248. Bonshey HA, Warnock DG, Smith LH Jr. New approaches to treating systemic lupus erythematosus. *West J Med* 1987;147:181.

249. Blaszczyk M, et al. Plasmapheresis in the treatment of systemic lupus erythematosus. *Arch Immunol Ther Exp* 1981;29:769.

250. Tsokos GC, et al. Effect of plasmapheresis on T and B lymphocyte functions in patients with systemic lupus erythematosus. *Clin Exp Immunol* 1982;48:449.

251. Lang PG. Sulfones and sulfonamides in dermatology today. *J Am Acad Dermatol* 1979;1:479.

252. Ruzicka T, Goerz G. Dapsone in the treatment of lupus erythematosus. *Br J Dermatol* 1981;104:53.

253. Kussmaul A, Maier R. Ober Eine bisher nicht beschriebene eigenthümiliche Arterienerkrankung (Periarteritis nodosa die mit Morbus Brighth and rapid fortschreitender allgemeiner Muskellahmung einhergeht). *Dtsch Arch Klin Med* 1866;1:484.

254. Zeek PM. Periarteritis nodosa and other forms of necrotizing angitis. *N Engl J Med* 1963;18:1764.

255. Rose GA, Spencer H. Polyarteritis nodosa. *Q J Med* 1957;26:43.

256. Citron BP, et al. Necrotizing angitis associated with drug abuse. *N Engl J Med* 1970;283:1003.

257. Gocke DJ, et al. Association between polyarteritis and Australian antigen. *Lancet* 1970;2:1149.

258. Sergent JS, et al. Vasculitis with hepatitis B antigenemia: Long-term observations in 9 patients. *Medicine* 1976;55:1.

259. Fye KH, et al. Immune complexes in hepatitis B antigen-associated periarteritis nodosa: detection by antibody-dependent cell-mediated cytotoxicity and the Raji cell assay. *Am J Med* 1977;62:783.

260. Gocke DJ, et al. Vasculitis in association with Australian antigen. *J Exp Med* 1971;134:330.

261. Trepo CG, et al. The role of circulating hepatitis B antigen/antibody immune complexes in the pathogenesis of vascular and hepatic manifestations in polyarteritis nodosa. *J Clin Pathol* 1964;27:863.

262. Fink CW. The role of the streptococcus in poststreptococcal reactive arthritis and childhood polyarteritis nodosa. *J Rheumatol* 1991;29:14.

263. Mader R, Keystone EC. Infections that cause vasculitis. *Curr Opin Rheumatol* 1992;4:35.

264. Redeker AG. Viral hepatitis: Clinical aspects. *Am J Med* Sci 1975;270:9.

265. Dixon FJ, et al. Pathogenesis of serum sickness. *Arch Pathol* 1958;65:18.

266. Juan JR, et al. The pathogenesis of arthritis associated with acute hepatitis B surface antigen-positive hepatitis. *Br J Clin Invest* 1975l;55:930.

267. Nordstoga K, Westbye K. Polyarteritis nodosa associated with nosematosis in blue foxes. *Acta Pathol Microbiol Scand* 1976;84:291.

268. Dillon MJ. Classification and pathogenesis of arteritis in children. *Toxicol Pathol* 1989;17:214.

269. Müller P. *Festschrift Surz Feier des fünfzigjährigen Bestehens des Stadtkrankenhauses zu Dresden-Friedrichstadt.* Dresden: W. Baensch, 1889:458.

270. Foster CS. Immunosuppressive therapy for experimental corneal ulceration. In: *Immunology of the eye. Workshop II: autoimmune phenomena and ocular disorders.* Arlington: Information Retrieval, 1981:91–102.

271. Foster CS, et al. Immunosuppression and selective inflammatory cell depletion in a guinea pig model of corneal ulceration after alkali burning. *Arch Ophthalmol* 1982;100:1820.

272. Foster CS. Systemic immunosuppressive therapy for progressive bilateral Mooren's ulcer. *Ophthalmology* 1985;92:1436.

273. Harbart F, McPherson SD. Scleral necrosis in periarteritis nodosa. *Am J Ophthalmol* 1947;30:727.

274. Moore JG, Sevel D. Corneoscleral ulceration in periarteritis nodosa. *Br J Ophthalmol* 1966;50:651.

275. Wise GN. Ocular periarteritis nodosa. *Arch Ophthalmol* 1952;48:1.

276. Brubaker R, Font RL, Shepherd EM. Granulomatous scleral uveitis: regression of ocular lesions with cyclophosphamide and prednisone. *Arch Ophthalmol* 1971;86:517.

277. Jampol LM, West C, Goldberg MF. Therapy of scleritis with cytotoxic agents. *Am J Ophthalmol* 1978;86:266.

278. Purcell JJ, Birkenkamp R, Tsai CC. Conjunctival lesions in periarteritis nodosa. *Arch Ophthalmol* 1984;102:736.

279. Foster CS, Forstot LS, Wilson LA. Mortality rate in rheumatoid arthritis patients developing necrotizing scleritis or peripheral ulcerative keratitis: Effects of systemic immunosuppression. *Ophthalmology* 1982;91:1253.

280. Klein BA. Ischemic infarcts of the choroid (Elschnig spots). *Am J Ophthalmol* 1968;66:1069.

281. Newman NM, Hoyt WF, Spencer WH. Macular sparring monocular blackouts: clinical and pathologic investigations of intermittent choroidal vascular insufficiency in a case of periarteritis nodosa. *Arch Ophthalmol* 1974;91:367.

282. Coppeto JR, Miller D. Polyarteritis nodosa diagnosed by temporal artery biopsy. *Am J Ophthalmol* 1986;102:541.

283. Cochrane CG, Koffler D. Immune complex disease in experimental animals and man. *Adv Immunol* 1973;16:186.

284. Fronert PP, Scheps FG. Long-term follow-up study of periarteritis nodosa. *Am J Med* 1967;43:8.

285. Pickering G, et al. Treatment of polyarteritis nodosa with cortisone; results after three years. Report to the Medical Research Counsel by the Collagen Diseases and Hypersensitivity Panel. *Br Med J* 1960;1:1399.

286. Fauci AS, Doppman JL, Wolff SM. Cyclophosphamide-induced remissions in advanced polyarteritis nodosa. *Am J Med* 1978;64:890.

287. Lieb ES, Restivo C, Paulus HE. Immunosuppressive and corticosteroid therapy for polyarteritis nodosa. *Am J Med* 1979;67:941.

288. Klinger H. Grenzformen der Periarteritis nodosa. *Z Pathol* 1931;42:455.

289. Wegener F. Uber generalisierte, septische Gefasserkrankungen. *Verh Dtsch Ges Pathol* 1936;29:202.

290. Wegener F. Uber eine eigenartige rhinogene Granulomotose mit besonderer Beteiligung des Arteriensystems und der Nieren. *Beitr Pathol Anat* 1939;102:36.

291. Fauci AS, Wolff SM. Wegener's granulomatosis: studies in 18 patients and a review of the literature. *Medicine* 1973;52:535.

292. Bondes P. Purely granulomatous Wegener's granulomatosis. *Semin Arthritis Rheum* 1990;19:365.

293. Roback SA, et al. Wegener's granulomatosis in a child: observations on pathogenesis and treatment. *Am J Dis Child* 1966;112:587.

294. Hu CH, O'Laughlin S, Winkleman RK. Cutaneous manifestations of Wegener's granulomatosis. *Arch Dermatol* 1977;113:175.

295. Howie SB, Epstein WV. Circulating immunoglobulin complexes in Wegener's granulomatosis. *Am J Med* 1976;60:259.

296. Fauci AS, et al. Wegener's granulomatosis. *Ann Intern Med* 1983;98:76.

297. Koyama T, et al. Wegener's granulomatosis with destructive ocular manifestations. *Am J Ophthalmol* 1984;98:736.

298. Austin P, et al. Peripheral corneal degeneration and occlusive vasculitis in Wegener's granulomatosis. *Am J Ophthalmol* 1978;85:311.

299. Ferry AP, Leopold IH. Marginal (ring) corneal ulcer as presenting manifestation of Wegener's granuloma. *Trans Am Acad Ophthalmol Otolaryngol* 1970;74:1276.

300. Frayer WC. The histopathology of perilimbal ulceration in Wegener's granulomatosis. *Arch Ophthalmol* 1960;64:58.

301. Leavitt JA, Butrus SI. Wegener's granulomatosis presenting as dacryoadenitis. *Cornea* 1991;10:542.

302. Cogan DG. Corneoscleral lesions in periarteritis nodosa and Wegener's granulomatosis. *Trans Am Ophthalmol Soc* 1955;53:321.

303. Haynes BF, et al. Ocular manifestations of Wegener's granulomatosis. *Am J Med* 1977;63:131.

304. Straatsma BR. Ocular manifestations of Wegener's granulomatosis. *Am J Ophthalmol* 1957;44:789.

305. Weiter J, Farkas CG. Situ tumor of the orbit as a presenting sign in Wegener's granulomatosis. *Surv Ophthalmol* 1972;17:106.

306. Bullen CL, et al. Ocular complications of Wegener's granulomatosis. *Ophthalmology* 1983;90:279.

307. Jaben SL, Norton EWD. Exudative retinal detachment in Wegener's granulomatosis. *Ann Ophthalmol* 1982;14:717.

308. Illum P, Thorling K. Otologic manifestations of Wegener's granulomatosis. *Laryngoscope* 1982;92:801.

309. Kalina PH, et al. Role of testing for anticytoplasmic autoantibodies in the differential diagnosis of scleritis and orbital pseudotumor. *Mayo Clin Proc* 1990;65:1110.

310. Pulido JS, et al. Ocular manifestations of patients with circulating antineutrophil cytoplasmic antibodies. *Arch Ophthalmol* 1990;108:845.

311. Soukiasian SH, et al. Diagnostic value of antineutrophil cytoplasmic antibodies in scleritis associated with Wegener's granulomatosis. *Ophthalmology* 1992;99:125.

312. Jennette JC, Falk RJ. Disease associations and pathogenic role of antineutrophil cytoplasmic autoantibodies in vasculitis. *Curr Opin Rheumatol* 1992;4:9.

313. Goeken JA. Antineutrophil cytoplasmic antibody. *J Clin Immunol* 1991;11:161.

314. Jennette JC, Falk RJ. Antineutrophil cytoplasmic autoantibodies and associated diseases. *Am J Kidney Dis* 1990;15:517.

315. Fauci AS. Vasculitis. In: Parker CW, ed. *Clinical immunology.* Philadelphia: Saunders, 1980:473–519.

316. Liebow AA. Pulmonary angitis and granulomatosis. *Am Rev Respir Dis* 1973;108:1.

317. Gonett GS, Amedee RG. Wegener's granulomatosis of the head and neck. *J La State Med Soc* 1990;142:13.

318. Harrison HL, et al. Bolus corticosteroid and cyclophosphamide for initial treatment of Wegener's granulomatosis. *JAMA* 1980;244:1599.

319. Curzio C. *Discussioni Anatomio-Pratiche di un Raro a Stravagante Morbo Cutaneo in Questo Grande Ospedale Degi Incurabili.* Naples: G. DiSiome, 1753.

320. Gintrac E. Note sur la sclerodermie. *Rev Med Chir* 1847;2:263.

321. Matsui S. Uber die Pathologie and Pathogenese von Sclerodermia universalis. *Mitt Med Fakult Kaiserl Univ Tokyo* 1924;31:55.

322. Goetz RH. The pathology of progressive systemic sclerosis (generalized scleroderma) with special reference to changes in viscera. *Clin Proc* 1945;4:337.

323. Rodnan GP, et al. The association of progressive systemic sclerosis (scleroderma) with coal miners' pneumoconiosis and other forms of silicosis. *Ann Intern Med* 1967;66:332.

324. Ercilla MG, et al. HLA antigens and scleroderma. *Arch Dermatol* Res 1981;271:381.

325. Claman HN. On scleroderma. *JAMA* 1989;262:1206.
326. Cormane RH, Hamerlinck F, Nunzi E. Antibodies eluted from lymphoid cell membrane. *Arch Dermatol* 1979;115:709.
327. Campbell PM, LeRoy EC. Pathogenesis of systemic sclerosis: A vascular hypothesis. *Semin Arthritis Rheum* 1975;4:351.
328. Alarcon-Segovia D, et al. Sjögren's syndrome and progressive systemic sclerosis (scleroderma). *Am J Med* 1974;57:78.
329. Kirkham TH. Scleroderma and Sjögren's syndrome. *Br J Ophthalmol* 1969;53:131.
330. Stucchi CA, Geiser JD. Manifestations oculares de la sclerodermie generalisee (points communs avec le syndrome de Sjögren). *Doc Ophthalmol* 1967;22:72.
331. Horan EC. Ophthalmic manifestations of progressive systemic sclerosis. *Br J Ophthalmol* 1969;53:388.
332. Arnett FC, Michels RG. Inflammatory ocular myopathy in systemic sclerosis (scleroderma). *Arch Intern Med* 1973; 132:740.
333. Manschot WA. Generalized scleroderma with ocular symptoms. *Ophthalmologica* 1965;149:131.
334. McWhae JA, Andrews DM. Transient corneal opacification induced by cold in Raynaud's disease. *Ophthalmology* 1991;98:666.
335. West RH, Barnett AJ. Ocular involvement in scleroderma. *Br J Ophthalmol* 1979;63:845.
336. Grennan DM, Forrester J. Involvement of the eye in SLE and scleroderma. *Ann Rheum Dis* 1977;36:152.
337. Ashton N, et al. Retinopathy due to progressive systemic sclerosis. *J Pathol Bacteriol* 1968;96:259.
338. Farkas TG, Sylvester V, Archer D. The choroidopathy of progressive systemic sclerosis (scleroderma). *Am J Ophthalmol* 1972;74:875.
339. D'Angelo WA, et al. Pathologic observations in systemic sclerosis (scleroderma): a study of 58 autopsy cases and 58 matched controls. *Am J Med* 1969;46:428.
340. Dau PC, Kahaleh MB, Sagebiel RW. Plasmapheresis and immunosuppressive drug therapy in scleroderma. *Arthritis Rheum* 1981;24:1128.
341. Shirley HH, et al. Lack of ocular changes with dimethyl sulfoxide therapy of scleroderma. *Pharmacotherapy* 1989;9:165.

24

MOOREN'S ULCER

C. STEPHEN FOSTER

Bowman first described what we now call Mooren's ulcer of the cornea (also known as *chronic serpiginous ulcer* and *ulcus rodens*) in 1849 (1). Mooren published cases describing the disorder in detail and establishing it as a distinct clinical entity in 1867 (1). Mooren's ulcer is a painful, relentlessly progressive chronic ulcerative keratitis that begins peripherally and progresses circumferentially and centrally. It is, by definition, idiopathic, occurring in the absence of any diagnosable systemic disorder associated with peripheral ulcerative keratitis (PUK). Its exact pathophysiology remains uncertain. Advances have been made in better understanding the etiopathogenesis and in the management of this disorder, but a significant percentage of cases remain refractory to available therapies and result in severe visual morbidity.

EPIDEMIOLOGY

Mooren's ulcer is uncommon. Lewallen and Courtright's (2) review of 20 published series of Mooren's ulcer numbered 187 patients. Some of the cases in the published series are probably cases of PUK in patients with occult systemic diseases such as rheumatoid arthritis (RA), Wegener's granulomatosis (WG), relapsing polychondritis (RP), or polyarteritis nodosa (PAN), judging from the scleral involvement of some of the cases (Mooren's does not result in necrotizing scleritis).

Wood and Kaufmann (3) have concluded, based on their review of the literature and a study of their own patients, that there were two distinct clinical types of Mooren's ulcer: unilateral, with mild to moderate symptoms, generally responding well to medical and surgical therapy, and often occurring in older patients (*typical* or *benign* Mooren's ulcer), and a more malignant, bilateral form with more pain and poor response to local medical and surgical therapy. This second type tends to occur in younger patients.

Mooren's ulcer is bilateral in 25% of the benign type and in 75% of the malignant type (4,5). Keitzman (6) published

a series of 37 cases of Mooren's ulcer primarily in Nigerian men in their 20s and 30s. A later report confirmed the frequent occurrence of the "malignant" form in young Nigerian men (7). As a result of these reports, it is commonly believed that the progressive and relentless atypical form of Mooren's ulcer has a predilection for young black men.

Lewallen and Courtright (2), however, in their review of the published series on Mooren's ulcer, suggest that these concepts about the epidemiology of Mooren's ulcer are not supported by the available data. For example, they found that 43% of older patients had bilateral disease, whereas bilateral disease was present in only one third of patients younger than 35 years. Also, whites were more than twice as likely to have bilateral disease than blacks. Although they found that men were 1.6 times more likely to have Mooren's ulcer than were women, the authors point out that this may be attributed to factors such as increased incidence of ocular trauma in men (an association with Mooren's ulcer is reported) or cultural patterns that discourage female clinic attendance in certain countries, and that this finding may not reflect a true biologic propensity for men.

Lewallen and Courtright (2) conclude that the available data are flawed by a collection period spanning more than 85 years, differences in the criteria for definition of the disease, poor documentation and follow-up, and problems inherent in non–population-based data collection, in 20 series from more than 14 different countries. Lewallen and Courtright do not suggest that their own statistical analysis is necessarily accurate either.

CLINICAL FEATURES

Patients with Mooren's ulcer complain of painful, red, tearing, photophobic eye. The pain is often incapacitating and may seem out of proportion to the inflammation noted on examination. Vision is affected secondary to associated iritis, central corneal involvement, or irregular astigmatism from peripheral corneal thinning.

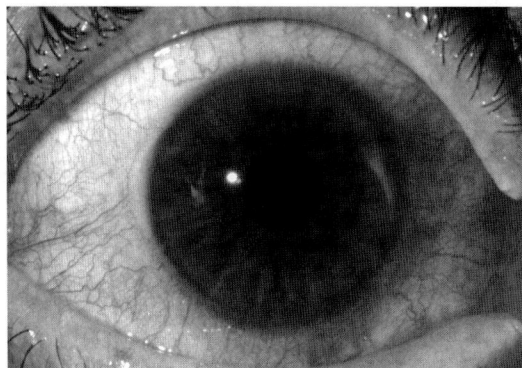

FIGURE 24-1. Early stage of Mooren's ulcer, with an inflammatory infiltrate in the anterior corneal stroma, 2 o'clock periphery, with associated conjunctival injection but without scleritis.

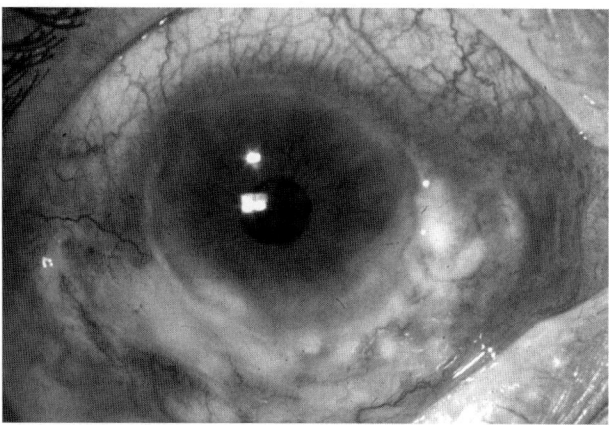

FIGURE 24-2. Example of peripheral ulcerative keratitis (PUK) in a patient with Wegener's granulomatosis, with associated adjacent scleritis, obviously very different from the characteristics of Mooren's ulcer shown in Fig. 24–1.

The first notable pathosis may be patchy, peripheral stromal infiltrates, which then coalesce, more often in the medial and lateral quadrants than in the superior and inferior ones. An epithelial defect and shallow furrow then develop. The tissue destruction extends to the limbus (unlike the keratitis infiltrate typical of staphylococcal hypersensitivity marginal keratitis) (Fig. 24-1), but not past the limbus, into the sclera (unlike the PUK so often seen in association with RA, PAN, WG, and RP) (Fig. 24-2) (5,8). The ulcer spreads circumferentially, posteriorly (deeper and deeper toward Descemet's membrane), and centrally to involve the entire cornea eventually. The anterior half, or more, of the stroma is involved, and one curious, semidiagnostic feature occurs early in the process: the undermined edge of the irregularly scalloped (as if eaten by a rat, hence ulcer rodens) central edge of the ulcer (Fig. 24-3). This same PUK morphology can occur in the eye as a consequence of RA, RP, PAN, or WG, and hence the importance of including these systemic (potentially lethal) diseases in the differential diagnosis of suspected Mooren's PUK. But these latter disorders generally (eventually) also produce significant scleral damage, and also (eventually) reveal other clinical or laboratory abnormalities that make clear the systemic diagnosis.

The extent of the corneal damage is almost always far greater than is obvious during slit-lamp biomicroscopy examination. The depth to which the matrix metalloproteinase enzymatic degradation of the corneal collagens and glycosaminoglycans has extended may be relatively obscured by the so-called overhanging lip or edge of the anterior-most cornea at the edge of the active PUK, with the anterior-most lamellae of the cornea infiltrated slightly with neutrophils, but not yet dissolved, and so "flopping" down onto and covering from view the deep gutter portion of the PUK. Indeed, even the application of 2% fluorescein dye to the ocular surface may produce the misleading finding of an "intact" surface, with simply a fine, thin line of fluorescein dye that has trickled into the gutter, fluorescing. But even more shocking, even to the corneal specialist who

has evaluated one or more patients with Mooren's ulcer previously, is the extraordinary extent of stromal digestion central to the PUK gutter, beginning at the gutter base. A fine probe (such as one tine of a Tubingen-Harms tying forceps) gently exploring the extent of damage central to the PUK gutter always discloses a cleavage plane in the stroma, with easy passage of the probe 1 to 4 mm into what clinically appeared to be normal cornea.

The damaged cornea peripheral to the advancing edge of the active, progressing ulcer is thinned as a consequence of the stromal digestion during the ulcer's active phase, but it reepithelializes, scars, and vascularizes, and generally (unless traumatized) does not perforate (although it can) (Figs. 24-4 and 24-5). This destructive inflammatory process progresses until (a) effective therapy stops it, or (b) the entire geographic extent of the cornea has been involved, at which

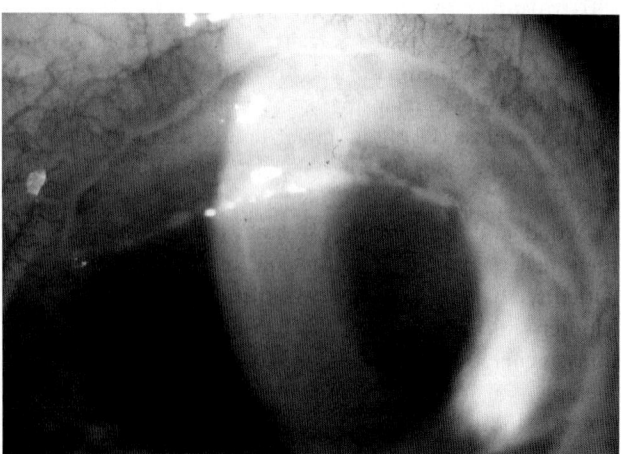

FIGURE 24-3. Mooren's ulcer with PUK extending from 10 o'clock to 2 o'clock, advancing approximately 3 mm into the cornea, with an infiltrated, shaggy, overhanging lip in advance of the ulcer, which is undermining otherwise normal-looking cornea central to the overhanging lip.

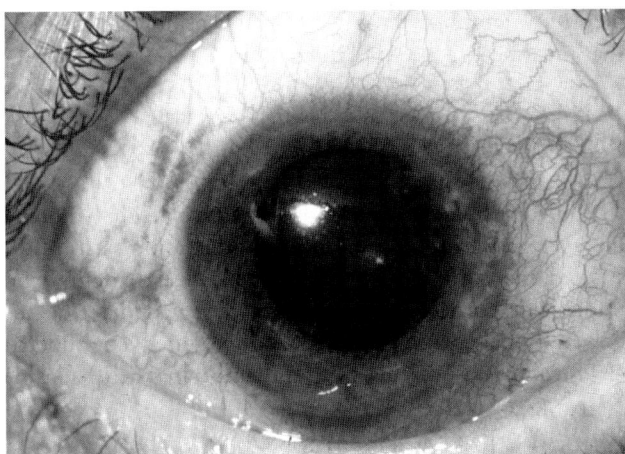

FIGURE 24-4. Vascularized, thinned peripheral bed of previously ulcerating cornea in a patient with PUK caused by Mooren's ulcer; note the area at approximately 2 o'clock.

point inflammation and pain subside, leaving the patient with a thinned, scarred, vascularized cornea and poor vision.

The conjunctiva, episclera, and sclera may be edematous and inflamed in areas adjacent to active corneal inflammation. Iritis may be present, but hypopyon is rare unless secondary infection occurs. Glaucoma and cataract may complicate matters. Perforation has been noted in up to 36% of cases, especially if there is minor trauma to the weakened cornea (8).

ASSOCIATIONS AND PROPOSED ETIOLOGIES

Various entities have been associated with Mooren's ulcer, often leading to conjecture that there may be a causal relationship. In Nigeria, there has been an association with

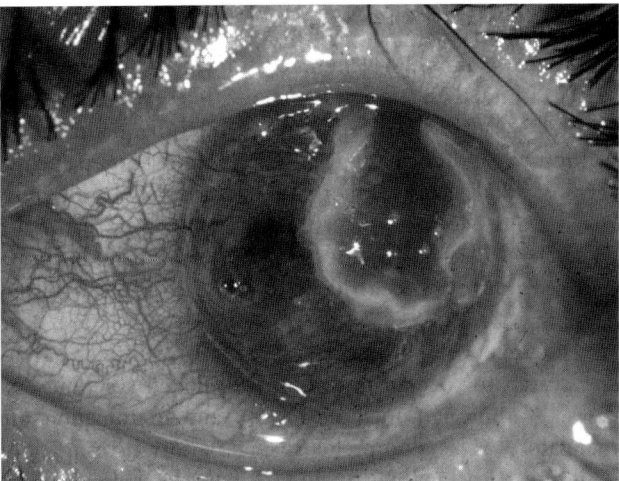

FIGURE 24-5. A more advanced example of progressive Mooren's ulcer, with only a small residual area of remaining full-thickness cornea, with the infiltrated edge of the overhanging lip, and a vascularized, thinned residuum of cornea left in the wake of the advancing ulcer.

helminthiasis; four of five cases were so associated in one series (7). Another study suggested that the progression of the ulcerative keratitis was arrested by local therapy in combination with systemic therapy for the parasitic infection (6). Schanzlin (9) has proposed a causal relationship, suggesting that helminth toxins or antigens deposited in the cornea may lead to antigen-antibody reactions or that infection may cause alteration of the host immune system, allowing the keratitis to occur. But helminthiasis is epidemic among the population involved in these studies and Mooren's ulcer is extremely rare, even in these populations.

Chronic hepatitis C infection was documented in two patients with bilateral Mooren's ulcers (12). The keratitis in both patients improved after treatment of the hepatitis with interferon-α2b. The authors propose that molecular mimicry may be involved, with the hepatitis C virus stimulating an autoimmune response to corneal antigens through cross-reacting epitopes. Alternately, they also propose that deposition of immune complexes in the limbal or peripheral corneal tissues may lead to an immune response and the release of proteolytic enzymes. Hepatitis C virus–associated vasculitis is a well-recognized entity, and careful analysis of biopsy specimens from conjunctiva and episclera adjacent to the PUK of patients with hepatitis C–associated Mooren's ulcer should settle the matter of this latter hypothesis. Chronic hepatitis C infection is not rare, and, if a causal relationship is present, Mooren's ulceration would be expected to be seen more frequently. Other infections that have been associated with Mooren's ulcer have included syphilis, tuberculosis, and salmonella (11).

Mooren's ulcer has also been reported following corneal disease. Specific associations include physical trauma (3), foreign body (12), chemical burn (15), herpes simplex infection (14), herpes zoster infection (15), and surgical procedures such as cataract extraction and penetrating keratoplasty (16,17). Some of these may not represent true cases of Mooren's ulcer; if they do, definitive associations and causal relationships have not been demonstrated.

PATHOPHYSIOLOGIC FEATURES

The exact pathophysiologic mechanism of Mooren's ulceration remains unknown, but there is much evidence to suggest that it is an autoimmune process, with both cell-mediated and humoral components. Plasma cells (18), neutrophils (19), mast cells, and eosinophils (18,20) have been found in the involved areas (21). Brown (18) demonstrated high levels of collagenase in the affected conjunctiva. And we found numerous activated neutrophils in the ulcerating cornea, and proposed that the neutrophils are the source of the proteases and collagenases (19).

Both we (19) and Mondino et al. (22) have shown cell-mediated immunity against corneal antigens; Mondino et al. elicited stimulated cytokine production (macrophage migration inhibition factor) response in response to corneal antigens presented to lymphocytes from Mooren's ulcer patients. And we demonstrated blastogenic transformation and lymphocyte proliferation in response to normal corneal stroma in a patient with the disease. Furthermore, Murray and Rahi (20) noted that, systemically, there is a decrease in the number of suppressor T cells relative to the number of helper T cells in Mooren's ulcer patients, proposing that unregulated helper T cells overproduce antibodies, resulting in the deposition of immune complexes, complement activation, inflammatory cell infiltration, and proteolytic enzyme release.

Schaap and associates (23) had, years earlier, used indirect immunofluorescent techniques to demonstrate circulating immunoglobulin G (IgG) antibodies to human corneal and conjunctival epithelium in patients with Mooren's ulcer. In addition, antibodies and complement have been demonstrated bound to the conjunctival epithelium in the affected areas (21,24). Patients have also been reported to have elevated serum IgA levels (22) and circulating immune complexes (25).

Gottsch and associates (26) have purified and partially characterized a corneal protein from bovine corneal stromal extracts to which antibodies in the serum of a patient with Mooren's ulcer bind. An enzyme-linked immunosorbent assay (ELISA) was developed using the corneal protein, and the serum of 15 other patients with Mooren's ulcer were tested on the ELISA. All 15 showed ELISA results greater than those of 14 normal individuals.

A similar target of the autoimmune attack on human cornea has not been identified, nor is the function or anatomic location in the cornea of the one isolated from bovine cornea known, although it may be a calcium binding protein of the S-100 family (27).

Martin and colleagues (28) have proposed a mechanism for the perpetuation of the ulcerative process, suggesting that systemic disease, infection, or trauma may alter corneal antigens, stimulating both humoral and cellular responses. In the process, complement activation leads to neutrophil chemotaxis and degranulation with release of matrix metalloproteinases that degrade collagen and proteoglycans, further altering and exposing altered corneal antigens, thus perpetuating the process. This cycle continues until the portion of the entire cornea containing the target autoantigen is consumed.

Replacement of the target autoantigen (e.g., through corneal transplantation) usually results in prompt resumption of the inflammatory immunologic process (i.e., recurrence of Mooren's PUK in the graft), indicating one of the most unique and diagnostic characteristics of an autoimmune process: anamnesis. The immune system never forgets. Despite the fact that the inflammatory attack subsided once all the target antigen had been destroyed, replenishment of a normal donor cornea (e.g., through lamellar grafting) is instantly recognized by the patient's immune system memory T lymphocytes as a fresh supply of "foreign" material that must be attacked and destroyed.

PATHOLOGIC FEATURES

The histopathologic features of tissue involved in Mooren's ulcer suggest an immune process. Young and Watson (29) studied the cornea of three Mooren's ulcer patients who underwent corneal grafting. They observed that the involved limbal cornea consisted of three zones. The superficial stroma was vascularized and infiltrated with plasma cells and lymphocytes. There was destruction of the collagen matrix in this region. Epithelium and Bowman's layer were absent. The midstroma showed hyperactivity of fibroblasts with disorganization of the collagen lamellae. The deep stroma was intact, but contained macrophages. Descemet's membrane and endothelium were spared. Neutrophil infiltration and dissolution of the superficial stroma was present at the leading edge of the ulcer (18,29). The neutrophils were degranulating (19). The adjacent conjunctiva revealed epithelial hyperplasia and a subconjunctival lymphocytic and plasma cell infiltration (18). Vasculitis was not present (19). During the course of healing, eosinophils were present in the conjunctiva adjacent to the healing PUK.

DIAGNOSIS

Mooren's ulcer is idiopathic, a diagnosis of exclusion. The differential diagnosis of PUK is extensive (Table 24-1).

Scrapings of the cornea for culture generally will establish an infectious origin for ulcerative keratitis. In those cases, there is also a characteristic discharge and a response to antibiotics. Mooren's ulcer is easily distinguished from the noninflammatory corneal degenerations, such as Terrien's or pellucid marginal degeneration, in which the epithelium remains intact and pain is absent. These degenerations generally begin in the superior and inferior quadrants, in contrast to Mooren's ulcer, which begins in the interpalpebral regions. Staphylococcal marginal keratitis may be differentiated from Mooren's ulcer by a lack of severe pain, the presence of blepharitis, a lucid zone between the infiltrate and the limbus, and a quick response to topical steroid therapy.

The presence of a Mooren's-like ulcer requires an extensive search for occult and potentially lethal systemic diseases. A thorough medical history and examination are mandatory, as is a comprehensive laboratory investigation. This investigation may include a complete blood count with evaluation of the differential count, platelet count, erythrocyte sedimentation rate, C-reactive protein, rheumatoid factor, complement components, antinuclear antibodies, antineutrophil cytoplasmic antibody (ANCA),

TABLE 24-1. DIFFERENTIAL DIAGNOSIS OF PERIPHERAL ULCERATIVE KERATITIS

Ocular Infectious	Bacterial (*Staphylococcus, Strep-tococcus, Gonococcus, Moraxella, Haemophilus*)
	Viral (herpes simplex, herpes zoster)
	Acanthamoeba
	Fungal
Noninfectious	Mooren's ulcer
	Traumatic or postsurgical
	Terrien's marginal degeneration
	Pellucid degeneration
	Exposure
	Dry eye
	Staphylococcal marginal keratitis
	Acne rosacea
	Neuroparalytic
Systemic Infectious	Tuberculosis
	Syphilis
	Varicella zoster
	Gonorrhea
	AIDS
	Bacillary dysentery
Noninfectious	Rheumatoid arthritis
	Systemic lupus erythematosus
	Wegener's granulomatosis
	Polyarteritis nodosa
	Relapsing polychondritis
	Progressive systemic sclerosis
	Sjögren's syndrome
	Adamantiades-Behçet's disease
	Sarcoidosis
	Inflammatory bowel disease
	Alpha$_1$-antitrypsin deficiency
	Leukemia

circulating immune complexes (by Raji cell and by C1q binding assays), liver function tests, fluorescent treponemal antibody absorption (FTA-ABS) tests, hepatitis B and C antigen and antibody studies, blood urea nitrogen, creatinine, serum protein electrophoresis, urinalysis and a chest roentgenogram. Additional testing is done as indicated by the review of systems. It is only after all other disorders are excluded that a diagnosis of Mooren's ulcer can be made.

MANAGEMENT

Mooren's ulcer is a progressive, relentless disease that often progresses to devastating visual loss despite all attempts at management and therapy. Many treatments have been espoused, but because the disorder is so rare, no placebo-controlled, masked, randomized clinical trial has been done. But, because of improvements in our understanding of the natural history and pathophysiology of this disorder, our ability to manage Mooren's ulcer has improved dramatically in the past 25 years.

Historically, a number of therapeutic agents for Mooren's ulcer have been tried and deemed unsuccessful. These have included subconjunctival bichloride of mercury (30), carbolic and nitric acid, formalin and tincture of iodine (29), trichloroacetic acid (31), subconjunctival heparin (32), and cyanide of mercury (33). In addition, a number of procedures, such as irradiation (34), galvanocautery (35), paracentesis (36), and delimiting keratotomy (37–39) have been attempted, with little success. More recently, case reports have been published in which Mooren's ulcer has been treated with plasma exchange (40), periosteal grafting (41), and Gore-Tex patch grafting (42). And there is nothing wrong with these approaches. But clearly, more study and experience are needed for these and other potential new therapies to be evaluated, especially for the more "malignant" bilateral form of the disease.

My approach to the management of a patient with Mooren's ulcer is initially driven by the laterality of the disease (43). If it is unilateral, I perform a generous conjunctival resection, remove obviously highly damaged, degraded, nonviable cornea, and prescribe a broad-spectrum antibiotic (such as fluoroquinolone) and extremely aggressive (e.g., every 15 minutes) topical 1% prednisolone acetate drops, as advocated by Brown and Mondino (14). I do this because of the compelling data suggesting that this form of Mooren's ulcer is truly different from the bilateral form in that it may not be an "autoimmune" problem yet, and many (or possibly most) such cases respond favorably to this approach, resolving and requiring nothing further (14).

Topical tetracycline or medroxyprogesterone may be used for the anticollagenolytic properties of each. A therapeutic soft contact lens or patching of the eye may be beneficial at this stage. Also, any concomitant eye disease, such as acne rosacea, meibomitis, blepharitis, dry eye, or eyelid abnormalities should be addressed at this time. If healing occurs, the steroids may be slowly tapered, over a period of months.

Tissue adhesive and a therapeutic soft contact lens may be necessary, depending on the depth of the corneal loss. Multiple conjunctival resections may be necessary, because excision of the conjunctiva interrupts the ulcerative process by removing the source of neutrophils and plasma cells, collagenolytic enzymes, complement, and immunoglobulin from areas adjacent to active ulceration, only temporarily (~6 weeks). Cryotherapy of limbal conjunctiva has been advocated by some authors and may have a similar effect (44). Brown (45) has reported that conjunctival excision is successful approximately 50% of the time. However, in one series, only two of 15 cases of simultaneous, bilateral ulcers were healed with this procedure (14), and hence my advice (below) regarding therapy for the bilateral form.

Systemic Immunosuppressives

Bilateral or progressive unilateral Mooren's ulcer cases that fail the preceding therapeutic attempts require systemic immunomodulatory therapy. The most commonly used agents are cyclophosphamide (3 mg/kg/day), methotrexate (7.5 to 25 mg/week), and azathioprine (3 mg/kg/day). Dosages are adjusted to control the inflammation while maintaining the white blood cell count above 3,500/dL by the trained chemotherapist in charge of this aspect of the patient's care. We reported arrest of the inflammatory process and preservation of ocular anatomy and function in eight of nine patients with bilateral involvement adequately treated with immunomodulatory agents for 6 to 24 months (46). The ninth patient, who went on to perforation, did not receive an adequate level of immunosuppression as measured by blood parameters. Agents such as cyclophosphamide may be effective by suppressing B lymphocytes, which produce autoantibodies and promote immune complex disease (47). Systemic cyclosporin has been successfully used to treat Mooren's ulcer (48,49). This agent may work by suppression of the helper T-cell population and stimulation of the depressed population of cytotoxic T cells present in patients with Mooren's ulcer (48,49).

Potential adverse effects of these medications include anemia, alopecia, nausea, nephrotoxicity, and hepatotoxicity; the administering physician must be vigilant about their onset. Systemic immunomodulatory therapy is best handled by close collaboration between the ophthalmologist and an oncologist.

The potentially serious side effects of systemic immunomodulatory agents have led several groups to investigate the efficacy of topically applied cyclosporin in treating Mooren's ulcer (50,51). In Holland et al.'s series (50) studying topical cyclosporin treatment of a variety of anterior segment inflammatory diseases, two patients had Mooren's ulcer. The first, with bilateral disease, showed reduced inflammation with minimal progression over 3 years, whereas the second, with unilateral disease, showed resolution of the ulcer on this medication. In Zhao and Jin's (51) series, 15 of 18 eyes with Mooren's ulcer improved, and 11 of these were cured with topical cyclosporin therapy. It is not clear how many of these cases were unilateral and how many bilateral.

Additional Surgical Procedures

Should these management steps fail, additional surgical procedures may be considered. Superficial lamellar keratectomy, in which the anterior corneal stroma is removed, has been shown to arrest the inflammatory process and allow healing (52). After refining the technique in previous series, Nian and colleagues (53) found 34 of 40 eyes to be successfully healed after lamellar keratectomy. Four of six eyes with recurrent ulcer healed with reoperation; the other patients refused any further intervention for the other two eyes. In this series, 32 patients were involved, eight bilaterally (38 eyes). The results were not stratified by unilateral or bilateral status. Martin and co-workers (28) logically suggest

that lamellar keratectomy effects a halt to the inflammation by removal of corneal antigenic targets of the attack on the cornea.

Some cases may progress to perforation despite management as just detailed. Small perforations may be treated with the application of tissue adhesive with the placement of a soft contact lens to provide comfort and prevent dislodging of the glue. Rarely, conjunctival flaps or even penetrating keratoplasty may be necessary. Corneal grafting procedures in the setting of acute inflammation in Mooren's ulcer have a very poor prognosis.

Rehabilitation

Even when the active disease has been arrested, or is "burned out," attempts at penetrating keratoplasty often are associated with recurrence and graft failure (54). Because of the immune system's remarkable memory, surgical attempts at rehabilitation in Mooren's ulceration should be done only with concurrent systemic immunosuppression, even in cases of apparent quiescence (43). In these instances, reparative attempts should be made first with a lamellar tectonic graft to add structural integrity to the thinned peripheral cornea, followed by a central penetrating graft. Some authors believe that the risk of recurrences is so great that patients are best served not by any intervention but by maintaining the current status, that is, the vision provided by their own thinned, scarred corneas (55).

CONCLUSIONS

Despite our still limited understanding of the etiology and pathophysiology of Mooren's ulcer, our gains in knowledge have allowed improved management of this difficult disorder. In some cases, particularly those of inadequate or failed therapy, hand-motions visual acuity or loss of the eye may still be the devastating result. However, even in those bilateral cases considered malignant, a useful final visual acuity— even 20/20—now is possible in a substantial percentage of cases (49).

REFERENCES

1. Nettleship E. Chronic serpiginous ulcer of the cornea (Mooren's ulcer). *Trans Ophthalmol Soc UK* 1902;98:383.
2. Lewallen W, Courtright P. Problems with current concepts of the epidemiology of Mooren's corneal ulcer. *Ann Ophthalmol* 1990; 22:52.
3. Wood T, Kaufman H. Mooren's ulcer. *Am J Ophthalmol* 1971;71:417.
4. Tabbara KF. Mooren's ulcer. *Int Ophthalmol Clin* 1986;26:91.
5. Frangieh T, Kenyon KR. Mooren's ulcer. In: Brightbill FS, ed. *Corneal surgery: theory, technique and tissue,* 2nd ed. St. Louis: Mosby, 1993.

6. Keitzman B. Mooren's ulcer in Nigeria. *Am J Ophthalmol* 1968;65:679.
7. Majekodunmi AA. Ecology of Mooren's ulcer in Nigeria. *Doc Ophthalmol* 1980;49:211.
8. Robin JB, Dugel R. Immunologic disorders of the cornea and conjunctiva. In: Kaufman HE, Barron BA, McDonald MB, et al., eds. *The cornea.* New York: Churchill Livingstone, 1988.
9. Schanzlin DJ. Mooren's ulceration. In: Smolin G, Thoft RA, eds. *The cornea.* Boston: Little, Brown, 1994.
10. Wilson SE, et al. Mooren-type hepatitis C virus associated corneal ulceration. *Ophthalmology* 1994;101:4.
11. Duke-Elder S. *System of ophthalmology: Part 2. Diseases of the outer eye.* St. Louis: Mosby, 1965.
12. Linn JG, Jr. Chronic serpiginous ulcer of the cornea (Mooren's ulcer): etiologic and therapeutic considerations. *Am J Ophthalmol* 1949;32:691.
13. Evans PJ. A case of Mooren's ulcer. *Trans Ophthalmol Soc UK* 1950;70:94.
14. Brown SI, Mondino BJ. Therapy of Mooren's ulcer. *Am J Ophthalmol* 1984;98:1.
15. Mondino BJ, Brown SI, Mondzelewski JP. Peripheral corneal ulcers with herpes zoster ophthalmicus. *Am J Ophthalmol* 1978; 86:611.
16. Mondino BJ, Hofbauer HD, Foos RY. Mooren's ulcer after penetrating keratoplasty. *Am J Ophthalmol* 1987;103:53.
17. Gottsch JD, Liu SH, Stark WJ. Mooren's ulcer and evidence of stromal graft rejection after penetrating keratoplasty. *Am J Ophthalmol* 1992;113:412.
18. Brown SI. Mooren's ulcer: histopathology and proteolytic enzymes of adjacent conjunctiva. *Br J Ophthalmol* 1975;59: 670.
19. Foster CS, et al. The immunopathology of Mooren's ulcer. *Am J Ophthalmol* 1979;88:2.
20. Murray PI, Rahi AHS. Pathogenesis of Mooren's ulcer. *Br J Ophthalmol* 1984;68:182.
21. Brown SI, Mondino BJ, Rabin BS. Autoimmune phenomenon in Mooren's ulcer. *Am J Ophthalmol* 1976;82:835.
22. Mondino BJ, Brown SI, Rabin BS. Cellular immunity in Mooren's ulcer. *Am J Ophthalmol* 1978;85:788.
23. Schaap OL, Feltkamp TEW, Bregbart AC. Circulating antibodies to corneal tissue in a patient suffering from Mooren's ulcer (ulcer rodens corneae). *Clin Exp Immunol* 1969;5:365.
24. Mondino BJ, Brown SI, Rabin BS. Autoimmune phenomena of the external eye. *Trans Am Acad Ophthalmol Otolaryngol* 1978;85:801.
25. Berkowitz PJ, et al. Presence of circulating immune complexes in patient's with peripheral corneal disease. *Arch Ophthalmol* 1983;101:242.
26. Gottsch J, Liu S, Minkovitz J, et al. Autoimmunity to a cornea-associated stromal antigen in patients with Mooren's ulcer. *Invest Ophthalmol Vis Sci* 1995;36:1541–1547.
27. Liu S, Gottsch J. Amino acid sequences of an immunogenic corneal stromal protein. *Invest Ophthalmol Vis Sci* 1996; 37:944–948.
28. Martin NF, Stark WJ, Maumenee AE. Treatment of Mooren's and Mooren's-like ulcer by lamellar keratectomy: report of six eyes and literature review. *Ophthalmic Surg* 1987;18:564.
29. Young RG, Watson PG. Light and electron microscopy of corneal melting syndrome (Mooren's ulcer). *Br J Ophthalmol* 1982;66:341.
30. Andrade E. Ulcus rodens corneae. *Ann Ophthalmol* 1900;29:654.
31. Stevens EW. Mooren's ulcer of the cornea. *Ophthalmol Rec* 1908;17:198.
32. Risley SD. Discussion of DeSchweinitz's paper. *Ann Ophthalmol* 1911;20:436.
33. Aronson SB, et al. Pathogenic approach to therapy of peripheral corneal inflammatory disease. *Am J Ophthalmol* 1970;70:65.
34. Jones EL. Simultaneous bilateral rodent ulcer of the cornea cured by combined curetting, thermocautery, and massive cyanide subconjunctival injection. *Br J Ophthalmol* 1976;18:187.
35. Ward R. Radium on ophthalmology with illustrative cases. *Proc R Soc Med* 1933;26:1515.
36. Cronquist S. Ulcus rodens corneae. *Nord Med* 1947;34:1449.
37. Mayou S. Chronic serpiginous ulceration of the cornea (Mooren's ulcer). *Ophthalmoscope* 1915;13:438.
38. Gifford SR. Rodent or Mooren's ulcer of the cornea. *Arch Ophthalmol* 1933;10:800.
39. Thygeson P. Marginal corneal infiltrates and ulcers. *Trans Am Acad Ophthalmol Otolaryngol* 1946;121:198.
40. Carmichael TR, et al. Plasma exchange in the treatment of Mooren's ulcer. *Ann Ophthalmol* 1985;17:311.
41. Dingeldein SA, et al. Mooren's ulcer treated with periosteal graft. *Ann Ophthalmol* 1990;22:56.
42. Huang WJ, Hu FR, Chang SW. Clinicopathologic study of Gore-Tex patch graft in corneoscleral surgery. *Cornea* 1994;13:82.
43. Foster CS. Immunologic disorders of the conjunctiva, cornea and sclera. In: Albert DA, Jakobiec FA, eds. *Principles and practice of ophthalmology.* Philadelphia: WB Saunders, 1994.
44. Aviel E. Combined cryoapplications and peritomy in Mooren's ulcer. *Br J Ophthalmol* 1972;56:48.
45. Brown SI. Mooren's ulcer. Treatment by conjunctival excision. *Br J Ophthalmol* 1975;59:675.
46. Foster CS. Systemic immunosuppressive therapy for progressive bilateral Mooren's ulcer. *Ophthalmology* 1985;92:1436.l
47. Lopez JS, et al. Immunohistochemistry of Terrien's and Mooren's corneal degeneration. *Arch Ophthalmol* 1991;109:988.
48. Hill JC, Potter P. Treatment of Mooren's ulcer with cyclosporin A: report of three cases. *Br J Ophthalmol* 1987;71:11.
49. Wakefield D, Robinson LP. Cyclosporin therapy in Mooren's ulcer. *Br J Ophthalmol* 1987;71:415.
50. Holland EJ, et al. Topical cyclosporin A in the treatment of anterior segment inflammatory disease. *Cornea* 1993;12:413.
51. Zhao JC, Jin XY. Immunological analysis and treatment of Mooren's ulcer with cyclosporin A applied topically. *Cornea* 1993;12:481.
52. Brown SI, Mondino BJ. Penetrating keratoplasty in Mooren's ulcer. *Am J Ophthalmol* 1980;89:255.
53. Nian ZD, et al. Mooren's ulcer treated by lamellar keratoplasty. *Jpn J Ophthalmol* 1979;23:257.
54. King JH. Destructive marginal ulceration. A saga of surgical therapy. *Trans Am Ophthalmol Soc* 1965;63:311.
55. Morris WR, Wood TO. Mooren's ulcer. In: Frauenfelder FT, Roy FH, eds. *Current ocular therapy,* vol 4. Philadelphia: WB Saunders, 1995.

SCLERITIS

MAITE SAINZ DE LA MAZA

The wall of the eyeball or sclera is an incomplete sphere averaging 22 mm in diameter that terminates anteriorly at the anterior scleral foramen surrounding the cornea and posteriorly at the posterior scleral foramen surrounding the optic nerve canal. It can be divided into three layer: the superficial one, the episclera; the middle one, the scleral stroma; and the deep one, the lamina fusca, which is adjacent to the uvea.

Inflammation of the wall of the eyeball ranges from benign and self-limiting disorders to severe and uncontrolled processes. Clinical differentiation of these conditions is important because they have different clinical, therapeutic, and prognostic considerations.

Based on the anatomic site of the inflammation and on the associated changes in the scleral vasculature, the classification proposed by Watson and Hayreh (1) differentiates two main categories: episcleritis and scleritis (Table 25-1). Episcleritis can be divided in simple and nodular forms and scleritis in anterior and posterior types. Anterior scleritis may be further subclassified into diffuse, nodular, necrotizing with inflammation (necrotizing), and necrotizing without inflammation (scleromalacia perforans).

Episcleritis is usually an acute, benign, self-limited disease involving the episclera, with symptoms usually limited to mild discomfort, and rarely accompanied by complications. It is infrequently associated with a systemic disease and rarely requires medical treatment. In contrast, scleritis is a chronic, painful, potentially blinding, destructive disease, involving the episclera and the sclera, and often accompanied by complications. It is commonly associated with potentially lethal systemic diseases and always requires systemic therapy. Whereas necrotizing scleritis presents a highly clinical characteristic picture, diffuse or nodular scleritis may be sometimes difficult to distinguish from simple or nodular episcleritis. The correct and rapid diagnosis and the subsequent appropriate treatment can improve both ocular and systemic prognoses.

STRUCTURAL CONSIDERATIONS OF THE SCLERA

The sclera, the dense connective tissue that covers about five sixths of the eye, is composed of a few fibroblasts and extracellular matrix components including dense bundles of collagen, a few elastic fibers, and a moderate amount of proteoglycans and glycoproteins (2,3). Cells and extracellular matrix components are functionally and metabolically interdependent in maintaining tissue homeostasis. The collagen bundles (75% of the sclera) strengthened by elastic fibers (2% of the sclera) give the sclera maximal rigidity and stability, which allows ocular rotations by the action of powerful muscles and fluctuations of intraocular pressure, without distortion in vision.

Because the sclera is richly innervated by branches from the short and long ciliary nerves, scleral inflammation may be a very painful process, mainly due to nerve stretching but also to direct damage.

The blood supply of the anterior segment of the eye is derived from the long posterior ciliary arteries and the anterior ciliary arteries. These arteries give off branches within the episclera that form three vascular arcades: the most superficial one, the conjunctival plexus; the middle one, the superficial episcleral plexus; and the deepest one, the deep episcleral plexus. Besides the scleral perforating vessels, which only traverse but do not supply directly, the scleral stroma is avascular, and therefore completely dependent for its nutrition on diffusion from the highly vascular episclera and to a lesser degree from the choroid. The conjunctival, the superficial episcleral, and the deep episcleral plexuses are visible on slit-lamp examination and can be imaged with different techniques such as videoangiography and high-speed, external, anterior segment, fluorescein angiography. The posterior sclera is supplied by a fine plexus of vessels derived from the short posterior ciliary arteries. Unlike elastic arteries (large-sized vessels), muscular arteries (medium-sized vessels), and arterioles (small-sized vessels), conjunctival and episcleral plexuses appear to be capillaries and postcapillary venules, and therefore, they do not possess a tunica media composed of smooth muscle cells; they only possess a simple wall composed of continuous endothelial cells and pericytes.

EPIDEMIOLOGY

Episcleritis

The prevalence of episcleritis is uncertain because of its self-limited nature and frequent management by general

TABLE 25-1. CLINICAL CLASSIFICATION OF EPISCLERAL AND SCLERAL INFLAMMATION

Episcleritis
  Simple
  Nodular
Scleritis
  Anterior
    Diffuse
    Nodular
    Necrotizing
      With inflammation
      Without inflammation (scleromalacia perforans)
  Posterior

physicians. Episcleritis occurs in all age groups but is most frequent in young and middle-aged adults, usually females, with a peak incidence in the fourth decade (3,4). Although episcleritis may occur in all parts of the world, there are no studies on racial predilection or genetic association.

Scleritis

Objective data on the prevalence of scleritis are difficult to obtain because they can vary greatly depending on the referral nature of the reporting institutions. Nevertheless it is rare. Approximately 0.08% of patients who were referred to the Department of Ophthalmology of Southern General Hospital and Victoria Infirmary of Glasgow during an 8-year period (5) and 2.6% of patients who were referred to the Ocular Immunology and Uveitis Service at the Massachusetts Eye and Ear Infirmary of Boston during an 11-year period (3) had scleritis.

Scleritis also may occur in all age groups but is most common in middle-aged and elderly individuals, usually women, with a peak incidence in the fifth decade (3,4). Scleritis in children is very rare. There is no known geographic or racial predisposition or genetic association.

PATHOGENESIS

Episcleritis and scleritis are both inflammatory diseases. The development of scleritis probably entails the interaction of genetically controlled mechanisms with environmental factors (infectious agents) or endogenous substances. This interaction gives rise to an autoimmune process that damages the episcleral and scleral perforating capillary and postcapillary venules causing inflammatory microangiopathy (a term equivalent to "vasculitis" in vessels that do not have a tunica media) through immune complex deposition, subsequent compliment activation, and neutrophil enzyme release (type III hypersensitivity). Persistent immunologic injury leads to a chronic granulomatous response (type IV hypersensitivity) mediated by

macrophages, epithelioid cells, multinucleated giant cells, and lymphocytes, mainly CD4 helper T (Th1) cells. Inflammatory microangiopathy and chronic granulomatous reaction interact as part of the immune network activated in scleritis, which can lead to scleral destruction (3).

The autoimmune nature of scleritis is also supported by the frequent association with systemic autoimmune disorders and by the favorable response to immunosuppressive therapy.

CLINICAL MANIFESTATIONS

Episcleritis

Episcleritis is abrupt in onset, mild in intensity, and recurrent in nature. The main symptom is mild discomfort, which can be described as a feeling of burning or irritation. Pain is uncommon, but if present, it is usually described as a slight ache localized to the eye (unlike scleritis, where it is usually referred to the forehead, the jaw, or the sinuses). Other symptoms include tearing (never true discharge) and mild photophobia. Unlike scleritis, there is no tenderness to globe palpation. If marked pain and/or tenderness to touch exist, the likelihood is considerable that in fact the patient has some component of occult scleritis. The main sign is redness, which may range from a mild red flush to fiery red, and can be localized in one sector or can involve the whole episclera.

Episcleritis is bilateral in about one third of cases, although not necessarily occurring simultaneously (3,4). Whether treated or not, the condition is self-limited after a few days or weeks, usually without therapy. Recurrences are frequent over a period of years and are not necessarily in the same location. The episodes become less frequent after the first 3 to 4 years until the problem no longer recurs; however, recurrences after as many as 30 years have been reported (1). In spite of these recurrences, episcleritis neither involves sclera nor leaves any residual tissue damage.

Vision is usually unaffected; extension of the inflammatory process to adjacent ocular structures (leading to keratitis, uveitis, glaucoma, cataract, or fundus abnormalities) is very uncommon (4).

Scleritis

Scleritis is insidious in onset, moderate to severe in intensity, and recurrent in nature. The main symptom is pain, which is moderate to severe in intensity, penetrating in character, only temporarily relieved by analgesics, and sometimes localized to the eye, but more frequently referred to the forehead, the jaw, or the sinuses. Patients with severe scleritis have difficulty sleeping because of the constant and severe nature of the pain. In patients with necrotizing scleritis, the pain may be so excruciating that it is totally disabling and a constant source of anxiety and depression. In some cases, the severity of pain may appear disproportionate to the clinical signs, and patients may undergo extensive neurologic evaluation prior to the diagnosis of scleritis. Other symptoms include tearing (never true discharge) and mild to moderate photophobia. Unlike episcleritis, there is tenderness to globe palpation. The main sign is redness, which gradually increases over several days. The redness has a bluish tinge and can be localized in one sector, most frequently to the interpalpebral area (followed by the superior quadrants) (6), or may involve the whole sclera. An exception to all of this is necrotizing scleritis without inflammation (scleromalacia perforans), in which neither pain nor redness is present.

About 34% to 50% of the cases are bilateral (1,3,6). Scleritis may recur involving the same or different eyes at different times, or both eyes at the same time. Recurrences of idiopathic uveitis may be frequent over a period of many years but the episodes become less frequent after the first 3 to 6 years until the problem no longer recurs (1).

Visual acuity may be decreased because of extension of the inflammation to adjacent structures (leading to keratitis, uveitis, glaucoma, cataract, or fundus abnormalities).

OCULAR EXAMINATION

The ocular examination in scleral diseases must include an episcleral and scleral examination and a general ophthalmologic examination. The episcleral and scleral examination should ideally be in daylight and with the slit-lamp light; the latter includes the white diffuse light, the white slit beam, and the red-free light.

Episcleritis

Episcleral Examination in Daylight

Examination in natural daylight may help to distinguish episcleritis from scleritis because slit-lamp light may not discriminate subtle color differences. The eye with episcleritis appears from mild pink to intense bright red. The congested area may be diffuse, involving the entire globe, or localized and sectorial.

Episcleral Examination with the Slit Lamp

Maximum vascular congestion is in the superficial episcleral plexus in patients with episcleritis, with no changes in the deep episcleral plexus. The edema is localized to the episcleral tissue.

White diffuse illumination helps to detect congestion of the superficial episcleral plexus and the presence of localized areas of inflammation or nodules. Congested vessels follow the usual radial pattern, unlike the situation in scleritis, where this pattern is altered and new, abnormal vessels are formed. With topical application of 10% phenylephrine, which only blanches the superficial episcleral plexus without

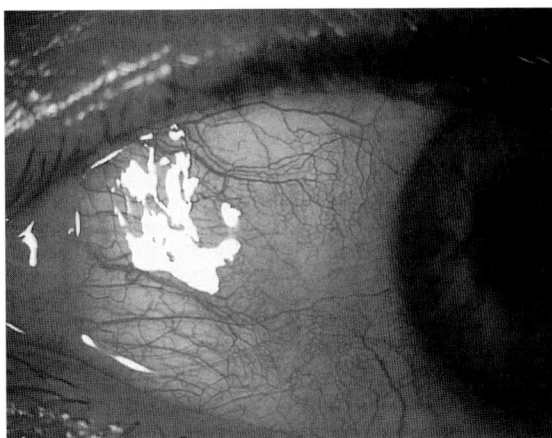

FIGURE 25-1. Nodular episcleritis. Note the vascular dilatation of conjunctival plexus and superficial episcleral plexus and the presence of a localized nodule over the sclera. Congested vessels follow the usual radial pattern. The edema is localized in the episcleral tissue.

significant effect on the deep plexus, the eye will appear white in patients with episcleritis (Figs. 25-1 and 25-2). And any nodules or localized areas of swelling can be moved freely over the sclera.

Slit-lamp white beam illumination serves mainly to detect the depth of inflammation. In episcleritis, the superficial episcleral plexus is displaced forward because of underlying episcleral edema, and the deep episcleral plexus remains flat against the sclera. The anterior edge of the slit-lamp beam is displaced forward because of underlying episcleral edema, whereas the posterior edge remains flat against the sclera, in its normal position.

Red-free light helps one study areas that have maximum vascular congestion and discloses lymphocytic infiltration of the episcleral tissue, manifested as yellow spots.

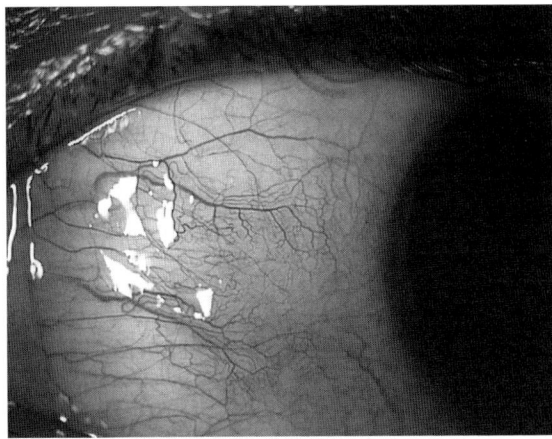

FIGURE 25-2. Same eye as in Fig. 25-1 after topical application of 10% phenylephrine. The eye appears white since phenylephrine blanches the superficial episcleral plexus.

General Ophthalmologic Examination

A general ophthalmologic examination should be performed for a patient with episcleritis, although extension of the inflammation to adjacent structures such as cornea, uvea, trabecular meshwork, ciliary body, lens, retina, choroid, optic disc, or macula is very uncommon (4).

Scleritis

Scleral Examination in Daylight

The eye of a patient with scleritis is red, but with a diffuse, deep bluish-red or violaceous hue. After several attacks of scleral inflammation, areas of scleral thinning and translucency appear, allowing the dark uvea to show. The congested area may be diffuse, involving the entire globe, or localized and sectorial. A black, gray, or brown area that is surrounded by active scleral inflammation indicates a necrotizing process. If tissue necrosis progresses, the scleral area may become avascular, producing a white sequestrum in the center that is surrounded by a well-defined black or dark brown circle. The slough may be gradually removed by granulation tissue, leaving the underlying uvea bare or covered by a thin layer of conjunctiva.

Scleral Examination with the Slit-Lamp

Maximum vascular congestion is in the deep episcleral plexus in an eye with scleritis, with also some congestion in the superficial episcleral plexus. The edema is localized to the scleral and episcleral tissues.

White diffuse illumination confirms the macroscopic impression of avascular areas with sequestra or uveal show. It also helps to detect new and abnormal vessels, congestion of the deep episcleral plexus (the key sign which differentiates scleritis from episcleritis), and the presence of localized areas of inflammation or nodules. With topical application of a vasoconstrictor such as 10% phenylephrine, which only blanches the superficial episcleral plexus without significant effect on the deep plexus, the eye remains congested and red in patients with scleritis (Figs. 25-3 and 25-4). Any nodules or localized areas of swelling are tender to touch and are nonmobile.

Slit-lamp white beam illumination discloses that both the deep and the superficial episcleral plexuses are displaced forward because of underlying scleral and episcleral edema. Both the posterior and the anterior edges of the slit-lamp beam are displaced forward because of underlying scleral and episcleral edema.

Red-free light is helpful in studying areas that have maximum vascular congestion, disclosing new vascular channels or avascular areas.

General Ophthalmological Examination

Evaluation of adjacent structures must always be performed at every follow-up visit of a patient with scleritis, because keratitis, uveitis, glaucoma, cataract, or fundus abnormalities are important reasons for vision loss and, in some cases, destruction of the eye.

CLASSIFICATION

Episcleritis

Episcleritis may be simple or nodular. It may differ in onset of the signs and symptoms, in localization of the inflammation, and in clinical course.

Simple Episcleritis

Simple episcleritis is more common than is nodular episcleritis (4). The onset of redness is usually rapid after the symptoms appear, reaching its peak in a few hours and gradually subsiding over a period usually between 5 and 10 days. Each

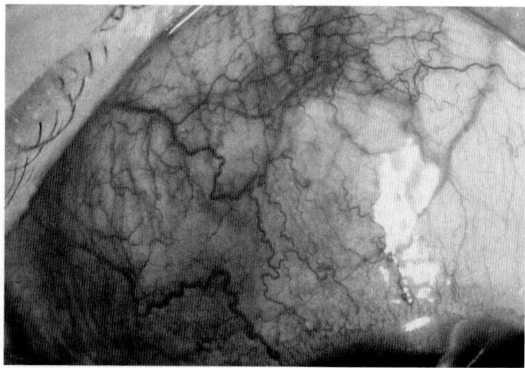

FIGURE 25-3. Diffuse scleritis. Note the vascular dilatation of conjunctival, superficial episcleral, and deep episcleral plexuses. The edema is localized in the episcleral and scleral tissues.

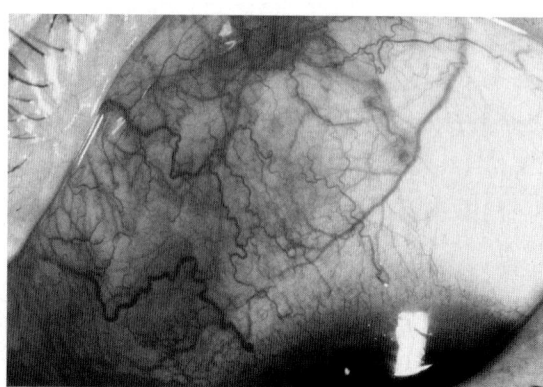

FIGURE 25-4. Same eye as in Fig. 25-3 after topical application of 10% phenylephrine. The eye remains congested since phenylephrine only blanches the superficial episcleral plexus without any effect on the deep episcleral plexus.

attack is self-limited, even without treatment. Recurrences in the same or opposite eye may occur. There is a specific subgroup of patients with a few prolonged episodes instead of multiple evanescent attacks. These patients are predominantly the ones who have some associated disease.

Nodular Episcleritis

In patients with nodular episcleritis, the inflammation is confined to a well-defined area, forming a round or oval nodule from 2 to 6 mm or larger in size, with little surrounding congestion. Nodular episcleritis can be differentiated from conjunctival phlyctenula because the overlying conjunctiva can be moved over the nodule. Nodular episcleritis can be differentiated from nodular scleritis because the episcleral nodule can be moved over the underlying sclera and it is not tender to touch. The onset of redness and the appearance of the nodule gradually increases over a period of 2 to 3 days. Following a chronic course of inflammation, the nodule slowly becomes paler and flatter after a period of 4 to 6 weeks, and then disappears entirely, leaving the underlying sclera normal. Recurrences in the same or opposite eye may occur, sometimes with more than one nodule at a time.

Scleritis

Scleritis can be divided into anterior and posterior categories. Even recognizing that posterior scleritis is underdiagnosed, anterior scleritis is much more frequent. Anterior scleritis may be further classified, depending on clinical appearance, into the subcategories of diffuse, nodular, necrotizing with inflammation and necrotizing without inflammation (scleromalacia perforans) (Table 25-1). This classification has been shown to be useful, because only 8% of Tuft and Watson's (7) patients progressed from one subcategory to another during the course of their scleral inflammation. Diffuse anterior scleritis is the mildest form, and necrotizing scleritis is the most severe form, with the majority of ocular complications.

Diffuse Anterior Scleritis

This is the most common form of anterior scleritis. The inflammation of diffuse anterior scleritis is generalized, involving either some small area or the whole anterior segment. The insidious onset, with gradual increase of signs and symptoms for 5 to 10 days, is characteristic. Without treatment it may last several months. It is the variety that may be misdiagnosed as simple episcleritis and therefore be undertreated. On slit-lamp examination the superficial and deep episcleral plexus are not only congested but also distorted and tortuous, losing the normal radial pattern of the vessels. New abnormal vascular channels may also appear. The anterior fluorescein angiogram usually shows a rapid although structurally normal flow pattern, with a decreased transit time for the dye (8); however, in some patients the flow pattern is distorted, with

the appearance of abnormal anastomoses between the larger vessels in the superficial or deep episcleral plexuses, which may show rapid early leakage. These anastomoses may persist and remain permeable for a prolonged period, even though the eye is uninflamed. There is no evidence of vascular closure. Although most of the patients diagnosed with diffuse scleritis maintain this category throughout the course of their scleral disease, a few may progress to a more severe categories such as nodular or necrotizing scleritis (7).

Nodular Anterior Scleritis

The inflammation of nodular scleritis is confined to a well-defined area, forming a deep red or violaceous scleral nodule (or nodules) which is extremely tender, firm to the touch, and totally immobile (Fig. 25-5). It is usually localized in the interpalpebral region about 3 to 4 mm from the limbus. As in diffuse anterior scleritis, the onset is insidious, gradually reaching its peak after 5 to 10 days, and if untreated, the nodules may last several months. Although it can be misdiagnosed as nodular episcleritis and be undertreated, detailed slit-lamp examination reveals the congestion and tortuosity of the superficial and deep episcleral plexuses overlying the nodule. The normal radial pattern is lost, and abnormal anastomosis due to the bypass from the arterial channels to the venous channels may appear. The anterior fluorescein angiography is similar to that of diffuse anterior scleritis. Although most of the patients diagnosed with nodular scleritis maintain this category throughout the course of their scleral disease, a few may progress to a more severe category such as necrotizing scleritis (7). The presence of an avascular center to the nodule that breaks down and circumferential progression of the nodular scleritis away from the original site of inflammation are physical signs that indicate that necrotizing changes are occurring.

Necrotizing Anterior Scleritis with Inflammation (Necrotizing Scleritis)

Necrotizing scleritis is the most severe form of scleritis and its presence is considered an ominous sign of the presence

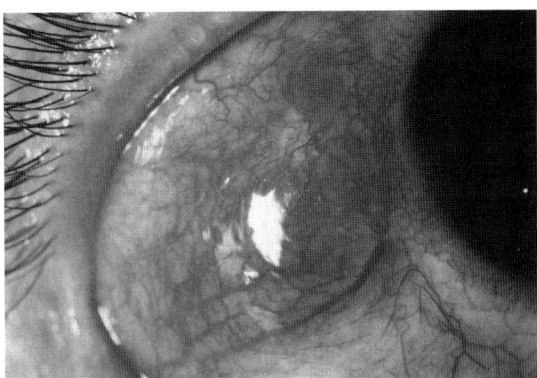

FIGURE 25-5. Nodular scleritis. As part of the sclera, the nodule is immobile as one tries to palpate and move it.

of occult, potentially lethal systemic vasculitic disease. Just how serious this condition is can be judged from the fact that 82% of our patients with necrotizing scleritis had a significant loss of visual acuity, 69% developed anterior uveitis, 41% developed peripheral ulcerative keratitis, 23% developed glaucoma, and 81% had an associated systemic connective tissue and/or vasculitic disease (4). Furthermore, Watson and Hayreh (1) reported that 29% of their patients with necrotizing scleritis died within 5 years of the onset of the scleritis; many of these deaths were caused by systemic vasculitic lesions. In another study performed by Foster et al. (9), seven of 20 patients with necrotizing scleritis died within 8 years of the onset of the scleritis; many of these deaths had been caused by vascular-related events. None had been treated with immunosuppressive therapy. Eleven of the 13 patients who remained alive had received immunosuppressive therapy.

The onset of pain and redness usually is insidious, reaching its peak in 3 or 4 days. The pain, always present without adequate medication for the scleritis, may be so intense and provoked by minimal touch to the scalp that it sometimes seems out of proportion to the physical signs. It usually worsens at night, keeping the patient awake and very anxious and distressed. The main characteristic is the presence of white avascular areas surrounded by swelling of the sclera and acute congestion of the abnormal vascular episcleral channels. The anterior fluorescein angiography shows hypoperfusion in the venous side of the capillary network, which may lead to nonperfusion or closure if the venules become thrombosed and permanently occluded. Because these venules rarely open, they are replaced by newly formed vessels that produce persistent leakage. Unlike in diffuse or nodular anterior scleritis, the transit time of the dye in necrotizing scleritis is markedly increased even when the eye is congested. If the inflammation is severe, vaso-occlusive changes in the conjunctival vessels also may occur.

The damaged area becomes thinned and translucent and shows the brown color of the underlying uvea (Fig. 25-6). If the process is allowed to continue, large areas of sclera may slough away, eventually leaving the choroid bare or covered only by a thin layer of conjunctiva. If there is elevation of the intraocular pressure, staphylomas may form in areas of thinned sclera. Spontaneous perforation can occur but more usually follows surgical or accidental trauma.

Necrotizing scleritis may appear for the first time after surgical trauma of the sclera following cataract extraction, transscleral suture fixation of an intraocular lens, retinal detachment repair, nonpenetrating and penetrating filtering procedures, strabismus repair, and pterygium excision (10–14). An associated systemic autoimmune condition is seen in 60% to 90% of the cases, the exception being pterygium surgery with the adjunctive use of mitomycin C. Surgically induced scleritis with or without peripheral ulcerative keratitis may develop after a latent period of a few weeks to many months. It may be the first manifestation of a potentially lethal systemic autoimmune vasculitic disease or may herald the onset of a vasculitis in a patient with an already-known systemic autoimmune disease, which was apparently in remission. Perioperative treatment with systemic steroids (prednisone 1 mg/kg/d beginning 3 days before and for 7 to 10 days after surgery) should be added to the usual treatment in patients with a history of scleritis undergoing ocular surgery.

Necrotizing Anterior Scleritis without Inflammation (Scleromalacia Perforans)

Scleromalacia perforans, a term coined by van der Hoeve in 1931 (15), is characterized by the appearance of yellow or grayish patches on the sclera that gradually develop a necrotic slough or sequestrum without surrounding inflammation; this sequestrum eventually separates from the underlying sclera, leaving the choroid bare or covered only by a thin layer of conjunctiva. Unless the intraocular pressure rises, no staphyloma is seen. Spontaneous perforation is rare but these eyes are quite susceptible to traumatic rupture. The condition has an insidious onset, slow progression and complete lack of symptoms. It is commonly bilateral, usually occurs in women, and is often found in association with severe, progressive, long-standing rheumatoid arthritis with extraarticular manifestations (46% of Watson and Hayreh's patients and 67% of ours patients) (1,16). The change in color of the sclera may often be detected by the patient while looking in the mirror, by the patient's family, by the rheumatologist by chance, or by the ophthalmologist in a routine eye examination.

On slit-lamp examination, a reduction in the number and size of vessels in the episclera surrounding the sequestrum may be seen, giving a porcelain-like appearance. These vessels anastomose with each other and sometimes cross the abnormal area to join with perilimbal vessels. Fluorescein angiography shows that the necrotic process in scleromalacia perforans appears to be caused by arteriolar obliteration,

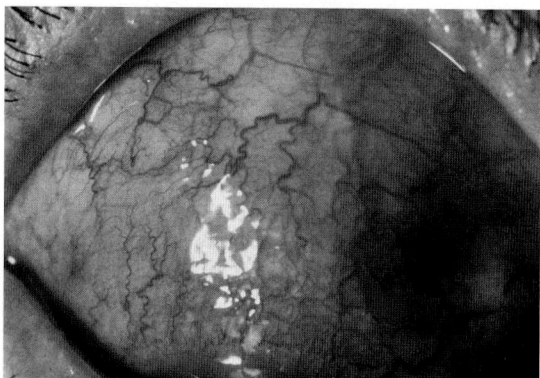

FIGURE 25-6. Necrotizing scleritis. The damaged area becomes thinned and translucent and shows the underlying uvea.

unlike in necrotizing scleritis, in which the necrotic process appears to be caused by venular obliteration (8,17).

Posterior Scleritis

Posterior scleritis is the inflammation involving the sclera posterior to the ora serrata, which may spread to the posterior segment of the eye, involving choroid, retina, and optic nerve; it also may extend outward, involving extraocular muscles and orbital tissues (18–22). Posterior scleritis is often associated with anterior scleritis; but it also may occur alone, in which case the absence of anterior scleral involvement makes the diagnosis difficult. And if the concomitant anterior scleritis is severe, posterior scleritis may be overlooked. Therefore, posterior scleritis is more prevalent than clinical recognition.

The most common presenting symptoms of posterior scleritis are decreased vision and pain. The reduction in vision may reflect, in some cases, a transient hyperopia, which is caused by a decrease in the axial length of the globe secondary to posterior scleral thickening and can be corrected with the addition of convex lenses. In other cases, the reduction in vision is not correctable because it is caused by severe complications such as choroidal or retinal detachment, distortion of the macula by an area of scleral inflammation, cystoid macular edema, and optic neuritis. These complications are often reversible, with a good visual outcome if adequate treatment for posterior scleritis is initiated shortly after its onset. If diagnosis and treatment are delayed, permanent damage may cause irreversible visual loss. The pain varies from mild to severe and often is referred to the brow, temple, face, or jaw. The pain is often correlated with the severity of the anterior involvement, and therefore patients with mild posterior scleritis alone have pain of a mild degree.

Diplopia and pain on eye movement are also frequent and are due to the extension of posterior scleral inflammation to the extraocular muscles.

The most common presenting sign is redness if there is anterior scleritis; conjunctival chemosis, proptosis, lid swelling, lid retraction, and limitation of ocular movements may also be detected and are due to the extension of posterior scleral inflammation to the orbit.

Choroidal folds, subretinal mass, disk edema, and macular edema are due to the extension of posterior scleral inflammation to the choroid, retina, and optic nerve. Annular ciliochoroidal detachment, serous retinal detachment, intraretinal deposits, and retinal striae may also appear.

Ultrasonography is the most useful test in the diagnosis of posterior scleritis because it shows the scleral and choroidal thickening and the presence of edema in Tenon's space (23,24). Computed tomography and magnetic resonance imaging may be needed to exclude orbital inflammatory diseases and orbital tumors (22). Fluorescein angiography may reveal choroidal folds, retinal pigment epithelial detachment, serous retinal detachment, disk edema, or cystoid

macular edema. The use of indocyanine green (ICG) may be helpful in the evaluation of choroidal involvement and in the assessment of disease evolution and response to therapy.

COMPLICATIONS

Episcleritis

Complications in episcleritis are rare. Mild peripheral corneal changes such as superficial and midstromal inflammatory cell infiltration may occasionally be observed in the area adjacent to the episcleral edema, but these infiltrates are small, localized, nonprogressive, and usually resolve without any sequelae. Cells in the anterior chamber and aqueous flare may rarely appear, but these are never severe. Glaucoma and cataract are not directly attributed to the episcleral inflammation; more often they are related to inappropriate steroid treatment.

Scleritis

Ocular complications associated with scleritis are more common, especially with necrotizing scleritis. They appear as a result of the extension of the scleral inflammation.

Significant visual loss may be caused by keratitis, cataract, macular edema, and less often, uveitis.

Keratopathy

Corneal complications are the most frequent and are localized in the corneal periphery. The different patterns of corneal involvement are related to the severity and type of scleral inflammation and they can be classified, depending on whether or not thinning (peripheral corneal thinning), infiltration (stromal keratitis), or ulceration (peripheral ulcerative keratitis) of the peripheral cornea occurs (25).

Peripheral corneal thinning is the most benign form and, although it may occur in young patients without any systemic condition, it is often found in middle-age and elderly individuals with long-standing rheumatoid arthritis. The peripheral cornea becomes grayish and thinned in one or more areas over a period of several years, eventually extending through the full circumference of the eye. The epithelium remains intact, but vascularization, lipid deposition, and further opacification and thinning may eventually involve the edematous stroma. Spontaneous perforation is rare, although trauma can rupture the thin cornea.

Stromal keratitis, typically acute in onset, is characterized by isolated or multiple white or gray nummular midstromal opacities. The lesions are usually in the periphery, in the same quadrant as the scleral inflammation, although they can involve the central cornea. If the treatment for the scleritis is delayed, they may eventually coalesce, resulting in large areas of diffuse corneal opacification, leading to an appearance resembling that of the sclera ("sclerosing" changes). Corneal vascularization may involve the superficial stroma, but vessels are always far behind the advancing edge of the opacity. Lipid deposition can be seen as crystalline deposits ("candy floss").

Peripheral ulcerative keratitis is the most severe form of keratitis associated with scleritis and is usually associated with necrotizing scleritis. It begins as a localized area of gray, swollen, infiltrated cornea adjacent to a region of scleral inflammation than in a few days may break down, leaving only some layers of deep stroma and/or Descemet's membrane with well-demarcated edges. An intrastromal yellow-white blood cell infiltrate may easily be seen at the advancing edge of the ulcer, which extends circumferentially rather than centrally and may involve 360 degrees of the cornea. If treatment is delayed, spontaneous corneal perforation may easily occur.

Uveitis

Uveitis in scleritis is also caused by extension of scleral inflammation. It is more frequently anterior, mild to moderate in intensity, and appears during the late course of the scleral inflammation (26). The chronicity of uveitis accompanying scleritis may allow the development of complications such as synechiae, glaucoma, and cataract that may cause progressive visual loss. Posterior uveitis is rare in patients with isolated anterior scleritis, and its presence usually signifies posterior scleritis. The presence of scleritis with uveitis, particularly when associated with glaucoma, should be considered a grave sign (Fig. 25-7).

Glaucoma

Increased intraocular pressure is caused by the accompanying scleral edema and uveal inflammation (27). It is essential

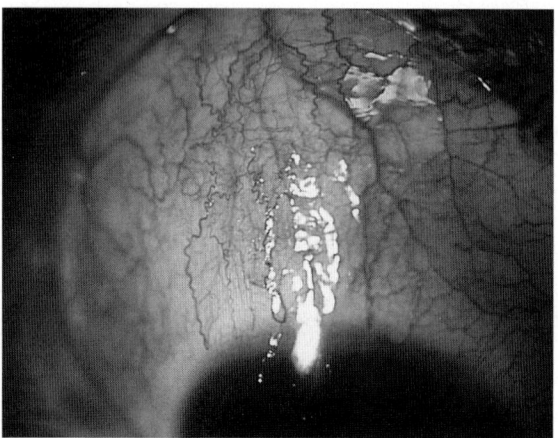

FIGURE 25-7. Diffuse scleritis with uveitis and ocular hypertension. The detection of uveitis and ocular hypertension accompanying scleritis requires early and aggressive therapy to control the inflammatory processes.

to monitor the intraocular pressure, the gonioscopic findings, and the optic disk regularly in patients with scleritis. Angle-closure glaucoma, open-angle glaucoma, and neovascular glaucoma are some of the possible mechanisms (3). The presence of scleritis with glaucoma, particularly when associated with uveitis, should be considered an ominous sign.

Cataract

Cataracts can develop because of the scleritis (mainly necrotizing scleritis), associated uveitis, or long-term steroid treatment, and is a significant cause of vision loss. When necessary, surgery should be attempted only in the absence of scleral inflammation. Perioperative systemic corticosteroids in a patient with a past history of scleritis is indicated to prevent relapse. Cataract removal through a corneal incision is advisable.

PATHOLOGY

Episcleritis

Light and electron microscopic studies of simple and nodular episcleritis show chronic, nongranulomatous inflammation with lymphocytes and plasma cells, vascular dilatation, and edema (3).

Scleritis

The sclera in nonnecrotizing scleritis, either diffuse or nodular, usually shows a nongranulomatous inflammatory reaction characterized by infiltration of mononuclear cells such as macrophages, lymphocytes, and plasma cells. In some cases, however, especially in the most severe ones, mononuclear cells organize into granulomatous lesions. Also, inflammatory microangiopathy, that is, neutrophilic infiltration in and around vessels, is present in some of these cases (28).

The sclera in necrotizing scleritis reveals a chronic granulomatous inflammation with epithelioid cells, multinucleated giant cells, lymphocytes, and plasma cells. Also, inflammatory microangiopathy is present in most of the cases.

ASSOCIATED DISEASES AND DIAGNOSTIC EVALUATION

Episcleritis

Connective tissue or vasculitic diseases, spondyloarthropathies, herpes zoster, rosacea, gout, syphilis, and atopy are the diseases most commonly associated with episcleritis; but the majority of patients have idiopathic disease (1,4,17). In our experience, 32% of patients with episcleritis had an associated disease.

The specific approach to episcleritis includes investigation of the illness (major complaint and history of present illness, past personal and family history), review of systems, and physical examination (head and extremities, eye). If the episcleritis attack is the first and evanescent one and medical review of systems and physical examination (head, extremities, other ocular structures besides episclera) are negatives, it is unnecessary to obtain complementary studies. Selective investigations should be performed to rule out specific diseases in patients with persistent or recurrent clinical course and symptoms suggestive of an associated systemic disease.

Scleritis

Connective tissue and vasculitic diseases are the main entities to be considered in the differential diagnosis of scleritis (1,4,17) (Table 25-2). Other diseases that should also be considered are the infections, atopy, rosacea, and gout. In our experience, 57% of patients with scleritis have an associated disease, including 48% with a connective tissue or vasculitic disease, 7% with an infectious cause, and 2% with atopy, rosacea, or gout (4). The specific diseases most commonly associated with scleritis are rheumatoid arthritis, Wegener's granulomatosis, relapsing polychondritis, and systemic lupus erythematosus (4,16,29–31). Scleritis can be a presenting clinical manifestation of a systemic disease. Necrotizing scleritis is most frequently identified with Wegener's

TABLE 25-2. ASSOCIATED DISEASES IN EPISCLERITIS AND SCLERITIS

Noninfectious
  Connective tissue diseases and other inflammatory conditions
    Rheumatoid arthritis
    Systemic lupus erythematosus
    Ankylosing spondylitis
    Reiter's syndrome
    Psoriatic arthritis
    Arthritis and inflammatory bowel disease
    Relapsing polychondritis
  Vasculitic diseases
    Polyarteritis nodosa
    Allergic angiitis of Churg-Strauss
    Wegener's granulomatosis
    Behçet's disease
    Giant cell arteritis
    Cogan's syndrome
    Associated with connective tissue diseases and other
    inflammatory conditions
  Miscellaneous
    Atopy
    Rosacea
    Gout
    Foreign-body granuloma
    Chemical injury
Infectious/immune-mediated from infectious agent
  Bacterial
  Fungal
  Viral
Parasitical

granulomatosis, rheumatoid arthritis, polyarteritis nodosa, or relapsing polychondritis, and it is unlikely to be seen with systemic lupus erythematosus, or in association with spondyloarthropathies.

The detection of a connective tissue or vasculitic disease in a patient with scleritis is a sign of poor general prognosis because it indicates potentially systemic complications that may be lethal unless managed with prompt and aggressive therapy. It is also a sign of poor ocular prognosis because patients with these systemic diseases frequently have more necrotizing scleritis, peripheral ulcerative keratitis, or decrease in vision than do patients without these diseases (31). In addition, the ocular prognosis of scleritis with connective tissue or vasculitic disease varies depending on the specific disease: scleritis associated either with spondyloarthropathies or with systemic lupus erythematosus is usually a benign and self-limiting condition, scleritis associated with rheumatoid arthritis or relapsing polychondritis is a disease of intermediate severity, and scleritis associated with Wegener's granulomatosis is a severe disease that can lead to permanent blindness or even loss of the eye.

The detection of scleritis, even if the attack is the first one, requires complementary studies. Based on the results obtained in the investigation of the illness (major complaint and history of present illness, past personal and family history), review of systems, and physical examination (head and extremities, eye), appropriate diagnostic tests can be selected to confirm or reject preliminary diagnoses. Sometimes, one series of diagnostic studies may be insufficient, and regular reinvestigations may be necessary to discover the diagnosis.

THERAPY

Episcleritis

Because episcleritis is a benign, self-limited process, it may be left untreated except for palliative therapy with cool compresses and iced lubrication. Topical nonsteroidal anti-inflammatory drugs (NSAIDs) are not effective (32). Topical steroids may speed the resolution; however, there are significant side effects, such as elevated intraocular pressure and cataracts, especially with prolonged use. Recurrences frequently occur with discontinuation of the steroids (rebound effect) (17).

A small number of patients, particularly those with nodular episcleritis with persistent episodes or frequent recurrences, require an oral NSAID (indomethacin, flurbiprofen, diflunisal, naproxen, etc.) to control the inflammation (3). Patients who do not respond to one NSAID may respond to another. The selective inhibitors of cyclooxygenase-2 (Cox-2 (celecoxib and rofecoxib) are the choice in cases with adverse effects or interactions with other medications (mainly anticoagulants). Episcleritis associated with rosacea, atopy, gout, or herpes, should be initially treated with specific therapy for each disease.

Scleritis

The treatment of scleritis always requires systemic therapy. Topical NSAIDs or topical steroids are insufficient (17). Scleritis associated with rosacea, atopy, gout, or herpes, should be initially treated with specific therapy for each disease.

In patients with noninfectious diffuse or nodular scleritis, oral NSAIDs (indomethacin, naproxen, diflunisal, flurbiprofen, ibuprofen, diclofenac, etc.) should be the initial choice (33). Response to therapy may not begin until up to 2 to 3 weeks after starting on NSAIDs. If one NSAID proves to be ineffective, another can be tried until a maximum of three have been tried. The selective inhibitors of Cox-2 (celecoxib and rofecoxib) can be selected in cases with adverse effects or interactions with other medications (mainly anticoagulants). In cases of therapeutic failure, oral steroids (prednisone 1 to 1.5 mg/kg/d) should be added or substituted as second-line therapy, tapering and discontinuing them as soon as possible while maintaining remission with continued NSAIDs. Intravenous pulse methylprednisolone (1 g/d three times for the first week and followed by a lower dose weekly thereafter) is recommended for refractory cases or in the event of an imminent potentially blinding process (34,35). Adjunctive periorbital, subconjunctival, and preseptal (36–40) steroid injections (triamcinolone acetonide) have been reported to be efficacious for non-necrotizing scleritis. However, although uncommon, scleral melting may occur after the injection, with severe and irreversible results (2,39). In cases of therapeutic failure, immunosuppressive drugs such as oral methotrexate (7.5 to 25 mg once a week), oral azathioprine (2–3 mg/kg/d), oral cyclophosphamide (2–3 mg/kg/d), or oral cyclosporine (2.5–5 mg/kg/d) should be added or substituted as third-line therapy. They may be initially supplemented by oral steroids, as response to therapy may take up to 6 weeks, with the latter being tapered and discontinued. Cyclophosphamide should be the first choice in treating patients with diffuse or nodular scleritis associated with Wegener's granulomatosis or polyarteritis nodosa.

In patients with noninfectious necrotizing scleritis, immunosuppressive drugs should be the initial choice, supplemented with steroids during the first month, with the latter slowly tapered, if possible. Cyclophosphamide is probably the most effective drug and can be used as a single daily oral dosage (2–3 mg/kg/d), or as intermittent, intravenous pulse therapy (10–20 mg/kg); the latter may be required for urgent cases and is followed by maintenance oral therapy. In cases of therapeutic failure, methotrexate, either 7.5 to 25 mg orally or intramuscularly once weekly; oral azathioprine 2 to 3 mg/kg/d; oral cyclosporine 2.5 to 5 mg/kg/d; or oral mycophenolate mofetil (1 g/twice daily) (41) may be used.

Preliminary reports with Daclizumab (Zenapax), an antibody directed against the interleukin-2 (IL-2) receptor that is expressed on activated but not resting T cells, show that the drug can be efficacious and safe in patients with conventional therapy-resistant scleritis (42). Infliximab and etanercept (43), the tumor necrosis factor inhibitors, have also shown some benefit in patients with refractory scleritis, although more experience is needed with respect to the efficacy and safety (44).

Because of the potential serious side effects, immunosuppressive drugs should be used in collaboration with a physician specifically trained in the early recognition and management of drug-induced complications of such treatment, such as an oncologist, hematologist, rheumatologist, internist, or ocular immunologist.

In cases of impending perforation, scleral patch grafting (using sclera from a fresh or frozen globe, glycerin preserved scleral tissue, pretibial periosteum, fascia lata, etc.) may be required to preserve the integrity of the globe; it should always be performed in association with immunosuppressive therapy to interrupt the destructive inflammatory process (45)

In patients with infectious scleritis, antimicrobial therapy should be instituted. It is important to differentiate infectious scleritis from noninfectious scleritis, because steroid therapy or immunosuppressive therapy (often used in noninfectious autoimmune scleritis) is contraindicated in active infection.

REFERENCES

1. Watson PG, Hayreh SS. Scleritis and episcleritis. *Br J Ophthalmol* 1976;60:163–191.
2. Watson PG, Hazleman BL. *The sclera and systemic disorders.* London: WB Saunders, 1976.
3. Foster CS, Sainz de la Maza M. *The sclera.* New York: Springer-Verlag, 1994.
4. Sainz de la Maza M, Jabbur NS, et al. Severity of scleritis and episcleritis. *Ophthalmology* 1994;101:389–396.
5. Williamson J. Incidence of eye disease in cases of connective tissue disease. *Trans Ophthalmol Soc UK* 1974;94:742–763.
6. McGavin DD, Williamson J, Forrester JV, et al. Episcleritis and scleritis: a study of their clinical manifestations and association with rheumatoid arthritis. *Br J Ophthalmol* 1976;60: 192–226.
7. Tuft SJ, Watson PG. Progression of scleral disease. *Ophthalmology* 1991;98:467–471.
8. Watson PG. Doyne Memorial Lecture, 1982. The nature and the treatment of scleral inflammation. *Trans Ophthalmol Soc UK* 1982;102:257–281.
9. Foster CS, Forstot SL, Wilson LA. Mortality rate in rheumatoid arthritis patients developing necrotizing scleritis or peripheral ulcerative keratitis. *Ophthalmology* 1984;91:1254–1263.
10. Sainz de la Maza M, Foster CS. Necrotizing scleritis after ocular surgery. A clinicopathologic study. *Ophthalmology* 1991;98: 1720–1726.
11. Glasser DB, Bellor J. Necrotizing scleritis of scleral flaps after transscleral suture fixation of an intraocular lens. *Am J Ophthalmol* 1992;113:529–532.

12. Scott JA, Clearkin LG. Surgically induced diffuse scleritis following cataract surgery. *Eye* 1994;8:292–297.

13. Galanopoulos A, Snibson G, O'Day J. Necrotizing anterior scleritis after pterygium surgery. *Aust N Z J Ophthalmol* 1994;22:167–173.

14. O'Donoghue, Lightman S, Tufts S, et al. Surgically induced necrotizing sclerokeratitis. *Br J Ophthalmol* 1992;76:17–21.

15. van der Hoeve J. Scleromalacia perforans. *Ned T Geneesk* 1931;75:4733–4735.

16. Sainz de la Maza M, Foster CS, Jabbur NS. Scleritis associated with rheumatoid arthritis and with other systemic immune-mediated diseases. *Ophthalmology* 1995;102:687–692.

17. Watson P. Diseases of the sclera and episclera. In: Tasman W, Jaeger EA, eds. *Duane's clinical ophthalmology,* rev ed., vol 4. Philadelphia: JB Lippincott, 1989:1–43

18. Calthorpe CM, Watson PG, McCartney ACE. Posterior scleritis: a clinical and histopathological survey. *Eye* 1988;2:267–277.

19. Cleary PE, Watson PG: Visual loss due to posterior segment disease in scleritis. *Trans Ophthalmol Soc UK* 1975;95:297–300.

20. Benson WE, Shields JA, Tasman W, et al. Posterior scleritis. A cause of diagnostic confusion. *Arch Ophthalmol* 1979;97:1482–1486.

21. Singh G, Guthoff R, Foster CS. Observations on long-term follow-up of posterior scleritis. *Am J Ophthalmol* 1986;101:570–575.

22. Benson WE. Posterior scleritis. *Surv Ophthalmol* 1988;32:297–316.

23. Cappaert WE, Purnell EW, Frank KE. Use of B-sector scan ultrasound in the diagnosis of benign choroidal folds. *Am J Ophthalmol* 1977;84:375–379.

24. Rochels R, Reis G. Echography in posterior scleritis. *Klin Monatsbl Augenheilk* 1980;177:611–613.

25. Sainz de la Maza M, Foster CS, Jabbur NS, et al. Ocular characteristics and disease associations in scleritis-associated peripheral keratopathy. *Arch Ophthalmol* 2002;120:15–19.

26. Sainz de la Maza M, Foster CS, Jabbur NS. Uveitis-associated scleritis. *Ophthalmology* 1997;104:58–63.

27. Wilhelmus KR, Grierson I, Watson PG. Histopathologic and clinical associations of scleritis and glaucoma. *Am J Ophthalmol* 1981;91:697–705.

28. Fong LP, Sainz de la Maza M, Rice BA, et al. Immunopathology of scleritis. *Ophthalmology* 1991;98:472–479.

29. Pavesio CE, Meier FM. Systemic disorders associated with episcleritis and scleritis. *Curr Opin Ophthalmol* 2001;12:471–478.

30. Jabs DA, Mudun A, Dunn JP, et al. Episcleritis and scleritis: clinical features and treatment results. *Am J Ophthalmol* 2000;130:469–476.

31. Sainz de la Maza M, Foster CS, Jabbur NS. Scleritis associated with systemic vasculitic diseases. *Ophthalmology* 1995;102:687–692.

32. Lyons CJ, Hakin KN, Watson PG. Topical flurbiprofen: an effective treatment for episcleritis? *Eye* 1990;4:521–525.

33. Sainz de la Maza M, Jabbur NS, Foster CS. An analysis of therapeutic decision for scleritis. *Ophthalmology* 1993;100:1372–1376.

34. McCluskey P, Wakefield D. Intravenous pulse methylprednisolone in scleritis. *Arch Ophthalmol* 1987;105:793–797.

35. Wakefield DE, McCluskey P, Penny R. Intravenous pulse methylprednisolone therapy in severe inflammatory eye disease. *Arch Ophthalmol* 1986;104:847–851.

36. Hakin KN, Ham H, Lightman SL. Use of orbital floor steroids in the management of patients with uniocular nonnecrotizing scleritis. *Br J Ophthalmol* 1991;75:337–339.

37. Tu EY, Culbertson WW, Pflugfelder SC, et al. Therapy of nonnecrotizing anterior scleritis with subconjunctival corticosteroid injection. *Ophthalmology* 1995;102:718–724.

38. Croasdale CR, Brightbill FS. Subconjunctival corticosteroid injections for nonnecrotizing anterior scleritis. *Arch Ophthalmol* 1999;117:966–968.

39. Zamir E, Read RW, Smith RE, et al. A prospective evaluation of subconjunctival injection of triamcinolone acetonide for resistant anterior scleritis. *Ophthalmology* 2002;109:798–807.

40. Sainz de la Maza M, Folch J. Transeptal steroids in necrotizing scleritis. *Arch Soc Esp Oftal* 2001;76:589–592.

41. Larkin G, Lightman S. Mycophenolate mofetil. A useful immunosuppressive in inflammatory eye disease. *Opthalmology* 1999;106:370–374.

42. Papaliodis GN, Chu D, Foster CS. Treatment of ocular inflammatory disorders with daclizumab. *Opthalmology* 2003;110:786–789.

43. Aeberli D, Oertle S, Mauron H, et al. Inhibition of the TNF-pathways: use of infliximab and etanercept as remission-inducing agents in cases of therapy-resistant chronic inflammatory disorders. *Swiss Med Wkly* 2002;132:414–422.

44. Smith JR, Levinson RD, Holland GN, et al. Differential efficacy of tumor necrosis factor inhibition in the management of inflammatory eye disease and associated rheumatic disease. *Arthritis Rheum* 2001;45:252–257.

45. Sainz de la Maza M, Tauber J, Foster CS. Scleral grafting for necrotizing scleritis. *Ophthalmology* 1989;96:306–310.

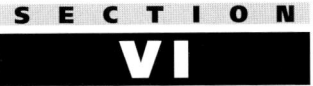

OCULAR SURFACE DISEASE

KERATOCONJUNCTIVITIS SICCA: INTRODUCTION

MICHAEL A. LEMP

Keratoconjunctivitis sicca (KCS) is a rubric to describe a variety of pathologic conditions characterized by abnormalities of the preocular tear film resulting in ocular surface damage (1). Our knowledge base concerning these disorders has grown substantially in the last three decades and has led to the recognition that the pathogenetic mechanisms operative in KCS are complex and interrelated. Far from being simply a matter of insufficient lacrimal fluid, it is now known that many factors involving the lacrimal glands, lids, ocular surface, lacrimal drainage ducts, medications, contact lens use, and environment affect the signs and symptoms. Various epithets have been used to characterize this group of conditions including dry eye, dry eye syndrome, blepharitis, meibomian gland dysfunction, and contact lens–induced dry eye. Some of these reflect an inclusive description, whereas others describe subtypes of KCS.

Although the presenting symptoms and signs of KCS are similar, an as yet unanswered question is whether there is a common underlying initial abnormality leading to a variety of changes in the morphology and function of the ocular surface and adnexal structures.

The preocular tear film has been previously thought of as a three-layered structure consisting of an innermost mucin layer, an intermediate aqueous layer, and an outer lipid layer (2). Recent research has elucidated this structure; there are two mucin-secreting systems, one produced by the corneal and conjunctival epithelial cells forming an outer glycocalyx cell-associated layer (MUC1) (3). In addition, a more highly hydrated form of mucin (MUC5AC), produced by the goblet cells of the conjunctiva, constitutes a loose mucin blanket dispersed within the aqueous layer (4). Both serve to protect the ocular surface. The aqueous layer produced primarily by the main and accessory lacrimal glands forms the bulk of the tear film. Its secretion is driven by neural stimulation and the previous distinction between "basal" and "stimulated" tears has largely been abandoned (5); as much as 10% of the aqueous tear component may come from transconjunctival flow. The outermost lipid layer is the product of the secretion of the meibomian glands of the eyelids.

These lipids form a bilayer structure that retards evaporative tear loss and stabilizes the film (6).

The tear film serves a number of important functions in maintaining a normal ocular surface in health and in the repair of the surface in response to injury. The tear film is the anterior refracting surface of the eye; breakdown in this principal optical element will degrade the visual image presented to the retina, compromising clear vision. In addition, the tear film is a source of essential nutrients and oxygen for the cornea and conjunctiva.

The ocular surface is supplied with dense sensory innervation. This neural array plays a central role in the maintenance of a healthy ocular surface. The lacrimal glands, meibomian glands of the eyelid, lacrimal outflow channels, and the ocular surface form an integrated functional unit that tightly regulates the turnover of cells of the ocular surface (7). Through the production of a large number of proteins (growth factors, cytokines, and chemokines), the lacrimal glands direct cellular activities at the ocular surface designed to maintain the regular formation, movement, and exfoliation of ocular surface epithelial cells and their recruitment in repair of the surface; the tear film is the conduit for this regulation. Sensory input from the surface informs the glandular structures directing the production of these various factors from the lacrimal glands, the meibomian glands of the lids, and the mucin-producing cells of the ocular surface. The tear film also provides hydration to corneal and conjunctival epithelium and lubrication to control the frictional forces between the upper lid and the ocular surface. Disruption in this exquisitely coordinated system can lead to a cascade of events resulting in symptoms ranging from irritation to incapacitating pain and signs of surface inflammation to breakdown of the ocular surface.

The National Eye Institute/Industry Workshop Report on Clinical Trials in Dry presented a classification of KCS eye in 1995 (Fig. 26-1). This schema identifies two main divisions of KCS: aqueous tear deficiency and evaporative tear deficiency. These categories describe two major pathogenetic mechanisms operative in ocular surface disease

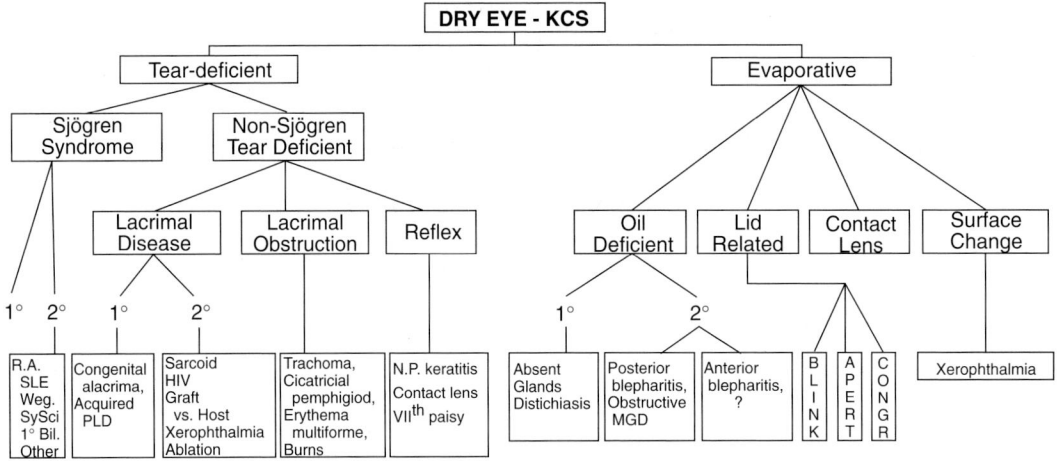

FIGURE 26-1. The National Eye Institute (NEI)/Industry Workshop on Clinical Trials in Dry Eye Classification

associated with dry eye. Although these are discrete mechanisms, they frequently coexist (and share common pathologic features); for example, over 60% of patients with Sjögren syndrome (SS)–associated KCS have both forms of dry eye (8). Another intriguing aspect of KCS is the relationship with SS. Many of the patients with more severe KCS have evidence of SS. It is not known whether patients with KCS but without SS represent a distinct pathologic category or rather a milder form of a similar immunologic abnormality (9).

Many factors are now known to contribute to the clinical picture of KCS. These factors include qualitative changes in tear composition (10), increased evaporative tear loss (11), immunologic abnormalities (12), age-related decreases in glandular function (13), hormonal dysfunction (14), changes in mucin production (15), inflammation of the glands and ocular surface (7), changes in epithelial cell turnover (16), abnormalities of tear flow, and decreased sensory function (7). Most of these factors are interactive; which of these are primary in the causation of KCS remains a subject of speculation.

Symptoms associated with KCS usually precede signs. Early complaints are usually those of ocular irritation; these range from intermittent mild symptoms to constant incapacitating pain. A number of different descriptors have been used to characterize the pain, including dryness, grittiness, stinging, foreign-body sensation, itching, burning, and photophobia. All of these reflect sensory impulses to the central nervous system signaling ocular surface distress. Integrative centers in the brain interpret these signals comparing them to prior experiences; differences in these processes probably reflect difference subjective descriptions of similar sensory signals. Recent studies of blink rates and tear film breakup have reported that patients with KCS have a tear film that breaks up prior to the new blink (17). This repeatedly disrupted tear film is thought to give rise to interblink desiccation, which may contribute to ocular surface damage.

A peculiar and frustrating aspect of the clinical presentation of KCS is the lack of correlation between symptoms and signs (18). Ocular irritation characteristically precedes the development of clinically apparent changes. This leads to difficulty in diagnosis of mild to moderate forms of KCS. Clinical signs such as staining and inflammation of the ocular surface occur more frequently in advanced cases. Paradoxically, some cases with severe surface disease are associated with a paucity of complaints; it has been suggested that this is due to downregulation of sensory receptors on the ocular surface by inflammation (19). Compromise of sensory input can result in a profound disruption of neurosensory control of tear production, cellular turnover, lid function, and tear flow. This can, in turn, give rise to a clinical picture seen in neurotrophic keratopathy. An example is the dry eye seen after LASIK surgery, in which approximately 60% of the nerve fibers to the cornea are severed, with resultant decrease in aqueous tear production, decreased blink rate, and a loss of trophic effects on corneal epithelial cells (20). Up to 50% of patients complain of ocular irritation after LASIK surgery and corneal staining is common (21). Symptoms and signs usually improve with recovery of sensation over a period of months.

One recently recognized feature of KCS is its subtle but profound effect on visual function. It has been demonstrated that between blinks, the tear film undergoes rapid breakup, degrading the visual image. This is not apparent with standard testing with a Snellen visual acuity chart, as more frequent blinking can temporarily reestablish the tear film and allow the patient to read the letters. Studies employing videokeratography (22) and wave front analysis (23), however, have documented these distressing and debilitating chronic changes.

Age-related changes in the functions of both the lacrimal and meibomian glands have been reported (24). Correlations with changes in hormonal status and advancing age suggest a role for circulating sex hormones in the maintenance of the secretion of both of these glands. Attention has been centered on the role of androgens in the maintenance of glandular function and the downregulation of inflammation. It has been proposed that androgen deficiency may play a leading role in the pathogenesis of KCS. This view is supported by animal models and the increased prevalence of KCS seen in patients with androgen abnormalities and in those undergoing antiandrogen therapy. In contrast, women on hormonal replacement therapy with estrogens are reported to be at increased risk for the development of KCS (25).

How prevalent is KCS? A number of studies have reported an increased prevalence of KCS in the elderly. Several studies have reported that about 15% of the elderly experience symptoms of KCS (18,26). A recent epidemiologic study, involving almost 40,000 women, reported a prevalence of moderate to severe KCS of 5.7% in those under 50 years of age to 9.8% in those 75 years and older (27). KCS is much more common in women than men but both sexes are affected. In addition, patients wearing contact lenses are thought to be at risk for developing KCS. Contact lens–induced dry eye is said to occur in 20% to 30% of soft lens wearers (28) and in up to 80% of hard lens wearers (29). This is related to increased evaporative tear loss. With the aging population, widespread contact lens use, the rise of LASIK surgery for ametropia, environmental and workplace stress on the tear film (e.g., the use of video display terminals and an associated decreased blink rate), it is estimated that the total number of patients suffering from mild to severe KCS might be as high as 40 million to 60 million in the U.S (30).

As knowledge of the multiple factors involved in the pathogenesis of KCS has increased, the opportunities to target specific pathologic features in the treatment of KCS has led to the advent of new therapies. Although palliative treatment with tear replacements has been the mainstay of therapy, the first truly therapeutic treatment [i.e., cyclosporin A (Restasis-Allergan)] has been approved by the U.S. Food and Drug Administration. Strategies currently under clinical investigation include other immunomodulating and inflammation- suppressing agents, mucin stimulators to protect the ocular surface, topically applied androgen agents, tear film stabilizers, and agents that protect surface cells from desiccation. In addition, systemic food supplements, such as flax seed oil and other supplements rich in omega-3 fatty acids, thought to suppress inflammation and contribute to the synthesis of the lipids of the meibomian glands, are in wide use.

This is an exciting time in dry eye research, with the promise of new, more effective measures to control the symptoms of KCS and intervene in the cellular abnormalities associated with this group of diseases. The challenges remaining include identifying early causative events and improving the clinical diagnosis of KCS. At present there is no single, reliable diagnostic test for KCS with high sensitivity and specificity. It has been suggested that tear osmolarity is a "gold standard." Indeed studies have demonstrated a high degree of sensitivity and specificity of tear osmolarity in the diagnosis of KCS. The lack of a commercially available low-cost instrument with demonstrated, reproducible results in dry eye patients has limited its use, however. The development of a single, disease-specific diagnostic tool should greatly aid in identifying patients with KCS. As the utility of each of the treatment strategies becomes clear, our ability to manage KCS should greatly improve; the path to a cure will await a greater fundamental understanding of the interactive roles of the pathologic events operative in KCS.

REFERENCES

1. Lemp MA. Report of the National Eye Institute/Industry Workshop on clinical trials in dry eyes. *CLAO J* 1995;21:221–232.
2. Holly FJ, Lemp MA. Tear physiology and dry eyes: a review. *Surv Ophthalmol* 1977;22:69–87.
3. Inatomi T, Spurr-Michaud S, Tisdale AS, et al. Human corneal and conjunctival epithelia express MUC1 mucin. *Invest Ophthalmol Vis Sci* 1995;36:1818–1827.
4. Jumblatt MM, McKenzie RW, Jumblatt JE. MUC5AC mucin is a component of the human precorneal tear film. *Invest Ophthalmol Vis Sci* 1999;41:703–708.
5. Jordan A, Baum JL. Basic tear flow, does it exist? *Ophthalmology* 1980;87:920–930.
6. McCulley JP, Shine WE. Meibomian gland and tear film lipids: structure, function and control. In: Sullivan D, et al., eds. *Lacrimal gland, tear film and dry eye syndromes 3*. New York: Kluwer Academic/Plenum Publishers, 2002.
7. Stern ME, Beuerman RW, Fox RI, et al. The pathology of dry eye: the interaction between ocular surface and the lacrimal glands. *Cornea* 1998;17:584–589.
8. Shimazaki J, Goto E, Ono M, et al. Meibomian gland dysfunction in patients with Sjögren's syndrome. *Ophthalmology* 1998;105:1485–1488.
9. Evaluation and differential diagnosis of keratoconjunctivitis sicca. *J Rheumatol Suppl* 2000;61:11–14.
10. Lemp MA, Dohlman CH, Kuwabara T, et al. Dry eye secondary to mucous deficiency. *Trans Am Acad Ophthalmol Otolaryngol* 1971;75(6):1223–1227.
11. Rolando M, Refojo MF, Kenyon KR. Increased tear evaporation in eyes with keratoconjunctivitis sicca. *Arch Ophthalmol* 1983;101:557–562.
12. Fox RI, Stern M, Michelson P. Update on Sjögren's syndrome. *Curr Opin Rheum* 2000;12:391–398.
13. Mathers WD, Lane JA, Zimmerman MB. Tear film changes associated with normal aging. *Cornea* 1996;15:229–234.
14. Sullivan DA Sex hormones and Sjögren syndrome. *J Rheumatol* 1997;24:17–23.
15. Gipson IK, Inatomi T. Mucin genes expression by the ocular surface epithelium. *Pro Ret Eye Res* 1997;16:81–98.
16. Lemp MA, Gold JB, Wong S, et al. An in vivo study of corneal surface morphologic features in patients with keratoconjunctivitis sicca. *Am J Ophthalmol* 1984;98:426–428.
17. Welch D, Ousler GW, Abelson MB. An approach to a more standardized method of evaluating tear film break-up time. *Invest Ophthalmol Vis Sci* (Suppl) 2003;44:2485.
18. Schein OP, Tielsch JM, Munoz B, et al. Relations between signs and symptoms in dry eye in the elderly. A population based perspective. *Ophthalmology* 1997;104:1395–1401.

19. Xu KP, Yagi Y, Tsubota K. Decrease in corneal sensitivity and change in tear function in dry eye. *Cornea* 1996;19:201–211.

20. Battat L, Macri A, Dursun D, et al. Effects of laser in situ keratomileusis on tear production, clearance, and the ocular surface. *Ophthalmology* 2001;108:1230–1235.

21. Duffey RJ, Leaming D. U.S trends in refractive surgery: 2001 International Society of Refractive Surgery Survey. *J Refract Surg* 2001;18:1885–1888.

22. Goto E, Yagi Y, Matsumoto MD, et al. Impaired functional visual acuity of dry eye patients. *Am J Ophthalmol* 2002;133:181–186.

23. Montes-Mico R, Alio JL, Munoz G, et al. Postblink changes in total and corneal ocular aberrations. *Ophthalmology* 2004;111(4):758–767.

24. Bron AJ, Tiffany JM. The meibomian glands and tear film lipids. In: Sullivan DA, Dartt DA, Meneray MA, eds. *Lacrimal gland, tear film, and dry eye syndromes 2*. New York: Plenum Press, 1998:281–295.

25. Schaumberg DA, Buring JE, Sullivan DA, et al. Hormone replacement therapy and dry eye syndrome. *JAMA* 2001;286:2114–2119.

26. Moss SE, Klein R, Klein BE. Prevalence of and risk factors for dry eye syndrome. *Arch Ophthalmol* 2000;118:1264–1268.

27. Schaumberg DA, Sullivan DA, Buring JE, et al. Prevalence of dry eye syndrome among US women. *Am J Ophthalmol* 2003 June;135(6):785–793.

28. Pascucci SE, Lemp MA, Cavanagh HD, et al. An analysis of age related morphologic changes of human meibomian glands. *Invest Ophthalmol Vis Sci* 1988;29(suppl):213.

29. Paugh JR, Knapp LL, Martinson JR, et al. Meibomian therapy in problematic contact lens wear. *Optom Vis Sci* 1990;67:803–806.

30. Morgan Stanley Equity Research. Dry Eye Market. No shedding tears over this opportunity. May 22, 2003. Research report available on the Internet at www.MorganStanley.com.

27

KERATOCONJUNCTIVITIS SICCA: PHYSIOLOGY AND BIOCHEMISTRY OF THE TEAR FILM

ROBIN R. HODGES AND DARLENE A. DARTT

FUNCTIONS OF THE TEAR FILM

The tear film is a complex fluid secreted by multiple adnexal glands surrounding the orbit as well as by the ocular surface epithelia. The tears form the first refractive surface encountered by light on its path to the retina. For clear vision, it is critical that the tears themselves are transparent. Tears, in addition, function to maintain the transparency of the second refractive surface that rays of light encounter, the cornea. Therefore, the key role of tears is to protect the ocular surface, the cornea, and conjunctiva, and to maintain their health and normal functions. The tear film protects the ocular surface from the external environment by responding dynamically to a wide range of external conditions and potentially damaging situations. These external stresses include desiccation, bright light, cold, mechanical stimulation, physical injury, noxious chemicals, and bacterial, viral, and parasitic infection. Tears also provide for a smooth and reflective surface and lubrication to avoid mechanical damage to the surface of the eye from the surprisingly high pressures generated by the blink. Tears transport oxygen and a limited number of other nutrients to the avascular cornea, regulate their electrolyte composition and pH, and function to remove waste products. Finally, tears contain a multitude of proteins and other molecules that not only protect the ocular surface but also can regulate a myriad of cellular functions of both the conjunctiva and cornea. Some of the main physical characteristics of tears are listed in Table 27-1. To respond to changes in the external environment and in the internal requirements of the cornea and conjunctiva, the volume, composition, and structure of the tears are exquisitely regulated. This control regulates the tear film primarily by coordinately regulating secretion from the adnexa, cornea, and conjunctiva, rather than by controlling tear drainage.

STRUCTURE OF THE TEAR FILM

The classical view of the tear film is as a stratified fluid consisting of three layers: an outer lipid layer, a middle aqueous layer, and an inner mucous layer. In addition there is a mucin-containing glycocalyx that extends from the apical membrane of the superficial cells of both the corneal and conjunctival epithelium, which acts as an interface between the ocular surface cells and the tears (Fig. 27-1). The different layers of the tear film have been measured; the lipid layer is 0.1 μm thick, the aqueous layer is 7 to 10 μm thick, and the mucous layer is 0.2 to 1.0 μm thick (1). Currently, there is controversy about the thickness and structure of the tear film. Measurements by Prydal and co-workers (2) indicated a far thicker mucous layer of about 30 μm and an aqueous layer that was 10 to 11 μm (2). Recent measurements, however, found a prelens tear film layer averages 2.7 μm (3,4). Still another hypothesis is that the mucous and aqueous layers are not distinct, but rather are a gradient of decreasing mucous and increasing aqueous content from the ocular surface to the lipid layer. Finally, McCulley and Shine (5) have suggested that the lipid layer is a monolayer consisting of two phases, a polar phase adjacent to the aqueous layer and a nonpolar phase at the tear film–air interface. The controversy over the structure and thickness of the tear film has yet to be resolved.

ADNEXA OF THE OCULAR SURFACE EPITHELIA THAT PRODUCE TEARS

Distinct tissues secrete the different layers of the tear film. The meibomian glands secrete the outer lipid portion of tears (Fig. 27-2). The glands of Zeis and Moll are minor contributors to this layer. The main lacrimal gland is the major gland that secretes the aqueous layer of tears. A minor amount of this layer is produced by the accessory lacrimal glands (the glands of Krause and Wolfring). There are two additional sources to the aqueous layer: the corneal and conjunctival epithelia. The cornea secretes a limited amount of electrolytes and water into tears, but the conjunctiva is a major source that has only recently been recognized. The conjunctival epithelium can additionally function to absorb specific components from the tears

TABLE 27-1. PHYSICAL CHARACTERISTICS OF TEARS

Characteristic	Value
pH	6.5–7.6
Osmolarity	302 ± 6.3 mOsm/L
Volume	6.5 ± 0.3 μL
Evaporation rate	10.1×10^{-7} g/cm^{-2}/sec^{-1}
Flow rate	1.2 μL/min^{-1}
Refractive index	1.336
Surface tension	40.1 ± 1.5 dyne/cm

From Lamberts DW. Physiology of the tear film. In: Smolin G, Thoft RA, eds. *The cornea*, 3rd ed. Boston: Little, Brown, 1994, 439–455.

(Fig. 27-2) (6,7). The goblet cells of the conjunctiva and the stratified squamous cells of the cornea and conjunctiva secrete the mucous layer of the tear film (Fig. 27-2). These stratified squamous cells also produce the glycocalyx. The lacrimal gland also secretes a soluble mucin.

Over the past few years, secretion from the individual ocular adnexa and the ocular surface epithelia has been extensively studied. This is in contrast to earlier studies of secretion from these tissues, especially from the main lacrimal gland, in which tear fluid was used. Tears are a mixture of secretions from multiple tissues, and analysis of tears does not present an accurate picture of secretion from any of the individual glands or other tissues. All the tissues that secrete tears respond to stimuli and thus need to be studied individually. Animal models to study lacrimal gland and corneal secretion have been available for many years and the majority of information on the secretion of tears has been derived from animals. Recently, cell cultures and immortalized cells of the individual cell types from the conjunctiva have been developed (8–12). Many of these cell types are of human origin. Culture of meibomian gland cells is ongoing (13). Study of the individual cells of the epithelia that secrete tears is elucidating the cellular mechanisms that control the secretion of the multiple components of the tear film.

LIPID LAYER

Meibomian Glands

The lipid layer is secreted primarily by the meibomian glands located in the upper and lower lids as described in Chapter 1. These glands secrete a complex fluid containing

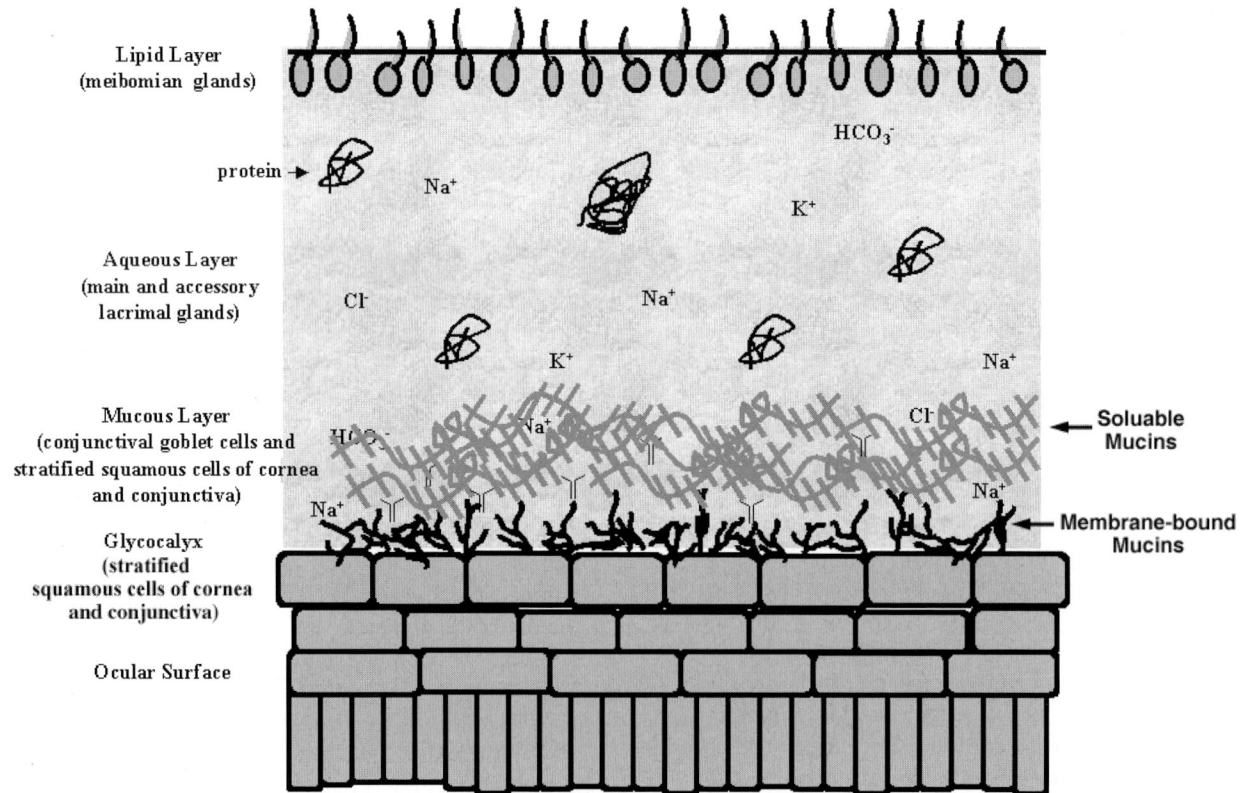

FIGURE 27-1. Schematic drawing of the three layers of the tear film. The tear film covers the cells of the ocular surface (cornea and conjunctiva). The upper lipid layer is secreted by the meibomian glands; the middle aqueous layer is secreted by the main and accessory lacrimal glands and the conjunctival epithelium; the inner mucous layer is secreted by conjunctival goblet cells and stratified squamous cells of the conjunctiva and cornea and the glycocalyx of the cornea and conjunctiva. (From Hodges and Dartt. Regulatory pathways in lacrimal gland epitheliom. *Int Rev Cytol* 2003;231:129–196.)

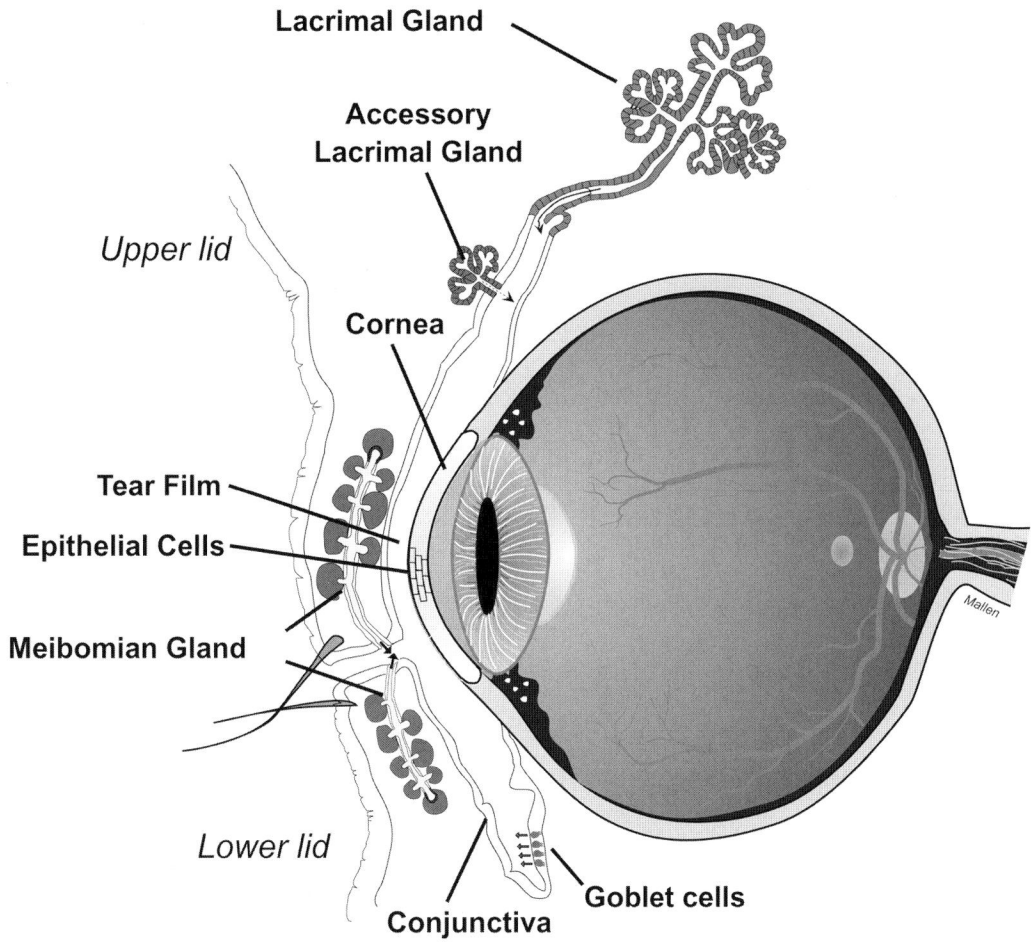

FIGURE 27-2. Schematic representation of the tear-producing glands. Cross section of the eye and the glands that produce the three layers of the tear film. (From Dartt DA. Regulation of mucin and fluid secretion by conjunctival epithelial cells. *Prog Retin Eye Res* 2002;21:555–576.)

a plethora of lipids, which melts at about 35°C and thus is always fluid in the living eye. The lipid layer behaves as a film essentially independent of the aqueous layer underneath. It is anchored at the orifices of the meibomian glands above and below and does not take part in the flow of tears from the lateral canthus to the lacrimal puncta (1). When the lids close during a blink, the lipid layer is compressed over the aqueous layer (14). When the lids open, the lipid layer begins to spread again over the aqueous layer. The spreading front can move faster than the opening lid, so the aqueous layer is never exposed (14). During lid closure the lipid layer thickens, and during eye opening it thins. This has been elegantly shown by Doane (15) using a specially designed interferometer that detects colors produced by interference patterns as the light passes through an oily layer whose thickness is changing.

Functional Anatomy of Meibomian Glands

Meibomian glands lie in a row in the superior and inferior eyelids. Each gland consists of a single, straight duct that

opens directly onto the inner margin of the eyelids adjacent to the mucocutaneous junction (Fig. 27-3). The duct is lined with four cell layers of ductal epithelial cells and branches off into smaller ducts that each terminate in an acinus (16). Each acinus is composed of several layers of epithelial cells with the outer single layer of cells consisting of germinal basal cells that do not contain lipid droplets (Fig. 27-3). As the cells mature they migrate toward the center of the acinus at a rate of 0.62 μm per day (17,18). During maturation the endoplasmic reticulum of each acinar cell develops and begins to synthesize lipids that are stored in secretory granules surrounded by a membrane. The closer the cell to the center of the acinus, the greater the number of lipid secretory granules. It takes an average of 4.1 days for the cells to mature and migrate (18). Secretion occurs when the mature cells in the center of the acinus disintegrate, known as holocrine secretion. The lipid content of the secretory granules as well as the secretory granule membranes and the remaining content of the cell is released into the duct. Thus meibomian gland fluid contains lipid secretory products as well as normal cellular contents.

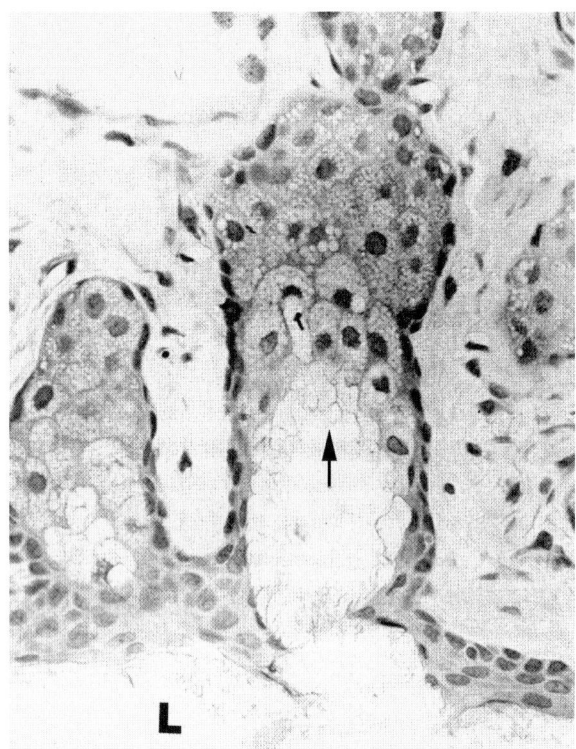

FIGURE 27-3. Light micrograph of alveoli of a rabbit meibomian gland. Cells in the outer layer *(arrow)* of the alveolus do not contain lipid droplets. Clear lipid droplets are visible in the middle layers of cells. Cells in the inner layer disintegrate into the alveolar duct, releasing the lipid droplets to form the secretory product that diffuses into the lumen (L) of the central duct. (H&E ×350.) (From Jester JV, Nicolaides N, Smith RE. Meibomian gland dysfunction. I: Keratin protein expression in normal human and rabbit meibomian glands. *Invest Ophthalmol Vis Sci* 1989;30:927.)

This accounts for the complex nature of the meibomian gland fluid. This fluid is stored in the ducts until released by the action of the blink.

Meibomian glands are richly innervated as described in Chapter 1. There is parasympathetic, sympathetic, and sensory innervation of these glands with parasympathetic innervation predominating (Fig. 27-4) (17,19–21). The parasympathetic nerves contain acetylcholine and vasoactive intestinal polypeptide (VIP) as neurotransmitters (20). The sympathetic nerves contain norepiephrine and the sensory nerves contain substance P and calcitonin gene-related peptide (CGRP). Although neuropeptide Y (NPY) is usually found in sympathetic nerves, in meibomian glands, it was found in nerves with a parasympathetic nerve–like distribution (21). Despite the fact that the meibomian gland is well innervated, the functional role of the nerves in this gland remains unknown.

The meibomian glands contain receptors for the sex hormones, which are important for the regulation of meibomian gland secretion. Androgen, progesterone, and estrogen receptors are present in the acinar cell nuclei of these glands (Fig. 27-5) (22–24). Androgens increase the size, activity, and lipid production in meibomian glands,

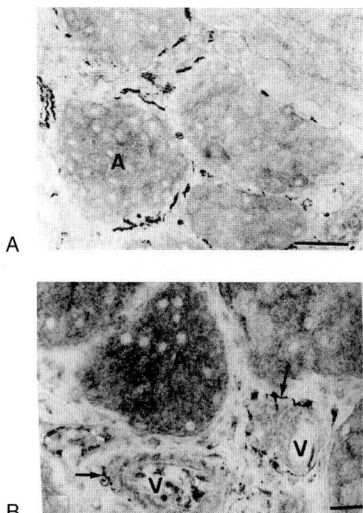

FIGURE 27-4. Innervation of the rat meibomian glands. Immunohistochemical microscopy showing localization of **(A)** sympathetic nerves using an antibody against tyrosine hydroxylase, which is one of the enzymes that coverts dopamine to norepinephrine, and **(B)** parasympathetic nerves using an antibody against choline acetyltransferase. (From Seifert P, Spitznas M. Immunocytochemical and ultrastructural evaluation of the distribution of nervous tissue and neuropeptides in the meibomian gland. *Graefes Arch Clin Exp Ophthalmol* 1996;234:648–656.)

whereas estrogens and progestins decrease them (25). Thus multiple functions of the meibomian glands are regulated by sex steroids and there are substantial gender-based differences between the meibomian glands of males and females.

Lipids Secreted by the Meibomian Glands

Meibomian glands secrete a complex fluid containing hydrocarbons, wax esters, triglycerides, diesters, free sterols,

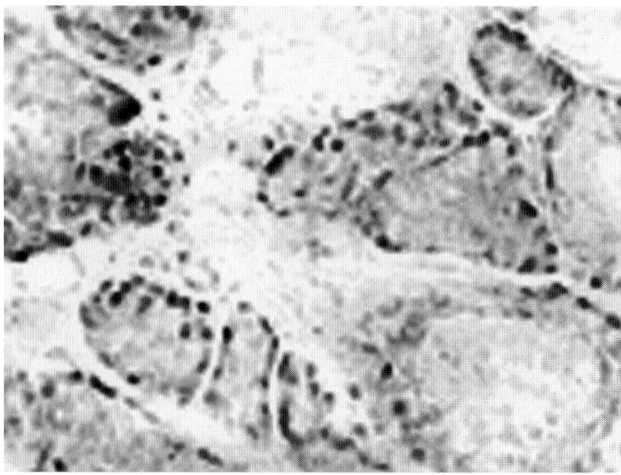

FIGURE 27-5. Presence of androgen receptor protein in acinar cells of the rat meibomian gland. Immunoperoxidase microscopy of meibomian gland showing the location of androgen receptor protein in acinar cells. (From Sullivan DA, Sullivan BD, Ullman MD, et al. Androgen influence on the Meibomian gland. *Invest Ophthalmol Vis Sci* 2000;41:3732–3742.)

sterol esters, free fatty acids, and polar lipids (for a review see ref. 26). The complexity of meibomian gland fluid reflects the products from the disintegrating cells as well as from the synthesized lipids. Meibomian gland lipids differ from cellular lipids in the acyl chain types and the sterol types. The major classes of lipids are the wax monoesters and sterol esters that make up about 60% to 70% of the meibomian gland fluid (26). A third type of lipid is the diesters that form ester linkages with fatty acids, fatty alcohols, or sterols. These diester compounds make up about 8% of the fluid.

Regulation of Meibomian Gland Secretion

The steps in the secretion of meibomian gland fluid include synthesis of lipids, release of lipids from the cells, and release of secretory fluid from the ducts. Synthesis of meibomian lipid is coordinated by differentiation of the acinar cells with the more differentiated cells having synthesized more lipid secretory product. Androgens control the differentiation of the acinar cells and their lipid production. A review by Sullivan et al. (22) summarizes this evidence. Androgens increase the transcription of genes that produce proteins to stimulate the synthesis and secretion of lipids. Androgen action is enhanced by the presence of an enzyme that converts testosterone into a more potent androgen. Furthermore, androgens modulate genes that induce fatty acid and cholesterol synthesis, the degree of fatty acid saturation and branching, incorporation of fatty acids into phospholipids and neutral lipids, the total amount of lipids, the secretion of wax esters and other lipids, and the metabolism of lipoproteins (22). Androgens also stimulate expression of transcription factors (sterol regulatory binding proteins) that coordinate regulation of the enzymes that regulate lipid synthesis. Meibomian gland lipids are secreted by disintegration of the acinar cells. The compounds that regulate this process are unknown. The final step in the secretion of meibomian gland fluid is the release of preformed meibomian gland fluid from the ducts where it has been stored. Evidence suggests that the blinking process itself regulates this step.

An additional candidate for the regulation of meibomian gland secretion is the nerves that innervate the gland and surround the acini at their basement membranes. Their role in regulating meibomian gland function is unknown. Nerves could potentially regulate the release of lipids stored in the secretory granules by stimulating fusion of the secretory granule membranes with the apical membrane or by inducing the disruption of the entire cell.

Functions of the Lipid Layer

As evaluated by Tiffany (26), the major functions of the lipid layer are to prevent the spillover of tears and contain the tears within the palpebral opening, prevent damage of the lid margin skin by tears, and form a seal over the exposed portion of the eye during sleep. The lipid layer may possibly reduce evaporation in the open eye, but opposing results have been obtained in studies of tear evaporation. Another possible function of the tear film was suggested by McCulley and Shine (5), who hypothesized that the lipid layer may protect the eye from microorganisms, pollen, and other organic matter by trapping these particles in the monolayer. There is no evidence for this function. Tiffany suggests that the lipid layer does not prevent sebaceous lipids from entering tears and does not increase the stability of the tear film.

AQUEOUS LAYER

Lacrimal Gland

Anatomy

The main lacrimal gland is the major contributor to the aqueous layer of the tear film and as such synthesizes, stores, and secretes proteins, water, and electrolytes. It is an almond-shaped gland located on the anterior and lateral parts of the roof of the orbit of the eye. This gland is a multilobed, tubuloacinar structure with ducts that terminate at the surface of the eye in front of the lateral portion of the superior fornix. The major cell type is the acinar cell, which composes about 80% of the gland. These cells appear as a ring in cross section in a structure termed an acinus (Fig. 27-6). The tubules containing the acinar cells converge into interlobular ducts, which empty into larger ducts, and eventually to the ocular surface.

Similar to other exocrine glands, lacrimal gland acinar cells are surrounded by tight junctions at the lumen dividing the plasma membrane into apical (lumen) and basolateral (blood) membranes (Fig. 27-6). This has the effect of generating a polarized secretory cell to allow for unidirectional secretion of proteins and secretion of electrolytes and water into the lumen. Nerves surround the acinar cells on the basolateral side. As a result, the basolateral membranes of acinar cells have receptors for the neurotransmitters and neuropeptides released from the nerves surrounding them.

In addition to acinar cells, the lacrimal gland also contains ductal cells, myoepithelial cells, and lymphocytes. Ductal cells line the ducts one to two cell layers thick. These cells secrete water and electrolytes and a small amount of protein. Myoepithelial cells surround the acinar and ductal cells on the basal side with multiple processes containing smooth muscle actin. Based on the similarities to myoepithelial cells in other tissues and studies in the lacrimal gland, it is believed that myoepithelial cells in the lacrimal gland are involved in contraction of the acinar and

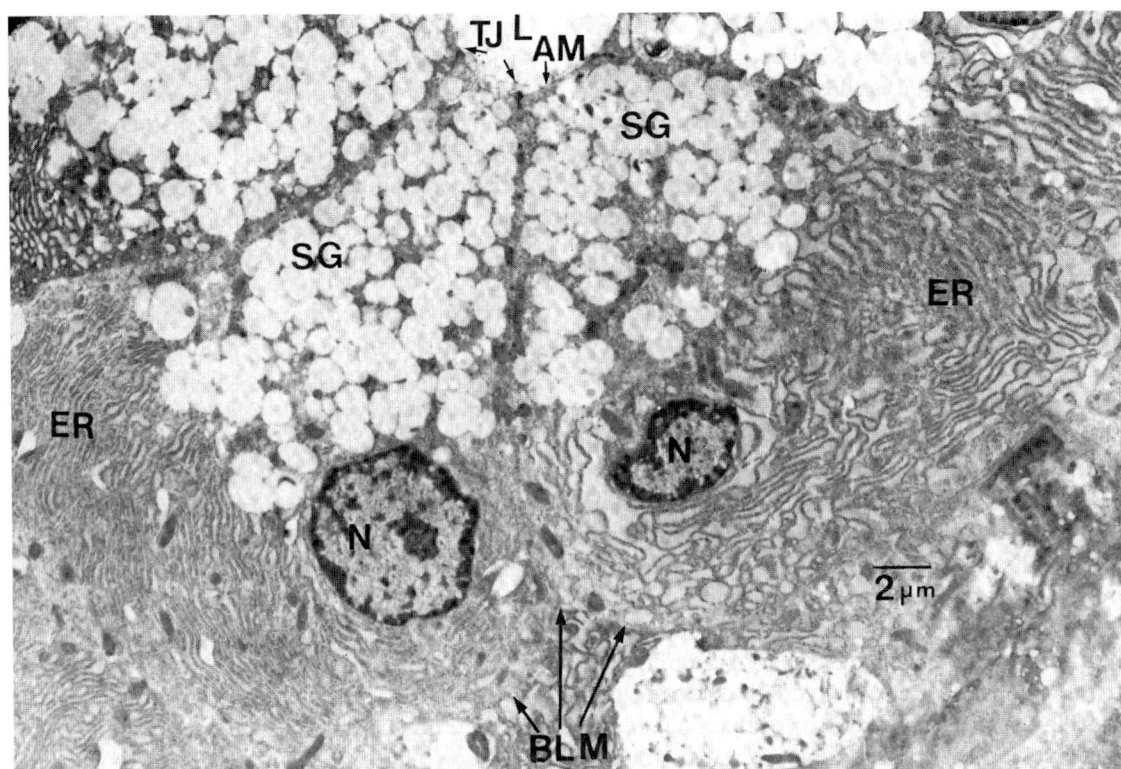

FIGURE 27-6. Electron micrograph of adjacent acinar cells from the rat lacrimal gland. The nucleus (N) lies in the basal portion of the cell and is surrounded by endoplasmic reticulum (ER). Secretory granules (SG) lie in the apical portion of the cell. Tight junctions (TJs) are present adjacent to the lumen (L) separate the apical membrane (AM) from the basolateral membrane (BLM). (From Dartt DA. Signal transduction and control of lacrimal gland protein secretion: a review. *Curr Eye Res* 1989;8:619–636.)

ductal cells to eject the secretory product (27). Many types of lymphocytes producing immunoglobulin (Ig) A, IgG, IgE, IgM, and IgD, plasma cells, mast cells, and macrophages are also present in the lacrimal gland.

Proteins Secreted by the Lacrimal Gland

Most of the proteins secreted by the lacrimal gland are antibacterial, antiviral, or otherwise involved in protection of the eye (Table 27-2). These proteins include lactoferrin, lysozyme, peroxidase, and group II secretory phospholipase A$_2$ as well as IgG, IgM, monomeric and polymeric IgA, secretory IgA (SIgA), and IgE. Other proteins such as cysteine-rich secretory proteins 1, 2, and 3, defensins, and convertase decay-accelerating factor are also secreted. In addition, the lacrimal gland produces many growth factors such as epidermal growth factor (EGF), transforming growth factor-α and -β, basic fibroblast growth factor, hepatocyte growth factor, and platelet-derived growth factor (28,29). The lacrimal gland has also been identified as the source of the retinol and retinal-binding protein found in tears (30,31). Recently, a novel protein has been detected in human tears that is secreted by the lacrimal gland. This protein, a glycoprotein, has been called lacritin and its function is unknown (32). Lacritin is expressed

at high levels in the lacrimal gland and at lower levels in the salivary glands, and is not expressed in any other tissue (32).

Gender Differences

Many hormones from the hypothalamic-pituitary-gonadal axis have significant effects on the lacrimal gland (Table 27-3). These effects include influencing the growth and differentiation of the gland as well as secretion from the gland. Disruption of this axis via either hypophysectomy or anterior pituitary ablation causes gland atrophy, a decrease in tissue protein and messenger RNA (mRNA) levels and a subsequent decrease in fluid and protein secretion. One of the major hormones to exert effects on the lacrimal gland is androgens. Androgens are known to stimulate the secretion of SIgA and cystatin-related protein and are responsible for many sex-related differences seen in the lacrimal gland (33). It has been shown that male rats secrete higher levels of secretory component (SC), IgA, and cystatin-related protein and peroxidase than female rats and in general secrete more tears (33). In all species studied thus far, lacrimal glands from males were larger than those from females. Major gender-related differences have also been observed in the morphology, histochemistry, and biochemistry of lacrimal glands (Table 27-3) (33).

TABLE 27-2. PROTEINS KNOWN TO BE SECRETED BY THE LACRIMAL GLAND

Apolipoprotein D

β-Amyloid protein precursor
Basic fibroblast growth factor

Convertase decay-accelerating factor
Cystatin
Cystatin-related protein

Defensins

Endothelin-1
Epidermal growth factor

Granulocyte-monocyte-colony stimulating factor
Group II phospholipase A$_2$

Hepatocyte growth factor

Immunoglobulin G
Immunoglobulin M
Interleukin-1α
Interleukin-1β

Lacritin
Lactoferrin
Lysozyme

Monomeric immunoglobulin A

Peroxidase
Plasminogen activator
Platelet-derived growth factors
Polymeric immunoglobulin A
Prolactin

Retinoic acid

Secretory component
Secretory immunoglobulin A

Tear lipocalins
Transforming growth factor-α
Transforming growth factor-β_1
Transforming growth factor-β_2
Tumor necrosis factor-α

Modified from Dartt DA and Sullivan DA. Wetting of the ocular surface. In: Albert D, Jakobiec F, eds. *Principals and practices of opthalmology.* Philadelphia: WB Saunders, 1994, 1043–1049.

Innervation of the Lacrimal Gland

It is well established that lacrimal gland protein secretion is under hormonal and neural control. Hormones play a major role in stimulation of constitutively secreted proteins, i.e., proteins that are secreted immediately upon synthesis. Nerves play a crucial role in the secretion of regulated protein secretion, i.e., proteins that are stored in secretory vesicles after synthesis and released upon the appropriate stimulus. Not surprisingly, stimuli of regulated and constitutive secretory proteins differ, as do the signaling pathways activated by these stimuli.

The lacrimal gland is innervated with parasympathetic, sympathetic, and sensory nerves (34). Parasympathetic nerves contain the neurotransmitter acetylcholine (ACh) and the neuropeptide VIP (Fig. 27-7A). Some VIP-containing nerves also contain pituitary adenylate cyclase activating peptide (35). There is additional evidence to suggest that parasympathetic nerves contain proenkephalin A–derived peptides (36).

Sympathetic nerves and sensory nerves are much less densely distributed than parasympathetic nerves (34) (Fig. 27-7B). Sympathetic nerves contain the neurotransmitter norepinephrine and may also contain the neuropeptide NPY (34). Sensory nerves originate from the trigeminal ganglion and contain substance P, galanin, and calcitonin gene-related protein (34). Sensory nerves do not participate in reflexes from the ocular surface, nor do their neurotransmitters stimulate protein secretion.

It is interesting to note that not all acinar cells are directly innervated. Gap junctions present within an acinus allow each cell to be electrically and chemically connected to adjacent cells. This allows for noninnervated cells to also be activated by neural stimulation (37).

Regulation of Lacrimal Gland Protein Secretion

Regulated Protein Secretion

Because the amount and composition of lacrimal gland fluid are critical to maintaining a healthy ocular surface, nerves tightly control the secretory process. Parasympathetic and sympathetic nerves are major stimuli of lacrimal gland protein secretion. The parasympathetic neurotransmitters ACh and VIP and the sympathetic neurotransmitter norepinephrine are potent stimuli of lacrimal gland secretion. The sympathetic neuropeptide NPY has a minor stimulatory effect on protein secretion.

Cholinergic Pathway

ACh released from parasympathetic nerves activates muscarinic receptors located on the basolateral membranes of acinar and the plasma membranes of myoepithelial cells (Fig. 27-8) (28). The M$_3$ or glandular subtype of muscarinic receptors is the only muscarinic receptor identified in the lacrimal gland (28). The activated M$_3$ receptor interacts with a G$\alpha_{q/11}$ G protein (28). Activated G proteins in turn activate phospholipase C (PLC) to breakdown phosphatidylinositolbisphosphate (PIP$_2$) into 1,4,5-inositol trisphosphate (1,4,5-IP$_3$) and diacylglycerol (DAG) (28). The 1,4,5-IP$_3$ released binds to and activates the IP$_3$ receptors located on intracellular Ca^{2+} (Ca$^{2+}_i$) stores such as the endoplasmic reticulum. This interaction releases Ca^{2+} into the cytosol (38). The Ca$^{2+}_i$ response is biphasic and includes a rapid peak followed by a slower sustained phase. It has been demonstrated that the rapid response is due to the release of Ca^{2+} from intracellular stores by 1,4,5-IP$_3$ whereas the slow, sustained phase is due to the entry of extracellular Ca^{2+} into the cell. Emptying of the Ca$^{2+}_i$ stores subsequently activates Ca^{2+} influx across the plasma membrane (38) (Fig. 27-8).

In addition to 1,4,5-IP$_3$, activation of PLC also produces DAG. DAG activates a family of enzymes known as protein kinase C (PKC). The role of PKC in lacrimal gland secre-

TABLE 27-3. GENDER-RELATED DIFFERENCES IN THE LACRIMAL GLAND AND TEAR FILM

	Male	Female
Morphology	Large acini Centrally located nucleus varying in size and shape Cell borders indistinct	Smaller acini Basally located nucleus uniform in size and shape Cell borders distinct
Biochemistry	Greater number of β-adrenergic receptors Greater level of androgen receptor protein Greater activity of carbonic anhydrase	Greater peroxidase activity Greater amounts of melatonin Greater amounts of *N*-acetyltransferase
Immunology	Increased synthesis of secretory component Greater production of immunoglobulin A (IgA)	Increased incidence of autoimmune disease
Secretion and tears	Greater amount of secretion Greater tear levels of **secretory component** (SC), IgA, and cystatin-related protein Higher tear levels of total protein Greater amounts of epidermal growth factor (EGF) and transforming growth factor-α (TGF-α)	Smaller amount of secretion Higher amounts of pancreatic lipase-related protein1

Modified from Dartt DA and Sullivan DA. Wetting of the ocular surface. In: Albert D, Jakobiec F, eds. *Principals and practices of opthalmology.* Philadelphia: WB Saunders, 1994, 1043–1049.

tion is complicated due to the fact that 11 different isoforms of PKC have been identified. The lacrimal gland contains PKC-α, δ, ε, and λ. In general, PKC isoforms have cell and tissue specific localizations, and the lacrimal gland is no exception (28). The PKC isoforms detected in the lacrimal gland have specific although somewhat overlapping distribution (28).

To determine the role of PKC isoforms in secretion, PKC isoform selective inhibitory peptides can be used. When such peptides were used, cholinergic agonist-stimulated secretion was inhibited the most by the PKC-α inhibitory peptide, followed by the PKC-ε inhibitory peptide with the least inhibition obtained using the PKC-δ inhibitory peptide. Confirming the role of these PKC isoforms in lacrimal gland secretion, treatment with phorbol esters downregulated PKC-α the most followed by PKC-δ and PKC-ε with

cholinergic agonist-stimulated secretion inhibited over 90% (28). Thus, these PKC isoforms play important, but differential, roles in lacrimal gland secretion stimulated by cholinergic agonists.

In addition to activating PLC, cholinergic agonists also activate phospholipase D (PLD) in the lacrimal gland. PLD hydrolyzes phospholipids preferring phosphatidylcholine as a substrate, which produces phosphatidic acid and free polar head group. The phosphatidic acid can be a signaling molecule itself or can be degraded to generate DAG. Cholinergic agonists, activation of PKC, and increasing the $[Ca^{2+}]_i$ all stimulated PLD activity in lacrimal gland acini (28). Because cholinergic agonists produced phosphatidic acid, but, surprisingly, activation of PKC and increasing the $[Ca^{2+}]_i$ did not, it appears that the lacrimal gland contained two different types of PLD activity.

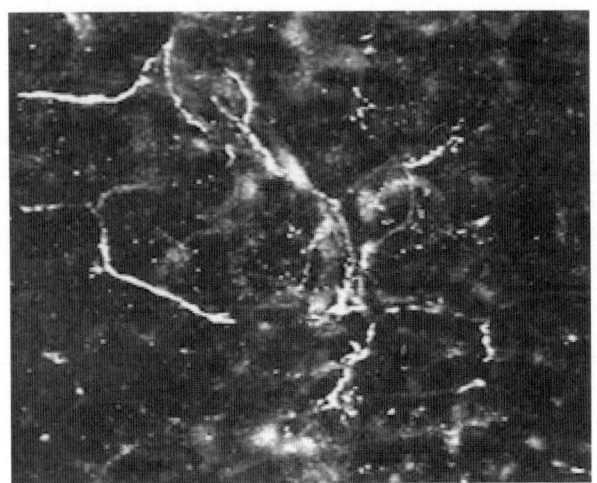
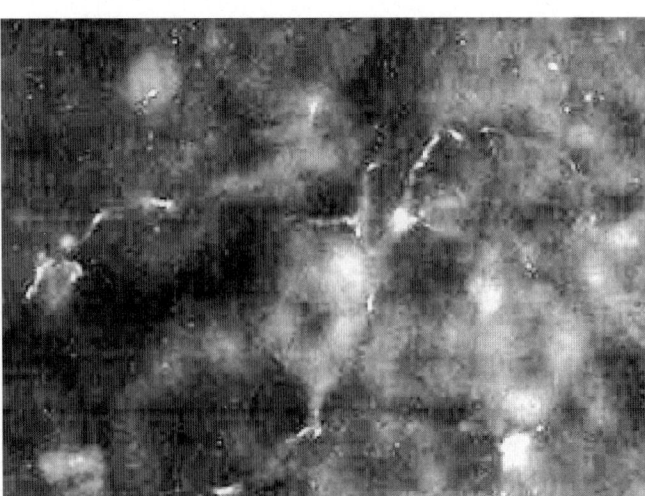

A   B

FIGURE 27-7. Innervation of the rat lacrimal gland. Immunofluorescent microscopy showing localization of **(A)** parasympathetic nerves using an antibody against vasoactive intestinal peptide (VIP). **B.** Sympathetic nerves using an antibody against dopamine β-hydroxylase which is the enzyme that coverts dopamine to norepinephrine.

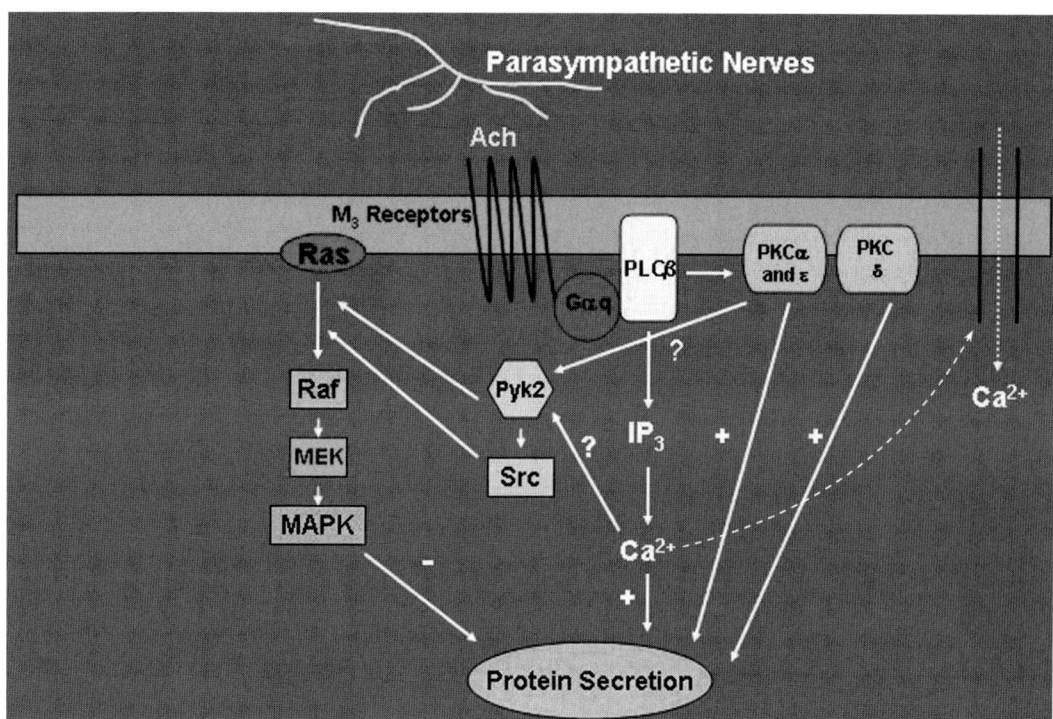

FIGURE 27-8. Schematic drawing of the signal transduction pathways activated by cholinergic agonists in the lacrimal gland. Ach, acetylcholine; M_3, muscarinic receptor subtype 3; $G\alpha q$, alpha subunit of Gq G protein; PLC, phospholipase C; Pyk2 and Src, nonreceptor tyrosine kinases; raf, mitogen-activated protein kinase kinase kinase; MEK, mitogen-activated protein kinase kinase; MAPK, p44/p42 mitogen-activated protein kinase; $InsP_3$, inositol trisphosphate; PKC, protein kinase C. (Modified from Dartt DA. Regulation of lacrimal gland secretion by neurotransmitters and the EGF family of growth factors. *Exp Eye Res* 2001;73:741–752.)

In summary, the lacrimal gland contains M_3 muscarinic receptors. Upon ligand binding, the receptor, through $G\alpha_{q/11}$ G proteins, activates PLC and PLD. The two second messengers, DAG and IP_3, are generated from PLC hydrolysis of PIP_2 and stimulate secretion, whereas the role of PLD is protein secretion is not known. DAG activates the PKC isoforms PKC-α, -δ, and -ε, whereas 1,4,5-IP_3 releases Ca^{2+} from intracellular stores. Both increasing $[Ca^{2+}]_i$ and activation of PKC-α, -δ, and -ε play integral roles in stimulation of cholinergic-induced protein secretion.

α_1-Adrenergic Pathway

In the lacrimal gland norepinephrine, released from sympathetic nerves, activates α_1-adrenergic receptors to stimulate lacrimal gland protein secretion (Fig. 27-9) (39,40). In fact stimulation by the α_1-adrenergic agonist phenylephrine was as potent and effective as cholinergic agonists in stimulating protein secretion. The types of α_1-adrenergic receptors ($\alpha_{1A, B,}$ or $_D$) present in the lacrimal gland are not known. α_1-Adrenergic agonists use the $G\alpha_{q/11}$ subunit G protein to stimulate about one third of its secretion (28). The G protein activating the remaining secretion remains unidentified.

The next step in the α_1-adrenergic agonist-signaling pathway, activation of a phospholipase, is unclear (Fig. 27-9). α_1-Adrenergic agonists in the lacrimal gland do not appear to activate either PLC or PLD in the lacrimal gland. The most likely candidate for α_1-adrenergic agonist activation is PLA_2, which generates arachidonic acid that can be converted to DAG. It is known that α_1-adrenergic agonists do cause a small increase in $[Ca^{2+}]_i$, which is about 20% of the cholinergic agonist response in isolated acini (28). In addition, activation of PKC isoforms plays a role in α_1-adrenergic agonist stimulated protein secretion. Although no translocation of any PKC isoforms was detected with stimulation of α_1-adrenergic agonists, when PKC isoforms were downregulated with a long-term phorbol ester treatment phenylephrine-induced secretion was increased (28). This suggests that activation of PKC inhibits α_1-adrenergic agonist-induced protein secretion. Using the PKC isoform selective inhibitor peptides, inhibition of PKC-α and -δ stimulated α_1-adrenergic agonist-induced protein secretion, whereas inhibition of PKC-ε blocked α_1-adrenergic agonist-stimulated protein secretion (28). It appears then that activation of PKC-α and -δ inhibits α_1-adrenergic agonist-induced protein secretion whereas activation of PKC-ε stimulates it. Thus cholinergic and α_1-adrenergic agonists are activating the same PKC isozymes PKC-α, -δ, and -ε, but are doing so differently. This suggests compartmentalization or targeting, because the same PKC isoforms either stimulate or inhibit secretion depending on the agonist. The targeting proteins in the lacrimal gland are unknown.

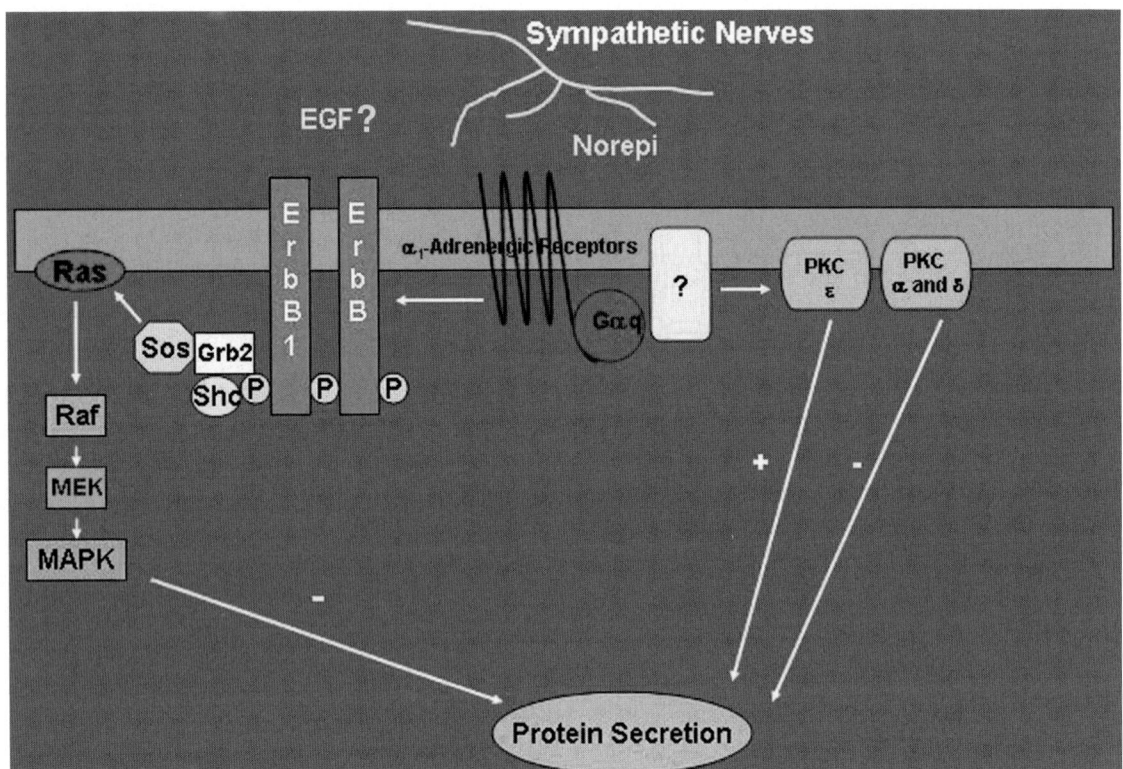

FIGURE 27-9. Schematic drawing of the signal transduction pathways activated by α_1-adrenergic agonists in the lacrimal gland. Norepi, norepinephrine; PKC, protein kinase C; ErbB1, the epidermal growth factor (EGF) receptor; ErbB, the EGF family of growth factor receptor; P, phosphorylated tyrosine residues on the ErbBs; SOS, Grb2 and Shc, adaptor proteins; raf, mitogen-activated protein kinase kinase kinase; MEK, mitogen-activated protein kinase kinase; MAPK, p44/p42 mitogen-activated protein kinase. (Modified from Dartt DA. Regulation of lacrimal gland secretion by neurotransmitters and the EGF family of growth factors. *Exp Eye Res* 2001;73:741–752.)

In summary, α_1-adrenergic agonists possibly activate PLA_2 that leads to production of DAG and activation of specific PKC isoforms. Activation of PKC-ϵ stimulates protein secretion, whereas activation of PKC-α and -δ inhibits secretion. These agonists also cause a small rise in $[Ca^{2+}]_i$, but the role of Ca^{2+}_i is secretion is unclear.

β-Adrenergic agonist pathway
Norepinephrine released from sympathetic nerves can stimulate both α- and β-adrenergic receptors. Activation of β-adrenergic receptors causes a small stimulation of protein secretion in the lacrimal gland (28). This response appears to be mediated by an increase in cellular cAMP levels (28). Activation of β-adrenergic receptors did not increase the $[Ca^{2+}]_i$ (28). It would appear that in the absence of an increase in $[Ca^{2+}]_i$ only a limited secretory response occurs.

VIP-dependent pathway
Parasympathetic nerves also release the bioactive peptide VIP. VIP causes a potent secretory response similar in magnitude to cholinergic and α_1-adrenergic agonists (28). In contrast to cholinergic and α_1-adrenergic agonists, VIP activates the cAMP-signaling pathway (Fig. 27-10). The components of the VIP-dependent signaling pathway have been identified in the lacrimal gland. Both of the two identified VIP receptors (VIPR), $VIPR_1$ and $VIPR_2$ have been localized in lacrimal gland (28). $VIPR_1$ is present on the basolateral membranes of acinar and ductal cells, whereas $VIPR_2$ is present on the plasma membrane of myoepithelial cells. Binding of VIP to its receptor activates the G protein $G\alpha_s$ (28). that in turn stimulates adenylyl cyclase.

There are six isoforms of adenylyl cyclase (ACI-VI), each of which has different, selective requirements for stimulation (41). Several types of Gα, as well as Gβα subunits stimulate AC isoforms. ACII, III, and IV have been found in the lacrimal gland, each with a different distribution (28). ACV/VI were not detected. Interestingly, none of the AC isoforms localized to the basolateral membranes of acinar and duct cells where they could interact with the VIPRs. Other AC isoforms could potentially have a basolateral membrane distribution or, alternatively, AC could be recruited from an internal membrane store upon stimulation (28).

AC stimulates an increase in intracellular cyclic adenosine monophosphate (cAMP) levels, which in turn activates protein kinase A (PKA). Using a membrane permeable inhibitor peptide based on protein kinase inhibitor

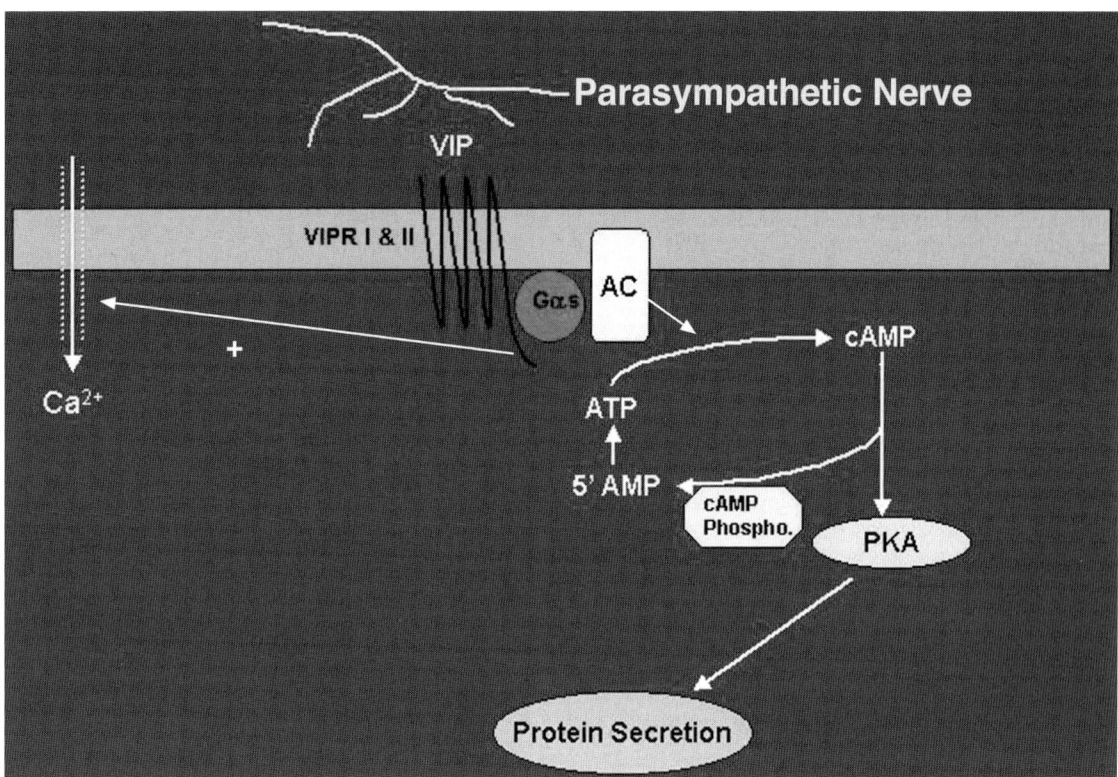

FIGURE 27-10. Schematic drawing of the signal transduction pathways activated by VIP in the lacrimal gland. Signal transduction pathways activated by VIP to stimulate protein secretion. Gαs, alpha subunit of Gs G protein; cAMP, 3',5'cyclic adenosine monophosphate; ATP, adenosine triphosphate; AMP, adenosine monophosphate. (Modified from Dartt DA. Regulation of lacrimal gland secretion by neurotransmitters and the EGF family of growth factors. *Exp Eye Res* 2001;73:741–752.)

(PKI), a known selective inhibitor of PKA, the role of PKA in VIP-induced protein secretion was determined. The PKA inhibitor peptide blocked most of the VIP-stimulated protein secretion from rat lacrimal gland acini, indicating that activation of PKA caused most, but not all, of VIP-induced secretion. An increase in $[Ca^{2+}]_i$ is the most likely mediator of the remainder of secretion as VIP increased the $[Ca^{2+}]_i$ by an amount that was approximately 25% of the carbachol response. This response was decreased substantially by the removal of Ca^{2+}_o (28). Because VIP did not increase cellular levels of IP_3, VIP apparently increases $[Ca^{2+}]_i$ by increasing Ca^{2+} influx rather than by releasing Ca^{2+}_i (28). Activated PKA stimulates secretion by phosphorylating specific protein substrates, none of which have yet been identified in the lacrimal gland.

Nitric Oxide

Nitric oxide (NO) is synthesized by the enzyme nitric oxide synthase from L-arginine in a reaction producing the gas NO and L-citrulline (42). There are three types of NO synthase (NOS), the enzyme responsible for the production of NO: neuronal (n), endothelial (e), and inducible (i). nNOS was identified by immunohistochemistry and is present predominantly in parasympathetic nerves in the cat and mouse lacrimal gland (43,44). nNOS was located in both the somata in the pterygopalatine (parasympathetic) ganglion and in the nerves surrounding the acini. The localization of nNOS in lacrimal gland parasympathetic nerves suggests that activation of these nerves stimulates release of NO, ACh, and VIP. The presence of eNOS or iNOS has not been investigated in the lacrimal gland.

NO appears to play a role in activating lacrimal gland function as elevation of NO by NO donors or NOS substrates increased the $[Ca^{2+}]_i$ in lacrimal gland acinar cells (45). In addition, an increase in NO levels stimulated protein secretion as a variety of NO donors and NOS substrates stimulated secretion (46). Elevation of NO stimulates secretion by increasing cellular cyclic guanosine monophosphate (cGMP) levels. Inhibition of guanylyl cyclase activity blocked secretion stimulated by NO producing compounds (46). Increasing the cellular NO level was as effective as the cholinergic agonist carbachol in stimulating protein secretion.

Growth Factors

A variety of growth factors have been identified in the lacrimal gland. These include EGF and its family of growth factors, fibroblast growth factor (FGF) 2, 7, and 10, hepatocyte growth factor (HGF), keratinocyte growth factor (KGF) (29), atrial natriuretic peptide, C-type natriuretic peptide, and growth factor-like glycerophosphate mediators of lysophosphatidic acid (28). Neurotrophins including nerve growth factor (NGF), brain-derived neurotrophic factor (BDNF), neurotrophin (NT)-3, and NT-4 (47) have also been identified in the lacrimal gland. Although multiple growth factors have been detected in the lacrimal gland, the EGF family of growth factors has been the most thoroughly characterized and the best studied.

The EGF family of growth factors consists of 11 members (28). These factors have a short cytoplasmic tail, a transmembrane domain, and an ectodomain with a single, 40 to 45 amino acid motif (6 kD) known as the EGF-like domain (28). The EGF family members are synthesized as transmembrane precursor molecules that are proteolytically cleaved to release soluble, mature growth factors. Unlike most other growth factors and biologically active peptides, both the membrane-anchored precursor molecules and the proteolytically cleaved forms are biologically active. After being inserted into the plasma membrane, the 170-kD EGF precursor is cleaved to release the ectodomain of 150 kD, known as pro-EGF. Not only is pro-EGF active because it contains the 6-kD EGF motif, it is also soluble, so it can diffuse to interact with neighboring cells. Furthermore, the 6-kD EGF can be released from the pro-EGF by proteolysis (28).

Of the EGF family of growth factors, EGF (6 kD and pro-EGF), transforming growth factor (TGF)-α, heparin binding (HB)-EGF, and heregulin have been identified in the lacrimal gland. EGF precursor mRNA, EGF precursor protein, and 6-kD EGF protein have all been detected in this gland (28) (112,113). TGF-α mRNA determined by reverse transcriptase polymerase chain reaction (RT-PCR) and protein have been found in the lacrimal gland, but the molecular weight of this growth factor has not been determined (28). HB-EGF and heregulin have been detected in the lacrimal gland by RT-PCR (28) (112).

In most tissues, the precursor form of EGF is inserted into the cell membrane. This form of EGF accumulates on the cell surface until a proteolytic process converts it to its soluble form and it is released from the cell surface in a process known as ectodomain shedding (28). The EGF family of growth factors released by ectodomain shedding could play a critical role in the regulation of a variety of functions of the lacrimal gland.

EGF family members bind to specific receptors known as erbB receptors. The erbB family consists of four members: erbB-1 (known as the EGF receptor), erbB-2 (also called HER2 or neu), erbB-3, and erbB-4. These receptors are tyrosine kinases consisting of an extracellular ligand-binding domain and an intracellular kinase domain (28). EGF family members bind to the extracellular domain inducing homo- and heterodimerization of the erbB receptors activating the intrinsic tyrosine kinase activity of the receptors and recruitment of adapter proteins. This receptor binding initiates a signaling pathway that culminates in the activation of a biologic process. Upon ligand binding erbB receptors can form 10 different homo- and heterodimers. These dimers have differential ligands, adapter proteins, biologic responses, and potency (28). All four erbB receptors were detected in the lacrimal gland by Western blot analysis (48) (Chen and Dartt, unpublished data).

After members of the EGF family of ligands bind to their receptors, the activated receptors phosphorylate each other on multiple tyrosine residues located within the cytoplasmic domain of the receptor (Fig. 27-11) (28). The phosphorylated tyrosine residues act as docking sites for adapter molecules that activate the three major, downstream signaling pathways: p44/p42 mitogen activated protein kinase (MAPK) or extracellular regulated kinase (ERK)-1 and -2, phosphoinositide-3 kinase (PI-3K), or PLC-γ (28). To stimulate the MAPK pathway, the adapter proteins Shc and Grb2 are recruited to the phosphorylated erbB receptors and are also tyrosine phosphorylated. This attracts SOS to Grb2. SOS catalyzes the exchange of guanosine diphosphate (GDP) for guanosine triphosphate (GTP) on Ras to activate it. Ras induces a cascade of serine-threonine kinases including Raf (MAPK kinase kinase), MEK (MAPK kinase), and MAPK. Activated MAPK translocates to the nucleus where it stimulates transcription factors to cause gene expression that can stimulate long-term processes such as cell proliferation, migration, differentiation, or apoptosis (28). Activated MAPK can also remain in the cytosol activating other signaling proteins that lead to short-term responses such as protein and electrolyte secretion (28). In the lacrimal gland, EGF binds to erbB receptors to activate the MAPK pathway (49). EGF also tyrosine phosphorylates Shc and Grb2 consistent with activation of this pathway (49) (Fig. 27-11). Other EGF family members, namely TGF-α, heregulin, and HB-EGF also activated MAPK (Chen and Dartt, unpublished data).

Binding of EGF family members to erbB receptors also activates PI-3K. This lipid kinase phosphorylates several lipids including phosphatidylinositol 4,5-bisphosphate, which is phosphorylated to produce phosphatidylinositol 3,4,5-trisphosphate. Phosphatidylinositol 3,4,5-trisphosphate production activates some PKC isoforms and Akt (also known as PKB). EGF does not use PI-3K to stimulate lacrimal gland protein secretion, as PI-3K inhibitors did not alter EGF-stimulated secretion (Fig. 27-8) (50). Activation of MAPK by EGF does not stimulate lacrimal gland secretion, as MEK inhibitors did not decrease EGF-stimulated secretion (Fig. 27-11).

The third signaling pathway activated by EGF family members is the PLC-γ pathway, which is similar to the PLC-β pathway activated by G-protein linked agonists. Activation of PLC-γ increases the $[Ca^{2+}]_i$ via IP_3 production and activates PKC by DAG production. In the lacrimal gland, EGF activates PLC as it increases the

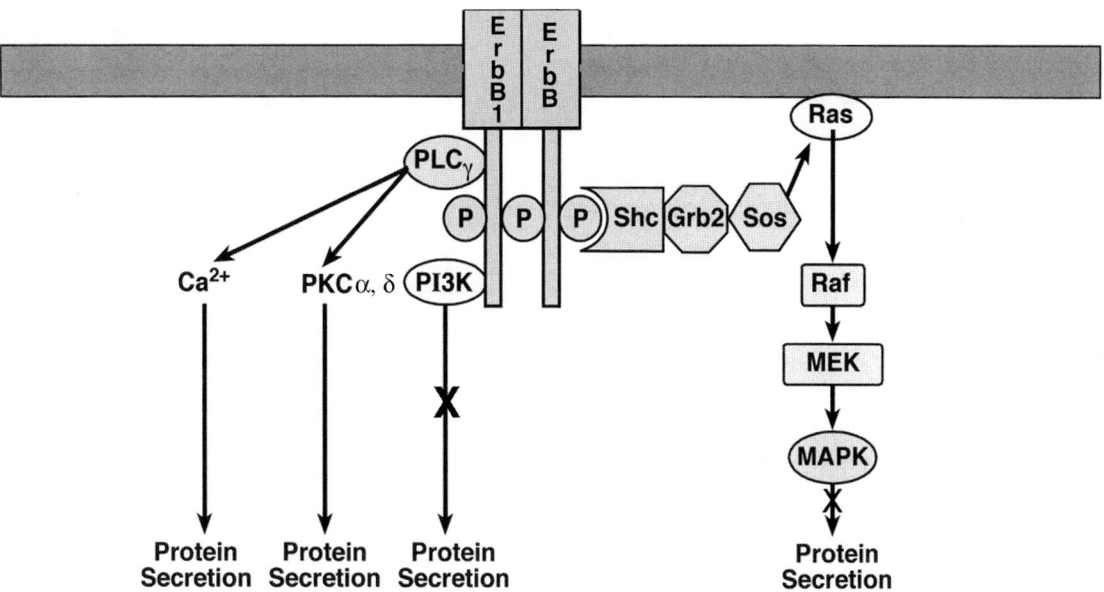

EGF

FIGURE 27-11. Schematic drawing of the signal transduction pathways activated by EGF in the lacrimal gland. Signal transduction pathways activated by EGF to stimulate protein secretion. ErbB1, the EGF receptor; ErbB, the EGF family of growth factor receptors; PLC, phospholipase C; PI₃K, phosphoinositide-3 kinase; P, phosphorylated tyrosine residue on the EGF receptor; raf, mitogen-activated protein kinase kinase kinase; MEK, mitogen-activated protein kinase kinase; MAPK, p44/p42 mitogen-activated protein kinase; PKC, protein kinase C. (From Hodges and Dartt. Regulatory pathways in lacrimal gland epithelium. *Int Rev Cytol* 2003;231:129–196.)

$[Ca^{2+}]_i$ to about one third the level of the cholinergic agonists (50) (Fig. 27-11). Chelation of Ca^{2+} blocked EGF-stimulated secretion as did downregulation of PKC by overnight incubation with phorbol esters implicating PLC-γ in EGF-stimulated secretion (50).

Crosstalk Between EGF- and Cholinergic- and α₁-Adrenergic Stimulated Signaling Pathways

The signaling pathways activated by the EGF family of growth factors and the G protein—linked agonists neurotransmitters are separate and distinct, but they can interact and have functional consequences (51). In the lacrimal gland, cholinergic and _₁-adrenergic agonists stimulate the EGF-dependent signaling pathway, which attenuates protein secretion stimulated by these two agonists (28). Use of an inhibitor of the MAPK pathway increased secretion stimulated by the cholinergic agonist carbachol and the α₁-adrenergic agonist phenylephrine. Consistent with cholinergic and α₁-adrenergic agonists using different G protein-linked pathways to stimulate secretion, they also use different mechanisms to interact with the EGF-dependent pathway (49). Cholinergic agonists, using PLC-β, increase the $[Ca^{2+}]_i$, and activate PKC. These two mediators increase MAPK activity and activate two nonreceptor tyrosine kinases, Pyk2 and Src, the former of which is Ca^{2+}-dependent (49). Carbachol caused phosphorylation of Pyk2 and Src in a time-dependent manner. By stimulating tyrosine phosphorylation, Pyk2 and Src activate a step in the EGF signaling pathway distal to the recruitment of Shc and Grb2 by the activated EGF receptor (Fig. 27-8).

α₁-Adrenergic agonists use a different mechanism to activate the EGF-dependent pathway (49). The α₁-adrenergic agonist phenylephrine does not activate Pyk2 or Src. Instead, phenylephrine transactivates the EGF receptor and phosphorylates it (Fig. 27-9). The mechanism by which phenylephrine transactivates the EGF receptor is not known, but might involve the stimulation of a metalloproteinase to cleave a membrane-bound EGF precursor. This releases EGF, which is then free to bind to the EGF receptor. Activation of the EGF receptor results in an increase in the amount of tyrosine phosphorylated Shc and Grb2 stimulating the remainder of the EGF-dependent pathway. The role of Ca^{2+} and PKC in the transactivation of the EGF receptor by α₁-adrenergic agonists has yet to be investigated.

If α₁-adrenergic agonist transactivation of the EGF receptor is mediated by ectodomain shedding of one the EGF family members leading to activation of MAPK and inhibition of secretion, the fact that the EGF itself can stimulate protein secretion seems contradictory. EGF itself stimulates protein secretion by a Ca^{2+}/PKC-dependent

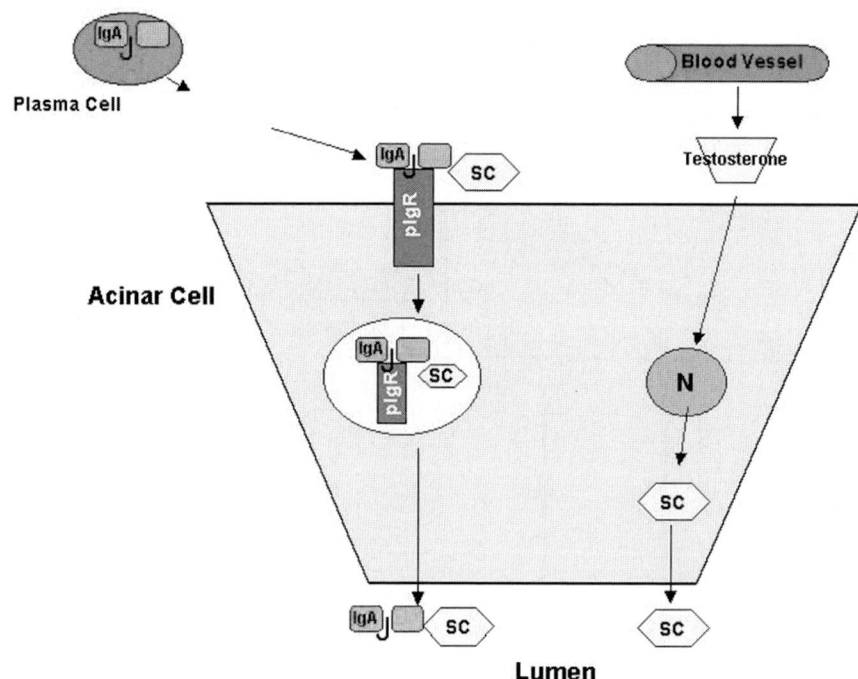

FIGURE 27-12. Schematic drawing of the signal transduction pathway for secretion of secretory component. Signal transduction pathway used to for the constitutively secreted protein, secretory component (SC). IgA, immunoglobulin A; J, J chain of immunoglobulin; pIgR, polymeric IgA receptor; N, nucleus. (Modified from Dartt DA and Sullivan DA. Wetting of the ocular surface. In: Albert D, Jakobiec F, eds. *Principals and practices of ophthalmology.* Philadelphia: WB Saunders, 1994, 1043–1049.)

pathway, but α_1-adrenergic agonist stimulation leads to inhibition of protein secretion by a MAPK-dependent pathway. This could be explained if activation of the EGF receptor by EGF phosphorylates distinct tyrosine residues, which then recruit different adapter proteins than those recruited occur during the transactivation of the receptor by α_1-adrenergic agonists. The molecular mechanism underlying the differential recruitment of adapter proteins to the EGF receptor remains unknown in the lacrimal gland.

Constitutive Protein Secretion and its Regulation by Androgens

Proteins secreted via the constitutive pathway are secreted shortly after synthesis and are not stored in secretory vesicles. Thus, regulation of their secretion occurs at the level of gene transcription and translation. Secretion of SIgA and SC are the best-studied examples of this type of secretory process (Fig. 27-12). SIgA consists of polymeric IgA and a J chain coupled to SC. IgA and the J chain are synthesized by the plasma cells present in the lacrimal gland, whereas the acinar and ductal cells synthesize SC. SC, which is synthesized as a precursor termed polymeric immunoglobulin (pIg) receptor, is inserted into the basolateral membrane of the acinar cell. Once IgA is bound to the pIg receptor, the complex is endocytosed and sorted directly to the apical membrane, where the vesicles fuse releasing SIgA into the

lumen to mix with the other secretory products. Androgens such as dihydrotestosterone increase synthesis and secretion of SC and are major regulators of this pathway. Androgens appear to regulate this secretion via diffusion of androgens to the nucleus where they bind to specific receptors, which interact with regulatory region on the SC gene (52).

Mechanism of Electrolyte and Water Secretion and its Control

Electrolyte and water secretion is regulated by activation of the ion channels and transport proteins located in the basolateral membranes (53). An increase in either $[Ca^{2+}]_i$ or cellular cAMP levels activates K^+ channels (BK channels) (Fig. 27-13) (53). The increase in $[Ca^{2+}]_i$ also activates Cl^- channels in the apical membranes. A Ca^{2+}-dependent K^+ channel in the apical membranes has also been identified. An increased $[Ca^{2+}]_i$ or cAMP causes Cl^- and K^+ efflux from acinar cells into the lumen. K^+ exits the cells into the extracellular space through activation of Ca^{2+} dependent channels and the $Na^+/K^+/Cl^-$ cotransporter (NKCC). This causes a negative potential difference that drives cations, especially Na^+, into the lumen. Secretion of water through aquaporins follows. The NKCC, Cl^-/HCO_3^- exchangers, and Na^+/H^+ exchangers in the basolateral membranes are then activated to replace the intracellular Cl^- that exited

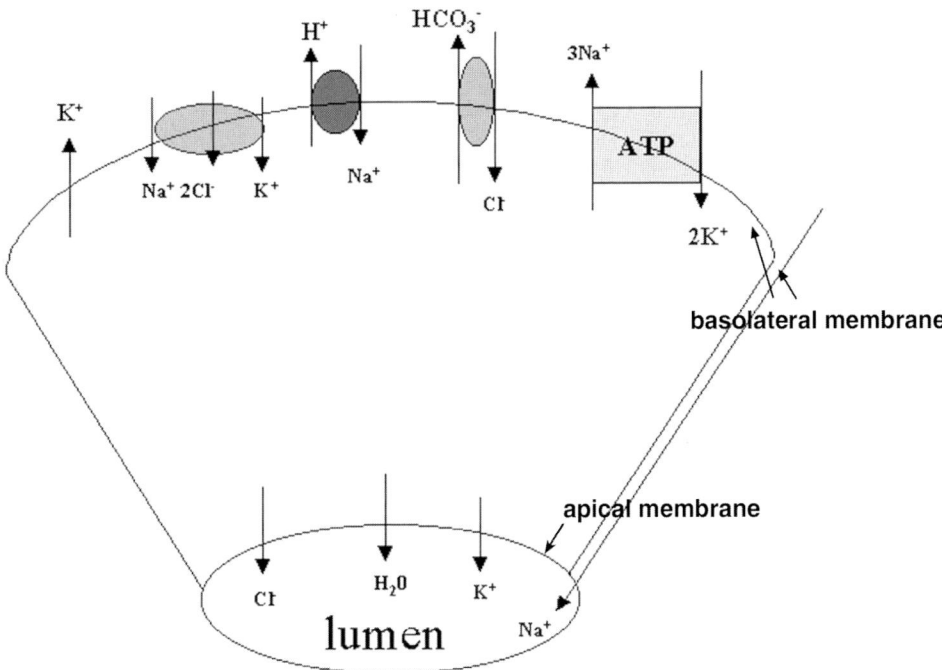

FIGURE 27-13. Schematic drawing of fluid secretion by rat lacrimal gland. Receptor activation stimulates K^+ channels that extrude K^+ across the basolateral membrane and Cl^- and K^+ across the apical membrane into the lumen. Water then follows. Movement of Cl^- into the lumen drives cations from paracellular spaces into the lumen. Because of the decreased cellular concentrations of K^+ and Cl^-, the $Na^+/K^+/2\ Cl^-$ cotransporter becomes active to replace intracellular K^+ and Cl^-. The Na^+/H^+ exchanger becomes active to extrude H^+. The Cl^-/HCO_3^- exchanger drives Cl^- uptake. Na^+-K^+ adenosine triphosphatase (ATPase) becomes active to extrude Na^+ and cause K^+ reuptake. (From Hodges and Dartt. Regulatory pathways in lacrimal gland epithelium. *Int Rev Cytol* 2003;231:129–196.)

the cell through the apical membrane. The increase in the intracellular Na^+ from the NKCC and Na^+/H^+ exchanger activity triggers the Na^+/K^+–adenosine triphosphatase (ATPase) in the basolateral membrane to extrude Na^+ from the cell and take up K^+. Cellular carbonic anhydrase replaces the H^+ and HCO_3^- extruded from the cell by the Cl^-/HCO_3^- and Na^+/H^+ exchangers. The net result of activation of these processes is the secretion of an isotonic fluid featuring Na^+, K^+, Cl^-, and HCO_3^- (Fig. 27-13).

Accessory Lacrimal Glands

Accessory lacrimal glands are located within the conjunctival epithelium and are about one tenth the size of the main lacrimal gland. The number of accessory lacrimal glands present in the human conjunctiva ranges from fewer than six in the inferior conjunctiva to as many as 42 in the superior conjunctiva. These glands contribute to the aqueous layer of the tear film by secreting proteins, water, and electrolytes.

The accessory lacrimal glands are very similar to the main lacrimal gland in that acinar cells, connected via tight junctions, surround a lumen. Multiple ducts run through the epithelium to empty onto the inner surface of the eyelid (Fig. 27-14) (54). Accessory lacrimal glands are innervated with nerve endings that morphologically appear to

be parasympathetic nerves with few sympathetic nerves (55). The presence of nerves implies that secretion from accessory lacrimal glands is regulated, similar to that of the main lacrimal gland. Indirect evidence also supports this hypothesis. Fluid secretion stimulated by topical application of cAMP analogs onto the cornea of a dry eye rabbit, in which the harderian and nictitans glands were removed and the main lacrimal gland excretory duct was blocked, was not inhibited by a topical anesthetic. This evidence suggests that activation of a cAMP-dependent pathway stimulates accessory lacrimal gland secretion. Many of the components of the aqueous layer secreted by the accessory lacrimal glands are also secreted by the main lacrimal gland. In fact, it has been shown that secretion from accessory lacrimal glands is sufficient to maintain a healthy, stable tear film after removal of the main lacrimal gland (56). These data have altered the original hypothesis that the accessory lacrimal glands contribute only to basal tears.

Corneal Epithelium

The corneal epithelium is a possible source of water and electrolytes secreted into the tears, though its contribution is minor compared to the main lacrimal gland. The apical layers of the corneal epithelium consist of three to four

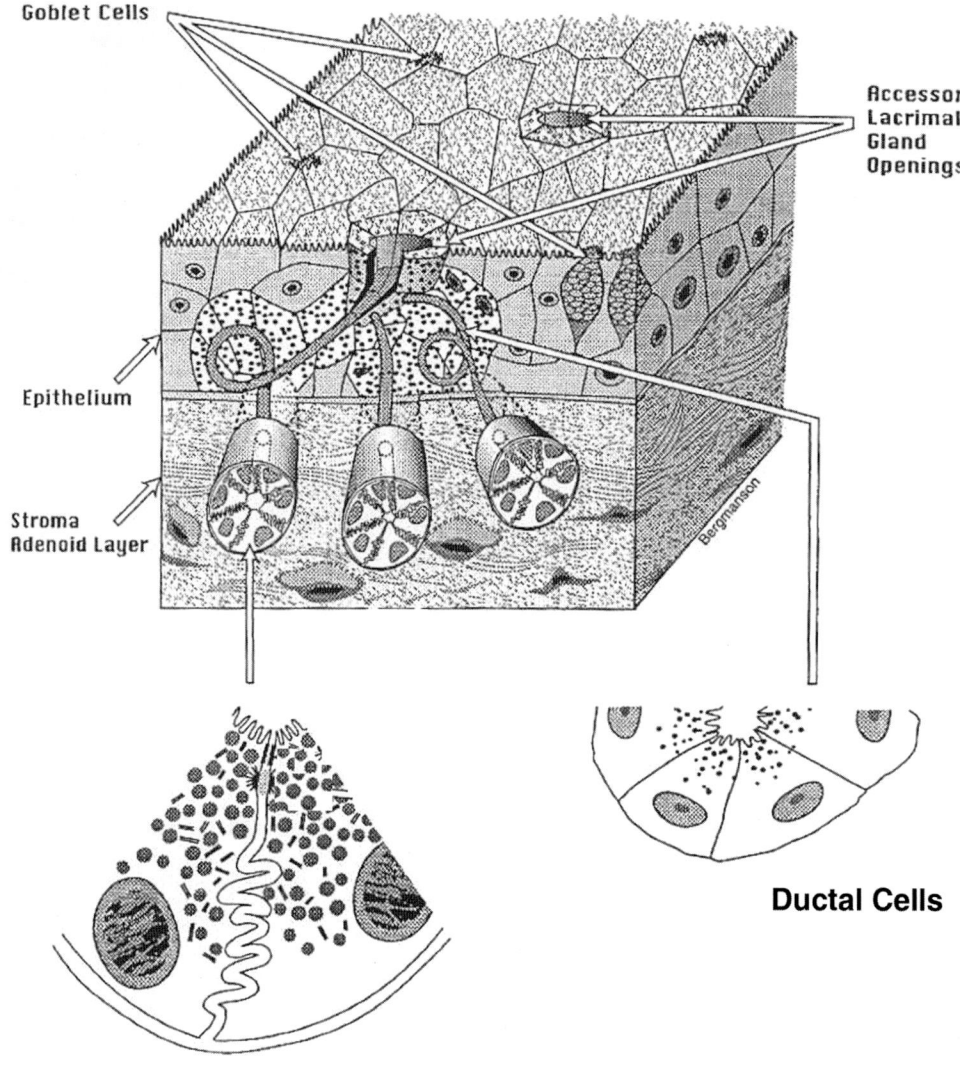

Acinar Cells

Ductal Cells

FIGURE 27-14. Schematic drawing of accessory lacrimal glands. Cross-sectional drawing of accessory lacrimal glands in the conjunctiva and their proposed excretory ductal system. (From Bergmanson JP, Doughty MJ, Blocker Y. The acinar and ductal organisation of the tarsal accessory lacrimal gland of Wolfring in rabbit eyelid. *Exp Eye Res* 1999;68:411–421.)

flattened stratified squamous cells. The midepithelial cell layer consists of one to three wing cells. At the bottom of the corneal epithelium is a single layer of columnar basal cells. A basement membrane and stroma are attached to the epithelium through hemidesmosomes (57).

Sensory nerves, containing substance P, CGRP, and gallanin, are present in the cornea in great abundance and a small number of sympathetic nerves. Sympathetic nerves are the main regulators of Na^+, Cl^-, and water secretion from the cornea via the release of the neurotransmitter norepinephrine (58). Norepinephrine binds to and activates primarily to β-adrenergic receptors though minor amount of secretion can also be attributed to α_1-adrenergic receptors.

β-Adrenergic receptors are located on the apical membranes of cells to activate the cAMP-dependent pathway via adenylate cyclase and increasing cAMP concentrations, as described for the lacrimal gland. The Na^+, Cl^-, and water transport mechanisms are present in the basolateral membranes. Cl^- secretion into tears occurs through channels located on the apical membrane, whereas water and Na^+ enter the tears through a paracellular pathway.

Conjunctival Epithelium

The human conjunctiva occupies 17 times more surface area than the cornea and thus is potentially a more significant source of electrolytes and water in the tear film than the cornea (59). The conjunctiva can modify the aqueous layer in two different ways: it can either secrete or absorb electrolytes and water (60,61). There are two possible sources for the fluid transport across the conjunctiva, the blood vessels and the epithelial cells of the conjunctiva. The blood vessels could contribute fluid to tears by an increase in vascular permeability that would induce plasma to leak into tears. An increase in plasma in tears occurs with pathologic conditions such as inflammation or topical application of drugs that increase vascular permeability. The second source of fluid transport in the conjunctiva is the conjunctival epithelial cells, i.e., the goblet cells and the stratified squamous cells. Under normal conditions, the conjunctival epithelial cells are the primary source of fluid transport in the conjunctiva. For a review of conjunctival fluid secretion see Dartt (62).

The conjunctiva also plays a role in absorption of drugs applied to the ocular surface (63). The conjunctiva is permeable to hydrophobic molecules up to 40 kD (7). The conjunctiva also actively transports drugs using nucleoside, monocarboxylate, dipeptide, and sodium-dependent transporters (64–66). Conjunctival epithelial cells can also absorb compounds by endocytosis (67).

Functional Anatomy of the Conjunctival Epithelium Related to Fluid Transport

As described in Chapter 1, the conjunctival epithelium contains two different cell types, stratified squamous cells and goblet cells. Goblet cells exist in the conjunctiva as single cells or clusters of cells interspersed between stratified squamous cells (Fig. 27-15) Intraepithelial clusters of cells known as the glands of Manz and the crypts of Henle are found in humans (68). Goblet cells are not evenly distributed throughout the conjunctiva. More goblet cell per unit area are found in the fornices compared to the tarsal and bulbar

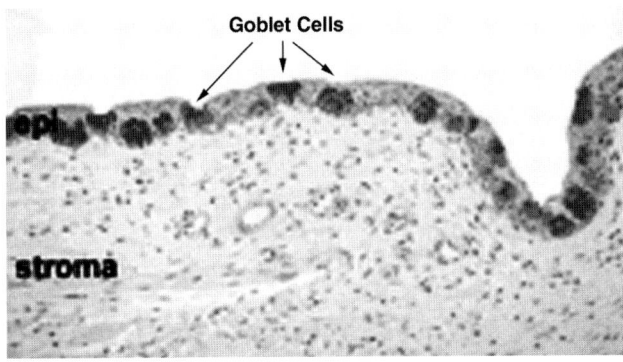

FIGURE 27-15. Histochemical reactivity of conjunctiva to Alcian blue/periodic acid-Schiff's (AB/PAS) reagent. Secretory products present in goblet cells of the conjunctiva reacted positively to AB/PAS, indicating the presence of both acidic (blue) and neutral (pink) glycoconjugates associated with the cells. epi, epithelium. (Magnification ×200.) (From Shatos MA, Rios JD, Tepavcevic V, et al. Isolation, characterization, and propagation of rat conjunctival goblet cells in vitro. Invest Ophthalmol Vis Sci 2001;42:1455–1464.)

conjunctiva, in the inferior compared to superior conjunctiva, and in the nasal compared to temporal conjunctiva (69). This finding complicates study of goblet cell function to be described in a subsequent section. It also has important implications for study of fluid transport by the intact conjunctiva. As no differences in electrolyte secretion were seen when investigators used different areas of the conjunctiva with different proportions of goblet cells, this suggests that goblet cells as well as stratified squamous cells transport electrolytes and water (70,71). Furthermore, ion transporters have been identified on goblet cells as well as on stratified squamous cells (70,71). The development of a cell line of pure goblet cells and stratified squamous cells will now allow the transport functions of these two cell types to be studied separately (9–12).

Sensory, sympathetic, and parasympathetic nerves innervate to conjunctiva (68,72,73). These are unmyelinated nerves that send free nerve endings onto blood vessels and into the epithelium around cells (68). The sensory nerves contain the neurotransmitters substance P, CGRP, and gallanin. Parasympathetic nerves contain acetylcholine and VIP. Sympathetic nerves contains norepinephrine and neuropeptide Y. External stimuli activating the sensory nerves in the cornea and conjunctiva could, by a local neural reflex, stimulate the parasympathetic and sympathetic nerves in the conjunctiva to release their neurotransmitters. These neurotransmitters could then activate conjunctival epithelial cells to increase electrolyte and water transport. Furthermore, irritation of the sensory nerves could cause antidromic release of sensory neurotransmitters from these nerves in the conjunctiva. Differential stimulation of stratified squamous compared to goblet cells could occur as parasympathetic and sympathetic nerve surround goblet cells, but sensory nerves do not (74).

Characterization of Conjunctival Epithelial Cell Electrolyte and Water Transport

Conjunctival fluid secretion into tears predominates over absorption and under basal conditions can account for a large portion of the volume of the tear film (75,76). Secretion of Cl^- and absorption of Na^+ are the ionic movements that drive conjunctival epithelial fluid transport. Cl^- secretion (basolateral to apical movement) accounts for about 60% of the ion transport and Na^+ absorption (apical to basolateral) for about 40% of the ion transport measured under short-circuit conditions (6,77). For Cl^- secretion, Na^+, K^+, and Cl^- enter the cell from the basolateral side using the NKCC transporter located on this membrane (Fig. 27-16) (6,70,77). Cl^- exits the cell through the apical membrane into the tears via a Cl^- channel. Na^+ is pumped out of the cell across the basolateral membrane via the Na^+,K^+-ATPase located there. K^+ exits the cell via a K^+ channel located in the basolateral membrane. Na^+ pumped out of the cell can diffuse into tears through the paracellular pathway as the counterion for Cl^- and maintain electroneu-

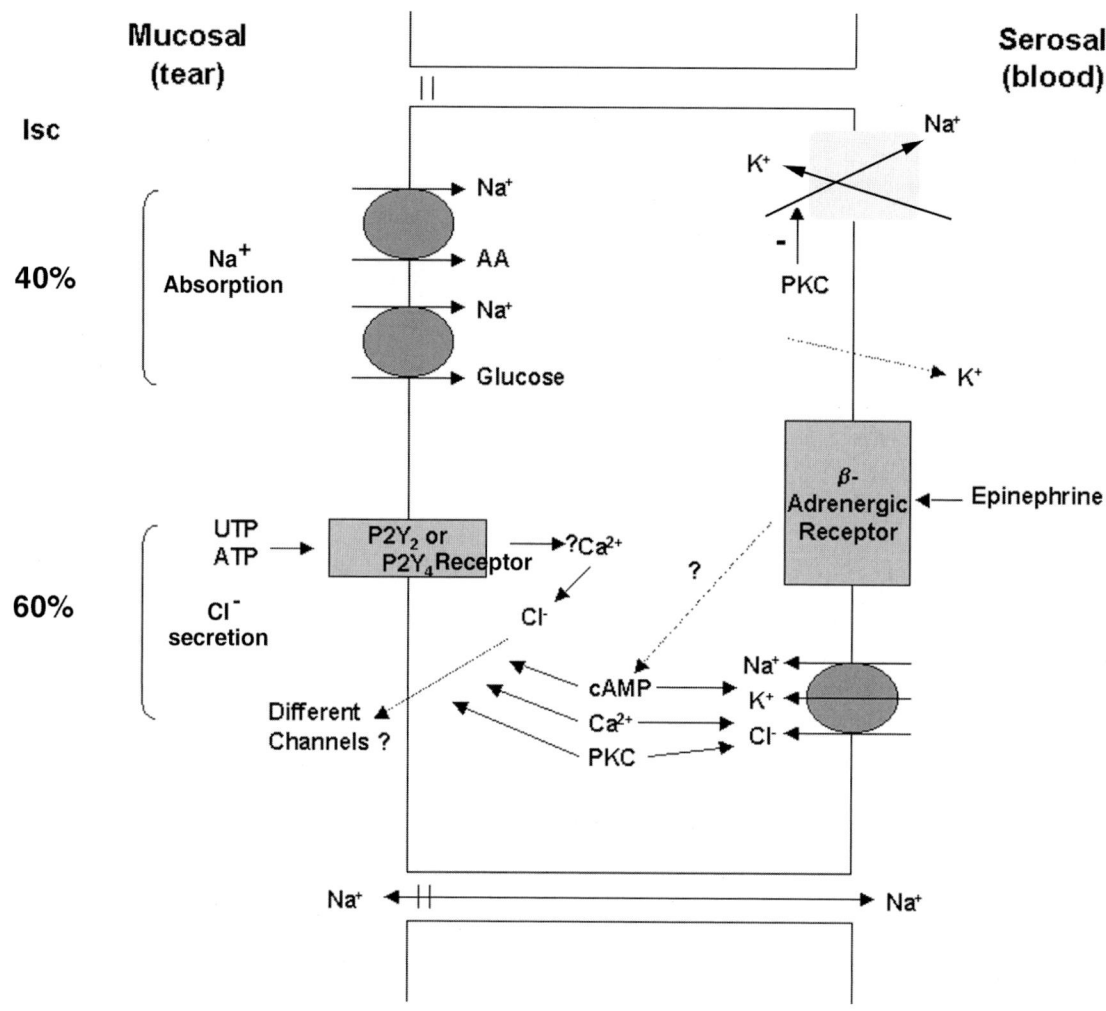

FIGURE 27-16. Schematic representation of ion transport in the conjunctiva. See text for further explanation. (From Dartt DA. Regulation of mucin and fluid secretion by conjunctival epithelial cells. *Prog Retin Eye Res* 2002;21:555–576.)

trality. Water enters tears following the ion movements and by both the paracellular and transcellular pathways, with transcellular fluxes predominating (75,76,78). Transcellular water movement is probably mediated by aquaporin type 3 (79).

The mechanisms responsible for Na^+ absorption have also been studied. The Na^+/H^+ exchanger does not play a role in conjunctival Na^+ absorption (6). In contrast, it is Na^+ coupled-glucose and amino acid–transport that are responsible for Na^+ absorption (7,80–82). These transporters are located on the apical membrane (Fig. 27-16). The Na^+ that enters the cell is pumped out of the cell on the basolateral side by the Na^+,K^+-ATPase located there.

All evidence to date indicates that the conjunctiva both secretes Cl^- and absorbs Na^+. Furthermore, the same cell type is both secretory and absorptive. It is unusual to find a tissue that both secretes and absorbs ions. It is also unique that the same cell type is both secretory and absorptive (70,71). This finding is based on evidence that the Na/glu-

cose transporter SGLUT1, NKCC, and Na^+, K^+-ATPase are all located on conjunctival stratified squamous cells and goblet cells.

Modulation of Conjunctival Epithelial Cell Electrolyte and Water Transport
Several types of neurotransmitters and other agonists can stimulate conjunctival fluid secretion. Release of norepinephrine from sympathetic nerves stimulates Cl^- secretion by activating β_2-adrenergic receptors (6,71,83). Receptors for β-adrenergic agonists have been localized in the mouse, rat, and human conjunctiva (74). All three species have β-adrenergic receptors on the basolateral membranes of conjunctival epithelial cells, although humans have β-, but not β_2-adrenergic receptors. Neither α-adrenergic nor cholinergic agonists stimulate conjunctival fluid secretion (71). α-Adrenergic receptors were not consistently found in the conjunctival epithelium, but, in contrast, several subtypes of muscarinic receptors (activated by cholinergic

agonists) were detected on both stratified squamous and goblet cells. To date only sympathetic nerves using β_2-adrenergic receptors stimulate conjunctival fluid secretion (Fig. 27-16).

Activation of purinergic receptors is another stimulus of conjunctival fluid secretion (75,84,85) (Fig. 27-16). Comparison of the rank order potency of a variety of nucleotides, including UTP and ATP, indicated that $P2Y_2$ or $P2Y_4$ receptors were activated.

In contrast to β_2-adrenergic, P2Y2, or P2Y4 agonists that stimulate conjunctival fluid secretion, serotonin [also known as 5-hydroxytryptamine (5-HT)] inhibits Cl^- secretion (86) (Fig. 27-16). This is an unusual effect of 5-HT as it usually stimulates secretion either by increasing Cl^- secretion or inhibiting Na^+ absorption. In the conjunctiva 5-HT downregulates apical Cl^- and basolateral K^+ channels to inhibit Cl^- secretion.

Signaling Pathways That Stimulate Conjunctival Electrolyte and Water Transport

The signaling pathway activated by β-adrenergic agonists to stimulate conjunctival fluid secretion is cAMP-dependent (6,71,83) (Fig. 27-16). Increasing the cellular cAMP level by activation of adenylyl cyclase, addition of permeable cAMP analogs, or by inhibiting cAMP phosphodiesterase activity stimulates Cl^- secretion. Furthermore, inhibition of adenylyl cyclase or of protein kinase A blocks secretion stimulated by epinephrine.

Activation of another signaling pathway, increasing Ca^{2+} and activating PKC also alters conjunctival electrolyte and water secretion. Shiue et al. (87) found that activation of these pathways gave a transient increase in Cl^- secretion, but Alvarez et al. (88) showed that the PKC effect was in fact followed by sustained decrease in secretion. This decrease was mediated by an inhibition of Na^+, K^+-ATPase.

Sympathetic nerves that release norepinephrine to activate β_2-adrenergic agonists and increase cellular cAMP levels are an important pathway that stimulates conjunctival fluid secretion (Fig. 27-16). 5-HT, which inhibits secretion, is most likely acting by decreasing cAMP levels (86), although there is conflicting evidence about the role of cAMP in this effect. Ca^{2+} is a second possible stimulus of conjunctival fluid secretion, although it is a less effective stimulus than cAMP (87). $P2Y_2$ agonists could potentially work by this signaling pathway. Finally, activation of PKC would inhibit secretion, but agonists that work via this pathway have yet to be identified.

Function of the Aqueous Layer of the Tear Film

The functions of the aqueous layer are extensive and varied. The aqueous layer of the tear film contains electrolytes, proteins, growth factors, and immune components. It is the main source of oxygen for the cornea and contains glucose and many electrolytes that are necessary to maintain optimal

health of the cells of the ocular surface (1). The concentrations of these ions are tightly regulated as a small change in osmolarity can cause significant damage to the ocular surface.

Many of the proteins identified as secreted by the lacrimal gland into the aqueous layer protect the eye by interfering with bacterial, viral, and parasitic adhesion. These proteins include lysozyme, lactoferrin, and peroxidase. Lysozyme destroys cell membranes of bacteria, whereas lactoferrin presumably exerts its antibacterial properties by complexing iron. In addition, lactoferrin may also suppress activation of the classical complement pathway to modulate the ocular inflammatory reactions. Thus the immune component of the aqueous layer is vital to the ocular surface.

The aqueous layer of the tear film also is the source for growth factors necessary for proliferation, migration of cornea and conjunctival epithelium and corneal wound healing. Indeed, many growth factors, including EGF, HB-EGF, KGF, HGF, TGF-α, TGF-β_1, TGF-β_2, interleukin (IL)-1α, IL-1β, and bFGF are all known to be present in tears. In addition, Wilson et al. (29) have shown that the mRNA levels of HGF, KGF, and EGF increase in the lacrimal gland after a corneal wound, implying that the lacrimal gland responds to changes on the ocular surface.

MUCOUS LAYER

Composition

The mucous layer consists of mucins, electrolytes, water, proteins including immunoglobulins, and lipids. This layer is secreted by the goblet cells of the conjunctiva and the stratified squamous cells of the corneal and conjunctival epithelia. The predominant component of this layer is the mucins. Mucins are highly glycosylated glycoproteins whose structure consists of a protein core and complex, heterogeneous side chains of oligosaccharides. Mucins have been classified according to the structure of their protein cores. Almost 20 different mucins, known as MUCs, have been cloned to date as described in chapter 1. Mucins can be either soluble or membrane bound. The soluble mucins can also be gel forming. The gel-forming mucins are large molecular weight molecules that form the scaffold for the mucous layer. They are stored in secretory granules in condensed form and secreted with the appropriate stimulus. Soluble mucins are smaller molecular weight than the gel-forming mucins, but are stored and secreted similarly to them. Membrane-bound mucins are also lower molecular weight than the gel-forming mucins. They have a cytoplasmic tail, transmembrane domain, and extracellular domain. Once synthesized the membrane bound mucins are inserted into cellular membranes and in particular the plasma membrane. These mucins form the glycocalyx of the apical surface of the ocular surface epithelia. Membrane-bound mucins can also become incorporated into the mucin layer when the extracellular domain is cleaved by the action of specific metalloproteases, a process known as ectodomain shedding. One type of membrane-bound mucin, MUC4 or asialoglycoprotein (ASPG), is cleaved intracellularly shortly after synthesis, to form a membrane-bound dimer and soluble portion (89). The soluble portion is stored in secretory granules and released into the tear film as are the gel-forming mucins.

Multiple mucins have been identified in tears and localized to corneal or conjunctival epithelial cells. The gel-forming mucin MUC5AC is secreted by the goblet cells (90). The membrane-bound mucins MUC1, MUC4, and MUC16 are produced in the stratified squamous cells of both the cornea and conjunctiva (91–93). In addition, the cornea and conjunctival epithelia also produce MUC2 and MUC7, other membrane bound mucins (94,95). As goblet cell mucins are secreted by different mechanisms than stratified squamous cell mucins, these two cell types will be discussed separately.

Goblet Cells

Functional Anatomy of Goblet Cells

Goblet cells, dispersed singly or in clusters throughout the conjunctival epithelium, are highly polarized cells (Fig. 27-17). They contain the synthetic enzymes for the unidirec-

tional synthesis and secretion of mucins. Mucins are stored in the apical portion of the cell in secretory granules that completely fill this portion of the cell. Mucin secretion occurs when the secretory granule membrane fuses with other secretory granule membranes and with the apical membrane of the cells. Once secretion has been induced the entire populations of granules in the stimulated cell are released, a mechanism known as apocrine secretion. The goblet cell body remains to resynthesize mucins and secrete again. It should be pointed out that many techniques used to identify goblet cells stain the secretory proteins in the granules. Once goblet cells have secreted, they can no longer be identified by these stains. Studies using this type of technique have the potential to underestimate the number of goblet cells in a given sample.

Regulation of Conjunctival Goblet Cell Secretion

Although the conjunctiva is innervated by sensory, sympathetic, and parasympathetic nerves, many studies suggested that goblet cells were not innervated (62). When care was taken to prevent activation of nerves and subsequent goblet cell secretion before removal of conjunctival tissue, nerves could be identified surrounding conjunctival goblet cells in rats, mice, and humans (74,96,97). Parasympathetic and sympathetic, but not sensory, nerves were detected surrounding conjunctival goblet cells (Fig. 27-18). Evidence that activation of nerves can stimulate conjunctival goblet cell secretion was obtained in rats in vivo. Kessler et al. (98) demonstrated that a strong sensory stimulus to the cornea caused goblet cell secretion in the conjunctiva that was blocked by local anesthetic. This suggests that activation of afferent sensory nerves, by induction of a local reflex,

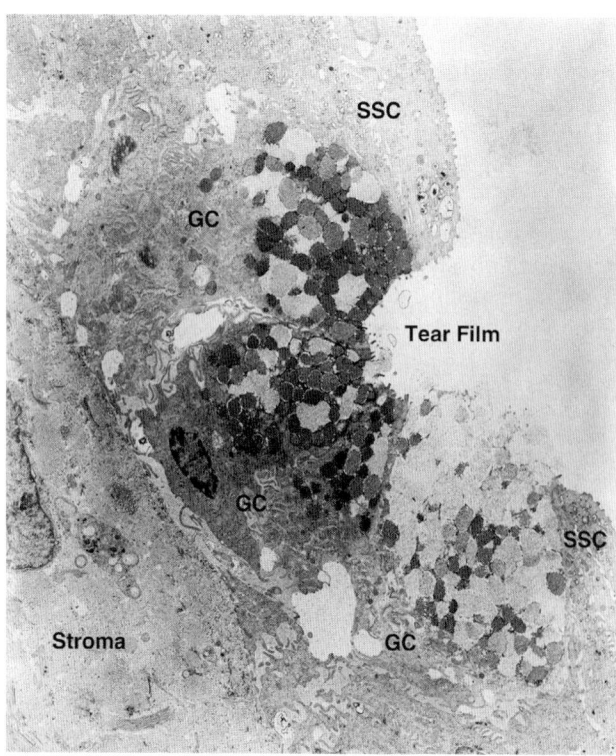

FIGURE 27-17. Electron micrograph of conjunctival goblet cells (GCs). Electron micrograph of a cluster of three goblet cells from rat conjunctiva. A large number of secretory vesicles can be seen filling most of the goblet cells. Goblet cells are surrounded by stratified squamous cells (SSCs). The nucleus can be seen in the lower, basal portion of the cell. (Magnification ×7,500.)

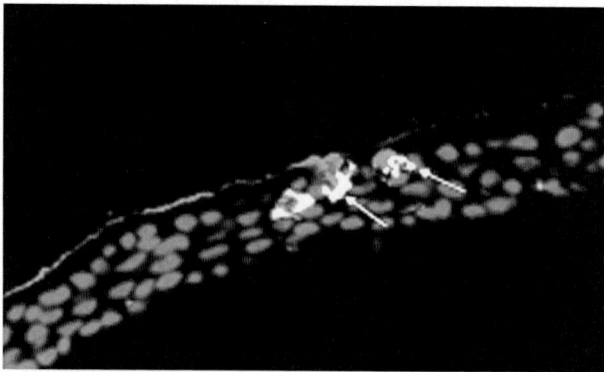

FIGURE 27-18. Immunolocalization of VIP in human goblet cells. Cryosections from human conjunctival biopsy were labeled with an anti-VIP antibody (*green*) to indicated parasympathetic nerves; HPA, *Helix pomatia* agglutin, (*red*) to indicate location of goblet cells and DAPI 4',6-diamidino-z-phenylindole to indicate the nucleus of the cells. Parasympathetic nerves were detected coursing through the conjunctival epithelium and adjacent to or surrounding goblet cells (*arrows*). (Magnification ×380.) (From Rios JD, Forde K, Diebold Y, et al. Development of conjunctival goblet cells and their neuroreceptor subtype expression. *Invest Ophthalmol Vis Sci* 2000;41:2127–2137.)

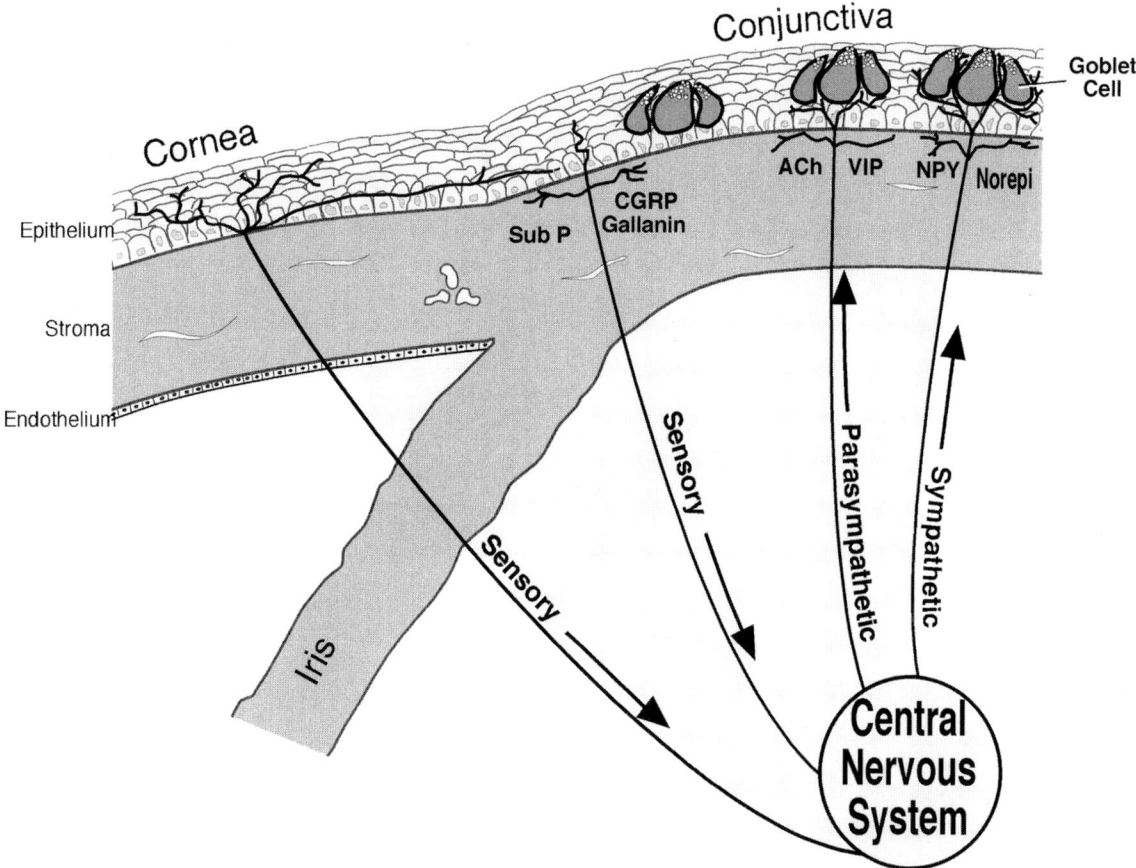

FIGURE 27-19. Schematic representation of neural innervation of conjunctival epithelium. Conjunctival goblet cells are surrounded by parasympathetic and sympathetic nerves, while sensory nerves innervate only stratified squamous cells. The cornea is innervated with sensory nerves, which can activate a neural reflex to stimulate conjunctival goblet cell secretion. (Modified from Dartt DA, McCarthy DM, Mercer HJ, et al. Localization of nerves adjacent to goblet cells in rat conjunctiva. *Curr Eye Res* 1995;14:993–1000.)

stimulates efferent parasympathetic or sympathetic nerves to stimulate secretion of the goblet cells that they surround (Fig. 27-19). Consistent with this hypothesis is the identification of neurotransmitter receptors on goblet cells. The following receptors have been identified on goblet cells: (a) three subtypes of muscarinic receptors (m1, m2, and m3) that are activated by the parasympathetic neurotransmitter acetylcholine, (b) VIP2 receptor that is activated by the parasympathetic neurotransmitter VIP, (c) one subtype of α-adrenergic receptor on human goblet cells that can be activated by the sympathetic neurotransmitter norepinephrine, and (d) three subtypes of β-adrenergic receptor (β1 and β2-adrenergic receptors in mice and rats and β3-adrenergic receptor on human goblet cells) that can also be activated by norepinephrine (74,97). Thus nerves surround goblet cells, stimulate these cells to secrete, and neurotransmitter receptors are present on goblet cells.

Select neurotransmitters can stimulate conjunctival goblet cell secretion. The parasympathetic neurotransmitters acetylcholine and VIP stimulate goblet cell secretion in rat, rabbits, and humans (99–101). In contrast, in unpublished data activators of α- and β-adrenergic receptors and

substance P did not stimulate goblet cell secretion. Thus parasympathetic nerves appear to be a major neural stimulus of conjunctival goblet cell secretion.

Another type of stimulus of goblet cells is the purinergic agonists (102). Nucleotides such as uridine triphosphate (UTP) and adenine triphosphate (ATP) stimulated goblet cell secretion. Determining the rank order of potency of a series of nucleotides implicated $P2Y_2$ receptors in activation of goblet cell secretion. The source of these agonists in the conjunctiva is unknown, but they could be released from nerve endings, platelets, or damaged cells.

Signaling Pathways that Regulate Conjunctival Goblet Cell Secretion

The signaling pathway activated by cholinergic agonists to stimulate goblet cell secretion has been characterized, (Figure 27-20) but that activated by VIP has not. Increasing the intracellular $[Ca^{2+}]$ either by ionomycin or the cholinergic agonist carbachol stimulates goblet cell secretion (101,103). Activation of PKC by phorbol esters also stimulates goblet cell secretion; however, activation of PKC by cholinergic agonists could not be determined as PKC inhibitors themselves stimulated goblet cell secretion (103).

Cholinergic agonists use an additional signaling pathway to stimulate conjunctival goblet cell secretion, that activated by EGF. Cholinergic agonists transactivate the EGF receptor and inhibitors of this process block cholinergic agonist stimulation of goblet cell secretion (104). Cholinergic agonists activate the nonreceptor tyrosine kinases Pyk2 and p60Src that function to transactivate the EGF receptor. Cholinergic agonists stimulate MAPK and inhibitors of the activation of MAPK block secretion. Stimulation of MAPK was dependent on Ca^{2+} and on activation of PKC. Using cultured human and rat goblet cells Horikawa et al. (105) found that cholinergic agonists similarly activated MAPK in both human and rat. Furthermore, EGF receptor as well as two other types of EGF receptors (erbB-2 and erbB-3) are present in the conjunctiva and in conjunctival goblet cells (10,106). A schematic illustrating this signaling pathway is presented in Fig. 27-20.

EGF is not the only growth factor present in the conjunctival goblet cells. Members of the neurotrophin family of growth factors, including HGF, BDNF, NT3, and NT4 as well as their receptors TRK-A, -B, and –C, are present in the conjunctiva. Finally, the vascular endothelial growth factor (VEGF) known as flt-1 was detected in goblet cells (107). Thus a wide variety of growth factors and their receptors are present in goblet cells or in the conjunctiva and could regulate goblet cell or conjunctival function.

Stratified Squamous Cells of the Conjunctiva and Cornea

Regulation of Stratified Squamous Cell Mucin Secretion

The stratified squamous cells of the conjunctiva contain the membrane-bound mucins MUC1 and MUC4. These two

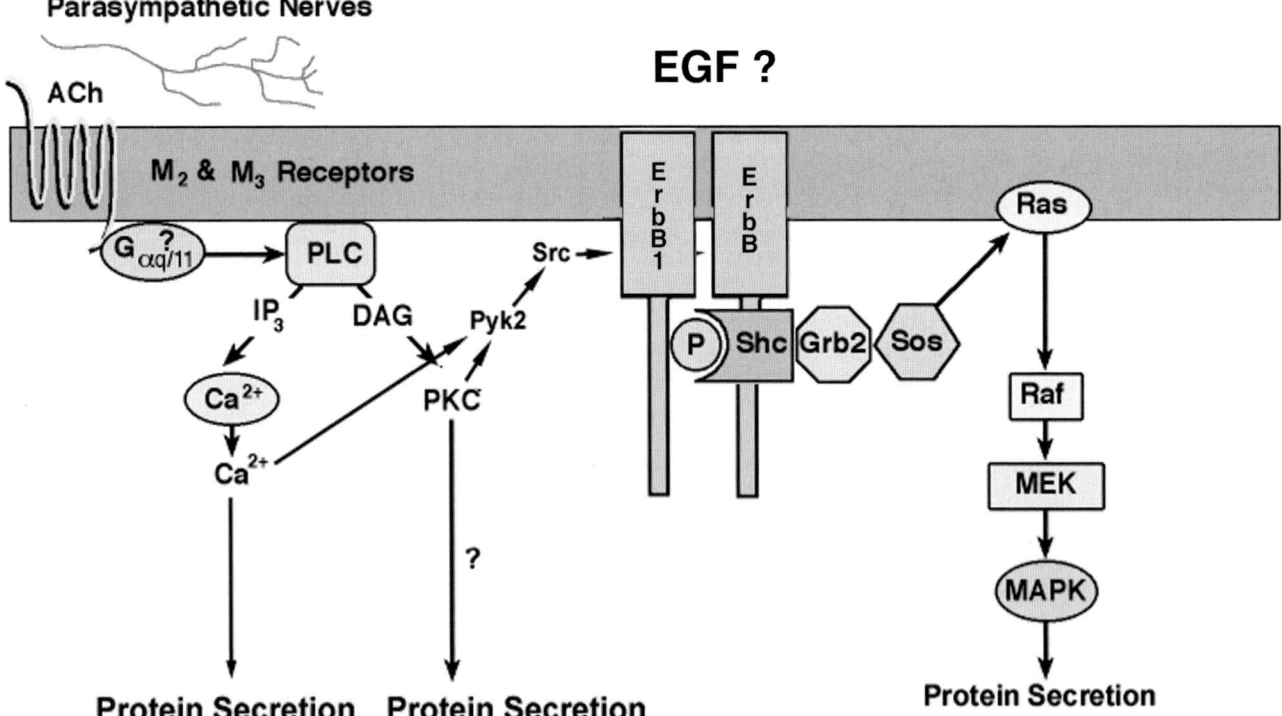

FIGURE 27-20. Schematic representation of signal transduction pathway utilized by cholinergic agonists and EGF in the conjunctival goblet cells. Muscarinic receptors (M_2 and M_3) activate G proteins ($G\alpha_{11}$), which in turn stimulate phospholipase C (PLC). PLC generates the production of the second messengers inositol trisphosphate (IP_3), which causes a rise in the concentration of intracellular Ca^{2+} and diacylglycerol (DAG), which activates protein kinase C (PKC). Both pathways potentially lead to secretion. The increase in Ca^{2+} and activation of PKC stimulated the nonreceptor tyrosine kinases, Pyk2 and Src, to transactivate the EGF receptor (ErbB). EGF binds to its receptor to activate its intrinsic tyrosine kinase activity. This stimulates the recruitment of the adaptor proteins Shc, Grb2, and Sos. This activates the protein kinase cascade of Ras, Raf (mitogen activated protein kinase kinase), MEK (mitogen activated protein kinase kinase), and ultimately p42/p44 MAPK (mitogen activated protein kinase). Activation of either pathway (Ca^{2+}/PKC or MAPK) leads to protein secretion from conjunctival goblet cells. (From Dartt DA. Regulation of mucin and fluid secretion by conjunctival epithelial cells. *Prog Retin Eye Res* 2002;21:555–576.)

mucins are inserted into the plasma membrane and released into the tear film by ectodomain shedding. Little is known about the regulation of release of these mucins. Gamache et al. (108) and Jumblatt et al. (109) showed that the eicosanoid 15(S)-hydroxyeicosatetraenoic acid (HETE) causes increased secretion of MUC1, but not MUC4 or MUC5AC into the tear film. The mucin specificity of the response is intriguing. Further investigation into the regulation of secretion of the membrane-bound mucins is warranted as no additional information has been produced on this subject.

MUC4 is also cleaved intracellularly to form a soluble mucin. MUC4 is likely to be stored in the small translucent vesicles in the stratified squamous cell, but this has yet to be demonstrated. Nerves, peptide hormones, or steroid hormones should regulate secretion of MUC4, but this has not been investigated to date. In fact no evidence on the regulation of soluble MUC4 secretion has been published.

The relative contribution of the goblet cells and stratified squamous cells to the mucin layer is not known. As goblet cells secrete, a gel-forming mucin, and stratified squamous cells secrete membrane-spanning mucins, it has been proposed that the two types of mucins have different roles to play on the ocular surface. Thus it is possible that their secretion is regulated differently, and secretion of either type mucin might depend upon the stimulus.

Functions of the Mucous Layer of the Tear Film

Lying adjacent to the ocular surface epithelia, the mucous layer is the last line of defense for the epithelia that form the anterior portion of the eye. The mucous layer has numerous mechanisms for preventing bacterial, viral, chemical, and mechanical insults. Antibacterial proteins such as defensins, trefoil peptides, and peroxidase are secreted by the conjunctival epithelium (110,111). Mucins contain carbohydrate moieties that mimic the binding sites for bacteria on the ocular surface epithelia (110,111). Bacteria bind to the mucins instead of the epithelial cells and thus are prevented from infecting the ocular surface. Mucus is extremely hydrophilic and thought to coat the ocular surface of the corneal epithelium and thus render it wettable by the aqueous layer. Mucus is also thought to maintain the stability of the tear film between blinks. It may prevent dry spot formation by preventing lipids from diffusing through the aqueous layer to the corneal epithelium.

Role of Tear Secretion in Ocular Surface Health and Disease

The amount and composition of the tear film plays a vital role in the maintenance of a healthy ocular surface. Tears act as a buffer between the external environment and the ocular surface and provide nutrients to these cells. Any change in amount or composition of tears results in diseases of the ocular surface. It appears then that secretion of the components of tears to form a multilayered tear film from numerous sources is tightly controlled and highly coordinated. Due to this complexity, it is not surprising that dry eye syndromes includes a large variety of ocular surface diseases.

ACKNOWLEDGMENTS

This work was funded by National Institutes of Health (NIH) grants EY06177 and EY09057 and Merit Award from Research to Prevent Blindness.

REFERENCES

1. Lamberts DW. Physiology of the tear film. In: Smolin G, Thoft RA, eds. *The cornea.* Boston: Little, Brown, 1994, 439–455.
2. Prydal JI, Artal P, Woon H, et al. Study of human precorneal tear film thickness and structure using laser interferometry. *Invest Ophthalmol Vis Sci* 1992;33:2006–2011.
3. Nichols JJ, King-Smith PE. Thickness of the pre- and post-contact lens tear film measured in vivo by interferometry. *Invest Ophthalmol Vis Sci* 2003;44:68–77.
4. King-Smith PE, Fink BA, Fogt N, et al. The thickness of the human precorneal tear film: evidence from reflection spectra. *Invest Ophthalmol Vis Sci* 2000;41:3348–3359.
5. McCulley JP, Shine WE. Meibomian gland and tear film lipids: structure, function and control. *Adv Exp Med Biol* 2002; 506:373–378.
6. Shi XP, Candia OA. Active sodium and chloride transport across the isolated rabbit conjunctiva. *Curr Eye Res* 1995;14:927–935.
7. Horibe Y, Hosoya K, Kim KJ, et al. Kinetic evidence for Na^+-glucose co-transport in the pigmented rabbit conjunctiva. *Curr Eye Res* 1997;16:1050–1055.
8. Shatos MA, Kano H, Rubin P, et al. Isolation and characterization of human goblet cells in vitro: regulation of proliferation and activation of mitogen-activated protein kinase by EGF and carbachol. *Adv Exp Med Biol* 2002;506:301–305.
9. Shatos MA, Rios JD, Tepavcevic V, et al. Isolation, characterization, and propagation of rat conjunctival goblet cells in vitro. *Invest Ophthalmol Vis Sci* 2001;42:1455–1464.
10. Shatos MA, Rios JD, Horikawa Y, et al. Isolation and characterization of cultured human conjunctival goblet cells. *Invest Ophthalmol Vis Sci* 2003;44:2477–2486.
11. Gipson IK, Spurr-Michaud S, Argueso P, et al. Mucin gene expression in immortalized human corneal-limbal and conjunctival epithelial cell lines. *Invest Ophthalmol Vis Sci* 2003;44:2496–2506.
12. Diebold Y, Calonge M, Fernandez N, et al. Characterization of epithelial primary cultures from human conjunctiva. *Graefes Arch Clin Exp Ophthalmol* 1997;235:268–276.
13. Sumida M, Kutsuna M, Kodama T, et al. Gene expression and fat deposit in primary cultures of rat meibomian gland cells. *Adv Exp Med Biol* 2002;506:489–493.
14. Holly FJ. Formation and rupture of the tear film. *Exp Eye Res* 1973;15:515–525.
15. Doane MG. An instrument for in vivo tear film interferometry. *Optom Vis Sci* 1989;66:383–388.
16. Jester JV, Nicolaides N, Smith RE. Meibomian gland studies: histologic and ultrastructural investigations. *Invest Ophthalmol Vis Sci* 1981;20:537–547.
17. Seifert P, Spitznas M. Immunocytochemical and ultrastructural evaluation of the distribution of nervous tissue and neuropeptides in the meibomian gland. Graefes *Arch Clin Exp Ophthalmol* 1996;234:648–656.

18. Olami Y, Zajicek G, Cogan M, et al. Turnover and migration of meibomian gland cells in rats' eyelids. *Ophthalmic Res* 2001; 33:170–175.

19. LeDoux MS, Zhou Q, Murphy RB, et al. Parasympathetic innervation of the meibomian glands in rats. *Invest Ophthalmol Vis Sci* 2001;42:2434–41.

20. Seifert P, Spitznas M. Vasoactive intestinal polypeptide (VIP) innervation of the human eyelid glands. *Exp Eye Res* 1999;68: 685–692.

21. Chung CW, Tigges M, Stone RA. Peptidergic innervation of the primate meibomian gland. *Invest Ophthalmol Vis Sci* 1996; 37:238–245.

22. Sullivan DA, Yamagami H, Liu M, et al. Sex steroids, the meibomian gland and evaporative dry eye. *Adv Exp Med Biol* 2002;506:389–399.

23. Wickham LA, Gao J, Toda I, et al. Identification of androgen, estrogen and progesterone receptor mRNAs in the eye. *Acta Ophthalmol Scand* 2000;78:146–153.

24. Esmaeli B, Harvey JT, Hewlett B. Immunohistochemical evidence for estrogen receptors in meibomian glands. *Ophthalmology* 2000; 107:180–184.

25. Suzuki T, Sullivan BD, Liu M, et al. Estrogen and progesterone effects on the morphology of the mouse meibomian gland. *Adv Exp Med Biol* 2002;506:483–488.

26. Tiffany JM. Physiological properties of the meibomian glands. *Prog Retin Eye Res* 1995;14:47–74.

27. Zelles T, Boros I, Varga G. Membrane stretch and salivary glands(facts and theories. *Arch Oral Biol* 1999;44:S67–S71.

28. Dartt DA. Regulation of lacrimal gland secretion by neurotransmitters and the EGF family of growth factors. *Exp Eye Res* 2001;73:741–752.

29. Wilson SE, Liang Q, Kim WJ. Lacrimal gland HGF, KGF, and EGF mRNA levels increase after corneal epithelial wounding. *Invest Ophthalmol Vis Sci* 1999;40:2185–2190.

30. Ubels JL, Foley KM, Rismondo V. Retinol secretion by the lacrimal gland. *Invest Ophthalmol Vis Sci* 1986;27: 1261–1268.

31. Lee SY, Ubels JL, Soprano DR. The lacrimal gland synthesizes retinol-binding protein. *Exp Eye Res* 1992;55:163–171.

32. Sanghi S, Kumar R, Lumsden A, et al. cDNA and genomic cloning of lacritin, a novel secretion enhancing factor from the human lacrimal gland. *J Mol Biol* 2001;310:127–139.

33. Sullivan DA. In: Freier S, ed. *The neuroendocrine-immune network.* Boca Raton, FL: CRC Press, 1990:199–238.

34. Dartt DA. Signal transduction and control of lacrimal gland protein secretion: a review. *Curr Eye Res* 1989;8:619–636.

35. Elsas T, Uddman R, Sundler F. Pituitary adenylate cyclase-activating peptide-immunoreactive nerve fibers in the cat eye. *Graefes Arch Clin Exp Ophthalmol* 1996;234:573–580.

36. Lehtosalo J, Uusitalo H, Mahrberg T, et al. Nerve fibers showing immunoreactivities for proenkephalin A-derived peptides in the lacrimal glands of the guinea pig. *Graefes Arch Clin Exp Ophthalmol* 1989;227:455–458.

37. Iwatsuki N, Petersen OH. Membrane potential, resistance, and intercellular communication in the lacrimal gland: effects of acetylcholine and adrenaline. *J Physiol* 1978;275:507–520.

38. Putney JW Jr. *Capacitative calcium entry.* Austin: Landes Bioscience, 1997.

39. Thorig L, Van Haeringen NJ, Timmermans PB, et al. Peroxidase secretion from rat lacrimal gland cells in vitro. I. Alpha-adrenergic stimulation in the absence of alpha-adrenoceptors. *Exp Eye Res* 1983;37:475–483.

40. Dartt DA, Rose PE, Dicker DM, et al. Alpha 1-adrenergic agonist-stimulated protein secretion in rat exorbital lacrimal gland acini. *Exp Eye Res* 1994;58:423–429.

41. Sunahara RK, Dessauer CW, Gilman AG. Complexity and diversity of mammalian adenylyl cyclases. *Annu Rev Pharmacol Toxicol* 1996;36:461–480.

42. Kiechle FL, Malinski T. Nitric oxide. Biochemistry, pathophysiology, and detection. *Am J Clin Pathol* 1993;100:567–575.

43. Ding C, Walcott B, Keyser KT. Neuronal nitric oxide synthase and the autonomic innervation of the mouse lacrimal gland. *Invest Ophthalmol Vis Sci* 2001;42:2789–2794.

44. Cheng SB, Kuchiiwa S, Kuchiiwa T, et al. Presence of neuronal nitric oxide synthase in autonomic and sensory ganglion neurons innervating the lacrimal glands of the cat: an immunofluorescent and retrograde tracer double-labeling study. *J Chem Neuroanat* 2001;22:147–155.

45. Looms DK, Tritsaris K, Dissing S. Nitric oxide-induced signaling in rat lacrimal acinar cells. *Acta Physiol Scand* 2002;174:109–115.

46. Beauregard C, Brandt PC, Chiou GC. Nitric oxide and cyclic GMP-mediated protein secretion from cultured lacrimal gland acinar cells. *J Ocul Pharmacol Ther* 2002;18:429–443.

47. Ghinelli E, Johansson J, Rios JD, et al. Presence and localization of neurotrophins and neurotrophin receptors in rat lacrimal gland. *Invest Ophthalmol Vis Sci* 2003;44:3352–3357.

48. Arango ME, Li P, Komatsu M, et al. Production and localization of Muc4/sialomucin complex and its receptor tyrosine kinase ErbB2 in the rat lacrimal gland. *Invest Ophthalmol Vis Sci* 2001;42:2749–2756.

49. Ota I, Zoukhri D, Hodges RR, et al. {alpha}1-Adrenergic and cholinergic agonists activate MAPK by separate mechanisms to inhibit secretion in lacrimal gland. *Am J Physiol Cell Physiol* 2002;284:C168–C178.

50. Tepavcevic V, Hodges RR, Zoukhri D, et al. Signal transduction pathways used by EGF to stimulate protein secretion in rat lacrimal gland. *Invest Ophthalmol Vis Sci* 2003;44:1075–1081.

51. Luttrell LM. Activation and targeting of mitogen-activated protein kinases by G-protein-coupled receptors. *Can J Physiol Pharmacol* 2002;80:375–382.

52. Sullivan DA. Ocular mucosal immunity. In: Ogra P, Mestecky J, Lamm M, eds. *Mucosal immunology.* Orlando: Academic Press 1998:1241–1281.

53. Dartt DA. Regulation of inositol phosphates, calcium, and protein kinase C in the lacrimal gland. *Prog Retin Eye Res* 1994;13:443–477.

54. Bergmanson JP, Doughty MJ, Blocker Y. The acinar and ductal organisation of the tarsal accessory lacrimal gland of Wolfring in rabbit eyelid. *Exp Eye Res* 1999;68:411–421.

55. Seifert P, Stuppi S, Spitznas M. Distribution pattern of nervous tissue and peptidergic nerve fibers in accessory lacrimal glands. *Curr Eye Res* 1997;16:298–302.

56. Maitchouk DY, Beuerman RW, Ohta T, et al. Tear production after unilateral removal of the main lacrimal gland in squirrel monkeys. *Arch Ophthalmol* 2000;118:246–252.

57. Gipson IK. Anatomy of the conjunctiva, cornea and limbus. In: Smolin G, Thoft RA, eds. *The Cornea.* Boston: Little, Brown, 1994:3–24.

58. Klyce SD, Crosson CE. Transport processes across the rabbit corneal epithelium: a review. *Curr Eye Res* 1985;4:323–331.

59. Watsky MA, Jablonski MM, Edelhauser HF. Comparison of conjunctival and corneal surface areas in rabbit and human. *Curr Eye Res* 1988;7:483–486.

60. Maurice DM. Electrical potential and ion transport across the conjunctiva. *Exp Eye Res* 1973;15:527–532.

61. Hosoya K, Horibe Y, Kim KJ, et al. Na$^+$-dependent L-arginine transport in the pigmented rabbit conjunctiva. *Exp Eye Res* 1997;65:547–553.

62. Dartt DA. Regulation of mucin and fluid secretion by conjunctival epithelial cells. *Prog Retin Eye Res* 2002;21:555–576.

63. Yang JJ, Ueda H, Kim K, et al. Meeting future challenges in topical ocular drug delivery: development of an air-interfaced primary culture of rabbit conjunctival epithelial cells on a permeable support for drug transport studies. *J Control Release* 2000;65:1–11.

64. Basu SK, Haworth IS, Bolger MB, et al. Proton-driven dipeptide uptake in primary cultured rabbit conjunctival epithelial cells. *Invest Ophthalmol Vis Sci* 1998;39:2365–2373.

65. Horibe Y, Hosoya K, Kim KJ, et al. Carrier-mediated transport of monocarboxylate drugs in the pigmented rabbit conjunctiva. *Invest Ophthalmol Vis Sci* 1998;39:1436–1443.

66. Gukasyan HJ, Kannan R, Lee VH, et al. Regulation of L-cystine transport and intracellular GSH level by a nitric oxide donor in primary cultured rabbit conjunctival epithelial cell layers. *Invest Ophthalmol Vis Sci* 2003;44:1202–1210.

67. Steuhl KP. Ultrastructure of the conjunctival epithelium. *Dev Ophthalmol* 1989;19:1–104.

68. Pepper JE, Ghuman T, Gill KS, et al. In: Jeager E, ed. *Duane's foundations of clinical ophthalmology*, vol. 1. Philadelphia: Lippincott Williams & Wilkins, 1996:1–30.

69. Lemp MA. *The dry eye: a comprehensive guide.* Heidelberg, Germany: Springer-Verlag, 1992.

70. Turner HC, Alvarez LJ, Bildin VN, et al. Immunolocalization of Na-K-ATPase, Na-K-Cl and Na-glucose cotransporters in the conjunctival epithelium. *Curr Eye Res* 2000;21:843–850.

71. Turner HC, Alvarez LJ, Candia OA. Cyclic AMP-dependent stimulation of basolateral K^+ conductance in the rabbit conjunctival epithelium. *Exp Eye Res* 2000;70:295–305.

72. Macintosh SR. The innervation of the conjunctiva in monkeys. An electron microscopic and nerve degeneration study. *Graefes Arch Klin Exp Ophthalmol* 1974;192:105–116.

73. Elsas T, Edvinsson L, Sundler F, et al. Neuronal pathways to the rat conjunctiva revealed by retrograde tracing and immunocytochemistry. *Exp Eye Res* 1994;58:117–126.

74. Diebold Y, Rios JD, Hodges RR, et al. Presence of nerves and their receptors in mouse and human conjunctival goblet cells. *Invest Ophthalmol Vis Sci* 2001;42:2270–2282.

75. Li Y, Kuang K, Yerxa B, et al. Rabbit conjunctival epithelium transports fluid, and P2Y2(2) receptor agonists stimulate Cl^- and fluid secretion. *Am J Physiol Cell Physiol* 2001;281:C595–602.

76. Shiue MH, Kulkarni AA, Gukasyan HJ, et al. Pharmacological modulation of fluid secretion in the pigmented rabbit conjunctiva. *Life Sci* 2000;66:L105–111.

77. Kompella UB, Kim KJ, Lee VH. Active chloride transport in the pigmented rabbit conjunctiva. *Curr Eye Res* 1993;12:1041–1048.

78. Zwick E, Daub H, Aoki N, et al. Critical role of calcium-dependent epidermal growth factor receptor transactivation in PC12 cell membrane depolarization and bradykinin signaling. *J Biol Chem* 1997;272:24767–24770.

79. Hamann S, Zeuthen T, La Cour M, et al. Aquaporins in complex tissues: distribution of aquaporins 1-5 in human and rat eye. *Am J Physiol* 1998;274:C1332–1345.

80. Candia OA, Shi XP, Alvarez LJ. Reduction in water permeability of the rabbit conjunctival epithelium by hypotonicity. *Exp Eye Res* 1998;66:615–624.

81. Hosoya K, Kompella UB, Kim KJ, et al. Contribution of Na^+-glucose cotransport to the short-circuit current in the pigmented rabbit conjunctiva. *Curr Eye Res* 1996;15:447–451.

82. Kompella UB, Kim KJ, Shiue MH, et al. Possible existence of Na^+-coupled amino acid transport in the pigmented rabbit conjunctiva. *Life Sci* 1995;57:1427–1431.

83. Kompella UB, Kim KJ, Shiue MH, et al. Cyclic AMP modulation of active ion transport in the pigmented rabbit conjunctiva. *J Ocul Pharmacol Ther* 1996;12:281–287.

84. Hosoya K, Ueda H, Kim KJ, et al. Nucleotide stimulation of Cl^- secretion in the pigmented rabbit conjunctiva. *J Pharmacol Exp Ther* 1999;291:53–59.

85. Murakami T, Fujihara T, Nakamura M, et al. $P2Y_2$ receptor stimulation increases tear fluid secretion in rabbits. *Curr Eye Res* 2000;21:782–787.

86. Alvarez LJ, Turner HC, Zamudio AC, et al. Serotonin-elicited inhibition of Cl^- secretion in the rabbit conjunctival epithelium. *Am J Physiol Cell Physiol* 2001;280:C581–592.

87. Shiue MH, Kim KJ, Lee VH. Modulation of chloride secretion across the pigmented rabbit conjunctiva. *Exp Eye Res* 1998;66:275–282.

88. Alvarez LJ, Candia OA, Turner HC, et al. Phorbol ester modulation of active ion transport across the rabbit conjunctival epithelium. *Exp Eye Res* 1999;69:33–44.

89. Komatsu M, Arango ME, Carraway KL. Synthesis and secretion of Muc4/sialomucin complex: implication of intracellular proteolysis. *Biochem J* 2002;368:41–48.

90. Argueso P, Gipson IK. Epithelial mucins of the ocular surface: structure, biosynthesis and function. *Exp Eye Res* 2001;73:281–289.

91. Argueso P, Spurr-Michaud S, Russo CL, et al. MUC16 mucin is expressed by the human ocular surface epithelia and carries the H185 carbohydrate epitope. *Invest Ophthalmol Vis Sci* 2003;44:2487–2495.

92. Inatomi T, Spurr-Michaud S, Tisdale AS, et al. Human corneal and conjunctival epithelia express MUC1 mucin. *Invest Ophthalmol Vis Sci* 1995;36:1818–1827.

93. Inatomi T, Spurr-Michaud S, Tisdale AS, et al. Expression of secretory mucin genes by human conjunctival epithelia. *Invest Ophthalmol Vis Sci* 1996;37:1684–1692.

94. Jumblatt MM, McKenzie RW, Steele PS, et al. MUC7 expression in the human lacrimal gland and conjunctiva. *Cornea* 2003;22:41–45.

95. McKenzie RW, Jumblatt JE, Jumblatt MM. Quantification of MUC2 and MUC5AC transcripts in human conjunctiva. *Invest Ophthalmol Vis Sci* 2000;41:703–708.

96. Dartt DA, McCarthy DM, Mercer HJ, et al. Localization of nerves adjacent to goblet cells in rat conjunctiva. *Curr Eye Res* 1995;14:993–1000.

97. Rios JD, Forde K, Diebold Y, et al. Development of conjunctival goblet cells and their neuroreceptor subtype expression. *Invest Ophthalmol Vis Sci* 2000;41:2127–2137.

98. Kessler TL, Mercer HJ, Zieske JD, et al. Stimulation of goblet cell mucous secretion by activation of nerves in rat conjunctiva. *Curr Eye Res* 1995;14:985–992.

99. Rios JD, Zoukhri D, Rawe IM, et al. Immunolocalization of muscarinic and VIP receptor subtypes and their role in stimulating goblet cell secretion. *Invest Ophthalmol Vis Sci* 1999;40:1102–1111.

100. Dartt DA, Kessler TL, Chung EH, et al. Vasoactive intestinal peptide-stimulated glycoconjugate secretion from conjunctival goblet cells. *Exp Eye Res* 1996;63:27–34.

101. Jumblatt JE, Jumblatt MM. Detection and quantification of conjunctival mucins. *Adv Exp Med Biol* 1998;438:239–246.

102. Jumblatt JE, Jumblatt MM. Regulation of ocular mucin secretion by P2Y2 nucleotide receptors in rabbit and human conjunctiva. *Exp Eye Res* 1998;67:341–346.

103. Dartt DA, Rios JR, Kanno H, et al. Regulation of conjunctival goblet cell secretion by Ca^{2+} and protein kinase C. *Exp Eye Res* 2000;71:619–628.

104. Kanno H, Horikawa Y, Hodges RR, et al. Cholinergic agonists transactivate the EGFR and stimulate MAPK to induce goblet cell secretion. *Am J Physiol Cell Physiol* 2003;284:C988–C998.

105. Horikawa Y, Shatos MA, Hodges RR, et al. Activation of mitogen-activated protein kinase by cholinergic agonists

and EGF in human compared with rat cultured conjunctival goblet cells. *Invest Ophthalmol Vis Sci* 2003;44:2535–2544.

106. Narawane MA, Lee VH. IGF-I and EGF receptors in the pigmented rabbit bulbar conjunctiva. *Curr Eye Res* 1995;14:905–910.

107. Joussen AM, Poulaki V, Mitsiades N, et al. VEGF-dependent conjunctivalization of the corneal surface. *Invest Ophthalmol Vis Sci* 2003;44:117–123.

108. Gamache DA, Wei ZY, Weimer LK, et al. Corneal protection by the ocular mucin secretagogue 15(S)-HETE in a rabbit model of desiccation-induced corneal defect. *J Ocul Pharmacol Ther* 2002;18:349–361.

109. Jumblatt JE, Cunningham LT, Li Y, et al. Characterization of human ocular mucin secretion mediated by 15(S)-HETE. *Cornea* 2002;21:818–824.

110. McNamara NA, Sack RA, Fleiszig SM. Mucin-bacterial binding assays. *Methods Mol Biol* 2000;125:429–437.

111. Fleiszig SM, Zaidi TS, Pier GB. Mucus and Pseudomonas aeruginosa adherence to the cornea. *Adv Exp Med Biol* 1994;350:359–362.

112. Chen L, Dartt DA. ARVO Abstract #3147, 2002.

113. Marechal H, Jammes H, Rossignol B, Mauduit P. EGF precursor mRNA and membrane-associated EGF precursor protein in rat exorbital lacrimal gland. *Am J Physiol* 1999;276:C734–C746.

114. Ghinelli E, Dartt DA. ARVO Abstract #3773, 2003.

115. Hodges RR, Dartt DA. Regulatory pathways in lacrimal gland epithelium. *Int Rev Cytol* 2003;231:129–196.

116. Dartt DA, Sullivan DA. Wetting of the ocular surface. In: Albert D, Jakobiec F, eds. *Principles and practices of ophthalmology.* Philadelphia: WB Saunders, 1994,1043–1049.

117. Sullivan DA, Sullivan BD, Ullman MD, Rocha EM, Krenzer KL, Cermak JM, Toda I, Doane MG, Evans JE, Wickham LA. Androgen influence on the Meibomian gland. *Invest Ophthalmol Vis Sci* 2000;41:3732–3742.

KERATOCONJUNCTIVITIS SICCA: CLINICAL ASPECTS

ABHA GULATI AND REZA DANA

Keratoconjunctivitis sicca (KCS) or dry-eye syndrome (DES) is composed of a variety of ocular surface disorders of diverse pathogenesis that share, as a common manifestation, signs and symptoms of ocular surface damage (1). According to the "global definition" of DES by the National Eye Institute/Industry Workshop on Clinical Trials in Dry Eyes, dry eye is a disorder of the tear film due to tear deficiency or excessive tear evaporation that causes damage to the interpalpebral ocular surface and is associated with symptoms of ocular discomfort (2). The healthy tear film and ocular surface form a complex and stable system that can lose its equilibrium through numerous disturbing factors. A sufficient quantity of tears, a normal composition of tear film, a normal lid closure, and regular blinking are the factors necessary for maintaining a stable preocular tear film. Disturbance in one or more of these factors leads to an unstable tear film, ocular surface damage, and dry eye disease. Most symptoms in patients with KCS result from an abnormal, nonlubricative ocular surface that increases shear forces under the eyelids, and diminishes the ability of the ocular surface to respond normally to environmental challenges. Increasingly, it has become apparent that KCS is associated with ocular surface inflammation and that the inflammatory component contributes to the symptoms as well as the disease process itself.

KCS is a chronic condition that currently has no cure. Early diagnosis and timely therapy usually helps in averting the complications, which may be severe and if inadequately treated, may lead to severe ocular surface damage and blindness (2). The use of artificial tears, which was the mainstay of therapy for dry eye disease in the past, is mainly palliative, resulting in a reduction of ocular surface eyelid shear forces and some transient symptomatic relief. Antiinflammatory therapies that target one or more of the components of the inflammatory response in dry eye are now increasingly being used in treating signs and symptoms of dry eye. Surgical intervention is required in treating end-stage dry eye disease and for visual rehabilitation in patients with severe corneal surface damage.

EPIDEMIOLOGY

An estimated 2.2 million women aged 55 and older have dry eye disease in the United States (3). In a community study by Jacobsson et al. (4) in Sweden, a prevalence rate of 15% was found among 705 members of the general population aged 55 to 72 years, based on the presence of dry eye symptoms and positive findings on Schirmer test, tear film breakup time, or rose bengal staining.

In the Salisbury Study (5), dry eye was assessed by questionnaire and clinical tests. The questionnaire queried subjects about six symptoms: dryness, grittiness/sandiness, burning, redness, crusting on the eyelashes, and eyes being stuck shut in the morning. Each subject was asked to describe the frequency with which he or she experienced each symptom as being "all of the time," "often," "sometimes," or "rarely." Based on the symptoms alone, a subject was considered to have DES if he or she experienced one of the six symptoms at least "often." In this study, 41% reported no symptoms, 45% reported one or more symptoms at least rarely or sometimes and 14% reported one or more symptoms at least often. According to the Melbourne Visual Impairment Project dry eye sub-study (6), the most commonly reported severe symptom of DES was photophobia.

Clinical dogma has long suggested that DES becomes more common with age, and some evidence suggests an age-related decrease in tear production (7). Schaumberg et al. (3) have summarized data on the relationship of dry eye prevalence with age in the four large epidemiologic studies (5,6,8,9) conducted to date. The results of these studies taken together were most consistent with a trend toward higher prevalence of DES in the older age groups. However, currently no information is available on the incidence, either generally or with regard to age, of dry eye in a population.

It has been observed that DES is more common in women, particularly after menopause. Androgens probably account for many gender-specific differences observed in lacrimal glands of numerous species (10). In the

Melbourne Study (6), women were nearly two times more likely to report severe symptoms of dry eye. In World Health Studies (WHS), 66% to 70% higher prevalence of severe dry eye symptoms or clinically diagnosed DES has been shown among postmenopausal women who use estrogen alone compared to women who never used hormone replacement therapy (11).

Various other factors that have shown statistically significant independent associations are arthritis history, cigarette smoking, caffeine use, thyroid disease, history of gout, and diabetes mellitus (9). Thus, to summarize, DES is a relatively common condition among middle-aged and older adults with higher prevalence among women than men.

ETIOLOGY

The etiology of KCS is multifactorial. Based on the concept of the "lacrimal functional unit" (12), which consists of the ocular surface, main and accessory lacrimal glands, interconnecting nerves, and neuroendocrine factors that regulate the function of these nerves, alterations at any of these levels that may disturb this functional unit can result in KCS.

The preocular tear film that covers the ocular surface consists of three layers. The superficial lipid layer, which is the outermost layer of the tear film, is believed to retard or decrease evaporation of tears. The middle aqueous layer is secreted by the main and accessory lacrimal glands and contains water-soluble factors and electrolytes, and helps to wet the conjunctival and corneal epithelial cells, causes mechanical flushing of debris and organisms, and its constituents help inhibit the growth of microorganisms on the ocular surface. It also serves as a permeability barrier and is essential for maintaining a smooth and regular optical surface. The deep mucinous layer is composed mainly of glycoproteins (mucin) secreted by goblet cells and epithelial cells of conjunctiva and cornea. It helps in lowering the surface tension of tears, thus enhancing its spreading and stability. Thus, integrity of the tear film can be affected by disorders involving epithelial cells, goblet cells, meibomian glands, lacrimal gland, and neuronal innervation.

Because the preocular tear film and the ocular surface exist in a state of equilibrium, broadly speaking, all those conditions that may directly or indirectly influence tear secretion or evaporation can result in an unstable tear film, ocular surface damage, and dry eye disease. For classification purposes, KCS is classified into (a) lacrimal- or tear-deficient dry eye, and (b) evaporative dry eye (2). However, in clinical practice, KCS is often seen as a combination of both tear-deficient and evaporative types. Various causes of KCS are enumerated in Table 28-1.

TABLE 28-1. ETIOLOGICAL CLASSIFICATION OF DRY-EYE SYNDROME

I. Tear-deficient dry eye
  A. Sjögren's syndrome dry eye
    1. Primary Sjögren's syndrome
    2. Secondary Sjögren's syndrome
      a. Rheumatoid arthritis
      b. Systemic lupus erythematosus
      c. Polyarteritis
      d. Wegener's granulomatosis
      e. Systemic sclerosis
      f. Primary biliary cirrhosis
      g. Mixed connective tissue disease
  B. Non-Sjögren's syndrome dry eye
    1. Congenital
      a. Familial dysautonomia (Riley-Day syndrome)
      b. Congenital alacrima
      c. Trigeminal nerve aplasia
      d. Ectodermal dysplasia
    2. Acquired
      a. Injury
        • Trauma
        • Lacrimal gland ablation
      b. Infections
        • Trachoma
        • Mumps
        • HIV
        • Mononucleosis
        • Other infections
      c. Immune mediated
        • Graft-versus-host disease
      d. Lacrimal obstructive
        • Cicatricial pemphigoid*
        • Burns*
        • Stevens-Johnson syndrome*
      e. Lymphoproliferative
        • Lymphoma
        • Leukemia
      f. Reflex hyposecretion
        • Neuropathic-neuroparalytic disorders
        • Contact lens wear
        • Diabetes
        • Aging
        • Corneal surgery
        • Herpetic keratitis
      g. Medications
        • Antihistamines
        • Antimuscarinics
        • Beta-adrenergic blockers
      h. Infiltrative
        • Sarcoidosis
        • Amyloidosis
        • Hemochromatosis
II. Evaporative dry eye
  A. Lipid deficiency
    1. Primary
      a. Absent meibomian glands
      b. Distichiasis
    2. Secondary
      a. Blepharitis
      b. Meibomian gland dysfunction (MGD)
      c. Medications: Accutane
  B. Lid abnormalities
    1. Blink abnormalities
      a. Parkinson's disease

TABLE 28-1. *(Continued)*

          b. Facial nerve palsy
          c. Leprosy
          d. Contact lens wear
       2. Aperture abnormalities
          a. Proptosis
          b. Lagophthalmos
       3. Lid surface abnormalities
          a. Coloboma
          b. Ectropion
          c. Entropion
    C. Ocular surface abnormalities
       1. Vitamin A deficiency
       2. Pterygium
       3. Symblepharon
       4. Scars and nodules

*Associated mucin deficiency.

Tear-Deficient Dry Eye

The aqueous layer forms the greatest bulk of the precorneal tear film. Aqueous tears are produced in the main lacrimal glands, with a lesser contribution from the accessory glands of Wolfring and Krause. Abnormalities of stimulation of tear secretion, destruction of lacrimal gland and accessory lacrimal glands, or scarring or occlusion of lacrimal gland secretory ducts may be responsible for the aqueous-deficient dry eye. Sjögren's syndrome, which is an immune-mediated disorder and the commonest type of aqueous tear deficient type of dry eye disease (see Chapter 29).

The most severe forms of KCS are due to the destruction, or rarely absence, of the lacrimal gland, and include Sjögren's syndrome, the acquired immune deficiency syndrome (AIDS) (13), graft-versus-host disease (GVHD) (14), and congenital and surgical removal of lacrimal gland. Less severe forms of KCS occur due to abnormalities of the regulation of tear secretion, such as that brought on by aging, alterations in hormone levels (menopause), and systemic medications. Ocular surface diseases such as ocular cicatricial pemphigoid, lichen planus, Stevens-Johnson syndrome, chemical burns, and GVHD can cause KCS through the scarring, narrowing, and obliteration of the lacrimal and accessory lacrimal gland secretory ducts.

Many systemic medications can cause dryness of eyes by altering tear flow and influencing production of natural tear substances, or by penetrating and combining with natural components of the tear film (15). Oral antihistamines, antihypertensives, antiemetics, antidepressants, and diuretics may cause DES (16). Antihistamines have antimuscarinic activity that may affect the aqueous layer by decreasing tear production, and the mucous layer by decreasing mucin output of the conjunctival goblet cells (15). Dry eye associated with long-standing contact lens wear is proposed to be due to decreased corneal sensation and blinking (17). Reduced sensory function facilitates drying by decreasing tear secretion and reducing the blink rate.

A similar mechanism is operative in dry eye following herpes infections and LASIK (18). Neurotrophic keratitis, caused by sensory loss in the distribution of the first division of the fifth cranial nerve, is associated with severe ocular surface disorder, which is also partly due to the loss of the trophic function of the trigeminal nerve.

Evaporative Dry Eye

A well-structured lipid layer of the tear film decreases evaporation of tears from the ocular surface (19) and also prevents the overflow from the aqueous-mucin layer, such as might occur during a blink. Deficiency of the lipid layer permits more rapid evaporation of moisture from the eye surface, and, in the absence of an adequate increase of tear production by the lacrimal glands, gives rise to evaporative form of dry eye (20).

Meibomian gland dysfunction (MGD) is believed to be a predominant cause of evaporative dry eye (21). MGD may result from local pathology (e.g., chronic blepharitis), from dermatologic disease (e.g., ocular rosacea), or from iatrogenic etiology such as drugs including isotretinoin (Accutane). Ocular rosacea produces blepharitis and MGD, which involves chronic inflammation of eyelids and ocular surface, with tear film, conjunctival, and occasional corneal impairment.

One of the most important functions of the lid is to resurface the eye with tears through blinking. Any break in the integrity of the lid or its close apposition to the ocular surface leads to increased tear evaporation and areas of dryness. Lid surface abnormalities including ectropion, entropion, and lid coloboma can cause dry eye due to excessive evaporation. The preocular tear film is dynamic such that it changes continuously and is thinned and disrupted after each blink, and blinking helps resurface and reestablish its integrity. Regular, frequent blinking prevents the formation of dry spots on the surface of the cornea and conjunctiva. Blink disorders such as seen in Parkinson's disease, in which there is infrequent blinking, can cause drying of the ocular surface.

An intact tear film, because it is very thin, is dependent on a smooth, uninterrupted epithelial surface. Any irregularity in the surface will cause an associated irregularity in the tear film. Such an irregular or elevated area will predispose the tear film to break up instantly at that spot, which may be one of the mechanisms involved in dry eye associated with pterygium and also vitamin A deficiency. Increased evaporation of tears can also occur secondary to increased palpebral fissure width. Palpebral fissure width may be large due to heredity, lid surgery, or thyroid eye disease. It has been recognized that tear film evaporation is proportional to the ocular surface area exposed (22). Indeed, increased rates of evaporation from the tear film can increase tear film osmolarity and create dry eye disease independent of abnormalities of aqueous tear secretion.

Combined-Mechanism Dry Eye

It has been seen that aqueous-deficient and evaporative types of dry eye usually occur in conjunction with one another, as lacrimal gland deficiency may often be accompanied by meibomian gland and goblet cell deficiency. For example, cicatricial conjunctival disease may cause dry eye both by occlusion of the lacrimal gland ductules, and by causing lid incongruity, which interferes with tear resurfacing with each blink. Additionally, studies have shown that in patients with Sjögren's syndrome, MGD may contribute to the ocular surface disease in addition to the aqueous tear deficiency (23).

Lack of aqueous tear secretion may predispose to blepharitis as a consequence of increased levels of bacterial flora resulting from decreased levels of tear immunoglobulin A (IgA), lactoferrin, and lysozyme. Blepharitis itself can also lead to abnormalities of meibomian gland secretion as well as disruption of the lipid layer, resultant tear film instability, and increased evaporation (24). Another explanation of the combined mechanism is that prolonged stimulation of enhanced secretion by the lacrimal gland, caused by the chronic increased evaporation of water from tear film, could result in neurogenically induced inflammation to the lacrimal gland itself, slowly transforming an evaporative dry eye into a tear deficient dry eye (20,25).

Mucin Deficiency and Dry Eye

The mucin layer lies immediately above the keratoconjunctival epithelium and plays an important role in helping spread the tear film over the anterior ocular surface and in providing the biophysical properties needed to interface with the hydrophobic epithelial layer of the eye surface. The ocular surface epithelium expresses at least three major mucin genes. In the conjunctiva, goblet cells are responsible for secreting gel-forming mucin MUC5AC, whereas the stratified epithelium produces the cell membrane-spanning mucins MUC1 and MUC4 (26–28).

Pathologies that damage the conjunctiva such as ocular cicatricial pemphigoid, and Stevens-Johnson syndrome, result in mucin deficiency due to loss of goblet cells, thereby causing increase in surface tension, increasing evaporation, ocular surface damage, and dry eye disease.

Alterations in the overall quantity and quality of ocular surface mucins may occur as a result of, as well as lead to, KCS (29,30). It has been suggested that elevated proinflammatory cytokine levels within the tear film, perhaps combined with reduced concentrations of essential lacrimal gland derived factors (i.e., epidermal growth factor, retinol), create an environment in which terminal differentiation of the ocular surface epithelium is impaired (30). As a consequence, the epithelium becomes hyperplastic, displaying increased mitotic activity, and loses the ability to express mature protective surface molecules including

the membrane-spanning mucin, MUC-1, which is secreted by epithelial cells to form the glycocalyx, deficiency of which will lead to an unstable tear film and dry eye disease. We have recently found a significant reduction of the goblet cell–specific mucin MUC5AC in the tears of patients with Sjögren's syndrome, corresponding to a decrease in the RNA transcripts of MUC5AC in the conjunctival epithelium (31). Thus, depletion of goblet cell MUC5AC mucin may be an additional mechanism contributing to tear film instability in Sjögren's syndrome (31).

PATHOGENESIS

Role of Immunity

Clinically significant KCS is associated with a variable degree of ocular surface inflammation characterized by the red eye. The first step in the generation of inflammation is an inciting stimulus, which may lead to expression of proinflammatory cytokines and a variety of other mediators (e.g., chemokines and adhesion factors) that in the aggregate signal the host that the normal physiology and microenvironment have been altered. In response to these signals, the second step in the cascade of events occurs when local (resident) tissue cells activate signal transduction pathways, e.g., NFκB (Nuclear factor Kappa B) that augment or down-modulate these cells' expression of cytokine gene and/or cytokine receptor genes, which in turn dictate the response of these resident cells to paracrine signals in the microenvironment by other cells in close proximity (32). The inflammatory immune response to ocular surface injury may be innate as well as adaptive. Adaptive (acquired) immunity is the more evolved arm of the immune response that is characterized by a delayed, stimulus-specific response. The generation of an adaptive immune response requires activation of local antigen-presenting cells to stimulate T cells (33,34).

Lymphocytic infiltration of the lacrimal gland by T cells has been described in both Sjögren's syndrome (35,36), and non-Sjögren's KCS (37,38). This infiltration is believed to be responsible for the dysfunction and/or destruction of normal secretory function. Immunopathologic studies of the lacrimal gland in patients with Sjögren's syndrome show that the lymphocytic infiltrate primarily consists of CD4+ T cells. Various studies have also shown that conjunctival inflammation is also present in more than 80% of patients with KCS (39,40). Certain proinflammatory cytokines, such as interleukin (IL)-1, IL-6, and tumor necrosis factor-α (TNF-α), have been detected at increased concentration in the tear fluid and conjunctival epithelium of patients with dry eye (41). Ocular rosacea, which is a prominent cause of KCS, has been found to be associated with differential increase in the levels of the proinflammatory cytokine IL-1α in the tear fluid (42), and an overexpression of immune inflammatory markers such as human leukocyte antigen (HLA)-DR and intercellular adhesion molecule-1 (ICAM-1) on conjunctival epithelium (43). All of these factors are thought to act in concert to promote the immunoinflammatory response in the ocular surface seen so commonly in severe DES.

Tear hyperosmolarity has been proposed as a possible mechanism of ocular surface inflammation in both tear-deficient (44) and evaporative forms of dry eye (45). It has been suggested that tear hyperosmolarity, together with the microabrasive effects of blinking in the dry eye state, leads to an upregulation of pro-inflammatory cytokines such as TNF-α, IL-1, and IL-6, which may be the critical intermediaries involved in maintaining and perpetuating the ocular surface inflammation seen in KCS (46). Finally, inflammatory cytokines have been implicated in the regulation of the expression of epithelial mucins (47).

Inflammation of the lacrimal gland and/or ocular surface leads to the anomalous production of secretory growth factors or cytokines that modulate gene expression within the conjunctival and lacrimal epithelium (48), leading to an altered cellular phenotype that can promote immune responsiveness. It has been shown that epithelial cells of the ocular surface or lacrimal glands overexpress major histocompatibility complex (MHC) class II antigens (40,49) in dry eye syndrome. A possible explanation of this phenomenon is that epithelial cells may acquire antigen-presenting capability, and that these immunologically activated epithelial cells may be the target of lymphocytes (49) or that they may directly participate in recruitment of inflammatory cells, thus perpetuating inflammation and immune responsiveness. However, to date, conclusive proof regarding the role of ocular surface epithelial cells in orchestrating T cell–mediated immunity has been lacking.

Role of Neuronal Regulation

The ocular surface is richly innervated, with the cornea having a density of free nerve endings approximately 60 times that of tooth pulp. It is well known that corneal stimulation results in a rapid reflex including immediate blinking, profuse reflex tearing, and withdrawal of the head. Sensory impulses from the cornea and conjunctiva travel via the ophthalmic branch of the trigeminal nerve. Efferent fibers from the pons extend (facial nerve) to the lacrimal gland, where they influence the secretomotor function of the gland (modulation of water and protein transport). The lacrimal gland is also densely innervated with parasympathetic nerves, and to a lesser extent with sympathetic and sensory nerves (50). Accessory lacrimal glands (51) and goblets cells are also innervated (52). Acetylcholine (parasympathetic mediator) acts through muscarinic receptors to stimulate secretion of water, proteins, and electrolytes from the lacrimal glands. Cholinergic stimulation also induces increased concentrations of lactoferrin and epidermal growth factor (EGF) in glandular tissues and

tears. The routes by which the signals from these various systems are transmitted are interconnected and closely related. An abnormality in any one of the steps in this complex cascade is likely to result in overall dysregulation of lacrimal function.

Parasympathetic neural transmission can be inhibited by cytokines (53). Studies by Zoukhri and associates (54) on the mouse model of Sjögren's syndrome led to the hypothesis that the impaired secretory function of lacrimal glands is most likely a functional blockage caused by inflammatory cytokines, either in neurotransmitter release from nerve endings, or in the cellular response to neuromediators, leading in both cases to a denervation-like supersensitivity. Recently, it has been demonstrated that there is upregulation of IL-1β in the lacrimal gland of the mouse model of Sjögren's syndrome, suggesting that proinflammatory cytokines such as IL-1β may be responsible for the impaired secretory function in the exocrine glands, in response to neuronal stimulation, as seen in Sjögren's syndrome (55).

Role of Hormones

There is evidence to support that the eye, like many other tissues, is a target organ for sex hormones, and that these hormones control certain trophic functions and homeostasis of the lacrimal system. The receptors of various steroid hormones have been identified in rat and human ocular tissues, particularly in the lacrimal gland, meibomian glands, conjunctiva, and cornea (56). In addition, messenger RNA (mRNA) for 5α-reductase, the key enzyme involved in the metabolism of androgens to their biologically active derivative 5α-dihydrotestosterone, has been found in these ocular structures (57).

Sex steroids have been implicated in the pathogenesis of Sjögren's syndrome through their action on the immune system (58). The mechanism of androgen action in lacrimal tissue appears to be mediated through hormone interaction with receptors in nuclei of epithelial cells (not lymphocytes) (59), which then leads to alterations in the expression of cytokines, proto-oncogenes, and apoptotic factors (60). These androgen-induced changes include enhancement of levels of transforming growth factor-β (TGF-β), a potent immunomodulatory and antiinflammatory cytokine, and suppression of mRNA content of proinflammatory cytokines (e.g., IL-1β and TNF-α) in the lacrimal glands (10). Moreover, apoptosis has been shown to occur in the lacrimal glands following withdrawal of androgen in the ovariectomized rabbits (61), which has led to the suggestion that these apoptotic fragments may be a source of potential autoantigens and could be subsequently presented by either interstitial antigen-presenting cells or acinar cells to initiate the autoimmune response.

The meibomian gland is also an androgen target organ, and androgens regulate this tissue's lipid profile (62,63).

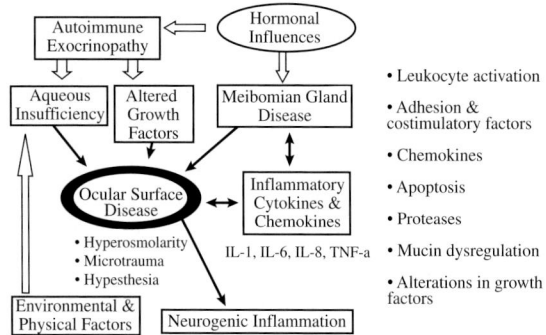

FIGURE 28-1. Paradigm for dry-eye pathogenesis.

Pathogenic Model for Dry Eye

The exact sequence of cellular and molecular events that leads to KCS remains unknown. It is possible that lacrimal dysfunction leads to decrease in tear volume and secretion of trophic factors with resultant ocular surface distress. The ocular surface distress and related hyperosmolarity and microabrasive effect of blinking on a surface that is not adequately protected by the proper mix of tear film constituents (mucins, lipids, etc.) leads to inflammation that can in turn add to the lacrimal insufficiency by affecting accessory lacrimal gland function. With reduced tear secretion, there is decreased tear clearance (64) that results in increased retention of inflammatory cytokines, released into the tear film from the ocular surface epithelium or lacrimal gland (65), thus perpetuating the inflammatory response. Additionally, with inflammation, there is abnormal lipid secretion onto the surface due to changes in the meibomian gland orifices, resulting in decreased tear film stability. Moreover, ocular surface changes as a result of the cytokine microenvironment may lead to relative hypesthesia and changes in blink rate that may in turn amplify the ocular surface disease by increasing exposure, evaporation, and altering the feedback to the lacrimal gland. Such a paradigm is illustrated in Fig. 28-1.

PATHOLOGY

Tears are necessary for the continued health of the ocular surface, maintaining the nonkeratinized surface essential for corneal transparency and lubrication required for movement of the lids on the globe. Morphologically, in KCS the conjunctiva is affected before the cornea is. Initially the conjunctival epithelium appears normal (66), but there is loss of conjunctival goblet cells (67), with subsequent edema in the conjunctival stroma (68). As the disease becomes more advanced, intracellular edema appears, manifested by decreased cytoplasmic density (69). Conjunctival epithelial cells with decreased cytoplasmic density demonstrate blunting and loss of cell surface

microplicae. As fluid moves between superficial conjunctival epithelial cells, there is an increase in conjunctival epithelial cell desquamation (66,68). With time, and as the disease progresses, squamous metaplasia of the conjunctiva develops (70), with further decrease in conjunctival goblet cell density (67), increase in the surface area and flattening of conjunctival epithelial cells (66), and eventually disappearance of intercellular and stromal edema (66).

The cornea is more resistant than the conjunctiva to disease in KCS. The corneal epithelium forms a protective barrier between the environment and underlying ocular structures. Using wide field color specular microscopy, a shift toward smaller superficial corneal epithelial cells has been shown in patients with KCS (71), a reflection of accelerated corneal desquamation.

CLINICAL FEATURES

In spite of their rather diverse origins, the clinical presentation of patients with dry eye diseases is similar. Tear film instability is a component of all forms of dry eye disease, and tear hyperosmolarity is a key mechanism for the ocular surface damage. Aqueous-deficient dry eye is associated with reduced lacrimal function, but lacrimal function may be reduced as part of the aging process without producing the signs or symptoms of dry eye. The various factors to be considered in the diagnosis of KCS are (a) presence or absence of inflammation, (b) assessment of the function of lacrimal tissues, (c) determination of causes that could lead to decreased reflex tearing, (d) assessment of meibomian glands, and (e) environmental factors.

History

The patient's history is extremely important in diagnosing dry-eye syndromes. Symptoms are a hallmark of the disease, and the most frequently encountered symptoms in patients with dry eyes are dryness, foreign-body or sandy sensation, burning, and photophobia. Patients may also complain of itching, excessive mucus secretions, heaviness of the eyelids, tight eyelids, inability to produce tears, pain, and redness. Moreover, as dry eye can coexist with other disorders (e.g., allergy), it is not unusual for patients to have symptoms due to multiple pathogenic mechanisms. The principal function of the tear film is to maintain a smooth, clear, refractive optical surface in a hostile external environment. Any adverse effect on the corneal regularity and clarity will interfere with vision and may cause symptoms. Patients often use the term "dryness" to describe their condition but will have difficulty defining exactly what this means. The term "discomfort" may be a more accurate summation of all the patient's symptoms. Various questionnaires have been developed (72–74) to assess symptoms in dry eye patients. These questionnaires are useful tools for clinical treatment trials in dry eye patients.

Dry eye patients are exquisitely sensitive to drafts and winds. Often they volunteer information regarding their intolerance to air conditioning or driving in the car with the windows down. Patients with KCS feel worse in a dry, cold environment and under conditions of increased evaporation. Reading is often difficult for dry eye sufferers. This probably occurs because the blink frequency decreases during tasks requiring concentration. Patients often complain that nighttime or awakening is the worst part of their day. Sleep (like general anesthesia) decreases tear production. If the eye is already compromised with regard to tear flow, further reduction during sleep may be enough to produce nocturnal symptoms. This is especially true if concurrent blepharitis or lagophthalmos is present. Smoke is almost universally intolerable to tear-deficient patients. Because smoke is actually a suspension of solids in air, the particulate bombardment of the ocular surface produces discomfort. Determining whether symptoms are worse or better indoors or out, at work or at home, will aid in identifying environments that need to be modified to improve the patient's symptoms.

Patients should be asked whether they are able to produce irritant and emotional tears. "Do you get tears when you peel onions? Can you cry when you feel sad or hurt? Affirmative responses suggest some lacrimal gland function remains, whereas negative answers suggest that the lacrimal gland is incapable of secreting tear fluid in response to any stimuli. In patients with KCS, the ability to generate irritant tears is lost before the ability to generate emotional tears.

"What medications do you take?" should also be asked. Systemic antihistaminics, antidepressants, anticholinergics, and diuretics are most responsible for decreased tear production. The use of systemic steroids and other immunosuppressives, such as hydroxychloroquine (Plaquenil), methotrexate, and cyclophosphamide (Cytoxan), which may be used in treating patients with Sjögren's syndrome and other collagen vascular diseases should be noted.

It is important to determine whether the patient has any associated systemic symptoms or diseases. Important questions should be directed toward detecting a history of dry mouth (xerostomia) or dental and gum disease. Patients with Sjögren's syndrome and xerostomia are at greater risk of dental and gum disease owing to lack of saliva. Questions that help in determining whether the patient has significant xerostomia include the following: "Can you feel saliva in your mouth?" "Can you swallow bread or meat without additional fluids?" Women should be asked whether they have experienced a noticeable decrease of vaginal secretions. Patients should be asked if they have ever been told they have Sjögren's syndrome, lupus, rheumatoid arthritis, systemic sclerosis, vasculitis, thyroid disease, lymphoma, or AIDS. If the patient has had a *Bone Marrow Transplant*, a history of rejection or graft-versus-host disease should be noted.

"Do you have any skin problems?" is a question that should always be asked. Although primary dermatologic illness is rarely the cause of dry eye, looking for such illnesses often provides useful clues. Examples are numerous: scleroderma, scurvy, thrombotic thrombocytopenic purpura, the facial rash in lupus (all these are seen in association with Sjögren's syndrome), skin lesions in pemphigoid, old scars from Stevens-Johnson syndrome, and acne rosacea (associated with lipid abnormalities). An equally important reason for exploring skin problems during history taking is to discover entities that may mimic tear deficiency. Many skin disorders are associated with superficial punctate keratopathy and may present a picture that could be confused with sicca. Some of these are seborrheic dermatitis, psoriasis, ichthyosis, and keratosis follicularis (Darier's disease). Family history should be elicited as to whether there is any blood relative with KCS, Sjögren's syndrome, collagen vascular disease, and other eye diseases.

Information should be obtained regarding use of lubricants and medications, including drops as well as ointments. Inquire about these specifically, as most patients will not consider topical treatment when asked generally about medications. "Are the topical lubricants preserved or unpreserved?" "How long have they been used and how often?" Most patients with KCS improve with topical lubricant therapy. The severity of a patient's KCS often can be determined by how frequently topical lubricants are used. Patients with severe KCS use topical lubricants more frequently than those with mild KCS. It is also important to remember that patients with moderate to severe KCS can be made worse by topical lubricants containing preservatives. Furthermore, any topical medication is potentially toxic due to the patient's inability to dilute it because of a lack of aqueous tear secretion. Patients should be asked whether they have had previous placement of temporary collagen plugs or silicone plugs, or whether previous permanent occlusion with laser or cautery has been performed. If so, then one should ask whether there was an improvement in symptoms and whether epiphora occurred.

Physical Examination

Nonocular Examination

A limited physical examination must be done before the eyes are examined. The facial skin must be examined for evidence of acne rosacea and for the malar rash of systemic lupus erythematosus (SLE). The parotid, submandibular, and submaxillary glands should be palpated for the presence of enlargement or masses. Salivary gland enlargement may be seen in patients with Sjögren's syndrome. The thyroid gland is palpated for enlargement and nodules. Thyroid disorders are commonly seen in patients with Sjögren's syndrome and with superior limbic keratitis. Exophthalmos and decreased blinking, which occur in Graves' disease, can cause symptoms and findings of dry eye due to increased evaporation. The mouth is examined for presence or absence of saliva and for oral candidiasis. The tongue is examined for evidence of dryness. The hands are assessed for joint inflammation and changes indicative of rheumatoid arthritis and scleroderma, in which case lacrimal insufficiency may be suspected. Petechial rashes and eczema must be looked for on extremities.

Ocular Examination

In early KCS, the eye may appear to be perfectly normal. Eyelids should be examined for presence and severity of dermatochalasis. Function of the eyelids, completeness of the blink, and blink rate must be assessed. The size of the lacrimal gland is evaluated by asking the patient to look down while the upper eyelid is retracted. Patients with Sjögren's syndrome, leukemia or sarcoidosis may show enlargement of the lacrimal glands.

The most characteristic finding on slit-lamp biomicroscopy examination is abnormality of the inferior tear meniscus. A height of 0.2 to 0.3 mm is most common, found in about 85% of normal subjects (75). Meniscus "floaters" are extremely common in dry eye patients. They can be seen as tiny bits of debris being carried along in the upper and lower tear menisci. These probably have two origins. Some are dead epithelial cells that have fallen off the surface of the cornea, and some are small fibrils of lipid-contaminated mucin. Although almost always present in dry eyes, they are not pathognomonic, because patients with conjunctival infections or blepharitis may also show these.

Mucous strands may be seen in some cases of dry eye syndrome. They are actually strings of lipid-contaminated mucus that have rolled up and been pushed into the cul-de-sac by the shearing action of the lids. Although common in aqueous-deficient states, they can become significant in the mucin-deficient diseases. If the aqueous layer of tears is thick enough to prevent diffusing lipid from contaminating the mucous layer before a blink, or if mucin is available in excess to absorb the lipid molecules before a blink, then mucous strands will not become a problem. On the other hand, if mucin and excess lipid become intermingled, mucous strands form.

Corneal filaments are commonly associated with dry eye conditions. Filaments are short (usually <2 mm long) "tails" that hang from the surface of the cornea (Fig. 28-2). Although the exact pathogenesis of filament formation is not known, it has been proposed that when the cornea dries to a point that is incompatible with a healthy epithelial layer, some surface cells become desiccated and are shed. This creates a small pit on the corneal surface that is hydrophobic compared with the mucus-coated normal surface. Lipid-contaminated mucus will become attached to these pits by hydrophobic bonding. Within a short time, surface epithelium will grow down these mucous cores,

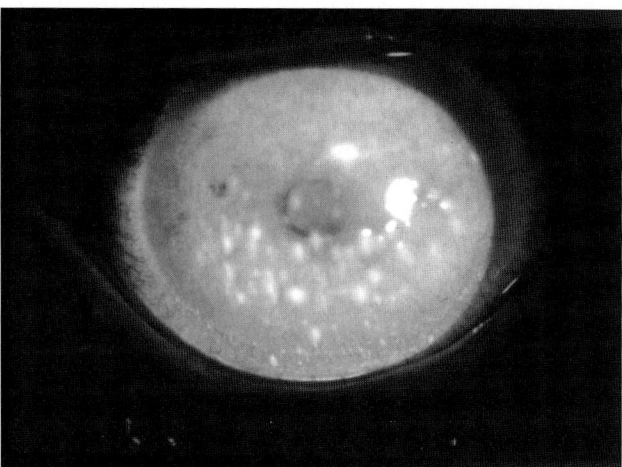

FIGURE 28-2. Filamentary keratopathy. Fluorescein staining of the cornea showing filaments that represent strands of epithelial cells attached to the surface of the cornea over a core of mucus.

and a true filament will thus be born. Because filaments are anchored to epithelial cells, pulling on them can be very painful. Unfortunately, this is exactly what happens during blinking, with the resultant symptoms not unlike those produced by a foreign body.

The eyelid margins should be examined for thickening, telangiectasia, and irregularity, which suggest chronic blepharitis. Broken and missing eyelashes are found in cases of chronic blepharitis. Trichiasis is seen in more severe form of eyelid inflammation. The health of meibomian glands must be assessed. Pouting, plugged, or missing meibomian gland orifices, toothpaste-like thick turbid secretions (Fig. 28-3), or the presence of oil or foam suggests MGD. Segmental inflammation of the posterior eyelid margin is seen in meibomianitis. The bulbar conjunctiva may lose its normal luster and may be thickened, edematous, and hyperemic, or show slight folding inferiorly. Papillary conjunctivitis, which is a nonspecific reaction of the conjunctiva to irritation, may also be seen in dry eye conditions.

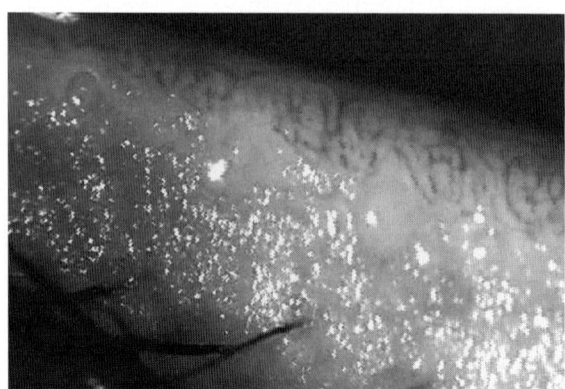

FIGURE 28-3. Meibomian gland dysfunction. Thick turbid secretions expressed at the mouth of meibomian glands.

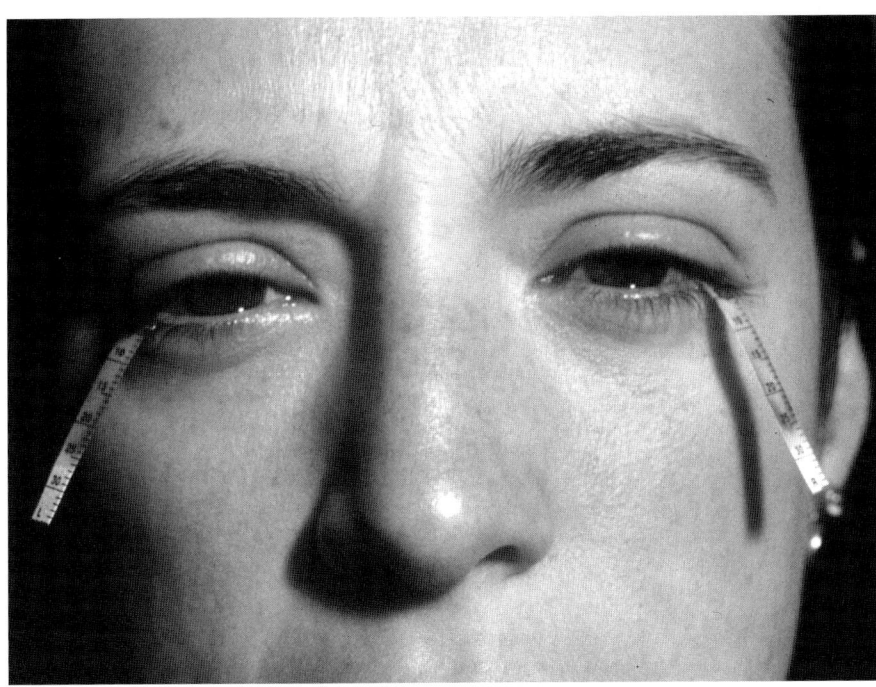

FIGURE 28-4. Schirmer test. The amount of wetting of the paper strip is a measure of tear flow.

Clinical Diagnostic Tests

Measurement of Tear Secretion

Schirmer and Jones's Test

The Schirmer I test without anesthetic is a test of tear secretion in response to conjunctival stimulation and basal, nonreflex secretion (76). It is by far the simplest test for assessing aqueous tear production. Less than 6 mm of wetting after 5 minutes indicates a diagnosis of tear deficiency, although the reliability of this test may be affected by environmental conditions such as temperature or humidity.

Historically, a wide variety of paper types (filter paper, litmus paper, cigarette paper, blotting paper) have been used for the Schirmer test. In 1961, Halberg and Berens (77) described their standardized Schirmer paper strip manufactured from No. 589 Black Ribbon filter paper (similar to Whatman No. 41 paper) and prepared in precut strips, 5 by 35 mm (SMP Division, Cooper Laboratories, San German, Puerto Rico). The test is performed without touching the paper strip directly with the finger to avoid contamination of skin oils. The strip is placed at the junction of the middle and lateral one third of the lower eyelid (Fig. 28-4). The patient is told to look forward and to blink normally. Strips are removed after 5 minutes and the wetting is recorded in millimeters. The Schirmer test may be done with the eyes open or closed.

Jones's basal secretion test after topical anesthesia is used to eliminate conjunctival reflex stimulation of tearing (78). The Schirmer I test is recommended to determine the amount of tear secretion without anesthesia; to determine the minimum (basal) amount of tear secretion using the Jones's basal secretion test. Therefore, for example, in patients with moderate

to severe KCS, where it is important to determine whether any functional lacrimal gland is present, Schirmer's test is preferred. In suspected mild cases or contact lens–induced dry eye, where it is important to determine the basal level of tear production, Jones's test is more appropriate.

Phenol Red Thread Test

In this test, a fine cotton thread that has been impregnated with phenol red, a pH-sensitive substance that color changes from yellow to red on contact with the near neutral pH of tears, is placed between the eye lid and the globe, and the amount of wetting over 15 seconds is measured (79) (Fig. 28-5). Normal values are 9 to 18 mm.

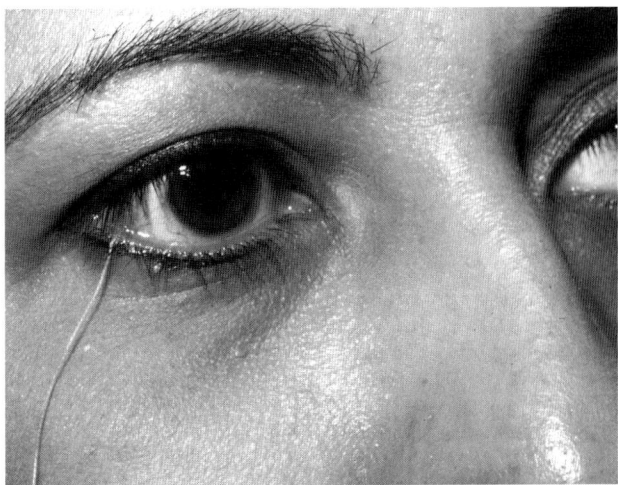

FIGURE 28-5. Phenol red thread test. It is a quick test used for diagnosing tear-deficient dry eye.

Tear Meniscometry

Tear meniscus volume is reduced in aqueous-deficient dry eye, as indicated by reduced height and radius of curvature. Radius of curvature can be measured by slit-image photography (80) or by the technique of reflective meniscometry (81) to provide a noninvasive method of diagnosis.

Measurement of Tear Film Stability

Tear Breakup Time

Tear breakup time (BUT) is the time elapsed from the blink to appearance of the first corneal dry spot, seen with the aid of fluorescein applied to the eye. BUT was originally described in 1969 by Norn (82), who referred to it as corneal wetting time. The concept of BUT was popularized in the United States in 1973 by Lemp and Hamill (83). Its measurement depends on the fact that with time, the undisturbed tear film thins and eventually ruptures (even in normal eyes). Measurement of BUT is accomplished as follows: fluorescein is instilled in the eye, the patient is asked to blink three times to distribute the dye, the patient is asked to stare straight ahead and not blink, while the examiner scans the cornea with the cobalt-blue light of the slit lamp, watching for an area of tear film rupture, manifested by the appearance of a black island within the green film of fluorescein. The BUT is the time in seconds between the last blink and the appearance of the dry spot. A mean of three trials is normally taken. A normal BUT is 10 seconds or more.

Noninvasive breakup line (NIBUT) is a test of tear stability that does not involve the instillation of fluorescein dye. Breakup time is measured as the time between the last blink and the breakup of a reflected image of a target on the tear film (84). A xeroscope or a keratometer is used. Normal NIBUT is greater than 20 seconds (85).

Measurement of Tear Film and Epithelial Integrity

Rose Bengal Stain

Rose bengal is a red aniline dye, a derivative of fluorescein but different from fluorescein in several important ways. Rose bengal stain is assumed to demonstrate ocular surface damage by being taken up into dead and degenerate cells (86). This assumption has been challenged by Feenstra and Tseng (87), who hypothesized that staining of the ocular surface by rose bengal is due to loss of the normal mucin layer in dry eye disease, allowing the dye to stain living epithelial cells that would normally be protected by mucin in the healthy eye. This theory, however, cannot explain the punctate nature of ocular surface staining with rose bengal, which appears to be confined to individual cells. Furthermore, removal of the mucin layer in the rabbit with acetyl cysteine does not cause dif-

fuse staining. Research has suggested that staining in dry eye is associated with an altered glycosylation of the surface mucin of apical conjunctival cells (29,88). Thus it appears that although stained cells are not necessarily degenerate, they may suffer from impaired expression of membrane-associated mucin.

Rose bengal application is quite valuable in the diagnosis of KCS. It has one disadvantage in that it causes irritation on instillation. The irritation seems to be directly related to the amount of epithelial damage present on the corneal surface and, to some extent, the amount of dye applied. A rose bengal–impregnated paper strip may be used to minimize the amount applied. A drop of anesthetic may also be instilled in the eye before the test to reduce irritation.

It is important to remember that in dry eye syndromes the pattern of the stain, not merely its presence, is important. Anything that can damage the epithelium (infection, trauma, toxic reactions) can cause rose bengal staining. Interpalpebral bulbar conjunctival and corneal staining is characteristic of KCS (Fig. 28-6). This area corresponds to the exposed surface of the eye within the palpebral fissure. Inferior corneal staining is seen in trauma, from factitious causes, lagophthalmos, and toxic keratitis. Superior corneal and limbic staining is seen in SLK. Staining of plica semilunaris and caruncle suggests mucus-fishing syndrome or eye rubbing. The entire cornea tends to stain in severe KCS, and in severe ocular surface diseases such as cicatricial pemphigoid and Stevens-Johnson syndrome and in keratitis medicamentosa. A small amount of stain over the body of a pterygium or pinguecula is common.

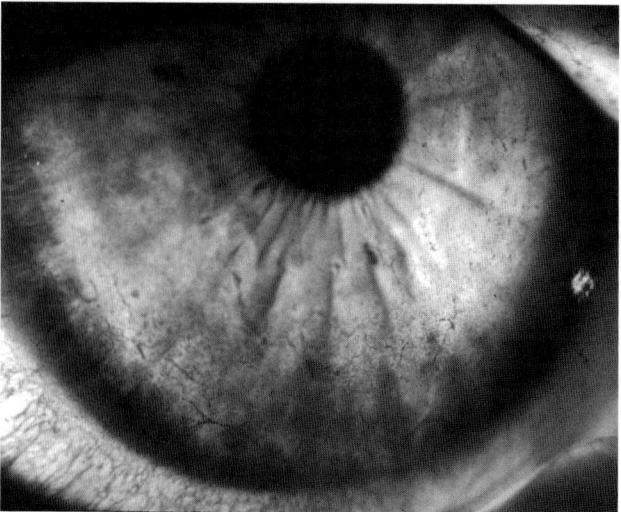

FIGURE 28-6. Keratoconjunctivitis sicca with typical epithelial erosions showing a characteristic pattern of distribution.

Fluorescein Staining

Fluorescein is a dye that is able to permeate through a disrupted epithelial layer and diffuse among the intercellular spaces (89). Fluorescein also stains the precorneal tear film, whereas rose bengal precipitates at the bottom of the meniscus. Fluorescein is an orange dye that fluoresces green when excited by blue light. It is typically applied to the eyes with a fluorescein–impregnated strip wetted with a drop of sterile saline; excess fluid is shaken from the strip prior to application. Fluorescein solution (1% to 2%) may also be used. Optimal results are obtained by viewing through a yellow barrier such as Kodak Wratten No. 12 absorption filter, used in combination with the standard blue exciter filter of the slit lamp. The cornea is best examined 2 to 3 minutes after instillation of the dye, an important fact often overlooked by examiners; premature examination of the surface underestimates the degree of epitheliopathy.

Conjunctival fluorescein staining occurs in mild to moderate KCS, and corneal staining in more severe KCS (Fig. 28-7). The staining usually has a characteristic distribution, confined to the exposed interpalpebral area of the ocular surface; but in severe dry eye, staining may extend to the unexposed surface of the globe, particularly the upper bulbar conjunctiva. Sometimes fluorescein staining can be seen in normal eyes and may be more prominent in the morning (89).

Other Dyes

Lissamine green is reported to stain dead and degenerated cells and mucus (90). The dyeing quality of lissamine green is the same as that of rose bengal. Both solutions can be made in 1% concentration. It may be advantageous to use lissamine green rather than rose bengal in diagnosing dry eye because it causes little to no stinging. However, lissamine green is not currently available commercially.

Sulphorhodamine B is a fluorescent dye that is viewed using a band-pass interference filter of 520 to 550 nm as an exciter and a Kodak Wratten No. 12 filter as a barrier. The staining properties of Sulphorhodamine B are similar to those of fluorescein (91). This dye is not available as a commercial preparation.

Laboratory Tests

Physical Characteristics of Tear Film

Tear Osmolarity

Considerable evidence suggests that tear hyperosmolarity plays a key role in the ocular surface damage in various forms of dry eye disease (92). There are various types of osmometers available for measuring tear osmolarity (93). Elevated tear osmolarity indicates an imbalance between the rate of tear secretion and the rate of evaporation in which a decrease in the former or an increase in the latter, or both, is sufficient to disturb the homeostatic mechanisms that normally keep tear osmolarity near 302 mOsmo/L (92). Reflex tear secretion at the time of sample collection can cause false-negative results.

Ocular Ferning Test

One of the interesting physical characteristics of mucus is its ability to crystallize and form "ferns" when observed on a dry slide with the microscope. Utilizing this characteristic, Tabbara and Okumoto (94) developed a new qualitative test for the study of conjunctival mucus. Microscopic arborization (ferning) is observed in normal eyes, whereas patients with cicatrizing conjunctivitis such as ocular pemphigoid, Stevens-Johnson syndrome, trachoma, or alkali burn may show decreased mucus production and absent or reduced ferning.

Tear Film Evaporation

Dry eye patients show an increased rate of evaporation compared to normals (0.43 mL/min vs. 0.14 mL/min) (95). The test is not specific for a particular type of dry eye; increased evaporation is seen in KCS and in many forms of MGD and ocular surface disease.

Tear Clearance

Tear secretion, stability, and evaporation affect tear clearance. Tear clearance is probably the best overall measure of the lacrimal gland, meibomian gland, and ocular surface as a functional unit. Measurement of tear clearance is helpful in the assessment and the follow-up of patients with KCS. When suboptimal tear clearance is accompanied by inflammation, a vicious cycle results, with increasing inflammation leading to further decreases in tear clearance and the retention of inflammatory cytokines on the ocular surface.

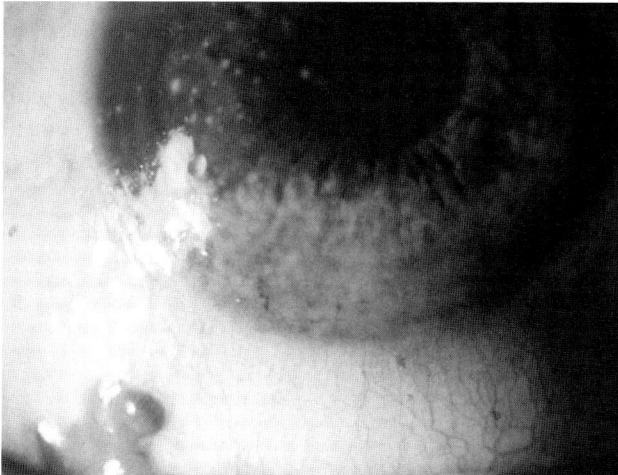

FIGURE 28-7. Superficial punctate keratopathy showing the exposed interpalpebral area of ocular surface, in keratoconjunctivitis sicca.

Tear clearance is measured by the change in the concentration of fluorescein in the tear film. Decreased tear clearance occurs when there is decreased tear secretion or blinking, increased evaporation, or following punctal occlusion. It is measured *in vivo* using fluorophotometric techniques (96,97).

Tests for Diagnosing Evaporative Dry Eye

Evaporative dry eye and tear-deficient dry eye are not mutually exclusive, as meibomian gland dysfunction is apparent in a majority of patients with significant aqueous-deficient dry eye. Precise diagnosis of evaporative dry eye requires demonstration of increased evaporation of tears in the presence of normal aqueous secretion. Diagnosis is based on the presence of extensive meibomian gland dysfunction in the context of normal aqueous tear production. Its relative contribution to the dry eye state is difficult to measure.

Diagnosis of lipid tear deficiency is mainly indirect. Obstructive meibomian gland disease is assessed by quantification of occluded gland orifices and grading the quality of expressed oil secretion (98). Morphological changes of the meibomian glands can be determined by meibography (99). Deficiency of oil delivery onto the lid margin can be measured quantitatively by meibometry, a technique in which samples of lid margin oil are taken from the lid with a strip of tape and quantified by densitometry (100). Tear interferometry is a noninvasive method in which a single static image of tear interference is obtained to semiquantify the lipid film thickness (101). Recently, a new method has been developed that utilizes direct digitization of sequential tear interference images for kinetic analysis (102). It is believed that kinetic analysis of tear interference will help in devising and monitoring future therapies directed to restoring meibomian gland functions.

Chemical Composition of Tear Film

Tear Lysozyme Measurements

Although lysozyme is normally found in human tears, it is absent in those of rodents. Patients with Sjögren's syndrome have decreased lysozyme production. Several assay systems can available to determine the level of lysozyme in tears. Normal tear lysozyme levels are between 2 and 4 mg/mL (103).

Tear Lactoferrin Measurements

Various methods have been described to measure tear lactoferrin levels (104,105). The Lactoplate test is an immunodiffusion assay performed in an agarose gel containing rabbit antisera to human lacroferrin (104). The Lactocard test is a solid-phase enzyme-linked immunosorbent assay (ELISA) that requires only 2 μL of tears in a rapid, simple test that is colorimetrically measured by a precise reflectance spectrometer (105).

Tear Protein Analysis

Tear protein analysis is based on the rationale that tears from dry eye patients may contain altered protein composition. Tear proteins can be measured using ELISA assay. Electrophoresis can be used to separate various proteins in tears. The electrophoretic pattern of tears from normal subjects and patients with KCS show qualitative differences (106). Recently, decreased levels of the goblet cell specific mucin MUC5AC have been demonstrated in tears of patients with Sjögren's syndrome (31).

Conjunctival Impression Cytology

Conjunctival impression cytology has been used to assay goblet cells in normal subjects and dry eye patients (107). Flow cytometry on conjunctival impression cytology is a technique that has been validated for quantitative analysis of fluorescence on cells, and has recently been utilized for analysis of various immune-inflammatory markers in KCS (108).

DIFFERENTIAL DIAGNOSIS
Keratoconjunctivitis Sicca

In mild DES, patients may have no signs of damage to corneal or conjunctival epithelial surfaces. In moderate and severe DES, fluorescein staining may reveal damage in the corneal epithelium. The staining pattern usually appears in the interpalpebral zone or inferiorly and shows punctate stippling. In severe DES, there may be keratinization over the conjunctiva, particularly over the exposed portion. Corneal filaments may occur, which are more prominent in the central anterior part of the cornea. Fluorescein stains of the cornea may be confluent as well as diffuse and punctate. Patients may also have an epithelial defect that may be slow to heal. Rapid sterile corneal ulceration may occur in the setting of a persistent epithelial defect due to enzymatic degradation of cornea. Secondary infection, especially with *Staphylococcus* species, may sometimes occur and result in indolent corneal ulceration.

Blepharitis

The lack of aqueous tear secretion may predispose to blepharitis as a consequence of increased levels of bacterial flora resulting from decreased levels of tear IgA, lactoferrin, and lysozyme. Patients with blepharitis present with symptoms of burning that are worse on awakening, better within an hour or so, and worse again later in the day. Patients may have rosacea or seborrheic dermatitis. There is minimal response of symptoms caused by blepharitis to artificial lubricants, but eyelid hygiene done on a regular basis improves symptoms. Oral tetracycline improves symptoms and signs, especially in patients with rosacea blepharitis. In posterior marginal blepharitis, there is meibomian gland dysfunction, with oil on the eyelid margins, plugged meibomian duct orifices, and inspissated glands. In anterior marginal blepharitis, there may be collarettes (staphylococcal) or scurf (seborrheic). There may be poor or incomplete blinking. There may also be inflammation of meibomian glands (meibomianitis), and increased tear film debris, as well as inferior punctate corneal staining with fluorescein. The BUT is usually abnormal (but can be normal in some cases). If there is coexistent tear-deficient KCS, interpalpebral staining will typically be present. Tear film osmolarity is also increased in blepharitis.

Toxic or Irritant Keratoconjunctivitis

The lack of aqueous tear secretion in KCS also results in an inability to dilute or wash out substances that come in contact with the eye, either purposely (topical lubricants or medications), or inadvertently (cosmetics to the face and eyelids). Inability to dilute or wash out potentially toxic substances can cause epithelial and tear film abnormalities. Patients present with symptoms of burning, foreign-body sensation, and photophobia, which are present constantly and worsen with continued use of the offending agent. There may be a history of KCS.

Allergic Keratoconjunctivitis

The primary symptom of allergic conjunctivitis is itching. Symptoms may follow a temporal pattern, as in seasonal hayfever or environmental exposure. A history of hayfever or atopic dermatitis can be present. Examination reveals papillary conjunctivitis. In some atopic eye diseases such as giant papillary conjunctivitis and vernal conjunctivitis, medium and large-sized papillae are present on the upper palpebral conjunctiva. Mucin debris may be seen in the tear film. There is usually no rose bengal or fluorescein staining present unless the papillae are large enough to cause mechanical injury to the cornea. But allergy and dry eye often coexist. In KCS, lack of tears and decreased tear turnover may result in an inability to dilute or wash out allergens, increasing the likelihood of allergic conjunctivitis. Conversely, systemic antiallergy medications can exacerbate dryness, and preservatives present in topical antiallergy medicines can also worsen the dry eye–related epitheliopathy. Inflammatory products released by allergic responses, as well as eye rubbing, can worsen clinical symptoms and findings.

Nocturnal Lagophthalmos

Patients commonly complain of burning in the eyes that is worse upon awakening. There is frequently a history of previous lid surgery, thyroid eye disease, or loose or floppy eyelids.

Superior Limbic Keratoconjunctivitis

Patients with superior limbic keratoconjunctivitis complain of burning and irritation and develop symptoms and remissions somewhat abruptly. A diurnal pattern to the symptoms, however, is usually not present. The factors initiating the development of exacerbations and remissions are not known. Episodes may last from days to years, and remissions may last for weeks or may be permanent. Vision is rarely affected. A history of thyroid dysfunction may be present. Importantly, some patients with classic superior limbic keratoconjunctivitis signs and thyroid disease also have lacrimal hyposecretion, as autoimmune thyroid and lacrimal gland disease can coexist.

COMPLICATIONS

Infectious Blepharitis and Conjunctivitis

Paralleling the decrease in tear secretion in the lacrimal glands, there is a decrease in certain enzymatic constituents of tears (e.g., lysozyme, lactoferrin, and beta-lysin). These enzymes can provide protection against infection; thus, there is decreased resistance of the external eye to infection especially with *Staphylococcus aureus* in keratoconjunctivitis sicca. Dry eye patients who wear contact lenses are especially high risk of developing contact lens-associated infections, presumably due to the higher propensity of bacteria to adhere to the drier, damaged ocular surface.

Keratinization

Any of the entities that are capable of harming the conjunctival goblet cells (vitamin A deficiency, cicatricial pemphigoid, alkali burns, Stevens-Johnson syndrome, trachoma) can lead to keratinization of the cornea and conjunctival epithelium. Keratinization results in discomfort, and if the lid margin tarsal conjunctival keratinization is severe enough, the cornea may be involved, with subsequent loss of vision. Keratinized epithelium has a peculiar pearly white sheen, unlike the normal pink and shiny epithelium. Keratinized epithelium also has a rough, slightly elevated surface that fluorescein does not cover because the surface does not wet well with tears. It is the rough surface that is irritating and abrasive, and so soft bandage lenses may be helpful, while simultaneously posing risk of infection. In the case of vitamin A deficiency, the keratinization process has been demonstrated to be reversible.

Band Keratopathy

In 1977, Lemp and Ralph (109) described the rapid development of band keratopathy within epithelial defects on dry corneas. Treatment is with ethylenediaminetetraacetic acid

(EDTA), along with attempts at therapy of the KCS in order to prevent recurrence of the band keratopathy.

Limbal Stem Cell Deficiency

Ocular surface disorders that can cause severe conjunctival inflammation and/or cicatrization (e.g., thermal and chemical burns, ocular cicatricial pemphigoid, Stevens-Johnson syndrome, chronic atopic keratoconjunctivitis), can result in limbal stem cell deficiency if the limbus is involved. The limbal stem cells are responsible for regeneration of the corneal epithelium. Thus stem cell deficiency can result in corneal epithelial breakdown, delayed epithelial healing, or vascularization.

Sterile Stromal Ulcers and Corneal Perforation

Stromal melting can occur in patients who have rheumatoid arthritis. The melt is typically an oval, noninfiltrated ulcer situated at, or just below, the visual axis, with its longest dimension horizontal. These lesions are usually initially sterile but tend to progress quickly and may perforate or even become secondarily infected. Sterile corneal ulcers in patients with severe Sjögren's syndrome can progress rapidly even though the eye appears white and "quiet."

Keratoconus-Like Changes

Inferior corneal steepening, with a keratoconus-like pattern, associated with nocturnal lagophthalmos and aqueous tear deficiency has been described (110). Chronic ocular desiccation and aqueous tear deficiency may be responsible for these changes. Lubricating and hydrating the regional corneal desiccation can reverse these topographic changes (110).

Psychological Effects

Dry eye is characterized by chronic symptoms of ocular dryness and discomfort that can be debilitating (111), and when severe may affect psychological health and ability to work. Even though many dry eye–related disorders are not directly sight threatening, the chronicity of the condition, as well as the fact that no cure currently exists for most forms of dry eye, renders the patients very frustrated. Some even develop a chronic pain syndrome and psychological features in which the symptoms of discomfort are significantly out of proportion to the objective findings. Because of the chronic nature of the problem, most patients go through periods of despondency and depression. Ophthalmologists must recognize this part of the illness and actively encourage their patients to continue to pursue their normal activities and maintain hope and

compliance with recommended treatments (and stay away from unproven "cures," many of which are touted over the Internet).

TREATMENT

The most basic principle that applies to the treatment of dry eye is the education of patients to help them to understand the rationale behind the recommended therapy, so as to encourage compliance. Lack of compliance is a predictor of failure for any treatment. Patients must also be alerted to the environmental conditions that aggravate dry eye (e.g., air-conditioning, airplane travel). They must also be told of the activities that provoke tear film instability (e.g., reading, computer use), so that they may alter behavioral patterns and environmental exposures in a way that can help with their treatment (112).

The major goal of therapy in dry eye syndrome is to reestablish, as much as possible, a qualitatively and quantitatively sufficient tear film in order to provide relief of symptoms, establish epithelial healing, and prevent serious complications related to tear film abnormalities, such as persistent epitheliopathy, sterile corneal ulceration, and secondary microbial infections.

Environmental Adjustments

Because blinking is essential for inducing tear secretion and spreading of the tear film over the cornea, any activity or occupation that requires particular visual concentration may result in reduced blinking, ocular fatigue, and dry eye symptoms. Certain ergonomic modifications such as placing video display terminals at a lower level so that workers do not have to keep their eyes open, may alleviate some of the symptoms (112).

Eliminating Aggravating Factors

Meibomian gland dysfunction (MGD) predisposes to increased tear film instability and evaporative dry eye. Its presence aggravates already-existing aqueous tear deficiency. MGD should be controlled with vigorous lid hygiene and lid massage regimens. Treatment of blepharitis often provides effective relief for the symptoms of dry eye, even in patients with aqueous deficiency. Oral doxycycline or other macrolide antibiotic therapy often adds to the success of lid massage (113).

Any abnormalities in eyelid blinking or nocturnal exposure that may cause inadequate tear film distribution or increased evaporation must be recognized. Use of lubricating ointments or taping the eyelid closed at night may help in such situations.

Certain systemic medications inhibit tear production and aggravate dry eye. The risk and benefit of each pharmacotherapy should be assessed. For example, although some diuretics or psychotropic medicines induce dry eye, terminating therapy is ill advised. However, understanding the role of medications in exacerbating dry eye is important. This information can be relayed to the other physicians in charge of patient care, and frequently alternate therapies can be selected.

Tear Substitution

Tear substitutes for KCS should provide an adequate amount of fluid for the ocular surface, to help in regular flushing and waste removal from the ocular surface, and allow adequate lubrication to the lid/globe system so as to reduce the shearing forces at the interfaces, and to facilitate the natural healing process of the ocular surface cells so that the glycocalyx can be rebuilt, and the ability of the ocular surface to retain water can be restored (114).

Tear replacement by topical artificial tears is the most widely used therapeutic modality in the treatment of KCS. This is a palliative therapy, but in many cases of mild to moderate dry eye syndrome it is the only modality that is required. The goal of using tear substitutes is to increase humidity at the ocular surface and to improve lubrication with subsequent secondary benefits. Artificial tears smooth the corneal surface of dye eye patients, an effect that contributes to improved vision (115).

The use of artificial tears has obvious limitations; they cannot duplicate the composition of natural tears. Natural tears have a complex composition of water, salts, hydrocarbons, proteins, and lipids. In addition, the integrity of the three-layered lipid, aqueous, and mucin structure, vital to the effective functioning of the tear film, cannot be reproduced by artificial components (116). The ideal tear substitute is the one that approximates the normal electrolyte composition of the tear film, has low surface tension, is well tolerated, is nonirritating, contains no toxic preservatives, and has a long residence time on the cornea and conjunctiva. A number of commercially marketed preparations are available that use a variety of components in an effort to meet the requirement of patients with dry eye of diverse etiology and severity.

Water makes up 98% to 98.5% of natural tears. Dry eye tear substitutes typically contain 97% to 99% water. Saline solutions are solutions of electrolytes designed to maintain the osmolarity of the nascent aqueous tear (approximately 300 mOsm/L) and the precorneal tear film (approximately 303 to 310 mOsm/L), or to a lower osmolarity without causing discomfort. Some electrolytes, besides their osmotic purpose, play an important role in corneal epithelial metabolism (e.g., potassium, bicarbonate). Some of the widely used electrolyte salts include sodium chloride, potassium chloride, calcium chloride, magnesium chloride, zinc chloride, sodium borate, sodium phosphate, and boric acid. Sodium bicarbonate is used to buffer the solutions, but also has an electrolytic effect.

Mucilages are made of cellulose or vegetable gums and have viscous and adhesive properties. They increase the viscosity of tears, and also provide moderate adsorptive properties to the corneal epithelium. The cellulose mucilages are used extensively in dry eye applications. Methylcellulose is the methyl derivative of cellulose. Methylcellulose increases the residence time of artificial tears (117). The refractive index of a 1% methylcellulose solution is 1.336, very similar to that of the natural tear.

Several water-soluble synthetic polymers are being used in artificial tear preparations that are basically vinyl derivatives of polyethylene glycol, forming a backbone to which different functional groups may be attached to confer the desired mucomimetic properties such as water solubility, and desirable oncotic pressure, surfactant qualities, and adsorption on the epithelial surface. Polyvinyl alcohol, pyrrolidone, and carbomers are some of the synthetic polymers that are commonly used in dry eye applications. Polyvinyl alcohol in a concentration of 1.4% remains in the lacrimal basin for 30 minutes because it is quite adsorptive. Polyvinyl pyrrolidone (povidone) in a concentration of 3% to 5% increases the viscosity of the solutions. Carbomers are used in ophthalmic hydrogels. It has been demonstrated that replacement of tears with a substance that prolongs the residence time improves the tear film breakup time and is superior to tear replacement fluids that are of low viscosity and are quickly washed away from the ocular surface after blinking (118).

Biologic fluids, such as autologous serum, colostrum, saliva, and egg whites, are not commercialized. Autologous serum drops (diluted 1% with saline) have been reported to improve ocular irritation symptoms and conjunctival and corneal dye staining in Sjögren's syndrome–associated KCS in several small clinical trials (119,120). Meaningful, randomized, controlled trials are required to validate the role of serum eyedrops in the management of severe ocular surface disease in KCS.

Lipids are typically formulated as ointments but can also be formulated as solution-based emulsions (121). However, there is no conclusive evidence of the utility of lipid containing eye drops to date (122). Because many patients with KCS develop problems during the night and upon awakening owing to decreased tear production during sleep, application of a lubricating ointment at night provides long-lasting relief during sleep. A new petrolatum ointment containing calcium carbonate, which is placed on the lower lid skin, and is based on the principle of supracutaneous drug delivery method (123), has also been shown to be helpful in dry eye patients (124).

Lacrisert, formerly known as the SR-AT (slow-releasing artificial tear), is a small, 5-mg pellet of hydroxypropyl cellulose. The pellet is placed in the inferior cul-de-sac with a plastic inserter. Within a short time, the Lacrisert absorbs tears and becomes a soft, gelatinous blob, and during the course of several hours it slowly dissolves and releases its polymer into the tear film. Patients generally use the insert once or twice daily. Common problems associated with Lacrisert use include inadvertent loss of the insert, blurred vision, and foreign-body sensation. Moreover, for Lacrisert to be effective, some degree of lacrimation is required; hence, this modality is not very effective in patients with severe lacrimal insufficiency.

Hyaluronic acid has been used to treat dry eye disease for several years (125). It has been reported that hyaluronic acid is effective in promoting wound healing of the corneal epithelium (126). Hyaluronic acid seems to be beneficial as a mucin substitute in dry eye management (127). It may also bind immunoreactive substances and thereby decrease the propensity for inflammation in the ocular surface of the dry eye patient. Hypotonic electrolyte-based formulations have also been developed, based on the recognition of the importance of tear osmolarity in ocular surface disease in DES. In one study, treatment with a hypotonic 0.4% hyaluronic acid tear substitute was shown to result in improvement of the epithelium in patients with KCS (128).

Some patients with KCS have highly viscous and stringy mucus that forms plaques and filaments on the ocular surface, and these are a major source of irritation and pain (129). The application of mucolytic solutions can be of help in these patients. Use of 10% acetylcysteine (Mucomyst) ophthalmic solution in an artificial tear base has been proposed; the major drawbacks include refrigeration and limited stability (130), features that preclude its commercialization.

Tear Substitutes and Preservatives

One of the most important drawbacks of many of the commercially available artificial tear substitutes and lubricants is the fact that they must contain preservatives, stabilizers, and other additives that supply stability and retard germ growth, thus ensuring the long shelf life required for commercialization. However, because of their high potential to provoke toxic and allergic reactions, some preservatives have been abandoned (e.g., thiomersal). The preservatives currently most commonly used in artificial tear preparations are benzalkonium chloride, chlorobutanol, and chlorhexidine. Preservatives have been shown to disrupt the precorneal tear film and damage the epithelial surface (131). Even though the concentration of preservatives in artificial tear preparations is generally low, their prolonged presence on an already-compromised ocular surface, such as that of a dry eye, can cause serious iatrogenic effects, worsening the ocular surface disease.

The introduction of preservative-free solutions is an important contribution to the formulation of tear substitutes. Preservative-free artificial tears are available in single-use vials. They are undoubtedly preferable to preserved tears, but affordability could become an issue, as preservative-free tears are more expensive. Another drawback with these formulations is that they can promote lack of compliance, as the patient has to carry numerous vials to maintain adequate dosage over 24 hours or more. Recently launched artificial tears are claimed to have gentler preservatives or preservatives that are broken down after contact with the eye surface.

Recommendations for Use of Tear Substitution Therapy for Dry Eye

Currently, the therapy of dry eye disease is determined by the severity of the condition. Mild cases of dry eye, in which there are no signs of damage to the conjunctiva or cornea, may be successfully managed with artificial tears applied up to four times per day. In moderate cases of dry eye, examination will reveal mild damage to the cornea, such as superficial punctate keratopathy (SPK). In these cases, more frequent treatment will be required (e.g., use of unpreserved artificial tears up to 12 times per day and an unpreserved lubricating ointment at bedtime). Severe dry eye is characterized by keratinization of the conjunctiva and moderate to severe corneal damage, including SPK, filaments, epithelial defects, and a subsequently higher risk of secondary infections. In addition to frequent instillation of unpreserved artificial tears and lubricating ointment at night, severe cases of dry eye require other treatment strategies, such as tear-conserving therapies as described below.

Preservation of Tears

Several methods of tear preservation have been described in the literature. They include punctal occlusion, moist chamber spectacles, swimmers' goggles, bandage contact lenses, clear food wrap shields, silicone rubber shields, and lid taping.

Punctal Occlusion

Use of punctal or canalicular occlusion as a treatment strategy in patients with KCS is based on the rationale that the tears drain into the nose via the tear ducts, and blocking this outflow will keep the tears on the eye surface for a longer time. This will help in reducing the tear film osmolarity, increasing tear volume, and prolonging residence time of externally applied tear substitutes. The use of punctal occlusion is an effective step in treating moderate to severe dry eye that is unresponsive to artificial tear substitutes (132). However, it should be remembered that punctal occlusion increases the possibility of toxicity associated with the use of preservative-containing tear substitutes by prolonging their residence time on the ocular surface. Therefore, in general, preservative-free tear substitutes should be used when punctal occlusion is employed.

Punctal or canalicular occlusion may be permanent or temporary.

Temporary Occlusion

Temporary punctal occlusion with collagen implants may be considered to ascertain if the punctal blockage will help reduce dry eye symptoms and also to rule out excessive tearing due to such blockage. Various methods of occlusion have been described that include temporary absorbable implants (e.g., collagen, gelatin, catgut) and semipermanent nonabsorbable implants (e.g., silicone, hydroethylmethacrylate, Teflon). Intracanalicular gelatin implants described by Foulds (133) in 1961 were long, slender rods of gelatin that were threaded down the canaliculus with forceps. In 1976, Patten (134) described the use of N-butyl cyanoacrylate tissue adhesive as a method of temporary punctal occlusion. Herrick (135) described a different approach to occlusive therapy. He invented a small collagen rod designed to be implanted into the canaliculus with jeweler's forceps. The implant is absorbable and provides temporary occlusion of the lacrimal system. In 1985, Hamano and colleagues (136) described a new punctum plug, which was made of a copolymer of polyvinylpyrrolidone and polymethylmethacrylate. The most striking feature of this new plug is that it shrinks to one-third its original volume when dried in air and is rehydrated to its original volume after insertion.

The method of temporary punctal occlusion most commonly used today is the Freeman (137) punctal plug. Most silicone punctal plugs are umbrella shaped, and the top part of the punctal plug rests on the eyelid surface. Either one punctum or both puncta may be closed in this manner. The obvious advantage of these devices is their ease of removal if epiphora ensues or if no improvement is noted. Complications have generally not been major, although in rare instances the plug can turn inward and rub on the nasal conjunctiva (Fig. 28-8). Spontaneous expulsion can occur and is not uncommon. In one study, we found that proportion of puncta still retaining plugs after 6 months was 53%, and there was a higher risk of loss of upper punctal plugs compared with lower punctal plugs (132). The risk of plug loss increases with each subsequent plug placed for a preceding expulsed plug. Additionally, patients with severe inflammatory and cicatrizing diseases such as pemphigoid and ocular graft-versus-host disease experience a higher rate of plug loss, likely due to the scarring at the punctum site. A few cases of permanent scarring of the punctum after removal of the plug (138) and a case of pyogenic granuloma (139) have been reported.

Punctal plug therapy is a simple treatment that can provide long-lasting punctal occlusion without significant surgical difficulties, expense, irreversibility, or discomfort associated with other punctal or canalicular occlusive procedures. Silicone punctal plugs are effective in aqueous

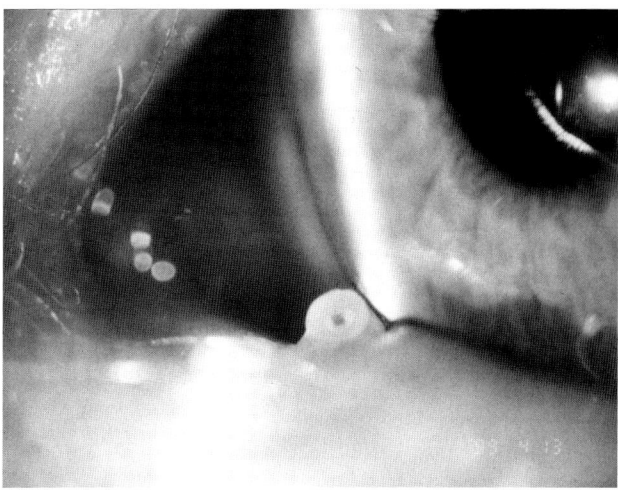

FIGURE 28-8. Displaced punctal plug. In rare cases, punctal plug can turn inward rubbing against conjunctiva and cornea.

deficient dry eye diseases and also as an adjunct therapy combined with other treatment modalities for complicated ocular surface diseases (140).

Permanent Occlusion

Permanent occlusion of the puncta or canaliculi can be accomplished with thermal or electric cauterization of puncta or canaliculi or by argon laser photocoagulation (141) of the punctal opening. Punctal laser cauterization has the advantage that the treatment may be "calibrated." For example, a patient may be encountered in whom one punctal occlusion is inadequate for therapy, and yet occlusion of both puncta leads to epiphora. In such a case, the laser can be used to produce just enough burns to cause stenosis, without total closure, of the second punctum (132). However, the tissue response with laser punctoplasty is not easy to predict. In one retrospective study of patients who had undergone laser punctal occlusion, only 14% of the puncta remained occluded at the time of the author's examination (13 to 21 months after treatment) (142). A case of acute dacryocystitis following laser occlusion of all four puncta has been reported (143). Surgical methods of permanent occlusion include dacrocystectomy, canalicular ligature, canalicular offset, canalicular excision, punctal tarsorrhaphy, and punctal patch.

In general, our approach when indicated is to use punctal plugs. In patients who experience multiple expulsions, or in those with very severe dryness, punctal cautery turns out to be more practical as the risk of plug loss is circumvented.

Moisture Chambers and Room Humidifiers

The concept behind moisture chambers is to enclose the eye so that evaporative loss of tears is reduced. The ability of high ambient humidity to retard evaporation and thereby preserve tear volume and reduce osmolarity can be achieved with the use of room humidifiers or with moisture chamber spectacles or goggles. To maximize the effectiveness of moisture-chamber spectacles, the device should contact the face and be airtight (144).

Hydrophilic Bandage Contact Lenses

A specific type of contact lens has been shown to produce a barrier to evaporation in dry eye disease (145). However, patients with dry eye disease may experience difficulty with contact lenses getting dry and falling off. Contact lenses will exacerbate the already increased risk of corneal infection in dry eye patients, and may worsen the already existing dry eye condition by acting as a "sponge," retaining the ocular surface moisture into the lens itself, rather than onto the ocular surface, a characteristic of particularly high water-content lenses. Thus, it is generally recommended that these lenses be used in only a small number of patients with intractable filamentary keratitis or in selected patients with nonhealing epithelial defects who cannot be managed by any other treatment modality. Vigilance in hygiene, and supplemental use of lubricants and antibiotics is required to minimize the risks of infection.

Antiinflammatory Therapy

It is now well recognized that inflammation plays a role in dry eye by the suppression of lacrimal secretion and by its damaging effect on the ocular surface. Artificial tears have been reported to decrease ocular irritation and blurred vision and to reduce the severity of ocular surface dye staining. However, they have no direct antiinflammatory effects, although they may secondarily decrease inflammation through their ability to lower tear osmolarity and to dilute the concentration of noxious and inflammatory factors, and flush them from the ocular surface. In contrast, antiinflammatory therapies that target one or more of the components of the inflammatory response to dry eye have been reported to have efficacy in treating the signs and symptoms of dry eye. Antiinflammatory therapies may be considered in those patients with KCS who continue to have symptoms on aqueous enhancement therapies.

Cyclosporin A

Cyclosporine is a naturally occurring fungal metabolite widely used as an immunosuppressant in human organ graft recipients. Immunosuppressive mechanisms of cyclosporine relate to binding of specific nuclear proteins required for initiation of T-cell activation, thus preventing T-cell production of inflammatory cytokines such as IL-2 and thereby disrupting immune mediated processes (146). More specifically, cyclosporine forms a complex with the cytosolic protein cyclophilin and inhibits the phosphatase activity of calcineurin, which regulates nuclear translocation and subsequent activation of nuclear factor of activated T-cells (NFAT) transcription factors (147). Cyclosporine also inhibits an initiating event in mitochondrial-mediated pathways of apoptosis by blocking the opening of the mitochondrial permeability pore (148). The potential of cyclosporin A (CsA) for treating dry eye–associated ocular surface disease was initially recognized in dogs that develop KCS (149).

Topical CsA received Food and Drug Administration (FDA) approval in December 2002 as Restasis (cyclosporine ophthalmic emulsion 0.05%, Allergan, Inc., Irvine, CA). Clinical trials investigating the safety and efficacy of topical cyclosporine have demonstrated safety in all trials (150,151). Patients treated with CsA, 0.05% or 1%, showed significantly ($p < .05$) greater improvement in two objective signs of dry eye disease (corneal fluorescein staining and Schirmer values) than those treated with vehicle. CsA 0.05% treatment also produced significantly greater improvements ($p < .05$) in three subjective measures of dry eye disease (blurred vision, need for concomitant artificial tears, and the global response to treatment). Although 17% of patients reported some stinging, only 6% of patients discontinued therapy as a result of the discomfort. Burning was noted with the same frequency in patients receiving the vehicle. The clinical improvement in these clinical trials have been accompanied by decreased expression of immune activation markers (i.e., HLA-DR), apoptosis markers, and inflammatory cytokine such as IL-6, by the conjunctival epithelial cells (108,152).

Corticosteroids

Corticosteroids are potent inhibitors of many inflammatory pathways. Activated corticosteroid receptors in the cell nucleus bind to DNA and regulate gene expression. They also interfere with transcriptional regulators (e.g., NFκB) of proinflammatory genes (153). Among their multiple biologic activities, corticosteroids inhibit inflammatory cytokine and chemokine production, and decrease synthesis of matrix metalloproteinases, and lipid mediators of inflammation (e.g., prostaglandins), decrease expression of cell adhesion molecules (e.g., ICAM-1), and stimulate lymphocyte apoptosis (154–157). Side chain substitutions on the corticosteroid ring structure alter their potency, free radical scavenging effects, and membrane stabilizing properties.

Corticosteroids have been reported to improve both signs and symptoms of dry eye in several clinical studies. In a retrospective clinical series, topical administration of a 1% solution of nonpreserved methylprednisolone, given three to four times daily for 2 weeks to patients with Sjögren's syndrome KCS, provided moderate or complete relief of symptoms in all patients (158). In addition, there was a decrease in corneal fluorescein staining and complete resolution of filamentary keratitis. This therapy was effective even for patients suffering from severe KCS who had no improvement with maximum aqueous enhancement therapies.

Unfortunately, the long-term side effects of corticosteroids, including cataract and steroid responsive glaucoma, preclude the use of steroids for long-term treatment of dry eye. Steroids nevertheless are useful in short-term treatment to suppress an acute flare-up of surface inflammation. A masked, placebo-controlled trial would be useful to further clarify the benefits and risks of corticosteroid therapy for dry eye.

Tetracyclines

Tetracyclines are compounds that have traditionally been used as antibiotics. More recently, they have been observed to have numerous antiinflammatory properties, including the abilities to decrease the production and activity of inflammatory cytokines, to decrease nitric oxide production, and to inhibit matrix metalloproteinase production and activation (159–161). With regard to the ocular surface, tetracyclines have been observed to decrease production of IL-1 and matrix metalloproteinases by human corneal epithelial cells (159,161). The semisynthetic tetracycline, doxycycline, has been reported to improve irritation symptoms, increase tear film stability, and decrease the severity of ocular surface disease in patients with ocular rosacea (162).

Recommendations for Use of Antiinflammatory Therapy for Dry Eye

Antiinflammatory therapies should be considered for patients with severe KCS who have intolerable irritation, blurred vision, or sight-threatening corneal complications (e.g., thinning, filamentary keratitis) despite maximum hydration and lubrication therapy. Because of their potential to raise intraocular pressure, cause posterior subcapsular cataracts, and increase the risk for infection, topical corticosteroids should be used in short pulses (1 to 4 weeks), followed by cessation or change to a low dose (once or twice daily) of an agent that carries less risk for glaucoma or cataract formation (e.g., loteprednol etabonate or fluorometholone). Patients on corticosteroids should be closely observed for steroid-related side effects. CsA and oral tetracyclines have excellent safety profiles and can be safely used for extended periods. Doxycycline can be used in lower and divided doses (40 to 50 mg/day) in order to reduce the gastrointestinal side effects.

EMERGING TREATMENTS
Stimulation of Tear Secretion

Various medications have been tried to stimulate tear production, but their side effects have limited the usefulness of such stimulants. Bromhexine and its derivatives do stimulate tear production, but adverse effects have discouraged their use in the United States. Oral pilocarpine (Salagen; MGI-Pharma Inc., Bloomington, MN) is available to treat the symptoms of dry eye and dry mouth. Improvement in symptoms has been documented in two studies (163,164). However, cholinergic side effects of sweating and diarrhea often limit tolerance to the medication. Cevimelin (Evoxac; Daiichi Pharmaceutical Co., Montvale, NJ) is approved in the United States for treatment of the symptoms of dry mouth, and although not approved for the treatment of dry eye, it is better tolerated than is pilocarpine, and appears effective in treating xerostomia and keratoconjunctivitis sicca at the 30-mg dose (165). Laboratory investigations have shown that topical agents that increase cyclic nucleotide levels can stimulate tear secretion, but none of these agents has advanced to clinical trials (166).

A promising medication to increase aqueous tear volume and stimulate mucin secretion is a novel P2Y2 receptor agonist (INS365; Inspire Pharmaceuticals Inc., Durham, NC). This topical agent has been shown to increase the flow of sodium and water across conjunctival membranes and to stimulate mucin production from goblet cells (167). Preliminary clinical trials demonstrate an amelioration of clinical symptoms and signs of surface staining in patients with dry eye (168). This agent is not yet approved for the treatment of dry eye disease.

The idea of developing stimulants of mucin production is based on therapies used in the treatment of gastritis and ulcers, some of which also stimulate mucin secretion. One such drug, gafarnate, has been studied for its effect on conjunctival goblet cells in rabbits, and a significant increase in goblet cells was found (169). Gafarnate-containing eyedrops may be a potential candidate for clinical use in dry eye.

Hormonal Supplementation

Hormonal supplementation is the most recent area of investigation in the clinical treatment of dry eye. The strong laboratory evidence associating decreased androgen levels with lacrimal gland inflammation and lacrimal insufficiency suggests that topical androgen supplementation may be a worthwhile therapy for dry eye disease (170). Clinical testing evaluating topical testosterone therapy for meibomian gland dysfunction and dry eye are currently planned for phase-3 trials in the United States.

Fatty Acid Derivatives

Anecdotal evidence suggests herbal or fish oil derivatives that contain omega-3 and omega-6 essential fatty acids may improve the symptoms of dry eye and tear film stability (Paul Honan, personal communication, 2001). One Scandinavian study suggested improvement in the inflammatory features of Sjögren's syndrome by oral administration of gamma-linolenic acid (GLA) from oil of primrose (171). It has been shown that GLA is a precursor of prostaglandin E_1 (PGE_1), a potent antiinflammatory agent successfully used in animal models of ocular inflammation (172). Recently, it has been shown that systemic therapy with linolenic acid and GLA reduces ocular surface inflammation and improves dry eye symptoms (173). Moreover, the prevalence of dry eye has been positively correlated with low ingestion of omega-3 fatty acid–rich foods (174). Prospective, randomized, masked clinical studies are needed to confirm the role of fatty acid derivatives in KCS therapy.

Topical Vitamin A

The use of topical vitamin A in the treatment of ocular disorders is controversial. Vitamin A is thought to be an essential factor for normal epithelial growth, and its deficiency can result in xerosis of the ocular surface and other organs (175). Retinol is present in tears (176) and the lacrimal gland seems to be its major provider to the ocular surface epithelium (177). It seems that although topical vitamin A derivatives are capable of reversing squamous metaplasia and keratinization at the ocular surface level, this condition is seen only in very severe dry eye conditions, typically those caused by cicatrizing conjunctivitis or GVHD (178).

Antiviral Agents

As viruses have been implicated in the pathogenesis of dry eye and dry mouth in patients with Sjögren's syndrome (179), some antiviral agents have been investigated for the treatment of dry eye conditions. Oral administration of 150 IU interferon-α three times a day in patients with primary Sjögren's syndrome has been reported to improve saliva production and relieve symptoms of xerostomia and xerophthalmia, and it was well tolerated by the patients (180).

Acupuncture

Acupuncture has shown beneficial effects in Sjögren's syndrome–related xerostomia (181), and non–Sjögren's syndrome–related dry eye (182). The mechanism of action is still speculative.

SURGICAL TREATMENT

Tarsorrhaphy

Tarsorrhaphy can substantially reduce the exposed surface area of the cornea, thus reducing evaporation of tears. In patients with severe ocular surface disease, particularly persistent epithelial defects, and noninfectious corneal ulcers, tarsorrhaphy can be extremely useful. A temporal tarsorrhaphy, closing half of the palpebral fissure, is usually adequate to protect the cornea and still provide a view of the globe. The procedure is reversible (183).

Parotid Duct and Salivary Gland Transplantation

Transplantation of parotid duct is a surgical procedure in which a duct leading from the parotid glands is transplanted to empty out to the conjunctival surface (184). The operation has for the most part been abandoned in the United States. Autologous transplantation of salivary glands is another procedure that has been employed in desperate dry eye conditions (183,185).

Amniotic Membrane Transplantation

Human amniotic membrane (AM) is composed of three layers: a single epithelial layer, a thick basement membrane, and an avascular stroma. Amniotic membrane has antiadhesive properties and is felt to promote epithelization and decrease inflammation, neovascularization, and fibrosis. Amniotic membrane transplantation has been shown to be effective in the reconstruction of the corneal surface in the setting of persistent epithelial defects, sterile corneal ulcerations, and partial limbal stem cell deficiency states, including those secondary to chemical or thermal burns (186). It is not clear, however, whether AM grafting is more effective than simple tarsorrhaphy in management of nonhealing surface defects associated with dry eye.

Stem Cell Transplantation

Schwab et al. (187) have described a technique in which cultured corneal epithelial stem cells seeded onto a matrix derived from amniotic membrane have been used to manage difficult ocular surface diseases including those with stem cell deficiency.

Conjunctival Transplantation

Cicatrizing ocular surface disorders associated with symblepharon, trichiasis, or cicatrizing lagophthalmos can be treated by conjunctival and/or limbal grafting and mucous membrane transplantation (188,189). Improved lid mobility provides better tear film distribution on the ocular surface.

Keratoprosthesis

Corneal prosthesis has been employed in the management of severe types of cicatricial disease such as ocular cicatricial pemphigoid, the Stevens-Johnson syndrome, severe trachoma, and chemical burns in which scarring has been excessive and the prognosis for corneal grafting very poor (190).

ACKNOWLEDGMENTS

We would like to thank Alan Sasai from Allergan Inc., Jerry Paugh, O.D., Ph.D., and the Southern California College of Optometry for contributing to the picture of meibomian gland dysfunction. We thank Dr. Roberto Pineda for the thread test picture.

REFERENCES

1. Holly FJ, Lemp MA. Tear physiology and dry eyes. *Surv Ophthalmol* 1977;22:69–87.
2. Lemp MA. Report of the National Eye Institute/Industry workshop on Clinical Trials in Dry Eyes. *CLAO J* 1995;21:221–232.
3. Schaumberg DA, Sullivan DA, Dana MR. Epidemiology of dry eye syndrome. *Adv Exp Med Biol* 2002;506:989–998.
4. Jacobsson LT, Axell TE, Hansen BU, et al. Dry eyes or mouth-an epidemiological study in Swedish adults, with special reference to primary Sjögren's syndrome. *J Autoimmun* 1989;2:521–527.
5. Schein OD, Munoz B, Tielsch JM, et al. Prevalence of dry eye among the elderly. *Am J Ophthalmol* 1997;124:723–728.
6. McCarty CA, Bansal AK, Livingston PM, et al. The epidemiology of dry eye in Melbourne, Australia. *Ophthalmology* 1998;105:1114–1119.
7. Mathers WD, Lane JA, Zimmerman MB. Tear film changes associated with normal aging. *Cornea* 1996;15:229–234.
8. Schaumberg DA, Sullivan DA, Buring JE, et al. Prevalence of dry eye syndrome among US women. *Am J Ophthalmol* 2003;36(2):318–326.
9. Moss SE, Klein R, Klein BE. Prevalence of and risk factors for dry eye syndrome. *Arch Ophthalmol* 2000;118:1264–1268.
10. Sullivan DA, Wickham LA, Rocha EM, et al. Influence of gender, sex steroid hormones, and the hypothalamic-pituitary axis on the structure and function of the lacrimal gland. *Adv Exp Med Biol* 1998;438:11–42.
11. Schaumberg DA, Buring JE, Sullivan DA, et al. Hormone replacement therapy and dry eye syndrome. *JAMA* 2001;286:2114–2119.
12. Stern ME, Gao J, Schwalb TA, et al. Conjunctival T-cell subpopulations in Sjögren's and non-Sjögren's patients with dry eye. *Invest Ophthalmol Vis Sci* 2002;43:2609–2614.
13. Lucca JA, Farris RL, Bielory L, et al. Keratoconjunctivitis sicca in male patients infected with human immunodeficiency virus type 1. *Ophthalmology* 1990;97:1008–1010.
14. Calissendorff B, el Azazi M, Lonnqvist B. Dry eye syndrome in long-term follow-up of bone marrow transplanted patients. *Bone Marrow Transplant* 1989;4:675–678.
15. Crandall DC, Leopold IH. The influence of systemic drugs on tear constituents. *Ophthalmology* 1979;86:115–125.
16. Jaanus SD. Ocular side effects of selected systemic drugs. *Optom Clin* 1992;2:73–96.
17. Meneray MA, Bennett DJ, Nguyen DH, et al. Effect of sensory denervation on the structure and physiologic responsiveness of rabbit lacrimal gland. *Cornea* 1998;17:99–107.
18. Chuck RS, Quiros PA, Perez AC, et al. Corneal sensation after laser in situ keratomileusis. *J Cataract Refract Surg* 2000;26:337–339.
19. McCulley JP, Shine WE. Meibomian gland and tear film lipids: structure, function and control. *Adv Exp Med Biol* 2002;506:373–378.
20. Rolando M, Refojo MF, Kenyon KR. Tear water evaporation and eye surface diseases. *Ophthalmologica* 1985;190:147–149.
21. Shimazaki J, Sakata M, Tsubota K. Ocular surface changes and discomfort in patients with meibomian gland dysfunction. *Arch Ophthalmol* 1995;113:1266–1270.
22. Rolando M, Refojo MF, Kenyon KR. Increased tear evaporation in eyes with keratoconjunctivitis sicca. *Arch Ophthalmol* 1983;101:557–558.
23. Shimazaki J, Goto E, Ono M, et al. Meibomian gland dysfunction in patients with Sjögren syndrome. *Ophthalmology* 1998;105:1485–1488.
24. Gilbard JP, Rossi SR, Heyda KG. Tear film and ocular surface changes after closure of the meibomian gland orifices in the rabbit. *Ophthalmology* 1989;96:1180–1186.
25. Stern ME, Beuerman RW, Fox RI, et al. The pathology of dry eye: the interaction between the ocular surface and lacrimal glands. *Cornea* 1998;17:584–589.
26. Inatomi T, Spurr-Michaud S, Tisdale AS, et al. Expression of secretory mucin genes by human conjunctival epithelia. *Invest Ophthalmol Vis Sci* 1996;37:1684–1692.
27. Inatomi, T, Spurr-Michaud S, Tisdale AS, et al. Human corneal and conjunctival epithelia express MUC1 mucin. *Invest Ophthalmol Vis Sci* 1995;36:1818–1827.
28. Pflugfelder SC, Liu A, Monroy D, et al. Detection of sialomucin complex (MUC4) in human ocular surface epithelium and tear fluid. *Invest Ophthalmol Vis Sci* 2000;41:1316–1326.
29. Danjo Y, Watanabe H, Tisdale AS, et al. Alteration of mucin in human conjunctival epithelia in dry eye. *Invest Ophthalmol Vis Sci* 1998;39:2602–2609.
30. Jones DT, Monroy D, Ji Z, et al. Alterations of ocular surface gene expression in Sjögren's syndrome. *Adv Exp Med Biol* 1998;438:533–536.
31. Argueso P, Balaram M, Spurr-Michaud S, et al. Decreased levels of the goblet cell mucin MUC5AC in tears of patients with Sjögren syndrome. *Invest Ophthalmol Vis Sci* 2002;43:1004–1011.
32. Cotran RS. Inflammation: historical perspectives. In: Gallin JI, Snyderman R, eds. *Basic principles and clinical correlates.* Philadelphia: Lippincott Williams & Wilkins, 1999:5–10.
33. Dana MR, Qian Y, Hamrah P. Twenty-five-year panorama of corneal immunology: emerging concepts in the immunopathogenesis of microbial keratitis, peripheral ulcerative keratitis, and corneal transplant rejection. *Cornea* 2000;19:625–643.
34. Geppert TD, Lipsky PE. Antigen presentation at the inflammatory site. *Crit Rev Immunol* 1989;9:313–362.
35. Matsumoto I, Tsubota K, Satake Y, et al. Common T cell receptor clonotype in lacrimal glands and labial salivary glands from patients with Sjögren's syndrome. *J Clin Invest* 1996;97:1969–1977.
36. Pepose JS, Akata RF, Pflugfelder SC, et al. Mononuclear cell phenotypes and immunoglobulin gene rearrangements in lacrimal gland biopsies from patients with Sjögren's syndrome. *Ophthalmology* 1990;97:1599–1605.
37. Damato BE, Allan D, Murray SB, et al. Senile atrophy of the human lacrimal gland: the contribution of chronic inflammatory disease. *Br J Ophthalmol* 1984;68:674–680.
38. Williamson J, Gibson AA, Wilson T, et al. Histology of the lacrimal gland in keratoconjunctivitis sicca. *Br J Ophthalmol* 1973;57:852–858.
39. Pflugfelder SC, Huang AJ, Feuer W, et al. Conjunctival cytologic features of primary Sjögren's syndrome. *Ophthalmology* 1990;97:985–991.
40. Baudouin C, Haouat N, Brignole F, et al. Immunopathological findings in conjunctival cells using immunofluorescence staining of impression cytology specimens. *Br J Ophthalmol* 1992;76:545–549.
41. Solomon A, Dursun D, Liu Z, et al. Pro- and anti-inflammatory forms of interleukin-1 in the tear fluid and conjunctiva of patients with dry-eye disease. *Invest Ophthalmol Vis Sci* 2001;42:2283–2292.
42. Barton K, Monroy DC, Nava A, et al. Inflammatory cytokines in the tears of patients with ocular rosacea. *Ophthalmology* 1997;104:1868–1874.
43. Pisella PJ, Brignole F, Debbasch C, et al. Flow cytometric analysis of conjunctival epithelium in ocular rosacea and keratoconjunctivitis sicca. *Ophthalmology* 2000;107:1841–1849.

44. Gilbard JP, Dartt DA. Changes in rabbit lacrimal gland fluid osmolarity with flow rate. *Invest Ophthalmol Vis Sci* 1982;23: 804–806.

45. Rolando M, Zierhut M. The ocular surface and tear film and their dysfunction in dry eye disease. *Surv Ophthalmol* 2001;45: S203–210.

46. Dana MR, Hamrah P. Role of immunity and inflammation in corneal and ocular surface disease associated with dry eye. *Adv Exp Med Biol* 2002;506:729–738.

47. Yoon JH, Kim KS, Kim HU, et al. Effects of TNF-alpha and IL-1 beta on mucin, lysozyme, IL-6 and IL-8 in passage-2 normal human nasal epithelial cells. *Acta Otolaryngol* 1999;119: 905–910.

48. Jones DT, Monroy D, Ji Z, et al. Sjögren's syndrome: cytokine and Epstein-Barr viral gene expression within the conjunctival epithelium. *Invest Ophthalmol Vis Sci* 1994;35:3493–3504.

49. Tsubota K, Fukagawa K, Fujihara T, et al. Regulation of human leukocyte antigen expression in human conjunctival epithelium. *Invest Ophthalmol Vis Sci* 1999;40:28–34.

50. Nikkinen A, Uusitalo H, Lehtosalo JI, et al. Distribution of adrenergic nerves in the lacrimal glands of guinea-pig and rat. *Exp Eye Res* 1985;40:751–756.

51. Seifert P, Spitznas M. Demonstration of nerve fibers in human accessory lacrimal glands. *Graefes Arch Clin Exp Ophthalmol* 1994;232:107–114.

52. Dartt DA, Kessler TL, Chung EH, et al. Vasoactive intestinal peptide-stimulated glycoconjugate secretion from conjunctival goblet cells. *Exp Eye Res* 1996;63:27–34.

53. Main C, Blennerhassett P, Collins SM. Human recombinant interleukin 1 beta suppresses acetylcholine release from rat myenteric plexus. *Gastroenterology* 1993;104:1648–1654.

54. Zoukhri D, Hodges RR, Rawe IM, et al. Ca2+ signaling by cholinergic and alpha1-adrenergic agonists is up-regulated in lacrimal and submandibular glands in a murine model of Sjögren's syndrome. *Clin Immunol Immunopathol* 1998;89: 134–140.

55. Zoukhri D, Hodges RR, Byon D, et al. Role of proinflammatory cytokines in the impaired lacrimation associated with autoimmune xerophthalmia. *Invest Ophthalmol Vis Sci* 2002;43: 1429–1436.

56. Wickham LA, Gao J, Toda I, et al. Identification of androgen, estrogen and progesterone receptor mRNAs in the eye. *Acta Ophthalmol Scand* 2000;78:146–153.

57. Rocha EM, Wickham LA, da Silveira LA, et al. Identification of androgen receptor protein and 5alpha-reductase mRNA in human ocular tissues. *Br J Ophthalmol* 2000;84:76–84.

58. Clark JH, Schrader, O'Malley WT. Mechanisms of action of steroid hormones. In: Wilson JD, Foster JW, eds. *Williams textbook of endocrinology.* Philadelphia: WB Saunders, 1992: 35–90.

59. Ono M, Rocha FJ, Sullivan DA. Immunocytochemical location and hormonal control of androgen receptors in lacrimal tissues of the female MRL/Mp-lpr/lpr mouse model of Sjögren's syndrome. *Exp Eye Res* 1995;61:659–666.

60. Toda I, Wickham LA, Sullivan DA. Gender and androgen treatment influence the expression of proto-oncogenes and apoptotic factors in lacrimal and salivary tissues of MRL/lpr mice. *Clin Immunol Immunopathol* 1998;86:59–71.

61. Azzarolo AM, Kaswan RL, Mircheff AK, et al. Androgen prevention of lacrimal gland regression after ovariectomy of rabbits. ARVO absracts. *Invest Ophthalmol Vis Sci* 1994;35:S1793.

62. Sullivan DA, Rocha EM, Ullman MD, et al. Androgen regulation of the meibomian gland. *Adv Exp Med Biol* 1998;438:327–331.

63. Tiffany JM. Physiological functions of the meibomian glands. *Prog Retinal Eye Res* 1995;14:47–74.

64. Prabhasawat P, Tseng SC. Frequent association of delayed tear clearance in ocular irritation. *Br J Ophthalmol* 1998;82: 666–675.

65. Pflugfelder SC, Jones D, Ji Z, et al. Altered cytokine balance in the tear fluid and conjunctiva of patients with Sjögren's syndrome keratoconjunctivitis sicca. *Curr Eye Res* 1999;19: 201–211.

66. Sjögren H. Keratoconjunctivitis sicca. In Ridley F, Sorsby A, eds. *Modern trends in ophthalmology.* London: Butterworth, 1940:403–413.

67. Abdel-Khalek LM, Williamson J, Lee WR. Morphological changes in the human conjunctival epithelium. II. In keratoconjunctivitis sicca. *Br J Ophthalmol* 1978;62:800–806.

68. Gilbard JP, Rossi SR, Gray KL, et al. Tear film osmolarity and ocular surface disease in two rabbit models for keratoconjunctivitis sicca. *Invest Ophthalmol Vis Sci* 1988;29:374–378.

69. Meyer E, Scharf Y, Schechner R, et al. Light and electron microscopical study of the conjunctiva in sicca syndrome. *Ophthalmologica* 1985;190:45–51.

70. Tseng SC. Staging of conjunctival squamous metaplasia by impression cytology. *Ophthalmology* 1985;92:728–733.

71. Lemp MA, Gold JB, Wong S, et al. An in vivo study of corneal surface morphologic features in patients with keratoconjunctivitis sicca. *Am J Ophthalmol* 1984;98:426–428.

72. McMonnies C, Ho A, Wakefield D. Optimum dry eye classification using questionnaire responses. *Adv Exp Med Biol* 1998;438:835–838.

73. Mangione CM, Lee PP, Pitts J, et al. Psychometric properties of the National Eye Institute Visual Function Questionnaire (NEI-VFQ). NEI-VFQ Field Test Investigators. *Arch Ophthalmol* 1998;116:1496–1504.

74. Schiffman RM, Christianson MD, Jacobsen G, et al. Reliability and validity of the Ocular Surface Disease Index. *Arch Ophthalmol* 2000;118:615–621.

75. Lamberts DW, Foster CS, Perry HD. Schirmer test after topical anesthesia and the tear meniscus height in normal eyes. *Arch Ophthalmol* 1979;97:1082–1085.

76. Schirmer O. Studien zur Physiologie und Pathologie der Tränenabsonderung und Tränenabfuhr. *Graefes Arch Clin Exp Ophthalmol* 1903;56:197–291.

77. Halberg GP, Berens C. Standardized Schirmer test kit. *Am J Ophthalmol* 1961;51:840.

78. Jones LT. The lacrimal secretory system and its treatment. *Am J Ophthalmol* 1966;62:47–60.

79. Hamano T. The clinical sigificance of the phenol red thread test. *Folia Ophthalmol Jpn* 1991;42:719–727.

80. Mainstone JC, Bruce AS, Golding TR. Tear meniscus measurement in the diagnosis of dry eye. *Curr Eye Res* 1996;15: 653–661.

81. Yokoi N, Bron A, Tiffany J, et al. Reflective meniscometry: a non-invasive method to measure tear meniscus curvature. *Br J Ophthalmol* 1999;83:92–97.

82. Norn MS. Desiccation of the precorneal film. I. Corneal wetting-time. *Acta Ophthalmol* 1969;47:865–880.

83. Lemp MA, Hamill JR Jr. Factors affecting tear film breakup in normal eyes. *Arch Ophthalmol* 1973;89:103–105.

84. Mengher LS, Bron AJ, Tonge SR, et al. Effect of fluorescein instillation on the pre-corneal tear film stability. *Curr Eye Res* 1985;4:9–12.

85. Mengher LS, Bron AJ, Tonge SR, et al. A non-invasive instrument for clinical assessment of the pre-corneal tear film stability. *Curr Eye Res* 1985;4:1–7.

86. Norn MS. Dead, degenerate, and living cells in conjunctival fluid and mucous thread. *Acta Ophthalmol (Copenh)* 1969;47: 1102–1115.

87. Feenstra RP, Tseng SC. What is actually stained by rose bengal? *Arch Ophthalmol* 1992;110:984–993.

88. Watanabe H, Tanaka M. Rose bengal staining and expression of mucin-like glycoprotein in cornea epithelium. *Invest Ophthalmol Vis Sci* 1996;37:S357.

89. Josephson JE, Caffery BE. Corneal staining characteristics after sequential instillations of fluorescein. *Optom Vis Sci* 1992;69:570–573.
90. Norn MS. Lissamine green. Vital staining of cornea and conjunctiva. *Acta Ophthalmol* 1973;51:483–491.
91. Eliason JA, Maurice DM. Staining of the conjunctiva and conjunctival tear film. *Br J Ophthalmol* 1990;74:519–522.
92. Gilbard JP, Farris RL, Santamaria J, 2nd. Osmolarity of tear microvolumes in keratoconjunctivitis sicca. *Arch Ophthalmol* 1978;96:677–681.
93. Farris RL, Stuchell RN, Mandel ID. Basal and reflex human tear analysis. I. Physical measurements: osmolarity, basal volumes, and reflex flow rate. *Ophthalmology* 1981;88:852–857.
94. Tabbara KF, Okumoto M. Ocular ferning test. A qualitative test for mucus deficiency. *Ophthalmology* 1982;89:712–714.
95. Mathers WD, Binarao G, Petroll M. Ocular water evaporation and the dry eye. A new measuring device. *Cornea* 1993;12:335–340.
96. Nelson JD. Simultaneous evaluation of tear turnover and corneal epithelial permeability by fluorophotometry in normal subjects and patients with keratoconjunctivitis sicca (KCS). *Trans Am Ophthalmol Soc* 1995;93:709–753.
97. Joshi A, Maurice D, Paugh JR. A new method for determining corneal epithelial barrier to fluorescein in humans. *Invest Ophthalmol Vis Sci* 1996;37:1008–1016.
98. Bron AJ, Benjamin L, Snibson GR. Meibomian gland disease. Classification and grading of lid changes. *Eye* 1991;5:395–411.
99. Robin JB, Jester JV, Nobe J, et al. In vivo transillumination biomicroscopy and photography of meibomian gland dysfunction. A clinical study. *Ophthalmology* 1985;92:1423–1426.
100. Yokoi N, Mossa F, Tiffany JM, et al. Assessment of meibomian gland function in dry eye using meibometry. *Arch Ophthalmol* 1999;117:723–729.
101. Yokoi N, Takehisa Y, Kinoshita S. Correlation of tear lipid layer interference patterns with the diagnosis and severity of dry eye. *Am J Ophthalmol* 1996;122:818–824.
102. Goto E, Tseng SC. Differentiation of lipid tear deficiency dry eye by kinetic analysis of tear interference images. *Arch Ophthalmol* 2003;121:173–180.
103. deLuise VP, Tabbara KF. Quantitation of tear lysozyme levels in dry-eye disorders. *Arch Ophthalmol* 1983;101:634–635.
104. Lucca JA, Nunez JN, Farris RL. A comparison of diagnostic tests for keratoconjunctivitis sicca: lactoplate, Schirmer, and tear osmolarity. *CLAO J* 1990;16:109–112.
105. McCollum CJ, Foulks GN, Bodner B, et al. Rapid assay of lactoferrin in keratoconjunctivitis sicca. *Cornea* 1994;13:505–508.
106. Boukes RJ, Boonstra A, Breebaart AC, et al. Analysis of human tear protein profiles using high performance liquid chromatography (HPLC). *Doc Ophthalmol* 1987;67:105–113.
107. Ralph RA. Conjunctival goblet cell density in normal subjects and in dry eye syndromes. *Invest Ophthalmol* 1975;14:299–302.
108. Brignole F, Pisella PJ, De Saint Jean M, et al. Flow cytometric analysis of inflammatory markers in KCS: 6-month treatment with topical cyclosporin A. *Invest Ophthalmol Vis Sci* 2001;42:90–95.
109. Lemp MA, Ralph RA. Rapid development of band keratopathy in dry eyes. *Am J Ophthalmol* 1977;83:657–659.
110. De Paiva CS, Harris LD, Pflugfelder SC. Keratoconus-like topographic changes in keratoconjunctivitis sicca. *Cornea* 2003;22:22–24.
111. McMonnies CW, Ho A. Patient history in screening for dry eye conditions. *J Am Optom Assoc* 1987;58:296–301.
112. Tsubota K, Nakamori K. Dry eyes and video display terminals. *N Engl J Med* 1993;328:584.
113. Dougherty JM, McCulley JP, Silvany RE, et al. The role of tetracycline in chronic blepharitis. Inhibition of lipase production in staphylococci. *Invest Ophthalmol Vis Sci* 1991;32:2970–2975.
114. Gipson IK, Yankauckas M, Spurr-Michaud SJ, et al. Characteristics of a glycoprotein in the ocular surface glycocalyx. *Invest Ophthalmol Vis Sci* 1992;33:218–227.
115. Liu Z, Pflugfelder SC. Corneal surface regularity and the effect of artificial tears in aqueous tear deficiency. *Ophthalmology* 1999;106:939–943.
116. Murube J, Paterson A, Murube E. Classification of artificial tears. I: Composition and properties. *Adv Exp Med Biol* 1998;438:693–704.
117. Swan KC. Use of methylcellulose in ophthalmology. *Arch Ophthalmol* 1945;33:378–381.
118. Al-Mansouri S, Tabbara KF. Carbomer gel in dry eye syndrome (abstract). *Ophthalmology* 1992;99:122.
119. Fox RI, Chan R, Michelson JB, et al. Beneficial effect of artificial tears made with autologous serum in patients with keratoconjunctivitis sicca. *Arthritis Rheum* 1984;27:459–461.
120. Tsubota K, Goto E, Fujita H, et al. Treatment of dry eye by autologous serum application in Sjögren's syndrome. *Br J Ophthalmol* 1999;83:390–395.
121. Rieger G. Lipid-containing eye drops: a step closer to natural tears. *Ophthalmology* 1990;201:206–212.
122. Tiffany JM. Lipid-containing eye drops. *Ophthalmologica* 1991;203:47–49.
123. MacKeen DL, Roth HW, Doane MG, et al. Supracutaneous treatment of dry eye patients with calcium carbonate. *Adv Exp Med Biol* 1998;438:985–990.
124. Tsubota K, Monden Y, Yagi Y, et al. New treatment of dry eye: the effect of calcium ointment through eyelid skin delivery. *Br J Ophthalmol* 1999;83:767–770.
125. Limberg MB, McCaa C, Kissling GE, et al. Topical application of hyaluronic acid and chondroitin sulfate in the treatment of dry eyes. *Am J Ophthalmol* 1987;103:194–197.
126. Nishida T, Nakamura M, Mishima H, et al. Hyaluronan stimulates corneal epithelial migration. *Exp Eye Res* 1991;53:753–758.
127. Tsubota K. New approaches to dry-eye therapy. *Int Ophthalmol Clin* 1994;34:115–128.
128. Iester M, Orsoni GJ, Gamba G, et al. Improvement of the ocular surface using hypotonic 0.4% hyaluronic acid drops in keratoconjunctivitis sicca. *Eye* 2000;14:892–898.
129. Lemp MA. Management of the dry-eye patient. *Int Ophthalmol Clin* 1994;34:101–113.
130. Anaizi NH, Swenson CF, Dentinger PJ. Stability of acetylcysteine in an extemporaneously compounded ophthalmic solution. *Am J Health Syst Pharm* 1997;54:549–553.
131. Gobbels M, Spitznas M. Influence of artificial tears on corneal epithelium in dry-eye syndrome. *Graefes Arch Clin Exp Ophthalmol* 1989;227:139–141.
132. Balaram M, Schaumberg DA, Dana MR. Efficacy and tolerability outcomes after punctal occlusion with silicone plugs in dry eye syndrome. *Am J Ophthalmol* 2001;131:30–36.
133. Foulds W. Intra-canalicular gelatin implants in the treatment of kerato-conjunctivitis sicca. *Br J Ophthalmol* 1961;45:625.
134. Patten JT. Punctal occlusion with n-butyl cyanoacrylate tissue adhesive. *Ophthalmic Surg* 1976;7:24–26.
135. Herrick RS. Canalicular occlusion. In: *Dacryon Dimensions* (Lubbock, TX). 1992;2:1.
136. Hamano T, Ohashi Y, Cho Y, et al. A new punctum plug. *Am J Ophthalmol* 1985;100:619–620.
137. Freeman JM. The punctum plug: evaluation of a new treatment for the dry eye. *Trans Am Acad Ophthalmol Otolaryngol* 1975;79:OP874–879.

138. Nelson CC. Complications of Freeman plugs. *Arch Ophthalmol* 1991;109:923–924.

139. Rapoza PA, Ruddat MS. Pyogenic granuloma as a complication of silicone punctal plugs. *Am J Ophthalmol* 1992;113:454–455.

140. Tai MC, Cosar CB, Cohen EJ, et al. The clinical efficacy of silicone punctal plug therapy. *Cornea* 2002;21:135–139.

141. Vrabec MP, Elsing SH, Aitken PA. A prospective, randomized comparison of thermal cautery and argon laser for permanent punctal occlusion. *Am J Ophthalmol* 1993;116:469–471.

142. Benson DR, Hemmady PB, Snyder RW. Efficacy of laser punctal occlusion. *Ophthalmology* 1992;99:618–621.

143. Glatt HJ. Acute dacryocystitis after punctal occlusion of keratoconjunctivitis sicca. *Am J Ophthalmol* 1991;111:769–770.

144. Davis RH, VanOrman EW. Making moisture-chamber spectacles. *Am J Ophthalmol* 1982;94:256–257.

145. Baldone JA, Kaufman HE. Extended wear contact lenses. *Ann Ophthalmol* 1983;15:595–596.

146. Hess AD. Mechanisms of action of cyclosporine: considerations for the treatment of autoimmune diseases. *Clin Immunol Immunopathol* 1993;68:220–228.

147. Matsuda S, Koyasu S. Mechanisms of action of cyclosporine. *Immunopharmacology* 2000;47:119–125.

148. Halestrap AP, McStay GP, Clarke SJ. The permeability transition pore complex: another view. *Biochimie* 2002;84:153–166.

149. Kaswan RL, Salisbury MA, Ward DA. Spontaneous canine keratoconjunctivitis sicca. A useful model for human keratoconjunctivitis sicca: treatment with cyclosporine eye drops. *Arch Ophthalmol* 1989;107:1210–1216.

150. Sall K, Stevenson OD, Mundorf TK, et al. Two multicenter, randomized studies of the efficacy and safety of cyclosporine ophthalmic emulsion in moderate to severe dry eye disease. CsA Phase 3 Study Group. *Ophthalmology* 2000;107: 631–639.

151. Stevenson D, Tauber J, Reis BL. Efficacy and safety of cyclosporin A ophthalmic emulsion in the treatment of moderate-to-severe dry eye disease: a dose-ranging, randomized trial. The Cyclosporin A Phase 2 Study Group. *Ophthalmology* 2000;107:967–974.

152. Turner K, Pflugfelder SC, Ji Z, et al. Interleukin-6 levels in the conjunctival epithelium of patients with dry eye disease treated with cyclosporine ophthalmic emulsion. *Cornea* 2000;19:492–496.

153. Almawi WY, Melemedjian OK. Negative regulation of nuclear factor-kappaB activation and function by glucocorticoids. *J Mol Endocrinol* 2002;28:69–78.

154. Dursun D, Kim MC, Solomon A, et al. Treatment of recalcitrant recurrent corneal erosions with inhibitors of matrix metalloproteinase-9, doxycycline and corticosteroids. *Am J Ophthalmol* 2001;132:8–13.

155. Liden J, Rafter I, Truss M, et al. Glucocorticoid effects on NF-kappaB binding in the transcription of the ICAM-1 gene. *Biochem Biophys Res Commun* 2000;273:1008–1014.

156. Brunner T, Arnold D, Wasem C, et al. Regulation of cell death and survival in intestinal intraepithelial lymphocytes. *Cell Death Differ* 2001;8:706–714.

157. Yoshida T, Tanaka M, Sotomatsu A, et al. Effect of methylprednisolone-pulse therapy on superoxide production of neutrophils. *Neurol Res* 1999;21:509–512.

158. Marsh P, Pflugfelder SC. Topical nonpreserved methylprednisolone therapy for keratoconjunctivitis sicca in Sjögren syndrome. *Ophthalmology* 1999;106:811–816.

159. Solomon A, Rosenblatt M, Li D, et al. Doxycycline inhibition of interleukin-1 in the corneal epithelium. *Am J Ophthalmol* 2000; 130:688.

160. Amin AR, Attur MG, Thakker GD, et al. A novel mechanism of action of tetracyclines: effects on nitric oxide synthases. *Proc Natl Acad Sci U S A* 1996;93:14014–14019.

161. Li DQ, Lokeshwar BL, Solomon A, et al. Regulation of MMP-9 production by human corneal epithelial cells. *Exp Eye Res* 2001;73:449–459.

162. Frucht-Pery J, Sagi E, Hemo I, et al. Efficacy of doxycycline and tetracycline in ocular rosacea. *Am J Ophthalmol* 1993;116:88–92.

163. Nelson JD, Friedlaender M, Yeatts RP, et al. Oral pilocarpine for symptomatic relief of keratoconjunctivitis sicca in patients with Sjögren's syndrome. The MGI PHARMA Sjögren's Syndrome Study Group. *Adv Exp Med Biol* 1998;438: 979–983.

164. Mathers WD, Dolney AM. Objective demonstration of stimulation with oral pilocarpine in dry eye patients. *Invest Ophthalmol Vis Sci* 2000;41:S60.

165. Petrone D, Condemi JJ, Fife R, et al. A double-blind, randomized, placebo-controlled study of cevimeline in Sjögren's syndrome patients with xerostomia and keratoconjunctivitis sicca. *Arthritis Rheum* 2002;46:748–754.

166. Gilbard JP, Rossi SR, Heyda KG, et al. Stimulation of tear secretion by topical agents that increase cyclic nucleotide levels. *Invest Ophthalmol Vis Sci* 1990;31:1381–1388.

167. Li Y, Kuang K, Yerxa B, et al. Rabbit conjunctival epithelium transports fluid, and P2Y2 receptor agonists stimulate C1(−) and fluid secretion. *Am J Physiol Cell Phys* 2001;281:C595–602.

168. Foulks G, Sall K, Greenberg M, et al. Phase 2 dose ranging efficacy trial of INS365 ophthalmic solution, a P2Y2 agonist, in patients with dry eye. ARVO abstract. *Invest Ophthalmol Vis Sci* 2001;42:S713.

169. Hamano T. Dry eye treatment with eye drops that stimulate mucin production. *Adv Exp Med Biol* 1998;438:965–968.

170. Sullivan DA, Wickham LA, Rocha EM, et al. Androgens and dry eye in Sjögren's syndrome. *Ann N Y Acad Sci* 1999;876:312–324.

171. Horrobin DF. Essential fatty acid and prostaglandin metabolism in Sjögren's syndrome, systemic sclerosis and rheumatoid arthritis. *Scand J Rheumatol Suppl* 1986;61:242–245.

172. Hoyng PF, Verbey N, Thorig L, et al. Topical prostaglandins inhibit trauma-induced inflammation in the rabbit eye. *Invest Ophthalmol Vis Sci* 1986;27:1217–1225.

173. Barabino S, Rolando M, Camicione P, et al. Systemic linoleic and gamma-linolenic acid therapy in dry eye syndrome with an inflammatory component. *Cornea* 2003;22:97–101.

174. Trivedi KA, Dana MR, Gilbard JP, et al. Dietary omega-3 fatty acid intake and risk of clinically diagnosed dry eye syndrome in women. *Invest Ophthalmol Vis Sci* 2003;44:E-Abstract 811.

175. Sommer A. Xerophthalmia and vitamin A status. *Prog Retin Eye Res* 1998;17:9–31.

176. Ubels JL, MacRae SM. Vitamin A is present as retinol in the tears of humans and rabbits. *Curr Eye Res* 1984;3:815–822.

177. Lee SY, Ubels JL, Soprano DR. The lacrimal gland synthesizes retinol-binding protein. *Exp Eye Res* 1992;55:163–171.

178. Murphy PT, Sivakumaran M, Fahy G, et al. Successful use of topical retinoic acid in severe dry eye due to chronic graft-versus-host disease. *Bone Marrow Transplant* 1996;18:641–642.

179. Tsubota K, Fujishima H, Toda I, et al. Increased levels of Epstein-Barr virus DNA in lacrimal glands of Sjögren's syndrome patients. *Acta Ophthalmol Scand* 1995;73: 425–430.

180. Khurshudian AV. A pilot study to test the efficacy of oral administration of interferon-alpha lozenges to patients with Sjögren's syndrome. *Oral Surg Oral Med Oral Pathol Oral Radiol Endod* 2003;95:38–44.

181. Blom M, Kopp S, Lundeberg T. Prognostic value of the pilocarpine test to identify patients who may obtain long-term relief from xerostomia by acupuncture treatment. *Arch Otolaryngol Head Neck Surg* 1999;125:561–566.

182. Nepp J, Derbolav A, Haslinger-Akramian J, et al. [Effect of acupuncture in keratoconjunctivitis sicca]. *Klin Monatsbl Augenheilkd* 1999;215:228–232.

183. Murube J. Surgical treatment of the dry eye. In: Boyd B, ed. *World Atlas Series of Ophthalmic Surgery,* Vol. 2. Panama, Highlights of Ophthalmology International, 1995:227–236.

184. Bennet JE. The management of total xerophthalmia. *Arch Ophthalmol* 1969;81:667–682.

185. Geerling G, Sieg P, Bastian GO, et al. Transplantation of the autologous submandibular gland for most severe cases of keratoconjunctivitis sicca. *Ophthalmology* 1998;105:327–335.

186. Tseng SC. Amniotic membrane transplantation for ocular surface reconstruction. *Biosci Rep* 200;21:481–489.

187. Schwab IR, Reyes M, Isseroff RR. Successful transplantation of bioengineered tissue replacements in patients with ocular surface disease. *Cornea* 2000;19:421–426.

188. Herman WK, Doughman DJ, Lindstrom RL. Conjunctival autograft transplantation for unilateral ocular surface diseases. *Ophthalmology* 1983;90:1121–1126.

189. Shore JW, Foster CS, Westfall CT, et al. Results of buccal mucosal grafting for patients with medically controlled ocular cicatricial pemphigoid. *Ophthalmology* 1992;99:383–395.

190. Barnham JJ, Roper-Hall MJ. Keratoprosthesis: a long-term review. *Br J Ophthalmol* 1983;67:468–474.

SJÖGREN'S SYNDROME

MURAT DOGRU AND KAZUO TSUBOTA

Sjögren's syndrome (SS) is a multifactorial autoimmune disorder, mainly affecting the salivary and lacrimal glands, which is influenced by genetic as well as environmental factors that are not yet completely understood. Henrik Sjögren described the syndrome in 1933 in the context we understand today. The evolution of historical issues related to the syndrome is shown in Table 29-1 (1). The manifestations of SS are generally the result of lymphocyte-mediated damage. Although dry eyes and dry mouth characterize the disease, the expression of clinical spectrum is diverse, extending from a solitary organ-specific autoimmune exocrinopathy to a systemic disorder affecting several organs (2) (Table 29-2). In the absence of an associated connective tissue disease, dry mouth and dry eye are referred to as the "sicca complex," or "primary SS." Secondary SS refers to the full triad of xerophthalmia, xerostomia, and a connective tissue or a collagen disease such as rheumatoid arthritis (RA), scleroderma, or systemic lupus erythematosus (SLE) (3).

EPIDEMIOLOGY

Sjögren's syndrome occurs worldwide and in people of all ages. However, the peak incidence is in the fourth and fifth decades of life, with a female-to-male ratio of 9:1. Prevalence studies have demonstrated that sicca symptoms and primary SS affect a considerable percentage of the population, with precise numbers dependent on the age group studied and on the criteria used. The incidence of primary SS reported in the literature varies from less than 1:1,000 to more than 1:100 (4). Fox and Saito (5) estimated the prevalence of primary SS at approximately 1 in 1,250 individuals based on a retrospective review of records using the San Diego criteria. Using the Copenhagen criteria to evaluate 705 randomly selected individuals in Sweden aged 52 to 72 years, Pillemer et al. found symptoms and signs of dry eyes in 15% and xerostomia in 8% of this general population (5a). SS, according to the Copenhagen criteria, was present in 2.7%, about 20-fold higher than estimates of SS using the San Diego criteria (5).

Bjerrum (6) reported that the frequency of keratoconjunctivitis sicca (KCS) in persons aged 30 to 60 years in Copenhagen was 11% according to the Copenhagen criteria and 8% according to the European criteria. The frequency of primary SS was estimated to be 0.2% to 0.8% according to the Copenhagen criteria and 0.6% to 2.1% according to the European criteria in that study. Other studies of the prevalence for primary SS in the healthy geriatric population have ranged from 2% to 4.8%. The prevalence of definite SS in a Greek population employing the European Community criteria was reported to be 0.59% (7). In studies of secondary SS, the prevalence of sicca symptoms among Greek patients with RA has been estimated to be at 31%, with systemic sclerosis at 20% and SLE at 8% (5). Approximately 17,000 new cases of SS are being diagnosed in Japan each year. The incidence of SS in Japan employing the Japanese diagnostic criteria is far lower than in other nations and is reported to be 0.026%, which may be due to racial differences (8). A cautious but realistic estimate from the studies presented thus far is that primary SS is a disease with prevalence not exceeding 0.6% of the general population (5).

PATHOGENESIS

Although generally considered a T-cell-mediated disease, potential mechanisms underlying SS range from disturbances in apoptosis on an inflammatory background to circulating autoantibodies against the ribonucleoproteins Ro and La or cholinergic muscarinic receptors. Others relate reduced salivary and tear flow to aberrant glandular aquaporin-5 water channels.

Inflammatory Background in Sjögren's Syndrome

Many exocrine glands, the ocular surface, and the lacrimal gland are affected by sex hormones, principally the androgens. It has been shown that androgen receptor protein exists within the epithelial cell nuclei of the human exocrine

TABLE 29-1. EVOLUTION OF HISTORICAL ISSUES RELATED TO SJÖGREN'S SYNDROME

Year	Scientist	First Description
1882	Leber	Filamentary keratitis (FK)
1888	Hadden	Dry eye–dry mouth association
1892	Mikulicz	Mikulicz's disease (salivary and lacrimal gland enlargement)
1919	Fuchs	FK and lacrimal hypofunction
1925	Gougerot	Dry eye: mouth, larynx, and vagina association
1933	Sjögren	Sjögren's syndrome
1955 and SS	Morgan and Castleman	Identical pathologic basis for Mikulicz's disease

TABLE 29-2. CLINICAL SPECTRUM OF SJÖGREN'S SYNDROME

Musculoskeletal
Arthralgias, Rheumatoid arthritis
Myalgias, polymyositis and myopathies

Cutaneous
Dry skin
Hyperglobulinemic purpura
Vasculitis (purple rash of lower legs with pale pink hive-like welts or ulcers)

Pulmonary
Xerotrachea
Pulmonary infiltrates with pneumonia and bronchitis

Gastrointestinal
Esophageal dysmotility
Gastric achlorhydria
Buccal membranes
Pancreatitis
Adult celiac disease
Oral ulcer and fissures
Hepatitis
Biliary cirrhosis
Dental caries

Renal
Renal tubular acidosis
Interstitial nephritis

Neurologic
Peripheral and cranial neuropathy
Central nervous system disease with cerebral vasculitis, paralysis, loss of speech, headaches and disorientation, multiple sclerosis, acute transverse myelopathy

Hematologic and vascular
Leucopenia
Hypergammaglobulinemia, cryoglobulinemia
Anemia
Polyarteritis nodosa

Oncologic
Lymphomas and pseudolymphomas

Otolaryngologic
Recurrent otitis media
Nasal dryness and epistaxis
Hoarseness
Parotid gland enlargement

Endocrinologic
Chronic thyroiditis
Hashimoto's thyroiditis

Gynecologic
Vaginal dryness, vaginitis, sexual dysfunction

glands, meibomian gland, conjunctiva, and cornea, suggesting that androgens influence their structural organization and functional activity, and have an especially profound impact on the immunology, molecular biology, and secretory capacity of the lacrimal gland (9). Such proven androgen effects have led to the idea that androgen deficiency states such as SS, SLE, RAs, aging, and the use of antiaging medications may be very important in the pathogenesis of dry eyes (10). The androgen binding to the receptors in the acinar nuclei of the exocrine glands (the lacrimal gland in the context of xerophthalmia) leads to an altered expression of numerous cytokines and proto-oncogenes. The activity of androgens in the exocrine glands is thought to induce the accumulation of antiinflammatory cytokines such as transforming growth factor-β (TGF-β) (10). The reduction of the androgen level below a certain threshold may result in the release of proinflammatory cytokines such as interleukin-1β (IL-1ß), IL-2, interferon-γ, and tumor necrosis factor-α (TNF-α) by the lymphocytes entering the gland (11). Experimental evidence has shown that progressive CD4$^+$ T-cell and B-cell infiltration occurs in lacrimal and salivary glands of patients with SS (12). Alterations of the nerve fibers among the glandular acini are superimposed on the inflammatory process in these patients. It is also possible that the central nervous system plays an important role in the cascade of events that occur in SS where the amount of tear flow is initially decreased through cellular infiltration of the tear gland. Increased friction between the lids dry cornea may cause exfoliation of the superficial corneal epithelium, resulting in constant repeated C-fiber nerve stimulation, which becomes dominant in time and acts in combination with central parasympathetic inhibition of tear flow. This could also explain the clinical and experimental discrepancies of the concept of infiltration and destruction of the lacrimal gland as a single cause of tear flow depression. In addition, central neural mechanisms may also explain those cases in which patients have subjective rather than objective improvement of complaints (13).

Under normal circumstances, lymphocytes entering the lacrimal or an exocrine gland are expected to undergo apoptosis. In the presence of inflammation, however, the apoptotic response is aborted, and the lymphocytes release proinflammatory cytokines and inflammatory cytokines such as IL-1β, IL-6, and IL-8 (14,15). The increased expression of human leukocyte antigen (HLA)-DR and intercellular adhesion molecule (ICAM) in the conjunctiva, for instance, has been reported to be associated with "homing" of more T cells and greater cytokine release within the lacrimal gland, increasing the level of inflammation (16).

Numerous investigators have attempted to analyze the association of primary SS with cytokine polymorphisms. Both human and animal studies indicate the involvement of IL-10 in the pathogenesis of primary SS, and mice transgenic for IL-10 develop a Fas-ligand mediated exocrinopathy that resembles SS (17,18). A recent study described an association between primary SS and IL-10 promoter polymorphisms in a cohort of Finnish individuals, and a specific haplotype was found to correlate with high plasma levels of IL-10 (19). Conversely, no association was found for IL-10 promoter polymorphism and primary SS or the presence of Ro autoantibodies in an Australian cohort of primary SS patients (20). The IL-1 receptor antagonist regulates IL-1 activity in inflammatory disorders by binding to the IL-1 receptor and thus, inhibiting its activity. The human IL-1 receptor antagonist gene *(IL1RN)* has a variable allelic polymorphism within intron 2. An increased frequency and carriage rate of the *ILRN*2* allele has been found in primary SS (21,22).

Inflammation-Ocular Surface Interactions

Solomon et al. (22a) reported that IL-1α and -1β, IL-6, IL-8, TGF-β1, and TNF-α were expressed at elevated levels in the conjunctival epithelia of patients with SS compared with dry eye controls. These investigators also demonstrated that the conjunctival epithelium of SS patients displayed increased numbers of S-phase cells; the authors formulated a model to explain the ocular surface pathology of SS: mechanical abrasion secondary to tear deficiency creates an inflammatory environment, with conjunctival epithelial cells and lymphocytes stimulated to produce and secrete various cytokines into the tear film. Elevated cytokine levels within the tear film, combined with reduced concentrations of essential lacrimal-gland derived factors such as epidermal growth factor (EGF) and retinol, create an environment in which terminal differentiation of the ocular surface epithelium is impaired. As a consequence, the epithelium becomes hyperplastic, displaying increased mitotic activity, and loses the ability to express mature surface protecting molecules, including membrane bound mucin, MUC-1. Indeed, conjunctival impression cytology supports this hypothesis, demonstrating "snake-like chromatin cells," increased squamous metaplasia, decreased goblet cell density and inflammatory cells in SS patients (24–26). The ocular surface changes in SS dry eyes are frequently associated with corneal hypoesthesia; this perpetuates a vicious cycle. These would all imply that antiinflammatory medications that suppress the inflammatory component of this cascade may ameliorate the ocular surface disease and discomfort experienced by SS patients.

The Role of Apoptosis in Sjögren's Syndrome

Autoimmune diseases are mostly characterized by tissue destruction and functional decline due to autoreactive T cells that escape self-tolerance. Although the specificity of cytotoxic T-lymphocyte function has been an important issue of organ-specific autoimmune responses, the mechanisms responsible for tissue destruction in SS remain to be elucidated. The histopathologic changes seen in minor salivary gland biopsies are characterized by focal and/or diffuse lymphoid cell infiltrates and parenchymal destruction. The majority of cells in glandular biopsy specimens are CD4$^+$ T cells, with a small proportion of CD8$^+$ T cells (27). These T cells express the $\alpha\beta$ receptor and cell surface antigens associated with mature memory T cells. When the repertoire of T-cell receptor (TCR) *Vβ* genes transcribed and expressed within the inflammatory infiltrates was analyzed in the animal model of primary SS, a preferential utilization of TCR *Vβ* genes was detected from the onset of the disease. A 120-kD organ-specific autoantigen was previously described from the salivary gland tissues of the animal model of SS [NFS/*sld* mutant mouse thymectomized 3 days after birth (3d-TX)]. The sequence of the first 20 NH$_2$-terminal residues is identical to that of the cytoskeletal protein human α-fodrin (27). And sera from patients with SS reacted positively with the purified 120-kD antigen, and induced a proliferative response of peripheral blood lymphocytes. Purified antigen was detected from SS patients, but not from SLE or RA patients and healthy controls. These results indicate that the anti-120-kD α-fodrin immune response may play a role in the development of primary SS. Recent reports have demonstrated evidence that caspase-3 is required for α-fodrin cleavage during apoptosis (27). It has been speculated that an increase in activity of apoptotic proteases is involved in the development of α-fodrin proteolysis during the development of SS. Fodrin cleavage by caspases can lead to cytoskeletal alterations. It is of interest to remember that α-fodrin binds to ankylin, which contains a cell death domain. It has been shown that cleavage products of α-fodrin inhibit adenosine triphosphate (ATP)-dependent glutamate and γ-aminobutyric acid accumulation into synaptic vesicles where a cleavage product can be a novel component of an unknown immunoregulatory network such as cytolinker proteins (28). It is now also clear that the interaction of Fas with FasL regulates a large number of pathophysiologic processes via apoptosis. Immunohistologic studies revealed that the majority of T cells infiltrating salivary glands bear FasL in the SS model, and epithelial duct cells express Fas antigen on their cell surface (29). CD4$^+$ T cells isolated from the affected glands bear a large proportion of FasL compared to CD8$^+$ cells (flow cytometry). Tsubota and associates (30) previously showed the presence of apoptosis of acinar cells, FasL expression in lacrimal glands (Fig. 29-1), and that the FasL expression highly correlated with glandular function, especially in those patients without glandular enlargement. FasL expression of infiltrating lymphocytes was low in the lacrimal glands of patients with SS with enlarged exocrine glands where the lacrimal gland function was well preserved even with massive lymphocyte invasion

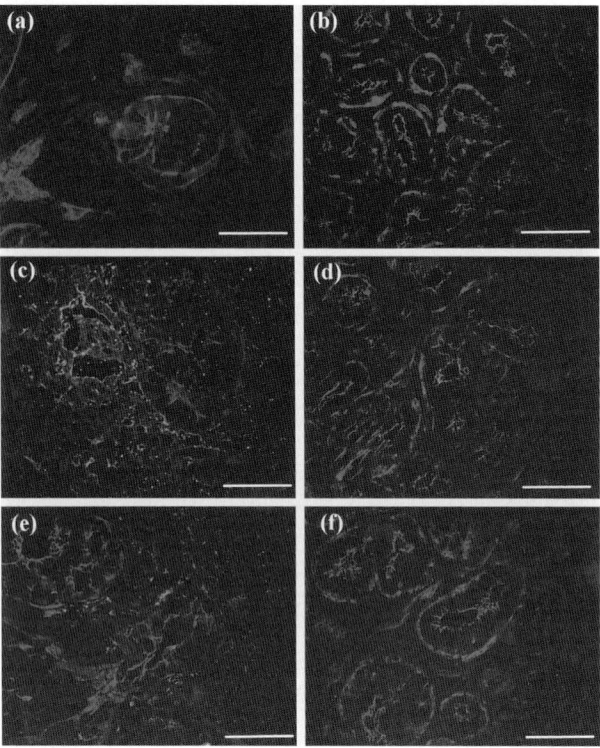

FIGURE 29-1. Quantitative evaluation and evidence of apoptotic mechanisms in Sjögren's syndrome (SS): double staining of actin and Apo2.7, Fas, or FasL in lacrimal gland. **A,C,E:** Lacrimal glands from SS. **B,D,F:** Lacrimal glands from non-SS were stained with Apo2.7 **(A,B)**, Fas **(C,D)**, and FasL **(E,F)** antibody followed by rhodamine-phalloidin. Bars: 50 μm. **A:** SS lacrimal gland. Note the (+) acinar cells. **B:** Non-SS lacrimal gland. No acinar cells are stained with Apo2.7 antibody. **C:** SS lacrimal gland. Note the (+) acinar cells, **D:** Non-SS lacrimal gland. Some acinar cells are stained with Fas antibody. **E:** SS lacrimal gland. Note (+) staining of infiltrating lymphocytes. **F:** Non-SS lacrimal gland. FasL antibody did not stain any cells. (From Tsubota K, Fujita H, Tsuzaka K, et al. Quantitative analysis of lacrimal gland function, apoptotic figures, Fas and Fas ligand expression of lacrimal glands in dry eye patients. *Exp Eye Res* 2003; 76:233–240. Copyright 2003, with permission from Elsevier.)

(30). In other words, the infiltration of lymphocytes alone did not cause glandular dysfunction. Apoptosis of acinar cells may explain the differences.

Infectious Background in Sjögren's Syndrome

Transgenic mice containing the human T-cell lymphotropic virus type-1 (HTLV-1) *ax* gene under the control of viral long terminal repeat develop an exocrinopathy that involves the salivary and lacrimal glands, resembling the pathology of SS (31). It has been suggested that the HTLV-1 infection might represent a primary event in the development of exocrinopathy by virally induced proliferation and perturbation of the function of the ductal epithelium. Sialadenitis and inflammation in lacrimal glands histologically resembling SS have been reported to be associated with hepatitis C viral infection (32). Epstein-Barr virus (EBV) has also long

been believed to play some role in the development of SS. Increased levels of EBV DNA in salivary glands of SS patients have been demonstrated by polymerase chain reaction technology, suggesting that viral reactivation or homing of EBV-infected circulating B cells may produce chronic autoimmune destruction of the salivary gland (33). Pflugfelder and associates (34) detected EBV DNA sequences in 80% of lacrimal glands from SS patients. SS has also been shown to develop after infectious mononucleosis, a condition caused by EBV. Crouse et al. (35) reported that EBV DNA was detected more in lacrimal glands compared to salivary glands. It has indeed been reported that, in any given individual with SS, lymphocytic infiltration of the lacrimal gland was far greater than that of the salivary gland (36). These findings corroborate the clinical evidence that dry eyes are more severe than dry mouth in SS. Pflugfelder et al. (37) have suggested that the conjunctival squamous metaplasia seen in SS may be primarily due to a dysfunctional immune system; the detection of EBV DNA in the conjunctival epithelium in their study was believed to support this hypothesis. It has been reported that 1% to 2% of the conjunctival cells from SS patients are T or B lymphocytes, with the latter serving as a possible source of EBV (38). It is not yet clear whether these EBV-infected B cells come from the lacrimal gland or subepithelial connective tissue. Like the lacrimal gland epithelial cells, conjunctival epithelium may have EBV receptors. Although further study is necessary, it seems likely that the conjunctiva is also primarily affected in SS.

Genetic Background in Sjögren's Syndrome

A genetic predisposition to SS appears to exist, and several families involving two or more cases of SS have been described. However, the extent of genetic contribution remains unknown (39–42). Large twin studies in SS are lacking, and the twin concordance rate cannot be estimated (43). A few available case reports reveal a very similar phenotype, with almost identical clinical presentation, including dry eyes and dry mouth, similar serologic data, with identical fine specificity in their immune responses to 60-kD Ro/SSA, and identical labial salivary gland focus scores (43). It is also common for an SS proband to have relatives with other autoimmune diseases (approximately 30% to 35%) (44,45). The major histocompatibility complex (MHC) genes are the best-documented genetic risk factors for the development of autoimmune disease (46–48). In European and American Caucasians, SS was found to be associated with the haplotypes B8, DRw52, and DR3 (49). The increased frequency of HLA-B8 was presumably due to an association (linkage disequilibrium) with the HLA class II allele HLA-DRB1*03 (50). However, a novel association of HLA class I alleles (HLA-A24) to susceptibility in primary SS was also recently described. An association with DR2 has been found in Scandinavians and with DR5 in Greeks (51). All of the haplotypes are in strong linkage disequilibrium, resulting in difficulties in establishing which of the genes contains the locus that confers the risk (52). It has been claimed that SS patients with DQ1/DQ2 alleles have a more severe autoimmune disease than do patients with any other allelic combination at HLA-DQ, and the DR3-DQ2 haplotype has been indicated as a possible marker for a more active immune response in Finnish patients with SS (53). Autoantibodies to Ro/SSA and La/SSB have been found to be associated with DR3, DQA, and DQB alleles (54–56). In Japan, HLA class II allele association has been reported to differ among anti-Ro/SSA (+) individuals according to the presence or absence of coexisting anti-La/SSB (8). The contribution of Ro/SSA and La/SSB in SS is not fully understood. It is not known how tolerance breakdown and autoantibody response to Ro/SSA and La/SSB is generated. The ribonucleoproteins are endogenous proteins that are normally hidden from the immune system and should not give rise to abnormal B-cell responses. However, stress, such as ultraviolet radiation, viral infections, and apoptosis have been suggested to lead to cell surface exposure of previously hidden autoantigens to the immune system (57). Genes that encode transporters associated with antigen processing (*TAP* genes) have also been associated with susceptibility to SS (58). Others have indicated a putative role for the cysteine-rich secretory protein 3 *(CRISP-3)* gene as an early response gene that may participate in the pathophysiology of the autoimmune disease in SS (59).

Background on Aberrant Glandular Water Transport

Aquaporins (AQPs) are water-specific membrane channel proteins that provide the molecular pathway for water permeability in many tissues (60–62). Among them, aquaporin 5 (AQP5) is normally expressed in the apical membranes of acinar cells in lacrimal and salivary glands, as well as the corneal epithelium and type-1 pneumocytes of the lung (60). At least five AQPs are expressed in the eye: AQP0 (MIP) in lens fiber; AQP1 in cornea endothelium, ciliary and lens epithelia, and trabecular meshwork; AQP3 in conjunctiva; AQP4 in ciliary epithelium and retinal Müller cells; and AQP5 in corneal and lacrimal gland epithelia. This cell-specific expression pattern suggests involvement of AQPs in corneal and lens transparency, intraocular pressure (IOP) regulation, retinal signal transduction, and tear secretion. Indeed, humans with mutant AQP0 develop cataracts. Mice lacking AQP1 have reduced IOP and impaired corneal transparency after swelling, and mice lacking AQP4 have reduced light-evoked potentials by electroretinography. There is evidence of impaired cellular processing of AQP5 in lacrimal glands of humans with SS (61). We carried out immunolabeling for AQP5 in biopsy samples from normal controls and patients with SS or non-SS type of dry eyes. An apical membrane-staining pattern was noted in normal subjects and in non-SS and Mikulicz's syndrome patients. In contrast, diffuse cytoplasmic staining was observed in the lacrimal gland biopsy samples of patients with SS, with almost no labeling at the apical membranes (63) (Fig. 29-2). Quantification of AQP5 by enzyme-linked immunosorbent assay (ELISA) in these three groups did not reveal significant differences of AQP5 expression, suggesting a defect in protein trafficking rather than synthesis. The cause of the defect remains unknown (Fig. 29-3). Additional immunohistochemical analyses showed that the sodium-potassium adenosine triphosphatase (ATPase) channels in the basolateral membranes and sodium channels in

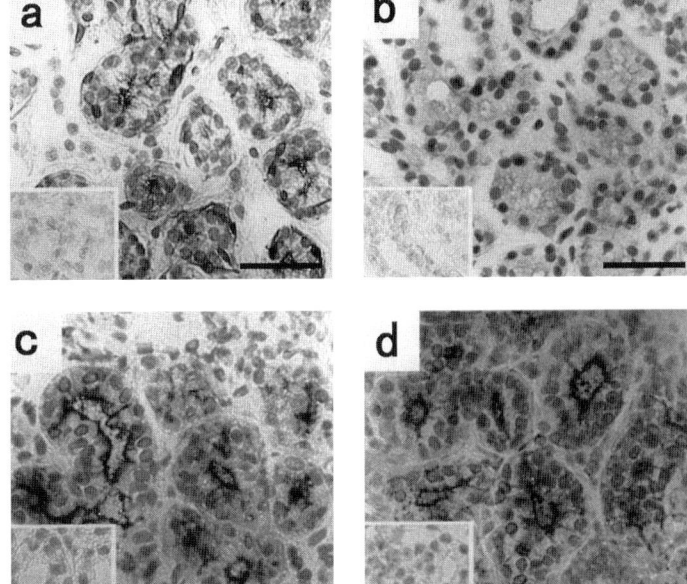

FIGURE 29-2. Immunolocalization of AQP5 in lacrimal glands. **A:** Normal control. **B:** Sjögren's syndrome (SS). **C:** Non-SS patient. **D:** Mikulicz's disease. All samples labeled with antibodies to human AQP5 and visualized with peroxidase conjugated secondary antibodies. Insets are (−) controls. Bars: 50 μm. (From Tsubota K, Hirai S, King LS, et al. Defective cellular trafficking of lacrimal gland aquaporin-5 in Sjögren's syndrome. Lancet 2001; 357:688–689, with permission from Elsevier.)

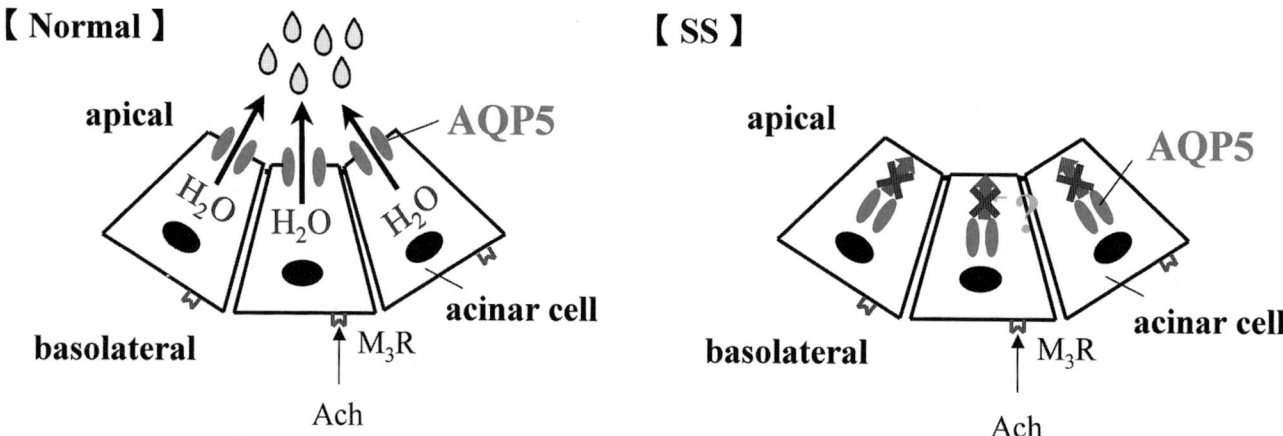

FIGURE 29-3. Aquaporin-5-mediated water transport in normal and SS eyes.

apical membranes were normally distributed in all patients (Table 29-3). In a recent study, we found that AQP5 increased in the tears of patients with severe SS compared with control subjects (64). This finding corresponds to a previous report that leakage of AQP5 in the tear was related to the lacrimal gland damage in experimental dacryoadenitis models. Although significant correlations exist between tear lactoferrin and EGF and clinical indices such as tear function index, Schirmer test and rose-Bengal staining scores, no correlation between AQP5 levels and clinical indices was observed. These differences suggest that lactoferrin and EGF produced by the lacrimal gland directly preserve ocular surface function, whereas AQP5 has not a direct but rather a secondary influence on the ocular surface disorder, caused by a decrease in the number of lacrimal gland cells (64).

The Role of Primary Sjögren's Syndrome Animal Models in the Current Pathophysiologic Concepts

Several animal models, both experimentally induced and spontaneous inflammatory reactions with features of SS, have been reported previously. The nonobese diabetic (NOD) mouse develops a disease that mimics human type 1 diabetes mellitus and also spontaneously develops sialadenitis and several other features of SS (65). Studies on

the importance of NOD non-MHC genes gave way to the creation of an H2^q congenic mouse, namely NOD.Q. A recent gene segregation experiment conducted on this mouse revealed one locus associated with sialadenitis on chromosome 4 (66). More recently, alleles from chromosomes 1 and 3 of NOD mice have been found to combine to influence SS-like autoimmune exocrinopathy. Also, chromosome 1 was reported to be a major susceptibility region for development of autoimmune sialadenitis (67).

The NZB, MKL/*lpr,* NOD, and NFS/*sld* strains are all experimental murine models that spontaneously develop salivary gland inflammation, of which the MSL/*lpr* and the NOD strains present with serum anti-Ro/SSA antibodies (68). A genome-wide scan of MSL/*lpr* mice revealed four susceptible loci, mapped on chromosomes 10, 18, 4, and 1, which were recessively associated with sialadenitis. Transgenic mice also proved to be good models to study the role of cytokines, especially IL-10 in the pathogenesis of SS (31).

DIAGNOSIS

Systemic Features

The criteria for diagnosis of SS remained controversial, and several sets of diagnostic criteria have been proposed. Among them, the San Diego criteria required evidence for an autoimmune process associated with severe destruction

TABLE 29-3. CLINICAL AND HISTOLOGICAL CHARACTERISTICS OF BIOPSY SAMPLES FROM NORMAL SUBJECTS AND DRY EYE PATIENTS

	Basal Tearing	Reflex Tearing	AOP5	Na$^+$ Channel	Na$^+$-K$^+$ ATP-ase
Controls	Normal	Normal	Normal	Normal	Normal
SS	Abnormal	Abnormal	Abnormal	Normal	Normal
Mikulicz	Abnormal	Normal	Normal	Normal	Normal
Non-SS	Abnormal	Normal	Normal	Normal	Normal

of salivary and lacrimal glands. On the other hand, the Copenhagen and European study groups have based their diagnostic criteria on clinical findings of dry eyes and mouth with no absolute requirement for gland biopsy or presence of autoantibodies (5). Recently, a consensus has been reached between the U.S. and European study groups, resulting in revised international classification criteria and revised rules for SS that have found wide acceptance (69) (Tables 29-4 and 29-5).

The proper diagnosis of SS depends on recognition of the characteristic clinical findings based on judgments made from the most commonly encountered clinical features such as dryness of the skin and pruritus, arthralgias (approximately 20% of patients with RA have secondary SS), cough (as the most frequent pulmonary symptom), xerostomia, problems of deglutition, mild hepatitis or pancreatitis diagnosed by routine laboratory testing, and KCS (2). Neurologic disease is perhaps the most common significant extraglandular manifestation of SS and can involve the cranial nerves and peripheral nerves, but rarely the central nervous system. One of the most common forms of cranial neuropathy in SS is trigeminal neuralgia. Glove and stocking

TABLE 29-4. REVISED INTERNATIONAL CLASSIFICATION CRITERIA FOR SJÖGREN'S SYNDROME

I. **Ocular symptoms:** (+) response to at least one of the following questions:
1. Have you had daily, persistent, troublesome dry eyes for more than 3 months?
2. Do you have a recurrent foreign-body sensation in the eyes?
3. Do you use tear substitutes more than three times a day?
II. **Oral symptoms:** (+) response to at least one of the following questions:
1. Have you had a daily feeling of dry mouth for more than 3 months?
2. Have you had recurrently/persistently swollen salivary glands as an adult?
3. Do you frequently drink fluids to aid in swallowing dry food?
III. **Ocular signs:** (+) result for at least one of the following two tests:
1. Schirmer's I test without anesthesia (5 mm in 5 minutes)
2. Rose-Bengal score (4 points in the Van Bijsterfeld scoring)
IV. **Histopathology:** Focal lymphocytic sialadenitis in minor salivary glands. Evaluated by an expert pathologist, with a focus score: 1 point, defined as a number of lymphocytic foci adjacent to normal appearing mucous acini and containing more than 50 lymphocytes per 4 mm^2 of glandular tissue.
V. **Salivary gland involvement:** (+) result for at least one of the following tests:
1. Unstimulated whole salivary flow (1.5 mL in 15 minutes)
2. Diffuse sialectasias in parotid sialography without obstruction in the ducts
3. Salivary scintigraphy showing delayed uptake, decreased concentration and/or delayed excretion of the tracer
VI. **Autoantibodies:** presence in the serum of autoantibodies to Ro (SSA) or La (SSB) antigens or both

TABLE 29-5. REVISED RULES FOR CLASSIFICATION OF SJÖGREN'S SYNDROME (SS)

For primary SS (in those without any potential disease associations):
1. Presence of any four of the six items listed in Table 29-4, as long as either item IV or VI is (+)
2. Presence of any three of the four objective criteria listed in Table 29-4 (items III to VI)

For secondary SS:
In patients with a potential disease association such as a well-defined connective tissue disease, the presence of item I or item II listed in Table 29-4, plus any two from items III, IV, and V listed in Table 29-4 may be considered as indicative of secondary SS

Exclusion criteria:
Past neck or head radiation treatment
Hepatitis C infection
AIDS
Preexisting lymphoma
Sarcoidosis
Graft-versus-host disease
Use of anticholinergic drugs

type peripheral neuropathy and (rarely) an ascending (Guillain-Barré) type of neuropathy can be seen. Progressive neuropathy with motor involvement (e.g., foot drop) may indicate the presence of necrotizing vasculitis, especially in the context of palpable purpura or cutaneous ulceration (70). Clinicians should also keep in mind that hepatitis C infection, AIDS, sarcoidosis, and primary or secondary amyloidosis may all resemble SS in presentation (2).

One of the major concerns in patients with SS for any clinician of any related specialty, including ophthalmology, is the potential for the development of lymphoma. It has been estimated that a primary SS patient has an approximately 40-fold increased risk of developing non-Hodgkin's lymphoma compared with age-matched controls (71). The clinician should be aware of signs suggestive of lymphoproliferation, such as an increase in the size of salivary and lacrimal glands, lymphadenopathy, splenomegaly, and pulmonary infiltrates. Development of a monoclonal protein, new-onset leukopenia and anemia, and loss of previously present antibody, such as antinuclear antibody (ANA) or SSA/B, have all been associated with the development of lymphoma (72). A laboratory evaluation for SS patients should always include a search for ANA and rheumatoid factor (RF), which are prevalent in but not specific for SS. The Sjögren antibodies SSA and SSB are more specific, but are seen in 30% and 15%, respectively, of SLE patients as well (2). Ophthalmologists taking care of pregnant patients with high SSA and SSB titers must be well aware of the risk of neonatal lupus, which can result in fatal congenital heart block. Therefore, relevant consultations before term are essential (2). Longitudinal monitoring of laboratory parameters is appropriate for SS patients. The recommended evaluation for SS is shown in Table 29-6.

TABLE 29-6. RECOMMENDED WORKUP FOR SJÖGREN'S SYNDROME

Ocular
Schirmer test (with and without nasal stimulation; no anesthesia)
Slit-lamp exam with ocular surface vital staining
Fluorescein staining and tear film break up time

Oral
Dental exam
Estimate of salivary flow
Salivary scintigram
Minor salivary gland biopsy

Systemic
Complete history and physical examination
CBC, ESR, LFTs, UA, BUN/Cr, ANA, RF, SSA, SSB, IgG, IgA, IgM, SPEP, TSH levels
Chest x-ray

Others (as indicated)
Salivary gland sonogram/MRI
Lymph node or bone marrow biopsy
Other rheumatologic testing (double-stranded DNA, complements, angiotensin-converting enzyme)
Organ specific antibodies (thyroid, liver, kidney, central nervous system)
Viral (hepatitis B and C, Epstein-Barr virus, HIV)

Diagnosis and Clinical Features of Keratoconjunctivitis Sicca (KCS)

The evaluation of a presumed SS patient should begin with a thorough history, with detailed information on symptomatology and patient's daily activities and lifestyle, so that initial decisions can be made on possible causes and to individualize the management and treatment according to the patient's needs. A medical history should also include information on medications in use, because antihistamines and decongestants, antihypertensives and diuretics, muscle relaxants, and psychotropic drugs can induce or aggravate dry eyes (3). SS is responsible for a wide range of symptoms, such as increased awareness of eye pain, heaviness of the eyelids, blurred vision, increased mucus secretions, burning, foreign-body sensation, photophobia, and tearing (73). Individuals who work in closed spaces, such as office buildings or airplanes, are especially susceptible to dry-eye symptoms (2,73). Infrequent blinking and prolonged staring at monitors result in worsening of symptomatology (2). The frequency of each symptom and the degree of interference with daily activities should be assessed. The symptoms can sometimes be severe enough to impair the daily routine. A recent report revealed that 60% of KCS patients with primary SS syndrome and 30% of those with non-Sjögren dry eyes felt that KCS interfered with their daily activities, and the patients had to close their eyes for relief several times a day (74). Indeed, dry eye symptoms have a considerable impact on the quality of life and impose a significant economic burden. It has been reported that the cost of dry-eye treatments for SS patients in the U.S. may exceed $150 million of "out of pocket" expenses

per year. Industry sources estimate that 40 million to 60 million people in the U.S. have dry-eye symptoms as of 2003, and the current therapeutic dry-eye U.S. market is estimated to grow to almost $450 million in 2008 (75,76). Proper selection of patients for treatment is an important issue, and we believe that it is important to use a currently available survey or a questionnaire such as McMonnies's Dry Eye Questionnaire, the National Eye Institute Visual Function Questionnaire, the Dry Eye Questionnaire, or the Ocular Surface Disease Index for diagnosis of dry eye when selecting patients for clinical trials (74,75).

Clinical signs of KCS are numerous and include decreased or fluctuating visual acuity, conjunctival hyperemia, low tear meniscus, and the presence of excess debris in the tear with occasional mucus strands, foam, and debris. Blepharitis and meibomianitis are commonly associated with KCS. Corneal findings consist of superficial punctate keratopathy (usually interpalpebral, variable), band keratopathy, corneal epithelial erosions, sterile or infectious corneal ulcers, peripheral corneal infiltrates or ulceration, stromal melting, and perforation (77).

Renowned practitioners in dry-eye clinics routinely use a diagnostic algorithm of multiple tests, an approach recognized as superior in identifying KCS than a single test alone. Most centers rely on patient history and questionnaires as the first-choice diagnostic tools and employ traditional diagnostic tests such as the Schirmer test, tear film breakup time, and ocular surface evaluation with fluorescein, rose Bengal, or lissamine green stains. In our experience, the routine Schirmer test without anesthesia should be performed first, followed by the measurement of reflex tears with the Schirmer II test, performed in conjunction with nasal stimulation in patients with values less than 5 mm (78). If the value found with the latter test is less than 5 mm, the patient is categorized as basic tearing (−) and reflex tearing (−). Lack of reflex tears can only differentiate between Sjögren and non-Sjögren dry eyes, because in the former type the lacrimal gland is incapable of producing either basic or reflex tears.

Most cases of severe graft-versus-host disease, ocular cicatricial pemphigoid, and Stevens-Johnson syndrome are considered by the authors as SS dry eyes, whereas milder cases of these conditions are categorized as non-SS dry eyes. We choose to divide our patients with KCS into two groups: those with good reflex tearing and those without. In the latter group, there seems to be a systemic immune deviation with increased soluble IL-2 receptor, ANA, and RF levels, which have been shown to correlate with lacrimal gland function (79,80).

To check ocular surface status, we use a mixture of 1% fluorescein, 1% rose Bengal, and saline applied to the conjunctival fornix with a micropipette. In our experience, the non-SS variant of dry eye involves less vital staining, squamous metaplasia, and ocular surface damage than does the usual SS type (81). Relatively newer diagnostic techniques with improved sensitivity and specificity include tear film osmolarity (usually in excess of 323 mOsm/kg in KCS of SS), tear fluid immunoassays measuring tear lactoferrin levels (decreased in SS), and tear fluorescein clearance rate (TCR) (<8×: suspicious KCS; <4×: definite KCS). We have shown that TCR strongly correlates with tear secretion and have proposed a useful new measure of tear dynamics, the tear function index (TFI) calculated as follows: Schirmer II value/TCR. A TFI lower than 34 was 78.9% sensitive and 91.8% specific for Sjögren dry eyes (82,83). A skillfully performed impression or brush cytology is an indispensable tool in the evaluation of the severity of ocular surface changes, associated inflammatory responses, assessment of the response to treatment, and definitely for research purposes. Impression cytology samples from SS patients would reveal snake-like chromatin cells, decreased cellular cohesion, increased grades of squamous metaplasia, decreased goblet cell density, and mucin pickup and inflammatory cells (84–86).

The value and safety of lacrimal gland biopsy has always been a concern, but it has been performed in Japan since the 1950s with proven efficacy and safety, and it contributes significantly to the potential diagnosis of SS. Although the biopsy itself can interfere with the already compromised lacrimal function, we have not observed serious complications in our series of patients. The lymphocytic infiltration of the exocrine glands is an important pathologic and diagnostic sign, and therefore biopsy can be considered in patients with dry eyes with poor reflex tearing (87). Biopsy in such patients would usually show extensive lymphocytic infiltration and acinar cell destruction (Fig. 29-4). Lacrimal gland biopsy specimens have a more evident histopathology than labial salivary gland specimens in our experience, and we recommend that both biopsies be performed in patients with suspected SS to reduce the false-negative results and improve diagnostic accuracy (88).

Meibomianitis, blepharitis, and blink disorders are frequently encountered in SS where the qualitatively and/or quantitatively altered lipids cannot interact with the mucin layer due to aqueous deficiency and fail to spread uniformly over the ocular surface of the Sjögren dry eye. The DR-1 tear interference camera (Kowa Co., Nagoya, Japan) for measuring tear film lipid layer interferometry can assist in analyzing the changes in composition and thickness and the structure of the tear lipid layer (Figs. 29-5 and 29-6) (89). Reflective meniscometry, measuring tear meniscus curvature, which is decreased in KCS and correlates well with ocular surface staining, is expected to find wide applications (90). The new tear stability analyses system (TSAS), which measures tear stability as functions of serial surface regularity index (SRI) and surface asymmetry index (SAI) topographic indices assessed with 1-second intervals within 10 seconds, has shown a decrease in stability with increase in SRI and SAI in SS dry eyes (91). The newly developed functional visual acuity meter, which presents Landolt optotypes every second within a defined time frame, has also shown, in our experience, that functional visual acuity continued to decline in SS dry eyes over 30 seconds despite normal acuity values measured by the conventional Landolt chart (92). We believe that both devices will change our understanding of KCS and our assessment of treatment outcomes as well.

MANAGEMENT OF SJÖGREN'S SYNDROME AND KERATOCONJUNCTIVITIS SICCA

The management of SS entails efforts spent in many areas. The ophthalmology specialist not only should focus on the ophthalmologic aspects of the disease, but also should ensure that all other aspects are managed well to increase the patient's quality of life. Initial efforts in the approach to the systemic disease must include referrals to rheumatology and dentistry subspecialties. An ophthalmologist can counsel the patient with regard to simple measures designed to

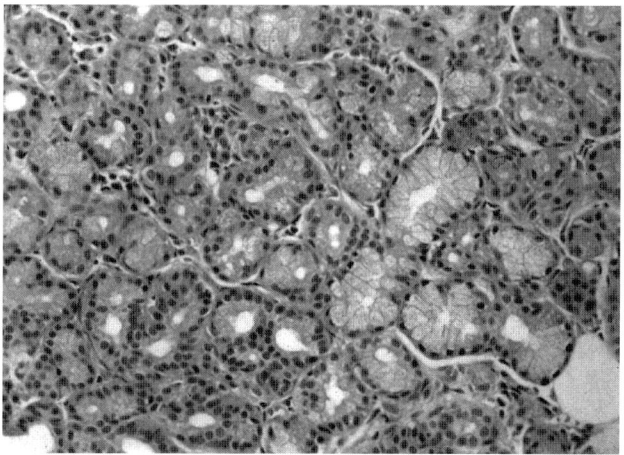
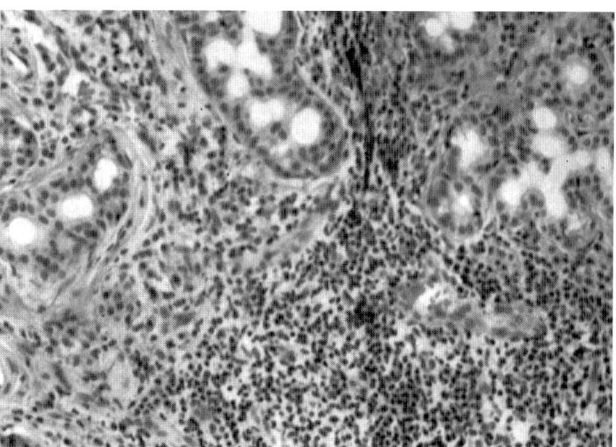

FIGURE 29-4. A: Normal lacrimal gland histology. **B:** Note the extensive lymphocytic infiltration and acinar cell destruction in SS lacrimal gland.

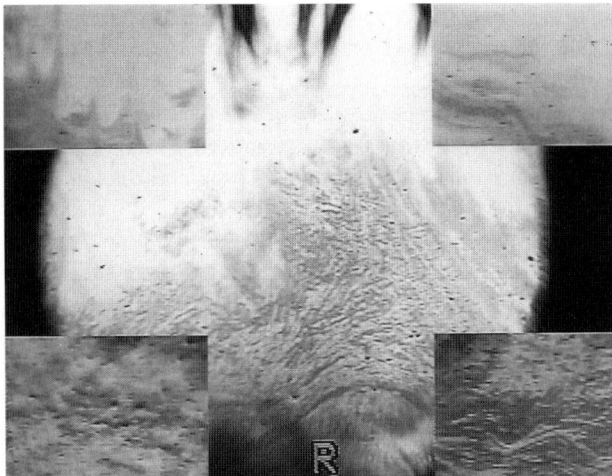

FIGURE 29-5. Tear film lipid layer interferometry in a patient with secondary Sjögren's syndrome revealed an irregular corneal surface with interference colors and numerous black dry spots, indicating a grade 4 change. **Upper left insert:** Grade 2 change, indicated by nonuniform distribution and normal pattern. **Upper right insert:** Grade 3 change, seen as having nonuniform distribution, and low-grade dry eye change. **Lower left insert:** Grade 4 change, indicated by nonuniform distribution and moderate dry eye change. **Lower right insert:** Grade 5 change, indicated by partially exposed corneal surface and severe dry eye change.

enhance moisture, such as the sufficient daily intake of fluids, avoidance of excessive alcohol, use of humidifiers, avoidance of excessive air conditioning and forced hot air heating systems, not allowing the skin to dry completely after daily baths, and use of skin moisturizers (2). More frequent instillations of tear substitutes or use of moisture chambers or dry-eye spectacles (Fig. 29-7) or warming the eyelids can be of help, especially during times of prolonged

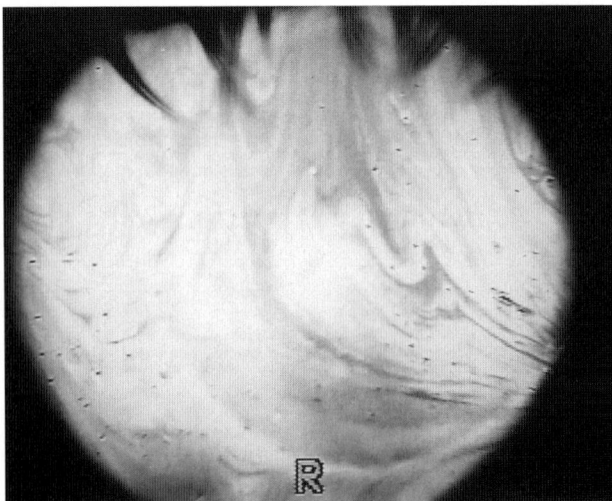

FIGURE 29-6. Tear film lipid layer interferometry in the same patient as in Fig. 29-5 showed the disappearance of interference colors after 2 months of autologous serum treatment (grade 2 change).

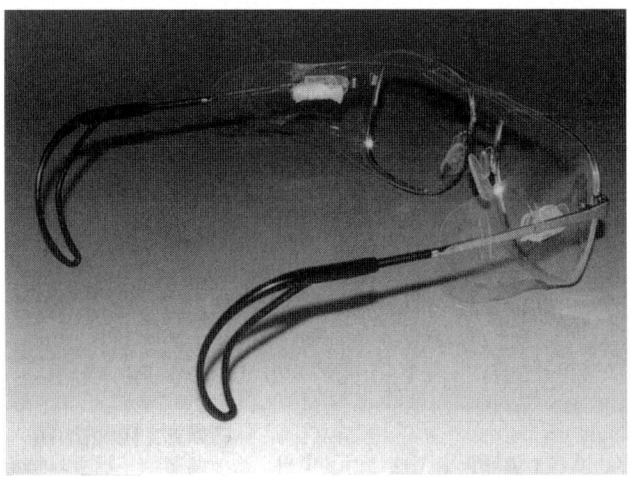

FIGURE 29-7. Dry-eye spectacles.

computer work or reading. Emphasis should be placed on fastidious dental care, including frequent examinations, and office and home tooth brushing. Patients can be advised to avoid keeping sugar-containing foods in the mouth for long periods of time, and to chew sugar-free gum (2). The ophthalmologist and dentist should diagnose signs and symptoms of intraoral candidiasis, which occurs frequently in patients with SS. In case of involvement of other organ systems, relevant consultations should be made without delay.

The Importance and Provision of Tears and Tear Components

Definitive treatment for SS dry eye is yet to be developed. Although trials for potent tear secretion-stimulating agents are going on, the alleviation of symptoms is the major aim of currently available treatments. The mainstay of dry-eye treatment regimens in SS has been and continues to be the use of artificial tear solutions and punctum plugs, and especially the use of unit-dose nonpreserved artificial tears in patients with significant keratopathy (93). Certain electrolyte compositions and the use of a bicarbonate buffering system in artificial teardrops have been shown to improve normal ocular surface homeostasis (94,95).

One of the electrolytes tested for the treatment of dry eyes is calcium, which is essential for the intercellular adhesions of the ocular surface epithelium mediated by cadherins or hemidesmosomes. Petrolatum-based ointment of calcium carbonate applied supracutaneously has been shown to produce statistically significant improvements in subjective symptoms, blink patterns, and vital staining of the ocular surface in SS dry eyes as well (96). In addition to these studies, we have investigated extensively whether the viscosity of eyedrops affects the distribution of the precorneal tear film (97). We found that aqueous artificial tears caused an uneven thickening of the tear film, with the inferior cornea benefiting less from the instillation of non-viscous solutions. We also tried sodium hyaluronate and hydroxypropyl methylcellulose (HPMC) as viscous preparations for the treatment of severe dry eyes in SS. Although sodium hyaluronate eyedrops were not shown to offer any advantages over the conventional tear substitutes in the improvement of subjective symptoms, they were effective in maintaining a healthy ocular surface epithelium. A solution of 0.5% HPMC was proven to improve the subjective scores and ocular surface damage of patients with dry eye due to SS (98,99).

Although artificial tear preparations have been reported to improve symptoms of irritation and to decrease the ocular surface vital dye staining in patients with KCS, their use may not improve ocular surface keratinization. This finding has stimulated increased research aimed at developing newer agents to supply tear components as well. The normal human tear fluid contains many biologically active proteins and growth factors that are essential for ocular surface health and are decreased in patients with lacrimal gland dysfunction. Autologous serum contains most of these components and has been recommended in the treatment of dry eye due to SS (100). It is not entirely clear why serum is of benefit to the ocular surface, but EGF in serum helps in the healing of epithelial erosions and facilitates epithelialization due to its antiapoptotic properties (100,101). Acidic and basic fibroblastic growth factors and fibronectin have been found to aid in epithelialization as well (102). Vitamin A is found in much higher concentrations in serum compared to tears and may decrease the overall ocular surface squamous metaplasia in KCS (100). Neural factors in the serum-like substance-P and insulin-like growth factor (IGF)-I are known to be important for epithelial migration (103). Autologous serum not only provides these essential substances but also increases MUC-1 expression by the ocular surface and improves the vital-staining scores (100). We found serum eyedrops to be very effective in the treatment of dry eye due to SS (Fig. 29-8), where we apply serum drops six to 10 times a day with the preexisting regimen of preservative-free artificial tears, hyaluronic acid drops, and the use of special dry-eye glasses with moist inserts for added humidity (100,104).

Making the Best of Remaining Tears with Lacrimal Punctal Occlusion

Punctal plug insertion is a simple, safe, effective, and reversible method to treat aqueous tear deficiency and ocular surface epitheliopathies not controlled with preservative-free lubricants. Lacrimal punctal occlusion may help by maximizing the time that essential tear components are in contact with the ocular surface epithelium. Indeed, punctal occlusion has been shown to be associated with a decrease in tear osmolarity, changes in corneal sensitivity, and improvements in both the ocular surface vital staining scores and the impression cytology parameters over the long term in SS patients as well (105). Punctal occlusion performed with collagen-rod, silicone, or plastic plugs seems to be very effective in patients with reflex tearing of 1 to 9 mm (Fig. 29-9) (106). Patients with no reflex tearing can receive both upper and lower puncta occlusion. We emphasize once again that it is very important to recognize the possibility of retention of deleterious components on the ocular surface longer with punctal occlusion. Thus, punctal occlusion should be performed only after or in conjunction with adequate management of local inflammatory conditions. Patients with these conditions must be instructed to wash their eyes with preservative-free drops three to four times a day, especially before going to sleep (106). The application and comparison of newer flow-controller plugs or atellocollagen plugs in different types of SS dry eyes remains another exciting area that needs to be studied. A study reported that botulinum toxin injection into the medial eyelids seemed to decrease lacrimal drainage and improve eye comfort in patients with dry eye and SS, but a randomized clinical trial is needed to determine the clinical potential of this treatment (107).

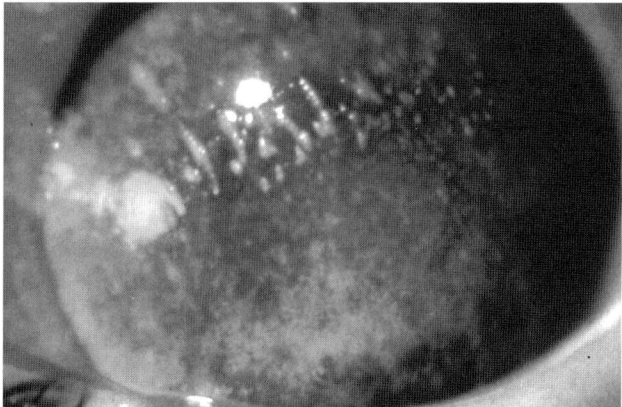
A

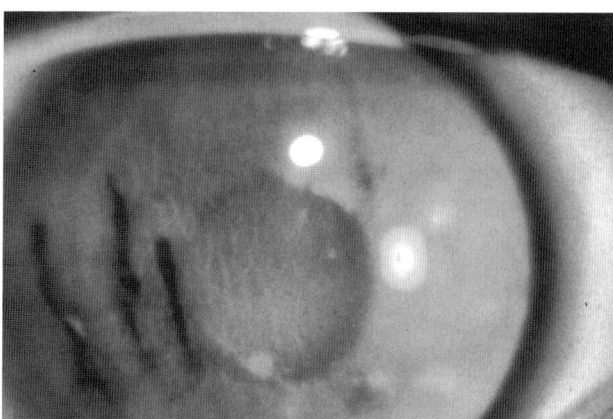
B

FIGURE 29-8. Ocular surface fluorescein staining before **(A)** and after **(B)** autologous serum treatment in a patient with SS.

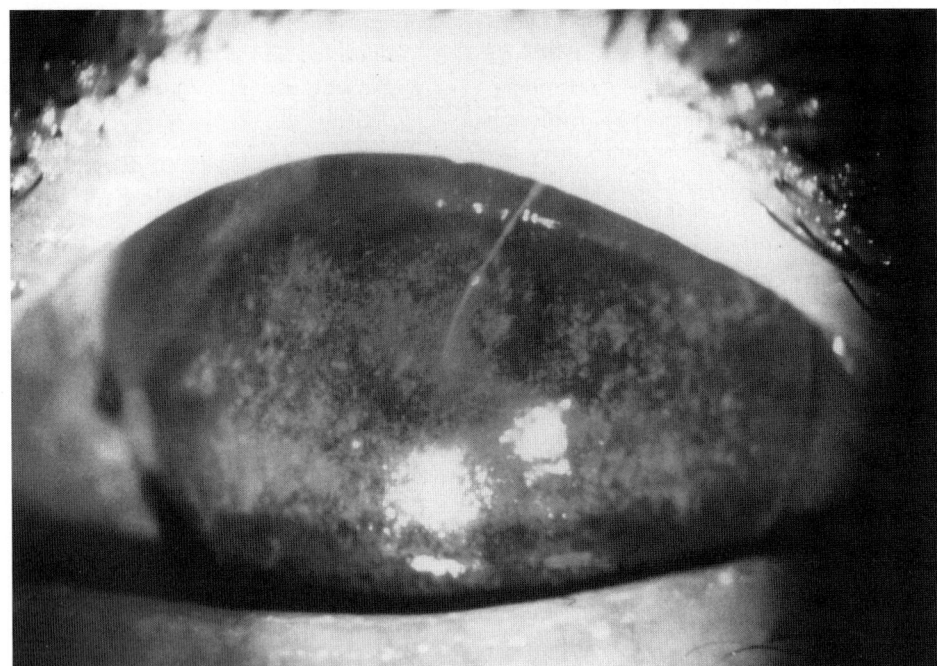

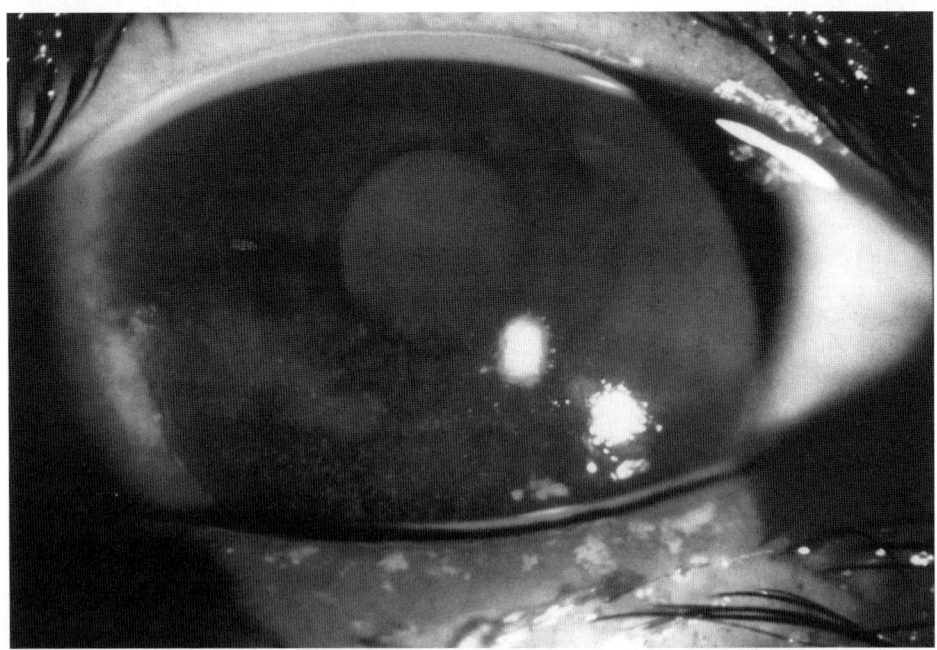

FIGURE 29-9. A: Ocular surface staining with fluorescein in a patient with Sjögren's syndrome prior to placement of punctum plugs. Note the very extensive epitheliopathy as evidenced by the extensive staining of the ocular surface with fluorescein dye. **B:** Same eye as shown in **A,** after placement of punctum plugs. Note the dramatic reduction in ocular surface uptake of fluorescein dye, indicative of very substantial improvement in ocular surface epithelial health as a consequence of tear preservation through the use of punctum plugs.

Antiinflammatory Treatments in KCS

One of the best known of antiinflammatory agents is 0.1% diclofenac sodium, which can be used for short-term therapy of dry eye and can be included in the clinician's armamentarium when considering prompt desired effect on subjective symptoms or on severe filamentary keratitis in patients with dry eye due to secondary SS (108). One immunomodulatory drug that has been the subject of many recent publications is cyclosporin A, which mediates its actions by binding to a specific cytosolic protein, cyclophilin, and inhibiting T-cell activities, e.g., the release of inflammatory cytokines such as IL-2 and IFN-γ. Phase II and III trials employing 0.05% and 0.1% topical cyclosporin A in SS patients have proven these formulations to be safe and effective in the treatment of moderate to severe KCS, yielding improvements in both subjective and objective measures, showing that patients were less prone to infection, and providing benefits that altered the patients' needs to use additional palliative treatment (109,110). Finally, Marsh and Pflugfelder (111) reported their experience that topical nonpreserved methylprednisolone decreased levels of the chemotactic cytokine IL-8 in the conjunctival epithelium in 21 SS patients and was efficacious for the treatment of severe aqueous deficiency refractory to preservative-free lubricants and punctal occlusion. Another study revealed that interferon-α_2, given as 2.3 million units three times a week for a mean period of 11 months in SS, could improve tear and salivary functions by 67% and 61% up from the baseline without causing significant side effects (112).

Ocular Surface and Lacrimal Gland Stimulation

The P2Y2 purinergic receptors expressed on human and rabbit ocular surfaces have been shown to mediate the regulation of mucin, Cl-secretion, and net fluid flux in the excised rabbit conjunctiva. Repetitive application of a uridine 5′-triphosphate (UTP) preparation called INS365 acts as a P2Y2 agonist and increases Schirmer scores in rabbits without decreasing protein and mucin-like glycoprotein concentrations in the tears of the rabbit dry eye model. P2Y2 receptor ligands may prove to be useful pharmacologic tools for therapeutic manipulation of lacrimal glands, ocular surface epithelia, and goblet cells (113). Experimental evidence suggested that topical gefarnate stimulated conjunctival goblet cell expression in experimental dry eye models (114). Another exciting development is the finding that topical applications of the eicosanoid 15-(S)-HETE causes the corneal epithelial cells to release a thick layer of mucin rapidly in moderately severe dry eyes and may be promising in stabilizing the tear film and inhibiting the progression of ocular surface disease (115). Topical retinoids and mucin ophthalmic solutions also await further controlled clinical trials and may be promising for the treatment of dry eyes (116,117). A well-recognized stimulatory agent is pilocarpine, a cholinergic parasympathomimetic agonist that binds to muscarinic M3 receptors in the lacrimal gland. A placebo-controlled multicenter trial showed that any patient with SS and some residual exocrine gland function benefited immensely from the administration of pilocarpine tablets (20 mg/day in divided doses) for the symptomatic treatment of dryness (118). The benefits of treatment outweighed the adverse effects of systemic treatment in that study. Likewise, treatment of SS patients with cevimeline, another muscarinic stimulant, given as 30 mg three times daily, resulted in substantial

improvement of tear and salivary flow rate with improvement of subjective symptoms of overall dryness (119). Diaphoresis, nausea, rhinitis, and diarrhea were the most common side effects of pilocarpine and cevimeline. In our experience, both drugs deserve a testing period on the suitable patient who can tolerate long-term use (119).

Surgery in and for Keratoconjunctivitis sicca

We believe that efficacy and safety of most ocular procedures will not be affected adversely by a preexisting dry-eye status (in the presence of reflex tearing) with a proper ocular surface management. The issue is especially important for refractive surgical procedures including laser *in situ* keratomileusis (LASIK) (120). Our recent data suggest that although the procedure is not affected, preexisting dry eye is a risk factor for severe postoperative dry eye with lower tear function, more vital staining of the ocular surface, and more severe symptomatology until 1 year and even longer alter LASIK. The pathogenesis and risk factors of such symptoms are now under investigation. Investigations on surgical treatment of dry eyes are being conducted. Geerling et al. (121) reported that autologous submandibular gland transplantation for medically refractive severe dry eyes in SS results in the production of salivary tears, which are similar to tears of lacrimal gland origin. However, the effects of such secretion on the ocular surface should be evaluated with further clinical and laboratory studies.

FUTURE EXPECTATIONS

There probably is no other area in the field of cornea and external eye disease in which more advances have been made in regard to the diagnosis, pathogenesis, and treatment of KCS. Future research hopes to define pathogenesis in much more detail and develop better diagnostic tools. On that front, we feel that further research on aquaporins will add to our understanding of the mechanisms involved in SS dry eyes and may provide opportunities for new treatment agents. We believe the functional visual acuity tester and TSAS will prove to be useful diagnostic tools and enjoy widespread acceptance in diagnosing and evaluating treatment outcome in several types of KCS. New color charts being developed for DR-1 tear film lipid layer interferometry, which can also assess tear thickness, will certainly broaden our knowledge on the pathogenesis of KCS. Further controlled trials on topical applications of newer medications such as antiinflammatory agents, immune suppressants such as cyclosporin A and FK-506, growth hormones, androgens, topical mucins, and ocular surface stimulating drugs like INS365, with potential therapeutic benefits for the ocular surface disease of patients with KCS, are definitely needed and will pave the way for newer treatment protocols in SS dry eyes. Indeed, the first topical cyclosporin prescription product was launched in April 2003. INS365 is expected to be launched in 2004,15-S-HETE in 2005, and androgen tears in 2006 (75).

We believe that the efforts of numerous talented dry-eye researchers with an interest in regenerative medicine coupled with efforts to overcome the autoimmune disease process will lead to the development of artificial lacrimal glands or at least the development of lacrimal gland stem cell cultures, which can be then transplanted to regenerate and/or replace the diseased gland in SS.

ACKNOWLEDGMENTS

This chapter is devoted to our loving families and to dry-eye patients all over the world. The authors would like to thank Mrs. Catherine Oshima and Mrs. Wendy Hanai for their secretarial assistance during the preparation of the chapter.

REFERENCES

1. Tojo T. Sjögren syndrome. In: Oguchi Y, Tsubota K, eds. *Diagnosis and treatment of ocular surface.* Tokyo: Medical Publishers, 1993:109–119. (Japanese language)
2. Carsons S. A review and update of Sjögren's syndrome: manifestations, diagnosis, and treatment. *Am J Manag Care* 2001; 7.S433–443.
3. Ferris RL. Sjögren's Syndrome. In: Gold DH, Weingeist TA, eds. *The eye in systemic disease.* Philadelphia: JB Lippincott, 1990:70–72.
4. Shearn MA. Sjögren's Syndrome. In: Smith LH, ed. Major problems in internal medicine. Philadelphia: Saunders, 1971, Vol. 2.
5. Fox RI, Saito I. Criteria for diagnosis of Sjögren's syndrome. *Rheum Dis Clin North Am* 1994;20:391–407.
5a. Pillemer SK, Matteson EL, Jacobsson LT, et al. Incidence of physician-diagnosed primary Sjögren's syndrome in residents of Olmsted County, Minnesota. 2001;76:593–599.
6. Bjerrum KB. Keratoconjunctivitis sicca and primary Sjögren's syndrome in a Danish population aged 30–60 years. *Acta Ophthalmol Scand* 1997;75:281–286.
7. Vitali C, Moutsopoulos HM, Bombardieri S. The European Community Study Group on diagnostic criteria for Sjögren's syndrome. Sensitivity and specificity of tests for ocular and oral involvement in Sjögren's syndrome. *Ann Rheum Dis* 1994;53: 637–647.
8. Eguchi K. *The manual of Sjögren's syndrome diagnosis by Japanese Medical Society for Sjögren's syndrome.* Nagasaki: Ryoin, 2000.
9. Stern ME, Beuerman RW, et al. The pathology of dry eye: the interaction between the ocular surface and lacrimal glands. *Cornea* 1998;17:584–589.
10. Sullivan DA, Wickham LA, Rocha EM, et al. Androgens and dry eye in Sjögren's syndrome. *Ann NY Acad Sci* 1999;876: 312–324.
11. Kroemer G, Martinez C. Cytokines and autoimmune disease. *Clin Immunol Immunopathol* 1991;61:275–295.
12. Pepose JS, Akata RF, Pflugfelder SC, et al. Mononuclear cell phenotypes and immunoglobulin gene rearrangements in lacrimal gland biopsies from patients with Sjögren's syndrome. *Ophthalmology* 1990;97:1599–1605.
13. van Bijsterveld OP, Kruize AA, Bleys RL. Central nervous system mechanisms in Sjögren's syndrome. *Br J Ophthalmol* 2003;87:128–130.
14. Jones DT, Monroy D, Ji Z, et al. Sjögren's syndrome: cytokine and Epstein-Barr viral gene expression within the conjunctival epithelium. *Invest Ophthalmol Vis Sci* 1994;35:3493–3504.
15. Baudouin C. The pathology of dry eye. *Surv Ophthalmol* 2001;45:S211–220.
16. Pflugfelder SC, Ji Z, Naqui R. Immune cytokine RNA expression in normal and Sjögren's syndrome conjunctiva. *Invest Ophthalmol Vis Sci* 1996;37:S358.
17. Halse A, Tengner P, Wahren-Herlenius M, et al. Increased frequency of cells secreting interleukin-6 and interleukin-10 in peripheral blood of patients with primary Sjögren's syndrome. *Scand J Immunol* 1999;49:533–538.
18. Saito I, Haruta K, Shimuta M, et al. Fas ligand-mediated exocrinopathy resembling Sjögren's syndrome in mice transgenic for IL-10. *J Immunol* 1999;162:2488–2494.
19. Hulkkonen J, Pertovaara M, Antonen J, et al. Genetic association between interleukin-10 promoter region polymorphisms and primary Sjögren's syndrome. *Arthritis Rheum* 2001;44: 176–179.
20. Limaye V, Lester S, Downie-Doyle S, et al. Polymorphisms of the interleukin 10 gene promoter are not associated with anti-Ro autoantibodies in primary Sjögren's syndrome. *J Rheumatol* 2000; 27:2945–2946.
21. Perrier S, Coussediere C, Dubost JJ, et al. IL-1 receptor antagonist (IL-1RA) gene polymorphism in Sjögren's syndrome and rheumatoid arthritis. *Clin Immunol Immunopathol* 1998;87: 309–313.
22. Jean S, Quelvennec E, Alizadeh M, et al. DRB1*15 and DRBl*03 extended haplotype interaction in primary Sjögren's syndrome genetic susceptibility. *Clin Exp Rheumatol* 1998;16: 725–728.
22a. Solomon A, Dursun D, Liu Z, et al. Pro- and anti-inflammatory forms of interleukin-1 in the tear fluid and conjunctiva of patients with dry-eye disease. *Invest Ophthalmol Vis Sci* 2001; 42:2283–2292.
23. Jones DT, Monroy D, Ji Z, et al. Alterations of ocular surface gene expression in Sjögren's syndrome. In: Sullivan DA, Dartt DA, Meneray MA, eds. *Lacrimal gland, tear film, and dry eye syndromes 2.* New York: Plenum Press, 1998:533–536.
24. Bjerrum KB. Snake-like chromatin in conjunctival cells of normal elderly persons and of patients with primary Sjögren's syndrome and other connective tissue diseases. *Acta Ophthalmol Scand* 1995;73:33–36.
25. Pflugfelder SC, Jones D, Ji Z, et al. Altered cytokine balance in the tear fluid and conjunctiva of patients with Sjögren's syndrome keratoconjunctivitis sicca. *Curr Eye Res* 1999;19: 201–211.
26. Pflugfelder SC, Tseng SC, Yoshino K, et al. Correlation of goblet cell density and mucosal epithelial membrane mucin expression with rose bengal staining in patients with ocular irritation. *Ophthalmology* 1997;104:223–235.
27. Hayashi Y, Arakaki R, Ishimaru N. The role of caspase cascade on the development of primary Sjögren's syndrome. *J Med Invest* 2003;50:32–38.
28. Ozkan ED, Lee FS, Ueda T. A protein factor that inhibits ATP-dependent glutamate and gamma-aminobutyric acid accumulation into synaptic vesicles: purification and initial characterization. *Proc Natl Acad Sci USA* 1997;94:4137–4142.
29. Tsubota K, Fujita H, Tadano K, et al. Abnormal expression and function of Fas ligand of lacrimal glands and peripheral blood

in Sjögren's syndrome patients with enlarged exocrine glands. *Clin Exp Immunol* 2002;129:177–182.

30. Tsubota K, Fujita H, Tsuzaka K, et al. Quantitative analysis of lacrimal gland function, apoptotic figures, Fas and Fas ligand expression of lacrimal glands in dry eye patients. *Exp Eye Res* 2003;76:233–240.

31. Green JE, Hinrichs SH, Vogel J, et al. Exocrinopathy resembling Sjögren's syndrome in HTLV-1 tax transgenic mice. *Nature* 1989;341:72–74.

32. Koike K, Moriya K, Ishibashi K, et al. Sialadenitis histologically resembling Sjögren syndrome in mice transgenic for hepatitis C virus envelope genes. *Proc Natl Acad Sci USA* 1997;94: 233–236.

33. Sixbey JW, Yao QY. Immunoglobulin A-induced shift of Epstein-Barr virus tissue tropism. *Science* 1992;255:1578–1580.

34. Pflugfelder SC, Crouse C, Pereira I, et al. Amplification of Epstein-Barr virus genomic sequences in blood cells, lacrimal glands, and tears from primary Sjögren's syndrome patients. *Ophthalmology* 1990;97:976–984.

35. Crouse CA, Pflugfelder SC, Cleary T, et al. Detection of Epstein-Barr virus genomes in normal human lacrimal glands. *J Clin Microbiol* 1990;28:1026–1032.

36. Tsubota K, Fujishima H, Toda I, et al. Increased levels of Epstein-Barr virus DNA in lacrimal glands of Sjögren's syndrome patients. *Acta Ophthalmol Scand* 1995;73:425–430.

37. Pflugfelder SC, Huang AJ, Feuer W, et al. Conjunctival cytologic features of primary Sjögren's syndrome. *Ophthalmology* 1990; 97:985–991.

38. Takamura E, Uchida Y, Tsubota K. Quantitative evaluation of conjunctival inflammatory cells in dry eye pr with circulating serum antibodies. *Invest Ophthalmol Vis Sci* 1991;32:S732.

39. Reveille JD, Wilson RW, Provost TT, et al. Primary Sjögren's syndrome and other autoimmune diseases in families. Prevalence and immunogenetic studies in six kindreds. *Ann Intern Med* 1984;101:748–756.

40. Koivukangas T, Simila S, Heikkinen E, et al. Sjögren's syndrome and achalasia of the cardia in two siblings. *Pediatrics* 1973;51:943–945.

41. Mason AM, Golding PL. Multiple immunological abnormalities in a family. *J Clin Pathol* 1971;24:732–735.

42. Sabio JM, Milla E, Jimenez-Alonso J. A multicase family with primary Sjögren's syndrome. *J Rheumatol* 2001;28:1932–1934.

43. Bolstad Al, Haga HJ, Wassmuth R, et al. Monozygotic twins with primary Sjögren's syndrome. *J Rheumatol* 2000;27:2264–2266.

44. Tanaka A, Igarashi M, Kakinuma M, et al. The occurrence of various collagen diseases in one family: a sister with ISSc, PBC, APS, and SS and a brother with systemic lupus erythematosus. *J Dermatol* 2001;28:547–553.

45. Reveille JD, Arnett FC. The immunogenetics of Sjögren's syndrome. *Rheum Dis Clin North Am* 1992;18:539–550.

46. Nepom GT. MHC and autoimmune diseases. *Immunol Ser* 1993;59:143–164.

47. Merriman TR, Todd JA. Genetics of autoimmune disease. *Curr Opin Immunol* 1995;7:786–792.

48. Tomlinson IP, Bodmer WF. The HLA system and the analysis of multifactorial genetic disease. *Trends Genet* 1995;11:493–498.

49. Loiseau P, Lepage V, Djelal F, et al. HLA class I and class II are both associated with the genetic predisposition to primary Sjögren syndrome. *Hum Immunol* 2001;62:725–731.

50. Manthorpe R, Morling N, Platz P, et al. HLA-D antigen frequencies in Sjögren's syndrome. Differences between the primary and secondary form. *Scand J Rheumatol* 1981;10:124–128.

51. Papasteriades CA, Skopouli FN, Drosos AA, et al. HLA-alloantigen associations in Greek patients with Sjögren's syndrome. *J Autoimmun* 1988;1:85–90.

52. Harley JB, Reichlin M, Arnett FC, et al. Gene interaction at HLA-DQ enhances autoantibody production in primary Sjögren's syndrome. *Science* 1986;232:1145–1147.

53. Kerttula TO, Collin P, Polvi A, et al. Distinct immunologic features of Finnish Sjögren's syndrome patients with HLA alleles DRB1* DQA1*0501, and DQB1*0201. Alterations in circulating T cell receptor gamma/delta subsets. *Arthritis Rheum* 1996;39:1733–1739.

54. Hadj Kacem H, Kaddour N, Adyel FZ, et al. HLA-DQB1 CAR1/CAR2, TNFa IR2/IR4 and CTLA-4 polymorphisms in Tunisian patients with rheumatoid arthritis and Sjögren's syndrome. *Rheumatology (Oxford)* 2001;40:1370–1374.

55. Rischmueller M, Lester S, Chen Z, et al. HLA class II phenotype controls diversification of the autoantibody response in primary Sjögren's syndrome (pSS). *Clin Exp Immunol* 1998; 111:365–371.

56. Fei HM, Kang H, Scharf S, et al. Specific HLA-DQA and HLA-DRB1 alleles confer susceptibility to Sjögren's syndrome and autoantibody production. *J Clin Lab Analysis* 1991;5: 382–391.

57. Ohlsson M, Jonsson R, Brokstad KA. Subcellular redistribution and surface exposure of the Ro52, Ro60 and La48 autoantigens during apoptosis in human ductal epithelial cells: a possible mechanism in the pathogenesis of Sjögren's syndrome. *Scand J Immunol* 2002;56:456–469.

58. Kumagai S, Kanagawa S, Morinobu A, et al. Association of a new allele of the TAP2 gene, TAP2*Bky2 (Val577), with susceptibility to Sjögren's syndrome. *Arthritis Rheum* 1997;40:1685–1692.

59. Tapinos NI, Polihronis M, Thyphronitis G, et al. Characterization of the cysteine-rich secretory protein 3 gene as an early-transcribed gene with a putative role in the pathophysiology of Sjögren's syndrome. *Arthritis Rheum* 2002;46:215–222.

60. King LS, Yasui M, Agre P. Aquaporins in health and disease. *Mol Med Today* 2000;6:60–65.

61. Verkman AS. Role of aquaporin water channels in eye function. *Exp Eye Res* 2003;76:137–143.

62. Raina S, Preston GM, Guggino WB, et al. Molecular cloning and characterization of an aquaporin cDNA from salivary, lacrimal, and respiratory tissues. *J Biol Chem* 1995;270: 1908–1912.

63. Tsubota K, Hirai S, King LS, et al. Defective cellular trafficking of lacrimal gland aquaporin-5 in Sjögren's syndrome. *Lancet* 2001;357:688–689.

64. Ohashi Y, Ishida R, Kojima T, et al. Abnormal protein profiles in tears with dry eye syndrome. *Am J Ophthalmol* 2003;136: 291–299.

65. Jonsson R, Skarstein K. Experimental models of Sjögren's Syndrome. In: Theofilopoulos AN, Bona CA, eds. *The molecular pathology of autoimmune diseases*, 2nd ed. New York: Taylor & Francis, 2002:437–452.

66. Johansson AC, Nakken B, Sundler M, et al. The genetic control of sialadenitis versus arthritis in a NOD.QxB10.Q F2 cross. *Eur J Immunol* 2002;32:243–250.

67. Brayer J, Lowry J, Cha S, et al. Alleles from chromosomes 1 and 3 of NOD mice combine to influence Sjögren's syndrome-like autoimmune exocrinopathy. *J Rheumatol* 2000;27: 1896–1904.

68. Nishihara M, Terada M, Kamogawa J, et al. Genetic basis of autoimmune sialadenitis in MRL/lpr lupus-prone mice: additive and hierarchical properties of polygenic inheritance. *Arthritis Rheum* 1999;42:2616–2623.

69. Vitali C, Bombardieri S, Jonsson R, et al. Classification criteria for Sjögren's syndrome: a revised version of the European criteria proposed by the American-European Consensus Group. *Ann Rheum Dis* 2002;61:554–558.

70. Alexander GE, Provost IT, Stevens MB, et al. Sjögren syndrome: central nervous system manifestations. *Neurology* 1981;31:1391–1396.

71. Skopouli FN, Dafni U, Ioannidis JP, et al. Clinical evolution, and morbidity and mortality of primary Sjögren's syndrome. *Semin Arthritis Rheum* 2000;29:296–304.

72. Kassan SS, Thomas TL, Moutsopoulos HM, et al. Increased risk of lymphoma in sicca syndrome. *Ann Intern Med* 1978;89:888–892.

73. Toda I. Symptoms of Dry Eye. In: Tsubota K, ed. *Dry eye clinic.* Tokyo: Igaku Shoin, 2000:25–30.

74. Begley CG, Caffery B, Chalmers RL, et al. Use of the dry eye questionnaire to measure symptoms of ocular irritation in patients with aqueous tear deficient dry eye. *Cornea* 2002;21:664–670.

75. Sullivan RM, Cermak JM, Papas AS, et al. Economic and quality of life impact of dry eye symptoms in women with Sjögren's syndrome. *Adv Exp Med Biol* 2002;506:1183–1188.

76. Goodman M, Nachman G, Bhalla A. Dry eye market: no shedding of tears over this opportunity. *Pharmaceuticals Specialty* 2003;5:1–44.

77. Ono M. Sjögren's syndrome. In: Watanabe N, Tano Y, eds. *Practical ophthalmology.* Tokyo: Bunkodo, 1998:82–88.

78. Tsubota K. Reflex tearing in dry eye not associated with Sjögren's syndrome. In: Sullivan DA, Dartt DA, Meneray MA, eds. *Lacrimal gland, tear film, and dry eye syndromes 2.* New York: Plenum Press, 1998:903–907.

79. Tsubota K, Fujihara T, Takeuchi T. Soluble interleukin-2 receptors and serum autoantibodies in dry eye patients: correlation with lacrimal gland function. *Cornea* 1997;16:339–344.

80. Tsubota K, Toda I, Yagi Y, et al. Three different types of dry eye syndrome. *Cornea* 1994;13:202–209.

81. Toda I, Tsubota K. Practical double vital staining for ocular surface evaluation. *Cornea* 1993;12:366–367.

82. Xu KP, Yagi Y, Toda I, et al. Tear function index. A new measure of dry eye. *Arch Ophthalmol* 1995;113:84–88.

83. Tsubota K. Tear dynamics and dry eye. *Prog Retin Eye Res* 1998;17:565–596.

84. de Rojas MV, Rodriguez MT, Ces Blanco JA, et al. Impression cytology in patients with keratoconjunctivitis sicca. *Cytopathology* 1993;4:347–355.

85. Rivas L, Oroza MA, Perez-Esteban A, et al. Morphological changes in ocular surface in dry eyes and other disorders by impression cytology. *Graefes Arch Clin Exp Ophthalmol* 1992;230:329–334.

86. Rivas L, Rodriguez JJ, Alvarez MI, et al. Correlation between impression cytology and tear function parameters in Sjögren's syndrome. *Acta Ophthalmol* 1993;71:353–359.

87. Tsubota K, Xu KP, Fujihara T, et al. Decreased reflex tearing is associated with lymphocytic infiltration in lacrimal glands. *J Rheumatol* 1996;23:313–320.

88. Xu KP, Katagiri S, Takeuchi T, et al. Biopsy of labial salivary glands and lacrimal glands in the diagnosis of Sjögren's syndrome. *J Rheumatol* 1996;23:76–82.

89. Danjo Y, Hamano T. Observation of precorneal tear film in patients with Sjögren's syndrome. *Acta Ophthalmol Scand* 1995;73:501–505.

90. Yokoi N, Bron AJ, Tiffany JM, et al. Reflective meniscometry: a new field of dry eye assessment. *Cornea* 2000;19:S37–43.

91. Goto T, Zheng X, Klyce SD, et al. A new method for tear film stability analysis using videokeratography. *Am J Ophthalmol* 2003;135:607–612.

92. Goto E, Yagi Y, Matsumoto Y, et al. Impaired functional visual acuity of dry eye patients. *Am J Ophthalmol* 2002;133:181–186.

93. Tsubota K, Dogru M. Changing perspectives for the treatment of dry eye. *Contemp Ophthalmol* 2002;1(18):1–8.

94. Gilbard JP, Rossi SR, Heyda KG. Ophthalmic solutions, the ocular surface, and a unique therapeutic artificial tear formulation. *Am J Ophthalmol* 1989;107:348–355.

95. Ubels JL, McCartney MD, Lantz WK, et al. Effects of preservative-free artificial tear solutions on corneal epithelial structure and function. *Arch Ophthalmol* 1995;113:371–378.

96. Tsubota K, Monden Y, Yagi Y, et al. New treatment of dry eye: the effect of calcium ointment through eyelid skin delivery. *Br J Ophthalmol* 1999;83:767–770.

97. Shimmura S, Goto E, Shimazaki J, et al. Viscosity-dependent fluid dynamics of eyedrops on the ocular surface. *Am J Ophthalmol* 1998;125:386–388.

98. Shimmura S, Ono M, Shinozaki K, et al. Sodium hyaluronate eyedrops in the treatment of dry eyes. *Br J Ophthalmol* 1995;79:1007–1011.

99. Toda I, Shinozaki N, Tsubota K. Hydroxypropyl methylcellulose for the treatment of severe dry eye associated with Sjögren's syndrome. *Cornea* 1996;15:120–128.

100. Tsubota K, Goto E, Fujita H, et al. Treatment of dry eye by autologous serum application in Sjögren's syndrome. *Br J Ophthalmol* 1999;83:390-395.

101. Pastor JC, Calonge M. Epidermal growth factor and corneal wound healing. A multicenter study. *Cornea* 1992;11:311–314.

102. Fredj-Reygrobellet D, Plouet J, Delayre T, et al. Effects of aFGF and bFGF on wound healing in rabbit corneas. *Curr Eye Res* 1987;6:1205–1209.

103. Nishida T, Nakamura M, Ofuji K, et al. Synergistic effects of substance P with insulin-like growth factor-1 on epithelial migration of the cornea. *J Cell Physiol* 1996;169:159–166.

104. Tsubota K, Yamada M, Urayama K. Spectacle side panels and moist inserts for the treatment of dry-eye patients. *Cornea* 1994;13:197–201.

105. Willis RM, Folberg R, Krachmer JH, et al. The treatment of aqueous-deficient dry eye with removable punctal plugs. A clinical and impression-cytologic study. *Ophthalmology* 1987;94:514–518.

106. Tsubota K. SS dry eye and non-SS dry eye: what are the differences? In: Homma M, Sugai S, Tojo T, et al, eds. *Sjögren's syndrome state of the art.* New York: Kugler, 1994:27–31.

107. Sahlin S, Chen E, Kaugesaar T, et al. Effect of eyelid botulinum toxin injection on lacrimal drainage. *Am J Ophthalmol* 2000;129:481–486.

108. Avisar R, Robinson A, Appel I, et al. Diclofenac sodium, 0.1% (Voltaren Ophtha), versus sodium chloride, 5%, in the treatment of filamentary keratitis. *Cornea* 2000;19:145–147.

109. Sall K, Stevenson OD, Mundorf TK, et al. Two multicenter, randomized studies of the efficacy and safety of cyclosporine ophthalmic emulsion in moderate to severe dry eye disease. CsA Phase 3 Study Group. *Ophthalmology* 2000;107:631–639.

110. Stevenson D, Tauber J, Reis BL. Efficacy and safety of cyclosporin A ophthalmic emulsion in the treatment of moderate-to-severe dry eye disease: a dose-ranging, randomized trial. The Cyclosporin A Phase 2 Study Group. *Ophthalmology* 2000;107:967–974.

111. Marsh P, Pflugfelder SC. Topical nonpreserved methylprednisolone therapy for keratoconjunctivitis sicca in Sjögren syndrome. *Ophthalmology* 1999;106:811–816.

112. Ferraccioli GF, Salaffi F, De Vita S, et al. Interferon alpha-2 (IFN alpha 2) increases lacrimal and salivary function in Sjögren's syndrome patients. Preliminary results of an open pilot trial versus OH-chloroquine. *Clin Exp Rheumatol* 1996;14:367–371.

113. Murakami T, Fujihara T, Nakamura M, et al. P2Y(2) receptor stimulation increases tear fluid secretion in rabbits. *Curr Eye Res* 2000;21:782–787.

114. Hamano T. Dry eye treatment with eye drops that stimulate mucin production. *Adv Exp Med Biol* 1998;438:965–968.

115. Jackson RS 2nd, Van Dyken SJ, McCartney MD, et al. The eicosanoid, 15-(S)-HETE, stimulates secretion of mucin-like glycoprotein by the corneal epithelium. *Cornea* 2001;20:516–521.

116. Kobayashi TK, Tsubota K, Takamura E, et al. Effect of retinol palmitate as a treatment for dry eye: a cytologjcal evaluation. *Ophthalmologica* 1997;211:358–361.

117. Shigemitsu T, Shimizu Y, Doi K, et al. Clinical evaluation of mucin ophthalmic solution on dry eye. *Cornea* 2000;19:S122.

118. Vivino FB, Al-Hashimi I, Khan Z, et al. Pilocarpine tablets for the treatment of dry mouth and dry eye symptoms in patients with Sjögren syndrome: a randomized, placebo-controlled, fixed-dose, multicenter trial. P92-01 Study Group. *Arch Intern Med* 1999;159:174–181.

119. Petrone D, Condemi JJ, Fife R, et al. A double-blind, randomized, placebo-controlled study of cevimeline in Sjögren's syndrome patients with xerostomia and keratoconjunctivitis sicca. *Arthritis Rheum* 2002;46:748–754.

120. Toda I, Asano-Kato N, Hori-Komai Y, et al. Laser-assisted in situ keratomileusis for patients with dry eye. *Arch Ophthalmol* 2002;120:1024–1028.

121. Geerling G, Honnicke K, Schroder C, et al. Quality of salivary tears following autologous submandibular gland transplantation for severe dry eye. *Graefes Arch Clin Exp Ophthalmol* 2000;238:45–52.

BLEPHARITIS AND MEIBOMIAN GLAND DYSFUNCTION

WILLIAM AYLIFFE

Blepharitis is, by definition, inflammation of the eyelids. Many clinical entities can cause blepharitis (1,2). This disorder is extremely common and several conditions can cause disease of the eyelids leading to blepharitis (3). Additionally, many patients with blepharitis also have dry eye symptoms and signs (4,5). Although it is often not serious, blepharitis may on occasion cause severe complications, including dry eyes, lid cicatrization and notching, trichiasis, marginal corneal ulceration, and corneal scarring.

Blepharitis may be broadly classified into anterior blepharitis, affecting the skin and lashes, and posterior blepharitis, involving the mucous membrane and meibomian glands. Anterior blepharitis is most often associated with staphylococcal infection or with seborrheic dermatitis. Seborrhea results from a functional overactivity of the sebaceous glands. It results in greasy skin, and blepharitis may also occur (3). Posterior blepharitis usually results from meibomian gland dysfunction.

Meibomian gland dysfunction describes a variety of changes in the tarsal meibomian glands that need not necessarily be inflammatory (6,7). However, there is a close relationship between these changes and blepharitis. Indeed, meibomian gland dysfunction may be found in up to 74% of patients with blepharitis (4,5). This is not surprising, because meibomian gland dysfunction is also associated with skin and sebaceous gland disorders (8,9). Furthermore, bacterial colonization of the lid margins can lead to inflammatory change either directly by infection, or indirectly by hypersensitivity (10) or by enzymatic degradation of lipids into inflammatory products (11).

Clearly there is much overlap between anterior and posterior blepharitis, so it is to be expected that confusion of terminology and classification will exist in the literature.

HISTORY AND TERMINOLOGY

The word *blepharitis* is derived from the Greek word βλέφχρον, for eyelid, and the condition is described in the Hippocratic collection (12).

Inflammation of lid became recognized as a separate clinical entity in the 19th century (13). John Dalrymple (1803–1852), surgeon at Moorfield's Eye Hospital, gave a detailed description of blepharitis in his illustrated textbook (14).

Traditionally blepharitis was divided into two types: squamous, characterized by inflamed lid border with dry or greasy scales (squames); or ulcerative, which had small pustules of the lid follicles leading to ulceration (2).

The importance of meibomian gland dysfunction in blepharitis was recognized in a few case reports, which attributed the inflammation to either bacteria or a direct chemical effect of the secretion (15). Blepharitis in acne rosacea was also noted to be associated with meibomianitis (2).

The tarsal glands were mentioned in ancient times by Galen, but were more fully described by Heinrich Meibom in 1666 (16). Because the meibomian glands were named after Meibom (Meibomius), the correct term for their secretion is meibomium, not meibum and inflammation of the gland should be called meibomianitis not meibomitis (16).

One of the earliest descriptions of meibomian gland dysfunction, called ophthalmia tarsi, was in Mackenzie's textbook (13). The oil glands were distended and filled with excessive amounts of thickened (puriform) secretion. Several terms were used to describe meibomian gland disease and blepharitis. These included puriform palpebral flux of Scarpa (1801), ophthalmia tarsi (13), conjunctivitis meibomianae (15), polyadenitis meibomiana chronica suppuritiva in the historical literature (17), and more recently blepharitis (2), chronic blepharo-conjunctivitis (18), meibomian keratoconjunctivitis (19), chronic meibomitis, seborrheic blepharo-kerato-conjunctivitis or seborrheic blepharitis (20).

The term *meibomian seborrhea* was coined by Cowper (21). Squeezing the normal tarsal plate produces a minute, clear, oily droplet at the orifice of the gland. In meibomian seborrhea, on the other hand, secretion could be abnormal in quantity and quality. Three types were described: thickened white material of cream cheese consistency, thin pus, or excess amounts of clear or mildly turbid yellowish oily fluid. Inflammation was not a feature. Other authors use the term to describe excess normal liquid oil contained in dilated ducts (3).

Meibomian gland dysfunction is increasingly the preferred term to describe the many changes observed in the tarsal glands and orifices, some of which are related to blepharitis.

Early in the 20th century, severe staphylococcal blepharitis was an intractable condition. The treatment with penicillin ointment developed by Ida Mann in Oxford was the beginning of modern management of the condition (22). It would seem that staphylococcal blepharitis is less frequently encountered and is less severe today than in the preantibiotic era. Increasingly important is the role of meibomian gland dysfunction. Nevertheless, blepharitis in all its different forms remains a common frustrating condition for patients and practitioners, and causes a myriad of problems from irritation and dry eye because of tear film instability (19) to contact lens intolerance (23).

Until recently, the etiological theories, classification, terminology, and management of blepharitis still owed more to historical dictum than rational science.

ANATOMY OF THE EYELID MARGIN

The normal adult lid margin, measured from the posterior lash line to the sharply curved posterior lid border, is 1.95 (±0.07) mm wide in the upper lid and 1.87 (±0.06) mm in the lower lid (24). The posterior quarter is lined with mucous membrane and ends with an abrupt right angle edge (Fig. 30-1A). This allows smooth contact with the globe, similar to a windscreen wiper, and change in conformation by rounding leads to ocular surface dysfunction. Increased rounding occurs in the upper lid with age and in the lower lid as a consequence of posterior blepharitis (24).

The anterior three quarters of the lid margin is composed of skin and the front edge is more rounded than the posterior lid margin. In young people, the lid margins are relatively avascular, although the papillary architecture of the mucosal vessels is easily identified. Cutaneous vessels become more obvious with age. A segmental venous drainage between the meibomian orifices has tributaries from the mucosa, which pass forward in the dermis (Fig. 30-1B) (7).

The mucocutaneous junction forms a curved line along the full length of the lid, parallel to its posterior edge. The lashes emerge in the anterior half of the skin-lined portion and the meibomian gland orifices are located just in front of the mucocutaneous junction in the cutaneous part (7).

The meibomian glands are modified, elongated sebaceous glands in the tarsal plates of the lids that open onto the lid margin. The main structure is the duct extending the full length of the gland. About 30 to 40 vertically orientated glands are found in the upper lid and slightly fewer in the lower lid. The concentration of these enlarged glands in the small area of the lids implies an important demand

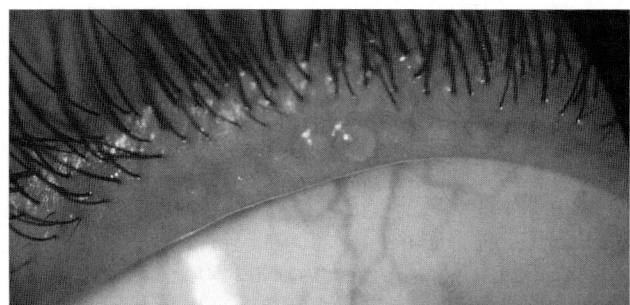

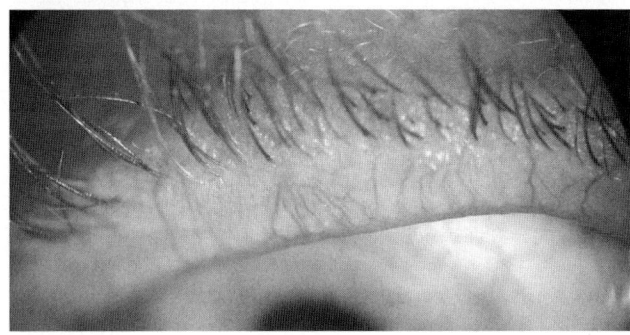

FIGURE 30-1. A: Normal eyelid in youth with capping of a meibomian gland orifice. Note the sharply curved posterior border and creamy cuffing surrounding normal meibomian gland orifices. **B:** Increased vascularization of the lid margin with age, showing segmental venous drainage between meibomian gland orifices passing forward into the dermis.

for lipid secretion to maintain a healthy ocular surface. They are tubular-acinar glands, composed of grape-like clusters of single or composite acinar lobules opening into lateral ductules on either side of the main duct. The duct is lined with partially keratinized epithelium (25). It terminates in an orifice flush with the surface of the lid margin. These orifices are visible with slit-lamp examination, which reveals a series of concentric zones, most easily identified in youth (Fig. 30-1A). There is a central punctum surrounded by an opaque cuff, presumably the keratinized lining of the duct. Around this is a translucent dark annulus of dermis. In nonpigmented skin, an outer cream colored, subepithelial cuff is seen that probably represents a deep structure such as the distal tip of the acinus or the muscle of Riolan, fine muscular extensions of the pars marginalis of orbicularis oculi (7,26).

MEIBOMIAN GLAND SECRETION

The secretion of the meibomian glands is holocrine, derived from lysis of the secretory cells. The acini are lined with glandular epithelium, cuboidal and fat-free peripherally and fat-laden centrally. The cells break down when mature and release their contents into the ductules. The main duct is filled with fat and can be seen as a yellow streak through the conjunctiva. Gentle pressure expresses a small dome of clear oily fluid over the gland orifices in normal individuals.

The composition of meibomian lipid is distinct from sebum, reflecting its different functions. Meibomian oil remains liquid at lid temperature (16). The melting point is a range with some components remaining semisolid until complete melting occurs.

The study of meibomian lipid chemistry is complex and affected by sampling and methods of analysis. Rancification of oils during preparation and problems with analysis of pooled samples should be considered in interpreting the results from the older literature (16). Indeed significant individual variation in the components of meibomian secretion exists in the normal population.

Wax, from the Anglo-Saxon word *weax,* meaning beeswax, is an important component of the surface covering of animals and plants. Waxes contain esters of long-chain fatty acids with long-chain fatty alcohols, usually of a similar length. In general, about 84% of meibomian lipid is composed of nonpolar lipid wax esters and sterol esters. The esters contain straight-chain, branched-chain, unsaturated, and hydroxy fatty acids with chain lengths of C_{12} to C_{34} (16,27). Smaller amounts of diesters, triesters, free sterols, triglycerides, and free fatty acids are also present (28). Triglycerides compose 6% of the total, and only 0.5% to 1% is free fatty acids (29).

The wax esters are composed of relatively short chain lengths (18 carbons or less). The major peak is a C_{42} ester containing 16:1 fatty acid and *iso*-C_{26} alcohol (30).

The major esterified sterol is cholesterol, but smaller amounts of others, including lathosterol, have been identified (30). The sterol esters use longer chains (20 carbons or more) than the wax esters (28).

Unsaturated fatty acids (containing a C=C double bond) in esters are particularly important because of their lower melting point compared to equivalent saturated fatty acids. Differences in the fatty acids esterified to waxes and sterols are found between patients with blepharitis and normal controls (31). Paste-like meibomian secretion obtained from blepharitis patients contains relatively low amounts of the 18-carbon unsaturated oleic acid (*cis*-9-octadecanoic acid) compared to more liquid meibomian lipid samples (32).

There are many types of lipid molecules in meibomian secretion. The combination of a variety of fatty acids with several fatty alcohols and sterols can generate an enormous number of different wax ester and sterol ester molecules (28,31).

Pure lipids are hydrophobic, and do not spread on the aqueous tear film. A surfactant of polar lipids is required, the hydrophilic end in the aqueous and a hydrophobic tail supporting the overlying lipid layer. The low amounts of polar lipids present in meibomian secretion, including phospholipids, sphingolipids, ceramides (fatty acids linked by an amide bond to the amine group of a long chain sphingoid base), cerebrosides, and polar unbranched saturated fatty acids, therefore, have an important functional role. It is likely that they form an extremely thin layer, one to three molecules thick, which acts as a surfactant between aqueous tears and the thicker nonpolar lipid layer (33). Low levels of two polar phospholipids, phosphatidylethanolamine (cephalin) and sphingolipid, are associated with keratoconjunctivitis sicca in patients with blepharitis, presumably due to increased tear evaporation (34).

The combination of all these molecular species gives the semisolid lipid mixture properties that allow its various functions. It must have the correct viscosity to flow out of the gland orifice and the correct range of melting points. The oily waxy meibomian substance is secreted onto the edge of the eyelid. Some of the secretion spreads onto the tear film forming the superficial lipid layer. The lipid layer component must have spreading characteristics that ensure coverage of the preocular tear film between blinks. This layer retards evaporation of tears and provides the optical qualities necessary for good image formation by the eye (35).

The remaining lipid on the lid forms a hydrophobic wall, preventing overspill of tears onto the skin, hindering contamination of the preocular tear film lipids with sebaceous lipids and ensuring a tight seal when the eyelids are closed.

Changes in the lipid secretion either endogenously or after modification by lipase enzymes derived from bacteria, can alter the properties of the oil. This can cause increased viscosity leading to stagnation in the glands, changes in rheology affecting tear film stability, and release of free fatty acids and other molecular species, which can directly cause irritation of the eye.

The control of secretion remains to be fully elucidated. Bundles of muscles of Riolan, or pars marginalis muscles, have been shown to form an ellipse around the ducts leading to the orifice of the gland (26). The interfascicular septa of the muscle continue around the ducts to become an integral part of the tarsal plate. Thus on contraction the muscle is pulled toward the tarsal plate and compresses the ducts preventing outflow of secretion. In contrast, the pars palpebrae of the orbicularis oculi has a milking action on the glands during blinks. Between blinks the muscle of Riolan is contracted, the orbicularis relaxed, and secretion in the duct cannot escape.

Hormonal, in particular androgenic, and nervous influences on secretion are also likely but not fully elucidated (36).

CHANGES IN THE LID MARGIN AND MEIBOMIAN SECRETION ASSOCIATED WITH BLEPHARITIS

Changes in lid margin anatomy (7) and meibomian gland secretion (27,31) occur in meibomian gland dysfunction. These changes may affect the lid margin morphology, the mucocutaneous junction, the meibomian glands (6), their orifices (19), and the quantity and quality of the excretion (7).

Patients with blepharitis have a lid margin that may become more thickened, rounded, and vascularized. In some, hyperkeratinization of the cutaneous border gives an eczematous appearance, occurring particularly in atopic lid disease. Irregularity of the margin is most commonly seen around obliterated meibomian gland orifices. More severe changes cause trichiasis and entropion (2).

The mucocutaneous junction becomes irregular in meibomian gland disease. It may migrate anterior to the orifices, or posteriorly with keratinized squamous metaplasia of the posterior lid margin. Mucosal absorption may occur without retroplacement of the mucocutaneous junction. This may lead to ridging of the junction.

Several changes in the gland orifice are seen in blepharitis. Elevation of the orifice, pouting, is an early sign of meibomian gland dysfunction. Some pouting glands may be blocked. The orifice may be dilated with inspissated (thickened) secretions or other material, such as keratin (Fig. 30-2A). It has been postulated that hyperkeratinization of the meibomian glands could be an initial stage of meibomian gland dysfunction, leading to blockage (27). The finding of typical epidermal lipids in a model of meibomian gland disease would support this contention (27). Histology of lids with meibomian gland dysfunction has confirmed

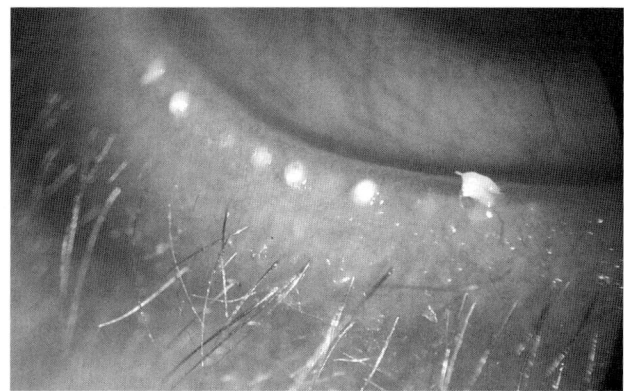

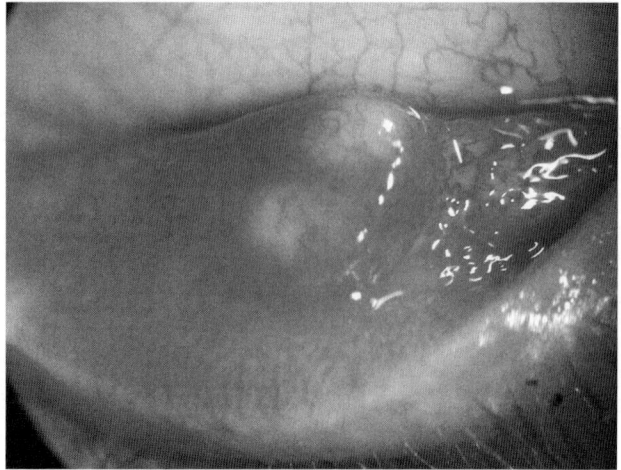

FIGURE 30-2. A: Expressed inspissated meibomian gland excretions. Thickened paste-like secretions expressed from inspissated gland orifices. **B:** Chalazion.

hyperkeratinization and sloughing of keratin into the ducts and ductules (6,20).

The involvement of keratinocytes may be more complicated than simple plugging of the orifices. When stimulated with lipopolysaccharide or ultraviolet light they can produce cytokines such as tumor necrosis factor-α (TNF-α), interleukin-1 (IL-1), IL-6, and IL-8, which in turn stimulate keratinocytes to produce proinflammatory lipids (5).

Occasional individual orifices may be capped by a dome of oil covered by a tough surface (20). The cap, which is easily punctured by a needle, may occur in otherwise normal lids (Fig. 30-1A) (7).

Retroplacement of the gland orifices by cicatricial changes in the tarsal mucosa leads to oval elongation of the orifices and exposure of the duct. Narrowing or occlusion of the gland orifices is seen with age and also in meibomian gland dysfunction. It is accompanied by increased vascularization. Dilatation and distortion of the glands in the tarsus may occur in meibomian gland disease as a consequence of duct narrowing and occlusion. Chalazia, secondary granulomatous inflammation to fat in the glands, may also develop (Fig. 30-2B).

Normal meibomian secretion is clear. In meibomian gland dysfunction, fluid may contain granular material, become cloudy or inspissated, thickened to toothpaste-like consistency (Fig. 30-2B). Foam formation at the lid margins is also seen in patients with meibomian gland dysfunction (37). Increased viscosity can lead to decreased secretion. Hypersecretion, true seborrhea, has not been clearly defined, to distinguish it from increased amount of stagnated fat expressed from dilated glands.

CLASSIFICATION OF BLEPHARITIS AND MEIBOMIAN GLAND DYSFUNCTION

Because the eyelid margin encompasses the junction of skin and mucous membrane, it may be affected by diseases of both components. Consequently, the classification of eyelid inflammations remains confused, and several different approaches are to be found in the literature.

Perhaps the simplest and most widely used classification is the division into anterior blepharitis, affecting the skin components, and posterior blepharitis, concerning the meibomian glands and adjacent mucous membrane (17). This close contact means that both types may occur together, so-called mixed, and broadly speaking this classification is helpful clinically.

Thygeson (2) in 1946 proposed three types of blepharitis: staphylococcic, seborrheic, and a rarer angular blepharitis attributed to *Haemophilus duplex* (*Moraxella*).

Seborrheic blepharitis was always associated with seborrheic dermatitis, was nonulcerative, and was associated with scales, and therefore it was also called squamous blepharitis.

Staphylococcic blepharitis was more often unilateral and characterized by ulceration and recurrent hordeolums and chalazions. It was associated with keratoconjunctivitis and in severe cases marginal corneal infiltrates and ulcers. A mixed type of blepharitis resembled seborrheic blepharitis except for more corneal and conjunctival complications.

Meibomian gland involvement was found in only a minority of cases, although it was present in all cases resistant to treatment. Hypersecretion of the glands and dilatation of their orifices was proposed to increase susceptibility to infection, and expression of secretions was recommended for palliation.

The importance of meibomian gland dysfunction in blepharitis became increasingly recognized. However, dysfunction of the meibomian glands may occur without inflammation, and classifications have been devised to account for this. An early proposal classified meibomian gland dysfunction into simple hypersecretion (with no inflammation), simple chronic meibomianitis, and chronic meibomianitis with hypertrophy and with chalazia (18).

A detailed biomicroscopic classification and grading system for meibomian gland dysfunction has been published (7). Although this is a useful description for meibomian gland dysfunction, it is not a classification of blepharitis per se.

McCulley et al. (3,8) subdivide chronic blepharitis into six major categories (as described in the following subsections) plus an extra group including patients with blepharitis caused by atopy, psoriasis, and other dermatologic conditions. The patients were evaluated by a dermatologist.

Staphylococcal Blepharitis

Patients with staphylococcal blepharitis were mostly female and relatively young (mean age 42 years). There was usually a short history of symptoms (mean 1.76 years) and the patients did not have dermatological disease.

The eyelids are inflamed along the ciliary portion of the lid, often extending onto the lid margin in staphylococcal blepharitis. Telangiectasis affecting the anterior lid margin is commonly seen (Fig. 30-3A). Collarettes surrounding individual eyelashes are found scattered among more nondescript lid and lash crusting (Fig. 30-3A). Madarosis, the loss of cilia, is common.

Conjunctival changes, including mild bulbar injection and mild papillary hypertrophy of the tarsal conjunctiva is uncommon. Keratitis, seen as punctate epithelial erosions, affects the lower one third of the cornea. Half of the patients have keratoconjunctivitis sicca.

Staphylococcus aureus was cultured from the lids in 46% of these patients compared to 15% of normal controls. It was hypothesized that *S. epidermidis* might play a role in the other patients with apparent staphylococcal blepharitis.

Seborrheic Blepharitis (Without Other Associated Lid Disease)

Patients with seborrheic blepharitis have only minimal or moderate inflammation along the anterior lid border

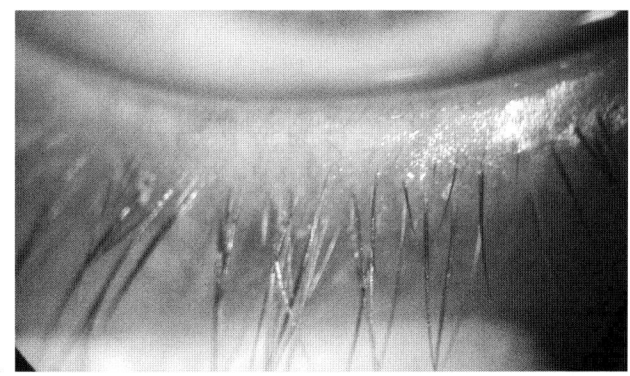
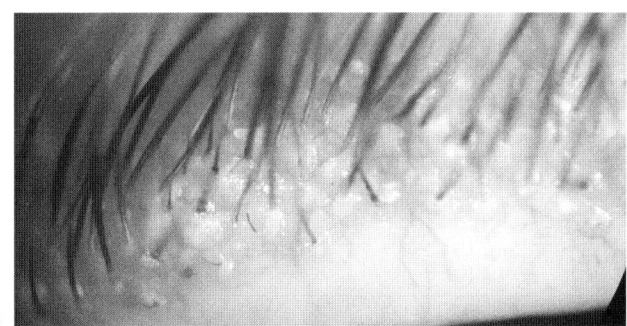

FIGURE 30-3. A: Staphylococcal blepharitis. There is erythema and edema along the anterior ciliary portion of the eyelid. Collarettes surround some lashes as well as nondescript crusting. **B:** Seborrheic blepharitis. There is greasy crusting of the anterior lid and lashes but minimal inflammation.

(Fig. 30-3B). Males and females were affected equally and the mean age was 50 years. This is a chronic condition with minimal inflammation of the anterior lid margin. An oily or greasy crusting is found on the lids and lashes. Keratoconjunctivitis sicca is present in a third of patients. Seborrheic dermatitis, which may be subtle, typically limited to retroauricular skin, glabella, eyebrows, scalp, and sternum, was found in all cases. Only 11% of lid cultures grew *S. aureus.*

Seborrheic-Staphylococcal Blepharitis

These patients are similar to the seborrheic blepharitis patients except that they have more inflammation, which also tends to involve the lid margin. The differentiating symptom is that of significant exacerbations superimposed on the chronic disease. When seen during these periods, the eyes were inflamed and there was eyelid and lash crusting of a mixed nature, oily or greasy scurf plus collarettes (Fig. 30-4A). Keratoconjunctivitis sicca was found in 35% of cases and 83% of lid cultures grew *S. aureus.*

Seborrheic Blepharitis with Meibomian Seborrhea

These patients have mild seborrheic blepharitis but with excessive meibomian secretions. They complain of burning,

652 *II. Clinical Topics*

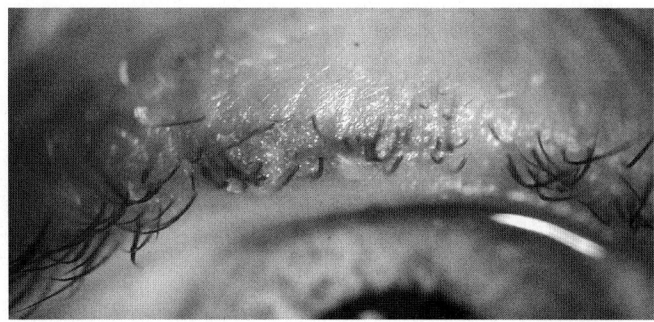
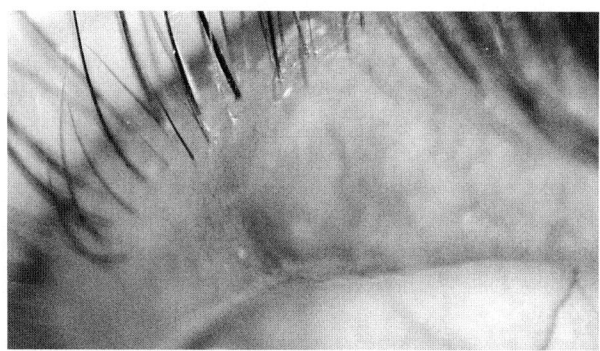

FIGURE 30-4. A: Mixed seborrheic and staphylococcal blepharitis. There is more inflammation than in seborrheic blepharitis and the crusting is mixed with greasy scales and collarettes around some cilia. **B:** Seborrheic blepharitis with secondary (spotty) meibomianitis, showing mild greasy scaling of the eyelashes and scattered patchy inflammation of groups of meibomian gland orifices.

most severe in the morning but persisting throughout the day. There is minimal anterior seborrheic blepharitis and the bulbar conjunctiva is mildly hyperemic. Foam in the tear film was commonly found. While the meibomian glands are not inflamed, they do show evidence of excessive secretion. The secretions can be seen in glands, which are dilated but do not exhibit plugging nor inspissation of the orifices, and are easily expressed.

Seborrheic Blepharitis with Secondary (Spotty) Meibomianitis (Fig. 30-4B)

Patients with this form of blepharitis describe a chronic history with exacerbations of the condition. In addition to the anterior eyelid changes of seborrheic blepharitis, scattered patches of inflammation of the lid margin around groups of meibomian glands, not a diffuse meibomianitis, is seen. The affected gland orifices are prominent and contain an inspissated plug that can be difficult or impossible to express. Keratoconjunctivitis is more common in this form of blepharitis than in patients with seborrheic blepharitis.

Primary Meibomianitis (Meibomian Keratoconjunctivitis)

In this group, the duration of symptoms, on average 2 to 3 years, was shorter than that in seborrheic blepharitis. The patients have prominent signs in the posterior part of the lid margin (Fig. 30-5A). Inflammation and pouting of the glands was noted with solidification of the lipid meibomian secretions. Inspissation near the gland orifice causes difficulty with expression of the gland contents. A significant conjunctivitis was typical, with bulbar injection and tarsal papillary hypertrophy. The unstable tear film was associated with interpalpebral superficial punctate keratitis and rose bengal staining of the interpalpebral bulbar conjunctiva. There was a predisposition to generalized seba-

ceous gland abnormality with either acne rosacea (Fig. 30-5B) in two thirds or seborrheic dermatitis in the remainder.

The above classification system has been used to generate an enormous literature on the causes of blepharitis, but it is not universally accepted. Other authors find it difficult to fit their patients into the above groups (38,39). Using cluster analysis, Mathers et al. (4) found that chronic blepharitis patients could be classified into four separate groups based on meibomian gland loss, quality of secretion, tear film osmolarity, and Schirmer's testing:

1. Seborrheic meibomian gland dysfunction: The commonest type of blepharitis was found to have higher than normal secretion of the meibomian glands and a low rate of gland drop out. The patients have normal

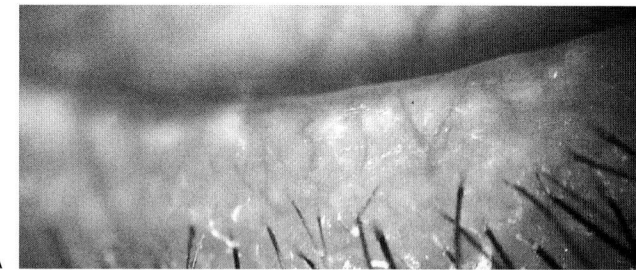
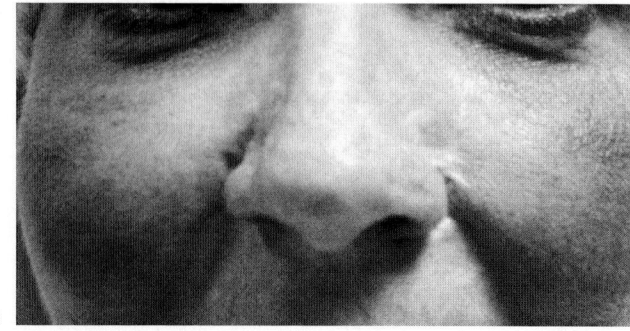

FIGURE 30-5. A: Primary meibomianitis. Inspissation of inflamed meibomian gland orifices in a patient with rosacea. **B:** Rosacea.

Schirmer's tests and low tear osmolarity. These patients are probably equivalent to patients described as seborrheic with meibomian gland seborrhea (3).

2. Obstructive meibomian gland dysfunction: These patients had low volumes of thickened meibomian secretions. Meibomian gland drop out was frequent. The Schirmer's test was normal but the tears had high osmolarity. This group may include patients classified as having staphylococcal blepharitis in other classification systems.

3. Obstructive with sicca: This cluster of patients had the highest meibomian gland drop out, very low secretion volume, and the highest thickness of secretion. The Schirmer's test was low and the tears had high osmolarity.

4. Sicca: These patients had normal meibomian glands and secretion. The Schirmer's test was low and tear osmolarity high. This suggests that some patients presenting with blepharitis may primarily have dry eye.

Although these systems that have been described are clearly useful, a universally agreed classification has yet to be accepted.

ETIOLOGY

Staphylococcal Infection

Staphylococcal colonization of the lid margin has been thought to be an important cause of blepharitis for a century or more (1–3,11). Ulcerative anterior blepharitis may well be due to staphylococcal infection of the lash follicles, and the condition improves with antibiotic therapy (22). However, the role of bacteria in nonulcerative blepharitis remains controversial. For example, pathogenic bacteria were not found in 88% of blepharitis patients and in no patients with meibomianitis (40). The failure to find *S. aureus* in cases with meibomianitis with greater frequency than in normals suggests that secondary meibomianitis is not primarily a bacterial disease. Furthermore, the punctate keratitis seen in some cases is unlikely to be due to staphylococcal exotoxins, as previously proposed. The keratitis could be due to instability of the tear film.

If infection is not the cause, then indirect effects from commensal bacteria could play a role in blepharitis. More *S. epidermidis* has been found on the lids of patients with primary meibomian disease than on the lids of normal controls (11). Particular attention has focused on the degradation of meibomian oil into toxic fatty acids, or lipids that are more viscous, both of which could perpetuate inflammation. The breakdown of major tear film lipid components to more polar lipids could further destabilize the tear film. Ocular flora has an enormous potential for modifying meibomian secretions (11). All *S. aureus* found in the ocular flora of both normal and inflamed eyes produce a triglyceride lipase (3), and a high percentage of *Propionibacterium* spp. make a

wax esterase, and 6% make a cholesterol esterase (11). It is possible that products generated by one species are utilized by another, further complicating the picture.

Hypersensitivity to Staphylococci

A rabbit model of ulcerative blepharitis required immunization with *S. aureus* cell walls (41). A study of 116 patients with blepharitis revealed enhanced cell-mediated immunity to *S. aureus* but not *S. epidermidis* (10). The hypersensitivity response was not found in normal subjects. Enhanced immunity correlated with eyelash folliculitis and the need for topical steroid use to control marginal ulceration.

Infestation

Demodex infestation of the lash follicles is common and is found in 22% to 60% of patients with blepharitis, but curiously not in cases with mixed seborrheic and staphylococcal blepharitis (3). Thygeson (2) failed to find *Demodex* in lid scrapings or meibomian secretion; but he did not examine the lash follicles. There is doubt as to whether this organism is causally related to blepharitis.

Irritation from lice infestation causes marginal blepharitis. The tell-tale tiny red excreta at the lash base should alert the clinician to the possibility of louse infection even if lice are not immediately seen.

In addition, a number of infections, such as molluscum contagiosum (Fig. 30-6), herpes viral infection, and dermatologic diseases may affect the eyelids and can present as blepharitis. Furthermore, malignant conditions such as sebaceous cell carcinoma can masquerade as chronic blepharitis.

Association of Blepharitis and Dry Eye

Keratoconjunctivitis sicca is commonly found in patients with blepharitis. Both problems are common conditions, and a causal association remains unproven, but several mechanisms can lead to dry eye in blepharitis patients (42).

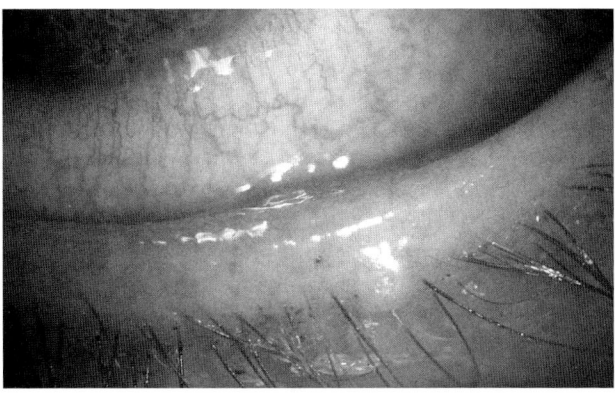

FIGURE 30-6. Molluscum contagiosum.

Stagnation of meibomian secretions may allow bacterial lipases to generate free fatty acids that destabilize the tear film, causing decreased tear film breakup time and sometimes paradoxical epiphora. Abnormal meibomian lipids can contribute to tear film instability because of altered spreading characteristics (5,43).

Objective evidence that meibomian gland dysfunction can lead to dry eye was obtained by closing the meibomian glands of rabbit eyes with light cautery. This led to increased tear osmolarity, despite normal lacrimal function, decreased conjunctival goblet cell density, and ocular surface changes of keratoconjunctivitis sicca (44).

The association of staphylococcal blepharitis with dry eye has not been fully explained. Possible causes include chronic inflammation causing obstruction of the main and accessory lacrimal ductules. Alternatively, patients with dry eye could be more susceptible to staphylococcal colonization of the eyelids and development of blepharitis (42).

TREATMENT

Physical Treatments

Massage of the eyelid is a traditional folk remedy for eyelid disorders, and Duke-Elder and MacFaul (1) quote Parson Woodforde (1791), who obtained relief by rubbing his eyelid with the tail of a black cat. Interestingly massage remains a cornerstone of management of blepharitis to this day. Mechanical expression of thickened meibomian secretions was advocated in the early literature (2,5,21) and is still an important component of management (9). The process is much easier if the secretions have been warmed, which reduces their viscosity. Warm compresses applied to the lid margins have traditionally been used to heat the lids and meibomian glands. A washcloth microwaved (45), or heated with hot tap water, is commonly employed. Alternatives such as a cotton stocking filled with dry rice heated to a comfortable temperature in a microwave are also advocated (9). The warm compress is applied to the closed eyelid for 2 to 10 minutes.

A variety of external devices have been developed for this purpose of lid warming over the years. None has gained widespread use. Recently, an infrared warm compress device has been shown to be efficacious (46).

The warm compress is followed by eyelid scrubs. One technique of expression is to hold the eyelid at the outer canthus with an index finger stretching the tarsus while the opposite index finger draped with a washcloth sweeps down the upper lid or up the lower lid, expressing the meibomian secretions (9). This massage is repeated 10 times on each lid.

It is important to explain the procedure carefully and preferably issue an illustrated handout to prevent patients innovating novel and potentially harmful variants, including scalding, bleach, and toothbrushes (45).

Cleaning of the eyelid margins with dilute soaps such as baby shampoo or proprietary cleansing solutions may help in cases with seborrhea (47).

Medical Therapy

Staphylococcal lid disease is treated with topical antibiotic ointments twice to four times a day. Bacitracin, erythromycin, fusidic acid, or chloramphenicol is applied to the lid margin and lash line after lid scrubs have removed the debris from the lashes.

The use of a topical steroid is generally discouraged, and its long-term use has predisposed to severe bacterial and fungal infections (42).

Systemic treatment with antibiotics is usually not required except for patients with meibomianitis. Oral tetracyclines reduce meibomian gland inflammation (48). The mechanism of tetracycline action could be by inhibition of bacterial lipases (49). This would inhibit the breakdown of meibomian lipids into potentially inflammatory fatty acids. Tetracycline and minocycline also inhibit production of nitric oxide and reactive oxygen species by white cells (5).

The effectiveness of tetracyclines is seen in smaller doses than required to treat bacterial infections. It is often prescribed as low-dose long-term therapy. Other authors prefer to start with a higher dose, such as tetracycline 250 mg orally four times a day, tapered over 3 months (42), or doxycycline 100 mg twice a day for up to 2 months before tapering to a maintenance dose of 100 mg a day for as long as needed (9). However, lower dose of oral doxycycline 100 mg for 1 month and then 50 mg a day for a further month followed by 50 mg on alternate days is effective in the management of ocular rosacea (50). Doxycycline is structurally similar to tetracycline hydrochloride but has some advantages. Doxycycline is absorbed better and is less affected by food; it has a longer half-life, does not have an anabolic effect, and can be used by patients with renal disease. It only needs to be given once a day, which may help compliance with long-term treatment. Tetracycline has a faster onset of action, and therapy can be initiated with this drug before switching to maintenance with doxycycline 50 mg once a day (50).

Nutritional Therapy

Animal models of meibomian gland dysfunction show a change in composition toward a more epidermal profile with increased free cholesterol and ceramides (27). The authors suggest that this reflects hyperkeratinization of the ductal epithelium. Linoleic and oleic acids are present in normal meibomian excretion and inhibit keratinocytes. Oil of evening primrose contains linoleic and gamma-linoleic fatty acids. These fatty acids are precursors of prostaglandins and could therefore modulate inflammation in the meibomian glands.

Controlled clinical trials are awaited. However, a small pilot study of eight patients with refractory meibomian gland dysfunction received dietary supplements of linoleic and linolenic fatty acids. Their symptoms improved, but slit-lamp examination found minimal change in the meibomian glands (51).

Flavonoid antioxidants, derived from plant sources such as bilberry extract, are also potentially useful supplements.

Hormonal Treatment

The meibomian gland may be modulated by androgens. In patients receiving antiandrogen therapy, there is a change in meibomian lipid composition compared to controls (36). However, the use of systemic androgens could induce virilization, so topical therapy is being investigated.

SUMMARY

Blepharitis describes a group of conditions with varying etiology that is chronic, difficult to treat, and frustrating for patients and their doctors. Severe bacterial infection of the lid margins and cilia is less common and less severe today than in the preantibiotic era. Blepharitis is no longer considered as a simple bacterial infection of the lids. The role of meibomian gland dysfunction in tear film instability and in lid margin inflammation is important. However, bacterial colonization of the lid margin may have a role by indirectly leading to inflammation. Alteration of meibomian gland secretion by bacterial lipase exoenzymes has the potential to generate inflammatory molecules from meibomian lipid.

Unesterified cholesterol, which can be metabolized by bacteria, stimulates growth of *S. aureus in vitro* and is present in meibomian gland dysfunction. Duct hyperkeratinization could be the origin of free cholesterol, or it could be released from cholesterol esters present in meibomian secretion by bacterial esterases. Thus, meibomian seborrhea, as a source of free cholesterol could encourage bacterial blepharitis. This mechanism could explain the mixed picture of blepharitis seen in many patients.

Skin diseases, such as rosacea and seborrheic dermatitis, and hormonal changes with age or drug use, lead to changes in meibomian gland composition. These changes can affect the melting point of the lipid mixture, leading to increased viscosity and inspissation of the gland orifices. The reduced clearance of this lipid may further encourage bacterial colonization.

The structural role of meibomian gland lipid in maintaining the tear film can be disrupted by these changes and dry eye symptoms result.

Inflammation of the lids can lead to thickening and rounding of the lid, which further aggravates the problem.

Later cicatricial changes cause notching, trichiasis, and entropion. Corneal involvement from blepharitis results from secondary dry eye or from corneal infiltration by leukocytes. On occasion severe corneal ulceration develops.

Newer therapies, including nutritional and hormonal supplements, hold some promise for the alleviation of these conditions.

REFERENCES

1. Duke-Elder S, MacFaul PA. System of ophthalmology. In: Duke-Elder S, ed. *The ocular adenexa*, part 1. London: Henry Kimpton, 1974;205–236.
2. Thygeson P. Etiology and treatment of blepharitis. A study in military personnel. *Arch Ophthalmol* 1946;36:445–477.
3. McCulley JP, Dougherty JM, Deneau DG. Classification of chronic blepharitis. *Ophthalmology* 1982;89:1173–1180.
4. Mathers WD, Sheilds WJ, Sachdev MS, et al. Meibomian gland dysfunction in chronic blepharitis. *Cornea* 1991;10:277–285.
5. McCulley JP, Shine WE. Changing concepts in the diagnosis and management of blepharitis. *Cornea* 2000;19:650–658.
6. Gutgesell VJ, Stern GA, Hood IA. Histopathology of meibomian gland dysfunction. *Am J Ophthalmol* 1982;94:383–387.
7. Bron AJ, Benjamin L, Snibson GR. Meibomian gland disease. Classification and grading of lid changes. *Eye* 1991;5:395–411.
8. McCulley JP, Dougherty JM. Blepharitis associated with acne rosacea and seborrheic dermatitis. *Int Ophthalmol Clin* 1985;25:159–172.
9. Paranjpe DR, Foulks GN. Therapy for meibomian gland disease. *Ophthalmol Clin North Am* 2003;16:37–42.
10. Ficker L, Ramakrishnan M, Seal D, et al. Role of cell-mediated immunity to Staphylococci in Blepharitis. *Am J Ophthalmol* 1991;111:473–479.
11. Dougherty JM, McCulley JP. Bacterial lipases and chronic blepharitis. *Invest Ophthalmol Vis Sci* 1986;27:486–491.
12. Albert MD, Edwards DD. *The history of ophthalmology.* Blackwell Science, 1996.
13. Mackenzie W. *A practical treatise of the eye*, 2nd ed. London: Longman, 1835.
14. Dalrymple J. *Pathology of the human eye*, 1st ed. London: Churchill, 1852.
15. Lydston JA. Conjunctivitis meibomianae. *JAMA* 1894;23:241–242.
16. Tiffany JM. The lipid secretion of the meibomian glands. *Adv Lipid Res* 1987;22:1–62.
17. Driver PJ, Lemp MA. Meibomian gland dysfunction. *Surv Ophthalmol* 1996;40:343–367.
18. Gifford SR. Meibomian Glands in chronic blepharo-conjunctivitis. *Am J Ophthalmol* 1921;4:489–494.
19. McCulley JP, Sciallis GF. Meibomian keratoconjunctivitis. *Am J Ophthalmol* 1977;84:788–793.
20. Keith CG. Seborrhoeic blepharo-kerato-conjunctivitis. *Trans Ophthalmol Soc UK* 1967;87:85–103.
21. Cowper HW. Meibomian seborrhea. *Am J Ophthalmol* 1922;5:25–30.
22. Florey ME, McFarley AM, Mann I. Report on 48 cases of marginal blepharitis treated with penicillin. *Br J Ophthalmol* 1945;29:333–338.
23. Henriquez AS, Korb DR. Meibomian gland and contact lens wear. *Br J Ophthalmol* 1981;65:108–111.
24. Hykin PG, Bron AJ. Age-related morphological changes in lid margin and meibomian gland anatomy. *Cornea* 1992;11:334–342.

25. Jester JV, Nicholaides N, Smith RE. Meibomian gland dysfunction. I. Keratin protein expression in normal human and rabbit meibomian glands. *Invest Ophthalmol Vis Sci* 1989;30:927–935.

26. Linton RG, Curnow DH, Riley WJ. The meibomian glands: an investigation into the secretion and some aspects of the physiology. *Br J Ophthalmol* 1961;45:718–723.

27. Nicholaides N, Santos EC, Smith RE, et al. Meibomian gland dysfunction III. Meibomian gland lipids. *Invest Ophthalmol Vis Sci* 1989;30:946–951.

28. Nicolaides N, Kaitaranta JK, Rowdah RN, et al. Meibomian gland studies: comparison of steer and human lipids. *Invest Ophthalmol Vis Sci* 1981;20:522–536.

29. Dougherty JM, McCulley JP. Analysis of the free fatty acid component of meibomian secretions in chronic blepharitis. *Invest Ophthalmol Vis Sci* 1986;27:52–56.

30. Harvey DJ, Duerden JM, Pandher KS, et al. Identification by combined gas chromatography-mass spectrometry of constituent long-chain fatty acids and alcohols from meibomian glands of the rat and a comparison with human meibomian lipids. *J Chromatogr* 1987;414:253–263.

31. Dougherty JM, Osgood JK, McCulley JP. The role of wax and sterol ester fatty acids in chronic blepharitis. *Invest Ophthalmol Vis Sci* 1991;32:1932–1937.

32. Shine WE, McCulley JP. Association of meibum oleic acid with meibomian seborrhea. *Cornea* 2000;19:72–74.

33. Shine WE, McCulley JP. Polar lipids in human meibomian gland secretions. *Curr Eye Res* 2003;26:89–94.

34. Shine WE, McCulley JP. Keratoconjunctivitis sicca associated with meibomian secretion polar lipid abnormality. *Arch Ophthalmol* 1998;116:849–852.

35. Mishima S, Maurice DM. The oily layer of the tear film and evaporation from the corneal surface. *Exp Eye Res* 1961;1: 39–45.

36. Sullivan BD, Evans JE, Krenzer KL, et al. Impact of antiandrogen treatment on the fatty acid profile of neutral lipids in human meibomian gland secretion. *J Clin Endocrinol Metab* 2000;85: 4866–4873.

37. Norn N. Expressibility of meibomian secretion. Relation to age, lipid precorneal film, scales, foam, hair and pigmentation. *Acta Ophthalmol* 1987;65:137–142.

38. Groden LR, Murphy B, Rodnite J, et al. Lid flora and blepharitis. *Cornea* 1991;10:50–53.

39. Huber-Spitzy V, Baumgartner I, Bohler-Sommeregger K, et al. Blepharitis-a diagnostic and therapeutic challenge. A report on 407 consecutive cases. *Graefes Arch Clin Exp Ophthalmol* 1991; 229:224–227.

40. Seal DV, McGill JI, Jacobs P, et al. Microbial and immunological investigations of chronic non-ulcerative blepharitis and meibomianitis. *Br J Ophthalmol* 1985;69:604–611.

41. Mondino BJ, Caster AI, Dethlefs B. A rabbit model of staphylococcal blepharitis. *Arch Ophthalmol* 1987;105:409–412.

42. Bowman RW, Dougherty JM, McCulley JP. Chronic blepharitis and dry eyes. Int Ophthalmol Clin 1987;27:27–35.

43. Lemp MA, Mahmood MA, Weiler HH. Association of rosacea and keratoconjunctivitis sicca. *Arch Ophthalmol* 1984;102: 556–557.

44. Gilbard PG, Rossi SR, Gray-Heyda K. Tear film and ocular surface changes after closure of the meibomian gland orifices in the rabbit. *Ophthalmology* 1989;96:1180–1186.

45. Harrison DA, Lawlor D. Experiences treating patients for blepharitis. *Arch Ophthalmol* 1998;116:1133–1134.

46. Goto E, Monden Y, Takano Y, et al. Treatment of non-inflamed obstructive meibomian gland dysfunction by an infrared warm compression device. *Br J Ophthalmol* 2002;86:1403–1407.

47. Leibowitz HM, Capino D. Treatment of chronic blepharitis. *Arch Ophthalmol* 1988;106:720.

48. Shine WE, McCulley JP. Meibomian gland in chronic blepharitis. *Adv Exp Med Biol* 1998;438:319–326.

49. Dougherty JM, McCulley JP, Silvaney RE, et al. The role of tetracycline in chronic blepharitis: inhibition of lipase activity in Staphylococci. *Invest Ophthalmol Vis Sci* 1991;32: 2970–2975.

50. Frucht-Perry J, Sagi E, Hemo I, et al. Efficacy of doxycycline and tetracycline in ocular rosacea. *Am J Ophthalmol* 1993;116: 88–92.

51. Lahners W, Palay D, Jones DC. Treatment of posterior blepharitis with essential fatty acids. ARVO abstracts. *Invest Ophthalmol Vis Sci* 1999;40:S541.

RECURRENT EROSION SYNDROME

ERIK LETKO AND C. STEPHEN FOSTER

Recurrent erosion syndrome (RES) is a corneal disorder characterized by recurrences of epithelial erosions that are typically associated with ocular pain, redness, watering, and photophobia. A set of symptoms consistent with RES was first described by Hansen (1) in 1872, who referred to the disorder as "intermittent neuralgic vesicular keratitis" Von Szily (2) described the principal features of RES in 1900. Paul Chandler (3), of the Massachusetts Eye and Ear Infirmary, and glaucoma fame, divided the syndrome into a macroform and a microform in 1945, with the macroform being associated more frequently with trauma. Later observations confirmed that the two forms can occur simultaneously and that there is no sharp distinction between the two (4).

ETIOLOGY

RES can be associated with trauma or anterior corneal dystrophies, including epithelial [Franceschetti type, epithelial rosette dystrophy, map, dot, fingerprint (Cogan's) dystrophy], basement membrane (Meesman's dystrophy, Reis-Bückler's dystrophy), and stromal (lattice, granular, and macular) dystrophies. RES provoked by trauma is also referred to as macroform RES, whereas spontaneous RES, more likely to be associated with a corneal dystrophy, is referred to as microform (4). The likelihood of recurrence of symptoms in patients with trauma induced RES was estimated to be 1:150 (5,6,7). Severity, frequency, and length of recurrences of corneal erosions varies widely. The symptoms may last from 1 to 4 hours in case of microform RES and from 1 to 21 days in case of macroform RES (4).

The exact etiology and pathogenesis of RES are not well understood, but several structural, biochemical, and functional abnormalities have been reported. The ultrastructural changes associated with RES include abnormal basal epithelial cell layer, abnormal epithelial basement membrane, absent or abnormal hemidesmosomes, and loss of anchoring fibrils (4,6,7). Binucleated cells and multinucleated giant cells have been found in the corneal epithelium (10). Tonofibrils, prominent in the abnormal epithelial cells, are probably responsible for forming these binucleated cells (8). Interestingly, all layers of the epithelium in patients with RES are infiltrated with neutrophils (8). Proteases released from lysozymes of these neutrophils are responsible for proteolytic degradation of the underlying basement membrane (9) and stroma (3). Additionally, matrix metalloproteinase-9, a collagenase produced by neutrophils as well as by corneal epithelial cells and macrophages (10), is overexpressed and is involved in degradation of the epithelial basement membrane (10,11).

Confocal microscopy in patients with RES associated with anterior membrane dystrophies discloses a spectrum of structural changes in the basal epithelium, basement membrane, Bowman's layer, anterior stroma, and corneal neurons (12,13). Whether these structural changes represent an abnormal matrix as a consequence of upregulated matrix metalloproteinase activity remains unclear (14). Interestingly, these abnormalities can be found on confocal microscopy even in eyes that do not present signs of anterior corneal dystrophy on slit-lamp examination (12).

In case of trauma, the initial injury causing corneal abrasion is commonly a slicing type injury, caused by a fingernail, edge of a paper, tree branch, or bush. The severity of the trauma is usually minor (15,16). Corneal injuries induced by fingernail are particularly at high risk of progressing to RES (4). It is noteworthy that the older ophthalmology literature refers to RES as "fingernail keratitis" (17). Injuries with paper, fingernails, or plant materials were estimated to be five times more likely to induce RES than injuries with harder and sharper objects such as metal, glass, or rock (18). On the other hand, corneal trauma involving penetration into deeper stroma is less likely to induce RES (19,20).

Following the injury, the corneal epithelial defect is filled rapidly by epithelial cells sliding from adjacent epithelial basal layers onto the surface of the epithelial defect. After the epithelial defect is completely covered with one layer of epithelium, the epithelial cells begin mitosis and production of suprabasal epithelial cell layers (21). Sliding of basal epithelial cells can occur over either preexisting basement membrane or bare stromal collagen (22). If the basement membrane remains intact after trauma, the new epithelial cell layer becomes firmly adherent within a week (22). However, if the injury involves removal of basement membrane, the strength of epithelial adherence can be altered for more than 2 months (22).

Patients with RES typically have a basement membrane problem (21). The absence of hemidesmosomes (and in some cases the absence of entire thickness of basement membrane) are the main electron microscopic characteristics of RES. Thinning and splitting of basement membrane can also be present (26,27). Collagen VII, another component of basement membrane, is one of the major components of the epithelial anchoring system (23,24). Not surprisingly, patients with epidermolysis bullosa, a mucocutaneous autoimmune disease characterized by autoantibodies to collagen VII, can develop RES (25).

An abnormally flat basal epithelial cell layer suggests that the epithelial cells may be responsible for abnormal production of and attachment to the basement membrane (21). The presence of a high number of mitochondria with abnormal shape in the basal epithelial cells, seen on electron microscopy as intracellular vacuoles, suggests an abnormal metabolic activity in these cells and supports the idea of the pathogenic role of basal epithelium in RES (21,22).

The epithelial defect in patients with RES is covered with epithelial cells within 1 to 3 days after injury, uneventfully, but several weeks later the attachment of the basal epithelial cell layer becomes loose. The loosely attached epithelium in this area can cause clinical symptoms, generally worse in the morning, upon awakening, with sudden pain, photophobia, and tearing. Alternatively, the tearing away of the epithelium may occur at the moment of transition from deep sleep to rapid-eye-movement (REM) sleep, with resultant pain that awakens the patient.

The appearance of the cornea on slit-lamp examination between the episodes of clinical symptoms may be normal. Sometimes, however, various degree of epithelial or subepithelial edema, located in the area of former erosion, may be seen during the asymptomatic intervals. This edema may be subtle (minimal bedewing) (21), discernible only with retroillumination. Alternatively, a fine linear subepithelial opacity in a shape of fine bubbles or a distinct subepithelial bulla may be visible (21).

TREATMENT

Although the therapy of RES is palliative rather than curative, it should be emphasized to the patient that although the disease and therapy may represent a considerable annoyance, it is typically not vision threatening (31). A spectrum of therapeutic interventions has been described for RES (Table 31-1), and some of these are widely accepted today. Typically, a stepladder approach, beginning

TABLE 31-1. SPECTRUM OF THERAPEUTIC INTERVENTIONS FOR RECURRENT EROSION SYNDROME

Intervention
Conservative
Topical
Hyperosmotic agents
Steroids
Epidermal growth factor
Fibronectin
Osmotic colloidal solutions
Digestive enzymes
Pyrimidine analogs
Bandage contact lens
Systemic
Tetracycline class antibiotics
Surgical
Chemical cauterization
Thermal cauterization
Nd:YAG laser
Superficial keratectomy
Anterior stromal puncture
Phototherapeutic keratectomy

Nd:YAG, neodymium:yttrium-aluminum-garnet.

with conservative measures and moving to invasive intervention, is followed. Adjuvant therapy added to a treatment program may provide significant benefit. For example, adding cycloplegics may offer additional relief of symptoms. And although keratoconjunctivitis sicca is not believed to be a cause of RES, it can be an important co-conspiracy factor that must be eliminated when successfully managing RES. Patients who do not respond favorably to preservative-free artificial tears may benefit from punctal occlusion (32). Simple elimination of dry eye may lead to a major improvement of RES in some cases (32). Topical steroids, another adjuvant to RES therapy, can be used to suppress the inflammatory component and reduce the epithelial infiltration with neutrophils (29). Systemic tetracycline antibiotic therapy and lid hygiene are indicated in patients with RES who also have meibomian gland dysfunction (29). In fact, meibomian gland dysfunction has been identified as a common disorder associated with RES (28,29). According to one report, 83% of patients with RES recalcitrant to conservative treatment had documented meibomian gland dysfunction, and 73% had acne rosacea (28). Most of these patients had the corneal abnormality located to the inferior and middle thirds of the cornea (28,30). A relationship of RES to menstruation further supports the role of meibomian gland dysfunction (4,30), because sex hormones have been shown to participate in regulation of sebaceous gland secretion (31).

Application of antibiotic ophthalmic ointment and pressure patching the eye, followed by daily application of a lubricant at bedtime, is generally considered the first step in treatment of RES (30,33). Relief of symptoms was reported in 90% of patients with RES treated with hypertonic saline ophthalmic ointment (34). However, according to one randomized prospective trial, there was no difference in success rate when ophthalmic lubricant or hypertonic saline ointment was used at bedtime after the initial epithelial defect healed in 117 patients with or without corneal abnormalities on slit-lamp examination (33). Forty-five percent of the patients became symptom free, and 50% improved but continued to have mild symptoms regardless of medication used at bedtime (33). A follow-up study performed 4 years later on this cohort of patients showed that 59% of them were symptomatic, and most of them (91%) experienced pain upon awakening (35). Patients with epithelial basement membrane dystrophy were more likely to have symptoms 4 years after the initial treatment, but the severity and frequency of their symptoms did not differ from those in patients without a history of epithelial basement membrane dystrophy.

Bandage contact lens application is generally the next step in treatment of RES for patients who fail to favorably respond to ophthalmic lubricants (31). The efficacy of bandage contact lens wear is reported to be higher in patients with visible anterior membrane dystrophies and spontaneous RES than in patients with posttraumatic RES (31). An arbitrary minimum length of 6 weeks of bandage contact lens wear was established as necessary for full regeneration of the basement membrane (22). Some individuals need to wear a bandage contact lens for as long as 18 months (31).

The invasive steps in treatment of recalcitrant RES include superficial keratectomy (17,36), anterior stromal puncture (17), microdiathermy (48), neodymium:yttrium-aluminum-garnet (Nd:YAG) keratectomy (36), and phototherapeutic keratectomy (PTK) with excimer laser (14,38,39). Unlike conservative methods, the invasive methods either alter or remove the abnormal epithelial basement membrane (45).

The success rate of stromal micropuncture for RES has been reported to be 80% (15,37). This technique is recommended particularly for patients with a localized rather than diffuse RES with or without epithelial basement membrane dystrophy (34). Some suggest employing stromal puncture earlier in the stepladder, prior to prolonged wear of bandage contact lens (40). The mechanisms by which stromal puncture works remain unknown. Some speculate that corneal epithelium invades and persists within the punctures of Bowman's membrane, creating firm epithelial anchors to the irregular lip of the stromal puncture (40). Histopathologic studies have shown that these "corneal epithelial plugs" persist in the anterior stroma for extended periods (41–44). This could explain the low likelihood of developing RES after radial keratectomy or other cornea trauma involving stroma.

The anterior stromal puncture is a relatively simple procedure that is generally performed at the slit lamp. A 20- to 27-gauge needle is used to create multiple anterior stromal punctures to a depth of no greater than 50% in the area of corneal abnormality through the loosely attached epithelium. The punctures should be spread 0.5 to 1.0 mm apart to minimize any effect on vision. Breaching Bowman's layer and the anterior stroma appears to be all that is mechanically required for anterior stromal puncture to initiate a successful healing of RES (41). Although some suggest that stromal puncture in the visual axis should be avoided, producing shallow punctures appears not to lead to visually significant scarring (41). The angle of attack between the needle and surface of the cornea should be perpendicular. Following the treatment a pressure patch is applied for 1 to 4 days (42). Patients who do not respond favorably to the first stromal puncture procedure may benefit from repeated stromal puncture extended to the area on the outside edge of the fluorescein staining (41). Stromal puncture has an excellent safety record. Only two cases of corneal perforation during stromal puncture have been reported (45). Paying attention to minimal invasion of the anterior stroma and use of a bent needle may prevent this rare complication (41).

Results of several studies employing PTK for RES have been reported. PTK is superior to surgical keratectomy for its precision and simplicity. The efficacy of PTK for RES seems to be at least equal to other methods. The reported success rate varies between 68% and 86% (49–55). According to one study as few as 13.8% of patients treated with PTK for RES had recurrence of corneal erosions during 1 year follow-up. All of these recurrences occurred within 6 months after PTK (47). The high success rate in this study suggests that PTK may be superior treatment for RES. Although the success rate of PTK for RES is comparable to conservative treatment and anterior stromal puncture, the fact that cases refractory to these therapeutic interventions were successfully treated with PTK (47,53,54) suggests that PTK may be superior to other treatments. The mechanisms by which PTK works in patients with RES remains unknown. Some speculate that removal of the anterior stroma by PTK eliminates abnormal extracellular matrix (56,57) and may strengthen the adhesion of basal epithelial cells to the underlying tissue by anchoring fibrils and hemidesmosomes (55,56).

Because of the diffuse nature of the abnormalities in epithelial basement membrane dystrophy, debridement of the entire corneal epithelium and treatment of the 7 to 9 mm central corneal epithelial defect with 50 to 75 pulses of excimer laser PTK is recommended (46). Despite the relatively large area of treatment and high number of pulses, best corrected visual acuity is generally preserved (46). The likelihood of inducing hyperopia, a major potential complication of phototherapeutic keratectomy (46,53,54), may be further reduced by decreasing the number of treatment pulses. Some suggest applying 50 or fewer treatment pulses in order to reduce the amount of induced hyperopia (46).

As few as 15 to 30 pulses are reported to be sufficient for localized phototherapeutic keratectomy (46,50). Bandage contact lens and a combination of topical antibiotics, steroids, and nonsteroidal antiinflammatory drugs is recommended in the postoperative period. Patients in whom symptoms of RES recur after initial PTK can be re-treated (57). PTK has an excellent safety record. A mild corneal haze that did not interfere with visual acuity was reported in two patients with RES treated by PTK (46). Interestingly, RES induced by laser *in situ* keratomileusis (LASIK) and photorefractive keratectomy (PRK) has also been reported. Such cases were reported in individuals who had no evidence of corneal dystrophies on preoperative slit-lamp biomicroscopy (5). A higher likelihood of developing RES and increased severity was associated with PRK rather than LASIK (7), particularly in patients diagnosed with dry eyes.

CONCLUSION

RES is a disorder that typically leads to significant discomfort of the affected individual. The natural course of RES is associated with recurrences of clinical symptoms that require repeated therapeutic interventions over the patient's life. However, despite the recurrences and repeated treatment, the visual acuity is preserved in the vast majority of patients. A spectrum of treatment methods with relatively high success rate is available. These vary in complexity and availability. Even though the safety and efficacy of these methods are well established, none of them treats the underlying etiology of RES.

The surgical interventions for RES may provide a higher success rate than conservative methods, but it is obvious that they do not represent a definitive answer to the issue of RES therapy.

REFERENCES

1. Hansen E. Om den intermittirende keratitis vesiculosa neuralgica af traumatisk oprindelse. *Hospitals-Tidende* 1872;15:201–203.
2. Von Szily. Ueber disjunction des Hornhautepithels. *Arch F Ophthalmol* 1900;51:486.
3. Chandler PA. Recurrent erosion of the cornea. *Am J Ophthalmol* 1945;28:355–363.
4. Brown N, Bron A. Recurrent erosion of the cornea. *Br J Ophthalmol* 1976;60:84–96.
5. Ti SE, Tan DTH. Recurrent corneal erosion after laser in situ keratomileusis. *Cornea* 2001;20:156–158.
6. Tripathi RC, Bron AJ. Ultrastructural study of non-traumatic recurrent erosion. *Br J Ophthalmol* 1972;56:73–85.
7. Goldman JN, Dohlman CH, Kravitt BA. The basement membrane of the human cornea in recurrent epithelial erosion syndrome. *Trans Am Acad Ophthalmol Otolaryngol* 1969;73:471–481.
8. Aitken DA, Beirouty ZA, Lee WR. Ultrastructural study of the corneal epithelium in the recurrent erosion syndrome. *Br J Ophthalmol* 1995;79:282–289.
9. Sugrue SP, Hay ED. The identification of extracellular matric (ECM) binding sites on the basal surface of embryonic corneal epithelium and the effect of ECM binding on epithelial collagen production. *J Cell Biol* 1986;102:1907–1916.
10. Matsubara M, Girard MT, Kublin CL, et al. Differential roles for two gelatinolytic enzymes of the matrix metalloproteinase family in the remodeling cornea. *Dev Biol* 1991;147:425–439.
11. Fini ME, Girard MT. Expression of collagenolytic/gelatinolytic metalloproteinases by normal cornea. *Invest Ophthalmol Vis Sci* 1990;31:1779–1788.
12. Rosenberg ME, Tervo TMT, Petroll WM, et al. In vivo confocal microscopy of patients with recurrent erosion syndrome or epithelial basement membrane dystrophy. *Ophthalmology* 2000;107:565–573.
13. Hernández-Quintela E, Mayer F, Dighiero P, et al. Confocal microscopy of cystic disorders of the corneal epithelium. *Ophthalmology* 1998;105:631–636.
14. Öhman L, Fogerholm P, Tengroth B. Treatment of recurrent corneal erosions with excimer laser. *Acta Ophthalmol* 1994;72:461–463.
15. McLean EN, MacRae SM, Rich LF. Recurrent erosion: treatment by anterior stromal puncture. *Ophthalmology* 1986;93:784–788.
16. Dohlman CN. Healing problems in the corneal epithelium. *Jpn J Ophthalmol* 1981;25:131–144.
17. Thygeson P. Observations on recurrent erosion of the cornea. *Am J Ophthalmol* 1959;47:48–52.
18. Weene LE. Recurrent corneal erosion after trauma: A statistical study. *Ann Ophthalmol* 1985;17:521.
19. Marmer RH. Radial keratotomy complications. *Ann Ophthalmol* 1987;19:409–411.
20. Nelson JD, Williams P, Lindstrom RL, et al. Map-fingerprint-dot changes in the corneal epithelial basement membrane following radial keratotomy. *Ophthalmology* 1985;92:199–205.
21. Goldman JN, Dohlman CH, Kravitt BA. The basement membrane of the human cornea in recurrent epithelial erosion syndrome. *Trans Am Acad Ophthalmol Otolaryngol* 1969;73:471–481.
22. Khodadoust AA, Silverstein AM, Kenyon KR, et al. Adhesion of regenerating corneal epithelium. *Am J Ophthalmol* 1968;65:339–348.
23. Keene DR, Sakai LY, Lunstrum GP, et al. Type VII collagen forms an extended network of anchoring fibrils. *J Cell Biol* 1987;104:611–621.
24. Gipson IK, Spurr-Michaud SJ, Tisdale AS. Anchoring fibrils form a complex network in human and rabbit cornea. *Invest Ophthalmol Vis Sci* 1987;28:212–220.
25. Woodley DT, Burgeson RE, Lunstrum G, et al. Epidermolysis bullosa acquisita antigen is the globular carboxyl terminus of type VII procollagen. *J Clin Invest* 1988;81:683–687.
26. Jakus MA. Further observations on the fine structure of the cornea. *Invest Ophthalmol* 1962;1:202–225.
27. Kayes J, Holmberg A. The fine structure of Bowman's layer and the basement membrane of the corneal epithelium. *Am J Ophthalmol* 1960;50:1013–1021.
28. Hope-Ross MW, Chell PB, Kervick GN, et al. Recurrent corneal erosion: clinical features. *Eye* 1994;373–377.
29. Hope-Ross MW, Chell PB, Kervick GN, et al. Oral tetracycline in the treatment of recurrent corneal erosions. *Eye* 1994;8:384–388.
30. William R, Buckley RJ. Pathogenesis and treatment of recurrent erosion. *Br J Ophthalmol* 1985;69:435–437.
31. Langston RHS, Machamer CJ, Norman CW. Soft lens therapy for recurrent erosion syndrome. *Ann Ophthalmol* 1978;?:875–878.
32. Tai MC, Cosar CB, Cohen EJ, et al. The clinical efficacy of silicone punctual plug therapy. *Cornea* 2002;21:135–139.

33. Hykin PG, Foss AE, Pavesio C, et al. The natural history and management of recurrent corneal erosion: a prospective randomized trial. *Eye* 1994;8:35–40.

34. Kenyon KR, Wagoner MD. Therapy of recurrent erosion and persistent defects of the corneal epithelium. In: American Academy of Ophthalmology. *Focal points,* vol 9, module 9 (section 3 of 3). San Francisco: AAO, 1991.

35. Heyworth P, Morlet N, Rayner S, et al. Natural history of recurrent erosion syndrome—a 4 year review of 117 patients. *Br J Ophthalmol* 1998;82:26–28.

36. Buxton JN, Fox ML. Superficial epithelial keratectomy in the treatment of epithelial basement membrane dystrophy. *Arch Ophthalmol* 1983;101:392–463.

37. Geggel HS. Successful treatment of recurrent corneal erosion with Nd:Yag anterior stromal puncture. *Am J Ophthalmol* 1990;110:404–407.

38. Fagerholm P, Fitzsimmons TD, Örndahl M, et al. Phototherapeutic keratectomy: Long-term results in 166 eyes. *Refract Corneal Surg Suppl* 1993;9:76–81.

39. Bernauer W, De Cock R, Dart JKG. Phototherapeutic keratectomy in recurrent corneal erosions refractory to other forms of treatment. *Eye* 1996;10:561–564.

40. Rubinfeld RS, Laibson PR, Cohen EJ, et al. Anterior stromal puncture for recurrent erosion: further experience and new instrumentation. *Ophthalmic Surg* 1990;21:318–326.

41. Stainer GA, Shaw EL, Binder PS, et al. Histopathology of a case of radial keratotomy. *Arch Ophthalmol* 1982;100:1473–1477.

42. Deg JK, Zavala EY, Binder PS. Delayed corneal wound healing following radial keratotomy. *Ophthalmology* 1985;92:734–740.

43. Binder PS, Nayak SK, Deg JK, et al. An ultrastructural and histochemical study of long-term wound healing after radial keratotomy. *Am J Ophthalmol* 1987;103:432–440.

44. Binder PS, Waring GO III, Arrowsmith PN, et al. Histopathology of traumatic corneal rupture after radial keratotomy. *Arch Ophthalmol* 1988;106:1584–1590.

45. Wood TO. Recurrent erosion. Presented at 14th Annual Meeting of the Castroviejo Corneal Society, Las Vegas, 1988.

46. Cavanaugh TB, Lind DM, Cutarelli PE, et al. Phototherapeutic keratectomy for recurrent erosion syndrome in anterior basement membrane dystrophy. *Ophthalmology* 1999;106:971–976.

47. Öhman L, Fagerholm P. The influence of excimer laser ablation on RCE: a prospective randomized study. *Cornea* 1998;17:349–352.

48. O'Brart DP, Muir MG, Marshall J. Phototherapeutic keratectomy for RCE. *Eye* 1994;8:378–383.

49. Morad Y, Haviv D, Zadok D, et al. Excimer laser phototherapeutic keratectomy for RCE. *J Cataract Refract Surg* 1998;24:451–455.

50. Ho CL, Tan DTH, Chan WK. Excimer laser PTK for RCE. *Ann Acad Med Singapore* 1999;28:787–790.

51. Jain S, Austin D. PTK for treatment of RCE. *J Cataract Refract Surg* 1999;25:1610–1614.

52. Kremer I, Blumenthal M. Combined PRK and PTK in myopic patients with RCE. *Br J Ophthalmol* 1997;81:551–554.

53. Algawi K, Goggin M, O'Keefe M. 193 mm excimer laser phototherapeutic keratectomy for recurrent corneal erosions. *Eur J Implant Refract Surg* 1995;7:11–13.

54. Dausch D, Landesz M, Klein R, et al. Phototherapeutic keratectomy in recurrent corneal epithelial erosion. *Refract Corneal Surg* 1993;9:419–424.

55. Wu WCS, Stark WJ, Green WR. Corneal wound healing after 193 mm excimer laser keratectomy. *Arch Ophthalmol* 1991;109:1426–1432.

56. SunderRaj N, Geiss M, Fantes F, et al. Healing of excimer laser ablated monkey corneas: an immunohistochemical evaluation. *Arch Ophthalmol* 1990;108:1604–1610.

57. Maini R, Loughnan MS. Phototherapeutic keratectomy retreatment for recurrent corneal erosion syndrome. *Br J Ophthalmol* 2002;86:270–272.

SUPERIOR LIMBIC KERATOCONJUNCTIVITIS

THANH HOANG-XUAN

Superior limbic keratoconjunctivitis (SLK) is characterized by chronic inflammation of the ocular surface, which can be easily overlooked (still too often the case) if one does not carefully examine the eye while keeping in mind the clinical suspicion of the possibility of SLK. The patient may then continue to suffer highly incapacitating symptoms unnecessarily (effective treatments are available) and be exposed to inappropriate drug therapy with its attendant adverse effects. The etiopathogenesis of SLK is unclear.

The initial description is attributed to Frederick Theodore (1), who in 1961 reported the first cases of an entity that, in 1963 (2), he named superior limbic kerato-conjunctivitis. His 11 patients had chronically recurrent lesions of the superior bulbar and palpebral conjunctivas and adjacent cornea, taking the form of superficial punctuate keratitis, which often was complicated by filamentary keratitis (2). A similar form of keratitis had in fact been described 8 years earlier by Braley and Alexander (3). At first, SLK and Thygeson's keratitis were considered to be different forms of the same entity (4,5), but Theodore subsequently completed the description of SLK on the basis of new cases (6,7).

EPIDEMIOLOGY

Although SLK can occur in both sexes and at all ages, it is most frequent in the middle-aged and in women, the latter accounting for 70% of cases (8). All cases reported so far have been sporadic, with the exception of affected twins (9). SLK is usually bilateral (70% of cases), but can be asymmetrical. Hyperthyroidism is found in 20% to 50% of patients with SLK (2,8,10–15).

CLINICAL ASPECTS

The diagnosis of SLK is often overlooked and thus delayed, yet the signs are highly evocative if one simply remembers to look for them. SLK is generally missed because the symptoms are often nonspecific and the nearly pathognomonic ocular lesions are hidden by the upper eyelid. The natural course of SLK is chronic, remitting/relapsing, and lasting many years; exacerbations are followed by increasingly lengthy remissions, and spontaneous recovery is the rule (2,6). Although SLK has a good visual prognosis (the central cornea is spared), the symptoms during exacerbations are too incapacitating to allow patients to wait, untreated, for spontaneous recovery.

The lack of specific ocular symptoms explains the frequent delay in diagnosis. The ocular manifestations generally consist of discomfort, foreign-body sensation, burning sensation, and photophobia. The intensity of symptoms is highly variable. Dry-eye syndrome and meibomian gland dysfunction are usually suspected. SLK should be suspected when the patient presents with superior bulbar conjunctival hyperemia that mainly affects the limbus and the adjacent bulbar conjunctiva. Blepharospasm and pseudoptosis can be found in severe cases with filamentous keratitis, in which mucous discharge is generally present.

The ocular lesions are remarkable since they are limited to the upper part of the eye. Typically, one finds moderate papillary hyperplasia of the superior tarsal conjunctiva (Fig. 32-1) and hyperemia of the superior bulbar conjunctiva, generally forming a large vertical band. The bulbar conjunctiva may appear corrugated, and it is excessively mobile as one rubs the globe through the upper lid; the redness fades gradually in intensity from the limbus to the superior bulbar conjunctiva, which appears thickened and redundant (Fig. 32-2). Raber (16) reported scarring of the palpebral conjunctiva in three patients. However, the eye can have a near-normal aspect in some cases. One major diagnostic feature of SLK is the uptake of fluorescein, rose bengal, or lissamine green dye by the superior limbal conjunctiva and the upper part of the cornea in a highly characteristic way, confined to a rectangular or trapezoidal area of the bulbar conjunctiva in a punctate pattern. There is usually a superior corneal micropannus associated with the epithelial keratitis. Severe forms are associated with corneal filaments in one-third to one-half of cases (Fig. 32-3)

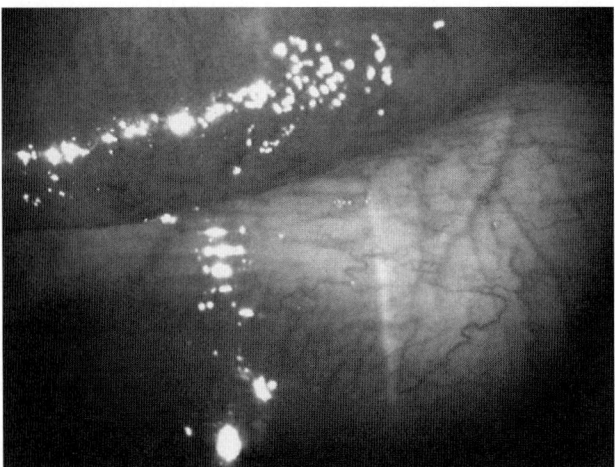

FIGURE 32-1. On instilling a drop of lissamine green in superior limbic keratoconjunctivitis, papillary hypertrophy of the superior tarsal conjunctiva is better seen, as well as the horizontal folds of the superior bulbar conjunctiva due to the poor adherence of the latter to the sclera. Also note the lucid appearance of the edematous superior limbal conjunctiva.

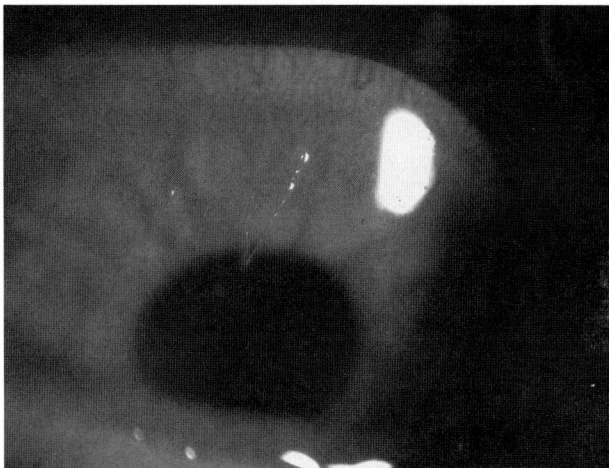

FIGURE 32-3. Filaments at the upper cornea in superior limbic keratoconjunctivitis.

(6,8,17). About one-quarter of patients have lacrimal deficiency (Schirmer's test) (8). One generally obvious feature is the lack of adherence between the superior bulbar conjunctiva and the sclera. This sign can be found by mobilizing the bulbar conjunctiva on the eyeball, either directly with a Merocel sponge after instilling an anesthetic eye drop, or indirectly with the finger through the upper eyelid (Figs. 32-1 and 32-4). This reveals conjunctival folds, parallel to the limbus, forming a sort of conjunctivochalasis. Some authors have also described concomitant inferior conjunctivochalasis (18).

PATHOLOGY

Histologic and ultrastructural examination of the conjunctiva shows squamous metaplasia of the superior bulbar conjunctival

epithelium, with a loss of goblet cells and acanthotic degeneration of epithelial cells (8,19–21). The latter have a condensed nuclear chromatin whose appearance on impression cytology is highly characteristic ("snake-like" chromatin) (22), together with cytoplasmic glycogen overload (21). The conjunctival stroma, which is edematous and contains abundant dilated lymphatics, is moderately infiltrated by inflammatory cells (23). Ultrastructurally, epithelial cells from the bulbar conjunctiva contain secondary intracytoplasmic lysosomes, keratohyalin granules, and increased numbers of condensed microfilaments that strangle the nucleus, conferring a polylobar or polynuclear aspect (21,23,24). In contrast, the palpebral conjunctiva is rich in goblet cells and its epithelium is normal. Its chorion contains abundant inflammatory cells (neutrophils, lymphocytes, and plasma cells) (15).

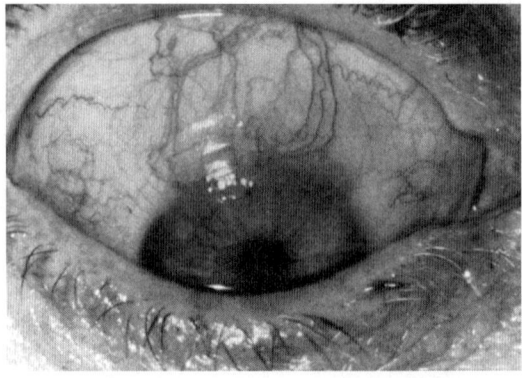

FIGURE 32-2. Hyperemia and thickening of the bulbar conjunctiva at the upper limbus in superior limbic keratoconjunctivitis.

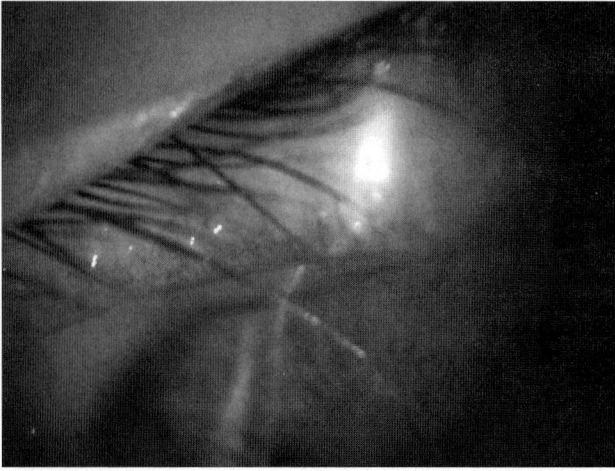

FIGURE 32-4. Downward pressure with the finger on the upper eyelid induces a conjunctival fold at the limbus due to loose adherence of the upper bulbar conjunctiva to the sclera.

DIFFERENTIAL DIAGNOSIS

Symptoms in patients with forms in which filamentary keratitis is absent can resemble those of miscellaneous disorders such as chlamydial conjunctivitis, Thygeson's superficial punctate keratitis, the limbal form of vernal keratoconjunctivitis, and phlyctenular keratoconjunctivitis. In contrast, there are almost no differential diagnoses when all the characteristic signs of SLK are present. Of note, a case of sebaceous carcinoma extending to the superior bulbar conjunctival epithelium and masquerading as SLK has been reported (25). In fact, only early-stage contact lens–induced keratoconjunctivitis resembles SLK, but filaments are extremely rare in the former condition. In advanced forms, contact lens–induced keratoconjunctivitis differs from SLK by its more severe epithelial keratitis, its more diffuse and severe conjunctival inflammation, and the decreased vision (26). Bloomfield and associates (20) reported a case of bilateral vascularized stromal opacification with pannus formation, necessitating keratoplasty (the patient refused to stop using her contact lenses). Generally, contact lens withdrawal leads to recovery (26–28). Contact lens–induced keratoconjunctivitis is attributed by some authors to an allergic hypersensitivity reaction to lipoprotein deposits on the lens or to the preservatives—especially thimerosal—contained in the contact lens care solutions (26). Fuerst et al. (27) reported finding no cases of hypersensitivity to preservatives in their patients with contact lens–induced keratoconjunctivitis. According to Carpel (29), contact lens–induced keratoconjunctivitis is due to the mechanical effect of the lens rubbing on the superior bulbar conjunctiva and cornea.

When filamentary keratitis is present, the main alternative diagnosis to SLK is keratoconjunctivitis sicca, in which filaments tend to predominate in the lower part of the cornea.

PATHOGENESIS

The etiopathogenesis of SLK is unknown. No culprit infectious agent has yet been found, either by culture or by histologic or ultrastructural examination (4,11,19,23,30). Some authors suspect an immunologic mechanism (13), but the sparse inflammatory component in conjunctival biopsy specimens, together with the absence of serologic and tear immunologic markers, and the poor therapeutic response to topical corticosteroids, all argue against this hypothesis (15,31). Another frequently incriminated cause is the dry-eye syndrome. Theodore (2) noted in his first published series that half his patients had tear deficiency. Yang et al. (32) also incriminated local ocular dryness, suggesting that it caused excessive friction between the upper bulbar and palpebral conjunctivas, leading to irritation and altered metabolic exchanges. However, other authors reported ocular dryness in only 25% of patients (8,15). In Wright's (15) hypothesis, chronic inflammation of the superior palpebral conjunctiva leads to defective maturation of its bulbar counterpart, thereby causing keratoconjunctivitis. Matsuda et al. (33) showed altered expression of cytokeratins in SLK, suggesting an abnormality of differentiation in the conjunctival epithelium. But some authors, including Donshik et al. (23), consider that the bulbar conjunctiva is the site from which the condition initially arises. An allergic stimulus has also been incriminated (34), a possibility supported by reports of an improvement in signs and symptoms on local antiallergic treatments (35–37).

The mechanical theory is currently most popular (38), and it explains the association of SLK with thyroid ophthalmopathy. Exophthalmos associated with thyroid diseases leads to inflammatory edema of the superior conjunctiva and then to laxity of the bulbar conjunctiva. Hypothyroidism has also been incriminated. A vicious circle would then occur, in which symptoms are maintained by friction between the superior bulbar and palpebral conjunctival surfaces. Tenzel was the first to forward the thyroid hypothesis, after observing serum abnormalities in his patients. The frequent association of SLK with dysthyroidism (20% to 50% of cases) (2,10–16), together with the disappearance of ocular symptoms during endocrine treatment (8,39), and the efficacy of treatments promoting adhesion of the superior bulbar conjunctiva all favor the mechanical theory. I recently examined a patient who developed bilateral SLK soon after eyelid cosmetic surgery aimed at reducing her interpalpebral aperture by stretching the external canthus. The patient, who had slightly protruded eyes, reported permanent sensation of friction of her superior eyelids on her eyeball. This case could represent iatrogenic SLK due to surgically induced mechanical rubbing between the palpebral and bulbar conjunctival surfaces.

TREATMENT

In his first reports, Theodore (2) recommended treating SLK with local applications of silver nitrate solution to the anesthetized superior palpebral conjunctiva (2). Some authors subsequently reported that a 0.5% to 1% solution could also be applied to the superior bulbar conjunctiva (8). However, this product, which acts by retracting the conjunctiva and inducing its adherence to the underlying sclera, has certain disadvantages. In particular, it must be freshly prepared and used immediately; and it must be applied with a cotton bud, avoiding any contact with the cornea (risk of tattooing by silver deposits). It is also an irritant and possibly corrosive for the cornea and necessitates abundant rinsing of the eye 2 minutes after application (2,19). Efficacy is irregular and can take some time to appear. If initial treatment fails, the application can be repeated a week later and then at variable intervals according to the frequency of symptom relapse (2,27).

Several other conservative treatments have been tried, but with very limited and inconsistent success. Antivirals, antibacterials, and corticosteroids have been tested, but with no immunohistopathologic rationale (17). Other treatments such as methylcellulose and the mucolytic agent *N*-acetylcysteine (15) have relieved symptoms in patients with SLK complicated by filamentary keratitis. Vitamin A eyedrops (retinol palmitate) were relatively effective in 10 out of 12 patients in a study by Ohashi et al. (12), for as long as it was administered. Mondino et al. (40) reported good results with pressure patching, usually followed by use of a therapeutic soft contact lens. Topical mast-cell stabilizers have also been tested with a certain degree of success; Confino and Brown (35) cured six of eight patients with cromolyn sodium, Grutzmacher et al. (36) cured three patients with 0.1% lodoxamide tromethamine solution, and Udell et al. (37) improved five patients (one durably) with ketotifen fumarate. However, the role of mast cells has never been proven in SLK, and the efficacy of these drugs remains to be explained. Some agents might act by interacting with other inflammatory cells or mediators.

In trials of therapeutic large hydrophilic soft lenses, they have been shown to alleviate the discomfort, especially in patients with filamentary keratitis. However, long-term tolerability in these latter patients is unclear, given the abundant conjunctival mucous discharge (15,40). The lens appears to act mechanically, by suppressing the friction between the superior bulbar and palpebral conjunctivas. However, these lenses can themselves induce conjunctival toxicity with clinical manifestations similar to those of SLK, and their use therefore requires close monitoring (20,26–28,41).

Treatment of dysthyroidism, and orbital decompression in severe forms, suppresses the keratoconjunctivitis (8,10,39).

Surgical alternatives can be considered if medical treatment fails, or even as a first-line approach, particularly as silver nitrate eyedrops are difficult to prepare and are highly toxic. Thermal cauterization of the inflamed superior bulbar conjunctiva, under local subconjunctival lidocaine anesthesia, can give good results. For example, Udell et al. (42) cured eight of 11 patients with this technique, of whom five had had a negative experience with silver nitrate. This surgery can lead to an improvement in squamous metaplasia of the superior conjunctiva and to an increase in goblet cell numbers, as shown by impression cytology. The mechanism of action of thermal cauterization could also involve a change in the mechanical interactions between the superior bulbar and palpebral conjunctivas. The authors, who reported ocular dryness in six of their patients, recommended punctal plugs as an adjuvant therapeutic measure in this situation. Yang et al. (32) and Katab (43) also obtained substantial symptom relief in 11 patients and one patient, respectively, after lacrimal punctal occlusion. As an alternative or an adjuvant to punctal occlusion, Goto et al. (44) recommended the instillation of 20% diluted autologous serum, obtaining improvement in nine of 11 patients.

However, the treatment that gives some of the best long-term results is resection of the superior bulbar conjunctiva: peritomy from 10 o'clock and 2 o'clock, and resection of a 5-mm large arcuate segment of conjunctiva and Tenon's capsule. Passons and Wood (11) thus cured eight of 10 patients (associated ocular dryness was implicated in the two failures). Anchoring the conjunctiva to the sclera with sutures does not seem to be beneficial (11,23). Adverse effects are very rare, consisting of pseudoptosis or scleral thinning in patients with a severe dry-eye syndrome (45). Yokoi et al. (18) cured six eyes of five patients using a surgical variant of these techniques that consisted of resecting the redundant bulbar conjunctiva, but distant from the rose bengal–stained area, and suturing the crescent conjunctival opening. In two eyes, this surgical procedure was performed together with surgery for inferior bulbar conjunctivochalasis (18).

REFERENCES

1. Theodore FH. *The Collected Letters of the International Correspondence Society of Ophthalmologists and Otolaryngologists* 1961(June 30):series 6:89.
2. Theodore FH. Superior limbic keratoconjunctivitis. *Eye Ear Nose Throat Month* 1963;42:25–28.
3. Braley AE, Alexander RC. Superficial punctate keratitis. *Arch Ophthalmol* 1953;50:147–154.
4. Thygeson P. Further observations on superficial punctate keratitis. *Arch Ophthalmol* 1961;66:158–167.
5. Thygeson P, Kimura S. Observations on chronic conjunctivitis and chronic keratoconjunctivitis. *Trans Am Acad Ophthalmol* 1963;67:494–517.
6. Theodore FH. Further observations on superior limbic keratoconjunctivitis. *Trans Am Acad Ophthalmol Otolaryngol* 1967;71:341–351.
7. Theodore FH. Superior limbic keratoconjunctivitis: a summary. *Mod Probl Ophthalmol* 1971;9:23–26.
8. Nelson JD. Superior limbic keratoconjunctivitis. *Eye* 1989;3:180–189.
9. Darrell RW. Superior limbic keratoconjunctivitis in identical twins. *Cornea* 1992;11:262–263.
10. Kadrmas EF, Bartley GB. Superior limbic keratoconjunctivitis. *Ophthalmology* 1995;102:1472–1475.
11. Passons GA, Wood TO. Conjunctival resection for superior limbic keratoconjunctivitis. *Ophthalmology* 1986;91:966–968.
12. Ohashi Y, Watanabe H, Kinoshita S. Vitamin A eye drops for superior limbic keratoconjunctivitis. *Am J Ophthalmol* 1988;105:523–527.
13. Cher I. Clinical features of superior limbic keratoconjunctivitis in Australia. *Arch Ophthalmol* 1969;82:580–586.
14. Tenzel RR. Comments on superior limbic filamentous keratoconjunctivitis. Part 2 (letter). *Arch Ophthalmol* 1968;79:508.
15. Wright P. Superior limbic keratoconjunctivitis. *Trans Ophthalmol Soc UK* 1972;92:555–560.
16. Raber IM. Superior limbic keratoconjunctivitis in association with scarring of the superior tarsal conjunctiva. *Cornea* 1996;15:12–16.

17. Theodore FH. Superior limbic keratoconjunctivitis (Theodore's SLK). In: Fraunfelder FT, Roy FH, eds. *Current ocular therapy.* Philadelphia: WB Saunders, 1980;387–388.

18. Yokoi N, Komuro A, Maruyama K, et al. New surgical treatment for superior limbic keratoconjunctivitis and its association with conjunctivochalasis. *Am J Ophthalmol* 2003;135: 303–308.

19. Theodore FH, Ferry AP. Superior limbic keratoconjunctivitis: clinical and pathologic correlations. *Arch Ophthalmol* 1970; 84:481–484.

20. Bloomfield SE, Jakobiec FA, Theodore FH. Contact lens-induced keratopathy. A severe complication extending the spectrum of keratoconjunctivitis in contact lens wearers. *Ophthalmology* 1984; 91:290–294.

21. Collin HB, Donshik PC, Foster CS. Keratinization of the superior bulbar conjunctival epithelium in superior limbic keratoconjunctivitis in humans. *Acta Ophthalmol* 1978;56:531–543.

22. Wander AH, Masukawa T. Unusual appearance of condensed chromatin in conjunctival cells in superior limbic keratoconjunctivitis. *Lancet* 1981;2:42–43.

23. Donshik PC, Collin HB, Foster CS. Conjunctival resection treatment and ultrastructural histopathology of superior limbic keratoconjunctivitis. *Am J Ophthalmol* 1978;85:101–110.

24. Collin HB, Donshik PC, Boruchoff SA, et al. The fine structure of nuclear changes in superior limbic keratoconjunctivitis. *Invest Ophthalmol Vis Sci* 1978;17:79–84.

25. Condon GP, Brownstein S, Codere F. Sebaceous carcinoma of the eyelid masquerading as superior limbic keratoconjunctivitis. *Arch Ophthalmol* 1985;103:1525–1529.

26. Sendele DD, Kenyon KR, Mobilia EF, et al. Superior limbic keratoconjunctivitis in contact lens wearers. *Ophthalmology* 1983;90: 616–622.

27. Fuerst DJ, Sugar J, Worobec S. Superior limbic keratoconjunctivitis associated with cosmetic soft contact lens wear. *Arch Ophthalmol* 1983;101:1214–1216.

28. Stenson S. Superior limbic keratoconjunctivitis associated with soft contact lens wear. *Arch Ophthalmol* 1983;101:402–404.

29. Carpel EF. Superior limbic keratoconjunctivitis. *Arch Ophthalmol* 1984;102:662–664.

30. Corwin ME. Superior limbic keratoconjunctivitis. *Am J Ophthalmol* 1968;66:338–340.

31. Eiferman RA, Wilkins EL. Immunologic aspects of superior limbic keratoconjunctivitis. *Can J Ophthalmol* 1979;14:85–87.

32. Yang HY, Fujishima H, Toda I, et al. Lacrimal punctal occlusion for the treatment of superior limbic keratoconjunctivitis. *Am J Ophthalmol* 1997;124:80–87.

33. Matsuda A, Tagawa Y, Matsuda H. Cytokeratin and proliferative cell nuclear antigen expression in superior limbic keratoconjunctivitis. *Curr Eye Res* 1996;15:1033–1038.

34. Corona R, Abraham JL. Superior limbic keratoconjunctivitis apparently related to particulate material from a ventilation system. *N Engl J Med* 1989;320:1354.

35. Confino J, Brown SI. Treatment of superior limbic keratoconjunctivitis with topical cromolyn sodium. *Am J Ophthalmol* 1987;19:129–131.

36. Grutzmacher RD, Foster RS, Feiler LS. Lodoxamide tromethamine treatment for superior limbic keratoconjunctivitis. *Am J Ophthalmol* 1995;120:400–402.

37. Udell IJ, Guidera AC, Madani-Becker J. Ketotifen fumarate treatment of superior limbic keratoconjunctivitis. *Cornea* 2002; 21:778–780.

38. Cher I. Superior limbic keratoconjunctivitis: multifactorial mechanical pathogenesis. *Clin Exp Ophthalmol* 2000;28:181–184.

39. Ostler HB. Superior limbic keratoconjunctivitis. In: Smolin G, Thoft RA, eds. *The cornea.* Boston: Little, Brown, 1987:295–298

40. Mondino BJ, Zaidman GW, Salamon SW. Use of pressure patching and soft contact lenses in superior limbic keratoconjunctivitis. *Arch Ophthalmol* 1982;100:1932–1934.

41. Wilson LA, McNatt J, Reitschel R. Delayed hypersensitivity to thimerosal in soft contact lens wearers. *Ophthalmology* 1981;88: 804–809.

42. Udell IJ, Kenyon KR, Sawa M. Treatment of superior limbic keratoconjunctivitis by thermocauterization of the superior bulbar conjunctiva. *Ophthalmology* 1986;93:162–166.

43. Kabat AG. Lacrimal occlusion therapy for the treatment of superior limbic keratoconjunctivitis. *Optom Vis Sci* 1998;75:714–718.

44. Goto E, Shimmura S, Shimazaki J, et al. Treatment of superior limbic keratoconjunctivitis by application of autologous serum. *Cornea* 2001;20:807–810.

45. Wander AH. Superior limbic keratoconjunctivitis (Theodore's SLK). In: Fraunfelder FT, Roy FH. *Current ocular therapy.* Philadelphia: WB Saunders, 1990:457–458.

LIGNEOUS CONJUNCTIVITIS

PETER C. DONSHIK, MELINDA L. RAMSBY,
AND GREGORY S. MAKOWSKI

BACKGROUND

Ligneous conjunctivitis is a rare form of chronic conjunctivitis first described in 1847 by Bouisson (1) as a case of pseudomembranous conjunctivitis. In 1933, Borel (2) described a young girl with bilateral membranous conjunctivitis and indurated eyelids. Borel was the first to use the term *ligneous* to describe the wood-like feeling of the indurated eyelids in this patient. In the last 70 years less than 150 cases have been reported. Ligneous conjunctivitis most commonly afflicts the upper eyelid, but can involve all palpebral surfaces. The course of ligneous conjunctivitis is typically one of recurrence and remission that persists for months, years, or throughout life.

EPIDEMIOLOGY

Ligneous conjunctivitis has a predilection for young children usually between the ages of 2 and 6 years but has been reported to occur as early as the first week of life (3) and as late as 85 years (4). In 119 reported cases, the average age of onset was 13.9 years whereas the median age of onset was 5 years (5). There is a female predilection (3:1), and familial cases suggest an autosomal-dominant transmission (6). In addition to the conjunctiva, ligneous lesions can involve other mucosal membranes including the mouth, nasopharynx, trachea, larynx, alveolar and tympanic membranes, vagina, cervix, and fallopian tubes (7–9). Cases also arise in association with antecedent infection, trauma, pinguecula, pterygium, cataract, and ptosis surgery (5,10–12), consistent with a role for injury in initiating the ligneous process.

CLINICAL

Ligneous conjunctivitis usually begins with an acute onset and then becomes chronic. It is unaffected by topical antibiotics or steroids. Lesions typically start with nonspecific indicators of mucosal irritation such as tearing and conjunctival hyperemia. Disease progression is characterized by the formation of friable pseudomembranes composed of loose fibrovascular tissue that is easily removed from the underlying conjunctiva but associated with profuse bleeding (Fig. 33-1). As the disease continues, a thick mass develops on top of the fibrovascular pseudomembrane and this new pseudomembrane is thick, firm, and "woody" (Fig. 33-2). These late stage lesions are tightly adherent to the underlying conjunctiva and are difficult to remove. Once removed, lesions tend to rapidly reoccur (Fig. 33-3). With continued inflammation the lid may become indurated.

The ligneous plaque can appear sessile or pedunculated, with a flat, smooth surface that is white or yellowish white in color (Fig. 33-4). The upper and lower (upper more common than lower) palpebral conjunctiva are the usual surfaces affected, but the bulbar conjunctiva can also be involved (Fig. 33-5). Although usually bilateral, the disease may present in an asymmetrical fashion with the first eye being more severely involved. The disease can progress for months or years, and approximately one third of cases undergo spontaneous regression.

Symptoms of discomfort, tearing, photophobia, and difficulty keeping the eye open can be mild or severe. Vision is usually unaffected. The chronic inflammation can cause ptosis of the lid (Fig. 33-6), and amblyopia can develop. Further, if the condition spreads to the limbus, the possibility of corneal complications such as opacification, neovascularization and perforation can arise (2). In the early stages, ligneous conjunctivitis can be confused with other pseudomembranous conjunctivitis. However, the chronic conjunctival inflammation, as well as recurrence of the pseudomembrane after removal, helps differentiate ligneous conjunctivitis from other conditions.

PATHOLOGY

Histologic examination of the ligneous pseudomembrane reveals acute and chronic fibrinous inflammation. Areas of

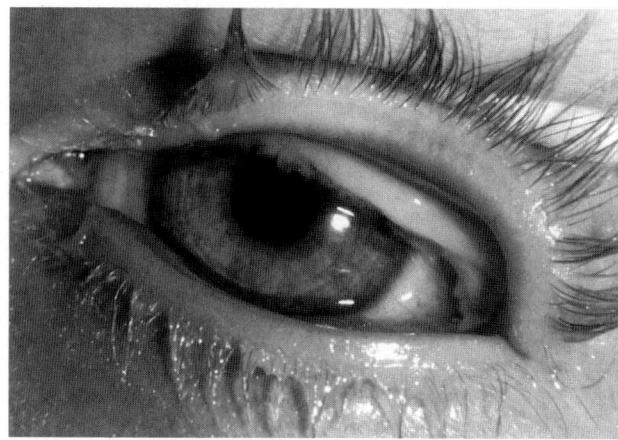

A

FIGURE 33-1. A: Thick pseudomembrane involving the upper lid in a 25-year-old woman. **B:** Everted upper lid showing the thick pseudomembrane attached to the upper tarsal surface. **C:** Removal of the pseudomembrane with associated bleeding.

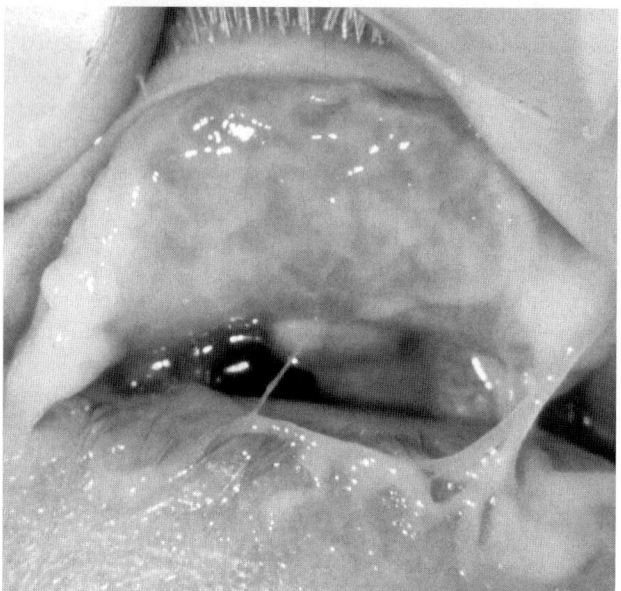

B

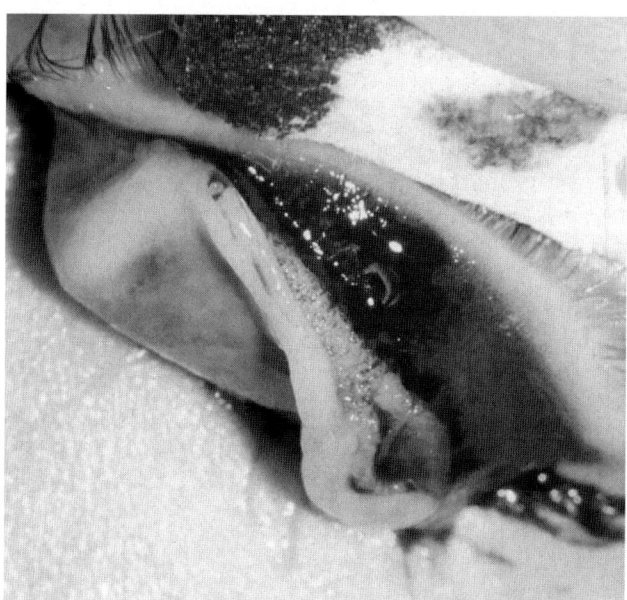

C

vascular and fibrinous organization are apparent, as are foci of granulation tissue exhibiting a variable cellular component of plasma cells, eosinophils, mast cells, lymphocytes, and neutrophils. Activated T cells and B lymphocytes have also been reported (13). Less consistent are the presence of focal epithelial degeneration, hypertrophy,

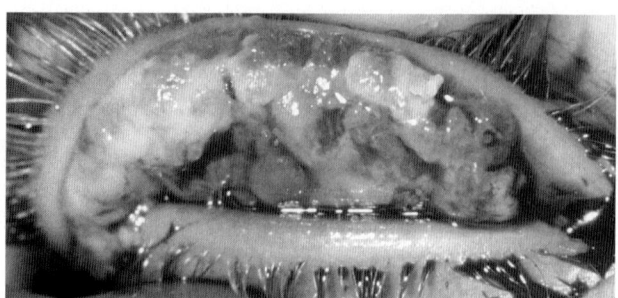

FIGURE 33-2. Thick firm woody appearance of the superior tarsal surface.

submucosa invasion, and vascular degeneration with endothelial gaps (14).

The hallmark of the ligneous lesion is the large, amorphous pools of relatively acellular, eosinophilic fibrils within the lamina propria and submucosa (Fig. 33-7). Electron microscopy of these amorphous deposits (Fig. 33-8) demonstrates tactoids of parallel filaments with cross striations and ultrastructural features characteristic of fibrin. Histochemical and immunochemical analyses reveal minor quantities of mucopolysaccharide, immunoglobulin G (IgG) and albumin (8), but unanimously confirm that fibrin is the major component of the ligneous plaque (7–9,14–16).

BIOCHEMISTRY

Biochemical analysis performed in our laboratory (17) demonstrate that the ligneous lesion is composed of mucoid and

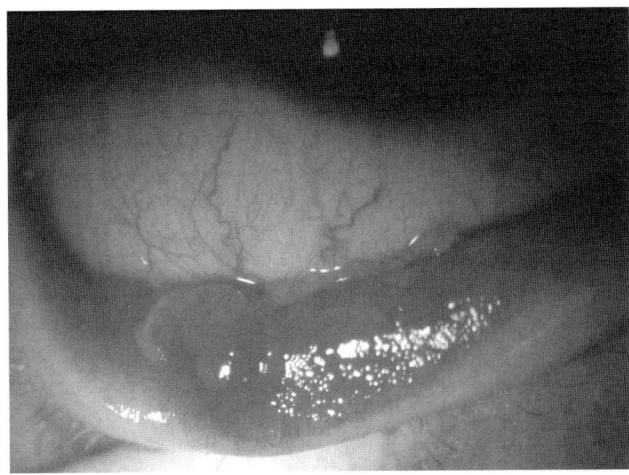

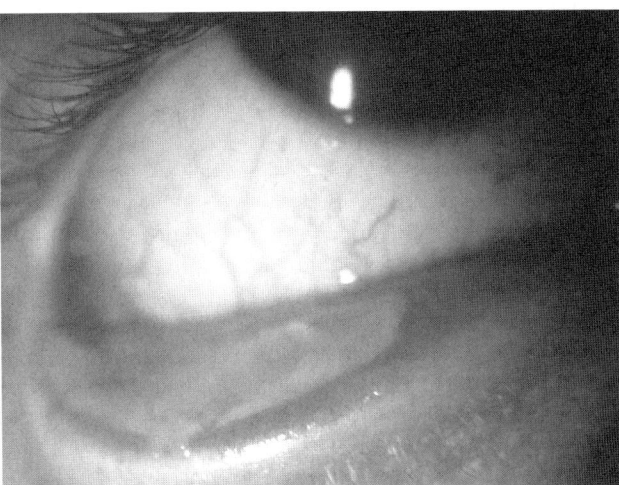

FIGURE 33-3. A: Lesion involving inferior tarsal surface before surgical removal. **B:** Recurrence of lesion 10 days after surgical removal, applications of cryotherapy, and subconjunctival injection of Decadron followed by topical treatment with α-chymotrypsin, hyaluronidase, and cromolyn.

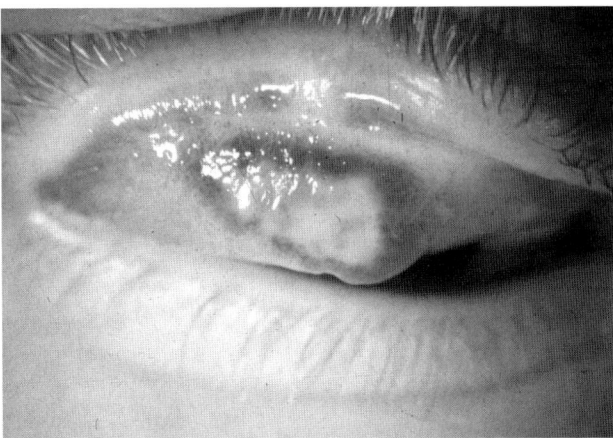

FIGURE 33-4. Pedunculated lesion with flat, smooth, whitish surface.

ligneous compartments. The mucoid fraction represents an exaggerated mucus thread and is easily harvested from the conjunctival cul-de-sac in affected eyes. The ligneous plaque is proteinaceous and not surprisingly, enriched in fibrin (Fig. 33-9): both intact β-monomers and γ-γ dimers (degradation-resistant cross-linked products of transglutaminase). The protease profile of mucoid and ligneous compartments is also distinct. Specifically, the ligneous compartment is selectively enriched in tissue plasminogen activator (tPA) (Fig. 33-10), and all three isoforms of matrix metalloproteinase-9 (MMP-9) (Fig. 33-11). In contrast, the mucoid compartment is relatively devoid of protein, and contains mostly inactive forms of MMP-9 and no tPA (Figs. 33-10 and 33-11).

MMP-9 is a neutrophil-derived type IV collagenase that degrades basement membranes; tPA is a serine protease that activates plasminogen and is the main regulator of fibrin degradation. Both MMP-9 and tPA bind fibrin and

are important for effective wound healing (18,19). The quantity of tPA in ligneous samples decreases with the depth of the lesion (17). Despite ample levels of tPA in superficial layers, fibrin degradation products are not detected. These observations are consistent with hypofibrinolysis in ligneous conjunctivitis.

ETIOLOGY

The etiology of ligneous conjunctivitis has been elusive, but with the recent developments in protein and molecular biology is beginning to be revealed. Findings of activated T cells, familial cases, and coexistence with other conditions suggest a systemic inflammatory disorder with a genetic predisposition. Onset following surgery, infection, or trauma identifies injury as a precipitating factor. The predominance of fibrin (14–17), the lack of fibrin degradation products, and the finding of engorged phagocytes (17) (Fig. 33-7) are consistent with hypofibrinolysis as a disease mechanism in ligneous conjunctivitis. Defects in fibrinolysis are well known to lead to impaired wound healing and promote formation of granulation tissue and chronic inflammation (20). Physiologically, fibrin degradation is a plasmin-dependent process regulated by tPA activation of plasminogen. Both tPA and plasminogen bind specific sites in the fibrin matrix and binding is required for efficient plasmin generation.

Evidence for defective fibrinolysis in ligneous conjunctivitis derives from a variety of case studies. Serendipitously, ligneous lesions were reported to develop in patients treated with tranexamic acid (21) and to resolve upon its removal. Tranexamic acid (ε-aminocaproic acid), a lysine analog, is a fibrinolytic inhibitor that prevents kringle domains in plasminogen from interacting with binding sites in fibrin, a step necessary for plasminogen activation by tPA (22). Further, concurrent reports found ligneous

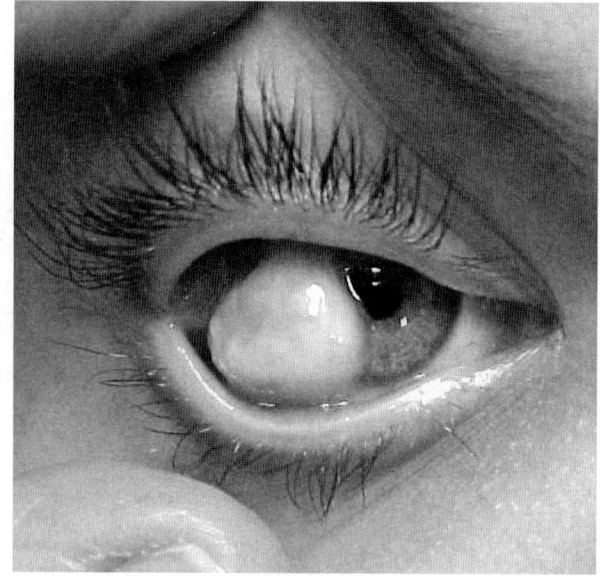

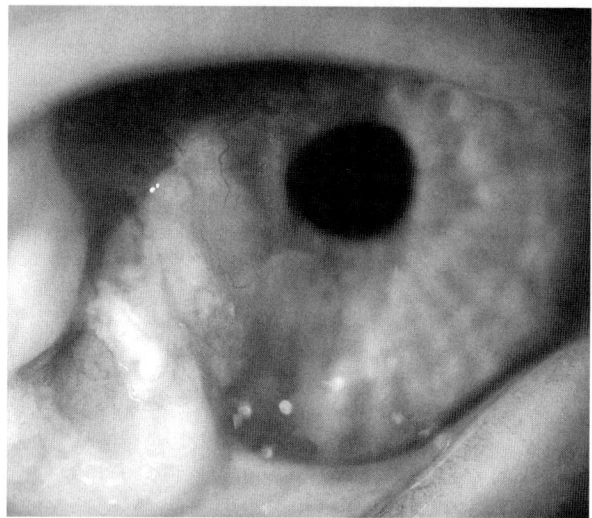

FIGURE 33-5. A: Bulbar conjunctival involvement. **B:** Bulbar conjunctival involvement with limbal corneal involvement. (Photos courtesy of Miroslav Dostalek, MD, Litomysll Hospital, Czech Republic.)

conjunctivitis to occur in unrelated girls with a homozygous defect in the plasminogen gene (23), and in plasminogen-deficient mice (24). Additional case studies confirm the association between ligneous conjunctivitis and plasminogen deficiency in humans (25–28). These studies demonstrate that inherited deficiency of type I plasminogen is the most common cause for this rare disease, and that a lys_{19} to glu mutation is the most common genetic defect (27,28). Severity of symptoms correlates with the levels of plasminogen functional activity. Thus, homozygous mutations produce the largest deficit, and are associated with the most severe disease as well as early age of onset. Heterozygous defects are milder. Surprisingly, homozygous deficiency of type I plasminogen is not associated with an increased risk of thromboembolic disease, and plasminogen functional activity can be affected by other variables that increase (oral contraceptives, hyperlipidemia) or decrease (liver disease, consumptive coagulopathies) plasminogen concentration (22).

Although defects in the type I plasminogen gene are most common, other causes of defective fibrinolysis can arise. Specifically, elevated homocysteine and lipoprotein(a) can induce a relative state of hypofibrinolysis by interfering with annexin II-mediated plasminogen binding to fibrin (22). Alternatively, aberrant transglutaminase activity can promote impaired fibrinolysis by increasing the degree of degradation-resistant γ-γ cross-links. Theoretically, defects at any site in the plasminogen-plasminogen activator pathway can impair fibrinolysis and should be suspect especially in late onset or transient cases of ligneous conjunctivitis.

In summary, the etiology of ligneous conjunctivitis centers on impaired fibrin degradation. Mutations in the type I plasminogen gene represent the most common defect, but other genetic and acquired defects are possible. Severity of symptoms and age of onset may correlate with the magnitude of the defect (homozygous versus heterozygous; genetic versus acquired). Overcoming the fibrinolytic defect by resolution of offending variables or recruitment of alter-

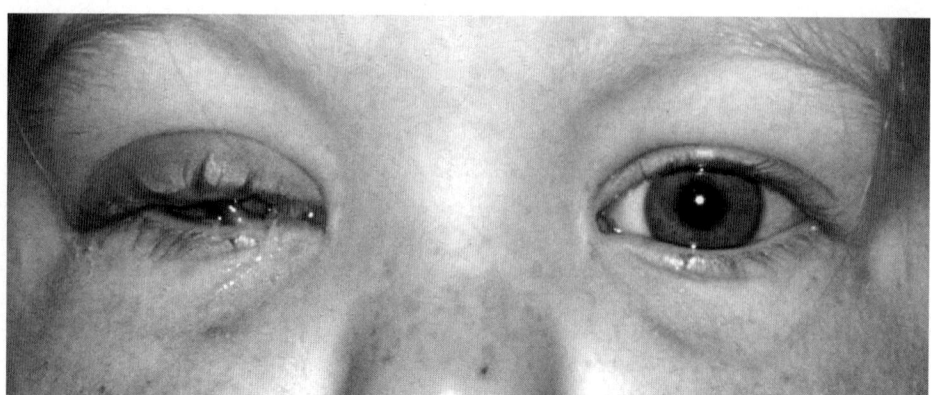

FIGURE 33-6. Active involvement of the upper lid with marked ptosis.

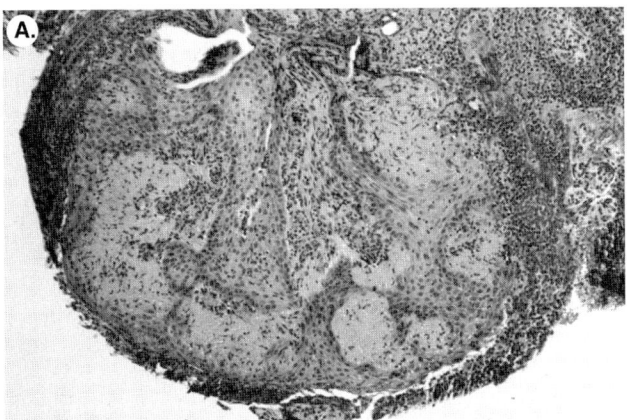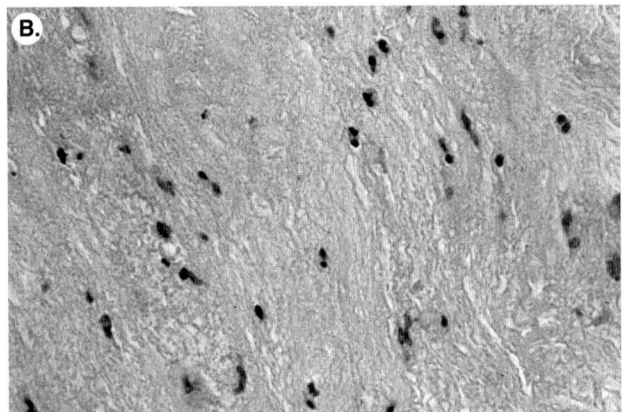

FIGURE 33-7. Histology of the ligneous lesion. Samples were formalin fixed and stained with hematoxylin-eosin. **A:** Light microscopy view of pedunculated lesion with submucosal amorphous (eosinophilic) masses, polymorphonuclear cells, and surface ulceration (4×). **B:** View of amorphous (eosinophilic) fibrils (40×). (From Ramsby ML, Donshik PC, Makowski GS. Ligneous conjunctivitis: biochemical evidence for hypofibrinolysis. *Inflammation* 2000;24:45–71, with permission.)

native proteolytic pathways may explain spontaneous disease resolution.

TREATMENT

There are no controlled studies as to the best treatment options for ligneous conjunctivitis, and both medical and surgical approaches have been reported. Early attempts to arrest lesions by injection of antidiphtheric serum or topical application of localized alcohol or silver nitrate proved ineffective. Subsequent reports of specific histologic abnormalities provided the rationale for a variety of topical medical approaches. Specifically, findings of increased hyaluronidase

led to use of hyaluronidase and α-chymotrypsin (29), whereas reposts of increased mast cells and activated T cells prompted use of cromolyn (30), a mast cell stabilizer, and cyclosporine (11,31,32), an immunosuppressant, respectively. These treatments produced variable results.

Combination surgical and medical treatment strategies have also been reported. One approach suggested by De Cock et al. (33) consisted of surgical resection of the pseudomembrane with instillation of heparin and topical corticosteroid therapy, and was found to be effective in 13 of 17 patients. Surgical excision with cryotherapy followed by medical management with hyaluronidase has also been advocated. These therapies, at best, afford only short-term effectiveness (34).

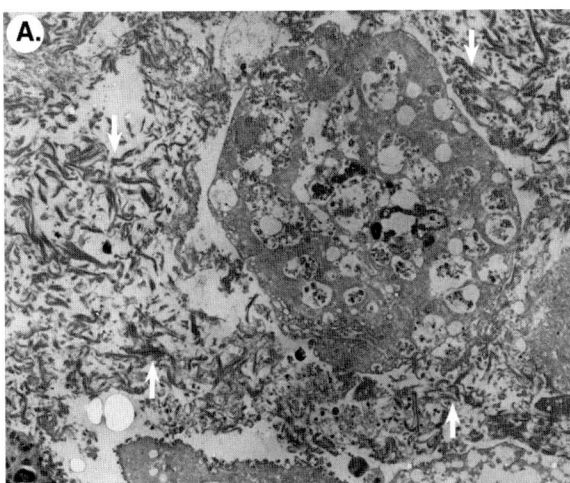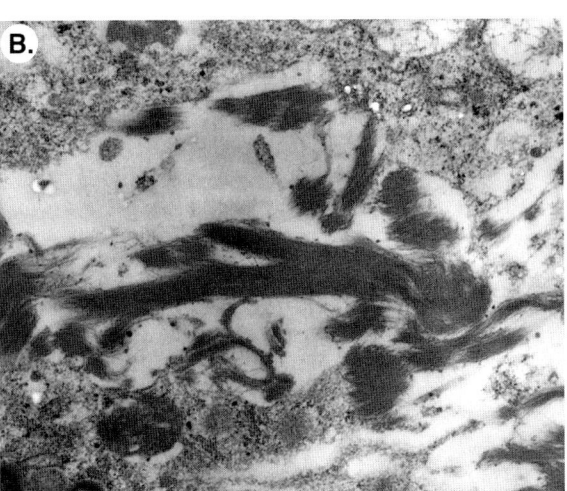

FIGURE 33-8. Electron microscopy of ligneous lesion. Samples were formalin fixed, embedded in paraffin blocks, and processed for transmission electron microscopy. **A:** Macrophage laden with phagocytic vacuoles amid a field of fibrin *(arrows)* (2,950×). **B:** Higher magnification of fibrin tactoids (15,500×). (From Ramsby ML, Donshik PC, Makowski GS. Ligneous conjunctivitis: biochemical evidence for hypofibrinolysis. *Inflammation* 2000;24:45–71, with permission.)

SDS – PAGE

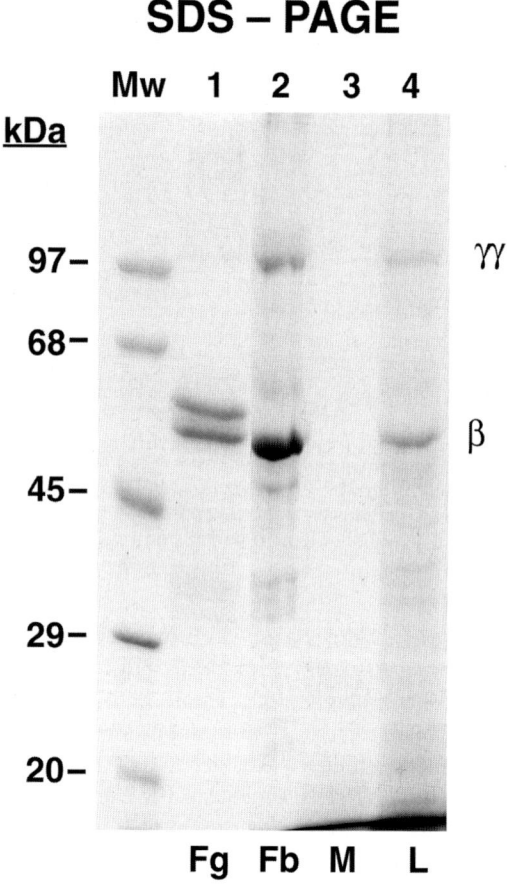

FIGURE 33-9. Protein composition of ligneous and mucoid samples. Mucoid (M) and ligneous (L) samples were electrophoresed on polyacrylamide gels in parallel with bovine fibrinogen (Fg), and human fibrin (Fb). Position of transglutaminase cross-linked product γ-γ dimers (g-g) and β-monomers (b) shown *(right)*. Position of molecular weight standards (Mw) shown *(left)*. (From Ramsby ML, Donshik PC, Makowski GS. Ligneous conjunctivitis: biochemical evidence for hypofibrinolysis. *Inflammation* 2000;24:45–71, with permission.)

The recent discoveries of type I plasminogen deficiency in ligneous conjunctivitis have led to treatment with topically administered plasminogen. Watts and co-workers (28) report this treatment was effective in three patients with ligneous conjunctivitis. All three of these patients had low or nonreportable plasminogen levels. The membranous lesions were excised and topical plasminogen drops were instituted. There were no recurrences during the 12-month follow up period. Alternatively, Kraft and co-workers (35) reported successful treatment of ligneous conjunctivitis in a girl with type I plasminogen deficiency using intravenous lys-plasminogen.

Thus, based on the current literature, the following treatment protocol is recommended: A patient with ligneous conjunctivitis should have a complete and thorough ocular examination. A thorough physical examination should also be undertaken, with special attention to the respiratory tract for associated disease. Plasminogen blood levels should be obtained: functional assay for primary assessment, and antigenic assay for dysplasminogenemia (21,22).

The ligneous lesions should be completely excised. If the lesions are not completely removed, the disease will rapidly reoccur. Bleeding can be controlled with cautery and topical epinephrine. Postoperatively, a course of topical corticosteroids (every 1 to 2 hours), hyaluronidase, acetylcysteine and broad-spectrum antibiotic (every 4 hours) are employed (5). Topical plasminogen drops should also be prescribed (28). The patient should be seen daily, and any recurrent lesions should be immediately debrided. If recurrences continue, then cyclosporin A can be added every hour to the tarsal surface with a sterile cotton-tip applicator (5). If the rate of reoccurrence of the lesions decreases, then the topical therapy can be slowly tapered. However, if the lesions progress despite this

Fibrin Zymography

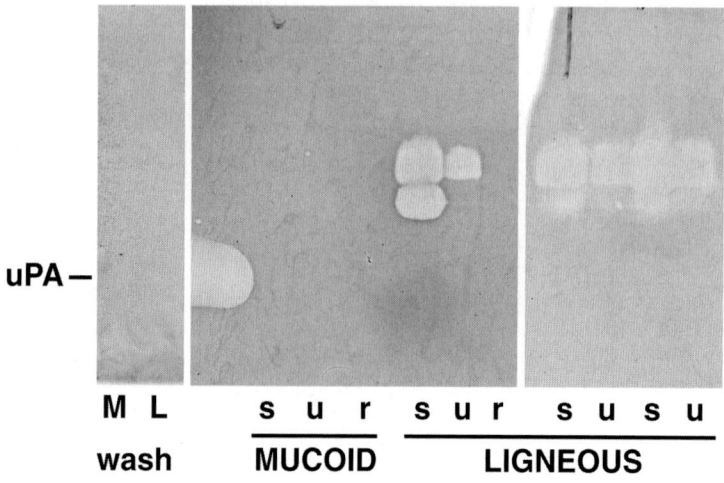

FIGURE 33-10. Plasminogen activator activity of ligneous and mucoid samples. Samples were saline washed and then extracted with 5M urea or sodium dodecyl sulfate (SDS) to disrupt protein-protein interactions and release associated enzymes. Samples were analyzed by fibrin zymography (16,17). Lytic zones of fibrin degradation were visualized by background staining. Saline washes of mucoid (M) and ligneous (L) samples were analyzed in parallel with SDS (s) and urea (u) extracts of mucoid and ligneous samples harvested at different occasions over a 2-month period. Residual material remaining after urea or SDS extraction was also analyzed (r). Urokinase standard (uPA) was loaded in the lane preceding the mucoid material. (From Ramsby ML, Donshik PC, Makowski GS. Ligneous conjunctivitis: biochemical evidence for hypofibrinolysis. *Inflammation* 2000;24:45-71, with permission.)

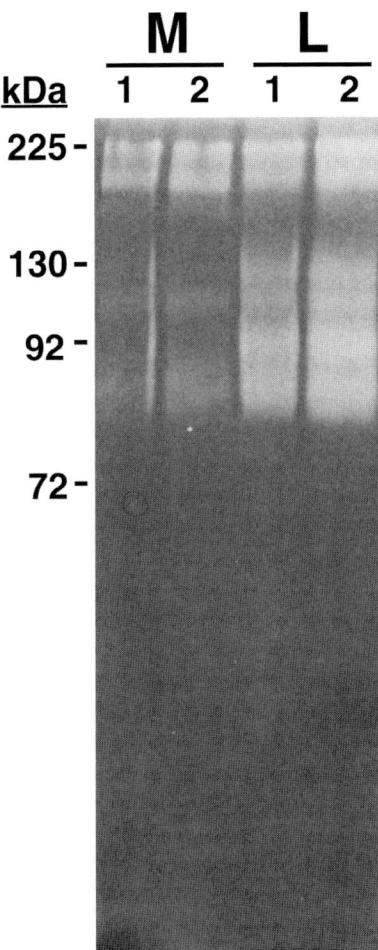

Gelatin Zymography

FIGURE 33-11. Matrix metalloproteinase (MMP) activity of ligneous and mucoid samples. SDS extracts of mucoid (M) and ligneous (L) samples were analyzed by gelatin zymography (16,18). Lytic zones of MMP activity was visualized by background staining. The position of MMP-2 (72-kD) and the MMP-9 complex (92-, 130-, and 225-kD) shown *(left).* (From Ramsby ML, Donshik PC, Makowski GS. Ligneous conjunctivitis: biochemical evidence for hypofibrinolysis. *Inflammation* 2000;24:45-71, with permission.)

therapy, then the patient is brought back to the operating room and surgical excision is repeated. Therapy may have to be continued for years before it can be discontinued without reoccurrence of the conjunctival lesions. In patients with plasminogen deficiency who have systemic manifestations in addition to the conjunctival lesions and are unresponsive to the previous mention of therapy, systemic therapy with purified plasminogen concentrate can be considered (3,35,36).

REFERENCES

1. Bouisson M. Ophthalmic sur-aigue avec de pseudomembranes a la surface de la conjonctive. *Ann Oculist* 1847;17:100–104.
2. Borel MG. Un nouvau syndrome palpebral. *Bull Soc Franc Ophthalmol* 1933;46:168–180.
3. Heinz C, Kremmer S, Externbrink P, et al. Ligneous conjunctivitis in a patient with plasminogen type I deficiency—a case report with review of literature. *Klin Monatsbl Augenheilkd* 2002; 3:156–158.
4. Weinstock SM, Kielar RA. Bulbar ligneous conjunctivitis after pterygium removal in an elderly man. *Am J Ophthalmol* 1975; 79:913–915.
5. Holland EJ, Schwartz GS. Ligneous conjunctivitis. In: Krachmer JH, Mannis MJ, Holland EJ, eds. *Cornea.* St. Louis: Mosby, 1997:863–889.
6. Bateman JB, Pettit TH. Ligneous conjunctivitis: an autosomal recessive disorder. *J Pediatr Ophthalmol Strabismus* 1986;23: 137–140.
7. Hidayat AA, Riddle PJ. Ligneous conjunctivitis. A clinicopathologic study of 17 cases. *Ophthalmology* 1987;94:949–959.
8. Marcus DMD, Walton D, Donshik PC, et al. Ligneous conjunctivitis with ear involvement. *Arch Ophthalmol* 1990;108: 514–519.
9. Scurry J, Planna R, Fortune DW, et al. Ligneous (pseudomembranous) inflammation of the female genital tract. *J Reprod Med* 1993;38:407–412.
10. Schwartz GS, Holland EJ. Induction of Ligneous conjunctivitis by conjunctival surgery. *Am J Ophthalmol* 1995;120:253–254.
11. Chambers JD, Blodi FC, Golden B, et al. Ligneous conjunctivitis. *Trans Am Ophthalmol Otolaryngol* 1969;73:996–1004.
12. Girard LT, Veselinovic A, Font AL. Ligneous conjunctivitis after pinqueculae removal in an adult. *Cornea* 1989;8:7–14.
13. Holland EJ, Chan CC, Kuwabara T, et al. Immunohistochemical findings and results of treatment with cyclosporine in ligneous conjunctivitis. *Am J Ophthalmol* 1989;107:160–166.
14. Kanai A, Polack FM. Histologic and electron microscopic studies of ligneous conjunctivitis. *Am J Ophthalmol* 1971;72:909–916.
15. Eagle RC, Brooks JJ, Ketowitz JA, et al. Fibrin as a major constituent of ligneous conjunctivitis. *Am J Ophthalmol* 1986;101: 493–494.
16. Kivela T, Tervo KE, Ravila A, et al. Pseudomembranous and membranous conjunctivitis: immunohistochemical features. *Acta Ophthalmol* 1992;70:534–542.
17. Ramsby ML, Donshik PC, Makowski GS. Ligneous conjunctivitis: biochemical evidence for hypofibrinolysis. *Inflammation* 2000; 24:45–71.
18. Ramsby ML, Kreutzer DL. Fibrin induction of tissue plasminogen activator in corneal endothelial cells in vitro. *Invest Ophthalmol Vis Sci* 1993;34:3207–3219.
19. Makowski GS, Ramsby ML. Binding of latent matrix metalloproteinase 9 to fibrin: activation via a plasmin-dependent pathway. *Inflammation* 1998;22:287–305.
20. Dvorak HF, Harvey VS, Estrella P, et al. Fibrin containing gels induce angiogenesis: implications for tumor stroma generation and wound healing. *Lab Invest* 1987;57:673–683.
21. Diamond JP, Chandra A, Williams C, et al. Tranexamic acid-associated ligneous conjunctivitis with gingival and peritoneal lesions. *Br J Ophthalmol* 1997;75:753–754.
22. Brandt JT. Plasminogen and tissue-type I plasminogen activator deficiency as risk for thromboembolic disease. *Arch Pathol Lab Med* 2002;126:1376–1381.
23. Schuster VA, Mingers AM, Seidenspinner S. et al. Homozygous mutations in the plasminogen gene of two unrelated girls with ligneous conjunctivitis. *Blood* 1997;90:958–966.
24. Drew AF, Kaufman AH, Kombrink KW, et al. Ligneous conjunctivitis in plasminogen deficient mice. *Blood* 1998;91:1616–1624.
25. Mingers AM, Heimburger H, Zeitler P, et al. Homozygous type I plasminogen deficiency. *Semin Thromb Hemost* 1997;23: 259–269.

26. Mingers AM, Philapitsch AP, Zeitler P, et al. Human homozygous type I plasminogen deficiency and ligneous conjunctivitis. *APMIS* 1999;107:62–72.

27. Schuster V, Zeitler P, Seregard S, et al. Homozygous and compound-heterozygous type I plasminogen deficiency is a common cause of ligneous conjunctivitis. *Thromb Haemost* 2001;85:1004–1010.

28. Watts P, Suresh P, Mezer E, et al. Effective treatment of ligneous conjunctivitis with topical plasmin. *Am J Ophthalmol* 2002;133:451–455.

29. Francois J, Victoria-Troncoso V. Treatment of ligneous conjunctivitis. *Am J Ophthalmol* 1968;65:674–678.

30. Friedlandaer MH, Ostler HB. Treatment of ligneous conjunctivitis with cromolyn: a case report. *Proctor Bull* 1978;1:3.

31. Holland EJ, Olsen HH, Sugar J. Topical cyclosporin A in treatment of anterior segment inflammatory diseases. *Cornea* 1993;12:413–419.

32. Rubin BI, Holland EJ, de Smet MD, et al. Response of reactivated ligneous conjunctivitis to topical cyclosporine. *Am J Ophthalmol* 1991;112:95–96.

33. De Cock R, Ficker LA, Dart JG, et al. Topical heparin in the treatment of ligneous conjunctivitis. *Ophthalmology* 1995;102:1654–1659.

34. Rao SK, Biswas J, Rajagopal R, et al. Ligneous conjunctivitis: a clinicopathologic study of 3 cases. *Int Ophthalmol* 1999;22:201–206.

35. Kraft J, Lieb W, Zeitler P, et al. Ligneous conjunctivitis in a girl with severe type I plasminogen deficiency. *Graefes Arch Clin Exp Ophthalmol* 2000;238:797–800.

36. Schott D, Dempfle C, Beck P, et al. Brief report: therapy with a purified plasminogen concentrate in an infant with ligneous conjunctivitis and homozygous plasminogen deficiency. *N Engl J Med* 1998;339;1679–1686.

34

ROSACEA

SONIA H. YOO AND ANDRE C. ROMANO

Rosacea is a chronic, idiopathic, inflammatory disorder affecting both the facial skin and the eye. The cutaneous manifestations include flushing, telangiectasia, and papules or pustules. The lesions are distributed in the flush areas (cheeks, forehead, nose, chin, and the upper chest). The typical facial feature of advanced rosacea is rhinophyma, or bulbous nose appearance caused by sebaceous gland hypertrophy.

Ocular involvement is less easily recognized than the skin changes seen in rosacea and often remains undiagnosed despite potentially serious sequelae. The most common symptoms of ocular rosacea are nonspecific and include a foreign body, gritty, or dry sensation, or burning, tearing, or redness (1). Ocular signs range from lid margin telangiectasia, meibomian gland dysfunction, and blepharoconjunctivitis, to vision-impairing corneal involvement such as neovascularization, thinning, and, in rare instances, perforation.

Cutaneous rosacea primarily affects adults between the ages of 40 and 50 years, but can also occur during childhood (2,3). It is reported to involve women twice as often as men (4), but cases with ocular manifestations are about evenly divided between the sexes, or show only a small female preponderance (5). Although there is a widespread clinical impression that rosacea affects fair-skinned people of northern European heritage, rosacea affects people of all races.

CLINICAL FEATURES

Dermatologic Findings

Flushing, telangiectasia, papules or pustules, and a later stage of sebaceous gland hypertrophy characterize skin involvement in rosacea. The lesions are distributed across the cheeks, forehead, nose, chin, and the upper chest. Initially, the hyperemia may be episodic and can be triggered by hot beverages, tobacco, alcohol, spicy foods, and emotional stress. Various mediators including substance P, histamine, serotonin, and prostaglandins have been implicated in this mechanism (6,7). The chronicity of this stage leads to dilation of small vessels and lymphatics (telangiectasia), followed by asymptomatic papular, and, less frequently,

pustular lesions resembling acne vulgaris. Rosacea is distinguished from acne vulgaris by the absence of comedones, by its confinement to flush areas, and by older age than those affected by acne vulgaris. In addition, hypertrophic changes seen in rosacea are not features of acne vulgaris. Rhinophyma, or bulbous nose, is the last stage of the disease, and is due to slowly progressive sebaceous gland hypertrophy (Fig. 34-1).

Ophthalmic Findings

The incidence of ocular involvement in rosacea varies widely from 3% to 58% in the literature (8,9). We believe that it is underappreciated and underreported because of mild cases going undiagnosed. The most frequent manifestations are meibomian gland dysfunction, telangiectasia of the lid margin, conjunctival hyperemia, and blepharoconjunctivitis.

Meibomian gland dysfunction may progress to obstructed gland orifices and lead to an irregular, hyperemic, thickened and telangiectatic lid margin (Fig. 34-2). Finally, hyperkeratinization of the ducts may displace glands posteriorly and make them less visible than in healthy subjects. The consequence is a quantitatively and qualitatively poor tear film.

Lemp et al. (10) reported that 36.7% of 60 rosacea patients had subnormal tear production compared to only 4.2% of 120 controls using Schirmer's test without anesthesia.

The altered lipid layer of the precorneal tear film leads to a rapid tear breakup time producing dry spots. These are demonstrated best with rose bengal or fluorescein staining, especially in the interpalpebral fissure where punctate keratitis may be seen (Fig. 34-3). The loss of the stabilizing effect on the tear film accounts for the most common complaints of ocular rosacea, which are burning, tearing, and foreign-body sensation.

Other frequent signs that affect the eyelids include chalasia and hordeolum. Posterior or internal hordeola often represent infection or inflammation in a meibomian gland. Fifty-seven percent of patients scheduled for excision of chalazia over 19 years of age and 64% of patients over the age of 29 were found to have rosacea (11).

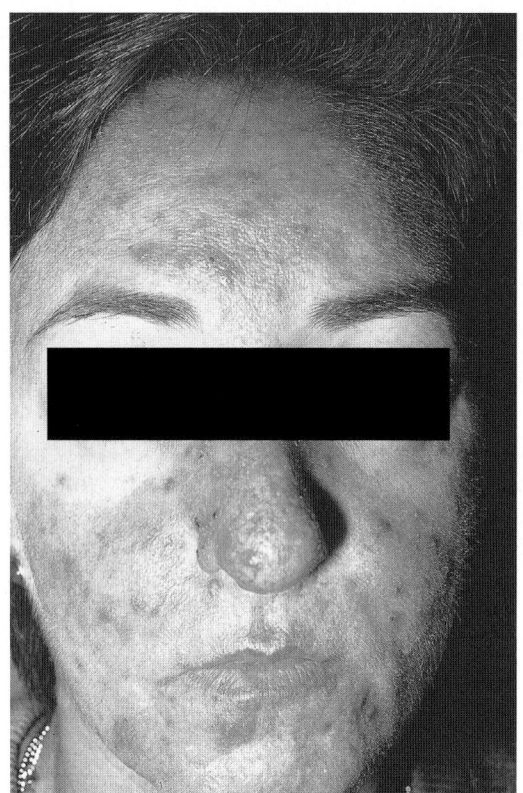

FIGURE 34-1. Rosacea dermatitis. Note the typical features of facial rosacea which include (1) facial erythema, (2) papules and pustules, and (3) rhinophyma.

Two types of conjunctivitis are associated with rosacea: diffuse hyperemia and a nodular conjunctivitis. In the diffuse form of conjunctivitis, the vessels of the tarsal and bulbar conjunctiva are engorged. A scant, watery secretion is usually found; a mucopurulent discharge suggests a superimposed bacterial conjunctivitis. The nodular conjunctivitis is much less common. Small, gray, highly vascularized nodules appear on the bulbar conjunctiva, especially near the limbus in the interpalpebral area. These phlyctenular lesions

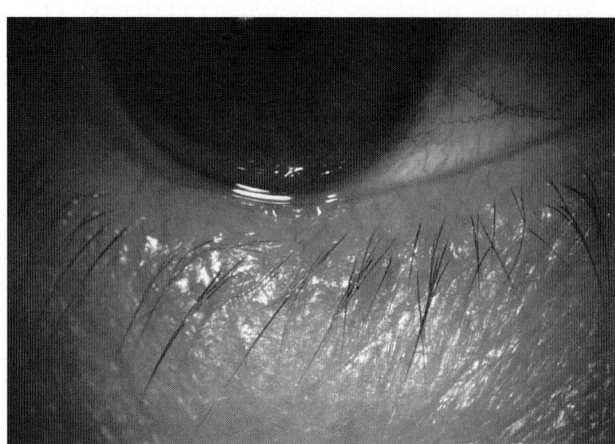

FIGURE 34-2. Thickened, hyperemic, telangiectatic lid margin.

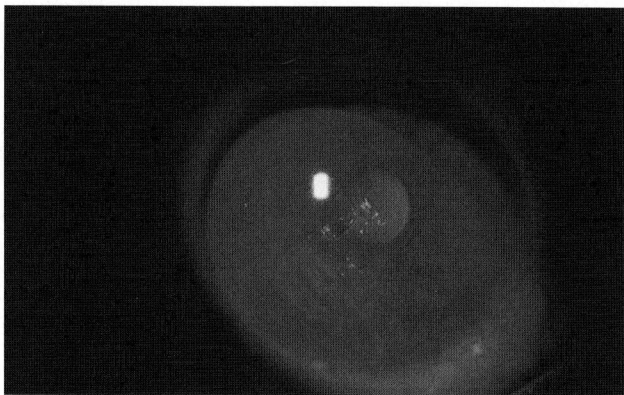

FIGURE 34-3. Superficial punctate keratitis and epithelial irregularity secondary to unstable tear film in rosacea. Sodium fluorescein dye helps to visualize punctate staining.

appear quickly, undergo superficial ulceration, and then disappear quickly. Fibrosis is the most serious conjunctival complication. It can lead to fornix foreshortening and symblepharon formation, can cause corneal complications, and can produce confusion by suggesting the possibility of ocular cicatricial pemphigoid (1).

Corneal changes in rosacea result from the combination of lid and conjunctival disease. The initial manifestation is a marginal vascular infiltration (12). Dilated vessels at the limbus advance into the superficial cornea predominantly inferiorly, which may be accompanied by punctate keratitis.

Subepithelial infiltrates are a more severe manifestation of rosacea keratitis (12). Small, round or oval, sharply delineated infiltrates may be seen near the limbus, and may appear larger toward the center of the cornea, mainly in the lower half. These infiltrates are highly vascularized with a spade- or wedge-shape (Fig. 34-4). Inflammatory episodes may lead to infiltrations of the deeper stroma, ulceration, thinning or, rarely, perforation (1,13). Scleritis, episcleritis,

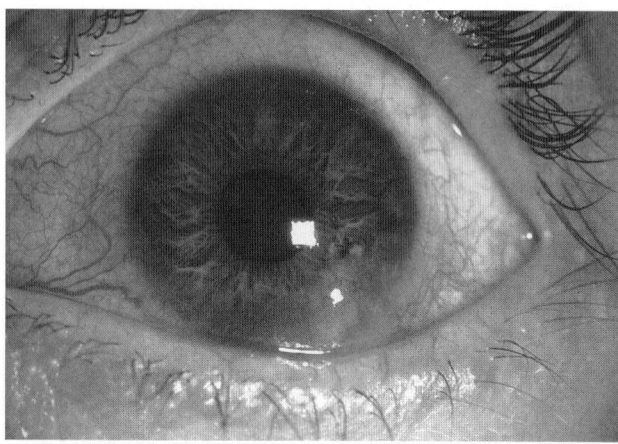

FIGURE 34-4. Vascularized corneal nodular infiltrate seen crossing the inferior limbal margin. Note the extensive corneal neovascularization that is present.

and conjunctival granulomas are less common findings in ocular rosacea (13).

PATHOGENESIS

The pathogenesis of rosacea is unknown, although several theories have been proposed. Hypotheses include climatic exposure, psychosomatic alterations, gastrointestinal disorders, bacterial infection, and immunologic causes (13).

The hypothesis that rosacea arises from exposure to the elements is based on surveys in which patients from either dermatologic (14) or ophthalmologic (15) clinics had marked preponderance of attacks during the spring. Marks and Harcourt-Webster (16) found extensive elastotic changes in 39 patients with rosacea compared to 39 control patients who had more sun exposure. However, some patients with rosacea had less elastotic changes in their skin than did the control patients. Similarly, a number of gastrointestinal disorders such as hypochlorhydria and jejunal mucosal atrophy have been inconsistently linked to rosacea. Marks (17), using interviews and psychiatric questionnaires, tried to establish a pattern of psychological traits in patients with rosacea. Although his data did not substantiate his psychosomatic hypothesis, individual case reports show that some patients' psychological state can affect disease severity (18).

Helicobacter pylori has also been postulated to play a role in the development of rosacea (22,23), but no clear evidence of an association of *H. pylori* infection of the gastric mucosa and rosacea exists. The presence of the mite, *Demodex folliculorum*, a normal inhabitant of human skin, has also been examined as a potential contributing factor to rosacea. Because these organisms feed on sebum and attract lymphocytes when they degenerate, it has been postulated that they may be responsible for meibomitis seen in patients with rosacea (24,25). In some cases, treatment of *Demodex* infestation has produced improvement in the rosacea (13,25). But in a review of 79 skin biopsies from patients with rosacea, Marks and Harcourt-Webster (16) noted *Demodex folliculorum* in only 19% of the specimens.

The colonization of certain bacteria on the eyelid margin and skin of patients with rosacea is a significant factor in the pathogenesis of ocular rosacea *Staphylococcus epidermidis*, *Propionibacterium acnes*, *Corynebacterium*, and *Staphylococcus aureus*, in decreasing order, produce lipases that appear to be indirectly responsible for meibomitis, by altering the meibomian gland secretions near the gland orifices. The lipases break down cholesterol esters present in the meibum (19,20) and release toxic free fatty acids that can destabilize the tear film. Direct lipase toxicity and a delayed cell-mediated hypersensitivity to exotoxin produced by commensal bacteria are thought to play a role in the inflammatory process associated with ocular rosacea (21).

HISTOLOGIC AND IMMUNOPATHOLOGIC FINDINGS

Histopathologic features in the skin of patients with rosacea include a marked vascular dilation with perivascular infiltration of inflammatory cells in the upper dermis (16). Papular rosacea is characterized by a more extensive and dense inflammatory cell infiltrate with numerous macrophages and a few giant cells. Most inflammatory infiltrates are predominantly lymphocytes, specifically CD4 helper T cells, which can also be seen infiltrating the conjunctiva (26).

Histologic and immunopathologic studies have been done in the conjunctiva of patients with ocular rosacea (26,27). An immunoenzymatic study showed an attenuated conjunctival epithelium infiltrated by inflammatory cells, mainly helper/inducer T cells, phagocytic cells, and antigen-presenting cells (26). The substantia propria contained clusters of chronic inflammatory cells and occasionally granuloma formation. Moreover, the helper-to-suppressor T-cell ratio was increased in both conjunctival epithelium and stroma. The mechanism involved in rosacea conjunctival inflammation resembles a type IV hypersensitivity reaction.

Other cell types such as neutrophils, macrophages, and inflammatory leukocytes have been reported to infiltrate the ocular surface in rosacea (26). They are the source of other inflammatory mediators and enzymes, for instance, interleukin-1 (IL-1) and elastase. The latter protease is known to degrade tissue inhibitor of metalloproteinase (TIMP)-1 and activate matrix metalloproteinase (MMP)-3 (28). TIMP-1 binds and inactivates the proenzyme MMP-9, which has been implicated as a causative factor in delayed corneal surface wound healing and reepithelialization (29). MMP-9 and TIMP-1 were detected at significantly higher concentrations in rosacea-affected than in normal tear fluids (30).

The high level of TIMP-1 detected in rosacea patients suggests an alternate mechanism of activation of MMP-9 in the ocular surface environment. One such mechanism could be a concomitant increase in the levels of both MMP-3 and elastase. Many events in this cascade may be mediated by inflammatory cytokines. Sobrin et al. (30) found greater concentrations of the mature form of IL-1β, which is a potent inflammatory factor that causes and promotes inflammation and neural activation.

TREATMENT

Management of rosacea is palliative; there is no cure available. Patients must be informed that ocular rosacea is a chronic disease and that reactivation/recurrences may occur. Nevertheless, improvement can be obtained with education regarding risk factors that may trigger the disease.

Appropriate general recommendations to patients include the following:

- Use of sunscreen with a protective factor (SPF) of 70 or higher;
- Avoidance of exposure to extremes of heat and cold and excessive sunlight;
- Avoidance of ingestion of hot beverages, alcohol, and spicy food.
- Daily eyelid hygiene with warm compresses, to dilate the meibomian ductules and to melt coagulated meibomium back to liquid, with subsequent massage of the lids to express the material from the glands and ductules (e.g., 10 strokes down on each upper lid and 10 strokes up on each lower lid). This should be performed a minimum of twice daily. Adjunctive use of a commercial lid scrub is appropriate for those patients with a seborrheic component to the problem, with scurf and collarettes of the lashes and lid margin.
- Short course of topical low-dose steroid (e.g., Alrex) to quiet acute exacerbations.

Antibiotic Treatment

Oral tetracyclines have been used for the treatment of rosacea by both ophthalmologists and dermatologists since the late 1960s (31). They are extremely effective if used correctly. Guidelines for treatment include the following:

- Tetracycline 250 mg four times daily for the first 6 weeks, tapering then to twice daily, *or*
- Minocycline or doxycycline 50 to 100 mg every 12 hours.

Treatment should be tailored to the individual patient based on clinical response. Tetracyclines appear to act by decreasing bacterial lipase production, thereby altering the fatty acid composition of the meibomian gland secretions and improving their solubility.

These medications also inhibit collagenase, decreasing the activity of pro-MMP-9. MMP-9 has been implicated as a causative factor in delayed corneal surface wound healing and reepithelialization (30). Tetracyclines, therefore, may protect the cornea from impending perforation secondary to inflammatory responses.

Potential adverse effects of the tetracyclines include diarrhea, rarely pancreatitis, candida vaginitis, sun sensitivity, and drug reaction. They should be avoided in patients less than 8 years of age, pregnant or breast-feeding women, and in patients with hepatic and renal failure, drug allergy, or chronic bronchitis.

Patients who are intolerant to the tetracyclines may benefit from the use of erythromycin or bacitracin, which may be used in the form of ointment applied to the lid margins once or twice daily. It reduces bacterial overgrowth contributing to lid margin disease. Systemic clindamycin and systemic erythromycin may also substitute for the tetracyclines.

Clarithromycin has been shown to exhibit antiinflammatory effects as well as activity against *H. pylori*. In a study comparing clarithromycin to doxycycline, clarithromycin showed milder side effects and found equivalent therapeutic responses (32).

Metronidazole 0.75% gel to the skin (ophthalmic preparations not yet available) has shown relative efficacy in combination with lid hygiene (33). It should be applied twice daily, substantially reducing inflammatory skin lesions after a minimum of 6 weeks of use. Long-term therapy is not advisable because it may cause atrophy, chronic vasodilation, and telangiectasia formation (34).

REFERENCES

1. Akpek EK, Merchant A, Pinar V, et al. Ocular rosacea: Patient characteristics and follow-up. *Ophthalmology* 1997;104:1863.
2. Drolet B, Paller AS. Childhood rosacea. *Pediatr Dermatol* 1992;9:22.
3. Erzurum SA, Feder RS, Greenwald MJ. Acne rosacea with keratitis in childhood. *Arch Ophthalmol* 1993;111:228.
4. Wise G. Ocular rosacea. *Am J Ophthalmol* 1943;26:591.
5. Borrie P. Rosacea with special reference to its ocular manifestations. *Br J Ophthalmol* 1953;65:458.
6. Powell FC, Corbally N, Powell D. Substance P and rosacea. *J Am Acad Dermatol* 1993;28:132.
7. Jansen T, Plewig G. The treatment of rosaceous lymphoedema. *Clin Exp Dermatol* 1997;22:57.
8. Borrie P. Rosacea with special reference to its ocular manifestations. *Br J Ophthalmol* 1953;65:458.
9. Starr PAH, McDonald A. Oculocutaneous aspects of rosacea. *Proc R Soc Med* 1969;62:9.
10. Lemp MA, Mahmood MA, Weiler HH. Association of rosacea and keratoconjunctivitis sicca. *Arch Ophthalmol* 1984;102:556.
11. Lempert SL, Jenkins MS, Brown SI. Chalazia and rosacea. *Arch Ophthalmol* 1979;97:1652.
12. Duke-Elder. *System of ophthalmology.* vol 8, part 1. *Diseases of the outer eye,* St. Louis: Mosby, 1965:498–527.
13. Browning DJ, Proia AD. Ocular rosacea. *Surv Ophthalmol* 1986;31:145.
14. Sobye P. Aetiology and pathogenesis of rosacea. *Acta Dermatovenereol* 1950;30:137.
15. Goldsmith AJB. The ocular manifestations of rosacea. *Br J Dermatol* 1953.
16. Marks R, Harcourt-Webster JN. Histopathology of rosacea. *Arch Dermatol* 1969;100:682.
17. Marks R. Concepts in the pathogenesis of rosacea. *Br J Dermatol* 1968;80:170.
18. Whitlock FA Psychosomatic aspects of rosacea. *Br J Dermatol* 1961;73:137.
19. Dougherty JM, McCulley JP. Comparative bacteriology of chronic blepharitis. *Br J Ophthalmol* 1984;68:524.
20. Groden LR, Murphy B, Rodnite J, et al. Lid flora in blepharitis. *Cornea* 1991;10:50.
21. Dougherty JM, McCulley JP. Bacterial lipases and chronic blepharitis. *Invest Ophthalmol Vis Sci* 1986;27:486.
22. Gurer MA, Erel A, Erbas D, et al. The seroprevalence of Helicobacter pylori and nitric oxide in acne rosacea. *Int J Dermatol* 2002;41:768.

23. Szlachcic A. The link between Helicobacter pylori infection and rosacea. *J Eur Acad Dermatol Venereol* 2002;16:328.
24. Shelley WB, Shelley ED, Burmeister V. Unilateral demodectic rosacea. *J Am Acad Dermatol* 1989;20:915.
25. Rufli T, Buchner SA. T-cell subsets in acne rosacea lesions and the possible role of Demodex folliculorum. *Dermatologica* 1984;169:1.
26. Hoang-Xuan T, Rodriguez A, Zaltas MM, et al. Ocular rosacea. A histologic and immunopathologic study. *Ophthalmology* 1990;97:1468.
27. Brown SI, Shahinian L Jr. Diagnosis and treatment of ocular rosacea. *Ophthalmology* 1978;85:779.
28. Itoh Y, Nagase H. Preferential inactivation of tissue inhibitor of metalloproteinase-1 that is bound to the precursor of matrix metalloproteinase 9 (progelatinase B) by human neutrophil elastase *J Biol Chem* 1995;270:16518.

29. Woessner JF. Matrix metalloproteinases and their inhibitors in connective tissue remodeling. *FASEB J* 1991;5:2145.
30. Sobrin L, Liu Z, Monroy DC, et al. Regulation of MMP-9 activity in human tear fluid and corneal epithelial culture supernatant. *Invest Ophthalmol Vis Sci* 2000;41:1703.
31. Sneddon IB. A clinical trial of tetracycline in rosacea. *Br J Dermatol* 1966;78:649.
32. Torresani C. Clarithromycin: a new perspective in rosacea treatment. *Int J Dermatol* 1998;37:347.
33. Aronson IK, Rumsfeld JA, West DP, et al. Evaluation of topical metronidazole gel in acne rosacea. *Drug Intell Clin Pharmacol* 1987;21:346.
34. Sneddon I. Adverse effect of topical fluorinated corticosteroids in rosacea. *Br Med J* 1969;1:671.

35

THYGESON'S SUPERFICIAL PUNCTATE KERATITIS

PARVEEN K. NAGRA AND PETER R. LAIBSON

The term *superficial punctate keratitis* was coined by Ernst Fuchs (1) to describe the corneal changes that he observed during an epidemic of acute conjunctivitis. The term still is used to describe many diverse, small discrete lesions of the epithelium, Bowman's membrane, and anterior stroma. In 1950, Phillips Thygeson (2) used the term to describe an entity in which the morphologic features are distinctive and quite appropriately described by the term *superficial punctate keratitis*. These features include multiple epithelial lesions limited to the corneal epithelium, without associated stromal involvement or corneal edema. The lesions, often referred to as *Thygeson's superficial punctate keratitis* (TSPK) are typically bilateral, transient, mildly to severely symptomatic, and not associated with conjunctivitis.

ETIOLOGY

The lesions of TSPK resemble the corneal lesions seen in measles during the convalescent stage of the infection, or in the early stages of epidemic keratoconjunctivitis before the subepithelial infiltrates appear. The morphologic similarity has led many to speculate that a virus may play a role in the etiology of the disease, and in fact Braley and Alexander (3) recovered a virus from one case of TSPK, and later Lemp and associates (4) reported the isolation of a varicella-zoster virus from a patient with this disease. Repeated attempts, by Thygeson and others, have been unsuccessful in isolating a virus through cultures or serologic studies, and epidemiologic studies have not shown a relationship to viral illnesses (5–8). The favorable response of the lesions to topical steroids also suggests that if the lesions are caused by a virus, they must at least in part represent an immunologic response to the virus.

Thygeson (5) observed that this entity was self-limited, and resolved within 4 years in all patients. More recent studies have demonstrated a more prolonged disease course

of decades, with the longest duration reported being 41 years (9). It has been speculated that the duration of the disease is prolonged by treatment with steroids. Topical steroids may have an adverse effect on the natural course of the disease, such as one would expect if it were a "slow virus" (7). Further research is warranted to confirm the role of a virus in this entity.

TSPK is reported to be associated with human leukocyte antigen (HLA)-DR3, suggesting a predisposition to the disease among some of the population (6). In addition, this association may imply an autoimmune component to the disease.

PATHOGENESIS

As the cause of TSPK is unknown, one can only speculate on the pathogenesis. As noted above, the lesions are similar to those seen during the convalescent period of measles and the coalescent phase of the corneal changes seen in epidemic keratoconjunctivitis between the first and second weeks of disease onset and before the subepithelial infiltrates appear, which suggests that the etiology may be a slow virus. In many slow viral infections, such as verruca and molluscum contagiosum, epidemiologic studies are unrewarding in explaining the source of the infections. In addition, the time between exposure to the agent and manifested clinical disease is so prolonged that there is little hope of determining the source of the infection. Moreover, serologic studies are unproductive for slow viral infections. The spontaneous healing of the lesions after 2 to 4 years in the early cases when steroids have not been used is also compatible with a slow viral infection, similar to the spontaneous resolution of most verruca and molluscum contagiosum nodules within that time frame. Conversely, the proposed prolongation of disease course with topical steroids may be similar to the prolongation of the duration of infections of verruca and molluscum contagiosum when immunosuppressive agents are used.

If the disease is caused by a slow virus, then the pathogenesis should be similar to other slow viral infections. Following exposure of a healthy or immunosuppressed host, the virus replicates in the epithelial cells of the cornea and gradually converts the cells' functions to its own use. The viral infection stimulates the cells to divide, and after many months the disease becomes manifest clinically. After a few days to several weeks, the lesions probably cause a nonspecific inflammatory reaction that leads to loss of the grossly infected cells and subsidence of the lesions. Subsequently, the entire process begins anew.

CLINICAL FEATURES

TSPK occurs in all areas of the world, affecting people of all races (10). There is no gender predilection. Patients of all ages have been affected, with the youngest reported patient being 2½ years old, and the oldest reported patient with active symptoms being 85 years old.

At onset, patients note the insidious onset of foreign-body sensation, photophobia, and tearing. Other symptoms include blurred vision, redness, and diplopia. Patients may be asymptomatic, with just one or two spots (11). Typically, the more spots seen, the more symptomatic patients are. The symptoms usually increase for 1 to 2 weeks, and then slowly subside. During a period of remission, the patients remain asymptomatic. Duration of remission can vary, but often lasts for 4 to 6 weeks, followed by the new onset of symptoms. Remissions and exacerbations may occur for years or decades.

On examination, there are discrete, slightly elevated, granular, white or gray dots in the corneal epithelium, usually less than one-quarter millimeter in size. The lesions may be located near the visual axis, and are less commonly near the limbus. They are best seen by broad slit-beam illumination (Fig. 35-1). Individual lesions are microscopic but tend to be grouped into larger macroscopic lesions that are oval in shape. The larger grouped lesions are readily seen with the slit lamp. The lesions are also apparent in retroillumination (Fig. 35-2) and may be visible on retinoscopy. The epithelium between the lesions appears normal.

During exacerbations, the lesions become slightly elevated, and small punctate foci overlying the lesions stain with fluorescein, lissamine green, or rose bengal. The number of lesions can vary from 1 to over 20 at any one time. As the disease subsides and disappears, the number of lesions during periods of exacerbation is often markedly reduced. During an exacerbation, the lesions may recur in the same area or may be found in other areas of the corneal epithelium.

At the time of remission, many or even all of the lesions may disappear completely. The remaining lesions flatten to

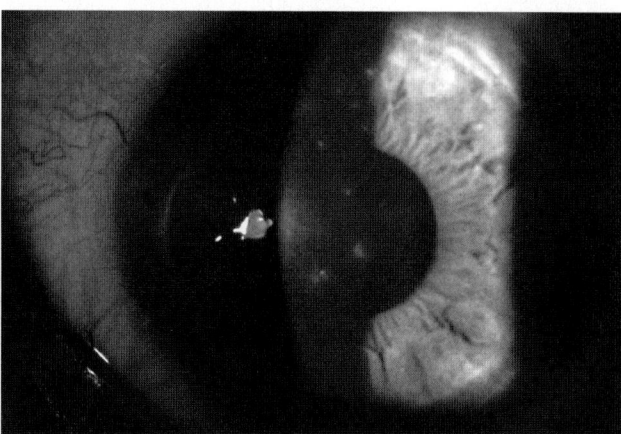

FIGURE 35-1. Thygeson's superficial punctate keratitis (TSPK) corneal lesions evident on broad slit illumination.

become even with the surface of the cornea, and overlying epithelium no longer stains with dye.

The lesions are entirely epithelial. However, during an exacerbation, mild edema of Bowman's layer or the very superficial stroma immediately beneath the lesions may develop. Topical idoxuridine (IDU) may damage this underlying Bowman's layer when used during active disease. A ghostlike image of the lesions that can persist for months to several years after the disease has completely subsided may occur after use of this topical medication (5,7).

The corneal sensation is usually normal. Corneal neovascularization is very unusual, but a few superficial vessels may develop in areas where recurrent lesions are located close the limbus. The disease is also unusual in that there is no associated conjunctivitis. Occasionally a mild limbal hyperemia may occur during exacerbations. Severe light sensitivity may occur, especially in children, when the corneal lesions are numerous. The ophthalmologist should be suspicious of this disease in children with severe intermittent light sensitivity who do not have conjunctival injection.

When corticosteroids are not used, the unaltered course of the disease is that of remissions and exacerbations, with

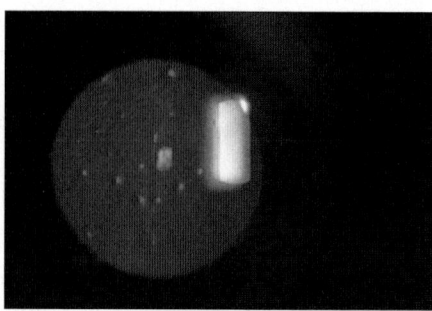

FIGURE 35-2. TSPK corneal lesions apparent on retroillumination.

eventual resolution within 2 to 4 years (2–5). During periods of exacerbations, the symptoms generally begin insidiously, gradually increasing in intensity over a 2-week period, and then slowly subside. Often, a remission lasts 4 to 6 weeks and is followed by exacerbation. The duration of the exacerbations and remissions varies from patient to patient and also with duration of the disease. In some instances, the exacerbations persist for only a few days, followed by remission of several months. In other cases, the exacerbation may persist for several months to be followed by only a very short period of remission. Normally as the disease subsides, the exacerbation become milder and shorter, and the remissions last longer and longer.

TREATMENT

Various modes of treatment have been employed, including removal of corneal epithelium, or use of antiviral agents, continuous-wear soft contact lenses, topical steroids, or topical cyclosporine.

Topical steroids have become many physicians' mainstay of therapy, resulting in relatively rapid, symptomatic relief as well as clinical improvement. Institution of a weak steroid, such as fluorometholone or loteprednol, four times a day, followed by a very slow taper over the course of months has been very effective in patients with TSPK. Some patients may require regular, infrequent use of these topical steroids (i.e., twice a week), to prevent exacerbations, whereas many can be tapered off steroids completely between episodes (11). Rarely, patients may require a stronger steroid, such as prednisolone acetate, if the weaker steroids do not lead to symptomatic relief. Potential side effects of topical steroid use should always be kept in mind, including increased intraocular pressure, cataract formation, and potentiation of infection, although some of these may be less frequent with the use of newer, low-dose steroids. In addition, as mentioned, although they are very effective in treating TSPK, topical steroids have been postulated to increase duration of disease.

Topical cyclosporine has also been used successfully in treating this entity (12–14). Reinhard and Sundmacher (14) found that more than two thirds of patients responded to topical cyclosporine 2%, although TSPK recurred in many of these patients during attempted tapering or shortly after the topical medication was discontinued. The greatest benefit of topical cyclosporine over topical steroids is the lack of the potential side effects of steroid. The main complaint with topical cyclosporine use has been a burning sensation during its application. In some cases, however, this burning sensation has been intolerable, leading to cessation of the medication. Because it probably acts through an antiinflammatory mechanism, similar to steroids,

cyclosporine may also lead to an increase in the duration of the disease.

Removal of corneal epithelium appears to have no effect on the disease course. The lesions recur at approximately the same interval as before and often in the same place on the cornea. A recent case report suggested improvement in TSPK following photorefractive keratectomy (PRK) for myopia, noting recurrent lesions in the periphery only, with sparing of the treated central cornea (15). The authors had also noted similar improvement in adenoviral subepithelial infiltrates (16). However, others have reported recurrence of lesions in the laser ablation zone following PRK, suggesting removal of anterior stroma alone may be insufficient to treat this condition.

IDU appears to frequently case ghostlike images in Bowman's layer in patients with TSPK. Even in patients who give no history of using IDU, further inquiry may indicate that the patient had used drops of an unknown type, which may have been IDU or a similar medication (7).

Nesburn and colleagues (17) reported resolution of TSPK with 1% trifluridine every 2 hours for varying periods of time, ranging from weeks to months. In some cases, the lesions did not recur after cessation of treatment. Symptomatic relief has also been achieved with the use of continuous-wear soft contact lenses (18). Patients may note a rapid relief in discomfort, although the corneal lesions may persist for months.

REFERENCES

1. Fuchs E. Keratitis punctate superficialis. *Wien Klin Wochenshr* 1889;2:837–841.
2. Thygeson P. Superficial punctate keratitis. *JAMA* 1950;144: 1544–1549.
3. Braley AE, Alexander RC. Superficial punctate keratitis: isolation of a virus. *Arch Ophthalmol* 1953;50:147–154.
4. Lemp MA, Chambers RW, Lundy J. Viral isolates in superficial punctate keratitis. *Arch Ophthalmol* 1974;91:8–10.
5. Thygeson P. Clinical and laboratory observation on superficial punctate keratitis. *Am J Ophthalmol* 1966;61:1344–1349.
6. Darrell R. Thygeson's superficial punctate keratitis: natural history and association with HLA-DR3. *Trans Am Ophthalmol Soc* 1981;79:486–516.
7. Tabbara KF, Ostler HB, Dawson C, et al. Thygeson's superficial punctate keratitis. *Ophthalmology* 1981;88:75–77.
8. VanBijsterveld OP, Mansour KH, Dubois FJ. Thygeson's superficial punctate keratitis. *Ann Ophthalmol* 1985;17:150–153.
9. Tanzier DJ, Smith RE. Superficial punctate keratitis of Thygeson's: the longest course on record? *Cornea* 1999;18: 729–730.
10. Quere MA, Diallo J, Rogez JP. Thygeson's superficial punctate keratitis. *Arch Ophthalmol (Paris)* 1968;28:497–506.
11. Nagra PK, Rapuano CJ, Cohen EJ, Laibson PR. Thygeson's superficial punctate keratitis: ten years' experience. *Ophthalmology* 2004;111:34–37.
12. Holsclaw DS, Wong IG, Sherman M. Masked trial of topical cyclosporine A in the treatment of refractory Thygeson's superficial punctate keratitis. *Invest Ophthalmol Vis Sci* 1994;35:1302.

13. Benitez Del Castillo JM, Benitez Del Castillo J, et al. Effect of topical cyclosporin A on Thygeson's superficial punctate keratitis. *Doc Ophthalmol* 1997;93:193–198.

14. Reinhard T, Sundmacher R. Topical cyclosporin A in Thygeson's superficial punctate keratitis. *Graefes Arch Clin Exp Ophthalmol* 1999;237:109–112.

15. Fite SW, Chodosh J. Photorefractive keratectomy for myopia in the setting of Thygeson's superficial punctate keratitis. *Cornea* 2001;20:425–426.

16. Fite SW, Chodosh J. Photorefractive keratectomy in the setting of adenoviral subepithelial infiltrates. *Am J Ophthalmol* 1998; 126:829–831.

17. Nesburn AB, Lowe GH, Lepoff NJ, et al. Effect of topical trifluridine on Thygeson's superficial punctate keratitis. *Ophthalmology* 1984;91:1188–1192.

18. Forstot SL, Binder PS. Treatment of Thygeson's superficial punctate keratopathy with soft contact lenses. *Am J Ophthalmol* 1979;88: 186–189.

36

FILAMENTARY KERATITIS

SHIGERU KINOSHITA AND NORIHIKO YOKOI

GENERAL FEATURES

Filamentary keratitis, first described by Leber (1) in 1882, is a chronic disorder of the cornea characterized by one or more filaments that hang from the surface of the cornea (2). Filamentary keratitis occurs secondary to various diseases or conditions (Table 36-1), but there are some cases in which no associated disease can be identified; these cases are then reported as cases of idiopathic essential filamentary keratitis (3,4).

Observation by a slit-lamp biomicroscope has disclosed that filaments appear as short tails, variable in length but usually less than 2 mm long, being connected to the surface of the cornea (Fig. 36-1) or, very rarely, to the conjunctiva. The location of filaments on the cornea varies in cases and may be related to the mechanism of the background disease. Filaments are stained with rose Bengal, or Lissamine green and less brightly, with fluorescein (3) (Fig. 36-1). At the base of each filament the superficial cells are observed to be elongated and stretched toward the filament (5). The superficial corneal epithelial cells between lesions are normal, but superficial punctate keratopathy is sometimes seen (Fig. 36-1), because filaments are the most common complication of tear-deficient dry eye. Beneath the attachment to the epithelium, there may be a gray subepithelial granular opacity (3), implying a possible association with inflammation due to the filament itself or its association with the background disease. Epithelial detachment is sometimes seen at the base of the filament, which can be detected by the diffusion of fluorescein into the detached subepithelial space (Fig. 36-2).

Histologically, filaments are known to be composed of a central mucin core, which is stained by a periodic acid-Schiff (PAS) or Alcian blue, and degenerated epithelial cells surrounding the core (Fig. 36-3). Also, a previous study reported that at the base of the filaments, just below the basal epithelium, scattered groups of inflammatory cells and fibroblasts were demonstrated, suggesting that filamentary keratitis occurs as a result of damage to either the basal epithelium, epithelial basement membrane, or both (6).

Filaments start out as quite small but grow larger, and in cases where filaments appear in the interpalpebral region, they are likely to be pulled off at the time of blinking. Because of their connection to the corneal surface, patients experience ocular pain, foreign-body sensation, photophobia, and lacrimation, not unlike those symptoms experienced in cases where a foreign body is present. Patients may also experience blepharospasm. (If they already suffer from this, there is the possibility of it becoming worse).

BACKGROUND DISEASE OR CONDITION

As summarized in Table 36-1, filamentary keratitis is related to dry eye, especially the tear-deficient type, and this association is most prevalent. Filamentary keratitis has also been associated with superior limbic keratoconjunctivitis, acute viral keratoconjunctivitis such as epidemic keratoconjunctivitis (Fig. 36-4), eye surgery such as penetrating keratoplasty (Fig. 36-5) or cataract surgery (Fig. 36-6), recurrent erosions, ocular trauma, vernal or atopic keratoconjunctivitis, neurotrophic keratitis, and prolonged closed eye conditions (ptosis, blepharospasm, or large angle strabismus) (3,7–9). Systemic diseases such as sarcoidosis, diabetes mellitus, and atopic dermatitis, or medications such as preservative-containing artificial tears, antiglaucoma eyedrops, and diphenhydramine hydrochloride (10) have also been reported as being connected to filamentary keratitis.

PATHOPHYSIOLOGY

In filamentary keratitis, long-term treatment is often ineffective and recurrences are common. It is therefore important to take the pathophysiology (Fig. 36-7) into consideration and treat any underlying disease, although the mechanism of filamentary keratitis remains obscure.

In the normal, healthy ocular surface, interaction between the tear film and the ocular surface epithelium is well maintained with a delicate balance. It is the case, however,

TABLE 36-1 (BACKGROUND DISEASE OR CONDITION)

Trauma/Surgery
- ocular trauma (chemical injury, foreign body, etc.)
- contact lens overwear
- penetrating keratoplasty
- cataract surgery
- refractive surgery

Eye disease
- dry eye (either evaporative, tear-deficient)
- superior limbic keratoconjunctivitis
- neurotrophic keratopathy
- prolonge eye patching
- ptosis
- starabisms
- recurrent corneal erosion
- vernal keratoconjunctivitis (atopic keratoconjunctivitis)
- epidemic keratoconjunctivitis
- conjunctivochalasis

Systemic disease
- diabetes mellitus
- sarcoidosis
- chronic rheumatoid arthritis

Medication
- benzalkonium chloride
- beta-blockers
- diclofenac
- diphenhydramine hydrochloride
- acyclovir
- aminoglycosides
- 5 fluouracil

that in eyes with filamentary keratitis, both major factors, the tear film and corneal epithelium, are disrupted and both of these abnormalities seem to be essential for the establishment of corneal filaments. Moreover, mucus glycoproteins in the tear film play an important role in maintaining the stability of tear film and thus keep the corneal surface intact. Alteration in the chemical composition of mucus, which occurs in dry eye, results in the change of

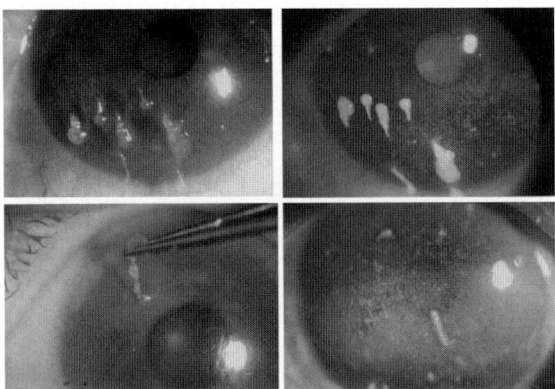

FIGURE 36-1. Various types of filamentary keratitis.

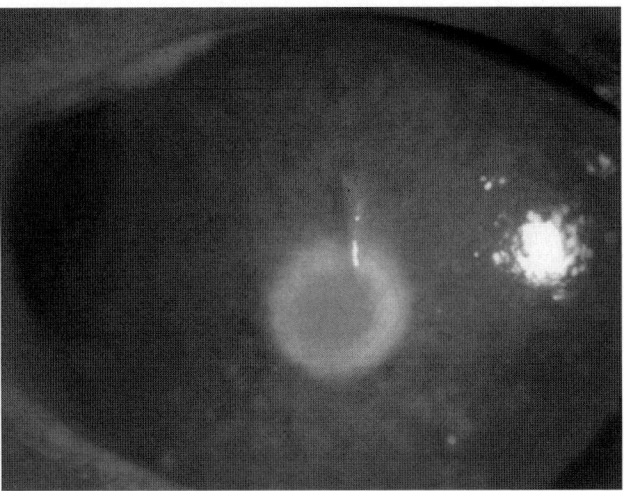

FIGURE 36-2. Epithelial detachment.

physical properties, with increased viscosity causing some of the distinctive clinical features seen in keratoconjunctivitis sicca, superior limbic keratoconjunctivitis, vernal keratoconjunctivitis, and neuroparalytic keratitis (11).

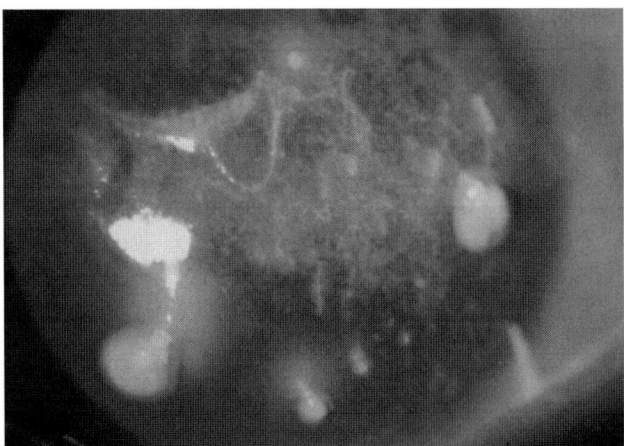

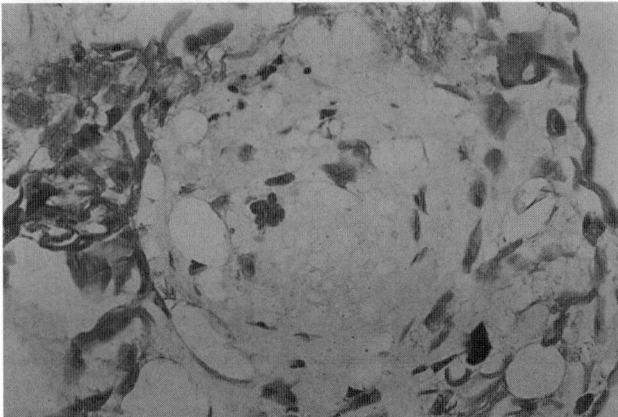

FIGURE 36-3. The large filament (*top*) taken for histologic examination is composed of a central mucin core and degenerated epithelial cells surrounding the core (*bottom*).

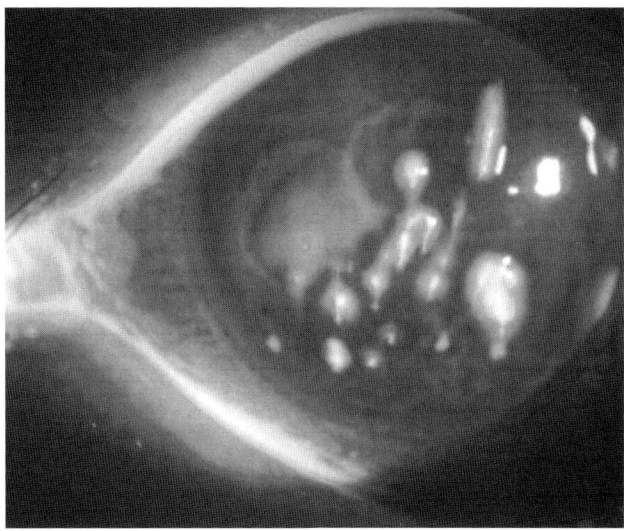

FIGURE 36-4. Filamentary keratitis in epidemic keratoconjunctivitis.

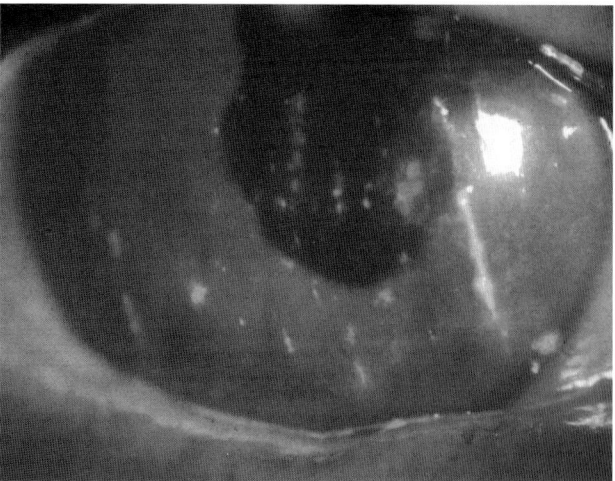

FIGURE 36-6. Filamentary keratitis after cataract surgery.

As in the tear film abnormality, which is one of the indispensable factors in the formation of filaments, an increase in the ratio of mucus to aqueous has been importantly proposed as an important factor (2). There are two instances where the mucus-to-aqueous ratio is increased: absolute or relative accumulation of mucus in the tears. Absolute accumulation of mucus occurs in cases with conjunctival inflammation, and this may explain the filaments seen in acute keratoconjunctivitis (Fig. 36-4). In general, conjunctival inflammation, whether from mechanical or microbial problems, chemical irritants, or allergies, is accompanied by increased goblet cell density, resulting in the increase of mucus-to-aqueous ratio (2).

Relative accumulation of mucus occurs mostly in patients with tear-deficient dry eye. In tear-deficient dry eye, due to diminished tear secretion, meniscus tear volume

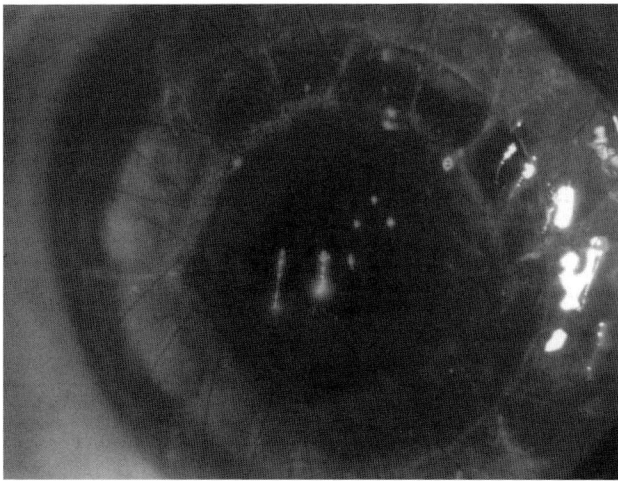

FIGURE 36-5. Filamentary keratitis on the graft after penetrating keratoplasty.

falls, resulting in decreased tear flow. As mucus turnover (12) is regulated by blinking and tear flow (13), decreased tear flow is accompanied by delayed mucus turnover, leading to relative accumulation of mucus on the cornea. This may explain the reason why filaments are most commonly associated with tear-deficient dry eye (11,12). It is also possible that dry eye-related hydrophobic alteration of the corneal surface may facilitate the adherence of mucus to the corneal surface (14), which may partly contribute to the formation of filaments.

As an abnormality of the ocular surface epithelium and one of the major factors responsible for the formation of filaments, a pathologic corneal epithelium in some systemic diseases may offer the substrates and attachment sites for filaments. An uncontrolled increase in blinking, as seen in blepharospasm, may also exert trauma to the epithelial cells acting as a risk factor for the formation of filaments (7). In blepharospasm, it is also possible that inefficient, short blinking may result in delayed mucus turnover.

In cases with tear-deficient dry eye, filamentary keratitis is likely to occur because both abnormalities in the tear film and the ocular surface epithelium are present. As the mechanism to the formation of filaments in tear-deficient dry eye, the following theory is very likely (Fig. 36-8): when the cornea dries to a point that is incompatible with a healthy epithelial layer, some surface cells will become desiccated and be shed, based on the dry-eye mechanism. This creates a small pit on the corneal surface that is hydrophobic compared with the mucus coated normal surface. Lipid contaminated normal mucus will become attached to these pits by hydrophobic bonding. Within a short time, the surface epithelium will grow down to these mucus cores based on the healing process of epithelial cells, and a true filament will thus be born *in situ*. This theory is applicable to the explanation of filamentary keratitis in various diseases. For example, superior limbic keratoconjunctivitis is caused by a friction between palpebral

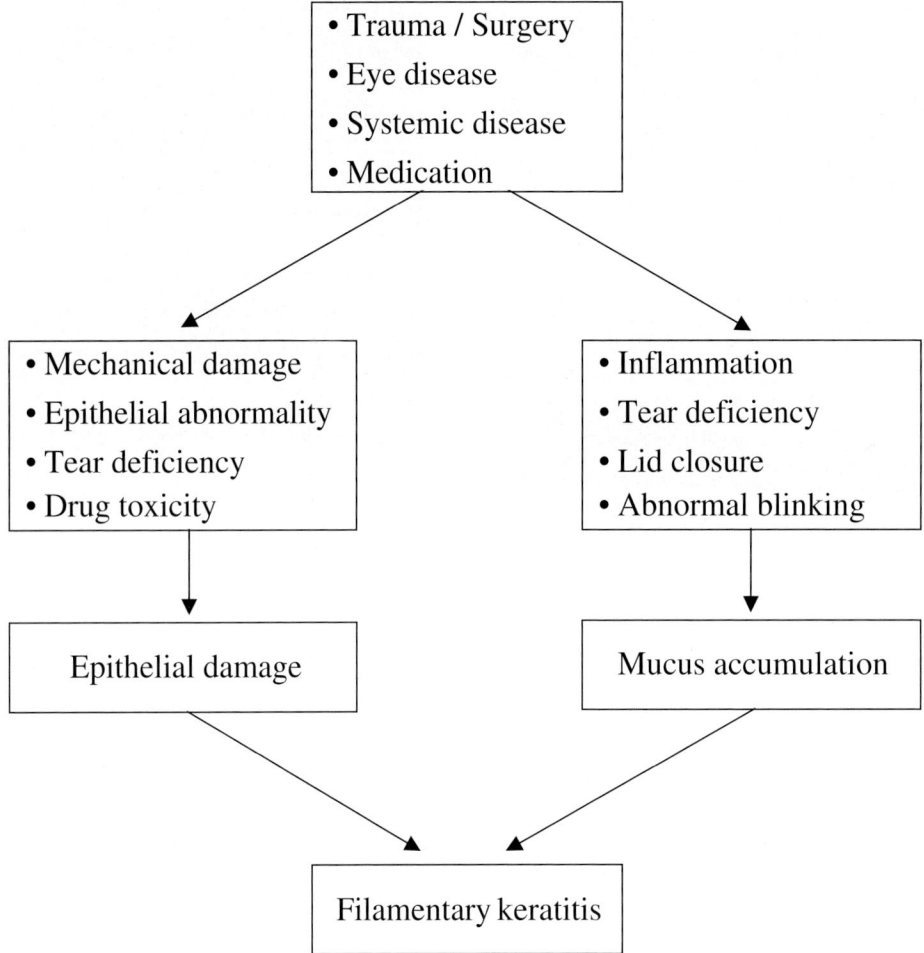

FIGURE 36-7. Schematic explanation of pathophysiology in filamentary keratitis.

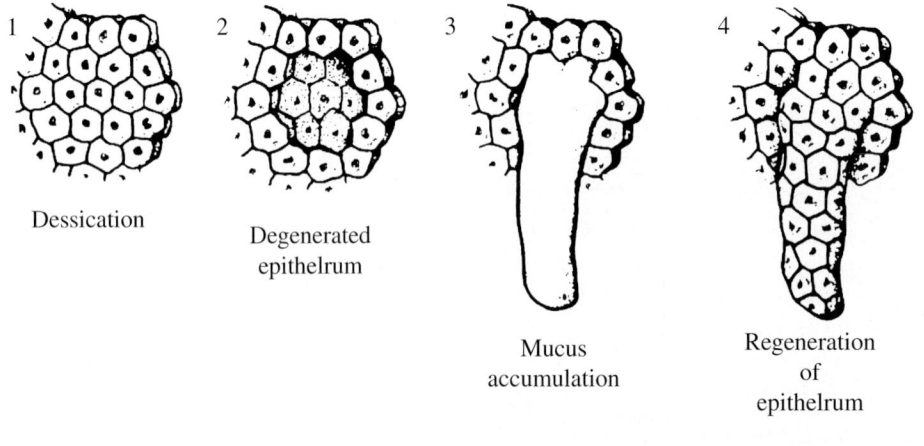

FIGURE 36-8. A theory of filament formation. As a normal epithelial surface degenerates due to desiccation (1), some cells die and fall off, leaving a defect (2). Mucin may adhere to this high-energy pit (3), and eventually epithelium may grow down over mucin to form a filament (4). (From DW Lamberts. Dry eye syndromes. In: CS Foster, ed. *Cornea and external disease.* Chicago: Year Book Medical Publishers, 1985. Copyrighted by Year Book Medical Publishers, with permission.)

and upper bulbar conjunctiva. Epithelial damage in the upper part of the cornea due to the friction and impaired blinking (which occurs as a reaction to the pain resulting from this disease) induces both epithelial damage and delayed mucus turnover, which may be accompanied by filamentary keratitis. Closed eye conditions, such as prolonged eye patching, also induce epithelial damage due to hypoxia and delayed mucus turnover because of a lack of blinking (15).

TREATMENT

For the mechanical removal of filaments, fine-tipped forceps, filter paper, or a glass rod with a smooth top is often used after the instillation of an anesthetic eyedrop. The glass rod is especially useful, because it is less harmful to the normal epithelium around the filaments. It must be noted that there is a danger of causing an epithelial defect, even rarely infection, after the mechanical removal of filaments, in those cases where filaments are accompanied by a loosened attachment of the epithelium to the basement membrane at the base of the filaments (Fig. 36-2). In such cases, fine-tip scissors to cut the filament from the base are safely used.

Because filamentary keratitis is generally a chronic disorder, and it is usually based on the complicated mechanism, being related to the malfunction of the lid, ocular surface epithelium, and/or tear film, the underlying pathophysiology must be considered in order to obtain a permanent resolution. Before the treatment, two important aspects regarding the formation of filaments, their acute or chronic and tear-deficient or -sufficient states, should be taken into account.

In the case of filaments produced during the acute phase of keratoconjunctivitis such as from viral or allergic origins, or after surgery, a spontaneous resolution would be expected in the course of the disease, when the treatment for the disease itself is properly maintained. For this group of filamentary keratitis, the control of ocular surface inflammation producing pain is most important, because a painful eye is accompanied by insufficient blinking as well as increased mucus production, resulting in absolute or relative mucus accumulation on the ocular surface, leading to the formation of filaments.

In cases with sufficient tears but with chronic recurrent filamentary keratitis, several medications are reportedly useful breaking the vicious cycle (Fig. 36-7) of the formation of filamentary keratitis, including a 5% sodium chloride eyedrop (3) that, as expected, draws conjunctival interstitial fluid osmotically, effectively delivering a greater amount of moisture to the cornea; acetylcysteine as a mucolytic agent to decrease the mucin-to-aqueous ratio; eledoisin as a tear stimulating agent; and diclofenac sodium, with antiinflammatory and analgesic effects (16–21). For this group, a bandage soft contact lens (together with the

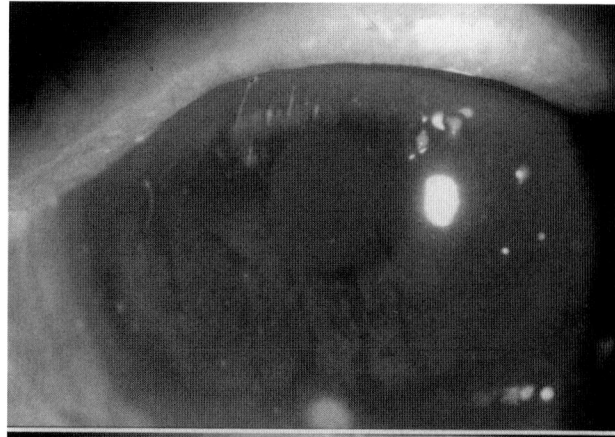
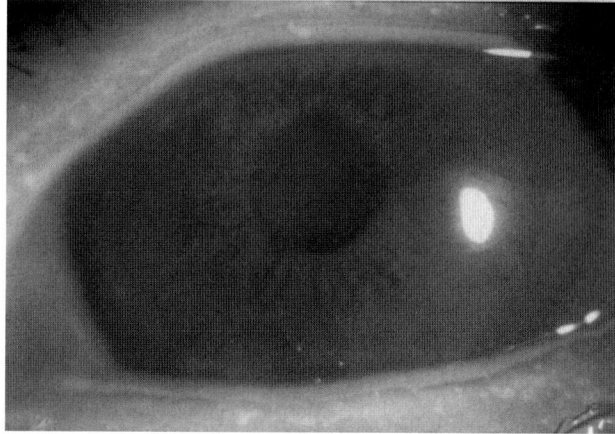

FIGURE 36-9. Filamentary keratitis in tear-deficient dry eye (*top*). Filaments disappear after punctal occlusion to both the upper and lower puncta (*bottom*).

instillation of preservative free artificial tears and/or steroid eyedrop) is the most effective form of treatment. It is presumed that a bandage soft contact lens can help avoid mechanical stress by the lid on the epithelium and facilitates epithelial healing by inhibiting the epithelial desquamation and stabilizing the attachment to the disrupted basement membrane (6), while delivering the full amount of water required under the lens. Also, temporal punctal occlusion using punctal plugs is successful by increasing tear volume in order to aid the interaction among the lid, epithelial surface, and tear film. When improvement of the interaction is obtained, permanent resolution is expected for this group.

In cases with dry eye either from tear-deficiency or evaporation, filaments are very commonly observed. Artificial tear eyedrops are often used for this group of patients, which are also helpful even for the treatment of underlying dry eye. However, to use tear substitutes that contain preservatives may be toxic to the epithelium and should be avoided. A mucolytic agent is also used for this group. Topical steroid or cyclosporine is effective in the control of dry-eye-related inflammation, and nonpreserved methylprednisolone is reportedly effective in keratoconjunctivitis sicca patients with filamentary keratitis (22). Dry eye with filaments generally correspond to relatively more severe forms of dry eye, or it accompanies relatively more severe cases of tear deficiency or evaporative state, and is often regarded as an indication of punctal occlusion to both the upper and lower puncta, and this fact will help in resolving the underlying dry eye as well as the chronic recurrence of filaments (Fig. 36-9). A bandage soft contact lens together with frequent instillation of preservative-free artificial tears may be considered as the treatment to relieve intractable pain for patients, when punctal occlusion has failed.

REFERENCES

1. Leber T. Praparate zu dem Vortag uber Entstehung der Netzhautablosung und uber verschiedene Hornhautaffecttionen. *Ber Ophthalmol Ges Heidelberg* 1882;14:165–166.
2. Wright P. Filamentary keratitis. *Trans Ophthalmol Soc UK* 1975; 95:260–266.
3. Hamilton W, Wood TO. Filamentary keratitis. *Am J Ophthalmol* 1982;93:466–469.
4. Bloomfield SE, Gasset AR, Forstot SL, et al. Treatment of filamentary keratitis with the soft contact lens. *Am J Ophthalmol* 1973;76:978–980.
5. Lohman LE, Rao GN, Aquavella JV. In vivo microscopic observations of human corneal epithelial abnormalities. *Am J Ophthalmol* 1982;93:210–217.
6. Zaidman GW, Geeraets R, Paylor RR, et al. The histopathology of filamentary keratitis. *Arch Ophthalmol* 1985;103:1178–1181.
7. Kim JC, Chung H, Tseng SCG. Botulinum toxin treatment for filamentary treatment keratitis associated with corneal occlusion by lids. In: Lass JH, ed. *Advances in corneal research.* New York: Plenum Press, 1977:105–115.
8. Rotkis WM, Chandler JW, Forstot SL. Filamentary keratitis following penetrating keratoplasty. *Ophthalmology* 1982;89: 946–949.
9. Good WV, Whitcher JP. Filamentary keratitis caused by corneal occlusion in large-angle strabismus. *Ophthalmic Surg* 1992;23:66.
10. Seedor JA, Lamberts D, Bergmann RB, et al. Filamentary keratitis associated with diphenhydramine hydrochloride (Benadryl). *Am J Ophthalmol* 1986;101:376–377.
11. Wright P, Mackie IA. Mucus in the healthy and diseased eye. *Trans Ophthalmol Soc UK* 1977;97:1–7.
12. Adams AD. The morphology of human conjunctival mucus. *Arch Ophthalmol* 1979;97:730–734.
13. Norn MS. Diagnosis of dry eye. In: Lemp MA, Marquardt R, eds. *The dry eye.* New York: Springer-Verlag, 1992:156–157.
14. Holly FJ. Biophysical aspects of epithelial adhesion to stroma. *Invest Ophthalmol Vis Sci* 1978;17:552–557.
15. Baum JL. The Castroviejo lecture. Prolonged eyelid closure is a risk to the cornea. *Cornea* 1997;16:602–611.
16. Arora I, Singhvi S. Impression debridement of corneal lesions. *Ophthalmology* 1994;101:1935–1940.
17. Tuberville AW, Frederick WR, Wood TO. Punctal occlusion in tear deficiency syndromes. *Ophthalmology* 1982;89:1170–1172.
18. Kowalik BM, Rakes JA. Filamentary keratitis—the clinical challenges. *J Am Optom Assoc* 1991;62:200–2004.
19. Jaeger W, Gotz ML, Kaercher T. Eledoisin—a successful therapeutic concept for filamentary keratitis. *Trans Ophthalmol Soc UK* 1985; 104:496.
20. Avisar R, Robinson A, Appel I, et al. Diclofenac sodium, 0.1% (Voltaren Ophtha), versus sodium chloride, 5%, in the treatment of filamentary keratitis. *Cornea* 2000;19:145–147.
21. Grinbaum A, Yassur I, Avni I. The beneficial effect of diclofenac sodium in the treatment of filamentary keratitis. *Arch Ophthalmol* 2001;119:926–927.
22. Marsh P, Pflugfelder SC. Topical nonpreserved methylprednisolone therapy for keratoconjunctivitis sicca in Sjogren syndrome. *Ophthalmology* 1999;106:811–816.

37

CLIMATIC KERATOPATHY

GARY N. FOULKS

The array of nonhereditary degenerative keratopathy related to geographic or climatic conditions or environmental exposure is vast. Climatic keratopathy is a rubric describing these various entities and presentations. Many of the names encompassed by this term are listed in Table 37-1. The conditions are degenerative corneal changes that share a common pathobiology consisting of elastotic degeneration related to chronic actinic exposure (1–28). Yellow, white, or gray lesions typically occur in the interpalpebral area of the superficial cornea, often associated with corresponding changes in the adjacent conjunctiva (21). One classification system divides spheroidal degeneration into three types: type 1 is primary, bilateral, and occurs without other evident ocular pathology; type 2 is secondary and occurs in conjunction with other ocular pathology; type 3 is the conjunctival expression of the disorder and commonly occurs in association with types 1 and 2 (10).

The incidence and severity of climatic keratopathy is geographically dependent, with a higher incidence in areas of high sun exposure. Rural areas usually have higher prevalence and increased severity of disease than metropolitan areas, probably due to differences in occupational sun exposure (17).

Familial occurrence of a similar clinical pattern of corneal deposits has been reported, particularly in Asian populations; but this disorder has a different dystrophic etiology as well as a different pathologic expression of amyloid deposits in the cornea (27–30).

CLINICAL DESCRIPTION

Climatic keratopathy is characterized by yellow, oily-appearing subepithelial deposits within the cornea in the interpalpebral area (Fig. 37-1). The changes are usually first visible in the periphery of the horizontal meridian of the cornea. The early appearance is that of minute droplets, appearing like oil, in both nasal and temporal edges of the cornea. Deposits increase in size and number with advancing age and exposure, and may extend across the cornea as a nontransparent band, prompting one description as noncalcific

band keratopathy (25,31). Similar deposits in the adjacent conjunctiva are also present but are sometimes less easily recognized (1,4,21). The condition usually occurs in association with pingueculae (1,4,20,21). The deposits initially occur superficially and may replace Bowman's zone. With advancing severity, the deposits lie deeper in the anterior cornea. Inflammation is usually absent unless secondary erosion or superinfection occur.

Symptoms are usually mild, particularly if only the periphery is involved with the deposits, but when the deposits occur centrally vision can be reduced (Fig. 37-2). Elevations of the deposits can result in desiccation of the corneal surface due to disturbance of the tear film, resulting in symptoms of foreign-body sensation and irritation. If aggravating local factors are present, the cornea may break down and ulceration can occur. Secondary infection also is a potential complication, and corneal perforation has been reported (32).

Clinical studies performed in several different parts of the world reveal that climatic keratopathy occurs most commonly in older men who have spent much time outdoors (12,26). It occurs less commonly in women, but occurs particularly in those women who spend much time outdoors (20). There is general agreement that the keratopathy is caused by exposure to environmental climatic factors (10,13,20,21). The incidence and severity vary considerably in different parts of the world, but it has been reported to occur in Africa, the Middle East, the Dahlak Islands, Australia, Newfoundland, Labrador, Italy, England, India and in various parts of North America (3,6,8,9,11,14,23,26,33–36). It is interesting to note that the frequency and severity of the disease is often greater in environments where reflection of sunlight from sand, ice, or water occurs, perhaps selecting the especially damaging wavelengths of incident actinic radiation.

PATHOLOGY

The elastoid deposits accumulating as extracellular concretions are the most striking histopathologic feature of climatic keratopathy (4,5,16,18,21,37). Figure 37-3 illustrates the

TABLE 37-1. TERMS ENCOMPASSED BY CLIMATIC KERATOPATHY

Bietti's nodular degeneration
Chronic actinic keratopathy
Climatic droplet keratopathy
Elastotic degeneration
Keratinoid degeneration
Labrador keratopathy
Non-calcific band keratopathy
Proteinaceous degeneration
Spheroidal degeneration

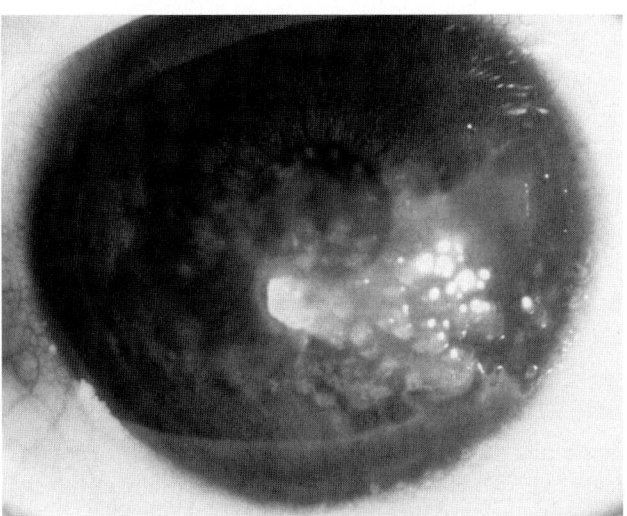

FIGURE 37-2. Extensive climatic keratopathy with yellowish discoloration of the limbal area, associated conjunctival changes, and irregular corneal surface with gray-white deposits.

morphology and yellow color of the deposits in an unstained thick section. The deposits display autofluorescence as illustrated in Fig. 37-4 when illuminated by ultraviolet light. Subepithelial location is demonstrated on the hematoxylin and eosin stained section in Fig. 37-5. Cytochemical studies reveal that the deposits are predominantly proteinaceous, with phenyl, indole, guanidyl, and sulfhydryl groups identified. Despite the oily appearance of the deposits on clinical examination, lipid is not a significant component of the concretions (21), and calcification is not a feature either. The deposits variably stain with methods that demonstrate elastin (Verhoff-Von Gieson stain). It has been suggested that the deposits represent denatured collagen that stains with elastin stains and resists digestion with elastase, but the technique of demonstrating such properties may not be reliable based on the fixation method employed (21,25). The deposits are identical to those occurring in pingueculae, in skin with actinic elastosis (solar elastosis), and at the limbus of eyes exhibiting sunlight-induced lesions (21). The deposits are ultrastructurally electron dense, appearing as extracellular, round to oval opacities of various sizes (1,16,20). Amyloid accumulation has been reported in association with the deposits (38) in one group of patients who also displayed lattice lines. Chemical analysis of the deposits has not been possible due to the small amount of material present in the cornea.

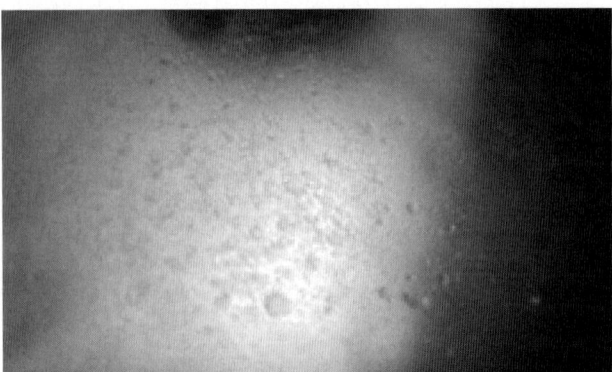

FIGURE 37-1. Early clinical appearance of deposits of climatic keratopathy. (Courtesy of George Michelson, University Eye Clinic, Erlangen, Germany, from *Atlas of Ophthalmology*, online atlas: *atlasophthalmology.com*.)

A separate form of climatic keratopathy has been identified in Saudi Arabia, with excess proteoglycan deposition and degeneration in the cornea. But the clinical appearance, although distributed in the interpalpebral area of the cornea, is more central and deeper in the stroma than the aforementioned entity (39). The condition can reduce vision. Some cases have shown amyloid deposits in addition to the presence of excess proteoglycans.

The fundamental pathobiologic process producing climatic keratopathy has been extensively discussed by Klintworth (27,28). The concretions are thought to contain derivatives of both collagen and elastin that have been denatured by chronic exposure to sunlight, particularly the ultraviolet wavelengths (24). The presence of sulfur-containing amino acid residues that are not a routine constituent of the collagen of the cornea suggest that diffusion or migration of the protein deposits could come from the breakdown of elastin fibers of the conjunctiva, which do contain sulfur-containing glycoproteins, or possibly from procollagens that also contain sulfur. It has also been suggested that the deposits could derive from the epithelium because there are histochemical similarities between the concretions and keratin (16,17). Because the chemical entities in the deposits are not normal components of the cornea, it is not likely that they represent an abnormal accumulation of a secreted native molecule. It bears emphasis that the chemical alterations occur in a chronic time course without the signs or symptoms of acute ultraviolet irradiation injury of the cornea. Lesions morphologically and histologically indistinguishable from the climatic keratopathy deposits can occur unilaterally, probably as a secondary change, in eyes with absolute glaucoma, phthisis bulbi, post-traumatic scarring and lattice dystrophy (21,25).

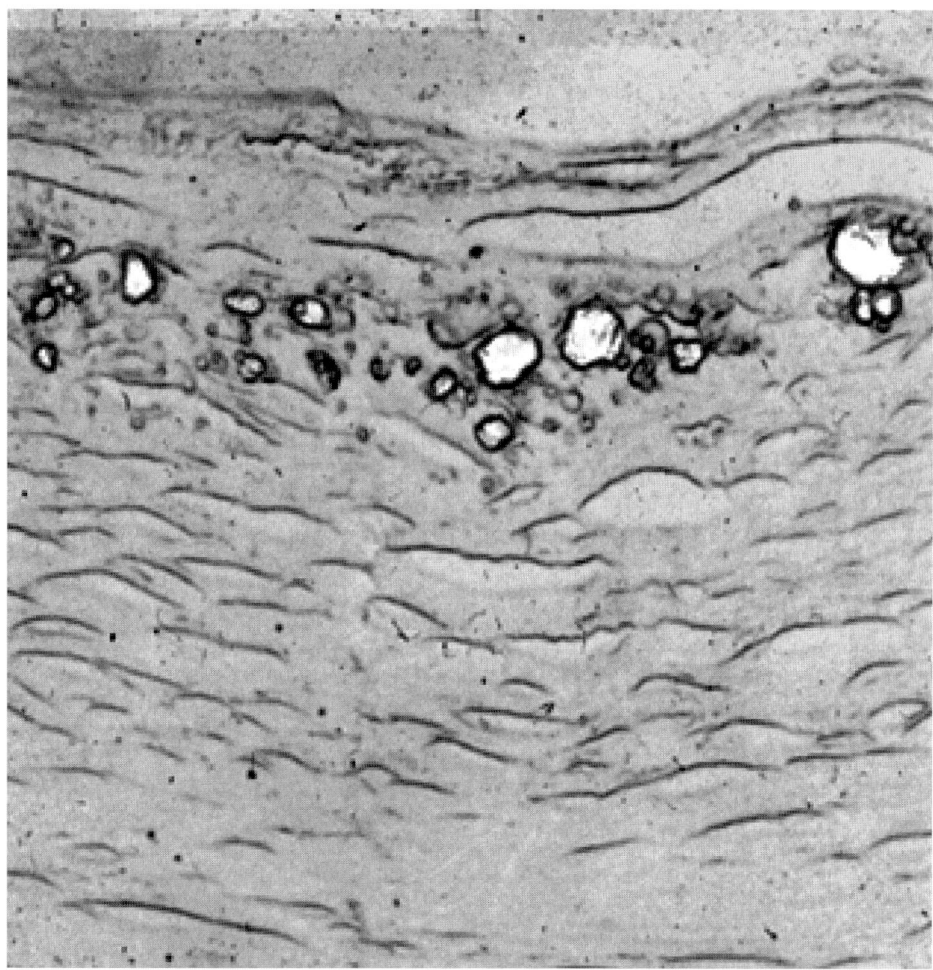

FIGURE 37-3. Unstained thick section of tissue with globular deposits. (Courtesy of Gordon K. Klintworth, MD, Duke University.)

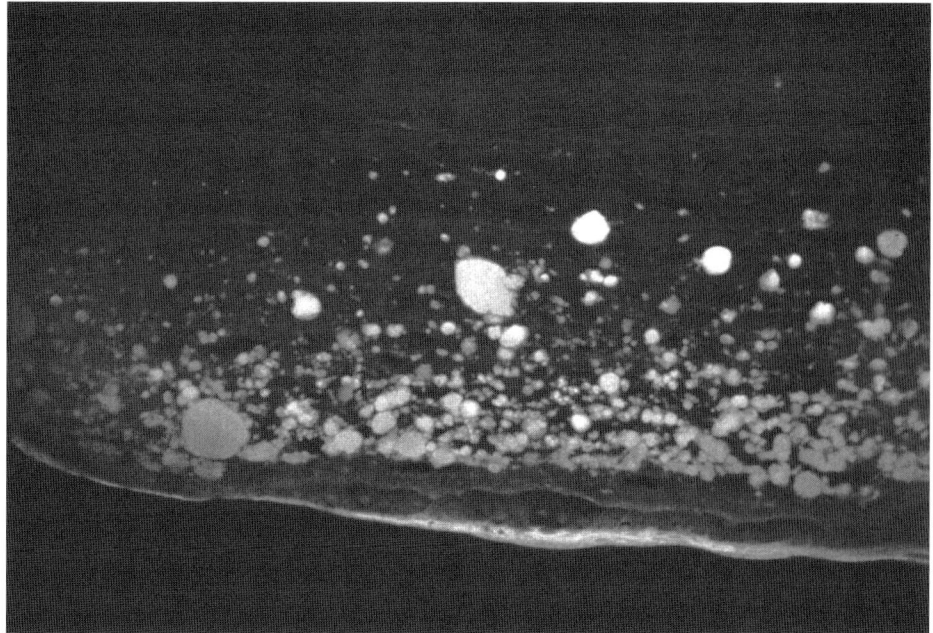

FIGURE 37-4. Autofluorescence of deposits in histologic section when viewed under ultraviolet light. (Courtesy of Gordon K. Klintworth, MD, Duke University.)

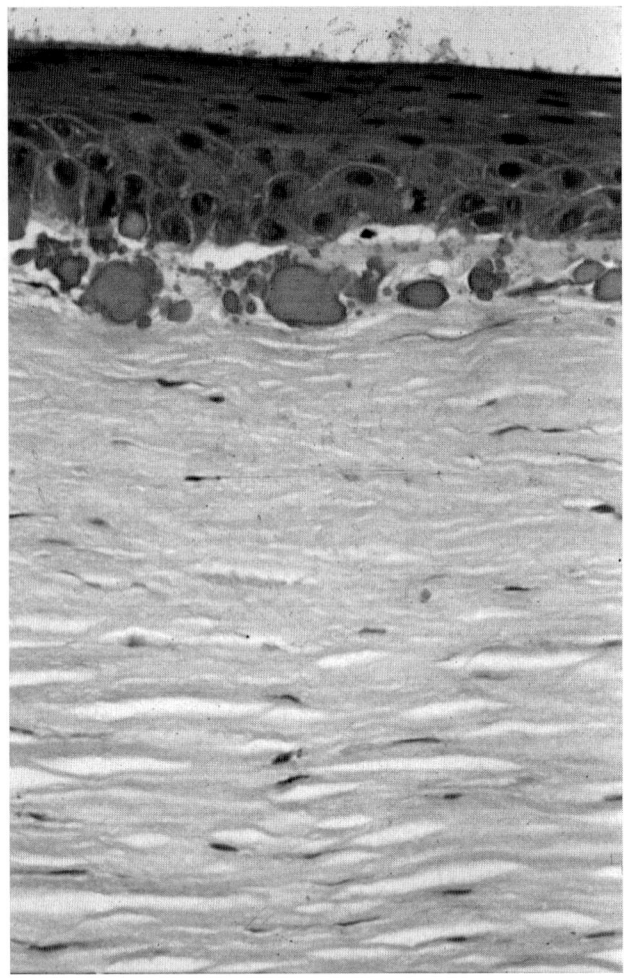

FIGURE 37-5. Hematoxylin and eosin section of tissue showing hyaline deposits.

TREATMENT

Mild involvement of the cornea with climatic keratopathy requires no treatment. If the peripheral deposits form elevated nodules that disturb the tear film resulting in punctate staining of the epithelium or corneal erosion, topical lubricants are indicated. If the lubrication therapy fails, superficial excision of the nodules is reasonable. If the central cornea is involved to the point of reducing visual acuity, superficial keratectomy is indicated. Excimer laser phototherapeutic keratectomy (PTK) has been advocated as treatment. One clinical trial demonstrated 98% success in reducing corneal opacification in patients with "smooth" climatic keratopathy, whereas "irregular" keratopathy had only an 80% success rate (40). The complication rates of delayed reepithelialization and secondary microbial keratitis were much higher in the "irregular" surface group, however, suggesting that PTK should be reserved for those corneas with a smooth opacification from the climatic keratopathy rather than an irregular surface. In severely diseased eyes, particularly if other scarring is also present, lamellar keratoplasty may be required.

REFERENCES

1. Ahmad A, Hogan M, Wood I, et al. Climatic droplet keratopathy in a 16- year old boy. *Arch Ophthalmol* 1977;95:149–151.
2. Alajmo A. Su di una forma non commune di degenerazione corneal. *Bass Ital Ottal* 1953;22:26–35.
3. Bietti GB, Guerra P, Ferraris de Gaspare PF. La dystrophie corneenne nodulair en ceinture des pays tropicaux a le sol aride: contributions cliniques et anatamo-pathologiques. *Bull Soc Fr Ophtalmol* 1955;68:101–129.
4. Brownstein S, Rodriguez MM, Fine BS, et al. The elastotic nature of hyaline corneal deposits: a histochemical, fluorescent, and electron microscopy examination. *Am J Ophthalmol* 1973;75:799–809.
5. Chrisensen GR. Proteinaceous corneal degeneration: a histochemical study. *Arch Ophthalmol* 1973;89:30–32.
6. D'Alena P, Wood IS. Labrador keratopathy: a microscopic study. *Am J Ophthalmol* 1972;74:430–435.
7. Falcone G. La distrofia corneale dei tropici. *Rav Ital Tracoma* 1954;6:3–17.
8. Falcone G. Tropical dystrophy. *East Afr Med J* 1954;31:471–475.
9. Fraunfelder FT, Hanna C, Parker JM. Spheroidal degeneration of the cornea and conjunctiva I: clinical course and characteristics. *Am J Ophthalmol* 1972;74:821–831.
10. Fraunfelder FT, Hanna C. Spheroidal degeneration of the cornea and conjunctiva III: incidence, classification, and etiology *Am J Ophthalmol* 1973;76:41–50.
11. Freedman A. Labrador keratopathy *Arch Ophthalmol* 1965;74:198–202.
12. Freedman A. Climatic droplet keratopathy I: clinical aspects *Arch Ophthalmol* 1973;89:193–197.
13. Freedman A. Labrador keratopathy and related diseases. *Can J Ophthalmol* 1973;8:286–290.
14. Freedman J. Nama keratopathy. *Br J Ophthalmol* 1973;57:688–691.
15. Gandolfi A. Osservazioni di distrofia corneale nodulare a bandellata dei paesi tropicali a suolo arido in Cirenaica (Libia). *Bull Oculist* 1962;41:129–134.
16. Garner A. Keratinoid corneal degeneration. *Br J Ophthalmol* 1970;54:769–780.
17. Garner A, Fraunfelder FT, Barras TC, et al. Spheroidal degeneration of cornea and conjunctiva. *Br J Ophthalmol* 1976;60:473–478.
18. Garner A, Morgan G, Tripathi RC. Climatic droplet keratopathy II: pathologic findings. *Arch Ophthalmol* 1973;89:198–204.
19. Hanna C, Fraunfelder FT. Spheroidal degeneration of the cornea and conjunctiva II: pathology. *Am J Ophthalmol* 1972;74:829–839.
20. Johnson CJ, Ghosh M. Labrador keratopathy: clinical and pathological findings. *Can J Ophthamol* 1975;10:119–135.
21. Klintworth GK. Chronic actinic keratopathy: a condition associated with conjunctival elastosis (pingueculae) and typified by extracellular concretions. *Am J Pathol* 1972;67:327–348.
22. Puglisi-Duranti G. Sulla degenerazione sferulare elaiode della cornea. *Bass Ital Ottalmol* 1935;4:752–766.
23. Rodger FC. Clinical findings, course, and progress of Bietti's corneal degeneration in the Dahlak islands. *Br J Ophthalmol* 1973;57:657–664.
24. Rodger FC, Cuthill JA, Fydelor PJ, et al. Ultraviolet radiation as a possible cause of corneal degenerative changes under certain

physiographic conditions. *Acta Ophthalmol (Copenh)* 1974;52: 777–785.

25. Rodriguez MM, Laibson PR, Weinreb S. Corneal elastosis: Appearance of band-like keratopathy and spheroidal degeneration. *Arch Ophthalmol* 1975;93:111–114.

26. Young YDH, Finlay RD. Primary spheroidal degeneration of the cornea in Labrador and Northern Newfoundland. *Am J Ophthalmol* 1975;79:129–134.

27. Klintworth GK. The cornea: structure and macromolecules in health and disease. *Am J Pathol* 1977;89:719–808.

28. Klintworth GK. Degeneration, depositions, and miscellaneous reactions of the cornea, conjunctiva and sclera. In: Garner A, Klintworth GK, eds. *The pathobiology of ocular disease.* New York: Marcel Dekker, 1999.

29. Nagataki S, Tanishima T, Sakamoto T. A case of primary gelatinous drop-like corneal dystrophy. *Jpn J Ophthalmol* 1972;16: 107–116.

30. Matsui M, Ito K, Akiya S. Histochemical and electron microscopic examinations on so called "gelatinous drop-like dystrophy of the cornea." *Folia Ophthalmol Jpn* 1973;23:466–473.

31. Cursino JW, Fine BS. A histological study of calcific and non-calcific band keratopathy. *Am J Ophthalmol* 1976;82: 395–404.

32. Ormerod LD, Dahan E, Hagele JE, et al. Serious occurrences in the natural history of advanced climatic keratopathy. *Ophthalmology* 1994;101:448–453.

33. Anderson J, Fuglsang H. Droplet degeneration of the cornea in North Cameroon: prevalence and clinical appearances. *Br J Ophthalmol* 1976;60:256–262.

34. Hill JC, Maske R, van der Walt S, et al. Corneal disease in rural Transkei. *S Afr Med J* 1989;75:469–472.

35. Hill JC. The prevalence of corneal disease in the coloured community of a Karoo town. *S Afr Med J* 1985;67:723–727.

36. Wyatt HT. Corneal disease in the Canadian North. *Can J Ophthalmol* 1973;8:298–305.

37. Johnson GJ, Overall M. Histology of spheroidal degeneration of the cornea in Labrador. *Br J Ophthalmol* 1978;62:53–61.

38. Matta CS, Tabbara KF, Cameron JA, et al. Climatic droplet keratopathy with corneal amyloidosis. *Ophthalmology* 1991;98: 192–195.

39. Waring GO, Mataly A, Grossnicklaus H. Climatic proteoglycan stromal keratopathy, a new corneal degeneration. *Ophthalmology* 1995;120:330–334

40. Badr IA, Al-Rajhi A, Wagoner MD, et al. Phototherapeutic keratectomy for climatic droplet keratopathy. *J Refract Surg* 1996; 12:114–122.

38

DACRYOADENITIS

**RAMZI K. HEMADY, ANH T. Q. NGUYEN, AND
SAJEEV S. KATHURIA**

INTRODUCTION AND BACKGROUND

The main lacrimal gland is an exocrine gland that contributes to the aqueous layer of the tear film. It consists of two major lobes, an orbital and a palpebral lobe, separated by the lateral extension of the levator aponeurosis. The orbital lobe is located in the lacrimal fossa of the orbit, and the palpebral lobe is located in the temporal portion of the superior fornix. Tears are excreted into the superior fornix via six to 12 lacrimal ductules that exit the palpebral lobe of the lacrimal gland. The lacrimal gland is highly vascularized and is innervated by sympathetic and parasympathetic nerves.

In his treatise on diseases of the lacrimal gland in 1803, Schmidt was the first to introduce the term *dacryoadenitis* in reference to inflammation of the main lacrimal gland (1). Dacryoadenitis is rare, with a reported incidence of approximately 1/10,000 ophthalmology visits (1–4). Males and females are equally affected, except for gonococcal dacryoadenitis, where males outnumber females (2). Dacryoadenitis may affect all age groups.

CLASSIFICATION

Dacryoadenitis may be acute or chronic, infectious or noninfectious, primary or associated with a systemic disease. Infectious causes of dacryoadenitis include viral, bacterial, fungal, and parasitic organisms. The infection may be local or systemic. Associated, noninfectious systemic conditions include Sjögren syndrome, sarcoidosis, Crohn disease, and Wegener granulomatosis. Additionally, pseudotumors of the orbit may involve the lacrimal gland.

CLINICAL MANIFESTATIONS

Acute dacryoadenitis is commonly unilateral and is usually caused by a local or systemic viral or bacterial infection. Patients present with acute pain and swelling of the lateral aspect of the upper eyelid. This may be accompanied by fever, malaise, and regional lymphadenopathy. Examination reveals eyelid edema, erythema, warmth, and occasionally proptosis and eyelid retraction (5). An S-shaped deformity of the upper lid is often noted. Induration, however, is characteristically absent. The lacrimal gland is usually enlarged and tender and the surrounding conjunctiva may be injected and chemotic. Abduction may be limited due to involvement of the lateral rectus muscle. Rarely, an abscess is detected (6,7). Vision is usually not affected.

Chronic dacryoadenitis is more commonly bilateral and may be caused by a noninfectious systemic disorder such as sarcoidosis or Sjögren syndrome. Less commonly, chronic dacryoadenitis is cased by a systemic viral infection such as mumps or the Epstein-Barr virus, or rarely by a granulomatous process such as tuberculosis or leprosy. Patients usually present with a painless mass in the superotemporal portion of the upper eyelid of several weeks' to several months' duration. Rarely, patients present with episodic upper eyelid swelling (8). Examination reveals ptosis if the lacrimal gland is significantly enlarged, and a firm, nontender mass in the area of the gland. Proptosis may be present, and the eye usually appears noninflamed.

ETIOLOGY

Dacryoadenitis may be due to local or systemic infection, noninfectious systemic disease, orbital pseudotumor, or it may be idiopathic. Infectious causes of dacryoadenitis include bacteria, viruses, fungi, and parasites. Infectious agents reach the lacrimal gland through the lacrimal ductules, nerves, blood supply, or directly after trauma (3,4).

Mumps used to be the most common cause of viral dacryoadenitis (1,3,4,9). However, widespread mumps immunization campaigns have led to a decrease in the incidence of mumps and consequently mumps-associated dacryoadenitis (4,9). Dacryoadenitis secondary to mumps is more commonly acute but may be chronic and is usually bilateral.

Several authors have reported dacryoadenitis in association with, or as the presenting sign of, Epstein-Barr virus (EBV) infections and infectious mononucleosis (1,3,4,9–12). Jones

(10) in 1955 deduced that one out of every 300 patients with infectious mononucleosis developed dacryoadenitis. In a more recent report by Rhem and colleagues (12), EBV accounted for approximately one third of all cases of dacryoadenitis seen over a 16-year period in a university practice. EBV dacryoadenitis is usually acute and bilateral. Chronic and unilateral cases have been reported, however. Clinical and laboratory evidence suggest a relationship between EBV infections and the development of primary Sjögren's syndrome (13–22).

In his manuscript on the etiology of dacryoadenitis published in 1955, Jones (10) reported a case of acute dacryoadenitis caused by herpes zoster infection. More recently, Obata and colleagues (23) reported a case of acute dacryoadenitis in a 30-year-old man associated with herpes zoster ophthalmicus. Herpes simplex viruses have also been associated with the development of acute dacryoadenitis (24). Herpes virus–related dacryoadenitis may be especially severe in immunocompromised patients.

A variety of bacteria have been associated with acute and chronic dacryoadenitis. *Staphylococcus* sp. are some of the most common bacterial cases of acute dacryoadenitis (1,3,4,9). Others include *Streptococcus* sp. and *Treponema pallidum.* Syphilitic dacryoadenitis may occur at any stage of the disease (3). Gonococcal infections of the lacrimal gland are usually acute, bilateral, and more common in males (2). The infectious agent reaches the lacrimal glands by direct extension from the conjunctiva, or by metastasis. Bekir and colleagues (25,26) from Turkey reported unilateral dacryoadenitis in a 16-year-old boy, and bilateral dacryoadenitis in a 34-year-old woman in association with systemic brucellosis. In a report published in 1997, Mawn and colleagues (27) described a case of pseudomonas dacryoadenitis secondary to a lacrimal ductule stone.

Chronic dacryoadenitis secondary to bacterial infections is rare. Tuberculosis is probably the most common bacterial cause of chronic dacryoadenitis (1,4,9,28). Sen (29) reported dacryoadenitis as the presenting manifestation of tuberculosis in one of 14 patients with tuberculosis orbital involvement. Madhukar and colleagues (30) reported a rare case of lacrimal gland abscess secondary to tuberculosis. The development of true dacryoadenitis secondary to trachoma is controversial (1). Fungal and parasitic infections of the lacrimal glands are exceedingly rare (1,4,9,31,32).

Acute dacryoadenitis may be the presenting manifestation of either the limited or the complete forms of Wegener's granulomatosis (33,34). The dacryoadenitis may be unilateral or bilateral. In a report by Spalton and colleagues (35), dacryoadenitis was present in one out of eight patients with the limited form of Wegener's granulomatosis. Dutt and colleagues (36) reported a 14-year-old boy with acute, bilateral dacryoadenitis associated with Crohn's disease.

Chronic dacryoadenitis is the most common orbital manifestation of sarcoidosis and has been reported in 7% to 69% of patients with sarcoidosis, and 16% to 37% of patients with ocular sarcoidosis (Fig. 38-1)(37). It is more

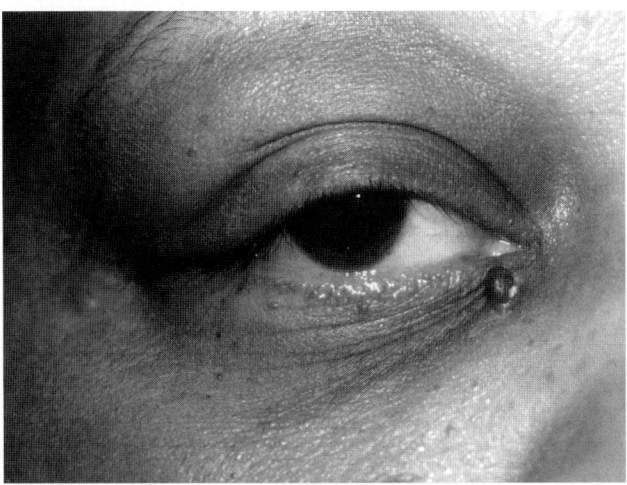

FIGURE 38-1. Enlarged right lacrimal gland in a patient with chronic dacryoadenitis secondary to biopsy-proven sarcoidosis.

common in black patients and may lead to dry eyes. Less commonly, sarcoidosis-associated dacryoadenitis has an acute onset. Chronic, progressive lacrimal gland enlargement with lymphoid cell infiltration may be seen in patients with primary or secondary Sjögren's syndrome.

Nonspecific enlargement of the lacrimal and salivary glands with xerostomia is referred to as Mikulicz syndrome (1). This may be associated with leukemia, lymphoma, tuberculosis, and sarcoidosis, among other conditions.

Pseudotumor of the orbit is defined as idiopathic, nonspecific orbital inflammation (38,39). The orbital inflammation may be generalized or focal. The lacrimal gland may be the site of focal inflammation (38–41). The orbital lobe of the lacrimal gland is more commonly affected than the palpebral lobe. The inflammation is usually unilateral and acute. Patients present in the third through the fifth decades of life with a palpable and tender mass in the superotemporal aspect of the upper eyelid with an S-shaped deformity. Inferonasal proptosis may be present. Less commonly, the presentation may be chronic with painless enlargement of the lacrimal gland evolving over several months. Males and females are equally affected.

Joussen and colleagues (42) reported a case of lymphocytic hypophysitis associated with acute, unilateral daryoadenitis. Pathologic examination revealed B- and T-cell infiltration.

Mouse models suggest a possible role for testosterone, T cells, adhesion molecules, and upregulation of local cytokines in the pathogenesis of autoimmune dacryoadenitis and primary Sjögren's syndrome (43–47). These findings may have future therapeutic implications in humans (48).

DIFFERENTIAL DIAGNOSIS

Benign and malignant tumors of the lacrimal gland must be included in the differential diagnosis of dacryoadenitis (49–51). Approximately half of all lacrimal gland masses are inflammatory, and the other half are neoplastic (50,51). The orbital lobe is more commonly involved in neoplastic lesions of the lacrimal gland than the palpebral lobe. Malignant tumors usually cause a diffuse and irregular enlargement of the lacrimal gland and may cause destruction of adjacent bone (49–51). The most common such tumor is adenoid cystic carcinoma (50,51). Benign tumors, such as the benign mixed tumors, may cause diffuse enlargement of the lacrimal gland, or may arise from the margin of the gland (50,51). Metastasis of distant malignancies to the lacrimal gland is rare.

Lymphoproliferative disorders may also affect the lacrimal glands. Lymphomatous invasion of the lacrimal gland is usually diffuse and may be bilateral. Patients usually present with a painless mass that may be fixed to the orbital rim and often has a characteristic salmon-pink color. Bone erosion is rare.

True lacrimal gland enlargement is rarely seen in patients with Graves' disease. Lacrimal gland prolapse, however, is not uncommon and may be mistaken for enlargement of the gland. Dermoid cysts often occur in the superolateral quadrant of the orbit and can simulate the appearance of an enlarged lacrimal gland.

DIAGNOSIS

In certain cases of infectious dacryoadenitis such as mumps or herpes zoster, the diagnosis may be clinically obvious. In most cases, however, a workup is necessary to establish the etiology.

Radiologic imaging studies are essential in the workup of patients with lacrimal gland lesions (38,50–54). Computed tomography (CT), magnetic resonance imaging (MRI), and B-scan ultrasonography may reveal the location and extent of the lesion (Fig. 38-2). CT scans are the most helpful imaging studies in evaluating lacrimal gland masses (38,50–54). Bone changes are best evaluated with CT scans (Fig. 38-3). In acute dacryoadenitis, the lacrimal gland is usually diffusely enlarged. Contrast may show associated lateral rectus myositis and scleritis. In chronic dacryoadenitis, the lacrimal gland may be massively enlarged, but scleral enhancement is rare. Bone compression or erosion is not a feature of acute or chronic dacryoadenitis.

CT scans of the lacrimal gland infiltrated with lymphoid tumors also reveal diffuse enlargement. In contrast to dacryoadenitis, however, the mass is oblong with contouring, molding, and draping of the gland around the globe. The mass tends to be bulkier and often shows evidence of anterior and posterior extension.

CT scans of pseudotumors of the lacrimal gland reveal findings typical for orbital inflammation including enhancement with contrast, a mass with indistinct borders and involvement of contiguous tissues such as the globe,

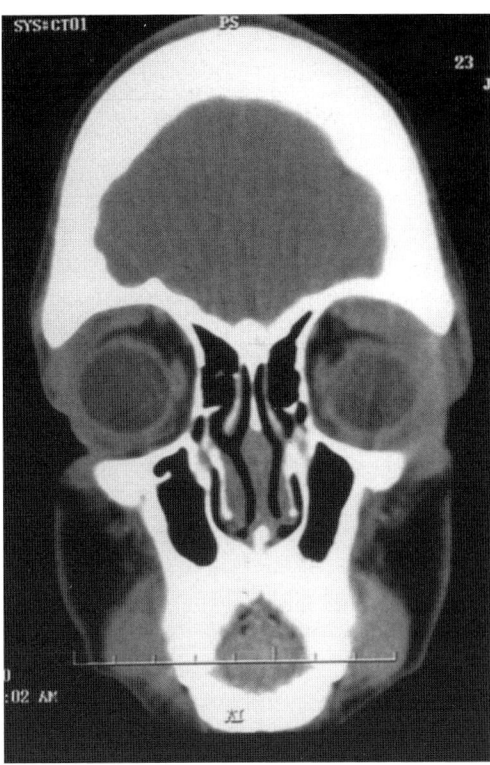

FIGURE 38-2. Computed tomography (CT) scan, coronal section, showing an enlarged left lacrimal gland in a patient with chronic dacryoadenitis secondary to sarcoidosis.

the lateral rectus muscle, and fat (38). Orbital bone involvement and extension outside the orbit are rare.

Benign mixed tumors of the lacrimal gland are round to oval and usually have a smooth contour due to their characteristic encapsulation. The orbital contents are usually displaced, and the globe is flattened contiguous to the tumor. Patients with benign mixed tumors typically present with painless masses of greater than 12 months' duration.

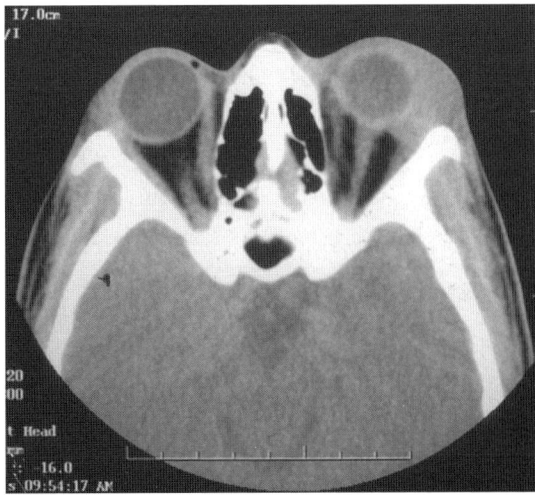

FIGURE 38-3. CT scan, cross section, showing absence of bone involvement in a patient with chronic dacryoadenitis.

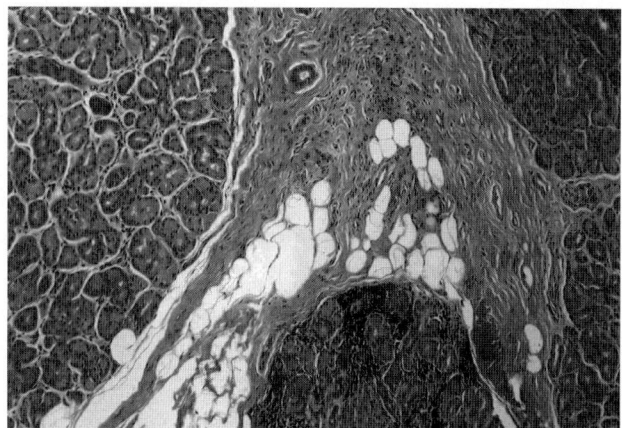

FIGURE 38-4. Histopathology of a lacrimal gland biopsy in a patient with chronic dacryoadenitis secondary to sarcoidosis showing lymphoid hyperplasia.

Malignant tumors often distort the globe and orbital contents, have irregular margins, and frequently show bone erosion. In contrast, bone erosion and compression are not features of inflammatory lesions of the lacrimal glands. Clinically, adenoid cystic carcinomas may be painful. The duration of symptoms is usually less than 12 months.

Ultrasonography reveals enlargement of the gland with a homogeneous acoustic pattern in cases of acute dacryoadenitis. Ultrasonography may also help differentiate lymphoproliferative lesions (lymphoma, pseudotumor) from epithelial tumors (benign mixed tumor, adenoid cystic carcinoma) involving the gland.

Open biopsy or fine-needle aspiration biopsy of the lacrimal gland may be especially helpful in the diagnosis of chronic dacryoadenitis (55). We prefer open biopsies to ensure a specimen of adequate size, and to enable marker studies for lymphoma if necessary (Fig. 38-4). If an open biopsy is performed, the palpebral lobe of the gland and the lacrimal ductules should be avoided due to the risk of inducing dry eyes. Any discharge should be cultured. Blood cultures are usually negative and are not necessary.

Laboratory investigations may be directed at the suspected etiology. These include mumps and EBV-specific antibody titers; angiotensin-converting enzyme (ACE), chest x-ray, gallium scan, purified protein derivative (PPD), and skin anergy panel for sarcoidosis and tuberculosis; salivary or lacrimal gland biopsy, antinuclear antibodies (ANA) and anti-SSA and anti-SSB titers for Sjögren's syndrome; cytoplasmic-staining antineutrophil cytoplasmic antibody (cANCA) and radiologic examination of the sinuses for Wegener's granulomatosis; human leukocyte antigen (HLA) typing, gastrointestinal imaging, colonoscopy, and biopsy for Crohn's disease; nonspecific [rapid plasma reagent (RPR), Venereal Disease Research Laboratory (VDRL)] and specific fluorescent treponema antibody (FTA) testing for syphilis; and radiologic studies and biopsy for pseudotumor, which is usually a diagnosis of exclusion.

Treatment

Treatment of dacryoadenitis depends on the etiology and the severity of symptoms. Dacryoadenitis due to mumps and EBV is usually self-limited, resolves in 4 to 6 weeks or less, and does not require therapy. Warm compresses and analgesics offer symptomatic relief and systemic corticosteroids may hasten recovery in more symptomatic cases. Severe viral dacryoadenitis in immunocompromised patients may respond well to a combination of systemic antiviral agents and corticosteroids. Bacterial dacryoadenitis requires treatment with systemic antibiotics; topical antibiotics do not penetrate lacrimal tissue adequately. The choice of antibiotic is based on the pathogen. Any abscess should be incised and drained. Dacryoadenitis secondary to tuberculosis, syphilis, or brucellosis should be treated with the appropriate systemic antimicrobials.

Dacryoadenitis associated with sarcoidosis and Crohn's disease usually responds well to systemic corticosteroids, whereas dacryoadenitis secondary to Wegener granulomatosis requires secondary immunosuppressive therapy.

Systemic corticosteroids are the traditional treatment for pseudotumors, including those that involve the lacrimal gland (39,41). Recurrences, however, are relatively common. The therapeutic response is especially poor in fibrotic and mass lesions. Alternative therapies include radiation and surgical excision. Radiation has been reported to be useful in cases of diffuse, nonfibrotic lesions of the lacrimal gland. In separate reports, Char and Miller (55), and Mombaerts and colleagues (56) reported successful outcomes after complete surgical tumor removal and debulking, especially in cases of discrete mass lesions. Dry eyes developed in 43% of patients, however. Dry eye was more common if the palpebral lobe was removed.

PROGNOSIS

The prognosis of dacryoadenitis is generally excellent regardless of the etiology (1,4,9). Some acute cases may progress to a subacute or chronic stage. EBV infections of the lacrimal gland have been implicated in the pathogenesis of Sjögren's syndrome and dry eyes. In separate reports, Pflugfelder et al. (15), Gaston et al. (17), and Merayo-Lloves et al. (21) reported the onset of primary Sjögren's syndrome after EBV infections. Additionally, Pflugfelder et al. (18,19) and others (13,16) detected chronic EBV infections in the lacrimal and salivary glands of patients with Sjögren's syndrome. Flescher and Talal (20), however, hypothesized that EBV was only a cofactor in the development of Sjögren's syndrome. Dry eyes may also result from inadvertent damage to the palpebral lobe or lacrimal ductules during a diagnostic biopsy of the lacrimal gland. One case of fatal meningitis has been reported secondary to untreated, acute, purulent dacryadenitis (1).

Rarely, a lacrimal cyst or fistula may develop as a consequence of dacryadenitis (1).

ACKNOWLEDGMENT

We would like to acknowledge the Department of Pathology at the University of Maryland School of Medicine, Baltimore, for providing the histopathology figure.

REFERENCES

1. Duke-Elder S, MacFaul PA. Inflammation of the lacrimal gland. In: Duke-Elder S, ed. *System of ophthalmology,* vol 13, *The ocular adnexa.* St Louis: CV Mosby 1974:601–624.
2. Richardson JM. Acute metastatic gonorrheal dacryoadenitis. A clinical and histologic study. *Arch Ophthalmol* 1942;28:93–133.
3. Jones BR. The clinical features and aetiology of dacryoadenitis. *Trans Ophthalmol Soc UK* 1955;75:435–450.
4. Fitzsimmons TD, Wilson SE, Kennedy RH. Infectious dacryoadenitis. In: Pepose JS, Holland GN, Wilhelmus KR, eds. *Ocular infection and immunity.* St Louis: CV Mosby, 1996:1341–1345.
5. Chang WJ, Goyal AK, Flanagan JC. Dacryoadenitis presenting with eyelid retraction. *Ophthalmic Surg* 1995;26:380–382.
6. Harris GJ, Snyder RW. Lacrimal gland abscess. *Am J Ophthalmol* 1987;104:193–194.
7. McNab A. Lacrimal gland abscesses: two case reports. *Aust NZ J Ophthalmol* 1999;27:75–78.
8. Gundiz K, Gunalp I, Ozden RG. Chronic dacryoadenitis misdiagnosed as eyelid edema and allergic conjunctivitis. *Jpn J Ophthalmol* 1999;43:109–112.
9. Tabbara KF. Infections of the lacrimal apparatus. In: Tabbara KF, Hyndiuk RA, eds. *Infections of the eye.* Boston: Little, Brown, 1986:543–545.
10. Jones BR. Lacrimal disease associated with infectious mononucleosis. *Trans Ophthalmol Soc UK* 1955;75:101–119.
11. Aburn NS, Sullivan TJ. Infectious mononucleosis presenting with dacryoadenitis. *Ophthalmology* 1996;103:776–778.
12. Rhem MN, Wilhelmus KR, Jones DB. Epstein-Barr virus dacryoadenitis. *Am J Ophthalmol* 2000;129:372–375.
13. Fox R, Pearson G, Vaughn J. Detection of Epstein-Barr virus-associated antigens and DNA in salivary gland biopsies from patients with Sjögren syndrome. *J Immunol* 1986;137:3162–3168.
14. Whittingham S, McNeilage J, Mackay IR. Epstein-Barr virus as an etiological agent in primary Sjögren syndrome. *Med Hypotheses* 1987;22:373–386.
15. Pflugfelder SC, Roussel TJ, Culbertson WW. Primary Sjögren's syndrome after infectious mononucleosis. *JAMA* 1987;257:1049–1050.
16. Crouse CA, Pflugfelder SC, Cleary T, et al. Detection Epstein-Barr virus genomes in normal human lacrimal glands. *J Clin Microbiol* 1990;28:1026–1032.
17. Gaston JSH, Rowe M, Bacon P. Sjögren's syndrome after infection by Epstein-Barr virus. *J Rheumatol* 1990;17:558–561.
18. Pflugfelder SC, Tseng SCG, Pepose JS, et al. Epstein-Barr virus infection and immunologic dysfunction in patients with aqueous tear deficiency. *Ophthalmology* 1990;97:313–323.
19. Pflugfelder SC, Crouse C, Pereira I, et al. Amplification of Epstein-Barr virus genomic sequences in blood cells, lacrimal glands and tears from primary Sjögren's syndrome patients. *Ophthlamology* 1990;97:976–984.
20. Flescher E, Talal N. Do viruses contribute to the development of Sjögren's syndrome. *Am J Med* 1991;90:283–285.
21. Merayo-Lloves J, Baltatzis S, Foster CS. Epstein-Barr virus dacryoadenitis resulting in keratoconjunctivitis sicca in a child. *Am J Ophthalmol* 2001;132:922–923.
22. Thomson J, Vassiliou G, Veys P, et al. Epstein-Barr virus dacryoadenitis as a complication of bone marrow transplant in a child with combined immunodeficiency. *Eye* 2001;15:815–816.
23. Obata H, Yamagami S, Saito S, et al. A case of acute dacryoadenitis associated with herpes zoster ophthalmicus. *Jpn J Ophthalmol* 2003;47:107–109.
24. Pierce PF. Infections of the orbit and orbital structures. In: Bosniak S, ed. *Principles and practice of ophthalmic and reconstructive surgery.* Philadelphia: WB Saunders, 1996:153.
25. Bekir NA, Gungor K, Namiduru M. Brucella melitensis dacryoadenitis: a case report. *Eur J Ophthalmol* 2000;10:259–261.
26. Bekir NA, Gungor K. Bilateral dacryoadenitis associated with brucellosis. *Acta Ophthalmol Scand* 1999;77:357–358.
27. Mawn LA, Sanon A, Conlon MR, et al. Pseudomonas dacryoadenitis secondary to a lacrimal gland ductule stone. *Ophthalmic Plast Reconstr Surg* 1997;13:135–138.
28. vanAssen S, Lutterman JA. Tuberculous dacryoadenitis: a rare manifestation of tuberculosis. *Neth J Med* 2002;60:327–329.
29. Sen DK. Tuberculosis of the orbit and lacrimal gland: a clinical study of 14 cases. *J Pediatr Ophthlamol Strabismus* 1980;17:232–238.
30. Madhukar K, Bhide M, Prasad CE. Tuberculosis of the lacrimal gland. *J Trop Med Hyg* 1991;94:150–151.
31. Jakobie FA, Gess L, Zimmerman LE. Granulomatous dacryoadenitis caused by Schistosoma haematobium. *Arch Ophthalmol* 1977;95:278–280.
32. Sen DK. Acute suppurative dacryoadenitis caused by a cysticercus cellulose. *J Pediatr Ophthalmol Strabismus* 1982;19:100–102.
33. Leavitt JA, Butrus SI. Wegener's granulomatosis presenting as dacryoadenitis. *Cornea* 1991;10:542–545.
34. Soheilian M, Bagheri A, Aletaha M. Dacryoadenitis as the earliest presenting manifestation of systemic Wegener's granulomatosis. *Eur J Ophthalmol* 2002;12:241–243.
35. Spalton DJ, Graham EM, Page NGR, et al. Ocular changes in limited form of Wegener's granulomatosis. *Br J Ophthalmol* 1981;65:553–563.
36. Dutt S, Cartwright MJ, Nelson CC. Acute dacryoadenitis and Crohn's disease: findings and management. *Ophthalmic Plast Reconstr Surg* 1992;8:295–299.
37. White VA, Rootman J. Orbital pathology. In: Albert DM, Jakobiec FA, eds. *Principles and practice of ophthalmology,* vol 4. Philadelphia: WB Saunders, 1994:2343.
38. Weber AL, Romo LV, Sabates NR. Pseudotumor of the orbit. Clinical, pathologic and radiologic evaluation. *Radiat Clin North Am* 1999;37:151–168.
39. Harms W. Pseudotumors. In: Bosniak S, ed. *Principles and practice of ophthalmic plastic and reconstructive surgery.* Philadelphia: WB Saunders, 1996:964–966.
40. Gunalp K, Gunduz K, Yazar Z. Idiopathic orbital inflammatory disease. *Acta Ophthalmol Scand* 1996;74:191–193.
41. Snebold NG. Orbital pseudotumor syndromes. *Curr Opin Ophthalmol* 1997;8:41–44.
42. Joussen AM, Sommer C, Flechtenmacher C, et al. Lymphocytic hypophysitis associated with dacryoadenitis. An autoimmunologically mediated syndrome. *Arch Ophthalmol* 1999;117:959–962.
43. Liu SH, Zhou DH, Hess AD. Adoptive transfer of experimental autoimmune dacryoadenitis in susceptible and resistant mice. *Cell Immunol* 1993;150:311–320.

44. Takahashi M, Mimura Y, Hayashi Y. Role of the ICAM-1/LFA-1 pathway during the development of autoimmune dacryoadenitis in an animal model for Sjögren's syndrome. *Pathobiology* 1996; 64:269–274.
45. Takahashi M, Mimura Y, Hamano H, et al. Mechanism of the development of autoimmune dacryoadenitis in the mouse model for primary Sjögren's syndrome. *Cell Immunol* 1996;170:54–62.
46. Takahashi M, Ishimaru N, Yanagi K, et al. High incidence of autoimmune dacryoadenitis in male non-obese diabetic (NOD) mice depending on sex steroids. *Clin Exp Immunol* 1997;109: 555–561.
47. Hunger RE, Carnaud C, Vogt I, et al. Male gonadal environment paradoxically promotes dacryoadenitis in nonobese diabetic mice. *J Clin Invest* 1998;101:1300–1309.
48. Liu SH, Zhou DH, Gottsch JD, et al. Treatment of experimental autoimmune dacryoadenitis with cyclosporin A. *Clin Immunol Immunopathol* 1993;67:78–83.
49. Harris GJ, Dixon TA, Haughton VM. Expansion of the lacrimal gland fossa by a lymphoid tumor. *Am J Ophthalmol* 1983;96: 546–547.
50. Sutula FC. Tumors of the lacrimal gland. In: Albert DM, Jakobied FA, eds. *Principles and practice of ophthalmology.* Philadelphia: WB Saunders, 1994:1952–1967.
51. Weber AL. Radiologic evaluation of the orbits and sinuses. In: Albert DM, Jakobied FA, eds. *Principles and practice of ophthalmology.* Philadelphia: WB Saunders 1994:3531–3533.
52. Mafee MF, Haik BG. Lacrimal gland and fossa lesions: role of computed tomography. *Radiat Clin North Am* 1987;25:767–779.
53. Milite JP, McCormich SA. The orbit. In: Bosniak S, ed. *Principles and practice of ophthalmic plastic and reconstructive surgery.* Philadelphia: WB Saunders, 1996:964.
54. Snebold NG. Noninfectious orbital inflammations and vasculitis. In: Albert DM, Jakobied FA, eds. *Principles and practice of ophthalmology.* Philadelphia: WB Saunders, 1994:1926.
55. Char DH, Miller T. Orbital pseudotumor. Fine-needle aspiration biopsy and response to therapy. *Ophthalmology* 1993;100: 1702–1710.
56. Mombaerts I, Schlingermann RO, Goldshmeding R, et al. The surgical management of lacrimal gland pseudotumors. *Ophthalmology* 1996;103:1619–1627.

SECTION

VII

METABOLIC AND
CONGENITAL DISEASE

CONGENITAL ABNORMALITIES AND METABOLIC DISEASES AFFECTING THE CONJUNCTIVA AND CORNEA

NADIA K. WAHEED AND NATHALIE AZAR

CONGENITAL ABNORMALITIES

Clinical Aspects

Congenital anomalies of the cornea are the result of abnormal corneal development and are evident as alterations in the morphology of the cornea at birth. This is in contrast to metabolic diseases of the cornea and to corneal dystrophies, which occur in previously normal tissue and appear clinically only some time after birth.

Absence of the Cornea and Agenesis of the Anterior Segment

Agenesis of the cornea is unknown as an isolated abnormality. In such cases, there is usually variable absence of other ocular structures derived from the surface ectoderm (1). The result is a scleral shell lined with choroid, retinal pigment epithelium, and retina, but lacking cornea, anterior chamber, iris, ciliary body, and lens. The affected eye is usually small. Ultrasonography may be used to distinguish this condition from true cryptophthalmos. Embryologically, this abnormality occurs when the optic vesicle forms and invaginates to form the optic cup, but the anterior segment fails to differentiate. This abnormality is a form of microphthalmos because it occurs after the formation of the optic vesicle and because the affected eye is usually small.

Cryptophthalmos

True cryptophthalmos (ablepharon) happens when the lids fail to form (1–3). The exposed cornea undergoes metaplasia to skin and so appears to be absent. Because the skin covering the eye is essentially metaplastic corneal tissue, the brows and lashes are absent, which allows for easy differentiation of cryptophthalmos from pseudocryptophthalmos (total ankyloblepharon), in which brows and lashes are present. In true cryptophthalmos, the lacrimal gland and puncta are likely to be missing as well, and the anterior segment of the globe is usually disorganized (4). Affected patients have a layer of skin extending from the forehead to the malar region. An *incomplete form* in which only the nasal aspect of the lid fold is involved is recognized. Still another presentation is the *abortive form,* in which the upper eyelid is replaced by a fold of skin that is adherent to the upper third of the cornea; the lower eyelid is normal (5). Even in the complete form, the underlying eye moves and may even show some reaction to bright light in the form of contractions of the periocular skin. However, attempts to treat it are futile, because any incision into the overlying skin will result in entry into the malformed eye. The only advantage of a cutaneous incision may be some slight cosmetic benefit. Embryologically, cryptophthalmos results from a failure of formation of the eyelid folds.

Cryptophthalmos is rare, with only about 50 cases reported. It is usually transmitted as an autosomal-recessive trait and may be unilateral or bilateral. When it is unilateral, the other eye may have symblepharon or coloboma of the eyelid. Males and females are affected equally.

When cryptophthalmos occurs in association with other systemic abnormalities, as it often does, the condition is described as cryptophthalmos syndrome. Associated systemic abnormalities include, most commonly, syndactyly, genitourinary anomalies, and craniofacial anomalies. Less commonly, spina bifida, deformed ears or teeth, cleft palate or lip, laryngeal or anal atresia, ventral hernias, cardiac anomalies, displacement of the nipples or umbilicus, basal encephaloceles, and mental retardation may also occur (2,5–7). Renal agenesis has been documented in siblings of patients with this syndrome.

Total Ankyloblepharon

In this condition, a fully formed eye is covered by skin. The lid folds are formed but fail to separate. Brows and lashes are present. Incision may be of some value, to expose the globe covered by the lid, although the newly formed lids tend to close again (1,8).

Abnormalities of Size

Megalocornea

Megalocornea is characterized by a primarily enlarged diameter of the cornea (more than 13 mm in horizontal diameter) in the absence of previous or concurrent elevated intraocular pressure (1–3). The corneal enlargement may occur as an isolated anomaly (*simple megalocornea*) or in association with enlargement of the ciliary ring and lens (*anterior megalophthalmos*) (9). Simple megalocornea is usually a nonprogressive, usually symmetric, inherited condition. Megalocornea is usually X-linked recessive, with 90% of cases in males, although all forms of inheritance have been reported, including occasionally dominant, less often recessive and germ-line mosaicism also reported (10).

Some patients with megalocornea are myopic because of increased corneal curvature, although the curvature may also be normal. With-the-rule astigmatism is often present when the corneal curvature is increased. Megalocornea can be differentiated from congenital glaucoma by the normal intraocular pressure, the clarity of the cornea, and the normal optic nerve in simple megalocornea. Moreover, megalocornea demonstrates normal endothelial cell population densities on specular microscopy, whereas in congenital glaucoma, these are diminished, ostensibly because of corneal distention (11). Studies have also suggested the use of A-scan ultrasonography to distinguish features of megalocornea that are not present in glaucoma, including increased anterior chamber depth, posterior lens and iris positioning, and short vitreous length (12). Some people believe megalocornea represents congenital glaucoma that has been arrested, but a histopathologic report on an eye with megalocornea did not show the angle abnormalities classically seen in congenital glaucoma. However, both megalocornea and congenital glaucoma have been reported in the same families and even in the same person (13,14).

Anterior megalophthalmos is associated with enlargement of the lens-iris diaphragm and ciliary body in addition to the cornea. This condition may be associated with a large myopic astigmatic error. The iris may demonstrate iris transillumination defects. The condition is usually harmless except for three complications that may appear later in life: ectopia lentis due to the abnormal architecture; glaucoma secondary to lens subluxation; and cataract, which is usually posterior subcapsular but may be nuclear or peripheral. Other associated abnormalities include Marfan's syndrome, Apert's syndrome, and mucolipidosis type II (1–3,14,15).

Megalocornea is probably the result of a failure of the anterior tips of the optic cup to grow sufficiently close to one another, the remaining space being taken up by the cornea. Other possible explanations are that it represents an exaggeration of the normal tendency for the cornea to be large, relative to the rest of the eye, from embryonic life to the age of 7 years; an atavistic regression to the tendency for nonhuman

TABLE 39-1. ABNORMALITIES ASSOCIATED WITH MEGALOCORNEA

Ocular
  Myopia
  Astigmatism
  Arcus juvenilis
  Krukenberg's spindle
  Mosaic corneal dystrophy
  Hypoplasia of iris stroma and pigment epithelium
  Miosis (hypoplasia of iris dilator)
  Prominent iris processes
  Pigmentation of trabecular meshwork
  Open-angle glaucoma
  Congenital glaucoma (rare)
  Cataract (usually posterior subcapsular)
  Ectopia lentis
Systemic
  Marfan's syndrome
  Craniosynostosis
  Lamellar ichthyosis
  Mental retardation (with recessive megalocornea)

mammals to have larger corneas relative to their globes; or spontaneously arrested congenital glaucoma.

Table 39-1 lists other abnormalities associated with megalocornea.

Microcornea

A microcornea is one that has an adult horizontal diameter of less than 11 mm (1,3). Note that the cornea usually reaches its adult size around 2 years of age. Microcornea can occur as an isolated anomaly, or the whole anterior segment may be small, in which case the term *anterior microphthalmos* applies. *Nanophthalmos* indicates an eye that is small but otherwise normal, and *microphthalmos* refers to a small eye that is also malformed in other ways.

Patients with microcornea are likely to be hyperopic because their corneas are relatively flat, but any kind of refractive error is possible owing to variations in length of the globe. Open-angle glaucoma develops later in life in 20% of patients, and some predisposition to narrow-angle glaucoma also exists because of the shallow anterior chamber with crowding of the anterior chamber structures seen in anterior microphthalmos. Congenital glaucoma coexists occasionally. An eye with microcornea (or microphthalmos) is sometimes misinterpreted as being normal in comparison to its fellow (actually normal) eye, which is thought erroneously to have corneal enlargement from congenital glaucoma. Certain somatic abnormalities have been described in conjunction with microcornea and anterior microphthalmos, including dwarfism and Ehlers-Danlos syndrome. Table 39-2 lists other problems that are sometimes associated with microcornea (1,16,17).

Microcornea is thought to be caused by an overgrowth of the anterior tips of the optic cup, leaving less than normal

TABLE 39-2. ABNORMALITIES ASSOCIATED WITH MICROCORNEA

Ocular
  Hyperopia (other refractive errors possible)
  Cornea plana
  Corneal leukoma
  Mesodermal remnants in angle
  Aniridia
  Uveal coloboma
  Corectopia
  Persistent pupillary membrane
  Congenital cataract
  Microphakia
  Open-angle glaucoma
  Angle-closure glaucoma
  Congenital glaucoma
  Retinopathy of prematurity
  Microblepharon
  Small orbit

Systemic
  Weill-Marchesani syndrome or similar habitus
  Ehlers-Danlos syndrome
  Meyer-Schwickerath and Weyers syndrome
  Rieger's syndrome
  Partial deletion of long arm of chromosome 18
  Nance-Horan (X-linked cataract-dental) syndrome

space for the cornea. It may be transmitted as a dominant or recessive trait, the former being more common.

Abnormalities of Shape

Horizontally Oval Cornea

The cornea is normally horizontally oval when viewed from in front, with the horizontal diameter approximately 1 mm larger than the vertical diameter (although it is round when seen from the back). The oval appearance is caused by greater scleral encroachment above and below than in the horizontal meridian. An exaggeration of the normal oval shape usually indicates the presence of some degree of sclerocornea (1,3).

A horizontally oval, bifid cornea attributed to maternal ingestion of large amounts of vitamin A throughout pregnancy has been reported (18). The condition was unilateral and manifested a cornea and iris having roughly the shape of an hourglass lying on its side. Reduplicated but clear crystalline lenses were also present.

Vertically Oval Cornea

A vertically oval cornea sometimes occurs in association with iris coloboma, Turner's syndrome (ovarian dysgenesis, XO karyotype), or intrauterine keratitis (usually from congenital syphilis) (1,13,16,19,20). It is interesting that the luetic interstitial keratitis can appear before or after the observation of the abnormal shape of the cornea.

Abnormalities of Curvature

Cornea Plana

Cornea plana (flat cornea) is seldom an isolated entity. It is more often seen in association with microcornea or sclerocornea (1,4,21). The sclerocornea is likely to be more prominent above and below, so that the cornea appears to be horizontally oval as well. The limbus in cornea plana is usually indistinct, whereas it is typically well defined in simple microcornea.

Cornea plana often produces hyperopia, but the refractive error is unpredictable because the length of the globe varies. The cornea itself must have a radius of curvature of less than 43 diopters if it is to be designated as a cornea plana, but measurements of 30 to 35 D are more common. A keratometry reading of as low as 23 D has been reported (4). A corneal curvature that is the same as that of the sclera is almost pathognomonic for cornea plana. The cornea is even flatter than the sclera in some cases. The anterior chamber is shallow, and angle-closure glaucoma is not uncommon. The incidence of open-angle glaucoma is also increased. Other possible abnormalities are listed in Table 39-3 (1,3,4,21).

Cornea plana is thought to be the result of a developmental arrest in the fourth month of fetal life, when the corneal curvature normally increases relative to that of the sclera. The heredity may be dominant or recessive. The recessive form is more severe and can be complicated by the presence of central corneal opacities. Cornea plana is especially likely to occur in patients of Finnish extraction (4).

TABLE 39-3. ABNORMALITIES ASSOCIATED WITH CORNEA PLANA

Ocular
  Hyperopia (other refractive errors possible)
  Blue sclera
  Sclerocornea
  Microcornea
  Arcus juvenilis
  Nonspecific corneal opacities
  Anterior segment dysgenesis
  Absence of normal iris markings and collarette
  Uveal and retinal coloboma
  Aniridia
  Congenital cataract
  Ectopia lentis
  Retinal and macular aplasia
  Angle-closure glaucoma
  Open-angle glaucoma
  Pseudoptosis (Streiff's sign)

Systemic
  Osteogenesis imperfecta
  Hurler's syndrome (mucopolysaccharidosis I-H)
  Maroteaux-Lamy syndrome (mucopolysaccharidosis VI)[a]
  Trisomy 13

[a]Personal observation.

Anterior Keratoconus and Keratoglobus

Anterior keratoconus usually develops during the first two decades of life and is only rarely evident at birth. Keratoglobus (globular cornea) is not infrequently congenital, but it, too, can appear after birth. Both of these corneal ectasias are usually classified as corneal dystrophies and so are not discussed here, although some of their features are summarized in Table 39-4.

Generalized Posterior Keratoconus

In this condition, the entire posterior surface of the cornea has an increased curvature, that is, it has a shorter radius of curvature and so is more strongly curved, whereas the contour of the anterior surface remains normal (1,22–24). The differential features of anterior keratoconus, keratoglobus, generalized posterior keratoconus, and circumscribed posterior keratoconus (discussed later) are given in Table 39-4 (1,22–24).

Generalized posterior keratoconus is the least common of the four disorders. It probably represents a developmental arrest, as the posterior surface of the cornea is normally more curved during fetal life (24). Generalized posterior keratoconus is usually unilateral. All examples have been in women, but there is no evidence of hereditary transmission. Central corneal thinning is present, but the condition is nonprogressive, and the vision is normal unless there is associated clouding of the cornea, which seldom occurs.

Keratectasia

Keratectasia is characterized by the presence of a bulging, opaque cornea that protrudes through the palpebral aperture (1,3,25). Most cases are unilateral and are probably the result of intrauterine keratitis; corneal perforation *in utero* causes the cornea to undergo metaplasia to tissue resembling skin (dermoid transformation). The metaplasia involves only the cornea and does not extend over the entire eye to the area of the lids, as occurs in cryptophthalmos.

Some examples of keratectasia may be caused by a failure of mesenchyme to migrate into the developing cornea, resulting in subsequent corneal thinning, bulging, and metaplasia, with or without preceding perforation.

Congenital Anterior Staphyloma

Congenital anterior staphyloma differs from keratectasia only in that the staphyloma is, by definition, lined by uveal tissue (1,3,25).

Corneal Astigmatism

Corneal astigmatism is usually just a variation, that is, a common and minor deviation from normality, although Duke-Elder considered radii of curvature of less than 6.75 mm or greater than 9.25 mm to be deformities (1,3,25).

Corneal astigmatism is nearly always dominant. Autosomal or X-linked recessive transmission is rare but may occur, especially with high degrees of astigmatism. The approximate amounts, and even the axes, of astigmatism are often remarkably similar in related individuals (3,21).

Abnormalities of Structure
Anterior Segment Dysgenesis

Anterior segment dysgenesis (ASD) was formerly called mesodermal dysgenesis (anterior chamber cleavage syndrome), but evidence indicates that the affected embryonic tissues probably originate from the neuroectoderm of the neural crest rather than from the mesoderm (26,27). These problems may be thought of as a spectrum in which any of several abnormalities may exist alone or in various combinations (1,14,22,25,28–30). Some of the more frequently

TABLE 39-4. COMPARATIVE FEATURES OF ANTERIOR KERATOCONUS, POSTERIOR KERATOCONUS, AND KERATOGLOBUS

Feature	Anterior Keratoconus	Generalized Posterior Keratoconus	Circumscribed Posterior Keratoconus	Keratoglobus
Frequency	Most common	Least common	Third most common	Second most common
Heredity	Uncertain	None	Usually none	Uncertain
Sex predilection	Slightly more females	All females	Mostly females	Uncertain
Laterality	Usually bilateral	Usually unilateral	Usually unilateral	Bilateral
Progression	Yes	No	No	Yes
Decreased acuity	Yes	Rarely	Sometimes	Yes
Corneal clouding	Sometimes	Seldom	Usually	Seldom
Anterior curve	Increased, distorted	Normal	Normal or distorted	Increased, distorted
Posterior curve	Increased	Increased	Increased locally	Increased
Corneal thinning	Central	Central	Variable	Peripheral
Acute hydrops	Occasionally	No	Seldom	Seldom

occurring combinations are given eponymic designations such as Rieger's anomaly, Peters' anomaly, and others.

In trying to understand this subject, it is helpful to review some of the embryology of the anterior segment of the eye (3,22,31). After separation of the lens vesicle, the surface ectoderm forms a layer that becomes corneal epithelium. Three waves of tissue then invade the primary mesenchyme that lies behind the surface ectoderm: the first wave gives rise to corneal endothelium, the second forms corneal stroma, and the third becomes the iris stroma. These waves of tissue (secondary mesenchyme) were once thought to be mesodermal, thus giving rise to the concept of mesodermal dysgenesis, but are now widely held to be of neural crest origin and the term most commonly used now is that of *anterior segment dysgenesis.*

During early development, there is no anterior chamber, the entire area being filled with primary or secondary mesenchyme. This gradually recedes, and its remnant in the form of the pupillary membrane begins to undergo atrophy at about the seventh month. The angle recess does not become fully opened until sometime during the first year after birth.

Three hypotheses have been proposed to explain the disappearance of mesenchyme and the consequent formation of the anterior chamber (25,26,28,32,33). The first idea was that the mesenchyme disappears by means of atrophy and absorption. The next explanation was that it is pulled apart passively as a result of different growth rates of the anterior tissues; there is no evidence to support this idea and so the term *anterior segment cleavage syndrome* is rarely used. The latest, and most plausible, explanation for the abnormalities that occur in conjunction with the development of the anterior chamber is that they represent abnormal migration, proliferation, or final differentiation of secondary mesenchymal cells that originate from the neural crest (26). This concept accounts also for the fact that associated abnormalities of the head and face are often present.

The various ASDs are now classified as follows: (a) abnormalities of neural crest cell migration (congenital glaucoma, posterior embryotoxon, Axenfeld's anomaly and syndrome, Rieger's anomaly and syndrome, Peters' anomaly, and sclerocornea); (b) abnormalities of neural crest cell proliferation (essential iris atrophy, Chandler's syndrome, and Cogan-Reese iris nevus syndrome); and (c) abnormalities of neural crest cell final differentiation (congenital hereditary endothelial dystrophy, posterior polymorphous corneal dystrophy, congenital cornea guttata, and Fuchs' corneal dystrophy). Other abnormalities such as prominent iris processes, dysgenesis of the iris, circumscribed posterior keratoconus (and, perhaps, generalized posterior keratoconus), goniodysgenesis with glaucoma, and iridogoniodysgenesis with cataract are probably also abnormalities of neural crest cell migration or differentiation.

Posterior Embryotoxon

Posterior embryotoxon is an exaggeration of the normal Schwalbe's ring. This structure is a collagenous band that encircles the periphery of the cornea on its posterior surface (34). The collagen fibers of Schwalbe's ring course circumferentially (parallel to the limbus), whereas the fibers elsewhere in the cornea run radially. Schwalbe's ring is bounded anteriorly by the termination of Descemet's membrane and posteriorly by the trabecular meshwork. Gonioscopically, it is seen just above the meshwork and is then referred to as Schwalbe's line. It may be flat and indistinct, or elevated and ridgelike.

In most persons, Schwalbe's ring is not visible biomicroscopically because it lies behind the opaque portion of the limbus; if it is sufficiently prominent and anteriorly displaced as to be visible, it is called a posterior embryotoxon and is present in 15% to 30% of normal eyes. It appears clinically as an arcuate or scalloped translucent membrane on the posterior surface of the cornea just inside the limbus. It is usually seen in the horizontal meridian, nasally and temporally, but may encircle the entire cornea.

Posterior embryotoxon is inherited as a dominant trait. The eye is usually otherwise normal unless Axenfeld's anomaly or syndrome (discussed below) is present. A prominent Schwalbe's line may be associated with other disorders, including primary congenital glaucoma, Alagille's syndrome (arteriohepatic dysplasia), megalocornea, aniridia, corectopia, and Noonan's syndrome.

Even a Schwalbe's ring that is not anteriorly displaced may be visible without gonioscopy if there is a sectoral deficiency of the normal extension of sclera into the superficial tissues of the limbus. This extremely rare anomaly is called the *partial limbal coloboma of Ascher* and exposes Schwalbe's ring and the meshwork to direct view (1).

Axenfeld's Anomaly and Syndrome

Axenfeld's anomaly is the combination of posterior embryotoxon with prominent iris processes. The iris processes extend across the angle and insert into the prominent Schwalbe's line. Axenfeld *syndrome* is the name given to Axenfeld anomaly occurring along with glaucoma (30,38). Both the anomaly and the syndrome are dominantly inherited. Hypertelorism is occasionally present. Systemic abnormalities are rare (10).

Rieger's Anomaly and Syndrome

Rieger's anomaly consists of the changes found in Axenfeld anomaly plus hypoplasia of the anterior iris stroma (28,30,33). Peripheral anterior synechiae, corectopia, and pseudopolycoria are often present also, as is glaucoma in 50% to 60% of cases. Rieger's syndrome is present when the Rieger's anomaly is accompanied by skeletal abnormalities, such as maxillary hypoplasia, microdontia, and other limb and spine malformations (35). Some patients are mentally retarded.

Rieger's anomaly and syndrome are usually dominant but are occasionally sporadic. One case showed a presumptive isochromosome of the long arm of chromosome 6 (36), and another had a pericentric inversion of chromosome 6 (37). Various systemic associations have been described, such as Down syndrome, Ehlers-Danlos syndrome, Franceschetti's syndrome, Noonan's syndrome, Marfan's syndrome, oculodentodigital dysplasia, and osteogenesis imperfecta.

Examination of these patients must include gonioscopy and tonometry: this not only helps make the differential diagnosis, it also helps direct treatment (especially if intraocular pressure is elevated). The pneumotonometer or Tonopen is preferable to the Perkins, or Schiötz tonometers because the presence of associated corneal abnormalities or small radius of corneal curvature may give false intraocular pressure readings. Also, a thorough assessment of the optic nerve is critical in determining the overall visual prognosis and deciding on the course of future treatment.

Medical therapy can be useful when intraocular pressure is high and needs to be decreased in an urgent manner. However, this disorder generally has a relatively poor surgical prognosis, both for glaucoma control and for corneal opacities, if present. Deciding on the correct balance between chronic administration of medications and performing surgery is difficult. The advent of effective use of antimetabolites for filtration in children may tip the balance in favor of surgery when the optic nerve is threatened significantly. However, this type of treatment in the maturing eye of a child is, itself, embryonic.

Goniodysgenesis with Glaucoma

Goniodysgenesis with glaucoma is probably just a minor form of Rieger's anomaly, lacking only posterior embryotoxon (30,38). Transmission is dominant.

Iridogoniodysgenesis with Cataract

Iridogoniodysgenesis with cataract differs from Rieger's anomaly in that cataract is present, posterior embryotoxon is absent, and the heredity is autosomal recessive (30,38). Iridogoniodysgenesis is not associated with systemic abnormalities, but Conradi's syndrome (congenital stippled epiphyses) sometimes manifests other forms of ASD in association with cataract.

Peters' Anomaly

Peters' anomaly is characterized by a central corneal opacity with corresponding defects in the stroma, Descemet's, and endothelium. Two variants of Peters' anomaly have been described: in the so-called *mesodermal form* (or, probably more properly, the *neuroectodermal form*) or type I Peter's anomaly, the central cornea has a congenital leukoma with strands of iris adherent to it (1,28,30,33,40–42). The adhesions usually, but not invariably, arise from the iris collarette and represent persisting remnants of the pupillary membrane. The lens, which is ectodermal in origin, is clear in the classic and purely mesodermal (neuroectodermal) form of the anomaly. It is most often sporadic but may be transmitted recessively or as an irregularly dominant trait (39). Approximately 80% of cases are bilateral, and about half include glaucoma. Other associated abnormalities such as microcornea and sclerocornea may be present, although they usually are not. This form of Peters' anomaly is caused by abnormal development of the tissues associated with the central portions of the iris, anterior chamber, and cornea. Descemet's membrane and endothelium are generally absent at the site of the leukoma, as is true also of the other two forms of the anomaly that are discussed below.

Peters' anomaly type II, or the *surface ectodermal form* of the anomaly, is the result of faulty separation of the lens vesicle from surface ectoderm. In addition to the features of the mesodermal (neuroectodermal) type, anterior cataract (polar, subcapsular, or reduplication) is present. This form is usually bilateral and is almost always associated with other more severe manifestations, both ocular and systemic. Fifty percent to 70% of patients have concomitant glaucoma, and other associated abnormalities include microcornea, microphthalmos, cornea plana, sclerocornea, colobomas, aniridia, and dysgenesis of the angle and iris.

The *inflammatory form* follows intrauterine inflammation and so is nonhereditary. The inflammation can interfere with surface ectodermal or neuroectodermal development or both. There is no definitive way to make the diagnosis, although signs of inflammation may still be present after birth, and the iris adhesions are extensive and do not arise only from the vicinity of the collarette. Cases of inflammatory Peters' anomaly nearly always fulfill the criteria for use of the term *von Hippel's posterior corneal ulcer*, namely inflammatory signs in association with congenital defects of Descemet's membrane and endothelium. We have already seen that some examples of circumscribed posterior keratoconus have these same features and so may also be referred to as cases of von Hippel's ulcer; in fact, there seems to be little, if any, difference between the inflammatory form of Peters' anomaly and the inflammatory form of circumscribed posterior keratoconus.

The management of patients with Peters' anomaly is complex, and the outcome of a keratoplasty depends on the ability to control the associated glaucoma.

Prominent Iris Processes

Although prominent iris processes are not corneal anomalies, they should be mentioned because they are part of the spectrum of ASD and because it is necessary to determine their relationship to the peripheral cornea in order to evaluate their pathologic importance (14).

It is normal for some slender processes (usually fewer than 100) to extend from the peripheral iris to the scleral roll (also known as the scleral spur) at the posterior edge of the trabecular meshwork or, occasionally, even to the central portion of the meshwork itself. Extensions to or beyond Schwalbe's ring are abnormal and are referred to as prominent iris processes. Abnormal processes are often more numerous, in addition to being more prominent and anteriorly displaced, than are normal processes.

Prominent iris processes can occur with any of the other manifestations of ASD. They are also seen in many cases of primary congenital glaucoma and in several systemic disorders that are associated with congenital glaucoma: phakomatosis; homocystinuria; rubella; and Marfan's, Lowe's, Pierre Robin, Hallermann-Streiff, Rubenstein-Taybi, and Turner's syndromes (14).

Anterior Segment Dysgenesis of the Iris

In addition to prominent iris processes, ASD may be associated with congenital peripheral anterior synechiae and a variety of abnormalities of the iris itself, including atrophy of the iris stroma, corectopia, pseudopolycoria, and congenital ectropion uveae.

Posterior Polymorphous Dystrophy

Posterior polymorphous dystrophy may be classified either as a dystrophy or as a congenital anomaly. Its histopathologic features suggest a relationship to ASD, and it not infrequently occurs with other forms of ASD (22,25,43,44). This entity is described in detail elsewhere in this book.

Congenital Cornea Guttata

Cornea guttata can occur, rarely, as a congenital anomaly. It is sometimes familial. A dominant pedigree with associated anterior polar cataract has been described, which suggests an abnormality in the secondary mesenchyme that helps to separate the lens from the surface ectoderm at about the sixth to eighth week of embryonic life (45). Congenital cornea guttata is also described elsewhere in this book.

Congenital Hereditary Endothelial Dystrophy

Congenital hereditary endothelial dystrophy (CHED) is now classified as an ASD. It is characterized by the presence, at birth or soon thereafter, of bilateral corneal edema that is often slightly worse centrally and that is not associated with vascularization or inflammation (44,46–49). Epithelial edema is not prominent, but the stroma may

be swollen to two or three times its normal thickness. Descemet's membrane, when visible, is seen to be thick and opaque, but guttate changes are not present. Intraocular pressures are normal. The corneas are not enlarged.

Two types of CHED with different modes of transmission are recognized (46,49,50). The recessive form is more common, and is usually more severe, than the dominant form. In the recessive disease, the corneas are cloudy at birth, and nystagmus is common. The condition is essentially nonprogressive and is asymptomatic except for severely decreased vision. Deafness is sometimes present; otherwise, there are no related systemic abnormalities (51).

Corneal edema in dominant CHED may not become apparent until sometime during the first or second year after birth (44,46,50). Nystagmus is absent. The edema is likely to progress slowly, and some patients develop pain, photophobia, and tearing.

Histopathologically, the anterior ("banded") portion of Descemet's membrane is normal, but the posterior nonbanded layer (which is formed later during development) is abnormal and consists of a variably thickened, or occasionally thinned, layer of aberrant collagen (47,52,53). Guttate excrescences do not form. Endothelial cells are absent or atrophic. The primary abnormality is presumed to be with the endothelial cells and must manifest itself during or after the fifth month of gestation, at which time the endothelial cells begin to form the posterior nonbanded portion of Descemet's membrane.

Asymptomatic relatives of patients with CHED may show corneal changes resembling posterior polymorphous dystrophy (54). An attempt should be made to identify such persons because their children seem to run a greater risk of having CHED.

Circumscribed Posterior Keratoconus

Circumscribed posterior keratoconus may be a localized form of Peter's anomaly. It is characterized by the presence of a localized, crater-like defect (convex toward the stroma) in the posterior surface of the cornea (22,30,40–42,55). Contrary to former belief, Descemet's membrane and endothelium are usually present in the area of the defect, although the collagen of Descemet's membrane may be thinned and abnormal in structure and configuration (22,40,42,55). More than one pit may be present. The overlying stroma often has nonspecific opacities. Most cases are in females, unilateral and sporadic, although familial examples have occurred. It is probably the result of abnormal migration or terminal induction of cells of neural crest origin in the area of involvement, perhaps secondary to some problem with separation of the lens vesicle. Some cases show evidence of being related to intrauterine inflammation: corneal infiltrates and vascularization, keratic precipitates, anterior synechiae, and uveitis; these cases often have defects in Descemet's membrane and endothelium and are

TABLE 39-5. ABNORMALITIES ASSOCIATED WITH CIRCUMSCRIBED POSTERIOR KERATOCONUS

Ocular
  Fleischer ring
  Aniridia
  Anterior segment dysgenesis
  Anterior lenticonus
Systemic
  Hypertelorism
  Poorly developed nasal bridge
  Brachydactyly
  Bull neck
  Mental retardation
  Growth retardation

TABLE 39-6. ABNORMALITIES ASSOCIATED WITH SCLEROCORNEA

Ocular
  High refractive errors
  Blue sclera
  Cornea plana
  Horizontally oval cornea
  Aniridia
  Anterior segment dysgenesis
  Uveal and retinal coloboma
  Cataract
  Open-angle glaucoma
  Angle-closure glaucoma
  Pseudoptosis
  Microphthalmos
Systemic
  Anomalies of skull and facial bones
  Deformities of the external ear
  Deafness
  Polydactyly
  Cerebellar dysfunction
  Testicular abnormalities
  Hereditary osteo-onychodysplasia
  Osteogenesis imperfecta
  Others (numerous and variable)

sometimes referred to as *von Hippel's posterior* (or *internal*) *corneal ulcer.*

The characteristics of circumscribed posterior keratoconus, as compared with generalized posterior keratoconus, anterior keratoconus, and keratoglobus, are summarized in Table 39-4. Associated ocular and systemic abnormalities are listed in Table 39-5 (22).

The anterior surface of the cornea is usually normal in these individuals, unless there is enough thinning to cause ectasia. Thus, although the posterior corneal surface may degrade vision to some extent, this is usually not enough to warrant a surgical procedure.

Sclerocornea

Sclerocornea is an abnormality in which the margins of the cornea are not well defined because scleral tissue with conjunctival vessels extends to the margins (56–58). The scleralization may be only peripheral or virtually complete. Even when it is complete, the central cornea is apt to be slightly less opaque than the periphery. Affected areas have fine, superficial vessels that are direct extensions of normal scleral, episcleral, and conjunctival vessels. Sclerocornea is usually bilateral (57).

Histopathologic studies reveal elastic fibers and collagen fibers of increased and variable diameter in the anterior corneal stroma. The deeper collagen fibers have smaller diameters than do the more anterior ones, as is typical of sclera; the reverse is true of normal cornea (58).

About 50% of cases of sclerocornea are sporadic, and the remainder can be dominant or recessive (57). The dominant forms are less severe than the recessive ones (58). Sclerocornea is occasionally caused by chromosomal aberrations. There is no sex predilection. The most common associated finding is cornea plana. Other ocular and systemic associations are given in Table 39-6 (7,57,59,60,61,62). In brief, sclerocornea is associated with cornea plana in about 80% of patients. Other associated ocular abnormalities include microphthalmos, iridocorneal synechiae, persistent

pupillary membrane, dysgenesis of angle and iris, congenital glaucoma, coloboma, and posterior embryotoxon of the fellow eye. Somatic abnormalities sometimes occur along with associated chromosomal abnormalities; they include mental retardation, deafness, and craniofacial, digital, and skin abnormalities.

Other Combined Forms of Anterior Segment Dysgenesis

Although the foregoing disorders are the most frequently encountered combined forms of ASD, it is worth reemphasizing that any combination of features is possible. This is illustrated well by the family reported by Grayson (43), in which some members had all of the following findings: cornea guttata, posterior polymorphous dystrophy, posterior embryotoxon, circumscribed posterior keratoconus, iris atrophy, peripheral anterior synechiae, prominent iris processes, and glaucoma. These patients also developed corneal edema and fibrocalcific band keratopathy.

Congenital Mass Lesions of the Cornea

Metaplasias

A metaplasia is a transformation of tissue from one type to another, usually in response to exposure, inflammation, or trauma (1,63). As mentioned earlier, the cornea can undergo metaplasia to skin (dermoid transformation) in the conditions of keratectasia, corneal staphyloma, and true cryptophthalmos. The metaplasia is at times of such proportions as to produce an apparent tumor of the cornea.

If the metaplasia is strictly ectodermal, the corneal epithelium is replaced by tissue resembling epidermis, sometimes with related derivatives such as hairs and glandular structures being present. Mesodermal metaplasia brings about the appearance in subepithelial stroma of the fibrofatty elements of dermis, and sometimes cartilage or bone. When the metaplasia consists primarily of a hypertrophic overgrowth of fibrous tissue, the term *corneal keloid* may be used (64).

Choristomas

A choristoma is a mass of tissue that has been displaced during prenatal development from its normal position to a location where it would not normally be found (63).

Corneal, Limbal, and Epibulbar Dermoids

Corneal, limbal and epibulbar dermoids consist of masses of tissue that were destined to become skin but were displaced to the surface of the eye (1,63). They can also occur in the orbit.

Choristomatous dermoids contain ectodermal elements (keratinizing epithelium, hair, sebaceous and sudoriferous glands, nerve, smooth muscle, and, rarely, teeth) and mesodermal derivatives (fibrous tissue, fat, blood vessels, and cartilage) in various combinations. They are called lipodermoids if fatty tissue predominates.

Clinically, an epibulbar dermoid is usually a round or ovoid, yellowish white, dome-like mass. Occasionally, a dermoid may be rather diffuse or may encircle the limbus or peripheral cornea. Hairs often protrude from the lesion. The surface may be pearly or clear and glistening, depending on the presence or absence of epithelial keratinization. The most common location is at the inferotemporal limbus, but dermoids can occur anywhere on the surface of the eye. The central cornea can be affected, although some of these lesions are probably the result of dermoid transformation (metaplastic dermoids) rather than being choristomatous malformations.

The second most common site for a dermoid is the superotemporal orbit. Dermoids usually exhibit little or no growth but do enlarge occasionally, especially at the time of puberty (65). They do not become malignant.

A limbal or corneal dermoid can cause decreased visual acuity by covering the visual axis or by causing astigmatism. An arcuate deposition of lipid often develops along the central (corneal) edge of a limbal dermoid and is another possible source of decreased vision. The lipid sometimes increases as long as the dermoid is present (65).

Limbal dermoids always involve some of the corneal stroma and can even extend into the anterior chamber. Any attempt at excision must be limited merely to shaving away the elevated portion of the lesion, unless one is willing to undertake a corneoscleral graft, which would seldom be

indicated. It is important to explain to the parents, or to the patient who is old enough to understand, that the shaving procedure can only eliminate the elevation and that the corneal opacity will remain. The surgery is not without some difficulty and risk. The cornea may be thin in the area of the dermoid, and perforation is possible. I have observed that if the dermoid covers the anterior portion of the sclera, the underlying extraocular muscles and their insertions may be anomalous and may inadvertently be transected if the surgeon is not careful.

Perhaps 30% of patients who have epibulbar dermoids have other abnormalities (65). These most often consist of some or all of the features of *Goldenhar's syndrome* (Goldenhar-Gorlin syndrome, facioauriculovertebral sequence, oculoauriculovertebral dysplasia) (2,16,65,66). Goldenhar's syndrome is the result of maldevelopment of the first and second branchial arches, which give rise to the maxilla, mandible, malar bone, auricle, and structures of the upper neck. The syndrome comprises a triad of findings: epibulbar (usually limbal) dermoid(s), abnormalities of the ear such as auricular appendages or pretragal fistulas, and anomalies of the vertebral column. Other abnormalities that sometimes occur are listed in Table 39-7 (2,16,65,66,68).

The cause of Goldenhar's syndrome is unknown. It is nearly always sporadic and nonhereditary, although familial examples have been reported twice (69,70). Most isolated epibulbar dermoids are also sporadic, but bilateral corneal dermoids can be hereditary, and dermoids that encircle the limbus (ring dermoid syndrome) can be dominantly transmitted (71,72).

Epibulbar dermoids are occasionally associated with systemic disorders other than Goldenhar's syndrome (Table 39-8) (65,67).

TABLE 39-7. ABNORMALITIES ASSOCIATED WITH GOLDENHAR'S SYNDROME[a]

Ocular
  Coloboma of upper eyelid
  Uveal coloboma
  Aniridia
  Miliary retinal aneurysms
  Duane's retraction strabismus syndrome
  Lacrimal stenosis
  Microphthalmos

Systemic
  Mandibular and malar hypoplasia
  Hemifacial microsomia
  Other facial and oral abnormalities
  Cardiac abnormalities
  Renal abnormalities
  Gastrointestinal abnormalities
  Genitourinary abnormalities
  Mental retardation

[a]In addition to the basic triad of epibulbar dermoid(s), anomalies of the ear, and anomalies of the vertebral column.

TABLE 39-8. SYSTEMIC MALFORMATION SYNDROMES SOMETIMES ASSOCIATED WITH EPIBULBAR DERMOIDS

Branchial arch syndromes
    Goldenhar's syndrome (oculoauriculovertebral dysplasia)
    Franceschetti (or Treacher Collins) syndrome
    (mandibulofacial dysostosis)

Congenital neurocutaneous syndromes
    Bloch-Sulzberger syndrome (incontinentia pigmenti)
    Encephalocraniocutaneous lipomatosis
    Linear sebaceous nevus syndrome

Chromosomal abnormalities
    Cri-du-chat syndrome (deletion of short arm of chromosome 5)

Abnormalities of Transparency

In a heterogeneous group of disorders, the clarity of the cornea is disturbed, but the cornea is not grossly malformed. Loss of transparency can be caused by edema, trauma, inflammation, biochemical depositions, or drying, as well as by any of the various mechanisms that have already been discussed. Many of these problems are not truly congenital anomalies and so are mentioned only briefly.

Edema

Birth Trauma

Mild trauma during birth can damage the corneal epithelium. More severe injury, usually from the use of forceps, can produce ruptures in Descemet's membrane and the endothelium. These ruptures tend to be linear and seem to occur more often in the left eye (when related to the use of forceps) because babies most commonly present in the left-occiput-anterior position; in such a case, the tears would run in an inferonasal-superotemporal axis. As healing ensues, a ridge of hypertrophic Descemet's membrane develops along the line of rupture. The edema may or may not clear and can recur later in life.

Primary or Secondary Congenital Glaucoma

Congenital glaucoma of any cause can produce corneal edema. The cornea enlarges, which causes ruptures of Descemet's membrane and endothelium (Haab's striae) and still more edema (14).

Congenital Hereditary Stromal Dystrophy

Congenital hereditary stromal dystrophy (CHSD) is a rare, dominant condition in which the superficial corneal stroma of both eyes has an ill-defined, feathery cloudiness (73). The haze is more prominent centrally and fades peripherally. There is no edema. CHSD is nonprogressive, but the opacity can be sufficiently dense as to cause substantial loss of vision. Searching nystagmus is usually present. The stromal collagen fibers are abnormal in form, size, and distribution.

Keratitis

Rubella

Rarely, rubella produces keratitis in the form of disciform stromal edema. It more often causes a cloudy cornea by virtue of its association with congenital glaucoma.

Syphilis

Luetic interstitial keratitis may occasionally be present at birth, although it characteristically appears during the first or second decade of life, as does the associated deafness.

Miscellaneous Infections

Many other infectious agents, including gonococcus, staphylococcus, and influenza virus (among others), can cause intrauterine keratitis. If the process is active, the presentation is with inflammatory signs in the cornea; if not, leukoma, keratectasia, or congenital anterior staphyloma may be seen.

Depositions

Arcus Juvenilis

Arcus juvenilis, a deposition of lipid in the peripheral cornea (also known as *anterior embryotoxon*), is the same as corneal arcus, except that the congenital variety is more often unilateral and sectoral in its distribution (3,74). The anomaly is of unknown etiology. When truly congenital, it is not related to elevated levels of serum cholesterol. However, the patient with juvenile arcus is often not seen until sometime after infancy, and it is then uncertain whether the finding was present at birth. In such a case, the serum cholesterol level should be checked because it can be elevated (and associated with premature atherosclerosis) in some cases of developmental juvenile arcus. Arcus juvenilis is sometimes found in association with megalocornea, aniridia, blue sclera, or osteogenesis imperfecta; hereditary nephritis and nerve deafness (Alport's syndrome); or corneal inflammation or malformation from any cause.

Other Depositions

Biochemical deposits can appear in the cornea early in life as a manifestation of any of several systemic diseases, but most of these deposits are not clinically apparent at birth. These diseases are listed in Table 39-9.

Neurotrophic Changes and Drying of the Cornea

The cornea may become dry soon after birth because of decreased corneal sensation, as happens with the Riley-Day syndrome (familial dysautonomia) or with isolated congenital dysfunction of the trigeminal nerve. Other causes of drying include congenital deficiency of tears (which may be idiopathic or may occur as another manifestation of the Riley-Day syndrome) and exposure from lagophthalmos.

TABLE 39-9. SYSTEMIC DISEASES THAT CAUSE CORNEAL OPACITIES EARLY IN LIFE[a]

Biochemical deposits
　Cystinosis
　Fabry's disease (angiokeratoma corporis diffusum)
　Mucopolysaccharidosis
　Mucolipidosis
　Tyrosinemia
　Tangier disease (high-density alpha-lipoprotein deficiency)
　Familial plasma lecithin-cholesterol acyltransferase deficiency
　Refsum's syndrome (heredopathia atactica polyneuritiformis)
　Schnyder's crystalline corneal dystrophy

Nonspecific (usually patchy or spotty) opacities
　Trisomy 13
　Trisomy 18
　Turner's syndrome (ovarian dysgenesis, XO karyotype)
　Phenylketonuria
　Chédiak-Higashi syndrome
　Genodermatoses

[a]Most of these opacities are not clinically apparent at birth.

Chromosomal Aberrations

Corneal anomalies are only occasionally caused by chromosomal aberrations, and most patients who have chromosomal disorders do not manifest corneal abnormalities. Nevertheless, some associations between the two groups of problems are known to exist. Patients who have a trisomy 21 (Down) syndrome have an increased incidence of keratoconus (75). The trisomy 18 (Edwards') syndrome is sometimes associated with abnormalities of the anterior cornea, whereas the chromosome 18 deletion syndromes are more likely to affect the posterior cornea.

No particular corneal anomaly constitutes, by itself, a need for chromosomal studies, but karyotyping may be indicated if some of the following features are also present: hypertelorism, epicanthus, pronounced mongoloid or antimongoloid slant of the palpebral fissures, ptosis, strabismus, ocular colobomas, peculiar facies, multiple systemic malformations, and especially, mental retardation.

The relationships between corneal anomalies and chromosomal aberrations are summarized in Table 39-10 (18,76–78).

METABOLIC DISEASES

Several of the inherited metabolic diseases may be associated with ocular manifestations. In this section, we discuss some of anterior segment manifestations of the metabolic diseases.

Carbohydrate

Diabetes

Until recently there was little awareness of corneal changes among diabetic patients. Slightly decreased corneal sensation has been noted in most diabetic corneas (79,80). This may be related to irregularities in the basal lamina of Schwann cells and axonal degeneration observed in diabetic animals (81). Punctate corneal staining (82) and neurotrophic corneal ulceration (81,83) have also been reported. Poor healing and persistent epithelial defects occur, most commonly after epithelial removal during vitrectomy (84,85). Poor epithelial healing, especially after vitrectomy, may be related to abnormal corneal innervation (82,85). Alternately reduced numbers of hemidesmosomes (86) and decreased penetration of anchoring fibrils into the stroma (87) have been suggested as contributory factors. Sorbitol accumulation from increased aldose reductase activity may play a role in diabetic corneal pathology as well. Studies of animal diabetic models have shown both structural (polymegathism, pleomorphism) and functional (increased permeability, slower recovery from induced edema) changes in the diabetic corneal epithelium and endothelium, although these have not always been borne out by studies on humans (88).

Oral aldose reductase inhibitor appears promising in the treatment of diabetic epithelial keratopathy, as does an inhibitor eye drop (CT-112) (89,90). Subtle irregularities and hypertrophy of diabetic corneal epithelium have been observed with specular microscopy (91). Increased corneal thickness and persistent stromal edema have occasionally been described, although the presence of increased central corneal thickness in these patients has been disputed by other studies (81,84,92). An abnormal diabetic endothelium, characterized by a decreased frequency of hexagonal cells but a normal age-related cell density, may be responsible for these observations (93). Diabetic corneal endothelium is more permeable to fluorescein and takes longer to recover from cataract surgery than nondiabetic endothelium (94,95). Others have been unable to detect any functional endothelial abnormality in the diabetic cornea (96). Interestingly, corneal autofluorescence has been noted to correlate with the presence of diabetic retinopathy (97).

Mucopolysaccharidoses

Mucopolysaccharide storage diseases (Table 39-11) are inborn errors of metabolism characterized by excessive storage of mucopolysaccharides due to deficiencies of lysosomal acid hydrolases, which degrade mucopolysaccharides. The normal cornea contains 4.0% to 4.5% mucopolysaccharides, of which 50% is keratan sulfate, 25% is chondroitin, and 25% is chondroitin 4-sulfate (98). In the mucopolysaccharidoses (MPSs), excess dermatan and keratan sulfate appear in the cornea, and heparan sulfate accumulates in the retina and central nervous system. This results in corneal opacity. The opacities usually appear during the neonatal period or later, reflecting the availability of maternal enzymes *in utero*. In some diseases, the corneal opacities appear within a few weeks to months of birth, raising the differentials of congenital glaucoma and CHED, and also

TABLE 39-10. CHROMOSOMAL ABERRATIONS THAT HAVE BEEN ASSOCIATED WITH CORNEAL ANOMALIES

Chromosomal Aberration	Corneal Anomaly [a]
Partial duplication of short arm of chromosome 2 (dup[2p21-2p25])	Microcornea, corneal opacities, anterior segment dysgenesis
Deletion of short arm of chromosome 4 (Wolf-Hirschhorn syndrome; 4p-)	Corneal opacities, sclerocornea, microcornea, megalocornea
Deletion of short arm of chromosome 5 (cri-du-chat syndrome; cat's cry syndrome; 5p-)	Megalocornea, epibulbar dermoid
Partial trisomy of short arm of chromosome B (trisomy Bp)	Patchy corneal opacities with vascularization
Isochromosome of long arm of chromosome 6	Rieger's syndrome
Pericentric inversion of chromosome 6	Rieger's syndrome
Trisomy of chromosome 8	Corneal opacity
Partial trisomy of long arm of chromosome 10 (trisomy 10q)	Sclerocornea
Ring chromosome D (Dr)	Retrocorneal mass or membrane
Deletion of long arm of chromosome D (Dq-)	Megalocornea
Deletion of short arm of chromosome 11 (Miller's syndrome; aniridia-Wilms' tumor syndrome; I lp-)	Aniridia [b] (with Wilms' tumor)
Deletion of long arm of chromosome 11 (11q-)	Peters' anomaly
Trisomy of chromosome 13 (Patau's or Bartholin-Patau syndrome)	Clinical anophthalmia, cyclopia, corneal dysgenesis, corneal opacities, sclerocornea
Partial trisomy of long arm of chromosome 16 (trisomy 16q)	Rieger's anomaly and glaucoma
Deletion of short arm of chromosome 18 (18p-)	Posterior keratoconus with deep corneal opacity
Deletion of long arm of chromosome 18 (18q-)	Microcornea, corneal opacities, Peters' anomaly, oval cornea, anterior segment "mesodermal" dysgenesis
Ring chromosome 18 (18r)	Corneal leukomas
Trisomy of chromosome 18 (Edwards' syndrome)	Anterior corneal opacities
Deletion of long arm of chromosome G (Gq-) or ring chromosome G (Gr)	Corneal opacities
Ring chromosome 21 (21r)	Peters' anomaly
Trisomy of chromosome 21 (Down's syndrome)	Keratoconus (occurs fairly often)
XO (Turner's syndrome; presence of only a single X1 sex chromosome)	Corneal opacities, microcornea, vertically oval cornea
Various translocations	Corneal opacities, Peters' anomaly, sclerocornea, megalocornea

[a]Most of these corneal anomalies have been reported very rarely, often only once or twice.
[b]Aniridia is not a corneal anomaly but is often associated eventually with the development of extensive opacification and vascularization (pannus) of the superficial cornea.

may be the first manifestation of the disease. Corneal opacities appear earlier in the MPS IH or Hurler's syndrome, Scheie syndrome, with G_{M1} gangliosidosis type I and in the mucolipidosis (where the opacities are mostly peripheral). In other forms of the MPS, the corneal opacities may appear later in life when the diagnosis is already established.

Hurler's Syndrome

Hurler's syndrome (mucopolysaccharidosis IH) or gargoylism is characterized by moderate dwarfism, protuberant abdomen, joint contractures, and mental retardation. A large head, hypertelorism, and thick lips with a large

TABLE 39-11. OCULAR MANIFESTATIONS OF MUCOPOLYSACCHARIDOSES

Mucopolysaccharidosis	Enzyme Deficiency	Corneal Clouding	RPE Degeneration	Optic Atrophy
Hurler (I-H)	α-L-iduronidase	+	+	+
Scheie (I-S)	α-L-iduronidase (partial)	+	+	+
Hurler-Scheie compound (I-H/S)	α-L-iduronidase (partial)	+	+	+
Hunter A (IIA) (severe phenotype)	Iduronate sulfatase	−	+	+
Hunter B (IIB) (mild phenotype)	Iduronate sulfatase	+	+	+
Sanfilippo A (IIIA)	Heparan sulfate sulfamidase	−	+	+
Sanfilippo B	N-acetyl-a-D-glucosaminidase	−	+	+
Morquio (IV)	N-acetyl-galactosamine sulfatase	+	−	+
Maroteaux-Lamy A (VIA) (severe phenotype)	Arylsulfatase B	+	−	+
Maroteaux-Lamy B (VIB) (mild phenotype)	Arylsulfatase B	+	−	−
Macular corneal dystrophy (Groenouw type II)	?	+	−	−

+, present; −, absent; RPE, retinal pigment epithelium.
(Modified from Kenyon KR. Lysosomal disorders affecting the ocular anterior segment. In: Nicholson DH, ed., *Ocular pathology update.* New York: Masson, 1980.)

tongue and hypertrophic gums are generally seen. The bridge of the nose is depressed, and the chest is usually enlarged with marked flaring of the lower ribs. The hands are broad and the fingers short and stubby. In the extreme cases, clawhand deformity may arise as well as bony changes in the feet. The skin is usually thickened, and there may be nodules over the scapular region. Hirsutism and deafness are often present. Respiratory disease results from deformity of the nasal and facial bones. Heart damage may be due to specific valvular lesions. Coronary artery and myocardial disease also occurs. Neurologic findings are variable, but spasticity and mental retardation have frequently been reported.

Corneal clouding, which occurs within a few days to months of birth, is a prominent feature of the disease (99) and helps to differentiate it from Hunter's syndrome. The opacities are located first in the anterior stroma and consist of fine gray punctate opacities. Later, the posterior stroma and endothelium become involved. Histologically, grossly ballooned macrophages are found in the cornea (100). Glaucoma has also been documented in these patients and is associated with the presence of the mucopolysaccharide-containing cells in the region of the aqueous drainage channels. Pigmentary retinopathy and optic atrophy are also commonly seen (101,102).

Scheie's Syndrome

Scheie's syndrome (mucopolysaccharidosis IS) is a variant of Hurler's syndrome, with the same enzymatic defect, a deficiency of α-L-iduronidase inherited as an autosomal-recessive trait. Increased amounts of dermatan sulfate and heparan sulfate are excreted in the urine (103). Scheie's syndrome does not have the typical features of Hurler's syndrome except for the clawhand deformity and bony changes in the feet. Physical growth is normal, and mental impairment is minimal or absent (104).

The most prominent ocular feature in Scheie's syndrome is a corneal haze that is often present at birth and very slowly progressive. The cornea appears thickened and somewhat edematous. The cloudiness is more marked in the corneal periphery. This is thought to occur because the stromal fibrils show a large range of sizes unlike normal corneal stroma where the sizes of the fibrils are remarkably similar, and by abnormally large stromal collagen. Mucopolysaccharide deposits are found in the keratocytes, and vacuoles or pleomorphic inclusions are found with electron microscopy (105,106,107). Corneal transplantation may be necessary later in life; however, transplants may do poorly (108).

Other ocular findings include pigmentary disease of the retina and optic nerve atrophy. Acute glaucoma has been reported (109), but the cause is unclear. It may be due to a narrow angle or possibly a thickening of the anterior ocular structures caused by abnormal acid mucopolysaccharide storage. A thickening and decrease in the elasticity of the conjunctiva have also been observed.

Hunter's Syndrome

Hunter's syndrome (mucopolysaccharidosis II) has clinical and biochemical features similar to those of Hurler's syndrome except Hunter's syndrome is less severe. It is inherited as an X-linked recessive trait and is seen more commonly than Hunter's syndrome. There is a failure to degrade dermatan sulfate and heparan sulfate. Lysosomal storage of these polymers leads to numerous clinical problems including skeletal abnormalities, limitation of joint motion, hepatomegaly, deafness, and cardiovascular disease (99,110). The gross facial features are similar to those in Hurler's syndrome. Mental retardation is less severe than in Hurler's syndrome, and lumbar gibbus does not usually occur. Deafness, however, is a common feature of Hunter's syndrome. Patients usually die in their 20s and 30s because of cardiac involvement with congestive heart failure.

Corneal clouding is generally not present in Hunter's syndrome, although exceptions have been recorded (111). Pathologic studies have also demonstrated the accumulation of mucopolysaccharides in the cornea, conjunctiva, and other ocular tissues (113–116). Two forms of Hunter's syndrome are said to exist. In the mild form, corneal opacities occur later in life but are mild and visually insignificant in contrast to those of other mucopolysaccharidoses. In the severe form, subclinical corneal clouding can be demonstrated histochemically. Thus, although the presence of corneal clouding has been used to distinguish Hurler's syndrome from Hunter's syndrome, this distinction is not always a reliable one. Some Hurler's patients have clear corneas up to the age of 14 years (115); other Hunter's patients have clear corneas until late in life. Retinal pigmentary changes and optic atrophy have been noted in Hunter's syndrome, and the sclera and cilia may also be affected (112,114).

Sanfilippo's Syndrome

Sanfilippo's syndrome (mucopolysaccharidosis III) is an autosomal-recessive disease in which patients excrete only heparan sulfate. It is seen less frequently than the Hurler or Hunter variant. It is characterized by severe mental retardation but fewer craniofacial changes than in Hurler's. Dwarfism is not a prominent feature. Joint movements are restricted, and neurologic symptoms including seizures and athetosis are quite prominent. Death usually occurs by age 14. Corneal cloudiness does not occur in Sanfilippo's syndrome. Retinal pigmentary degeneration and optic atrophy have been observed.

Morquio's Syndrome

Morquio's syndrome (mucopolysaccharidosis IV) is inherited as an autosomal-recessive trait and is associated with the accumulation of keratan sulfate in the tissues. The patients have a dwarf appearance, with knock-knee, barrel chest with pigeon breast, short neck, and osteoporosis. The facial appearance is characteristic, with a broad mouth, short nose, widely spaced teeth with defective enamel, and a prominent maxilla. Hepatosplenomegaly, deafness, and metachromatic granulation of leukocytes has also been noted. Intelligence is normal, but neurologic symptoms may result from deformity of the spine, and cardiac complications may result from malformation of the chest. Corneal clouding may occur but may not be grossly evident until after the age of 10 years. Cloudiness may consist of a mild stromal haze, or it may be severe (116). Retinopathy and optic nerve changes are not present.

Maroteaux-Lamy Syndrome

Maroteaux-Lamy syndrome (mucopolysaccharidosis VI) is an autosomal-recessive disease in which dermatan sulfate accumulates in the tissues. Skeletal changes are a prominent feature of the syndrome. Lumbar kyphosis, protrusion of the sternum, and genu valgum are found. The facial appearance is abnormal, but not as striking as in Hurler's syndrome. Intellectual function is normal. Corneal opacities occur in all patients, but may be subtle, and a slit-lamp examination may be necessary to see them (117). Histology on a penetrating keratoplasty specimen has shown degenerated epithelial cells with apoptotic nuclei. Proteoglycans were present in epithelial cells, intercellular spaces, swollen desmosomes, and throughout the stroma. Keratocytes showed no cell organelles, were vacuolated, and contained a large quantity of abnormal proteoglycans. Hydrocephalus, papilledema, and optic atrophy may also be seen (117). The accumulation of lipid-like material in the stroma in addition to glycosaminoglycans (118,119) suggests a relationship between Maroteaux-Lamy syndrome and the mucolipidoses.

In one patient, the affected cornea around a penetrating keratoplasty cleared (120,121).

β-Glucuronidase Deficiency

β-glucuronidase deficiency (mucopolysaccharidosis VII) is an autosomal-recessive trait in which dermatan sulfate accumulates in the tissues. Skeletal dysplasia, hepatosplenomegaly, and mental retardation are known to occur, but no ocular complications have been reported.

Glucose 6-Phosphatase Deficiency

Glucose 6-phosphatase deficiency (von Gierke's disease) is an autosomal-recessive glycogen storage disease caused by the deficiency of glucose-6-phosphatase. Like the other glycogen storage diseases, it is characterized by enlargement of the liver and kidneys and bouts of severe hypoglycemia.

Liver tissue is needed for diagnosis. If patients survive the initial hypoglycemia, the prognosis is good. Xanthomas with prominent lipemia are characteristic. Seizures and vomiting also occur. The cornea may show a faint brown peripheral clouding, and discrete yellow perimacular lesions have also been observed. Although no treatment exists for this disease, early diagnosis and recognition have led to an increased life expectancy.

Lipid

Mucolipidoses

The mucolipidoses are inherited metabolic diseases characterized by abnormal accumulation of acid mucopolysaccharides, sphingolipids, and glycolipids. Corneal opacities as well as psychomotor retardation and other systemic abnormalities are associated with this group of diseases.

Clinical Features: General

Mucolipidosis I is recessively inherited, but the specific enzymatic defect is unknown.

In this condition, physical growth is normal in the first years of life but slows after the age of 10. Hepatosplenomegaly and hernias are sometimes seen. Mental development is slow and patients usually have a moderate degree of mental retardation.

Mucolipidosis II is also recessively inherited with a deficiency of β-galactosidase. The disease is characterized by severe growth and psychomotor retardation, hepatomegaly, gargoyle-like facies, and thickened skin. The disease is also known as I-cell disease because of the cytoplasmic inclusions in fibroblasts and macrophages of affected persons (122).

Mucolipidosis III, also known as pseudo-Hurler, is a recessively inherited disease with an unknown enzymatic defect. Musculoskeletal abnormalities including small stature, short neck, scoliosis, hip dysplasia, and restricted joint mobility are seen. Moderate mental retardation is present, and gargoyle-like facies sometimes appear. Neither hepatosplenomegaly, severe psychomotor retardation, nor excessive excretion of mucopolysaccharides in the urine occurs in this disorder.

Mucolipidosis IV is probably a recessive disorder with an unknown enzymatic defect affecting mainly Ashkenazic Jews. It is characterized clinically by corneal clouding and profound psychomotor retardation but no skeletal or facial deformity, organomegaly, gross neurologic abnormalities, or mucopolysacchariduria.

Clinical Features: Ocular

In mucolipidosis I, corneal opacities are rarely seen, but when they occur, they are associated with a cherry red spot on the macula (123,124). Corneal opacities have been seen in association with spokelike cataracts, tortuous retinal and conjunctival vessels, and strabismus (124). Histologically, inclusion vacuoles are seen in the conjunctival and corneal epithelium.

Mucolipidosis II may be associated with bilateral corneal haziness, early cortical cataracts, and bilateral prominence of the eyes (123,125,126). Glaucoma, megalocornea, optic atrophy, absent retinal blood vessels, and severe retinal degeneration have also been described (127). Mucolipidosis III can be associated with fine corneal opacities, which are presumably abnormal storage material around stromal keratocytes (128).

Mucolipidosis IV is characterized by severe corneal clouding, ocular pain, and corneal surface irregularities seen at birth or early infancy (129–132). The severe and early corneal involvement distinguishes type IV from the other mucolipidoses. Light microscopy reveals swollen corneal and conjunctival cells containing foamy cytoplasm and vacuolated keratocytes. This material may represent phospholipids (120). Cataract, outer retinal degeneration, and optic atrophy may also be found. A case report described removal of the affected corneal epithelium and conjunctival transplantation from a related donor resulting in corneal clarity in a 28-month-old patient (133).

Fabry's Disease

Fabry's disease is a sphingolipidosis caused by a lack of alpha-galactosidase, transmitted as an X-linked recessive trait. The hemizygous male is most seriously affected. Female carriers may be asymptomatic or exhibit mild symptoms. High-performance liquid chromatography is a sensitive method for analyzing the urinary sediment for glycolipids and detecting asymptomatic heterozygotes (134). The skin is affected with clusters of punctate lesions that vary from purple to maroon to brownish but have a very characteristic distribution over the genitalia and lumbosacral area. The genitourinary, central nervous, musculoskeletal, and cardiovascular systems may all be involved. Common neurologic changes include hemiplegia, aphasia, cerebellar disorders, and stroke. Pain in the fingers and toes is common.

Ocular

Ocular findings are frequent and quite characteristic. The most typical ocular feature is cornea verticillata, a fine, whorl-like superficial corneal opacity caused by the accumulation of sphingolipids in the corneal epithelium (135–137). This corneal change can be found in both the affected male patient and the female carrier, and resembles the corneal opacities found after administration of chloroquine and amiodarone. Corneal opacities have been seen as early as the age of 6 months.

Other ocular alterations include dilatation and tortuosity of the conjunctival vessels, sometimes associated with aneurysms. Spoke-like posterior sutural cataracts consisting of nine to 12 spokes are seen in 50% of patients. Cream-colored anterior capsular deposits, sometimes in a propeller distribution, are also noted (138). Periorbital and retinal edema, optic atrophy and papilledema, and dilatation and tortuosity of the retinal vessels may be present.

The visual prognosis in Fabry's disease is excellent, although severe visual loss caused by central retinal artery occlusion has been reported (138). Internuclear ophthalmoplegia may rarely occur (139).

Without treatment, the disease is compatible with long life; deaths related to cardiovascular, renal, and gastrointestinal complications occur in midlife (140). The Food and Drug Administration (FDA) recently approved a drug for Fabry's disease (Fabrazyme) that works to reduce fat buildup in organs of patients with this condition.

Hyperlipoproteinemias

Five types of hyperlipoproteinemias have been distinguished (141). All the hyperlipoproteinemias may be associated with corneal arcus, xanthelasma, conjunctival xanthomas, and lipid keratopathy, except type I hyperlipoproteinemia, which is not usually associated with corneal arcus (142).

Familial Plasma Cholesterol Ester Deficiency

Familial plasma cholesterol ester deficiency [lecithin-cholesterol acyltransferase (LCAT) deficiency] is characterized by a marked reduction of plasma cholesterol esters and lysolecithin, and an increase in the level of unesterified cholesterol, triglycerides, and phospholipids. The deficiency of LCAT prevents the maintenance of a normal balance between cholesterol and cholesterol esters in cell membranes (143). The cornea shows a nebulous cloudiness and a pronounced annular opacity near the limbus. The opacity, found in the stroma, is composed of innumerable tiny dots and resembles a corneal arcus, but the peripheral border is not as sharply demarcated. It is believed that the corneal opacity is due to lipid deposits as a consequence of abnormal plasma lipid and glycoprotein deposition (144). Occasionally, crystals appear near Descemet's membrane peripheral to the opacity.

Tangier Disease

Tangier disease is an autosomal-recessive disease associated with the complete absence of plasma high-density α-lipoproteins. Corneal involvement consists of stromal clouding caused by deposition of cholesterol esters (145) and many small dots in the posterior stroma, sometimes in a whorl-like distribution. A haze in the peripheral horizontal meridian may be seen, but no arcus is present. Sometimes, visual impairment due to corneal clouding may be significant (146).

Histiocytosis X

In histiocytosis X (Hand-Schüller-Christian disease, Letterer-Siwe disease), large xanthomas or xanthelasma may be present on the lids. Infrequently a peripheral yellow-white infiltration may be present in all layers of the cornea. Similar corneal lesions may rarely be seen in juvenile xanthogranuloma.

Protein

Porphyria

The term *porphyria* embraces a group of diseases characterized by abnormalities in the enzymes involved in the biosynthesis of heme, resulting in the accumulation of one or more intermediate fluorescent pigments, known as porphyrins. Porphyria can be divided into two general groups: *erythropoietic porphyria,* in which excessive quantities of porphyrins accumulate in red blood cells, and *hepatic porphyria,* in which porphyrins accumulate in the liver. The latter may be subdivided into at least four different types: acute intermittent porphyria, porphyria variegata, porphyria cutanea tarda, and hereditary coproporphyria. Although there is some overlap between the erythropoietic and hepatic groups, specific inherited enzymatic defects have been identified in at least three of the porphyrias (erythropoietic uroporphyria, acute intermittent porphyria, and porphyria cutanea tarda). The enzymatic defects are present in many tissues; however, the resulting metabolic derangements are most prominent in either the liver or erythroid tissue.

Clinical Features

None of the erythropoietic porphyrias have ocular manifestations; the eyelids, however, may be involved as part of the involvement of the skin of the face. In erythropoietic uroporphyria, the skin manifestations take the form of blisters occurring on the skin surfaces exposed to light, especially the face and the hands, starting in childhood. With time, scarring and mutilation occur, with loss of fingers and facial tissues. In erythropoietic protoporphyria, there is skin photosensitivity with intense itching, edema, and erythema of the exposed skin. The disease is usually benign, consisting of chronic skin changes on the hands and face. Oral β-carotene provides effective protection against sun sensitivity but the reason for this is not known.

Of the hepatic porphyrias, acute intermittent porphyria is a rare autosomal-dominant disease, which is not usually associated with ocular manifestations, but which presents with gastrointestinal and neuropsychiatric manifestations.

Porphyria variegata is an autosomal-dominant condition characterized by cutaneous lesions and attacks of colic. It is also associated with ocular manifestations and is therefore discussed in greater detail here. Coproporphyrins and protoporphyrins are excreted in the feces in large amounts. The skin is unusually sensitive to light, and it blisters and abrades easily. Jaundice, colic, and psychosis may occur during acute attacks. Between attacks, there may be no symptoms.

Porphyria cutanea tarda is the most common form of porphyria; it is also associated with ocular manifestations. It is an autosomal-dominant disease and is characterized by photosensitive dermatitis, hyperpigmentation of the skin, liver disease, and hypertrichosis. The skin is sensitive to light and trauma, and blisters, ulcers, and scars may occur on areas exposed to light. Porphyria cutanea tarda may remain latent for several years, only to be precipitated by alcoholic cirrhosis or exposure to drugs or toxins.

Hereditary coproporphyria is an autosomal-dominant disease characterized by increased excretion of coproporphyrin in the urine and feces. Acute attacks may be precipitated by ingestion of barbiturates and other drugs. Symptoms consist of psychiatric crises and skin abnormalities.

Ocular

Acute intermittent porphyria has no ocular manifestations. Ocular involvement tends to occur in porphyria variegata and coproporphyria. The ocular findings in coproporphyria are variable and may affect all tissues of the eye. The eyebrows may be thinned or thickened and may meet in the midline (147). Bullous lesions of the eyelids may be followed by pigmentation and scarring. Ocular manifestations are similar to those of ocular pemphigoid, with blisters developing on the exposed area of the conjunctiva, resulting in symblepharon and shrinkage of the conjunctival sac, and possible stenosis of the punctum and canaliculus (148). Lacrimation, photophobia, and blepharospasm are common features (149). The conjunctiva becomes infiltrated by chronic inflammatory cells and forms adhesions to the underlying sclera, typically in the second or third decade of life.

Corneal complications are the result of cicatricial ectropion or vesiculation of the cornea. Vesicles occur in exposed areas of the cornea and heal forming nebulae or leukomas. Occasionally, the vesicles may lead to perforation (149). The cornea may be thin peripherally, contain numerous crystals in Bowman's layer, and have deep stromal lamellar opacification (150). Lesions resembling phlyctenules may precede corneal ulceration. Exposure keratitis and corneal opacification may result from severe ectropion.

Scleromalacia perforans may occur, with punched-out scleral ulcers occurring most commonly temporally (150). These ulcers may sometimes extend over the limbus onto the cornea. Scleritis is sometimes seen, and red fluorescence has been observed in the sclera, vitreous, and retina. The tissue damage that is seen is probably the result of oxidative or fluorochemical reactions.

Ophthalmoscopic changes include brown cotton-wool patches of edema. After 3 weeks, these become dense, black globular patches. Retinal hemorrhages and discrete annular choroidal lesions are sometimes observed (150). Atrophy of the ganglion cell and nerve fiber layer of the retina has also been described (151). Optic atrophy has been reported (152).

Diagnosis

The conjunctival changes of porphyria must be differentiated from those of cicatricial pemphigoid. The scleral and corneal changes must be distinguished from keratomalacia associated with vitamin A deficiency and peripheral corneal degenerations associated with local and systemic immunologic diseases. The retinal and choroidal lesions of porphyria can be confused with various types of uveitis. The systemic features of porphyria, the excretion of porphyrins, and the fluorescence of skin and ocular tissues will help in making a definitive diagnosis.

Treatment

If ultraviolet exposure causes damage, sunlight should be avoided. β-carotene, 30 mg/day orally, may be of value in reducing dermal sensitivity to sunlight. Crystalline retinopathy does not occur after long-term therapy with β-carotene as it does with canthaxanthin (153,154). Splenectomy and phlebotomy to remove the excess iron load from the liver are effective treatments for certain kinds of porphyria. Slow subcutaneous infusion of desferrioxamine may be helpful when phlebotomy is contraindicated. For acute attacks, a liberal intake of glucose orally or intravenously is the most effective treatment. Supportive therapy, including analgesics, fluids, and respiratory support, is also important for acute attacks.

Treatment of ocular lesions begins with proper medical management of systemic porphyria. Protection from the sun and abstention from alcohol seem to be helpful. Corticosteroids have been recommended for the scleritis of porphyria (150), but surgical treatment with scleral grafting may be necessary.

Gout

Gout is an abnormality of uric acid metabolism characterized by hyperuricemia, that results in the deposition of sodium urate crystals in the joints, soft tissues, and urinary tract. Primary gout occurs due to an inborn error of metabolism. Secondary gout occurs when hyperuricemia occurs as a result of some acquired metabolic derangement (and not an inherited metabolic disorder). Myeloproliferative disorders, high purine intake, alcohol consumption, cytotoxic chemotherapy, obesity, and hypertriglyceridemia can lead to hyperuricemia. The prevalence varies from approximately 0.2% in the United States and Western Europe to 10% in the adult male Maori of New Zealand. One third of patients with gout give a positive family history, and at least 50% are regular alcohol drinkers. Over 90% of gout is found among adult men, but 3% to 7% may occur in postmenopausal women. Secondary gout constitutes 5% to 10% of all cases and usually is a complication of myeloproliferative disorders or hypertensive cardiovascular disease.

Uric acid is formed by oxidation of purine bases, which may be of dietary or biosynthetic origin. In most cases with primary gout, the major cause of the hyperuricemia is the overproduction of uric acid, but there is also increased excretion. Not all cases of hyperuricemia are associated with the clinical syndrome of gout. Idiopathic hyperuricemia is 10 times more common than gout.

Clinical Features

The natural history of gout consists of three phases: asymptomatic hyperuricemia, acute gouty arthritis, and chronic gouty arthritis. Fifty percent of initial acute attacks involve the great toe (podagra), and 90% of gout patients experience podagra during the course of their disease. Attacks may be precipitated by many kinds of stress. Dietary, physical, and emotional factors have been implicated. Chronic gouty arthritis is associated with a progressive inability to dispose of urate and deposition of urate crystals in the cartilage, synovial membranes, tendons, and soft tissues. Tophaceous deposits may produce irregular swelling over the joints or the helix of the ear. Eventually, destruction of the joints ensues. The incidence of permanent joint change is considerably less now that drugs are available to control uric acid levels.

Ocular

Acute ocular inflammation in gout is characterized by a conjunctivitis and episcleritis adjacent to the limbus. There is marked hyperemia and scanty discharge. The conjunctival vessels are dilated and tortuous (155) and the patient experiences a burning, hot, prickly sensation. This has been referred to by Hutchinson (156) as the "hot eye of gout." Conjunctival tophi have also been reported (157). The inflammation is episodic and associated with acute attacks of gouty arthritis. True scleritis may rarely be associated with gout, and urate crystals occasionally are found in the sclera (157). Clinical gout is present in about 2% of patients with scleritis. Acute iritis has also been reported but is extremely rare (155). The cornea may be affected with the uric acid crystals deposited in the interpalpebral limbal area adjacent to the episcleral blood vessels. Pinguecula-like limbal masses of urate have been described and band keratopathy has also been observed with gout (158); it may be impossible to distinguish this condition from calcific band keratopathy by slit-lamp examination. Monosodium urate crystals may be deposited in the superficial stroma and epithelium of both the conjunctiva and the cornea (159). Corneal scraping reveals urates that can be demonstrated by colorimetry and spectrophotometry (158). Urate crystals occur within the nuclei of the corneal epithelial cells (159). The crystals are needle-like and demonstrate negative birefringence.

Diagnosis

Ocular gout should be distinguished from keratitis urica (160), a localized dystrophic disease of the cornea having an uncertain cause but unassociated with gout. Uric acid levels, a history of typical attacks of gouty arthritis, and the presence of tophi help in making a correct diagnosis. It must be noted, though, that only 2% of cases with scleritis and 7% with episcleritis may have clinical gout. In the absence of hyperuricemia and the characteristic clinical features of gout, corneal urate deposits must be differentiated from the deposits of other metabolic corneal diseases as well as certain drug depositions. Rheumatoid arthritis, acute rheumatic fever, and osteoarthritis may need to be distinguished from gouty arthritis.

Treatment

Treatment of gouty arthritis is aimed at terminating the acute attack and preventing new recurrences, as well as preventing and reversing uric acid deposition in the joints and kidneys. Colchicine, indomethacin, naproxen, and phenylbutazone are effective in treating the acute gouty arthritis attack. Hydrocortisone may be injected intraarticularly for prompt relief of pain. Drugs that lower the serum level of uric acid include probenecid, salicylates, sulfinpyrazone, and allopurinol (161,162). Allopurinol is a potent inhibitor of xanthinoxidase and has been associated with the development of cataracts (163). In some cases, surgical removal of urate deposits may be necessary. Tophaceous deposits can also be surgically removed from the conjunctiva. Superficial keratectomy may be necessary to remove the urate band keratopathy. Purified uricase may supplement the scraping of the superficial deposits.

Cystinosis

Cystinosis (Lignac-Fanconi syndrome) is a rare autosomal-recessive disorder of cystine storage. French Canada has the highest incidence of cystinosis in the world. The lysosomal cystine transport system is thought to be defective (164), and cystine is found in lipid-storing membranes of circulating leukocytes, fibroblasts, and macrophages (165). Cystinosis usually occurs in childhood in association with Fanconi's syndrome, which is a descriptive term for a group of physiologic abnormalities that include proximal renal tubular dysfunction, notably glucosuria; generalized aminoaciduria; phosphaturia; and renal tubular acidosis. Occasionally, ocular and systemic cystine storage occurs in the adult in the absence of renal disease.

Cystinosis results from the intracellular deposition of crystalline cystine in the reticuloendothelial cells of the bone marrow, liver, spleen, lymphatic system, and kidney.

Clinical Features

Three clinical forms of cystinosis are recognized. The infantile form with Fanconi's syndrome is a severe disorder usually leading to death by the age of 10. Severe rickets with stunting of growth and failure to thrive is evident in the first few months of life and the disorder may be associated with secondary hyperparathyroidism and frequent pyelonephritis with consequent renal failure. An intermediate form presents in early young adulthood with fever and renal problems. The third, adult form, is benign.

Ocular

Ocular manifestations of cystinosis are characterized by the deposition of cystine crystals in the cornea. These crystals, which are glistening, polychromatic, and needle-like to rectangular, are distributed throughout the anterior stroma with a slight predilection for the periphery. Mild photophobia is the most common ocular symptom and patients may also complain of increased glare sensitivity, decreased contact sensitivity, and decreased vision. In infantile cystinosis, the corneal crystals may appear as early as 6 months of age and can cause intense photophobia. In adult cystinosis, they may be the only manifestation of the disease. Crystals may be found throughout the entire thickness of the corneal stroma (166); if they are extensive, visual acuity may be reduced. The corneal thickness is increased, possibly reflecting subclinical corneal edema (167). Corneal sensitivity is decreased (168).

Intracellular crystals have also been demonstrated within cells of the iris, ciliary body, choroid, and retinal pigment epithelium (165–169). Retinopathy associated with extensive degeneration and loss of the pigment epithelium has also been described (170). These peripheral fundus abnormalities may precede the corneal deposits and prove helpful in making an early diagnosis of cystinosis. Crystalline macular changes may occur as a result of cystine crystals in the choroid or pigment epithelium (171). Retinoschisis and retinal detachment have been reported in conjunction with adult cystinosis (172). In the adolescent form of cystinosis, corneal crystals and nephropathy may be present, but retinopathy is absent (173).

Diagnosis

Cystinosis must be differentiated from other types of corneal depositions, including the paraproteinemias. Conjunctival biopsy is a useful technique in which cystine can be extracted and analyzed by column chromatography (174). In addition, the characteristic retinal lesions may be very useful in making a proper diagnosis (175).

Treatment

Dietary restriction is not successful, because cystine is synthesized from the essential amino acid methionine. Renal transplantation has been carried out successfully in a number of patients. Potassium replacement to reverse chronic acidosis and vitamin D therapy to promote normal calcification of bone are important.

The mainstay of therapy, however, is cysteamine administration (176), which may prevent the development of the complications of cystinosis and remove crystals after they have developed (177,178). The major problem with the drug is its taste and odor. The phosphorothioester of cysteamine, which is tasteless and odorless, is presently being tested (179). Cysteamine eyedrops prevent the deposition of crystals in the cornea. The adult form of the disease is benign and requires no treatment.

Type II Hypertyrosinemia

Type II hypertyrosinemia is caused by a deficit of the enzyme tyrosine aminotransferase. A dendritic lesion may develop in the cornea (180,181), which must be differentiated from a healing wound and herpetic disease. Other ocular changes include conjunctival plaques, strabismus, and cataracts. A chronic keratitis may develop (182). The systemic findings include hyperkeratotic skin lesions and mental retardation (183,184).

Alkaptonuria

This hereditary metabolic disease is caused by an absence of the enzyme homogentisic acid oxidase, which results in an accumulation of homogentisic acid, a normal intermediary in the metabolism of phenylalanine and tyrosine, in the urine and other tissues including the eye. Oxidation of homogentisic acid produces a form of degenerative arthritis and a dark pigmentary change in connective tissues known as ochronosis.

Clinical Features
The first description of alkaptonuria was by Garrod in 1902 (185). The disease occurs in about 1 in 200,000 births. In the infant, darkening of the urine on a wet diaper may be the first sign. Alkaptonuria is a benign disorder until midlife, when degenerative joint changes begin to take place in the majority of patients, primarily in the large joints and the spine. Ochronotic pigmentation of the ear, nose, and sclera is often seen. Internal structures such as the costochondral junctions, joints, and ligaments have also been noted to have ochronotic pigmentation. A diagnosis is usually made on the basis of the triad of arthritis, ochronotic pigmentation, and urine that darkens on the addition of a strong alkali.

Ocular
Ocular pigmentation is found in the interpalpebral sclera at the insertion of the recti muscles (186). In addition, a more diffuse pigmentation may also be found in the conjunctiva and cornea. The pigmentation may be gray to bluish black but microscopically appears ochre. Corneal pigment is located in the deep epithelium and in Bowman's layer. Pigmentation of the tarsal plates and lids may also be seen.

Treatment
Attempts to treat alkaptonuria with vitamin C and cortisone may delay the onset of arthritis (187). Dietary restriction of phenylalanine and tyrosine is not practical except for brief periods, and there is no conclusive evidence that it is of benefit. Enzyme replacement and gene transfer therapies are also not available at present.

Amyloidosis

Amyloid is an eosinophilic hyaline material that can be deposited in various tissues of the body, including the eye, as part of a localized or systemic disease. There are at least two different types of amyloid. Type A amyloid (also known as AA) is a nonimmunoglobulin protein of unknown origin. Type B amyloid has been shown to be identical to a fragment of the light chain of immunoglobulin. Amyloid deposits are associated with a structural protein known as P or AP (188).

Amyloidosis is sometimes classified as primary or secondary. Either type A or type B amyloid can occur in both forms. Amyloidosis may also be defined as systemic or localized. A third type of amyloid, known as type C, may be seen adjacent to tumors of neuroectodermal origin and in aging.

Several mechanisms may account for the deposition of amyloid in the tissues of the body, including catabolism by macrophages of deposited antigen-antibody complexes, de novo synthesis of whole immunoglobulins or light chains with reduced solubility, genetic deletions in the light-chain gene producing an anomalous protein of reduced solubility, and separate synthesis of discrete regions of the light chain. Other types of amyloid may be formed by complexing precursors of polypeptide hormones. The reason for amyloid deposition is unknown. It may be a disorder of protein metabolism, an abnormality of the reticuloendothelial system, the result of chronic immunologic stimulation, a disorder of delayed hypersensitivity, or a combination of these defects (189).

Clinical Features
Many classifications of amyloidosis exist. The most widely used classification divides amyloidosis into the following: (a) Primary amyloidosis occurs in the absence of a preexisting disease. (b) Secondary amyloidosis usually follows chronic diseases such as neoplasms, infections, and connective tissue disorders. (c) Tumor-forming amyloid is an isolated mass of amyloid that appears in the skin, eye, or urinary tract. (d) Familial types of amyloidosis affect different organ systems and have different patterns of inheritance. The most common is associated with familial Mediterranean fever, seen mostly in Sephardic Jews.

Virtually any organ system can be affected in amyloidosis. Kidney involvement is usually the main cause of death. Renal involvement is the preponderant manifestation in secondary amyloidosis and in approximately half the patients with primary amyloidosis. Cardiac deposition of amyloid may be asymptomatic or lead to congestive heart failure. Amyloid may be deposited in any portion of the gastrointestinal tract, from the tongue to the anus. Diagnosis can sometimes be made by biopsy of the rectum, conjunctiva, or gingivae. Amyloid infiltration may also be seen in nearly every other tissue of the body. Involvement is often limited to the walls of small blood vessels, and clinical manifestations may be absent.

Ocular

The skin of the eyelid is a frequent site of amyloid deposition. Small papules with a waxy, yellowish appearance are typical. Conjunctival amyloid nodules, although rarely seen, may mimic various forms of conjunctivitis, including trachoma. Occasionally, large tumor-like conjunctival nodules may be seen in the absence of any apparent predisposing condition (190).

Amyloid may be deposited in the cornea as the result of preexisting chronic inflammation (e.g., in interstitial keratitis patients). Amyloid has been demonstrated in the corneal epithelium of a patient with retinopathy of prematurity (191). It has also been detected in the corneas in seven unsuspected cases of amyloidosis showing corneal scarring and opacification (192). Corneal involvement is characterized by the presence of cobblestone masses of yellowish pink material, which stain bright salmon pink with 0.2% Congo red (193). A gelatinous or drop-like change in the cornea has been described in primary corneal amyloidosis, especially in Japan (194–197). Familial amyloidosis of the cornea has also been described (198) and may be associated with cataracts (which do not contain amyloid). Lattice dystrophy of the cornea is considered a localized form of amyloidosis (199,200), but it may be associated with systemic amyloidosis as well, or with the Meretoja syndrome (201). Type A amyloid has been identified in the cornea of a patient with lattice corneal dystrophy (202).

Amyloid may be deposited in the iris secondary to chronic infection (203), or it may be found in the vitreous where it has a characteristic glass-wool appearance. Most patients with vitreous amyloid have familial amyloidosis, although some have no family history of the disease. Vitreous opacities can be unilateral or bilateral. They may be in contact with the posterior lens surface. Pupillary abnormalities are not uncommon in familial amyloidosis. The irides may show segmented paralysis (204), pupillary dissociation (205), inequality (206), or heterochromia (207). Scalloped pupils are a characteristic feature of familial amyloidosis and may be a helpful clue in making a correct diagnosis (207,208). This pupillary abnormality may be due to infiltration of the sphincter of nonadjacent ciliary nerves with amyloid.

Orbital involvement may be seen in amyloidosis and may lead to proptosis (209,210). Lacrimal gland and extraocular muscle involvement has also been described (209).

Histopathology

Homogeneous amyloid consists of characteristic long fibrils, which measure 80 Å. It is not known whether these fibrils are synthesized as such or whether they are the result of degradation of intact protein molecules. Clinically suspected amyloidosis must be confirmed by biopsy of appropriate tissues. Amyloid stains with hematoxylin and eosin. It is periodic acid-Schiff (PAS)-positive and stains mahogany brown with iodine, changing to blue with the addition of sulfuric acid. Amyloid stains brown with Congo red and exhibits dichroism and birefringence with polarized light. Amyloid fluoresces yellow green with thioflavine T.

Treatment

In amyloidosis associated with plasma cell tumors, treatment is directed at the tumor; however, regression of the amyloid lesions may be slow or imperceptible. Treatment of an infection or an inflammatory process may cause mobilization of systemic amyloid. Colchicine may abort the febrile episodes of familial Mediterranean fever, a disease often accompanied by amyloidosis. This drug can also prevent the development of amyloidosis in mice (211) and may be useful in far-advanced human disease. Various other agents including steroids, ascorbic acid, and immunosuppressive agents have also been tried, but without clear-cut benefit.

The vitreous deposits associated with amyloidosis may be removed by vitrectomy (212); however, redeposition tends to occur. Corneal transplantation may be necessary in advanced lattice corneal dystrophy or for the localized forms of corneal amyloidosis.

Graves' Disease

Among the metabolic disorders that affect the eye, Graves' disease (thyroid exophthalmopathy) is one of the most common and potentially severe. In this disorder, lymphocytes and plasma cells infiltrate the thyroid gland and retro-orbital tissues. This infiltration may lead to mild or severe exophthalmos and corneal exposure.

Graves' disease is an autoimmune condition. Antibodies to thyroid and other tissues are found in virtually all patients with Graves' disease (213). Other immunoglobulin-containing substances have also been identified in the serum of patients with Graves' disease, and there is evidence of cellular immunity to thyroid antigens in patients with Graves' disease and Hashimoto's thyroiditis (214).

Deposition of mucopolysaccharides, fat hypertrophy, and soft tissue edema lead to exophthalmos in Graves' disease. The exophthalmos may occur in the acute stage of the disease, or may occur while the patient is euthyroid.

Clinical Features

The signs and symptoms of Graves' disease are due to the overproduction of thyroid hormone. Tissue metabolism is increased, and the patient experiences restlessness, heat intolerance, weight loss, and palpitations. The skin is warm, moist, and smooth, and sweating is excessive. A diffusely enlarged thyroid gland may be found on physical examination.

A fine tremor, tachycardia, wide pulse pressure, and muscle weakness are also characteristic.

Ocular

Half the patients with hyperthyroidism have no ocular abnormalities. Common findings include widening of the palpebral fissures owing to retraction of the upper eyelid (the cause remains unknown), lid lag on downward gaze, and infrequent blink. About 20% of patients with Graves' disease exhibit proptosis. This is thought to reflect retro-orbital infiltration and soft tissue swelling. If proptosis and lid retraction are severe enough, exposure keratitis may result. The earliest change is punctate staining of the inferior cornea and conjunctiva. This may indicate nocturnal lagophthalmos. More severe exposure will lead to frank epithelial cell loss and sometimes a persistent epithelial defect. If the exposure is not corrected, corneal stromal ulceration and even corneal perforation may result. This may or may not be accompanied by secondary microbial keratitis. Because the progression of events may be rapid, early recognition of exposure keratitis is important.

The most severe complication associated with Graves' ophthalmopathy is irreversible optic nerve damage caused by pressure on the optic nerve or its blood supply resulting from orbital congestion. Milder forms of this syndrome may result in diplopia, papillitis, retrobulbar neuritis, or papilledema.

Treatment

The treatment of hyperthyroidism associated with Graves' disease may involve removal of the thyroid gland, administration of radioactive iodine, or therapy with antithyroid drugs (215).

Mild ophthalmopathy is relatively easy to treat by keeping the cornea well hydrated with lubricants and preventing exposure keratitis. It may be helpful to tape the lids closed at night after lubricants are instilled. Fishing goggles that create a humidity chamber may be useful. More severe cases may require lid surgery. Tarsorrhaphy or surgical procedures designed to decrease upper eyelid retraction, such as recession of the levator and Müller's muscle, may be effective. However, eyelid procedures are undertaken only after the orbital and muscle issues have been addressed, if surgical decompression of the orbits and muscle surgery is needed.

High-dose systemic steroids may in some instances be successful in reducing exophthalmos. Supervoltage orbital radiation may also be used in acute cases of optic nerve compression (216). Surgical decompression of the orbit is highly effective for severe ophthalmopathy.

Minerals

Calcium

Calcium deposition can occur in the cornea under a wide variety of circumstances ranging from local ocular inflammation to widespread systemic metabolic abnormalities. The most frequent pattern of corneal calcification is band keratopathy. However, diffuse corneal calcification, sometimes accompanied by conjunctival calcification, is known to occur (217).

Band keratopathy begins in the peripheral cornea in the interpalpebral zones. A clear interval is usually present between the band and the limbus. If severe, the deposit may extend across the visual axis. In many cases, the band simply remains in the periphery. Tiny Swiss cheese-like holes are usually present in the deposit. These are thought to be located in areas where corneal nerves penetrate Bowman's layer.

Histologically, the calcium is deposited in and around Bowman's layer. The early histologic change consists of a basophilic stippling of the epithelial basement membrane followed by deposition and fragmentation within Bowman's layer.

When calcific deposits in the cornea impair visual acuity, they can be removed by a variety of methods (218).

Hyperparathyroidism

Corneal calcification has been studied extensively in both primary and secondary hyperparathyroidism (219,220). Calcium, in the form of hydroxyapatite crystals, is found intracellularly in both the conjunctiva and the cornea. In other cases of band keratopathy, calcium spherules and conglomerates are usually found extracellularly. It has been suggested that parathyroid hormone may have an effect on the intracellular deposition of calcium (219,220).

Hypophosphatasia

Hypophosphatasia is a rare familial disease characterized clinically by multiple skeletal abnormalities, pathologic fractures of long bones, malformation of the skull and orbits, early loss of teeth, failure to thrive, and often early death caused by nephrocalcinosis and the other sequelae of hypercalcemia. Band keratopathy and conjunctival calcification have been noted in this syndrome and may be associated with blue sclera, harlequin orbits, pathologic lid retraction, papilledema, and increased intracranial pressure (221,222).

Dietary Causes

Excessive vitamin D intake in a range of 100,000 to 500,000 IU daily may lead to band keratopathy and nephrocalcinosis in a few months to a few years. Excessive ingestion of antacids, a condition known as the milk-alkali syndrome, has been associated with similar changes.

Renal Failure

Patients with renal failure may demonstrate uremia, hypercalcemia, and band keratopathy. In some cases, renal damage may result from high calcium and alkali intake. Red eyes and conjunctival irritation are sometimes associated with renal failure (223,224). The conjunctival injection and granular appearance of the conjunctiva are due to a deposition of microcrystals of calcium phosphate salts in the conjunctiva and cornea. Over 80% of severely uremic patients will have corneal and conjunctival calcific deposits. Most of these patients are asymptomatic, and chronic hemodialysis does not seem to have any influence on the deposits (225). Typical conjunctival and corneal changes associated with chronic renal failure consist of diffuse opacification of the peripheral limbal area and the interpalpebral zone (226). Such deposits may regress after kidney transplantation.

Neoplastic and Inflammatory Diseases

Diffuse or bandlike calcific changes may be associated with sarcoidosis and with various malignancies with and without bone metastases. Multiple myeloma and Paget's disease of bone may also lead to band keratopathy.

Corneal Scars

Band keratopathy is frequently associated with chronic ocular inflammation such as trachoma and interstitial keratitis (227). The severity of the band reflects the duration of the inflammation.

Iridocyclitis

Band keratopathy is a well-known complication of chronic iridocyclitis, especially cases occurring in children. The exact mechanism of this deposition is unknown. It has been suggested that gaseous exchange at the surface of the exposed cornea with loss of carbon dioxide and a localized elevation of pH may be an important factor (228). Experimental band keratopathy can regularly be induced in rabbits with immunogenic uveitis that have been given systemic calciferol (229). Lid closure may prevent the development of these calcific deposits.

Dry-Eye Syndrome

Rapid development of band keratopathy has been reported in dry-eye patients with corneal inflammation who use artificial tears frequently (230). Whether this corneal change is due to some component of the artificial tears or another mechanism is still unclear.

Mercurial Compounds

Atypical band keratopathy has been reported in glaucoma patients using pilocarpine with the preservative phenylmercuric nitrate (231,232). The reason for this deposition is unclear, and this preservative is no longer used in eye drops.

Copper

Copper deposition in the eye may be the result of metabolic diseases or intraocular foreign bodies composed of copper or copper alloys. Hepatolenticular degeneration or Wilson's disease is a deficiency of the copper-binding serum protein ceruloplasmin. This condition is characterized by deposition of free copper in nearly all the body's tissues,

especially the liver, basal ganglia of the brain, kidney, and cornea. Patients with Wilson's disease have ataxia, hepatosplenomegaly, cirrhosis of the liver, and progressive neurologic impairment. The disease is inherited as an autosomal-recessive trait. Copper excretion is high, but serum copper is low because the copper is deposited in the tissues. The most characteristic ocular feature of Wilson's disease is the Kayser-Fleischer ring in the peripheral cornea. This ring is a deposition of copper 1 to 3 mm wide in the peripheral cornea. It is green, blue, red, yellow, brown, or a mixture of any of these colors. There is no lucid interval unless an anterior embryotoxon is present. The ring is at the level of Descemet's membrane. It may be absent before the age of 10, and it may also disappear on treatment with chelating agents and restricted copper intake. Anterior subcapsular cataracts, sometimes called sunflower cataracts, may be part of the ocular picture of Wilson's disease.

Copper may also be deposited in the cornea in primary biliary cirrhosis, progressive intrahepatic cholestasis of childhood, and chronic active hepatitis (233).

Intraocular foreign bodies of pure copper produce a marked suppurative reaction and loss of the eye. Copper alloys containing less than 85% copper result in less severe reactions (234,235). Intraocular copper produces a blue-green discoloration between the endothelium and Descemet's membrane, especially in the peripheral cornea. The iris, vitreous, and lens may also be affected. If electroretinographic changes develop, the copper foreign body should be removed and medical treatment with a chelating agent instituted. Penicillamine, 250 mg, can be taken orally four times each day for extended periods.

Gold

Intramuscular gold therapy has been used in the treatment of rheumatoid arthritis and other collagen vascular diseases. The exact therapeutic mode of action is uncertain; however, gold may be capable of inhibiting lysosomal hydrolases. With continued therapy, gold is deposited in various tissues including the kidney, liver, spleen, and eye (236).

Two forms of gold deposition have been reported in the cornea. Corneal chrysiasis consists of numerous, minute, yellowish brown to violet, glistening deposits that are distributed irregularly throughout the cornea at various depths (236–238). Sometimes, the deposits are described as dustlike and are gold to purple violet (239). Deposits may be seen in the deep stroma or in the epithelium (240). Occasionally, a vortex distribution can be seen. Most patients receiving an excess of 1,500 mg of gold or 25 mg/wk for 6 months will demonstrate corneal chrysiasis. Other ocular features include deposition of gold in bulbar conjunctiva and anterior lens capsule. Dermatitis and stomatitis are signs of gold toxicity. Ocular chrysiasis does not usually produce any symptoms, and visual acuity is not ordinarily impaired. A second form of

TABLE 39-12. ADDITIONAL METABOLIC DISEASES THAT AFFECT THE CORNEA

Disease	Enzyme Deficiency	Corneal Findings	Other Ocular Findings	Systemic Findings
Alport's syndrome	Unknown	Lenticonus, cataract, retinal flecks	Arcus, posterior polymorphous dystrophy, granular stroma	Nephritis, deafness
Fish eye syndrome	Unknown	Clouding	None	Hyperlipoproteinemia
Goldberg-Cotlier disease	β-Galactosidase	Clouding	Macular cherry red spot	Gargoylism, skeletal. abnormalities, mental retardation, seizures, hearing loss
Lowe's syndrome	Unknown	Keloids	Cataract, glaucoma, miotic pupil	Mental retardation, aminoaciduria
Norrie's disease	Unknown	Band keratopathy	Cataract, retrolental membrane, microphthalmos, retinal folds	Hearing loss, mental retardation
Phenylketonuria	Hepatic phenylalanine hydroxylase	Opacities	Strabismus, cataract, albinoid fundus	Seizures, mental retardation, melanin abnormality, gait alteration, microcephaly
Riley-Day syndrome	Dopamine-β-hydroxylase	Anesthesia, epithelial erosion	Dry eye	Familial dysautonomia

ocular disease caused by gold is a possibly allergic response consisting of marginal ulceration and keratitis (240). Painful, white, crescent-shaped ulcers bordering the limbus are seen. Distinct, flat, white, superficial opacities have also been noted.

Corneal gold deposition is not necessarily an indication for discontinuing gold therapy. Deposits tend to resolve when gold treatment is stopped, and penicillamine appears to be effective for the toxic reactions.

Silver

Silver deposition in the cornea, conjunctiva, and lens has been observed during the use of topical silver preparations, such as mild silver protein (Argyrol), and after industrial exposure to organic silver salts. Argyrosis is rare today, although a number of cases have been reported (241–244).

The conjunctiva develops a slate-gray appearance. The nasal portion where the tear pool accumulates may be nearly black. The cornea may contain fine, blue-gray, green, or gold deposits. These are found in the deep stroma and in Descemet's membrane, especially inferiorly. Electron microscopic examination has shown that minute silver deposits are located intracellularly in the connective tissue of the conjunctiva and extracellularly in Descemet's membrane (243). Ocular argyrosis produces only cosmetic changes; it does not impair vision. The skin and the eyelids may develop a slate-gray hue. Argyrosis of the nasolacrimal sac has been reported (244), and iridescent cataracts have been described as well. Severe silver nitrate injury to the cornea has been reported after use of the concentrated applicator sticks (242). Obviously, these applicators should not be used around the eye.

Rare Metabolic Disorders

Parathyroid and thyroid tumors as well as those in the pancreas and adrenal cortex can be associated with the multiple endocrine neoplasia (MEN) syndrome. MEN type I consists of an aggregation of tumors of parathyroid, pancreatic, and pituitary glands. MEN type II consists of medullary carcinomas of the thyroid and pheochromocytoma. Type III includes type II tumors plus mucosal neuromas, intestinal ganglioneuromatosis, marfanoid habitus, thickened eyelids, subconjunctival neuromas, and prominent corneal nerves (245). Refsum's disease, a rare metabolic disorder, can also be associated with prominent corneal nerves.

Corneal abnormalities may be found in several other rare metabolic disorders. For the sake of completeness, some of these are listed in Table 39-12.

ACKNOWLEDGMENTS

Dr. Fred M. Wilson II and Mitchell H. Friedlaender were the original authors of this chapter. Their comprehensive work, with only minimal revision, was the framework for this chapter.

REFERENCES

1. Duke-Elder S. *Normal and abnormal development: congenital deformities. System of ophthalmology series.* St. Louis: Mosby, 1964.
2. Bergsma D. *Birth defects: atlas and compendium.* Baltimore: Williams & Wilkins, 1973.

3. Mann I. *Developmental abnormalities of the eye.* London: Cambridge University Press, 1937.

4. Erikkson AW, Lehmann W, Forsius H. Congenital cornea plana in Finland. *Clin Genet* 1973;4:301.

5. Codère F, Brownstein S, Chen MF. Cryptophthalmos syndrome with bilateral renal agenesis. *Am J Ophthalmol* 1981; 91:737.

6. Goldhammer Y, Smith JL. Cryptophthalmos syndrome with basal encephaloceles. *Am J Ophthalmol* 1975;80:146.

7. Ide CH, Wollschlaeger PB. Multiple congenital abnormalities associated with cryptophthalmia. *Arch Ophthalmol* 1969;81:638.

8. Reinecke RD. Cryptophthalmos. *Arch Ophthalmol* 1971;85:376.

9. Vail DT Jr. Adult hereditary anterior megalophthalmos sine glaucoma: a definite disease entity. With special reference to the extraction of cataract. *Arch Ophthalmol* 1931;6:39.

10. Pearce WG. Autosomal dominant megalocornea with congenital glaucoma: evidence for germ-line mosaicism. *Can J Ophthalmol* 1991;26:21.

11. Skuta GL, Sugar J, Ericson ES. Corneal endothelial cell measurements in megalocornea. *Arch Ophthalmol* 1983;101:51.

12. Meire FM, Delleman JW. Biometry in X-linked megalocornea: pathognomonic findings. *Br J Ophthalmol* 1994;78:781.

13. Malbran E, Dodds R. Megalocornea and its relation to congenital glaucoma. *Am J Ophthalmol* 1960;49:908.

14. Shaffer RN, Weiss DI. *Congenital and pediatric glaucomas.* St. Louis: Mosby, 1970.

15. Young AI. Megalocornea and mosaic dystrophy in identical twins. *Am J Ophthalmol* 1968;66:734.

16. Geeraets WJ. *Ocular syndromes,* 3rd ed. Philadelphia: Lea & Febiger, 1976.

17. Lewis RA, Nussbaum RL, Stambolian D. Mapping X-linked ophthalmic diseases. IV Provisional assignment of the locus for X-linked congenital cataracts and microcornea (the Nance-Horan Syndrome) to X. p. 22.2-p. 22.3. *Ophthalmology* 1990;97:110.

18. Evans D, Hickey-Dwyer MU. Cleft anterior segment with maternal hypervitaminosis A. *Br J Ophthalmol* 1991;75:691.

19. Thomas C, Cordier J, Reny A. Les manifestations ophthalmologiques du syndrome de Turner. *Arch Ophthalmol* 1969; 29:565.

20. Wilkins L. *The diagnosis and treatment of endocrine disorders in childhood and adolescence.* Springfield, IL: Thomas, 1950.

21. Waardenburg PJ, Franceschetti A, Klein D. *Genetics and ophthalmology.* Assen, Netherlands: Royal van Gorcum, 1961.

22. Arffa RC. *Grayson's diseases of the cornea,* 3rd ed. St. Louis: Mosby, 1991.

23. Jacobs HB. Posterior conical cornea. *Br J Ophthalmol* 1957; 41:31.

24. Ross JVM. Keratoconus posticus generalis. *Am J Ophthalmol* 1950;33:801.

25. Laibson PR, Waring GO. Diseases of the cornea. In: Harley RD, ed. *Pediatric ophthalmology.* Philadelphia: Saunders, 1975.

26. Balm CF, et al. Classification of corneal endothelial disorders based on neural crest origin. *Ophthalmology* 1984;91:558.

27. Spencer H. Cornea. In: Spencer WH, ed. *Ophthalmic pathology: an atlas and textbook,* 3rd ed. Philadelphia: Saunders, 1985:248.

28. Alkemade PPH. *Dysgenesis mesodermalis of the iris and cornea: a study of Rieger's syndrome and Peters' anomaly.* Assen, Netherlands: Thomas and Royal van Gorcum, 1969.

29. Reese AB, Ellsworth RM. The anterior chamber cleavage syndrome. *Arch Ophthalmol* 1966;75:307.

30. Waring GO III, Rodrigues MM, Laibson PR. Anterior-chamber cleavage syndrome: a stepladder classification. *Surv Ophthalmol* 1975;20:3.

31. Duke-Elder S, Cook C. *Normal and abnormal development: embryology. System of ophthalmology series.* St. Louis: Mosby, 1963.

32. Allen L, Burian HM, Braley AE. New concept of development of anterior chamber angle. *Arch Ophthalmol* 1955;53:783.

33. Henkind P, Siegel I, Carr RE. Mesodermal dysgenesis of the anterior segment: Rieger's anomaly. *Arch Ophthalmol* 1965; 73:810.

34. Ferguson JG, Hicks EL. Rieger's anomaly and glaucoma associated with partial trisomy 16q. *Arch Ophthalmol* 1987;105:323.

35. Brear DR, Insler MS. Axenfeld's syndrome associated with systemic abnormalities. *Ann Ophthalmol* 1985;17:291.

36. Tabbara KF, Khouri FP, der Kaloustian VM. Rieger's syndrome with chromosomal anomaly (report of a case). *Can J Ophthalmol* 1973;8:488.

37. Heinemann M, Breg R, Cother E. Rieger's syndrome with pericentric inversion of chromosome 6. *Br J Ophthalmol* 1979; 63:40.

38. Henkind P, Friedman AH. Iridogoniodysgenesis with cataract. *Am J Ophthalmol* 1971;72:949.

39. Stone DL, et al. Congenital central corneal leukoma (Peters' anomaly). *Am J Ophthalmol* 1976;81:173.

40. Townsend WM. Congenital corneal leukomas: I. Central defect in Descemet's membrane. *Am J Ophthalmol* 1974;77:80.

41. Townsend WM, Font RL, Zimmerman LE. Congenital corneal leukomas: II. Histopathologic findings in 19 eyes with central defect in Descemet's membrane. *Am J Ophthalmol* 1974; 77:192.

42. Townsend WM, Font RL, Zimmerman LE. Congenital corneal leukomas: III. Histopathologic findings in 13 eyes with noncentral defect in Descemet's membrane. *Am J Ophthalmol* 1974; 77:400.

43. Grayson M. The nature of hereditary deep polymorphous dystrophy of the cornea: its association with iris and anterior chamber dysgenesis. *Trans Am Ophthalmol Soc* 1974;72:516.

44. Waring GO III Rodrigues MM, Laibson PR. Corneal dystrophies: II. Endothelial dystrophies. *Surv Ophthalmol* 1978; 23:147.

45. Dohlman CH. Familial congenital cornea guttata in association with anterior polar cataract. *Acta Ophthalmol* 1951; 29:445.

46. Judisch GF, Maumenee IH. Clinical differentiation of recessive congenital hereditary endothelial dystrophy and dominant congenital hereditary endothelial dystrophy. *Am J Ophthalmol* 1978; 85:606.

47. Kenyon KR, Maumenee AE. Further studies of congenital hereditary endothelial dystrophy of the cornea. *Am J Ophthalmol* 1973;76:419.

48. Maumenee AE. Congenital hereditary corneal dystrophy. *Am J Ophthalmol* 1960;50:1114.

49. Pearce WG, Tripathi RC, Morgan G. Congenital endothelial corneal dystrophy. Clinical, pathological and genetic study. *Br J Ophthalmol* 1969;53:477.

50. Waring GO III, Rodrigues MM, Laibson PR. Corneal dystrophies. I. Dystrophies of the Bowman's layer, epithelium and stroma. *Surv Ophthalmol* 1978;23:71.

51. Harboyan G, et al. Congenital corneal dystrophy: progressive sensorineural deafness in a family. *Arch Ophthalmol* 1971; 85:27.

52. Antine B. Histology of congenital hereditary corneal dystrophy. *Am J Ophthalmol* 1970;69:964.

53. Kenyon KR, Maumenee AE. The histological and ultrastructural pathology of congenital hereditary corneal dystrophy: a case report. *Invest Ophthalmol* 1968;7:475.

54. Levenson JE, Chandler JW, Kaufman HE. Affected asymptomatic relatives in congenital hereditary endothelial dystrophy. *Am J Ophthalmol* 1973;76:967.

55. Wolter JR, Haney WP. Histopathology of keratoconus posticus circumscriptus. *Arch Ophthalmol* 1963;69:357.

56. Friedman AH, et al. Sclero-cornea and defective mesodermal migration. *Br J Ophthalmol* 1975;59:683.

57. Howard RO, Abrahams IW. Sclerocornea. *Am J Ophthalmol* 1971;71:1254.

58. Kanai A, et al. The fine structure of sclerocornea. *Invest Ophthalmol* 1971;10:687.

59. Rodrigues MM, Calhoun J, Weinreb S. Sclerocornea with an unbalanced translocation (17p, 10q). *Am J Ophthalmol* 1974; 78:49.

60. Fenske HD, Spitalny LA. Hereditary osteoonychodysplasia. *Am J Ophthalmol* 1970;70:604.

61. Goldstein JE, Cogan DG. Sclerocornea and associated congenital anomalies. *Arch Ophthalmol* 1962;67:99.

62. March WF, Chalkley THF. Sclerocornea associated with Dandy-Walker cyst. *Am J Ophthalmol* 1974;78:54.

63. Yanoff M, Fine BS. *Ocular pathology: a text and atlas.* Hagerstown, MD: Harper & Row, 1975.

64. O'Grady RB, Kirk HQ. Corneal keloids. *Am J Ophthalmol* 1972;73:206.

65. Benjamin SN, Allen HF. Classification for limbal dermoid choristomas and branchial arch anomalies: presentation of an unusual case. *Arch Ophthalmol* 1972;87:305.

66. Baum JL, Feingold M. Ocular aspects of Goldenhar's syndrome. *Am J Ophthalmol* 1973;75:250.

67. Gellis SS, Feingold M. *Atlas of mental retardation syndromes: visual diagnosis of facies and physical findings.* Washington, DC: U.S. Government Printing Office, 1968.

68. Mansour AM, et al. Ocular findings in the facioauriculovertebral sequence (Goldenhar-Gorlin syndrome). *Am J Ophthalmol* 1985;100:555.

69. Krause U. The syndrome of Goldenhar affecting two siblings. *Acta Ophthalmol* 1970;48:494.

70. Summitt RL. Familial Goldenhar syndrome. *Birth Defects* 1969;5:106.

71. Henkind P, et al. Bilateral corneal dermoids. *Am J Ophthalmol* 1973;76:972.

72. Mattos J, Contreras F, O'Donnell FE Jr. Ring dermoid syndrome: a new syndrome of autosomal dominantly inherited, bilateral, annular limbal dermoids with corneal and conjunctival extension. *Arch Ophthalmol* 1980;98:1059.

73. Witschel H, et al. Congenital hereditary stromal dystrophy of the cornea. *Arch Ophthalmol* 1978;96:1043.

74. Duke-Elder S, Leigh AG. *Diseases of the outer eye: cornea and sclera. System of ophthalmology series.* St. Louis: Mosby, 1965.

75. Shapiro MB, France TD. The ocular features of Down's syndrome. *Am J Ophthalmol* 1985;99:659.

76. Cibis GW, Waeltermann J, Harris DJ. Peters' anomaly in association with ring 21 chromosomal abnormality. *Am J Ophthalmol* 1985;100:733.

77. Jay M. *The eye in chromosome duplications and deficiencies. Ophthalmology series.* New York: Dekker, 1977.

78. Kivlin JD, et al. Peters' anomaly as a consequence of genetic and nongenetic syndromes. *Arch Ophthalmol* 1986;104:61.

79. Schwartz DE. Corneal sensitivity in diabetics. *Arch Ophthalmol* 1974;91:174.

80. Scullica L, Proto F. Rilievi clinici e statistici sulla sensibilita corneale nei diabetici. *Boll Ocul* 1965;44:944.

81. Olson T, et al. Corneal thickness in diabetes mellitus. *Lancet* 1980;1:883.

82. Schultz RO, et al. Diabetic keratopathy as a manifestation of peripheral corneal neuropathy. *Am J Ophthalmol* 1983;96:368.

83. Hyndiuk R, et al. Neurotrophic corneal ulcers in diabetes mellitus. *Arch Ophthalmol* 1977;95:2193.

84. Foulks GN, et al. Factors related to corneal epithelial complications after closed vitrectomy in diabetics. *Arch Ophthalmol* 1979;97:1076.

85. Ishida I, et al. Corneal nerve alterations in diabetes mellitus. *Arch Ophthalmol* 1984;102:1380.

86. Tabatabay CA, et al. Reduced number of hemidesmosomes in the corneal epithelium of diabetics with proliferative vitreoretinopathy. *Graefes Arch Clin Exp Ophthalmol* 1988;226:389.

87. Azar DT, et al. Decreased penetration of anchoring fibrils into the diabetic cornea. A morphometric analysis. *Arch Ophthalmol* 1989;107:1520.

88. Cisarik-Fredenburg P. Discoveries in research on diabetic keratopathy. *Optometry* 2001;72:691–704.

89. Fujishima H, Tsubota K. Improvement of corneal fluorescein staining in post cataract surgery of diabetic patients by an oral aldose reductase inhibitor, ONO-2235. *Br J Ophthalmol* 2002; 86:860–863.

90. Ohashi Y, et al. Aldose reductase inhibitor (CT-112) eyedrops for diabetic corneal epitheliopathy. *Am J Ophthalmol* 1988;105:233.

91. Tsubota K, et al. Corneal epithelium in diabetic patients. *Cornea* 1991;10:156.

92. Inoue K, Kato S, Inoue Y, et al. The corneal endothelium and thickness in type II diabetes mellitus. *Jpn J Ophthalmol* 2002; 46:65–69.

93. Schultz RO, et al. Corneal endothelial changes in type I and type II diabetes mellitus. *Am J Ophthalmol* 1984;98:401.

94. Goebbels M, Spiznas M. Endothelial barrier function after phacoemulsification: a comparison between diabetic and nondiabetic patients. *Graefes Arch Clin Exp Ophthalmol* 1991;229:254.

95. Lass JH, et al. A morphologic and fluorophotometric analysis of the corneal endothelium in the type I diabetes mellitus and cystic fibrosis. *Am J Ophthalmol* 1985;100:783.

96. Keoleian GM, et al. Structural and functional studies of the corneal endothelium in diabetes mellitus. *Am J Ophthalmol* 1992;113:64.

97. Stolwizk TR, et al. Corneal autofluorescence: an indicator of diabetic retinopathy. *Invest Ophthalmol Vis Sci* 1992;33:92.

98. Cother E. The cornea. In: Moses RH, ed. *Adler's physiology of the eye.* St. Louis: Mosby, 1966.

99. McKusick VA. *Heritable disorders of connective tissue,* 3rd ed. St. Louis: Mosby, 1966.

100. Kenyon KR, et al. The systemic mucopolysaccharidoses. *Am J Ophthalmol* 1972;73:811.

101. Spellacy E, Bankes JL, Crow J, et al. Glaucoma in a case of Hurler disease. *Br J Ophthalmol* 1980;64:773–778.

102. Gills PJ, et al. Electroretinography and fundus oculi findings in Hurler's disease and allied mucopolysaccharidoses. *Arch Ophthalmol* 1965;74:596.

103. Kajii T, et al. Hurler/Scheie genetic compound (mucopolysaccharidosis IH/IS) in Japanese brothers. *Clin Genet* 1974;6:394.

104. McKusick VA, et al. The genetic mucopolysaccharidoses. *Medicine* 1965;44:445.

105. Quantock AJ, Meek KM, Fullwood NJ, et al. *Can J Ophthalmol* 1993;28:266–272. Scheie's syndrome: the architecture of corneal collagen and the distribution of corneal proteoclycans.

106. Tabone E, et al. Ultrastructural aspects of corneal fibrous tissue in Scheie syndrome. *Virchows Arch B Cell Pathol* 1978;27:63.

107. Tremblay M, Dube L, Gagne R. Alterations de la cornée dans la maladie de Scheie. *J Fr Ophtalmol* 1979;2:193.

108. Sugar J. Corneal manifestations of the systemic mucopolysaccharidoses. *Ann Ophthalmol* 1979;11:531.

109. Quigley HA, MaumeneE AE, Stark WJ. Acute glaucoma in systemic mucopolysaccharidosis I-S. *Am J Ophthalmol* 1975; 80:70.

110. Dorfman A, Matalon R. The mucopolysaccharidoses. In: Stanbury JB, Wyngaarden JB, Fredrickson DS, eds. *The metabolic basis of inherited disease,* 3rd ed. New York: McGraw-Hill, 1972.

111. Van Pelt JF, Huizinga J. Some observations on the genetics of gargoylism. *Acta Genet* 1962;12:1.

112. Goldberg MF, Duke JR. Ocular histopathology in Hunter's syndrome. *Acta Ophthalmol* 1967;77:503.

113. McDonnell JM, Green RW, Maumenee IH. Ocular histopathology of systemic mucopolysaccharidosis type II-A. *Ophthalmology* 1985;92:1772.

114. Topping TM, et al. Ultrastructural ocular pathology of Hunter's syndrome. *Arch Ophthalmol* 1971;86:164.

115. Gardner RJM, Hay JR. Hurler's syndrome with clear cornea. *Lancet* 1974;2:845.

116. Von Noorden G, Zellweger H, Ponseti IV. Ocular findings in Morquio-Ullrich's disease. *Arch Ophthalmol* 1960;64:137.

117. Goldberg MF, Scott CI, McKusick VA. Hydrocephalus and papilledema in the Maroteaux-Lamy syndrome (mucopolysaccharidosis type VI). *Am J Ophthalmol* 1970;69:969.

118. Akhtar S, Tullo A, Caterson B, et al. Clinical and morphological features including expression of beta ig-h3 and keratan sulphate proteoglycans in Maroteaux-Lamy syndrome type B and in normal cornea. *Br J Ophthalmol* 2002;86:147–151.

119. Süveges I. Histological and ultrastructural studies of the cornea in Maroteaux-Lamy syndrome. *Graefes Arch Clin Exp Ophthalmol* 1979;212:29.

120. Naumann G. Clearing of cornea after perforating keratoplasty in mucopolysaccharidosis type VI. *N Engl J Med* 1985;312:995.

121. Sly WS, et al. (3-Glucuronidase deficiency: report of clinical, radiologic, and biochemical features of a new mucopolysaccharidosis. *J Pediatr* 1973;82:249.

122. DeMars R, Leroy JG. The remarkable cells cultured from a human with Hurler's syndrome. *In Vitro* 1967;2:107.

123. Libert J, et al. Ocular findings in I-cell disease (mucolipidosis type II). *Am J Ophthalmol* 1977;83:617.

124. Cibis GW, et al. Mucolipidosis I. *Arch Ophthalmol* 1983;101:933.

125. Borit A, Sugarman GI, Spencer WH. Ocular involvement in I-cell disease (mucolipidosis II): light and electron microscopic findings. *Graefes Arch Clin Exp Ophthalmol* 1976;198:25.

126. Kenyon KR, Sensenbrenner JA. Mucolipidosis II (I-cell disease): ultrastructural observation of conjunctiva and skin. *Invest Ophthalmol* 1971;10:555.

127. Newell FW, Matalon R, Meyer S. A new mucolipidosis with psychomotor retardation, corneal clouding, and retinal degeneration. *Am J Ophthalmol* 1975;80:440.

128. Quigley HA, Goldberg MF. Conjunctival ultrastructure in mucolipidosis III (pseudo-Hurler polydystrophy). *Invest Ophthalmol* 1971;10:568.

129. Kenyon KR, et al. Mucolipidosis IV: Histopathology of conjunctiva, cornea, and skin. *Arch Ophthalmol* 1979;97:1106.

130. Merin S, et al. The cornea in mucolipidosis IV. *J Pediatr Ophthalmol* 1976;13:289.

131. Newman NJ. Corneal surface irregularities and episodic pain in a patient with mucolipidosis IV. *Arch Ophthalmol* 1990;108:251.

132. Philipson BT. Fish eye disease. *Birth Defects* 1982;18:441

133. Dangel ME, et al. Treatment of corneal opacification in mucolipidosis IV with conjunctival transplantation. *Am J Ophthalmol* 1985;99:137.

134. Cable WJL, et al. Fabry's disease. *Neurology (ICY)* 1982;32:1139.

135. François J, Hanssens M, Teuchy H. Corneal ultrastructural changes in Fabry's disease. *Ophthalmologica* 1978;176:313.

136. Spaeth GL, Frost P. Fabry's disease. *Arch Ophthalmol* 1965;74:760.

137. Weingeist TA, Blodi FD. Fabry's disease: Ocular findings in a female carrier. *Arch Ophthalmol* 1971;85:169.

138. Sher NA, Letson RD, Desnick RJ. The ocular manifestations in Fabry's disease. *Arch Ophthalmol* 1979;97:671.

139. Ho PC, Feman SS. Internuclear ophthalmoplegia in Fabry's disease. *Ann Ophthalmol* 1981;13:949.

140. Karr WJ Jr. Fabry's disease (angiokeratoma corporis diffusum universale). *Am J Med* 1959;27:829.

141. Fredrickson DS, Levy RI, Lees FS. Fat transport in lipoproteins—An integrated approach to mechanisms and disorders. *N Engl J Med* 1967;276:34.

142. Vinger PF, Sachs BA. Ocular manifestations of hyperlipoproteinemia. *Am J Ophthalmol* 1970;70:563.

143. Gjone E, Bergaust B. Corneal opacity in familial plasma cholesterol ester deficiency. *Acta Ophthalmol* 1969;47:222.

144. Barchiesi BJ, et al. The cornea and disorders of lipid metabolism. *Surv Ophthalmol* 1991;36:1.

145. Hoffman H II, Fredrickson DS. Tangier disease (familial high-density lipoprotein deficiency): clinical and genetic features in two adults. *Am J Ophthalmol* 1965;39:582.

146. Pressly TA, et al. Ocular complications of Tangier disease. *Am J Med* 1987;83:991.

147. Barnes HD, Boshof FPA. Ocular lesions in patients with porphyria. *Arch Ophthalmol* 1952;48:567.

148. Sober AJ, Grove AS Jr, Muhlbauer JE. Cicatricial ectropion and lacrimal obstruction with porphyria cutanea tarda. *Am J Ophthalmol* 1984;91:396.

149. Sevel D, Burger D. Ocular involvement in cutaneous porphyrias. *Arch Ophthalmol* 1971;85:580.

150. Chumbley LC. Scleral involvement in symptomatic porphyria. *Am J Ophthalmol* 1977;84:729.

151. Wolter JR, Clark RL, Kallet HA. Ocular involvement in acute intermittent porphyria. *Am J Ophthalmol* 1972;74:666.

152. DeFrancisco M, Savino PJ, Schatz NJ. Optic atrophy in acute intermittent porphyria. *Am J Ophthalmol* 1979;87:221.

153. Poh-Fitzpatrick MB, Barbera LG. Absence of crystalline retinopathy after long-term therapy with β-carotene. *J Am Acad Dermatol* 1984;11:111.

154. Gibertini P, et al. Advances in the treatment of porphyria cutanea tarda. *Liver* 1984;4:280.

155. Ferry AP, Safir A, Melikian HE. Ocular abnormalities in patients with gout. *Ann Ophthalmol* 1985;17:632.

156. Hutchinson J. The relation of certain diseases of the eye to gout. *Br Med J* 1884;2:995.

157. McWilliams JR. Ocular findings in gout. *Am J Ophthalmol* 1952;35:1778.

158. Fishman RS, Sunderman FW. Band keratopathy in gout. *Arch Ophthalmol* 1966;75:367.

159. Slansky HH, Kuwabara T. Intranuclear urate crystals in corneal epithelium. *Arch Ophthalmol* 1969;80:338.

160. Weve HJM. *Uric acid keratitis and other ocular findings in gout.* Rotterdam: Van Hengel, 1924.

161. Edwards NL. The diagnosis and management of gouty arthritis. *Compr Ther* 1983;9:14.

162. O'Connor JP, Emmerson BT. The treatment of hyperuricemia and gout. *Aust Fam Physician* 1985;14:193.

163. Lerman S, Megaw J, Fraunfelder FT. Further studies on allopurinol therapy and human cataractogenesis. *Am J Ophthalmol* 1984;97:205.

164. Johnston SS, et al. Norrie's disease. *Birth Defects* 1982;18:729.

165. Sanderson PO, et al. Cystinosis: a clinical, histopathologic and ultrastructural study. *Arch Ophthalmol* 1974;91:270.

166. Yamamoto GK, et al. Long-term ocular changes in cystinosis: Observations in renal transplant recipients. *J Pediatr Ophthalmol* 1979;16:21.

167. Katz B, et al. Corneal thickness in nephrotic cystinosis. *Br J Ophthalmol* 1989;73:665.

168. Katz B, et al. Corneal sensitivity in nephrotic cystinosis. *Am J Ophthalmol* 1987;104:413.

169. Kenyon KR, Sensenbrenner JA. Electron microscopy of cornea and conjunctiva in childhood cystinosis. *Am J Ophthalmol* 1974;78:68.

170. Wong VG, Schulman JD, Seegmiller JE. Alterations of pigment epithelium in cystinosis. *Arch Ophthalmol* 1967;77:361.

171. Read J, et al. Nephropathic cystinosis. *Am J Ophthalmol* 1973; 76:791.

172. Dodd MJ, Pusin SM, Green WR. Adult cystinosis. *Arch Ophthalmol* 1978;96:1054.

173. Zimmerman TJ, Hood I, Gasset AF. "Adolescent" cystinosis. *Arch Ophthalmol* 1974;92:265.

174. Wong VG, Schulman JD, Seegmiller JE. Conjunctival biopsy for the biochemical diagnosis of cystinosis. *Am J Ophthalmol* 1970;70:278.

175. Schneider JA, Wong V, Seegmiller JE. The early diagnosis of cystinosis. *J Pediatr* 1969;74:114.

176. Theone JG, et al. Cystinosis. *J Clin Invest* 1976;58:180.

177. Da Silva R, et al. Long-term treatment of infantile nephropathic cystinosis with cysteamine. *N Engl J Med* 1985;313:1460.

178. Kaiser-Kupfer MI, et al. A randomized placebo-controlled trial of cysteamine eye drops in neuropathic cystinosis. *Arch Ophthalmol* 1990;108:689.

179. Schneider JA. Therapy of cystinosis. *N Engl J Med* 1985;313: 1473.

180. Baum JL, Tannenbaum M, Kolodny EH. Refsum's syndrome with corneal involvement. *Am J Ophthalmol* 1965;60:699.

181. Sammaritino AG, et al. Familial Richner-Hanhart syndrome. *Ann Ophthalmol* 1984;16:1069.

182. Herre F, et al. Incurable keratitis and chronic palmoplantar hyperkeratosis with hypertyrosinemia. Cure using a tyrosine-restricted diet. *Arch Fr Pediatr* 1986;43:19.

183. Burn RP. Soluble tyrosine aminotransferase deficiency. *Am J Ophthalmol* 1972;73:400.

184. Charlton KH, et al. Pseudodendritic keratitis and systemic tyrosinemia. *Ophthalmology* 1981;88:355.

185. Garrod AE. The incidence of alkaptonuria: a study in chemical individuality. *Lancet* 1902;2:1616.

186. Smith JW. Ochronosis of the sclera and cornea complicating alkaptonuria: Review of the literature and report of four cases. *JAMA* 1942;120:1282.

187. La Du BN. Alkaptonuria. In: Stanbury JB, Wyngaarden JB, Fredrickson DS, eds. *The metabolic basis of inherited disease,* 3rd ed. New York: McGraw-Hill, 1972:308–324.

188. Spark ED, et al. The identification of amyloid P-component (protein AP) in normal cultured human fibroblasts. *Lab Invest* 1978;38:556.

189. Scheinberg MA, Cathcart ES. Casein-induced experimental amyloidosis. III. Responses to mitogens, allogeneic cells and graft versus host reactions in the murine model. *Immunology* 1974;27:953.

190. Blodi FC, Apple DJ. Localized conjunctival amyloidosis. *Am J Ophthalmol* 1979;88:346.

191. Stafford WR, Fine BS. Amyloidosis of the cornea. Report of a case without conjunctival involvement. *Arch Ophthalmol* 1966;75:53.

192. McPherson SD, Kiffney TG Jr, Freed CC. Corneal amyloidosis. *Am J Ophthalmol* 1966;62:1025.

193. Ramsey MS, Fine BS, Cohen SW. Localized corneal amyloidosis. *Am J Ophthalmol* 1972;73:560.

194. Garner A. Amyloidosis of the cornea. *Br J Ophthalmol* 1969;53:73.

195. Kirk HQ, et al. Primary familial amyloidosis of the cornea. *Trans Am Acad Ophthalmol Otolaryngol* 1973;77:411.

196. Nagataki S, Tanishima T, Sakimoto T. A case of primary gelatinous drop-like corneal dystrophy. *Jpn J Ophthalmol* 1972; 16:107.

197. Weber FL, Babel J. Gelatinous drop-like dystrophy. *Arch Ophthalmol* 1980;98:144.

198. Stock EL, Kielar R. Primary familial amyloidosis of the cornea. *Am J Ophthalmol* 1976;82:266.

199. Boysen G, et al. Familial amyloidosis with cranial neuropathy and corneal lattice dystrophy. *J Neurol Neurosurg Psychiatry* 1979;42:1020.

200. Meretoja J. Comparative histopathological and clinical findings in eyes with lattice corneal dystrophy of two types. *Ophthalmologica* 1972;165:15.

201. Wong IG, Oskvig RM. Immunofluorescent detection of antibodies to ocular melanomas. *Arch Ophthalmol* 1974;92:98.

202. Mondino BJ, et al. Protein AA and lattice corneal dystrophy. *Am J Ophthalmol* 1980;89:377–380.

203. Ratnaker KS, Mohan M. Amyloidosis of the iris. *Can J Ophthalmol* 1976;11:256–257.

204. Walsh FB, Hoyt WF. *Clinical neuroophthalmology,* 3rd ed. Baltimore: Williams & Wilkins, 1969:811.

205. Konigstein H, Spiegel EA. Muskelatrophie bei Amyloidose. *Neurol Psychiatr* 1924;88:220.

206. Falls HF, et al. Ocular manifestations of hereditary primary systemic amyloidosis. *Arch Ophthalmol* 1955;54:660.

207. Andrade C. A peculiar form of peripheral neuropathy: familial atypical generalized amyloidosis with special involvement of peripheral nerves. *Brain* 1952;75:408.

208. Lessell S, et al. Scalloped pupils in familial amyloidosis. *N Engl J Med* 1975;293:914.

209. Knowles DM, et al. Amyloidosis of the orbit and adnexa. *Surv Ophthalmol* 1975;19:367.

210. Sarino PJ, Schat NJ, Rodrigues MM. Orbital amyloidosis. *Can J Ophthalmol* 1976;11:252.

211. Kedar I, et al. Colchicine inhibition of casein induced amyloidosis in mice. *Isr J Med Sci* 1974;10:787.

212. Kasner D, et al. Surgical treatment of amyloidosis of the vitreous. *Trans Am Acad Ophthalmol Otolaryngol* 1968;72:410.

213. Volpe R, et al. The pathogenesis of Graves' disease in Hashimoto's thyroiditis. *Clin Endocrinol* 1974;3:239.

214. Lamki L, Auerbach PS, Hayes EC. A blood test for multiple sclerosis based on the adherence of lymphocytes to measles-infected cells. *N Engl J Med* 1976;294:1423.

215. Barbosa J, Wong E, Doe RP. Ophthalmology of Graves' disease: Outcome after treatment with radioactive iodine, surgery or antithyroid drugs. *Arch Intern Med* 1972;130:111.

216. Donaldson SS, Bagshaw MA, Kriss JP. Super-voltage orbital radiotherapy for Graves' ophthalmopathy. *J Clin Endocrinol Metab* 1973;37:276.

217. Cogan DG, Henneman PH. Diffuse calcification of the cornea in hypercalcemia. *N Engl J Med* 1957;257:451.

218. Wood TO, Walker GG. Treatment of band keratopathy. *Am J Ophthalmol* 1975;80:553.

219. Berkow JW, Fine BS, Zimmerman LE. Unusual ocular calcification in hyperparathyroidism. *Am J Ophthalmol* 1968;66:812.

220. Jensen OA. Ocular calcifications in primary hyperparathyroidism. *Acta Ophthalmol (Copenh)* 1975;53:173.

221. Brenner RL, et al. Eye signs of hypophosphatasia. *Arch Ophthalmol* 1969;81:614.

222. Cogan DG, Albright F, Bartter FC. Hypercalcemia and band keratopathy. *Arch Ophthalmol* 1948;40:624.

223. Berlyne GM. Microcrystalline conjunctival calcification in renal failure. *Lancet* 1968;2:366.

224. Berlyne GM, Shaw AB. Red eyes in renal failure. *Lancet* 1967;1:4.

225. Harris LS, et al. Conjunctival and corneal calcific deposits in uremic patients. *Am J Ophthalmol* 1971;72:130.

226. Demco TA, McCormick AG, Richard JSF. Conjunctival and corneal changes in chronic renal failure. *Can J Ophthalmol* 1974;9:208.

227. Friedlaender MH, Smolin G. Corneal degeneration. *Ann Ophthalmol* 1974;11:1485.

228. O'Connor GR. Calcific band keratopathy. *Trans Am Ophthalmol Soc* 1972;70:58.

229. Doughman DJ, et al. Experimental band keratopathy. *Arch Ophthalmol* 1969;81:264.

230. Lemp MA, Ralph RA. Rapid development of band keratopathy in dry eyes. *Am J Ophthalmol* 1977;83:657.

231. Kennedy RE, Roca PD, Landers PH. Atypical band keratopathy in glaucomatous patients. *Am J Ophthalmol* 1972;72:917.

232. Kennedy RE, Roca PD, Platt DS. Further observations on atypical band keratopathy in glaucoma patients. *Trans Am Ophthalmol Soc* 1974;72:107.

233. Fleming CR, et al. Pigmented corneal rings in non-Wilsonian liver disease. *Ann Intern Med* 1977;86:285.

234. Oae NA, Tso MOM, Rosenthal AR. Chalcosis in the human eye: A clinicopathologic study. *Arch Ophthalmol* 1976;94:1379.

235. Rosenthal AR, Appleton B, Hopkins JL. Intraocular copper foreign bodies. *Am J Ophthalmol* 1974;78:671.

236. Bron AJ, McLendon BF, Camp AV. Epithelial deposition of gold in the cornea of patients receiving systemic therapy. *Am J Ophthalmol* 1979;88:354.

237. Gottlieb NL, Major JC. Ocular chrysiasis correlated with gold concentrations in the crystalline lens during chrysotherapy. *Arthritis Rheum* 1978;21:704.

238. Hashimoto A, et al. Corneal chrysiasis: a clinical study in rheumatoid arthritis patients receiving gold therapy. *Arthritis Rheum* 1972;15:309.

239. Roberts WH, Wolter JR. Ocular chrysiasis. *Arch Ophthalmol* 1956;56:48.

240. Grant WM. *Toxicology of the eye*. Springfield, IL: Thomas, 1974:530.

241. Bartlett RE. Generalized argyrosis with lens involvement. *Am J Ophthalmol* 1954;38:402.

242. Grayson M, Pieroni D. Severe silver nitrate injury to the eye. *Am J Ophthalmol* 1970;70:227.

243. Hanna C, Fraunfelder FT, Sanchez J. Ultrastructural study of argyrosis of the cornea and conjunctiva. *Arch Ophthalmol* 1974;92:18.

244. Yanoff M, Scheie HG. Argyrosis of the conjunctiva and lacrimal sac. *Arch Ophthalmol* 1964;72:57.

245. Spector B, Klintworth GK, Wells SA. Histologic study of ocular lesions in multiple endocrine neoplasia syndrome type IIB. *Am J Ophthalmol* 1981;91:204.

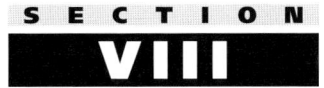

SECTION VIII

CONJUNCTIVAL CORNEAL DYSPLASIA AND MALIGNANCY

OVERVIEW OF TUMORS OF THE CONJUNCTIVA AND CORNEA

CAROL L. SHIELDS AND JERRY A. SHIELDS

GENERAL CONSIDERATIONS

Tumors of the conjunctiva and cornea occupy a large spectrum of conditions ranging from benign inflammatory lesions such as pingueculitis or episcleritis to aggressive, life-threatening malignancies such as melanoma or Kaposi's sarcoma (1–3). The clinical differentiation of these tumors is based on the patient's medical background as well as certain typical clinical features of the tumor. The recognition and proper management of such tumors requires an understanding of the anatomy of the conjunctiva and cornea and knowledge of general principles of tumor management, both of which are described below. The specific clinical and histopathologic features as well as the management of each tumor is discussed, based on the authors' personal experience with over 1,500 patients with conjunctival tumors during a 30-year period (3).

Anatomy

The conjunctiva is a continuous mucous membrane that covers the anterior portion of the globe. It extends from the eyelid margin onto the back surface of the eyelid (palpebral portion), into the fornix (forniceal portion), onto the surface of the globe (bulbar portion), and up to the corneoscleral limbus (limbal portion). The conjunctiva is composed of epithelium and stroma. The epithelium consists of both stratified squamous and columnar epithelium. The squamous pattern is found near the limbus and the columnar pattern is found near the fornix. The stroma is composed of fibrovascular connective tissue that thickens in the fornix and thins at the limbus.

Special regions of the conjunctiva include the plica semilunaris and caruncle. The plica semilunaris is a vertically oriented fold of conjunctiva, located in the medial portion of the bulbar conjunctiva. It is speculated that the plica semilunaris represents a remnant of the nictitating membrane found in certain animals. The caruncle is located in the medial canthus between the upper and lower punctum. It contains both conjunctival and cutaneous structures such as nonkeratinized stratified squamous epithelium overlying the stroma of fibroblasta, melanocytes, sebaceous glands, hair follicles, and striated muscle fibers.

The conjunctiva can spawn neoplasms from both its epithelial and stromal structures. These are similar clinically and histopathologically to tumors that arise from other mucous membranes in the body. Similarly, the cornea can develop epithelial tumors, but stromal tumors are extremely rare from this structure. The caruncle, with its unique composition of both mucous membrane and cutaneous structures, can generate tumors found both in mucosa and skin.

Diagnostic Approaches

Unlike many other mucous membranes in the body, the conjunctiva is readily visible. Thus, tumors and related lesions that occur in the conjunctiva are generally recognized at a relatively early stage. Since many of these tumors have typical clinical features, an accurate diagnosis can often be made by external ocular examination and slit-lamp biomicroscopy, provided that the clinician is familiar with their clinical characteristics. A diagnostic biopsy is not usually necessary in cases of smaller tumors that appear benign. If a smaller tumor does require a biopsy, it is often better to completely remove the lesion in one operation (excisional biopsy). In cases of larger lesions, however, it may be appropriate to remove a portion of the tumor (incisional biopsy) to obtain a histopathologic diagnosis prior to embarking upon more extensive therapy. Because conjunctival tumors are readily accessible to incisional biopsy, it is rarely necessary to do exfoliative cytology or fine-needle aspiration biopsy, both of which provide less material than incisional biopsy.

In addition to evaluation of the conjunctival lesion, meticulous slit-lamp examination of the cornea is essential in patients with suspected conjunctival tumors. Invasion of squamous cell carcinoma and melanoma into the peripheral cornea may appear as a subtle, gray surface opacity. It is important to completely outline such corneal involvement prior to surgery, because it is often less visible through the operating microscope than it is with slit-lamp biomicroscopy in the office.

Management

Depending on the presumptive diagnosis and the size and extent of the lesion, management of a conjunctival tumor can consist of serial observation, incisional biopsy, excisional biopsy, cryotherapy, chemotherapy, radiotherapy, modified enucleation, orbital exenteration, or various combinations of these methods (4–7). If large areas of conjunctiva are removed, mucous membrane grafts from the conjunctiva of the opposite eye, buccal mucosa, or amniotic membrane may be necessary (8,9).

Observation

Observation is generally the management of choice for most benign, asymptomatic tumors of the conjunctiva. Selected examples of lesions that can be observed without interventional treatment include pingueculum, dermolipoma, and nevus. External or slit-lamp photographs are advisable to document all lesions and are critical to follow-up of the more suspicious lesions. Most patients are examined every 6 to 12 months looking for evidence of growth, malignant change, or secondary effects on normal surrounding tissues.

Incisional Biopsy

Incisional biopsy is reserved for extensive suspicious tumors that are symptomatic or suspected to be malignant. Examples include large squamous cell carcinoma, primary acquired melanosis, melanoma, and conjunctival invasion by sebaceous gland carcinoma. It should be understood that if such tumors occupy four clock hours or less on the bulbar conjunctiva, excisional biopsy is generally preferable to incisional biopsy. However, larger lesions can be approached by incisional wedge biopsy or punch biopsy. Further definitive therapy would then be planned based on the results of biopsy. Incisional biopsy is also appropriate for conditions that are ideally treated with radiotherapy, chemotherapy, or other topical medications. Such lesions include lymphoid tumors, metastatic tumors, extensive papillomatosis, and some cases of squamous cell carcinoma and primary acquired melanosis.

Excisional Biopsy

Primary excisional biopsy is appropriate for intermediate and small tumors that are symptomatic or suspected to be malignant. In such situations, excisional biopsy is preferred over incisional biopsy to avoid inadvertent tumor seeding. Examples of benign and malignant lesions that are ideally managed by excisional biopsy include symptomatic limbal dermoid, epibulbar osseous choristoma, steroid-resistant pyogenic granuloma, squamous cell carcinoma, and melanoma. When such lesions are located in the conjunctival

fornix they can be completely excised and the conjunctiva reconstructed primarily with absorbable sutures, sometimes with fornix deepening sutures or symblepharon ring to prevent adhesions. If the defect cannot be closed primarily, then a mucous membrane graft can be inserted.

Most primary malignant tumors of the conjunctiva, such as squamous cell carcinoma and melanoma, arise in the interpalpebral area near the limbus, and the surgical technique for limbal tumors is different than that for forniceal tumors (4–6). Limbal neoplasms have a propensity to invade through the corneal epithelium and sclera into the anterior chamber and also through the soft tissues into the orbit. Thus, it is often necessary to remove a thin lamella of sclera to achieve tumor-free margins and to decrease the chance for tumor recurrence. In this regard, we employ a partial lamellar sclerokeratoconjunctivectomy with primary closure in for such tumors (Fig. 40-1). Because cells from these friable tumors can seed into adjacent tissues, a gentle technique without touching the tumor (no touch technique) is mandatory. Additionally, the surgery should be performed using microscopic technique, and the operative field should be left dry so that cells adhere to the resected tissue. It is wise to avoid wetting the field with balanced salt solution until after the tumor is completely removed to minimize seeding of cells.

The technique for resection of limbal tumors is shown in Fig. 40-1. Using retrobulbar anesthesia and the operating microscope, the corneal epithelial component is approached first and the conjunctival component is dissected second, with the goal of excising the entire specimen completely in one piece. Absolute alcohol soaked on an applicator is gently applied to the entire corneal component. This causes epithelial cellular devitalization and allows easier release of the tumor cells from Bowman's layer. A beaver blade is used to microscopically outline the malignancy within the corneal epithelium using a delicate epithelial incision or epitheliorhexis technique 2 mm outside the corneal component. The beaver blade is then used to sweep gently the affected corneal epithelium from the direction of the central cornea to limbus, into a scroll that rests at the limbus. Next, a pentagonal or circular conjunctival incision based at the limbus is made 4 to 6 mm outside the tumor margin. The incision is carried through the underlying Tenon's fascia until the sclera is exposed so that full-thickness conjuctiva and Tenon's fascia is incorporated into the excisional biopsy. Cautery is applied to control bleeding. A second incision is then outlined by a superficial scleral groove approximately 0.2 mm in depth and 2.0 mm outside the base of the overlying adherent conjunctival mass. This groove is continued anteriorly to the limbus. The area outlined by the scleral groove is removed by flat dissection of 0.2-mm thickness within the sclera in an attempt to remove a superficial lamella of sclera, overlying Tenon's fascia and conjunctiva with tumor, and the scrolled corneal epithelium. In this way, the entire tumor with

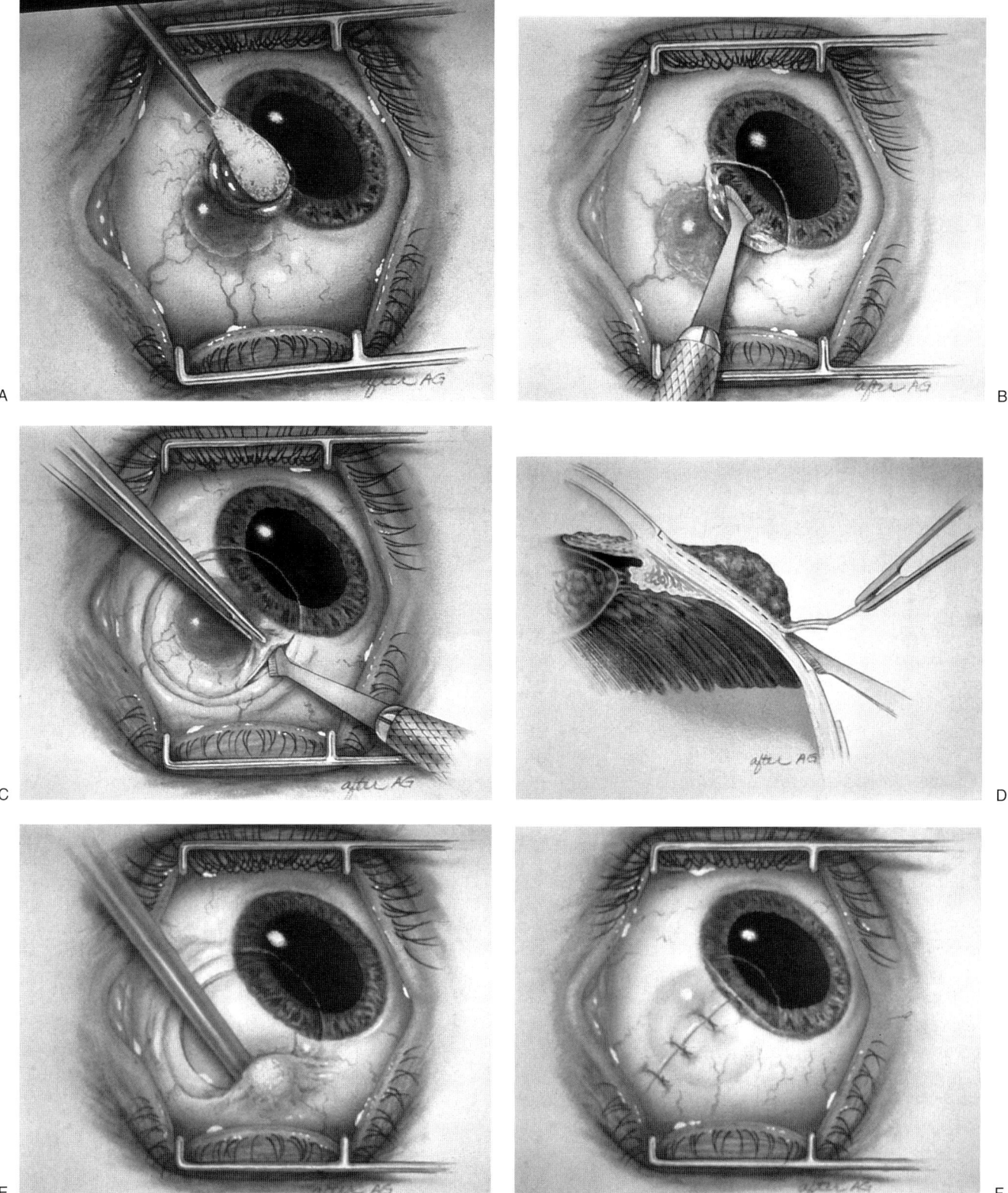

FIGURE 40-1. Surgical excision of conjunctival malignancy using the "no touch" technique. **A:** Absolute alcohol is applied by a cotton-tip applicator to the involved cornea to allow for controlled corneal epitheliectomy. **B:** The corneal epithelium is scrolled off using a controlled sweeping motion with a beaver blade. **C:** The conjunctival incision is made approximately 4 mm outside the tumor margin. A beaver blade is used to create a thin lamella of tumor-free sclera underlying the limbal portion of the tumor. **D:** The conjunctival malignancy is removed, along with tumor-free margins, including underlying sclera and limbal corneal epithelium. **E:** Cryotherapy is applied to the conjunctiva at the site of resection. **F:** Closure of the conjunctiva with absorbable sutures is performed.

tumor-free margins is removed in one piece without touching the tumor itself (no-touch technique). The removed specimen is then placed flatly on a piece of thin cardboard from the surgical tray and then placed in fixative and submitted for histopathologic studies. This step prevents the specimen from folding and allows better assessment of the tumor margins histopathologically. The used instruments are then replaced with fresh instruments for the subsequent steps, to avoid contamination of healthy tissue with possible tumor cells.

After excision of the specimen, cryotherapy is applied to the margins of the remaining bulbar conjunctiva. This is performed by freezing the surrounding bulbar conjunctiva as it is lifted away from the sclera using the cryoprobe. When the ice ball reaches a size of 4 to 5 mm, it is allowed to thaw and the cycle repeated once. The cryoprobe is then moved to an adjacent area of the conjunctiva and the cycle is repeated until all of the margins have been treated by this method. It is not necessary to treat the corneal margins with cryoapplication. The tumor bed is treated with absolute alcohol wash on cotton-tip applicator and bipolar cautery, avoiding cryotherapy directly to the sclera.

Using clean instruments, the conjunctiva is mobilized for closure of the defect by loosening the intermuscular septum with Steven's scissors spreading and creation of transpositional conjunctival flaps. Closure is completed with interrupted absorbable 6–0 or 7–0 sutures. If the surgeon prefers, an area of bare sclera can be left near the limbus, but we prefer complete closure as this promotes better healing and allows for facility of further surgery if the patient should develop recurrence. The patient is treated with topical antibiotics and corticosteroids for 2 weeks and then followed at 3- to 6-month intervals.

Cryotherapy

In the management of conjunctival tumors, cryotherapy can be used as a supplemental treatment to excisional biopsy as described above. In such cases it can eliminate microscopic tumor cells and prevent recurrence of malignant tumors such as squamous cell carcinoma and melanoma. It can also be used as a principal treatment for primary acquired melanosis and pagetoid invasion of sebaceous gland carcinoma. If cryotherapy can devitalize the malignant or potentially malignant cells in such instances, radical surgery such as orbital exenteration can often be delayed or avoided.

Chemotherapy

Recent evidence has revealed that topical eyedrops composed of mitomycin C, 5-fluorouracil, interferon, or cidofovir are effective in treating epithelial malignancies such as squamous cell carcinoma, primary acquired melanosis, and pagetoid invasion of sebaceous gland carcinoma (10–19).

TABLE 40-1. PROTOCOL FOR USE OF MITOMYCIN C FOR CONJUNCTIVAL SQUAMOUS CELL NEOPLASIA AND PRIMARY ACQUIRED MELANOSIS

Time	Medication and Frequency
Week 1	Slit-lamp biomicroscopy
	Place upper and lower punctal plugs
	Cycle 1: mitomycin C 0.04% q.i.d. to the affected eye
Week 2	No medication
Week 3	Cycle 2: mitomycin C 0.04% q.i.d. to the affected eye
Week 4	No medication
	Slit-lamp biomicroscopy
	Prescribe more cycles if residual tumor exists
	Remove punctal plugs after all medication complete

Mitomycin C or 5-fluorouracil are employed most successfully for squamous cell carcinoma, especially after tumor recurrence following previous surgery. This medication is prescribed topically four times daily for a 1-week period followed by a 1-week hiatus to allow the ocular surface to recover (Table 40-1). This cycle is repeated once again so that most patients receive a total of 2 weeks of the chemotherapy topically. Both mitomycin C and 5-fluorouracil are most effective for squamous cell carcinoma and less effective for primary acquired melanosis and pagetoid invasion of sebaceous gland carcinoma. Toxicities include most commonly dry-eye findings, superficial punctate epitheliopathy, and punctal stenosis. Corneal melt, scleral melt, and cataract can develop if these agents are used with open conjunctival wounds or used excessively. Topical interferon can be effective for squamous epithelial malignancies and is less toxic to the surface epithelium, but this medication may require many months of use to effect a result (16). Other topical antiviral medications including cidofovir can be employed with little toxicity for squamous epithelial tumors (17).

Radiotherapy

Two forms of radiotherapy are employed for conjunctival tumors, namely external beam radiotherapy and custom-designed plaque radiotherapy. External beam radiotherapy to a total dose of 3000 to 4000 cGy is used to treat conjunctival lymphoma and metastatic carcinoma when such lesions are too large or diffuse to excise locally. Side effects of dry eye, punctate epithelial abnormalities, and cataract should be anticipated.

Custom-designed plaque radiotherapy (20) to a dose of 3,000 to 4,000 cGy can be used to treat conjunctival lymphoma or metastasis. A higher dose of 6,000 to 8,000 cGy can be employed to treat the more radiation-resistant melanoma and squamous cell carcinoma. In general, plaque radiotherapy is reserved for those patients who have diffuse tumors that are incompletely resected and for those who display multiple recurrences. The two designs for conjunctival custom plaque radiotherapy include a conformer plaque technique with six fractionated treatment sessions as an outpatient or a reverse plaque technique with the device sutured onto the episcleral as an inpatient. In unique instances, plaque radiotherapy to a low dose of 2,000 cGy is employed for benign conditions such as steroid resistant pyogenic granuloma that show recurrence after surgical resection (21). Such treatment should be performed by experienced radiation oncologists and ocular oncologists.

Modified Enucleation

Modified enucleation is a treatment option for primary malignant tumors of the conjunctiva that have invaded through the limbal tissues into the globe, producing secondary glaucoma. Such an occurrence is quite rare but can occasionally occur with squamous cell carcinoma and melanoma. The uncommon mucoepidermoid variant of squamous cell carcinoma of the conjunctiva has a greater tendency for such invasion (22,23). At the time of enucleation, it is necessary to remove the involved conjunctiva intact with the globe so as to avoid spreading tumor cells. Thus, the initial peritomy should begin at the limbus, but when the tumor is approached, the incision should proceed posteriorly from the limbus to surround the tumor-affected tissue by at least 3 to 4 mm. The tumor will remain adherent to the globe at the limbus. Occasionally, a suture is employed through the surrounding conjunctiva into the episclera to secure the tumor to the globe so that it will not be displaced during subsequent manipulation. The remaining steps of enucleation are gently performed and the globe is removed with tumor adherent after cutting the optic nerve from the nasal side. The margins of the remaining, presumed unaffected conjunctiva are treated with double freeze-thaw cryotherapy. Often this surgical technique leaves the patient with a limited amount of residual unaffected conjunctiva for closure. In these instances, a mucous membrane graft or amniotic membrane graft may be necessary for adequate closure and to provide fornices for a prosthesis. In some instances, a simple horizontal inferior forniceal conjunctival incision from canthus to canthus may suffice, as long as the conformer is constantly worn as a template so the new conjunctival fornix grows deep and around this structure.

Orbital Exenteration

Orbital exenteration is probably the treatment of choice for primary malignant conjunctival tumors that have invaded the orbit or that exhibit complete involvement of the conjunctiva (7,24,25). Either an eyelid-removing or eyelid-sparing exenteration is employed, depending on the extent of eyelid involvement. The eyelid-sparing technique is preferred in that patients have a better cosmetic appearance and they heal within 2 or 3 weeks. Specifically, if the anterior lamella of the eyelid is uninvolved with tumor, an eyelid-sparing (eyelid-splitting) exenteration may be accomplished (4,7,25).

Mucous Membrane Graft

Mucous membrane grafts are occasionally necessary to replace vital conjunctival tissue after removal of extensive conjunctival tumors. The best donor sites include the forniceal conjunctiva of the ipsilateral or contralateral eye and buccal mucosa from the posterior aspect of the lower lip or lateral aspect of the mouth. Such grafts are usually removed by a freehand technique, fashioned to fit the defect, and secured into place with cardinal and running absorbable 6–0 or 7–0 sutures. Currently, in most instances, we employ a donor amniotic membrane graft to replace lost conjunctiva (8,9). The tissue is delivered frozen and must be defrosted for 20 minutes. The fine, transparent material is carefully peeled off its cardboard surface, laid basement membrane side up, and sutured into place with absorbable sutures. Topical antibiotic and steroid ointments are applied following all conjunctival grafting procedures.

It is important that the surgeon use a minimal manipulation technique for tumor resection. For graft harvest and placement, the surgeon should always use clean, sterile instruments at both the donor and the recipient sites. Free tumor cells can rest on instrument tips and later implant and grow in previously uninvolved areas if such precautions are not taken.

CONGENITAL LESIONS

A variety of tumors and related conditions may be present at birth or become clinically apparent shortly after birth (26,27). Most of the lesions to be considered here are choristomas, consisting of tissue elements that are not normally present at the involved site. Despite their presence at a young age, all of the conjunctival choristomas discussed herein are sporadic, without hereditary tendency.

Dermoid

Conjunctival dermoid is a congenital well-circumscribed yellow-white solid mass that involves the bulbar conjunctiva or at the corneoscleral limbus (26–29). It characteristically occurs near the limbus inferotemporally, and often this tumor has fine white hairs, best seen with slit-lamp biomicroscopy (Fig. 40-2). In rare cases, it can extend to the central cornea or be located in other

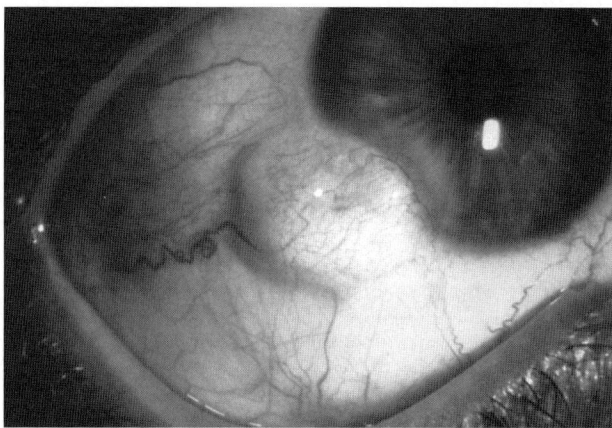
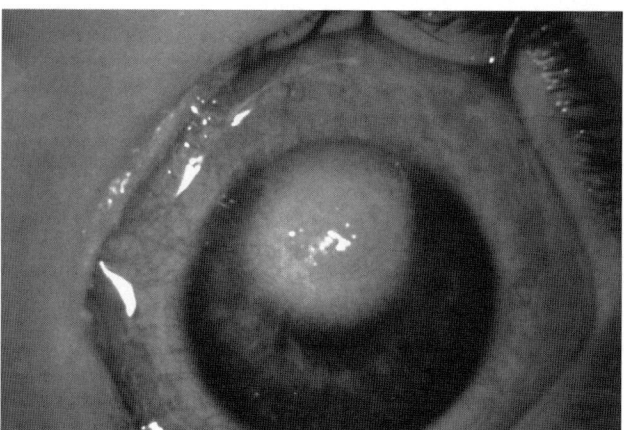

A   B

FIGURE 40-2. Epibulbar dermoid. **A:** Limbal dermoid. **B:** Central corneal dermoid.

quadrants on the bulbar surface. It may occur as an isolated lesion or it can be associated with Goldenhar's syndrome. Hence, the patient should be evaluated for ipsilateral or bilateral preauricular skin appendages, hearing loss, eyelid coloboma, and orbitoconjunctival dermolipoma, and cervical vertebral anomalies that comprise this nonheritable syndrome. Histopathologically, the conjunctival dermoid is a simple choristomatous malformation that consists of dense fibrous tissue lined by conjunctival epithelium with deeper dermal elements such as hair follicles and sebaceous glands.

The management of an epibulbar dermoid includes simple observation if the lesion is small and visually asymptomatic. It is possible to excise the lesion for cosmetic reasons, but the remaining corneal scar is sometimes cosmetically unacceptable. Larger or symptomatic dermoids can produce visual loss from astigmatism. These can be approached by lamellar keratosclerectomy with primary closure of overlying tissue if the defect is superficial or closure using corneal graft if the defect is deep or full thickness. It has been reported that the cosmetic appearance may improve, but the refractive and astigmatic error and visual acuity may not change (29). When the lesion involves the central cornea, a lamellar or penetrating keratoplasty may be necessary and long-term amblyopia can be a problem. Occasionally, extensive dermoids involve the lateral canthus, and carefully planned excision with lateral canthal repair is necessary.

Dermolipoma

Dermolipoma is believed to be congenital and present at birth, but it typically remains asymptomatic for years and may not be detected until adulthood, when it protrudes from the orbit through the conjunctival fornix superotemporally (Fig. 40-3). It appears as a pale yellow, soft, fluctuant, fusiform mass below the palpebral lobe of the lacrimal gland, best visualized with the eye in inferonasal gaze.

It usually extends for a variable distance into the orbital fat and onto the bulbar conjunctiva, and occasionally it can extend anteriorly to reach the limbus. Unlike herniated orbital fat, dermolipoma can contain fine white hairs on its surface and it cannot be reduced with digital pressure into the orbit.

With computed tomography (CT) or magnetic resonance imaging (MRI), dermolipoma has features similar to orbital fat from which it may be indistinguishable. Histopathologically, it is lined by conjunctival epithelium on its surface and the subepithelial tissue has variable quantities of collagenous connective tissue. Pilosebaceous units and lacrimal gland tissue may occasionally be present. The majority of dermolipomas require no treatment, but larger symptomatic ones or those that are cosmetically unappealing can be managed by excision of the entire orbitoconjunctival lesion through a conjunctival forniceal approach or by simply removing the anterior portion of the lesion in a manner similar to that used to remove prolapsed orbital fat.

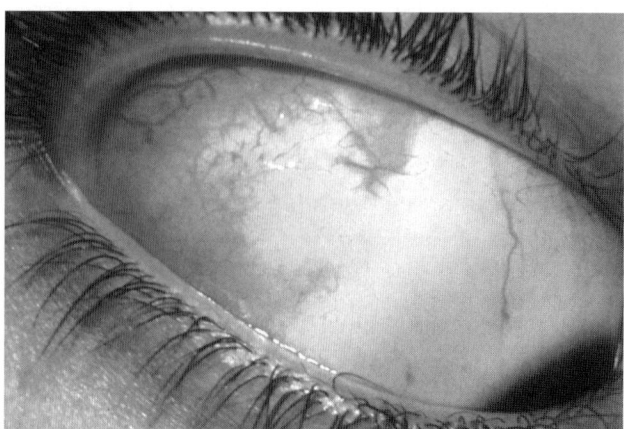

FIGURE 40-3. Dermolipoma in superotemporal conjunctival fornix.

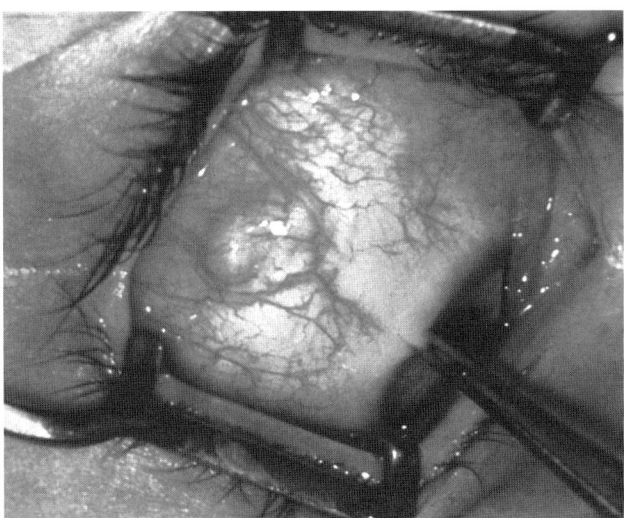

FIGURE 40-4. Epibulbar osseous choristoma on bulbar conjunctiva superotemporally, presenting as a firm, palpable mass.

Epibulbar Osseous Choristoma

Epibulbar osseous choristoma is a rigid deposit of bone generally located in the bulbar conjunctiva superotemporally (30) (Fig. 40-4). It is believed to be congenital and typically remains undetected until personally palpated by the patient in the preteen years. It is clinically suspected due to its rock-hard consistency on palpation, although fibrous tissue tumors can feel similar. The diagnosis can be confirmed with ultrasonography or CT to illustrate the calcium component. This tumor is generally best managed by periodic observation. Occasionally patients report a foreign-body sensation, and such symptomatic lesions can be excised with a circumtumoral conjunctival incision followed by dissection to bare sclera for full-thickness conjunctival resection. For those tumors that might be adherent to the sclera, a superficial sclerectomy might be warranted (30).

Lacrimal Gland Choristoma

Lacrimal gland choristoma is a congenital lesion often discovered in young children as an asymptomatic pink stromal mass, most often in the inferior bulbar or forniceal conjunctiva. It is speculated that this lesion presents in such location due to the pathway that the lacrimal gland takes during embryogenesis from the inferior to the superotemporal region. The lacrimal gland choristoma can masquerade as a focus of inflammation due to its pink color. Rarely, a cystic appearance ensues from this secretory mass if there is no connection to the conjunctival surface. Excisional biopsy is usually performed to confirm the diagnosis.

Respiratory Choristoma

In unique instances, a cystic choristoma, appearing as congenital sclerocorneal ectasia, is found. In one report, such a case was found to manifest respiratory mucosa (31).

Complex Choristoma

The conjunctival dermoid and epibulbar osseous choristoma are termed simple choristomas as they contain one tissue type, such as skin or bone. A complex choristoma contains a greater variety of tissue, such as dermal appendages, lacrimal gland tissue, cartilage, bone, and occasionally other elements. It is quite variable in its clinical appearance and may cover much of the epibulbar surface or it may form a circumferential growth pattern around the limbus (Fig. 40-5). For example, such tumor with extensive lacrimal tissue appears as a lobular pink mass, whereas one with dermal tissue appears yellow and thick and one with cartilage displays a smooth blue-gray hue. The complex choristoma has a peculiar association with the linear nevus sebaceous of Jadassohn (32–34). The nevus sebaceous of Jadassohn includes cutaneous features such as sebaceous nevus in the facial region and neurologic features such as seizures, mental retardation, arachnoid cyst, and cerebral atrophy. The ophthalmic features of this syndrome include epibulbar complex choristoma and posterior scleral cartilage (32).

The management of the complex choristoma depends on the extent of the lesion. Observation and wide local excision with mucous membrane graft reconstruction are options. In the rare case of a very extensive lesion, where the lesion causes dense amblyopia with no hope for visual acuity, modified enucleation with ocular surface reconstruction may be necessary.

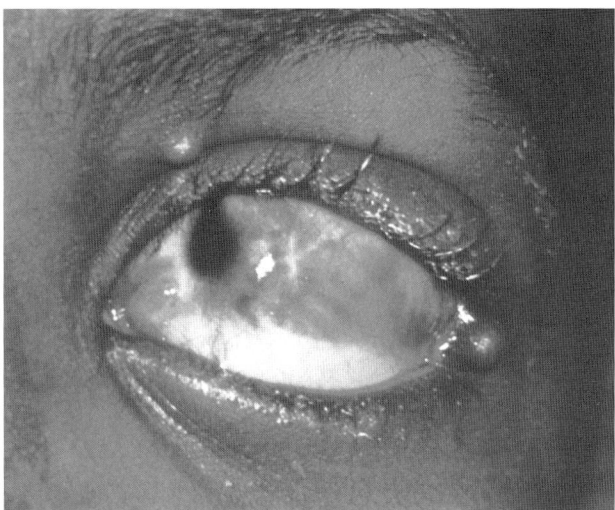

FIGURE 40-5. Epibulbar complex choristoma that was found histopathologically to have cartilage and ectopic lacrimal gland.

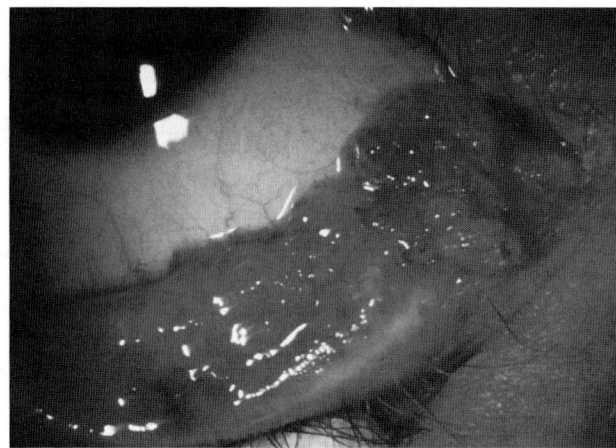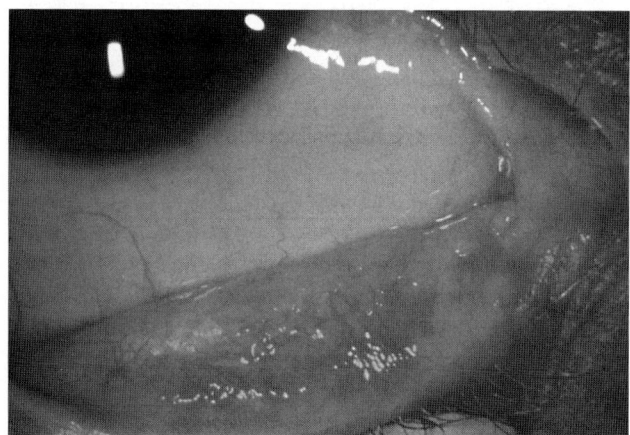

FIGURE 40-6. Recurrent conjunctival papilloma in a child. **A:** The fibrovascular mass caused bloody tears. **B:** Following 3 months of oral cimetidine, the mass resolved.

BENIGN TUMORS OF SURFACE EPITHELIUM

Several benign tumors and related conditions can arise from the squamous epithelium of the conjunctiva. The more common of these lesions are discussed in more detail in Chapter 41.

Papilloma

Squamous papilloma is a benign tumor, documented to originate from human papillomavirus infection of the conjunctiva (35,36). This tumor can occur in both children and adults, and appears as a pink fibrovascular frond of tissue arranged in a sessile or pedunculated configuration. In children, the lesion is usually small, multiple, and located in the inferior fornix (Fig. 40-6). In adults, it is usually solitary, more extensive, and can often extend to cover the entire corneal surface simulating malignant squamous cell carcinoma.

Keratoacathoma

The conjunctiva can give rise to benign reactive inflammatory lesions that simulate carcinoma such as pseudocarcinomatous hyperplasia and its variant, keratoacanthoma (37). In some instances a distinct nodule is found. This lesion appears gelatinous or leukoplakic, similar to squamous cell carcinoma of the conjunctiva, but its onset may be more rapid. Massive acanthosis, hyperkeratosis, and parakeratosis are found histopathologically (37).

Hereditary Benign Intraepithelial Dyskeratosis

Hereditary benign intraepithelial dyskeratosis (HBID) is a peculiar condition seen in an inbred isolate of Caucasians,

African Americans, and American Indians (Haliwa Indians). It is an autosomal-dominant disorder characterized by bilateral elevated fleshy plaques on the nasal or temporal perilimbal conjunctiva (38) (Fig. 40-7). Similar plaques can occur on the buccal mucosa. It can remain relative asymptomatic or it can cause severe redness and foreign-body sensation. In some instances it can extend onto the cornea.

Epithelial Inclusion Cyst

Conjunctival cysts can occur spontaneously or following inflammation, surgery, or nonsurgical trauma. Histopathologically, they are lined by conjunctival epithelium and are filled with clear fluid that often contains desquamated cellular debris (Fig. 40-8). Such cysts can be simply observed or they can be excised completely with primary closure of the conjunctiva.

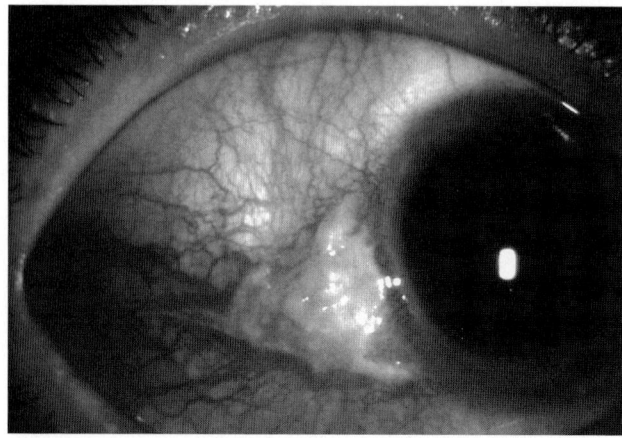

FIGURE 40-7. Hereditary benign intraepithelial dyskeratosis in a young woman who was a descendent of a Haliwa Indian. The opposite eye had a similar lesion.

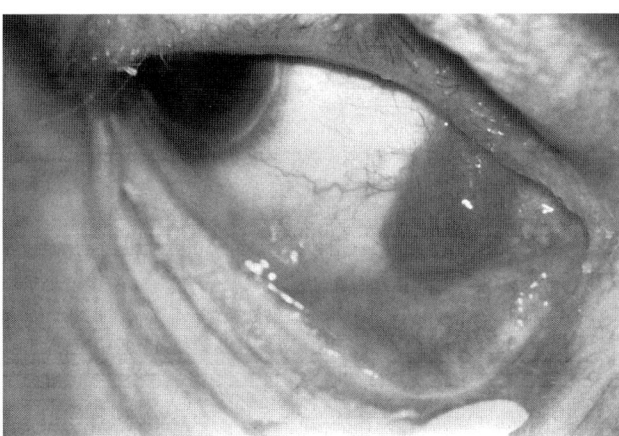

FIGURE 40-8. Epibulbar inclusion cyst with thick mucous from conjunctival glands.

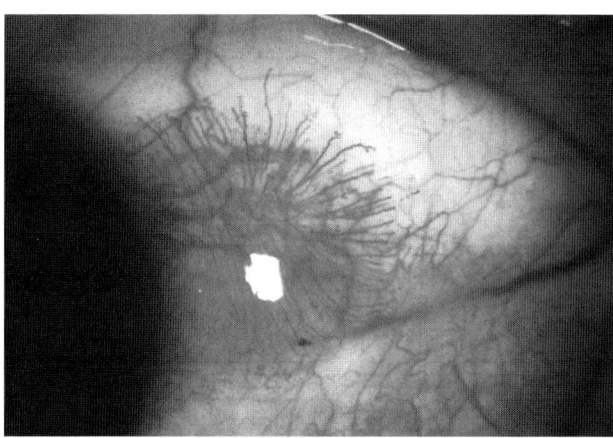

FIGURE 40-9. Conjunctival intraepithelial neoplasia (CIN, carcinoma-in-situ) with corneal involvement, displaying leukoplakia on both the conjunctiva and cornea.

Dacryoadenoma

Dacryoadenoma is a rare conjunctival tumor, noted in children or young adults as a pink mass in the inferior bulbar or palpebral region (39). It is uncertain if the lesion is congenital or acquired. This benign tumor appears to originate from the surface epithelium and proliferate into the stroma, forming glandular lobules similar to the lacrimal gland.

Keratotic Plaque

Keratotic plaque is a white limbal or bulbar conjunctival mass, usually in the interpalpebral region (1). It is composed of acanthosis and parakeratosis with keratinization of the epithelium. It appears similar to squamous cell carcinoma with leukoplakia.

Actinic Keratosis

Actinic keratosis is a frothy, white lesion usually located over a chronically inflamed pingueculum or pterygium (1). Histopathologically, it is composed of a proliferation of surface epithelium with keratosis. Clinically, it resembles squamous cell carcinoma of the conjunctiva.

MALIGNANT LESIONS OF SURFACE EPITHELIUM

Squamous cell neoplasia can occur as a localized lesion confined to the surface epithelium (conjunctival intraepithelial neoplasia, Fig. 40-9) or as a more invasive squamous cell carcinoma that has broken through the basement membrane and invaded the underlying stroma (Fig. 40-10) (21,22,40–44). The former has no potential to metastasize but the latter can gain access to the conjunctival lymphatics

and occasionally metastasize to regional lymph nodes. It has been found that most squamous cell neoplasia is related to human papillomavirus infection of the conjunctival epithelium, and this is most certain in those patients with bilateral squamous cell neoplasia and those immunosuppressed patients who develop this disease (45,46). These lesions are covered in detail in Chapter 41.

MELANOCYTIC TUMORS

Several clinically important tumors arise from the melanocytes of the conjunctiva and episclera (47–63). Benign pigmented lesions include conjunctival nevus (Fig. 40-11) and racial melanosis (Fig. 40-12). Ocular melanocytosis, a benign pigmentation of the sclera, is occasionally misdiagnosed as a pigmented lesion of the conjunctiva (Fig. 40-13), and is therefore often included in a discussion of these lesions. Malignant or potentially malignant pigmented lesions include primary acquired melanosis (Fig. 40-14) and malignant melanoma (Fig. 40-15). Pigmented tumors of the conjunctiva are covered in detail in Chapter 42, but a summary of their important clinical features is included in Table 40-2.

VASCULAR TUMORS

Pyogenic Granuloma

Pyogenic granuloma is a proliferative fibrovascular response to prior tissue insult by inflammation, surgery, or nonsurgical trauma. It is sometimes classified as a polypoid form of acquired capillary hemangioma (64). It appears clinically as an elevated red mass, often with a florid blood supply. Microscopically, it is composed of granulation tissue with chronic inflammatory cells and numerous small

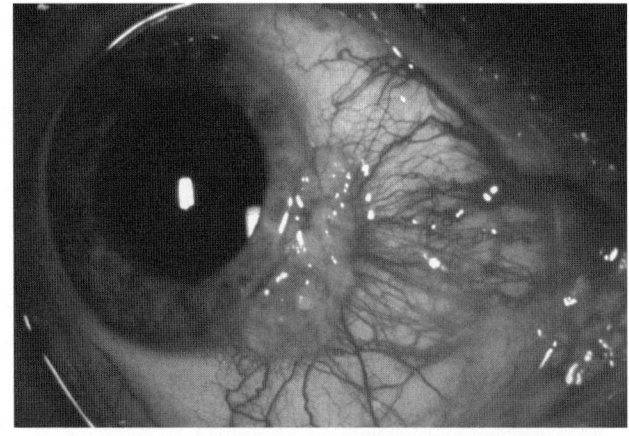

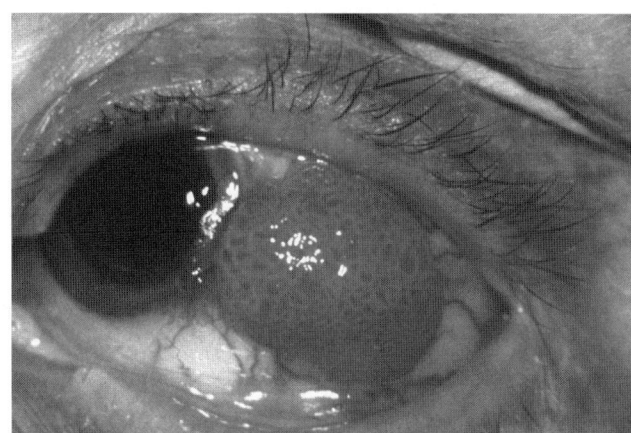

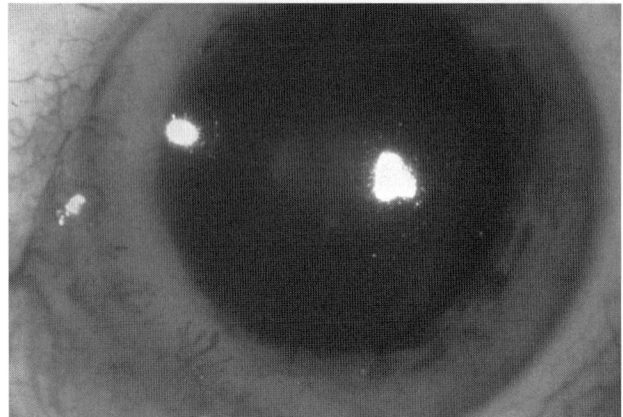

FIGURE 40-10. Invasive squamous cell carcinoma of the conjunctiva. **A:** Gelatinous limbal squamous cell carcinoma. **B:** Nodular squamous cell carcinoma. **C:** Flat diffuse squamous cell carcinoma.

caliber blood vessels (Fig. 40-16). Because the lesion is neither pyogenic nor granulomatous, the term *pyogenic granuloma* is a misnomer. Pyogenic granuloma will sometimes respond to topical corticosteroids, but many cases ultimately require surgical excision. In bothersome recurrent cases, low-dose plaque radiotherapy can be applied (20).

Capillary Hemangioma

Capillary hemangioma of the conjunctiva generally presents in infancy, several weeks following birth, as a red stromal mass, sometimes associated with cutaneous or orbital capillary hemangioma (Fig. 40-17). Similar to its cutaneous counterpart, the conjunctival mass might

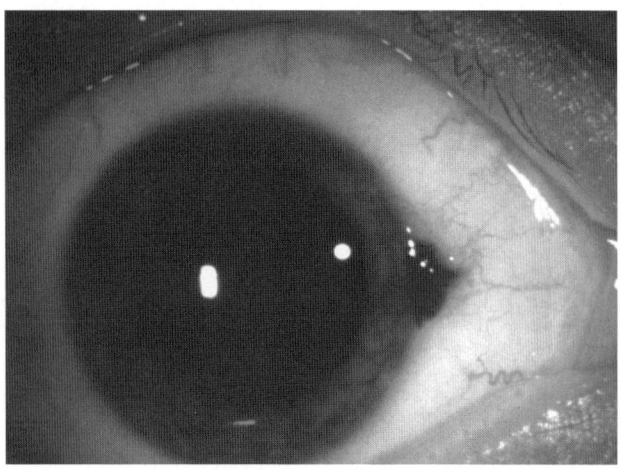

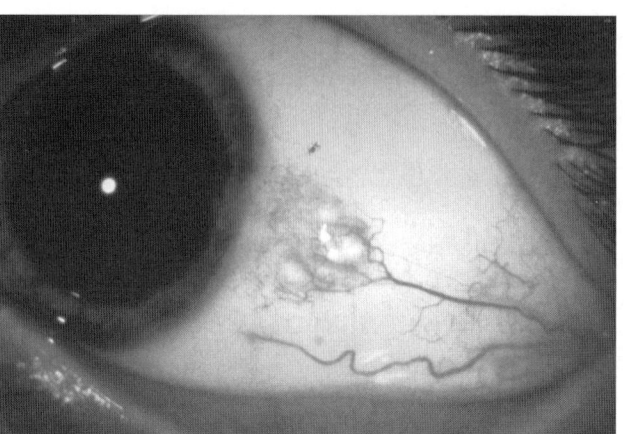

FIGURE 40-11. Conjunctival nevus. **A:** Pigmented conjunctival nevus. **B:** Nonpigmented conjunctival nevus.

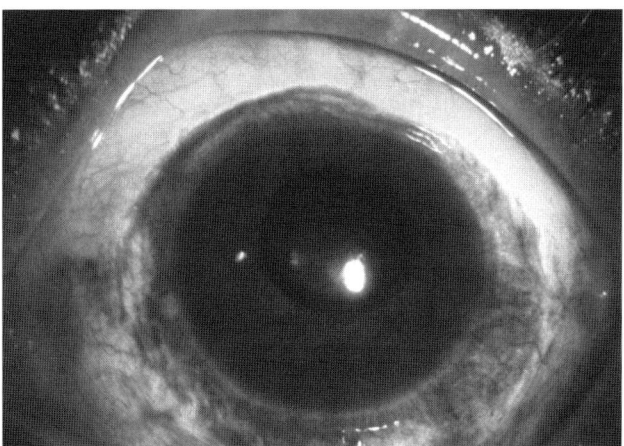

FIGURE 40-12. Racial melanosis found bilaterally in patient with dark skin complexion.

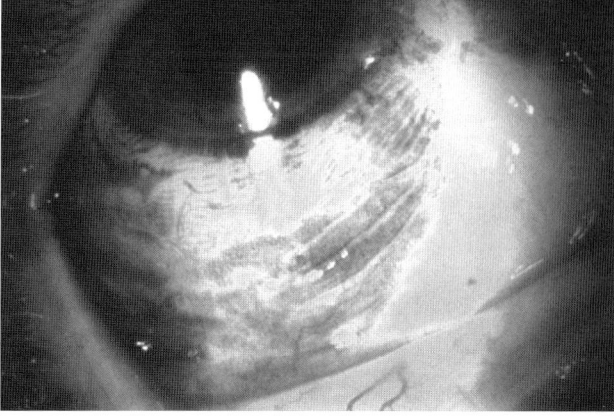

FIGURE 40-14. Primary acquired melanosis of the conjunctiva, showing the characteristic irregular patchy flat pigmentation.

enlarge over several months and then spontaneously involute. Management includes observation most commonly, but surgical resection or local or systemic prednisone can be employed.

Cavernous Hemangioma

Cavernous hemangioma of the conjunctiva is rare (65). This benign tumor appears as a red or blue lesion usually in the deep stroma in young children (Fig. 40-18). It may be similar to the orbital cavernous hemangioma that is generally diagnosed in young adults. It can be managed by local resection.

Racemose Hemangioma

Occasionally, dilated arteriovenous communication without intervening capillary bed (racemose hemangioma) is found in the conjunctiva. This appears as a loop or neatly

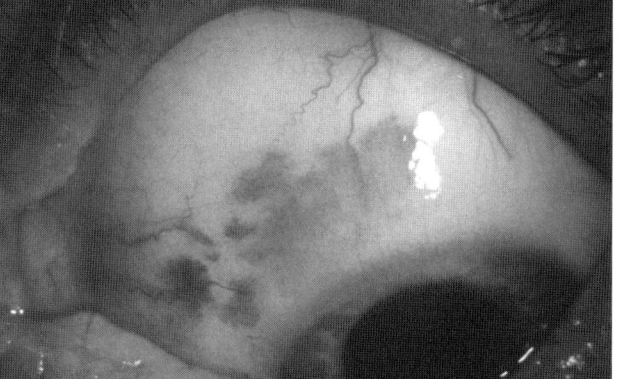

FIGURE 40-13. Ocular melanocytosis with heavy uveal pigment and little conjunctival pigment.

wound monolayer of a dilated, noncrossing vessel in the stroma with no evident stimulus or planned direction. It can remain stable for years and is generally monitored conservatively. It is important to rule out Wyburn-Mason syndrome in such cases.

Lymphangioma

Conjunctival lymphangioma can occur as an isolated conjunctival lesion or, more often, represents a superficial component of a deeper diffuse orbital lymphangioma (66). It usually becomes clinically apparent in the first decade of life and appears as a multiloculated mass containing variable-sized clear dilated cystic channels (Fig. 40-19). In most instances, one sees blood in many of the cystic spaces. These have been called "chocolate cysts." The treatment of conjunctival lymphangioma is often extremely difficult because surgical resection or radiotherapy cannot completely eradicate the mass.

Varix

Varix is a venous malformation that can be found in the orbit and rarely the conjunctiva. It is a mass of dilated venous channels that can enlarge with the Valsalva maneuver. Some authorities believe that this condition is in the spectrum of lymphangioma. Treatment involves cautious observation. If clotted and painful, cold compresses and aspirin may be useful. Surgical resection should be cautiously employed due to the risk for prolonged bleeding at surgery (67).

Hemangiopericytoma

Hemangiopericytoma is a tumor composed of the pericytes that surround blood vessels. It can show both benign and malignant cytologic features. It appears as a red conjunctival

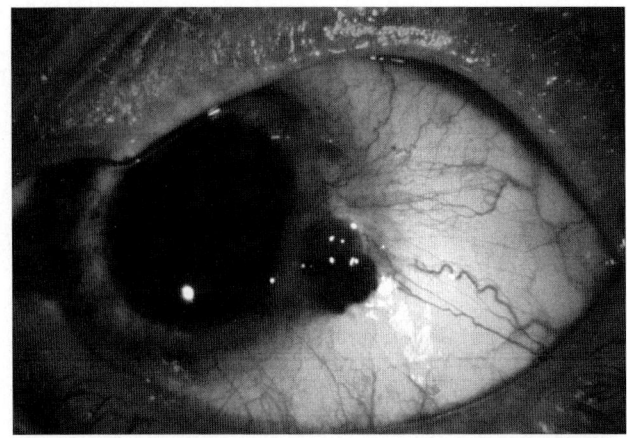
A

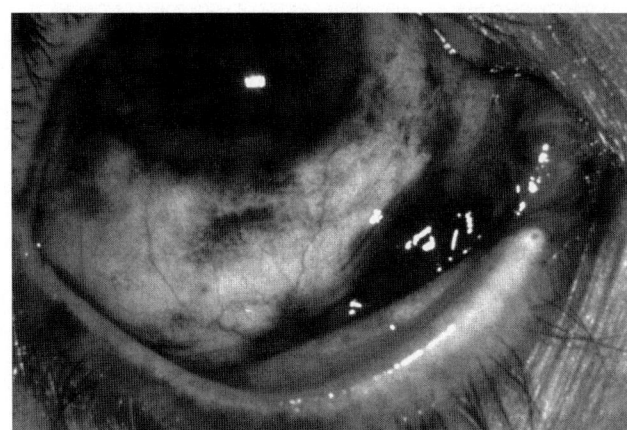
B

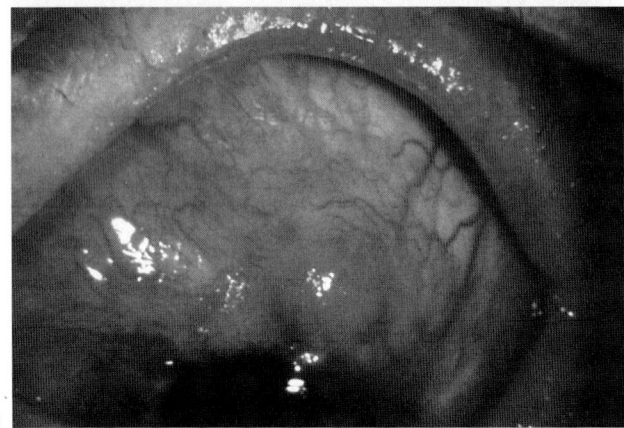
C

FIGURE 40-15. Conjunctival melanoma. **A:** Pigmented melanoma that arose de novo. **B:** Pigmented melanoma that arose from primary acquired melanosis *(left arrow).* Note the flat extension of the melanoma into the cornea. **C:** Nonpigmented melanoma, recurrent following previous excisions.

TABLE 40-2. DIFFERENTIAL DIAGNOSIS OF PIGMENTED EPIBULBAR LESIONS[a]

Condition	Anatomic Location	Color	Depth	Margins	Laterality	Other Features	Progression
Nevus	Interpalpebral limbus usually	Brown or yellow	Stroma	Well defined	Unilateral	Cysts	<1% progress to conjunctival melanoma
Racial melanosis	Limbus >bulbar >palpebral conjunctiva	Brown	Epithelium	Ill defined	Bilateral	Flat, no cysts	Very rare progression to conjunctival melanoma
Ocular melanocytosis	Bulbar conjunctiva	Gray	Episclera	Ill defined	Unilateral more so than bilateral	Congenital, usually 2 mm from limbus, often with periocular skin pigmentation	<1% progress to uveal melanoma
Primary acquired melanosis (PAM)	Anywhere, but usually bulbar conjunctiva	Brown	Epithelium	Ill defined	Unilateral	Flat, no cysts	Progresses to conjunctival melanoma in nearly 50% cases that show cellular atypia
Malignant melanoma	Anywhere	Brown or pink	Stroma	Well defined	Unilateral	Vascular nodule, dilated feeder vessels, may be non pigmented	32% develop metastasis by 15 years

[a] See Figs. 40-11 through 40-15 for clinical illustrations.

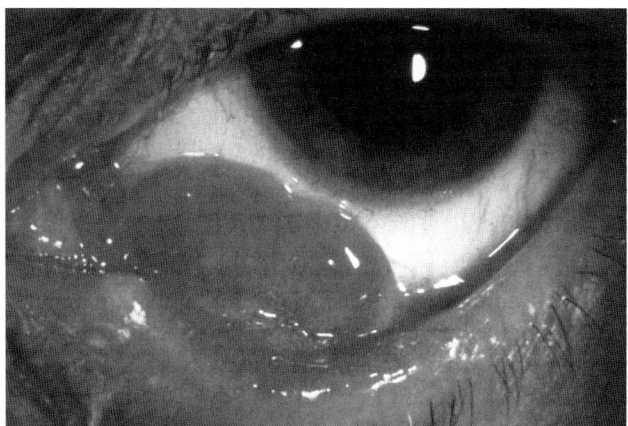

FIGURE 40-16. Pyogenic granuloma.

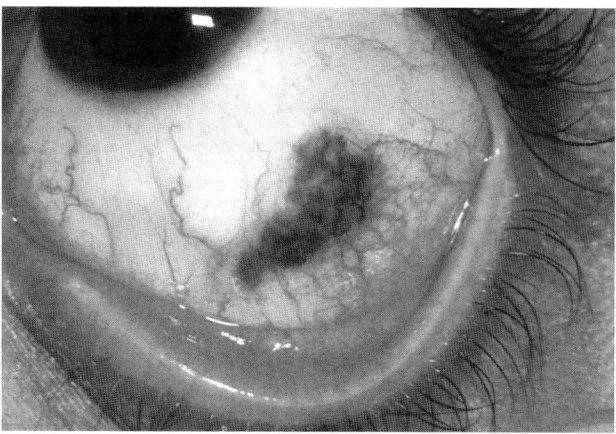

FIGURE 40-18. Cavernous hemangioma of the conjunctiva in a young child.

mass originating from the stroma. Wide surgical resection with tumor-free margins is advised.

Kaposi's Sarcoma

Kaposi's sarcoma is best known as a cutaneous malignancy that occurs in elderly immunosuppressed patients. With the advent of acquired immune deficiency syndrome (AIDS), this tumor has become more common and often affects mucous membranes, such as conjunctiva. Clinically it appears as one or more reddish vascular masses that may resemble a hemorrhagic conjunctivitis (Fig. 40-20). It is moderately responsive to chemotherapy and markedly responsive to low-dose radiotherapy (68).

FIBROUS TUMORS

Fibroma

Fibroma is a rare conjunctival tumor that appears as a white stromal mass, either unifocal or multifocal. Surgical resection is advised.

Fibrous Histiocytoma

Fibrous histiocytoma is a rare mass of the conjunctiva and is composed of fibroblasts and histiocytes. Clinically and histopathologically it resembles many other amelanotic stromal tumors. In the conjunctiva it can be benign, locally invasive, or malignant. Wide excision with tumor-free margins is advised.

Nodular Fasciitis

Nodular fasciitis is a benign proliferation of connective tissue that most commonly occurs in the skin and less commonly in the eyelid, orbit, and conjunctiva. Clinically and histopathologically it can resemble fibrosarcoma. The lesion appears as a solitary white mass in Tenon's fascia. Complete excision is advised as the lesion can recur.

NEURAL TUMORS

Neural tumors of the conjunctiva are rare. They tend to manifest a more yellow appearance than the fibrous tumors.

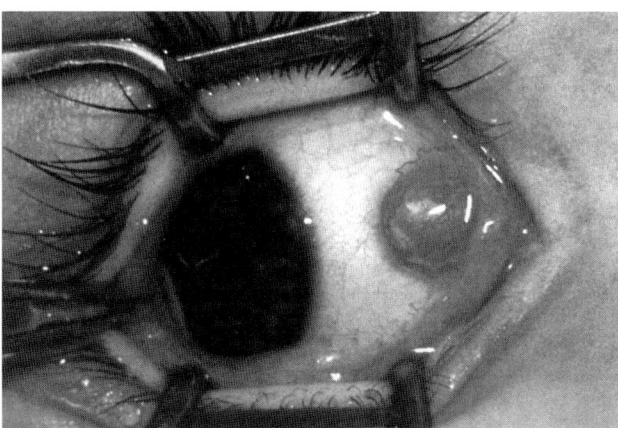

FIGURE 40-17. Capillary hemangioma of the conjunctiva in a newborn infant.

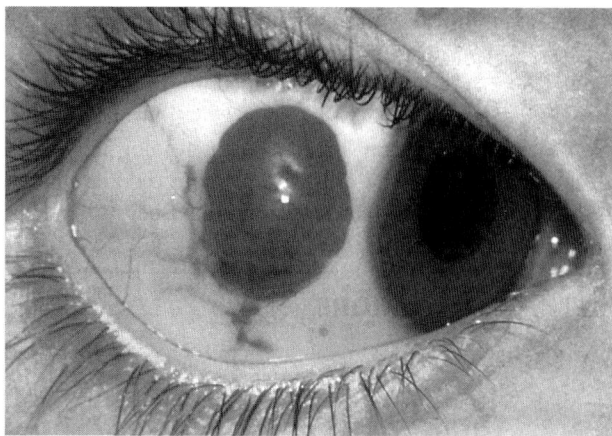

FIGURE 40-19. Lymphangioma of the conjunctiva.

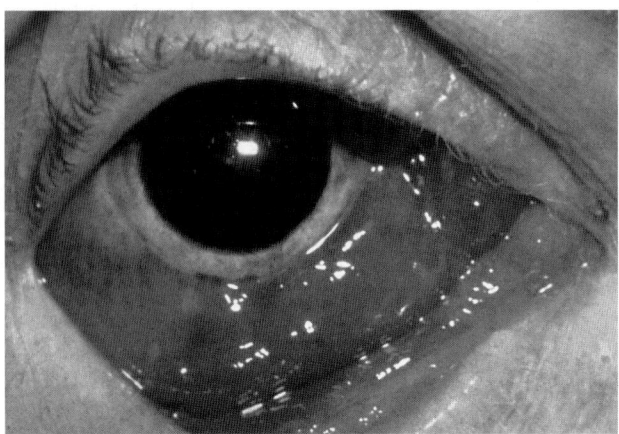

FIGURE 40-20. Kaposi's sarcoma of the conjunctiva with typical surrounding hemorrhage.

Neurofibroma

Neurofibroma can occur in the conjunctiva as a solitary mass or as a diffuse or plexiform variety. The former is not usually associated with systemic conditions and the latter is generally a part of von Recklinghausen's neurofibromatosis (33,34). The solitary tumor is a slowly enlarging elevated stromal mass that is best managed by complete surgical resection. The plexiform type is more difficult to surgically excise, and debulking procedures are often necessary.

Neurilemoma

Neurilemoma, also known as schwannoma, is a benign proliferation of Schwann cells that surround the peripheral nerves. This tumor more commonly arises in the orbit, but there are reports of such rare tumor in the conjunctiva (69). Clinically, this lesion is a yellowish-pink, nodular mass in the stroma. Complete excision is warranted to minimize recurrence.

Granular Cell Tumor

Granular cell tumor is a rare tumor and of disputed origin, but currently, most authorities speculate that it is of Schwann cell origin (1). This benign tumor clinically appears smooth, vascular, and pink, and is located in the stroma or within Tenon's fascia. Histopathologically, it is composed of large round cells with pronounced granularity to the cytoplasm. Complete excision is advised.

HISTIOCYTIC TUMORS

Xanthoma

Xanthoma most often occurs within the cutaneous dermis, near extensor surfaces and its location on the conjunctiva is exceptionally rare. Conjunctival xanthoma appears as a

yellow subepithelial smooth mass affecting one or both epibulbar surfaces. Bilateral conjunctival involvement has been found in a condition termed xanthoma disseminatum. Histopathologically, subepithelial infiltrate of lipidized histiocytes, eosinophils, and Touton giant cells are seen.

Juvenile Xanthogranuloma

Juvenile xanthogranuloma is a relatively common cutaneous condition that presents as painless, pink skin papules with spontaneous resolution, generally in children under the age of 2 years. Rarely, conjunctival, orbital, and intraocular involvement is noted. In the conjunctiva, the mass appears as an orange-pink stromal mass, typically in young adults (Fig. 40-21). If the classic skin lesions are noted, the diagnosis is established clinically and treatment with observation or topical steroid ointment is provided. Otherwise, biopsy is suggested, and recognition of the typical histopathologic features of histiocytes admixed with Touton's giant cells confirms the diagnosis.

Reticulohistiocytoma

Reticulohistiocytoma is a rare tumor, often found as part of a systemic multicentric reticulohistiocytosis. Clinically, the tumor appears as a pink, vascular limbal mass in an adult. Histopathologically, it is composed of large histiocytes with granular cytoplasm (70).

MYXOID TUMORS
Myxoma

Myxoma is a rare conjunctival tumor that appears as an orange-pink mass within the stroma. This tumor can be associated with Carney complex, a syndrome of cardiac myxomas, systemic myxomas, cutaneous lentigines, and Sertoli cell tumor of the testicle (71,72). Histopathology reveals slender stellate and spindle cells interspersed in a loose stroma.

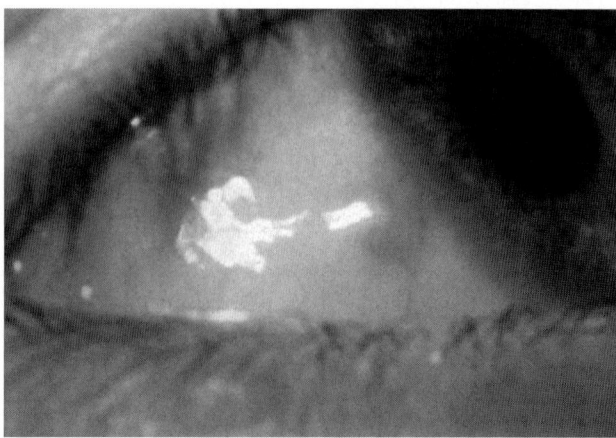

FIGURE 40-21. Juvenile xanthogranuloma of the conjunctiva in a child.

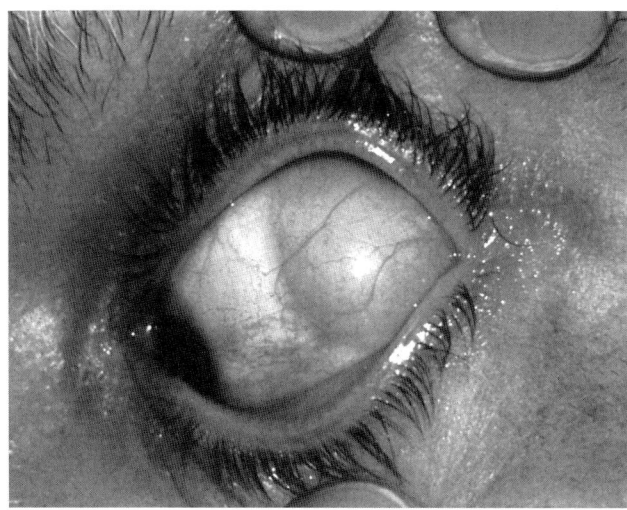

FIGURE 40-22. Herniated orbital fat.

LIPOMATOUS TUMORS

Lipoma

Conjunctival lipoma is quite rare and generally is found in adults as a yellowish-pink stromal mass (71,72). Most are of the pleomorphic type with large lipid vacuoles surrounded by stellate cells.

Herniated Orbital Fat

Occasionally, orbital fat presents in the conjunctiva as a herniation from the superotemporal orbit. The condition is often bilateral and represents deficiency in the orbital connective tissue to maintain the proper location of the normal orbital fat. Clinically, the mass is deep to Tenon's fascia and is most prominent on inferonasal gaze (Fig. 40-22). Digital reposition of the fat into the orbit can be performed, but is only temporary. Management is observation, unless the condition causes symptoms of dry eye from

eyelid malposition. In such cases, resection of the herniated fat and resuspension of the orbit position of the fat is advised. Histopathologically, the tissue is composed of large lipid cells.

Liposarcoma

Liposarcoma of the conjunctiva has been rarely recognized and shows clinical features similar to lipoma. Histopathologically, neoplastic stellate lipid cells and signet-ring type cells have been observed (72).

LYMPHOID TUMORS

Lymphoid tumors can occur in the conjunctiva as isolated lesions or they can be a manifestation of systemic lymphoma (73–76). Clinically, the lesion appears as a diffuse, slightly elevated pink mass located in the stroma or deep to Tenon's fascia, most commonly in the forniceal region (Fig. 40-23). This appearance is similar to that of smoked salmon; hence it is termed the "salmon patch" (75). It is not usually possible to differentiate clinically between a benign and malignant lymphoid tumor. Therefore, biopsy is necessary to establish the diagnosis, and a systemic evaluation should be done in all affected patients to exclude the presence of systemic lymphoma (Table 40-3). Histopathologically, sheets of lymphocytes are found and classified as reactive lymphoid hyperplasia or malignant lymphoma. Most are B-cell lymphoma (non-Hodgkin's type). Rarely T-cell lymphoma is noted (77). Treatment of the conjunctival lesion should include chemotherapy if the patient has systemic lymphoma or external beam irradiation (2,000 to 4,000 cGy) if the lesion is localized to the conjunctiva. Other options include excisional biopsy and cryotherapy (78), local interferon injections, or observation.

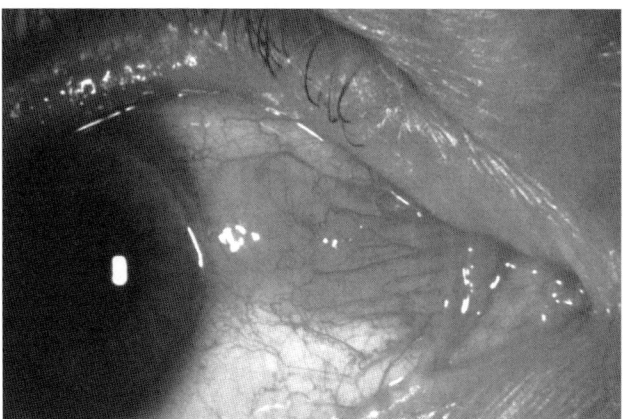
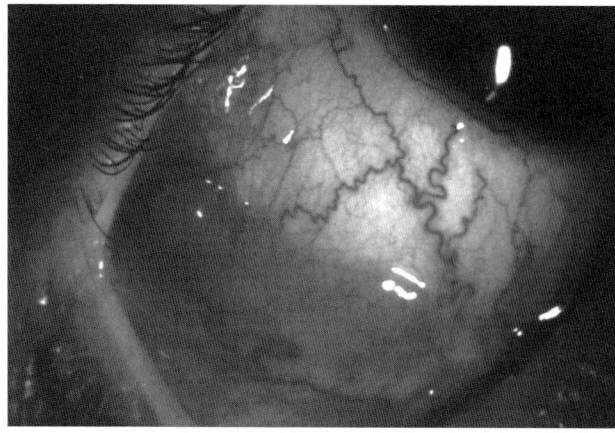

A   B

FIGURE 40-23. Conjunctival lymphoma. **A:** Limbal tumor. **B:** Forniceal tumor.

TABLE 40-3. RISKS FOR THE DEVELOPMENT OF SYSTEMIC LYMPHOMA IN PATIENTS WHO PRESENT WITH CONJUNCTIVAL LYMPHOID INFILTRATE AND NO SIGN OF SYSTEMIC LYMPHOMA

	Development of systemic lymphoma		
	@ 1 years	@ 5 years	@ 10 years
Generally, if conjunctival lymphoid tumor	7%	15%	28%
Specifically, if conjunctival lymphoma	12%	38%	79%

From Shields CL, Shields JA, Carvalho C, et al. Conjunctival lymphoid tumors: clinical analysis of 117 cases and relationship to systemic lymphoma. *Ophthalmology* 2001;108:979–984.

LEUKEMIA

Leukemia generally manifests in the ocular region as hemorrhages from associated anemia and thrombocytopenia rather than leukemic infiltration. However, leukemic infiltration can be found with chronic lymphocytic leukemia. In such cases, the tumor appears as a pink smooth mass within the conjunctival stroma either at the limbus or the fornix, similar to a lymphoid tumor. Biopsy reveals sheets of large leukemic cells. Treatment of the systemic condition is advised with secondary resolution of the conjunctival infiltration.

METASTATIC TUMORS

Metastatic tumors rarely occur in the conjunctiva but conjunctival metastasis can occur from breast carcinoma, cutaneous melanoma, and other primary tumors (79). Metastatic carcinoma appears as one or more fleshy pink vascularized conjunctival stromal tumors (Fig. 40-24). Metastatic melanoma to the conjunctiva usually is pigmented (79).

SECONDARY CONJUNCTIVAL INVOLVEMENT FROM ADJACENT TUMORS

The conjunctiva can be secondarily involved by tumors of adjacent structures, particularly by direct extension from tumors of the eyelids. The most important tumor to exhibit such behavior is sebaceous gland carcinoma of the eyelid (80,81). This tumor can exhibit pagetoid invasion and extend directly into the conjunctival epithelium. This can result in a clinical picture compatible with chronic unilateral blepharoconjunctivitis. Uveal melanoma in the ciliary body region can extend extrasclerally into the subconjunctival tissues, simulating a primary conjunctival tumor. Rhabdomyosarcoma of the orbit, a tumor typically found in children, occasionally presents first with its conjunctival component before the mass is discovered in the orbit (82,83).

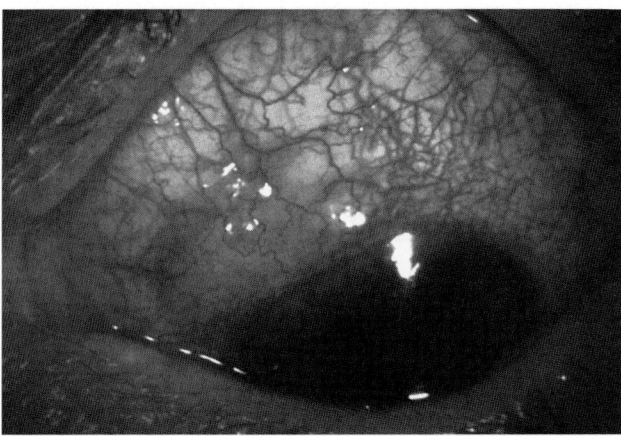

FIGURE 40-24. Metastatic breast carcinoma to the conjunctiva.

CARUNCULAR TUMORS AND CYSTS

The caruncle is a unique anatomic structure that contains elements of both conjunctiva and skin. The tumors and re-

TABLE 40-4. TYPES AND FREQUENCY OF TUMORS OF THE CARUNCLE: COMPARISON OF TWO MAJOR SURVEYS

Lesions	Luthra et al. (84) (*n* = 112)	Shields et al. (85) (*n* = 57)
Papilloma	13%	32%
Nevus	43%	24%
Pyogenic granuloma	3%	9%
Epithelial inclusion cyst	4%	7%
Chronic inflammation	4%	7%
Oncocytoma	4%	4%
Normal caruncle	0	4%
Sebaceous gland hyperplasia	8%	2%
Sebaceous gland adenoma	0	2%
Lipogranuloma	0	2%
Seborrheic keratosis	1%	2%
Lymphangiectasia	0	2%
Histiocytic lymphoma	0	2%
Squamous cell carcinoma	0	2%
Basal cell carcinoma	0	2%
Reactive lymphoid hyperplasia	4%	0
Foreign-body granuloma	3%	0
Malignant melanoma	2%	0
Capillary hemangioma	2%	0
Senile keratosis	1%	0
Freckle	1%	0
Adrenochrome pigment	1%	0
Cavernous hemangioma	1%	0
Dermoid	1%	0
Granular-cell myeloblastoma	1%	0
Plasmacytoma	1%	0
Apocrine hydrocystoma	1%	0
Pilar cyst	1%	0
Sebaceous gland carcinoma	1%	0
Ectopic lacrimal gland	1%	0

From Luthra CL, Doxanas MT, Green WR. Lesions of the caruncle. A clinicopathologic study. *Surv Ophthalmol* 1978;23:183–195; and Shields CL, Shields JA, White D, et al. Types and frequency of lesions of the caruncle. *Am J Ophthalmol* 1986;102:771–778.

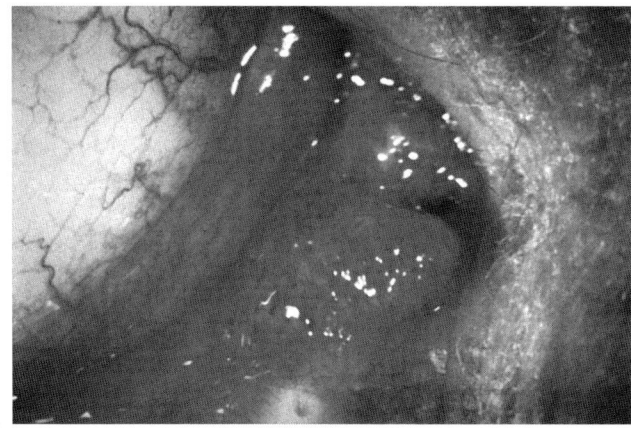

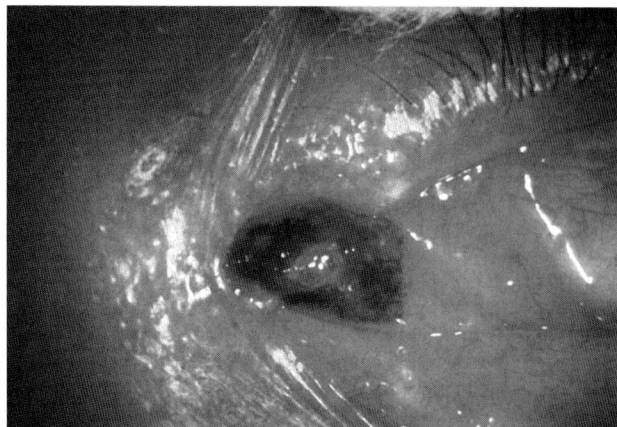

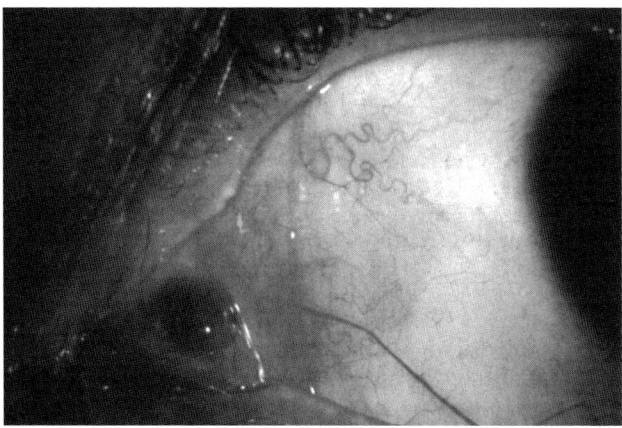

FIGURE 40-25. Caruncular tumors. **A:** Papilloma of the caruncle. **B:** Nevus of the caruncle. **C:** Oncocytoma of the caruncle.

lated lesions that develop in the caruncle are similar to those that occur in mucous membranes and cutaneous structures. By histopathologic analysis, 95% of caruncular tumors are benign and 5% are malignant (84). The most common lesions include papilloma and nevus (84,85) (Table 40-4) (Fig. 40-25). Other caruncular lesions include pyogenic granuloma, inclusion cyst, sebaceous hyperplasia, and sebaceous adenoma, and oncocytoma (86). Malignant tumors such as squamous cell carcinoma, melanoma, lymphoma, and sebaceous carcinoma are relatively rare in the caruncle. The oncocytoma is a benign tumor that occurs more commonly in the lacrimal or salivary glands. In the caruncle it probably arises from accessory lacrimal gland tissue and often has a blue cystic appearance (Fig. 40-25). The treatment of most caruncular masses is either observation or local resection, depending on the final diagnosis.

MISCELLANEOUS LESIONS THAT CAN SIMULATE CONJUNCTIVAL NEOPLASMS

A number of nonneoplastic conditions can simulate neoplasms. These include pingueculum, pterygium, foreign body, inflammatory granuloma, amyloidosis, and others (1). In most instance, the history and clinical findings should make the diagnosis obvious. In some instances, however, excision of the mass may be necessary in order to exclude a neoplasm.

ACKNOWLEDGMENT

This work is supported by the Eye Tumor Research Foundation, Inc., Philadelphia, PA.

REFERENCES

1. Shields JA, Shields CL. Tumors and pseudotumors of the conjunctiva. In: *Atlas of eyelid and conjunctival tumors.* Philadelphia: Lippincott Williams & Wilkins, 1999:199–334.
2. Grossniklaus HE, Green WR, Luckenbach M, et al. Conjunctival lesions in adults. A clinical and histopathologic review. *Cornea* 1987;6:78–116.
3. Shields CL, Demirci H, Karatza KC, et al. Survey of 1500 eyes with conjunctival tumors and pseudotumors. *In press.*
4. Shields JA, Shields CL. Management of conjunctival tumors. In: *Atlas of eyelid and conjunctival tumors.* Philadelphia: Lippincott Williams & Wilkins, 1999:332–334.
5. Shields JA, Shields CL, De Potter P. Surgical management of circumscribed conjunctival melanomas. *Ophthalmic Plast Reconstr Surg* 1998;14:208–215.
6. Shields JA, Shields CL, De Potter P. Surgical management of conjunctival tumors. The 1994 Lynn B. McMahan Lecture. *Arch Ophthalmol* 1997;115:808–815.

7. Shields JA, Shields CL, Suvarnamani C, et al. Orbital exenteration with eyelid sparing: indications, technique and results. *Ophthalmic Surg* 1991;22:292–297.

8. Shields CL, Shields JA, Armstrong T. Management of conjunctival and corneal melanoma with combined surgical excision, amniotic membrane allograft, and topical chemotherapy. *Am J Ophthalmol* 2001;132:576–578.

9. Paridaens D, Beekhuis H, van Den Bosch W, et al. Amniotic membrane transplantation in the management of conjunctival malignant melanoma and primary acquired melanosis with atypia. *Br J Ophthalmol* 2001;85:658–661.

10. Frucht-Pery J, Rozenman Y. Mitomycin C therapy for corneal intraepithelial neoplasia. *Am J Ophthalmol* 1994;117:164–168.

11. Frucht-Pery J, Sugar J, Baum J, et al. Mitomycin C treatment for conjunctival-corneal intraepithelial neoplasia: a multicenter experience. *Ophthalmology* 1997;104:2085–2093.

12. Shields CL, Naseripour M, Shields JA. Topical mitomycin C for extensive, recurrent conjunctival-corneal squamous cell carcinoma. *Am J Ophthalmol* 2002;133(5):601–606.

13. Yeatts RP, Engelbrecht NE, Curry CD, et al. 5-Fluorouracil for the treatment of intraepithelial neoplasia of the conjunctiva and cornea. *Ophthalmology* 2000;107:2190–2195.

14. Midena E, Angeli CD, Valenti M, et al. Treatment of conjunctival squamous cell carcinoma with topical 5-fluorouracil. *Br J Ophthalmol* 2000;84:268–272.

15. Yamamoto N, Ohmura T, Suzuki H, et al. Successful treatment with 5-fluorouracil of conjunctival intraepithelial neoplasia refractive to mitomycin-C. *Ophthalmology* 2002;109:249–252.

16. Karp CL, Moore JK, Rosa RH Jr. Treatment of conjunctival and corneal intraepithelial neoplasia with topical interferon alpha-2b. *Ophthalmology* 2001;108:1093–1098.

17. Sherman M, Feldman K, Farahmand S, et al. Treatment of conjunctival squamous cell carcinoma with topical cidofir. *Am J Ophthalmol* 2002;134:432–433.

18. Shields CL, Demirci H, Shields JA, et al. Dramatic regression of conjunctival and corneal acquired melanosis with topical mitomycin C. *Br J Ophthalmol* 2002;86:244–245.

19. Shields CL, Naseripour M, Shields JA, et al. Topical Mitomycin C for conjunctival pagetoid invasion of sebaceous gland carcinoma. *Ophthalmology* 2002 Nov;109:2129–2133.

20. Shields CL, Shields JA, Gunduz K, et al. Radiation therapy for uveal malignant melanoma. *Ophthalmol Surg Lasers* 1998;29:397–409.

21. Gunduz K, Shields CL, Shields JA, et al. Plaque radiotherapy for recurrent conjunctival pyogenic granuloma. *Arch Ophthalmol* 1998;116:538–539.

22. Brownstein S. Mucoepidermoid carcinoma of the conjunctiva with intraocular invasion. *Ophthalmology* 1981;88:1126–1130.

23. Gunduz K, Shields CL, Shields JA, et al. Intraocular neoplastic cyst from mucoepidermoid carcinoma of the conjunctiva. *Arch Ophthalmol* 1998;116:1521–1523.

24. Shields CL, Shields JA, Gunduz K, et al. Conjunctival melanoma: risk factors for recurrence, exenteration, metastasis, and death in 150 consecutive patients. *Arch Ophthalmol* 2000;118:1497–1507.

25. Shields JA, Shields CL, Gunduz K, et al. Clinical features predictive of orbital exenteration for conjunctival melanoma. *Ophthalmic Plast Reconstr Surg* 2000;16:173–178.

26. Cunha RP, Cunha MC, Shields JA. Epibulbar tumors in childhood. A survey of 283 biopsies. *J Pediatr Ophthalmol* 1987;24:249–254.

27. Shields JA, Shields CL. Pediatric ocular and periocular tumors. *Pediatr Ann* 2001;30:491–501.

28. Dailey EB, Lubowitz RM. Dermoids of the limbus and cornea. *Am J Ophthalmol* 1962;53:661–665.

29. Scott JA, Tan DT. Therapeutic lamellar keratoplasty for limbal dermoids. *Ophthalmology* 2001;108:1858–1867.

30. Shields JA, Eagle RC, Shields CL, et al. Epibulbar osseous choristoma. Computed tomography and clinicopathologic correlation. *Ophthalmic Pract* 1997;15:110–112.

31. Young TL, Buchi ER, Kaufman LM, et al. Respiratory epithelium in a cystic choristoma of the limbus. *Arch Ophthalmol* 1990;108:1736–1739.

32. Shields JA, Shields CL, Eagle RC Jr, et al. Ophthalmic features of the organoid nevus syndrome. *Ophthalmology* 1997;104:549–557.

33. Shields JA, Shields CL. Systemic hamartomatoses ("phakomatoses") In: Shields JA, Shields CL. *Intraocular tumors. A text and atlas.* Philadelphia: WB Saunders, 1992:513–539.

34. Shields CL, Shields JA. Phakomatoses. In: Regillo CD, Brown GC, Flynn HW Jr, eds. *Vitreoretinal disease. The essentials.* New York: Thieme Medical Publishers, 1999:377–390.

35. Sjo NC, Heegaard S, Prause JU, et al. Human papillomavirus in conjunctival papilloma. *Br J Ophthalmol* 2001;85:785–787.

36. Shields CL, Lally MR, Singh AD, et al. Oral cimetidine (Tagamet) for recalcitrant, diffuse conjunctival papillomatosis. *Am J Ophthalmol* 1999;128:362–364.

37. Munro S, Brownstein S, Liddy B. Conjunctival keratoacanthoma. *Am J Ophthalmol* 1993;116:654–655.

38. Shields CL, Shields JA, Eagle RC. Hereditary benign intraepithelial dyskeratosis. *Arch Ophthalmol* 1987;105:422–423.

39. Jakobiec FA, Perry HD, Harrison W, et al. Dacryoadenoma. A unique tumor of the conjunctival epithelium. *Ophthalmology* 1989;96:101410–101420.

40. Tunc M, Char DH, Crawford B, et al. Intraepithelial and invasive squamous cell carcinoma of the conjunctiva: analysis of 60 cases. *Br J Ophthalmol* 1999;83:98–103.

41. Cha SB, Shields CL, Shields JA, et al. Massive precorneal extension of squamous cell carcinoma of the conjunctiva. *Cornea* 1993;12:537–540.

42. McKelvie PA, Daniell M, McNab A, et al. Squamous cell carcinoma of the conjunctiva: a series of 26 cases. *Br J Ophthalmol* 2002;86:168–173.

43. Iliff WJ, Marback R, Green WR. Invasive squamous cell carcinoma of the conjunctiva. *Arch Ophthalmol* 1975;93:119–122.

44. Shields JA, Shields CL, Gunduz K, et al. The 1998 Pan American Lecture. Intraocular invasion of conjunctival squamous cell carcinoma in five patients. *Ophthalmic Plast Reconstr Surg* 1999;15(3):153–160.

45. Scott IU, Karp CL, Nuovo GJ. Human papillomavirus 16 and 18 expression in conjunctival intraepithelial neoplasia. *Ophthalmology* 2002;109:542–547.

46. Shelil AE, Shields CL, Shields JA, et al. Aggressive conjunctival squamous cell carcinoma in a liver transplant patient. *Arch Ophthalmol* 2003 Feb;121:280–282.

47. Gerner N, Norregaard JC, Jensen OA, et al. Conjunctival naevi in Denmark 1960–1980. A 21-year follow-up study. *Acta Ophthalmol Scand* 1996;74:334–337.

48. Shields CL, Fasiuddin A, Mashayekhi A, et al. Conjunctival nevi: Clinical features and natural course in 410 consecutive patients. *Arch Ophthalmol* 2004 Feb;122:167–175.

49. Crawford JB, Howes EL Jr, Char DH. Combined nevi of the conjunctiva. *Arch Ophthalmol* 1999;117:1121–1127.

50. Singh AD, DePotter P, Fijal BA, et al. Lifetime prevalence of uveal melanoma in white patients with oculo(dermal) melanocytosis. *Ophthalmology* 1998;105:195–198.

51. Folberg R, McLean I W, Zimmerman LE. Primary acquired melanosis of the conjunctiva. *Hum Pathol* 1985;16:136–143.

52. Folberg R, McLean IW. Primary acquired melanosis and melanoma of the conjunctiva; terminology, classification, and biologic behavior. *Hum Pathol* 1986;17:652–654.

53. Gloor P, Alexandrakis G. Clinical characterization of primary acquired melanosis. *Invest Ophthalmol Vis Sci* 1995;36:1721–1729.

54. Seregard S. Conjunctival melanoma. *Surv Ophthalmol* 1998;42:321–350.

55. Paridaens AD, Minassian DC, McCartney AC, et al. Prognostic factors in primary malignant melanoma of the conjunctiva: a clinicopathological study of 256 cases. *Br J Ophthalmol* 1994;78: 252–259.

56. Paridaens AD, McCartney AC, Minassian DC, et al. Orbital exenteration in 95 cases of primary conjunctival malignant melanoma. *Br J Ophthalmol* 1994;78:520–528.

57. Strempel I, Kroll P. Conjunctival malignant melanoma in children. *Ophthalmologica* 1999;213:129–132.

58. Tuomaala S, Aine E, Saari KM, et al. Corneally displaced malignant conjunctival melanomas. *Ophthalmology* 2002;109:914–919.

59. Esmaeli B, Eicher S, Popp J, et al. Sentinel lymph node biopsy for conjunctival melanoma. *Ophthalmic Plast Reconstr Surg* 2001;17:436–442.

60. Shields CL. Conjunctival melanoma (editorial). *Br J Ophthalmol* 2002;86:127.

61. Anastassiou G, Heiligenhaus A, Bechrakis N, et al. Prognostic value of clinical and histopathological parameters in conjunctival melanomas: a retrospective study. *Br J Ophthalmol* 2002;86: 163–167.

62. Shields JA, Shields CL, Demirci H, et al. Experience with eyelid-sparing orbital exenteration. The 2000 Tullos O. Coston Lecture. *Ophthalmic Plast Reconstr Surg* 2001;17:355–361.

63. Shields JA, Shields CL, Eagle RC Jr, et al. Pigmented conjunctival squamous cell carcinoma simulating a conjunctival melanoma. *Am J Ophthalmol* 2001;132:104–106.

64. Ferry AP. Pyogenic granulomas of the eye and ocular adnexa: a study of 100 cases. *Trans Am Ophthalmol Soc* 1989;87:327–347.

65. Ullman SS, Nelson LB, Shields JA, et al. Cavernous hemangioma of the conjunctiva. *Orbit* 1988;6:261–265.

66. Krema H. Shields CL, Shields JA. Orbital and conjunctival lymphangioma. Analysis of 45 patients. *Ophthalmology (in press).*

67. Shields JA, Eagle RC Jr, Shields CL, et al. Orbital varix presenting as a subconjunctival mass. *Ophthalmic Plast Reconstr Surg* 1995;11(1):37–38.

68. Shields JA, De Potter P, Shields CL, et al. Kaposi's sarcoma of the eyelids: response to radiotherapy. *Arch Ophthalmol* 1992;110:1689.

69. Perry HD. Isolated episcleral neurofibroma. *Ophthalmology* 1982;89:1095–1098.

70. Eagle RC Jr, Penne RA, Hneleski IS Jr. Eyelid involvement in multicentric reticulohistiocytosis. *Ophthalmology* 1995;102:426–430.

71. Shields JA. Lipomatous and myxomatous tumors. In: Shields JA. *Diagnosis and management of orbital tumors.* Philadelphia: WB Saunders, 1989:236–238.

72. Shields JA, Shields CL. Lipomatous and myxomatous tumors. In: Shields JA, Shields CL. *Atlas of orbital tumors.* Philadelphia: Lippincott Williams & Wilkins, 1999:143–152.

73. Knowles DM II, Jakobiec FA. Ocular adnexal lymphoid neoplasms: clinical, histopathologic, electron microscopic, and immunologic characteristics. *Hum Pathol* 1982;123:148–162.

74. Cockerham GC, Jakobiec FA. Lymphoproliferative disorders of the ocular adnexa. *Int Ophthalmol Clin* 1997;37:39–59.

75. Shields CL, Shields JA, Carvalho C, et al. Conjunctival lymphoid tumors: clinical analysis of 117 cases and relationship to systemic lymphoma. *Ophthalmology* 2001;108:979–984.

76. McKelvie PA, McNab A, Francis IC, et al. Ocular adnexal lymphoproliferative disease: a series of 73 cases. *Clin Exp Ophthalmol* 2001;29:387–393.

77. Shields CL, Shields JA, Eagle RC. Rapidly progressive T-cell lymphoma of the conjunctiva. *Arch Ophthalmol* 2002;120: 508–509.

78. Eichler MD, Fraunfelder FT. Cryotherapy for conjunctival lymphoid tumors. *Am J Ophthalmol* 1994;118:463–467.

79. Kiratli H, Shields CL, Shields JA, et al. Metastatic tumours to the conjunctiva: report of 10 cases. *Br J Ophthalmol* 1996;80: 5–8.

80. Chao AN, Shields CL, Krema H, et al. Outcome of patients with periocular sebaceous gland carcinoma with and without conjunctival intraepithelial invasion. *Ophthalmology* 2001;108(10): 1877–1883.

81. Honavar SG, Shields CL, Maus M, et al. Primary intraepithelial sebaceous gland carcinoma of the palpebral conjunctiva. *Arch Ophthalmol* 2001;119:764–767.

82. Shields CL, Shields JA, Honavar SG, et al. Clinical spectrum of primary ophthalmic rhabdomyosarcoma. *Ophthalmology* 2001;108: 2284–2292.

83. Shields JA, Shields CL. Ocular rhabdomyosarcoma: Review. *Surv Ophthalmol (in press).*

84. Luthra CL, Doxanas MT, Green WR. Lesions of the caruncle. A clinicopathologic study. *Surv Ophthalmol* 1978;23:183–195.

85. Shields CL, Shields JA, White D, et al. Types and frequency of lesions of the caruncle. *Am J Ophthalmol* 1986;102:771–778.

86. Shields CL, Shields JA, Arbizo V. Oncocytoma of the caruncle. *Am J Ophthalmol* 1986;102:315–319.

EPITHELIAL TUMORS INVOLVING THE OCULAR SURFACE

**GLENN C. COCKERHAM AND
KIMBERLY P. COCKERHAM**

The ocular surface, consisting of the cornea, limbus, conjunctiva and caruncle, is covered by a continuous lining of nonkeratinizing epithelium. The epithelial phenotype varies according to location and function. Bulbar and tarsal conjunctiva contains columnar epithelium with mucus-producing goblet cells, whereas squamous epithelium covers the corneal surface. Epithelial stem cells found in the crypts of Vogt at the corneal limbus proliferate rapidly and are responsible for a large percentage of squamous neoplasia.

Abnormal cellular differentiation may lead to nonspecific changes in ocular surface epithelium, as in epithelial tissues elsewhere. Proliferation of normal cells with thickening of the epithelial layer is *acanthosis*. *Hyperkeratosis* is the production of surface keratin by normally nonkeratinizing cornea or conjunctiva. Keratinized epithelium has a crusty white surface, which is commonly known as *leukoplakia*. *Dyskeratosis* is the histologic presence of keratin deeper within the epithelium. All of the processes above may be found in benign as well as malignant tumors. *Dysplasia* is loss of cellular differentiation, manifest by abnormal size and shape of epithelial cells and nuclei. Biopsy with histopathologic examination is required for definitive diagnosis of suspicious epithelial lesions.

HEREDITARY BENIGN INTRAEPITHELIAL DYSKERATOSIS

Hereditary benign intraepithelial dyskeratosis (HBID) is an inherited disorder of epithelial maturation of the oral mucosa and bulbar conjunctiva. Autosomal-dominant transmission with high penetrance has been reported (1). HBID affects a population of triracial heritage (African, native American, and Caucasian) located in northeastern North Carolina in Halifax and Washington counties, and therefore known as Haliwa Indians. A family with identical phenotype but no known relationship to Haliwa Indians has also been described (2).

Dilated superficial vessels are associated with elevated keratotic plaques in the nasal and temporal perilimbal regions

of the bulbar conjunctiva (Fig. 41-1). Vision may be affected if plaques affect the central cornea. The chronic conjunctival hyperemia is recognized as the "red eye" in the endemic community (3). HBID may be initially mistaken for limbal vernal keratoconjunctivitis. Tearing and photophobia are common. Oral lesions, varying from spongy areas to thick plaques, have been found in all cases. No malignant transformation of ocular or oral lesions has been reported (4).

Pathologic examination reveals the benign nature of the lesion. Acanthosis and hyperkeratosis are seen, as well as a characteristic inclusion of keratin within individual cells (dyskeratosis). No cellular atypia is present. Treatment consists of ocular lubrication for mild irritation. Topical corticosteroids may be helpful for exacerbations of inflammation and irritation. Lesions will recur after excision, but removal of plaques affecting vision is helpful (5).

SQUAMOUS PAPILLOMAS

Squamous papillomas are benign proliferations of conjunctival surface epithelium. Conjunctival papillomas may occur at any age, but are most common between the ages of 20 and 39 years (6). Papilloma accounted for 7% of 302 epibulbar tumors in children under age 15 (7). The predominant growth pattern is exophytic and may be exuberant, involving a large portion of the ocular surface (Fig. 41-2). Limbal papillomas may extend into corneal epithelium (8). Inverted papillomas of the conjunctiva, with downward growth, are rare (9). Pedunculated multiple papillomas are usually of viral origin, whereas sessile papillomatous lesions in elderly patients may represent an intraepithelial neoplasm.

Human papilloma virus (HPV) is an oncogenic double-stranded DNA papovirus implicated in verrucae (skin warts), condylomata acuminata (venereal warts) and mucocutaneous papillomas. Conjunctival inoculation with HPV may occur with delivery through an infected birth canal, through sexual contact, or by autoinoculation (10). Sjo and colleagues (6) identified the DNA of HPV type 6 or 11 in over 80% of

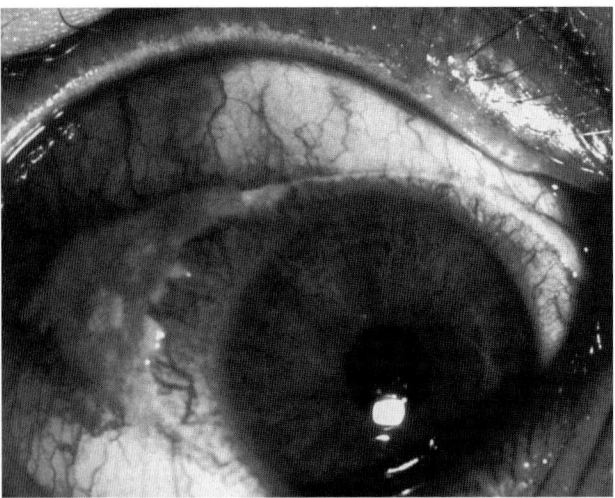

FIGURE 41-1. Hereditary benign intraepithelial dyskeratosis (HBID). Raised, vascular hyperkeratotic lesion is located on the temporal interpalpebral conjunctiva. (Courtesy of the Armed Forces Institute of Pathology).

conjunctival papilloma samples tested by polymerase chain reaction (PCR). Eng and colleagues (11) demonstrated HPV 6 or 11 in 58% of conjunctival papillomas.

Standard therapy of papillomas consists of surgical excision, with cautery or cryotherapy of the base (12,13). Despite thorough destruction of the lesions and adjacent epithelium, papillomas may recur. Vaporization of lesions with a carbon dioxide laser may be beneficial in the treatment of recurrent papillomas (14). Mitomycin-C 0.3 mg/mL on a cellulose sponge applied to the epithelial defect for 3 minutes after excision has proven helpful in preventing recurrence (15). Topical mitomycin C 0.02% applied four times daily for 2 weeks, beginning 1 week after excision, has also been employed successfully in the management of recurrent papillomas (16). Caution should be employed in treating an

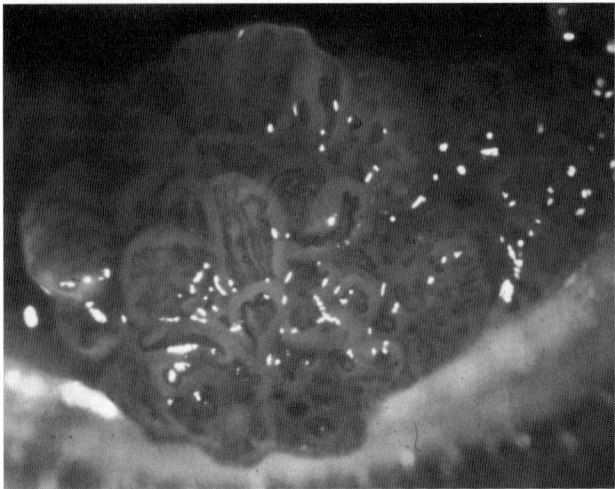

FIGURE 41-2. Squamous papilloma. Exuberant proliferation of benign conjunctiva is present in the inferior fornix.

area of conjunctival excision with topical mitomycin C, because of reports of scleral thinning and perforation in bare sclera pterygium excision treated with mitomycin C (17).

Intramuscular interferon-alfa-N1 given daily for 1 month suppressed the recurrence of papillomas after excision, but was not felt to be curative (18). Topical interferon-alfa-2b 1 million units/mL four times daily has resulted in resolution of papillomas by 3 months without surgical excision (19). Four months of oral therapy with liquid cimetidine 30/mg/kg was successful in resolving recalcitrant, diffuse conjunctival papillomatosis in a child (20). Cimetidine is a histamine-2 receptor antagonist, which also has immunomodulation properties, such as inhibition of suppressor T-cell function.

Microscopically, papillomas consist of multiple branching fronds, emanating from a pedunculated base. Acanthotic nonkeratinizing epithelium surrounds a vascularized core of connective tissue, often with light inflammation. Koilocytes, viral inclusions within the epithelium, are a variable finding within papillomas.

CONJUNCTIVAL-INTRAEPITHELIAL NEOPLASIA (CIN) AND SQUAMOUS CELL CARCINOMA

Epithelial neoplasia of the ocular surface is considered a disease complex, comprising a spectrum of changes originating within the epithelial layers. Previously used terms for this condition include Bowen's disease and ocular surface squamous neoplasia. Pizzarello and Jakobiec suggested the currently used term, *conjunctival intraepithelial neoplasia* (CIN), similar to cervical intraepithelial neoplasia used in gynecologic pathology (21). *Conjunctival-corneal intraepithelial dysplasia* (CCIN) is appropriate if the cornea is also involved (22). The earliest change is dysplasia, confined by the underlying epithelial basement membrane. Increasing degrees of dysplasia occur if the process is not arrested, culminating in transgression of the basement membrane with invasion of the underlying space and structures. This invasion of subjacent tissue is the hallmark of squamous cell carcinoma (Fig. 41-3). Histologic examination is required for definitive diagnosis.

Incidence and Etiology

CIN occurs primarily in elderly, lightly-complexioned men with extensive actinic exposure. In a review of 26 cases of squamous cell carcinoma of the conjunctiva in an Australian population, 77% of the patients were male and 69% were older than 60 years of age (23). The incidence of squamous cell carcinoma of the eye has been calculated to increase 49% for each 10-degree decrease in latitude (24). The incidence of CIN in African tribal peoples in Uganda was 0.13 cases/100,000 between 1961 and 1966. In the pre-

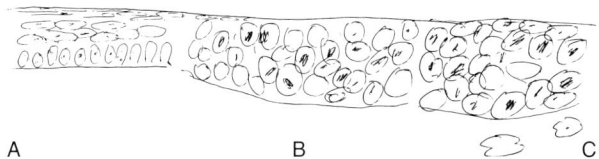

FIGURE 41-3. Conjunctival epithelium. Diagram demonstrates **(A)** normal epithelium, **(B)** dysplasia confined to the epithelium, and **(C)** squamous cell carcinoma, with invasion of the underlying tissue.

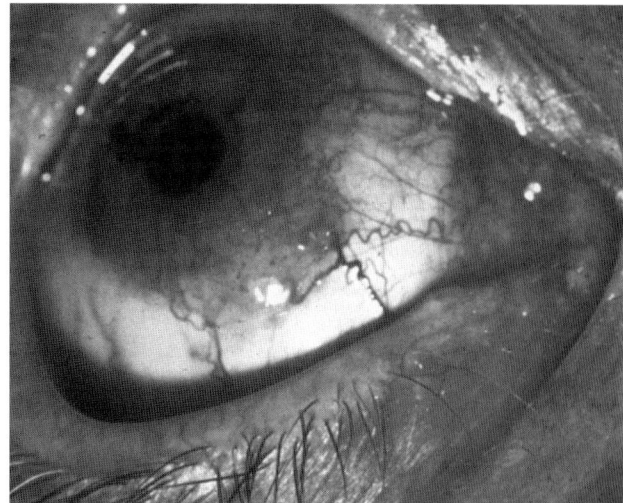

FIGURE 41-4. Conjunctival intraepithelial neoplasia (CIN). A thickened, gelatinous lesion with increased vascularity is noted at the limbus. (Courtesy of the Armed Forces Institute of Pathology).

dominantly Caucasian population of Australia, the incidence of CIN in the period 1980 to 1989 was 1.9/100,000 (21). Previous history of skin cancer is a positive prognosticator for CIN. In addition to ultraviolet light, other reported risk factors include previous history of skin cancer, smoking, ocular trauma, and petroleum derivative exposure (25, 26).

Human papilloma virus (HPV), especially types 16 and 18, has been identified in conjunctival epithelial neoplasia by immunohistochemical and molecular analysis (27–29). However, the role of HPV in the etiology of CIN remains unclear. Karcioglu and Issa (30) identified the DNA of HPV types 16 and 18 in 57% of CIN specimens, 55% of invasive squamous cell carcinoma of the conjunctiva, and in 32% of normal conjunctiva obtained during cataract surgery. Eng and colleagues (11) were unable to demonstrate the DNA of HPV 16 or 18 in any of 20 specimens of CIN.

Atypical, rapidly progressive CIN occurring in younger patients has been associated with human immunodeficiency virus (HIV) (31–33). CIN has been reported in younger organ transplant patients treated with long-term cyclosporine therapy (34). Xeroderma pigmentosum is an autosomal-recessive disorder characterized by inadequate repair of DNA damage caused by ultraviolet radiation. Affected patients are predisposed to epithelial cancers, including those of the conjunctiva and cornea (35).

The limbus is the transitional zone from columnar conjunctival epithelium to stratified squamous corneal epithelium. Within its crypts of Vogt are the progenitor cells of the corneal epithelium, the limbal stem cells. This area is analogous to the uterine cervix. Similar to cervical tissue, the corneal limbus is the site of origin for the vast majority of dysplastic and neoplastic changes of the ocular surface.

Clinical Presentation

The patient with CIN most commonly presents with ocular irritation or complaints of redness or a "growth on the eye." Vision is typically not affected. Lesions are readily accessible to slit-lamp biomicroscopy; however, differentia-

tion of benign from malignant surface tumors is difficult, even for the experienced observer. Examination may reveal a vascular limbal mass, usually located within the interpalpebral area. The affected area is thickened, and may appear gelatinous or velvety. Gelatinous thickening, with discrete superficial blood vessels, is most common (Fig. 41-4) (21).

CIN may present as diffuse chronic conjunctivitis with minimal thickening (36, 37). Other less common presentations include necrotizing scleritis with scleral perforation (38) or sclerokeratitis, described as focal corneal or scleral thinning and inflammation without a tumor mass (39). Sclerokeratitis may mimic interstitial keratitis or Mooren's ulceration. Biopsy should be performed in cases of atypical or chronic scleritis or conjunctivitis unresponsive to standard therapy.

Hyperkeratosis is a feature of CIN and may manifest as a white surface plaque, or leukoplakia (Fig. 41-5). Leukoplakia has no diagnostic significance, and is not helpful in distinguishing benign from malignant tumors. Neoplastic cells may invade corneal epithelium, usually as a continuation of limbal CIN. Isolated squamous cell carcinoma of the central cornea without limbal attachment has been reported (40). It is possible that neoplastic cells in these cases originated at the limbus and migrated centrally. Affected epithelium is translucently gray, with sharply demarcated borders (Fig. 41-6). Finger-like extensions, as well as isolated islands may be found on the leading edge. The epithelium within the lesion is thickened, and blood vessels may be present, especially near the limbus. Spontaneous regression of the corneal process has been reported (22).

Squamous cell carcinoma is a progression of dysplasia, with invasion through the basement membrane of the epithelium.

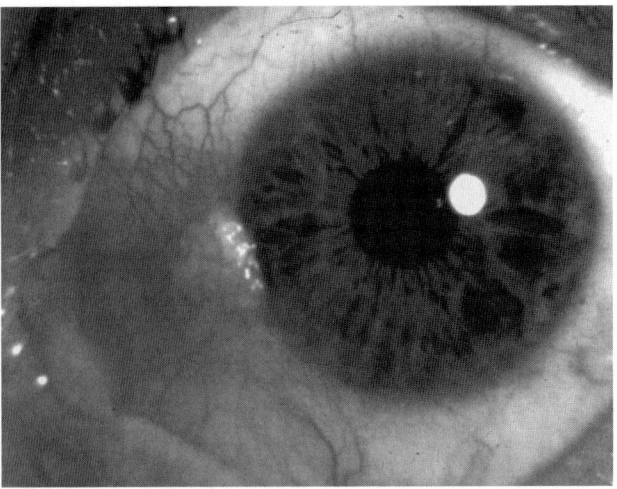

FIGURE 41-5. CIN. Hyperkeratosis (proliferation of surface keratin) gives this lesion a white appearance (leukoplakia). Keratin is not normally present in the conjunctiva. The presence of surface keratin has no diagnostic significance. (Courtesy of the Armed Forces Institute of Pathology).

Marked thickening of a limbal lesion, as well as fixation of the mass to underlying tissue, suggests squamous cell carcinoma (Fig. 41-7).

The study of representative cells from a lesion may yield helpful diagnostic information. In both exfoliative cytology and impression cytology, superficial cells are removed from a suspicious area, fixed and stained with a Papanicolaou technique, and studied by a cytopathologist. In exfoliative cytology cells are removed with a sterile platinum spatula, whereas in impression cytology cells are retained on cellulose acetate paper strips, which are pressed against the area in question. Cells are graded on degree of atypia, including size, shape, nuclear and nucleolar characteristics,

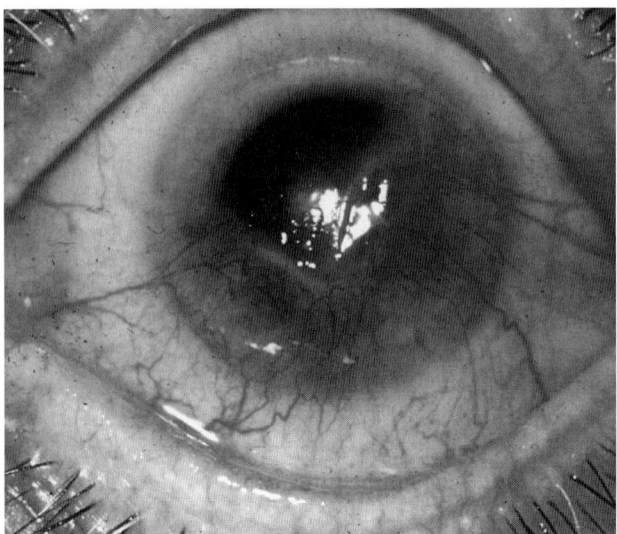

FIGURE 41-6. CIN. Extension of translucent dysplastic epithelium into the cornea. This degree of limbal involvement causes limbal stem cell deficiency. (Courtesy of the Armed Forces Institute of Pathology).

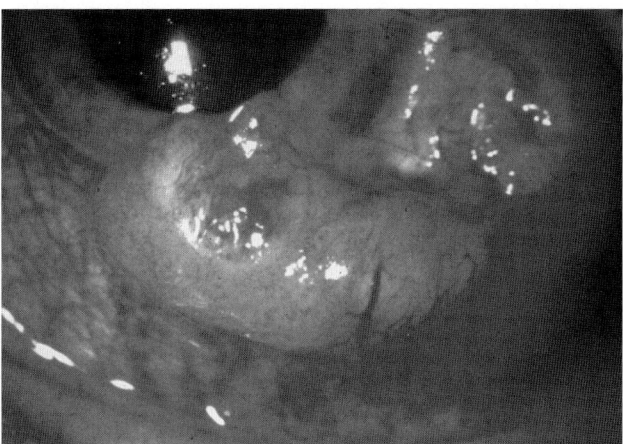

FIGURE 41-7. Squamous cell carcinoma. A markedly thickened conjunctival tumor originates at the limbus. (Courtesy of the Armed Forces Institute of Pathology).

and mitotic figures. Cytology has been reported to be positive in 77% of biopsy-proven cases (41).

Differential Diagnosis

Benign epithelial lesion–associated thickening and surface keratin are often clinically indistinguishable from CIN. Irritation caused by stromal inflammation or by pinguecula or pterygia may lead to *pseudoepitheliomatous hyperplasia*, with thickening of the epithelium and leukoplakia. This appearance suggests a neoplastic process. Biopsy will reveal the benign histologic appearance of acanthosis and hyperkeratosis without dysplasia. Simple excision is curative.

Actinic keratosis of the ocular surface is felt to be related to ultraviolet radiation. As such, these lesions occur in older, lightly complexioned people with extensive previous exposure to sunlight, the same population at higher risk for CIN. Thickening of the lesion with hyperkeratosis is usually present. Histopathologic examination may demonstrate a spectrum of change, from mild acanthosis with hyperkeratosis and inflammation, to marked acanthosis with cellular pleomorphism.

Benign conjunctival papillomas, chronic conjunctivitis, and inflammation of a pingueculum or pterygium may resemble CIN.

Pathology

Histologic examination is required for definitive diagnosis. If the lesion is small, excisional biopsy with removal of the entire mass is performed. Incisional biopsy of the most atypical area is performed for larger lesions. Routine staining with hematoxylin-eosin and periodic acid-Schiff is sufficient for the diagnosis of most CIN lesions. Biopsy allows determination of the depth of the lesion, as well as whether the margins are free of tumor. The transition from normal to abnormal epithelium is relatively abrupt (Fig. 41-8).

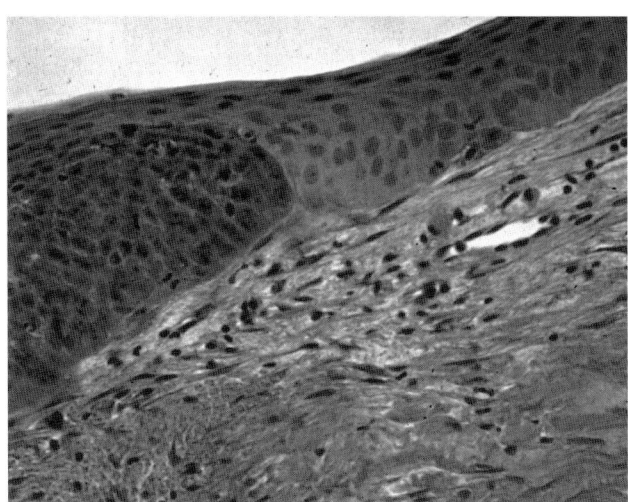

FIGURE 41-8. CIN. Full-thickness intraepithelial dysplasia is seen. Note the abrupt transition between dysplastic and normal epithelium. (Courtesy of the Armed Forces Institute of Pathology).

Specimens are graded on location and degree of atypia. Full-thickness dysplasia corresponds to carcinoma-in-situ. Extension of tumor cells into the subepithelial space (substantia propria, sclera, or cornea) constitutes squamous cell carcinoma. Advanced tumors may extend into ciliary body, iris, and trabecular meshwork.

Mucoepidermoid carcinoma is unusual in the conjunctiva. Clinically it is indistinguishable from CIN. Histopathologic examination demonstrates epidermoid cells and mucus-secreting cells. Special stains for mucin, such as Alcian blue or mucicarmine are helpful in the diagnosis. Because mucoepidermoid carcinoma of the conjunctiva tends to be more locally aggressive than CIN, this diagnosis should prompt heightened vigilance for invasion and recurrence (42).

Spindle cell carcinoma is another aggressive variant of conjunctival squamous cell carcinoma that may arise on the ocular surface. Clinical differentiation of this tumor from other forms of CIN is not possible. Pathologically, pleomorphic spindle cells are seen, sometimes arranged in fascicles. Morphologically, it may be difficult to distinguish spindle cell carcinoma from other spindle cell tumors, such as spindle cell melanoma, leiomyoma, rhabdomyosarcoma, or other sarcomas. Immunohistochemical analysis with cytokeratin stains will demonstrate the epithelial origin of spindle cell carcinoma. Transmission electron microscopy may be helpful in difficult cases (43,44).

Treatment

Surgical excision of the suspicious area is the standard approach to therapy, especially if the entire lesion can be removed in toto. Staining of the tumor with rose bengal will highlight abnormal epithelium. A wide surgical margin of 2 to 3 mm around the visible tumor is recommended.

Frozen section control can assess the lateral surgical margins, but is not helpful with the deep margins.

Cryotherapy with a nitrous oxide probe performed after surgical excision lowers the recurrence rate of CIN. Frauenfelder et al. (45) demonstrated the feasibility of this modality in external ocular lesions. After removal of the lesion with 2- to 3-mm margins, freezing of the remaining conjunctival margins and the sublesional base is accomplished with formation of an ice ball for 6 seconds, followed by a slow thaw. A double freeze-thaw technique is usually performed; however, three cycles are recommended if inadequate removal of tumor is suspected. Cryotherapy can destroy tumor cells by thermal disruption as well as resultant local ischemia. Peksayar et al. (46) reported recurrence in 1 of 19 (5%) eyes with primary CIN, including squamous carcinoma, treated with excision and cryotherapy. Adverse effects of cryotherapy include elevation or decrease in intraocular pressure, corneal scarring, iris atrophy, and destruction of retina.

Local application of beta-irradiation has been utilized as primary treatment of squamous epithelial tumors, as well as treatment of incompletely excised squamous epithelial tumors. In a study of 15 patients treated with radioactive strontium and yttrium, total surface doses ranging from 10,000 to 18,000 rads were dispensed in daily doses of 1,000 rads. In general, epithelial neoplasia resolved within in 1 to 2 months. Ten patients had squamous cell carcinoma, four had carcinoma-in-situ, and one patient had "epidermalization." One patient had recurrence after treatment, leading to enucleation (47). Jones and colleagues (48) employed strontium 90 with epithelial removal to treat recurrent CIN of the cornea after excision and cryotherapy (three cases) and multiple excisions (one case). No recurrence was seen with follow-up in all cases of at least 3 years. Undesirable effects of irradiation are dose related and include cataract, secondary glaucoma, local scarring, dry eye, and loss of cilia. The threshold cataractogenic dose of surface strontium 90 is estimated to be 5,000 rads (48).

Therapy with antimetabolite agents has proven beneficial in the adjunctive treatment of partially excised corneal epithelial neoplasia, as well as initial therapy in recurrent disease. Other possible uses include extensive disease with ill-defined borders, or situations in which excessive conjunctiva would be removed, causing a severe dry eye or limbal stem cell deficiency. The rationale is to use the highest possible dose against the smallest amount of tumor. Both mitomycin C and 5-fluorouracil have a selective effect on rapidly growing tumor cells. Because of dose-related local toxicity, cycles of topical chemotherapy with intervening rest periods are employed. Rest intervals may spare the limbal stem cells. Punctal plugs are useful to protect the nasolacrimal system during therapy and reduce systemic absorption. Alternatively, manual punctal occlusion may be performed after each dose of medication. The ability of topical therapy to eradicate nests of tumor cells located in the subepithelial space remains an area of concern, especially in possible squamous cell carcinoma with scleral invasion. Reports suggest that small islands of tumor cells underneath the basement membrane may respond to topical therapy (49,50). Long-term observation is necessary, as squamous cell carcinoma may recur years after excision.

Mitomycin C (MMC) is a chemotherapeutic antibiotic derived from *Streptomyces caespitosus*, which functions as an alkylating agent and inhibits DNA synthesis. Alkylating agents are radiomimetic, simulating radiation effects in their mechanism of action. As expected, rapidly dividing cells are the most sensitive (51). In addition to effects on epithelial cells, MMC has a pronounced effect on fibroblasts and stem cells. Therapeutic applications include 0.02% or 0.04% MMC four times daily for 14-day courses (52,53); 0.02% MMC three times daily for 14 days (54); and 0.04% MMC four times daily for 1 week cycles (55). A combination of excision, cryotherapy, and topical MMC has proven effective in recurrent CIN (56). Clinical and, in some cases, histologic tumor regression was noted in each series, with follow-up periods as long as 50 months. In a large study of 17 patients, 10 remained disease-free after one course of therapy; others responded to additional courses. In two patients, regrowth occurred with return of CCIN to original size (50). Adverse reactions to topical treatment range from mild hyperemia and tearing to photophobia, hyperemia, punctuate epithelial keratopathy, and blepharospasm. Severe pain occurs if used continuously more than 14 days; cessation of therapy leads to resolution of pain (50). More severe side effects, including scleral ulceration and perforation, have been described. Adverse effects of this magnitude were associated with bare sclera techniques and may be less likely if the epithelium is intact (17).

5-Fluorouracil (5-FU) inhibits DNA formation by blocking thymidylate synthetase, an essential enzyme. As such, it functions as a cytostatic drug with antimetabolite properties. Rapidly growing cells accumulate lethal amounts of 5-FU. 5-FU has been reported useful as an adjunct in recurrent or incompletely excised squamous cell carcinoma. Reported series have used 1% 5-FU in artificial tear base three to four times daily for 2- to 3-week cycles, until sloughing of the epithelium occurs. A rest period then follows to allow regeneration of epithelium, followed by additional courses of therapy if neoplastic disease remains. Clinical improvement or resolution of intraepithelial neoplasia has been reported in all cases. In one series, three patients treated with 5-FU had recurrences, of which two responded to additional cycles, and one required treatment with MMC (57). In another series, of six patients treated, one required reexcision and one required orbital exenteration for squamous cell carcinoma (58). Follow-up has been as long as 30 months (58). Toxic keratoconjunctivitis was seen in all cases (59). Both MMC and 5-FU inhibit epithelial wound healing in rabbit eyes, with MMC exerting a much more potent effect (60).

Recombinant interferon-alfa-2b has been used successfully in the treatment of corneal and conjunctival intraepithelial neoplasia, with an initial injection of 3 million international units (IU), followed by topical interferon-alfa-2b drops (1 million IU/mL) four times daily. If clinical response was noted by 1 week, topical therapy was continued until resolution of the CIN. If minimal response was seen at 1 week, subconjunctival and perilesional injections were performed three times weekly until clinical resolution. Vann and Karp (61) reported complete resolution in six patients with biopsy-proven CIN treated in this manner, with average follow-up of over 7 months. No complications were noted with topical therapy, although fever and myalgia may occur with subconjunctival injection. Intralesional interferon-alfa-2b has also proven successful in the treatment of squamous cell carcinoma and basal cell carcinoma of the skin. The mechanism of action is unknown.

Regression of biopsy-proven conjunctival CIN has been reported after 6 weeks of topical therapy with cidofovir (2.5 mg/mL), one drop every 2 hours initially, with a weekly taper in frequency over the next 6 weeks. A residual focus of tumor required excision, followed by cryotherapy (62).

If spread to the regional lymph nodes occurs, radical neck dissection may help prevent distant metastases.

Prognosis

Conjunctival CIN, including squamous cell carcinoma, is considered to be a low-grade malignancy. Recurrence is influenced by the integrity of surgical margins, reinforcing the need for wide margins and histopathologic examination. The degree of histologic atypia and presence of subepithelial neoplastic cells (squamous cell carcinoma) also corresponds to the recurrence rate. Erie and associates (63) found a recurrence rate for intraepithelial neoplasia of 24% versus a rate of 41% for squamous cell carcinoma. Lee and Hirst (21) found a recurrence rate for intraepithelial neoplasia of 17% versus a rate of 30% for squamous cell carcinoma. In an analysis of 60 cases, Tune and associates (64) reported recurrence rates of 4.5% and 5.3%, respectively, for intraepithelial neoplasia and squamous cell carcinoma, with a mean follow-up of 56 months. The differences in reported recurrence rates may reflect differences in patient population, treatment, or classification. The majority of neoplasia recur within 2 years, although recurrences have occurred as late as 5 years after excision (21).

Intraocular invasion has been reported in 3% to 11% of patients with conjunctival squamous cell carcinoma (64,65). The mucoepidermoid variant of conjunctival squamous cell carcinoma is aggressive and more likely to invade adjacent tissues. Rao and Font (42) reported intraocular involvement in two of three patients (67%) with limbal mucoepidermoid squamous cell carcinoma, and orbital invasion in two of two (100%) patients with extralimbal disease. Extension of squamous cell carcinoma most commonly affects the sclera, anterior chamber, trabecular meshwork, ciliary body, and choroid. Signs of globe invasion include iridocyclitis, ciliary body elevation, and secondary glaucoma (65). Orbital invasion has been noted in 11% to 15% of invasive squamous cell carcinoma of the conjunctiva (23,64). Exenteration is recommended in cases involving the orbit. Conjunctival squamous cell carcinoma metastasizes to the preauricular and cervical lymph nodes, with a reported incidence of 0 to 4% (66). Metastases to the parotid gland, lungs and bone have occurred.

SEBACEOUS CARCINOMA

Etiology and Incidence

Sebaceous carcinomas may arise from the adnexal epithelium of sebaceous glands throughout the body. Sebaceous glands, like hair and apocrine glands, arise from the embryonal stratum germinativum (basal cell layer). The ocular adnexa accounts for 25% of sebaceous carcinoma and is the most common locale for these tumors (67). Sebaceous carcinomas may originate in the meibomian glands of the tarsus, the glands of Zeiss at the lid margin, and sebaceous glands of the caruncle or surrounding skin and eyebrow (68). The most common adnexal site is within the meibomian glands of the upper and lower eyelids. Meibomian glands are larger than sebaceous glands elsewhere and are not associated with hair follicles (69). Boniuk and Zimmerman (70) originally reported a series of 88 cases from the Registry of Ophthalmic Pathology at the Armed Forces Institute of Pathology. This series was later extended to 104 cases by Rao et al. (68). In that review the authors found that 51% of adnexal sebaceous carcinoma arose from meibomian glands, 10% from the glands of Zeiss, and 7% from the caruncle. Eyebrow involvement has been reported in 2% of cases in (71). Simultaneous occurrence in both eyelids has been reported in 6% to 8% (69–71). Other sites of sebaceous carcinoma in decreasing frequency include external genitalia, parotid and submandibular glands, external auditory canal, and the trunk and upper extremity (67).

The incidence of sebaceous carcinoma among all eyelid tumors is 0.2% to 0.7% and 1% to 5.5% of malignant eyelid tumors (69). Rao and associates (68) found sebaceous carcinoma second only to basal cell carcinoma in frequency of eyelid malignancies. Other reviews rank it fourth in frequency, behind basal cell carcinoma, squamous carcinoma, and malignant melanoma (67). Sebaceous carcinoma of the ocular adnexa is more common in women than in men (57% and 77% in large studies). Older patients are more commonly afflicted, with diagnosis usually between the fifth and ninth decade of life, although cases in children have been reported (69,72). Two cases of sebaceous carcinoma in younger patients with human immunodeficiency virus have been reported (73).

Sebaceous carcinoma may occur after radiation treatment for other tumors (70,72). Kivela and associates (72) describe sebaceous carcinoma developing within the radiation field of 11 children treated for hereditary retinoblastoma, with a median age of 14 years. Two patients with a history of hereditary retinoblastoma without radiation therapy also developed sebaceous carcinoma, although much later in life, at ages 32 and 54 years. Rumelt et al. (74) reported four-eyelid sebaceous carcinoma in a 74-year-old man with a prior history of whole face radiation for eczema.

Sebaceous adenomas and sebaceous carcinomas are associated with malignant visceral disease in the Muir-Torre syndrome. Most sebaceous tumors in this syndrome involve the head and neck, with the ocular adnexa affected less frequently. Associated malignancies include the colon and rectum (47%) genitourinary tract (21%) and breast (12%) (75). A family history of visceral cancer is present in 70% of patients.

Clinical Presentation

Sebaceous carcinoma may present in a variety of ways, mimicking common conditions and delaying diagnosis. The usual presentation is that of a painless, slowly progressive mass arising within the eyelid. The upper lid is involved two to three times more frequently than the lower, perhaps because of the greater number of meibomian glands in the upper eyelid. Ulceration of the eyelid skin typically occurs late, unlike basal cell or squamous cell carcinomas, although ulceration may occur earlier in cases originating near the lid margin. Sebaceous carcinoma may cause atrophy and loss of cilia. A yellow tint is present in some cases.

The eyelid tumor may remain relatively small, whereas intraepithelial spread of tumor cells leads to inflammation of the ocular surface. Thus, sebaceous carcinoma may mimic benign conditions such as conjunctivitis, blepharoconjunctivitis, blepharitis, superior limbic keratoconjunctivitis, and keratitis (Fig. 41-9) (76–80). Foster and Allansmith (80) described symblepharon formation and corneal neovascularization in a case of sebaceous carcinoma masquerading as chronic blepharoconjunctivitis. Treatment of "chronic conjunctivitis" for as long as 10 years before the correct diagnosis of sebaceous carcinoma has been reported (78). Sebaceous carcinoma presenting as a papillary growth of the palpebral conjunctiva has been described (81).

Sebaceous carcinoma of the eyelid may be mistaken for a chalazion. Chalazia tend to occur rapidly, whereas sebaceous carcinoma is slowly progressive. Helpful differentiating signs in carcinoma include adhesion of the skin to a firm underlying mass, erythema, trichiasis, destruction of the cilia, and conjunctival cicatrization. Growth or spread of a localized carcinoma may conceivably be facilitated by inappropriate incision and curettage. A longstanding

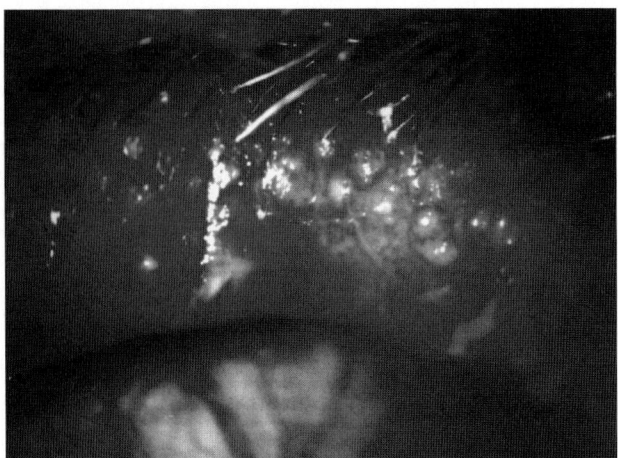

FIGURE 41-9. Sebaceous carcinoma. The eyelid is thickened and inflamed. Sebaceous carcinoma is often mistaken for recurrent chalazion or chronic blepharitis.

recommendation has been to perform a full-thickness eyelid biopsy for all recurrent eyelid masses originally felt to be a chalazion. Clear communication by the surgeon of any suspicion or concern for sebaceous carcinoma to the ophthalmic pathologist is important.

Differential Diagnosis

As described above, the main considerations include chronic conjunctivitis, chronic keratitis and recurrent chalazion.

Pathology

Sebaceous carcinoma requires biopsy for definitive diagnosis. Any suspicion of sebaceous carcinoma by the surgeon should be communicated to the ophthalmic pathologist, as special preparation of the specimen is required. Routine

processing of formalin-fixed tissue will remove intracellular lipid; fresh frozen sections, however, will preserve this lipid, which can then be stained with oil red-O or other fat stains to facilitate diagnosis.

Difficulties may arise in pathologic diagnosis of sebaceous carcinoma, as well as in clinical diagnosis. It is most frequently misdiagnosed as basal cell carcinoma or squamous cell carcinoma. Unlike these epithelial tumors, sebaceous carcinoma will often have an identifiable site of origin deeper within the eyelid. Well-differentiated tumors are composed of pleomorphic cells with foamy or vacuolated cytoplasm (Fig. 41-10). Fresh frozen sections stained with oil red-O or other fat stains will demonstrate lipid within the cytoplasm. Less differentiated neoplasms contain less lipid and a more basophilic cytoplasm, as well as mitotic figures. These cells may be mistaken for basal cell carcinoma. Because meibomian gland ducts normally show squamous differentiation as they approach the surface, sebaceous carcinomas may have squamous differentiation and contain keratin. Such tumors may simulate squamous cell carcinoma (68).

Intraepithelial carcinomatous change may occur in either eyelid skin or conjunctiva, or in both. Individual cells or small clusters may be found within epithelium (Fig. 41-11). This pattern is called pagetoid spread, as it resembles intraepithelial spread in Paget disease of the breast. Intraepithelial involvement may also resemble severe dysplasia or squamous carcinoma-in-situ, replacing the entire epithelium with malignant sebaceous cells. Diagnosis of carcinoma-in-situ of the palpebral conjunctiva without a contiguous limbal lesion should alert the clinician to the possibility of underlying sebaceous carcinoma (82). Intraepithelial involvement was noted in 44% of 104 specimens (68) and in 50% of 40 specimens (71). Severe chronic inflammation is usually present, correlating with the clinical inflammation seen in cases mimicking chronic blepharitis,

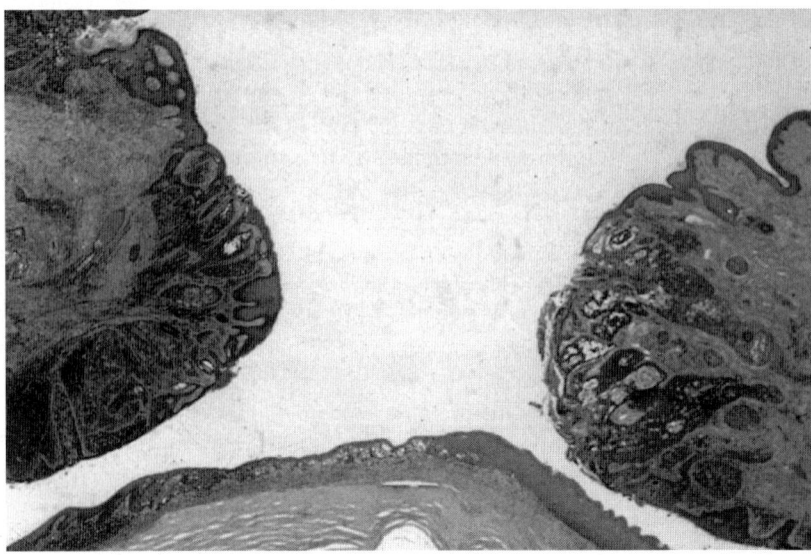

FIGURE 41-10. Sebaceous carcinoma. Pleomorphic cells with foamy cytoplasm representing lipid. (Courtesy of Ahmed A. Hidayat, M.D.)

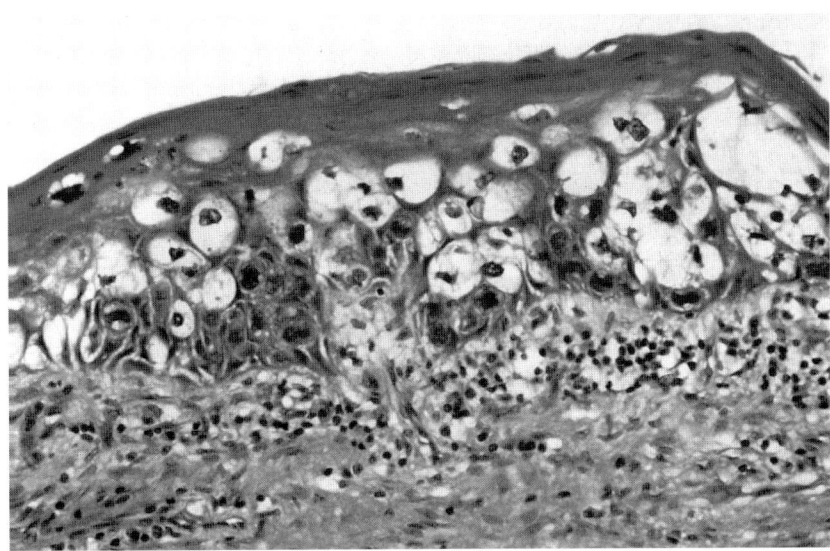

FIGURE 41-11. Sebaceous carcinoma. Neoplastic cells are found within conjunctival epithelium. Infiltration of the conjunctival or corneal epithelium is termed pagetoid spread. (Courtesy of Ahmed A. Hidayat, M.D.)

conjunctivitis, or keratitis. The various clinical and pathologic presentations of intraepithelial sebaceous carcinoma illustrate the necessity of full-thickness eyelid biopsy to find the underlying tumor. Excision of skin or conjunctiva only may lead to erroneous diagnosis. Cases of sebaceous pagetoid spread without underlying eyelid tumor have been reported. One possible reason for this phenomenon is regression of the original tarsal tumor. Residual nests of sebaceous carcinoma in areas of tarsus with fibrosis and inflammation seen in some cases lend support to this explanation (83).

EVALUATION OF A PATIENT WITH SEBACEOUS CARCINOMA

If sebaceous carcinoma is confirmed by biopsy, a complete history, family history, physical examination, and complete eye examination is indicated. The family history should inquire about benign or malignant skin lesions, as well as internal malignancies that characterize Muir-Torre syndrome. Complete evaluation of the skin for other cutaneous tumors as well as palpation of the lymph nodes should be performed. Baseline studies include chest x-ray, liver function tests, and complete blood count. If the clinician suspects the possibility of Muir-Torre syndrome, further testing includes rectal examination, colonoscopy, and barium enema. Mammography may be indicated (67,84,85).

Treatment

Wide surgical excision with eyelid reconstruction is the primary treatment for sebaceous carcinoma of the eyelid. The goal is to obtain 5- to 6-mm surgical margins clear of tumor by fresh frozen tissue control (86,87). The surgical excision must extend past any conjunctival involvement,

including follicular changes (88). If the conjunctiva is involved, map biopsies to determine the presence and extent of pagetoid spread is useful. As originally described by Putterman (89), local anesthesia of the eyelids as well as palpebral and bulbar conjunctiva is achieved with 2% lidocaine with epinephrine. Biopsies of conjunctiva and underlying tarsus are obtained from the temporal, central, and nasal areas of the upper and lower eyelids, as well as temporal, central, and nasal bulbar conjunctiva. Full-thickness excision of the eyelid in any involved area is then performed under frozen section control, with 5-mm normal margins.

Adjunctive cryotherapy to areas of affected conjunctiva has been described in six patients. In each case wide resection of the eyelid was followed by cryotherapy to affected conjunctiva as determined by mapping. The patients remained free of recurrence with follow-up ranging from 12 to 50 months (90). A concern of any technique using representative biopsies is failure to diagnose clinically inapparent areas of involvement.

Mohs micrographic surgery (MMS) of eyelid sebaceous carcinoma has been described, with primary repair of the ensuing eyelid defect by an oculoplastic surgeon. Spencer and colleagues (91) reported a recurrence rate of 11% in 18 patients with an average follow-up of 37 months. Snow et al. (92) reported a recurrence rate of 12% with 1 to 4 years of follow-up in nine patients treated by MMS.

Radiation therapy is considered palliative and not curative in sebaceous carcinoma. Pardo and colleagues (93) reported local control at the primary site in four patients treated with 4500 to 6300 rads over 4 to 7 weeks. Nunery and Welsh (94) reported recurrence within 2 years in six patients treated with external beam radiation of 3,300 to 11,900 rads as initial therapy of sebaceous carcinoma. Rao and associates (68) report a 4-year mortality of 78% for patients undergoing radiation treatment, versus 7% for those treated with wide surgical excision.

Shields and associates (95) reported resolution of conjunctival intraepithelial sebaceous carcinoma in three patients treated with topical 0.04% mitomycin C four times daily for 1-week cycles, interspersed with rest cycles of 1 week. Pretreatment map biopsies revealed intraepithelial involvement ranging from 25% to 90% of the conjunctival surface, including the cornea in one case. No tumor deeper in the conjunctiva or eyelid was present.

If diffuse spread into both eyelids is found, or extension into the orbit, orbital exenteration is recommended. A limited orbital exenteration with removal of eyelid, conjunctival sac, globe, and tenonectomy has been described for sebaceous carcinoma with pagetoid spread to conjunctiva and cornea (79). Biopsy should be performed if the ipsilateral parotid or cervical lymph nodes are enlarged, because inflammation alone may cause this change. If the lymph nodes contain tumor cells, radical neck dissection, superficial parotidectomy, and postoperative radiation have been recommended (69). Chemotherapy has also been used for recurrent sebaceous carcinoma.

Prognosis

Boniuk and Zimmerman (70) reported a 5-year mortality rate of 30% for death attributable to sebaceous carcinoma in 30 patients. A number of factors, including delay in diagnosis, tumor location and size, and pathologic features, have been associated with a poorer prognosis. Rao and associates (68) reported a mortality rate of 38% with delays in diagnosis of greater than 6 months, versus a mortality rate of 14% if the tumor was diagnosed before 6 months. In their series of 104 patients, mortality was 83% if both upper and lower eyelids were involved; 28% for the upper eyelid only; 14% for the caruncle; and 0% for the lower eyelid only. Increase in the largest dimension of the tumor correlated with increasing mortality; tumors less than 6 mm had a mortality rate of 0%, 6 to 10 mm had a mortality rate of 18%, 11 to 20 mm had a mortality of 50%, and tumors greater than 20 mm had a mortality of 60%. Pathologic features associated with a poor prognosis included multicentric origin, poor degree of differentiation, highly infiltrative pattern, intraepithelial carcinoma, invasion of vascular or lymphatic channels, and extension into the orbit (68). Metastases may occur in the ipsilateral parotid and cervical lymph nodes, as well as in the lungs, brain, liver, and bone (70).

SUMMARY

A variety of disorders may arise within the epithelium of the ocular surface. Differentiation of benign versus malignant epithelial proliferations is often not possible by clinical examination alone. Cytopathologic or histopathologic examination is recommended for definitive diagnosis. Numerous modalities are available for the treatment of epithelial neoplasia, including wide excision with frozen section control, cryotherapy, local irradiation, topical antimetabolites, and topical and intralesional interferon. Sebaceous carcinoma may mimic many ocular disorders, and should always be considered in the differential diagnosis of chronic blepharoconjunctivitis or recurrent chalazion. Long-term follow-up is necessary to detect recurrence of malignancies of the ocular surface.

REFERENCES

1. Witkop CJ, Shankle DH, Graham JB, et al. Hereditary benign intraepithelial dyskeratosis: oral manifestations and hereditary transmission. *Arch Pathol Lab Med* 1960;70:696–711.
2. McLean IW, Riddle PL, Scruggs JH, et al. Hereditary benign intraepithelial dyskeratosis. *Ophthalmology* 1981;88:164–168.
3. Reed JW, Cashwell LF, Klintworth GK. Corneal manifestations of hereditary benign intraepithelial dyskeratosis. *Arch Ophthalmol* 1979;97:297–300.
4. Haisley-Royster CA, Allingham RR, Klintworth GK, et al. Hereditary benign intraepithelial dyskeratosis: report of two cases with prominent oral lesions. *J Am Acad Dermatol* 2001;45:634–636.
5. Shields LC, Shields JA, Eagle RC. Hereditary benign intraepithelial dyskeratosis. *Arch Ophthalmol* 1987;105:422–423.
6. Sjo NC, Heegaard S, Prause JU, et al. Human papillomavirus in conjunctival papilloma. *Br J Ophthalmol* 2001;85:785–787.
7. Elsas FJ, Green WR. Epibulbar tumors in childhood. *Am J Ophthalmol* 1975;79:1001–1007.
8. Chaudhuri Z, Das JC, Arora R, et al. Limbal papilloma with massive corneal extension. *Ophthalmic Surg Lasers* 2000;31:73–75.
9. Streeten BW, Carrillo R, Jamison R, et al. Inverted papilloma of the conjunctiva. *Am J Ophthalmol* 1979;88:1062–1066.
10. Buggage RR, Smith JA, Shen D. Conjunctival papillomas caused by human papillomavirus type 33. *Arch Ophthalmol* 2002;120:202–203.
11. Eng HL, Lin TM, Chen SY, et al. Failure to detect human papillomavirus DNA in malignant neoplasms of conjunctiva by polymerase chain reaction. *Am J Clin Pathol* 2002;117:429–436.
12. Harkey ME, Metz HS. Cryotherapy of conjunctival papillomata. *Am J Ophthalmol* 1968;66:872–874.
13. Omohundro JM, Elliott JH. Cryotherapy of conjunctival papilloma. *Arch Ophthalmol* 1970;84:609–610.
14. Bosniak SL, Novick NL, Sachs ME. Treatment of recurrent squamous papillomata of the conjunctiva by carbon dioxide laser vaporization. *Ophthalmology* 1986;93:1078–1082.
15. Hawkins AS, Yu J, Hamming NA, et al. Treatment of recurrent conjunctival papillomatosis with mitomycin-C. *Am J Ophthalmol* 1999;128:638–640.
16. Yuen HKL, Yeung EFY, Chan NR, et al. The use of postoperative topical mitomycin C in the treatment of recurrent conjunctival papilloma. *Cornea* 2002;21:838–839.
17. Rubinfeld RS, Pfister RR, Stein RM, et al. Serious complications of topical mitomycin-C after pterygium surgery. *Ophthalmology* 1992;99:1647–1654.
18. Lass JH, Foster CS, Grove AS, et al. Interferon-alpha therapy of recurrent conjunctival papillomas. *Am J Ophthalmol* 1987;103:294–301.
19. Schechter BA, Rand WJ, Velazquez GE. Treatment of conjunctival papillomata with topical interferon alfa-2b. *Am J Ophthalmol* 2002;34:268–270.

20. Shields CL, Lally MR, Singh AD, et al. Oral cimetidine (Tagamet) for recalcitrant, diffuse conjunctival papillomatosis. *Am J Ophthalmol* 1999;128:362–364.
21. Lee GA, Hirst L. Ocular surface squamous neoplasia. *Surv Ophthalmol* 1995;39:429–450.
22. Waring GO III, Roth AM, Ekins MB. Clinical and pathologic description of 17 cases of corneal intraepithelial neoplasia. *Am J Ophthalmol* 1984;97:547–559.
23. McKelvie PA, Daniell M, McNab A, et al. Squamous cell carcinoma of the conjunctiva: a series of 26 cases. *Br J Ophthalmol* 2002;86:168–173.
24. Newton R. A review of the aetiology of squamous cell carcinoma of the conjunctiva. *Br J Ophthalmol* 1996;74:1511–1513.
25. Farah S, Baum TD, Conlon MR, et al. Tumors of the Cornea and Conjunctiva. In: Albert DM, Jakobiec FA, eds. *Principles and practice of ophthalmology,* 2nd ed, vol 2. Philadelphia: WB Saunders, 2000:1002–1019.
26. Yang J, Foster CS. Squamous cell carcinoma of the conjunctiva. *Int Ophthalmol Clin* 1997;37:73–85.
27. Nakamura Y, Mashima Y, Kameyama K, et al. Detection of human papillomavirus infection in squamous tumours of the conjunctiva and lacrimal sac by immunohistochemistry, in situ hybridization and polymerase chain reaction. *Br J Ophthalmol* 1997;81:308–313.
28. McDonnell J, McDonnell P, Mounts P, et al. Demonstration of papillomavirus capsid antigen in human conjunctival neoplasia. *Arch Ophthalmol* 1986;104:1801–1805.
29. Scott IU, Karp CL, Nuovo GJ. Human papillomavirus 16 and 18 expression in conjunctival intraepithelial neoplasia. *Ophthalmology* 2002;109:542–547.
30. Karcioglu ZA, Issa TM. Human papilloma virus in neoplastic and non-neoplastic conditions of the external eye. *Br J Ophthalmol* 1997;81:595–598.
31. Winward KE, Curtin VT. Conjunctival squamous cell carcinoma in a patient with human immunodeficiency virus infection. *Am J Ophthalmol* 1989;107:554–555.
32. Margo CE, Mack W, Guffey JM. Squamous cell carcinoma of the conjunctiva and human immunodeficiency virus infection. *Arch Ophthalmol* 1996;114:349.
33. Muccioli C, Belfort R Jr, Burnier M, Rao N. Squamous cell carcinoma of the conjunctiva in a patient with the acquired immunodeficiency syndrome. *Am J Ophthalmol* 1996;121:94–96.
34. Macarez R, Bossis, Robinet A, et al. Conjunctival epithelial neoplasia in organ transplant patients receiving cyclosporine therapy. *Cornea* 1999;18:495–497.
35. Spencer WH, Zimmerman LE. Conjunctiva. In: Spencer WH, ed. *Ophthalmic pathology: an atlas and textbook,* 3rd ed, vol 1. Philadelphia: WB Saunders, 1985:109–228.
36. Irvine AR. Diffuse epibulbar squamous cell epithelioma. *Am J Ophthalmol* 1967;64:550–554.
37. Akpek EK, Polcharoen W, Chan R, et al. Ocular surface neoplasia masquerading as chronic blepharoconjunctivitis. *Cornea* 1999;18:282–288.
38. Lindenmuth KA, Sugar A, Kincaid MC, et al. Invasive squamous cell carcinoma of the conjunctiva presenting as necrotizing scleritis with scleral perforation and uveal prolapse. *Surv Ophthalmol* 1988;33:50–54.
39. Mahmood MA, Al-Rajhi A, Riley F, et al. Sclerokeratitis: An unusual presentation of squamous cell carcinoma of the conjunctiva. *Ophthalmology* 2001;108:553–558.
40. Cameron JA, Hidayat AA. Squamous cell carcinoma of the cornea. *Am J Ophthalmol* 1991;111:571–574.
41. Nolan GR, Hirst LW, Bancroft BJ. The cytomorphology of ocular surface neoplasia by using impression cytology. *Cancer Cytopathol* 2001;93:60–67.
42. Rao NA, Font RL. Mucoepidermoid carcinoma of the conjunctiva: a clinicopathologic study of five cases. *Cancer* 1976;38:1699–1709.
43. Cohen BH, Green WR, Iliff NT, et al. Spindle cell carcinoma of the conjunctiva. *Arch Ophthalmol* 1980;98:1809.
44. Wise AC. A limbal spindle cell carcinoma. *Surv Ophthalmol* 1967;12:244.
45. Frauenfelder FT, Wallace TR, Farris HE, et al. The role of cryosurgery in external ocular and periocular disease. *Trans Am Acad Ophthalmol Otol* 1977;83:713–724.
46. Peksayar G, Soyturk MK, Demiryunt M. Long term results of cryotherapy on malignant epithelial tumors of the conjunctiva. *Am J Ophthalmol* 1989;107:337–349.
47. Lommatzsch P. Beta-ray treatment of malignant epithelial tumors of the conjunctiva. *Am J Ophthalmol* 1976;81:198–206.
48. Jones DB, Wilhelmus KR, Font RL. Beta radiation of recurrent corneal intraepithelial neoplasia. *Trans Am Ophthalmol Soc* 1991;89:285–301.
49. Heigle TJ, Stulting RD, Palay DA. Treatment of recurrent conjunctival epithelial neoplasia with topical mitomycin C. *Am J Ophthalmol* 1997;124:397–399.
50. Frucht-Pery J, Sugar J, Baum J, et al. Mitomycin C treatment for conjunctival-corneal intraepithelial neoplasia: a multicenter experience. *Ophthalmology* 1997;104:2085–2093.
51. Wilson MW, Hungerford JL, George SM, et al. Topical mitomycin C for the treatment of conjunctival and corneal epithelial dysplasia and neoplasia. *Am J Ophthalmol* 1997;124:303–311.
52. Frucht-Pery J, Rozenman Y. Mitomycin C therapy for corneal intraepithelial neoplasia. *Am J Ophthalmol* 1994;117:164–168.
53. Frucht-Pery J, Rozenman Y, Pe'er J. Topical mitomycin-C for partially excised conjunctival squamous cell carcinoma. *Ophthalmology* 2002:109:548–552.
54. Akpek EK, Ertoy D, Kalayci D, et al. Postoperative topical mitomycin-C in conjunctival cell neoplasia. *Cornea* 1999;18:59–62.
55. Shields CL, Naseripour M, Shields JA. Topical mitomycin-C for extensive, recurrent conjunctival-corneal squamous cell carcinoma. *Am J Ophthalmol* 2002;133:601–606.
56. Khokhar S, Soni A, SinghSethi H, et al. Combined surgery, cryotherapy and mitomycin-C for recurrent ocular surface squamous neoplasia. *Cornea* 2002;21:189–191.
57. Yeatts RP, Engelbrecht NE, Curry CD, et al. 5-Fluorouracil for the treatment of intraepithelial neoplasia of the conjunctiva and cornea. *Ophthalmology* 2000;107:2190–2195.
58. Yeatts RP, Ford JG, Stanton CA, et al. Topical 5-Fluorouracil in treating epithelial neoplasia of the conjunctiva and cornea. *Ophthalmology* 1995;102:1338–1344.
59. Midena E, Angeli CD, Valenti M, et al. Treatment of conjunctival squamous cell carcinoma with topical 5-fluorouracil. *Br J Ophthalmol* 2000;84:268–272.
60. Ando H, Ido T, Kawai Y, et al. Inhibition of corneal epithelial wound healing. *Ophthalmology* 1992;99:1809–1814.
61. Vann RR, Karp CL. Perilesional and topical interferon alfa-2b for conjunctival and corneal neoplasia. *Ophthalmology* 1999;106:91–97.
62. Sherman MD, Feldman KA, Farahmand SM, et al. Treatment of conjunctival squamous cell carcinoma with topical Cidofovir. *Am J Ophthalmol* 2002;134:432–433.
63. Erie JC, Campbell RJ, Liesegang J. Conjunctival and corneal intraepithelial and invasive neoplasia. *Ophthalmology* 1986;93:176–183.
64. Tune M, Char DH, Crawford B, et al. Intraepithelial and invasive squamous cell carcinoma of the conjunctiva: Analysis of 60 cases. *Br J Ophthalmol* 1999;83:98–103.
65. Shields JA, Shields CL, Gunduz K, et al. Intraocular invasion of conjunctival squamous cell carcinoma in five patients. *Ophthalmic Plast Reconstr Surg* 1999;15:153–160.

66. Bhattacharyya N, Wenokur RK, Rubin PA. Metastasis of squamous cell carcinoma of the conjunctiva: Case report and review of the literature. *Am J Ophthalmol* 1997;18:217–219.

67. Nelson BR, Hamlet KR, Gillard M, et al. Sebaceous carcinoma. *J Am Acad Dermatol* 1995;33:1–15.

68. Rao, NA, Hidayat AA, McLean IW, et al. Sebaceous carcinoma of the ocular adnexa: a clinicopathologic study of 104 cases, with five-year follow-up data. *Hum Pathol* 1982;13:113–122.

69. Kass LG, Hornblass A. Sebaceous carcinoma of the ocular adnexa. *Surv Ophthalmol* 1989;33:477–490.

70. Boniuk M, Zimmerman LE. Sebaceous carcinoma of the eyelid, eyebrow, caruncle and orbit. *Trans Am Acad Ophthalmol Otolaryngol* 1968;72:619–641.

71. Doxanas MT, Green WR. Sebaceous gland carcinoma: Review of 40 cases. *Arch Ophthalmol* 1984;102:245–249.

72. Kivela T, Asko-Seljavaara S, Pihkala U, et al. Sebaceous carcinoma of the eyelid associated with retinoblastoma. *Ophthalmology* 2001;108;1124–1128.

73. Yen MT, Tse DT. Sebaceous cell carcinoma of the eyelid and human immunodeficiency virus. *Ophthalmic Plast Reconstr Surg* 2000;16:206–210.

74. Rumelt S, Rubin PAD, Jakobiec FA. Four-eyelid sebaceous cell carcinoma following irradiation. *Arch Ophthalmol* 1998;116:1670–1672.

75. Cohen PR, Kohn SR, Kurzrock R. Association of sebaceous gland tumors and internal malignancy: the Muir-Torre syndrome. *Am J Med* 1991;90:606–613.

76. Gloor P, Ansari I, Sinard J. Sebaceous carcinoma presenting as a unilateral papillary conjunctivitis. *Am J Ophthalmol* 1999;127:458–459.

77. Honavar SG, Shields CL, Maus M, et al. Primary intraepithelial sebaceous gland carcinoma of the palpebral conjunctiva. *Arch Ophthalmol* 2001;119:764–767.

78. Margo CE, Lessner A, Stern GA. Intraepithelial sebaceous carcinoma of the conjunctiva and skin of the eyelid. *Ophthalmology* 1992;99;227–231.

79. Wolter JR, Bromley WC. Intraepithelial sebaceous epithelioma of lids, conjunctiva and cornea treated with minimal orbital exenteration. *Ophthalmic Surg* 1991;22;341–344.

80. Foster CS, Allansmith MR. Chronic unilateral blepharoconjunctivitis caused by sebaceous carcinoma. *Am J Ophthalmol* 1978;86:218–220.

81. Miyagawa M, Hayasaka S, Hagaoka S. Sebaceous gland carcinoma of the eyelid presenting as a conjunctival papilloma. *Ophthalmologica* 1994;208:46–48.

82. Leibsohn J, Bullock J, Waller R. Full thickness eyelid biopsy for presumed carcinoma-in-situ of the palpebral conjunctiva. *Ophthalmic Surg* 1982;13:840–842.

83. Margo CE, Grossniklaus HE. Intraepithelial sebaceous neoplasia without underlying invasive carcinoma. *Surv Ophthalmol* 1995;39:293–301.

84. Stockl FA, Dolmetsch AM, Codere F, et al. Sebaceous carcinoma of the eyelid in an immunocompromised patient with Muir-Torre syndrome. *Can J Ophthalmol* 1995;30:324–326.

85. Jakobiec FA, Zimmerman LE, La Piana F, et al. Unusual eyelid tumors with sebaceous differentiation in the Muir-Torre syndrome. *Ophthalmology* 1988;95:1543–1548.

86. Epstein GA, Putterman AM. Sebaceous adenocarcinoma of the eyelid. *Ophthalmic Surg* 1983;14:935–940.

87. Piest KL. Malignant lesions of the eyelids. *J Dermatol Surg Oncol* 1992;18:1056–1059.

88. Tenzel RR, Stewart WB, Boynton JR, et al. Sebaceous adenocarcinoma of the eyelid: definition of surgical margins. *Arch Ophthalmol* 1977;95:2203–2204.

89. Putterman AM. Conjunctival map biopsy to determine pagetoid spread. *Am J Ophthalmol* 1986;102:87–90.

90. Lisman RD, Jakobiec FA, Small P. Sebaceous carcinoma of the eyelids: The role of adjunctive cryotherapy in the management of conjunctival pagetoid spread. *Ophthalmology* 1989;96:1021–1026.

91. Spencer JM, Nossa R, Tse DT, et al. Sebaceous carcinoma of the eyelid treated with Moh's micrographic surgery. *J Am Acad Dermatol* 2001;44:1004–1009.

92. Snow SN, Larson PO, Lucarelli MJ, et al. Sebaceous carcinoma of the eyelids treated by Mohs micrographic surgery: Report of nine cases with review of the literature. *Dermatol Surg* 2002;28:623–631.

93. Pardo FS, Wang CC, Albert D, et al. Sebaceous carcinoma of the ocular adnexa: radiotherapeutic management. *Int J Radiat Oncol Biol Phys* 1989;17:643–647.

94. Nunery WR, Welsh MG. Recurrence of sebaceous carcinoma of the eyelid after radiation therapy. *Am J Ophthalmol* 1983;96:10–15.

95. Shields CL, Naseripour M, Shields JA, et al. Topical mitomycin-C for pagetoid invasion of the conjunctiva by eyelid sebaceous gland carcinoma. *Ophthalmology* 2002;109:2129–2133.

42

PIGMENTED TUMORS OF THE CORNEA AND CONJUNCTIVA

ANH T. Q. NGUYEN AND KATHRYN COLBY

Pigmented lesions of the conjunctiva may be divided into melanocytic or nonmelanocytic lesions. Melanocytic lesions of the conjunctiva can be due to disorders either of melanocyte proliferation (melanocytosis) or of melanin production. The melanocytic lesions may be further subdivided into primary and secondary lesions, which may be congenital or acquired, and benign or malignant. In this chapter, the primary melanocytic lesions of the conjunctiva including conjunctival melanosis and its two subsets epithelial (racial) melanosis and subepithelial (congenital) melanocytosis are reviewed. Conjunctival nevi, primary acquired melanosis (PAM), and malignant melanoma are also discussed.

Melanocytes are cells of neural crest origin that migrate to mucus membranes, including the conjunctiva, and to the skin during embryogenesis (1). They reside in the basal layers of the conjunctival epithelium near the basement membrane. Conjunctival melanocytes closely resemble the dendritic melanocytes of the skin. Melanocytes contain melanosomes, which synthesize and store melanin and are therefore responsible for mucus membrane and skin pigmentation. Melanin may be released from melanocytes and taken up by epithelial cells. Skin and mucous membrane pigmentation in individuals with darker complexions is usually due to increased synthesis and release of melanin, rather than to an increase in the number of melanocytes. Conjunctival melanocytes are divided into three main types: dendritic cells that are located in the basal layer of the epithelium, intraepithelial nevus cells, and subepithelial fusiform melanocytes (2).

MELANOSIS
Epithelial Melanosis
Clinical Presentation

Epithelial or racial melanosis of the conjunctiva is a primary melanotic condition affecting blacks more commonly than whites (3,4). Racial melanosis first appears in early childhood and stabilizes in early adulthood. Typically, flat patches of pigment are scattered in the conjunctival epithelium, most commonly in the interpalpebral and perilimbal areas (Fig. 42-1). Both eyes are usually affected, although the amount of pigment may be asymmetric. The lesions commonly fade near the fornices. Because of their intraepithelial location, these pigmented lesions are freely mobile over the globe. The pigmentation may extend into the peripheral cornea and may be especially pronounced around the perforating branches of the anterior ciliary nerves.

Histopathology

Histopathologic examination of epithelial melanosis reveals an increased deposition of melanin granules in the basal layer of the conjunctival epithelium (3,4). The conjunctival epithelium shows normal morphology and maturation. The pigment does not extend further than the basal epithelium and there is no cellular atypia.

Treatment and Prognosis

Epithelial melanosis is a benign condition. Treatment consists of periodic observation. Care should be taken to distinguish racial melanosis from primary acquired melanosis, especially in darkly pigmented patients, where this distinction may be difficult (3). Biopsies maybe useful to confirm the histopathologic diagnosis if there is any concern.

Subepithelial Melanocytosis
Clinical Presentation

Subepithelial (congenital) melanocytosis of the deep conjunctiva, episclera or superficial sclera is a congenital condition that is more common in African Americans, Asians, and Hispanics (3,4). On examination, the pigmented lesions appear bluish or slate-gray and are usually unilateral (Fig. 42-2). Unlike epithelial melanosis, these lesions are deep and immobile. The overlying conjunctiva is not pigmented.

The melanocytosis may also affect the uvea, meninges, and soft tissues of the orbit. Ipsilateral dermal melanocytosis

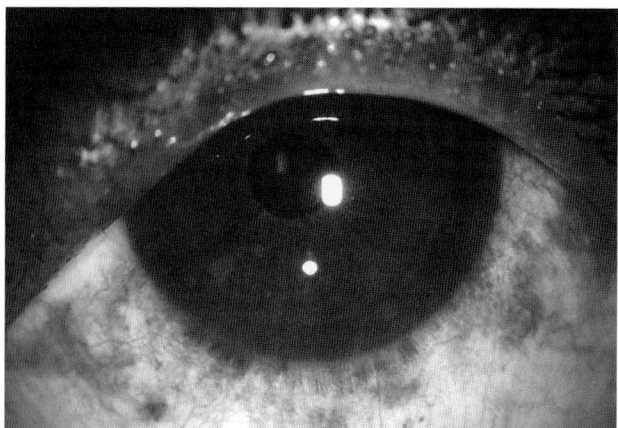

FIGURE 42-1. Racial melanosis in a 45-year-old black woman with neurofibromatosis. Lisch nodules are an incidental finding.

in the distribution of the ophthalmic and maxillary branches of the trigeminal nerve may be found in approximately 50% of patients with congenital melanocytosis. This is referred to as oculodermal melanocytosis or nevus of Ota (4).

Histopathology

The classic histopathologic finding in this condition is focal proliferation of subepithelial melanocytes (3,4). These melanocytes are more elongated and fusiform with more prominent branching processes than the melanocytes found in nevi (5).

Treatment and Prognosis

The overall prognosis is good. However, white patients with the lesion have an increased risk of developing uveal melanoma (3,4). Glaucoma associated with hyperpigmentation of the trabecular meshwork develops in up to 10% of patients. Yearly ophthalmic evaluation is recommended.

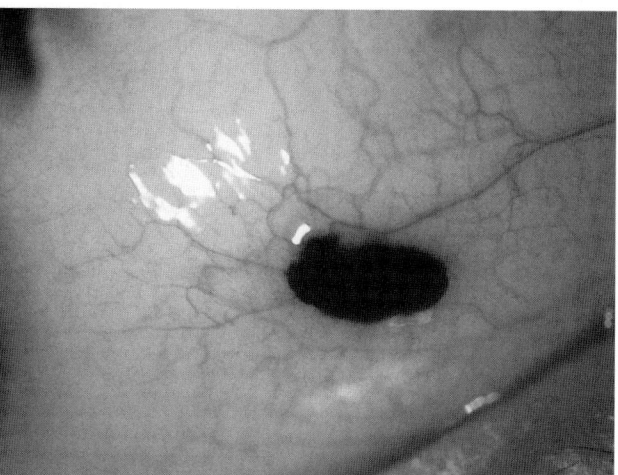

FIGURE 42-3. Small localized pigmented conjunctival nevus in a 12-year-old boy.

Conjunctival Nevi

Classification and Clinical Presentation

Nevi are common lesions of the conjunctiva. Their color ranges from tan to dark brown (Figs. 42-3 and 42-4). As many as 30%, however, may be lightly pigmented or even nonpigmented (Fig. 42-5). Pigmentation may increase during puberty, and previously nonpigmented lesions can become pigmented, making it seems as if the lesion has grown.

Nevi may be congenital, but more commonly arise during childhood or early adulthood. Similar to skin nevi, conjunctival nevi are classified by the layer in which they are found into intraepithelial (junctional), compound, or subepithelial nevi (2,4,5). It is difficult to distinguish the layer involved on clinical exam only. Nevi have little or no malignant potential.

Conjunctival nevi are usually solitary, well-circumscribed, flat to slightly elevated, brown, pigmented, freely mobile lesions most commonly found near the limbus (2,4,5).

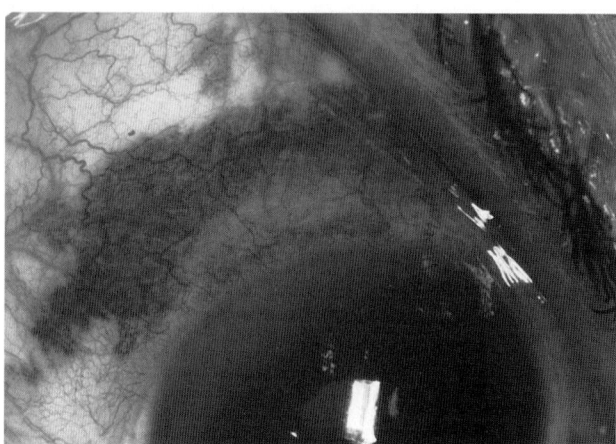

FIGURE 42-2. Ocular melanocytosis revealing deep flat, slate gray pigment. The overlying conjunctiva is not pigmented. (Photo courtesy of Frederick A. Jakobiec, M.D., with permission.)

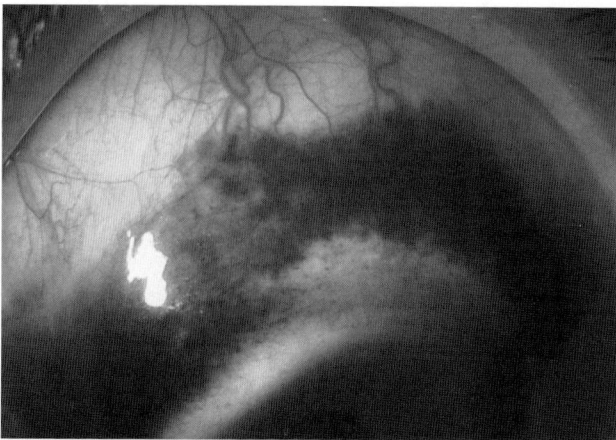

FIGURE 42-4. Diffuse pigmented conjunctival nevus in a 30-year-old Hispanic man. The lesion is brown rather than slate gray (cf. Fig. 42-2). The superficial location of the pigment is the conjunctiva is confirmed by the fact that the lesion is freely mobile with a surgical sponge.

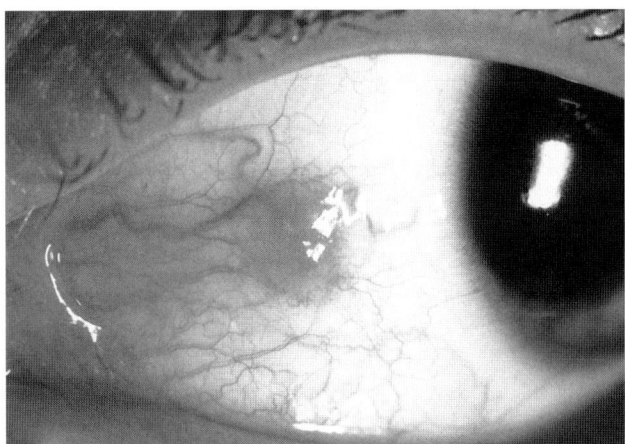

FIGURE 42-5. Nonpigmented conjunctival nevus. (Photo courtesy of Frederick A. Jakobiec, M.D.)

Nevi may be focal or diffuse, but are almost never multifocal. Many nevi contain small cysts (Fig. 42-6).

Blue nevi differ from the more common nevi described above in that they are deeper, more localized, have a palpable thickness, and are more cellular (5,6). They are characteristically gray or blue in color and usually appear early in childhood. Blue nevi are usually benign, but have malignant potential if they are hypercellular (6,7).

Split nevus of the eyelid, a rare entity, has been reported in association with malignant melanoma of the conjunctiva (8).

Histopathology

Histopathologic examination of conjunctival nevi typically reveals spindle-shaped or multipolar dendritic cells full of fine melanin granules (nevus cells). The location of these cells determines if the nevus is junctional, subepithelial, or compound. In junctional nevi, nests of nevus cells are found at the junction between the epithelial and subep-

ithelial tissues. Junctional nevi may occasionally be difficult to differentiate from PAM with atypia or melanomas due to histopathologic similarities. In contrast to PAM and melanomas, however, junctional nevi usually occur during childhood and pagetoid (intraepithelial) spread is rare.

Compound nevi of the conjunctiva show nevus cells both within and beneath the epithelium. In subepithelial nevi, the cells are located beneath the epithelium. Another variant, the combined nevus, is contains both a blue nevus and a junctional, compound, or subepithelial nevus (9,10). The blue nevus part of a combined nevi is usually smaller and deeper than the other component (9,10). Less common conjunctival nevus variants include the balloon cell nevus, the nevus of Spitz, and the pigmented spindle cell nevus of Reed (11).

Treatment and Prognosis

Nevi are benign lesions and most do not require treatment or surgical excision. Occasionally, nevi may become inflamed and may exhibit periods of rapid growth leading to the clinical suspicion of malignancy (12). The rapid growth typically occurs around puberty and is most commonly seen in compound nevi near the limbus. Patients with a history of allergies can also be prone to this phenomenon. Histopathology confirms the benign, inflammatory nature of these nevi.

Nevi of the palpebral conjunctiva, fornix, caruncle, and cornea are rare. Pigmented lesions in these locations, therefore, should be suspected of being malignant and an excisional biopsy performed.

Primary Acquired Melanosis

Clinical Presentation

PAM of the conjunctiva consists of unilateral, multiple, flat, indistinct areas of golden to dark brown coloration with irregular margins (1,2,4,13) (Fig. 42-7). The size and color of PAM lesions may change over time. The lesions are

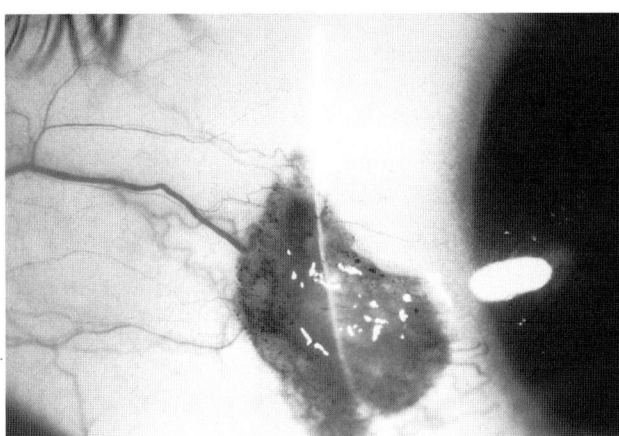

FIGURE 42-6. Conjunctival nevus illustrating characteristic clear cysts. (Photo courtesy of Frederick A. Jakobiec, M.D.)

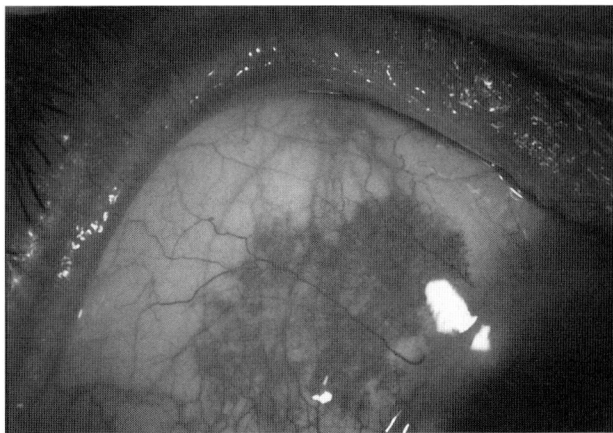

FIGURE 42-7. Primary acquired melanosis (PAM) in a 65-year-old Caucasian man showing characteristic golden brown color. The lesion is localized, flat, and freely mobile.

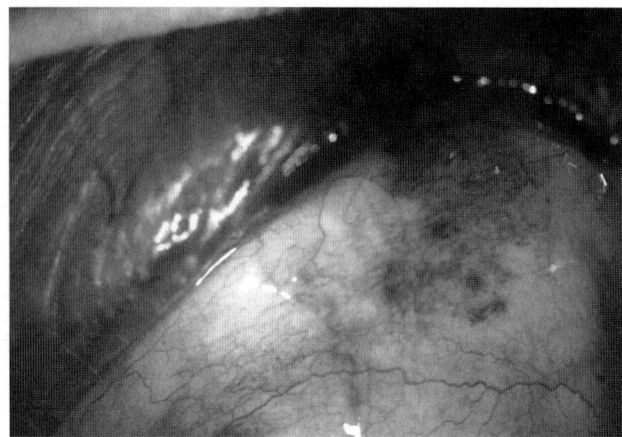
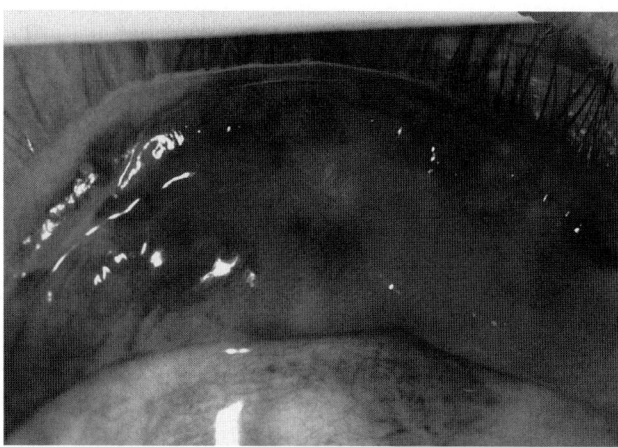

FIGURE 42-8. A: Diffuse PAM with atypia on the bulbar conjunctiva of a 75-year-old man. There is pigment at the mucocutaneous junction of the upper lid. **B:** Lid eversion demonstrates involvement of the upper palpebral conjunctiva. Examination of the entire conjunctiva is essential for appropriate management of patients with pigmented conjunctival tumors.

usually freely mobile and may involve any part of the conjunctiva (1,5,13). Slit-lamp biomicroscopy, therefore, should include lid eversion with careful inspection of the palpebral conjunctiva (Fig. 42-8). Double eversion of the upper lid may be needed to inspect the entire upper fornix. The lacrimal gland and lacrimal sac are rarely involved by PAM (1,13).

PAM is relatively common in middle-aged or elderly whites and is extremely rare in blacks of all ages (1,13). The reported prevalence of PAM in the general population ranges from 10% to 36% (1). The melanosis in PAM is caused by an increase in melanin production with or without melanocytosis.

Malignant transformation of PAM lesions is common when histologic atypia is present (1–5,13,14). Overall, almost one half of patients with PAM with atypia will progress to melanoma. This rate approaches 90% for lesions that show epithelioid cells or a pagetoid growth pattern (13). Malignant transformation should be suspected in enlarging, highly vascularized lesions, lesions greater than 7.5 × 10 mm, or in lesions with patchy pigmentation (1,13). Development of one or more nodules in a previously flat lesion is an ominous sign.

Histopathology

Clinical features alone cannot distinguish precancerous PAM (with histologic atypia) from benign PAM without atypia (1,4). Suspicious lesions, therefore, should undergo an excisional biopsy, as this is the only way to determine the presence or absence of atypia.

Lesions without histologic atypia almost never become malignant (1,2,4,13). Histologically, PAM lesions without atypia may exhibit increased melanin production with or without melanocytosis (2). The melanocytosis in these lesions is usually restricted to the basilar regions of the conjunctival epithelium. Nuclear hyperchromasia is usually

absent and the nucleoli are not prominent. Patients with PAM without atypia tend to be younger than patients with PAM with atypia (13). PAM without atypia may progress to PAM with atypia.

PAM with atypia has a significantly increased chance of malignant transformation. Five different patterns of atypical cells have been described with varied rates of progression to melanoma (1,13). These include small polyhedral cells, spindle cells, large dendritiform melanocytes, epithelioid cells, or polymorphous (mixture). The degree of atypia increases with the size of the nucleus and prominence of the nucleoli. These cells may remain in the basilar epithelial layer, form nests throughout the epithelium, spread to all levels of the epithelium in a pagetoid fashion, or proliferate in a sheetlike fashion. Lesions composed primarily of epithelioid cells or exhibiting pagetoid spread have the highest rate of malignant transformation (1,13).

Immunohistostaining with the monoclonal antibodies MIB-1 and PC-10 that stain for the proliferation markers Ki-67 and the proliferating cell nuclear antigen (PCNA) respectively, may help differentiate between PAM with and without atypia (15). It is still unclear, however, if staining with these proliferation markers is better at predicting the potential for malignant transformation than traditional histologic criteria (15–21).

Treatment and Prognosis

Complete excision of all lesions with atypia should be the goal of treatment, with special attention given to obtaining tumor-free margins (1). Clearly this is more difficult in diffuse disease. In the setting of diffuse PAM, excision of any nodular areas is critical. Multiple map biopsies of the remaining conjunctiva, even in areas where there is no pigment, will help in assessing the extent of the disease.

Cryotherapy, radiotherapy, or topical mitomycin C are useful adjunctive therapies (1,22–27). Topical mitomycin

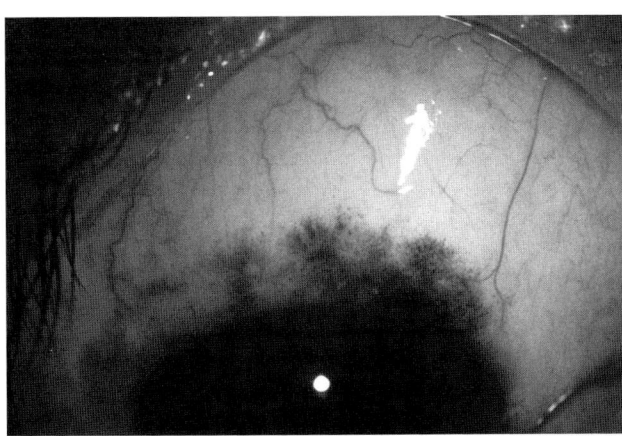
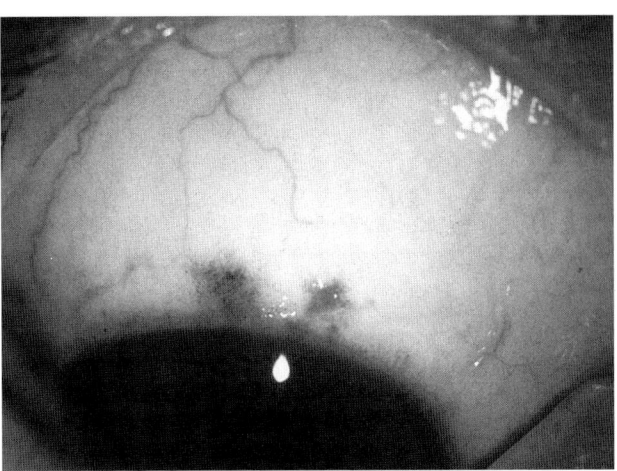

FIGURE 42-9. A: PAM without atypia in a 45-year-old Hispanic woman before treatment with topical mitomycin C. **B:** Appearance following three cycles of mitomycin C. Note marked reduction in conjunctival pigment.

C is particularly appealing in patients with diffuse disease, as it treats the entire ocular surface, as opposed to cryotherapy, which acts only at the site of application.

Jakobiec and colleagues (22) treated 10 patients who had PAM with atypia with a combination of surgical excision and cryotherapy. Four required re-treatment for recurrent PAM but none progressed to malignant melanoma after an average of 3.3 years of follow-up. Complications of this approach include conjunctival scarring, loss of lashes, ptosis, lid laxity and floppiness, symblepharon, and pseudopterygium. Extensive cryotherapy to the limbus can compromise the stem cell population to the point of creating an unstable ocular surface. One elderly patient with diffuse PAM developed anterior segment necrosis syndrome after extensive cryotherapy.

Shields et al. (27) reported dramatic regression of an extensive biopsy-proven PAM lesion with atypia in an elderly man treated primarily with six weekly cycles of topical mitomycin C 0.04%. Similar favorable experiences with mitomycin C have been reported by others without serious complications (23–27) (Fig. 42-9). Salomao and colleagues (28), however, reported cytologic changes in the conjunctiva mimicking malignancy after topical treatment of PAM with 0.02% to 0.04% mitomycin C drops. These changes were localized to the superficial layers of the conjunctival epithelium and include nuclear enlargement, chromatin smudging-hyperchromasia, cytoplasmic eosinophilia, single cell necrosis, and subepithelial chronic inflammation.

Primary acquired melanosis can recur after surgical excision, and new lesions may develop elsewhere on the conjunctiva. Because of the potential for malignant transformation and the possibility of recurrences after excision, patients with PAM should undergo careful ocular examination and photographic documentation several times each year. At each follow-up visit, we also perform a head and neck exam to determine the status of cervical lymph nodes.

CONJUNCTIVAL MELANOMA

Clinical Presentation

The term *melanoma* was first introduced by Carswell in 1838 (1). These uncommon lesions make up less than 1% of all ocular malignancies and only 2% to 5% of all ocular melanomas (1,29). Conjunctival melanomas are less common than uveal and skin melanomas. The annual incidence in a Western population ranges between 0.02 to 0.05 cases per 100,000 inhabitants. Based on data collected from the Surveillance, Epidemiology and End Results (SEER) program database, and the National Cancer Institute (NCI), Yu and colleagues (30) determined that the incidence of conjunctival melanomas is increasing for white men above the age of 60 years. A similar increase in the incidence of skin melanomas has been noted. The authors speculate that the increased incidence of conjunctival melanomas may be due to increased sun exposure.

Malignant melanomas of the uvea and conjunctiva are histopathologically and clinically different and therefore should be considered separate entities (1,13). In fact, melanomas of the conjunctiva have more in common with melanomas of the skin than with melanomas of the uveal tract (1,13,30).

Conjunctival melanomas are extremely rare in blacks and Asians. They usually develop after the third decade of life (1,13,32). The mean age at diagnosis is 52 to 60 years (1,13,31). In most series, males and females are equally affected.

Conjunctival melanomas in children are also very rare (1,13). Croxatto and colleagues (33) reported an 11-year-old

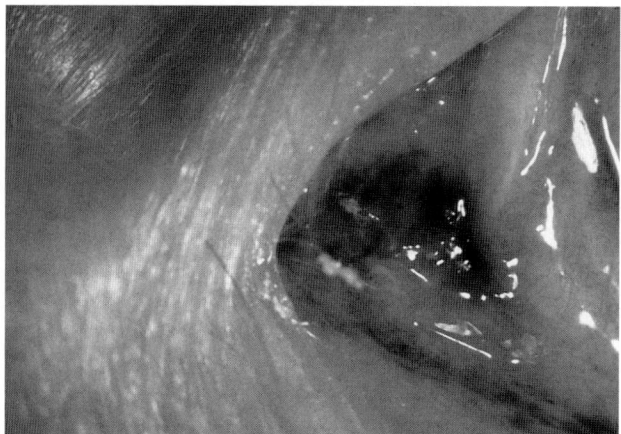

FIGURE 42-10. Invasive malignant melanoma of the caruncle. The tumor is nodular and multifocal.

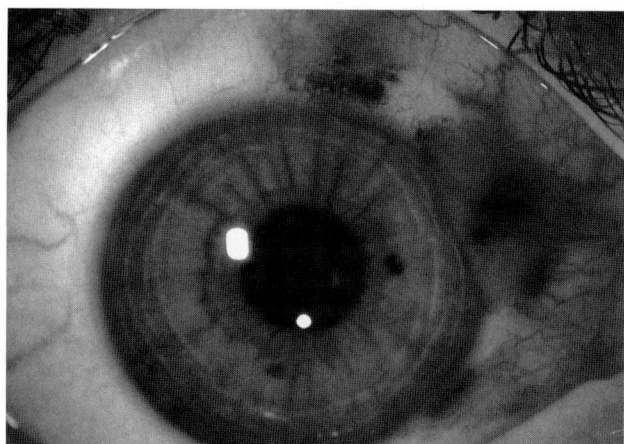

FIGURE 42-11. Multifocal invasive conjunctival melanoma in a 23-year-old white woman. Note variations in pigment and prominent vasculature. Conjunctival melanomas are extremely rare in young adults.

boy with conjunctival malignant melanoma and regional metastasis who underwent exenteration. Strempel and Kroll (34) reported three cases of conjunctival melanoma in children 14 years of age or younger.

Approximately 75% of conjunctival melanomas arise from preexisting PAM (1,5,13,14). The rest occur de novo, from a nevus or a blue nevus, or secondary to metastasis from a melanoma elsewhere (1,5,13,35). A rare aggressive form of amelanotic melanoma arises from PAM without pigmentation (sine pigmento) (36). Chronic exposure to ultraviolet radiation has been implicated in the etiology of conjunctival melanomas.

Several case reports have described conjunctival and uveal melanomas in patients with the dysplastic nevus syndrome of the skin, suggesting an association between these malignancies (1). The dysplastic nevus syndrome consists of atypical cutaneous nevi, which may be sporadic or familial. This skin nevus has a typical clinical appearance, but nuclear atypia is found on histologic exam.

Conjunctival malignant melanoma lesions tend to be nodular. They may invade the globe or extend posteriorly into the orbit (1,13). Some lesions are pedunculated. Multicentric cases have been reported. Pigmentation is variable and they tend to be heavily vascularized (Figs. 42-10–42-12). The bulbar conjunctiva and limbus are the most commonly involved sites (1).

Primary malignant melanoma of the cornea is extremely rare (1,37). Romaniuk and colleagues (37) reported a case of malignant melanoma of the cornea without limbal or conjunctival involvement in a 59-year-old white woman. Histopathologic examination revealed nodular malignant melanoma. Most melanomas of the cornea, however, are secondary to extension from the neighboring conjunctiva and usually involve the superficial layers of the cornea anterior to the basement membrane.

Histopathology

Histopathology of malignant melanomas of the conjunctiva reveals four different cell types (1,13): small polyhedral

cells, spindle cells, balloon cells, and round epithelioid cells. Lesions composed mostly of spindle cells have the lowest potential for metastasis.

Prognosis and Metastatic Potential

The overall survival rate following conjunctival melanoma varies from 70% to 87% at 10 years (1,29,31). Risk factors for death from tumor metastasis include a lump as the presenting symptom, a melanoma arising de novo, and the technique of initial surgery (1,13,29,31,38,39). Prognosis also depends in part on the location of the lesion and its cytologic characteristics. Bulbar conjunctival melanomas have a more favorable prognosis than palpebral conjunctival tumors or tumors involving the fornix or caruncle. Large, multicentric, thick, or recurrent tumors, pagetoid growth pattern, and lymphatic invasion are risk factors for

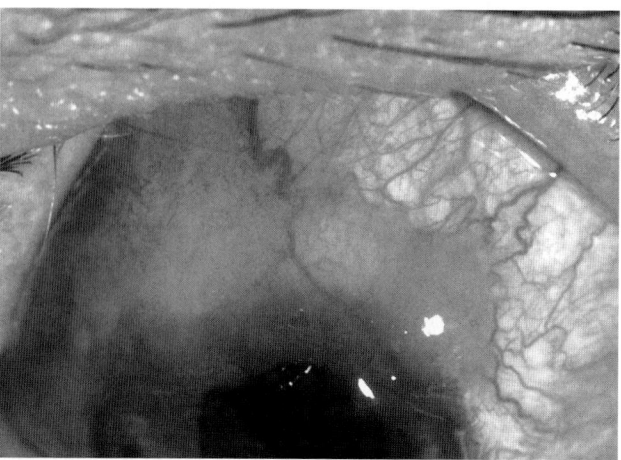

FIGURE 42-12. Recurrent amelanotic malignant melanoma. The original tumor was pigmented. (Photo courtesy of Frederick A. Jakobiec, M.D.)

metastasis (1,13,29,31,38,39). Tumors composed mostly of spindle cells have a better prognosis than those composed of mixed cell types (1,13). Hitzer and colleagues (17) found that tumor markers could not reliably differentiate between benign and malignant melanocytic lesions of the conjunctiva, and positive tumor markers did not correlate with local recurrence or metastasis. Sharara et al. (19), however, found that the HMB45 antigen could help differentiate benign from malignant conjunctival lesions.

Up to 30% to 40% of tumors metastasize at an average of 3.2 years after initial diagnosis (1,29,40). Risk factors for metastasis include tumor location away from the limbus and lateral tumor margin involvement on pathologic examination (29). Jakobiec and colleagues (13) determined that metastasis was related to the presence of PAM sine pigmento, forniceal, palpebral, or caruncular location, lesion thickness of more than 2 mm, and histologic evidence of intralymphatic spread. Unlike the hematogenous metastasis characteristic of uveal melanomas, metastasis of conjunctival melanomas occurs via the lymphatics to regional lymph nodes especially the parotid (preauricular) and submandibular nodes (1,40). Palpation of these areas is an important part of the follow up of patients with conjunctival melanoma. Once metastasis has occurred, the survival rate declines markedly. Sentinel lymph node mapping and selective lymphadenectomy may help detect early metastasis (40–42).

Local intraocular extension of tumor may occur, although this is infrequent. Wenkel and co-workers (43) reported a case of intraocular extension of a recurrent, loculated malignant melanoma of the conjunctiva in a 75-year-old white man. The authors postulated that this was possibly due to tumor cell seeding during surgical excision of the tumor. Similarly, Lommatzsch et al. (44) reported intraocular extension of a conjunctival melanoma in a 71-year-old woman after multiple attempts at surgical excision.

Treatment

In the past, melanomas of the conjunctiva were considered so malignant, and their behavior so unpredictable, that orbital exenteration was commonly performed even for small lesions (1). Currently, therapy involves less drastic approaches. Suspicious lesions should be removed via an excisional biopsy. If a melanoma is confirmed on histopathologic analysis, complete excision with cryotherapy of the conjunctival margins and scleral base should be performed. In Jakobiec et al.'s (22) series, 27 of 30 patients with histopathologically diagnosed unifocal conjunctival melanoma treated with a combination of surgical excision and cryotherapy were free of recurrence an average of 3.5 years after treatment. Two patients had recurrences that were successfully treated, and one developed metastatic disease. Twenty-three of the 30 patients had preexisting PAM. Patients with multifocal melanomas faired much more poorly: 45% developed

metastasis after treatment and only two of the 22 patients treated did not develop recurrences.

The surgical technique used to manage conjunctival melanomas is important, as incomplete tumor removal increases the risk of recurrence (29,45). In general, one should avoid incisional biopsies when a lesion is suspicious for malignant melanoma as this can lead to "seeding" of tumor cells onto the conjunctival surface. Complete surgical excision of nodular or vascularized conjunctiva with superficial lamellar dissection of underlying sclera for adherent tumors, using the "no-touch" technique described in Chapter 40 decreases recurrences, tumor cell seeding, and metastasis (45). A 3- to 5-mm tumor-free margin is ideal (46). Cryotherapy, using a double freeze-thaw approach, can be applied to the cut edges of conjunctiva and to the scleral base at the time of excision. Clean instruments should be used for subsequent surgical maneuvers (i.e., amniotic membrane grafting), once the tumor has been removed from the operative field.

Extension of tumor cells onto the cornea, which is usually superficial and does not penetrate Bowman's membrane, can be managed using alcohol-assisted epithelial removal. One should avoid penetrating Bowman's layer during surgery, as this layer serves as a natural barrier against tumor extension into the corneal stroma (13).

Map biopsies of surrounding PAM and even of uninvolved conjunctiva should be done at the time of tumor excision to determine the extent of the disease and the degree of histologic atypia.

Amniotic membrane transplantation may be used to restore the conjunctival surface following tumor excision, especially for large tumors in which the conjunctival defect is too large to close primarily (47,48). Amniotic membrane grafting reduces scarring and symblepharon formation, thereby improving postoperative cosmesis and ocular motility.

Adjunct treatments are very useful postoperatively, especially for conjunctival melanoma in the setting of diffuse PAM with atypia. Cryotherapy, the historical standard of care for extensive PAM that cannot be completely removed surgically, can cause significant ocular surface morbidity when applied over a large area. Topical chemotherapy using mitomycin C has been shown to be effective, and in general, is well tolerated. It has the added advantage of treating the entire ocular surface, as opposed to cryotherapy, which treats only the areas to which it is applied. The optimal strength and duration of mitomycin C treatment has not been established in clinical trials. However, 0.02% to 0.04% eyedrops applied four times daily for 1- to 2-week cycles have been used with good success and minimal side effects (23–26,49).

Serious complications from mitomycin C use have occurred in other settings (50) and one should approach this medication with caution. We wait until the ocular surface is completely healed following surgical manipulations before starting mitomycin C drops. Patients are cautioned to avoid contact of the medication with their skin, as it can cause

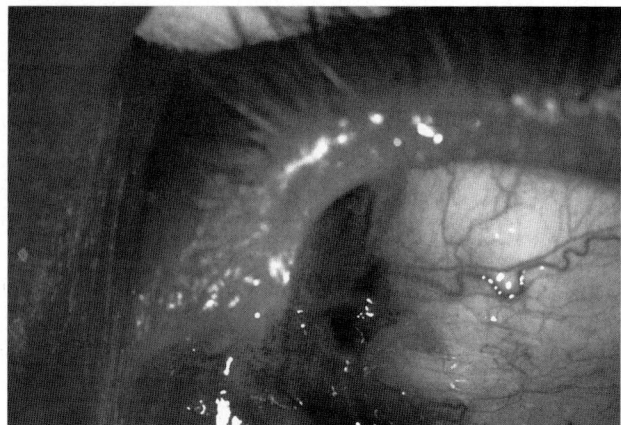

A

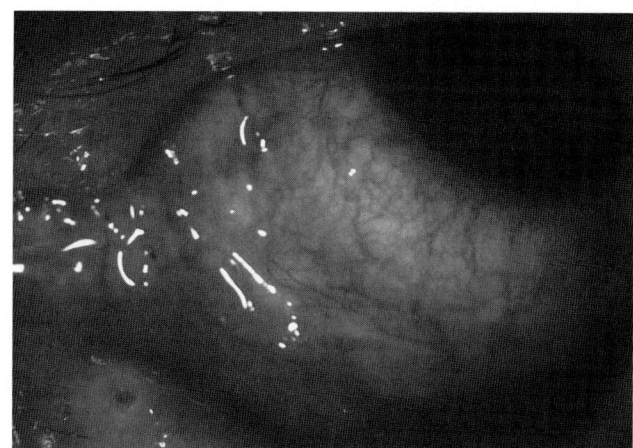

B

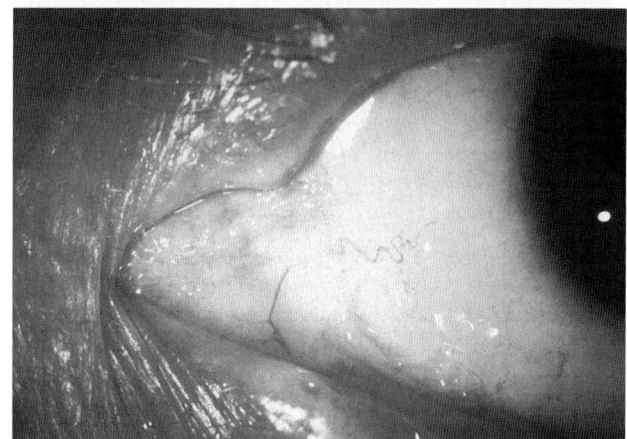

C

FIGURE 42-13. A, Conjunctival melanoma of the plica semilunaris in a 72-year-old Caucasian woman. The superior aspect of the tumor is obscured by the upper eyelid. Tumor excision, cryotherapy, and amniotic membrane grafting was performed. **B,** Appearance 3 weeks following surgery. Adjuvant treatment with topical mitomycin C was given. One year postoperative appearance shows excellent cosmesis and no motility restriction or residual tumor, which was confirmed with map biopsies.

contact dermatitis. Punctal plugs are placed in both the upper and lower punctum before beginning a course of mitomycin C and are replaced as needed during treatment to reduce systemic absorption. Manual punctal occlusion following each application of medication is an alternative to punctal plugs. We typically give 0.04% mitomycin C drops for times daily for 1 week, followed by a 3-week holiday. Patients are examined prior to beginning the next course of mitomycin C. Usually two to three cycles are needed to see a reduction in conjunctival pigment. Conjunctival injection occurs almost universally, especially during later treatment courses. A bland ophthalmic ointment such as erythromycin or a steroid-antibiotic ointment combination can be given to soothe the eye. Refrigerated artificial tears and cold compresses may also be suggested. Map biopsies are repeated several months after the last course of mitomycin C to assess for residual disease (Fig. 42-13).

Orbital exenteration may be considered in aggressive, advanced, or bulky tumors especially if the eyelids and/or orbit are involved (1). This procedure, however, does not improve survival (51). Exenteration should not be performed in the elderly because of the associated morbidity in this population, or in cases in which distant metastasis have already occurred (1,52). Shields and colleagues (52) reported their experience with exenteration for conjunctival melanomas over a 23-year period. In their series, 20 of 151 (13%) patients with conjunctival melanoma underwent exenteration. Risk factors for exenteration included poor vision, amelanotic or red colored tumor, and extralimbal tumor location.

Conjunctival melanomas are not very radiosensitive (1). Iodine-125 brachytherapy, however, may be a useful alternative in patients who might otherwise require exenteration, or as an adjunct to surgical excision (1,53). In a series of 14 patients reported by Stannard and colleagues (53), good local control was achieved with an average dose of 37 Gy. All 14 patients had undergone previous debulking or resection. Proton beam therapy and beta irradiation are also other alternatives (1).

Recurrence

Recurrences after treatment have been estimated to occur in 35% of patients, at an average of 3.5 to 4.5 years after primary treatment (1,29). Patients with a history of conjunctival melanoma, therefore, should be examined several times each year. Tumor recurrence is more common in melanomas arising from preexisting PAM, in extralimbal lesions, and in multifocal tumors (29). In a study of 150 patients, Shields et al. (29) reported an overall local recurrence rate of 35%, with a recurrence rate of 26% at 5 years,

51% at 10 years, and 65% at 15 years. Major risk factors for recurrence included nonlimbal location of the tumor and tumor cells at the margin after excision. Adjunctive cryotherapy decreases the chance of recurrences after surgical excision (1,29). Treatment of recurrent conjunctival melanoma is similar to the treatment of the primary tumor. Recurrent tumors may occasionally be nonpigmented, even if the original tumor was pigmented (Fig. 42-12).

Metastatic spread occurs in 16% of patients at 5 years, 26% at 10 years, and 32% at 15 years (29). Metastasis occurs more commonly following recurrent melanoma. The prognosis is extremely poor after metastasis. These sobering statistics underscore the importance of accurate diagnosis and meticulous surgical and medical management of patients with conjunctival melanoma and primary acquired melanosis.

DIFFERENTIAL DIAGNOSIS

The differential diagnosis of primary melanocytic lesions of the conjunctiva includes secondary melanocytic lesions and nonmelanocytic pigmentary lesions (1–5). The clinical history and histopathologic features of these entities differentiate them from the primary melanocytic lesions discussed in this chapter.

Addison's disease and pregnancy may lead to conjunctival melanosis due to hormonal changes. Topical medications containing epinephrine products or silver and systemic medications such as the phenothiazines may lead to pigmentary deposits in the conjunctiva. New-onset pigmentary deposits in the conjunctiva and uveal tissue prolapse may be noted after ocular surgical procedures (54). Congenital blue sclera and areas of scleral thinning from any cause may mimic primary pigmentary conjunctival lesions. Very rarely, intraocular melanomas may extend to the conjunctiva or cornea, or conjunctival metastasis from the skin or other melanomas may occur.

Other lesions may rarely simulate conjunctival melanomas. Tseng and colleagues (55) reported a case of a benign seborrheic keratosis that involved the limbus in a 66-year-old man, simulating a malignant melanoma. The correct diagnosis was established after impression cytology and histopathologic examination of a biopsy specimen. Laquis and colleagues (56) reported a case of conjunctival mycosis involving the limbus mimicking a melanoma in a 75-year-old white man. Histopathologic examination after an excisional biopsy established the correct diagnosis and no further treatment was required.

CONCLUSION

Pigmented lesions of the conjunctiva and cornea are relatively common clinical findings. These lesions run the gamut from completely benign (racial melanosis, nevi) to potentially lethal (conjunctival melanoma and PAM with atypia). Table 40-2 in Chapter 40 summarizes the clinical characteristics of these lesions.

Appropriate diagnosis is essential for optimal outcomes. Management of malignant pigmented tumors of the conjunctiva has advanced greatly in recent years, aided by the introduction of topical chemotherapy and amniotic membrane grafting. Disease control, while maintaining good cosmesis and ocular surface function, is an obtainable goal for most patients.

REFERENCES

1. Seregard S. Conjunctival melanoma. *Surv Ophthalmol* 1998;42: 321–350.
2. Farber M, Schutzer P, Mihm MC. Pigmented lesions of the conjunctiva. *J Am Acad Dermatol* 1998;38:971–978.
3. Rodrigues-Sians RS. Pigmented conjunctival neoplasms. *Orbit* 2002;21:231–238.
4. Grin JM, Grant-Kels JM, Grin CM, et al. Ocular melanomas and melanocytic lesions of the eye. *J Am Acad Dermatol* 1998;38: 716–730.
5. Weiss JS. Conjunctival and corneal pathology. In: Albert DM, Jakcobiec FA, eds. *Principles and practice of ophthalmology,* vol 4. Philadelphia: WB Saunders, 1994:2127–2145.
6. Kabukcuoglu S, McNutt NS. Conjunctival melanocytic nevi of childhood. *J Cutan Pathol* 1999;26:248–252.
7. Demorici H, Shields CL, Shields JA, et al. Malignant melanoma arising from unusual conjunctival blue nevus. *Arch Ophthalmol* 2000;118:1581–1584.
8. Nawa Y, Hara Y, Saishin M. Conjunctival melanoma associated with extensive congenital conjunctival nevus and split nevus of eyelid. *Arch Ophthalmol* 1999;117:269–271.
9. Crawford JB, Howes EL, Char DH. Combined nevi of the conjunctiva. *Trans Am Ophthalmol Soc* 1999;67:171–185.
10. Crawford JB, Howes EL, Char DH. Combined nevi of the conjunctiva. *Arch Ophthalmol* 1999;117:1121–1127.
11. Seregard S. Pigmented spindle cell naevus of Reed presenting in the conjunctiva. *Acta Ophthalmol Scand* 2000;78:104–106.
12. Zamir E, Mechoulam H, Micera A, et al. Inflamed juvenile conjunctival naevus: clinicopathological characterisation. *Br J Ophthalmol* 2002;86:28–30.
13. Jakobiec FA, Folberg R, Iwamoto T. Clinicopathologic characteristics of premalignant and malignant melanocytic lesions of the conjunctiva. *Ophthalmology* 1989;96:147–166.
14. Meyer A, D'Hermies F, Schwartz L, et al. Malignant melanoma on primary acquired conjunctival melanosis. *J Fr Ophtalmol* 1999; 22(9):983–986.
15. Chowers I, Livni N, Solomon A, et al. MIB-1 and PC-10 immunostaining for the assessment of proliferative activity in primary acquired melanosis without and with atypia. *Br J Ophthalmol* 1998; 82:1316–1319.
16. Chowers I, Livni N, Frucht-Perry J, et al. Immunostaining of the estrogen receptor in conjunctival primary acquired melanosis. *Ophthalmic Res* 1999;31:210–212.
17. Hitzer S, Bialasiewicz AA, Richard G. Immunohistochemical markers for cytoplasmic antigens in acquired melanoses, malignant melanoses, and nevi of the conjunctiva. *Klin Monatsbl Augenheilkd* 1998;213:230–237.
18. Abe T, Ohashi T, Tamai M. Expression of cytokine genes in a patient with conjunctival melanoma compared with other pigment cells. *Ophthalmic Res* 1998;30:255–262.

19. Sharara NA, Alexander RA, Luthert PJ, et al. Differential immunoreactivity of melanocytic lesions of the conjunctiva. *Histopathology* 2000;39:426–431.

20. Wilson MW, Schelonka LP, Siegel D, et al. Immunohistochemical localization of NAD(P)H: quinone oxidoreductase in conjunctival melanomas and primary acquired melanosis. *Curr Eye Res* 2001; 22:348–352.

21. Lee WR. Towards a more accurate assessment of the malignant potential in conjunctival melanosis. *Br J Ophthalmol* 1998;82: 1227.

22. Jakobiec FA, Rini FJ, Fraunfelder FT, et al. Cryotherapy for conjunctival primary acquired melanosis and malignant melanoma. *Ophthalmology* 1988;95:1058–1070.

23. Kemp EG, Harnett AN, Chatterjee S. Preoperative topical and intraoperative local mitomycin C adjuvant therapy in the management of ocular surface neoplasias. *Br J Ophthalmol* 2002;86: 31–34.

24. Finger PT, Czechonska G, Liarikos S. Topical mitomycin C chemotherapy for conjunctival melanoma and PAM with atypia. *Br J Ophthalmol* 1998;82:476–479.

25. Werschnik C, Lommatzsch PK. Mitomycin C in the treatment of conjunctival melanoma and primary acquired melanosis. *Klin Monatsbl Augenheilkd* 1998;212:465–468.

26. Demirci H, McCormick SA, Finger PT. Topical mitomycin chemotherapy for conjunctival malignant melanoma and primary acquired melanosis with atypia. Clinical experience with histopathologic observations. *Arch Ophthalmol* 2000;118:885–891.

27. Shields CL, Demirci H, Shields JA, et al. Dramatic regression of conjunctival and corneal acquired melanosis with topical mitomycin C. *Br J Ophthalmol* 2002;86:244–245.

28. Salomao DR, Mathers WD, Sutphin JE, et al. Cytologic changes in the conjunctiva mimicking malignancy after topical mitomycin C chemotherapy. *Ophthalmology* 1999;106:1756–1761.

29. Shields CL, Shields JA, Gunduz K, et al. Conjunctival melanoma. Risk factors for recurrence, exenteration, metastasis, and death in 150 consecutive patients. *Arch Ophthalmol* 2000;118:1497–1507.

30. Yu GP, Hu DN, McCormick S, et al. Conjunctival melanoma: is it increasing in the United States? *Am J Ophthalmol* 2003;135: 800–806.

31. Tuomaala S, Eskelin S, Tarkaanen A, et al. Population-based assessment of clinical characteristics predicting outcome of conjunctival melanoma in whites. *Invest Ophthalmol Vis Sci* 2002; 43:3399–3408.

32. Singh AD, Campso OE, Rhatigan RM, et al. Conjunctival melanoma in the black population. *Surv Ophthalmol* 1998;43:127–133.

33. Croxatto JO, Iribarren G, Ugrin C. Malignant melanoma of the conjunctiva. Report of a case. *Ophthalmology* 1987;94:1281–1285.

34. Strempel I, Kroll P. Conjunctival malignant melanoma in children. *Ophthalmologica* 1999;213:129–132.

35. Dhar-Munshi S, Ameen M, Wilson RS. Simultaneous metastases of cutaneous malignant melanoma to conjunctiva and choroids. *Br J Ophthalmol* 2000;84:930–931.

36. Jay V. Font RL. Conjunctival amelanotic malignant melanoma arising in primary acquired melanosis sine pigmento. *Ophthalmology* 1998;105:191–194.

37. Romaniuk W, Koziol H, Muskalski K, et al. A unique case of primary corneal melanoma. *Jpn J Ophthalmol* 2002;46:114–116.

38. Desjardins L, Poncet P, Levy C, et al. Prognostic factors in primary malignant melanoma of the conjunctiva. Clinicopathologic study of 56 cases. *J Fr Ophtalmol* 1999;22:315–321.

39. Bobic-Radovanovic A, Latkovic Z, Marinkovic J, et al. Predictors of survival in malignant melanoma of the conjunctiva: a clinicopathological and follow-up study. *Eur J Ophthalmol* 1998;8:4–7.

40. Esmaili B, Wang X, Yuossef A, et al. Patterns of regional and distant metastasis in patients with conjunctival melanoma. Experience at a cancer center over four decades. *Ophthalmology* 2001; 108:2101–2105.

41. Esmaili B, Eicher S, Popp J, et al. Sentinel lymph node biopsy for conjunctival melanoma. *Ophthalmic Plast Reconstr Surg* 2001; 17:436–442.

42. Esmaili B. Sentinel lymph node mapping for patients with cutaneous and conjunctival malignant melanoma. *Ophthalmol Plast Reconst Surg* 2000;16:170–172.

43. Wenkel H, Rummelt V, Naumann GOH. Malignant melanoma of the conjunctiva with intraocular extension. *Arch Ophthalmol* 2000;118:557–560.

44. Lommatzsch PK, Werschnik C, Gutz W. Intraocular invasion of a conjunctival melanoma. *Klin Monatsbl Augenheilkd* 1999;215: 370–372.

45. Shields JA, Shields CL, De Potter P. Surgical management of circumscribed conjunctival melanomas. *Ophthalmic Plast Reconstr Surg* 1998;14:208–215.

46. De Potter P, Shields CL, Shields JA. Malignant melanoma of the conjunctiva. *Int Ophthalmol Clin* 1993;33:25–30.

47. Paridaens D, Beekhuis H, van den Bosch W, et al. Amniotic membrane transplantation in the management of conjunctival melanoma and primary acquired melanosis with atypia. *Br J Ophthalmol* 2001;85:658–661.

48. Shields CL, Shields JA, Armstrong T. Management of conjunctival and corneal melanoma with surgical excision, amniotic membrane allograft, and topical chemotherapy. *Am J Ophthalmol* 2001;132:576–578.

49. Majmudar PA, Epstein RJ. Antimetabolites in ocular surface neoplasia. *Curr Opin Ophthalmol* 1998;9:35–39.

50. Rubinfeld RS, Pfister RR, Foster CS, et al. Serious complications of topical mitomycin-C after pterygium surgery. *Ophthalmology* 1992;99:1647–1654.

51. Parideans ADA, McCartney ACE, Minassian DC, et al. Orbital exenteration in 95 cases of primary conjunctival malignant melanoma. *Br J Ophthalmol* 1994;78:520–528.

52. Shields JA, Shields CL, Gunduz K, et al. Clinical features predictive of orbital exenteration for conjunctival melanoma. *Ophthalmic Plast Reconst Surg* 2000;16:173–178.

53. Stannard CE, Sealy RH, Hering ER, et al. Malignant melanoma of the eyelid and palpebral conjunctiva treated with Iodine-125 brachytherapy. *Ophthalmology* 2000;107:951–958.

54. Kiratli H, Irkec M. Acquired anterior ocular melanocytosis following cataract extraction. *Ophthalmic Surg Lasers* 2002;33:71–73.

55. Tseng SH, Chen YT, Huang FC, et al. Seborrheic keratosis of the conjunctiva simulating a malignant melanoma. An immunocytochemical study with impression cytology. *Ophthalmology* 1999; 106:1516–1520.

56. Laquis SJ, Wilson MW, Haik BG, et al. Conjunctival mycosis masquerading as melanoma. *Am J Ophthalmol* 2002;134:117–118.

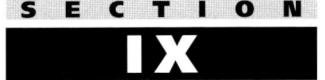

TRAUMA

CHEMICAL TRAUMA

ROSWELL R. PFISTER

INTRODUCTION AND HISTORICAL BACKGROUND

Humans have encountered a variety of naturally occurring powerful chemicals from the dawn of civilization. As industry evolved, so did the requirement for a greater variety and strength of chemicals to meet the needs of developing civilizations. Chemical injuries of the eye have had poor outcomes, particularly since the age of the industrial revolution, when large numbers of workers first became exposed to a wide variety of powerful chemicals in the production of manufactured items from raw materials. It was natural for physicians to employ mechanistic, animal, or vegetable therapies to what seemed to be an inevitable conclusion: pain, blindness, and often, loss of the eye. Until relatively recently this outcome was still common. Progress has been made toward delineating the nature of the destructive inflammatory process and the subsequent repair of many tissues crucial to ocular stability. In many cases there is now the realistic prospect of return of considerable vision, following chemical trauma.

EPIDEMIOLOGY

Injury by a chemical occurs in the workplace, in the home or its environs, or as a direct result of an assault. In the past the concept of safety for workers was not a consideration taken seriously, nor were there any safety engineers to guard against accidental injuries. In many parts of the world this unsafe situation still exists.

There are profound psychological, social, and economic repercussions that occur after chemical injury. Injury of one eye often results in costly medical care dependency, loss of job, interpersonal conflicts, and isolation for the period of time necessary to stabilize the injured eye. Blindness resulting from bilateral injury severely restricts job and economic opportunities, with an additional burden placed on the family and social systems for subsidence and loss of taxable income.

Chemical injury can be acidic, alkaline, or toxic. Strong acids causing injury include sulfuric, hydrochloric, nitric, and hydrofluoric. Alkalis causing eye injury include ammonium hydroxide, sodium hydroxide, potassium hydroxide, magnesium hydroxide, and calcium hydroxide (1). Toxic agents include a huge variety of chemicals that are destructive to biologic tissues, but that are not particularly acidic or alkaline. Table 43-1 summarizes the sources and relevant comments pertaining to the commonest types of acid and alkali injury. In addition, a comprehensive review of chemical injuries is presented by Wagoner (2).

Data gathered from a large urban hospital show that young black men are at greatest risk of a severe alkali-injury assault, usually in a domestic setting, where there is low income, high-density housing, and a record of alcoholism and prior assaults (3). In the industrial sector, approximately 10% of 52,142 cases of ocular trauma reported from 16 states were chemical injuries (1.6% acid and 0.6% alkali). Safety monitors have reduced the incidence of job-related eye injuries, but despite such programs, the storage and use of powerful chemicals, under extreme pressure and high temperature, continue to pose serious threats even to the properly attired worker wearing protective clothing and goggles.

Of 221 chemical injuries reported in 180 patients at the Croyden Eye Unit, United Kingdom, there were nearly twice as many alkali as acid injuries. Males comprised 75.6% and females 24.4% of all injuries. Most patients were between the ages of 16 and 25 (4). Accidental injuries accounted for 89.4%, and the remainder assaults. Work-related accidents accounted for 63%, and 33% occurred at home and 3% at school.

Two large series of chemical injuries were reported by Kuckelkorn et al. (5) in Aachen, Germany, in 1990 to 1991. In the first report 236 injuries occurred in 171 patients of whom 70% were males. Industrial accidents accounted for 61%, 37% were household accidents, and 2% unknown. Most injuries were classified as mild (88%). In Kuckelkorn et al. (6) second series, they evaluated 42 patients sustaining severe alkali injuries occurring over a 7-year period. The industrial sector contributed 73.8%, and the rest were sustained at home.

Farmers using liquid ammonia as fertilizer in remote areas, and homeowners using powerful cleansing agents, without eye protection, continue to be at special risk.

TABLE 43-1. CHEMICALS COMMONLY USED IN INDUSTRY OR IN THE HOME

Class	Compound	Common Source/Uses	Comments
Alkali	Ammonia [NH_3]	1. Fertilizers 2. Refrigerants 3. Cleaning agents (7% solution)	1. Combines with water to form NH_4OH fumes 2. Very rapid penetration
	Lye [NaOH]	1. Drain cleaners	1. Penetrates almost as rapidly as ammonia
	Potassium hydroxide [KOH]	1. Caustic potash	1. Severity similar to that of lye
	Magnesium hydroxide [$Mg(OH)_2$]	1. Sparklers	1. Produces combined thermal and alkali injury
	Lime [$CA(OH)_2$]	1. Plaster	1. Most common cause of chemical injury in work place
		2. Mortar	2. Poor penetration
		3. Cement	3. Toxicity increased by retained particulate matter
		4. Whitewash	
Acid	Sulfuric acid [H_2SO_4]	1. Industrial cleaners	1. Combines with water to produce corneal thermal injury
		2. Battery acid	2. May have associated foreign body or laceration from battery acid
	Sulfurous acid [H_2SO_3]	1. Formed from sulfur dioxide (SO_2) by combination with corneal water 2. Fruit and vegetable preservatives 3. Bleach 4. Refrigerants	1. Penetrates more easily than other acids
	Hydrofluoric acid [HF]	1. Glass polishing 2. Glass frosting 3. Mineral refining 4. Gasoline alkylation 5. Silicon production	1. Penetrates easily 2. Produces severe injury
	Acetic acid [CH_3COOH]	1. Vinegar 4–0%	1. Mild injury with less than 10% contamination
		2. Essence of vinegar 80% 3. Glacial acetic acid 90%	2. Severe injury with higher concentration
	Chromic acid [Cr_2O_3]	1. Used in the chrome plating industry	1. Chronic exposure produces chronic conjunctivitis with brown discoloration
	Hydrochloric acid [HCL]	1. Used as a 31–38% solution	1. Severe injury only with high concentration and prolonged exposure

(Reproduced, with permission, from Wagoner M and Kenyon K. 1994. Chemical injuries of the eye. In: Albert D, Jakobiac F, eds. *Principles and practice of ophthalmology: clinical practice*, vol. 1. Philadelphia: WB Saunders.)

Last, the deployment of certain types of automobile airbags occasionally releases sodium hydroxide as part of the chemically driven, rapid inflation process, causing corneal abrasions and mild alkali injuries. Although these cases make up 21.6% of eye injury cases caused by airbags, in most cases they heal readily (7).

MAJOR CHEMICAL DIFFERENCES AMONG ALKALI, ACID, AND TOXIC INJURY OF THE EYE

Alkali

The pain, lacrimation, and blepharospasm following an ocular alkali injury result from direct injury of free nerve endings located in the epithelium of the cornea, conjunctiva, and eyelids. Depending on the severity of the injury, a wave of hydroxyl ions rapidly advance through ocular tissues causing saponification of cellular membranes with massive cell death and extensive hydrolysis of the corneal matrix consisting of glycosaminoglycans and collagen.

Ammonia

Ammonia (NH_3) is encountered as a fertilizer and a refrigerant as well as in the manufacturing of other chemicals. The most common form is household ammonia, a 7% solution used as a cleaning agent. Ammonia fumes stimulate the eye to secrete tears, which tends to dilute the chemical, reducing its potential for major ocular damage. However, the gas is soluble in water and tears. With prolonged exposure to the eye, ammonia gas forms ammonium hydroxide (NH_4OH), capable of causing major ocular damage. The lipid solubility and high penetrability of ammonia allow it to pass through the cornea and into the eye almost instantaneously (8). Such rapid penetration makes the injury very difficult to ameliorate by subsequent irrigation.

Lye

Lye [i.e., sodium hydroxide (NaOH), caustic soda, sodium hydrate] penetrates into the interior of the eye in 3 to 5 minutes (8). Solid sodium hydroxide, often used as a drain cleaner, can cause pressure to develop within the drain pipe, with resultant explosion of lye into the face and eyes of the unprepared. Warmed lye is also commonly used to straighten kinky hair. Lye injuries rank second in severity to those produced by ammonium hydroxide.

Other Hydroxides

Potassium hydroxide (KOH, caustic potash) and magnesium hydroxide [MG(OH)$_2$] are less usual causes of chemical injuries of the eye. Potassium hydroxide penetrates the eye slightly less rapidly than sodium hydroxide but the injuries are of similar severity. Magnesium hydroxide is found in sparklers and flares; the combination of thermal injury and chemical injury accounts for more severe injury than that occurring as a result of heat alone (9).

Lime

Injuries from lime [Ca(OH)$_2$], fresh lime, quicklime [CaO + H$_2$O = Ca(OH)$_2$], calcium hydrate, slaked lime, hydrated lime, plaster, mortar, cement, and whitewash, used primarily in the building industry, are common sources of ocular injuries. It penetrates the eye less rapidly because it reacts with epithelial cell membranes, forming calcium soaps that precipitate and hinder further penetration.

Despite that, these injuries can be quite severe with the corneal opacity visible before the opacities seen as a result of ammonium or sodium hydroxide (10).

Methyl Ethyl Ketone Peroxide

Methyl ethyl ketone peroxide is a catalyst commonly used in various industries. Immediate and delayed corneal injury can occur. Exacerbations and remissions of limbal and corneal disease lasting more than 20 years have been reported (11).

Acid

Weak acidic compounds contacting the outer eye precipitate proteins within the corneal and conjunctival epithelium, thus acting as a partial barrier to further ingress of the chemical. In their wake is left a grayish-white epithelium, often obscuring all tissues posterior to it. Stripping off this opacified epithelial layer often reveals a relatively clear underlying corneal stroma (Fig. 43-1). As long as the corneal stem cells ringing the cornea are not damaged, then epithelial recovery is likely with little or no stromal cloudiness.

Very strong acids, however, overcome this precipitated proteinaceous obstacle handily and progress through tissue much as alkali. The end result of a very severe acid injury is often indistinguishable from that of an alkaline injury. For that reason this chapter deals with alkaline and acid injuries as one entity, unless otherwise specified.

Sulfuric Acid

Sulfuric acid (H$_2$SO$_4$) is a commonly used industrial chemical as well as the acid used in batteries. The great

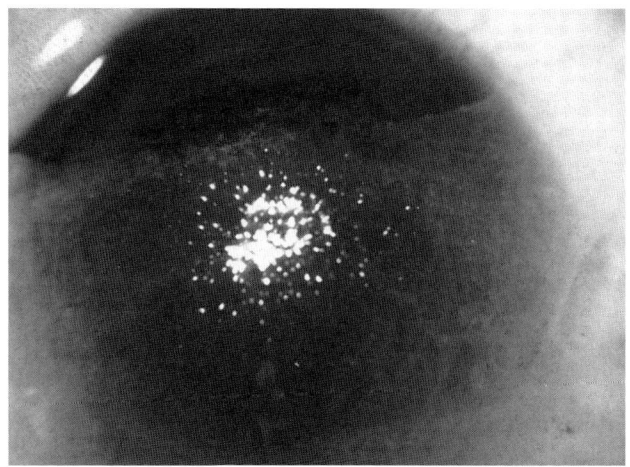 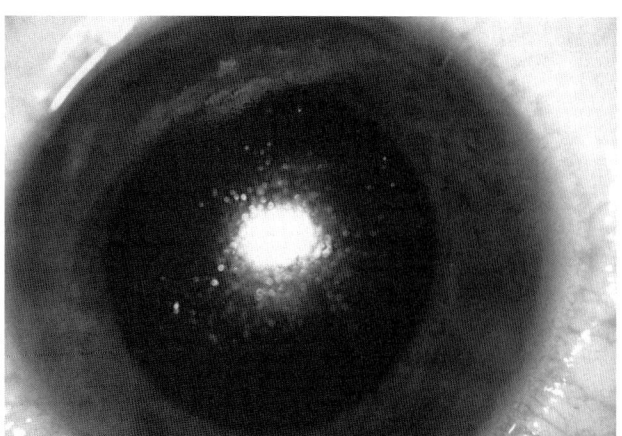

FIGURE 43-1. A: Acid injury of the cornea and adjacent conjunctiva. Note the opalescent surface, a consequence of protein denaturation of the full thickness of the affected epithelium. **B:** Stripping off the cloudy epithelial layer uncovers the underlying crystal clear corneal stroma. Healing can take place without scarring or with very mild superficial nebulae.

avidity of concentrated sulfuric acid for water results in the release of heat, the cause of tissue charring. Sulfuric acid produces injuries ranging from mild to very severe. Most of the injuries, especially the more severe ones, occur as the result of battery explosions. Hydrogen and oxygen are produced by electrolysis when sulfuric acid combines with water in the battery. This gaseous mixture explodes on contact with flame. Matches or cigarette lighters used as illumination sources or sparks produced by jumper cables are the most common modes of ignition. Injuries that result from battery explosions commonly are combinations of acid burn and contusion from particulate matter but might also show laceration or intraocular foreign body penetration.

Sulfurous Acid

Sulfur dioxide (SO_2) forms sulfurous acid (H_2SO_3) when it combines with water in ocular tissue. It might be encountered as sulfurous anhydride or sulfurous oxide, a fruit and vegetable preservative, bleach, and refrigerant. When used as a refrigerant, it is mixed with oil. Tissue injury is more severe in patients damaged from SO_2 mixed with oil because the hydrocarbon prolongs contact. Ocular and tissue damage are severe when a direct jet of the gas or liquid and oil hits the skin or eye. The initial injury damages the corneal nerves, resulting in relative tissue anesthesia and little discomfort. At first, visual acuity is not severely affected but it worsens greatly over hours to days as the ocular condition deteriorates. It is not the sulfur dioxide's freezing effect on the tissue that produces the injury but rather sulfurous acid itself, denaturing protein, and inactivating numerous enzymes. Because of its high lipid and water solubility, sulfurous acid penetrates the tissues easily.

Hydrofluoric Acid

Hydrofluoric acid (HF, hydrogen fluoride) is a weak inorganic acid but a strong solvent. It has been used for centuries, but in current industry use it is found either in its pure form (in solutions ranging from 0.5% to 70.0% in strength) or mixed with other agents such as nitric acid, ammonium difluoride, and acetic acid. Hydrofluoric acid is used in etching and polishing glass and silicone and in frosting glass. It is also used in the pickling or chemical milling of metals, as well as in the refining of uranium, tantalum, and beryllium. It is also used in the alkylation of high-octane gasoline, the production of elemental and inorganic fluoride, and the preparation of organic fluorocarbons. It has found a new use in the semiconductor industry where it is essential technology in the manufacture of silicon chips for computers and other devices controlled by digital technology. It is so highly toxic that as little as 7 mL or a 2.5% burn of the body is sufficient to cause death from uncontrolled hypocalcemia (12).

Much has been written on skin burns caused by hydrofluoric acid; however, the literature is sparse relative to that for ocular injuries. Hydrofluoric acid produces a severe ocular injury because of its high degree of activity in dissolving cellular membranes. In addition, the low molecular weight and small size of the hydrofluoric acid molecule allow it to penetrate the tissues readily.

Other Acids

Chromic acid is a strong caustic derived from chromic oxide and chromium trioxide (Cr_2O_3). Rare cases of severe ocular injury have occurred after direct instillation of the liquid in the eye. However, ocular injuries caused by chromic acid are more often associated with exposure to droplets of the acid in the chrome-plating industry, resulting in chronic conjunctival inflammation and a brown discoloration of the epithelium in the interpalpebral fissure.

Hydrochloric acid is commonly used as a 32% to 38% solution. Hydrogen chloride gas is irritating to the eye; thus, the profuse tearing serves to limit ocular damage.

At high concentrations and with prolonged exposure, liquid hydrochloric acid produces severe ocular damage.

Injuries produced by nitric acid (HNO_3) are similar to those produced by hydrochloric acid, except that the epithelial opacity produced by nitric acid is yellowish rather than white as it is in the other acid burns.

Acetic acid (CH_3COOH), a relatively weak organic acid, is also known as ethanoic acid, ethylic acid, methane carboxylic acid, vinegar acid, and glacial acetic acid. The various forms of acetic acid, especially vinegar acid (4% to 10% acetic acid) typically produce only minor ocular damage, unless exposure is prolonged. Exposure to a solution greater than 10% produces a severe injury unless the time of exposure is exceedingly short. "Essence of vinegar" (80% acetic acid) and glacial acetic acid (90%) are the most concentrated forms of acetic acid likely to produce severe ocular injury.

Toxic

Other types of chemical injuries of the eye are usually less severe than alkali and acid injuries. The reader is referred to Grant's (13) *Toxicology of the Eye* for a detailed discussion of the adverse ocular effects of petroleum products and other organic chemicals.

Chemical mace and similar compounds can cause minor to severe ocular injury, depending on a number of factors. These tear gas compounds are not under government regulatory control; hence considerable variability exists in commercially available products. Ocular injury associated with the original chemical mace is caused by the lacrimator chloroacetophenone. When possible, the exact product formulation should be obtained to determine if other toxic substances have been added. The degree of severity of reported injuries is related to proximity of the spray can to the eye, quantity of chemical entering the eye, duration of exposure, state of normal reflex mechanisms, and the mechanism of propelling the chemical, for example, solvent spray, pressurization, or explosion.

Police recommend directing the spray away from the eyes or at the eyes of unconscious individuals, and from a distance greater than 6 feet. Under these conditions only minor injury is likely to occur (13). If a larger quantity of the chemical is applied directly to the surface of the eye, especially in the absence of normal reflexes, severe injury may occur. Loss of ocular surface epithelium, severe persistent stromal edema, presumably secondary to endothelial damage, stromal clouding, and corneal neovascularization are among the resultant injuries.

The reader is referred to a comprehensive review of mustard gas injuries inflicted during military campaigns (14).

THE NATURAL SEQUENTIAL COURSE OF CHEMICAL INJURIES

Strong chemicals exert their destructive effect directly by damaging cellular and extracellular matrices and indirectly by initiating an inflammatory process that is not necessarily time-limited.

Some alkali can penetrate into the anterior chamber in 5 to 15 seconds, reaching a maximum in 2 to 3 minutes. The poor buffering capacity of anterior segment tissues and aqueous humor is rapidly overcome. There is a sudden, spiking rise in the intraocular pressure up to 20 to 40 mm Hg above normal lasting about 10 minutes, caused primarily by shrinkage of the collagenous envelope of the eye. A more prolonged rise in pressure quickly follows, secondary to prostaglandin release (15). Within 1 minute, the severe rise in aqueous humor pH causes lysis of corneal cells as well as those lining and adjacent to the anterior chamber, compromising the blood–aqueous barrier and releasing necrotic debris into the aqueous humor. This leads to a severe fibrinous inflammatory reaction in the entire anterior segment of the eye.

Glaucoma may ensue from inflammatory products accumulating in the aqueous humor and chamber angle, promoting closure by anterior synechiae, especially inferiorly. The travecular meshwork and ciliary body may be injured directly by penetration of alkali through the sclera or by contact with alkalotic aqueous humor percolating through the meshwork. Ocular hypertension or hypotension, or both, may occur at different time periods, depending on the predominance of one or more factors. Chemical injury to the iris, crystalline lens, and ciliary body may produce mydriasis, cataract, and even phthisis bulbi, respectively. Externally, this inflammatory reaction may be so profound as to lead to extensive symblephara and even ankyloblepharon from the apposition of raw conjunctival folds and

the inexorable scarring process, severely contracting the total conjunctival surface area.

REPAIR PROCESSES

Self-repair of the eye after a severe chemical injury is a complex process that involves both cellular and extracellular components of each tissue layer, including the eyelids, corneal and conjunctival epithelium, fibroblasts, collagen and glycosaminoglycans, endothelium, and all other tissues contiguous to the anterior chamber. The repair of each tissue is interdependent on other tissues, both contiguous and noncontiguous.

Epithelium

Destruction of the corneal epithelium alone in a mild injury might lead, at most, to a recurrent corneal erosion, resulting from injury to the basal lamina and anterior corneal stroma. When a portion of the limbal stem cells is destroyed, the remaining stem cell population heals first by the propagation of pluripotential epithelial stem cells around the corneal periphery and then by centripetal growth of transitional and daughter cells phenotypic for cornea. If the injury destroys the full thickness of the limbal palisades of Vogt, then the phenotypic source of corneal epithelium is lost. Under these circumstances, resurfacing the cornea requires that the remaining conjunctival epithelial cells must first spread over the collagenous tissues of Tenon's capsule or the subjacent episclera and then continue over corneal stroma. On the cornea, this rate of spread is initially similar to epithelial recovery occurring after a simple abrasion (16,17).

When the injury to the cornea is very severe, but the corneal epithelial stem cell population is left intact, then initial epithelial healing still usually proceeds at a rate similar to that when the stem cell population has been destroyed (16). An experimental alkali-injury of 12 mm, which did not destroy the limbal stem cells, showed substantial epithelial adhesion problems leading to persistent epithelial defects. At 84 hours, epithelial movement usually stops when the leading edge loses its adherence and then subsequently peels back from the stroma as a sheet (96 hours), thereafter maintaining a persistent epithelial defect. It has been suggested that this loss of epithelial adhesion might result from accelerated degradation of fibrinogen by plasminogen activator, a substance probably secreted in excessive amounts by the basal epithelial cells in the alkali-injured eye (18). Therefore, in the alkali-injured cornea, the presence of a normal corneal stem cell population does not necessarily imply that epithelial healing is assured. In fact, persistent epithelial defects might result from the consequences of a denatured framework of the stroma. Clearly, epithelial-stromal interaction plays an important role in the adhesion of epithelium to stroma.

Stroma

Healing of the corneal stroma in a timely manner is the key to avoidance of ulceration and perforation of the globe. Two events proceed simultaneously in the repair process: (a) degradation and removal of necrotic debris, and (b) replacement of portions of the fixed cells, collagenous matrix, and glycosaminoglycans (GAGs). Concentrated alkali exposure strips the cornea of its vital cells and GAG, leaving behind the skeletal framework of the collagen in a partially denatured form. Direct alkali hydrolysis of cellular and extracellular proteins yields inflammatory mediators, which are chemotactic to neutrophils (19). At high concentrations, these simple tripeptides, consisting of acetylated or methylated proline-glycine-proline, constitute powerful attractive agents that diffuse to the limbus where they initiate and promote neutrophilic invasion into the cornea within hours of the injury. This might represent one of the signals from the wound inducing the secretion of adhesion molecules from the vascular endothelium (E-selectin) and the intravascular leukocytes (L-selection) to incite leukocyte rolling, leading to adhesion to the vascular endothelium.

Once neutrophils accumulate they release leukotrienes, and the presence of interleukin-1α and -6 serves to recruit successive waves of inflammatory cells (20). These inflammatory components serve to perpetuate surface inflammation, with continued release of a variety of degradative enzymes including *N*-acetylglucosaminidase and cathepsin-D into the tissues and tear film. The positive side of neutrophil presence is the finding that they seem to stimulate epithelial proliferation when examined by their proliferative cellular nuclear expression (21). In this study neutrophils appear to act as the initiating messenger promoting the process of corneal vascularization.

Alkali-injury of collagen also releases a second inflammatory mediator (respiratory burst factor) that metabolically stimulates the neutrophils to undergo a respiratory burst. Prodigious oxygen utilization by the stimulated neutrophils results in the by-product superoxide radicals, an unstable form of oxygen that is highly destructive of tissues. When the mediator is present in excess there is extreme stimulation, causing neutrophil lysis with the release of granules containing a wide variety of enzymes. The release and activation of degrader enzymes from the specific and azurophilic granules of neutrophils act to destroy tissue by cleaving proteins and other molecular species. These responses serve to promote dissolution of the remaining corneal stroma, tipping the scales toward corneal ulceration and perforation.

Fibroblasts invading the cornea after severe alkali injuries are immature, with their polysomal systems in disarray. Collagen produced from these cells is underhydroxylated, preventing them from winding into the triple helical structure of normal collagen. The individual strands of amino acids are as vulnerable to enzymatic lysis as is the alkali-denatured collagen. These tissue characteristics are the sine qua non of localized tissue scorbutus (22). As a result of this ascorbate deficiency, the repair process is faulty, with the destruction-repair equation shifted in the direction of tissue disappearance, and hence corneal ulceration. In very severe injuries fibroblasts are slow to repopulate the cornea, or do not do so at all, resulting in rapid conversion of corneal stroma into a necrotic sequestrum.

Endothelium

In mild injuries, penetration of alkali is minimal and the endothelium is relatively unscathed. Moderate injuries probably cause some endothelial cell death but mostly interfere with the pump mechanism, leading to a variable degree of reversible corneal edema and endothelial cell loss. Severe injuries destroy endothelium, which leads to severe corneal thickening. The gain in corneal thickness from loss of endothelial cells might be counterbalanced by the simultaneous loss of GAG water binding capacity in the cornea, for little net gain or loss of thickness during the early stages.

ASSESSMENT OF CHEMICAL INJURIES: CLINICAL TECHNIQUE

Understanding and documenting the salient features of an alkali-injury of the eye permits proper classification so that appropriate immediate treatment can be initiated and accurate prognostication adduced. Documentation of the following physical data is recommended in the form of a labeled drawing:

1. Epithelial defect: Instill fluorescein and measure the size and draw the shape of the defect. It is critical to include any conjunctival epithelial defects, particularly with reference to the palisades of Vogt (stem cells). Document all defects including into the fornices.
2. Stromal opacity: Gradations are made on the basis of a penlight examination: grade 0, clear cornea; grade 1, mild corneal haze; grade 2, mild to moderate opacity; grade 3, moderate opacity; grade 4, moderate to severe opacity, details of iris trabeculae cannot be seen but pupil visible; grade 5, severe corneal opacity, pupil not visible with penlight.
3. Perilimbal ischemia: Document the clock hours where the conjunctiva is whitened. In these areas the conjunctiva and episclera are devoid of blood vessels. This whitening is not to be confused with less severe injury where there is chemosis and thrombosed blood vessels but some of the conjunctiva is still viable. Although not originally understood when the criteria were formulated,

perilimbal whitening has proved to be a useful parameter by which to judge the extent of corneal stem cell damage and, indirectly, injury of the underlying ciliary body and trabecular meshwork. Documentation of these findings allow for a later, more accurate determination of the necessity for corneal stem cell transplantation.

4. Adnexa: The blinking pattern, exposure, and/or lagophthalmos should be measured and documented.

These measurements and findings can then be applied to the classification of alkali-injuries as described by Hughes and modified by Pfister and Koski (23). This classification, with accompanying drawings and photographs, represents the span of damage encountered after alkali-injury (Fig. 43-2). The accuracy of early assessment becomes very important in subsequent evaluation and treatment plans.

Regarding terminology, the literature is replete with allusions to alkali "burns," potentially confusing the alkali-injury terminology with a thermal component that often does not exist. Herein we recommend the designation *alkali injury* or *acid injury of the eye* to distinguish chemical from true thermal burns. When both injuries occur simultaneously, then the term *alkali-thermal injury* or *thermal-alkali injury* might be used, with what is thought to be the most prominent injurious agent stated first. Acid injuries should be referred to in a similar way.

TREATMENT OPTIONS AFTER CHEMICAL INJURY

Emergency Medical Treatment

The harm caused by alkali-injury is predicated on the concentration of the cation, in the case of acid, the anion, the duration of exposure, the pH of the solution, and both the extent and specific areas of ocular tissue exposure. Although it may be helpful to determine the pH in the inferior cul-de-sac by using litmus paper before irrigation, under no circumstances should irrigation be delayed to accomplish this. To remove the chemical agent from the external eye, immediate irrigation of the eye with available water at the scene of the accident and in the medical aid station or emergency room for 1 to 2 hours is thereafter wise. The value of litmus paper to monitor the effectiveness of irrigation has never been subjected to scientific inquiry. If available, litmus paper might be used to give a rough estimate of the pH value, bearing in mind that pH levels of less than 10 are reported to be compatible with cell survival (10). The effectiveness of this technique alone to reduce the alkali concentration in the corneal stroma and aqueous humor after a severe alkali injury is open to question. Studies on the effect of 90 minutes of external irrigation on intraocular pH in an animal model have shown only a 1.5-pH-unit reduction from an elevated pH (8). Removal of the aqueous by paracentesis lowers the pH by 1.5 pH units. Reformation of the aqueous humor with

buffered phosphate solution lowers the pH by an additional 1.5 pH units. It is premature to suggest that all severe alkali-injuries should undergo paracentesis. However, in the absence of strict scientific information, it is reasonable to suggest that in severe injuries, occurring 1 to 2 hours previously, that paracentesis and removal of an aliquot of aqueous humor be performed if specialized facilities and personnel are available. This can be accomplished at the slit lamp or in the minor operating room suite. Under topical anesthesia, a razor blade fragment or commercially available supersharp blade can create a partial-thickness, self-sealing tunnel at the limbus down which a 25-gauge needle is inserted, finally penetrating into the anterior chamber. If available, it is preferable to replace the aqueous humor with a buffered phosphate solution or balanced salt solution to reduce the intraocular pH to near normal levels.

There are several chemical injuries that require special treatment. For example the pultaceous character of lime used in cement compounds clings to the conjunctiva. The bulk of material can be removed with a cotton-tip applicator, but the sticky paste in contact with the conjunctiva can be removed with greater ease by irrigation with a solution of ethylenediaminetetraacetic acid (EDTA) of 0.01 M.

The intraocular pressure rise after alkali injury can usually be treated by topical alpha and/or beta blockers, prostaglandin analogs, and topical or systemically administered carbonic anhydrase inhibitors. Rarely are intravenous hyperosmotic agents required. If the pressure fails to respond, immediate control of an acute pressure rise can be achieved by paracentesis at the limbus, under topical anesthesia, followed by periodic release of aqueous humor, for 1 or 2 days, through a beveled incision made at the slit lamp or in the minor surgical suite.

The presence of necrotic tissue in the eye gives rise to inflammatory mediators that attract neutrophils into the damaged cornea and stimulate the full range of enzyme and metabolic products destructive to even the remaining normal tissues. To avert some of these devastating consequences, careful excision of necrotic tissues might be carried out to reduce the mediator load encouraging this process (19).

The degree of eyelid dysfunction after alkali injury is usually dependent on the severity of orbital and periorbital skin and conjunctival injury. Immediately after injury and for several days, eyelid edema makes eye observations difficult. The eyelid position and periodic blinking required to resurface the exposed cornea and conjunctiva with tears is usually disturbed, at least temporarily, even in the mildest injuries. More often, the intense blepharospasm and photophobia induced by a more severe injury persist until the inflammatory or ulcerative process has subsided, sometimes only after years. Some injuries can render the skin white or resemble third-degree thermal burns with surface crusting and eventual sloughing of eyelid tissue.

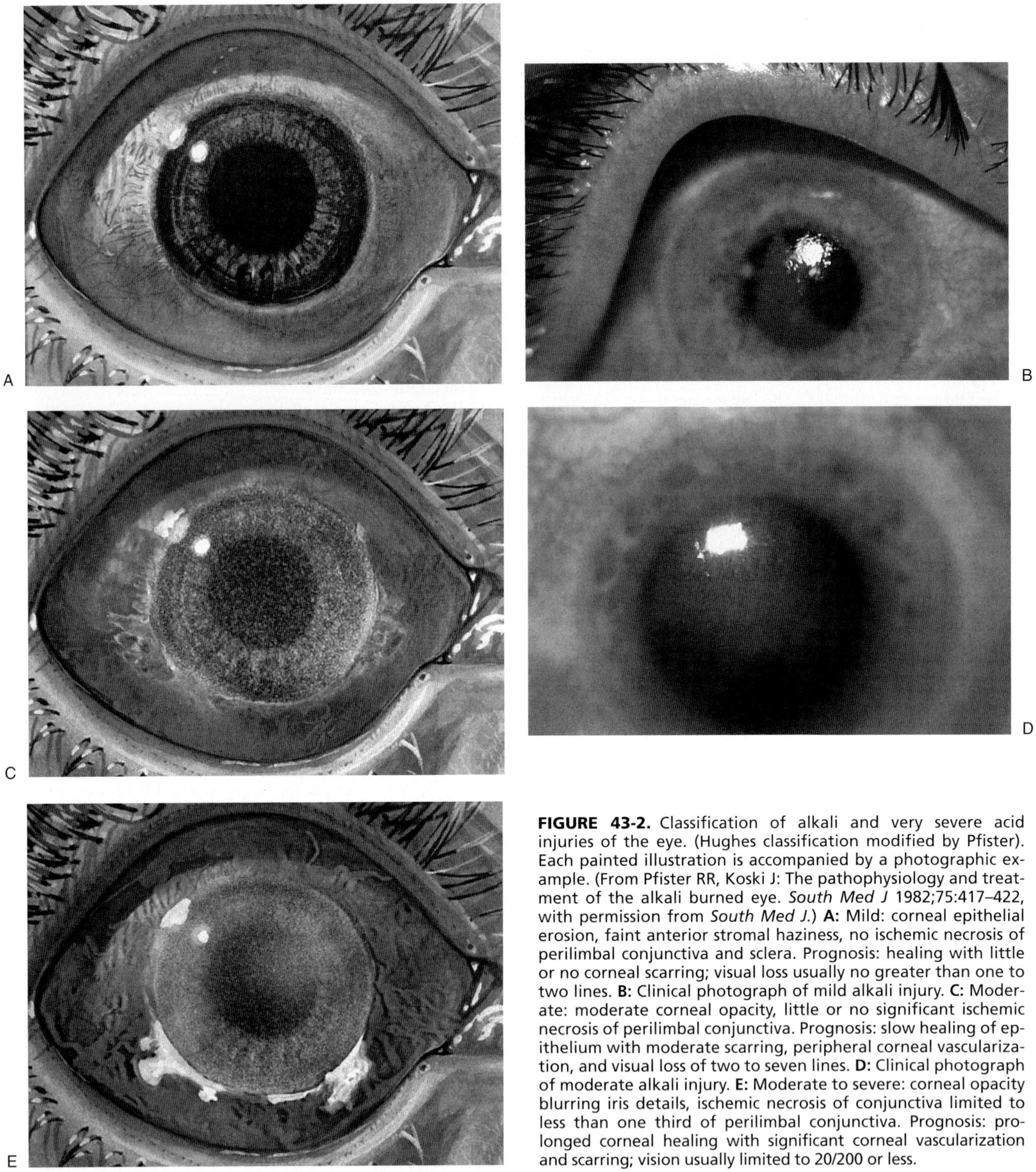

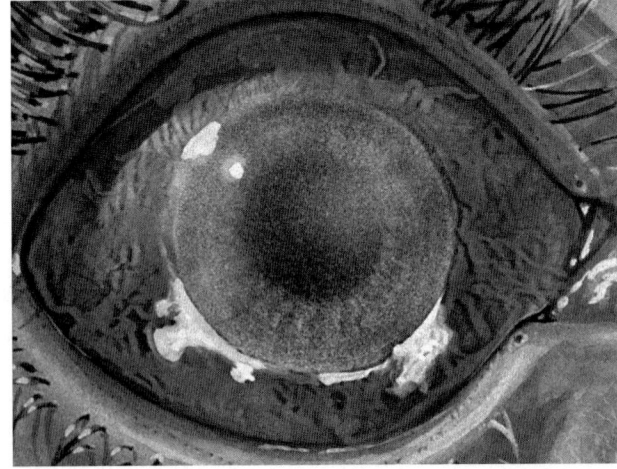

FIGURE 43-2. Classification of alkali and very severe acid injuries of the eye. (Hughes classification modified by Pfister). Each painted illustration is accompanied by a photographic example. (From Pfister RR, Koski J: The pathophysiology and treatment of the alkali burned eye. *South Med J* 1982;75:417–422, with permission from *South Med J*.) **A:** Mild: corneal epithelial erosion, faint anterior stromal haziness, no ischemic necrosis of perilimbal conjunctiva and sclera. Prognosis: healing with little or no corneal scarring; visual loss usually no greater than one to two lines. **B:** Clinical photograph of mild alkali injury. **C:** Moderate: moderate corneal opacity, little or no significant ischemic necrosis of perilimbal conjunctiva. Prognosis: slow healing of epithelium with moderate scarring, peripheral corneal vascularization, and visual loss of two to seven lines. **D:** Clinical photograph of moderate alkali injury. **E:** Moderate to severe: corneal opacity blurring iris details, ischemic necrosis of conjunctiva limited to less than one third of perilimbal conjunctiva. Prognosis: prolonged corneal healing with significant corneal vascularization and scarring; vision usually limited to 20/200 or less.

Alkali destruction of conjunctival epithelium, in combination with the inflammatory reaction, causes fibrinous adhesions that must be opened periodically under topical anesthesia. A glass rod or a cotton-tip applicator, wet in saline, helps to separate these tissues and remove fibrinous membranes. When extensive damage of the conjunctiva has occurred, fibrous proliferation in the subconjunctival tissues shrinks the surface area of the conjunctiva and promotes the formation of symblephara, particularly by contact between the raw surfaces of naturally apposed conjunctiva. In the most severe cases the eyelids become scarred to the globe (ankyloblepharon), causing the exposed cornea to dry with resultant epithelial defects, leading to neutrophilic infiltration, ulceration, and eventually perforation.

Prophylactic approaches to maintain eyelid mobility and limit conjunctival and fornical contracture are of unproven

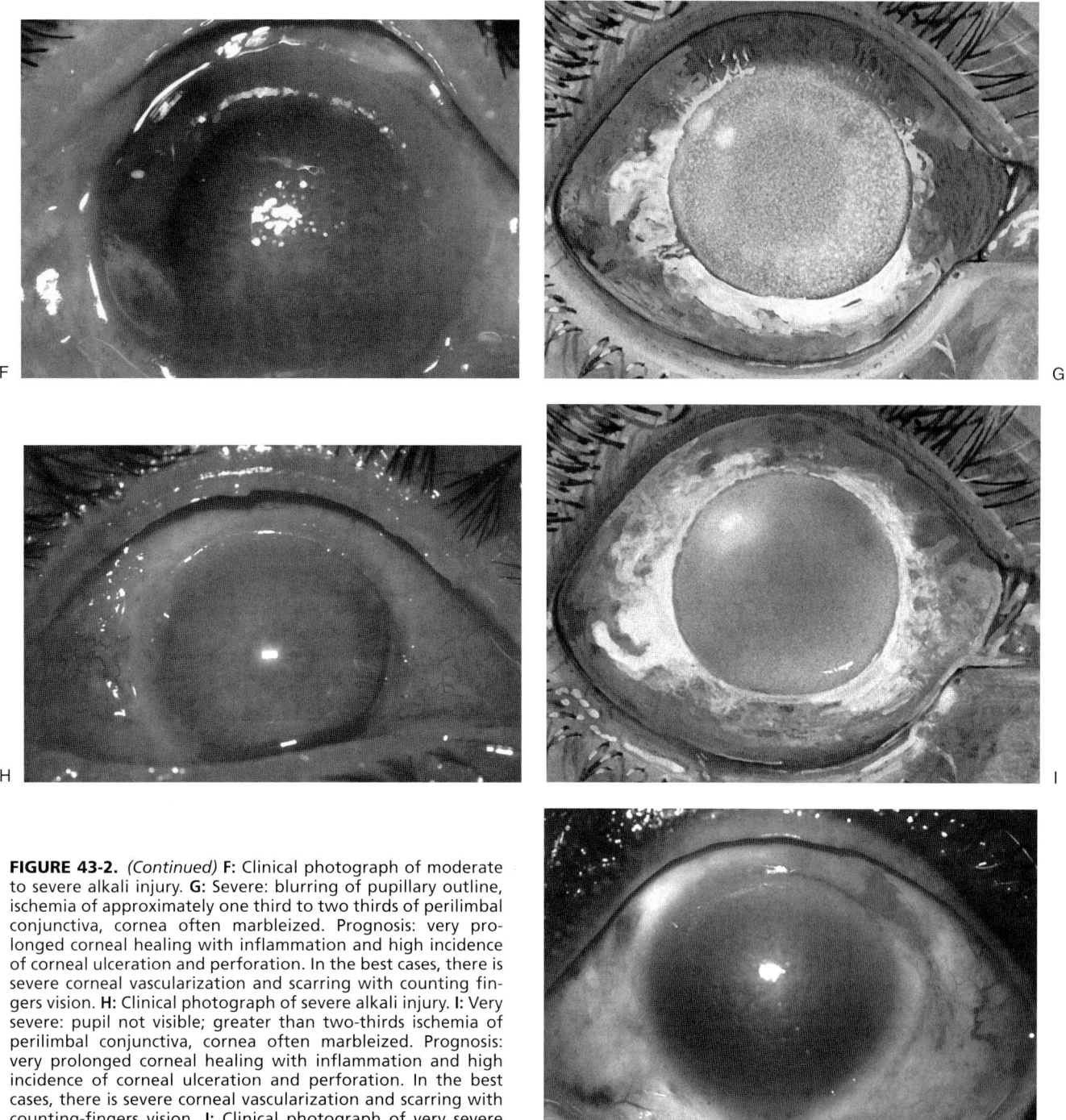

FIGURE 43-2. *(Continued)* **F:** Clinical photograph of moderate to severe alkali injury. **G:** Severe: blurring of pupillary outline, ischemia of approximately one third to two thirds of perilimbal conjunctiva, cornea often marbleized. Prognosis: very prolonged corneal healing with inflammation and high incidence of corneal ulceration and perforation. In the best cases, there is severe corneal vascularization and scarring with counting fingers vision. **H:** Clinical photograph of severe alkali injury. **I:** Very severe: pupil not visible; greater than two-thirds ischemia of perilimbal conjunctiva, cornea often marbleized. Prognosis: very prolonged corneal healing with inflammation and high incidence of corneal ulceration and perforation. In the best cases, there is severe corneal vascularization and scarring with counting-fingers vision. **J:** Clinical photograph of very severe alkali injury.

value. These consist of lining the palpebral conjunctiva with a thin plastic wrap, which is secured by sutures passing through the upper and lower fornices. When lid mobility has already been compromised by scarring, re-created tissue planes can seldom be covered by rearrangement of existing conjunctiva. In the absence of natural conjunctiva, coverage of these raw areas with split-thickness mucus membrane, obtained from the mouth, might have a better chance of remaining open. Unfortunately the phenotype of buccal

mucosal epithelium is not conducive to any subsequent efforts to rehabilitate the eye by corneal transplantation. Most recently the use of amniotic membrane has found use in expanding the conjunctival surface. When ankyloblepharon is present, any known effort to reconstitute a semblance of the natural conjunctival environment, for the purpose of preparation for corneal transplantation, has been unsuccessful.

Pain management during this stage of the disease is not complicated. The pain at the time of injury is excruciating but usually short-lived. Pain receptors are destroyed by the alkali, hence they do not continue to transmit a pain response. When necessary, pain control might be required for several days, rarely longer than 1 week. Photophobia, however, can be extreme, creating a painful environment that can be improved only with UV protective, dark, wraparound sunglasses or complete exclusion of ambient light.

New Concepts of Treatment

Transitional-Stage Medical Treatment

The transitional-stage treatment of the alkali-injured eye begins as early as 1 to 2 weeks in milder injuries and as late as 1 to 2 months in more severe cases. Problems such as epithelial defects, inflammation and ulceration, glaucoma, symblephara, and eyelid dysfunction might appear or continue from the acute stage through the subacute to the chronic stage imperceptibly and without interruption.

Epithelium

The healing of a corneal epithelial defect after alkali injury is largely predicated upon the severity of the injury and the extent of perilimbal injury. Part of the significance of perilimbal injury is the finding that the stem cell phenotype for corneal epithelial cells resides deep within a narrow band of cells located on, and partially straddling, the limbus. Loss of some portion of the stem cells requires that corneal epithelium be repopulated from the geographically distant remaining stem cells. If all corneal stem cells have been destroyed, then corneal reepithelialization proceeds from the viable edge of the conjunctival epithelium with cells phenotypic for conjunctiva. If the conjunctival stem cells, located, in part, in the fornices, are also destroyed, then the de-epithelialized and inflamed conjunctival surfaces are likely to result in extensive symblephara or ankyloblepharon. At this time there are no data regarding conjunctival stem cell replacement.

The formulation and frequency of applied medications used during this period can be toxic to fresh epithelium covering the alkali-injured cornea. Preservatives, such as benzalkonium chloride and ointments, especially containing lanolin, can perpetuate or create epithelial defects. It is wise to avoid topical treatment with multiple medications in the hope of preventing corneal ulceration when there is no clear-cut indication to do so. At most, initial treatment with an antibiotic (q.i.d.) and cycloplegic (b.i.d.) is indicated.

Soft contact lenses are of limited benefit in chemical injuries. The expectation that these lenses would promote epithelial healing in persistent defects has not been fully realized. Much of this failure is traceable to corneal stem cell destruction and the consequent invasion of conjunctival epithelial cells on to the cornea. The solution here is to repopulate the cornea with corneal stem cells, placed surgically. There are some instances, however, when a soft contact lenses might combat persistent drying effects or exposure from improper blinking, and hence encourage epithelial migration onto the corneal surface. Soft contact lenses, therefore, can act to facilitate epithelialization but prove inadequate to solve basic epithelial problems. After fitting the lens, evaluation of its effectiveness in promoting epithelial healing and integrity may be difficult to accomplish. The lens can be taken off briefly, and fluorescein can be used to determine the size of the residual defect. In general, the therapeutic soft lens must be left in place for at least 6 to 8 weeks after the epithelium has healed to ensure adequate adhesion between the epithelium and its underlying substrate. Frequent tear supplementation with preservative free fluid helps to maintain lens hydration and hence movement.

Inflammation and Corneal Ulceration

Alkali injury of the cornea has been shown to trigger the release of inflammatory mediators, which are believed to be responsible for chemoattraction and subsequent activation of neutrophils within the corneal stroma. The density of the neutrophil infiltrate appears to be directly related to the severity of the injury and to the likelihood of subsequent ulceration. Although all cells of the cornea have been shown to be capable of releasing a broad spectrum of enzymes destructive of collagen and glycosaminoglycans, the presence of enormous numbers of neutrophils and absence of any other cells in significant numbers suggest that neutrophils and their products are the major cellular elements associated with ulceration.

Historically, treatment of ulcers resulting from alkali injuries has been directed at the inhibition of type I collagenase, produced by keratocytes, and capable of cleavage of the collagen molecule into one-quarter, three-quarter fragments. Newer data have identified the collagenases as a family of enzymes, referred to as matrix metalloproteinases (MMPs) and consisting of collagenase type I (MMP-1 degrades type I, II, and III collagen), stromelysin (MMP-3 degrades casein, proteoglycan, and fibronectin, and to a limited extent laminin, elastin, gelatin, and type IV collagen), and gelatinase (MMP-9 degrades gelatin, type IV, V, and VI collagen and fibronectin) (21). When activated, this full array of enzymes is available to degrade both the residual normal cornea as well as denatured corneal matrix (24).

Although controversy still exists, acetylcysteine, L-cysteine, and EDTA all have been reported to inhibit mammalian collagenase *in vitro* and significantly reduce the incidence of ulceration in animal corneas after alkali injuries. In contrast, one study in extreme alkali-injured animal eyes showed no favorable effect of acetylcysteine when compared to control eyes (81% versus 75%) (25). In an open clinical study, L-cysteine (0.2 M solution) was begun on the seventh day after a "total" alkali injury in 33 human eyes, and only one eye perforated (26). An alkali injury study including 28 human eyes substantiated the favorable effect of L-cysteine in the acute stage, in the presence of an ulcer, and before or after corneal transplantation. In 35 patients with corneal ulceration (diseases unspecified) treated with 0.2 M EDTA, 86% healed or remained unchanged compared to 46% of the 26 control eyes (27). Cysteine and acetylcysteine (20%) are both effective inhibitors of collagenase, but the latter has the advantage of greater stability and is already marketed as a mucolytic agent used in intermittent positive breathing apparatus. Although it is suspected that acetylcysteine has a favorable effect in some human alkali-injured corneas, this has not yet been proven by clinical trial.

The use of topical steroids after chemical injury is controversial. If used for the first 7 days after injury, it is believed to decrease the inflammatory reaction of the entire anterior segment, possibly reducing some of the late side effects, such as glaucoma (28). This article reported that if used for longer than 10 days, topical steroids might interfere with the repair process and therefore enhance the opportunity for corneal ulceration and perforation. Subsequent research in human eyes by Davis et al. (29) has confirmed that when topical steroids are accompanied by simultaneous use of 10% topical ascorbate hourly and 1 g of ascorbate orally per day, ulceration is statistically diminished if used up to the time of corneal reepithelialization. Oral steroids pose potential systemic complications as well as providing comparatively poor corneal and intraocular steroid levels when compared to topical administration. Their use, therefore, is inadvisable.

A surgical emergency arises when a leaking descemetocele or frank perforation supervene. If the perforation is smaller than 1.0 mm in diameter (the ulcer bed itself is usually much larger) and relatively free of blood vessels, then adhesive closure with isobutylcyanoacrylate is the least invasive and the most effective way of reestablishing the integrity of the eye (30). A soft contact lens diminishes the discomfort of the adhesive. The adhesive remains in place for 2 to 10 weeks after which it falls off, or is loosened enough to be picked off with a jeweler's forceps. Large corneal ulcerations and perforations require a fresh corneal patch graft to replace tissue lost from ulceration. The ulcer bed and edges are cleaned of epithelium and inflammatory debris. Necrotic tissue is excised from the edges and base to create a viable bed of stroma into which the transplanted tissue is positioned. The donor patch graft is trephined about 0.5 mm larger than the greatest diameter of the recipient bed, trimmed during the suturing procedure to fit the contours of the ulcer bed, and fastened to the edges of the ulcer with interrupted sutures of 10-0 nylon with their knots buried into the stroma (31).

Glaucoma

Any chemical agent might damage the trabecular meshwork directly, or necrotic and inflammatory debris can clog the outflow channels. Organization of this inflammatory sediment in the anterior chamber results in fibroproliferation, collagen retraction, and the formation of anterior synechiae, further embarrassing outflow facility.

Treatment of this type of glaucoma consists mainly of diminishing aqueous production. Topical or oral carbonic anhydrase inhibitors and topical beta blockers continue to form the mainstay of intraocular pressure control. Alpha blockers and prostaglandin analogs are also likely to control pressure in alkali injuries, but reports of their success have not yet surfaced. Severe scarring of the perilimbal and bulbar conjunctiva, combined with foreshortening of the fornices, makes filtration surgery problematical. Cautious use of fibroblast inhibiting agents such as mitomycin C can improve success significantly. If one or more filtration surgeries fail, or are doomed to failure, then the use of translimbal intraocular setons, linked to equatorial filtration plates, offers an effective way to siphon aqueous humor from an intractably glaucomatous eye.

Surgical Treatment

Tenon-plasty

Alkali injured eyes and anterior segment necrosis share a similar fate of vascular insufficiency. To improve vascular support of the anterior segment in alkali-injured eyes, Reim et al. (32) have popularized excision of necrotic conjunctiva and advancement of viable Tenon's capsule, the latter obtained by careful dissection to preserve the posterior vascular supply. The procedure, referred to as tenonplasty, prevented or arrested corneal ulceration in 24 eyes of 21 patients sustaining severe alkali injury.

Amniotic Membrane

The use of amniotic membrane in ocular surface disease, and ophthalmic operations in general, has expanded considerably. Its longevity is variable but its presence, even for a temporary period, can materially improve the outcome. When spread on the inflamed ocular surface, amniotic membrane significantly decreases inflammation in the underlying tissues and provides a new substratum for the growth of epithelial cells over its surface. Amniotic membrane does not take the place of stem cells of the cornea or conjunctiva after a severe chemical injury where all corneal stem cells are destroyed (33). When living donors provide corneal stem cell tissue, 68.75% success is achieved. Covering the cornea with amniotic membrane in partial stem cell deficiency gave 100% success in four cases. Amniotic membrane and autologous stem cell tissue, obtained from the other healthy eye, reestablished a normal ocular surface in five patients (83.3%). It is best used as an adjunctive procedure in stem cell deficiency by covering the cornea and any adjacent raw areas with amnion, even those created after synechialysis. Stem cell replacements can then be surgically placed into the limbal niche where they can actively proliferate. That the corneal epithelial phenotype of the donor is maintained after 6 months has recently been demonstrated by immunohistochemical methods (34).

Corneal Epithelial Stem Cell Replacement

Replacement of the corneal stem cells lost from disease or injury is a new and exciting surgical procedure (35–37). If the injury is monocular, then autotransplantation of corneal limbal stem cells from the uninjured eye offers an opportunity to replenish the stem cell supply autogenously (Fig. 43-3). The use of lenticular grafts, pioneered by Thoft (35) at the Massachusetts Eye and Ear Infirmary in Boston, led the way to a variety of surgical approaches to replenish the corneal stem cell population from related or unrelated donors. When the injury is bilateral, research by Pfister (37) indicated that allografted limbal tissue was capable of restoring the stem cell population from an unrelated donor (Fig. 43-4). Replacement of the entire cornea and adjacent stem cells by penetrating keratoplasty has been performed successfully and reported in two different series. Kuckelkorn et al. (38) replaced the entire cornea in sterile, ulcerating, alkali-injured eyes, preserving an intact epithelium and absence of ulceration over a 1-year period. Redbrake et al. (39) reported nine eyes operated this way, preserving the epithelium but maintaining clarity in only two. Nevertheless, under the circumstances, these results should be considered a success. One potential danger might be that such large transplants might interfere with the trabecular outflow channels and hence increase the likelihood of glaucoma. In a separate study the use of a 12- or 13-mm lamellar corneal transplant, including the limbal epithelial stem cell population, managed to restore the epithelial integrity, without complications, in an average of 5.2 days (40). Lamellar keratoplasty performed in this way, an average of 29.5 months after injury, might gain all the advantages of replacement of the cornea and associated stem cells but reduce the chance of consequent glaucoma by preserving some of the outflow channels. An alternative approach in the case of deep corneal ulceration, desmetocele, or frank corneal perforation would be to suture a piece of cornea into the ulcerated bed to reestablish integrity of the globe.

The optimal medical and surgical conditions necessary to promote allografted corneal stem cell growth and to protect them from the immune process is currently being investigated. It is clear, however, that immunosuppression of some type is required to sustain the vitality of these allografted tissues. As an adjunct, amniotic membrane stretched over the alkali-injured cornea has proved to be useful when transplanting corneal stem cells by replacing the abnormal surface of the cornea with a new surface tending to quiet the inflammatory process (41,42). Amniotic membrane alone does not substitute for corneal stem cells in a severe alkali injury where there is a stem cell deficiency or loss. The advent of *in vitro* techniques to culture and expand corneal stem cells might soon provide a new and immunologically more suitable source of corneal stem cells (43).

REHABILITATION OF VISION

General

The prospects for restoration of vision after chemical injury have been substantially improved over the past decade. To achieve success, it is imperative that the intraocular and extraocular *milieu* be favorable to support the special conditions required for corneal transplantation. Success in any type of restorative surgery will be governed by (a) lid–globe congruity with normal blinking and the absence of corneal exposure; (b) sufficient resurfacing of the tear film layer to which a transplanted cornea can adapt; (c) the presence of epithelial stem cells

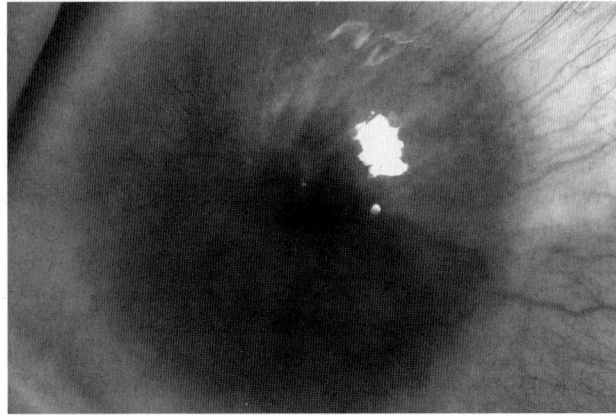
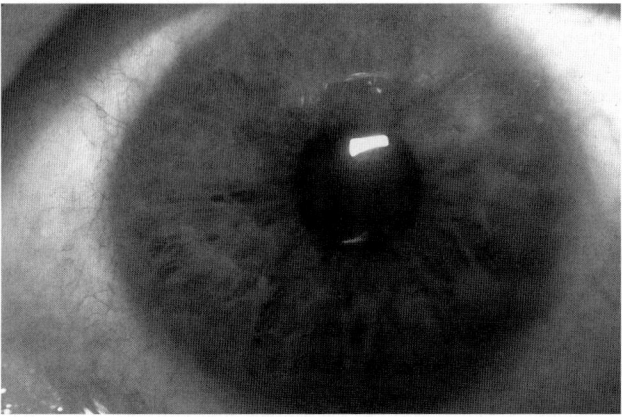

A

B

FIGURE 43-3. A: A moderate alkali-injury caused corneal stem cell deficiency, resulting in vascular overgrowth of the cornea. The underlying corneal stroma was seen to be clear. **B:** Corneal stem cell replacement from the other eye reestablished the corneal phenotype; resulting in a clear cornea.

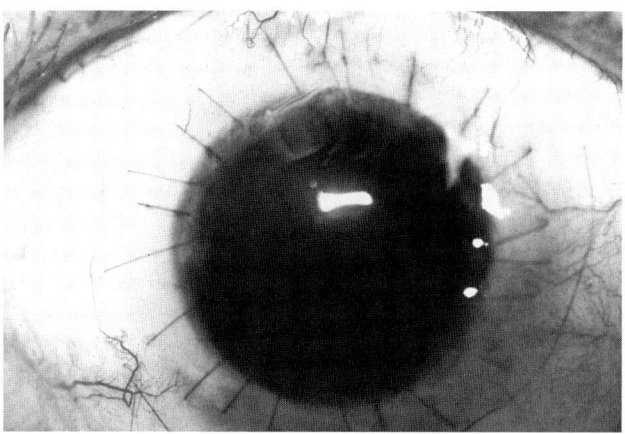

FIGURE 43-4. The patient has undergone corneal stem cell replacement after an alkali injury that left him stem cell deficient. A ring of phenotypically corneal stem cells, of donor origin, has been sutured around the limbus. Note the continuous vertical mattress suture placed circumferentially in the perilimbal zone. Four months after corneal stem cell replacement a successful corneal transplant was performed and then photographed at 10 months postoperatively.

phenotypic for cornea; (d) the absence of any current ulceration, inflammation, or uncontrolled glaucoma; (e) flawless surgical technique; and (f) fresh corneal transplant tissue.

Preparatory procedures to lyse symblephara, expand cul-de-sacs, and eliminate lagophthalmos are often required to reestablish normal lid physiology and anatomy. Secondary glaucoma must also be controlled with medications, cyclocryothermy, or filtration surgery. Laser of large feeder vessels at the limbus may be done preoperatively to reduce vascular supply and to reduce bleeding at the time of surgery.

If corneal surgery is delayed 18 months to 2 years after a chemical burn, it increases the chances of success, especially without preexisting ulceration, perforation, or glaucoma (44). Corneal surgery is indicated for the worse eye in bilateral burns when serviceable vision is not available. In some patients with severe monocular injuries, if a definite need for binocularity does not exist, corneal transplantation might not be contemplated, because transplantation in chemically burned eyes is fraught with numerous potential complications.

If corneal transplantation is indicated, it is important to pay meticulous attention to the rigorous protocol of fine corneal surgery. A few points of importance will be mentioned. Trephination with a vacuum cutter and vertical section of remaining attachments with scissors improves the quality of the wound architecture. If suction cannot be achieved due to surface irregularity, layering a ring of viscoelastic on the peripheral cornea usually assists vacuum adherence. Absorb fresh blood from the wound edges with cellulose sponges, applying pressure to active bleeders by squeezing with fine-toothed forceps until it stops or until

suture placement closes the vessel. Even light applications of wet-field cautery cause wound retraction, hence it should be used sparingly, if at all.

The donor cornea should be fresh, with intact epithelium, cut 0.50 to 0.75 mm larger than the recipient bed. Oversizing the donor corneal button by 0.5 mm or even 0.75 mm compensates for retraction of the scarred and vascularized recipient bed. Donor tissue is age-matched but human leukocyte antigen (HLA) or blood typing is not usually done for the first transplant. A single continuous 10-0 nylon suture might be used if the recipient corneal tissue is firm and of near-normal thickness with mild vascularity. When the quality of the recipient bed is soft or friable, then it is generally safer to use 24 interrupted sutures, eight more than the number usually employed. This is especially true for more extensively vascularized or thin corneas. The knots must be buried to avoid epithelial defects and limit portals for infection. Occasionally it is necessary to thicken the recipient bed by a lamellar graft in preparation for penetrating keratoplasty, approximately 3 to 6 months later.

When a cataract is present, it is usually wisest to remove it at the time of corneal surgery. Cataract surgery should follow modern techniques with special emphasis on the approach to the open eye. If preoperative pressure devices reduce the vitreous volume such that the crystalline lens has no tendency to prolapse forward, then a curvilinear capsulorhexis (CCR) can be performed. Efforts to create a CCR, in the presence of positive vitreous pressure, usually results in a radial tear that, if it crosses the equator, can result in zonular dehiscence, posterior capsular tear, and possibly vitreous loss. To avert this, if positive vitreous pressure is noted, a "can-opener" technique should be employed. In either case, hydrodissection of the lens usually prolapses the lens nucleus for easy removal. Cortical cleanup with irrigation and aspiration and intracapsular placement of an intraocular lens can then be accomplished. Choice of the intraocular lens should be dictated by haptic design, namely torsional strength, slight anterior angulation (15 degrees), easy collapsability, and null anteroposterior movement on linear collapse. The B&L model 122uv fulfills these requirements and can be used in the anterior as well as the posterior chamber.

In the immediate postoperative period, my own preference is to patch the eye continuously for 3 to 4 weeks and allow progressive air exposure while monitoring the quality of corneal surface. Later, if epithelial defects are noted, a soft contact lens can be fitted for continuous wear or a one- or two-pillar tarsorrhaphy performed. It is critical to remove interrupted sutures that become loose or break through the epithelium as soon as it occurs.

In the most severe cases, implantation of a keratoprosthesis might afford the only means by which vision can be restored (45) (Fig. 43-5). Corneas exhibiting exuberant vascularity, repeated failures of fresh transplanted corneal

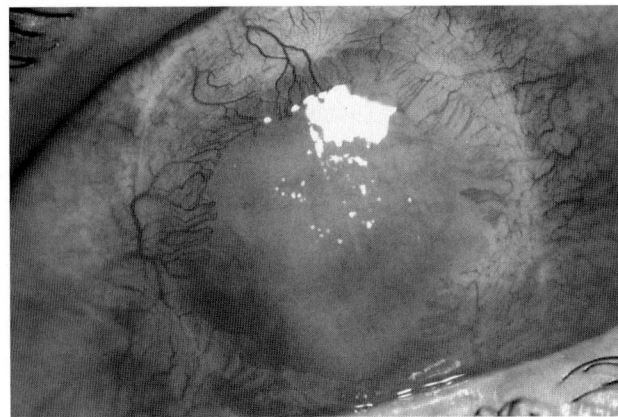
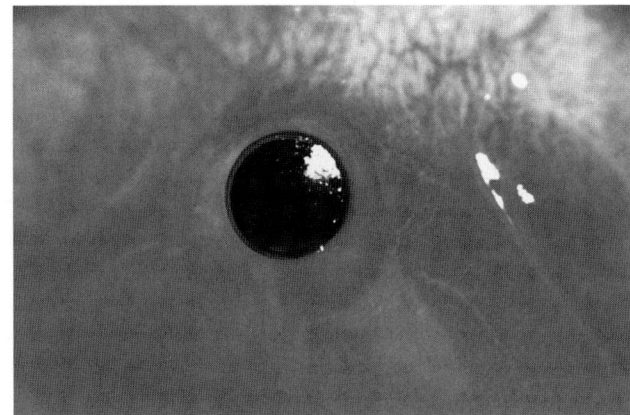

A

B

FIGURE 43-5. **A:** Repeated corneal transplants failed to restore vision to this severe alkali-injured eye with extensive scarring and vascularization. **B:** Keratoprosthesis implantation resulted in 20/50 visual acuity.

tissue, and the inability to restore normal lid anatomy are potential indications for this procedure. The operation is advisable only in those with severe bilateral injuries where serviceable vision is not present in either eye. All currently available devices are investigational and are difficult to implant. Despite this a surprising degree of success has been achieved, but this must be balanced against the sometimes serious and untreatable complications that can occur.

THE FUTURE OF CHEMICAL TRAUMA TREATMENT

Our concept of the basic biochemical, physiologic, and anatomic changes in the anterior segment of the eye after alkali injury has matured substantially in recent years. This has been driven by the evolution of the disciplines of molecular biology and biochemistry as applied to ocular disease. As a result, we are now employing orthomolecular approaches to supplement our traditional treatment.

Ascorbate Treatment

The ascorbic acid level is depressed to one third of normal in the rabbit model of severe alkali injury to the eye. Topical (hourly for 12 hours a day or subcutaneously (once daily) administered ascorbate (10%) significantly decreased the incidence of corneal ulcerations and perforations. If the aqueous humor ascorbate level was elevated to 15 mg/dL or greater, then corneal ulceration or perforation was abolished (22). Light and electron microscopy and radioactive tracer experiments showed that the mechanism by which ascorbate accomplished this was to replenish ascorbic acid to the scorbutic fibroblasts of the cornea. Among its many roles ascorbate is required by fibroblasts to act as a reducing agent, converting proline to hydroxyproline, while the collagen molecule is being fabricated in

the rough endoplasmic reticulum. Ascorbate deficiency results in the production of underhydroxylated collagen, which collects within these immature cells and, if discharged from the cell, fails to form into the normal triple helical structure of collagen. In this state it is also very vulnerable to the plenitude of degradative enzymes. Replenishing these corneal fibroblasts with ascorbate allows collagen synthesis to proceed, promoting healing of damaged corneal tissues, and reducing the incidence of corneal ulceration.

Citrate Treatment

Citrate (10%), applied topically as drops, has been shown to be extremely effective in decreasing the incidence of corneal ulceration after alkali-injury of the animal eye (25). Citrate-treated eyes encountered ulceration in 21% of eyes, whereas control eyes suffered an 80% ulceration incidence. To understand this phenomenon, recognize that virtually all the activities of the neutrophil require calcium acting as an important intracellular second messenger within the cell. The major stores of calcium in the neutrophil are maintained on the plasma membrane. In this location the cell is uniquely vulnerable to calcium depletion from its environment. Citrate is a powerful chelator of extracellular calcium; hence it is capable of stripping calcium off the neutrophil plasma membrane. Inhibition of the neutrophils, through calcium depletion, may be caused by interference with calcium-calmodulin microfilament or microtubule interfaces in the plasma membrane (46). Hence, topical treatment with citrate can entirely halt neutrophil activities.

Citrate also inhibits the efferent limb of the inflammatory response by interfering with the adherence of neutrophils to vascular endothelium. If neutrophils fail to adhere to vascular endothelium, then the process of neutrophil extravasation is halted. In essence this effect decreases the migration of neutrophils from the perilimbal arcades into the damaged cornea, thus diminishing the load of hydrolytic enzymes potentially discharged into the corneal stroma.

Combination Ascorbate and Citrate Treatment

Ascorbate and citrate, when used separately, reduce the incidence of corneal ulceration in alkali-injured eyes by radically different mechanisms. This accounts for the substantial further reduction in corneal ulceration in alkali-injured animals when ascorbate (10%) and citrate (10%) topical drops are used on alternate hours. Corneal ulcers from an untreated control was 80% compared to a transitory 4.6%, consisting of very superficial ulcers, when citrate and ascorbate eye drops were alternated concurrently throughout a 12-hour day (47).

The strategy of combined therapy with ascorbate and citrate has been subjected to a human clinical trial. Using the Roper-Hall modification of Hughes classification of alkali-injuries Brodovsky et al. (48) showed that grade III injuries treated with a combination of ascorbate, citrate, and fluorometholone (FML) attained vision of 20/40 or better in the treated group including 27 of 29 eyes (93%), compared to three of six eyes in the control group. There was also a trend toward shorter hospital stays in the treatment group. Specific topical treatment consisted of 10% ascorbate, 10% citrate, and FML every 2 hours, day and night, 1% atropine t.i.d., and chloramphenicol q.i.d. To this was added 500 mg ascorbate q.i.d. and 4 g of a proprietary urinary alkalinizer containing 720 mg of citric acid anhydrous and 620 mg of sodium citrate anhydrous t.i.d. In none of the other groups is there any statistical differences between the treated and control groups. The power of this combination treatment was clearly evident in this study.

Other Treatments

Other putative treatments to prevent corneal ulceration in severe alkali injury, such as oral tetracycline, subconjunctival progesterone, intramuscular nortestosterone, and thiol dipeptides have all shown favorable effects in animal models of alkali injuries. However, a clinical trial will be needed before any of these approaches can be considered for routine human use.

Fibronectin has been implicated as a key element in wound healing for its involvement in cell-to-cell and cell-to-matrix adhesion and cell spreading. Eye trauma causes exudation of large proteins such as fibrinogen from conjunctival blood vessels, reaching the bare basement membrane where polymerization and deposition take place. Epithelial defects occurring in herpetic keratitis, trophic corneal ulcers, and after cataract surgery have responded to fibronectin drops when used in an open-label study. However, albumin eye drops were as effective as fibronectin in the treatment of persistent epithelial defects after alkali injuries in rabbits (49). This suggests a nonspecific response. The determination of the value of fibronectin in persistent epithelial defects again can only be gleaned from a prospective, randomized clinical trial.

Epidermal growth factor (EGF) enhances the rate of healing and induces hyperplasia in corneal epithelium (50). EGF stimulated complete epithelial healing after alkali injury in two studies, but in each instance recurrent erosions reestablished the defect (51,52). Epithelial proliferation is clearly stimulated by EGF, but its utility in corneal diseases is unknown. Its use may be limited to certain types of persistent epithelial defects where adhesion problems are least significant. Growth factors might find a more favored place in the acceleration of wound strength by enhancement of macromolecular synthesis.

The devastating nature of alkali injuries of the eye that result in severe personal, social, and economic loss attract the attention of researchers, ophthalmologists, occupational medicine practitioners, and employers. The impact of the medical and surgical solutions found for the problems of chemically injured patients might well find uses in other broad areas of inflammation in the body.

REFERENCES

1. Wagoner M, Kenyon K. Chemical injuries of the eye. In: Albert D, Jakobiac F, eds. *Principles and practice of ophthalmology: clinical practice,* vol 1. Philadelphia: WB Saunders, 1994:234–245.
2. Wagoner M. Chemical injuries of the eye: current concepts in pathophysiology and therapy. *Surv Ophthalmol* 1997;41:275–313.
3. Klein R, Lobes LA. Ocular alkali burns in a large urban area. *Ann Ophthalmol* 1976;8:1185–1189.
4. Morgan S. Chemical burns of the eye: causes and management. *Br J Ophthalmol* 1987;71:854–857.
5. Kuckelkorn R, Luft I, Kottek A, et al. Chemical and thermal eye burns in the residential area of RWTH Aachen. Analysis of accidents in 1 year using a new automated documentation of findings. *Klin Monatsbl Augenheikd* 1993;203:34–42.
6. Kuckelkorn M, Makropoulos W, Kotteck A, et al. Retrospective study of severe alkali burns of the eyes. *Klin Monatsbl Augenheikd* 1993;203:397–402.
7. Pearlman J, Au Eong K, Kuhn F. Airbags and eye injuries: epidemiology, spectrum of injury, and analysis of risk factors. *Surv Ophthalmol* 2001;46:234–243.
8. Paterson CA, Pfister RR, Levinson RA. Aqueous humor pH changes after experimental alkali burns. *Am J Ophthalmol* 1975;79:414–419.
9. Harris LS, Cohn K, Galin MA. Alkali injury from fireworks. *Ann Ophthalmol* 1971;3:849.
10. Grant WM, Kern HL. Action of alkalies on the corneal stroma. *Arch Ophthalmol* 1955;54:931.
11. Fraunfelder FT, et al. Ocular injury induced by methyl ethyl ketone peroxide. *Am J Ophthalmol* 1990;110:635.
12. Kirkpatrick J, Enion D, Burd D. Hydrofluoric acid burns: a review. *Burns* 1995;21:483–493.

13. Grant WM. *Toxicology of the eye,* 2nd ed. Springfield, IL: Charles C Thomas, 1974.

14. Pfister R. *Ocular effects of mustard agents and lewisite in veterans at risk: the health effects of mustard gas and lewisite.* Washington, DC: National Academy Press, 1993:131–147.

15. Paterson CA, Pfister RR. Intraocular pressure changes after alkali burns. *Arch Ophthalmol* 1974;91:211–218.

16. Pfister R, Burstein N. The alkali-burned cornea. I. Epithelial and stromal repair. *Exp Eye Res* 1976;23:519–535.

17. Dua HS, Forrester JV. The corneoscleral limbus in human corneal epithelial wound healing. *Am J Ophthalmol* 1990;110:646–656.

18. Berman M, Leary R, Gage G. Evidence for a role of the plasminogen activator—plasmin system in corneal ulceration. *Invest Ophthalmol Vis Sci* 1980;19:1201–1221.

19. Pfister RR, et al. Identification and synthesis of chemotactic tripeptides from alkali-degraded whole cornea: a study of N-acetyl-Proline-Glycine-Proline and N-methyl-Proline-Glycine-Proline. *Invest Ophthalmol Vis Sci* 1995;36:1306–1316.

20. Sotozono C, He J, Matsumoto Y, et al. Cytokine expression in the alkali-burned cornea. *Curr Eye Res* 1997;16:670–676.

21. Gan L, Fagerholm P, Kim H-J. Effect of leukocytes on corneal cellular proliferation and wound healing. *Invest Ophthalmol Vis Sci* 1999;40:575–581.

22. Pfister RR, Paterson C. Additional clinical and morphological observations on the favorable effect of ascorbate in experimental ocular burns. *Invest Ophthalmol Vis Sci* 1977;16:478–487.

23. Pfister RR, Koski J. The pathophysiology and treatment of the alkali burned eye. *South Med J* 1982;75:417–422.

24. Werb Z, Aggeler J. Proteases induce secretion of collagenase and plasminogen activator by fibroblasts. *Proc Natl Acad Sci USA* 1978;75:1839–1843.

25. Pfister RR, Nicolaro ML, Paterson CA. Sodium citrate reduces the incidence of corneal ulcerations and perforations in extreme alkali-burned eyes—acetylcysteine and ascorbate have no favorable effect. *Invest Ophthalmol Vis Sci* 1981;21:486–490.

26. Brown S, Akiya S, Weller CA. Prevention of the ulcers of the alkali-burned cornea: preliminary studies with collagenase inhibitors. *Arch Ophthalmol* 1969;82:95–97.

27. Slansky HH, Dohlman CH, Berman MB. Prevention of corneal ulcers. *Trans Am Acad Ophthalmol Otolaryngol* 1971;75:1208–1211.

28. Donshik PC, Berman MB. Donlman CH, et al. Effect of topical corticosteroids on corneal ulceration in alkali-burned corneas. *Arch Ophthalmol* 1978;96:2117–2120.

29. Davis A, Ali Q, Aclimandos W. Topical steroid use in the treatment of ocular alkali burns. *Br J Ophthalmol* 1997;81:732–734.

30. Fogle J, Kenyon K, Foster C. Tissue adhesive arrests stromal melting in the human cornea. *Am J Ophthalmol* 1980;89:795–802.

31. Abel R, Binder P, Polack F, et al. The results of penetrating keratoplasty after chemical burns. *Trans Am Acad Ophthalmol Otolaryngol* 1975;79:584–595.

32. Reim M, Overkamping B, Kuckelkorn R. 2 years experience with tenon-plasty. *Ophthalmologe* 1992;89:524–530.

33. Gomes JA, dos Santos MS, Cunha C, et al. Amniotic membrane transplantation for partial and total limbal stem cell deficiency secondary to chemical burn. *Am Acad Ophthalmol* 2003;110:466–473.

34. Espana EM, Grueterich M, Ti SE, et al. Phenotypic study of a case receiving a keratolimbal allograft and amniotic membrane for total limbal stem cell deficiency. *Am Acad Ophthalmol* 2003;110:481–486.

35. Thoft R. Indications for conjunctival transplantation. *Ophthalmology* 1982;89:335–339.

36. Kenyon KR. Conjunctival autograft transplantation for advanced and recurrent pterygium. *Ophthalmology* 1985;92:1461–1470.

37. Pfister RR. Stem cell disease. *CLAO J* 1993;20:64–72.

38. Kukelkorn R, Redbrade C, Scharage N, et al. Keratoplasty with 11–12 mm diameter for management of severely chemically-burned eyes. *Ophthalmologe* 1993;90:683–687.

39. Redbrake C, Buchal V, Reim M. Keratoplasty with a scleral rim after most severe eye burns. *Klin Monatsbl Augenheilkd* 1996;208:145–151.

40. Vajpayee R, Thomas S, Sharma N, et al. Large-diameter lamellar keratoplasty in severe ocular alkali burns. *Ophthalmology* 2000;107:1765–1768.

41. Tsai R, Tseng S. Human allograft limbal transplantation for corneal surface reconstruction. *Cornea* 1994;13:389–400.

42. Meller D, Pires R, Mack R, et al. Amniotic membrane transplantation for acute chemical or thermal burns. *Invest Ophthalmol Vis Sci* 2000;107:980–990.

43. Grueterich M, Espana E, Touhami A, et al. Phenotypic study of a case with successful transplantation of ex vivo expanded human limbal epithelium for unilateral total limbal stem cell deficiency. *Ophthalmology* 2002;109:1547–1552.

44. Kramer S. Late numerical grading of alkali burns to determine keratoplasty prognosis. *Trans Am Ophthalmol Soc* 1983;81:97–106.

45. Dohlman C, Doane M. Keratoprosthesis in end stage dry eye. *Adv Exp Med Biol* 1994;350:561–564.

46. Pfister R, Haddox J, Dodson B. Polymorphonuclear leukocytic inhibition by citrate, other metal chelators and trifluoperazine: evidence to support calcium binding protein involvement. *Invest Ophthalmol Vis Sci* 1984;25:955–970.

47. Pfister R, Haddox J, Barr D. The combined effect of citrate/ascorbate treatment in alkali-injured rabbit eyes. *Cornea* 1991;10:100B–104.

48. Brodovsky S, McCarty C, Snibson G. Management of alkali burns: an 11-year retrospective review. *Ophthalmology* 2000;107(10):1829–1835.

49. Boisjoly H, et al. The effect of fibronectin compared to albumin on rabbit epithelial wound healing. *Invest Ophthalmol Vis Sci* 1987;28(suppl):52.

50. Ho P, et al. Kinetics of corneal epithelial regeneration and epidermal growth factor. *Invest Ophthalmol Vis Sci* 1974;13:804.

51. Eiferman R, Schultz G. Treatment of alkali burns in rabbits with epidermal growth factor. *Invest Ophthalmol Vis Sci* 1987;28:52.

52. Singh G, Foster CS. Epidermal growth factor in alkali-burned corneal epithelial wound healing. *Am J Ophthalmol* 1987;103:802–807.

44

PHYSICAL INJURIES OF THE CORNEA

PUWAT CHARUKAMNOETKANOK, MAHNAZ NOURI, AND ROBERTO PINEDA II

Physical injury to the cornea can have potentially devastating consequences to the vision and health of the eye. However, a poorly prepared plan to repair the injury without careful evaluation and initiation of appropriate treatments can lead to a suboptimal outcome that is equally visually unsatisfying. This chapter discusses important considerations in the evaluation of corneal blunt trauma and perforating injuries, highlights appropriate treatment recommendations directed by theoretical or evidence-based support, and discusses other physical injuries of the cornea including thermal injuries, phacoemulsification-related corneal trauma, and traumatic injuries related to corneal refractive surgery.

BLUNT TRAUMA OF THE ANTERIOR SEGMENT

Blunt Corneal Trauma

Severe intraocular damage to the eye can occur even when the force of injury is insufficient to rupture the globe (open-globe injury). Fortunately, the effects of blunt trauma on the healthy cornea are usually transient (1). For example, a direct, focal, concussive force from BB pellet or paint ball results in mechanical injury to the surrounding endothelium manifesting as a ring of corneal edema (2).

Blunt trauma with severe corneal contusion may result in a rupture of Descemet's membrane. The resultant breach of the endothelial barrier leads to acute hydrops, characterized by marked corneal edema similar to that seen with keratoconic hydrops. However, healthy endothelium is capable of healing such ruptures by sliding or migrating over the area of retracted Descemet's membrane. This mechanism restores the normal endothelial pump and barrier functions necessary to maintain corneal deturgescence, and usually occurs over 3 months. Routinely, on clinical slit-lamp examination, a footprint of parallel striae or a fishmouth break in Descemet's membrane can be found. These lesions are visual indicators of previous traumatic events but seldom result in significant visual impairment of vision. Numerous treatment modalities have been proposed including patching, bandage soft contact lens, topical corticosteroids, topical glaucoma medications, hypertonic sodium chloride preparations, anterior chamber air or expansible gases, as well as thermokeratoplasty, however their usefulness remains unproven (1).

Corneal rupture is uncommon following blunt trauma unless the eye has predisposing risk factors including corneal ectatic pathology such as keratoconus, pellucid marginal degeneration, Terrien's marginal degeneration, or prior corneal surgery such as penetrating keratoplasty (3), or incision surgery such as radial or astigmatic keratotomy.

Corneal Abrasions

Corneal abrasions, partial or complete removal of the corneal epithelium, are one of the most common ocular injuries. Studies have estimated that corneal abrasions account for 10% of new patient visits to the eye emergency room (4) and occur in 3.5% of the population (5). Tangential impact from foreign bodies, including fingernails, paper, plants, or brushes, is the most frequent cause of corneal abrasions. It is also frequently encountered in ocular chemical or thermal injuries.

The basal cells of the corneal epithelium rest on a basement membrane and are anchored to the stroma by hemidesmosomes (6). Corneal scarring does not occur with traumatic epithelial abrasions. However, if the abrasion extends beyond the epithelial basement membrane and the underlying Bowman's layer and corneal stroma are violated, corneal keratocytes are activated, resulting in new collagen deposition and cicatrix formation. Scarring will occur if Bowman's layer is violated or the underlying corneal stroma is involved in the trauma.

Clinically, patients often present with symptoms of pain, photophobia, foreign-body sensation, and tearing. An irregular or denuded ocular surface may result in decreased vision that may not improve with pinhole visual acuity testing. The presence of an abrasion can be confirmed by application of fluorescein dye, which highlights the epithelial defect in apple green when viewed with a cobalt blue light.

Examination of a corneal abrasion should focus on the extent of abrasion, the degree of stromal involvement, and the presence of other associated injuries. As in all eye trauma, the examiner must be mindful of the possibility of occult ocular injuries such as an open globe or retained intraocular foreign body. A corneal abrasion may be the only clue of a high-velocity foreign object that may pass completely through the cornea with minimal disturbance of the corneal anatomy (7,8).

Most corneal abrasions resolve without long-term complications within 24 to 72 hours (9). Therefore, the aims of therapy are to maximize the patient comfort, promote epithelial healing, and prevent complications. Common treatment modalities include topical antibiotics, cycloplegic agents, and ocular patching or a bandage soft contact lens.

The corneal epithelium provides a principal barrier against harmful organisms, and because the mechanism of injury is usually a dirty foreign body, a major concern regarding corneal abrasion is the risk of microbial keratitis. Patients should be considered at high risk for corneal infection until re-epithelialization is complete. Instillation of broad-spectrum antibiotics is recommended for microbial prophylaxis. There is no study to date that demonstrates that any one antibiotic is better than another. However, it is important to note that almost all topical medications retard epithelial healing to some degree due to the presence of preservatives in the solution (10).

To alleviate patients' pain, cycloplegic agents should be used to minimize ciliary spasm. Physicians should select agents with appropriate duration of action according to the extent of the injuries. A randomized, double-masked, placebo-controlled study demonstrated that when used as adjunctive therapy, ketorolac tromethamine 0.5% ophthalmic solution provided increased patients' comfort without adverse effects (11).

Due to the risk of promoting infection, patching is clearly not recommended when corneal abrasion involves vegetable matter, wood, contact lens use, or other "dirty" materials. The efficacy of patching in relieving pain or promoting reepithelialization is controversial. A randomized clinical trial suggests that eye patching in children (aged 3 to 17 years) with isolated corneal abrasions makes no difference in the rate of healing (9). Gregersen et al. (12) reported faster epithelial healing and less subjective symptoms in patients with double eye patches for 24 hours than those patched for 6 hours. However, numerous studies have contradicted this finding, and have questioned the effectiveness of patching in support of no patching (13–16).

Kaiser (14) conducted a large-scale, randomized, controlled trial in patients with noninfected, non-contact lens-related traumatic corneal abrasions. The patients were treated with topical antibiotics and mydriatics and were randomized to receive either a pressure patch or no patch (14). The authors concluded that for small abrasion (<10 mm²), patients treated with antibiotic ointment and

mydriatics alone had significantly faster healing times and lower pain level scores. The authors noted that pressure patching was not a benign treatment because it removed binocular vision and could be uncomfortable for the patient.

However, for large traumatic abrasions (>10 mm²), the study by Kaiser (14) found that the patched group had a faster healing time. The abrasion took 3.45 days to heal in the patch group, compared with 4.20 days in the nonpatch group. Due to the small number of patients with large abrasions, this study was not powered to detect a statistically significant difference. Nonetheless, the author recommends that, unless contraindicated, abrasions larger than 10 mm² should continue to be patched until the effectiveness of pressure patching is established in this subset of patients by additional studies.

Alternatively, bandage soft contact lenses have been thought to be an attractive alternative to patching. It protects the epithelium from eyelids friction and promotes healing and reduces patient discomfort (17). Treating physicians must be careful of complications from contact lens such as an increased risk of infection and reduced oxygen permeability. Therefore, these patients may require closer attention for this form of therapy.

In summary, most corneal abrasion heals uneventfully within 24 to 48 hours. Common complications include infection and development of recurrent erosion syndrome (18–20), which has been reported to occur in 7.7% of traumatic abrasions (21).

Corneal Foreign Body

Corneal foreign bodies are one of the most frequently encountered urgencies seen in ophthalmic practice. Patients with corneal foreign bodies are usually motivated to seek prompt medical attention because of ocular discomfort. Many particles may cause injury including glass, plastic, insect parts, plant debris, wood splinters, paint chips, and cinders (8). However, metal objects represent the most hazardous material to the eye.

Patients often present with pain, photophobia, excessive tearing, redness, and blurred vision. Particles that are hot and projected at high speed may become embedded in the stroma and not initially produce ocular discomfort. Patients often seek care when the eye becomes inflamed hours later and may not recognize that the foreign body is the cause of their symptoms. A detailed history is important for high-quality patient care and for medicolegal reasons. Transparent materials such as fiberglass and glass, which may be difficult to locate, can be more readily identified when the physician anticipates their presence. Furthermore, high-speed projectile objects may penetrate the eye with minimal evidence of entry (7). Careful slit-lamp examination is essential to observe location, depth, and type of particles. The globe should be assessed for signs of perforation such as hypotony, shallow anterior chamber, altered pupil size, and a positive Seidel's test. The upper and lower lid should always be everted to ensure that all debris has been removed. Treating physicians must be sure to ask about the patient's tetanus status if metallic material is suspected and a tetanus booster administered if indicated.

Metallic corneal foreign bodies must be removed. Particles lodged near the visual axis should be removed with care to minimize further injury to the cornea. Foreign bodies located at the level of Bowman's layer or in the stroma will produce scarring regardless of the physician's skill. However, not all foreign bodies require removal. Small inert materials such as glass may be left in the cornea.

Irrigation may be attempted to dislodge superficial foreign bodies by using sterile irrigating solution pointed at a slight angle to avoid further embedding the particle more posteriorly into the cornea. If irrigation is not successful, mechanical instrumentation should be used to dislodge the foreign body at the slit lamp. A stainless steel spud, shaped like a golf club or hockey stick, is very effective. Alternatively, the beveled tip of a sterile disposable small gauge needle can also be utilized. To prevent inadvertent penetration, the instrument should be held tangential to the cornea rather than perpendicular to it. Epithelial damage, either during the initial trauma or after removal of foreign body, is unavoidable. Patients should receive treatment for the corneal abrasion as well as the foreign body.

Iron-containing foreign bodies often produced rust rings that delay healing and may be a continuous source of irritation (22). Within hours of the corneal injury, rust stains adjacent epithelial cells and Bowman's membrane, eventually diffusing into the corneal stroma.

Various instruments, including battery-powered drills (e.g., Alger brush) or needle tip, may be used to remove the rust ring (Fig. 44-1). These instruments are equally effective, although using a needle is generally more

time-consuming (23). Extraction of the rust ring may be difficult in a fresh corneal injury. The clinician may have to wait a few days and repeat the procedure when the surrounding tissue becomes softened and the rust has solidified. Every trace of the rust ring need not be removed because the retained particles will eventually extrude over time.

When multiple foreign bodies exist, removal of particles individually may result in excessive scarring. The debridement of the corneal epithelium may be a more appropriate approach to remove foreign bodies without excessively disrupting the integrity of Bowman's layer (24).

Removal of deep corneal foreign bodies may be impossible if the size, contrast, or location precludes visualization by slit-lamp or surgical biomicroscopy. Au et al. (25) described a lamellar pocket technique for removal of a deep intrastromal corneal foreign body. In this technique, the foreign body was removed through a peripheral corneal incision minimizing unwanted distortion of the corneal topography. Yang (26) described a simple technique using the suture needle for removal of corneal foreign bodies that project into the anterior chamber. A 6-mm needle (10-0, micropoint spatula, Ethicon, United Kingdom) was used to pass just beneath the corneal foreign bodies, slightly lifting the cornea, and everting the anterior opening of the wound. The use of a suture needle enhanced visualization by providing reflection of light from the back, maintaining the anterior chamber, exposing the corneal foreign bodies, and stabilizing the globe. After removing the foreign body, the suture could then be tied as a temporary suture before placement of permanent suture(s).

Organic foreign bodies, such as those from plants and insects, pose an additional challenge due to increased risk of infection and inflammation (27). Patients should be followed closely, and if an infection does develop, the treating physician must maintain a high suspicion for the possibility of a

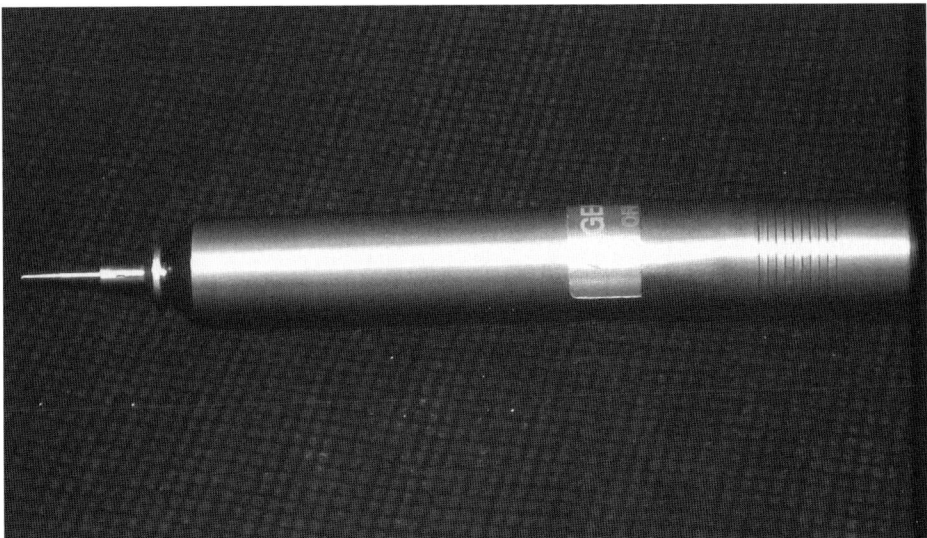

FIGURE 44-1. Battery-powered drills (Alger brush II) used to remove the rust ring from metallic foreign bodies.

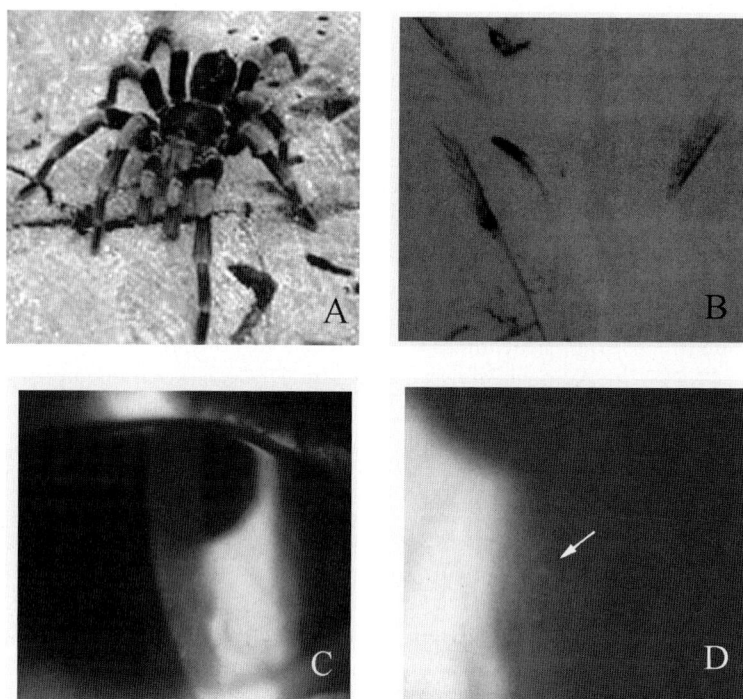

FIGURE 44-2. Tarantula keratits. **A:** Tarantula spider. **B:** High magnification examination of the tarantula hairs. **C:** Corneal edema. **D:** Higher magnification of the cornea demonstrating embedded tarantula's hair *(arrow).*

mycotic organism. Exposure to tarantula spiders demonstrates how insect parts can result in a significant inflammatory reaction of the cornea (28–30) (Fig. 44-2). Cooke et al. (31) classified tarantulas' hairs into four types. Of these, type III (long, thin, with sharp points and multiple barbs) can embed and penetrate skin or cornea. Typical ocular responses to insect foreign bodies, termed ophthalmic nodosa, include conjunctival granulomas, corneal stromal infiltrate, and anterior chamber reaction (32). The goals of therapy are removal of the tarantula hairs and control of ocular inflammation. Long-term suppression of inflammation may be necessary until the hairs are resorbed (33).

Laser *in situ* keratomileusis (LASIK) has been associated with decreased corneal sensation. The increasing number of patients having LASIK suggests that corneal foreign bodies may become more common in this population. Porges et al. (34) reported nine eyes of eight patients who presented with corneal foreign bodies after LASIK. The removal was carried out with a 27-gauge needle with no flap-related complications. The authors recommended avoidance of antibiotic ointment to prevent a possible penetration of oily material beneath the flap. Interestingly, half of the patients did not realize that they had the corneal foreign bodies. Transient post-LASIK corneal hypoesthesia might explain this phenomenon. Protective eyewear should be an integral part of postoperative precaution in patients who have undergone refractive surgery.

After removal of corneal foreign bodies, the cornea will usually heal quickly without sequelae. However, if the basement membrane has been damaged, it may take up to 6 weeks or more to restore secure cellular attachments of the epithelium to the underlying basement membrane. Rarely, recurrent corneal erosions may complicate the post-traumatic injury and may occur weeks, months, or even years after the event (35).

Airbag Injuries

Because of mandatory installation of automotive airbags on all 1998 and later vehicle models, airbags have undoubtedly reduced the incidence of fatal and severe injuries in automobile collisions (36). However, numerous case reports of airbag-related eye injuries have been published (36–39). Airbags are rubber-lined nylon bags folded into the steering column and dashboard. Upon deployment, combustion of sodium azide-generated nitrogen gas fills the 50-L volume of the airbags in 0.05 seconds, and propels it toward the automobile occupant at speeds of 100 to 200 mph (40). In addition, airbag deployment also generates heat, alkaline aerosols, and carbon dioxide.

Injuries related to automotive airbags constitute two major categories: mechanical injuries and chemical burns. The types of corneal injuries described with airbags include corneal abrasion, contusion, edema, corneal blood staining, and corneal laceration (41–45) (Fig. 44-3). At least one case of permanent bullous keratopathy after airbag trauma has been documented (46). In another case report, alkali burn of the eye was associated with airbag deployment (47).

Duma et al. (48) investigated 22,236 individual crashes in the United States from the National Automotive Sampling System database from January 1993 through December 1999. The authors proposed a new four-level eye injury severity

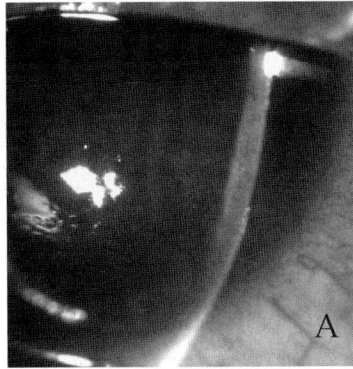

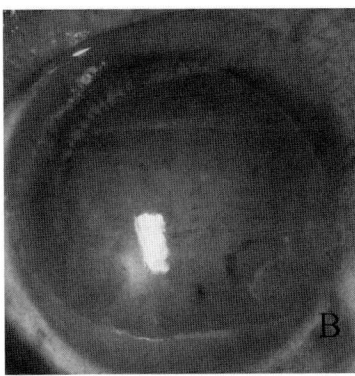

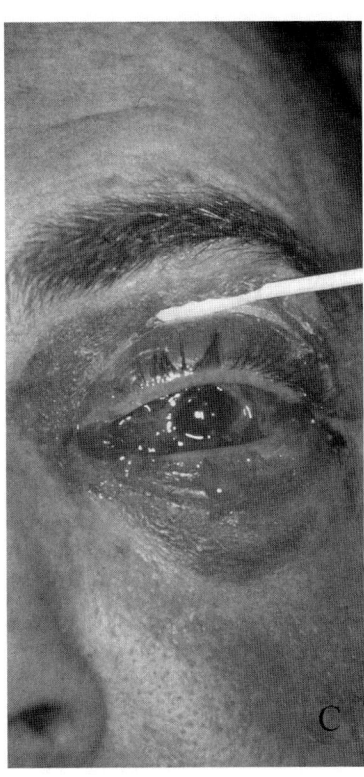

FIGURE 44-3. Consequences of airbag injuries. **A:** Corneal edema, which may result from chemical irritation or from the contusion injury. **B:** The impact can be severe enough to cause subluxation of crystalline lens. **C:** Blunt globe rupture presents with conjunctival injection and chemosis.

scale that quantifies injuries based on recovery time, need for surgery, and possible loss of sight. Three percent of automotive occupants who encountered airbag deployment sustained an eye injury compared with 2% of those who did not. This difference, however, was not found to be statistically significant. A closer examination of the type of eye injuries demonstrated a statistically significant increased risk of corneal abrasions for occupants exposed to airbag deployment. However, occupants from car crashes without airbag deployment sustained a greater number of severe ocular injuries. Characteristics of occupants and crashes, such as eyeglasses, contact lens, or seat belt uses, age, height, and crash velocity, were not significantly correlated with the risk of airbag-induced eye injury.

Lehto et al. (49) performed a retrospective observational case series (*n* = 378) from data collected between 1993 and 1997 in Finland to evaluate the risk of eye injuries from airbag deployment and the relationship between eye injuries and eyewear. The authors reported a risk of 2.5% for any airbag-related eye injury and 0.4% for severe eye injuries. There was no significant difference in the risk for eye injury between survivors in accidents involving airbag deployment and those not involving airbags. Furthermore, eyeglasses or contact lens did not contribute to a greater risk of eye injuries. However, the power of this study was low because of the small number of individuals with ocular injuries.

The rising proportion of airbag-equipped cars as well as the increasing percentage of the population electing for corrective vision surgery are two converging trends that may increase the risk and severity of airbag-induced ocular injuries. Thus, innovation of airbag and eyewear protection designs is particularly needed. One such innovation is the development of airbags that would inflate at different speeds depending on the severity of the collision and the physical characteristics of the occupants.

PERFORATING INJURIES OF THE ANTERIOR SEGMENT

Corneal and Corneoscleral Lacerations

This section reviews important concepts related to corneal lacerations, including partial-thickness lacerations, simple full-thickness lacerations, angular and intersectional lacerations, and stellate lacerations. It also explores various issues pertaining to complicated anterior segment traumas, including corneoscleral lacerations with uveal prolapse or iris incarceration, corneoscleral laceration repair, and cataract extraction, as well as anterior segment intraocular foreign bodies. The fundamentally important mission of corneal laceration repair is complete watertight wound closure with restoration of corneal sphericity. Moreover, goals of wound repair should always include release of uveal and vitreous incarceration, prevention and management of infections, and preparation for secondary anterior segment reconstruction.

Keratorefractive Principles

Understanding of the micromechanical effects of penetrating injury and its repair is crucial for facilitating primary corneal restoration and maximizing ultimate visual outcome by managing astigmatism and corneal scarring (50). The corneal laceration itself along with its subsequent surgical repair as well as the tissue wound healing responses exert significant influence on residual astigmatism after the recovery.

Effect of the Laceration

Corneal incisions produce keratometric flattening over the affected region of the cornea due to wound gaping (51,52). Circumferential incisions (transverse or arcuate incisions) flatten the cornea along the meridian parallel to the incision while steepening the axis 90 degrees away. On the other hand, radial incisions flatten the cornea along both the axis of incision and the axis 90 degrees away (53).

The anatomy of the lacerations [vertical (perpendicular) or oblique (shelved or beveled)] affects gaping of the incision differently (Fig. 44-4). The valve rule of Eisner (54) states, "Incisions through the wall of the globe produce valves whose margin of watertightness is equal to the projection of the surface of the incision onto the surface of the globe." Thus, vertical corneal lacerations gape more than shelved corneal lacerations. Moreover, incisions perpendicular to the cornea open spontaneously and require sutures for coaptation. By contrast, shelved incisions tend to close spontaneously.

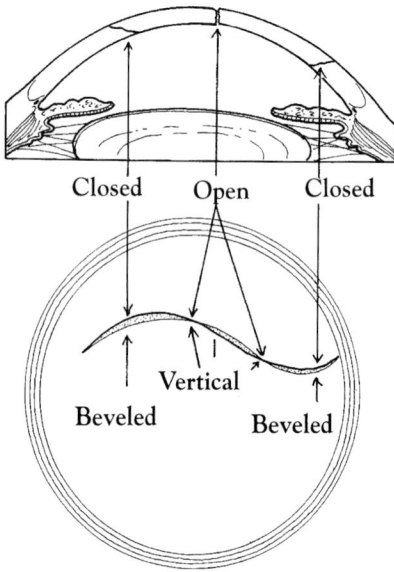

FIGURE 44-4. Beveled incisions gape less and may close spontaneously, whereas vertical corneal incisions and lacerations gape and open spontaneously. (From Pineda R II. Four pearls for suturing corneal incisions and lacerations. In: Melki SA, Azar DT, eds. *One hundred one pearls in refractive, cataract, and corneal surgery.* Thorofare, NJ: SLACK Inc., 2001:131–137, with permission.)

Effect of Sutures

Both radially and circumferentially sutured incisions flatten the cornea directly under the suture but steepen the area closer to the cornea center or visual axis (i.e., similar to tight sutures in extracapsular cataract surgery). Eisner (54) has discussed in detail the five components of suture effects: (a) compression factors, (b) torquing, (c) splinting, (d) tissue eversion, and (e) tissue inversion.

Concerning the compression factors, the zone of tissue compression along the incision is roughly equal to the length of the suture (Fig. 44-5). Thus, fewer long sutures are needed for wound closure because they have greater lateral zones of tissue compression. However, longer sutures are associated with greater tissue distortion (i.e., astigmatism), particularly when placed close to the visual axis (Fig. 44-6).

Because nonradial sutures produce tissue torque that leads to wound gaping and leakage, it is important to place interrupted sutures precisely perpendicular to the corneal laceration itself. This concept is equally important when utilizing a running suture. The intrastromal portion of a running suture provides splinting (resistance to lateral movement of the tissues), whereas the overlying running suture tends to produce tissue torque (lateral movement). The torque occurs in the direction that produces the shortest distance between neighboring exit and entry sites.

Single interrupted sutures produce equal everting and inverting wound forces; thus, there is no tendency toward tissue elevation or depression. In contrast, a running suture produces a wound eversion tendency over the intrastromal suture bite while creating an inverting force beneath the overlying bite.

Wound override is the result of unequal entrance and exit suture passage from the wound margin or uneven depth on both sides of the corneal laceration. Tissue override produces a microwedge resection effect, flattening the surrounding cornea and creating an irregular corneal surface. Closure of an oblique corneal laceration, however, requires a different approach. When closing oblique wounds, placement of the suture should be centered on the posterior aspect and not the anterior side of the corneal laceration as is routinely done to prevent tissue distortion (Fig. 44-7).

Partial-Thickness Lacerations

Not all ocular trauma leads to a full-thickness corneal laceration. Important clues can be used to help determine whether a corneal laceration is a full- or partial-thickness injury. Close examination of Descemet's membrane may help to rule out occult perforation. Seidel's evaluation with 2% fluorescein should be performed. Careful provocative testing with gentle pressure may reveal microscopic leaks in an otherwise self-sealing wound.

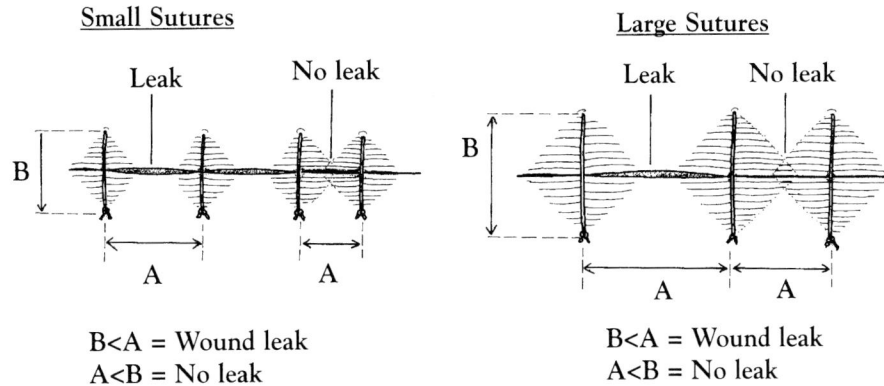

FIGURE 44-5. The "zone of compression" is equal to the length of the suture placed to close the incision. To prevent wound leak, longer sutures can be spaced further apart, while shorter sutures need to be close together. (From Pineda R II. Four pearls for suturing corneal incisions and lacerations. In: Melki SA, Azar DT, eds. *One hundred one pearls in refractive, cataract, and corneal surgery.* Thorofare, NJ: SLACK Inc., 2001:131–137, with permission.)

Treatment goals in a partial-thickness corneal laceration include promoting reepithelialization, stromal healing, and prevention of infection. All efforts should focus on minimizing corneal scarring and surface irregularity.

Simple superficial wounds with nonoverriding edges and without significant wound gape may be treated with pressure patching and topical ophthalmic antibiotics. For deeper wounds, a bandage soft contact lens may be used to support the wound and shield the cornea from eyelid contact. Thicker and larger contact lenses (i.e., Permalens or Kontur) are generally preferred for their ability to splint the cornea. The contact lens must be properly fitted to ensure wound stabilization, adequate oxygenation, as well as patient comfort. Antibiotic prophylaxis is recommended for the duration of bandage contact lens use. The contact lens should remain in place until epithelialization is complete and the stromal wound has become relatively stable (3 to 6 weeks). If corneal epithelialization is a problem, a contact lens can be used for up to 2 months to ensure sufficient formation of epithelial-basement membrane adhesion complexes and to minimize the risk of recurrent erosion. Sutures may be necessary in long wounds, particularly in those cases with avulsion of corneal tissue, and in wounds with significant wound override or gape (55).

Simple Full-Thickness Lacerations

A simple corneal laceration is one that does not violate the limbus and has neither iris nor vitreous incarceration, nor traumatic damage to the lens (55). Any lacerations extending beyond the limbus require meticulous exploration to delineate the full extent of the trauma.

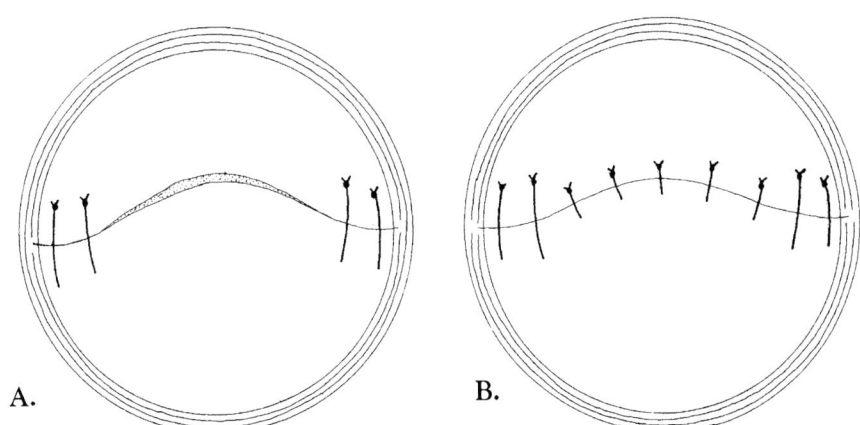

FIGURE 44-6. Corneal laceration repair. **A.** Longer compression sutures are placed peripherally near the limbus. **B.** Shorter appositional sutures are placed centrally to minimize flattening and restore sphericity of the cornea. (From Pineda R II. Four pearls for suturing corneal incisions and lacerations. In: Melki SA, Azar DT, eds. *One hundred one pearls in refractive, cataract, and corneal surgery.* Thorofare, NJ: SLACK Inc., 2001:131–137, with permission.)

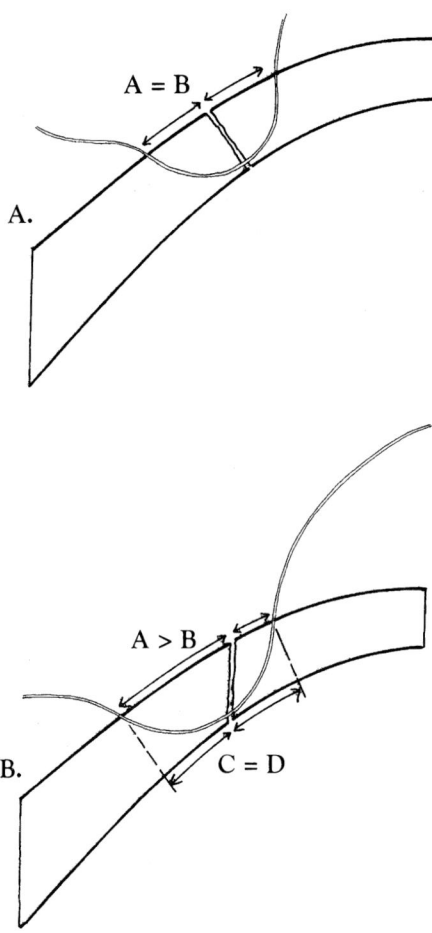

FIGURE 44-7. A. In perpendicular incisions and lacerations, the suture must be placed equidistance and equal depth (approximately 90%) to prevent tissue override. **B.** In oblique incisions and lacerations, the suture should be centered over the posterior aspect of the wound and not over the anterior aspect as in perpendicular lacerations. (From Pineda R II. Four pearls for suturing corneal incisions and lacerations. In: Melki SA, Azar DT, eds. *One hundred one pearls in refractive, cataract, and corneal surgery.* Thorofare, NJ: SLACK Inc., 2001:131–137, with permission.)

One may consider not suturing small simple full-thickness corneal lacerations that satisfy all of the following six requirements (56): (a) the laceration length is 3 mm or less (57,58); (b) there is no intraocular tissue to the wound; (c) there are no other ocular structures involved; (d) there is no foreign material in the laceration; (e) the wound is a self-sealing or Seidel positive only with provocation; and (f) patients are not children or uncooperative adults. Nonsurgical treatments such as bandage contact lenses or tissue adhesive are two of the effective treatment modalities.

A bandage contact lens may be sufficient to protect and support the wound as it heals. The contact lens should be kept in place, about 3 to 6 weeks, until the wound has stabilized. The patient should be encouraged to wear a protective metal shield or eyewear at all times. Topical antibiotic prophylaxis and cycloplegia are recommended while the lens is in place. However, if the anterior chamber fails to reform within 24 hours, and if aqueous leakage persists, or

if iris or lens incarceration occurs, further surgical intervention is warranted.

Cyanoacrylate tissue adhesive (59) is useful for selected small (<2 mm) lacerations that do not self-seal, those that would require excessive suture placement in the visual axis, puncture wounds with small amounts of central tissue loss, and stellate wounds with poor central apposition. Currently available commercial brands include Dermabond (Ethicon, Sommerville, NJ), MSI-EpiDermGlu (Medisave Services, Inc., Ontario, Canada), and Histacryl (B. Braun, Tuttlingen, Germany). The length of carbon side chains differentiates the available cyanoacrylate glues. Medical grade isobutyl-2-cyanoacylate (4 carbon side chain) offers excellent adhesive properties with negligible harmful side effects. Despite its proven effectiveness for this purpose, cyanoacrylate is not currently approved for clinical use by the U.S. Food and Drug Administration (55).

Stellate, Angular, and Intersectional Lacerations

Techniques useful for closure of challenging stellate lacerations include multiple interrupted sutures, bridging sutures, and purse-string sutures. Adjunctive treatment with bandage lens application, tissue adhesive, or patch grafting may be necessary for closure of central stellate lacerations that are difficult to appose and leak persistently. In the case of an angulated pedicle flap of tissue resulting from an avulsive injury, sutures should be angled toward the apex of the wound to bring the avulsed corneal tissue back into proper position.

Corneoscleral Lacerations with Uveal Prolapse and Iris Incarceration

The decision to redeposit uveal tissue versus excision should be made only after meticulous examination of the injury. Devitalized, macerated, feathery, or depigmented iris should be excised. Exposed uveal tissue incarcerated for more than 24 hours should be removed to reduce the risks of infection and epithelial ingrowth. However, if the incarcerated tissue is not exposed and is not necrotic, it may cautiously be reposited after 24 hours. The possible risk from preserving damaged tissues should be carefully weighed against the benefit of tissue conservation for subsequent reconstruction and maintenance of a normal iris diaphragm.

Corneal Lacerations with Vitreous Involvement

Vitreous incarceration in traumatic wounds may lead to many complications including infection, cystoid macular edema, chronic inflammation, vitreous fibrosis, and retinal detachment. Vitreous in the anterior chamber can also damage the corneal endothelium. Thus, vitreous incarceration of the corneal wound should be managed with amputation, and preferably complete removal of vitreous from the anterior chamber. Ideally, postoperatively, the pupil should be round without peaking, and the vitreous maintained behind the iris.

Corneoscleral Laceration Repair and Cataract Extraction

After an ocular injury, the crystalline lens can immediately lose its transparency by either direct or indirect trauma. In general, lens extraction can be deferred until the eye has recovered from the primary surgical repair. In particular, lens extraction is inadvisable in the setting of poor visualization through an edematous cornea and in the presence of a marked fibrinous anterior chamber reaction or pupillary membrane (58). However, one can consider primary removal of the lens in the following settings: (a) a disruption of capsule with flocculent lens material to prevent phacogenic inflammation (60); (b) the opaque lens prohibits proper management of intraocular foreign bodies or posterior segment injury (61); or (c) the ocular trauma is limited to the anterior segment, and keratometry and A-scan echography can be obtained in the fellow eye (61). Crystalline lens extraction should be performed only with good visualization, appropriate equipment, and under controlled circumstances. The appropriateness of intraocular lens (IOL) placement during initial trauma surgery is controversial (62,63). One must consider the integrity of capsular support when placing a posterior chamber IOL (64,65). Iris or transscleral sutures should be considered when capsular support is inadequate or absent.

Anterior Segment Intraocular Foreign Bodies (IOFBs)

Gonioscopy should not be performed in the acute setting unless there is a strong suspicion for anterior segment IOFBs. Intraoperative gonioscopy may be helpful when performed in a gentle and controlled fashion. Anterior segment IOFBs can be removed through the wound or through a limbal corneoscleral shelved incision. Rarely, a lenticular IOFBs can be left in place with close observation (61).

Thermal Burns

The effect of thermal energy to the cornea varies throughout the different cellular layers. The corneal epithelium will regenerate if intact limbal stem cells exist. However, the corneal endothelium is incapable of mitosis and therefore may suffer permanent damage. The primary effect of thermal energy on the corneal stromal layer is on the collagen matrix, in a biphasic manner, with reversible and irreversible components. The initial insult in thermal corneal injuries is the reversible contraction of the collagen fibril alpha helix while preserving the triple helix structure and the covalent bond. This is seen clinically as corneal striae. With increased thermal exposure, irre-

versible corneal collagen changes occur, including lysis of the interhelix covalent bonds and triple helix destruction of the collagen fibril (66).

As surgeons perform more complicated phacoemulsification cases, an increasingly recognized potential complication is corneal and scleral thermal wound injuries during nuclear cataract removal because of increased phacoemulsification power and duration. Postoperatively, diffuse corneal edema occurs and may become visually significant long term. Steepening in the axis of incision may result in irregular astigmatism and loss of best spectacle corrected visual acuity (67). Moreover, inadvertent filtering blebs may also occur resulting in reduced intraocular pressure due to wound fistula formation. Davison (68,69) reported development of temporary filtering blebs in two patients with thermal injury (due to phacoemulsification) as well as induced astigmatism. Paraxial scarring of the cornea has been reported by Majid et al. (70), where uncorrected visual acuity was reduced to 20/200 three months postoperatively.

One principle reason for phacoemulsification thermal injuries is the decreased flow around the needle tip of the phacoemulsification hand piece in addition to the increased tip exposure with friction of the sleeve, and high phacoemulsification power. This has become more pertinent in recent years with modified surgical techniques such as the utilization of clear cornea incisions as well as smaller phacoemulsification needles. The increased number of cataract extractions performed by phacoemulsification (71) may explain the increased incidence of phacoemulsification-related thermal injuries to the wound (66).

Dense cataract nuclei as well as high phacoemulsification power has been reported to be associated with increased incidence of phacoemulsification wound burns as noted by Singh et al. (72) in cases of brunescent nuclear cataract. In these cases, mechanical breakage of the nucleus into smaller sections as well as use of pulse/burst mode have been shown to decrease the total amount of phacoemulsification power required for nuclear disassembly (66).

The thermal injury during phacoemulsification may occur rapidly, often within 1 to 3 seconds (73). Preventative measures to reduce the risk of phacoemulsification thermal injuries include increasing flow around the tip by raising the bottle height, noting an empty bottle early, and verification of fluid in the irrigation tubing. Also, the flow of fluid through the irrigation hand piece should be verified prior to entry into the eye. Adequate wound size may prevent increased friction of the devices at the anterior lip of the wound, allowing appropriate flow of fluid around the sleeve. Aspiration flow may also be affected by occlusion of the tip by lens particles, viscoelastic material, or inadequate vacuum levels.

The key to avoiding thermal phacoemulsification injury is prevention and awareness. Once a thermal injury to the cornea or sclera has occurred, the wound can be repaired with sutures to assure closure of the fish-mouthed wound as a result of gaping of the anterior and posterior lips of the incision. A horizontal mattress suture has been reported to be effective for wound closure in phacoemulsification thermal burns (66). Alternatively, phacoemulsification thermal burns can also be managed conservatively with a bandage contact lens, corticosteroid drops, and potentially oral nonsteroidal antiinflammatory medications (67,70). Astigmatism secondary to shrinkage of tissue may improve with time (67,74). One technique that has been helpful in some patients has been the use of astigmatic keratotomy in cases of debilitating residual astigmatism postoperatively (75). This approach should be guided by the use of corneal topography.

CORNEAL TRAUMA AFTER REFRACTIVE SURGERY

As the number of patients undergoing laser vision correction exceeds more than 1 million per year, there is increasing awareness of ocular trauma in the immediate postoperative period as well as potential long-term risks. Although demographic data on refractive surgery trauma is lacking in the current ophthalmic literature, this section reviews pertinent complications of corneal trauma after refractive surgery.

Refractive surgical techniques have expanded enormously, and corrections may be done utilizing several different procedures including: radial keratotomy (RK), photorefractive keratectomy (PRK), LASIK, and astigmatic keratotomy (AK).

In a study by Peacock et al. (76), the ocular integrity of the human eye was evaluated in whole human globes undergoing eight-incision RK, ALK, PRK, and LASIK. The eyes were then subjected to increasing trauma until the globes ruptured. They found that all operated eyes "required less energy to rupture the globe compared to control eyes." But they stated, "The energy required to rupture ALK, PRK, LASIK eyes is not significantly different from that for normal eyes." All RK eyes ruptured at the incision site, whereas the PRK and LASIK eyes ruptured near the edge of the flap or limbus.

Lee et al. (77) reported a case of AK and RK separation of a wound 91 months after blunt trauma with no extension beyond the corneal scleral limbus. Another study in 1997 compared the strength of RK versus PRK incision in a 25-year-old man who had undergone eight-incision RK in the left eye and PRK in the right eye. He sustained trauma to both eyes in an explosion 22 months later; there was full-thickness rupture of four RK incisions and full-thickness laceration due to mineral projection in the PRK eye. However, the authors pointed out that in other animal models "healthy eyes or eyes that have PRK rupture at the sclera and that those that have RK rupture at the cornea" (78).

Uchio et al. (79) analyzed a computer simulation to assess the impact of an airbag injury causing corneal rupture after four-, six-, or eight-incision RK. The airbag was pro-

grammed to hit the surface of post-RK eyes at different velocities. At a medium velocity of 30 m/sec, corneal rupture was likely, whereas at 40 m/sec air-bag impact velocity, three of four, five of six, and eight of eight RK incisions had a likely chance of rupture, resulting in open-globe injuries in all cases. At 40 m/sec, the investigators noted that lacerations extended beyond the incisions to involve an intact cornea (79).

Vinger et al. (80) reported 28 cases of globe perforation due to blunt trauma after refractive surgery; 27 occurred in RK incisions and one through hexagonal keratotomy incisions. Twelve percent occurred 6 weeks after surgery, 8% occurred before 6 months, and 81% after 6 months. Fifteen percent of the open-globe injuries occurred along the RK incisions 5 years postoperatively. There was no correlation found between the postoperative time period and extent of the injury. In 31% of cases, vision recovered to 20/40 or better, 23% had best corrected visual acuity (BCVA) of 20/40 to 20/100, whereas 23% were legally blind, and 23% were completely blind.

Blunt trauma after incisional surgery such as RK has been shown to predispose to open-globe rupture at energy levels less than that required for an intact normal globe. Delayed and incomplete wound healing in RK studies has been shown to exist up to 47 months postoperatively; complete healing by histologic studies were observed at 66 months postoperatively (81,82). Tangential AK incisions were found to heal faster, by 9 to 10 months (83). However, in one case report, the rupture of the RK incisions occurred 13 years after the original surgery (80).

Panda et al. (84) reported three cases of blunt trauma resulting in open globes 10 to 13 years after RK. The globes ruptured through the keratotomy incision sites, one due to daily living activities, another due to assault, and one during sports. Two eyes recovered 20/30 or better vision, whereas one eye was lost (84).

One of the major risk factors for incisional rupture is the depth and length of the corneal incision (85–87). Pinheiro et al. (86) reported decreased corneal rupture in incisional surgery due to increased intraocular pressure, and reduced length of the RK incision ("mini-RK," limiting the radial incisions to within 3.5 mm from center of the central clear zone, instead of "conventional RK," where the incisions extend in proximity of the limbus) as with cases of blunt trauma (86).

Binder and associates (92) reported a histopathologic study of traumatic corneal rupture after RK in two patients involved in motor vehicle accidents. A 24-year-old woman had undergone 16-incision RK in the left eye in 1981. Two years later she suffered head trauma in a motor vehicle accident with loss of consciousness. Vision in the left eye was found to be light perception on the day of injury. A stellate corneal-scleral rupture was seen with the main rupture in the center of the cornea in the vertical axis with 1.5 mm extensions into the sclera on both sides, connecting the two RK incision sites in that axis. A horizontal rupture of the cornea in the RK site at the 9 o'clock position also extended to the center and connected with the oblique rupture. Complete avulsion of the lens and iris was seen, with vitreous beyond the wound. The corneal-scleral lacerations were repaired the same day with anterior vitrectomy. One month later the vision remained at light perception. The patient subsequently developed ghost cell glaucoma, and a posterior vitrectomy was done to control intraocular pressure. A penetrating keratoplasty was performed for corneal edema, and 1 month postoperatively vision was corrected to 20/50 with a contact lens. The second patient was a 27-year-old man who underwent eight-incision RK on the left eye and four-incision RK on the right eye. One year after surgery on the left eye, the patient was involved in a motor vehicle accident causing head trauma. He died 7 days later and a traumatic corneoscleral laceration was seen at the time of autopsy. Histologic studies showed incomplete wound healing at the RK incisions (92).

Interestingly, there have also been reports in the literature of ocular trauma cases without rupture in post-RK eyes (84,88–91). Casebeer et al. (88) reported two cases of severe ocular trauma (airplane crash with facial bone fractures and blunt trauma due to high-speed racquetball) without rupture of the RK incisions.

In another report of ocular trauma occurring 2 weeks to 53 months after RK surgery in eight eyes of seven patients, two eyes had dehiscence of the radial incisions and were treated with bandage contact lens, whereas in the other six eyes, the RK incisions remained intact. In this small series, all the eyes regained pretraumatic vision (91). The authors note that although some cases may heal spontaneously, others may need a bandage contact lens and some may require surgical repair.

As RK incisions are prone to gaping, entry of foreign bodies into the incisions during trauma may result in foreign-body corneal stromal entrapment. Soong (93) described a case of a 41-year-old man who has had undergone eight-incision RK. He was struck in the eye with a tree branch 6 years later, with tree bark embedding in the anterior stroma of three of the RK incisions. The embedded foreign bodies were removed and the incisions irrigated with balanced salt solution. Subconjunctival cephalosporin was administered and the patient received 1 week of topical ofloxacin four times a day. Best spectacle corrected visual acuity (BSCVA) 5 weeks after the injury was 20/25 (93). A similar scenario in the military literature of a soldier who sustained ocular trauma after RK surgery during field training exercises has also been reported. This injury resulted in a full-thickness corneal perforation through an RK incision. Fortunately, the visual outcome was excellent (94).

Unlike incisional refractive surgery, eyes that have undergone PRK or LASIK have not been shown to require energy levels significantly different to cause globe rupture compared to unoperated eyes (95–97). In one animal study, the depth of corneal laser ablation in pigs was not shown to compromise the integrity of the cornea until a depth of 40% total corneal thickness (corneal rupture in lateral incision) was achieved (95).

It is well recognized in LASIK that during the immediate postoperative period flap displacement and folds can occur. This can be best appreciated on retroillumination or with negative staining using fluorescein. Both micro- and macrostriae may be visually significant, requiring elevation and reposition of the LASIK flap often in conjunction with corneal stretching or ironing depending on the time interval after the procedure or injury. A bandage contact lens should be placed over the cornea after treatment for corneal striae. In cases of macrostriae or long-standing microstriae, corneal suture placement may be necessary. Both interrupted and running suture techniques have been described. Extensive manipulation during surgery or epithelial defects in the immediate postoperative days may predispose to diffuse lamellar keratitis (DLK) (97).

Traumatic displacement of the LASIK flap has also been reported as a late complication occurring weeks to months after the surgery. Early flap dislocation has been reported by some to be due to early flap slippage with loss of BSCVA of no more than two lines due to separation of the flap. Melki et al. (98) reported four cases of late traumatic flap dislocation after LASIK. They noted flap susceptibility to trauma 2 months after LASIK and the ease of lifting the LASIK flap after the initial surgery up to 1 year for enhancements.

Several other case reports have described corneal flap dislocation due to trauma. These include flap dislocation 10 months post-LASIK secondary to a fingernail (99), a tree branch accident causing flap dehiscence 6 months after LASIK (100), trauma due to a flying stone 10 months after LASIK (resulting in a 10-mm horizontal laceration across the stromal bed) (101), late flap dislocation at 3 months (direct blow to the eye due to a pecan falling from a tree), 11 months (hit with a cable at work), and 38 months (motor vehicle accident with deployed airbag causing knuckles to be forced into the eye) after LASIK due to direct trauma (102), and complete subtarsal flap dislocation 1 day post-superior hinge LASIK due to eye rubbing in a patient with history of mental illness and epilepsy (103).

Displaced LASIK flaps should be repaired emergently in order to prevent fixed folds, epithelial ingrowth, or DLK (Diffuse Lamellar Keratitis), and to provide the best chance for visual recovery. Removal of the epithelial cells and debris on the LASIK stromal bed and the underside of the LASIK flap should be performed prior to repositioning of the flap. This can be done using a No. 15 Bard Parker blade or dry Murocel sponge. A contact lens should be placed on the cornea after the procedure. If a flap is completely dislocated, positioning of the flap without surgical marks may become a challenge, resulting in improper seating and resultant irregular astigmatism. Additional repositioning with suturing of the flap may be necessary. If the flap is lost, healing epithelium often causes a hyperopic shift due to overall flattening of the cornea (98).

A report by Tumbocon et al. (104) in 2003 reviewed the management of flap displacement after bilateral LASIK in two patients. A 25-year-old man who was struck with a dog's paw 26 months after bilateral LASIK and was seen 4 hours after the trauma with a dehisced and folded LASIK flap with adjacent striae. He underwent a flap unfolding, repositioning, stretching, and irrigation as well as epithelial mechanical scraping of the underside of the flap with bandage contact lens placement. He was noted to have DLK the next day and was treated with increasing topical steroids. Six weeks later, his vision stabilized to 20/20 without correction. In the second case, a 35-year-old man had bilateral LASIK 7 months earlier prior to being struck with a rock to the left side of his face in a kayaking accident. He was seen 2 days later and noted to have a displaced flap with a central epithelial defect and macrofolds as well as a left orbital floor fracture. The flap was lifted, repositioned, and stretched after irrigation with gentle scraping of the stromal bed and underside of the flap. A bandage contact lens was placed. He was found to have DLK the next day, which was treated with topical steroids. The LASIK flap was relifted 3 days later, and again 2 weeks later to smooth microstria present centrally. Two weeks after the final surgical treatment, uncorrected visual acuity (UCVA) was 20/40+.

Aldave et al. (105) summarized several reported cases of late flap displacements in the literature and their management. They also reported on their own institution's experience with a displaced LASIK flap 18 months after surgery and 14 months after enhancement when the patient was struck in the eye by a finger during a basketball game. The patient was seen an hour later and the flap repositioned and bandage contact lens was placed. The next day epithelial ingrowth was present and the flap relifted. Epithelial cells were removed, copious irrigation under the flap was performed, the flap was repositioned, and the bandage contact lens replaced. The next day DLK was noted and treated with topical steroids. Three weeks after the injury, uncorrected visual acuity was 20/20 and remained stable 7 months later on examination.

Both infectious keratitis and diffuse lamellar keratitis have been described postoperatively following traumatic ocular injury. DLK is reported in 0.2% to 1.8% of patients who present within a week of primary LASIK or an enhancement procedure. Late-onset cases have also been noted from 2 to 12 months after LASIK with traumatic spontaneous epithelial defects (105). DLK has been reported due to both traumatic flap displacement from a dog's paw (98) and metallic foreign-body removal from a flap (106). These cases were treated with frequent steroids followed by a tapering schedule with full visual recovery in 1 to 2 weeks.

Many patients undergo laser vision correction to relieve themselves of eyeglasses, especially while engaging in sports, which in itself is a risk factor for ocular trauma. It is necessary for patients to understand the risks involved before undergoing a refractive surgery procedure. This is particularly true for those in law enforcement, the military, or participating in contact sports. The choice of surgery as well as the postoperative care should be reviewed at length with all patients. A special consideration should be given to recommending protective eyewear during high-risk activities (military, sports), with polycarbonate, shatter-resistant, eye wear that meet the American Society for Testing and Material E803-88a Standard. Helmets may also be necessary for face and eye safety for some activities (107).

In summary, trauma after refractive surgery can have severe visual consequences. The occurrences of traumatic flap dislocation in cases of LASIK surgery or rupture of corneal incisions following RK or AK surgery are infrequent but well documented. All refractive surgery-related injuries should be considered emergencies and treated immediately and appropriately. Informed consent and patient education in the preoperative period are essential so patients undergoing corneal refractive surgery procedures can take a proactive approach to protect their corneas.

REFERENCES

1. Kenyon KR, Wagoner MD. Conjunctival and corneal injuries. In: Shingleton BJ, Hersh PS, Kenyon KR, eds. *Eye trauma.* St. Louis: Mosby-Year Book, 1991:63–78.
2. Slingsby JG, Forstot SL. Effect of blunt trauma on the corneal endothelium. *Arch Ophthalmol* 1981;99:1041–1043.
3. Topping TM, Stark WJ, Maumenee E, et al. Traumatic wound dehiscence following penetrating keratoplasty. *Br J Ophthalmol* 1982;66:174–178.
4. Chiapella AP, Rosenthal AR. One year in an eye casualty clinic. *Br J Ophthalmol* 1985;69:865–870.
5. Carter K, Miller KM. Ophthalmology inpatient consultation. *Ophthalmology* 2001;108:1505–1511.
6. Fujikawa LS, Foster CS, Gipson IK, et al. Basement membrane components in healing rabbit corneal epithelial wounds: immunofluorescence and ultrastructural studies. *J Cell Biol* 1984;98:128–138.
7. Potts AM, Distler JA. Shape factor in the penetration of intraocular foreign bodies. *Am J Ophthalmol* 1985;100:183–187.
8. Augeri PA. Corneal foreign body removal and treatment. *Optom Clin* 1991;1:59–70.
9. Michael JG, Hug D, Dowd MD. Management of corneal abrasion in children: a randomized clinical trial. *Ann Emerg Med* 2002;40:67–72.
10. Pfister RR, Burstein N. The effects of ophthalmic drugs, vehicles, and preservatives on corneal epithelium: a scanning electron microscope study. Invest Ophthalmol 1976;15:246–259.
11. Kaiser PK, Pineda R 2nd. A study of topical nonsteroidal anti-inflammatory drops and no pressure patching in the treatment of corneal abrasions. Corneal Abrasion Patching Study Group. *Ophthalmology* 1997;104:1353–1359.
12. Gregersen PL, Ottovay E, Kobayashi C, et al. [Treatment of corneal abrasion]. *Ugeskr Laeger* 1991;153:2123–2124.
13. Easty DL. Is an eye pad needed in cases of corneal abrasion? *BMJ* 1993;307:1022.
14. Kaiser PK. A comparison of pressure patching versus no patching for corneal abrasions due to trauma or foreign body removal.

Corneal Abrasion Patching Study Group. *Ophthalmology* 1995; 102:1936–1942.

15. Patterson J, Fetzer D, Krall J, et al. Eye patch treatment for the pain of corneal abrasion. *South Med J* 1996;89:227–229.

16. Arbour JD, Brunette I, Boisjoly HM, et al. Should we patch corneal erosions? *Arch Ophthalmol* 1997;115:313–317.

17. Ali Z, Insler MS. A comparison of therapeutic bandage lenses, tarsorrhaphy, and antibiotic and hypertonic saline on corneal epithelial wound healing. *Ann Ophthalmol* 1986;18:22–24.

18. Sabri K. High prevalence of recurrent symptoms following uncomplicated traumatic corneal abrasion (reply). *Br J Ophthalmol* 1998;82:850.

19. Sabri K, Pandit JC, Thaller VT, et al. National survey of corneal abrasion treatment. *Eye* 1998;12(pt 2):278–281.

20. Kenyon KR. Recurrent corneal erosion: pathogenesis and therapy. *Int Ophthalmol Clin* 1979;19:169–195.

21. Weene LE. Recurrent corneal erosion after trauma: a statistical study. *Ann Ophthalmol* 1985;17:521–522,524.

22. Zuckerman BD, Leiberman TW. Corneal rust ring. *Arch Ophthalmol* 1960;63:254–265.

23. Sigurdsson H, Hanna I, Lockwood AJ, et al. Removal of rust rings, comparing electric drill and hypodermic needle. *Eye* 1987;1(pt 3):430–432.

24. Pavan-Langston D. Burns and trauma. In: Pavan-Langston D, ed. *Manual of ocular diagnosis and therapy,* 5th ed. Philadelphia: Lippincott Williams & Wilkins, 2002:37–38.

25. Au YK, Libby C, Patel JS. Removal of a corneal foreign body through a lamellar corneal pocket. *Ophthalmic Surg Lasers* 1996;27:471–472.

26. Yang X. Removal of corneal foreign bodies that project into the anterior chamber: use of a suture needle. *Am J Ophthalmol* 2000;129:801–802.

27. Steahly LP, Almquist HT. Corneal foreign bodies of coconut origin. *Ann Ophthalmol* 1977;9:1017–1021.

28. Watts P, McPherson R, Hawksworth NR. Tarantula keratouveitis. *Cornea* 2000;19:393–394.

29. Stulting RD, Hooper RJ, Cavanagh HD. Ocular injury caused by tarantula hairs. *Am J Ophthalmol* 1983;96:118–119.

30. Chang PC, Soong HK, Barnett JM. Corneal penetration by tarantula hairs. *Br J Ophthalmol* 1991;75:253–254.

31. Cooke JA, Miller FH, Grover RW, et al. Urticaria caused by tarantula hairs. *Am J Trop Med Hyg* 1973;22:130–133.

32. Hered RW, Spaulding AG, Sanitato JJ, et al. Ophthalmia nodosa caused by tarantula hairs. *Ophthalmology* 1988;95:166–169.

33. Waggoner TL, Nishimoto JH, Eng J. Eye injury from tarantula. *J Am Optom Assoc* 1997;68:188–190.

34. Porges Y, Landau D, Douieb J, et al. Removal of corneal foreign bodies following laser in situ keratomileusis. *J Refract Surg* 2001;17:559–560.

35. Brown N, Bron A. Recurrent erosion of the cornea. *Br J Ophthalmol* 1976;60:84–96.

36. Stein JD, Jaeger EA, Jeffers JB. Air bags and ocular injuries. *Trans Am Ophthalmol Soc* 1999;97:59–82; discussion 82–86.

37. Vichnin MC, Jaeger EA, Gault JA, et al. Ocular injuries related to air bag inflation. *Ophthalmic Surg Lasers* 1995;26:542–548.

38. Duma SM, Kress TA, Porta DJ, et al. Airbag-induced eye injuries: a report of 25 cases. *J Trauma* 1996;41:114–119.

39. Ghafouri A, Burgess SK, Hrdlicka ZK, et al. Air bag-related ocular trauma. *Am J Emerg Med* 1997;15:389–392.

40. Kuhn F, Morris R, Witherspoon CD. Eye injury and the air bag. *Curr Opin Ophthalmol* 1995;6:38–44.

41. Larkin GL. Airbag-mediated corneal injury. *Am J Emerg Med* 1991;9:444–446.

42. Bhavsar AR, Chen TC, Goldstein DA. Corneoscleral laceration associated with passenger-side airbag inflation. *Br J Ophthalmol* 1997;81:514–515.

43. Baker RS, Flowers CW Jr, Singh P, et al. Corneoscleral laceration caused by air-bag trauma. *Am J Ophthalmol* 1996;121:709–711.

44. Chialant D, Damji KF. Ultrasound biomicroscopy in diagnosis of a cyclodialysis cleft in a patient with corneal edema and hypotony after an air bag injury. *Can J Ophthalmol* 2000;35:148–150.

45. Fukagawa K, Tsubota K, Kimura C, et al. Corneal endothelial cell loss induced by air bags. *Ophthalmology* 1993;100:1819–1823.

46. Geggel HS, Griggs PB, Freeman MI. Irreversible bullous keratopathy after air bag trauma. *CLAO J* 1996;22:148–150.

47. White JE, McClafferty K, Orton RB, et al. Ocular alkali burn associated with automobile air-bag activation. *Can Med Assoc J* 1995;153:933–934.

48. Duma SM, Jernigan MV, Stitzel JD, et al. The effect of frontal air bags on eye injury patterns in automobile crashes. *Arch Ophthalmol* 2002;120:1517–1522.

49. Lehto KS, Sulander PO, Tervo TM. Do motor vehicle airbags increase risk of ocular injuries in adults? *Ophthalmology* 2003;110:1082–1088.

50. Rowsey JJ. Corneal laceration repair: topographic considerations and suturing techniques. In: Shingleton BJ, Hersh PS, Kenyon KR, eds. *Eye trauma.* St. Louis: Mosby-Year Book, 1991:159–168.

51. Rowsey JJ. Ten caveats in keratorefractive surgery. *Ophthalmology* 1983;90:148-55.

52. Rowsey JJ. Topographical analysis of the cornea: ten caveats in keratorefractive surgery. *Int Ophthalmol Clin* 1983;23:1–32.

53. Rowsey JJ, Balyeat HD, Rabinovitch B, et al. Predicting the results of radial keratotomy. *Ophthalmology* 1983;90:642–654.

54. Eisner G. *Eye surgery: an introduction to operative technique,* 1st ed. New York: Springer-Verlag, 1980.

55. Hersh PS, Shingleton BJ, Kenyon KR. Management of corneoscleral lacerations. In: Shingleton BJ, Hersh PS, Kenyon KR, eds. *Eye trauma.* St. Louis: Mosby-Year Book, 1991:143–158.

56. Pineda R 2nd. Four pearls for suturing corneal incisions and lacerations. In: Melki SA, Azar DT, eds. *One hundred and one pearls in refractive, cataract, and corneal surgery.* Thorofare, NJ: SLACK Incorporated, 2001:131–137.

57. Barr CC. Prognostic factors in corneoscleral lacerations. *Arch Ophthalmol* 1983;101:919–924.

58. Eagling EM. Perforating injuries of the eye. *Br J Ophthalmol* 1976;60:732–736.

59. Refojo MF, Dohlman CH, Ahmad B, et al. Evaluation of adhesives for corneal surgery. *Arch Ophthalmol* 1968;80:645–656.

60. Muga R, Maul E. The management of lens damage in perforating corneal lacerations. *Br J Ophthalmol* 1978;62:784–787.

61. MacCumber MW, Zanger MW. Open-globe injuries. *Focal Points* 2001;19:1–14.

62. Rubsamen PE, Irvin WD, McCuen BW 2nd, et al. Primary intraocular lens implantation in the setting of penetrating ocular trauma. *Ophthalmology* 1995;102:101–107.

63. Anwar M, Bleik JH, von Noorden GK, et al. Posterior chamber lens implantation for primary repair of corneal lacerations and traumatic cataracts in children. *J Pediatr Ophthalmol Strabismus* 1994;31:157–161.

64. Apple DJ, Price FW, Gwin T, et al. Sutured retropupillary posterior chamber intraocular lenses for exchange or secondary implantation. The 12th annual Binkhorst lecture, 1988. *Ophthalmology* 1989;96:1241–1247.

65. Stark WJ, Gottsch JD, Goodman DF, et al. Posterior chamber intraocular lens implantation in the absence of capsular support. *Arch Ophthalmol* 1989;107:1078–1083.

66. Sippel KC, Pineda R Jr. Phacoemulsification and thermal wound injury. *Semin Ophthalmol* 2002;17:102–109.

67. Sugar A, Schertzer RM. Clinical course of phacoemulsification wound burns. *J Cataract Refract Surg* 1999;25:688–692.

68. Davison JA. Acute intraoperative suprachoroidal hemorrhage in capsular bag phacoemulsification. *J Cataract Refract Surg* 1993;19:534–537.

69. Davison JA. Acute intraoperative suprachoroidal hemorrhage (letter). *J Cataract Refract Surg* 1994;20:107–108.

70. Majid MA, Sharma MK, Harding SP. Corneoscleral burn during phacoemulsification surgery. *J Cataract Refract Surg* 1998;24:1413–1415.

71. Leaming DV. Practice styles and preferences of ASCRS members—1994 survey. *J Cataract Refract Surg* 1995;21:378–385.

72. Singh R, Vasavada AR, Janaswamy G. Phacoemulsification of brunescent and black cataracts. *J Cataract Refract Surg* 2001;27:1762–1769.

73. Wirt H, Heisler JM, von Domarus D. Experimental study of the temperature during phacoemulsification. *Ophthalmologe* 1995;92:339–345.

74. Ernest P, Rhem M, McDermott M, et al. Phacoemulsification conditions resulting in thermal wound injury. *J Cataract Refract Surg* 2001;27:1829–1839.

75. Davis PL. Phaco transducers: basic principles and corneal thermal injury. *Eur J Implant Ref Surg* 1993;5:109–112.

76. Peacock LW, Slade SG, Martiz J, et al. Ocular integrity after refractive procedures. *Ophthalmology* 1997;104:1079–1083.

77. Lee BL, Manche EE, Glasgow BJ. Rupture of radial and arcuate keratotomy scars by blunt trauma 91 months after incisional keratotomy. *Am J Ophthalmol* 1995;120:108–110.

78. Schmitt-Bernard CF, Villain M, Beaufrere L, et al. Trauma after radial keratotomy and photorefractive keratectomy. *J Cataract Refract Surg* 1997;23:803–804.

79. Uchio E, Ohno S, Kudoh K, et al. Simulation of air-bag impact on post-radial keratotomy eye using finite element analysis. *J Cataract Refract Surg* 2001;27:1847–1853.

80. Vinger PF, Mieler WF, Oestreicher JH, et al. Ruptured globes following radial and hexagonal keratotomy surgery. *Arch Ophthalmol* 1996;114:129–134.

81. Deg JK, Zavala EY, Binder PS. Delayed corneal wound healing following radial keratotomy. *Ophthalmology* 1985;92:734–740.

82. Binder PS, Nayak SK, Deg JK, et al. An ultrastructural and histochemical study of long-term wound healing after radial keratotomy. *Am J Ophthalmol* 1987;103:432–440.

83. Deg JK, Binder PS. Wound healing after astigmatic keratotomy in human eyes. *Ophthalmology* 1987;94:1290–1298.

84. Panda A, Sharma N, Kumar A. Ruptured globe 10 years after radial keratotomy. *J Refract Surg* 1999;15:64–65.

85. Luttrull JK, Jester JV, Smith RE. The effect of radial keratotomy on ocular integrity in an animal model. *Arch Ophthalmol* 1982;100:319–320.

86. Pinheiro MN Jr, Bryant MR, Tayyanipour R, et al. Corneal integrity after refractive surgery. Effects of radial keratotomy and mini-radial keratotomy. *Ophthalmology* 1995;102:297–301.

87. Steinemann TL, Baltz TC, Lam BL, et al. Mini radial keratotomy reduces ocular integrity. Axial compression in a postmortem porcine eye model. *Ophthalmology* 1998;105:1739–1744.

88. Casebeer JC, Shapiro DR, Phillips S. Severe ocular trauma without corneal rupture after radial keratotomy: case reports. *J Refract Corneal Surg* 1994;10:31–33.

89. Spivack L. Radial keratotomy incisions remain intact despite facial trauma from plane crash. *J Refract Surg* 1987;3:59–60.

90. John ME Jr, Schmitt TE. Traumatic hyphema after radial keratotomy. *Ann Ophthalmol* 1983;15:930–932.

91. Forstot SL, Damiano RE. Trauma after radial keratotomy. *Ophthalmology* 1988;95:833–835.

92. Binder PS, Waring GO 3rd, Arrowsmith PN, et al. Histopathology of traumatic corneal rupture after radial keratotomy. *Arch Ophthalmol* 1988;106:1584–1590.

93. Soong K. Foreign body entrapment in radial keratotomy incisions. *Arch Ophthalmol* 1999;117:836–837.

94. Nolan BT. Perforation by a foreign body through a pre-existing radial keratotomy wound. *Mil Med* 1991;156:151–154.

95. Burnstein Y, Klapper D, Hersh PS. Experimental globe rupture after excimer laser photorefractive keratectomy. *Arch Ophthalmol* 1995;113:1056–1059.

96. Campos M, Lee M, McDonnell PJ. Ocular integrity after refractive surgery: effects of photorefractive keratectomy, phototherapeutic keratectomy, and radial keratotomy. *Ophthalmic Surg* 1992;23:598–602.

97. Shah MN, Misra M, Wihelmus KR, et al. Diffuse lamellar keratitis associated with epithelial defects after laser in situ keratomileusis. *J Cataract Refract Surg* 2000;26:1312–1318.

98. Melki SA, Talamo JH, Demetriades AM, et al. Late traumatic dislocation of laser in situ keratomileusis corneal flaps. *Ophthalmology* 2000;107:2136–2139.

99. Patel CK, Hanson R, McDonald B, et al. Case reports and small case series: late dislocation of a LASIK flap caused by a fingernail. *Arch Ophthalmol* 2001;119:447–449.

100. Geggel HS, Coday MP. Late-onset traumatic laser in situ keratomileusis (LASIK) flap dehiscence. *Am J Ophthalmol* 2001;131:505–506.

101. Lombardo AJ, Katz HR. Late partial dislocation of a laser in situ keratomileusis flap. *J Cataract Refract Surg* 2001;27:1108–1110.

102. Iskander NG, Peters NT, Anderson Penno E, et al. Late traumatic flap dislocation after laser in situ keratomileusis. *J Cataract Refract Surg* 2001;27:1111–1114.

103. Maldonado MJ, Juberias JR. Subtarsal flap dislocation after superior hinge laser in situ keratomileusis in a patient with borderline mental illness. *J Refract Surg* 2003;19:169–171.

104. Tumbocon JAJ, Paul R, Slomovic A, et al. Late traumatic displacement of laser in situ keratomileusis flaps. *Cornea* 2003;22:66–69.

105. Aldave AJ, Hollander DA, Abbott RL. Late-onset traumatic flap dislocation and diffuse lamellar inflammation after laser in situ keratomileusis. *Cornea* 2002;21:604–607.

106. Lam DS, Leung AT, Wu JT, et al. Management of severe flap wrinkling or dislodgment after laser in situ keratomileusis. *J Cataract Refract Surg* 1999;25:1441–1447.

107. Vinger PF. Prescribing for contact sports. *Optom Clin* 1993;3:129–143.

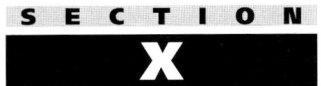

CORNEAL DYSTROPHIES AND DEGENERATIONS

ANTERIOR CORNEAL DYSTROPHIES: DYSTROPHIES OF THE EPITHELIUM, EPITHELIAL BASEMENT MEMBRANE, AND BOWMAN'S LAYER

PUWAT CHARUKAMNOETKANOK, SUHAS TULI, AND DIMITRI T. AZAR

Corneal dystrophies are noninflammatory, hereditary disorders that principally involve the central cornea and appear to have little or no relationship to systemic or environmental factors. They are classified according to the anteroposterior localization of the major pathologic alteration in the cornea: epithelial, stromal, and posterior dystrophies (Table 45-1) (1). This chapter focuses on the anterior dystrophies affecting the epithelium, epithelial basement membrane, and Bowman's layer. The study of the pathogenesis of corneal dystrophies at the molecular level has increased our understanding of the genetic basis of corneal dystrophies. A gene-based reclassification of corneal dystrophies may be possible in the near future (2). At present, however, the current classification scheme, based on the clinical and histologic findings, remains useful for the management of patients suffering from these potentially blinding corneal disorders.

JUVENILE HEREDITARY EPITHELIAL DYSTROPHY (MEESMANN'S DYSTROPHY)

Meesmann's dystrophy is a bilateral, diffuse, symmetric corneal dystrophy involving accumulation of intracytoplasmic deposits in the corneal epithelium and manifesting as uniformly sized epithelial cysts.

The disorder was first described clinically by Pameijer (3) in 1935 and histopathologically by Meesmann and Wilke (4) in 1939. This rare autosomal-dominant dystrophy (5) has incomplete penetrance (as low as 60%) and variable expressivity (3–9). However, Stocker and Holt (5) also reported a recessive form in 20 individuals in a group of 200 descendants of Moravian settlers. The molecular basis of Meesmann's epithelial corneal dystrophy has been attributed to mutations in two causative genes, the cornea specific keratin genes *KRT3* (chromosome 12q13) and *KRT12* (chromosome 17q12), which encode cytoskeletal proteins K3 and K12, respectively (10–12). The mechanisms by which these mutations cause the Meesmann's phenotype remain to be elucidated.

Clinical Features

Corneal involvement is bilateral and is most prominent in the interpalpebral zone. Clusters of tiny round cysts in the epithelium appear as discrete white spots on focal illumination and as refractile, clear, cystlike structures on retroillumination (Fig. 45-1) (8). These myriad fine round cysts of uniform size and shape usually become visible by 12 months of age and increase in number throughout life. Coalescence of cysts may form refractile lines. Patients remain asymptomatic until the fourth or fifth decades of life, when photophobia, redness, and pain occur because of recurrent erosions due to rupture of cysts. Subepithelial gray opacities appear at the late stage of the disease. In general, visual acuity remains functionally good, but patients may complain of blurred vision (5).

Histopathology

The primary pathosis in Meesmann's dystrophy is in the basal epithelium, with accumulation of an abnormal, electron-dense, intracytoplasmic material described as a "peculiar substance" (Fig. 45-2). This fibrillogranular material, whose exact composition is unknown, causes cell death. Cysts are actually areas of cellular degeneration and contain periodic acid-Schiff (PAS)-positive material (Fig. 45-3). Increased cell turnover results in thickening of the basement membrane and increased glycogen content of the basal epithelial cells (6,13,14). Bowman's layer and the superficial stroma are unaffected.

TABLE 45-1*: CORNEAL DYSTROPHIES

Dystrophies	Inheritance	Gene	Locus
Epithelium and Basement Membrane Dystrophies			
Epithelium:			
Meesmann's dystrophy	AD	KRT3 and KRT12	12q13 and 17q12
Epithelium Basement Membrane:			
Map/dot/fingerprint dystrophy	Sporadic/AD		
Stromal Dystrophies			
Bowman's layer:			
Reis-Bucklers dystrophy	AD	βig-h3	5q31
Anterior membrane dystrophy of Grayson-Wilbrandt	AD		
Honeycomb dystrophy of Thiel and Behnke	AD		10q23-q24
Subepithelial mucinous corneal dystrophy	AD		
Stroma:			
Granular dystrophy	AD	βig-h3	5q31
Avellino's dystrophy	AD	βig-h3	5q31
Lattice dystrophy (Type I, III, IIIA, and IV)	AD	βig-h3	5q31
Meretoja syndrome (Lattice Type II)	AD	Gelsolin	9q34
Macular dystrophy	AR		16q21
Gelatinous droplike dystrophy	AD	M1S1	1p
Fleck dystrophy	AD		
Central crystalline dystrophy of Schnyder	AD	MTHFR, galactose 4-epimerase	1p36-p34.1
Marginal crystalline dystrophy of Bietti	AD		4q35ter
Central cloudy dystrophy of Francois	AD		
Parenchymatous dystrophy of Pillat	AD		
Posterior amorphous dystrophy	AD		
Pre-Descemet:			
Typical pre-Descemet's dystrophy associated with ichthyosis	AD/XR	STS	Xp22.32
Polymorphic stromal dystrophy			
Cornea farinata			
Endothelial Dystrophy			
Endothelium:			
Fuchs' endothelial dystrophy	AD	COL8A2, ?Mitochondria	1p34.3-p32
Congenital hereditary endothelial dystrophy	AD/AR		20p, 20tel
Posterior polymorphous dystrophy	AD		20q11

* Modified from Ref 1.
KRT: keratin genes
βig-h3: human TGF beta induced gene, keratoepithelin
M1S1: membrane component, chromosome 1, surface marker 1.
MTHFR: methylene tetrahydrofolate reductase

Management

Because the patients are usually asymptomatic or have minimal symptoms, treatment is rarely required. Debridement of the epithelium is usually followed by reappearance of symptoms. Although curative, superficial keratectomy is rarely warranted (15). Excimer laser phototherapeutic keratectomy (PTK) has emerged as an alternative treatment of recalcitrant recurrent erosions. With PTK the epithelial defect sites are ablated to a depth of 3 to 4 μm with reportedly promising results (16–24). Lamellar and penetrating keratoplasty are seldom indicated (5,13). Although the dystrophy can recur in grafts, the recurrent disease is often less severe.

EPITHELIAL BASEMENT MEMBRANE DYSTROPHY (COGAN'S MICROCYSTIC DYSTROPHY)

Epithelial basement membrane dystrophy (EBMD) is a corneal disorder characterized by recurrent epithelial erosion as a result of abnormal epithelial turnover, maturation, and production of basement membrane. The lesions are bilateral but can be asymmetric. The findings are variable and may change with time.

This dystrophy is also known by many other names: fingerprint/map/dot dystrophy, fingerprint dystrophy, anterior basement dystrophy, and dystrophic recurrent erosion. The

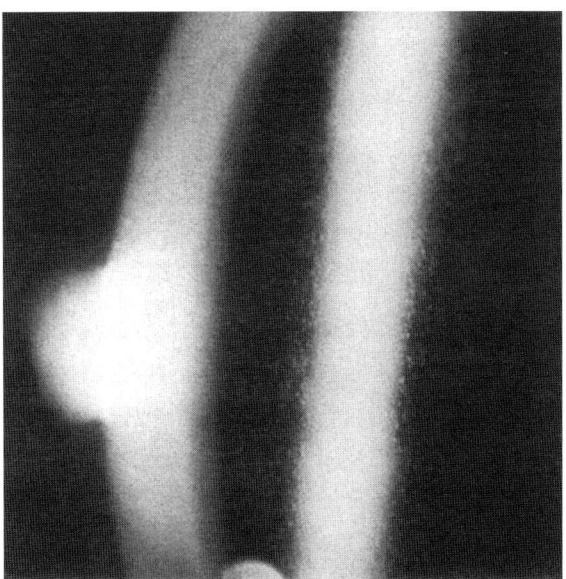

FIGURE 45-1. Meesmann's dystrophy. Retroillumination views of characteristic multiple small uniform cysts seen on slit-lamp examination. (From Irvine AD, Coleman CM, Moore JE, et al. A novel mutation in KRT12 associated with Meesmann's epithelial corneal dystrophy. *Br J Ophthalmol* 2002;86:729–732, with permission.)

underlying pathology is localized to the abnormal epithelial–basement membrane adhesion complex and manifests clinically as recurrent erosions. The primary alteration in the epithelial–basement membrane adhesion complex could be due to a defect of the epithelium, the epithelial basement membrane, or Bowman's membrane, in combination with or without production of abnormal substances.

Clinical Features

EBMD is the most frequently encountered anterior corneal dystrophy in clinical practice (15,25–28). Although autosomal-dominant forms have been reported (29–31),

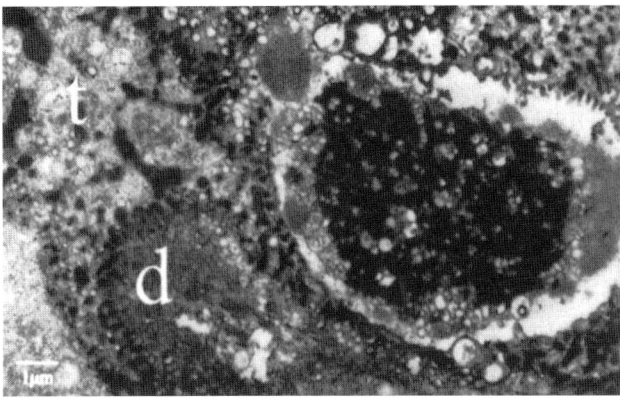

FIGURE 45-2. Meesmann's dystrophy. Electron microscopic detail of the electron-dense "peculiar substance." T, tonofilament; d, desmosomes. (From Irvine AD, Coleman CM, Moore JE, et al. A novel mutation in KRT12 associated with Meesmann's epithelial corneal dystrophy. *Br J Ophthalmol* 2002;86:729–732, with permission.)

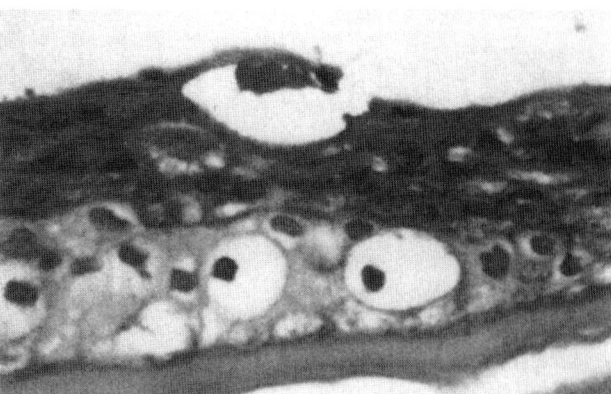

FIGURE 45-3. Meesmann's dystrophy. Light microscopy showing abnormal corneal epithelium that appears acanthotic and disordered. Many keratinocytes contain periodic acid-Schiff (PAS)-positive fibrillar material. (From Irvine AD, Coleman CM, Moore JE, et al. A novel mutation in KRT12 associated with Meesmann's epithelial corneal dystrophy. *Br J Ophthalmol* 2002; 86:729–732, with permission.)

many cases do not have a definite hereditary pattern. Changes similar to fingerprint/map/dot dystrophy are seen in about 6% of the normal population above the age of 50 years (32).

Cogan et al. (25) first described microcystic dystrophy of the cornea in five unrelated women at the Massachusetts Eye and Ear Infirmary in Boston, who had bilateral grayish-white spherical lesions of varying sizes. Maplike dystrophy was described by Guerry in 1965 (33), who had earlier reported fingerprint lines (34).

The patients with EBMD are predominantly white women above 30 years of age. But EBMD can become manifest as early as 4 to 8 years of age in familial cases. In nonfamilial cases, recurrent erosions occur for a few years, improve spontaneously, and do not leave significant residual visual acuity loss (35). Maps are geographic circumscribed gray lesions best seen with broad oblique illumination. They appear in varying shapes and sizes and do not stain with fluorescein (Fig. 45-4). Dots are cysts or fine blebs seen as gray-white intraepithelial opacities of various sizes in close proximity to the maplike patches (Fig. 45-5). Fingerprint lines are branching refractile lines with club-shaped terminations (Fig. 45-6) (31). Retroillumination will strikingly highlight these lesions. Leashes of long, thick fingerprint lines are called "mares tails." Combinations of map and dots are encountered most frequently, followed by maps alone. Dots are the least frequently encountered of the three lesions. It is rare that fingerprints are present along with maps and dots, whereas dots alone are never seen. Visual acuity is usually minimally affected. However, irregular astigmatism or higher-order aberration may lead to visual loss.

Histopathology and Pathogenesis

The basic pathology in EBMD is the synthesis of abnormal basement membrane that is responsible for the whole spectrum of clinical manifestations. Erosions are due to absence

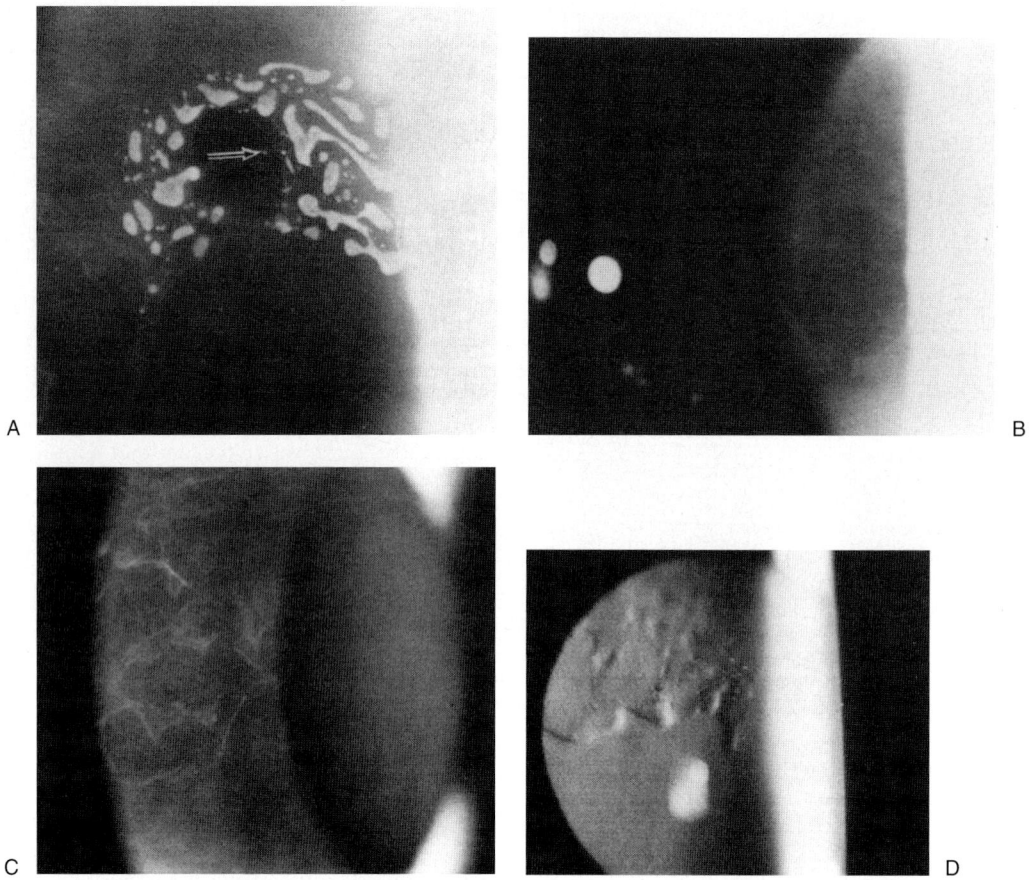

FIGURE 45-4. Epithelial basement membrane dystrophy. Map lines are thick irregular linear opacity surrounded by a faint haze. They resemble geographic borders on the maps. (From Laibson PR. Microcystic corneal dystrophy. *Trans Am Ophthalmol Soc* 1976;74:488–531, with permission.)

of hemidesmosomal connections of the epithelial cells in areas with abnormal basement membrane. Maps are projections of abnormal multilaminar basement membrane into the epithelium (Fig. 45-7) (36). Dots are pseudocysts filled with lipid and cytoplasmic and nuclear debris (Fig. 45-8). Cysts form in areas with intraepithelial exten-

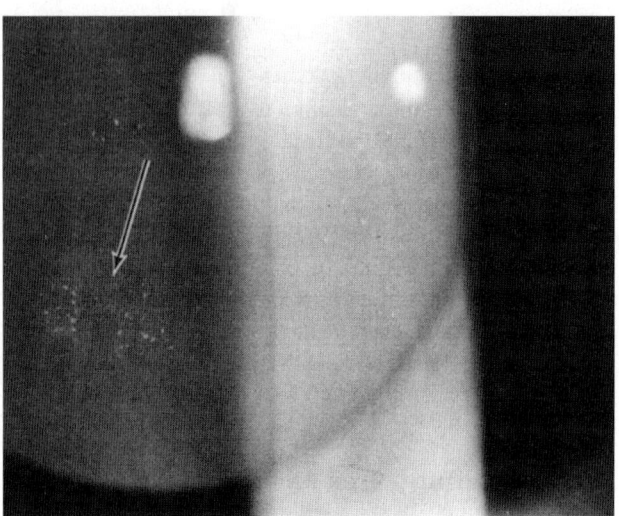

FIGURE 45-5. Epithelial basement membrane dystrophy. Fine clear dots are seen in retroillumination. (From Laibson PR. Microcystic corneal dystrophy. *Trans Am Ophthalmol Soc* 1976; 74:488–531, with permission.)

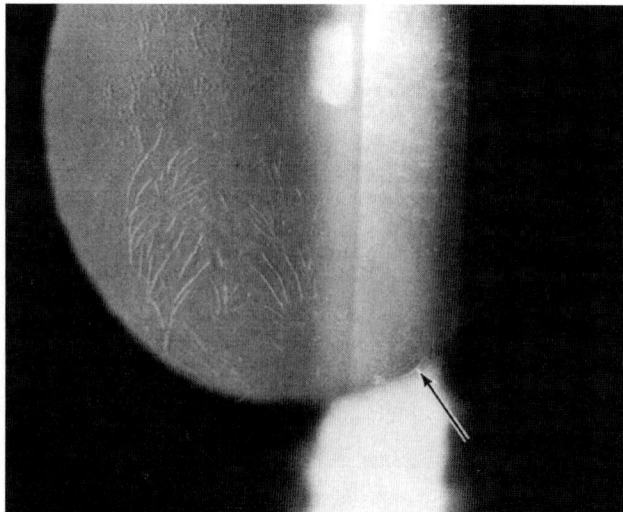

FIGURE 45-6. Epithelial basement membrane dystrophy. Fingerprint lines are thin hairliked lines. Several of them are often arranged in clusters resembling fingerprints. (From Laibson PR. Microcystic corneal dystrophy. *Trans Am Ophthalmol Soc* 1976;74:488–531, with permission.)

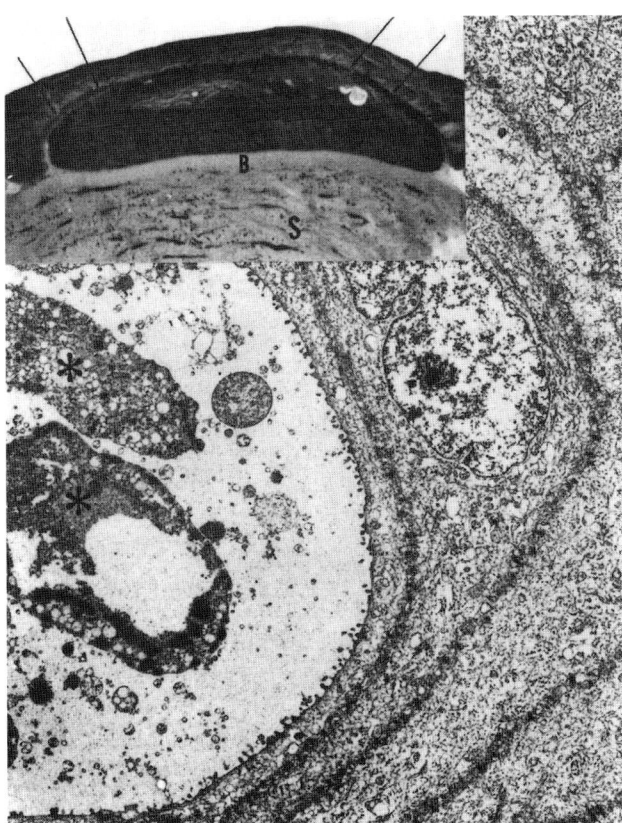

FIGURE 45-7. Epithelial basement membrane dystrophy. A histologic specimen from patient with map and microcysts. The *inset* shows detached intraepithelial basement membrane. B, Bowmen's layer; S, superficial stroma. The electron micrograph shows degenerated epithelial cell remnants (*) within an epithelial microcyst (×5,760). (From Laibson PR. Microcystic corneal dystrophy. *Trans Am Ophthalmol Soc* 1976;74:488–531, with permission.)

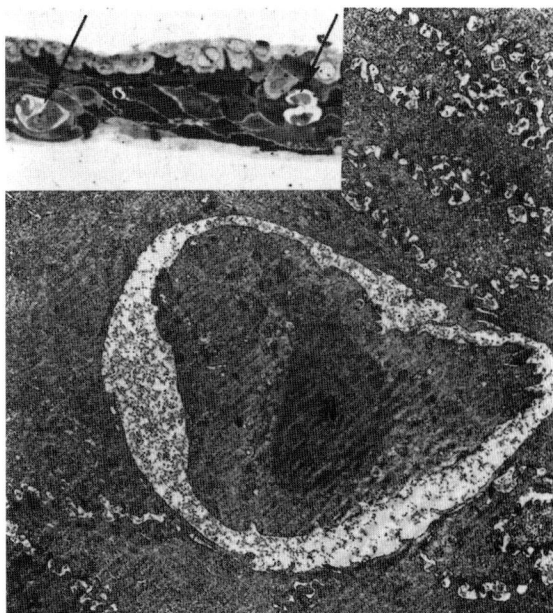

FIGURE 45-8. Epithelial basement membrane dystrophy. The *inset* demonstrates intraepithelial microcysts of varying size *(arrows)*. Electron micrograph shows an abnormal desquamated epithelial cell with pyknotic nucleus (N) with in an epithelial cyst (×6,120). (From Laibson PR. Microcystic corneal dystrophy. *Trans Am Ophthalmol Soc* 1976;74:488–531, with permission.)

sions of aberrant basement membrane. Epithelial cells beneath the aberrant basement membrane become vacuolated and liquefied. Rupture of these cysts causes recurrent erosions. Fingerprints represent linear projections of fibrillogranular material into the epithelium with thickening of the basement membrane (Fig. 45-9).

Management

Two major indications for treatment are debilitating recurrent erosions and visual loss due to irregular astigmatism. In the early stages, treatment consists of symptomatic management of recurrent erosions with hypertonic saline and double patching, and a thin, loosely fitting, high water content soft contact lens. Epithelial debridement has been reported to be successful in severe cases (37). In recalcitrant cases superficial keratectomy and a soft contact lens relieve symptoms (38). Diamond burr superficial keratectomy has been shown to be an effective and safe method of treating recurrent erosions (39). Anterior stromal puncture with a 23- to 25-gauge needle to a 0.1-mm depth induces new basement membrane formation and a fibrocytic reaction and may help decrease recurrences (40). There are several

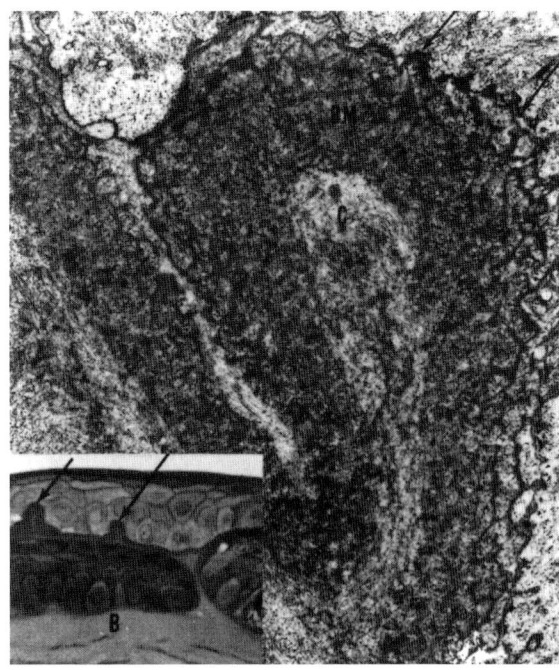

FIGURE 45-9. Epithelial basement membrane dystrophy. A specimen from a patient with fingerprint lines. The *inset* shows basement membrane excrescences *(arrows)* in the basal epithelium. Noted an intact Bowman's layer (B). Electron micrograph shows severely thickened multilaminar basement membrane (BM). The hemidesmosomes are detached and the basement membrane is separated from Bowman's layer by collagen (C). (From Laibson PR. Microcystic corneal dystrophy. *Trans Am Ophthalmol Soc* 1976;74:488–531, with permission.)

reports of treatment of recalcitrant recurrent erosions with excimer laser phototherapeutic keratectomy with success rates ranging from 74% to 100% (16–19,23,24). Hard contact lens effectively treats epithelial irregularity and may also decrease the severity of basement membrane changes.

REIS-BÜCKLERS DYSTROPHY

Reis-Bücklers dystrophy is a bilateral disorder characterized by superficial pleomorphic deposits in Bowman's layer secondary to generalized replacement of Bowman's layer by irregular collagen fibrils.

This condition was first reported by Reis (41) in 1917 as a superficial corneal annular dystrophy with geographic opacities. Later, Bücklers (42) gave a more detailed description in another family. The mode of inheritance is autosomal dominant with variable expressivity. Kuchle and colleagues (43) studied corneal dystrophy of the Bowman's layer (CDB) by light and electron microscopy and reviewed the literature. They concluded that two distinct autosomal-dominant CDBs exist and proposed the designation CDB type I (geographic or true Reis-Bücklers dystrophy) and CDB type II (honeycomb-shaped or Thiel-Behnke dystrophy). This proposal is supported by the discovery that CDB type I is the result of mutation in keratoepithelin gene on chromosome 5q31 (44), whereas CDB type II is linked to chromosome 10q23-q24 (45).

Clinical Features

Reis-Bücklers dystrophy manifests in the first decade of life with recurrent episodes of ocular irritation, photophobia, and tearing. The episodes are due to recurrent erosions that decrease in frequency with time as Bowman's layer is progressively replaced with scar tissue (41,46). Attacks typi-

cally occur four to five times a year and stabilize after the third decade of life, around which time visual acuity is reduced. The diffuse opaque irregular surface contributes to the decrease in visual acuity (Fig. 45-10).

Superficial gray-white opacities develop at the level of Bowman's layer. These opacities are linear, geographic, honeycombed, or ringlike and cause progressive corneal clouding (41,47,48) and are best seen with broad oblique illumination. The lesions are located in the central and the midperipheral cornea, giving an annular or ring-shaped appearance. The peripheral cornea is spared and the intervening areas are essentially normal, although a diffuse haze that extends to the limbus can be seen by retroillumination. Corneal sensations are decreased (49–51) and prominent corneal nerves (46) may be seen.

Etiology

The structural alterations in Reis-Bücklers dystrophy could be caused by (a) anomalous fibrous tissue production by anterior stromal keratocytes causing destruction of Bowman's layer; (b) abnormal basal epithelium causing activation of anterior stromal keratocytes, which leads to scar formation and secondary destruction of Bowman's layer; or (c) primary dystrophy of Bowman's layer causing secondary alterations in the epithelium and stroma. Immunolocalization of laminin and bullous pemphigoid antigen favors an epithelial defect as the primary cause for this dystrophy (52). Basement membrane collagens have been localized in the anterior stroma, further implicating an epithelium problem (53) in the pathogenesis of this dystrophy.

Histopathology

Bowman's layer is almost completely replaced by masses of disoriented collagen fibrils and smaller electron-dense fibrils

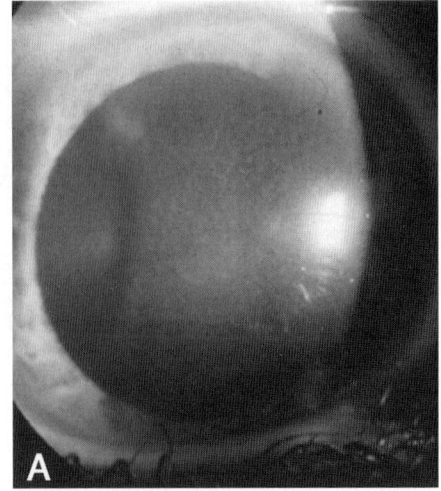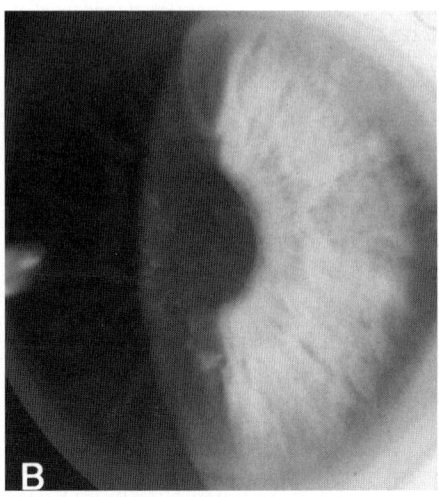

FIGURE 45-10. A,B: Reis-Bücklers's corneal dystrophy. Irregular subepithelial elevation formed a net-like pattern in the central cornea. (From Charukamnoetkanok P, Dohlman CH. Corneal dystrophies in the age of the human genome project. *MEJO* 2002;10:112–128, with permission.)

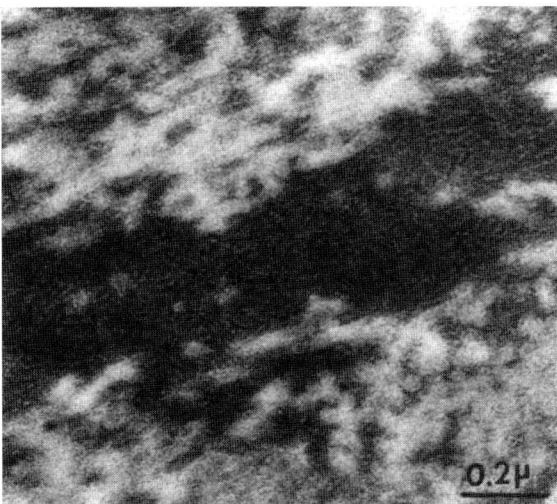

FIGURE 45-11. Reis-Bücklers's corneal dystrophy. Electron micrograph shows curly dense collagen fibrils of the superficial layer. The fibrils are aggregated and tangled (×48,468). (From Yamaguchi T, Pollack FM, Valenti J. Electron microscopic study of recurrent Reis-Bücklers's corneal dystrophy. *Am J Ophthalmol* 1980;90:95–101, with permission.)

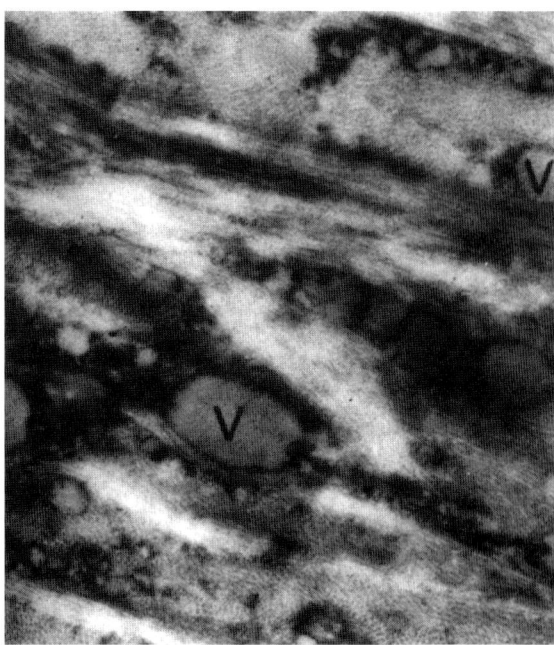

FIGURE 45-12. Reis-Bücklers's corneal dystrophy. Higher magnification of the electron microscopic study demonstrates oval-shaped vacuoles (V) in degenerated keratocytes. These vacuoles are filled with a lipid-like substance (×8,871). (From Yamaguchi T, Pollack FM, Valenti J. Electron microscopic study of recurrent Reis-Bücklers's corneal dystrophy. *Am J Ophthalmol* 1980;90:95–101, with permission.)

whose composition and origin have not been determined (Fig. 45-11) (46,49–51,54–60). In places where Bowman's layer remains intact, this material accumulates between the Bowman's layer and epithelium. Almost all epithelial cells, but especially the basal cells, and anterior stromal keratocytes show degenerative changes, such as swollen mitochondria, large vacuoles, swelling, and disruption of the endoplasmic reticulum (Fig. 45-12). The posterior epithelial layer demonstrates a sawtooth configuration. The basement membrane breaks down and is absent in places. The posterior stroma, Descemet's membrane, and endothelium are unaffected.

Ultrastructurally, the fibrocellular material consists of large collagen fibrils (diameter 250 to 400 Å) with a regular periodicity interspersed with short curly filaments with a diameter of 100 Å. There is disorganization of the epithelial basement membrane adhesion structures with loss of hemidesmosomes (54). The epithelial basement membrane of the bulbar conjunctiva may occasionally show reduplication (60).

Genetic Studies

In 1965, Duke-Elder and Leigh (61) suggested that some of the corneal dystrophies are not independent entities but rather phenotypic variations in the expression of a single gene. Other findings support this suggestion at the molecular level. Reis-Bücklers corneal dystrophy (62) along with granular dystrophy of Groenouw type I (CDGG1) (63), lattice corneal dystrophy type I (CDL1) (64), and Avellino corneal dystrophy (ACD) (65) have been mapped to the same chromosomal region on 5q31.

Munier and associates (44) generated a YAC contig of the linked area and, following cDNA selection, recovered

the gene, *beta-ig-h3* (human TGF-β–induced gene), that encodes keratoepithelin. This observation established a molecular common origin of the four 5q31-linked corneal dystrophies (44). Keratoepithelin is constitutively expressed in numerous tissues. In the human eye, it is detected predominantly on the external surface of the corneal epithelial cells and is expressed in both the epithelium layer and stromal keratocytes of rabbits (66).

Management

Treatment of Reis-Bücklers dystrophy includes treatment of recurrent erosions in the early stages. Debridement can be done in cases with recalcitrant erosions. PTK with the excimer laser has been shown to be very effective (23,24,67–71) for the treatment of this disorder. PTK is performed to a depth ranging from 18 to 100 μm following epithelial debridement or ablation. Superficial keratectomy and keratoplasty (46,49,59,72) are warranted when visual acuity is significantly reduced or if the symptoms are debilitating. Recurrences may occur after keratectomy or keratoplasty (60,73,74).

ANTERIOR MEMBRANE DYSTROPHY OF GRAYSON-WILBRANDT

Anterior membrane dystrophy of Grayson-Wilbrandt is a bilateral disorder of the central cornea characterized by accumulation of abnormal material in the basement membrane

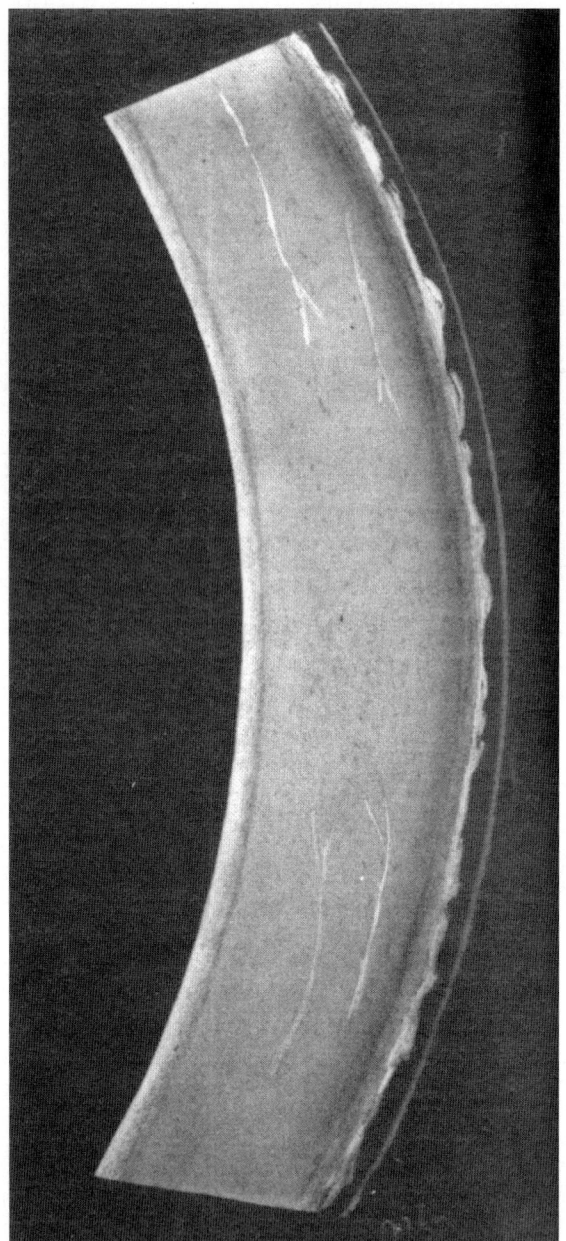

FIGURE 45-13. Grayson-Wilbrandt dystrophy. A sketch of optical section shows irregular opacities in Bowman's layer extend into and involve the epithelium. (From Grayson M, Wilbrandt H. Dystrophy of the anterior limiting membrane of the cornea [Reis-Bücklers type]. *Am J Ophthalmol* 1966;61:345–349, with permission.)

that disrupts the Bowman's layer. The intact corneal sensation and later onset distinguish this disorder from Reis-Bücklers dystrophy.

Grayson and Wilbrandt (75) described a corneal dystrophy similar to Reis-Bücklers dystrophy in two generations of one family. The onset of this disease occurs at 10 to 11 years of age. Recurrent erosions are infrequent and visual acuity is not generally affected. Slit-lamp examination reveals gray-white moundlike opacities at the level of Bowman's layer protruding into the epithelium (Fig. 45-13). The intervening

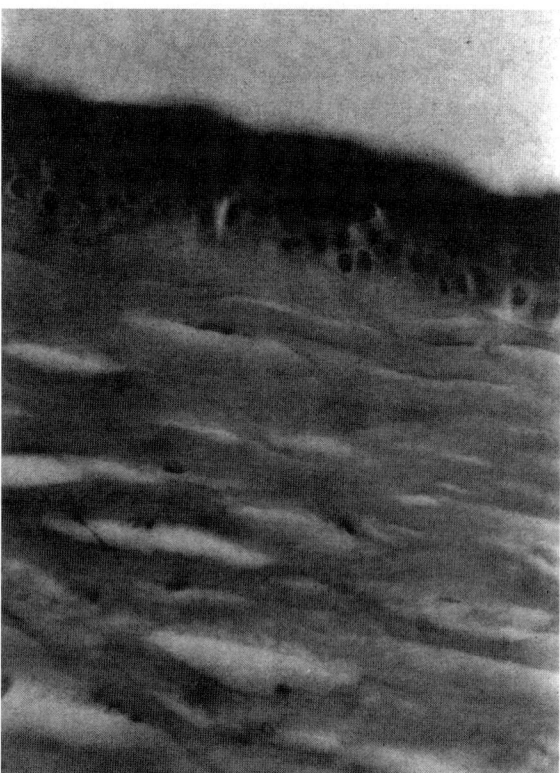

FIGURE 45-14. Grayson-Wilbrandt dystrophy. PAS-positive material locates beneath and extends into the epithelium. There is also vacuolization of the basal cells of the epithelium. (From Grayson M, Wilbrandt H. Dystrophy of the anterior limiting membrane of the cornea. [Reis-Bücklers type]. *Am J Ophthalmol* 1966;61:345–349, with permission.)

areas are clear and the peripheral cornea is spared. The corneal sensation is normal. Some authors consider Grayson-Wilbrandt dystrophy to be a variant of Reis-Bücklers dystrophy. The differentiating features are its later onset, normal corneal sensations, and relatively preserved visual acuity.

Histopathology

There are interruptions of Bowman's layer and PAS-positive material at the level of the basement membrane (Fig. 45-14). In one patient (76), ultrastructural examination revealed accumulation of fibrocellular material above an intact Bowman's layer and thickening of the basement membrane. Grayson-Wilbrandt dystrophy has also been described in members of a Japanese family who developed bilateral ring-shaped corneal opacities in adolescence (77).

HONEYCOMB DYSTROPHY OF THIEL AND BEHNKE

This disorder is a progressive dystrophy consisting of a honeycomb-like subepithelial opacity developing in the central cornea, with sparing of the peripheral cornea. The

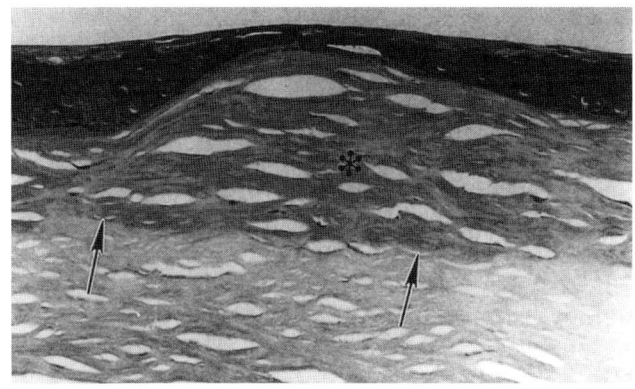

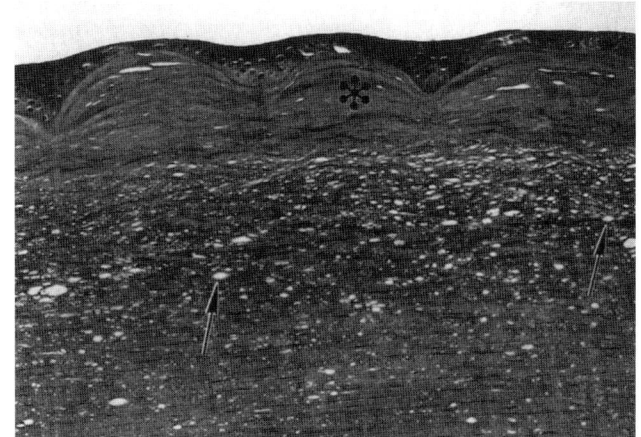

FIGURE 45-15. Thiel-Behnke dystrophy. Light microscopy shows a fibrocellular tissue *(asterisk)* that has a sawtooth-like configuration and is interposed between epithelium and underlying stroma. Arrows point to sharp demarcation between interposed tissue and underlying stroma. (From Kuchle M, Green WR, Volcker HE, et al. Reevaluation of corneal dystrophies of Bowman's layer and the anterior stroma [Reis-Bücklers and Thiel-Behnke types]: a light and electron microscopic study of eight corneas and a review of the literature. *Cornea* 1995;14:333–354, with permission.)

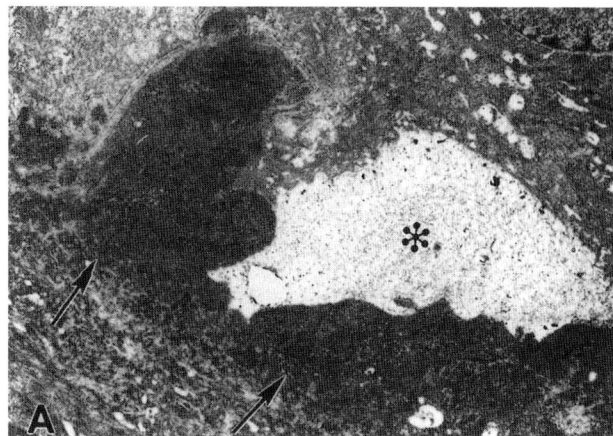

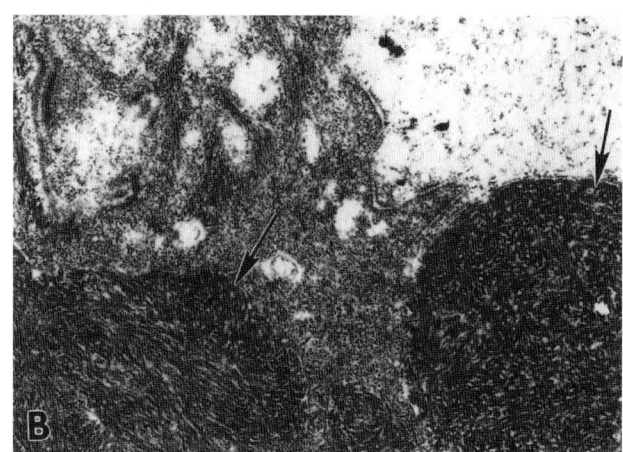

FIGURE 45-16. Thiel-Behnke dystrophy. Electron microscopy reveals mound-like extensions of "curly" collagen fibers *(arrows)* that indent overlying epithelium. Asterisk indicates an area of bollous detachment of epithelium from the underlying electron-dense material. (×30,000). (From Kuchle M, Green WR, Volcker HE, et al. Reevaluation of corneal dystrophies of Bowman's layer and the anterior stroma [Reis-Bücklers and Thiel-Behnke types]: a light and electron microscopic study of eight corneas and a review of the literature. *Cornea* 1995;14:333–354, with permission.)

corneal surface remains smooth, and corneal sensations are normal.

Thiel and Behnke (78,79) described a bilateral autosomal-dominant disorder with onset in childhood. Patients suffer from progressive recurrent erosions that cease later in life and are followed by a decrease in visual acuity. Previously thought to be a variant of Reis-Bücklers dystrophy (80), the Thiel-Behnke form of corneal dystrophy was mapped to chromosome 10q23-q24. Designations of CDB type I and CDB type II were proposed (43).

Histopathology

A fibrillogranular material is deposited under the epithelium with projections into the overlying cells in a "sawtooth" configuration (Fig. 45-15). The epithelial basement membrane is thickened, split, or duplicated (80). Reis-Bücklers dystrophy differs from this disease in that Bowman's layer is primarily affected in the former. Electron microscopy demon-

strates "curly fibers" instead of "rod-shaped bodies" seen in Reis-Bücklers dystrophy (Fig. 45-16). Wittebol-Post and associates (82) reexamined the family reported to have the corneal dystrophy of Waardenburg and Jonkers (81), and their biomicroscopical and histopathologic examination revealed findings similar to those of honeycomb dystrophy.

SUBEPITHELIAL MUCINOUS CORNEAL DYSTROPHY

Subepithelial mucinous corneal dystrophy is a diffuse, bilateral disorder that demonstrates homogeneous subepithelial haze, most dense centrally and fading toward the limbus.

Feder and colleagues (83) described a dystrophy in a family in which patients ranged in age from 45 to 78 years.

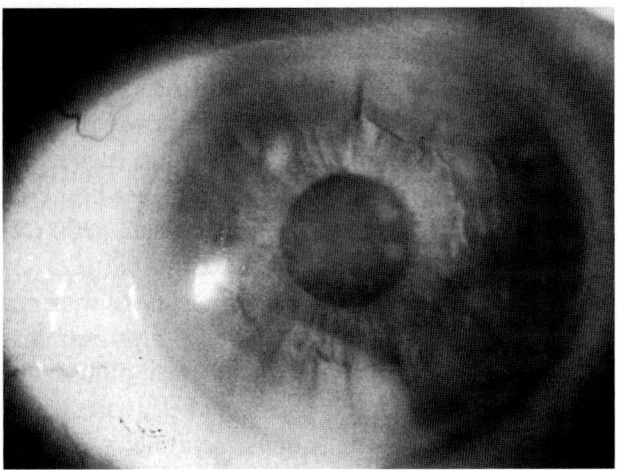

FIGURE 45-17. Subepithelial mucinous corneal dystrophy. Slit-lamp examination shows a dense central haze with gray-white nodular lesions. (From Feder RS, Jay M, Yue BY, et al. Subepithelial mucinous corneal dystrophy. Clinical and pathological correlations. *Arch Ophthalmol* 1993;111:1106–1114, with permission.)

Recurrent erosions begin in early childhood with progressively decreasing visual acuity. The visual acuity varied from 20/25 to 20/400. The central and paracentral parts of the cornea exhibit irregularly shaped, dense, gray-white, subepithelial patches (Fig. 45-17). Some of these patches are elevated, causing distortion of the anterior corneal contour. The epithelium is intact and the cornea is of normal thickness.

Histopathology

Light microscopic examination reveals degeneration of the epithelium without evidence of pseudocysts. A homogeneous eosinophilic layer is present anterior to Bowman's layer (Fig. 45-18). There is thinning of the overlying epithelium, and the deposits are elevated above the level of the basement membrane. The material shows a positive PAS reaction and stains with Masson's trichrome and Alcian blue. It does not stain positively for hyalin or Congo red. Immunohistochemical staining is positive for chondroitin-

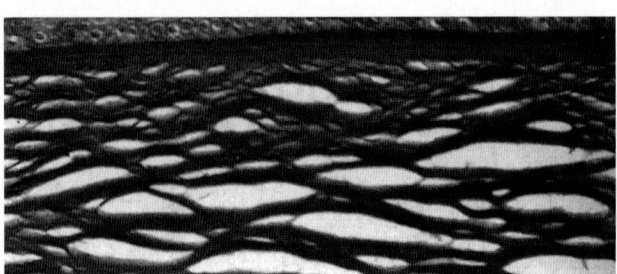

FIGURE 45-18. Subepithelial mucinous corneal dystrophy. Light microscopy reveals normal epithelium and stroma. A layer of PAS-positive material is seen anterior to Bowman's layer. (From Feder RS, Jay M, Yue BY, et al. Subepithelial mucinous corneal dystrophy. Clinical and pathological correlations. *Arch Ophthalmol* 1993;111:1106–1114, with permission.)

4-sulfate and dermatan sulfate.

Electron microscopy demonstrates irregular deposits of a fine fibrillar material consistent with proteoglycan, which is the main component of connective tissue mucins. The epithelial adhesion structures are absent in places where the basement membrane is disrupted. This dystrophy is similar to the Grayson-Wilbrandt variant of Reis-Bücklers corneal dystrophy clinically, but differs from it histochemically. Corneas of patients with Grayson-Wilbrandt disease do not stain with Alcian blue or Masson's technique.

Management

Treatment includes management of recurrent erosions in the early stages. Penetrating keratoplasty and superficial keratectomy can be performed if vision is reduced. Because the disease is superficial, PTK with the excimer laser has potential as an effective treatment.

SUMMARY

Three general trends emerge from the study of corneal dystrophy on a molecular level. First, some disorders that were previously thought to be unrelated are caused by the same genetic defect. For instance, the keratoepithelin gene on chromosome 5 is responsible for Reis-Bücklers, lattice dystrophy, Avellino dystrophy, and granular dystrophy. Second, disorders grouped together based on morphologic studies may have different genetic bases. Previously thought to be a variant of Reis-Bücklers dystrophy (80) (which maps to chromosome region 5q31), the Thiel-Behnke form of corneal dystrophy maps to chromosome 10q23-q24. New designations of corneal dystrophy CDB type I (geographic or true Reis-Bücklers dystrophy) and CDB type II (honeycomb-shaped or Thiel-Behnke dystrophy) have been proposed (43). Third, with time, some conditions not conventionally considered to be dystrophies might be reclassified as such. For example, genetic tools may allow for more sensitive and extensive genealogies of polymorphic amyloid degeneration that may demonstrate heritability (84).

PTK offers the ability to precisely control the ablation of the cornea and allows for the preservation of useful visual function of the patients with corneal dystrophies for a significant amount of time, delaying the need for penetrating keratoplasty. It is exciting to hope that new insights gained from molecular elucidation of their pathogenesis will lead to novel and effective treatments of corneal dystrophies.

REFERENCES

1. Chang SW, Tuli S, Azar DT. Corneal Dystrophies. In: Traboulsi ET, ed. *Genetic diseases of the eye.* Oxford: Oxford University

Press, 1997:217–266.

2. Gupta SK, Hodge WG. A new clinical perspective of corneal dystrophies through molecular genetics. *Curr Opin Ophthalmol* 1999;10:234–241.

3. Pameijer JK. Ueber eine Fremdarige Familiere Obrflεchliche HornhautverEnderung (German). *Klin Monatsbl Augenheilkd* 1935;95:516.

4. Meesmann A, Wilke F. Klinische und Anatomische Untersuchungen Ueber eine Bisher Unbekannte, Dominant Vererbte Epithldystrophie de Hornhaut (German). *Klin Monatsbl Augenheilkd* 1939;103:361.

5. Stockeer FW, Holt LB. Rare form of hereditary epithelial dystrophy. *Arch Ophthalmol* 1955;53:536.

6. Kuwabara R, Ciccarelli EC. Meesman's corneal dystrophy. *Arch Ophthalmol* 1964;71:676.

7. Meesmann A. Ueber eine Bisher Nicht Beschriebene Dominant Vererbte Dystrophia alis Corneae (German). *Beer Dtsch Ophthalmol Bes* 1938;52:154.

8. Snyder WB. Hereditary epithelial corneal dystrophy. *Am J Ophthalmol* 1963;55:56.

9. Burki E. Kenntnis des erblichen Epitheldystrophie der Hornhaut. *Ophthalmolica.* 1946;111:134–139.

10. Irvine AD, Corden LD, Swensson O, et al. Mutations in cornea-specific keratin K3 or K12 genes cause Meesman's corneal dystrophy. *Nature Genet* 1997;16:184–187.

11. Irvine AD, Coleman CM, Moore JE, et al. A novel mutation in KRT12 associated with Meesmann's epithelial corneal dystrophy. *Br J Ophthalmol* 2002;86:729–732.

12. Corden LD, Swensson O, Swensson B, et al. Molecular genetics of Meesmann's corneal dystrophy: ancestral and novel mutations in keratin 12 (K12) and complete sequence of the human KRT12 gene. *Exp Eye Res* 2000;70:41–49.

13. Burns RP. Meesmann's corneal dystrophy. *Trans Am Ophthalmol Soc* 1968;66:531–635.

14. Fine BS, et al. Meesman's epithelial dystrophy of the cornea. *Am J Ophthalmol* 1977;83:633.

15. Cogan DG, et al. Microcystic dystrophy of the corneal epithelium. *Trans Am Ophthalmol Soc* 1964;62:213.

16. Dausch D, Landesz M, Klein R, et al. Phototherapeutic keratectomy in recurrent corneal erosion. *Refract Corneal Surg* 1993;9:419–424.

17. Fagerholm P, Fitzsimmons TD, Orndahl M, et al. Phototherapeutic keratectomy: long-term results in 166 eyes. *Refract Corneal Surg* 1993;9(2 suppl):76–81.

18. Foster W, Grewe S, Atzleer U, et al. Phototherapeutic keratectomy in corneal diseases. *Refract Corneal Surg* 1993;9(2 suppl):85–90.

19. John ME, Karr Van D, et al. Excimer laser phototherapeutic keratectomy for treatment of recurrent corneal erosion. *J Cataract Refract Surg* 1994;20:179–180.

20. Niesen U, Thomann U, Schipper I. Phototherapeutic keratectomy (German). *Klin Monatsbl Augenheilkd* 1994;205:187–195.

21. Ohman L, Fagerholm P, Tengroth B. Treatment of recurrent corneal erosions with the excimer laser. *Acta Ophthalmol (Copenh)* 1994;72:461–463.

22. Poirier C, Coulan P, Williamson W, et al. Results of therapeutic photokeratectomy using the excimer laser. Apropos of 12 cases (review) (French). *J Fr Ophthalmol* 1994;17:262–270.

23. Dinh R, Rapuano CJ, Cohen EJ, et al. Recurrence of corneal dystrophy after excimer laser phototherapeutic keratectomy. *Ophthalmology* 1999;106:1490–1497.

24. Sher NA, Bowers RA, Zabel RW, et al. Clinical use of the 193-nm excimer laser in the treatment of corneal scars. *Arch Ophthalmol* 1991;109:491–499.

25. Cogan DG, et al. Microcystic dystrophy of the cornea. *Arch Ophthalmol* 1974;92:470.

26. King RG JR, Geeraets R. Cogan-Guerry microcystic corneal epithelial dystrophy. *Med Coll Va Q* 1972;8:241.

27. Trobe JD, Laibson PR. Dystrophic changes in the anterior cornea. *Arch Ophthalmol* 1972;87:378.

28. Wolter JR, Franlick FB. Microcystic dystrophy of the corneal epithelium. *Arch Ophthalmol* 1966;75:380.

29. Bron AJ, Buriless SEP. Inherited recurrent corneal erosion. *Trans Ophthalmol Soc UK* 1981;101:239.

30. Franceschetti A. Hereditdre Rezidivierende Erosion der Homhaut (German). *Z Agenheilkd* 1928;66:309.

31. Laibson PR, Krachmer JH. Familial occurrence of dot, map, and fingerprint dystrophy of the cornea. *Invest Ophthalmol* 1975;14:397.

32. Laibson PR. Microcystic corneal dystrophy. *Trans Am Ophthalmol Soc* 1976;74:488–531.

33. Guerry DUP III. Observations on Cogan's microcystic dystrophy of the corneal epithelium. *Trans Am Ophthalmol Soc* 1965;63:320.

34. Guerry D III. Fingerprint-like lines in the cornea. *Am J Ophthalmol* 1950;33:724.

35. Waring GO III, Rodrigues MM, Laibson PR. Corneal dystrophies I. Dystrophies of the epithelium, Bowman's layer and stromal. *Surv Ophthalmol* 1978;23:71–122.

36. Broderick JD, Dark AJ, Pearce GW. Fingerprint dystrophy of the cornea. *Arch Ophthalmol* 1974;92:483.

37. Nirankari VS, et al. An unusual case of epithelial basement membrane dystrophy. *Am J Ophthalmol* 1989;107:552.

38. Buxton JN, Fox ML. Superficial epithelial keratectomy in the treatment of epithelial basement membrane dystrophy. *Arch Ophthalmol* 1983;101:392.

39. Soong HK, Farjo Q, Meyer RF, et al. Diamond burr superficial keratectomy for recurrent corneal erosions. *Br J Ophthalmol* 2002;86:296–298.

40. Katsev DA, et al. Recurrent corneal erosion: pathology of corneal puncture. *Cornea* 1991;10:418.

41. Reis W. Familidre, Fleckige Homhautentartung (German). *Dtsch Med Wochenschr* 1917;43:575.

42. Bucklers M. gber eine weitere familiare Hornhautdystrophie (German). *Klin Monatsbl Augenheilkd* 1949;114:386.

43. Kuchle M, Green WR, Volcker HE, et al. Reevaluation of corneal dystrophies of Bowman's layer and the anterior stroma (Reis-Bucklers and Thiel-Behnke types): a light and electron microscopic study of eight corneas and a review of the literature. *Cornea* 1995;14:333–354.

44. Munier FL, Korvatska E, Djemai A, et al. Kerato-epithelin mutations in four 5q31-linked corneal dystrophies. *Nature Genet* 1997;15:247–251.

45. Yee RW, Sullivan LS, Lai HT, et al. Linkage mapping of Thiel-Behnke corneal dystrophy (CDB2) to chromosome 10q23-q24. *Genomics* 1997;46:152–154.

46. Jones ST, Stauffer LH. Reis-Bucklers corneal dystrophy. *Trans Am Acad Ophthalmol Otolaryngol* 1970;74:417.

47. Johnson BL, Brown SI, Zaidman GW. A light and electron microscopic study of recurrent granular dystrophy of the cornea. *Am J Ophthalmol* 1981;92:49.

48. Paufique L, Bonnet M. La dystrophie corneenne Heredito-familiale de Reis-Bucklers (French). *Ann Oculist* 1966;199:14.

49. Hall P. Reis-Bucklers dystrophy. *Arch Ophthalmol* 1974;91:170.

50. Kaufman HG, Clowe FW. Irregularities of Bowman's membrane. *Am J Ophthalmol* 1966;62:227.

51. Wittehol-Post D, van Bijsterveld OP, Delleman JM. The honeycomb type of Reis-Bucklers dystrophy of the cornea: Biometrics and interpretation. *Ophthalmologica* 1987;194:65.

52. Lohse E, Stock EL, Jones JC, et al. Reis-Bucklers corneal dystrophy: Immunofluorescent and electron microscope studies. *Cornea* 1989;8:200.

53. Chan CC, Cogan DG, Bucci FS, et al. Anterior corneal dystrophy with dyscollagenosis. (Reis-Buckler type?). *Cornea* 1993;12:51–460.

54. Akiya S, Ito I, Matsui M. Gelatinous drop-like dystrophy of the cornea. *Jpn J Clin Ophthalmol* 1972;56:815.
55. Griffith DG, Fine BS. Light and electron microscopic observations in a superficial corneal dystrophy. *Am J Ophthalmol* 1967;62:1659.
56. Hoizan M, Wood I. Reis-Bucklers corneal dystrophy. *Trans Ophthalmol Soc UK* 1971;91:41.
57. Kanai A, Kaufman HE, Polack FM. Electron microscopic studies of Reis-Bucklers dystrophy. *Ann Ophthalmol* 1973;5:953.
58. Perry HD, Fine BS, Caldwell CR. Reis-Bucklers dystrophy. *Arch Ophthalmol* 1979;97:664.
59. Rice NSC, et al. Reis-Bucklers dystrophy. *Br J Ophthalmol* 1968;52:577.
60. Yamaguchi T, Polack F, Valenti J. Reis-Bucklers corneal dystrophy. *Am J Ophthalmol* 1980;90:95.
61. Duke-Elder S, Leigh AG. Diseases of the outer eye. Part 2. In: Duke-Elder S, ed. *System of ophthalmology*, vol 8. St. Louis: CV Mosby 1965:921–976.
62. Okada M, Yamamoto S, Tsujikawa M, et al. Two distinct kerato-epithelin mutations in Reis-Bucklers corneal dystrophy. *A J Ophthalmol* 1998;126:535–542.
63. Eiberg H, Moller HU, Berendt I, et al. Assignment of granular corneal dystrophy Groenouw type I (CDGG1) to chromosome 5q. *Eur J Hum Genet* 1994;2:132–138.
64. Stone EM, Mathers WD, Rosenwasser GOD, et al. Three autosomal dominant corneal dystrophies map to chromosome 5q. *Nature Genet* 1994;6:47–51.
65. Folberg R, Alfonso E, Croxatto JO, et al. Clinically atypical granular corneal dystrophy with pathologic features of lattice-like amyloid deposits: a study of three families. *Ophthalmology* 1988;95:46–51.
66. Escribano J, Hernando N, Ghosh S, et al. cDNA from human ocular ciliary epithelium homologous to beta ig-h3 is preferentially expressed as an extracellular protein in the corneal epithelium. *J Cell Physiol* 1994;160:511–521.
67. Chamon W, Azar DT, Stark WJ, et al. Phototherapeutic keratectomy. *Ophthalmol Clin North Am* 1993;6:399–413.
68. Hahn TW, Sah WJ, Kim JH. Phototherapeutic keratectomy in nine eyes with superficial corneal diseases. *Refract Corneal Surg* 1994;9(2 suppl):115–118.
69. McDonnell PJ, Seiler T. Phototherapeutic keratectomy with excimer laser for Reis-Buckler corneal dystrophy. *Refract Corneal Surg* 1992;8:306–310.
70. Orndahl M, Fagerholm P, Fitzsimmons T, et al. Treatment of corneal dystrophies with excimer laser. *Acta Ophthalmol (Copenh)* 199;72:235–240.
71. Rogers C, Cohen P, Lawless M. Phototherapeutic keratectomy for Reis-Bucklers corneal dystrophy. *Aust NZ J Ophthalmol* 1993; 21:247–250.
72. Wood TO, et al. Treatment of Reis-Bucklers corneal dystrophy by removal of subepithelial fibrous tissue. *Am J Ophthalmol* 1978; 85:360.
73. Caldwell DR. Postoperative recurrence of Reis-Bucklers corneal dystrophy. *Am J Ophthalmol* 1978;85:567.
74. Olson RJ, Kaufman HE. Recurrence of Reis-Bucklers corneal dystrophy in a graft. *Am J Ophthalmol* 1978;85:349.
75. Grayson M, Wilbrandt H. Dystrophy of the anterior limiting membrane of the cornea (Reis-Bucklers type). *Am J Ophthalmol* 1966;63:345.
76. Fogle JA, Green WR, Kenyon KR. Anterior corneal dystrophy. *Am J Ophthalmol* 1974;77:529.
77. Kurome H, Noda S, Hayasaka S, et al. A Japanese family with Grayson-Wilbrandt variant of Reis-Bucklers corneal dystrophy. *Jpn J Ophthalmol* 1993;37:143–147.
78. Behnke H, Thiel HJ. Ueber die hereditaere Epitheldystrophie der Hornhaut (Typ Meesman-Wilke) in Schleswig-Holstein (German). *Klin Monatsbl Augenheilkd* 1965;147:662–672.
79. Thiel HJ, Behnke H. Eine Bisher Unbekannte Subepitheliale Hereditaire Hornhautdystrophie (German). *Klin Monatsbl Augenheilkd* 1967;150:862.
80. Yamaguchi T, Polack FM, Rowsey JJ. Honeycomb-shaped corneal dystrophy: A variation of Reis-Bucklers dystrophy. *Cornea* 1982; 1:71.
81. Waardenburg PJ, Jonkers GH. A specific type of dominant progressive dystrophy of the cornea, developing after birth. *Acta Ophthalmol (Copenh)* 1961;39:919.
82. Wittebol-Post D, Van Schooneveld MJ, Pel V. The corneal dystrophy of Waardenburg and Jonkers. *Ophthalmic Paediatr Genet* 1989;10:249–255.
83. Feder RS, Jay M, Yue BYJT, et al. Subepithelial mucinous corneal dystrophy: Clinical dn pathological correlations. *Arch Ophthalmol* 1993;111:1106–1114.
84. Mannis MJ, Krachmer JH, Rodrigues MM, et al. Polymorphic amyloid degeneration of the cornea. A clinical and histopathologic study. *Arch Ophthalmol* 1981;99:1217–1223.

STROMAL AND PRE-DESCEMET'S DYSTROPHIES

PUWAT CHARUKAMNOETKANOK, SHU-WEN CHANG, DIMITRI T. AZAR

Stromal and pre-Descemet's dystrophies are characterized by the appearance of deposits within or between the stromal keratocytes. The most common stromal dystrophies (granular, lattice, and macular dystrophies) often result in progressive visual loss (1). In contrast, pre-Descemet's dystrophy and other less common stromal dystrophies (such as fleck dystrophy and central cloudy dystrophy) seldom result in decreased vision. The classification of stromal dystrophies was traditionally based on the clinical appearance of the stromal deposits and on the immunohistological and ultrastructural findings. Recent advances in molecular genetics have better clarified the similarities among various dystrophies (2). For example, granular, lattice, Avellino, and Reis-Bücklers dystrophies result from defects in the same gene on chromosome 5q31 (keratoepithelin gene). New technologic advances also lead to new treatment options for anterior stromal dystrophies. For example, superficial variants and recurrent dystrophies after penetrating keratoplasty may lend themselves to treatment with excimer laser phototherapeutic keratectomy (PTK).

GRANULAR DYSTROPHY (GROENOUW TYPE I)

Clinical Features

Granular dystrophy, also called Groenouw type I dystrophy, is inherited as an autosomal-dominant dystrophy, with 100% penetrance (3–6). The clinically obvious corneal lesions develop in early adolescence. These lesions are bilateral, symmetric, sharply demarcated grayish-white opacities of variable size and shape, or radial lines in the superficial stroma with intervening clear areas (Fig. 46-1 A,B). Opacities may vary in extent but rarely reach the limbus. Visual acuity is minimally affected in the early stages. Photophobia may occur due to scattering of light by the opacities. The opacities slowly progress, coalesce, and involve the deeper stroma. The overlying epithelium and the corneal sensations are intact.

Several variants of granular dystrophy are recognized. These include the progressive corneal dystrophy of Waardenburg and Jonkers (7) in which the onset is the first decade of life. Broad, oblique illumination on slit-lamp biomicroscopy offers the best visualization of the snowflake-like opacities. Retroillumination and indirect illumination reveal the fine granularity of a myriad punctate opacities. Visual acuity is severely affected by the fourth decade of life due to stromal opacification. Wittebol-Post and associates (8) have considered this dystrophy a variant of Reis-Bücklers' dystrophy.

Rodrigues and colleagues (10) described another variant of granular dystrophy with onset in infancy. The deposits are superficial and cause painful recurrent erosions that require early surgical intervention. There are numerous deposits in the region of Bowman's layer. The presence of classic granular dystrophy in parents or siblings may indicate that they are expressions of the same genotype (9,10).

In another variant of granular dystrophy, corneal opacities appear later in life. This alternative form of granular dystrophy is less severe and slower in progression than the other variants (8,11). The opacities have a breadcrumb-like appearance, and patients do not usually suffer from recurrent erosions.

Histopathology

The stroma contains hyaline eosinophilic deposits that stain intensely with Masson trichrome, weakly with periodic acid-Schiff (PAS) stain, and negatively with Verhoeff stain (Fig. 46-2). Congo red may stain the peripheral portions of the deposits (12,13). The epithelial basement membrane and Bowman's layer may have area of thinning or may be absent in places (14).

Ultrastructurally, electron-dense rodlike deposits (100 to 500 μm wide) are present in the subepithelial region between the stromal lamellae and intracytoplasmically in keratocytes (9,15,16) (Fig. 46-3). The exact source of these deposits is unknown (17). Degenerative changes are

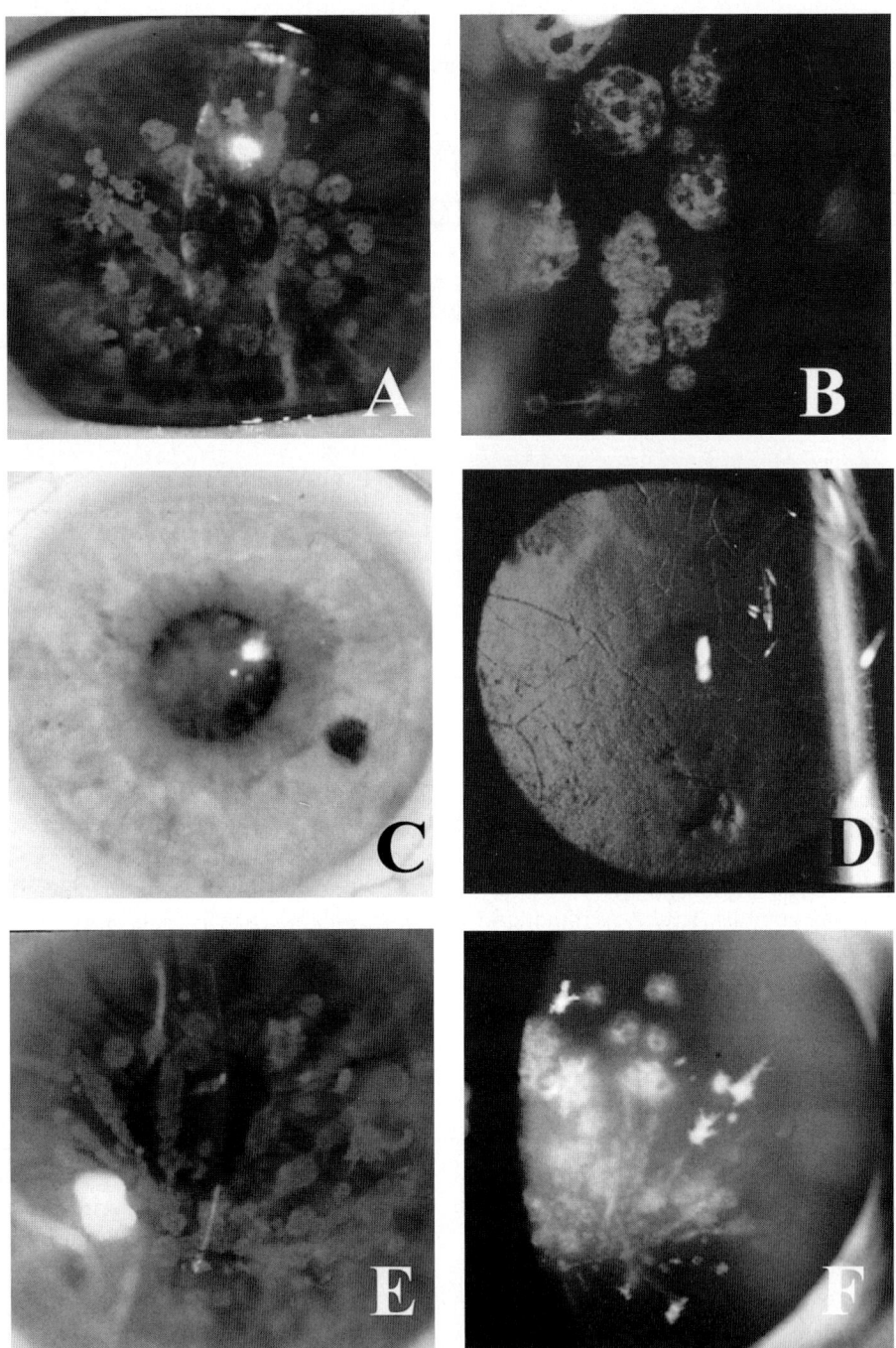

FIGURE 46-1. A,B: Granular dystrophy. Slit-lamp photograph demonstrates discrete, white, round-to-oval, bread crumblike opacities with intervening clear areas that do not reach the limbus. **C,D:** Lattice dystrophy. Notice subepithelial opacity in the central cornea. Retroillumination shows branching, ropy lesions. **E,F:** Avellino dystrophy. (From Charukamnoetkanok P, Dohlman CH. Corneal dystrophies in the age of the human genome project. *MEJO* 2002;10:112–128, with permission.)

apparent in keratocytes, with cytoplasmic vacuolization and dilatation of endoplasmic reticulum (18). The deposits are either filamentous, homogeneous, or have a moth-eaten pattern (16,18). Tubular microfibrils can be seen surrounding these lesions. Histochemically, they contain tyrosine, tryptophan, and sulfur-containing amino acids (12). Moller and associates (19) demonstrated the presence

of kappa and lambda light chains of immunoglobulin G in the lesions.

Genetic Studies

Granular dystrophy (20) is one of the four dystrophies that have been mapped to the same chromosomal region on

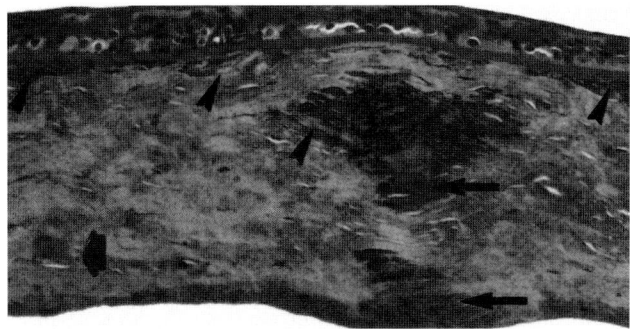

FIGURE 46-2. Granular dystrophy. Masson trichrome staining of a corneal button from a patient with granular dystrophy shows granular hyaline deposits at the level of superficial and midstroma. (From Santo RM, et al. Clinical and histopathologic features of corneal dystrophies in Japan. *Ophthalmology* 1995; 102:557–567, with permission.)

5q31 (21). The other dystrophies are Reis-Bücklers corneal dystrophy (22), lattice corneal dystrophy type I (CDL1) (21), and Avellino corneal dystrophy (ACD) (23). Munier and associates (24) generated a YAC contig of the linked area, and following cDNA selection, recovered the *BIG-H3* gene, which encodes the structural protein keratoepithelin. This observation established a common molecular origin of the four 5q31-linked corneal dystrophies (24).

Treatment

Intervening clear areas between the opacities allow unobstructed vision. Thus, patients are asymptomatic in the early stages. As the disease progresses, visual acuity is reduced and superficial keratectomy may be visually beneficial (25). In the superficial variant, treatment with the excimer laser (PTK) may be an attractive alternative to lamellar keratectomy. The goal of PTK is to remove the anterior corneal opacity and smooth the anterior refractive surface. PTK is performed after removal of the epithelium

either mechanically or by ablation with the excimer laser. If the epithelial surface is rough, application of a smoothing or modulating agent may be necessary to create a more regular surface prior to laser ablation of the cornea.

Variable success rates ranging from 66% to 100% have been reported (26). Recurrences after keratectomy have been reported as early as 1 year (27,28) and are more frequent in the superficial variant. It is believed that in this disease, homozygous patients present earlier, have a more severe form, and have earlier recurrences following surgical intervention (6,29). Penetrating keratoplasty is required in the more advanced cases. Recurrences of granular dystrophy in the graft manifest as diffuse haze in the peripheral graft or as granular lesions in the stroma. The diffuse haze occurs due to growth of fibrous tissue between the epithelium and Bowman's layer and it can be stripped by superficial keratectomy.

AVELLINO CORNEAL DYSTROPHY

In 1988, Folberg and associates (23) first reported three families with histologic features of both granular and lattice dystrophies (Figs. 46-4–46-6). Because all of these patients traced their origins to Avellino, Italy, it was later named Avellino corneal dystrophy by Holland and colleagues (30).

Clinical Features

Avellino dystrophy is inherited as an autosomal-dominant trait with very high penetrance (greater than 90%) and moderately variable expressivity. Males and females are equally affected. The dystrophy usually appears in the first or second decade of life. Three clinical signs characterize Avellino corneal dystrophy: (a) discrete anterior stromal, gray-white granular deposits; (b) mid to posterior stromal lattice lesions; and (c) anterior stromal haze.

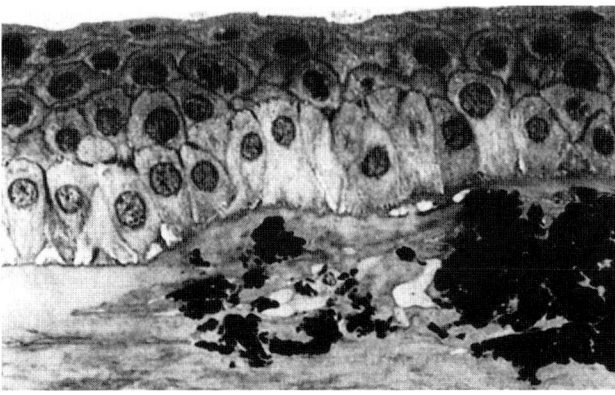

FIGURE 46-3. Semifine micrograph of the cornea from a patient with granular dystrophy shows deposits in the anterior stromal layer. (From Werner LP, et al. Confocal microscopy in Bowman and stromal corneal dystrophies. *Ophthalmology* 1999;106: 1697–1704, with permission.)

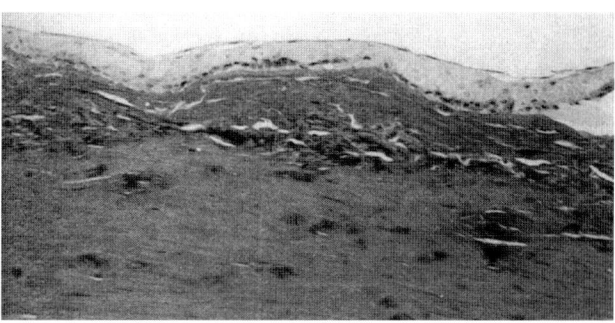

FIGURE 46-4. Avellino dystrophy. Masson trichrome stain of the patient with clinical finding of lattice dystrophy shows negative staining. (From Folberg R, et al. The relationship between granular, lattice type 1, and Avellino corneal dystrophies. A histopathologic study. *Arch Ophthalmol* 1994;112:1080–1085, with permission.)

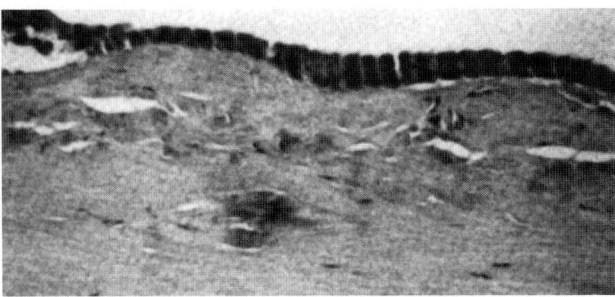

FIGURE 46-5. Avellino dystrophy. (From Folberg R, et al. The relationship between granular, lattice type 1, and Avellino corneal dystrophies. A histopathologic study. *Arch Ophthalmol* 1994; 112:1080–1085, with permission.)

The earliest clinical evidence of this condition is discrete granular deposits, predominantly in the anterior third of the corneal stroma. Granules reach their mature size early and remain nearly stationary in size. They often coalesce to form linear opacities, especially in the inferior cornea. Lattice changes appear later in life and increase proportionally as the patient ages. They are located initially in the mid- and deep stroma and later involve the entire stroma (Fig. 46-1E,F). The lattice rods are thicker than those in lattice corneal dystrophy type I (LCD I) and bear a resemblance to lattice corneal dystrophy type IIIA (31). The last clinical sign to emerge is diffuse, ground-glass stromal haze located between the granular deposits.

Visual acuity is minimally affected, and depends on the predominant location of the deposits, which may be either central or peripheral. Patients complain of glare and decreased night vision. Recurrent erosions occur in the third and fourth decades of life, and the granular deposits that are superficial seem to be the cause of these erosions (32). Recurrent erosions are more common in patients with Avellino corneal dystrophy than in patients with typical granular dystrophy.

Histopathology

Granular deposits demonstrate both a hyaline appearance by hematoxylineosin staining and bright-red staining with Masson trichrome (Fig. 46-6). Numerous fusiform stromal deposits of amyloid that stain with Congo red and demonstrate birefringence and dichroism with the cross-polarization that is typical of lattice dystrophy are also present (30,33,34). The superficial granular deposits are ultrastructurally homogeneous and electron dense (Fig. 46-7). Microfilaments suggestive of amyloid can be seen in some of these deposits (Fig. 46-8).

Genetic Studies

Earlier reports had suggested that there may be a close relationship between lattice type I and granular dystrophy (12,25). Evidence illustrated that mutations in the *BIG-H3* gene are the common molecular origin of the Avellino dystrophy, lattice type I dystrophy, granular dystrophy, and Reis-Bücklers dystrophy (24).

Treatment

Treatment is conservative and includes hypertonic saline and bandage contact lenses for recurrent erosions. PTK has been used to treat corneal erosions and to clear the central cornea of granular and lattice deposits (36). Treatment for decreased visual acuity also includes penetrating keratoplasty, which is generally required late in the course of the disease. Recurrences have been reported following keratoplasty as late as 9 years after the graft (30). The pattern

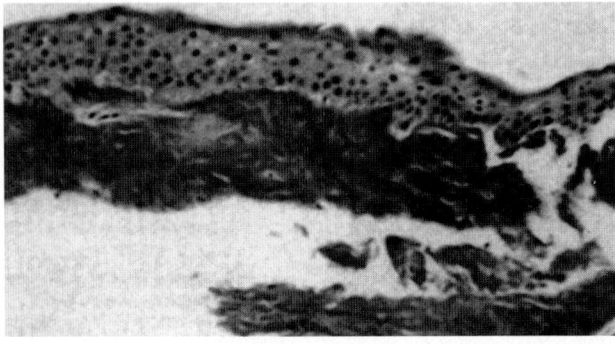

FIGURE 46-6. Avellino dystrophy. Superficial keratectomy specimen from a patient shows bright red granular deposit underneath the epithelium by Masson trichrome stain. (From Folberg R, et al. The relationship between granular, lattice type 1, and Avellino corneal dystrophies. A histopathologic study. *Arch Ophthalmol* 1994;112:1080–1085, with permission.)

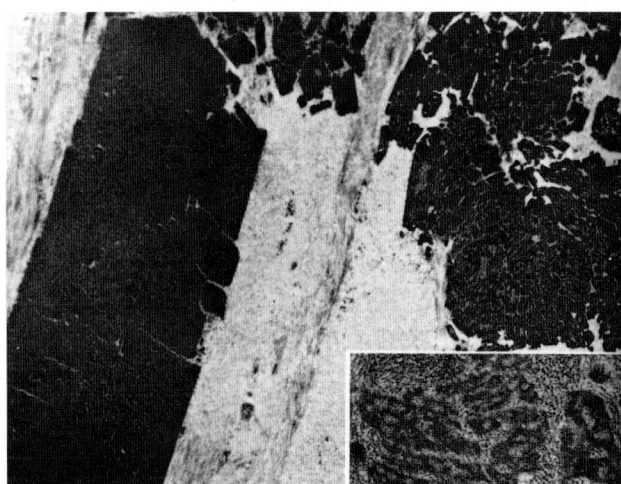

FIGURE 46-7. Avellino dystrophy. Electron micrograph shows electron dense deposits *(left)* and deposits that are apertured *(right)*. Randomly oriented fibrils are located at the periphery of the apertured deposits *(inset)*. (From Folberg R. Clinically atypical granular dystrophy with pathologic features of lattice-like amyloid deposits: study of these families. *Ophthalmology* 1988;95:46–51, with permission.)

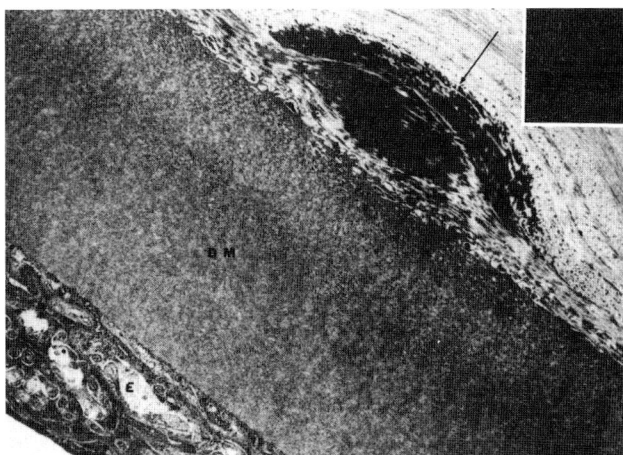

FIGURE 46-8. Avellino dystrophy. Electron micrograph demonstrates a fusiform deposit *(arrow),* composed of densely packed filaments *(inset)* is located anterior to Descemet's membrane (DM). E = endothelium. (From Folberg R. Clinically atypical granular dystrophy with pathologic features of lattice-like amyloid deposits: study of these families. *Ophthalmology* 1988; 95:46–51, with permission.)

of recurrence seems to follow the natural history of the disease, with granular lesions being the first to appear.

LATTICE DYSTROPHY

There are four known types of lattice dystrophies: type I, Meretoja's syndrome (type II), type III, and type IIIA.

Lattice Type I Corneal Dystrophy

Lattice dystrophy type I, also named Biber-Haab-Dimer dystrophy, was first described by Biber in the 1890s. The mode of inheritance is autosomal dominant with variable penetrance and expressivity. The disease may be detected in only a few members of the affected family. Other members may show only recurrent erosions with minimal stromal opacification (37).

Clinical Features

Lattice dystrophy appears in the first decade of life. Rarely does it appear after age 30 years (37,38). Corneal involvement is usually bilaterally symmetrical. However, unilateral cases have been reported in which the onset occurs later and the clinical course is less severe (39–41). In the early stages, the lesions appear as irregular lines and dots in the anterior axial stroma with clear intervening stroma or as a diffuse haze in the center. The faint central haze becomes denser with time, and it is this central disk-shaped opacity that eventually causes reduced visual acuity and may obscure the underlying lattice pattern (Fig. 46-1C). The dots and lines increase in size and number with time to

become comma-shaped specks, thick ropy cords, and small nodules.

On direct illumination, gray opacities with irregular margins are seen, and on retroillumination, refractile rods with a clear core and double contour are obvious (Fig. 46-1D). The lines extend to the periphery, and go deeper in the stroma and toward the epithelium. As the opacities coalesce, a diffuse haze appears, involving the anterior and midstroma (Fig. 46-1C). At this stage the lattice dystrophy may be difficult to distinguish from granular or macular dystrophies, but careful examination usually reveals the typical branching lattice lines. The lattice filaments range from fine lines to coarse bands with nodular dilations. The lattice lines branch dichotomously near their central terminations and overlap one another at various stromal levels to create a lattice pattern. In advanced cases the lattice lines fluoresce under cobalt-blue slit-lamp illumination. Pseudofilaments may form due to the linear configuration of dots.

Epithelial erosions secondary to involvement of the subepithelial area and Bowman's layer occur later in life and are the cause of discomfort and decreased visual acuity due to irregular astigmatism. They remain a serious problem until the third or fourth decade of life, after which they diminish in frequency. The corneal sensations decrease with concomitant symptomatic improvement. Vascularization rarely occurs.

An association between vestibulocochleopathy and lattice corneal dystrophy has been reported in a case of nonfamilial amyloidosis (42). Coexistence of progressive external ophthalmoplegia and corneal lattice dystrophy was seen in a family pedigree of 33 patients (43).

Lattice dystrophy should be differentiated from a nonprogressive, nonhereditary condition, polymorphic amyloid degeneration (parenchymatous dystrophy of Pillat) (44), in which stromal amyloid deposits are seen in patients above 60 years of age. Lattice lines can also be produced by hydroxyethylmethacrylate (HEMA) contact lenses but these disappear on removal of the contact lens.

Histopathology

Involvement of the epithelial or Bowman's layer can be confirmed by polarization microscopy. Descemet's membrane and the endothelium are unaffected. The deposits in lattice dystrophy are composed of amyloid, which has been confirmed by immunofluorescence (45), Congo red, PAS, and Masson's trichrome staining. The deposits exhibit dichroism and manifest green birefringence (46,47). Dichroism is demonstrated by alternate red and green color when viewed through a rotating polarizing filter; and green birefringence is demonstrated by an intermittent yellowish-green against a black background when the lesion is viewed through two rotating polarizing filters. The deposits show a greenish-yellow fluorescence on staining with thioflavine T. Crystal violet staining shows metachromasia.

The amyloid protein is probably related to transthyretin (48,49).

Ultrastructurally, the epithelium is of variable thickness, with degeneration of the basal epithelium. The basement membrane is thickened and continuous but without normal hemidesmosomes (50,51). Bowman's membrane and superficial stroma contain amyloid structures, collagen fibrils, and fibroblasts. The stroma contains large irregular deposits that distort the normal configuration of the corneal lamellae. They contain highly aligned short, delicate, nonbranching electron-dense fibrils with diameters of 80 to 100 Å (52,53). There is a decrease in the number of keratocytes, with evidence of degeneration (46–48,54).

Amyloid is a complex of chondroitin, sulfuric acid, and protein found extracellularly. The amyloid seen in lattice dystrophy is distinct from amyloid in systemic amyloidosis or in primary or secondary amyloid degeneration of the cornea.

Genetic Studies

Linkage analysis and further studies revealed that the genetic mutation in patients with lattice dystrophy type I involves the *BIG-H3* gene on chromosome 5q. Missense mutations occur at the CpG dinucleotide of two arginine codons: R124C in lattice dystrophy type I, R555W in granular dystrophy, R555Q in Reis-Bücklers' dystrophy, and R124H in Avellino dystrophy (24).

Treatment

Managing lattice dystrophy in the early stages includes treatment of recurrent erosions. PTK is emerging as an attractive alternative to treat superficial corneal opacities and surface irregularities. The goal is to avoid or delay more invasive procedures such as lamellar and penetrating keratoplasty. PTK has been reported to be very successful for the treatment of lattice dystrophy (26). Penetrating keratoplasty is indicated when there is a decrease in visual acuity or, rarely, when the recurrent erosions become incapacitating. This is generally required in the third or fourth decade of life. Among major stromal dystrophies, recurrences after penetrating keratoplasty are more frequent in patients with lattice dystrophy. Recurrence of lattice dystrophy in the graft occurs as soon as 3 years postoperatively and is seen as dotlike filamentous subepithelial opacities or as a diffuse stromal haze (76).

Lattice Type II Corneal Dystrophy

Originally described by Meretoja (55,56) in the early 1970s, this systemic amyloidosis, also known as familial amyloid polyneuropathy type IV and amyloidosis V, is inherited as an autosomal-dominant disorder. The corneal changes appear in the third to fourth decade of life.

Systemic involvement of the skin, peripheral nerves, and cranial nerves occurs later. This corneal dystrophy is less severe than is lattice type I dystrophy. Dots and lattice lines extend to the limbus and are fewer, thicker, and more radial. Erosions are less frequent and vision is unaffected until the seventh decade of life (57).

Histopathology

In type II lattice corneal dystrophy, amyloid deposits replace corneal nerves. Meretoja syndrome can be retrospectively diagnosed from corneal buttons based on the fact that monoclonal antibody to gelsolin labels almost all the deposits in contrast to the faint labeling of only some of the deposits in corneas from patients with type I lattice corneal dystrophy (58,59).

Genetic Studies

Lattice corneal dystrophy type II is caused by a specific mutation (asp187-to-asn) in the gelsolin gene on chromosome 9q34 (60). The amyloid protein found in patients with familial amyloidosis of the Finnish type (FAF) has been found to be an internal degradation fragment of gelsolin, with substitution of asparagine for aspartic acid at position 15, which is due to a guanine-to-adenine transversion in the gene. This mutation co-segregates with the disease phenotype and can be used as a diagnostic assay, including in prenatal evaluation (61).

Lattice Type III and Type IIIA Corneal Dystrophies

Reported in two families in Japan (62,63), type III lattice dystrophy manifests as thick translucent lattice lines and diffuse subepithelial opacities in the cornea. Lattice dystrophy type III may be autosomal recessive. The onset occurs after age 40, and vision is not affected until 70 years of age. Corneal erosions do not occur (31,62). A variant of this dystrophy (lattice type IIIA) has a similar clinical appearance. However, later age of onset (70 to 90 years), the occurrence of recurrent erosions, and an autosomal-dominant inheritance pattern differentiate it from lattice type III (64). Unilateral occurrence of type III lattice dystrophy has been reported in two cases and was confirmed by electron microscopy based on the presence of typical amyloid fibrils (65,66).

Histopathology

Both lattice dystrophy type I and type III deposits contain protein AA and protein AP (31,62,63) (Fig. 46-9). Fluorescent staining for immune deposits such as kappa chains, lambda chains, immunoglobulin C (IgC), IgM, and IgA are negative (67,68), unlike the findings in primary or secondary systemic amyloidosis in which these

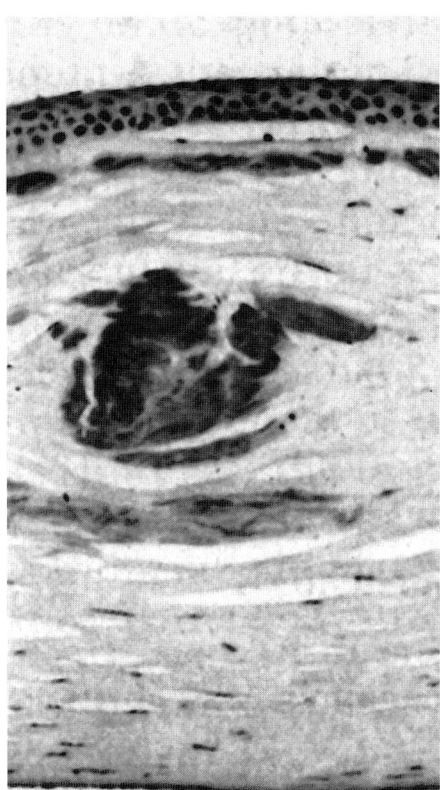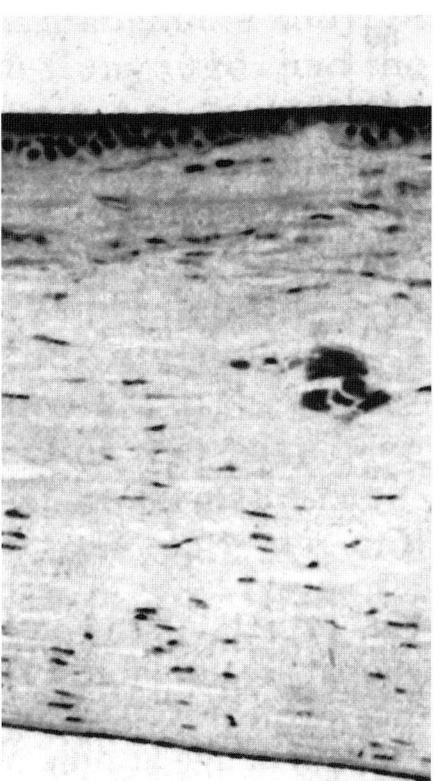

FIGURE 46-9. Comparison of lattice corneal dystrophy type III *(left)* and type I *(right).* Lattice dystrophy type III has uniform epithelium with a band of amyloid beneath intact Bowman's layer, and had much larger amyloid stromal deposit than type I. (From Hida T, et al. Histopathologic and immunochemical features of lattice corneal dystrophy type III. *Am J Ophthalmol* 1987;104:249–254, with permission.)

proteins are present. The deposition of amyloid occurs either due to release of lysosomal enzymes by abnormal keratocytes (69,70) or by abnormal keratocyte synthesis (71,72). It is believed that sequestration of glycoprotein in the corneal stroma from plasma membranes of epithelial cells may stimulate amyloid deposition. Elastotic degeneration within amyloid deposits has been reported (73). Antibodies to C-reactive protein in the epithelium of corneas affected by lattice dystrophy has been reported, although the significance of this is uncertain (74).

Genetic Studies

Yamamoto and colleagues (64) found that the mutation in type IIIA lattice corneal dystrophy was the missense change Pro501Thr in the keratoepithelin gene.

MACULAR DYSTROPHY (GROENOUW TYPE II)

Macular corneal dystrophy (MCD; also known as Groenouw type II) is divided into three subgroups on the basis of immunohistochemical studies (75–78) and serum analysis of antigenic keratan sulfate (AgKS). In MCD type I, the more common subgroup, there is a virtual absence of AgKS in the serum and cornea. MCD type IA is differentiated from type I by the presence, in the former, of highly sulfated AgKS within corneal keratocytes in patients with undetectable amount of this form of AgKS in serum (78,79). In MCD type II, the AgKS is present in cornea and serum (75).

Clinical Features

Macular corneal dystrophy is transmitted as an autosomal-recessive trait. It is the least common of the three classic stromal dystrophies (granular, lattice, and macular), but it is the most severe. The corneal changes usually are first noted between 3 and 9 years of age, when a diffuse clouding is seen in the central superficial stroma (Fig. 46-10). Unlike granular dystrophy, the macular opacities have indistinct edges, and the intervening stroma is not clear. The clouding extends peripherally to the limbus and into the deeper stoma as the disease progresses.

By the teens, the opacification involves the entire thickness of the cornea and may extend out to the limbus. Within this sea of haziness are gray-white, denser opacities with

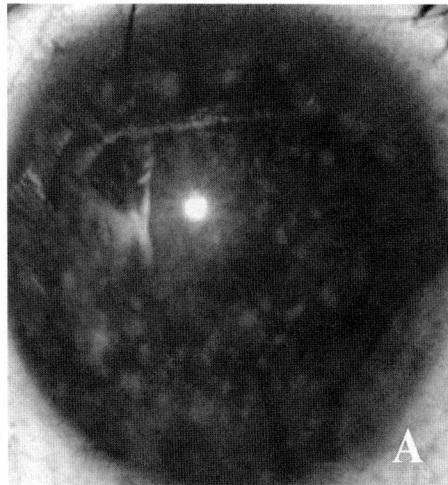
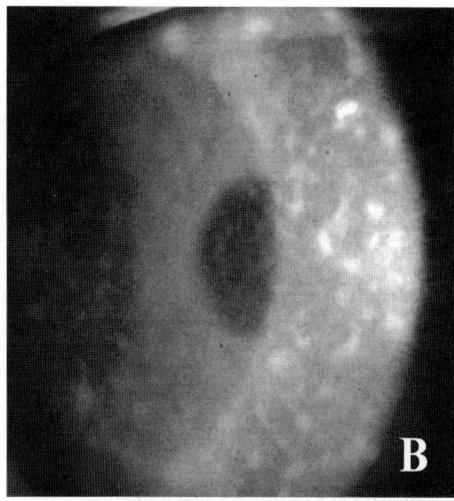

FIGURE 46-10. A,B: Macular dystrophy. The opacities have indistinct edges, the intervening stroma is not clear, and the clouding extends peripherally to the limbus. (From Charukamnoetkanok P, Dohlman CH. Corneal dystrophies in the age of the human genome project. *MEJO* 2002; 10:112–128, with permission.)

ill-defined borders. These denser, macular opacities can protrude anteriorly, resulting in irregularity of the epithelial surface, or posteriorly, causing irregularity, grayness, and guttate appearance of Descemet's membrane. This may result in progressive loss of vision, irritation, and photophobia. These opacities can enlarge with time and coalesce. Corneal thinning, confirmed by central pachymetry, has been documented (80,81). In most cases, vision is severely impaired by age 20 or 30. Recurrent erosions are seen, but they are less frequent than in patients with lattice dystrophy. Heterozygous carriers do not manifest corneal abnormalities.

Biochemical studies have shown decreased α-galactosidase in keratocytes from cornea with macular dystrophy (82), and that the primary defect is in the synthetic pathway of the KS proteoglycans (82–84). The pathogenesis of macular dystrophy was thought to result from incomplete glycosaminoglycan sulfation (85). This view was supported by the fact that monoclonal antibodies demonstrated the absence of sulfated KS in the cornea and serum of patients with macular dystrophy (type I) (84). However, a new subtype of macular dystrophy was immunohistochemically identified in 1988, in which KS is present in the cornea and serum (type II) (75,76). Type I macular dystrophy is most prevalent in Europe and in North America. It is characterized by the absence of KS in the cornea as well as in the serum, and it may represent a more widespread systemic disorder of KS metabolism (86). Type II macular dystrophy may be more prevalent in Japan, based on a limited study by Santo and associates (87).

Histopathology

In macular dystrophy, the cornea synthesizes chondroitin/dermatan sulfate proteoglycans that are larger than normal and oversulfated (85). Histologically, macular dystrophy is characterized by the accumulation of glycosaminoglycans (52,88) (acid mucopolysaccharide) between the stromal lamellae, underneath the epithelium, within stromal keratocytes, and within the endothelial cells (52,88–91). The glycosaminoglycans stain intensely with Alcian blue and with colloidal iron, minimally with PAS, and not at all with Masson's trichrome. Birefringence is decreased. Proteoglycan-specific cuprolinic blue staining has revealed that these proteoglycans accumulate and aggregate in both type I and type II macular dystrophy corneas (Fig. 46-11). Degeneration of the basal epithelial cells and focal epithelial thinning is seen over the accumulated

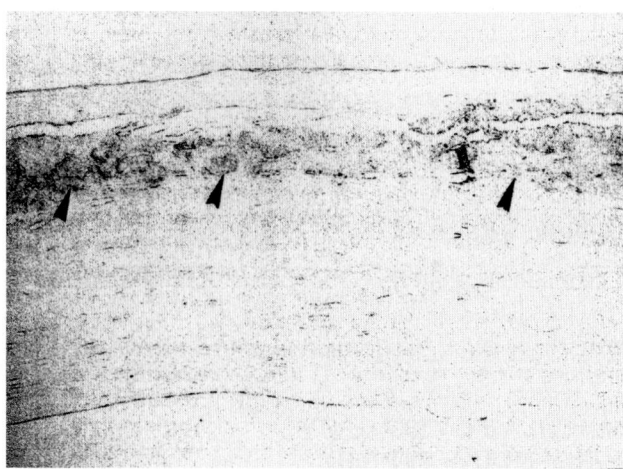

FIGURE 46-11. Macular dystrophy. The histologic section illustrates positive staining of the deposits *(arrowheads)* with a monoclonal antibody to keratan sulfate (KS). (From Santo RM, et al. Clinical and histopathologic features of corneal dystrophies in Japan. *Ophthalmology* 1995;102:557–567, with permission.)

material (92). Bowman's layer is thinned or absent in some areas. The accumulated material varies; its staining by different anti-KS antibodies varies among patients (75,76).

Using synchrotron x-ray diffraction, Quantock and colleagues (93) found that the interfibrillar spacing of collagen fibrils was significantly lower in type I macular dystrophy as compared to that of normal adult human corneas. The authors suggested that this close-packing of collagen fibrils was responsible for the reduced thickness of the central cornea in macular dystrophy.

Electron microscopy shows accumulation of mucopolysaccharide within stromal keratocytes (89,94–97). The keratocytes are distended by numerous intracytoplasmic vacuoles, which appear to be the dilated cisternae of the rough endoplasmic reticulum. Some of these vacuoles are clear, but many contain fibrillar or granular material, and occasionally membranous lamellar material.

The corneal pathology of macular corneal dystrophy differs from that of the systemic mucopolysaccharidoses in several respects (98). In the systemic mucopolysaccharidoses, the abnormal material accumulates in lysosomal vacuoles, whereas in macular dystrophy it accumulates in endoplasmic reticulum. Also, epithelial involvement is more prominent in the systemic mucopolysaccharidoses, and Descemet's membrane usually is not affected.

Genetic Studies

Linkage analysis of American and Icelandic families suggest the two phenotypically distinct forms of MCD are due to mutation at the same genetic locus on chromosome 16 (99,100).

Akama and associates (101) identified a novel carbohydrate sulfotransferase gene *(CHST6)* encoding an enzyme designated corneal *N*-acetylglucosamine-6-sulfotransferase (c-GlnNAc6ST). In MCD type I, they discovered seven mutations that were predicted to lead to inactivation of the enzyme. In MCD type II, they found large deletions and/or replacements caused by homologous recombination in the upstream region of the *CHST6* gene. *In situ* hybridization analysis failed to detect *CHST6* transcripts in corneal epithelium in an MCD type II patient, suggesting that the mutations found in type II lead to loss of cornea-specific expression of *CHST6*.

GlcNAc6ST activity in the extracts from MCD-affected corneas was much lower than in those corneas with keratoconus and in normal control corneas. The decrease in GlcNAc6ST activity in the cornea with MCD might result in the occurrence of low- or nonsulfated KS and thereby cause the corneal opacity (102).

Treatment

Penetrating keratoplasty for macular dystrophy results in good outcomes. Recurrences can occur in both lamellar and penetrating grafts, but they usually are delayed for many years (103,104). Host keratocytes invade the graft and produce abnormal glycosaminoglycan. The periphery of the graft is most affected, particularly the superficial and deep layers. Surprisingly, the endothelium and Descemet's membrane also are affected.

SCHNYDER'S CRYSTALLINE CORNEAL DYSTROPHY (SCCD)

Central crystalline dystrophy is an autosomal-dominant dystrophy characterized clinically by bilateral central corneal opacities that are sometimes associated with premature corneal arcus and limbal girdle of Vogt (105–107). It occurs early in life and may be seen as early as 2 months of age (106). Xanthelasmas can also be seen in some cases. Congenital cases are seen sporadically. Visual acuity usually is not affected, but occasionally it is moderately reduced.

The main feature of the dystrophy is the presence of bilateral, axial, ring-shaped, or disciform opacities (105,107–111). The opacities usually consist of fine, polychromatic, needle-shaped crystals, but in some cases a disciform opacity is present without evidence of crystals (106,112).

Schnyder's dystrophy is probably a spectrum of disease, and the distribution of the corneal opacities could be subdivided into five morphologic types (Fig. 46-12): type A, disk-shaped amorphous opacity without distinct crystals (Fig. 46-12A); type B, disk-shaped opacity composed of many small, bright crystals in the form of needles and small iridescent plates with indistinct borders; type C, disk-shaped opacity composed of crystals, without a clear center, and with a garland-like outline (Fig. 46-12B); type D, ring-shaped amorphous opacity, with local crystal accumulation and with a clear center (Fig. 46-12C); and type E, ring-shaped opacity, composed of crystals and with a clear center (Fig. 46-12D). On rare occasions, clouding extends to the arcus (113), but usually a clear cornea persists between the central opacification and the surrounding arcus (Fig. 46-12C) (114). The yellow-white opacity primarily involves Bowman's layer and anterior stroma but may extend into the deeper layers. The epithelium is normal and the intervening stroma usually is clear, but punctate white opacities can be scattered in the stroma (Fig. 46-12E), or the stroma can develop a milky opalescence (108,109). Corneal sensation is normal and this is a feature that distinguishes Schnyder's dystrophy from lipid neurotropic deposits (Fig. 46-12F). The opacities progress slowly and usually stabilize later in life. Progression is more frequent in patients with diffuse opacities (types A and D) than in those with crystalline deposits (115).

The severity of dyslipidemia, which may (105, 116–118) or may not (119–122) be associated with Schnyder's dystrophy, usually does not correlate with the extent of opacification or the progression of the disease (115). A significant number of patients with Schnyder's dystrophy

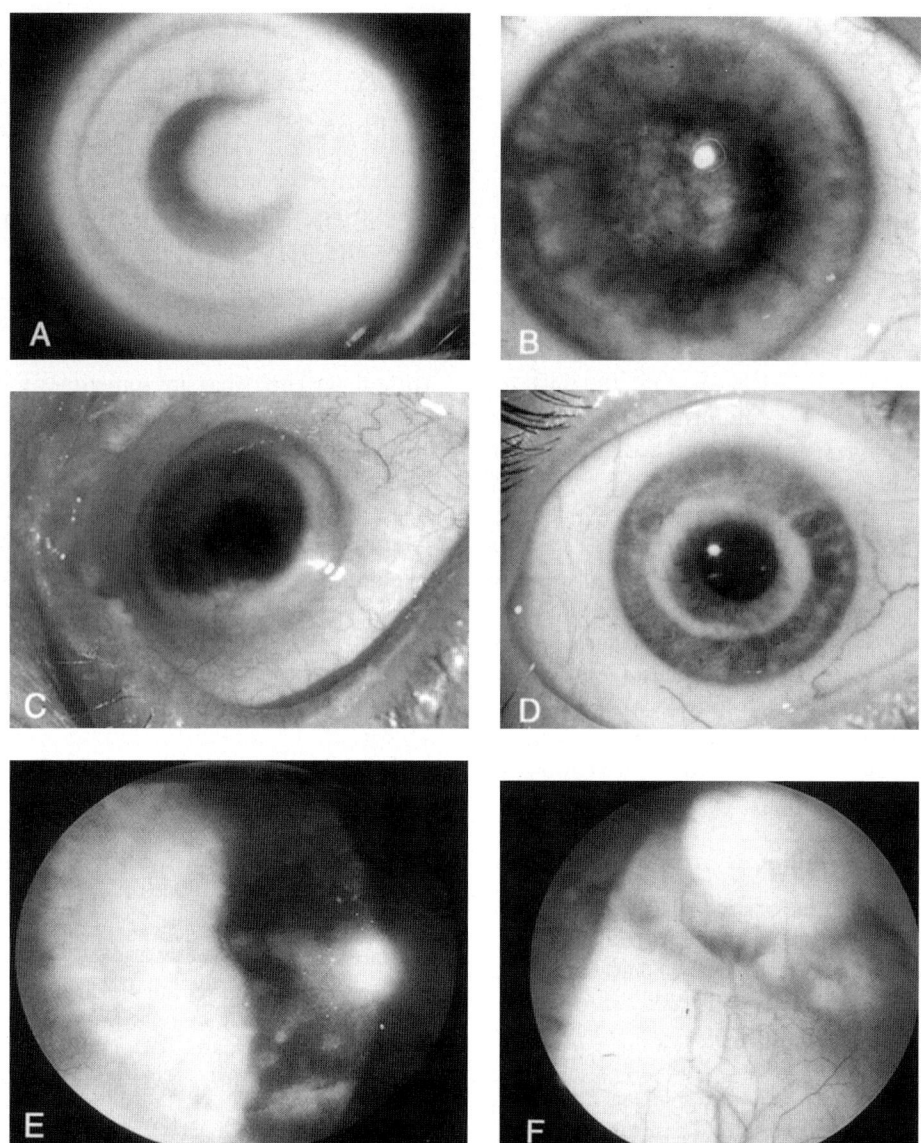

FIGURE 46-12. A: Clinical appearance of a patient with type A Schnyder's crystalline dystrophy. **B:** Disk-shaped crystalline deposits in type C Schnyder's dystrophy. **C:** Ring-shaped amorphous opacity of type D Schnyder's dystrophy. **D:** Type E Schnyder's dystrophy shows a ring-shaped opacity composed of crystals with a clear central area. This is similar to the corneal lipid deposits of Bietti's dystrophy. **E:** Scattered early lipid deposits. **F:** Neurotrophic lipid deposition having a similar appearance of type A Schnyder's dystrophy. Decreased corneal sensation and the presence of peripheral feeder vessel(s) differentiate the former from the latter. (From Chang SW, Tuli S, Azar DT. Corneal dystrophies. In: Traboulsi ET, ed. *Genetic diseases of the eye.* Oxford: Oxford University Press, 1997:217–266, with permission.)

have hyperlipidemia, but the type and severity of the hyperlipidemia vary (108,109). Some individuals within a single family may have only crystalline dystrophy, others may have hyperlipidemia and crystalline dystrophy, and others have only hyperlipidemia. Chondrodystrophy and genu valgum also are associated with Schnyder's dystrophy in some families (105,108,109,123).

Bietti's crystalline corneoretinal dystrophy is a form of Schnyder's dystrophy associated with crystalline retinopathy. In 1937, Bietti first described crystalline fundus dystrophy with crystalline changes in the marginal cornea (124–126)

in three patients (145). In the majority of patients with Bietti's dystrophy (124–127), the first symptoms are noticed during the third decade of life and take the form of visual loss and decreased night vision. The corneal deposits are numerous, tiny, yellowish-white, and are concentrated in the superficial layers of the cornea near the limbus (127). They are morphologically similar to Schnyder's dystrophy type E. These punctate deposits can be found in the upper and lower areas or for 360 degrees. The corneal deposits remains unchanged, whereas the retinal crystals diminish with time (125,128).

Because Bietti's dystrophy showed familial clustering, an autosomal-recessive mode of inheritance was assumed to be involved (128). Later reports suggested that there may be an autosomal-dominant variant of Bietti's dystrophy (129–131). The reports published to date cover several ethnic groups. Bietti's dystrophy is a relatively rare disease in the West but a relatively common one in China (132).

The clinical picture of a marginal corneal dystrophy and crystalline retinopathy provides little latitude with regard to the differential diagnosis, as few conditions show refractile bodies in both cornea and retina. The crystals of cystinosis are found throughout the entire cornea, not solely at the limbus, and appear in the choroid and retinal pigment epithelium but not the neuroretina (133).

Histopathology

The main histopathologic feature of Schnyder's dystrophy is the presence of phospholipid, cholesterol crystals, noncrystalline cholesterol, cholesterol esters, and neutral fats in the stroma (109,111,120,122) (Fig. 46-13). The clinically

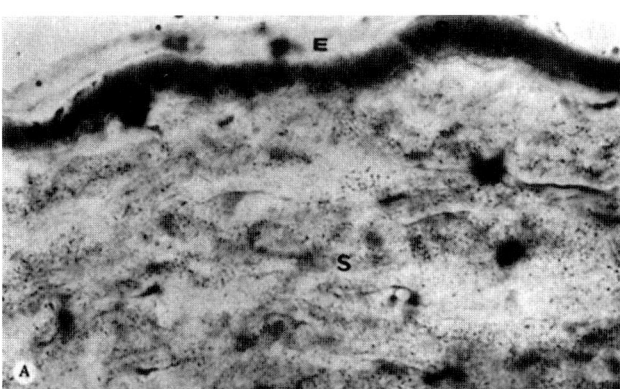

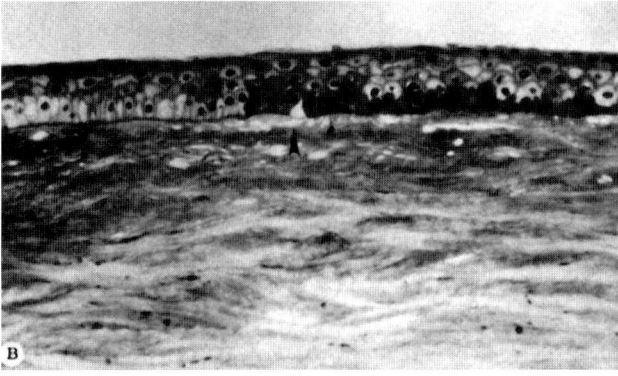

FIGURE 46-13. Schnyder's crystalline dystrophy. **A:** Oil red O stained frozen specimen of superficial cornea demonstrates unstained epithelium (E). Bowman's layer (B) has very heavy deposit of stain. Anterior stoma (S) has scattered granular stain. **B:** Light micrograph stained with toluidine blue shows numerous dark and light cells in the epithelium. There are many optically empty spaces *(arrow)* in Bowman's zone. (From Burns RP, et al. Cholesterol turnover in hereditary crystalline corneal dystrophy of Schnyder. *Trans Am Ophthalmol Soc* 1978; 76:184–196, with permission.)

apparent crystals correspond to cholesterol accumulations, both extracellulary and within keratocytes. Occasionally similar deposits have been noted in basal epithelial cells (119). The deposits are most numerous in the anterior stroma, but they can extend posteriorly to Descemet's membrane (134). Destruction of Bowman's layer and superficial stroma with disorganization of collagen has often been observed.

The pathogenesis of Schnyder's dystrophy is unclear but is thought to involve a primary disorder of corneal lipid metabolism (105,114,117), the severity of which may be altered by systemic hyperlipidemia. Burns and colleagues (135) administered radiolabeled cholesterol intravenously to a patient with crystalline dystrophy 2 weeks before keratoplasty. The radioactivity in the cornea was higher than that in the blood, suggesting active deposition of cholesterol in the cornea.

Phospholipid and unesterified cholesterol are important constituents of cell membranes. The increase of these lipids in Schnyder's dystrophy suggests the possibility of a primary disorder of corneal lipid metabolism, resulting in the accumulation of abnormal and subsequently unstable cell membranes. The primary abnormality could involve excess production or diminished breakdown of phospholipids, unesterified cholesterol, or other constituents of cell membranes. This concept can be supported by the findings that keratocytes and their membranes are abnormal in Schnyder's dystrophy (105,116) and the characteristic membrane-bound vacuoles appearing to bud from degenerating keratocytes (116). Both the vacuoles and keratocytes were noted to have similar trilamellar membranes (112) (Fig. 46-14). Such budding could represent breakdown of unstable cell membranes in part composed of excess phospholipid and unesterified cholesterol (Fig. 46-15).

Mirshahi and associates (136) showed a much lower secretion of plasminogen activators by corneal fibroblasts from Schnyder's dystrophy cornea than that secreted by normal corneal fibroblasts. Because plasminogen activators are involved in extracellular matrix remodeling, the deficiency may be responsible for diminished breakdown of cell membranes in corneal dystrophy.

A metabolic storage disease has been suggested as a cause of crystalline corneal-retinal dystrophy in Bietti crystalline corneoretinal dystrophy (126,128). Cholesterol, cholesterol esters, complex lipid inclusions, and immunoproteins (137) have been reported in corneal fibroblasts and circulating lymphocytes in the limbus (126,128).

Genetic Studies

Shearman and colleagues (138) performed a genome-wide linkage analysis in two large families with Schnyder's crystalline corneal dystrophy living in central Massachusetts (both kindreds were of Swedish-Finnish descent and

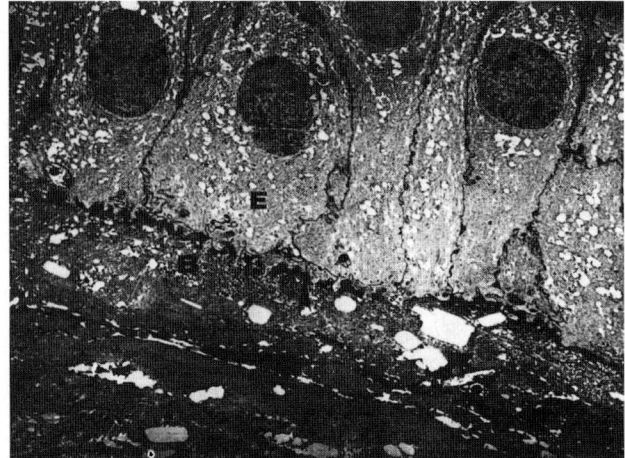

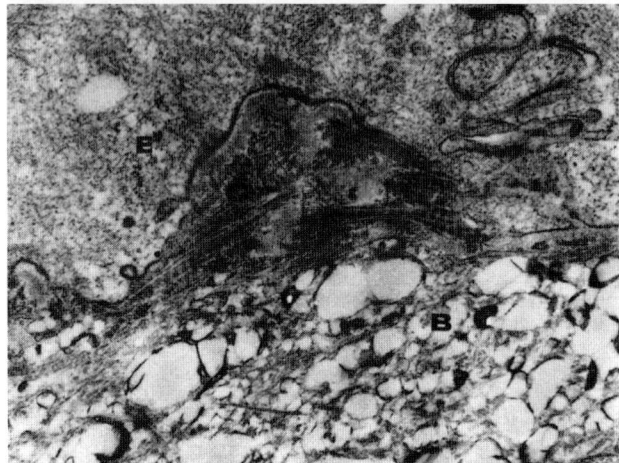

FIGURE 46-14. Schnyder's crystalline dystrophy. **A:** Electron micrograph of basal epithelium and Bowman's layers illustrates vacuolated corneal epithelium (E), thickened basement membrane *(arrow),* and distorted, vacuolated Bowman's zone (B). **B:** High magnification of the area of basal epithelial cell (C) and almost unrecognizable Bowman's zone (B) with numerous vacuoles. (From Burns RP, et al. Cholesterol turnover in hereditary crystalline corneal dystrophy of Schnyder. *Trans Am Ophthalmol Soc* 1978;76:184–196, with permission.)

traced their ancestry to the same region of the southwest coast of Finland), and assigned the *SCCD* gene in both families to 1p36-p34.1. Two candidate genes lie in that region: galactose 4-epimerase and methylene tetrahydrofolate reductase (MTHFR). Three uncharacterized expressed sequence tags had also been mapped to the 1p36-p34.1 interval. Interestingly, galactose 4-epimerase-deficient hamster cells grown in the absence of exogenous galactose and galactosamine lack normal posttranslational processing of low-density lipoprotein (LDL) receptors and other glycoproteins and have an LDL receptor-deficient phenotype. Variants of the MTHFR gene are associated with atherosclerotic changes and thromboembolism.

Genetic studies of Bietti's crystalline corneoretinal dystrophy showed that this condition is linked to another gene on chromosome 4 (4q35-qter) (139).

Treatment

In most cases of crystalline dystrophy the corneal disease requires no treatment. Serum lipid profiles should be obtained because elevated serum lipid levels and concomitant cardiovascular disease are associated features in some patients (105), and the severity of a systemic lipid abnormality does not necessarily correlate with the severity of the corneal disease. Patients with abnormal systemic lipid profiles should be evaluated and treated by a cardiologist.

Efforts directed at visual improvement through such means as reduction of cholesterol intake have proven beneficial in only one case report (140). Penetrating or lamellar keratoplasty can be performed for visual rehabilitation, but the dystrophy can recur (105,117). Recurrence of crystalline deposits occurs sooner and in larger amounts in lamellar grafts than in full-thickness grafts (106). Postoperative changes in the posterior layers of the cornea in Schnyder's crystalline dystrophy may contribute to the comparatively poorer surgical outcomes obtained with lamellar grafts as compared to full-thickness grafts (134).

FLECK DYSTROPHY (FRANÇOIS-NEETENS)

Fleck dystrophy, also called speckled dystrophy or mouchetee dystrophy, is a rare dystrophy that is transmitted as an autosomal-dominant trait (141–148). The cornea in fleck dystrophy is characterized by numerous tiny, small opacities scattered throughout the entire corneal stroma. The lesions are semiopaque, flattened opacities that may be oval, round, comma-shaped, granular, or stellate. The condition usually is detectable very early during the first decade of life and, in some patients, is congenital. It is stationary, with no loss of visual acuity and is usually noted during a routine examination. Some degree of photophobia may be present (141,142).

The lesions usually are bilateral, although they can be asymmetric or even unilateral. Small opacities are present in all layers of the corneal stroma except Bowman's layer, and they involve the peripheral as well as the central stroma. Many have a doughnut-like appearance with a relatively clear center. These small opacities are well demarcated, and the intervening stroma is clear. They are best demonstrated by retroillumination. Corneal sensation is normal in most cases, but in some families sensation is decreased (143).

Fleck dystrophy has been noted in association with a variety of disorders such as keratoconus (143), limbal dermoids, central cloudy dystrophy, angioid streaks, papillitis, and punctate cortical lens opacities (143,144, 148–150). It is unclear whether the relationship is more than coincidental.

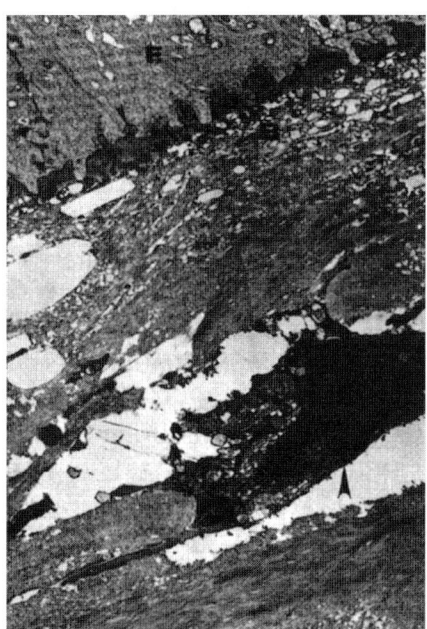
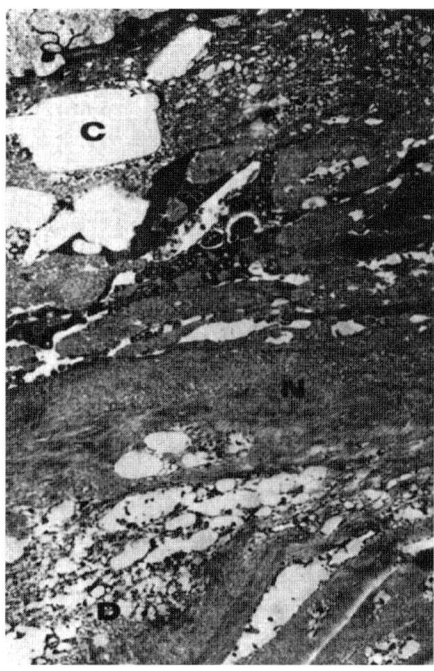

FIGURE 46-15. Schnyder's crystalline dystrophy. **A:** Region of cornea shows basal epithelium (E) with thickened basement membrane *(small arrow)*, disorganized Bowman's layer (B), and vacuolated keratocyte *(large arrow)*. **B:** Electron micrograph of Bowman's layer illustrates the notch at the end of the empty space (C), suggesting that the structure is the ghost of a cholesterol crystal. There are bundles of normal-appearing collagen (N) alternated with disorganized collagen (D). (From Burns RP, et al. Cholesterol turnover in hereditary crystalline corneal dystrophy of Schnyder. *Trans Am Ophthalmol Soc* 1978;76:184–196, with permission.)

Histopathology

Histopathologic studies reveal abnormal and distended keratocytes throughout the stroma. Bowman's layer, epithelium, Descemet's membrane, and endothelium are normal. The keratocytes stain with oil red O and Sudan black B, indicating the presence of lipid, and Alcian blue and colloidal iron, indicating the presence of mucopolysaccharide (151,152).

On electron microscopy, the keratocytes are seen to contain varying numbers of membrane-lined intracytoplasmic vacuoles containing a fibrillogranular material (152,153) (Fig. 46-16). Some of these vacuoles also contain membranous inclusions or pleomorphic, electron-dense deposits (Fig. 46-17). The vacuoles appear to arise from the Golgi apparatus and therefore are lysosomal vacuoles (Fig. 46-18). Because of this, fleck dystrophy seems to be a storage disorder of glycosaminoglycans and complex lipids that is limited to the cornea.

CENTRAL CLOUDY DYSTROPHY (OF FRANÇOIS)

Central cloudy dystrophy is transmitted as an autosomal-dominant trait, with an early onset and no progression with age (154,155). It is characterized by axial clouding of the cornea, densest posteriorly and fading anteriorly and peripherally (Fig. 46-19). The cloud is broken into segments by an interlacing network of clear lines, creating a mosaic pattern. Sometimes the opacification extends to, or in rare cases involves, Bowman's layer; in this location the opacities are smaller and less numerous. There is a pool of extracellular mucopolysaccharide in the corneal stroma (Fig. 46-20).

Ultrastructurally, the affected area shows degenerated keratocytes with numerous vacuoles in (Fig. 46-21). Vision is not affected, and there are no other symptoms, so the diagnosis often is not made until late in life. Most likely, the pathologic mechanism of this condition is the same as that of posterior mosaic (crocodile) shagreen. It has been noted in association with fleck dystrophy (156), pseudoxanthoma elasticum (157), and pre-Descemet's dystrophy.

PARENCHYMATOUS DYSTROPHY (OF PILLAT)

This very rare corneal dystrophy has only been described in a few case reports (158–160). Thomsitt and Bron (160) also coined the term polymorphic stromal dystrophy. Deep stromal opacities are seen, which are gray-white on focal illumination and clear on retroillumination. The deposits are punctate and filamentous and can be central, peripheral, or annular in distribution, and usually are noted in patients in the sixth decade. Progression of the disorder has not been

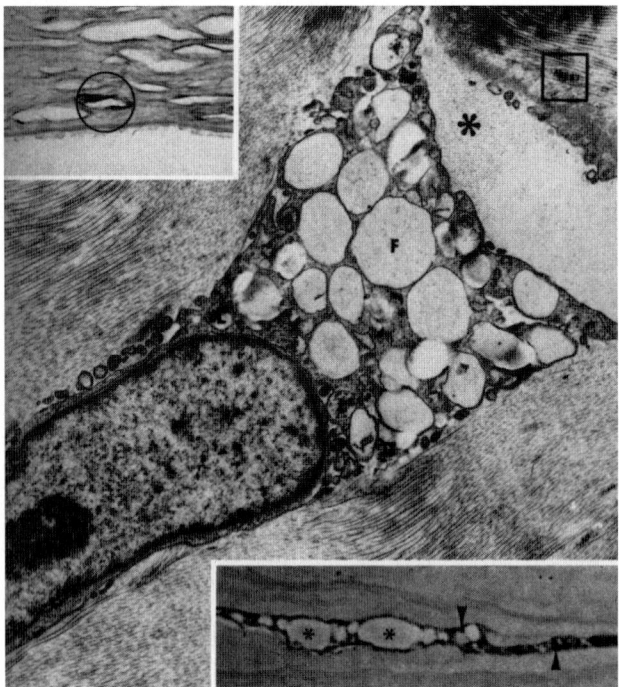

FIGURE 46-16. Fleck dystrophy. Electron micrograph of a markedly vacuolated keratocyte filled with fibrillogranular (F) or lipid (L) substances. The only extracellular abnormalities are an accumulation of fine granular material *(asterisk)* and occasional foci of long-spacing collagen *(square)*. *Bottom inset* is a phase-contrast photomicrograph of a severely damaged keratocyte demonstrating foamy cytoplasm with larger clear vacuoles *(asterisks)* and small refractile inclusions *(arrowheads)*. *Top inset* shows positive staining for acid mucopolysaccharide limited to a swollen keratocyte *(circled)*. (From Nicholson DH, et al. A clinical and histopathological study of François-Neetens speckled corneal dystrophy. *Am J Ophthalmol* 1977;83:554–560, with permission.)

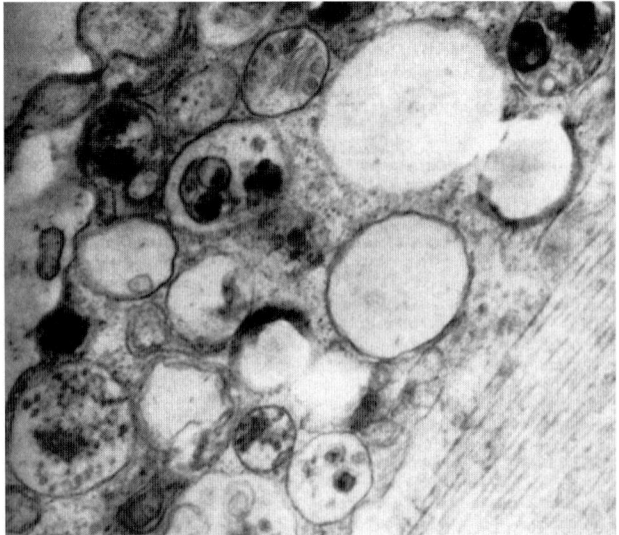

FIGURE 46-17. Fleck dystrophy. Electron micrograph reveals limiting vacuoles with sparse fine granular contents and pleomorphic, electron-dense lamellar substances. (From Nicholson DH, et al. A clinical and histopathological study of François-Neetens speckled corneal dystrophy. *Am J Ophthalmol* 1977; 83:554–560, with permission.)

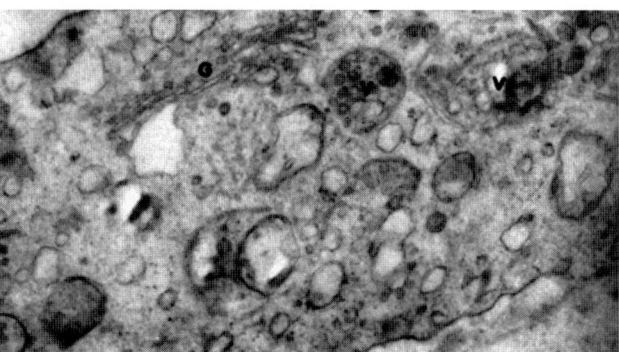

FIGURE 46-18. Fleck dystrophy. Electron micrograph of a less involved keratocytes demonstrates vacuoles (V) with pleomorphic contents in close association with prominent Golgi complex (G) from which a clear vacuole appears to be emanating. (From Nicholson DH, et al. A clinical and histopathological study of François-Neetens speckled corneal dystrophy. *Am J Ophthalmol* 1977;83:554–560, with permission.)

demonstrated. The punctate opacities are polymorphic flecklike, stellate, linear, or guttate. The filaments are identical to those seen in lattice dystrophy; they can have beading, striations, or dichotomous branching. Vision and corneal sensation are not affected. Although the condition has been noted in two siblings, no heritability has been demonstrated. Most likely this is a degenerative change and is the same as polymorphic amyloid degeneration (44).

POSTERIOR AMORPHOUS DYSTROPHY

Clinical Manifestations

An autosomal-dominant posterior amorphous dystrophy has been described in only five families (134,161–164). Changes have been noted as early as 16 weeks of age and thus may be present at birth. Visual acuity is only mildly affected and is rarely worse than 20/40, and progression has not been documented. Gray, amorphous sheetlike opacities can involve any portion of the stroma but are most prominent posteriorly. These sheetlike opacities may be irregular and broken with clear intervening stroma. They can affect the central or peripheral portions of the cornea or both. Descemet's membrane may show posterior bowing and distortion of the endothelial mosaic. Central corneal thinning, flattening, and hyperopia may be present (Fig. 46-22).

Various iris and angle abnormalities have been noted, including a prominent Schwalbe ring, with numerous fine iris processes, pupillary remnants, corectopia, iridocorneal adhesions, and anterior stromal tags. It is important to differentiate this type of dystrophy from interstitial keratitis, because both can show posterior corneal opacification. However, no vascularization or inflammation is seen in posterior amorphous dystrophy. In view of the early onset, lack of progression, and association with iris abnormalities, this condition may be a dysgenesis rather than a dystrophy (161).

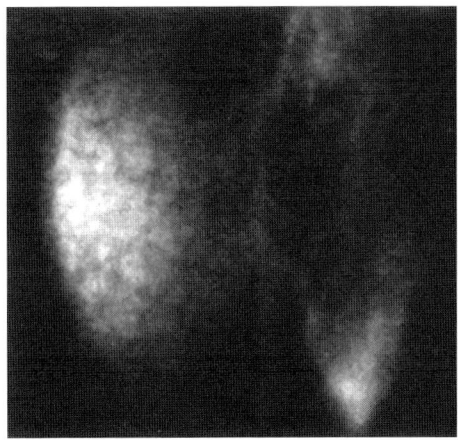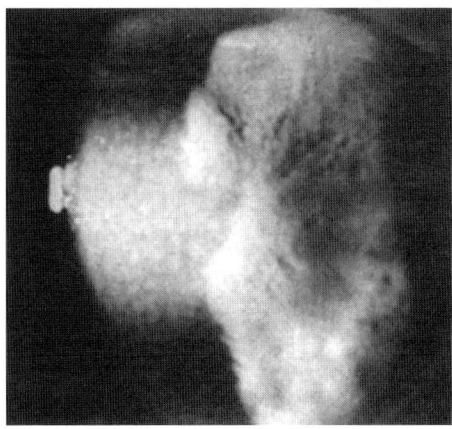

A   B

FIGURE 46-19. A,B: Central cloudy cornea dystrophy of François. Slit-lamp examination demonstrates symmetric, polygonal, stromal opacities separated by clear cracklike zones in a mosaic pattern in the central corneas. (From Karp CL, et al. Central cloudy cornea dystrophy of François. *Arch Ophthalmol* 1997;115:1058–1062, with permission.)

Histopathology

Johnson and colleagues (163) described the keratoplasty specimen from a 5-year-old child, which demonstrated fracturing of the posterior stromal collagen lamellae, a thin Descemet's membrane, and focal attenuation of endothelial cells (Fig. 46-23). Ultrastructural studies showed disorganization of the posterior stromal collagen (Fig. 46-24).

GELATINOUS DROPLIKE DYSTROPHY (PRIMARY FAMILIAL AMYLOIDOSIS OF THE CORNEA)

Clinical Manifestation

Gelatinous droplike dystrophy (GDLD) is a rare familial disorder of the cornea, which is more common in Japan (92,165–169). It accounted for the greatest number of

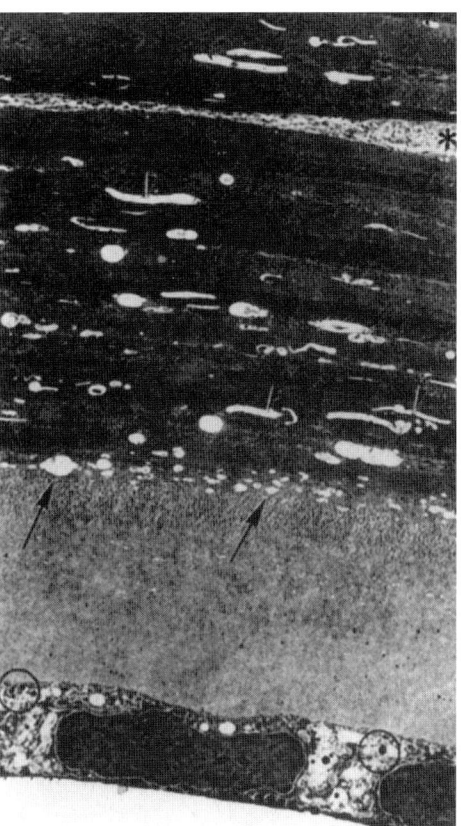

FIGURE 46-21. Central cloudy cornea dystrophy of François. Electron micrograph demonstrates a posterior portion of the cornea with a degenerated keratocyte *(asterisk)* and numerous vacuoles in stroma *(arrowheads)* concentrated just anterior to Descemet's membrane *(arrows)*. The endothelium has numerous vacuoles that contain electron-dense globules *(circles)*. (From Karp CL, et al. Central cloudy cornea dystrophy of François. *Arch Ophthalmol* 1997;115:1058–1062, with permission.)

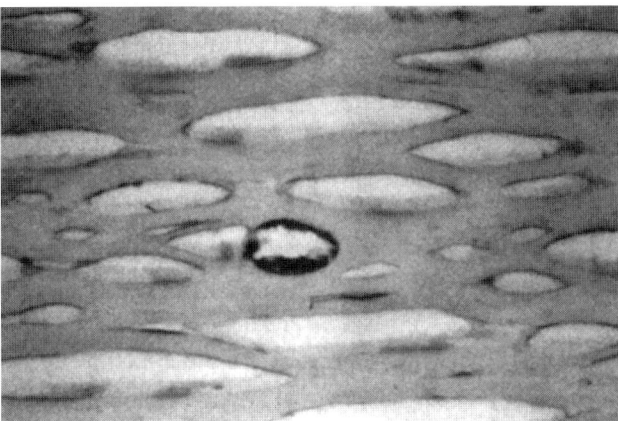

FIGURE 46-20. Central cloudy cornea dystrophy of François. Alcian blue stain shows a pool of extracellular mucopolysaccharide in the corneal stroma. (From Karp CL, et al. Central cloudy cornea dystrophy of François. *Arch Ophthalmol* 1997;115: 1058–1062, with permission.)

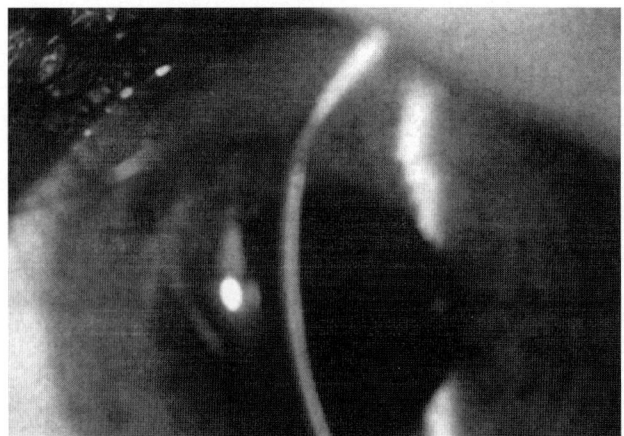
A

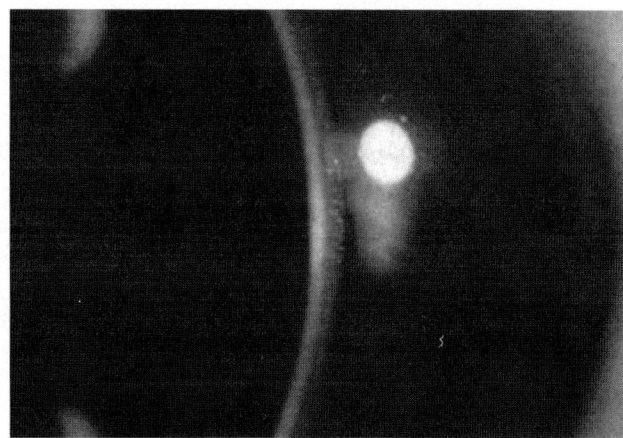
B

FIGURE 46-22. Posterior amorphous corneal dystrophy. **A:** Slit-lamp photograph shows gray-white sheetlike posterior stroma opacity with clear zones presenting superior to corneal thinning. **B:** The posterior stroma opacity with clear zones without corneal thinning. (From Branco BC, et al. Posterior amorphous corneal dystrophy: ultrasound biomicroscopy findings in two cases. *Cornea* 2002;2:220–222, with permission.)

specimens in one Japanese study of corneal dystrophies (87). Early investigators in the United States termed the condition primary familial amyloidosis of the cornea (170,171). A similar condition was described in the European literature in 1930 (172). The pattern of inheritance is unclear but is most likely autosomal recessive (170).

The disorder usually appears in the first decade, with photophobia, lacrimation, and decreased visual acuity. Early in the dystrophy, the deposits are fairly flat and can resemble band-shaped keratopathy (15). Examination shows bilateral, central, raised, multinodular, subepithelial mounds of amyloid. These are white on direct illumination and transparent on illumination but can become yellow and milky with time (Fig. 46-25). Flat subepithelial opacities can be seen surrounding the mounds. The opacities increase in number and depth with age. In the late stages, the cornea can have a diffuse, mulberry-like appearance. Vascularization, if present, is usually minimal. Anterior and posterior cortical lens changes may be associated (170).

Histopathology

The amyloid nature of these deposits has been demonstrated histologically and ultrastructurally (14,165,167,170,171) (Fig. 46-26). Bowman's layer usually is absent, and amyloid

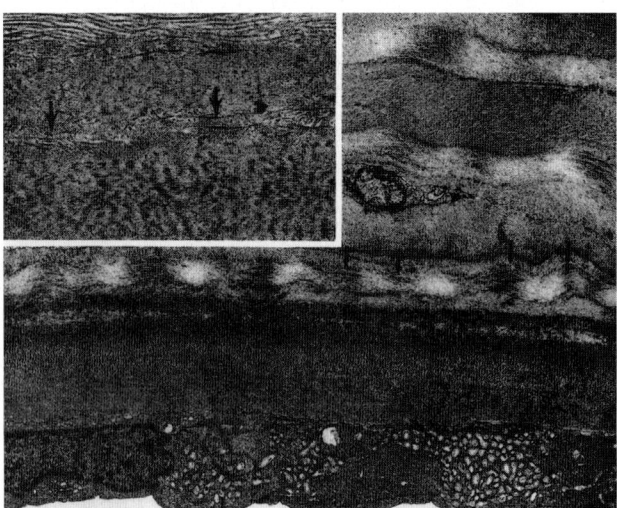

FIGURE 46-23. Posterior amorphous corneal dystrophy. Electron micrograph shows alternating longitudinal *(arrows)* and cross-sectional profiles of collagen fibrils in several of the lamellae. A region of collagen fibrils resembling those of the stroma *(arrowheads)* interrupts the anterior-banded portion of Descemet's membrane. The nonbanded portion of Descemet's membrane *(asterisk)* appears normal. *Inset* illustrates a higher magnification electron micrograph at the boundary between stroma and Descemet's membrane. The broad-banded collagen of Descemet's membrane is interrupted by randomly arranged fibrils that appear similar to stromal collagen *(arrows)*. (From Johnson AT, et al. The pathology of posterior amorphous corneal dystrophy. *Ophthalmology* 1990;97:104–109, with permission.)

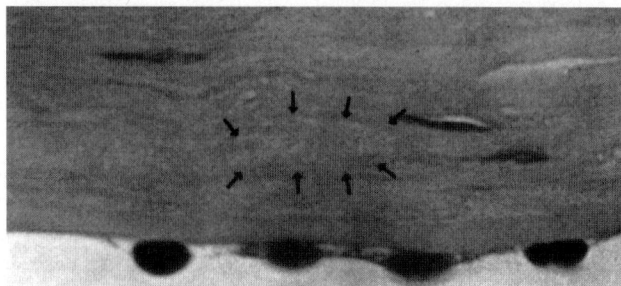

FIGURE 46-24. Posterior amorphous corneal dystrophy. Light micrograph shows several areas where the stromal lamellae adjacent to Descemet's membrane are fractured and disrupted *(arrows)*. The endothelium is focally attenuated. (From Johnson AT, et al. The pathology of posterior amorphous corneal dystrophy. *Ophthalmology* 1990;97:104–109, with permission.)

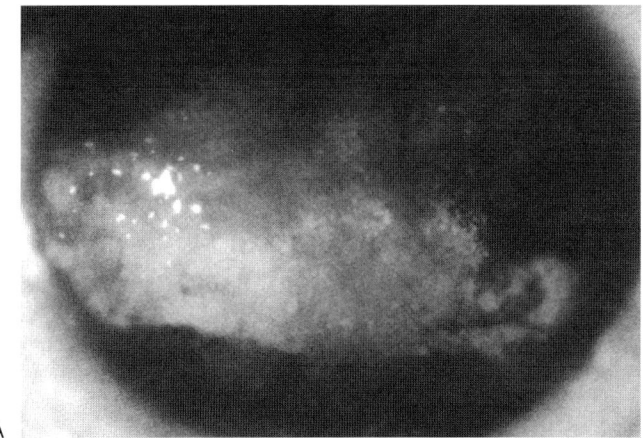
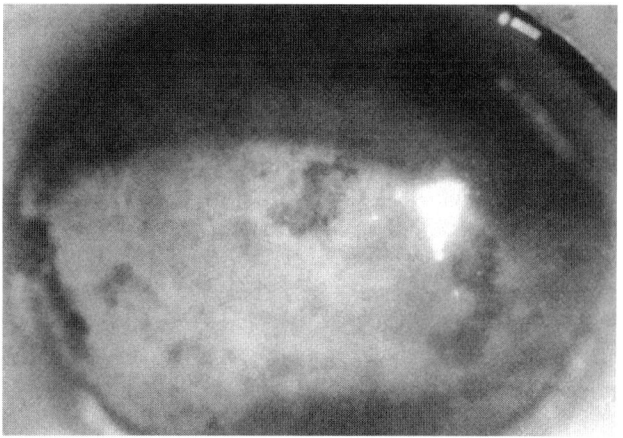

A

B

FIGURE 46-25. Gelatinous droplike corneal dystrophy. Clinical pictures show the corneas of two patients before penetrating keratoplasty. (From Kinoshita S, et al. Epithelial barrier function and ultrastructure of gelatinous drop-like corneal dystrophy. *Cornea* 2000;19:551–555, with permission.)

is deposited in the basal epithelial cells, and fusiform deposits similar to lattice dystrophy occur in the deeper stroma. A flat, more uniform layer of a similar material may surround the nodular masses. Amyloid can also deposit in the deep stroma (87) (Fig. 46-27). The type of corneal amyloid deposits containing protein AP but not protein AA or immunoglobulins may be different from that found in lattice dystrophy (173).

The specimens obtained from the perilimbal conjunctiva showed amyloid deposits in the stroma (87). This may support the idea that the epithelial cells, more precisely the limbal cells, are involved in the synthesis of amyloid fibrils and might have a role in the recurrence process. This also would explain the success observed when lamellar keratoplasty is combined with keratoepithelioplasty around the limbal area after a 360-degree peritomy (27).

However, the finding of stromal deposits suggests that keratocytes may participate in some way in the pathogenesis of this disease. Gelatinous droplike dystrophy and lattice dystrophy might be two facets of the same basic disorder, with the former representing the epithelial expression and the latter the stromal expression (92).

Genetic Studies

Tsujikawa and colleagues (174) performed linkage analysis of 10 consanguineous Japanese families with a total of 13 affected members and defined the disease locus within a region of approximately 2.6 centimorgan (cM) between D1S2890 and D1S2801 on chromosome 1p. In 1999, they mapped GDLD to a 400-kilobase critical region that included M1S1 (membrane component, chromosome 1, surface marker 1)

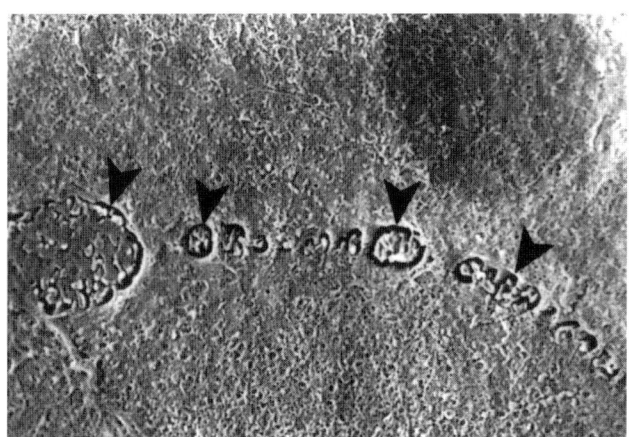
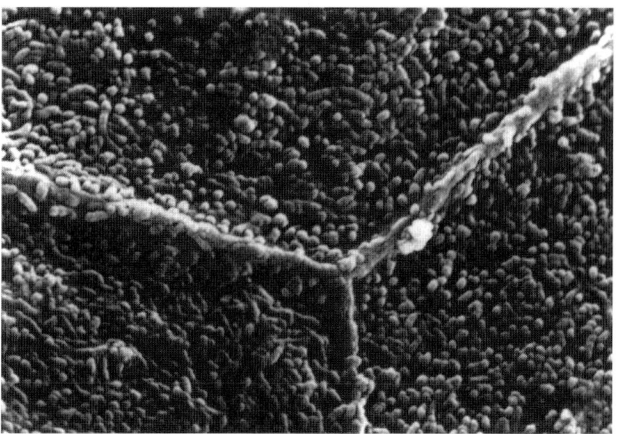

A

B

FIGURE 46-26. Gelatinous droplike corneal dystrophy (GDLD). Scanning electron micrographs of the epithelial cell borders from the patient **(A)** and normal cornea **(B)**. The junction between the GDLD epithelial cells is rounded and the adjacent cells have only intermittent contact *(arrowheads)*. In contrast, adjacent normal epithelial cells have straight, continuous junctions. (From Kinoshita S, et al. Epithelial barrier function and ultrastructure of gelatinous droplike corneal dystrophy. *Cornea* 2000;19:551–555, with permission.)

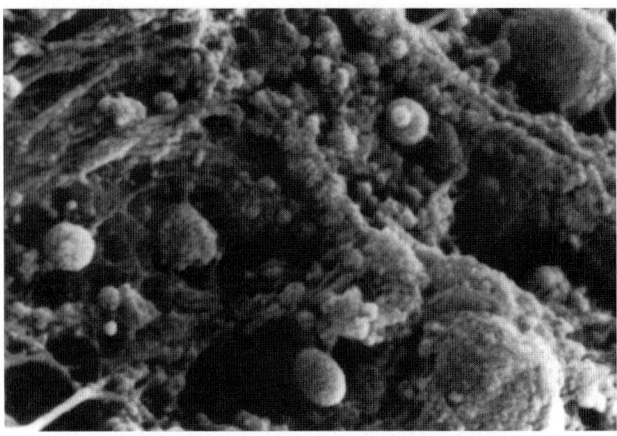

FIGURE 46-27. Gelatinous droplike corneal dystrophy. Scanning electron micrographs demonstrate that amyloid material closely associated with the collagen fibrils and aggregated into spherical clumps. (From Kinoshita S, et al. Epithelial barrier function and ultrastructure of gelatinous droplike corneal dystrophy. *Cornea* 2000;19:551–555, with permission.)

(175). They found four mutations in 26 affected members of 20 Japanese GDLD families: gln118 to ter (Q118X), gln207 to ter (Q207X), ser170 to ter (S170X), and 632delA. Expression analysis indicated that M1S1 is expressed in the cornea as well as in kidney, lung, placenta, pancreas, and prostate. Protein expression analysis revealed aggregation of the mutated, truncated protein in the perinuclear region, whereas the normal protein was distributed diffusely in the cytoplasm with a homogeneous or fine granular pattern.

Ren and colleagues (176) extended molecular studies of GDLD to patients with diverse ethnic backgrounds by performing linkage analyses in eight unrelated GDLD families from India, the United States, Europe, and Tunisia. In seven of these families, the disease locus mapped to a 16-cM interval on the short arm of chromosome 1 that included the region of the M1S1 gene.

Treatment

Treatment may include either superficial keratectomy or keratoplasty. Recurrence is seen after penetrating keratoplasty (87,166,172). In fact, in one series, recurrences in a graft accounted for more than half the patients undergoing penetrating keratoplasty (87).

PRE-DESCEMET'S DYSTROPHY

Pre-Descemet's dystrophy has several very rare subgroups. A variety of fine posterior stromal opacities have been described in patients in the fourth decade or older. Many of these may represent degenerative diseases rather than dystrophies (113). A clear pattern of heredity is not always obvious. However, some of these conditions have been reported in a number of family members, over two to four generations (156,157,177–179). The vision is usually not affected and the patients usually do not feel discomfort. These subgroups may be considered variants of one diagnosis (pre-Descemet's dystrophy), similar to how the map, dots, and fingerprints lesions are grouped together under the diagnosis of anterior basement membrane dystrophy.

The pathologic condition of pre-Descemet's dystrophy is limited to the keratocytes of the posterior stroma (157,179). The keratocytes contained lipid-like material in their cytoplasmic vacuoles (secondary lysosomes). Ultrastructural study of these vacuoles reveals fibrillogranular and electron-dense lamellar inclusions, suggesting that the accumulated material most likely was lipofuscin, a degenerative "wear and tear" lipoprotein associated with aging. There is no extracellular deposition of such material.

Similar opacities have been noted in association with the other ocular or systemic abnormalities, and these have been called secondary pre-Descemet's dystrophies, which also have been reported in patients with epithelial basement membrane dystrophy (178), ichthyosis (deep punctate dystrophy of Franceschetti and Maeder) (180), central cloudy corneal dystrophy (157), pseudoxanthoma elasticum (157), and in female carriers of sex-linked ichthyosis.

GRAYSON-WILBRANDT DYSTROPHY

Grayson and Wilbrandt (179) described primary pre-Descemet's dystrophies that consisted of mixtures of opacities: (a) dendritic or stellate, (b) boomerang, (c) circular or dot, (d) comma, (e) linear, and (f) filiform. The opacities resemble those in cornea farinata, but they are larger and more polymorphous. The deposits could be axial, peripheral, or diffuse.

PUNCTIFORM AND POLYCHROMATIC PRE-DESCEMET'S DOMINANT DYSTROPHY

A pedigree with more uniform, polychromatic deep stromal filaments in a diffuse pattern extending to the limbus (144) was described, affecting 46 family members from four generations, and the inheritance appeared to be autosomal dominant. No particular aggregations or annular patterns were appreciated, and Descemet's membrane and the endothelium were not clinically affected. No histopathologic specimens are available from this clinical variant.

DEEP FILIFORM DYSTROPHY

Deep filiform dystrophy of Maeder and Danis (181) has been reported in association with keratoconus. The lesions consist of multiple filiform, gray opacities in the pre-Descemet's area that affect the entire width of the cornea except for a perilimbal region. Yassa and colleagues (182) reported a case with bilateral optically dense linear striae of variable lengths and a crisscross pattern forming a lacy network. The opacities lie between the deep stromal lamellae immediately anterior to Descemet's membrane. Both corneas showed immunoglobulin deposited extracellularly in the posterior third of the stroma and intracellularly in the keratocytes of the posterior two thirds. Although the results of serum protein electrophoresis were within normal limits, the possibility of a dysproteinemia undetectable by currently available methods could not be excluded. Thus, in all cases diagnosed clinically as pre-Descemet's dystrophy, one may consider examining the patient's serum for the possibility of dysproteinemia.

The collagen fibrils appeared to be both mechanically displaced and replaced by the accumulating material in the posterior third. Morphologically, the intracellular and extracellular material were similar. Ultrastructurally, the immunoglobulins were located within dilated cisternae of the rough endoplasmic reticulum in the keratocytes, rather than phagocytosis.

CORNEA FARINATA

Cornea farinata is sometimes classified with pre-Descemet's dystrophies, but is more often considered an age-related degeneration. It consists of tiny, punctate, gray opacities in the deep stroma immediately anterior to Descemet's membrane. Sometimes larger and more polymorphous types of comma-shaped, circular, linear, filiform, and dotlike opacities are located in the pre-Descemet's area. The opacities may be distributed axially or annularly. Visual acuity is usually not affected.

REFERENCES

1. Chang SW, Tuli S, Azar DT. Corneal dystrophies. In: Traboulsi ET, ed. *Genetic diseases of the eye.* Oxford: Oxford University Press, 1997:217–266.
2. Klintworth GK. Advances in the molecular genetics of corneal dystrophies. *Am J Ophthalmol* 1999;128:747–754.
3. Akiya S, Brown S. Granular dystrophy of the cornea. *Arch Ophthalmol* 1970;84:179.
4. Andersen IL. Granular corneal dystrophy or Groenouw's diseases type I. A challenge to Norwegian biochemists, geneticists and ophthalmologists (Norwegian). *Tidsski Nor Laegeforen* 1995;115:355–356.
5. Moller HU, Ridgway AEA. Granular corneal dystrophy Groenouw type I: a report of a probable homozygous patient. *Acta Ophthalmol (Copenh)* 1990;68:97–101.
6. Schutz S. Hereditary corneal dystrophy. *Arch Ophthalmol* 1943;29:523.
7. Waardenburg PJ, Jonkers GH. A specific type of dominant progressive dystrophy of the cornea, developing after birth. *Acta Ophthalmol (Copenh)* 1961;39:919.
8. Wittebol-Post D, Van Schooneveld MJ, Pel V. The corneal dystrophy of Waardenburg and Jonkers. *Ophthalmic Paediatr Genet* 1989;10:249–255.
9. Haddad R, Front RL, Fine BS. Unusual superficial variant of granular dystrophy of the cornea. *Am J Ophthalmol* 1977; 83:213.
10. Rodrigues MM, Gaster RN, Pratt MV. Unusual superficial confluent form of granular corneal dystrophy. *Ophthalmology* 1983;90:1507.
11. Forsius H, Eriksson AW, Karna J, et al. Granular corneal dystrophy with late manifestation. *Acta Ophthalmol (Copenh)* 1983;61:514–528.
12. Garner A. Histochemistry of corneal granular dystrophy. *Br J Ophthalmol* 1969;53:799.
13. Iwamoto T, Stuart JC, Srinivasan BD, et al. Ultrastructural variation in granular dystrophy of the cornea. *Graefes Arch Klin Exp Ophthalmol* 1975;194:1–9.
14. Matsui M, Ito K, Akiua S. Histochemical and electron microscopic examinations on so-called gelatinous drop-like dystrophy of the cornea. *Folia Ophthalmol Jpn* 1972;23:466.
15. Kannai A, Kaufman HE. Electron microscopic studies of primary band-shaped keratopathy and gelatinous drop-like corneal dystrophy in two brothers. *Ann Ophthalmol* 1982; 1:535.
16. Wittebol-Post D, van der Want JJ, van Bijsterveld OP. Granular dystrophy of the cornea (Groenouw type I): Is the keratocyte the primary source after all? *Ophthalmologica* 1987;195:169.
17. Lyons CJ, McCartney AC, Kirkness CM, et al. Granular corneal dystrophy. Visual results and pattern of recurrence after lamellar or penetrating keratoplasty. *Ophthalmology* 1994;101: 1812–1817.
18. Somson E. Granular dystrophy of the cornea: an electron microscopic study. *Am J Ophthalmol* 1965;59:1001.
19. Moller HU, Bojsen-Moller M, Schroder HD, et al. Immunoglobulins in granular corneal dystrophy Groenouw type I. *Acta Ophthalmol (Copenh)* 1993;71:548–551.
20. Eiberg H, Moler HU, Berendt I, et al. Assignment of granular corneal dystrophy Groenouw type I (CDGG1) to chromosome 5q. *Eur J Hum Genet* 1994;2:132–138.
21. Stone EM, Mathers WD, Rosenwasser GO, et al. Three autosomal dominant corneal dystrophies map to chromosome 5q. *Nature Genet* 1994;6:47–51.
22. Okada M, Yamamoto S, Tsujikawa M, et al. Two distinct kerato-epithelin mutations in Reis-Bucklers corneal dystrophy. *Am J Ophthalmol* 1998;126:535–542.
23. Folberg R, Alfonso E, Croxatto JO, et al. Clinically atypical granular corneal dystrophy with pathologic features of lattice-like amyloid deposits. A study of three families. *Ophthalmology* 1988;95:46–51.
24. Munier FL, Korvatska E, Djemai A, et al. Kerato-epithelin mutations in four 5q31-linked corneal dystrophies. *Nature Genet* 1997;15:247–251.
25. Moller HU, Ehlers N. Early treatment of granular dystrophy (Groenouw type I). *Acta Ophthalmol (Copenh)* 1985;63:597.
26. Campos M, Nielsen S, Szerenyi K, et al. Clinical follow-up of phototherapeutic keratectomy for treatment of corneal opacities. *Am J Ophthalmol* 1993;115:433–440.
27. Sakuma A, Yokoyama T, Katou K, et al. Lamellar keratoplasty combined with keratoepithelioplasty in four cases for recurrent gelatinous drop-like corneal dystrophy (in Japanese). *Rinsho Ganka* 1991;45:527–530.
28. Tripathi R, Garner A. Corneal granular dystrophy: a light and electron microscope study of its recurrence in a graft. *Br J Ophthalmol* 1970;54:361.
29. Diaper CJ. Severe granular dystrophy: a pedigree with presumed homozygotes. *Eye* 1994;8:448–452.

30. Holland EJ, Daya SM, Stone EM, et al. Avellino corneal dystrophy. Clinical manifestations and natural history. *Ophthalmology* 1992;99:1564–1568.

31. Stock EL, Feder RS, O'Grady RB, et al. Lattice corneal dystrophy type IIIA: clinical and histopathologic correlations. *Arch Ophthalmol* 1991;109:354–358.

32. Rosenwasser GOD, Sucheski BM, Rosa N, et al. Phenotypic variation in combined granular-lattice (Avellino) corneal dystrophy. *Arch Ophthalmol* 1993;111:1546–1552.

33. Folberg R, Stone EM, Sheffield VC, et al. The relationship between granular, lattice type 1, and Avellino corneal dystrophies. A histopathologic study. *Arch Ophthalmol* 1994;112:1080–1085.

34. Sassani JW, Smith SG, Rabinowitz YS. Keratoconus and bilateral lattice-granular corneal dystrophies. *Cornea* 1992;11:343–350.

35. Yanoff M, Fine BS, Colosi NJ, et al. Lattice corneal dystrophy. Report of an unusual case. *Arch Ophthalmol* 1977;95:651–655.

36. Cennamo G, Rosa N, Rosenwasser GOD, et al. Phototherapeutic keratectomy in the treatment of Avellino dystrophy. *Ophthalmologica* 1994;208:198–200.

37. Dark AJ, Thompson DS. Lattice dystrophy of the cornea. A clinical and microscopic study. *Br J Ophthalmol* 1960;44:257.

38. Ramsey RM. Familial corneal dystrophy lattice type. Trans *Am Ophthalmol Soc* 1957;60:701.

39. Mehta RF. Unilateral lattice dystrophy of the cornea. *Br J Ophthalmol* 1980;64:53.

40. Raab MF, Blodi F, Boniuk M. Unilateral lattice dystrophy of the cornea. *Trans Am Acad Ophthalmol Otolaryngol* 1974;78:440.

41. Reschmi CS, English FP. Unilateral lattice dystrophy of the cornea. *Med J Aust* 1971;1:966.

42. Tsunoda I, Awano H, Kayama H, et al. Idiopathic AA amyloidosis manifested in autonomic neuropathy, vestibulocochleopathy and lattice corneal dystrophy. *J Neurol Neurosurg Psychiatry* 1994;57:635–637.

43. Petroutsos G, Kitsos G, Asproudis I, et al. Association of progressive external ophthalmoplegia and lattice corneal dystropy. *J Fr Ophthalmol* 1992;15:592–595.

44. Mannis MJ, Krachmer JH, Rodrigues MM, et al. Polymorphic amyloid degeneration of the cornea. A clinical and histopathologic study. *Arch Ophthalmol* 1981;99:1217–1223.

45. Bowen RA, Hassard DT, Wong VG, et al. Lattice dystrophy of the cornea as a variety of amyloidosis. *Am J Ophthalmol* 1970;70:822–825.

46. Francois J, Feh Jr J. Light microscopical and polarization optical study of lattice dystrophy of the cornea. *Ophthalmologica* 1972;164:1.

47. Hogan M, Alvarado S. Ultrastructure of lattice dystrophy of the cornea: a case report. *Am J Ophthalmol* 1967;64:656.

48. Julien J. Familial amyloid neuropathies (review) (French). Rev Neurol (Paris) 1993;149:517–523.

49. Maury CP, Teppo AM, Karinemi AL, et al. Amyloid fibril protein in familial amyloidosis with cranial neuropathy and corneal lattice dystrophy (FAP type IV) is related to transthyretin. *Am J Clin Pathol* 1988;89:359–364.

50. Fogle JA, Kenyon KR, Stark WJ, et al. Defective epithelial adhesion in anterior corneal dystrophies. *Am J Ophthalmol* 1975;79:925–940.

51. Zechner EM, Croxatto JO, Malbran ES. Superficial involvement in lattice corneal dystrophy. *Ophthalmologica* 1986;193:193–199.

52. Francois J, Hanssens M, Teuchy H. Ultrastructural changes in lattice dystrophy of the cornea. *Ophthalmic Res* 1975;7.

53. McTigue JW, Fine BS. The stromal lesion in lattice dystrophy of the cornea. A light and electron microscopic study. *Invest Ophthalmology* 1964;3:355.

54. Klintworth GK. Lattice corneal dystrophy: an inherited variety of amyloidosis restricted to the cornea. *Am J Pathol* 1967;50:371.

55. Meretoja J. Comparative histopathological and clinical findings in eyes with lattice corneal dystrophy of two different types. *Ophthalmologica* 1972;165:15–37.

56. Meretoja J. Genetic aspects of familial amyloidosis with corneal lattice dystrophy and cranial neuropathy. *Clin Genet* 1973;4:173–185.

57. Asaoka T, Amano S, Sunada Y, et al. Lattice corneal dystrophy type II with familial amyloid polyneuropathy type IV. *Jpn J Ophthalmol* 1993;37:426–431.

58. Kivela T, Tarkkanen A, McLean I, et al. Immunohistochemical analysis of lattice corneal dystrophies types I and II. *Br J Ophthalmol* 1993;77:799–804.

59. Rodrigues MM, Rajgopalan S, Jones K, et al. Gelsolin immunoreactivity in corneal amyloid, wound healing and macular and granular dystrophies. *Am J Ophthalmol* 1993;115:644–652.

60. de la Chapelle A, Tolvanen R, Boysen G, et al. Gelsolin-derived familial amyloidosis caused by asparagine or tyrosine substitution for aspartic acid at residue 187. *Nature Genet* 1992;2:157–160.

61. Haltia M, Levy E, Meretoja J, et al. Gelsolin gene mutation—at codon 187—in familial amyloidosis. (Finnish): DNA-diagnostic assay. *Am J Med Genet* 1992;42:357–359.

62. Hida T, Tsubota K, Kigasawa K, et al. Clinical features of a newly recognized type of lattice corneal dystrophy. *Am J Ophthalmol* 1987;104:241–248.

63. Hida T, Proia AD, Kigasawa K, et al. Histopathologic and immunochemical features of lattice corneal dystrophy type III. *Am J Ophthalmol* 1987;104:249–254.

64. Yamamoto S, Okada M, Tsujikawa M, et al. A kerato-epithelin (betaig-h3) mutation in lattice corneal dystrophy type IIIA. *Am J Hum Genet* 1998;62:719–722.

65. Akiya S, Nagaya K, Fukui A, et al. Inherited corneal amyloidosis predominantly manifested in one eye. *Ophthalmologica* 1991;203:204–207.

66. Seitz B, Weidle E, Naumann GO. Unilateral type III (Hida) lattice stromal corneal dystrophy. *Klin Monatsbl Augenheilkd* 1993;203:279–285.

67. Mondino BJ, Raj CV, Skinner M, et al. Protein AA and lattice corneal dystrophy. *Am J Ophthalmol* 1980;89:377–380.

68. Wheeler GE, Eiferman RA. Immunohistochemical identifications of the AA protein in lattice dystrophy. *Exp Eye Res* 1983;36:181.

69. Francois J, Hanssens M, Stockmans L. Pellucid marginal degeneration of the cornea. *Ophthalmologica* 1968;155:337–356.

70. Francois J, Neetans A. Nouvelle dystrophie heredofamiliare du parenchyma cornee (French). *Bull Soc Belge Ophthalmol* 1956;114:641.

71. Klintworth GK. Current concepts on the ultrastructural pathogenesis of macular and lattice corneal dystrophies. *Birth Defects Orig Art Ser* 1971;7:27.

72. Pouliquen Y, Dhermy P, Taillebourg O. Electron microscopic study of a Haab-Dimmer lattice dystrophy. *Arch Ophthalmol Rev Gen Ophthalmol* 1973;33:485–499.

73. Pe'er J, Fine BS, Dixon A, et al. Corneal elastosis within lattice dystrophy lesions. *Br J Ophthalmol* 1988;72:183–188.

74. Rodrigues MM, Robey PG. C-reactive protein in human lattice corneal dystrophy. *Curr Eye Res* 1983;2:721.

75. Yang CJ, SundarRaj N, Thonar EJ-MA, et al. Immunohistochemical evidence of heterogeneity in macular corneal dystrophy. *Am J Ophthalmol* 1988;106:65–71.

76. Edward DP, Yue BY, Sugar J, et al. Heterogeneity in macular corneal dystrophy. *Arch Ophthalmol* 1988;106:1579–1583.

77. Warren JF, Aldave AJ, Srinivasan M, et al. Novel mutations in the CHST6 gene associated with macular corneal dystrophy in southern India. *Arch Ophthalmol* 2003;121:1608–1612.

78. Cursiefen C, Hofmann-Rummelt C, Schlotzer-Schrehardt U, et al. Immunohistochemical classification of primary and recurrent macular corneal dystrophy in Germany: subclassification of immunophenotype I A using a novel keratan sulfate antibody. *Exp Eye Res* 2001;73:593–600.

79. Klintworth GK, Oshima E, al-Rajhi A, et al. Macular corneal dystrophy in Saudi Arabia: a study of 56 cases and recognition of a new immunophenotype. *Am J Ophthalmol* 1997;124:9–18.

80. Donnenfeld ED, Cohen EJ, Ingraham HJ, et al. Corneal thinning in macular corneal dystrophy. *Am J Ophthalmol* 1986;101:112–113.

81. Ehlen N, Bramsen T. Central thickness in corneal disorders. *Acta Ophthalmol (Copenh)* 1978;56:412.

82. Bruner WE, Dejak TR, Grossniklaus HE, et al. Corneal alpha-galactosidase deficiency in macular corneal dystrophy. *Ophthalmic Paediatr Genet* 1985;5:179–183.

83. Hassell JR, Newsome DA, Krachmer JH, et al. Macular corneal dystrophy: failure to synthesize a mature keratin sulfate proteoglycan. *Proc Natl Acad Sci USA* 1980;77:3705–3709.

84. Klintworth GK, Meyer R, Dennis R, et al. Macular corneal dystrophy. Lack of keratan sulfate in serum and cornea. *Ophthalmic Paediatr Genet* 1986;7:139–143.

85. Nakazawa K, Hassell JR, Hascall VC, et al. Defective processing of keratin sulfate in macular corneal dystrophy. *J Biol Chem* 1984;259:13751–13757.

86. Edward DP, Thonar EJ, Srinivasan M, et al. Macular dystrophy of the cornea. A systemic disorder of keratan sulfate metabolism. *Ophthalmology* 1990;97:1194–1200.

87. Santo RM, Yamaguchi T, Kanai A, et al. Clinical and histopathologic features of corneal dystrophies in Japan. *Ophthalmology* 1995;102:557–567.

88. Jones ST, Zimmerman LE. Histopathologic differentiation of granular, macular, and lattice dystrophies of the cornea. *Am J Ophthalmol* 1961;51:394.

89. Garner A. Histochemistry of corneal macular dystrophy. *Invest Ophthalmol* 1969;9:473.

90. Snip RC, Kenyon DR, Green RD. Macular corneal dystrophy: ultrastructural pathology of the corneal endothelium and Descemet's membrane. *Invest Ophthalmol* 1973;12:88.

91. Teng CC. Macular dystrophy of the cornea: a histochemical and electron microscopic study. *Am J Ophthalmol* 1966;62:436.

92. Weber FL, Babel J. Gelatinous drop-like dystrophy. *Arch Ophthalmol* 1980;98:144.

93. Quantock AJ, Meek KM, Ridgway AEA, et al. Macular corneal dystrophy: reduction in both corneal thickness ana collagen interfibrillar spacing. *Curr Eye Res* 1990;9:393–398.

94. Klintworth GK, Vogel FS. Macular corneal dystrophy: an inherited acid mucopolysaccharide storage disease of corneal fibroblasts. *Am J Pathol* 1964;45:565.

95. Livni N, Abraham FA, Zauberman H. Groenouw's macular dystrophy: histochemistry and ultrastructure of the cornea. *Doc Ophthalmol* 1974;37:327.

96. Morgan G. Macular dystrophy of the cornea. *Br J Ophthalmol* 1966;50:57.

97. Quantock AJ, Meek KM, Thonar EJMA, et al. Synchrotron X-ray diffraction in atypical macular dystrophy. *Eye* 1993;7:779–784.

98. Klintworth GK, Smith CF. Macular corneal dystrophy. Studies of sulfated glycosaminoglycans in corneal explant and confluent stromal cell cultures. *Am J Pathol* 1977;89:167–182.

99. Jonasson F, Oshima E, Thonar EJMA, et al. Macular corneal dystrophy in Iceland: a clinical, genealogic, and immunohistochemical study of 28 patients. *Ophthalmology* 1996;103:1111–1117.

100. Vance JM, Jonasson F, Lennon F, et al. Linkage of a gene for macular corneal dystrophy to chromosome 16. *Am J Hum Genet* 1996;58:757–762.

101. Akama TO, Nishida K, Nakayama J, et al. Macular corneal dystrophy type I and type II are caused by distinct mutations in a new sulphotransferase gene. *Nature Genet* 2000;26:237–241.

102. Hasegawa N, Torii T, Kato T, et al. Decreased GlcNAc 6-O-sulfotransferase activity in the cornea with macular corneal dystrophy. *Invest Ophthalmol Vis Sci* 2000;41:3670–3677.

103. Klintworth GK, Reed J, Stainer GA, et al. Recurrence of macular corneal dystrophy within grafts. *Am J Ophthalmol* 1983;95:60–72.

104. Robin AL, Green WR, Lapsa TP, et al. Recurrence of macular corneal dystrophy after lamellar keratoplasty. *Am J Ophthalmol* 1977;84:457–461.

105. Bron AJ, Williams HP, Carruthers ME. Hereditary crystalline stromal dystrophy of Schnyder: clinical features of a family with hyperlipoproteinemia. *Br J Ophthalmol* 1973;56:383.

106. Delleman JW, Winkelman JE. Degeneratio corneae cristallinea hereditaria: a clinical, genetical, and histological study. *Ophthalmologica* 1968;155:409–426.

107. Grop K. Clinical and histologic findings in crystalline corneal dystrophy. *Acta Ophthalmol (Copenh)* 1973;51:52.

108. Ehlers N, Mathiessen M. Hereditary crystalline dystrophy of Schnyder. *Acta Ophthalmol (Copenh)* 1967;51:1.

109. Kaseras A, Price A. Central crystalline corneal dystrophy. *Br J Ophthalmol* 1970;54:659.

110. Luxenburg M. Hereditary crystalline dystrophy of the cornea. *Am J Ophthalmol* 1967;63:507.

111. Van Went JM, Wilbaut F. Een Zeldzane erfelijke hoornvliesaandoening (German). *Ned Tijdschr Geenskd* 1924;68:2996.

112. McCarthy M, Innis S, Dubord PJ, et al. Panstromal Schnyder corneal dystrophy. *Ophthalmology* 1994;101:895–901.

113. Waring GO III, Rodrigues MM, Laibson PR. Corneal dystrophies. I. Dystrophies of the epithelium, Bowman's layer and stroma. *Surv Ophthalmol* 1978;23:71–122.

114. Barchiesi BJ, Eckel RH, Ellis PP. The cornea and disorder of lipid metabolism. *Surv Ophthalmol* 1991;36:1–22.

115. Lisch W, Weidle EG, Lisch C, et al. Schnyder's dystrophy. Progression and metabolism. *Ophthalmic Paediatr Genet* 1986;7:45–56.

116. Brownstein S, Jackson WB, Onerheim RM. Schnyder's crystalline corneal dystrophy in association with hyperlipoproteinemia: histopathological and ultrastructural findings. *Can J Ophthalmol* 1991;26:273–279.

117. Garner A, Tripathi RC. Hereditary crystalline stromal dystrophy of Schnyder. II. Histopathology and ultrastructure. *Br J Ophthalmol* 1972;56:400–408.

118. Williams HP, Bron AJ, Tripathi RC, et al. Hereditary crystalline corneal dystrophy with an associated blood lipid disorder. *Trans Ophthalmol Soc UK* 1971;91:31–41.

119. Ghosh M, McCulloch C. Crystalline dystrophy of the cornea: a light and electron microscopic study. *Can J Ophthalmol* 1977;12:321.

120. Rodrigues MM, Kruth HS, Krachmer JH, et al. Unesterified cholesterol in Schnyder's corneal crystalline dystrophy. *Am J Ophthalmol* 1987;104:157–163.

121. Rodrigues MM, Kruth HS, Krachmer JH, et al. Cholesterol localization in ultrathin frozen sections in Schnyder's corneal crystalline dystrophy. *Am J Ophthalmol* 1990;110:513–517.

122. Weller RO, Rodger FC. Crystalline stromal dystrophy: histochemistry and ultrastructure of the cornea. *Br J Ophthalmol* 1986;64:46–52.

123. Fry WE, Pickett WE. Crystalline dystrophy of the cornea. *Trans Am Ophthalmol Soc* 1950;48:220.

124. Bernauer W, Daicker B. Bietti's corneal-retinal dystrophy. A 16-year progression. *Retina* 1992;12:18–20.

125. Harrison RJ, Acheson RR, Dean-Hart JC. Bietti's tapetoretinal degeneration with marginal corneal dystrophy (crystalline retinopathy): case report. *Br J Ophthalmol* 1987;71:220–223.

126. Wilson DJ, Weleber RG, Klein ML, et al. Bietti's crystalline dystrophy. A clinicopathologic correlative study. *Arch Ophthalmol* 1989;107:213–221.

127. Bagolini B, Ioli-Spada G. Bietti's tapetoretinal degeneration with marginal corneal dystrophy. *Am J Ophthalmol* 1968; 65:53–60.

128. Welch RB. Bietti's tapetoretinal degeneration with marginal corneal dystrophy crystalline retinopathy. *Trans Am Ophthalmol Soc* 1977;75:164–179.

129. Mauldin WM, O'Connor PS. Crystalline retinopathy (Bietti's tapetoretinal degeneration without marginal corneal dystrophy). *Am J Ophthalmol* 1981;92:640–646.

130. Richards BW, Brodstein DE, Nussbaum JJ, et al. Autosomal dominant crystalline dystrophy. *Ophthalmology* 1991;98:658–665.

131. Weber U, Owzarek J, Kluxen G, et al. Klinischer Verlauf bei Biettischer kristalliner tapetoretinaler Degeneration. *Klin Monatsbl Augenheilkd* 1983:259–261.

132. Hu DN. Ophthalmic genetics in China. *Ophthalmol Paediat Genet* 1983;2:39–45.

133. Sanderson PO, Kuwabara T, Stark WJ, et al. Cystinosis: a clinical, histopathologic, and ultrastructural study. *Arch Ophthalmol* 1974;91:270–277.

134. Freddo RF, Polack FM, Leibowitz HM. Ultrastructural changes in the posterior layers of the cornea in Schnyder's corneal crystalline dystrophy. *Cornea* 1989;8:170–177.

135. Burns RP, Connor W, Gipson I. Cholesterol turnover in hereditary crystalline corneal dystrophy of Schnyder. *Trans Am Ophthalmol Soc* 1978;76:184–196.

136. Mirshahi M, Mirshahi SS, Soria C, et al. Secretion of plasminogen activators and their inhibitors in corneal fibroblasts. Modification of this secretion in Schnyder's lens corneal dystrophy. *CR Acad Sci III* 1990;311:253–260.

137. Klein ML, Green WR. In: *Spencer ophthalmic pathology II.* Philadelphia: WB Saunders, 1984:1168.

138. Shearman AM, Hudson TJ, Andresen JM, et al. The gene for Schnyder's crystalline corneal dystrophy maps to human chromosome 1p34.1-p36. *Hum Mol Genet* 1996;5:1667–1672.

139. Jiao X, Munier FL, Iwata F, et al. Genetic linkage of Bietti crystallin corneoretinal dystrophy to chromosome 4q35. *Am J Hum Genet* 2000;67:1309–1313.

140. Sysi R. Xanthoma corneae as hereditary dystrophy. *Br J Ophthalmol* 1950;34:369–374.

141. Akova YA, Unla N, Duman S. Fleck dystrophy of the cornea: a report of cases from three generations of a family. *Eur J Ophthalmol* 1994;4:123–125.

142. Aracena T. Hereditary fleck dystrophy of the cornea: report of a family. *J Pediatr Ophthalmol* 1975;12:223.

143. Birndoft LA, Ginsberg SP. Hereditary fleck dystrophy associated with decreased corneal sensitivity. *Am J Ophthalmol* 1972;73:670.

144. Collier M. Dystrophie naugeuse centrale et dystrophie ponctiforme predescemetique (French). *Bull Soc Ophthalmol Fr* 1964; 64:1034.

145. Goldberg MF, Krimmer B, Sugar J, et al. Variable expression in flecked (speckled) dystrophy of the cornea. *Ann Ophthalmol* 1977;9:889–896.

146. Patten JT, Hyndiuk RA, Donaldson DD, et al. Fleck (Mouchetee) dystrophy of the cornea. *Ann Ophthalmol* 1976; 8:25–32.

147. Purcell JJ Jr, Krachmer JH, Weingeist TA. Fleck corneal dystrophy. *Arch Ophthalmol* 1977;95:440.

148. Streeten BW, Falls HF. Hereditary fleck dystrophy of the cornea. *Am J Ophthalmol* 1961;51:275.

149. Franceschetti A. Hereditdre Rezidivierende Erosion der Homhaut. *Z Agenheilkd* 1928;66:309.

150. Gellespie F, Covelli B. Fleck (Mouchetee) dystrophy of the cornea: report of a family. *South Med J* 1963;56:1265.

151. Kiskaddon BM, et al. Fleck dystrophy of the cornea: case report. *Ann Ophthalmol* 1980;12:700.

152. Nicholson DH, Green WR, Cross HE. A clinical and histopathological study of Francois-Neetens speckled corneal dystrophy. *Am J Ophthalmol* 1977;83:554.

153. Stankovic I, Stojanovic D. L'heredodystrohie Mouchetee du parenchyma cornee (French). *Ann Oculist (Paris)* 1964;197:52.

154. Bramsen T, Ehlers N, Baggesen KH. Central cloudy corneal dystrophy of Francois. *Acta Ophthalmol (Copenh)* 1976;54:221.

155. Strachan IM. Central cloudy corneal dystrophy of Francois: five cases in the same family. *Br J Ophthalmol* 1969;53:192.

156. Collier MT. Dystrophie mouchete du parenchyma corneen avec dystrophie nuageuse centrale. *Bull Soc Ophtalmol Fr* 1964;4:608.

157. Collier MT. Elastorrhexie systee et dystrophies corneenees chez deux soerus (French). *Bull Soc Ophthalmol Fr* 1965;65:301.

158. Pillat A. Zur frage der familiuaren Hornhautentartung: Unber eine einzigartige tiefe scholige und periphere gitterformige familire Hornhautdystrophie (German). *Klink Monatsbl Augenheilkd* 1939;104:571.

159. Strachan IM. Pre-Descemetic corneal dystrophy. *Br J Ophthalmol* 1968;52:716.

160. Thomsitt J, Bron AJ. Polymorphic stromal dystrophy. *Br J Ophthalmol* 1975;59:125.

161. Carpel EF, Sigelman RJ, Doughman DJ. Posterior amorphous corneal dystrophy. *Am J Ophthalmol* 1977;83:629.

162. Dunn SP, Krachmer JH, Ching SS. New findings in posterior amorphous corneal dystrophy. *Arch Ophthalmol* 1984;102:236–239.

163. Johnson AT, Folberg R, Vrabec MP, et al. The pathology of posterior amorphous corneal dystrophy. *Ophthalmology* 1990; 97:104–109.

164. Roth SI, Millelman D, Stock EL. Posterior amorphous corneal dystrophy. An ultrastructural study of a variant with histopathological features of an endothelial dystrophy. *Cornea* 1992;11:165–172.

165. Akiya S, Ito I, Matsui M. Gelatinous drop-like dystrophy of the cornea. *Jpn J Clin Ophthalmol* 1972;56:815.

166. Gartry DS, Falcon MG, Cox RW. Primary gelatinous drop-like keratopathy. *Br J Ophthalmol* 1989;73:661.

167. Nagataki S, Tanishima T, Sakomoto T. A case of primary gelatinous drop-like corneal dystrophy. *Jpn J Ophthalmol* 1972; 16:107.

168. Nakaizmi K. A rare case of corneal dystrophy. *Nippon Ganka Gakkai Zasshi* 1914;18:949.

169. Ramsey MS, Fine BS. Localized corneal amyloidosis. *Am J Ophthalmol* 1972;75:560.

170. Kirk HQ, Rabb M, Hattenhauer J, et al. Primary familial amyloidosis of the cornea. *Trans Am Acad Ophthalmol Otolaryngol* 1973;77:OP411–417.

171. Stock EI, Kielar RA. Primary familial amyloidosis of the cornea. *Am J Ophthalmol* 1976;82:266.

172. Lewkojewa EF. Uber einen Fall primarer Degenerationamyloidose der Kornea (German). *Klin Monatsbl Augenheilkd* 1930;85:117.

173. Mondino BJ, Rabb MF, Sugar J, et al. Primary familial amyloidosis of the cornea. *Am J Ophthalmol* 1981;92:732–736.

174. Tsujikawa M, Kurahashi H, Tanaka T, et al. Identification of the gene responsible for gelatinous drop-like corneal dystrophy. *Nature Genet* 1999;21:420–423.

175. Fornaro M, Dell'Arciprete R, Stella M, et al. Cloning of the gene encoding Trop-2, a cell-surface glycoprotein expressed by human carcinomas. *Int J Cancer* 1995;62.

176. Ren Z, Lin PY, Klintworth GK, et al. Allelic and locus heterogeneity in autosomal recessive gelatinous drop-like corneal dystrophy. *Hum Genet* 2002;110:568–577.

177. Collier M. Caracre heredo-familial de la dystrophie ponctiforme predescemetique (French). *Bull Soc Ophthalmol Fr* 1964; 64:731.

178. Fernandez-Sasso D, Acosta JEP, Malbran E. Punctiform and polychromatic pre-Descemet's dominant corneal dystrophy. *Fr J Ophthalmol* 1979;64:336.

179. Grayson M, Wilbrandt H. Pre-Descemet dystrophy. *Am J Ophthalmol* 1967;64:276.

180. Franceschetti A, Schlaeppi V. Degenerescence en bandelettes et dystophie predescemetique de la cornee dans un cas d'ichyhyose congenitale (French). *Dermatologica* 1957;115:217.

181. Maeder G, Danis P. Surune nouvelle forme de dystrophie corneene (dystrophia filiformis profunda corneae) associe a un keratocone (French). *Ophthalmologica* 1947;114:246.

182. Yassa NH, Font RL, Fine BS, et al. Corneal immunoglobulin deposition in the posterior stroma: a case report including immunohistochemical and ultrastructural observations. *Arch Ophthalmol* 1987;105:99–103.

CORNEAL ENDOTHELIAL DYSTROPHIES

PATRICK C. YEH AND KATHRYN COLBY

The posterior surface of the cornea is lined by the corneal endothelium, a monolayer of closely interdigitated hexagonal cells arranged in a mosaic (Fig. 47-1). This pattern of endothelial cells minimizes individual cell perimeter, thus reducing surface tension energy (1–3). The endothelium maintains corneal deturgescence and, thereby, corneal clarity, passively by functioning as a barrier to the influx of aqueous into the stroma and actively by pumping excess fluid out of the stroma via Na/K-adenosine triphosphatase (ATPase) pumps (4).

Human corneal endothelial cells are arrested in G1-phase and typically do not proliferate *in vivo* (5–7), although they can be stimulated to divide in *ex vivo* conditions (8). Specular microscopy, developed approximately 30 years ago (9), is currently the most commonly used technique to estimate endothelial cell density. Endothelial cell density is highest at birth (6,000 cells/mm^2) (10). Cell density decreases in a nonlinear fashion during the first 2 years of life as a result of rapid growth in corneal size. Thereafter, the rate of cell loss is linear at about 0.5% to 10% per year (10,11). Average adult endothelial cell density is 2,400 cells/mm^2, with a range of 1,500 to 3,500 cells/mm^2 (12). Endothelial cell density is a gauge of endothelial functional reserve, although it does not always correlate with corneal thickness (13–15), suggesting that cell density is not the only determinant of endothelial cell function.

As endothelial cells die, from either normal attrition or injury, neighboring cells enlarge and migrate in an attempt to maintain the endothelial cell monolayer (16). Consequently, endothelial cells *in vivo* display not only a tendency toward decreasing density, but also increasing pleomorphism (variation in cell shape) and polymegethism (variation in cell size). Specular microscopy data suggest that endothelial cell density in the peripheral and paracentral cornea may be higher than central cell density (17). The peripheral endothelial cells may serve as a reservoir to repopulate the central cornea.

As endothelial cell density decreases, the risk of developing corneal edema increases (18). When the endothelial cell density decreases to a critical threshold, the cornea swells, and eventually decompensates into bullous keratopathy. Interestingly, the minimum endothelial cell density needed to maintain corneal deturgescence varies from patient to patient. Most corneas will become edematous with cell counts less than 500 cells/mm^2. However, some corneas remain clear with as few as 300 cells/mm^2 (15). Corneas with cell counts from 500 to 1,000 cells/mm^2 are typically not edematous, but are at high risk for decompensation following intraocular surgery (19). Similarly, corneas with abnormal endothelial cell morphology are more susceptible to surgical trauma (20).

Diverse factors influence endothelial cell density and morphology. Various types of surgery including radial keratotomy (21), penetrating keratoplasty (22,23), cataract extraction (24,25), and intraocular lens implantation (26) are known to affect the endothelium. Chemical agents such as benzalkonium chloride (27) and epinephrine (28) have been shown to cause endothelial changes. Both ultraviolet (29) and infrared radiation (30), as well as the neodymium: yttrium-aluminum-garnet (Nd:YAG) laser (31), can have adverse effects on the endothelium. Endothelial changes are the hallmark of primary endothelial disorders such as cornea guttae (32) and Fuchs' dystrophy (33). Similar changes can be secondary to diabetes (34), glaucoma (35), inflammation (36), or contact lens wear (37,38).

The corneal endothelial dystrophies encompass three major entities: (a) Fuchs' endothelial dystrophy (FED), (b) congenital hereditary endothelial dystrophy (CHED), and (c) posterior polymorphous dystrophy (PPMD). These primary diseases of the corneal endothelium are not associated with ocular inflammation or systemic diseases. These diseases have a heritable component. These dystrophies share three characteristic features: thickening of Descemet's membrane, disruption of normal endothelial mosaic pattern, and dysfunction of endothelial pumps (39). The diseased endothelial cells produce fibrillar collagenous tissue that is deposited between the original Descemet's membrane and the endothelial layer. This ultrastructural change is associated with a decrease in pump function by a mechanism that is not yet understood. There may be concomitant breakdown of the passive endothelial barrier as well.

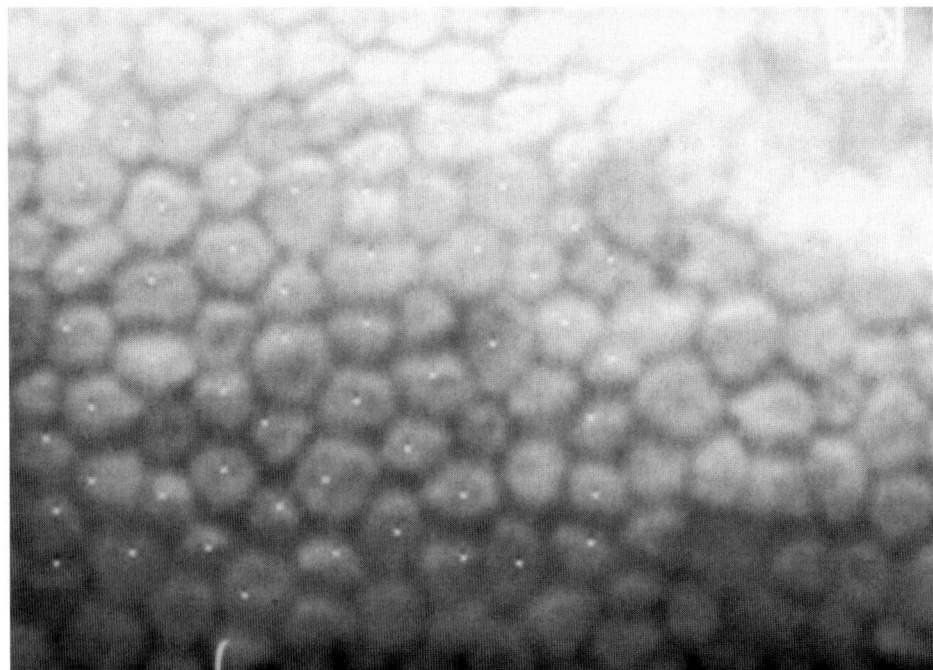

FIGURE 47-1. Specular microscopy of normal corneal endothelium. Cells are relatively uniform in size and shape.

The corneal endothelium is derived from the neural crest, and this fact has been exploited in another classification system of the corneal endothelial dystrophies (40,41). In this scheme, the endothelial dystrophies listed above result from abnormalities in neural crest cell final differentiation. Iridocorneal endothelial (ICE) syndrome, another primary disorder of the corneal endothelium, is proposed to result from abnormal crest cell proliferation. ICE syndrome is not, strictly speaking, a dystrophy, as it is acquired and unilateral. However, ICE syndrome shares many overlapping clinical features with PPMD. Therefore, ICE syndrome is included in this chapter and considered with the classic corneal endothelial dystrophies as part of a more inclusive disease category: corneal endotheliopathies.

FUCHS' ENDOTHELIAL DYSTROPHY

Fuchs' endothelial dystrophy (FED) is a bilateral, slowly progressive, primary disorder of the corneal endothelium that causes corneal edema and eventually painful blindness (42). End-stage FED currently accounts for up to 29% of penetrating keratoplasties in the United States (43,44).

The disorder was first described in 1910 by the Viennese ophthalmologist, Ernst Fuchs (45), who reported 13 cases of bilateral central clouding in elderly patients, nine of whom were women. Although he initially referred to it as "dystrophia epithelialis corneae," Fuchs speculated that "an alteration of the posterior endothelial covering" may underlie the "increased passage of the aqueous humor into the cornea." With the newly introduced biomicroscope,

Koeppe (46) noted focal "dimples" in the endothelial layer in patients with corneal edema. The term *gutta* (Latin: noun; pl., *guttae*; meaning "droplet"; adjective *guttata*) was first coined by Vogt (47) to describe the endothelial changes as observed under the slit lamp. In 1920, Kraupa (48) first correctly deduced the progression from the endothelial changes to epithelial edema, although others soon followed suit (49–51). Thereafter, FED was referred to as "endothelial dystrophy of the cornea." Ultrastructural studies in the 1970s provided evidence that the pathologic changes of the epithelium and stroma in FED were the direct result of primary dysfunction of the corneal endothelium (52–54).

There is a hereditary component to FED. In our population, approximately 30% of patients have a known family history of the disease (55). An autosomal-dominant pattern of inheritance has been suggested for FED (56–59), although several characteristics of the disorder make determination of the exact inheritance pattern challenging. Specifically, FED is asymptomatic in its early stages and therefore may go undiagnosed. Clinically significant manifestations of the disease occur late in life when it may be difficult to obtain complete pedigrees due to death of older family members.

Most studies suggest that FED is more common in women, with as high as a 4:1 female-to-male ratio in some series (56–59). The penetrance and disease expression may vary from family to family. Women appear to be more severely affected, for unclear reasons. Epigenetic factors are likely to play a role in the expression of the disease, but these have not been well defined as of yet.

The female-to-male ratio of Fuchs' endothelial dystrophy patients undergoing penetrating keratoplasty is about 3 to 4:1 (60,61).

FED has been associated with other conditions. It may occur more frequently in patients with cardiovascular disease (62). It also has been associated with keratoconus (63,64), age-related macular degeneration (65), and short axial length with a narrow anterior chamber angle (66). The relationship between FED and open-angle glaucoma is controversial, as some studies report decreased aqueous outflow in patients with FED (67), whereas others have not (68).

Clinical Features

Fuchs' dystrophy is a slowly progressive disorder, typically progressing over several decades. Although clinically evident in the fourth to fifth decade of life, it usually does not cause visual disturbance until patients are in their 50s or 60s. The corneal changes are usually bilateral, but often asymmetric. The disease has four stages (42,55,69).

The first stage is asymptomatic. Slit-lamp examination discloses central corneal guttae, but vision and corneal thickness are normal. Guttae, irregularly scattered excrescences in the posterior cornea, are often associated with fine pigment dusting (Fig. 47-2). Descemet's membrane may appear opaque and thickened. At this stage, one cannot diagnose Fuchs' dystrophy, as the vast majority of individuals with corneal guttae will not progress to corneal edema (70).

The diagnosis of FED can be made once stroma edema occurs in the setting of corneal guttae, most typically in the fifth decade of life (Fig. 47-3). In this second stage, patients have painless decreased vision, especially upon awakening. Vision may improve as the day progresses as evaporation promotes corneal deturgescence. Glare and haloes may be noted. As the disease progresses, the entire stroma becomes edematous, giving the cornea a ground-glass

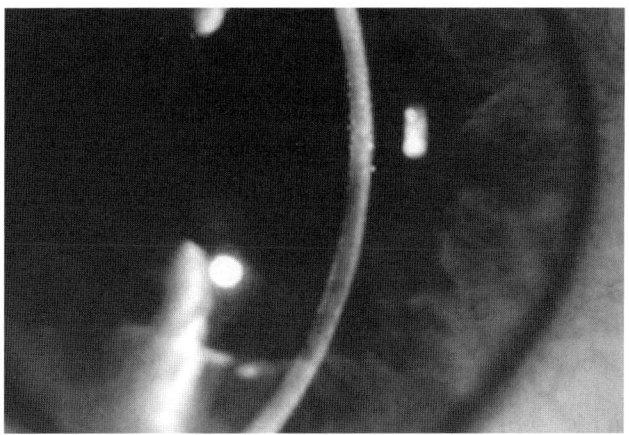

FIGURE 47-2. Central corneal guttae without stromal thickening.

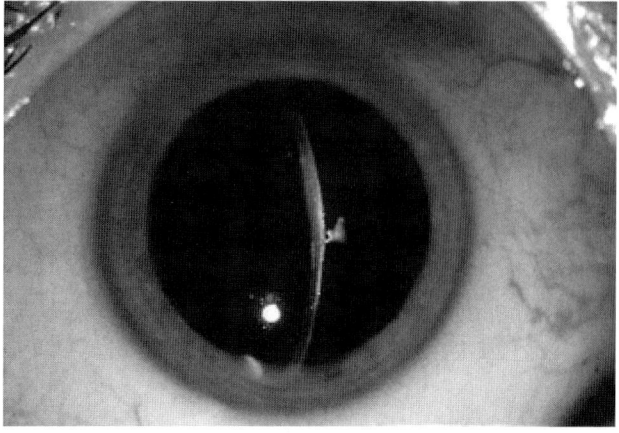

A

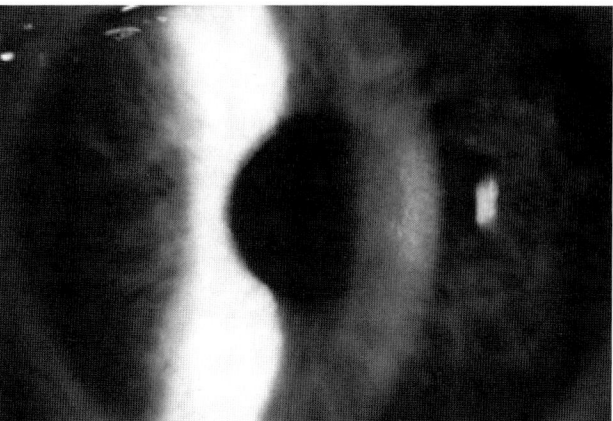

B

FIGURE 47-3. A: Stage 2 Fuchs' endothelial dystrophy. Corneal guttae with pigmentary dusting create a beaten metal appearance. Note the stromal edema in central cornea; peripheral cornea is of normal thickness. **B:** Late stage 2 Fuchs' endothelial dystrophy. The cornea has diffuse stromal edema with haze. No epithelial edema is noted.

appearance. Specular microscopy demonstrates reduced endothelial cell density with abnormal morphology (pleomorphism and polymegathism), although advancing edema may make it difficult to obtain adequate specular images (Fig. 47-4). Ultrasonic pachymetry, which measures corneal thickness, may also be used to determine if the endothelial dysfunction is advancing (increasing pachymetry readings) or remaining stable. Normal central corneal thickness is approximately 500 to 550 μm. When pachymetry readings exceed 700 μm, the likelihood of eventual corneal decompensation requiring penetrating keratoplasty is high.

Epithelial edema characterizes the third stage (Fig. 47-5). Initially, fine epithelial microcysts are noted. The epithelial surface is roughened, with an irregular surface texture. Vision invariably deteriorates during this stage and marked fluctuations in vision are common. Occasionally, erosive symptoms are the presenting complaint. Anterior basement membrane changes may be noted on exam. As the endothelial dysfunction worsens, epithelial cysts coalesce to form large intraepithelial and subepithelial bullae (Fig. 47-6). These bullae may rupture, resulting in

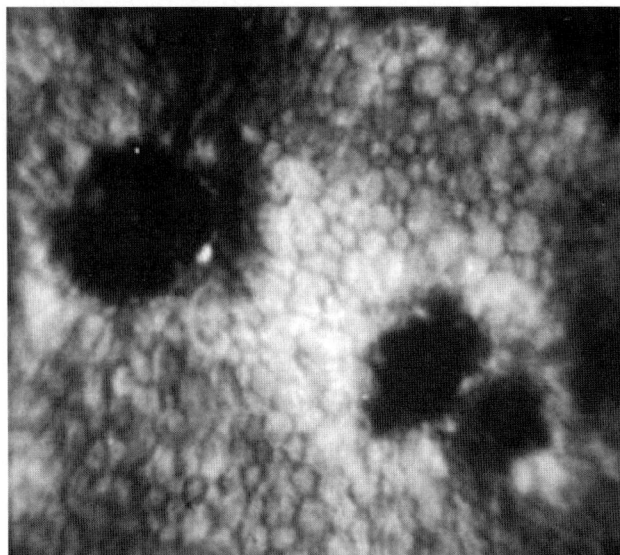

FIGURE 47-4. Specular microscopy of Fuchs' endothelial dystrophy. The endothelial mosaic is disrupted by irregular dark areas devoid of endothelial cells (guttae). The remaining endothelial cells show increases in size (polymegathism) and variations in shape (pleomorphism).

severe eye pain and rendering the patient susceptible to infection.

In the fourth stage, growth of avascular subepithelial connective tissue occurs, causing reduced vision from scarring. The cornea is opaque and compact (Fig. 47-7). Pain is decreased, but vision is severely reduced to the hand motions level. Corneal sensation is decreased or absent. With time, peripheral corneal vascularization may occur (42).

Histopathology

Normal Descemet's membrane has two discernible layers identified by electron microscopy: an anterior banded layer and a posterior nonbanded layer. The anterior layer is only produced during fetal development. It is approximately 3 μm thick and consists of 110 nm banded collagen. The posterior nonbanded layer is deposited continuously throughout life at an average rate of about 1 to 2 μm per decade. As a result, the thickness of the posterior layer increases on average from 3 μm at age 20 to 10 μm at age 80 (71).

In FED, the anterior banded layer is normal; however, the posterior nonbanded layer is attenuated or absent (52,72). In its place is an abnormal banded layer, which thickens Descemet's membrane to 20 μm or more (39,69). This abnormal layer consists of 110 nm collagen banded fibrils similar to those in the anterior banded layer, but which are arranged in a patchy and disorderly fashion. The abnormal posterior layer also contains spindle-shaped bundles of collagen, microfibrils, and amorphous ground material (72,73). Oxytalan fibers, not a normal constituent of the posterior cornea, are also present (74). Endothelial cells that have undergone fibroblastic transformation may

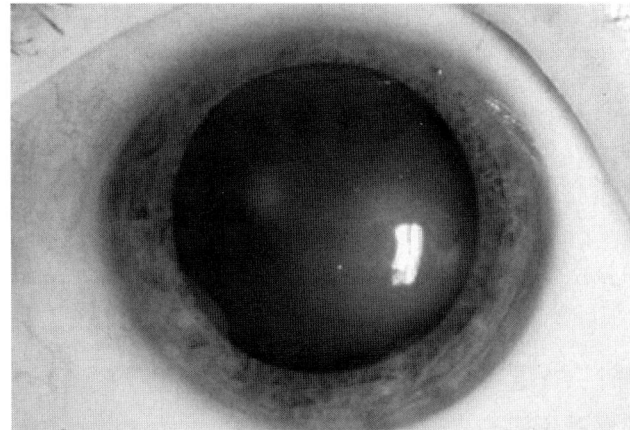

A

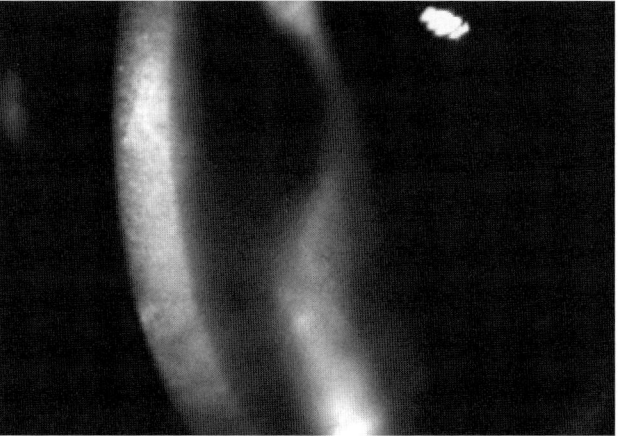

B

FIGURE 47-5. A: Stage 3 Fuchs' endothelial dystrophy localized to a small area of the cornea. When endothelial cell density reaches a critical level, epithelial edema occurs, manifested by the irregular corneal light reflex. **B:** Stage 3 Fuchs' endothelial dystrophy showing diffuse stromal and epithelial edema with microcystic changes.

be responsible for the deposition of abnormal material into the posterior layer of Descemet's membrane (75).

Microscopically, Descemet's membrane thickening can manifest four patterns: (a) discrete excrescences, or guttae,

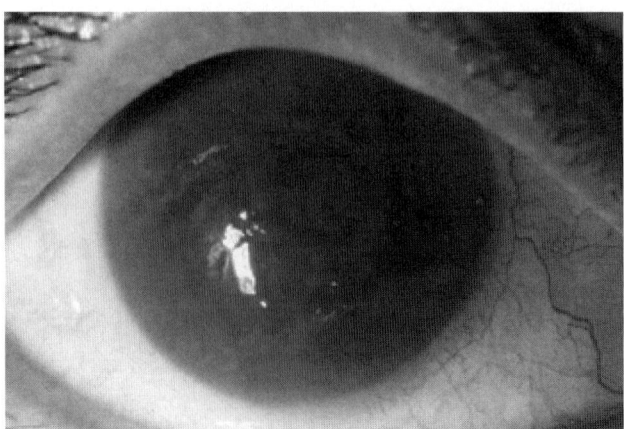

FIGURE 47-6. Bullous keratopathy. Diffuse stromal and epithelial edema are seen. The eye becomes painful with increased risk of infection when bullae rupture.

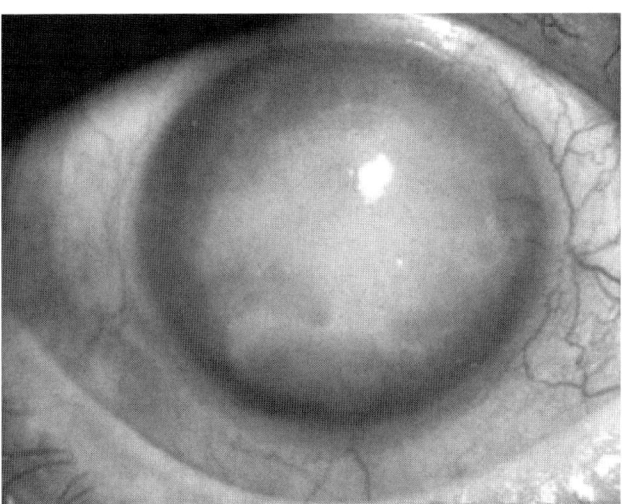

FIGURE 47-7. Stage 4 Fuchs' endothelial dystrophy. The vision is severely diminished by the dense corneal opacification with avascular subepithelial fibrosis. However, the eye is generally comfortable.

protruding into the anterior chamber; (b) multilamellar excrescences; (c) excrescences buried within the multilamellar collagen tissue; or (d) multilamellar collagen tissue without excrescences (76). The excrescences cause thinning and morphologic changes in the overlying endothelial cells. As a result, the endothelial cells appear attenuated, with widely spaced nuclei, especially over the apices of the excrescences. Areas of marked thickening of Descemet's membrane and endothelial cell attenuation have been shown histologically to correspond to areas of severe corneal edema seen clinically (73).

Ultrastructural studies of Fuchs' dystrophy corneas have demonstrated numerous changes. Although endothelial cell morphology is largely maintained, loss of mitochondrial cristae has been noted (55). Nonspecific degenerative changes such as vacuoles, swollen organelles, myelin figures, dilated endoplasmic reticulum, clumps of pigment, and increased cytoplasmic filaments also occur (52,73,76,77). Cell size is increased to approximately 1,000 μm^2, from a normal of 400 μm^2. As the disease progresses, the endothelial cells lose their characteristic hexagonal shape (32). Junctional complexes between the cells are loosened, with resulting discontinuity within the endothelial cell monolayer. Scanning electron microscopy has confirmed the irregular posterior corneal surface in FED, showing severely degenerated endothelial cells with patches of cell loss exposing a fibrous network of collagen tissue underneath (75). These changes are localized to areas of corneal edema. Endothelial cells in nonedematous areas and at the corneal periphery display a relatively normal ultrastructure (73).

Specular microscopy provides *in vivo* assessment of endothelial cell morphology and can be used to follow the progression of FED (Fig. 47-4). Early in the disorder, specular microscopy reveals reduced endothelial count with disruption of the endothelial mosaic by hyporeflective spots. These spots, corresponding to guttae, appear dark because the endothelial cells over the excrescences are displaced posteriorly out of the plane of focus (69). When the guttae become numerous, it is usually not possible to observe the endothelial tessellation. The increasing polymegathism (increase in cell size) and pleomorphism (variability in cell shape) that characterizes progression of the disease is also easily demonstrated by specular microscopy (78).

The stroma in FED is affected secondarily as a result of the endothelial changes, but the changes in the stroma are less distinctive. In the early stages, the stroma can appear normal under the light microscope. When stromal edema ensues, there is disruption of the normal architecture of the collagen lamellae, with widened interfibrillar spaces and areas of granular filamentous material laid down by the activated keratocytes. Bowman's layer remains intact for the most part except for occasional focal defects filled with connective tissue (53). In the advanced stage of the disease, thick, subepithelial avascular connective tissue may be observed between Bowman's layer and the epithelial basement membrane. This fibrocellular layer contains active fibroblasts, collagen fibrils, and basement membrane–like material, and may accumulate a thickness up to 350 μm, about seven times the normal epithelial thickness (53). Vascularization of this layer may occur with time (42).

The epithelium is also passively affected as the edema spreads anteriorly. Initially, intraepithelial cysts are noted in the basal layer of the epithelium (intracellular edema). As more fluid accumulates, the cells may rupture, leading to intercellular edema. With time, the basal epithelial cells may become focally detached from the basement membrane, resulting in subepithelial bullae (53,79,80).

Pathophysiology

The underlying pathology of Fuchs' dystrophy resides in the corneal endothelium. Abnormal production of collagenous material by the affected endothelial cells causes marked thickening of Descemet's membrane, which becomes studded with excrescences (guttae). Changes in endothelial cell morphology and function eventually result in corneal edema.

Corneal deturgescence is primarily maintained by active transport of electrolytes (with secondary transport of water down the osmotic gradient) from the stroma to the anterior chamber via adenosine triphosphate (ATP)-requiring Na-K pumps. Both pump density (81,82) and rate (32) can be increased in early FED, potentially representing a compensatory mechanism for the decreasing number of functional endothelial cells. As the disease progresses, there is a gradual decline in the number of functional Na-K pumps (81,82). Eventually the remaining endothelial cells can no longer maintain corneal deturgescence and corneal edema ensues.

The intact endothelial monolayer also serves as a passive barrier to diffusion of water and solutes from the aqueous humor. It is not clear whether this barrier function is compromised in FED. Several studies have demonstrated increased endothelial permeability in patients with central cornea guttae, suggesting that a breakdown in the endothelial barrier function may be an early finding in FED (32,83,84). However, these results were not supported by measurements made using two-dimensional scanning fluorophotometry (85).

Although there is a reasonably good understanding of the site of the primary pathology and of the natural history of FED, the etiology of its characteristic endothelial dysfunction remains an enigma. Numerous hypotheses regarding the pathogenesis of FED have been proposed, but none has as yet been proven.

A role for the fibrinolytic system in the pathogenesis of FED has been suggested, based on a report of increased fibrinogen degradation products in serum and aqueous humor of patients with FED (86). Immunofluorescence staining localized fibrinogen/fibrin antigens to abnormal Descemet's membrane in FED, but not in normal eyes (87). Finally, a single study noted improvement in central corneal thickness and visual acuity in patients with bullous keratopathy secondary to FED treated with a systemic antifibrinolytic drug, tranexamic acid (88). Although intriguing, the significance of this finding is unclear.

Some studies have investigated the possibility that primary abnormalities in the composition of the aqueous humor may play a role in the pathogenesis of FED. Alterations in anterior chamber concentrations of multiple amino acids have been noted in FED patients (89). However, these differences may simply be a by-product of the abnormal endothelial transport mechanism.

The increased incidence and more severe phenotypic expression of FED in women have led to the speculation of a possible hormonal role in its pathogenesis (42), although there is a paucity of data supporting this hypothesis. Interestingly, though, it has been shown that the posterior nonbanded layer of Descemet's membrane is twice as thick in normal women above age 70 as it is in age-matched men (71).

The corneal endothelium is of neuroectodermal origin. FED, along with other hereditary corneal endothelial dystrophies, may result from abnormal terminal induction or final differentiation of neural crest cells (40). Recently, missense mutations in the *COL8A2* gene, which encodes the $\alpha2$ chain of type VIII collagen, a component of endothelial basement membranes, were identified in familial and sporadic cases of FED (90). Similar findings in a family with PPMD led the authors to hypothesize that abnormalities in type VIII collagen may perturb the terminal differentiation of corneal endothelial cells in these diseases.

Several lines of evidence suggest that apoptosis or its regulation may play a role in FED (91,92). The average percentage of apoptotic endothelial cells is significantly higher in FED patients than in controls, although transmission electron microscopy did not show conclusive evidence of increased endothelial apoptosis in FED (91). Marked differences in keratocyte apoptosis have been found in normal and FED corneas (92). Keratocytes participate in the turnover of the extracellular matrix, and more importantly, in the maintenance of normal endothelial function by providing physical and growth factor support (93). Growth of corneal endothelial cells in culture shows a twofold increase when keratocytes are included, suggesting that keratocytes secrete factors that are involved in endothelial cell maintenance and proliferation (94). Excessive apoptosis of keratocytes, with subsequent loss of their supportive factors, could potentially represent the primary event that leads to endothelial dysfunction. The temporal relationship between keratocyte apoptosis and endothelial dysfunction has not yet been established, however.

Several lines of evidence suggest that mitochondrial abnormalities may play a role in Fuchs' dystrophy (55). Endothelial Na-K pumps use a tremendous amount of ATP to maintain corneal deturgescence. Thus, any process that disturbs energy production or utilization will adversely affect endothelial cells function. The activity of cytochrome oxidase, a key enzyme in ATP production, is reduced in edematous areas of FED corneas, believed to reflect a decrease in either the number or the metabolic activity of endothelial mitochondria in the dysfunctional endothelial cells (95). Marked abnormalities in mitochondrial ultrastructure have been seen in corneal endothelial cells from patients with Fuchs' dystrophy (55).

Mitochondria possess a number of unique features (96). They contain their own extrachromosomal DNA, which is inherited maternally and is distinct from nuclear DNA. The mitochondrial genome, 16.6 kilobases of circular, double-stranded DNA, codes for structural RNAs and proteins involved in oxidative phosphorylation. Mitochondria replicate, transcribe, and translate their DNA independently. Effective energy production, however, requires coordinated interactions among the mitochondrially encoded gene products and those imported from the nucleus.

The mutation rate of mitochondria DNA is 10-fold higher than that of nuclear DNA. Not only is the mitochondrial DNA bathed in the free-radical byproducts of oxidative phosphorylation, but it also lacks both protective histones and a sophisticated DNA repair system. Because mitochondrial DNA has no introns, mutations are more likely to affect coding regions. Inherited germ mutations in the mitochondrial DNA accumulate sequentially through maternal lineages. In addition to heritable mutations, nonheritable mitochondrial DNA mutations or deletions occur within somatic cells. Accumulation of somatic cell mutations may contribute to the pathogenesis of age-related diseases such as Parkinson's disease (55). Normal and mutant mitochondrial DNA often coexist within the same cell, a condition known as heteroplasmy. There is a threshold effect, where the proportion of mutant mitochondrial DNA required to cause clinical expression of the deficit in ATP production varies among individuals, organ systems, and within a given tissue.

Mitochondrial DNA abnormalities cause a diverse group of disorders, collectively referred to as the mitochondrial encephalomyopathies. These disorders, which include diseases such as Leber's hereditary optic neuropathy and chronic progressive external ophthalmoplegia, have protean manifestations, primarily affecting cells and tissues with high energy requirements (97). The postmitotic nature of corneal endothelial cells and their tremendous metabolic demands make them a likely site to manifest mitochondrial DNA damage, either inherited or acquired. Several cases of primary corneal endothelial abnormalities in patients with mitochondrial disorders have been reported (98–101). These clinical associations, combined with the unique features of mitochondrial DNA and the biologic nature of corneal endothelial cells, suggest that defects in mitochondrial DNA, either inherited or acquired, might underlie the endothelial dysfunction of Fuchs' dystrophy (55).

Management

Early Fuchs' dystrophy is asymptomatic and requires no treatment. Patients may wish to avoid contact lens use, as the relative hypoxia may unduly stress the compromised endothelium (102,103). Similarly, topical carbonic anhydrase inhibitors are best avoided in this population, as irreversible corneal edema has been linked to these agents (104).

Topical hyperosmotic agents, which act by temporarily increasing the osmolality of the precorneal tear film, may be used with variable success once corneal edema occurs. Some patients may benefit from using topical 5% sodium chloride solution several times upon awakening or throughout the day; ointment form may also be used prior to sleep to help reduce morning visual blurring. A hair dryer held at arms length from the cornea may also be used to facilitate corneal dehydration. Alternatively, lowering the intraocular pressure may reduce the hydrostatic pressure, which acts to push fluid into the cornea and thereby decrease corneal edema. Unfortunately, none of the currently available treatments are particularly efficacious, especially for stromal edema. In patients with bullous keratopathy and/or recurrent erosion symptoms, a loosely fit, high-water-content soft contact lens, e.g., Kontur lens, may be used to reduce the irritation and pain. Cycloplegic agents can be added to relieve the discomfort associated with ciliary spasm. There is no clear role for the use of topical corticosteroids to treat stromal edema in patients with FED (105). A conjunctival flap may reduce pain in patients with advanced bullous keratopathy who are not candidates for corneal transplantation.

Penetrating keratoplasty is indicated for patients whose reduced vision or eye pain interferes with their daily activities. Although variability exists in the literature about the long-term results after penetrating keratoplasty for FED, the graft survival and visual outcome are in general favorable. The long-term (with at least 1 year of follow-up) rate of graft clarity ranges from 61% to 98% (106–111). Visual acuity stabilization following keratoplasty in FED is comparable to that in keratoconus and faster than that in pseudophakic or aphakic corneal edema, with 50% of patients achieved a visual acuity of better than 20/40 at 3 months (112). Nonetheless, the lifetime prognosis for corneal transplants in FED is still guarded, as progressive loss of endothelial cells always occurs and there is no source of healthy host endothelium to repopulate the graft, the way there is in keratoconus (113,114). Graft rejection, a major cause of graft failure, occurs in 5% to 29% of transplants performed for FED (108,115). Early recognition and aggressive treatment of rejection episodes can reduce the chance of ensuing graft failure (110). Patient education regarding the symptoms of graft rejection (blurred vision, eye redness, prolonged foreign-body sensation) is a key component in the management of any postkeratoplasty patient.

Many of the patients who require penetrating keratoplasty for FED are elderly and have preexisting lens opacities (107,116). Management of the cataract in FED patients undergoing keratoplasty may be approached in several ways. There appears to be no statistically significant difference in the final visual outcome between combined and nonsimultaneous procedures for FED and coexistent cataract (117). Patient age, medical health, and status of the other eye should all be considered when deciding which procedure to perform.

In patients with stage 2 Fuchs' dystrophy with stromal edema and a visually significant cataract, phacoemulsification alone can be attempted, if the corneal view allows it. The surgeon should use liberal amounts of viscoelastic and minimal amounts of ultrasound power during cataract extraction in this setting. It is important to counsel patients preoperatively that corneal decompensation may occur following cataract surgery, but if it does not, then corneal transplantation can be delayed.

In the setting of bullous keratopathy with cataract, the decision is whether to perform a triple procedure (penetrating keratoplasty, cataract extraction, and intraocular lens implantation) or a corneal transplant alone, followed by cataract extraction after the corneal transplant has stabilized. Each approach has advantages. Simultaneous surgery allows quicker visual rehabilitation and requires only one surgery. This may be desirable for older patients and those with significant medical issues. Sequential surgeries allows for more accurate intraocular lens power calculations (118) and allows for small incision cataract surgery, which is safer than the open-sky approach required in the setting of a triple procedure for advanced bullous keratopathy.

Despite its relatively high success rate in FED, penetrating keratoplasty is not risk-free. Postoperative astigmatism, suture-related problems, and ineffective wound healing remain as significant issues that prolong the visual recovery period (119,120). Recently, several innovative surgical techniques for selective endothelial transplantation have been described with promising early results (121–128).

Selective transplantation of a disk of posterior stroma and endothelium through a large scleral incision (deep lamellar endothelial keratoplasty) minimizes surgically induced astigmatism, as the anterior surface of the cornea remains intact (123,127). However, this technically demanding approach currently requires manual lamellar dissection, therefore creating interface irregularities that reduce best-corrected postoperative vision. This technique also theoretically reduces the risk of wound dehiscence, as the wound is created in the vascularized sclera, rather than the avascular cornea.

In microkeratome-assisted endokeratoplasty (121,122), an anterior corneal flap is created mechanically. The flap is reflected in the operating room and a corneal button of posterior stroma and endothelium is transplanted, as in a full-thickness keratoplasty. Infant donor cornea, which has very high cell counts but lacks the tensile strength to support a full-thickness graft, has been used with this technique with good success (124). Because endothelial loss is a major factor in graft failure in FED patients, the ability to use infant tissue may represent a significant advance in the management of this disease.

Finally, successful *in vitro* transplantation of a thin scroll of Descemet's membrane carrying viable endothelium through a small scleral incision has been described (126). These novel techniques are still in their infancy, but have the potential to revolutionize the surgical management of Fuchs' dystrophy.

Although corneal endothelial cells do not divide *in vivo*, they can be stimulated to proliferate in culture (8,129–139). Their growth can be modulated by diverse factors including fibroblast growth factor, epidermal growth factor, and endothelial cell growth factor (129,130,132–134,138,139). The recent demonstration that cultured human corneal endothelial cells can form a high cell density monolayer following *ex vivo* transplantation to recipient human cornea provides a foundation for the future advancement of endothelial replacement techniques (8), especially in combination with the surgical techniques described above. Future work may enable us to enhance the cell density of donor tissue prior to surgery. Ultimately, it may be possible to stimulate *in situ* repair and controlled proliferation of the corneal endothelial cells with exogenous growth factors or with gene therapy.

CONGENITAL HEREDITARY ENDOTHELIAL DYSTROPHY

Congenital hereditary endothelial dystrophy (CHED) was first described in 1863 as "corneitis interstitialis in utero" (140). It was initially classified as a variant of intrauterine interstitial keratitis (140), and subsequently as a stromal dystrophy (141–144). In 1960, Maumenee (145) was the first to hypothesize that CHED resulted from a primary dysfunction of the corneal endothelium, which was later confirmed by histopathologic and electron microscopy data (146–149). In 1971, the name congenital hereditary endothelial dystrophy was suggested (149).

CHED can be inherited in either an autosomal-dominant (AD) or an autosomal-recessive (AR) pattern (150,151). Linkage analysis had localized the dominant form (CHED1) to chromosome 20, near the locus for PPMD (152,153). Recessive CHED (CHED2) is not linked to this region, suggesting that it is a genetically distinct entity (154–156).

Clinical Features

Congenital hereditary endothelial dystrophy is characterized by diffuse, noninflammatory corneal opacity with edema (Fig. 47-8). The disease is bilateral and tends to be symmetric. Marked impairment of vision is characteristic. CHED typically presents at birth or in early infancy, and is a common cause of childhood corneal opacification (39,157). The two forms of CHED have different clinical characteristics (157).

Children with dominant CHED (CHED1) have clear corneas at birth. Corneal clouding is first noted during the first or second year of life and slowly progresses over 5 to 10 years. Photophobia and epiphora are common and may be the presenting signs of the disease. As corneal opacification increases, however, these signs may actually decrease. Nystagmus is uncommon in CHED1. Vision tends to be better (in the range of 20/40 to 20/400) than in recessive CHED (39,157). Some authors have suggested that CHED1 is more appropriately termed infantile hereditary endothelial dystrophy, given its clinical characteristics (157).

In contrast, corneal clouding is present at birth or within the neonatal period in patients with recessive CHED (CHED2). Corneal opacification is dense at the time of diagnosis, and does not tend to progress. There is no associated photophobia or epiphora. Nystagmus is invariably present, presumably the result of severe corneal opacification at an early age (39,157).

The clinical findings in CHED include corneal opacification, which extends to the limbus without an intervening clear zone. The opacification can vary in severity from mild haze to a milky, ground-glass appearance. Extensive bilateral corneal edema, with corneal thickness up to three times normal, is common. Fine epithelial edema creates a

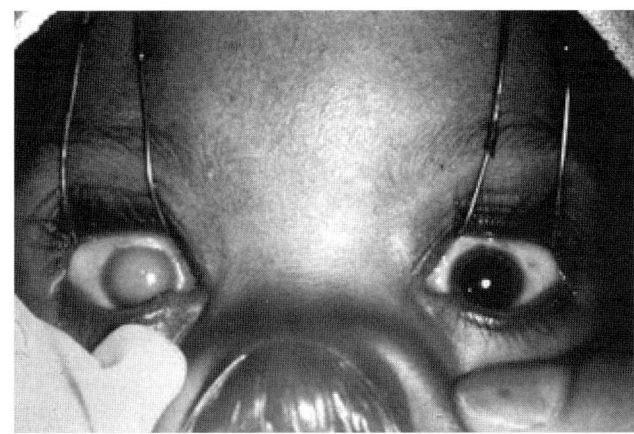

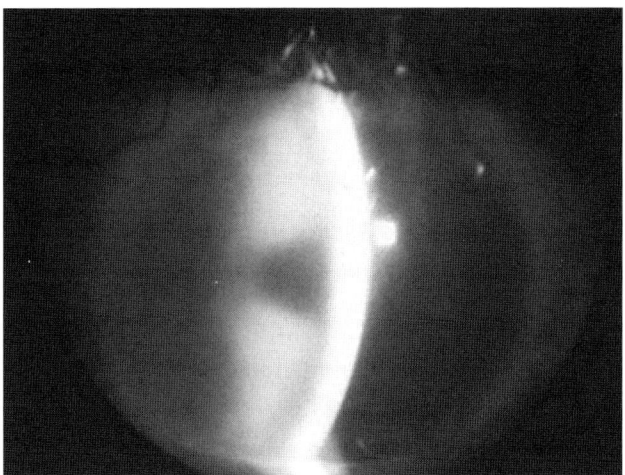

FIGURE 47-8. A: Congenital hereditary endothelial dystrophy (CHED). Note the diffuse corneal opacification that creates a ground-glass appearance in the right eye. The left eye has a clear corneal transplant with hazy host corneal rim. **B:** CHED. Diffuse corneal clouding extends to the limbus without an intervening clear zone. Marked stromal thickening is noted. (Photo courtesy of Claes H. Dohlman, M.D., with permission.)

roughened corneal surface and distorts the light reflex. Descemet's membrane is thickened, but no guttae are present. Secondary changes such as band keratopathy, subepithelial fibrosis, and spheroidal degeneration may accompany the extensive edema, more commonly in the dominant variant (39,149,147,157). Subepithelial amyloid deposits resembling gelatinous droplike keratopathy have been reported in CHED2 (158,159). Painful epithelial erosion rarely occurs in CHED because bullous keratopathy is not characteristic, in contrast to Fuchs' dystrophy.

CHED has been associated with congenital glaucoma (160–162). Congenital glaucoma is postulated to be a result of abnormal neural crest cell migration (163), whereas CHED may result from deficient terminal differentiation (40). Abnormalities in the neural crest could theoretically cause both entities in a single patient. Because both conditions can present with corneal opacification and edema, accurate diagnosis may be difficult (160). False elevations

of intraocular pressure (IOP) caused by stromal edema can compound this problem. Other clinical characteristics must often be considered to distinguish the two diseases. For example, progressively enlarging corneal diameter is more characteristic of congenital glaucoma. Corneal edema from congenital glaucoma should resolve after the IOP is lowered. Finally, other causes of corneal opacification, such as posterior polymorphous dystrophy, also need to be considered in the differential diagnosis. In contrast to CHED, the corneal thickness is usually normal in PPMD.

CHED has not been consistently associated with systemic diseases. However, there have been isolated case reports with associated sensory neural deafness (164), and agenesis of the corpus callosum (165).

Histopathology

Histopathologic changes in CHED are concentrated in the endothelium and Descemet's membrane (166,167). There is often a complete absence of endothelial cells in the central cornea. Unlike Fuchs' dystrophy, CHED does not manifest guttae (147).

Descemet's membrane may be either thickened (168) or thinned (169–171) in CHED, possibly related to the degree and timing of endothelial dysfunction (149,162,167). Thinned or attenuated Descemet's membrane may be the sequela of endothelial dysfunction *in utero*, so that only the fetal anterior banded zone is produced. Thickened Descemet's membrane, on the other hand, is the result of persistent dystrophic or dysfunctional endothelium that secretes a reactive posterior collagenous layer or an exaggerated, but structurally normal, posterior nonbanded layer (167).

In general, the anterior layer of Descemet's membrane appears normal in CHED (39). In contrast, posterior Descemet's has markedly abnormal ultrastructure, which varies between the two forms of CHED. In dominant CHED (CHED1), there is deposition of an abnormal posterior collagenous layer containing disorganized collagen fibrils of varying diameters with interspersed basement membrane-like material (39,146). The abnormal material is thought to be secreted by metaplastic, fibroblast-like endothelial cells. In recessive CHED (CHED2), basement membrane-like material is mixed with fine fibrillary collagen in an orderly matrix to form a thickened nonbanded zone, which retains the structure of normal posterior Descemet's membrane (167).

The endothelial cells of the peripheral cornea in CHED have a relatively normal appearance. The endothelium becomes attenuated in the midperiphery and is completely absent from the central cornea (146–149). In the transition zone, cells are irregularly shaped, with pleomorphism and polymegathism. The normal hexagonal pattern is lost (168). Multinucleated cells may be present. Endothelial organelles are abnormal, including dilated mitochondria (168). Corneal endothelial permeability is significantly increased, as is expected with a dysfunctional endothelial barrier (168).

Nonspecific changes in the corneal epithelium and stroma occur secondary to the endothelial dysfunction. Stromal collagen fibrils may have a relatively normal diameter and periodicity (149) or may become swollen (145,146,172). Homogeneous granular materials with fluid pockets may accumulate in between the stromal collagen fibrils, resulting in marked thickening of the stroma and severely disorganized lamellae. These alterations cause light scattering, giving the cornea its ground-glass appearance. Stromal keratocytes have normal ultrastructure with normal cytoplasmic organelles, despite an increase in vacuolization. Stromal inflammation and neovascularization are generally not found (146,147,172,173).

Irregular thickening and fragmentation of Bowman's layer has been noted in CHED, but this is not a consistent finding (167,172). Subepithelial fibrosis with calcification has been seen in dominant CHED, whereas subepithelial amyloid deposition has been noted in the recessive variant (158,159).

The epithelium also becomes thickened in CHED, increasing from 5 to 15 cell layers. There can be focal loss of epithelial cell polarity. Intracellular or intercellular edema occurs, especially in the basal epithelium (149,168,172). Fluid clefts and vacuoles may separate the basal epithelium from Bowman's layer. Electron micrographs reveal a slight decrease in the number of mitochondria in the basal cells, as well as numerous vacuoles surrounding the nuclei of the basal cells (172). Despite focal absence of basement membrane, recurrent erosions are rare as the basal epithelial cells are adherent to the cornea (39,145–147,167,173).

Pathophysiology

CHED is a primary dysfunction of the endothelial cells. Progressive stromal and epithelial edema is accompanied by secondary structural changes resulting from chronic edema. The normal appearance of the anterior banded zone of Descemet's membrane suggests that the endothelium is most likely functionally normal up to the fifth month *in utero*. Degeneration starting with the central cornea occurs thereafter (39,149,162,167,168,172), believed to arise from an abnormality in the terminal differentiation of neural crest cells (40,162).

The mechanisms underlying the two forms of CHED remain unknown. Significant differences in the age of onset, disease course, and hereditary, along with the involvement of different gene loci, suggest that CHED1 and CHED2 may have different etiologies. Apoptosis or a genetic defect in cell metabolism may underlie endothelial cell degeneration and production of an abnormal posterior collagenous layer that more typically characterizes dominant CHED. Persistent loss of growth regulation, on the other hand, might lead to accumulation of the thickened

but structurally normal posterior nonbanded layer that is found in the recessive form of the disease (167). The rarity of these conditions makes elucidation of their etiologies difficult.

Management

Penetrating keratoplasty is currently the only option for visual rehabilitation in children with CHED. Corneal transplantation for CHED has a better prognosis than do other pediatric indications because eyes with CHED typically lack corneal neovascularization, inflammation, and concomitant intraocular pathology (174). However, the decision to operate is complex and should not be undertaken lightly (175). Pediatric penetrating keratoplasty poses greater technical challenges and, in general, is less successful than is corneal transplantation in adults (176). Effective visual rehabilitation in patients with CHED is time-consuming for all involved—parents, child, and surgeon. Aggressive amblyopia management is critical for optimal visual recovery.

Assessment of the risk-benefit ratio of penetrating keratoplasty for an individual patient is challenging (175). Estimation of preoperative visual acuity, especially in preverbal children, may be inaccurate because the degree of corneal opacification does not always correlate with visual acuity (169). It can be surprising how little visual development is impaired, even with significant corneal clouding from birth (169).

Pediatric keratoplasty is technically challenging, due the small size of the infant eye and its low scleral rigidity. However, the rigors of postoperative management make the surgery itself seem somewhat trivial. Rapid and exuberant inflammatory responses in children predispose to graft rejection, glaucoma and cataract formation. Early corneal neovascularization, early loosening of sutures, and irregular astigmatism can also arise from vigorous wound healing (175). Frequent postoperative visits, even daily during the first postoperative week, are crucial for success. Regular, repeated examinations under anesthesia are a key component in management of pediatric grafts (175). Early suture removal may improve graft survival by decreasing the incidence of suture-related problems (174,177). Family members must be willing to commit the extensive amount of time needed for postoperative medications, office visits, exams under anesthesia, and amblyopia management. The wise surgeon is very cautious about undertaking corneal transplantation in a child if there is any doubt about the family's commitment to its success.

Results from early studies of penetrating keratoplasty in CHED were poor (147,149). Graft failure was common, with only 15% of grafts remaining clear at 2 years (147). Later studies have shown more promising results, likely due in part to advances in surgical techniques and suture materials (162,169,174,177). A multicenter, retrospective study of 164 pediatric corneal transplantations showed that 67% of grafts were clear at 2 years, with a median survival time of more than 9 years (174). Several other series have demonstrated a 90% graft survival rate with a mean follow-up of approximately 3 years (169,177). One study found the graft survival rate to be higher in delayed-onset CHED (96%) than in CHED present at birth (56%), although there was no correlation between age at the time of surgery and graft survival (178).

The optimal timing of corneal transplantation in CHED is still controversial, although there is a trend toward earlier surgery (175). There appears to be no decrease in graft survival with early surgery, which may reduce the risk of amblyopia, nystagmus, and strabismus (178). Others, however, recommended that surgery be delayed as long as the patient demonstrates good fixation and the eyes have normal alignment (177).

Substantial improvements in vision following keratoplasty in CHED can occur even when surgery is delayed into adolescence or adulthood (169). Some degree of amblyopia is virtually universal, but only a small percentage of eyes (16%) have dense amblyopia (visual acuity less than 20/100), even when surgery is delayed (177).

Keratoprosthesis has been suggested as a "temporary" measure in younger patients in whom the risk of amblyopia is the highest (175). Keratoprosthesis provides immediately clear vision without the problem of astigmatism and the risk of graft rejection. In theory, this would make the management of amblyopia easier and more effective. Traditional keratoplasty can then be done when the child is older.

Future advances in the surgical management of CHED may include one or more of the selective endothelial transplantation techniques described above for Fuchs' dystrophy. These techniques have the theoretical advantage of replacing only the diseased part of the cornea, with reduction in postoperative astigmatism and wound healing issues. High cell-count infant donor material, which lacks the tensile strength necessary to support a full-thickness graft, may eventually be useful in this management of this challenging condition (124).

POSTERIOR POLYMORPHOUS DYSTROPHY

PPMD, a slowly progressive disease of the cornea, was first described in 1916 by Koeppe (179). He named the condition "keratitis bullosa interna" to describe the characteristic bullous lesions he noted in the posterior cornea.

A wide spectrum of corneal changes can be seen in PPMD, ranging from a few vesicular lesions to total opacification of the cornea with edema (180). In PPMD, dystrophic endothelial cells exhibit epithelial features, and produce secondary abnormalities in Descemet's membrane

(181). Iris and anterior chamber angle structures may also be affected in some patients with PPMD (182–186).

Posterior polymorphous dystrophy typically has an autosomal-dominant inheritance pattern, although penetrance of the disease is low (180). In addition, the clinical expression of the disease can vary considerably, even within affected families (182). For example, one member of the family may only be minimally affected with asymptomatic corneal lesions, whereas a sibling may have severe peripheral synechiae with glaucoma and corneal decompensation.

Clinical Features

PPMD is a dystrophy of the corneal endothelium. Most often it is asymptomatic and is noted incidentally during slit-lamp examination. The disease can be slowly progressive, but in many cases the findings are static. PPMD can rarely cause visual dysfunction from corneal edema, iridocorneal adhesions, corectopia, and glaucoma (185). The precise age of onset of PPMD is difficult to determine because most patients have no symptoms. However, a majority of patients are diagnosed in the second or third decade of life. There appears to be a congenital variant, which exhibits corneal edema at birth similar to the recessive variant of CHED (180).

Corneal changes in PPMD are usually bilateral but may show marked asymmetry, and typically assume one of three basic configurations: vesicular lesions, band lesions, and diffuse opacities (39) (Fig. 47-9). One study found that vesicles and bands were twice as common in women as in men, and that vesicles were mostly bilateral (94%) whereas bands were usually unilateral (85%) (184). The significance of these findings is not known.

Vesicles may appear in isolation or in clusters throughout the posterior cornea. With the slit lamp, the vesicles appear as small blisters on Descemet's membrane. Clinically, the vesicles are surrounded by a diffuse gray halo. In general, they do not affect visual acuity, and may remain stationary, regress, or increase in number with time. Grouped vesicles may aggregate to form larger geographic lesions. Specular microscopy reveals that vesicles are composed of abnormal pleomorphic cells with indistinct borders, creating black areas in the endothelial mosaic that are surrounded by enlarged endothelial cells (184). Geographic lesions are often surrounded by a more normal-appearing endothelial mosaic (Fig. 47-10) (185). Band lesions extend across the posterior corneal surface as two scalloped, raised ridges that run roughly parallel to each other. Like the vesicular lesions, band lesions may be present anywhere in the posterior cornea, although they are most commonly found just inferior to the central cornea. Finally, diffuse opacities present as irregular thickening of Descemet's membrane with grayish opacities in a swirled pattern. Patchy corneal edema often accompanies diffuse PPMD.

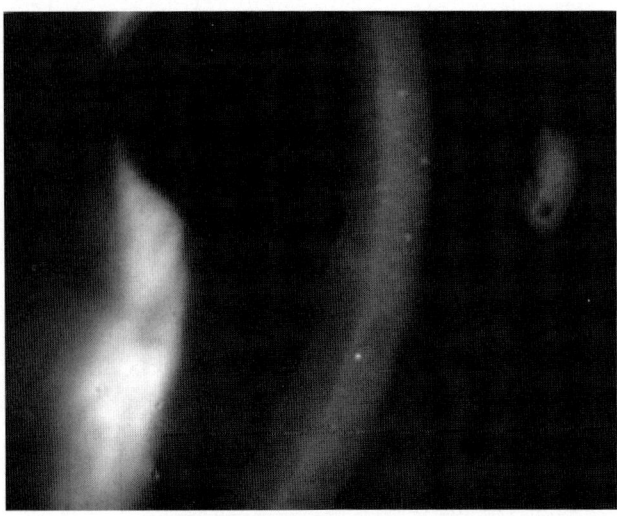
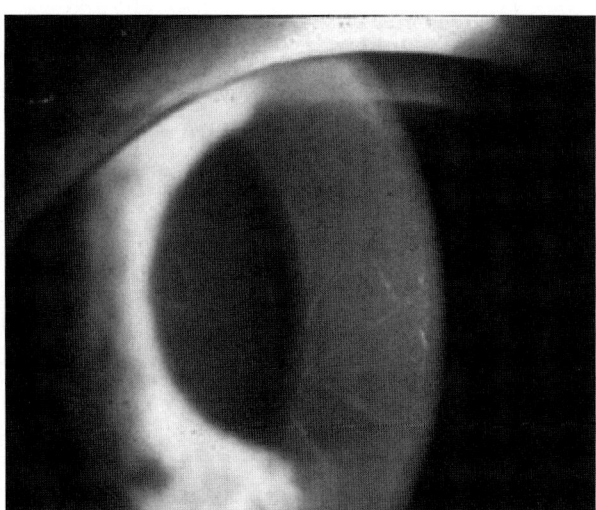

A   B

FIGURE 47-9. A: Posterior polymorphous dystrophy (PPMD). Endothelial vesicular lesions with scalloped edges are seen in the paracentral cornea. (Photo courtesy of Claes H. Dohlman, M.D., with permission) **B:** PPMD. Irregular endothelial bands are present throughout the central cornea.

In retroillumination, the posterior cornea has the appearance of beaten metal or peau d'orange (39,182).

Corneal edema is not common in PPMD. However, vision can be reduced if the edema progresses to involve the epithelium. Corneal edema can appear at any age, and may be rapidly progressing or remain stable. Lipid deposition or band keratopathy may be seen in advanced cases (186). Keratoplasty is rarely needed in PPMD.

Iridocorneal adhesions with associated pupillary ectropion and corectopia can also be seen in PPMD (186–188). Iris changes range from subtle peripheral anterior synechiae

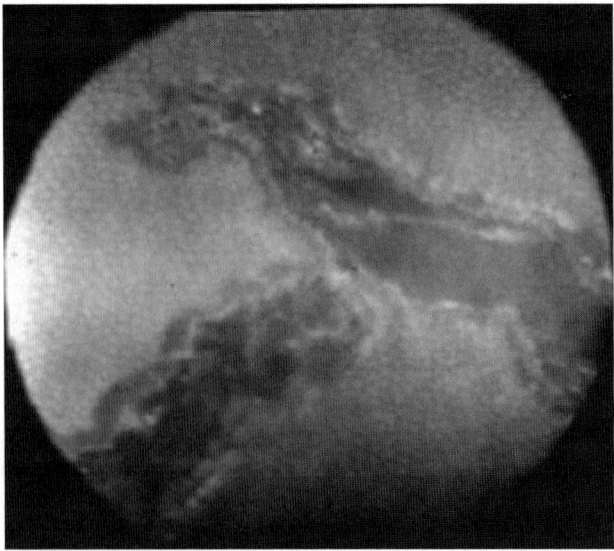

FIGURE 47-10. Specular microscopy of PPMD. Grouped vesicles with indistinct borders coalesce to create black areas in the endothelial mosaic. The surrounding endothelium has a normal appearance. (Photo courtesy of Claes H. Dohlman, M.D., with permission.)

visible only with gonioscopy to broad-based peripheral iridocorneal adhesions. Glaucoma is common in patients with symptomatic PPMD and is often difficult to manage, especially after a penetrating keratoplasty (186).

Histopathology

Corneal endothelium abnormalities are the hallmark of PPMD. The primary event is believed to be "epithelialization" of the corneal endothelium (39,153,189–195). The stimulus for this transformation is not known. The epithelial-like endothelial cells exhibit many morphologic and growth features of the normal epithelium, including a multilaminar pattern, desmosomal junctions, microvilli, cytoplasmic keratin, sparse mitochondria, and rapid growth in tissue culture (186,191,192,195). They also stain with antisera prepared against human epidermal keratin (195). The transition between endothelial and epithelial-appearing cells can be abrupt (192).

The epithelial-like cells are capable of migrating over the endothelial cells without adhering to them and can grow to cover the trabecular meshwork and iris, leading to intractable glaucoma (182,186,188). The "epithelialized" cells secrete a thick membrane that resembles an abnormal Descemet's membrane. These cells may even regenerate after corneal transplantation (186). Descemet's membrane is absent or markedly attenuated in the areas covered by the epithelial-like cells. The description of slit-like spaces in the posterior stroma that are lined by epithelial-like endothelium and open to the anterior chamber through defects in Descemet's membrane is an addition to the ultrastructural spectrum of PPMD (196).

In addition to the characteristic epithelial-like cells, many other changes in the endothelium have been noted.

Metaplastic fibroblast-like endothelial cells can be seen (190,192,197–199). Pleomorphism and degeneration of endothelial cells are common findings in PPMD (185,190, 192,197,198). Attenuated endothelial cells with disorganized organelles, large vacuoles, phagosomal inclusions, and disrupted cell membranes have been described using transmission electron microscopy. Areas of hypertrophic endothelial cells coexist with areas of focal endothelial cell loss, suggesting competing degenerative and regenerative processes (190,192,198).

Alterations in Descemet's membrane, including deposition of abnormal collagen, guttae, and pits, are a common finding in PPMD (189–192,197,198,200). The changes are believed to be secondary to the primary alterations in the endothelium, similar to Fuchs' dystrophy. The proportion of dystrophic endothelial cells may determine the extent of abnormalities seen in Descemet's membrane (192). The timing of the endothelial dysfunction can also affect the severity of structural changes in Descemet's membrane (181).

Thickening of Descemet's membrane is the typical finding, although attenuation of this layer has occasionally been noted (188,201). The posterior collagenous layer can be interrupted by irregular excrescences, which resemble the cornea guttae observed in FED (192,195). The anterior banded zone of Descemet's usually has normal structure. However, in the rare PPMD patients with corneal clouding and edema at birth, the anterior banded zone may be partially absent or thinned, suggesting that endothelial dysfunction occurs before the 12th week of gestation (181). In contrast, the posterior nonbanded layer is abnormal in virtually all patients with PPMD. This layer is irregularly thickened by a mixture of collagenous fibrils, basement membrane-like material, and cellular debris with multiple laminations. The characteristic vesicular lesions seen clinically are believed to represent irregularities and craters in the collagenous tissue. Infolding of Descemet's membrane causes stromal pits within the posterior cornea (192).

Stromal changes are also believed to be secondary to the underlying endothelial dysfunction, and are primarily localized to the posterior cornea. Keratocytes in the posterior cornea show cytoplasmic enlargement and electrolucency with a prominent rough endoplasmic reticulum under electron microscopy, consistent with cornea edema (181). The collagen fibrils in the anterior and mid-stroma have a normal banding pattern and diameter. The interfibrillar space is enlarged with random orientation of the fibrils.

The epithelium may also show secondary changes from low-grade edema. Bowman's layer is typically intact (181). Rarely, the epithelium may be thinned with irregularities in Bowman's layer. In severe cases, there may be subepithelial fibrosis, calcification, or lipid degeneration (170,186).

Given the considerable differences in the clinical and pathologic findings of PPMD from those of FED and CHED, some have suggested that they should not be considered together, even though PPMD is also primarily an endothelial dystrophy (186).

Pathophysiology

The pathogenesis of PPMD likely involves abnormal transformation and migration of the endothelial cells with secondary alterations in Descemet's membrane, but the stimulus for these events is unclear.

The concept of metaplasia has been proposed to explain the endothelial changes in PPMD. Epithelial or fibroblastic transformation in PPMD may represent a metaplastic response of endothelial cells, although the trigger is not known (190,197,202). Differential staining patterns with specific epithelial and endothelial antibodies support the idea that endothelial cell transformation occurs in PPMD (203). Some endothelial cells stain only with the endothelial antibody, some stain with both types of antibodies, and others stain only with the epithelial antibody, suggesting that endothelial cells progress from a normal phenotype to a transitional phenotype, and finally to an abnormal epithelial phenotype.

Classifications of endothelial disorders based on neural crest cell development and differentiation have traditionally grouped PPMD, CHED, and FED together as disorders of terminal differentiation (40). Under this scheme, ICE syndrome typically stands alone, resulting from abnormal neural crest cell proliferation. Similarities among these syndromes may help provide clues about etiology. Despite differences in heredity, disease course, and histology in ICE and PPMD (Table 47-1), studies have suggested that these diseases may have more in common than previously thought. Epithelioid changes in the endothelium in ICE syndrome have been demonstrated in several studies (204–208), suggesting that ICE syndrome and PPMD may be part of a similar spectrum. Clinically these diseases have considerable overlap, as both can exhibit peripheral synechiae, ectropion, corectopia, and glaucoma (188,190), findings not typically seen in FED or CHED.

A "two-hit" theory, similar to that of retinoblastoma, has been suggested as a unifying hypothesis for pathogenesis of ICE (sporadic and unilateral) and PPMD (autosomal dominant and bilateral) (209). According to this theory, the predisposition for either condition is inherited as an inactive germline allele, the so-called "first hit." Inactivation of the second allele, or "second hit," either in embryogenesis (PPMD) or later in corneal development (ICE syndrome), could cause disease expression. The timing and nature of the "hits" would produce various clinical patterns. Although this hypothesis potentially unifies several of the endotheliopathies, it remains speculative.

Some progress has been made toward uncovering the genetic basis of PPMD. Linkage of PPMD to the long arm of chromosome 20 (20q11) has been shown (210). This is

TABLE 47-1. MAIN CLINICAL CHARACTERISTICS OF THE CORNEAL ENDOTHELIAL DYSTROPHIES

Feature	FED	CHED	PPMD	ICE
Onset	40–50 years	10–20 years (CHED 1) Infancy (CHED 2)	20–30 years	30–50 years
Inheritance	Probably AD with variable Penetrance; women may be More severely affected	AD (CHED 1) or AR (CHED 2)	Typically AD with low penetrance and considerably variable expression	Sporadic, although rarely familial
Laterality	Bilateral, often asymmetric	Bilateral, usually symmetric	Bilateral with marked asymmetry	Unilateral, rarely bilateral
Corneal findings	Corneal guttae with stromal edema in early stage, Epithelial edema with cystic changes in later stage, Avascular subepithelial fibrosis in end stage	Severe corneal edema with opacification extending to limbus *CHED 1:* clear cornea at birth, corneal clouding in first/second decade, photophobia, epiphora, better vision *CHED 2:* dense corneal clouding at birth/neonatal period, poor vision with nystagmus	Endothelial vesicular lesions, band lesions, diffuse opacities Corneal edema uncommon, but may progress to involve epithelium and affect vision	Variable from "hammered-silver" appearance in iris nevus and iris atrophy variants to stromal edema and occasional bullous keratopathy in Chandler's variants
Other ocular findings	May be associated with narrow angles, short axial lengths, and keratoconus	May be associated with congenital glaucoma	Variable degree of peripheral anterior synechiae, pupillary ectropion, corectopia, glaucoma	Peripheral anterior synechiae, iris atrophy, pseudopolycoria, pupillary ectropion, corectopia, iris nodules, glaucoma
Specular microscopy	Decreased endothelial cell density with polymorphism, polymegethism, and variable dark areas within endothelial mosaic (guttae)	Not visible	Vesicles composed of abnormal pleomorphic cells	Large, pleomorphic "ICE" cells with dark/light reversal
Progression	Slowly progressive	*CHED 1:* minimal to slowly progressive *CHED 2:* stationary	Minimal	Severe
Pathology	Primary endothelial cell dysfunction with thickened Descemet's membrane	Primary endothelial cell dysfunction with complete absence of endothelial cells in central cornea	Epithelialization of corneal endothelium	Aberrant proliferation of abnormal corneal endothelial cells over cornea, iridocorneal angle, and iris
Prognosis for graft	Favorable in general, although lifelong prognosis may be guarded due to progressive endothelial loss without source of replenish	Better than other pediatric indications in general, but still technically challenging with rigorous postoperative management course	Favorable in general unless concomitant iris adhesions and glaucoma	Favorable in general, but adequate glaucoma control is the major determinant of long term success

FED, Fuchs' endothelial dystrophy; CHED, congenital hereditary endothelial dystrophy; PPMD, posterior polymorphous dystrophy; ICE, iridocorneal endothelial syndrome.

close to the region assigned to CHED1 (152). The establishment of a common location for these phenotypically distinct disorders is intriguing.

Other syndromes have been loosely associated with PPMD. Endothelial vesicles and patchy areas of attenuated endothelium similar to PPMD have been described in Alport syndrome (211,212), and some patients with PPMD also have hematuria, sensorineural hearing loss, and Alport-like renal abnormalities (211). An association with keratoconus has also been observed in a number of cases (209,213–215). It is unclear whether the clinical association is coincidental or relates to a common pathogenesis. However, various mutations in the *VIX1* homeobox gene have recently been identified to be associated with keratoconus and PPMD (216).

Management

Most patients with PPMD remain asymptomatic. This disease is only rarely progressive or visually impairing. Therapeutic intervention is not typically required. If epithelial edema occurs, it may be treated with hypertonic agents. Glaucoma management is challenging in patients with PPMD. Continued growth of the abnormal endothelium over the angle impedes aqueous outflow and can even clog trabeculectomy sites (186).

Penetrating keratoplasty may be required in patients with severe disease. In a series of 120 PPMD cases from a tertiary care cornea practice, approximately 10% of patients required penetrating keratoplasty for corneal edema (186). The proportion of patients with severe disease who need keratoplasty may be higher in this referral-based practice than in the general population.

Overall, the prognosis for surgery is good, unless iris adhesions or glaucoma are present. In one series, 50% of all patients undergoing penetrating keratoplasty achieved 20/40 vision or better, and 55% of patients maintained clear grafts (186). Outcomes were less successful in the setting of preoperative glaucoma and iris adhesions. Postoperative glaucoma occurred universally in eyes with preoperative glaucoma. Despite aggressive management, postkeratoplasty glaucoma was associated with a less successful outcome. The extent of preoperative iridocorneal adhesions also influenced postkeratoplasty prognosis. Eyes with iridocorneal adhesions had a lower transplant success rate (31% achieving 20/40 vision or better) compared to eyes without iridocorneal adhesions (78%). In patients with iridocorneal adhesions visible with a slit lamp, only 18% had 20/40 or better visual acuity, whereas 82% of the patients with iridocorneal adhesions visible only by gonioscopy achieved 20/40 or better vision (186).

Recurrence of PPMD following corneal transplantation has been reported, typically manifesting as a retrocorneal membrane or thick fibrous deposits between the epithelialized cells and Descemet's membrane (186,199,217). Graft failure typically ensues as the donor endothelium is damaged or replaced by the abnormal host cells. This is a serious complication and must be considered when recommending keratoplasty. Some authors recommend delaying keratoplasty in the second eye as long as the first eye is doing well, to minimize the chance of this complication (217).

IRIDOCORNEAL ENDOTHELIAL SYNDROME

Iridocorneal endothelial (ICE) syndrome encompasses a spectrum of diseases that includes iris nevus (Cogan-Reese) syndrome, Chandler's syndrome, and essential iris atrophy (218). Essential iris atrophy, consisting of concurrent unilateral iris abnormalities and glaucoma, was first reported in the late 19th century (219). Chandler's syndrome, predominantly characterized by corneal edema with minimal iris changes, was described in 1956 at the Massachusetts Eye and Ear Infirmary (220). It was subsequently suggested that essential iris atrophy and Chandler's syndrome represented different manifestations of the same disease (221). A third related entity, whose unique feature was pigmented nodules on the anterior surface of the iris, was termed Cogan-Reese syndrome (222,223). Because these three entities share many common clinical and histopathologic features, the term iridocorneal endothelial syndrome was proposed to unify all three conditions as a clinical spectrum of one disease process (224). An abnormality in the corneal endothelium is believed to underlie all of these manifestations.

ICE syndrome is an uncommon, typically sporadic, nonfamilial, unilateral disorder with a predilection for middle-aged women (224,225). However, familial or bilateral cases are occasionally seen (226–228). The disease occurs predominantly in whites. Only a few cases of ICE syndrome have been described in black or Asian patients (227,229,230).

Clinical Features

ICE syndrome is characterized by a progressive proliferation of abnormal corneal endothelium. The aberrant endothelium grows in a sheetlike fashion over the cornea, iridocorneal angle, and surface of the iris, causing peripheral anterior synechiae, glaucoma, and corneal edema. Contraction of the membrane results in progressive pupillary distortion and iris stromal abnormalities.

ICE syndrome typically manifests clinically between the ages of 30 and 50 (221), although pediatric cases have been rarely reported (227). Pupillary distortion is the most common presenting symptom in patients with the iris nevus or essential iris atrophy form of the disease (220) (Fig. 47-11). Patients with Chandler's syndrome are more likely to complain of decreased or distorted vision, usually worse in the early morning. Peripheral anterior synechiae are present almost universally in all types of ICE syndrome. Increased

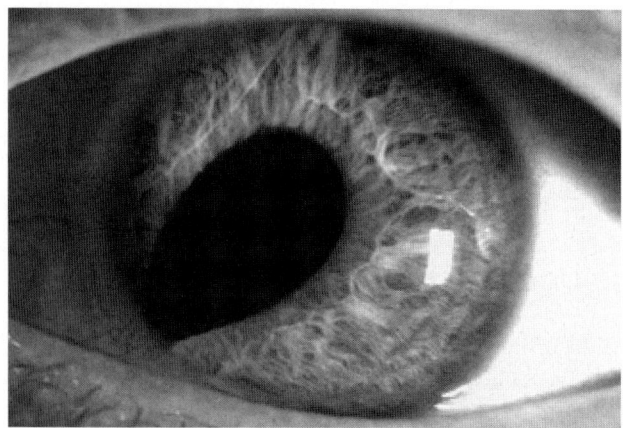

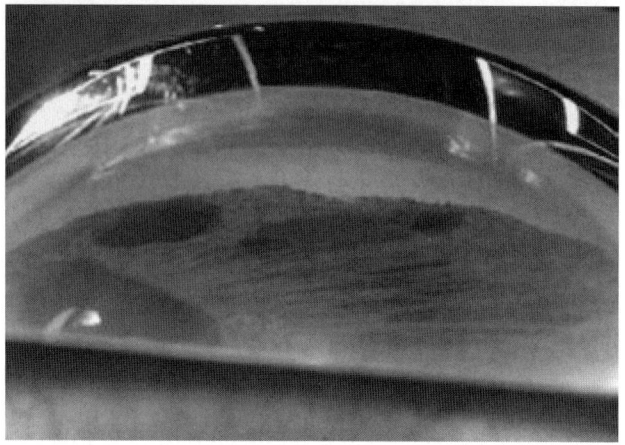

FIGURE 47-11. A: Essential iris atrophy variant of iridocorneal endothelial (ICE) syndrome. Extensive iris abnormalities include corectopia and iris stromal thinning with hole formation. Diffuse peripheral anterior synechiae are present. **B:** Gonioscopic photograph of ICE syndrome shows extensive peripheral anterior synechiae associated with corectopia, ectropion uveae, iris stretching, and atrophy. Multiple iris holes are present.

intraocular pressure is more common in essential iris atrophy or iris nevus syndrome than in Chandler's syndrome (218,231). Pain is uncommon until late in the disease. Although ICE syndrome is typically unilateral, abnormalities in the contralateral, clinically uninvolved eye have also been described, including iris transillumination defects and corneal endothelial pleomorphism (228,232,233).

Specular microscopy is helpful for diagnosis of ICE syndrome, as this technique reveals a population of abnormal endothelial cells whose appearance is unique to this syndrome. These so-called "ICE cells" are a pathognomonic finding (234) (Fig. 47-12). They are present in all patients with ICE syndrome, although they cannot be demonstrated in those whose corneal edema precludes specular examination. ICE cells are larger and more pleomorphic than normal endothelium. They have dark cell surfaces (instead of light) and light intercellular borders (instead of dark). This dark/light reversal is diagnostic for ICE cells, and is believed to result from their tall, conical

shape, which causes disruption of the specular reflex from the sloping sides of these cells (235). A central light reflex is often present (234). ICE cells can completely replace the normal endothelium (total ICE). In other cases, both ICE cells and normal-appearing endothelial cells are observed (subtotal ICE) (234).

The most obvious clinical finding in the essential iris atrophy variant of ICE syndrome is structural abnormalities of the iris. Early in the disease the iris changes may be subtle. Pupillary abnormalities including corectopia, pseudopolycoria, and ectropion uveae occur with thinning of the iris stroma as the disease advances. Iris ischemia or vascular abnormalities may contribute to progression of the iris defects (236,237). Peripheral anterior synechiae are common. Initially they may be subtle and only visualized with gonioscopy. More advanced synechiae may be seen with the slit lamp. The extent of peripheral anterior synechiae usually correlates with reduction in outflow facility and thereby elevation of intraocular pressure. Angle-closure glaucoma may result from progressive synechialization or endothelialization of the angle (218,238). The cornea may be normal or may show changes in the posterior layers giving it a fine "hammered-silver" appearance (218,220). Corneal edema is occasionally present (236,239).

The primary finding in Chandler's syndrome is corneal edema, which ranges from asymptomatic stromal edema to painful bullous keratopathy (Fig. 47-13). Specular microscopy demonstrates characteristic ICE cells. The remaining endothelial cells have abnormal shape and size and increased intracellular spacing. Iris atrophy is minimal and typically limited to the stroma, without formation of iris holes (218,240). Peripheral anterior synechiae may also occur later in the course of the disease. Intraocular pressure may be normal or only slightly elevated. Trabeculectomy specimens from eyes with Chandler's syndrome have demonstrated Descemet's membrane extending across the trabecular meshwork, as seen in essential iris atrophy (240).

The last disease in the ICE syndrome, iris nevus syndrome, shows elevated, pigmented nodules of varying sizes on the anterior iris surface. The disease is misnamed, as there are actually no nevus cells within the iris nodules. The nodules usually occur late in the disease after changes of essential iris atrophy have been present for years (241). Endothelialization of the iris leads to loss of normal iris crypts and gives the underlying iris stroma its characteristic matted appearance (218). The nodules, which initially appear as fine, light-tan protrusions on the iris surface, are composed of iris stromal melanocytes that project through fenestra in the membrane produced by the abnormal endothelium, simulating nevi (242). Early lesions have been misdiagnosed as malignant melanoma, resulting in enucleation (243). The nodules eventually increase in number and assume a dark brown color. Because the appearance of the nodules coincides with extension of the endothelium over the iris surface,

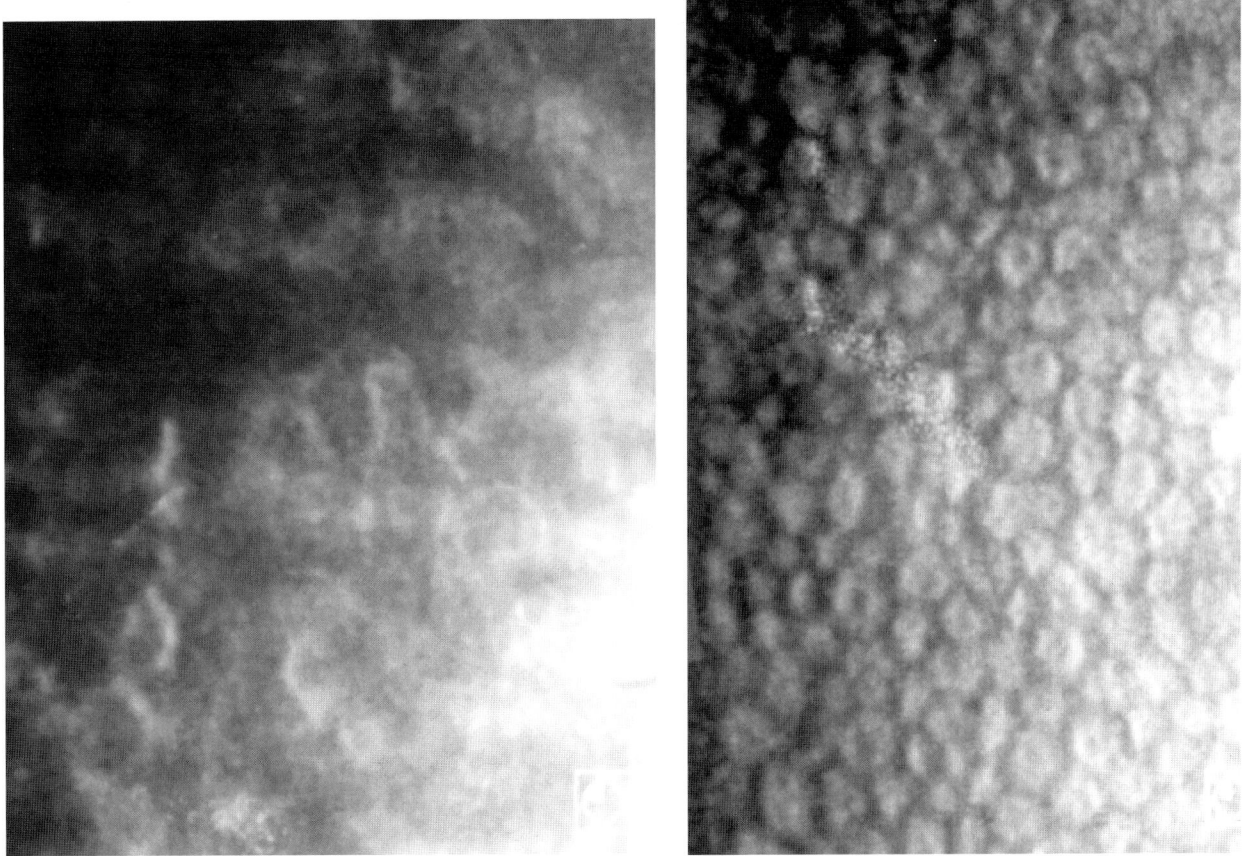

FIGURE 47-12. A: Specular micrograph of ICE syndrome showing dark-light reversal diagnostic for ICE cells. The endothelial mosaic is markedly disrupted. **B:** Contralateral (uninvolved) eye of patient in **(A)** showing normal endothelial mosaic.

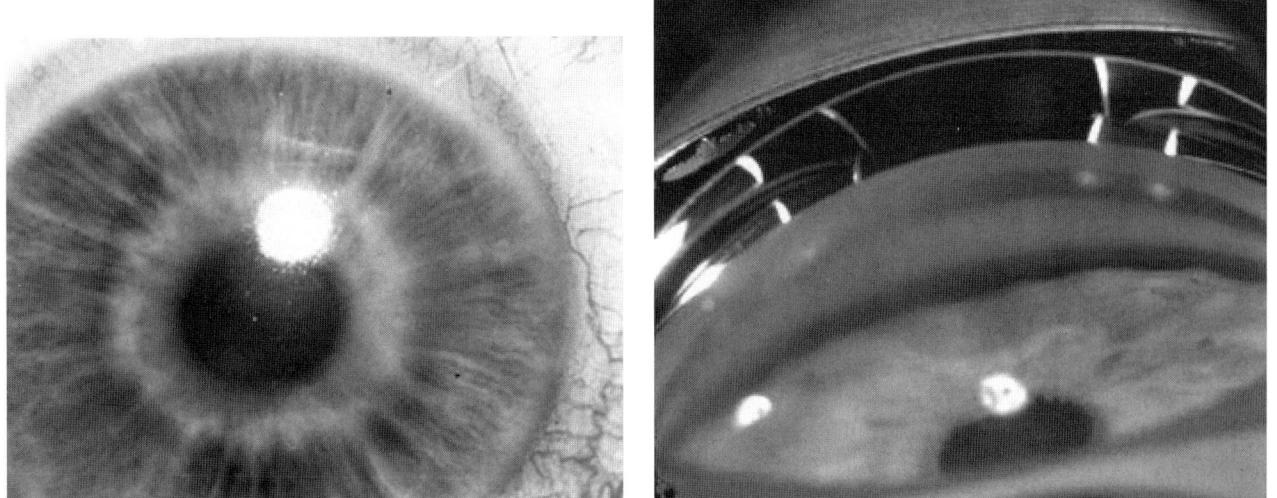

FIGURE 47-13. A: Chandler's variant of ICE syndrome. Patients may complain of decreased vision from corneal edema. Iris abnormalities are typically minimal. **B:** Chandler's syndrome. Peripheral anterior synechiae are usually subtle and visible only with gonioscopy.

one can monitor the abnormal growth of the endothelium by noting the topographic progression of the iris nodules and the effacement of normal iris architecture (238,244).

Although the three forms of the ICE syndrome vary in their degree of corneal, angle, and iris abnormalities, they share many common features. Although it is important to distinguish ICE syndrome from other conditions, such as PPMD or iris melanoma, it is less important to differentiate among the three ICE syndrome subgroups. In contrast, it is of greater importance to try to predict those cases likely to develop glaucoma. Clearly, eyes with large amounts of synechial angle closure have a higher risk of glaucoma. Another potential risk factor is the degree of corneal endothelial abnormality. Elevation in intraocular pressure eventually almost always accompanies diffuse involvement of the endothelium. On the other hand, if only a portion of the endothelium has the characteristic abnormal hammered-silver appearance, the IOP is more likely to remain normal (234).

Histopathology

Histopathologic findings in ICE syndrome overlap with those seen in the other diseases of the corneal endothelium. Endothelial atrophy and degeneration are predominant features (224,239,235). Extensive endothelial cell loss is found in advanced cases of ICE with irreversible corneal edema (245,246). Abnormal endothelial cells assume epithelial features, such as surface microvilli, desmosomes, and loss of contact inhibition (204,208,224,235,246,247). Sheets of these epithelial-like endothelial cells have been found in the anterior chamber (235). These cells are believed to be the histologic equivalent of the ICE cells demonstrated by the specular microscopy (235,248). Cellular pleomorphism is common. The abnormal cells are more conical than normal endothelial cells. They lack tight junctions, but do have numerous desmosomal connections in the intercellular junctions. The lateral intercellular borders have much more complex interdigitations than normal endothelial cells (235). These interlocking "fingerlike" processes at the apical intercellular borders are more prominent in Chandler's syndrome than in the other ICE variants. This feature may inhibit the migration of the abnormal endothelium over the angle, and may underlie the decreased incidence of glaucoma in Chandler's syndrome (231).

Other cell types are present in ICE syndrome endothelium, including cells with normal endothelial morphology, fibroblast-like cells, and inflammatory cells (239,235,249). Abnormal necrotic cells, inflammatory cells, and fibroblast-like cells can be seen interspersed throughout areas that contain endothelial cells with normal morphology (235). Fibroblast-like cells likely result from a nonspecific metaplastic transformation, similar to that observed in end-stage FED and after corneal endothelial injury (54,235,250). Corneal guttae are not found in ICE syndrome (251).

Descemet's membrane is often abnormal in ICE syndrome (249,251). Several distinct morphologic patterns have been identified. In the most common pattern, both the anterior banded and the posterior nonbanded layers appear normal. However, an abnormal posterior collagenous layer is found posterior to Descemet's membrane. The posterior collagenous layer is a bilayer composed of widely spaced collagen and microfibrils (251). The overall thickness of Descemet's membrane is increased because of the presence of the posterior collagenous layer. In the second pattern, the anterior banded zone is abnormal, with marked disruption or absence of its widely spaced collagen (251). This pattern, in which only one layer of Descemet's membrane is missing, is unique and may result from abnormal turnover and removal of the widely spaced collagen, possibly secondary to abnormal secretion of proteolytic enzymes (193,251). Finally, some ICE specimens retain normal Descemet's membrane morphology (251).

Pathophysiology

ICE syndrome, a primary disorder of the corneal endothelium, is characterized by proliferation and migration of abnormal endothelium onto the trabecular meshwork and iris, with secondary secretion of abnormal extracellular material. Several lines of evidence support this mechanism. First, the endothelial cells in affected eyes shows marked morphologic abnormalities, including pleomorphism and polymegathism. Second, ectopic endothelium has been found on the trabecular meshwork and anterior iris in histology specimens from patients with ICE syndrome (246). However, the underlying stimulus for these endothelial changes remains a mystery. A variety of hypotheses have been proposed to explain the pathogenesis of ICE syndrome, including neural crest cell abnormalities, embryonic ectopia, metaplasia, and infection with either herpes simplex or Epstein-Barr virus (40,252–255).

Neural crest–derived cells give rise to the connective tissues between the lens and the corneal epithelium, including the iris (41). During embryogenesis, these neural crest cells form a continuous layer extending from the corneal endothelium to the trabecular meshwork and onto the anterior iris surface (256). This continuity is lost between the seventh and eighth month of gestation (256). It has been proposed that ICE syndrome may result from abnormal neural crest cell proliferation during embryogenesis (40). During embryogenesis, some of these neural crest–derived cells may persist as "nests" of undifferentiated, inactive mesenchymal cells on the corneal endothelium, trabecular meshwork, or anterior iris (252). With appropriate stimulation, these nests of cells become activated and begin to proliferate, migrate, and produce abnormal basement membrane. The location of the activated cells might determine which clinical manifestation is seen, thus accounting for the different forms of ICE syndrome (252).

Another theory suggests that ICE cells arise as a result of embryonic ectopia or metaplasia (207). ICE cells are known to possess epithelial qualities (235,248). They express cytokeratin (CK) 19, a marker that is strongly expressed by limbal epithelium, but is not typically found in normal corneal epithelium or endothelium (207). Heterotopia or misplacement of limbal epithelium during anterior segment morphogenesis might explain these observations. The delayed onset of clinical disease in ICE syndrome may be secondary to the small number or low mitotic rate of the ectopic cells. A precipitating factor, such as viral infection, might be the stimulus required to trigger proliferation (207). Alternatively, ICE cells may result from metaplastic transformation of corneal endothelial cells to an epithelial phenotype, initiated by some insult, possibly viral infection (207). Metaplasia is consistent with the adult onset, predominant unilateral, and acquired nature of the disease.

ICE syndrome has been associated with herpes simplex virus-1 (HSV-1). HSV DNA has been localized within endothelial cells in ICE syndrome by polymerase chain reaction, whereas it was not detected in normal corneas or in other chronic nonviral corneal diseases (254). HSV DNA has also been found in the aqueous humor of a patient with ICE syndrome (255). Other disease findings that support a viral etiology include occasional chronic iridocyclitis (239) and inflammatory cells within the endothelium (246). A significant number of patients have documented conjunctival hyperemia before the onset of ICE syndrome (254). Although suggestive, none of these findings provides definitive evidence that herpes simplex causes the ICE syndrome (257).

High titers of antibodies to Epstein-Barr virus (EBV) antigens have been found in patients with ICE syndrome (253). These elevated titers likely represent EBV reactivation, which may be either a marker for cellular immune dysfunction or a representation of a role for EBV in the pathogenesis of the syndrome. A viral etiology for the ICE syndrome is consistent with the acute onset with rapid progression, occasional signs of mild inflammation, and the characteristic unilateral expression of the disease. As evidenced by the diversity of hypothesized etiologies for the ICE syndrome, the true cause of these diseases has yet to be defined.

Management

The management of ICE syndrome depends on the disease manifestations and an individual patient's symptoms. Glaucoma is common and often difficult to treat in all variants of ICE syndrome. Medical management succeeds only temporarily. Surgical intervention is often required (258). Laser trabeculoplasty is not effective in ICE syndrome mainly due to progressive angle closure with continued endothelialization of the trabecular meshwork. Trabeculectomy outcomes vary from poor to nearly comparable to that of age-matched controls with primary open-angle glaucoma (259). Bleb failure is a common sequela of disease progression. Use of intraoperative mitomycin C may help improve the success rate of filtering surgery in ICE patients (260). Glaucoma drainage implants have been used with some success in patients with ICE syndrome, although revisions and tube repositionings are common (261).

When mild corneal edema occurs in ICE syndrome, topical hyperosmotics may be used. Lowering of the intraocular pressure can also facilitate corneal deturgescence if some endothelial function still exists. The pressure can be lowered either medically or surgically (220). In the setting of complete endothelial dysfunction, however, edema can persist even at a low intraocular pressure (239). Penetrating keratoplasty then becomes the treatment of choice. In general, penetrating keratoplasty is a safe and effective means to improve vision and relieve pain in ICE syndrome, although some patients may require multiple corneal and glaucoma procedures.

The overall prognosis for keratoplasty in ICE syndrome is favorable, with graft survival rates ranging from 83% to 100% (262–265). Extensive iris disease and glaucoma reduce the chance of successful transplantation (263,265). Postoperative vision better than 20/40 has been achieved in a majority of patients in most reported series (262,264,265). Penetrating keratoplasty is very successful in relieving painful bullous keratopathy (262). Although a hammered-silver endothelial appearance had been observed postoperatively, no definitive evidence of recurrence of ICE syndrome has been reported (262,264).

As expected, glaucoma is a prominent feature in many ICE patients requiring penetrating keratoplasty (262–265). The importance of aggressive pressure control to ensure long-term graft clarity cannot be overstated. Glaucoma surgery should precede corneal transplantation if objective glaucomatous changes are present. Adequate control of glaucoma is often the major factor in determining final visual outcome in patients with ICE syndrome undergoing keratoplasty.

The efficacy of peripheral anterior synechialysis at the time of penetrating keratoplasty is not proven, as it has not been shown to prevent the progression of synechial angle closure (218,262,265). Similarly, the effect of posterior chamber intraocular lens implantation on the abnormal endothelialization in the anterior chamber has not been studied, although no adverse effect was observed in one patient who underwent a corneal triple procedure (263). It would seem inherently prudent to avoid anterior chamber intraocular lenses in patients with ICE syndrome. It is usually not necessary to treat iris atrophy or corectopia. However, if pupillary distortion is sufficiently severe to interfere with vision, a surgical or Nd:YAG laser iridoplasty may be considered to close the peripheral iris defect or to create a pupillary opening within the visual axis.

CONCLUSIONS

The endotheliopathies are a diverse group of disorders with a wide variety of clinical manifestations. A primary dysfunction of the corneal endothelium underlies all of these conditions. Similarities and differences in the characteristic features of these diseases are summarized in Table 47-1. Despite the fact that several of these disorders were described almost 100 years ago, little is known about the etiology of any of the corneal endotheliopathies. Surgical treatment of these conditions has an overall good success rate, although glaucoma can complicate their management. Novel surgical techniques for selective endothelial replacement hold promise for future treatment, as do basic science advances into the underlying causes of these enigmatic diseases.

REFERENCES

1. Thompson DW. The forms of tissues on cell-aggregates. In: Bonner JT, ed. *On growth and form.* Cambridge: Cambridge University Press, 1982:88–119.
2. Rao GN, Lohman LE, Aquavella JV. Cell-size-shape relationships in corneal endothelium. *Invest Ophthalmol Vis Sci* 1982; 22:271–274.
3. Honda H. Geometrical models for cells in tissues. Int Rev Cytol 1983;81:191–248.
4. Hodson S. Evidence for a bicarbonate-dependent sodium pump in corneal endothelium. *Exp Eye Res* 1971;11:20–29.
5. Egan CA, Saver-Train I, Shay JW, et al. Analysis of telomere lengths in human corneal endothelial cells from donors of different ages. *Invest Ophthalmol Vis Sci* 1998;39: 648–653.
6. Senoo T, Joyce NC. Cell cycle kinetics in corneal endothelium from old and young donors. *Invest Ophthalmol Vis Sci* 2000;41: 660–667.
7. Joyce NC, Meklir B, Joyce SJ, et al. Cell cycle protein expression and proliferative status in human corneal cells. *Invest Ophthalmol Vis Sci* 1996;37:645–755.
8. Chen KH, Azar D, Joyce NC. Transplantation of adult human corneal endothelium ex vivo: a morphologic study. *Cornea* 2001;20:731–737.
9. Laing RA. In vivo photomicrography of the corneal endothelium. *Arch Ophthalmol* 1975;93:143–145.
10. Murphy C, Alvarado J, Juster R, et al. Prenatal and postnatal cellularity of the human corneal endothelium. *Invest Ophthalmol Vis Sci* 1984;25:312–322.
11. Laule A, Cable MK, Hoffman CE, et al. Endothelial cell population changes of human cornea during life. *Arch Ophthalmol* 1978;96:2031–2035.
12. Hoffer KJ, Kraff MC. Normal endothelial cell count range. *Ophthalmology* 1980;87:861–865.
13. Waltman SR. Penetrating keratoplasty for pseudophakic bullous keratopathy. *Arch Ophthalmol* 1981;99:415–416.
14. Laing RA, Sandstrom M, Berrospi AR, et al. Morphological changes in corneal endothelial cells after penetrating keratoplasty. *Am J Ophthalmol* 1976;82:459–464.
15. Hoffer KJ. Corneal decompensation after corneal endothelium cell count. *Am J Ophthalmol* 1979;87:252–253.
16. Treffers WF. Human corneal endothelial wound repair. *In vitro* and *in vivo. Ophthalmology* 1982;89:605–613.
17. Amann J, Holley GP, Lee SB, et al. Increased endothelial cell density in the paracentral and peripheral regions of the human cornea. *Am J Ophthalmol* 2003;135:584–590.
18. Olsen T. On the significance of a low endothelial cell density in Fuchs' endothelial dystrophy. A specular microscopic study. *Acta Ophthalmol* 1980;58:111–116.
19. American Academy of Ophthalmology. Ophthalmic procedures assessment: corneal endothelial photography. *Ophthalmology* 1991;98:1464–1468.
20. Rao GN, Aquavella JV, Goldberg SH, et al. Pseudophakic bullous keratopathy: relationship to preoperative corneal endothelial status. *Ophthalmology* 1984;91:1135–1140.
21. Bergmann L, Hartmann C, Renard G, et al. Damage to the corneal endothelium caused by radial keratotomy. *Fortschr Ophthalmol* 1991;88:368–373.
22. Bourne WM, O'Fallon WM. Endothelial cell loss during penetrating keratoplasty. *Am J Ophthalmol* 1978;85:760–766.
23. Liesegang TJ. The response of the corneal endothelium to intraocular surgery. *Refract Corneal Surg* 1991;7:81–86.
24. Sobottka Ventura AC, Walti R, et al. Corneal thickness and endothelial density before and after cataract surgery. *Br J Ophthalmol* 2001;85:18–20.
25. Inoue K, Tokuda Y, Inoue Y, et al. Corneal endothelial cell morphology in patients undergoing cataract surgery. *Cornea* 2002;21:360–363.
26. Olsen T, Eriksen JS. Corneal thickness and endothelial damage after intraocular lens implantation. *Acta Ophthalmol* 1980;58: 773–786.
27. Eleftheriadis H, Cheong M, Sandeman S, et al. Corneal toxicity secondary to inadvertent use of benzalkonium chloride preserved viscoelastic material in cataract surgery. *Br J Ophthalmol* 2002;86:299–305.
28. Hull DS, Chemotti MT, Edelhauser HF, et al. Effect of epinephrine on the corneal endothelium. *Am J Ophthalmol* 1975; 79:245–250.
29. Karai I, Matsumura S, Takise S, et al. Morphological changes in the corneal endothelium due to ultraviolet radiation in welders. *Br J Ophthalmol* 1984;68:544–548.
30. Doughty MJ, Oriowo OM, Cullen AP. Morphometry of the corneal endothelium in glassblowers compared to non-glassblowers. *J Photochem Photobiol B Biol* 2002;67:130–138.
31. Meyer KT, Pettit TH, Straatsma BR. Corneal endothelial damage with neodynium–YAG laser. *Ophthalmology* 1984;91: 1022–1027.
32. Burns RR, Bourne WM, Brubaker RF. Endothelial function in patients with cornea guttata. *Invest Ophthalmol Vis Sci* 1981; 20:77–85.
33. Brooks AMV, Grant G, Gillies WE. A comparison of corneal endothelial morphology in cornea guttata, Fuchs' dystrophy and bullous keratopathy. *Aust N Z J Ophthalmol* 1988;16:93–100.
34. Schultz RO, Matsuda M, Yee RW, et al. Corneal endothelial changes in type I and type II diabetes mellitus. *Am J Ophthalmol.* 1984;98:401–410.
35. Gagnon MM, Boisjoly HM, Brunette I, et al. Corneal endothelial cell density in glaucoma. *Cornea* 1997;16:314–318.
36. Waring GO, Font RL, Rodrigues MM, et al. Alternations of Descemet's membrane in interstitial keratitis. *Am J Ophthalmol* 1976;81:773–785.
37. Nieuwendaal CP, Odental MTP, Kok JHC, et al. Morphology and function of corneal endothelium after long term contact lens wear. *Invest Ophthalmol Vis Sci* 1994;35:3071–3077.
38. Chang SW, Hu FR, Lin LL. Effects of contact lenses on corneal endothelium–a morphological and functional study. *Ophthalmologica* 2001;215:197–203.
39. Waring GO III, Rodrigues MM, Laibson PR. Corneal dystrophies. II. Endothelial dystrophies. *Surv Ophthalmol* 1978;23: 147–168.
40. Bahn CF, Falls HF, Varley BS, et al. Classification of corneal endothelial disorders based on neural crest origin. *Ophthalmology* 1984;91:558–563.
41. Johnston MC. The neural crest in abnormalities of the face and brain. *Birth Defects* 1975;11:1–18.

42. Adamis AP, Filatov V, Tripathi BJ, et al. Fuchs' endothelial dystrophy of the cornea. *Surv Ophthalmol* 1993;38:149–167.

43. Brady SE, Rapuano CJ, Arentsen JJ, et al. Clinical indications for and procedures associated with penetrating keratoplasty, 1983–1988. *Am J Ophthalmol* 1989;108:118–122.

44. Lindquist TD, McGlothan JS, Rotkis WM, et al. Indications for penetrating keratoplasty: 1980–1988. *Cornea* 1991;10:210–216.

45. Fuchs E. Dystrophia epithelialis corneae. *Graefes Arch Klin Exp Ophthalmol* 1910;76:478–508.

46. Koeppe L. Klinische Beobachtungen mit der Nernstspaltlampe und dem Hornhautmikroskop (German). *Graefes Arch Klin Exp Ophthalmol* 1916;91:363–379.

47. Vogt A. Weitere Ergebnisse der Spaltlampenmikroskopie des vordern Bulbusabschnittes (German). *Graefes Arch Klin Exp Ophthalmol* 1921;106:63–103.

48. Kraupa E. Pigmentierung der Hornhauthinterflache bei "Dystrophia epithelialis (Fuchs)" (German). *Z Augenheilkd* 1920;44:247–250.

49. Graves B. A bilateral chronic affection of the endothelial face of the cornea of elderly persons with an account of the technical and clinical principles of its slit-lamp observation. *Br J Ophthalmol* 1924;8:502–544.

50. Kirby DB. Excrescences of the central area of Descemet's membrane. *Arch Ophthalmol* 1925;54:588–591.

51. Friedenwald H, Friedenwald JS. Epithelial dystrophy of the cornea. *Br J Ophthalmol* 1925;9:14–20.

52. Iwamoto T, DeVoe AG. Electron microscopic studies on Fuchs' combined dystrophy. I. Posterior portion of the cornea. *Invest Ophthalmol* 1971;10:4–28.

53. Iwamoto T, DeVoe AG. Electron microscopic studies on Fuchs' combined dystrophy. II. Anterior portion of the cornea. *Invest Ophthalmol* 1971;10:29–40.

54. Pollack FM. The posterior corneal surface in Fuchs' dystrophy. Scanning electron microscope study. *Invest Ophthalmol* 1974;13:913–922.

55. Borboli S, Colby K. Mechanisms of disease: Fuchs' endothelial dystrophy. *Ophthalmol Clin North Am* 2002;15:17–25.

56. Cross HE, Maumenee AE, Cantolino SJ. Inheritance of Fuchs' endothelial dystrophy. *Arch Ophthalmol* 1971;85:268–272.

57. Krachmer JH, Purcell JJ, Young CW, et al. Corneal endothelial dystrophy. *Arch Ophthalmol* 1978;96:2035–2039.

58. Magoven M, Beauchamp GR, McTigue JW, et al. Inheritance of Fuchs' combined dystrophy. *Ophthalmology* 1979;86:1897–1923.

59. Rosenblum P, Stark WJ, Maumenee IH. Hereditary Fuchs' dystrophy. *Am J Ophthalmol* 1980;90:455–462.

60. Dobbins KRB, Price FW, Whitson WE. Trends in the indications for penetrating keratoplasty in the Midwestern United States. *Cornea* 2000;19:813–816.

61. Maeno A, Naor J, Lee HM, et al. Three decades of corneal transplantation: indications and patient characteristics. *Cornea* 2000;19:7–11.

62. Olsen T. Is there an association between Fuchs' endothelial dystrophy and cardiovascular disease? *Graefes Arch Clin Exp Ophthalmol* 1984;221:239–240.

63. Lipman RM, Rubenstein JB, Torcznski E. Keratoconus and Fuchs' corneal endothelial dystrophy in a patient and her family. *Arch Ophthalmol* 1990;108:993.

64. Orlin SE, Raber IM, Eagle RC, et al. Keratoconus associated with corneal endothelial dystrophy. *Cornea* 1990;9:299.

65. Rao GP, Kaye SB, Agius-Fernandez A. Central corneal endothelial guttae and age-related macular degeneration: is there an association? *Indian J Ophthalmol* 1998;46:601–604.

66. Pitts JF, Jay JL. The association of Fuchs' corneal endothelial dystrophy with axial hypermetropia, shallow anterior chamber, and angle closure glaucoma. *Br J Ophthalmol* 1990;74:601.

67. Buxton JN, Preson RW, Riechers R, et al. Tonography in cornea guttata: a preliminary report. *Arch Ophthalmol* 1967;77:602–603.

68. Roberts CW, Steinert RF, Thomas JV, et al. Endothelial guttata and the facility of aqueous outflow. *Cornea* 1984;3:5.

69. Wilson SE, Bourne WM. Fuchs' dystrophy. Cornea 1988;7:2–18.

70. Lorenzetti DWC, Votila MH, Parikh N, et al. Central cornea guttata. *Am J Ophthalmol* 1967;64:1155–1158.

71. Johnson DH, Bourne WM, Campbell RJ. The ultrastructure of Descemet's membrane. I. Changes with age in normal corneas. *Arch Ophthalmol* 1982;100:1942–1947.

72. Bourne WM, Johnson DH, Campbell RJ. The ultrastructure of Descemet's membrane. III. Fuchs' dystrophy. *Arch Ophthalmol* 1982;100:1952–1955.

73. Rodrigues MM, Krachmer JH, Hackett J, et al. Fuchs' corneal dystrophy. A clinicopathologic study of the variation in corneal edema. *Ophthalmology* 1986;93:789.

74. Alexander RA, Grierson I, Garner A. Oxytalan fibers in Fuchs' endothelial dystrophy. *Arch Ophthalmol* 1981;99:1622–1627.

75. Polack FM. The posterior corneal surface in Fuchs' dystrophy. Scanning electron microscope study. *Invest Ophthalmol* 1974;13:913.

76. Hogan MJ, Wood I, Fine M. Fuchs' endothelial dystrophy of the cornea. *Am J Ophthalmol* 1974;78:363–383.

77. Kayes J, Holmberg A. The fine structure of the cornea in Fuchs' endothelial dystrophy. *Invest Ophthalmol* 1964;3:47–67.

78. Bigar F. Specular microscopy of the corneal endothelium. Optical solutions and clinical results. *Dev Ophthalmol* 1982;6:1–94.

79. Bron AJ, Tripathi RC. Cystic disorders of the corneal epithelium. I. Corneal aspects. *Br J Ophthalmol* 1973;57:361–375.

80. Tripathi RC, Bron AJ. Cystic disorders of the corneal epithelium. II. Pathogenesis. *Br J Ophthalmol* 1973;57:376–390.

81. Geroski DH, et al. Pump function of the human corneal endothelium. *Ophthalmology* 1985;92:759.

82. McCartney MD, Wood TO, McLaughlin BJ. Moderate Fuchs' endothelial dystrophy ATPase pumpsite density. *Invest Ophthalmol Vis Sci* 1989;30:1560.

83. Stanley JA. Water permeability of the human cornea. *Arch Ophthalmol* 1972;87:568.

84. Waltman SR, Kaufman HE. *In vivo* studies of human corneal endothelial permeability. *Am J Ophthalmol* 1970;70:45.

85. Wilson SE, Bourne WM, O'Brien PC, et al. Endothelial function and aqueous humor flow rate in patients with Fuchs' dystrophy. *Am J Ophthalmol* 1988;106:270–278.

86. Bramsen T, Stenbjerg S. Fibrinolytic factors in aqueous humor and serum from patients with Fuchs' dystrophy and patients with cataract. *Acta Ophthalmol* 1979;57:470–476.

87. Kenney MC, Labermeier U, Hins D, et al. Characterization of the Descemet's membrane/posterior collagenous layer isolated from Fuchs' endothelial dystrophy corneas. *Exp Eye Res* 1984;39:267–277.

88. Bramsen T, Ehlers N. Bullous keratopathy (Fuchs' endothelial dystrophy) treated systemically with 4-trans-aminocyclohexano-carboxylic acid. *Acta Ophthalmol* 1977;55:665–673.

89. Rosenthal WN, Blitzer M, Insler MS. Aqueous amino acid levels in Fuchs' corneal dystrophy. *Am J Ophthalmol* 1986;102:570–574.

90. Biswas S, Munier FL, Yardley J, et al. Missense mutations in *COL8A2*, the gene encoding the alpha2 chain of type VIII collagen, cause two forms of corneal endothelial dystrophy. *Hum Mol Genet* 2001;10:2415–2423.

91. Borderie VM, Baudrimont M, Vallee A, et al. Corneal endothelial cell apoptosis in patients with Fuchs' dystrophy. *Invest Ophthalmol Vis Sci* 2000;41:2501–2505.

92. Li QJ, Ashraf F, Shen DF, et al. The role of apoptosis in the pathogenesis of Fuchs endothelial dystrophy of the cornea. *Arch Ophthalmol* 2001;119:1597–1604.

93. Thalmann-Goetsch A, Engelmann K, Bednarz J. Comparative study on the effects of different growth factors on migration of bovine corneal endothelial cells during wound healing. *Acad Ophthalmol Scand* 1997;75:490–495.

94. Senoo T, Takahashi K, Chiba K, et al. Stimulation of corneal endothelial cell proliferation by interleukins, complete mitogens and corneal parenchymal cell-derived factors. *Nippon Gakkai Zasshi* 1996;100:845–852.

95. Tuberville AW, Wood TO, McLaughlin BJ. Cytochrome oxidase activity of Fuchs' endothelial dystrophy. *Curr Eye Res* 1986;5:939–947.

96. Johns DR. Mitochondrial DNA and disease. *N Engl J Med* 1995;333:638–644.

97. DiMauro S, Moraes CT. Mitochondrial encephalomyopathies. *Arch Neurol* 1993;50:1197–1208.

98. Ohkoshi K, Ishida N, Yamaguchi T, et al. Corneal endothelium in a case of mitochondrial encephalomyopathy (Kearns–Sayre syndrome). *Cornea* 1989;8:210–214.

99. Kosmorsky GS, Meisler DM, Sheeler LR, et al. Familial ophthalmolplegia-plus syndrome with corneal endothelial disorder. *Neuro–Ophthalmology* 1989;9:271–277.

100. Chang TS, Johns DR, Walker D, et al. Ocular clinicopathologic study of the mitochondrial encephalomyopathy overlap syndromes. *Arch Ophthalmol* 1993;111:1254–1262.

101. Albin RL. Fuchs' corneal dystrophy in a patient with mitochondrial DNA mutations. *J Med Genet* 1998;35:258–259.

102. Liesegang TJ. Physiologic changes of the cornea with contact lens wear. *CLAO J* 2002;28:12–27.

103. Nguyen T, Soni PS, Brizendine E, et al. Variability in hypoxia-induced corneal swelling is associated with variability in corneal metabolism and endothelial function. *Eye Contact Lens* 2003;29:117–125.

104. Konowal A, Morrison JC, Brown SV, et al. Irreversible corneal decompensation in patients treated with topical dorzolamide. *Am J Ophthalmol* 1999;127:403–406.

105. Wilson SE, Bourne WM. Effect of dexamethasone on corneal endothelial function in Fuchs' dystrophy. *Invest Ophthalmol Vis Sci* 1987;28(suppl):326.

106. Fine M, West CE. Late results of keratoplasty for Fuchs' dystrophy. *Am J Ophthalmol* 1971;72:109–114.

107. Payant JA, Gordon LW, VanderZwaag R, et al. Cataract formation following corneal transplantation in eyes with Fuchs' endothelial dystrophy. *Cornea* 1990;9:286–289.

108. Olsen T, Ehlers N, Favini E. Long–term results of corneal grafting in Fuchs' endothelial dystrophy. *Acta Ophthalmol* 1984;62:445–452.

109. Sharif KW, Casey TA. Penetrating keratoplasty for keratoconus: complications and long–term success. *Br J Ophthalmol* 1991;75:142–146.

110. Pineros O, Cohen EJ, Rapuano CJ, et al. Long–term results after penetrating keratoplasty for Fuchs' endothelial dystrophy. *Arch Ophthalmol* 1996;114:15–18.

111. Price FW, Whitson WE, Marks RG. Graft survival in four common groups of patients undergoing penetrating keratoplasty. *Ophthalmology* 1991;98:322–328.

112. Price FW, Whitson WE, Marks RG. Progression of visual acuity after penetrating keratoplasty. *Ophthalmology* 1991;98:1177–1185.

113. Langenbucher A, Seitz B, Nguyen NX, et al. Corneal endothelial cell loss after nonmechanical penetrating keratoplasty depends on diagnosis: a regression analysis. *Graefes Arch Clin Exp Ophthalmol* 2002;240:387–392.

114. Reinhard T, Bohringer D, Huschen D, et al. Chronic endothelial cell loss of the graft after penetrating keratoplasty: influence of endothelial cell migration from graft to host. *Klin Monatsbl Augenheilkd* 2002;219:410–416.

115. Arentsen JJ. Corneal transplant allograft rejection: possible predisposing factors. *Trans Am Ophthalmol Soc* 1983;81:361–402.

116. Martin TP, Reed JW, Legault C, et al. Cataract formation and cataract extraction after penetrating keratoplasty. *Ophthalmology* 1994;101:113–119.

117. Pineros OE, Cohen EJ, Rapuano CJ, et al. Triple vs. nonsimultaneous procedures in Fuchs' dystrophy and cataract. *Arch Ophthalmol* 1996;114:525–528.

118. Shimmura S, Ohashi Y, Shiroma H, et al. Corneal opacity and cataract: triple procedure versus secondary approach. *Cornea* 2003;22:234–238.

119. Riddle H, Parker D, Price F. Management of post-keratoplasty astigmatism. *Curr Opin Ophthalmol* 1998;9:15–28.

120. VanRooij J, Christo G, Geerards A. Long term follow-up and suture related complications after penetrating keratoplasty with nylon sutures. *Invest Ophthalmol Vis Sci* 1998;40:S633.

121. Azar DT, Jain S, Sambursky R, et al. Microkeratome-assisted posterior keratoplasty. *J Cataract Refract Surg* 2001;27:353–356.

122. Busin M, Arffa RC, Sebastinani A. Endokeratoplasty as an alternative to penetrating keratoplasty for the surgical treatment of diseased endothelium. *Ophthalmology* 2000;107:2077–2082.

123. Melles GR, Lander F, van Dooren BT, et al. Preliminary clinical results of posterior lamellar keratoplasty through a sclerocorneal pocket incision. *Ophthalmology* 2000;107:1850–1856.

124. Shiuey Y, Moshirfar M. Use of infant donor tissue for endokeratoplasty. *J Cataract Refract Surg* 2001;27:1915–1918.

125. Melles GRJ, Lander F, Nieuwendaal C. Sutureless, posterior lamellar keratoplasty: a case report of a modified technique. *Cornea* 2002;21:325–327.

126. Melles GRJ, Lander F, Rietveld FJR. Transplantation of Descemet's membrane carrying viable endothelium through a small scleral incision. *Cornea* 2002;21:415–418.

127. Terry MA, Ousley PJ. Replacing the endothelium without corneal surface incisions or sutures: the first United States clinical series using the deep lamellar endothelial keratoplasty procedure. *Ophthalmology* 2003;110:755–764.

128. Guell JL, Velasco F, Guerrero E, et al. Preliminary results with posterior lamellar keratoplasty for endothelial failure. *Br J Ophthalmol* 2003;87:241–243.

129 Yue BYJT, Sugar J, Gilboy JE, et al. Growth of human corneal endothelial cells in culture. *Invest Ophthalmol Vis Sci* 1989;30:248–253.

130. Engelmann K, Bohnke M, Friedl P. Isolation and long-term cultivation of human corneal endothelial cells. *Invest Ophthalmol Vis Sci* 1988;29:1656–1662.

131. Blake DA, Yu H, Young DL, et al. Matrix stimulates the proliferation of human corneal endothelial cells in culture. *Invest Ophthalmol Vis Sci* 1997;38:1119–1129.

132. Engelmann K, Friedl P. Optimization of culture conditions for human corneal endothelial cells. *Invest Ophthalmol Vis Sci* 1989;25:1065–1072.

133. Engelmann K, Friedl P. Growth of human corneal endothelial cells in a serum-reduced medium. *Cornea* 1995;14:62–70.

134. Samples JR, Binder PS, Nayak SK. Propagation of human corneal endothelium in vitro effect of growth factors. *Exp Eye Res* 1991;52:121–128.

135. Schultz G, Cipolla L, Whitehouse A, et al. Growth factors and corneal endothelial cells: III. Stimulation of adult human corneal endothelial cell mitosis *in vitro* by defined mitogenic agents. *Cornea* 1992;11:20–27.

136. Engelmann K, Drexler D, Bohnke M. Transplantation of adult human or porcine corneal endothelial cells onto human recipients in vitro. Part I: cell culturing and transplantation procedure. *Cornea* 1999;18:199–206.

137. Bohnke M, Eggli P, Engelmann K. Transplantation of adult human or porcine corneal endothelial cells onto human recipients in vitro. Part II: evaluation in the scanning electron microscope. *Cornea* 1999;18:207–213.

138. Woost PG, Jumblatt MM Eiferman RA, et al. Growth factors and corneal endothelial cells. I. Stimulations of bovine corneal endothelial cell DNA synthesis by defined growth factors. *Cornea* 1992;11:1–10.

139. Hoppenreijs VPT, Pels E, Vrensen GFJM, et al. Corneal endothelium and growth factors. *Surv Ophthalmol* 1996;41:155–164.

140. Laurence GZ. *Klin Monatsbl Augenheilkd* 1863:351 (cited by Pearce [147]).

141. Armaignac M. Almost complete congenital opacities of both corneas in two children of the same family. *Arch Ophthalmol* 1911;31:468.

142. Komoto J. Congenital hereditary opacities of the cornea. *Klin Monatsbl Augenh* 1909;47:445–446.

143. Fischer FP, Ancona S. Familial congenital opacities of the cornea. *Acta Ophthalmol* 1936;14:406.

144. Turpin R, Tisserand M, Serane J. Hereditary and congenital corneal opacities divided on three generations and involving two monozygotic twins. *Arch Ophthalmol* 1939;3:109.

145. Maumenee AE. Congenital hereditary corneal dystrophy. *Am J Ophthalmol* 1960;50:1114–1124.

146. Kenyon KR, Maumenee AE. The histological and ultrastructural pathology of congenital hereditary corneal dystrophy: a case report. *Invest Ophthalmol* 1968;7:475.

147. Pearce WG, Tripathi RC, Morgan G. Congenital endothelial corneal dystrophy: clinical, pathological, and genetic study. *Br J Ophthalmol* 1969;53:577–591.

148. Antine B. Histology of congenital corneal dystrophy. *Am J Ophthalmol* 1970;69:964.

149. Kenyon KR, Antine B. The pathogenesis of congenital hereditary endothelial dystrophy of the cornea. *Am J Ophthalmol* 1971;72:787–795.

150. Goldberg MF. *Genetic and metabolic eye disease.* Boston: Little, Brown, 1974:305–306.

151. McKusick VA. *Mendelian inheritance in man*, 4th ed. Baltimore: Johns Hopkins University Press 1975:67,387.

152. Toma NMG, Ebenezer ND, Inglehearn CF, et al. Linkage of congenital hereditary endothelial dystrophy to chromosome 20. *Hum Mol Gen* 1995;4:2395–2398.

153. Witshcel H, Sundmacher R, Theopold H, et al. Posterior polymorphous dystrophy of the cornea: an unusual clinical variant. *Graefes Arch Clini Exp Ophthalmol* 1980;214:15–25.

154. Callaghan M, Hand CK, Kennedy SM, et al. Homozygosity mapping and linkage analysis demonstrate that autosomal recessive congenital hereditary endothelial dystrophy (CHED) and autosomal dominant CHED are genetically distinct. *Br J Ophthalmol* 1999;83:115–119.

155. Kanis AB, Al-Rajhi AA, Taylor CM, et al. Exclusion of AR-CHED from the chromosome 20 region containing the PPMD and AD-CHED loci. *Ophthalmic Genet* 1999;20:243–249.

156. Hand CK, Harmon DL, Kennedy SM, et al. Localization of the gene for autosomal recessive congenital hereditary endothelial dystrophy (CHED2) to chromosome 20 by homozygosity mapping. *Genomics* 1999;61:1–4.

157. Judisch GF, Maumenee IH. Clinical differentiation of recessive congenital hereditary endothelial dystrophy and dominant hereditary endothelial dystrophy. *Am J Ophthalmol* 1978;85:606–612.

158. Mahmood MA, Teichmann KD. Corneal amyloidosis associated with congenital hereditary endothelial dystrophy. *Cornea* 2000;19:570–573.

159. Vemuganti GK, Sridhar MS, Edward DP, et al. Subepithelial amyloid deposits in congenital hereditary endothelial dystrophy. *Cornea* 2002;21:524–529.

160. Keates RH, Cvintal T. Congenital hereditary corneal dystrophy. *Am J Ophthalmol* 1965;60:892–894.

161. Pedersen O, Rushood A, Olsen EG. Anterior mesenchymal dysgenesis of the eye. Congenital hereditary endothelial dystrophy and congenital glaucoma. *Acta Ophthalmol* 1989;67:470–476.

162. Mullaney PB, Risco JM, Teichmann K, et al. Congenital hereditary endothelial dystrophy associated with glaucoma. *Ophthalmology* 1995;102:186–192.

163. Cibis GW. Congenital glaucoma. *J Am Optom Assoc* 1987;58:728–733.

164. Harboyan G, Mamo J, Der Kaloustian V, et al. Congenital corneal dystrophy: progressive sensorineural deafness in a family. *Arch Ophthalmol* 1971;85:27–32.

165. Akhtar S, Bron AJ, Meek KM, et al. Congenital hereditary endothelial dystrophy and band keratopathy in an infant with corpus callosum agenesis. *Cornea* 2001;20:547–552.

166. Ehlers N, Modis L, Moller-Pedersen T. A morphological and functional study of congenital hereditary endothelial dystrophy. *Acta Ophthalmol Scand* 1998;76:314–318.

167. Moller-Pedersen T. A comparative study of human corneal keratocytes and endothelial cell density during aging. *Cornea* 1997;16:333–338.

168. Chan CC, Green WR, Barraquer J, et al. Similarities between posterior polymorphous and congenital hereditary endothelial dystrophies: a study of 14 buttons of 11 cases. *Cornea* 1982;1:155–172.

169. Kirkness CM, McCartney A, Rice NSC, et al. Congenital hereditary corneal edema of Maumenee: its clinical features, management, and pathology. *Br J Ophthalmol* 1987;71:130–144.

170. McCartney ACE, Kirkness CM. Comparison between posterior polymorphous dystrophy and congenital hereditary endothelial dystrophy of the cornea. *Eye* 1988;2:63–70.

171. Stainer GA, Akers PH, Binder PS, et al. Correlative microscopy and tissue culture of congenital hereditary endothelial dystrophy. *Am J Ophthalmol* 1982;93:456–465.

172. Kenyon KR, Maumenee AE. Further studies of congenital hereditary endothelial dystrophy of the cornea. *Am J Ophthalmol* 1973;76:419–439.

173. Kanai A, Waltman S, Polack F, et al. Electron microscopic study of hereditary corneal edema. *Invest Ophthalmol Vis Sci* 1971;10:89–99.

174. Dana MR, Moyes AL, Gomes JAP, et al. The indications for and outcome in pediatric keratoplasty: a multicenter study. *Ophthalmology* 1995;102:1129–1138.

175. Graham MAR, Azar NF, Dana MR. Visual rehabilitation in children with congenital hereditary endothelial dystrophy. *Int Ophthalmol Clin* 2001;41:9–18.

176. Frueh BE, Brown SI. Transplantation of congenitally opaque corneas. *Br J Ophthalmol* 1997;83:115–119.

177. Sajjadi H, Javadi MA, Hemmati R, et al. Results of penetrating keratoplasty in CHED: congenital hereditary endothelial dystrophy. *Cornea* 1995;14:18–25.

178. Al-Rajhi AA, Wagoner MD. Penetrating keratoplasty in congenital hereditary endothelial dystrophy. *Ophthalmology* 1997;104:956–961.

179. Koeppe L. Klinische Beobachtungen mit der Nernstspaltlampe und dem Hornhautmikroskop. *Graefes Arch Ophthalmol* 1916;91:375–379.

180. Levy SG, Moss J, Noble BA, et al. Early-onset posterior polymorphous dystrophy. *Arch Ophthalmol* 1996;114:1265.

181. Sekundo W, Lee WR, Kirkness CM, et al. An ultrastructural investigation of an early manifestation of the posterior polymorphous dystrophy of the cornea. *Ophthalmology* 1994;101:1422–1431.

182. Cibis GW, Krachmer JH, Phelps CD, et al. The clinical spectrum of posterior polymorphous dystrophy. *Arch Ophthalmol* 1977;95:1429–1537.

183. Pardos GJ, Krachmer JH, Mannis MJ. Posterior corneal vesicles. *Arch Ophthalmol* 1981;99:1573.

184. Laganowski HC, Sherrard ES, Kerr Muir MG. The posterior corneal surface in posterior polymorphous dystrophy: a specular microscopical study. *Cornea* 1991;10:224–232.

185. Hirst LW, Waring GO III. Clinical specular microscopy of posterior polymorphous endothelial dystrophy. *Am J Ophthalmol* 1983;95:143.

186. Krachmer JH. Posterior polymorphous corneal dystrophy: a disease characterized by epithelial-like endothelial cells which influence management and prognosis. *Trans Am Ophthalmol Soc* 1985;83:413–475.

187. Cibis GW, Krachmer JH, Phelps CD, et al. Iridocorneal adhesions in posterior polymorphous corneal dystrophy. *Trans Am Acad Ophthalmol Otolaryngol* 1976;81:770–777.

188. Rodrigues MM, Phelps CD, Krachmer JH, et al. Glaucoma due to endothelialization of the anterior chamber angle: a comparison of posterior polymorphous dystrophy of the cornea and Chandler's syndrome. *Arch Ophthalmol* 1980;98:688–696.

189. Boruchoff SA, Kuwabara T. Electron microscopy of posterior polymorphous degeneration. *Am J Ophthalmol* 1971;72:879–887.

190. Grayson M. The nature of hereditary deep polymorphous dystrophy of the cornea: its association with iris and anterior chamber dysgenesis. *Trans Am Ophthalmol Soc* 1974;72:516–559.

191. Rodrigues MM, Sun TT, Krachmer JH, et al. Epithelialization of the corneal endothelium in posterior polymorphous dystrophy. *Invest Ophthalmol Vis Sci* 1980;19:832–835.

192. Henriquez AS, Kenyon KR, Dohlman CH, et al. Morphologic characteristics of posterior polymorphous dystrophy: a study of nine corneas and review of the literature. *Surv Ophthalmol* 1984;29:139–147.

193. De Felice GP, Braidotti P, Viale G, et al. Posterior polymorphous dystrophy of the cornea: an ultrastructural study. *Graefes Arch Clin Exp Ophthalmol* 1985;223:265–272.

194. Matsumoto K, Weber PA, Makley TA. Posterior polymorphous dystrophy: a histopathologic presentation. *Ann Ophthalmol* 1988;20:388–393.

195. Rodrigues MM, Newsome DA, Krachmer JH, et al. Posterior polymorphous dystrophy of the cornea: cell culture studies. *Exp Eye Res* 1981;33:535–544.

196. Feil SH, Barraquer J, Howell DN, et al. Extrusion of abnormal endothelium into the posterior corneal stroma in a patient with posterior polymorphous dystrophy. *Cornea* 1997;16:439–446.

197. Johnson BL, Brown SI. Posterior polymorphous dystrophy: a light and electron microscopic study. *Br J Ophthalmol* 1978; 62:89–96.

198. Polack FM, Bourne WM, Forstot SL, et al. Scanning electron microscopy of posterior polymorphous corneal dystrophy. *Am J Ophthalmol* 1980;89:575–584.

199. Boruchoff SA, Weiner MJ, Albert DM. Recurrence of posterior polymorphous dystrophy after penetrating keratoplasty. *Am J Ophthalmol* 1990;109:323–328.

200. Rodrigues MM, Sun TT, Krachmer JH, et al. Posterior polymorphous corneal dystrophy: recent developments. *Birth Defects* 1982;18:479–491.

201. Hanna C, Fraunfelder FT, McNair JR. An ultrastructure study of posterior polymorphous dystrophy of the cornea. *Ann Ophthalmol* 1977;9:1371–1378.

202. Johnson BL, Brown SI. Congenital epithelialization of the posterior cornea. *Am J Ophthalmol* 82:83–89.

203. Ross JR, Foulks GN, Sanfilippo FP, et al. Immunohistochemical analysis of the pathogenesis of posterior polymorphous dystrophy. *Arch Ophthalmol* 1995;113:340–345.

204. Hirst LW, Green WR, Luckenbach M, et al. Epithelial characteristics of the endothelium in Chandler's syndrome. *Invest Ophthalmol Vis Sci* 1983;24:603–611.

205. Howell DN, Damms T, Burchette JL, et al. Endothelial metaplasia in the iridocorneal endothelial syndrome. *Invest Ophthalmol Vis Sci* 1997;38:1896–1901.

206. Hirst LW, Bancroft J, Yamauchi K, et al. Immunohistochemical pathology of the corneal endothelium in iridocorneal endothelial syndrome. *Invest Ophthalmol Vis Sci* 1995;36:820–827.

207. Levy SG, McCartney AC, Baghai MH, et al. Pathology of the iridocorneal endothelial syndrome: the ICE-cell. *Invest Ophthalmol Vis Sci* 1995;36:2592–2601.

208. Chiou AGY, Kaufman SC, Beuerman RW, et al. Confocal microscopy in the iridocorneal endothelial syndrome. *Br J Ophthalmol* 1999;83:697–702.

209. Blair SD, Seabrooks D, Shields WJ, et al. Bilateral progressive essential iris atrophy and keratoconus with coincident features of posterior polymorphous dystrophy: a case report and proposed pathogenesis. *Cornea* 1992;11:255–261.

210. Heon E, Mathers WD, Alward WL, et al. Linkage of posterior polymorphous corneal dystrophy to 20q11. *Hum Mol Genet* 1995;4:485–488.

211. Teekhasaenee C, Nimmanit S, Wutthiphan S, et al. Posterior polymorphous dystrophy and Alport syndrome. *Ophthalmology* 1991;98:1207–1215.

212. Sabates R, Krachmer JH, Weingeist TA. Ocular findings in Alport's syndrome. *Ophthalmologica* 1983;186:204–210.

213. Gassett AR, Zimmerman TJ. Posterior polymorphous dystrophy associated with keratoconus. *Am J Ophthalmol* 1974; 78:535.

214. Weissman BA, Ehrlich M, Levenson JE, Pettit TH. Four cases of keratoconus and posterior polymorphous corneal dystrophy. *Optom Vis Sci* 1989;66:243.

215. Bechara SJ, Grossniklaus NE, Waring GO, et al. Keratoconus associated with posterior polymorphous dystrophy. *Am J Ophthalmol* 1991;112:729.

216. Heon E, Greenberg A, Kopp KK, et al. VSX1: a gene for posterior polymorphous dystrophy and keratoconus. *Hum Mol Genet* 2002;11:1029–1036.

217. Sekundo W, Lee WR, Aitken DA, et al. Multirecurrence of corneal posterior polymorphous dystrophy: an ultrastructural study. *Cornea* 1994;13:509–515.

218. Shields MB. Progressive essential iris atrophy, Chandler's syndrome, and the iris nevus (Cogan–Reese) syndrome: a spectrum of disease. *Surv Ophthalmol* 1979;24:3–20.

219. Johnson GL. Atrophy of the iris. *Ophthalmol Rev* 1886;5: 57–58.

220. Chandler PA. Atrophy of the stroma of the iris. Endothelial dystrophy, corneal edema, and glaucoma. *Am J Ophthalmol* 1956;41:607–615.

221. Chandler PA, Grant WM. *Lectures on glaucoma.* Philadelphia, Lea & Febiger 1965;276–285.

222. Kline BA. Pseudomelanomas of the iris. *Am J Ophthalmol* 1941;24:133–138.

223. Cogan DG, Reese AB. A syndrome of iris nodules, ectopic Descemet's membrane, and unilateral glaucoma. *Doc Ophthalmol* 1969;26:424–433.

224. Eagle RC, Font RL, Yanoff M, et al. Proliferative endotheliopathy with iris abnormalities. The iridocorneal endothelial syndrome. *Arch Ophthalmol* 1979;97:2104–2111.

225. Wilson MC, Shields MB. A comparison of the clinical variations of the iridocorneal endothelial syndrome. *Arch Ophthalmol* 1989;107:1465–1468.

226. Hemady RK, Patel A, Blum S, et al. Bilateral iridocorneal endothelial syndrome: case report and review of the literature. *Cornea* 1994;13:368–372.

227. Blum JV, Allen JH, Holland MG. Familial bilateral essential iris atrophy (group 1). *Trans Am Acad Ophthalmol Otolaryngol* 1962;66:493–500.

228. Kupfer C, Kaiser-Kupfer MI, Datiles M, et al. The contralateral eye in the iridocorneal endothelial (ICE) syndrome. *Ophthalmology* 1983;90:1343–1350.

229. Yamaguchi M, et al. A case of Chandler's syndrome. *Folia Ophthalmol Jpn* 1992;43:862–865.

230. Teekhasaenee C, Ritch R. Iridocorneal endothelial syndrome in Thai patients: clinical variations. *Arch Ophthalmol* 2000;118:187–192.

231. Wilson MC, Shields MB. A comparison of the clinical variations of the iridocorneal endothelial syndrome. *Arch Ophthalmol* 1989;107:1465–1468.

232. Kaiser-Kupfer M, Kuwabara T, Kupfer C. Progressive bilateral essential iris atrophy. *Am J Ophthalmol* 1977;83:340–346.

233. Lucas-Glass TC, Baratz KH, Nelson LR, et al. The contralateral corneal endothelium in the iridocorneal endothelial syndrome. *Arch Ophthalmol* 1997;115:40–44.

234. Sherrad ES, Frangoulis MA, Muir MG, et al. The posterior surface of the cornea in the iridocorneal endothelial syndrome: a specular microscopical study. *Trans Ophthalmol Soc UK* 1985;104:766–774.

235. Levy SG, Kirkness CM, Moss J, et al. The Histopathology of the iridocorneal–endothelial syndrome. *Cornea* 1996;15:46–54.

236. Shields MB, Campbell DG, Simmons RJ. The essential iris atrophies. *Am J Ophthalmol* 1978;85:749–759.

237. Mitsui Y, Matsubara M, Kanagawa M. Fluorescein iridocorneal photography. *Br J Ophthalmol* 1969;53:505–512.

238. Campbell DG, Shields MB, Smith TR. The corneal endothelium and the spectrum of essential iris atrophy. *Am J Ophthalmol* 1978;86:317–324.

239. Shields MG, McCracken JS, Klintworth GK, et al. Corneal edema in essential iris atrophy. *Ophthalmology* 1979;86(8):1533–1550.

240. Hetherington J Jr. The spectrum of Chandler's syndrome. *Ophthalmology* 1978;85:240–244.

241. Shields MB, Campbell DG, Simmons RJ, et al. Iris nodules in essential iris atrophy. *Arch Ophthalmol* 1976;94:406–410.

242. Eagle RC, Font RL, Yanoff M, et al. The iris naevus (Cogan-Reese) syndrome: light and electron microscopic observations. *Br J Ophthalmol* 1980;64:446–452.

243. Klein BA. Pseudomelanomas of the iris. *Am J Ophthalmol* 1941;24:133–138.

244. Tester RA, Durcan FJ, Mamalis N, et al. Cogan-Reese syndrome: progressive growth of endothelium over iris. *Arch Ophthalmol* 1998;116:1126–1127.

245. Quigley HA, Forster RF. Histopathology of cornea and iris in Chandler's syndrome. *Arch Ophthalmol* 1978;96:1878–1882.

246. Patel A, Kenyon KR, Hirst LW, et al. Clinicopathologic features of Chandler's syndrome. *Surv Ophthalmol* 1983;27:327–344.

247. Kramer TR, Grossniklaus HE, Vigneswaran N, et al. Cytokeratin expression in corneal endothelium in the iridocorneal endothelial syndrome. *Invest Ophthalmol Vis Sci* 1992;33:3581–3585.

248. Levy SG, Kirkness CM, Moss J, et al. On the pathology of the iridocorneal endothelial syndrome: the ultrastructural appearances of "subtotal ICE." *Eye* 1995;9:318–323.

249. Alvarado JA, Murphy CG, Maglio M, et al. Pathogenesis of Chandler's syndrome, essential iris atrophy and the Cogan-Reese syndrome: I. alterations of the corneal endothelium. *Invest Ophthalmol Vis Sci* 1986;27:853–872.

250. Matsuda H, Smelser GK. Endothelial cells in alkali-burned corneas: ultrastructural alterations. *Arch Ophthalmol* 1973;89:402–409.

251. Levy SG, McCartney ACE, Sawada H, et al. Descemet's membrane in the iridocorneal-endothelial syndrome: morphology and composition. *Exp Eye Res* 1995;61:323–333.

252. Kupfer C, Chan CC, Burnier M Jr, et al. Histopathology of the ICE syndrome. *Trans Am Ophthalmol Soc* 1992;149–156.

253. Tsai CS, Ritch R, Straus SE, et al. Antibodies to Epstein–Barr virus in iridocorneal endothelial syndrome. *Arch Ophthalmol* 1990;108:1572–1576.

254. Alvarado JA, Underwood JL, Green WR, et al. Detection of herpes simplex viral DNA in the iridocorneal endothelial syndrome. *Arch Ophthalmol* 1994;112:1601–1609.

255. Groh MJM, Seitz B, Schumacher S, et al. Detection of herpes simplex virus in aqueous humor in iridocorneal endothelial (ICE) syndrome. *Cornea* 1999;18:359–360.

256. Kupfer C, Ross K. The development of outflow facility in human eyes. *Invest Ophthalmol* 1971;10:513–515.

257. Hooks JJ, Kupfer C. Herpes simplex virus in iridocorneal endothelial syndrome. *Arch Ophthalmol* 1995;113:1226–1227.

258. Laganowski HC, Kerr-Muir MG, Hitchings RA. Glaucoma and the iridocorneal endothelial syndrome. *Arch Ophthalmol* 1992;110:346–350.

259. Kidd M, Hetherington J, Magee S. Surgical results in iridocorneal endothelial syndrome. *Arch Ophthalmol* 1988;106:199–201.

260. Lanzl IM, Wilson RP, Dudley D, et al. Outcome of trabeculectomy with mitomycin–C in the iridocorneal endothelial syndrome. *Ophthalmology* 2000;107:295–297.

261. Kim DK, Aslanides IM, Schmidt CM, et al. Long-term outcome of aqueous shunt surgery in ten patients with iridocorneal endothelial syndrome. *Ophthalmology* 1999;106:1030–1034.

262. Crawford GJ, Stulting RD, Cavanagh HD, et al. Penetrating keratoplasty in the management of iridocorneal endothelial syndrome. *Cornea* 1989;8:34–40.

263. Alvim PTS, Cohen EJ, Rapuano CJ, et al. Penetrating keratoplasty in iridocorneal endothelial syndrome. *Cornea* 2001;20:134–140.

264. Buxton JN, Lash RS. Results of penetrating keratoplasty in iridocorneal endothelial syndrome. *Am J Ophthalmol* 1984;98:297–301.

265. Chang PC, Soong HK, Couto MF, et al. Prognosis for penetrating keratoplasty in iridocorneal endothelial syndrome. *Refract Corneal Surg* 1993;9:129–132.

48

CORNEAL AND CONJUNCTIVAL DEGENERATIONS

FINA CAÑAS BAROUCH AND KATHRYN COLBY

Corneal dystrophies are usually bilateral, inherited, symmetric conditions with onset early in life. In contrast, corneal degenerations can be unilateral or bilateral, are often asymmetric, with findings typically located peripherally and not associated with any inheritance pattern or genetic predisposition. The onset of the degenerations is often in middle life or later, and is characterized by slow progression. We describe in this chapter the corneal and conjunctival degenerations. Ectatic degenerations are discussed in Chapter 49.

PINGUECULA/PTERYGIUM

A pinguecula is an elevated, grayish yellow, horizontally oriented, triangular area of thickened bulbar conjunctiva adjacent to the limbus within the interpalpebral fissure. A pinguecula can encroach toward the cornea, but if it crosses onto the cornea it then becomes, by definition, a pterygium. Pingueculae are most frequently found nasally and are usually bilateral (1). They are pathologically characterized by elastotic degeneration, with hyalinization of the conjunctival stroma.

The incidence of pingueculae increases with age. Most individuals over the age of 80 have some degree of pinguecula formation (2). Their etiology is unknown but may be related to ultraviolet (UV) light exposure (3). It is thought that the nasal location may be due to actinic damage that preferentially occurs in this area from reflection of sunlight from the nose onto the nasal limbus (4). Other possible etiologic factors for pingueculae include trauma, wind, or drying. Pingueculae rarely cause symptoms, but if they become inflamed they can be treated with lubricants or topical antiinflammatory medications.

A pterygium is a growth of horizontally oriented wing-like, fibrovascular tissue onto the cornea. Like pingueculae, pterygia are found within the interpalpebral fissure and are more commonly located nasally than temporally (Fig. 48-1). Although pterygia and pingueculae are similar clinically and histopathologically, it is unclear if pingueculae give rise to pterygia. Pterygia are associated with UV exposure and are more common in warmer climates, particularly in equatorial countries (5–7). Histopathologically, pterygia are characterized by fibrovascular proliferation and elastotic degeneration of collagen with the destruction of Bowman's layer of the cornea (8).

Pterygia are often bilateral and progressive. When they involve the visual axis, reduced vision, induced astigmatism, irritation, and tearing can occur. The cosmetic appearance of the pterygium may also be the presenting complaint. True pterygia are considered conjunctival degenerations. In contrast, pseudopterygia, characterized by connections of the conjunctiva to the cornea that are not adherent at the limbus, often develop in response to trauma or inflammation. True pterygia are always located horizontally within the palpebral fissure, whereas pseudopterygia may be located in any axis. A probe cannot be passed beneath a true pterygium because of its adherence to the limbus.

Medical treatments for pterygia include lubrication and vasoconstrictors. Patients may be counseled to avoid sun, wind, and dust. When a pterygium approaches the visual axis or induces significant astigmatism, surgical excision should be considered. Simple excision leaving bare sclera is associated with a 30% to 70% recurrence rate, whereas excision with primary closure of the conjunctiva is associated with a 5% to 10% recurrence rate (9,10). Further reductions in recurrence rate have been noted following excision with a conjunctival autograft or an amniotic membrane graft (9–11). Adjuvant mitomycin C may also be used to discourage recurrence, although serious side effects can occur if this agent is used postoperatively on bare sclera as opposed to a single intraoperative application (12).

CALCIFIC BAND KERATOPATHY

Calcific band keratopathy is characterized by calcium deposition within the anterior cornea, most typically in the interpalpebral fissure. The calcium, primarily in the form of hydroxyapatite, deposits in the epithelial basement

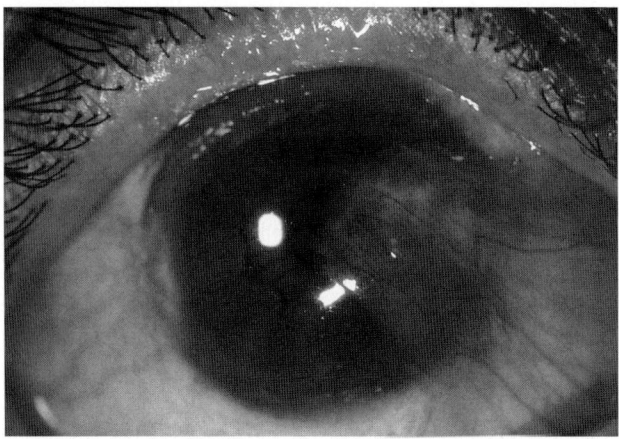

FIGURE 48-1. Right eye with pterygia. The larger nasal and smaller temporal pterygia are within the interpalpebral fissure.

membrane, Bowman's layer, and the anterior stroma. The overlying epithelium is sometimes involved and may be disrupted, leading to symptoms of recurrent erosion. Band keratopathy typically begins in the peripheral cornea at the 3 and 9 o'clock positions (Fig. 48-2A). The central cornea is affected last. In advanced cases, the calcium deposits traverse the entire cornea (Fig. 48-2B). The peripheral edge is usually sharply demarcated and separated from the limbus by a clear zone. The clear zone may be due to the buffering capacity of the limbal vessels that prevents the precipitation of calcium. Alternatively, it may be due to the termination of Bowman's layer in the peripheral cornea (13). The central edge of the deposit tends to be less sharply demarcated with a feathered appearance. Early calcium deposition is hazy and gray. As the disease progresses, the deposits become chalky white and opaque. Holes scattered throughout the band keratopathy represent the corneal nerves penetrating Bowman's layer, giving the deposit a "Swiss cheese" appearance.

Deposition of basophilic granules in Bowman's layer is the earliest change detected on histology (14). Eventually the granules coalesce and Bowman's layer becomes calcified. The calcium deposition is primarily extracellular. In cases of hypercalcemia, however, the calcium deposition is also found within the basal epithelial cells. Calcified Bowman's layer can break into small plaques and disrupt the overlying epithelium. Hyaline material deposits between the fragments of calcified Bowman's layer and the overlying epithelium giving the appearance of reduplication of Bowman's layer (13,14).

The pathogenesis of band keratopathy has not been well defined. Calcium and phosphate are present in tears at concentrations that are barely soluble. Precipitation of calcium can occur easily with an alteration in tear osmolality, elevation of the pH from corneal tissue metabolism, increase in the concentration of either calcium or phosphate, or tear evaporation from exposure within the interpalpebral fissure. The pH of the interpalpebral fissure is higher than that of the rest of the ocular surface because of carbon dioxide release from the exposed zone. This also enhances calcium precipitation. In an experimental model in which animals with induced ocular inflammation were given overdoses of vitamin D, band keratopathy developed only in animals with open eyelids but did not develop if the eyelids were kept closed (15). In addition, band keratopathy can occur rapidly in patients with dry eyes, further suggesting a role for tear evaporation in the pathogenesis of this process (16).

Calcific band keratopathy is associated with hypercalcemic states, chronic ocular disease, and repeated ocular injury (Table 48-1). Band keratopathy is often seen in patients with chronic keratitis, long-standing glaucoma, or chronic uveitis (e.g., children with juvenile idiopathic arthritis). Interestingly, band keratopathy can be seen in cases of chronic uveitis that begin in childhood but rarely in chronic uveitis of adult onset. It is also seen in patients with systemic hypercalcemia or hyperphosphatemia such as in chronic renal failure, hyperparathyroidism, milk-alkali syndrome, sarcoidosis, vitamin D toxicity, and metastatic

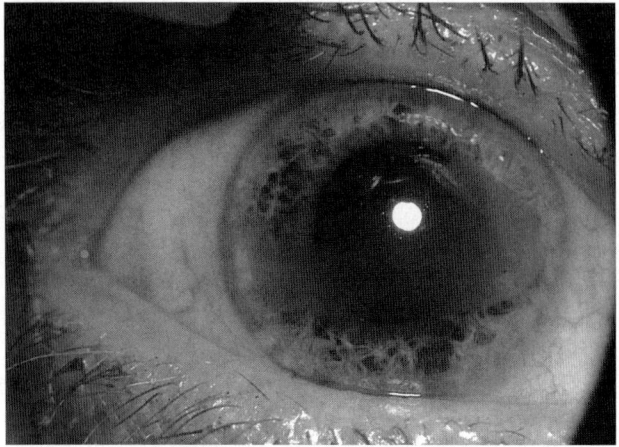

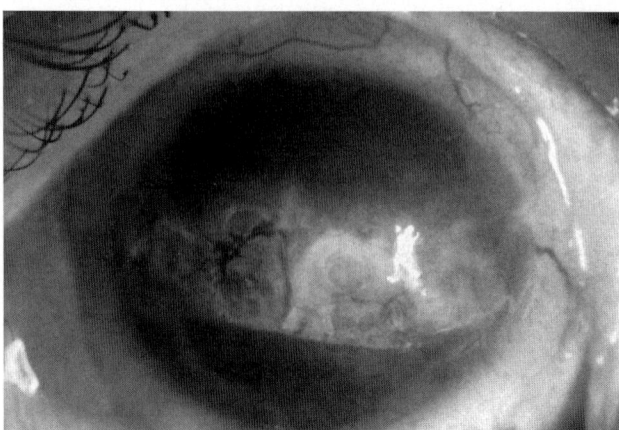

FIGURE 48-2. Early **(A)** and advanced **(B)** calcific band keratopathy.

TABLE 48-1. CONDITIONS ASSOCIATED WITH BAND KERATOPATHY

Hypercalcemia
    Hyperparathyroidism
    Excessive vitamin D (e.g., oral intake, sarcoidosis, osteoporosis)
    Renal failure (e.g., Fanconi's syndrome)
    Hypophosphatasia
    Milk-alkali syndrome
    Paget's disease
    Multiple myeloma
    Metastatic carcinoma to bone
    Idiopathic

Chronic ocular diseases
    Chronic uveitis
    Phthisis bulbi
    Long-standing glaucoma
    Interstitial keratitis
    Dry eye and corneal exposure syndromes
    Spheroidal keratopathy
    Keratoprosthesis

Chemicals
    Mercury fumes
    Phosphate-containing drops
    Intraocular silicone oil
    Viscoelastics
    Thiazides

Inherited diseases
    Norrie's disease
    Congenital band keratopathy

Systemic diseases
    Discoid lupus
    Gout
    Tuberous sclerosis

neoplastic disease (17–21). Band keratopathy has also been associated with the use of pilocarpine with mercurial preservatives, intraocular silicone oil, older viscoelastics with high phosphate concentrations, and phosphate forms of corticosteroids (22–26). Hereditary forms occur in hypophosphatasia, Norrie's disease, and autosomal-recessive congenital band keratopathy.

Patients with band keratopathy are typically asymptomatic and do not require treatment. In cases in which vision is reduced or there is discomfort and foreign-body sensation when the band breaks through the epithelium or the deposits irritate the eyelids, the central deposits can be removed. The mainstay of treatment is chelation of the calcium with ethylenediaminetetraacetic acid (EDTA) (27,28). The epithelium is removed with a sponge or a blade to allow penetration of the EDTA. EDTA (0.35%) can be applied to the subepithelial calcification via surgical sponges or directly using a reservoir such as a corneal trephine or a photorefractive keratectomy (PRK) well to hold the solution. The chemical reaction takes several minutes to occur (at least 5 minutes). Mechanical scraping following application of EDTA facilitates removal. Multiple EDTA applications are typically needed to remove all of the calcium. The excimer laser has also been used to remove calcification

within the visual axis (29,30). Phosphate-containing drops are avoided to prevent recalcification. Amniotic membrane transplantation after the surgical removal of calcium deposits has been shown to help facilitate resurfacing of the epithelial defect with corneal epithelium, although a bandage contact lens is generally sufficient to accomplish the same goal (31).

LIMBAL GIRDLE OF VOGT

Limbal girdle of Vogt is a narrow, arcuate, chalky white opacity in the nasal and temporal limbal areas of the cornea within the interpalpebral fissure (32). It occurs more frequently in the nasal limbus than in the temporal limbus but is often symmetric. There are two types of limbal girdle: Type 1 is thought to represent early calcific band keratopathy and is characterized by a white band that contains multiple holes separated from the limbus by a clear area. Type 2 is the more common true limbal girdle. It is a chalky band without holes that is contiguous to the conjunctiva. No lucent zone is present. Fine white lines that run radially in type 2 limbal girdle are best seen using retroillumination and sclerotic scatter. Histopathologically, limbal girdle is composed of hyperelastotic degeneration at the level of Bowman's layer similar to that seen in pingueculae. The prevalence of limbal girdle increases with age (32). It is present in normal eyes in 55% of those ages 40 to 60 and in 100% of those over 80 years of age (32). It does not cause any symptoms or decreased vision and thus does not require treatment.

CALCAREOUS DEGENERATION

Calcareous degeneration is characterized by calcium deposition within the deep and anterior layers of cornea. It is similar to calcific band keratopathy but also involves the posterior corneal stroma. Calcium deposition can be full thickness or can spare Bowman's layer and the corneal epithelium. The calcification typically occurs more rapidly than in band keratopathy and may develop as quickly as within a 24-hour period (33). Calcareous degeneration is usually seen in seriously diseased or injured eyes with an epithelial defect and exposed stroma or with anterior segment vascular compromise. It can be a complication of severe dry eye, recurrent corneal ulcerations, chronic ocular inflammation, or multiple surgical procedures (33–36). It is also seen in phthisis bulbi and can be associated with bone formation elsewhere in the globe. Primary calcareous degeneration can occur in patients with normal calcium and phosphate levels. It has been reported in a case of a failed corneal graft and following the use of topical steroid-phosphate therapy in a patient with chronic keratoconjunctivitis after Stevens-Johnson syndrome (37,38). Chelation with EDTA is ineffective in treating this condition because the calcium deposition is deeper than in band keratopathy. Penetrating keratoplasty is often required for visual rehabilitation (39).

SALZMANN'S NODULAR DEGENERATION

Salzmann's nodular degeneration, first described in 1925, is characterized by elevated gray to blue-gray, fibrous nodules in the superficial corneal stroma just beneath the epithelium (Fig. 48-3) (40). The nodules elevate the epithelium. There are usually one to nine discrete paracentral lesions, often in a circular array at areas of corneal scarring or at the junction of old corneal scars and clear cornea. Each nodule is separated from other nodules by clear cornea, and iron lines may outline each nodule (41). The nodules are not vascularized but the underlying stroma may be (42). Salzmann's nodular degeneration is associated with past corneal inflammation, but the onset of the lesions is gradual and often occurs many years after the keratitis. It may follow phlyctenular keratitis, vernal keratitis, trachoma, interstitial keratitis, exposure keratopathy, keratitis sicca, Thygeson's superficial punctate keratitis, and other forms of chronic keratitis (42–44). It can also be associated with recurrent corneal erosions (45). It occurs more often in women than in men, and the nodules can be bilateral or unilateral.

Histopathologically, Bowman's layer is replaced by eosinophilic material. There is thinning and flattening of the epithelium with degeneration of the basal cells and disorganization of the underlying stromal collagen. The nodule itself is not vascularized and consists of dense collagenous tissue. In addition, residua of old keratitis may be seen in the surrounding stroma.

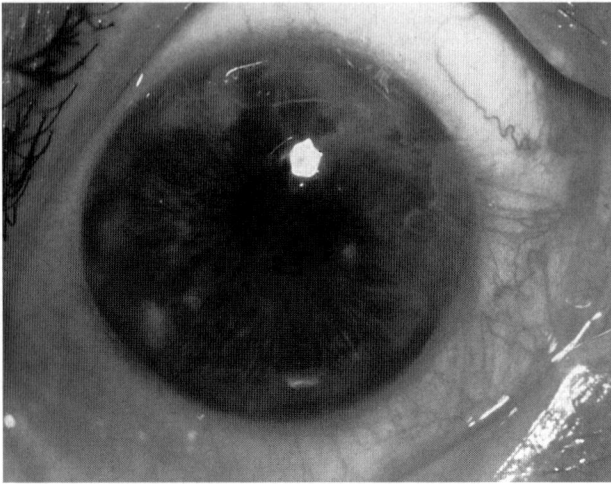

FIGURE 48-3. Multiple elevated nodules in the cornea of a patient with Salzmann's nodular degeneration.

Many patients with Salzmann's nodular degeneration are asymptomatic. Patients may complain of reduced vision if the nodules are located in the central cornea. Elevated nodules can cause discomfort and epithelial erosions. Treatment by simple excision of the nodule, lamellar keratectomy, or excimer laser phototherapeutic keratectomy is indicated if vision is decreased or if recurrent erosions occur (46–48). Recurrences are common but take many years to develop.

IRON DEPOSITIONS

Iron deposits in the deep corneal epithelium can assume a variety of configurations including lines, rings, or diffuse depositions. The most common iron deposition is the Hudson-Stähli line (49,50). Hudson-Stähli lines are located in the deep corneal epithelium at the line of eyelid closure at the junction of the middle and lower thirds of the cornea. The line curves downward at its center, is approximately 0.5 mm wide, 1 to 2 mm long, and is usually yellow, green, brown, or white in color. It is best visualized as a black line when cobalt blue light is used. Hudson-Stähli lines occur most commonly in patients over the age of 50, but decrease in frequency after the age of 70 (50,51). There is no sex predilection. Histologic evaluation shows intracellular iron deposition in the form of ferritin-like material, possibly hemosiderin, in the basal epithelial cells of the cornea (50). The cause of Hudson-Stähli lines is unknown, but the tear film may be the source of iron (49). Other possible sources of iron include the aqueous humor, limbal vessels, and cellular or blood breakdown.

Other iron lines include Fleischer rings around a cone in keratoconus (50), Ferry lines near filtering blebs (52), and Stocker-Busacca lines in front of pterygia (53). Iron lines can occur in association with superficial corneal scars, after corneal transplants (54), and surrounding refractive corneal procedures (e.g., after radial keratotomy and laser *in situ* keratomileusis) (55,56). They may also be seen with Salzmann's nodules (57), in congenital spherocytosis (58), and in association with iron foreign bodies. Alterations in corneal shape with secondary pooling of tears are thought to contribute to the formation of iron lines (54,55). In addition, migration of corneal epithelial cells may contribute to the location and shape of iron lines (59). Iron lines are asymptomatic and do not require treatment.

Coats's white ring is an iron deposition that occurs at the level of Bowman's layer (60). The overlying epithelium remains intact. It is usually located in the inferior cornea and is 1 mm or less in diameter. It appears as a small ring made up of discrete white dots that can coalesce. The rings are secondary to corneal trauma and may in fact represent remnants of old metallic foreign bodies (61). Coats's rings are incidental findings and do not require treatment.

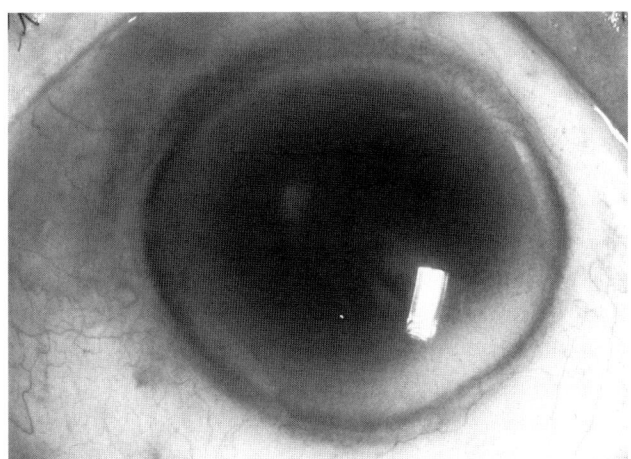

FIGURE 48-4. Arcus senilis is characterized by a whitish yellow ring in the peripheral cornea.

ARCUS SENILIS

Arcus senilis (corneal arcus) is a circumferential deposit of extracellular lipid in the corneal stroma that appears as a yellowish white ring in the peripheral cornea (Fig. 48-4). It first appears in the inferior cornea, followed by the superior cornea, and then encircles the entire cornea (62,63). There is a clear interval between the sharply demarcated peripheral edge of the arcus and the limbus that is approximately 0.3 to 1.0 mm (lucid interval of Vogt). The central edge of the arcus is usually indistinct and the central cornea is never involved. Typically arcus occurs symmetrically and bilaterally but can also occur unilaterally. Unilateral arcus senilis has been described in patients with unilateral carotid artery occlusion (64,65). The eye on the side of the occlusion does not develop arcus due to the reduced blood flow to the eye and subsequent decrease in corneal temperature, whereas a normal arcus develops on the unaffected side. Unilateral arcus has also been described in ocular hypotony due to surgery or trauma. Increased blood flow within the anterior segment in the hypotonous eye results in a warmer ocular temperature and in an exaggerated arcus (66). Any patient with unilateral arcus without hypotony should be referred to an internist for further evaluation.

Lipid deposits occur in the deep stroma initially and later in the superficial stroma. Less dense deposits are present in the mid-stroma, giving the lipid hourglass configuration on cross section (67,68). In advanced cases there is heavy lipid deposition throughout the entire stroma including Bowman's layer and Descemet's membrane. The deposits are composed of extracellular cholesterol, cholesterol esters, phospholipids, and triglycerides (67,69). These lipids, particularly low-density lipoproteins (LDL) of vascular origin, leak across the limbal capillaries into the cornea (70).

Corneal arcus preferentially forms in areas of increased vascularity (71). In the warmer regions of the cornea there is increased vascular permeability resulting in preferential lipid deposition. Because the inferior and superior portions of the cornea are the warmest regions of the cornea, whereas the central cornea is the coolest, arcus preferentially forms peripherally. In addition, a functional barrier to the flow of large molecules may exist, preventing the deposits from reaching the central cornea (72). The clear interval of Vogt may be due to the ability of the limbal blood vessels to reabsorb lipid in this area before it precipitates in the cornea.

Arcus senilis is the most common corneal opacity. Its prevalence is between 20% and 35% and its incidence increases with age (71,73,74). The prevalence of arcus senilis ranges from 40% to 69% in people in their eighties and is approximately 100% in people older than 90 (73,75,76). It is found more commonly in men than in women, and is more common in blacks than in any other race (71,73).

Patients with arcus senilis are asymptomatic and do not require treatment. Arcus senilis is generally a consequence of aging. However, it may be associated with hyperlipidemia and may be clinically significant in patients under 40 years of age (71). The amount of arcus correlates with plasma concentration of LDL (77). Patients under the age of 40 with arcus are at an increased risk for coronary artery disease, hypercholesterolemia, and hyperlipoproteinemia types 2 and 3, and should be referred to an internist to undergo lipid and cardiovascular evaluation (71).

LIPID KERATOPATHY

Lipid keratopathy (lipid degeneration, fatty degeneration of the cornea) is characterized by the deposition of lipids in the posterior corneal stroma, typically around abnormal blood vessels. The infiltrate is usually dense and yellowish white with feathery edges (Fig. 48-5). It can be similar to

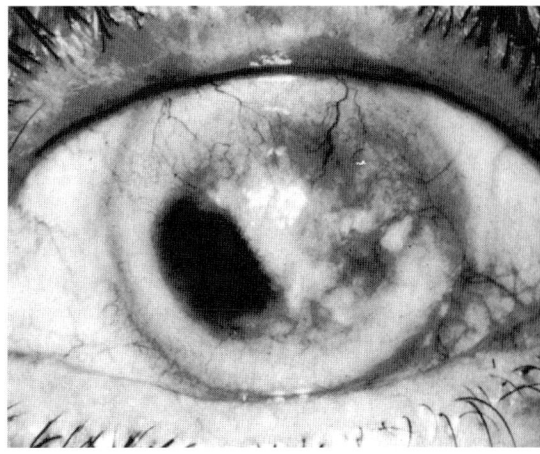

FIGURE 48-5. Lipid keratopathy with dense lipid deposition in the peripheral and central portions of the cornea.

arcus senilis or may occur as a single discoid mass. The lipid deposit tends to follow the distribution of vessels within the cornea and often has a fan-shaped appearance. The lipids are similar to those seen in arcus senilis and consist of intracellular and extracellular cholesterol, cholesterol esters, phospholipids, and triglycerides (78,79). The cause of lipid keratopathy is unknown. Increased permeability of the newly formed vessels and altered metabolic activity of dying keratocytes may result in the release of lipids into the stroma.

Lipid keratopathy occurs in two forms: primary and secondary. Primary lipid keratopathy is rare and is not associated with trauma or corneal neovascularization (80,81). Primary lipid keratopathy is bilateral and is thought to be an extension of arcus senilis into the central cornea, decreasing vision when it extends into the visual axis. Patients with primary lipid keratopathy have serum lipids in the normal range. Secondary lipid keratopathy can be seen with any condition that causes corneal neovascularization, including trauma, interstitial keratitis, herpetic keratitis, corneal hydrops, corneal ulceration, and diffuse anterior scleritis (79,82,83). Several rare autosomally inherited diseases such as apoprotein A-1 deficiency, Tangier disease, fish-eye disease, and familial lecithin-cholesterol acyltransferase (LCAT) deficiency can also result in lipid deposition in the cornea (71). Patients with primary lipid keratopathy should be referred for screening of these disorders.

In cases of secondary lipid keratopathy, corticosteroids can be used to suppress corneal inflammation and neovascularization to help slow lipid deposition. Argon green laser photocoagulation of the feeder vessels identified by fluorescein angiography has been shown to help reduce lipid deposition in a small series of patients, but this treatment can be associated with bleeding, corneal thinning, and iris atrophy (84–86). Photodynamic therapy has been shown to be effective in closing corneal neovascularization in animal models, but has not been proven in humans (87). Penetrating keratoplasty can be used for visual rehabilitation but recurrence in the graft has been reported (79,88).

SPHEROIDAL DEGENERATION

Spheroidal degeneration is known by many names, including climatic droplet keratopathy, Labrador keratopathy, Bietti's nodular corneal degeneration, fisherman's keratitis, chronic actinic keratopathy, oil droplet degeneration, keratinoid corneal degeneration, elastoid degeneration, degeneration sphaerularis elaiodes, and hyaline degeneration (89,90). Spheroidal degeneration has been classified into three types: Type 1 is a primary corneal degeneration that occurs bilaterally in corneas without ocular pathology. Type 2 is a secondary corneal degeneration that occurs in association with other ocular pathology. Type 3 is the conjunctival form that may coexist with either type 1 or 2 disease (90,91). Clinically it is often difficult to categorize the condition into these types.

Primary spheroidal degeneration has been further classified into three grades (89). Asymptomatic, fine shiny droplets in the peripheral cornea, best seen with retroillumination, characterize grade 1. These golden yellow droplets occur within the interpalpebral fissure in areas of exposure and are found beneath the conjunctival and corneal epithelium, within Bowman's layer in the cornea, or in the superficial corneal stroma. Initially the droplets appear clear but later become opaque. Grade 2 has central corneal involvement with larger deposits in the anterior stroma and concomitant decreased vision to the 20/100 level. Large corneal nodules that elevate the epithelium and reduce vision to the 20/200 level or worse characterize grade 3. Secondary spheroidal degeneration generally does not follow this grading system and tends to occur only in areas of scarring. Type 2 spheroidal degeneration occurs in patients with ocular disease such as chronic corneal edema, traumatic corneal scars, herpetic keratitis, glaucoma, and lattice corneal dystrophy. The conjunctival form of spheroidal degeneration develops within the interpalpebral fissure and is generally associated with pingueculae (91,92).

Histopathologic specimens show that the spherules are extracellular amorphous globules made of proteinaceous material with elastotic features that coalesce to form larger masses in Bowman's layer. The etiology of this material is unknown, but it may be produced as a by-product of the effects of ultraviolet light on proteins that diffuse into the cornea and conjunctiva from limbal blood vessels (89,93,94).

Spheroidal degeneration occurs most commonly in areas with extreme climates, such as deserts and the arctic. Risk factors associated with spheroidal degeneration include ultraviolet radiation, aging, low humidity, welding, prior corneal inflammation, extremes of temperature, and microtrauma from wind, sand, or ice (95,96). Its incidence increases with age. A high incidence of open-angle glaucoma has been reported in type 1 spheroidal degeneration (92).

Treatment is not typically necessary, although spheroidal degeneration does progress as long as patients are continuously exposed to the risk factors cited above. In patients with advanced disease limiting vision or causing significant foreign-body sensation, lamellar or penetrating keratoplasty or direct excision of conjunctival lesions may be indicated.

AMYLOIDOSIS

Amyloidosis is a heterogeneous group of disorders in which fibrillar hyaline proteins including amyloid P protein (AP), prealbumin or transthyretin (AF), immunoglobulin light chains (AL), and acute phase reactants (AA) are deposited in a variety of target tissues (97). Amyloid stains metachromatically with crystal violet or methyl violet, produces secondary fluorescence with thioflavine, and shows red-green birefringence following Congo red staining when viewed under a polarizing microscope.

Amyloidosis can be primary or secondary, each of which can be systemic or localized. Primary systemic amyloidosis typically involves amyloid deposition in the tongue, heart, gastrointestinal tract, peripheral nerves, and kidney, leading to macroglossia, cardiomyopathy, malabsorption, neuropathy, and nephrotic syndrome. Amyloid deposits in ocular muscles can lead to ophthalmoplegia, neuropathy can result in ptosis, and vitreous veil-like opacities can occasionally be found. Meretoja syndrome, an example of a familial form of primary systemic amyloidosis, presents with lattice corneal dystrophy and cranial neuropathies.

Secondary systemic amyloidosis is the most commonly encountered form of amyloidosis. It is typically found in association with malignancies, tuberculosis, syphilis, rheumatoid arthritis, and other chronic inflammatory conditions (98). In secondary systemic amyloidosis, amyloid deposits accumulate in the liver, spleen, and kidney. Ocular involvement is rare, but can include immunoglobulin deposits in the cornea and conjunctiva in association with multiple myeloma and paraproteinemia (99).

In contrast to systemic amyloidosis, localized amyloidosis commonly has ocular manifestations. Localized amyloidosis can also be primary or secondary. Primary localized amyloidosis encompasses disorders such as lattice corneal dystrophy, polymorphic amyloid degeneration (PAD), and gelatinous drop-like corneal dystrophy. Amyloid is typically deposited beneath the corneal epithelium in the anterior stroma. Lattice dystrophy can present with opaque masses on the anterior cornea. Penetrating keratoplasty for visual rehabilitation or relief of recurrent erosions has shown short-term efficacy, although amyloid deposits typically recur in the graft. PAD is a common condition in elderly individuals in which bilateral amyloid deposition occurs in the central posterior corneal stroma and causes indentation of Descemet's membrane (100,101). The deposits appear as punctate or filamentous opacities in the stroma that appear gray with direct illumination and may look crystalline on retroillumination. The lesions may branch with intervening clear stroma, similar in appearance to the deposits of lattice dystrophy. PAD deposits are usually not associated with any other conditions, are not inherited, do not affect vision, and do not require treatment. Primary localized amyloidosis can be manifested yellow-pink masses located on the palpebral conjunctiva.

Secondary localized amyloidosis can also be found in the cornea, most commonly occurring in association with local eye disease such as ocular trauma, uveitis, keratoconus, retinopathy of prematurity, and trachoma (Fig. 48-6) (98,102,103). Diagnosis is typically made pathologically rather than clinically. In pathologic series, the incidence of

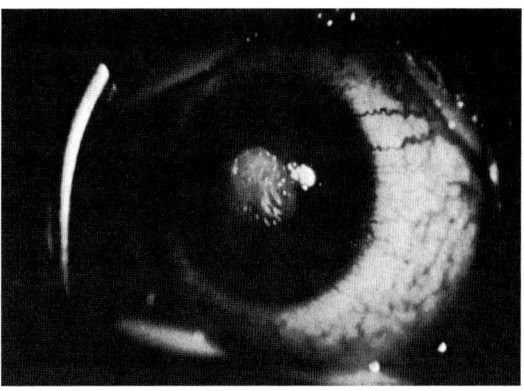

FIGURE 48-6. Amyloid deposition in a cornea.

amyloid corneal deposition was 3.5%, although the clinical significance of this finding is uncertain (98). In patients with chronic keratitis or inflammation, large amyloid deposits can accumulate in the subepithelial anterior cornea and cause a foreign-body sensation or interfere with vision. Such "cobblestone" amyloid degeneration can result in thinning of the epithelium and destruction of Bowman's layer. Treatment usually requires a penetrating keratoplasty.

CORNEAL VERTICILLATA

Corneal verticillata (vortex keratopathy) was first described by Fleischer in 1910 as a whorl-shaped corneal dystrophy characterized by stippling of the corneal epithelium in patients with Fabry's disease (104). Corneal verticillata consist of fine lines that swirl from a point below the center of the cornea and radiate to the peripheral cornea in a vortex-like pattern. Corneal verticillata consist of deposits at the level of the epithelium that usually do not alter visual acuity. They are usually seen as a side effect of certain medications and as corneal manifestations of sphingolipidoses. They have also been reported in a patient with multiple myeloma (105).

Medications known to cause corneal verticillata include chloroquine, hydroxychloroquine, amiodarone, chlorpromazine, indomethacin, tamoxifen, and atovaquone. Deposits from the antimalaria drug chloroquine develop with no relationship to the dose or duration of treatment. The deposits are generally reversible and disappear on discontinuation of the medication. Rarely, patients complain of halos around lights. Amiodarone, used for cardiac arrhythmias, causes verticillata in a dose-dependent fashion (Fig. 48-7). On low doses up to 200 mg per day, affected corneas are typically clear or only mildly cloudy. Keratopathy develops with doses in the range of 400 to 1,400 mg per day (106,107). Microscopic studies of the cornea from a patient with amiodarone keratopathy revealed complex lipid deposits within lysosomal intracytoplasmic inclusions in both corneal and conjunctival epithelium (108). Tamoxifen, an

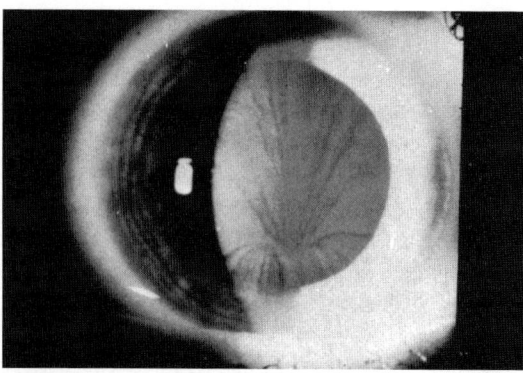

FIGURE 48-7. Corneal verticillata in a patient with amiodarone keratopathy.

antiestrogen used in the treatment of certain types of breast cancer, also causes dose-related corneal verticillata.

Corneal verticillata are also seen in the sphingolipidoses such as Fabry's disease, multiple sulfatase deficiency, and generalized gangliosidosis (GM_1 gangliosidosis type 1). Multiple sulfatase deficiency and GM_1 gangliosidosis type 1 are both autosomal-recessive disorders associated with subtle diffuse corneal opacities. In Fabry's disease there is an accumulation of ceramide trihexoside in the renal and cardiovascular systems due to a deficiency of α-galactosidase A (104). Fabry's disease is X-linked recessive and typically begins in childhood with angiokeratomata (hyperkeratotic red papules on the skin), abdominal cramps, and fevers. By the ages of 20 to 30, patients develop progressive renal insufficiency. Detection of ceramide trihexoside in the urine of affected patients is diagnostic. Corneal verticillata develop in approximately 90% of affected patients and are typically bilateral, symmetrical, and restricted to the corneal epithelium. Female carriers are usually systemically asymptomatic, but typically show corneal verticillata. Histologic examination shows a thickened corneal epithelium and an intact Bowman's layer (109,110). Other ocular manifestations of Fabry's disease include periorbital edema, conjunctival vessel tortuosity and dilatation, papilledema, retina edema, optic atrophy, and spokelike posterior cataracts (111).

CORNEAL KELOIDS

Corneal keloids are rare and occasionally form in scarred corneas. They have been described in association with Lowe's syndrome and after corneal trauma, and they rarely occur congenitally (112–114). Keloids appear as white nodules similar to those seen clinically in Salzmann's nodular degeneration, and are usually superficial but may extend deep into the corneal stroma. Histopathologic examination shows fibroblastic proliferation of the corneal stroma (115). Symptoms from corneal keloids include irritation and reduced visual acuity. Treatment in the form of lamellar or penetrating keratoplasty is usually reserved for symptomatic individuals.

ANTERIOR/POSTERIOR CROCODILE SHAGREEN

Crocodile shagreen, manifested as a mosaic pattern within the cornea, consists of grayish, white, polygonal opacities separated by clear spaces that resemble the skin of a crocodile (Fig. 48-8) (116). Crocodile shagreen is typically bilateral. The opacities are most commonly seen in the anterior cornea but can also be seen in the posterior cornea. Both forms are usually seen in elderly patients.

Histopathologically, the stroma is folded either at the level of Bowman's layer in anterior crocodile shagreen or at the level of Descemet's membrane in posterior crocodile shagreen. The mosaic pattern seen in anterior crocodile shagreen is a result of the collagen structure of the anterior cornea with collagen fibers inserting obliquely into Bowman's layer. Ridges form, indenting the epithelium and producing the mosaic pattern. Calcium may be deposited in these ridges. This mosaic pattern can also be seen when the normal tension of Bowman's layer is relaxed, as in hypotony, with aging, and in keratoconus patients wearing hard contact lenses. In posterior crocodile shagreen there is an irregular sawtooth configuration of the collagen lamellae that results in alternating clear and opaque areas (117).

Anterior crocodile shagreen is primarily an age-related degeneration. It has also been associated with hypotony, trauma, band keratopathy, X-linked megalocornea, and in patients with keratoconus wearing hard contact lenses (118). Usually anterior crocodile shagreen is visually insignificant, but rarely can reduce visual acuity.

Posterior crocodile shagreen is always age-related. It is similar to anterior crocodile shagreen but the opacities are at the level of the deep corneal stroma. Central cloudy dystrophy of François has an autosomal-dominant inheritance pattern and is clinically similar to posterior crocodile shagreen (119). Although the opacities in posterior shagreen

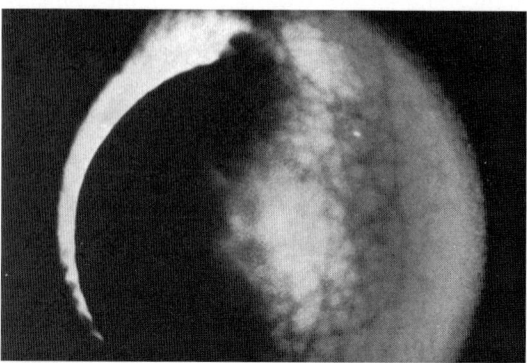

FIGURE 48-8. Crocodile shagreen is characterized by polygonal gray opacities in the corneal stroma.

are mainly central, when peripherally located they may resemble arcus senilis. These opacities are usually visually insignificant and do not require treatment.

CORNEA FARINATA (FLOURED)

Cornea farinata appears with fine tiny, grayish white, dust-like, flour-like opacities scattered in the posterior corneal stroma near Descemet's membrane. Cornea farinata has an appearance similar to pre-Descemet's dystrophies, but the opacities are smaller and occur later in life (120). These opacities occur bilaterally in elderly patients, are usually in the pupillary area, and are seen best on retroillumination. Familial cases with dominant inheritance have been reported (121). Histologic studies have shown that the deposits may be composed of lipofuscin within stromal keratocytes (120). Lipofuscin is a degenerative pigment that accumulates in old cells and is also seen in pre-Descemet's dystrophies. The etiology of these deposits is unknown. The opacities do not cause any symptoms and are usually incidental findings.

CORNEAL GUTTAE

Corneal guttae, also known as Hassall-Henle bodies or Descemet's warts, occur normally with aging in the peripheral cornea. The posterior nonbanded layer of Descemet's membrane progressively thickens with age (122). Guttae, localized nodular excrescences of Descemet's membrane produced by degenerating endothelial cells, are due to an overproduction of hyaline. They can be seen best with specular microscopy as small, dark, round areas within the normal endothelial mosaic pattern. Central corneal guttae are identical to Hassall-Henle bodies. Central guttae increase with age and are associated with Fuchs' endothelial dystrophy. This entity is discussed in Chapter 47.

CORNEAL DELLEN

Dellen are depressions in the peripheral corneal surface that occur most often at the temporal limbus. Dellen are usually transient, lasting only 24 to 48 hours, but in rare cases can last several weeks and lead to scarring. They usually occur adjacent to areas of conjunctival elevation but may also be idiopathic (Fig. 48-9). They may be found adjacent to areas of conjunctival chemosis from pterygia, episcleritis, conjunctivitis, or after cataract, glaucoma filtering, or strabismus surgery. Dellen are also seen after anesthetic use, particularly with cocaine. Histopathologically there is thinning of the corneal epithelium, Bowman's layer, and the superficial stroma. Treatment of dellen is with the use of ocular lubricants or pressure patching.

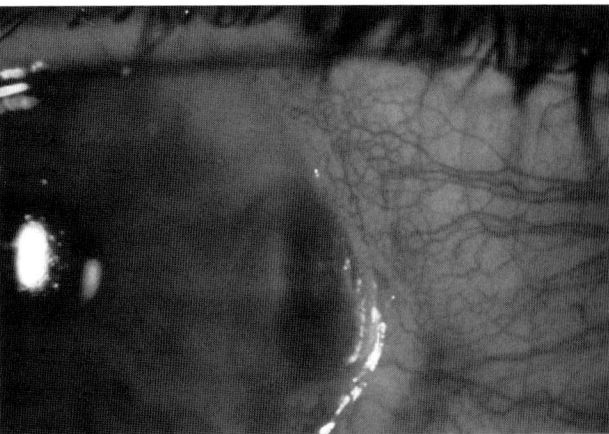

FIGURE 48-9. Corneal dellen adjacent to an inflamed pinguecula.

TERRIEN'S MARGINAL DEGENERATION

Terrien's marginal degeneration is a rare peripheral corneal disorder of unknown etiology. It can occur at any age but is most common between the ages of 20 and 40 (123). Men are affected three times more commonly than are women (123). It is bilateral in 86% of cases but may be asymmetric, occurring in the second eye many years after the first eye is affected (124).

The lesion usually begins in the superior corneal limbus but can occur at any location around the limbus. Initially it appears as fine, punctate stromal opacity separated from the limbus by a lucent zone similar to that of corneal arcus senilis. The area then becomes superficially vascularized from extension of vessels from the limbus. Gradually the peripheral cornea thins, forming an indentation parallel to the limbus, bounded centrally by an area of yellow-white lipid infiltration (Fig. 48-10A). The thinning usually causes flattening in the involved area, which leads to secondary irregular astigmatism (125). The area of thinning spreads circumferentially. The corneal epithelium remains intact, but hydrops or perforation may occur spontaneously or with minor trauma because the involved area may bulge ectatically (126). Terrien's marginal degeneration is associated with a pseudopterygium in 20% of the cases (Fig. 48-10B) (124). Histopathologically, Terrien's marginal degeneration is characterized by subepithelial connective tissue and vessels with fibrillar degeneration of collagen (127). The lipid deposits consist of cholesterol crystals.

Patients may present with decreased vision from the induced astigmatism or with episodes of painful inflammation, episcleritis, or scleritis (Fig. 48-11A,B). Although there is no treatment to prevent the progression of the disease, patients are treated with rigid gas-permeable contact lenses for the astigmatism or with tectonic corneal grafts if severe thinning is present (Fig. 48-11C) (125).

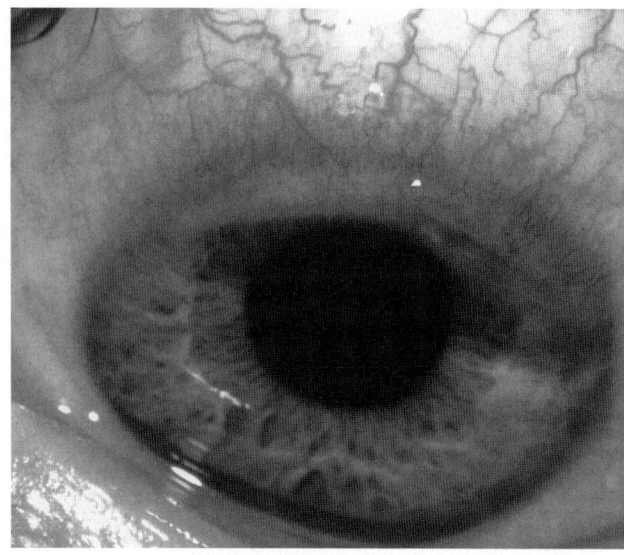
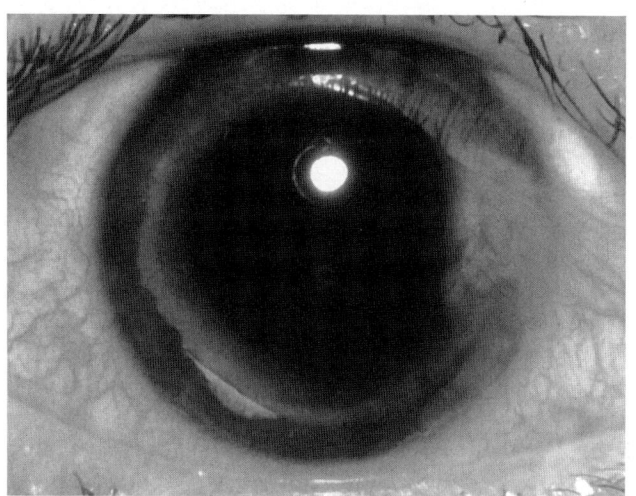

FIGURE 48-10. A: Terrien's marginal degeneration in the superior cornea. **B:** Terrien's marginal degeneration associated with a pseudopterygium.

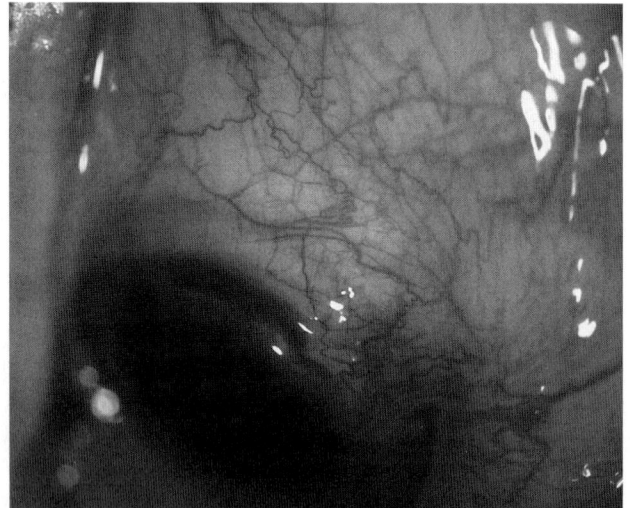
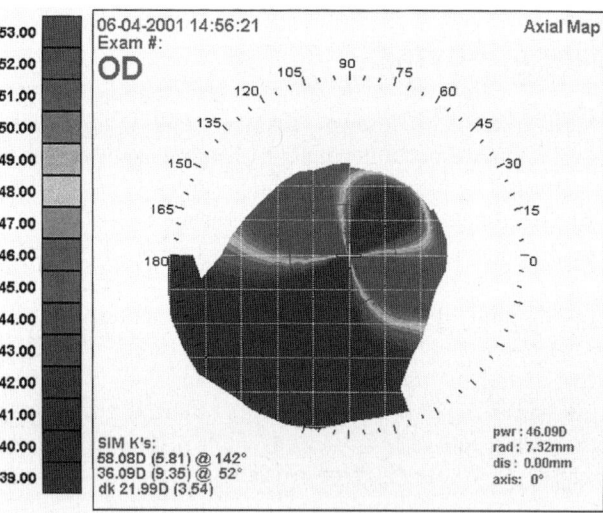
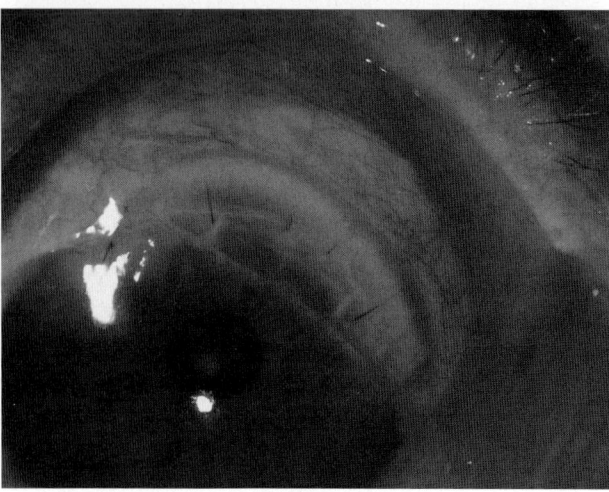

FIGURE 48-11. A: A 70-year-old patient presented with a history of decreased visual acuity of the right eye since the age of 47. Examination of the cornea revealed extensive corneal thinning superiorly and an adjacent conjunctival cyst. **B:** Corneal topography of the cornea in Fig. 48-11A showed induced high oblique astigmatism. **C:** The patient underwent excision of the conjunctival cyst and tectonic corneal grafting to reinforce the eye.

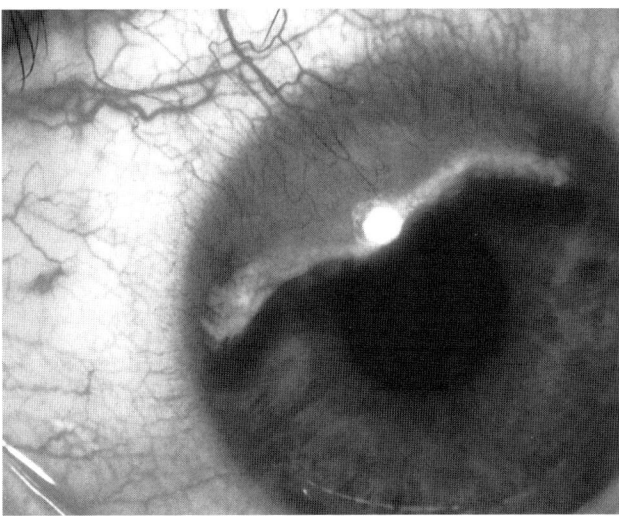

FIGURE 48-12. Marginal furrow.

FURROW DEGENERATION

Furrow degeneration is a rare condition found in elderly individuals in which the lucent area peripheral to corneal arcus senilis (lucid interval of Vogt) undergoes minimal thinning (Fig. 48-12). Generally there is no associated inflammation or neovascularization, and furrow degeneration does not lead to corneal perforation. Patients are typically asymptomatic and do not require treatment.

REFERENCES

1. Taylor HR, West SK, Rosenthal FS, et al. Corneal changes associated with chronic UV irradiation. *Arch Ophthalmol* 1989; 107:1481–1484.
2. Hinnen E. Die Altersveranderungen des vorderen bulbusabschnittes. *Z Augenheilkd* 1921;45:129–134.
3. Klintworth GK. Chronic actinic keratopathy: a condition associated with conjunctival elastosis (pingueulae) and typified by characteristic extracellular concretions. *Am J Pathol* 1972; 67:327.
4. Perkins ES. The association between pinguecula, sunlight, and cataract. *Ophthalmic Res* 1985;17:325–330.
5. Taylor HR, West S, Munoz B, et al. The long-term effects of visible light on the eye. *Arch Ophthalmol* 1992;110:99–104.
6. Mackenzie FB, Hirst LW, Battistutta D, et al. Risk analysis in the development of pterygia. *Ophthalmology* 1992;99:1056–1060.
7. Saw SM, Tan D. Pterygium: prevalence, demography, and risk factors. *Ophthalmic Epidemiol* 1999;6:219–228.
8. Austin P, Jakobiec A, Iwamoto T. Elastodysplasia and elastodystrophy as the pathologic bases of ocular pterygia and pinguecula. *Ophthalmology* 1983;90:96–109.
9. Gibson JBG. Brisbane survey of pterygium. *Trans Ophthalmol Soc Aust* 1956;16:125.
10. Hoffman RS, Power WJ. Current options in pterygium management. *Int Ophthalmol Clin* 1999;39:15–26.
11. Kenyon KR, Wagoner MD, Hettinger ME. Conjunctival autograft transplantation for advanced and recurrent pterygium. *Ophthalmology* 1985;92:1461.
12. Rubinfeld RS, Pfister RR, Stein RM, et al. Serious complications of topical mitomycin-C after pterygium surgery. *Ophthalmology* 1992;99:1647–1654.
13. O'Connor GR. Calcific band keratopathy. *Trans Am Ophthalmol Soc* 1972;70:58.
14. Cursino JW, Fine BS. A histologic study of calcific and noncalcific band keratopathies. *Am J Ophthalmol* 1976;82:395–404.
15. Doughman DJ, Olson GA, Nolan S, et al. Experimental band keratopathy. *Arch Ophthalmol* 1969;81:264.
16. Lemp MA, Ralph RA. Rapid development of band keratopathy in dry eye. *Am J Ophthalmol* 1977;83:657–659.
17. Cogan DG, Albright F, Bartter FC. Hypercalcemia and band keratopathy. *Arch Ophthalmol* 1948;40:624.
18. Porter R, Crombie AL. Corneal and conjunctival calcification in chronic renal failure. *Br J Ophthalmol* 1973;57:339.
19. Porter R, Crombie AL. Corneal calcification as a presenting and diagnostic sign in hyperparathyroidism. *Br J Ophthalmol* 1973;57:655–658.
20. Klaassen-Broekema N, van Bijsterveld OP. Limbal and corneal calcification in patients with chronic renal failure. *Br J Ophthalmol* 1993;77:569–571.
21. Allen SH. Shah JH. Calcinosis and metastatic calcification due to vitamin D intoxication. A case report and review. *Horm Res* 1992;37:68–77.
22. Kennedy RE, Roca PD, Landers PH. Atypical band keratopathy in glaucomatous patients. *Am J Ophthalmol* 1971;72:917.
23. Brazier DJ, Hitchings RA. Atypical band keratopathy following long-term pilocarpine treatment. *Br J Ophthalmol* 1989;73:294.
24. Bennett SR, Abrams GW. Band keratopathy from emulsified silicone oil. *Arch Ophthalmol* 1990;108:1387.
25. Nevyas AS, Raber IM, Eagle RC, et al. Acute band keratopathy from intracameral viscoat. *Arch Ophthalmol* 1987;105:958–964.
26. Taravella MJ, Stulting RD, Mader TH, et al. Calcific band keratopathy associated with the use of topical steroid-phosphate preparations. *Arch Ophthalmol* 1994;112:608–613.
27. Bokosky JE, Meyer RF, Sugar A. Surgical treatment of calcified band keratopathy. *Ophthalmic Res* 1985;16:645–647.
28. Wood TO, Walker GG. Treatment of band keratopathy. *Am J Ophthalmol* 1975;80:553.
29. O'Brart DPS, et al. Treatment of band keratopathy by excimer laser phototherapeutic keratectomy: surgical techniques and long term follow up. *Br J Ophthalmol* 1993;77:702–708.
30. Maloney RK, Thompson V, Ghiselli G, et al. A prospective multicenter trial of excimer laser phototherapeutic keratectomy for corneal vision loss. *Am J Ophthalmol* 1996;122:144–160.
31. Anderson DF, Prabhasawat P, Alfonso E, et al. Amniotic membrane transplantation after the primary surgical management of band keratopathy. *Cornea* 2001;20:354–361.
32. Sugar HS, Kobernick S. The white limbus girdle of Vogt. *Am J Ophthalmol.* 1960;50:101–107.
33. Freddo T, Leibowitz H. Bilateral acute corneal calcification. *Ophthalmology* 1985;92:537–542.
34. Bloomsfield S, David D, Rubin A. Acute corneal calcification. *Ann Ophthalmol* 1978;10:355–360.
35. Brodrick J. Keratopathy following retinal detachment surgery. *Arch Ophthalmol* 1978;96:2021–2026.
36. Grossniklaus H, Wood W, Bargeron C, et al. Sulfur and calcific keratopathy associated with retinal detachment surgery and vitrectomy. *Ophthalmology* 1986;93:260–264.
37. Duffey RJ, LoCascio JA 3rd. Calcium deposition in a corneal graft. *Cornea* 1987;6:212–215.
38. Schlotzer-Schrehardt U, Zagorski A, Holbach LM, et al. Corneal stromal calcification after topical steroid-phosphate therapy. *Arch Ophthalmol* 1999;117:1414–1418.
39. Sharif KW, Casey TA, Casey R, et al. Penetrating keratoplasty for bilateral acute corneal calcification. *Cornea* 1992;11:155–162.

40. Salzmann M. Über eine Abart der knotchenformigen Hornhautdystrophie. *Z Augenheilkd* 1925;57:92.

41. Reinach NW, Baum J. A corneal pigmented line associated with Salzmann's nodular degeneration. *Am J Ophthalmol* 1981;91:677.

42. Vannas A, Hogan MJ, Wood I. Salzmann's nodular degeneration of the cornea. *Am J Ophthalmol* 1975;79:211–219.

43. Abbott RL, Forster RK. Superficial punctate keratitis of Thygeson associated with scarring and Salzmann's nodular degeneration. *Am J Ophthalmol* 1979;87:296.

44. Katz D. Salzmann's nodular corneal dystrophy. *Acta Ophthalmol (Copenh)* 1953;31:377.

45. Wood TO. Salzmann's nodular degeneration. *Cornea* 1990;9:17–22.

46. Maloney RK, Thompson V, Ghiselli G, et al. A prospective multicenter trial of excimer laser phototherapeutic keratectomy for corneal vision loss. *Am J Ophthalmol* 1996;122:144–160.

47. Severin M, Kirchof B. Recurrent Salzmann's corneal degeneration. *Graefes Arch Clin Exp Ophthalmol* 1990;222:101–104.

48. Steinert RF, Puliafito CA. Excimer laser phototherapeutic keratectomy for a corneal nodule. *Refract Corneal Surg* 1990;6:352.

49. Norn MS. Hudson-Stähli line of the cornea. *Acta Ophthalmol (Copenh)* 1968;46:106.

50. Gass JDM. The iron lines of the superficial cornea. *Arch Ophthalmol* 1964;71:348–358.

51. Rose GE, Lavin MJ. The Hudson–Stähli line. I. An epidemiologic study. *Eye* 1987;1:466.

52. Ferry AP. A "new" line of the superficial cornea: occurrence in patients with filtering blebs. *Arch Ophthalmol* 1968;79:142–145.

53. Stocker FW. Demonstrationen: eine pigmentierte Hornhautlinie bei Pterygium. *Schweiz Med Wochenschr* 1939;20:19.

54. Mannis MJ. Iron deposition in the corneal graft. Another corneal iron line. *Arch Ophthalmol* 1983;101:1858–1861.

55. Koenig SB, Mc Donald MB, Yamaguchi T, et al. Corneal iron lines after refractive keratoplasty. *Arch Ophthalmol* 1983;101:1862–1865.

56. Vongthongsri A, Chuck RS, Pepose JS. Corneal iron deposits after laser in situ keratomileusis. *Am J Ophthalmol* 1999;127:85–86.

57. Reinach NW, Baum J. A corneal pigmented line associated with Salzmann's nodular degeneration. *Am J Ophthalmol* 1981;91:677.

58. Dalgleish R. Ring-like corneal deposits in a case of congenital spherocytosis. *Br J Ophthalmol* 1965;49:40.

59. Rose GE, Lavin MJ. The Hudson-Stähli line. III. Observations on morphology, a critical review of aetiology and a unified theory for the formation of iron lines of the corneal epithelium. *Eye* 1987;1:475–479.

60. Nevins RC, Davis WH, Elliott JH. Coats' white ring of the cornea- unsettled metal fettle. *Arch Ophthalmol* 1968;80:145–146.

61. Miller EM. Genesis of white rings of the cornea. *Am J Ophthalmol* 1966;61:904–907.

62. François J, Feher J. Arcus senilis. *Doc Ophthalmol* 1973;34:165–182.

63. Rifkind BM. Corneal arcus and hyperlipoproteinemia. *Surv Ophthalmol* 1972;16:295–304.

64. Kaptein EM. Unilateral corneal arcus without carotid artery stenosis. *JAMA* 1977;238:303.

65. Smith JL, Susac JO. Unilateral arcus senilis. Sign of occlusive disease of the carotid artery. *JAMA* 1973;226:676.

66. Naumann GOH, Kuchle M. Unilateral arcus lipoides corneae with traumatic cyclodialysis in two patients. *Arch Ophthalmol* 1989;107:1121–1122.

67. Cogan DG, Kuwabara T. Arcus senilis: Its pathology and histochemistry. *Arch Ophthalmol* 1959;61:553–560.

68. Cogan DG. The corneal arcus. *N Engl J Med* 1974;291:1156.

69. Andrews JS. The lipids of arcus senilis. *Arch Ophthalmol* 1962;68:264–266.

70. Walton KW. Studies on the pathogenesis of corneal arcus formation: the human corneal arcus and its relation to atherosclerosis as studied by immunofluorescence. *J Pathol* 1973;111:263–274.

71. Barchiesi BJ, Eckel RH, Ellis PP. The cornea and disorders of lipid metabolism. *Surv Ophthalmol* 1991;36:1–22.

72. Green K, DeBarge LR, Cheeks L, et al. Centripetal movement of fluorescein dextrans in the cornea. Relevance to arcus. *Acta Ophthalmol* 1987;65:538–544.

73. Cooke NT. Significance of arcus senilis in Caucasians. *J R Soc Med* 1981;74:201–204.

74. McAndrew GM, Ogston D. Arcus senilis in middle-aged men. *Br Med J* 1965;1:425–427.

75. Macareg PVJ, Lasagna L, Synder B. Arcus not so senilis. *Ann Intern Med* 1968;345–354.

76. Friedlaender MH, Smolin G. Corneal degenerations. *Ann Ophthalmol* 1979;11:1486–1495.

77. Pe'er J, Vidaurri J, Halfon St, et al. Association between corneal arcus and some of the risk factors for coronary artery disease. *Br J Ophthalmol* 1983;67:795–798.

78. Jack RL, Lase SA. Lipid keratopathy, an electron microscopic study. *Arch Ophthalmol* 1970;83:678.

79. Friedlaender MH, Cavanagh HD, Sullivan WR, et al. Bilateral central lipid infiltrates of the cornea. *Am J Ophthalmol* 1977;84:781.

80. Fine BS, Townsend WM, Zimmerman LE, et al. Primary lipoidal degeneration of the cornea. *Am J Ophthalmol* 1974;78:12.

81. Baum JL. Cholesterol keratopathy. *Am J Ophthalmol* 1969;67:372.

82. Shapiro LA, Farkas TG. Lipid keratopathy following corneal hydrops. *Arch Ophthalmol* 1977;95:456.

83. Morisawa M, Yamagami S, Inoki T, et al. Bilateral centripetal lipid keratopathy with diffuse anterior scleritis. *Acta Ophthalmol Scand* 2003;81:202–203.

84. Marsh RJ, Marshall J. Treatment of lipid keratopathy with the argon laser. *Br J Ophthalmol* 1982;66:127–135.

85. Marsh RJ. Argon laser treatment of lipid keratopathy. *Br J Ophthalmol* 1988;72:900–904.

86. Gordon YJ, Mann RK, Mah TS, et al. Fluorescein-potentiated argon laser therapy improves symptoms and appearance of corneal neovascularization. *Cornea* 2002;21:770–773.

87. Gohto Y, Obana A, Kanai M, et al. Photodynamic therapy for corneal neovascularization using topically administered ATX–S10 (Na). *Ophthalmic Surg Lasers* 2000;31:55–60.

88. Sullivan WR. Bilateral central lipid infiltrates of the cornea. *Am J Ophthalmol* 1977;84:781–787.

89. Gray RH, Johnson GJ, Freedman A. Climatic droplet keratopathy. *Surv Ophthalmol* 1992;36:241.

90. Fraunfelder FT, Hanna C. Spheroidal degeneration of the cornea and conjunctiva. 3. Incidence, classification, and etiology. *Am J Ophthalmol* 1973;76:41.

91. Fraunfelder FT, Hanna C, Parker JM. Spheroidal degeneration of the cornea and conjunctiva. 1. Clinical course and characteristics. *Am J Ophthalmol* 1972;74:821–828.

92. Hanna C, Fraunfelder FT. Spheroidal degeneration of the cornea and conjunctiva. 2. Pathology. *Am J Ophthalmol* 1972;74:829–839.

93. Ormerod LD, Dahan E, Hagele JE, et al. Serious occurrences in the natural history of advanced climatic keratopathy. *Ophthalmology* 1994;101:448–453.

94. Johnson GJ, Overall M. Histology of spheroidal degeneration of the cornea in Labrador. *Br J Ophthalmol* 1978;62:53–61.

95. Garner A, Fraunfelder FT, Barras TC, et al. Spheroidal degeneration of the cornea and conjunctiva. *Br J Ophthalmol* 1976;60:473.

96. Norn M, Franck C. Long-term changes in the outer part of the eye in welders. *Acta Ophthalmol (Copenh)* 1991;69:382.
97. Blodi FC, Apple DJ. Localized conjunctival amyloidosis. *Am J Ophthalmol* 1979;88:346–350.
98. McPherson SD, Kiffney GT. Corneal amyloidosis. *Am J Ophthalmol* 1966;62:1025–1033.
99. Gorevic PE, et al. Lack of evidence for protein AA reactivity in amyloid deposits of lattice corneal dystrophy and amyloid corneal degeneration. *Am J Ophthalmol* 1984;98:216–224.
100. Mannis MJ, Krachmer JH, Rodrigues MM, et al. Polymorphic amyloid degeneration of the cornea: a histopathologic study. *Arch Ophthalmol* 1981;99:1217–1223.
101. Nirankari V, Rodrigues MM, Rajagopalan S, et al. Polymorphic amyloid degeneration. *Arch Ophthalmol* 1989;107:595.
102. Collyer RT. Amyloidosis of the cornea. *Can J Ophthalmol* 1968;3: 35–38.
103. Garner A. Amyloidosis of the cornea. *Br J Ophthalmol* 1969;53: 73–81.
104. Francois J. Cornea verticillata. *Doc Ophthalmol* 1969;27:235–251.
105. Chong EM, Campbell RJ, Bourne WM. Vortex keratopathy in a patient with multiple myeloma. *Cornea* 1997;16:592–594.
106. Wilson FM, Schmitt TE, Grayson M. Amiodarone-induced cornea verticillata. *Ann Ophthalmol* 1980;12:657.
107. Nielsen CE, Andreasen F, Bjerregaard P. Amiodarone induced cornea verticillata. *Acta Ophthalmol (Copenh)* 1983;61:474–480.
108. D'Amico DJ, Kenyon KR, Ruskin JR. Amiodarone keratopathy: drug-induced lipid storage disease. *Arch Ophthalmol* 1981; 99:257–261.
109. Colley JR, Miller DL, Hutt MSR, et al. The renal lesion in angiokeratoma corporis diffusum. *Br Med J* 1958;1:1266–1268.
110. Francois J, Hanssens M, Teuchy H. Corneal ultrastructural changes in Fabry's disease. *Ophthalmologica* 1978;176:313.
111. Sher NA, Letson RD, Desnick RJ. The ocular manifestations of Fabry's disease. *Arch Ophthalmol* 1979;97:671.
112. Mejia LF, Acosta C, Santamaria JP. Clinical, surgical, and histopathologic characteristics of corneal keloid. *Cornea* 2001;20: 421–424.
113. McElvanney AM, Adhikary HP. Corneal keloid: aetiology and management in Lowe's syndrome. *Eye* 1995;9:375–376.
114. Weiner MJ, Albert DM. Congenital corneal keloid. *Acta Ophthalmol Suppl* 1989;192:188–196.
115. Shoukrey NM, Tabbara KF. Ultrastructural study of a corneal keloid. *Eye* 1993;7:379–387.
116. Vogt A. *Textbook and atlas of slit lamp microscopy of the living eye.* Bonn: Wayenborgh Editions, 1981.
117. Meyer JC, Quantock AJ, Thonar EJ-MA, et al. Characterization of a central corneal cloudiness sharing features of posterior crocodile shagreen and central cloudy dystrophy of Francois. *Cornea* 1996;15:347.
118. Dangel ME, Krachmer GP, Stark WJ. Anterior corneal mosaic in eyes with keratoconus wearing hard contact lenses. *Arch Ophthalmol* 1984;102:888–890.
119. Bramsen T, Ehlers N, Braggesen LH. Central cloudy corneal dystrophy of François. *Acta Ophthalmol (Copen)* 1976;54: 221–226.
120. Curran RE, Kenyon KR, Green WR. Pre-Descemet's membrane corneal dystrophy. *Am J Ophthalmol* 1974;77:711–716.
121. Grayson M, Wilbrandt H. Pre-Descemet dystrophy. *Am J Ophthalmol* 1967;64:276–282.
122. Johnson DH, Bourne WM, Campbell RJ. The ultrastructure of Descemet's membrane. I. Changes with age in normal corneas. *Arch Ophthalmol* 1982;100:1942.
123. Beauchamp GR. Terrien's marginal corneal degeneration. *J Pediatr Ophthalmol Strabismus* 1982;19:97–99.
124. Etzine S, Friedmann A. Marginal dystrophy of the cornea with total ectasia. *Am J Ophthalmol* 1963;55:150.
125. Wilson SE, Lin DTC, Klyce SD, et al. Terrien's marginal degeneration: corneal topography. *Refract Corneal Surg* 1990; 6:15.
126. Soong HK, Fitzgerald J, Boruchoff SA, et al. Corneal hydrops in Terrien's marginal degeneration. *Ophthalmology* 1986; 93:340.
127. Suveges I, Levai G, Alberth B. Pathology of Terrien's disease. *Am J Ophthalmol* 1972;74:1191.

49

ECTATIC DISORDERS OF THE CORNEA

YARON S. RABINOWITZ

DESCRIPTION

Keratoconus is a clinical term used to describe a condition in which the cornea assumes a conical shape as a result of noninflammatory thinning. The corneal thinning in keratoconus induces irregular astigmatism, myopia, and protrusion, resulting in mild to marked impairment in the quality of vision (1,2). It is a progressive disorder ultimately affecting both eyes, although only one eye may be affected at the initial encounter with the patient (3,4).

Keratoconus classically has its onset at puberty and is progressive until the third to fourth decade of life, when it usually arrests. It may, however, commence later in life and progress or arrest at any age. It is most commonly an isolated condition, although it is frequently linked with other disorders in isolated cases (1).

Commonly reported associations include Down's syndrome, Leber's congenital amaurosis, and connective tissue disorders. Several reports have shown a high incidence of mitral valve prolapse (58%) in patients with advanced keratoconus (3,5). Atopy, eye rubbing, and hard contact lenses are also reported to be highly associated with this disorder. From 6% to 14% of cases reported to date have a positive family history or show evidence of familial transmission (1–3,6).

The incidence of keratoconus is variable, with most estimates ranging between 50 and 230 per 100,000 (approximately 1 in 2,000), with a prevalence rate of 54.5 per 100,000 (1,7–10). The variability in the reported incidence reflects the subjective criteria often used to establish the diagnosis, with subtle forms often being overlooked. Keratoconus occurs in all ethnic groups, with no male or female preponderance.

SYMPTOMS AND SIGNS

Symptoms are highly variable and are in part dependent on the stage of the disorder. Early in the disease there may be no symptoms, and the only sign may be an inability to refract the patient to a clear 20/20. In advanced disease there is significant distortion of vision accompanied by a profound decrease in vision (1,2). Patients with keratoconus fortunately never become totally blind as a result of their corneal disease.

Clinical signs also differ depending on the severity of the disease at the time of presentation (Table 49-1). In moderate to advanced disease, any one or combination of the following signs may be detectable by slit-lamp examination of the cornea: conical protrusion (Fig. 49-1), stromal thinning (centrally or paracentrally) (Figs. 49-2 and 49-3), an iron line partially or completely surrounding the cone (Fleischer's ring), and Vogt's striae, which are fine vertical lines in the deep stroma and Descemet's membrane that parallel the axis of the cone and disappear transiently on gentle digital pressure (Figs. 49-4 and 49-5). Other accompanying signs can include epithelial nebulae, anterior stromal scars (Fig. 49-6), enlarged corneal nerves, increased intensity of the corneal endothelial reflex, and the presence of subepithelial fibrillary lines (2,3,11).

Munson's sign and Rizutti's sign are useful external signs associated with keratoconus (11). Munson's sign is a V-shaped conformation of the lower lid produced by the ectatic cornea in downgaze (Fig. 49-7). Rizutti's sign is a sharply focused beam of light near the nasal limbus, produced by lateral illumination of the cornea in patients with advanced keratoconus.

Early in the disease the cornea may appear normal on slit-lamp biomicroscopy. However, there may be slight distortion or steepening of keratometry mires centrally or inferiorly. In such instances it is useful to dilate the pupil. Retroillumination may reveal scissoring of the retinoscopic reflex or the "Charleaux" oil droplet sign, which may confirm the diagnosis in suspicious cases (12). In these early cases, where the cornea appears normal but keratoconus is suspected, videokeratography of the cornea is the best means for confirming the diagnosis (1).

Ultrasonic pachymetry may be used to document corneal thinning in patients with suspected keratoconus. It cannot be solely relied on to make the diagnosis because of

TABLE 49-1. SIGNS OF KERATOCONUS

External signs:
Munson's sign
Rizzuti phenomenon

Slit-lamp findings:
Stromal thinning
Posterior stress lines (Vogt's striae)
Iron ring (Fleischer ring)
Scarring: epithelial or subepithelial

Retroillumination signs:
Scissoring on retinoscopy
Oil droplet sign ("Charleaux")

Photokeratoscopy signs:
Compression of mires inferotemporally (egg-shaped mires)
Compression of mires inferiorly or centrally

Videokeratography signs:
Localized increased surface power
Inferior-superior dioptric asymmetry
Relative skewing of the steepest radial axes above and below
the horizontal meridian (Fig. 49-6)

Videokeratography indices:
K value greater than 47.2 (with an AB/SRAX pattern)
I-S value greater than 1.6 (with an AB/SRAX pattern)
KISA% greater than 100

the large range and variation of pachymetry readings both centrally and paracentrally in the normal population (13).

TOPOGRAPHIC DIAGNOSIS

Several devices are currently available for detecting keratoconus by measuring the anterior corneal topography. These range from simple inexpensive devices such as a hand-held

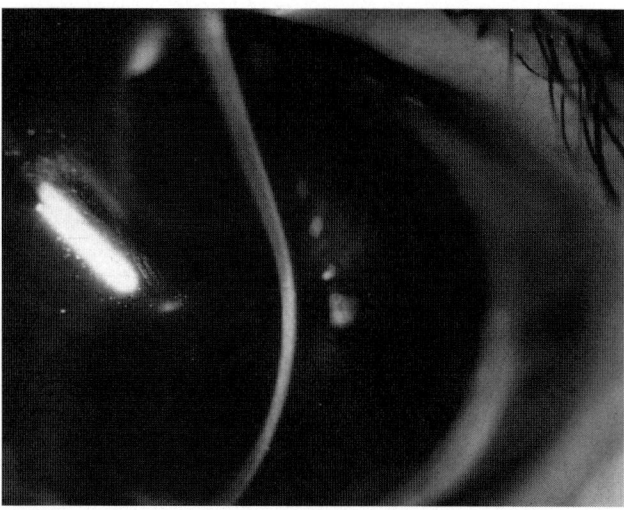

FIGURE 49-2. Slit-lamp photograph illustrating paracentral corneal thinning in a patient with an oval cone.

keratoscopes (Placido disks) to expensive sophisticated devices such as computer-assisted videokeratoscopes. With hand-held keratoscopes, such as the Klein keratoscope, early keratoconus is characterized by a downward deviation of the horizontal axis of the Placido disk reflection (14,15). In the past, nine-ring photokeratoscopes, such as the Corneascope (Kera Corp., Santa Clara, CA) were commonly used by cornea specialists. With this device early keratoconus is characterized by compression of the mires inferiorly or inferotemporally (16).

Computer-assisted videokeratoscopes that generate color-coded maps and topographic indices are currently the most sensitive technique for confirming the diagnosis of keratoconus. Videokeratography in keratoconus has three characteristic features: an increased area of corneal

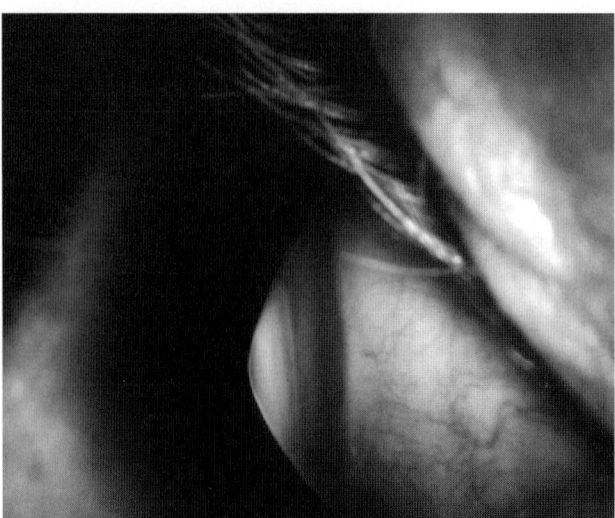

FIGURE 49-1. Slit-lamp photograph demonstrating conical shape of the cornea in keratoconus.

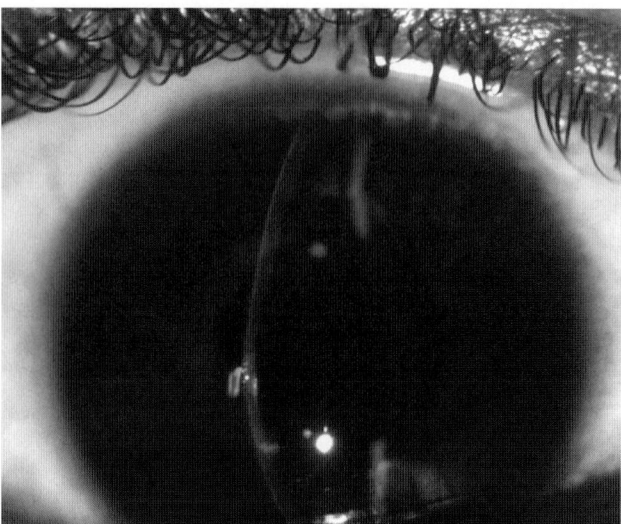

FIGURE 49-3. Slit-lamp photograph illustrating central thinning in a patient with a nipple-type cone.

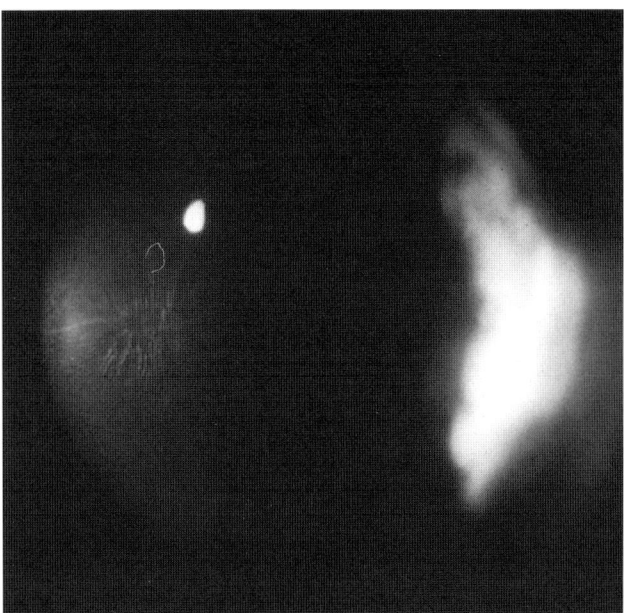

FIGURE 49-4. Slit-lamp photograph demonstrating Vogt's striae at the level of Descemet's membrane.

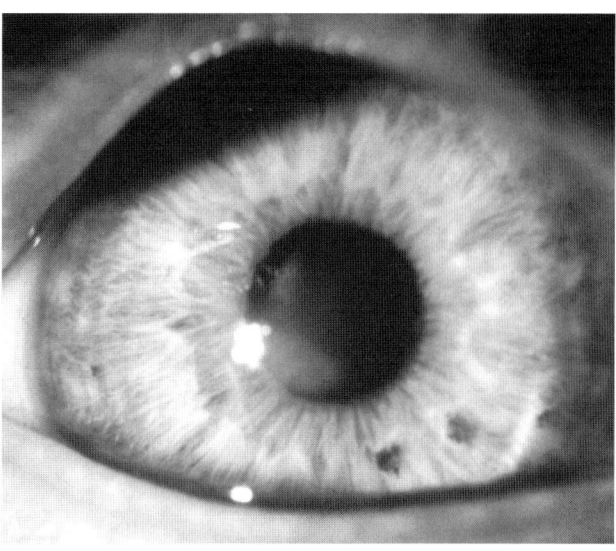

FIGURE 49-6. Stromal scarring in keratoconus.

power surrounded by concentric areas of decreasing power, inferior-superior power asymmetry, and skewing of the steepest radial axes above and below the horizontal meridian (Fig. 49-8).

Several studies have characterized the topographic patterns of clinically detectable keratoconus (17,18). The pattern found is usually the same in the two eyes of an individual patient, although it may be more advanced in one eye relative to the other.

The majority of patients have peripheral cones, with steepening extending into the periphery. In this group, corneal steepening is usually confined to one or two quadrants.

A smaller group of patients has central topographic alterations. Many central cones have a bow-tie configuration similar to that found in naturally occurring astigmatism. In the keratoconus patient, however, the bow-tie pattern is asymmetric, with the inferior loop being larger in the majority of cases. In contrast to patients who have with-the-rule astigmatism, in keratoconus the steep radial axes above and below the horizontal meridian appear skewed, giving the bow-tie a lazy-eight configuration. Another pattern found in central cones is more symmetric steepening without a bow-tie appearance. These peripheral and central cones probably correspond roughly to the oval-sagging and nipple-shaped cones described by Perry et al. (19).

FIGURE 49-5. Magnified view of Vogt's striae or stress lines in the cornea.

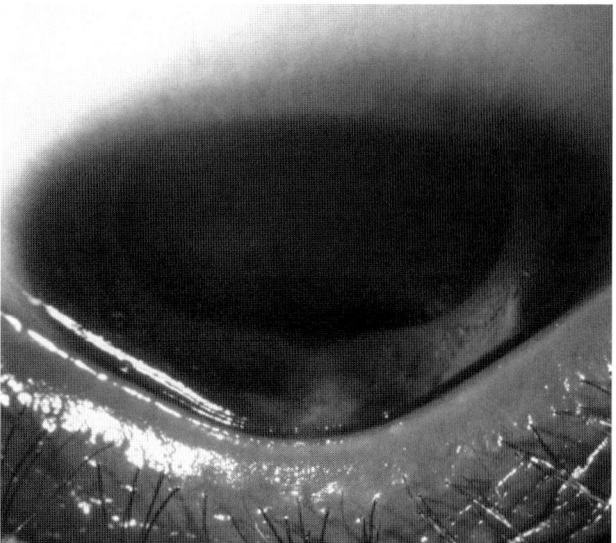

FIGURE 49-7. Munson's sign, showing overhanging of the cone over the lower eyelid.

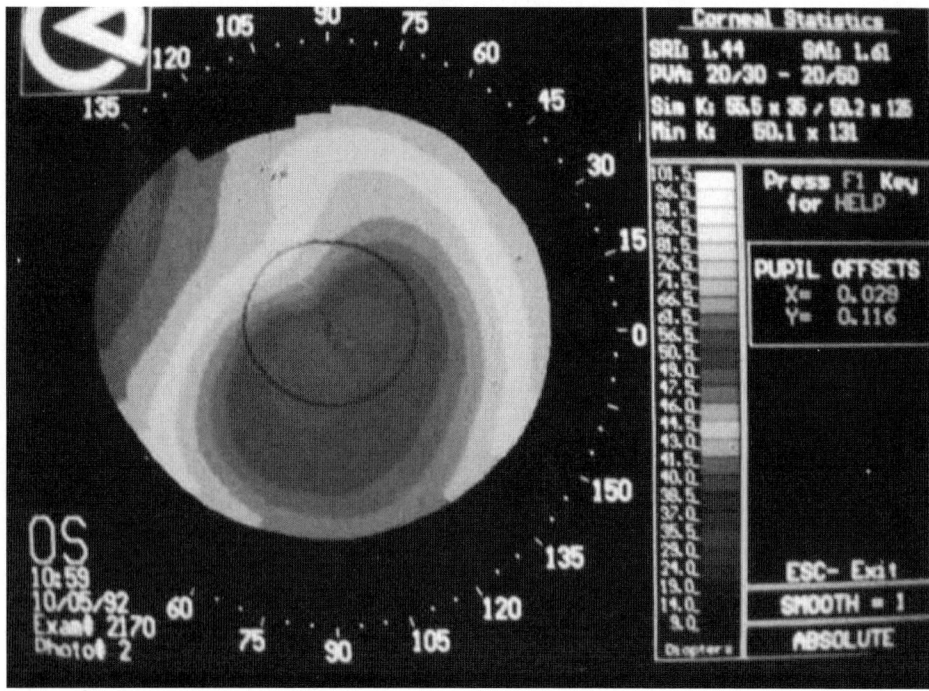

FIGURE 49-8. Videokeratograph of an oval cone in keratoconus.

Similar patterns have been noted in clinically normal family members of patients with keratoconus and in the clinically normal fellow eye of patients with clinically unilateral keratoconus (20–22). These patterns are less pronounced (as measured by dioptric power) than the patterns noted in clinically obvious keratoconus (20,21).

HISTOPATHOLOGY

Thinning of the corneal stroma, breaks in Bowman's membrane, and deposition of iron in the basal layers of the corneal epithelium (Fig. 49-9) are the classical histopathologic features of keratoconus. Depending on the stage of

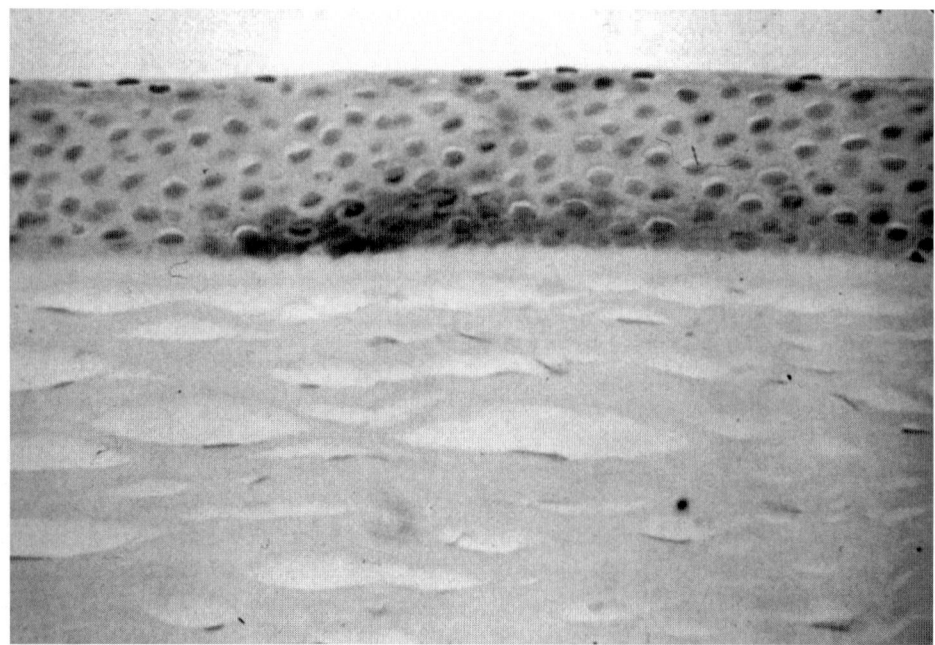

FIGURE 49-9. Histopathologic micrograph illustrating iron deposition at the basal epithelial layer seen in keratoconus.

the disease, every layer of the cornea can become involved in the pathologic process. Fine details of these processes are most clearly appreciated by electron microscopy.

The epithelium may show degeneration of its basal cells, breaks within and downgrowth of epithelium into Bowman's membrane, particles within a thickened subepithelial basement membrane-like layer and between basal epithelial cells, and accumulation of ferritin particles within and between epithelial cells most prominently in the basal layer of the epithelium. Changes in Bowman's layer may include breaks filled by eruptions of underlying stromal collagen, periodic acid-Schiff (PAS)-positive nodules, z-shaped interruptions possibly due to separation of collagen bundles, and reticular scarring. Compaction and derangement of fibrillar architecture in the anterior stroma may occur, along with a decrease in the number of collagen lamellae. Normal and degenerating fibroblasts and keratocytes may be seen. A fine granular and microfibrillar material may be associated with the keratocytes (2).

Descemet's membrane is rarely affected except for breaks seen in acute hydrops. The corneal endothelium is also usually normal. Reported endothelial abnormalities include intracellular "dark structures," pleomorphism, and elongation of cells with their long axis toward the cone.

Gross histopathologic analysis of corneal buttons from patients undergoing penetrating keratoplasty for keratoconus has revealed the presence of two types of cone morphology: nipple-type cones, which are located centrally, and oval-type (sagging) cones, which are located inferiorly or inferotemporally (19).

Histopathologic examination of corneal buttons in patients with a history of acute hydrops reveals stromal edema (Fig. 49-10). During acute hydrops, Descemet's membrane separates from the posterior corneal surface and retracts into scrolls, ledges, or ridges. During the repair process, corneal endothelium extends over the anterior and posterior surfaces of the detached Descemet's membrane and denuded stroma. Endothelial integrity is usually reestablished 3 to 4 months after the acute event (23).

ASSOCIATED DISORDERS

Keratoconus has been reported as an isolated sporadic disorder, and in association with other rare genetic disorders, Down's syndrome, Leber's congenital amaurosis, and connective tissue disorders. It has also been associated with hard contact lens wear and eye rubbing. Small but significant proportions of patients have a positive family history of the disorder (2,24–26) (Table 49-2). These associations, however, require further critical evaluation.

By far the most common presentation of keratoconus is as an isolated sporadic disorder with no other systemic or ocular disease detectable by clinical evaluation. To put this in perspective, of 1,200 consecutive keratoconus patients screened in a genetic research study at the Cedars-Sinai Medical Center in Los Angeles, 98% had keratoconus with no associated genetic disease.

A list of reported associations with keratoconus is presented in Table 49-3. For the most part these associations should be regarded to have occurred by chance. For example, if the incidence of keratoconus is 1 in 2,000 and the incidence of neurofibromatosis is 1 in 4,000, then there is a 1 in 8,000,000 chance that these two disorders could occur together by chance alone (30 potential cases in the United States). Rare associations with keratoconus are important, however, particularly if they occur as a result of a chromosomal translocation and the disorder cosegregates with keratoconus. This may provide clues as to the chromosomal location of the inherited form of keratoconus. As such, it is worthwhile to perform cytogenetic studies in patients with keratoconus who have mental retardation or other rare known genetic disorders that result from chromosomal translocations.

Down's syndrome has been reported to have a high association with keratoconus. The incidence of keratoconus in patients with Down's syndrome ranges from 0.5% to 15% (2,27,28). This is 10 to 300 times more frequent than in the general population. Similarly, a high incidence of keratoconus has been reported in patients with Leber's congenital amaurosis, with up to 30% of patients with amaurosis above the age of 15 manifesting keratoconus (29). Both of

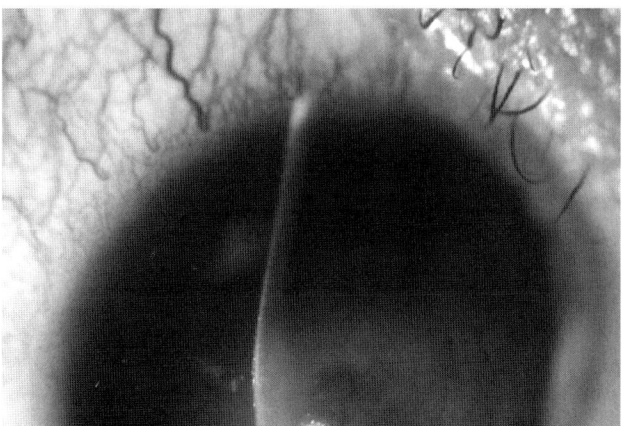

FIGURE 49-10. Stromal opacity as a result of corneal edema in a patient with acute hydrops.

TABLE 49-2. CLINICAL SETTINGS IN WHICH ISOLATED KERATOCONUS MAY OCCUR

Contact lens wear
Eye rubbing
Atopy
Leber's congenital amaurosis
Mitral Valve prolapse
Positive family history

TABLE 49-3. DISEASES REPORTED IN ASSOCIATION WITH KERATOCONUS

Multisystem
Alagille's syndrome
Albers-Schönberg's syndrome
Anetoderma
Angelman's syndrome
Apert's syndrome
Autographism
Bardet-Biedl's syndrome
Crouzon's syndrome
Down's syndrome
Ehlers-Danlos's syndrome
Goltz-Gorlin's syndrome
Hyperornithemia
Ichthyosis
Kurz's syndrome
Laurence-Moon-Biedl's syndrome
Marfan's syndrome (see ref. 6)
Mulvihil-Smith's syndrome
Nail patella's syndrome
Neurocutaneous angiomatosis
Neurofibromatosis
Noonan's syndrome
Oculodentodigital's syndrome
Osteogenesis imperfecta
Pseudoxanthoma elasticum
Rieger's syndrome
Rothmund's syndrome
Tourette's syndrome
Turner's syndrome
Xeroderma pigmentosa

Ocular
Anetoderma and bilateral subcapsular cataracts
Aniridia
Ankyloblepharon
Bilateral macular coloboma
Blue sclerae

Congenital cataracts
Ectodermal and mesodermal anomalies
Floppy eyelid syndrome
Gyrate atrophy
Iridoschisis
Leber's congenital amaurosis
Microcornea
Persistent pupillary membrane
Posterior lenticonus
Retinitis pigmentosa
Retinopathy of prematurity
Retrolental fibroplasia
Vernal conjunctivitis

Corneal
Atopic keratoconjunctivitis
Avellino dystrophy
Axenfeld's anomaly
Chandler's syndrome
Corneal amyloidosis
Deep filiform corneal dystrophy
Essential iris atrophy
Fleck corneal dystrophy
Fuchs' corneal dystrophy
Iridocorneal dysgenesis
Lattice dystrophy
Pellucid marginal degeneration
Posterior polymorphous dystrophy
Terrien's marginal degeneration

Other
Congenital hip dysplasia
False chordae tendineae of left ventricle
Joint hypermobility
Measles retinopathy
Mitral valve prolapse
Ocular hypertension
Thalasselis syndrome

these associations, however, have been attributed to a higher incidence of eye rubbing in these two disorders (due to increased blepharitis in Down's syndrome and the oculodigital sign in Leber's congenital amaurosis). Elder's (30) study of children in a school for the blind contradicts this theory and suggests the association with keratoconus might be due to genetic factors rather than eye rubbing.

Several reports suggest an association between keratoconus and connective tissue disorders (31–35). Case reports have linked keratoconus with disorders of collagen metabolism such as osteogenesis imperfecta and subtypes of Ehlers-Danlos. Another study reported joint hypermobility in 22 of 44 (50%) of keratoconus patients. Two recent studies dispute the association of joint hypermobility and keratoconus (36,37). In the latter study, 34/218 (16%) of keratoconus versus 10/183 (5%) of normal age-matched controls had joint hypermobility (not statistically significant (Table 49-4). Other compelling evidence in support of a connective tissue abnormality in keratoconus does exist, however. Several reports have suggested an association between advanced keratoconus and mitral valve prolapse

(38,39). In one study, mitral valve prolapse was found in 58% of keratoconus patients requiring surgery and only 7% of normal controls (39).

Many studies report a high association of eye rubbing in patients with keratoconus, but a cause-and-effect relationship is difficult to prove (2). A preliminary study suggests that keratoconus patients do rub their eyes more often than normal controls (Table 49-4) (37).

Another form of mechanical trauma implicated in the pathogenesis of keratoconus is caused by contact lenses (2,40,41). In early keratoconus, patients have mild myopic

TABLE 49-4. ETIOLOGIC FACTORS (RESPONSE TO QUESTIONNAIRE)

	Normal Controls (n = 183)	Keratoconus (n = 218)
Allergy	66 (36%)	96 (44%) $p <.105$ (N.S.)
Joint hypermobility	10 (5%)	34 (16%) $p <.305$ (N.S.)
Eye rubbing	106 (58%)	174 (80%) $p <.001$
Positive family history	1 (0.05%)	22 (10%) $p <.001$

astigmatism with clinically normal corneas. Vision is typically best corrected with rigid contact lenses. Thus, it is extremely difficult to determine which came first, the keratoconus or the contact lens wear. In none of the reports citing these associations were topographic studies done prior to contact lens fitting. There is no way to determine whether these patients had early keratoconus prior to wearing contact lenses. However, it is theoretically possible that mechanical trauma induced by eye rubbing and or hard contact lens wear might act as environmental factors enhancing the progression of the disorder in genetically predisposed individuals.

Although atopy is often cited as being highly associated with keratoconus, a review of the literature suggests conflicting data regarding this association (2,42–44). In a study conducted at Cedars-Sinai Medical Center in Los Angeles, 96/218 (44%) of keratoconus patients had a history or symptoms of allergic disorders, compared with 66/183 (36%) of normal age-matched controls (Table 49-4). This difference was not statistically significant (37).

ETIOLOGY AND PATHOGENESIS: BIOCHEMICAL STUDIES

Despite intensive biochemical investigation into the pathogenesis of keratoconus, its etiologic basis remains poorly understood. Corneal thinning appears to result from loss of structural components in the cornea, but why this occurs is not clear. Theoretically the cornea can thin for the following reasons: fewer collagen lamellae, less collagen fibrils per lamella, closer packing of collagen fibrils, or various combinations of the above. This may result from defective formation of extracellular constituents of corneal tissue, destruction of previously formed components, increased distensibility of corneal tissue with sliding collagen fibers or collagen lamellae, or a combination of these mechanisms (45).

Biochemical and immunohistologic studies of keratoconus corneas suggest that the loss of corneal stroma after digestion by proteolytic enzymes could follow either increased levels of proteases and other catabolic enzymes (46) or decreased levels of proteinase inhibitors (47). Observations of the corneal proteinase inhibitors, α_1-proteinase inhibitor and α_2-macroglobulin, confer further support on the hypothesis that the degradation process may be aberrant in keratoconus (48). Both inhibitors can be demonstrated throughout normal human corneas and corneas with diseases other than keratoconus using immunohistochemistry. However, the staining intensity in corneal epithelium from keratoconus corneas was markedly diminished. The decrease in α_2-macroglobulin was confirmed by Western dot blot assays (48).

Tissue inhibitor of metalloproteinase–1 (TIMP-1), another proteinase inhibitor that inhibits matrix metalloproteinases, was not found to be implicated in the increased levels of gelatinolytic activity noted in prior biochemical studies of keratoconic corneas (49–51). These proteases and inhibitors require further study to clarify their precise role in the pathogenesis of keratoconus.

Increasing attention to the communication between the corneal epithelial and stromal cells has given rise to an attractive new concept of keratoconus etiology. Wilson and co-workers (52) have shown that the loss of anterior stromal keratocytes, which accompanies corneal epithelial abrasion or subepithelial ablation, is likely due to apoptotic cell death. Both the corneal epithelium and endothelium produce interleukin-1 (IL-1). Stromal keratocytes express the IL-1 receptor. IL-1 induces keratocyte death *in vitro*, inhibits keratocyte chemotaxis, and can upregulate hepatocyte and keratinocyte growth factors (52). It can also regulate the expression of keratocyte metalloproteinases, collagenases, and complement factors. IL-1 is postulated to be a modulator of epithelial-stromal interactions, with a role in the regulation of corneal cell proliferation, differentiation, and death. The IL-1 system has been hypothesized to play a role in the pathogenesis of keratoconus (52). Previous work has demonstrated that keratocytes from keratoconus corneas have a fourfold greater number of IL-1 receptors than normal corneas (53). Wilson and co-workers have suggested that the increased expression of the IL-1 receptor sensitizes the keratocytes to IL-1 released from the epithelium or endothelium, causing a loss of keratocytes through apoptosis and a decrease in stromal mass over time. This hypothesis makes sense in light of the relationship of keratoconus to eye rubbing, contact lens wear, and atopy, as the epithelial microtrauma associated within these conditions may lead to an increased release of IL-1 from the epithelium (54).

EARLY DETECTION
Historical Perspective

Marc Amsler was the first to describe early corneal topographic changes in keratoconus patients using a photographic placido disk. His classic studies on the natural history of keratoconus documented its progression from minor corneal surface distortions to clinically detectable keratoconus. He classified keratoconus into clinically recognizable stages and an earlier latent stage recognizable only by placido disk examination of corneal topography. The early stages were subdivided into two categories: "keratoconus fruste," which entailed a 1- to 4-degree deviation of the horizontal axis of the placido disk, and "early or mild keratoconus," which entailed a 5- to 8-degree deviation of the horizontal axis. Only slight degrees of asymmetric oblique astigmatism could be detected in these early forms of keratoconus. Similar findings were absent in patients with regular astigmatism (14,15).

In Amsler's study of 600 patients, 22% had clinically obvious keratoconus in both eyes, 26% had clinical keratoconus in one eye and latent keratoconus in the other, and 52% had latent keratoconus bilaterally. Progression was highly variable and typically asymmetric. The cone could remain stationary, progress rapidly over 3 to 5 years, and arrest or progress intermittently over an extended period of time. When Amsler reexamined 286 eyes 3 to 8 years after the diagnosis, only 20% of the entire group, including 66% of the latent cases, had progressed. Progression was most likely to occur in patients between 10 and 20 years of age, decreased slightly between 21 and 30, and was less likely to occur after age 30 (14,15).

Videokeratography Studies

In the past two decades, computer-assisted videokeratoscopes have gained rapid acceptance in clinical practice (55). There are many videokeratoscopes currently available, most of which use placido disk principles, although other technologies such as wavefront analysis are rapidly emerging. A detailed discussion of these devices and how they operate is beyond the scope of this chapter. Interested readers may wish to refer to a publication by Merlin and Cantera (55).

One such device used primarily in topography studies of keratoconus is the Topographic Modeling System (TMS-1; Computed Anatomy, New York, NY). This device consists of a placido disk-type nose cone, which captures the placido disk image into a computer-based system. Data can then be rapidly analyzed in an accurate and reproducible manner. Both the central and paracentral cornea can be measured in one sitting. This device uses spherically biased algorithms ("sagittal topography"), which have been shown to be highly accurate and reproducible on spherical surfaces and in the central two thirds of normal human corneas (56–59).

Topographic data points in polar coordinates using 256 radial lines scanning across 25 rings are examined and approximately 7,000 data points are generated. A color-coded map is generated, which allows easy appreciation of changes in the corneal curvature. The 25-ring photokeratoscope mires can be superimposed on the maps for qualitative interpretation, and a series of quantitative indices including simulated keratometry readings are part of the data output (60).

Because placido disk-based computer videokeratoscopes, such as the TMS-1, have the combined features of both a keratometer and photokeratoscope, and can record curvature changes in both the central and paracentral cornea, they are ideally suited for detecting the subtle topographic changes present in early keratoconus. They are also valuable for documenting disease progression by serial topographic analysis. Using videokeratography, there are two means of differentiating subtle keratoconus topography from the normal population: pattern recognition and differentiation through quantitative descriptors.

Videokeratography Pattern Recognition

Although pattern recognition with color-coded maps is relatively easy for an experienced observer, the minimal topographic criteria needed to assign a diagnosis of keratoconus can be challenging until one has viewed many topographic images. Videokeratography maps that look suspicious for keratoconus in the presence of a clinically normal eye should be labeled "keratoconus suspect" until progression to keratoconus can be documented (61). One way to become proficient in recognizing subtle pathology is to print maps of all patients examined in the absolute scale (in the TMS-1 this scale divides the cornea into 1.5-D intervals between 35 and 50 D and 5-D intervals outside of this range) (62). Using a single scale allows the clinician to get used to normal pattern variations, allowing earlier recognition of subtle abnormal topography. The normalized scale in the TMS-1 that divides the cornea into 11 equal colors can be confusing. Many clinically normal patients with slight inferior steepening might inadvertently be labeled as "keratoconus suspects" using this scale. A database of videokeratography patterns of 195 normal individuals using the absolute scale has been described in detail and is accurate and reproducible even among inexperienced users (Fig. 49-11) (63,64). This database of videokeratography patterns has been a useful baseline reference for longitudinal topographic studies of keratoconus family members. It is also useful to help the clinician determine whether subtle deviations in corneal topography exist in a particular patient observed at any point in time.

Analysis of these patterns suggest that only 1/195 (0.5%) of normal patients have topographic features similar to, but

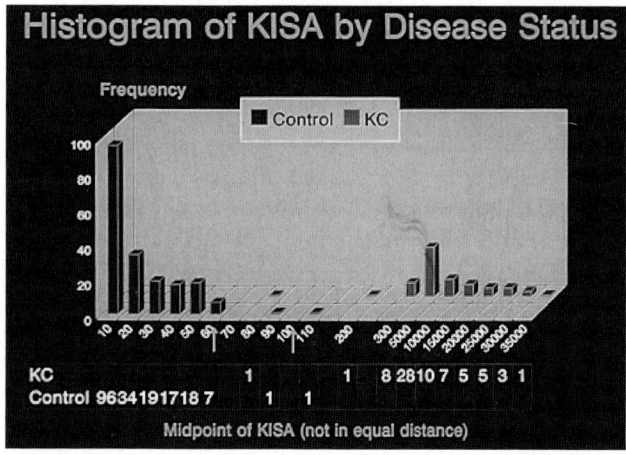

FIGURE 49-11. Classification scheme for normal corneas using the absolute scale with the Topographic Modeling System (TMS) videokeratoscope.

milder than, those seen in clinically detectable keratoconus (asymmetric bowtie with skewed radial axis [AB/SRAX]; Fig. 49-11) (65,66). Long-term follow-up of normal fellow eyes of patients with unilateral keratoconus shows that a significant number of patients with the AB/SRAX pattern in their clinically normal eye ultimately progress to keratoconus (66).

Clear, consistent definitions of keratoconus are essential for accurate genetic pedigree analyses. Therefore, we have devised a classification scheme using clinical signs and videokeratography based on our observation of the topographic progression of keratoconus "suspects" and "early" keratoconus to clinically significant keratoconus over a 10-year period. The classification is as follows: (a) keratoconus: one or more of the following clinical signs: stromal thinning, Vogt's striae, Fleischer ring, scissoring of the retinoscopic reflex with a fully dilated pupil, and an AB/SRAX videokeratography pattern; (b) "early keratoconus": no slit-lamp findings but scissoring of the retinoscopic reflex with a fully dilated pupil with an AB/SRAX videokeratography pattern; and (c) keratoconus "suspect": no clinical or retroillumination signs of keratoconus but an AB/SRAX videokeratography pattern.

Several reports in the literature suggest that to better understand the genetics of keratoconus and its modes of heredity, patients with subtle forms of the disorder detectable only by corneal topography should be included in family pedigree analysis (1,14,15). The topographic patterns described in the preceding paragraph have now proven useful for constructing family pedigrees for molecular genetic analyses and for predicting which "keratoconus suspect" eyes ultimately progress to keratoconus.

Pseudokeratoconus

A confounding issue in assigning minimal topographic criteria for the diagnosis of keratoconus is videokeratography patterns that simulate keratoconus (videokeratographic pseudokeratoconus) (67). The most common culprit is contact lens wear. Both hard and soft contact lenses induce patterns of inferior steepening that may be very difficult to distinguish from keratoconus (67). These patterns, however, disappear with time as contact lens wear is discontinued. Videokeratographic pseudokeratoconus can also result from technical errors including inferior eyeball compression or misalignment of the eye with inferior or superior rotation of the globe during image capture. Dry spot formation with incomplete digitization of mires can also cause an image that appears steep inferiorly. Early pellucid marginal degeneration, inflammatory corneal thinning, and previous ocular surgery can all induce patterns that simulate keratoconus by videokeratography (68). An awareness of these pitfalls will allow for a better appreciation of the true topographic changes occurring in the earliest stages of keratoconus (108).

Quantitative Descriptors

Videokeratoscopes generate numeric indices as part of their output. Developing accurate quantitative descriptors of videokeratography patterns in keratoconus would allow for easier recognition of patterns and would enable us to develop a quantitative phenotype that could be universally used for formulating minimal topographic criteria for diagnosing keratoconus. This has particular application in screening patients for refractive surgery, because unpredictable results and patient dissatisfaction have been attributed to refractive surgery performed on myopic patients with undiagnosed early keratoconus (70–73). Quantitative indices are also useful for genetic analyses of keratoconus.

In a preliminary study comparing videokeratographs from keratoconus patients to those from normal controls, we developed three indices that distinguished keratoconus from normals: central K (descriptive of central steepening), I-S values (inferior-superior dioptric asymmetry; Fig. 49-12), and right versus left (difference between right and left central corneal power). Videokeratography studies on 28 family members of five patients with keratoconus revealed that 50% of the subjects had mild topographic abnormalities and at least one index greater than 2 standard deviations from their control group (21,74). These abnormalities were similar to, but less severe than, those found in the patients with keratoconus. This work has been duplicated by several other investigators in family studies and on studies of fellow eyes of keratoconus patients (21,75,76). These studies suggest that these indices might be diagnostic of the earliest stages of keratoconus in clinically normal eyes, before disease progression occurs. These indices quantified two early phenotypic features of keratoconus, i.e., central steepening and inferior-superior dioptric asymmetry. The SRAX index, used to quantify the irregular astigmatism in keratoconus, was also developed to increase the sensitivity

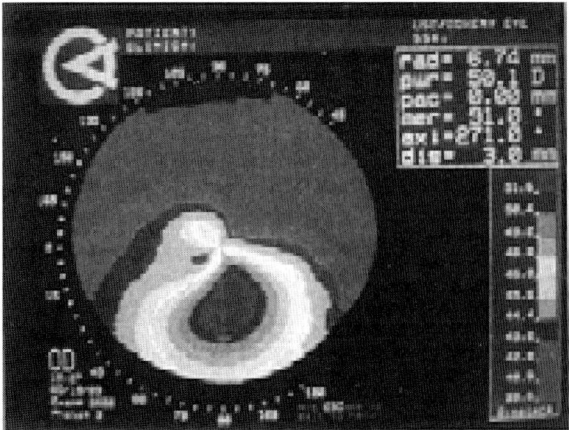

FIGURE 49-12. Topographic phenotypic features of keratoconus and calculation of the I-S value (inferior-superior dioptric asymmetry).

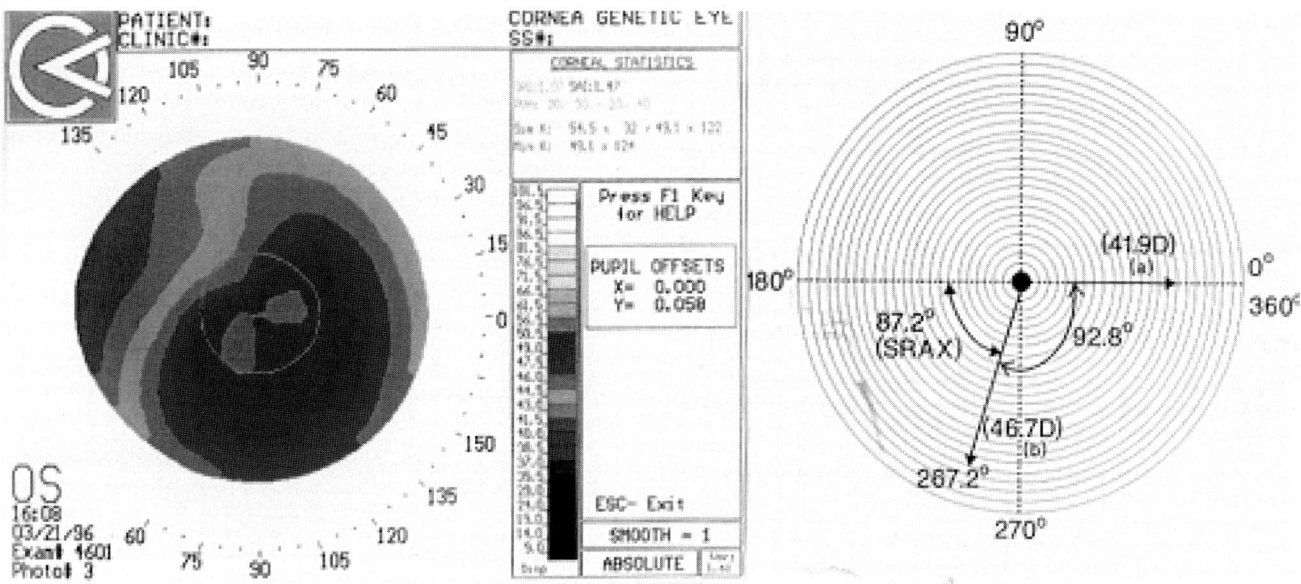

FIGURE 49-13. Topographic phenotypic features of keratoconus and calculation of the SRAX index, used in calculating the KISA% index.

and specificity of these descriptors (Fig. 49-13) (77). Subsequent to this, a new single index incorporating all the videokeratographic phenotypic features of keratoconus, the KISA% index, was developed (78). This index is the product of all previously developed indices descriptive of keratoconus (the K value, I-S value, SRAX value, and the regular astigmatism as measured by K readings). This formula produces a percent index whereby any patient who has clinical keratoconus has a KISA% index of greater than 100 (Fig. 49-14 and Table 49-5). In a study using this index to study normal controls and clinically obvious keratoconus, a cutoff point of 100% correctly classified 280 of 281 participants (99.6%) (Fig. 49-15). Six of eight eyes with "keratoconus suspect" topography had a KISA% between 60% and 100% and 11 of 12 eyes with early keratoconus had a KISA% of greater than 100% (78).

This index has been extremely useful in longitudinal analysis of "suspect" patients over time. Figure 49-16 illustrates eyes that have been followed for 5 years that have evolved from normal to suspect to early keratoconus, and then subsequently to clinically obvious keratoconus. As the patterns have changed over time, the KISA% index allowed us to quantify this progression in an accurate and reproducible manner.

This single numeric value has allowed us to make significant advances in our understanding of the genetics of keratoconus. We are now able to provide minimal topographic criteria for accurately assigning status to keratoconus family members for use in formal pedigree analyses. In addition, the KISA% index has allowed us to perform complex segregation analyses that have demonstrated that genes play a major role in the pathogenesis of keratoconus. Finally, this index may allow us to identify genes

causing keratoconus using techniques such as genomewide screens.

GENETICS

Keratoconus is a very heterogeneous disorder and not all keratoconus is the same. To clearly understand the genetics of keratoconus, this disease should be divided into three broad categories: (a) isolated keratoconus associated with rare genetic disorders (Table 49-2), (b) keratoconus in the setting of commonly reported associations (Table 49-3), and (c) isolated keratoconus with no associations.

Isolated keratoconus with no associations is by far the most common presentation (1). The genetics of this common form of keratoconus is discussed in this chapter.

Several lines of evidence suggest that genetic factors play a role in the pathogenesis of isolated keratoconus. These include twin studies (79–90), the bilaterality of the disorder (91–93), reports of familial aggregation (94–96), and formal genetic analyses (97).

Twins have a special place in human genetics as they allow comparison of the effects of both genes and environment. The importance of twin studies for comparison of the effects of "nature and nurture" was originally observed by Galton in 1875 (98). Diseases caused wholly or partly by genetic factors have a higher concordance rate in monozygotic twins than in dizygotic twins. Even if a condition does not show a simple genetic pattern, comparison of its incidence in monozygotic and dizygotic twin pairs can reveal that heredity is involved. Moreover, if monozygotic twins are not fully concordant for a given condition, then nongenetic factors must also play a part in its etiology.

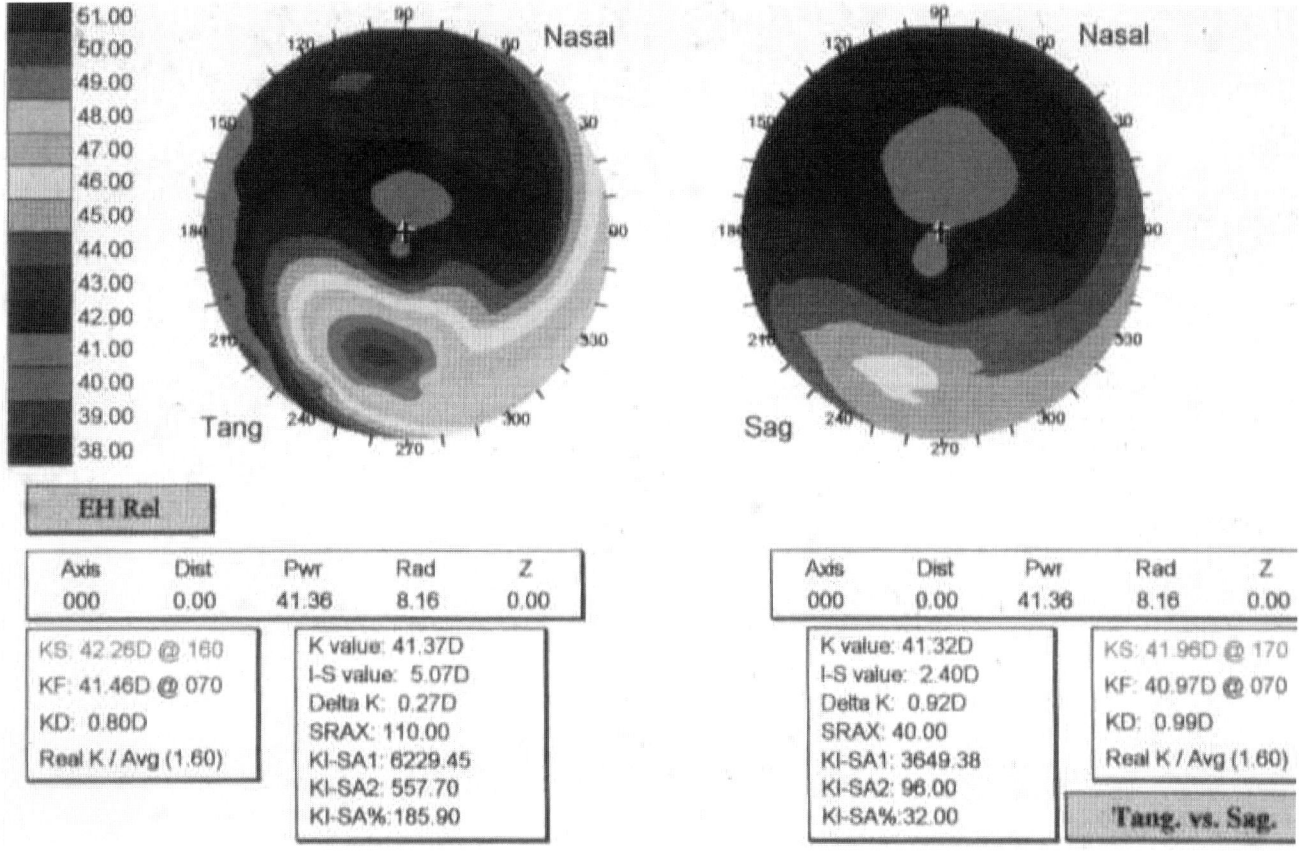

FIGURE 49-14. Calculation of the KISA% index, the K value, and I-S value in the fellow eye of a patient with keratoconus both in the sagittal and tangential mode, showing increased sensitivity of tangential topography for detecting keratoconus.

TABLE 49-5. CALCULATION OF THE KISA% INDEX

The KISA% index quantifies the topographic features seen in patients with clinical keratoconus. It is the product of four indices: the K value, an expression of central corneal steepening; the I-S value, an expression of inferior-superior dioptric asymmetry; the AST index, which quantifies the degree of regular corneal astigmatism (Sim K1 − Sim K2); and the SRAX index, an expression of the irregular astigmatism occurring in keratoconus. These individual indices and the methods by which they are calculated have previously been described in detail (10). The method for calculating the SRAX index is repeated as an illustration for the purposes of this paper.

The algorithm for calculating the KISA% index was initially derived as follows: KISA% = (K) × (I-S) × (AST) × (SRAX) × 100. Because each individual index quantifies a topographic feature of keratoconus, when they are multiplied by each other any abnormality in one amplifies the resultant product. In addition to the above, the following rules apply: (a) The value of 1 was substituted in the equation whenever any index calculated index had a value of less than 1. The purpose of this is to amplify any abnormality. (b) Only absolute values are used (for example, if the I-S value is −2, this is corrected to 2; therefore, there can be no negative values for the KISA%). (c) The K value used is that which is in excess of 47.2 D (which is greater than 2 standard deviations of normal controls). For values less than 47.2 D, the value of 1 is substituted in the calculation. This index was calculated for all 86 keratoconus patients in our database.

The eye with the lowest KISA% value, but which still had the most minimal clinical signs of keratoconus, i.e., scissoring of the red reflex, and a topographic pattern consistent with keratoconus, had a KISA% of 30,900. Because our goal was to have an index where a patient with the minimal clinical features of keratoconus was as close to 100% as possible we divided this index by 300, to give this patient a KISA% value of 103%. The KISA% index is thus calculated as follows:

$$\text{KISA\%} = \frac{(K) \times (I\text{-}S) \times (AST) \times (SRAX) \times 100}{300}$$

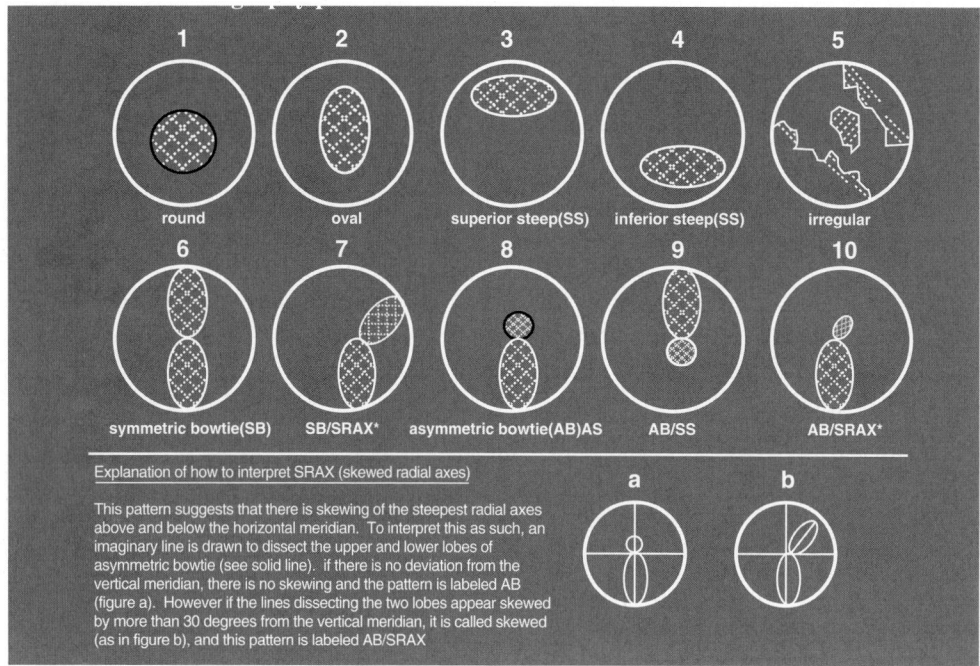

FIGURE 49-15. Histogram of KISA% index showing spread between keratoconus and normal controls.

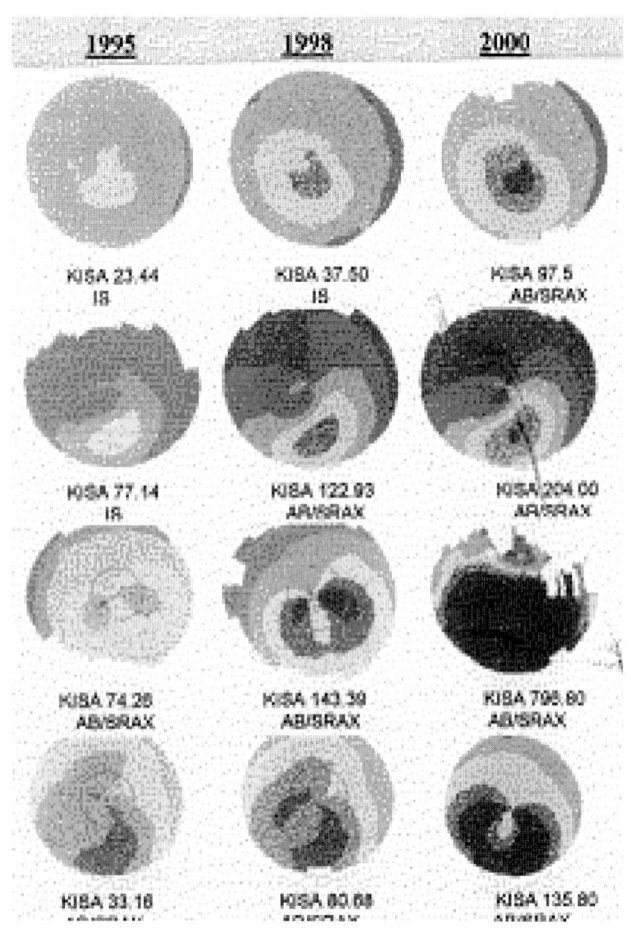

FIGURE 49-16. Examples of eyes that progressed from normal and keratoconus suspect to keratoconus over time, illustrating accompanying pattern analyses and KISA% quantitative indices.

In the published literature, there are at least 18 sets of monozygotic twins in which one or both of the pair show some degree of keratoconus. Thirteen of these pairs were described without the use of videokeratography: seven were concordant and six were discordant for keratoconus (99). The majority of twin reports currently in the literature strongly support a genetic etiology for keratoconus.

Corneal dystrophies, all of which have a genetic basis, are almost universally bilateral. There can be little doubt that the preponderance of patients with keratoconus have bilateral disease. Although the disease may start unilaterally, over time the other eye typically becomes involved, although in many instances the involvement may be subclinical. Over 90% of patients have evidence of bilateral changes when they are evaluated with videokeratography (91–93). The bilateral nature of keratoconus, similar to that of corneal dystrophies, also strongly suggests that it has a genetic basis.

Familial aggregation of a disease is one of the most commonly recognized bases for genetic influences in a disease. Though keratoconus is most commonly reported as sporadic, the incidence of familial aggregation reported in the literature ranges from 6% to 23.5% (2,37,79,100). In our center, 10% of keratoconus patients have a positive family history. It could be argued that because we are recruiting patients specifically for genetic studies, our numbers may be slightly higher than in the general population, as patients with a positive family history would naturally gravitate to our studies. However, the Collaborative Longitudinal Evaluation of Keratoconus (CLEK) Study reported a positive family history in 14% of subjects (94). This

TABLE 49-6. SEGREGATION ANALYSIS RESULTS

		Using Clinical Criteria Only	Using Topographic Indices
		Keratoconus (*n* = 218)	Normal Controls (*n* = 183)
Rejected	No major gene	$p < .05$	$p < .001$
	Sporadic	$p < .05$	$p < .005$
	Environment	$p < .025$	$p < .005$
	Additive	$p < .05$	$p < .010$
	Dominant	$p < .05$	***
Not rejected	Major gene	$p > .25$	$p > .10$
	Recessive	$p > .50$	$p > .90$
	Dominant	***	$p > .90$

study was a multicenter longitudinal study to observe the natural history of keratoconus without the ascertainment bias that could be attributed to our genetic studies. Both our study and the CLEK study enrolled a very broad and ethnically diverse group of patients. In more homogeneous populations such as those certain parts of Finland, New Zealand, and Tasmania the incidence of familial disease is much higher, on the order of 19% to 23% (79,100). Pronounced gene pooling from larger families with common ancestry is implicated in these unusual populations.

Most studies on the heredity of keratoconus probably underreport the true incidence of a positive family history, because subtle degrees of keratoconus may remain undetected in family members who are asymptomatic. Most reports in the literature suggest an autosomal-dominant mode of inheritance with variable expression, with emphasis being placed on subtle forms of the disorder, such as keratoconus fruste or mild irregular astigmatism in order to resolve the mode of inheritance (21,95,101–104). In 10 of the 52 families reported by Hammerstien (102), keratoconus was detected in two or more relatives. The degree of penetrance was approximately 20% with variable expressivity. In a report of seven pedigrees, Redmond (103) suggested that keratoconus fruste and high degrees of astigmatism represent incomplete expression of the keratoconus gene and should be taken into account in pedigree analysis. Rabinowitz et al. (21) used videokeratography to detect abortive forms of keratoconus in five families of patients with keratoconus. In all five families, hereditary patterns were consistent with autosomal-dominant transmission with variable expressivity. Videokeratographic abnormalities were found in at least one parent of seven sets of clinically normal parents of patients with keratoconus in another study (104).

Although several reports have suggested a recessive inheritance pattern in some families, none of these reports examined three generations or included subtle forms of the disorder in the pedigree analysis (105). Failure to include subclinical forms of keratoconus detectable only by videokeratography will lead to an underestimation of the true familial aggregation rate of keratoconus (1,14,15).

The strongest evidence for a genetic basis for keratoconus to date are the formal genetic studies (segregation analysis)

performed at Cedars-Sinai Medical Center on 95 keratoconus families recruited as part of our Keratoconus Genetics Research program. This study by Wang and co-workers (97) demonstrated that keratoconus prevalence in first-degree relatives of affected patients was 3.34%, 15 to 67 times higher than in the normal population. Videokeratography indices (I-S values and KISA% index) were significantly higher in sibling and parent–offspring pairs than in marital pairs, whereas those in marital pairs were no different from the normal population. Segregation analyses rejected both sporadic and environmental models and suggest a major gene effect using both clinical criteria and topographic indices (Table 49-6). This study, which was in part dependent on videokeratography descriptors of keratoconus, demonstrates that genes play a major role in the development of keratoconus and its subclinical manifestations (97).

MOLECULAR GENETIC STUDIES

The genetics of keratoconus are extremely complex. Because keratoconus is very heterogeneous, it is likely that this disease can be caused by multiple genes. In many instances, it may result from complex interactions between genes and environmental factors. It is also likely that in different families keratoconus may be caused by different gene defects or different gene–environment interactions. All of the factors make it difficult to clearly identify a single gene defects. The best opportunity for identifying genes for keratoconus is in rare populations with high concentrations of keratoconus because of a common founder. In these families heterogeneity is significantly minimized so that results of linkage analysis become more valid.

Though such families are rare, some progress has been made using the linkage approach to identify potential gene loci for keratoconus. To date, three studies have been performed on families with isolated autosomal-dominant keratoconus (and no other associated disease). Tyynismaa and co-workers (107) studied 20 families with autosomal-dominant keratoconus. All families originated from a common founder in a specific area in Finland with a high incidence of keratoconus. Using a genome-wide screen approach linkage was demonstrated to 16q22.3-q23.1, between markers D16S2624 and D16S3090, with a maximum parametric logarithm of odds (LOD) score of 4.10 and a nonparametric score of 3.27 (nonparametric linkage analyses [NPL], p = .00006). The authors suggest that this single locus for familial autosomal-dominant keratoconus without heterogeneity is the location of the causative gene for keratoconus. Unfortunately, there appear to be no genes in this region that could explain the development of keratoconus.

Fullerton and co-workers (100) used a novel "identity by descent" approach to study eight individuals with keratoconus from northwest Australia. These patients were from a coastal town in Tasmania where the incidence of keratoconus is five times that found in the general population. It was assumed that the individuals studied were likely related through a founder effect. Only seven or eight generations separated this population from its founders. A genome-wide search of the eight unrelated individuals was conducted. An association between marker D20S119 at 20q12 and keratoconus was suggested. Again, no genes have been identified in this region that might play a role in keratoconus.

Zhu's group (106) studied a large family from Utah with autosomal-dominant keratoconus using markers on chromosome 21. This area was chosen because of the known association between Down syndrome and keratoconus. Linkage has been demonstrated to a small 6.8-centimorgan (cM) section of chromosome 21 adjacent to its centromere, between markers D21S1905 and D21S409. Currently no known genes have been identified in this region. This family is being studied with other markers on the rest of the human genome to determine whether linkage is confined to this area or whether there might be other regions of stronger linkage in this and other families.

Another study has suggested that mutations in the *VSX1* homeobox gene (mapped to chromosomal region 20p11-q11) may play a role in up to 4.7% of patients with isolated keratoconus (107). However, this gene plays a role only in the embryonic retina and is not present in the adult human cornea. Further work is needed to determine what role, if any, the *VSX1* gene may play in the pathogenesis of keratoconus.

There is a strong association with keratoconus and retinal disease, in particular Leber's congenital amaurosis (30). Gene loci for families with keratoconus and Leber's have been identified on chromosome 17. There is no evidence that any genes in these regions play a role in isolated keratoconus (109,110). The chromosomal loci described in this section are summarized in Table 49-7.

DIFFERENTIAL DIAGNOSIS

It is important to distinguish keratoconus from other ectatic and thinning disorders such as pellucid marginal degeneration, Terrien's marginal degeneration, and keratoglobus

TABLE 49-7. POTENTIAL LOCI FOR KERATOCONUS GENES

Loci	Reference
Loci for isolated keratoconus	
16q22.3-q23	Tyynismaa et al., 2002 (107)
20q12	Fullerton et al., 2002 (100)
21p	Rabinowitz et al., *Invest Ophthalmol and Vis Sci* abstr, 1999 (106)
Loci for keratoconus associated with other disorders	
20p11-q11(VSX1 gene)	Heon et al., 2002 (108)
17p13 Leber's congenital amaurosis (LCA4)	Hameed et al., 2000 (109)
17p Leber's congenital amaurosis *AIPL-1* gene	Damji KF et al., 2001 (110)

because the management and prognosis in these disorders differ markedly from that in keratoconus. The distinction can usually be made by careful slit-lamp evaluation. Corneal topography is a useful adjunct to differentiate these disorders in subtle or early cases (72).

Pellucid marginal degeneration is characterized by a peripheral band of thinning of the inferior cornea from the 4 to the 8 o'clock position. There is 1- to 2-mm uninvolved area between the thinning and the limbus (Fig. 49-17). The corneal protrusion is most marked above the area of thinning, and the central cornea is usually of normal thickness. Pellucid marginal degeneration is a progressive disorder affecting both eyes, though findings may be asymmetric. In moderate cases, pellucid marginal degeneration can easily be differentiated from keratoconus by slit-lamp evaluation because of the classical location of the thinning. In early cases the cornea may look relatively normal.

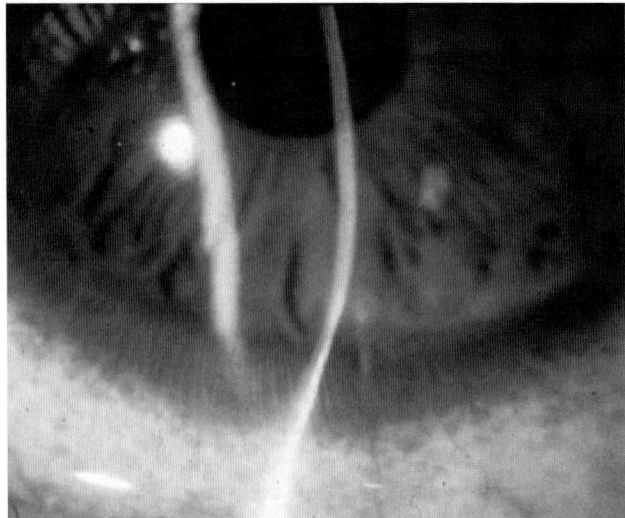

FIGURE 49-17. Slit-lamp photograph in a patient with pellucid marginal degeneration demonstrating thinning from the 4 to 8 o'clock position approximately 2 mm from the inferior limbus.

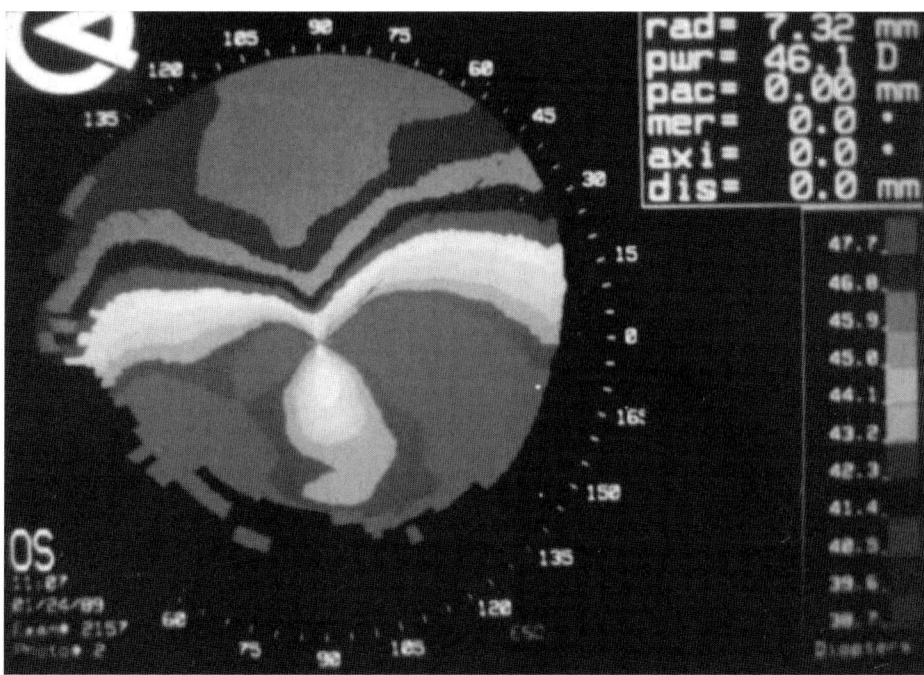

FIGURE 49-18. Videokeratograph of pellucid marginal degeneration showing typical "crab claw" appearance and against-the-rule astigmatism.

Advanced pellucid marginal degeneration may be difficult to distinguish from keratoconus because the thinning may progress to involve most, if not all, of the inferior cornea. In both early and advanced disease, videokeratography is very useful to make the distinction. The videokeratograph of pellucid marginal degeneration has a classical "butterfly" appearance (Fig. 49-18) and demonstrates large amounts of against-the-rule astigmatism as measured by simulated keratometry (72,111).

Pellucid marginal degeneration can be differentiated from other peripheral corneal thinning disorders such as Terrien's marginal degeneration in that the area of thinning is always epithelialized, clear, avascular, and without lipid deposition. Terrien's corneal degeneration affects a similar age group and results in high astigmatism. However, it may affect both the superior and inferior cornea and is accompanied by lipid deposition and vascular invasion (Fig. 49-19). Videokeratography can also be used to differentiate these two disorders because they have distinctly different topographic patterns (112).

Patients with pellucid marginal degeneration are much more difficult to fit with contact lenses than patients with keratoconus because of the large amounts of against-the-rule astigmatism. Large overall diameter spherical or aspheric contact lenses should initially be attempted in early to moderate cases. In patients in whom contact lenses do not adequately correct vision or in patients who are contact lens intolerant, surgery may be considered.

Pellucid patients are typically poor candidates for penetrating keratoplasty for two reasons. First, thinning occurs very peripherally, so that removing the ectatic cornea results in the donor being placed very close to the corneal limbus, thus increasing the chances of graft rejection. Second, penetrating keratoplasty in these patients typically induces large amounts of postoperative astigmatism because of the extreme thinning and its location. Postoperative

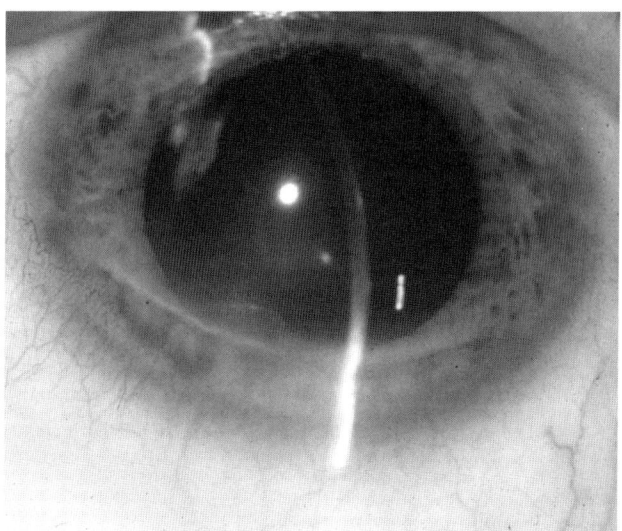

FIGURE 49-19. Slit-lamp photograph of a patient with Terrien's marginal degeneration.

astigmatism is often difficult to correct in pellucid patients because of disparity in graft–host thickness.

Crescentic lamellar keratoplasty is a useful initial surgical procedure in patients with pellucid marginal degeneration. This procedure involves removing a crescentic inferior layer of ectatic tissue by lamellar dissection and replacing it with a thicker lamellar donor graft (113). This approach often reduces the astigmatism and in some instances makes the patient contact lens tolerant, thus bypassing the need for a full-thickness procedure. In contact lens failures, penetrating keratoplasty can subsequently be performed, encompassing part of the lamellar graft, and significantly reducing the risk of graft rejection and postkeratoplasty astigmatism (114).

Keratoglobus is a rare disorder in which the entire cornea is thinned most markedly near the corneal limbus, as opposed to the localized central or paracentral thinning noted in keratoconus (115). In keratoglobus, thinning can approach up to 20% of corneal thickness, causing the cornea to assume a globular shape. In advanced keratoconus, the entire cornea can also become so thinned that it assumes a globular shape, making it difficult to distinguish these two entities. Invariably, however, even in very advanced keratoconus there may be a small area of uninvolved cornea superiorly that approaches normal corneal thickness. Keratoglobus is also bilateral, but is usually present from birth and tends to be nonprogressive. It can be distinguished from megalocornea and congenital glaucoma by the fact that the cornea is usually of normal diameter. It is a recessive disorder and is often associated with blue sclerae and other systemic features, in contrast to keratoconus, which is most commonly an isolated disorder (115). Keratoglobus corneas are prone to rupture from even minimal trauma. This is not the case with keratoconus. As such, hard contact lenses are contraindicated and protective spectacles should be strongly encouraged. If the cornea is extremely thin, a tectonic limbus-to-limbus lamellar keratoplasty should be considered to provide strength to the cornea and prevent it from rupturing. A subsequent central penetrating keratoplasty may be considered if adequate visual rehabilitation cannot be achieved with glasses.

MANAGEMENT

The management of keratoconus varies depending on the stage of the disease. Contact lenses are the mainstay of therapy in this disorder and are the treatment modality of choice in 90% of patients (116–119). In very early cases, patients may be satisfied with glasses for visual correction. More commonly, however, vision is best corrected with contact lenses, as glasses do not compensate for the unusual shape of the cornea and the resultant induced irregular astigmatism.

The type of contact lens used varies depending on the stage of the disease. Early in the disease, soft toric lenses are often adequate. As the disease progresses, more complex rigid gas-permeable lenses are used, including multicurve spherical-based lenses, aspheric lenses, and bispheric lenses. A hybrid lens that has a rigid central portion for obtaining best optics and a soft hydrophilic peripheral skirt is also popular with some practitioners (118,119). Contact lens fitting in keratoconus is a complex task embraced by few contact lens practitioners. The challenge is to keep the patient contact lens tolerant with good visual acuity despite a cornea that may be changing in shape over time. Common complications from contact lens use include induced corneal abrasions, apical scarring, neovascularization from induced hypoxia, lens discomfort, and lenses not staying on the cornea for adequate periods of time. Although some reports suggest that rigid contact lenses induce keratoconus, and anecdotal reports contend that keratoconus can be arrested by good contact lens fitting, there is no good evidence to support either of these contentions. It is my feeling that no keratoconus patient who can tolerate contact lenses should be denied the good visual rehabilitation afforded by them because of fear that they may enhance the progression of the disease.

Cornea transplantation (penetrating keratoplasty) is the best and most successful option for keratoconus patients not adequately visually rehabilitated by contact lenses. Because of the avascular nature of the cornea, this procedure carries over a 93% to 96% success rate (120–122). A patient with keratoconus has an approximately 10% to 20% risk over his lifetime of needing a cornea transplant. Due to improvements in both eye banking and surgical technique, this procedure can be done on an outpatient basis with minimal downtime to the patient. Complete visual recovery, however, may take as long as 6 months. Indications for cornea transplants include contact lens failures or intolerance, central scarring precluding good vision from contact lenses, and poor visual acuity despite tolerating contact lenses. Keratoconic corneas almost never perforate, and as such, advanced thinning by itself is not necessarily an indication for surgery.

Some surgeons have suggested that because of improved corneal transplant techniques and new and improved modalities to correct refractive error subsequent to corneal transplantation, patients whose best corrected spectacle visual acuity is suboptimal should be offered corneal transplantation in lieu of contact lens fitting (55). With the new contact lenses now available and with good fitting techniques, many patients with 20/40 spectacle correction may enjoy stable 20/20 to 20/25 contact lens corrected vision for many years without having to assume the risks inherent in cornea transplantation (118,119,123).

Patients with advanced disease may occasionally present with a sudden onset of visual loss accompanied by pain. On slit-lamp examination the conjunctiva may be injected and a diffuse stromal opacity is noted in the cornea. This condition, referred to as acute hydrops, is caused by breaks in Descemet's membrane with stromal imbibition of aqueous through these breaks (Fig. 49-10). The edema may persist for weeks or months, usually diminishing gradually, with relief of pain and resolution of the redness. Corneal edema is ultimately replaced by scarring. Acute hydrops is not an indication for penetrating keratoplasty because in many instances the hydrops will resolve with the resultant scar outside of the visual axis. The scarring may flatten the cornea, making the patients more contact lens tolerant, with improved visual acuity with contact lenses. Patients with hydrops can be treated initially with cycloplegics, steroids, or nonsteroidal antiinflammatory agents, and 5% sodium chloride solution (Muro128). A bandage contact lens may be needed in rare instances (124). Once the hydrops resolves, appropriate surgical or contact lens management can be undertaken.

Patients who are candidates for penetrating keratoplasty should be counseled that despite the high success rate of surgery, there is still a 50% chance that they may need contact lenses, because of either residual myopia or postkeratoplasty astigmatism. To decrease the amount of postoperative myopia, some surgeons perform keratoplasties using equal-size donor and host trephines (125,126). Typically this is 7.5 mm, as the incidence of rejection is slightly higher with larger size grafts. Although this approach, in many instances, does reduce the amount of myopia, patients who are axial myopes to begin with may still be left with large amounts of residual myopia (127). Despite significant advances in surgical techniques, patients with keratoconus may still end up with high amounts of postkeratoplasty

astigmatism even after all the sutures are removed. A combination of relaxing incisions and compression sutures, guided by videokeratography, can be used to correct large amounts of postkeratoplasty astigmatism, resulting in small residual amounts that are well corrected with rigid gas permeable lenses (72). Following these procedures, it is better to leave the patient with a small amount of with-the-rule astigmatism, because it is better tolerated and allows for easier contact lens fitting than against-the-rule astigmatism.

LASIK may also be considered to treat postkeratoplasty myopia and astigmatism. LASIK should be done only on patients with stable refractions and less than 4 D of cylinder who are at least 6 months postremoval of all corneal sutures. Patients with high astigmatism can be initially treated with astigmatic cuts and countertraction sutures to reduce the cylinder prior to LASIK (Figs. 49-20 to 49-23).

Postkeratoplasty LASIK is typically done in two stages (72). The flap, which is created during the first stage, is then put back in place and left for 6 weeks without any further treatment, because cutting through the graft–host junction will influence the amount of residual astigmatism left to be treated. After 6 weeks, a refraction is done and the flap is lifted for the final treatment. It is not uncommon for these patients to regress and require an enhancement. Posttransplant photorefractive keratectomy (PRK) commonly produces significant scarring and is therefore probably inadvisable.

In compliant patients, complications following penetrating keratoplasty are rare, but include graft rejection, postoperative astigmatism, a fixed dilated pupil (Urrets-Zavalia's syndrome),

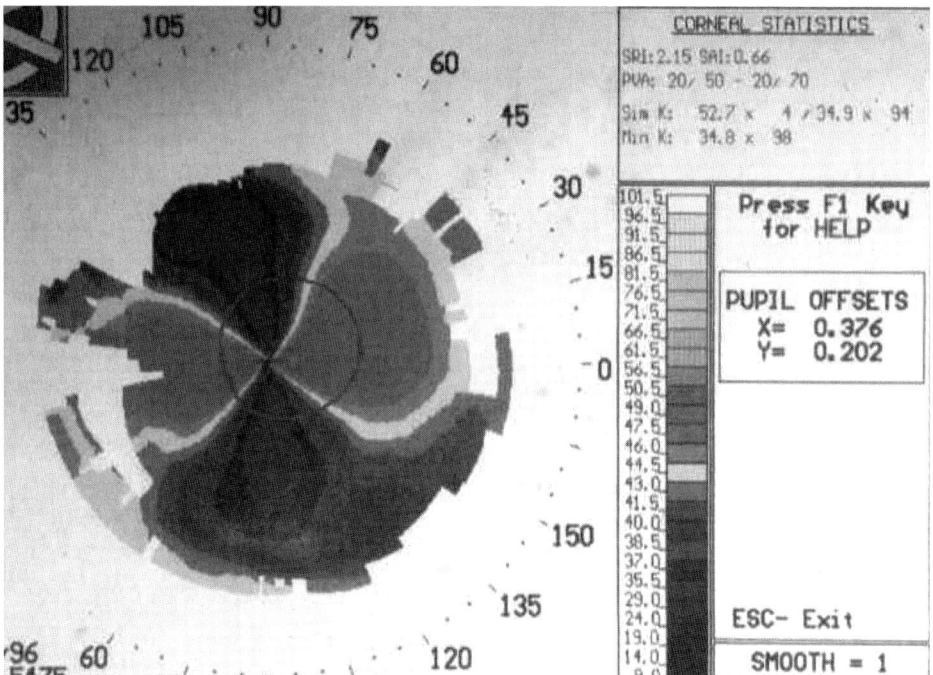

FIGURE 49-20. Videokeratograph showing large amount of astigmatism following penetrating keratoplasty not correctable with glasses or contact lenses.

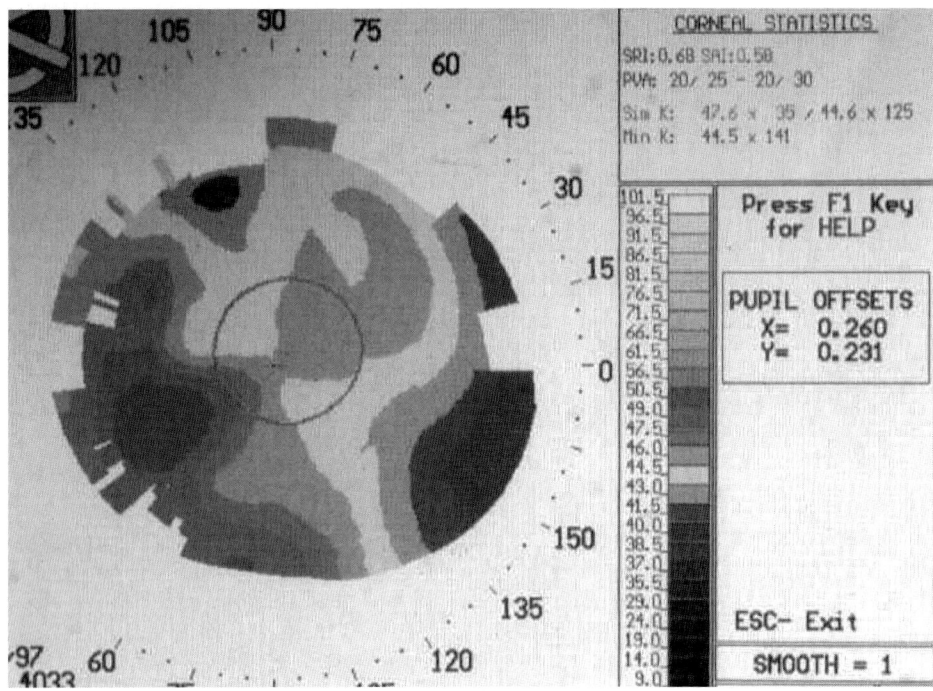

FIGURE 49-21. Videokeratograph showing reduction of astigmatism following arcuate astigmatic keratotomy and compression sutures.

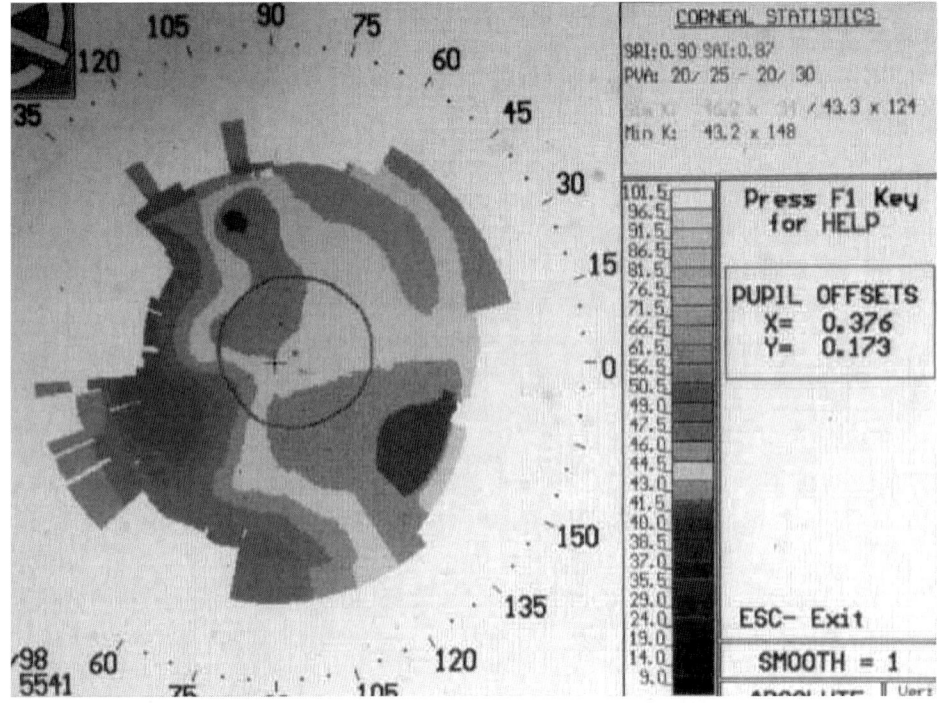

FIGURE 49-22. Videokeratograph showing further reduction of astigmatism and myopia after LASIK; uncorrected vision of 20/30.

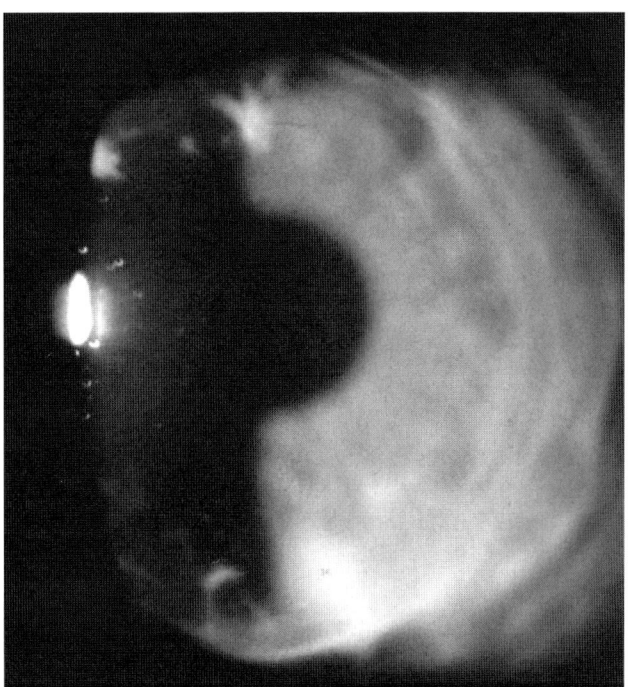

FIGURE 49-23. Slit-lamp photograph of the same patient as in Fig. 49-22 with a clear visual axis after cornea transplant, astigmatic keratotomy, and LASIK procedure. Scars from the transplant and astigmatic keratotomy are visible, but the LASIK scar at the 9.5-mm optical zone is not seen.

a femtosecond laser. The segments flatten the cornea, thus reducing the amount of myopia and making patients more contact lens tolerant. These segments can be removed at any time and patients can still undergo a cornea transplant without any harmful effects should the INTACS fail to achieve the desired effect. In the United States, INTACS are currently only approved for the correction of myopia. Their use in patients with keratoconus is regarded as an off-label procedure.

Recent studies suggest that in addition to making patients more contact lens tolerant, there may be other beneficial effects of implanting INTACS in patients with keratoconus. These include improving both uncorrected acuity and best corrected acuity, as well as decreasing higher order aberrations as measured by wavefront analysis (134,135).

Not infrequently, patients with suspicious topographies present for refractive surgery evaluation. Often these patients are unable to obtain 20/20 vision with spectacles. It behooves all refractive surgeons to carefully screen patients for "forme fruste" or early keratoconus. LASIK is contraindicated in all patients with clinically apparent or early keratoconus. It is probably best to avoid LASIK in patients with "keratoconus suspect" topography. Multiple reports of corneal decompensation and progression of keratoconus and early keratoconus have been published (Fig. 49-24) (136,137). Disease progression in patients who were keratoconus "suspects" prior to their LASIK surgery has resulted in significant litigation in the United States. This underscores the need for refractive surgeons to pay careful attention and become proficient with the minimal topographic criteria for diagnosing keratoconus. Unusual topographies should be considered to represent keratoconus "suspect" when the guidelines outlined earlier in this chapter are met and LASIK should be deferred in these patients. Excimer laser PRK should also be avoided in patients with pellucid marginal degeneration, because significant corneal scarring has been demonstrated even in patients with extremely mild disease (Fig. 49-25).

On the other hand, excimer laser phototherapeutic keratectomy (PTK) has been demonstrated to be useful in the management of patients with keratoconus who have nodular subepithelial corneal scars causing contact lens intolerance. This technique provides a smooth corneal surface, allowing patients to regain contact lens tolerance. Such nodules may also be removed at the slit lamp with a sharp hand-held blade potentially achieving a similar result, albeit with less precision (138).

One small study, with short-term data only, suggests that the excimer laser may provide an improved refractive effect and delay the need for penetrating keratoplasty in patients with advanced keratoconus who are scheduled to undergo penetrating keratoplasty (139). This mode of treatment for keratoconus is not currently commonly accepted and should be approached with extreme caution until long-term

and recurrence of keratoconus (128–130). Graft rejection rates in keratoconus are low and may be reversed with medication if treated early. There have been isolated reports of keratoconus recurring in the graft decades after surgery. These reports are extremely rare and it is not entirely clear whether keratoconus resulted from the disease recurring in the graft or from transplanted donor buttons with mild undetected disease (131,132). Patients may ask about recurrence, and these isolated reports should be mentioned within this context.

Epikeratoplasty gained acceptance in the past as a mode of treatment for patients with keratoconus with a clear visual axis. Good long-term results have been reported (133). However, epikeratoplasty has been largely abandoned in favor of penetrating keratoplasty because of the superior quality of vision afforded by the latter procedure. There still is a role for epikeratoplasty in select high-risk circumstances, such as patients with Down's syndrome in whom an extraocular procedure might be preferable because of reduced risk of wound rupture and graft rejection.

In patients who are contact lens intolerant with a clear visual axis, intrastromal corneal rings (INTACS) are a potential option to avoid the need for a cornea transplant. Two polymethylmethacrylate (PMMA) arcuate segments are inserted into the midstroma of the cornea. The channels are created either with a mechanical keratome or with

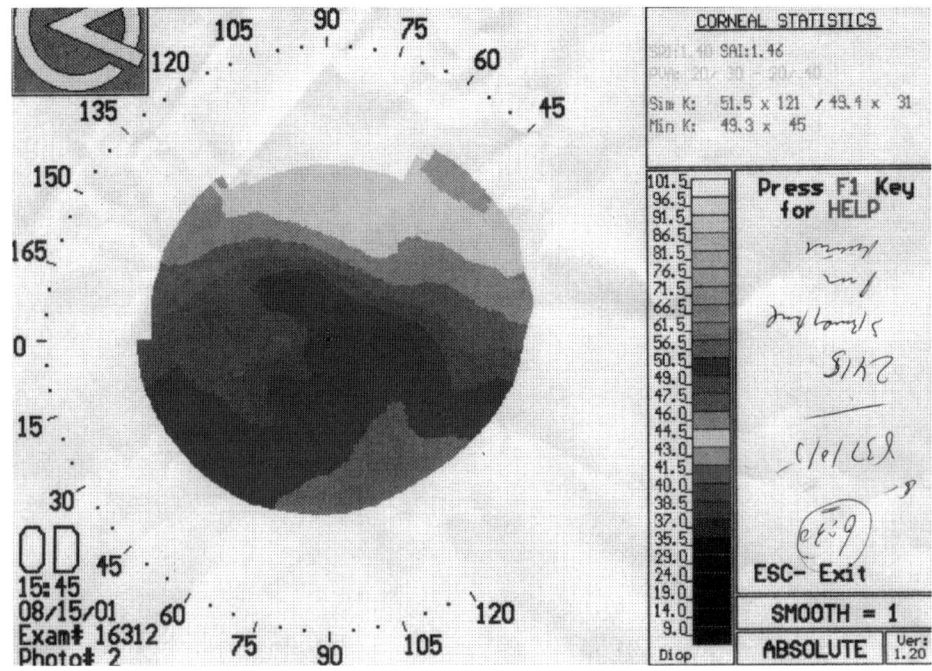

FIGURE 49-24. Ectasia in a patient who had LASIK with undiagnosed early keratoconus.

data on outcomes become available. Performing this procedure on an already thinned and irregular cornea could be hazardous, with the potential for immediate complications exceeding the long-term therapeutic effect.

Clinical trials of PRK using custom cornea excimer laser software on patients with mild keratoconus whose disease has stabilized (i.e., over age 45) are to commence soon. This might prove useful in select cases where the irregular

astigmatism can be treated to improve the refractive effect without thinning the cornea excessively (140).

REFERENCES

1. Rabinowitz YS. Keratoconus: update and new advances. *Surv Ophthalmol* 1998;42:297–319.
2. Krachmer JH, Feder RS, Belin MW. Keratoconus and related noninflammatory corneal thinning disorders. *Surv Ophthalmol* 1994;28:293–322.
3. Smolin G. Dystrophies and degenerations. In: Smolin G, Thoft RA, eds. *The cornea scientific foundations and clinical practice.* Boston: Little, Brown, 1987:448.
4. Rabinowitz YS, Nesburn AB, McDonnell PJ. Videokeratography of the fellow eye in unilateral keratoconus. *Ophthalmology* 1993;100:181–186.
5. Sharif KW, Casey TA, Colart J. Prevalence of mitral valve prolapse in keratoconus patients. *J R Soc Med* 1992;85:446–448.
6. Hallerman W, Wilson EJ. Genetische betrachtungen uber den keratoconus (German). *Klin Monatsbl Augenhlkd* 1977;170:906–908.
7. Duke-Elder S, Leigh AG. *System of ophthalmology. Diseases of the outer eye,* vol 8, part 2. London: Henry Kimpton, 1965:964–976.
8. Franceschetti A. Keratoconus. In: King JH, McTigue JW, eds. *The cornea. World Congress.* Washington: Butterworths, 1965:152–168.
9. Hofstetter H. A keratoscopic survey of 13,395 eyes. *Am J Optom Acad Optom* 1959;36:3–11.
10. Kennedy RH, Bourne WM, Dyer JA. A 48-year clinical and epidemiologic study of keratoconus. *Am J Ophthalmol* 1986;101:267–273.
11. Maguire LJ, Meyer RF. Ectatic corneal degenerations. In: Kaufman H, ed. *The cornea.* 1988:485–510.
12. Rabinowitz YS, Klyce SD, Krachmer JH, et al. Videokeratography, keratoconus, and refractive surgery. *Opin Refract Corneal Surg* 1992;5:403–407.

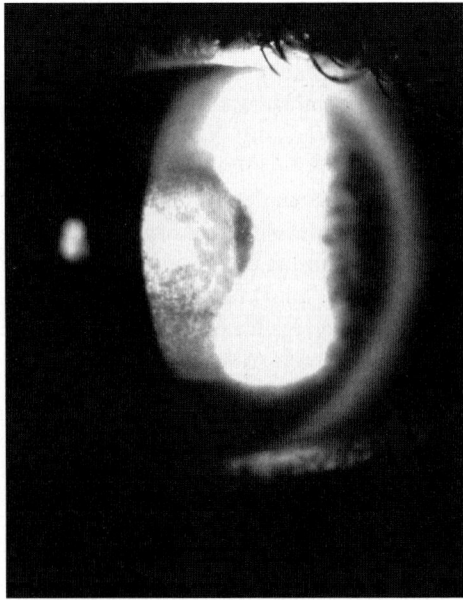

FIGURE 49-25. Central scarring following photorefractive keratectomy (PRK) in a patient with undiagnosed early pellucid marginal degeneration.

13. Rabinowitz YS, Rasheed K, Yang H, et al. Accuracy of ultrasonic pachymetry and videokeratography in detecting keratoconus. *J Cataract Refract Surg* 1998;24:196–200.

14. Amsler M. Le keratocone fruste au javal (French). *Ophthalmologica* 1938;96:77–83.

15. Amsler M. Keratocone classique et keratocone fruste, arguments unitaires. *Ophthalmologica* 1946;111:96–101.

16. Rowsey JJ, Reynolds AE, Brown R. Corneal topography. Corneascope. *Arch Ophthalmol* 1981;99:1093–1100.

17. Rabinowitz YS, McDonnell PJ. Computer-assisted corneal topography in keratoconus. *Refract Corneal Surg* 1989;56:400–406.

18. Wilson SE, Lin DTC, Klyce SD. The topography of keratoconus. *Cornea* 1991;10:2–8.

19. Perry HD, Buxton JN, Fine BS. Round and oval cones in keratoconus. *Ophthalmology* 1980;87:905–909.

20. Maguire LJ, Bourne W. Corneal topography of early keratoconus. *Am J Ophthalmol* 1989;108:107–112.

21. Rabinowitz YS, Garbus J, McDonnell PJ. Computer-assisted corneal topography in family members of keratoconus. *Arch Ophthalmol* 1990;108:365–371.

22. Klyce SD. Computer-assisted corneal topography. High resolution graphic presentation and analysis of keratoscopy. *Invest Ophthalmol Vis Sci* 1984;25:1426–1435.

23. Stone DL, Kenyon KR, Stark WJ. Ultrastructure of keratoconus with healed hydrops. *Am J Ophthalmol* 1976;82:450–458.

24. Hartstien J. Keratoconus that developed in patients wearing corneal contact lenses. *Arch Ophthalmol* 1968;80:345–346.

25. McKusick VA. *Heritable diseases of connective tissue.* St. Louis: CV Mosby, 1966:56.

26. McKusick VA. Inherited disorders of connective tissue. In: Harrison TR, ed. *Principles of internal medicine.* New York: McGraw-Hill, 1974:2015–2020.

27. Cullen JF, Butler HG. Mongolism (Down's syndrome) and keratoconus. *Br J Ophthalmol* 1963;47:321–330.

28. Shapiro MB, France T. The ocular features of Down's syndrome. *Am J Ophthalmol* 1985;99:659.

29. Alstrom CH, Olson O. Heredo-retinopathia congenitalis. Monohybride recessiva autosomalis. *Hereditas Genttiskt* 1957;43:1–177.

30. Elder MJ. Leber congenital amaurosis and its association with keratoconus and keratoglobus. *J Pediatr Ophthalmol Strabismus* 1994;31:38–40.

31. Judisch F, Wariri M, Krachmer J. Ocular Ehlers-Danlos syndrome with normal lysyl hydrolase activity. *Arch Ophthalmol* 1976;94:1489.

32. Kirkham TH, Werner EB. The ophthalmic manifestations of Rothmund's syndrome. *Can J Ophthalmol* 1975;10:1–14.

33. McKusick VA. *Heritable diseases of connective tissue.* St. Louis: CV Mosby, 1966:56.

34. McKusick VA. Inherited disorders of connective tissue. In: Harrison TR, ed. *Principles of internal medicine.* New York: McGraw-Hill, 1974:2015–2020.

35. Robertson I. Keratoconus and Ehlers Danlos syndrome. A new aspect of keratoconus. *Med J Aust* 1975;1:571–573.

36. Street DA, Vinokur ET, Waring GO III, et al. Lack of association between keratoconus, mitral valve prolapse and joint hypermobility. *Ophthalmology* 1991;98:170–176.

37. Tretter T, Rabinowitz YS, Yang H, et al. Aetiological factors in keratoconus. *Ophthalmology* 1995;102A:156.

38. Beardsley TL, Foulks GN. An association of keratoconus and mitral valve prolapse. *Ophthalmology* 1982;89:35–37.

39. Sharif KW, Casey TA, Colart J. Prevalence of mitral valve prolapse in keratoconus patients. *J R Soc Med* 1992;85:446–448.

40. Gasset AR, Houde WI, Garcia-Bengochea H. Contact lens wear as an environmental risk factor for keratoconus. *Am J Ophthalmol* 1978;85:339–341.

41. Hartstien J. Keratoconus that developed in patients wearing corneal contact lenses. *Arch Ophthalmol* 1968;80:345–346.

42. Negris R. Floppy eyelid syndrome associated with keratoconus. *J Am Optom Assoc* 1992;63:316–319.

43. Rahi A, Davies P, Ruben M, et al. Keratoconus and coexisting atopic disease. *Br J Ophthalmol* 1977;61:761.

44. Wachmeister L, Ingemannsson SO, Moller E. Atopy and HLA antigens in patients with keratoconus. *Acta Ophthalmol (Copenh)* 1982;60:113.

45. Klintworth GK, Damms T. Corneal dystrophies and keratoconus. *Curr Opin Ophthalmol Curr Sci* 1995;6:44–56.

46. Sawagamuchi S, Yue BYT, Sugar J, et al. Lysosomal abnormalities in keratoconus. *Arch Ophthalmol* 1989;107:1507–1510.

47. Fukuchi T, Yue B, Sugar J, et al. Lysosomal enzyme activities in tissues of patients with keratoconus. *Arch Ophthalmol* 1994;112:1368–1374.

48. Sawagamuchi S, Twinning SS, Yue BY, et al. Alpha 2 macroglobulin levels in normal human and keratoconus corneas. *Invest Ophthalmol Vis Sci* 1994;35:4008–4014.

49. Kenney MC, Chwa M, Opbroek AJ, et al. Increased gelatinolytic activity in keratoconus keratocyte cultures. A correlation to an altered matrix metalloproteinase-2/tissue inhibitor of metalloproteinase ratio. *Cornea* 1994;13:108–113.

50. Opbroek A, Kenney MC, Brown D. Characterization of a human corneal metalloproteinase inhibitor (TIMP-1). *Curr Eye Res* 1993;12:877–883.

51. Smith VA, Hoh VB, Littleton L, et al. Overexpression of gelatinase A activity in keratoconus. *Eye* 1995;9:429–433.

52. Wilson SE, He YG, Weng J, et al. Epithelial injury induces keratocyte apoptosis; hypothesized role for the interleukin 1 system in the modulation of corneal tissue organization and wound healing. *Exp Eye Res* 1996;62:325–337.

53. Bereau J, Fabre EJ, Hecquet C, et al. Modification of prostaglandin E2 and collagen synthesis in keratoconus fibroblasts associated with an increase of interleukin 1 alpha receptor number. *CR Acad Sci Paris* 1993;316:425–430.

54. Bron A, Rabinowitz YS. Corneal dystrophies and keratoconus. *Curr Opin Ophthalmol* 1996;7:71–82.

55. Merlin U, Cantera E. In: Burrato L, ed. *Corneal topography. The clinical atlas.* New Jersey: Slack, 1996:9–93.

56. Gormley DJ, Gersten M, Koplin RS, et al. Corneal modeling. *Cornea* 1988;7:30.

57. Hannush SB, Crawford SL, Waring GO III, et al. Accuracy and precision of keratometry, photokeratoscopy, and corneal modeling on calibrated steel balls. *Arch Ophthalmol* 1989;107:1235–1239.

58. Maguire LJ, Wilson SE, Camp JJ, et al. Evaluating the reproducibility of topography systems on spherical surfaces. *Arch Ophthalmol* 1993;111:259–262.

59. Wilson SE, Verity SM, Conger DL. Accuracy and reproducibility of the corneal analysis system and topographic modeling system. *Cornea* 1992;11:28–35.

60. Wilson SE, Klyce SD. Quantitative descriptors of corneal topography. A clinical study. *Arch Ophthalmol* 1991;109:349–353.

61. Waring GO, Rabinowitz YS, Sugar J, et al. Nomenclature for keratoconus suspects. *Opin Refract Corneal Surg* 1993;9:3:219–221.

62. Wilson SE, Klyce SD, Husseini MD. Standardized color coded maps for corneal topography. *Ophthalmology* 1993;100:1723–1727.

63. Rabinowitz YS, Yang H, Akkina J, et al. Videokeratography of normal human corneas. *Br J Ophthalmol* 1996;80:610–616.

64. Rasheed K, Rabinowitz YS, Remba M, et al. Inter- and intra-observer reliability of a classification scheme for corneal topographic patterns. *Br J Ophthalmol* 1998;82:1401–1406.

65. Rabinowitz YS. Videokeratographic indices to aid in screening for keratoconus. *J Refract Surg* 1995;11:371–379.

66. Li X, Rabinowitz YS, Yang H. Longitudinal analysis of the normal eyes in unilateral keratoconus. *Ophthalmology (in press)*.

67. Wilson SE, Lin DTC, Klyce SD, et al. Topographic changes in contact lens-induced corneal warpage. *Ophthalmology* 1990;97:734–744.

68. Maguire LJ, Klyce SD, McDonald ME, et al. Corneal topography of pellucid marginal degeneration. *Ophthalmology* 1987;94:519–524.

69. Rabinowitz YS. Tangential vs sagittal videokeratographs in the "early" detection of keratoconus. *Am J Ophthalmol* 1996;122:888–889.

70. Durand L, Monot JP, Burillon C, et al. Radial keratotomy in a patient with keratoconus. *Refract Corneal Surg* 1991;7:374–376.

71. Mammilis N, Montgomery S, Anderson C, et al. Radial keratotomy in a patient with keratoconus. *Refract Corneal Surg* 1991;7:374–376.

72. Rabinowitz YS, Wilson SE, Klyce SD. *Corneal topography: interpreting videokeratography.* New York: Igaku Shoin Medical Publishers, 1993:63.

73. Nesburn AB, Bahri S, Salz J, et al. Keratoconus in photorefractive keratectomy candidates detected by computer–assisted videokeratography. *Refract Corneal Surg* 1995;11:194–201.

74. Rabinowitz YS, McDonnell PJ. Computer-assisted corneal topography in keratoconus. *Refract Corneal Surg* 1989;5,6:400–406.

75. Morrow GL, Stein RM, Racine JS, et al. Computerized videokeratography of keratoconus kindreds. *Can J Ophthalmol* 1997;32:233–243.

76. Salabert D, Cochener B, Mage F, et al. Keratoconus and familial topographic corneal anomalies. *J Fr Ophthalmol* 1994;17:646–656.

77. Rabinowitz YS. Videokeratographic indices to aid in screening for keratoconus. *Refract Corneal Surg* 1995;11:371–379.

78. Rabinowitz YS, Rasheed K. KISA% system a new videokeratography system for the early detection of keratoconus. *J Cataract Refract Surg* 1999;25:1327–1336.

79. Ihalainen A. Clinical and epidemiological features of keratoconus: genetic and external factors in the pathogenesis of the disease. *Acta Ophthalmol* 1986;178:1–64.

80. Etzine S. Conical cornea in identical twins. *S A Med J* 1954;28:154–155.

81. Hammerstien W. Keratoconus concurrent in identical twins. *Ophthalmologica* 1972;165:449–452.

82. Franccceschetti A, Lisch K, Klein D. Two pairs of identical twins concordant for keratoconus. *Klin Monatsbl Augenberld* 1958;33:15–30.

83. Woilez M, Razemon P, Constantinides G. A recent case of keratoconus and univitteline twins. *Bull Soc Ophthalmol* 1976;76:279–281.

84. Zadnik K, Mannis MJ, Johnson CA. An analysis of contrast sensitivity in identical twins with keratoconus. *Cornea* 1984;3:99–103.

85. Bourne WM, Michaelis W. Keratoconus in one identical twin. *Cornea* 1982;1:35–37.

86. Iwaskzkiewcz E, Czubak M, Galecki K, et al. Keratoconus and coexisting diseases in monozygotic twins. *Klin Oczna* 1992;94:345–346.

87. Owens H, Watters GA. Keratoconus in monozygotic twins in New Zealand *Clin Exp Optom* 1995;78:125–129.

88. Bechara SJ, Waring GO 3rd, Insler MS. Keratoconus in two pairs of identical twins. *Cornea* 1996;15:90–93.

89. Parker J, Ko WW, Pavlopoulos G, et al. Videokeratography of keratoconus in monozygotic twins. *J Refract Surg* 1996;12:180–183.

90. McMahon TT, Shin JA, Newlin A, et al. Discordance for keratoconus in two pairs of monozygotic twins. *Cornea* 1999;18:444–451.

91. Rabinowitz YS, Nesburn AB, McDonnell PJ. Videokeratography of the fellow eye in unilateral keratoconus. *Ophthalmology* 1993;100:181–186.

92. Lee LR, Hirst LW, Readshaw G. Clinical detection of unilateral keratoconus. *Aust N Z J Ophthalmol* 1995;23:129–133.

93. Holland DR, Maeda N, Hannush SB, et al. Unilateral keratoconus. Incidence and quantitative topographic analysis. *Ophthalmology* 1997;104:1409–1413.

94. Zadnik K, Barr J, Edrington TB, et al. Baseline findings in the Collaborative Longitudinal Evaluation of Keratoconus (CLEK) Study. *Invest Ophthalmol Vis Sci* 1998;39:2537–2546.

95. Ihalainen A. Clinical and epidemiological features of keratoconus genetic and external factors in the pathogenesis of the disease. *Acta Ophthalmol Suppl* 1986;178:1–64.

96. Owens H, Gamble G. A profile of keratoconus in New Zealand. *Cornea* 2003;2:122–125.

97. Wang Y, Rabinowitz YS, Rotter JI, et al. Genetic epidemiological study of keratoconus: evidence for major gene determination. *Am J Med Genet* 2000;93:403–409.

98. Thompson JS, Thompson MW. Twins in medical genetics. In: Thompson JS, Thompson MW, eds. *Genetics in medicine.* Philadelphia: WB Saunders, 1986.

99. Edwards M, McGhee CN, Dean S. The genetics of keratoconus. *Clin Exp Ophthalmol* 2001;29:345–351.

100. Fullerton J, Paprocki P, Foote S, et al. Identity-by-descent approach to gene localisation in eight individuals affected by keratoconus from north-west Tasmania, Australia. *Hum Genet* 2002;110:462–470.

101. Falls HF, Allen AW. Dominantly inherited keratoconus. *J Genet Hum* 1969;17:317–324.

102. Hammerstien W. Keratoconus concurrent in identical twins. *Ophthalmologica* 1972;165:449–452.

103. Redmond K. The role of heredity in keratoconus. *Trans Ophthalmol Soc Aust* 1968;27:52–54.

104. Gonzalez V, McDonnell PJ. Computer-assisted corneal topography in parents of patients with keratoconus. *Arch Ophthalmol* 1992;110:1413–1414.

105. Francois J. Afflictions of the cornea. In: Francois J, ed. *Heredity in ophthalmology.* St. Louis: CV Mosby, 1961:297–298.

106. Rabinowitz YS, Zhu H, Yang H, et al. Keratoconus. Nonparametric linkage analysis suggests a gene near the centromere of chromosome 21. *Invest Ophthalmol Vis Sci* 1999;40:2975.

107. Tyynismaa H, Sistonen P, Tuupanen S, et al. A locus for autosomal dominant keratoconus: linkage to 16q22.3–q23.1 in Finnish families. *Invest Ophthalmol Vis Sci* 2002;43:3160–3164.

108. Heon E, Greenberg A, Kopp KK, et al. Related VSX1: a gene for posterior polymorphous dystrophy and keratoconus. *Hum Mol Genet* 2002;11:1029–1031.

109. Hameed A, Khaliq S, Ismail M, et al. A novel locus for Leber congenital amaurosis (LCA4) with anterior keratoconus mapping to chromosome 17p13. *Invest Ophthalmol Vis Sci* 2000;41:629–633.

110. Damji KF, Sohocki MM, Khan R, et al. Leber's congenital amaurosis with anterior keratoconus in Pakistani families is caused by the Trp278X mutation in the AIPL1 gene on 17p. *Can J Ophthalmol* 2001;36:252–259.

111. Maguire LJ, Singer DE, Klyce SD. Graphic presentation of computer-analyzed keratoscope photographs. *Arch Ophthalmol* 1987;105:223–230.

112. Wilson SE, Lin DTC, Klyce SD, et al. The corneal topography of Terrien's marginal degeneration. *Refract Corneal Surg* 1990;6:15–20.
113. Schanzlin DJ, Samo EM, Robin JB. Crescentic lamellar keratoplasty in pellucid marginal degeneration. *Am J Ophthalmol* 1983;96:253.
114. Rasheed K, Rabinowitz YS. Surgical treatment of advanced pellucid marginal degeneration. *Ophthalmology* 2000;2:1: 17–20.
115. Verrey F. Keratoglobe aigu. *Ophthalmologica* 1947;114:284.
116. Buxton JN. Contact lenses in keratoconus. *Contact Intraocular Lens Med J* 1978;4:74.
117. Rabinowitz YS, Garbus JJ, Garbus C, et al. Contact lens selection for keratoconus using a computer-assisted videophotokeratoscope. *CLAO J* 1991;17:88–93.
118. Rosenthal P, Cotter JM. Clinical performance of a spline-based apical vaulting keratoconus corneal contact lens design. *CLAO J* 1995;21:42–46.
119. Yeung K, Egbahli F, Weissman BA. Clinical experience with piggyback contact lens systems on keratoconic eyes. *J Am Optom Assoc* 1995;66:539–543.
120. Price FW, Whitson WE, Marks RG. Graft survival in four common groups of patients undergoing penetrating keratoplasty. *Ophthalmology* 1991;98:322–328.
121. Sharif KW, Casey TA. Penetrating keratoplasty for keratoconus: complications and long term success. *Br J Ophthalmol* 1991;75:142–146.
122. Williams KA, Muehlberg SM, Lewis RF, et al. How successful is corneal transplantation? A report from the Australian Corneal Graft Register. *Eye* 1995;9:219–227.
123. Buzard KA, Fundingsland BR. Cornea transplants for keratoconus. Results in early and late disease. *J Refract Surg* 1997;23:398–496.
124. Smolin G. Dystrophies and Degenerations. In: Smolin G, Thoft RA, eds. *The cornea scientific foundations and clinical practice.* Boston: Little, Brown, 1987:449.
125. Tuft SJ, Gregory WM, Davison CR. Bilateral penetrating keratoplasty for keratoconus. *Ophthalmology* 1995;102:462–468.
126. Goble RR, Hardman Lea SJ, Falcon MG. The use of the same size host and donor trephine in penetrating keratoplasty for keratoconus. *Eye* 1994;8:311–314.
127. Tuft SJ, Fitzke FW, Buckley RJ. Myopia following penetrating keratoplasty for keratoconus. *Br J Ophthalmol* 1992;76: 642–645.
128. Kirkness C, Ficker L, Steele A, et al. Refractive surgery for graft-induced astigmatism after penetrating keratoplasty for keratoconus. *Ophthalmology* 1991;98:1786–1792.
129. Tuft SJ, et al. Iris ischaemia following penetrating keratoplasty for keratoconus (Urets-Zavalia syndrome). *Cornea* 1995;14:618–622.
130. Kremer I, Eagle RC, Rapuano CJ, et al. Histologic evidence of recurrent keratoconus seven years after keratoplasty. *Am J Ophthalmol* 1995;119:511–512.
131. Nirankari VS, Karesh J, Bastion F, et al. Recurrence of keratoconus in a donor cornea 22 years after successful keratoplasty. *Br J Ophthalmol* 1983;67:32.
132. Lass JH, Stocker EG, Fritz ME, et al. Epikeratoplasty. The surgical correction of aphakia, myopia, and keratoconus. *Ophthalmology* 1987;94:912–925.
133. Waller SG, Steinert RF, Wagoner MD. Long-term results of epikeratoplasty for keratoconus. *Cornea* 1995;14:84–88.
134. Colin J, Cochener B, Savary G, et al. INTACS inserts for treating keratoconus: one-year results. *Ophthalmology* 2001;108: 1409–1414.
135. Siganos D, Ferrara P, Chatzinikolas K, et al. Management of keratoconus with Intacs. *Am J Ophthalmol* 2003;135:64–70.
136. Rao SN, Epstein RJ. Early onset ectasia following laser *in situ* keratomileusus: case report and literature review. *J Refract Surg* 2002;18:177–184.
137. Kohnen T. Iatrogenic keratectasia: current knowledge, current measurements. *J Cataract Refract Surg* 2002;28:2065–2066.
138. Ward MA, Artunduaga G, Thompson KP, et al. Phototherapeutic keratectomy for the treatment of nodular subepithelial corneal scars in patients with keratoconus who are contact lens intolerant. *CLAO J* 1995;21:130–132.
139. Mortensen J, Ohrstrom A. Excimer laser photorefractive keratectomy for treatment of keratoconus. *J Refract Corneal Surg* 1994;10:368–372.
140. Tamayo Fernandez GE, Serrano MG. Early clinical experience using custom excimer laser ablations to treat irregular astigmatism. *J Cataract Refract Surg* 2000;26:1442–1450.

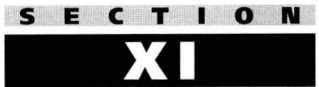

SECTION XI

CORNEAL AND CONJUNCTIVAL MANIFESTATIONS OF DIETARY DEFICIENCIES

CORNEAL AND CONJUNCTIVAL MANIFESTATIONS OF DIETARY DEFICIENCIES

PETER C. DONSHIK

Dietary deficiencies rarely produce clinical disease in developed countries; however, they are an important factor in the production of systemic and ocular disease in other parts of the world. Ocular problems associated with vitamin A deficiency and protein-energy malnutrition are the most common. Hundreds of thousands of preschool-age children may be afflicted each year with potentially blinding consequences of poor nutrition. The clinical disease, together with limited or poor access to preventive and curative health services, leads to enhanced ophthalmic disease. Although there is wide variability in the prevalence of the ocular manifestation of vitamin A deficiency (1), an example of the potential magnitude of the problem is indicated by a study performed in Aborigine children in Malaysia. In this study, night blindness was found in 16% of the children, conjunctival xerosis in 57.3%, Bitot's spot in 2.8%, and corneal xerosis in 0.5% (2). It is estimated that in Africa, Asia, and South America, 10 million new cases of xerophthalmia occur per year, of which 280,000 to 500,000 result in blindness (3). Worldwide vitamin A deficiency is probably the leading cause of blindness in children, with approximately 228 million children affected (4).

TYPES OF MALNUTRITION

Two categories of malnutrition have been associated with specific clinical syndromes in children. These are marasmus, a generalized protein-energy deficiency, and kwashiorkor, which is associated primarily with protein deficiency. Both of these conditions are seen most frequently in those between weaning and 6 years of age. Ocular manifestations of vitamin A deficiency are seen in both conditions.

Marasmus

When environmental factors, such as widespread famine, lead to chronic deficiency of all food categories, marasmus

results. This manifestation of starvation is illustrated in Fig. 50-1, which shows the small and poorly developed child. Body fat does not develop, muscles waste away, the muscle tone is significantly deceased, skin elasticity is lost, and there is mental dullness. The eyes are staring, with a decreased blink rate. There is little animation or response to stimulation, and if the child does cry, it is usually a very weak cry.

The prognosis for children with marasmus is guarded. It is estimated that 40% of children who are treated for marasmus will ultimately die of starvation. One of the main factors for the poor prognosis is that even if the child is treated in the hospital, once he or she returns home, the underlying problems that caused the condition in the first place have not changed. These children are at high risk for development of vitamin A deficiency, and they are also more vulnerable to the complications of routine childhood diseases such as measles or herpes simplex infection.

Kwashiorkor

Kwashiorkor occurs when an infant is placed on a diet high in carbohydrate and low in protein. There is an insufficient supply of essential amino acids, which affects normal protein synthesis. This results in an inability to maintain the usual intravascular volume, which results in edema. Clinically, a child with kwashiorkor has edema of the abdomen and extremities with wastage of the musculature (Fig. 50-2). A change in the color and texture of the hair with a loss of the usual pigmentation as well as coarsening of the hair strands can also occur. In addition, because vitamin A is transported on protein carriers, the abnormalities of protein synthesis can have a direct effect on the transport of vitamin A.

Nonspecific Protein-Energy Malnutrition

When malnutrition in children and adults does not result in either marasmus or kwashiorkor, the nutritional deficiencies

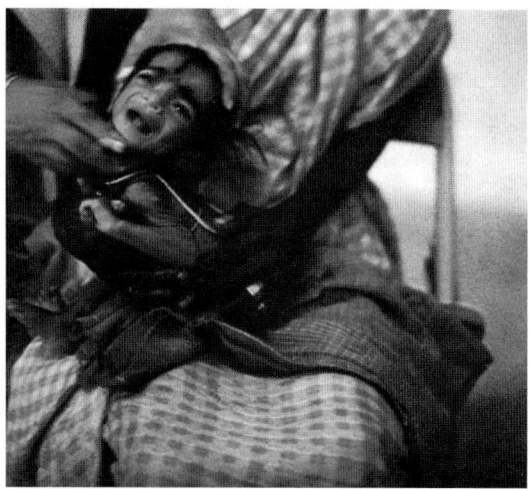

FIGURE 50-1. Marasmus. This disease is caused by a chronic deficiency of all food categories.

may be classified under a more general term of *protein-energy malnutrition*. In these conditions, replacement therapy should include a wide variety of nutrients (5). The tissues and organs usually affected are those in which cells are constantly turning over and being replaced. Thus, the skin and mucous membranes, hematopoietic tissue, and the gastrointestinal tract are commonly affected. The effect

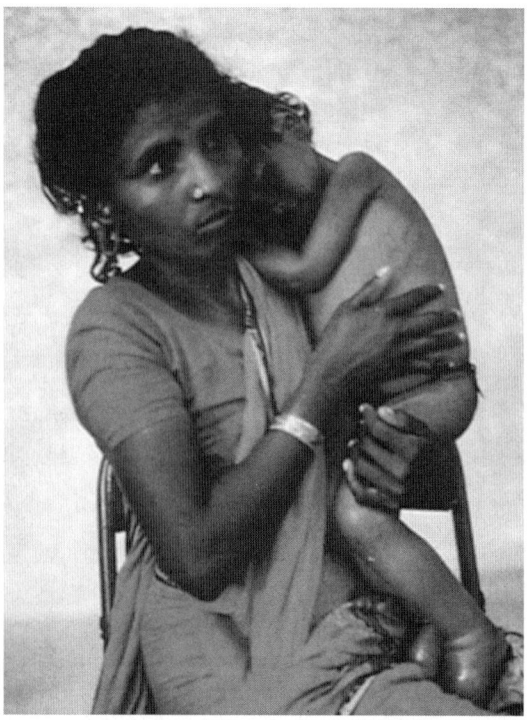

FIGURE 50-2. Kwashiorkor. The manifestations of this clinical entity are due largely to protein deficiency. A characteristic feature is massive edema of the abdomen and extremities, concurrent with muscle wastage.

on the gastrointestinal tract reduces absorption, which compounds the inadequate intake of food with malabsorption. Vitamin A deficiency is frequently associated with nonspecific protein-energy malnutrition.

VITAMIN A DEFICIENCY

Vitamin deficiencies occur in the presence of protein-energy malnutrition, and it is often impossible to separate them. However, of the vitamin deficiencies, vitamin A deficiency is the most important cause of ocular diseases, and a number of clinical conditions are ascribed specifically to vitamin A deficiency. In addition, many of these conditions can be reproduced in a vitamin A–deficient animal model (6,7).

Vitamin A is found in foods such as milk, eggs, fish, meat, and liver. It is fat soluble, ingested in the form of retinol. In the mucosal cells of the small intestine, it is esterified to palmitic acid. Vitamin A can also be obtained from its precursors, the carotenes. These substances are found in yellow fruits, green leafy vegetables, and red palm oils (8). In the small intestine, they are metabolized into retinol and absorbed. However, the carotenes are not active biologically, and it requires six times by weight to achieve the same metabolic effect as ingestion of retinol (9). After retinol is esterified to palmitic acid, the retinyl palmitate then travels to the liver through the lymphatic system. When metabolic demands require vitamin A, retinyl palmitate is hydrolyzed to retinol, released from the liver, attached to retinol-binding protein (RBP), a carrier protein produced by the liver, and transported by the bloodstream to the required tissue, such as the conjunctiva or cornea. Vitamin A is important in conjunctival cell RNA and glycoprotein synthesis, which are necessary in maintaining the health of the conjunctival mucosa and corneal stroma. Both zinc and protein are required for the production of RBP, without which vitamin A cannot be transported (10).

In the neonatal period, the child depends on the mother's milk for vitamin A. The levels of vitamin A in breast milk are similar to plasma levels (40 μg/100 mL) (11). Thus, if the mother is deficient in vitamin A, the child's supply of vitamin A is also deficient. This is one of the reasons why vitamin A–deficient ocular surface diseases are more prevalent in young children. They are born with low vitamin A stores, get little from breastfeeding, yet have the demands of rapid growth and the added complication of infectious childhood diseases that increase the body's requirements for vitamin A (10).

Abnormalities involving the ocular surface secondary to vitamin A deficiency are referred to as *xerophthalmia*. In 1976, the World Health Organization (WHO) published a classification for xerophthalmia (12), which was modified in 1982 (13).

Classification	Primary Sign
X1A	Conjunctival xerosis
X1B	Bitot's spot with conjunctival xweosis
X2	Corneal xerosis
X3A	Corneal ulceration with xerosis
X3B	Keratomalacia
XN	Night blindness
XS	Corneal scars
Biochemical criterion	Plasma vitamin A 0.35 umol/L (10 µg/dl) or Less

Ocular Manifestations of Vitamin A Deficiency

X1A: Conjunctival Xerosis

Dryness, lack of wettability, loss of transparency, thickening, wrinkling, and pigmentation are features of conjunctival xerosis. The dry patches often stand out "like sandbanks at receding tide" (14) and usually stain with rose bengal or lissamine green. The bulbar conjunctiva, especially the temporal interpalpebral areas, is usually involved. Histologically, there is a change in the conjunctival epithelium. The epithelium changes from its normal columnar appearance to a stratified squamous appearance. There is a loss of goblet cells and the epithelium becomes keratinized. The severity of these findings depends on the severity of the condition. Conjunctival disease is more common in children between 3 and 6 years of age. This sign can easily be overdiagnosed, especially because there is often observer variability. In addition, conjunctival thickening, wrinkling, and pigmentation can be seen in chronic ultraviolet light, smoke, and dust exposure, and eye infections (15). As a result, this is considered a "soft sign" in evaluating nutritional eye disease in a population. However, the dry patches, especially if they extend to and involve the inferior conjunctiva, are a fairly reliable sign of vitamin A deficiency (16).

X1B: Bitot's Spot with Conjunctival Xerosis

A Bitot's spot is a small, light-gray plaque with a foamy surface that appears on the bulbar conjunctiva in the temporal or nasal quadrants, and is frequently bilateral (Fig. 50-3). Histologically, an inflammatory infiltration of the subepithelial tissue is present. The conjunctival epithelium is keratinized and shows acanthotic thickening and loss of goblet cells (signs of xerosis). The Bitot's spot is a mixture of keratin, bacteria (often *Corynebacterium xerosis* is present), and occasionally fungi (17). The "foamy" appearance is thought to be due to the mixture of bacteria and mucus (18). Although the foamy spots can be removed, the underlying base remains and the foamy spots reform in a few days.

There has been some question as to whether Bitot's spots are always associated with vitamin A deficiency

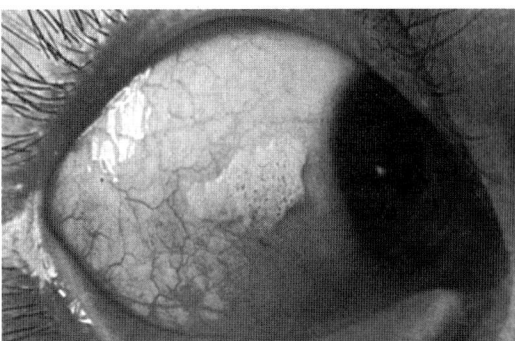

FIGURE 50-3. Bitot's spot, a foamy, light-gray area of conjunctiva frequently found in vitamin A deficiency in humans. (From Sommer A. *Nutritional blindness: xerophthalmia and keratomalacia.* New York: Oxford University Press, 1982, with permission.)

because there are cases in which the Bitot's spot does not respond to vitamin A therapy. Sommer has reported that nasally located Bitot's spots are a more reliable sign of vitamin A deficiency than temporally located lesions. In addition, he found that in children younger than 6 years of age, 97% of the lesions were responsive to vitamin A therapy, whereas 60% of the lesions in children older than 10 years were unresponsive to therapy. Thus, the presence of Bitot's spot accompanied by conjunctival xerosis in a child younger than 6 years of age is strong evidence of vitamin A deficiency (10). However, serious eye disease can occur in vitamin A deficiency without the presence of a Bitot's spot. The disease does not necessarily progress through the stages of the WHO classification.

X2: Corneal Xerosis

Corneal involvement can first appear as superficial punctate staining involving the inferior-inferonasal corneal surface. It can then progress to involve the entire corneal surface. As the corneal involvement progresses, a roughened, lusterless, dull appearance of the cornea develops, with keratinization and stromal edema (19) (Fig. 50-4). The corneal

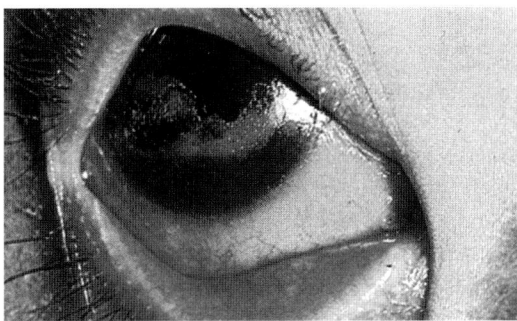

FIGURE 50-4. Corneal xerosis. Keratinization and superficial punctate keratitis are characteristic of epithelial involvement in nutritional disease. (From Sommer A. *Field guide to the detection and control of xerophthalmia.* Geneva: World Health Organization, 1978, with permission.)

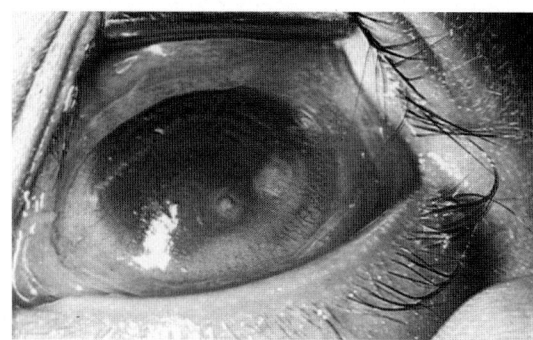

FIGURE 50-5. Corneal ulceration with xerosis. (From Sommer A, Tjakrasudjatma S. Corneal xerophthalmia and keratomalacia. *Arch Ophthalmol* 1982;100:404, with permission.)

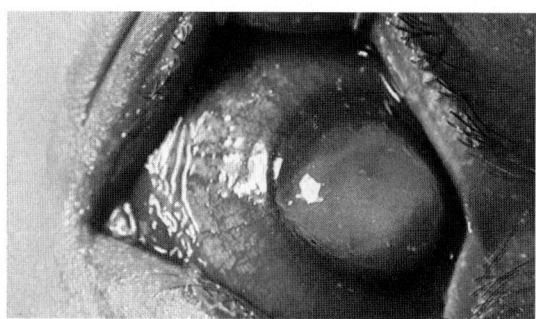

FIGURE 50-6. Keratomalacia. Rapid melting of cornea accompanies advanced starvation in children. (From Sommer A. *Nutritional blindness: xerophthalmia and keratomalacia.* New York: Oxford University Press, 1982, with permission.)

surface becomes less wettable and the tear breakup time is significantly reduced as a result of corneal surface changes. This leads to desiccation of the corneal epithelial cells. The accumulation of keratin debri and bacteria can form lesions that resemble Bitot's spots (20).

Although vitamin A deficiency has been shown to reduce aqueous tear production (21), the composition of the tear film has not been studied. However, because vitamin A has an important role in maintaining goblet cells, abnormalities in tear film mucin probably occur in vitamin A deficiency. This can lead to corneal drying and epithelial cell loss (22).

Vitamin A supplements can reverse corneal xerosis, with no permanent damage to the corneal or conjunctival surface, in both humans as well as in animal models (23).

X3A: Corneal Ulceration with Xerosis

The exact role of vitamin A deficiency in corneal ulceration is unknown. The ulcers usually appear as small, sharply demarcated defects in the epithelium and anterior stroma (Fig. 50-5). They often involve the peripheral nasal cornea and have the clinical appearance of being noninfectious. They can vary in size, but to be classified as X3A they can involve no more than one third of the corneal surface. Superficial ulcers can heal with small scars; however, deeper ulcers have the propensity to perforate. They are frequently, but not always, found in association with marked protein-energy malnutrition. However, isolated vitamin A therapy does appear to reverse ulceration of the corneal stroma in humans (10).

Because epithelial loss in other conditions does not always lead to stromal ulceration, it is possible that the stroma in vitamin A deficiency is particularly vulnerable. In animal studies, stromal ulceration is rare in severe vitamin A deficiency, but trauma can precipitate the ulceration in these animals (24), suggesting that the stroma is in some way susceptible to ulceration when the epithelium is damaged.

X3B: Keratomalacia

Corneal ulceration involving more than one third of the cornea is classified as X3B. This is usually associated with stromal necrosis and dissolution of the cornea (Fig. 50-6). With minimal inflammatory reaction, the cornea can very quickly melt away in part or entirely. This is associated with extrusion or prolapse of intraocular contents, with loss of vision, if not the eye. Deep stromal ulcers can lead to descemetoceles, which can rupture easily. They are often sealed with iris plugs and form anterior staphylomata. Their effect on vision depends on the location of the scar. Keratomalacia is usually seen in young children (between 6 months and 3 years of age) with chronic severe malnutrition. The condition can be aggravated by systemic infection such as measles or gastrointestinal, respiratory, or parasitic infections. Local bacterial infections may also play a role in hastening the ulceration in an already compromised cornea. If keratomalacia is untreated, the mortality rate is between 50% to 90%, with pneumonia or diarrhea and dehydration as the cause of death (25).

XN: Night Blindness

This is considered a secondary sign of vitamin A deficiency. Retinal function requires an adequate source of vitamin A because retinol is necessary for the production of rhodopsin by the rod photoreceptors. Night blindness has been produced in volunteers subjected to a diet deficient in vitamin A (26). Night blindness is thought to be an early sign of vitamin A deficiency and rapidly responds to systemic vitamin A supplementation. It has been used as a sensitive and specific screening tool for vitamin A deficiency (10). Night blindness during pregnancy is strongly associated with low serum and breast milk vitamin A concentration, abnormal conjunctival impression cytology, and impaired dark adaptation. It therefore can be considered a valid indicator of vitamin A deficiency (27).

XF: Xerophthalmic Fundus

This is also considered a secondary sign of vitamin A deficiency. A characteristic appearance of the fundus associated with chronic night blindness consists of whitish-yellow changes in pigment epithelium that appear to be window defects on fluorescein angiography and may correspond to areas of temporary visual field loss (28,29). Usually both eyes are affected, but not necessarily to the same degree. These lesions respond to vitamin A therapy with fading of the retinal lesions and normalization of the visual field. There has been no attempt to use fundus changes as either a survey parameter or for assessing the severity of vitamin A deficiency in individual cases.

XS: Corneal Scars

By a process of exclusion, it seems reasonable to attribute otherwise nonspecific scars to nutritional deficiencies in appropriate populations. The clinical picture is that of a healed ulcer in a child known to have had an episode of severe malnutrition. If other causes (measles, bacterial infection, herpes simplex, trachoma, trauma) have been ruled out, the scar may be due to vitamin A deficiency. The danger in such diagnosis by exclusion is apparent.

NUTRITIONAL EYE DISEASE IN DEVELOPED COUNTRIES

In adults, protein-energy malnutrition can be a manifestation of decreased dietary intake or reduced absorption. In developed counties, the most common forms of dietary deficiencies are those in alcoholism, liver disease, malabsorption, and self-imposed bizarre diets.

Malnutrition is a problem frequently associated with alcoholism. Usually, deficiencies of specific vitamins such as folic acid, thiamine, niacin, and vitamin B_6 are found, leading to a variety of clinical signs. Ethanol administration can depress hepatic levels of vitamin A, even in patients receiving large amounts of the vitamin (30). The fatty liver of alcoholism is morphologically indistinguishable from that seen in childhood protein-energy malnutrition. Although it has been suggested that the liver damage may be the result of nutritional deficiencies seen when much of the dietary intake is confined to alcohol, there also appear to be direct hepatotoxic effects of ethanol. In addition to the possible lack of nutrients in the alcoholic patient's diet, the altered hepatic metabolism in the alcoholic patient influences the uptake and storage of nutrients and may interfere with the synthesis of carrier proteins (31, 32).

Descriptions of possible nutritional eye disease in seemingly well-nourished populations have been limited to case reports with a variety of dietary and pathologic observations, as well as documentations of response to therapy (33–35). One report describes two cases of ocular abnormalities in alcoholic patients (35); vitamin A levels were abnormally low in both patients. An important observation was made regarding the conjunctiva in these cases. Initially, biopsy specimens of conjunctival tissue showed

virtually no goblet cells, although the specimens were taken from the inferonasal location, the area with the highest proportion of goblet cells under normal circumstances. In addition, there was loss of nuclei, and keratinization of the superficial cells, which was interpreted as epidermidalization. After 3 weeks of vitamin A therapy coupled with improvement in the general nutritional status, the biopsy specimen from the one patient who could be followed showed a restoration of the normal cuboidal basal cells, with loss of most of the superficial keratinization and reappearance of a few goblet cells. After 6 weeks of nutritional therapy, the conjunctival biopsy specimen was essentially normal. In addition to these histologic changes, the blood levels of vitamin A in this patient promptly rose into the normal range. The clinical appearance changed dramatically also, from an irregular surface of both the conjunctiva and the cornea to the normal lustrous appearance. It is notable that there was no demonstrable deficiency of aqueous tears, as judged by normal Schirmer test values in both patients.

Another series of two patients highlights the difficulty in separating specific vitamin deficiencies from generalized starvation (33). In two cachectic hospitalized patients, ocular signs consistent with stage X2 (corneal xerosis) were observed. In these patients, serum protein levels were quite abnormal, evidenced by very low albumin and globulin, but the vitamin A levels were normal (not below 40 μg/mL). Such cases suggest that the nutritional eye disease may exist in the absence of vitamin A deficiency.

TREATMENT OF VITAMIN A DEFICIENCY

Once vitamin A deficiency is suspected, serum should be drawn for protein and vitamin A levels to confirm the diagnosis. Other diagnostic tests that can be considered include the Mancini-type immunoassay for circulating RBP (36), holo-RBP determination (37), and conjunctival impression cytology (38,39). The diagnosis of xerophthalmia should be considered a medical emergency and therapy with vitamin A should be instituted. Vitamin A supplementation can be given orally or parenterally, or both; studies have shown that oral dosage is as effective as parenteral (40). The initial dose is 200,000 IU of vitamin A in oil (110 mg of retinol palmitate or 66 mg retinol acetate) or, if necessary, 200,000 IU of water-soluble vitamin A intramuscularly. The next day an additional 200,000 IU of vitamin A should be given. One to 2 weeks later, an additional 200,000 IU of vitamin A should be administered. For children younger than 1 year of age, half of these doses should be given (9). If severe protein deficiency is present, it is probably useful to repeat the doses every 2 weeks until the protein status returns to normal (41). Children who are at high risk may require a repeat dose of vitamin A at 4 to 6 months. In the presence of normal intestinal absorption, no more than 195 IU/kg of body weight in children to 36 IU/kg of body weight in adults must be supplied daily to maintain adequate stores of the vitamin after the initial deficiency is eliminated. Because the liver can store vitamin A for 6 months, daily dosing is not necessary, but rather the required maintenance dose should be given at 4 to 6 months. In addition, strategies to remove the risk factors such as measles and prevention of diarrhea should be undertaken, as well as education about proper nutrition with foods rich in vitamin A.

Larger doses of vitamin A are contraindicated because vitamin A toxicity should be avoided. In one study, a dosing regimen of 300,000 IU resulted in 4% of the population experiencing symptoms of vitamin A toxicity (42). Factors influencing chronic hypervitaminosis A include dosing regimen; the physical form of the vitamin; general health status; dietary factors, such as ethanol and protein intake; and interactions with vitamins C, D, E, and K. Hypervitaminosis A can cause diarrhea, vomiting, weight loss, fatigue, anorexia, bone and joint pain, osteoporosis, bone fractures, hepatosplenomegaly, dryness and fissuring of the lips, headache, anemia, and thrombocytopenia (43–45). Vitamin A supplementation should be avoided during pregnancy, but once the child is born, supplementation can be given to the mother. There may be a relationship between vitamin A supplementation and acute lower respiratory tract infections (46), which may be due to an immunosuppressive effect of vitamin A (47).

Topical Vitamin A

Topical retinoic acid in a petrolatum ointment reversed ocular surface keratinization in vitamin A–deficient animals (48), and topical vitamin A palmitate eye drops reversed the superficial punctate keratitis and increased the goblet cells in the conjunctiva, as well as increased the serum retinol concentration in rabbits (49).

Topical vitamin A is not helpful in severe ocular vitamin A–deficient diseases. It may help in healing corneal ulcers (23), but it has been associated with an increase in vascularization as well as in the density of the resulting scar (50). In no cases should children or adults with clinical systemic vitamin A deficiency be treated with topical retinoids alone. If used, topical applications of these compounds should be considered only when systemic levels of vitamin A are normal (20 μg/dL).

A more general use of vitamin A compounds was suggested by Tseng and coworkers (51). These authors noted the presence of squamous metaplasia in a number of ocular surface diseases, including not only systemic vitamin A deficiency but ocular cicatricial pemphigoid, drug-induced pseudopemphigoid, Stevens-Johnson syndrome, and keratoconjunctivitis sicca (17). The squamous metaplasia changes were reversible by the topical application of 0.015% or 0.10% all-trans retinoic acid ointment applied one to three times a day. Although improvements were noted in impression cytology with evidence of restoration of goblet cells, there was no significant change in aqueous tear restoration. Further clinical studies have shown that topical vitamin A is not helpful in keratoconjunctivitis sicca or conjunctival cicatricial diseases, but may be useful in the treatment of certain selected patients with surface keratinization (1).

PREVENTION OF NUTRITIONAL EYE DISEASE

With 228 million children affected by moderate to severe vitamin A deficiency and the high morbidity and mortality associated with this condition, this is indeed a serious public health concern. National and world attention has been directed on how best to achieve adequate nutrition in the developing nations to alleviate this problem. Although the best method would be the provision of adequate quantities of all the essential foodstuffs, the magnitude and difficulty of such a solution have led to the proposal that vitamin A supplementation per se might be effective in reducing the prevalence of blinding diseases.

Several techniques have been suggested for vitamin A supplementation. These include linking to immunization programs, fortifying common foods, periodic dosing, and nutritional education in an effort to increase the intake of red, orange, and green leafy vegetables (52). Research is being conducted to genetically engineer "golden rice" that contains both iron and beta-carotene (53). In addition, it is necessary to address the problems of protein malnutrition, childhood illness such as measles, and diarrhea. Until all children receive adequate protein, calories, and vitamins as part of their regular diet, the search will continue for effective methods of supplementation.

REFERENCES

1. Soon HK, Martin NF, Wagoner MD, et al. Topical retinoid therapy for squamous metaplasia of various ocular surface disorders: a multicenter, placebo-controlled double masked study. *Ophthalmology* 95: 1442,1988.
2. Ngah NT, et al. Ocular manifestation of vitamin A deficiency among Orang asli (Aborigine) children in Malaysia. *Asia Pac J Clin Nutr* 2002;11:88.
3. Maurin JF, Renard JP. Ocular manifestations of vitamin A deficiency and their prevention. *Rev Int Trach Pathol Ocul Trop Subtrop Sante Publique* 1977;74:21.
4. World Health Organization. *Prevention of childhood blindness.* Geneva: World Health Organization, 1994.
5. Milner RDG. Protein-calorie malnutrition. In: *Present knowledge in nutrition*, 4th ed. Nutrition Review Series. Washington, DC: Nutrition Foundation, 1976.
6. Pirie A. Xerophthalmia. *Invest Ophthalmol* 1976;15:417.
7. Pirie A. Effects of locally applied retinoic acid on corneal xerophthalmia in the rat. *Exp Eye Res* 1977;27:297.

8. Marks J. *The vitamins: their role in medical practice.* Lancaster, United Kingdom: MTP Press, 1985.
9. Steinkuller PG. Nutritional blindness in Africa. *Soc Sci Med* 1983;17:1775.
10. Sommer A. *Nutritional blindness: xerophthalmia and keratomalacia.* New York: Oxford University Press, 1982.
11. Thanangkul O, et al. Comparison of the effects of a single high dose of vitamin A given to mother and infant upon the plasma levels in the infant. Presented at the Joint/WHO/UUSAMD Meeting on the Control of Vitamin A Deficiency: Priorities for Research and Action Programmes, Jakarta, Indonesia, November 25–29, 1974.
12. World Health Organization. *Vitamin A deficiency and xerophthalmia.* WHO Technical Series Report no. 590. Geneva: World Health Organization, 1978.
13. World Health Organization. *Report of a joint WHO/UNICEF/USAID/HKI/IVACG meeting: Control of Vitamin A Deficiency.* Technical Series Report no. 672. Geneva: World Health Organization, 1982.
14. Sommer A, et al. Incidence, prevalence and scale of blinding malnutrition. *Lancet* 1981;1:1407.
15. McLaren DS. *Nutritional ophthalmology*, 2nd ed. London: Academic Press, 1980.
16. Sommer A, Emran N, Tjokrasudjatma S. Clinical characteristics of vitamin A-responsive and nonresponsive Bitot's spots. *Am J Ophthalmol* 1980;90:160.
17. Sommer A, Green R, Kenyon KR. Clinical histopathologic correlations of vitamin A responsive and nonresponsive Bitot's spots. *Arch Ophthalmol* 1981;99:2014.
18. Roger FC, et al. A reappraisal of the ocular lesions known as Bitot's spots. *Br J Nutr* 1963;17:475.
19. Sommer A, Emran N, Tamba T. Vitamin A-responsive punctate keratopathy in xerophthalmia. *Am J Ophthalmol* 1979;87:330.
20. Sommer A. *Field guide to the detection and control of xerophthalmia and keratomalacia.* New York: Oxford University Press, 1982.
21. Sommers A, Emran N. Tear production in vitamin A response xerophthalmia. *Am J Ophthalmol* 1982;93:84.
22. Sommer A, Green WR. Goblet cell response to vitamin A treatment for corneal xerophthalmia. *Am J Ophthalmol* 1982;94:213.
23. Sommer A, Emran N. Topical retinoic acid in the treatment of corneal xerophthalmia. *Am J Ophthalmol* 1978;86:615.
24. Seng WL, et al. The effect of thermal burns on the release of collagenase from corneas of vitamin A-deficient rats. *Invest Ophthalmol Vis Sci* 1980;19:1461.
25. Tielech JM, Sommer A. The epidemiology of vitamin A deficiency and xerophthalmia. *Annu Rev Nutr* 1984;4:183.
26. Hume EM, Krebs HA. *Vitamin A requirement of human adults: an experimental study of vitamin A deprivation in man.* Medical Research Council Special Report Series no. 264. London: Her Majesty's Stationery Office, 1949.
27. Christian P. Recommendations for indicators: night blindness during pregnancy—a simple tool to assess vitamin A deficiency in a population. *J Nutr* 2002;132:2884s.
28. Hing TK. Fundus changes in hypovitaminosis A. *Ophthalmologica* 1959;137:81.
29. Sommer A, et al. Vitamin-responsive panocular xerophthalmia in a healthy adult. *Arch Ophthalmol* 1978;96:1630.
30. Leiber CS. Alcohol, liver and nutrition. *J Am Coll Nutr* 1991;10:602.
31. Halsted CH. Nutritional implications of alcohol. In: *Present knowledge in nutrition*, 4th ed. Nutrition Review Series. Washington, DC: Nutrition Foundation, 1976.
32. Sebrell WH. Malnutrition. In: Moxey-Rosenau JF, Sartwell PF, eds. *Preventive medicine and public health.* New York: Appleton Century-Crofts, 1973.
33. Baum J, Rao G. Keratomalacia in the cachectic hospitalized patient. *Am J Ophthalmol* 1976;82:435.
34. Smith R, Farrell T, Bailey TA. Keratomalacia. *Surv Ophthalmol* 1975;20:213.
35. Sullivan WR, McCulley JP, Dohlman CH. Return of goblet cells after vitamin A therapy in xerosis of the conjunctiva. *Am J Ophthalmol* 1973;75:720.
36. Smith FR, Roy A, Goodman DS. Radio-immunoassay of human plasma retinol-binding protein. *J Clin Invest* 1970;49:1754.
37. Glover J, Moxley L, Muhilal H, et al. Micro-method for fluorometric assay of retinol-binding protein in blood plasma. *Clin Chim Acta* 1974;50:371.
38. Natadisastra G, Wittpenn JR, Muhilal H, et al. Impression cytology: a practical index of vitamin A status. *Am J Clin Nutr* 1988;48:695.
39. Polizza A, et al. Role of impression cytology during hypovitaminosis A. *Br J Ophthalmol* 1998;82:303.
40. Sommer A, et al. Oral vs. intramuscular vitamin A in the treatment of xerophthalmia. *Lancet* 1980;1:557.
41. Sommers A. *Nutritional Blindness: Xerophthalmia and Ketatomalacia.* New York: Oxford University Press, 1982.
42. Swaminathan MC, et al. Field prophylactic trial with a single annual oral dose of vitamin A. *Am J Clin Nutr* 1970;23:119.
43. Brinklry N, Krueger D. Hypervitaminosis A and bone. *Nutr Rev* 2000;58:138.
44. Chiu TK, Lai MS, Ho JC, et al. Acute fish liver intoxication: report of three cases. *Changgeng Yi Xue Zhi* 1999;22:468.
45. Perrotta S, Nobili B, Rossi F, et al. Infant hypervitaminosis A causes severe anemia and thrombocytopenia: evidence of a retinol-dependent bone marrow cell growth inhibition. *Blood* 2002;99:2017.
46. Standsfield SK, et al. Vitamin A supplementation and increased prevalence of childhood diarrhea and acute respiratory infections. *Lancet* 1993;342:578.
47. Friedman A, et al. Decreased resistance and immune response to *Escherichia coli* in chicks with low and high intakes of vitamin A. *J Nutr* 1991;121:395.
48. Ubels JL, Edelhouser HF, Austin KH. Healing of experimental corneal wounds treated with topically applied retinoids. *Am J Ophthalmol* 1983;95:353.
49. Kubo Y, et al. Effect of vitamin A palmitate on vitamin A deficient rabbits. *Jpn J Ophthalmol* 2000;44:189.
50. Sommer A. Treatment of corneal xerophthalmia with topical retinoic acid. *Am J Ophthalmol* 1983;95:349.
51. Tseng SCG, et al. Topical retinoid treatment for various dry eye disorders. *Ophthalmology* 1985;92:717.
52. Sommer A, Muhilal H, Tarwotjo I. Protein deficiency and treatment of xerophthalmia. *Arch Ophthalmol* 1982;100:785.
53. Friedrich MJ. Genetically enhanced rice to help fight malnutrition. *JAMA* 1999;282:1508.

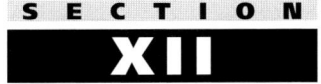

SECTION XII

CONTACT LENSES

THE ROLE OF CONTACT LENSES IN THE MANAGEMENT OF CORNEAL DISORDERS

PERRY ROSENTHAL* AND JANIS COTTER

HISTORY AND INTRODUCTION

Contact lenses are an important but underused tool in the management of many corneal disorders. Conceived by Leonardo da Vinci in 1508, as outlined in three of his sketches (1), proof of principle of the ability of rigid (glass) scleral contact lenses to neutralize irregular corneal astigmatism was provided by Fick and Kalt in 1888 (2). Scleral lenses were revived in 1936 by Feinbloom, a New York optometrist, who was the first to use plastic in their construction. However, their usefulness was limited by the rapid development of microcystic corneal edema (Sattler's veil) in the short term and the development of corneal neovascularization that accompanied their longer-term use. In a seminal paper, Smelser and Ozanics in 1952 established the importance of ambient air as the primary source of oxygen needed to maintain the metabolism of corneal tissue, and scleral lens–induced corneal edema was shown to be a consequence of corneal oxygen deprivation (3). Efforts to avoid this complication by increasing the transport of oxygen-saturated tears to the underlying cornea through the introduction of fenestrations, slots, and channels were unsuccessful, and scleral lenses were virtually abandoned when rigid corneal and soft contact lenses became available.

Contact lenses are classified as rigid (hard) and flexible (soft). Their designs are described as corneal (supported entirely on the cornea), corneoscleral (supported by the cornea and sclera), and scleral (supported entirely by the sclera).

Rigid contact lenses have the unique capability to improve the optics of the damaged corneal surface by neutralizing irregular corneal astigmatism. However, exploiting their optical benefits in eyes with damaged corneas has posed significant obstacles. Because their fitting characteristics depend on the distorted geometries of diseased corneas on which they rest, it is often not possible to achieve a satisfactory result.

The inability of soft contact lenses to neutralize irregular corneal astigmatism relegates their non-cosmetic use to protecting damaged corneal surfaces from desiccation and the friction of blinking. However, this function depends on the availability of an adequate supply of tears to maintain their hydration and avoid lens adhesion that can create shearing forces at the corneal surface during blinking.

PHYSICAL PROPERTIES OF CONTACT LENS POLYMERS: CLINICAL IMPLICATIONS

The physiologic tolerance of contact lenses depends on their ability to maintain an adequate supply of corneal oxygen (estimated to be in the order of 75 mm Hg) (4) and avoid the accumulation of carbon dioxide. The rate of gas transmission through a contact lens is directly related to the Dk (gas permeability constant) of the contact lens material and inversely to its average thickness (L) (5). Their ratio, Dk/L, is known as the gas transmissibility of a particular lens and reflects the respiratory constraints that it places on the cornea. If the gas transmissibility of a contact lens is insufficient, corneal edema will result owing to the toxic effects of the resulting acidosis (6,7). The edema threshold of Dk/L varies among normal corneas, and is significantly lower in those with impaired endothelial function (8). Prolonged lid closure, as occurs during sleep, imposes an additional hypoxic burden on the cornea and requires a significantly greater oxygen transmissibility to avoid increasing the incremental corneal swelling that normally occurs during sleep.

*Dr. Rosenthal is founder and president of the Boston Foundation for Sight, a 501(C)3 nonprofit foundation that receives financial support from Bausch & Lomb and Johnson & Johnson, and is an unpaid consultant for Bausch & Lomb.

Chronic corneal hypoxia can induce corneal neovascularization and endothelial polymegethism (9). Moreover, it is believed that a hypoxic corneal environment increases the risk of bacterial keratitis (10).

The surface properties of contact lenses also have important clinical implications. Although the surfaces of rigid gas-permeable (RGP) and hydrogel lenses are inherently wettable, it is more accurate to describe them (and that of the mucin layer of the cornea) as transitional. Such surfaces are hydrophilic (water-attracting) when exposed to an aqueous medium and become hydrophobic (water-repellant) when in contact with air. Most contact lenses, including soft lenses (Holden BA, personal communication), become adherent during overnight wear because of the accumulation of a sticky mucinous material that binds them to the cornea. It can be reasoned that during periods of lens immobility and stagnation of the fluid compartment between the lens and cornea, the corneal mucin layer fills the space between these two surfaces. In the absence of tear flow, the lipid content and hydrophobicity of the mucin increase. This is accompanied by the expelling of its aqueous component and, as it shrinks, this gluelike material pulls the lens against the cornea. When the adherent lens breaks free as blinking and normal tear production is reestablished on awakening, shear forces are generated at the corneal surface that can detach loosely bound epithelium (11). This phenomenon is accelerated in dry eyes and, most likely, in the presence of silicon-containing polymers.

SOFT CONTACT LENSES AS A CORNEAL BANDAGE

This role has been traditionally been limited to hydrogel contact lenses. The goals are to protect the corneal epithelial surface from the desiccating effects of exposure to air and the shearing forces of blinking, and to provide relief from pain. However, their effectiveness as a corneal bandage requires an adequate tear supply to maintain lens hydration and avoid corneal adhesion. This limits their usefulness in dry eyes. Although soft lenses that have a greater bulk and lower water content are more resistant to dehydration, lower oxygen transmissibility compromises their physiologic tolerance during extended wear.

A new generation of silicon-containing hydrogel polymers offers higher gas transmissibility and better physiologic tolerance during extended wear (12). It is unclear whether their hydrophilic coating is effective in reducing the incidence of overnight adhesion.

Use of soft bandage lenses in corneal disorders requires close monitoring. The extended wear of soft contact lenses has been shown to increase the risk of microbial keratitis (13), which is probably further increased in the presence of epithelial defects.

Indications

Acute Corneal Abrasions

A soft contact lens used as a clear patch for 24 hours has been shown to be as effective in wound healing and pain reduction as traditional procedures (14).

After Ocular Surgery

Corneal epithelial defects after ocular surgery may be effectively treated with the short-term continuous wear of a soft contact lens to reduce the postoperative pain that follows laser refractive procedures (15). Large soft bandage contact lenses are used to secure amniotic membrane grafts and limbal allografts after surgery and to reduce postoperative discomfort (16).

Recurrent Corneal Erosion

The extended wear of a hydrogel contact lens can be helpful in the treatment of recurrent corneal erosions by protecting the loosely bound epithelium from the shearing force of the first blinks on awakening. However, this may require the lens to be worn for several months after resolution of symptoms (17).

Persistent Corneal Epithelial Defect

Chronic epithelial defects threaten the integrity of the globe by increasing the risk for microbial keratitis and progressive stromal thinning. Bandage soft lenses can be effective in treating persistent epithelial defects. However, the increased risk for infection with extended contact lens wear, especially in the presence of an epithelial defect, and the requirement of adequate tear production to maintain lens hydration, limit their usefulness.

Bullous Keratopathy

Continuous wear of soft bandage contact lenses is especially helpful in managing pain in chronic bullous keratopathy (18,19). Because corneal edema is intensified under a soft lens worn for extended periods and its long-term use may provoke corneal neovascularization (which can eliminate bullous formation and obviate the continued need for a bandage lens), the long-term use of a soft bandage lens is appropriate only for eyes that have no potential for useful vision.

Filamentary Keratitis

Soft bandage contact lens therapy may be useful in filamentary keratitis that is not responsive to other therapies (20). The author has had similar success with daily-wear RGP corneal and scleral contact lenses.

Corneal Perforations and Wound Leaks

When the corneal perforation is small and the wound edges are well opposed, the application of a soft lens can seal the gap, thereby enabling the wound to heal. In the presence of tissue loss, a soft bandage lens is applied over the plug of tissue adhesive that has been used to seal the perforation to protect it from the shearing forces of blinking and to minimize lid discomfort (21).

Eyelid Abnormalities

In the presence of an adequate tear supply, soft bandage lenses can be helpful in protecting the cornea from the mechanical effects of entropion, trichiasis, distichiasis, and lid margin keratinization.

RIGID GAS-PERMEABLE CORNEAL CONTACT LENSES

Because the refractive indices of the cornea and tears are similar, the smooth anterior surface of the fluid compartment created by a rigid contact lens masks most of the irregular corneal astigmatism. However, these lenses do not correct high-order aberrations that are associated with keratoconus (22) and those in eyes subjected to unsuccessful radial keratotomy and laser *in situ* keratomileusis (LASIK) procedures.

Indications

Corneal Ectasia

Exploiting the optical benefits of corneal RGP contact lenses for eyes with ectatic corneal disease has been, for many patients, an unmet promise. This is exemplified by keratoconus, in which the inferior decentration of the cone poses an obstacle to achieving the lens centration and blink-induced excursion patterns necessary to provide adequate vision correction and wearing comfort. Although there have been many attempts to overcome the challenge of fitting these eyes with proprietary designs, the fitting process remains time-consuming and the results are often disappointing, even when the disease is mild. The goal of achieving the classic three-point touch to minimize apical compression, while providing sufficient peripheral lens clearance, is often not achievable in more advanced disease (23). In many of these eyes, the only means of providing an acceptable degree of wearing comfort is to use the apex of the cone as a pivot to lever the lens in a high riding position. However, excessive apical compression that creates whorl-shaped apical erosions can lead to nodular apical scars (Fig. 51-1). The epithelium overlying these hypertrophic scars is often extremely fragile and easily eroded, resulting in further loss of contact lens–wearing tolerance. The benefits of excising or

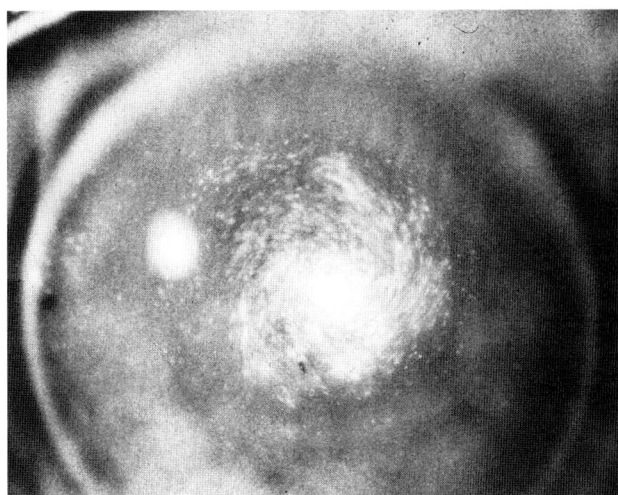

FIGURE 51-1. Typical whorl-shaped staining pattern caused by contact lens apical compression.

ablating the elevated portion of the nodular scars to reestablish contact lens tolerance are rarely permanent unless the lens can be redesigned to provide apical clearance. Combination systems can be helpful in some cases, the hybrid permalens may be useful in the short term.

Anecdotal experience indicates that the quality of vision correction provided by RGP contact lenses can sometimes be improved by apical compression. Presumably this reduces high-order aberrations. Because the improvement of vision is limited to the reduction of irregular astigmatism, higher-order aberrations associated with decentered cones, especially coma and trefoil (24), are not corrected by RGP lenses, especially in dim ambient light. This explains the often disappointing quality of vision correction achieved with rigid contact lenses in this disease. Correcting the residual astigmatism with spectacles when present, can be helpful.

Fitting corneal RGP contact lenses on corneas deformed by pellucid degeneration (25) and keratoglobus is even more challenging, and rarely successful.

After Penetrating Keratoplasty

Corneal grafts often become tilted and warped because of the uneven circumferential healing of the graft–host junction and graft decentration. This can create excessive astigmatism, both regular and irregular, that cannot be corrected with spectacle lenses. The best visual results after keratoplasty were found in keratoconus (26). Yet, in one series, 14% of patients achieved less than 20/40 best tolerated spectacle-corrected vision, and of the 86% who enjoyed better vision, only 67% were correctable with spectacle lenses (27). This underscores the importance of rigid contact lenses in rehabilitating the vision of eyes after successful keratoplasty. However, the trial-and-error corneal contact lens fitting process of these eyes is time-consuming, and failure to achieve adequate contact lens positional stability is common.

After Radial Keratotomy

Conventional RGP corneal contact lens designs are generally unsatisfactory because of their inability to achieve a stable and comfortable fitting result. Reverse-geometry lenses in which the intermediate zone is steeper than the central optic zone are more useful, but they too have significant limitations (28,29). The quality of vision provided by RGP contact lenses in these cases largely depends on the degree to which the incisions encroach on the pupillary zone and on the presence of high-order aberrations. Moreover, their failure adequately to vault the elevated cornea adjacent to the flattened central zone is a significant limitation of traditional methods of mathematically defining contact lens surfaces.

Post-LASIK Corneas

The obstacles to fitting these corneas with rigid corneal lenses are similar to those posed by corneas that have undergone radial keratotomy (30).

Irregular Astigmatism Due to Other Causes

Patients with anterior corneal dystrophies may also benefit from the use of a rigid contact lens in the absence of a history of recurrent erosions (31). Rigid contact lenses can also be helpful in masking the astigmatism resulting from the traction created by pterygia (32) and scars resulting from corneal laceration (33) and infectious keratitis (34). The contribution to visual impairment of irregular astigmatism and loss of transparency caused by a central corneal scar cannot be evaluated by slit-lamp examination alone. Before keratoplasty is recommended, the potential benefit offered by an RPG contact lens should be determined by refracting over a large trial contact lens.

GAS-PERMEABLE SCLERAL LENSES

By vaulting the distorted topography of damaged corneas, scleral lenses avoid the limitations of rigid corneal lenses that rest on the corneal surface. They are especially useful for eyes in which the distorted corneal surface is an unsuitable platform for corneal RGP contact lenses.

Scleral lenses consist of a central zone (optic) that is designed to vault the cornea, a peripheral haptic that forms the scleral bearing surface, and a transitional zone that joins the optic and haptic and vaults the limbus (Fig. 51-2). Contemporary scleral lenses are lathe-cut from highly oxygen-permeable polymers.

The major challenge to the successful use of gas-permeable scleral lenses is avoiding suction. If the posterior haptic

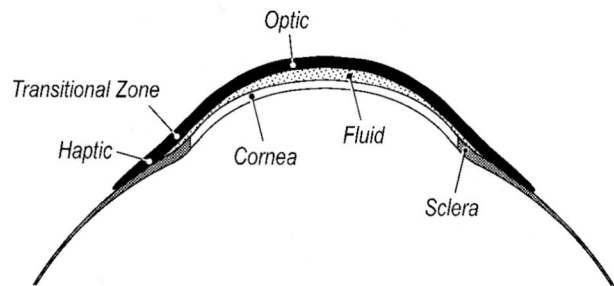

FIGURE 51-2. Scleral contact lens design.

bearing surface creates a complete ring of scleral compression, it will block the influx of tears necessary to replace the volume of fluid that is squeezed out of the precorneal compartment during blinking and eye movements. Under these circumstances, the lens acts as a one-way valve generating increasing suction that can cause intense corneal edema and challenge the atraumatic removal of the lens. Therefore, these devices must incorporate a safety valve to prevent the development of negative hydrostatic pressure behind the lens.

Air-Ventilated Scleral Lenses

Ezekiel was the first to report the use of gas-permeable polymers in the fabrication of scleral lenses (35). His strategy of avoiding lens suction is to drill a hole (fenestration) into the peripheral optic that enables air to be aspirated into the fluid compartment as the means of preventing the development of negative hydrostatic pressure. However, corneal desiccation caused by the presence of air bubbles is especially harmful in the presence of severe ocular surface disease. Moreover, the back surface of the central zone must be hand-adjusted to control the position of air bubbles to avoid their intrusion into the visual axis, a process that requires skill, experience, and time.

Fluid-Ventilated Scleral Lenses

These devices are designed to aspirate tears into the fluid compartment to abort the development of suction. The scleral bearing surface (haptic) is designed to create radial channels over the sclera sufficient to facilitate the transit of tears while excluding air bubbles.

THE BOSTON SCLERAL LENS PROSTHETIC DEVICE

The Boston Scleral Lens is a fluid-ventilated, gas-permeable scleral lens device that uses the precision and flexibility of spline functions in its design process to address two challenges that practitioners face in fitting scleral lenses designed by traditional methodology. By incorporating a vault

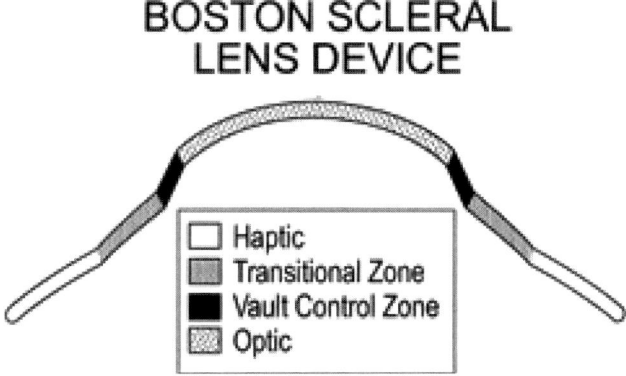

FIGURE 51-3. The Boston Scleral Lens: mechanism of vault control.

control zone in the periphery of the optic (Fig. 51-3), the central zone can be elevated or depressed in micrometer steps to control precisely the thickness of the fluid compartment independently of the back surface optic radius. This enables the fitter to create a more uniform fluid compartment and control its thickness.

The haptic bearing surface incorporates a series of radial channels to facilitate tear fluid exchange. It is also defined by spline functions that provide the design flexibility required to adapt the posterior haptic surface to the underlying scleral topography to avoid obstructing the venting channels. The functionality of the channels is confirmed in each case by placing fluorescein on the external surface of the lens and observing its passage under the haptic and into the fluid compartment after the lens has been worn a minimum of 2 hours. The fitting process uses a series of diagnostic lenses to determine the optimal diameter, vault, power, and haptic design.

The fluid compartment enclosed by the device has two functions: It creates a smooth artificial (aqueous) optical surface over the damaged cornea that neutralizes irregular astigmatism, and it functions as a liquid bandage to protect the corneal surface from the effects of exposure to air and the friction of blinking.

Indications

Correction of Irregular Astigmatism

This device is indicated for disorders in which corneal RGP lenses have the potential to provide significantly superior vision correction than spectacle lenses, but are not tolerated (36). These include pellucid degeneration, keratoglobus, keratoconus, Terrien's marginal degeneration, corneal scars, and certain anterior corneal dystrophies, as well as after radial keratotomy and laser ablation. Typically, scleral lenses provide excellent vision correction for eyes with postkeratoplasty astigmatism and should be considered as the method of choice in rehabilitating the vision of these eyes when spectacle lenses are inadequate or are not tolerated and RGP corneal lenses have failed.

Management of Severe Ocular Surface Disease

The corneal liquid bandage provided by fluid-ventilated, gas-permeable scleral lenses represents a unique and powerful tool in the management of severe ocular surface disease (37,38). Because the liquid reservoir maintained by these devices does not depend on the availability of an adequate supply of tears, they are effective when soft bandage contact lenses have failed. By protecting the corneal surface from desiccation and the friction and shearing forces created during blinking, fluid-ventilated, gas-permeable scleral lenses are especially useful for eyes in which the corneal epithelial reparative process is impaired, as in stem cell–deficient and neurotrophic corneas and in severe dry eyes. Eyes with exposure keratopathy can also benefit from this device.

The most dramatic benefits are found in patients suffering from the ocular sequelae of Stevens-Johnson's syndrome and draft versus host disease. In addition to providing a nurturing environment that better maintains the integrity of the corneal surface, these lenses greatly attenuate the disabling symptoms of ocular pain and photophobia. Although they can be effective in healing persistent epithelial defects when all other measures fail (39), the requirement of continuous wear until the defect has healed and the concurrent use of topical antibiotics and steroids increase substantially the risks of bacterial keratitis. However, the new generation of fluoroquinolones placed in the fluid reservoir of the lens may reduce the incidence of this complication. In general, fluid-ventilated, gas-permeable scleral lenses should be considered in patients for whom a partial (or complete) tarsorrhaphy is being considered. Fitting of these devices is especially challenging in eyes in which the fornices are compromised by symblepharon, and extensive customization of the design is often required in these cases.

The presence of corneal edema or transplants with borderline endothelial function are contraindications to the use of scleral contact lenses because stromal and epithelial edema will become intensified and limit their usefulness.

LARGE-DIAMETER CORNEAL/ CORNEOSCLERAL RIGID GAS-PERMEABLE CONTACT LENSES

The recent interest in large-diameter rigid lenses that approach or overlap the limbus circumferentially is driven by the desire to improve the stability and wearing comfort of this modality. However, there are two major obstacles that limit their usefulness. The stagnation of the precorneal tear compartment and the close proximity of the lens and corneal surfaces promote lens adhesion. This is not a benign phenomenon. As the gluelike mucinous material fills the space between the lens and cornea and shrinks in volume, it can pull the lens against the cornea with a force sufficient to damage the integrity of the cornea at the junction of the optic and peripheral zone of the lens. This is a concern when it occurs at the limbus and may be a factor in the anecdotal reports of acute iritis associated with these lenses. The use of peripheral fenestrations can be helpful by enabling air bubbles to be aspirated under the lens periphery.

Overcoming the adhesion phenomenon would open the door to the use of this design platform in developing a new generation of RGP contact lenses for a variety of corneal disorders, including keratoconus, after unsuccessful radial keratotomy and LASIK, postkeratoplasty astigmatism, central corneal scars, and certain anterior corneal dystrophies. However, achieving this requires these lenses to create an adequate space over the corneal surface while maintaining tear flow in the absence of lens movement. This is not possible with the traditional method of designing contact lens surfaces by linking a series of conics.

THE BOSTON MINISCLERAL LENS DEVICE

This large (14- to 15.5-mm) lens is designed to rest on the peripheral cornea and drape over the adjacent limbus and sclera. It incorporates a vault control mechanism (similar to that of the Boston Scleral Lens) that enables the fitter precisely to elevate or depress the central zone (base curve) over a wide range. This feature is capable of providing apical clearance for many ectatic corneas. Tear exchange sufficient to avoid lens adhesion is maintained by the pumping action actuated by blinking and eye movement and facilitated by the presence of a series of radial channels that function as fluid conduits.

However, the maximum vault offered by this device is significantly less than that of scleral lenses, and it is not useful for eyes with advanced keratoconus, pellucid marginal degeneration, keratoglobus, and certain cases of postkeratoplasty astigmatism. Moreover, it is not indicated in the management of severe ocular surface disease.

REFERENCES

1. da Vinci L. Codex of the eye, Manuscript D (ca. 1508). Translation and illustrations by Hofstetter HW, Graham R. Leonardo and contact lenses. *Am J Optom* 1953;30:41.
2. Fick AE. A contact lens [translation by May CH]. *Arch Ophthalmol* 1888;19:215.
3. Smelser GK, Ozanics V. Importance of atmospheric oxygen for maintenance of the optical properties of the human cornea. *Science* 1952;115:140.
4. Holden BA, Sweeney DF, Sanderson G. The minimal precorneal oxygen tension to avoid corneal edema. *Invest Ophthalmol Vis Sci* 1984;25:476.
5. Efron N, Brennan NA. Simple measurement of oxygen transmissibility. *Aust J Optom* 1985;68:27.
6. Polse KA, Brand RJ, Cohen SR, et al. Stromal acidosis affects corneal hydration control. *Invest Ophthalmol Vis Sci* 1990;31:1542.
7. Bonanno JA. Contact lens induced corneal acidosis. *CLAO J* 1996;22:70.
8. Sweeney DF, Holden BA, Vannas A, et al. The clinical significance of corneal endothelial polymegathism. ARVO Abstracts. *Invest Ophthalmol Vis Sci* 1985;26[3 Suppl]:53(abstr).
9. Carlson KH, Bourne WM, Brubaker RF. Effect of long-term contact lens wear on corneal endothelial cell morphology and function. *Invest Ophthalmol Vis Sci* 1988;29:185.
10. Ren DJ, Petroll WM, et al. The relationship between contact lens oxygen finding of *Pseudomonas aeruginosa* to human corneal epithelial cells after overnight and extended wear. *CLAO J* 1999;25:80.
11. Swarbrick HA, Holden BA. Rigid gas-permeable lens binding: significance and contributing factors. *Optom Physiol Opt* 1987;64:815.
12. Lim L, Tan DTH, Chan WK. Therapeutic use of Bausch & Lomb PureVision contact lenses. *CLAO J* 2001;27:179.
13. Schein OD, Glynn RJ, Poggio EC, et al. The relative risk of ulcerative keratitis among users of daily-wear and extended-wear soft contact lenses. *N Engl J Med* 1989;321:773.
14. Sabri K, Pandit JC, Thaller VT, et al. National survey of corneal abrasion treatment. *Eye* 1998;12:278.
15. Stein R, Stein H, Cheskes A, et al. Photorefractive keratectomy and post-operative pain. *Am J Ophthalmol* 1994;117:403.
16. John T. Human amniotic membrane transplantation: past, present, and future. *Ophthalmol Clin North Am* 2003;16:43.
17. Liu C, Buckley R. The role of the therapeutic contact lens in the management of recurrent corneal erosions: a review of treatment strategies. *CLAO J* 1996;22:81.
18. Leibowitz HM, Rosenthal P. Hydrophilic contact lenses in corneal disease. *Arch Ophthalmol* 1971;85:163.
19. Andrew NC, Woodward EG. The bandage lens in bullous keratopathy. *Ophthalmic Physiol Opt* 1989;9:66.
20. Bloomfield SE, Gasset AR, Forstot SL, et al. Treatment of filamentary keratitis with the soft contact lens. *Am J Ophthalmol* 1973;76:978.
21. Moschos M, Droutsas D, Boussalis P, et al. Clinical experience with cyanoacrylate tissue adhesive. *Doc Ophthalmol* 1996;93:237.
22. Maeda N, Fujikado T, Mihashi T, et al. Wavefront aberrations measured with Hartmann-Shack sensor in patients with keratoconus. *Ophthalmology* 2002;109:1996.
23. Rosenthal P, Cotter JM. Clinical performance of a spline-based apical vaulting keratoconus corneal contact lens design. *CLAO J* 1995;21:42.
24. Kompella VB, Aasuri MK, Rao GN. Management of pellucid marginal degeneration with rigid gas permeable contact lenses. *CLAO J* 2002;28:140.
25. Karchmer JH, Feder RS, Belin MW. Keratoconus and related noninflammatory corneal thinning disorders. *Surv Ophthalmol* 1984;28:314.
26. Claesson M, Armitage WJ, et al. Visual outcome in corneal grafts: a preliminary analysis of the Swedish Corneal Transplant Register. *Br J Ophthalmol* 2002;86:174.
27. Lim L, Pesudovs K, Coster DJ. Penetrating keratoplasty for keratoconus: visual outcome and success. *Ophthalmology* 2000;107:1125.
28. Lim L, Siow KL, Sakamoto R, et al. Reverse geometry contact lens wear after photorefractive keratectomy, radial keratotomy, or penetrating keratoplasty. *Cornea* 1999;19:320.
29. Hjortdal JO, Olsen H, Ehlers N. Prospective randomized study of corneal aberrations 1 year after radial keratotomy or photorefractive keratectomy. *J Refract Surg* 2002;18:23.
30. Yeung KK, Olson MD, Weissman BA. Complexity of contact lens fitting after refractive surgery. *Am J Ophthalmol* 2002;133:607.
31. Waring GO, Rodrigues M, Laibson P. Corneal dystrophies: I. Dystrophies of the epithelium, Bowman's layer, and stroma. *Surv Ophthalmol* 1978;23:74.
32. Smith RJ, Hallak J, Vogel M, et al: Visually debilitating pterygium: surgical and contact lens treatment. *CLAO J* 1996;22:83.

33. Smiddy WE, Hambburg TR, Kracher GP, et al. Contact lenses for visual rehabilitation after corneal laceration repair. *Ophthalmology* 1989;96:293.

34. Lois N, Cohen EJ, Rapuano CJ, et al. Contact lens use after contact lens-associated infectious ulcers. *CLAO J* 1997;23:192.

35. Ezekiel DF. Gas permeable haptic lenses. *J Br Contact Lens Assoc* 1983;6:158.

36. Schein OD, Rosenthal P, Ducharme C. A gas-permeable scleral contact lens for visual rehabilitation. *Am J Ophthalmol* 1990;109:318.

37. Kok JHC, Visser R. Treatment of ocular surface disorders and dry eyes with high gas-permeable scleral lenses. *Cornea* 1992;11:518.

38. Romero-Rangel T, Stavrou P, Cotter JM, et al. Gas permeable scleral lens therapy in ocular surface disease. *Am J Ophthalmol* 2000;130:41.

39. Rosenthal P, Cotter JM. Treatment of persistent epithelial defect with extended wear of a fluid-ventilated gas permeable scleral contact lens. *Am J Ophthalmol* 2000;130:25.

CORNEAL, SCLERAL, AND CONJUNCTIVAL SURGERY

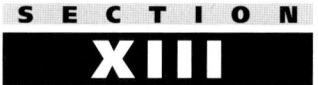

SECTION
XIII

SUPPORTIVE AND PROTECTIVE

TISSUE ADHESIVES

C. STEPHEN FOSTER

Coover and associates, studying the chemistry and characteristics of cyanoacrylate adhesives, published, in 1959, a seminal paper on the basic characteristics of these chemical compounds, including their adhesive properties (1). Carton and associates quickly exploited the first commercially available cyanoacrylate adhesive, Eastman 910 (methyl 2-cyanoacrylate monomer), modified with a plasticizer (a sebacate), a thickening agent (polymethylmethacrylate), and an inhibitor (SO_2) for joining blood vessels in dogs (2). This began then the series of experiments in the use of cyanoacrylate adhesives and their interaction with tissues, and the exploitation of this "tissue glue" in medicine (particularly surgery) and dentistry. And although the original Eastman 910 product (indeed, all lower alkyl cyanoacrylate derivatives) proved to have considerable secondary toxic effects (all polycyanoacrylates release formaldehyde and other breakdown products as they interact with water and degrade), the search for less toxic tissue glues involved not only experimentation with higher-alkylated cyanoacrylates, but the potential medical utility of other adhesives of other categories, including epoxy adhesives, polyurethane adhesives, fibrin "glue," and marine products.

As far as I can judge, Steve Bloomfield, an ophthalmologist in New York City, was the first to explore the potential utility of cyanoacrylate tissue adhesive for ocular use, engaging in a series of experiments in rabbit eyes using the Eastman 910 product in 1963 (3,4). Additional derivatives, particularly higher-alkylated forms of cyanoacrylate, were then prepared and studied, most notably by Lehman and associates at the Walter Reed Army Medical Center (5–10). By 1969, higher-alkylated derivatives of cyanoacrylate were commercially available, and these were then systematically tested by Claes H. Dohlman of the Harvard Medical School, and his associates at the Massachusetts Eye and Ear Infirmary and, most notably, by his research colleague, Miguel Refojo of the Eye Research Institute in Boston (11–15). Researchers determined that the alkyl cyanoacrylate derivatives with four or more carbon atoms in the side chain, known to degrade very slowly, were much better tolerated by living tissues than the lower derivatives,

such as methyl derivatives of cyanoacrylate. Refojo classified the tolerance level of the available cyanoacrylate adhesives in the following order: 1-decyl, N-octyl, N-atptyl, N-hexyl, N-butyl, and isobutyl 2-cyanoacrylate (16). N-butyl cyanoacrylate quickly became the standard against which all other tissue adhesives were compared. Robert Webster and Harvey Slansky and the rest of the Dohlman team at the Massachusetts Eye and Ear Infirmary were the first to report on the use of cyanoacrylate tissue adhesive for the closure of corneal perforations, reporting two cases in the *Archives of Ophthalmology* in 1968 (17). The same group, a year later, reported on an expanded series in which adhesives had been used in various applications in corneal surgery (18). Many others subsequently confirmed these early promising results (19–21), and the potential uses of tissue adhesive began to expand, to include not only the original indications of impending or actual corneal perforations, but leaking conjunctival filtering blebs, scleral defects, punctal occlusion, and temporary tarsorrhaphy.

INDICATIONS AND TECHNIQUES

The preeminent indication for the use of tissue adhesive in ophthalmology has been for impending or actual corneal perforation. This use alone of tissue adhesive in ophthalmology revolutionized the care of patients with corneal perforation or impending perforation, and actually set the standard of care for management of such problems, obviating the need for the so-called "*keratoplasty à chaud*" and allowing the surgeon to maintain the integrity of the globe, definitively deal with the underlying cause of the corneal ulcer, and allow the inevitably present inflammation of the eye to quiet. This in turn set the stage for elective keratoplasty for attempted visual rehabilitation, a strategy vastly superior, in terms of outcomes achieving the desired goal of successful grafting with improved vision, compared with keratoplasty *à chaud*.

Gluing the descemetocele or otherwise impending perforation is considerably easier than gluing a frank perforation, and the technique for managing these two problems is strikingly different. Descemetoceles or deep ulcers can typically be managed very successfully through the following series of steps, which can be performed either at the slit lamp or under the operating microscope in the minor surgery room; I prefer the patient supine, so that I can work under an operating microscope with the benefit of gravity helping me to get the adhesive precisely where I wish it to be. I find the following steps to be particularly helpful in achieving the desired goal: firm adhesion of an extremely thin layer of adhesive that seals the corneal defect but does not produce a bump or bulge above the normal contour of the cornea. Adhesive adheres best to corneal basement membrane, less well to corneal stroma, less well still to conjunctiva, and least well to sclera and corneal epithelium. Therefore, I typically remove epithelium from an area surrounding the corneal ulcer, searching for normal basement membrane, approximately 1 mm in width, circling the ulcer, which will provide the primary point of adhesion for the tissue adhesive (Fig. 52-1). I remove debris from the ulcer crater, and dry the basement membrane. I then apply adhesive to the area, in very small (microdrop) aliquots, beginning with the denuded basement membrane, either with the supplied applicator of the product used or with a 23-gauge Angiocath catheter, needle removed, having used capillary attraction to "load" adhesive into the Angiocath from the supply source (Fig. 52-2). I try to ensure that all the ring of bared basement membrane is coated with an ultrathin layer of the adhesive, and then begin to apply tiny amounts of adhesive onto the naked stroma, making no specific effort to fill the divot, down to Descemet's membrane. Packing the ulcer crater with glue can actually be counterproductive because ultimately one would like to have fibroblast proliferation, with good wound healing characteristics, new collagen production, and so forth. And although it may seem counterintuitive that the less glue used, the better the outcome, in fact the primary function of the glue is not to provide structural support for the cornea, but rather to prevent further proteoglycan and collagen degradation by excluding from the ulcerating area the source of such degradation: matrix metalloproteinases, including the "classic" collagenase delivered to the area through neutrophils, the primary source of which is the preocular tear film (22). I use a Weck cell sponge in the event that an inadvertent excess amount of glue, during any one attempt at glue application, appears, which can be, with very rapid movement, removed with Weck cell sponge; failure to be extremely rapid with the maneuver, however, can result in the Weck cell sponge becoming glued to the cornea, clearly a result that is not very desirable.

After the desired adhesive result has been obtained, irrigation of the surface with balanced salt solution or physiologic saline provides assurance that all polymerization of the adhesive has occurred, after which a large bandage soft contact lens [e.g., the 18-mm Kontur (Kontur Kontact Lens Co., Richmond, CA)] must be applied, in an effort to ensure patient comfort; the glue surface is always extremely rough, no matter how elegant the adhesive application has been, and the wiping action of the upper lid with each blink produces the sensation of the eyelid wiping over sandpaper if a barrier, such as a contact lens, in not used. Glue that is properly applied in the previously described manner may remain in place indefinitely; I have patients with glue that has remained in place for 3 or more years (Fig. 52-3).

The technique appropriate for the cornea with a frank perforation differs from the preceding description in several important ways. The preparation of the site of most importance for glue adhesion (corneal basement membrane) remains the same, but because of the continual egress of aqueous from the site of perforation, it is virtually impossible to apply glue into the ulcer crater without instant polymerization of a bubble-type dome of glue. Therefore, unless specifically contraindicated, positioning a small air bubble into the anterior chamber, such that it occludes, by its surface tension, the site of perforation, preventing continual aqueous egress from the perforation site, can eliminate this problem, allowing the surgeon then to apply the glue in the manner described previously. Obviously, larger air bubbles would be required for larger perforations, and larger air bubbles then pose a risk of pupillary occlusion and high intraocular pressure. If for no other reason, we suggest that perforations larger than 1 mm not be managed with tissue adhesive, but rather with a blowout patch graft, amniotic membrane packing of the crater, or some other technique. Intraocular Healon for accomplishing this same goal may also be attempted, but one then also runs the risk of retained Healon producing significant spikes in intraocular pressure.

Tissue adhesive may also be used to close microperforations or leaks in conjunctiva, with the most notable example of the need for such a strategy being a leaking glaucoma filtration bleb. Maintaining glue on the site for a very long period of time is usually not necessary, and therefore preparation of the site of application need not be as meticulous and extensive as that described previously for the cornea. I simply have the patient massage the eye, softening it, and of course ballooning the bleb in the process. Five minutes later, the rate of egress of aqueous from the bleb leak site is usually less than before the massage, and after drying of the site of with a Weck cell sponge, one tiny drop from the applicator onto the site of the leak is usually sufficient for coverage of the leak. Application of the 18-mm Kontur soft contact lens then ensures stability of the glue, free from the rubbing action of the blinking upper lid, and also patient comfort.

The opportunity to deal with a scleral pathologic process is not common for the vast majority of the world's ophthalmologists, and hence dealing with this problem when it does arise is usually extremely daunting. Even the

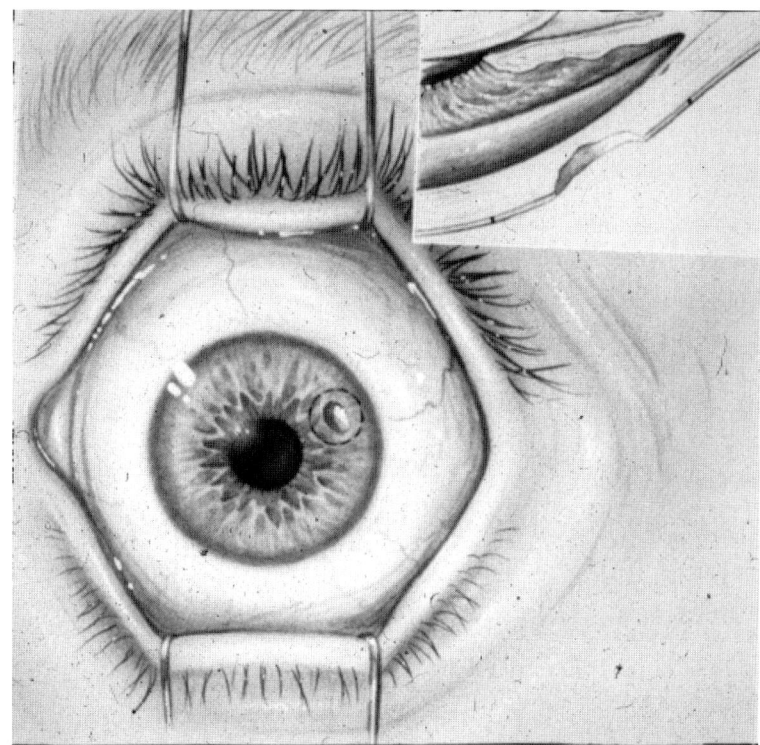

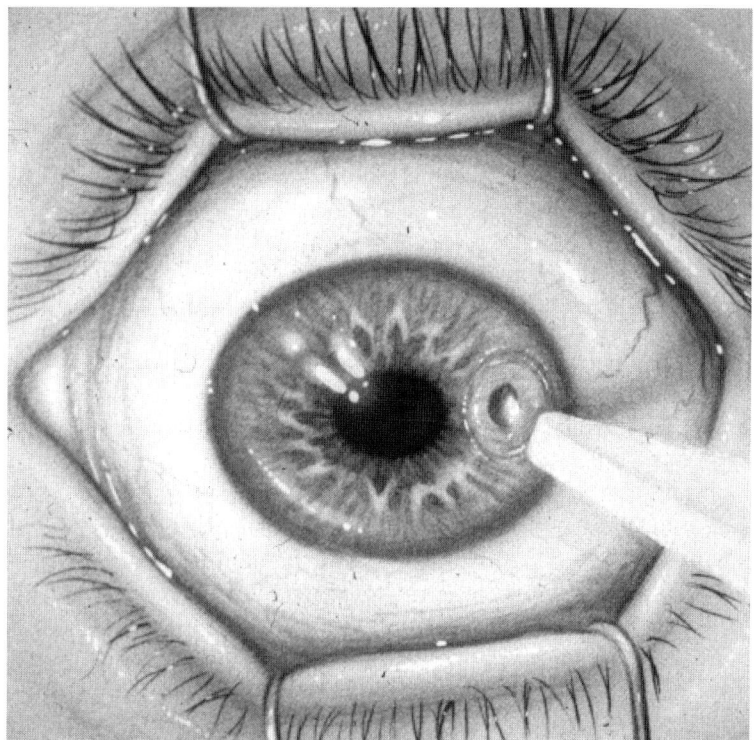

FIGURE 52-1. A: A paracentral corneal ulcer. **B:** Ulcer shown in **(A)** being prepared for glue application with epithelium being removed from basement membrane in a 1-mm zone around the ulcer.

decision regarding whether anything need be done can be challenging. Not every patient with scleral loss and uveal "show" must have this problem addressed. For example, patients with scleromalacia perforans rarely need structural support, and hence rarely need surgery or tissue adhesive for their problem. On the other hand, patients with necrotizing

scleritis with frank scleral perforation and herniation of uvea out of the perforated site clearly must have something done, or the globe is almost inevitably going to be lost. Should that patient be managed with attempts at support through tissue adhesive? Should that patient be managed with scleral grafting? Neither! At least neither in isolation

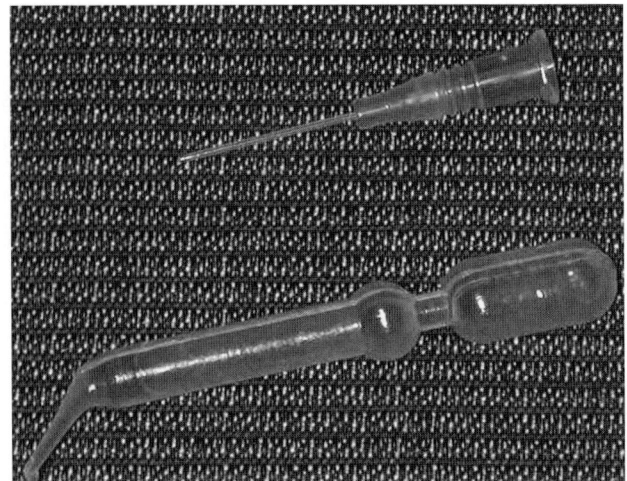

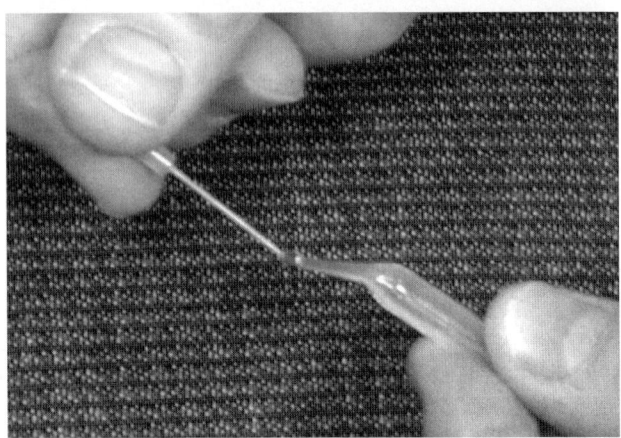

FIGURE. 52-2. A: Adhesive in its container, along with catheter part of a 25-gauge Angiocath to be used for application instead of the container itself. **B:** Adhesive being taken up, by capillary attraction, into a 25-gauge Angiocath catheter, which will be used as the applicator for distributing the glue onto the prepared surface.

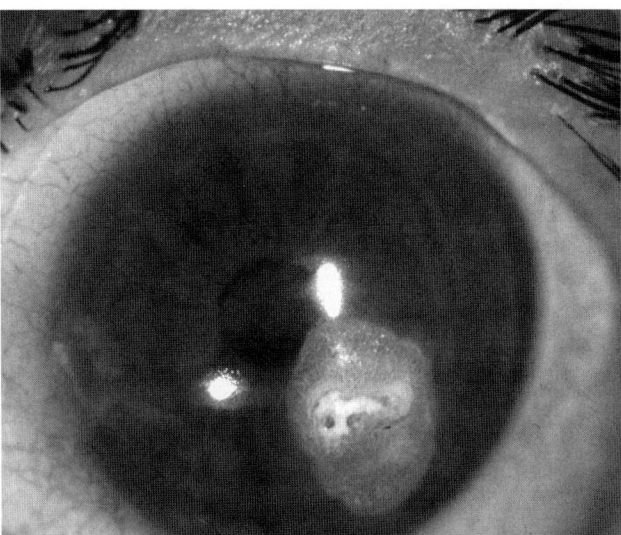

FIGURE. 52-3. Tissue adhesive on a paracentral corneal ulcer.

from an infinitely more important management technique: immunosuppressive chemotherapy in the event that the necrotizing scleritis has occurred in the context of a diagnosable systemic autoimmune disease such as rheumatoid arthritis, Wegener's granulomatosis, relapsing polychondritis, or polyarteritis nodosa. Failure to deal definitively with the underlying cause of the initial necrotizing problem in the first place guarantees not only that the battle for retaining the eye will be lost, but usually that the patient will die because of failure to induce a durable remission in the underlying, potentially lethal systemic disorder. And it can even be that the necrotizing scleritis is on an infectious basis, most particularly herpes simplex or varicella zoster virus. Hence, the decision making can be exceptionally complicated in the patient with scleral loss and uveal show. I reserve the application of tissue adhesive for scleral defect problems, for those cases clearly in need of structural support, in whom the defect is quite small (2 mm or less).

I use a technique identical to that described previously for the cornea, that is, exposing the area in need of attention, applying the adhesive in the way described, and applying a large contact lens (the Kontur lens comes in diameters up to 24 mm).

Probably one of the most underexploited areas of utility of tissue adhesive for management of corneal and external disease problems is with the eyelids. Punctal occlusion can easily be accomplished, temporarily or semipermanently, through the application of a small amount of glue just inside and at the opening of the lacrimal puncta. The adhesive will remain longer if epithelium is depleted from the area of application before applying the glue, or more briefly if the epithelium is left intact.

Temporary tarsorrhaphies can be easily accomplished, by one of two techniques, with tissue adhesive. This exercise carries with it some risk (i.e., that inadvertent application of glue to the cornea will occur), with the obvious consequences of that (i.e., before removal of same, creation of an epithelial defect/abrasion as a consequence, possible need for a bandage soft contact lens, and the like).

The two potential techniques for temporary glue tarsorrhaphy include gluing of eyelashes together (23) or, alternatively, applying the glue to the anterior portion of the lid margin. Each of these techniques has its advantages and disadvantages. The advantage of a lash gluing technique is that it is more remote from the cornea and hence carries with it less risk of inadvertent glue application to the cornea, and it is more readily reversible simply because of the trimming of eyelashes proximal to the point of application of the glue that has been used to glue upper to lower eyelashes. The disadvantage of the technique is that it is less permanent than gluing of lid margins, and reversing it is associated with the temporary cosmetic blemish associated with having a portion of the eyelashes trimmed.

Applying glue to the lid margin to accomplish temporary tarsorrhaphy is technically more difficult than is the gluing of upper to lower eyelashes, and must be done with great care if one is to reduce to the lowest extent possible the potential risk of inadvertent glue application to the cornea. The duration of the temporary tarsorrhaphy will be longer if the epithelium from the anterior lamellae of the lid margins, both upper and lower, is removed before application of a thin layer of glue to one margin, followed by a purposeful bringing together of the two lid margins. The adhesion is nearly instantaneous, so one need not hold the lids together longer than 2 or 3 seconds for the goal to be accomplished.

TISSUE ADHESIVES

Cyanoacrylates

N-*Butyl Cyanoacrylate*

Leahey and associates (24) investigated the outcomes and complications of the use of *N*-butyl cyanoacrylate tissue adhesive [Nexacryl; Tripoint Medical, LP, Raleigh, NC (another product is Tissue Glue; Elman International Manufacturing, Hewlett, NY)] in 44 patients with corneal perforations or impending perforations, ulcers, leaking filtering blebs, wound leaks, and exposure keratopathy. They found that this product was highly effective for stabilization of the globe and was well tolerated, and predicted that the material would soon be available for ophthalmologists in the United States to use for indications such as those in their report. Indeed, this tissue glue for ocular use is now on the market, and extensive experience has been gained in its use in ophthalmology. That experience has confirmed the early experience of Leahey and associates in terms of the efficacy and tolerability of this material.

N-*Butyl Ester Cyanoacrylate*

Vetbond (3M Company, St. Paul, MN) is available for animal use, and has been studied by Olliver and associates in intracorneal injection in rabbits (25). These investigators determined that only a mild inflammatory response developed after intrastromal and surface application of this product to a corneal defect, with no interference in the reparative process, indicating, in their view, that this surgical adhesive "would be acceptable for treating corneal ulcerations in animals."

N-*Butyl-2-Cyanoacrylate*

Histoacryl (B. Braun Melsungen AG, Melsungen, Germany) was the preeminent tissue adhesive used throughout the 1970s and 1980s by cornea and external disease experts in their management of patients with impending or frank corneal perforations. In countries in which the product was not commercially available, it was frequently "bootlegged" into these countries by various ophthalmologists for use in the care of their patients with the aforementioned problems. The German company producing this medical-grade adhesive chose never to go through the procedures required by the U.S. Food and Drug Administration (FDA) for approval for sale in the United States.

Fibrin Glue

Tisseel VH Fibrin Sealant (Baxter Healthcare Corp., Glendale, CA) is commercially available in the United States, with FDA approval for use in hemostasis in cardiopulmonary bypass surgery and in the treatment of splenic injuries. It does not have FDA approval for ocular use, but several studies have indicated that it is safe and effective as an adhesive for use in ophthalmology, including adherence of a lamellar graft into the recipient bed without the use of sutures, and the attachment of amniotic membrane to the ocular surface similarly without the use of sutures. It consists of fibrinogen derived from pooled human plasma, and thrombin. Collin and Watts used fibrin glue successfully, instead of sutures, in full-thickness mucous membrane grafting for fornix reconstruction, and published these findings in 1992 (26). Fibrin glue can also be prepared from autologous sources, using a cryoprecipitate method for harvesting fibrinogen (approximately 450 mL of blood is needed). Fibrin glue can be used to seal corneal perforations, with preparation of the area essentially identical to that described for the application of cyanoacrylate tissue adhesive (i.e., deepithelialization, drying with Weck cell sponges, and so forth). The two components of the "glue," fibrinogen and thrombin, are applied simultaneously in equal amounts (one drop each) at the site of perforation. The glue must be left undisturbed for approximately 3 minutes while it transforms from a gel into a white plug. Multiple applications may be required, depending on the depth of the corneal ulcer (27). Fibrin glue has been used over the past 30 years for closing conjunctiva after glaucoma filtering surgery (28), closure of wounds after cataract surgery (29), and closure of conjunctiva after strabismus surgery (30). Sharma and associates demonstrated that, compared with *N*-butyl-2-cyanoacrylate, fibrin glue provided faster healing and induced significantly less corneal vascularization in humans, but did require significantly longer for the adhesive plug to form and to be stable (27).

Katzin first proposed using fibrin for wound closure in rabbit corneal transplants in 1945 (31), and Tassman reported its use clinically for keratoplasty in 1949 (32).

A slight twist in the fibrin as adhesive story developed in 1999, when Goins and associates, from the University of Chicago, reported the results of their animal experiments (rabbits), in which radial keratotomy incisions were made and wound healing was assessed sequentially, and compared in those eyes that had received radial keratotomy alone and in those that had had radial keratotomy plus photodynamic biologic tissue glue treatment (33). This photodynamic biologic tissue glue treatment involved the use of fibrinogen mixed with riboflavin-biphosphate, placed into radial keratotomy wounds and then exposed to argon glue-green laser, 0.6 W, 2-mm spot-size, for 2 minutes. The wounds so treated were stronger than the wounds not receiving this treatment, and the authors hypothesized that photodynamically induced cross-linkage of fibrinogen to collagen led to more rapid stromal wound healing. The authors extended their studies on this technique to human cadaver eyes, publishing the results in 1998 (34) and demonstrating that photodynamic biologic tissue glue treatment was comparable with sutures in providing adequate corneal wound strength in penetrating keratoplasties performed in the human cadaveric model. The authors speculated that wound closure with this system "may reduce the number of sutures required in corneal transplantation and decrease the incidence of suture-related complications and allograft rejection." Additional efforts in the use of laser activation of tissue adhesive, aimed at a more controlled rate of polymerization (thereby avoiding the "instant" polymerization one sees with application of the commercially available cyanoacrylate adhesives), by Miki and associates involved the use of methacrylated modified hyaluronic acid, with subsequent argon laser applications (35). The photopolymerizable polymer was prepared with a 2% weight/volume solution of sodium hyaluronate, in an excess of methacrylic anhydride, kept together for 24 hours at 5°C, after which the methacrylated modified hyaluronic acid was precipitated in excess ethanol. This photo–cross-linkable polymer was then applied to lacerations made in rabbit corneas, and photo–cross-linked with three 10-second applications of low-intensity argon laser radiation (200 mW; 1- to 2-mm area) to produce a clear hyaluronic acid–methacrylated hydrogel seal. Clinical and histopathologic studies were performed at 6 hours, and at days 1, 4, 7, 14, 21, and 28 after surgery. No toxicity was clinically observed, and all anterior chambers had reformed by 6 hours of application of the glue. There was no evidence of leakage at any point in 37 of the 38 eyes treated, and the intraocular pressure was near normal by day 7. Histopathologic studies disclosed minimal inflammatory cell infiltration and excellent fibroblast proliferation and wound healing. The authors concluded that this methacrylated hyaluronan polymer may prove useful for sealing corneal lacerations and for other sutureless ophthalmic surgical procedures.

Indeed, Kaufman and associates (36) demonstrated, in 2003, that a fibrin adhesive proved satisfactory in attaching, without sutures, lamellar corneal grafts and amniotic membrane grafts in six patients, five of whom underwent lamellar keratoplasty and one of whom received an amniotic membrane graft. The fibrin glue used was Tisseel VH Fibrin Sealant.

Marine Glue

Several marine species produce adhesive substances, with barnacles and mussels being preeminent among them. Robin and associates (37) evaluated Histoacryl and a biologic (marine) adhesive in a tissue tolerance model in the corneas of New Zealand rabbits. The marine adhesive studied was a mussel-derived polyphenolic protein combined with an enzyme polymerizer (COX). The MAP is a repeating decapeptide derived from the common blue mussel (*Mytilus edulis*), and is known as mussel adhesive protein (MAP). Both MAP and COX were obtained from BioPolymers, Inc. (Farmington, CT), and the MAP was used at a concentration of 5 mg/mL whereas the COX was used at a concentration of 324 μg/mL. Intrastromal injections were performed, clinical observations were made, and histopathologic studies were done. The investigators concluded that the marine adhesive produced less tissue reaction than did the histoacrylate, suggesting that the marine adhesive could eventually be developed into an effective biologic glue for ocular use.

Other Bioadhesives

Bloom and associates (38) investigated the utility of a bioadhesive composed of a poly(L-lactic-co-glycolic acid) (PLGA) porous scaffold doped with a protein solder mix composed of serum albumin and indocyanine green, which was then activated with a diode laser. The laser application was with 808-nm diode laser focused through a fiberoptic cable with a radiance of 15.9 W/cm^2. The authors then measured tensile strength of extraocular rectus muscle–to–extraocular rectus muscle, sclera-to-sclera, and extraocular rectus muscle–to–sclera adhesions using a calibrated material strength-testing machine (858 Table Top System; MTS, Eden Prairie, MN) interfaced with the computer. The repaired tissue specimens were clamped to the tensiometer with pneumatic grips attached to a 100-N load cell and pulled apart along an axis in the plane of adhesion between the tissue and the adhesive, at a rate of 1 gravitational force per second, until the repair failed. The authors concluded that sutureless surgery using this bioadhesive appeared feasible.

Alio and associates (39) studied a different bioadhesive, an acrylic copolymer tissue adhesive, ADAL (Adhesives of Alicante; SN 75489630.USA, 2000), which is an acrylic copolymer composed of *N*-butyl cyanoacrylate cyclohexyl ethyl maleate. *N*-butyl cyanoacrylate and cyclohexyl ethyl maleate are stored in separate containers at 5°C and mixed in a polypropylene or glass syringe shortly before use.

After experiments in corneal incisions in rabbits, the authors concluded that wounds sealed with the ADAL adhesive had a tensile strength that was greater than that of wounds closed with 10-0 nylon suture in the first week after surgery. The tensile strength of the wounds in the following weeks was not significantly different between the groups. The ADAL adhesive was well tolerated.

The development of tissue adhesives revolutionized the care of certain problems in ophthalmology and certain aspects of the practice of ophthalmology. Further developments in this area may very well additionally revolutionize our care of patients with ocular wounds and those requiring ocular surgery—obviating the need, for example, for suturing lamellar or penetrating grafts or even the sclerostomy sites for a vitrectomy.

REFERENCES

1. Coover HW Jr, Joyner FB, Shearer NH Jr, et al. Chemistry and performance of cyanoacrylate adhesives. *Soc Plast Eng* 1959; 15:413–417.
2. Carton CA, Kessler LA, Seidenberg B, et al. A plastic adhesive method of small blood vessel surgery. *World Neurol* 1960;1:356–362.
3. Bloomfield S, Barnert AH, Kanter P. The use of Eastman-910 monomer as an adhesive in ocular surgery: I. Biologic effects on ocular tissues. *Am J Ophthalmol* 1963;55:742–748.
4. Bloomfield S, Barnert AH, Kanter P. The use of Eastman-910 monomer as an adhesive in ocular surgery: II. Effectiveness in closure of limbal wounds in rabbits. *Am J Ophthalmol* 1963; 55:946–953.
5. Lehman RAW, Hayes GJ, Leonard F. Toxicity of alkyl 2-cyanoacrylates: I. Peripheral nerve. *Arch Surg* 1966;93:441–446.
6. Lehman RAW, West RL, Leonard F. Toxicity of alkyl 2-cyanoacrylates. *Arch Surg* 1966;93:447–450.
7. Leonard F. The N-alkylalphacyanoacrylate tissue adhesives. *Ann NY Acad Sci* 1968;146:203–13.
8. Leonard F. The N-alkylalphacyanoacrylate tissue adhesives. In: Stark L, Agarwal G, eds. *Biomaterials.* New York: Plenum Press, 1969:15–30.
9. Leonard F, Collins JA, Porter HJ. Interfacial polymerization of N-alkyl alpha-cyanoacrylate homologs. *J Appl Polymer Sci* 1966; 10:1617–1623.
10. Leonard F, Kulkarni RK, Brandes G, et al. Synthesis and degradation of poly (alkyl alpha-cyanoacrylates). *J Appl Polymer Sci* 1966; 10:259–272.
11. Refojo MF. Glyceryl methacrylate hydrogels. *J Appl Polymer Sci* 1965;9:3161–3170.
12. Refojo MF. Surgical adhesives in ophthalmology. *J Macromol Sci Chem* 1970;A4:667–674.
13. Refojo MF. Adhesives in ophthalmology. In: Polack FM, ed. *Cornea and external diseases of the eye: First Inter-American Symposium.* Springfield, IL: Charles C Thomas, 1970:183–189.
14. Refojo MF, Dohlman CH. The tensile strength of adhesive joints between eye tissues and alloplastic materials. *Am J Ophthalmol* 1969;68:248–255.
15. Refojo MF, Dohlman CH, Ahmad B, et al. Evaluation of adhesives for corneal surgery. *Arch Ophthalmol* 1968;80:953–955.
16. Refojo MF, Dohlman CH, Koliopoulos J. Adhesives in ophthalmology: a review. *Surv Ophthalmol* 1971;15:217–236.
17. Webster RG Jr, Slansky HH, Refojo MF, et al. The use of adhesives for the closure of corneal perforations: report of two cases. *Arch Ophthalmol* 1968;80:705–709.
18. Boruchoff SA, Refojo M, Slansky HH, et al. Clinical applications of adhesives in corneal surgery. *Trans Am Acad Ophthalmol Otolaryngol* 1969;73:499–504.
19. Malaev AA. MK-2 cyanoacrylate glue in penetrating wounds of the cornea and sclera (preliminary report). *Vestn Oftalmol* 1969;4:17–19.
20. Straatsma BR, Allen RA, Hale PN, et al. Experimental studies employing adhesive compounds in ophthalmic surgery. *Trans Am Acad Ophthalmol Otolaryngol* 1963;67:320–333.
21. Ellis RA, Levine AM. Experimental sutureless ocular surgery. *Am J Ophthalmol* 1963;55:733–741.
22. Fogle JA, Kenyon KR, Foster CS. Tissue adhesive arrests stromal melting in the human cornea. *Am J Ophthalmol* 1980;89:795–802.
23. Donnenfeld ED, Perry HD, Nelson DB. Cyanoacrylate temporary tarsorrhaphy in the managements of corneal epithelial defects. *Ophthalmic Surg* 1991;22:591–593.
24. Leahey AB, Gottsch JD, Stark WJ. Clinical experience with N-butyl cyanoacrylate (Nexacryl) tissue adhesive. *Ophthalmology* 1993;100:173–180.
25. Ollivier F, Delverdier M, Regnier A. Tolerance of the rabbit cornea to an N-butyl-ester cyanoacrylate adhesive (Vetbond®). *Vet Ophthalmol* 2001;4:261–266.
26. Collin R, Watts MT. The use of fibrin glue in mucous membrane grafting of the fornix. *Ophthalmic Surg* 1992;23:689–690.
27. Sharma A, Kaur R, Kumar S, et al. Fibrin glue versus N-butly-2-cyanoacrylate in corneal perforations. *Ophthalmology* 2003;110: 291–298.
28. Gammon RR, Prum BE Jr, Avery N, et al. Rapid preparation of small-volume autologous fibrinogen concentrate and its same day use in bleb leaks after glaucoma filtration surgery. *Ophthalmic Surg Lasers* 1998;29:1010–1012.
29. Henrick A, Gaster RN, Silverstone PJ. Organic tissue glue in the closure of cataract incisions. *J Cataract Refract Surg* 1987;13: 551–553.
30. Buschmann W. Fibrinogen concentrate and topical antifibrinolytic treatment for conjunctival wounds and fistulas. In: Schlag C, Redl H, eds. *Fibrin sealant in operative medicine*, vol 2. New York: Springer-Verlag, 1986:68–69.
31. Katzin HM. Aqueous fibrin fixation of corneal transplants in the rabbit. *Arch Ophthalmol* 1945;35:415.
32. Tassman IS. The use of fibrin coagulum fixation in ocular surgery: keratoplasty. *Trans Am Acad Ophthalmol Otolaryngol* 1949;53:134.
33. Goins KM, Khadem J, Majmudar PA, et al. Photodynamic biologic tissue glue to enhance corneal wound healing after radial keratotomy. *J Cataract Refract Surg* 1997;23:1331–1338.
34. Goins KM, Khadem J, Majmudar PA. Relative strength of photodynamic biologic tissue glue in penetrating keratoplasty in cadaver eyes. *J Cataract Refract Surg* 1998;24:1566–1570.
35. Miki D, Dastgheib K, Kim T, et al. A photopolymerized sealant for corneal lacerations. *Cornea* 2002;21:393–399.
36. Kaufman HE, Insler MS, Ibrahim-Elzembely HA, et al. Human fibrin tissue adhesive for sutureless lamellar keratoplasty and scleral patch adhesion. *Ophthalmology* 2003;110:2168–2172.
37. Robin JB, Lee CF, Riley JM. Preliminary evaluation of two experimental surgical adhesives in the rabbit cornea. *Refract Corneal Surg* 1989;5:302–306.
38. Bloom JN, Duffy MT, Davis JB, et al. A light-activated surgical adhesive technique for sutureless ophthalmic surgery. *Arch Ophthalmol* 2003;121:1591–1595.
39. Alio JL, Mulet ME, Cotlear D, et al. Evaluation of a new bioadhesive copolymer (ADAL®) to seal corneal incisions. *Cornea* 2004;23:180–189.

TECTONIC CORNEAL TRANSPLANTATION

BEATRICE E. FRUEH

Tectonic (from Latin *tectum,* "roof") grafts, also called *patch grafts,* are either lamellar or perforating, and cover corneal stromal defects, restoring the structure of the cornea or sclera.

INDICATIONS

Indications for tectonic keratoplasty include infectious and sterile stromal defects, with perforation or impending perforation. Patch grafts can be used temporarily (for a later penetrating keratoplasty with better donor material and when there is less inflammation) or permanently to repair peripheral or central descemetoceles and perforations (1,2). Local and systemic autoimmune diseases, like rheumatoid arthritis, Sjögren's syndrome, Wegener's granulomatosis, polyarteritis nodosa, Stevens-Johnson syndrome, systemic sclerosis, and Mooren's ulcer can cause stromal ulceration (3–6). In developed countries, herpes simplex virus and varicella zoster virus are the most frequent causes of infectious stromal melting, whereas in developing countries fungal and bacterial keratitis are more frequent. Thinning disorders, like Terrien's marginal degeneration, pellucid marginal degeneration, and keratoglobus, can also be improved with tectonic grafts. Corneal ulceration can also be caused by secondary changes resulting from other diseases, such as conjunctival cicatrization, lid abnormalities, keratoconjunctivitis sicca, and trichiasis. The correct diagnosis of the etiology of the melting process is extremely important to treat underlying disease before and after the corneal surgery.

SURGICAL TECHNIQUE AND POSTOPERATIVE CARE

Depending on the clinical situation, a patch graft can be performed with cornea, sclera, tissue adhesive, amniotic membrane, or polytetrafluoroethylene (Gore-Tex). In general, cyanoacrylate tissue adhesive can seal only small perforations and is rather unsuitable for use in the visual axis (less transparent than a patch graft with corneal tissue). In case of larger or central perforations, penetrating keratoplasty may be a better option.

In cases of Mooren's ulcer, conjunctival excision should be performed before the melting process becomes too severe, or at the time of tectonic grafting (7). Application of tissue adhesive can stop the melting process (8) or, in case of perforation, reform the anterior chamber and also allow one to wait for suitable donor tissue. Before surgery, a bandage soft contact lens can be fitted to reform the anterior chamber.

Surgery is preferably done with general anesthesia after mannitol infusion for reduction of intraocular pressure. After placing a speculum, a paracentesis is performed and a viscoelastic is injected into the anterior chamber. Usually the paracentesis can be done even if the anterior chamber is flat and the eye is soft. If this is not possible, viscoelastic agents can be injected directly through the perforation site. All necrotic tissue should be removed from the area of the stromal melt to assess the real size of the ulceration and decide on the size and shape of the trephination. The goal of the dissection should be to remove all affected corneal tissue but to preserve as much healthy host tissue as possible. When possible, the visual axis should be spared from wound margins or sutures. Peripheral ulcers may require conjunctival peritomy and scleral dissection. If the ulceration or thinned area is peripheral and not too irregular in shape, a small, standard hand-held trephine can be used (9). A partial-thickness trephination of the recipient bed is performed: In most cases, the trephination will be superficial because of the hypotony. Deepening of the trephination with a sharp blade or diamond knife and lamellar dissection are then performed. A donor button of the same size or slightly oversized, full or partial thickness, is then sutured in place using interrupted 10-0 nylon sutures. Running sutures are contraindicated because of the greater risk for suture loosening in inflamed eyes. In cases of irregular or crescentic ulcerations, the patch graft should match the ulceration shape and therefore cannot be achieved with a simple round trephination. In such instances, one side of the trephination can be achieved with an hand-held trephine and the rest must be cut freehand. It is advisable to use a caliper to measure exactly the size of the lesion before cutting the donor tissue. A template exactly matching the area to be removed can be cut from a surgical drape and can be helpful in cutting the donor tissue. In perforated corneas or when the iris adheres firmly to the cornea, an iridectomy is performed.

At the end of surgery, the viscoelastic agent is removed, and antibiotic (gentamicin 40 mg/mL) and steroid are injected subconjunctivally. We refrain from injecting steroids in cases of fungal or severe bacterial infections. An ointment (tobramycin and dexamethasone) is applied and systemic antibiotics are administered. The postoperative topical regimen depends on the etiology of the melt: For sterile ulcerations, prednisolone acetate 1% is given four times daily. For infectious ulcers, the further use of fortified antibiotics (according to sensitivity tests) or antifungal agents may be needed, and the use of corticosteroids is contraindicated, despite a higher risk for rejections. The eradication of the infection in the perioperative period is more important than a possible rejection of the patch graft. In viral ulcers, antivirals locally and systemically are indicated. The treatment of underlying autoimmune diseases, with appropriate systemic immunosuppression, is of eminent importance (10,11).

Secondary glaucoma, because of synechia formation, intraocular inflammation, or steroid dependence, is not uncommon. I prefer not to prescribe prostaglandin agonists or prostamides as first-line therapy because of their potential for causing increased inflammation.

A not uncommon problem of patch grafts is nonhealing epithelial defects, leading to stromal melt and loosening of sutures. Aggressive lubrication, punctum plugs, serum drops, and bandage contact lens or tarsorrhaphy should be used. All loose sutures must be removed and replaced. If the epithelial defect is persistent, amniotic membrane transplantation or conjunctival flap should be considered before the melting process resumes. After the first 6 to 8 postoperative weeks, long-term care usually does not differ from that in standard keratoplasty.

RESULTS

Results vary depending on the initial diagnosis, and a comparison of technique outcomes is difficult owing to the relative paucity of patch grafts compared with standard lamellar or penetrating keratoplasties, the variety of shapes and sizes of the melting processes and their medical management, and the severity of systemic disease.

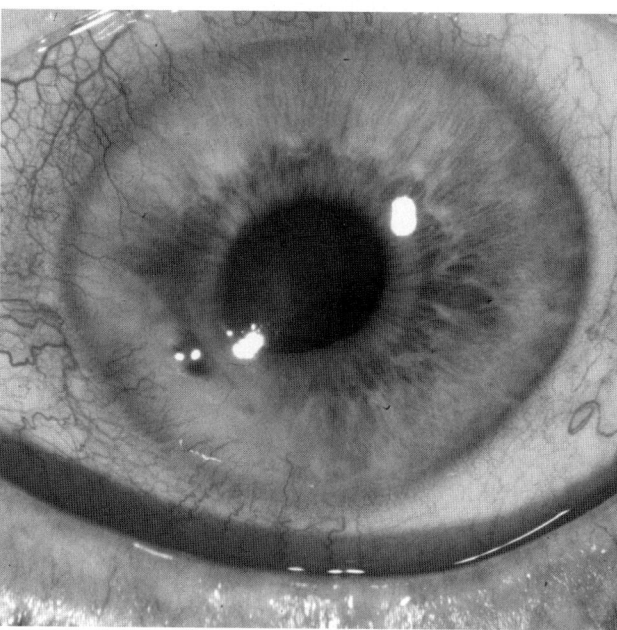

FIGURE 53-1. Peripheral ulcerative sterile keratitis in an 84-year-old patient without an underlying immunologic disorder.

Visual results of tectonic keratoplasties are in general inferior to elective penetrating keratoplasties in nonmelting situations (12,13).

Mooren's ulcer, as a special entity, appears to do favorably after lamellar keratectomy or lamellar keratoplasty. The possible mechanism is the removal of a corneal antigen stimulus to a self-perpetuating autoimmune process (14).

Crescentic lamellar keratoplasties or two-step annular tectonic lamellar keratoplasties have been proven to be effective in severe Terrien's marginal degeneration, improving the against-the-rule astigmatism (15–17).

In case of peripheral ulcerative keratitis, tectonic keratoplasty, either lamellar or perforating, combined with systemic immunosuppression could preserve most eyes and maintain or gain vision (18) (Figs. 53-1 through 53-3).

OTHER TECHNIQUES

Several authors have refined the techniques of tectonic grafting. In nonvascularized corneas, some groups have successfully used the excimer laser to trephine host and donor tissues (19,20). Glycerin-preserved and cryopreserved corneas have been used as patch grafts for infectious keratitis, mostly fungal (21, 22). Lamellar dissection of the donor cornea can be achieved with a microkeratome and an artificial anterior chamber system as well as with blunt dissection from a whole globe (23,24). Lamellar corneal autograft alone or with keratoplasty has occasionally been tried for perforations, providing both tectonic and optical functions (25,26). Tectonic epikeratoplasty is

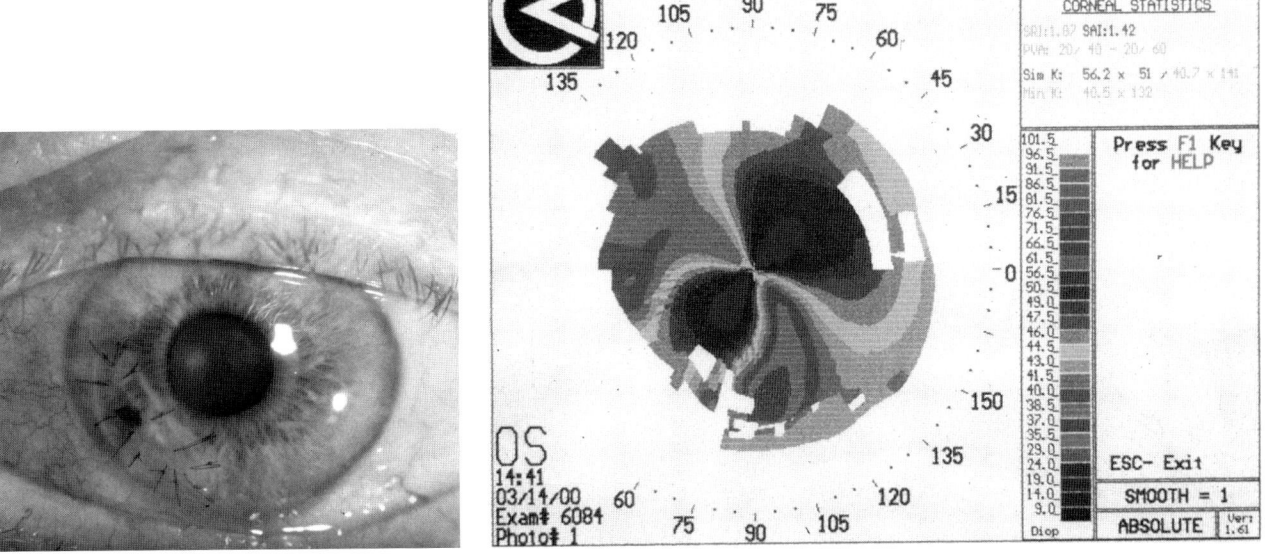

FIGURE 53-2. Same patient as in Fig. 53-1. **A:** One month after tectonic keratoplasty and iridectomy. **B:** Corneal topography shows 16 diopters of astigmatism.

an alternative in the attempt to preserve globe integrity, but has worse results than penetrating keratoplasty *à chaud* (27,28).

When extensive surgery is contraindicated and the corneal perforation is too big to be closed by cyanoacrylate tissue adhesive, a combination of free tissue scleral patch with tissue adhesive can be performed (29,30). In emergency situations, the use of Gore-Tex has also been advocated (31). Amniotic membrane has been shown to be ineffective as a patch graft for near-perforated or perforated corneas (32). Amniotic membrane can successfully be used instead of a conjunctival flap over a scleral graft for scleromalacia repair (33).

For ulcers in the vicinity of the graft–host junction of a penetrating keratoplasty, a small overlapping tectonic keratoplasty is a safe and effective procedure with fewer risks than a repeat keratoplasty, especially if oversized (34) (Fig. 53-4).

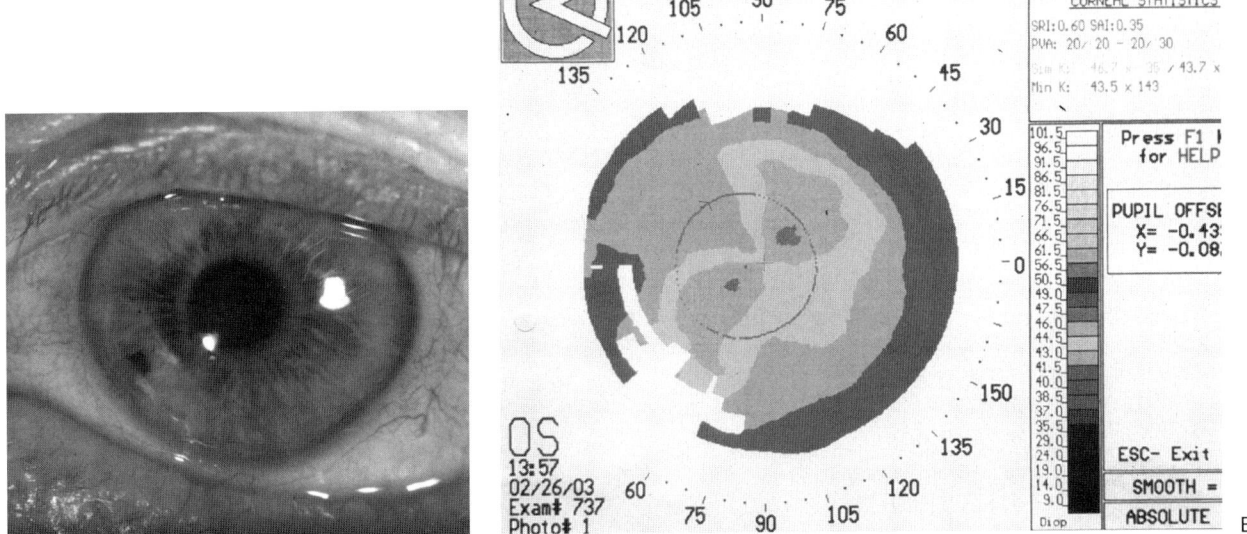

FIGURE 53-3. Same patient as in Fig. 53-1. **A:** Three years after tectonic keratoplasty. **B:** After suture removal, the topographic astigmatism has decreased to 3 diopters.

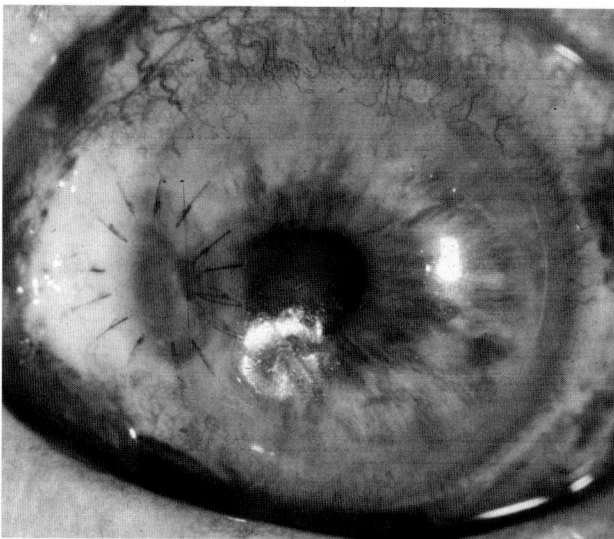

FIGURE 53-4. Peripheral minikeratoplasty for perforated rheumatoid ulcer in a 75-year-old patient.

Mushroom grafts have been proposed in cases of perforation with a circumferential flange of cornea at the edge of the corneal perforation (35).

Tectonic sclerokeratoplasty can be a valid alternative to keratoplasty for perilimbal corneal ulcers (36).

REFERENCES

1. Paufique L. Indications for the therapeutic lamellar corneal graft. *Am J Ophthalmol* 1950;33:24–25.
2. Terry MA. The evolution of lamellar grafting techniques over twenty-five years. *Cornea* 2000;19:611–616.
3. Messmer EM, Foster CS. Destructive corneal and scleral disease associated with rheumatoid arthritis: medical and surgical management. *Cornea* 1995;14:408–417.
4. Austin P, Green WR, Sallyer DC, et al. Peripheral corneal degeneration and occlusive vasculitis in Wegener's granulomatosis. *Am J Ophthalmol* 1978;85:311–317.
5. Krachmer JH, Laibson RR. Corneal thinning and perforation in Sjögren's syndrome. *Am J Ophthalmol* 1974;78:917–920.
6. Wood TO, Kaufman HE. Mooren's ulcer. *Am J Ophthalmol* 1971;71:417–421.
7. Brown SI. Mooren's ulcer: treatment by conjunctival excision. *Br J Ophthalmol* 1975;59:675–682.
8. Fogle JA, Kenyon KR, Foster CS. Tissue adhesive arrests stromal melting in the human cornea. *Am J Ophthalmol* 1980;89:795–802.
9. Völker HE, Naumann GOH. Exzentrische tektonische Mini-Keratoplastik bei kornealen, korneoskleralen und skleralen Prozessen. *Klin Monatsbl Augenheilkd* 1984;185:158–166.
10. Foster CS, Forstot SL, Wilson LA. Mortality rate in rheumatoid arthritis patients developing necrotizing scleritis or peripheral ulcerative keratitis: effects of systemic immunosuppression. *Ophthalmology* 1984;91:1253–1263.
11. Tauber J, Saiz de la Maza M, Hoang-Xuan T, et al. An analysis of therapeutic decision making regarding immunosuppressive chemotherapy for peripheral ulcerative keratitis. *Cornea* 1990;9:66–73.
12. Soong HK, Farjo AA, Katz D, et al. Lamellar corneal patch grafts in the management of corneal melting. *Cornea* 2001;19:126–134.
13. Killingsworth DW, Stern GA, Driebe WT, et al. Results of therapeutic penetrating keratoplasty. *Ophthalmology* 1993;100:534–541.
14. Martin NF, Stark WJ, Maumenee AE. Treatment of Mooren's and Mooren's-like ulcer by lamellar keratectomy: report of six eyes and literature review. *Ophthalmic Surg* 1987;18:564–569.
15. Schanzlin DJ, Sarno EM, Robin JB. Crescentic lamellar keratoplasty for pellucid marginal degeneration. *Am J Ophthalmol* 1983;96:253–254.
16. Pettit TH. Corneoscleral freehand lamellar keratoplasty in Terrien's marginal degeneration of the cornea: long term results. *Refract Corneal Surg* 1991;7:28–32.
17. Hahn TW, Kim JH. Two-step annular tectonic lamellar keratoplasty in severe Terrien's marginal degeneration. *Ophthalmic Surg* 1993;24:831–834.
18. Raizman MB, Sainz de la Maza M, Foster CS. Tectonic keratoplasty for peripheral ulcerative keratitis. *Cornea* 1991;10:312–316.
19. Küchle M, Seitz B, Langenbucher A, et al. Nonmechanical excimer laser penetrating keratoplasty for perforated or predescemetal corneal ulcers. *Ophthalmology* 1999;106:2203–2209.
20. Schmitz K, Behrens-Baumann W. Perforierende Keratoplastik in freier Form unter Einsatz des Excimer-Lasers: Erste Anwendung am Patienten. *Klin Monatsbl Augenheilkd* 2003;220:247–252.
21. Sharma A, Gupta P, Narang S, et al. Clear tectonic penetrating graft using glycerine-preserved donor corneas. *Eye* 2001;15:345–347.
22. Yao Y-F, Zhang P, Zho P, et al. Therapeutic penetrating keratoplasty in severe fungal keratitis using cryopreserved donor corneas. *Br J Ophthalmol* 2003;87:543–547.
23. Wiley LA, Joseph MA, Springs CL. Tectonic lamellar keratoplasty utilizing a microkeratome and an artificial anterior chamber system. *Cornea* 2002;2:661–663.
24. Bessant DAR, Dart JKG. Lamellar keratoplasty in the management of inflammatory corneal ulceration and perforation. *Eye* 1994;8:22–28.
25. Lam S, Rapuano CJ, Krachmer JH, et al. Lamellar corneal autograft for corneal perforation. *Ophthalmic Surg* 1991;22:716–717.
26. Titiyal JS, Ray M, Sharma N, et al: Intralamellar autopatch with lamellar keratoplasty for paracentral corneal perforations. *Cornea* 2002;21:615–618.
27. Lifshitz T, Oshry T. Tectonic epikeratoplasty: a surgical procedure for corneal melting. *Ophthalmic Surg Lasers* 2001;32:305–307.
28. Bull H, Behrens-Baumann W. Tektonische Epikeratoplastik als Alternative zur Keratoplastik à chaud? *Klin Monatsbl Augenheilkd* 1997;210:78–81.
29. Mizuano K, Hayasaka S. Penetrating keratoplasty with use of adhesive and scleral strip in acute corneal perforations. *Ophthalmic Surg* 1982;13:475–477.
30. Hyndiuk RA, Hull DS, Kinyoun JL. Free tissue patch and cyanoacrylate in corneal perforations. *Ophthalmic Surg* 1974;5:50–55.
31. Legeais JM, Renard G, D'Heries F, et al. Surgical management of corneal perforation with expanded polytetrafluoroethylene (Gore-Tex®). *Ophthalmic Surg* 1991;22:213–217.
32. Blanco Azura A, Pillai CT, Dua HS. Amniotic membrane transplantation for ocular surface reconstruction. *Br J Ophthalmol* 1999;83:399–402.
33. Oh JH, Kim JC. Repair of scleromalacia using preserved scleral graft with amniotic membrane transplantation. *Cornea* 2003;22:288–293.
34. Soong HK, Meyer RF, Sugar A. Small, overlapping tectonic keratoplasty involving graft-host junction of penetrating keratoplasty. *Am J Ophthalmol* 2000;129:465–467.
35. Vanathi M, Sharma N, Titiyal JS. Tectonic grafts for corneal thinning and perforations. *Cornea* 2002;21:792–797.
36. Jonas JB, Rank RM, Budde WM. Tectonic sclerokeratoplasty and tectonic penetrating keratoplasty as treatment for perforated or predescemetal corneal ulcers. *Am J Ophthalmol* 2001;132:14–18.

CONJUNCTIVAL FLAPS

MARTIN FILIPEC

The creation of conjunctival flaps is a surgical procedure used in the management of corneal surface diseases when other medical or surgical therapy is not successful or available. Conjunctiva is used to cover part or all of the corneal surface to heal and stabilize the corneal surface. Conjunctival flaps as a therapeutic modality were first described at the end of 19th century (1,2), but the procedure did not gain widespread popularity until the second half of the 20th century, when Gundersen, at the Massachusetts Eye and Ear Infirmary in Boston, described the technique of fashioning a very thin conjunctival flap (3). The major innovation of Gundersen was to use conjunctiva split from Tenon's capsule, thereby decreasing the common tendency for flap retraction often seen with earlier, thicker flaps.

Although the mechanism of a conjunctival flap's effect on corneal healing is not fully understood, several possible explanations exist. The flap does not promote epithelial cell proliferation, but it does enhance healing by the apposition of vascularized conjunctival substantia propria to the corneal surface (4). Conjunctiva contains not only blood but lymphatic vessels. Bringing them into close contact with the diseased cornea may provide a source of cells and growth factors helpful in the process of infection resolution and corneal wound healing. The corneal surface is protected from the deleterious action of enzymes such as collagenases, metalloproteinases, and other proteases responsible for corneal melting after conjunctival flap surgery. Mechanical protection may also promote corneal wound healing.

With the enlargement of our armamentarium in the conservative medical treatment of infectious and immune-mediated diseases and dry-eye conditions, and with improved (corneal grafting, glue, contact lenses, amniotic membrane) and new (limbal stem cell transplantation) strategies for surgical treatment, the role of the conjunctival flap in the care of patients with ocular surface disease has decreased. But conjunctival flaps are still very useful, and probably are underused today in the management of corneal diseases (4–6). Just as every cornea specialist must know how to perform a tarsorrhaphy expertly, so too should he or she know how to perform a conjunctival flap.

The use of a conjunctival flap at the right time may solve an otherwise difficult problem and may prevent disastrous consequences related to the loss of globe integrity from corneal perforation and loss of the eye from endophthalmitis. It can also improve the overall quality of the patient's life through pain control and a decreased frequency of medication and visits to the ophthalmologist's office (6).

INDICATIONS

Conjunctival flaps are the last resort in the treatment of resistant infectious corneal diseases, eye surface diseases threatening the loss of corneal integrity, painful corneal disorders, and injuries (Table 54-1). Conjunctival flaps can be used when other means of treatment are not successful, available, or indicated. However, the decision to perform a conjunctival flap should be made early enough to preserve the integrity of the cornea. Conjunctival flaps are not appropriate for the care of corneal perforations. They might be used in this indication only in situations in which other, more appropriate methods of treatment are not available. A conjunctival flap may serve as a temporary measure to treat inflammation and stabilize the cornea before other surgery (e.g., penetrating keratoplasty) is undertaken. Flaps may also be used as a permanent measure when visual rehabilitation of the eye is not contemplated in the near future, or the probability of improving the underlying pathologic process through other techniques is low.

Therapeutic Indications

In the management of infectious keratitis, when medical therapy is failing and the situation is not under control in the long term, the use of a conjunctival flap is an option. Successful use of conjunctival flaps was reported in the treatment of infectious keratitis caused by many types of pathogens (7). From the technical point of view, it is important to

TABLE 54-1. INDICATIONS FOR CONJUNCTIVAL FLAP SURGERY

1. *Therapeutic indications*—to manage corneal infection resistant to conventional medical therapeutic strategies
   Necrotic stromal herpes simplex virus and herpes zoster virus keratitis
   Fungal keratitis
   Bacterial keratitis
   Acanthamoeba keratitis

2. *Tectonic indications*—to prevent or halt corneal stromal melting and disintegration of the cornea
   Neurotrophic keratitis
   Noninfectious and infectious melting corneal ulcers
   Corneal graft melting
   Exposure keratitis
   Trauma

3. *Palliative indications*—to control pain
   Bullous keratopathy
   Dry eye

perform concomitant keratectomy to remove as much necrotic and infected corneal tissue as possible.

Conjunctival flaps usually do not have a role in the management of bacterial keratitis. However, the successful use of a conjunctival flap in the therapy of bacterial keratitis has been reported in seven patients (8), and in *Pseudomonas* keratitis, success was reported in three of four patients (9).

The most common indication for the use of a conjunctival flap in the treatment of infectious diseases is in herpetic keratitis. Metaherpetic and stromal keratitis are the most common indications for a conjunctival flap (3,5,6,8,10,11).

Good results of a partial conjunctival flap associated with keratectomy were reported in the management of peripheral fungal keratitis when medical therapy failed (12).

The treatment of *Acanthamoeba* keratitis with conjunctival flaps in patients with failed medical treatment has been shown to be ineffective as a single procedure (13). The use of a conjunctival flap and deep lamellar keratectomy was successfully used in three eyes (14).

Tectonic Indications

Conjunctival flaps are used as an eye-saving procedure in cases of primary corneal melting or recurrent melting when medical and surgical treatment such as amniotic membrane transplantation, patch grafting, or penetrating keratoplasty failed. A conjunctival flap may be used in association with lamellar or perforating keratoplasty.

A lack of corneal sensitivity and decreased lacrimation is typical in neurotrophic ulcerations. This condition can be very difficult to manage, and a conjunctival flap may help to maintain corneal integrity and is more cosmetically acceptable than tarsorrhaphy (15). Metaherpetic keratitis is sometimes difficult to manage, and a conjunctival flap may

be a good solution. Also, in children with the rare Riley-Day syndrome, a conjunctival flap may be used.

Conjunctival flaps were used in the past quite often to cover leaking corneal wounds after perforating injury, but their success rate in permanently restoring corneal integrity is not more than 30% (16). Flaps are no longer used for this indication because refined microsurgical technique gives better results. Conjunctival flaps can be used in cases of descemetocele or corneal perforation when other therapy is unavailable (17).

In peripheral ulcerative keratitis of autoimmune origin, conjunctival resection at the place of inflammation is indicated together with appropriate systemic immunosuppressive therapy (18). A conjunctival flap may be considered in cases of central and paracentral ulcerations in rheumatoid arthritis.

Palliative Indications

A conjunctival flap may be used to relieve pain.

The most common corneal disease associated with pain in which a conjunctival flap can be useful is bullous keratopathy due to Fuchs' dystrophy or related to cataract surgery (5,8,10). The flap is indicated only in cases in which other procedures, such as contact lens fitting, penetrating keratoplasty, endothelial replacement, anterior stromal puncture, or amniotic membrane transplantation, are not available, successful, or indicated.

The use of a conjunctival flap can also be helpful in severe keratoconjunctivitis sicca when other treatments, such as tear substitution, punctal occlusion, and tarsorrhaphy, are not helpful. A flap may substantially relieve pain and stop the occurrence of filamentary keratitis, continual epithelial breakdowns, and frank ulcerations. A conjunctival flap may also be used in patients with dry eye when tectonic keratoplasty *à chaude* was necessary.

CONTRAINDICATIONS

Conjunctival flap surgery is contraindicated as a primary procedure in most instances of active corneal infection, descemetocele, and corneal perforation, and is used only when other therapeutic strategies have failed.

Conjunctival flap surgery has no place in the treatment of peripheral ulcerative keratitis associated with systemic vasculitis in autoimmune diseases and in Mooren's ulcer (10). Conjunctival resection at the location of corneal melting and systemic immunosuppressive therapy are recommended (18).

TECHNIQUES

There are two general types of conjunctival flap used in different pathologic processes. In conditions involving the whole corneal surface, *total conjunctival flaps* are used.

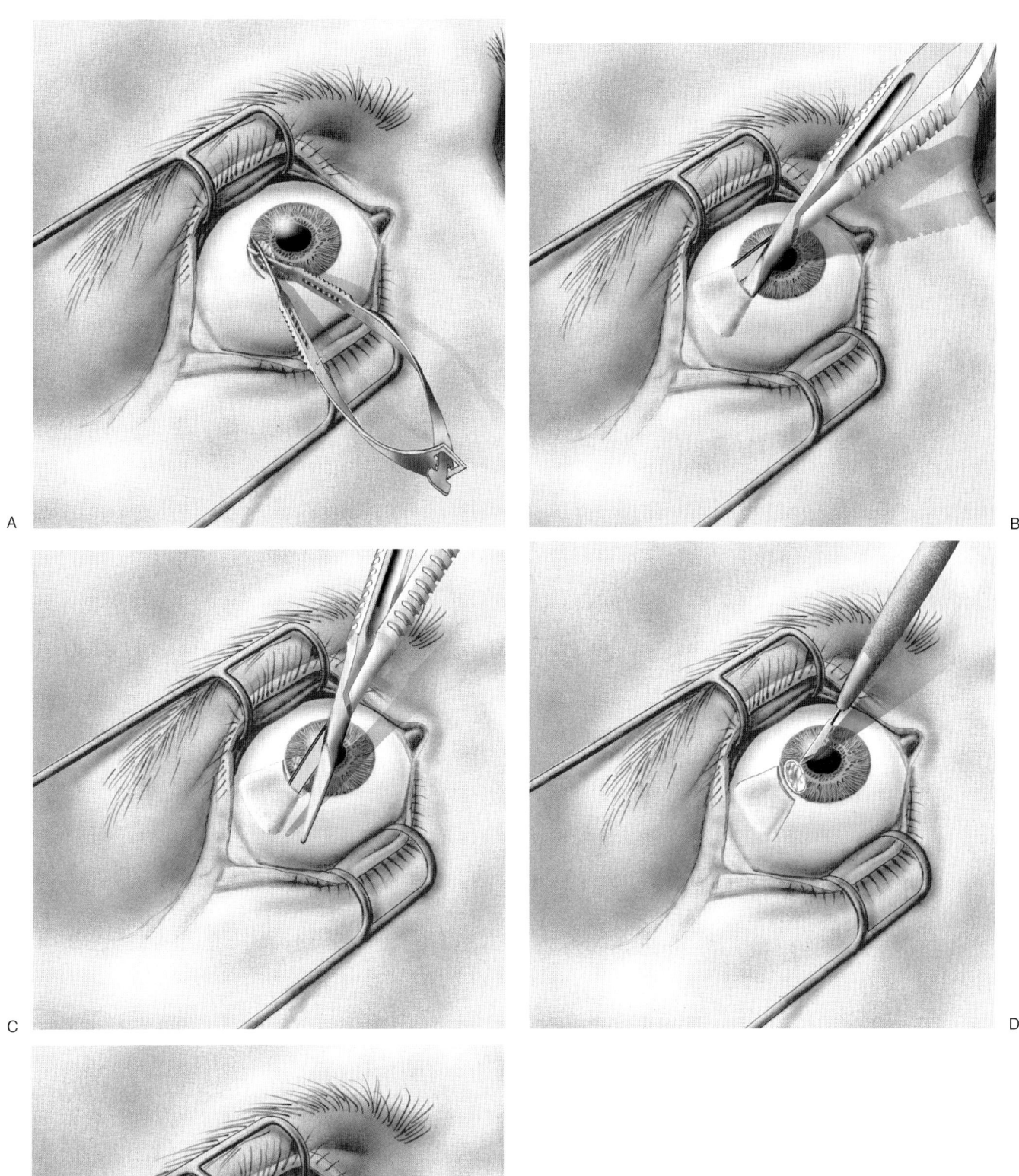

FIGURE 54-1. Partial peripheral conjunctival flap—surgical technique. **A:** Perilimbal conjunctival incision. **B:** After subconjunctival separation by anesthetic solution, conjunctiva is dissected from Tenon's capsule. **C:** Radial incision of the conjunctiva. **D:** Excision of necrotic corneal tissue. **E:** Conjunctival flap is sutured by interrupted sutures.

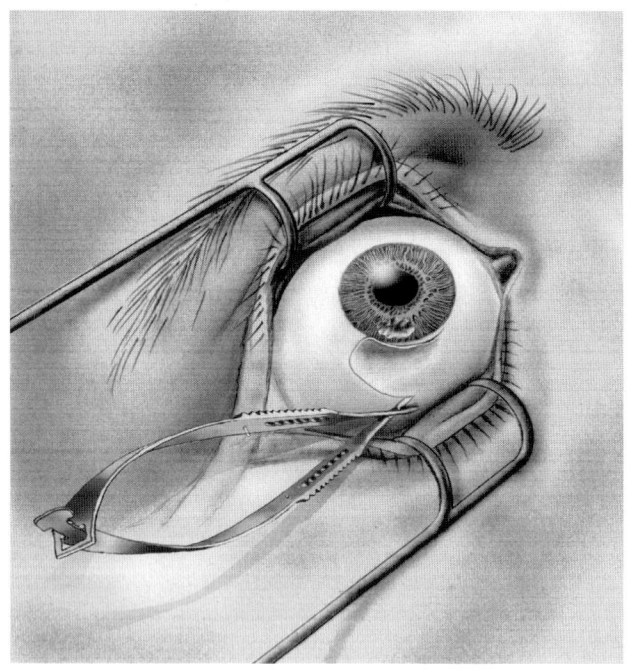

A

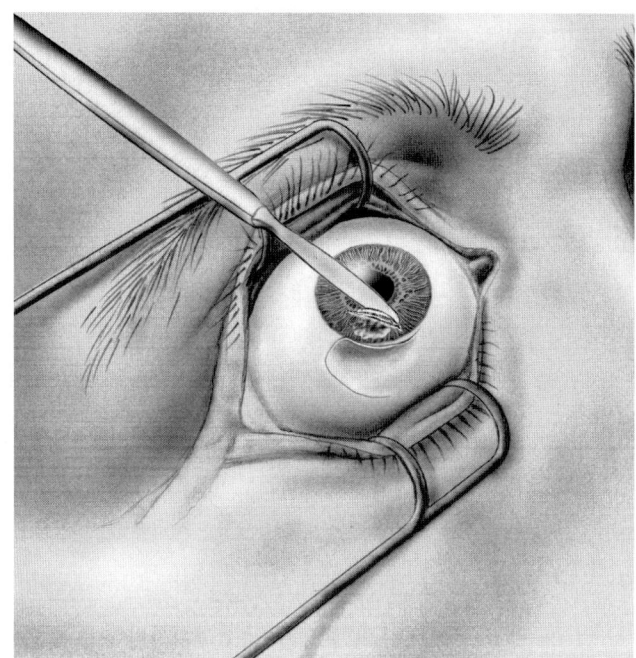

B

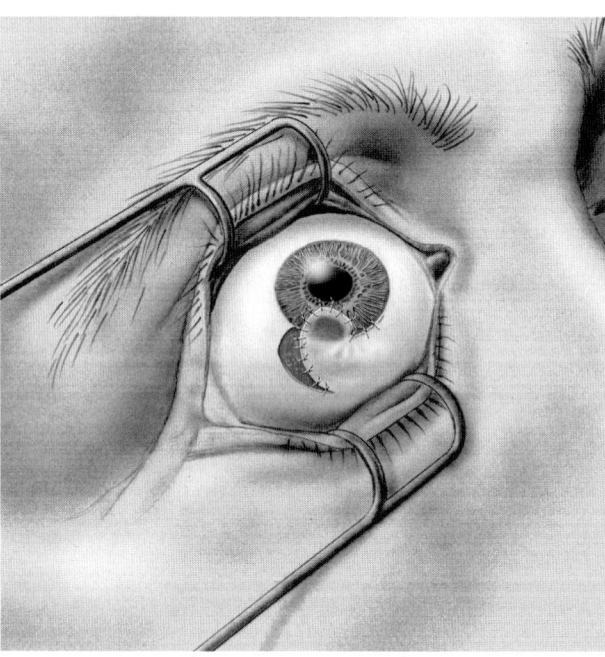

C

FIGURE 54-2. Partial pedicle conjunctival flap—surgical technique. **A:** Incision of the conjunctiva after subconjunctival injection of the anesthetic. **B:** Debridement of epithelium under the flap. **C:** Conjunctival flap is sutured by interrupted sutures.

In conditions involving just a part of the cornea, *partial conjunctival flaps* are indicated.

For both techniques, there are four major principles that make the procedure successful:

1. The flap should be large enough to cover the diseased area; tension on the flap should be avoided to prevent retraction.
2. The conjunctival flap should not contain Tenon's membrane.
3. The flap must be integral; any hole in the flap compromises the success of the procedure.

4. The cornea under the flap should be thoroughly mechanically debrided of epithelium or accompanied by lamellar keratectomy of necrotic or infected tissue to enhance the adhesion of the flap and thus prevent its retraction.

When preoperatively adherent or scarred conjunctival tissue is found, the use of a flap should be reconsidered.

The procedure can be performed under retrobulbar or periocular anesthesia. Before the instillation of the anesthetic, the diameter of the partial conjunctival flap should be marked by a pen. The flap should be at least 1 mm larger than the lesion on the cornea that is to be covered. In a total flap, the conjunctival flap should be as large as possible.

The injection of anesthetic (lidocaine 2% with epinephrine 1:100,000 to prevent bleeding) is used to balloon the conjunctiva and split it from Tenon's membrane. It is important to put the anesthetic solution in the current plane between the conjunctiva and Tenon's membrane, and at the same time not compromise the integrity of the flap by placing the needle into the area of the intended flap. Multiple injections of anesthetic from the limbal peritomy may facilitate the sometime tedious and (especially for an inexperienced surgeon) difficult preparation of the thin conjunctival flap (19). For separation of conjunctiva from Tenon's membrane, a combination of gentle blunt and sharp dissection is used, with particular attention to avoidance of excessive grasping of the conjunctiva, especially with toothed forceps, and careful observation of the scissor tips, both directly and indirectly, through the anterior surface of the flap. We usually mobilize a 14-mm flap for total coverage, after performing a 360-degree peritomy, and we make certain that it lies without tension from its attachments temporally and nasally before suturing.

Mattress or interrupted 8-0 vicryl sutures are used to secure the conjunctival flap. If the flap is sutured to the cornea, 10-0 nylon is used. Absorbable sutures may also be used.

Postoperative care consists of topical antibiotic. Combining this care with steroids or nonsteroidal antiinflammatory drugs is possible, depending to the underlying pathologic process. The penetration of drugs under the flap is low (4).

Partial Flap

Partial flaps are used for limited corneal disease. When the lesion is in the corneal periphery, the peripheral conjunctival flap (van Lint hood) (3,20,21) can be used (Fig. 54-1). Another alternative, used especially in the case of a more centrally located lesion, is the pedicle (racquet) flap (22) (Figs. 54-2 and 54-3). When the lesion is larger or there is not enough conjunctiva in the area, a bipedicle (bucket handle) flap (23) can be used (Fig. 54-4). In contrast to a total flap, pedicle flaps allow one to observe the anterior chamber, and the cornea not covered by the flap.

The technical principles for the preparation of partial and total flaps are the same. Because the partial flap is mostly sutured to the cornea, 10-0 nylon interrupted sutures are preferable. Partial flaps should be 1.3 to 1.5 times larger than the lesion (24).

Total Conjunctival Flap (Gundersen Flap)

The goal of a total conjunctival flap is to cover the entire cornea (3). A 360-degree peritomy is performed. A 7-0

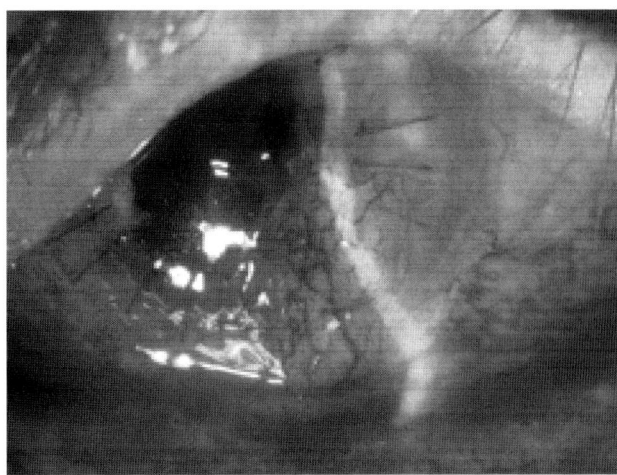

FIGURE 54-3. Corneal graft melting in patient with rheumatoid arthritis treated succesfully with partial pedicle conjunctival flap.

silk or vicryl traction suture is placed at 12 o'clock deep in the limbus (Fig. 54-5a). The globe is than rotated downward, and the conjunctiva is separated from the underlying Tenon's membrane by a subconjunctival injection of lidocaine 2% with epinephrine 1:100,000 introduced in a location outside of the area of the future flap, with a 30-gauge needle, in order not to create a hole in the flap (Fig. 54-5b). The incision of the conjunctiva in the upper fornix should be 2.5 to 3 cm long, and the entry should be as far as possible from the limbus (Fig. 54-5c,d). The conjunctiva is then separated from Tenon's membrane, exercising great care not to perforate the flap (Fig. 54-5e).

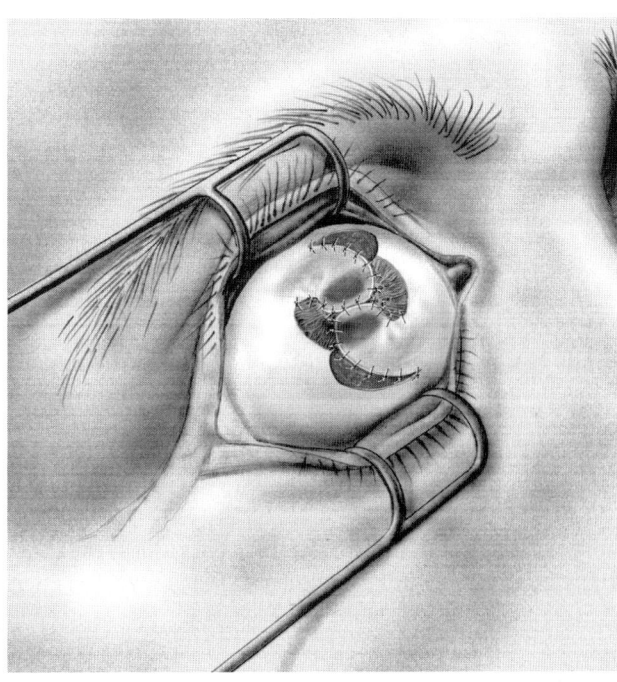

FIGURE 54-4. Partial bipedicle conjunctival flap.

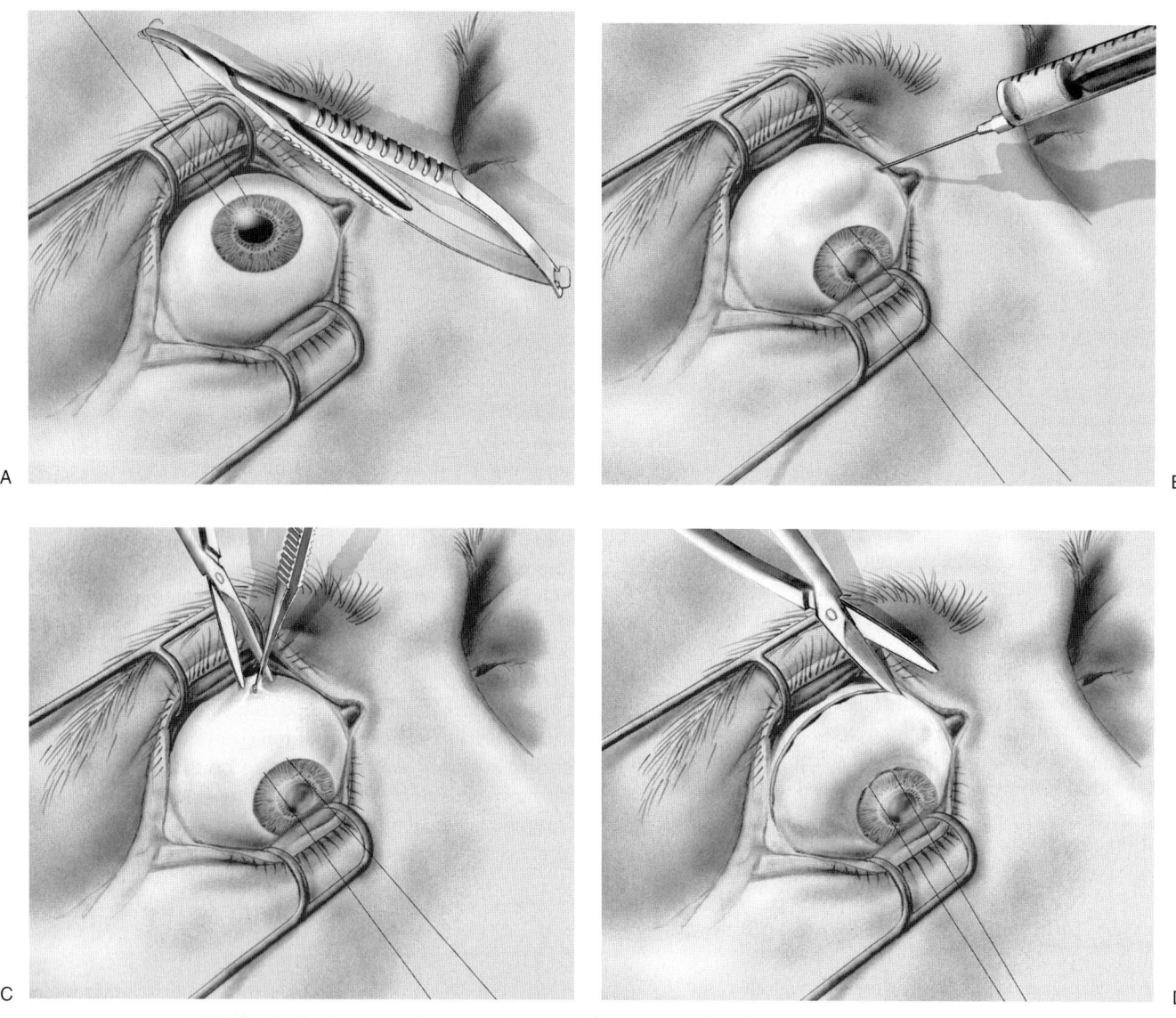

FIGURE 54-5. Total Gundersen conjunctival flap—surgical technique. **A:** Traction suture is placed deep through the limbus at 12 o'clock. **B:** Anesthetic injection is used to balloon the conjunctiva and separate it from Tenon's capsule. **C,D:** Conjunctival incision in the upper fornix. *(Continued)*

The upper fornix is deeper than the lower one (25), and the distance from the limbus to the limit of the upper fornix is usually 16 to 18 mm (3). Thus, there is usually enough conjunctiva to cover the cornea. When this is not the case, the technique of ballooning the conjunctiva after upper eye lid eversion can increase the amount of tissue available for the surgery (26). If more tissue is available, it is better to make a larger flap. An assistant is needed to hold the tissue with forceps, alternately exposing the inner and the outer side of the conjunctiva for the surgeon's better orientation and viewing of the scissor tips. Cautery of the conjunctiva is to be avoided. The epithelium is removed from the corneal surface (Fig. 54-5g). The flap is

then sutured to the sclera by single or mattress sutures (Fig. 54-5h and Fig. 54-6). The area above the upper limbus can be left uncovered; its epithelialization is usually very rapid and uncomplicated (3).

Fornix-Based Conjunctival Flap

In special circumstances, such as during war when an emergency procedure is needed to cover an injured or infected cornea, a fornix-based conjunctival flap can be performed (27,28). The conjunctiva is sutured starting from the inner and outer canthus toward the center of the cornea, pulling down the conjunctiva from the upper

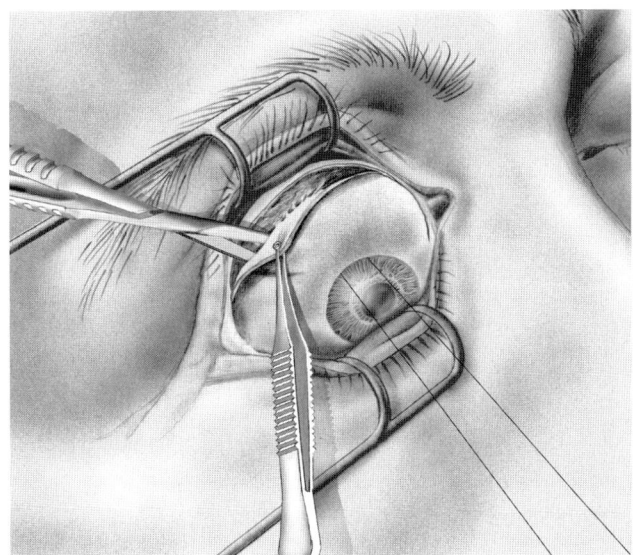

E

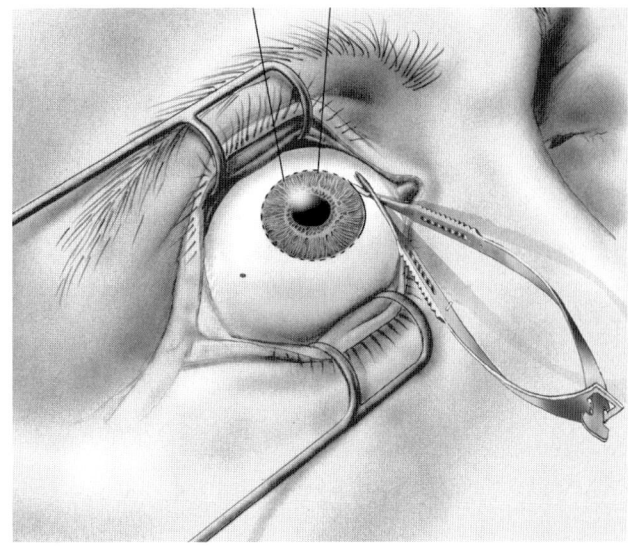

F

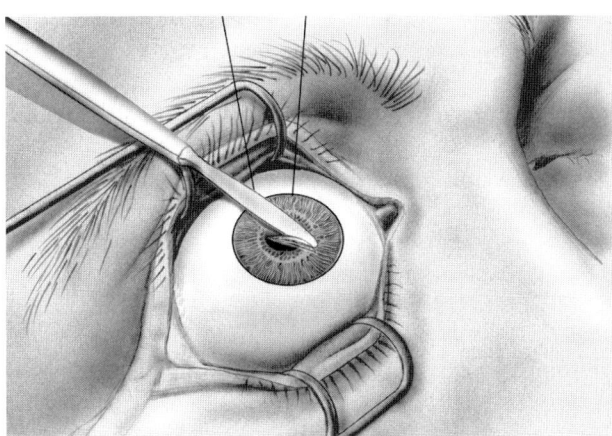

G

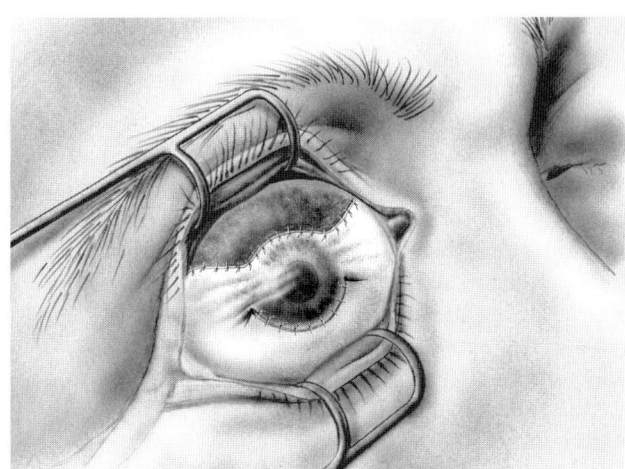

H

FIGURE 54-5. E: Surgical preparation of the conjunctival flap. **F:** Peritomy. **G:** Debridement of the epithelium. **H:** Conjunctival flap is sutured by interrupted sutures.

fornix and pulling up the conjunctiva from the lower fornix without any dissection.

RESULTS

The results of conjunctival flap surgery depend mainly on the indication and the timing and technical precision of the surgery. The results are usually very good, leading to permanent stabilization of the cornea, a reduction of inflammation and pain, and even (in some patients) visual acuity improvement up to 20/200 if the flap is sufficiently thin (3,6,10). The improved quality of the patient's life is probably the most important benefit, related to a substantial decrease in the need for medication and the frequency of visits to the ophthalmologist, as well as pain relief (6).

The eye usually becomes quiet and the conjunctiva transparent within 8 weeks; the cosmetic effect is usually negligible for the patient.

COMPLICATIONS AND DISADVANTAGES

The major operative complication related to the surgery is the creation of a buttonhole in the flap. This buttonhole will enlarge and compromise the results of the entire procedure. Therefore, any hole in the flap should be repaired with a 10-0 or 11-0 nylon suture passing through the edges of the hole and underlying cornea if possible (7). Another, usually early postoperative complication is retraction of the flap. This complication is often related to improper surgical technique. A flap that is too thick (containing some

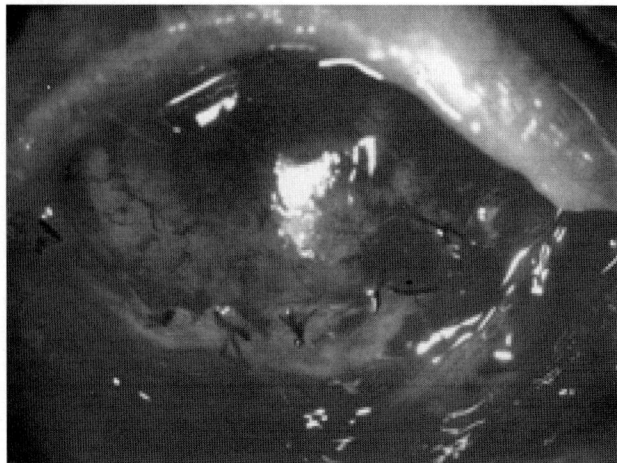

FIGURE 54-6. Gundersen flap 2 weeks after the surgery in patient with central corneal melting in primary Sjögren's syndrome.

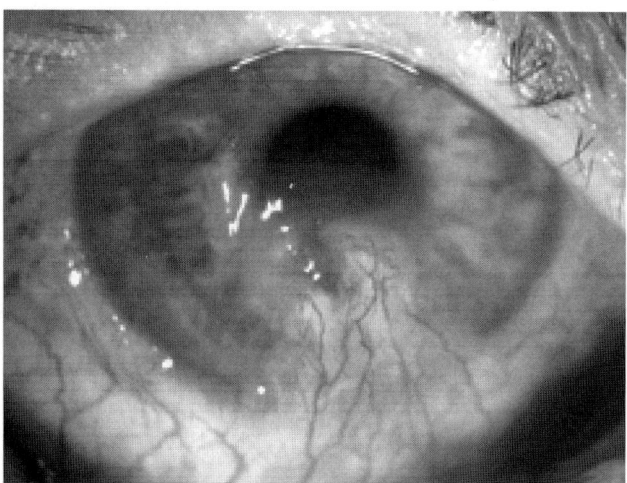

FIGURE 54-8. Corneal melting on the central margin of partial conjunctival flap in patient with stromal herpetic keratitis.

Tenon's membrane), a flap that is too narrow, and incomplete debridement of the corneal epithelium are major reasons for subsequent flap retraction.

Necrosis of the conjunctival flap is rare but possible. It may occur in cases of a narrow pedicle flap with compromised vascular supply or if the conjunctival tissue is abnormal (e.g., in cicatricial pemphigoid) (Fig. 54-7).

Conjunctival cyst formation is a rare and nonserious complication resulting from the proliferation of conjunctival epithelium under the flap (29). If large, it may need surgical excision. Corneal melting and perforation under the conjunctival flap is a rare complication described in patients with herpetic stromal keratitis (30,31) (Fig. 54-8).

A total conjunctival flap, at least for the first weeks after the surgery, precludes any possibility of examining the cornea or anterior chamber. The underlying disease might progress undetected. Endophthalmitis or a flat anterior chamber due to corneal perforation may be recognized by ultrasonographic examination. Intraocular pressure can be measured only by pneumotonometry or estimated by digital palpation. Reoperation in conjunctival flap surgery due to a buttonhole or flap retraction is difficult and often impossible.

Ptosis is usually transient and is a minor potential complication (3).

CONCLUSIONS

Despite its decreased frequency of use, conjunctival flap surgery should not be considered as an obsolete procedure. It remains a last resort but an important tool in the management of corneal diseases. It is often not considered or offered because of cosmetic reasons. But when it is accepted by a long-suffering patient, it is extraordinarily rewarding for both the patient and the ophthalmologist. Performed correctly, it solves the stubborn underlying problem, relieving pain and breaking the vicious circle of repeated problems, treatments, and office visits. And it can even be acceptable cosmetically after several months, and the patient can have useful visual acuity.

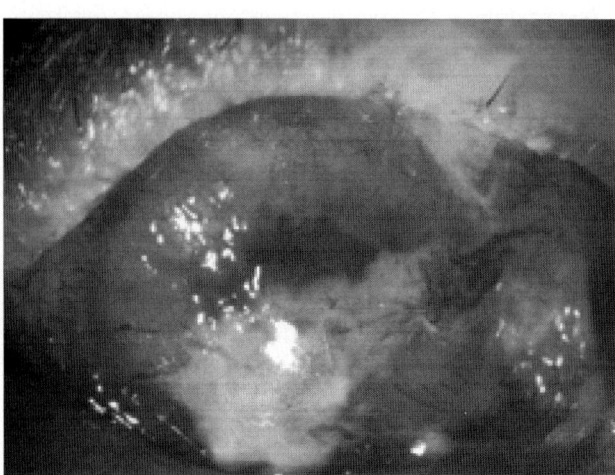

FIGURE 54-7. Partial conjunctival flap necrosis in patient with ocular cicatricial pemphigoid 6 weeks after surgery.

REFERENCES

1. Scholer KW. *Jahresberichte uber die Wirksamkeit der Augenklinik, in den Jahren 1874-1880.* Berlin: H. Peters, 1875–1881.
2. Kuhnt H. *Beitrage zur operativen Augen-heilkunde.* Jena: G. Fischer, 1883:69, 87.
3. Gundersen T. Conjunctival flaps in treatment of corneal diseases. *Arch Ophthalmol* 1958;6:880–888.
4. Thoft RA. Conjunctival and limbal surgery for corneal diseases. In: Smolin G, Thoft RA, eds. *The cornea: scientific foundations and clinical practice,* 3rd ed. Boston: Little, Brown, 1994: 711–714.

5. Gundersen T, Pearlson HR. Conjunctival flaps for corneal disease: their usefulness and complications. *Trans Am Ophthalmol Soc* 1969;67:78–95.
6. Alino AM, Perry HD, Kanellopoulos AJ, et al. Conjunctival flaps. *Ophthalmology* 1998;105:1120–1123.
7. Gardner PB. Conjunctival flaps. In: Kaufman H, Barron B, Kaufman HE, Barron BA, McDonald MB, Kaufman SC, eds. *The Cornea*, 2nd ed [on CD]. St. Louis, MO: Butterworth-Heinemann, 1999.
8. Insler MS, Pechous B. Conjunctival flaps revisited. *Ophthalmic Surg* 1987;18:455–458.
9. Buxton JN, Fox ML. Conjunctival flaps in the treatment of refractory *Pseudomonas* corneal abscess. *Ann Ophthalmol* 1986;18:315–318.
10. Paton D, Milauskas AT. Indications, surgical technique, and results of thin conjunctival flaps on the cornea: a review of 122 consecutive cases. *Int Ophthalmol Clin* 1970;10:329–345.
11. Brown DD, McCulley JP, Bowman RW, et al. The use of conjunctival flaps in the treatment of herpes keratouveitis. *Cornea* 1992;11:44–46.
12. Sanitato JJ, Kelley CG, Kaufman HE. Surgical management of peripheral fungal keratitis (keratomycosis). *Arch Ophthalmol* 1984;102:1506–1509.
13. Auran JD, Starr MB, Jakobiec FA. *Acanthamoeba* keratitis: review of the literature. *Cornea* 1987;6:2–26.
14. Cremona G, Carrasco MA, Tytiun A, et al. Treatment of advanced *Acanthamoeba* keratitis with deep lamellar keratectomy and conjunctival flap. *Cornea* 2002;21:705–708.
15. Lugo M, Arentsen JJ. Treatment of neurotrophic ulcers with conjunctival flaps. *Am J Ophthalmol* 1987;103:711–712.
16. Saini JS, Sharma A, Grewal SP. Chronic corneal perforations. *Ophthalmic Surg* 1992;23:399–402.
17. Webster RG Jr. Corneal injuries. In: Smolin G, Thoft RA, eds. *The cornea: scientific foundations and clinical practice*, 2nd ed. Boston: Little, Brown, 1987:517–527.
18. Tauber J, Sainz de la Maza M, Hoang-Xuan T, et al. An analysis of therapeutic decision making regarding immunosuppressive chemotherapy for peripheral ulcerative keratitis. *Cornea* 1990;6:66–73.
19. Maguire LJ, Shearer DR. A simple method of conjunctival dissection for Gunderson flap. *Arch Ophthalmol* 1991;109:1168–1169.
20. van Lint A. The sliding flap operation in the removal of cataract. *Ophthalmoscope* 1912;10:563–568.
21. King JH Jr, Wadsworth JAC. Surgery of the cornea. In: *An atlas of ophthalmic surgery*, 2nd ed. Philadelphia: JB Lippincott, 1970:249–330.
22. Cies WA, Odeh-Nasrala N. The racquet conjunctival flap. *Ophthalmic Surg* 1976;7:31–32.
23. Reinhart WJ. Conjunctival flap surgery. In: Bruner WE, Stark WJ, Maumenee AE, eds. *Manual of corneal surgery*. New York: Churchill Livingstone, 1987.
24. Nichols BD. Conjunctival flaps. In: Krachmer JH, Mannis MJ, Holland EJ, eds. *Cornea: surgery of the cornea and conjunctiva*. St. Louis: Mosby-Year Book, 1997:1903–1909.
25. Ehlers N. On the size of the conjunctival sac. *Acta Ophthalmol* 1965;43:205–210.
26. Lauring L, Wergeland FL. Total conjunctival flap with a modification of the Gundersen operation. *Am J Ophthalmol* 1973;76:953–956.
27. Haik GM. A fornix conjunctival flap as a substitute for the dissected conjunctival flap: a clinical and experimental study. *Trans Am Ophthalmol Soc* 1954;52:497–524.
28. Taylor RP. Fornix-based conjunctival flap in the treatment of corneal ulcers. *Am J Ophthalmol* 1969;67:754–756.
29. Cammarosano CA, Thoft RA. Complications of conjunctival surgery. *Int Ophthalmol Clin* 1992;32:41–48.
30. Lesher MP, Lohman LE, Yeakley W, et al. Recurrence of herpetic stromal keratitis after a conjunctival flap surgical procedure [letter]. *Am J Ophthalmol* 1992;114:231–233.
31. Rosenfeld SI, Alfonso EC, Gollamudi S. Recurrent herpes simplex infection in conjunctival flap [letter]. *Am J Ophthalmol* 1993;116:242–244.

SCLERAL TRANSPLANTATION

WILLIAM J. POWER AND ANDRA S. BOBART

The sclera has been successfully used for transplantation in dental, nasal, plastic-reconstructive, and ocular surgeries. Sclera may be transplanted for scleral ectasia, staphyloma, scleral perforation, glaucoma implant surgery, and patch graft repair of leaking filtering blebs (1).

Scleral tissue loss occurs secondary to inflammatory, necrotizing, traumatic, infective, iatrogenic, or idiopathic mechanisms. Recurrent scleritis leads to scleral thinning, which may eventually result in uveal prolapse and full-thickness scleral perforation. This tissue loss can be reinforced, repaired, or replaced with human sclera.

HISTORY

Historically, enucleation was performed in eyes with very severe uveal ectasia to avoid the risk of imminent rupture of the globe. Many materials have been used for scleral repair, including fascia lata, auricular cartilage, periosteum, autologous sclera, and preserved sclera (2–6). The use of autologous donor sclera was described at least as early as 1948 by Larsson for repair of a corneal perforation, and in 1953 homologous donor sclera was used by Paufique for the repair of scleromalacia perforans (5,6). It has been suggested by Curtin et al. that the use of homologous sclera may be better than autologous sclera in cases of scleromalacia perforans because the entire body collagen may be affected by the rheumatoid disease (7). The use of autologous sclera has largely been replaced with preserved human sclera from eye bank donor eyes. The use of sclera from an older donor may be preferable because it has greater rigidity and higher tensile strength.

HISTOLOGY AND IMMUNOLOGY

The sclera is relatively avascular, with blood vessels traversing it rather than supplying it directly. It is also relatively acellular, with up to 75% of its dry weight being collagen and up to 70% of its intact weight being water. The remainder of the sclera is made up of noncollagenous protein, proteoglycans, and mucopolysaccharides (8–10). Although collagen has been shown to induce specific humoral and cell-mediated immune reactions in experimental animals, the sclera itself has been repeatedly shown to have low antigenicity. Iacono et al. confirmed this in 1980 after testing the reactivity of human peripheral blood leukocytes to extracts of sclera (11–15). Scleral homograft rejection, therefore, is rarely encountered.

Necrotizing scleritis is the main cause of extreme scleral thinning requiring scleral transplantation. Histopathologic studies on patients with necrotizing scleritis demonstrate a mixed mononuclear and neutrophil infiltrate and fibrinoid necrosis of vessel walls. Immune complex deposition and a perivasculitis may also be seen (16).

Two main types of histopathosis have been described in necrotizing scleritis (17). The first is zonal necrotizing granulomatous inflammation, which surrounds a central necrotic area and is associated with vasculitis. This is mainly associated with rheumatoid arthritis, relapsing polychondritis, Goodpasture's syndrome, Wegener's granulomatosis, collagen vascular disease, and previous herpes zoster ophthalmicus. The second main type is necrotizing inflammation with multiple microabscesses. This may be associated with either positive or negative cultures for microorganisms. Proteoglycans are absent in areas of active necrotizing scleritis, even though the collagen fibers themselves are initially intact. This may be due to proteoglycan resorption by the products of inflammatory cells, by cytokines, and by active resident fibroblastic cells. The latter are most likely largely responsible for the extracellular degradation of collagen (18,19). Matrix metalloproteinase-3 (stromelysin) has been identified as one of the collagen-degrading enzymes in scleritis (20). A combination of the proinflammatory cytokines tumor necrosis factor-α and interleukin-1α may be responsible for enhanced matrix metalloproteinase-3 expression, thereby leading to increased tissue destruction (21). After scleral allografting, there is a severe immune reaction of edema, hyperemia, and a cellular infiltrate around the graft. After approximately 20 days, there is a reduction in this immune reaction that coincides with the extraction of glycosaminoglycans from the collagen fibers of the allograft. It has been shown that the partially extracted glycosaminoglycans are gradually replaced by the recipient tissue, and a no-scar regenerate develops. There is fourfold less scarring where there is at least a 70% structural similarity between the donor and host tissue (13).

CAUSES OF SCLERAL TISSUE LOSS

The sclera was described by Duke-Elder as being "inert and purely supportive in function" (22). Loss of this support due to progressive collagen destruction and thinning can cause the underlying choroid to bulge and cause scleral ectasia. The uvea may even break through the overlying thin covering of sclera and the conjunctiva. Thin sclera is blue in color, and with progressive thinning the affected area becomes dark because of the color of the underlying uvea.

Scleral thinning may be inherited in conditions such as in Marfan's syndrome, osteogenesis imperfecta, or Ehlers-Danlos syndrome (23–25). It may also be acquired in conditions such as pathologic myopia, iron-deficiency anemia, perilimbic scleromalacia, and after surgery (26–31). In staphyloma secondary to glaucoma, Thale et al. demonstrated a loss of the normal rhombic collagenous alignment of the inner sclera with scleral protrusion between parallel collagen bundles (8). And although scleritis rarely leads to frank perforation of the globe, postsurgical scleritis and scleral inflammation secondary to granulomatous, nongranulomatous, infective, and vasculitic disease have all been shown to lead to extreme scleral thinning, ectasia, and subsequent perforation.

Necrotizing scleritis is characterized as either necrotizing scleritis with inflammation (Fig. 55-1) or necrotizing scleritis without inflammation (scleromalacia perforans; Fig. 55-2). Necrotizing scleritis is frequently associated with the development of peripheral keratopathy (Fig. 55-3). The presence of scleritis with peripheral ulcerative keratopathy has a poor prognosis (32). Both types of necrotizing scleritis can lead to spontaneous or traumatic perforation and are associated with rheumatoid arthritis and with other autoimmune or systemic diseases. In one case series described by Sainz de la Maza et al., approximately 95% of patients with necrotizing scleritis had an associated systemic disease. Necrotizing scleritis was also seen in this study to be the most common type of scleritis when presenting as the first manifestation of systemic disease (33). Rheumatoid arthritis is the disease most commonly associated with scleromalacia perforans and with bilateral scleritis. Wegener's granulomatosis is also associated with necrotizing scleritis with inflammation. Other associated systemic diseases include relapsing polychondritis, polyarteritis nodosa, and inflammatory bowel disease. Necrotizing scleritis is

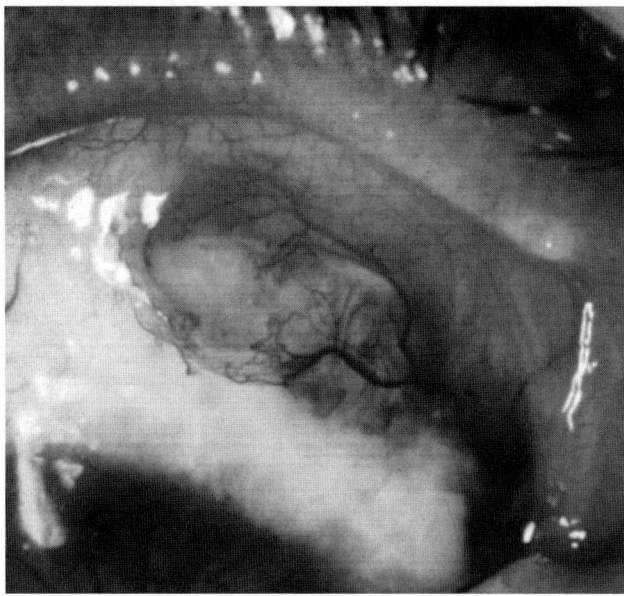

FIGURE 55-1. Necrotizing scleritis with inflammation.

uncommon in patients with juvenile idiopathic arthritis, Behâet's disease, the spondyloarthropathies, and systemic lupus erythematosus. Up to 10% of patients with necrotizing scleritis require some form of surgical intervention (32,33). Watson and Hayreh reported systemic or ocular complications in 60% of their patients with necrotizing scleritis and a mortality rate of 29% within 5 years (34). The presence of vasculitis with necrotizing scleritis can be associated with significant systemic morbidity (35).

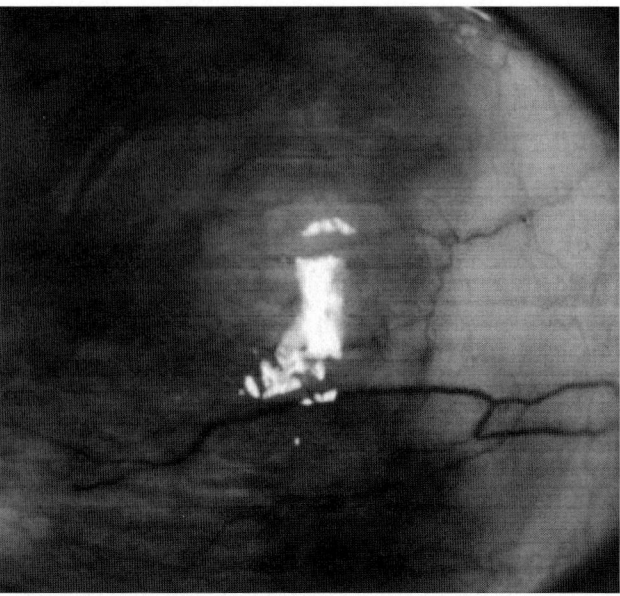

FIGURE 55-2. Necrotizing scleritis without inflammation (scleromalacia perforans).

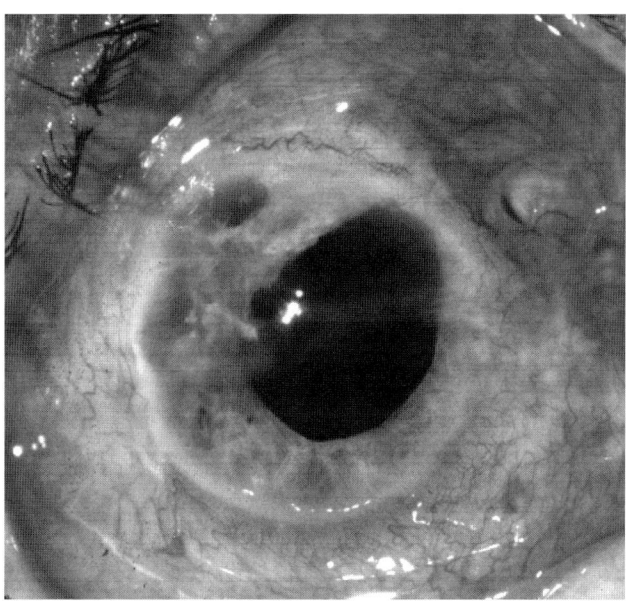

FIGURE 55-3. Necrotizing scleritis with associated peripheral corneal ulceration.

DONOR MATERIAL

Preserved human sclera is for single-case use only. Glycerin and ethanol are the two media that are most commonly used to store sclera. Neither appears to alter the structural integrity of the preserved sclera (36). Sclera preserved in glycerin becomes thin, translucent, and yellowish-brown because of dehydration. It can be stored for 12 months without refrigeration, or alternatively stored at 5°C. Histologically, the arrangement of the lamellae, the elastic fiber content, and the number of fixed cells are unchanged by this method of preservation (37). The scleral white color is usually restored within 30 minutes when it is rehydrated. Grafts preserved in absolute or 95% ethanol must be rinsed in balanced salt solution. If this is done for longer than 20 minutes in the material preserved in 95% ethanol, there may be less than 2% residual ethanol left in the donor tissue (38). Most eye banks use either 70% or absolute ethanol. Other storage methods used by eye banks include formalin, freezing in antibiotic solution at −20°C, and freeze-drying. The same criteria for serology/donor selection apply for sclera as for cornea because the risk of disease transmission is thought to be comparable for "living" cornea and fixed, "vascularized" sclera. A donor may not test positive for human immunodeficiency virus (HIV) as long as 6 months after infection, and therefore a negative test is not an absolute guarantee against HIV positivity (39). The unused tissue and remaining solutions should be treated as hazardous waste and should be appropriately disposed of. Creutzfeldt-Jakob disease (classic or variant forms) may rarely be contracted by tissue transplantation. There have been three reported cases of possible transmission of the Creutzfeldt-Jakob disease prion through corneal transplantation, but not with scleral transplantation to date (40–42). The relatively rich innervation of the cornea, which is much greater than that of the sclera, may be relevant in this matter.

Microorganisms can survive in glycerin-preserved sclera for at least 8 days, but the same is not true for ethanol-preserved sclera because of its greater antibacterial and antiviral activity (36,43). Resistant microorganisms were shown to survive in both glycerin- and ethanol-preserved scleral tissue by an *in vitro* study by Lucci et al. They showed that benzalkonium chloride diluted in 70% alcohol to be the best disinfectant for human sclera after 24 hours (44). The presence of bacterial infection in donors appears to have no effect, however, on the incidence of endophthalmitis in recipients.

SURGERY: TECHNIQUE AND POTENTIAL COMPLICATIONS

Anesthesia

Scleral grafting can be carried out under local anesthesia with sedation, or under general anesthesia if it is thought the patient may not be capable of remaining stationary for the duration of the procedure. The anesthesiologist should be made aware of the patient's previous immunosuppressant therapy because many of these elderly patients can have significant adrenal suppression.

Surgical Technique

The initial step is preparation of the surgical bed. This involves dissection of conjunctiva, Tenon's capsule, and any underlying episcleral tissue to expose the area of disease. A very thorough inspection of the surgical bed is then carried out. In many cases the involved area at the time of surgery is surprisingly larger than that estimated on clinical examination. It is also important to inspect all adjacent areas because there may be more than one area of disease. If the lesion involves the sclera at the base of insertion of one of the rectus muscles, it may be necessary to detach the insertion of the muscle and reattach it at the end of the procedure.

The ulcerated area of cornea is next removed, followed by necrotic conjunctiva and, last, by very careful removal of the necrotic sclera. Great care is needed at this stage to prevent inadvertent uveal perforation and subsequent intraocular hemorrhage. It is useful to undermine the edge of the remaining healthy recipient sclera because this facilitates easier placement of the subsequent sutures.

A template for the graft is fashioned using a marking pen and a sterile surgical plastic drape. The template is then used to determine the size and shape of the graft needed to be excised from the donor material. The graft is secured to the recipient bed using 9-0 nylon sutures with all knots buried. If prominent ectasia is present with significant uveal bulge, a prior anterior chamber paracentesis can be useful to decompress the eye. Gentle pressure over the center of the graft with an iris repositor now facilitates a better placement of the graft and also helps to reposition the prolapsing uvea. As much healthy conjunctiva as possible should be mobilized to cover the graft because this will help with the subsequent epithelialization and vascularization of the graft (45).

Complications

The most devastating intraoperative complication is choroidal perforation with subsequent intraocular hemorrhage. A slow and careful scleral bed dissection should help in preventing this potentially blinding complication. The most common postoperative complication is progressive melting of the scleral graft, which occurs most frequently owing to inadequate immunosuppressive treatment (Fig. 55-4). A second grafting procedure may be attempted once adequate immunosuppression is achieved. Other reported complications include infectious keratitis and endophthalmitis (45).

The scleral graft is not a cure when there is an underlying disease process affecting the sclera, but rather is a method to remove and replace the diseased area, or to reinforce it. Scleral rejection is uncommon after transplantation. An inherent T-cell suppressor mechanism, which may be triggered by scleral collagen, may provide immunologic tolerance to human donor allografts (46). The donor sclera may also stimulate tissue regeneration during resorption of the allograft (Figs. 55-5 through 55-7).

POSTOPERATIVE TREATMENT

After scleral transplantation, it is very important that a thorough histologic evaluation of the resected tissue be performed, with particular reference to the presence of any vasculitis. When necrotizing scleritis or vasculitis is present, the use of immunosuppressants should commence before the transplantation and continue into the postoperative period (45). Where the offending cause is infective, the appropriate antiinfective agents must also be prescribed in the same manner. Scleral grafting for noninflammatory causes of scleral thinning may be treated during and after surgery with topical antibiotics and steroids.

Immunosuppressive drugs as first-choice drugs in necrotizing scleritis have been shown to dampen the inflammation successfully in 74% of patients in one case series by Sainz de la Maza et al. (47). In that series, 89% of the patients had an underlying connective tissue or vasculitic disease. They found the use of nonsteroidal antiinflammatory drugs and steroids to be ineffective. Tuft and Watson reported that 67% of patients in their study required systemic immunosuppression to control their disease (48). Foster et al. reported that none of the 17 patients on immunosuppression in a case series of 34 patients with rheumatoid arthritis had progression of necrotizing scleritis or keratopathy (49).

Immunosuppressants prescribed in necrotizing scleritis may be subgrouped into the antimetabolites, T-cell inhibitors, or alkylating agents. Agents in the first group include azathioprine, methotrexate, and mycophenolate

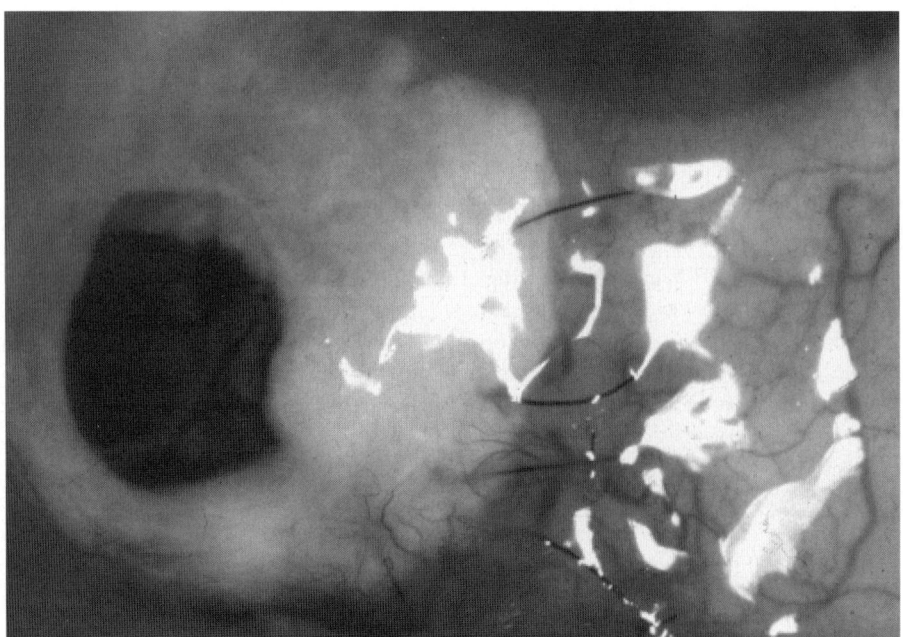

FIGURE 55-4. Recurrence of scleral necrosis in a scleral transplant in a patient who discontinued systemic immunosuppression.

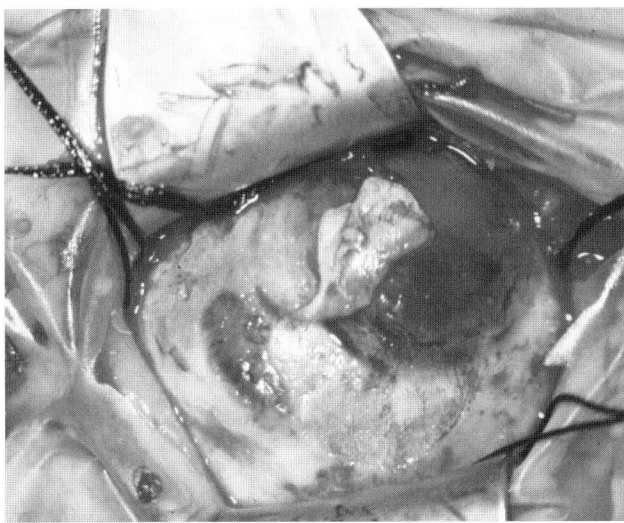

FIGURE 55-5. Intraoperative photograph of a patient with necrotizing scleritis and peripheral ulcerative keratitis secondary to relapsing polychondritis. Vast amounts of tissue damage were revealed during surgery.

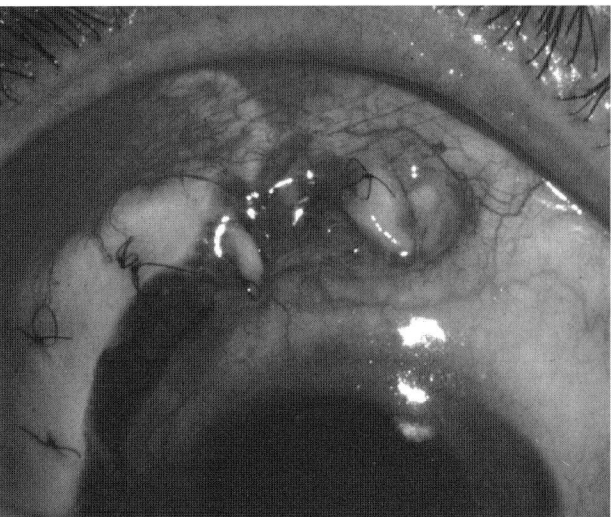

FIGURE 55-7. Recurrence of necrotizing scleritis in a patient with rheumatoid arthritis who was not immunosuppressed, but whose necrotizing scleritis was simply treated with scleral grafting, a strategy guaranteed to have this outcome.

mofetil. Azathioprine may be used for rheumatoid arthritis and combined with steroids or cyclosporine in transplantation; methotrexate is prescribed for arthritis- and systemic lupus erythematosus related-scleritis and is relatively safe to use in children (50). Mycophenolate mofetil has shown promising results when used in conjunction with other agents for scleritis. Only 1 of the 11 patients treated for ocular disease in a study by Larkin et al. experienced mild side effects of nausea and headache (51). Cyclosporine, a T-cell inhibitor, blocks T-cell replication and the production of interleukin-2 and may be prescribed for both the prevention and the treatment of graft rejection. Cyclophosphamide is

an alkylating agent that may be used as a steroid-sparing agent. It is the most commonly prescribed drug for both necrotizing systemic scleritis and refractory necrotizing scleritis, and is often prescribed in conjunction with steroids (49,52).

Immunosuppressants may be prescribed as monotherapy, or as combination therapy with steroids and other immunosuppressants. There are no long-term, randomized, controlled clinical studies to compare the effect of monotherapy versus combination therapy in the treatment of necrotizing scleritis and vasculitis in scleral transplantation. Tamesis et al. have advocated cessation of immunosuppressants after a minimum of 1 year of clinically stable ocular inflammatory disease, to minimize the side effects (53).

The type and duration of immunosuppression after scleral transplantation are variable and depend on the underlying disease. The early introduction of immunosuppressants in the presence of a histopathologic vasculitis has been shown by Sainz de la Maza et al. to be an important prognostic factor in a scleral graft study of 12 patients (45). The mean follow-up time for this study was 11 months, and the duration of the immunosuppression varied according to the disease. Ten of the 12 patients had histologic evidence of vasculitis, and 8 of these received immunosuppression either before or immediately after grafting. Six of these eight immunosuppressed patients with vasculitis had stable grafts. The other two of these eight patients had graft necrosis. In one patient, this occurred 10 months after discontinuing a year of systemic therapy, and in the other patient this graft necrosis was due to infective keratitis and endophthalmitis. The two patients with histologic evidence of vasculitis who received no immunosuppression both had graft necrosis within 2 months of surgery. The authors demonstrated scleral graft

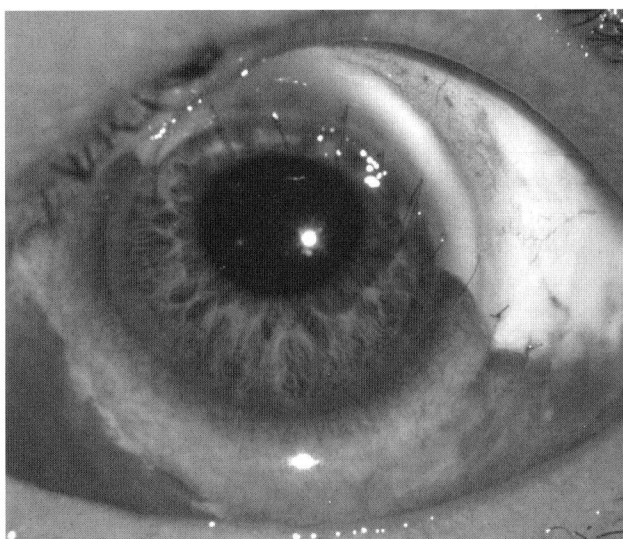

FIGURE 55-6. Same patient as in Fig. 55-5, after the hand-fashioning and suturing of the corneoscleral graft required to fill the areas of tissue damage exposed in the course of the surgery.

stability in the two patients without vasculitis who were not immunosuppressed (45,54).

ALTERNATIVES TO SCLERAL GRAFTING

There are limited reports of alternatives to scleral tissue for grafting. Preserved amniotic membrane, as well as being good for ocular surface reconstruction, has antiinflammatory, antiproteolytic, and antimicrobial activity (55–57). It has been used in uncontrolled case studies for both nonimmune sterile and nonimmune infectious scleral ulceration (58,59). Gore-Tex patch grafting for one case of necrotizing scleritis was described in a human study by Huang et al. in 1994 (60). It may be suitable for tectonic grafting because it has a high tensile strength and is resistant to degradation. However, in this report the overall result was poor. The tissue showed no fibrovascular invasion and there was little adhesion of the graft to the host tissue. Another alternative to sclera is the use of the microporous Neuro-Patch, which is made of purified polyurethane. This has been successfully used in the past for neurosurgical repair of dural defects. It has low antigenicity and is biostable. It was successfully used in a single case report to cover a dehisced and degraded scleral wound in a nonautoimmune perforation (61).

Scleral grafting with human donor sclera is a useful and effective procedure for the treatment of scleral destructive disease. In those subgroups of patients with immune-mediated disease, the adjunctive use of immunosuppression is indicated. The development of synthetic scleral tissue alternatives in the future may further improve this potentially sight-saving procedure.

REFERENCES

1. Melamed S, Ashkenazi I, et al. Donor scleral graft patching for persistent filtration bleb leak. *Ophthalmic Surg* 1991;22: 164–165.
2. Torchia RT, Dunn RE, Pease PJ. Fascia lata grafting in scleromalacia perforans with lamellar corneal-scleral dissection. *Am J Ophthalmol* 1968;66:705–709.
3. Renard G, Lelievre P, Mazel J. Scleromalacie perforante. *Bull Soc Ophthalmol Fr* 1953;66:243–251.
4. Breslin CW, Katz JI, et al. Surgical management of necrotizing scleritis: scleral reinforcement with autogenous periosteum. *Arch Ophthalmol* 1977;95:2038–2040.
5. Larsson S. Treatment of perforated corneal ulcer by autoplastic scleral transplantation. *Br J Ophthalmol* 1948;32:54.
6. Paufique L, Moreau PG. La scleromalacia perforante: aspect histologique traitement par greffe sclerale. *Ann Doculistique* 1953;186:1068–1076.
7. Curtin BJ. Surgical support of the posterior sclera: Part I. Experimental results. *Am J Ophthalmol* 1960;49:1341.
8. Thale A, Tillmann B, Rochels R. Scanning electron-microscopic studies of the collagen architecture of the human sclera: normal and pathological findings. *Ophthalmologica* 1996;210:137–141.
9. Keeley FW, Morin JD, Vesely S. Characterization of collagen from normal human sclera. *Exp Eye Res* 1984;39:533–542.
10. Rada JA, Achen VR, Perry CA, et al. Proteoglycans in the human sclera: evidence for the presence of aggrecan. *Invest Ophthalmol Vis Sci* 1997;38:1740–1751.
11. Seiffert KE. Biological aspects of collagenous homografts. *Acta Otorhinolaryngol Belg* 1970;24:27–33.
12. Iacono VJ, Gomes BC, et al. Clinical and laboratory studies on human sclera allografts. *J Periodontol* 1980;51:211–216.
13. Muldashev ER, Muslimov SA, et al. Basic research conducted on alloplant biomaterials. *Eur J Ophthalmol* 1999;9:8–13.
14. Trentham DE, Townes AS, et al. Humoral and cellular sensitivity to collagen in type II collagen-induced arthritis in rats. *J Clin Invest* 1978;61:89–96.
15. Whiteside TL, Hamada S, Manski WJ. Immunochemical analysis of tissue antigens in different corneal layers and sclera. *Exp Eye Res* 1973;16:413–420.
16. Fong LP, Sainz de la Maza M, et al. Immunopathology of scleritis. *Ophthalmology* 1991;98:472–9.
17. Rao NA, Marak GE, Hidayat AA. Necrotizing scleritis: a clinicopathologic study of 41 cases. *Ophthalmology* 1985;92:1542–1549.
18. Young RD, Powell J, Watson PG. Ultrastructural changes in scleral proteoglycans perceived destruction of the collagen fibril matrix in necrotizing scleritis. *Histopathology* 1988;12:75–84.
19. Young RD, Watson PG. Microscopical studies of necrotising scleritis: II. Collagen degradation in the scleral stroma. *Br J Ophthalmol* 1984;68:781–789.
20. Di Girolamo N, McCluskey PJ, et al. Stromelysin (matrix metalloproteinase-3) and tissue inhibitor of metalloproteinase (TIMP-1) mRNA expression in scleritis. *Ocul Immunol Inflamm* 1995;3:181–194.
21. Di Girolamo N, Lloyd A, et al. Increased expression of matrix metalloproteinases *in vivo* in scleritis tissue and *in vitro* in cultured human scleral fibroblasts *Am J Pathol* 1997;150:653–666.
22. Duke-Elder S. *System of ophthalmology*, vol 8, part II. London: CV Mosby, Henry Kimpton, 1965:995.
23. Allen RA, Straatsma BR, et al. Ocular manifestations of the Marfan syndrome. *Trans Am Acad Ophthalmol Otol* 1967;71:18–38.
24. Ruedeman AD. Osteogenesis imperfecta congenita and blue sclerotics. *Arch Ophthalmol* 1953;49:6.
25. Stein R, Lazar M, Adam A. Brittle cornea: a familial trait associated with blue sclera. *Am J Ophthalmol* 1968;66:67.
26. Curtin BJ, Teng CC. Scleral changes in pathological myopia. *Trans Am Acad Ophthalmol* 1958;62:777–790.
27. Agnoletto A. Blue sclerotics in iron deficiency. *Lancet* 1971;2:1160.
28. Pope FM. Blue sclerotics in iron deficiency. *Lancet* 1971;2:1160.
29. Hall GH. Blue sclerotics in iron deficiency. *Lancet* 1971;2:1377.
30. Duke-Elder S. *System of ophthalmology*, vol 8, part II. London: CV Mosby, Henry Kimpton, 1965:1042.
31. Sainz de la Maza M, Foster CS, et al. Necrotizing scleritis after ocular surgery: a clinicopathologic study. *Ophthalmology* 1991; 98:1720–1726.
32. Sainz de la Maza M, Foster CS et al. Ocular characteristics and disease associations in scleritis-associated peripheral keratopathy. *Arch Ophthalmol* 2002;120:15–19.
33. Sainz de la Maza M, Jabbur NS, Foster CS. Severity of scleritis and episcleritis. *Ophthalmology* 1994;101:389–396.
34. Watson PG, Hayreh SS. Scleritis and episcleritis. *Br J Ophthalmol* 1976;60:163–191.
35. Sainz de la Maza M, Foster CS, Jabbur NS. Scleritis associated with systemic vasculitic disease. *Ophthalmology* 1995;102:687–692.
36. Dailey JR, Rosenwasser GOD. Viability of bacteria in glycerin and ethanol preserved sclera. *Refract Corneal Surg* 1994;10:38–40.
37. El-Refaii A, El-Naggar AB, Sheta A. Evaluation of different methods of preservation of the sclera. *Bull Ophthalmol Soc Egypt* 1971;64:105–115.

38. Enzenauer RW, Sieck EA, et al. Residual ethanol content of donor sclera after storage in 95% ethanol and saline rinse of various durations. *Am J Ophthalmol* 1999;128:522–524.

39. Horsburgh CR, Ou CY, Jason J, et al. Duration of human immunodeficiency virus infection before detection of antibody. *Lancet* 1989;2:637.

40. Duffy P, et al. Possible person-to-person transmission of Creutzfeldt-Jakob disease. *N Engl J Med* 1974;290:692–693.

41. Uchiyama K, Ishida C, et al. An autopsy case of Creutzfeldt-Jakob disease associated with corneal transplantation. *Dementia* 1994;8:466–473.

42. Heckmann JG, Lang CJG, et al. Transmission of Creutzfeldt-Jakob disease via a corneal transplant. *J Neurol Neurosurg Psychiatry* 1997;63:388–390.

43. Rosenwasser GOD, Jones RL, Greene WH. Recovery of herpes simples virus from preserved sclera. *Invest Ophthalmol Vis Sci* 1993;34:1494.

44. Lucci LMD, Yu MCZ, Höfling-Lima AL. Decontamination of human sclera: an in vitro study. *Cornea* 1999;18:595–598.

45. Sainz de la Maza M, Tauber J, Foster CS. Scleral grafting for necrotizing scleritis. *Ophthalmology* 1989;96:306–310.

46. Felts C, Engel D, et al. Immunologic tolerance to collagen and glycosaminoglycan components of scleral allografts in humans: evidence for T cell suppression. *J Periodontol* 1981;52:603–608.

47. Sainz de la Maza M, Jabbur NS, Foster CS. An analysis of therapeutic decision for scleritis. *Ophthalmology* 1993;100:1372–1376.

48. Tuft SJ, Watson PG. Progression of scleral disease. *Ophthalmology* 1991;98:467–471.

49. Foster CS, Forstot SL, Wilson LA. Mortality rate in rheumatoid arthritis patients developing necrotizing scleritis or peripheral ulcerative keratitis: effects of systemic immunosuppression. *Ophthalmology* 1984;91:1253–1263.

50. Wallace CA. The use of methotrexate in childhood rheumatic disease. *Arthritis Rheum* 1998;41:381–391.

51. Larkin G, Lightman S. Mycophenolate mofetil: a useful immunosuppressive in inflammatory eye disease. *Ophthalmology* 1999;106:370–374.

52. Gerber DA, Bonham CA, Thomson AW. Immunosuppressive agents: recent developments in molecular action and clinical application. *Transplant Proc* 1998;30:1573–1579.

53. Tamesis RR, Rodriguez A, et al. Systemic drug toxicity trends in immunosuppressive therapy of immune and inflammatory ocular disease. *Ophthalmology* 1996;103:768–775.

54. Sainz de la Maza M, Foster CS, Tauber J. Value of scleral homografting in necrotizing scleritis management. Ocular Immunology Today: Proceedings of the 5th International Symposium on the Immunology and Immunopathology of the Eye, Tokyo, March 13–15, 1990. *Int Congress Ser* 1990;918:455–458.

55. Na BK, Hwang JH, Jim JC, et al. Analysis of human amniotic membrane components as proteinase inhibitors for development of therapeutic agent for recalcitrant keratitis. *Trophoblast Res* 1999;13:453–466.

56. Kim JS, Kim JC, Na BK, et al. Amniotic membrane patching promotes healing and inhibits proteinases activity on wound healing following acute corneal alkali burn. *Exp Eye Res* 2000;70:329–337.

57. Talmi YP, Sigler L, Inge E, et al. Antibacterial properties of human amniotic membranes. *Placenta* 1991;12:285–288.

58. Rodríguez-Ares MT, Touriño R, Capeans C, et al. Repair of scleral perforation with preserved scleral and amniotic membrane in Marfan's syndrome. *Ophthalmic Surg Laser* 1999;30:485–487.

59. Ma DHK, Wang SF, Su WY, et al. Amniotic membrane graft for the management of scleral melting and corneal perforation in recalcitrant infectious scleral and corneoscleral ulcers. *Cornea* 2002;21:275–283.

60. Huang WJ, Fung-Rong H, Chang SW. Clinicopathologic study of Gore-Tex patch graft in corneoscleral surgery. *Cornea* 1994;13:82–86.

61. Dori D, Beiran I, Carmi R, et al. Synthetic patch for scleral tissue loss. *Eur J Ophthalmol* 1997;7:105–107.

SECTION
XIV

REHABILITATIVE

OCULAR SURFACE REHABILITATION

C. STEPHEN FOSTER

Ocular surface rehabilitation efforts may be appropriate in a variety of circumstances, either with relatively limited goals, such as stabilization of the ocular surface or improved patient comfort, or with grander goals, such as improvement of vision. But failure to identify the cause of the ocular surface problem in the first place, and failure to eliminate that cause before proceeding with attempts at ocular surface rehabilitation virtually guarantees failure to achieve the desired goal. The first two, most essential elements in the quest toward ocular surface rehabilitation are (a) to identify the cause of the ocular surface pathologic process, and (b) to eliminate that cause so that it will not continue to produce the pathologic process. For example, it has been obvious to all ophthalmologists for approximately four decades that corneal transplantation, in an effort to rehabilitate the ocular surface in a patient who has had corneal scarring and neovascularization as a consequence of active ocular cicatricial pemphigoid, is the height of folly, because failure to control the underlying cause of the ocular surface disorder (active pemphigoid) ensures that the new cornea will be damaged by the same inflammatory process that damaged the patient's original cornea.

Similarly, it is critical to identify sources of ongoing damage even once the original cause of the ocular surface problem has been identified and eliminated. For example, even in that same patient with pemphigoid, once the active pemphigoid has been completely controlled with immunomodulatory therapy, damage to lid and adnexal structures from the previously active pemphigoid may result in sources of ongoing sabotage to the ocular surface, such as trichiatic lashes, profound sicca syndrome, profound meibomian gland dysfunction, entropion, lagophthalmos, keratinization of the posterior lid margin, incomplete blink, and so forth. Placing a corneal transplant into an environment possessing one or more of these saboteurs will result in damage to the ocular surface epithelium of the transplant. Therefore, all such identifiable sources of ongoing damage must be treated, or corrected, before proceeding with attempts at rehabilitation of the ocular surface. Thus, medications toxic to the ocular surface epithelium must be eliminated; dry eye must be treated with topical cyclosporine or artificial tears and with conservation methods, such as punctal occlusion and partial tarsorrhaphy; exposure and surface sensibility problems must be treated with the same strategies, with heavy emphasis on tarsorrhaphy; trichiatic lashes should be permanently destroyed through electrolysis or cryopexy; keratinization of the posterior lid margin should be treated with amniotic membrane or with mucous membrane grafting; and meibomian gland dysfunction should be treated with warm compresses with lid massage twice daily and systemic doxycycline.

Once these steps have been accomplished—that is, the cause of the ocular surface problem has been identified and eliminated and any sources of ongoing damage have been identified and eliminated—then one can embark on the effort at rehabilitation of the ocular surface through limbal stem cell grafting or simple amniotic membrane strategies, through lamellar or penetrating keratoplasty, and the like.

57

EYE PLASTICS CONSIDERATIONS FOR THE ANTERIOR SEGMENT SURGEON: INDICATIONS AND TECHNIQUES

C. ROBERT BERNARDINO AND PETER A. D. RUBIN

EXPOSURE KERATOCONJUNCTIVITIS

Exposure keratoconjunctivitis is one of the most common anterior segment problems related to eyelid dysfunction. Common signs include conjunctival injection and chemosis in the interpalpebral zone, superficial punctate keratopathy, and, in advanced cases, corneal ulceration. Eyelid malposition, eyelid retraction or ectropion, and poor eyelid closure lead to lagophthalmos and subsequent ocular surface exposure. Involutional changes can lead to lateral canthal instability and ectropion (1). Eyelid retraction may occur secondary to cicatricial changes (Fig. 57-1), solar dermal changes, chronic inflammation from infections or ocular medications, or malignancies. And, of course, poor eyelid closure from facial nerve palsy can also cause lagophthalmos (2) (Fig. 57-2). Proptosis from an orbital mass or thyroid eye disease can also cause relative eyelid retraction and secondary exposure (Fig. 57-3). Conjunctival chemosis can cause persistent lagophthalmos and exposure keratopathy (Fig. 57-4A). Of note, the chemosis often does not resolve (Fig. 57-4B) until the exposure is eliminated.

Correcting the eyelid malposition leads to resolution of the anterior segment pathologic process in most cases of exposure keratoconjunctivitis. Eyelid retraction often resolves when the inflammation abates. Repair of ectropion with lateral canthal surgery improves exposure symptoms. Gold weight placement can address paralytic eyelid issues (2). Reduction of proptosis with decompression surgery or removal of intraorbital masses reduces the relative eyelid retraction.

Office-based procedures can temporarily treat exposure. Besides aggressive ocular lubrication, temporary tarsorrhaphies with glue (3) or sutures (4) are helpful, and botulinum toxin A has also been used to induce ptosis for exposure keratopathy (5).

Cyanoacrylate glue (medical grade) is used to create a temporary adhesion between either the eyelashes or the eyelid margins for a glue tarsorrhaphy. The eyelids are held together and the glue is carefully applied to the anterior lamellar surface only (Fig. 57-5). Care is taken not to allow the glue to seep posteriorly. If a lateral glue tarsorrhaphy is performed, the handle of a smooth instrument can be slid behind the eyelid as a backstop to protect the ocular surface. The eyelids should be held together for about 30 seconds to allow the glue to set. This type of tarsorrhaphy lasts approximately 4 weeks. If the tarsorrhaphy needs to be opened sooner, warm compresses help release the tarsorrhaphy, or the eyelashes can be cut if the lashes have been exploited for the gluing.

Suture tarsorrhaphy is a more definitive procedure than glue tarsorrhaphy. This can be accomplished in the cooperative patient under local anesthesia. This form of eyelid closure can be placed in a slipknot fashion, so as to allow opening of the eyelids for examination of the underlying globe (6). The main complication of this technique is premature release of the suture, usually from the suture cheese-wiring through the eyelid; this is most likely due to improper placement of the sutures through the tarsus. Bolsters also help distribute the tension of the sutures evenly across the eyelid surface.

To perform this procedure, local anesthetic is first administered in both eyelids, with care taken to anesthetize the eyelid margin. Permanent, nonbraided sutures (e.g., nylon) are preferable, single or double armed; double-armed sutures allow the surgeon to pass all the sutures in the same direction. We prefer sutures that are supplied in a foam container, so that bolsters can be fashioned from the packing material.

Both arms of a double-armed 5-0 nylon suture are first passed through a foam bolster, approximately 5 mm in width by 3 mm in height. One arm of the suture is then passed through the skin of the lower eyelid 5 mm below the eyelid margin. The tarsus is engaged and the suture is advanced until it exits through a meibomian gland orifice; this ensures that a proper bite of tarsus was taken. The upper eyelid is then engaged at the opposite meibomian gland orifice and the suture advanced until it exits the skin of the upper eyelid. The suture is then placed through a

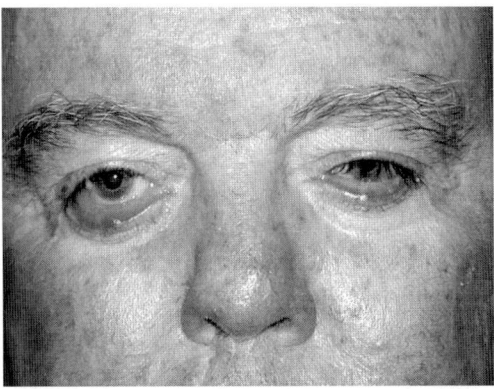

FIGURE 57-1. Bilateral cicatricial ectropion in a patient with marked actinic changes of the skin.

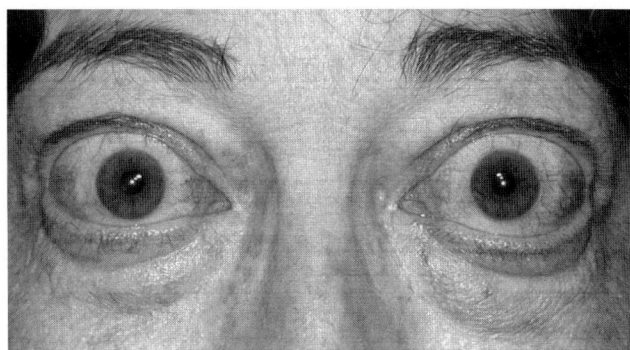

FIGURE 57-3. A patient with marked proptosis and eyelid retraction secondary to thyroid-related ophthalmopathy.

second foam bolster. The other arm of the suture is passed in a similar fashion.

The choice of location of the suture tarsorrhaphy is based on the clinical situation. A patient may need minimal closure assistance of the eyelids, in which case a laterally placed tarsorrhaphy is appropriate. However, in patients with extremely poor closure, central tarsorrhaphies are appropriate. In patients with massive proptosis or chemosis, multiple tarsorrhaphies across the eyelid reduce the tension across any individual suture. In cases of massive chemosis, the edematous conjunctiva may be deposited behind the eyelid with the handle of an instrument during placement of the tarsorrhaphy. Once the chemosis resolves, the tarsorrhaphy is often not needed.

A more permanent solution is needed for eyelid closure in some cases. Intermarginal adhesions must then be surgically created to ensure that a permanent adhesion will last. Most failures of this procedure occur because of the improper creation of these adhesions (7); skin closure is not sufficient for retention of a permanent tarsorrhaphy, and adhesion between the two tarsal plates, orbicularis, and skin is needed to ensure a lasting closure.

Local anesthetic is infiltrated into the eyelids, including the eyelid margins. Eyelid margin epithelium in the area of the tarsorrhaphy is excised; this bares underlying tarsus.

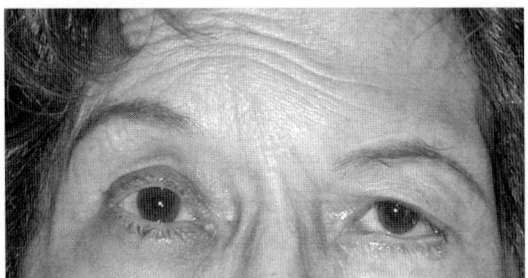

FIGURE 57-2. A left facial nerve palsy causes orbicularis weakness and secondary lower eyelid retraction. Note the lack of forehead wrinkles and brow ptosis on the left secondary to the paralysis.

The skin and pretarsal orbicularis are undermined to create a skin/muscle flap (Fig. 57-6A). It may be advisable to excise the lashes during this dissection. The skin/muscle flap is further divided into an orbicularis layer and the superficial eyelid skin layer. A similar procedure is performed on the opposite eyelid.

Layered closure is performed to form the permanent tarsorrhaphy. Tarsus is approximated to the opposite tarsus with 5-0 polyglactin suture in a partial-thickness fashion (Fig. 57-6B); full-thickness sutures can rub on the underlying ocular surface and so should obviously be avoided. The orbicularis is then closed in a second layer, and finally the skin is closed. This three-layered closure ensures that the tarsorrhaphy will not open.

KERATOPATHY SECONDARY TO EYELID MALPOSITION

Lower eyelid malpositions (ectropion and entropion) can cause keratopathy. Keratopathy is typically secondary to exposure keratopathy as well as decreased lacrimal pump function (Fig. 57-7) in patients with ectropion, and to direct contact of the eyelashes and the keratinized eyelid skin with the ocular surface (Fig. 57-8) in entropion.

Most lower eyelid malpositions are caused by involutional changes based around the lateral canthal tendon. Depending on the forces generated by the orbicularis and the eyelid retractors, an eyelid with a lax lateral canthal tendon will either turn in or out (8). Therefore, the definitive repair of these malpositions is based around the lateral canthal tendon: the lateral tarsal strip procedure.

However, before repair of the lateral canthal tendon, it is often desirable to perform a temporizing procedure. Most cases of ectropion are temporized with aggressive lubrication. However, if severe lagophthalmos is present, a suture tarsorrhaphy is appropriate. A Quickert suture can redirect the eyelid until permanent repair is performed in patients with entropion (9). This technique is quite useful, particularly in

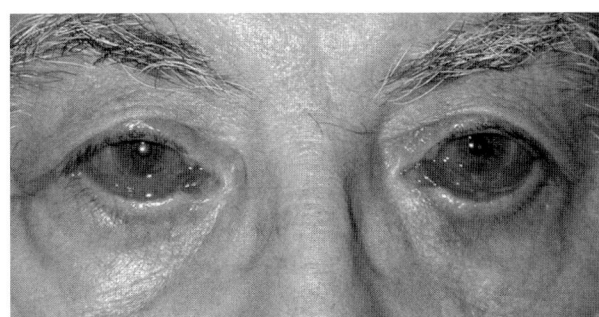
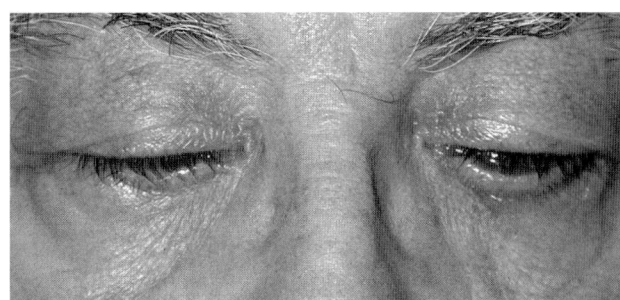

FIGURE 57-4. A, Marked chemosis secondary to an allergic reaction to topical antibiotics. **B,** Chemosis induces lagophthalmos, which can cause worsening exposure and chemosis.

spastic entropion; the Quickert procedure allows the inflammation associated with the entropion to resolve and may allow the entropion to resolve without further intervention.

To perform a Quickert suture, a double-armed, monofilament suture is essential; use of a single-armed suture necessitates the passing of the needle toward the globe, risking perforation. Like the suture tarsorrhaphy, we also prefer suture contained in a foam insert so the foam can be used to create a bolster to pass the suture through. Anesthesia is infiltrated into the lower eyelid, including the margin and fornix. The suture (5-0 nylon, double armed) is passed from the conjunctival fornix and directed anterior to tarsus to exit 3 mm inferior to the eyelid margin (Fig. 57-9A). The suture is passed through the bolster. The other arm of the suture is placed in a similar fashion. When the sutures are pulled taut, the eyelid should be slightly everted (Fig. 57-9B).

A lateral tarsal strip is performed to address permanently the lower eyelid malposition (10). In essence, the lower eyelid is shortened horizontally and sutured to Whitnall's tubercle. A suture with a tight-curving needle (P-2) must be used to fasten the lower eyelid to the inner aspect of the lateral orbital rim.

Local anesthetic is infiltrated into the lateral aspect of the lower and upper eyelid. The needle of the anesthetic is

then directed toward the inner aspect of the lateral orbital rim; the bone is engaged and the needle is retracted slightly to anesthetize this region. A lateral canthotomy and cantholysis is then performed. A #15 Bard Parker blade is used to make a 1-cm horizontal incision lateral to the lateral commisure; for cosmesis, the incision should be placed in a preexisting rhytid. Westcott scissors are used to incise the lateral commisure and dissection is continued to the lateral orbital rim periosteum. The cut edge of the lower eyelid is elevated with toothed forceps, and the inferior crus of the lateral canthal tendon is palpated and incised with the scissors.

The eyelid is distracted laterally to measure the amount of shortening desired; typically the eyelid is shortened between 5 and 10 mm. This determined length will be the length of the tarsal strip created. Overshortening will cause the puncta to be overly lateralized. The scissors are used to undermine the skin and orbicularis along the lateral aspect of the eyelid. An incision is made just posterior to the lash line for the length of the strip. Lid margin epithelium is excised with scissors. The conjunctiva and lower eyelid retractors are also incised at the inferior border of tarsus (Fig. 57-10A). Finally, the posterior aspect of this strip is scraped with the scalpel to remove conjunctival epithelium.

We use 5-0 polyglactin suture on a small, tightly curved needle (e.g., Ethicon P-2) for this procedure. A small tissue rake is used to expose the lateral orbital rim periosteum. A malleable retractor or the handle of a pair of forceps to used to push the globe medially. The suture is then passed in a lateral-to-medial fashion along the inner aspect of the lateral orbital rim; the periosteum is engaged at the region of Whitnall's tubercle. The suture is then passed in an anterior-to-posterior fashion through the tarsal tab at the medial border of the strip, along its inferior margin. The suture is then passed in a posterior-to-anterior fashion along the strip's superior margin. This allows the tarsal strip to lie flat along the lateral orbital rim. Excess tarsus is excised, with care taken not to cut the sutures. The suture is directed superiorly to the first suture of the lateral orbital rim periosteum, in a medial-to-lateral fashion

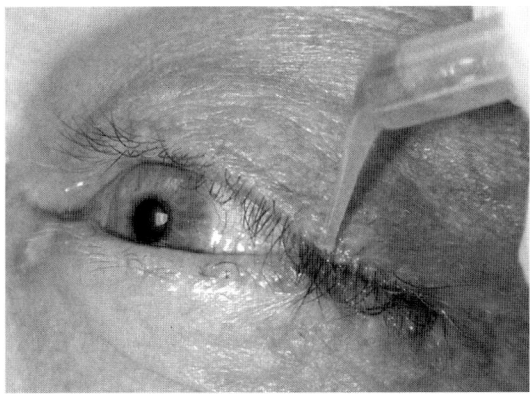

FIGURE 57-5. Cyanoacrylate glue is applied to the lateral eyelid margin to form a temporary tarsorrhaphy.

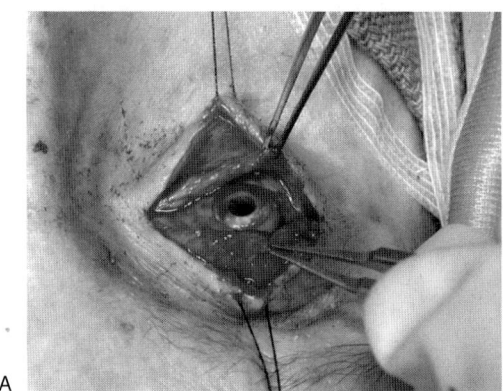
A

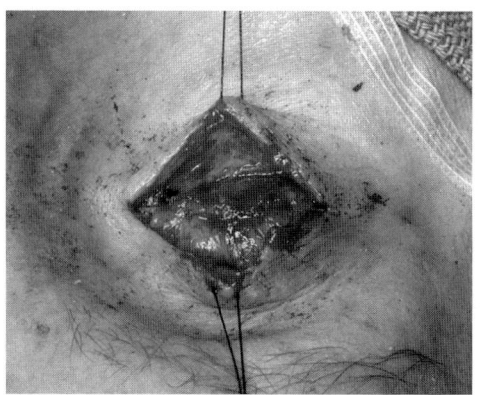
B

FIGURE 57-6. A: The tarsus and orbicularis/skin flap are separated in preparation for a complete permanent tarsorrhaphy in this patient with a keratoprosthesis. **B:** The tarsus is closed in a single layer with 5-0 polyglactin suture. The orbicularis and skin will also be closed in two additional layers.

(Fig. 57-10B). Pulling both ends of the suture approximates the final result of the tarsal strip procedure.

The lateral edge of the upper lid epithelium is excised with scissors to allow reformation of the commisure. The commisure is reformed with 5-0 polyglactin suture placed at the edge of both upper and lower eyelid tarsus in a horizontal mattress fashion (Fig. 57-10C). The sutures of the tarsal strip are pulled taut and secured. Excess lower eyelid skin is excised with a #15 Bard Parker blade. Orbicularis is closed in a separate layer if permanent sutures are used for the tarsal strip; if an absorbable deep suture is used, the skin can be approximated primarily.

If this procedure fails, it usually fails for one of two reasons: either the tarsal strip fixation was not placed along the inner aspect of the lateral orbital rim periosteum, or these sutures were not placed high enough along the lateral orbital rim. In the first case, the lid does not rest against the eyelid, and this decreases the efficiency of the blink and lacrimal pump. In the second example, the sutures are placed too low along the lateral orbital rim, giving the eyelid an antiMongoloid slant, which also decreases the eyelid closure efficiency. The goal of surgery should be overcorrection in lateral eyelid height (Fig. 57-10D); this contour relaxes to a normal position during the postoperative period (Fig. 57-10E).

KERATOPATHY SECONDARY TO EYELASH MALPOSITION

Misdirected eyelashes independent of eyelid malposition can cause significant ocular surface problems (11). Epiblepharon, in which skin and orbicularis override the eyelid margin, can push the eyelashes against the cornea, causing epithelial defects; this is more common in Asian children who have a poorly developed lower eyelid crease (12). The eyelid crease is formed by projections from the lower eyelid. Distichiasis is the abnormal growth of lashes from the meibomian gland orifices; this can be congenital or acquired, of which the latter variety is associated with inflammation. Trichiasis is the abnormal growth of eyelashes that are misdirected toward the globe, also associated with inflammation or trauma (Fig. 57-11).

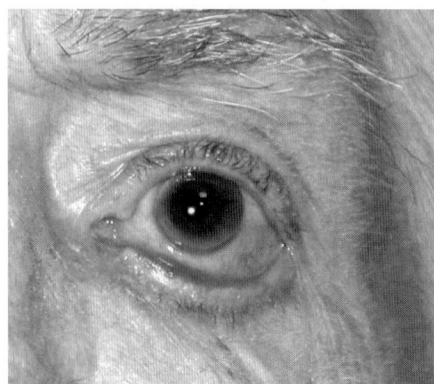

FIGURE 57-7. Involutional ectropion secondary to lateral canthal dystopia.

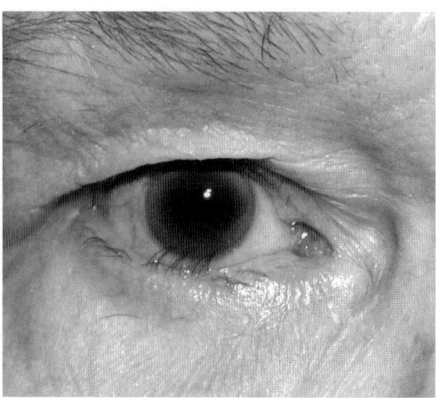

FIGURE 57-8. Involution entropion secondary to lateral canthal laxity and lower eyelid retractor instability.

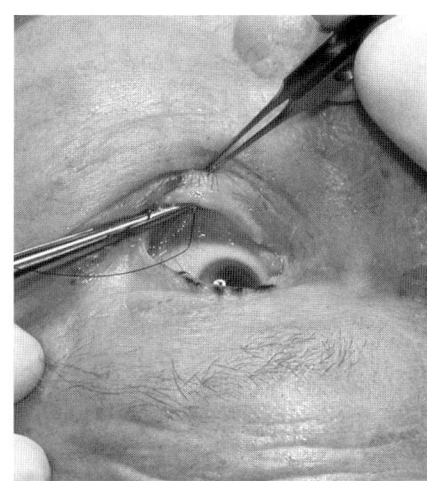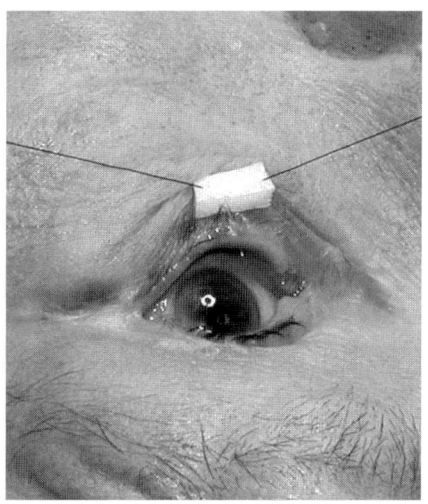

FIGURE 57-9. A: A 5-0 nylon suture is passed through the fornix and externalized along the anterior surface of tarsus below the eyelid margin in the Quickert suture technique. **B:** Both arms of the 5-0 nylon suture are placed through a foam bolster. Tightening of the suture causes out-turning of the eyelid.

Keratopathy secondary to epiblepharon is treated by excising the overriding orbicularis and skin and reforming a lower eyelid crease. A subciliary incision is made at the location where the final eyelid crease will lie (2 to 4 mm below the eyelid margin). The surgeon should err on placing this incision closer to rather than further away from the eyelid margin; although an eyelid crease further from the eyelid margin may increase the success of outward rotation of the eyelashes, the more prominently formed crease would be incongruous with the overall Asian aesthetic ideal, particularly if the upper eyelid lacked an eyelid crease. At first, a skin flap is raised down to the level of the inferior tarsal border (4 to 5 mm below the lower eyelid margin), preserving the pretarsal orbicularis. A small strip of the superior preseptal orbicularis is excised. In selected cases, the lower eyelid retractors are identified and sutured to the inferior tarsal border. A small crescent of lower eyelid skin (maximal height approximately 2 mm) is marked and excised. Care is taken not to excise too much of the anterior lamellae; this can induce postoperative ectropion or eyelid retraction. The lower eyelid crease is formed by the suture closure in which the skin suture is passed from upper skin edge to the underlying capsulopalpebral fascia, followed by the lower skin edge. The success of this procedure depends most on the fixation to the deeper structures with wound closure, not the excision of skin and muscle. In fact, many mild cases of epiblepharon are typically managed with a nonexcisional, full-thickness mattress suture (13). Thus, the goal of intervention is to form an adhesion between the skin and the capsulopalpebral fascia, analogous to the fibers that form the lower eyelid crease in the white eyelid. The end point of surgery is outward rotation of the eyelashes away from the globe (Fig. 57-12).

Eyelashes must be removed for treating trichiasis or distichiasis. Manual epilation with forceps is a simple procedure to remove a lash, but this, of course, is not a permanent solution. A permanent solution requires ablating the hair follicle at the time of epilation with electrocautery, cryotherapy (14), or laser ablation (15). An alternative to hair follicle ablation is complete extirpation through surgery.

With electroepilation, the patient is grounded and a monopolar electrode is inserted into each individual hair shaft (Fig. 57-13). The cautery, at the lowest effective setting, is applied until a small bubble is seen at the surface of the follicle; the electrode is then retracted. This procedure is performed under local anesthesia. At completion, the lash should easily slip out of the pore; a bulb from the follicle is often seen at the end of the hair shaft.

Multiple hair follicles are treated with each application of cryoepilation (14). After local anesthetic is instilled into the eyelid and margin, the eyelid should be lightly lubricated with surgical jelly; this helps the probe couple to the treatment area. The probe is applied at the base of the hair shafts, just adjacent to the eyelid margin. The probe is applied for 30 to 45 seconds, during which time an ice ball should adhere the probe to the eyelid skin. The ice ball is allowed to thaw slowly, and then a second freezing is performed. Although cryotherapy is effective at treating a large area of lash follicles, it can be associated with prolonged eyelid pain and edema, eyelid notching, and depigmentation.

Focal trichiasis associated with eyelid notching from previous trauma is amenable to full-thickness resection of the eyelid margin; this procedure can remove the eyelashes, along with restoring eyelid contour. Direct surgical

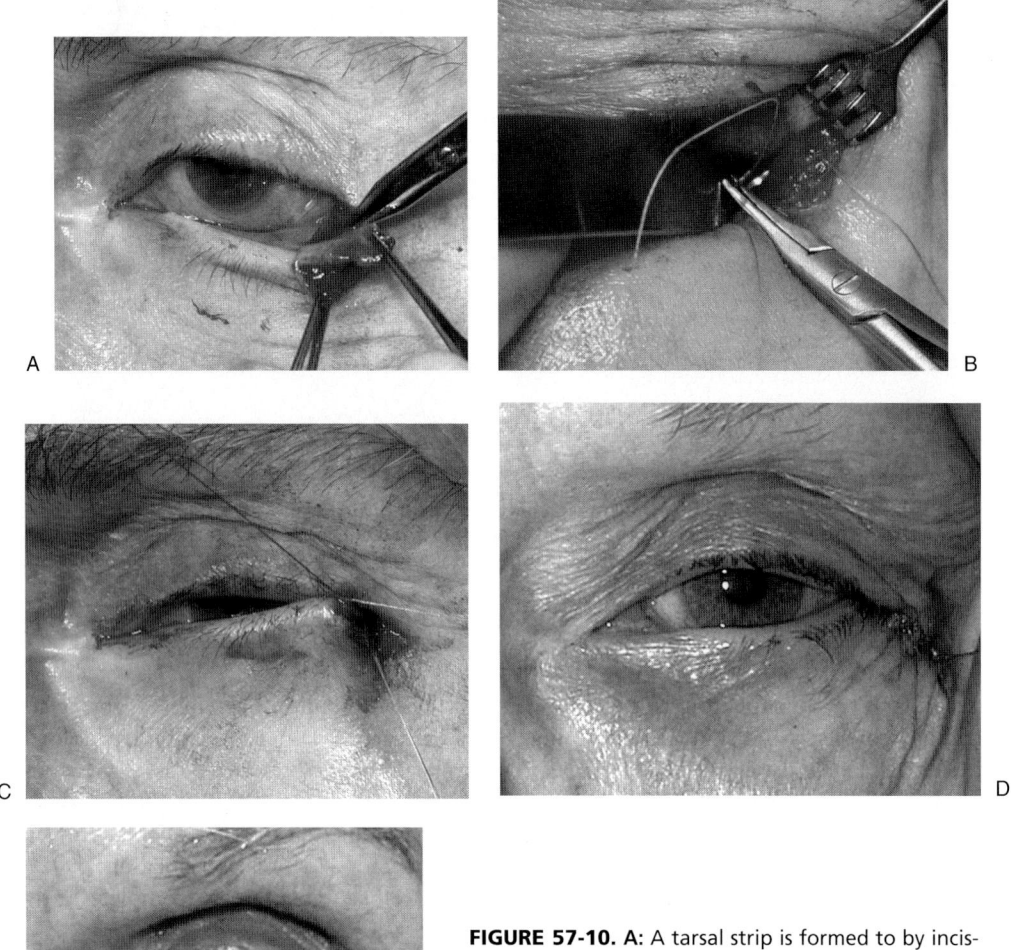

FIGURE 57-10. A: A tarsal strip is formed to by incising lower eyelid retractors, conjunctiva, and eyelid margin epithelium. **B:** Tarsal fixation suture is passed into the periosteum along the inner aspect of the lateral orbital rim periosteum. **C:** The lateral commissure is reformed with a horizontal mattress suture through the cut edges of tarsus. **D:** Immediate postoperative result of lateral tarsal strip. Note the overcorrected appearance of the lateral canthal height. **E:** Three months after lateral tarsal strip procedure. Note the natural appearance of the lateral canthal height.

excision of follicles can be performed under microscopic guidance for follicles resistant to electroepilation or cryotherapy.

KERATOPATHY SECONDARY TO CONJUNCTIVAL DYSFUNCTION

Conjunctival scarring can cause significant eyelid malposition and secondary keratopathy. Furthermore, this posterior lamellar disease is often progressive, making effective management very difficult. In addition, posterior lamellar surgery can even reactivate quiescent disease or make active disease much worse (e.g., in Stevens-Johnson syndrome and in ocular cicatricial pemphigoid).

Debridement of Keratin

The eyelid margin can become keratinized from squamous metaplasia in mild cases of cicatrizing disease. This roughed surface can cause significant discomfort and corneal epitheliopathy independent of trichiasis (15). Areas of keratinization can be debrided or excised, or overgrafted with amniotic membrane or mucous membrane grafts.

Anterior Lamellar Recession (Eyelid Margin Rotation)

Recession of the anterior lamella causes outward rotation of the eyelid margin and eyelashes (16) in mild to moderate cases of cicatricial entropion. This involves

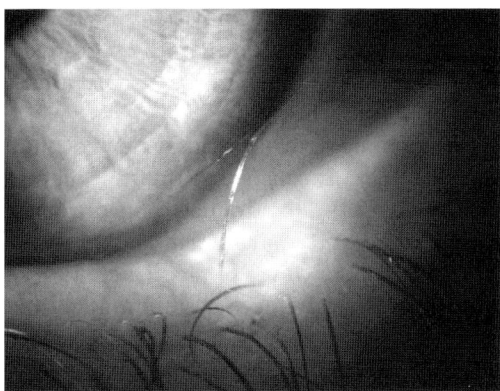

FIGURE 57-11. Misdirected lashes in a patient with trichiasis.

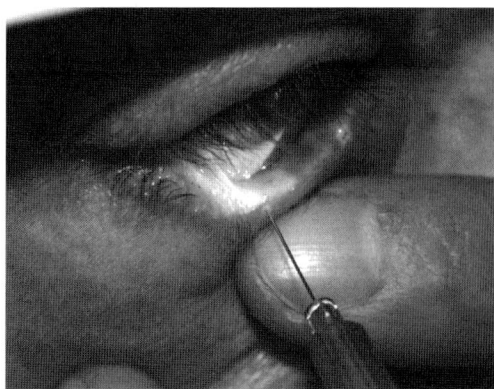

FIGURE 57-13. Monopolar electrode is inserted into the hair follicle of a patient with ocular cicatricial pemphigoid and trichiasis.

separating the anterior lamella (skin and orbicularis) from underlying tarsus and levator through a lid crease incision. The dissection is carried along the anterior surface of tarsus. Everting sutures (6-0 silk, double armed) are placed, partial thickness, through the upper edge of tarsus in a horizontal fashion and then externalized inferiorly through the skin. These sutures should initially induce overcorrection, and may be left in place for up to 6 weeks. For extra margin eversion, a horizontal tarsotomy should be performed to allow free rotation of the margin. Care is taken not to violate the posterior lamella in either instance. These procedures may not be as successful on the lower eyelid because of the shorter height of the lower tarsus.

Posterior Lamellar Surgery with Grafting

In cases of severe entropion, in which marked posterior lamellar scarring and foreshortening exist, the scar must be

released and the posterior lamella lengthened. Because surgery is to be performed on the posterior lamella, care must be taken to ensure that inflammation is maximally suppressed.

It is important to attempt to excise any scar bands causing the eyelid malposition during surgery on the posterior lamella. Tarsal release to allow maximal rotation through full-thickness tarsotomies may also be necessary. Whether amniotic membrane (17) or mucous membrane is used, use of an oversized graft is critical because of inevitable postoperative graft shrinkage. We prefer mucous membrane because it is thicker than amnion, and so may resist contraction better. The eyelid should be immobilized in the immediate postoperative period, either with Frost sutures or with suture tarsorrhaphies, to ensure graft integration.

KERATOPATHY SECONDARY TO TEAR FILM DYSFUNCTION

Although there are many promising therapies for tear film deficiency, including various lubricating formulations, nutritional supplementation, and immunomodulary therapy, the mainstay of therapy is increasing ocular lubrication, both with external placement of tears and ointments and with the occlusion of the puncta (18).

Punctal Occlusion

The goal of punctual occlusion is to limit tear escape through the nasolacrimal duct system (19). Theoretically, occlusion can be performed anywhere along this drainage system: the two puncta, the canaliculi, common canaliculi, and even the lacrimal sac and nasolacrimal duct. The puncta and canaliculi are the common locations chosen for occlusion. Occlusive devices are designed specifically both for the location of deployment and the duration of the

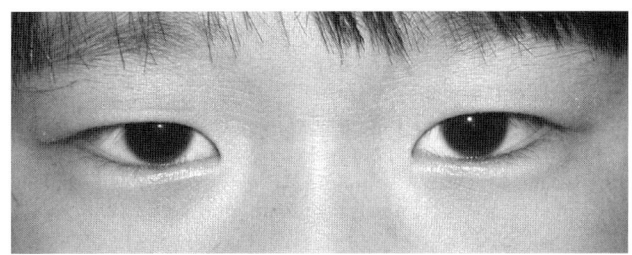

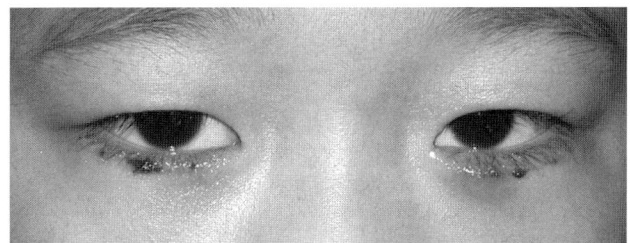

FIGURE 57-12. A: A young Chinese girl with ocular irritation secondary to epiblepharon. **B:** One week after epiblepharon repair. Note the outward turning of the eyelashes.

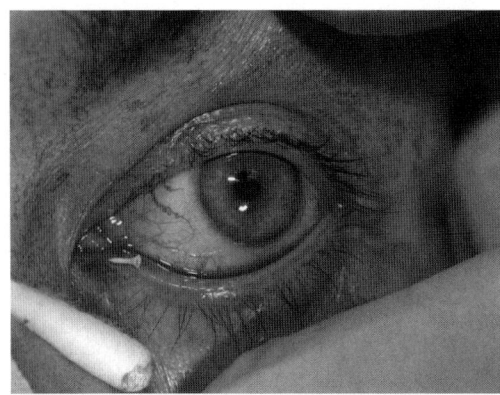

FIGURE 57-14. This Herrick intracanalicular plug was removed after causing chronic conjunctivitis.

occlusion; occlusion can be temporary, semipermanent/reversible, and permanent/nonreversible.

Temporary occlusion is typically used for diagnostic measures to determine whether a patient will benefit from and tolerate lacrimal drainage occlusion. Temporary plugs are dissolvable and are usually made of hydroxypropyl cellulose, gelatin, collagen, or catgut. These are inserted into the puncta and lodged at the level of the vertical canaliculus; they last for approximately 1 week. Because they rest at the level of the vertical canaliculus, there is little risk for extrusion or foreign-body sensation.

If a patient finds benefit with temporary occlusion, a form of semipermanent/reversible plugs or permanent procedure may be chosen. There are two classes of permanent plugs; one is designed specifically to be deployed into the puncta and the other into the canaliculus. The punctual plugs have the advantage of being readily reversible because they sit at the entrance of the puncta they can be grasped and removed with forceps. The main disadvantage is that because they sit flush against the puncta, they can rub on the ocular surface and cause discomfort (20). Rarely, they can also fall out or migrate into the canaliculus.

Canalicular plugs are designed to be inserted into the puncta and deployed into the horizontal canaliculus. The advantage of these is that they rest inside the eyelid, away from the ocular surface. Theoretically, they are reversible by forcible irrigation through the canalicular system into the lacrimal sac. However, their use has been associated with chronic conjunctivitis (Fig. 57-14), canaliculitis, and dacryocystitis (21). Therefore, the use of these products should probably be avoided.

The puncta can also be closed on a more permanent basis. A simple method involves cauterizing the puncta under local anesthesia. A low-temperature cautery is used; high-temperature cautery will burn through the puncta and eyelid. The cautery tip is inserted down to the vertical portion of the canaliculus (2 mm), and then cautery is applied while the tip is retracted from the puncta. This ensures that the entire length of the puncta and vertical canaliculus is burned; the inflammation from healing scars the canaliculus closed. A cutdown onto the scarred puncta could be performed and the scar tissue excised if this procedure must to be reversed.

Other methods of permanent closure include suturing of the puncta (22) and canaliculus or full-thickness excision of the canaliculus (23). The advantage of permanent closure is there is no risk of infection, foreign-body reaction of the tear drainage system, or ocular surface irritation.

A protocol for tear drainage occlusion might include a trial of occlusion with either an absorbable or a silicone punctal plug (24). If a cellulose plug were used and the effect desirable, a silicone plug can be tried next. If the patient liked the effect of occlusion but had plug intolerance, permanent closure could be offered.

CONCLUSION

Many ocular surface problems can be attributed to eyelid pathologic processes. With an understanding of the intimate relationship between the eyelids and the conjunctiva and cornea, many eye plastics problems can be diagnosed and managed by the anterior segment specialist.

REFERENCES

1. Nichols KK, Zadnik K. The repeatability of diagnostic test and surveys in dry eye. *Adv Exp Med Biol* 2002;506:1171–1175.
2. Faraj HG, Hoang-Xuan T. Chronic cicatrizing conjunctivitis. *Curr Opin Ophthalmol* 2001;12:L250–L257.
3. Balent A. An accidental tarsorrhaphy caused by acrylic adhesive. *Am J Ophthalmol* 1976;82:501.
4. Westfall CT, Shore JW, Netland PA. Bolster material for suture tarsorrhaphy. *Ophthalmology* 1990;97:1579–1580.
5. Kirkness CM, Adam GW, Dilly PN, et al. Botulinum toxin A–induced protective ptosis in corneal disease. *Ophthalmology* 1988;95:473–480.
6. Rapoza PA, Harrison DA, Bussa JJ, et al. Temporary sutured tube-tarsorrhaphy: reversible eyelid closure technique. *Ophthalmic Surg* 1993;24:328–330.
7. Cosar CB, Cohen EJ, Rapuano CJ, et al. Tarsorrhaphy: clinical experience from a cornea practice. *Cornea* 2002;20:787–791.
8. Bashour M, Harvey J. Causes of involutional ectropion and entropion: age-related tarsal changes are key. *Ophthal Plast Reconstr Surg* 2000;16:131–141.
9. Quickert MH, Rathbun E. Suture repair of entropion. *Arch Ophthalmol* 1971;85:304–305.
10. Anderson RL, Gordy DD. The tarsal strip procedure. *Arch Ophthalmol* 1979;97:2192–2196.
11. Choo PH. Distichiasis, trichiasis, and entropion: advances in management. *Int Ophthalmol Clin* 2002;42:75–87.
12. Jeong S, Park H, Park YG. Surgical correction of congenital epiblepharon: low eyelid crease reforming technique. *J Pediatr Ophthalmol Strabismus* 2001;38:356–358.
13. Quickert MH, Wilkes TD, Dryden RM. Nonincisional correction of epiblepharon and congenital entropion. *Arch Ophthalmol* 1983;101:778–781.

14. Sullivan JH. The use of cryotherapy for trichiasis. *Trans Am Acad Ophthalmol Otolaryngol* 1977;83:708–712.

15. Maumenee AE. Keratinization of the conjunctiva. *Trans Am Ophthalmic Soc* 1979;77:133.

16. Kemp EG, Collins JRO. Surgical management of upper eyelid entropion. *Br J Ophthalmol* 1986;70:575–579.

17. Ti SE, Tow SL, Chee SP. Amniotic membrane transplantation in entropion surgery. Ophthalmology 2001;108:1209–1217.

18. Foulks GN. The evolving treatment of dry eye. *Ophthalmol Clin North Am* 2003;16:29–35.

19. Murube J, Murube E. Treatment of dry eye by blocking the lacrimal canaliculi. *Surv Ophthalmol* 1996;40:463–480.

20. Tai MC, Cosar CB, Cohen EJ, et al. The clinical efficacy of silicone punctal plug therapy. *Cornea* 2002;21:135–139.

21. White WL, Bartley GB, Hawes MJ, et al. Iatrogenic complications related to the use of Herrick lacrimal plugs. *Ophthalmology* 2001;108:1835–1837.

22. Liu D, Sadhan Y. Surgical punctal occlusion: a prospective study. *Br J Ophthalmol* 2002;86:1031–1034.

23. Putterman AM. Canaliculectomy in the treatment of keratitis sicca. *Ophthalmic Surg* 1991;22:478–480.

24. Glatt HJ. Failure of collagen plugs to predict epiphora after permanent punctal occlusion. *Ophthalmic Surg* 1992;23:292–293.

AMNIOTIC MEMBRANE TRANSPLANTATION

ERIK LETKO AND C. STEPHEN FOSTER

Amniotic membrane transplantation (AMT) is indicated for numerous ocular surface disorders, the spectrum of which has been expanding recently (Table 58-1). The first written report on the use of amniotic membrane graft (AMG) in clinical medicine was made after Davis used both chorion and amnion in skin transplantation cases in 1910 (1). Since then, living (rather than preserved) amniotic membrane has been used for various purposes (2). The first report on the use of amniotic membrane for ocular disorders was by DeRoth in 1940; he used both amnion and chorion in the treatment of conjunctival defects (3). After a half century of lack of written reports on amnion use for ocular surface disorders, Battle and Perdomo introduced, in 1993, the idea of amniotic membrane transplantation to North America (4). Two years later, Kim and Tseng published their observations that preserved amniotic membrane facilitated corneal surface healing in rabbits after epithelial removal and limbal lamellar keratectomy (5). Since then, the use of amniotic membrane has been explored in a growing number of ocular surface disorders.

BASIC SCIENCE

Human amnion is the innermost layer of the placenta. It is composed of five layers that can be distinguished histologically (6). These include a single epithelial layer, a basement membrane, and an avascular connective tissue that is composed of three layers: the compact layer attached to the basement membrane, the fibroblast layer, and the spongy layer (6). The thickness of human amnion is approximately 0.02 to 0.50 mm (6). The epithelium consists of one layer of cells, the shape of which varies between cuboidal in the amnion reflectum, to columnar over the placental surface, and squamous over the cord amnion (7). The basement membrane consists of reticular fibers with processes to the basal region of the epithelial cells (6). The compact layer is thought to be the strongest layer, with significant tensile strength (6). The fibroblast layer is the thickest layer of the amnion and contains a loose fibroblast network and reticulum (6).

The spongy layer is the outermost layer of the amnion. It contains wavy bundles of reticulin and scattered fibroblasts (6).

The mechanisms by which amniotic membrane promotes healing of the ocular surface are not fully understood. The previously proposed mechanism of action through oxygen permeability, epithelial hydration, and mechanical protection (8) may be too simplistic because soft contact lenses have these characteristics, too (9), yet there are numerous reports on cases where AMT resulted in epithelialization of epithelial defects after bandage soft contact lens therapy failed. There is growing evidence that biologic factors, including collagens and cytokines, may make a major difference between a soft contact lens and amniotic membrane. The amniotic membrane is believed to provide a superior substrate for migration of epithelial cells (10), reinforce adhesion of basal epithelial cells (11,12), promote epithelial differentiation (13–16), prevent apoptosis of epithelial cells (17,18), and reduce neovascularization and fibrosis by reduction of inflammatory cell infiltration (19–21).

Both collagens IV and VII, components of corneal and conjunctival epithelial basement membrane, are present in the basement membrane of amniotic membrane (22). In addition, amniotic membrane contains collagen III (another collagen component of conjunctival epithelial basement membrane), collagens I, II, and V, fibronectin, and laminin (22–25). The composition of amniotic basement membrane may be closer to conjunctival than to corneal basement membrane based on the presence of type IV collagen and laminin subchains (22).

The presence of cytokines expressed in the amniotic membrane has been investigated recently. The experiments show that cytokines that promote epithelialization and reduce inflammation, scarring, and neovascularization are present in preserved (26) as well as epithelium-denuded amniotic membrane (27). These cytokines are found in both the epithelium and stroma of the amniotic membrane, but are believed to be synthesized predominantly by the epithelium (28). The cytokines are present in cryopreserved amniotic membrane (26) and, surprisingly, approximately 50% of the epithelial cells of amniotic membrane

TABLE 58-1. EXAMPLES OF CLINICAL APPLICATION OF AMNIOTIC MEMBRANE GRAFTING

Surgical Technique	Indication	Underlying Diagnosis
Corneal epithelial defect type (with or without stromal ulcer)	Descemetocele Excision of epithelial/stromal lesion Partial limbal stem cell deficiency Perforation (corneal or scleral) Persistent epithelial defect Removal of the epithelium	Aniridia Atopic keratoconjunctivitis Band keratopathy Bullous keratopathy Chemical burn Contact lens–induced keratopathy Dellen Diabetes mellitus Exposure keratopathy Graft-versus-host disease Keratoconjunctivitis sicca Melanosis Mooren's ulcer Neoplasia Neurotrophic ulcer Postinfectious Radiation keratopathy Recurrent erosion syndrome Rheumatoid arthritis Sjögren's syndrome Stevens-Johnson syndrome Thermal burn Thyroid ophthalmopathy Toxic epidermal necrolysis Vernal keratoconjunctivitis
Fornix reconstruction type	Ankyloblepharon Symblepharon	Atopic keratoconjunctivitis Chemical burn Ocular cicatricial pemphigoid Stevens-Johnson syndrome Strabismus surgery Thermal burn Toxic epidermal necrolysis
Conjunctival lesion/pterygium excision type	Excision of conjunctival lesion	Conjunctival chalasis Conjunctival filtering bleb leak Granuloma Melanosis Neoplasia Pterygium

cryopreserved for several months can still be viable (29). Hence, it is possible that the amnion epithelial cells continue production of cytokines after transplantation. Nerve growth factor, epidermal growth factor, keratocyte growth factor, and hepatocyte growth factor, all present in the amnion, may play a role in promoting the epithelialization of the ocular surface after AMT (27,28).

The mechanisms by which amniotic membrane may reduce scarring, inflammation, and angiogenesis are more complex. Amniotic membrane matrix uniquely suppresses transforming growth factor-β signaling, resulting in reduction in fibroblasts and scarring (30). The AMGs trap inflammatory cells of monocyte–macrophage lineage that show signs of apoptosis (31). Fresh human amniotic epithelial and mesenchymal cells express potent antiangiogenic agents, interleukin-1 receptor antagonist, all four matrix metalloproteinase inhibitors, collagen XVIII, interleukin-10, and

thrombospondin-1 (26). Similar observations were made in residual epithelial cells and stroma of cryopreserved amniotic membranes (26).

Unlike other allograft transplantations, AMT does not require administration of systemic immunosuppressive therapy to prevent immune rejection. The amniotic membrane typically dissolves within 3 to 5 weeks. It is not clear whether alloreactive immune mechanisms are involved in the process of amniotic graft dissolution after placement onto the ocular surface. The earlier hypotheses about lack of immune rejection response proposed that this phenomenon is a result of lack of human leukocyte antigens (HLA) in a cryopreserved amniotic membrane, but recent studies suggest that the issue is more complex. It is believed that amnion is an immune-privileged tissue (29). The epithelium, stroma, and fibroblasts of cryopreserved amniotic membrane contain HLA class I and II antigens, but the amnion does have the ability to suppress alloreactive T cells *in vitro* (32). Furthermore, amnion expresses HLA-G, a nonclassic major histocompatibility complex class I molecule expressed in the extravillous cytotrophoblast at the fetomaternal interface, that protects the fetus from maternal cellular immunity. This antigen, along with some other immunoregulatory molecules (e.g., Fas ligand), plays a role in suppressing the infiltration of CD4+ and CD8+ T cells into amnion (29).

PREPARATION AND STORAGE OF AMNION

The vast majority of clinical experience comes from the use of cryopreserved AMGs, but the use of fresh amniotic membrane has been previously reported (33–36). Both *in vivo* and *in vitro* studies suggest that there is very little or no difference between fresh and cryopreserved amniotic membranes. The amniotic membrane shows little morphologic change after cryopreservation in 50% glycerol (37). Fresh amnion may be a good source of AMGs in countries where preserved tissue is not accessible, but the risk of blood-borne infections seems to be elevated (33,34). The cryopreserved amniotic membrane is typically stored in −80°C on a nitrocellulose paper in 50% glycerol with the epithelium side up. The epithelium side is smooth and can be distinguished from the sticky stromal side by touching it with a Weck-cel sponge (Edward Weck & Co, Inc., Research Triangle Park, NC). The AMGs can be stained before removal from the nitrocellulose paper with lissamine green B 1% that is not toxic to corneal epithelium and allows for better visualization of edges and folds or wrinkles during the surgical procedure. The color of the amniotic membrane returns to normal within 120 minutes of application of the dye.

The preparation and preservation techniques for AMGs were first described by Lee and Tseng (38). Amnion is obtained from placentas of donors undergoing elective caesarean section to eliminate contamination from vaginal delivery (39). Donor screening to exclude the presence of human immunodeficiency virus (HIV)-1 and HIV-2 (HIV-1 and HIV-2 antibodies), hepatitis B (surface antigen and core antibody), hepatitis C (antibody), human T-lymphocyte virus 1 and 2 (antibodies), and syphilis (rapid plasma reagin) in the donor's serum are performed before harvesting placenta, and this is repeated 6 months later to guard against transmission of blood-borne pathogens. The placenta is transported under sterile conditions to a lamellar-flow hood and cleaned of blood clots with sterile Earle's balanced saline solution (Life Technologies, Inc., Gaithersburg, MD) containing 50 μg/mL of penicillin, 50 μg/mL of streptomycin, 100 μg/mL of neomycin, and 2.5 μg/mL of amphotericin (Bio-Tissue Form #H-005.0, Miami, FL). The amnion is separated from chorion by blunt dissection and placed onto nitrocellulose paper with

a pore size of 0.45 μm (Bio-Rad, Gainesville, FL) with the epithelium side up. The nitrocellulose paper with amnion is then cut into pieces typically not larger than 4 cm × 4 cm and stored at −80°C in a sterile vial containing Dulbecco's modified Eagle medium (Life Technologies, Inc.) and glycerol (Baxter Healthcare Corporation, Stone Mountain, GA) at the ratio of 1:1.

Preserved human AMGs can be prepared as previously described, provided the availability of trained personnel, access to the ingredients, equipment necessary for processing the tissue, and storage equipment exist. Preserved amnion is also commercially available, either cryopreserved (Bio-Tissue, Miami, FL) or low-heat–dehydrated and sterilized (OKTO Ophtho, Costa Mesa, CA). Unlike low-heat–dehydrated amnion, cryopreserved amnion requires storage at −80°C if stored longer than 4 weeks. It can be stored at −20°C for as long as 4 weeks before use (Bio-Tissue, AmnioGraft Information Summary). The cryopreserved amnion is thawed before its use in the operating room. The low-heat–dehydrated amnion is stored at room temperature and is rehydrated with saline solution minutes before use. Unlike cryopreserved amnion, low-heat–dehydrated amnion is supplied without a carrier sheet.

SURGICAL TECHNIQUE
Corneal Epithelial Defect (with or without Stromal Ulcer)

After retrobulbar anesthesia, the base of epithelial defect or stromal ulcer is debrided with a microsponge and the surrounding poorly adherent epithelium is removed. The cryopreserved amniotic membrane is peeled from the nitrocellulose paper and placed on the surface of the defect in an overlay or inlay fashion.

Overlay Technique

In the overlay technique (Fig. 58-1), the amniotic membrane is placed epithelium side down to cover the entire corneal, limbal, and perilimbal surfaces. The graft is secured with interrupted 9-0 polyglactin sutures to the conjunctiva. A running 10-0 nylon suture can be added at the surgeon's discretion to secure the AMG to the corneal stroma. It is preferable that the knots not be buried to prevent tears in the AMG.

Inlay Technique

The inlay technique (Fig. 58-2) can be used in the presence of stromal ulcer. One or multiple layers of the amniotic membrane, depending on the depth of the stromal defect, can be applied. In this case the amniotic membrane is placed epithelium side up onto the surface of stromal bed and secured by interrupted 10-0 nylon sutures to the edge

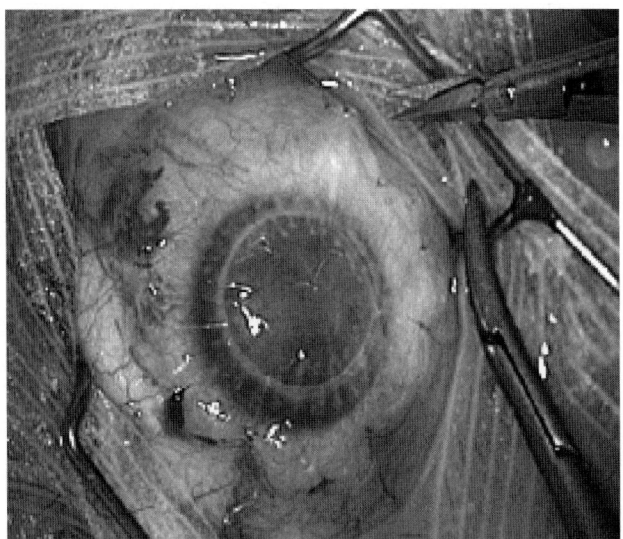

FIGURE 58-1. Overlay amniotic membrane graft.

of the ulcer. The knots are then buried into the corneal stroma. The overlay technique can be added to cover the inlay AMG at the surgeon's discretion (Fig. 58-3).

Fornix Reconstruction

After retrobulbar anesthesia, a 4-0 silk can be sutured to the tarsal plate of the eyelid to apply traction. The scarred conjunctiva is cut with scissors to release adhesions from the perilimbal area and then dissected from the underlying sclera towards the fornix. Excessive bleeding is controlled by Gelaspon (Chauvin Ankerpharm GmbH, Rudolstadt, Germany) or epinephrine applied subconjunctivally or topically. The amniotic membrane is removed from the nitrocellulose paper and placed epithelium side up onto the surface of bulbar and palpebral conjunctiva. The amniotic membrane is trimmed to fit the area of defect. The margin

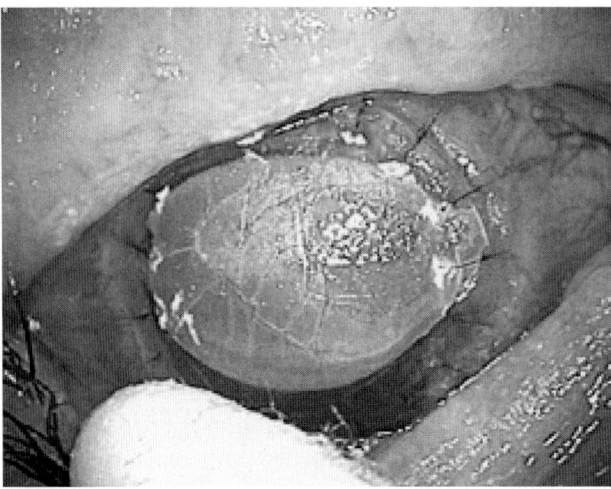

FIGURE 58-2. Inlay amniotic membrane graft.

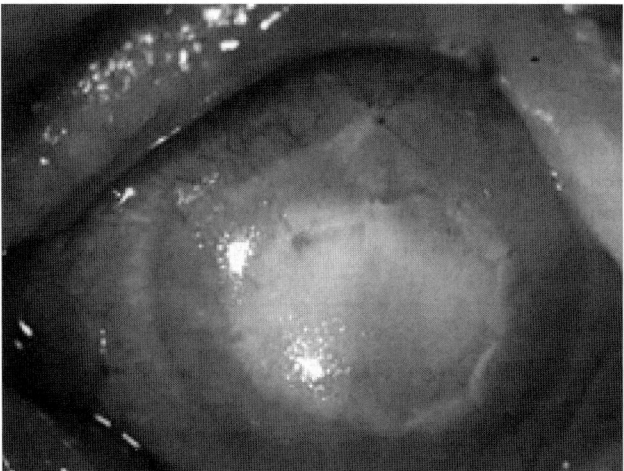

FIGURE 58-3. Overlay and inlay amniotic membrane grafts.

of the amniotic membrane is placed under the edge of conjunctiva and secured with 9-0 polyglactin sutures (Fig. 58-4). The amniotic membrane is then pulled and secured to the apex of the fornix with 9-0 polyglactin sutures. Alternatively, the amniotic membrane can be pulled and secured to the fornix through the eyelid with two or three double-armed 6-0 polyglactin using silicone bolsters or a symblepharon ring secured through the eyelid with 7-0 silk suture with bolsters.

Conjunctival or Corneal Lesion/Pterygium Excision

After retrobulbar anesthesia, the lesion is dissected to bare sclera or corneal stroma. Application of mitomycin C at a concentration of 0.02% the surface for 3 minutes, followed by irrigation with balanced saline solution, may be used. The amniotic membrane is placed on the area of dissection with the epithelium side up and trimmed to the size of defect. The membrane is secured with 8-0 polyglactin suture to the sclera and with 10-0 nylon suture to the corneal stroma. After AMT, a limbal autologous transplant (3 × 5 mm) or autologous limbal stem cell transplant (5 × 5 mm), obtained from the upper bulbar conjunctiva or from the fellow eye, may be placed on the amniotic membrane and secured with 10-0 and 8-0 polyglactin sutures to the corneal stroma and sclera, respectively.

POSTOPERATIVE CARE

A hydrophilic bandage contact lens is placed on the ocular surface at the end of procedure. Alternatively, a central tarsorrhaphy can be performed in cases with poor fit of the bandage contact lens. Leaving the ocular surface without a bandage contact lens may lead to an early detachment of the amniotic membrane and lack of epithelialization (40). A combination

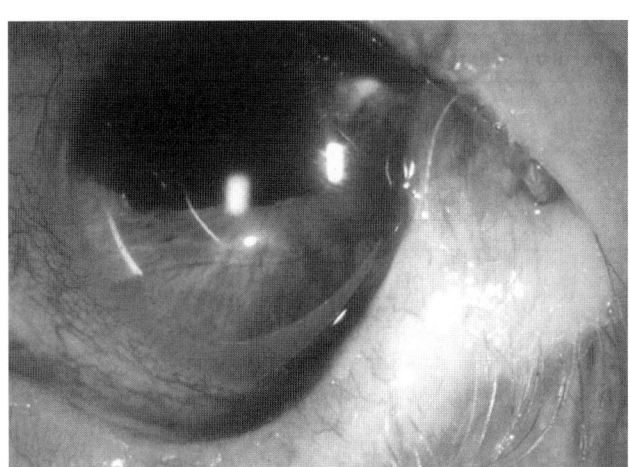
A

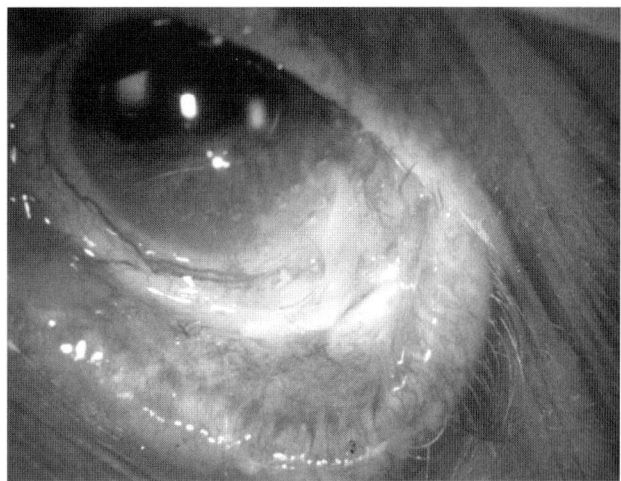
B

FIGURE 58-4. Symblepharon in a patient with ocular cicatricial pemphigoid before **(A)** and 1 month after **(B)** conjunctival fornix reconstruction with amniotic membrane graft.

of topical antibiotics and corticosteroid drops is used over the period of 4 weeks after the surgery. The amniotic membrane typically dissolves within 3 to 6 weeks. The bandage contact lens is preferably kept in place until the AMG is completely dissolved. The use of topical antibiotics is discontinued after removal of the bandage contact lens, provided that the epithelium is healed. Topical corticosteroids are used until the inflammation subsides. The 10-0 nylon suture, if used, can be removed after complete dissolution of the AMG.

CLINICAL EXPERIENCE

Corneal Epithelial Defect (with or without Stromal Ulcer)

The amniotic membrane became yet another tool in treatment of persistent epithelial defects of the cornea associated with a spectrum of ocular and systemic conditions. The reports show that AMT is effective and safe in treatment of persistent epithelial defects of the cornea (19,20,38,40–53) (Table 58-2). Although the efficacy of AMT has not been compared in controlled studies with other therapeutic interventions, amniotic membrane was

shown to be able to promote healing of persistent epithelial defects in cases where other treatments, including topical lubricants, bandage contact lens, and tarsorrhaphy, failed. The success rate measured by the percentage of eyes with epithelialization of corneal defects after AMT ranges between 58% and 100%, according to the different reports that vary greatly in number of cases studied, spectrum of patient population, etiologic factors, size and severity of epithelial defects, stromal thinning, comorbid factors, and duration of follow-up period. Patients whose epithelial defect does not heal after the first AMT may benefit from repeated grafting (41). The success rate in treatment of persistent epithelial defects seems to be unrelated to the technique used (41). Multiple layers of amnion transplanted using the inlay technique may be superior to single-layer graft in case of deep stromal ulcers (1,20). The disadvantage of placing the amnion in an inlay fashion is a decrease in corneal transparency that may persist for many months. Once the amniotic membrane is reabsorbed, it is replaced by a new fibrotic stroma (54). The rate of recurrences of epithelial defects after successful AMT has been reported as between 0% and 29%. The success rate in cases with persistent epithelial defects associated with an underlying

TABLE 58-2. PREVIEW OF RESULTS OF AMNIOTIC MEMBRANE TRANSPLANTATION FOR CORNEAL DEFECTS

Indication	N (Eyes)	Success Rate (%)	Recurrence Rate (%)	Follow-up (mo)	Reference
Corneal epithelial	30	70	29	8	41
defect with or without	11	91	0	9	38
stromal thinning	16	76	–	18	19
	11	82	18	12	20
	24	58	–	–	47
	11	100	–	19	48
	28	82	–	11	44
	30	90	15	6	49
	140	75	–	6	50

TABLE 58-3. PREVIEW OF RESULTS OF AMNIOTIC MEMBRANE GRAFTING FOR PTERYGIUM EXCISION

Indication	N (Eyes)	Success Rate (%)	Recurrence Rate (%)	Follow-up (mo)	Reference
Primary pterygium	33	97	3	12	55
	28	89	10	14	58
	46	89	10	11	57
Recurrent pterygium	21	90	9	14	55
	8	62	37	11	57

systemic autoimmune disease is lower compared with those with persistent epithelial defects associated with a condition limited to the eye (41,43).

Pterygium

The use of AMGs for pterygium excision has been reported by several authors (55–60) (Table 58-3). If AMT is added to pterygium excision as a single procedure, the recurrence rate over a follow-up period of approximately 1 year varies between 3% and 10% for primary (55,57,58) and between 9% and 27% for recurrent (55,57) pterygium excision. The AMT combined with bare sclera excision seems to be superior to bare sclera excision alone for primary pterygium (58). The rate of pterygium recurrence can be decreased when autologous limbal stem cell or autologous conjunctival transplantation are used concurrently with AMT (56).

Conjunctival Lesion/Defect

The conjunctiva may heal with clinically significant chronic inflammation and scar formation after surgical trauma, even in individuals with no history of underlying ocular or systemic disorder that would lead to excessive fibrosis and inflammation. Although the benefit of amniotic membrane for conjunctival lesion excision has not been established in randomized, controlled trials, reports in the literature indicate that fibrosis and inflammation are reduced if amniotic membrane is used. The success of conjunctival surface reconstruction correlates with recovery of the conjunctival epithelial phenotype (61). AMGs were used after excision of a spectrum of conjunctival lesions (57,62,63) and symptomatic conjunctivochalasis refractory to medical treatments (64). The use of AMGs after removal of neoplastic lesions such as melanoma, conjunctival intraepithelial neoplasm, or conjunctival mucosa–associated lymphoid tissue lymphoma and acquired melanosis was associated with no scar formation, but a cyst or conjunctival inflammation surrounding the amniotic graft was present during the follow-up period in half of these cases (62,65). Similar observations were made in a group of patients who had AMT for symptomatic conjunctivochalasis refractory to medical treatments (64). Focal conjunctival inflammation or scar formation were seen in approximately 25% of eyes. The amniotic membrane may not be able to prevent granuloma formation or recurrence of carcinoma *in situ* in all patients (66).

Fornix Reconstruction

Amniotic membrane transplantation was used for fornix reconstruction in patients with symblepharon formation associated with systemic autoimmune conditions, such as ocular cicatricial pemphigoid (62,63,67), atopic keratoconjunctivitis (62,67,68), and Stevens-Johnson syndrome or toxic epidermal necrolysis, as well as for fornix reconstruction in patients with symblepharon formation associated with disorders limited to the eye, including trauma due to ocular surgeries, recurrent pterygium (62,67), and thermal or chemical burns. Five of 9 eyes with ocular cicatricial pemphigoid (63) and 9 of 10 eyes with Stevens-Johnson syndrome were symblepharon free 7 and 13 months, respectively, after fornix reconstruction with AMT (63,68). Even more encouraging results were reported when amniotic membrane was used for fornix reconstruction in disorders limited to the eye (62,67). Interestingly, the conjunctival epithelium can be repopulated with goblet cells after AMT in patients with advanced ocular cicatricial pemphigoid (63,69).

Symptomatic Bullous Keratopathy

Patients with ocular pain due to bullous keratopathy in whom penetrating keratoplasty is not indicated may benefit from AMT (70,71), an alternative to conjunctival flap or long-term bandage contact lens wear. Complete pain relief was reported in approximately 90% of patients during the follow-up period of as long as 25 months (70,71). The epithelial edema and bullae recurred in only 10% of patients within 2 years after AMT (71).

Band Keratopathy

Ocular pain associated with band keratopathy resolved and remained absent over a 14-month follow-up period in 14 of 15 patients who underwent surgical removal of calcific deposits with or without ethylenediaminetetraacetic acid followed by AMT (72).

Glaucoma Filtering Bleb Leak

Amniotic membrane transplantation can be used successfully to repair late-onset glaucoma filtering bleb leak (73,74), but a prospective, randomized trial in a larger cohort of patients disclosed a success rate of only 46% with AMG, as opposed to a 100% success rate with conjunctival advancement, 2 years after the repair, suggesting that conjunctival advancement is superior to amniotic membrane for filtering bleb leak repair (73). AMT, however, may be a good alternative in cases where anatomic factors prevent conjunctival advancement.

Emergency Indications

Unlike most other transplantations, in which procedures are performed after maximum reduction of inflammation to reduce likelihood of immune rejection reaction and other postoperative complications, amniotic membrane can be therapeutically useful for reduction of inflammation because of its unique antiinflammatory intrinsic properties and for maintaining the integrity of ocular surface.

Multilayered AMG with (75,76) or without (1,43–46) application of tissue adhesive was successfully used to restore and maintain the anterior chamber and the integrity of the ocular surface in a limited number of patients with corneal or scleral perforation or descemetocele. Application of multiple layers of amniotic membrane in patients with deep stromal ulcers with or without descemetocele and perforation is more effective than single-layer AMG in corneal reepithelialization and preventing recurrence of perforation (1,20). The AMT needed to be repeated for recurrence of corneal perforation in some cases (1,41,44). Although AMT was reported to restore the integrity of ocular surface for a relatively long follow-up period of up to 1 year (1,43–46) in some patients, tectonic keratoplasty is not always avoidable (1,45). Others may require corneal graft for vision rehabilitation later during the follow-up after AMT.

AMT can be used for acute ocular inflammatory conditions such as chemical or thermal burns (77,78) and Stevens-Johnson syndrome or toxic epidermal necrolysis (79,80). Covering the ocular surface and eyelid skin lesions with amnion during the acute episode of toxic epidermal necrolysis may reduce the severity of ocular sequelae and likelihood of blindness later (80). Similar benefits of AMT were seen in patients with acute chemical or thermal burns (36,81,82). The amnion was shown to be capable of altering the complex pathogenic mechanisms in the corneal stroma after burn trauma that lead to tissue damage and neovascularization (83). The use of amniotic membrane alone during the acute stage of burn trauma to suppress inflammation and tissue damage, followed by an attempt to rehabilitate the ocular surface with limbal stem cell grafting combined with another AMT during the chronic stages of burn trauma, seems to be a good approach in the management of acute injuries to the ocular surface (84).

Adjunct to Limbal Stem Cell Transplantation

Results of limbal stem cell transplantation combined with AMT were reported in several clinical studies (85–90).

AMG has a good success rate in restoring corneal epithelium in partial limbal stem cell deficiency (85–87,89), but it is insufficient in case of total limbal stem cell deficiency (85,89). In such cases, limbal stem cell transplantation with or without AMT is required. The amniotic membrane and limbal stem cell transplantation may result in good vision restoration. Additional surgical procedures, such as penetrating or lamellar keratoplasty, may be required (88).

The amnion can affect the environment of the limbal stem cell graft; the intrinsic properties of amnion, including reduction of alloreactive T-cell infiltration (32), may (hypothetically) discourage limbal stem cell graft rejection, but this has not been shown in an experimental model (91). Data from an *in vitro* study suggest that AMG denuded of epithelial cells may be more efficient in signal transmission to the migrating epithelial cells and inducing their differentiation from stem cells into transient amplifying cells compared with amniotic membrane with epithelium (92). The clinical significance of this observation is not yet clear.

Ex Vivo Limbal Stem Cell Transplants

The use of human amniotic membrane as a substrate for *ex vivo* cultured limbal stem cells opened a new avenue to ocular surface reconstruction (93). The principle lies in culturing corneal limbal epithelial cells obtained from a donor eye on the surface of epithelium-denuded amniotic membrane and then transplanting the prepared limbal grafts onto the ocular surface. The source of limbal epithelial cells can be either a cadaver donor eye or a living fellow or donor eye. Systemic immunosuppressive therapy is required in case of allografting (94). The amniotic membrane is capable of maintaining and expanding limbal epithelial stem cells that retain their *in vivo* properties of slow cycling and undifferentiation (95,96). The phenotype of the resultant epithelium is limbal, but the architecture is similar to that of the corneal epithelium (97). Although the results of clinical and experimental studies (93–100) on *ex vivo* expanded limbal stem cells on amniotic membrane seem to be similar to the ones using conventional single-donor limbal stem cell grafts, the major benefit of *ex vivo* prepared grafts probably lies in minimal invasion of the donor limbal stem cells, or no invasion if *in vitro* bioengineered limbal stem cell lines are used. This fact may account for rapid expansion of the novel technique in clinical practice in the future.

COMPLICATIONS

AMT has an excellent safety profile. Few postoperative complications have been reported in the literature thus far. Ocular infection, although relatively rare, is the most common complication after nonpreserved AMT (33,34). Whether washing the amnion with antibiotics before transplantation would prevent ocular infection in such cases is unknown.

Postoperative complications after transplantation of preserved amniotic membrane are very rare. Hypopyon formation in the absence of infection after AMT is documented in three cases (101,102). All of these patients had hypopyon after repeated AMT from the same donor. This fact became the basis for a hypothesis that noninfectious hypopyon after AMT represents a local immune reaction after sensitization to foreign antigens of the previous AMG from the same donor. Using the amnion from a different donor for repeated AMT may reduce the likelihood of hypopyon formation.

Corneal calcification was reported in some cases of AMT. Avoiding the use of phosphate-containing eye drops in the postoperative period may prevent this phenomenon (103).

Bacterial keratitis with *Staphylococcus aureus* was documented in one case after preserved AMT (52). *S. aureus* was not detected in either sample of the amnion obtained by caesarean section (39). These observations suggest that the contamination of amnion with *S. aureus* is secondary and occurs most likely while handling the AMG.

CONCLUSION

Clinical experience and results of experimental studies provide growing evidence that human amniotic membrane is effective and safe in the treatment of ocular surface disorders. The spectrum of mechanisms of action through which amniotic membrane alters epithelialization exceeds those involved in other treatments. Whether the amniotic membrane application is clinically superior to the other methods has not been established. Although controlled, randomized trials comparing the effects of amniotic membrane with other therapeutic interventions are lacking, success has been recorded in some cases where other methods failed. The idea that multiple, controlled, randomized trials will be conducted in the near future is probably unrealistic, given the complexity of factors and processes involved in the pathogenesis of ocular surface disorders and the lack of widely accepted criteria for assessment of their severity. It is more likely, given the availability of AMGs, the simplicity of the surgical techniques, and its exceptionally good safety profile, that amnion will be used for an expanding variety of indications.

REFERENCES

1. Davis JW. Skin transplantation with a review of 550 cases at The Johns Hopkins Hospital. *Johns Hopkins Med J* 1910; 15:307.
2. Trelford JD, Trelford-Sauder M. The amnion in surgery, past and present. *Am J Obstet Gynecol* 1979;134:833–845.
3. De Roth A. Plastic repair of conjunctival defects with fetal membrane. *Arch Ophthalmol* 1940;23:522–525.
4. Battle JF, Perdomo FJ. Placental membranes as a conjunctival substitute. *Ophthalmology* 1993;100:107(abstr).
5. Kim JC, Tseng SCG. Transplantation of preserved human amniotic membrane for surface reconstruction in severely damaged rabbit corneas. *Cornea* 1995;14:473–484.
6. Bourne GL. The microscopic anatomy of the human amnion and chorion. *Am J Obstet Gynecol* 1960;79:1070–1073.
7. van Herendael BJ, Oberti C, Brosens I. Microanatomy of the human membranes: a light microscopic, transmission, and scanning electron microscopic study. *Am J Obstet Gynecol* 1978;131: 872–880.
8. Baum J. Amniotic membrane transplantation: why is it effective? *Cornea* 2002;21:339–341.
9. John T. Human amniotic membrane transplantation: past, present, and future. *Ophthalmol Clin North Am* 2003;16:43–65.
10. Terranova VP, Lyall RM. Chemotaxis of human gingival epithelial cells to laminin: a mechanism for epithelial cell apical migration. *J Periodontol* 1986;57:311–317.
11. Khodadoust AA, Silverstein AM, Kenyon KR, et al. Adhesion of regenerating corneal epithelium: the role of basement membrane. *Am J Ophthalmol* 1968;65:339–348.
12. Sonnenberg A, Calafat J, Janssen H, et al. Integrin a6/b4 complex is located in hemidesmosomes, suggesting a major role in epidermal cell-basement membrane adhesion. *J Cell Biol* 1991;113: 907–917.
13. Barcellos-Hoff MH, Aggeler J, Ram TG, et al. Functional differentiation and alveolar morphogenesis of primary mammary cultures on reconstituted basement membrane. *Development* 1989;105:223–235.
14. Guo M, Grinnel F. Basement membrane and human epidermal differentiation *in vitro*. *J Invest Dermatol* 1989;93:372–378.
15. Streuli CH, Bailey N, Bissell MJ. Control of mammary epithelial differentiation: basement membrane induces tissue-specific gene expression in the absence of cell-cell interaction and morphological polarity. *J Cell Biol* 1991;115:1383–1395.
16. Tseng SCG, Prabhasawat P, Lee SH, et al. Amniotic membrane transplantation for conjunctival surface reconstruction. *Am J Ophthalmol* 1997;124:765–774.
17. Boudreau N, Sympson CJ, Werb Z, et al. Suppression of ICE and apoptosis in mammary epithelial cells by extracellular matrix. *Science* 1995;267:891–893.
18. Boudreau N, Werb Z, Bissell MJ. Suppression of apoptosis by basement membrane requires three-dimensional tissue organization and withdrawal from the cell cycle. *Proc Natl Acad Sci U S A* 1996;93:3500–3513.
19. Chen HJ, Pires RTF, Tseng SCG. Amniotic membrane transplantation for severe neurotrophic corneal ulcers. *Br J Ophthalmol* 2000;84:826–833.
20. Kruse FE, Rohrschneider K, Volcker HE. Multilayer amniotic membrane transplantation for reconstruction of deep corneal ulcers. *Ophthalmology* 1999;106:1504–1510.
21. Choi YS, Kim JY, Wee WR, et al. Effect of the application of human amniotic membrane on rabbit corneal wound healing after excimer laser photorefractive keratectomy. *Cornea* 1998;17:389–395.
22. Fukuda K, Chikama T, Nakamura M, et al. Differential distribution of subchains of the basement membrane components type IV collagen and laminin among the amniotic membrane, cornea, and conjunctiva. *Cornea* 1999;18:73–79.
23. Kurpakus-Wheater M. Laminin-5 is a component of preserved amniotic membrane. *Curr Eye Res* 2001;22:353–357.
24. Polzin WJ, Lockrow EG, Morishige WK. A pilot study identifying type V collagenolytic activity in human amniotic fluid. *Am J Perinatol* 1997;14:103–106.
25. Modesti A, Scarpa S, D'Orazi G. Localization of type IV and V collagens in the stroma of human amnion. *Prog Clin Biol Res* 1989;296:459–463.

26. Hao Y, Ma DH, Hwang DG, et al. Identification of antiangiogenic and antiinflammatory proteins in human amniotic membrane. *Cornea* 2000;19:348–352.

27. Touhami A, Grueterich M, Tseng SC. The role of NGF signaling in human limbal epithelium expanded by amniotic membrane culture. *Invest Ophthalmol Vis Sci* 2002;43:987–994.

28. Koizumi NJ, Inatomi TJ, Sotozono CJ, et al. Growth factor mRNA and protein in preserved human amniotic membrane. *Curr Eye Res* 2000;20:173–177.

29. Kubo M, Sonoda Y, Muramatsu R, et al. Immunogenicity of human amniotic membrane in experimental xenotransplantation. *Invest Ophthalmol Vis Sci* 2001;42:1539–1546.

30. Lee SB, Li DQ, Tan DT, et al. Suppression of TGF-beta signaling in both normal conjunctival fibroblasts and pterygial body fibroblasts by amniotic membrane. *Curr Eye Res* 2000;20:325–334.

31. Shimmura S, Shimazaki J, Ohashi Y, et al. Antiinflammatory effects of amniotic membrane transplantation in ocular surface disorders. *Cornea* 2001;20:408–413.

32. Ueta M, Kweon MN, Sano Y, et al. Immunosuppressive properties of human amniotic membrane for mixed lymphocyte reaction. *Clin Exp Immunol* 2002;129:464–70.

33. Khokhar S, Sharma N, Kumar H, et al. Infection after use of nonpreserved human amniotic membrane for the reconstruction of the ocular surface. *Cornea* 2001;20:773–774.

34. Mejia LF, Acosta C, Santamaria JP. Use of nonpreserved human amniotic membrane for the reconstruction of the ocular surface. *Cornea* 2000;19:288–291.

35. Panda A. Amniotic membrane transplantation in ophthalmology (fresh vs preserved tissue). *Br J Ophthalmol* 1999;83:1410–1411.

36. Ucakhan OO, Koklu G, Firat E. Nonpreserved human amniotic membrane transplantation in acute and chronic chemical eye injuries. *Cornea* 2002;21:169–172.

37. Kruse FE, Joussen AM, Rohrschneider K, et al. Cryopreserved human amniotic membrane for ocular surface reconstruction. *Graefes Arch Clin Exp Ophthalmol* 2000;238:68–75.

38. Lee SH, Tseng SCG. Amniotic membrane transplantation for persistent epithelial defects with ulceration. *Am J Ophthalmol* 1997;123:303–312.

39. Adds PJ, Hunt C, Hartley S. Bacterial contamination of amniotic membrane. *Br J Ophthalmol* 2001;85:228–230.

40. Gris O, Campo Z, Wolley-Dod C, et al. Amniotic membrane implantation as a therapeutic contact lens for the treatment of epithelial disorders. *Cornea* 2002;21:22–27.

41. Letko E, Stechschulte SU, Kenyon KR, et al. Amniotic membrane inlay and overlay grafting for corneal epithelial defects and stromal ulcers. *Arch Ophthalmol* 2001;119:659–663.

42. Sridhar MS, Sangwan VS, Bansal AK, et al. Amniotic membrane transplantation in the management of shield ulcers of vernal keratoconjunctivitis. *Ophthalmology* 2001;108:1218–1222.

43. Hanada K, Shimazaki J, Shimmura S, et al. Multilayered amniotic membrane transplantation for severe ulceration of the cornea and sclera. *Am J Ophthalmol* 2001;131:324–331.

44. Prabhasawat P, Tesavibul N, Komolsuradej W. Single and multilayer amniotic membrane transplantation for persistent corneal epithelial defect with and without stromal thinning and perforation. *Br J Ophthalmol* 2001;85:1455–1463.

45. Azuara-Blanco A, Pillai CT, Dua HS. Amniotic membrane transplantation for ocular surface reconstruction. *Br J Ophthalmol* 1999;83:399–402.

46. Solomon A, Meller D, Prabhasawat P, et al. Amniotic membrane grafts for nontraumatic corneal perforations, descemetoceles, and deep ulcers. *Ophthalmology* 2002;109:694–703.

47. Gabric N, Mravicic I, Dekaris I, et al. Human amniotic membrane in the reconstruction of the ocular surface. *Doc Ophthalmol* 1999;98:273–283.

48. Ivekovic B, Tedeschi-Reiner E, Petric I, et al. Amniotic membrane transplantation for ocular surface reconstruction in neutrophic corneal ulcera. *Coll Antropol* 2002;26:47–54.

49. Ferreira De Souza R, Hofmann-Rummelt C, Kruse FE, et al. Multilayer amniotic membrane transplantation for corneal ulcers not treatable by conventional therapy: a prospective study of the status of cornea and graft during follow-up. *Klin Monatsbl Augenheilkd* 2001;218:528–534.

50. Prabhasawat P, Kosrirukvongs P, Booranapong W, et al. Amniotic membrane transplantation for ocular surface reconstruction. *J Med Assoc Thai* 2001;84:705–718.

51. Gris O, Guell JL, Lopez-Navidad A, et al. Application of the amniotic membrane in ocular surface pathology. *Ann Transplant* 1999;4:82–84.

52. Dogru M, Yildiz M, Baykara M, et al. Corneal sensitivity and ocular surface changes following preserved amniotic membrane transplantation for nonhealing corneal ulcers. *Eye* 2003;17:139–148.

53. Dua HS, Azuara-Blanco A. Amniotic membrane transplantation. *Br J Ophthalmol* 1999;83:748–752.

54. Gris O, Wolley-Dod C, Guell JL, et al. Histologic findings after amniotic membrane graft in the human cornea. *Ophthalmology* 2002;109:508–512.

55. Solomon A, Pires RTF, Tseng SCG. Amniotic membrane transplantation after extensive removal of primary and recurrent pterygia. *Ophthalmology* 2001;108:449–460.

56. Shimazaki J, Kosaka K, Shimmura S, et al. Amniotic membrane transplantation with conjunctival autograft for recurrent pterygium. *Ophthalmology* 2003;110:119–124.

57. Prabhasawat P, Barton K, Burkett G, et al. Comparison of conjunctival autografts, amniotic membrane grafts, and primary closure for pterygium excision. *Ophthalmology* 1997;104:974–985.

58. Tekin NF, Kaynak S, Saatci AO, et al. Preserved human amniotic membrane transplantation in the treatment of primary pterygium. *Ophthalmic Surg Lasers* 2001;32:464–469.

59. Schimazaki J, Shinozaki N, Tsubota K. Transplantation of amniotic membrane and limbal autograft for patients with recurrent pterygium associated with symblepharon. *Br J Ophthalmol* 1998;82:235–240.

60. Ti SE, Tseng SC. Management of primary and recurrent pterygium using amniotic membrane transplantation. *Curr Opin Ophthalmol* 2002;13:204–212.

61. Prabhasawat P, Tseng SC. Impression cytology study of epithelial phenotype of ocular surface reconstructed by preserved human amniotic membrane. *Arch Ophthalmol* 1997;115:1360–1367.

62. Tseng SCG, Prabhasawat P, Lee SH. Amniotic membrane transplantation for conjunctival surface reconstruction. *Am J Ophthalmol* 1997;124:765–774.

63. Barabino S, Rolando M, Bentivoglio G, et al. Role of amniotic membrane transplantation for conjunctival reconstruction in ocular-cicatricial pemphigoid. *Ophthalmology* 2003;110:474–480.

64. Meller D, Maskin SL, Pires RTF, et al. Amniotic membrane transplantation for symptomatic conjunctivochalasis refractory to medical treatments. *Cornea* 2000;19:796–803.

65. Kobayashi A, Takahira M, Yamada A, et al. Fornix and conjunctiva reconstruction by amniotic membrane in a patient with conjunctival mucosa-associated lymphoid tissue lymphoma. *Jpn J Ophthalmol* 2002;46:346–348.

66. Espana EM, Prabhasawat P, Gruterich M, et al. Amniotic membrane transplantation for reconstruction after excision of large ocular surface neoplasias. *Br J Ophthalmol* 2002;86:640–645.

67. Solomon A, Espana EM, Tseng SCG. Amniotic membrane transplantation for reconstruction of the conjunctival fornices. *Ophthalmology* 2003;110:93–100.

68. Honavar SG, Bansal AK, Sangwan VS, et al. Amniotic membrane transplantation for ocular surface reconstruction in Stevens-Johnson syndrome. *Ophthalmology* 2000;107:975–979.

69. Barabino S, Rolando M. Amniotic membrane transplantation elicits goblet cell repopulation after conjunctival reconstruction in a case of severe ocular cicatricial pemphigoid. *Acta Ophthalmol Scand* 2003;81:68–71.

70. Espana EM, Grueterich M, Sandoval H, et al. Amniotic membrane transplantation for bullous keratopathy in eyes with poor visual potential. *J Cataract Refract Surg* 2003;29:279–284.

71. Pires RTF, Tseng SCG, Prabhasawat P, et al. Amniotic membrane transplantation for symptomatic bullous keratopathy. *Arch Ophthalmol* 1999;117:1291–1297.

72. Anderson DF, Prabhasawat P, Alfonso E, et al. Amniotic membrane transplantation after the primary surgical management of band keratopathy. *Cornea* 2001;20:354–361.

73. Budenz DL, Barton K, Tseng SC. Amniotic membrane transplantation for repair of leaking glaucoma filtering blebs. *Am J Ophthalmol* 2000;130:580–588.

74. Kee C, Hwang JM. Amniotic membrane transplantation for late-onset glaucoma filtering blebs. *Am J Ophthalmol* 2002; 133:834–835.

75. Duchesne B, Tahi H, Galand A. Use of human fibrin glue and amniotic membrane transplant in corneal perforation. *Cornea* 2001;20:230–232.

76. Su CY, Lin CP. Combined use of an amniotic membrane and tissue adhesive in treating corneal perforation: a case report. *Ophthalmic Surg Lasers* 2000;31:151–154.

77. Meller D, Pires RTF, Mack RJS, et al. Amniotic membrane transplantation for acute chemical or thermal burns. *Ophthalmology* 2000;107:980–989.

78. Shimazaki J, Yang HY, Tsubota K. Amniotic membrane transplantation for ocular surface reconstruction in patients with chemical and thermal burns. *Ophthalmology* 1997;104:2068–2076.

79. Tsubota K, Satake Y, Ohyama M, et al. Surgical reconstruction of the ocular surface in advanced ocular cicatricial pemphigoid and Stevens-Johnson syndrome. *Am J Ophthalmol* 1996;122: 38–52.

80. John T, Foulks GN, John ME, et al. Amniotic membrane in the surgical management of acute toxic epidermal necrolysis. *Ophthalmology* 2002;109:351–360.

81. Meller D, Pires RTF, Mack RJS, et al. Amniotic membrane transplantation for acute chemical or thermal burns. *Ophthalmology* 2000;107:980–990.

82. Sridhar MS, Bansal AK, Sangwan VS, et al. Amniotic membrane transplantation in acute chemical and thermal injury. *Am J Ophthalmol* 1997;124:765–774.

83. Rigal-Sastourne JC, Tixier JM, Renard JP, et al. Corneal burns and matrix metalloproteinases (MMP-2 and -9): the effects of human amniotic membrane transplantation. *J Fr Ophtalmol* 2002;25:685–693.

84. Espana EM, Grueterich M, Ti SE, et al. Phenotypic study of a case receiving a keratolimbal allograft and amniotic membrane for total limbal stem cell deficiency. *Ophthalmology* 2003;110: 481–486.

85. Tseng SCG, Prabhasawat P, Barton K, et al. Amniotic membrane transplantation with or without limbal allografts for corneal surface reconstruction in patients with limbal stem cell deficiency. *Arch Ophthalmol* 1998;116:431–441.

86. Pires RT, Chokshi A, Tseng TS. Amniotic membrane transplantation or conjunctival limbal autograft for limbal stem cell deficiency induced by 5-fluorouracil in glaucoma surgeries. *Cornea* 2000;19:284–287.

87. Anderson DF, Ellies P, Pires RT, et al. Amniotic membrane transplantation for partial limbal stem cell deficiency. *Br J Ophthalmol* 2001;85:567–575.

88. Stoiber J, Ruckhofer J, Muss W, et al. Amniotic membrane transplantation with limbal stem cell transplantation as a combined procedure for corneal surface reconstruction after severe thermal or chemical burns). *Ophthalmologe* 2002;99: 839–848.

89. Gomes JA, dos Santos MS, Cunha MC, et al. Amniotic membrane transplantation for partial and total limbal stem cell deficiency secondary to chemical burn. *Ophthalmology* 2003;110:466–473.

90. Dekaris I, Gabric N, Karaman Z, et al. Limbal-conjunctival autograft transplantation for recurrent pterygium. *Eur J Ophthalmol* 2002;12:177–182.

91. Marinho D, Hofling-Lima AL, Kwitko S, et al. Does amniotic membrane transplantation improve the outcome of autologous limbal transplantation? *Cornea* 2003;22:338–342.

92. Grueterich M, Espana E, Tseng SC. Connexin 43 expression and proliferation of human limbal epithelium on intact and denuded amniotic membrane. *Invest Ophthalmol Vis Sci* 2002;43: 63–71.

93. Koizumi N, Inatomi T, Quantock AJ, et al. Amniotic membrane as a substrate for cultivating limbal corneal epithelial cells for autologous transplantation in rabbits. *Cornea* 2000;19:65–71.

94. Koizumi N, Inatomi T, Suzuki T, et al. Cultivated corneal epithelial stem cell transplantation in ocular surface disorders. *Ophthalmology* 2001;108:1569–1574.

95. Grueterich M, Tseng SC. Human limbal progenitor cells expanded on intact amniotic membrane ex vivo. *Arch Ophthalmol* 2002;120:783–790.

96. Meller D, Pires RT, Tseng SC. Ex vivo preservation and expansion of human limbal epithelial stem cells on amniotic membrane cultures. *Br J Ophthalmol* 2002;86:463–471.

97. Grueterich M, Espana EM, Touhami A, et al. Phenotypic study of a case with successful transplantation of ex vivo expanded human limbal epithelium for unilateral total limbal stem cell deficiency. *Ophthalmology* 2002;109:1547–1552.

98. Ti SE, Anderson D, Touhami A, et al. Factors affecting outcome following transplantation of ex vivo expanded limbal epithelium on amniotic membrane for total limbal deficiency in rabbits. *Invest Ophthalmol Vis Sci* 2002;43:2584–2592.

99. Shimazaki J, Aiba M, Goto E, et al. Transplantation of human limbal epithelium cultivated on amniotic membrane for the treatment of severe ocular surface disorders. *Ophthalmology* 2002;109:1285–1290.

100. Cohen EJ. Use of autologous limbal epithelial cells cultured on amniotic membranes for unilateral stem cell deficiency. *Arch Ophthalmol* 2001;119:123–124.

101. Bernhard G, Lohman CP. Hypopyon after repeated transplantation of human amniotic membrane onto the corneal surface. *Ophthalmology* 2000;107:1344–1346.

102. Messmer EM. Hypopyon after amniotic membrane transplantation. *Ophthalmology* 2001;108:1714–1715.

103. Anderson SB, de Souza RF, Hofmann-Rummelt C, et al. Corneal calcification after amniotic membrane transplantation. *Br J Ophthalmol* 2003;87:587–591.

59

LIMBAL STEM CELL TRANSPLANTATION

ERIK LETKO AND C. STEPHEN FOSTER

The objective of limbal stem cell transplantation is to restore the corneal surface with normal corneal epithelium. Normal corneal epithelium is maintained in the state of homeostasis by balancing epithelial shedding from the surface with centripetal movement of stem cell-derived epithelial cells from the limbus and proliferation of the basal cells (1,2). This so-called XYZ hypothesis of Thoft and Friend, where X represents proliferation of basal cells, Y proliferation and centripetal migration of limbal cells, and Z represents epithelial cell loss from the surface of the cornea, was first proposed in 1983 (3). Cotsarelis et al. were the first to report on the existence of slow-cycling corneal epithelial cells located in the basal cell layer of the limbus (2). These cells were later referred to as *corneal limbal stem cells*.

The limbal stem cells have several distinct biologic and morphologic characteristics. Their life span is believed to be lifelong. They do not have direct cell-to-cell communication by gap junctions and therefore they must maintain a distinct intracellular environment with a substantial degree of metabolic autosufficiency that enables them to survive isolated from their neighbors (4). The absence of expression of the cornea-specific 64-kD protein K3 and expression of keratin-19 are unique features of limbal stem cells. The stem cells have a capacity to self-renew and generate transient amplifying cells that are positioned in the basal cell layer of the corneal epithelium. Unlike suprabasal corneal epithelial cells, both stem cells and transient amplifying cells are characterized by prolonged retention of H-labeled thymidine under stimulation by a tumor promoter (1,2,5). The transient amplifying cells maintain a high capacity for proliferation, but unlike stem cells, their life span is reduced to several months. Stem cells and transient amplifying cells form the proliferative tissue compartment (6). The remaining corneal epithelial cells, located in suprabasal layers, are terminally differentiated cells with a life span of approximately 1 week. Unlike limbal grafts that contain stem cells, penetrating and lamellar corneal grafts contain only transient amplifying and terminally differentiated cells (7). Limbal epithelial cells (but not conjunctival epithelial cells) inhibit fibroblast-stimulated angiogenesis and may therefore play a role in the maintenance of corneal avascularity (8).

Corneal surface reconstruction by transplanting a graft from other ocular surface epithelium was first reported in 1977 by Thoft, who used autologous contralateral conjunctiva in patients with severe unilateral alkali burn (9). Six years later, Thoft proposed transplantation of limbal corneal epithelium from fresh cadaver eyes and called this procedure *keratoepithelioplasty* (10). Kenyon and Tseng then described a series of patients with "limbal stem cell transplantation" in 1989 (11), and since then, many others have used this procedure successfully in patients with a spectrum of disorders characterized by limbal stem cell deficiency (Table 59-1).

Limbal stem cell deficiency can present with clinical signs of persistent corneal epithelial defect, neovascularization, "conjunctivalization," scarring, stromal ulcer, calcification, and band keratopathy (12–17). The most common symptoms of limbal stem cell deficiency are decreased vision, photophobia, tearing, blepharospasm, recurrent pain, and redness.

Chronic inflammation of the conjunctiva, conjunctival scarring, symblepharon formation, trichiasis, distichiasis, meibomian gland dysfunction, and lacrimal gland inflammation are all factors that can lead to tear film abnormalities and ultimately to damage to limbal stem cells and corneal epithelium that can present as persistent epithelial defect, corneal scarring, and neovascularization (18). These factors can compromise limbal stem cells and exacerbate limbal stem cell insufficiency. Therefore, they need to be identified and eliminated to the maximum possible extent before limbal stem cell grafting to increase the graft survival time. The data indicating that success rates of limbal stem cell transplantation performed several months after burn injury may be higher compared with earlier transplantation (19) further support the idea that limbal stem cell transplantation in inflamed eyes should be avoided.

TABLE 59-1. INDICATIONS FOR LIMBAL STEM CELL TRANSPLANTATION

Aniridia
Chemical burns
Chronic keratoconjunctivitis
Chronic limbitis
Contact lens-induced epitheliopathy
Cryotherapy
5-Fluorouracil-induced limbal stem cell deficiency
Multiple surgeries
Neurotrophic keratopathy
Ocular cicatricial pemphigoid
Radiation
Severe microbial keratitis
Squamous cell carcinoma
Stevens-Johnson's syndrome
Subepithelial amyloidosis
Systemic cytotoxic therapy (hydroxyurea)
Thermal burns
Trachoma

SURGICAL TECHNIQUE AND PERIOPERATIVE MANAGEMENT

Chronic inflammation of the conjunctiva, conjunctival scarring, symblepharon formation, trichiasis, distichiasis, meibomian gland dysfunction, and lacrimal gland inflammation are all factors that can lead to tear film abnormalities and ultimately to a damage to limbal stem cells and corneal epithelium that can present as persistent epithelial defect, corneal scarring and neovascularization (18). These factors can compromise limbal stem cells and exacerbate limbal stem cell insufficiency. Therefore, such factors must be identified and eliminated to the maximum possible extent prior to limbal stem cell grafting; otherwise, the grafted tissue will be damaged and will probably not survive. The data indicating that success rate of limbal stem cell transplantation performed several months after burn injury may be higher compared to earlier transplantation (19) further support the idea that limbal stem cell transplantation in inflamed eyes should be avoided.

After peribulbar anesthesia, a 360-degree peritomy is performed on the recipient eye. Abnormal epithelium is removed from the cornea, and a superficial keratectomy is performed to ensure a smooth surface.

Attention is then paid to the donor eye. After peribulbar anesthesia, a 15 degree supersharp blade is used to outline the corneal portion of donor lenticle approximately 1 mm from the limbus and spanning 2 clock hours circumferentially. Vannas scissors are used to dissect the conjunctival portion of the lenticle, approximately 2 mm posterior to the limbus. One edge of the lenticle is lifted with forceps and dissected, as a lamellar dissection, from its remaining attachment at the limbus and cornea, and the donor graft is immediately placed in balanced salt solution. After harvesting one to three lenticles (a maximum of 6 clock hours), an antibiotic and steroid ointment is applied onto

the surface of the donor eye and the eye is pressure patched until the following day.

The donor lenticles are then placed onto the limbal area of the recipient eye and secured to the cornea with 10–0 nylon sutures and to the episclera using 10–0 polyglactin sutures. An amniotic membrane graft may be placed to cover the entire corneal surface at the surgeon's discretion and sutured to the episclera and conjunctiva with 10–0 polyglactin sutures. An 18-mm hydrophilic bandage contact lens is placed onto the ocular surface at the end of the procedure.

Topical steroids and antibiotics are applied regularly in the postoperative period. The antibiotic drops are discontinued after the epithelium has healed and the bandage contact lens has been removed. The steroid drops, administered every hour for the first week after surgery, are tapered gradually and discontinued when inflammation has subsided. Systemic immunosuppressive therapy to prevent graft rejection is indicated in patients with limbal stem cell allograft. Additional use of autologous serum drops in the postoperative period may enhance corneal reepithelialization (20) (Fig. 59-1).

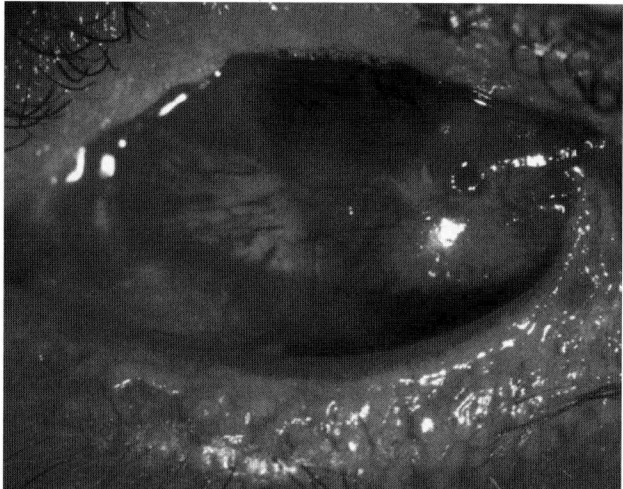

A

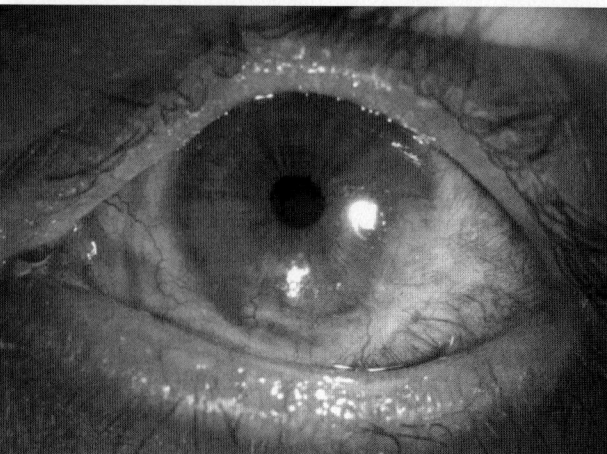

B

FIGURE 59-1. A patient with history of toxic epidermal necrolysis before **(A)** and 6 months after **(B)** limbal stem cell allotransplantation.

COMPLICATIONS

Limbal stem cell transplantation has an excellent safety record. Only scattered intraoperative and postoperative complications have been reported. Immune rejection reaction and limbal stem cell graft failure are the most common postoperative complications in the recipient eye. Increased intraocular pressure after limbal stem cell transplantation, believed to be related to the use of steroids in the postoperative period, was reported in up to 37% of patients after limbal stem cell transplantation (21). This observation suggests an early institution of steroid-sparing therapy to prevent the immune rejection reaction. An infectious keratitis complicating the postoperative period may compromise limbal stem cells and lead to a permanent limbal stem cell failure (22). Corneal epithelial cells differentiated from donor-derived limbal stem cells repopulate the corneal surface after limbal stem cell transplantation (23). Donor-derived epithelial cells are present on the corneal surface much longer after limbal stem cell transplantation than after penetrating keratoplasty alone (23). The size of the donor graft may play a role in graft sufficiency (24). Although reepithelialization of the corneal surface with total limbal stem cell deficiency can occur with limbal stem cell grafts 5 mm long or smaller (24), these grafts are less efficient than 7- to 10-mm limbal grafts (24,25). However, even with larger limbal grafts, graft function can be compromised over time (26,27). The duration of postoperative limbal stem cell survival is limited by several factors, such as persistent inflammation, dry eye, and progressive rejection of the limbal stem cell graft (28). A limbal stem cell graft is considered to have failed if signs of stem cell deficiency are present.

Few cases of intraoperative or postoperative complications have been reported in donor eyes. These include microperforation (29), donor filamentary keratitis (30), epitheliopathy in a patient with history of contact lens wear (31), pseudopterygium (32,33), "abnormal epithelium" (25), and "corneal depression" (34).

AUTOLOGOUS LIMBAL STEM CELL TRANSPLANTATION

Autologous limbal stem cell grafts can be used in patients with unilateral limbal stem cell deficiency or in patients with limbal stem cell deficiency limited to a small portion of the limbus (e.g., pterygium). The autologous graft can be obtained either from the healthy fellow eye or from the affected eye. The choice of donor eye is made according to the extent and etiology of limbal stem cell deficiency. Three clock hours of limbal stem cell autograft were successfully removed and transplanted to a different area of the limbus of the same eye in a patient with recurrent pterygium (30) (Fig. 59-2). The major advantage of autologous grafting is

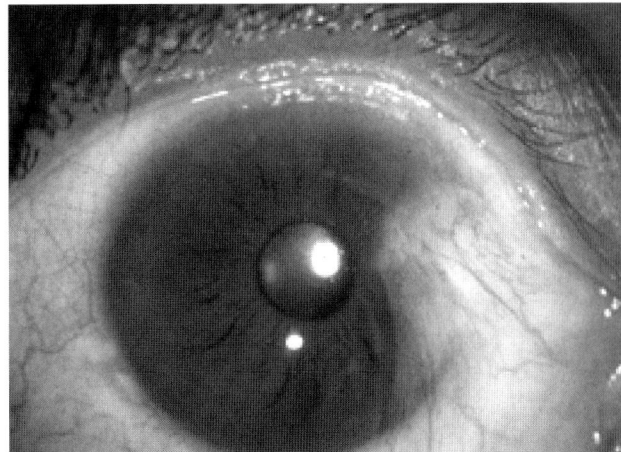

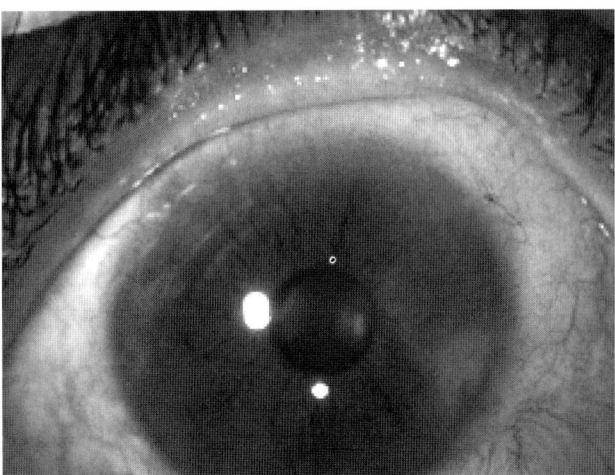

FIGURE 59-2. A patient with recurrent pterygium before **(A)** and 6 months after **(B)** limbal stem cell autotransplantation from the same eye.

avoidance of immunosuppressive therapy to prevent the immune rejection reaction. When total limbal stem cell deficiency is present only in one eye, limbal stem cell grafts can be obtained from the fellow eye (11).

ALLOGENIC LIMBAL STEM CELL TRANSPLANTATION

If limbal stem cell deficiency involves both eyes, corneal surface reconstruction depends on an allogenic source of limbal stem cells. The allogenic graft can be obtained either from living donors (35,36) or from cadaveric donors (20,25,35,37). It is generally accepted that harvesting of up to 6 clock hours of limbal stem cells is considered to be safe in a normal, healthy living donor eye. Special attention needs to be paid to the donor eye during the preoperative slit-lamp examination. Subtle signs such as alteration or loss of palisades of Vogt from the inferior limbus may be indicative of damage to the limbus (14). Preoperative impression cytology of the donor corneal epithelium is recommended in cases suspect for limbal stem cell deficiency (19). The presence of goblet cells on the cornea is a sign of compromised limbal stem cell function, and harvesting limbal stem cells from such a donor eye should be avoided (38). The advantage of using a cadaver donor eye is that all limbal stem cells can be harvested.

Because the conjunctiva and limbus are vascularized and the content of antigen-presenting cells is high in these tissues, human leukocyte antigen (HLA) matching (three-locus HLA-A, HLA-B, and HLA-C match and two-locus HLA-D match) plays an important role in graft survival (7,39). The allograft is preferably harvested from a patient's relative (especially brother or sister) with the closest HLA match. Data indicate that even an unmatched limbal stem cell graft from an HLA-matched living relative can provide some level of immune histocompatibility (39), which may reduce the dose of immunosuppressive drugs required to prevent immune rejection reaction of the graft. The 18-month survival rate of limbal stem cell grafts obtained from a living related donor is between 77.8% (24) and 91.6% (39) if no immunosuppressive agents are used. The limbal stem cell graft survival rate can be increased by use of systemic immunosuppressive agents (36). Interestingly, the rate of immune rejection reaction when no prophylactic cyclosporine is used in the postoperative period is between 25% (39) and 33.3% (24), and does not differ if cyclosporine is used as monotherapy (36). The immune rejection reaction is typically treated with high-dose systemic and topical corticosteroids and an increase in the dose of immunosuppressive agents. Successful reconstruction of the ocular surface with limbal stem cell graft obtained from an HLA-matched donor without subsequent immunosuppressive therapy has been reported (25), but data obtained during a long-term follow-up indicate that even if HLA-matched living related limbal allografts are used, immunosuppressive therapy is recommended because such therapy does prolong allograft survival (23,24). Using an HLA-unmatched limbal stem cell graft typically leads to failure to reconstruct the ocular surface (24).

Despite the use of systemic immunosuppression, the graft survival rate after allogenic limbal stem cell transplantation declines from 75% to 80% (20,25,37) 1 year after transplantation to 50% (21), 5 years after the surgery. An additional penetrating keratoplasty performed at the time of limbal stem cell transplantation may further compromise the outcome (21,35,40–42). The survival rate of limbal stem cell grafts in such cases declines even more, from 70% to 80%, 1 to 2 years after surgery (25,28,35,37,40,43) to 47.4%, 3 years after surgery (28).

Recognizing the clinical signs of limbal stem cell graft rejection is difficult. Limbal ischemia and presence of engorged limbal vessels were described as early signs of limbal stem cell graft rejection (20,24). Although these signs may be reversible with the use of topical and systemic immunosuppressive therapy, their clinical relevance remains controversial (44). Often, however, the therapeutic intervention for presumed immune rejection reaction needs to be empirical to prevent stem cell graft failure.

The primary advantage of using a cadaver donor eye is that one may harvest a 360-degree circular limbal stem cell graft. The circular limbal stem cell graft prevents invasion of conjunctival epithelium onto the corneal surface more efficiently than do segmental limbal stem cell grafts (23). Some data suggest that transplantation of limbal stem cell grafts from a cadaver donor may be associated with reduction in graft survival to 49% (21) compared with 55% (22), 3 years after surgery when a limbal stem cell graft from a living related donor is used. Limbal stem cell transplantation may be capable of restoring corneal clarity and satisfactorily increasing the visual acuity in some cases, but in others subsequent or concurrent procedures for vision rehabilitation, such as penetrating or lamellar keratoplasty, are required. Patients who are likely to require penetrating or lamellar keratoplasty after limbal stem cell transplantation and who are receiving the limbal stem cell graft from a cadaver donor may benefit from a one-stage procedure that obtains both the limbal stem graft and corneal graft from the same donor (41). However, the likelihood of endothelial immune rejection reaction if limbal stem cell grafting is performed at the same time as lamellar or penetrating keratoplasty from the same donor may be higher (40,44,45): approximately 35.6% (44) to 64.3% (40) compared with rejection rates after sequential limbal stem cell grafting and penetrating keratoplasty despite the use of topical corticosteroids and cyclosporine and systemic immunosuppressive therapy (44). In addition, these patients may require higher doses or a combination of systemic immunosuppressive drugs.

When penetrating keratoplasty is performed at the same session with limbal stem cell transplantation, the survival of both grafts appears to be shorter compared with performing these procedures in two sessions (28,44). If penetrating keratoplasty is performed simultaneously with limbal stem cell transplantation, endothelial immune rejection reaction develops in 36% to 46% (21,44). One study showed that none of the corneal grafts survived 5 years after surgery if the two procedures were performed simultaneously (28). The poor prognosis of central corneal graft survival is speculated to be caused by increased exposure of the host immune system to the donor antigens. Moreover, the penetrating keratoplasty may enhance the wound healing response and inflammation, which may alter stem cell survival (28). For these reasons, some propose waiting at least 3 months after limbal stem cell transplantation before performing penetrating keratoplasty (28,47). Interestingly, the survival rate of a second limbal stem cell graft can be 2.5-fold greater than that of the first limbal stem cell graft combined with penetrating keratoplasty (28). The disadvantage of performing penetrating keratoplasty later after limbal stem cell transplantation is additional antigenic stimulation (41) associated with an increased risk of immune rejection and removal of transient amplifying cells (24).

The mechanisms by which limbal stem cell grafts maintain an intact corneal surface remain unclear (48). The amount of donor-derived cells in the suprabasal epithelial cell layers was found to be very limited despite the use of immunosuppressive therapy and a stable corneal surface (48). These data suggest that success of limbal stem cell transplantation may not directly correlate with the number of donor-derived suprabasal corneal epithelial cells. It is also noteworthy that, according to one report, immunohistologic studies from corneas after limbal stem cell graft rejection were not able to detect any epithelial cells with the corneal phenotype (49).

Failure of primary epithelialization of the corneal surface and severe ocular inflammation are poor prognostic factors for limbal stem cell graft survival (36). Hence, the factors that contribute to the pathogenesis of corneal epithelial disease should be eliminated to the greatest possible extent before attempting to restore the corneal surface with limbal stem cell grafts.

The limbal stem cell graft survival rate in patients with Stevens-Johnson syndrome is particularly diminished (22,24,28,35,36,39). A higher frequency of immune rejection reaction, probably secondary to recurrent or chronic immune-driven inflammation of the ocular surface, may account for the decreased survival rate in this group of patients (50).

LIMBAL STEM CELL TRANSPLANTATION WITH AMNIOTIC MEMBRANE TRANSPLANTATION

Results of limbal stem cell transplantation combined with amniotic membrane grafting were reported in several clinical studies (40,51–54). Amniotic membrane graft may help restore corneal epithelium in partial limbal stem cell deficiency (40,53–55), but amniotic membrane graft is insufficient in case of total limbal stem cell deficiency (40,55). In such cases, limbal stem cell transplantation with or without amniotic membrane grafting is required. Combined amniotic membrane and limbal stem cell transplantation may result in vision restoration. Additional surgical procedures, such as penetrating or lamellar keratoplasty, also may be required (52).

The amnion theoretically may affect the environment of the limbal stem cell graft by reducing alloreactive T-cell infiltration (56), but the *in vivo* benefit has not been shown in an experimental model (57). The data suggest that amniotic membrane denuded of epithelial cells may be more efficient in transmitting signals to the migrating epithelial cells and enhancing their differentiation from stem cells into transient amplifying cells compared with amniotic membrane with epithelium (58). The clinical significance of this observation is yet to be established. At the very least, however, amnion functions well as a biologic bandage, protecting freshly transplanted limbal stem cells.

EX VIVO LIMBAL STEM CELL EXPANSION

The use of *ex vivo* limbal stem cell transplants cultured on human amniotic membrane as a substrate opened a new avenue in ocular surface reconstruction (59). The principle of this procedure lies in culturing corneal limbal epithelial cells obtained from a donor eye on the surface of amniotic membrane, thereby expanding the number of cells to be transplanted onto the ocular surface. The source of limbal epithelial cells can be either a cadaver donor eye or a living fellow or donor eye. Systemic immunosuppressive therapy is required in the case of allografting (60). The amniotic membrane is capable of maintaining and expanding limbal epithelial stem cells that retain their *in vivo* properties of slow cycling and undifferentiation (61,62). The phenotype of the resultant epithelium is limbal, but the architecture is similar to that of the corneal epithelium (63). Although the results of clinical and experimental studies (59–66) of *in vivo* limbal stem cells expanded on amniotic membrane seem to be similar to the ones using conventional single-donor limbal stem cell grafts, the major benefit of *in vivo* grafts probably lies in minimal trauma to the donor limbal stem cells, or no trauma if *in vitro* bioengineered limbal stem cell lines are used. This fact may account for rapid expansion of the novel technique in clinical practice in the future.

CONCLUSION

Limbal stem cell transplantation is a safe and effective technique for reconstruction of the corneal epithelium in patients with limbal stem cell deficiency. The success rate of this technique depends on limbal stem cell survival, which is limited not only by the well-being of the ocular surface, but also by immune system-mediated graft rejection. The data suggest that autologous limbal stem cell grafts should be used whenever possible. If allotransplantation is unavoidable, the donor, preferably a close relative, should be selected based on HLA match results. Allograft survival can be increased by long-term immunosuppressive therapy.

Perforating keratoplasty represents an additional risk factor for immune rejection reaction that typically leads to a decrease in limbal stem cell graft survival. Therefore, it should be avoided in cases when limbal stem cell grafting results in good corneal clarity and satisfactory vision rehabilitation.

The data suggest that if limbal stem cell grafting alone does not provide good vision rehabilitation and perforating keratoplasty is required, a two-step rather than simultaneous procedure is preferred. After successful limbal stem cell allografting in one eye, allografting in the second eye, although very tempting, should be avoided. A limbal stem cell allograft in the second eye will most likely induce immune rejection, typically leading to failure of both allografts.

Some patients require one or more additional limbal stem cell transplantations during their lifetime. The availability of donor tissue with a good HLA match is a major limiting factor in such cases. The recent development and transplantation of *in vitro* bioengineered limbal stem cell grafts represents a promising source of donor tissue in the future.

REFERENCES

1. Schermer A, Galvin S, Sun TT. Differentiation-related expression of a major 64K corneal keratin *in vivo* and in culture suggests limbal location of corneal epithelial stem cells. *J Cell Biol* 1986;103:49–62.
2. Cotsarelis G, Cheng SZ, Dong G, et al. Existence of slow-cycling limbal epithelial basal cells that can be preferentially stimulated to proliferate: implications on epithelial stem cells. *Cell* 1989;57:201–209.
3. Thoft RA, Friend J. The X, Y, Z hypothesis of corneal epithelial maintenance. *Invest Ophthalmol Vis Sci* 1983;24:1442–1443.
4. Matic M, Petrov IN, Chen S, et al. Stem cells of the corneal epithelium lack connexins and metabolite transfer capacity. *Differentiation* 1997;61:251–260.
5. Kasper M, Moll R, Stosiec P, et al. Patterns of cytokeratin and vimentin expression in the human eye. *Histochemistry* 1988;89:369–373.
6. Jensen PKA, Pedersen S, Bolund L. Basal-cell subpopulations and cell cycle kinetics in human epidermal explant cultures. *Cell Tissue Kinet* 1985;18:201–215.
7. Holland E, Schwartz G. The evolution of epithelial transplantation for severe ocular surface disease and a proposed classification system. *Cornea* 1996;15:549–556.
8. Ma DH, Tsai RJ, Chu WK, et al. Inhibition of vascular endothelial cell morphogenesis in cultures by limbal epithelial cells. *Invest Ophthalmol Vis Sci* 1999;40:1822–1828.
9. Thoft RA. Conjunctival transplantation. *Arch Ophthalmol* 1977;95:425–427.
10. Thoft RA. Keratoepithelioplasty. *Am J Ophthalmol* 1984;97:1–6.
11. Kenyon KR, Tseng SCG. Limbal autograft transplantation for ocular surface disorders. *Ophthalmology* 1989;96:709–723.
12. Kruse EF. Stem cells and corneal regeneration. *Eye* 1994;8:170–183.
13. Nishida K, Kinoshita S, Ohashi Y, et al. Ocular surface abnormalities in aniridia. *Am J Ophthalmol* 1995;120:368–375.
14. Chen JJY, Tseng SCG. Corneal epithelial wound healing in partial limbal deficiency. *Invest Ophthalmol Vis Sci* 1990;31:1301–1314.
15. Huang AJW, Tseng SCG. Corneal epithelial wound healing in the absence of limbal epithelium. *Invest Ophthalmol Vis Sci* 1991;32:96–105.
16. Kenyon KR, Bulusoglu G, Ziske JD. Clinical pathologic correlations of limbal autograft transplantation. *Am J Ophthalmol* 1990;31:1.
17. Kinoshita S, Kiorpes T, Friend J, et al. Limbal epithelium in ocular surface wound healing. *Invest Ophthalmol Vis Sci* 1982;23:73–80.
18. Chan RY, Foster CS. A step-wise approach to ocular surface rehabilitation in patients with ocular inflammatory diseases. *Int Ophthalmol Clin* 1999;39:83–108.
19. Basti S, Rao S. Current Status of limbal conjunctival autograft. *Curr Opin Ophthalmol* 2000;11:224–232.
20. Tsai RJF, Tseng SCG. Human allograft limbal transplantation for corneal surface reconstruction. *Cornea* 1994;13:389–400.
21. Tsubota K, Satake Y, Kaido M, et al. Treatment of severe ocular surface disorders with corneal epithelial stem-cell transplantation. *N Engl J Med* 1999;340:1697–1703.
22. Samson CM, Nduaguba C, Baltatzis S, et al. Limbal stem cell transplantation in chronic inflammatory eye disease. *Ophthalmology* 2002;109:862–868.
23. Shimazaki J, Kaido M, Shinozaki N, et al. Evidence of long-term survival of donor-derived cells after limbal allograft transplantation. *Invest Ophthalmol Vis Sci* 1999;40:1664–1668.
24. Rao SK, Rajagopal R, Sitalakshmi G, et al. Limbal allografting from related live donors for corneal surface reconstruction. *Ophthalmology* 1999;106:822–828.
25. Tan DTH, Ficker LA, Buckley RJ. Limbal transplantation. *Ophthalmology* 1996;103:29–36
26. Shimazaki J, Yang HY, Tsubota K. Amniotic membrane transplantation for ocular surface reconstruction in patients with chemical and thermal burns. *Ophthalmology* 1997;104:2068–2076.
27. Henderson TRM, McCall SH, Taylor GR, et al. Do transplanted corneal limbal stem cells survive in vivo long-term? Possible techniques to detect donor cell survival by polymerase chain reaction with the amelogenin gene and Y-specific probes. *Eye* 1997;11:779–785.
28. Solomon A, Ellies P, Anderson DF, et al. Long-term outcome of keratolimbal allograft with or without penetrating keratoplasty for total limbal stem cell deficiency. *Ophthalmology* 2002;109:1159–1166.
29. Morgan S, Murray A. Limbal auto-transplantation in the acute and chronic phases of severe chemical injuries. *Eye* 1996;10:349–354.
30. Dua HS, Azuara-Blanco A. Autologous limbal transplantation in patients with unilateral corneal stem cell deficiency. *Br J Ophthalmol* 2000;84:273–278.
31. Jenkins C, Tuft S, Liu C, et al. Limbal transplantation in the management of chronic contact lens-associated epitheliopathy. *Eye* 1993;7:629–633
32. Gris O, Güell JL, del Campo Z. Limbal-conjunctival autograft transplantation for the treatment of recurrent pterygium. *Ophthalmology* 2000;107:270–273.
33. Basti S, Mathur U. Unusual intermediate-term outcome in three cases of limbal autograft transplantation. *Ophthalmology* 1999;106:958–963.
34. Shimazaki J, Shinozaki N, Tsubota K. Transplantation of amniotic membrane and limbal autograft for patients with recurrent pterygium associated with symblepharon. *Br J Ophthalmol* 1998;82:235–240.
35. Holland EJ. Epithelial transplantation for the management of severe ocular surface disease. *Trans Am Ophthalmol Soc* 1996;94:677–743.
36. Daya SM, Ilari L. Living related conjunctival limbal allograft for the treatment of stem cell deficiency. *Ophthalmology* 2001;108:126–134.
37. Tsubota K, Toda I, Saito H, et al. Reconstruction of the corneal epithelium by limbal allograft transplantation for severe ocular surface disorders. *Ophthalmology* 1995;102:1486–1496.
38. Prabhasawat P, Tseng SC. Impression cytology study of epithelial phenotype of ocular surface reconstructed by preserved human amniotic membrane. *Arch Ophthalmol* 1997;115:1360–1367.

39. Kwitko S, Marinho D, Barcaro S, et al. Allograft conjunctival transplantation for bilateral ocular surface disorders. *Ophthalmology* 1995;102:1020–1025.

40. Tseng SCG, Prabhasawat P, Barton K, et al. Amniotic membrane transplantation with or without limbal allografts for corneal surface reconstruction in patients with limbal stem cell deficiency. *Arch Ophthalmol* 1998;116:431–441.

41. Theng JTS, Tan DTH. Combined penetrating keratoplasty and limbal allograft transplantation for severe corneal burns. *Ophthalmic Surg Lasers* 1997;28:765–768.

42. Tsubota K, Shimazaki J. Surgical treatment of children blinded by Stevens-Johnson's syndrome. *Am J Ophthalmol* 1999;128: 573–581.

43. Tsubota K, Satake Y, Ohyama M, et al. Surgical reconstruction of the ocular surface in advanced ocular cicatricial pemphigoid and Stevens-Johnson's syndrome. *Am J Ophthalmol* 1996;122: 38–52.

44. Shimazaki J, Maruyama F, Shimmura S, et al. Immunological rejection of the central graft following combined limbal allograft transplantation and penetrating keratoplasty. *Cornea* 2001;20: 149–152.

45. Maguire MG, Stark WJ, Gottsch JD, et al. Risk factors for corneal graft failure and rejection in the Collaborative Corneal Transplantation studies. *Ophthalmology* 1994;101:1536–1547.

46. Hill JC. Systemic cyclosporine in high-risk keratoplasty: long-term results. *Eye* 1995;9:422–428.

47. Croasdale CR, Schwartz GS, Malling JV, et al. Keratolimbal allograft: recommendations for tissue procurement and preparation by eye banks, and standard surgical technique. *Cornea* 1999;18:52–58.

48. Henderson TRM, Coster DJ, Williams KA. The long term outcome of limbal allografts: the search for surviving cells. *Br J Ophthalmol* 2001;85:604–609.

49. Daya SM, Bell RWD, Habib NE, et al. Clinical and pathologic findings in human keratolimbal allograft rejection. *Cornea* 2000; 19:443–450.

50. Foster CS, Fong LP, Azar DT, et al. Episodic conjunctival inflammation after Stevens-Johnson syndrome. *Ophthalmology* 1988; 95:453–462.

51. Meallet MA, Espana EM, Grueterich M, et al. Amniotic membrane transplantation with conjunctival limbal autograft for total limbal stem cell deficiency. *Ophthalmology* 2003;110: 1585–1592.

52. Stoiber J, Ruckhofer J, Muss W, et al. Amniotic membrane transplantation with limbal stem cell transplantation as a combined procedure for corneal surface reconstruction after severe thermal or chemical burns). *Ophthalmologe* 2002;99: 839–848.

53. Anderson DF, Ellies P, Pires RT, et al. Amniotic membrane transplantation for partial limbal stem cell deficiency. *Br J Ophthalmol* 2001;85:567–575.

54. Pires RT, Chokshi A, Tseng TS. Amniotic membrane transplantation or conjunctival limbal autograft for limbal stem cell deficiency induced by 5-fluorouracil in glaucoma surgeries. *Cornea* 2000;19:284–287.

55. Gomes JA, dos Santos MS, Cunha MC, et al. Amniotic membrane transplantation for partial and total limbal stem cell deficiency secondary to chemical burn. *Ophthalmology*. 2003;110: 466–473.

56. Ueta M, Kweon MN, Sano Y, et al. Immunosuppressive properties of human amniotic membrane for mixed lymphocyte reaction. *Clin Exp Immunol* 2002;129:464–470.

57. Marinho D, Hofling-Lima AL, Kwitko S, et al. Does amniotic membrane transplantation improve the outcome of autologous limbal transplantation? *Cornea* 2003;22:338–342.

58. Grueterich M, Espana EM, Touhami A, et al. Phenotypic study of a case with successful transplantation of ex vivo expanded human limbal epithelium for unilateral total limbal stem cell deficiency. *Ophthalmology* 2002;109:1547–1552.

59. Koizumi N, Inatomi T, Quantock AJ, et al. Amniotic membrane as a substrate for cultivating limbal corneal epithelial cells for autologous transplantation in rabbits. *Cornea* 2000;19:65–71.

60. Koizumi N, Inatomi T, Suzuki T, et al. Cultivated corneal epithelial stem cell transplantation in ocular surface disorders. *Ophthalmology* 2001;108:1569–1574.

61. Grueterich M, Tseng SC. Human limbal progenitor cells expanded on intact amniotic membrane ex vivo. *Arch Ophthalmol* 2002;120:783–790.

62. Meller D, Pires RT, Tseng SC. Ex vivo preservation and expansion of human limbal epithelial stem cells on amniotic membrane cultures. *Br J Ophthalmol* 2002;86:463–471.

63. Grueterich M, Espana EM, Touhami A, et al. Phenotypic study of a case with successful transplantation of ex vivo expanded human limbal epithelium for unilateral total limbal stem cell deficiency. *Ophthalmology* 2002;109:1547–1552.

64. Ti SE, Anderson D, Touhami A, et al. Factors affecting outcome following transplantation of ex vivo expanded limbal epithelium on amniotic membrane for total limbal deficiency in rabbits. *Invest Ophthalmol Vis Sci* 2002;43:2584–2592.

65. Shimazaki J, Aiba M, Goto E, et al. Transplantation of human limbal epithelium cultivated on amniotic membrane for the treatment of severe ocular surface disorders. *Ophthalmology* 2002;109:1285–1290.

66. Cohen EJ. Use of autologous limbal epithelial cells cultured on amniotic membranes for unilateral stem cell deficiency. *Arch Ophthalmol* 2001;119:123–124.

PTERYGIUM AND ITS SURGERY

GURINDER SINGH

DEFINITION

Pterygium (From the Greek *pterygos*, meaning "wing"; plural, "pterygia") is a triangular, wing-shaped, degenerative, fibrovascular, hyperplastic proliferative tissue actively growing from the conjunctival limbal area onto the cornea (Fig. 60-1). Usually it is preceded by pinguecula (from the Latin *pinguis*, "fat"; plural, "pingueculae"), which itself is a degenerative tissue involving conjunctiva and underlying episclera. Pterygium is usually a raised leash of fibrovascular conjunctival tissue that grows very gradually onto cornea in the interpalpebral area. It continues to grow toward the center of the cornea, mostly from the nasal side, but it can come from the temporal side; it rarely grows from both nasal and temporal sides simultaneously.

HISTORY

According to Bidyadhar (1,2), Rosenthal (3), Thomas (4), and Jaros and DeLuise (5), the first recorded description of pterygium and the surgical procedure to treat it was by Susruta, the world's first surgeon-ophthalmologist, who lived in India around 1000 B.C. Since then, Celsus (29 A.D.), Vagblat (third to fourth century), Paul (600 A.D.), Rhazes (932 A.D.), Avicenna (1037 A.D.), Chakradatta (1060 A.D.), and others have described it in detail (3,6). Almost all of these authors suggested surgical treatment for the condition with modifications to the original procedure recommended by Susruta.

Numerous practitioners, including Merigot de Teigny, Coirre, Aëtius, Hippocrates, Celsus, Galen, Archigenes, Saint-Yves, Maitre Jean, Desmarres, Gonin, and others, attempted medical treatment of pterygium. They tried various forms of collyrium of lead, zinc, copper, iron, bile, urine, women's milk, white wine, vinegar, candied sugar, water of Euphrasia, cuttlefish bone, silver nitrate, lead acetate, mercuric lanoline, and others (3,4,6).

Similarly, many surgical procedures have been described, tried, and advocated since the time of Susruta. Many surgeons have warned of the dangers of the procedures, and have advised temporizing as long as vision was not impaired. Some have recommended surgery only if the patient was "esthetically tormented" (3). Celsus of Rome (around 1 A.D.) used a scalpel to remove pterygium from the cornea after lifting it from the sclera with a thread passed beneath it. Paul of Aegineta used horsehair to saw it from its attachments. Ali bin Isa, of Baghdad, recognized two types of pterygia, and recommended surgery only for the hard, red type and not for the soft, delicate type (3). Ali bin Isa recommended putting the patient to sleep for the surgery, which suggests that Arabs may have been the first to use general anesthesia. Acrel (1771) was the first to perform total removal of the head of pterygium from the cornea and circumscribe it with the bistoury (3).

It seems that Scarpa in 1802 was the first to perform a kind of bare-sclera excision of pterygium, later performed by Travers (1805), Westhoff, Peterquin, Pellier de Opinsy, and Rubio. Bell (1813), Woolhouse, and Beer recommended cauterization and scarification of the pterygium. Grandelement used chromic acid, McCallan used carbonic snow, Ajily-Bay-Haydar used silver nitrate, and Shaugnessy used nitric acid to treat pterygia (3). Coccius, and later Arlt, successfully closed the conjunctival resection baresclera area with sutures in an attempt to prevent recurrence of the pterygium. Weller (1832) and Walton (1853) transfixed the neck of the pterygium with a thread passed underneath, and then cut the corneal attachment and the base of the growth, extirpating the growth. Arlt (1850) removed a rhomboid of tissue and closed the wound in a cruciate manner (3).

The elder Desmarres (7) devised the procedure of transplantation of the pterygium for the purpose of diverting the growth from the cornea into the adjacent lower fornix. He mobilized a small flap of conjunctiva that was sutured between the mobilized pterygium and the corneal margin. The pterygium atrophied after this procedure, and that established a principle used in all transplantation operations. Terrien brought the pterygium growth upward to the upper fornix. Knapp (1868) bisected the growth and pulled the upper half superiorly and the lower half inferiorly. Hobbs (1894) introduced the use of galvanocautery

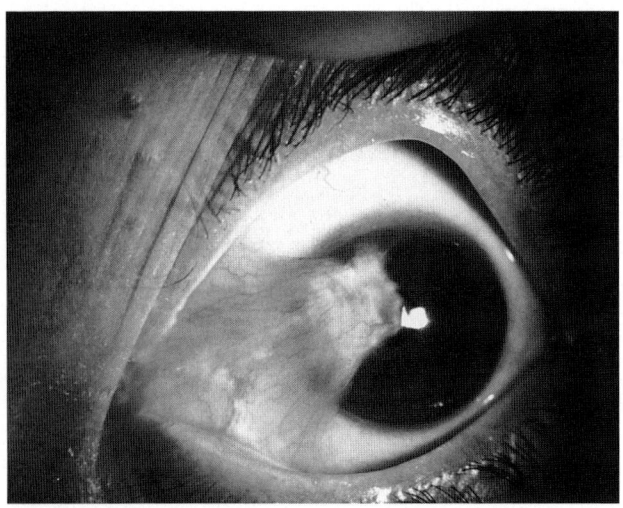

FIGURE 60-1. Primary nasal pterygium growing into visual axis.

(52 V) for cutting across the neck of the pterygium, and Coe (1896) and Loring advocated the use of thermal cautery with a heated platinum wire (3).

Free tissue grafts to cover the bare sclera after pterygium excision were introduced by Klein in 1876. He used mucous membrane grafts in cases in which insufficient bulbar conjunctiva was left after pterygium excision to cover bare sclera (3). Gifford (1909), Cozalis (1920), Duverger (1926), Green (1937), and Dosorova (1942) also used these grafts. In 1888, Hobby mobilized adjacent conjunctiva to cover bare sclera. Elschnig covered the bare sclera with a pedicle conjunctival flap graft. Hotz (1892) used the Thiersh grafts with success (3). Gifford used these grafts in recurrent pterygia. Autografting with free fragments of conjunctiva was used by de Gama Pinto, Gomez-Marques, and de Paula Xavier. In 1931, Mata covered the denuded area after pterygium excision with buccal mucous membrane (8). Hawley, in 1911, introduced the use of superficial thin skin grafts from behind the ear or from the thigh, and reaffirmed his procedure in 1937 (9,10). Morax and Magitot, in 1911, tried the use of artificially preserved homografts from the corneas of fetuses and adults, the early forms of corneal grafting. Terson of Paris first referred to the use of radiation treatment after pterygium excision in 1911(11). Burnam and Neill, in 1940, described their use of radon to prevent pterygium recurrence. Since then, Ruedemann, Iliff, Swanberg, Hughes, and many others have used radium, radon, and beta irradiation as adjunctive treatment to pterygium excision (3).

The procedure of "subvolution" was devised by Galezowski in 1880, tried by Numar, and named by Bettman in 1894 (12). It involved freeing the head and neck of the pterygium and folding it under the body of the pterygium and suturing the edges. Avulsion of a pterygium head from the cornea with a muscle hook occurred accidentally while Prince in 1885 was performing another procedure. A similar

accident happened to Wright in 1888. Wright has recorded a case of a patient who pulled his own pterygium from his cornea with "eye tweezers," without anesthesia, and with excellent results (3). Boeckman, in 1885, suggested recession of conjunctival edges after excision of the head to the pterygium and suturing the conjunctival edges to their new position, leaving behind bare sclera to reepithelialize by itself (13).

Rosenthal has concluded his article on the chronology of pterygium therapy by saying

> down through history were many who practiced and reported upon various operative techniques without making any outstanding contributions. They number in hundreds and their names may be found in the literature of all nations and all ages. And so it appears that for about 30 centuries man has tried to conquer this little growth called pterygium. It had been incised, removed, split, transplanted, excised, cauterized, grafted, inverted, galvanized, heated, dissected, rotated, coagulated, repositioned, and irradiated. It has been analyzed statistically, geographically, etiologically, microscopically, and chemically—yet it grows onward primarily and secondarily. We look with interest to its future (3).

With this background, I venture to discuss what is known about pterygium and its current treatment.

EPIDEMIOLOGY

Geographic Distribution

The prevalence of pterygium has been directly related with proximity to the equator: the nearer to the equator, the greater the prevalence. Most commonly seen on either side of the equator, pterygium has been endemic in the Indian subcontinent, Southeast Asia, Hawaii, the Samoan Islands, the Middle East, Mexico, the Caribbean, Australia, Northern and Western Africa, and the sunbelt states of the United States. Cameron's world map summarizes the prevalence rates of pterygium (14). Generally rare in the cooler climates of Europe and the northern states in the United States, its prevalence, oddly, is high among the Inuit (Eskimos).

Prevalence

Prevalence rates of pterygium have been as high as 22.5% on the island of Aruba (15 degrees latitude from the equator), 18% in Puerto Rico (18 degrees latitude), and 5% to 15% in Texas, Florida, California, Arizona, and New Mexico in the United States (latitude 28 to 36 degrees from the equator). The prevalence rate drops to 2% or less in geographic areas more than 40 degrees from the equator. A true pterygium is a condition found chiefly in the sunny, hot, dusty regions in the world and in people more exposed to these climatic conditions, such as fishermen, farmers, construction workers, roofers, beachgoers, and Inuit. The

Inuit are probably exposed to ultraviolet (UV) light reflected from snow.

Age

Pterygium is most common in the elderly, but the appearance of new cases per annum is higher in the younger age group. Pterygium is uncommon in individuals younger than 20 years of age and in people wearing glasses (14). The incidence rises suddenly in the age groups between 20 and 40 years. It has been reported in three relatives in a family in whom the onset occurred when the patients were at 4, 6, and 20 years of age (15).

Interestingly, this difference in incidence and prevalence rates related to age, geography, environmental exposure, or all, does not exist in patients with pinguecula (discussed later). Both the incidence and prevalence of pinguecula increase with age.

Sex

In general, pterygium is twice as common in male as in female patients, except in Aruba, where it is equally common in both sexes.

Heredity

Pterygium has a dominant inheritance with low penetrance. It is not the actual lesion that is transmitted, but rather the tendency of the eye to react in this special way to environmental factors. It is a commonly seen condition among the Hispanic population in the northern United States that left the geographic confines of Mexico and the sunbelt states of the United States many generations ago.

Involvement of the Second Eye

Pterygium is mostly a bilateral condition (Fig. 60-2). Like many other conditions, one eye may follow the other by months to years. The second eye, almost always, has a pinguecula that evolves into a pterygium. Most commonly, the nasal pterygia are seen in both eyes, but cases have been recorded in which one eye had a nasal and the second one had a temporal pterygium, double pterygia (Fig. 60-3), or other combinations.

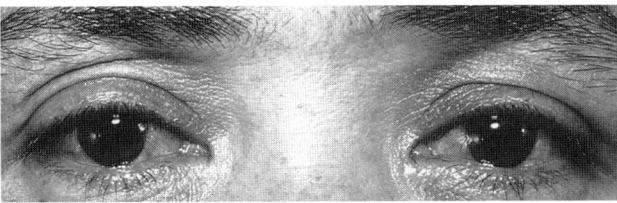

FIGURE 60-2. Bilateral primary nasal pterygia (in both eyes), and a temporal pterygium in the right eye.

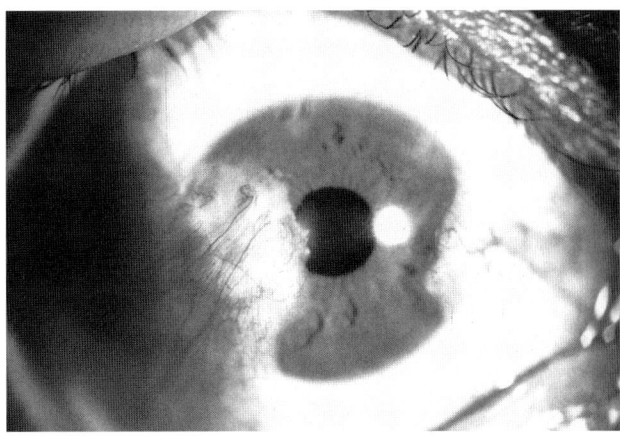

FIGURE 60-3. Double (nasal and temporal) pterygia in an eye; the temporal pterygium is growing into the papillary area, causing visual symptoms.

ETIOLOGY AND PATHOGENESIS

The etiology of pterygium is still unknown. Its incidence related to definite geographic areas compels one to assume that certain environmental factors or agents must contribute to its development. Heat, dry climate, high winds, and abundance of dust in these geographic areas led many authors incriminate these factors as etiologic. But these fail to explain the common occurrence of pterygium in the Caribbean islands, with humid conditions year round. Desiccation from climatic conditions and a decrease of basic lacrimal secretions, with genetic predisposition, have been postulated as potent etiologic factors.

An association with exposure to UV type B (UVB) light in solar radiation has been found to be the most significant environmental factor contributing to pterygium development (14,16–28). Factors like a dry, dusty climate and genetic predisposition probably contribute to the development of pterygium. The geographic distribution of pterygium can be easily explained by the exposure to UV rays of the sun in the dry, dusty climates of deserts, in the humid conditions of the Caribbean, in Inuit from sun snow-glare, and in fishermen and beachgoers. In an investigation of more than 100,000 Australian Aborigines, researchers found a significant positive correlation between climatic UV radiation and pterygium prevalence (20). Pterygium was also significantly associated with UV radiation among fishermen on Chesapeake Bay (26,27). Similarly, the infrared spectrum of sunlight has also been blamed (28). Involuntary partial closure of the interpalpebral fissure, mostly confined to the temporal side, to avoid glare from bright sun, might explain the predominance of pterygia on the nasal side.

In a risk analysis study recently conducted in Australia, Mackenzie et al. (25) showed a several hundred-fold higher risk for development of pterygium in subjects who worked mainly on sand, and almost a 20-fold higher risk in subjects who worked in an environment that was mainly concrete, compared with those who worked indoors. According to this study, those subjects who spent their first 5 years of life at latitudes less than 30 degrees had almost 40 times the risk of pterygium growth than those living at latitudes greater than 40 degrees, and had a 20-fold increased risk for development of pterygium if they had spent most of their time outdoors during these earliest years of life. They also found that wearing regular spectacle eyeglasses and, more important, dark sunglasses, or even wearing hats to protect eyes from exposure to sunlight had a very strong protective effect against pterygium growth (25).

Pinguecula

A pinguecula is a yellowish triangular patch formed by elastotic degeneration of the connective tissue, situated in the bulbar conjunctiva on either side of the cornea. It is the combined expression of changes due to age and exposure to UV light. It affects first the nasal and then the temporal side. A pinguecula appears as a roughened, raised yellowish area in the bulbar conjunctiva in the palpebral aperture near the limbus. Gradually it develops into a triangular patch with its base abutting against the cornea. Most commonly it grows to a moderate size and then ceases growing. Occasionally, nasal and temporal pingueculae may grow along the inferior limbus to meet below the cornea.

Pinguecula as a Precursor of Pterygium

Zehender, in 1869, introduced the idea that pinguecula was the precursor of pterygium (29). This hypothesis was reaffirmed by Fuchs, Parsons, and Alt, who proposed that proliferation of hyaline and elastic tissue in the connective tissue of the conjunctiva along with degenerative changes in its bulk progressed to invade the cornea and developed into a pterygium. Once pterygium has grown to a certain extent, it is impossible to locate the position of the supposed precursor or pinguecula, although it is supposed to be in the head of pterygium. This has not been confirmed histologically. This hypothesis may be acceptable for primary pterygium; however, it is known that pinguecula has no relationship to growth of recurrent pterygium.

Sugar (30) proposed that degenerative changes in pingueculae incite hyperplasia and hypertrophy of the elastic tissue and deposition of hyaline material that elevates the epithelium away from Bowman's layer. This process causes changes at the limbus and adjoining cornea and leads to the laying down of connective tissue that contracts and pulls this fascial layer onto the cornea. D'Ombrain (31) was of the opinion that pinguecula and pterygium both are degenerative processes. If the pinguecula grew close to the limbus it would grow onto the cornea to form a pterygium; if it stayed away from the limbus, it would continue to stay as pinguecula.

Overall, it is accepted that pinguecula and primary pterygium are somehow related to each other (similar degenerative changes in response to similar environmental factors). However, recurrent pterygium is not preceded by pinguecula.

Numerous other theories have been proposed and refuted for the pathogenesis of pterygium. These include choline deficiency (32), inflammation (6,33–36), allergic basis (34), degeneration (30,37–39), tissue angiogenesis factor (40), elastic tissue changes (41,42), and immune mechanisms (43). Theories to explain the development of pterygium on neoplastic, inflammatory, episcleritis, chlamydial, and allergic bases have not been well accepted. Both direct and reflected UVB radiation has been implicated in the causation of pterygium (14,16–23). Mackenzie et al. (25), in a risk analysis study conducted in Australia, has suggested that the exposure of formative ocular tissue to UV radiation in the first 5 years of life probably either sensitizes or initiates a genetic, biochemical, or morphologic change that is reflected in later years of life by the development of a pterygium. This early exposure to UV light might initiate a tissue change, probably at the "putative" stem cells at the corneal limbus (25), that requires the later promoting effect of cumulative UV radiation to the ocular surface.

It is believed that UV radiation denatures corneal proteins and induces an antigen–antibody reaction that triggers fibrovascular proliferation (34). Some unidentified etiologic factor initiates a row of fibroblasts to advance into limbal cornea and penetrate the tissue in its superficial layers between Bowman's layer and the basement membrane of the overlying corneal epithelium. Accumulation of these fibroblasts is thought to prepare a path for the head of the pterygium to enter the cornea, and on their way, the fibroblasts push Bowman's membrane posteriorly. Gradually, Bowman's membrane gets fragmented and the pterygium tissue grows through these fragmented areas into underlying stroma and becomes firmly adherent to the corneal tissue.

It remains unclear at this time if the invasion of cornea by pterygium tissue is initiated/triggered by degenerative changes in the basal cell layer or induced by solar radiation, by an immunologic response to altered basement membrane material, or by an inflammatory process with possible involvement of a type 1 hypersensitivity response to antigenic pollens and dust particles (40,43).

Barraquer (44) proposed a hypothesis that limbal elevation by a pinguecula, causing tear film disruption, desiccation of corneal tissue, and microulceration of adjoining corneal epithelium, was the etiopathologic factor that induced conjunctival fibrovascular proliferation to invade cornea. Dellen formation or microulceration of the corneal epithelium has been documented, but neither is a consistent finding in an active pterygium. This pathogenetic theory has lost ground because, contrary to this hypothesis, others have suggested that there is an accumulating iron line from the pooling of tears at the apex of the head of pterygium.

Recently, it has been proposed that pterygium is a growth disorder in which mutation of the *p53* tumor suppressor gene plays a vital role (45,46). Dushku and Reid (45) and Tan et al. (46) have demonstrated high p53 protein expression in the epithelium overlying the pterygium and have speculated on the existence of a *p53* gene mutation in pterygia. The hypothesis that pterygium is a benign neoplastic lesion has been further supported by the finding of microsatellite instability and loss of heterozygosity in human pterygia, two common findings in tumorous tissues (47). This theory has not been well received because Onur et al. (48) found only 3 of 38 pterygia and Chowers et al. (49) found only half of the primary and recurrent pterygia had *p53* immunoreactivity in their studies. Also, *p53* gene mutation has not yet been demonstrated in pterygium. To refute further the theory that pterygium is a tumorous growth, Karukonda et al. (50) found proliferative activity to be similar among primary and recurrent pterygium and normal conjunctiva by using flow cytometry; another common finding in tumorous tissues. Chowers et al. (49) did not find a difference in *p53* immunoreactivity between eyes with primary pterygium that did not recur and primary pterygium that was followed by recurrence of pterygium. In addition, proliferative activity of primary pterygia that recurred was similar to that of primary pterygia without recurrence, indicating that proliferative activity was not a reliable marker for recurrence (49). The results of an immunohistochemical study of human pterygium suggest that an immunopathogenetic mechanism is responsible for the pathogenesis of pterygium. It is postulated that this mechanism is perhaps triggered by preexisting conjunctivitis or microtrauma in combination with the patient's predisposition (51).

PATHOLOGY AND HISTOPATHOLOGY

Histopathologically, pterygium is a fibrovascular proliferation of conjunctival tissue onto clear cornea. Anatomically, pterygium is divided into a head, neck, and body. The head is the part on the cornea, the neck is at the limbus, and the body of the pterygium is on the sclera. An epithelial layer that histologically resembles atrophic conjunctival epithelium covers all these layers. It extends beyond its confines onto cornea. It covers the mass of pterygium that is formed by the thickened, hypertrophied, and degenerative connective tissue. Redslob (52) and Austin et al. (41) have suggested that the subepithelial tissue is fibroblastic dysplasia. Histologically it is hyperplasia, and not dysplasia. The abnormal collagen tissue is aggregated into a coiled and fibrillated pattern, similar to elastic tissue. This denatured collagen shows basophilia and can be stained with elastic tissue stains. Unlike elastic tissue, it is not digested by elastase (53) and therefore is called *elastotic degeneration*. Congested new blood vessels that are dispersed between hypertrophied collagen fibers richly supply this degenerative tissue.

The body of the pterygium incorporates the underlying Tenon's capsule but spares the episcleral tissue; therefore, it is not adherent to sclera and can be easily mobilized. But, at the limbus, the absence of Tenon's capsule makes the neck of the pterygium adherent to underlying episclera and sclera. The head of the pterygium grows in a plane between Bowman's layer and the basement membrane of the overlying corneal epithelium. A row of fibroblasts advances in front of the apex of the head of the pterygium at this plane and "prepares" a path for the head of the pterygium to invade the cornea. In this process, Bowman's layer is pushed posteriorly and eventually fragments and makes openings for the fibrovascular tissue of the pterygium to grow into the underlying superficial stroma of cornea. That makes the head of the pterygium firmly adherent to cornea.

In the body of the pterygium are also some tubular glands and larger spaces lined with epithelium. Both of these may result in the formation of cysts in the body of the pterygium. Histologic examination of excised pterygia also reveals a lymphocytic infiltration consisting predominantly of T cells (54).

Ultrastructural studies have revealed that both pinguecula and pterygia are composed of degenerative, basophilic, subepithelial tissue with fibers that enhance with elastic stains. Hogan and Alvarado (38) found that some fibers were sensitive to elastase, whereas others were not, concluding that the resistant fibers arose from degeneration of collagen. Austin et al. (41) found that the elastin was immature and abnormal, perhaps explaining its partial insensitivity to elastase.

The apex of the pterygium causes pooling of tears at the leading edge of slow-growing or stationary pterygia, and iron deposits settle in the form of a line central to the apex of pterygium, called *Stocker's line* (55). It usually implies chronicity because rapidly growing pterygium does not allow pooling of tears in one area for periods sufficient for iron to deposit. Stocker's line is usually not seen in active and fast-growing pterygia.

Histopathologically, primary and recurrent pterygia are two distinct entities. Recurrent pterygium is composed only of fibrovascular tissue in the absence of elastotic degeneration. It involves underlying episclera, sclera, rectus muscle sheath, and corneal stroma, and is firmly adherent to the underlying structures throughout its extent. It is highly vascularized tissue.

CLINICAL CHARACTERISTICS
Primary Pterygium

A pterygium appears as a triangular, fleshy growth almost invariably found on the nasal side slightly below the horizontal meridian (Fig. 60-1). Usually both eyes are affected on the nasal side, although unequally. Almost always it starts over the area of a preexisting pinguecula. The first change is the appearance of gray, circumscribed opacities in the cornea near the limbus. The conjunctiva opposite these opacities shows shrinkage that is apparent by its tenseness and a displacement of the semilunar fold. As the conjunctiva encroaches on the cornea, it is preceded by the appearance of the same gray infiltrates in this tissue, at first as small islands, which gradually fuse. When fully developed, the head of the pterygium looks triangular with a blunt apex. Central to the apex are the small irregular opacities that can be seen with the slit lamp at the level of Bowman's layer. More central to these changes, Stocker's line may be seen, a pigmented line at the level of this membrane containing iron deposits (55). Toward the limbus, the conjunctival fold runs backward to the sclera in a tightly drawn triangular wing. At the limbal area it is referred to as the neck of the pterygium, and the fleshy mass spreading out into a fan shape on sclera is the body of the pterygium. The upper and lower borders of the body are folded; a probe can be slipped under the folds for a very short distance, and not through the full thickness because the area of adhesion is always smaller than its total breadth. These folds merge imperceptibly into the bulbar conjunctiva at the base of the pterygium and usually have considerable tension, which is manifested by the straight course of the vessels, the numerous folds, and the gross displacement of the plica semilunaris.

CLASSIFICATION AND STAGING OF PTERYGIUM

Progressive pterygium: An actively growing, fleshy, vascular, and inflamed-looking pterygium is called progressive pterygium. This fleshy and vascular pterygium has also been called pterygium crassum, vasculosum, or carnosum (4,6). Progressive pterygium has a very fleshy, succulent appearance and usually does not have Stocker's line ahead of it.

Stationary pterygium: At some stage the pterygium may still look vascular, but the head of the pterygium looks pale and sparsely vascularized and stops growing and is called stationary pterygium. Stationary pterygium loses its vascular appearance and develops a Stocker's line because of tears pooling at its apex and depositing iron into Bowman's membrane.

Regressive pterygium: A pale, thin, papery, gray, anemic, and membranous pterygium appears to be regressing, but in reality the pterygium never gets smaller or disappears. Regressive pterygium has a gray apex resembling a corneal opacity. It is usually seen in the elderly and may represent age-related degenerative changes, as seen in other parts of the body.

Gerundo classified these three stages as: (a) proliferative papillomatous, (b) fibromatous, and (c) atrophic-sclerotic, respectively (56). Recently, Townsend (57) has classified pterygium into five groups depending on their risk of

recurrence: (a) actively growing, (b) fleshy, (c) slowly growing, (d) stationary, and (e) atrophic pterygia.

Nasal

Nasal pterygium is by far the most common, representing 60% of total pterygia (Fig. 60-1).

Temporal

The next most common is the pterygium growing from the temporal side onto the clear cornea, representing approximately 20% of total pterygia (Fig. 60-3).

Double

Nasal and temporal pterygia presenting in the same eye are called *double pterygia* (Fig. 60-3) and represent approximately 20% of total pterygia.

Bilateral

Pterygia in both eyes are called *bilateral pterygia*; pterygia are usually bilateral (Fig. 60-2). The presence of a nasal pterygium in one eye and a temporal pterygium in the other eye, or double pterygia in one eye and a nasal or temporal pterygium in the second eye, is common (Fig. 60-2).

Recurrent

Regrowth of the pterygium after primary excision is called *recurrent pterygium*. Pathologically, recurrent pterygium differs from primary pterygium; it is fibrovascular tissue growing onto the cornea without elastotic degeneration. It involves the underlying sclera, episclera, and Tenon's capsule and grows onto corneal stroma, where it is very firmly adherent to the underlying tissues (Fig. 60-4). Recurrent

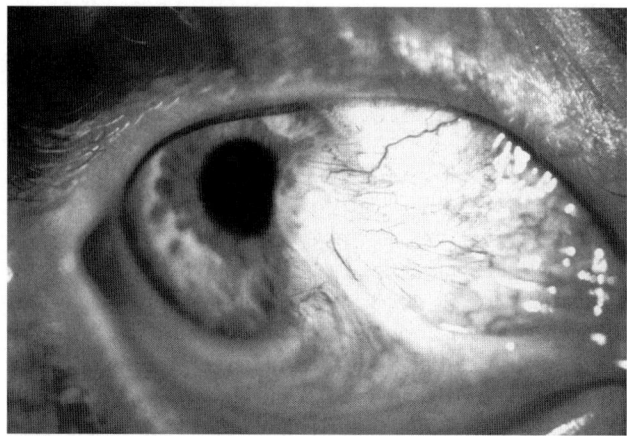

FIGURE 60-4. Recurrent nasal pterygium adherent to the underlying episclera/sclera and cornea can restrict ocular motility.

pterygium can cause restriction of ocular motility because of scar tissue or involvement of the horizontal rectus muscle sheaths.

Pseudopterygium

A pseudopterygium is the result of an inflammatory process wherein a fold of inflamed conjunctiva becomes adherent to denuded cornea near the limbus or more centrally. Marginal corneal ulceration, traumatic epithelial defects, or peripheral corneal degenerations can involve the chemotic conjunctival fold in the healing process, dragging conjunctiva across the cornea. Pseudopterygium does not respect the interpalpebral location and can be seen at any meridian on the eye. It makes a bridge of tissue growing from conjunctiva onto the corneal denuded area over limbus; a probe can be passed under its full breadth (6). It is usually unilateral and does not tend to regrow after primary breaking of the adhesions.

SYMPTOMS

Both pingueculae and small pterygia are asymptomatic. A small pterygium gives rise to no symptoms; its only disadvantage is a cosmetic blemish. A pinguecula or a pterygium may become inflamed, causing episodic inflammation, pain, and tenderness. Inflammation of pinguecula is called *pingueculitis*, and may resemble episcleritis. It is very rare to see inflammation of the pterygium itself.

A pterygium of significant size induces flattening of the corneal curvature in its horizontal meridian, producing with-the-rule astigmatism of up to 1.5 D. When it grows large enough to encroach on the papillary aperture, however, it obstructs peripheral vision first and eventually central vision as well. A large pterygium may cause binocular diplopia by limiting eye movements away from the pterygium body because of traction on the conjunctiva. Binocular diplopia is more common with recurrent pterygium because of its adherence to underlying sclera and episclera and sometimes because of involvement of the rectus muscle itself.

Pterygium has commonly been blamed for eye irritation, foreign-body sensation, dryness, photophobia, epiphora, and pruritus. Pinguecula has also been associated with these symptoms. These symptoms in reality are caused by the underlying dry-eye condition. UV exposure, dry climate, genetic predisposition, or any similar factor singly or in combination can cause dry-eye syndrome before the appearance of a pinguecula or pterygium. Some surgeons have recommended not operating on a pterygium in eyes with associated dryness. These symptoms start before the growth of a pinguecula or pterygium, and inadequately treated dry eye itself is believed to induce the growth of pingueculae and pterygia. These symptoms can be treated successfully with treatment of dry eye in the presence of a pinguecula or pterygium.

DIFFERENTIAL DIAGNOSIS

Pinguecula and "early" pterygium may mistakenly appear clinically similar. We emphasize that either it is a pinguecula or a pterygium. The growth on the sclera is a pinguecula; when it grows to involve cornea, it is pterygium. Clinically these are two distinct entities.

An atypical location of a pterygium in an oblique axis should suggest an alternate diagnosis, such as Terrien's marginal corneal degeneration (5), pseudopterygium (57), tumor (57), or traumatic pannus.

TREATMENT

Prophylaxis

Because the etiology and pathogenesis of pterygium growth are unclear, the role of prophylaxis is also uncertain. Theoretically, preventing or limiting exposure to UV light might be of some help. A change of environment might not be feasible or practical. Protection of the eyes by regular spectacles, dark sunglasses, or hats when exposed to the sun or irritating environmental conditions could certainly do some good, as suggested by Cameron (14), Rosenthal et al. (58,59), and Mackenzie et al. (25). Cameron (14) found in Australia that the rate of incidence of pterygium was reduced from an average of 15% to 3% among those who had worn glasses constantly from before the age of 15 years. Mackenzie et al. (25) found that the normal population that did not wear regular spectacles was at a threefold higher risk for development of pterygium compared with the population that wore regular spectacles. The population that wore dark sunglasses when exposed to the sun was fivefold better protected than the general population against pterygium growth. This association has also been found with wearing a hat in the sun. Mackenzie et al. (25) has recommended avoidance of exposure to UV light, especially in the first 5 years of life.

Medical Treatment

Since the time of Susruta, approximately 1000 years B.C., medical treatment has been tried and found unsatisfactory. In the 20th century, local applications of solid choline chloride (32) or of topical steroids (6), or subconjunctival injection of hyaluronidase (6) have proved of little value (6).

Surgical Treatment

The only effective treatment for pterygium is surgery. However, none of the surgical procedures is perfect and universally accepted because of high recurrence rates. Since the time of Susruta, mankind has tried almost every imaginable procedure to remove pterygia with the hope that there would be no recurrence. Even in ancient times the problems of pterygium management were recognized. Susruta wrote, "Any remnant of the pterygium should be removed with a scarifying ointment to prevent recurrence" (3). According to Rich et al. (60), "to manage pterygia, we can incise, excise, bury, transplant, graft, freeze, burn, cauterize, diathermize, divulse, evulse, chemically assault, irradiate or simply leave them to fate." The many therapeutic options available to manage pterygia imply that no single one is completely effective. Almost all (91.6%) recurrences appear by 360 days after surgery. It has been suggested that 1 year is the optimal follow-up time to identify recurrence of pterygium (61).

Indications for Surgery

The primary indication for pterygium excision is decreased visual acuity because of encroachment of the pterygium into the visual axis or the irregular astigmatism induced by the growth. Surgery may also be indicated because of the breakup of the precorneal tear film. Other reasons for surgical intervention include ocular irritation and discomfort unresponsive to lubrication, restricted ocular motility, binocular diplopia (mostly due to recurrent pterygium), or the progression of the pterygium toward the visual axis. Surgery may also be indicated in cases where the pterygium, or even pinguecula, restricts wearing of contact lenses. Difficulty in performing corneal refractive surgery has also been added to the list of surgical indications for pterygium excision. Most patients seek surgical excision of the pterygium for cosmetic reasons, but they need to be informed of the high recurrence rate and the scarring left after pterygium excision.

Current Surgical Procedures for Pterygium Treatment

Bare-Sclera Excision

The bare-sclera method involves surgical dissection of the pterygium, either starting from the head of the pterygium with lamellar keratectomy and extending to remove the body of the pterygium, or starting from the body and removing the head by keratectomy or simply peeling it off the cornea. Castroviejo (62) recommended the use of a very superficial keratectomy, no deeper than necessary, to prevent corneal thinning. Most surgeons begin at the apex of the pterygium in clear cornea, and with sharp dissection perform a superficial lamellar keratectomy up to the neck of the pterygium at the limbus. The body of the primary pterygium is lifted away from the underlying episclera. There are loose adhesions to underlying episclera that are

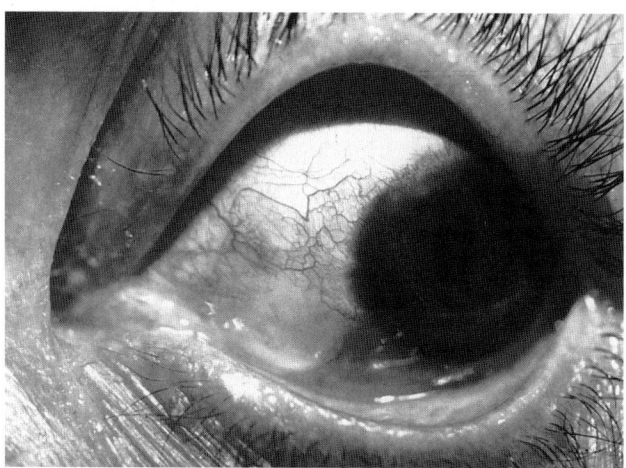

FIGURE 60-5. Bare-sclera excision of a nasal pterygium.

cut. Two radial incisions are placed on either side of the body of the pterygium for 5 to 7 mm, depending on its size. These incisions are united by another incision running parallel to the limbus. The head, neck, and body of the pterygium are removed in one piece, leaving behind bare sclera. The conjunctival edges retract a little, leaving behind a bare scleral area slightly bigger than the body of the removed pterygium (Fig. 60-5). Hemostasis is achieved with unipolar or bipolar thermal cautery. Care must be taken not to overtreat the episclera and the sclera with thermal cautery, especially if that tissue is to be subsequently exposed to irradiation, thiotepa (triethylenethiophosphoramide), or mitomycin C. Similarly, during removal of the body of a recurrent pterygium that is firmly adherent to sclera, the surgeon must be careful not to perform a deep dissection into the sclera. The adhesions are removed with sharp dissection, avoiding the sclera. Kasner (5) has recommended meticulous removal of all pterygium tissue, followed by polishing the area with a diamond-burr polisher. I see no advantage to such polishing in preventing pterygium recurrence.

Sugar (30) believed that the subconjunctival tissue and Tenon's capsule served as a medium enabling the regrowth of conjunctiva over the cornea in pterygium recurrence. By excising the subconjunctival episcleral tissue at the limbus, the conjunctiva is allowed to become adherent to underlying sclera, preventing its migration over the cornea (5,30). But histopathologic investigation of recurrent pterygium demonstrates that this is not true. Despite strong adhesions to underlying sclera, the recurrent pterygium keeps growing onto the cornea.

The bare-sclera method has a very high recurrence rate of 23% to 75% (6,28,57,63–66). The conjunctival healing process after bare-sclera excision is usually very invasive, more so than the original pterygium, and frequently seen as postoperative conjunctival granuloma formation that grows onto the cornea to form a recurrent pterygium. Recurrent pterygium grows much more quickly and into a bigger pterygium than the primary pterygium.

At present, only a few surgeons perform the bare-sclera technique as the primary procedure, but this procedure forms the basis for all adjunct treatments used to prevent pterygium recurrence. The results of a survey conducted in Australia disclosed that for primary pterygium, 29% of ophthalmologists performed bare-sclera excision, nearly one fourth of the respondents added adjunctive therapies such as beta irradiation or mitomycin C, and approximately half the respondents used a swinging conjunctival flap. For recurrent pterygium, one third of ophthalmologists preferred adjunctive therapies such as mitomycin C and beta irradiation, and 57% used conjunctival autografting to prevent pterygium recurrence (67). Successful use of the chemotherapeutic agent daunorubicin has been reported (68), but 5-fluorouracil as adjunctive treatment after pterygium excision has yielded less predictable results. Pikkel et al. (69) found 5-fluorouracil efficacious, but Maldonado et al. (70) found it inefficacious in preventing pterygium recurrence. 5-Fluorouracil induced inflammation after pterygium excision to cause a recurrence rate of 60%, compared with 35% seen with placebo (70).

Adjunctive Use of Beta Irradiation

Terson in Paris (11) was probably the first to refer to radiation therapy for pterygium (3). It was established that irradiation was ineffective on an established pterygium without surgical removal of the bulk of the tissue first (71). Castroviejo was especially optimistic that a combination of adequate surgical removal and adjunct beta irradiation could solve the problem of pterygium recurrence (62). Initially, nonstandardized irradiation was administered in variable amounts with radon bulbs, radium plaques, Grenz rays, and x-rays, causing confusion and an inability to compare results among studies. Gradually, beta irradiation as an adjunct therapy was determined to be the safest and most effective radiation method to reduce recurrences to a range of 0.5% to 16% (65). Pico observed a recurrence rate of 3% with and 8% without beta irradiation (28), Hilgers found recurrence rates of 8% with and 23% without beta irradiation (34), whereas Cameron found a recurrence rate of 16% with and more than 50% without beta irradiation (14). Simsek et al. (72) found a recurrence rate of 6.4% after a 1,000- to 7,000-cGy dose of beta irradiation with Sr-90 in eyes treated for primary and recurrent pterygia after a mean follow-up of 7 years. Amano et al. reported a 23% recurrence rate in 61 eyes treated with a total dose of 21.6 Gy of beta irradiation after primary pterygium excision, with a mean follow-up of 31 months (73).

Radiation causes ionization changes in both the nucleus and cytoplasm of cells. Tissues with neovascularization and fibroblasts, which are responsible for pterygium recurrence, physiologically and radiobiologically, are the most susceptible to irradiation during their peak of mitotic activity, division, and proliferation. Irradiation induces obliterative endarteritis and arrest of fibroblast proliferation (5,74). Beta irradiation has a beneficial effect only on the immature tissue that grows rapidly after surgery (75). The use of Sr-90, applied in controlled amounts, is the safest and most effective mode of applying beta irradiation to the surface of the eye (75,76). The amount of radiation delivered by the active surface of the Sr-90 applicator, which delivers only beta and no gamma emissions (77), varies according to the applicator's strength. A standard applicator, with shield, usually delivers approximately 3,000 reps (roentgen-equivalent physical) per minute over its entire radiation surface (78). The unit for the Sr-90 applicator is the rep (1 rep = 1.08 rad). Strontium-90 beta irradiation has a distinct advantage in that it delivers irradiation in a depth dose pattern. Beta rays expend their energy (ionize) maximally in the superficial 2 mm of tissue. The dose falls from 100% on the surface to 41% at 1 mm, 19% at 2 mm, 9% at 3 mm, and 1% at 5 mm (78). Lemp improved on dose delivery to the surface area by raising the tip of the applicator by 1 mm. He covered the bare sclera with two soft contact lenses placed on top of each other, each having 0.5 mm thickness and 70% water content to provide a water interface and allow the beta irradiation to be focused at the outermost 1 mm of ocular tissue (5).

It has been recommended that beta irradiation be applied immediately after surgical excision of the pterygium for a better chance of inhibiting neovascularization and controlling later proliferation of vasculature because of the prolonged effects of irradiation (77,79–81).

Controversy exists in the literature over the most effective regimen for beta irradiation in preventing pterygium recurrence (81). Pinkerton has used Sr-90 in managing pterygium since 1954. He recommends using approximately 1,500 reps of Sr-90 per area (77). Overlap occurs in certain areas of irradiation because it is impossible to place the applicator exactly adjacent to the previously treated area. To prevent complications, caution should be taken not to exceed 3000 reps of irradiation even in these overlapped areas (77). The irradiation regimens have varied from 1,500 to 2,500 reps as a single dose to total of 3,000 reps in three divided doses over 3 weeks. Beta irradiation can be applied immediately after pterygium excision while the area is still anesthetized and expert personnel are available for radiation therapy (77,80).

Limitations, Side Effects, and Complications of Beta Irradiation

Only trained personnel certified by the Nuclear Regulatory Commission to handle and apply beta irradiation after pterygium excision can perform the treatment. In most institutions, radiologists or radiotherapists administer the radiation, and their involvement obviously must be coordinated.

Cataract formation after beta irradiation has been a well-documented complication (65,82–85). Penetrating ionizing radiation at the limbal area injures the equatorial cells of the lens epithelium, which in turn causes changes in the lens fibers and posterior subcapsular region (85). Cataract formation is dose related; the incidence and extent of cataracts increase with increasing radiation dose. New lens fibers are laid in the equatorial region, and these cells are most vulnerable to radiation toxicity. Doses of 1,500 to 3,000 reps have been demonstrated to cause cataract formation in the periphery, but doses up to 8,000 to 10,000 reps cause significant central cataractous changes involving the visual axis, resulting in decreased visual acuity (85). After 5-year follow-up, Hilgers found no cataract formation after a fractionated dose of 3,000 reps, but found cataract developing in 6% of eyes after 3,000 to 5,000 reps (71). Approximately one third of his patients had progressive lens opacities when examined after 8 years (71).

Other serious complications of excessive Sr-90 irradiation include chronic conjunctival hyperemia persisting for many months, keratitis sicca, episcleritis, iritis, corneal thinning, ulceration, and perforation, scleral ulceration (Fig. 60-6) and atrophy, and *Pseudomonas* endophthalmitis (65,86). These complications have been associated with excessive dosage or repeated dosage of beta irradiation to the same area. In a study of 63 eyes, after a mean follow-up of 12 years, almost 81% eyes had scleral ulceration with an irradiation dose of approximately 3500 rads. In four of these patients, *Pseudomonas* endophthalmitis developed (65,86). Distinct cellular changes, including polymorphism, giant cell formation, and chromatin abnormalities, have

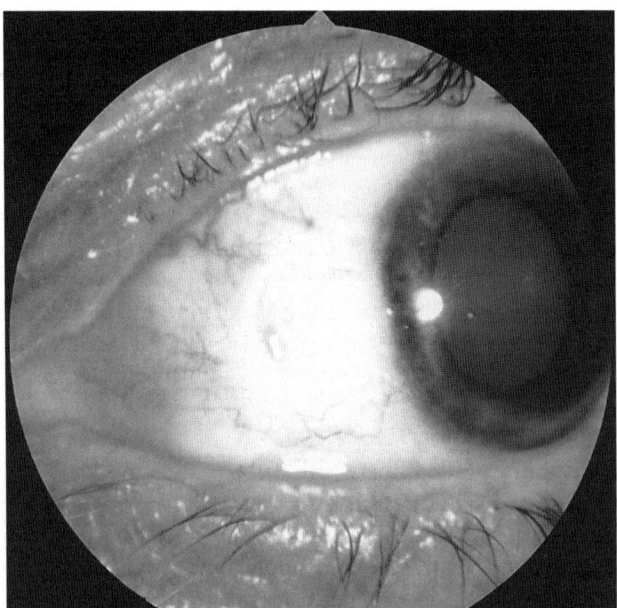

FIGURE 60-6. Scleral thinning seen 2 years after beta irradiation of the bare sclera as adjunctive treatment after excision of a nasal pterygium. There are no signs of pterygium recurrence.

been observed in conjunctiva irradiated with 3,000 reps in three divided doses (81,82).

Substitution of 20-kV soft x-ray irradiation for Sr-90 beta irradiation has been suggested, with no severe side effects and a low recurrence rate of 9% in recurrent pterygium management (87).

Adjunctive Use of Thiotepa

Thiotepa (triethylenethiophosphoramide) is a radiomimetic drug of the nitrogen mustard family. The mode of action is believed to be due to the release of ethylenimine radicals and their effect on actively dividing cells. Thiotepa inhibits capillary endothelial proliferation, thereby preventing neovascularization and pterygium recurrence. Systemic use inhibits the hematopoietic system, but topical use has not been demonstrated to cause any systemic complications.

Langham first used thiotepa topically in 1960 (88) on rabbits to prevent capillary endothelial proliferation and vascularization of corneas. In 1962, Meacham (89) used topical thiotepa as an adjunct to pterygium surgery in human eyes. After 1 year of follow-up, he did not see any recurrence. Mori (90) and Cassady (91) used this topical adjunct treatment with 16% and 0% recurrence rates, respectively. Liddy and Morgan (92) used a topical 1:2000 (0.5 mg/mL) solution of thiotepa after bare-sclera excision of pterygium with a 4% recurrence rate of pterygium, compared with a 50% recurrence rate in a control group. They used two drops of thiotepa every 3 hours while the patient was awake, for 6 weeks. Joselson and Muller had a 2% recurrence rate after primary pterygium excision and thiotepa use (93). With these success rates, thiotepa was considered the solution to pterygium management until Howitt and Karp (94) reported serious and irreversible complications of poliosis and periorbital skin depigmentation, especially in dark-skinned people. Similar complications, including postoperative conjunctival injection and hypertrophy (93), chronic conjunctivitis, and scleral ulceration, seen by others (95) made this modality for treating pterygia fall from favor. Thiotepa is rarely used now.

Adjunctive Use of Mitomycin C

Mitomycin is an antibiotic–antineoplastic and antimetabolite agent isolated from the fermentation filtrate of *Streptomyces caespitosus* (96–98). It selectively inhibits DNA replication by forming covalent bonds between adenine and guanine, and it is non–cell-specific, exerting its actions primarily during the late G1 and S phases of cell division. However, rapidly dividing cells are preferentially sensitive to the effects of mitomycin C. It also inhibits cellular RNA synthesis and protein synthesis and inhibits collagen production by fibroblasts, thus preventing pterygium recurrence (99).

Mitomycin C was originally used as a systemic chemotherapeutic agent for gastric and pancreatic carcinomas. Kunitomo and Mori were the first to use it in treating pterygium (100), and we introduced this modality to the Western world in 1987 and 1988 (98,101). Others have since then also successfully used it as adjunctive treatment in pterygium surgery to prevent recurrences (102–107). Mitomycin C also gained popularity in other selected ophthalmic procedures, such as glaucoma filtering surgery for better bleb survival (108), in the treatment of conjunctival and corneal intraepithelial neoplasia (109–111), in the adjunctive treatment of ocular cicatricial pemphigoid (112), as a potential modulator of wound healing after photorefractive keratectomy (113–115), and during nasolacrimal duct probing (116), silicone nasolacrimal intubation (117), and dacryocystorhinostomy (118) for nasolacrimal duct obstruction.

Postoperative Topical Mitomycin C Application

We studied postoperative adjunctive application of topical mitomycin C dissolved into 1 mg/mL (0.1%) concentration after primary and recurrent pterygium excision in 1987 and 1988 (98,101,119–124). We observed a 5% (1 of 20 pterygia) recurrence rate after a 5-month follow-up (98,101,119). This concentration instilled four times a day for 10 days was found to be locally irritating. It induced lower lacrimal punctal occlusion in one eye, and caused excessive lacrimation, mild superficial punctate keratitis, iritis, and chronic inflammation in other eyes. Another late complication observed with the 0.1% concentration was scleral melt seen 22 months after surgery (98,119–121). I assumed that the scleral melt was induced by the exposure of scleral lamellae to mitomycin C because of intraoperative damage to sclera during pterygium excision (119). These results led us to suggest that a lower concentration of mitomycin C be used after surgery (98,101,119–124).

We studied a lower concentration of 0.4 mg/mL (0.04%) mitomycin C after primary and recurrent pterygium excision for a few years (98,101,119–124). This concentration was observed to be safe and effective in preventing pterygium recurrences without complications (Figs. 60-7 and 60-8). Postoperative follow-up for the eyes treated with mitomycin C eyedrops ranged from 3 to 34 weeks (mean, 23 weeks). During this period, 1 of 44 pterygia recurred after 5 months (recurrence rate of 2.3%), and that eye was treated with a 1 mg/mL (0.1%) concentration. We did not see any recurrence (recurrence rate, 0%) in eyes treated with 0.4 mg/mL (0.04%) mitomycin C (98,101,119,124). A similar efficacy of mitomycin C eyedrops instilled after surgery has been observed by subsequent studies using even lower concentrations of mitomycin C.

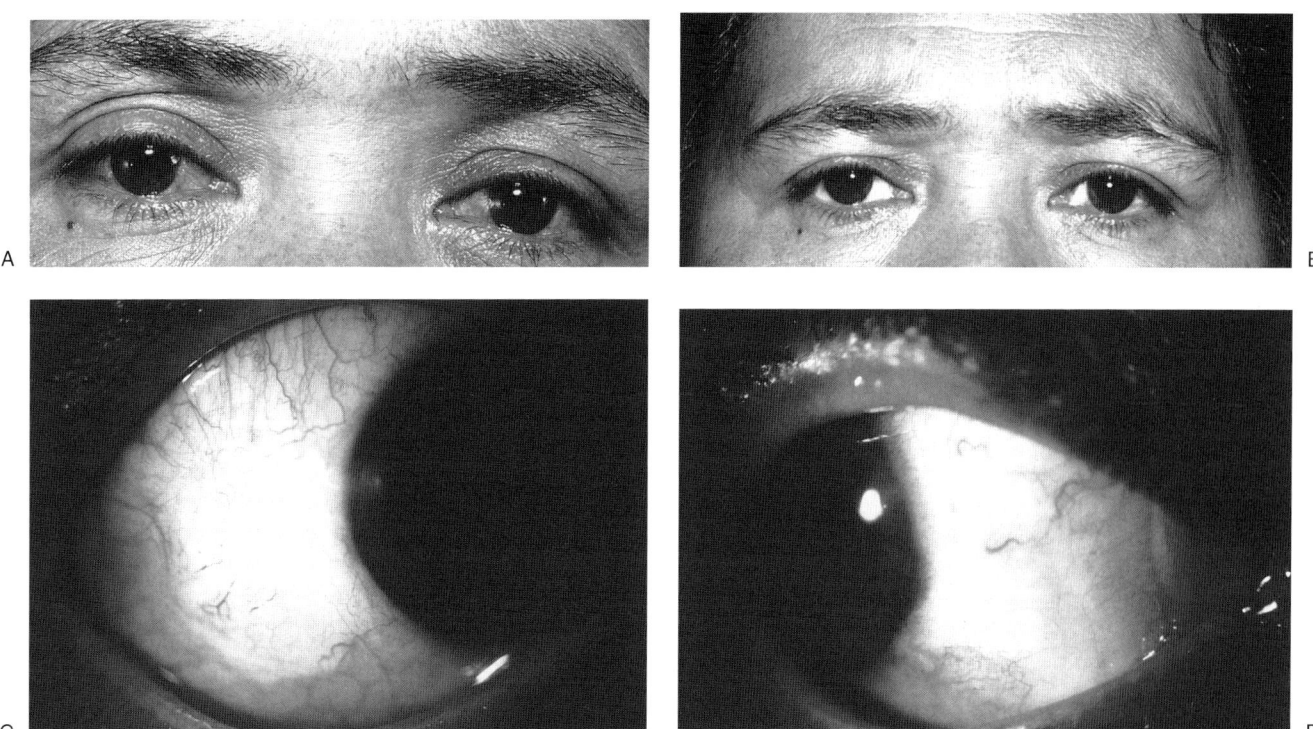

FIGURE 60-7. A, Preoperative *primary* double pterygia in the right eye and a primary nasal pterygium in the left eye. **B,** Same patient without pterygium recurrence in either eye and excellent cosmetic results seen 2 years after surgery with adjunctive use of 0.4 mg/mL (0.04%) mitomycin C. **C,** Close-up appearance of the temporal area of the right eye. **D,** Close-up appearance of the nasal area of the right eye.

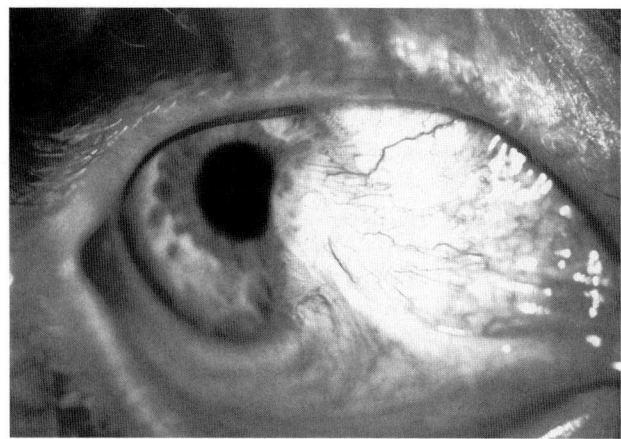
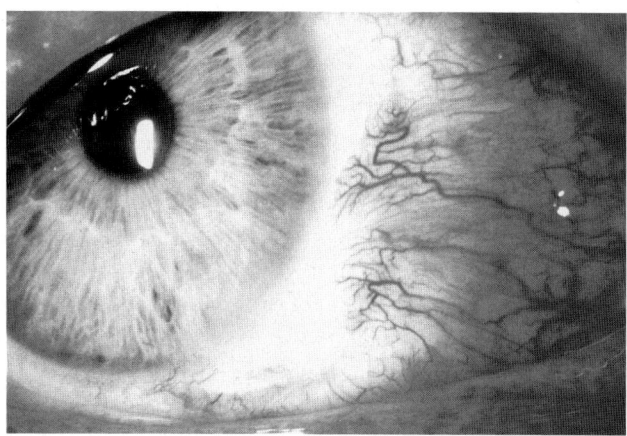

FIGURE 60-8. A: Preoperative appearance of recurrent nasal pterygium that had been operated four times previously with conjunctival autografting. **B:** Same eye without any recurrence 9 months after pterygium excision and adjunctive use of 0.4 mg/mL (0.04%) mitomycin C.

Postoperative adjunct application of topical mitomycin C in a 0.02% dilution used twice daily for 5 days lowered the recurrence rate to 2.6% in patients with primary pterygium seen at 6- to 11-month follow-up (125). The side effects encountered for this group included avascularized sclera in almost one third, ocular discomfort and lacrimation in 13%, superficial punctate keratopathy in 8%, and pyogenic granuloma in 2.6% patients. These were all mild, self-limiting, and easily treated side effects (125). Topical postoperative application of 0.02% (0.2 mg/mL) mitomycin C four times a day for 7 days resulted in a recurrence rate of 21.1% (4 of 19 eyes) after a mean follow-up time of 16 months (126).

Intraoperative Mitomycin C Application

Conflicting results have been obtained after intraoperative application of mitomycin C as adjunct treatment to bare-sclera pterygium excision. The reason for these disparate results could be that different studies had adopted different treatment protocols. Intraoperative application of 0.02% mitomycin C for 30 seconds to bare sclera after pterygium excision lowered the pterygium recurrence rate to 7.9% in primary pterygium surgery and to 19.2% in recurrent pterygium surgery after follow-up of over 2 years (127). Intraoperative application of 0.05% (0.5 mg/mL) mitomycin C for 1 minute along with 20-mg depot steroid subconjunctival injection after primary pterygium excision resulted in no recurrences after 4 to 14 months of follow-up (128). Adjunct intraoperative application of 0.02% (0.2 mg/mL) mitomycin C for 5 minutes to bare sclera after excision of primary and recurrent pterygia lowered the recurrence rate to 4% (2 of 49 patients) after a follow-up ranging from 12 to 28 months (129); the recurrence rate in the control group was 46.7% (15 of 32 patients). Intraoperative application of 0.04% (0.4 mg/mL) mitomycin C for 3 minutes decreased the recurrence rate from 33.3% in the control group (without mitomycin C) to 6.7% in the eyes treated

with intraoperative mitomycin C (130). Similarly, intraoperative application of 0.04% (0.4 mg/mL) mitomycin C for 3 minutes after excision of primary pterygia had a 10.5% recurrence rate after a mean follow-up time of 16 months (126). In a prospective, randomized clinical trial, intraoperative application of 0.02% (0.2 mg/mL) mitomycin C for 5 minutes, of 0.04% (0.4 mg/mL) mitomycin C for 5 minutes, of 0.02% (0.2 mg/mL) mitomycin C for 3 minutes, and of 0.04% (0.4 mg/mL) mitomycin C for 3 minutes resulted in recurrence rates of 8.3%, 8.6%, 42.9%, and 22.9%, respectively, compared with a recurrence rate of 75% in the control group of eyes treated with placebo (131). A high recurrence rate (23.8%) was observed after 6 months' follow-up in patients treated with 0.025% (0.25 mg/mL) mitomycin C for 2 minutes in another study (132). A review of 870 patients with primary and recurrent pterygia in the Virgin Islands who were treated with a small conjunctival flap and a single application of 0.04% mitomycin C to bare sclera revealed a very low recurrence rate of 0.35% (133).

Preoperative Intralesional Mitomycin C Injection

Mitomycin C has been injected into the head of pterygia before surgery in an effort to destroy the fibroblasts and prepare the area for prevention of recurrence. A single 0.1- to 0.15-mL injection of 0.01% (0.1 mg/mL) of mitomycin C has been given into the head of the pterygium and the pterygium excised 1 month later (134,135). Both of these reports demonstrated serious side effects using this strategy. In a more recent study, 0.1 mL of 0.15 mg/mL mitomycin C was injected into the head of the pterygium and it was excised with bare-sclera technique 1 month later. These 36 patients were followed from 6 to 42 months after surgery (mean follow-up, 24.4 months), and there was a recurrence rate of 6% over this period (136). Besides preventing pterygium recurrence, the advantages sought by preoperative intralesional mitomycin C injection were to destroy the fibroblasts before surgery and to prevent corneal epithelial damage from topical mitomycin C.

Side Effects and Complications Associated with Topical Mitomycin C

Scleral thinning has been observed as a complication of postoperative or intraoperative mitomycin C application. This must be distinguished from a dellen effect because of excessive dissection or because of localized dry spot formation after pterygium excision. Dellen formation is common after pterygium surgery during the early phase of healing and has been mistaken for scleral thinning caused by topical mitomycin C. Singh et al. and Tsai et al. each have reported such a case in which conservative treatment led to filling up of the thinned sclera and resolution without problems (119,137).

The long-term use or use of high concentrations of topical mitomycin C has been associated with ocular toxicity (98,101,120). Fujitani et al. reported corneoscleral thinning and perforation after use of 0.04% (0.4 mg/mL) topical mitomycin C three times a day for 10 days after surgery (138), and Rubinfeld et al. (140) reported 10 cases of serious and vision-threatening ocular complications after adjunctive topical use of mitomycin C in the treatment of pterygium. These complications included secondary glaucoma, corneal edema, corneal perforation, iritis, photophobia, and pain. However, these adverse outcomes were seen after prolonged and unsupervised topical administration of mitomycin C, and in some cases the concentration of mitomycin C was much higher than the recommended concentration (139). There have also been reports of toxicity after a single dose of mitomycin C. Dougherty et al. reported one case of corneoscleral melt in their series of intraoperative applications of 0.02% (0.2 mg/mL) mitomycin C for 3 minutes to bare sclera during pterygium surgery. There were no other adverse effects in this series (140). Frucht-Pery and Ilsar demonstrated

that a lower concentration of mitomycin C administrated over a short time increases safety without compromising efficacy (141). In our original report and subsequently, we strongly recommended lower-dose mitomycin C for pterygium surgery (98,101,119,120).

Conjunctival Transplantation

Elschnig and Spaeth separately performed pedicle flap conjunctival grafts to prevent pterygium recurrence in 1926 (6). Campodonico in 1922 and Bangerter in 1943 performed movable conjunctival flap grafting (6). Jacobi et al. in Germany and Said et al. in Egypt separately successfully performed this procedure in 1975 (138). Kenyon et al. revisited the procedure of conjunctival autografting in preventing pterygium recurrence (138), using essentially the same procedure, with some modifications, that Barraquer (44) had described. We studied this procedure and compared its results with use of topical mitomycin C (118,120) (Fig. 60-9). The recurrence rates for pterygium after conjunctival autografting have been as low as 5.3% (142) and 7.7% (143). Our recurrence rate with this procedure was 6.6% (124). Cheng et al. found a recurrence rate of 6.3% after 3.5-year follow-up in patients who had recurrent pterygia excised and had received conjunctival autografting (127). Manning et al. reported a recurrence rate of 22.2% (4 of 18 eyes) after a mean follow-up of 16 months (126).

In a preliminary report of conjunctival miniautografting in eight patients, there were no recurrences after follow-up periods ranging from 5 to 9 years (144). Akura et al. observed similar results after primary pterygium excision and adjunct miniflap conjunctival transpositioning technique, with a 1-year follow-up (145). Their technique differed in that they used additional adjunct application of intraoperative mitomycin C to the bare sclera. They reported a 4.2% recurrence rate after large flap conjunctival transpositioning along with intraoperative mitomycin C application,

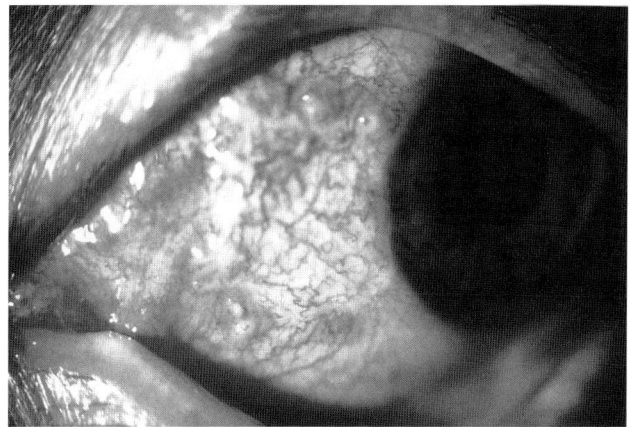
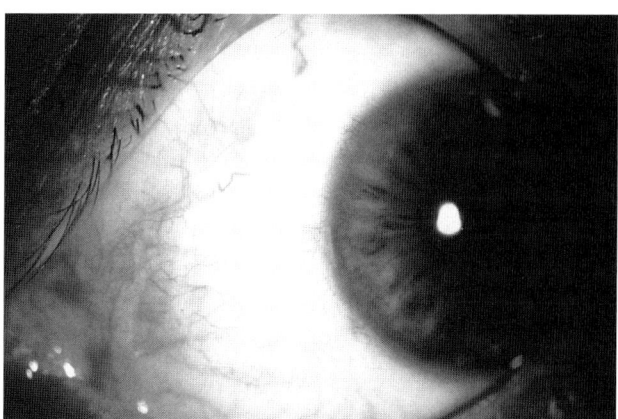

FIGURE 60-9. A: Conjunctival autograft 2 weeks after primary nasal pterygium excision. **B:** Same eye with excellent results 1 year after conjunctival autografting.

compared with a 15.5% recurrence rate if the large flap conjunctival transpositioning was performed without adjunctive use of mitomycin C (145). Others have also used intraoperative mitomycin C with conjunctival autograft in pterygium surgery (146).

Limbal Stem Cell Transplantation

Strampelli first described autologous limbal transplantation in 1960 and Barraquer popularized it in the management of ocular surface disorders in 1964 (147). Corneal epithelial stem cells are located in the deep layer of limbal epithelial cells. It has been suggested that healthy limbal epithelium acts as a junctional barrier to conjunctival cells migrating onto the corneal surface (148,149). Tseng et al. have speculated that pterygium represents "local limbal stem cell deficiency" (150). Based on this idea, it has been suggested that limbal stem cells be included in any conjunctival autograft used to prevent pterygium recurrence. This would theoretically restore the barrier function of the limbus and would achieve better anatomic and functional reconstruction after pterygium removal (151). Limbal conjunctival autograft transplantation has been effective in preventing recurrence of pterygium (152,153).

The surgical technique resembles the basic technique used for conjunctival autografting after bare sclera pterygium excision, with the difference being the harvesting of the conjunctival graft. The limbal-conjunctival graft includes 0.5 mm of the limbus/peripheral cornea. A superficial circumferential incision is made in the cornea 0.5 mm from the limbus, equal in length to the resected limbus at the time of pterygium excision. The conjunctival graft is mobilized from the distal end of this corneal incision, and dissection is continued forward to join the corneal incision and remove 0.5 mm of peripheral limbal cornea along with the conjunctiva. This free graft is placed in the correct orientation onto the scleral recipient bed. The corneal limbal side of the graft is sutured in place with interrupted 10/0 nylon and the conjunctival side is sutured with 10/0 vicryl sutures. Postoperative care is the same as for conjunctival autografting.

The recurrence rates of pterygium after limbal autografting have been variable, from zero to 15%. Gris et al. reported no recurrences after limbal conjunctival autografting in seven patients who had recurrent pterygia (154), and Pulte et al. reported a 2.85% recurrence rate (2 recurrences of a total of 70 pterygia, 62 primary and 8 recurrent) with a mean follow-up of 45 months (155). Rao et al. reported a 3.8% recurrence rate after a mean follow-up of 19 months, with 2 recurrences in a group of 53 (36 primary, 17 recurrent) pterygia (156). But Shimazaki et al. recorded a recurrence rate of 7.9% with advanced and recurrent pterygia after a mean follow-up of 11 months after limbal conjunctival autografting (157), and similar results (7.4% recurrence rate) were recorded after limbal stem cell transplantation

at 10.5 months' follow-up by Ivekovic et al. (132). Kmiha et al. recorded a recurrence rate of 10% with limbal conjunctival autografting after primary and recurrent pterygia excision with a mean follow-up of 14 months (158). Ozer et al. documented a 13.7% recurrence rate after marginal conjunctival autografting, compared with a 37.8% recurrence rate after bare-sclera pterygium excision (159). Mutlu et al. reported a 14.6% recurrence rate with a minimum follow-up of 15 months after limbal stem cell conjunctival autografting to prevent pterygium recurrences (160), and Wong et al. experienced an 18.2% recurrence rate (2 of 11 eyes) after a mean follow-up of 16.2 months in patients who had recurrent pterygium removed with adjunctive inferior limbal conjunctival autograft transplantation (161).

Clearly, limbal-conjunctival autograft transplantation has its limitations. It is technically demanding and time-consuming, requiring excellent attention to surgical details such as complete removal of episcleral scar tissue, harvesting a graft of proper size and free of Tenon's capsule tissue, and meticulous dissection and handling of the graft tissue. Several authors have attributed pterygium recurrences and graft failure to lack of surgical experience in performing combined limbal and conjunctival grafting (160,162,163). Others have attributed failure to inadequate postoperative antiinflammatory therapy (157).

Amniotic Membrane Allograft Transplantation

Panzardi first performed amniotic membrane grafting after pterygium excision in 1947 (6). Recent advances in our understanding of postsurgical fibrosis and pterygium recurrence have rekindled interest in amniotic membrane transplantation in pterygium management. The hyperproliferative nature of subconjunctival fibroblasts can result in fibrosis with accelerated growth of recurrent pterygium after primary pterygium removal. It is hypothesized that if the underlying disorder of subconjunctival fibrosis is not addressed, pterygia will recur. Transplantation of preserved human amniotic membrane suppresses postsurgical fibrosis and fibroblast proliferation, lowering the rate of recurrence of pterygium (164–167).

Amnion is the innermost layer of the placenta. It consists of a thick basement membrane and an avascular stroma. Placenta is obtained at the time of elective cesarean section from a willing donor who has been shown, by all the appropriate testing, to be free of potentially transmittable infections, such as human immunodeficiency virus, hepatitis B, hepatitis C, and syphilis. Amnion is manually separated from chorion and washed with physiologic saline containing an antibiotic. The amniotic membrane is cut into small pieces, which are immersed in sequential concentrations (0.5 M, 1.0 M, and 1.5 M) of dimethylsulfoxide. These pieces are stored at $-80°C$ until they are used. This tissue is thawed and washed with physiologic saline immediately before use (168).

In 1940, de Rötth was the first to use live fetal membrane, amnion, and chorion together in the management of symblepharon (169). It is hypothesized that live cells and chorion transplanted with amnion in his technique induced graft rejection in a large number of patients. With recent advances in preserving pure amnion in Dulbecco's modified Eagle's culture medium and glycerol, with storage at a temperature of $-80°C$, the amnion is rendered a substrate without live cells, and the problem of graft rejection is solved. Amniotic membrane is commercially available as dehydrated, sterilized, and lyophilized tissue packaged for room-temperature storage. After bare-sclera pterygium excision and hemostasis, the graft is cut to cover that area, and sutured in the recipient bed.

It has been shown that amniotic membrane stromal matrix suppresses transforming growth factor-β signaling, proliferation, and myofibroblastic differentiation of normal human corneal and limbal fibroblasts (170) and normal conjunctival and pterygium body fibroblasts (171). This mechanism of action probably helps reduce scar formation after conjunctival reconstruction (172) and prevents fibroblast activation and pterygium recurrence. The amniotic membrane stromal matrix also suppresses the expression of certain inflammatory cytokines that originate from the ocular surface epithelia (173). It has been demonstrated that inflammatory cytokines activate the pterygium body fibroblasts to overexpress metalloproteinases types 1 and 3 (174). Suppression of inflammation is a key element in the prevention of further fibrovascular proliferation and scar formation after pterygium removal. Therefore, it is important extensively to remove the fibrovascular tissue in recurrent pterygia in an effort to prevent inflammatory reaction and to promote the success of amniotic membrane transplantation (167). It has been recommended that intraoperative and postoperative long-acting corticosteroids be used to suppress the ongoing inflammation in an effort to reduce the recurrence rate for both primary and recurrent pterygia after amniotic membrane transplantation (167). Furthermore, amniotic membrane supports the normal phenotype of a nongoblet conjunctival epithelium in culture (175,176), and amniotic membrane transplantation maintains a normal conjunctival epithelium with goblet cell differentiation *in vivo* (175). This makes amniotic membrane grafts theoretically superior to buccal or other mucous membrane grafts, whose epithelia are different from that of the conjunctiva (173).

A recurrence rate of pterygia of 15.4% (2 of 13 patients) has been recorded after 4 months of follow-up by Ivekovic et al. in patients treated with amniotic membrane transplantation (132). The recurrence rate of primary pterygium after bare-sclera excision and adjunctive use of preserved human amniotic membrane transplant was 10.7% (3 of 28 eyes), compared with a recurrence rate of 64.5% (20 of 31 eyes) after simple bare-sclera pterygium excision by Tekin and associates, with a mean follow-up of 15 months (177).

It has been suggested that amniotic membrane transplantation is more successful in preventing pterygium recurrence if the graft is covered with either limbal or conjunctival autograft transplants (168). The success rate of these newer procedures has been approximately 80% in preventing pterygium recurrence (168).

Lamellar Keratoplasty

Lamellar keratoplasty has been performed to replace the thinned and scarred corneal tissue after pterygium excision and has been used as a barrier against the regrowth of pterygium. It is performed as an adjunctive procedure to treat only recurrent pterygium. Magitot was the first to recommend keratoplasty in the treatment of pterygium, in 1916 (178). He prepared a conjunctival flap to secure the lamellar corneal graft in place. Pierse and Casey treated nine patients with rectangular keratoplasty, without any recurrences (179). Mohan et al. successfully used the keyhole-shaped lamellar corneoscleral graft in pterygium treatment (180). Laughrea and Arentsen used circular corneoscleral lamellar grafts sutured with 10/0 nylon sutures after pterygium excision (181). Busin and associates treated 13 eyes with recurrent pterygia with lamellar keratectomy followed by placement of a precarved, lyophilized donor corneal tissue in the recipient bed (182). The corneal graft was sutured in the bed with 10/0 nylon sutures and the bare sclera was covered with pedunculated or free conjunctival autograft.

The recurrence rates of pterygium after different lamellar keratoplasty procedures have ranged from no recurrence (179,183,184) to 100% recurrence (63,64). Overall, the use of lamellar keratoplasty for recurrent pterygium resulted in recurrence rates of 5% (180), 30% (181), 31% (185), and 55% (186). Use of lyophilized donor tissue in lamellar keratoplasty did not have any distinct advantage because the recurrence rate was 23% (3 of 13) after these procedures (182).

Lamellar keratoplasty has no special advantage in preventing pterygium recurrence and has not been a favored procedure in treating primary pterygium. It has been mostly used in treating recurrent pterygium to restore the structural integrity of the globe in patients with thinned corneas by providing a new Bowman's layer in the affected area. In certain cases, multiple attempts to remove recurrent pterygia might lead to so much thinning of cornea that penetrating keratoplasty would be needed to restore the integrity of the cornea. An advantage of lyophilized donor tissue over fresh tissue is that the preserved tissue can be stored for up to 2 months and used in event of emergency.

CONCLUSION

Despite recent advances in our understanding of the etiopathology of pterygium and in its treatment with the adjunctive use of mitomycin C, conjunctival transplantation, limbal stem cell transplantation, amniotic membrane allograft transplantation, or different combinations of these treatment modalities, management of pterygium remains a challenge because of its tendency to recur. Adjunctive use of mitomycin C is toxic to the eye with prolonged use or in high concentrations, but if used within safe guidelines, it definitely has a role in preventing pterygium recurrence. Limbal stem cell and amniotic membrane transplantation procedures have demonstrated encouraging results but are still being investigated for long-term results. For a comprehensive ophthalmologist, these procedures are time-consuming and need meticulous handling of the tissue, and for those reasons still are not well accepted.

ACKNOWLEDGMENT

Malika G. Singh and Annie-Claire Binoche have been very supportive and inspirational in the completion of this chapter.

REFERENCES

1. Bidyadhar NK. Susruta and his operations. *Arch Ophthalmol* 1939;22:550–574.
2. Bidyadhar NK. Pterygium: ancient and modern concepts. *Antiseptic* 1941;38:282–286.
3. Rosenthal JW. Chronology of pterygium therapy. *Am J Ophthalmol* 1953;36:601–616.
4. Thomas CI. Pterygium. In: Thomas CI, ed. *The cornea.* Springfield, IL: Charles C Thomas, 1955:775–807.
5. Jaros PA, DeLuise VP. Pingueculae and pterygia. *Surv Ophthalmol* 1988;33:41–49.
6. Duke-Elder S. Diseases of the outer eye. In: Duke-Elder S, ed. *System of ophthalmology*, vol VIII, part 1: *Conjunctiva.* St. Louis: CV Mosby, 1965:573–582.
7. Desmarres LA. *Traite theorique et pratique des maladies des yeux*, 2nd ed. Paris: G. Baillere, 1866:168.
8. Mata P. Surgical treatment of pterygium with mucous autoplasty. *Arch Oftal Hispanoam* 1931;31:177.
9. Hawley CW. Transplantation of skin for pterygium. *Ann Ophthalmol* 1911;20:451.
10. Hawley CW. A pterygium operation. *Ill Med J* 1937;71:489.
11. Terson A. Structure and pathogenesis of pterygium: with a modified operation. *Arch Ophthalmol* 1911;31:161.
12. Bettman B. Subvolution: a new pterygium operation. *Chicago Med Rec* 1894;6:1.
13. Boeckman E. The operative treatment of pterygium. *JAMA* 1897;28:97.
14. Cameron ME. *Pterygium throughout the world.* Springfield, IL: Charles C Thomas, 1965:141, 171.
15. Islam SI, Wagoner MD. Pterygium in young members of one family. *Cornea* 2001;20:708–710.
16. Kerkenezov N. A pterygium survey of the far north coast of New South Wales. *Trans Ophthalmol Soc Aust* 1956;16:110–119.
17. Darrell RW, Bachrach CA. Pterygium among veterans: an epidemiologic study showing a correlation between frequency of pterygium and degree of exposure of ultraviolet in sunlight. *Arch Ophthalmol* 1963;70:158–169.
18. Elliot R. The aetiology and pathology of pterygium. *Trans Ophthalmol Soc Aust N Z* 1966;25:71–74.
19. Taylor HR. Aetiology of climate droplet keratopathy and pterygium. *Br J Ophthalmol* 1980;64:154–163.
20. Moran DJ, Hollows FC. Pterygium and ultraviolet radiation: a positive correlation. *Br J Ophthalmol* 1984;68:343–346.
21. Karai I, Horiguchi S. Pterygium in welders. *Br J Ophthalmol* 1984;68:347–349.
22. Rojas JR, Malaga H. Pterygium in Lima, Peru. *Ann Ophthalmol* 1986;18:147–149.
23. Wharton KR, Yolton RL. Visual characteristics of rural Central and South Americans. *J Am Optom Assoc* 1986;57:426–430.
24. Serra A. An epidemiological study on actinic effect of light in Sardinia. *Bull Soc Belg Ophthalmol* 1987;224:139–146.
25. Mackenzie FD, Hirst LW, Battistutta D, et al. Risk analysis in the development of pterygium. *Ophthalmology* 1992;99:1056–1061.
26. Taylor HR. Ultraviolet radiation and the eye: an epidemiological study. *Trans Am Ophthalmol Soc* 1989;87:802–853.
27. Taylor HR, West SK, Rosenthal FS, et al. Corneal changes associated with chronic UV irradiation. *Arch Ophthalmol* 1989;107:1481–1484.
28. Pico G. Pterygium: current concept of etiology and management. In: King JH, McTigue JW, eds. *The cornea: First World Congress on the Cornea.* Washington, DC: Butterworths, 1965:280–291.
29. Zehender. Cited by Parsons JHL. *Pathology of the eye.* London: GP Putnam's Sons, 1904:107.
30. Sugar HS. Surgical treatment of pterygium. *Am J Ophthalmol* 1949;32:912–916.
31. D'Ombrian A. The surgical treatment of pterygium. *Br J Ophthalmol* 1948;32:65–71.
32. Beard HH, Dimitry TJ. Some observations upon the chemical nature of pterygium. *Am J Ophthalmol* 1945;28:303–305.
33. Detels R, Dhir SP. Pterygium: a geographical study. *Arch Ophthalmol* 1967;78:485–491.
34. Hilgers JHC. Pterygium: its incidence, heredity and etiology. *Am J Ophthalmol* 1960;50:635–644.
35. Kamel S. Pterygium: its nature and a new line of treatment. *Br J Ophthalmol* 1946;30:549–564.
36. King JH. The pterygium: brief review of certain methods of treatment. *Arch Ophthalmol* 1950;44:854–858.
37. Vass Z, Tapaszto I. The histochemical examination of the fibers of pterygium by elastase. *Acta Ophthalmol* 1964;42:849–854.
38. Hogan MJ, Alvarado J. Pterygium and pinguecula: electron microscopic study. *Arch Ophthalmol* 1967;78:174–186.
39. Ansari MW, Rahi AHS, Shukla BR. Pseudoelastic nature of pterygium. *Br J Ophthalmol* 1970;54:473–476.
40. Wong WW. A hypothesis on the pathogenesis of pterygium. *Ann Ophthalmol* 1978;10:303–308.
41. Austin P, Jakobiec FA, Iwamoto T. Elastodysplasia and elastodystrophy as the pathologic basis of ocular pterygia and pinguecula. *Ophthalmology* 1983;90:96–109.
42. Cameron ME. Histology of pterygium: an electron microscopic study. *Br J Ophthalmol* 1983;67:604–608.
43. Pinkerton OD, Hokama Y, Shigemura LA. Immunologic basis for the pathogenesis of pterygium. *Am J Ophthalmol* 1984;98:225–228.
44. Barraquer JI. Etiology, pathogenesis, and treatment of the pterygium. In: *Symposium on medical and surgical diseases of the cornea: transactions of the New Orleans Academy of Ophthalmology.* St. Louis: CV Mosby, 1980:167–178.
45. Dushku N, Reid TW. P53 expression in altered limbal basal cells of pingueculae, pterygia, and limbal tumors. *Curr Eye Res* 1997;16:1179–1192.
46. Tan DTH, Lim ASM, Goh HS, et al. Abnormal expression of the p53 tumor suppressor gene in the conjunctiva of patients with pterygium. *Am J Ophthalmol* 1997;123:404–405.

47. Spandidos DA, Sourvinos G, Kiaris H, et al. Microsatellite instability and loss of heterozygosity in human pterygia. *Br J Ophthalmol* 1997;81:493–496.

48. Onur CA, Orhan D, Orhan M, et al. Expression of p53 protein in pterygium. *Eur J Ophthalmol* 1998;8:157–161.

49. Chowers I, Pe'er J, Zamir E, et al. Proliferative activity and p53 expression in primary and recurrent pterygia. *Ophthalmology* 2001;108:985–988.

50. Karukonda SRK, Thompson HW, Beuerman RW, et al. Cell cycle kinetics in pterygium at three latitudes. *Br J Ophthalmol* 1995;79:313–317.

51. Perra MT, Maxia C, Zucca I, et al. Immunohistochemical study of human pterygium. *Histol Histopathol* 2002;17:139–149.

52. Redslob E. Contribution a l'étude de la nature du pterygion (French). *Ann Oculist* 1933;170:42.

53. Cogan DG, Kuwabara T, Howard J. The nonelastic nature of pingueculas. *Arch Ophthalmol* 1959;61:388.

54. Hill JC, Maske R. Pathogenesis of pterygium. *Eye* 1989;3:218–226.

55. Stocker FW. Eine pigmentierte Hornhautlinie beim Pterygium (German). *Klin Monatsbl Augenheilkd* 1939;102:384–388.

56. Gerundo M. On the etiology and pathology of pterygium. *Am J Ophthalmol* 1951;34:851–856.

57. Townsend WM. Pterygium. In: Kaufman HE, McDonald MB, Barron BA, et al., eds. *The cornea*. New York: Churchill Livingstone, 1988:461–483.

58. Rosenthal FS, Bakalian AE, Taylor HR. The effect of prescription eyewear on ocular exposure to ultraviolet radiation. *Am J Public Health* 1986;76:1216–1220.

59. Rosenthal FS, Bakalian AE, Lou CQ, et al. The effect of sunglasses on ocular exposure to ultraviolet radiation. *Am J Public Health* 1988;78:72–74.

60. Rich AM, Keitzman B, Payne T, et al. A simplified way to remove pterygia. *Ann Ophthalmol* 1974;6:739–741.

61. Avisar R, Arnon A, Avisar E, et al. Primary pterygium recurrence time. *Isr Med Assoc J* 2001;3:836–837.

62. Castroviejo: Symposium on the cornea. *Trans Am Acad Ophthalmol Otolaryngol* 1972;76:165–172.

63. Youngson RM. Recurrence of pterygium after excision. *Br J Ophthalmol* 1972;56:120–125.

64. Youngson RM. Pterygium in Israel. *Am J Ophthalmol* 1972;74:954–959.

65. Tarr KH, Constable IJ. Late complications of pterygium treatment. *Br J Ophthalmol* 1980;64:496–505.

66. Gibson JBG. Brisbane survey of pterygium. *Trans Ophthalmol Soc Aust* 1956;16:125.

67. Troutbeck R, Hirst L. Review of treatment of pterygium in Queensland: 10 years after a primary survey. *Clin Exp Ophthalmol* 2001;29:286–290.

68. Dadeya S, Kamlesh. Intraoperative daunorubicin to prevent the recurrence of pterygium after excision. *Cornea* 2001;20:172–174.

69. Pikkel J, Porges Y, Ophir A. Halting pterygium recurrence by postoperative 5-fluorouracil. *Cornea* 2001;20:168–171.

70. Maldonado MJ, Cano-Parra J, Navea-Tejerina A, et al. Inefficacy of low-dose intraoperative fluorouracil in the treatment of primary pterygium. *Arch Ophthalmol* 1995;113:1356–1357.

71. Hilgers JHC. Strontium 90 β-irradiation, cataractogenicity, and pterygium recurrence. *Arch Ophthalmol* 1966;76:329–333.

72. Simsek T, Gunalp I, Atilla H. Comparative efficacy of beta-irradiation and mitomycin-C in primary and recurrent pterygium. *Eur J Ophthalmol* 2001;11:126–132.

73. Amano S, Motoyama Y, Oshika T, et al. Comparative study of intraoperative mitomycin C and beta irradiation in pterygium surgery. *Br J Ophthalmol* 2000;84:618–621.

74. Bahrassa F, Datta R. Postoperative beta radiation treatment of pterygium. *Int J Radiat Oncol Biol Phys* 1983;9:679–684.

75. Friedell HL, Thomas CI, Krohmer JS. An evaluation of the clinical use of a strontium 90 beta-ray applicator with a review of the underlying principles. *Radiology* 1954;71:25–39.

76. Cooper JS. Post-operative irradiation of pterygia: ten more years of experience. *Radiology* 1978;128:733–756.

77. Pinkerton OD. Post-op strontium 90 treatment lowers pterygium recurrence. *Ophthalmol Times* 1986;(May):15:54.

78. Pinkerton OD. Strontium barriers in pterygium surgery. *Trans Am Acad Ophthalmol Otolaryngol* 1975;79:613–614.

79. Alaniz-Camino F. The use of post-operative beta radiation in the treatment of pterygia. *Ophthalmic Surg* 1982;13:1022–1025.

80. Thommy CP, Abiose A. Beta irradiation in the management of pterygium. *J Ocular Ther Surg* 1983;60:236–241.

81. van den Brenk HAS. Results of prophylactic post-operative irradiation in 1,300 cases of pterygium. *AJR Am J Roentgenol* 1968;103:723–733.

82. Merriam GR. The effects of beta radiation on the eye. *Radiology* 1956;66:240–245.

83. Merriam GR, Focht EF. A clinical study of radiation cataracts and the relationship to dose. *AJR Am J Roentgenol* 1957;77:739.

84. Haik GM, Lyda W, Waugh RL Jr, et al. Cataract formation following beta-ray radium therapy. *Am J Ophthalmol* 1954;38:465.

85. Thomas CI, Storaasli JP, Friedell HL. Lenticular changes associated with beta radiation of the eye and their significance. *Radiology* 1972;79:588–595.

86. Hughes WF. Beta radiation sources, uses and dangers in treatment of the eye. *JAMA* 1959;170:2096.

87. Willner J, Flentje M, Lieb W. Soft X-ray therapy of recurrent pterygium: an alternative to 90Sr eye applicators. *Strahlenther Onkol* 2001;177:404–409.

88. Langham ME. Inhibition of corneal vascularization by triethylene thiophosphoramide. *Am J Ophthalmol* 1960;49:1111–1125.

89. Meacham CT. Triethylene thiophosphoramide in the prevention of pterygium recurrence. *Am J Ophthalmol* 1962;54:751–753.

90. Mori S. Studies on the pterygium. Report III: a new treatment of the pterygium. *Acta Soc Ophthalmol Jpn* 1962;66:990–1000.

91. Cassady JR. The inhibition of pterygium recurrence by Thiotepa. *Am J Ophthalmol* 1966;61:886–888.

92. Liddy BSL, Morgan JF. Triethylene thiophosphoramide (Thiotepa) and pterygium. *Am J Ophthalmol* 1966;61:888–890.

93. Joselson GA, Muller P. Incidence of pterygium recurrence in patients treated with Thio-tepa. *Am J Ophthalmol* 1966;61:891–892.

94. Howitt D, Karp EJ. Side-effect of topical Thio-tepa. *Am J Ophthalmol* 1969;68:473–474.

95. Asregadoo ER. Surgery, Thio-tepa, and corticosteroids in the treatment of pterygium. *Am J Ophthalmol* 1972;74:960–963.

96. Wakaki S, Marumo H, Tomioka K. Isolation of new fractions of anti-tumor mitomycins. *Antibiot Chemother* 1958;8:228–240.

97. Verweij J, Stoter G. Severe side effects of the cytotoxic drug mitomycin-C. *Neth J Med* 1987;30:43–50.

98. Singh G, Wilson MR, Foster CS. Mitomycin eye drops as treatment for pterygium. *Ophthalmology* 1988;95:813–821.

99. Hardman JG, Limbird LE, Molinoff PB, et al., eds. *Goodman & Gilman's the pharmacological basis of therapeutics*, 9th ed. New York: McGraw-Hill, 1996:1268.

100. Kunitomo N, Mori S. Studies on the pterygium. Report IV: Treatment of the pterygium by mitomycin C instillation. *Nippon Ganka Gakkai Zasshi* 1963;67:601–607.

101. Singh G, Wilson MR, Foster CS. Mitomycin eye drops as treatment for pterygium. *Ophthalmology* 1987;94[Suppl]:76.

102. Choon LK, Fong CY. The pterygium and mitomycin-C therapy. *Med J Malaysia* 1976;31:69–72.

103. Chayakul V. Prevention of recurrent pterygium by mitomycin-C. *Fortschr Ophthalmol* 1987;84:422–424.

104. Hayasaka S, Noda S, Yamamoto Y, et al. Postoperative instillation of low-dose mitomycin C in the treatment of primary pterygium. *Am J Ophthalmol* 1988;106:715–718.

105. Mahar PS, Nwokora GE. Role of mitomycin C in pterygium surgery. *Br J Ophthalmol* 1993;77:433–435.

106. Kraut A, Drnovsek-Olup B. Instillation of mitomycin C after recurrent pterygium surgery. *Eur J Ophthalmol* 1996;6:264–267.

107. Helal M, Messiha N, Amayem A, et al. Intraoperative mitomycin-C versus postoperative topical mitomycin-C drops for the treatment of pterygium. *Ophthalmic Surg Lasers* 1996;27:674–678.

108. Palmer SS. Mitomycin as adjunct chemotherapy with trabeculectomy. *Ophthalmology* 1991;98:317–321.

109. Frucht-Pery J, Rozenman Y. Mitomycin C therapy for corneal intraepithelial neoplasia. *Am J Ophthalmol* 1994;117:164–168.

110. Wilson MW, Hungerford JL, George SM, et al. Topical mitomycin C for the treatment of conjunctival and corneal epithelial dysplasia and neoplasia. *Am J Ophthalmol* 1997;124:303–311.

111. Heigle TJ, Stulting RD, Palay DA. Treatment of recurrent conjunctival epithelial neoplasia with topical mitomycin C. *Am J Ophthalmol* 1997;124:397–399.

112. Donnenfeld ED, Perry HD, Wallerstein A, et al. Subconjunctival mitomycin C for the treatment of ocular cicatricial pemphigoid. *Ophthalmology* 1999;106:72–79.

113. Majmudar PA, Forstot SL, Dennis RF, et al. Topical mitomycin-C for subepithelial fibrosis after refractive corneal surgery. *Ophthalmology* 2000;107:89–94.

114. Talamo JH, Gollamudi S, Green WR, et al. Modulation of corneal wound healing after excimer laser keratomileusis using topical mitomycin C and steroids. *Arch Ophthalmol* 1991;109:1141–1146.

115. Schipper I, Suppelt C, Gebbers JO. Mitomycin C reduces scar formation after excimer laser (193 nm) photorefractive keratectomy in rabbits. *Eye* 1997;11:649–655.

116. Tsai CC, Kau HC, Kao SC, et al. Efficacy of probing the nasolacrimal duct with adjunctive mitomycin-C for epiphora in adults. *Ophthalmology* 2002;109:172–174.

117. Liu D, Bosley TM. Silicone nasolacrimal intubation with mitomycin-C: a prospective, randomized, double masked study. *Ophthalmology* 2003;110:306–310.

118. Liao SL, Kao SCS, Tseng JHS, et al. Results of intraoperative mitomycin C application in dacryocystorhinostomy. *Br J Ophthalmol* 2000;84:903–906.

119. Singh G. Postoperative instillation of low-dose mitomycin C in the treatment of primary pterygium [letter]. *Am J Ophthalmol* 1989;107:570.

120. Singh G, Wilson MR, Foster CS. Effectivity and late complications of mitomycin in treatment of pterygium. *Ophthalmology* 1989;96[Suppl]:120.

121. Singh G. Toxicity of mitomycin eye drops as a treatment for pterygium. In: *Proceedings of the 72nd Annual Meeting of the Pacific Coast Oto-Ophthalmol Soc, Coronado, CA.* 1988;69:82–83.

122. Singh G, Wilson MR, Foster CS. Comparison of mitomycin treatment after pterygium excision with conjunctival autograft transplantation. *Ophthalmology* 1988;95[Suppl]:146.

123. Singh G. Pterygium in the tropics [letter]. *Ophthalmology* 1990;97:542.

124. Singh G, Wilson MR, Foster CS. Long-term follow-up study of mitomycin eye drops as adjunctive treatment for pterygia and its comparison with conjunctival autograft transplantation. *Cornea* 1990;9:331–334.

125. Rachmeil R, Leiba H, Levartovsky S. Results of treatment with topical mitomycin C 0.02% following excision of primary pterygium. *Br J Ophthalmol* 1995;79:233–236.

126. Manning CA, Kloess PM, Diaz MD, et al. Intraoperative mitomycin in primary pterygium excision: a prospective, randomized trial. *Ophthalmology* 1997;104:844–848.

127. Cheng HC, Tseng SH, Kao PL, et al. Low-dose intraoperative mitomycin-C as chemoadjuvant for pterygium surgery. *Cornea* 2001;20:24–29.

128. Mypet C, Oko H. Results of intra-operative 0.5mg/ml mitomycin-C with 20mg depo steroid in the treatment of primary pterygium. *Cent Afr J Med* 2000;46:330–332.

129. Frucht-Pery J, Siganos CS, Ilsar M. Intraoperative application of topical mitomycin C for pterygium surgery. *Ophthalmology* 1996;103:674–677.

130. Mastropasqua L, Carpineto P, Ciancaglini M, et al. Effectiveness of intraoperative mitomycin C in the treatment of recurrent pterygium. *Ophthalmologica* 1994;208:247–249.

131. Lam DSC, Wong AKK, Fan DSP, et al. Intraoperative mitomycin C to prevent recurrence of pterygium after excision: a 30-month follow-up study. *Ophthalmology* 1998;105:901–905.

132. Ivekovic R, Mandic Z, Saric D, et al. Comparative study of pterygium surgery. *Ophthalmologica* 2001;215:394–397.

133. Anduze AL. Pterygium surgery with mitomycin-C: ten-year results. *Ophthalmic Surg Lasers* 2001;32:341–345.

134. Donnenfeld ED, Perry HD, Kornstein A, et al. Subconjunctival mitomycin C in the management of recurrent pterygia. Presented at The Castroviejo Cornea Society Annual Meeting, New Orleans, LA, November 7, 1998.

135. Carrasco MA, Rapuano CJ, Cohen EJ, et al. Scleral ulceration after preoperative injection of mitomycin C in the pterygium head. *Arch Ophthalmol* 2002;120:1585–1586.

136. Donnenfeld ED, Perry HD, Fromer S, et al. Subconjunctival mitomycin C as adjunctive therapy before pterygium excision. *Ophthalmology* 2003;110:1012–1016.

137. Tsai YY, Lin JM, Shy JD. Acute scleral thinning after pterygium excision with intraoperative mitomycin-C: a case report of scleral dellen after bare sclera technique and review of literature. *Cornea* 2002;21:227–229.

138. Fujitani A, Hayasaka S, Shibuya Y, et al. Corneoscleral ulceration and corneal perforation after pterygium excision and topical mitomycin C therapy. *Ophthalmologica* 1993;207:162–164.

139. Dougherty PJ, Hardten DR, Lindstrom RL. Corneoscleral melt after pterygium surgery using a single intraoperative application of mitomycin-C. *Cornea* 1996;102:537–540.

140. Rubinfeld RS, Pfister RR, Stein RM, et al. Serious complications of topical mitomycin-C after pterygium surgery. *Ophthalmology* 1992;99:1647–1654.

141. Frucht-Pery J, Ilsar M. The use of low-dose mitomycin C for prevention of recurrent pterygium. *Ophthalmology* 1994;101:759–762.

142. Kenyon KR, Wagoner MD, Hettinger ME. Conjunctival autograft transplantation for advanced and recurrent pterygium. *Ophthalmology* 1985;92:1461–1470.

143. Dowlut MS, Laflamme MY. Les ptérygions récidivants: fréquence et correction par autogreffe conjonctivale (French). *Can J Ophthalmol* 1981;16:119–120.

144. John T. Pterygium excision and conjunctival mini-autograft: preliminary report. *Eye* 2001;15:292–296.

145. Akura J, Kaneda S, Matsuura K, et al. Measures for preventing recurrence after pterygium surgery. *Cornea* 2001;20:703–707.

146. Wong VA, Law FCH. Use of mitomycin C with conjunctival autograft in pterygium surgery in Asian-Canadians. *Ophthalmology* 1999;106:1512–1515.

147. King JH Jr, McTigue JW. *The cornea: world congress.* Baltimore: Butterworths, 1965:354.

148. Dushku N, Reid TW. Immunohistochemical evidence that human pterygia originate from an invasion of vimentin-expressing altered limbal epithelial basal cell. *Curr Eye Res* 1994;13:473–481.

149. Tseng SCG. Concept and application of limbal stem cells. *Eye* 1989;3:141–157.
150. Tseng SCG, Chen JJY, Huang AJW, et al. Classification of conjunctival surgeries for corneal diseases based on stem cell concept. *Ophthalmol Clin North Am* 1990;3:595–610.
151. Al Fayez MF. Limbal versus conjunctival autograft transplantation for advanced and recurrent pterygium. *Ophthalmology* 2002;109:1752–1755.
152. Koch JM, Mellin KB, Waubke TN. The pterygium, autologous conjunctiva-limbus transplantation as treatment [in French]. *Ophthalmologe* 1992;89:143–146.
153. Guler M, Sobaci C, Ilker S, et al. Limbal-conjunctival autograft transplantation in cases with recurrent pterygium. *Acta Ophthalmol (Copenh)* 1994;72:721–726.
154. Gris O, Guell JL, del Campo Z. Limbal-conjunctival autograft transplantation for the treatment of recurrent pterygium. *Ophthalmology* 2000;107:270–273.
155. Pulte P, Heilingenhaus A, Koch J, et al. Long-term results of autologous conjunctiva-limbus transplantation in pterygium [in German]. *Klin Monatsbl Augenheilkd* 1998;213:9–14.
156. Rao SK, Lekha T, Mukesh BN, et al. Conjunctival-limbal autografts for primary and recurrent pterygia. *Indian J Ophthalmol* 1998;46:203–209.
157. Shimazaki J, Yang HY, Tsubota K. Limbal autograft transplantation for recurrent and advanced pterygia. *Ophthalmic Surg Lasers* 1996;27:917–923.
158. Kmiha N, Kamoun B, Trigui A, et al. Effectiveness of conjunctival autograft transplantation in pterygium surgery [in French]. *J Fr Ophtalmol* 2001;24:729–732.
159. Ozer A, Yildirim N, Erol N, et al. Results of autografting of marginal conjunctiva in pterygium excision. *Ophthalmologica* 2002;216:198–202.
160. Mutlu FM, Sobaci G, Tatar Y, et al. A comparative study of recurrent pterygium surgery: limbal conjunctival autograft transplantation versus mitomycin C with conjunctival flap. *Ophthalmology* 1999;106:817–821.
161. Wong AK, Rao SK, Leung AT, et al. Inferior limbal-conjunctival autograft transplantation for recurrent pterygium. *Indian J Ophthalmol* 2000;48:21–24.
162. Ti SE, Chee SP, Dear KB, et al. Analysis of variation in success rates in conjunctival autografting for primary and recurrent pterygium. *Br J Ophthalmol* 2000;84:385–389.
163. Starc S, Knorr M, Steuhl KP, et al. Autologous conjunctival-limbus transplantation in treatment of primary and recurrent pterygium [in French]. *Ophthalmologe* 1996;93:219–223.
164. Shimazaki J, Shinozaki N, Tsubota K. Transplantation of amniotic membrane and limbal autograft for patients with recurrent pterygium associated with symblepharon. *Br J Ophthalmol* 1998;82:235–240.
165. Prabhasawat P, Barton K, Burkett G, et al. Comparison of conjunctival autografts, amniotic membrane grafts, and primary closure for pterygium excision. *Ophthalmology* 1997;104:974–985.
166. Ma DHK, See LC, Liau SB, et al. Amniotic membrane graft for primary pterygium: comparison with conjunctival autograft and topical Mitomycin C treatment. *Br J Ophthalmol* 2000;84:973–978.
167. Solomon A, Pires RTF, Tseng SCG. Amniotic membrane transplantation after extensive removal of primary and recurrent pterygia. *Ophthalmology* 2001;108:449–460.
168. Shimazaki J, Kosaka K, Shimmura S, et al. Amniotic membrane transplantation with conjunctival autograft for recurrent pterygium. *Ophthalmology* 2003;110:119–124.
169. de Rötth A. Plastic repair of conjunctival defects with fetal membrane. *Arch Ophthalmol* 1940;23:522–525.
170. Tseng SCG, Li DQ, Ma X. Suppression of transforming growth factor-beta isoforms, TGF-beta receptor type II, and myofibroblast differentiation in cultured human corneal and limbal fibroblasts by amniotic membrane matrix. *J Cell Physiol* 1999;179:325–335.
171. Lee SB, Li DQ, Tan DTH, et al. Suppression of TGF-beta signaling in both normal conjunctival fibroblasts and pterygial body fibroblasts by amniotic membrane. *Curr Eye Res* 2000;20:325–334.
172. Tseng SCG, Prabhasawat P, Lee SH. Amniotic membrane transplantation for conjunctival surface reconstruction. *Am J Ophthalmol* 1997;124:765–774.
173. Solomon A, Espana EM, Tseng SCG. Amniotic membrane transplantation for the reconstruction of the conjunctival fornices. *Ophthalmology* 2003;110:93–100.
174. Solomon A, Li DQ, Lee SB, et al. Regulation of collagenase, stromelysin, and urokinase-type plasminogen activator in primary pterygium body fibroblasts by inflammatory cytokines. *Invest Ophthalmol Vis Sci* 2000;41:2154–2163.
175. Meller D, Tseng SCG. Conjunctival epithelial cell differentiation on amniotic membrane. *Invest Ophthalmol Vis Sci* 1999;40:878–886.
176. Cho BJ, Djalilian AR, Obritsch WF, et al. Conjunctival epithelial cells cultured on human amniotic membrane fail to transdifferentiate into corneal epithelial-type cells. *Cornea* 1999;18:216–224.
177. Tekin NF, Kaynak S, Saatci AO, et al. Preserved human amniotic membrane transplantation in the treatment of primary pterygium. *Ophthalmic Surg Lasers* 2001;32:464–469.
178. Magitot A. Etude critique sur certaines proprietes biologiques due tissue corneen et sur la keratoplastie humaine (French). *Ann Oculist* 1916;153:417.
179. Pierse D, Casey TA. Lamellar keratoplasty. *Br J Ophthalmol* 1959;43:733–743.
180. Mohan M, Panda A, Goyal JL. Surgical management of recurrent pterygium (Mohan's technique). In: Cavanagh HD, ed. *The cornea: transactions of the World Congress on the Cornea III.* New York: Raven Press, 1988:377–381.
181. Laughrea PA, Arentsen JJ. Lamellar keratoplasty in the management of recurrent pterygium. *Ophthalmic Surg* 1986;17:106–108.
182. Busin M, Halliday BL, Arffa RC, et al. Precarved lyophilized tissue for lamellar keratoplasty in recurrent pterygium. *Am J Ophthalmol* 1986;102:222–227.
183. Jacobi KW, Krey H. Lamelläre Keratoplastik und Bindehauttransposition bei Pterygium. *Klin Monatsbl Augenheilkd* 1975;167:206–209.
184. Poirier RH, Fish JR. Lamellar keratoplasty for recurrent pterygium. *Ophthalmic Surg* 1976;7:38–41.
185. Hallermann W, Schroeder GM, Salehi AN. Ergebnisse der lamellaren Keratoplastik bei rezidivierenden Pterygien. *Klin Monatsbl Augenheilkd* 1977;171:191.
186. Pearlman G, Susal AL, Hushaw J, et al. Recurrent pterygium and treatment with lamellar keratoplasty with presentation of a technique to limit recurrences. *Ann Ophthalmol* 1970;2:763.

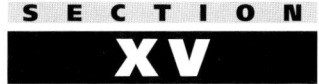

SECTION
XV

CORNEAL VISUAL REHABILITATION SURGERY

61

PENETRATING KERATOPLASTY

MICHELE MABON AND HELENE BOISJOLY

Penetrating keratoplasty (PK) is the surgical removal of diseased cornea with replacement by full-thickness corneal donor tissue. The procedure is performed for either optical reasons (restoration of corneal clarity) or tectonic reasons (restoration of structural integrity). At present, PK addresses both endothelial and stromal failures in either structure or function. With current and future developments, posterior lamellar keratoplasty with endothelial replacement may become an alternative to PK for cases of endothelial failure with a clear, healthy stroma. Most surgeons favor a PK over an anterior lamellar keratoplasty for deep stromal diseases because the visual acuity results appear to be better with PK. Deep anterior lamellar keratoplasty is, however, being revisited. Anterior and posterior lamellar keratoplasties are discussed in Chapters 62 and 63.

In 1838, Kissam performed a xenograft from the pig to a human, which failed (1). Zirm, however, is the first to have performed a successful human corneal PK in 1905, in Eastern Europe. In Prague, Elschnig emphasized the use of PK soon after 1910 (2). Tudor-Thomas popularized keratoplasty in Great Britain two decades later (3). An increased interest in PK arose with the arrival of corticosteroids in the 1950s, with the development of improved microsurgical techniques in the 1970s, including operative microscopes and fine sutures, and with improvements in availability and preservation of corneal tissue (4,5) (Fig. 61-1). PK has become the most frequently performed solid tissue transplantation, with over 46,949 corneal donor grafts obtained from the Eye Bank Association of America in 2000 used for transplantation in the United States (71% of donor grafts) or exported internationally (6).

When low- and high-risk PK cases are combined, corneal transplantation is as successful as kidney transplantation, with a 75% success rate at 5 years (7). In low-risk clinical situations, PK is one of the most successful transplantations, with a 10-year success rate, defined as corneal clarity, of 72% to 80% (8–10). This very high success rate in uncomplicated cases is despite the fact that tissue matching is not routinely performed and that systemic immunosuppression is rarely used unless required by high-risk clinical indications. Repeat corneal transplantation (10–13) and other high-risk

cases, in particular recipients with significant corneal vessels (10,11,14), carry a poor 40% to 50% success rate, comparable with that of liver transplantation (7).

A successful outcome after PK should, however, be measured not only by corneal clarity (Fig. 61-2). A clear cornea does not always correspond to improved visual acuity in the grafted eye, mostly because of residual regular and irregular astigmatism (15). Also, daily-life functional improvement after PK is greater if the level of vision is low in the other eye (16–18).

This chapter reviews donor and recipient preoperative considerations, the PK surgical procedure, surgical complications and their management, and immunologic rejection and tissue matching.

DONOR CONSIDERATIONS

Although there are anecdotal reports of xenografts, human donor corneas with a viable endothelial layer are required for corneal allografts. At present, one of the most important determinants of a successful corneal transplant program is high-quality eye bank screening and processing of human donor corneal tissue. Artificial corneas made of 2-hydroxyethyl methacrylate (PHEMA) with porous skirts are being developed (19). Similar to a keratoprosthesis, these artificial corneas can be associated with wound healing problems at the recipient–artificial cornea interface (20). Although promising, there is no indication that artificial corneas will substantially replace human donor tissue in the next few years.

Donor screening for infectious diseases is essential to protect recipients from severe or life-threatening illnesses by donor tissue transmission of human immunodeficiency virus (HIV) (21) and prions (22–24). Donor serology is used to screen for syphilis, hepatitis, and HIV (25). Eye bank staff aim to detect donor risk behaviors for HIV with a detailed sociobehavioral history. They also screen for Creutzfeld-Jakob disease, searching for the quadrate clinical prodrome of cognitive changes, speech abnormalities, cerebellar findings, and myoclonus or a history of recent travel to countries

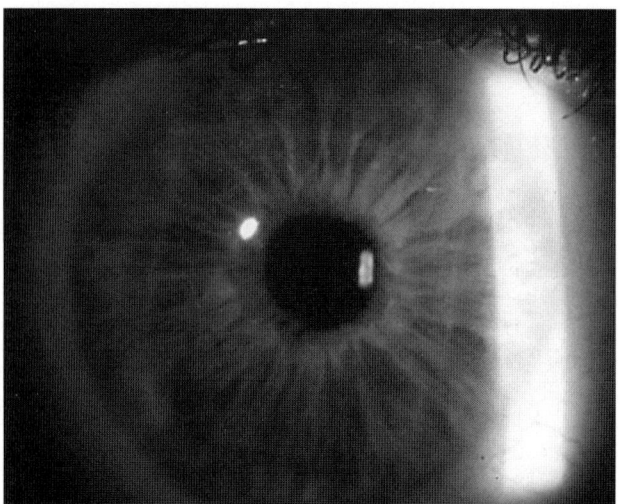

FIGURE 61-1. Square graft as performed by Castroviejo.

with reported prion encephalitis. There is no proven laboratory test yet available to eliminate the presence of prions in ocular tissue. The only available experimental marker testing for the presence of prions is the protease-resistant isoform of the prion protein. It has been detected in the human retina and optic nerve, but not yet in the cornea (26). It therefore is theoretically probably safer to procure the donor cornea with a scleral rim directly from the donor than to enucleate the donor before cutting out a corneoscleral button. There are other factors that bear on the decision about the suitability of donor tissue for transplantation. The Eye Bank Association of America has an ongoing committee that periodically reviews available data and sets

criteria for donor tissue selection and eye banking in the United States. Its most recent exclusion criteria, which are followed in many other countries, are reproduced in Table 61-1.

In our experience, donor corneas obtained from infants younger than 18 months of age should be avoided for transplantation because corneal ectasia and high myopia tend to develop in recipients after PK. Although it is common for surgeons to refuse corneal tissue from older donors, the scientific literature is not conclusive about this matter (27–36). There are reports suggesting that, given a normal endothelial cell count, older tissue performs equally as well as younger tissue. A 5-year prospective, masked trial designed to determine the safety and efficacy of using older donor tissue for keratoplasty is currently underway: the Cornea Donor Study. Specular microscopy with corneal endothelial cell count on donor tissue of all ages is an important preventive measure against primary donor failure.

Adequate donor cornea preservation before PK is essential because PK requires a viable donor endothelial layer that can sustain the surgical trauma and future cellular changes and cell loss (37). A variety of methods have been developed to ensure endothelial cell viability since the earlier methods of storage at 4°C and the first storage media introduced by McCarey and Kaufman (4) (Fig. 61-3). Most surgeons now use storage in nutrient media such as Optisol for up to several days (38) from the time of donor cornea procurement to the time of surgery. Other surgeons, mostly in Europe, have developed methods of long-term incubation at 37°C for several weeks before transplantation (39–41). Cryopreservation (42) is an alternative rarely used today because the local need for corneal tissue exceeds the supply.

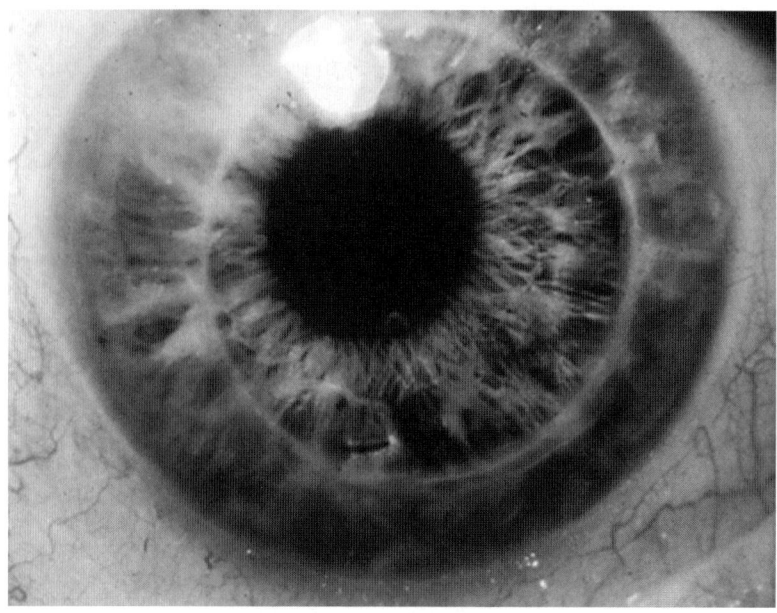

FIGURE 61-2. A clear corneal graft does not always confer a successful outcome.

TABLE 61-1. EYE BANK ASSOCIATION OF AMERICA MEDICAL STANDARDS (NOVEMBER 2002)

Exclusion criteria for donor material for penetrating keratoplasty:
1. Death of unknown cause.
2. Death with neurologic disease of unestablished diagnosis.
3. Dementia, unless due to cerebrovascular disease, brain tumor, or head trauma. Donors with toxic or metabolic-induced dementia may be acceptable pending documentation of consultation with the Medical Director. The approval of the Medical Director is required.
4. Subacute sclerosing panencephalitis.
5. Progressive multifocal leukoencephalopathy.
6. Congenital rubella.
7. Reye's syndrome.
8. Active viral encephalitis or encephalitis of unknown origin or progressive encephalopathy.
9. Active septicemia (bacteremia, fungemia, viremia).
10. Active bacterial or fungal endocarditis.
11. Active viral hepatitis.
12. Rabies.
13. Intrinsic eye disease:
    a. Retinoblastoma.
    b. Malignant tumors of the anterior ocular segment or known adenocarcinoma in the eye of primary or metastatic origin.
    c. Active ocular or intraocular inflammation: conjunctivitis, scleritis, iritis, uveitis, vitreitis, choroiditis, retinitis.
    d. Congenital or acquired disorders of the eye that would preclude a successful outcome for the intended use (e.g., a central donor corneal scar for an intended penetrating keratoplasty, keratoconus, and keratoglobus).
    e. Pterygia or other superficial disorders of the conjunctiva or corneal surface involving the central optical area of the corneal button.
14. Prior intraocular or anterior segment surgery:
    a. Refractive corneal procedures (e.g., radial keratotomy, lamellar inserts).
    b. Laser photoablation surgery is allowed to be used in cases of tectonic grafting and posterior lamellar procedures.
    c. Corneas from patients with anterior segment (e.g., cataract, intraocular lens, glaucoma filtration surgery) may be used if screened by specular microscopy and meet the Eye Bank's endothelial standards.
    d. Laser surgical procedures such as argon laser trabeculoplasty retinal and panretinal photocoagulation do not necessarily preclude use for penetrating keratoplasty but should be cleared by the Medical Director.
15. Leukemias.
16. Active disseminated lymphomas.
17. Hepatitis B surface antigen positive donors (as specified in Section G1.230).
18. Recipients of human pituitary-derived growth hormone (pit-hGH) during the years from 1963–1985 (2).
19. Human T-lymphotrophic virus (HTLV)-I or HTLV-II infection.
20. Recipient of nonsynthetic dura mater graft.
21. Hepatitis C seropositive donors.
22. Human immunodeficiency virus (HIV) seropositive donors (as specified in Section G1.220).
23. HIV or high risk for HIV: Persons meeting any of the following criteria should be excluded from donation (Behavioral/History Exclusionary Criteria, FDA Guidance for Industry, July 1997):
    a. Men who have sex with another man in the preceding 5 years.
    b. Persons who have injected drugs for a nonmedical reason in the preceding 5 years, including intravenous, intramuscular, or subcutaneous injection of drugs.
    c. Persons with hemophilia or related clotting disorders who have received human-derived clotting factor concentrates.
    d. Men and women who have engaged in sex for money or drugs in the preceding 5 years.
    e. Persons who have had sex in the preceding 12 months with any person described in items a–d above or with a person known or suspected to have HIV, hepatitis B virus, or hepatitis C virus infection.
    f. Persons who have been exposed in the preceding 12 months to known or suspected HIV-, hepatitis B virus–, or hepatitis C virus–infected blood through percutaneous inoculation or through contact with an open wound, nonintact skin, or mucous membrane.
    g. Inmates of correctional systems (including jail and prisons) and individuals who have been incarcerated for more than 72 consecutive hours during the previous 12 months.
    h. Persons who have had close contact with another person having viral hepatitis within 12 months of donation or who have undergone tattooing, acupuncture, ear or body piercing in which shared instruments are known to have been used.

TISSUE MATCHING

The benefits of donor–recipient tissue matching to prevent allograft immune rejection and ultimate graft failure are still controversial. The normal cornea enjoys a relative immune privilege well described by Streilein (43), with a low antigen load, few antigen-presenting cells, and a donor-specific anterior chamber (AC)–associated immune deviation that develops after transplantation. The suppression of the delayed-type hypersensitivity immune reaction is elicited by the intracameral inoculation of allogeneic antigens (44). This immune privilege is nonetheless relative. Both major

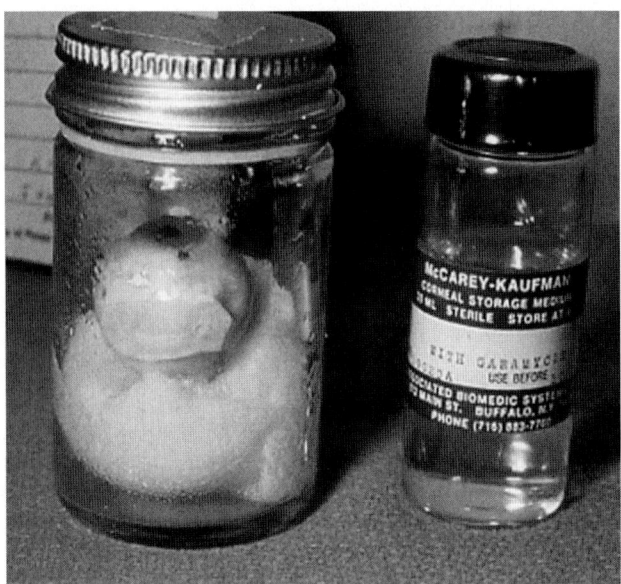

FIGURE 61-3. Donor eye and storage medium.

and minor histocompatibility antigens present in the donor cornea can activate lymphokines as well as donor and recipient antigen-presenting cells to trigger lymphocyte proliferation in the draining lymph node (Fig. 61-4). If activated, these lymphocytes will return to the eye to destroy donor corneal cells.

Major histocompatibility complex (MHC) antigens, known in humans as human leukocyte antigens (HLA), are genetically determined protein antigens. Class I MHC antigens such as HLA-A and HLA-B are present on all human living cells, including corneal cells. The class II MHC antigen (HLA-DR) phenotype is expressed on circulating cells and antigen-presenting cells, as in inflamed or vascularized corneas, and on Langerhans dendritic cells (Fig. 61-5).

In the rat animal model, class I MHC and nonMHC (i.e., minor histocompatibility antigens) antigen mismatching is associated with significantly lower rejection-free graft survival rates (45,46). This is probably also the case in humans. The large prospective cohort studies on class I HLA-A and HLA-B matching were based on serologic specificities, with variable reproducibility of laboratory data from one institution to another. This may in part explain why the Collaborative Corneal Transplantation Studies (CCTS) did not confirm the association of good donor–recipient HLA-A and HLA-B matching and improved graft survival with less frequent immunologic rejection episodes (47–50). Furthermore, the CCTS protocol probably used enough topical corticosteroids to obscure some effects of tissue compatibility. Class II HLA-DR matching does not appear to be associated with improved graft survival (47,51). Some reports have even suggested that a perfect HLA-DR match can be deleterious (52).

With molecular biology technology, the great polymorphism of the HLA system is now better recognized. For example, the 21 HLA-A antigens determined as serologic specificities are now known to correspond to 225 alleles determined as nucleotide sequences (53). The HLA polymorphism may theoretically be limited by race matching (53), which limits the pool of different possible alleles. Until revisited with cheaper HLA matchmakers based on

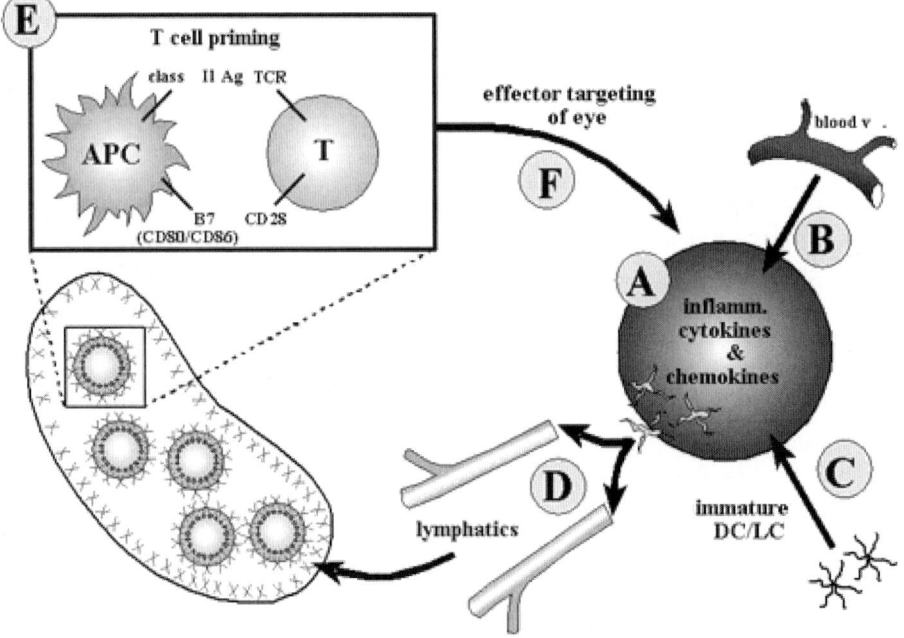

FIGURE 61-4. Diagrammatic representation of anterior chamber–associated immune deviation. APC, antigen-presenting cell; TCR, T-cell receptor. (Courtesy Reza Dana, M.D.)

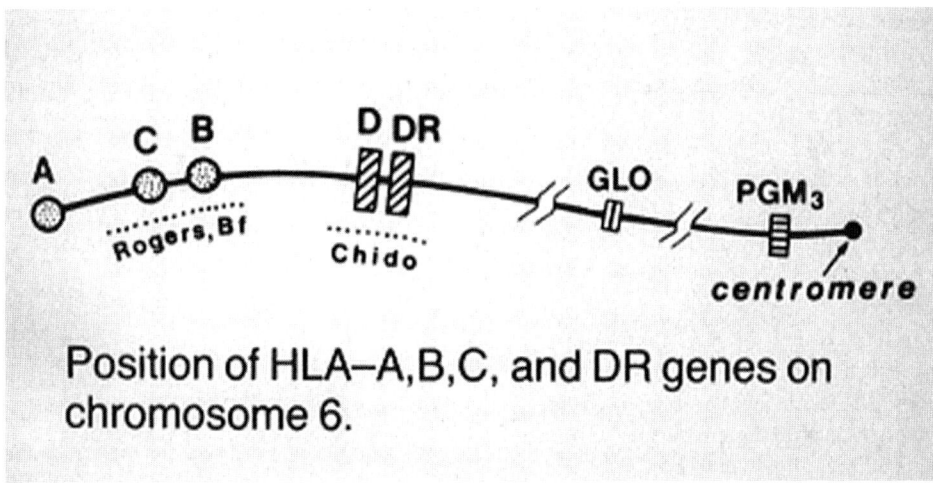

FIGURE 61-5. Human leukocyte antigen (HLA)-A, B, C, and DR genes on chromosome 6.

nucleotide sequence allele determination and large cohort studies, class I HLA-A and HLA-B matching is probably not more cost-efficient than using systemic or intensive topical immunosuppression. Avoiding, whenever possible, corneal donor grafts of 8 mm or larger is probably a good preventive measure for decreasing the antigenic load and rate of immune rejection and failure (47).

Minor histocompatibility antigens are small sugar antigens that can be attached to MHC antigens (54). ABO blood group and male sex Y-antigens are such minor histocompatibility antigens. ABO blood group matching prevents early allograft rejection and failure in vascularized corneas in high-risk patients (12,55,56). The current state of knowledge about tissue matching for corneal transplantation programs is that ABO blood group matching prevents graft failure at a currently acceptable cost in high-risk patients.

RECIPIENT CONSIDERATIONS

The most common indication for PK is pseudophakic corneal edema, although there is a decreasing trend for this indication (6), which accounted for 20% of cases in 2000 according to Eye Bank Association of America survey statistics. Fuchs' dystrophy, repeat corneal transplantation, and keratoconus are the next most frequent indications. Their order of frequency and the percentage of cases for these three indications vary from one study to another (57–60). Corneal opacity as the end result of trauma or inflammatory or infectious conditions (herpes simplex virus [HSV], in particular) and hereditary stromal dystrophies are other conditions that may benefit from PK. The surgeon should, however, have exhausted all medical measures (antiinfectious, antiinflammatory, and hypertonic agents) and should have attempted visual correction by optical means (e.g., contact lenses) before recommending a PK procedure for these conditions.

There is a trend toward increasing numbers of repeat corneal transplantation in the United States and certain parts of Canada (6,57,60,61). This may in part be due to the fact that corneal donor tissue is more readily available in these locations. Repeat PK has a poorer outcome compared with primary PK (11,13,61–64). The recipient with a previous history of graft failure has often been exposed to poor prognostic factors such as presence of corneal vessels, peripheral anterior synechiae, and prior immune allograft reaction mediators (13,65).

Restoration of optical clarity for the aforementioned indications is therefore the most frequent goal of PK. Tectonic PK is also indicated for those situations in which lamellar keratoplasty would not be expected to alleviate the situation. Corneal perforations, ongoing diffuse inflammatory processes in which medical measures have failed to halt stromal loss, might be indications for tectonic PK. The surgeon should consider a tectonic lamellar keratoplasty for cases with marked variations in stromal thickness.

The surgeon must be convinced that the patient will benefit from PK. The macular and optic nerve function should be assessed to ensure a reasonable visual potential. Pupillary reflexes to light, visual fields, B-scan ultrasonography, optical coherence tomography, and electrophysiology testing should be performed as needed. Intraocular pressure control in patients with glaucoma before or at the time of surgery is essential because a preoperative diagnosis of glaucoma comorbidity is the primary risk factor for corneal graft failure. Although high pressure itself can usually be controlled after surgery by a combination of medical and surgical means, there is a fourfold increased risk of graft failure for recipients with a preoperative diagnosis of glaucoma or increased intraocular pressure (11,65,66). Preoperative glaucoma is frequently made worse after PK by partial loss of the filtration angle. The chronic use of steroids after PK may also induce glaucoma in patients who are steroid responders. Abnormally low preoperative intraocular pressure, such as in patients with chronic uveitis, may be further aggravated by the surgery, causing macular edema and poor visual outcome.

Any intraocular inflammation must be controlled before PK unless surgery is required in an emergency situation (e.g., corneal perforation). The outcome of a PK is much poorer for patients with active corneal herpetic inflammation than for patients with a quiet herpetic corneal scar (67,68). The presence of deep corneal vessels is associated with a twofold increased risk of allograft immune reaction and failure (10,50,69).

Ocular surface conditions such as cicatricial conjunctival diseases (e.g., ocular cicatricial pemphigoid and the Stevens-Johnson's spectrum of diseases), severe dry eye (e.g., Sjögren's syndrome), or limbal stem cell deficiency conditions (e.g., congenital aniridia, chemical burn) all carry with them a dire prognosis for PK because epithelial healing is very poor in such conditions. Limbal stem cell transplantation alone for congenital aniridia keratopathy (70,71) should be considered. For cicatricial conjunctival diseases with corneal scarring, either a two-step procedure with limbal stem cell transplantation followed by PK or a keratoprosthesis is preferable to PK. Persistent epithelial defects, stromal melting, and corneal perforation may well develop after PK in these patients.

Major mechanical or inflammatory lid abnormalities must be noted and corrected before surgery. Lid notching and malposition or incomplete lid closure may all produce localized or generalized areas of inadequate corneal epithelial wetting, causing corneal melting. Patients with severe chronic blepharitis and atopic blepharitis are at high risk for graft infection and melt (72). These conditions must be under control at the time of and after PK.

The level and expectation of improvement in quality of life after PK depend on the best eye corrected visual acuity (17,18,73). Consideration of the vision in the other eye is therefore important. Patient satisfaction is better predicted by subjective outcomes than by objective outcomes such as visual acuity (74). The needs of the patient as defined by age, occupation, and preferred activities of daily living must also be taken into account. The patient's and family's compliance with postoperative care and safety recommendations must be taken into consideration, particularly for PK in the pediatric age group and in patients with mental retardation. One must also consider the general health status of the patient. Severe obesity is also associated with intraoperative complications (75).

SURGICAL PROCEDURE

Preoperative Considerations

Surgical Setting

In the present era, the procedure of PK is safely performed in an outpatient surgical setting under monitored anesthesia care. General anesthesia, still the preferred anesthesia technique by many surgeons, is now more commonly reserved for difficult clinical settings such as the perforated globe or other conditions including deafness, aphasia, extreme anxiety, inability to remain still, and young patient age.

Patient Positioning

As in all ocular surgery, it is best to have the patient's head positioned so as not inadvertently to increase intraocular pressure by Valsalva maneuver. All patients with truncal obesity should be in slight reverse Trendelenburg position.

Preoperative Drops

Either myotic or mydriatic agents, or both, are used concurrently when performing PK, depending on the phakic status of the eye or whether a combined procedure such as phacoemulsification or extracapsular cataract extraction with intraocular lens (IOL) implantation, lens repositioning, secondary lens implantation, or vitrectomy is planned.

Pilocarpine 2% to 4% is typically applied three times at 5-minute intervals, 1 hour before surgery. This ensures a constricted lens–iris diaphragm, therefore reducing potential damage to the lens, IOL, lens capsule, and vitreous face.

Mydriatic agents used to ensure adequate pupillary dilation include 1% tropicamide, 2.5% phenylephrine, and 1% cyclopentolate. These agents are used when prior phacoemulsification, open-sky cataract extraction, or posterior lens repositioning or lens suturing is planned.

Osmotic Agents

The use of an osmotic agent, such as mannitol, aids in decreasing positive pressure by lowering intraocular pressure (76) and possibly by shrinking the vitreous jelly. A 20% solution (20 g/100 mL) can be administered at a dosage of 1 to 2 g/kg, usually not to exceed 300 mL (60 g) given in the hour before surgery. It is to be used cautiously in the elderly. Disadvantages, however, include a diuretic effect and bladder discomfort if the patient cannot void in a supine position. All patients should therefore be instructed to void before entering the surgical suite.

Asepsis, Akinesia, and Intraocular Pressure Control

In attempt to decrease the risk of endophthalmitis, the use both of povidone–iodine (77–79), which is bactericidal, and topical antibiotics alone (80–82) or in combination (83) is advocated to decrease or eradicate bacterial flora on the ocular surface. Targeted bacteria include those known to be normal commensals of the ocular surface, most notably gram-positive organisms, often implicated in postoperative endophthalmitis (78,84–86).

Ocular akinesia is attained by retrobulbar injection of a mixture of local anesthetic, usually a 50/50 mixture of 1%

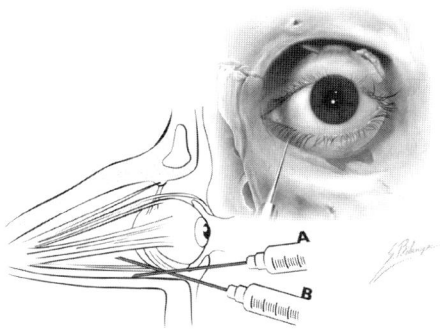

FIGURE 61-6. Retrobulbar injection showing intraconal positioning of needle.

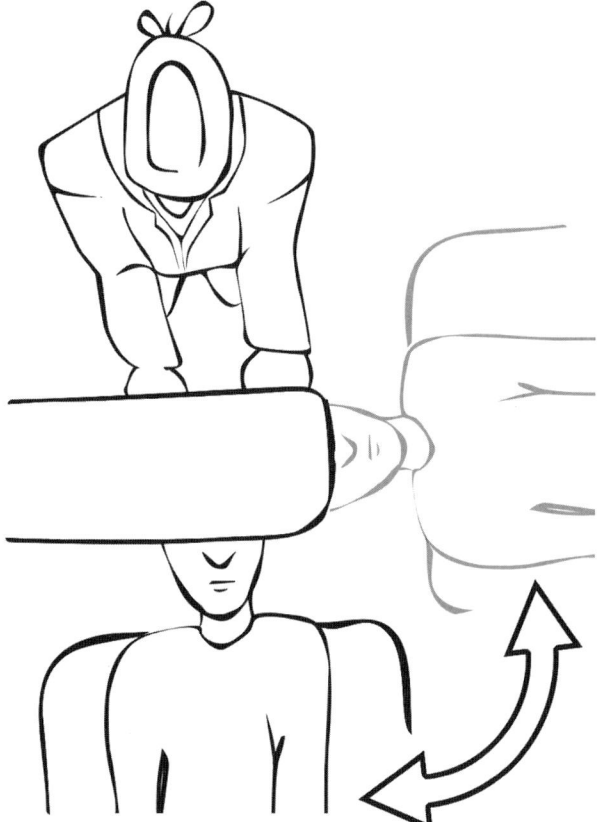

FIGURE 61-7. Diagram of traditional and alternate surgeon positioning.

to 2% lidocaine and 0.5% bupivacaine. Akinesia of the lids can also be performed using either the O'Brien or Nadbath technique if pronounced blepharospasm or discomfort is induced by the chosen lid speculum (Fig. 61-6).

Intraoperative control of intraocular pressure is paramount before performing PK because AC penetration must be done in a controlled fashion. The use of a Honan balloon reduces intraocular pressure after both retrobulbar and peribulbar injection of anesthetic (87,88). The Honan balloon is commonly positioned for 5 to 10 minutes after retrobulbar injection of anesthetics. If a Honan balloon is not available, simple ocular massage can also be done. Objective endothelial cell count measurements after PK have been shown to be higher when simple ocular massage was used before the surgical procedure to decrease intraocular pressure and decrease subsequent endothelial contact by the iris and lens (89).

Surgeon Positioning

Although it is traditional for the surgeon to perform PK from a superior approach, this position often creates difficult and challenging surgical exposure problems owing to the presence of a prominent orbital rim and crowding due to a large nose. A temporal approach to PK can alleviate these problems and can be a useful alternative to the traditional superior approach in the patient who presents with such physiognomy (90) (Fig. 61-7).

Procedure-Related Instruments

The surgeon should be intimately acquainted with all instruments required in performing PK. Personal preferences do apply to numerous instruments, as indicated by hand size and personal whim.

Scissors
A pair of blunt-tip, Westcott, both straight and curved Vannas scissors, as well as right- and left-going corneal scissors are required during the PK procedure. Both the blunt-tip and Westcott scissors may be used for cutting drapes,

large bridal sutures, and scleral fixation sutures, but it is to be stressed that Vannas scissors are to be used to cut only fine 10-0 and 11-0 sutures as well as intraocular adhesions, membranes, iris, and an uneven corneal bevel.

Forceps
Anterior segment surgery requires the use of 0.12-mm forceps. These forceps are designed for tissue handling and not needle handling. They often have a tying platform, therefore precluding the use of additional tying forceps.

The Polack double corneal forceps allows for better grasping of the donor corneal tissue, especially the first and second cardinal sutures in the 12 and 6 o'clock positions. Additional forceps required during the procedure include MacPherson or Kelman straight and angled forceps for manipulation of the IOL.

Needle-Drivers
Two types of needle-drivers, both locking and nonlocking, are required for the procedure. A large locking or nonlocking needle-driver is used for bridal suture placement and a large nonlocking holder is used for scleral fixation suture placement. A fine-jawed, curved needle-driver is used for all other components of the procedure.

Spatulas, Hooks, Blades, and Cannulae

Both iris and cyclodialysis spatulas are useful during the procedure for lysis of synechiae. A Paton spatula is useful for the donor cornea transfer. A selection of IOL and iris hooks should be available, as well as both a 15- and 30-degree disposable blade. Numerous cannulae are required and usually include both 27- and 30-gauge cannulae. The viscoelastic cannula is often useful as an additional instrument, as well as a manual Simcoe cannula for manual irrigation–aspiration during a combined cataract extraction procedure.

Intraoperative Keratometers

A variety of instruments exist to project a circle onto the cornea, therefore allowing the surgeon to assess corneal asphericity. Any marked degree of asphericity can then be ascertained and corrected by cutting the tight suture and resuturing.

Host Preparation

Lid Speculum Insertion and Scleral Fixation

The most important feature of a lid speculum is that it provides adequate exposure without causing pressure on the globe. A lateral canthotomy can also be performed to free the interpalpebral fissure should it be narrow or tight after retrobulbar injection of anesthetic. The addition of a bridal suture on both the superior and inferior rectus muscles not only stabilizes the globe, but can provide additional exposure when it is suboptimal. A 4-0 silk suture provides adequate tension for this purpose.

Scleral fixation provides support to the globe, thereby avoiding scleral collapse and secondary posterior pressure. The most commonly used scleral ring is the Flieringa ring. It is most commonly used before pediatric grafting, in aphakic PK, and before open-sky extracapsular cataract extraction. The most commonly used sizes are the 17- and 18-mm rings, which allow adequate space for suture placement onto the sclera and the use of a suction-assisted trephine system. Experimental data support placement of scleral ring fixation sutures between the muscles in an attempt to decrease induced astigmatism (91). The chosen ring is sutured in place using a spatulated needle to avoid intraocular penetration.

Graft Centration

The geometric and optical axes of the cornea must be considered before marking the center of the corneal. The geometric axis is found by bisecting both the vertical and horizontal meridians of the cornea, whereas the optical axis is found by centering on the anatomic nasally positioned pupil (Fig. 61-8). Most surgeons position the center of the graft on the pupil, thereby slightly displacing the corneal graft nasally. Gentian violet is used to mark the

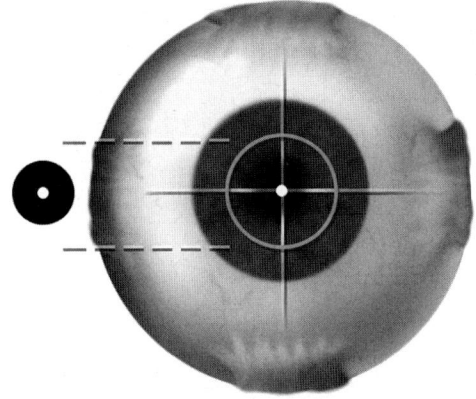

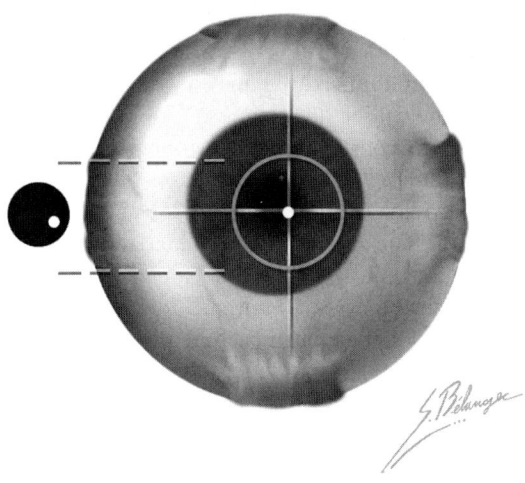

FIGURE 61-8. Diagram of graft centration.

center of the cornea and the appropriate graft size is then determined. A radial marker can then be positioned using the chosen center to help with symmetric suture placement.

Graft Size Determination

Before handling the donor cornea, the recipient graft size should be decided and both donor and recipient trephine blades should be examined under the operative microscope to ascertain the indicated correct size and quality of the blades.

Graft size determination is based on three main factors: the size of the recipient cornea, the targeted disease, and the known increased risk of rejection with increasing graft size. Most adult corneas measure slightly greater in the horizontal meridian compared with the vertical meridian because the superior limbus descends slightly superiorly. White-to-white measurements for an adult cornea in the horizontal meridian are on average 12.5 mm. A normal-sized cornea with endothelial disease such as Fuchs' endothelial dystrophy, iridocorneal endothelial syndrome, or pseudophakic bullous keratopathy would typically be trephinated with a

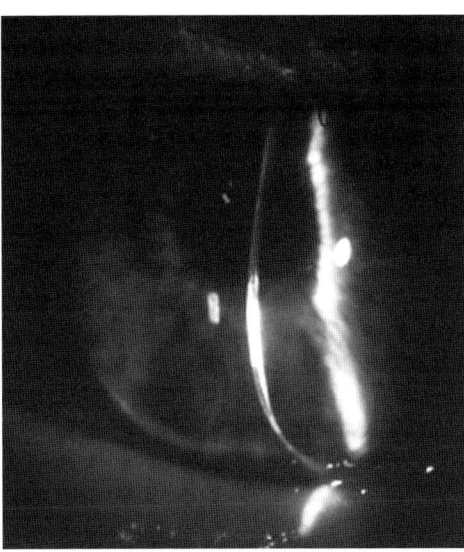

FIGURE 61-9. Pellucid marginal degeneration with inferior corneal ectasia.

7.5-mm trephine. Although a larger recipient size trephination would supply a larger quantity of healthy endothelial cells, larger donor corneal size (> 8 to 8.5 mm) is associated with a higher risk of rejection (69,92). Ectatic corneal pathologic processes, including keratoconus and pellucid marginal degeneration, require prior recipient donor size measurements at the slit lamp because the area of corneal thinning is often larger than that seen under the operating microscope. It is paramount that the area of thinning be encompassed in the trephinated tissue to avoid tissue disparity and wound mismatch (Fig. 61-9). These large, eccentric grafts unfortunately are subject to a higher risk of rejection and astigmatism (93) (Fig. 61-10).

Most surgeons use a 0.25-mm oversize in the donor button to counteract the 0.2-mm difference in size produced by endothelial trephination of the donor cornea. This essentially counteracts the disparity to give an equivalent donor and recipient trephination.

Trephines

Many types of trephines and punches exist to cut both recipient and donor corneas. Each has advantages and disadvantages (Fig. 61-11 and Table 61-2) The main goal remains to allow for a central, uniform cut, therefore avoiding damage to intraocular structures and donor endothelium.

Recipient corneas are trephinated with either a suction-assisted trephine or free-standing, nonguarded, or handle-mounted disposable trephines. Suction-assisted trephines include the Hanna, Hessburg-Barron, Krumeich, and Liebermann trephine systems.

To minimize the postoperative refractive error, tissue disparity and wound mismatch between the donor and recipient cornea must be limited (94). In an ideal setting, the surgeon would perform a well-centered, circular graft with perfectly geometrically matched—that is, epithelial, stromal, and endothelial matched—margins. It has been shown experimentally that this is a very difficult task (95,96). Numerous factors implicated in the geometry of corneal buttons include trephine pressure on the globe, variable corneal thickness and elasticity, trephine centration, intraocular pressure, and the ability to hold the trephine perpendicular to the corneal tissue (97,98). Photogrammetric analysis of host corneal trephination reveals that the Hanna microkeratotrephine shows the greatest precision and produces a vertical cut (96).

The donor corneal tissue is typically cut from the endothelial surface on a cutting block of Teflon, or through the epithelial surface, using an artificial AC such as with the Hanna, Krumeich, or Lieberman systems. Advantages of

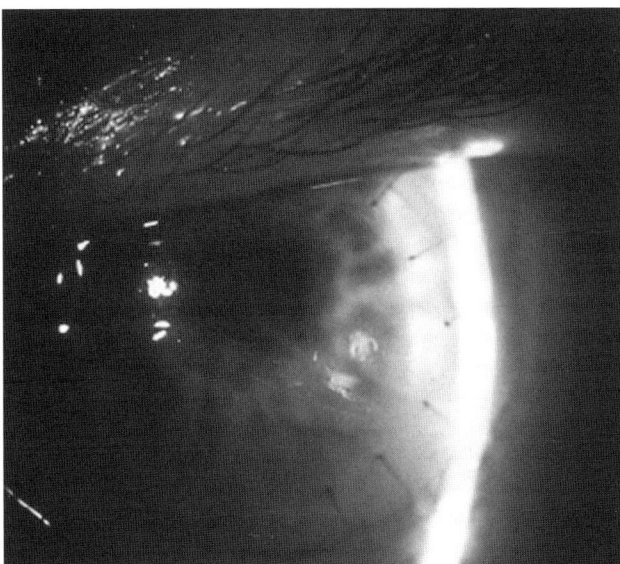

FIGURE 61-10. Khodadoust endothelial rejection line in a large excentric graft for pellucid marginal degeneration.

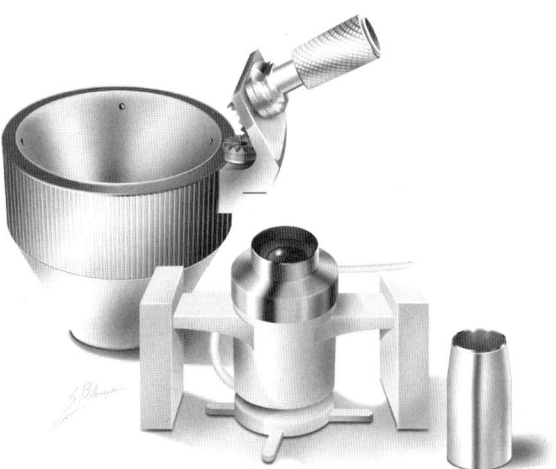

FIGURE 61-11. Hanna trephine (*left*); Baron Hessburg trephine (*middle*); and open disposable trephine (*right*).

TABLE 61-2. TREPHINES USED IN PENETRATING KERATOPLASTY

Trephine Type	Advantages	Disadvantages
Open, disposable trephine	Small, least cumbersome	Even trephination challenging
Baron-Hessburg suction-assisted trephine	Small, uncomplicated No assembly required Rotation of 360 degrees advances blade 250 μm	No stop for calibration depth
Hanna suction-assisted trephine	Precise depth calibration Each turn of the knob advances blade 88 μm controlled trephination	Slightly cumbersome Assembly required

the artificial AC include better donor and recipient tissue matching because the cut is performed in the same direction, therefore decreasing tissue disparity between both donor and recipient. Disadvantages of the artificial AC are few, but include the need for a wider donor scleral rim. This is not always possible because donor corneas are often provided from different eye banks with different harvesting techniques, including whole-globe or simple corneoscleral harvesting.

Trephination

It is customary first to trephinate the donor cornea before the recipient trephination, thereby avoiding any error in sizing and an incomplete or aborted donor cornea trephination. Any error in donor cornea trephination precludes continuing with the procedure. A paracentesis is performed and a viscoelastic agent is injected into the AC to inflate slightly the recipient chamber. Many surgeons prefer, however, to trephinate without the use of a prior viscoelastic injection. It has been shown that the use of a viscoelastic agent decreases the mean endothelial cell loss at 4 and 6 months (99). The chosen trephine is centered on the previously marked center of the cornea and trephination is then done (Fig. 61-12). It is best not to enter the AC with the trephine to avoid damaging intraocular structures, although prior viscoelastic installation

often provides a buffer against this situation. A 30-degree disposable blade can then be used to enter the AC vertically in a controlled fashion and the corneal button can then be removed with the corneal scissors. A meticulous bed must be present after corneal scissor dissection, and Vannas scissors are used to correct the presence of a residual posterior lip.

A small amount of viscoelastic is then applied to the recipient cornea bed and pupil area to protect the previously cut donor cornea as it is placed into the recipient bed, as well as to protect the crystalline lens.

Suturing

Many methods of suturing exist, including single interrupted or single continuous running sutures, a combination of the two, double continuous running sutures, and a deep suturing technique using either a combination of single interrupted and continuous running suture or a double running suture. Regardless of the chosen technique, the goal remains to obtain good apposition of the donor and recipient tissue with the smallest degree of wound mismatch, thus creating the least degree of postoperative astigmatism. The four cardinal sutures placed initially remain the most important sutures because they ensure equal distribution of tissue (Fig. 61-13). These sutures are placed deeply in the cornea, to 90% depth (100), and, ideally, a closed system is ob-

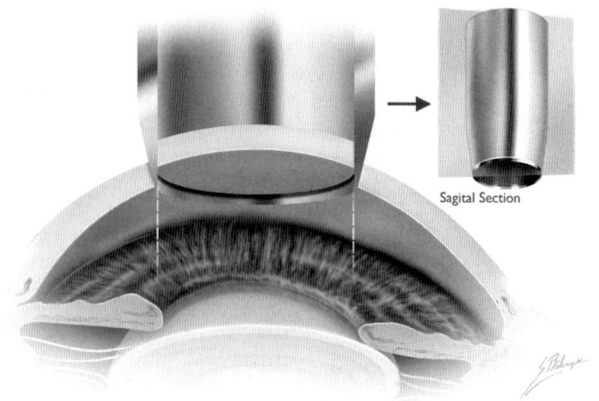

FIGURE 61-12. Trephination, centered with prior viscoelastic injection into the anterior chamber.

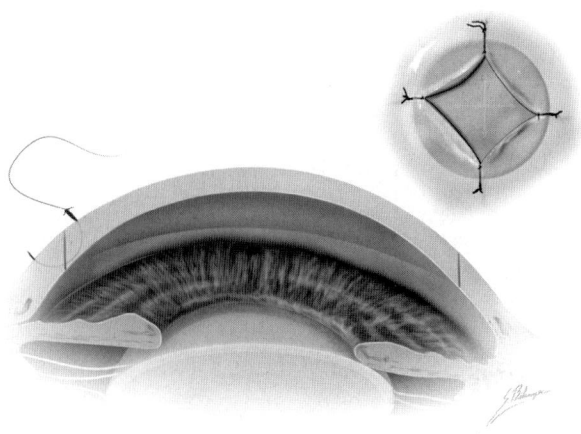

FIGURE 61-13. Four cardinal sutures with inset showing depth.

tained. It is important to bury the suture knots because they otherwise become an irritative focus and can cause secondary neovascularization and possibly contribute to infection. The AC is maintained when possible by injection of balanced salt solution throughout the procedure, and wound integrity is verified with a Weck cell sponge at the end of the procedure. All wound leaks should then be corrected.

COMPLICATIONS

Intraoperative Complications

All surgical steps in performing PK have possible complications. Most of these can, however, be avoided if meticulous attention is paid to each detail. When they do occur, they are usually corrected at the time of the initial procedure.

Scleral Perforation

Bridal suture placement as well as scleral ring placement can result in inadvertent scleral perforation. Adequate muscle traction is usually sufficient to avoid this complication, as well as the use of a spatulated needle. The anatomic placement of a scleral ring is usually well within the anatomic borders of the pars plana and therefore in theory retinal perforation can be avoided.

Damage to Donor Cornea

It is necessary to trephinate the donor cornea before recipient trephination. Any damage to the donor cornea, whether contamination or improper or incomplete trephination, warrants cancellation of the surgery. Should the donor corneal button remain within the trephine after punching, care should be taken not to use instrumentation to tweak it to fall back in the well. Rather, balanced salt solution or Optisol from the corneal transport container dripped into the trephine can be used to coax the button to fall back on its own. Any confusion as to the direction of the button is impossible to confirm visually, and therefore a "no touch" approach to the donor corneal button is the best approach.

Recipient Trephination

All trephine sizes should be double checked by a second observer, thereby avoiding the disastrous complication of trephine reversal. Because most surgeons still oversize donor buttons by 0.25 mm, a trephine reversal would cause unwanted hyperopia and difficulty in closing the wound.

Retained Descemet's Membrane

Inadvertent retention of Descemet's membrane is surprisingly easy in edematous corneas because it is transparent.

This occurs when incomplete penetration into the AC has occurred and the corneal scissors remains above the membrane during cutting. The iris should be inspected and gently touched with a Weck sponge to ensure the absence of Descemet's membrane. Retention of Descemet's membrane causes primary graft failure by diffuse endothelial failure of the corneal button. The presence of a double AC on postoperative day 1 suggests the retention of Descemet's membrane and the need for regrafting.

Iris–Lens Damage

The advent of viscoelastics has greatly decreased the prevalence of intraocular damage during trephination. Any iris damage can be repaired using 10-0 polypropylene suture. Should damage occur to the anterior lens capsule, a combined cataract extraction with IOL placement must be done. Fortunately, this is a rare event with the use of calibrated trephines.

Anterior Chamber Hemorrhage

In the presence of iris damage, either iatrogenic or traumatic, slight bleeding usually stops spontaneously on its own with closure of the eye and return of adequate intraocular pressure. Closed-loop IOLs must be removed with care to avoid bleeding, and when complete removal is thought to be impossible, it is safer to leave small pieces of the haptics in place.

Suprachoroidal Expulsive Hemorrhage

The most dreaded and visually devastating complication during PK is suprachoroidal expulsive hemorrhage (SEH; Fig. 61-14). All of the modalities previously discussed,

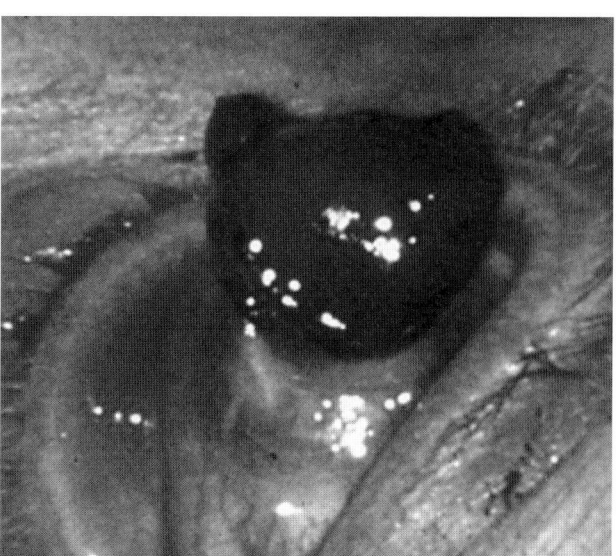

FIGURE 61-14. Expulsive hemorrhage.

including proper positioning of the patient, patient comfort, adequate globe and lid akinesia and anesthesia, adequate intraocular pressure control, and a controlled surgical setting, may aid in decreasing its occurrence. Few reports exist of its occurrence in PK (101,102), but prevention and anticipation of its occurrence are probably the best preventive measures. Increased axial length, glaucoma, generalized atherosclerosis, and intraoperative tachycardia have been shown to increase the risk of suprachoroidal expulsive hemorrhage (103).

Postoperative Complications

Early Complications

A host of complications may arise in the early postoperative period in PK. It is important to initiate treatment rapidly because this may prevent early graft failure. Wound-related problems, epithelial complications (including persistent epithelial defects), filamentary keratitis, suture-related problems (including infection, endophthalmitis, and immune infiltrates), glaucoma, pupillary block, the fixed-dilated pupil, and primary graft failure can all be encountered in this early period.

Wound Leaks

The best method for preventing wound leaks is to have meticulous wound apposition at the end of the surgical procedure. Leaks are still seen when the wound is checked on the first postoperative day using the Seidel test. It is best to use a fluorescein strip to perform the Seidel test to be able to see best very small as well as larger leaks.

A shallow AC does not necessarily indicate a wound leak, but its presence should strongly suggest it. A loose interrupted suture must be removed to avoid a wick effect and increased risk of infection. Should the leak be controlled with a bandage contact lens, resuturing is not necessary. It is, however, most prudent to replace any broken sutures, and this can safely be done in a treatment room using a surgical microscope under topical anesthesia and antibiotic coverage.

Any large degree of wound dehiscence or wound step should be repaired in the operating room (Fig. 61-15).

Epithelial Defects

The donor epithelium sloughs off the donor button with time, and a complete epithelial defect can be seen on the first postoperative day, especially if it has been removed at the end of the procedure. Preoperative donor factors increasing the risk for the presence of an epithelial defect on postoperative day 1 include a longer time interval from death to preservation (104) and diabetes in the donor (105). This initial epithelial defect usually heals within the first postoperative week, but attention should be paid to

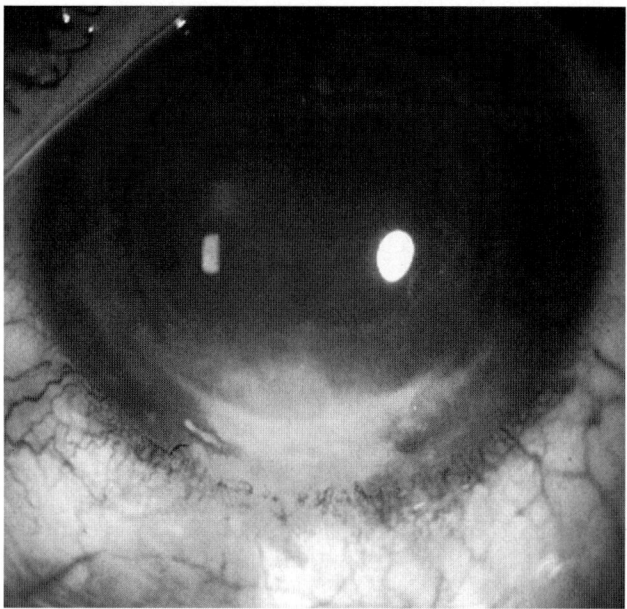

FIGURE 61-15. Large wound dehiscence.

the presence of blepharitis, inadequate lid closure, older patient age, and inadequate eye hydration to avoid it becoming a persistent defect. The presence of an epithelial defect on day 1 has not been shown to correlate with its presence at 1 or 3 months (106).

The treatment of a persistent epithelial defect in the grafted patient should be performed with a degree of urgency (Fig. 61-16). The use of a partial tarsorrhaphy (Fig. 61-17) is not to be overlooked as a treatment modality, as well as adequate hydration with ointments and drops or the use of a bandage contact lens. A whorl-like keratopathy, also referred to as *hurricane keratitis*, is sometimes seen as a toxic side effect of many topical medications (107), including benzalkonium chloride and neomycin. In addition,

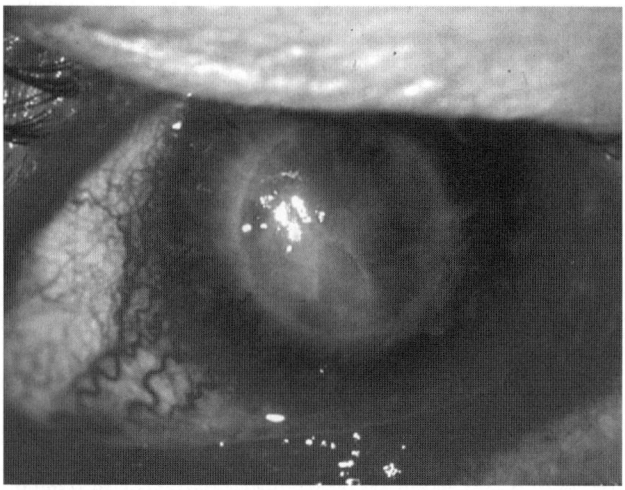

FIGURE 61-16. A persistent epithelial defect.

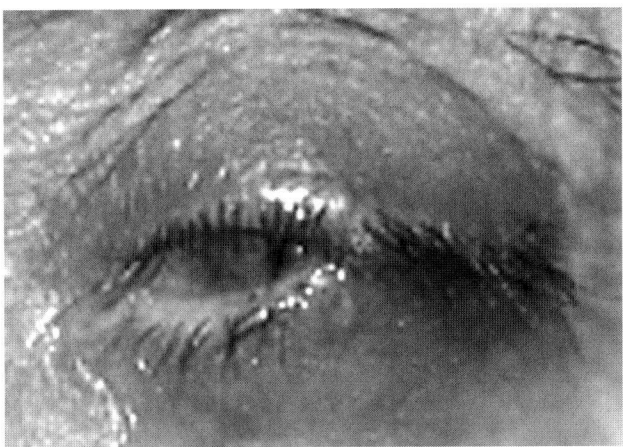

FIGURE 61-17. Tarsorrhaphy.

topical corticosteroids inhibit corneal healing (108); therefore, in the presence of a large epithelial defect, the application of topical corticosteroids should be decreased.

Filamentary Keratitis

Many causes of filamentary keratitis are present in the grafted patient (109). These include relative ptosis, dry eye, neurotrophic keratopathy, and the presence of sutures. The filaments, composed of dead epithelial cells and mucus, are often seen at a suture site. Intensive lubrication or removal are often warranted (Fig. 61-18).

Suture-Related Complications

Infection

Both gram-positive and gram-negative organisms have been implicated in suture-related infections in the grafted patient (110,111). These infections are sometimes related

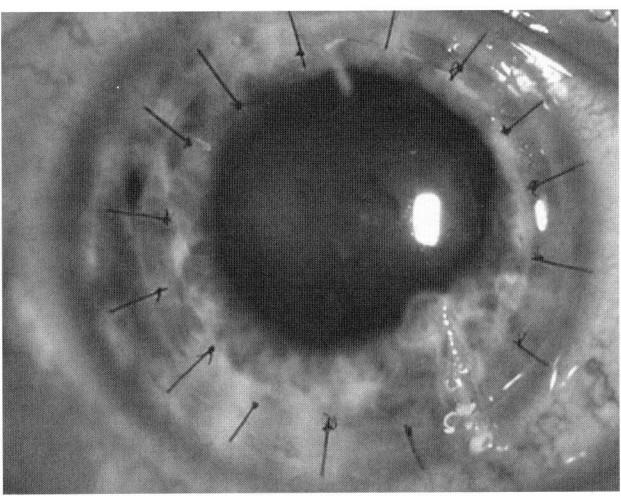

FIGURE 61-18. A corneal filament composed of desquamated epithelial cells and mucus.

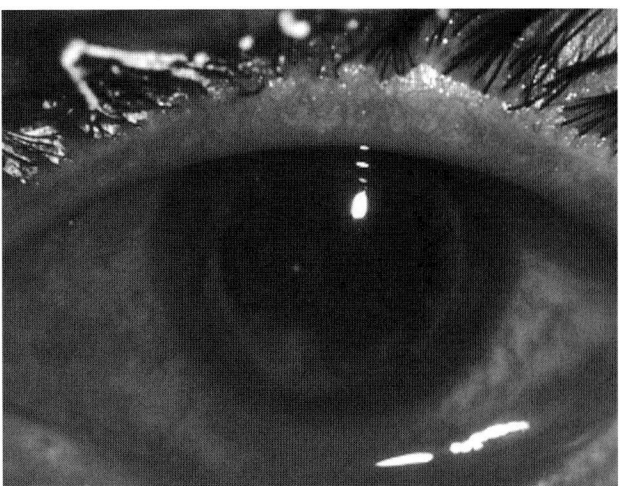

FIGURE 61-19. Suture-related infectious keratitis.

to exposed sutures, but the concomitant use of long-term corticosteroids and antibiotics probably contributes to their occurrence (112). Suture infections must be managed as an emergency, in the same fashion as any serious infectious keratitis (Fig. 61-19). They can lead to wound dehiscence, endophthalmitis, and corneal scarring and thinning, which all can contribute to eventual graft failure.

Infectious crystalline keratopathy is a distinctive clinical entity first described by Gorovoy and colleagues (113); often seen in the grafted patient, it is a pauciinflammatory infiltrate in the corneal stroma associated with gram-positive bacteria, most notably nutrient-variable *Streptococcus* (114,115), *Streptococcus pneumoniae* (116), gram-negative rods and yeasts (117), as well as nontuberculous mycobacteria (118). This arborescent, crystal-like keratitis is indolent in nature and is associated with long-term topical steroid use and epithelial defects (Fig. 61-20). The nonturbid, normal state of deturgescence of the cornea has been shown experimentally to be required for formation of the distinctive crystalline appearance (119).

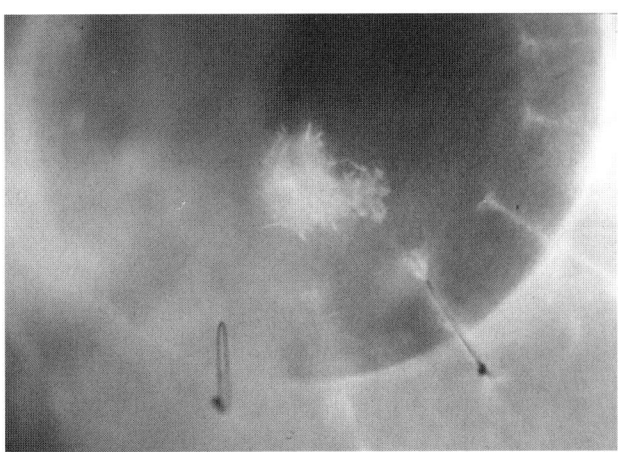

FIGURE 61-20. Infectious crystalline keratopathy.

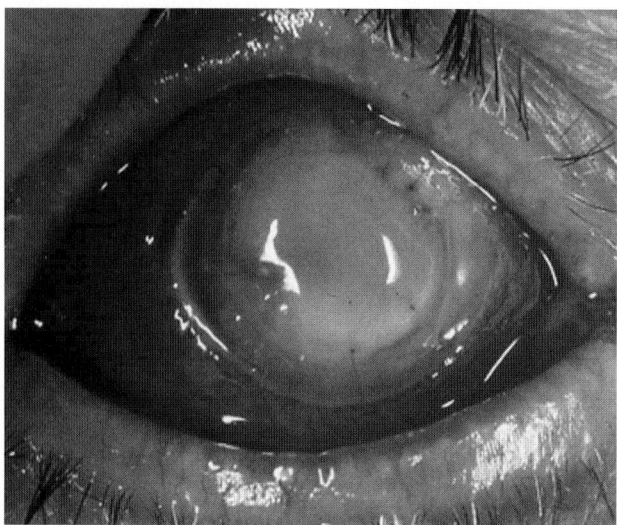

FIGURE 61-21. Postoperative endophthalmitis after penetrating keratoplasty.

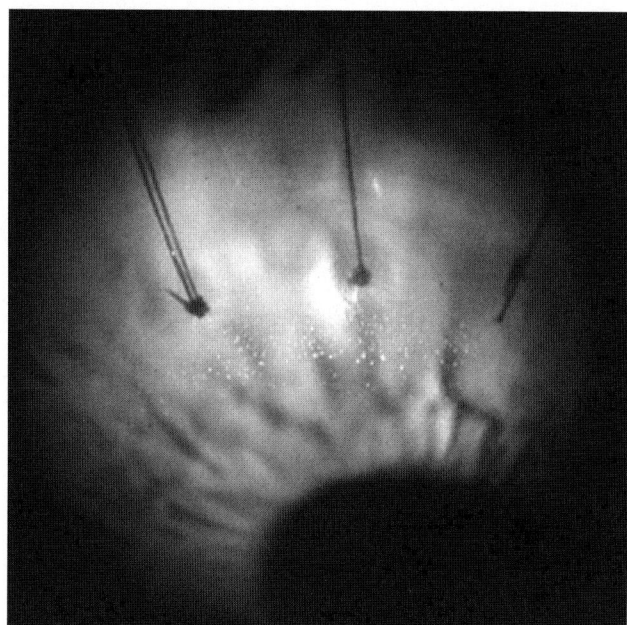

FIGURE 61-22. Kaye dots are a short distance from sutures and are nonpathologic.

Endophthalmitis

Endophthalmitis is a potentially devastating complication after PK (Fig. 61-21). The 6-month incidence of endophthalmitis is approximately 0.77% (120) after PK. Other studies with fewer total patients have calculated the endophthalmitis rate to be from 0.20% to 2.02% (121–124). This is considerably higher than that associated with cataract extraction alone, where the risk is approximately 0.08% (120,124). Aseptic technique is therefore of utmost importance when performing PK.

Immune Infiltrates

Immune infiltrates tend to be multiple, on the recipient side of the cornea, and are often seen in patients who have other risk factors for immunologic reaction. It is thought that perhaps these multiple immune reactions are secondary to the suture material because they usually are found along the suture tract. Intensive topical corticosteroid therapy is often required, with eventual removal of the sutures.

Kaye Dots

Small epithelial dots may be seen a short distance from sutures on the donor side, and these are referred to as *Kaye dots* (125) (Fig. 61-22). They are not pathologic and usually disappear after suture removal. They are thought to be epithelial in origin.

Glaucoma

Early postoperative glaucoma, first described in 1969 by Irvine and Kaufman (126), is best treated to avoid endothelial damage. It is especially important to avoid retained viscoelastic at the end of the procedure and to inflate the AC with balanced salt solution. Other factors implicated in

early glaucoma include the presence of anterior synechiae and pupillary block. A steroid response can also be the cause of early glaucoma, and topical antiglaucomatous agents should be used judiciously to avoid long-standing high pressure and glaucomatous optic neuropathy.

Anterior Synechiae

The presence of anterior synechiae has been shown experimentally in the rat to increase the prevalence of allograft rejection (127). Patients with anterior synechiae also show a higher prevalence of graft edema (128). Postoperative dilation does increase AC depth, but it should be used cautiously in keratoconus, where a fixed, dilated pupil can result (129).

Pupillary Block

The presence of a shallow AC, a high intraocular pressure, and an intact wound would suggest pupillary block caused by either aqueous misdirection or marked choroidal detachment. The appropriate treatment of dilation with mydriatic and cycloplegic drops and fundus examination reveals the cause. Aqueous misdirection is rarely treated alone medically, and a partial vitrectomy is often required to break the misdirection.

Urrets-Zavalia Pupil

The Urrets-Zavalia syndrome, also known as *mydriasis acuta iridoatrophicans*, is essentially the presence of an irregular pupil occuring a few days after PK for keratoconus (129). The syndrome includes iris stromal atrophy, ectropion uvea, multiple posterior synechiae, and discrete disseminated subcapsular opacities. The cause for this syndrome is unknown, and its frequency seems to have decreased significantly, as described by the author. The use of viscoelastics perhaps has contributed to its decreased prevalence.

Unusual Transmission of Infection

Although donor screening is performed to prevent transmission of systemic infections, ophthalmic diseases, and malignancies, there have been seven reports of rabies transmission after PK. The first case, in 1978, was in the United States (130), the second case, in 1979, in France (131), the third and fourth cases in Thailand (132), the fifth and six in 1988 in India (133), and the seventh case in Iran (134). All recipients died of rabies. There is one case of survival in a recipient having received a cornea from a donor who had died of rabies (135).

There is also one case in the literature of neoplastic transmission of papillary adenocarcinoma to the iris in a young patient who underwent PK for keratoconus (136). At present, donors who have died of cancer are not refused for corneal donation.

Late Postoperative Complications

Immunologic Rejection

The use of the term *rejection* refers to the immunologic response of the recipient to the donor tissue without regard to the effect of the response on graft survival.

Although immunologic graft rejection is the most common cause of graft failure, graft endothelial failure can be the result of other situations. Early primary donor failure (Fig. 61-23) can result from poor donor quality. Intraoperative trauma to the donor endothelium and prolonged flat chamber in the immediate postoperative period can also result in irreversible corneal graft edema. In the late postoperative period, some grafts fail. These late graft endothelium failures can be due to the natural attrition of endothelial cells that occurs with age. Uncontrolled increased intraocular pressure and excessive inflammation can also contribute to corneal endothelial cell failure. Increasing corneal thickness measured by pachymetry is a very good means to document progressing graft failure. Intensive topical steroids should immediately be instituted for newly documented corneal graft failures. If the corneal thickness is unchanged or worse after a few weeks with such treatment, it is unlikely that the failed graft will clear. As recommended by Wilson and Kaufman in their comprehensive review of graft failure after PK (137), to avoid ambiguity, actual failure of the graft due to immunologic processes is best described by the phrase *graft failure due to rejection*.

The diagnosis of immunologic rejection can be made only in a technically successful graft that has remained clear for a few weeks after PK. The risk of an immunologic rejection episode is constant over the first 3 years after transplantation, as shown by a straight rejection-free survival slope in (47). Classic endothelial rejection lines have been observed 10 and 20 years after PK.

Many types of corneal graft rejection have been described: epithelial rejection lines, subepithelial infiltrates, stromal rejection haze, endothelial rejection lines, and diffuse endothelial rejection (137,138). Epithelial rejection (Fig. 61-24) is a benign situation characterized by an elevated epithelial rejection line that stains with fluorescein or rose bengal. It is often asymptomatic and responds to mild steroid therapy, as do the subepithelial white infiltrates (Fig. 61-25) that are thought to be an immune reaction because they are seen only in the donor tissue. Although stromal haze, often appearing as an immunologic arc, commonly occurs simultaneously with endothelial rejection in rabbit experimental models of corneal allograft rejection (139), human stromal rejection is very rarely encountered in our experience. On the contrary, an endothelial rejection line, referred to as the *Khodadoust*

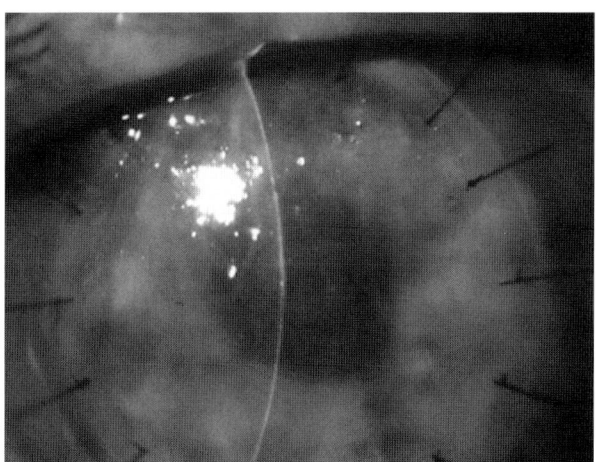

FIGURE 61-23. Primary graft failure.

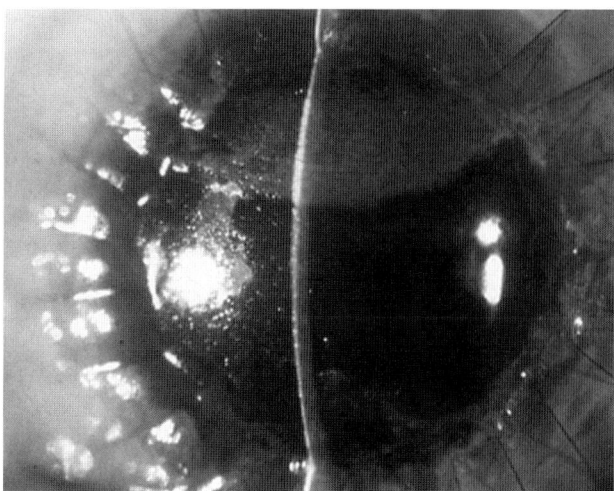

FIGURE 61-24. Epithelial rejection line, which is often asymptomatic.

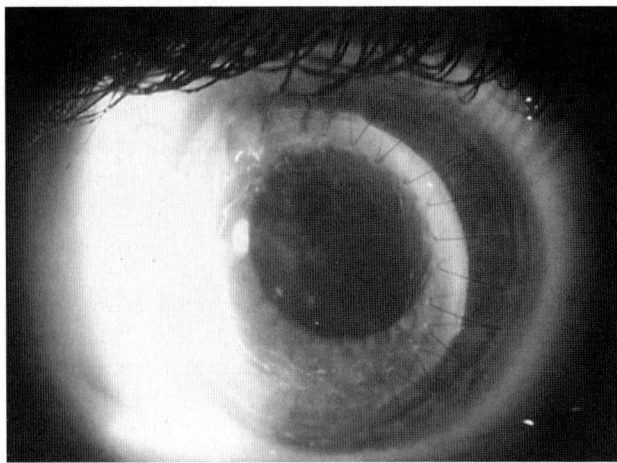

FIGURE 61-25. Subepithelial infiltrates respond to topical corticosteroids.

line (139) (Fig. 61-26), is present and usually symptomatic at one time or another in 20% of patients (69). If left untreated, the endothelial rejection line, composed of lymphoid cells, usually proceeds across the donor endothelium from a point of origin at the graft wound, like an advancing forest fire line, leaving damaged endothelium behind it. In the more diffuse type of endothelial rejection, isolated or diffuse keratic precipitates composed of lymphoid cells are scattered across the endothelium. They are limited to the donor endothelium and are often associated with an AC reaction. Damage to the endothelium, if left unattended, results in disruption of the regulation of corneal hydration and, subsequently, localized or diffuse corneal edema.

Several potential risk factors for corneal immunologic rejection episodes have been described. The factor most commonly associated with an increased risk of allograft rejection is corneal vascularization. Several prospective cohort studies with actuarial analysis have demonstrated either an increased incidence of immunologic rejection episodes or a

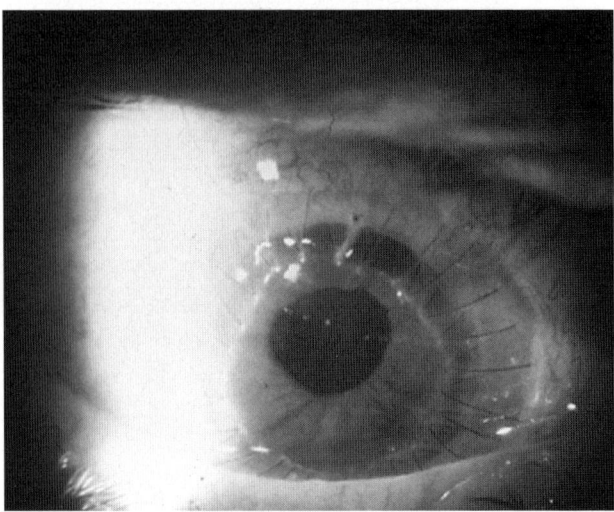

FIGURE 61-26. Khodadoust line.

decreased graft survival in eyes with deep stromal corneal vascularization (11,50,67,69,140). These vessels probably provide a route for allogeneic antigens to reach lymphatic tissue. This is substantiated by the recent discovery of lymphatic endothelium markers in the cornea (141). Previous graft failure also increases the probability of an immunologic rejection episode in repeat PK (13,49,50,69,140). Large graft size and eccentric grafts may also increase the risk of immunologic rejection (69).

Treatment of corneal allograft immunologic rejection is more likely to be effective if begun early. Approximately 50% of rejection episodes respond to treatment. Patient education about potential rejection symptoms is therefore very important. Decrease in visual acuity, irritation, redness, photophobia, and tearing are the most frequently reported symptoms. Suspected endothelial rejection episodes must be treated aggressively. The basic approach is to give topical 1% prednisolone acetate or 0.1% dexamethasone sodium phosphate drops every hour while the patient is awake, and 0.05% dexamethasone sodium phosphate ointment at bedtime for a few days. This corticosteroid regimen is then tapered slowly over a period of several weeks to a few months after observing improvement of the AC reaction, disappearance of some keratic precipitates, and normalization of pachymetric readings. Patients with repeated episodes of immunologic rejection or pseudophakic and aphakic patients without elevated intraocular pressures are often kept on topical corticosteroids at one drop per day, indefinitely. Several clinicians give corticosteroids by a route other than the topical at the time of diagnosis of an immunologic rejection episode, either an intravenous bolus of methylprednisolone, oral prednisolone for a few days, or subconjunctival dexamethasone. There is no study to prove or disprove that these therapeutic modalities are superior to intensive topical therapy alone.

To prevent rejection in high-risk patients or to treat patients with recurrent immunologic rejection episodes, topical 1% cyclosporine is an excellent alternative. It must, however, be given for several months up to 1 or 2 years. Discontinuing this topical immunosuppressant can be difficult because immunologic rejection signs and symptoms tend to manifest themselves after its discontinuation. Cyclosporine inhibits T cells. It can also be given orally, but systemic secondary effects are significant (142–144). There are reports of the use of oral tacrolimus (145), also a T-cell inhibitor, and of mycophenolate mofetil (146), a purine synthesis inhibitor. However, they also result in significant systemic side effects.

Postoperative Astigmatism

As previously mentioned, success in PK is not based on corneal clarity alone. Despite numerous advances in microsurgical technique, including suction-assisted trephines, corneal astigmatism remains a vexing postoperative problem and one that contributes greatly to patient and surgeon dissatisfaction. Factors contributing to significant postoperative astigmatism in PK include trephination disparity between donor and recipient, central versus eccentric trephination, disparity between donor and recipient tissue thickness, suturing technique, donor and recipient diameter disparity, recipient wound healing, timing of suture removal, and wound disparity or override (147). The use of a suction-assisted trephine decreases the amount of recipient tissue vaulting in the trephine and therefore decreases the potential for an oval trephination (95). Eccentric PK is associated with severe astigmatism (93), and therefore a well-centered graft is often the aim in PK. Belmont et al. (148) suggested rotating the donor tissue and using an intraoperative keratometer before suturing to reduce the final sutures-out astigmatism. Innumerable suturing techniques have been described with and without suture adjustment to reduce postoperative astigmatism (147,149–153). Despite this, the average keratometric postoperative astigmatism is approximately 4D (154,155).

A recently described suturing technique consisting of deep suture placement to decrease visual rehabilitation time and refractive error has been described in keratoconus (156). The future of this suturing technique has yet to be ascertained. As previously mentioned, the new technique of deep lamellar endothelial keratoplasty would address the vexing problem of postoperative astigmatism related to the anterior cornea by completely avoiding trephination. This exciting new technique will be evaluated in the future.

CONCOMITANT REQUIRED SURGERY

Phacoemulsification of a Cataract

Whenever PK is considered, cataract extraction must be entertained if a cataract is present. The indication for its removal is determined by its significance and contribution to diminished visual acuity. One must also take into account the fact that PK hastens cataract formation. With this in mind, a combined procedure is often performed. The goal of a combined procedure of cataract extraction and PK is to perform two procedures in one surgical setting. This is done, however, with the final goal of safety in mind. All surgeons who perform open-sky cataract extraction and PK are fully acquainted with the inherent difficulties of performing a continuous capsulorrhexis in an open setting, as well as the possibility of encountering excessive positive pressure after nucleus expulsion. For this reason, phacoemulsification is now favored by many if adequate visualization through the pathologic cornea is possible (157). Because the cornea will be trephinated after the cataract procedure, phacoemulsification can be performed in the AC to avoid complications.

Intraocular Lens Exchange

The most common indication for PK in North America remains pseudophakic bullous keratopathy (6), and therefore the surgeon is confronted with the decision as to whether to perform AC IOL exchange should the IOL be unstable. Open-loop AC IOLs are often stable and best left untouched.

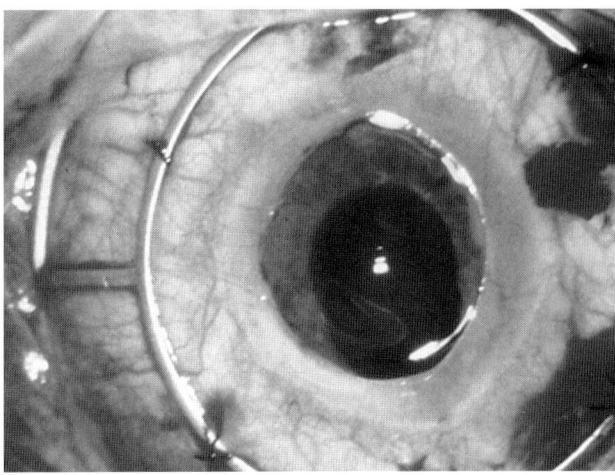

FIGURE 61-27. Before open-sky pupilloplasty.

Closed-loop AC IOLs are often the cause of the pseudophakic bullous keratopathy and are therefore removed during a combined procedure (158,159). They are often tricky to remove, and the surgeon must become familiar with adequate pictorial descriptions of these lenses before planning their explantation. It is often best to amputate the haptic segment in a large segment to decrease the potential for bleeding (160).

Iris-fixated posterior chamber IOLs (161) and transscleral fixation of posterior chamber IOLs (162) remain alternatives to AC IOLs, with the advantage of diminishing endothelial risk. However, they are technically more difficult to perform.

Anterior Segment Reconstruction

At the time of PK, the surgeon is often called on to reestablish a more normal configuration of the iris by performing a pupilloplasty (Figs. 61-27 and 61-28). This is done with 10-0 Prolene suture after the recipient cornea has been trephinated.

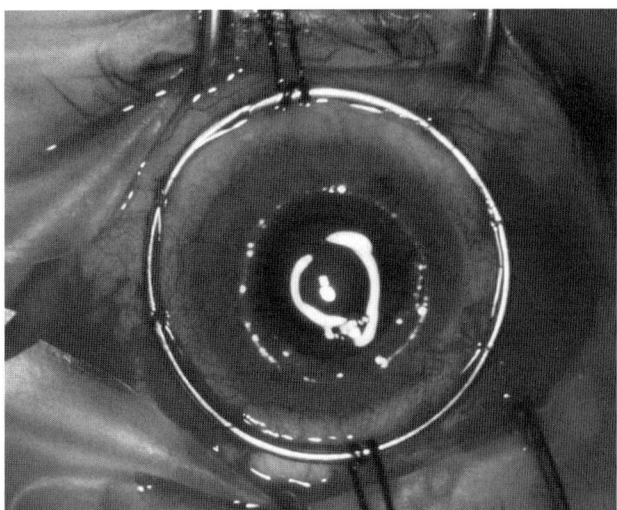

FIGURE 61-28. Open-sky pupilloplasty.

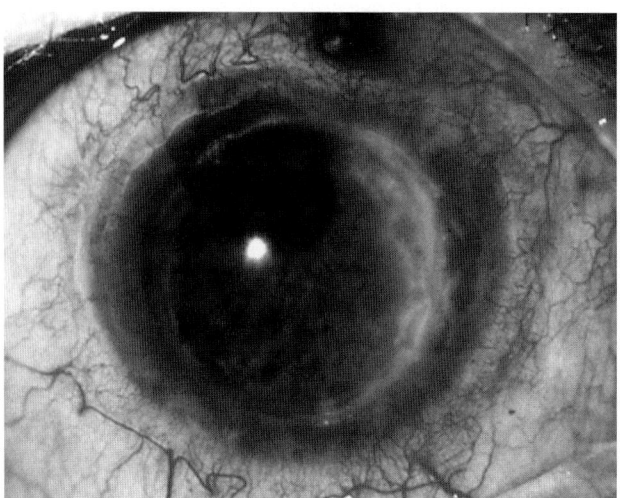

FIGURE 61-29. Herpes simplex virus disease epithelial recurrence in graft.

SPECIAL CIRCUMSTANCES

Penetrating Keratoplasty in Herpes Simplex Virus Keratitis

Recurrence of disease (Fig. 61-29) and allograft rejection are common causes of graft failure in HSV infection (163–165). For this reason, PK in patients with herpes simplex is considered a high-risk procedure (Fig. 61-30). The use of postoperative systemic acyclovir has been shown to influence graft survival favorably (166,167). The potential for emergence of resistance (168) must be considered when using oral antivirals for a prolonged period.

Pediatric Penetrating Keratoplasty

Pediatric PK is a high-risk procedure with a complex postoperative course. Graft survival and prognosis are

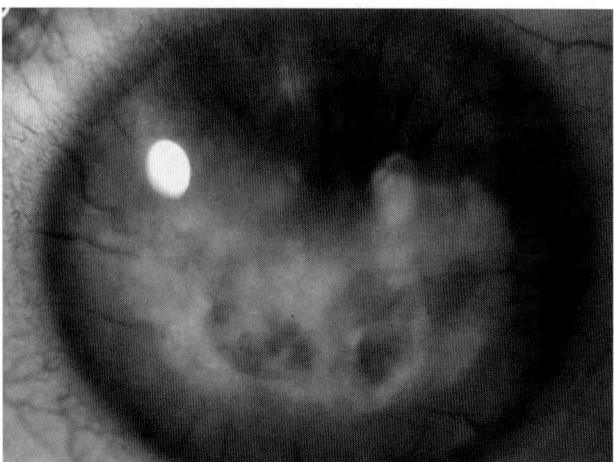

FIGURE 61-30. Corneal leukoma secondary to herpes simplex virus infection, with marked neovascularization.

influenced by the preoperative diagnosis, which includes congenital opacities, such as congenital hereditary endothelial dystrophy (CHED), acquired nontraumatic opacities, and acquired traumatic opacities. Best results are obtained in those with acquired opacities and in older patient age (169,170). The success in CHED is variable, described as reasonable (171) to excellent (172). A conservative approach is suggested by Javadi et al. (173) in patients with CHED. Variables, including preoperative vascularization, the presence of epithelial defects, and performance of vitrectomy (174,175), are associated with poor survival. Many cases of failure are secondary to infectious keratitis, allograft rejection, and secondary glaucoma.

REFERENCES

1. Niederkorn JY. Mechanisms of corneal graft rejection: the sixth annual Thygeson Lecture, presented at the Ocular Microbiology and Immunology Group meeting, October 21, 2000. *Cornea* 2001;20:675–679.
2. Elschnig A. On keratoplasty. *Parg Med Wochenschr* 1914;39:30.
3. Tudor-Thomas JW. Corneal transplantation on an opaque cornea. *Proc R Soc Med* 1936.
4. McCarey B, Kaufman H. Improved corneal storage. *Invest Ophthalmol Vis Sci* 1974;13:165–173.
5. Troutman R. In: *Microsurgery of the eye*, vol 2. St. Louis: CV Mosby, 1977.
6. Aiken-O'Neill P, Mannis MJ. Summary of corneal transplant activity Eye Bank Association of America. *Cornea* 2002;21: 1–3.
7. Waldock A, Cook SD. Corneal transplantation: how successful are we? *Br J Ophthalmol* 2000;84:813–815.
8. Ing JJ, Ing HH, Nelson LR, et al. Ten-year postoperative results of penetrating keratoplasty. *Ophthalmology* 1998;105: 1855–1865.
9. Inoue K, Amano S, Oshika T, et al. A 10-year review of penetrating keratoplasty. *Jpn J Ophthalmol* 2000;44:139–145.
10. Thompson RW Jr, Price MO, Bowers PJ, et al. Long-term graft survival after penetrating keratoplasty. *Ophthalmology* 2003;110: 1396–1402.
11. Boisjoly HM, Tourigny R, Bazin R, et al. Risk factors of corneal graft failure. *Ophthalmology* 1993;100:1728–1735.
12. Maguire MG, Stark WJ, Gottsch JD, et al. Risk factors for corneal graft failure and rejection in the collaborative corneal transplantation studies. Collaborative Corneal Transplantation Studies Research Group. *Ophthalmology* 1994;101:1536–1547.
13. Weisbrod D, Sit M, Naor J, et al. Outcomes of repeat penetrating keratoplasty and risk factors for graft failure. *Cornea* 2003;22: 429–434.
14. Vail A, Gore S, Bradley B, et al. Corneal graft survival and visual outcome: a multicenter study. Corneal Transplant Follow-up Study Collaborators. *Ophthalmology* 1994;101:120–127.
15. Riddle H, Parker D, Price F. Management of postkeratoplasty astigmatism. *Curr Opin Ophthalmol* 1998;9:15–28.
16. Boisjoly H, Gresset J, Fontaine N, et al. The VF-14 index of functional visual impairment in candidates for a corneal graft. *Am J Ophthalmol* 1999;128:38–44.
17. Boisjoly H, Gresset J, Charest M, et al. The VF-14 index of visual function in recipients of a corneal graft: a 2-year follow-up study. *Am J Ophthalmol* 2002;134:166–171.

18. Mendes F, Schaumberg D, Navon S, et al. Assessment of visual function after corneal transplantation: the quality of life and psychometric assessment after corneal transplantation (Q-PACT) study. *Am J Ophthalmol* 2003;135:785–793.
19. Chirila T. An overview of the development of artificial corneas with porous skirts and the use of PHEMA for such an application. *Biomaterials* 2001;22:3311–3317.
20. Hicks C, Crawford G, Lou X, et al. Corneal replacement using a synthetic hydrogel cornea, AlphaCor device: preliminary outcomes and complications. *Eye* 2003;17:385–392.
21. Caron M, Wilson R. Review of the risk of HIV infection through corneal transplantation in the United States. *J Am Optom Assoc* 1994;65:173–178.
22. Hogan R, Brown P, Heck E, et al. Risk of prion disease transmission from ocular donor tissue transplantation. *Cornea* 1999;18:2–11.
23. Lang C, Heckmann J, Neundorfer B. Creutzfeldt-Jakob disease via dural and corneal transplants. *J Neurol Sci* 1998;160:128–139.
24. Lueck C, McIlwaine G, Zeidler M. Creutzfeldt-Jakob disease and the eye: I. Background and patient management. *Eye* 2000;14:263–290.
25. Glasser D. Serologic testing of cornea donors. *Cornea* 1998;17:123–128.
26. Head MW, Northcott V, Rennison K, et al. Prion protein accumulation in eyes of patients with sporadic and variant Creutzfeldt-Jakob disease. *Invest Ophthalmol Vis Sci* 2003;44:342–346.
27. Armitage WJ, Easty DL. Factors influencing the suitability of organ-cultured corneas for transplantation. *Invest Ophthalmol Vis Sci* 1997;38:16–24.
28. Beck RW, Gal RL, Mannis MJ, et al. Is donor age an important determinant of graft survival? *Cornea* 1999;18:503–510.
29. Chipman M, Basu P, Willett P, et al. The effects of donor age and cause of death on corneal graft survival. *Acta Ophthalmol (Copenh)* 1990;68:537–542.
30. Gain P, Rizzi P, Thuret G, et al. Corneal harvesting from donors over 85 years of age: cornea outcome after banking and grafting [in French]. *J Fr Ophtalmol* 2002;25:274–289.
31. Inoue K, Amano S, Oshika T, et al. Risk factors for corneal graft failure and rejection in penetrating keratoplasty. *Acta Ophthalmol Scand* 2001;79:251–255.
32. Kuchle M, Cursiefen C, Nguyen N, et al. Risk factors for corneal allograft rejection: intermediate results of a prospective normal-risk keratoplasty study. *Graefes Arch Clin Exp Ophthalmol* 2002;240:580–584.
33. Musch DC, Meyer RF, Sugar A. Predictive factors for endothelial cell loss after penetrating keratoplasty. *Arch Ophthalmol* 1993;111:80–83.
34. Palay D, Kangas T, Stulting R, et al. The effects of donor age on the outcome of penetrating keratoplasty in adults. *Ophthalmology* 1997;104:1576–1579.
35. Redbrake C, Becker J, Salla S, et al. The influence of the cause of death and age on human corneal metabolism. *Invest Ophthalmol Vis Sci* 1994;35:3553–3556.
36. Yamagami S, Suzuki Y, Tsuru T. Risk factors for graft failure in penetrating keratoplasty. *Acta Ophthalmol Scand* 1996;74:584–588.
37. Bourne WM. Cellular changes in transplanted human corneas. *Cornea* 2001;20:560–569.
38. Kaufman HE, Beuerman RW, Steinemann TL, et al. Optisol corneal storage medium. *Arch Ophthalmol* 1991;109:864–868.
39. Borderie VM, Scheer S, Touzeau O, et al. Donor organ cultured corneal tissue selection before penetrating keratoplasty. *Br J Ophthalmol* 1998;82:382–388.
40. Ehlers H, Ehlers N, Hjortdal J. Corneal transplantation with donor tissue kept in organ culture for 7 weeks. *Acta Ophthalmol Scand* 1999;77:277–278.
41. Frueh BE, Bohnke M. Prospective, randomized clinical evaluation of Optisol vs organ culture corneal storage media. *Arch Ophthalmol* 2000;118:757–760.
42. Brunette I, Le Francois M, Tremblay M, et al. Corneal transplant tolerance of cryopreservation. *Cornea* 2001;20:590–596.
43. Streilein J. Immunobiology and immunopathology of corneal transplantation. *Chem Immunol* 1999;73:186–206.
44. Niederkorn J, Streilein J. Alloantigens placed into the anterior chamber of the eye induce specific suppression of delayed-type hypersensitivity but normal cytotoxic T lymphocyte and helper T lymphocyte responses. *J Immunol* 1983;131:2670–2674.
45. Nicholls S, Williams N. MHC matching and mechanisms of alloactivation in corneal transplantation. *Transplantation* 2001;72:1491–1497.
46. Katami M. Corneal transplantation: immunologically privileged status. *Eye* 1991;5:528–548.
47. Boisjoly HM, Roy R, Bernard PM, et al. Association between corneal allograft reactions and HLA compatibility. *Ophthalmology* 1990;97:1689–1698.
48. The Collaborative Corneal Transplantation Studies (CCTS) Research Group. Effectiveness of histocompatibility matching in high-risk corneal transplantation. The Collaborative Corneal Transplantation Studies Research Group. *Arch Ophthalmol* 1992;110:1392–403.
49. Sanfilippo F, MacQueen J, Vaughn W, et al. Reduced graft rejection with good HLA-A and B matching in high-risk corneal transplantation. *N Engl J Med* 1986;315:29–35.
50. Volker-Dieben H, D'Amaro J, Kok-van Alphen C. Hierarchy of prognostic factors for corneal allograft survival. *Aust N Z J Ophthalmol* 1987;15:11–18.
51. Bradley BA, Vail A, Gore SM, et al. Negative effect of HLA-DR matching on corneal transplant rejection. *Transplant Proc* 1995;27:1392–1394.
52. Gore S, Vail A, Bradley B, et al. HLA-DR matching in corneal transplantation: systematic review of published evidence. Corneal Transplant Follow-up Study Collaborators. *Transplantation* 1995;60:1033–1039.
53. Tiercy J. Molecular basis of HLA polymorphism: implications in clinical transplantation. *Transplant Immunol* 2002;9:173–180.
54. Batchelor JR. The laws of transplantation: a modern perspective. *Eye* 1995;9:152–154.
55. Borderie VM, Lopez M, Vedie F, et al. ABO antigen blood-group compatibility in corneal transplantation. *Cornea* 1997;16:1–6.
56. Inoue K, Tsuru T. ABO antigen blood-group compatibility and allograft rejection in corneal transplantation. *Acta Ophthalmol Scand* 1999;77:495–499.
57. Cosar C, Sridhar M, Cohen E, et al. Indications for penetrating keratoplasty and associated procedures, 1996–2000. *Cornea* 2002;21:148–151.
58. Dobbins K, Price F, Whitson W. Trends in the indications for penetrating keratoplasty in the midwestern United States. *Cornea* 2000;19:813–816.
59. Legeais J, Parc C, d'Hermies F, et al. Nineteen years of penetrating keratoplasty in the Hotel-Dieu Hospital in Paris. *Cornea* 2001;20:603–606.
60. Liu E, Slomovic A. Indications for penetrating keratoplasty in Canada, 1986–1995. *Cornea* 1997;16:414–419.
61. Patel NP, Kim T, Rapuano CJ, et al. Indications for and outcomes of repeat penetrating keratoplasty, 1989–1995. *Ophthalmology* 2000;107:719–724.
62. Bersudsky V, Blum-Hareuveni T, Rehany U, et al. The profile of repeated corneal transplantation. *Ophthalmology* 2001;108:461–469.

63. Dandona L, Naduvilath TJ, Janarthanan M, et al. Survival analysis and visual outcome in a large series of corneal transplants in India. *Br J Ophthalmol* 1997;81:726–731.

64. Williams K, Roder D, Esterman A, et al. Factors predictive of corneal graft survival: report from the Australian Corneal Graft Registry. *Ophthalmology* 1992;99:403–414.

65. Wilson S, Kaufman H. Graft failure after penetrating keratoplasty. *Surv Ophthalmol* 1990;34:325-56.

66. Ayyala R. Penetrating keratoplasty and glaucoma. *Surv Ophthalmol* 2000;45:91–105.

67. Cobo LM, Coster DJ, Rice NS, et al. Prognosis and management of corneal transplantation for herpetic keratitis. *Arch Ophthalmol* 1980;98:1755–1759.

68. Larkin DFP. Corneal transplantation for herpes simplex keratitis. *Br J Ophthalmol* 1998;82:107–108.

69. Boisjoly HM, Bernard PM, Dube I, et al. Effect of factors unrelated to tissue matching on corneal transplant endothelial rejection. *Am J Ophthalmol* 1989;107:647–654.

70. Holland EJ, Djalilian AR, Schwartz GS. Management of aniridic keratopathy with keratolimbal allograft: a limbal stem cell transplantation technique. *Ophthalmology* 2002;110:125–130.

71. Tiller A, Odenthal M, Verbraak F, et al. The influence of keratoplasty on visual prognosis in aniridia: a historical review of one large family. *Cornea* 2003;22:105–110.

72. Ghoraishi M, Akova Y, Tugal-Tutkun I, et al. Penetrating keratoplasty in atopic keratoconjunctivitis. *Cornea* 1995;14:610–613.

73. Brown G. Vision and quality-of-life. *Trans Am Ophthalmol Soc* 1999;97:473–511.

74. Uiters E, van den Borne B, van der Horst F, et al. Patient satisfaction after corneal transplantation. *Cornea* 2001;20:687–694.

75. Johansen T, Mannis M, Macsai M, et al. Obesity as a factor in penetrating keratoplasty. *Cornea* 1999;18:12–18.

76. Mauger T, Nye C, Boyle K. Intraocular pressure, anterior chamber depth and axial length following intravenous mannitol. *J Ocul Pharmacol Ther* 2000;16:591–594.

77. Apt L, Isenberg S, Yoshimori R, et al. Chemical preparation of the eye in ophthalmic surgery: III. Effect of povidone-iodine on the conjunctiva. *Arch Ophthalmol* 1984;102:728–729.

78. Speaker MG, Menikoff JA. Prophylaxis of endophthalmitis with topical povidone-iodine. *Ophthalmology* 1991;98:1769–1775.

79. Boes DA, Lindquist TD, Fritsche TR, et al. Effects of povidone-iodine chemical preparation and saline irrigation on the perilimbal flora. *Ophthalmology* 1992;99:1569–1574.

80. Snyder-Perlmutter LS, Katz HR, Melia M. Effect of topical ciprofloxacin 0.3% and ofloxacin 0.3% on the reduction of bacterial flora on the human conjunctiva. *J Cataract Refract Surg* 2000;26:1620–1625.

81. Donnenfeld ED, Perry HD, Snyder RW, et al. Intracorneal, aqueous humor, and vitreous humor penetration of topical and oral ofloxacin. *Arch Ophthalmol* 1997;115:173–176.

82. Callegan MC, Booth MC, Gilmore MS. In vitro pharmacodynamics of ofloxacin and ciprofloxacin against common ocular pathogens. *Cornea* 2000;19:539–545.

83. Isenberg SJ, Apt L, Yoshimori R, et al. Chemical preparation of the eye in ophthalmic surgery: IV. Comparison of povidone-iodine on the conjunctiva with a prophylactic antibiotic. *Arch Ophthalmol* 1985;103:1340–1342.

84. Microbiologic factors and visual outcome in the endophthalmitis vitrectomy study. *Am J Ophthalmol* 1996;122:830–846.

85. Callegan MC, Engelbert M, Parke DW II, et al. Bacterial endophthalmitis: epidemiology, therapeutics, and bacterium-host interactions. *Clin Microbiol Rev* 2002;15:111–124.

86. Speaker MG, Milch FA, Shah MK, et al. Role of external bacterial flora in the pathogenesis of acute postoperative endophthalmitis. *Ophthalmology* 1991;98:639–649; discussion, 650.

87. Chang BY, Hee WC, Ling R, et al. Local anaesthetic techniques and pulsatile ocular blood flow. *Br J Ophthalmol* 2000;84:1260–1263.

88. Quist LH, Stapleton SS, McPherson SD Jr. Preoperative use of the Honan intraocular pressure reducer. *Am J Ophthalmol* 1983;95:536–538.

89. Bourne WM. Reduction of endothelial cell loss during phakic penetrating keratoplasty. *Am J Ophthalmol* 1980;89:787–790.

90. Smith RJ, Chayet AS, Mondino BJ. Penetrating keratoplasty from a temporal approach. *Am J Ophthalmol* 2000;130:517–519.

91. Rudd J, Weis J, Connors R, et al. Introduction of corneal astigmatism through placement of a scleral fixation ring in eye bank eyes. *Cornea* 2001;20:864–865.

92. Sharif KW, Casey TA. Penetrating keratoplasty for keratoconus: complications and long-term success. *Br J Ophthalmol* 1991;75:142–146.

93. van Rij G, Cornell FM, Waring GO III, et al. Postoperative astigmatism after central vs eccentric penetrating keratoplasties. *Am J Ophthalmol* 1985;99:317–320.

94. Swinger CA. Postoperative astigmatism. *Surv Ophthalmol* 1987;31:219–248.

95. van Rij G, Waring GO III. Configuration of corneal trephine opening using five different trephines in human donor eyes. *Arch Ophthalmol* 1988;106:1228–1233.

96. Pflugfelder SC, Roussel TJ, Denham D, et al. Photogrammetric analysis of corneal trephination. *Arch Ophthalmol* 1992;110:1160–1166.

97. Olson RJ. Variation in corneal graft size related to trephine technique. *Arch Ophthalmol* 1979;97:1323–1325.

98. Krumeich J, Binder PS, Knulle A. The theoretical effect of trephine tilt on postkeratoplasty astigmatism. *CLAO J* 1988;14:213–219.

99. Alpar J. The use of Healon in corneal transplant surgery with and without intraocular lenses. *Ophthalmic Surg* 1984;15:757–760.

100. Eve F, Troutman R. Placement of sutures used in corneal incisions. *Am J Ophthalmol* 1976;82:786–789.

101. Purcell JJ Jr, Krachmer JH, Doughman DJ, et al. Expulsive hemorrhage in penetrating keratoplasty. *Ophthalmology* 1982;89:41–43.

102. Taylor D. Expulsive hemorrhage: some observations and comments. *Trans Am Ophthalmol Soc* 1974;72:157–169.

103. Speaker MG, Guerriero PN, Met JA, et al. A case-control study of risk factors for intraoperative suprachoroidal expulsive hemorrhage. *Ophthalmology* 1991;98:202–209; discussion, 210.

104. Kim T, Palay D, Lynn M. Donor factors associated with epithelial defects after penetrating keratoplasty. *Cornea* 1996;15:451–456.

105. Chou L, Cohen E, Laibson P, et al. Factors associated with epithelial defects after penetrating keratoplasty. *Ophthalmic Surg* 1994;25:700–703.

106. Machado R, Mannis M, Mandel H, et al. The relationship between first postoperative day epithelial status and eventual health of the ocular surface in penetrating keratoplasty. *Cornea* 2002;21:574–577.

107. Blanchard D. Hurricane keratitis in penetrating keratoplasty. *Cornea* 1984;3:75–76.

108. Gasset AR, Lorenzetti DW, Ellison EM, et al. Quantitative corticosteroid effect on corneal wound healing. *Arch Ophthalmol* 1969;81:589–591.

109. Rotkis W, Chandler J, Forstot S. Filamentary keratitis following penetrating keratoplasty. *Ophthalmology* 1982;89:946–949.

110. Sonavane A, Sharma S, Gangopadhyay N, et al. Clinico-microbiological correlation of suture-related graft infection following penetrating keratoplasty. *Am J Ophthalmol* 2003;135:89–91.

111. Leahey A, Avery R, Gottsch J, et al. Suture abscesses after penetrating keratoplasty. *Cornea* 1993;12:489–492.

112. Fong L, Ormerod L, Kenyon K, et al. Microbial keratitis complicating penetrating keratoplasty. *Ophthalmology* 1988;95: 1269–1275.

113. Gorovoy MS, Stern GA, Hood CI, et al. Intrastromal noninflammatory bacterial colonization of a corneal graft. *Arch Ophthalmol* 1983;101:1749–1752.

114. Meisler D, Langston R, Naab T, et al. Infectious crystalline keratopathy. *Am J Ophthalmol* 1984;97:337–343.

115. Ormerod L, Ruoff K, Meisler D, et al. Infectious crystalline keratopathy: role of nutritionally variant streptococci and other bacterial factors. *Ophthalmology* 1991;98:159–169.

116. Matoba A, O'Brien T, Wilhelmus K, et al. Infectious crystalline keratopathy due to *Streptococcus pneumoniae*: possible association with serotype. *Ophthalmology* 1994;101:1000.

117. Khater T, Jones D, Wilhelmus K. Infectious crystalline keratopathy caused by gram-negative bacteria. *Am J Ophthalmol* 1997;124:19–23.

118. Labalette P, Maurage C, Jourdel D, et al. Nontuberculous mycobacterial keratitis: report of two cases causing infectious crystalline keratopathy [in French]. *J Fr Ophtalmol* 2003;26:175–181.

119. Butler TKH, Dua HS, Edwards R, et al. *In vitro* model of infectious crystalline keratopathy: tissue architecture determines pattern of microbial spread. *Invest Ophthalmol Vis Sci* 2001;42:1243–1246.

120. Aiello LP, Javitt JC, Canner JK. National outcomes of penetrating keratoplasty: risks of endophthalmitis and retinal detachment. *Arch Ophthalmol* 1993;111:509–513.

121. Leveille AS, McMullan FD, Cavanagh HD. Endophthalmitis following penetrating keratoplasty. *Ophthalmology* 1983;90:38–39.

122. Guss RB, Koenig S, De La Pena W, et al. Endophthalmitis after penetrating keratoplasty. *Am J Ophthalmol* 1983;95:651–658.

123. Cameron JA, Antonios SR, Cotter JB, et al. Endophthalmitis from contaminated donor corneas following penetrating keratoplasty. *Arch Ophthalmol* 1991;109:54–59.

124. Aaberg TM Jr, Flynn HW Jr, Schiffman J, et al. Nosocomial acute-onset postoperative endophthalmitis survey: a 10-year review of incidence and outcomes. *Ophthalmology* 1998;105: 1004–1010.

125. Kaye D. Epithelial response in penetrating keratoplasty. *Am J Ophthalmol* 1980;89:381–387.

126. Irvine A, Kaufman H. Intraocular pressure following penetrating keratoplasty. *Am J Ophthalmol* 1969;68:835–844.

127. Yamagami S, Tsuru T. Increase in orthotopic murine corneal transplantation rejection rate with anterior synechiae. *Invest Ophthalmol Vis Sci* 1999;40:2422–2426.

128. Tragakis M, Brown S. The significance of anterior synechiae after corneal transplantation. *Am J Ophthalmol* 1972;74:532–533.

129. Urrets-Zavalia A. Acute iridoatrophying mydriasis: status of the matter at the present time [in French]. *Bull Mem Soc Fr Ophtalmol* 1986;97:166–168.

130. Houff SA, Burton RC, Wilson RW, et al. Human-to-human transmission of rabies virus by corneal transplant. *N Engl J Med* 1979;300:603–604.

131. Centers for Disease Control. Human to human transmission of rabies via a corneal transplant: France. *MMWR Morb Mortal Wkly Rep* 1980;29:25–26.

132. Centers for Disease Control. Human to human transmission of rabies via corneal transplant. Thailand. *MMWR Morb Mortal Wkly Rep* 1981;30:473–474.

133. Gode G, Bhide N. Two rabies deaths after corneal grafts from one donor. *Lancet* 1988;2:791.

134. Javadi M, Fayaz A, Mirdehghan S, et al. Transmission of rabies by corneal graft. *Cornea* 1996;15:431–433.

135. Sureau P, Portnoi D, Rollin P, et al. Prevention of inter-human rabies transmission after corneal graft [in French]. *C R Seances Acad Sci III* 1981;293:689–692.

136. McGeorge AJ, Vote BJ, Elliot DA, et al. Papillary adenocarcinoma of the iris transmitted by corneal transplantation. *Arch Ophthalmol* 2002;120:1379–1383.

137. Wilson SE, Kaufman HE. Graft failure after penetrating keratoplasty. *Surv Ophthalmol* 1990;34:325–356.

138. Alldredge OC, Krachmer JH. Clinical types of corneal transplant rejection: their manifestations, frequency, preoperative correlates, and treatment. *Arch Ophthalmol* 1981;99:599–604.

139. Khodadoust A, Silverstein A. Transplantation and rejection of individual cell layers of the cornea. *Invest Ophthalmol Vis Sci* 1969;8:180–195.

140. Volker-Dieben H, Kok-van Alphen C, Lansbergen Q, et al. Different influences on corneal graft survival in 539 transplants. *Acta Ophthalmol (Copenh)* 1982;60:190–202.

141. Cursiefen C, Chen L, Dana M, et al. Corneal lymphangiogenesis: evidence, mechanisms, and implications for corneal transplant immunology. *Cornea* 2003;22:273–281.

142. Poon AC, Forbes JE, Dart JKG, et al. Systemic cyclosporin A in high risk penetrating keratoplasties: a case-control study. *Br J Ophthalmol* 2001;85:1464–1469.

143. Reinhard T, Moller M, Sundmacher R. Penetrating keratoplasty in patients with atopic dermatitis with and without systemic cyclosporin A. *Cornea* 1999;18:645–651.

144. Young A, Rao S, Cheng L, et al. Combined intravenous pulse methylprednisolone and oral cyclosporine A in the treatment of corneal graft rejection: 5-year experience. *Eye* 2002;16:304–308.

145. Sloper CML, Powell RJ, Dua HS. Tacrolimus (FK506) in the management of high-risk corneal and limbal grafts. *Ophthalmology* 2001;108:1838–1844.

146. Reinhard T, Reis A, Bohringer D, et al. Systemic mycophenolate mofetil in comparison with systemic cyclosporin A in high-risk keratoplasty patients: 3 years' results of a randomized prospective clinical trial. *Graefes Arch Clin Exp Ophthalmol* 2001;239: 367–372.

147. Binder PS. Selective suture removal can reduce postkeratoplasty astigmatism. *Ophthalmology* 1985;92:1412–1416.

148. Belmont SC, Troutman RC, Buzard KA. Control of astigmatism aided by intraoperative keratometry. *Cornea* 1993;12:397–400.

149. Serdarevic O, Renard G, Pouliquen Y. Randomized clinical trial comparing astigmatism and visual rehabilitation after penetrating keratoplasty with and without intraoperative suture adjustment. *Ophthalmology* 1994;101:990–999.

150. Van Meter WS, Gussler JR, Soloman KD, et al. Postkeratoplasty astigmatism control: single continuous suture adjustment versus selective interrupted suture removal. *Ophthalmology* 1991;98: 177–183.

151. Musch DC, Meyer RF, Sugar A, et al. Corneal astigmatism after penetrating keratoplasty: the role of suture technique. *Ophthalmology* 1989;96:698–703.

152. Lin DT, Wilson SE, Reidy JJ, et al. An adjustable single running suture technique to reduce postkeratoplasty astigmatism: a preliminary report. *Ophthalmology* 1990;97:934–938.

153. Davison JA, Bourne WM. Results of penetrating keratoplasty using a double running suture technique. *Arch Ophthalmol* 1981;99:1591–1595.

154. Perlman EM. An analysis and interpretation of refractive errors after penetrating keratoplasty. *Ophthalmology* 1981;88:39–45.

155. Stainer GA, Perl T, Binder PS. Controlled reduction of postkeratoplasty astigmatism. *Ophthalmology* 1982;89:668–676.

156. Busin M, Arffa R. Deep suturing technique for penetrating keratoplasty. *Cornea* 2002;21:680–684.

157. Rao S, Padmanabhan P. Combined phacoemulsification and penetrating keratoplasty. *Ophthalmic Surg Lasers* 1999;30:488–491.

158. Speaker M, Lugo M, Laibson P, et al. Penetrating keratoplasty for pseudophakic bullous keratopathy: management of the intraocular lens. *Ophthalmology* 1988;95:1260–1268.

159. Kornmehl E, Steinert R, Odrich M, et al. Penetrating keratoplasty for pseudophakic bullous keratopathy associated with closed-loop anterior chamber intraocular lenses. *Ophthalmology* 1990;97:407–412.

160. Koenig S, Solomon J. Removal of closed-loop anterior chamber intraocular lenses during penetrating keratoplasty. *Cornea* 1987;6:207–208.

161. Price F Jr, Whitson W. Visual results of suture-fixated posterior chamber lenses during penetrating keratoplasty. *Ophthalmology* 1989;96:1234–1239.

162. Davis R, Best D, Gilbert G. Comparison of intraocular lens fixation techniques performed during penetrating keratoplasty. *Am J Ophthalmol* 1991;111:743–749.

163. Fine M, Cignetti FE. Penetrating keratoplasty in herpes simplex keratitis: recurrence in grafts. *Arch Ophthalmol* 1977;95:613–616.

164. Moyes AL, Sugar A, Musch DC, et al. Antiviral therapy after penetrating keratoplasty for herpes simplex keratitis. *Arch Ophthalmol* 1994;112:601–607.

165. Foster C, Duncan J. Penetrating keratoplasty for herpes simplex keratitis. *Am J Ophthalmol* 1981;92:336–343.

166. Barney N, Foster C. A prospective randomized trial of oral acyclovir after penetrating keratoplasty for herpes simplex keratitis. *Cornea* 1994;13:232–236.

167. Tambasco FP, Cohen EJ, Nguyen LH, et al. Oral acyclovir after penetrating keratoplasty for herpes simplex keratitis. *Arch Ophthalmol* 1999;117:445–449.

168. Sonkin P, Baratz K, Frothingham R, et al. Acyclovir-resistant herpes simplex virus keratouveitis after penetrating keratoplasty. *Ophthalmology* 1992;99:1805–1808.

169. Cowden J. Penetrating keratoplasty in infants and children. *Ophthalmology* 1990;97:324–328.

170. Erlich C, Rootman D, Morin J. Corneal transplantation in infants, children and young adults: experience of the Toronto Hospital for Sick Children, 1979–88. *Can J Ophthalmol* 1991;26:206–210.

171. Schaumberg D, Moyes A, Gomes J, et al. Corneal transplantation in young children with congenital hereditary endothelial dystrophy. Multicenter Pediatric Keratoplasty Study. *Am J Ophthalmol* 1999;127:373–378.

172. Frueh BE, Brown SI. Transplantation of congenitally opaque corneas. *Br J Ophthalmol* 1997;81:1064–1069.

173. Javadi M, Baradaran-Rafii A, Zamani M, et al. Penetrating keratoplasty in young children with congenital hereditary endothelial dystrophy. *Cornea* 2003;22:420–423.

174. Stulting R, Sumers K, Cavanagh H, et al. Penetrating keratoplasty in children. *Ophthalmology* 1984;91:1222–1230.

175. Aasuri M, Garg P, Gokhle N, et al. Penetrating keratoplasty in children. *Cornea* 2000;19:140–144.

LAMELLAR KERATOPLASTY

JOHN D. GOOSEY AND
CHRISTOPHER W. STURBAUM

The history of lamellar keratoplasty covers more than 100 years, beginning with the first successful lamellar corneal transplantation performed by Arthur von Hippel at the end of the 19th century (1). Lamellar keratoplasty represents a more conservative surgical approach than penetrating keratoplasty in that only the diseased portions of a compromised cornea are removed, whereas the healthy structures remain intact. Traditionally, lamellar keratoplasty replaces abnormal anterior corneal tissue from the host with healthy tissue from the anterior portion of a donor cornea while maintaining the integrity of the recipient's Descemet's membrane and endothelium. The advantages of such a technique have long been recognized. The most obvious advantage is that sparing the host endothelium eliminates the possibility of endothelial rejection, which is the leading cause of graft failure with penetrating keratoplasty. Other advantages of anterior lamellar keratoplasty result from it being an extraocular procedure, which mitigates complications such as endophthalmitis, expulsive hemorrhage, glaucoma, and cataract formation. In spite of these advantages, most corneal surgeons have eschewed lamellar keratoplasty because of its perceived technical difficulty and the widely held belief that penetrating keratoplasty gives superior visual outcomes. Recent microsurgical techniques and instrumentation have led to increased interest in lamellar keratoplasty. One of the largest factors contributing to this increased interest is the growing popularity of the refractive lamellar procedure, laser-assisted *in situ* keratomileusis (LASIK). As corneal surgeons have gained more familiarity with microkeratomes and the lamellar aspects of LASIK, the overall interest in lamellar keratoplasty has grown.

Recently, the lamellar surgical philosophy of conservatively sparing healthy host tissue and removing diseased corneal tissue has been applied to the posterior layers of the cornea (2). Posterior lamellar endothelial keratoplasty involves the removal of posterior stroma, Descemet's membrane, and unhealthy endothelium, followed by replacement with similar healthy donor corneal tissue (3,4). The advantages of posterior lamellar endothelial keratoplasty are derived from maintaining the anterior corneal surface

of the recipient, with resultant improved control of postoperative astigmatism. This evolving technique offers the hope of faster visual rehabilitation for those patients with a compromised endothelium than the currently used penetrating keratoplasty techniques. However, the long-term efficacy of deep lamellar endothelial keratoplasty remains to be determined (5).

Lamellar keratoplasty can now be used to replace any specific part of the cornea. The indications, techniques, outcomes, and complications of both anterior lamellar keratoplasty and posterior lamellar keratoplasty are covered in this chapter.

ANTERIOR LAMELLAR KERATOPLASTY

Anterior lamellar keratoplasty is defined as the removal and replacement of deformed or diseased anterior corneal tissue (epithelium, Bowman's layer, and stroma) while sparing the host Descemet's membrane and endothelium. The depth of the lamellar dissection is determined by the depth of the anterior corneal pathologic process. Complete removal of stromal tissue to the level of Descemet's membrane is seldom indicated and carries the risk of penetrating into the anterior chamber. Anterior lamellar keratoplasty can be divided into two major categories: optical and tectonic. Optical lamellar grafts are often large in diameter, and tectonic grafts vary in shape and can be fashioned into specific shapes depending on the indication (Fig. 62-1).

Indications

Anterior lamellar keratoplasty is indicated for the treatment of corneas that have a healthy endothelium but have structural or pathologic changes anterior to Descemet's membrane. Optical anterior lamellar keratoplasty is very useful for visual rehabilitation of patients with anterior stromal scars after infectious keratitis or trauma. A growing indication for optical lamellar keratoplasty is the treatment of complications after refractive surgery. Visually significant haze after photorefractive keratectomy or scarring of

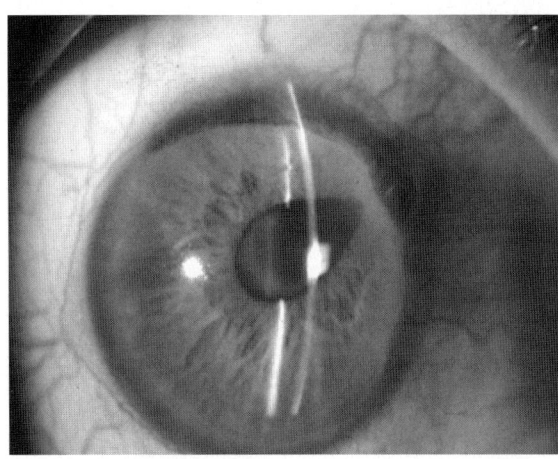
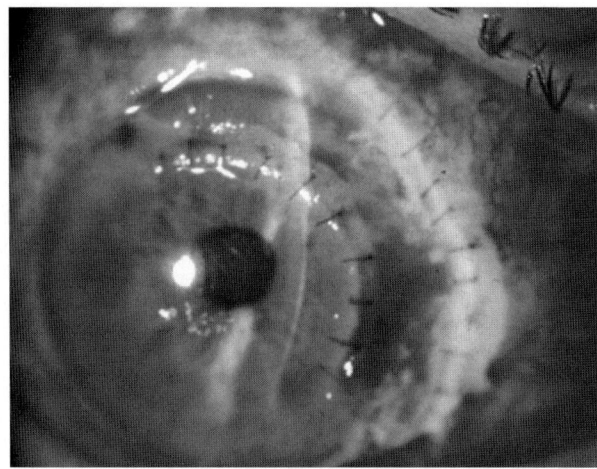

FIGURE 62-1. Tectonic lamellar keratoplasty for the treatment of a perforated Terrien's marginal degeneration after trauma. **A:** Peripheral corneal perforation is shown with iris incarceration in the corneal wound and a peaked pupil. **B:** Corneal integrity is restored by a tectonic horseshoe-shaped lamellar graft. (Courtesy of Jeffrey D. Lanier, M.D., with permission)

the anterior cornea following LASIK or radial keratotomy can be successfully managed with optical lamellar keratoplasty (Figs. 62-2 and 62-3). Other optical indications include corneal dystrophies such as Reis-Bückler, Salzmann's nodular dystrophy, and lattice, granular, or macular dystrophy. Because macular corneal dystrophy can involve both the stroma and endothelium, anterior lamellar keratoplasty should be restricted to those cases of macular corneal dystrophy that have no significant endothelial involvement (Fig. 62-4). Reis-Bückler dystrophy commonly recurs in lamellar grafts, but this problem is safely and easily managed by replacing the graft (6).

Tectonic anterior lamellar keratoplasty is useful for reestablishing the structural integrity of the cornea from peripheral, noninflammatory thinning disorders such as Terrien's marginal degeneration or pellucid marginal degeneration. Tectonic grafts can also be used to treat peripheral ulcerative keratitis in autoimmune disorders such as Mooren's ulcer. The inflammatory condition must be resolved to ensure graft survival (7). Structural integrity of a neurotrophic corneal melt from herpes zoster or diabetes can also be managed with a tectonic graft. If the underlying or associated reason for the corneal melt is not recognized and treated, the tectonic graft will fail secondary to stromal melting. In the case of herpes zoster, inferior corneal melting is almost always associated with lagophthalmos, so a tectonic graft combined with a lateral tarsorrhaphy may give the optimal result.

Combined optical and tectonic indications for anterior lamellar keratoplasty include keratoconus, pellucid marginal degeneration and iatrogenic keratoectasia after refractive surgery. LASIK surgery performed on patients with subclinical keratoconus or pellucid marginal degeneration leads to accelerated corneal ectasia with high levels of irregular astigmatism. Such corneas are ideally managed with lamellar keratoplasty because the patient can be visually rehabilitated without future concerns for endothelial graft

reactions. The treatment of advanced keratoconus in which the patient is contact lens intolerant is another indication for anterior lamellar keratoplasty (8,9).

Surgical Procedure

A basic understanding of the morphology and biomechanical properties of the corneal stroma is necessary to develop an optimal surgical approach to lamellar keratoplasty. The stroma comprises approximately 90% of the total corneal thickness and is made up of 300 to 500 lamellae (10). Anteriorly, the lamellae are significantly interwoven and often oriented obliquely to the corneal surface. In the posterior two thirds of the stroma, the lamellae are stacked parallel to the corneal surface (11). These features explain why shearing corneal lamellae is much more difficult anteriorly than posteriorly. Collagen interweaving is also more extensive in the corneal periphery than in its center (12). This explains the finding that cohesive strength is greater in the corneal periphery than in the central cornea (13). Cohesive strength is defined as the force required to separate a stromal sample along a cleavage plane parallel to the lamellar axis by pulling in a direction perpendicular to the cleavage plane. Knowing the relative cohesive strength of different areas of the stroma is useful when performing lamellar surgery.

Preparation of the Host Bed

Optical Lamellar Keratoplasty (Malbran's "Peeling Off" Technique)

The first step in the procedure is to center a trephine over the host corneal tissue to be removed (14,15). Most disorders requiring an optical lamellar keratoplasty can be treated with an 8- to 9-mm diameter trephine. Popular trephines include the Hessburg-Barron vacuum trephine (Jedmed Instrument Co., St. Louis, MO; Katena Products,

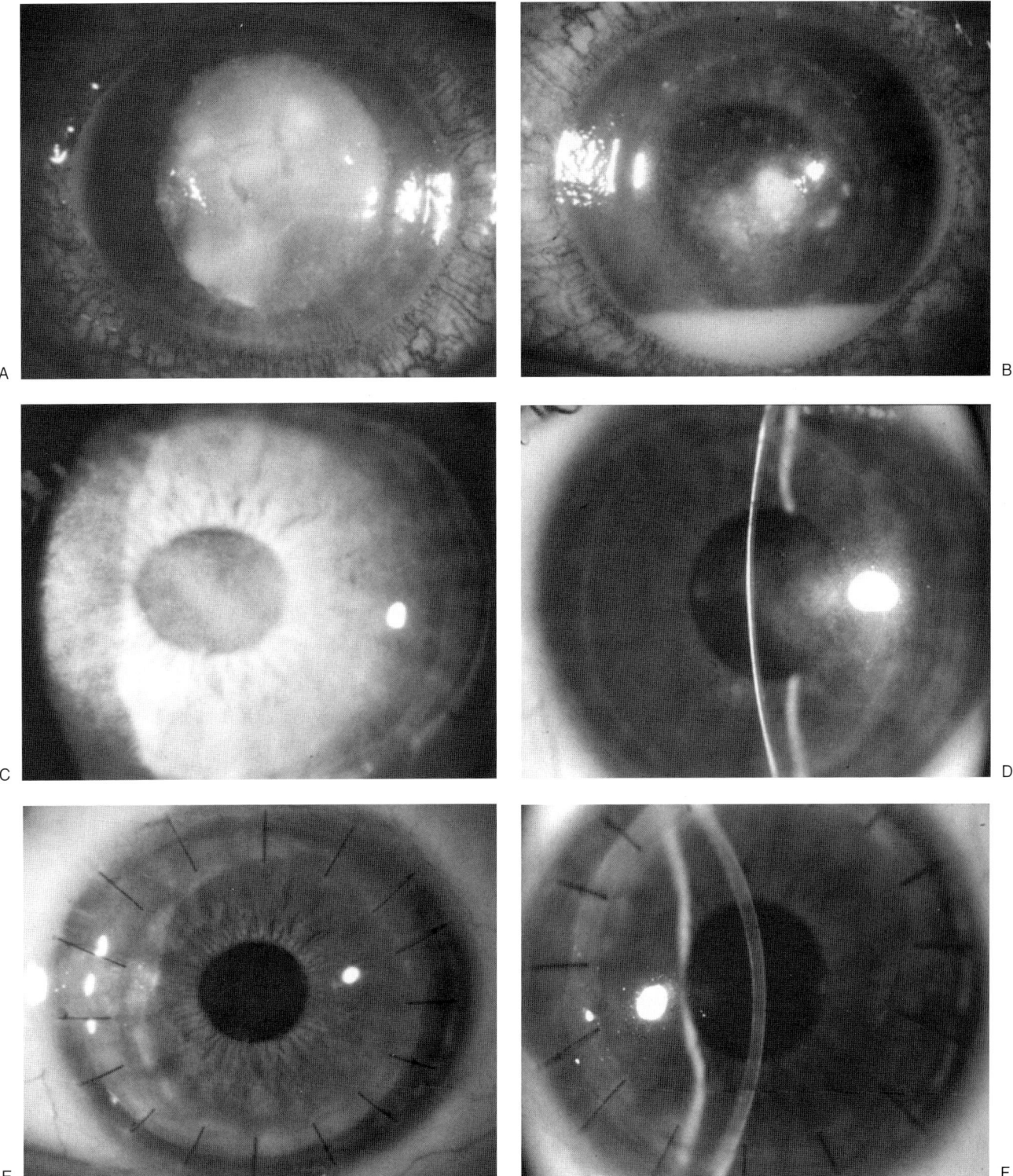

FIGURE 62-2. Infectious keratitis after laser-assisted *in situ* keratomileusis (LASIK) resulting in a superficial scar that was subsequently treated with lamellar keratoplasty. **A:** *Staphylococcus aureus* abscess under a LASIK flap. **B:** The necrotic LASIK flap was removed and the remaining corneal ulcer with hypopyon was treated with antibiotics. **C:** Corneal scar after removal of LASIK flap and antibiotic treatment. **D:** Slit-lamp view of corneal scar showing moderate depth of scar. **E:** Postoperative lamellar graft 2 weeks after surgery. **F:** Slit-lamp view showing clear lamellar graft with non discernible interface.

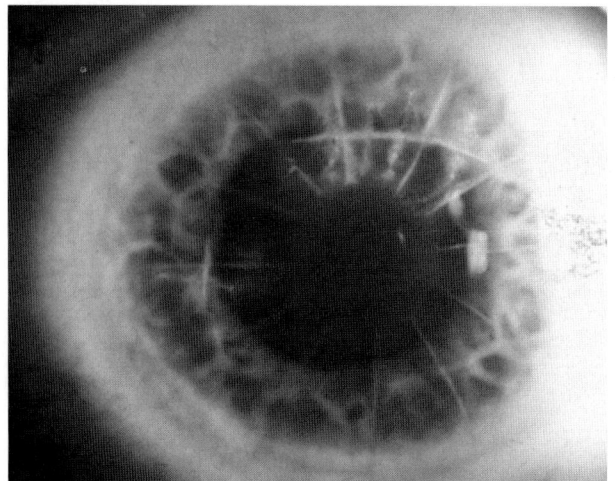

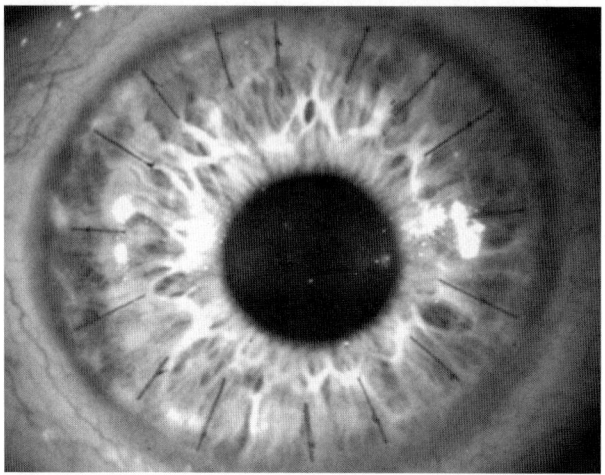

FIGURE 62-3. Irregular astigmatism with fluctuating vision after radial keratotomy (RK). **A:** Multiple RK incisions deforming the cornea, resulting in distorted vision that could not be corrected with a contact lens. **B:** Lamellar graft showing removal of RK scars. The patient's myopia returned, but he was correctable to 20/25.

Denville, NJ), the Hanna trephine (Moria, Antony, France), and the Krumeich trephine system (Rhein Medical, Tampa, FL). The Hessburg-Barron trephine is easy to use and is disposable, but an exact trephination depth can only be approximated. Because the blade of the Hessburg-Barron vacuum trephine spirals downward, the depth of the annular keratotomy created by this trephine is not uniform. One complete revolution of the blade of this trephine incises an annular keratotomy depth of approximately 250 to 300 μm. The desired depth of the trephination is determined by the depth of the corneal lesion, keeping in mind that too deep a trephination could result in entering the anterior chamber and require aborting the procedure. Regardless of the depth of the corneal lesion, a minimum trephination depth of a at least 300 μm is recommended to ensure that the lamellar dissection is started within the posterior stromal lamellae. Lamellar dissection within the anterior stroma is very difficult because of the interlacing nature of these lamellae.

Once the trephination is completed to the desired depth, a 0.12 forceps is used to grasp the inner edge of the annular keratotomy at the 12 o'clock position and, after pulling the inner edge of the trephine cut centrally, the depth is visually inspected. A microsurgical blade (Grieshaber 681.21) is then positioned at the base of the keratotomy incision and lamellar dissection is initiated at the 12 o'clock position by gently cutting the deep lamellae immediately anterior to the base of the trephination. Keeping the microsurgical blade just anterior to the base of the trephination minimizes the risk of inadvertently entering the anterior chamber. The lamellar dissection is then extended for approximately 3 mm centrally from the inner edge of the trephine incision. This 3-mm peripheral dissection should extend along the perimeter of the inner

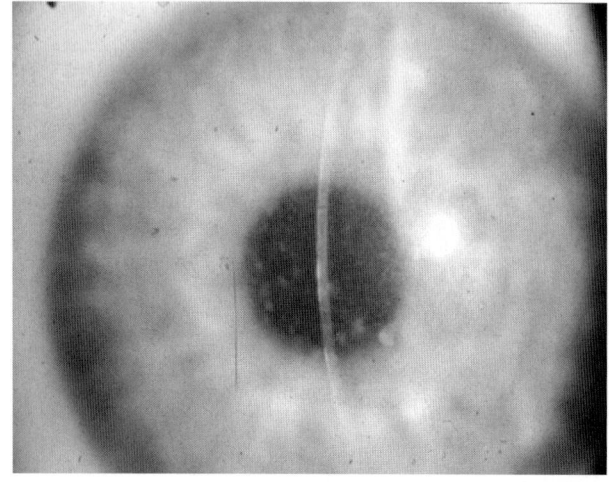

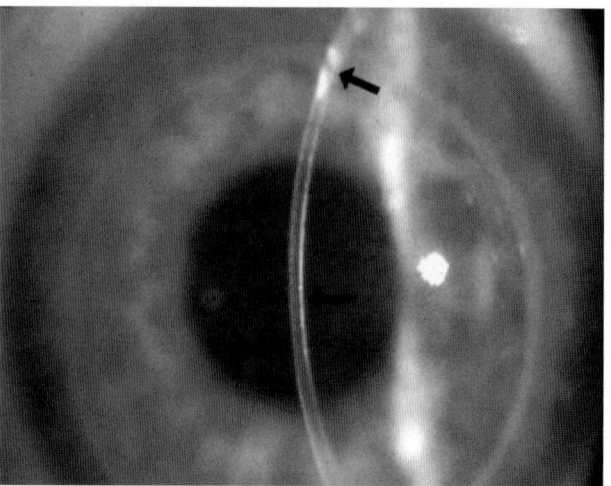

FIGURE 62-4. Macular corneal dystrophy. **A:** Preoperative photograph showing diffuse stromal opacities consistent with macular dystrophy. **B:** Clear lamellar graft 3 months after surgery. *Top arrow* shows the perforation site, which required closure with a 10 nylon suture to complete the procedure. *Bottom arrow* shows slight interface haze, but patient has 20/25 acuity.

edge of the keratotomy incision for 270 degrees. Before extending the lamellar keratectomy centrally, the interlacing peripheral corneal lamellae are dissected, thereby reducing the biomechanical forces that resist shearing of the corneal lamellae. This surgical maneuver allows for a much easier and safer dissection of the central posterior lamellae. Some surgeons start the lamellar dissection centrally and omit the initial peripheral dissection. However, if one takes time to perform this peripheral dissection, the central lamellae peel away with mechanical traction applied by pulling the host tissue with a 0.12 or Pollack forceps, obviating the need to cut the central lamellae with the microsurgical blade. Upward traction is applied to the inner edge of the keratectomy at the 12 o'clock position and then the tissue is pulled both upward and axially (centrally). As the posterior lamellae begin to shear, air appears in the fibers at the base of the lamellar keratectomy, making the lamellar fibers appear snow-white (Fig. 62-5). By keeping the microsurgical blade angled slightly upward, a fine sweeping motion just anterior to the base of the keratectomy is used to tease these white fibers away from the stromal bed and extend the lamellar

keratectomy centrally. As the central point of the dissection is reached, the cohesive forces of the posterior lamellae are easily overcome by mechanical traction applied with the 0.12 or the Polack forceps. In Malbran's original description of this technique, two forceps were used to apply traction with firm and sustained movement, always working from the periphery to the center. The safety advantage of not using a knife over the central cornea is obvious, but an additional advantage of using this peeling method is the natural tendency of the dissection to stay in the same lamellar plane so that a very smooth dissection is obtained. As the dissection passes the central cornea and moves toward the inferior edge of the trephination, some additional peripheral dissection with the microsurgical blade may be required. Once the inferior edge is reached, Vannas scissors can be used to complete the removal of the lamellar keratectomy tissue. Using this dissection approach greatly reduces the risk of inadvertent entry into the anterior chamber when performing lamellar keratoplasty for deep stromal scars or advanced keratoconus. With advanced keratoconus, it is not unusual to bare Descemet's membrane as one peels the central

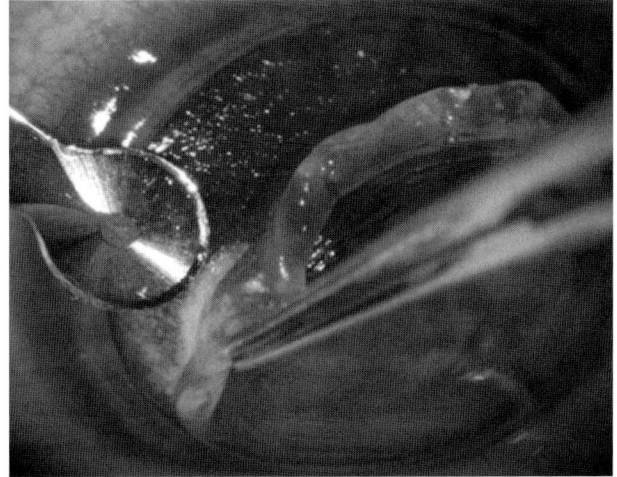

A

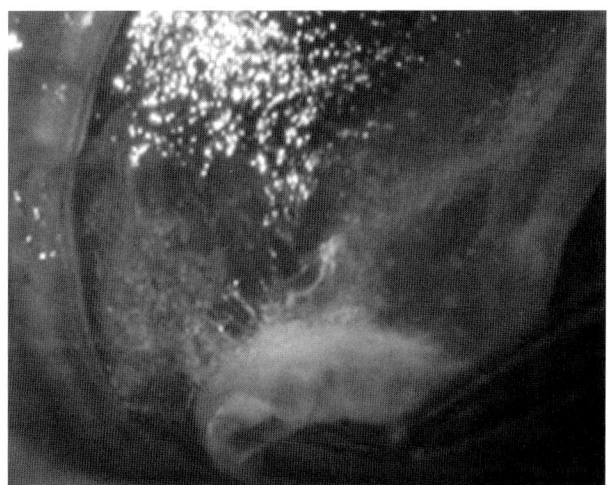

B

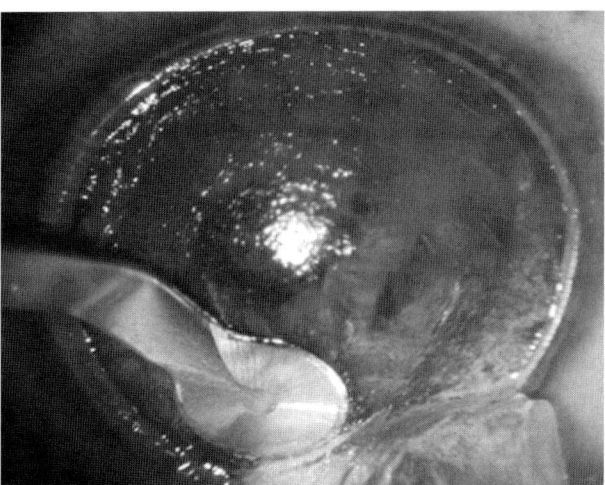

C

FIGURE 62-5. Intraoperative lamellar keratectomy using Malbran's technique on a patient with advanced keratoconus. **A:** Peripheral lamellar dissection keeping blade slightly upward just anterior to white stromal fibers, which form when air enters the dissection plane. **B:** After peripheral dissection, the central lamellae peel away with mechanical traction without the need to use a microsurgical blade. **C:** As the peripheral aspect of the inferior edge is reached, the microsurgical blade is used to complete the lamellar keratectomy. Note the glassy, smooth appearance of the central stromal bed, which was safely created without the use of the lamellar blade.

stroma away from the host bed. At this point in the dissection, the use of a blade is both unnecessary and unsafe.

After the lamellar dissection is completed, the recipient bed is inspected. If additional tissue requires removal, a deeper lamellar dissection can be performed by first scratching down on the peripheral edge of the recipient bed with a supersharp knife, and then a second pass at a deeper lamellar plane can be completed. This maneuver is risky and is rarely needed.

In summary, for optimal results, always start each lamellar dissection with a 270-degree peripheral dissection and keep the depth of the dissection at the level of the parallel posterior lamellae. This approach reduces the cohesive forces that naturally resist separation of corneal lamellae and allows for the safe and consistent creation of a smooth lamellar bed.

Air Dissection Technique

Intrastromal air injection can facilitate deep lamellar dissection along a plane in the posterior stroma immediately above or at the level of Descemet's membrane (16,17). The cornea is trephined to access the deep lamellar tissue. A 30-gauge needle is bent approximately 5 mm from the tip so that the terminal segment angles upward 60 degrees and the bevel faces down. The needle is placed on a 3-mL air syringe. Then the needle is introduced bevel down into the base of the keratotomy incision and advanced obliquely 3 to 4 mm from the keratotomy edge in a plane parallel and just anterior to Descemet's membrane. The needle is advanced bevel down to avoid penetrating Descemet's membrane, and obliquely to avoid the thinner central part of the cornea. Approximately 1 mL of air is injected into the posterior stroma to create a plane of tissue separation. If the cannula is accurately placed just above Descemet's membrane, a large bubble will fill the space between the posterior stroma and Descemet's membrane. A successful dissection results in a white, semiopaque disk with a near-circular outline. An unsuccessful attempt yields a fuzzy region of white, opaque cornea. If the first attempt fails, the needle is withdrawn and the procedure may be repeated at another point on the perimeter of the trephine groove. The needle tip should be visible and bevel down at all times to avoid perforation. Because each attempt leaves part of the cornea opaque, only three or four tries are possible. Accurate needle placement is enhanced by using intraoperative ultrasonic pachymetry and a microcalibrated trephine to create an annular keratotomy at the pre-Descemet's level (Hanna or Krumeich trephine).

After creating a large bubble separation of Descemet's membrane from posterior stroma, a paracentesis is made at a site peripheral to the edge of the large air bubble, but no aqueous is drained at this time. A partial-thickness anterior keratectomy is manually performed, leaving a layer of posterior stroma in place anterior to the bubble. Then aqueous is drained through the paracentesis. A sharp-tipped blade held nearly parallel to the corneal surface is used to penetrate the remaining stromal layers near the center of the cornea. The knife should be held in one plane because if it is tilted after entering the bubble, air may escape prematurely. The opening is made large enough to insert a wire spatula (Anwar spatula; Katena Products). The spatula is advanced in the cleavage plane that was created by the air until its tip reaches the trephination groove. The spatula is lifted anteriorly to tent slightly the residual stromal layers. The layers are then dissected by cutting down on the spatula with a supersharp knife. This maneuver is repeated in other directions either at a 180-degree angle or in any other radial direction to enlarge Descemet's membrane exposure. Then the deepest stromal layers are circularly excised with a blunt-tipped microscissors to leave a bare Descemet's membrane recipient bed.

Hydrodissection Technique

After trephination to the appropriate depth, a 30-gauge needle is used to inject balanced salt solution (BSS) into the four quadrants of the partially trephined disk. The disk is converted into a completely opaque and swollen area relative to the area of the recipient cornea outside the area of trephination. Lamellar dissection is then completed in layers and is guided by removal of opacified and swollen stromal fibers. Lamellar dissection is carried to the level of Descemet's membrane with its glistening, clear surface or to the clear deep stromal layers adjacent to it (8).

Hydrodelamination Technique

A partial trephination is followed by an anterior lamellar keratectomy using a Paufique knife. The stroma is lifted and cut in the area of whiteness at the edge of the incision that is the result of air infiltrating between the collagen fibers. Deeper lamellar dissection is then continued with hydrodelamination. The remaining stromal fibers in the host bed are carefully cut across with a supersharp microsurgical blade to create a depression in the stromal bed. BSS is then injected with a blunt 27-gauge needle at the bottom of the depression. The BSS penetrates between the fibers, which whiten and swell. A fine 0.25 spatula is then inserted through a small incision in the hydrodelaminated tissue and the spatula is moved fanlike in different directions to loosen residual stroma, which is then dissected from the host bed until Descemet's membrane is exposed (18).

Viscoelastic Dissection Technique

This technique relies on the precise placement of a 30-gauge needle into the central cornea to a visually controlled depth just above Descemet's membrane (19). Accurate placement of the 30-gauge needle to the pre-Descemet's level requires filling the anterior chamber with air. At the air-to-endothelium interface, a specular light reflex is created by the indentation of the stroma as the needle enters the cornea. The portion of the cornea posterior to the needle is seen as a dark band between the needle tip and the light reflex. The width of this dark band is the distance the needle must travel to reach the endothelium. If the needle is placed just anterior to the air-to-endothelium light reflex, it will be at the pre-Descemet's level. Once this level is reached, viscoelastic material is injected into the cornea to separate Descemet's membrane from the overlying stroma, creating a pseudo-anterior chamber. Once Descemet's membrane has been pushed posteriorly by the viscoelastic, the recipient central stoma is excised by routine trephination, leaving Descemet's membrane as the remaining recipient bed.

Microkeratome Technique

With the evolution of modern refractive surgery, microkeratomes have become reliable instruments for creating very smooth lamellar dissections. Unfortunately, microkeratome lamellar resections cannot be used for disorders with variable corneal thickness or surface irregularities. Microkeratomes are designed to cut a corneal disc with parallel faces. Therefore, if the corneal thickness or surface is not uniform, these irregularities will be transferred to the host bed (20). Use of a microkeratome to prepare a lamellar bed in moderate to advanced keratoconus is contraindicated because the apical thinning in such corneas could result in the perforation of Descemet's membrane and entry into the anterior chamber, with disastrous consequences.

Several refractive microkeratomes are available with 160- to 180-μm heads that can be used to create smooth anterior lamellar keratectomies in corneas with anterior stromal opacities of uniform thickness. Deeper stromal opacities with uniform thickness can be removed with the Moria microkeratome, which has heads that resect up to 425 μm of lamellar tissue. One of the main difficulties encountered when using a microkeratome for lamellar resection is obtaining a consistent diameter of resected tissue. To overcome this problem, Barraquer described a combination technique in which a central microkeratome resection was circumscribed by a larger trephination with a uniform depth. Manual lamellar dissection is then performed from the edge of the microkeratome resection to the edge of the trephination incision. This technique offers the advantage of a smooth central host bed created by a microkeratome and a consistent and controlled bed diameter, which can be matched with donor tissue obtained by applying a similar technique to a donor globe or corneal scleral rim on an artificial chamber (10).

Lamellar Pocket Technique

After trephination, a three-pocket dissection is performed. The first pocket defines the depth of the lamellar keratoplasty and is created by blunt dissection to split and cut the lamellae at the inner edge of the trephine keratotomy. This can be done by using the back (dull) part of a supersharp knife to dissect to the desired depth. Using a Thornton

ring to pressurize the eye, a second pocket is dissected with a Paufique knife. This pocket runs parallel to the posterior lamellae, approximately 2 to 3 mm central to the edge of the keratotomy incision, with a width of approximately 4 mm. The third and last pocket is developed using Troutman corneal splitters. These are large spatulated splitters with a serrated leading edge. With the eye pressurized by the Thornton ring, the corneal splitters are passed through the posterior lamellae in a rocking, fanlike motion, taking care to maintain the dissection in a uniform horizontal plane until the entire area in the trephination has been dissected. Additional undercutting peripheral to the edge of the trephination for 1 to 2 mm in the same lamellar plane creates a pocket to aid in dovetailing the donor graft to the recipient bed. The lamellar bottom is removed with Vannas scissors to expose the recipient bed. Occasionally it is necessary to repeat this process to remove additional abnormal tissue from the recipient bed.

Lamellar Dissection for Tectonic Grafts

Lamellar dissection of abnormal tissue for tectonic purposes often requires a creative approach that is dictated by the extent and the location of the corneal lesion. Usually the size and the shape of the recipient bed is determined only after the abnormal tissue has been completely resected. A convenient approach for lamellar tissue resection is to outline the area to be excised with a diamond knife set to an appropriate depth. To ensure an adequate recipient bed with secure margins, the lamellar resection of abnormal tissue should extend approximately 1 mm into the healthy recipient tissue. Additional undermining of the peripheral margins of the recipient bed aids in securing the donor graft.

Preparation of Donor Material

Because the primary goal of anterior lamellar keratoplasty is to replace deformed or diseased anterior lamellae, the main requirement for donor tissue is a clear and healthy Bowman's layer and stroma. No viable epithelial or endothelial cells or keratocytes are necessary. This allows for a broader selection of donor tissue that would not be used for penetrating keratoplasty. Lamellar donor tissue is screened for potentially transmissible diseases using the same criteria required for penetrating keratoplasty donor tissue.

Preparation of donor material can involve a number of techniques: free hand dissection using a whole globe, manual removal of endothelium and Descemet's membrane from corneal scleral rim, microkeratome preparation using either a whole globe or artificial anterior chamber, or processing tissue on a Barraquer cryolathe. Free-hand dissection using a whole globe is facilitated by increasing the intraocular pressure of the donor globe. This is readily achieved with the injection of air through the optic nerve. A diamond knife preset to obtain the desired thickness of the lamellar tissue is used to cut a 120-degree arc along the limbus of a whole donor globe. Then an anterior lamellar dissector or a cyclodialysis spatula is inserted into the base of the limbal incision and is gently swept back and forth in a horizontal plane to create a lamellar dissection from limbus to limbus at a depth necessary to achieve the desired thickness. A trephination of the appropriate diameter is then performed in an anterior–posterior direction to obtain a donor graft with the desired diameter and thickness. If a horseshoe- or crescent-shaped graft is needed, it is best to remove the entire diameter of donor cornea (12-mm diameter) and then place the donor material over the host recipient bed, and free-hand cut the appropriate shape of donor tissue needed to fit in the recipient bed.

Donor material may also be prepared by manual removal of Descemet's membrane and endothelium from a corneal scleral rim. This technique is facilitated by using the vital dye trypan blue. Manual removal of endothelium cells with a Weck cell sponge is followed by the application of the trypan blue dye, which stains the remaining endothelium cells and Descemet's membrane. Descemet's membrane can then be completely removed with a nontoothed forceps and brisk rubbing with a Weck cell sponge, resulting in a full-thickness stromal lamellar graft. The graft can then be trephined to the desired diameter (21).

Preparation of donor tissue with a microkeratome can be done with any of the currently available microkeratomes for LASIK if a whole globe is available and the manufacturer of the microkeratome makes a head for the microkeratome with a fixed blade gap that will cut the appropriate thickness of donor tissue. The Moria microkeratome is available with a range of microkeratome heads that cut tissue ranging from 100 to 450 μm in thickness. In addition, the Moria microkeratome can also be used with an artificial chamber device so that corneal scleral rims can be used in lieu of whole globes when preparing lamellar tissue (Fig. 62-6). Matching host and recipient tissue diameters can present a problem when using a microkeratome. One solution to this problem has been described by Barraquer (10) and has already been discussed in the section describing the microkeratome technique for preparation of the host bed.

The Barraquer cryolathe can be used to shape parallel-faced, smooth lamellar donor corneal tissue of precise thickness and diameter (22). Use of a corneal press to obtain uniform corneal hydration and thickness before cryolathing enhances the quality and precision of the lathed tissue. The donor tissue can be frozen for long-term storage or placed in tissue culture media if surgery is planned within 1 week. Cryolathed lamellar tissue is available through Cryo-Optics, Inc. (Houston, TX).

Suturing

Several options are available for suturing the lamellar donor tissue into the host bed. Multiple interrupted

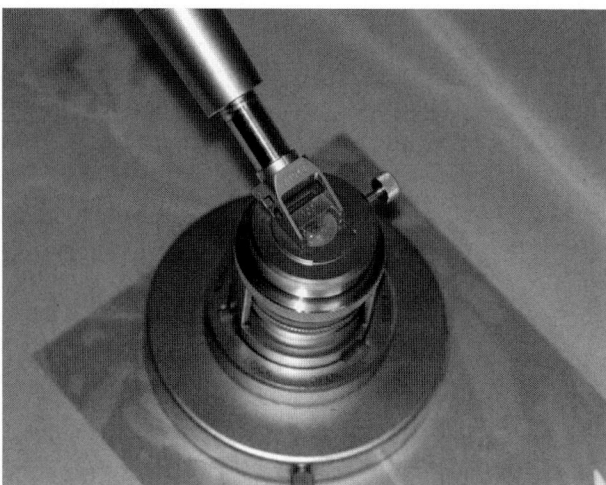

FIGURE 62-6. Artificial anterior chamber. The device shown is a Moria artificial anterior chamber that allows the use of corneal scleral rims to prepare donor tissue to be used in either anterior or posterior lamellar keratoplasty.

sutures or interrupted sutures combined with a running suture is recommended for lamellar keratoplasty to treat keratoconus. These grafts must be placed under a lot of tension to flatten the cone, so interrupted sutures are required. The use of adjustable interrupted sutures allows control of intraoperative astigmatism (23). Single continuous running sutures have been used to control astigmatism after lamellar keratoplasty (24). Using corneal topography, postoperative astigmatism is measured and then the tension of the single continuous running suture is adjusted with a smooth tying forceps to tighten the suture in the flat meridian and loosen it in the steep meridian until a more spherical result is obtained.

Outcomes

Optical Lamellar Keratoplasty

Excellent visual rehabilitation has been reported with the various techniques for optical lamellar keratoplasty. Using Malbran's lamellar keratoplasty technique and cryolathed donor tissue, 91% of 23 eyes with contact lens–intolerant keratoconus obtained 20/30 or better corrected vision (9). No intraoperative complications were encountered, which was consistent Malbran's early experience. Using his "peeling off" technique, 115 keratoconic eyes were treated with no perforations of Descemet's membrane (25). Hydrodissection or fluid-assisted lamellar keratoplasty was reported to achieve a corrected vision of 20/30 or better in 96% of 26 eyes with moderate to advanced keratoconus. Unfortunately, two eyes in this study required conversion to penetrating keratoplasty because of perforation of Descemet's membrane (8). When the hydrodelamination technique was used to treat 120 eyes with various anterior corneal lesions, an average postoperative acuity of

20/30 was obtained (18). However 39.2% of the eyes in this study had a perforation of Descemet's membrane. All the perforated eyes were successfully treated with lamellar keratoplasty, and after 1 year no differences in visual acuity or endothelial cell counts were noted in the punctured versus nonpunctured group. Mixed results have been reported for the air dissection technique, which is complicated by incomplete dissection involving the area of most stromal scarring (26). When Price evaluated this technique, 3 of 10 patients experienced a perforation of Descemet's membrane requiring conversion to penetrating keratoplasty (27). Refinements of the air dissection technique by Anwar and Teichmann may enhance its usefulness (17). Reports on viscodissection have been limited. Manche et al. reported excellent vision (20/25 and 20/30) in two patients using sodium hyaluronate–assisted lamellar keratoplasty (28). Melles and colleagues used hydroxypropylmethylcellulose for viscodissection and reported rupture of Descemet's membrane in 5 of 25 eye bank eyes, and 1 of 3 patients undergoing his technique required conversion to penetrating keratoplasty because of a Descemet's tear (21).

Panda and Singh reported a comparison of various agents used to facilitate intralamellar dissection (29). Four groups of 10 eyes underwent lamellar keratoplasty, with group 1 receiving air dissection, group 2 receiving hydrodissection, group 3 viscodissection, and group 4 standard lamellar dissection with no agent. The visual outcomes were similar in all four groups, but fluid-assisted lamellar keratoplasty resulted in less operating time because of more efficient preparation of the host bed. Incomplete lamellar dissection was encountered with the air and viscodissection techniques. The study concluded that each surgeon should adopt the surgical technique with which he or she is most comfortable.

Based on the outcomes reported in the literature, each of the various techniques for performing lamellar keratoplasty has its merits, but a risk–benefit analysis would favor Malbran's technique as the safest procedure with the easiest learning curve. Proper application of Malbran's technique almost completely eliminates the risk of perforating Descemet's membrane, which can be as high as 8% to 39% with other techniques. Using Malbran's technique for keratoconus, the shiny, glasslike appearance of Descemet's membrane at the apex of the cone is frequently observed during lamellar dissection. Because the posterior lamellae are peeled and not cut away from Descemet's membrane, perforation at this stage in the procedure does not occur. Baring of Descemet's membrane is never intentional with Malbran's technique, but occurs when the posterior lamellar dissection plane naturally follows a level at or above Descemet's membrane as the keratectomy specimen is peeled off the recipient bed. The main focus of the lamellar keratectomy should be to obtain a smooth host bed and not complete removal of posterior lamellae to the level of Descemet's membrane. Deep lamellar dissection to the level of Descemet's membrane may sometimes be necessary to remove all diseased cornea, but this need not be the goal in every lamellar keratoplasty. Final visual results with deep lamellar keratoplasty compared with the results obtained with Malbran's technique do not justify the risk of perforation. In the case of keratoconus treated with lamellar keratoplasty, inferior visual results are usually attributed to fixed folds in Descemet's membrane and not to interface haze. These folds occur regardless of the depth of the lamellar dissection and are due to the loss of elasticity in Descemet's membrane in advanced or mature keratoconus rather than to surgical technique.

Tectonic Lamellar Keratoplasty

A successful outcome with tectonic lamellar keratoplasty begins with restoration of the cornea's structural integrity. The continual success of these grafts often requires identification and treatment of the inflammatory or autoimmune disorder that led to the loss of corneal structure or a corneal melt. Systemic immunosuppressive therapy may be necessary to preserve the cornea in the case of Mooren's ulcer and the systemic disorders associated with peripheral ulcerative keratitis (7,30).

Restoration of tectonic strength in cases of Terrien's marginal degeneration is often accompanied by a reduction in preoperative astigmatism. This is also observed with the crescent-shaped lamellar graft or resection used to treat pellucid marginal degeneration (31,32).

Complications

The most serious intraoperative complication with lamellar keratoplasty is perforation of Descemet's membrane or entry into the anterior chamber. This may occur during trephination, but usually occurs during deep lamellar dissection. If the perforation site is small, the procedure is continued by reforming the anterior chamber with air. Sometimes suturing the perforation site is needed to maintain the anterior chamber. If air is left in the anterior chamber at the conclusion of the procedure, the pupil should be pharmacologically dilated or constricted. Air can enter the posterior chamber, and when the pupil is mid-dilated, pupillary block results in high intraocular pressure. When perforation of Descemet's membrane occurs, the lamellar procedure can usually be completed with minimal difficulty. In such cases, aqueous fluid sometimes enters the space between the lamellar graft and the host recipient bed, creating a pseudo-anterior chamber. Management of this complication requires filling the anterior chamber with air and draining the aqueous fluid between the donor graft and recipient bed by gently opening the anterior wound with a 30-gauge cannula. This technique can be performed with the patient sitting at the slit lamp.

The most commonly observed early postoperative complication is failure of the graft to epithelialize. This is usually due to a preexisting ocular surface disorder. Aggressive treatment of the lid margins with lid scrubs and oral tetracycline may be needed. If lagophthalmos is present, it needs to be treated by taping the lids shut or with a lateral tarsorrhaphy. The use of preservative-free artificial tears is helpful. The use of topical steroids should be avoided until the graft has completely epithelialized. Reepithelialization of the graft is an important goal in the postoperative course. Failure to reepithelialize can result in a corneal melt. If a graft has not reepithelialized within 2 to 3 weeks, a temporary tarsorrhaphy to control this complication should be considered.

Other complications are seen when sutures are not removed at the appropriate time and include suture abscesses and vascularization of the bed. This is managed by suture removal and topical antibiotic or steroid treatment. Graft reaction rarely or never occurs. If a stromal reaction occurs, it presents as subepithelial opacities similar to the subepithelial infiltrates that occur with an adenovirus infection, but without any history of conjunctivitis. Stromal graft reactions are not sight-threatening and are managed by topical steroids.

POSTERIOR LAMELLAR KERATOPLASTY

Posterior lamellar keratoplasty involves the transplantation of diseased or damaged endothelial cells by placement of a posterior lamellar graft that contains healthy endothelial cells (Fig. 62-7). There are two novel approaches to posterior lamellar surgery (2). One approach involves a using microkeratome to create a deep lamellar flap. The flap is retracted and the posterior stroma, Descemet's membrane, and endothelium are trephined, removed, and replaced with a posterior lamellar graft containing healthy endothelium. The flap is then sutured back into position. In the other technique, a limbal incision is made and a deep lamellar pocket is created. The posterior stroma with attached diseased endothelium is then removed through the limbal incision and replaced with a donor posterior lamellar graft that has healthy endothelial cells. The limbal incision is then closed with sutures.

Indications

Posterior lamellar keratoplasty is indicated for the treatment of corneal disease arising from unhealthy or poorly functioning endothelium. Such conditions include Fuchs' endothelial corneal dystrophy and aphakic or pseudophakic bullous keratopathy.

Surgical Procedure

Microkeratome-Assisted Technique

This technique has been referred to as *endothelial lamellar keratoplasty* by Jones and Culbertson (33), *endokeratoplasty* by Busin et al. (34), and *microkeratome-assisted posterior keratoplasty* by Azar et al. (35). The procedure involves the use of a microkeratome to create a 160-μm thick, 9.5-mm

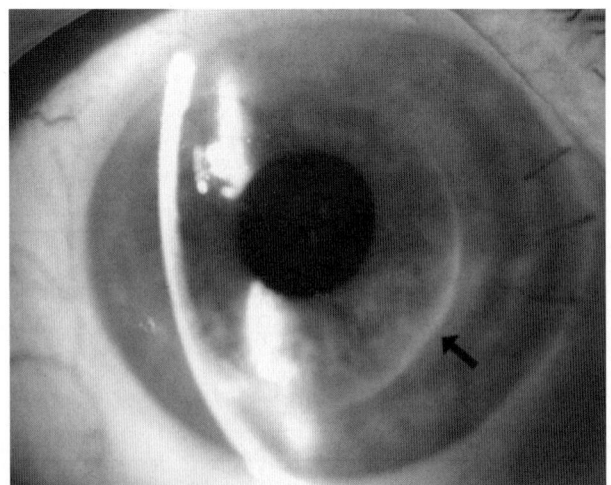
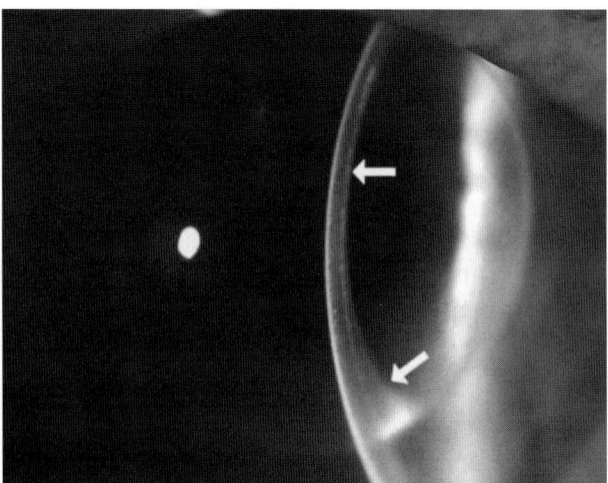

FIGURE 62-7. Posterior lamellar keratoplasty for the treatment of pseudophakic bullous keratopathy. **A:** Posterior lamellar graft created using the limbal pocket approach, 1 month after surgery. Note the three limbal sutures used to close the temporal limbal incision. The central cornea is clear and has a healthy epithelial surface. The inferior cornea remains edematous but is clearing with time. The *arrow* denotes white donor tissue from an inadvertent eccentric donor trephination. **B:** Slit-lamp view showing normal-thickness cornea centrally with negligible interface haze (*top arrow*). *Bottom arrow* shows residual corneal edema in the area of the donor that was eccentrically trephined.

diameter hinged flap. The flap is retracted and a 6.5-mm diameter trephine is used to make a penetrating keratotomy through the remaining layers of the posterior cornea. The donor tissue is prepared using an artificial anterior chamber; this involves resecting a 160-μm cap with a microkeratome and trephining a 7-mm posterior lamellar disk with healthy endothelium. The 7-mm donor button is sutured into the recipient bed with a running suture. Then the flap is repositioned and sutured into place. Recent modifications of this technique omit suturing of the donor tissue and secure it into position by placing air into the anterior chamber (34).

Limbal Pocket Technique

This technique has been called *posterior lamellar keratoplasty* (4,36) or *deep lamellar endothelial keratoplasty* (5). The surgical procedure begins with a 9-mm, one-half–depth limbal incision. Air is then placed in the anterior chamber and used to determine the depth of the posterior lamellar pocket by observing the specular reflex created by the air-to-endothelial interface (19). A total posterior lamellar pocket is created by blunt dissection. Then an intralamellar trephine is placed in the intralamellar pocket and a 7.5-mm trephination of the posterior cornea is performed. The recipient disk is excised with microscissors and removed through the limbal incision. A same-diameter donor disk with healthy endothelium and stroma is then prepared from a donor corneal scleral rim placed on an artificial anterior chamber. The donor disk is inserted through the limbal incision and positioned against the posterior recipient bed by placing air in the anterior chamber. The donor tissue adheres without sutures. Finally, the limbal incision is closed with sutures. Recent modifications of this procedure include using microscissors to resect the recipient tissue instead of a trephine and folding the donor tissue so it can be inserted through a 5-mm limbal incision.

Outcomes

Terry and Ousley reported on results of eight eyes undergoing posterior lamellar keratoplasty with the limbal pocket approach (5). They referred to the procedure as deep lamellar endothelial keratoplasty. All eight patients had corneal edema from Fuchs' dystrophy and were pseudophakic. Corrected visual acuity at 6 months ranged from 20/30 to 20/70 for the eight eyes. The average change in astigmatism from before surgery was only +1.13 ± 1.5 diopters. The average change in corneal power from before surgery was only −4 ± 1.7 diopters, and the quality and the smoothness of the corneal topography was excellent. The endothelial cell density averaged 2290 ± 372 cell/mm² and represented a 21% average endothelial cell loss from preoperative eye bank measurements of the donor tissue. One patient originally entered in the study

had a microperforation during the initial recipient lamellar pocket dissection, and the operation was converted to penetrating keratoplasty.

Melles and colleagues reported on seven eyes that underwent posterior lamellar keratoplasty through a limbal pocket incision (36). Best corrected spectacle visual acuity was limited by maculopathy in two eyes and ranged from 20/80 to 20/20. Postoperative astigmatism average 1.54 ± 0.81 diopters. Postoperative endothelial cell density averaged 2520 ± 340 cells/mm². A microperforation during stromal pocket dissection in one patient required conversion to penetrating keratoplasty.

The results of microkeratome-assisted posterior lamellar keratoplasty were reported on seven patients with corneal edema from Fuchs' dystrophy or pseudophakic bullous keratopathy. Corrected visual acuity ranged from 20/40 to 20/200 after 1-month follow-up and remained stable at the 4-month visit. One patient required flap removal because of epithelial ingrowth. The authors believe that this technique provides more rapid visual rehabilitation than conventional penetrating keratoplasty (34).

Complications

Intraoperative complications with the limbal pocket technique include perforation of Descemet's membrane during posterior lamellar dissection, which may require conversion to penetrating keratoplasty. Additional problems may arise if the donor tissue is not properly centered in the area of the recipient bed created by the trephination of the posterior recipient cornea. If the donor tissue is not centered in this posterior recipient bed, it may dislodge into the anterior chamber and require repositioning.

Early postoperative complications include a pseudo-anterior chamber created by the presence of aqueous humor between the donor button and the recipient posterior stroma. This may result from failure properly to position the donor tissue in the recipient bed and is remedied by repositioning the donor graft so that is does not overlap with recipient tissue outside the perimeter of the recipient bed. Pseudo-anterior chambers can readily be corrected by filling the anterior chamber with air if the donor tissue is properly centered.

Because of the lack of corneal sutures, few surface problems are observed with the limbal pocket approach. Delayed visual recovery with interface haze sometimes occurs. This is probably the result of irregular posterior astigmatism resulting from an irregular posterior lamellar dissection.

The microkeratome-assisted posterior lamellar keratoplasty procedure suffers from many of the problems seen with conventional penetrating keratoplasty. The suturing of the donor tissue into the deep lamellar bed as well as flap suturing cause irregular astigmatism (37). Central corneal power surprises can occur after microkeratome-assisted posterior lamellar keratoplasty. Azar et al. reported 16 diopters of induced hyperopia in one case (35). This resulted from excessive flattening of the flap when it was sutured onto the posterior donor tissue. Epithelial ingrowth under the flap can lead to flap melting if not detected early and treated by lifting the flap and debriding (34).

LAMELLAR KERATOPLASTY VERSUS PENETRATING KERATOPLASTY

In spite of many advances with lamellar surgery, the visual results after penetrating keratoplasty are usually better than those after lamellar keratoplasty. Visual results after lamellar keratoplasty for the treatment of stromal scars in children often equal those after penetrating keratoplasty. In addition, the visual results of lamellar keratoplasty for the treatment of keratoconus patients between the ages of 20 and 30 years approach those found with penetrating keratoplasty (9). When one considers the documented progressive endothelial cell loss over time after penetrating keratoplasty (38) and the negligible endothelial cell loss over time after lamellar keratoplasty (39), a reasonable argument can be made for favoring lamellar keratoplasty over penetrating keratoplasty in these younger individuals. Conversely, the relatively high risk for development of fixed Descemet's membrane folds in patients with keratoconus undergoing lamellar keratoplasty argues in favor of the initial treatment of these patients with penetrating keratoplasty because these folds can limit the visual outcome.

The use of posterior lamellar keratoplasty for the management of endothelial cell decompensation offers many theoretical advantages over penetrating keratoplasty. The potential for rapid rehabilitation and more predictable postoperative corneal curvatures compared with standard penetrating keratoplasty has created much excitement regarding this procedure. However, some patients experience a slow visual recovery similar to that with penetrating keratoplasty. This is thought to be due to the current methods used to perform the lamellar dissections. Technique refinements such as the use of the femtosecond laser for creating lamellar dissections may help to realize these theoretical advantages (40).

REFERENCES

1. von Hippel A. Eine neue Methode der Hornhaut Transplantation (German). *Graefes Arch Ophtalmol* 1888;34:108–130.
2. Terry MA. The evolution of lamellar grafting techniques over twenty-five years. *Cornea* 2000;19:611–616.
3. Ko W, Freuh B, Shield C, et al. Experimental posterior lamellar transplantation of the rabbit cornea. *Invest Ophthalmol Vis Sci* 1993;34:1102.
4. Melles G, Eggink F, Lander F, et al. A surgical technique for posterior lamellar keratoplasty. *Cornea* 1998;17:618–626.
5. Terry MA, Ousley PJ. Replacing the endothelium without corneal surface incisions or sutures: the first United States clinical series using deep lamellar endothelium keratoplasty procedure. *Ophthalmology* 2003;110:755–764.
6. Olsen RJ, Kaufman HE. Recurrence of Reis-Bückler's corneal dystrophy in a graft. *Am J Ophthalmol* 1978;85:349.
7. McDonnell P. Recurrence of Mooren's ulcer after lamellar keratoplasty. *Cornea* 1989;8:191–194.
8. Amayen AF, Anwar M. Fluid lamellar keratoplasty in keratoconus. *Ophthalmology* 2000;107:76–79.
9. Benson W, Goosey C, Prager T, et al. Visual improvement as a function of time after lamellar keratoplasty for keratoconus. *Am J Ophthalmol* 1993;116:207–211.
10. Maurice DM. The cornea and sclera. In: Davson H, ed. *The eye*, vol 16: *Vegetative physiology and biochemistry*. Orlando, FL: Academic Press, 1984:1–158.
11. Komai Y, Ushiki T. The three-dimensional organization of collagen fibers in the human cornea and sclera. *Invest Ophthalmol Vis Sci* 1991;32:2244–2258.
12. Polack FM. Morphology of the cornea: I. Study with silver stains. *Am J Ophthalmol* 1961;51:179.
13. Smolek MK, McCarey BE. Interlamellar adhesive strength in human eye bank corneas. *Invest Ophthalmol Vis Sci* 1990;31:1087–1095.
14. Polack FM. Lamellar keratoplasty: Malbran's "peeling off" technique. *Arch Ophthalmol* 1971;86:293–295.
15. Malbran E, Stephani C. Lamellar keratoplasty in corneal ectasias. *Ophthalmologica* 1972;164:50–58.
16. Archila E. Deep lamellar keratoplasty dissection of host tissue with intrastromal air injection. *Cornea* 1985;3:217–218.
17. Anwar M, Teichmann KD. Big-bubble technique to bare Descemet's membrane in anterior lamellar keratoplasty. *J Cataract Refract Surg* 2002;28:398–403.
18. Suguita J, Kondo M, Monden Y, et al. Deep lamellar keratoplasty with complete removal of pathological stroma for vision improvement. *Br J Ophthalmol* 1997;81:184–188.
19. Melles G, Rietveld F, Remeijer L, et al. A technique to visualize corneal incision and lamellar dissection depth during surgery. *Cornea* 1999;18:80–86.
20. Barraquer J. Lamellar keratoplasty (special techniques). *Ann Ophthalmol* 1972;4:437–469.
21. Melles G, Remeijer L, Geerards A. A quick surgical technique for deep, anterior lamellar keratoplasty using visco-dissection. *Cornea* 2000;19:427.
22. Barraquer J. Basis of refractive keratoplasty. *Arch Soc Am Ophthalmol Optom* 1967;6:21–68.
23. Benson W, Goosey J. Lamellar keratoplasty. In: Krachmer J, Mannis M, Holland E, eds. *Cornea: surgery of the cornea and conjunctiva*. St. Louis: Mosby-Year Book, 1997:1833–1842.
24. Tsubota K, Kaido M, Monden Y, et al. A new surgical technique for deep lamellar keratoplasty with single running suture adjustment. *Am J Ophthalmol* 1998;126:1–8.
25. Malbran E, Stephani C. Lamellar keratoplasty in corneal ectasias. *Ophthalmologica* 1972;164:59–70.
26. Chau G, Dilly S, Sheard C, et al. Deep lamellar keratoplasty with complete removal of pathological stroma for vision improvement. *Br J Ophthalmol* 1997;81:184–188.
27. Price F. Air lamellar keratoplasty. *Refract Corneal Surg* 1989;5:240–243.
28. Manche EE, Holland GN, Maloney RK. Deep lamellar keratoplasty using viscoelastic dissection. *Arch Ophthalmol* 1999;117:1561–1565.
29. Panda A, Singh R. Intralamellar dissection techniques in lamellar keratoplasty. *Cornea* 1999;117:1561–1565.
30. Foster CS. Systemic immunosuppressive therapy for progressive bilateral Mooren's ulcer. *Ophthalmology* 1985;92:1436.

31. Schanzlin DJ, Sarno EM, Robin JB. Crescentic lamellar keratoplasty for pellucid marginal degeneration. *Am J Ophthalmol* 1983;96:253.

32. Cameron J. Results of lamellar crescentic resection for pellucid marginal corneal degeneration. *Am J Ophthalmol* 1992;113:296–302.

33. Jones DT, Culbertson WW. Endothelial lamellar keratoplasty (ELK). ARVO Abstracts. *Invest Ophthalmol Vis Sci* 1998;39 [4 Suppl]:S76(abstr).

34. Busin M, Arffa RC, Sebastian A. Endokeratoplasty as an alternative to penetrating keratoplasty for the surgical treatment of diseased endothelium: initial results. *Ophthalmology* 2000;107: 2077–2082.

35. Azar DT, Jain S, Sambursky, et al. Micro-keratome assisted posterior keratoplasty. *J Cataract Refract Surg* 2001;27:353–356.

36. Melles GRJ, Lander F, van Dooren BTH, et al. Preliminary clinical results of posterior lamellar keratoplasty through a sclerocorneal pocket incision. *Ophthalmology* 2000;107:1850–1856.

37. Ehlers N, Ehlers H, Hjortdal, et al. Grafting of the posterior cornea: description of a new technique with 12-month clinical results. *Acta Ophthalmol Scand* 2000;78:543–546.

38. Bourne WM. Cellular changes in transplanted human corneas. *Cornea* 2001;20:560–569.

39. Morris E, Kirwon J, Sujatha S, et al. Corneal endothelial specular microscopy following deep lamellar keratoplasty with lyophilized tissue. *Eye* 1998;12:612–622.

40. Sletten KR, Yen KG, Sayegh S, et al. An in vivo model of femtosecond, laser intrastromal refractive surgery. *Ophthalmic Surg Lasers* 1999;30:742.

POSTERIOR LAMELLAR ENDOTHELIAL KERATOPLASTY

NICOLETTA FYNN-THOMPSON AND DIMITRI T. AZAR

Posterior lamellar endothelial keratoplasty refers to the removal of the diseased posterior corneal layers and their replacement by partial-thickness donor tissue. A clear advantage of this form of lamellar keratoplasty over penetrating keratoplasty is that it replaces only the diseased portion of the cornea, leaving the uninvolved anatomic layers of the recipient cornea intact.

Anterior lamellar keratoplasty is discussed in another chapter. It is used for tectonic support of the globe in patients with corneal thinning disorders (such as peripheral ulcerative keratitis, Mooren's ulceration, and Terrien's marginal degeneration) and for replacement of anterior stromal tissue, caused by such conditions as keratoconus, corneal stromal dystrophies, and stromal scarring after resolved corneal ulcers. The recipient's Descemet's membrane and endothelium are in retained anterior lamellar keratoplasty (1).

Posterior lamellar keratoplasty is performed when the corneal endothelium is not functioning properly, such as in cases of Fuchs' endothelial dystrophy and aphakic and pseudophakic bullous keratopathy. Theoretically, lamellar keratoplasty reduces the amount of corneal resection and provides greater visual benefit.

Compared with full-thickness penetrating keratoplasty, there are several theoretical advantages to performing posterior lamellar keratoplasty. These include lower risk of intraoperative complications and astigmatism, faster visual recovery, less frequent follow-up visits for suture adjustment, elimination of suture-induced corneal neovascularization, less risk of wound dehiscence, and fewer side effects of topical steroid therapy. In addition, donor tissue may be used more efficiently, for example by using the remaining tissue for the management of complicated photorefractive keratectomy (2).

There are drawbacks to posterior lamellar keratoplasty. The surgical techniques may be more demanding than penetrating keratoplasty. Meticulous dissection of the corneal lamellae is required. Also, perforation may occur. In this situation, the procedure may have to be converted to penetrating keratoplasty. In addition, patients with postoperative astigmatism cannot benefit from suture adjustment, as used in penetrating keratoplasty. There is also a risk of interface haze, which occurs in varying degrees (3).

SURGICAL TECHNIQUES

Posterior lamellar endothelial keratoplasty is used for corneal decompensation secondary to endothelial dysfunction. There are currently two surgical approaches: the scleral incision approach and the microkeratome flap approach. The first involves posterior corneal disk transplantation by scleral incision and trephination using an intrastromal trephine. The second approach uses an automated microkeratome to create a hinged anterior stromal flap and trephination of the diseased posterior stroma using a standard trephine (4).

Scleral Incision Approach

Early reports and the surgical technique for this approach for posterior lamellar keratoplasty were described in patients with Fuchs' dystrophy or deep stromal opacities (5,6). This surgical technique was slightly altered by Melles et al. (7) for transplantation of posterior corneal tissue through a scleral incision and deep stromal pocket. It was initially performed on cadaveric human eyes and *in vivo* animal models. Melles and colleagues used same-size recipient cornea and donor disk in a sutureless technique. Postoperative examination revealed well-positioned posterior implants, and complete apposition of host and donor stromal edges in the cadaveric specimens. They later reported treating a total of eight patients with sighted eyes suffering from Fuchs' endothelial dystrophy or bullous keratopathy (pseudophakic or aphakic) (8,9). Terry et al. introduced the Melles technique to the United States and described the results in the first two

U.S. patients who had endothelial dysfunction from Fuchs' endothelial dystrophy (10).

Melles' Original Surgical Technique

The donor eye is mounted on an eye holder (8). Through a paracentesis site, the anterior chamber is completely filled with air. A 4-mm peripheral corneal incision is made. A stromal pocket is dissected with a custom-made spatula blade (D.O.R.C. International, Zuidland, the Netherlands) across the cornea at 60% stromal depth using the air-to-endothelial interface as a guide for dissection depth (11). In the mirror effect, the air bubble in the anterior chamber acts as a convex mirror, such that a blade held at the anterior corneal surface is reflected at the posterior corneal surface (Fig. 63-1). The indentation effect describes the specular light reflex created near the tip of the blade by the indentation of the tissue. The amount of nonincised tissue between the light reflex and blade is seen as a dark band (Fig. 63-2). The folding effect describes the increased number in small folds that develop in the posterior corneal tissue as the blade approaches the posterior surface (Fig. 63-3). Once the stromal pocket is dissected, a plastic strip is inserted into the

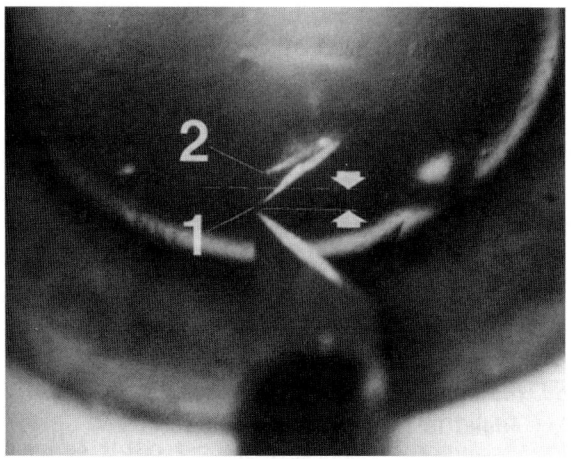

FIGURE 63-1. Mirror effect. In an eye that has the anterior chamber completely filled with air, two mirror images of the blade are visible, one a reflection from the anterior corneal surface [1] and one from the posterior surface [2]. The *dotted line* indicates the approximate location of the plane of reflection (i.e., the posterior surface). Thus, the estimated corneal thickness (*arrows*) is half the distance between the blade tip and its reflection from the posterior corneal surface [2]. (From Melles GRJ, Rietveld FJR, Beekhuis WH, et al. A technique to visualize corneal incision and lamellar dissection depth during surgery. *Cornea* 1999;18:80-86.)

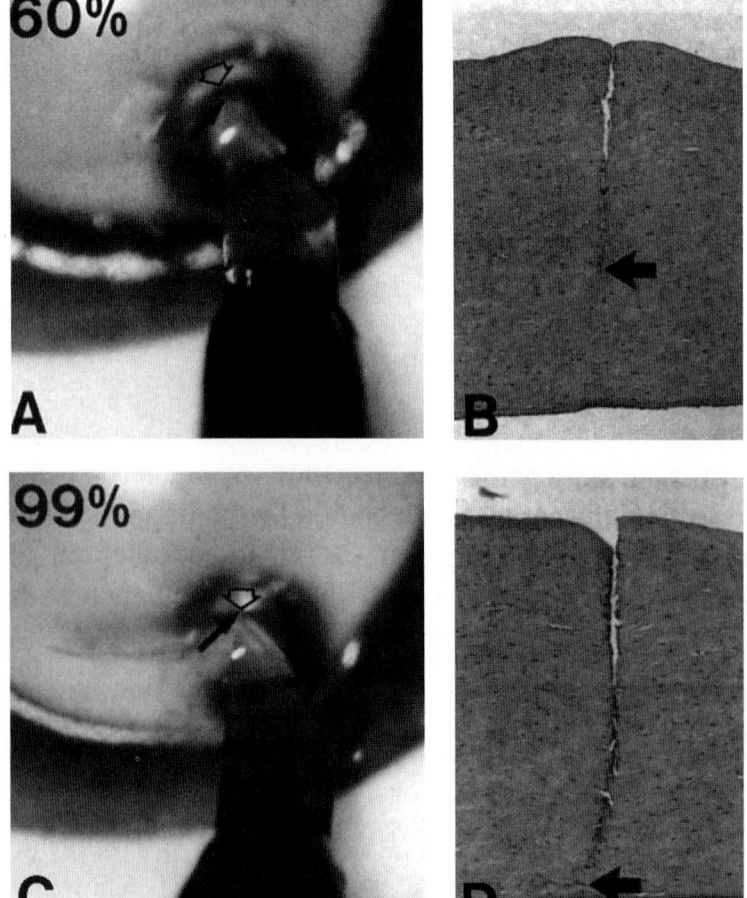

FIGURE 63-2. Indentation effect. Clinical and light-microscopic pictures of incisions made at intended corneal depths of 60% **(A, B)** and 99% **(C, D)**. A dark band is visible between the blade tip (*arrow*) and the semicircular light reflex at the air-to-endothelium interface (*open arrow*). Note how the amount of nonincised tissue underneath the blade tip in **A** and **C** compares with the incision depth in **B** and **D**. Thus, the achieved incision depth (*thick arrow*) can be estimated by the thickness of the dark band adjacent to the blade tip. (From Melles GRJ, Rietveld FJR, Beekhuis WH, et al. A technique to visualize corneal incision and lamellar dissection depth during surgery. *Cornea* 1999;18:80-86.)

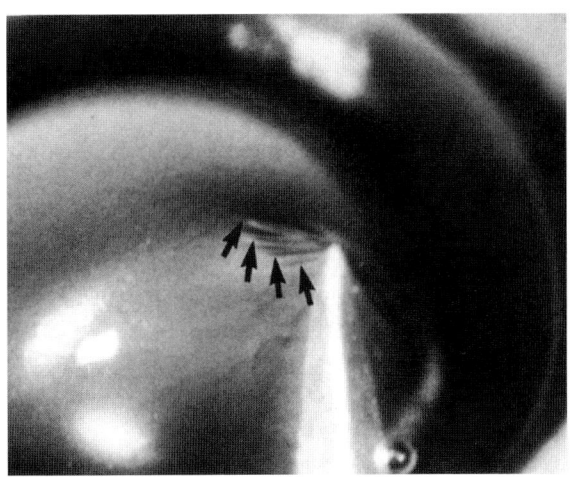

FIGURE 63-3. Folding effect. Small folds (*arrows*) in the posterior corneal tissue are visible adjacent to the tip of a dissection blade that approaches the posterior corneal surface. (From Melles GRJ, Rietveld FJR, Beekhuis WH, et al. A technique to visualize corneal incision and lamellar dissection depth during surgery. *Cornea* 1999;18:80-86.)

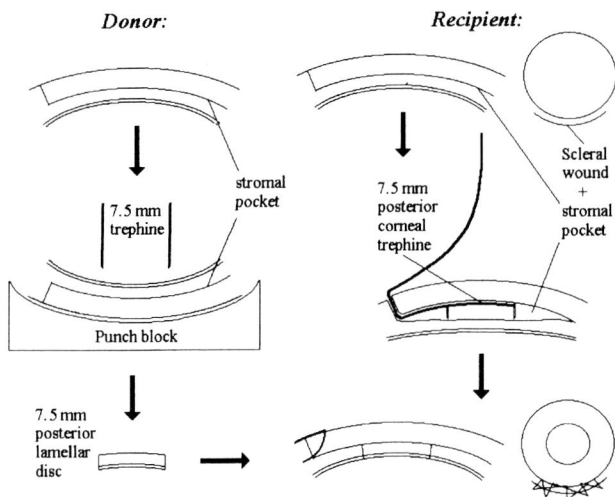

FIGURE 63-4. Diagrammatic representation of the posterior lamellar keratoplasty procedure. After dissection of a stromal pocket through a scleral incision, a posterior lamellar disk is trephinated from the donor cornea. In the recipient cornea, a stromal pocket is made and a flat trephine is inserted in it to excise a posterior disk. The donor disk is implanted into the recipient opening, and the scleral wound is sutured. (From Melles GRJ, Lander F, van Dooren BTH, et al. Preliminary clinical results of posterior lamellar keratoplasty through a sclerocorneal pocket incision. *Ophthalmology* 2000;107:1850-1856.)

pocket and the corneoscleral rim is excised and mounted endothelial side up on a punch block (Medical Workshop, De Meern, the Netherlands). A full-thickness corneal button is excised with a 7- to 7.5-mm punch trephine (Ophtec, Groningen, the Netherlands). The donor button is placed endothelial side down onto a custom-made spoon-shaped glide (D.O.R.C. International). It is covered with viscoelastic substance [hydroxypropylmethylcellulose (Ocucoat); Storz, Clearwater, FL]. The anterior lamella and plastic glide are then removed (Fig. 63-4).

The recipient eye's anterior chamber is completely filled with air through a paracentesis site. A 9-mm partial-thickness scleral incision is made after the superior conjunctiva is opened. A stromal pocket is dissected across the cornea at 80% depth with a dissection spatula, using the air-to-endothelium interface (11). A custom-made 7- to 7.5-mm diameter flat trephine (D.O.R.C. International) is inserted into the stromal pocket and the posterior lamellar disk is excised. Remaining attachments of the corneal tissue may be removed with custom-made microscissors (D.O.R.C. International; Fig. 63-5). The spoon-shaped glide containing the "same-size" donor posterior disk is introduced into the recipient stromal pocket and positioned into the recipient's posterior opening. The scleral incision is closed with 10-0 monofilament nylon sutures (Alcon, Gorinchem, the Netherlands; Fig. 63-5).

Deep Lamellar Endothelial Keratoplasty

Terry et al. (12) described his technique of deep lamellar endothelial keratoplasty for the treatment of endothelial dysfunction. This procedure is based on the original technique of Melles et al. Refinements on this technique continue to

evolve including the small incision approach and the use of the femtosecond laser. Hence we describe the standard technique of DLEK (12). A 9-mm limbal-scleral incision is made by a trifaceted guarded diamond knife 1 mm posterior to the superior limbus. The knife is set at a depth of 350 μm. An angled crescent tunnel blade (Wilson Ophthalmics, Mustang, OK) is used to make the deep lamellar dissection from the incision into clear cornea, approximately 3 mm centrally. A special semisharp dissector spatula (Bausch and Lomb, St. Louis, MO) extends the lamellar pocket over the entire cornea (Fig. 63-6). A paracentesis is made at the 2 o'clock position with a supersharp blade (Katena, Denville, NJ) at the limbus, and air is injected in the anterior chamber with a 30-gauge cannula. The air bubble is maintained at all times. A low-profile intralamellar trephine (Terry Trephine; Bausch and Lomb) with a cutting diameter of 7 mm, along with an external knurled circular handle, is used to trephinate the posterior lamellar recipient tissue (Fig. 63-7). When the anterior chamber is entered, air escapes into the deep lamellar plane. The remaining stromal fibers are cut with intralamellar corneal scissors and the stromal disk is grasped with angled Kelman forceps (Storz, St. Louis, MO) and removed. The anterior chamber depth is maintained with repeated injections of air.

The donor corneoscleral cap is placed onto a modified artificial anterior chamber device (Ophthalmic Specialties, San Gabriel, CA) with sodium hyaluronate (Healon; Pharmacia and Upjohn, Kalamazoo, MI) placed on the endothelial surface. The artificial anterior chamber is maintained with

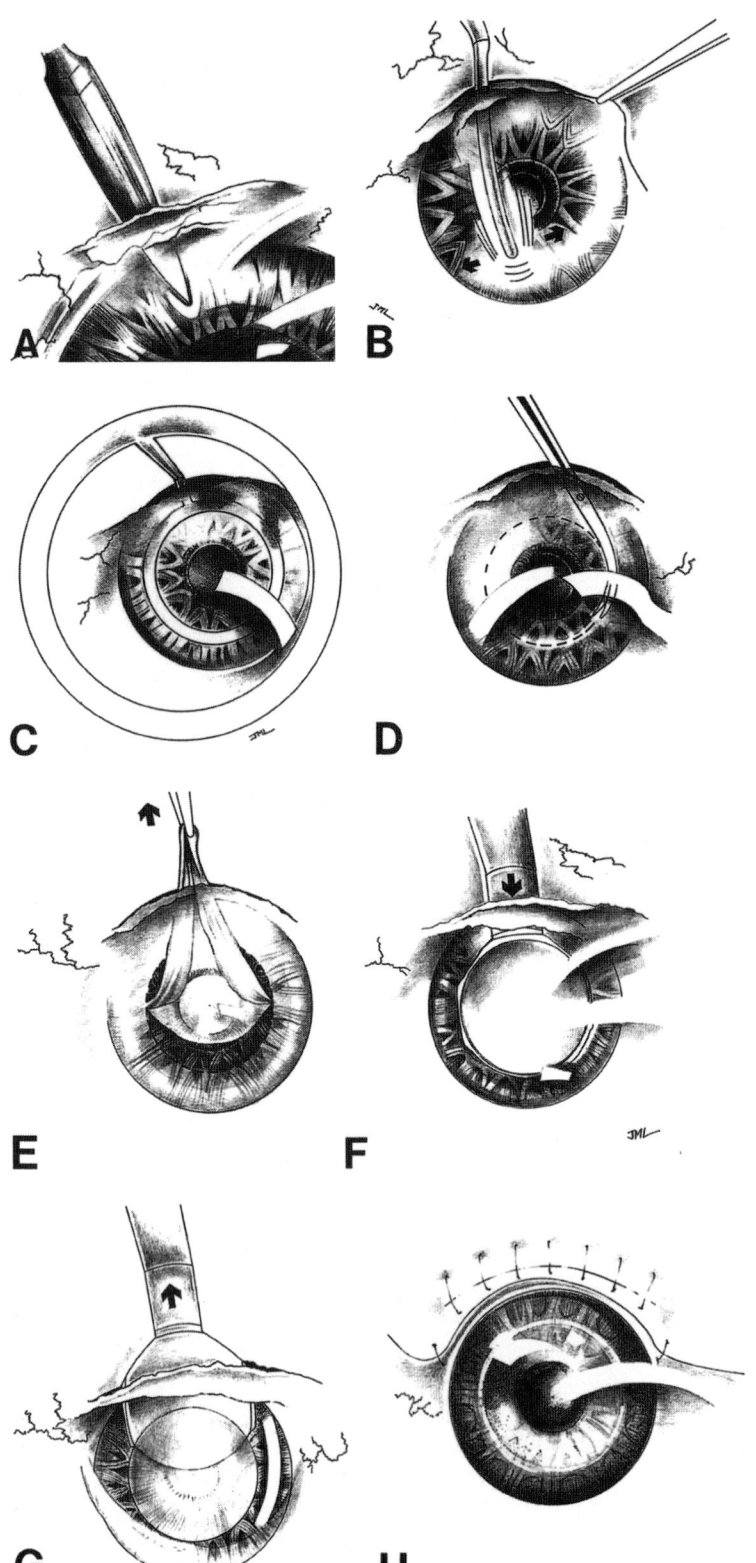

FIGURE 63-5. Preliminary clinical results of posterior lamellar keratopathy through a sclerocorneal pocket incision. **A:** Using the optical effects of the air bubble in the anterior chamber, the dissection is started at approximately 80% corneal depth. **B:** The dissection is then extended across the cornea. **C:** A posterior corneal trephine is inserted into the pocket to excise a posterior lamellar disk. **D:** Remaining stromal attachments are cut with microscissors. **E:** The posterior disk is removed from the recipient cornea. **F:** On a glide, the donor posterior disk is inserted into the stromal pocket. **G:** The spoon is then withdrawn after positioning of the donor tissue. **H:** The scleral incision is sutured, and the anterior chamber is filled with air to push the donor posterior disk against the anterior recipient cornea. (From Melles GRJ, Lander F, van Dooren BTH, et al. Preliminary clinical results of posterior lamellar keratoplasty through a sclerocorneal pocket incision. *Ophthalmology* 2000;107: 1850-1856.)

Healon and Optisol-GS solution. The tissue is secured and intraocular pressure raised to greater than 30 mm Hg. The deep lamellar pocket plane is created in a fashion similar to that in the recipient's cornea. The donor corneoscle-ral cap is removed from the artificial anterior chamber and placed on a Brightbill Teflon block (Storz) with the epithelial side down. A 7- to 8-mm disposable trephine (Katena) is used to cut a central donor disk. Fine forceps

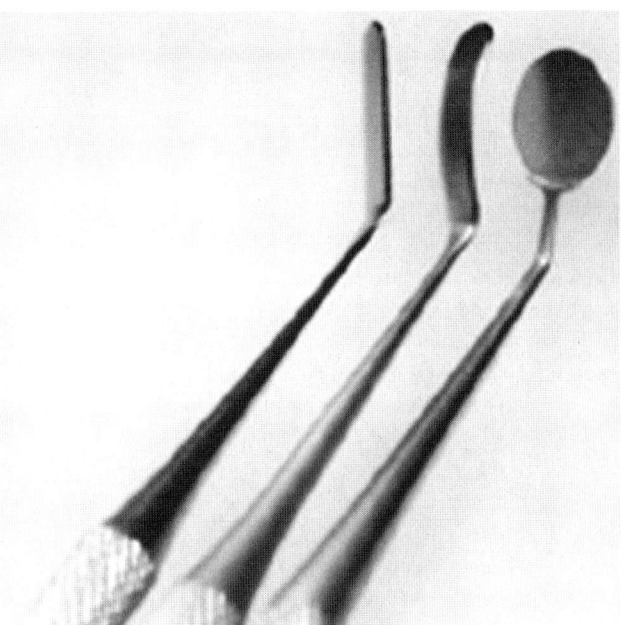

FIGURE 63-6. *Left*, Straight stromal dissection spatula. *Middle*, Curved stromal dissection spatula. *Right*, Donor disk insertion spatula. (From Terry MA, Ousley PJ. Endothelial replacement without surface incisions or sutures: topography of the deep lamellar endothelial keratoplasty procedure. *Cornea* 2001; 20: 14–18.)

are used to grasp the stromal disk of tissue with donor endothelium and gently transfer it endothelial side down to a specially designed, Healon-coated transfer spatula (Bausch and Lomb; Fig. 63-6).

The transfer spatula with the donor disk is inserted through the recipient's pocket wound, dropped down into the anterior chamber (which remains filled with air), and then lifted upward to place the donor disk into the recipient's bed. The transfer spatula is retracted, leaving the donor tissue disk self-adhering to the central posterior recipient bed. Adjustments to the edges of the donor disk and recipient bed are made with a Sinskey hook (Stephens

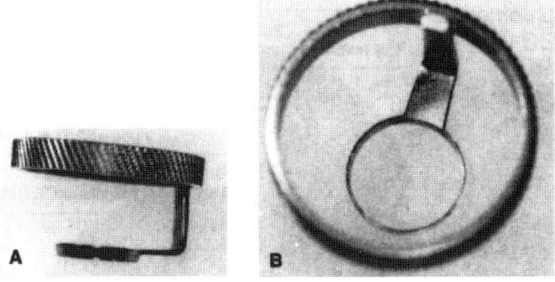

FIGURE 63-7. A, Terry trephine seen from above. B, Terry trephine seen in profile. Note the knurled circular handle and the low profile of the intralamellar trephine cutting edge. (From Terry MA, Ousley PJ. Endothelial replacement without surface incisions or sutures: topography of the deep lamellar endothelial keratoplasty procedure. *Cornea* 2001;20:14–18.)

Instruments, Lexington, KY) through the paracentesis. The superior pocket wound is closed with 10-0 nylon sutures, and the anterior chamber bubble is replaced with balanced salt solution through the side port.

Melles' Sutureless Technique

This technique describes the transplantation of the posterior donor lamellar disk through a small scleral incision, without the use of sutures (13). A 5-mm scleral tunnel incision is made, and a stromal pocket is dissected across the cornea in the fashion described previously. Using trypan blue 0.06% (VisionBlue; D.O.R.C. International) diluted 1:6 with balanced salt solution, the stromal interface is stained by injecting the solution into the stromal pocket. An 8.5-mm punch trephine is used to mark the corneal surface epithelium to outline the size of the posterior lamellar disk to be excised. Using custom-made curved microscissors, an 8.5-mm diameter recipient posterior lamellar disk is excised. An 8.5-mm donor disk is trephinated from the corneoscleral rim after dissecting a deep corneal pocket at 80% stromal depth from the donor globe. The endothelium is covered with viscoelastic (Ocucoat). The donor disk is folded with the endothelium to the inside using a custom inserter (D.O.R.C. International). The air is removed from the recipient's eye, and the donor disk is positioned into the recipient anterior chamber. It is then unfolded and positioned without suture fixation. The anterior chamber is filled with air for 5 minutes, followed by exchanging the air with balanced salt solution.

Microkeratome Flap Approach

Several groups have investigated the use of a microkeratome to create a corneal flap, followed by transplantation of the posterior stroma and repositioning of the anterior stromal flap (14–18).

Using human cadaveric eyes, Jones and Culbertson (14) described a technique they termed *endothelial lamellar keratoplasty*, in which a 9.5-mm hinged superficial corneal flap measuring 480 μm in thickness was created and a 7.2-mm diameter donor button measuring 250 μm in thickness was transplanted into a 7-mm opening in the recipient's bed.

Busin et al. (15) described a similar surgical technique, which they termed *endokeratoplasty*, performed on seven patients with either pseudophakic or aphakic bullous keratopathy or Fuchs' endothelial dystrophy. Nonradial marks are made on the recipient's inferior limbal cornea with a marking pen. An automated keratome (Hansatome; Chiron, Irvine, CA) is used to create a 9.5-mm diameter and 160-μm thick hinged flap. The flap is retracted superiorly. A 6.5-mm trephine and corneal scissors are used to excise the central posterior lamellae. The donor cornea is prepared by simple trephination through the endothelial side of corneoscleral rim with a 7-mm hand-held trephine. The corresponding amount of tissue is removed from the anterior lamella of the donor button and is transplanted into the recipient bed. The recipient anterior chamber is filled with viscoelastic and the donor button is placed in the recipient bed. The donor button is sutured into place using four 10-0 nylon cardinal sutures and a running eight-bite antitorque 8-0 polygalactin suture. The donor epithelium is removed with 70% alcohol and a methylcellulose sponge, if the entire stroma is transplanted. The cardinal sutures are removed. The corneal hinged flap is replaced and sutured into position with a running eight-bite antitorque 10-0 nylon suture (Fig. 63-8).

Azar et al. (4,17) described a similar technique in which a hinged anterior corneal flap is created using a microkeratome. The posterior stroma and endothelium are resected. A donor button of posterior stroma and endothelium is transplanted and the anterior stromal hinged flap is repositioned. The donor stromal button is prepared on a dedicated artificial anterior chamber (Bausch and Lomb). A microkeratome (Automated Corneal Shaper or Hansatome; Bausch and

Lomb) creates an 8.5- to 9.5-mm diameter, 180-μm thick anterior corneal cap without a hinge, and it is discarded. The donor cornea is then placed on a Teflon block endothelial side up. A 6- to 8-mm trephine is used to punch the donor button.

The recipient's cornea is marked for alignment to allow accurate repositioning of the tissue once the anterior corneal flap is reposed. A hinged anterior corneal flap 180 μm thick and 8.5 to 9.5 mm in diameter is created using the microkeratome. The suction ring is centered on the recipient's cornea and over the pupil. It is activated, and intraocular pressure is raised to 80 mm Hg. The hinged flap is created and elevated using a flat spatula. A 6- to 8-mm trephine is used to remove a full-thickness disk of the dissected posterior layers. Viscoelastic is placed into the anterior chamber. The donor button is placed into the recipient bed and secured with interrupted 10-0 nylon sutures or a running eight-bite antitorque 8-0 polygalactin suture. The hinged flap is refloated into position and allowed to seal into place. Sutures or a bandage contact lens may be used to secure the flap, if necessary (Fig. 63-9). A similar

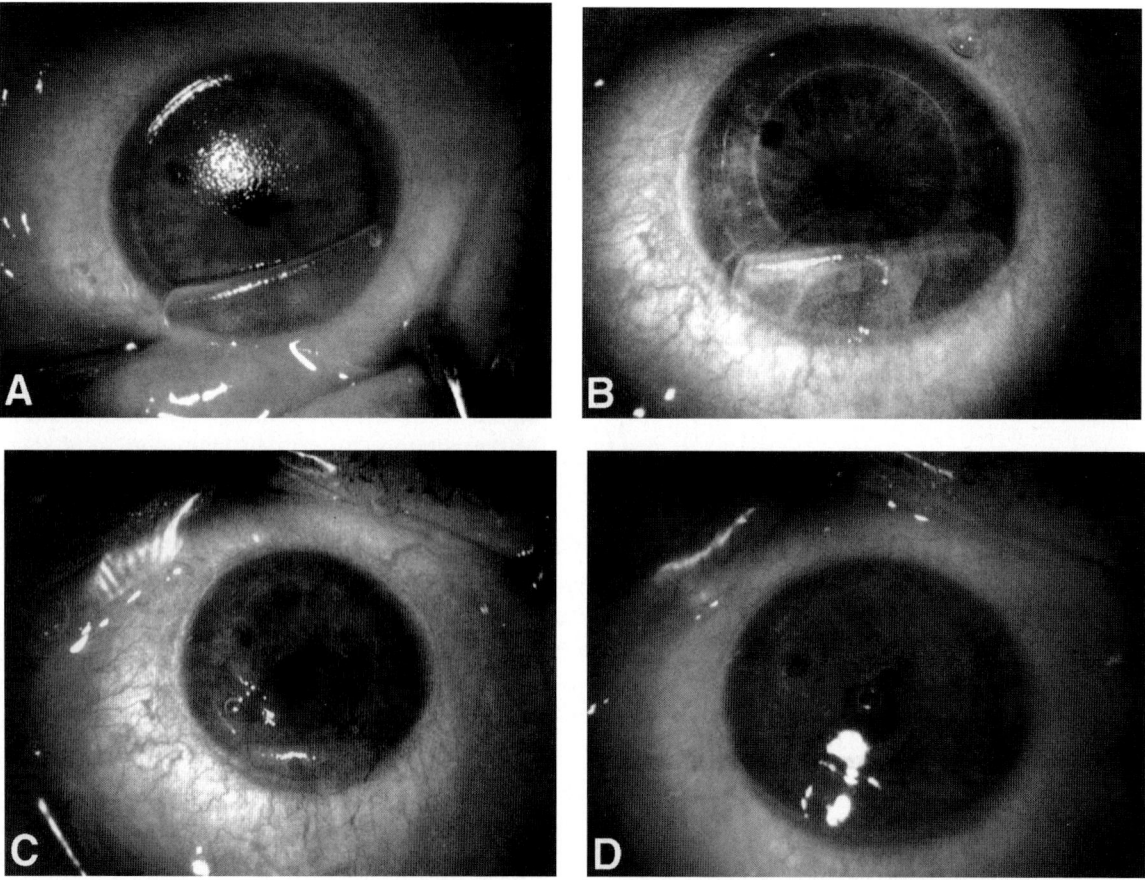

FIGURE 63-8. A: Hinged flap, 9.5 mm in diameter, retracted superiorly. **B:** Exposure of the anterior chamber after removal of a 6.5-mm recipient button, including deep stroma and endothelium. **C:** Donor button sutured in place using a running 8-0 polygalactin suture. The four 10-0 nylon cardinal sutures are removed after tying the running suture. **D:** Corneal flap sutured back into position using a running 10-0 nylon suture. (From Busin M, Arffa RC, Sebastiani A. Endokeratoplasty as an alternative to penetrating keratoplasty for the surgical treatment of diseased endothelium: initial results. *Ophthalmology* 2000;107:2077-2082.)

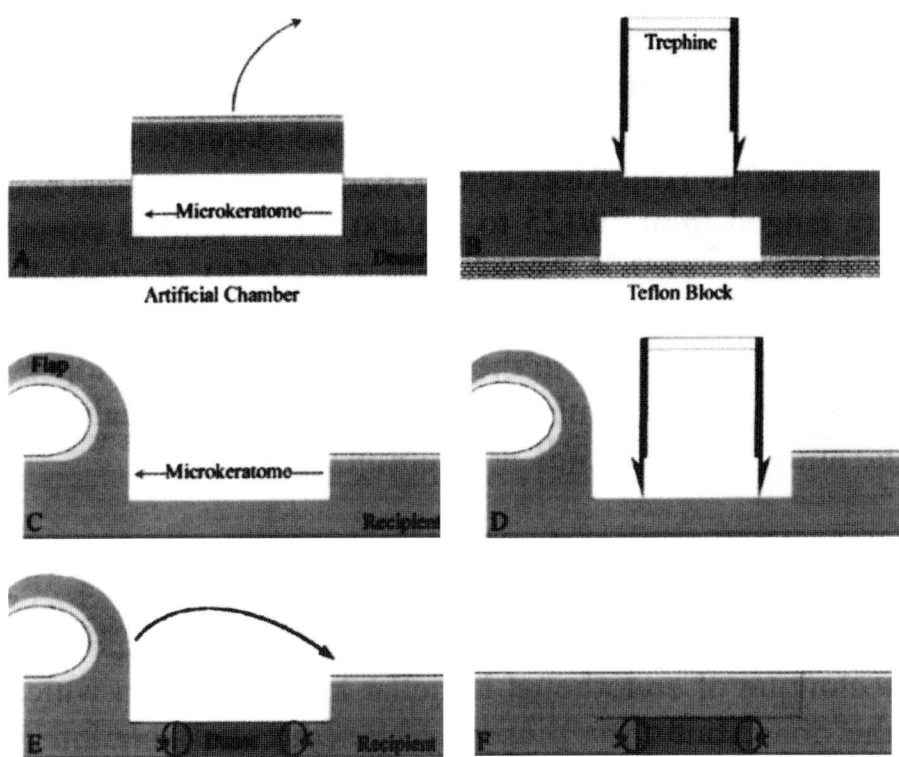

FIGURE 63-9. Microkeratome-assisted posterior keratoplasty technique. Schematic drawing showing donor preparation **(A, B)**, recipient bed preparation **(C, D)**, and transplantation **(E, F)**. **A:** Donor lenticule is excised using a microkeratome and a dedicated artificial anterior chamber and discarded. **B:** Donor cornea is placed endothelial side up on a Teflon block and a trephine is used to excise a donor stromal button (*red*). **C:** Hinged anterior stromal flap is created in the host cornea using a microkeratome and lifted. **D:** A trephine is used to excise the posterior host stroma and endothelium. **E:** The donor stromal button (*red*) is transplanted onto the host bed (*green*) and secured using sutures (*black*). **F:** The host corneal flap is refloated over the transplanted donor button. (From Jain S, Azar DT. New lamellar keratoplasty techniques: posterior keratoplasty and deep lamellar keratoplasty. *Curr Opin Ophthalmol* 2001;12:262-268.)

technique was reported by Ehlers et al. (18) on four eyes of three patients with pseudophakic and aphakic bullous keratopathy.

CLINICAL RESULTS

All six patients with bullous keratopathy or Fuchs' endothelial dystrophy who underwent uneventful surgery in the study by Melles et al. (8) had transplants that remained *in situ* in the postoperative period. One patient had a perforation during stromal dissection. All transplants were clear, with a normal, transient degree of postoperative inflammation. Biomicroscopy showed minimal scarring at the interface. Follow-up at 6 to 12 months demonstrated visual acuity from 20/80 to 20/20 (two eyes had maculopathies); astigmatic error was 1.54 D, average pachymetry was 0.49 mm, and endothelial cell count was 2520 cells/mm^2. Postoperative complications included increased intraocular pressure in one patient with a history of uveitis-glaucoma-hyphema before the posterior keratoplasty, development of peripheral anterior synechiae in one patient

with positive vitreous pressure, and a microperforation during dissection of the stromal pocket in one patient, thus converting the operation to a penetrating keratoplasty.

Terry et al. (12) reviewed preoperative and postoperative astigmatism and central corneal diopter power from their eight recipient eyes. The mean change in net corneal astigmatism was 0.4 ± 0.5 D, showing no significant difference. The axis of the steep meridian showed an insignificant shift from a mean axis of 103 to 115 degrees. There was no significant change in the corneal power before or after surgery. The net change was 0.2 ± 0.4 D. In addition, the disk in the recipient bed remained in good position despite attempts with blunt trauma and vigorous shaking to dislodge it. In a report on *in vivo* transplantation in two patients, Terry et al. (10) reported at 1 week a clear central cornea overlying the graft with persistent edematous recipient peripheral cornea. This contrast was more apparent at 1 month. Central corneal pachymetry was reduced by 65 μm and 157 μm, respectively, in patients 1 and 2. Regularity of surface corneal topography was remarkable. The lamellar interface was still detectable, although less apparent. At 6 months, uncorrected visual acuities were 20/60 and

20/70, respectively, for patients 1 and 2. Manifest refraction improved vision to 20/40+2 and 20/40−2, respectively. The graft centrally was clear, although the peripheral ungrafted corneal edema persisted (Fig. 63-10). Topography was smoother at 6 months. UltraPac pachymetry at 6 months showed the area of central thinning posttransplantation to be from 690 μm to 573 μm, and 814 μm to 618 μm, respectively, for patients 1 and 2. Endothelial cell count at 6 months after surgery were 1692 cells/mm² and 2631 cells/mm², respectively.

In the modified "sutureless" technique of Melles et al. (13), the best corrected visual acuity (BCVA) was 20/25 after 1 year in the single case reported. Keratometer readings were 42.25 D × 80°/44.25 D × 10°. There was minimal scarring between the donor and recipient stromal surfaces. This modified technique requires folding of the donor disk after a drop of viscoelastic is placed on the endothelial surface. They reported minimal endothelial damage, except for a straight line of dead cells at the fold. This loss is compensated for by the larger donor disk diameter compared with that of standard penetrating keratoplasty, thus increasing the total number of living endothelial cells transplanted. However, at 1 year, the modified sutureless technique has a lower endothelial count than the unmodified technique.

Results from the microkeratome-assisted technique by Busin et al. (15) in seven patients with either aphakic or pseudophakic bullous keratopathy or Fuchs' endothelial dystrophy show one postoperative case complication of interface epithelial ingrowth observed at 3 months. This patient had extensive melting of the flap and received a full-thickness donor graft. Within 14 days of surgery in the six uncomplicated cases, complete epithelialization of the corneal flap was achieved. The BCVA ranged from 20/40 to 20/100 in the seven patients, with a postoperative follow-up time of at least 4 months. BCVAs were less than 20/60 in

three patients because of a previous history of retinal detachment in one patient, and cystoid macular edema in two. At 1 month, the myopic spherical equivalent was between −1.00 D and −4.00 D by refraction. Mean keratometric readings ranged from 45.25 to 48.5 D. The astigmatic error was within 4.00 D for all patients. Topography showed regular morphology of the astigmatism. The 8-0 polygalactin suture dissolved by the end of the second postoperative month from the donor graft, and the 10-0 nylon suture from the flap was removed at 3 to 4 months after surgery.

Azar and colleagues' (4) report of the first U.S. case, treated in 1996, showed that corneal topography was flat at 6 months, leading to +16.0 D of hyperopia. The BCVA was 20/50. At 2 years, uncorrected visual acuity was 20/100 and the graft–host interface showed mild haze.

Ehlers et al. (18) reported that all four grafts were clear at 12 months. There was no wound dehiscence, the anterior chambers were of appropriate depths, and intraocular pressures were normal in all four cases. After 12 months, the total thickness of the cornea was increased in one of the four corneas. Endothelial cell counts ranged from 1200 to 2300 cells/mm². *In vivo* confocal microscopy revealed normal epithelium, but activated keratocytes in the anterior flap with particles visible in the interface. Donor keratocytes and endothelium appeared normal.

CONCLUSION

Posterior lamellar endothelial keratoplasty involves several evolving lamellar techniques for treating corneal disorders associated with endothelial dysfunction. Several approaches have been described with varying surgical, technical, topographic, and visual outcomes. With newer surgical techniques, modifications of old techniques, and better use

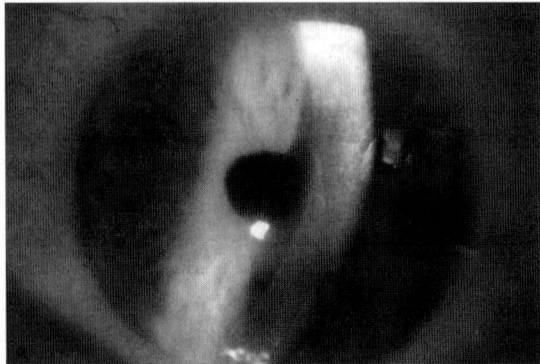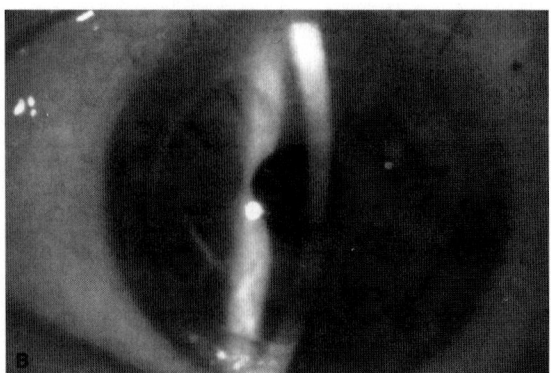

FIGURE 63-10. A, Preoperative photograph of edematous cornea due to Fuchs' dystrophy. **B,** Postoperative photograph of grafted cornea after months. Note the clarity of the central grafted cornea and the persistent edema of the nongrafted peripheral cornea. (From Terry MA, Ousley PJ. Deep lamellar endothelial keratoplasty in the first United States patient: early clinical results. *Cornea* 2001;20:239-243.)

of corneal topography and refractive surgery, these procedures offer a promising alternative to the use of penetrating keratoplasty for restoring useful vision in patients with endothelial dysfunction. The use of DLEK has been increasing worldwide. Future advances in femtosecond laser applications may allow for greater safety and improved clinical outcomes.

REFERENCES

1. Terry MA. The evolution of lamellar grafting techniques over twenty-five years. *Cornea* 2000;19:611–616.
2. Melles GRJ, Remeijer L, Geerards AJM, et al. The future of lamellar keratoplasty. *Curr Opin Ophthalmol* 1999;10:253–259.
3. Melles GRJ. Posterior lamellar keratoplasty. *Arch Soc Esp Oftalmol* 2002;77:175–176.
4. Azar DT, Jain S, Sambursky R, et al. Microkeratome-assisted posterior keratoplasty. *J Cataract Refract Surg* 2001;27:353–356.
5. Rodriguez-Barrios R. The treatment of Fuchs' dystrophy with posterior lamellar keratoplasty. In: Pollack FM, ed. *First Inter-American Symposium on Corneal and External Diseases of the Eye*. Springfield, IL.: Charles C Thomas, 1970:247–257.
6. Barraquer JI. *Microsurgery of the cornea: an atlas and textbook*. Barcelona: Ediciones Scriba, 1984:289–294.
7. Melles GRJ, Eggink FAGJ, Lander F, et al. A surgical technique for posterior lamellar keratoplasty. *Cornea* 1998;17:618–626.
8. Melles GRJ, Lander F, van Dooren BTH, et al. Preliminary clinical results of posterior lamellar keratoplasty through a sclerocorneal pocket incision. *Ophthalmology* 2000;107:1850–1856.
9. Melles GRJ, Lander F, Beekhuis WH, et al. Posterior lamellar keratoplasty for a case of pseudophakic bullous keratopathy. *Am J Ophthalmol* 1999;127:340–341.
10. Terry MA, Ousley PJ. Deep lamellar endothelial keratoplasty in the first United States patients: early clinical results. *Cornea* 2001;20:239–243.
11. Melles GRJ, Rietveld FJR, Beekhuis WH, et al. A technique to visualize corneal incision and lamellar dissection depth during surgery. *Cornea* 1999;18:80–86.
12. Terry MA, Ousley PJ. Endothelial replacement without surface corneal incisions or sutures: topography of the deep lamellar endothelial keratoplasty procedure. *Cornea* 2001;20:14–18.
13. Melles GRJ, Lander F, Nieuwendaal C. Sutureless, posterior lamellar keratoplasty: a case report of a modified technique. *Cornea* 2002;21:325–327.
14. Jones DT, Culbertson WW. Endothelial lamellar keratoplasty (ELK). ARVO Abstracts. *Invest Ophthalmol Vis Sci* 1998;39 [4 Suppl]:S76(abstr).
15. Busin M, Arffa RC, Sebastiani A. Endokeratoplasty as an alternative to penetrating keratoplasty for the surgical treatment of diseased endothelium: initial results. *Ophthalmology* 2000;107: 2077–2082.
16. Alio JL, Shah S, Barraquer C, et al. New techniques in lamellar keratoplasty. *Curr Opin Ophthalmol* 2002;13:224–229.
17. Jain S, Azar DT. New lamellar keratoplasty techniques: posterior keratoplasty and deep lamellar keratoplasty. *Curr Opin Ophthalmol* 2001;12:262–268.
18. Ehlers N, Ehlers H, Hjortdal J, et al. Grafting of the posterior cornea: description of a new technique with 12-month clinical results. *Acta Ophthalmol Scand* 2000;78:543–546.

INTRASTROMAL IMPLANTS FOR KERATOCONUS

JOSEPH COLIN

Keratoconus is a noninflammatory, progressive, ectatic, and thinning disease of the cornea that has been studied extensively, but the underlying mechanisms of stromal thinning are not well understood. Recent work suggests that the loss of corneal stromal tissue may be caused by increased levels and activity of proteases or decreased levels of inhibitors of protease activity. Epithelial injury resulting from trauma or refractive surgery may also cause loss of anterior stromal keratocytes through apoptosis modulated by interleukin-1 (1,2).

Noninvasive treatment modalities such as spectacles and contact lenses can provide functional vision in the early stages of this progressive disease (3–5). These modalities are less effective in correcting severe corneal irregular astigmatism and stromal opacities. Penetrating keratoplasty (PK) may be needed to restore visual function, particularly in the presence of marked central opacities (6–9). Patients suffering from irregular astigmatism without corneal opacities may be reluctant to pursue PK, and may seek less invasive interventions to improve best corrected spectacle visual acuity (BCVA) or uncorrected visual acuity (UCVA). These include lamellar keratoplasty, epikeratoplasty, phakic intraocular lenses (IOLs), and intrastromal corneal rings.

Incisional and excimer laser refractive surgery keratorefractive procedures are contraindicated in keratoconus. Incisional surgery (radial keratotomy and astigmatic keratotomy) and ablative corneal procedures [photorefractive keratectomy (PRK) and laser-assisted *in situ* keratomileusis (LASIK)] may induce intraoperative complications and may have an unacceptably high rate of unpredictability and instability (10–23).

TREATMENT OPTIONS

PK provides good visual outcomes for most patients with keratoconus. However, visual rehabilitation is slow, there is constant endothelial cell loss, and keratoconus may recur 15 to 20 years later. In patients with Down's syndrome, known to have a high frequency of keratoconus, the risk of serious complications after PK is considerably increased because of poor cooperation and extensive eye rubbing.

Deep lamellar keratoplasty can be used to decrease the incidence of graft rejection after PK (24). Air is injected into the corneal stroma, expanding its normal thickness as much as threefold. Lamellar dissection is performed as deeply as possible, close to Descemet's membrane. The rehydrated donor button is sutured in place with interrupted monofilament sutures. The surgical technique is more demanding than PK. The advantages compared with PK include preservation of the endothelium, no graft rejection, more rapid wound healing, and short duration of topical corticosteroid regimen.

Plano epikeratoplasty adds healthy donor tissue, thereby flattening the ectatic cornea and supporting the bulged corneal dome (14,17–19,25,26). Krumeich et al. used epikeratoplasty for the treatment of mild and moderate keratoconus, and reported that progression of the disease was arrested in some cases (26). If epikeratoplasty is unsuccessful, the patient may safely undergo PK at a later date.

Wagoner et al. compared the results of 443 eyes that received PK with 161 eyes treated with epikeratoplasty (19). With at least 2 years of postoperative follow-up data, the study showed PK provided better visual outcomes, but the results with epikeratoplasty were sufficiently good to recommend its use as a surgical alternative in cases when PK was not desirable (certain lifestyle demands and Down's syndrome).

A retrospective study compared the results of epikeratophakia with PK and LP for patients with keratoconus. Epikeratophakia was recommended as the grafting procedure of choice in most patients; however, in selected cases, PK may be performed with better functional results, if uncomplicated (4).

Phakic refractive IOLs are easily implanted and provide predictable refractive and visual results in myopic patients. The implantation of a refractive IOL is a refractive surgical option in patients with early keratoconus, high myopia, and minimal astigmatism. The surgery is facilitated by the greater anterior chamber in keratoconus.

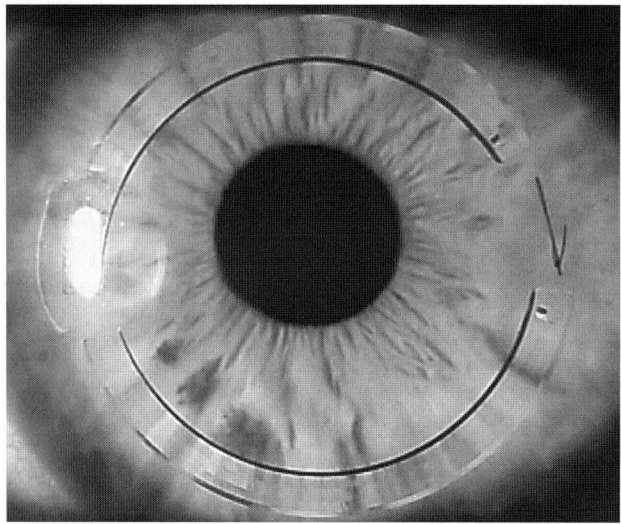

FIGURE 64-1. Slit-lamp aspect of the keratoconic cornea after Intacs implantation.

TABLE 64-1. A STUDY CONDUCTED BY COLIN ET AL. SHOWED THAT INTACS IMPLANTATION CAN IMPROVE VISUAL ACUITY IN KERATOCONIC EYES

UCVA	Preoperatively	6 months Postoperatively
≥0.1	46%	95%
≥0.5	0	48%
≥0.8	0	19%

BCVA	Preoperative RGPL	Postoperative 6 months spectacles
≥0.2	100%	100%
≥0.4	100%	90%
≥0.5	74%	82%
≥0.8	22%	41%

Intrastromal corneal rings were initially used for the correction of low myopia (22,27–30). They act as passive spacing elements that shorten the arc length of the anterior corneal surface, flattening the central cornea (23,31). This biomechanical effect is expected to be greater in keratoconic eyes, which have thinner corneas.

Now supplied by Addition Technology of Fremont, California, Intacs prescription inserts are delivered in boxes containing two segments of the same thickness. In Europe, Intacs intrastromal corneal rings are available in 11 sizes, ranging from 0.21 to 0.45 mm. In the United States, the rings are available in five sizes, from 0.25 mm to 0.35 mm.

The major objective is to reshape keratoconic corneas with two Intacs inserts of differing thickness. Intacs inserts are applied to lift the inferior ectasia and flatten the soft keratoconic corneal tissue in an attempt to decrease the asymmetric astigmatism induced by keratoconus, without removing any corneal tissue or touching the central cornea (Fig. 64-1). The rings may be explanted if needed.

Intacs inserts do not eliminate the corneal disease but they may improve visual acuity, and delay or eliminate the need for corneal transplantation. The best candidates are keratoconic patients with contact lens intolerance and a clear central cornea. In patients with apical and superficial opacities, phototherapeutic ablation may be performed before Intacs implantation.

EARLY INTACS STUDIES

Research indicates that Intacs implantation is safe and effective for keratoconic eyes. Most patients experience improved BCVA and UCVA, with a very low risk of complications.

Colin et al. performed the first Intacs implantation into keratoconic eyes in June 1997 (20). The surgery was performed in patients with clear central corneas and contact lens intolerance. The spherical equivalent error and refractive astigmatism were significantly reduced after surgery, topographic regularity was increased, and UCVA was improved in almost all patients, at all postoperative time points examined ($p \leq .05$). BCVA and UCVA values are presented in Table 64-1. Topographic corneal shape (size and height of the cone) was improved for all subjects compared with baseline measurements. Average postoperative mean keratometry was reduced by approximately 3 diopters (D), and mean keratometric astigmatism decreased steadily over postoperative time points (Figs. 64-2 and 64-3).

Stability of outcomes is a critical issue in keratoconus. Four of 20 eyes were followed for 24 months or more after Intacs insertion. During this time, keratometry readings were stable in all eyes, with progressive improvement of UCVA and BCVA.

Another study of Intacs inserts concluded that asymmetric implantation can improve UCVA and BCVA, and reduce irregular astigmatism in keratoconic corneas with and without corneal scarring (32,33). Boxer-Wachler et al. treated 74 keratoconic eyes, ranging from forme fruste to advanced keratoconus with scarring (which were awaiting PK). All patients enrolled had keratoconus with clear central corneas and were contact lens intolerant. Patients had BCVAs of 20/100 or better in the treatment eye and a corneal thickness of 400 μm or more at the location where Intacs were placed.

Except for the location of the incision (usually temporal), the surgical technique was similar to the standard technique used for low myopia. Pachymetry was used at the incision site and the incision was made to 66% of corneal thickness. Patients received either a 0.3-mm or a 0.35-mm ring segment in the inferior cornea. All patients had a thinner segment (0.25 mm) placed superiorly. Thicker segments induce greater local flattening immediately central

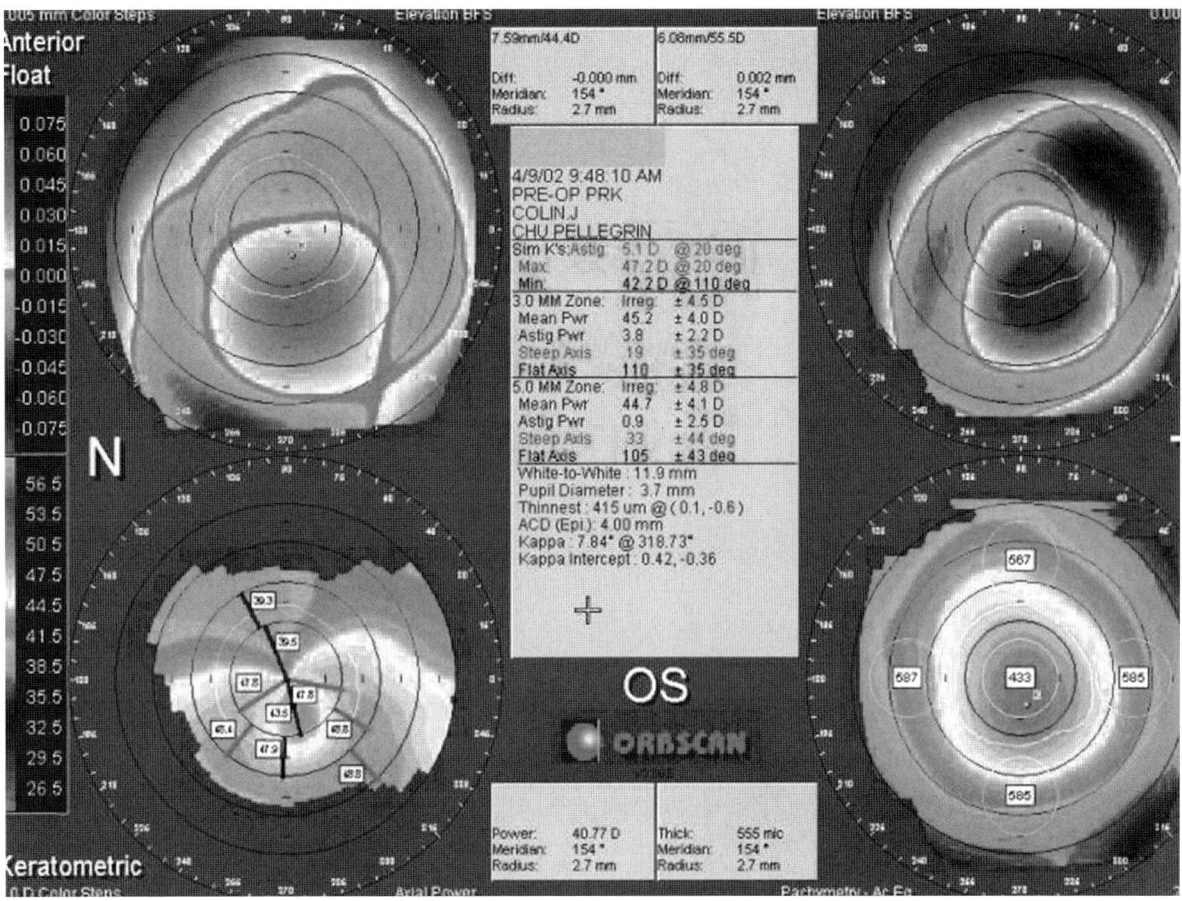

FIGURE 64-2. Corneotopographic image of a keratoconus case before surgery.

to the segment itself, resulting in larger, statistically significant changes in spherical equivalent.

Significant refractive flattening was achieved with the 0.25/0.35 mm group, whereas no refractive change was seen in the 0.25/0.30 mm group. BCVA improved for both ring sizes, with the greater change in the larger ring combinations. The 0.25/0.35 mm group gained five lines of UCVA, whereas the 0.25/0.30 mm group gained one line of UCVA (the 0.25/0.35 mm group had better postoperative UCVAs than the 0.25/0.30 mm group, even though their preoperative degrees of keratoconus and myopia were higher). There was a trend toward better improvement in UCVA with lower degrees of preoperative cylinder. Average inferior-superior values (1.4 is considered keratoconic) were reduced from a preoperative level of 25.62 to 6.60 after surgery.

After surgery, 41% of eyes experienced two lines of improvement in BCVA and 66% achieved a similar improvement in UCVA. Better preoperative BCVA corresponded with better postoperative BCVA, although eyes with worse preoperative acuity often had greater improvements in postoperative acuity. A functional improvement of four lines of acuity is notably more dramatic in patients with a BCVA of counting fingers compared with patients with a baseline BCVA of 20/40. Postoperative UCVA significantly improved in all eyes, although eyes with 6 D of cylinder or less had better UCVA than eyes with more than 6 D of cylinder.

Even though corneal scarring is clinically evident before surgery, it does not preclude significant improvement of BCVA and UCVA. Eyes with corneal scarring had the most improvement in BCVA (five lines) of all the subgroups analyzed.

RECENT STUDIES

More recent studies of Intacs inserts for keratoconus and post-LASIK corneal ectasia support the earlier reports of corneal flattening or regularization, and improved visual acuity.

Siganos et al. implanted 33 keratoconic eyes with Intacs inserts (34). All subjects had clear central corneas and were contact lens intolerant. To achieve maximum corneal flattening, each eye was implanted with two Intacs inserts of 0.45-mm thickness. Follow-up ranged from 1 to 24 months, with a mean of 11 months.

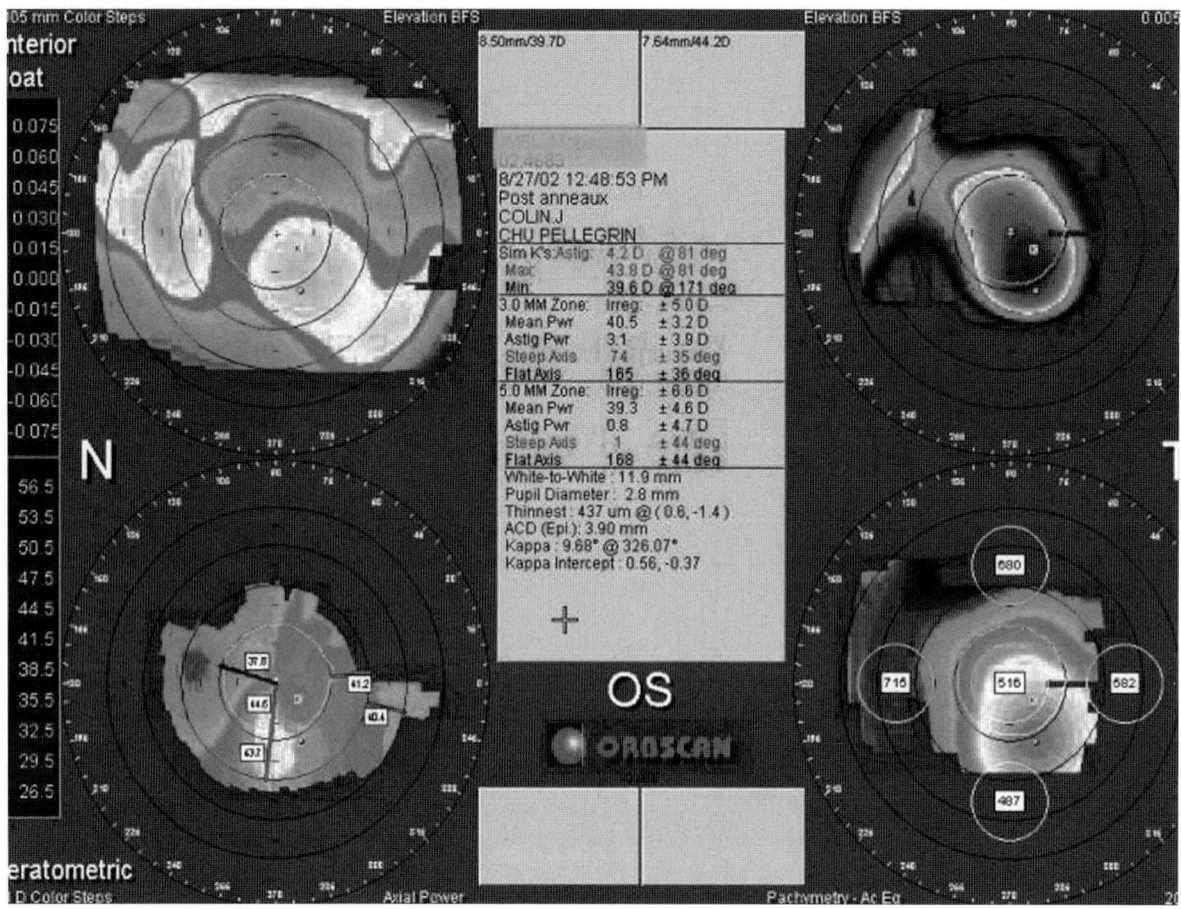

FIGURE 64-3. Same eye as in Fig. 64-2 after Intacs implantation.

UCVA significantly improved in 28 eyes, which gained 1 to 10 lines of visual acuity. Two eyes lost one line of UCVA, and three eyes maintained the preoperative UCVA. BCVA improved in 25 eyes, which experienced a 1- to 6-line gain in acuity. Four eyes lost one or two lines of BCVA, whereas four eyes maintained the preoperative BCVA. Intacs inserts were explanted in three eyes, and one of these eyes underwent successful PK.

Although acknowledging the benefits to the majority of subjects, these researchers expressed some caution regarding the results: "Even though the results are encouraging, concern still exists regarding the predictability as well as the long-term effect of such an approach for the management of keratoconus."

Colin et al. published similar results for 10 keratoconic patients who had received Intacs inserts and were followed for 12 months (21). In these eyes, Intacs inserts of 0.45 mm were placed in the inferior cornea to lift the cone, and 0.25-mm inserts were placed superiorly to counterbalance and flatten the overall anterior corneal surface. The mean postoperative UCVA was 20/50, compared with 20/200 for the preoperative UCVA. Mean postoperative BCVA was 20/32, compared with 20/50 before surgery. Topo-

graphic corneal shape (size and height of the cone) was improved for all subjects.

It is unclear how long Intacs inserts will stave off progression of keratoconus, or whether placement will totally eliminate the need for PK. Should keratoconus progress after placement of Intacs inserts and PK become necessary, Intacs inserts can be removed before performing PK. The scar induced by the channels will not alter the 8-mm graft. Performing PK at the time of Intacs inserts removal may induce some degree of undesirable postoperative astigmatism.

Intacs inserts appear to be a viable and minimally invasive method for treating clear corneal keratoconus for patients who are contact lens intolerant. After surgery, corneal steepening and astigmatism associated with keratoconus were reduced and UCVA was improved in almost all cases.

Future studies are needed to evaluate outcome measures, including contrast sensitivity, contact lens tolerance, and best corrected contact lens visual acuity. The response of keratoconic corneal tissue to the intrastromal corneal ring segment is not the same as that of normal corneal tissue. Although the use of more expanded ranges of implant thickness may improve efficacy and adjustability, the predictability of the procedure remains suboptimal. Soft contact lenses may be fitted after surgery to correct the residual spherical and cylindrical refractive error. In some cases, combined surgical options may be used, including a combination of Intacs and phakic IOLs or PRK (for keratoconus associated with myopia), or Intacs and phototherapeutic keratectomy (in case of apical corneal scar).

Ferrara Rings

South American surgeons have implanted Ferrara's ring segments (FRS), supplied by Mediphacos, Brazil. These polymethylmethacrylate implants differ from Intacs in several ways:

- A single radius of curvature of 2.5 mm
- Variable thickness from 150 to 350 μm
- Triangular anterior shape
- Prism format with the flat posterior surface implanted facing corneal endothelium
- Require two corneal incisions to be implanted at an 80-degree depth, with a virtually free-hand technique.

In a study of 36 severely keratoconic eyes that were wait-listed for PK, BCVA was improved in more than 90% of eyes (34). UCVA improved in 86% of eyes. None of the patients lost any lines of preoperative visual acuity. Mean central corneal curvature was reduced from 60.94 ± 8.65 D before surgery to 54.09 ± 8.0 D at the last postoperative examination.

During the procedure, FRS thickness and arc length were selected according to a previous nomogram. Two 1-mm radial incisions were performed at the steep corneal meridian based on preoperative corneal topography, separated by 180 degrees from each other, between optical zones of 5 and 7 mm, with a double-faced guided refractive keratectomy diamond knife. Two concentric stromal corneal tunnels, with an internal radius of curvature of 2.5 mm and an extension of 170 degrees, were constructed with an appropriate curved spatula. The FRS were implanted in these tunnels.

The study results suggest that FRS have a definite place in the treatment of keratoconus, especially in keratoconic patients who are contact lens intolerant and candidates for PK.

INTACS: SURGICAL TECHNIQUE AND COMPLICATIONS

Author's Technique for Intacs Implantation in Keratoconus

Preoperative evaluation included complete ophthalmologic evaluation, including UCVA and BCVA, keratometry, biomicroscopic examination with accurate description of the corneal opacities and folds, topography (location and height of the cone), corneal pachymetry with Orbscan and

TABLE 64-2. AUTHOR'S NOMOGRAM FOR INTACS FOR KERATOCONUS: TYPE OF KERATOCONUS

Type of Keratoconus	Ring Pattern
Asymmetric cone	One thin superior/one thick inferior
Global cone	Two rings of the same thickness
Central cone	Two rings of the same thickness

ultrasonography, contact lens fitting evaluation, and subjective tolerance of contact lenses.

In all patient eyes, a 0.45-mm Intacs insert was placed inferiorly to lift the conus. A 0.35-mm Intacs insert was placed superiorly to flatten the cornea and decrease baseline keratoconic asymmetric astigmatism. The goal of the treatment was to reshape keratoconic corneas with two Intacs inserts of different thickness. Intacs inserts were applied to lift the inferior ectasia and flatten the soft keratoconic corneal tissue in an attempt to decrease the asymmetric astigmatism induced by keratoconus.

The suggested current nomograms (Tables 64-2 and 64-3) are based on:

- The preoperative spherical equivalent (<3 D or >3 D of myopia)
- The location of the cone
- The asymmetric astigmatism induced by the keratoconus.

The surgical procedure was similar to that used for the correction of low myopia, except for location of incision site. After the patient was prepared for normal anterior segment surgery and placed under topical anesthesia, a small corneal incision (~1.8 mm) was made temporally with a diamond knife at the edge of the 7-mm optical zone, at two thirds of the corneal thickness at that location (the location of the incision depends on the morphology of the keratoconus). Two intrastromal tunnels (clockwise and counterclockwise) were created using the same specialized instruments developed for the placement of Intacs inserts for myopia. Special care was taken when making the inferior tunnel, where the cornea is relatively thinner.

Postoperative care included steroid and antibiotic ointment combination, plastic shield for 2 days, topical

TABLE 64-3. AUTHOR'S NOMOGRAM FOR INTACS FOR KERATOCONUS: TYPE OF CONE

Type of Cone	Preoperative Spherical Equivalent <3 D	Preoperative Spherical Equivalent >3 D
Asymmetric cone:		
Moderate asymmetry	0.35/0.40 mm	0.40/0.45 mm
High asymmetry	0.25/0.40 mm	0.25/0.45 mm
Global cone	0.40/0.40	0.45/0.45 mm
Central cone	0.40/0.40	0.45/0.45 mm

corticosteroids, and antibiotics and lubricants for 2 weeks. The suture was removed 10 to 15 days after surgery. Patients were instructed not to rub their eyes.

Complications of Intacs for Keratoconus

The following are complications seen after Intacs implantation for keratoconus:

1. Undercorrection: After the implantation of the two segments, the shape of the cornea may still be too asymmetric. In those cases, an adjustment may be considered, if thicker rings are available. If the corneal shape has improved, but the patient still has some degree of myopia, a phakic refractive IOL may be implanted. In most cases, the anterior chamber depth is optimal for refractive phakic IOLs (>3 mm)
2. Overcorrection: If the patient becomes hyperopic, ring exchange with thinner segments should be performed. If the surgery produces an increase in the corneal asymmetry (too flat superior cornea) with increased astigmatism, the superior segment should be removed.
3. Neovascularization toward the incision: This condition may occur when the incision is performed at the 12 o'clock position, in patients with a history of long-standing contact lens wear and new limbal vessels. When the incision is performed on the temporal meridian, vessels are very uncommon, and because of the dimensions of the cornea, the incision is located further from the limbus.
4. Migration of segment toward the wound: This complication may occur when one or two segments were left too close to the wound during surgery. The natural tendency of the synthetic ring is then to move toward the incision, with a risk of corneal stromal melting at this point. The segment(s) may be repositioned 3 to 6 months later, if the corneal melting is minimal or moderate.
5. Extrusion: Progressive stromal thinning and melting may occur if the rings are implanted too superficially in thin corneas, especially when the rings are implanted vertically. In such cases, the segments must be removed.
6. Unacceptable visual side effects such as glare or haloes: Topical brimonidine tartrate (Alphagan; Allergan, Irvine, CA) eyedrops, which reduce the pupil size, may help the patient; if the side effects are severe, the patient may request segment removal.

INTACS FOR POSTLASIK ECTASIA

Among refractive surgeons, there has been increasing concern regarding the occurrence of postoperative keratectasia, which may be caused by tectonic changes and weakening of the cornea, leading to corneal instability (35–39). Excessive thinning of the stromal bed, together with the action of intraocular pressure, may cause a progressive keratectasia manifesting months after the LASIK procedure. The pathogenesis seems multifactorial, although a posterior remaining stromal bed with a thickness of less than 250 μm appears to be a major causative factor. Preoperative, undiagnosed forme fruste keratoconus may also be a common cause of postLASIK corneal ectasia.

Clinical suspicion of keratectasia arises when a patient post-LASIK develops unstable vision associated with regression of the laser effect and the appearance of irregular astigmatism. In the past, contact lenses, lamellar keratoplasty, or PK were the only options to treat this complication.

LASIK weakens the biomechanics of the cornea. According to stress–strain measurements comparing normal and keratoconic corneas, a reduction in thickness of the normal stroma by approximately 50% yields values comparable with those in keratoconus. There have been reports of iatrogenic keratectasia after LASIK in which less than 250 μm of stromal bed was left after ablation, and in cases of forme fruste keratoconus. Ectasia has also occurred when more than 250 μm was left in the bed, suggesting that the phenomenon may be tissue dependent.

Kymionis et al. implanted 10 eyes with post-LASIK corneal ectasia with Intacs inserts (40). Intacs inserts were successfully implanted in all eyes. Before receiving Intacs inserts, UCVA was 20/100 or worse in all eyes; after receiving Intacs inserts, 90% of eyes had UCVA of 20/40 or better. Seven of 10 eyes gained 1 to 2 lines of BCVA, whereas the remaining 3 maintained pre-Intacs BCVA.

Lovisolo and Fleming implanted Intacs inserts in 10 eyes with keratectasia 12 to 44 months after LASIK or PRK (41). With pre-Intacs UCVA of no better than 20/100, nine patients achieved UCVA of 20/40 or better with Intacs inserts. BCVA improved by one to two lines for seven patients, and stayed the same for three patients.

Alio et al. evaluated whether Intacs can correct or stabilize ectasia after LASIK and provide an alternative to keratoplasty (42). They observed marked improvement of posterior anterior corneal surface steepening (ectasia), and the corneal topography became more regular. In addition, they observed significant enlargement of the optical zones.

THE FUTURE

Expanded therapeutic uses for intrastromal corneal rings are likely. Wavefront analysis of keratoconic eyes may allow a better understanding of corneal aberrations and promote improved visual outcomes. Use of segments of different lengths will allow customized corrections according to the specific corneal topography and will offer a more effective reshaping of the cornea. Creating the channels with the femtosecond laser will offer more precision compared with manual dissection because the laser beam can be focused in the stroma at an accuracy of 5 to 10 μm.

A study of 62 procedures, presented at the 2003 American Association of Cataract and Refractive Surgeons meeting, indicates that use of the Intralase femtosecond laser to create the implantation channel is easier than mechanical implantation, provides improved visual acuity, and reduces the rate of intrastromal corneal ring segment explantation (43).

REFERENCES

1. Rabinowitz YS. Keratoconus. *Surv Ophthalmol* 1998;42:297–319.
2. Brierly SC, Isquierdo L, Mannis MJ. Penetrating keratoplasty for keratoconus. *Cornea* 2000;19:329–332.
3. Coombes AG, Kirwan JF, Rostron CK. Deep lamellar keratoplasty with lyophilized tissue in the management of keratoconus. *Br J Ophthalmol* 2001;85:788–791.
4. Haugen OH, Hovding G, Eide GE, et al. Corneal grafting for keratoconus in mentally retarded patients. *Acta Ophthalmol Scand* 2001;79:609–615.
5. Lahners WJ, Russel B, Grossniklaus HE, et al. Keratolysis following excimer laser phototherapeutic keratectomy in a patient with keratoconus. *J Refract Surg* 2001;17:555–558.
6. Mortensen J, Ohrstrom A. Excimer laser photorefractive keratectomy for treatment of keratoconus. *J Refract Corneal Surg* 1994;10:368–372.
7. Colin J, Cochener B, Bobo C. Myopic photorefractive keratectomy in eyes with atypical inferior corneal steepening. *J Cataract Refract Surg* 1996;22:1423–1426.
8. Moodaley L, Lin C, Woodward EG. Excimer laser superficial keratectomy for proud nebulae in keratoconus. *Br J Ophthalmol* 1994;78:454–457.
9. Kremer I, Shochot Y, Kaplan A, et al. Three year results of photoastigmatic refractive keratectomy for mild and atypical keratoconus. *J Cataract Refract Surg* 1998;24:1581–1588.
10. Bilgihan K, Ozdek SC, Konuk O, et al. Results of photorefractive keratectomy in keratoconus suspects at 4 years. *J Refract Surg* 2000;16:438–443.
11. Vinciguerra P, Camasasca FI. Prevention of corneal ectasia in laser *in situ* keratomileusis. *J Refract Surg* 2001;17:S187–S189.
12. Lafond G, Bazin R, Lajoie C. Bilateral severe keratoconus after LASIK in a patient with forme fruste keratoconus. *J Cataract Refract Surg* 2001;27:1115–1118.
13. Buzart KA, Tuengler A, Febbraro JL. Treatment of mild to moderate keratoconus with laser in situ keratomileusis. *J Cataract Refract Surg* 1999;25:1600–1609.
14. Kaufman HE, Werblin TP. Epikeratophakia for the treatment of keratoconus. *Am J Ophthalmol* 1982;93:342–347.
15. McDonald MB, Kaufman HE, Durrie DS. Epikeratophakia for keratoconus: the nationwide study. *Arch Ophthalmol* 1986;104:1294–1300.
16. Krumeich JH, Daniel J, Knulle A. Live-epikeratophakia for keratoconus. *J Cataract Refract Surg* 1998;24:456–463.
17. Vajpayee RB, Sharma N. Epikeratoplasty for keratoconus using manually dissected fresh lenticules: 4-year follow-up. *J Refract Surg* 1997;13:659–662.
18. Buratto L, Belloni S, Valeri R. Excimer laser lamellar keratoplasty of augmented thickness for keratoconus. *J Refract Surg* 1998;14:517–525.
19. Wagoner MD, Smith SD, Rademaker WJ, et al. Penetrating keratoplasty vs. epikeratoplasty for the surgical treatment of keratoconus. *J Refract Surg* 2001;17:138–146.
20. Colin J, Cochener B, Savary G, et al. Correcting keratoconus with intracorneal rings. *J Cataract Refract Surg* 2000;26:1117–1122.
21. Colin J, Cochener B, Savary G, et al. Intacs inserts for treating keratoconus: one year results. *Ophthalmology* 2001;108:1409–1414.
22. Schanzlin DJ, Asbell PA, Burris TE, et al. The intrastromal corneal ring segments: phase II results for the correction of myopia. *Ophthalmology* 1997;104:1067–1078.
23. Burris TE, Baker PC, Ayer CT, et al. Flattening of central corneal curvature with intrastromal corneal rings of increasing thickness: an eye-bank eye study. *J Cataract Refractive Surg* 1993;19[Suppl]:182–187.
24. Edrington TB, Szczotka LB, Barr JT, et al. Rigid contact lens fitting relationships in keratoconus. *Optom Vis Sci* 1999;76:692–699.
25. McDonald MB, Kaufman HE, Durrie DS, et al. Epikeratophakia for keratoconus: the nationwide study. *Arch Ophthalmol* 1986;104:1294–1300.
26. Krumeich JH, Daniel J, Knulle A. Live-epikeratophakia for keratoconus. *J Cataract Refract Surg* 1998;24:456–463.
27. Nose W, Neves RA, Burris TE, et al. Intrastromal corneal ring: 12 months sighted myopic eyes. *J Refract Surg* 1996;12:20–28.
28. Fleming JF, Wan WL, Schanzlin D. The theory of corneal curvature change with the ICR. *CLAO J* 1989;2:146–150.
29. Cochener B, Le Floch G, Colin J. Intracorneal rings for the correction of low myopias. *J Fr Ophtalmol* 1998;21:191–208.
30. Asbell PA, Ucakhan OO, Durrie DS, et al. Adjustability of refractive effect for corneal ring segments. *J Refract Surg* 1999;15:627–631.
31. Burris TE, Ayer CT, Evensen DA, et al. Effects of Instrastromal corneal ring size and thickness on corneal flattening in human eyes. *Refract Corneal Surg* 1994;7:45–50.
32. Chou B, Boxer Wachler BS. Intacs: a promising new option for a keratocone. *Rev Optom* 2000;137:97–98.
33. Boxer Wachler BS, Chandra NS, Chou B, et al. Intrastromal corneal ring segments for keratoconus. *Ophthalmology* 2003;110:1031–1040.
34. Siganos CS, Kymionis GD, Kartakis N, et al. Management of keratoconus with Intacs. *Am J Ophthalmol* 2003;135:64–70.
35. Hori-Komai Y, Toda I, Asano-Kato N, et al. Reasons for not performing refractive surgery. *J Cataract Refract Surg* 2002;28:795–797.
36. Seiler T, Koufala K, Richter G. Iatrogenic keratectasia after laser in situ keratomileusis. *J Refract Surg* 1998;14:312–317.
37. Pallikaris IG, Kymionis GD, Astyrakakis NI. Corneal ectasia induced by laser *in situ* keratomileusis. *J Cataract Refract Surg* 2001;27:1796–1802.
38. McLeod SD, Kisla T, Caro NC, et al. Iatrogenic keratoconus: cornea ectasia following laser *in situ* keratomileusis for myopia. *Arch Ophthalmol* 2000;118:282–284.
39. Haw WW, Manche EE. Iatrogenic keratectasia after a deep primary keratotomy during laser *in situ* keratomileusis. *Am J Ophthalmol* 2001;132:920–921.
40. Kymionis GD, Siganos CS, Kounis G, et al. Management of post-LASIK corneal ectasia with Intacs inserts: one-year results. *Arch Ophthalmol* 2003;121:322–326.
41. Lovisolo CF, Fleming JF. Intracorneal ring segments for iatrogenic keratectasia after laser *in situ* keratomileusis or photorefractive keratectomy. *J Refract Surg* 2002;18:535–541.
42. Alio JL, Salem TF, Artola A, et al. Intracorneal rings to correct corneal ectasia after laser *in situ* keratomileusis. *J Cataract Refract Surg* 2002;28:1568–1574.
43. Neatrour G, Lipton M, Zook A. Intacs: a comparison of results with Intralase vs. mechanical techniques. Presented at the meeting of the American Association of Cataract and Refractive Surgeons, Virginia Beach, VA, April, 2003.

65

PHOTOTHERAPEUTIC KERATECTOMY

**LEE A. SNYDER, AALEYA F. KOREISHI,
CHRISTOPHER STARR, AND WALTER J. STARK**

The advent of the 193-nm argon-fluoride (ArF) excimer laser has provided corneal surgeons with a major therapeutic tool in the management of anterior corneal disease. Its potential for precise corneal ablations was demonstrated by Trockel and coworkers, who performed an ablation of a bovine cornea in 1983 (1). Seiler et al., in 1985, performed the first human excimer laser phototherapeutic keratectomy (PTK) in a sighted eye (2). The ability to ablate tissue with submicron accuracy, without damage to surrounding tissue, lends the excimer laser well to the removal of diseased layers of the anterior cornea and to the smoothing of its surface (1,3). In addition, the management of certain corneal diseases with PTK may delay or obviate the need for penetrating or lamellar keratoplasty and its associated risk and expense. The mechanism of action involves the use of high-energy ultraviolet radiation with a wavelength of 193 nm to break molecular bonds of proteins in the cornea. Tissue fragments are ejected at a high speed, minimizing transfer of energy to adjacent corneal structures (4,5).

CORNEAL WOUND HEALING

As the excimer laser is incorporated into the armamentarium of therapies used to treat corneal disease, its effect on corneal wound healing must be understood, for the complex manner in which the cornea heals plays a significant role in the final visual outcome of the procedure (6). The cornea is an intricate tissue that serves both to add structural support to the globe and to transmit and reflect light. The goals of laser therapy should include preservation of both its integrity and transparency.

After removal of the epithelium, reepithelialization typically occurs within 1 week, although reestablishment of the desmosomes and hemidesmosomes to the underlying stroma occurs 1 to 3 months later (1,7–13). There is some evidence for the formation of a pseudomembrane that covers the exposed ablated surface almost immediately after the procedure and may aid in reepithelialization (9,14,15). Stromal deposition occurs after epithelial regrowth, and may depend on the epithelium for the initiation of connective tissue synthesis (10).

Laser-induced scarring may be related to depth of ablation. Goodman et al. showed that ablations of less than 50 μm on rabbit corneas did not induce scarring, epithelial hyperplasia, or new collagen deposition (15). Wu et al., however, reported anterior stromal scarring with ablation depths of 50 to 113 μm on four eyes that underwent PTK followed by penetrating keratoplasty (PK) (3). Loss of endothelial cells has not been demonstrated in ablations that are within 40 μm of Descemet's membrane (11,16–18).

PTK has also been shown to improve the health of the ocular surface. Dogru et al. recently reported that variables such as corneal sensitivity, tear function, and impression cytology parameters improve after PTK for granular/Avellino dystrophy and corneal scars (19,20). These improvements are maintained until the primary corneal dystrophy recurs (21).

PREOPERATIVE ASSESSMENT

Careful patient selection and surgical planning are crucial to successful outcomes in PTK. A thorough preoperative evaluation (Table 65-1) consists of a comprehensive review of the patient's ocular and systemic history. Specific attention should be given to aspects of the history, including collagen vascular disorders, uncontrolled diabetes, or active inflammation, because they may adversely affect wound healing and represent contraindications to PTK (6). PTK should be avoided in eyes with severe keratoconjunctivitis sicca and stem cell deficiencies because they are prone to persistent epithelial defects that can, in turn, stimulate more scarring. Herpes simplex virus may be reactivated in the setting of PTK, and it is recommended that eyes with prior herpes infection be disease free for at least 1 year before PTK is attempted. In addition, prophylactic acyclovir or valacyclovir and topical trifluridine should be added to the PTK regimen (22–24).

TABLE 65-1. RECOMMENDED PREOPERATIVE EVALUATION OF PATIENTS UNDERGOING PHOTOTHERAPEUTIC KERATECTOMY

History (ocular and systemic)
Visual acuity (uncorrected and best corrected)
Manifest refraction
Hard contact lens overrefraction (if necessary)
Pupillary examination
Extraocular motions
Confrontation visual fields
Intraocular pressure
Slit-lamp examination (corneal lesion size, depth, location)
Corneal sensation
Schirmer's test (if necessary)
Keratometry
Topography
Pachymetry (ultrasonographic or optical)
Dilated funduscopic examination
Ultrasonography (if necessary)

TABLE 65-2. CORNEAL PATHOLOGIC PROCESSES TREATABLE WITH PHOTOTHERAPEUTIC KERATECTOMY

Anterior corneal dystrophies
  Map-dot-fingerprint
  Reis-Buckler
  Meesman's
  Lattice
  Granular
  Avellino
  Fuchs' endothelial
  Salzmann's nodular
  Schnyder's
Recurrent epithelial erosions
Corneal scars
  Infectious
  Herpetic
  Trachomatous
  Traumatic
  Pterygium
  Stevens-Johnson syndrome
  Contact lens related
Other irregularities
  Band keratopathy
  Apical scars in keratoconus
  Shield ulcers
Corneal intraepithelial dysplasia

A detailed ophthalmic examination, including uncorrected and best corrected visual acuity, manifest refraction with hard contact lenses if indicated, pupillary examination, tonometry, slit-lamp examination, keratometry and topography, as well as a dilated fundus examination, is an important part of preoperative planning. All layers of the cornea should be evaluated. PTK should be avoided in eyes with irregularities resulting from endothelial decompensation (6). Blepharitis should be treated before PTK is performed. If dry eye is suspected, Schirmer's test should be performed. Patients should be informed that they may need to wear rigid gas-permeable (RGP) lenses after surgery to achieve their best corrected acuity, and therefore a trial of RGP contact lenses is recommended before embarking on PTK. If poor preoperative visual acuity is due to irregular astigmatism, RGP lenses may neutralize these corneal aberrations and obviate the need for PTK. Potential acuity can be assessed with hard contact lens overrefraction, pinhole acuity, or the Guyton-Minkowski potential acuity meter. Corneal topography is a helpful tool in planning surgical technique and in comparing preoperative with postoperative data. Finally, although altering refractive error is not the primary goal of PTK, the ablation can have significant effects on refractive error, and this should be kept in mind as the procedure is planned (25).

To qualify for PTK, the patient's symptoms should be explained by the observable corneal pathologic process (Table 65-2). Furthermore, the lesion amenable to PTK should be located within the anterior 5% to 20% of the cornea. Depth can be estimated at the slit lamp with additional information obtained by optical pachymetry or ultrasonic biomicroscopy, both of which can be useful in planning for PTK (26–30). Pathologic processes limited to Bowman's layer may be more amenable to mechanical epithelial debridement before attempted PTK. Treatment should be limited to areas of disease that are visually significant.

It may not be necessary to remove all clinically observable opacities to achieve acceptable visual rehabilitation. As with other excimer laser procedures, the remaining stromal bed should be at least 250 μm thick to avoid the development of postoperative ectasia (6). Informed consent can be tailored to the specific PTK technique used based on the preoperative indications.

The protocol for PTK should include laser calibration before use of the excimer laser. An adequate supply of gases needed for surgery, as well as calibration of laser fluence, must be ensured. This is usually accomplished by ablating a standardized material such as polymethylmethacrylate to ensure a flawless and homogeneous ablation (6). Proper centration of the beam and reticle alignment should be checked before each procedure. Pulse rate and spot size are chosen by the surgeon according to type of correction desired. Although these tasks may be delegated to a technician, the surgeon must verify results of the laser calibration.

Immediately before the procedure, the patient should be reexamined at the slit lamp to finalize the ablation strategy. Techniques vary depending on the location, diffuseness, and elevation of the underlying lesion. A topical anesthetic is applied to both eyes and the patient is positioned on the chair and centered under the operating microscope. A speculum is placed into the operative eye and focus is achieved under high magnification. The patient is then asked to stare at the red blinking light during the ablation.

SURGICAL TECHNIQUES

Because of the wide variety of pathologic processes amenable to phototherapeutic ablation, the surgeon must individualize the approach for each patient. Techniques of epithelial removal and patterns of stromal ablation vary depending on characteristics of the corneal lesion and treatment goals, but certain guidelines can be taken into account (Table 65-3).

Smooth Corneal Opacities

PTK can be a highly effective therapy for a central corneal pathologic process arising beneath a relatively smooth epithelial surface, as in many anterior stromal dystrophies (31). When the anterior corneal surface is smooth, or the lesion in Bowman's membrane or anterior stroma is not causing significant surface irregularity, the goal of PTK is twofold. The first aim is to translate this smooth surface to a level deeper than the corneal lesion, and the second is to minimize the induced refractive error (6). In these cases, epithelial removal is best accomplished by the laser rather than by mechanical debridement. The epithelium itself acts as a masking agent to allow irregularities in Bowman's layer and the superficial stroma to be differentially ablated. Some surgeons prefer to use a masking fluid on intact epithelium, ablating until the blue fluorescence disappears, signifying the point at which all epithelium has been ablated and stromal ablation begins (32,33). Manual epithelial debridement has been shown to be problematic for corneal dystrophies such as Reis-Buckler. Lawless et al. noted that manual epithelial removal in an eye with Reis-Buckler dystrophy was often patchy and the end point for complete removal difficult to assess (34–36).

Because corneal dystrophies usually manifest as a diffuse pathologic area, a large spot size, measuring 6 to 7 mm, centered on the entrance pupil, can be used to ablate both epithelium and underlying anterior stroma. Initial depth of ablation should be 75% of the estimated depth of the corneal lesion. After the initial ablation, the surgeon examines the patient at the slit lamp to evaluate the effect, and to assess if further ablation should be done. The "ablate and check" method is performed until the desired bulk of diseased cornea is removed (31). The depth of the opacity can be difficult to assess with this technique, and care should be taken not to exceed the planned preoperative depth of ablation as determined by careful slit-lamp examination and optical pachymetry.

The surgeon must remember that as ablation depth increases, the change in refractive error also increases, and care should be taken to ablate the minimal amount of lesion needed to alleviate patient symptoms (6,37). Undertreatment is preferable to overtreatment because the procedure can be repeated.

Mechanical debridement is the preferred method for epithelial removal when treating recurrent epithelial erosions or any disorder in which the epithelium is deemed irregular compared with the underlying Bowman's membrane. This can be accomplished manually with a Bard-Parker blade (38). The epithelium is removed over the area of erosion. If the visual axis is involved, it may be wise to include this area so as not to induce irregularities into the ablation profile. Masking fluid, such as 1% hydroxymethylcellulose, 0.5% tetracaine, or Tears Naturale, may be applied after manual debridement to smooth the surface before ablation (6). The ablation zone is chosen to encompass the area of debrided epithelium. A depth of 3 to 10 μm is usually sufficient to remove a portion of Bowman's layer (6,31,37).

TABLE 65-3. SUGGESTED SURGICAL TECHNIQUES FOR PHOTOTHERAPEUTIC KERATECTOMY OF SINGLE OR MULTIPLE LESIONS

Single Lesion	Multiple Lesions

IF elevated/calcific/fibrous:
  Initial mechanical debridement
	IF sparse:
	  Treat per single lesion protocol

THEN	IF dense lesions AND IF elevated/calcific/fibrous: Initial mechanical debridement
IF peripheral: Focal ablation to level of surrounding tissue with aggressive masking agent (moderate viscosity)	THEN

IF central:
  Focal ablation just short of level of surrounding tissue with aggressive masking agent (moderate viscosity)
THEN
  Complete ablation with large spot size and masking agent (moderate viscosity)
	Initial ablation with high-viscosity masking agent, large spot size, low pulse rate
	THEN
	  Complete ablation with moderate-viscosity masking agent
	THEN
	  Taper ablation at border using 2-mm spot size to 20 μm depth

Modified from Azar DT, Steinert RF, Stark WJ, eds. *Excimer laser phototherapeutic keratectomy: management of scars, dystrophies and PRK complications.* Baltimore: Williams & Wilkins, 1997.

To smooth the resultant stromal bed for epithelialization and to reduce the magnitude of induced hyperopia after performing a large central ablation, a transition zone can be created. Approximately 1 D of hyperopic shift is induced for every 20 μm of stromal ablation (6). Sher et al. used a circular motion of the eye to perform a "smoothing technique" (34). The Summit excimer laser trials used a related "polish technique" whereby the patient's head was moved in a brisk circular manner under the laser (39,40). Subsequently, Stark et al. described a "modified taper technique" whereby the surgeon moves the eye in a circular fashion under the laser, treating the periphery of the ablation zone with a 20-μm deep, 2-mm diameter spot size. The additional peripheral ablation limits induced hyperopia by approximately 2 to 4 D (7,40). Alternatively, a hyperopic photorefractive keratectomy (PRK) ablation may be used after PTK to minimize induced hyperopia. In this circumstance, epithelial ablation should be carried out to 8 mm. Combining PTK with PRK is technically easier and potentially more precise than the polish techniques; however, it requires additional costs for the hyperopic card and removes additional central as well as peripheral tissue. From previous studies, it is known that approximately 1 D of hyperopic shift is induced for every 20 μm of stromal ablation (6), and the depth of both the PTK and PRK ablations should be considered in the total tissue removed. Care should be taken to avoid too much thinning of the peripheral cornea because a corneal transplantation may be considered at a later time. PTK combined with PRK can also be considered for PTK candidates who have concurrent myopia.

Scars and Nodules

Allowing the precise removal of a predefined amount of corneal tissue, PTK is well suited for ablation of elevated scars and nodules. Such lesions can be seen in keratoconus, Salzmann's degeneration, and posttraumatic or infectious scars. Decreased vision may be secondary to opacification, surface irregularities, or associated refractive errors (6). Again, disease limited to the anterior stroma is most amenable to PTK. Unlike ablation of smooth corneal lesions, with the treatment of elevated nodules or scars, the goal is to smooth the lesion selectively, while simultaneously limiting refractive change. It is best to measure the densest portion of the scar in the optical zone using the optical pachymeter, and to limit ablation to the depth determined before surgery. Because the excimer laser removes surface tissue and does not automatically smooth contour irregularities, any preexisting irregularities will be duplicated at a deeper level if ablation rate and spot size stay constant (41). In addition, scars or calcific lesions may ablate more slowly than normal corneal tissue, and the excimer laser can induce respective peaks and valleys in the contour that were not present before treatment (42–44).

Finally, selective ablation of central lesions can lead to large hyperopic shifts, whereas ablation of peripheral lesions can induce myopia (6).

The importance of surface modulators in these circumstances to aid in smoothing the contour of the areas to be treated cannot be overestimated. The smooth contour created by these modulators can be translated to the new postablation surface (6). Fluid masking agents, which fill valleys in the corneal surface, are probably the most commonly used type of surface modulator. These fluids include 0.9% saline (Unisol), 1% carboxymethylcellulose sodium (Celluvisc), and 0.3% hydroxypropylmethylcellulose 2910 with 0.01% dextran 70 (Tears Naturale II). These solutions all exhibit sufficient absorbance by the 193-nm ArF laser, although 0.3% hydroxypropylmethylcellulose 2910 and a 0.1% dextran 70 solution showed greater absorbance than 0.9% saline (41). The viscosity of a masking fluid should be high enough to remain in surface depressions without runoff and low enough to coat the surface uniformly. A thin layer of fluid should be applied with a damp cellulose sponge. A "sight and sound" method can be used to assess the adequacy of the application. Because the excimer laser turns many masking fluids white, a white area overlying a peak indicates that too thick a layer of fluid has been applied. Because ablation of the fluid emits a soft "click" versus the loud "snap" of naked cornea, a louder treatment than predicted signifies deficient coverage of fluid on the cornea (39). The fluid may need to be reapplied several times to attain the desired layering throughout the procedure.

Another type of surface modulator of more recent interest consists of a collagen gel molded by a rigid lens with a desired contour and radius of curvature. The laser preferentially ablates the gel until the protruding areas of elevated corneal tissue are encountered (45,46). One drawback of this method, as opposed to a liquid masking agent, is that it cannot be altered for dynamic management of induced irregularities. If the corneal epithelium is smooth in relation to the underlying Bowman's layer or anterior stromal surface, the epithelium itself may also be used as a surface modulator (33). Finally, the use of a low ablation rate, through lengthening the ablation time, has been shown to improve posttreatment corneal regularity, perhaps by allowing the masking fluid more time to redistribute over corneal depressions (47).

To manage all of these issues effectively, the surgeon plays an active role not only in the preoperative planning, but in making treatment decisions during the procedure. The approach to these types of cases can be tailored based on the number and distribution of anterior corneal lesions. The initial step of the procedure is focused on attaining a relatively smooth pretreatment surface. In isolated nodules, Talamo et al. suggested "preparatory surgical keratectomy" before ablation in lesions elevated over 20 μm, and only local epithelial removal in those elevated less than 20 μm (48). Azar et al. further proposed that removing epithelium overlying the elevated area, as well as a small area of surrounding epithelium, followed by the application of masking fluid, may aid in selective ablation of such nodules (38). If the lesion is particularly calcific or dense, it should be mechanically debulked before ablation. The focal ablation is carried out using a spot size that includes the lesion (1 to 3 mm). While the patient is fixating on the target, the head is gently rotated in a circular manner. Masking fluid is used generously throughout the ablation, with frequent pauses of the laser to reapply the masking agent. If the elevated lesion is peripheral, it is ablated to the level of the surrounding epithelium. Both direct illumination and sclerotic scatter may be used to provide adequate illumination of the lesion to be eliminated (49). If it is central, the ablation is performed just short of the surrounding epithelium, and then a larger spot size (6 mm) is used to smooth the corneal surface (6). The goal is to ablate just enough tissue to alleviate patient symptoms because a conservative treatment can always be augmented at a later date.

If multiple elevated lesions are present, they can be treated individually using the aforementioned protocol if there is adequate intervening space between the lesions. Again, lesions that are significantly elevated or that contain calcific or dense fibrotic scars can be mechanically debulked before ablation. If, however, the lesions are clustered, they should initially be ablated using a large spot size (6 mm), high-viscosity masking fluid, and a low pulse rate (2 to 5 Hz) (6). Then, a small additional ablation can be performed with a moderate-viscosity masking solution. Finally, to limit hyperopia and even out a sharp treatment edge, the "modified taper technique" can be applied to the ablation border using a 2-mm spot size, ablation depth of 20 μm, and gentle circular movements of the patient's head (7).

POSTOPERATIVE CARE

The goal in the early postoperative period is to hasten reepithelialization and decrease pain (Table 65-4). Collagen

plugs can be placed at the end of the procedure to improve tear function and facilitate epithelial healing If the treatment entailed the removal of a small nodule, an antibiotic ointment alone may be used (6). Although treatment regimens vary, standard therapies include a well-fitting bandage contact lens and an antibiotic drop four times a day. A cycloplegic agent may be instilled in the presence of a large epithelial defect. Alternatively, an antibiotic or combination antibiotic–steroid ointment may be given and a pressure patch placed. A nonsteroidal antiinflammatory agent and cold compresses can often ease postoperative pain. Patients are seen every 1 to 2 days until complete reepithelialization occurs, which is usually complete within 1 week. The contact lens need not be removed until the epithelial defect resolves completely. The antibiotic drops may then be discontinued, but an antibiotic ointment can be given at bedtime for added lubrication. The nonsteroidal drops can be substituted with a mild topical steroid such as fluorometholone 0.1%, which is tapered over the next 2 to 6 months.

Patients are typically seen at 1, 3, 6, 12, and 24 months, at which time visual acuity, intraocular pressure, and a detailed biomicroscopic examination are repeated. Corneal haze should be graded separately for each corneal layer: 0 = clear; 0.5 = barely detectable; 1.0 = mild, not affecting refraction; 1.5 = mildly affecting refraction; 2 = moderate, refraction possible but difficult; 3.0 = opacity preventing refraction, anterior chamber easily viewed; 4.0 = impaired view of anterior chamber; and 5.0 = inability to see anterior chamber (7). Keratometry and topography should be obtained to monitor the patient's progress and to serve as a feedback mechanism for the corneal surgeon.

CLINICAL RESULTS

Analysis of the early major clinical studies on PTK reveals that the treatment of corneal disease such as basement membrane and anterior corneal stromal dystrophies generates more successful and consistent results than treatment of corneal scars and calcifications (38). Stark et al. reported improved visual acuity in 78% of eyes with lesions ranging from lattice, granular, macular, and Reis-Buckler dystrophies to corneal scars and Salzmann's degeneration (7). Campos et al. reported that 50% of 18 eyes with superficial corneal opacities were improved, but suggested long-standing scars may not be as amenable to treatment with PTK (50). A study by Rapuano et al. of 20 eyes with anterior corneal disease unresponsive to medical treatment found that 45% of patients experienced improvement in visual acuity after PTK and 75% were judged to have "functional improvement" (51). Fagerholm et al., in a study of 166 eyes with varying pathologic processes, achieved an 84% success rate, defined as improvement in visual acuity, contact lens fit, wound healing, or cosmesis (52).

TABLE 65-4. MANAGEMENT OF PATIENTS AFTER PHOTOTHERAPEUTIC KERATECTOMY

Before Reepithelialization	After Reepithelialization
Antibiotic drops and bandage contact lens	Antibiotic ointment at night
OR	Mild steroid with slow taper
Antibiotic ointment and pressure patch	
Nonsteroidal antiinflammatory drops	Artificial tears, as needed
Cycloplegic drops	

Modified from Azar DT, Steinert RF, Stark WJ, eds. *Excimer laser phototherapeutic keratectomy: management of scars, dystrophies and PRK complications.* Baltimore: Williams & Wilkins, 1997.

More recent studies of large numbers of eyes have corroborated these results. Starr et al. found that of 45 eyes, most of which had postinfectious, posttraumatic, or postsurgical scars, 47.5% had improved best spectacle-corrected visual acuity, and 72.5% had improved visual acuity if contact lens correction was included (53). In a prospective study of 232 eyes, Maloney et al. demonstrated that 45% experienced increased vision and 5% had decreased vision. Treatment was most effective for those with corneal dystrophies and elevated opacities and least effective for those with band keratopathy and scars associated with corneal thinning (54).

Because of the diverse range of indications for PTK, no one parameter such as visual acuity can serve as the single measure of success in all cases. It is helpful to divide the clinical results into subsections of corneal disorders treated by PTK.

Recurrent Epithelial Erosions and Corneal Dystrophies

Recurrent epithelial erosions can occur secondary to trauma or dystrophy, or can be idiopathic. The presence of blepharitis or dry eyes should be excluded before eyes with recurrent erosion are treated with PTK (37). PTK is generally viewed as a successful method of treating eyes with recurrent erosions for which more conservative treatments, such as topical lubrication, hypertonic solutions, therapeutic contact lenses, epithelial debridement, or anterior stromal puncture, have been documented to have failed. Dausch et al. found that 74.4% of 74 eyes with posttraumatic recurrent erosions were recurrence free at a follow-up period of 6 months to 4 years (55). Another study found that 86.2% of 48 eyes with recurrent erosion in anterior basement membrane dystrophy were asymptomatic at 12 months. All recurrences presented within 6 months (56). In 30 eyes with map-dot-fingerprint dystrophy treated with PTK for recurrent erosions, reduced visual acuity, or other visual symptoms, Orndahl et al. found that 82% achieved the goal of improved visual acuity, 100% of eyes with bothersome visual symptoms improved, and 90% of eyes with recurrent erosion were free of symptoms with a mean follow-up of 30 months (57). The only prospective study evaluated 56 eyes randomized either to manual epithelial ablation alone versus manual ablation followed by excimer laser ablation, and found that the additional laser ablation significantly reduced symptoms and episodes of recurrence (58). Reis-Buckler dystrophy has also been shown to be particularly amenable to PTK, although recurrences are known to occur after the first postoperative year (32,59–62).

Treatment of corneal stromal dystrophies with PTK has also proven to be effective, especially in eyes with more superficial opacities. Success rates as high as 90% to 100% have been demonstrated in treating lattice dystrophy (7,33,35,50,63).

Granular dystrophy has also been treated with PTK with an efficacy of 66% to 100% (7,34,35,50,51,61,63,64). Although Sher et al. did not achieve improvement in vision in two patients with granular dystrophy, glare symptoms were reduced in both eyes (34). PTK studies have included only small numbers of eyes with Schnyder's dystrophy, but these have shown success in improving vision and symptoms of glare, with lengthy recurrence-free intervals and preserved visual acuity (35,51,64–67). Treatment with PTK may prevent or delay the need for PK in many of these patients. A recent study by Koreishi and colleagues compared the treatment of lattice and granular corneal dystrophies with PK versus PTK. Visual acuity outcomes at 2 years were similar, and time to recurrence was 6.7 years after PK and 4 years after PTK. Their study concluded that, because recurrences do occur after both PK and PTK, PTK is a preferred alternative to PK in appropriate patients with anterior stromal dystrophies because PTK can be repeated even on grafted corneas, and PTK avoids the potential complications of PK (68).

Scars and Nodules

Much of the literature shows variability of results for PTK in management of corneal scars. Sher and coworkers had improvement in five of eight posttraumatic and three of five postinfectious scars (34), whereas Campos et al. reported no improvement in three eyes with posttraumatic scars, but significant improvement in two of six eyes with postinfectious scars (50). More recently, Migden et al. reported on 22 eyes with corneal scars and found that posttraumatic scars had the most successful outcomes, with 4 of 8 showing visual improvement at 3 months, whereas none of the 5 postinfectious scars demonstrated significant visual improvement at three months (69). Scars secondary to herpetic keratitis are also amenable to PTK, although recurrence has been reported in up to 25% of patients, and pretreatment with a systemic antiviral medication is recommended (34,52,70). The differing depth and composition of each scar may alter the rate of ablation and result in outcome variability. The surgeon must therefore tailor the treatment to the preoperative appearance and postoperative goals in these cases.

Treatment of elevated nodules can be accomplished by PTK alone, or in conjunction with mechanical debulking. Salzmann's nodular degeneration has been treated with high rates of success (7,33,34,51,64). Topical mitomycin C as an adjuvant to PTK has been used in a recurrent nodule with a good 6-month result (71). Although some studies have shown efficacy using PTK to treat band keratopathy, ethylenediaminetetraacetic acid chelation has in general been considered the preferred method for treating band keratopathy. In also avoids the refractive change and the risk of scarring that may occur with PTK. A combination approach can be used, using the chelating agent first with supplemental PTK for residual lesions (40,72). PTK has proven useful in treating keratoconus nodules that can render patients unable to tolerate contact lenses, and may even help to delay PK (34,51,52,64,72,73). However, one case of keratolysis after PTK for a protuberant nodule has been reported (74).

Other indications for which PTK has been attempted include scarring after pterygium removal (33,34,51,52,55,64) and recurrent corneal intraepithelial dysplasia and intraepithelial corneoconjunctival carcinoma (75,76). Literature on PTK and these disorders is limited, and PTK should be undertaken with caution. Another realm of management for which PTK has been proposed includes management of PRK complications such as central islands, decentrations, and subepithelial haze, where a combined PTK-PRK approach may be best suited (77,78). Recently, PTK has been proposed to treat persistent post–laser *in situ* keratomileusis macrostriae and microstriae.

COMPLICATIONS

Postoperative complications after PTK are minimal, but have been reported in the literature (Table 65-5).

Pain

Most patients experience discomfort of varying degrees after removal of the epithelium owing to release of arachidonic acid metabolites that may stimulate pain fibers in the ciliary nerves (79). Typically, the pain starts 30 to 60 minutes after PTK and peaks at 4 to 6 hours. This can be treated with a postoperative pressure patch or a bandage contact lens and nonsteroidal antiinflammatory drops (6,80–82). Some patients also require oral pain medications such as ibuprofen or narcotics.

Persistent Epithelial Defects and Recurrent Erosions

Although most patients experience complete epithelial regrowth and diminished pain within 1 week of PTK, some

TABLE 65-5. REPORTED COMPLICATIONS AFTER PHOTOTHERAPEUTIC KERATECTOMY

Complication	References
Delayed reepithelialization	7, 35, 57, 86, 94
Herpes simplex keratitis recurrence	23, 25, 56, 57, 72, 86
Elevated intraocular pressure	7, 56
Bacterial keratitis	57, 85
Iritis	57
Graft rejection	57, 90, 91, 94
Episcleritis	86
Angle closure after cycloplegics	86

investigators report delayed wound healing as a complication. Stark et al. reported two patients in whom corneal reepithelialization was complete in 3 to 4 weeks (7,33,83). Sher et al. reported one patient for whom delayed epithelial healing took place who eventually required a PK and tarsorrhaphy (34). Commonly, other risk factors for delayed wound healing such as dry eye, diabetes, collagen vascular disease, or poor diet are present. Delayed healing can lead to haze and recurrent erosions, and can place patients at risk for corneal ulcers and persistent epithelial defects (7).

Corneal Infiltrates

Discerning among the many possible causes of postoperative corneal infiltrates may be complicated. Infectious sources should always be ruled out and appropriate cultures taken (84). Bacterial keratitis is quite rare and has been reported in a patient who was not treated with antibacterial drops after surgery (54,85). Reactivation of herpetic keratitis should also be in the differential diagnosis (22,24,53,54,70,86), and therefore it is recommended that patients be recurrence free for at least 1 year before PTK. Patients with such a history should be treated with preoperative and postoperative oral antivirals (acyclovir 400 mg orally at least twice daily), as well as a topical antiviral medication. Noninfectious corneal infiltrates can rarely be seen in patients using topical nonsteroidal agents, but they usually resolve after changing to topical corticosteroids (87).

Refractive Change

Although the goal of PTK is to treat corneal disease without inducing a refractive change, hyperopia is the most common and predictable refractive side effect of PTK. Possible reasons for the hyperopic shift include the following: (a) centrifugal plumes of debris may shield the peripheral cornea from deeper ablation; (b) decreased angle of incidence of the laser beam to the peripheral cornea may decrease laser effectiveness; and (c) increased corneal wound healing and epithelial and stromal hyperplasia at the peripheral treatment margin may create a myopic lens effect (3,15,83,88).

Undesirable hyperopia can be anticipated and minimized if the surgeon is aware that the depth of ablation correlates to the amount of induced refractive error (83). Therefore, ablation of the least amount of anterior corneal tissue needed to achieve satisfactory results should be performed. Surface-modulating agents can help by allowing elevated areas of disease to be ablated without removing surrounding tissue. The modified taper technique described by Stark et al. has been shown to result in substantially lower magnitudes of hyperopia (7). Sher et al. described both a modified taper technique of moving the patient's head under a beam of varying size, as well as a combined ablation technique where the PTK treatment was supplemented with a hyperopic ablation to the peripheral cornea (34). A combined hyperopic PRK ablation may be a promising and more accurate way to minimize induced hyperopia after PTK treatment.

Irregular astigmatism may be caused by incomplete epithelial debridement, ablation of scars with components of varying densities and ablation rates, or selective treatment of paracentral lesions. The surgeon can anticipate and minimize such potential pitfalls by mechanically debulking elevated scars, and, in some cases, completing a central PTK treatment of a paracentral lesion with the use of a masking agent.

Haze

Subepithelial scarring and stromal haze can occur because of abnormal collagen deposition after PTK. After an initial increase during the first 3 months, it usually subsides after 6 months (6,10). Visually significant corneal haze after PTK is rare after 6 months and is most often a result of deeper ablations. The role of mitomycin C in minimizing or treating haze has not yet been fully elucidated, but initial investigations are promising (89,90). Because haze is often more prominent when PTK is performed on corneal grafts, the use of mitomycin C may have a more beneficial effect. Concern about unreported or late complications suggests caution when considering the use of mitomycin C.

Graft Rejection

PK graft rejection is a rare but reported side effect of PTK (54,91–93). As a result, Epstein et al. have changed their protocol to consist of the use of 1% prednisolone every 2 hours instead of 0.1% fluorometholone after PTK in patients with a previous graft (91).

CONCLUSIONS

PTK can be an effective tool for treating a wide variety of anterior corneal disease, but it requires the surgeon to be familiar with individual patient goals and the ability of the excimer laser to achieve these goals. The best results have been demonstrated for lattice and granular corneal dystrophies, and PTK should be preferred over PK because dystrophies tend to recur in grafts. Whether ablating diffuse opacities or focal scars, improvement in functional visual acuity may be achieved with a conservative approach. Removing only the anterior portion of the lesion and limiting the depth of ablation, rather than attempting to ablate all visible opacities, minimizes haze and induced hyperopia. The rule should be to treat less rather than more because the eye can always be retreated at a later time.

In the future, additional experience will allow surgeons to manage refractive error and achieve more predictable results. Exciting technologies such as wavefront ablation may enable surgeons to combine PRK and PTK in the treatment of problematic disorders such as irregular astigmatism. For those patients whose only other option is PK, PTK may be a reasonable alternative and can be repeated for recurrence of disease. Proper patient selection, careful presurgical planning, and reasoned intraoperative and postoperative decision making can lead to highly successful results.

REFERENCES

1. Trokel SL, Srinivasan R, Braren B. Excimer laser surgery of the cornea. *Am J Ophthalmol* 1983;96:710–715.
2. Seiler T, Kahle G, Kriegerowski M. Excimer laser (193 nm) myopic keratomileusis in sighted and blind human eyes. *Refract Corneal Surg* 1990;6:165–173.
3. Wu WC, Stark WJ, Green WR. Corneal wound healing after 193-nm excimer laser keratectomy. *Arch Ophthalmol* 1991;109:1426–1432.
4. Waring GO. Development of a system for excimer laser corneal surgery. *Trans Am Ophthalmol Soc* 1989;78:854–983.
5. Krauss JM, Puliafito CA. Lasers in ophthalmology. *Lasers Surg Med* 1995;17:102–159.
6. Azar DT, Steinert RF, Stark WJ, eds. *Excimer laser phototherapeutic keratectomy: management of scars, dystrophies, and PRK complications.* Baltimore: Williams & Wilkins, 1997.
7. Stark WJ, Chamon W, Kamp MT, et al. Clinical follow-up of 193-nm ArF excimer laser photokeratectomy. *Ophthalmology* 1992;99:805–812.
8. Salz JJ, Maguen E, Macy JI, et al. One-year results of excimer laser photorefractive keratectomy for myopia. *Refract Corneal Surg* 1992;8:269–273.
9. Gaster RN, Binder PS, Coalwell K, et al. Corneal surface ablation by 193 nm excimer laser and wound healing in rabbits. *Invest Ophthalmol Vis Sci* 1989;30:90–98.
10. Tuft SJ, Zabel RW, Marshall J. Corneal repair following keratectomy: a comparison between conventional surgery and laser photoablation. *Invest Ophthalmol Vis Sci* 1989;30:1769–1777.
11. Marshall J, Trokel SL, Rothery S, et al. Photoablative reprofiling of the cornea using an excimer laser: photorefractive keratectomy. *Lasers Ophthalmol* 1986;1:21–48.
12. Hanna KD, Pouliquen Y, Waring GO III, et al. Corneal stromal wound healing in rabbits after 193-nm excimer laser surface ablation. *Arch Ophthalmol* 1989;107:895–901.
13. Fountain TR, de la Cruz Z, Green WR, et al. Reassembly of corneal epithelial adhesion structures after excimer laser keratectomy in humans. *Arch Ophthalmol* 1994;112:967–972.
14. Marshall J, Trokel SL, Rothery S et al. Long-term healing of the central cornea after photorefractive keratectomy using an excimer laser. *Ophthalmology* 1988;95:1411–1421.
15. Goodman GL, Trokel SL, Stark WJ, et al. Corneal healing following laser refractive keratectomy. *Arch Ophthalmol* 1989;107:1799–1803.
16. Dehm EJ, Puliafito CA, Adler CM, et al. Corneal endothelial injury in rabbits following excimer laser ablation at 193 and 248 nm. *Arch Ophthalmol* 1986;104:1364–1368
17. Bende T, Seiler T, Wollensak J. Side effects in excimer corneal surgery: corneal thermal gradients. *Graefes Arch Clin Exp Ophthalmol* 1988;226:277–280.
18. Ozler SA, Liaw LH, Neev J, et al. Acute ultrastructural changes of cornea after excimer laser ablation. *Invest Ophthalmol Vis Sci* 1992;33:540–506.

19. Dogru M, Katakami C, Miyashita M, et al. Visual and tear function improvement after superficial phototherapeutic keratectomy (PTK) for mid-stromal corneal scarring. *Eye* 2000;14: 779–784.
20. Dogru M, Katakami C, Miyashita M, et al. Ocular surface changes after excimer laser phototherapeutic keratectomy. *Ophthalmology* 2000;107:1144–1152.
21. Dogru M, Katakami C, Nishida T, et al. Alteration of the ocular surface with recurrence of granular/Avellino corneal dystrophy after phototherapeutic keratectomy: report of five cases and literature review. *Ophthalmology* 2001;108:810–817.
22. Vrabec MP, Anderson JA, Rock ME, et al. Electron microscopic findings in a cornea with recurrence of herpes simplex keratitis after excimer laser phototherapeutic keratectomy. *CLAO J* 1994;20:41–44.
23. Tervo T, Tuunanen T. Excimer laser and reactivation of herpes simplex keratitis. *CLAO J* 1994;20:152–153, 157.
24. Pepose JS, Laycock KA, Miller JK, et al. Reactivation of latent herpes simplex virus by excimer laser photokeratectomy. *Am J Ophthalmol* 1992;114:45–50.
25. Thompson VM. Excimer laser phototherapeutic keratectomy: clinical and surgical aspects. *Ophthalmic Surg Lasers* 1995;26: 461–472.
26. Stark WJ, Gilbert ML, Gottsch JD, et al. Optical pachometry in the measurement of anterior corneal disease: an evaluative tool for phototherapeutic keratectomy. *Arch Ophthalmol* 1990;108: 12–13.
27. Reinstein DZ, Silverman RH, Trokel SL, et al. High-frequency ultrasound digital signal processing for biometry of the cornea in planning phototherapeutic keratectomy. *Arch Ophthalmol* 1993;111:430–431.
28. Allemann N, Chamon W, Silverman RH, et al. High-frequency ultrasound quantitative analyses of corneal scarring following excimer laser keratectomy. *Arch Ophthalmol* 1993;111:968–973.
29. Pavlin CJ, Harasiewicz K, Foster FS. Ultrasound biomicroscopic assessment of the cornea following excimer laser photokeratectomy. *J Cataract Refract Surg* 1994;20[Suppl]:206–211.
30. Silverman RH, Rondeau MJ, Lizzi FL, et al. Three-dimensional high-frequency ultrasonic parameter imaging of anterior segment pathology. *Ophthalmology* 1995;102:837–843.
31. Rapuano CJ. Excimer laser phototherapeutic keratectomy. *Int Ophthalmol Clin* 1996;36:127–136.
32. Rogers C, Cohen P, Lawless M. Phototherapeutic keratectomy for Reis Bucklers' corneal dystrophy. *Aust N Z J Ophthalmol* 1993;21:247–250.
33. Hersh PS, Spinak A, Garrana R, et al. Phototherapeutic keratectomy: strategies and results in 12 eyes. *Refract Corneal Surg* 1993;9[2 Suppl]:S90–S95.
34. Sher NA, Bowers RA, Zabel RW, et al. Clinical use of the 193-nm excimer laser in the treatment of corneal scars. *Arch Ophthalmol* 1991;109:491–498.
35. Orndahl M, Fagerholm P, Fitzsimmons T, et al. Treatment of corneal dystrophies with excimer laser. *Acta Ophthalmol (Copenh)* 1994;72:235–240.
36. Lawless MA, Cohen PR, Rogers CM. Retreatment of undercorrected photorefractive keratectomy for myopia. *Refract Corneal Surg* 1994;10[Suppl]:S174–S177.
37. Fagerholm P. Phototherapeutic keratectomy: 12 years of experience. *Acta Ophthalmol Scand* 2003;81:19–32.
38. Azar DT, ed. *Refractive surgery.* Stamford, CT: Appleton & Lange, 1997.
39. Thompson V, Durrie DS, Cavanaugh TB. Philosophy and technique for excimer laser phototherapeutic keratectomy. *Refract Corneal Surg* 1993;9[2 Suppl]:S81–S85.
40. Salz JJ, McDonnell PJ, McDonald MB, eds. *Corneal laser surgery.* St. Louis: Mosby-Year Book, 1995.
41. Kornmehl EW, Steinert RF, Puliafito CA. A comparative study of masking fluids for excimer laser phototherapeutic keratectomy. *Arch Ophthalmol* 1991;109:860–863.
42. O'Brart DP, Gartry DS, Lohmann CP, et al. Treatment of band keratopathy by excimer laser phototherapeutic keratectomy: surgical techniques and long term follow up. *Br J Ophthalmol* 1993;77:702–708.
43. McDonnell JM, Garbus JJ, McDonnell PJ. Unsuccessful excimer laser phototherapeutic keratectomy: clinicopathologic correlation. *Arch Ophthalmol* 1992;110:977–979.
44. Binder PS, Anderson JA, Rock ME, et al. Human excimer laser keratectomy: clinical and histopathologic correlations. *Ophthalmology* 1994;101:979–989.
45. Stevens SX, Bowyer BL, Sanchez-Thorin JC, et al. The BioMask for treatment of corneal surface irregularities with excimer laser phototherapeutic keratectomy. *Cornea* 1999;18:155–163.
46. Kremer F, Aronsky M, Bowyer B et al. Treatment of corneal surface irregularities using BioMask as an adjunct to excimer laser phototherapeutic keratectomy. *Cornea* 2002;21:28–32.
47. Fasano AP, Moreira H, McDonnell PJ, et al. Excimer laser smoothing of a reproducible model of anterior corneal surface irregularity. *Ophthalmology* 1991;98:1782–1785.
48. Talamo JH, Steinert RF, Puliafito CA. Clinical strategies for excimer laser therapeutic keratectomy. *Refract Corneal Surg* 1992;8: 319–324.
49. Hayashi H, Maeda N, Ikeda Y, et al. Sclerotic scattering illumination during phototherapeutic keratectomy for better visualization of corneal opacities. *Am J Ophthalmol* 2003;135:559–561.
50. Campos M, Nielsen S, Szerenyi K, et al. Clinical follow-up of phototherapeutic keratectomy for treatment of corneal opacities. *Am J Ophthalmol* 1993;115:433–440.
51. Rapuano CJ, Laibson PR. Excimer laser phototherapeutic keratectomy for anterior corneal pathology. *CLAO J* 1994;20:253–257.
52. Fagerholm P, Fitzsimmons TD, Orndahl M, et al. Phototherapeutic keratectomy: long-term results in 166 eyes. *Refract Corneal Surg* 1993;9[2 Suppl]:S76–S81.
53. Starr M, Donnenfeld E, Newton M, et al. Excimer laser phototherapeutic keratectomy. *Cornea* 1996;15:557–565.
54. Maloney RK, Thompson V, Ghiselli G, et al. A prospective multicenter trial of excimer laser phototherapeutic keratectomy for corneal vision loss. The Summit Phototherapeutic Keratectomy Study Group. *Am J Ophthalmol* 1996;122:149–160.
55. Dausch D, Landesz M, Klein R, et al. Phototherapeutic keratectomy in recurrent corneal epithelial erosion. *Refract Corneal Surg* 1993;9:419–424.
56. Cavanaugh TB, Lind DM, Cutarelli PE, et al. Phototherapeutic keratectomy for recurrent erosion syndrome in anterior basement membrane dystrophy. *Ophthalmology* 1999;106:971–976.
57. Orndahl MJ, Fagerholm PP. Phototherapeutic keratectomy for map-dot-fingerprint corneal dystrophy. *Cornea* 1998;17: 595–599.
58. Ohman L, Fagerholm P. The influence of excimer laser ablation on recurrent corneal erosions: a prospective randomized study. *Cornea* 1998;17:349–352.
59. McDonnell PJ, Seiler T. Phototherapeutic keratectomy with excimer laser for Reis-Buckler's corneal dystrophy. *Refract Corneal Surg* 1992;8:306–310.
60. Lawless MA, Cohen P, Rogers C. Phototherapeutic keratectomy for Reis-Buckler's dystrophy. *Refract Corneal Surg* 1993;9[2 Suppl]: S96–S98.
61. Hahn TW, Sah WJ, Kim JH. Phototherapeutic keratectomy in nine eyes with superficial corneal diseases. *Refract Corneal Surg* 1993;9[2 Suppl]:S115–S118.
62. Dinh R, Rapuano CJ, Cohen EJ, et al. Recurrence of corneal dystrophy after excimer laser phototherapeutic keratectomy. *Ophthalmology* 1999;106:1490–1497.

63. Nassaralla BA, Garbus J, McDonnell PJ. Phototherapeutic keratectomy for granular and lattice corneal dystrophies at 1.5 to 4 years. *J Refract Surg* 1996;12:795–800.

64. Rapuano CJ, Laibson PR. Excimer laser phototherapeutic keratectomy. *CLAO J* 1993;19:235–240.

65. Paparo LG, Rapuano CJ, Raber IM, et al. Phototherapeutic keratectomy for Schnyder's crystalline corneal dystrophy. *Cornea* 2000;19:343–347.

66. Herring JH, Phillips D, McCaa CS. Phototherapeutic keratectomy for Schnyder's central crystalline dystrophy. *J Refract Surg* 1999;15:489.

67. Orndahl MJ, Fagerholm PP. Treatment of corneal dystrophies with phototherapeutic keratectomy. *J Refract Surg* 1998;14:129–135.

68. Koreishi A, Starr C, Stark WJ. Phototherapeutic keratectomy versus penetrating keratoplasty in the treatment of lattice and granular corneal dystrophies. The Association for Research in Vision and Ophthalmology, 2003.

69. Migden M, Elkins BS, Clinch TE. Phototherapeutic keratectomy for corneal scars. *Ophthalmic Surg Lasers* 1996;27[5 Suppl]:S503–S507.

70. Fagerholm P, Ohman L, Orndahl M. Phototherapeutic keratectomy in herpes simplex keratitis: clinical results in 20 patients. *Acta Ophthalmol (Copenh)* 1994;72:457–460.

71. Marcon AS, Rapuano CJ. Excimer laser phototherapeutic keratectomy retreatment of anterior basement membrane dystrophy and Salzmann's nodular degeneration with topical mitomycin C. *Cornea* 2002;21:828–830.

72. Rapuano CJ. Excimer laser phototherapeutic keratectomy: long-term results and practical considerations. *Cornea* 1997;16:151–157.

73. Ward MA, Artunduaga G, Thompson KP, et al. Phototherapeutic keratectomy for the treatment of nodular subepithelial corneal scars in patients with keratoconus who are contact lens intolerant. *CLAO J* 1995;21:130–132.

74. Lahners WJ, Russell B, Grossniklaus HE, et al. Keratolysis following excimer laser phototherapeutic keratectomy in a patient with keratoconus. *J Refract Surg* 2001;17:555–558.

75. Dausch D, Landesz M, Schroder E. Phototherapeutic keratectomy in recurrent corneal intraepithelial dysplasia. *Arch Ophthalmol* 1994;112:22–23.

76. Spadea L, Petrucci R, Balestrazzi E. Excimer laser phototherapeutic keratectomy for recurrent intraepithelial corneoconjunctival carcinoma. *J Cataract Refract Surg* 2002;28:2062–2064.

77. Majmudar PA, Forstot SL, Dennis RF, et al. Topical mitomycin-C for subepithelial fibrosis after refractive corneal surgery. *Ophthalmology* 2000;107:89–94.

78. Rachid MD, Yoo SH, Azar DT. Phototherapeutic keratectomy for decentration and central islands after photorefractive keratectomy. *Ophthalmology* 2001;108:545–552.

79. Phillips AF, Szerenyi K, Campos M, et al. Arachidonic acid metabolites after excimer laser corneal surgery. *Arch Ophthalmol* 1993;111:1273–1278.

80. Arshinoff SA, Mills MD, Haber S. Pharmacotherapy of photorefractive keratectomy. *J Cataract Refract Surg* 1996;22:1037–1034.

81. Arshinoff S, D'Addario D, Sadler C, et al. Use of topical nonsteroidal anti-inflammatory drugs in excimer laser photorefractive keratectomy. *J Cataract Refract Surg* 1994;20[Suppl]:216–222.

82. Sher NA, Frantz JM, Talley A, et al. Topical diclofenac in the treatment of ocular pain after excimer photorefractive keratectomy. *Refract Corneal Surg* 1993;9:425–436.

83. Chamon W, Azar DT, Stark WJ, et al. Phototherapeutic keratectomy. *Ophthalmol Clin North Am* 1993;6:399–418.

84. Trudo EW, Stark WJ, Azar DT. Phototherapeutic keratectomy. In: Kaufman HE, Barron BA, McDonald MB, eds. *The cornea*, 2nd ed. Boston: Butterworth-Heinemann, 1998:749–759.

85. Fulton JC, Cohen EJ, Rapuano CJ. Bacterial ulcer 3 days after excimer laser phototherapeutic keratectomy. *Arch Ophthalmol* 1996;114:626–666.

86. Zuckerman SJ, Aquavella JV, Park SB. Analysis of the efficacy and safety of excimer laser PTK in the treatment of corneal disease. *Cornea* 1996;15:9–14.

87. Sher NA, Krueger RR, Teal P, et al. Role of topical corticosteroids and nonsteroidal antiinflammatory drugs in the etiology of stromal infiltrates after excimer photorefractive keratectomy. *Refract Corneal Surg* 1994;10:587–588.

88. Azar DT, Spurr-Michaud SJ, Tisdale AS, et al. Reassembly of the corneal epithelial adhesion structures following human epikeratoplasty. *Arch Ophthalmol* 1991;109:1279–1284.

89. Talamo JH, Gollamudi S, Green WR, et al. Modulation of corneal wound healing after excimer laser keratomileusis using topical mitomycin C and steroids. *Arch Ophthalmol* 1991;109:1141–1146.

90. Jain S, McCally RL, Connolly PJ, et al. Mitomycin C reduces corneal light scattering after excimer keratectomy. *Cornea.* 2001;20:45–49

91. Epstein RJ, Robin JB. Corneal graft rejection episode after excimer laser phototherapeutic keratectomy. *Arch Ophthalmol* 1994;112:157.

92. Hersh PS, Jordan AJ, Mayers M. Corneal graft rejection episode after excimer laser phototherapeutic keratectomy. *Arch Ophthalmol* 1993;111:735–736.

93. Hersh PS, Burnstein Y, Carr J, et al. Excimer laser phototherapeutic keratectomy: surgical strategies and clinical outcomes. *Ophthalmology* 1996;103:1210–1222.

KERATOPROSTHESIS SURGERY

CLAES H. DOHLMAN AND MAHNAZ NOURI

Why should we attempt to develop keratoprostheses (KPro) for corneal opacity when standard corneal transplantation is so well established and relatively safe? If the latter procedure were uniformly successful, there certainly would be no need for a KPro, with its even higher risks and greater demands on health resources. The answer lies in the stubborn failure rate of keratoplasty, in spite of a century of development. The outcome of keratoplasty varies markedly with underlying disease, geography, availability of donor tissue, health budget, and other factors, and it is still poorly documented. Some statistics are beginning to emerge, however, even if they are not population based but instead drawn from individual surgeons' office practices—which automatically excludes the "inoperable" cases. For instance, the Eye Bank Association of America's report for 2002 indicates that of a total of 33,000 transplants in the United States, more than 13% were done for failed grafts (1). (It is not known how many graft failures were *not* reoperated.) In a large outcome study, only 20% of regrafts for all causes remained clear for 5 years (2). In another group of first regrafts, again only 20% survived 5 years, whereas all *repeat* regrafts failed within the same time period (3). Moreover, on a world-wide basis, a large number of people with corneal blindness have no access to corneal surgery. The World Health Organization reports that approximately 6 million people are bilaterally blind from trachoma alone (4). Few of these patients receive a corneal transplant, and when it is performed, the failure rate is reportedly high.

The fact that standard keratoplasties have failed or have been deemed hopeless in such a large cohort of corneal patients does not automatically mean that a KPro is the immediate next step. In spite of efforts by fearless surgeons over 200 years, progress in developing long-lasting and safe KPro techniques has been slow. Creation of meaningful animal models has been difficult, and the long delay in the development of postoperative complications, many of them catastrophic, has made changes in technique and design slow in coming and hard to interpret. In spite of these impediments, however, very substantial progress has been made, especially during the past few decades. Rapid rehabilitation and sometimes spectacular vision in KPro eyes after corneal graft failures is now no longer a rarity. The long history of KPro development will not be detailed here—the reader is referred to earlier reviews (5,6).

The current KPro effort is maintained primarily in approximately a dozen centers worldwide and encompasses diverse approaches. One technique has been inspired by Strampelli (7), and a number of followers have modified the original principles further [Falcinelli et al. (8), Marchi et al. (9), Temprano (10), Grabner et al. (11), Liu et al. (12), Hille (13), and others]. This technique involves harvesting a tooth from the patient and preparing a slice of osteodental lamina to be used as a skirt for a cylinder of polymethylmethacrylate (PMMA), which is to be inserted (in two steps) into the patient's cornea and covered by lid skin or buccal mucosal graft. The procedure is somewhat invasive but it has a reputation for stability and low rate of infection. Pintucci et al. (14), Girard et al. (15), Legeais et al. (16), and others have replaced the autologous tooth-derived skirt with "biocolonizable" porous plastic materials. In Russia, a large number of patients, especially with chemical burns, have been implanted with devices of different designs, but the optical core is still being made of PMMA (17,18). Yet another approach has been to develop a hydrogel sheet with porous edges to serve as an "artificial cornea." It is implanted intrastromally and covered by a conjunctival flap. The center of the device is exposed later. This technique appears to be of value for graft failures in less inflamed eyes (19). Many smaller-scale efforts, some ingenious, are also currently under way (20).

In Boston, we have for a number of years used a PMMA KPro of a double-plated "collar button" design (21). Such a general configuration has been suggested in the past (22,23), and has been modified by us as described in the following section. Design and material of KPros are undoubtedly important in themselves, but it should be emphasized that the health of the surrounding tissue is vitally important. Without claiming superiority, we devote this chapter to the devices, surgical techniques, and follow-up routines that we have gradually developed.

DEVICES

The double-plated, or "collar button"–shaped devices we currently use come in two main designs (Fig. 66-1). The simple collar button (type I) is the most frequently used and is favored in eyes with reasonable blink and tear secretion mechanisms. Made of medical-grade PMMA, it consists of an anterior part with a 6-mm diameter front plate with an attached 3.35-mm stem with screw threads. A separate back plate is 7 mm in diameter and has eight holes, each 1.3 mm in diameter. The holes facilitate nutrition and hydration of the corneal graft, which is sandwiched between the two plates on completion (Fig. 66-1). Different modifications have been used in the past.

The type II device is similar except that it has a 2-mm long anterior nub designed to penetrate the skin or buccal mucosa in end-stage dry eyes (Fig. 66-1). The diameter of the front plate is now 6 mm. A posterior plate of 8.5-mm diameter is usually chosen. It has eight holes, each 1.5 mm in diameter.

The latest type I KPro has an anterior–posterior length of 3.7 mm and allows a maximum field of vision of 60 degrees. Type II is 4.7 mm long and can give a 40-degree field of vision. Details of the fabrication of these KPros have been described elsewhere (24).

PROGNOSTIC CATEGORIES AND INDICATIONS

Analysis of our KPro results has clearly shown the detrimental role that inflammation, past and present, has on the long-term outcome. Severe inflammatory diseases carry a much worse prognosis for the KPro than after graft failures in noninflammatory conditions. This means that presumed autoimmune diseases such as pemphigoid, Stevens-Johnson syndrome, uveitis, and so forth, as well as past severe chemical burn, have a quite guarded prognosis. On the other hand, graft failures in relatively noninflammatory situations, such as when the initial condition was a corneal dystrophy or other edematous condition, or trauma, have good prognosis. Also, after infectious keratitis (bacterial, viral, fungal), long-term success is likely (25).

In more specific terms, we believe that a KPro type I is indicated in the nonautoimmune graft failure group, where blink and tear mechanisms are reasonably normal, and when visual acuity is less than 20/400. Also, the opposite eye should have suboptimal vision, such as 20/80 or less. When survival time is uncertain, old age strengthens this indication.

End-stage dry eyes (e.g., pemphigoid, Stevens-Johnson syndrome, some chemical burns) need a type II device,

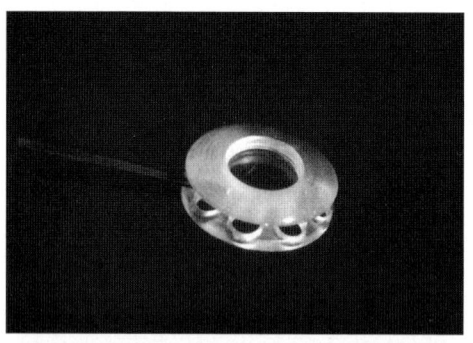
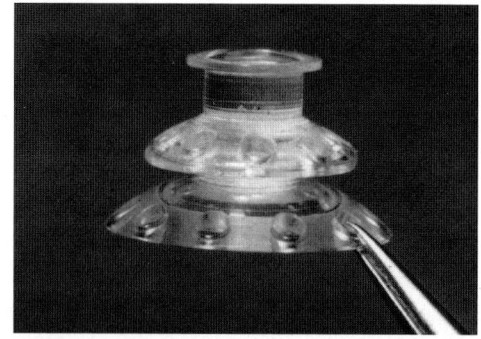
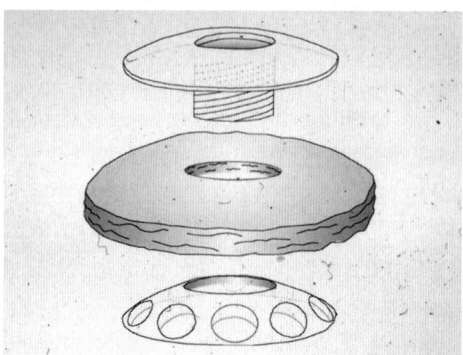
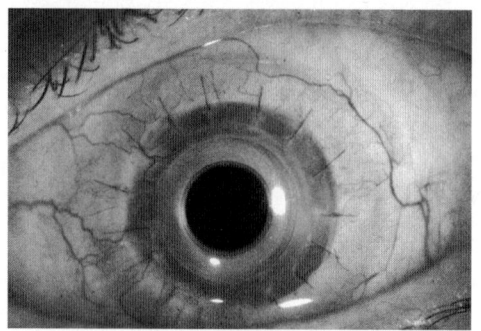

FIGURE 66-1. *Upper left*: The type I double-plated keratoprosthesis (KPro), the type most commonly used. It requires reasonably intact tear secretion and blink frequency. *Upper right*: The type II KPro, with a nub, is reserved for through-the-lid placement in end-stage dry eyes. *Lower left*: Principle of assembly of a type I KPro. A fresh corneal graft, with a punched 3-mm hole, is slid over the stem and the back plate is screwed on. The graft–KPro combination is then sutured in place like a standard corneal graft. The holes in the back plate facilitate nutrition and hydration of the overlying graft tissue. *Lower right*: Large-diameter soft contact lenses, worn indefinitely (with replacements), have proven highly protective of the corneal surface around the KPro.

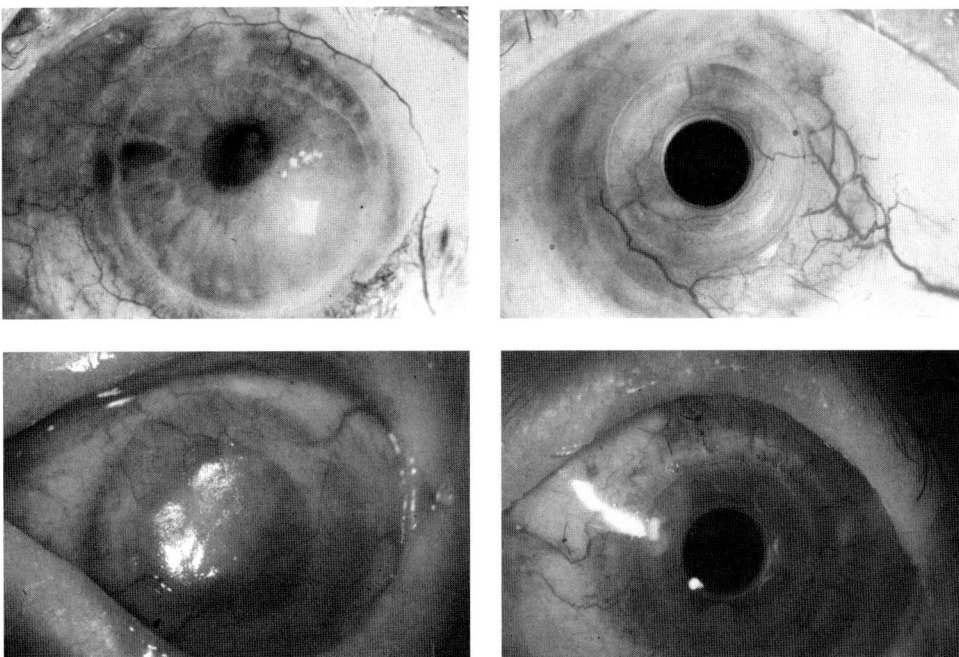

FIGURE 66-2. *Upper left*: Eye with repeated graft failures in lattice dystrophy. *Upper right*: Same patient as in *upper left*, 10 years after type I keratoprosthesis (KPro) insertion with a conjunctival flap. Vision is 20/20. *Lower left*: Long-standing Stevens-Johnson syndrome. *Lower right*: Same patient as in *lower left*; the KPro type I has been followed for 1 year and vision is 20/40.

which involves not only more complicated surgery, but a closer follow-up regimen and more frequent need for revision (26). The surgeon taking on this type of KPro surgery must be prepared to follow the patient for a lifetime.

PATIENT EVALUATION

History

Documenting a detailed history of the ocular condition, as well as any important systemic disease, is mandatory. Duration of ocular symptoms (episodic, such as in herpes simplex, or steadily progressive), unilateral or bilateral, and status of the opposite eye should be explored in detail. Precise knowledge about previous surgery (e.g., cataract extraction, keratoplasty, glaucoma surgery, retina repair) is obviously crucial. A history of glaucoma is extremely important to solicit, especially after chemical burns, because the extent of optic nerve damage at the time of the examination is often very difficult to evaluate.

Visual Acuity

Standard refraction using a Snellen chart is usually sufficient to evaluate the degree of visual impairment. The next step, to ascribe relative contributions to the cornea, cataract, retina, or optic nerve disease, is not always easy in eyes that are so severely damaged that they are candidates for KPro. The corneal influence can be due to irregular surface or to stromal opacities, a question that can be solved by hard contact lens refraction. A visual field is rarely possible in these cases, but gross projection of a strong light source can be revealing. If nasal projection is absent and, particularly, if central fixation is uncertain, end-stage glaucoma with only finger-counting potential must be suspected.

Intraocular Pressure

Evaluation of the pressure in eyes with severely damaged cornea can be difficult and unreliable. The pneumotonometer is of more help than the applanation device, but both can give grossly erroneous readings. The phosphene tonometer is rarely of use when lids are thickened or when the visual field is restricted. Simple digital palpation gives only an approximate impression, but it is frequently the most reliable approach.

Blink Rate and Tear Secretion

Because evaporative damage to the corneal tissue around a KPro type I can be very detrimental, especially if a soft contact lens cannot be retained, tear film stability is very important. Therefore, poor blink rate and chronic exposure, as well as low tear secretion, must be taken into consideration. Blink rate and completeness should be noted before surgery when the patient does not feel he or she is being observed. Tear secretion should be evaluated with a standard Schirmer's test. Quantifying breakup time is of little preoperative value.

Slit-Lamp Examination

This procedure is the cornerstone of the patient evaluation. The corneal surface should be judged for irregularity, keratinization, epithelial defects, and subepithelial vascularization. Stromal opacities, thickness, edema, and deep blood vessels should be evaluated separately, and drawings made. The lid structures should be inspected for lid surface incongruities, and the conjunctiva may show inflammation, important fornix shortening, or frank symblephara. Anterior chamber depth, appearance of pupil and iris, angle (narrow, closed?), the status of the lens or intraocular lens, all merit detailed notes in the record. The fundus is rarely seen well in KPro candidates, but an effort should be made to examine it with a 78- or 90-D lens and, if possible, the disk appearance recorded. Gross macular changes, such as massive age-related macular degeneration, may be observable. Indirect ophthalmoscopy of the peripheral retina should at least be attempted. During these maneuvers, special attention should be given to signs of inflammation, past or present, because of its importance for the prognosis of the contemplated KPro surgery.

Special Examinations

Ultrasonographic examination is necessary in most cases being evaluated for KPro. A retinal detachment must be ruled out with B-scan ultrasonography. This mode can also illuminate presence and degree of vitreous debris, but it cannot measure a glaucomatous optic nerve cupping with precision. Absence of a visible cup on the ultrasonogram does not guarantee a healthy nerve. If a glaucoma shunt has been previously implanted, a fluid cleft over the plate can usually be identified and, if present, it ensures patency of the intraocular tube. However, a visible cleft does not rule out existence of a dense capsule that has formed around the plate and which can obstruct flow enough to cause an unacceptably high intraocular pressure. Also, a B-scan can reveal the presence or absence of an intraocular lens. An A-scan measurement of the axial length of the eye is also mandatory to allow the selection of a KPro with the appropriate dioptric power. In our experience, electroretinography and visual evoked response are not of much value in KPro preoperative evaluation.

Documentation

External photography and detailed drawings, before and after surgery, are very important for documentation of outcome, including complications. A brief sketch should be made in the record at every visit, ideally using easily identifiable color-coding (e.g., blue for edema, green for epithelial defect, pencil for opacity, red for vessels).

PREPARATION FOR SURGERY

Preparation for KPro surgery includes the following:

1. A KPro, type I or II, with dioptric power for pseudophakia or aphakia (to match axial length of recipient eye), as well as back plate, should be obtained from the Massachusetts Eye and Ear Infirmary (243 Charles Street, Boston, MA 02114). Included with the KPro is a 3-mm punch (Acuderm Inc., Fort Lauderdale, FL), a wrench for the back plate and, for type I, an adhesive patch for stabilizing assembly, as well as a soft contact lens (Kontur Lens, 16-mm diameter, 9.8-mm base curve, plano; Kontur Contact Lens Co., Richmond, CA), and, for type II, dried pericardium (New World Medical, Inc., Rancho Cucamonga, CA, or other source).

2. Standard keratoplasty instruments should include a Troutman punch (Pilling Weck Surgical, Fort Washington, PA) or similar instrument. Fine bipolar cautery is mandatory. Katzin scissors (Storz #E3232 and E3233) are recommended for excision of the patient's cornea.

3. Trephine blades (Storz-long) and a universal handle (Storz #E3095). If the front plate of the KPro has a diameter of 6 mm, a blade of 8.5-mm diameter should be used for trephining of the graft, and an 8-mm blade should be selected for the patient's eye. If the KPro front plate is 7 mm, trephine blades of 1-mm larger diameters are required, thus 9.5 and 9 mm. A Hessberg-Barron vacuum trephine (Barron Precision Instruments, Grand Blanc, MI) is rarely usable on the patient's eye owing to surface irregularities.

4. Irrigation/aspiration unit, vitrector, and light pipe.

5. Dexamethasone phosphate solution (4 mg/mL) or triamcinolone acetonide (40 mg/mL), tuberculin syringe, and 27- or 30-gauge cannula or needle; fluoroquinolone drops (avoid sulfa-containing antibiotics); viscoelastics optional.

6. If needed, glaucoma valve shunt (Ahmed S-2) and dried pericardium (see earlier).

7. Video (optional).

8. Preoperative medical clearance.

9. General anesthesia preferred, when medically safe.

10. Prophylactic intravenous antibiotic (e.g., cefazolin 1 g, if no allergy) is recommended at the start of surgery.

TYPE I SURGERY

Assembly of the Keratoprosthesis

The first step of the operation consists of the implantation of the KPro into a fresh corneal graft (Fig. 66-1). Preferably on a small side table, the donor cornea is brought out and placed in the well of a Troutman punch loaded with an 8.5-mm trephine blade (9.5-mm blade if the KPro front plate is 7 mm in diameter instead of 6 mm). After the trephination, the center of the endothelial side is briefly blotted with a cellulose sponge and marked with a dye pen. Using the 3-mm punch, a hole is made in the graft as central as possible.

The KPro front part and back plate (they are usually packaged separately) are brought out and sterility indicators checked. The adhesive patch, included in the package, has the bottom cover layer removed and is pressed against a hard surface such as the Troutman plate. The top cover is then peeled off, exposing the adhesive surface. The KPro front part is now pressed to the adhesive, front plate down, facilitating subsequent assembly. The corneal graft is placed on top and slid over the stem, a step that is completed by gentle pressure with the hollowed end of the white wrench pin. Excessive pressure should be avoided. Finally, the back plate is placed on the stem, the wrench is applied to the holes of the plate, and the latter is screwed on until resistance is encountered. To avoid damage to the screw threads, it is advisable first to rotate the wrench briefly *counterclockwise* until the threads feel engaged, and then rotate clockwise until firm resistance is met. If the adhesive patch should become wet and slippery, thereby making the tightening of the back plate difficult, the surgeon must grasp the front plate edge by the fingernails and apply reasonable pressure. The very unlikely possibility of the posterior plate slowly unscrewing in the eye after surgery can be prevented with a locking ring, supplied with the device. The hibanium ring is snapped into a groove in the stern behind the back plate, locking it in position. The fully assembled graft–KPro combination is finally placed back into the storage solution to await the preparatory work on the recipient eye.

The Recipient Eye

The patient's eye should be prepared in the standard manner by cleaning lids and lid margins with 10% povidone–iodine solution (harmless if reaching the ocular surface), and application of drapes. We prefer a Weiner speculum to expose the eye. Canthotomy or lysing of symblepharons may be necessary. A trephine blade of appropriate diameter is chosen (1 mm larger diameter than the front plate of the KPro, hence usually 8 mm). The blade is attached to the hand-held trephine handle. A vacuum trephine is preferable but is often unusable because of the irregular surface of the cornea, which can prevent sustainable vacuum. If the recipient cornea is vascularized—and it usually is—it is advisable initially to trephine only half-way through the cornea and to cauterize the groove before proceeding. This is important to prevent later infiltration of the vitreous with blood. The cautery is most effectively done with fine bipolar jewelry forceps cautery, and the groove should be dry at the end. This unavoidably causes some tissue shrinkage, but this is harmless because the graft

is prepared with a 0.5-mm larger diameter. Application of epinephrine in a 1:10,000 dilution can also augment hemostasis. Finally, the wound is opened with a sharp knife and the excision is completed with cornea scissors in standard manner.

The status of the iris is assessed next. The iris and pupil should be left intact, if possible, to prevent excessive postoperative glare. This may in the long run result in angle-closure glaucoma, but that problem will then have to be addressed with glaucoma medication or a valve shunt. In addition, removal of the iris by the root can result in postoperative bleeds, especially in the presence of intraocular steroids. Large iridectomies may have to be closed with 10-0 nylon sutures, again to prevent glare. A small sphincterotomy may be necessary if the pupil appears eccentric.

The lens issue is then addressed. In fact, it will have been decided before surgery so that the appropriate KPro is made available. If the eye is pseudophakic, it is advisable to leave the intraocular lens in place and have a KPro with the optical power to match, that is, with a back focal length in air of approximately 20 mm. If the natural lens is in place, it is recommended that it be removed, regardless of whether cataractous. Later cataract extraction could be complicated and risky. We advise extracapsular extraction, leaving the posterior capsule to constrain the vitreous. Should the capsule opacify later, a yttrium-aluminum garnet (YAG) laser capsulotomy is usually easy to perform. In an aphakic eye, the anterior vitreous surface is rarely unbroken, but if it is, it can be left intact. Otherwise, a moderate open-sky core vitrectomy should be done, avoiding getting too close to the ciliary body or a region where tugging on poorly visible strands may lead to retinal detachment. It is particularly important to remove any heme that may have seeped down during the procedure. If a more extensive open-sky vitrectomy should be necessary, an experienced vitreoretinal specialist should be co-surgeon.

For the eye ending up aphakic, it is important to select a KPro with dioptric power to match the axial length of the eye. A-scan ultrasonography provides the surgeon with the necessary information before ordering the device.

The final step is to transfer the graft–KPro combination from its storage solution to the eye. The oversized graft (0.5 mm larger than the trephine opening) is sutured in place in the standard manner with 16 10-0 nylon interrupted sutures, burying the knots. The anterior chamber is temporarily deepened with saline to ensure that the iris has not been inadvertently incorporated into the wound. We follow with injection of 400 μg dexamethasone into the anterior chamber, using a tuberculin syringe with a 30-gauge cannula. The steroids reduce postoperative inflammatory reaction but threaten immediate wound healing, and therefore discretion is advised. A few drops of antibiotics (e.g., a fluoroquinolone) are applied to the eye, followed by application of a soft contact lens (see earlier).

Permanent use of a soft contact lens is usually highly desirable in a KPro type I eye, but loss of lens or need for replacement is fairly frequent, and therefore somewhat expensive (Fig. 66-1). A total conjunctival flap at the time of KPro surgery can have the same protective effect as a soft contact lens, and this approach can be more practical in developing countries. A wide, fairly thick flap is mobilized from above or the temporal side of the eye and anchored securely with 10-0 nylon. All corneal and conjunctival epithelium beneath the flap must have been removed, by scraping or alcohol, to allow the connective tissue surfaces to adhere well. A central 3-mm opening is done at the end of surgery—this opening later slowly expands to the edge of the front plate. In general, although mobilization of a conjunctival flap substantially prolongs surgery time, it has a very protective effect, and it is of special value in patients with tear or blink deficiencies or in a dry climate (27). In extreme exposure situations, permanent tarsorrhaphies may be necessary to protect the ocular surface tissues. This can be arranged in such a way that only the plastic is exposed to air, although the ability to blink in such cases has usually been sacrificed.

For further details on type I KPro surgery, see a recent review by Dohlman et al. (28).

TYPE II SURGERY

Assembly of the Keratoprosthesis

The principle of assembly of a type II device is very similar to that of type I. A corneal graft, usually 9.5 mm in diameter, is trephined and a central 3-mm hole is punched. The graft is slid over the stem and the back plate is screwed on tightly. The surgeon facilitates this maneuver by holding the nub between his or her fingers. The KPro–graft combination is then stored in the storage solution until ready for transfer.

The Patient

In this through-the-lid approach, the KPro and the cornea will be covered with lid skin, although another alternative is to use buccal mucosa. Our experience has dealt primarily with the skin coverage method, which is briefly described here.

The lid skin of the upper and lower lids are separated from underlying tissue (lid margin, tarsus, some orbicularis, tarsal conjunctiva). This is done by making a lid-long incision approximately 2 mm distal to the lash line down to the tarsus and dissecting the skin approximately 10 mm toward the lid base. The remaining portion of the lid is clamped with a hemostat and sliced off using a #15 Bard-Parker blade. Next, all bulbar conjunctiva and corneal pannus is dissected away completely so that no epithelium is left. This is in principle straightforward, but in practice

quite tedious. In situations where a type II KPro is indicated, such as end-stage dry eye in pemphigoid or Stevens-Johnson syndrome, bleeding during dissection can be profuse and prolonged and take prolonged cautery to still. In the end, the lid skin above and below will be held back by 4-0 silk stay sutures, baring the now deepithelialized, nonbleeding ocular surface. The rest of the procedure on the eye itself is the same as in type I surgery. The corneal stroma in these conditions is usually so heavily vascularized that heavy cautery of the preliminary nonpenetrating trephining is often required to prevent subsequent bleeding into the eye. Steroids and antibiotics are given as in the type I procedure.

When the graft with its KPro is finally sutured in place (9-0 nylon interrupted sutures, knots need not be buried), we sometimes apply a layer of dried pericardium (see earlier) over the KPro front plate to increase the eventual lid thickness. A disk of the pericardium is cut to approximately 15-mm diameter and a central 3-mm hole is punched. This disk, aided by a short radial cut from the hole, is slid over the nub and left unsutured. The lid skin edges are now approximated and sutured together with 6-0 nylon or 8-0 nylon, covering the KPro completely. The wound will end up below the KPro nub, which can be felt through the skin.

The final step is to expose the nub. A mark is made where it is felt and a small horizontal incision is made into the skin and the subcutaneous tissue, with care taken not to scratch the soft plastic with the knife. When the nub is totally exposed, the skin edges must be sutured to the level of the front flange, otherwise the edematous edges have a tendency quickly to grow over the nub, requiring skin revision later. This fixation can be done by tying a loop of 8-0 nylon around the nub, passing the needle twice through the upper lid skin edge, and tying tightly. The same procedure is repeated for the lower skin edge, and finally skin-to-skin sutures (tight) are placed on both sides of the nub. In this way, the position is stabilized until the skin has lost its postoperative edema and begun to fall back. This suturing procedure is quite effective but also time-consuming. The whole operation usually takes approximately 4 hours.

GLAUCOMA SURGERY

Glaucoma is a major problem after KPro surgery. A substantial percentage of the eyes that have corneas so damaged by disease that they are candidates for a KPro also have preoperative glaucoma. After surgery, the glaucoma often worsens. Also, many patients with initially normal pressure suffer pressure complications after surgery. The problem is aggravated by the difficulty in assessing the intraocular pressure in the presence of the rigid plate in the cornea. No standard tonometer can be used accurately, and a phosphene tonometer has limited value. Palpation by fingers is, in spite of its great imprecision, a very valuable, in fact crucial, method. Disk appearance and visual fields should obviously be followed whenever possible. Medical treatment also has its limitations after KPro. Glaucoma drops are effective after type I surgery (enough medication passes through the peripheral cornea), but not after type II. Here, only systemic carbonic anhydrase inhibitors are available. All these circumstances have emphasized the frequent need of glaucoma shunts in KPro recipients (29).

The shunt we use is primarily the Ahmed S-2 valve shunt. This device can obviously be implanted before, during, or after KPro surgery. If the shunt is part of the KPro procedure, it should be implanted before opening the eye, hence after the nonpenetrating trephination of the patient's cornea and cautery of the groove. We now realize that the tube should end up centrally, close to the KPro, with its opening visible through the stem. This way, any blockage of the tube opening becomes visible and it is possible to clear it with YAG laser. A centrally located tube does not decrease vision, contrary to expectations.

POSTOPERATIVE CARE

Type I Keratoprosthesis

The patient should be seen on the first postoperative day and symptoms, such as pain during the night, should be registered. The visual acuity is recorded in the standard way and the intraocular pressure estimated by finger palpation. After cleaning the lid margins, a detailed slit-lamp examination should include observation of the position of the soft contact lens, the graft wound, the degree of inflammation in the anterior chamber, the presence of blood or vitreous, and the position of iris and pupil. If possible, the fundus should be examined using a 78- or 90-D lens. Especially important are the signs of inflammation because their degree dictates the level of postoperative steroid treatment. Subsequent visits are routinely scheduled after 1 week, another 2 weeks, then monthly for the first half year. Subsequent intervals are typically 2 to 3 months (Fig. 66-2).

Standard postoperative medication include fluoroquinolone drops and prednisolone acetate 1% suspension, initially four times daily, but after a week or two the frequency can be reduced to twice a day. This level of medication, with some modifications, should be kept up *for life*, a point that would have been stressed to the patient already before surgery. Antibiotics can be alternated in the future, and the steroid medication should be adjusted according to signs of inflammation or concomitant glaucoma. If postoperative inflammation is excessive, an occasional peribulbar injection of 40 mg triamcinolone is indicated. Alternatively, oral prednisone, starting at 60 mg/day, can be given, but excessive steroid doses too early can jeopardize graft wound healing and result in aqueous leak. Systemic antibiotics are recommended, such as cephalexin 500 mg two or three times a day for a week after the surgery, unless penicillin allergy dictates a substitute.

If elevation of the intraocular pressure is suspected, standard glaucoma drops are effective. Enough medication diffuses into the eye around the plastic plates, as witnessed by the effect of dilating drops on the pupil. Oral carbonic anhydrase inhibitors have the usual effect on the pressure. Inspection of the optic disk should be performed at every visit, if possible, and visual field examination done when needed. If glaucoma is present, it may be advisable to have a glaucoma subspecialist follow the patient at regular intervals.

Type II Keratoprosthesis

This type of surgery requires observation and follow-up similar to that with type I, with some differences. A type II through-the-lid procedure is done only in end-stage dry eyes in autoimmune diseases, or after very severe chemical burns. Therefore, a more severe inflammatory response is to be expected, requiring larger doses of postoperative steroids. A retroprosthesis membrane is more apt to form in this situation (see later). Skin retraction away from the nub is also a complication peculiar to the type II KPro, and should be looked for at every visit. The 8-0 nylon sutures around the nub can be removed after a month, but they are not easily cut because of their position. Cleaning of the nub surface can be easily performed using Johnson & Johnson baby shampoo on a cellulose sponge, followed by irrigation with balanced salt solution.

KPros in autoimmune diseases (e.g., pemphigoid, Stevens-Johnson syndrome, graft-versus-host disease, Sjögren's syndrome) are much more subject to infection and endophthalmitis than in nonautoimmune patients. Our experience has been that fluoroquinolone drops alone are not sufficient to protect against endophthalmitis (30). Therefore, we now routinely add vancomycin drops (14 mg/mL) to the nub, initially four times a day, later twice daily (31). In addition, we give medroxyprogesterone 1% suspension twice daily, which we believe retards skin retraction around the nub (32) (Fig. 66-3).

COMPLICATIONS

Loss of the Soft Contact Lens in Type I

Addition of a soft contact lens after KPro type I surgery and keeping it (or replacements) in place for an indefinite time has been a remarkable boon to the health of the tissue around the device. Epithelial defects, drying, dellen, and other surface complications have been markedly reduced. It seems that the soft lens effectively diffuses the evaporative forces and allows the tissue to remain hydrated and healthy (33).

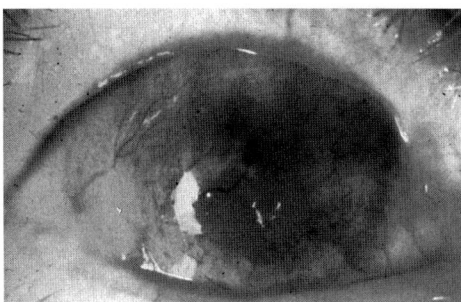 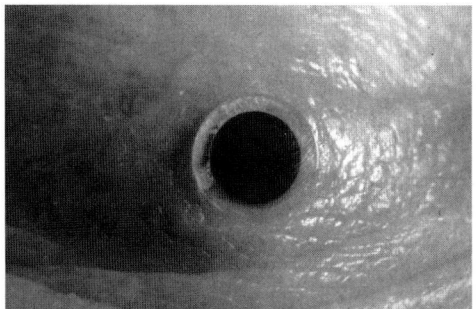

FIGURE 66-3. Before and after type II keratoprosthesis insertion in ocular pemphigoid. Observation time was 6 years until the patient's death, and vision was 20/30.

At surgery we usually use a Kontur lens (see earlier) with a 16-mm diameter and a 9.8-mm base curve. Later, with steepening of the corneal–KPro surface, a larger lens with an 18- or 20-mm diameter and 7-mm base curve may be substituted. If the lens is lost repeatedly and the condition of the ocular surface seems to require its presence, a small temporal tarsorrhaphy may be required. If the patient has lost much iris tissue during previous disease processes, postoperative glare may be bothersome, and even intolerable in chemical burn cases. In such situations, a tinted lens with central clear zone can be highly effective.

Inflammation

Many eyes that end up with KPro surgery have had numerous previous interventions and episodes of inflammation. This can result in chronic post-KPro inflammation that in turn may result in glaucoma, retroprosthetic membrane, or even epiretinal membrane. As mentioned previously, particularly severe autoimmune diseases, as well as chemical burn, fall into this category. Corticosteroids are the standard treatment to suppress such developments. In the type I KPro, topical prednisolone drops (see earlier) are routine, sometimes augmented by peribulbar injections of triamcinolone, 20 to 40 mg. Systemic steroids are used uncommonly because of a less favorable risk–benefit ratio. After type II surgery, no antiinflammatory drops can reach the anterior chamber, and therefore peribulbar/subtenon injections or systemic steroids are the only means to influence intraocular events. Other types of systemic immunosuppression are rarely indicated, but if the patient has an active systemic immune process, treatment may be indicated, although it should preferably be directed by a colleague with special expertise in this field.

Retroprosthesis Membrane

Such membranes are rare after KPro in previously noninflamed cases. In patients whose history includes longstanding preoperative inflammation, however, a gradually developing membrane often occurs adjacent to the back KPro surface. Usually they can be opened by YAG laser (34). Energy higher than 2 mJ should be avoided, however, because the plastic can become pockmarked or cracked. Also, a posterior lens capsule often opacifies, requiring the same treatment. A peribulbar injection of 40 mg triamcinolone is recommended afterward (Fig. 66-4).

If the retroprosthesis membrane has become very thick and leathery, it requires surgical breaking up, using a 25-gauge needle or a Ziegler (or Haab) knife. When blood vessels have clearly invaded the membrane, it is necessary to resort to a three-port membranectomy under high infusion pressure to close the vessels (by a vitreoretinal surgeon) (35). In some cases, it is preferable to repeat the whole KPro procedure, this time prepared to give higher doses of postoperative steroids.

Endophthalmitis–Sterile Vitreitis

Sudden, disastrous bacterial endophthalmitis was in the past not uncommon after KPro surgery and was the main obstacle to more widespread use of the procedure. Even more recently, endophthalmitis could occur in Stevens-Johnson syndrome and pemphigoid, even while on prophylactic fluoroquinolone drops or polymyxin B/trimethoprim drops (30). In our experience, the infectious agents were all gram-positive organisms. However, after adding vancomycin drops 4 years ago to the fluoroquinolone regimen, no bacterial endophthalmitis has occurred (31). Therefore, we consider this combination mandatory in autoimmune diseases and burns (mostly type II)—for life. No vancomycin resistance has emerged. In the much more common type I procedures in nonautoimmune situations, fluoroquinolone drops alone twice daily should be enough. These regimens require strict compliance, however, or the risk of infection is not eliminated.

Should ocular pain, redness, and decreased vision suddenly occur, and fibrin be visible in the anterior chamber, the standard diagnostic and therapeutic measures for endophthalmitis should be undertaken immediately. Aqueous or vitreous tap for smear and culture, followed by injection of 1 mg vancomycin, 0.4 mg amikacin, and 0.4 mg

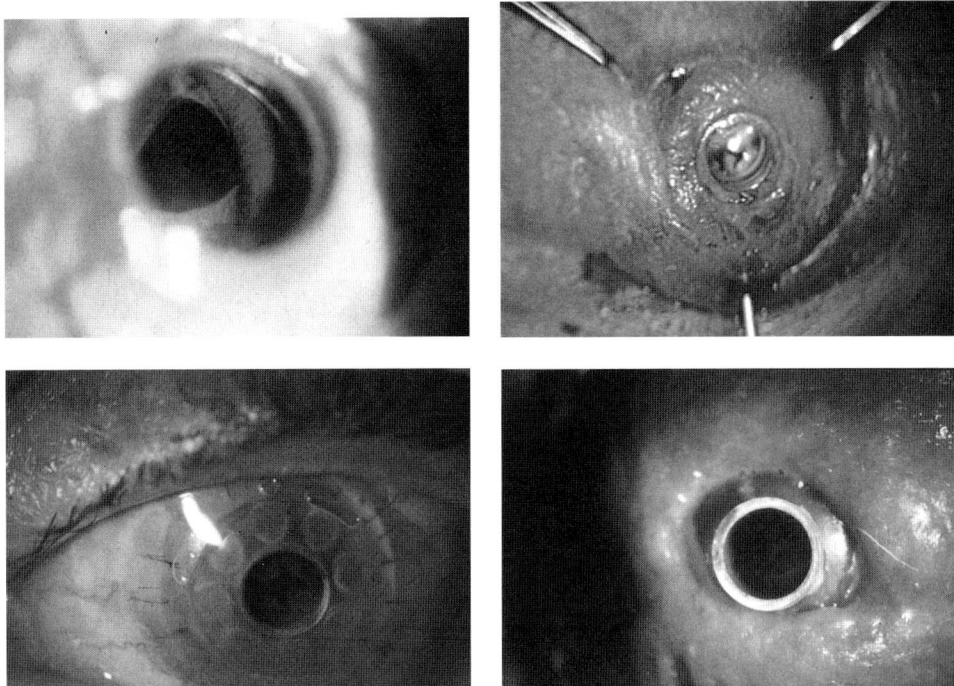

FIGURE 66-4. *Upper left*: In cases with prolonged postoperative inflammation, a retroprosthesis membrane can form. If thin, it can be readily broken up with the YAG laser. *Upper right*: In more severely inflamed cases, laser treatment may be difficult. *Lower left*: If a thick membrane with blood vessels has formed, only a three-part membranectomy under pressure is effective (35). *Lower right*: Skin retraction around a type II nub is not uncommon and may require revision. Prophylactic antibiotics drops are effective in preventing infection.

dexamethasone is our preferred approach. The patient should be hospitalized with hourly topical as well as intravenous antibiotics. Prognosis is poor once a bacterial endophthalmitis has developed.

The possibility of fungal colonization on a soft contact lens or plastic surface, even leading to keratitis or endophthalmitis, is very rare and seems to occur primarily in pemphigoid or Stevens-Johnson syndrome. Suspect deposits should be cultured and drops of amphotericin B 0.15% be administered according to clinical severity.

A peculiar phenomenon of sudden, severe vitreitis, with a benign course, can be found in a small percentage of KPro recipients who have adhered to their antibiotic drop regimen. There is little redness or pain and cultures have been equivocal. They have been treated as for bacterial endophthalmitis, for safety. They have rapidly cleared up and regained the vision they had before the event. It is quite possible that this phenomenon is due to an immune reaction.

Glaucoma

With the drastic reduction in incidence of endophthalmitis after KPro, glaucoma has emerged as the greatest problem in severe cases. As discussed previously, any preexisting glaucoma can be expected to worsen and new glaucoma can appear after surgery, especially in chemically burned or autoimmune eyes. The mechanism is most likely inflammation leading to angle closure. The difficulty in arriving at exact pressure measurements adds to the problem.

As mentioned earlier, standard glaucoma drops are effective in type I, but not after type II KPro insertion. Oral carbonic anhydrase inhibitors have the usual effect but should be used with caution in patients with Stevens-Johnson syndrome, and obviously not at all in patients with sulfa allergy. Because of these restrictions, we have frequently resorted to glaucoma shunts (Fig. 66-5). In most cases, an Ahmed S-2 valve shunt works well, but in cicatrizing conditions (burn, autoimmunity), the capsule forming around the shunt plate can become very thick, severely impeding the flow of aqueous. A new experimental shunt device has been developed (with the help of Dr. Ahmed) in which the valve is totally enclosed and a distal tube attached, which allows us to lead the aqueous to an adjacent epithelialized cavity (36). There, a restricting capsule is unlikely to form. The cavity can be the maxillary sinus, the ethmoid sinuses, or the lacrimal sac. The unidirectionality of the valve makes retrograde infection very unlikely; in fact, no endophthalmitis has occurred in up to 2 years of observation. We now routinely implant such a device, leading to the maxillary sinus, approximately a month before KPro surgery in cases in which we suspect severe glaucoma will develop (Fig. 66-5). Further

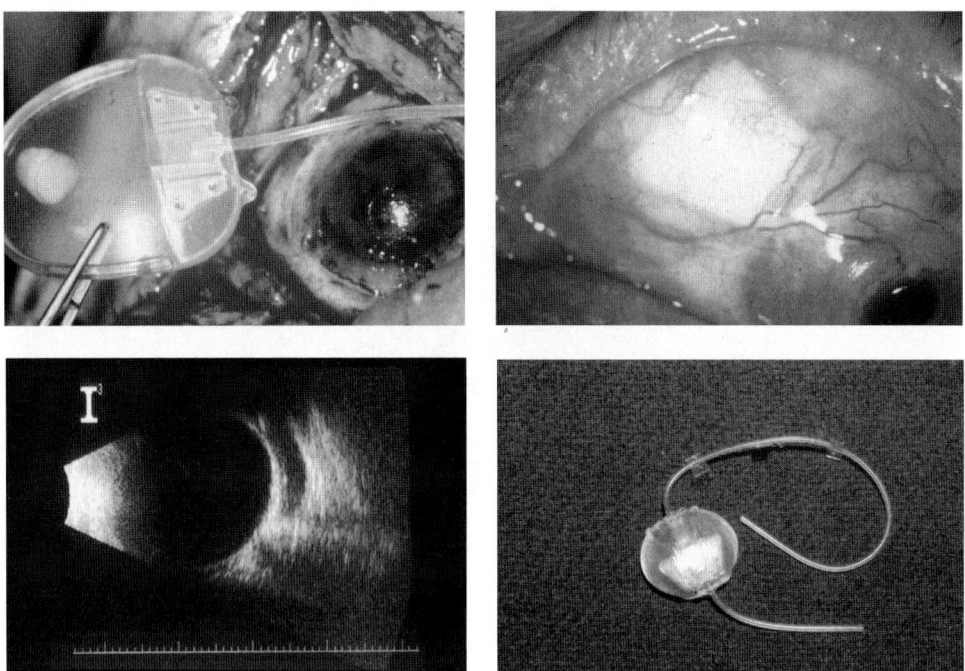

FIGURE 66-5. *Upper left*: Patients receiving a keratoprosthesis often need glaucoma shunts. An Ahmed S-2 shunt is being inserted. *Upper right*: Pericardium is placed to protect the tube. *Lower left*: On B-scan ultrasonography, a clear cleft is visible over the shunt plate, indicating a patent tube. Still, a thick capsule can result in a too high intraocular pressure. *Lower right*: An experimental shunt with an enclosed Ahmed valve and a distal tube. This tube is inserted into the maxillary sinus, where a fluid-restricting capsule is less likely to form (36).

developments in the registering of pressure and keeping it within normal limits are needed, however, to allow more safe and widespread use of KPro surgery.

CONCLUSIONS

A number of centers around the world have contributed to very substantial progress in KPro surgery during the last few decades. The approach will undoubtedly continue to spread owing to generally rapid rehabilitation and, when successful, unsurpassed visual acuity. On the other hand, standard corneal transplantation can be expected to become more refined as well, and therefore the borderline between the indications for the two procedures will always be a fluent one. In the individual case of severe corneal opacity, there can always be a question of doing a standard graft or doing a KPro—or neither for the moment.

Under any circumstances, because KPro will assume an expanded role, it is important that a few cornea surgeons in most countries take a serious long-term interest. It is not advisable to do just an occasional KPro and hope for the best. Life-long follow-up is important for these patients, and therefore the surgeon should be prepared to keep up interest for a very long time. In this way, the outcome can be very rewarding for patients and surgeon alike.

REFERENCES

1. Eye Bank Association of America. *2002 Eye banking statistical report*. Washington, DC: Eye Bank Association of America, 2002.
2. Dandona L, Naduvilath TJ, Janarthanan M, et al. Survival analysis and visual outcome in a large series of corneal transplants in India. *Br J Ophthalmol* 1997;81:726–731.
3. Bersudsky V, Blum-Hareuveni T, Rehany U, et al. The profile of repeated corneal transplantation. *Ophthalmology* 2001;108:461–469.
4. Thylefors B, Negrel AD, Pararajasegaram R, et al. Global data on blindness: reviews/analyses. *Bull World Health Org* 1995;73:115–121.
5. Cardona H. Plastic keratoprostheses: human application. In: King H Jr, McTigue JW, eds. *The cornea world congress*. Washington, DC: Butterworths, 1965:672–684.
6. Mannis MJ, Dohlman CH. The artificial cornea: a brief history. In: Mannis MD, ed. *Corneal transplantation: a history in profiles*. 1999:321.
7. Strampelli B. Osteo-odontocheratoprotesi. *Ann Ottalmol Clin Ocul* 1963;89;1039–1041.
8. Falcinelli G, Missiroli A, Pettiti V, et al. Osteo-odonto-keratoprosthesis up to date. In: *Acta XXV Concilium Ophthalmologicum*. Milano: Kugler & Ghedini, 1987.
9. Marchi V, Ricci R, Pecorella I, et al. Osteo-odonto-keratoprosthesis: description of surgical technique with results in 85 patients. *Cornea* 1994;13:125–130.
10. Temprano J. Resultados a largo plazo de osteo-odonto-queratoprotesis y queratoprotesis tibial. *An Inst Barraquer* 1998;27[Suppl]:53–65.

11. Stoiber J, Csaky D, Schedle A, et al. Histopathologic findings in explanted osteo-odontokeratoprosthesis. *Cornea* 2002;21: 400–404.
12. Liu C, Herold J, Sciscio A, et al. Osteo-odonto-keratoprosthesis surgery. *Br J Ophthalmol* 1999;83:127.
13. Hille K. Keratoprothesen. *Klin Aspekt Ophthalmol* 2002;99: 523–531.
14. Pintucci S, Pintucci F, Caiazza S, et al. The Dacron felt colonizable keratoprosthesis: after 15 years. *Eur J Ophthalmol* 1996;6: 125–130.
15. Girard LJ, Hawkins RS, Nieves R, et al. Keratoprosthesis: a 12 year follow-up. *Ophthalmol Trans Am Acad Ophthalmol Otolaryngol* 1977;83:252–267.
16. Legeais JM, Renard G, Parel JM, et al. Keratoprosthesis with biocolonizable microporous fluorocarbon haptic: preliminary results in a 24-patient study. *Arch Ophthalmol* 1995;113: 757–763.
17. Yakimenko S. Results of a PMMA/titanium keratoprosthesis in 502 eyes. *Refract Corneal Surg* 1993;9:197–198
18. Moroz ZI. Artificial cornea. In: Fyodorov SN, ed. *Microsurgery of the eye: main aspects.* Moscow: Mir, 1987.
19. Crawford GJ, Hicks CR, Lou X, et al. The Chirila keratoprosthesis: phase I human clinical trial. *Ophthalmology* 2002;109: 883–889.
20. Kim MK, Lee JL, Wee WR, et al. Seoul-type keratoprosthesis: preliminary results of the first 7 human cases. *Arch Ophthalmol* 2002;120:761–766.
21. Dohlman CH, Schneider HA, Doane MG. Prosthokeratoplasty. *Am J Ophthalmol* 1974;77:694–700.
22. Dorzee MJ. Kératoprothèse en acrylique. *Bull Soc Belg Ophtalmol* 1955;108:582–592.
23. Barraquer J. Keratoplasty and keratoprosthesis. Pocklington Memorial Lecture delivered at the Royal College of Surgeons of England on 5th May, 1966. *Ann R Coll Surg Engl* 1967;40(2): 71–81.
24. Doane MG, Dohlman CH, Bearse MG. Fabrication of keratoprosthesis. *Cornea* 1996;15:179–184.
25. Yaghouti F, Nouri M, Abad JC, et al. Keratoprosthesis: preoperative prognostic categories. *Cornea* 2001;20:19–23.
26. Dohlman CH, Terada H. Keratoprosthesis in pemphigoid and Stevens-Johnson syndrome. *Adv Exp Med Biol* 1998;438: 1021–1025.
27. Al-Merjan J, Sadeq N, Dohlman CH. Temporary tissue coverage in keratoprosthesis. *Mideast J Ophthalmol* 2000;8:12.
28. Dohlman CH, Abad JC, Dudenhoefer EJ, et al. Keratoprosthesis: beyond corneal graft failure. In: Spaeth GL, ed. *Ophthalmic surgery: principles and practice.* Philadelphia: WB Saunders, 2003:199–207.
29. Netland PA, Terada H, Dohlman CH. Glaucoma associated with keratoprosthesis. *Ophthalmology* 1998;105:751–757.
30. Nouri M, Terada H, Alfonso EC, et al. Endophthalmitis after keratoprosthesis: incidence, bacterial causes, and risk factors. *Arch Ophthalmol* 2001;119:484–489.
31. Dohlman CH, Nouri M, Barnes S, et al. Prophylactic antibiotic regimens in keratoprosthesis. *Invest Ophthalmol Vis Sci* 2003; 1455–B351. ARVO abstract.
32. Dohlman CH, Doane MG. Some factors influencing outcome after keratoprosthesis surgery. *Cornea* 1994;13:214–218.
33. Dohlman CH, Dudenhoefer EJ, Khan BF, et al. Protection of the ocular surface after keratoprosthesis surgery: the role of soft contact lenses. *CLAO J* 2002;28:72–74.
34. Bath PE, McCord RC, Cox KC. Nd:YAG laser discission of retroprosthetic membrane: a preliminary report. *Cornea* 1983;2: 225–228.
35. Ray S, Khan BF, Dohlman CH, et al. Management of vitreoretinal complications in eyes with permanent keratoprosthesis. *Arch Ophthalmol* 2002;120:559–566.
36. Dohlman CH, Grosskreutz CL, Dudenhoefer EJ, et al. Connecting Ahmed valve shunt to the lacrimal sac or nasal sinuses in severe glaucoma. *Am Acad Ophthalmol* 2002;258. Poster.

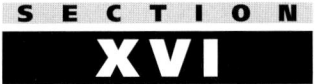

KERATOREFRACTIVE SURGERY

67

THE BIOLOGY OF CORNEAL REFRACTIVE SURGERY

STEVEN E. WILSON, MARCELO NETTO, AND RENATO AMBRÓSIO, JR.

The results of corneal refractive surgical procedures are influenced by the biologic responses to the surgical injury, including corneal wound healing and biomechanics. Intensive research has provided a relatively complete understanding of the healing response, complications associated with wound healing and tissue changes, and the possibility of using pharmacologic agents to modulate the response to corneal refractive surgery. Understanding the biology of the cornea and the interactions between its cellular components allows for better appreciation of anomalous results and complications that may occur after laser *in situ* keratomileusis (LASIK), photorefractive keratectomy (PRK), and other refractive surgical procedures. In the absence of such knowledge, it is possible to attribute these outcomes incorrectly to external factors.

This chapter outlines our understanding of the relevant cells and structures that are involved in corneal wound healing and biomechanics. In addition, the biology of specific corneal refractive surgical procedures is described, along with the biologic mechanisms that underlie surgical outcomes and complications.

CORNEAL STRUCTURES INVOLVED IN WOUND HEALING AFTER REFRACTIVE SURGERY

The systems that orchestrate the response to refractive surgical procedures evolved to maintain and restore vision after mechanical injury and infection. The cellular elements of the cornea that participate in responses to refractive surgical procedures include the epithelium, stroma, and nerves (1,2). The epithelium is stratified squamous. Epithelial stem cells are thought to reside in the limbus (3). The normal stroma is populated by keratocytes. These cells differ in density from the anterior to the posterior stroma, with the density being higher in the anterior stoma (4,5). Keratocytes may differ in differentiated characteristics from the anterior to the posterior and the center to the peripheral stroma.

The endothelium may participate in some types of injuries, such as deep incisions or laser burns. Inflammatory cells from the immune system also contribute to the response to all injuries (6–9).

Structural elements include the basement membrane of the epithelium, Bowman's layer (in humans and some other species), corneal lamellae, proteoglycans, and other extracellular matrix components. Bowman's layer is the acellular anterior layer of the stroma that lies below the epithelial basement membrane. Bowman's layer has a different arrangement of collagen fibers compared with deeper layers of the stroma.

The cornea–sensory nerve–central nervous system–motor nerve–lacrimal gland–tear film axis also participates in the corneal wound healing response (10). Tears contain many components that modulate the epithelial and stromal wound healing responses, including cytokines and growth factors (11–13).

CORNEAL WOUND HEALING

The corneal wound healing response comprises a complex cascade of processes involving the corneal epithelium, stroma, nerves, inflammatory cells, lacrimal gland, tears, and their components. The overall response is similar after various types of injuries, but important variations occur in different surgical procedures that may affect refractive outcomes and complications.

The earliest corneal event noted after traumatic or surgical injury to the corneal epithelium is keratocyte apoptosis (7,14,15) (Fig. 67-1). The disappearance of keratocytes after epithelial injury was first noted by Dohlman and co-workers (16) and rediscovered several times by other investigators. Many years passed before it became clear that the disappearance of keratocytes was mediated by apoptosis or programmed cell death, occurring in every species examined to date, including rabbits, rats, mice, chickens, monkeys, and humans (15,17).

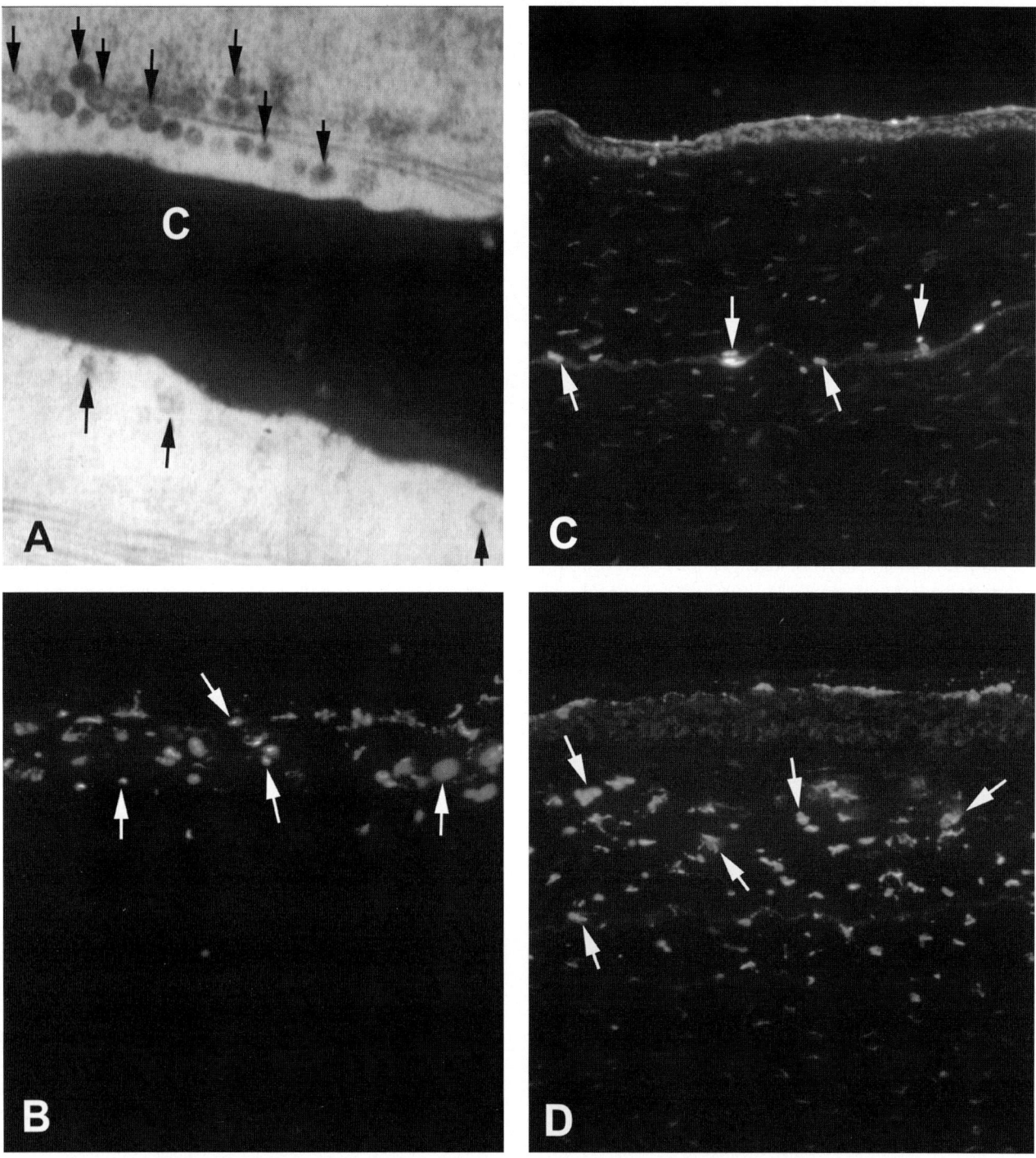

FIGURE 67-1. Keratocyte apoptosis. **A:** Keratocyte apoptosis is the earliest stromal event after epithelial injury. Superficial keratocytes undergoing apoptosis can be detected by transmission electron microscopy immediately after injury to the epithelium. Chromatin condensation (C) is present in this keratocyte, along with formation of hundreds of apoptotic bodies (*arrows*) containing cellular contents (original magnification × 18,000). **B:** At 4 hours after photorefractive keratectomy, most of the keratocytes in the anterior stroma are staining with the TUNEL assay (*arrows*), indicating apoptosis (original magnification × 200). **C:** In laser *in situ* keratomileusis (LASIK), there are typically fewer keratocytes that undergo apoptosis at 4 hours after surgery, and those that do are located both anterior and posterior to the lamellar interface (*arrows*; original magnification × 200). **D:** The level of keratocyte apoptosis after LASIK varies from eye to eye. In this eye, there are a large number of keratocytes undergoing apoptosis at 4 hours after LASIK (original magnification × 200).

The initial keratocyte apoptosis response to epithelial injury is surprisingly rapid. If the epithelium of a freshly enucleated eye is scraped with a scalpel and the eye is then immersed into an electron microscopy fixative, cellular changes characteristic of apoptosis can be seen by transmission electron microscopy (15). The terminal deoxyribonucleotidyl transferase–mediated dUTP-digoxigenin nick and labeling (TUNEL) assay for fragmented DNA characteristic of apoptosis peaks at approximately 4 hours after epithelial injury, when nuclear DNA degradation has peaked (7,15) (Fig. 67-1). TUNEL-positive stromal cells can be detected for approximately 1 week after PRK or LASIK (7,18). Transmission electron microscopy demonstrates that almost all cells dying in the stroma at 4 hours after epithelial injury are undergoing apoptosis, with cell shrinkage, chromatin condensation, and formation of apoptotic bodies (7,14,15) (Fig. 67-1). At time points later than 4 hours, an increasing proportion of dying cells in the stroma undergo necrosis (7). These cells include keratocytes, wound healing fibroblasts, myofibroblasts, and inflammatory cells.

Localization of the keratocyte undergoing apoptosis varies with the surgical procedure (Fig. 67-1). For example, with PRK and laser subepithelial keratomileusis (LASEK), it occurs in the anterior subepithelial stroma. In uncomplicated LASIK, it occurs just anterior and posterior to the lamellar interface in the deeper stroma. After a LASIK buttonhole flap, it occurs along the superficial lamellar interface and in the anterior stromal region where the blade perforates the epithelium. With incisional procedures it is noted along the depth of the stromal incision (Wilson SE, unpublished data, 1995). Reports of stromal cell death after collagen shrinkage procedures, corneal rings, or stromal inlays are lacking. The localization of the early apoptosis response may be important in determining the localization of later events in the wound healing process (7). The location of the stromal wound healing response relative to the epithelium is probably a critical determinant of differences in regression, haze, and other complications between PRK and LASIK (7).

The mechanism through which epithelial injury induces keratocyte apoptosis remains controversial. Many studies have demonstrated that cytokines expressed by the corneal epithelial cells trigger keratocyte apoptosis *in vitro* and after *in vivo* microinjection. For example, interleukin (IL)-1 is expressed at high levels in the corneal epithelium and can be released only through death of, or injury to, the epithelial cells (Fig. 67-2). Microinjection of mouse IL-1α into the quiescent central stromal of the mouse cornea induces keratocyte apoptosis (15). Many other cytokines produced by the corneal epithelium can trigger keratocyte apoptosis. These include tumor necrosis factor-α (TNF-α), Fas ligand, and bone morphogenic proteins 2 and 4 (19–22). Importantly, the effect of a cytokine such as IL-1 depends on the concentration of the cytokine and the

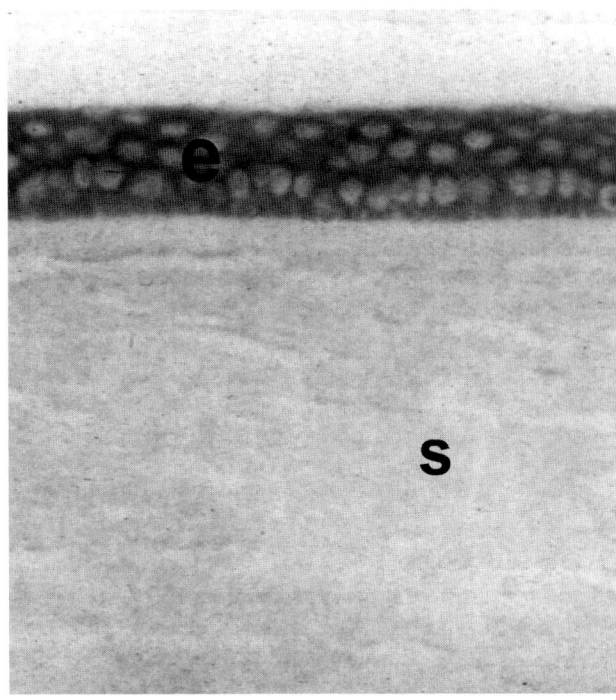

FIGURE 67-2. Interleukin-1α (IL-1α) is expressed constitutively (continually) in corneal epithelium (e). This immunocytochemical assay for IL-1α shows high levels (brown stain) in the epithelial cells of the unwounded human cornea. The IL-1α is released only with injury or death of the epithelial cells. Once it is released, it diffuses into the stroma (s) and binds receptors on keratocyte cells. There, depending on the concentration and the cellular milieu, it modulates cellular functions such as apoptosis, production of growth factors like hepatocyte growth factor and keratinocyte growth factor, and modulates production of metalloproteinases and collagenases (original magnification ×400).

milieu of the cell. Thus, IL-1 may trigger apoptosis in a quiescent keratocyte in the normal stoma, whereas it upregulates metalloproteinase production and secretion of keratinocyte growth factor (KGF) in a myofibroblast during wound healing. A possible mechanism of keratocyte apoptosis thus would be active stimulation of cell death by the epithelium or by epithelial-derived factors (23,24).

A potential mechanism through which keratocyte apoptosis may be mediated is autocrine suicide. Keratocytes constitutively produce the cell death receptor Fas, but not the Fas ligand in the unwounded cornea (22). Fas ligand is expressed in corneal epithelium (22). However, Fas ligand is a membrane-associated cytokine and requires cell–cell (juxtacrine) contact between the cells for induction of apoptosis. This contact does not appear to be the predominant mechanism of keratocyte apoptosis. However, when corneal fibroblasts in culture are exposed to IL-1, they begin expressing Fas ligand (19). This induction of Fas ligand could trigger keratocyte cell death through autocrine suicide because the keratocytes would be producing the Fas ligand and receptor. This mechanism has been found to function in several other cells (19).

Zhao and coworkers (25) suggested that the tears contain the factors that trigger keratocyte apoptosis. Keratocyte apoptosis, however, still occurs in the enucleated eye washed free of tears, and many tear factors are themselves derived from the epithelium (26). Intentional introduction of corneal epithelium beneath a LASIK flap increases keratocyte apoptosis (23). In addition, an epithelial defect is not required for induction of keratocyte apoptosis. Viral infection of intact epithelium (24) or even pressure on the cornea with a cloning cylinder (27) induces keratocyte apoptosis underlying the site of epithelial injury. So although tear factors derived from corneal or lacrimal gland epithelium could contribute to induction of keratocyte apoptosis, they do not appear to be the only factors involved in mediating this process.

Epithelial healing starts almost immediately after epithelial injury. It is regulated by autocrine cytokine networks in the epithelial cells; cytokines produced by stromal cells like keratocytes and wound healing fibroblasts (2,11,13,28–30); and lacrimal gland–derived factors secreted into tears (11,13,28). Early after surface ablation procedures like PRK, the anterior stroma is devoid of cells (15). Tear cytokines derived from the lacrimal glands probably regulate early corneal epithelial cell proliferation and migration. The stromal cells probably become the most important regulators of epithelial healing as this layer is repopulated with keratocytes, corneal fibroblasts, and myofibroblasts. Important cytokines likely include hepatocyte growth factor (HGF) and KGF produced by the stromal cells and lacrimal gland (11,13,30). HGF and KGF are classic mediators of stromal–epithelial interactions. They are produced by the stromal cells and regulate proliferation, migration, and differentiation of the receptor-bearing epithelial cells. Autocrine, paracrine, and juxtacrine (requiring cell–cell contact) epidermal growth factor, transforming growth factor (TGF)-α, and TGF-β are also likely among the complex array of cytokines that modulate corneal epithelial proliferation, migration, and differentiation during corneal wound healing (31). Healing of the epithelium can be accompanied by epithelial hyperplasia that can persist indefinitely.

Inflammatory cells invade the corneal stroma as early as 8 to 12 hours after epithelial injury (7,8). These cells include monocytes (Fig. 67-3), granulocytes, T cells, and other inflammatory cells (32) (Wilson SE, Huang J, Possin D, et al., unpublished data, 2002). These cells function to eliminate microorganisms and debris produced by the injury and wound healing response. They persist for up to several weeks after PRK and LASIK (7).

Inflammatory cells are drawn into the cornea by chemokines such as monocyte chemotactic and activating factor (MCAF) and granulocyte colony-stimulating factor produced keratocytes in response to cytokines like IL-1 and TNF-α released from injured corneal epithelial cells (6,9). Other chemokines are derived from epithelial cells and possibly other sources.

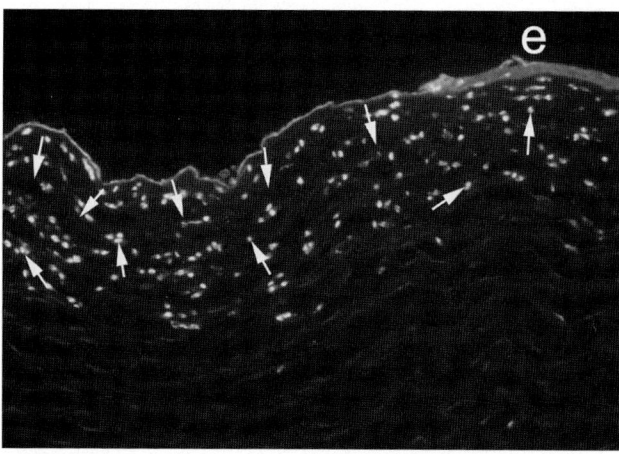

FIGURE 67-3. At 24 hours after epithelial scrape, there are numerous CD11b-positive monocytes detected by immunocytochemistry in the anterior stroma of the rabbit cornea. Intact epithelium (e) is present to the right and monocytes (*arrows*) are present in the anterior stroma (original magnification ×250).

Beginning 12 to 24 hours after epithelial injury, proliferation of residual keratocytes can be detected in the stroma by immunocytochemistry for the mitosis-specific antigen Ki67 (7,33). In PRK and LASEK, this proliferation occurs in a band of peripheral and posterior stroma surrounding the zone of earlier keratocyte apoptosis (7,33) (Fig. 67-4A). In LASIK, it occurs surrounding the lamellar interface (34) (Fig. 67-4B). Currently it is thought that these proliferating keratocytes give rise to all activated keratocytes, myofibroblasts, and corneal fibroblasts that repopulate the depleted stroma. However, investigations are ongoing to determine whether infiltrating monocytes could also give rise to some of the stromal participants in the wound healing process, analogous to monocyte differentiation into osteoclasts in bone (Wilson SE, Mohan RR, unpublished data, 2002). The same cytokines that regulate the transformation from monocyte to osteoclast are also expressed in the corneal stroma. Our working hypothesis is that monocytes give rise to fibroblastic cells that participate in stromal remodeling in the cornea during wound healing (keratoclasts).

Many changes occur in the corneal stroma in the weeks after corneal injury. Most of the changes are poorly characterized at the molecular and cellular level. Stromal cells called *myofibroblasts* (express alpha smooth muscle actin) may appear immediately beneath the epithelium a week or two after PRK (7). These cells are presumably derived from proliferating keratocytes under the influence of TGF-β (35–37). They become most prominent approximately 1 month after PRK (Fig. 67-5). Whether they appear depends on the level of correction in PRK (7). In LASIK, myofibroblasts are usually detected only in the periphery of the cornea, where the lamellar interface intersects the epithelium (7). However, they may be detected in the central cornea along the lamellar interface

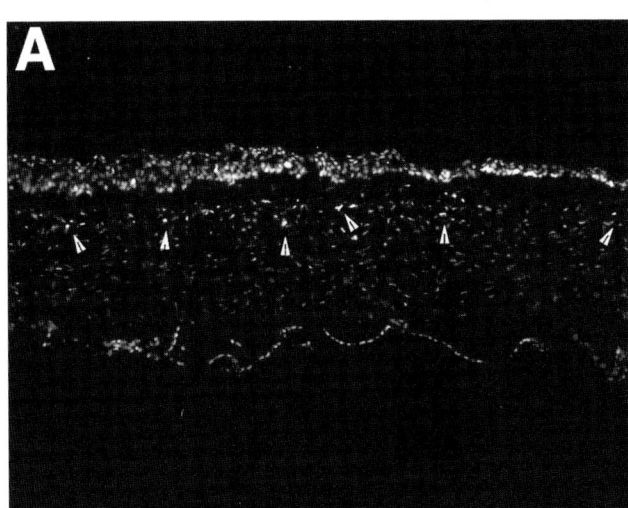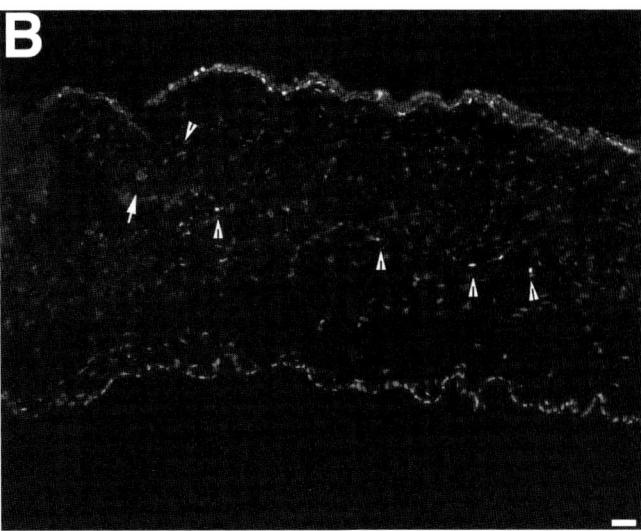

FIGURE 67-4. Keratocyte proliferation at 72 hours after photorefractive keratectomy (PRK) **(A)** and 72 hours after laser *in situ* keratomileusis (LASIK) **(B)** in rabbits. Keratocytes undergoing mitosis were detected using immunocytochemistry by expression of the Ki-67 mitosis-specific antigen (7). Note that keratocytes undergoing mitosis are more superficial in PRK (*arrows* in **A**) than in LASIK (*arrows* in **B**). There are epithelial cells undergoing mitosis in both the eye that had PRK and the eye that had LASIK. There is epithelial hyperplasia in the eye that had PRK (original magnification ×400). (Courtesy of Audrey E. K. Hutcheon and James D. Zieske, with permission.)

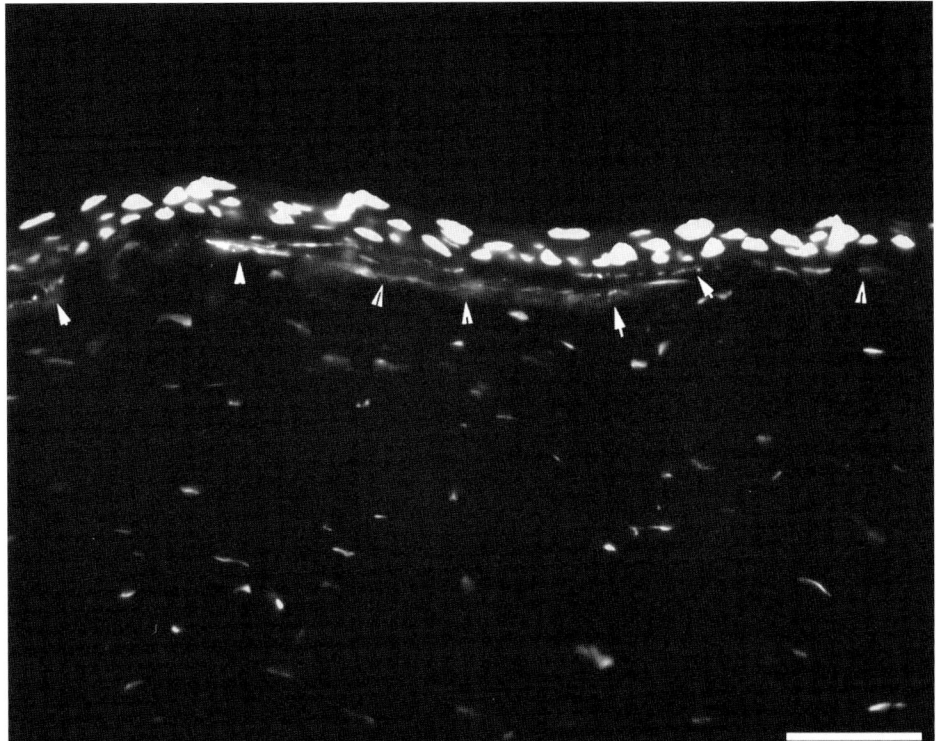

FIGURE 67-5. Myofibroblasts that stain for alpha smooth muscle actin (*arrowheads*) in the subepithelial stroma at 1 month after photorefractive keratectomy for 9 diopters of myopia in the rabbit. Red nuclear staining is DAPI (original magnification ×400). (Courtesy of Audrey E. K. Hutcheon and James D. Zieske, with permission.)

if epithelial debris is retained in the intralamellar space at the time of surgery (21). Myofibroblasts are important in contraction of the wound in incisional procedures (35,36). Their function in a broad wound like PRK is not apparent, although on immunohistologic studies they produce high levels of growth factors like HGF that modulate proliferation and differentiation of the overlying epithelial cells (2,30,38). They contribute to haze (opacity) in procedures like PRK because the myofibroblasts themselves are opaque and produce disordered collagen (35,36). Recent studies have demonstrated that these cells are generated after PRK for high myopia, but not PRK for low myopia, in the rabbit (7). They are rarely seen in the central cornea in LASIK, even in LASIK for high myopia (7), in the absence of epithelial debris or inflammation. Myofibroblasts do appear on both sides of the lamellar interface if epithelial debris is retained beneath the flap in LASIK (23).

Quantitative studies in rabbits have demonstrated a correlation between the level of keratocyte apoptosis, keratocyte proliferation, and myofibroblast generation in PRK and LASIK (7). In high PRK corrections (−9 diopters of myopia), there were higher levels of all three wound healing parameters than in lower PRK corrections (−4.5 diopters). The levels of keratocyte apoptosis, keratocyte proliferation, and myofibroblast generation were still lower in LASIK, even when comparing high correction for −9 diopters of myopia in LASIK with lower correction of −4.5 diopters in PRK.

It remains to be determined whether there is a cause-and-effect relationship between early keratocyte apoptosis and later events such as keratocyte mitosis and myofibroblast generation. If pharmacologic agents that inhibit keratocyte apoptosis without triggering keratocyte necrosis can be developed, it should be possible to determine whether these relationships are casual.

At present, little information is available regarding the wound healing response after LASEK. It is likely to be similar to PRK, but further study will be needed to determine if parameters like keratocyte apoptosis, keratocyte proliferation, and myofibroblast generation are different in PRK and LASEK for the same level of correction.

One study suggested that the level of haze after PRK was determined by the volume of stromal tissue removed (39). It remains to be determined, however, whether the volume of stromal tissue or other cellular response variables that would also be increased with higher levels of correction are the more important factors.

In vivo confocal microscopy is a valuable method for monitoring the effect of PRK and LASIK on corneal nerves, overall opacity, flap thickness, and the density of stromal cells over time. It, however, cannot reliably distinguish live from dead cells, apoptosis from necrosis, or even specific cell types such as keratocyte, corneal fibroblasts, myofibroblasts, monocytes, or polymorphonuclear cells.

Thus, its utility in understanding the cellular changes that contribute to the wound healing response is limited.

Epithelial hyperplasia may occur after PRK (40–42) or LASIK (43–46). Epithelial hyperplasia can cause regression of the effect of correction of myopia, hyperopia, and astigmatism. It also will likely influence the custom corneal ablation with LASIK, LASEK, or PRK because the features that will be applied to correct higher-order aberrations will often be measured in microns (47).

The factors leading to epithelial hyperplasia are complex. An abrupt change in corneal contour or a rough surface can be associated with epithelial hyperplasia. However, epithelial hyperplasia can occur in corneas with a smooth surface and may occur when there is epithelial scrape injury without refractive ablation (48). In some eyes, the hyperplasia may be related to production of high levels of cytokines like HGF and KGF by keratocytes, corneal fibroblasts, or myofibroblasts. There could be genetic factors that regulate the response of the epithelium to these cytokines in a particular eye. HGF and KGF are candidate modulators of epithelial hyperplasia because these growth factors stimulate proliferation and inhibit terminal differentiation of epithelial cells (2,11,29,30).

Another late event that occurs after refractive surgical procedures is stromal remodeling. This includes deposition and resorption of disorganized collagen laid down in the stroma by keratocytes, corneal fibroblasts, or myofibroblasts (49–51). Disorganized collagen may be replaced by ordered collagen characteristic of clear corneas. Remodeling could also include changes in glysosaminoglycans in the corneal stroma (44,45,52,53). Such stromal remodeling could also be associated with regression of the effect of all refractive surgery procedures.

Some procedures have greater tendency to trigger epithelial hyperplasia. For example, there appears to be more epithelial hyperplasia associated with PRK for high myopia compared with LASIK for high myopia. Different eyes having the same procedure can also have differing levels of epithelial hyperplasia. These procedure and individual differences are also noted for stromal remodeling. In turn, the levels of epithelial hyperplasia and stromal remodeling affect refractive affect regression after a procedure. These factors are discussed later in this chapter as they relate to the individual procedures.

Over time, there is a slow return toward normal in eyes that have had refractive surgical procedures. Keratocyte apoptosis, necrosis, and proliferation diminish markedly approximately 1 week after surgery. Most immune cells disappear from the cornea through apoptosis or necrosis at 1 to 2 weeks after surgery. Myofibroblasts diminish over weeks to years. Disappearance of myofibroblasts is likely mediated by apoptosis or transdifferentiation back to keratocytes.

Corneal remodeling, including resorption of disorganized collagen, occurs over a period of several months to years after any type of injury (54,55), including surgical injury. Epithelial hyperplasia may take years to resolve (41,43). These changes can result in refractive instability.

An example will serve to illustrate these possible effects. An eye with high myopia that has PRK or LASIK could have regression due to epithelial hyperplasia. Early enhancement, typically 3 to 6 months after the original procedure, might be used to provide additional correction to overcome the effects of the hyperplasia. If, however, the epithelial hyperplasia resolves over time, the eye could end up overcorrected to hyperopia a year or two later. The effect of enhancement could be different, however, if the regression was secondary to stromal remodeling. Rapid and accurate methods to measure preoperative and postoperative epithelial thickness and stromal thickness could provide important insights into the cause of regression in individual eyes and guide appropriate treatment.

CORNEAL BIOMECHANICS

Recently, there has been increasing interest in the biomechanical effects of refractive surgery procedures and how changes in biomechanical properties of the cornea induced by surgery affect the outcome (56–59). Biomechanical parameters include tensile strength, stress–strain relationship, and stress–relaxation properties. There is overlap between the wound healing process and biomechanics. For example, epithelial hyperplasia is a wound healing response that may have biomechanical effects on surgical outcomes. Another example of potential biomechanical effects would be if there was a mechanical effect of ablation of Bowman's layer in PRK or cutting through Bowman's layer in LASIK on the corneal contour. Very little has been reported regarding biomechanical changes that occur with surgery, and more study is needed to establish the importance of purely biomechanical changes induced by PRK, LASIK, and other procedures relative to the changes resulting from the wound healing response.

BIOLOGIC RESPONSES TO SPECIFIC REFRACTIVE SURGICAL PROCEDURES

Photorefractive Keratectomy

Effect of Ablation of Bowman's Layer

Bowman's layer is an acellular layer of connective tissue positioned between the epithelial basement membrane and the stroma that is present in some species, including humans, but absent in others (60). The organization of collagen in Bowman's layer is different from that in the underlying stroma. The collagen forms a finely woven mesh rather than the more precise lamellar structure of the underlying stroma.

Despite the multiple properties that have been attributed to Bowman's layer (61), there is no conclusive evidence of

a specific function associated with maintenance of corneal shape or barrier to microorganisms. We hypothesize that Bowman's layer represents a buffer between the basal epithelium and stroma that is formed during embryogenesis as a result of cytokine-mediated negative chemotactic influences of the epithelium on primordial keratocyte cells derived from neural crest (61). These cytokine-mediated cellular interactions may persist in the adult as a part of mechanisms involved in the maintenance of tissue organization. Breakdown of these interactions in diseases such as advanced bullous keratopathy after progression to epithelial edema and dysfunction results in destruction of Bowman's layer and movement of stromal fibroblastic cells to a position beneath the epithelium to form pannus (Fig. 67-6). In situations where epithelial plugs are retained in the stroma, such as in astigmatic keratotomy (AK) or radial keratotomy (RK), a Bowman's-like layer accumulates gradually adjacent to the epithelium (62,63). Bowman's-like layers may be noted years after PRK, although related studies are limited.

The hypothesis that Bowman's layer does not have a critical function is supported by the hundreds of thousands of patients who have undergone PRK since 1988. It has been suggested that development of significant corneal haze in PRK is a result of ablation of Bowman's layer. However, visually significant haze is very rare in eyes that have undergone PRK to treat myopia of less than 5 diopters,

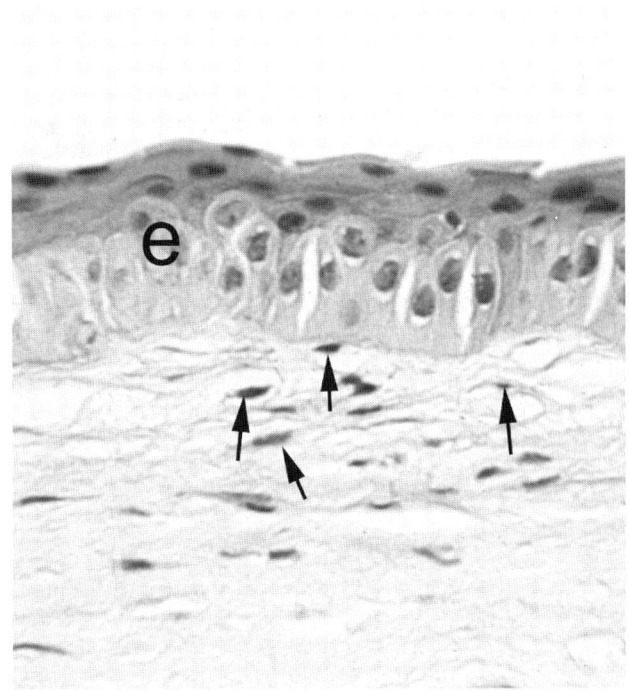

FIGURE 67-6. Destruction of Bowman's layer in bullous keratopathy with chronic edema of the epithelium. Notice that Bowman's layer is no longer present and fibroblastic cells that are thought to be derived from keratocytes now lie immediately beneath the epithelium.

despite the fact that Bowman's layer is removed. This suggests that other factors are more important in the development of clinically significant haze after PRK.

Undercorrection and Overcorrection Attributable to Wound Healing

PRK is a stromal surface ablation procedure. The levels of anterior stromal keratocyte apoptosis, keratocyte proliferation, and myofibroblast generation depended on the level of correction (7). This could indicate some influence by shock waves or other laser-related factors on keratocyte apoptosis or subsequent wound healing processes. Alternatively, there could be a difference in the response when more posterior keratocytes proliferate and give rise to myofibroblasts and other stromal cell types. There is a higher tendency for regression of the effect of PRK with higher levels of correction. The regression could result from stromal remodeling or epithelial hyperplasia (40–42). However, assuming that the technical aspects of surgery are preformed correctly, both overcorrection and undercorrection related to diminished or increased wound healing, respectively, are more common after higher levels of PRK correction. This likely is attributable to variable wound healing, resulting in differences in epithelial hyperplasia or stromal remodeling.

In the case of epithelial hyperplasia, higher levels of keratocyte proliferation and increased numbers of myofibroblasts may trigger increased production of HGF and KGF cytokines by the activated stromal cells.

Epithelial hyperplasia that varies in eyes that have PRK and LASIK will likely confound efforts to improve results through custom corneal ablation directed by wavefront analysis (47). Some of the custom features are measured in terms of just a few microns of thickness, and epithelial hyperplasia will tend to mask these subtle variations in corneal contour.

It is important to realize that epithelial hyperplasia can be induced by epithelial scrape injury without application of excimer laser ablation (48).

Previous studies have demonstrated that transepithelial PRK, in which the excimer laser is used to ablate both the overlying epithelium and the stroma, is associated with lesser keratocyte apoptosis (14,64). This corresponds to an increase in refractive correction for each diopter of laser applied to the stroma and a need for algorithm adjustment (65).

Stromal Opacity (Haze)

Haze is a term that has been accepted by surgeons and patients to describe stromal opacity occurring after excimer laser procedures. It is most common after PRK, but is clinically significant in only a small proportion of eyes. Almost all eyes treated with PRK have some level of haze. Clinically significant corneal haze is typically localized in the subepithelial anterior stroma.

Increased opacity of the activated stromal keratocytes and myofibroblasts and diminished corneal crystalin production by the cells (35) are important contributing factors to haze. Crystalins are proteins present in high concentration that lend clarity to the corneal cells, similar to crystalins in the lens. That the opacity has a cellular basis follows from the observation that treatment of the exposed stroma with mitomycin C often improves severe haze (66–68). Mitomycin C triggers cell death (69) and, therefore, probably has its effect on haze through induction of death of the opaque myofibroblasts and activated keratocytes in the anterior stroma. Some of the haze may also be attributable to increased deposition of disorganized collagen and other stromal components (45,49–51,53). The incidence and severity of haze in PRK have been shown to increase with the level of attempted correction (39). This is likely related to increased generation of myofibroblasts and the matrix materials they produce with increasing levels of correction (7). The authors have never noted (in more than 2,000 eyes that had lower corrections) clinically significant haze in eyes that had less than 6 diopters of PRK for myopia, unless there was a delay in closure of the epithelial defect lasting for more than 1 week (Wilson SE, unpublished data, 2002).

There also seems to be a correlation between the smoothness of the stromal surface after PRK and the incidence of haze (70). It is also the authors' experience that haze was more common in eyes treated with the Summit Apex laser, which produced visible surface irregularity, compared with those treated with the VISX S3 or Alcon-Autonomous laser (Wilson SE, unpublished data, 2001). We hypothesize, based on recent observations regarding the effect of epithelium (7,23), that this is attributable to an increase in stromal surface area available for stromal–epithelial interactions and, therefore, increased myofibroblast generation in eyes with rough surfaces after PRK.

There may be at least two types of corneal haze that occur after PRK. The more common type ("typical haze") occurs in all eyes that have PRK. It is typically noted at 1 month after surgery and peaks between 1 and 3 months after surgery. It usually disappears within the first year after surgery. This type of haze is rarely associated with clinical symptoms. Another, less common, type of haze is referred to as *late haze* (71). This type of haze tends to be a more significant clinical problem than the early haze that is noted in a high proportion of eyes that have PRK. Late haze typically occurs in eyes that have more than 6 diopters of correction for myopia and increases in frequency with greater attempted correction. Late haze typically occurs at 2 to 4 months after an otherwise normal PRK procedure and is accompanied by severe, reticulated, subepithelial haze associated with severe regression of correction (Fig. 67-7). It is nearly always bilateral. The incidence of late haze varies from 0.1% to more than 2% (71) (Wilson SE, unpublished data, 1998). Late haze typically requires 1 to 3 years

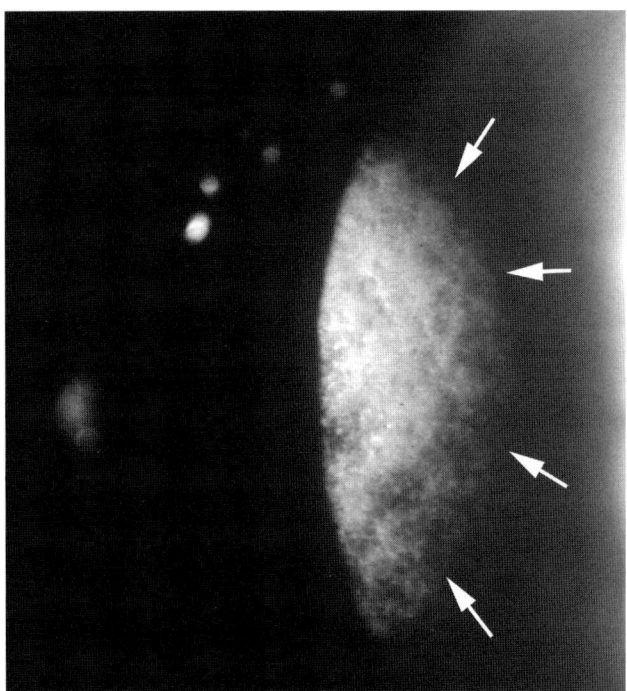

FIGURE 67-7. Slit-lamp photograph of late haze (*arrows*) that occurred in the subepithelial stroma at 3 months after photorefractive keratectomy for 9 diopters of myopia in the human.

to resolve. There is a very high recurrence rate with retreatment. Late haze also responds to mitomycin C treatment, suggesting that myofibroblasts and other activated stromal cells are major contributors. We hypothesize that late haze is brought on by some sort of defect(s) in the wound healing process that could be identified through molecular genetic investigations. This would require an appropriately large family in which some members had late haze after PRK and others did not.

Neurotrophic Epitheliopathy

Neurotrophic epitheliopathy is much less common after PRK than it is after LASIK. Presumably, this is attributable to only the nerve endings being ablated in PRK. Thus, regenerating nerve endings would be in close proximity to the overlying epithelial surface and a shorter time would be required for complete reinnervation of the epithelial cells (72). In addition, the nerves are affected over a smaller corneal diameter in PRK for myopia than they are with the flap in LASIK. Thus, the epithelial cells likely have better access to neurotrophic factors released from the nerves during the early postoperative period after PRK compared with LASIK, where the nerves are cut at the flap edge.

Laser Subepithelial Keratomileusis

In the LASEK procedure, dilute (typically 20%) alcohol is applied (typically for 20 to 30 seconds) to loosen the epithelium. Instruments are used to displace the epithelium from the central cornea to allow photoablation to be performed. The epithelium is subsequently repositioned and protected with a bandage contact lens.

Several methods have been used to displace the epithelium after alcohol exposure. In the first method developed, the epithelium is trephined at a diameter of 7 to 8.5 mm and the sheet remains attached by a hinge (73,74). Vinciguerra and Camesasca (75) subsequently developed the alternative butterfly LASEK, in which the epithelium is incised paracentrally after alcohol exposure and the two sheets of epithelium are pushed peripherally. The potential advantage of the butterfly technique is that the repositioned epithelium retains attachment to the peripheral epithelial tissue with higher proliferative potential. McDonald (76) recently reported gel-assisted LASEK. In this procedure, gel is used to displace the epithelium after alcohol exposure.

A critical issue regarding LASEK is whether the epithelium retains viability after displacement and repositioning. Azar and coworkers (73) demonstrated that epithelial viability after alcohol exposure varied with the concentration of ethanol and the duration of exposure. In their studies, 20-second exposure of cultured, immortalized human cells to various concentrations of ethanol resulted in a significant reduction in viable cells when the concentration exceeded 25%. Increasing the duration of application of 20% ethanol beyond 30 seconds also resulted in a significant reduction in viable cells. Importantly, these authors demonstrated that there was great variability between different eyes with regard to whether all or part of the basement membrane remained attached to the epithelial sheet after displacement. When epithelial cells are removed from their basement membrane, they typically undergo apoptosis (77). This alone would therefore result in variability in epithelial flap viability between different eyes that had LASEK, and even within a single epithelial flap, regardless of the toxic effects of the alcohol itself.

Clinical studies have reported varying results with regard to retention and healing of the epithelium after LASEK. This could be attributable, at least in part, to variability in the surgical techniques and the method used to monitor epithelial viability. There have been anecdotal reports of smaller epithelial defect detected with fluoroscein staining the first few days after LASEK compared with PRK, with larger epithelial defects in LASEK eyes at 3 to 6 days. This suggests the epithelial sheet was not viable in some eyes after LASEK and that the presence of the sheet may have inhibited epithelial healing. It is possible that the presence of an epithelial eschar alone could alter the wound healing response, even if the epithelial cells are not viable.

There are other sources of variability between LASEK and PRK that could affect the laser ablation or the subsequent wound healing response. For example, LASEK requires more time than PRK to perform and there tends to be greater variability in the time required to displace the epithelium after alcohol exposure in different eyes. This could result in differences in hydration of the ablated anterior stroma that may affect the ablation and clinical outcome. Another example is the effect of the alcohol on the keratocytes in LASEK. Exposure to alcohol in LASEK induces early necrosis of anterior keratocytes. This would contrast with the keratocyte apoptosis that occurs in PRK (7,64). The potential effects these differences have on factors such as the algorithm used in LASEK and the wound healing response have not been well characterized.

At present, there are insufficient data to determine whether the incidence of important clinical parameters such as regression and haze are lower in LASEK than PRK, especially for higher levels of correction of myopia and hyperopia. Only large, randomized studies directly comparing LASEK and PRK are likely to detect these differences if they are present because the incidence of regression and clinically significant haze is relatively low after PRK performed with modern lasers that produce smooth ablations.

Laser *in Situ* Keratomileusis

Formation of a flap in routine LASIK procedures results in retention of the central epithelium. This is associated with lower keratocyte apoptosis and necrosis, as well as decreases in other important parameters of the wound healing response such as keratocyte proliferation and myofibroblast differentiation (7). The localization of these processes is also altered, with keratocyte apoptosis, necrosis, and proliferation tending to be deeper in the stroma, away from the epithelium, in LASIK compared with PRK. The thinner the flap in an eye that has LASIK, the greater are the similarities in localization of the wound healing response between LASIK and PRK (7).

Regression

Regression in LASIK is likely attributable to epithelial hyperplasia (43,44,78). Epithelial hyperplasia associated with LASIK can induce regression of the effect of correction of myopia, hyperopia, or astigmatism. It is possible that stromal remodeling contributes to regression in some eyes, although there are limited data confirming this. The tendency for regression is minimal in most eyes that have LASIK. In the eyes of some individuals, however, significant regression is noted, even after lower corrections. This variability could be related to differences in the overall wound healing response between individuals or differences in factors such as flap thickness and, thus, localization of the wound healing response (79,80).

Some variables occurring with LASIK, such as epithelial defects (Oliva MS, Ambrósio R, Periman L, et al., unpublished data, 2002) and diffuse lamellar keratitis (DLK) (81), increase the likelihood that significant regression will occur. These factors increase the overall wound healing response. Epithelial defects also trigger apoptosis and the subsequent

wound healing events in the subepithelial stroma. In these LASIK eyes, wound healing occurs both in the subepithelial stroma and at the level of the lamellar interface. In this case, the overall wound healing response is much greater and regression necessitating enhancement is likely to occur.

Haze

Haze is noted only at the edge of the flap in normal LASIK procedures. This is related to the requirement for epithelial participation in the generation of opaque myofibroblast cells associated with the haze (7,23). However, haze can be noted in the central interface under certain circumstances. The most common situations where haze may be noted after LASIK include DLK, buttonhole flaps, and retention of epithelial debris in the interface.

Haze commonly develops at the level of the interface in eyes affected by severe DLK. This haze is often accompanied by surface irregularity that compromises spectacle-corrected visual acuity. This opacity could be attributable to deposition of disorganized collagen or generation of opaque myofibroblast cells. At present, it is uncertain which of these processes makes the greater contribution.

Buttonhole flaps or irregular flaps/caps are commonly associated with stromal haze at the sites of perforation of the epithelium (Fig. 67-8). Epithelial perforation triggers the typical wound healing cascade, including the generation of myofibroblast cells, at the site of epithelial injury.

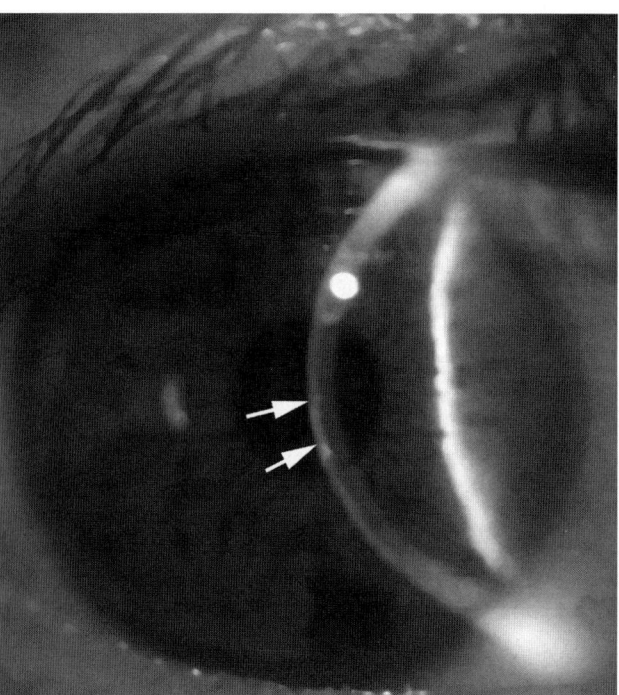

FIGURE 67-8. Slit-lamp photograph of superficial haze (*arrows*) 3 months after a buttonhole flap in laser *in situ* keratomileusis. No excimer laser ablation was applied.

This haze usually persists for many years, but may eventually fade completely in some eyes.

Retention of epithelial debris in the interface or epithelial ingrowth can be associated with the development of interface haze. Presumably, this is attributable to the epithelium participating in the generation of myofibroblast cells at the level of the interface (23).

LASIK-Induced Neurotrophic Epitheliopathy

Most "LASIK-induced dry eye" is probably not dry eye. Rather, it is likely a LASIK-induced neurotrophic epitheliopathy (LINE) attributable to loss of neurotrophic factors from the sensory nerves cut during flap formation (82,83). These soluble factors contribute to normal epithelial physiology and viability. It has not been elucidated which specific factor or factors released by the nerves are important in the pathophysiology of LINE. Blinking rates and other functions related to exposure may also have a role.

Many patients in whom LINE develops have no symptoms or signs of dry eye before surgery (83,84). The typically have onset of dry-eye–like symptoms, associated with punctate epithelial erosions (Fig. 67-9) and rose bengal staining of the epithelium of the flap, from 1 day to a few weeks after surgery. The symptoms often improve with artificial tear treatment, but the signs typically persist until 6 to 8 months after surgery. This correlates with the time required for the nerves to regenerate into the flap (85).

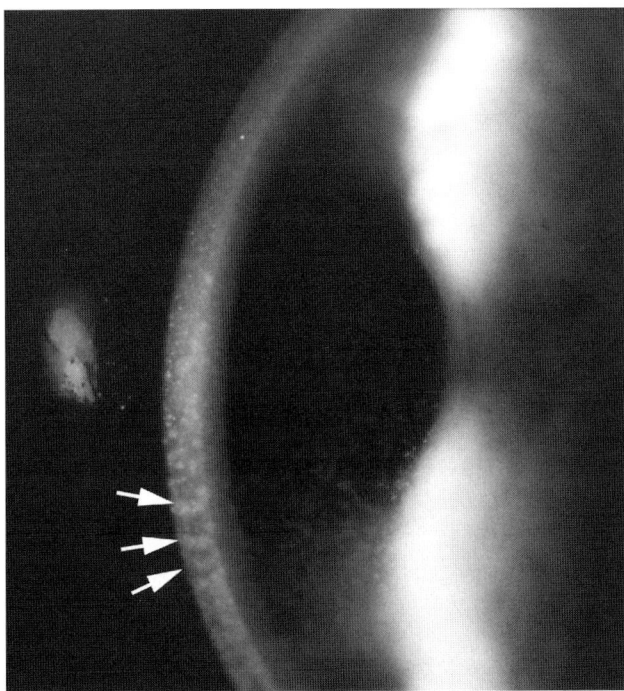

FIGURE 67-9. Slit-lamp photograph of punctate epithelial erosions (*arrows*) of the cornea in an eye at 1 week after laser *in situ* keratomileusis (LASIK). The patient had no symptoms or signs of dry eye before LASIK.

Diffuse Lamellar Keratitis

DLK is an inflammatory condition associated with ocular redness, pain, and decreased vision (81,86,87). At the histologic level, DLK is related to inflammatory cell influx along the lamellar interface.

Epidemic and sporadic DLK likely differ in their pathophysiologic processes (81,88). In epidemic DLK, an exogenous toxic material like detergent from instrument cleaning or exotoxin from improper sterilization (89) probably acts as a direct or indirect chemoattractant to inflammatory cells. These cells migrate into the interface because it is a potential space of least resistance (88). Some sporadic cases could also involve a toxic substance, but many are associated with epithelial defects or blood in the interface. The epithelial defects that precipitate DLK can occur at the time of primary surgery, during retreatment, or months to years after surgery (88). These sporadic cases are likely endogenous and result from activation of systems involving the production of chemokines like MCAF by epithelial and keratocyte cells (6,88). These endogenous chemokines attract inflammatory cells into the potential space of least resistance represented by the lamellar interface.

Epithelial Ingrowth in the Interface

Epithelial growth in the interface is a complication of LASIK that varies in incidence from less than 1% to more than 10%, depending on the study (78,90–93). This section focuses on the sources of epithelial ingrowth in the interface and the biologic effects of the ectopic epithelial tissue on corneal physiology.

Epithelial growth in the LASIK interface can be derived from ingrowth from the periphery at the edge of the flap, downgrowth from the central surface when there are breaks in the flap (i.e. buttonhole flaps), or implantation by the microkeratome blade (91,92). The extent of epithelial growth typically depends on the source of epithelium.

The limbal stem cells are thought to be the ultimate source of the stratified corneal epithelium (3). Progeny of the limbal stem cells with high proliferative capacity are referred to as *transient amplifying cells* (3). These cells are thought to reside at higher density in the peripheral cornea. They may have tremendous proliferative capacity, to the extent that large epithelial defects may be healed with no proliferation of the stem cells themselves. It has been suggested that central corneal epithelial cells have limited proliferative capacity, although an important study that received little attention demonstrated that central basal corneal epithelial cells retain significant potential for mitosis (94).

Epithelial ingrowth beneath the flap edge retains a connection to the peripheral corneal epithelium. Thus, this source of ingrowth has high capacity for progressive extension into the interface. However, even downgrowth from a

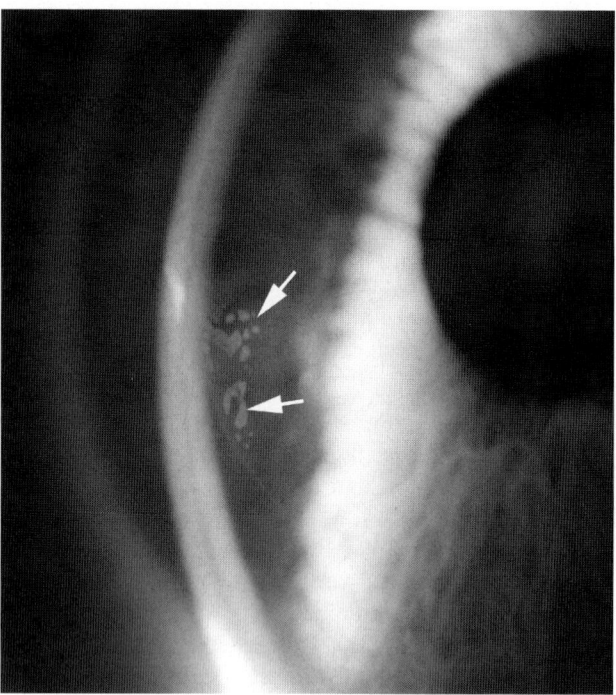

FIGURE 67-10. Slit-lamp photograph of peripheral nests of epithelium at one month after laser *in situ* keratomileusis (LASIK).

central buttonhole flap has the capacity for marked extension into the interface owing to the proliferative capacity of the central basal epithelial cells. In contrast, most epithelial growth in the interface derived from implantation is limited. In these cases, the epithelial cells proliferate to a limited degree and produce islands of epithelial tissue (Fig. 67-10). These islands typically stop expanding when the proliferative capacity of the implanted cells is exhausted. The epithelial islands tend to remain stable for varying periods and then degenerate over time. These nests are usually peripheral and rarely produce symptoms or signs that dictate removal (Fig. 67-10). Rarely, epithelial nests that appear to be produced by implantation undergo a surprising level of extension in the interface. Presumably, this indicates the implanted seed cells included transient amplifying cells.

What is the effect of the ectopic epithelial tissue in the stromal interface? In most cases, especially when the ectopic cells have limited proliferative potential, there is little effect on the physiology of the cornea. The resulting peripheral nests can merely be observed and typically degenerate over time. Ectopic epithelial cells can, however, rarely produce clinically significant complications. One example is DLK initiated by interface epithelial cells or debris (82,88,90). Chemokines from the ectopic epithelial tissue may trigger keratocytes to produce chemokines that attract inflammatory cells (6). Epithelial tissue may also trigger localized stromal remodeling that results in changes to the stroma anterior and posterior to the ectopic epithelium. This stromal remodeling may produce interface irregularity that persists after the epithelium is removed.

This is one reason it is important to intervene early if epithelial ingrowth encroaches on the entrance pupil. Prolonged retention of the epithelium may generate interface irregularity that is projected to the corneal surface.

Epithelial ingrowth in the interface may also trigger stromal melting or necrosis. Most commonly this occurs at the edge of the flap, but it may occur centrally in cases with extensive epithelial ingrowth. There are at least three potential etiologies for stromal melting or necrosis associated with epithelial ingrowth.

First, stromal necrosis can result from deprivation of nutritional support to stromal cells. The cells of the cornea derive energy and molecular building blocks from the aqueous humor. The corneal endothelium maintains a leaky barrier. Under homeostatic conditions, there is a balance between the leak of aqueous humor (with nutrients) through the endothelial layer into the stroma and pumping of water by endothelial cells in the opposite direction. If an impermeable barrier is placed in the stroma, keratocytes anterior to the barrier are deprived of the nutrients. Eventually, the stroma undergoes necrosis (91,93). The first sign of this type of stromal necrosis would be inflammation in the stroma anterior to the ectopic epithelium.

This nutritional deprivation mechanism is usually cited as the cause of stromal melt associated with epithelial ingrowth. There are, however, other mechanisms that may contribute to stromal melting in these cases.

A second mechanism is a chronic loss of keratocytes due to apoptosis. Cytokines such as IL-1, TNF-α, or Fas ligand derived from ectopic corneal epithelium may trigger ongoing apoptosis of keratocytes and other stromal cells (23). Prolonged depletion of keratocytes from an area of stroma could result in melting or necrosis.

A third mechanism is stromal degradation by upregulated collagenases and metalloproteinases. IL-1 released from the ectopic epithelium stimulates production of collagenases, gelatinases, metalloproteinases, and other enzymes by stromal cells (95–97).

One or more of these mechanisms likely has a role in the pathophysiologic process of stromal necrosis associated with epithelial ingrowth. The dominant mechanism in a particular case probably depends on factors such as the location and extent of the ectopic epithelium.

Ectasia

Progressive iatrogenic ectasia that occurs after LASIK has long been attributed to biomechanical factors related to the effect of intraocular pressure on a cornea with insufficient residual posterior stromal bed (<250 μm) (98). However, progressive ectasia has been documented in cases in which the posterior stromal bed appears more than 300 μm with no signs of keratoconus (99). Conversely, many corneas were left with posterior stromal beds of 200 μm or less in the early days of LASIK (Stulting D, personal communication, 2001), without development of ectasia. Thus, although intraocular pressure undoubtedly has an influence on corneal shape, it likely that other factors underlie the progressive nature of ectasia.

One possibility is that LASIK permanently alters normal cellular physiology in some corneas. For example, studies have suggested that the corneal nerves do not fully regenerate in some eyes after LASIK (85). Several studies have also demonstrated that there is a persistent decrease in keratocyte density in the flap after LASIK (100,101). This decrease may be present years after surgery. It is not known whether corneal nerves have trophic influences on keratocytes similar to those documented for epithelial cells. Progressive loss of stromal volume could be related to lack of sufficient keratocytes to maintain stromal integrity. This type of mechanism would be more likely to contribute to ectasia when the relatively acellular stroma makes up a larger proportion of the total stroma. Thus, an eye with a thick flap in a cornea with normal thickness or a normal flap in a relatively thin cornea could be at risk. There could also be genetic factors that predispose some eyes to the development of progressive ectasia, even when there was no evidence of keratoconus or forme fruste keratoconus before surgery. Further research is needed to evaluate the effect of keratocyte density on the development of LASIK-induced ectasia.

Collagen Shrinkage Procedures (Laser Thermokeratoplasty and Conductive Keratoplasty)

Laser thermokeratoplasty (LTK) (102–104) and conductive keratoplasty (CK) (34) are procedures that produce changes in corneal curvature by shrinking tissue in the peripheral cornea. LTK uses energy from a holmium:yttrium-aluminum garnet (YAG) laser and CK uses radio waves. Both denature and shrink the affected stromal collagen. These procedures are commonly used to correct hyperopia or to induce myopia to produce monovision. There are likely differences between the two procedures, but it remains to be determined whether these distinctions will be reflected in clinically significant differences in long-term biologic responses to the procedures.

Regression

Refractive instability and regression are common complications of LTK (102–104). This is not surprising, given that a primary function of keratocytes is to monitor and repair collagen molecules that make up the lamellae of the cornea. Remodeling of collagen and a return of stromal clarity occur over a long period of time after any insult that damages stromal collagen (54,55).

It has been hypothesized that the tendency for regression may be less after CK than after LTK. This remains to be ascertained. However, based on the procedure producing its change by altering collagen structure, it seems likely that long-term stability will also be an issue after CK. The only report on CK with follow-up for at least 1 year shows that there is continued regression in at least some eyes at 1 year after surgery (34).

Induced Astigmatism

Induced astigmatism has also been a common complication in studies of LTK (104). This is likely attributable to differences in the wound healing responses at the multiple lesions applied around the circumference of the cornea. If the initial contraction were greater in a particular meridian, then greater corneal curvature would be induced in this meridian relative to others. Alternatively, if late stromal remodeling is more efficient in one meridian, then astigmatism is likely to develop in the meridian 90 degrees away.

Retreatment in Laser Thermokeratoplasty and Conductive Keratoplasty

Is it safe to reapply LTK or CK in eyes that have regression after the primary procedure or subsequent retreatments? There are no data to address this question. Care, however, should be taken in repeatedly reapplying either LTK or CK. Surface irregularity overlying the entrance pupil associated with localized peripheral ectasia over sites of reapplication of burns is a concern.

Incisional Procedures (Radial Keratotomy and Astigmatic Keratotomy)

Incisional procedures work by weakening corneal structure and producing anterior surface gape that increases anterior corneal surface volume. Both RK and AK include nearly full-thickness incisions, with partial-thickness incisions having far less refractive effect. In RK, radial incisions are used for correction of myopia. In AK, peripheral tangential or circumferential incisions are used for correction of astigmatism.

Myofibroblasts have an important role in healing of incisional wounds in the cornea (105). These contractile cells likely mediate normal healing and strong healing associated with regression of the refractive effect of RK or AK. Studies have suggested that tension in the wound is generated through the formation of intracellular stress fibers and interactions between stress fibers and the extracellular matrix (105). Specific membrane receptor molecules likely act as transducers between the intracellular contractile components and elements of the extracellular matrix. Interestingly, it has been shown that the actin filament–fibronectin–integrin assembly associated with wound contraction in myofibroblasts is aligned parallel with the incision rather than perpendicular in the cat RK model (106).

Histologic studies have demonstrated that many RK and AK incisions retain epithelial plugs (62,63,107). The epithelial plugs extend into the stroma and may contribute to certain complications associated with incisional surgery (Fig. 67-11). Examples include central corneal scarring (possibly due to ongoing stromal–epithelial interactions in the incisions), neurotrophic keratitis (possibly due to blockage of nerve regeneration by epithelial plugs), and progressive hyperopia and fluctuation of vision (possibly due to lack of complete healing of the stroma in areas where epithelial plugs persist in the stroma).

The variability of the wound response in RK and AK is a major determinant of the accuracy and precision of these procedures. The greater accuracy and precision of PRK and LASIK have diminished the role of incisional procedures in refractive surgery.

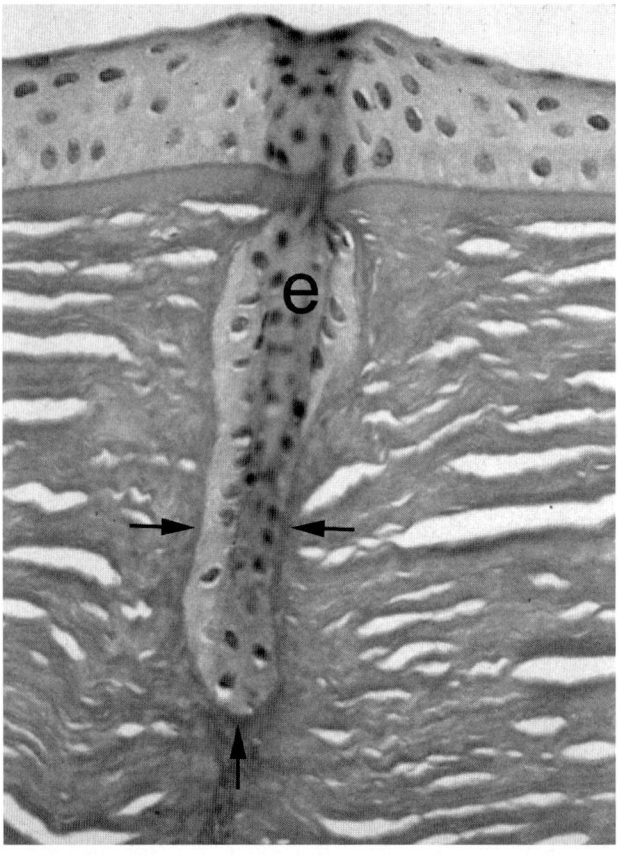

FIGURE 67-11. Human cornea that had radial keratotomy many years before histologic analysis. Note retained epithelial plug (e) extending deep into the stroma. Also note the acellular Bowman's like layer (*arrows*) extending around the epithelial plug. This layer is likely derived and maintained through ongoing epithelial–stromal interactions (hematoxylin and eosin stain, original magnification ×250). (Courtesy of Perry S. Binder, with permission.)

Intrastromal Corneal Ring Segments

Intrastromal corneal ring segments (ICRS) are polymethylmethacrylate (PMMA) inlays placed into circumferential channels in the peripheral cornea to correct low to moderate myopia (108,109). The rings tend to flatten the central cornea to provide refractive effect. Studies have indicated that stability is reasonably good in the intended range of correction.

An advantage of the ICRS is the lack of epithelial or stromal healing in the central cornea. Thus, complications such as central corneal haze are rarely associated with this procedure. Long-term refractive changes due to stromal remodeling around the rings have not been noted, but longer-term studies are needed.

Lamellar channel haze and deposits develop around the segments in some eyes months after implantation. This material may be chalky or gelatinous (Fig. 67-12). One study suggested that some deposits are lipid (cholesterol ester, triglyceride, and unesterified cholesterol) (109). This material is likely produced by keratocytes. The significance of these deposits to long-term corneal physiology and health remains unknown, although they do not appear to affect vision in most patients with several years observation.

Corneal Inlays

The use of corneal inlays to correct myopia or hyperopia involves creation of a lamellar flap and placement of clear synthetic material in the stroma. Various types of synthetic inlays have been tested, including polysulfone (110–112), PMMA (112), and hydrogel (113–115). The contour of the implant determines the correction of refractive error. Inlays that can be modified by laser ablation have also been proposed.

Two of the major issues with inlays are stromal opacities and necrosis. These may be related complications. Stromal and epithelial cells in the cornea obtain energy and nutrients from aqueous humor that leaks through the endothelium. Any type of barrier that blocks the flow of the nutrients can lead to abnormal function of the corneal stromal and epithelial cells. One complication noted is the appearance of stromal deposits. In one study of PMMA intrastromal implants, this material was found to stain positively with oil red 0 and filipin, indicating the presence of neutral fat, as well as unesterified cholesterol (112). In some cases, necrosis or opacification of the overlying cornea can occur. These complications are more commonly noted with polysulfone and PMMA intrastromal lenses (110–112). Hydrogel lenses appear to be better tolerated (113,114).

Regression of the refractive effect has been noted with intracorneal inlays (113). This may result from changes of the lens material or stromal remodeling over time. Further

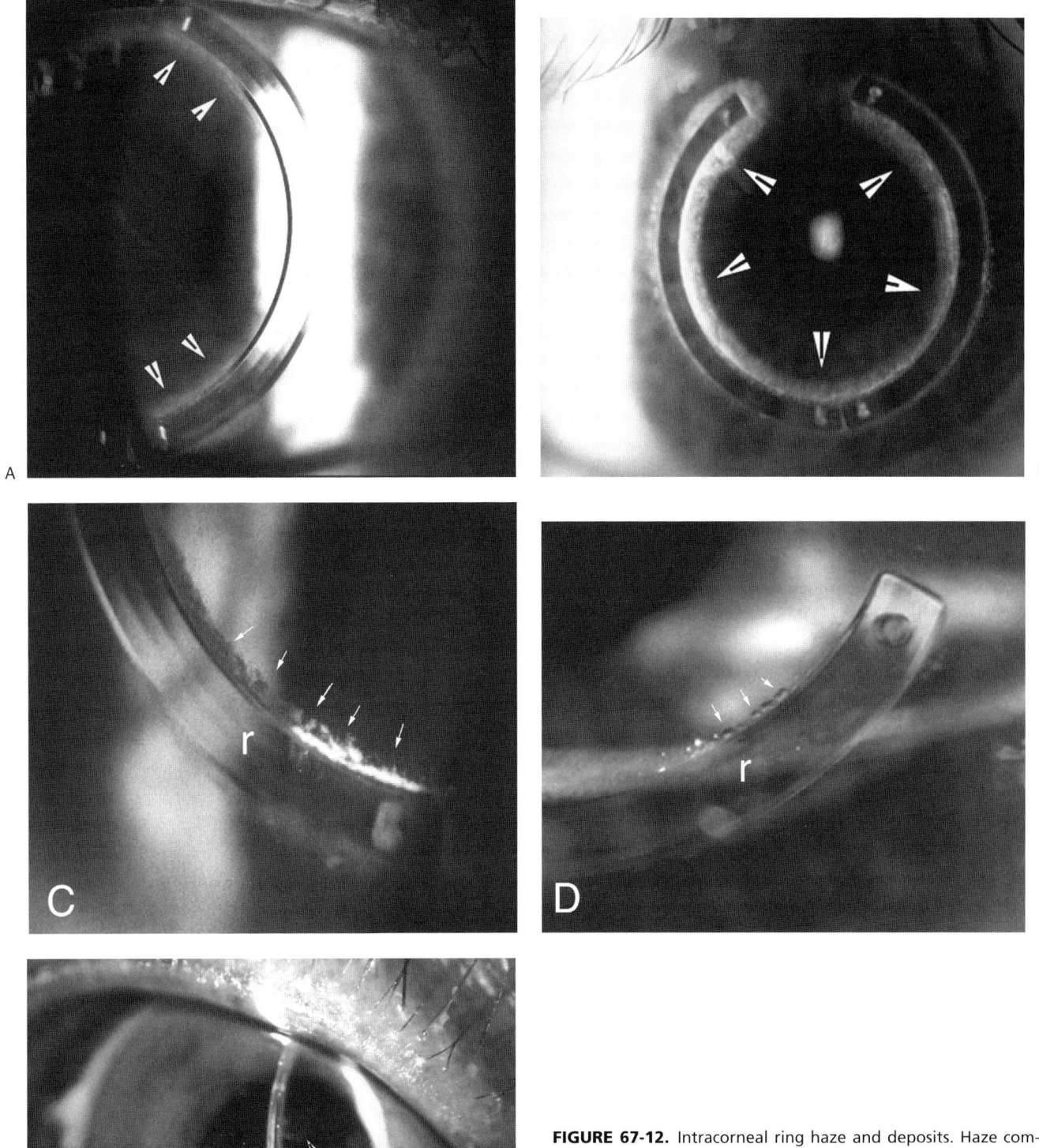

FIGURE 67-12. Intracorneal ring haze and deposits. Haze commonly develops surrounding corneal rings. It can be minimal, moderate **(A)**, or marked **(B)**, depending on the patient. Deposits also occur in some patients. There are several variations of deposits. Chalky **(C)** and gelatinous **(D)** deposits are shown here. The intracorneal ring is indicated by an "r." Stromal deposits **(E)** may develop after implantation of an intrastromal lens. In this example, the lens was placed in the stroma of a monkey cornea. (**A, B, C,** and **D** courtesy of R. Doyle Stulting, with permission; **E** courtesy of Bernard McCarey, from Parks RA, McCarey BE, Knight PM, et al. Intrastromal crystalline deposits following hydrogel keratophakia in monkeys. *Cornea* 1993;12:29, with permission.)

studies are needed to determine whether synthetic inlays can be used to provide stable refractive changes with high optical quality.

REFERENCES

1. Alio JL, Perez-Santonja JJ, Tervo T, et al. Postoperative inflammation, microbial complications, and wound healing following laser in situ keratomileusis. *J Refract Surg* 2000;16:523.
2. Wilson SE, Mohan RR, Mohan RR, et al. The corneal wound healing response: cytokine-mediated interaction of the epithelium, stroma, and inflammatory cells. *Prog Retin Eye Res* 2001; 20:625.
3. Lehrer MS, Sun TT, Lavker RM. Strategies of epithelial repair: modulation of stem cell and transit amplifying cell proliferation. *J Cell Sci* 1998;111:2867.
4. Patel SV, McLaren JW, Camp JJ, et al. Automated quantification of keratocyte density by using confocal microscopy in vivo. *Invest Ophthalmol Vis Sci* 1999;40:320.
5. Petroll WM, Boettcher K, Barry P, et al. Quantitative assessment of anteroposterior keratocyte density in the normal rabbit cornea. *Cornea* 1995;14:3.
6. Hong J-W, Liu JJ, Lee J-S, et al. Pro-inflammatory chemokine induction in keratocytes and inflammatory cell infiltration into the cornea. *Invest Ophthalmol Vis Sci* 2001;42:2795.
7. Mohan RR, Hutcheon AEK, Choi R, et al. Apoptosis, necrosis, proliferation, and myofibroblast generation in the stroma following LASIK and PRK. *Exp Eye Res* 2003;76:71.
8. O'Brien T, Li Q, Ashraf MF, et al. Inflammatory response in the early stages of wound healing after excimer laser keratectomy. *Arch Ophthalmol* 1998;116:1470.
9. Tran MT, Tellaetxe-Isusi M, Elner V, et al. Proinflammatory cytokines induce RANTES and MCP-1 synthesis in human corneal keratocytes but not in corneal epithelial cells: beta-chemokine synthesis in corneal cells. *Invest Ophthalmol Vis Sci* 1996;37:987.
10. Stern ME, Beuerman RW, Fox RI, et al. A unifying theory of the role of the ocular surface in dry eye. *Adv Exp Med Biol* 1998;438:643.
11. Li Q, Weng J, Mohan RR, et al. Hepatocyte growth factor (HGF) and HGF receptor protein in lacrimal gland, tears, and cornea. *Invest Ophthalmol Vis Sci* 1996;37:727.
12. Tuominen I, Vesaluoma M, Teppo AM, et al. Soluble Fas and Fas ligand in human tear fluid after photorefractive keratectomy. *Br J Ophthalmol* 1999;83:1360.
13. Wilson SE, Liang Q, Kim W-J. Lacrimal gland HGF, KGF, and EGF mRNA levels increase after corneal epithelial wounding. *Invest Ophthalmol Vis Sci* 1999;40:2185.
14. Helena MC, Baerveldt F, Kim WJ, et al. Keratocyte apoptosis after corneal surgery. *Invest Ophthalmol Vis Sci* 1998;39:276.
15. Wilson SE, He Y-G, Weng J, et al. Epithelial injury induces keratocyte apoptosis: hypothesized role for the interleukin-1 system in the modulation of corneal tissue organization. *Exp Eye Res* 1996;62:325.
16. Dohlman CH, Gasset AR, Rose J. The effect of the absence of corneal epithelium or endothelium on stromal keratocytes. *Invest Ophthalmol Vis Sci* 1968;7:520.
17. Ambrósio R Jr, Kalina R, Mohan RR, et al. Early wound healing response to epithelial scrape injury in the human cornea. ARVO Abstracts. *Invest Ophthalmol Vis Sci* 2002;43[4 Suppl]:4206(abstr).
18. Gao J, Gelber-Schwalb TA, Addeo JV, et al. Apoptosis in the rabbit cornea after photorefractive keratectomy. *Cornea* 1997; 16:200.
19. Mohan RR, Liang Q, Kim W-J, et al. Apoptosis in the cornea: further characterization of Fas/Fas ligand system. *Exp Eye Res* 1997;65:575.
20. Mohan RR, Mohan RR, Kim WJ, et al. Modulation of TNF-alpha-induced apoptosis in corneal fibroblasts by transcription factor NF-κb. *Invest Ophthalmol Vis Sci* 2000;41:1327.
21. Wilson SE. Analysis of the keratocyte apoptosis, keratocyte proliferation, and myofibroblast transformation responses after photorefractive keratectomy and laser *in situ* keratomileusis. *Trans Am Ophthalmol Soc* 2002;100:411.
22. Wilson SE, Li Q, Weng J, et al. The Fas/Fas ligand system and other modulators of apoptosis in the cornea. *Invest Ophthalmol Vis Sci* 1996;37:1582.
23. Wilson SE, Mohan RR, Hutcheon AEK, et al. Effect of ectopic epithelial tissue within the stroma on keratocyte apoptosis, mitosis, and myofibroblast transformation. *Exp Eye Res* 2003;76:193.
24. Wilson SE, Pedroza L, Beuerman R, et al. Herpes simplex virus type-1 infection of corneal epithelial cells induces apoptosis of the underlying keratocytes. *Exp Eye Res* 1997;64:775.
25. Zhao J, Nagasaki T, Maurice DM. Role of tears in keratocyte loss after epithelial removal in mouse cornea. *Invest Ophthalmol Vis Sci* 2001;42:1743.
26. Wilson SE. Activation of keratocyte apoptosis in response to epithelial scrape injury does not require tears [electronic letter to the editor]. *Invest Ophthalmol Vis Sci* April 2002. Available at http://www.iovs.org/cgi/eletters/42/8/1743.
27. Wilson SE. Keratocyte apoptosis in refractive surgery: Everett Kinsey Lecture. *CLAO J* 1998;24:181.
28. Tervo T, Vesaluoma M, Bennett GL, et al. Tear hepatocyte growth factor (HGF) availability increases markedly after excimer laser surface ablation. *Exp Eye Res* 1997;64:501.
29. Weng J, Mohan RR, Li Q, et al. IL-1 upregulates keratinocyte growth factor and hepatocyte growth factor mRNA and protein production by cultured stromal fibroblast cells: interleukin-1 beta expression in the cornea. *Cornea* 1996; 16:465.
30. Wilson SE, He Y-G, Weng J, et al. Effect of epidermal growth factor, hepatocyte growth factor, and keratinocyte growth factor, on proliferation, motility, and differentiation of human corneal epithelial cells. *Exp Eye Res* 1994;59:665.
31. Zieske JD, Takahashi H, Hutcheon AE, et al. Activation of epidermal growth factor receptor during corneal epithelial migration. *Invest Ophthalmol Vis Sci* 2001;41:1346.
32. Huang J, Kwon R, Possin D, et al. Characterization of inflammatory cell infiltration in rabbits following PRK and LASIK. ARVO Abstracts. *Invest Ophthalmol Vis Sci* 2002;43[4 Suppl]: 4235(abstr).
33. Zieske JD, Guimaraes SR, Hutcheon AE. Kinetics of keratocyte proliferation in response to epithelial debridement. *Exp Eye Res* 2001;72:33.
34. McDonald MB, Davidorf J, Maloney RK, et al. Conductive keratoplasty for the correction of low to moderate hyperopia: 1-year results on the first 54 eyes. *Ophthalmology* 2002; 109:637.
35. Jester JV, Moller-Pedersen T, Huang J, et al. The cellular basis of corneal transparency: evidence for corneal crystallins. *J Cell Sci* 1999;112:613.
36. Jester JV, Petroll WM, Cavanagh HD. Corneal stromal wound healing in refractive surgery: the role of myofibroblasts. *Prog Retin Eye Res* 1999;18:311.
37. Masur S, Dewal HS, Dinh TT, et al. Myofibroblasts differentiate from fibroblasts when plated at low density. *Proc Natl Acad Sci USA* 1996;93:4219.
38. Wilson SE, Chen L, Mohan RR, et al. Expression of HGF, KGF, EGF, and receptor messenger RNAs following corneal epithelial wounding. *Exp Eye Res* 1999;68:377.

39. Moiler-Pedersen T, Cavanagh HD, Petroll WM, et al. Corneal haze development after PRK is regulated by volume of stromal tissue removal. *Cornea* 1998;17:627.

40. Gatry DS, Kerr Muir MG, Marshall J. Excimer laser photorefractive keratectomy: 18-month follow-up. *Ophthalmology* 1992;99:1209.

41. Gauthier CA, Holden BA, Epstein D, et al. Role of epithelial hyperplasia in regression following photorefractive keratectomy. *Br J Ophthalmol* 1996;80:545.

42. Gauthier CA, Holden BA, Epstein D, et al. Factors affecting epithelial hyperplasia after photorefractive keratectomy. *J Cataract Refract Surg* 1997;23:1042.

43. Erie JC, Patel SV, McLaren JW, et al. Effect of myopic laser in situ keratomileusis on epithelial and stromal thickness. *Ophthalmology* 2002;109:1447.

44. Lohmann CP, Guell JL. Regression after LASIK for the treatment of myopia: the role of the epithelium. *Semin Ophthalmol* 1998;13:79.

45. Lohmann CP, Patmore A, O'Brart D, et al. Regression and wound healing after excimer laser PRK: a histopathological study on human corneas. *Eur J Ophthalmol* 1997;7:130.

46. Soadea K, Fasciani R, Necozione S, et al. Role off the corneal epithelium in refractive changes following laser in situ keratomileusis for high myopia. *J Refract Surg* 2000;16:133.

47. Wilson SE, Mohan RR, Hong J-W, et al. The wound healing response after laser *in situ* keratomileusis and photorefractive keratectomy: elusive control of biological variability and effect on custom laser vision correction. *Arch Ophthalmol* 2001;119:889.

48. Kim W-J, Helena MC, Mohan RR, et al. Changes in corneal morphology associated with chronic epithelial injury. *Invest Ophthalmol Vis Sci* 1999;40:35.

49. Anderson NJ, Edelhauser HF, Sharara N, et al. Histologic and ultrastructural findings in human corneas after successful laser in situ keratomileusis. *Arch Ophthalmol* 2002;120:288.

50. Kaji Y, Obata H, Usui T, et al. Three-dimensional organization of collagen fibrils during corneal stromal wound healing after excimer laser keratectomy. *J Cataract Refract Surg* 1998;24:1441.

51. Nakayasu K, Watanabe Y, Gotoh T, et al. Long-term healing of excimer laser ablated rabbit corneas. *Nippon Ganka Gakkai Zasshi* 1999;103:99.

52. Kato T, Nakayasu K, Ikegami K, et al. Analysis of glycosaminoglycans in rabbit cornea after excimer laser keratectomy. *Br J Ophthalmol* 1999;83:609.

53. Weber BA, Gan L, Fagerholm PP. Short-term impact of corticosteroids on hyaluronan and epithelial hyperplasia in the rabbit cornea after photorefractive keratectomy. *Cornea* 2001;20:321.

54. Cintron C, Gregory JD, Damle SP, et al. Biochemical analyses of proteoglycans in rabbit corneal scars. *Invest Ophthalmol Vis Sci* 1990;31:1975.

55. Cintron C, Hassinger LC, Kublin CL, et al. Biochemical and ultrastructural changes in collagen during corneal wound healing. *J Ultrastruct Res* 1978;65:13.

56. Bohm A, Kohlhaas M, Lerche RC, et al. Biomechanical study of corneal stability after photorefractive keratectomy. *Ophthalmologe* 1997;94:109.

57. Dupps WJ, Roberts C. Effect of acute biomechanical changes on corneal curvature after photokeratectomy. *J Refract Surg* 2001;17:658.

58. Roberts C. The cornea is not a piece of plastic. *J Refract Surg* 2000;16:407.

59. Zeng Y, Yang J, Huan K, et al. A comparison of biomechanical properties between human and porcine cornea. *J Biomech* 2001;34:533.

60. Hayashi S, Osawa T, Tohyama K. Comparative observations on corneas, with special reference to Bowman's layer and Descemet's membrane in mammals and amphibians. *J Morphol* 2002;254:247.

61. Wilson SE, Hong JW. Bowman's layer structure and function: critical or dispensable to corneal function? A hypothesis. *Cornea* 2000;19:417.

62. Melles GR, Binder PS, Anderson JA. Variation in healing throughout the depth of long-term, unsutured, corneal wounds in human autopsy specimens and monkeys. *Arch Ophthalmol* 1994;112:100.

63. Melles GR, Binder PS, Moore MN, et al. Epithelial-stromal interactions in human keratotomy wound healing. *Arch Ophthalmol* 1995;113:1124.

64. Kim W-J, Shah S, Wilson SE. Differences in keratocyte apoptosis following transepithelial and laser-scrape photorefractive keratectomy. *J Refract Surg* 1998;14:526.

65. Johnson DG, Kezirian GM, George S, et al. Removal of corneal epithelium with phototherapeutic technique during multizone, multipass photorefractive keratectomy. *J Refract Surg* 1998;14:38.

66. Jain S, McCally RL, Connolly PJ, et al. Mitomycin C reduces corneal light scattering after excimer keratectomy. *Cornea* 2001;20:45.

67. Majmudar PA, Forstot SL, Dennis RF, et al. Topical mitomycin-C for subepithelial fibrosis after refractive corneal surgery. *Ophthalmology* 2000;107:89.

68. Raviv T, Majmudar PA, Dennis RF, et al. Mytomycin-C for post-PRK corneal haze. *J Cataract Refract Surg* 2000;26:1105.

69. Kim T, Tchah H, Lee SA, et al. Apoptosis in keratocytes caused by mitomycin C. *Invest Ophthalmol Vis Sci* 2003;44:1912.

70. Vinciguerra P, Azzolini M, Airaghi P, et al. Effect of decreasing surface and interface irregularities after photorefractive keratectomy and laser *in situ* keratomileusis on optical and functional outcomes. *J Refract Surg* 1998;14:S199.

71. Lipshitz I, Loewenstein A, Varssano D, et al. Late onset corneal haze after photorefractive keratectomy for moderate and high myopia. *Ophthalmology* 1997;104:369.

72. Perez-Santonja JJ, Sakla HF, Cardona C, et al. Corneal sensitivity after photorefractive keratectomy and laser *in situ* keratomileusis for low myopia. *Am J Ophthalmol* 1999;127:497.

73. Chen CC, Chang JH, Lee JB, et al. Human corneal epithelial cell viability and morphology after dilute alcohol exposure. *Invest Ophthalmol Vis Sci* 2002;43:2593.

74. Kornilovsky IM. Clinical results after subepithelial photorefractive keratectomy (LASEK). *J Refract Surg* 2001;17:S222.

75. Vinciguerra P, Camesasca FI. Butterfly laser epithelial keratomileusis for myopia. *J Refract Surg* 2002;18:S371.

76. McDonald M. American Academy of Ophthalmology, 2001.

77. Boudreau N, Werb Z, Bissell MJ. Suppression of apoptosis by basement membrane requires three-dimensional tissue organization and withdrawal from the cell cycle. *Proc Natl Acad Sci USA* 1996,93:3509.

78. Stulting RD, Carr JD, Thompson KP, et al. Complications of laser in situ keratomileusis for the correction of myopia. *Ophthalmology* 1999;106:13.

79. Behrens A, Seitz B, Langenbucher A, et al. Evaluation of corneal flap dimensions and cut quality using the Automated Corneal Shaper microkeratome. *J Refract Surg* 2000;16:83.

80. Yildirim R, Aras C, Ozdamar A, et al. Reproducibility of corneal flap thickness in laser in situ keratomileusis using the Hansatome microkeratome. *J Cataract Refract Surg* 2000;26:1729.

81. Johnson JD, Harissi-Dagher M, Pineda R, et al. Diffuse lamellar keratitis: incidence, associations, outcomes, and a new classification system. *J Cataract Refract Surg* 2001;27:1560.

82. Wilson SE. LASIK: management of common complications. *Cornea* 1998;17:459.

83. Wilson SE. Laser *in situ* keratomileusis-induced (presumed) neurotrophic epitheliopathy. *Ophthalmology* 2001;108:1082.

84. Wilson SE, Ambrósio R Jr. Laser *in situ* keratomileusis-induced neurotrophic epitheliopathy. *Am J Ophthalmol* 2001;132:405–406.

85. Linna TU, Vesaluoma MH, Perez-Santonja JJ, et al. Effect of myopic LASIK on corneal sensitivity and morphology of subbasal nerves. *Invest Ophthalmol Vis Sci* 2000;41:393.

86. Linebarger EJ, Hardten DR, Lindstrom RL. Diffuse lamellar keratitis: diagnosis and management. *J Cataract Refract Surg* 2000;26:1072.

87. Smith RJ, Maloney RK. Diffuse lamellar keratitis: a new syndrome in lamellar refractive surgery. *Ophthalmology* 1998;105:1721.

88. Wilson SE, Ambrósio R Jr. Sporadic diffuse lamellar keratitis (DLK) following LASIK. *Cornea* 2002;21:560.

89. Holland SP, Mathias RG, Morck DW, et al. Diffuse lamellar keratitis related to endotoxins released from sterilizer reservoir biofilms. *Ophthalmology* 2000;107:1227.

90. Ambrósio R Jr, Wilson SE. Complications of laser *in situ* keratomileusis: etiology, prevention, and treatment. *J Refract Surg* 2001;17:350.

91. Helena MC, Meisler DM, Wilson SE. Epithelial growth within the lamellar interface following laser *in situ* keratomileusis (LASIK). *Cornea* 1997;16:300.

92. Walker MB, Wilson SE. Incidence and prevention of epithelial growth within the interface after laser *in situ* keratomileusis. *Cornea* 2000;19:170.

93. Wang MY, Maloney RK. Epithelial ingrowth after laser *in situ* keratomileusis. *Am J Ophthalmol* 2000;129:746.

94. Haddad A. Renewal of the rabbit corneal epithelium as investigated by autoradiography after intravitreal injection of 3H-thymidine. *Cornea* 2000;19:378.

95. Girard MT, Matsubara M, Fini ME. Transforming growth factor-beta and interleukin-1 modulate metalloproteinase expression by corneal stromal cells. *Invest Ophthalmol Vis Sci* 1991; 32:2441.

96. Li DQ, Lokeshwar BL, Solomon A, et al. Regulation of MMP-9 production by human corneal epithelial cells. *Exp Eye Res* 2001;73:449.

97. West-Mays JA, Strissel KJ, Sadow PM, et al. Competence for collagenase gene expression by tissue fibroblasts requires activation of an interleukin 1 alpha autocrine loop. *Proc Natl Acad Sci U S A* 1995;92:6768.

98. Pallikaris IG, Kymionis GD, Astyrakakis NI. Corneal ectasia induced by laser *in situ* keratomileusis. *J Cataract Refract Surg* 2001;27:1796.

99. Amoils SP, Deist MB, Gous P, et al. Iatrogenic keratectasia after laser in situ keratomileusis for less than −4.0 to −7.0 diopters of myopia. *J Cataract Refract Surg* 2000;26:967.

100. Mitooka K, Ramirez M, Maguire LJ, et al. Keratocyte density of central human cornea after laser in situ keratomileusis. *Am J Ophthalmol* 2002;133:307.

101. Vesaluoma M, Perez-Santonja J, Petroll WM, et al. Corneal stromal changes induced by myopic LASIK. *Invest Ophthalmol Vis Sci* 2000;41:369.

102. Brinkmann R, Radt B, Flamm C, et al. Influence of temperature and time on thermally induced forces in corneal collagen and the effect on laser thermokeratoplasty. *J Cataract Refract Surg* 2000;26:744.

103. Geerling G, Koop N, Tungler A, et al. Dioden-Laserthermokeratoplastik. *Erste Klin Erfahr Ophthalmol* 1999;96:306.

104. Tutton MK, Cherry PM. Holmium:YAG laser thermokeratoplasty to correct hyperopia: two years follow-up. *Ophthalmic Surg Lasers* 1996;27:S521.

105. Garana RM, Petroll WM, Chen WT, et al. Radial keratotomy: II. Role of the myofibroblast in corneal wound contraction. *Invest Ophthalmol Vis Sci* 1992;33:3271.

106. Petroll WM, Cavanagh HD, Jester JV. Assessment of stress fiber orientation during healing of radial keratotomy wounds using confocal microscopy. *Scanning* 1998;20:74.

107. Melles GR, Sundar Raj N, Binder PS, et al. Immunohistochemical analysis of unsutured and sutured corneal wound healing. *Curr Eye Res* 1995;14:809.

108. Asbell PA, Ucakhan OO. Long-term follow-up of Intacs from a single center. *J Cataract Refract Surg* 2001;27:1456.

109. Ruckhofer J. Clinical and histological studies on the intrastromal corneal ring segments (ICRS). *Klin Monatsbl Augenheilkd* 2002;219:557.

110. Horgan SE, Fraser SG, Choyce DP, et al. Twelve year follow-up of unfenestrated polysulfone intracorneal lenses in human sighted eyes. *J Cataract Refract Surg* 1996;22:1045.

111. Kirkness CM, Steele AD, Garner A. Polysulfone corneal inlays. Adverse reactions: a preliminary report. *Trans Ophthalmol Soc UK* 1985;104:343.

112. Rodrigues MM, McCarey BE, Waring GO, et al. Lipid deposits posterior to impermeable intracorneal lenses in rhesus monkeys: clinical, histochemical, and ultrastructural studies. *Refract Corneal Surg* 1990;6:32.

113. Barraquer JI, Gomez ML. Permalens hydrogel intracorneal lenses for spherical ametropia. *J Refract Surg* 1997;13:342.

114. Steinert RF, Storie B, Smith P, et al. Hydrogel intracorneal lenses in aphakic eyes. *Arch Ophthalmol* 1996;114:135.

115. Werblin TP, Patel AS, Barraquer JI. Initial human experience with Permalens myopic hydrogel intracorneal lens implants. *Refract Corneal Surg* 1992;8:23.

PREOPERATIVE CONSIDERATIONS: PATIENT SELECTION AND EVALUATION

SANDEEP JAIN AND MARGARET CHANG

Preoperative evaluation for refractive surgery follows a structured sequence that includes patient interview followed by a complete ophthalmologic examination (Table 68-1). The aim of preoperative evaluation is to answer three broad questions in addition to generating specific refractive data for the actual treatment:

1. Is it possible safely to perform refractive surgery in the patient?
2. What is the risk of possible complications, given the patient specifics?
3. Is it possible to meet the expectations that the patient has from the surgery?

Patients are advised to discontinue wearing contact lenses at least two weeks before the preoperative evaluation and to schedule up to 2 hours for the preoperative evaluation examination. Because cycloplegic refraction is performed as part of the examination, patients are advised that they may be unable to read for 6 to 12 hours and are advised against driving by themselves during this time.

A detailed history forms an important part of the patient selection process. The purpose is to identify patients who either are not expected to have a good postoperative outcome or not expected to be satisfied with the procedure.

PATIENT CHARACTERISTICS

Patients younger than 18 years of age and women who are pregnant or breast-feeding cannot have refractive surgery. Patients engaged in sports in which blows to the face and eyes are a common occurrence (boxing, wrestling, or martial arts), or in occupations that have a greater likelihood of producing trauma or injuries (armed forces, police, or secret service), may have refractive surgery but are usually offered photorefractive keratectomy (PRK) or laser subepithelial keratomileusis (LASEK) as alternatives to laser *in situ* keratomileusis (LASIK). Because refractive surgery may cause loss of best corrected visual acuity, loss in contrast sensitivity, or higher-order aberrations (if the treatment is decentered),

patients should check with their prospective employers about the qualifying refractive criteria. Some employers require contrast sensitivity testing and glare disability measurement in addition to determining uncorrected Snellen visual acuity.

Expectation from the Surgery

The goal of refractive surgery is to reduce the dependence on eyeglasses and contact lenses. Postoperative vision invariably can be improved further with additional optical correction. In presbyopic patients, additional near-vision correction is required after adequate distance-vision correction. Patients who expect perfect distance vision or presbyopic patients who expect equally good distance and reading vision are poor candidates for refractive surgery. If monovision is suggested as an option, then a 2-week trial of contact lens monovision is given to determine if the patient accepts the compromises inherent in the monovision strategy. One in four patients fails to adapt to monovision (1,2).

Refractive Stability

The refraction should be stable over at least 1 year. Patients in whom refraction has changed considerably over the past 1 year (more than 0.5 D), are poor candidates for surgery.

Ocular and Medical History

Refractive surgery is contraindicated in patients with history of herpes simplex or herpes zoster ophthalmicus. Reactivation of herpes virus infection has been reported in the postoperative period (3). Refractive surgery is not performed in patients who have keratoconus and in those who are on Accutane therapy. Relative contraindications to refractive surgery include patients who have glaucoma, patients who are glaucoma suspect or have ocular hypertension, or those who have a history of uveitis. If the patient has a history of prior refractive surgeries, particularly radial or astigmatic keratotomy, then additional refractive procedures (PRK or

TABLE 68-1   PREOPERATIVE TESTS FOR REFRACTIVE SURGERY

Examination	Value	Consider These Additional Tests
Pachymetry	<500 μm	Orbscan, intraoperative pachymetry
	>600 μm	Specular microscopy
Keratometry	<40 D or >48 D	Topography: simulated keratometry (Sim K), Orbscan
Tonometry	≥21 mm Hg	Visual field test and glaucoma consultation
Funduscopy	C:D ≥ 0.5	Glaucoma consultation
	Lattice	Retina consultation
Topography	Inferior-superior (I-S) value ≥ 1.4	Repeat topography in 2 wk to rule out contact lens warpage or keratoconus
Schirmer's test	≤5 mm wetting	Temporary collagen plugs

*CD, cup: disk

LASIK) are associated with unpredictable refractive outcomes and greater potential complications.

Certain medical conditions, such as autoimmune diseases (e.g., lupus, rheumatoid arthritis), immunodeficiency states (e.g., human immunodeficiency virus infection), and diabetes, may prevent proper healing after a refractive procedure and therefore also are considered relative contraindications. If the patient has a history of keloid formation, then PRK or LASEK is to be avoided. Although safety with PRK has been reported in keloid formers, LASIK seems to be safer in such patients given the minimal wound healing response (4).

EYE EXAMINATION

A complete ophthalmic examination is performed. This includes recording uncorrected Snellen visual acuity, visual acuity with current eyeglasses, dry manifest refraction, and wet manifest refraction (after cycloplegia with 1% cyclopentolate eye drops). Based on the currently approved indications, the extent of myopia and astigmatism determines the choice of excimer laser as well as whether wavefront-guided surgery is an option (Table 68-2).

The pupil size is measured with room lights as well as in darkness (with an infrared pupillometer such as the Colvard pupillometer). If the pupil dilates to more than 7 mm in the dark, then the patient may be at a higher risk for postoperative glare and haloes. This is especially true for patients who have high astigmatism (because of the elliptical shape of the treatment) or high refractive error, and who are young (5).

The intraocular pressure is measured using applanation tonometry (Goldmann tonometer or pneumotonometer). If the patient has ocular hypertension, a baseline glaucoma workup should be performed. This includes a visual field test and optic nerve pictures as well as glaucoma service consultation. After refractive surgery, the intraocular pressure measurement is lower than the real measurement. It is possible to miss patients with ocular hypertension who may progress to development of glaucoma because the falsely lower pressure may not be subjected to the same degree of glaucoma suspicion and testing as a higher-than-normal pressure (6,7).

Ultrasonographic pachymetry is performed to measure the corneal thickness. If the cornea is unusually thick (>600 μm) or thin (<500 μm), topographic analysis using the Orbscan (Bausch & Lomb, Rochester, NY) could be per-

TABLE 68-2   U. S. FOOD AND DRUG ADMINISTRATION-APPROVED LASERS FOR LASIK

Laser and Model	Approval Date	Approved Indications
Alcon LADARVision	10/18/02	Wavefront-guided LASIK: myopia up to −7 D with or without astigmatism <0.5 D
	5/9/00	LASIK: myopia < −9 D with or without astigmatism from −0.5 to −3 D
Bausch & Lomb	5/15/02	Myopia < −11 D with or without astigmatism < −3 D
Technolas 217a	2/25/03	Hyperopia between 1 and 4 D with or without astigmatism up to 2 D
VISX		
Star S2 and S3	11/19/99	Myopia < −4 D with or without astigmatism between −0.5 and −5 D
	4/27/01	Hyperopia between +0.5 and +5 D with or without astigmatism up to +3 D
	11/16/01	Mixed astigmatism up to 6 D
Star S4 and WaveScan	5/23/03	Wavefront-guided LASIK: myopia up to −6 D with or without astigmatism up to −3 D
Nidek EC5000	4/14/00	Myopia from 1 to −14 D with or without astigmatism <4 D
LaserSight LaserScan LSX	9/28/01	Myopia from −0.5 to −6 D with or without astigmatism up to 4.5 D

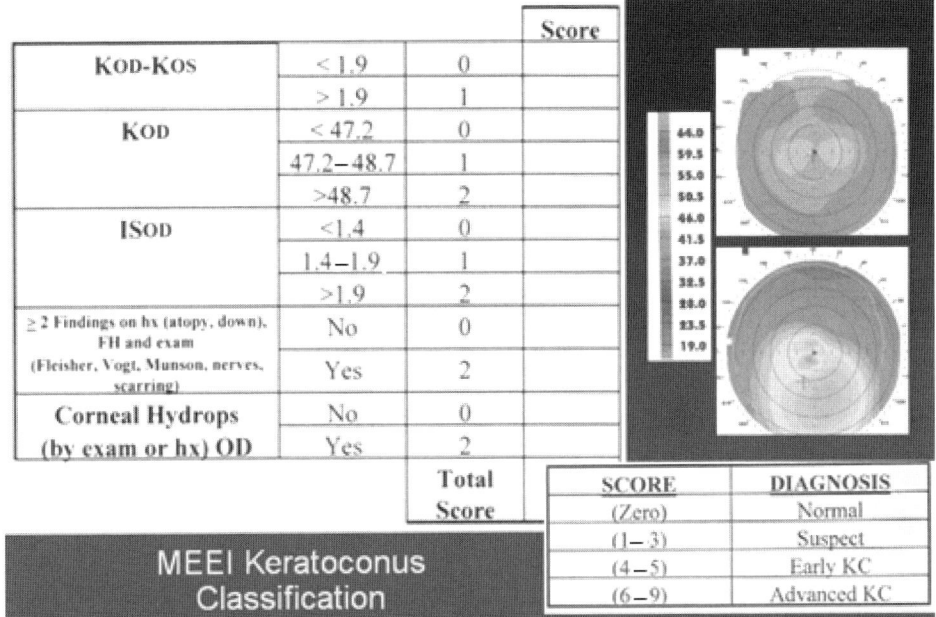

		Score			
KOD–KOS	< 1.9	0			
	> 1.9	1			
KOD	< 47.2	0			
	47.2–48.7	1			
	>48.7	2			
ISOD	<1.4	0			
	1.4–1.9	1			
	>1.9	2			
≥ 2 Findings on hx (atopy, down), FH and exam	No	0			
(Fleisher, Vogt, Munson, nerves, scarring)	Yes	2			
Corneal Hydrops	No	0			
(by exam or hx) OD	Yes	2			
	Total Score				

SCORE	DIAGNOSIS
(Zero)	Normal
(1–3)	Suspect
(4–5)	Early KC
(6–9)	Advanced KC

MEEI Keratoconus Classification

FIGURE 68-1. Massachusetts Eye and Ear Infirmary keratoconus classification. Based on history, clinical examination, and corneal topography findings a score is generated to diagnose keratocomy.

formed to confirm the measurements. Although slit-lamp examination of the endothelium using specular reflection reveals presence of guttata, specular microscopy may be performed to assess endothelial cell morphology and density. If the cornea is thin (<500 μm), PRK or LASEK may be preferable to LASIK. Given that at least 250 μm of bed is left untreated to prevent the possibility of postoperative ectasia, and given that the corneal flap is approximately 160 to 180 μm in thickness, only a limited extent of treatment is possible in patients with thin corneas. In addition, there may be buttonholes or other flap-cutting complications. Because the actual flap thickness after a microkeratome cut may vary, the patient is advised that intraoperative pachymetry performed after the corneal flap is fashioned will provide a better estimate of how much treatment can be performed.

Eye dominance is determined by the hole-in-the-card test or by viewing a distant object through a gap between the outstretched hands. Usually the nondominant eye is operated first. The second eye (dominant eye) may be operated either on another day (usually within a week) or on the same day as the first eye. If the patient requests both eyes to be operated on the same day, then counseling regarding the additional potential risk is provided. Although sequential surgery allows assessment of complications in the first eye, it probably does not in general reduce the risk of a complication in the second eye. Simultaneous bilateral LASIK has been reported to be as safe and effective as sequential surgery.

Slit-lamp examination of the anterior and posterior segments of the eye is performed. Specifically, the presence of blepharitis is noted and treated if present before surgery. The presence of superficial punctuate keratitis may be due to dry eyes. Schirmer's test is performed. Wetting less than 5 mm in 5 minutes is consistent with severe dry-eye disease. Because after the refractive surgery the dry-eye disease will most likely worsen, the patient is counseled about this possibility (8). A punctal plug may be placed before or immediately after surgery. The presence of clinical signs of keratoconus is noted. These include corneal thinning, Fleischer's ring, and Vogt's striae. The Massachusetts Eye and Ear Infirmary method of keratoconus classification is a useful method to detect patients with suspected keratoconus (Fig. 68-1). The presence of corneal guttata is noted and, if present, specular microscopy is requested for endothelial cell count and morphology.

Dilated fundus examination is performed using slit-lamp biomicroscopy (using a +78 D or +90 D lens) to examine the central fundus and indirect ophthalmoscopy (using a +20 D lens) to examine the retinal periphery. If peripheral retinal degenerations (lattice degeneration or atrophic retinal holes) are present, retina consultation may be sought. Retinal detachment has been reported in a few cases 2 to 9 months after LASIK (9,10).

CORNEAL TOPOGRAPHY AND WAVEFRONT ANALYSIS

Computed corneal topography examination is an important part of the preoperative evaluation. The average simulated keratometry (Sim K) value is noted. This number is used to choose the diameter of the flap cut (9.5 mm if ≤40 D and 8.5 mm if ≥48 D). If the inferior-superior (I-S) value is more than 1.4, keratoconus is suspected and should be ruled out. Any inferior steepening should raise the suspicion of forme fruste keratoconus. Refractive surgery in such patients may lead to keratectasia (11,12). To exclude the possibility that the inferior steepening may be due to contact lens warpage, a repeat topography is performed after 2 weeks. Contact lens warpage-induced steepening will reduce on subsequent topography examinations. Wavefront analysis is performed to determine the extent of higher-order aberrations.

PATIENT EDUCATION AND INFORMED CONSENT

An important part of the preoperative evaluation concerns informing the patient about potential risks and limitations of the surgery, as well as providing a copy of the consent form for the patient to read, understand, and sign.

Complications of refractive surgery are infrequent, occurring in general in less than 5% patients, but nonetheless can cause permanent vision sequelae (13). Some of the potential complications include undercorrection, overcorrection, additional surgeries, glare, haloes, flap complications (in LASIK) (14), infection, inflammation, need for eyeglasses after surgery, loss of best corrected vision, and loss of vision and eye. The likely risk of these complications based on the results of the eye examination are discussed with the patient. A video demonstration of the procedure helps to provide further clarity about these issues.

It is important to maintain records of preoperative refractive data. If the patient needs cataract surgery in the future, it becomes very difficult to calculate the correct power of intraocular lens needed if data from before refractive surgery are unavailable (15).

Refractive surgery is an elective surgery that is performed to enhance the quality of life in patients who depend on eyeglasses or contact lenses. A carefully performed preoperative examination helps to select individuals in whom a satisfactory outcome can be reasonably expected. Patients who have a high risk for development of potential complications or who have unrealistic expectations for the surgery are advised against having refractive surgery.

REFERENCES

1. Jain S, Ou R, Azar DT. Monovision outcomes in presbyopic individuals after refractive surgery. *Ophthalmology* 2001; 108:1430–1433.
2. Jain S, Arora I, Azar DT. Success of monovision in presbyopes: review of the literature and potential applications to refractive surgery. *Surv Ophthalmol* 1996;40:491–499.
3. Perry HD, Doshi SJ, Donnenfeld ED, et al. Herpes simplex reactivation following laser *in situ* keratomileusis and subsequent corneal perforation. *CLAO J* 2002;28:69–71.
4. Tanzer DJ, Isfahani A, Schallhorn SC, et al. Photorefractive keratectomy in African Americans including those with known dermatologic keloid formation. *Am J Ophthalmol* 1998; 126:625–629.
5. Lee YC, Hu FR, Wang IJ. Quality of vision after laser in situ keratomileusis: influence of dioptric correction and pupil size on visual function. *J Cataract Refract Surg* 2003; 29:769–777.
6. Shaikh NM, Shaikh S, Singh K, et al. Progression to end-stage glaucoma after laser *in situ* keratomileusis. *J Cataract Refract Surg* 2002;28:356–359.
7. Duch S, Serra A, Castanera J, et al. Tonometry after laser *in situ* keratomileusis treatment. *J Glaucoma* 2001;10:261–265.
8. Ang RT, Dartt DA, Tsubota K. Dry eye after refractive surgery. *Curr Opin Ophthalmol* 2001;12:318–322.
9. Aras C, Ozdamar A, Karacorlu M, et al. Retinal detachment following laser *in situ* keratomileusis. *Ophthalmic Surg Lasers* 2000;31:121–125.
10. Wilkinson CP. Retina and vitreous pathology after LASIK. *Ophthalmology* 2001;108:2157.
11. Lafond G, Bazin R, Lajoie C. Bilateral severe keratoconus after laser in situ keratomileusis in a patient with forme fruste keratoconus. *J Cataract Refract Surg* 2001;27:1115–1118.
12. Schmitt-Bernard CF, Lesage C, Arnaud B. Keratectasia induced by laser *in situ* keratomileusis in keratoconus. *J Refract Surg* 2000;16:368–370.
13. Melki SA, Azar DT. LASIK complications: etiology, management, and prevention. *Surv Ophthalmol* 2001;46:95–116.
14. Knorz MC. Flap and interface complications in LASIK. *Curr Opin Ophthalmol* 2002;13:242–245.
15. Randleman JB, Loupe DN, Song CD, et al. Intraocular lens power calculations after laser *in situ* keratomileusis. *Cornea* 2002;21:751–755.

PREOPERATIVE CONSIDERATIONS: CORNEAL TOPOGRAPHY

DOUGLAS D. KOCH AND LI WANG

Detailed examination of corneal curvature is an essential part of the workup before refractive surgery. Computerized videokeratography (CVK) plays several critical roles in the preoperative considerations of refractive surgery, including: (a) providing general information regarding the corneal shape; (b) detecting corneal warpage and monitoring the topographic stability after discontinuation of contact lens wear; and (c) detecting ectatic corneal disorders, such as keratoconus or keratoconus suspects, pellucid marginal degeneration (PMD), keratoglobus, or other topographic abnormalities.

ASSESSMENT OF CORNEAL SHAPE

Two principles of CVK exist: the reflection-based system and the projection-based system. Placido disk technology is based on the reflection principle and has been most widely accepted, used, and understood. The Placido target is projected onto the cornea and reflected off the tear film, which is in turn captured and analyzed to reconstruct the corneal shape. The Orbscan slit-scanning topography system (Bausch & Lomb, Rochester, NY) is the only commercially available device that uses the principle of projection to measure directly the corneal elevation.

Display of Corneal Shape

There are several ways in which the shape of the cornea can be measured and represented by color-coded maps.

Radius of Curvature

Radius of curvature can be calculated by two means:

- *Axial radius of curvature*: Axial radius of curvature is calculated by measuring the perpendicular distance from the tangent at a point to the optical (or sagittal) axis. Although the axial map is the most commonly used CVK display, it has a spherical bias because each measured curvature is referred to the optical axis (1) (Fig. 69-1A).

- *Tangential (instantaneous/local) radius of curvature*: Tangential radius of curvature is calculated at each point with respect to its neighboring points by fitting the best-fit sphere (BFS). Tangential radius of curvature shows more marked changes over smaller regions and provides more accurate measurements of corneal curvature, and certainly better representation of local irregularity, than axial radius of curvature (Fig. 69-1B).

Corneal Power

The radius of curvature (r, in meters) can be converted to power (P, in diopters) using a simplified paraxial formula by assuming that the rays of light striking the cornea are paraxial:

$$P = (n' - 1)/r \; [1]$$

where n' is the standardized value for keratometric index of refraction; 1.3375 is used for most CVK devices. The standardized value for keratometric index of refraction, n', is not the true refractive index of the cornea but is an approximated index to yield the total corneal power as a single refracting surface by compensating for the negative power of the posterior surface. Corneal power relates to the patient's refractive status, and is therefore frequently used in clinical practice; however, it is less accurate than the tangential curvature map when representing the corneal shape because of the paraxial assumption made during its derivation.

Corneal Height or Elevation

Corneal height or elevation is defined by the distance of each of point on the corneal surface from a reference plane. The reference plane is determined using a least-squares method, and the elevation display depends on reference surface size, shape, alignment, and fitting zone. Positive elevation measurements indicate that the corneal surface falls above the reference plane and are represented as warm colors, whereas negative values indicate that the corneal surface falls below the reference plane and are represented

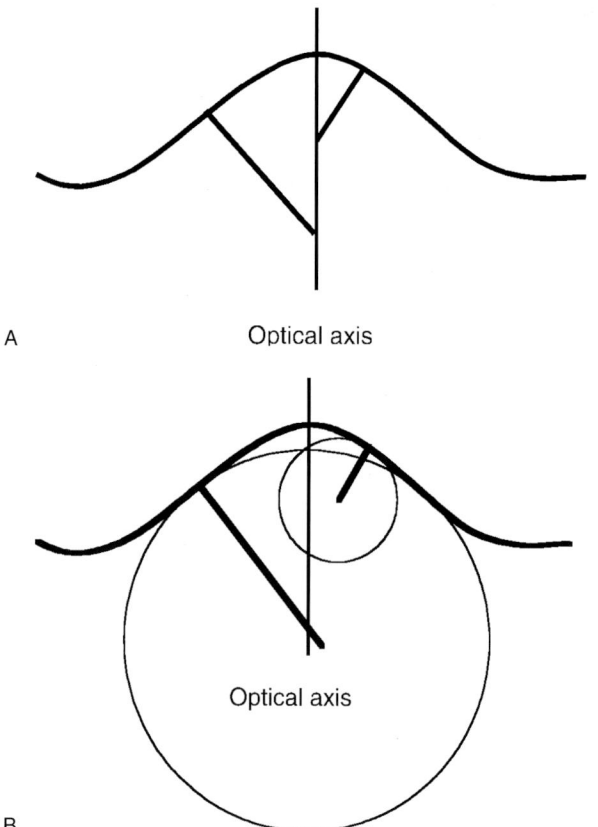

FIGURE 69-1. Two approaches for the calculation of corneal radius of curvature. **A,** Axial radius of curvature. **B,** Tangential radius of curvature.

as cool colors on the elevation maps (Fig. 69-2). Elevation maps have particular value in assessing postoperative visual problems and guiding topography-based ablation.

Color-Coded Maps

A number of different dioptric intervals have been recommended for standardized scales of color-coded maps. Scales with intervals greater than 0.5 D are useful for corneas with large dioptric ranges, and a 0.5-D scale is required to obtain sufficient detail regarding nuances that affect visual performance. Most topographers offer some type of standardized absolute scale and adjustable scales that allow the clinician to customize the information for maximal clinical value. It is critical first to check the scale and step interval when viewing a color-coded topographic map.

Numeric and Statistical Indices

CVK devices provide a number of numeric and statistical indices that can tremendously enhance analysis of topographic maps. The cursor can be moved to any position on the map and the information regarding its radius of curvature, power or elevation, and its distances and axis from the corneal center or the entrance pupil center are displayed.

Most of the devices provide some type of numeric display, which gives numeric values along certain meridians and annular zones (Fig. 69-3). Statistical indices summarize particular features of the cornea:

- *Simulated keratometry (Sim K):* Sim K is provided by all devices; this value attempts to mimic conventional keratometry readings and represents orthogonal curvatures at the 3-mm zone.
- *Mean values at central zone:* Some systems display the mean values in certain central zones. For example, the effective refractive power (EffRP) from the Holladay Diagnostic Summary Display of the EyeSys Corneal Analysis System (EyeSys Technologies, Houston, TX) represents the mean refractive power of the cornea over the central 3-mm zone, taking into account the Stiles Crawford effect (2).
- *Surface regularity index (SRI):* The SRI is a measure of the local regularity of the corneal surface in the central 4.5-mm diameter. SRI values increase with increasing irregular astigmatism and approach zero for a smooth corneal surface. Studies have demonstrated that the SRI is highly correlated with best spectacle-corrected visual acuity (BCVA) (3–6).
- *Surface asymmetry index (SAI):* The SAI measures the difference in corneal powers at each ring 180 degrees apart as a measure of symmetry. The SAI value would be zero for a perfect sphere, a surface with perfectly spherocylindrical regular astigmatism, and for any surface with power values that are radially symmetric (3).
- *Potential visual acuity (PVA) or predicted corneal acuity (PCA):* PVA or PCA is an estimation of predicted visual acuity if the cornea is the only factor limiting vision. A study reported that the PCA appears to be most useful in predicting the BCVA in patients with normal corneas, but is less precise in patients with corneal abnormalities (7).
- *Asphericity:* Asphericity is usually quantitatively described by the Q value. For a sphere, $Q = 0$. For prolate surfaces, $Q < 0$, and for oblate surfaces, $Q > 0$. Mean reported Q values ranges from -0.15 to -0.30 (8–10). Related parameters include eccentricity of the equivalent conic section (e), and shape factor (P), where $Q = -e^2$, and $P = Q + 1$, respectively.
- *Keratoconus detection indices:* A number of keratoconus detection indices are displayed by certain devices to estimate the likelihood of the presence of keratoconus; these are discussed in detail later.

Pattern Recognition

There are a variety of corneal topographic patterns in a normal population with good vision. Using the Corneal Modeling System, Bogan et al. (11) described five CVK patterns in normal corneas: round, oval, symmetric bow tie, asymmetric bow tie, and irregular. Naufal et al. (12)

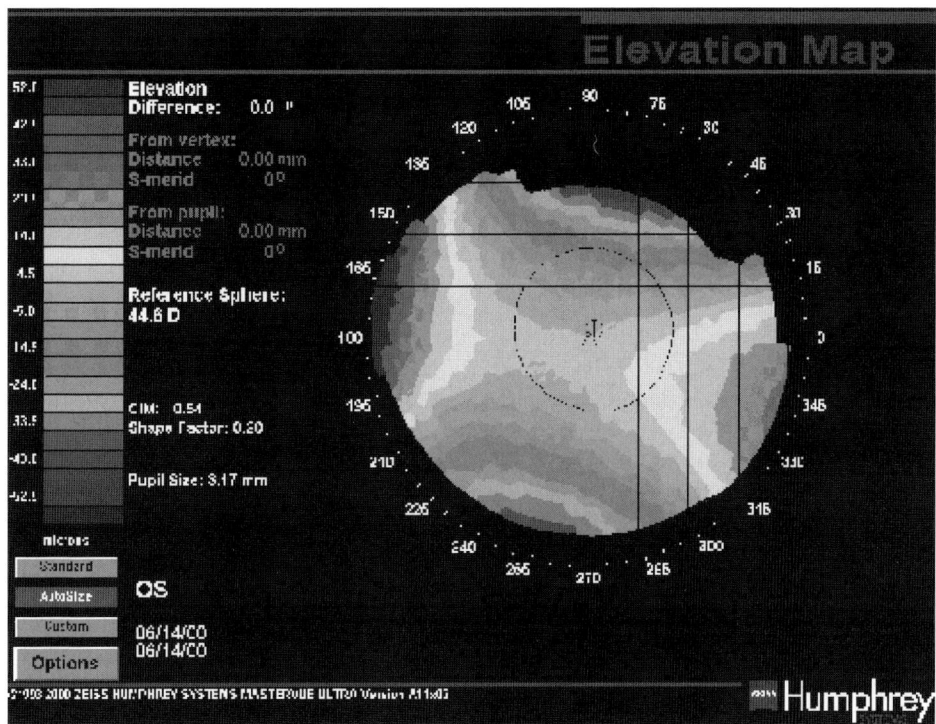

FIGURE. 69-2. Elevation map of a cornea with regular astigmatism. The elevated portion represents the flatter meridian of the cornea.

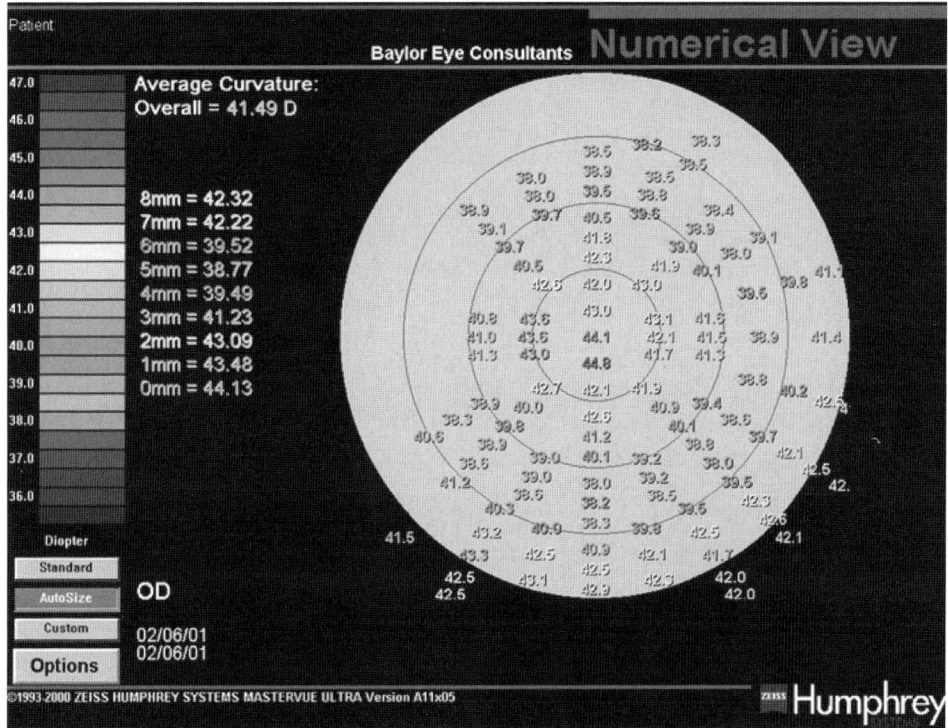

FIGURE 69-3. Numeric display from Humphrey Atlas.

defined rasterstereography-based classification of normal corneas: island, regular ridge, incomplete ridge, irregular ridge, and unclassified. Using the EyeSys Corneal Analysis System, Budak and colleagues (13) provided a corneal topographic classification of myopic eyes based on axial, instantaneous, refractive, and profile difference maps. They defined six types of patterns for axial, instantaneous, and refractive maps: circular, circular with central bow tie, circular with central irregularity, symmetric bow tie, asymmetric bow tie, and irregular pattern.

Although there is large range of topographic appearances of a normal cornea, a pattern outside this spectrum should be classified as abnormal cornea only after careful investigation to rule out artifacts, such as improper alignment and focusing or tear film irregularities. Inspection of the videokeratoscopic ring image is often useful in this regard.

Role of Corneal Curvature Measurement in Surgical Planning

Although corneal curvature can be determined by standard keratometry, automated keratometry, and corneal topography, corneal topographic measurement offers the advantage of providing curvature values over the entire measured surface. As such, it can detect focal areas of steepening or flatness that could affect surgical planning, including the suitability of the patient for refractive surgery and the selection of the microkeratome. Overly flat or steep corneas may pose an increased risk for flap complications with certain microkeratomes. For example, buttonholes may be more likely to occur in eyes with corneas steeper than 46 D. Conversely, free caps may occur more frequently in corneas flatter than 40 D. Clinicians have suggested that corneas steeper than 48 to 50 D or flatter than 35 D may result in poor quality of vision, but we are unaware of any peer-reviewed data supporting these contentions.

MONITORING TOPOGRAPHIC STABILITY AFTER DISCONTINUATION OF CONTACT LENS WEAR

Contact lens wear can alter the shape of the cornea and induce corneal warpage from direct mechanical pressure of the lens and perhaps from hypoxic corneal damage. Liu and Pflugfelder (14) reported that long-term contact lens wear (≥5 years) increased corneal curvature and surface irregularity. Corneal topographic patterns of warpage include some combination of central irregular astigmatism, loss of radial symmetry, and reversal of the normal topographic pattern of progressive flattening of corneal contour from the center to the periphery (15). Superior-riding lenses produce flattening superiorly and result in a relatively steeper contour inferiorly that simulates the topography of early keratoconus.

It is important to monitor corneal topographic changes after discontinuation of contact lens wear to ascertain stability before surgery (Fig. 69-4). Using the EyeSys Corneal Analysis System, Budak and colleagues (16) reported that, for patients whose manifest refraction and CVK maps were within 0.5 D of earlier values, discontinuation of soft contact lens wear for 2 weeks and rigid gas-permeable contact lens wear for 5 weeks were adequate for the cornea to return to its baseline topographic state. A much longer time, up to 5 months, was required for a return of a stable corneal topography in eyes with contact lens–induced corneal warpage caused by rigid lenses (15).

DETECTING ECTATIC CORNEAL DISORDERS

Keratoconus, PMD, and keratoglobus are noninflammatory corneal disorders characterized by progressive corneal thinning, protrusion, and scarring. These disorders are considered contraindications to laser *in situ* keratomileusis (LASIK) because of the iatrogenic keratectasia that may result from the procedure (17). The role of photorefractive keratectomy (PRK) in treating corneas with these disorders is as yet undefined. Mortensen and colleagues (18) have shown improvement in vision with no evidence of accelerated ectasia in keratoconic eyes treated with PRK, and Bilgihan and coauthors (19) reported safe results of PRK with 4 years of follow-up in keratoconus suspects detected by videokeratography. We are unaware of any peer-reviewed reports documenting ectasia from PRK performed in eyes with or without ectatic disorders; the only exception is one eye reported by Lovisolo and Fleming (20), in which the patient underwent multiple surface ablative procedures. However, follow-up of 10 years or longer may be required to validate fully the safety of PRK in ectatic corneas. Therefore, detection of these corneal disorders is a critical issue in patients who are potential candidates for LASIK and PRK.

Keratoconus

Patients with moderate to advanced keratoconus are easily diagnosed clinically and topographically. The challenge is to detect keratoconus in its early stages before obvious clinical and topographic signs are present. Corneas with subtle topographic abnormalities suggestive of early keratoconus are referred to as forme fruste keratoconus or keratoconus suspects. Several quantitative corneal indices and detection programs have been designed to aid in the topographic diagnosis of keratoconus.

Patterns and Indices Based on Placido Disk Systems

The most characteristic finding in the color-coded curvature maps of a keratoconic cornea is abnormal localized

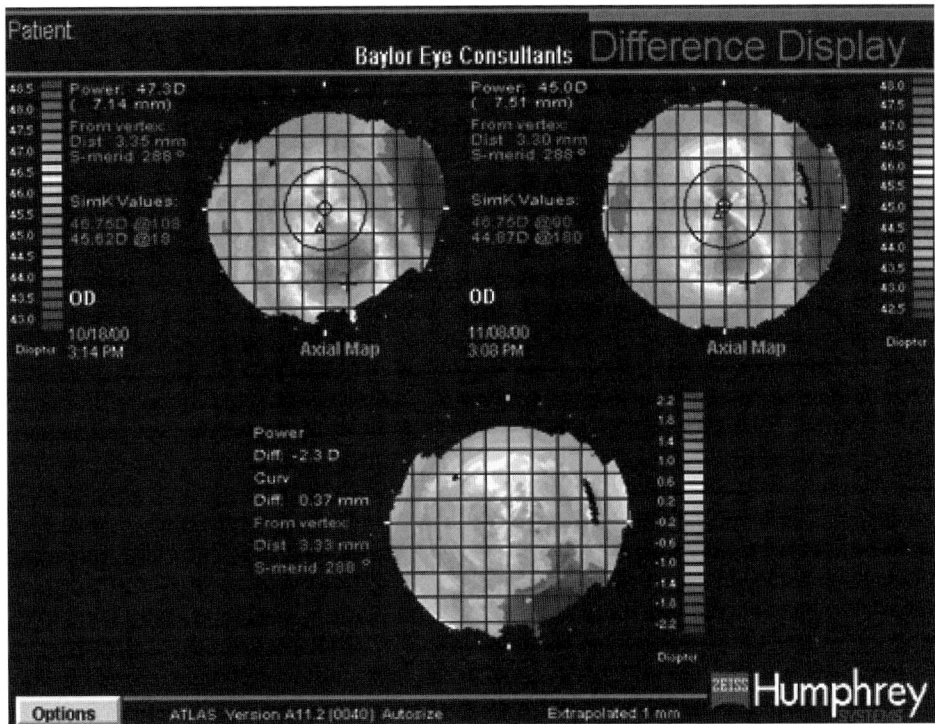

FIGURE 69-4. Contact lens–induced corneal warpage (*upper left*) that reversed 1 month after discontinuation of contact lens wear (*upper right*). Difference map (*bottom*) shows the inferior flattening that occurred after contact lens wear was stopped.

steepening (Fig. 69-5). For most patients with keratoconus, the steepening occurs inferotemporally or inferiorly. In patients with a central cone, central steepening with or without a skewed bow tie pattern can be seen. Indices based on the Placido disk devices included:

- *Inferior–superior value (I-S) and central corneal power:* Rabinowitz and McDonnell first described these

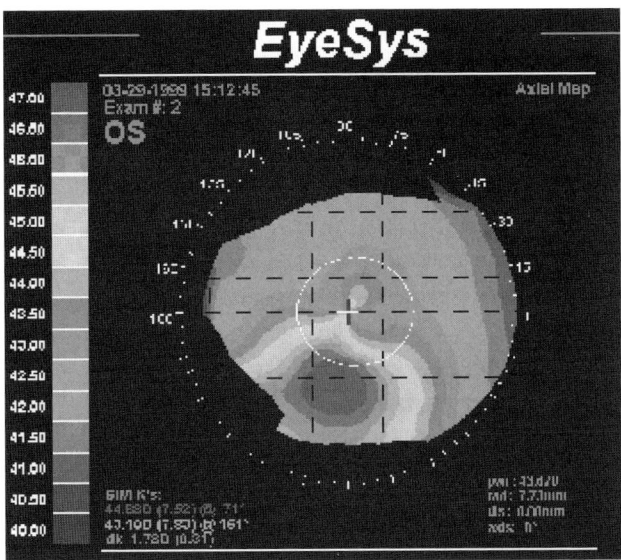

FIGURE 69-5. Classic pattern of keratoconus as displayed on an axial radius of curvature map.

keratoconus detection indices (21). The I-S value is designed to detect clinically significant inferior corneal steepening. It is defined as corneal power difference between the averages of five inferior points and five superior points 3 mm from the center at 30-degree intervals; an I-S value greater than 1.4 D is suggestive of keratoconus. Central corneal power is an index that quantifies the central steepening in keratoconic eyes with central cones. Central corneal power of greater than 47.2 D is indicative of keratoconus. These two diagnostic features should be used with caution, and subjective interpretation is necessary (22).

- *Keratoconus predictability index (KPI):* Maeda and colleagues developed the KPI, which is a single value derived by linear discriminant analysis of eight quantitative topographic indices that represent specific topographic features of keratoconus (23). A KPI value greater than 0.23 is indicative of keratoconus.

- *Keratoconus index (KCI):* In addition to the discriminant analysis classifier, Maeda et al. (23) also developed the KCI with the artificial intelligence method known as the expert system. The degree of the keratoconus-like pattern is determined and expressed as a percentage, KCI%. A value of zero is normal, with greater values describing an increasing likelihood of the presence of keratoconus.

- *Keratoconus severity index (KSI):* KSI was proposed by applying a neural network, which is another type of artificial intelligence, to the automated detection of keratoconus (24). Keratoconus suspect is interpreted when the

KSI reaches 0.15. A KSI of 0.3 or higher indicates clinical keratoconus.

- *KISA% index*: The KISA% index is derived from the product of four indices: central K-reading (K-value), inferior-superior value (I-S value), AST index (astigmatism as measured by Sim K reading), and skewed radial axis (SRAX) index (25). At a cutoff point for KISA% of 100, 280 of 281 participants (99.6%) were correctly classified. The KISA% index set at 100 is highly sensitive and specific for diagnosing keratoconus, and a range of 60% to 100% is useful for designating suspects.

- *Highest rate of steepening (HRS)*: The HRS is the highest rate of corneal power changes (in diopters per millimeter) away from the apex (the point of maximum curvature) to the periphery measured along its semimeridian (26). A cutoff value of 1.40 D/mm has a sensitivity of 95.7% (67/70), a specificity of 96.4% (16 false-positive results), and an accuracy of 96.3% for detection of keratoconus.

- *SDSD and Asph*: Chastang and colleagues (27) described a method using binary decision trees with two indices (SDSD and Asph) from the EyeSys videokeratoscope data for automated keratoconus screening. The SDSD is the standard deviation of the standard deviations of the radii of curvature of each ring in the central 4-mm zone, and the Asph index is a measure of the asphericity of the corneal surface within the 4.5-mm pupil. They reported that the sensitivity was 88.5% and specificity was 94.9% for detection of keratoconus.

- *Corneal wavefront Zernike index*: A keratoconus detection scheme with wavefront parameters based on topography height data has been developed (28,29). Corneal topography height data were decomposed into orthogonal Zernike polynomials. This index was found to perform at least as well as keratoconus detection schemes based on the Klyce-Maeda and the Rabinowitz-McDonnell indices.

Patterns and Indices Based on the Slit-Scanning System

The slit-scanning Orbscan topography system can measure both anterior and posterior surfaces of the cornea. In keratoconic cornea, the cone on the anterior or posterior elevation BFS map appears as an area of increased elevation surrounded by concentric zones of decreasing elevation (30). Indices based on the elevation of anterior or posterior surface have been developed:

- *Posterior elevation*: Rao and colleagues (31) proposed a screening criterion of 40 μm of posterior elevation. If the posterior elevation is greater than 40 μm, posterior ectasia is suggested, and the patient is counseled not to undergo corneal refractive surgery. If the posterior elevation is less than 40 μm, in the absence of other risk factors, the surgery can proceed. Using this screening scheme on 966 eyes, they reported that there were no cases of post-LASIK ectasia with a minimum of 10 months of follow-up.

- *Discriminant color number within central 3-mm area*: With the 10- and 20-μm interval color scales for the anterior and posterior elevation maps, respectively, Tanabe and colleagues (32) suggested that the presence of four or more colors in the central 3-mm area in anterior or posterior elevation BFS maps indicated abnormality in screening. If the anterior and posterior elevation maps are used in combination, sensitivity and specificity for the detection of keratoconus can be improved to 96% and 100%, respectively.

Longer follow-up for more eyes based on the Orbscan topography elevation criteria is needed to assess the performance of these keratoconus detection schemes. The accuracy of posterior corneal surface measurements also needs further validation.

Classification Based on Clinical Examination and Topographic Indices

Azar and Lu (33) reported an Massachusetts Eye and Ear Infirmary (MEEI) keratoconus scoring system, which combines history, examination, and topographic indices to establish criteria for distinguishing healthy control subjects, keratoconus suspects, and early and advanced keratoconus:

- If corneal hydrops is present on examination or obtained from history, 2 points are assigned; otherwise, 0 points are assigned.

- If at least two findings on examination (Fleischer ring, Vogt's striae, Munson's sign, scarring) or history (atopy, Down's syndrome family history) are present, 2 points are assigned; if fewer than two findings are present, 0 points are assigned.

- If asymmetric anterior central corneal power between right and left eyes is 1.9 D or less, 0 points are assigned to both eyes; if asymmetry greater than 1.9 D is present, the eye with the higher corneal power receives 1 point and the other eye receives 0 points.

- Anterior central corneal power K < 47.2 D, 47.2 to 48.7 D, or >48.7 D is assigned 0, 1, or 2 points, respectively.

- Inferior–superior asymmetry (I-S value) <1.4 D, 1.4 to 1.9 D, or >1.9 D is assigned 0, 1, or 2 points, respectively.

Total scores of 0, 1 to 3, 4 or 5, or 6 to 9 points are interpreted as normal cornea, keratoconus suspect, early keratoconus, or advanced keratoconus, respectively.

Pellucid Marginal Degeneration and Keratoglobus

Histopathologically, PMD is considered a variant of keratoconus, and PMD may indeed be part of the clinical spectrum of keratoconus. However, classic PMD has distinct clinical features consisting of a zone of inferior corneal thinning within 2 to 3 mm of the inferior limbus. Likewise, the classic topographic pattern of PMD is the

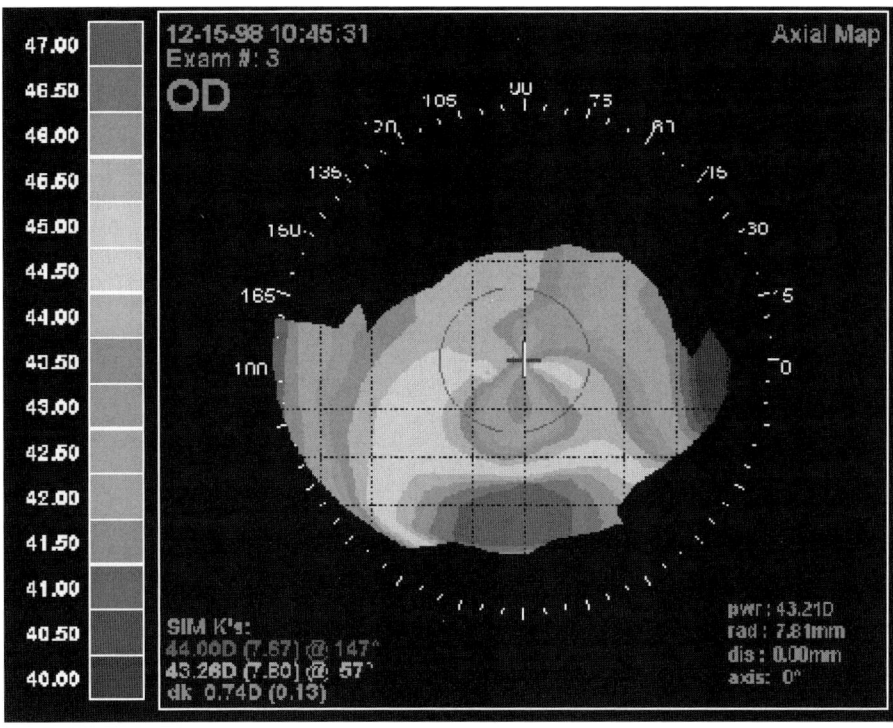

FIGURE 69-6. Classic pattern of pellucid marginal degeneration as displayed on an axial radius of curvature map.

"butterfly" appearance, demonstrating large amounts of against-the-rule astigmatism and inferior corneal steepening, which creates the appearance of a "C" lying on its back (34,35) (Fig. 69-6). Rare cases of superior corneal thinning in PMD have been reported (36,37). Commonly used keratoconus screening indices may not detect PMD because these indices are generated from more central regions of the cornea, whereas the corneal steepening in PMD occurs more peripherally adjacent to the limbus.

Keratoglobus is a rare disorder characterized by limbus-to-limbus corneal thinning and a globular protrusion of the cornea evident on profile examination (38). The topographic appearance is generalized corneal steepening with irregular astigmatism.

SUMMARY

CVK is important for preoperative screening of candidates for corneal refractive surgery. When an abnormal topographic pattern is suspected, the clinician should first rule out any artifacts, such as misalignment or tear film irregularies. Contact lens–induced corneal warpage may mimic a keratoconus topographic pattern, and surgery should be considered only after the cornea has stabilized in its baseline topographic state.

For the crucial step of ruling out forme fruste keratoconus or other ectatic disorders, clinicians may use one of the several options noted previously. If the topographer has specific keratoconus screening software, this may be used.

In the absence of validated screening software, clinicians can manually calculate the I-S differences in central corneal curvature. The Azar system can then be applied as a method of screening these eyes. There is no approach, however, that guarantees correct discrimination of all normal and ectatic corneas. For detection of PMD, pattern recognition is currently the best option because current keratoconus indices may not detect this abnormality.

If an ectatic disorder is suspected, we recommend that LASIK not be performed. As previously noted, the role of PRK in these eyes is less clear, but the decision to undertake surgery in this setting should be taken with caution and only after extensive discussions with the patient. Continued use of spectacles or contact lenses, or perhaps implantation of a phakic intraocular lens, may be preferable for these eyes.

REFERENCES

1. Roberts C. Characterization of the inherent error in a spherically-biased corneal topography system in mapping a radially aspheric surface. *J Refract Corneal Surg* 1994;10:103–111.
2. Holladay JT. Corneal topography using the Holladay Diagnostic Summary. *J Cataract Refract Surg* 1997;23:209–221.
3. Wilson SE, Klyce SD. Quantitative descriptors of corneal topography: a clinical study. *Arch Ophthalmol* 1991;109:349–353.
4. Lin DT. Corneal topographic analysis after excimer photorefractive keratectomy. *Ophthalmology* 1994;101:1432–1439.
5. Smolek MK, Oshika T, Klyce SD, et al. Topographic assessment of irregular astigmatism after photorefractive keratectomy. *J Cataract Refract Surg* 1998;24:1079–1086.

6. Shiotani Y, Maeda N, Inoue T, et al. Comparison of topographic indices that correlate with visual acuity in videokeratography. *Ophthalmology* 2000;107:559–564.

7. Weiss JS, Oplinger NL. An analysis of the accuracy of predicted corneal acuity in the Holladay diagnostic summary program. *CLAO J* 1998;24:141–144.

8. Kiely PM, Smith G, Carney LG. The mean shape of the human cornea. *Optica Acta* 1982;29:1027–1040.

9. Townsley M. New knowledge of the cornea contour. *Contacto* 1970;14:38–43

10. Guillon M, Lydon DPM, Wilson C. Corneal topography: a clinical model. *Ophthalmol Physiol Optom* 1986;6:47–56.

11. Bogan SJ, Waring GO III, Ibrahim O, et al. Classification of normal corneal topography based on computer-assisted videokeratography. *Arch Ophthalmol* 1990;108:945–949.

12. Naufal SC, Hess JS, Friedlander MH, et al. Rasterstereography-based classification of normal corneas. *J Cataract Refract Surg* 1997;23:222–230.

13. Budak K, Hamed AM, Friedman NJ, et al. Corneal topography classification in myopic eyes based on axial, instantaneous, refractive, and profile difference maps. *J Cataract Refract Surg* 1999;25:1069–1079.

14. Liu Z, Pflugfelder SC. The effects of long-term contact lens wear on corneal thickness, curvature, and surface regularity. *Ophthalmology* 2000;107:105–111.

15. Wilson SE, Lin DT, Klyce SD, et al. Topographic changes in contact lens-induced corneal warpage. *Ophthalmology* 1990;97:734–744

16. Budak K, Hamed AM, Friedman NJ, et al. Preoperative screening of contact lens wearers before refractive surgery. *J Cataract Refract Surg* 1999;25:1080–1086.

17. Seiler T, Quurke AW. Iatrogenic keratectasia after LASIK in a case of forme fruste keratoconus. *J Cataract Refract Surg* 1998;24:1007–1009.

18. Mortensen J, Carlsson K, Ohrstrom A. Excimer laser surgery for keratoconus. *J Cataract Refract Surg* 1998;24:893–898.

19. Bilgihan K, Ozdek SC, Konuk O, et al. Results of photorefractive keratectomy in keratoconus suspects at 4 years. *J Refract Surg* 2000;16:438–443.

20. Lovisolo CF, Fleming JF. Intracorneal ring segments for iatrogenic keratectasia after laser in situ keratomileusis or photorefractive keratectomy. *J Refract Surg* 2002;18:535–541.

21. Rabinowitz YS, McDonnell PJ. Computer-assisted corneal topography in keratoconus. *Refract Corneal Surg* 1989;5:400–406.

22. Koch DD, Husain SE. Corneal topography to detect and characterize corneal pathology. In: Gills JP, et al., eds. *Corneal topography: the state of the art.* Thorofare, NJ: Slack, 1995:159–169.

23. Maeda N, Klyce SD, Smolek MK, et al. Automated keratoconus screening with corneal topography analysis. *Invest Ophthalmol Vis Sci* 1994;35:2749–2757.

24. Smolek MK, Klyce SD. Current keratoconus detection methods compared with a neural network approach. *Invest Ophthalmol Vis Sci* 1997;38:2290–2299.

25. Rabinowitz YS, Rasheed K. KISA% index: a quantitative videokeratography algorithm embodying minimal topographic criteria for diagnosing keratoconus. *J Cataract Refract Surg* 1999;25:1327–1335.

26. Dastjerdi MH, Hashemi H. A quantitative corneal topography index for detection of keratoconus. *J Refract Surg* 1998;14:427–436.

27. Chastang PJ, Borderie VM, Carvajal-Gonzalez S, et al. Automated keratoconus detection using the EyeSys videokeratoscope. *J Cataract Refract Surg* 2000;26:675–683.

28. Schwiegerling J, Greivenkamp JE. Keratoconus detection based on videokeratoscopic height data. *Optom Vis Sci* 1996;73:721–728.

29. Langenbucher A, Gusek-Schneider GC, Kus MM, et al. Keratoconus screening with wave-front parameters based on topography height data. *Klin Monatsbl Augenheilkd* 1999;214:217–223.

30. Auffarth GU, Wang L, Volcker HE. Keratoconus evaluation using the Orbscan Topography System. *J Cataract Refract Surg* 2000;26:222–228.

31. Rao SN, Raviv T, Majmudar PA, et al. Role of Orbscan II in screening keratoconus suspects before refractive corneal surgery. *Ophthalmology* 2002;109:1642–1646.

32. Tanabe T, Oshika T, Tomidokoro A, et al. Standardized color-coded scales for anterior and posterior elevation maps of scanning slit corneal topography *Ophthalmology* 2002;109:1298–1302.

33. Lu PC, Azar DT. Preoperative considerations: diagnosis, classification, and avoidance of keratoconus complications. In: Azar DT, Koch DD, eds. *LASIK: fundamentals, surgical techniques, and complications.* New York: Marcel Dekker, 2003:153–162.

34. Maguire LJ, Klyce SD, McDonald MB, et al. Corneal topography of pellucid marginal degeneration. *Ophthalmology* 1987;94:519–524.

35. Karabatsas CH, Cook SD. Topographic analysis in pellucid marginal corneal degeneration and keratoglobus. *Eye* 1996;10:451–455.

36. Cameron JA, Mahmood MA. Superior corneal thinning with pellucid marginal corneal degeneration. *Am J Ophthalmol* 1990;109:486–487.

37. Taglia DP, Sugar J. Superior pellucid marginal corneal degeneration with hydrops. *Arch Ophthalmol* 1997;115:274–275.

38. Cavara V. Keratoglobus and keratoconus: a contribution to the nosological interpretation of keratoglobus. *Br J Ophthalmol* 1950;34:621–626.

70

RADIAL KERATOTOMY

CLÁUDIA M. FRANCESCONI

Radial keratotomy (RK) is one of several surgical procedures for flattening to central corneal used, thus correcting myopia by decreasing the refractive power of the eye to match its axial length. It relies on the weakening effect of deep (80% to 90%) radial stromal incisions to alter the central corneal curvature indirectly. This chapter provides an overview of radial keratotomy including patient selection, instrumentation, techniques, complications, and their management.

HISTORY OF RADIAL AND ASTIGMATIC KERATOTOMY

During the 19th century, Snellen (1869) (1), Schiötz (1885) (2), Bates (1894) (3), and Lans (1898) (4) described methods to reduce astigmatism. In 1939, Sato (5) described spontaneous breaks in Descemet's membrane in keratoconus that caused flattening of the cornea and reduction of myopia. In 1953, Sato and colleagues (6) suggested that by making radial incisions in the posterior as well as the anterior cornea, astigmatism and myopia could be treated. Sato's surgical technique required entry into the anterior chamber at three to four different sites. Incisions were then made using a "free hand" technique through the endothelial surface, from the edge of a 6-mm central optical zone through 50% of the corneal thickness. Additional anterior incisions, placed in between the posterior ones, were then made at approximately the same depth. There is no indication that pachymetry was performed. Yamaguchi and associates (7) have estimated that 40% to 50% of the endothelial surface was damaged at the time of surgery. Approximately 75% to 80% of the 200 patients who underwent Sato's procedure developed visually significant corneal edema an average of 20 years after the operation.

In the early 1970s, in the former Soviet Union, Yenaliev (8), Fyodorov, Agranorsky, and Durnev (8–11) modified Sato's technique, performing anterior radial incisions in the peripheral cornea and sclera. In 1978, Bores, Myers, and Cowden (12,13) reported the outcomes of the first RK procedure in the United States, using Fyodorov's techniques (8,10).

In 1980, the National Eye Institute funded the Prospective Evaluation of Radial Keratotomy (PERK) Study to assess the efficacy, safety, predictability, and stability of RK (14). The PERK study used rigid, standardized, surgical protocols, data collection by independent observers, and a multicenter design. It was a collaborative effort among university-based and private ophthalmologists in nine clinical centers. The protocol did not allow corrections for astigmatism. The surgical plan was based on the amount of myopic error and no other preoperative factors such as age, sex, or intraocular pressure were addressed (14–16).

The surgical protocol of the PERK Study required eight freehand centrifugal incisions (clear zone to limbus) made with the length of a 45-degree diamond blade set using ultrasonic pachymetry at 100% of the thinnest paracentral corneal measurement (16). Preoperatively, optical zones were limited to 3, 3.5, or 4 mm, corresponding to low-, medium-, or high-myopia levels (range −2 to −8 D). Repeat surgery for enhancement (eight additional incisions were made between the initial eight) was carried out under specific guidelines (15,17).

The RK postoperative outcome in the PERK study showed a decrease in myopia in all patients: 88% of patients achieved uncorrected visual acuity of 20/40 or better; 90% of patients with myopia of 6 D or less achieved visual acuity of 20/40 or better. Reduction of best-corrected visual acuity (20/25) was noted in 0.8% of patients.

Throughout the decade following the initiation of the PERK study, numerous advances were introduced through the work of various surgeons (Table 70-1) (18–26). Two principal techniques for RK evolved: (a) American style (centrifugal), or backcutting, in which incisions are made from center to periphery; and (b) Russian style (centripetal), or frontcutting, in which incisions are made from the limbus to the edge of the desired optical zone. It has been shown that centrifugal incisions inherently yield a diminished range of corneal flattening, because incision depth for a given diamond setting is less reliable than that with a centripetal incision (27–29).

TABLE 70-1. STUDY OUTCOMES OF RADIAL KERATOTOMY

	Deitz (21)	Werblin (103)	Verity (25)	Lindstrom (26)	PERK (15)	PERK (95)
Number of patients/eyes	458/972	128/241	238/375	50/100	435/793	374/693
Follow-up	1 yr	3 yrs	1 yr	6 m	5 yrs	10 yrs
Preoperative myopia range	−1.5–11.9	+0.25*–9.62	−1.0–9.0	−1.5–6.0	−1.5–8.0	−1.5–8.75
Postoperative refraction percentage						
> 1.0 D myopic	12	NR	13	8	19	38
− 1.0 to + 1.0 D	76	84	85	92	64	60
> 1.0 hyperopic	12	NR	1.3	0	17	NR
Uncorrected visual acuity						
% 20/20 or better	47	52	NR	72	60	53
% 20/40 or better	88	96	95	94	88	85
BSCVA % losing ¶ 2 lines	0.5	2.9	0.3	0	3	3
Postoperative result within 1.0 D of predicted, grouped by preoperative refraction (%)						
Low**	90	94	93	NR	76	NR
Moderate**	76	95	88	NR	61	NR
High**	53	90	74	NR	46	NR
Postoperative uncorrected visual acuity 20/40 or better, grouped by preoperative refraction (%)						
Low**	96	97	NR	NR	92	92
Moderate**	89	100	NR	NR	86	86
High**	77	94	NR	NR	72	77
Reoperations (%)	0.5	36	27	8	12	NR

BSCVA, best-spectacle-corrected visual acuity.
* Spherical equivalent with positive cylinder.
** For PERK and Deitz, low (1.5–3.0 D), moderate (3.12–6.0 D), and high (6.12 D or more).
For Werblin, low (+0.25–3.12 D), moderate (−3.25–4.37 D), and high (−4.5–9.62 D).

From these two approaches evolved the Genesis and Duotrack (or "combined") techniques, which combined the safety of the centrifugal incision with the efficacy of the centripetal incision (24,30). In the combined technique, the centrifugal component provided the surgeon with a relatively shallow and linear safety groove. The centripetal component further deepened the incision groove and undercut the deep stroma adjacent to the optical zone, increasing the range of corneal flattening (Fig. 70-1) (30,31). The diamond knife blade employed for the combined technique enabled the surgeon to begin the incision at the optical (clear) zone, extend out toward the limbus, and then reverse direction back toward the central optical zone without optical zone invasion. The angled edge on the back surface (centrifugal cutting component) is sharpened along the entire length, and the vertical edge of the front surface is ground sharp to a cutting edge for a distance of only 200 to 250 μm from the blade tip (Fig. 70-2). The blunt upper portion of the vertical knife edge reduced the chance of unwanted invasion of the central optical zone when the blade tip is initially inserted into the cornea at the optical zone margin (32). In a comparative study using donor eyes (31), the combined (Genesis) technique demonstrated greater corneal flattening than the centrifugal (American) method of incision and reduced variability when compared with the centripetal (Russian) method.

As experience with RK increased, a tendency for shorter incisions developed (26,33–36). In a cadaver eye study, Jester and associates (34) found that incisions extending beyond the limbus reduced the efficacy of RK. Salz and colleagues (35) found a small decrease in efficacy when using a shorter incision, but a significant effect was maintained. This is consistent with the results from Lindstrom's (26) modified technique for low to moderate myopes, known as *minimally invasive* RK ("mini-RK"), which reduces the length of cornea incised. In a cadaver eye study, eight short incisions were performed from the 3-mm to the 7-mm optical zone (Fig. 70-3), producing 92% of the efficacy of full-length incisions made to the 11-mm optical zone. Pinheiro and co-workers' (36) eye bank study also showed that reducing the incision length reduced the likelihood of corneal rupture as intraocular pressure is increased.

PATIENT EVALUATION

Approximately 25% of the adult population in the United States is myopic (37,38). It has been reported that the majority of candidates seeking keratorefractive surgery state their goal as good visual function without physical dependence on spectacles or contact lenses (39,40). Occasionally, patients may have medical (e.g., contact lens intolerance),

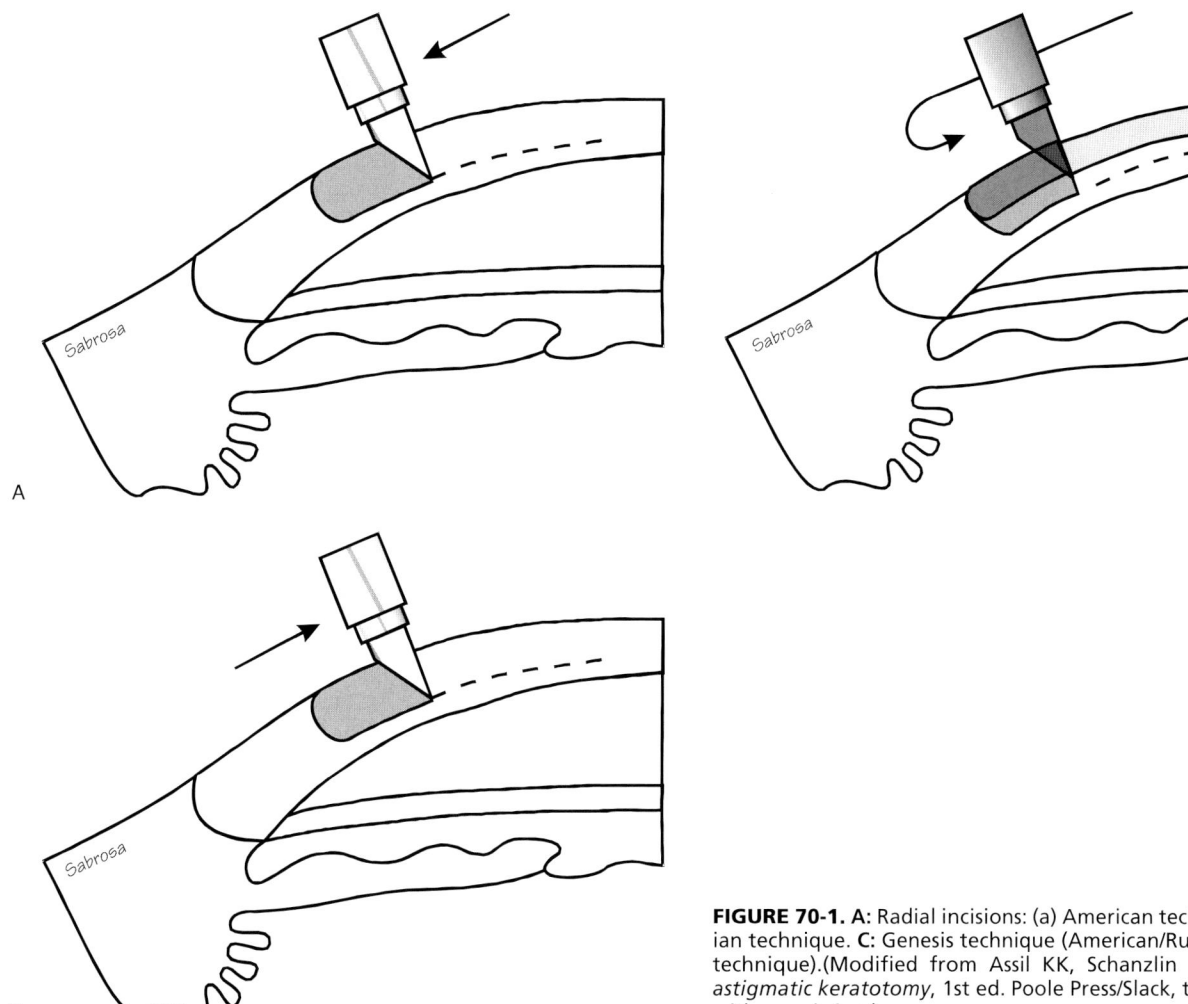

A

B

C

FIGURE 70-1. A: Radial incisions: (a) American technique. **B:** Russian technique. **C:** Genesis technique (American/Russian combined technique).(Modified from Assil KK, Schanzlin DJ. *Radial and astigmatic keratotomy*, 1st ed. Poole Press/Slack, therefore, 1994, with permission.)

occupational, recreational, or cosmetic reasons for seeking surgery.

RK should be limited to patients with low to moderate myopia and an otherwise normal eye examination (24,41,42). Higher degrees of myopia have variable responses to RK, and procedures such as photorefractive keratectomy and laser-*in-situ* keratomileusis (LASIK) may yield better and more stable results. For extreme high myopes, clear lens extraction or phakic intraocular lens implantation may be more appropriate. In the case of the RK candidate, myopia, and astigmatism must be stable and nonprogressive (43). Postoperative corneal transplant and cataract surgery patients with residual myopic astigmatism may benefit from incisional keratotomy after all sutures are completely removed and refractive stability documented. Table 70-2 outlines the appropriate surgical procedures for the levels of severity of ametropia.

Patient History

A complete patient history should be taken, including a medical and ocular history, a family history, a list of medications, the refractive stability, as well as a relevant social and occupational history.

Absolute Contraindications (Table 70-3)

1. Scleritis: A history of scleritis disqualifies patients from all keratorefractive surgeries because of the potential for associated systemic disease, corneal melting, and perforation.
2. Delayed epithelial wound healing: Patients considered ineligible for RK because of delayed epithelial wound healing are those with a history of neurotrophic corneal ulcers, herpes zoster ophthalmicus, or nonhealing epithelial defects.
3. Corneal ectasias: Corneal ectasias such as keratoconus are absolute contraindications to incisional keratotomy (44–46). Keratoconus is a progressive corneal ectasia that can cause wide variations and fluctuations in pre- and postoperative refractions (46–49). Refractive surgery may accelerate the progression of this disease. Other corneal ectasias include keratoglobus, Terrien's, and pellucid marginal degeneration.

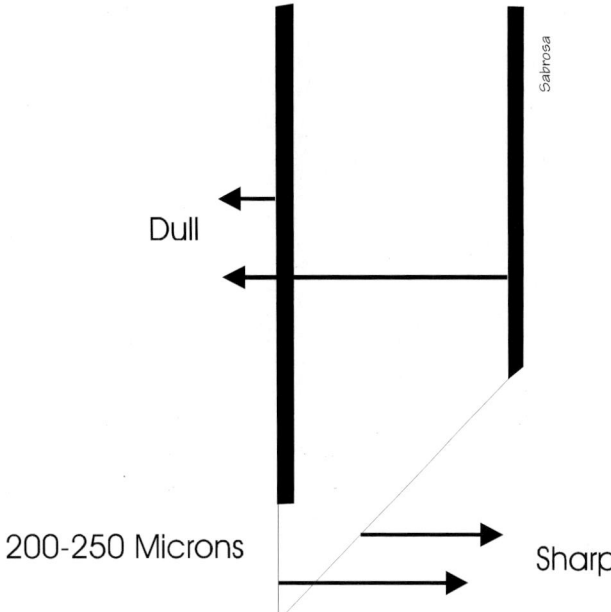

FIGURE 70-2. Diamond knife design for combined (Genesis) radial incision technique. (Modified from Assil KK, Schanzlin DJ. *Radial and astigmatic keratotomy*, 1st ed. Thorofare, NJ: Poole Press/Slack, 1994, with permission.)

4. Cataracts: Cataracts are an absolute contraindication to RK surgery, as refractive shifts and loss of best-corrected visual acuity frequently occur as a result of progression. However, patients with stable, visually insignificant congenital lens opacities are reasonable candidates for keratorefractive surgery.

5. Retinal diseases: Retinal diseases such as macular degeneration, diabetic retinopathy or other vasculopathy, and progressive retinal degenerations are absolute contraindications, because of the potential for loss of low-contrast

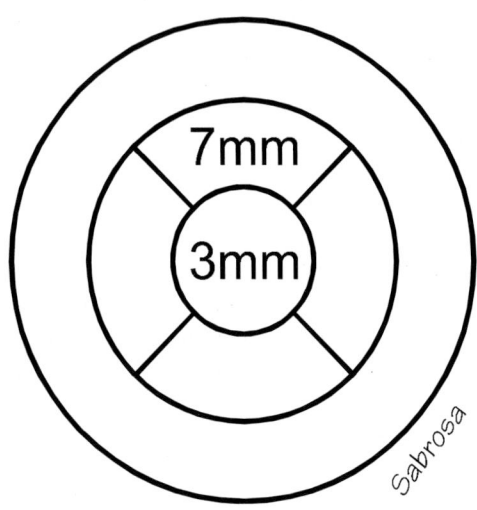

FIGURE 70-3. Mini-RK technique. Incisions extending from 3.0 to 7.0 mm optical zone.

TABLE 70-2. SURGICAL PROCEDURES FOR AMETROPIA CORRECTION

Myopia
Low (< 6 D)
  Radial keratotomy (1–4D)
  Photorefractive keratectomy
  LASIK **
  Intracorneal ring segments (1–4)

Moderate (6–15 D)
Excimer	Multipass multizone
	Scanning lasers **
Keratomileusis	Cryolathe *
	Automated lamellar keratoplasty (ALK)
	Excimer laser-in-situ (LASIK)
Intrastromal	Hydrogel
implants	
Phakic IOL **	

High (>15 D)
  Epikeratoplasty *
  Clear lens extraction
  Phakic intraocular lens

Hyperopia
Low to moderate
Thermokeratoplasty	Infrared lasers
	Direct heating probes *
Keratomileusis	Excimer (LASIK)
	Automated lamellar keratoplasty (ALK)
Hexagonal keratotomy *	
Photorefractive keratectomy (PRK)	

Aphakia/high hyperopia
  Epikeratoplasty
  Keratophakia
  Hydrogel inlay
  Polysulfone inlay *

Astigmatism
Transverse keratotomy
Arcuate keratotomy ± compression sutures
Ruiz procedure *
Postkeratoplasty relaxing incisions with or without compression sutures
Photoastigmatic refractive keratectomy (PARK)

  * Included for historical purposes only.
 ** Investigational.

acuity, which may accelerate loss of best-corrected acuity in these patients.

6. Connective tissue disease: Connective tissue diseases, including rheumatoid arthritis and Sjögren's syndrome, affect corneal wound healing and therefore are contraindications for RK. Patients with history of inflammatory bowel diseases (e.g., Crohn's disease, ulcerative colitis, or Wegener's granulomatosis) have the potential for corneal melting and are poor candidates for this surgery.

7. Immunosuppression: Patients with history of immunosuppression due to acquired immunodeficiency syndrome or chronic active hepatitis, as well as those who are pharmacologically immunosuppressed from systemic

TABLE 70-3. CONTRAINDICATION OF RADIAL KERATOTOMY

Absolute contraindications
Age <18 years
Refractive instability
Rheumatoid arthritis
Connective tissue disease
Scleritis
Severe ocular surface disorders
Neurotrophic corneal disease
AIDS, other immunosuppression
Keratoconus
Pregnancy
Cataracts

Relative contraindications
Moderately dry eye
Diabetes mellitus
Herpes simplex virus
Blepharitis, rosacea
Glaucoma

corticosteroids or other cytotoxic agents are poor candidates for refractive surgery.

8. Pregnancy: Pregnancy is an absolute contraindication to RK because of the changes in corneal curvature and refraction that can occur during this time. Incisional keratotomy should be delayed until stability of refraction is documented after delivery. The effects of RK in nursing mothers have not been well documented, but in general it is advisable to defer surgery until lactation has ceased and a stable refractive state documented.

Relative Contraindications

1. Keratoconjunctivitis sicca: Keratoconjunctivitis sicca resulting from Sjögren's syndrome, alkali burns, or ocular cicatricial pemphigoid is an absolute contraindication, but moderate to severe primary dry-eye syndromes resulting in surface abnormalities are considered relative contraindications to keratorefractive surgery. These patients should be treated with punctal occlusion and tear replacement before surgery to normalize the ocular surface. If a normal ocular surface cannot be achieved with such interventions, it is best to avoid surgery.

2. Herpes simplex keratitis: In general, refractive surgery in patients with a documented history of ocular herpes simplex keratitis should be approached with extreme caution. Patients without a history of stromal disease who have been free from herpes simplex keratitis for at least 1 year may be reasonable surgical candidates, particularly if corneal sensation is normal, but it should be considered that they may be at reserved risk for herpes simplex-related ocular morbidity if they undergo surgery. Oral acyclovir given in the perioperative period may also be beneficial in preventing recurrence of the disease (50).

3. Blepharitis, ocular rosacea, and meibomitis: These conditions can also be relative contraindications to refractive surgery and need to be treated preoperatively with lid hygiene, and in some cases with oral tetracycline, doxycycline, or minocycline. Moreover, medical treatment of these disorders must be continued after surgery to minimize the chances of abnormal corneal wound healing. In the presence of corneal pannus, RK should be deferred until the underlying cause is controlled, because these eyes are at higher risk of developing vascularization within the incisions, resulting in subsequent refractive instability.

4. Glaucoma: A history of glaucoma is a relative contraindication to incisional keratotomy. The use of topical steroids in the postoperative period of incisional keratotomy may increase the intraocular pressure, and fluctuations in intraocular pressure may affect the refractive state of the eye as well.

5. Diabetes mellitus: Diabetes mellitus is a relative contraindication. This is due to concerns about delayed wound healing and abnormal immune responses, although there have been no specific complications reported in diabetic patients undergoing RK. Certainly a diabetic patient with documented ocular complications of diabetes is not a good candidate for refractive surgery.

6. Atopic disease: Atopic patients with severe lid abnormalities, cataracts, keratoconus, or severe eye rubbing are poor candidates for surgery. Eye rubbing can lead to an increased incidence of infection, a delay in wound healing, and postoperative refractive instability. Antihistamines and behavior modification may be beneficial in preventing and treating ocular itching and eye rubbing, respectively.

Family History

The family history should include documentation of corneal dystrophies, keratoconus, glaucoma, retinal detachment, retinal dystrophies, optic nerve abnormalities, diabetes mellitus, collagen vascular disease, early cardiovascular disease, and any other hereditary diseases.

Medications

A complete list of past and current systemic and ophthalmic medications should be obtained from the patient. This list can provide clues to the existence of diseases that may have been overlooked or forgotten by patients during the medical and ocular history.

Refractive Stability

Patients younger than 18 and those who have had a 0.5 D or greater change in sphere or cylinder per year over the preceding 2 years are not eligible for surgery. In general, waiting until at least 21 years of age before attempting refractive surgery is preferable.

Contact Lens Wear Considerations

Candidates for keratorefractive surgery should discontinue soft contact lens wear 2 weeks before surgical evaluation. Rigid, gas-permeable lens wearers must discontinue lenses for a minimum of 3 weeks before surgical evaluation. Manifest and cycloplegic refractions, along with corneal topography, should be used to monitor and confirm stabilization of the corneal curvature of refraction before the surgery can be planned. The existence of corneal warping due to contact lens wear (usually rigid, gas permeable lenses) is a contraindication to keratorefractive surgery until the condition has stabilized. It may take months or years for some corneas to recover from warping due to contact lens wear (51). If corneal topography or refraction is unstable at the time of evaluation, repeat testing after 2 to 3 weeks is usually performed.

Social and Occupational History

Patients of presbyopic age may benefit from refractive correction of monovision, whereas younger patients (35 to 40 years of age or younger) are usually not tolerant of this approach. Patients involved in contact sports clearly should not be considered good candidates for RK. When applicable, patients should be made aware that some airlines and branches of the military do not recognize refractive surgery as a valid means of visual correction.

Patient Expectations

Patients with unrealistic expectations for surgical outcomes, such as those who expect an improvement in best-corrected acuity or better vision than that achievable with corrective contact lenses, should be considered poor candidates for refractive surgery unless properly educated about realistic expectations of RK.

Patient Evaluation

A complete ophthalmologic examination is performed, including measurements of ocular dominance and motility, pupil size (in light and dim illumination), corneal sensitivity, and intraocular pressure. Examination procedures should include retinoscopy, manifest and cycloplegic refractions as well as external slit-lamp and dilated funduscopic examinations. Funduscopic examination should include posterior pole examination for the presence of myopic degeneration and examination of the periphery to check for presence of lattice degeneration or evidence of other myopic vitreoretinal abnormality.

Preoperative testing usually includes corneal topography and screening pachymetry. For corneal topography, computed videokeratography (CVK) can be used to detect regular and irregular astigmatism, corneal warping from contact lens wear, or compressive lid lesions, as well as evidence of keratoconus (44,45,52–55), or pellucid marginal degeneration. For astigmatic keratotomy (AK), topography helps to refine placement of arcuate or tangential incision or incisions, although it should be kept in mind that the correlation between refractive and topographic astigmatism is sometimes poor (56).

Patient Education

It is crucial that the prospective patient demonstrate reasonable comprehension of the potential risks and benefits of the primary surgery and possible enhancement procedures as well as reasonable surgical and nonsurgical alternatives. It should be stressed that additional corrective optical aids (i.e., glasses or contact lenses) may still be necessary to improve vision postoperatively. Changes in corneal shape may, in some cases, make contact lens wear more difficult or impossible. Furthermore, it should be stressed that corneal surgery will not change the normal aging process of the crystalline lens, whereby most individuals at or near emmetropia require reading glasses by their mid-40s.

Preoperatively the patient must read and sign an informed consent document after discussing the planned procedure and the postoperative instructions with the keratorefractive surgeon. It is preferable to conduct the informed consent discussion at a visit separate from the day of surgery. This allows the patient time to digest the information received and ask further questions, if necessary.

INSTRUMENTS FOR INCISIONAL KERATOTOMY

Operating Microscope

Keratorefractive surgery is performed under a microscope with adequate illumination. An illuminated target is often used to help with proper centration.

Diamond Knife

A variety of diamond micrometer knives are available for radial, astigmatic, and enhancement keratotomy, each consisting of a handle, footplate, and a blade. For the combined technique, a diamond knife with a blunt upper portion to its vertical edge is used (Fig. 70-2). This decreases the chance of unwanted invasion of the optical zone margin during the initial (centrifugal) incision, and most importantly at the conclusion of the centripetally directed trajectory of the incision. The diamond knife also includes a footplate designed to maintain the diamond blade at a uniform depth within the stroma, over a broad range of angular excursion with respect to the corneal surface. The knife footplate should be relatively broad so as to provide maximal lateral support while allowing the blade to maintain constant and uniform stromal penetration and should generate minimal resistance against the corneal epithelium over the course of the incision.

The trifaceted diamond and 15 degree arc-T blades facilitate the execution of arcuate incisions (57). A 45-degree diamond blade with a front cutting double-edge for astigmatic incisions may also be used.

Micrometer Calibration Microscope

A micrometer calibration microscope is used for setting and inspection of the diamond-blade and the alignment of the footplate.

Ultrasonic Pachymeter

An ultrasonic pachymeter should be used intraoperatively to measure the thickness of the cornea: in the optical zone of 3.0 mm, at four to eight points in the meridians, where incisions are planned, and at the corneal apex (Fig. 70-4). For astigmatic keratotomy, pachymetry is performed over the quadrant of interest at the predetermined optical zone.

Optical Zone and Incision Markers

Optical zone and incision markers with cross-hairs (3.0 to 5.0 mm, in 0.25-mm increments) are utilized for centralization and definition of the surgical central clear zone for RK. The smaller the diameter of the clear zone, the greater

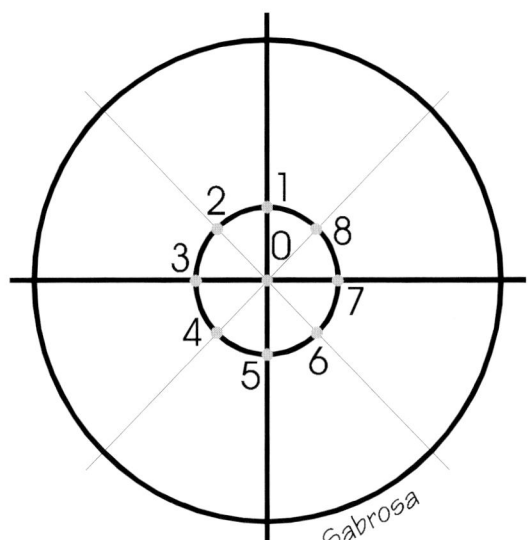

FIGURE 70-4. Pachymetry. Corneal thickness measured on the apex of the cornea and eight points in the meridians.

the corneal flattening will be. An optical zone smaller than 3.0 mm will increase glare symptoms (58); an optical zone greater than 5.0 mm will be ineffective in most cases. For correction of astigmatism, markers are used to delineate the axis, length, and orientation of the transverse or arcuate incisions. The axis of the incision can be oriented with a hand-held reticule (Mendez gauge). Individual arcuate markers in 30-, 45-, 60-, 75-, or 90-degree arcs are available to make arcuate impressions on the epithelium of the steep axis. The diameters of these markers range between 5.0 and 9.0 mm, in 1.0-mm increments.

RADIAL KERATOTOMY SURGICAL TECHNIQUES AND NOMOGRAMS

Although there is no universal consensus on RK technique among ophthalmologists (59), comprehensive statements on the subject have been published to help guide surgeons and patients considering the procedure (60–62). When planning the surgery, the optical zone, number of incisions, depth of incisions, and orientation of radial incisions are selected.

Preoperative Medications, Preparation, Positioning

Preoperative sedation is optional (e.g., Valium 5 to 10 mg PO or similar agent). Topical anesthesia with 0.5% proparacaine, tetracaine, or 4% Xylocaine is administered using two to three drops over 10 to 15 minutes. Some surgeons use weak miotics and prophylactic topical antibiotics as well. A povidone-iodine solution is applied around the operative eye, and a small sterile drape is placed over the eyelashes.

The patient is positioned under the microscope with his/her head perpendicular to the microscope optics. An eyelid speculum is inserted, and the patient is instructed to fixate on the microscope light while the pupil/visual axis, optical zone and incision marks are placed.

Marking Incisional Sites/Optical Zones

As a reference point for centration, the center of the miotic or physiologic pupil should be used. Some surgeons advocate the use of the corneal light reflex for centration (as in the PERK Study), which they feel is an approximation of the corneal intercept of the visual axis, but this approach is now used by a minority of refractive surgeons. Coaxial fixation light sources, which are either mounted onto surgical microscopes or aligned within the microscope optical system, make localization of the pupil center simpler. These coaxial targets enable the patient to stare at a light source other than the light filament of the operating microscope. Some surgeons believe that a reference point for determination of the astigmatic keratotomy axis should be marked at the slit lamp, thus avoiding real or apparent position-dependent cyclotorsion of the globe, which may occur when the axis is marked in the supine position (32,63). Although it is likely that the cylinder axis does not change significantly or predictably when most subjects move from a seated position to a supine position, axis misalignment is still quite possible, and marking the patient upright is a worthwhile practice (64,65). A Sinskey hook or similar instrument is then used to indent the epithelium overlying the pupil center or presumed visual axis.

A Mendez axis marker or similar device is then positioned and preoperative anatomy is carefully lined up at the previously defined axis. For an astigmatic procedure, an arcuate or transverse (T cut) marker is then positioned in the steep axis of the astigmatism, as per the surgical plan, and is centered over the pupil or visual axis mark. Because studies of incisional techniques for treating compound myopic astigmatism show no advantage to staging the surgery, it is usually preferable to perform both the radial and arcuate incisions at the same procedure (25,66,67).

A preselected optical zone marker with cross-hairs is then taken and centered on the visual axis mark, and a small indentation is made in the epithelium. The radial incision marker should be centered with respect to the optical zone marker and placed in contact with the corneal epithelium, using moderate pressure.

Intraoperative ultrasonic pachymetry is then performed in the 3.0-mm optical zone as previously described. The diamond knife is set based on the thinnest paracentral reading, adjusting for desired depth (generally 100% or 100% minus 10 to 20 μm) under the calibrating microscope. For radial incisions, the angle formed by the tip of the knife should be 35 to 45 degrees.

Incisional Techniques

Radial incisions are made depending on the technique used: (a) from the optical zone mark to the corneal periphery (centrifugal—American); (b) from the periphery to the optical zone mark (centripetal—Russian); a centripetal approach provides reliably deeper incision depth than the centrifugal approach, whereas a centrifugal approach decreases the risk of violating the central optical zone; (c) combined Genesis or Duotrack technique, where an initial centrifugal (up to 1 mm from the limbus) incision is made, followed by a centripetal incision as described above. A variant of these techniques is mini-RK performed from the central clear (optical) zone of approximately 3 mm to the 7-mm outer zone (26). With all techniques, the blade must be held constantly perpendicular to the corneal surface (Fig. 70-1). It is advisable to order the incision placement, because the cornea thickness decreases during the procedure. Incise the thinnest zone first (usually inferior-temporal), then proceed to the thicker locations in a

graded fashion. Fixation of the globe in RK is achieved with forceps or a circular footed fixation ring. An effective technique utilizes the fixation forceps to counteract the motion of the knife by grasping the globe 180 degrees away from the incision. A "no-touch" technique has been advocated by some (68), but seems inadvisable given the potential for loss of control with invasion of the central optical zone.

After completion of the incisions, the incisions may or may not be irrigated. Broad-spectrum antibiotic, nonsteroidal anti-inflammatory (e.g., diclofenac sodium 0.1% or Ketorolac), and steroid drops are usually applied. The eye may be lightly patched for no more than several hours after the surgery. The recommended interval for surgery on the fellow eye varies from several days to 6 weeks. Simultaneous bilateral surgery is advocated by some surgeons, but we feel this approach is inadvisable due to the small but real possibility of a devastating complication such as infectious keratitis or endophthalmitis, whose presence may not be evident at the time of surgery or in the immediate postoperative period (69,70).

Nomograms for Incisional Keratotomy

Numerous nomograms have been published, and there is currently no unanimity regarding a preferred nomogram or cutting style. The nomograms serve to direct the placement, number, length (as measured by optical-zone and limbal clear zone size) and depth of incisions, thus influencing the amount of myopic (or astigmatic) correction to be achieved (20,71–74). The nomograms usually take into account variables such as age and degree of myopia. Keratometry, intraocular pressure, and patient gender are also thought to be important by some investigators (71,73); however, there are no published results indicating that these factors would favorably affect the outcome of astigmatism-correction surgery (75).

The spherical equivalent (SE) may be used for determining the extent of radial incisions. If a large (e.g., >0.50 D) discrepancy exists between manifest and cycloplegic SE, it is best to use the cycloplegic value. In general, nomograms for centrifugal incisions tend to predict lower degrees of correction than do those for centripetal or combined incisions. Many nomograms incorporate options for four, six, or eight radial keratotomy incisions, which in turn vary the optical zone size. Some surgeons have constructed nomograms that produce an intentional undercorrection (staged procedures) in a large percent of eyes, preventing overcorrections in the vast majority and protecting against progressive hyperopic shifts that are known to occur with radial keratectomy (76). Each surgeon must refine his/her individual approach to incisional keratotomy. This is best accomplished via the use of regression analysis of one's clinical data, keeping in mind the relative instability of the procedure. Nomograms of incisional techniques for radial and astigmatic keratotomy are presented in Figs. 70-5 through 70-10.

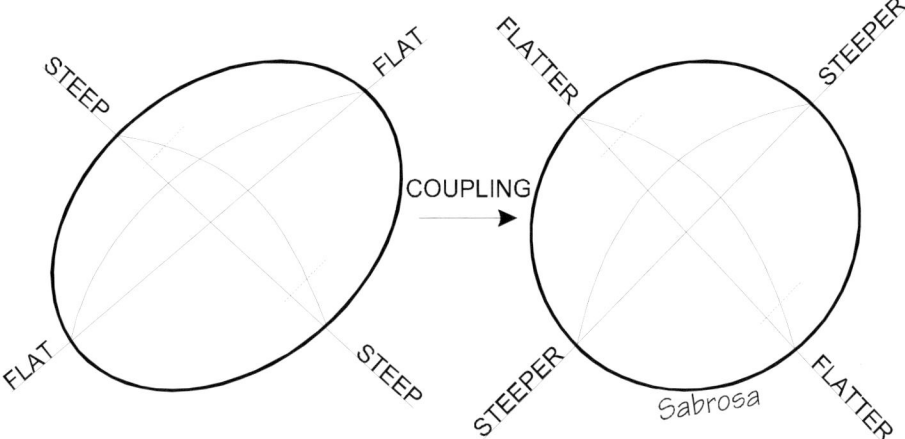

FIGURE 70-5. Coupling effect. Steeping the cornea 90 degrees away from the arcuate transverse incision.

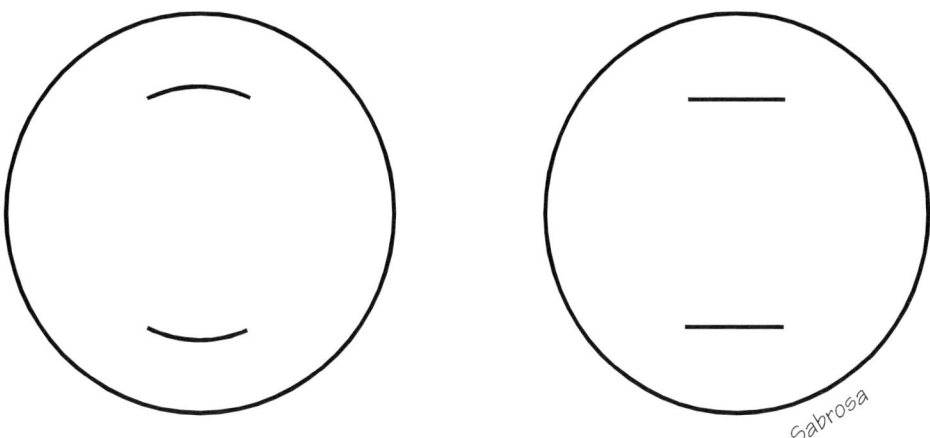

FIGURE 70-6. Arcuate incision/transverse incision.

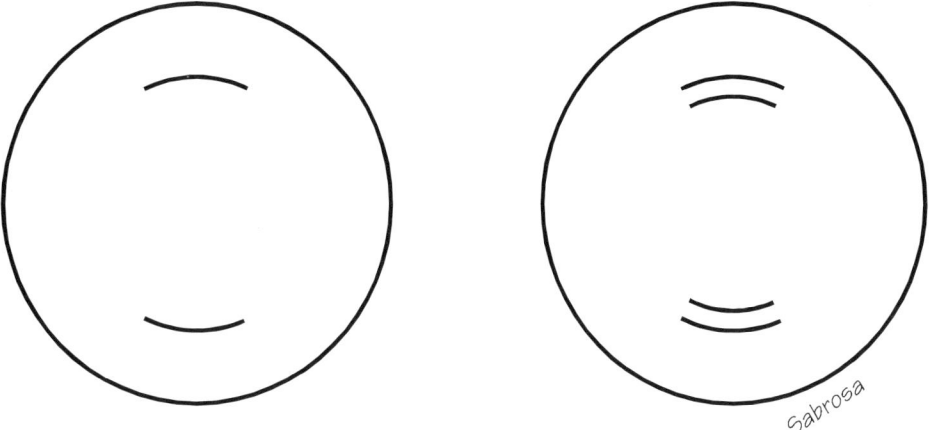

FIGURE 70-7. Arcuate incisions maintain a constant distance from the visual axis.

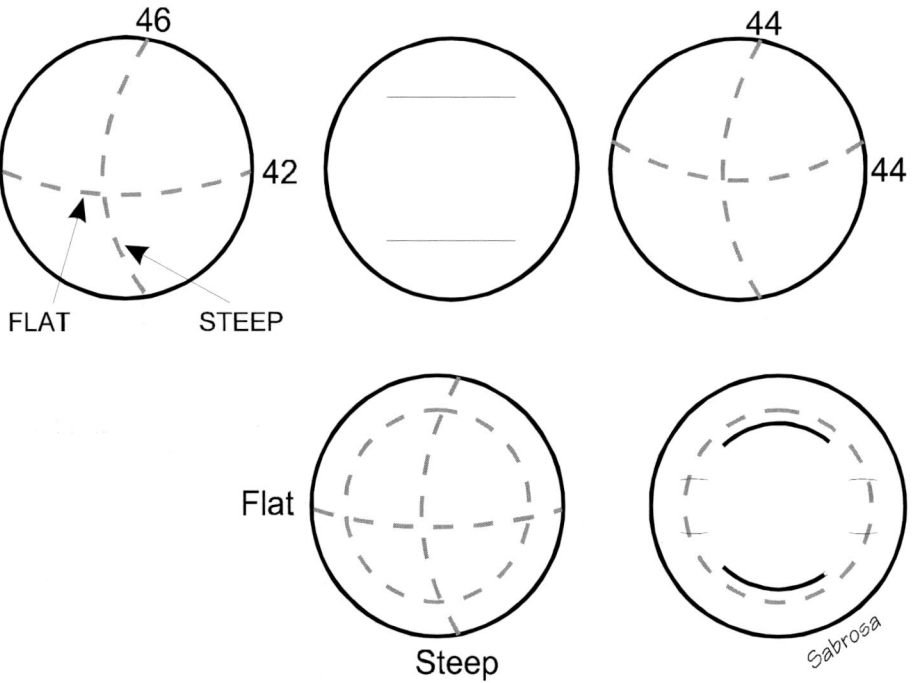

FIGURE 70-8. Astigmatic keratotomy. **A:** Transverse keratotomy incision made on the plus cylinder axis flattens the steeper meridian. **B:** Arcuate keratotomy combined with compression sutures to treat postkeratoplasty astigmatism. The use of arcuate incisions within the donor button avoids the variable wound thickness encountered at the graft-host interface.

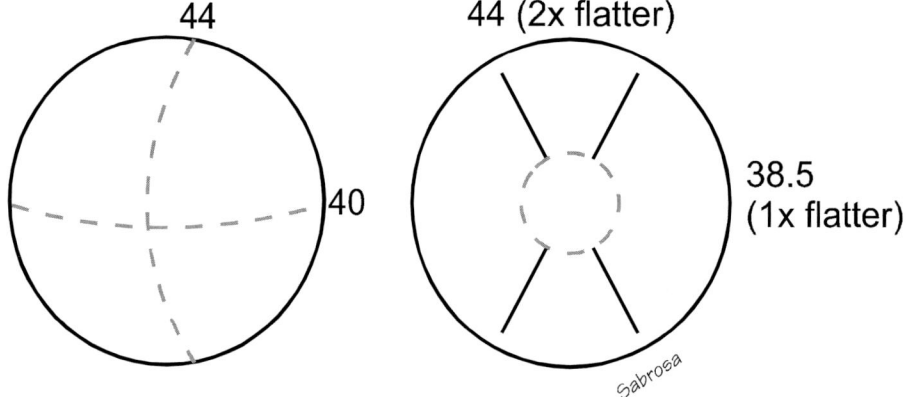

FIGURE 70-9. Semiradial incisions have twice as much flattening effect in the principal meridian of the incisions when compared with 90 degrees away. This permits concomitant correction of myopia and small degrees of astigmatism.

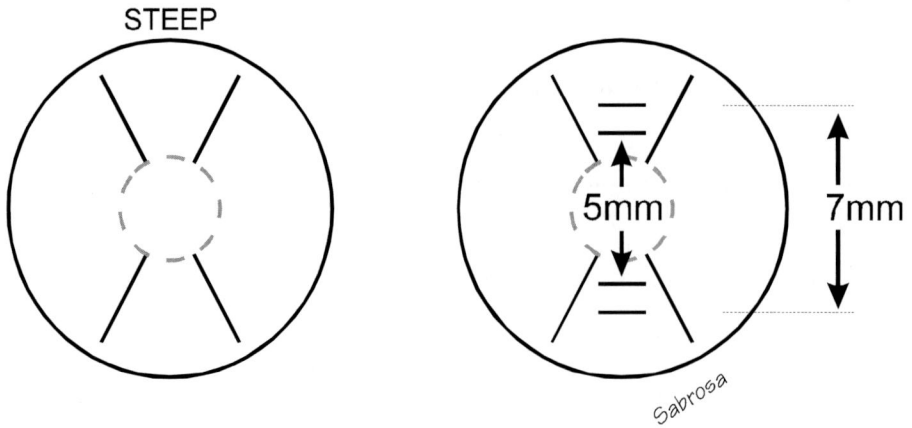

FIGURE 70-10. Trapezoidal keratotomy utilizes a combination of transverse cuts and semiradial incisions.

POSTOPERATIVE CARE AND ENHANCEMENTS FOR RADIAL KERATOTOMY CARE

Topical corticosteroids, and broad-spectrum topical antibiotics, are applied four times a day for 4 to 7 days. Topical nonsteroidal antiinflammatory drugs (NSAIDs) should be limited to the first 24 to 48 hours only. Oral analgesic agents are rarely needed.

Postoperative follow-up examinations are usually made on days 2 and 7; at 4 to 6 weeks; and at months 6 and 12 months following radial keratotomy surgery. On day 2, visual acuity without correction is checked and slit-lamp examination is performed. At subsequent follow-up visits, visual acuity without correction, refraction, applanation tonometry, and slit-lamp examination should be performed. If significant under- or overcorrection is noted or suspected, cycloplegic manifest refraction should be performed. If additional surgery is planned, CVK data may be helpful.

Enhancement rates vary with each surgeon but are generally in the range of 15% to 25% for RK. It is advisable to perform no more than two surgical enhancements per eye (77) at no sooner than 6 weeks between procedures (25). A surgical enhancement method is applied only if cycloplegic refraction reveals the degree of residual myopia to be greater than 0.5 D below the target correction. Correction of residual refractive error after RK is commonly accomplished by adding incisions (cumulative total not greater than eight incisions), deepening the primary incisions (as guided by refraction, slit-lamp exam and topography), reducing the size of the central clear zone (to no smaller than 3-mm), or reducing the limbal clear zone (to no smaller than 0.5-mm). As predictability can be less than satisfactory, a conservative approach should be utilized. Moreover, peripheral redeepening is of minimal benefit in the opinion of many surgeons (78,79).

Excimer laser photorefractive keratectomy (PRK) provides an alternative approach to improving the refractive result in patients with residual refractive error (80–87). It is suggested that results after PRK are less predictable than the above corrective procedures and that the post-RK eyes respond with more haze than normal eyes (88,89). Myopic keratomileusis (both ALK and LASIK) has also been used to correct residual refractive error after RK (90–92), and LASIK may be the enhancement procedure of advice if significant residual myopia exists (i.e., ≥3 D) and the corneal incisions are well healed.

Nonsurgical enhancement methods may be applied if the degree of residual myopia at the 1-week follow-up is greater than 0.5 D. A mechanical pressure patch should be applied at night for the first week following the procedure, continuing for 6 weeks thereafter, to compress the corneal apex, maintaining incision gape during the corneal wound healing process. Alternatively, some surgeons advocate manual compression. Steroid treatment may be prolonged in an attempt to increase the refractive correction. It should be noted that peer-reviewed data to confirm the efficacy of such nonsurgical enhancement techniques is lacking.

CLINICAL RESULTS FOLLOWING RADIAL KERATOTOMY

The PERK study, a multicenter clinical trial to evaluate a standardized technique (centrifugal, or "American") of radial keratotomy (15,74,93–102), has evaluated the results of the procedure at 6 months and at 1, 3, 5, 6, and 10 years following RK. Verity et al. (25) reported a multicenter study using a combined technique with better results than those obtained by PERK, as did Werblin and Stafford (103), who reported 3-year follow-up data on 128 patients who had undergone radial/astigmatic keratotomy. This study differs from PERK and Verity et al. because it used nomograms that employed a centripetal ("Russian") rather than combined technique. The mean target refraction was plano in most patients, and the number of average enhancements greater than the other two studies.

PERK Study Results

In the PERK study, uncorrected visual acuity (UCVA) of 20/40 or better was achieved in 92% of patients in the lower myopia group (−1.50 to −3.12 D) immediately following surgery and remained unchanged over a period of 10 years. In the moderate myopia group (−3.25 to −4.37 D), UCVA of 20/40 or better was attained by 81% of patients at 1 year postoperatively, increasing to 86% at 10 years, as a result of hyperopic shift following initial undercorrection. Similarly, in the high myopia group (−4.50 to −8.87 D), UCVA of 20/40 or better increased from 63% of postoperative eyes at 1 year to 77% at 10 years following RK.

One year after surgery, best-spectacle-corrected visual acuity (BSCVA) was unchanged in 61% of patients, decreased by one Snellen chart line in 13%, decreased by two to three lines in 0.7%, increased by one line in 24%, and increased by two to three lines in 1.7%. BSCVA remained fairly stable over a 10-year period. There was a slight increase in the percentage of patients who lost two to three lines of BSCVA (0.7% at 1 year to 1.4% at 3 years to 3% at 4 years after RK), but remained unchanged at 3% from 4 to 10 years following RK. Ten years after RK, BSCVA was 20/20 or better in 98%, 20/25 in 1.6%, and 20/30 in 0.4% of eyes in the PERK study. No patient had BSCVA worse than 20/30 10 years after RK.

In normal corneas, diurnal refractive fluctuation is minimal. In one study, nearly two thirds of patients had stable vision throughout the day. In the remaining third, daily vision varies by one Snellen line loss due to steepening of the cornea and increase in the minus power of their refraction during the day (96). Following RK, diurnal fluctuation is common for the first several months, but appears to be infrequent thereafter. However, in a small subgroup of PERK patients who complained of visual fluctuation 1 year following RK, only 24% had stable vision throughout the day (74,94,97,98). The major change in refraction occurred within the first hour after awakening and continued for a few hours. After this a small drift persisted in some patients (159). In general, gradual corneal steepening occurred during the day, with a resultant increase in myopia. Diurnal myopic shift of 0.5 to 1.0 D was observed in 33% of postoperative eyes, compared with 8% of unoperated eyes. The maximum myopic fluctuation observed in postoperative RK patients was 1.25 D.

Ten years following surgery, results of the PERK study demonstrated that this technique of RK effectively reduces but does not completely eliminate myopia. Thirty-eight percent of eyes had a final refractive error within ± 0.5 D, and 60% within ±1.0 D (95). This 10-year study found a long-term instability or a mean hyperopic shift of 1.0 D, leading to a less predictable long-term outcome. The mean rate of change was approximately 0.10 D per year. The duration and maximum amount of these trends toward hyperopic shift remains unknown. Other studies have also identified this hyperopic shift (Table 70-4). There is no published evidence that the hyperopic shift will stop at an identifiable time after surgery, suggesting that patients are best left slightly undercorrected. Notwithstanding the issue of refractive instability, RK as performed in the PERK study has a reasonable margin of safety, and sight-threatening complications were rare.

TABLE 70-4. HYPEROPIC SHIFT IN STUDIES OF RADIAL KERATOTOMY

Study	No. of Eyes	Follow-Up Interval	Hyperopic Shift ≤ 1 D, % of Eyes
Waring GO et al. (95)	310	6 mo to 10 y	43
Deitz et al. (105)	143	1 to 8.5 y	54
Arrowsmith and Marks (106)	156	1 to 5 y	22
Sawelson and Marks (19)	198	1.5 to 5 y	17
Neumann et al. (107)	118	1 to 5 y	26
Werblin and Stafford (103)	182	3 y	21.7

Modified from Waring GO, et al. Results of prospective evaluation of radial keratotomy (PERK) study 10 years after surgery. *Arch Ophthalmol* 1994;112:1298–1308.

Results of More Recent RK/AK Studies

The PERK results of 17% undercorrection by 1.0 D or more at 10 years following RK falls within the spectrum of results from other studies, where 11% to 46% of patients were undercorrected by 1.0 D or more. Verity et al. (25) reported undercorrection by −1.0 D in 6%, 10%, and 25% of patients in the low (1.0 to 3.12 D), moderate (3.25 to 4.25 D), and high (4.50 to 9.5 D) myopia groups, respectively.

Like undercorrection, overcorrection by 1.0 D or more in the PERK study 10 years after RK (23%) was not inconsistent with the results of some other studies, where the range of patients overcorrected by 1.0 D or more varied between 3% and 33%.

Radial keratotomy induced 0.5 to 2.75 D astigmatism in 34% of eyes. From those, 24% increased 0.50 to 0.75 D of astigmatism, 3 years following RK (108). In 10% of eyes, the amount of induced astigmatism 3 years after RK, exceeded 1 D. A greater increase in astigmatism was associated with small-diameter optical zones. The association of small-diameter optical zone and induced astigmatism was also found 1 year after RK in a study utilizing the combined Genesis technique (25).

A study performed by Lindstrom (26) stated that a 1% increase in central corneal flattening was achieved when incisions were extended from the mini-RK configuration (7 mm) to full length (11 mm), further confirming that mini-RK is a useful alternative to reduce the invasiveness of RK while retaining its efficacy in eyes with low to moderate myopia.

INCISIONAL KERATOTOMY SIDE EFFECTS AND COMPLICATIONS

RK incisions, like any corneal incisions, permanently weaken the cornea (109–112), and this structural weakening can cause several complications and side effects (66,113–116) (Table 70-5).

The complications of incisional keratotomy may be divided into self-limited, intraoperative, and postoperative.

Self-Limited Side Effects (15,93,94)

These adverse effects are also present following other refractive procedures during the early postoperative period.

Halos and Starburst Effects

Irregular astigmatism or small zones of central corneal flattening induced by incisional keratotomy may produce these symptoms, principally when the pupil dilates. These complications may be reduced in patients with large pupils

TABLE 70-5. COMPLICATIONS OF RADIAL AND ASTIGMATIC KERATOTOMY

Transient
    Pain
    Photophobia

Permanent: best-corrected visual acuity unchanged
    Overcorrection/undercorrection
    Diurnal fluctuation of visual acuity
    Mild glare
    Poor contact lens fit

Permanent: best-corrected visual acuity decreased
    Disabling glare
    Irregular astigmatism
    Corneal perforation
    Corneal neovascularization
    Infectious keratitis
    Endothelial damage
    Cataract
    Endophthalmitis
    Traumatic ruptured globe

by designing an incisional keratotomy procedure to maximize incision number, thereby minimizing the need for a small central clear zone (58). Moreover, removing epithelial cysts or debris from the incisions following surgery can sometimes lessen visual aberrations.

Diurnal Visual Fluctuation and Early Regression (117–119)

Immature wound architecture, sometimes coupled with stromal corneal edema adjacent to the radial incisions, is the principal cause of visual fluctuation over the course of a day during the first several postoperative weeks. Edema develops overnight while the eyelids are closed and results in relatively increased corneal flattening. As the day progresses, the cornea deturgesces and tends to re-steepen, with regression of the refractive result. Stabilization occurs in most cases by 4 to 8 weeks postoperatively. The amplitude of diurnal fluctuation decreases over time, as the wounds "mature" and stabilize. Eye rubbing following incisional keratotomy and chronic postoperative contact lens wear may destabilize the wounds, leading to progressive hyperopia, chronic diurnal fluctuation and refractive instability.

Intraoperative Complications (120,121)

Inaccurate marking of the visual axis can result in incisions invading the optical zone, potentially leading to increased glare and significant, irregular astigmatism. Irregular astigmatism often responds only to rigid gas permeable contact lens correction. Another intraoperative complication is the extension of incisions into the corneoscleral limbus and limbal vascular arcades. Peripheral extension of incisions may lead to contact lens intolerance,

due to associated deep neovascularization of the incisions, or may result in corneal destabilization, diurnal fluctuation, and progression of refractive effect. Central clear zone invasion by incisions represents one of the more worrisome potential complications of centripetal cutting techniques (i.e., "Russian" style). Patient education and globe fixation may reduce, but not entirely eliminate, the potential for optical-zone invasion. Combined incision (Genesis or Duotrak) techniques may help to avoid this complication. Another intraoperative complication is intersecting incisions, which may lead to wound gape and poor healing. Interrupted 10-0 or 11-0 nylon sutures may be necessary to reapproximate the gaped wound margins. Corneal perforation is another possible intraoperative complication. A microperforation is a self-sealing perforation and does not continue to leak, even when challenged using an instrument such as a Weck cell sponge. Microperforations seal spontaneously as the adjacent corneal stroma becomes edematous and acts as a tamponade. Instillation of cycloplegic eye drops, as well as an aqueous suppressant (beta-blocker) may be helpful in this situation. With careful attention given to the possible causes of perforation, the surgeon may be able to complete the surgery. It is important to recheck blade depth under a calibrating microscope and then retract the blade 20 to 30 μm before proceeding. When resetting the blade, it is usually best to retract slightly using the micrometer handle and re-advance (i.e., to shorten 30 μm retract 50, then advance 20). A shield should be placed over the eye, without patching, until the next day.

Macroperforation will leak spontaneously or upon gentle compression using a Weck cell sponge. Operating in a dry field increases the likelihood of early detection of a microperforation and preventing macroperforations. Macroperforations should be sutured with interrupted 10-0 nylon sutures. Excessive suture tension should be avoided. Suture removal within a few weeks postoperatively can avoid persistent irregular astigmatism and lead to a good refractive result (177).

In summary, intraoperative complications of RK may be minimized if the surgeon does not cross incisions, incise to the limbus, redeepen the periphery, ignore microperforation, or operate on a wet field.

Postoperative Complications (Sight-Threatening and Non-Sight-Threatening)

Non-Sight-Threatening Complications

Although some postoperative keratotomy patients experience a regression of 1 D or more toward myopia at 5 years, 43% of patients experience progressive change of μ 1 D toward hyperopia 10 years following RK. The incidence and magnitude of hyperopic shift is thought to increase linearly with the magnitude of attempted myopic correction, and hence is directly related to the number and length of radial incisions (95).

Non-sight-threatening complications resulting from refractive changes include undercorrections and overcorrections. Undercorrections are not always undesirable, and may in fact be the primary goal of the surgical procedure (123–125). Undesired undercorrection has been reported in 20% (18) to 30% (24) of patients following RK, either because the incisions were not sufficiently deep or because of poor biologic response. In patients with unsatisfactory uncorrected visual acuity, a second surgical procedure may be performed to enhance the refractive effect (see section on postoperative care and enhancement for RK care).

Induced hyperopia (overcorrection) is a serious potential complication of radial keratotomy and has few effective treatments (123,124,126–130). Pilocarpine, a miotic, is thought to reduce overcorrections after RK when applied postoperatively. It is possible that pilocarpine may stimulate corneal wound healing, but steepening of corneal curvature may not be permanent (131,132). The PERK study reported an 11% incidence of overcorrections greater than +1.0 D 1 year after surgery (16), which increased to 17% 4 years after the procedure (15) and 43% at 10 years after the procedure (95). Arrowsmith and Marks (106) reported 33% of postkeratotomy patients showed overcorrections of more than 1.0 D at 5 years after surgery. Deitz et al. (126) noted that overcorrections of greater than 1.0 D occurred in 31% of patients 4 years after surgery. Factors that may contribute to initial or delayed overcorrections include improper selection of the central clear zone, an excessive number of radial incisions, elevated intraocular pressure, undetected keratoconus, poor wound healing, age, diabetes, and use of corticosteroids (132,133). As previously stated, because RK surgery results in progressive hyperopic shifts over time, surgeons should intentionally undercorrect the initial RK (22,170).

Numerous approaches have been used to treat overcorrection (133–138). The medical management of eyes overcorrected by RK includes pilocarpine, contact lens wear, and topical hypertonic solutions. Other antiglaucoma medications, such as timolol and acetazolamide, have been advocated to decrease overcorrections (136), but no published data documents their usefulness. Experimental studies show that elevations in intraocular pressure, within a physiologic range, have little effect on the keratometric readings after RK (139–141). Contact lens fitting following RK is more difficult than in normal eyes. After surgery, there is a substantial change in corneal topography, with flattening of the central cornea and steepening of the paracentral cornea, often referred to as the "peripheral knee" (133). Hofmann et al. (134) reported a 56% success rate in fitting rigid gas permeable contact lenses after RK. Surgeons must be aware, however,

that the incidence of neovascularization in eyes fitted with contact lenses following RK may be as high as 33% (135), leading to contact lens intolerance. However, neovascularization may be minimized by shortening the incisions so as not to avoid extension to the limbus and by careful monitoring of contact lens wearers. Hypertonic agents may be useful if there is significant edema around the incisions after surgery (133). Overcorrections may also be managed by using a secondary surgical procedure, such as wound suturing or hyperopic LASIK (142). The incisions can be closed with interrupted sutures or continuous purse-string suture (137,138,143–145). If interrupted sutures are used, great care should be taken to fully reopen and clean the full length of the incision(s), as full reapproximation of stromal wound edges can occur only after all residual epithelial cells have been removed. Nonbiodegradable suture material with minimal elasticity (such as Mersilene) should be used. Disadvantages of the interrupted and purse-string suture techniques are the loss of effect over time, approximately 70% (137), and persistent nonmicrobial keratitis (145). It is possible that progression of effect over time may be reduced after RK techniques that maximize central clear zone diameter, minimize incision number, and do not extend to the limbus (74,146,147).

Regression of effect is a consequence of the early wound-healing process and shows variability between patients. It is more likely to be accompanied by more aggressive scarring of the RK incisions.

Irregular and induced astigmatism may occur if incisions are placed asymmetrically about the visual axis, invade the central cornea, are of variable depths, are nonradial, or are decentered with respect to the visual axis or pupil center (148,149).

Occasionally, recurrent erosions may be present in the first 6 postoperative weeks, before the reformation of new epithelial basement membrane is complete. Symptoms may persist, if excessive epithelial debris accumulates within incisions. Treatment in such cases requires reopening and thoroughly debriding the material from the incisions. In the absence of such abnormalities, conventional graded therapy for recurrent corneal erosion may be necessary, including lubricants, hypertonics, bandage contact lens, stromal micropuncture, and superficial keratectomy (manual or excimer phototherapeutic keratectomy).

Epithelial inclusion cysts (150) and foreign particles such as cosmetics may also appear within the incisions. These are generally expelled over time, but should be removed if evidence of ongoing inflammation is present. In the case of crossed incisions, epithelial cysts may become more problematic.

There have been several studies evaluating endothelial cell loss following RK, reporting a slight decrease in cell density (i.e., 1.6%) (151) with or without progression over time (151,152). Microperforations and small central clear zone diameter appear to be the two greatest risk factors. PERK study data indicate that endothelial cell loss does not lead to corneal edema 10 years after RK (150).

Sight-Threatening Complications

Stromal melting (153) often develops in patients with crossed incisions. This may be prevented by avoiding crossing incisions during the surgical procedure. However, it is also often associated with patients having collagen vascular disease such as rheumatoid arthritis concomitant with severe keratoconjunctivitis sicca.

Infectious keratitis (68,154–159) (Fig. 70-11) is another complication that may occur in the perioperative period, although delayed cases can usually be associated with contact lens wear. Sterile operation technique and application of prophylactic, broad-spectrum antibiotic drops before and at the end of the surgery are prudent. Be aware that although gram-positive organisms are most prevalent in acute post-RK infection, gram-negative organisms such as *Serratia* sp. and *Pseudomonas* sp. have also been documented, so antibiotic coverage should be tailored to address both possibilities. Moreover, postoperative keratotomy patients should be instructed to avoid wearing eye makeup or exposing themselves to contaminated water for at least 2 weeks following surgery. Hot tubs and fresh water lakes are particularly dangerous. In the event of an infection, early detection and treatment is important. Cultures should be taken and intensive broad-spectrum antibiotic therapy prescribed. Close follow-up is mandatory, as an infected RK incision provides easy access to Descemet's membrane and poses an increased risk of endophthalmitis over more superficial corneal infections.

Approximately 28 cases (160) of ruptured corneas following blunt trauma in eyes previously subjected to radial (113,114), hexagonal, or arcuate transverse keratotomies have been reported (114,120,161,162), even as long as 10 years after the procedure (163). Pinheiro et al. (36) have reported that the rupture threshold of mini-RK incisions is not significantly different from that of normal eyes under experimental conditions, adding yet another theoretical advantage to this approach to incisional/keratotomy.

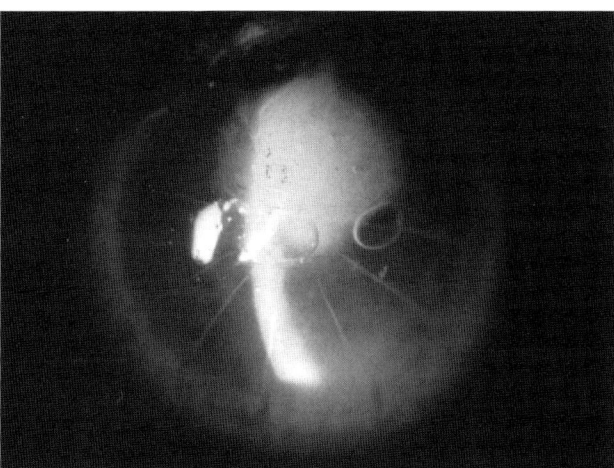

FIGURE 70-11. Infectious keratitis. (Incisional keratotomy complication.)

REFERENCES

1. Snellen H. Die Richtung der Hauptmeridiane des astigmatischen Auges (German). *Graefes Arch Clin Exp Ophthalmol* 1869; 15:199–207.
2. Schiötz HJ. Ein Fall von hochgradigem Hornhautastigmatismus nach Staarextraction. Besserung auf operativem Wege (German). *Arch Augenhd* 1885;15:178–181.
3. Bates WH. A suggestion of an operation to correct astigmatism. *Arch Ophthalmol* 1894;23:9–13.
4. Lans LJ. Experimentelle Untersuchungn über Entstehung von Astigmatismus durch nicht-perforirend Corneawunden (German). *Graefes Arch Clin Exp Ophthalmol* 1898;45:117–152.
5. Sato T. Treatment of conical cornea (incision of Descemet's membrane) [in Japanese]. *Nippon Ganka Gakkai Zasshi* 1939; 43:544–555.
6. Sato T, Akiyama K, Shibata H. A new surgical approach to myopia. *Am J Ophthalmol* 1953;36:823–829.
7. Yamaguchi T, Kanai A, Tanaka M, et al. Bullous keratopathy after anterior-posterior radial keratotomy for myopia. *Am J Ophthalmol* 1982;93:600–606.
8. Yenaliev. Experience in surgical treatment of myopia. *Vestn Ophthalmol* 1978;3:52–56.
9. Fyodorov SN, Agronovsky AA. Long-term results of radial keratotomy. *J Ocul Ther Surg* 1982;1:217–223.
10. Fyodorov SN, Durnev VV. Operation of dosaged dissection of corneal circular ligament in cases of myopia of mild degree. *Ann Ophthalmol* 1979;11:1885–1889.
11. Durnev V. Decrease of corneal refraction by anterior keratotomy method with the purpose of surgical correction of myopia of mild to moderate degree. Proceedings of the first Congress of Ophthalmology of Transcaucasia, Tbilisi, Georgia, 1976: 129–132.
12. Bores LD, Myers W, Cowden J. Radial keratotomy: an analysis of the American experience. *Ann Ophthalmol* 1981;13:941–948.
13. Bores LD. Historical review and clinical results of radial keratotomy. *Int Ophthalmol Clin* 1983;23:93–118.
14. Waring GO, Moffitt S, Gelender H, et al. Rationale for and design of the National Eye Institute Prospective Evaluation of Radial Keratotomy (PERK) Study. *Ophthalmology* 1983;90: 40–58.
15. Waring GO, Lynn M, Nizam A, et al. Results of the Prospective Evaluation of Radial Keratotomy (PERK) Study five years after surgery. *Ophthalmology* 1991;98:1164–1176.
16. Waring GO, Lynn M, Gelender H, et al. Results of the Prospective Evaluation of Radial Keratotomy (PERK) Study one year after surgery. *Ophthalmology* 1985;92:177–198.
17. Cowden J, Lynn M, Waring GO, et al. Repeated radial keratotomy in the Prospective Evaluation of Radial Keratototmy (PERK) Study. *Am J Ophthalmol* 1987;103:423–431.
18. Waring GO, Lynn M, Fielding B, et al. Results of the Prospective Evaluation of Radial Keratotomy (PERK) Study four years after surgery for myopia. *JAMA* 1990;263:1083–1091.

19. Sawelson H, Marks RG. Five-year results of radial keratotomy. *Refract Corneal Surg* 1989;5:8–20.
20. Arrowsmith PN, Marks RG. Visual, refractive and keratometric results of radial keratotomy: a two-year follow-up. *Arch Ophthalmol* 1987;105:76–80.
21. Deitz MR, Sanders DR, Raanan MG. A consecutive series (1982–1985) of radial keratotomy performed with the diamond blade. *Am J Ophthalmol* 1987;103:417–422.
22. Salz JJ, Salz JM, Salz M, et al. Ten years experience with a conservative approach to radial keratotomy. *Refract Corneal Surg* 1991;7:12–22.
23. Thornton SP. Thornton guide for radial keratotomy incisions and optical zone size. *J Refract Surg* 1985;1:29–33.
24. Werblin TP, Stafford GM. The Casebeer system for predictable keratorefractive surgery: one-year evaluation of 205 consecutive eyes. *Ophthalmology* 1993;100:1095–1102.
25. Verity SM, Talamo JH, Chayet A, et al. The combined (Genesis) technique of radial keratotomy: a prospective multicenter trial. *Ophthalmology* 1995;102:1908–1917.
26. Lindstrom RL. Minimally invasive radial keratotomy: mini-RK. *J Cataract Refract Surg* 1995;21:27–34.
27. Melles GRJ, Binder PS. Effect of radial keratotomy incision direction on wound depth. *Refract Corneal Surg* 1990;6:394–403.
28. Melles GRJ, Wijdh RHJ, Cost B, et al. Effect of blade configuration knife action and intraocular pressure on keratotomy incision depth and shape. *Cornea* 1993;12:299–309.
29. Flanagan GW, Binder PS. Effect of incision direction on refractive outcome after radial keratotomy. *J Cataract Refract Surg* 1996;22:915–923.
30. Berkeley RG, Sanders DR, Piccolo MG. Effect of incision direction on radial keratotomy outcome. *J Cataract Refract Surg* 1991;17:819–823.
31. Assil KK, Kassoff J, Schanzlin DJ, et al. A combined incision technique of radial keratotomy. A comparison to centripetal and centrifugal incision techniques in human donor eyes. *Ophthalmology* 1994;101:746–754.
32. Assil KK, Schanzlin DJ. Astigmatic keratotomy surgical technique and protocol. In: Assil KK, Schanzlin DJ, eds. *Radial and astigmatic keratotomy,* vol I. Thorofare, NJ: Poole Press/Slack, 1994:126.
33. Schachar RA, Black TD, Huang T. A physicist view of radial keratotomy with practical surgical implications. In: Schachar RA, Levy NS, Schachar L, eds. *Keratorefraction. Proceedings of the Keratorefractive Society Meeting.* Denison, TX, 1980:195–219.
34. Jester JV, Venet T, Lee J, et al. A statistical analysis of radial keratotomy in human cadaver eyes. *Am J Ophthalmol* 1981;92: 172–177.
35. Salz J, Lee JS, Jester JV, et al. Radial keratotomy in fresh human cadaver eyes. *Ophthalmology* 1981;88:742–746.
36. Pinheiro MN, Bryant MR, Tayyanipour R, et al. Corneal integrity after refractive surgery: effects of radial keratotomy and mini-radial keratotomy. *Ophthalmology* 1995;102:297–301.
37. Sperduto R, Seigel D, Roberts J, et al. Prevalence of myopia in the United States. *Arch Ophthalmology* 1983;101:405–407.
38. Kraff MC, Sanders DR, Karcher D, et al. Changing practice patterns in refractive surgery: results of a survey of the American Society of Cataract and Refractive Surgery. *J Cataract Refract Surg* 1994;20:172–178.
39. Borque LB, Cosand BB, Drews C, et al. Reported satisfaction, fluctuation of vision and glare among patients one year after surgery in the Prospective Evaluation of Radial Keratotomy (PERK) study. *Arch Ophthalmol* 1986;104:356–363.
40. Powers MK, Meyerowitz BE, Arrowsmith PN, et al. Psychological findings in radial keratotomy patients two years after surgery. *Ophthalmology* 1984;91:1193–1198.
41. Assil KK, Barrett AM, Fouraker BD et al. One-year results of the intrastromal corneal ring in non-functional human eyes. *Arch Ophthalmol* 1995;113:159–167.
42. Percival SPB, Vyas AV. Radial keratotomy for myopia from 5.00 to 13.00 diopters two years after surgery. *J Refract Surg* 1996;12:86–90.
43. Price FW Jr, Grene RB, Marks RG, et al. Arcuate transverse keratotomy for astigmatism followed by subsequent radial or transverse keratotomy. *J Refract Surg* 1996;12:68–76.
44. Nesburn AB, Bahri S, Berlin M, et al. Computer-assisted corneal topography (CACT) to detect mild keratoconus in candidates for photorefractive keratectomy. *Invest Ophthalmol Vis Sci* 1992;33(suppl):995.
45. Waring GO. Nomenclature for keratoconus suspects. J *Refract Corneal Surg* 1993;9:219–222.
46. Rabinowitz YS. Keratoconus, videokeratography and refractive surgery. *Refract Corneal Surg* 1992;8:403–407.
47. Durand L, Monnot JP, Burillon C, et al. Complications of radial keratotomy: eyes with keratoconus and late wound dehiscence. J *Refract Corneal Surg* 1992;8:311–314.
48. Mamalis N, Montgomery S, Anderson C, et al. Radial keratotomy in a patient with keratoconus. *Refract Corneal Surg* 1991;7:374–376.
49. Ellis W. Radial keratotomy in a patient with keratoconus. *J Cataract Refract Surg* 1992;18:406–409.
50. Barney NP, Foster CS. A prospective randomized trial of oral acyclovir after penetrating keratoplasty for herpes simplex keratitis. *Cornea* 1994;13:232–236.
51. Wilson SE, Klyce SD. Screening for corneal topographic abnormalities before refractive surgery. *Ophthalmology* 1994; 101:147–152.
52. Maguire LJ, Lowry JC. Identifying progression of subclinical keratoconus by serial topography analysis. *Am J Ophthalmol* 1991;112:41–45.
53. Rabinowitz YS, Nesburn AB, McDonnell PJ. Videokeratography of the fellow eye in unilateral keratoconus. *Ophthalmology* 1993;100:181–186.
54. Rabinowitz YS, Garbus J, McDonnell PJ. Computer-assisted corneal topography in family members of patients with keratoconus. *Arch Ophthalmol* 1990;108:365–371.
55. Gangadhar DV, Talamo JH. Corneal topography: adjunctive use in keratorefractive surgery. In: Azar D, ed. *Refractive surgery,* vol 1. Stamford, CT: Appleton & Lange, 1996: 169–183.
56. Bogan SJ, Waring GO, Ibrahim O, et al. Classification of normal corneal topography based on computer-assisted videokeratography. *Arch Ophthalmol* 1990;108:945–949.
57. Pulaski JP. Transverse incisions for mixed and myopic idiopathic astigmatism. *J Cataract Refract Surg* 1996;22: 307–312.
58. Grimmett MR, Holland EV. Complications of small clear-zone radial keratotomy. *Ophthalmology* 1996;103:1348–1356.
59. The PERK study group. Radial keratotomy for simple myopia. Diagnostic and Therapeutic Technology Assessment (DATTA). *JAMA* 1988;260:264–267.
60. The PERK study group. Ophthalmic procedures assessment. *Ophthalmology* 1989;96:671–687.
61. Aron-Rosa D, Binder PS, Deitz MR, et al. Statement on radial keratotomy in 1988. *J Refract Surg* 1988;4:80–90.
62. American Academy of *Ophthalmology.* Ophthalmic Procedures Assessment. Radial Keratotomy for Myopia. *Ophthalmology* 1993;100:1103–1115.
63. Chavez S, Chayet A, Celikkol L, et al. Analysis of astigmatic keratotomy with a 5.0–mm optical clear zone. *Am J Ophthalmol* 1996;121:65–76.

64. Smith EM, Talamo JH, Assil KK, et al. Comparison of astigmatic axis in the seated and supine positions. *J Refract Corneal Surg* 1994;10:615–620.

65. Smith EM, Talamo JH. Cyclotorsion in the seated and supine patient. *J Cataract Refract Surg* 1995;21:402–403.

66. Lindstrom RL. The surgical correction of astigmatism: a clinician's perspective. *Refract Corneal Surg* 1990;6:441–454.

67. Thornton SP, Sanders DR. Graded non-intersecting transverse incisions for correction of idiopathic astigmatism. *J Cataract Refract Surg* 1987;13:27–31.

68. Casebeer JC. Surgical procedures for correcting myopia and astigmatism. In: *Casebeer: incisional keratotomy,* 1st ed. Thorofare, NJ: Slack, 1995:116.

69. Szerenyi K, McDnnell JM, Smith RE, et al. Keratitis as a complication of bilateral, simultaneous radial keratotomy. *Am J Ophthalmol* 1994;117:462–467.

70. McLeod SD, Flowers CW, Lopez PF, et al. Endophthalmitis and orbital cellulitis after radial keratotomy. *Ophthalmology* 1995;102:1902–1907.

71. Arrowsmith PN, Marks RG. Evaluating the predictability of radial keratotomy. *Ophthalmology* 1985;92:331–338.

72. Arrowsmith PN, Marks RG. How predictable is radial keratotomy? *Cataract* 1986;3:7–14.

73. Deitz MR, Sanders DR. Marks RG. Radial keratotomy: an overview of the Kansas City study. *Ophthalmology* 1984;91:467–478.

74. Lynn MJ, Waring GO, Sperduto RD, et al. Factors affecting outcome and predictability of radial keratotomy in the PERK study. *Arch Ophthalmol* 1987;105:42–51.

75. Price FW, Grene RB, Marks RG, et al. Astigmatism reduction clinical trial: a multicenter prospective evaluation of the predictability of arcuate keratotomy. *Arch Ophthalmol* 1995;113:277–282.

76. Waring GO, Gordon JF, Lee PA, et al. A comparison of the Duotrak™ blade technique and the Russian technique in prospective multicenter clinical studies of refractive keratotomy for myopia and astigmatism. *Invest Ophthalmol Vis Sci* 1994;35(suppl):1637.

77. Talley AR, Assil KK, Schanzlin DJ. Patient selection and evaluation. In: Talamo JH, Krueger RR, eds. *The excimer manual,* 1st ed. Boston: Little, Brown, 1996:50.

78. Poirier L, Coulon P, Williamson W, et al. Effect of peripheral deepening of radial keratotomy incisions. *J Refract Corneal Surg* 1994;10:621–624.

79. Coulon P, Poirier L, Williamson, et al. Value and complications of peripheral deepenings in radial keratotomies. (French) *J Fr Ophthalmol* 1993;16:103–107.

80. McDonnell PJ, Garbus JJ, Salz JJ. Excimer laser myopic photorefractive keratotomy after undercorrected radial keratectomy. *Refract Corneal Surg* 1991;7:146–150.

81. Seiler T, Jean B. Photorefractive keratectomy as a second attempt to correct myopia after radial keratotomy. *Refract Corneal Surg* 1992;8:211–214.

82. Hahn TW, Kim JH, Lee YC. Excimer laser photorefractive keratectomy to correct residual myopia after radial keratotomy. *J Refract Corneal Surg* 1993;9:S25–29.

83. Frangie JP, Park SB, Kim J, et al. Excimer laser keratectomy after radial keratotomy. *Am J Ophthalmol* 1993;115 634–639.

84. Durrie DS, Schumer DJ, Cavanaugh TB. Photorefractive keratectomy for residual myopia after previous refractive keratotomy. J *Refract Corneal Surg* 1994;10(suppl):S235–238.

85. Maloney RK, Steinert RF, Hersh PS, et al. A multi-center trial of photorefractive keratectomy for residual myopia following previous ocular surgery. *Ophthalmology* 1994;101(suppl):74.

86. Kwitko ML, Gow JA, Bellavance F, et al. Excimer photorefractive keratectomy after undercorrected radial keratotomy. *J Refract Surg* 1995;11:S280–283.

87. Lee YC, Park CK, Sah WJ, et al. Photorefractive keratectomy for undercorrected myopia after radial keratotomy: two-year follow up. *J Refract Surg* 1995;11(3 suppl):S274–279.

88. Ribeiro JC, McDonald MB, Lemos MM, et al. Excimer laser photorefractive keratectomy after radial keratotomy. *J Refract Surg* 1995;11:165–169.

89. Burnstein Y, Hersh PS. Photorefractive keratectomy following radial keratotomy. *J Refract Surg* 1996;12:163–170.

90. Swinger CA, Barker BA. Myopic keratomileusis following radial keratotomy. *J Refract Surg* 1985;1:53–55.

91. Nordan LT, Harvins WE. Undercorrected radial keratotomy treated with myopic keratomileusis. *J Refract Surg* 1985;1:56–58.

92. Forseto AS, Nose RA, Francesconi CM, et al. Laser *in situ* keratomileusis for undercorrection after radial keratotomy. *J Refract Surg* 1999;15:424–428.

93. Waring GO, Lynn MJ, Strahlman ER, et al. Stability of refraction during four years after radial keratotomy in the Prospective Evaluation of Radial Keratotomy Study. *Am J Ophthalmol* 1991;111:133–144.

94. Bourque LB, Cosand BB, Drews C, et al. Reported satisfaction, fluctuation of vision, and glare among patients one year after surgery in the Prospective Evaluation of Radial Keratotomy (PERK) Study. *Arch Ophthalmol* 1986;104:356–363.

95. Waring GO, Lynn MJ, McDonnell PJ, et al. Results of the Prospective Evaluation of Radial Keratotomy (PERK) study 10 years after surgery. *Arch Ophthalmol* 1994;112:1298–1308.

96. Schanzlin DJ, Santos VR, Waring GO, et al. Diurnal changes in refraction, corneal curvature, visual acuity, and intraocular pressure after radial keratotomy in the PERK study. *Ophthalmology* 1986;93:167–175.

97. Santos VR, Waring GO, Lynn MJ, et al. Relationship between refractive error and visual acuity in the prospective evaluation of radial keratotomy (PERK) study. *Arch Ophthalmol* 1987;105:86–92.

98. Holladay JT, Lynn MJ, Waring GO, et al. The relationship of visual acuity, refractive error, and pupil size after radial keratotomy. *Arch Ophthalmol* 1991;109:70–76.

99. Binder PS. Four-year postoperative evaluation of radial keratotomy. *Arch Ophthalmol* 1985;103:779–780.

100. Lynn MJ, Waring GO, the PERK study group, et al. Symmetry of refractive and visual acuity outcome in the prospective evaluation of radial keratotomy (PERK) study. *Refract Corneal Surg* 1989;5:75–81.

101. Ginsburg AP, Waring GO, Steinberg EB, et al. Contrast sensitivity under photopic conditions in the prospective evaluation of radial keratotomy (PERK) study. *Refract Corneal Surg* 1990;6:82–91.

102. Rowsey JJ, Balyeat HD, Monlux R, et al. Prospective evaluation of radial keratotomy. Photokeratoscope corneal topography. *Ophthalmology* 1988;95:322–334.

103. Werblin TP, Stafford GM. Three year results of refractive keratotomy using the Casebeer System. *J Cataract Refract Surg* 1996;22:1023–1029.

104. Applegate RA, Howland HC. Magnification and visual acuity in refractive surgery. *Arch Ophthalmol* 1993;111:1135–1142.

105. Deitz MR, Sanders DR, Raanan MG, et al. Long-term (5- to 12-year) follow-up of metal-blade radial keratotomy procedure. *Arch Ophthalmol* 1994;112:614–620.

106. Arrowsmith PN, Marks RG. Visual refractive and keratometric results of radial keratotomy: five-year follow-up. *Arch Ophthalmol* 1989;107:506–511.

107. Neumann AC, Oster RH, Fenzl RE. Radial keratotomy: a comprehensive evaluation. *Doc Ophthalmol* 1984;56:275–301.

108. Waring GO, Lynn MJ, Culbertson W, et al. Three-year results of the prospective evaluation of radial keratotomy (PERK) study. *Ophthalmology* 1987;94:1339–1354.

109. Ingraham HJ, Guber D, Green WR. Radial keratotomy: Clinicopathologic case report. *Arch Ophthalmol* 1985;103:683–688.

110. Yamaguchi T, Tamaki K, Kaufman HE, et al. Histologic study of a pair of human corneas after anterior radial keratotomy. *Am J Ophthalmol* 1985;100:281–292.

111. Luttrull JK, Jester JV, Smith RE. The effect of radial keratotomy on ocular integrity in an animal model. *Arch Ophthalmol* 1982;100:319–320.

112. McKnight SJ, Fitz J, Giangiacomo J. Corneal rupture following radial keratotomy in cats subjected to BB gun injury. *Ophthalmic Surg* 1988;19:165–167.

113. Simons KB, Linsalata RP. Ruptured globe following blunt trauma after radial keratotomy: a case report (abstract). *Ophthalmology* 1987;94(suppl):148.

114. Binder PS, Waring GO III, Arrowsmith PN, et al. Histopathology of traumatic corneal rupture after radial keratotomy. *Arch Ophthalmol* 1988;106:1584–1590.

115. Spigelman AV, Williams PA, Nichols BD, et al. Four incision radial keratotomy. *J Cataract Refract Surg* 1988;14:125–128.

116. Spigelman AV, Williams PA, Lindstrom RL. Further studies of four incision radial keratotomy. *Refract Corneal Surg* 1989;5:292–295.

117. McDonnell PJ, Nizam A, Lynn MJ, et al. Morning-to-evening change in refraction, corneal curvature, and visual acuity 11 years after radial keratotomy in the Prospective Evaluation of Radial Keratotomy Study. *Ophthalmology* 1996;103:233–239.

118. Santos VR, Waring III GO, Lynn MJ, et al. Morning-to-evening change in refraction, corneal curvature, and visual acuity 2 to 4 years radial keratotomy in the PERK study. *Ophthalmology* 1988;95:1487–1493.

119. MacRae S, Rich L, Phillips D, et al. Diurnal variation in vision after radial keratotomy. *Am J Ophthalmol* 1989;107:262–267.

120. Rashid ER, Waring GO III. Complications of radial and transverse keratotomy. *Surv Ophthalmol* 1989;34:73–106.

121. Leroux les Jardins S, Bertrand I, Massin M. Intraoperative and early postoperative complications in 466 radial keratotomies. *Refract Corneal Surg* 1992;8:215–216.

122. MacRae S, Cox W, Bedrossian R, et al. The treatment of persistent wound leak after radial keratotomy. *Refract Corneal Surg* 1993;9:62–64.

123. Werblin TP, Stafford GM. Hyperopic shift after refractive keratotomy using the Casebeer system. *J Cataract Refract Surg* 1996;22:1030–1036.

124. Sawelson H, Marks RG. Ten-year refractive and visual results of radial keratotomy. *Ophthalmology* 1995;102:1892–1901.

125. Waring GO, FRCOphth, Casebeer JC, et al. One-year results of a prospective multicenter study of the Casebeer system of refractive keratotomy. *Ophthalmology* 1996;103:1337–1347.

126. Deitz MR, Sanders DR. Progressive hyperopia with long-term follow-up of radial keratotomy. *Arch Ophthalmol* 1985;103:782–784.

127. Richmond RD. Special report: radial keratotomy as seen through operated eyes. *J Refract Surg* 1987;3:22–27.

128. Richmond RD. Radial keratotomy as seen through operated eyes. Part II. *J Refract Surg* 1988;4:91–95.

129. Wyzinski P, O'Dell L. Diurnal cycle of refraction after radial keratotomy. *Ophthalmology* 1989;94:120–124.

130. Wyzinski P, O'Dell L. Subjective and objective findings after radial keratotomy. *Ophthalmology* 1989;96:1608–1611.

131. Laranjeira E, Buzard KA. Pilocarpine in the management of overcorrection after radial keratotomy. *J Refract Surg* 1996;12:382–390.

132. Troutman RC, Buzard KA. *Corneal astigmatism: etiology, prevention and management.* St. Louis: Mosby Yearbook, 1992:64–91.

133. Waring GO. *Refractive keratotomy for myopia and astigmatism.* St. Louis: Mosby Yearbook, 1992:878–881.

134. Hofmann RF, Starling JC, Masler W. Contact fitting after radial keratotomy: one year results. *J Refract Surg* 1986;2:155–162.

135. Shivitz IA, Arrowsmith PN, Russel BM. Contact lenses in the treatment of patients with overcorrected radial keratotomy. *Ophthalmology* 1987;94:899–903.

136. Busin M, Suarez H, Bieber S, et al. Overcorrected visual acuity improved by antiglaucoma medication after radial keratotomy. *Am J Ophthalmol* 1986;101:374–375.

137. Lindquist TD, Williams PA, Lindstrom RL. Surgical treatment of overcorrection following radial keratotomy: evaluation of clinical effectiveness. *Ophthalmic Surg* 1991;22:12–15.

138. Hofmann RF. Reoperations after radial and astigmatic keratotomy. *J Refract Surg* 1987;3:119–128.

139. Maloney RK, Stark WJ, McCally RL, et al. The refractive change induced by radial keratotomy is not affected by intraocular pressure. *Ophthalmology* 1987;94(suppl):128.

140. Maloney RK. Effect of corneal hydration and intraocular pressure on keratometric power after experimental radial keratotomy. *Ophthalmology* 1990;97:927–933.

141. Busin M, Arffa RK, McDonald MB, et al. Change in corneal curvature with elevation in intraocular pressure after radial keratotomy in the primate eye. *CLAO J* 1988;14:110–112.

142. Francesconi CM, Nosé RA, Nosé W. Hyperopic laser-assisted in situ keratomileusis for radial keratotomy induced hyperopia. *Ophthalmology* 2002;109:602–605.

143. Lyle WA, Jin GJ. Long-term stability of refraction after intrastromal suture correction of hyperopia following radial keratotomy. *J Refract Surg* 1995;11:485–489.

144. Alio J, Ismail M. Management of radial keratotomy overcorrections by corneal sutures. *J Cataract Refract Surg* 1993;19:595–599.

145. Lyle WA, Jin JC. Circular and interrupted suture technique for correction of hyperopia following radial keratotomy. *Refract Corneal Surg* 1992;8:80–83.

146. Sanders D, Deitz M, Gallagher. Factors affecting predictability of radial keratotomy. *Ophthalmology* 1985;92:1237–1243.

147. Smith RS, Cutro J. Computer analysis of radial keratotomy. *CLAO J* 1984;10:241–248.

148. Parmley V, Ng J, Gee B, et al. Penetrating keratoplasty after radial keratotomy. A report of six patients. *Ophthalmology* 1995;102:947–950.

149. McDonnell PJ, Caroline PJ, Salz J. Irregular astigmatism after radial keratotomy. *Am J Ophthalmol* 1989;107:42–46.

150. Vila-Coro AA, Bonafonte S, del Cotero JNF. Epithelial inclusion cysts after radial keratotomy. *Ann Ophthalmol* 1988;20:367–370.

151. Chiba K, Oak SS, Tsubota K, et al. Morphometric analysis of corneal endothelium following radial keratotomy. *J Cataract Refract Surg* 1987;13:263–267.

152. Ganem S, Galle P, Loisance D, et al. Endothelial effects of radial keratotomy in a non-human primate (French). *Ophtalmologie* 1989;3:13–15.

153. Hersh PS, Kalevar V, Kenyon KR. Penetrating keratoplasty for severe complications of radial keratotomy. *Cornea* 1991;10:170–174.

154. Gussler JR, Miller D, Jaffe M, et al. Infection after radial keratotomy. *Am J Ophthalmol* 1995;119:798–799.

155. Gelender H, Flynn HW, Mandelbaum SH. Bacterial endophthalmitis resulting from radial keratotomy. *Am J Ophthalmol* 1982;93:323–326.

156. Jain S, Azar DT. Eye infection after refractive keratotomy. *J Refract Surg* 1996;12:148–155.

157. Heidemann DG, Dunn SP, Watts JC. Aspergillus keratitis after radial keratotomy. *Am J Ophthalmol* 1995;120:254–256.

158. Duffey RJ. Bilateral Serratia marcescens keratitis after simultaneous bilateral radial keratotomy. *Am J Ophthalmol* 1995;119:233–236.

159. Matoba AY, Torres J, Wilhelmus KR, et al. Bacterial keratitis after radial keratotomy. *Ophthalmology* 1989;96:1171–1175.

160. Vinger PF, Mieller WF, Oestreicher JH, et al. Ruptured globes following radial and hexagonal keratotomy surgery. *Arch Ophthalmol* 1996;114:129–134.

161. Pearlstein ES, Agapitos, PJ, Cantrill HL, et al. Ruptured globe after keratotomy (letter). *Am J Ophthalmol* 1988;106:755–756.

162. Bloom HR, Sands J, Schneider D. Corneal rupture from blunt trauma 22 months after radial keratotomy. *Refract Corneal Surg* 1990;6:197–199.

163. McDermott ML, Wilkinson WS, Tukel DB, et al. Corneoscleral rupture ten years after radial keratotomy (letter). *Am J Ophthalmol* 1990;110:575–577.

INCISIONAL SURGERY FOR NATURAL AND SURGICALLY-INDUCED ASTIGMATISM

ROGER F. STEINERT

Regular and irregular astigmatism cause impairment of uncorrected visual acuity and, in moderate to large amounts, loss of best corrected visual acuity. Spectacle correction of higher amounts of astigmatism induces distortion that can be reduced with the use of rigid gas permeable contact lenses or toric soft contact lenses. Surgical intervention to reduce astigmatism provides a permanent alternative solution. In general, the goal of surgical intervention is not the complete elimination of the astigmatism, a goal difficult to achieve because of the variability of the corneal response to astigmatic correction. Rather, the appropriate goal is to reduce the amount of astigmatism to a level that has less functional impact on uncorrected visual acuity and allows a satisfactory correction of the residual smaller astigmatism through the use of spectacles or contact lenses.

HISTORICAL PERSPECTIVE

The first successful surgical intervention for astigmatism occurred in 1885, when Schiotz placed a 3.5-mm limbal penetrating incision in a steep meridian, reducing astigmatism after cataract surgery from 19.5 D to 7 D (1). Lucciola was the first surgeon to employ nonperforating incisions to correct astigmatism (2). Lans (3) first appreciated that the flattening that occurs in a corneal meridian after placing a transverse incision was associated with steepening in the opposite meridian.

He also demonstrated that deeper and longer incisions had more effect. Refinement of astigmatic keratometry has occurred through many investigations, often employing cadaver eye models (4–10).

Introduction of excimer laser ablation into clinical practice offers the surgeon the ability to directly address astigmatism by reshaping the corneal surface, either with photorefractive keratectomy (PRK) or laser *in-situ* keratomileusis (LASIK).

CHOOSING A SURGICAL PROCEDURE

Choosing between the surgical alternatives for astigmatism correction begins with the preoperative assessment of the patient. In addition to quantifying the amount of astigmatism and documenting the corresponding corneal topographic change, the surgeon must evaluate the etiology of the astigmatism and the impact of each of the surgical alternatives on the patient's overall optical balance.

In the case of naturally occurring astigmatism, corneal topography is essential to differentiate between regular astigmatism and astigmatism due to corneal ectasias, principally keratoconus and pellucid marginal degeneration. Astigmatic incisions in the presence of corneal ectasia generally do poorly, with unpredictable and unstable results. Excimer laser ablation will thin an already abnormally weakened cornea, and is generally regarded as contraindicated in the presence of corneal ectasia. In some cases, patients are motivated to seek reduction in astigmatism as an independent procedure. More commonly, surgery for naturally occurring astigmatism becomes a consideration when a patient is undergoing cataract surgery, as surgeons and patients elevate their expectations for high levels of uncorrected visual acuity postoperatively.

Postoperative induced astigmatism is best separated into the separate categories of limbal incision surgically induced astigmatism and postkeratoplasty astigmatism.

Limbal incisions at the time of cataract surgery have been a troublesome cause of astigmatism for the entire history of cataract surgery, until the recent introduction of incisions in the range of 3 mm or less. With phacoemulsification cataract extraction, and the implantation of foldable intraocular lenses, the induction of a functionally troublesome amount of astigmatism is now infrequent. Because some patients still require a larger incision for extracapsular cataract extraction or management of some operative complications, however, cataract surgery remains a major cause of surgically induced astigmatism. In addition, astigmatism is seen not infrequently in conjunction with glaucoma filtration surgery, particularly if the filtration site is combined with a larger incision for simultaneous cataract surgery.

Postkeratoplasty astigmatism typically includes a combination of regular and irregular astigmatism. Treatment of postkeratoplasty astigmatism is complicated by this combination; surgical intervention for irregular astigmatism is difficult at best. Moreover, the etiology of postkeratoplasty astigmatism resides in the junction of the graft and host, which usually is at a diameter between 7 and 9 mm.

Residing closer to the optical zone, this keratoplasty wound has a much larger impact on the central corneal optics than a limbal incision. Moreover, because a corneal transplant incision occupies the full 360 degrees, the opportunity for optically significant distortion is greatly magnified compared to a surgical limbal wound. In addition, centration of corneal transplants relative to the visual axis is often suboptimal for a number of reasons, not the least of which is that the visual axis cannot be directly measured. Lessons learned from laser vision correction as well as radial keratotomy emphasize the deleterious impact of decentration of the treatment zone relative to the visual axis.

From these starting points, the surgeon must then determine several other components of the treatment plan. Is the needed correction primarily the reduction of astigmatism, or is it also a major shift in residual hyperopia or myopia? Incisional keratotomy has a modest impact, at most, on the spherical equivalent, particularly with arcuate keratotomy, which is the most commonly employed form of incisional keratotomy. A major shift in the spherical equivalent is better addressed with PRK or LASIK, or, in addition to the astigmatic incision, placement of a secondary intraocular lens or intraocular lens exchange to alter the spherical equivalent.

A second critical component in the treatment plan is to determine whether the principal astigmatic component is excessive flattening in one meridian, or excessive steepening in another. In examining the corneal topography, excessive flattening is readily determined, typically heralded by hemimeridian dioptric values below 40 diopters. A flat hemimeridian suggests significant wound slippage.

It is better to surgically remedy the surgical wound first, before resorting to secondary astigmatic surgery. For example, if a large cataract incision is associated with flattening, the incision should be carefully inspected to see if there is visible wound separation, in which case, the surgeon should evaluate the ability to expose the incision, freshen the wound margins, and resuture the defect. This is particularly prominent when there is an accompanying inadvertent filtering bleb.

In the case of penetrating keratoplasty, excessive flattening is often associated with override of the graft–host junction. The contour of the graft relative to the host can be appreciated not only through the color maps of the typical corneal topography representation but, sometimes more strikingly,

in viewing the placido mires of the corneal topography and direct examination of the cornea three-dimensionally at the slit lamp. The placido mires often have a dramatic "teardrop" distortion toward an area of graft-host override. If this type of deformity is a major contributor to the patient's postoperative astigmatism, the misalignment of the graft and host should be addressed through opening of the defective wound area and repositioning the graft with multiple interrupted 10-0 nylon sutures. Attempting to correct the astigmatism through other measures, while leaving the graft-host junction abnormality, invariably results in a poor outcome.

ASTIGMATIC KERATOTOMY

Patient Selection and Evaluation

Peripheral corneal relaxing incisions (PCRIs), commonly known as *limbal relaxing incisions*, have the advantage of more reliable wound healing, particularly in elderly individuals where clear corneal incisions heal variably and sometimes poorly, and less potential of inducing irregular astigmatism because of their more peripheral location. PCRIs have less effective power than more centrally located incisions in the clear cornea, however. Decision about the location of the incision, therefore, is driven by an evaluation of the patient's likely wound healing capability and the amount of astigmatic correction desired. In many cases, adequate improvement in visual function can be obtained with only a partial correction of the full astigmatic error. It is not necessary to target zero residual cylinder, which risks an overcorrection in some patients.

In addition to a comprehensive examination, particular attention should be given to corneal topography and pachymetry. Any areas of previous surgery also need careful inspection to assess the potential that wound slippage is the underlying problem that needs to be addressed rather than superimposing astigmatic surgery.

Surgical Technique

The surgeon must be equipped with surgical markers in order to lay down the pattern of the desired correction, an intraoperative pachymeter to determine the corneal thickness at the time of treatment, a diamond knife designed for astigmatic surgery, and an operating microscope.

With the patient upright, the limbus should be marked with a gentian violet sterile surgical marking pen in order to correct for any cyclotorsion or head malposition that may occur with a patient in the supine position. Some surgeons prefer to make marks at the 3 and 9 o'clock positions, whereas others make marks at the 6 and 12 o'clock positions. If a slit lamp is available that allows rotation of the light beam to a specific setting in degrees, it is possible to directly mark the meridian for the surgery.

Anesthesia is achieved typically with topical 0.5% proparacaine or tetracaine with three or four applications every 5 minutes. More profound anesthesia can be obtained with lidocaine jelly, but the residual gel on the ocular surface is undesirable at the time of performing the surgery, and the extra anesthesia is generally unnecessary. Many surgeons apply one to two drops of 0.5% povidone-iodine solution and employ a sterile small lid speculum such as a Barraquer wire lid speculum. Draping the skin and lashes is preferred by some surgeons; others feel that the drape becomes an encumbrance as well as causing patient anxiety.

The surgical incisions are usually centered relative to the entrance pupil. The apical light reflex is not necessarily the visual axis, and the center of the pupil is a more reliable guide for centration in the absence of an abnormal pupil.

With a patient fixating on the coaxial light of the operating room microscope, the surgeon places the appropriate marks depending on the desired treatment pattern (see below). If the cornea is relatively dry, the impression of the marker on the corneal epithelium may be sufficient. Some surgeons prefer to place gentian violet ink from a sterile surgical marker on the corneal marking device in order to leave a readily visible guide for the incisions. Pachymetry is then performed immediately prior to the incisions. In clear corneal incisions, a calibrated diamond knife is usually set at 90% to 100% of the pachymetry value, depending on the surgeon's experience. The goal is to achieve an incision as deep as possible without perforating through Descemet's membrane. In the case of PCRIs, most surgeons use a standard setting of either 600 or 650 μm for the periphery.

While the patient is fixating on the operating microscope light, the surgeon fixates the limbus with a forceps and the knife is inserted at the beginning of the incision. The surgeon should pause at this point to allow the blade to penetrate to the full depth, and then slowly and steadily advance the knife along the incision.

Most surgeons prefer a front-cutting knife in order to obtain good visibility.

At the completion of the procedure, a drop of a broad-spectrum antibiotic and a nonsteroidal antiinflammatory drug are typically applied. Routine patching, application of a bandage contact lens, and cycloplegia are usually not necessary. If a perforation has occurred, the cornea should be observed for sealing. If a slow, spontaneous leak persists, an interrupted 10-0 nylon suture should be placed.

Choice of Astigmatic Keratotomy Pattern

Clear corneal incisions are typically either straight (transverse keratotomy) or curved parallel to the limbus (arcuate keratotomy). Peripheral corneal relaxing incisions are always in an arc parallel to the limbus, just inside the vascular arcade. In the past, transverse incisions were sometimes applied with the addition of radial keratotomy incisions, but now this is rarely employed. These different patterns of incisions

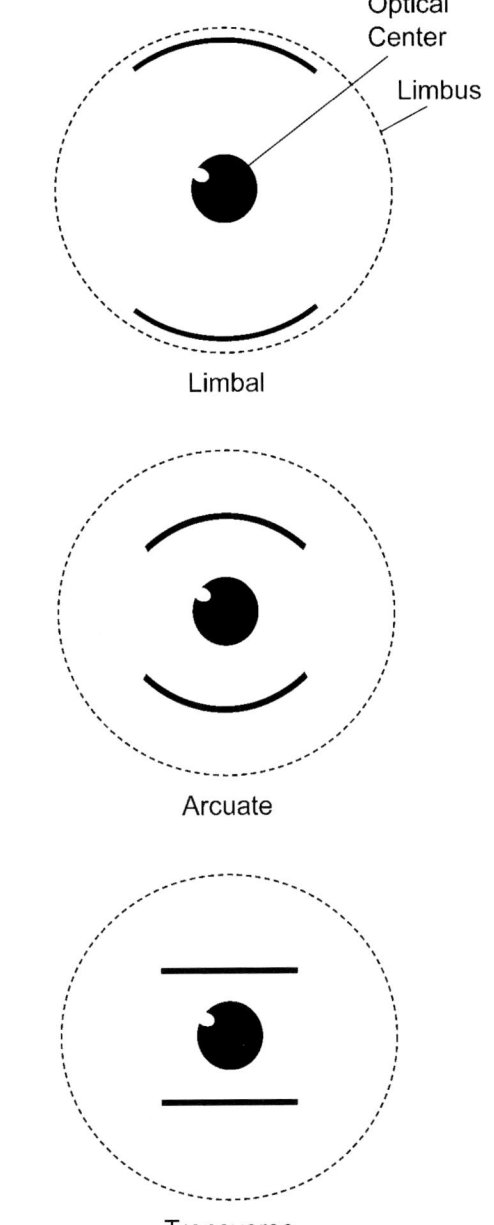

FIGURE 71-1. Patterns of astigmatic keratotomy.

are illustrated in Figure 71-1. Transverse incisions have increasingly fallen out of favor relative to arcuate incisions. The effect of a transverse incision is maximal at its center, where the incision is closest to the optical center of the cornea, with less effect in the periphery, where the straight incision becomes more distant from the optical zone. In contrast, an arcuate keratotomy incision maintains the same distance from the optical zone throughout its length. Surgical experience has led many surgeons to favor arcuate keratotomy for all clear corneal incisions, with a feeling that a longer arcuate keratotomy and a larger optical zone are preferable to a shorter transverse keratotomy closer to the optical zone.

Coupling refers to the phenomenon that placement of the incision in the steep meridian leads to flattening of the steep meridian, but accompanied by some degree of steepening of the untreated flat meridian 90 degrees away from the incision.

If there is an equal amount of steepening of the flat meridian compared to the flattening of the steep meridian, the coupling ratio is 1:1, and there is no change in the spherical equivalent. In most applications of astigmatic keratotomy, the coupling ratio is close to 1:1. At most, there is a mild hyperopic shift amounting to between 0.5 and 1 D. In the past, transverse keratotomies were sometimes combined with adjacent radial incisions to either side, which was reported to achieve a coupling ratio as high as 5:1. This degree of flattening of the steep meridian with markedly less steepening of the flat meridian 90 degrees away would achieve a more dramatic hyperopic shift, and could be used to manipulate a patient's spherical equivalent to reduce myopia. Lack of predictability of this procedure, however, has largely caused it to be abandoned. In most cases where a large shift in the spherical equivalent is desired, consideration should be given to PRK or LASIK.

In principle, a reversed coupling ratio, where there is a net myopic shift, can be achieved with arcuate incisions greater than 90 degrees in length. The instability of such a large incision makes it inadvisable under most circumstances, however.

Variables Effecting Outcome

An increased effect occurs with incisions closer to the visual axis, longer incisions, arcuate rather than straight incisions, increased number of incisions, increased depth of incision, increasing patient age, and male gender.

Typical nomograms for arcuate, transverse, and peripheral corneal relaxing incisions are given in Tables 71-1 to 71-4.

Complications

Irregular Astigmatism

Irregular astigmatism occurs more commonly with incisions closer to the visual axis, decentered incisions, and poor wound healing. For example, an asymmetrical overresponse, where one hemimeridian flattens more than the other due to excessive wound separation, should be recognized and treated immediately with placement of 10-0 nylon sutures to reappose the excessively separated incision. When there is a choice, a conservative surgeon will choose the surgical technique that places the incision as peripheral as possible, but not exceeding a maximum of 75 to 90 degrees in arc length.

Overcorrection

Symmetrical overcorrection should be treated by cleaning out the incision and resuturing with interrupted 10-0 nylon sutures. If at all possible, the surgeon should avoid attempting

TABLE 71-1. NOMOGRAM FOR PERIPHERAL CORNEAL RELAXING INCISIONS TO CORRECT KERATOMETRIC ASTIGMATISM DURING CATARACT SURGERY (TEMPORAL 3.2- TO 3.5-mm CLEAR-CORNEAL INCISION)

Preoperative Astigmatism (D)	Age (year)	Number	Length (Degrees)
WTR			
0.75-1	<65	2 (or 1 × 60 degrees)	45
	≥65	1	45
1.01-1.50	<65	2	60
	≥65	2 (or 1 × 60 degrees)	45
>1.50	<65	2	80
	≥65	2	60
ATR			
1-1.25[a]	–	1	35
1.26-2	–	1	45
≥2	–	2	45

[a]Especially if cataract incision is not directly centered on steep meridian.
From Koch D, Lindstrom RL, Wang L, Osher RH. Control of astigmatism in the cataract patient. In: Steinert RF, ed. *Cataract surgery*, 2nd ed. New York: Elsevier, 2004, with permission.

to treat overcorrection by placing further astigmatic incisions in the meridian 90 degrees opposite the original meridian. The combination of astigmatic incisions in multiple meridians commonly leads to irregular astigmatism.

Undercorrection

Undercorrection can be treated by redeepening the original incisions (utilizing a blade with sharp edges only at the depth of the blade in order to stay within the original incision track), lengthening the original incision, or placing a new set of incisions closer to the optical zone.

Infectious Keratitis

An opportunistic infection may occur in the corneal incisions. For that reason, use of povidone-iodine to prepare the globe immediately preoperatively and use of a broad-spectrum antibiotic postoperatively until wound healing occurs is advisable. Even then, breakdown in the epithelial barrier may allow a late-onset opportunistic infection. The patient should be advised to report the onset of redness, pain, or a shift in vision immediately.

Corneal Perforation

A small perforation may spontaneously seal, or respond well to simple pressure patching or a bandage soft contact lens. If in doubt, however, one or more interrupted 10-0 nylon sutures should be placed immediately. Rare cases of endophthalmitis or epithelial ingrowth into the anterior chamber have been reported after perforations following radial keratotomy and/or astigmatic keratotomy.

TABLE 71-2. ARCUATE KERATOTOMY 6-mm OPTICAL ZONE NOMOGRAM

		Surgical Option				
Age (y)	1 × 30 Degrees	2 × 30 Degrees or 1 × 45 Degrees	1 × 60 Degrees	2 × 45 Degrees or 1 × 90 Degrees	2 × 60 Degrees	2 × 90 Degrees
20	0.60	1.20	1.80	2.40	3.60	4.80
21	0.62	1.23	1.85	2.46	3.69	4.92
22	0.63	1.26	1.89	2.52	3.78	5.04
23	0.65	1.29	1.94	2.58	3.87	5.16
24	0.66	1.32	1.98	2.64	3.96	5.28
25	0.68	1.35	2.03	2.70	4.05	5.40
26	0.69	1.38	2.07	2.76	4.14	5.52
27	0.71	1.41	2.12	2.82	4.23	5.64
28	0.72	1.44	2.16	2.88	4.32	5.76
29	0.74	1.47	2.21	2.94	4.41	5.88
30	0.75	1.50	2.25	3.00	4.50	6.00
31	0.77	1.53	2.30	3.06	4.59	6.12
32	0.78	1.56	2.34	3.12	4.68	6.24
33	0.80	1.59	2.39	3.18	4.77	6.36
34	0.81	1.62	2.43	3.24	4.86	6.48
35	0.83	1.65	2.48	3.30	4.95	6.60
36	0.84	1.68	2.52	3.36	5.04	6.72
37	0.86	1.71	2.57	3.42	5.13	6.84
38	0.87	1.74	2.61	3.48	5.22	6.96
39	0.89	1.77	2.66	3.54	5.31	7.08
40	0.90	1.80	2.70	3.60	5.40	7.20
41	0.92	1.83	2.75	3.66	5.49	7.32
42	0.93	1.86	2.79	3.72	5.58	7.44
43	0.95	1.89	2.84	3.78	5.67	7.56
44	0.96	1.92	2.88	3.84	5.76	7.68
45	0.98	1.95	2.93	3.90	5.85	7.80
46	0.99	1.98	2.97	3.96	5.94	7.92
47	1.01	2.01	3.02	4.02	6.03	8.04
48	1.02	2.04	3.06	4.08	6.12	8.16
49	1.04	2.07	3.11	4.14	6.21	8.28
50	1.05	2.10	3.15	4.20	6.30	8.40
51	1.07	2.13	3.20	4.26	6.39	8.52
52	1.08	2.16	3.24	4.32	6.48	8.64
53	1.10	2.19	3.29	4.38	6.57	8.76
54	1.11	2.22	3.33	4.44	6.66	8.88
55	1.13	2.25	3.38	4.50	6.75	9.00
56	1.14	2.28	3.42	4.56	6.84	9.12
57	1.16	2.31	3.47	4.62	6.93	9.24
58	1.17	2.34	3.51	4.68	7.02	9.36
59	1.19	2.37	3.56	4.74	7.11	9.48
60	1.20	2.40	3.60	4.80	7.20	9.60
61	1.22	2.43	3.65	4.86	7.29	9.72
62	1.23	2.46	3.69	4.92	7.38	9.84
63	1.25	2.49	3.74	4.98	7.47	9.96
64	1.26	2.52	3.78	5.04	7.56	10.08
65	1.28	2.55	3.83	5.10	7.65	10.20
66	1.29	2.58	3.87	5.16	7.74	10.32
67	1.31	2.61	3.92	5.22	7.83	10.44
68	1.32	2.64	3.96	5.28	7.92	10.56
69	1.34	2.67	4.01	5.34	8.01	10.68
70	1.35	2.70	4.05	5.40	8.10	10.80
71	1.37	2.73	4.10	5.46	8.19	10.92
72	1.38	2.76	4.14	5.52	8.28	11.04
73	1.40	2.79	4.19	5.58	8.37	11.16
74	1.41	2.82	4.23	5.64	8.46	11.28
75	1.43	2.85	4.28	5.70	8.55	11.40

Find patient age, then move right to find result closest to refractive cylinder without going over.
(From Koch D, Lindstrom RL, Wang L, Osher RH. Control of astigmatism in the cataract patient. In: Steinert RF, ed. *Cataract surgery*, 2nd ed. New York: Elsevier, 2004, with permission.)

TABLE 71-3. ARCUATE KERATOTOMY NOMOGRAM FOR MALES WITH 7-mm OPTICAL ZONE

	Surgical Option						
Age (y)	1 × 45 Degrees	2 × 30 Degrees	1 × 60 Degrees	1 × 90 Degrees	2 × 45 Degrees	2 × 60 Degrees	2 × 90 Degrees
20	0.32	1.62	0.92	2.02	2.22	2.72	3.82
21	0.36	1.66	0.96	2.06	2.26	2.76	3.86
22	0.39	1.69	0.99	2.09	2.29	2.79	3.89
23	0.40	1.73	1.03	2.13	2.33	2.83	3.93
24	0.46	1.76	1.06	2.16	2.36	2.86	3.96
25	0.50	1.80	1.10	2.20	2.40	2.90	4.00
26	0.54	1.84	1.14	2.24	2.44	2.94	4.04
27	0.57	1.87	1.17	2.27	2.47	2.97	4.07
28	0.61	1.91	1.21	2.31	2.51	3.01	4.11
29	0.64	1.94	1.24	2.34	2.54	3.04	4.14
30	0.68	1.98	1.28	2.38	2.58	3.08	4.18
31	0.72	2.02	1.32	2.42	2.62	3.12	4.22
32	0.75	2.05	1.35	2.45	2.65	3.15	4.25
33	0.79	2.09	1.39	2.49	2.69	3.19	4.29
34	0.82	2.12	1.42	2.52	2.72	3.22	4.32
35	0.86	2.16	1.46	2.56	2.76	3.26	4.36
36	0.90	2.20	1.50	2.60	2.80	3.30	4.40
37	0.93	2.23	1.53	2.63	2.83	3.33	4.43
38	0.97	2.27	1.57	2.67	2.87	3.37	4.47
39	1.00	2.30	1.60	2.70	2.90	3.40	4.50
40	1.04	2.34	1.64	2.74	2.94	3.44	4.54
41	1.08	2.38	1.68	2.78	2.98	3.48	4.58
42	1.11	2.41	1.71	2.81	3.01	3.51	4.61
43	1.15	2.45	1.75	2.85	3.05	3.55	4.65
44	1.18	2.48	1.78	2.88	3.08	3.58	4.68
45	1.22	2.52	1.82	2.92	3.12	3.62	4.72
46	1.26	2.56	1.86	2.96	3.16	3.66	4.76
47	1.29	2.59	1.89	2.99	3.19	3.69	4.79
48	1.33	2.63	1.93	3.03	3.23	3.73	4.83
49	1.36	2.66	1.96	3.06	3.26	3.76	4.86
50	1.40	2.70	2.00	3.10	3.30	3.80	4.90
51	1.44	2.74	2.04	3.14	3.34	3.84	4.94
52	1.47	2.77	2.07	3.17	3.37	3.87	4.97
53	1.51	2.81	2.11	3.21	3.41	3.91	5.01
54	1.54	2.84	2.14	3.24	3.44	3.94	5.04
55	1.58	2.88	2.18	3.28	3.48	3.98	5.08
56	1.62	2.92	2.22	3.32	3.52	4.02	5.12
57	1.65	2.95	2.25	3.35	3.55	4.05	5.15
58	1.69	2.99	2.29	3.39	3.59	4.09	5.19
59	1.72	3.02	2.32	3.42	3.62	4.12	5.22
60	1.76	3.06	2.36	3.46	3.66	4.16	5.26
61	1.80	3.10	2.40	3.50	3.70	4.20	5.30
62	1.83	3.13	2.43	3.53	3.73	4.23	5.33
63	1.87	3.17	2.47	3.57	3.77	4.27	5.37
64	1.90	3.20	2.50	3.60	3.80	4.30	5.40
65	1.94	3.24	2.54	3.64	3.84	4.34	5.44
66	1.98	3.28	2.58	3.68	3.88	4.38	5.48
67	2.01	3.31	2.61	3.71	3.91	4.41	5.51
68	2.05	3.35	2.65	3.75	3.95	4.45	5.55
69	2.08	3.38	2.68	3.78	3.98	4.48	5.58
70	2.12	3.42	2.72	3.82	4.02	4.52	5.62
71	2.16	3.46	2.76	3.86	4.06	4.56	5.66
72	2.19	3.49	2.79	3.89	4.09	4.59	5.69
73	2.23	3.53	2.83	3.93	4.13	4.63	5.73
74	2.26	3.56	2.86	3.96	4.16	4.66	5.76
75	2.30	3.60	2.90	4.00	4.20	4.70	5.80

Subtract 0.37 from each predicted value for females.
(From Koch D, Lindstrom RL, Wang L, Osher RH. Control of astigmatism in the cataract patient. In: Steinert RF, ed. *Cataract surgery*, 2nd ed. New York: Elsevier, 2004, with permission.)

TABLE 71-4. NOMOGRAM FOR 3-mm T-CUTS

Cylinder (D)	Optical Zone (mm)
1.5	8.5
2	8
2.5	7-7.5
3	6-6.5
3.5	2 pair: 6 and 8.5

From Koch D, Lindstrom RL, Wang L, Osher RH. Control of astigmatism in the cataract patient. In: Steinert RF, ed. *Cataract surgery*, 2nd ed. New York: Elsevier, 2004, with permission.

Cataract Surgery and Astigmatism

Correction of astigmatism at the time of small-incision cataract surgery can be achieved through PCRIs or implantation of a toric intraocular lens. Clear corneal midperipheral incisions are generally best avoided due to the variability in wound healing, particularly in an elderly population. If a small amount of astigmatism is present, simply orienting the cataract incision in the steep meridian, sometimes with an accompanying large peripheral groove, is adequate to address the bulk of the astigmatism. Otherwise, an astigmatically neutral small incision should be employed for the cataract surgery. One or two PCRI incisions are then placed in the steep meridian. Some surgeons prefer to place these at the beginning of the procedure; others firm the eye at the end of the procedure and place the astigmatic incisions as a last step.

Correction of astigmatism after the completion of the cataract surgery is performed in a manner essentially identical to correction of astigmatism in nonpostsurgical corneas as outlined earlier.

POSTKERATOPLASTY ASTIGMATISM

As reviewed earlier, assessment of a patient with unacceptable postkeratoplasty astigmatism begins with inspection of the graft-host junction and examination of the corneal topography. Excessive flattening in a hemimeridian suggests wound slippage, and slit-lamp examination should be directed to that zone. If any discontinuity of the graft-host Bowman layer apposition is detected, or if separation of the incision can be seen, heralded by a broad incision and/or epithelial cysts in the incision, then the incision should be taken down, cleaned, and resutured with multiple interrupted 10-0 nylon sutures (Fig. 71-2). The surgeon must take special care to press the central donor cornea posteriorly, as the needle passes across the graft-host junction, in order to reverse the forward protrusion of the graft.

In the past, techniques have been described for wedge resection of a crescent of donor cornea in an effort to reverse

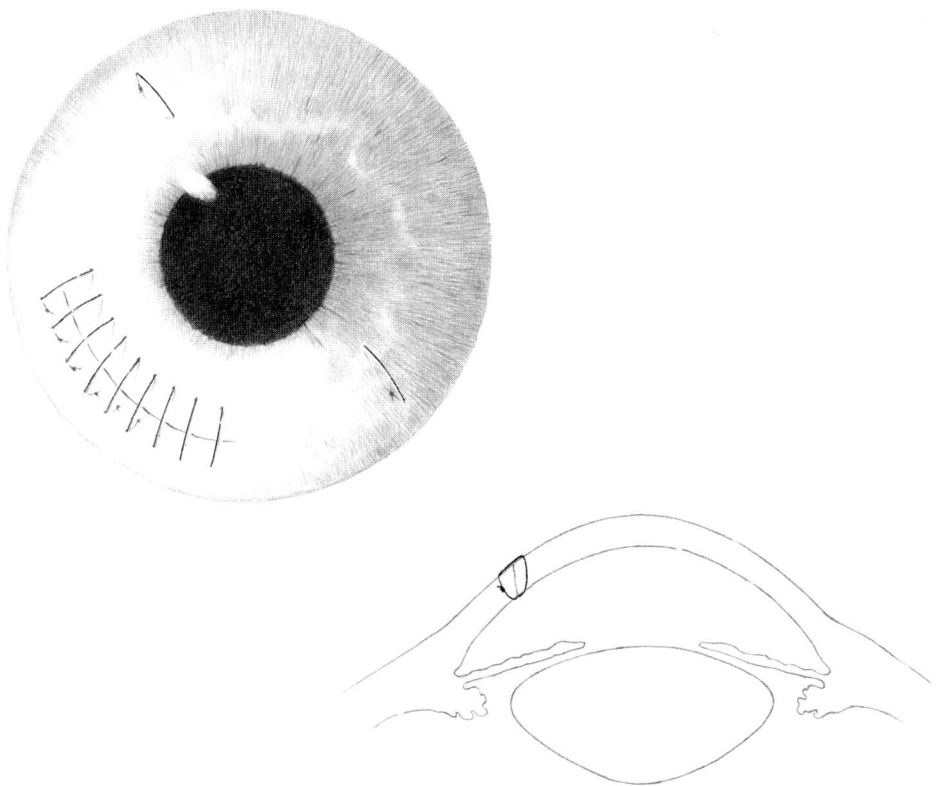

FIGURE 71-2. Poor penetrating keratoplasty wound apposition is repaired by cleaning the incision and resuturing with multiple 10-0 nylon sutures.

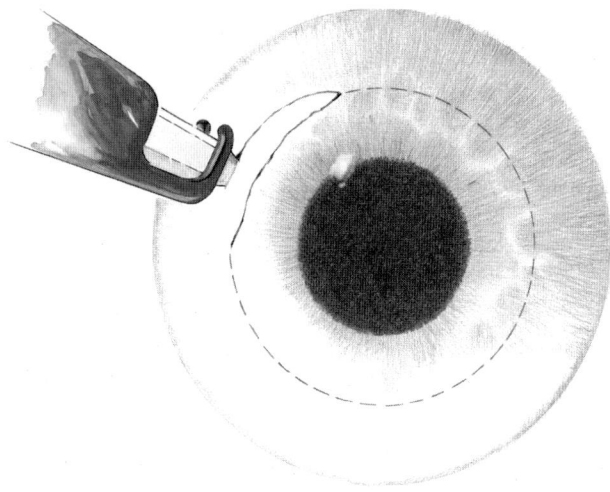

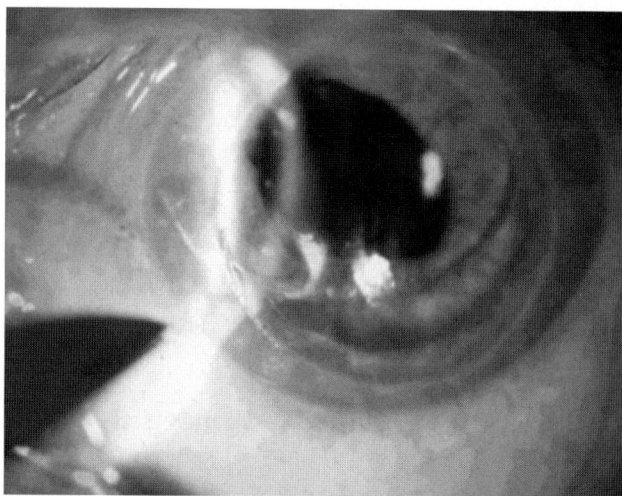

FIGURE 71-4. A blade breaks down the scar at Bowman's layer to create a relaxing incision in the keratoplasty incision.

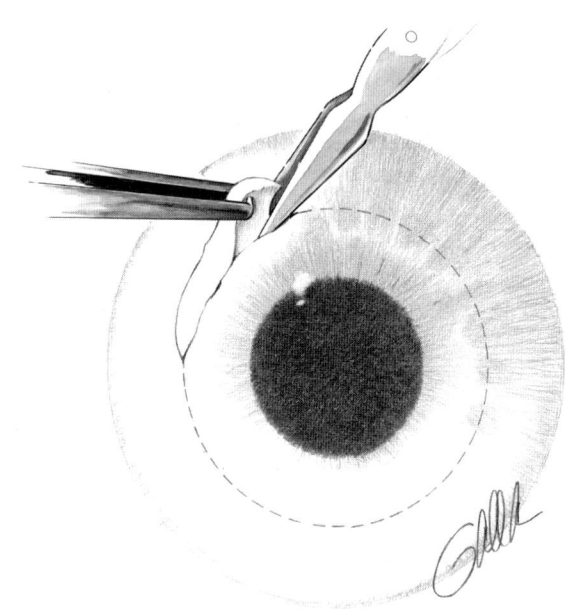

FIGURE 71-3. Wedge resection to steepen a flat meridian.

excessive flattening (Fig. 71-3). Wedge resections are difficult to perform well. If attempted, a diamond knife should be employed because of its sharpness. Even so, the excised wedge is usually irregular, and may be excessive, resulting in excessive steepening and/or induction of irregular astigmatism.

Astigmatic keratometry can be helpful in selected cases. Arcuate incisions are placed just inside the graft-host junction or within the incision. Arcuate incisions peripheral to the graft-host junction have little effect. In addition, the disadvantage of causing distortion of the host rim may lead to ongoing astigmatism difficulties if the patient is subsequently regrafted. Alternatively, instead of using an incisional knife, a surgeon can obtain an effect similar to arcuate keratotomy in the incision by breaking down the scar at the level of Bowman's layer with a blade or with sharp pointed

forceps, and expand the incisional separation down to the level of Descemet's membrane (Fig. 71-4).

The nomograms for arcuate keratotomy can be a guide to the amount of astigmatic change to be expected from an incision in penetrating keratoplasty patients. However, because the graft is frequently under larger tension than the native cornea, a significantly larger correction can occur. Many surgeons use a guide of anticipating a double correction in corneal transplants compared to natural corneas. It is preferable to go back and enhance an undercorrection with expansion of the original incision than to try to reverse an overcorrection with placement of sutures.

Arcuate keratotomies can address some degree of asymmetry in the astigmatism by being placed centered on each of the steep hemimeridians. This may not be exactly 180 degrees apart, such as in a "sagging bowtie" pattern. However, a highly asymmetric cornea is unlikely to respond well to arcuate keratotomy.

Care must also be taken to avoid sequential arcuate keratotomies due to an evolving and shifting pattern of astigmatism. A shift in the position of the steep meridian after an initial arcuate keratotomy often does not respond well to a second, third, and even more sequential arcuate keratotomies. This phenomenon is presumably due to the exaggerated and invisible corneal tension present in a grafted cornea.

LASIK AND PRK

Excimer laser principles, techniques, and outcomes are discussed extensively in other chapters.

A special application of the excimer laser is the treatment of astigmatism in patients who have had previous penetrating keratoplasty.

Several special considerations apply to performing excimer laser treatment of postkeratoplasty astigmatism. Because the laser is capable of correcting spherical error as well as astigmatism, it offers the surgeon the opportunity to address a broader range of refractive error than possible with astigmatic keratotomy.

PRK performed on postkeratoplasty corneas disappointed most surgeons, and no large series was published. Haze and unpredictability were viewed as unacceptable by most surgeons who attempted this technique. More recently, however, anecdotal reports have suggested that the adjunctive use of topical mitomycin C at the completion of PRK may result in a better response to PRK in postkeratoplasty eyes.

LASIK has the potential advantage of avoiding the surface healing response seen with PRK. However, the creation of the LASIK flap after prior penetrating keratoplasty poses several challenges. The cornea must have healed adequately to allow full suture removal, and, even then, the surgeon has the difficult task of assessing whether the keratoplasty wound is adequately healed not only to withstand the elevated intraocular pressure during the creation of the flap, but also to maintain integrity as the LASIK flap is cut. Typically the cornea will have an abrupt topographic shift at the keratoplasty wound, and the LASIK flap edge accordingly tends to be either at the keratoplasty wound or to cut across it. As a result, the healing of the keratoplasty incision at the level of Bowman's membrane will be incorporated in the flap, and will no longer provide wound integrity for the underlying remaining keratoplasty stroma. Many patients have weak healing at the stroma-to-stroma interface, and therefore may lose wound integrity with the LASIK flap cut across Bowman's layer. The surgeon needs to err on the side of caution, therefore, in assessing the appearance of scar formation within the wound and the amount of time that has occurred for wound healing postkeratoplasty. The more edematous the peripheral cornea and the older the patient, the slower this healing process takes place.

In addition, steep corneas are prone to thin flaps and frank buttonhole formation. The surgeon should be mindful of this tendency in assessing a candidate patient preoperatively and selecting the microkeratome head. If the stromal thickness is adequate, the surgeon should select a microkeratome designed to create a relatively thick flap in order to avoid difficulties with an unexpected thin flap.

The creation of the flap alone may impact the optics of the postkeratoplasty cornea. A study by Busin and co-workers (11) examined the impact of creating a hinged flap alone, in the absence of any excimer laser ablation, on nine postkeratoplasty eyes with high astigmatism. They found that a superior hinged corneal flap with an intended thickness of 160 μm and diameter of 9 mm resulted in a mean flattening of 1 D and a mean decrease in astigmatic cylinder of 1.5 D. Most of the effect on the spherical equivalent was

present at 1 day but there was a small ongoing progression through 1 month. No patient lost acuity, and some patients gained between one and four lines of Snellen uncorrected visual acuity. The mean preoperative myopia in these patients was −5.4 D, and thus the flattening would be expected to improve uncorrected acuity through the reduction of the myopia.

Two major studies have examined LASIK for the correction of myopia and astigmatism in postkeratoplasty eyes. Donnenfeld et al. (12) reported on the results of LASIK in 23 eyes of 22 patients who were spectacle or contact lens intolerant after penetrating keratoplasty. In that study, three surgeons performed the procedures and all patients had 12 months of follow-up. All eyes were within 3 D of attempted spherical equivalent, with a tendency toward undercorrection, and the mean cylinder was reduced from 3.64 D preoperatively to 1.29 D at 12 months postoperation. Undercorrection of cylinder occurred in all eyes. Procedures were performed with the Hansatome microkeratome and the VISX Star broad-beam laser. Two patients lost best corrected visual acuity (one line in one patient and three lines in another patient) and 21 of the 23 eyes either maintained or gained best corrected acuity; 21 of the 23 eyes experienced between one and nine lines of improvement in uncorrected visual acuity. Anisometropia was reduced from a preoperative mean of 6.3 D to a postoperative mean of 1.42 D. No LASIK or corneal transplant complications occurred.

A smaller series by Kwitko et al. (13) reported on the results of 14 eyes of 13 patients who were a minimum of 1 year after penetrating keratoplasty and had at least 12 months' follow-up after subsequent LASIK, performed by four surgeons utilizing the Meditec Aesculap MEL 60 laser and the Chiron ACS microkeratome with a 160-μm plate. At 12 months follow-up, their myopic patients improved from a preoperative mean of −5.33 D to a postoperative mean of +0.19 D, and their hyperopic patients improved from an average of +5.04 D to a postoperative refraction of 0.42 D. The correction of the astigmatism was less predictable, with a preoperative mean of 5.37 D reducing to a postoperative mean of 2.82 D. They reported a re-treatment rate of 42.9%, all being performed for undercorrected cylinder. Best spectacle-corrected visual acuity (BSCVA) improved in six eyes and was stable in four eyes. Five eyes lost one line of BSCVA. A flap buttonhole complication occurred in one eye.

Surgical opinion remains divided about whether it is advisable to perform the LASIK flap first and reassess the optics, or whether to perform LASIK treatment immediately after creating the flap, even though the flap itself is documented to result in an optical shift. The surgeon should be aware that relifting a healed LASIK flap is more difficult in the presence of penetrating keratoplasty because the scar reaction where the flap intersects the penetrating keratoplasty incision will be stronger and therefore more

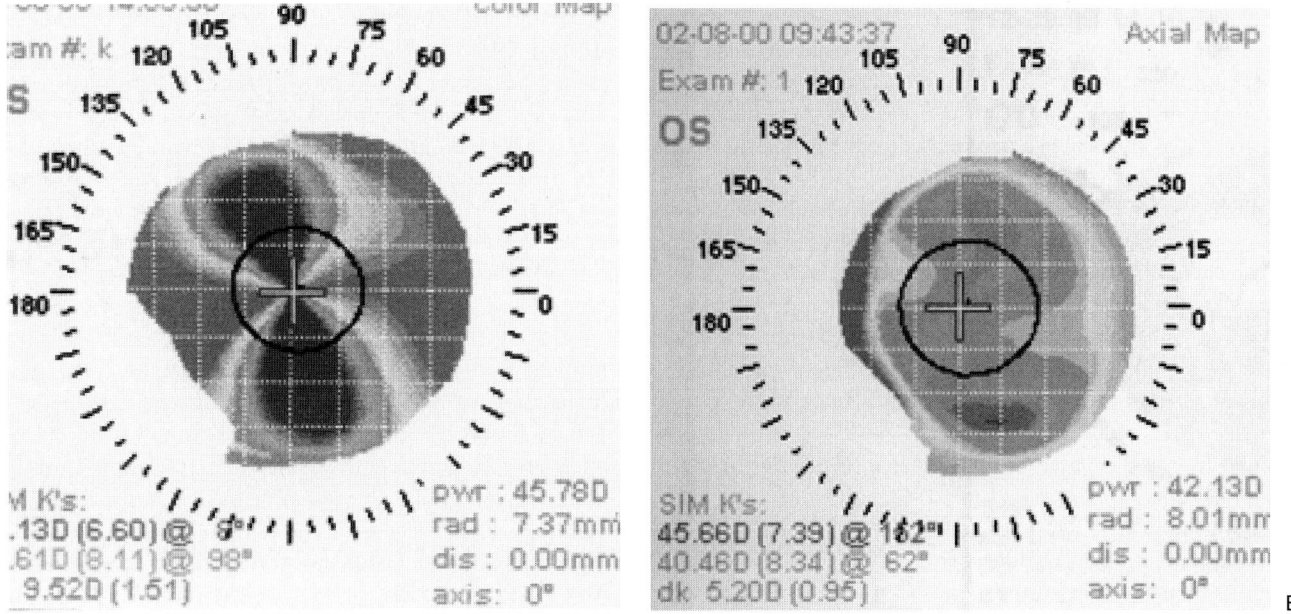

FIGURE 71-5. Case 1. **A:** A high degree of astigmatism is present after keratoplasty with a regular pattern. **B:** After LASIK, a marked reduction in the astigmatism is evident.

difficult to cleanly reopen. In addition, because the refractive results obtained from LASIK are less predictable in penetrating keratoplasty than they are in native eyes, many surgeons accept that a high retreatment rate will be necessary, and do not wish to subject the patient to the potential of three procedures (one to create the flap, one original later LASIK treatment, and a high rate of a third procedure for enhancement).

Irregular astigmatism is a remaining unaddressed challenge in the optical correction of these patients. Current techniques address only the regular component of the astigmatism. The following case studies illustrate this challenge.

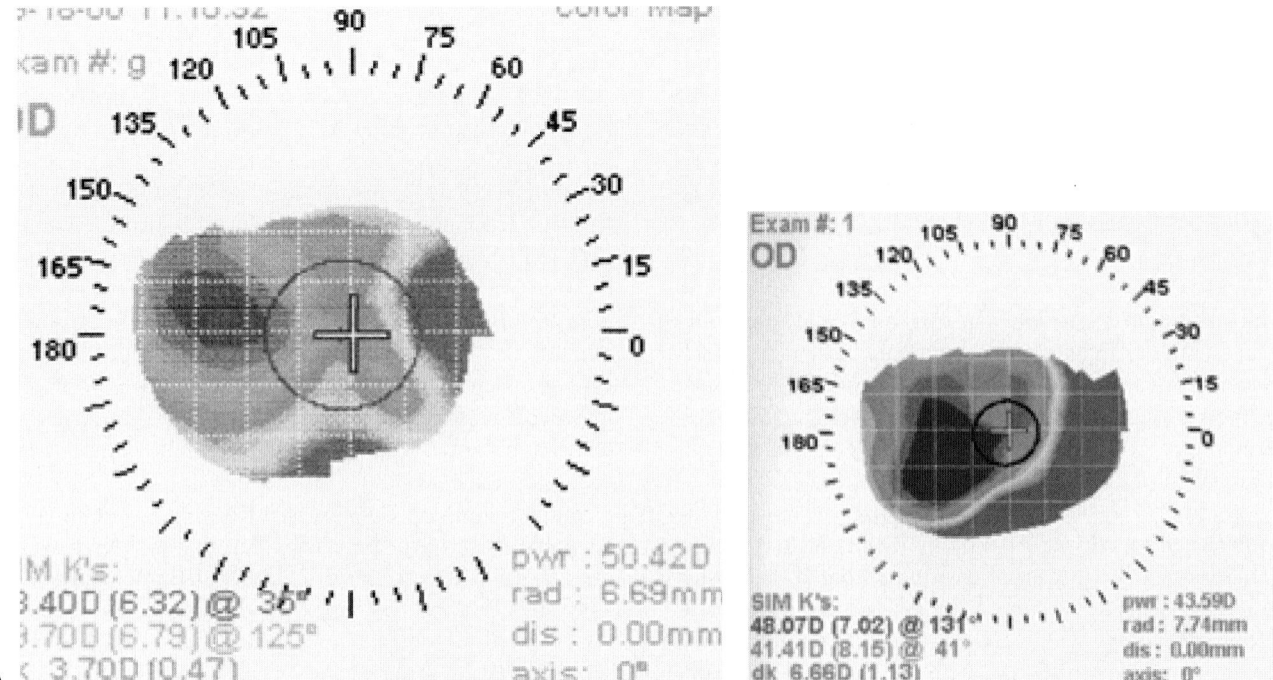

FIGURE 71-6. Case 2. **A:** The astigmatism is highly irregular, with a steep zone visible to the down and right. **B:** After LASIK with a conventional treatment for astigmatism, the total astigmatism is reduced but the pattern remains highly irregular with reduced best-corrected visual acuity.

CASE 1

A 60-year-old man with keratoconus had penetrating keratoplasties performed initially in 1970 accompanied by high astigmatism. The original transplants had high astigmatism, and therefore the patient had a repeat larger penetrating keratoplasty in the left eye in December 1996. Three years later, with all sutures removed, he had a refractive error of +1 − 8 × 120 (Fig. 71-5A). An uncomplicated LASIK procedure was performed and the residual refractive error was −1 − 1.25 × 90 with 20/25 acuity. Figure 71-5B shows the marked improvement in the topographic pattern.

CASE 2

A 68-year-old man experienced corneal edema and cystoid macular edema after cataract surgery with implantation of an anterior chamber intraocular lens. In August 1997 a penetrating keratoplasty accompanied by a vitrectomy and an intraocular lens exchange for a transscleral suture fixated posterior chamber intraocular lens was performed. Three years later, the running suture was removed. The residual refractive error was −2 − 4 × 176, causing both anisometropic symptoms and poor spectacle corrected visual acuity of 20/70, due partially to the longstanding preoperative cystoid macular edema but also due to irregular astigmatism (Fig. 71-6A). A LASIK was performed, with the laser programmed to correct only the 4 D of cylinder, in the anticipation that a hyperopic shift would occur with the creation of the LASIK flap. Despite programming a correction of zero sphere and 4 D of astigmatism, the treatment with the broad beam laser resulted in a postoperative refraction of +3.25 − 2.50 × 140. In addition, the BSCVA remained 20/70, and, as seen from the corneal topography, the difficulty of the irregular astigmatism remains evident postoperatively (Fig. 71-6B).

New technology, particularly with the advent of wavefront-guided ablation, and perhaps in conjunction with topographic-guided ablation, may result in effective therapeutic correction of these challenging cases.

REFERENCES

1. Shiotz LJ. Hin Fall von hochgradigem Hornhautsastigmatismus nach Staarextraction. *Besserung auf operativem Wege Arch Augenheilkd* 1885;15:178.
2. Waring GO III. History of radial keratotomy. In: Sanders DR, Hoffmann RF, Salz JJ, eds. *Refractive corneal surgery.* Thorofare, NJ: Slack, 1985.
3. Lans LJ. Experimentelle Untersuchungen uber Entstehung von Astigmatismus durch nich-perforirende Corneawunden. *Graefes Arch Ophthalmol* 1998;45:117.
4. Duffey RJ, et al. Paired arcuate keratotomy. A surgical approach to mixed and myopic astigmatism. *Arch Ophthalmol* 1988;106:1130.
5. Duffey RJ, Tchah H, Lindstrom, RL. Spoke keratotomy in the human cadaver eye. *J Refract Surg* 1988;4:9.
6. Franks JB, Binder PS. Keratotomy procedures for the correction of astigmatism. *J Refract Surg* 1985;1:11.
7. Lavery GW, Lindstrom RL. Trapezoidal astigmatic keratotomy in human cadaver eyes. *J Refract Surg* 1985;1:18.
8. Lindquist TD, et al. Trapezoidal astigmatic keratectomy: Quantification in human cadaver eyes. *Arch Ophthalmol* 1986;104:1534.
9. Lindstrom RL. The surgical correction of astigmatism: a clinician's perspective. *Refract Corn Surg* 1990;6:441.
10. Alz JJ, et al. Radial keratotomy in fresh human cadaver eyes. *Ophthalmology* 1981;88:472.
11. Busin M, Arffa RC, Zambianchi L, et al. Effect of hinged lamellar keratotomy on post-keratoplasty eyes. *Ophthalmology* 2001;108:1845–1851.
12. Donnenfeld ED, Kornstein HS, Amin A, et al. Laser-in-situ keratomileusis for correction of myopia and astigmatism after penetrating keratoplasty. *Ophthalmology* 1999;106:1966–1975.
13. Kwitko S, Marinho DR, Rymer S, et al. Laser-in-situ keratomileusis after penetrating keratoplasty. *J Cataract Refract Surg* 2001;27:374–379.

72

EPIKERATOPLASTY

MICHAEL D. WAGONER AND ALI A. AL-RAJHI

Epikeratoplasty was originally introduced by Dr. Herbert Kaufman (1) at the Jackson Memorial Lecture at the American Academy of Ophthalmology as an extension of the pioneering work of Joaquin Barraquer (2) in the development of keratophakia for aphakia and keratomileusis for myopia. Both of the Barraquer procedures require dissection and removal of a portion of the central cornea, technically challenging cryolathing, and expensive equipment (2). Epikeratoplasty is performed by suturing a commercially cryolathed corneal "lenticule" with specific dioptric power onto de-epithelialized central cornea without disturbance of the anterior stroma (3,4). It provides the refractive benefits of the Barraquer procedures, but with less technical complexity, cost, and risk of central corneal scarring.

Epikeratoplasty was originally introduced for contact lens intolerant, monocularly aphakic adults, in whom secondary intraocular lens implantation was contraindicated (1). The indications were later expanded to include the correction of keratoconus (5,6), pediatric aphakia (7,8), adult aphakia (9–12), and myopia (13). Between 1985 and 1988 a nationwide study involving 234 ophthalmologists was conducted to evaluate prospectively the safety and efficacy of epikeratoplasty for each of these indications (13–17).

SURGICAL TECHNIQUE

Epikeratoplasty lenticules are prepared from corneal tissue that meet the criteria of the Eye Bank Association of America for transplantation, but do not qualify for use for penetrating keratoplasty due to factors such as poor endothelial cell counts, long death-to-preservation times, or excessive length of storage. The tissue is treated with a water-soluble green dye to aid in visualization and cryolathed to a specific dioptric power based on the patient's spherical equivalent corrected to the corneal plane (with the exception of keratoconus, which was lathed to plano power). It may then be placed in standard corneal storage media or lyophilized prior to shipment to the operating surgeon. The lenticules are processed under environmental conditions similar to other donor corneal tissue and are not sterile. They may be obtained from Cryo-Optics (Houston, TX) or the Keratec Eye Bank (St. George's Hospital Medical School, London, UK).

Epikeratoplasty may be performed with general anesthesia, retrobulbar or peribulbar anesthesia, or topical anesthesia (in extremely cooperative adults). The central corneal epithelium is debrided at least l to 1.5 mm beyond the edge of the anticipated trephination with a dull spatula, facilitated by topically applied 4% cocaine, if necessary. The use of topical alcohol should be avoided because it may contribute to poor postoperative epithelial healing, especially if limbal stem cells are damaged. All epithelia should be removed from the surgical field and fornices to prevent accidental retention of epithelial nests in the interface during lenticular suturing.

After epithelial removal, a Hessburg-Barron trephine is centered on the visual axis, and trephination is performed approximately 200 to 225 μm into the corneal stroma. A 7-mm trephine is used for aphakia and myopia, and an 8.5-mm trephine is used for keratoconus. For eyes with aphakia or myopia a 1-mm lamellar "pocket" is dissected from the base of the trephination into peripheral cornea. No lamellar dissection is required for eyes with keratoconus. Many surgeons perform an annular keratectomy of approximately 0.5 mm in diameter on the inner aspect of the trephine incision, although this is not mandatory.

Nonlyophilized tissue that has been stored in standard corneal storage media containing antibiotics may be transferred directly to the recipient eye. Lyophilized tissue is rehydrated in balanced salt solution to which an appropriate antibiotic, such as gentamicin, has been added for at least 20 minutes before use. A "refractively neutral" suture technique is used to suture an 8.5-mm donor lenticule in eyes with myopia (13) and aphakia (15–17). A 10-0 nylon needle is passed through the 130-μm thick wing of the lenticule and then into the apex of the peripheral lamellar dissection pocket. The sutures are loosely tied to avoid excessive tension on the graft and minimize risk of undercorrection of myopia and overcorrection of aphakia. Although several different sutures techniques have been tried, the use of 16 interrupted 10-0 nylon sutures has become the preferred technique. Some surgeons advocated a "no-stitch" technique

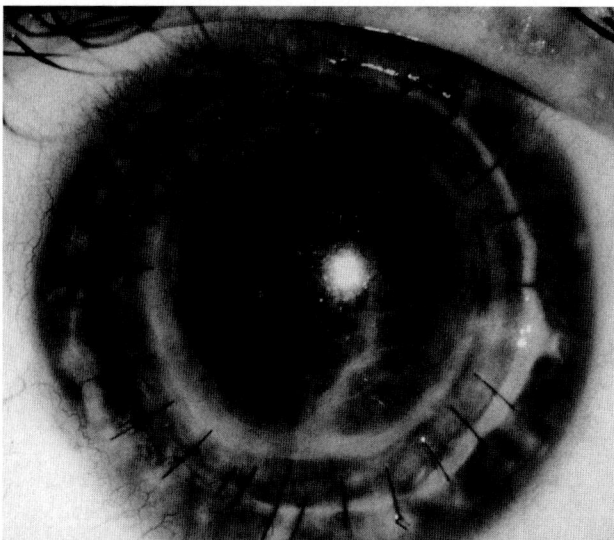

FIGURE 72-1. Epikeratoplasty for keratoconus, 1 day postoperative. Twenty-four tight 10-0 nylon sutures have been used to maximize corneal flattening, as demonstrated by the marked folds in Descemet's membrane.

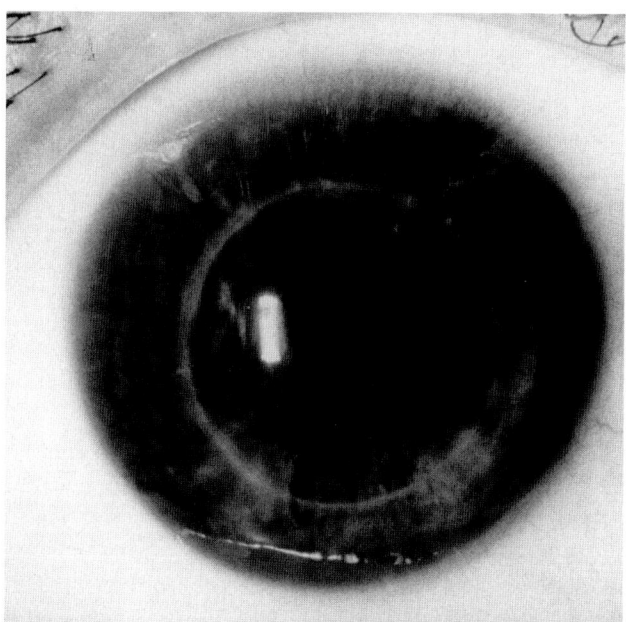

FIGURE 72-2. Epikeratoplasty for keratoconus, 2 year postoperatively. Excellent flattening of the cone has been achieved and maintained, with excellent interface clarity. The folds in Descemet's membrane have completely disappeared.

for myopic and aphakic epikeratoplasty (18), but this did not gain popular acceptance.

A "corneal flattening" suture technique is used to tightly suture a 9-mm, plano donor lenticule of approximately 0.3 mm thickness in eyes with keratoconus (14). A total of 16 or 24 sutures interrupted 10-0 nylon sutures are placed, using edge-to-edge approximation. To obtain maximum flattening of the cone, some surgeons utilize a 9-0 silk suture for the four cardinal sutures and replace them with 10-0 nylon sutures at the conclusion of the case. These sutures are tied as securely as possible while the assistant flattens the cone with a flat spatula. Folds should be present in Descemet's membrane at the conclusion of the procedure, indicating that the cone has been flattened significantly (Fig. 72-1). They vanish after suture removal (Fig. 72-2).

POSTOPERATIVE MANAGEMENT

The success of epikeratoplasty is highly dependent on facilitating prompt reepithelialization of the lenticule, especially when lyophilized tissue is used. Despite the use of pressure patching or soft contact lens therapy, epithelial defects persisting more than 2 weeks are not uncommon after epikeratoplasty. In 405 cases of epikeratoplasty performed at the King Khaled Eye Specialist Hospital (KKESH) between 1987 and 1997, persistent epithelial defects occurred in 4 (2.5%) of 161 eyes with keratoconus, 5 (4.1%) of 123 children with aphakia, and 6 (5%) of 121 adults with aphakia. A study from the Massachusetts Eye and Ear Infirmary demonstrated that placement of a temporary tarsorrhaphy at the conclusion of the surgical procedure reduced the

mean time of reepithelialization to 4.61 days, compared to 8.03 days with pressure patching ($p < .01$) and 13.2 days with bandage soft contact lenses ($p < .005$) (19). Because delayed reepithelialization of 2 weeks or longer is often associated with irreversible loss of lenticular clarity, prophylactic placement of a temporary suture tarsorrhaphy at the conclusion of every epikeratoplasty procedure has now become routine practice.

Removal of the epikeratoplasty lenticule is occasionally necessary in the early postoperative period (13–17,20–29). Graft removal is highly recommended when delayed reepithelialization results in loss of graft clarity and a poor visual result. In almost every case, lenticule removal under these circumstances is associated with complete reversal of the original status of the recipient cornea. Graft removal is mandatory when delayed reepithelialization is associated with sterile ulceration or secondary microbial keratitis, which may extend into the recipient cornea and produce permanent scarring (24–27).

Fortunately, secondary microbial keratitis is rare with an overall incidence of 1.5% in children (15) and less than 1% in adults (22). Only 2 (0.5%) of the 405 eyes in the KKESH series developed secondary microbial keratitis and only 1 (0.2%) eye developed sterile corneal ulceration (27).

All sutures are removed 2 to 3 weeks after epikeratoplasty for pediatric aphakia (15,16) and at 8 weeks for myopia (13) and adult aphakia (17). Suture removal was originally recommended at 3 months after epikeratoplasty for keratoconus (14). It is now known that better results are obtained when suture removal is delayed for at least 6 months (20–22).

Topical corticosteroids are recommended in eyes with keratoconus to prevent premature suture vascularization and loosening, thereby reducing the desired objective of flattening the cone and reducing irregular astigmatism.

Edema may persist in the lenticle for a period of time that is proportional to the health of the recipient endothelium. Graft edema usually resolves sufficiently in children to permit initiation of occlusive and optical therapy within 1 month of surgery (15,16). Many aphakic adult patients require 3 to 6 months to reach preoperative levels of best corrected visual acuity. Full resolution of graft edema may be delayed for 6 to 12 months in some elderly patients (17,20).

Late lenticular removal may be necessary if there is an unsatisfactory visual result due to insufficient lenticular clarity or an unacceptable refractive outcome. The highest rates of removal of epikeratoplasty lenticles for loss of clarity are in children under the age of 8 where approximately 10% of lenticles were removed in the nationwide study (15) and 8% were removed in the large series from KKESH. These results contrast sharply with the nationwide study of epikeratoplasty in older children where no lenticles were removed from 65 eyes (16) and the KKESH series where only 1 (1.6%) lenticle was removed. The overall rate of removal of lenticles for keratoconus is approximately 5%, with an equal distribution between those removed for loss of graft clarity related to delayed reepithelialization and those removed for unsatisfactory refractive outcome (14,20–22). The highest rate of removal was for eyes with myopia where refractive regression, proportional to the original degree of myopia, occurred during the first year after suture removal. Some series have reported removal rates of more than 50% in eyes with moderate and high myopia (13,20).

RESULTS

Keratoconus

When epikeratoplasty was introduced, there was optimism that epikeratoplasty would provide visual results comparable to penetrating keratoplasty but offer the advantages of lamellar keratoplasty. Unfortunately, the initial nationwide study and subsequent studies have not completely met these expectations (14,21–23,31–33).

The nationwide study of epikeratoplasty for keratoconus reported the results of 82 patients in whom more than 30 days of follow-up was available following suture removal (14). Uncorrected visual acuity improved in all but two patients. Whereas only 9% of eyes had an uncorrected visual acuity of 20/100 or better preoperatively, 64% had an uncorrected visual acuity of 20/100 or better postoperatively. All but two patients achieved a best corrected visual acuity within one line of the preoperative best corrected contact lens visual acuity. In most cases, the reduction in

irregular astigmatism allowed this outcome to be achieved with spectacle correction. For patients who chose to continue contact lens wearing, the flattening of the cone permitted more satisfactory fitting, comfort, and wearing time.

The largest comparative study came from Saudi Arabia where 161 eyes with keratoconus treated with epikeratoplasty at KKESH were compared to 443 eyes treated contemporaneously with penetrating keratoplasty at the same institution by the same surgeons (22). A minimum of 24 months of follow-up was available on every case, with a mean follow-up period of 54 months for epikeratoplasty and 52 months for penetrating keratoplasty. Among patients who chose either spectacle or contact lens rehabilitation, the median visual acuity was 20/50 for 77 eyes treated with epikeratoplasty compared to 20/40 for 209 eyes treated with penetrating keratoplasty ($p = .0003$). Among patients who did not choose to use optical correction postoperatively, the median visual acuity was 20/60 in 84 eyes treated with epikeratoplasty and 234 eyes treated with penetrating keratoplasty.

Several other studies have compared the results with epikeratoplasty and penetrating keratoplasty. Frontiere and Portesani (30) reported similar mean uncorrected visual acuity (20/63 vs. 20/52), spectacle corrected visual acuity (20/23 vs. 20/22), and contact lens corrected visual acuity (20/21 vs. 20/20) in a comparison with epikeratoplasty and penetrating keratoplasty, respectively. Steinert and Wagoner (21) reported a mean best corrected spectacle acuity of 20/32 vs. 20/27 after 2 years with epikeratoplasty and penetrating keratoplasty, respectively, although no eyes with epikeratoplasty achieved 20/20 acuity. Goosey et al. (31) observed that although 93% of eyes achieve best corrected acuity of 20/40 or better after either epikeratoplasty or penetrating keratoplasty, only 23% with epikeratoplasty obtained 20/20 vision, compared to 73% with penetrating keratoplasty. Contrast sensitivity is reduced with or without glare after epikeratoplasty when compared with both rigid gas permeable hard contract lenses or penetrating keratoplasty (32).

The Food and Drug Administration (FDA) approved epikeratoplasty for clinical use in keratoconus in the United States. There has been limited enthusiasm about using this procedure as an alternative to penetrating keratoplasty because of the poorer visual results and reduced contrast sensitivity. Epikeratoplasty may be still considered as a reasonable alternative to penetrating keratoplasty, however, there are concerns about postoperative patient compliance. The large series of patients treated at KKESH was generated, in part, because of logistic concerns about the ability of many of the patients to have access to prompt intervention for graft related complications due to long distances required to travel to the surgical center. Only two (1.2%) of the eyes in this series required subsequent penetrating keratoplasty. Epikeratoplasty should also be considered as an option if there are concerns about self-induced trauma from rubbing (e.g., Down syndrome) or external trauma related to professional or athletic activities, especially if the alternative is withholding surgical therapy.

Epikeratoplasty may be performed as part of a "staged" procedure in the treatment of keratoglobus, pellucid marginal degeneration, or other peripheral thinning disorders (34–36). Large custom-made lenticules, approximately 0.3 mm in thickness, may be ordered and used to reinforce the entire cornea in the first stage. If the postoperative improvement in corneal contour affords acceptable visual acuity with spectacles or contact lens, no additional therapy is needed. If the visual acuity remains inadequate, a standard size, central penetrating keratoplasty can be performed to complete visual rehabilitation. There is no evidence that previous epikeratoplasty compromises the result of subsequent penetrating keratoplasty.

Pediatric Aphakia

Epikeratoplasty was introduced as a means of aphakic rehabilitation of children in an era when primary and secondary intraocular lens placement was seldom performed. In the nationwide study for epikeratoplasty for pediatric aphakia for children under the age of 8 years, 89% of eyes maintained a clear lenticule and 73% were within three diopters of emmetropia, thereby facilitating subsequent optical correction and amblyopia therapy (15). The major shortcoming of the study was a lack of visual data in a substantial proportion of the patients, many of whom were preverbal at the time of the surgery and many of whom were and remained densely amblyopic. Nonetheless, the procedure did offer an acceptable alternative to abandoning amblyopia therapy altogether due to noncompliance with the other available alternatives.

In the nationwide study of epikeratoplasty for pediatric aphakia in children over the age of 8 years, 100% of eyes maintained a clear lenticule and 73% of eyes were within 3 diopters of emmetropia (16). Eyes with congenital cataracts gained an average of one line of best corrected visual acuity, whereas eyes with traumatic cataracts lost an average of one line of best corrected visual acuity.

The FDA approved epikeratoplasty for clinical use in children in the U.S. Since that time, the near-universal placement of primary intraocular lenses at the time of cataract surgery (37), as well as excellent safety record of secondary intraocular lenses in children (38), has largely eliminated the need for pediatric aphakic epikeratoplasty. Posterior chamber intraocular lens placement is associated with more rapid visual rehabilitation, better visual acuity, and superior refractive accuracy than epikeratoplasty (15,16,37,38). Epikeratoplasty should be offered only in the rare situation when intraocular lens insertion is contraindicated and optical noncompliance compromises amblyopia therapy.

Adult Aphakia

Epikeratoplasty was introduced as a means of rehabilitation of adult aphakia in an era when primary and secondary intraocular lens implantation was not universally practiced (1). In the nationwide study of epikeratoplasty for adult aphakia, 95% of eyes had a postoperative improvement in uncorrected visual acuity, 78% had a postoperative best corrected visual acuity within two lines of the best preoperative corrected visual acuity, and 75% were within 3 D of emmetropia (17). In the KKESH series of 121 adult eyes with aphakia, visual acuity of 20/40 or better was obtained in 55%, 20/50 to 20/100 was obtained in 37%, and worse than 20/100 was obtained in 8%. Visual rehabilitation was often slow due to delayed clearing of graft edema, especially in elderly patients (17,20). Patients under the age of 70 were much more likely to achieve best corrected visual acuity within two lines of preoperative best corrected visual acuity than those over the age of 70 (98% vs. 54%, respectively). Contrast sensitivity is significantly decreased in eyes rehabilitated with aphakic epikeratoplasty compared to the use of either intraocular or contact lenses (39).

The FDA approved aphakic epikeratoplasty for clinical use in aphakic adults in the U.S. The near-universal placement of primary intraocular lenses at the time of cataract surgery, as well as excellent safety record of secondary intraocular lenses (40), has largely eliminated the demand for aphakic epikeratoplasty. Secondary intraocular lens placement with anterior chamber, iris-sutured posterior chamber, or scleral-sutured posterior chamber intraocular lenses is associated with more rapid visual rehabilitation, better visual acuity, better contrast sensitivity, and superior refractive accuracy than epikeratoplasty (17,20,39,40). Epikeratoplasty may still be offered in the rare situation when intraocular lens insertion is contraindicated.

Myopia

Initial optimism regarding refractive predictability and stability of myopic epikeratoplasty was short-lived (13,20). In the nationwide study of epikeratoplasty for myopia, only 33% of treated eyes achieved uncorrected visual acuity of 20/40 or better, whereas 31% were 20/200 or worse (14). Many patients experienced significant loss of refractive correction during the first postoperative year (13,20). There was a direct correlation between the amount of attempted correction and the amount of regression (13), with many patients experiencing the loss of 50% to 100% of the attempted correction (20). The results of surgical modification of myopic undercorrection or regression with epithelial debridement (41), retrephination of the groove at the graft-host junction (42), and excimer laser photorefractive keratectomy (43) were disappointing. Contrast sensitivity, in the presence and absence of a glare source, is worse after myopic epikeratoplasty than it is after with spectacles, contact lenses, or radial keratotomy (44). In response to these poor results, the FDA did not approve myopic epikeratoplasty for clinical use in the U.S. There is no currently accepted indication for myopic epikeratoplasty.

REFERENCES

1. Kaufman HE. The correction of aphakia. *Am J Ophthalmol* 1980;89:1–10.
2. Barraquer JI. Keratomileusis and keratophakia. In: Rycroft PV, ed. *Corneoplastic surgery: Proceedings of the 2nd International Cornea-Plastic Conference.* New York: Pergamon, l969.
3. McDonald MB. Onlay lamellar keratoplasty. In: Kaufman HE, Barron BA, McDonald MB, et al. *The cornea.* New York: Churchill Livingstone, l988:697–711.
4. McDonald MB, Morgan KS. Epikeratophakia for aphakia and myopia. In: Kaufman HE, Barron BA, McDonald MB, et al. *The cornea.* New York: Churchill Livingstone, l988:823–847.
5. Kaufman HE, Werblin TP. Epikeratophakia for the treatment of keratoconus. *Am J Ophthalmol* 1982;93:342–347.
6. McDonald MB, Koenig SB, Safir A, et al. Onlay lamellar keratoplasty for the treatment of keratoconus. *Br J Ophthalmol* 1983;67: 615–618.
7. Morgan KS, Werblin TP, Asbell PA, et al. The use of epikeratophakia grafts in pediatric monocular aphakia. *J Pediatr Ophthalmol Strabismus* 1981;18: 23–29.
8. Morgan KS, Asbell PA, McDonald MB, et al. Preliminary visual results of pediatric epikeratophakia. *Arch Ophthalmol* 1983;101: 1540–1544.
9. McDonald MB, Koenig SB, Safir A, et al. Epikeratophakia: the surgical correction of aphakia. Update l982. *Ophthalmology* 1983;90: 668–672.
10. Werblin TP, Kaufman HE, Friedlander MH, et al. A prospective study of the use of hyperopic epikeratophakia grafts for the correction of aphakia in adults. *Ophthalmology* 1981;88:1137–1140.
11. Werblin TP, Kaufman HE, Friedlander MH, et al. Epikeratophakia: the surgical correction of aphakia. III. Preliminary results of a prospective clinical trial. *Arch Ophthalmol* 1981;99: 1957–1960.
12. Werblin TP, Kaufman HE, Friedlander MH, et al. Epikeratophakia: the surgical correction of aphakia. Update l981. *Ophthalmology* 1982;89:916–920.
13. McDonald MB, Kaufman HE, Aquavella JV. The nationwide study of epikeratophakia for myopia. *Am J Ophthalmol* 1987;103: 375–383.
14. McDonald MB, Kaufman HE, Durrie DS, et al. Epikeratophakia for keratoconus: the nationwide study. *Arch Ophthalmol* 1986;104: 1294–1300.
15. Morgan KS, McDonald MB, Hiles DA, et al. The nationwide study of epikeratophakia for aphakia in children. *Am J Ophthalmol* 1987;103:366–374.
16. Morgan KS, McDonald MB, Hiles DA, et al. The nationwide study of epikeratophakia for aphakia in older children. *Ophthalmology* 1988;95:526–531.
17. McDonald MB, Kaufman HE, Aquavella JV, et al. The nationwide study of epikeratophakia for aphakia in adults. *Am J Ophthalmol* 1987;103:358–365.
18. Cotter JB. No-suture aphakic epikeratoplasty. *Refract Corneal Surg* 1992;8:27–32.
19. Wagoner MD, Steinert RF. Temporary tarsorrhaphy enhances re-epithelialization following epikeratoplasty. *Arch Ophthalmol* 1988;106:13–14.
20. Wagoner MD, Steinert RF. Epikeratoplasty for adult and pediatric aphakia myopia, and keratoconus: the Massachusetts Eye and Ear Infirmary experience. *Acta Ophthalmol* 1989;67(suppl 192): 38–45.
21. Steinert RF, Wagoner MD. Long term comparison of epikeratoplasty and penetrating keratoplasty for keratoconus. *Arch Ophthalmol* 1988;106:493–496.
22. Wagoner MD, Smith SD, Rademaker WJ, et al. Penetrating keratoplasty vs. epikeratoplasty for the surgical treatment of keratoconus. *J Refract Surg* 2001;17:138–146.
23. Fronterre A, Portesani GP. Epikeratoplasty for keratoconus. Report of 40 cases. *Cornea* 1989;8:236–239.
24. Bechara SJ, Grossniklaus HE, Waring GO. Sterile stromal melt of epikeratoplasty lenticule. *Arch Ophthalmol* 1992;110:1528–1529.
25. Frangieh GT, Kenyon KR, Wagoner MD, et al. Epithelial abnormalities and sterile stromal ulceration in epikeratoplasty grafts. *Ophthalmology* 1988;95:213–227.
26. Price FW, Binder PS. Scarring of a recipient cornea following epikeratoplasty. *Arch Ophthalmol* 1987;105:1556–1560.
27. Teichmann KT, Wagoner MD. Mooren ulcer after epikeratoplasty for keratoconus. *Arch Ophthalmol* 1998;116:1381–1382.
28. Hemady RK, Bajart AM, Wagoner MD. Interface abscess after epikeratoplasty. *Am J Ophthalmology* 1990;109:735–736.
29. Al-Rajhi AA, Al-Kharashi S. Epithelial inclusion cysts following epikeratoplasty. *J Refract Cataract Surg* 1996;12:515–518.
30. Fronterre A, Portesani GP. Comparison of epikeratoplasty and penetrating keratoplasty for keratoconus. *Refract Corneal Surg* 1991;7:167–173.
31. Goosey JD, Prager TC, Goosey CB, et al. A comparison of penetrating keratoplasty to epikeratoplasty in the management of keratoconus. *Am J Ophthalmol* 1991;111:145–151.
32. Carney LG, Lembach RG. Management of keratoconus: comparative visual assessment. *CLAO J* 1991;17:52–58.
33. Kirkness CM, Ficker LA, Steele AD, et al. The success of penetrating keratoplasty for keratoconus. *Eye* 1990;4:673–688.
34. Cameron JA. Epikeratoplasty for keratoglobus associated with blue sclera. *Ophthalmology* 1991;98:446–452.
35. Cameron JA. Keratoglobus. *Cornea* 1993;12:124–130.
36. Fronterre A, Portesani GP. Epikeratoplasty for pellucid marginal degeneration. *Cornea* 1991;10:450–453.
37. Zwaan J, Mullaney PB, Awad A, et al. Pediatric intraocular lens implantation. *Ophthalmology* 1998;105:112–118.
38. Awad AH, Mullaney PB, Al-Hamad A, et al. Secondary posterior chamber intraocular lens implantation in children. *J AAPOS* 1998;2:269–273.
39. Carney LG, Kelley CG. Visual performance after aphakic epikeratoplasty. *Curr Eye Res* 1991;10:939–945.
40. Wagoner MD, Cox TA, Ariyasu RG, et al. Intraocular lens implantation in the absence of capsular support. *Ophthalmology* 2003; 110:840–859.
41. Suarez E, Arffa RC, Salmeron B, et al. Efficacy of surgical modifications in myopic epikeratophakia. *J Refract Surg* 1985;l:156.
42. Choi YS, Choi SK. Trephination with a vacuum trephine in undercorrection of myopic epikeratoplasty. *Korean J Ophthalmol* 1993;7:16–19.
43. Colin J, Sangiuolo B, Malet F, et al. Photorefractive keratectomy following undercorrected myopic epikeratoplasties. *J Fr Ophthalmol* 1992;15:384–388.
44. Carney LG, Kelley CG. Visual losses after myopic epikeratoplasty. *Arch Ophthalmol* 1991;109:499–502.

KERATOMILEUSIS AND AUTOMATED LAMELLAR KERATOPLASTY

STEPHEN U. STECHSCHULTE AND
JOHN F. DOANE

The concept of lamellar refractive corneal surgery, or keratomileusis, originated with J. I. Barraquer (1,2) in 1949. Using a manual keratome (Fig. 73-1) he created a thin, free cap of corneal tissue that could be reshaped to alter its curvature and refraction. The cap was frozen and the underside was lathed to predictably flatten the curvature before replacing the cap on the stromal bed (Fig. 73-2). In Barraquer's (3) hands, results of keratomileusis with a cryolathe were encouraging; however, the technique was complex and the equipment was costly to maintain.

A consistent and accurate manual free cap keratectomy is dependent on the speed at which the keratome passes over the eye. Moving too quickly results in an uneven and thin cap, whereas too slow of a pass creates an abnormally thick flap. Corneal cap irregularities can translate into irregular astigmatism and loss of acuity (4). Similarly, any irregularity in the lathing process can result in irregular astigmatism and loss of best corrected visual acuity. Additionally, the cryolathe was a very difficult instrument to maintain and master. The lack of consistent results with the manual keratome coupled with the complexities of the cryolathe led to a decline in popularity of keratomileusis and stalled its widespread adoption.

Although keratomileusis as conceived by Barraquer never gained popularity, his vision inspired the continuing evolution of lamellar refractive surgery. Krawawicz (5) and Pureskin (6) described a central stromal keratectomy, keratomileusis *in situ,* where tissue was removed from the corneal bed after a free cap had been created. Ruiz, working in Bogota, developed a microkeratome with gears that automatically advanced the microkeratome across a geared-track. This automation and the adjustable height suction ring made an automated lamellar keratoplasty technique possible. The motorized advancement of the microkeratome at a constant velocity created a predictably thick corneal cap, a predictable depth lamellar keratectomy, and a smoother corneal stromal bed. This instrumentation breakthrough made lamellar corneal surgery appealing to a larger number of surgeons.

SURGICAL TECHNIQUE: AUTOMATED LAMELLAR KERATOPLASTY FOR MYOPIA (ALK-M)

Automated lamellar keratoplasty (ALK) is done in an outpatient setting under topical anesthesia. As with all refractive surgery, extensive patient education and counseling is required. The patient must have an adequate knowledge of the procedure and its risks, and realistic expectations. Oral sedation may be used but is not mandatory. Prior to prepping and draping the patient the conjunctival cul-de-sacs are irrigated to remove debris and eyelid glandular secretions. It is important during the draping to create a clear path for microkeratome passage. The patient is instructed to look at the microscope light and an inked marker is used to delineate the optical center, a pararadial line for orientation of the flap and a 9-mm optical zone circle to center the circular suction ring. A spacer device, or depth plate, is placed in the microkeratome to determine the thickness of the cut. The first keratectomy in the current ALK technique is typically suggested to have a 160-μm depth plate. An adjustable suction ring is placed on the eye and engaged. The suction ring fixates the globe, provides a geared path for the microkeratome, and raises the intraocular pressure so that a smooth keratectomy may be obtained. A stopper device is often used to ensure the creation of a hinge in the corneal flap. Just prior to passage of the microkeratome the intraocular pressure is checked to make certain it is greater than 65 mm Hg with a hand-held Barraquer tonometer or a pneumotonometer. After the first cut, which has a planned diameter of 7.5 to 8 mm, the suction ring is removed. The adjustable suction ring is reset to resect a 4.2-mm-diameter piece of stromal tissue. A second depth plate is placed, which corresponds to the planned myopic correction. The suction ring is then replaced and a

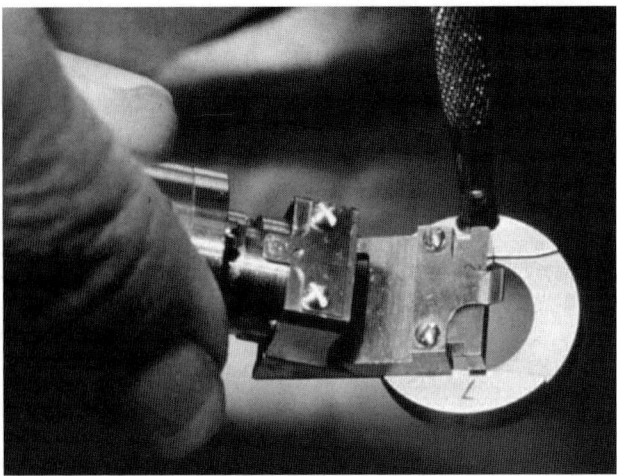

FIGURE 73-1. Manual keratome as used by J. I. Barraquer.

second cut is made after checking the diameter and the intraocular pressure. The flap is then replaced and positioned, usually without sutures. The patient's eye is not patched, and the patient is released from the clinic on antibiotic drops. The eye is examined the next day.

SURGICAL TECHNIQUE: AUTOMATED LAMELLAR KERATOPLASTY FOR HYPEROPIA (ALK-H)

The treatment of hyperopia with ALK is an ectasia procedure and may be used to treat up to 6.5 diopters of intended correction. A thick flap is cut allowing the basal stromal bed of cornea to bow forward and increase the central corneal diopteric power. Typically, this single cut must be at least 60% to 70% of corneal thickness. The effect is graded by altering the diameter of the keratectomy. The same complications such as centration, epithelium in the interface, and displaced caps may occur. Hyperopic ALK has also been used in the treatment of consecutive hyperopia

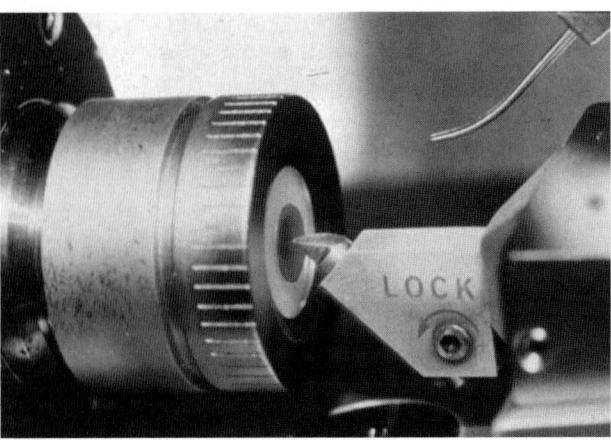

FIGURE 73-2. Cryolathe engaging frozen corneal cap.

after RK. This should be approached with considerable caution. An operation that induces ectasia can result in a keratoconus-like condition.

RESULTS

Manual Myopic Keratomileusis *In Situ*

Despite a long manual history of lamellar surgery, few published data exist for myopic keratomileusis *in situ*. In the available reports that do exist refractive results appear to be improving. In 1991, Bas and Nano (7) reported on the first large series of myopic keratomileusis *in situ* and experienced the unpredictable nature of the technique as previously reported by Barraquer 20 years earlier. Arenas-Archila et al. (8) reported that keratomileusis *in situ* with manual keratomes as not being technically safe, precise, or predictable.

Automated Lamellar Myopic Keratoplasty (ALK-M) for Myopia

Between 1995 and 1996 several groups reported their results with ALK (9-11). In general the results showed a moderate degree of accuracy with standard deviation for the procedure between one and two diopters. Irregular astigmatism was a significant problem, and several incidents of epithelial ingrowth were also noted. Mastering the technical difficulties of the procedure was anecdotally reported to create a significant learning curve for the novice lamellar corneal surgeon.

Automated Lamellar Keratoplasty for Hyperopia (ALK-H)

Between 1995 and 1996 at least three groups of authors reported results for the ALK for hyperopia technique (12-14). Accuracy of about plus or minus one diopter was reported. In one study (13), applanation lens diameter and resection depth accounted for 54% of the variability in outcome. Inaccuracies in the nomogram were also reported as a significant problem (14). Ghiselli et al. (13) reported a mean undercorrection of 1.26 ± 0.91 diopters at 3 months postoperatively, whereas Manche et al. (14) reported a mean undercorrection of 1.4 ± 0.8 diopters 6 months postoperatively. Longer-term studies and the incidence of progressive ectasia are not available.

Neither manual keratomileusis nor ALK constitutes a significant percentage of cases in a modern refractive surgery practice. Shortcomings of ALK, specifically the relatively wide predictability range for myopic ALK, prompted researchers to substitute lasers for the keratome in the refractive correction step of the myopic ALK procedure (16–18). This change led to the development of laser-assisted *in situ* keratomileusis (LASIK) (15). LASIK, the topic of the following chapter, remains, in 2004, the primary modality of refractive surgery.

REFERENCES

1. Barraquer JI. Oueratoplastia refractiva. *Estudios Inform Oftal Inst Barraquer* 1949;10:2–21.
2. Barraquer JI. Keratomileusis. *Int Surg* 1967;48:103–117.
3. Barraquer JI. Results of myopic keratomileusis. *J Refract Surg* 1987;3:98–101.
4. Maguire LJ, Klyce SD, Sawelson H, et al. Visual distortion after myopic keratomileusis: computer analysis of keratoscope photographs. *Ophthalmic Surg* 1987;18:352–356.
5. Krwawicz T. Lamellar corneal stromectomy. *Am J Ophthalmol* 1964;57:828–833.
6. Pureskin N. Weakening ocular refraction by means of partial stromectomy of cornea under experimental conditions. *Vestnik Oftalmologii* 1967;80:19–24.
7. Bas AM, Nano HD Jr. In situ myopic keratomileusis results in 30 eyes at 15 months. *Refract Corneal Surg* 1991;7:223–231.
8. Arenas-Archila E, Sanchez-Thorin JC, Naranjo-Uribe JP, et al. Myopic keratomileusis *in situ*: a preliminary report. *J Cataract Refract Surg* 1991;17:424–435.
9. Lyle WA, Jin GJC. Initial results of automated lamellar keratoplasty for correction of myopia: one year follow-up. *J Cataract Refract Surg* 1996;22:31–43.
10. Manche EE, Elkins B, Maloney R. Keratomileusis *in situ* (ALK) for high myopia. Abstract, International Society of Refractive Surgery Annual Meeting, Atlanta, October 27, 1995.
11. Price FW, Whitson WE, Gonzales JS, et al. Automated lamellar keratomileusis *in situ* for myopia. *J Refract Surg* 1996;12:29–35.
12. Kezirian GM, Germillion CM. Automated lamellar keratoplasty for the correction of hyperopia. *J Cataract Refract Surg* 1995;21:386–392.
13. Ghiselli G, Manche E, Maloney R. Factors that influence the outcome of hyperopic automated lamellar keratoplasty. Abstract, International Society of Refractive Surgery Annual Meeting, Atlanta, October 27, 1995.
14. Manche EE, Judge A, Maloney RK. Lamellar keratoplasty for hyperopia. *J Refract Surg* 1996;12:42–49.
15. Burrato L, Ferrari M, Genisi C. Myopic keratomileusis with the excimer laser: one-year follow-up. *Refract Corneal Surg* 1993;9:12–19.
16. Eyman GA, Badaro RM, Khoobehi B. Corneal ablation in rabbits using an infrared (2.9 microns) erbium:YAG laser. *Ophthalmology* 1989;96:1160–1169.
17. Pallikaris IG, Papatzanaki ME, Stathi EZ, et al. Laser *in situ* keratomileusis. *Lasers Surg Med* 1990;10:463–468.
18. Brint SF, Ostrick DM, Fisher C, et al. Six-month results of the multicenter phase I study of excimer laser myopic keratomileusis. *J Cataract Refract Surg* 1994;20:610–615.

74

INTRASTROMAL CORNEAL IMPLANTS

JONATHAN H. TALAMO, MAHNAZ NOURI, AND AZHAR N. RANA

HISTORY AND BACKGROUND

Additive keratorefractive surgery has undergone many changes since the early efforts of Barraquer (1), Stone and Herbert (2), Belau et al. (3), and Choyce (4) in the 1940s, 1950s, and 1960s. As technology and understanding have progressed, a variety of materials have been evaluated for implantation within the corneal stroma to correct refractive errors, and have included synthetic materials (2-4) as well as autologous donor tissue (1). New refractive techniques are being developed for the treatment of corneal ectasia and presbyopia with corneal implants. This chapter addresses the use of intrastromal implants for myopia, hyperopia, and corneal ectatic conditions.

Synthetic Materials

Belau (3) studied the use of several materials for implantation within corneal stroma, experimenting with polysulfone, polymethymethacrylate (PMMA), polyprolene, and silicone oil. Polysulfone is a thermoplastic compound first synthesized and for use as a corneal inlay (4,5). Due to the very high refractive index of polysulfone, thin lenses can be made to allow correction of large refractive errors. Unfortunately, clinical trials of polysulfone implants resulted in corneal haze and degenerative changes with thinning and necrosis of the overlying corneal stroma and epithelium (6,7). Years later, hydrogel (hydroxyethyl methacrylate) lenses were developed (8). Hydrogel lenses are permeable to water, oxygen, glucose, and other metabolites. Although hydrogel is well tolerated by the human cornea, early refractive results were not very predictable (9,10). Revised models of these inlays are currently in clinical trials.

Animal studies showed that use of impermeable corneal implants such as PMMA blocked the flow of metabolites and water, thus causing thinning and necrosis of corneal stroma (11). It was later discovered that reducing the diameter and increasing the depth of placement for impermeable inlays would improve the diffusion of metabolites to the adjacent corneal tissue. Thus, the diameter and depth

of a stromal implant appeared to be of critical importance if an impermeable material was to be used. These insights resulted in the development of intrastromal ring segments (Intacs), conceived by Reynolds in 1978 and first studied in the late 1980s (12). Although originally conceived and studied as a 360-degree implant, this device has evolved into two 150-degree arcuate segments that are easier to implant and manipulate within the peripheral cornea and cause fewer healing problems.

Autologous Donor Corneal Tissue

Keratophakia was introduced by Barraquer (1) in 1949. Keratophakia (*kera:* cornea; *phacos:* lens) refers to the placement of donor lenticules with refractive power within the stromal lamellae to correct either myopia or hyperopia. The lenticule is a piece of autologous donor corneal stroma that is frozen and shaped by a cryolathe (13) or harvested fresh by a microkeratome (14). Once implanted within the central stroma, the lenticule alters the anterior corneal curvature and thus its dioptric power (Fig. 74-1).

The keratophakia procedure as performed by Barraquer in the 1970s with cryolathe techniques or with early microkeratomes was skill-intensive and technically complex, and as a result was never widely adopted. With the advent of safer, more flexible microkeratome systems and artificial anterior chambers, autologous keratophakia may in the future claim a place within the practice of mainstream refractive surgery.

CURRENT APPROACHES

There are many strategies for the correction of myopia, hyperopia, and astigmatism via the alteration of corneal shape using additive surgical procedures. As with any elective refractive surgery, such procedures should be safe, effective, predictable, and stable. The potential adjustability and reversibility of corneal implant surgery are additional positive attributes. We will describe the procedures currently

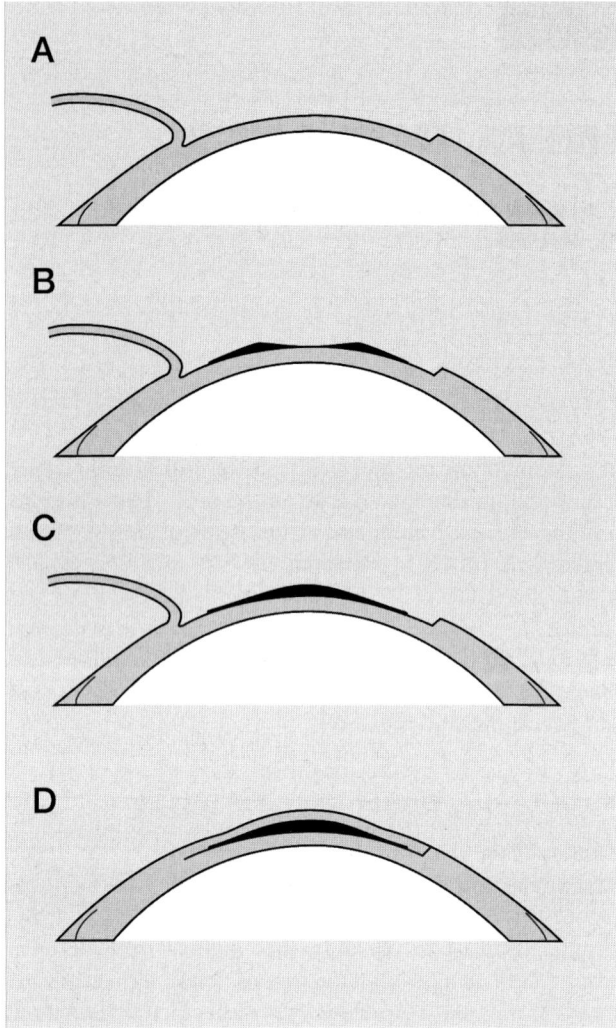

FIGURE 74-1. Keratophakia. **A:** A partial-thickness corneal flap or cap is created with a microkeratome. **B,C:** A stromal lenticule of the appropriate shape is placed on the stromal bed to correct either myopia **(B)** or hyperopia **(C)**. **D:** The corneal flap or cap is then replaced.

used in clinical practice to correct myopia and hyperopia along with clinical indications, surgical techniques, published results, and future directions.

Space does not permit an extensive discussion of patient selection and preoperative evaluation, and these issues are discussed at length elsewhere in this text. However, important components of any elective keratorefractive presurgical evaluation include a complete past medical and ocular history with specific attention to the history of the refractive state of the eye as well as ocular and systemic conditions that may be contraindications to corneal surgery in general. The complete preoperative ophthalmic exam should include as a minimum the following: visual acuity [uncorrected visual acuity (UCVA) and best spectacle-corrected visual acuity (BSCVA)], manifest and cycloplegic refraction, slit-lamp examination (with particular attention to the health of the ocular surface and adnexa), intraocular pressure measurement, and fundus examination. Corneal

topography and pachymetry are important adjunctive studies, as they help exclude corneal ectatic conditions and are important for surgical planning. If there is any question as to the health of the corneal endothelium, analysis by specular microscopy is mandatory.

Intrastromal Corneal Ring and Ring Segments (ICR/ICRS-Intacs)

The 360-degree intrastromal corneal ring (ICR) and the 150-degree intrastromal corneal ring segment (ICRS) implants (Intacs, Addition Technology, Inc., Des Plaines, IL) are made of PMMA and may be used for the correction of low to moderate myopia of −1 to −4 D, although their optimal range seems to be from −1 to −3 D. The use of the 360-degree ring was abandoned after early clinical trials, as it became apparent that it was difficult to implant and more prone to healing problems near the incision site. The use of multiple, small peripheral segments is being investigated for the treatment of low hyperopia up to 2 D.

Myopic ICRS (Fig. 74-2) have an arc length of 150 degrees, an inner diameter of 7 mm, an outer diameter of 8.1 mm, and thickness in the range of 0.25 mm to 0.45 mm with increments of 0.05 mm. A 0.21-mm segment is also available for corrections of less than −1 D. Only the 0.25-, 0.30-, and 0.35-mm rings are approved for use in the United States. Table 74-1 describes the recommended prescribing range for Intacs and summarizes the refractive effects achieved with each segment diameter in the larger U.S. and European multicenter clinical trials.

When implanted within the peripheral cornea, ICRS flatten the anterior surface of the cornea by increasing the arc length curvature of the central cornea, with resultant flattening (Fig. 74-3). The advantage of ICRS over the other myopic keratorefractive procedures include surgery that spares the central cornea, maintenance of prolate asphericity of the cornea (15–17), and the reversibility of surgical effect with removal of segments (18–20).

Patient Selection

Implantation of ICRS is indicated for stable myopia of a mild degree (−1 to −3 diopters spherical equivalent), and a stable refraction. Good candidates have refractive cylinder of 0.5 D or less, as astigmatism is not readily correctable with this procedure. ICRS are contraindicated for individuals with autoimmune disorders, collagen vascular disease, and pregnant or nursing women. Ocular contraindications include the conditions described for other keratorefractive procedures, including recurrent corneal erosion syndrome and some corneal dystrophies, history of herpetic eye disease, and uncontrolled ocular surface disorders. Patients using such medications as amiodarone, sumatriptan, and isotretinoin are also not considered candidates for ICRS. Select patients with mild to moderate keratoconus may benefit from implantation of Intacs or

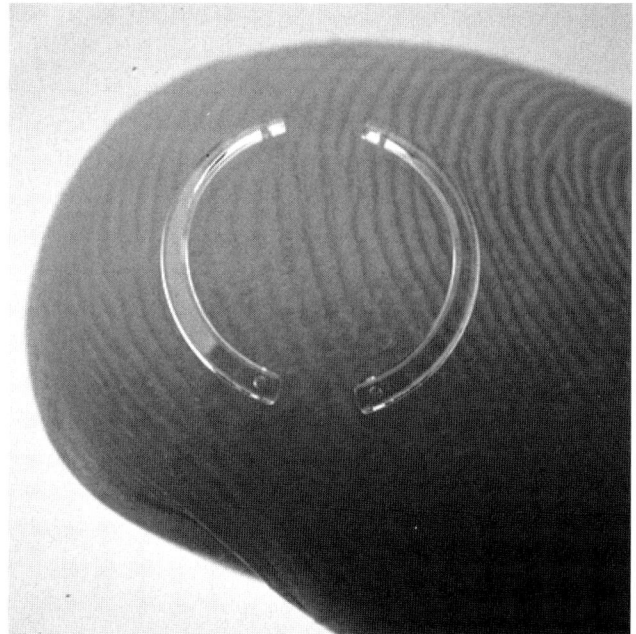

A

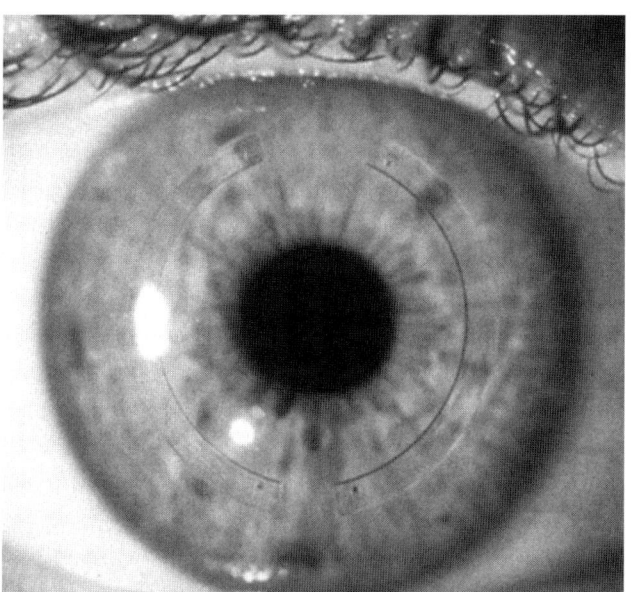

B

FIGURE 74-2. Intrastromal corneal ring segment (Intacs) 150-degree segments for myopia *ex vivo* **(A)** and *in vivo* **(B)**.

Ferrara rings (another type of ICRS), and this topic is discussed further below.

Surgical Technique: Intacs for Myopia

Intacs implantation can be done using topical anesthesia with mild oral sedation under sterile conditions. A 0.9- to 1.2-mm radial incision is typically made at the 12 or 3 o'clock position, 7 to 8 mm from the geometric center of the cornea, using a diamond knife set at 68% of the pachymetric reading at the incision site. Corneal thickness should be at least 600 μm in the regions of the planned incision site and stromal channel dissections. The corneal tissue is then separated with a Suarez Spreader (Storz, St Louis, MO). This allows easy introduction of a blunt curved stromal separator under high suction, which is used to create stromal channels for the implant of ICRS. The separator is rotated 180 degrees clockwise and then withdrawn and reintroduced on the other side of the incision and rotated. Alternatively, a femtosecond yttrium-aluminum-garnet (YAG) laser such as the Intralase FS (Intralase, Irvine, CA) may be used to create both the incision in the cornea and the stromal channels. A laser dissection allows easier centering of the stromal channels as well as the potential to create a beveled or tunneled incision, which may allow development of larger segments or even a 360-degree ring again in the future.

The ICRS are slid in a rotating fashion through the keratotomy incision into the channels until they are at an equal and sufficient distance from the incision site. The wound is either closed with 11-0 nylon or left sutureless if no corneal gap is seen. A bandage contact lens and topical nonsteroidal antiinflammatory drug (NSAID) are frequently used for 1 to 3 days to promote postoperative comfort. The patient is maintained on topical steroids and antibiotics for 5 to 10 days.

Complications

Complications after ICRS surgery may relate to the incision, the stromal channels, or the implant itself, and include stromal thinning and necrosis anterior to the segments,

TABLE 74-1. INTRASTROMAL RING SEGMENTS (INTACS) FOR MYOPIA: CLINICAL RESULTS AND PRESCRIBING INFORMATION

| | U.S. FDA Trials (21) | | European Multicenter Trial (28) | | |
Intacs Thickness (mm)	Predicted Nominal Correction (D)	Recommended Prescribing Range (D)	ICRS Size	Preoperative CRSE Mean ± SD	Predicted Correction
0.250	−1.30	−1 to −1.50	0.25	−1.17 ± 0.29	1.3
0.275	−1.70	−1.625 to −1.75	0.30	−1.83 ± 0.49	2
0.300	−2	−1.875 to −2.125	0.35	−2.59 ± 0.42	2.7
0.325	−2.30	−2.25 to −2.50	0.40	−3.27 ± 0.51	3.4
0.350	−2.70	−2.65 to −3	0.45	−4.32 +/−0.53	4.1

CRSE, cycloplagic refractive spherical equivalent; ICRS, intrastromal corneal ring segment.

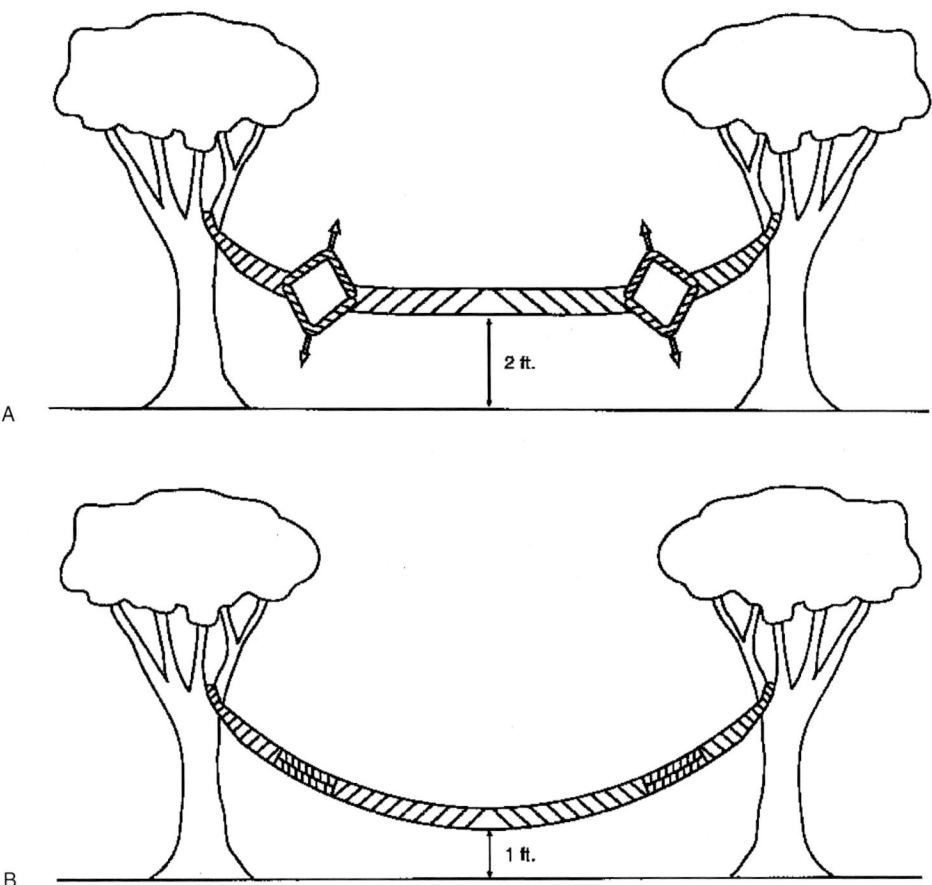

FIGURE 74-3. Mechanism of myopia correction with intrastromal ring segments (Intacs).

epithelial plug formation and ingrowth, wound dehiscence, neovascularization, induced astigmatism, segment extrusion, refractile deposits within the Intacs channels, infectious keratitis, and anterior or posterior corneal perforation. Glare and loss of best spectacle-corrected visual acuity may result from segment decentration. These problems have been shown to resolve with segment removal (21–26).

Intacs seem to be well tolerated by the endothelium, and serial specular microscopy examinations found no sign of significant changes in cell density 2 years after Intacs implantation in 102 eyes (27).

Clinical Results

The results from the Food and Drug Administration (FDA) trials of Intacs for low myopia show excellent efficacy, predictability, stability, and safety data on a par with those reported after PRK and laser-assisted *in situ* keratomileusis (LASIK) for patients with low myopia during the 1990s. Schanzlin et al. (21) reported 2-year results after Intacs implantation for correction of myopia; 452 eyes at 11 investigational sites were enrolled and 24-month follow-up was completed for 358 patients (79%). At month 24, 328 of 354 patients (93%) were within ±1 D of predicted

refractive outcome. Stability analysis showed that refraction changed by 1 D or less in 97% of eyes (421/435) between 3 and 6 months after implantation and in 96% (343/358) between 18 and 24 months. Before surgery, 87% (390/448) of eyes saw worse than 20/40 uncorrected. Twenty-four months after surgery, 55% of eyes (196/358) saw 20/16 or better, 76% (271/358) saw 20/20 or better, and 97% (346/358) saw 20/40 or better. Uncorrected visual acuity results were best in eyes receiving the two thinnest ring segments. Although two eyes (2/358; 0.56%) lost two or more lines at 24 months, visual acuity in both of these eyes was 20/20 or better. Intraoperative complications included anterior corneal surface perforation (three eyes) and anterior chamber perforations (two eyes, one during an attempted exchange procedure): all healed spontaneously without suturing or loss of BSCVA. Intacs were repositioned in five eyes to adjust the refractive effect. Postoperative complications in one eye each were infectious keratitis and shallow anterior chamber (resolved).

European studies examining a wider range of correction (−1 to −4 D) revealed comparable results, although the incidence of induced astigmatism was increased in eyes receiving 0.4- and 0.45-mm segments (28). Despite these promising data, Intacs have not achieved the widespread acceptance experienced by PRK and LASIK. This phenomenon is perhaps explained by the more limited range of correction treatable with these devices, the unique set of instruments and surgical skills required, and the slower visual rehabilitation of these patients compared to those undergoing LASIK surgery.

Intacs for Residual Myopia After PRK and LASIK

Intacs are a useful adjunct procedure for myopic patients with corneas too thin to safely utilize optimal ablation depth and diameter for LASIK or PRK (29). Intacs may be placed as either part of a staged primary treatment or in place of excimer laser enhancement surgery (30).

Intacs for Hyperopia

Small Intacs segments (0.5 to 0.8 mm wide, 1.8 to 2 mm long) placed within radial incisions of the peripheral cornea at two-thirds depth in corneal stroma are being evaluated for the correction of hyperopia up to 2 D (Fig. 74-4) (31). The mechanism of action is thought to be central corneal steepening. Change in device thickness alters the refractive effect. The procedure is still under investigation and is not used outside of clinical trials. The device can reportedly correct up to three diopters of hyperopia and refractive stability was achieved by 3 months, with 6 to 12 months' follow-up obtained for all eyes (32).

Intacs for Astigmatism

Short arc-length segments are currently being evaluated for treatment of myopic astigmatism, but few data are available at the present time (33).

Intracorneal Ring Segments for Keratoconus and Iatrogenic Keratectasia After LASIK

Colin (34,35) was the first to report the results of intracorneal ring placement in patients with keratoconus, finding that the flattening effect of Intacs on keratoconic tissue was greater and more asymmetric than that observed in normal corneas. The majority of eyes treated experienced some improvement in UCVA and BSCVA as well as reduced refractive astigmatism and improved corneal topographic regularity, often reflected by reduced size and improved centration of the cone (Fig. 74-5). Our unpublished experience with approximately 20 eyes supports Colin's data and conclusions. The best clinical results are achieved in mild to moderate cases with clear central corneas and BSCVA of 20/40 or better, and we recommend reserving this procedure for patients who fit these criteria and who are rigid contact lens intolerant, as the refractive effect of Intacs is seldom exact in this setting.

Siganos et al. (36) reported clinical improvement in keratoconus patients after insertion of smaller diameter Ferrara rings. In contrast to Intacs, Ferrara rings are implanted around the center of the cone rather than the pupil or geometric center of the cornea, and the more triangular shape of this device may create a prismatic effect that may reduce the glare noted by some patients with Intacs, but the evidence remains anecdotal to date.

Clinical improvement of LASIK-induced keratectasia has also been reported following Intacs implantation (37–39), and in some cases may provide at least a short-term satisfactory solution to this serious and difficult problem. A recent publication by Siganos et al. (37) reports successful Intacs implantation in three eyes of two patients with ectasia after

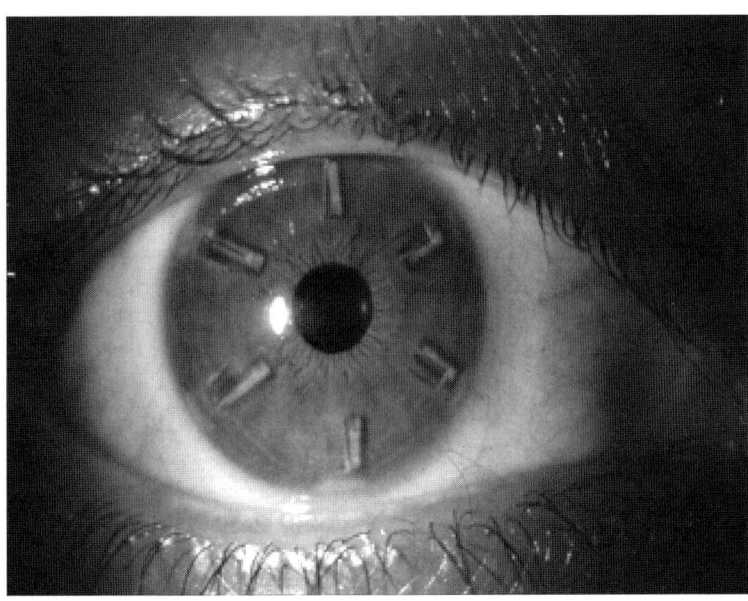

FIGURE 74-4. Intacs segments for correction of hyperopia.

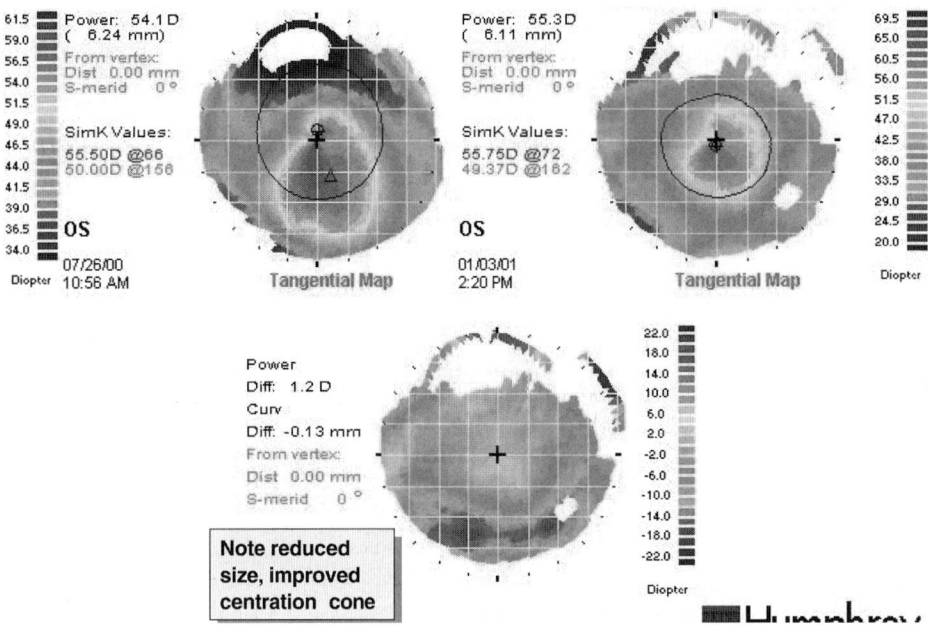

FIGURE 74-5. Topographic effect of Intacs for Keratoconus.

LASIK with 8 to 10 months' follow-up. Best corrected visual acuity improved in all cases. One of us (J.H.T.) has obtained 2-year follow-up on three eyes of three patients with post-LASIK keratectasia, and found a stable refractive effect along with improvement of two lines of BSCVA in two eyes (20/40 to 20/25; 20/30 to 20/20) and no change in one eye (20/30). All patients reported subjective improvement in their uncorrected and best corrected vision.

Synthetic Keratophakia Lamellar Hydrogel Implants

Hydrogel is a material of high water content that is permeable to corneal nutrients. Its refractive index (1.385) is similar to that of the cornea (1.376) and therefore achieves its effect through alteration of anterior curvature. Several devices are currently being investigated in FDA-sanctioned clinical trials and are being manufactured for both myopia and hyperopia (Permavision Lens, Anamed Inc., Irvine, CA; Permalens, Alcon Labs, Ft. Worth, TX; Keratogel, Allergan Medical Optics, Irvine CA). Two small-diameter corneal inlays (SDCI, Bausch and Lomb, Rochester, NY; Paraxial adaptive optic implant, Acufocus, Boston, MA) are undergoing clinical evaluation for correction of presbyopia. Although limited clinical data have been presented at scientific meetings, no peer-reviewed publications exist for any of the devices that are currently in clinical trials.

Surgical Technique and Complications

Hydrogel lens implants can be performed under local anesthesia with mild oral or intravenous sedation implantation.

For myopic and hyperopic correction, three surgical approaches have been used: creation of free corneal flap with a microkeratome, creation of a lamellar pocket within the stroma, and placement of the lens under a hinged corneal flap without suturing after surgical lamellar dissection with a microkeratome. When these implants are placed within the stroma, they must conform to the shape of the lamellar bed. At present, the simplest and most promising approach seems to be the hinged flap (Fig. 74-6). For this approach, a microkeratome is used to create a corneal flap that is 180 to 250 μm thick and at least 9.5 mm in diameter. The resultant effect is that the anterior corneal curvature conforms to the shape of the implant, thus altering the anterior corneal radius

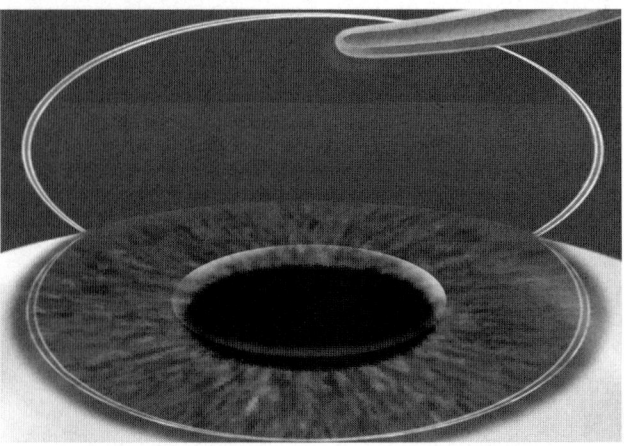

FIGURE 74-6. Synthetic keratophakia under a hinged corneal flap.

and dioptric power. For the presbyopic small-diameter intracorneal inlay lens (SDCI), an intrastromal pocket is created through a small circumferential peripheral incision.

These procedures can have complications related to the microkeratome, incision for pocket creation, suturing (if used), lens placement (particularly centration), and abnormal wound healing resulting in inflammation around the implant and/or tissue melting/necrosis.

Hydrogel Lenses: Laboratory and Clinical Results

A study of rhesus monkeys with hydrogel intracorneal implants was reported by Parks et al. (40) with 4 years of follow-up. Eleven of 49 monkeys developed intrastromal crystals from 21 to 151 days after implantation. Stromal edema was seen postoperatively (within 3 weeks) in all of these cases. It was postulated that these stromal crystals may be lipid deposits ("unesterified cholesterol and neutral fat"), with "thin, fibrillar or needle-like crystals" seen via specular microscopy. In this study the lipid deposits were postulated to be produced de novo.

Another theory was that the production of lipid by the stromal keratocytes occurred in response to stress, such as surgical trauma. This finding is likely similar to the "channel deposits" observed after Intacs, and its long-term clinical significance is unknown.

Werblin et al. (9) reported the first human experiments with hydrogel lens implants. Five myopic patients (spherical equivalent -9.50 to -19 D) were followed up for 18 months. Visual acuity recovered in 1 month, but significant undercorrection (-2.50 to -8 D) relative to the attempted correction was noted. There was loss of refractive effect with time in two of five patients. In a later study by Barraquer and Gomez (10), results in five myopic and five aphakic patients also suggested that hydrogel lenses were well tolerated. Myopic eyes showed some regression postoperatively, which was thought to be due to corneal steepening over time. The average keratometric power change from 1 to 72 months was $+4.86 \pm 2.23$ D. The aphakic patients were stable with overall change in keratometric power of $+8.56 \pm 0.60$ D.

Steinert and colleagues (41) reported results from 35 aphakic eyes implanted with the Kerato-Gel lens (Allergan Medical Optics, Irvine, CA), a glucose-permeable hydrogel with an equilibrium water content of 68%. Nineteen of 35 patients were followed for 2 years, at which time the average refractive spherical equivalent was -0.63 ± 2.07 D, 50% of eyes were within 1 D of emmetropia, and 88% were within 3 D. A mean loss of 3.25 lines of best corrected visual acuity (Snellen) was observed in this patient cohort. The authors concluded that the implant material was well tolerated, but felt that further progress in surgical technique was necessary to achieve results that would warrant the use of this device in widespread clinical practice.

The effective optical zone achieved by newer hyperopic implants (such as the Anamed Permavision lens, with lens diameters of 5 and 6 mm) is slightly larger than the implant size due to the "draping" effect of the corneal flap anterior to the implant. These newer lenses are made up of microporous hydrogel with properties that closely mimic natural corneal stroma. In the case of the Anamed Permavision, the refractive index is 1.376 and the water content 78%, making it more permeable to glucose and oxygen than prior hydrogel implants. As for previous hydrogel lenses, animal studies suggest the material has long-term biocompatibility. In a recent study by Ismail (42), Anamed Permavision lenses were implanted in 20 Albino rabbits and followed using confocal microscopy. Six-month follow-up showed excellent compatibility with no fibrocytic activity or intralamellar deposits. This device is currently in clinical trials internationally, with phase II FDA trials to begin soon in the U.S. No peer-reviewed data have been published.

Future Directions

Intracorneal hydrogel lenses have been shown to be biocompatible and relatively stable. The main problem with large lenses may be related to the surgical procedure, where optimal parameters for the keratectomy depth and methods to maintain centration of the lens must be determined and achieved reproducibly to obtain improved refractive accuracy. The small-diameter intracorneal inlay lens (SDCI) and the paraxial adaptive focus lens may be easier to insert due to their reduced thickness and diameter, but again there are no peer-reviewed data available at this time.

NEW APPLICATIONS OF AUTOLOGOUS KERATOPHAKIA

Due to its surgical complexity and the variable clinical outcomes, autologous keratophakia was largely abandoned after the 1970s. After the failure of epikeratophakia and automated lamellar keratoplasty to gain widespread acceptance in the 1980s and early 1990s due to similar reasons, interest in this approach was not rekindled until improved microkeratome technology became available, driven by the popularity of LASIK surgery in the middle to late 1990s. The marriage of the modern microkeratome with the artificial anterior chamber (43) and the ready availability of fresh or frozen human corneal tissue through improved eye banking laws and techniques has again made keratophakia a potentially viable approach, and the literature has described its use to correct complications of automated lamellar keratoplasty (44) and LASIK (45).

Corneal Augmentation Lamellar Keratoplasty

Corneal augmentation lamellar keratoplasty (CALAK) is a term proposed by Vidaurri et al. (46) for a new procedure that combines keratophakia and LASIK. CALAK is a surgical alternative for patients with high myopia who are not suitable candidates for LASIK due to inadequate corneal thickness. Keratophakia, as mentioned earlier, uses human donor cornea lenticules to produce a change in curvature and thickness in the recipient cornea. To achieve a predetermined refractive effect using traditional keratophakia, the donor lenticule must be lathed frozen and thawed before placing it on the recipient stromal bed or within a lamellar pocket. The procedure may correct large amounts of ametropia (up to 16 to 17 diopters). CALAK (Fig. 74-7) involves two procedures: (a) At the time of primary surgery, a donor lenticule of undetermined refractive power but predetermined thickness is harvested from fresh donor tissue with a microkaratone and placed under a LASIK flap following partial treatment of the baseline refraction by excimer photoablation to the stromal bed (Fig. 74-7A,B). (b) Two months later, after the lenticule has healed in place and the refractive state of the eye has stabilized, the LASIK flap is elevated and excimer photoablation is performed to achieved the full desired refractive effect (Fig. 74-7C,D).

Clinical Results

Vidaurri et al. (46) treated 26 eyes of 16 patients with manifest refractive spherical equivalents from −8.25 to −17.25 diopters (D) with up to −6 D of cylinder. Mean manifest refractive spherical equivalent (MRSE) measured −13.94 ± 3.08 D. Best spectacle-corrected visual acuity (BSCVA) before surgery ranged from 20/20 to 20/60.

Before treatment 80.7% of eyes had UCVA of CF at 3 feet and 19.2% CF at 6 feet. At 6 months following ablation of the donor lenticule, 7 of 26 (27%) of the cases had 20/40 or better UCVA, and 22 of 26 (85%) had 20/60 or better UCVA. At 1 year, 7 of 15 eyes (47%) had 20/40 or better and 13 of 15 (87%) had 20/60 or better UCVA. At 1 year, 33% of the eyes achieved an UCVA equal to or better that their preoperative BSCVA.

SUMMARY

The use of both autologous and synthetic lamellar implants to correct refractive error is likely to grow in the coming years. Although intracorneal ring procedures have been clearly shown to meet acceptable criteria to warrant routine clinical usage, much more research is needed to establish the efficacy, predictability, stability, and safety of synthetic lamellar inlays. As the limitations of tissue subtraction procedures such as PRK and LASIK become better

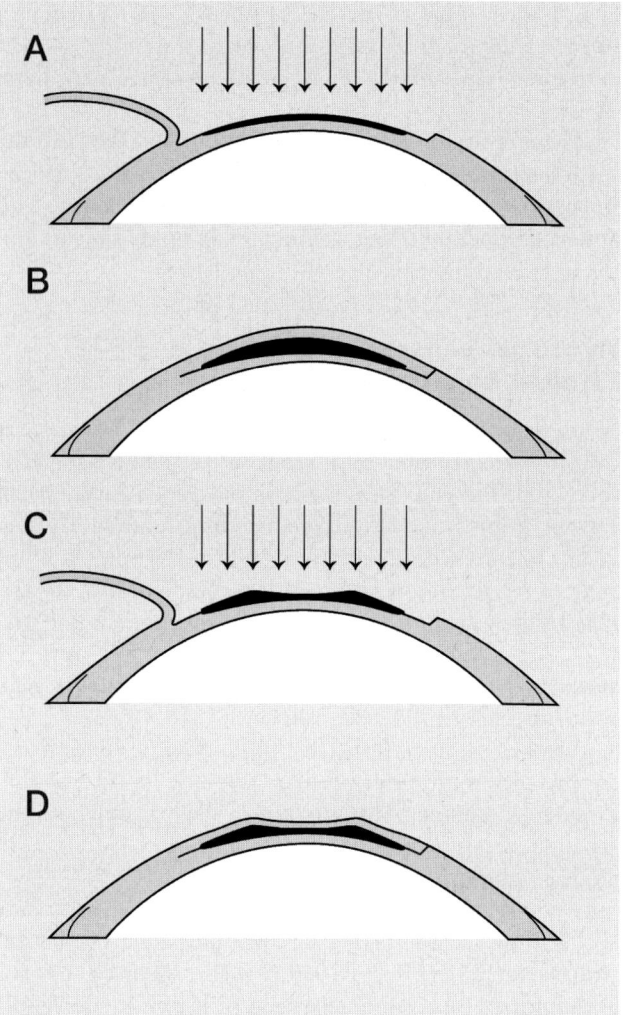

FIGURE 74-7. Corneal augmentation laser-assisted keratophakia (CALAK). **A:** Approximately 20% of the total intended myopic refractive correction is delivered to the stromal bed after creation of a lamellar keratectomy flap using excimer photoablation. **B:** A fresh autologous stromal lenticule is harvested from donor cornea and placed within the previously ablated stromal bed and the flap replaced. **C:** After allowing the lenticule to heal into the stromal bed for 2 months, the flap is relifted and the remaining myopic/astigmatic correction is administered with the excimer laser to the lenticule. **D:** The flap is replaced over the newly ablated myopic lenticule, thus achieving full refractive effect.

defined and technology to refine surgical approaches for additive keratorefractive procedures continue to improve, procedures such as CALAK and synthetic lamellar implant could become a more important part of the refractive surgeon's armamentarium.

REFERENCES

1. Barraquer JI. Modification of refraction by means of intracorneal inclusions. *Int Ophthalmol Clin* 1966;1:53–78.

2. Stone W, Herbert E. Experimental study of plastic material as a replacement for the cornea: a preliminary report. *Am J Ophthalmol* 1953;36(part II):168–173.

3. Belau PG, Dyer JA, Ogle KN, et al. Correction of ametropia with intrastromal lenses: an experimental study. *Arch Ophthalmol* 1964;72:541–549.

4. Choyce DP. The correction of the refractive errors with polysulfone corneal inlays. *Trans Ophthalmol Soc UK* 1985;104:332.

5. Deg JK, Binder PS. Histopathology and clinical behavior of polysulfone intracorneal implants in the baboon model. Polysulfone lens implants. *Ophthalmology* 1988;95(4):506–515.

6. Horgan SE, Fraser SG, Choyce DP, et al. Twelve year follow-up of unfenestrated polysulfone intracorneal lenses in human sighted eyes. *J Cataract Refract Surg* 1996;22(8):1045–1051.

7. Lane SL, Lindstrom RL, Cameron JD, et al. Polysulfone corneal lenses. *J Cataract Refract Surg* 1986;12(1):50–60.

8. McCarey BE, Andrews DM. Refractive keratoplasty with intrastromal hydrogel lenticular implants. *Invest Ophthalmol Vis Sci* 1981;21:107–115.

9. Werblin TP, Patel AS, Barraquer JI. Initial human experience with hydrogel intracorneal lens implants. *Refract Corneal Surg* 1992;8(1):23–26.

10. Barraquer JI, Gomez ML. Permalens hydrogel intracorneal lenses for spherical ametropia. *J Refract Surg* 1997;13(4):342–348.

11. McCarey BE. Alloplastic refractive keratoplasty. In: Sanders DR, ed. *Refractive corneal surgery.* Thorofare, NJ: Slack, 1986:551–563.

12. Fleming J, Reynolds A, Kilmer L. The intrastromal corneal ring: two cases in rabbits. *J Refract Surg* 1987;3:227–232.

13. Friedlander MH, Rich LF, Werblin TP, et al. Keratophakia using preserved lenticules. *Ophthalmology* 1980;87:687–692.

14. Krumeich JH, Swinger CA. Non-freeze keratophakia for the correction of myopia. *Am J Ophthalmol* 1987;103:397–403.

15. Burris TE, Baker PC, Ayer CT, et al. Flattening of central corneal curvature with intrastromal corneal rings of increasing thickness: an eye-bank eye study. *J Cataract Refract Surg* 1993;19(suppl):182–187.

16. Burris TE. Intrastromal corneal ring technology: results and indications. *Curr Opin Ophthalmol* 1998;9(4):9–14.

17. Holmes-Higgin DK, Baker PC, Burris TE, et al. Characterization of the aspheric corneal surface with intrastromal corneal ring segments. *Refract Surg* 1999;15(5):520–528.

18. Asbell PA, Ucakhan OO, Abbott RL, et al. Intrastromal corneal ring segments: reversibility of refractive effect. *J Refract Surg* 2001;17(1):25–31.

19. Chan SM, Khan HN. Reversibility and exchangeability of intrastromal corneal ring segments *J Cataract Refract Surg* 2002;28(4):676–681.

20. Clinch TE, Lemp MA, Foulks GN, et al. Removal of INTACS for myopia. *Ophthalmology* 2002;109(8):1441–1446.

21. Schanzlin DJ, Abbott RL, Asbell PA, et al. Two-year outcomes of intrastromal corneal ring segments for the correction of myopia: *Ophthalmology* 2001;108(9):1688–1694.

22. Rapuano CJ, Sugar A, Koch DD, et al. Intrastromal corneal ring segments for low miopia: a report by the American Academy of Ophthalmology. *Ophthalmology* 2001;108:1922–1928.

23. Ruckhofer J, Stoiber J, Alzner E, et al. One year results of European multicenter study of intrastromal corneal ring segments part 2: complications, visual symptoms, and patient satisfaction. *J Cataract Refract Surg* 2001;27:287–296.

24. Twa MD, Ruckhofer J, Shanzlin DJ. Surgically induced astigmatism after implantation of Intacs intrastromal corneal ring segments. *J Cataract Refract Surg* 2001;27(3):411–415.

25. Assil KK, Quantock AJ, Barrett AM, et al. Corneal iron lines associated with the intrastromal corneal ring. *Am J Ophthalmol* 1993;116(3):350–356.

26. Ruckhofer J, Twa M, Schanzlin DJ. Clinical characteristics of lamellar channel deposits after implantation of Intacs. *J Cataract Refract Surg* 2000;26:1473–1479.

27. Azar RG, Holdbrook MJ, Lemp M, et al. Two-year corneal endothelial cell assessment following Intacs implantation. *J Refract Surg* 2001;17:542–548.

28. Ruckhofer J, Stoiber J, Alzner E, et al. One year results of European multicenter study of intrastromal corneal ring segments. Part 1: refractive outcomes. *J Cataract Refract Surg* 2001;27:277–286.

29. Fleming JF, Lovisolo CF. Intrastromal corneal ring segments in a patient with previous Laser *in situ* keratomileusis. *J Refract Surg* 2000;16:365–367.

30. Primack JD, Azar DT. Laser *in situ* keratomileusis and intrastromal corneal ring segments for high myopia. Three-step procedure. *J Cataract Refract Surg* 2003;869–874.

31. Ruckhofer J. Clinical and histological studies on the intrastromal corneal ring segments (ICRS(R), Intacs(R)). *Klin Monatsbl Augenheilkd* 2002;219:557–74

32. Verity SM. *Intacs for myopia and hyperopia.* American Academy of Ophthalmology, 2001 Subspecialty Day—Refractive Surgery, pp. 83–87.

33. Ruckhofer J, Stoiber J, Twa MD, et al. Correction of astigmatism with short arc-length intrastromal corneal ring segments. Preliminary results. *Ophthalmology* 2003;110(3):516–524.

34. Colin J, Cochener B, Savary G, et al. Correcting keratoconus with intracorneal rings. *J Cataract Refract Surg* 2000;16:438–443.

35. Colin J, Cochener B, Savary G, et al. INTACS inserts for treating keratoconus. *Ophthalmology* 2001;108:1409–1414.

36. Siganos D, Ferrara P, Chatznikolas K, et al. Ferrara intrastromal corneal rings for the correction of keratoconus. *J Cataract Refract Surg* 2002;28:1947–1951.

37. Siganos CS, Kymionis GD, Astyrakakis N, et al. Management of corneal ectasia after laser *in situ* keratomileusis with Intacs. *J Refract Surg* 2002;18:43–46.

38. Lovisolo CF, Fleming JF. Intracorneal ring segments for iatrogenic keratectasia after laser *in situ* keratomileusis or photorefractive keratectomy. *J Refract Surg* 2002;18:535–541.

39. Alio, Salem TF, Artola A, et al. Intracorneal rings to correct corneal ectasia after laser in situ keratomileusis. *J Cataract Refract Surg* 2002;28:1568–1574.

40. Parks RA, McCarey BE, Knight PM, et al. Intrastromal crystalline deposits following hydrogel keratophakia in monkeys. *Cornea* 1993;12(1): 29–34.

41. Steinert RF, Storie B, Smith P, et al. Hydrogel intracorneal implants in aphakic eyes. *Arch Ophthalmol* 1996;11:135–141.

42. Ismail MM. Correction of hyperopia with intracorneal implants. *J Cataract Refract Surg* 2002;28(3):527–530.

43. Maguen E, Villasenor RA, Ward DE, et al. A modified anterior chamber for use in refractive keratoplasty. *Am J Ophthalmol* 1980;89:742–744.

44. Chan WK, Maloney RK. Autologous keratophakia for the correction of consecutive hyperopia after automated lamellar keratoplasty for myopia. *J Refract Surg* 1996;12(4):513–515.

45. Jankov M, Mrochen MC, Bueler M, et al. Experimental results of preparing laser-shaped stromal implants for laser-assisted intrastromal keratophakia in extremely complicated laser in situ keratomileusis cases. *J Refract Surg* 2002;18(5):S639–643.

46. Vidaurri JV, Talamo JH, Rodriguez M, et al. CALK (Corneal augmentation lamellar keratoplasty) for Extreme Myopia. Presented in part at the International Society of Refractive Surgery Annual Meeting, October, 2002, Orlando, FL. *(Submitted for publication.)*

EXCIMER LASER SURFACE ABLATION: PHOTOREFRACTIVE KERATECTOMY (PRK) AND LASER SUBEPITHELIAL KERATOMILEUSIS (LASEK)

SCOTT BARNES AND DIMITRI T. AZAR

The field of refractive surgery has been greatly impacted by the development of the excimer laser. This high-energy ultraviolet (UV) laser has been employed in various industrial and medical applications. The term *excimer* is a contraction of *exc*ited di*mer*, which was a term first used by photochemists in 1960 to describe an energized molecule with two identical components. However, rather than two identical components, most excimer lasers involve a high-energy complex ("excited complex") of halogen and inert atoms of noble gases, achieved under a very high voltage electrical field (1,2). Such excited dimers are molecules that have minimal binding in the ground state but are more closely bound in a higher energy ("excited") state. Various combinations of halogens and gases can produce dimers in wavelengths between 193 and 351 nm. This high-energy complex, being unstable, decays and releases energy in the form of a photon of UV radiation. These photons are then amplified, phased, and collimated to form a laser beam (1–3).

Originally developed in 1975 (4), the excimer laser was employed for research in physical chemistry and for various industrial uses, precisely etching a number of polymers (5–8). This process was originally called *ablative photodecompensation* but has evolved into the term *photoablation* (3,9,10). The energy of a UV photon, excited between 193 and 351 nm, exceeds the covalent bond strength of many molecules; ablative photodecompensation directs this UV energy toward a specific molecule, breaking chemical bonds, which increases pressure in a confined volume thus ejecting the molecular fragments into the atmosphere (5,9,11,12).

Taboda and colleagues (13,14) reported the first use of an excimer laser on corneal tissue in 1981 at the U.S. Air Force School of Aerospace Medicine. In 1983, Trokel and colleagues (15) reported that UV light could predictably ablate corneal tissue while producing minimal damage to surrounding structures (16,17). Kruger and associates (18) evaluated four excimer generated wavelengths in their interaction with corneal tissue: argon-fluoride (193 nm), krypton-fluoride (248 nm), xenon-chloride (308 nm), and xenon-fluoride (351 nm). The 193-nm wavelength gave more precise and smoother results compared to the increased surrounding thermal damage noted with the longer wavelengths.

EXCIMER LASER ABLATION

The property of the excimer laser beam that makes its interaction with the stromal surface of the cornea unique compared to other lasers, such as those driven by yttrium-aluminum-garnet (YAG) or CO_2, is the ability to impart very high energy to such tissue without a correspondingly high thermal component (1–3,19). This is due to the ability of the mixture of a rare gas (argon, krypton, or xenon) and a halogen (fluoride, chloride, or bromide) to produce a wavelength (especially ArF = 193 nm), which is extremely well absorbed by the covalent bonds (carbon-nitrogen and carbon-carbon) found supporting the corneal epithelium and stroma (1–3).

Direct bond breakage with a high-energy photon is a photochemical interaction. Although the laser energy is largely converted to heat with typical thermal effects seen in the ejected fragments (20), minimal thermal injury to the adjacent tissue is seen, presumably due to both the highly specific and effective photon absorption and the rapid photoablation process (21). Measurements of intrastromal thermal gradients show that local temperature elevation increases with laser repetition rate, drops exponentially with increasing distance from the edge of the ablation zone, and does not exceed 5°C at the edge of the keratectomy (22). There is some controversy regarding the degree of photochemical versus photothermal mechanism with laser ablation (23); shorter wavelengths such as 193 nm may involve a total photochemical process, whereas longer wavelengths, such as 248 to 308 nm, may involve a photothermal process. At any rate, short wavelength pulses delivered at a low repetition rate may help limit local heating, thereby producing less coagulation of protein adjacent to the ablation zone.

As energy density increases above threshold, each pulse of laser light removes a constant amount of corneal tissue proportional to the amount of energy striking the cornea. The amount varies with the wavelength used to produce the light. Kruger et al. (18), Kruger and Trokel (24), and Puliafito et al. (25) studied ablation rates. They observed that in wavelengths greater than 193 nm, the threshold for corneal ablation increased as the laser repetition rate decreased. However, at 193 nm, the threshold was constant regardless of variance in repetition rate. This observation supports the photochemical theory of excimer ablation at 193 nm, with thermal mechanisms becoming a greater issue only at longer wavelengths.

Puliafito et al. (22) used high-speed photography to analyze excimer laser ablation and noted that fragments are ejected from the corneal surface in a mushroom-shaped smoke plume for several hundred nanoseconds after the laser exposure. Increases in plume size and initial ejection velocity are seen with increasing exposure energy.

EXCIMER LASER SURFACE ABLATION: ANALYSIS OF LASER-CORNEAL INTERACTIONS

Use of UV radiation brings a concomitant concern of mutagenesis and carcinogenesis. Most carcinogens have been shown to be mutagens as well (26). UV radiation–induced mutation increased proportionally with DNA absorption (27). Due to the low density of keratocytes in the stroma, carcinogenesis resulting from stromal photoablation may be unlikely. Several studies have failed to show cellular mutations or carcinogenic changes associated with 193-nm irradiation. Nuss et al. (28) evaluated the repair of damaged pyrimidine dimers by observing unscheduled DNA synthesis after photoablation. Such DNA synthesis did not increase after 193 nm linear ablation compared to that seen following diamond knife incisions as a control. Interestingly, there was a statistically significant increase in such DNA synthesis after 248 nm irradiation. Theories for decreased toxicity with 193 nm include a general lack of cytotoxic breakdown products at that wavelength, damage that can be repaired by the molecule's cellular environment, absorption of the wavelength by some type of protective protein coat, or that mutagenic repair processes are not possible due to the extent of tissue destruction caused by 193 nm energy (29).

Skin and corneal models further illustrate the influence of such high-energy irradiation. Skin irradiation with 193 nm light produced the least DNA damage and cytotoxicity, 248 nm energy produced the greatest damage, and 308-nm exposure resulted in a moderate degree of toxicity (29). Further, 193 nm irradiation of the cornea produces fluorescence between 295 and 425 nm, levels at which mutations or cataract development would be likely (30). However, the highly attenuated energy of such fluorescence makes the level of exposure 10,000 times lower than the minimum average annual exposure to solar UVB radiation. Trokel et al. (15) examined the results of 193 nm excimer ablation of the cornea in 1983. Puliafito and colleagues (31) observed the histopathology of linear corneal ablation using 193 and 248 nm. Both reports confirmed preservation of normal corneal microstructure adjacent to the ablation zone with 193 nm, and Puliafito's study showed disorganization of such microstructure at least 10 μm into the adjacent stroma after exposure to 248 nm pulses. Further, electron microscopy revealed a submicrometer zone of electron density adjacent to the ablation site. Kerr-Muir and associates (32) postulated that this may represent a type of "pseudomembrane" that may "seal" cells and material transected by 193 nm ablation. This may account for the optically clear cornea adjacent to the 193-nm ablation zone and the loss of transparency in the cornea adjacent to the 248 nm ablation. Additionally, Peyman and colleagues (33) reported a significant coagulative effect, corneal necrosis, stromal opacification, and endothelial cell damage with 308 nm irradiation. Based on this and other supporting studies, argon-fluoride (193 nm) has become the most common gas mixture used in clinical lasers.

ENDOTHELIUM AND SURFACE ABLATION

Given the well-known findings of late-onset corneal edema following the initial Japanese technique of radial keratotomy involving incisions in the endothelium, such endothelial damage from excimer laser refractive surgery remains a major concern.

In spite of the near complete absorption of 193 nm photons within 1 μm of tissue, minor endothelial effects have been noted. Dehm and colleagues (34) reported minimal endothelial effects with 193 nm linear "incisions" to the same corneal depth used with diamond knife radial keratotomy (RK); the endothelial effects were similar to those seen in standard RK incisions. Interestingly, significant loss of endothelial cells was noted with 248 nm "incisions." After surface ablation with 193 nm light, Hanna and associates (35) reported the presence of electron dense granules in rabbit endothelium, which migrated through Descemet's membrane and eventually dissipated over several weeks. This phenomenon may be a transient pressure-induced injury experienced during ablation. The impact of the excimer laser energy on the cornea produces an acoustic shock wave resulting in an audible snap. The resultant shock wave has been photographed in the air above the eye (36) and recorded underneath the cornea using piezoelectric transducers. Zabel and colleagues (37) have shown that this shock wave can generate up to 100 atm of pressure on the endothelium. However, no obvious disruption of the endothelium has been noted. In fact, acute morphologic studies of primate and human endothelium have failed to show endothelial changes unless the laser beam approaches Descemet's membrane (38,39). Clinically significant endothelial cell loss after excimer laser photorefractive keratectomy (PRK) has not been recorded (39–41), and in fact, endothelial morphology seems to improve after PRK in contact lens wearers, perhaps reflecting the elimination of the lens.

EXCIMER LASER RADIAL KERATOTOMY

Clinical excimer laser refractive surgery involved application within the known framework of RK. Although incisions are produced with diamond knives, laser RK actually involves excisions, as the tissue is actually removed through ablation. In 1985, Cotliar and co-workers (42) obtained approximately 5 diopters (D) of corneal flattening on enucleated human eyes with laser radial excisions. They showed that the excision depth and amount of flattening was proportional to the amount of laser energy. Steinert and Puliafito (43) developed a system to perform RK laser excisions on rabbit eyes *in vivo*. Aron-Rosa and colleagues (44) were the first to report outcomes of laser RK in a series of human eyes scheduled for enucleation; 2 to 4 D of flattening was attained with the central corneas remaining clear up to 3 weeks after ablation. Interestingly, to achieve similar degrees of corneal flattening, excimer linear excisions needed to be less deep than incisions with a knife, perhaps due to the ablation's removal of tissue rather than the tissue splitting of standard RK.

The advantage of excimer laser versus standard RK was in the increased precision and reproducibility. Depending on delivery systems, laser RK could be an office-based procedure, with the patient in either the supine or upright position, under topical anesthesia. The potential for customized treatment patterns for individual refractive errors combined with possible real-time adjustments via corneal topography during the course of the treatment held great appeal. However, several concerns arose regarding the width of the excisions and their effect on the structural and optical integrity of the cornea. The expected epithelial plug filling the laser RK excisions would be present for months or years. The cornea would remain weakened as the epithelium gradually converted to a fibroblastic scar. Such scars may be more dense and produce more glare than those associated with standard RK. These concerns led to the

abandonment of the excimer laser RK procedure in favor of a more novel approach to refractive ablation.

EXCIMER LASER PHOTOREFRACTIVE KERATOTOMY

The goal of direct ablation of the superficial central cornea over a wide area is to maintain clarity and optical function while creating a new anterior corneal curvature. Although this might more precisely be called *laser anterior keratomileusis*, it has become known as *photorefractive keratectomy* (PRK). To treat myopic refractive errors, corneal tissue is ablated centrally with progressively less removal toward the periphery, resulting in corneal flattening. Conversely, to treat hyperopic refractive errors, more corneal tissue is removed in an annular pattern in the periphery, resulting in corneal steepening. More complex patterns of preferential tissue removal are employed to address correction of astigmatism.

LASER DELIVERY SYSTEMS FOR PRK

Broad-beam delivery models generally employ a diaphragm system, which places a movable circular aperture in the laser path (45). This diaphragm operates similarly to that of a camera system, which can either expand or contract during the exposure. The central cornea receives ablation with every pulse, whereas the successive peripheral areas receive correspondingly less ablation. Combining the diaphragm with moving parallel slit blades can achieve elliptical or cylindrical ablations depending on the type of astigmatism. Treatment times are much faster with such systems, thereby lessening the chance of corneal dehydration, patient discomfort, and the tendency to drift from fixation. However, the resulting "step-like" ablations with broad-beam lasers may be a disadvantage. Although this can be minimized by moving the diaphragm with each pulse, the significance of this ablation pattern is debated. It is theorized that a step-like ablation may stimulate a more aggressive healing response.

A variant of the diaphragm system employs a series of fixed apertures (46). Moving the apertures, which range from small to large, through the beam with successive pulses will cause central corneal flattening in a similar manner as the expanding diaphragm system.

Another delivery model involves the use of an ablatable mask on or near the cornea (47). The mask is made of a synthetic material that is gradually ablated by the laser beam. The shape of the mask could be thought of as similar to a spherical or toric hard contact lens. As the laser pulses gradually break through the polymer, the underlying cornea will be ablated in a pattern mirroring the shape of the mask. The different shapes of the mask (myopic, hyperopic, cylindrical) are responsible for the different refractive changes in the ablated cornea. Most mask systems are used in conjunction with a broad-beam system and therefore have the attendant advantages and disadvantages.

Scanning spot or scanning beam delivery models (48,49) use small spots (0.2 to 1 mm) or a small rectangular beam to rapidly move across the corneal surface in a variety of patterns depending on the capabilities of the motor and computer control mechanisms. The main advantage of such systems centers on the potential for a smoother ablation due to the overlapping beam and multidirectional scanning. Another advantage is the possibility of large treatment zones with multiple ablation profiles without the need for masks or apertures. The flying spot system is particularly suited for customized ablations by microprocessor-controlled "pixel-by-pixel" corneal ablations (50). However, the scanning system (particularly the flying spot) ablates such a small area of the cornea with each pulse that much longer treatment times are necessary as compared to the broad-beam systems. This longer treatment time may be associated with corneal dehydration and increased patient drift; however, active eye tracking devices, infrared or video-based, have been and are being developed for use in such systems.

SURFACE ABLATION: EARLY ANIMAL STUDIES OF PRK

The difficulty in finding a suitable and practical animal model to simulate the human cornea has hindered the study of the optical changes induced by excimer ablation. Of the animals available for practical laboratory evaluations, only primate and cat corneas have a Bowman's layer visible on light microscopy, and this is markedly thinner than in the human. The aggressive wound healing response demonstrated by most animal species, as compared to humans, has made direct laboratory comparison with, and prediction of, human responses questionable.

Marshall and colleagues (51,52) ablated 7-mm disks from monkey and rabbit corneas; smoother ablation surfaces and borders were found with 193 nm than those seen with 248 nm. The rabbit corneas developed much more haze than seen in the single monkey cornea studied. The average time for reepithelialization was 4 days. Krauss et al. (3) summarized unpublished data from Mandel and co-workers, who found opacification in the relatively deep ablation zone of monkey corneas within 1 week after exposure. Partial regression of the initial flattening as well as progressive corneal thinning was noted over several months. When using 3 mm disk ablations in monkeys, Marshall et al. (52) noted that although all ablation zones were initially clear, all but the shallowest ablations showed some degree of opacification by 1 month. However, by 6 months, all but the deepest ablations were free of haze. In these monkeys, the reepithelialization was complete by 1 to

2 days. Pathology analysis showed a stromal reaction with an increase in keratocytes and vacuole formation. However, by 8 months, the only evidence of disorganization was found in the stromal fibers under the epithelium. Marshall's group theorized that these disorganized stromal fibers acted as a "substitute" Bowman's membrane capable of supporting reepithelialization.

Hanna et al. (35,48,49) used a moving slit-laser system with rabbit corneas. Variable amounts of corneal haze were noted on pathology examination. Hanna et al. attributed this effect to variations in laser technique or uncontrolled differences in wound healing. Del Pero and colleagues (53) performed 4- to 7-mm myopic and hyperopic ablations in monkey corneas. All corneas were noted to have some degree of anterior stromal haze but this had diminished in all cases by the 12th month. An initial, unintended overcorrection was noted with gradual regression observed over a number of months. Fantes et al. (54) and McDonald and colleagues (45) confirmed the previously observed healing effects including the regression of the initial overcorrection, the rapid reepithelialization, the appearance and regression of stromal haze, and the increased activity of keratocytes within the ablation zone.

Tuft and colleagues (55) examined their results after ablations with rabbit corneas. A specific fluorescent dye was used to demonstrate new connective tissue at the stromal base with accompanying epithelial hyperplasia. The development of the connective tissue was reduced with the use of topical steroids after the ablation; however, the epithelial hyperplasia appeared unchanged. Goodman and co-workers (56) reported very different results with their contoured myopic ablations in rabbit corneas. No evidence of epithelial hyperplasia or new collagen formation was found in ablation depths under 50 μm. However, corneal opacification was noted in all ablations to 100 μm.

SURFACE ABLATION: EARLY HUMAN TRIALS OF PRK

With the nearly universal finding of at least some degree of corneal haze and resultant opacification in the animal studies, the human trials of PRK understandably focused on the incidence and time course of haze and permanent scarring. Cintron (57) asserted that in contrast to rabbit corneas, known to respond vigorously to wounds by synthesizing scar tissue, higher vertebrates, such as humans and monkeys, are more sluggish in healing. Although this might address some concerns related to the rabbit corneas, it did not help explain the haze and scarring that was seen in the studies involving monkeys.

In general, corneal clarity after PRK in humans is significantly better than that which was seen in the animal studies, including the nonhuman primates. The improved lasers and delivery methods of the commercial ophthalmic laser systems, compared to using scientific excimer systems in an optical research bench or even a prototype ophthalmic laser system, may contribute to this favorable observation.

L'Esperance et al. (58) and Taylor and colleagues (59,60) reported their results with the first PRK ablations on humans in the United States. The 5-mm ablations in 1987 were limited to blind eyes or eyes scheduled for enucleation. The initial results were similar to those seen in the animal studies with a 3-day reepithelialization, no recurrent erosions, minimal inflammation, and a mild anterior haze noted by the second week. The initial refractive correction was noted to regress by about 33%, and the histopathology on the enucleated eyes suggested new collagen formation. McDonald and co-workers' (61) initial myopic PRK in humans involved nine blind eyes whose range of refractive error was −1.74 to −11 D. Rapid reepithelialization was attained by the fifth day with no recurrent erosions. A third of the corneas were clear at the 6-month follow-up examination, whereas two thirds had only minimal haze. Once again, the initial refractive results in the 5-mm ablations were followed by a regression proportional to the degree of applied ablation.

Seiler and colleagues (62) published their results with PRK in blind and normally sighted humans. Reepithelialization occurred within 3 days and the initial overcorrection was followed by subsequent regression. The 3-month follow-up revealed that 12 of the 13 sighted eyes achieved correction within 1 D of that intended; 10 of those 13 eyes kept that level of correction at the 6-month exam. Stromal haze was present in most eyes at the 6-month exam but judged to be clinically insignificant. One patient's complaint of halos around lights at night after his 3.5-mm-diameter ablation illustrates the possible benefit of a larger ablation zone. Although large ablation zones would tend to reduce some of the glare or halos, the size of ablation is dictated by the mechanics of the laser delivery system and the concern of corneal effects with wider and deeper ablations.

CORNEAL HAZE AFTER PRK

The depth of the ablation for myopic correction increases linearly for the dioptric power but as a square exponential function of the diameter of the optical zone (63). Most of the early clinical studies indicated that the frequency and severity of corneal haze increased proportionally to the degree of attempted correction, especially over −6 D (64–67). Taylor and colleagues (68) reported an essentially linear relationship with mild corneal haze and attempted correction; however, more severe haze (grade II or higher) was uncommon in corrections under −10 D.

Although animal studies and early clinical observations in humans supported the idea that haze was correlated with ablation depth, problems with smaller optical zones began to surface. Halos and glare in dim light combined with the

lack of margin for error in centration with small optical zones led researchers to increase the ablation zone to 6 mm. Interestingly, the human corneas not only tolerated the increased ablation zone and resultant increased depth but actually showed a reduced incidence of haze, greater predictability of outcomes, and less tendency of regression in refractive effect (69–76). Anecdotal as well as published evidence has suggested that a large optical zone in conjunction with an aspheric peripheral "blend" zone will give improved results (73); however, other reports fail to confirm a beneficial effect from a multizone peripheral contour (76). At any rate, in the human cornea there appears to be a serendipitous effect of less corneal haze and improved predictability and stability associated with a 6-mm treatment zone in spite of the increased ablation depth (Fig. 75-1)

OBJECTIVE ANALYSIS OF CORNEAL HAZE AFTER PRK

Lohmann and co-workers (77,78) reported their observations using techniques for quantifying light scattering based on the Scheimpflung principle. Excellent visual function was demonstrated in PRK patients compared with spectacle- or contact lens-wearing controls. Their report further identified the importance of differentiating "back-scattering," which is visible to the observer, from "forward scattering," which may be noticed by the patient. Harrison and colleagues (79) found no evidence of forward scatter in 24 PRK patients 1 month after treatment; however, no patient had a haze score greater than 0.5. This was in contrast to Lohmann's findings of significant forward scatter 1 month after treatment, but their study used 4-mm optical zones compared to 6-mm zones used in the Harrison study.

Braunstein and co-workers (80) measured the backscatter and noted that such light was well correlated with the degree of clinical haze. It was further noted that ablations of less than 80 μm have much less backscatter than those with greater depths. Schallhorn and colleagues (81) used the stray-light meter developed by van den Berg and Ijspeert (82) to objectively measure the forward-scattered light falling on the macula in patients after PRK with 6-mm ablation zones. There was a 5% average increase in forward scatter at 1 month, but the measurements at 3, 6, 9, and 12 months were unchanged from preoperative levels. When measured after pupil dilation, however, the forward scatter was increased compared to the preoperative levels through the sixth month, but had returned to baseline by the 12-month exam.

Maldonado and associates (83) examined slit-lamp photographs of 40 eyes after PRK utilizing computerized digital analysis. Backscattered light showed a weak but positive correlation with the amount of haze and the degree of correction ranging from −6 to −22 D. Although the ini-

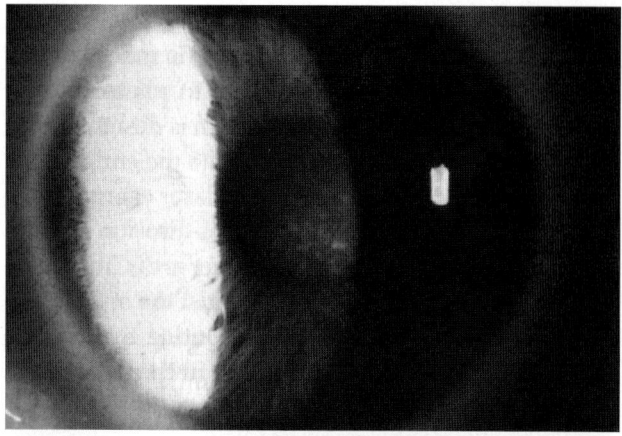

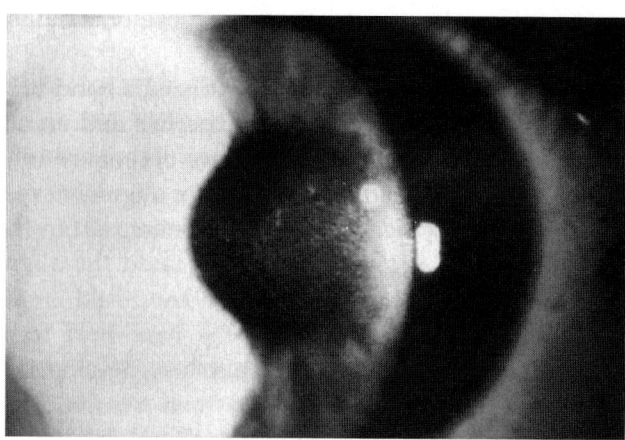

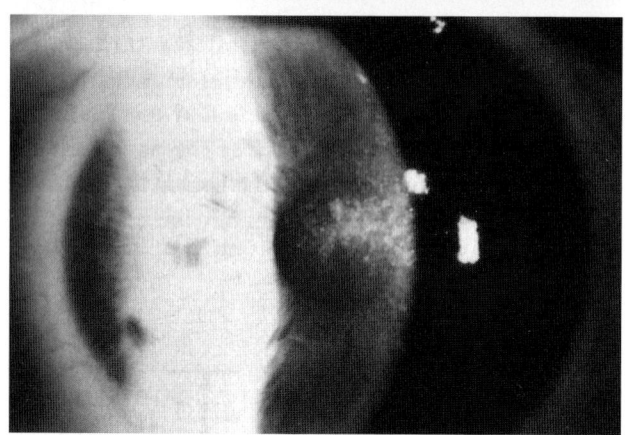

FIGURE 75-1. Postoperative haze formation. Subepithelial haze may present by 1 month postoperatively, peak between 3 and 6 months, and gradually subside by 12 to 18 months. The slides represent trace **(A)**, mild **(B)**, and moderate haze **(C)**. (From Thompson V, Seiler T. Excimer laser photorefractive keratectomy for myopia. In: Azar DT, ed. *Refractive surgery.* Stamford, CT: Appleton and Lange, 1997:427, with permission.)

tial appearance of haze appeared quite uniform throughout the ablation zone, there was a significantly greater reduction in central as compared to peripheral haze throughout the postoperative course.

BASIC TECHNIQUES FOR EXCIMER LASER PRK

Mechanical Epithelial Removal

To alter the refractive shape of the cornea, the stroma must be ablated. There are numerous methods of removing the overlying epithelium. One common method employs either a blunt or sharp surgical blade (Fig. 75-2A). The epithelium is manually removed, exercising caution not to nick Bowman's layer. The periphery is removed first, preserving the central epithelium until later in order to prevent dehydration of this critical area of ablation.

A variant of the manual debridement involves the use of a small, battery-operated rotating brush (Fig. 75-2B). This modification of an "electric toothbrush" used a brush head slightly larger than the desires ablation zone. The brush is designed to initially remove the peripheral epithelium, occasionally leaving a small central zone that can be easily removed with a blunt instrument (Fig. 75-2C,D).

Chemical Epithelial Removal

The desmosomes and hemidesmosomes of the epithelium can be loosened or broken with various chemical agents. Local application over the desired area of ablation may be accomplished through pledgets or cellulose sponges. Chemical leakage has led to the development of numerous "wells" that maintain the agent within the desired boundaries. Topical anesthetics (proparacaine and tetracaine) are effective but take 5 to 10 minutes to loosen the epithelium. Lidocaine, cocaine, and aminoglycosides have also been used but have largely been supplanted by ethanol. A 15% to 20% dilution can rapidly loosen the epithelium, often in 15 to 20 seconds.

Laser Epithelial Removal

The excimer laser itself can be used to remove the epithelium. This process, termed *transepithelial ablation*, involves ablating the epithelium over an area slightly larger than the desired stromal treatment zone. The technique employs the visualization of a slight cobalt blue fluorescence seen with ablation of epithelium but not stroma. The earlier, broad-beam laser systems were better suited for this approach as they could easily create a planar ablation also known as PTK. As epithelium can vary in thickness over the surface of the

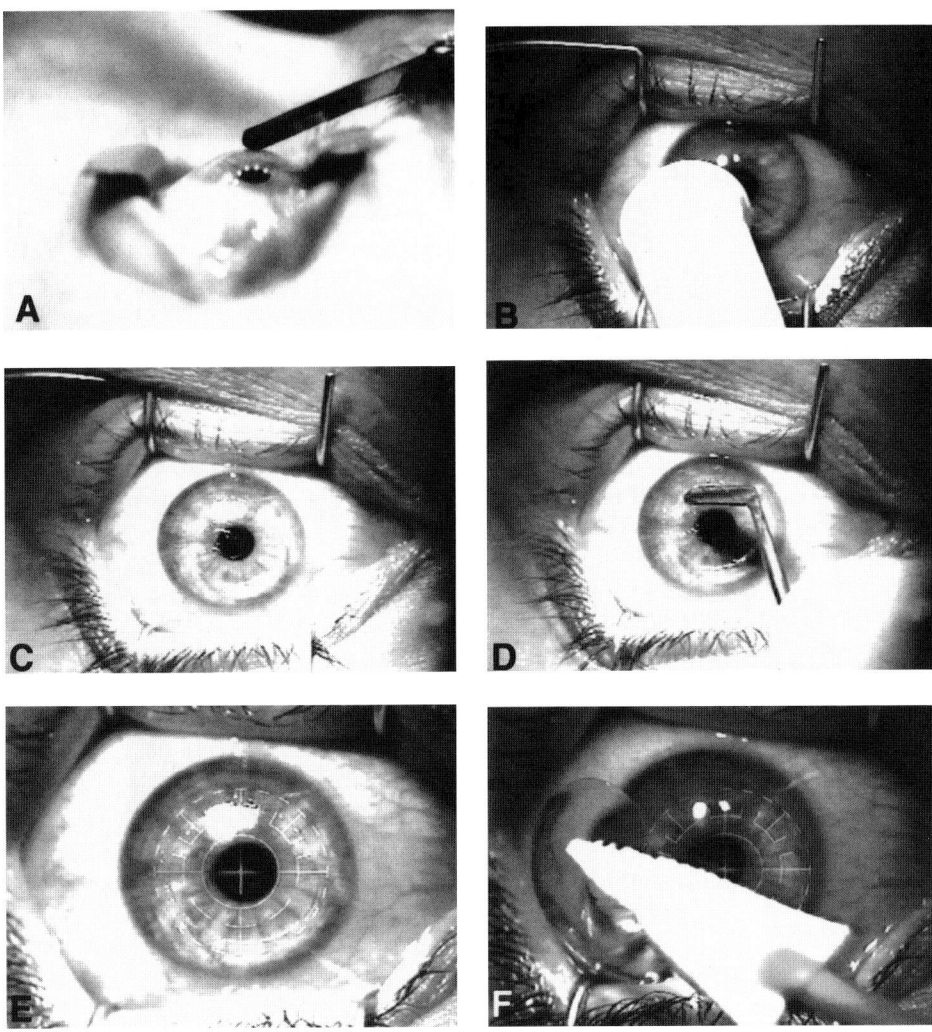

FIGURE 75-2. Technique of photorefractive keratectomy (PRK). Epithelium may be manually removed using a sharp blade **(A)** in a gentle "pulling" fashion or by using a rotating soft brush **(B)** similar to an "electric toothbrush." The brush technique often leaves a residual central portion of epithelium **(C)**, which can easily be removed with a blunt "hockey-stick" blade **(D)**. The exposed Bowman's membrane, and underlying stromal bed, is then ablated **(E)**. A bandage contact lens is placed over the ablated surface during the initial phase of reepithelialization **(F)**. (Fig. 75-2A from Thompson V, Seiler T. Excimer laser photorefractive keratectomy for myopia. In: Azar DT, ed. *Refractive surgery.* Stamford, CT: Appleton and Lange, 1997:423, with permission.)

cornea, a modification of the laser removal has emerged. Stopping the ablation just prior to, or at the moment of first penetration through the epithelium and then manually removing the residual basal layer has been termed *laser-scrape.* This technique avoids placing an irregular ablation pattern on the stroma as the laser "breaks" through a nonuniform epithelial layer. Flying spot laser systems and increasingly large treatment zones without accompanying large PTK options have limited the usefulness of this technique.

Laser Ablation

After Bowman's layer is exposed, the excimer laser is applied directly to the surface in order to remove the appropriate tissue (Fig. 75-2E). In recent years, numerous modifications

have been made regarding the actual mechanics of laser ablation, some of which were previously covered in the section on laser delivery systems. Myopic ablations involve primarily the central cornea, hyperopic ablations are more peripheral-based, and astigmatic ablations involve a combination. More precise applications of laser ablation have been accomplished through various eye-tracking systems (i.e., video based, radar based, or infrared based).

Postablation Treatment

The ablated surface is then covered with a bandage contact lens and postoperative medications are begun (Fig. 75-2F). Topical steroids and antibiotics are mainstays of treatment. Nonsteroidal antiinflammatory drops are to be used with caution. Oral narcotics may be necessary in the first few days. The epithelial defect resolves over 3 to 7 days, at which time the contact lens is removed. The antibiotics are discontinued after the epithelial defect heals and a slow taper of the steroids is thought to reduce the incidence of visually significant subepithelial haze.

RESULTS OF HUMAN PRK TRIALS

In the United States, about 2000 patients were treated with the excimer laser as part of the clinical studies supervised by the Food and Drug Administration (FDA). In the Summit phase III study (84), 90.7% of patients had uncorrected visual acuity of 20/40 or better, 66.3% achieving 20/20 or better, and less than 1% of eyes lost two lines of best corrected acuity. In the VISX FDA study (85), 85% of eyes had an uncorrected acuity of 20/40 or better, with only 1% losing two lines of best corrected visual acuity. Several other studies have followed eyes for at least 12 months after PRK (86–107). The number of eyes with uncorrected acuity of 20/40 or greater varied from 27% to 100%, with 34% to 100% of eyes within 1 D of emmetropia. Eyes losing two or more lines of best corrected acuity varied from 0 to 22%.

The primary motivation for patients seeking refractive surgery is to decrease their dependence on corrective optical devices (90,108). Achieving this goal depends on the patient's activities and daily visual requirements. Most patients with 20/25 or better visual acuity can easily function without corrective eyewear (109). The Summit phase III trial (84) demonstrated that 77% of patients achieved 20/25 or better uncorrected acuity after PRK, with the VISX FDA trial (85) achieving a similar level.

Dioptric refractive outcome is a less meaningful measure of successful outcome after PRK as corneal asphericity caused by PRK results in better visual acuity than expected simply based on the refractive outcome. For this reason, uncorrected visual acuity, as well as other measures of visual function, should be the primary parameters used in determining the outcome after PRK; however, 78% and 79% of the eyes evaluated in the Summit (84) and VISX FDA (85) trials were found to be within 1 D of emmetropia at 1 year. The refractive outcome, which was quite good early on, achieved stabilization by the sixth month after surgery for most patients other than the high myopes and by the ninth month in all patients.

Several important conclusions can be drawn from these studies. Initial attempts to avoid stromal haze and scarring led early investigators to use small treatment zones in order to avoid greater ablation depths. An increase in the incidence and severity of haze as well as loss of best corrected visual acuity appears to occur in increasing order when treating higher amounts of myopia (68). Greater amounts of attempted correction are also associated with decreased

predictability and less likelihood of attaining 20/40 or better uncorrected vision (68).

Succeeding studies demonstrated that haze and scarring were not as strongly correlated with ablation depth for the low and moderate degrees of myopia (72,76,77). Increasing the diameter of the ablation zone has not resulted in an increased incidence and severity of haze, and has actually reduced the initial overcorrection and subsequent regression seen in the first month (72). Focal irregularities of the corneal epithelium have been found at the edges of the treatment zone 6 months or more after PRK (78). Central epithelial hyperplasia may be caused by the smaller treatment zone combined with the steep edge of the ablation margin, which in turn may reduce the initial flattening of the central cornea, thus causing a greater regression. The broader profile in the larger ablation zones may be less likely to stimulate such an aggressive healing response. Therefore, it appears that using a 6-mm ablation diameter in PRK has reduced haze formation and increased refractive predictability (72). Another benefit of the larger treatment zone appears to be the reduction of complaints of poor night vision, glare, and halos (72,76–78,107,108, 110,111).

Overall, the effectiveness of PRK has markedly improved from 1987 to the present. During this time, the initial two excimer systems have gone through a number of upgrades and improvements, although quite a number of other excimer laser systems have been developed. The numerous studies have documented this progression in improved and predictable outcomes.

Therefore, PRK appears highly successful in achieving its stated objective. However, there are some patient concerns. Because the central cornea has to reepithelialize and then continue to smooth, vision may be affected for some weeks. Those over 40 may particularly be bothered by a degree of initial overcorrection in the first 1 to 3 months, which was the most common reason given in one study as to why patients did not seek PRK in their second eye (112). The next most common complaints in patients who were disappointed with PRK involved poor night vision, glare, and halos (113).

Despite the aforementioned drawbacks, patient acceptance of PRK is high. Further refinement in techniques, improvements in the contour/edges of the ablation zone leading to better visual outcomes, advances in or elimination of the need for pharmacologic manipulation in wound healing, and improved postoperative pain control could lead to improved refractive outcomes and even greater acceptance of PRK.

LASER-ASSISTED *IN-SITU* KERATOMILEUSIS (LASIK) AND SURFACE ABLATION: PROS AND CONS

PRK is quite a safe procedure; however, major concerns center on the associated postoperative discomfort, variable subepithelial haze, and a prolonged visual recovery period.

Epithelial removal, along with some variety of inflammatory cytokines, which may be produced during ablation in PRK, are theorized to be major factors in the development of such concerns. The desire to avoid some of PRK's drawbacks has led to LASIK's becoming the most common procedure for laser correction of ammetropia. In fact, LASIK is one of the most commonly performed of all surgical procedures (114,115). This procedure has enjoyed several advantages over PRK for a number of reasons. By ablating under a 160- to 180-μm flap of epithelium and stroma, LASIK boasts rapid visual recovery, almost negligible postoperative discomfort, minimal postoperative haze, and a relatively easy route to enhance residual refractive errors (lifting rather than recutting a LASIK flap).

But LASIK is not without its complications and possible contraindications. Recent reports have noted a number of drawbacks, primarily related to the surgically induced flap. Free caps (116), epithelial defects (116), incomplete or irregular flaps created by the microkeratome (116,117), flap wrinkles (Fig. 75-3) (118), microbial keratitis (117, 119–124), epithelial ingrowth (125–128), flap melt (129), interface debris (116), diffuse lamellar keratitis (130–133), corneal ectasia (134–138), and postsurgical traumatic flap dislocations (139–148) are among the notable concerns with LASIK.

In addition to the flap-related complications, LASIK may be relatively unsafe in a number of medical conditions. Anterior basement membrane dystrophies and recurrent erosions may be aggravated with LASIK, whereas surface ablation is one of the therapeutic treatment modalities for such conditions (149). Those with retinal pathology may be at greater risk with LASIK compared to surface ablation (150). Lee and colleagues (151) suggested that moderate to severe dry-eye patients may do worse after LASIK than with surface ablation.

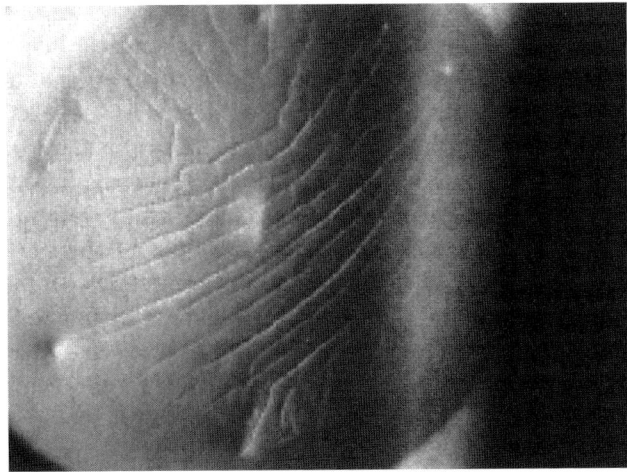

FIGURE 75-3. Wrinkles seen in LASIK flap on day 1 examination. (From Buratto L, Brint S. Complications of LASIK. In: Buratto L, Brint S, eds. *LASIK, surgical techniques and complications.* Thorofare, NJ: SLACK, 2000:227, with permission.)

A patient's corneal shape/thickness may be a relative contraindication for LASIK. Those patients with irregular astigmatism who do not fit the rigid criteria for keratoconus may want to avoid refractive surgery altogether; however, a surface ablation may provide a safer and more predictable option for those desiring laser correction (152–154). Corneas too thin to safely permit LASIK (generally require 250 to 300 μm remaining under flap after ablation) may do better with surface ablation.

Ocular anatomy and/or previous surgery may impact the type of refractive procedure. Patients with flat corneas (40 to 42 D), poor exposure, or deep-set orbits may be more likely to experience keratome-related complications. Anteriorly positioned scleral buckles may not allow the suction ring of LASIK to be correctly positioned. Some studies have even suggested that PRK may be better than LASIK in treating residual refractive error after phakic intraocular lens (IOL) surgery (155,156) as well as in some types of re-treatments after previous refractive surgery (RK, LASIK) (157,158), although there is substantial debate particularly regarding PRK after LASIK.

Another factor in the choice of refractive procedure may be the surgeon's ability. Yo and co-workers (159) concluded that the inexperienced and/or occasional refractive surgeon may do better with the less complicated PRK than with LASIK.

Lastly, a recommendation for PRK over LASIK may be due to the patient's lifestyle or profession: military personnel, athletes involved in contact sports, other professions with a high likelihood of ocular trauma, and low degrees of myopia with the attendant lower risk of haze formation may do better with PRK.

The benefits of PRK are many. In addition to avoiding all microkeratome-related complications, surface ablation may be more versatile regarding the above-mentioned medical conditions, most anatomic anomalies, many situations involving prior surgery, in cases with lesser experienced surgeons, and with most patient lifestyles/professions in which ocular trauma is to be expected. Moreover, with regard to visual acuity, recent clinical studies have failed to show any significant superiority of LASIK over PRK other than during the first few weeks after surgery (115, 160–166). However, some clinicians and patients would prefer an alternative to PRK.

AN ALTERNATIVE SURFACE-BASED ABLATION

Laser subepithelial keratomileusis (LASEK) may be just such a reasonable alternative for patients in whom PRK might have been the recommended procedure. With the advent and popularity of LASIK, some predicted that surface-based ablation (PRK) would eventually disappear. However, it has continued to survive and, with the rising popularity of LASEK, it has been revisited as a viable alternative for laser vision correction. Although PRK and LASEK require more initial follow-up, many clinicians performing these procedures are pleased with the excellent results obtained with the newer-generation lasers as well as the avoidance of a number of major complications associated with LASIK (167–169).

A number of the attractive benefits of LASIK are potentially being accomplished through LASEK, including reduced postoperative discomfort, rapid visual recovery (often within 24 hours), minimal stromal haze, and a more rapid stabilization of refractive effect. As previously mentioned, studies using more modern generation laser systems have failed to demonstrate any significant superiority for LASIK over PRK or LASEK other than in the first few weeks after surgery (115,160–166).

Techniques of LASEK

With any rapidly evolving technology, texts and atlas entries may appear outdated by the time of publication. That is the case with refractive surgery in general, and LASEK in particular. At present, there appear to be two major techniques for performing LASEK. Azar and colleagues (170) described the evolution of their technique, first performed in 1996. Based on the literature support for alcohol-assisted epithelial removal in PRK (171–174), the epithelium under a semisharp circular well is exposed to 18% alcohol for 25 seconds. The cornea receives a number of positioning marks prior to alcohol exposure. A jeweler's forceps or modified Vannas scissors is inserted under the epithelium and traced around the delineated margin, leaving two to three clock-hour positions of intact margin. The resulting loosened epithelium is then peeled back as a single sheet using a Merocel sponge. After standard laser ablation, a 30-gauge irrigating cannula with balanced salt solution (BSS) is used to hydrate the stroma and epithelial flap. The epithelial sheet is then gently repositioned using the cannula with intermittent irrigation. The epithelium is carefully realigned using the preplaced positioning marks and allowed to dry for 5 minutes.

In 2000, Camellin and Cimberle (175) reported on their experience after 1 year of performing LASEK. This technique involves an epithelial preincision using a specialized trephine with a 70-mm-deep calibrated blade designed to leave an 80-degree hinge at the 12 o'clock position (Fig. 75-4A). A silicone irrigator sleeve or metal "well" is used for a 30-second exposure using 20% alcohol (Fig. 75-4B). After alcohol removal (Fig. 75-4C) and irrigation with BSS, an epithelial microhoe is used to gently detach and fold the epithelial sheet back at the 12 o'clock position (Fig. 75-4D,E). Standard laser ablation is then completed, after which a repositioning spatula is used to reapproximate the position of the epithelial sheet (Fig. 75-4F,G). A bandage contact lens is placed at the completion of the epithelial repositioning (Fig. 75-4H).

Along with the two major techniques, several others are gaining popularity. Vinciguerra and McDonald's (176) butterfly technique involves cutting the epithelium in the paracentral meridian and reflecting outwardly toward the limbus, thus preserving the connection to the stem cells for 360 degrees. Vinciguerra and McDonald's viscoelastic dissection uses a standard microkeratome suction ring to help detach and reflect the epithelium without any alcohol exposure. Pallikaris (177) has described epi-LASIK, in which he modified his original LASIK microkeratome to create a flap that only involves the epithelium. Claringbold (178) has been involved with the first U.S. clinical trials of LASEK using the epithelial microkeratome. The initial reports are quite positive and may be due to the decreased operating time, lack of alcohol-assisted epithelial removal, and more predictive consistency between patients.

Perioperative medications are generally similar in all the various techniques. Topical nonsteroidal antiinflammatory, antibiotic, and steroid drops are applied at the completion of the procedure. Oral pain medication is prescribed and patients are instructed to use artificial tears on an as-needed basis. The contact lens is generally removed between days 3 and 7 based on the patient's progress. Antibiotic medication is usually continued for 1 week and steroid drops are often tapered over the first 2 to 4 weeks.

Viability of Epithelial Cells After LASEK

Whether this epithelial flap is viable tissue that reintegrates into the surface epithelium or is simply a nonviable biologic "bandage" continues to be a source of substantial debate. Specimens of LASEK for pathologic examination are understandably difficult or impossible to obtain. Azar and co-workers (170) used transmission electron microscopy to analyze specimens obtained from patients undergoing alcohol-assisted epithelial removal associated with PRK (Fig. 75-5). Intact epithelial cells were found without accompanying edematous cells or abnormal vacuoles. Discontinuities and irregularities were noted in the basement membrane; however, fragments of the basement membrane were found attached to basal epithelial cells. No evidence of Bowman's layer or corneal stromal cells was found in the specimens. Of note, no irregularity in the ultrastructure of the desmosomes and hemidesmosomes was observed.

The basement membrane is believed to provide stability and support to the epithelium. This support helps keep the epithelium intact during manipulation, thus maintaining the integrity and viability of the corneal epithelium. Therefore, the finding of the basement membrane adherent to the basal epithelial cells after alcohol-assisted removal would appear significant. Epithelial readherence to the ablated stroma may be enhanced through the presence of the desmosomes, which might act as an anchoring device.

Chen and associates (179) analyzed the response of cultured human epithelial cells after exposure to alcohol for

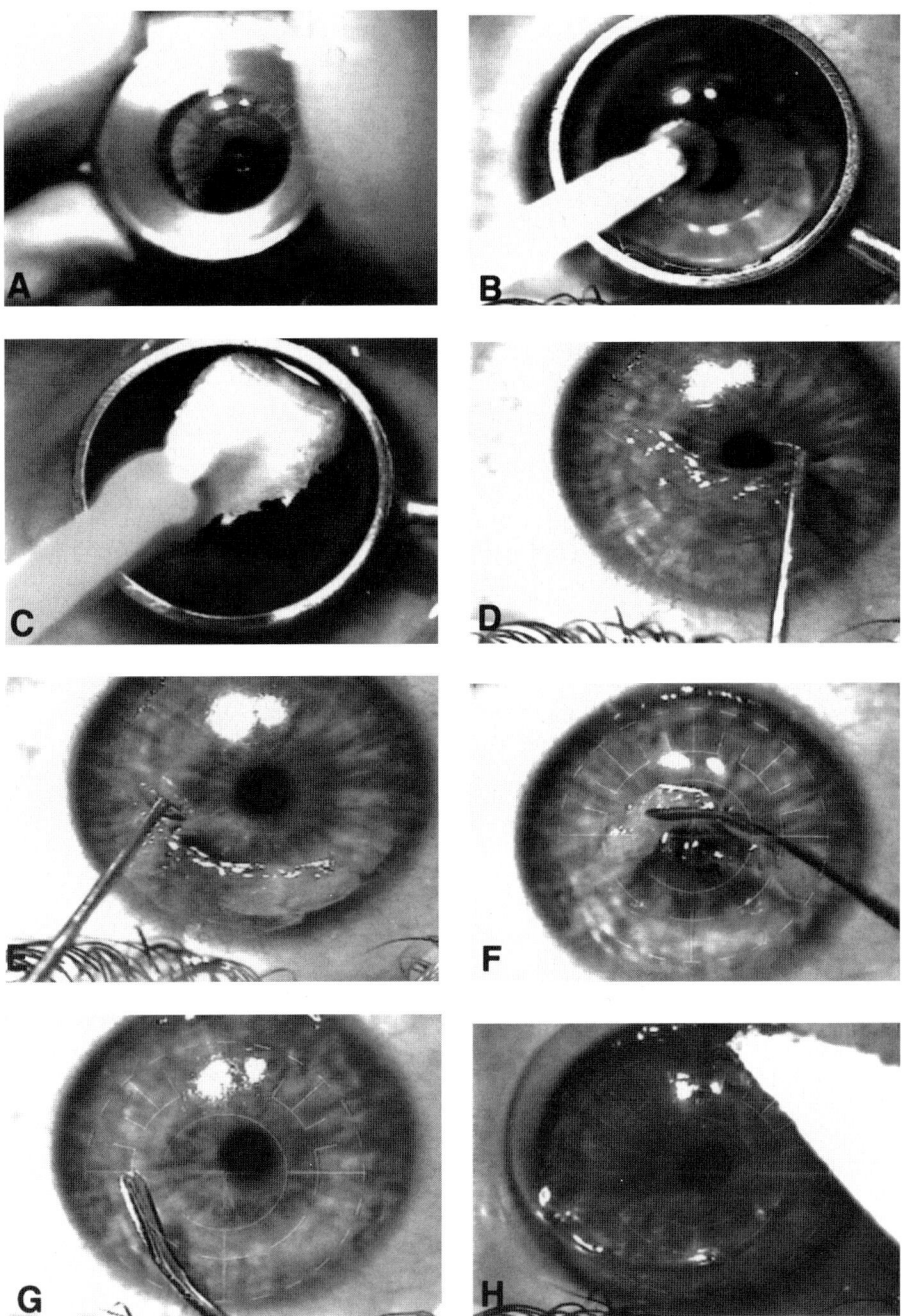

FIGURE 75-4. Technique of LASEK. An initial incision is made with a guarded 75-μm epithelial trephine **(A)**. A well is filled with dilute ethanol in order to weaken the intraepithelial bonds **(B)**. The ethanol is removed after 20 to 30 seconds using a methylcellulose sponge **(C)**. The epithelial flap is manually reflected away from the periphery **(D)**, eventually toward a hinged location outside of the ablation zone **(E)**. After the surface ablation, the epithelium is repositioned toward the center **(F)**, eventually being smoothed back into its original position **(G)**. A bandage contact lens is placed at the end of the procedure **(H)**.

varying lengths of time and concentrations (Fig. 75-6). Cell viability, determined by epithelial migration and attachment, was significantly reduced with alcohol concentrations above 20% and with exposure times greater than 30 seconds (70% viable after 30 second exposure, 10.45% viable after 40 seconds). These cultured cells were in a monolayer; thus the actual human multilayered LASEK flap may exhibit even greater degrees of viability *in vivo*.

Gabler's group (180) examined corneal epithelial flaps in recently obtained human cadaver eyes; 20% alcohol produced a cleavage plane between the lamina densa and Bowman's layer. If exposure times were held to 30 seconds or

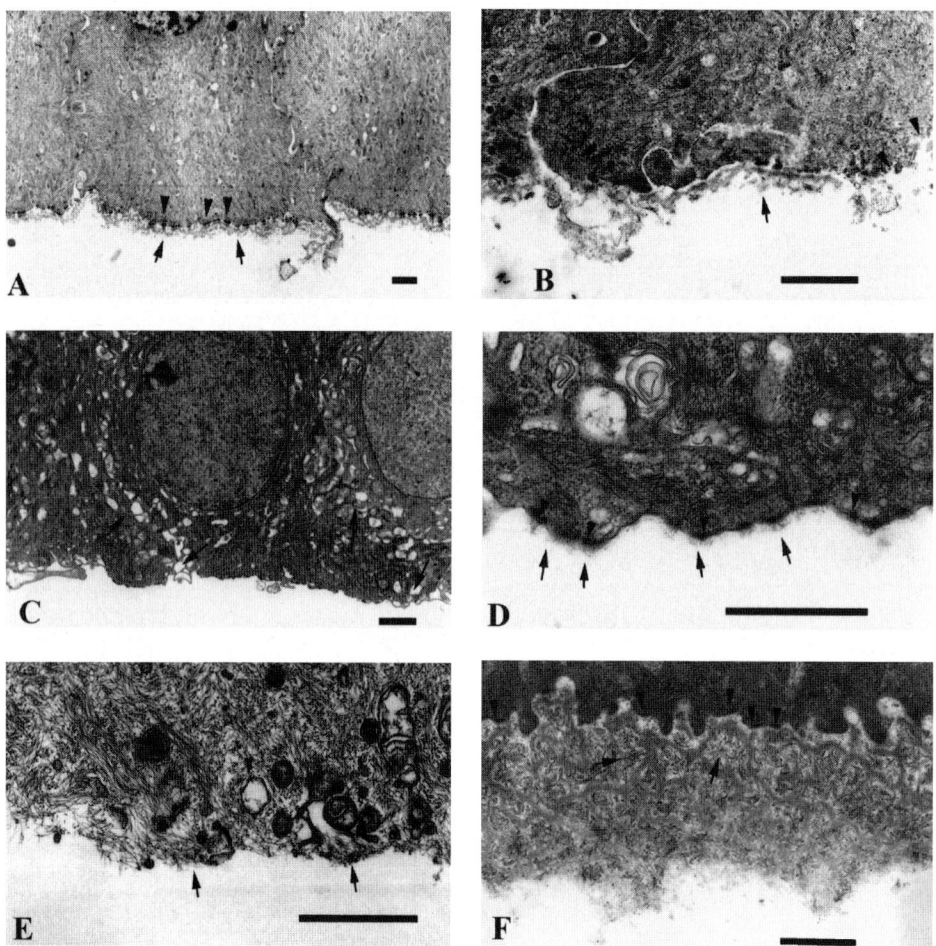

FIGURE 75-5. Transmission electron micrographs of human epithelium removed after 25-second application of 20% ethanol. The basement membrane (BM) is shown in various degrees of separation. Basal epithelial cells with an intact BM *(arrows)* and hemidesmosomal attachments *(arrowheads)* can be seen **(A).** The same specimen at higher magnification **(B)** reveals a focal area of irregular BM *(arrow)* and basal cell membrane disruption *(arrowheads).* Autophagic vacuoles *(arrows)* can be seen in some slides **(C).** Less electron-dense hemidesmosomes *(arrowheads)* were found in areas where disruption of the BM *(arrows)* occurred under the basal cell layer **(D).** Some specimens revealed disrupted basal cell and basement membranes *(arrows);* autophagic vacuoles *(arrowhead)* were present throughout the cytoplasm **(E).** A duplicated BM was present in some specimens **(F).** A network of anchoring fibrils is present between layers of basal lamina *(arrows).* The basal cell membrane shows numerous electron-dense hemidesmosomal attachments *(arrowheads).* (From Chen CC, Chang JH, Lee JB, et al. Human corneal epithelial cell viability and morphology after dilute alcohol exposure. *Invest Ophthalmol Vis Sci* 2002;43:2595, with permission.)

less, 80% of epithelial cells demonstrated viability. Exposure times up to 45 seconds led to viability in 46% of cells. The 46% viability compared to Chen's 11% may represent the multilayered nature of the cadaver "flaps." Gabler's group's overall findings suggested the alcohol produced viable epithelium with cleavage of the anchoring fibrils between Bowman's layer and the epithelial basement membrane.

Potential Advantages of LASEK

LASEK has been increasingly associated with many of the healing advantages previously only seen with LASIK. The advantages, actual and theoretical, are numerous: potentially less pain and a more rapid visual recovery than seen

with PRK, elimination of the microkeratome complications/effects seen with LASIK, and no postoperative flap trauma seen months and even years after LASIK (139–148). A reduction in postoperative haze, with LASEK as compared to PRK, has been noted anecdotally but will require further investigation regarding statistical significance.

LASEK may be a reasonable alternative for those patients for whom PRK might have been the recommended procedure. Although LASEK and PRK generally require more initial follow-up than LASIK, many clinicians performing these procedures are pleased with the excellent results obtained with the newer generation lasers while avoiding a number of complications associated with LASIK (168–170). Some clinicians have been so impressed with this procedure that

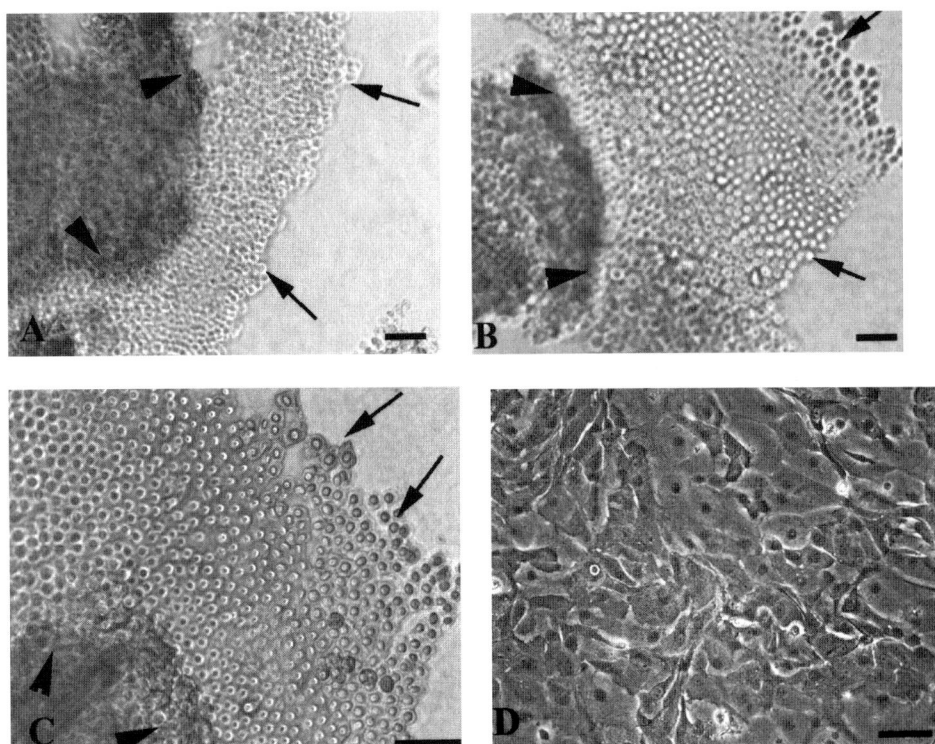

FIGURE 75-6. Micrographs of tissue culture generated from epithelial specimens exposed to 20% ethanol for 25 seconds **(A-C)** and one specimen derived from primary epithelial cell culture **(D)**. The *arrows* represent the outer edge of epithelial proliferation, and the *arrowheads* demonstrate the original border. Epithelial proliferation was noted at day 1 **(A)**, increasing in cellular attachment and outgrowth until day 15 **(B)**. Higher magnification at day 15 highlights the epithelial cell contours and adherence to the culture plate **(C)**. The epithelial cells from the primary culture show a more elongated appearance **(D)**. (From Chen CC, Chang JH, Lee JB, et al. Human corneal epithelial cell viability and morphology after dilute alcohol exposure. *Invest Ophthalmol Vis Sci* 2002;43:2595, with permission.)

LASEK is their preferred alternative in some or all of their patients originally considering LASIK (178).

Results of LASEK Surgery

No technique will replace another unless the outcome is similar and/or the benefits outweigh the risk. Although PRK lost favor when LASIK demonstrated early healing advantages, LASEK is increasingly seen as a reasonable alternative to LASIK.

Camellin and Cimberle (175) provided some of the earliest reports on LASEK outcomes with 249 eyes. No pain was experienced by 44% of cases during the first 24 hours after surgery. By the 10th postoperative day, 90% of patients had achieved at least 80% of their preoperative best corrected visual acuity. Intraoperative flap management was reportedly easy in 60% of cases, average in 28%, and difficult in 12%.

Azar and colleagues (170) found that epithelial defects were present in 63% and 9% of eyes on days 1 and 3, respectively. Postoperative pain was reported by 53% on day 1 and only 18% by day 3. All eyes examined at 1 week had uncorrected visual acuity of 20/40 or better, with 64% at 20/25 or better. At the 1 month exam, 92% of eyes examined had uncorrected visual acuity of 20/25 or better.

A spherical equivalent within 0.50 D of intended was measured in 58% of eyes at 1 month and in 100% of eyes measured at 12 months. Postoperative pain and recurrent erosions were not reported after the 1-week examination.

Kornilovsky (181) reported on LASEK in one eye of 12 patients compared to having PRK or LASIK on the second eye. Flap management was reportedly easy in 42%, average in 33%, and difficult in 25%. No pain was reported in 50% of the LASEK eyes, mild discomfort in 33%, and frank pain in 17%. The authors further reported that the visual and refractive results after LASEK were similar to those seen in the PRK- and LASIK-treated eyes.

Lohmann and co-workers (182) performed LASEK on 21 eyes between −2 and −15 D of myopia. Up to 6 months of follow-up revealed that all eyes were within 1 D of emmetropia and no haze was noted in any cornea on slit-lamp biomicroscopy.

Rouweyha and colleagues (183) reported their results with 58 eyes treated for myopia between −1.50 and −14.75 D compared to randomly selected LASIK-treated eyes as controls. Patients were followed up to 6 months. Uncorrected visual acuity of 20/40 or better was seen in 45%, 83%, 85%, and 89% of eyes at 1 day, 1 week, 2 weeks, and 1 month, respectively. At 6 months, 97% of eyes achieved an uncorrected visual acuity of 20/40 or better, with 73% at 20/20 or better. Visually significant haze was noted in four eyes at 6 months. The authors concluded that LASEK was a safe, effective, and comparable alternative to LASIK, even for higher amounts of myopia. However, given the potential for late-onset scarring after PRK in high myopia, many investigators may avoid the routine use of LASEK in higher myopes until further studies indicate a safety profile.

Condon (184) presented the results of 122 LASIK-treated eyes, 61 PRK-treated eyes, and 38 LASEK-treated eyes. LASIK was found to produce slight undercorrections, whereas LASEK was associated with slight overcorrections. Condon concluded that LASEK avoided a number of the drawbacks of PRK and was a reasonable alternative to LASIK in low degrees of myopia.

Claringbold (185) reported on 222 consecutive eyes treated with LASEK for myopia between −1.25 and −11.25 D. The uncorrected visual acuity was 20/40 or better in 84% and 98% at day 4 and 2 weeks, respectively. Twelve-month follow-up was noted on 84 eyes, showing uncorrected visual acuity (UCVA) of 20/25 or better in 100%, 20/20 or better in 81%, and 20/15 or better in 19%. There was no loss in best spectacle-corrected acuity and no eye required re-treatment.

Lee and co-workers (186) detailed their results in 27 patients (54 eyes) having LASEK in one eye and PRK in the other. The epithelium was completely healed by day 5 in the LASEK eyes and day 4 in the PRK eyes, with a mean of 3.64 and 3.18 days, respectively (not statistically significant). A statistically significant difference was noted in pain scores of 1.63 and 2.36 for LASEK and PRK, respectively; 59% of LASEK eyes and 37% of PRK eyes had achieved 20/25 or better UCVA by the first week; at 3 months, this level was achieved in 63% of LASEK and 56% of PRK eyes. The mean spherical refraction showed no statistically significant differences during the 1 week, 1 month, and 3 month examinations.

Although Sher and colleagues (187) reported that corneal haze peaked 3 months after PRK, Lee found that such haze was less at 3 months than that observed at 1 month in both PRK and LASEK. The statistically significant difference in haze found at 1 month with LASEK (score of 0.46) compared to PRK (score of 0.86) was no longer evident at 3 months. Interestingly, 63% of the patients preferred the LASEK procedure due to a more rapid visual recovery, decreased postoperative discomfort, and better visual acuity.

The vast majority of reports and studies have found LASEK quite favorable, even with higher refractive errors, when compared directly to PRK and LASIK. However, Litwak et al. (188) published contrary findings 1 month after 25 patients had PRK in one eye and LASEK in the other. Although there was no difference in corneal haze (none found in any patient), the patients' subjective responses overwhelmingly favored PRK to LASEK due to subjectively better visual acuity and less discomfort. Of note is the fact that the 20%

ethanol was left in place for 45 seconds rather than the 30 seconds used in most of the literature reports. Whether this had a contributory effect on the patient's response is uncertain; however, Chen et al. (179) and Gabler's group (180) noted epithelial cell survival rates of 70% to 80% with a 30-second exposure, but between 11% and 54% viability when the exposure was extended to 45 seconds.

The specific events responsible for the reduced haze in LASEK are not known at this time, but theories center on the role of matrix metalloproteinases, tear fluid transforming growth factor-β (189), or some other cellular agent. The reason for the decreased discomfort is not altogether clear either; however, the epithelial flap may act as a better tolerated biologic "bandage lens," which serves to reduce the mechanically abrasive action of the eyelid.

WAVEFRONT-GUIDED ABLATIONS

Wavefront-based corneal analysis has become increasingly popular. In early 2003, the FDA began approving the use of wavefront-guided ablations. Wavefront-guided refractive surgery allows for very fine differential adjustments to the ablated surface and has thus raised the question of which surgical approach takes the greatest advantage of this technology.

McDonald (190) presented her initial experience with wavefront-guided ablations in 1999, suggesting that results were better with PRK than with LASIK. A number of factors may be responsible for such results. Theoretically, the fine adjustments (often only a few micrometers different from the surround) are more likely to be diminished with a 160- to 180-μm flap repositioned over the ablated surface than with an epithelial covering. The absence of a LASIK flap may contribute to the advantages of LASEK in achieving customized laser ablations. It is likely that the predictability of wavefront-guided laser ablations may be greater with surface-based procedures than with LASIK; however, it is uncertain whether these differences would be better appreciated by allowing the surface to reepithelialize, as with PRK, or by repositioning the much thinner epithelial "flap," as with LASEK.

These questions require further observation and, indeed, several clinical trials are underway. However, in the absence of results from prospective, randomized studies of wavefront-guided (or custom) LASIK versus LASEK, one may hypothesize that the surface ablation is the ideal procedure for customized refractive surgery.

CONCLUSION

Although LASEK involves longer surgical times than PRK and more involved follow-up than LASIK, it is a fairly straightforward, inexpensive, reproducible technique that may offer less discomfort, faster visual recovery, and less subepithelial haze.

TABLE 75-1. SAMPLE SUMMARIES OF PHOTOREFRACTIVE KERATECTOMY (PRK) STUDIES FOR MYOPIA

Author of Study	Year of Report	No. of Eyes	Range (SE in D)	UCVA ≥20/20 (%)	UCVA ≥20/25 (%)	CVA ≥20/40 (%)	Loss of ≥2 Lines BCVA (%)
Tengroth et al. (99)	1993	420	−1.5 to −7.5	NR	NR	87	NR
Talley et al. (193)	1994	91	−1 to −7.5	NR	72	92	0
Hardten et al. (194)	1994	134	−1.6 to −14.3	NR	49	81	4
Thompson et al. (FDA Summit) (84)	1995	576	−1.5 to −6	66	NR	91	<1
Seiler and McDonnell (FDA VISX) (85)	1995	691	−1 to −6	NR	NR	85	1
Hamburg-Nystom et al. (105)	1996	456	−1.25 to −7.5	NR	NR	91	NR
Schallhorn et al. (81)	1996	60	−2 to −5.5	100	100	100	<1
Shah and Hersh (195)	1996	45	−1.5 to −6	62	NR	100	0
Pop and Payette (196)	2000	107	−1 to −9.5	86	NR	NR	0
Stevens et al. (197)	2002	198	−0.5 to −5.9	82	NR	97	0
Dausch et al. (198)	2003	30	−1.9 to −8	83	NR	NR	0

D, diopters; UCVA, uncorrected visual acuity; BCVA, best corrected visual acuity; NR, not reported; SE, spherical equivalent.

The benefits of this technique may outweigh the risks, especially given the fact that if one cannot complete the creation of the flap, the surgery can be converted to the already proven safe and predictable PRK (Table 75-1), whose increased postoperative discomfort may be decreased through the use of dilute topical proparacaine (191). LASEK may extend the therapeutic possibilities in the numerous cases where LASIK may be contraindicated. The safety, efficacy, predictability, and epithelial adhesion mechanism of this surgical technique must be confirmed through more extensive, long-term evaluations with greater patient populations (192).

REFERENCES

1. Seiler T, Fantes FE, Waring GO, et al. Laser corneal surgery. In: Waring GO, ed. *Refractive keratotomy.* St. Louis: CV Mosby 1992:669–745.
2. Waring GO. *Refractive keratotomy for myopia and astigmatism.* St. Louis: CV Mosby 1992:830–859.
3. Krauss JM, Puliafito CA, Steinert RF. Laser interactions with the cornea. *Surv Ophthalmol* 1986;31:37–53.
4. Searles SK, Hart GA. Stimulated emission at 281.8 nm from XeBr. *Appl Phys Lett* 1975;27:243–245.
5. Srinivasan R, Leigh WJ. Ablative photodecompensation on poly(ethylene teraphthalate) films. *J Am Chem Soc* 1982;104:6784–6785.
6. Deutsch TF, Geis MW. Self-developing UV photoresist using excimer laser exposure. *J Appl Phys* 1983;54:7201–7204.
7. Koren G, Yeh JT. Emission spectra, surface quality, and mechanism of excimer laser etching of polyimide films. *Appl Phys Lett* 1984;44:1112–1114.
8. Srinivasan R, Mayne-Banton V. Self-developing photoetching of poly(ethylene teraphthalate) films by far-ultraviolet excimer laser radiation. *Appl Phys Lett* 1983;41:576–578.
9. Srinivasan R. Kinetics of ablative photodecompensation of organic polymers in the far-ultraviolet (193 nm). *J Vac Sci Tech B* 1983;1:923–926.

10. Keyes T, Clarke RH, Isner JM. Theory of photoablation and its implications for laser phototherapy. *J Phys Chem* 1985;89:4194–4196.
11. Garrison BJ, Srinivasan R. Microscopic model for the ablative photodecompensation of polymers by far-ultraviolet radiation (193 nm). *Appl Phys Lett* 1984;44:849–851.
12. Jellinek HHG, Srinivasan R. Theory of etching of polymers by far-ultraviolet, high-intensity pulsed laser and long-term irradiation. *J Phys Chem* 1984;88:3048–3051.
13. Taboada J, Mikesell GW, Reed RD. Response of the corneal epithelium to KrF excimer laser pulses. *Health Phys* 1981;40:677–683.
14. Taboada J, Archibald CJ. An extreme sensitivity in the corneal epithelium to far UV ArF excimer laser pulses. Proceedings of the Scientific Program of the Aerospace Medical Association, San Antonio, TX, 1981.
15. Trokel SL, Srinivasan R, Braren B. Excimer laser surgery of the cornea. *Am J Ophthalmol* 1983;96:710–715.
16. Seiler T, Wollensak J. *In vivo* experiments with the excimer laser—Technical parameters and healing processes. *Ophthalmologica* 1986;192:65–70.
17. Srinivasan R, Sutcliffe E. Dynamics of the ultraviolet laser ablation of corneal tissue. *Am J Ophthalmol* 1987;103:470–471.
18. Kruger RR, Trokel SL, Schubert HD. Interaction of ultraviolet laser light with the cornea. *Invest Ophthalmol Vis Sci* 1985;26:1455–1464.
19. Seiler T, McDonnell PJ. Excimer laser photorefractive keratectomy. *Surv Ophthalmol* 1995;40:89–118.
20. Kahle G, Stadter H, Seiler T, et al. Gas chromatographic and mass spectroscopic analysis of excimer and erbium:yttrium aluminum garnet laser-ablated human cornea. *Invest Ophthalmol Vis Sci* 1992;33:2180–2184.
21. Bende T, Seiler T, Wollensak J. Side effects in excimer corneal surgery: corneal thermal gradients. *Graefes Arch Clin Exp Ophthalmol* 1988;226:277–280.
22. Puliafito CA, Stern D, Krueger RR, et al. High-speed photography of excimer laser ablation of the cornea. *Arch Ophthalmol* 1987;105:1255–1259.
23. Gorodetsky G, Kazyaka TG, Melcher RL, et al. Calorimetric and acoustic study of ultraviolet laser ablation of polymers. *Appl Phys Lett* 1985;46:828–830.

24. Kruger RR, Trokel SL. Quantitation of corneal ablation by ultraviolet laser light. *Arch Ophthalmol* 1985;103:1741–1742.

25. Puliafito CA, Wong K, Steinert RF. Quantitative and ultrastructural studies of excimer laser ablation of the cornea at 193 and 248 nanometers. *Lasers Surg Med* 1987;7:155–159.

26. McCann J, Ames BN. Detection of carcinogens as mutagens in the salmonella/microsome test: assay of 300 chemicals: discussion. *Proc Natl Acad Sci USA* 1976;73:950–954.

27. Smith KC. Ultraviolet radiation effects on molecules and cells. In: Smith KC, ed. *The science of photobiology.* New York: Plenum 1985:113–141.

28. Nuss RC, Puliafito CA, Dehm EJ. Unscheduled DNA synthesis following excimer laser ablation of the cornea *in vivo*. *Invest Ophthalmol Vis Sci* 1987;28:287–294.

29. Kochevar IE. Cytotoxicity and mutagenicity of excimer laser radiation. *Lasers Surg Med* 1989;9:440–445.

30. Muller-Stolzenburg NW, Schrumder S, Buchwald HJ, et al. UV exposure of the lens during 193nm excimer laser corneal surgery. *Arch Ophthalmol* 1990;108:915–916.

31. Puliafito CA, Steinert RF, Deutsch TF, et al. Excimer laser ablation of the cornea and lens: experimental studies. *Ophthalmology* 1985;92:741–748.

32. Kerr-Muir MG, Trokel SL, Marshall J, et al. Ultrastructural comparison of conventional surgical and argon fluoride excimer laser keratectomy. *Am J Ophthalmol* 1987;103:448–453.

33. Peyman GA, Kuszak JR, Weckstrom K, et al. Effects of XeCl excimer laser on the eyelid and anterior segment structures. *Arch Ophthalmol* 1986;104:118–122.

34. Dehm EJ, Puliafito CA, Adler CM, et al. Corneal endothelial injury following excimer laser ablation at 193 and 248 nm. *Arch Ophthalmol* 1986;104:1364–1368.

35. Hanna KD, Pouliquen Y, Waring GO, et al. Corneal stromal wound healing in rabbits after 193nm excimer laser surface ablation. *Arch Ophthalmol* 1989;107:895–901.

36. Krueger RR, Krasinski JS, Radzewicz C, et al. Photography of shock waves during excimer laser ablation of the cornea: effect of helium gas on propagation velocity. *Cornea* 1993;12:330–334.

37. Zabel R, Tuft S, Marshall J. Excimer laser photorefractive keratectomy: endothelial morphology following area ablation of the cornea. *Invest Ophthalmol Vis Sci* 1988;29:390.

38. Asano Y, Mizuno K. The effect of ultraviolet irradiation on the corneal endothelium. *Acta Soc Ophthalmol Jpn* 1988;92:578–583.

39. Isager P, Guo S, Hjortdal JO, et al. Endothelial cell loss after photorefractive keratectomy for myopia. *Acta Ophthalmol Scand* 1998;76:304–307.

40. Carones F, Brancato R, Venturi E, et al. The corneal endothelium after myopia excimer photorefractive keratectomy. *Arch Ophthalmol* 1994;112:920–924.

41. Stulting RD, Thompson KP, Lynn MJ (Summit PRK Endothelial Cell Investigator Group). The effect of excimer laser photorefractive keratectomy (PRK) on the human corneal endothelium. *Invest Ophthalmol Vis Sci* 1995;36:S710.

42. Cotliar AM, Schubert HD, Mandel ER, et al. Excimer laser radial keratotomy. *Ophthalmology* 1985;92:206–208.

43. Steinert RF, Puliafito CA. Corneal incisions with the excimer laser. In: Sanders DR, Hofmann RF, Salz JJ, eds. *Refractive corneal surgery.* Thorofare, NJ: Slack 1986:401–410.

44. Aron-Rosa DS, Beorner C, Gross M, et al. Wound healing following excimer laser radial keratotomy. *J Cataract Refract Surg* 1988;14:173–179.

45. McDonald MB, Frantz JM, Klyce SD, et al. One-year refractive results of central photorefractive keratectomy for myopia in the nonhuman primate cornea. *Arch Ophthalmol* 1990;108:40–47.

46. Missotten L, Boving R, Francois G, et al. Experimental excimer laser keratomileusis. *Bull Soc Belge Ophtalmol* 1986;220:103–120.

47. Waring GO III. Development of a system for excimer laser corneal surgery. *Trans Am Ophthalmol Soc* 1989;87:854–983.

48. Hanna KD, Chastang JC, Pouliquen Y, et al. Excimer laser keratectomy for myopia with a rotating-slit delivery system. *Arch Ophthalmol* 1988;106:245–250.

49. Hanna KD, Chastang JC, Asfar L, et al. Scanning slit delivery system. *J Cataract Refract Surg* 1989;15:390–396.

50. Cutarelli PE, Durrie DS, Boxer Wachler BS. Laser systems for excimer laser refractive surgery. In: Wu HK, Thompson VM, Steinert RF, et al, eds. *Refractive surgery.* New York: Thieme, 1999;247–262.

51. Marshall J, Trokel SL, Rothemy S, et al. Long-term healing of the central cornea after photorefractive keratectomy using an excimer laser. *Ophthalmology* 1988;95:1411–1421.

52. Marshall J, Trokel SL, Rothemy S, et al. Photoablative reprofiling of the cornea using an excimer laser. Photorefractive keratectomy. *Lasers Ophthalmol* 1986;1:21–48.

53. Del Pero RA, Gigstad J, Roberts A, et al. A refractive and histopathologic study of excimer laser keratectomy in primates. *Am J Ophthalmol* 1990;109:419–429.

54. Fantes FE, Hann D, Waring GO III, et al. Wound healing after excimer laser keratomileusis (photorefractive keratectomy) in monkeys. *Arch Ophthalmol* 1990;108:665–675.

55. Tuft SJ, Zabel RW, Marshall J. Corneal repair following keratectomy: a comparison between conventional surgery and laser photoablation. *Invest Ophthalmol Vis Sci* 1989;30:1769–1777.

56. Goodman GL, Trokel SL, Stark WJ, et al. Corneal healing following laser refractive keratectomy. *Arch Ophthalmol* 1989;107:1799–1803.

57. Cintron C. Corneal epithelial and stromal reactions to excimer laser photorefractive keratectomy. II. Unpredictable corneal cicatrisation. *Arch Ophthalmol* 1990;108:1540–1541.

58. L'Esperance FA, Taylor DM, Warner JW. Human excimer laser keratectomy: short-term histopathology. *Refract Corneal Surg* 1988;4:118–124.

59. Taylor DM, L'Esperance FA, Del Pero RA, et al. Human excimer laser lamellar keratectomy: a clinical study. *Ophthalmology* 1989;96:654–664.

60. Taylor DM, L'Esperance FA, Warner JW, et al. Experimental corneal studies with the excimer laser. *J Cataract Refract Surg* 1989;15:384–389.

61. McDonald MB, Frantz JM, Klyce SD, et al. Central photorefractive keratectomy for myopia: the blind eye study. *Arch Ophthalmol* 1990;108:799–808.

62. Seiler T, Kahle G, Kriegerowski M. Excimer laser (193 nm) myopic keratomileusis in sighted and blind human eyes. *Refract Corneal Surg* 1990;6:165–173.

63. Colliac JP, Shammas HJ. Optics for photorefractive keratectomy. *J Cataract Refract Surg* 1993;19:356–363.

64. Seiler T, Derse M, Pham T. Repeated excimer laser treatment after photorefractive keratectomy. *Arch Ophthalmol* 1992;110:1230–1233.

65. Ehlers N, Hjortdal JO. Excimer laser refractive keratectomy for high myopia: 6–month follow-up of patients treated bilaterally. *Acta Ophthalmol* 1992;70:578–586.

66. Caubert E. Cause of subepithelial corneal haze over 18 months after photorefractive keratectomy for myopia. *Refract Corneal Surg* 1993;9:65–70.

67. Kim JH, Hahn TW, Lee YC, et al. Photorefractive keratectomy in 202 myopic eyes: one year results. *Refract Corneal Surg* 1993;9:11–16.

68. Taylor HR, McCarty CA, Aldred GF, and the Melbourne Excimer Laser Group. Predictability of excimer laser treatment of myopia. *Arch Ophthalmol* 1996;114:248–251.

69. Sher NA, Barak M, Daya S, et al. Excimer laser photorefractive keratectomy in high myopia: a multicenter study. *Arch Ophthalmol* 1992;110:935–943.

70. Sher NA, Chen V, Bowers RA, et al. The use of the 193–nm excimer laser for myopic photorefractive keratectomy in sighted eyes: a multicenter study. *Arch Ophthalmol* 1991;109: 1525–1530.

71. Salz JJ, Maguen E, Macy JI, et al. One-year results of excimer laser photorefractive keratectomy for myopia. *Refract Corneal Surg* 1992;8:269–273.

72. O'Brart DPS, Corbett MC, Lohmann CP, et al. The effects of ablation on the outcome of excimer laser photorefractive keratectomy. *Arch Ophthalmol* 1995;113:438–443.

73. Pop M, Aras M. Multizone/multipass photorefractive keratectomy: six month results. *J Cataract Refract Surg* 1995;21: 633–643.

74. Kalski RS, Sutton G, Bin Y, et al. Comparison of 5–mm and 6–mm ablation zones in photorefractive keratectomy for myopia. *J Cataract Refract Surg* 1996;12:61–67.

75. Morris AT, Ring CP, Hadden OB. Comparison of photorefractive keratectomy for myopia using 5–mm and 6–mm diameter ablation zones. *J Refract Surg* 1996;12:S275–277.

76. O'Brart DPS, Corbett MC, Verma S, et al. Effects of ablation diameter, depth, and edge contour on the outcome of photorefractive keratectomy. *J Refract Surg* 1996;12:50–60.

77. Lohmann CP, Timerlake GT, Fitzke FW, et al. Corneal light scattering after excimer laser photorefractive keratectomy: the objective measurement of haze. *Refract Corneal Surg* 1992;8: 114–121.

78. Lohmann CP, Fitzke FW, O'Brart DPS, et al. Corneal light scattering and visual performance in myopic individuals with spectacles, contact lenses, or excimer laser photorefractive keratectomy. *Am J Ophthalmol* 1993;115:444–453.

79. Harrison JM, Tennant TB, Gwin MC, et al. Forward light scatter at month after photorefractive keratectomy. *J Refract Surg* 1995;11:83–88.

80. Braunstein RE, Jain S, McCally RI, et al. Objective measurement of corneal light scattering after excimer laser keratectomy. *Ophthalmology* 1996;103:439–443.

81. Schallhorn SC, Blanton CL, Kaupp SE, et al. Preliminary results of photorefractive keratectomy in active-duty United States Navy personnel. *Ophthalmology* 1996;103:5–22.

82. van den Berg TJTP, Ijspeert JK. Clinical assessment of intraocular stray light. *Appl Optics* 1996;31:3694–3696.

83. Maldonado MJ, Arnau V, Nevea A, et al. Direct objective quantification of corneal haze after excimer laser photorefractive keratectomy for high myopia. *Ophthalmology* 1996;103:1970–1978.

84. Thompson KP, Steinert RF, Stulting RD. Photorefractive keratectomy with the Summit excimer laser: The phase III U.S. results. In: Salz JJ, ed. *Corneal laser surgery.* St. Louis: CV Mosby, 1995:57–63.

85. Seiler T, McDonnell PJ. Excimer laser photorefractive keratectomy. *Surv Ophthalmol* 1995;40:89–118.

86. Dutt S, Steinert RF, Raizman MB, et al. One-year results of excimer laser photorefractive keratectomy for low to moderate myopia. *Arch Ophthalmol* 1994;112:1427–1436.

87. Durrie DS, Lesher MP, Cavanaugh TB. Classification of variable clinical response after photorefractive keratectomy for myopia. *J Refract Surg* 1995;11:341–347.

88. Gartry DS, Kerr-Muir MG, Lohmann CP, et al. The effect of topical corticosteroids on refractive outcome and corneal haze after photorefractive keratectomy: a prospective, randomized, double-blind trial. *Arch Ophthalmol* 1992;110:944–952.

89. McCarty CA, Aldred GF, Taylor HR, et al. Comparison of excimer laser correction of all degrees of myopia at 12 months postoperatively. *Am J Ophthalmol* 1995;121:372–383.

90. Gimbel HV, Van Westenbrugge JA, Johnson WH, et al. Visual, refractive, and patient satisfaction results following bilateral photorefractive keratectomy for myopia. *Refract Corneal Surg* 1993;9:5–10.

91. Kim JH, Hahn TW, Lee YC, et al. Photorefractive keratectomy in 2020 myopic eyes: one year results. *Refract Corneal Surg* 1993;9:11–16.

92. Lavery FL. Photorefractive keratectomy in 472 eyes. *Refract Corneal Surg* 1993;9:98–100.

93. Talley AR, Hardten DR, Sher NA, et al. Results one year after using the 193–nm excimer laser for photorefractive keratectomy in mild to moderate myopia. *Am J Ophthalmol* 1994;118:304–311.

94. Goes FJ. Photorefractive keratectomy for myopia of −8.00 to −24.00 diopters. *J Refract Surg* 1996;12:91–97.

95. Chan W, Heng WJ, Tseng P, et al. Photorefractive keratectomy for myopia of 6 to 12 diopters. *J Refract Surg* 1995;11: S286–292.

96. Siganos DS, Pallikaris IG, Margaritis VN. Photorefractive keratectomy with a transition zone for myopia from −7 to −14 diopters. *J Refract Surg* 1996;12:S261–263.

97. Menezo JL, Martinez-Costa R, Navea A, et al. Excimer laser photorefractive keratectomy for high myopia. *J Cataract Refract Surg* 1995;21:393–397.

98. Williams DK. Excimer laser photorefractive keratectomy for extreme myopia. *J Cataract Refract Surg* 1996;22:910–914.

99. Tengroth B, Epstein D, Fagerholm P, et al. Excimer laser photorefractive keratectomy for myopia: clinical results in sighted eyes. *Ophthalmology* 1993;100:739–745.

100. Piebenga LW, Matta CS, Deitz MR, et al. Excimer photorefractive keratectomy for myopia. *Ophthalmology* 1993;100: 1335–1345.

101. Brancato R, Tavola A, Carones F, et al. Excimer laser photorefractive keratectomy for myopia: results in 1165 eyes. *Refract Corneal Surg* 1993;9:95–104.

102. Kim JH, Sah WJ, Kim M, Lee Y, et al. Three year results of photorefractive keratectomy for myopia. *J Refract Surg* 1995; 11:S248–252.

103. Amano S, Shimizu K. Excimer laser photorefractive keratectomy for myopia: two year follow-up. *J Refract Surg* 1995;11: S253–260.

104. Maguen E, Salz J, Nesburn A, et al. Results of excimer laser photorefractive keratectomy for the correction of myopia. *Ophthalmology* 1994;101:1548–1557.

105. Hamburg-Nystom H, Fagerholm P, Tengroth B, et al. Thirty-six month follow-up of excimer laser photorefractive keratectomy for myopia. *Ophthalmic Surg Lasers* 1996;27:S418–420.

106. Epstein D, Fagerholm P, Hamberg-Nystrom H, et al. Twenty-four month follow-up of excimer laser photorefractive keratectomy for myopia. Refractive and visual acuity results. *Ophthalmology* 1994;101:1558–1563.

107. O'Brart DP, Gartry DS, Lohmann CP, et al. Excimer laser photorefractive keratectomy of 4.00– and 5.00–millimeter ablation zones. *J Refract Corneal Surg* 1994;10:87–94.

108. Corbett MC, Verma S, O'Brart DP, et al. Effect of ablation profile on wound healing and visual performance 1 year after excimer laser photorefractive keratectomy. *Br J Ophthalmol* 1996;80:224–234.

109. Rosa N, Cennamo G, Pasquariello A, et al. Refractive outcome and corneal topographic studies after photorefractive keratectomy with different sized ablation zones. *Ophthalmology* 1996; 103:1130–1138.

110. Bourque LB, Rubenstein R, Cosand BB, et al. Psychosocial characteristics of candidates for the Perspective Evaluation of Radial Keratotomy (PERK) study. *Arch Ophthalmol* 1984; 102:1187–1192.

111. Waring GO III, Lynn MJ, McDonnell PJ, et al. Results of the prospective evaluation of radial keratotomy (PERK) study 10 years after surgery. *Arch Ophthalmol* 1994;112:1298–1308.

112. Quah BL, Wong EYM, Tseng PSF, et al. Analysis of photorefractive keratectomy patients who have not had PRK in their second eye. *Ophthalmic Surg Lasers* 1996;27:S429–434.

113. Halliday BL. Refractive and visual results and patient satisfaction after excimer laser photorefractive keratectomy for myopia. *Br J Ophthalmol* 1995;79:881–887.

114. Pallikaris IG, Siganos DS. Excimer laser *in situ* keratomileusis and photorefractive keratectomy for correction of high myopia. *J Refract Corneal Surg* 1994;10:498–510.

115. Hersh PS, Brint SF, Maloney RK, et al. Photorefractive keratectomy versus laser *in situ* keratomileusis for moderate to high myopia: randomized prospective study. *Ophthalmology* 1998;105:1512–1523.

116. Doane JF, Slade SG. Complications of lamellar refractive surgery. In: Wu H, Steinert R, Slade S, et al., eds. *Refractive surgery.* New York: Thieme 1999:419–428.

117. Lin RT, Maloney RK. Flap complications associated with lamellar refractive surgery. *Am J Ophthalmol* 1999;127:129–136.

118. Gutierrez AM. Treatment of flap folds and striae following LASIK. In: Burrato L, Brint SF, eds. *LASIK.* Thorofare, NJ: Slack, 2000:557–562.

119. Perez-Santoja JJ, Sakia HF, Abad JL, et al. Nocardial keratitis after laser *in situ* keratomileusis [case report]. *J Refract Surg* 1997;13:314–317.

120. Reviglio V, Rodriguez ML, Picotti GS, et al. Mycobacterium chelonae keratitis following laser *in situ* keratomileusis. *J Refract Surg* 1998;14:357–360.

121. Stulting DR, Carr JD, Thompson KP, et al. Complications of laser *in situ* keratomileusis for the correction of myopia. *Ophthalmology* 1999;106:13–20.

122. al-Reefy M. Bacterial keratitis following laser *in situ* keratomileusis for hyperopia. *J Refract Surg* 1999;15:216–217.

123. Kim HM, Song JS, Han HS, et al. Streptococcal keratitis after myopic laser *in situ* keratomileusis. *Korean J Ophthalmol* 1998;12:108–111.

124. Fulcher SFA, Fader RC, Rosa RH, et al. Delayed-onset mycobacterial keratitis after LASIK. *Cornea* 2002;21:546–554.

125. Haw WW, Manche EE. Treatment of progressive or recurrent epithelial ingrowth with ethanol following laser *in situ* keratomileusis. *J Refract Surg* 2001;17:63–68.

126. Linebarger EJ, Hardten DR, Lindstrom RL. Epithelial ingrowth treated with alcohol. In: Probst LE, ed. *Complex cases with LASIK: advanced techniques and complication management.* Thorofare, NJ: Slack, 2000:214–218.

127. Lumba JD, Hersh PS. Topography changes associated with sublamellar epithelial ingrowth after laser *in situ* keratomileusis. *J Cataract Refract Surg* 2000;26:1413–1416.

128. Wright JD Jr, Neubaur CC, Stevens G Jr. Epithelial ingrowth in a corneal graft treated by laser *in situ* keratomileusis: light and electron microscopy. *J Cataract Refract Surg* 2000;26:49–55.

129. Castillo A, Diaz-Valle D, Gutierrez AR, et al. Peripheral melt of flap after laser *in situ* keratomileusis. *J Refract Surg* 1998;14:61–63.

130. Kaufman SC, Maitchouk DY, Chiou AG, et al. Interface inflammation after laser *in situ* keratomileusis: Sands of Sahara syndrome. *J Cataract Refract Surg* 1998;24:1589–1593.

131. Haw WW, Manche EE. Late onset diffuse lamellar keratitis associated with an epithelial defect in six eyes. *J Cataract Refract Surg* 2000;16:744–748.

132. Chang-Godinich A, Steinert RF, Wu HK. Late occurrence of diffuse lamellar keratitis after laser *in situ* keratomileusis. *Arch Ophthalmol* 2001;119:1074–1076.

133. Weisenthal RW. Diffuse lamellar keratitis induced by trauma 6 months after laser *in situ* keratomileusis. *J Refract Surg* 2000;16:749–751.

134. Seiler T, Koufala K, Richter G. Iatrogenic keratectasia after laser *in situ* keratomileusis. *J Refract Surg* 1998;14:312–317.

135. Seiler T, Quurke AW. Iatrogenic keratectasia after LASIK in case of forme fruste keratoconus. *J Cataract Refract Surg* 1998;24:1007–1009.

136. Geggel HS, Talley AR. Delayed onset keratectasia following LASIK. *J Cataract Refract Surg* 1999;25:582–586.

137. Koch DD. The riddle of iatrogenic keractectasia. *J Cataract Refract Surg* 1999;25:453–454.

138. Seitz B, Torres F, Langenbucher A, et al. Posterior corneal curvature changes after myopic laser *in situ* keratomileusis. *Ophthalmology* 2001;108:666–673.

139. Iskander NG, Peters NT, Anderson-Penno E, et al. Late traumatic flap dislocation after laser *in situ* keratomileusis. *J Cataract Refract Surg* 2001;27:1111–1114.

140. Kim EK, Lee DH, Lee K, et al. Nocardia keratitis after traumatic detachment of a laser *in situ* keratomileusis flap. *J Refract Surg* 2000;16:467–469.

141. Lombardo AJ, Katz HR. Late partial dislocation of a laser *in situ* keratomileusis flap. *J Cataract Refract Surg* 2001;27:1108–1110.

142. Lemly HL, Chodosh J, Wolf TC, et al. Partial dislocation of laser *in situ* keratomileusis flap by air bag injury. *J Refract Surg* 2000;16:373–374.

143. Chaudhry NA, Smiddy WE. Displacement of corneal cap during vitrectomy in a post-LASIK eye. *Retina* 1998;18:554–555.

144. Geggel HS, Coday MP. Late-onset traumatic laser *in situ* keratomileusis (LASIK) flap dehiscence. *Am J Ophthalmol* 2001;131:505–506.

145. Leung AT, Rao SK, Lam DS. Traumatic partial unfolding of laser *in situ* keratomileusis flap with severe epithelial ingrowth. *J Cataract Refract Surg* 2000;26:135–139.

146. Melki SA, Talamo JH, Demetriades AM, et al. Late traumatic dislocation of laser *in situ* keratomileusis corneal flaps. *Ophthalmology* 2000;107:2136–2139.

147. Patel CK, Hanson R, McDonald B, et al. Case reports and small case series: late dislocation of a LASIK flap caused by a fingernail. *Arch Ophthalmol* 2001;119:447–449.

148. Schwartz GS, Park DH, Schloff S, et al. Traumatic flap displacement and subsequent diffuse lamellar keratitis after laser *in situ* keratomileusis. *J Cataract Refract Surg* 2001;27:781–783.

149. Jain S, Austin DJ. Phototherapeutic keratectomy for treatment of recurrent corneal erosion. *J Cataract Refract Surg* 1999;25:1610–1614.

150. Arevalo JF, Freeman WR, Gomez L. Retina and vitreous pathology after laser-assisted *in situ* keratomileusis: Is there a cause-effect relationship? *Ophthalmology* 2001;108:839–840.

151. Lee JB, Ryu CH, Kim J, et al. Comparison of tear secretion and tear film instability after photorefractive keratectomy and laser *in situ* keratomileusis. *J Cataract Refract Surg* 2000;26:1326–1331.

152. Sun R, Gimbel HV, Kaye GB. Photorefractive keratectomy in keratoconus suspects. *J Cataract Refract Surg* 1999;25:1461–1466.

153. Bilgihan K, Ozdek SC, Konuk O, et al. Results of photorefractive keratectomy in keratoconus suspects at 4 years. *J Refract Surg* 2000;16:438–443.

154. Dausch D, Schroder E, Dausch S. Topography-controlled excimer laser photorefractive keratectomy. *J Refract Surg* 2000;16:13–22.

155. Sanchez-Galeana CA, Smith RJ, Rodriguez X, et al. Laser *in situ* keratomileusis and photorefractive keratectomy for residual refractive error after phakic intraocular lens implantation. *J Refract Surg* 2001;17:299–304.

156. Pop M, Payette Y, Amyor M. Clear lens extraction with intraocular lens followed by photorefractive keratectomy or laser *in situ* keratomileusis. *Ophthalmology* 2001;108:104–111.

157. Kohnen T. Retreating residual refractive errors after excimer surgery of the cornea: PRK versus LASIK. *J Cataract Refract Surg* 2000;25:625–626.

158. Gimbel HV, Stoll SB. Photorefractive keratectomy with customized segmental ablation to correct irregular astigmatism after laser *in situ* keratomileusis. *J Refract Surg* 2001;17: S229–232.

159. Yo C, Vroman D, Ma S, et al. Surgical outcomes of photorefractive keratectomy and laser *in situ* keratomileusis by inexperienced surgeons. *J Cataract Refract Surg* 2000;26:510–515.

160. El Danasoury MA, Maghraby AE, Klyce SD, et al. Comparison of photorefractive keratectomy with excimer laser *in situ* keratomileusis in correcting low myopia {from −2.00 to −5.50 diopters}. A randomized study. *Ophthalmology* 1999;106:411–421.

161. Pop M, Payette Y. Photorefractive keratectomy versus laser *in situ* keratomileusis. *Ophthalmology* 2000;107:251–257.

162. Fraunfelder FW, Wilson SE. Laser in situ keratomileusis versus photorefractive keratectomy in the correction of myopic astigmatism. *Cornea* 2001;20:385–387.

163. Walker MB, Wilson SE, Fraufelder F. Recovery of uncorrected visual acuity after laser *in situ* keratomileusis or photorefractive keratectomy for low myopia. *Cornea* 2001;20:153–155.

164. Tole DM, McCarty DJ, Couper T, et al. Comparison of laser *in situ* keratomileusis and photorefractive keratectomy for the correction of myopia of −6.00 diopters or less. Melbourne Excimer Laser Group. *J Refract Surg* 2001;17:46–54.

165. el-Agha M, Johnston E, Bowman RW, et al. Excimer laser treatment of spherical hyperopia: PRK or LASIK? *Trans Am Ophthalmol Soc* 2000;98:59–69.

166. Scerrati E. Laser *in situ* keratomileusis vs. laser epithelial keratomileusis (LASIK vs. LASEK). *J Refract Surg* 2001;17:S219–221.

167. Jackson WB. Photorefractive keratectomy: Indications, surgical techniques, complications, and results. *Ophthalmic Practice* 2001;19:18–30.

168. Stein R. Photorefractive keratectomy. *Int Ophthalmol Clin* 2000;40:35–56.

169. Brunette I, Gresset J, Boivin JF, et al. Functional outcome and satisfaction after photorefractive keratectomy. Part 2: survey of 690 patients. *Ophthalmology* 2001;107:1790–1796.

170. Azar DT, Ang RT, Lee JB, et al. Laser subepithelial keratomileusis: Electron microscopy and visual outcomes of flap photorefractive keratectomy. *Curr Opin Ophthalmol* 2001;12: 323–328.

171. Abad JC, An B, Power WJ, et al. A prospective evaluation of alcohol-assisted versus mechanical epithelial removal before photorefractive keratectomy. *Ophthalmology* 1997;104:1566–1575.

172. Abad JC, Talamo JH, Vidaurri-Leal J, et al. Dilute ethanol versus mechanical debridement before photorefractive keratectomy. *J Cataract Refract Surg* 1996;22:1427–1433.

173. Stein HA, Stein RM, Price C, et al. Alcohol removal of the epithelium for excimer laser ablation: outcomes analysis. *J Cataract Refract Surg* 1997;23:1160–1163.

174. Shah S, Doyle SJ, Chatterjee A, et al. Comparison of 18% ethanol and mechanical debridement for epithelial removal before photorefractive keratectomy. *J Refract Surg* 1998;14: S212–214.

175. Camellin M, Cimberle M. LASEK technique promising after 1 year of experience. *Ocular Surg News* 2000;18:1,14–17.

176. Vinciguerra P, McDonald MB. Presented at the 1st LASEK Congress [unpublished data], Houston, March 2002.

177. Pallikaris I. Presented at American Society of Cataract and Refractive Surgeons' Annual Meeting [unpublished data], Philadelphia, May 2002.

178. Claringbold TV. LASIK Instructional Course. American Academy of Ophthalmology Annual Meeting, Anaheim, CA, November 2003.

179. Chen CC, Chang JH, Lee JB, et al. Human corneal epithelial cell viability and morphology after dilute alcohol exposure. *Invest Ophthalmol Vis Sci* 2002;43:2593–2602.

180. Dreiss AK, Winkler von Mohrenfels C, Gabler B, et al. Laser epithelial keratomileusis (LASEK): histological investigation for vitality of corneal epithelial cells after alcohol exposure. *Klin Monatsbl Augenheilkd* 2002;219:365–369.

181. Kornilovsky IM. Clinical results after subepithelial photorefractive keratectomy (LASEK). *J Refract Surg* 2001;17: S222–223.

182. Lohmann CP, von Mohrenfels W, Gabler B, et al. LASEK: a new surgical procedure to treat myopia. *Invest Ophthalmol Vis Sci* 2001;42:S599.

183. Rouweyha RM, Chuang AZ, Mitra S, et al. Laser epithelial keratomileusis for myopia with the autonomous laser. *J Refract Surg* 2002;18:217–224.

184. Condon PI. LASEK: an alternative to LASIK and PRK. American Society of Cataract and Refractive Surgeons' Symposium, San Diego, CA. May 2001.

185. Claringbold TV. Laser-assisted subepithelial keratectomy for the correction of myopia. *J Cataract Refract Surg* 2002;28: 18–22.

186. Lee JB, Seong GL, Lee JH, et al. Comparison of laser epithelial keratomileusis and photorefractive keratectomy for low to moderate myopia. *J Cataract Refract Surg* 2001;27:565–570.

187. Sher NA, Hardten DR, Fundingsland B, et al. 193–nm excimer photorefractive keratectomy in high myopia. *Ophthalmology* 1994;101:1575–1581.

188. Litwak S, Zadok D, Garcia-de Quevedo V, et al. Laser-assisted subepithelial keratectomy versus photorefractive keratectomy for the correction of myopia. A prospective comparative study. *J Cataract Refract Surg* 2002;28:1330–1333.

189. Lee JB, Choe CM, Kim HS, et al. Comparison of TGF-beta 1 in tears following laser subepithelial keratomileusis and photorefractive keratectomy. *J Refract Surg* 2002;18:130–134.

190. McDonald MB. New Innovations in Refractive Surgery. Presented at the American Academy of Ophthalmology Subspecialty Day. Dallas, TX. 1999.

191. Shahinian LJ, Jain S, Jager RD, et al. Dilute topical proparacaine for pain relief after photorefractive keratectomy. *Ophthalmology* 1997;104:1327–1332.

192. Dudenhoefer EJ, Azar DT. In: Melki SA, Azar DT, eds. *101 Pearls in refractive, cataract, and corneal surgery.* Thorofare, NJ: Slack, 2001:34–36.

193. Talley AR, Sher NA, Kim MS, et al. Use of the 193 nm excimer laser for photorefractive keratectomy in low to moderate myopia. *J Cataract Refract Surg* 1994;20:S239–242.

194. Hardten DR, Lindstrom RL. Treatment of low, moderate, and high myopia with the 193–nm excimer laser. *Klin Monatsbl Augenheilkd* 1994;205:259–265.

195. Shah SI, Hersh PS. Photorefractive keratectomy for myopia with a 6–mm beam diameter. *J Refract Surg* 1996;12:341–346.

196. Pop M, Payette Y. Photorefractive keratectomy versus laser in situ keratomileusis: a control-matched study. *Ophthalmology* 2000;107:251–257.

197. Stevens J, Giubilei M, Ficker L, et al. Prospective study of photorefractive keratectomy for myopia using the VISX StarS2 excimer laser system. *J Refract Surg* 2002;18:502–508.

198. Dausch D, Dausch S, Schroder E. Wavefront-supported photorefractive keratectomy: 12–month follow-up. *J Refract Surg* 2003;19:405–411.

LASIK INSTRUMENTATION: MICROKERATOMES, EXCIMER LASERS, AND WAVEFRONT ANALYZERS

RAYMOND S. LOH AND DAVID R. HARDTEN

At the onset of the 21st century, the basic requirements of any refractive surgery remain unchanged with the primary goals of safety, reproducibility, accuracy and, stability being foremost in the surgeons' mind. With advances in microkeratome design, laser technology, and eye-tracking, the accuracy and reproducibility of laser refractive surgery has improved. The development of commercially available wavefront-sensing devices and the improvements in laser technology have paved the way for potential treatments of lower and higher order optical aberrations, not only in normal eyes but also in decentered ablations, central islands, and postpenetrating keratoplasty irregular astigmatism (1–8). Advances in these technologies have led to both wavefront and topographically guided laser surgery in an effort to treat the preexisting aberrations and the aberrations induced by the refractive treatment itself (9–15).

Laser *in-situ* keratomileusis (LASIK) remains the most common form of laser refractive procedure, although the onset of wavefront driven corrective surgery has led to renewed interest and study of surface ablation procedures, laser subepithelial keratomileusis (LASEK), and photorefractive keratomileusis (PRK) (10,16). However the most important instruments in laser refractive surgery remain, arguably, the microkeratome and laser.

This chapter provides an overview of the microkeratome and guidelines for use. (Analysis of individual instrument designs is beyond the scope of this chapter due to the continuing evolution of various manufacturer specifications.) This chapter also provides a brief overview of the femtosecond laser and its applications with regard to lamellar flap creation. With the onset of custom ablation, the requirement for the surgeon to be familiar with the nuances and eccentricities of the particular wavefront analyzer becomes even more important. The principles of the excimer laser and guidelines for laser settings as well as a brief discussion on factors affecting refractive outcome reproducibility and construction of nomograms are also provided. The methods and minimal requirements of eye tracking are then

discussed in relation to eye movements during surgery. Finally, we discuss wavefront sensing and the technological requirements for wavefront and topographical driven ablation.

MICROKERATOMES: PRINCIPLES AND SETTINGS

Jose I. Barraquer (17) designed the first manual microkeratome. The basic components of current microkeratomes have remained relatively unchanged: suction ring, keratome head with putative depth or variable depth plate, blade control and variables, mechanism for travel across the cornea, and the control unit providing vacuum for suction and drive for the keratome. The main variables with regard to the microkeratome are as follows:

1. Suction ring size and flap diameter
2. Flap thickness/head plate depth and hinge location
3. Vacuum setting
4. Blade selection, control and variables.

Suction Ring Size

The suction ring diameter determines how much of the cornea protrudes into the microkeratome and is the primary determinant of flap diameter. In general, a large diameter suction ring results in a larger diameter flap. Preoperative keratometry values influence the diameter of the flap (18,19). As the cornea becomes steeper, more of the cornea passes through the ring resulting in a larger diameter flap. Conversely, a flat cornea does not protrude into a given suction ring as much, and would produce a flap of reduced diameter.

In patients with steep corneas, use of a large diameter suction ring, such as a 9.5-mm ring, can produce a flap that exceeds the clear cornea diameter, potentially injuring the limbus and causing unnecessary bleeding especially in patients with a history of long-term soft contact lens wear and peripheral corneal neovascularization. Steep corneas can also produce buttonhole complications during the microkeratome pass (Fig. 76-1). This is most likely due to buckling of the cornea against the microkeratome footplate. A larger diameter ring size may increase the potential for this phenomenon. If available, we recommend a smaller diameter ring size for significantly steep corneas. With myopic or smaller optical zone ablations, various keratometry (K) values varying from 43 to 46 diopters (D) have been used as cut off values. Using the 8.5-mm Hansatome microkeratome ring for K equal to or larger than the cutoff value, and the 9.5 mm ring for K less than the cutoff values, provided there is adequate corneal diameter. For hyperopic, or large optical zone ablations, a higher K reading is used as the cutoff point, using the 8.5-mm ring for K equal to or larger than the cutoff value and the 9.5-mm ring for K less than the cut off value.

Flatter corneas present less tissue through a given ring size, producing smaller diameter flaps and are at risk of producing a free cap during flap creation. This occurs when relatively less of the corneal dome protrudes above the level of the ring, producing a flap that is so small that it is completely excised. For these reasons, the authors prefer a relatively high cutoff value. When performing myopic ablations, the authors recommend a larger ring size, a 9.5-mm or 10.0-mm ring, for corneas with K <46 D. A small flap from flatter corneas creates a potential problem, as such patients commonly present for hyperopic correction, which requires a larger ablation zone. When attempting large ablations for hyperopia or mixed astigmatism, the authors utilize the 9.5-mm suction ring in patients with K values below 49 D. Other authors, including one of the editors, use a cutoff value closer to 43.5 D.

The guidelines used by the authors typically allow creation of a flap that is significantly larger than the diameter needed for the ablation zone. The advantages and disadvantages are listed in Table 76-1. In short, the advantages of a large flap, especially the ability to perform the larger ablation zones required for wavefront-guided treatment, has to be balanced against the problems of causing bleeding from limbal vessels and the higher likelihood of striae and buttonhole formation or dry eye.

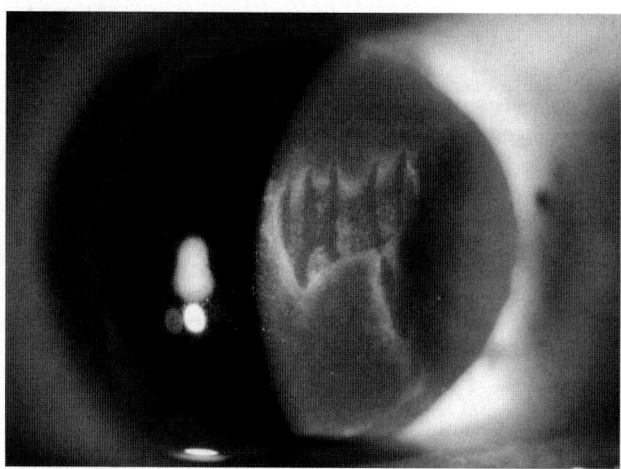

FIGURE 76-1. Button-hole formation with secondary scarring.

Flap Thickness, Head Plate Depth, and Hinge Location

Most microkeratomes designed for LASIK on the market today offer multiple footplate depths to produce a range of flap thickness. Factors that affect flap thickness are choice of head-plate depths, corneal thickness, preoperative refractive error, blade sharpness, blade length, translational speed across the cornea, and intraocular pressure.

The two most important patient factors to be considered in the choice of keratome head plates are corneal thickness and the preoperative refractive error. Preoperative pachymetry can be one of the biggest determinants of flap thickness (19,20). Thinner corneas tend to produce thinner flaps, and thicker corneas yield thicker flaps. Intraocular pressure can affect flap thickness as well, with lower pressures resulting in thinner flaps.

Another important factor to consider when choosing head plate depth is that the actual flap depth produced by different microkeratome heads of the same putative plate depth can vary substantially (20,21). In microkeratomes with replaceable depth plates, incorrect plate insertion can result in a deeper than intended cut with possible entry into the anterior chamber. Newer microkeratomes with a fixed depth plate are less likely to cause this complication.

Several factors influence the choice of the site of hinge placement including the risks of subsequent laser-associated

TABLE 76-1. FLAP SIZE: ADVANTAGES AND DISADVANTAGES

	Advantages	Disadvantages
Large flap	Larger area for ablation	Increased fluid under flap
	Decentered flap unlikely to interfere with ablation	Increased risk of epithelial defects
	Flap hinge further from treatment area	Increased risk of striae
	Reduces potential of previous incision separation	Edge closer to limbus: possible increased risk of epithelial in-growth
	Increase area for flap adhesion	
	Edges closer to limbus: aid epithelial wound healing	Increased risk of limbal vessel hemorrhage/damage

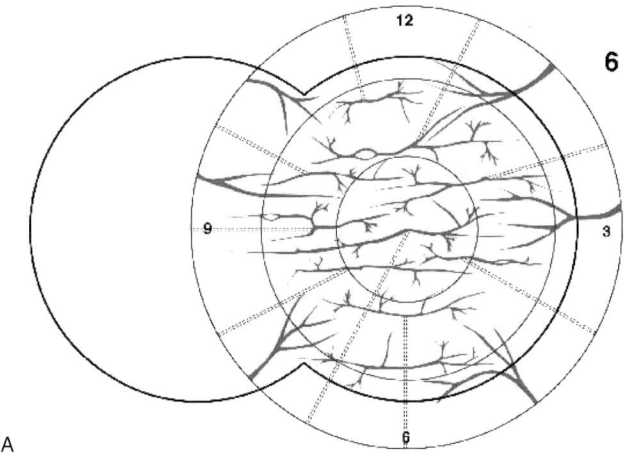

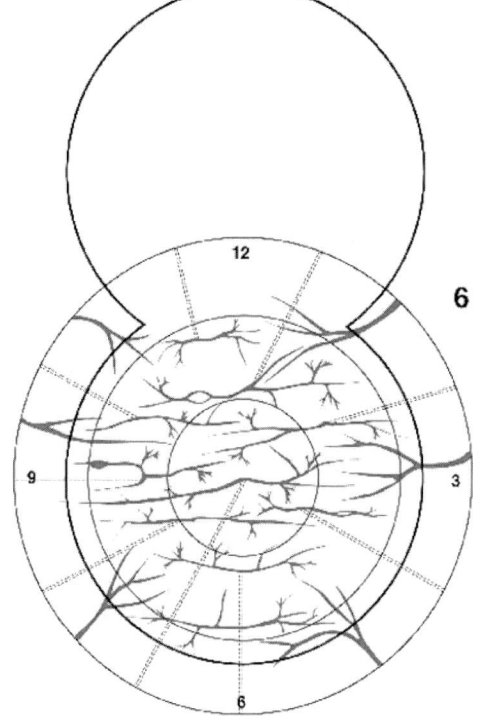

FIGURE 76-2. Nerve plexus of the cornea illustrating main innervations from nasal and temporal nerve branches demonstrating the potential effects of **(A)** nasal hinge and **(B)** superior hinge. (Courtesy of Eric D. Donnenfeld, M.D.)

dry eye/epitheliopathy, relationship to astigmatic treatment, and reducing the risk of the flap truncating the ablation zone causing irregular astigmatism (22). Superior hinge placement has been proposed to have the advantages of vertical lid movement/upper lid compression maintaining flap position, distention, and centration. In contrast, corneal hypoesthesia lasts approximately 6 to 9 months, appearing to be greater with a superior than a nasal lamellar hinge (Fig. 76-2) in a prospective, randomized self-controlled trial, although there appears to be confounding reports of greater reduction in corneal sensation with a nasal hinge (23,24). In comparing hinge location and the effects on dry-eye symptoms/signs, superior hinge locations were associated with greater dry-eye symptoms (Fig. 76-3) (23).

Residual Posterior Stromal Thickness

One of the most important factors to consider when choosing flap depth is the limitation imposed by the patient's central corneal thickness and level of ametropia. It is not known exactly how much residual posterior stromal thickness (RPST) is required to prevent consecutive ectasia following LASIK (Fig. 76-4). An RPST of 250 μm is adequate in most cases, but there probably will be rare cases where ectasia can occur even with a RPST of greater than 250 μm (25,26). Thus, 250 μm and the flap thickness are subtracted from the lowest central pachymetry reading to determine how much ablation can be performed. The ablation depth can be approximated using the Munnerlyn formula (depth of ablation = diopters of correction $\times$ (ablation diameter)^2/3).

Blend zones and aspheric treatments as well as patient biomechanical response to treatment may alter these calculations (Fig. 76-5) (27). In corneas where the computation is close, the safest approach is to measure the residual thickness with ultrasonic pachymetry after the flap is lifted,

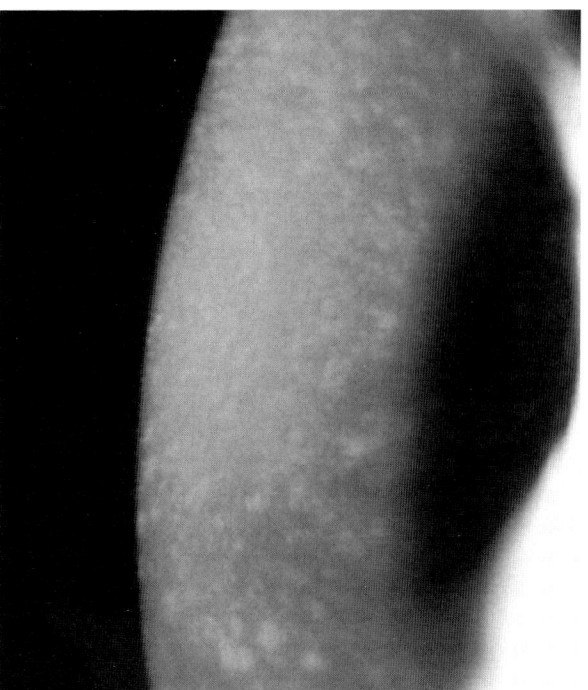

FIGURE 76-3. LASIK-induced corneal hypoesthesia with corneal punctate staining in a patient with nasal flap hinge.

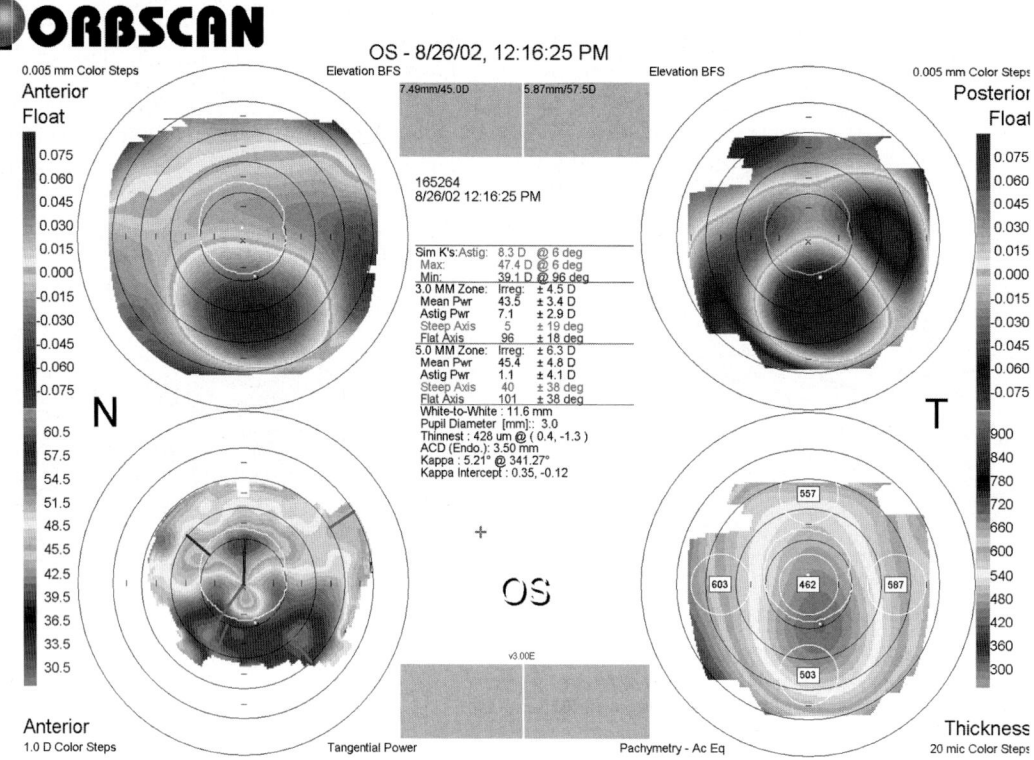

FIGURE 76-4. Orbscan of corneal ectasia secondary to myopic LASIK. The minimum post-LASIK corneal thickness is 428 μm. Calculated residual stromal bed was 300 μm after myopic ablation depth of 50 μm and presumed flap thickness of 180 μm.

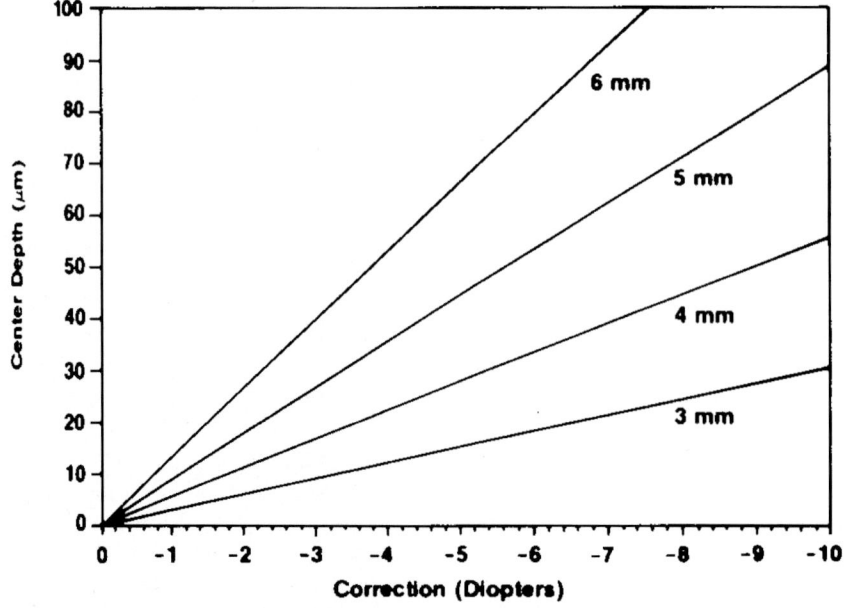

FIGURE 76-5. Maximum depth of cut for myopic correction. Each line represents the depth of cut on the optical axis for a given size of treatment. (From Munnerlyn CR, Koons SJ, Marshall J. Photorefractive keratectomy: a technique for laser refractive surgery. *J Cataract Refract Surg* 1988;14(1):49, with permission.)

eliminating the unknown factor of flap thickness, and alerting the surgeon to a flap that may be thicker than expected.

The decision to use a lower footplate setting, and thus a thinner flap, is probably only advantageous in a setting where there is a risk of exceeding the minimum safe residual stromal bed thickness of 250 μm. The decision to electively create a thinner flap without exceeding the parameters of minimum RPST is balanced by the disadvantages of a thin flap (potentially higher risk of flap folds/irregular astigmatism, buttonhole formation, increased difficulty handling thinner flaps/lifting flaps for enhancements, and less margin of error when cutting the flap) or using an alternative treatment such as LASEK, PRK, or phakic intraocular lens.

Vacuum Setting

Accurate and consistent flap creation is dependent on achieving and maintaining appropriate vacuum levels in any conventional microkeratome system. The suction system, therefore, should be checked prior to every procedure. Suction should be sufficient to raise the intraocular pressure to at least 65 mm Hg for most microkeratomes, with the newer systems allowing a degree of adjustment for variations in altitude. When using the Hansatome, the vacuum level required to achieve this intraocular pressure is approximately 20 to 27 inches Hg, depending on altitude. Lower pressures can produce thinner, less consistent or irregular flaps, whereas higher pressures increase the risk of chemosis, subconjunctival hemorrhages, and optic nerve injury. The intraocular pressure should be checked after the suction is activated to make certain that it is high enough to proceed with the microkeratome pass. Use of a pneumotonometer increases the accuracy of intraocular pressure measurements; if proper suction is not achieved or lost during the cut, the cut should not be performed or forward progress should be stopped immediately, as transection of the flap is possible. Newer microkeratomes have safety features that stop blade oscillation and forward progress if there is loss of suction.

Blade Selection, Control, and Variables

Blade assembly and inspection are critical to the success of the procedure. The surgeon should inspect the blade assembly, even if performed by trained personnel, in every case. An examination under the microscope should be done looking for smooth finish, good edge quality with no pitting, and no residue or metal shavings. Any blade irregularities can seriously affect flap quality and final visual outcome (Fig. 76-6). Blade quality can vary from unit to unit, and poor-quality blades should be rejected and replaced. It has been shown that dull blades produce thinner flaps and increase the risk of irregular flaps (28). Many centers utilize the same blade on both eyes of the same pa-

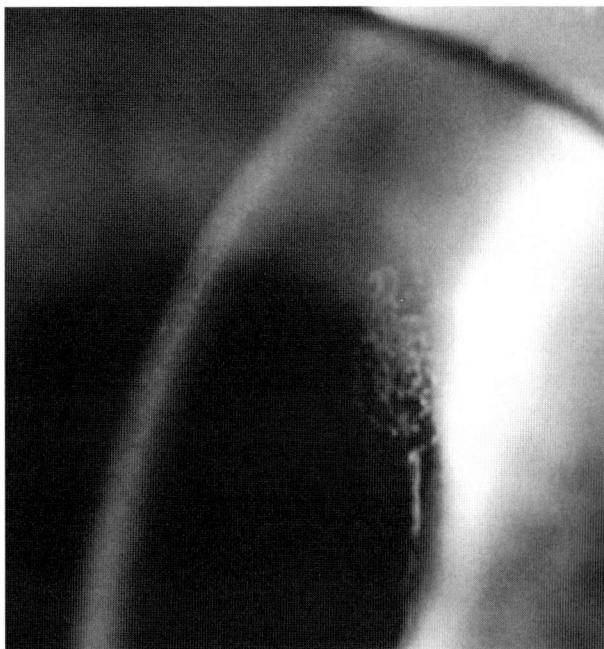

FIGURE 76-6. Postoperative photograph of an irregular flap secondary to a nick in the microkeratome blade.

tient, but not more than this. Even in this usage it has been demonstrated that the second flap cut is somewhat thinner than the first (29).

The microkeratome blade oscillates in a horizontal manner across the axis of travel by the keratome. The forward travel of the microkeratome along guided rails, track, or around a pinion is by either automated or manual means, i.e., mechanically driven or pushed forward by the surgeon. Blade entry angles vary from 25 to 30 degrees in the majority of keratomes. A steeper angle of blade entry enables the prescribed depth to be reached earlier, theoretically allowing easier alignment of the flap after the laser treatment. Horizontal blade oscillations of most keratomes vary between 12,000 and 18,000 oscillations/second. Translation, or forward progress, across the cornea may occur in a linear or rotational manner. Studies on the effects of translational speed and blade oscillations have reported that both have a significant effect on both flap thickness and smoothness of the stromal bed (30,31). Some commercially available units have independent engines for blade oscillation and head translation, allowing greater torque and independence of one from the other. An independent motor for blade oscillations allows blade movement to stop once the forward movement is complete.

FEMTOSECOND LASER

In contrast to the excimer laser with its ability to ablate tissue to a submicrometer level, approximately 0.3 μm per pulse, the relative inaccuracy of mechanical keratomes (with a standard deviation of 20 to 30 μm) has led to the search for new technologies that could improve the precision and reproducibility of this surgical step in LASIK while reducing the complication rates of lamellar creation (32,33). These include water jet and short pulse lasers (34,35).

With a short pulse of laser in the femtosecond (10^{-15} second) pulse length, the energy required to produce sufficient power (energy/time) for photodisruption is very small, such that the size of the cavitation bubbles and the secondary shockwave are minimal (36,37).

The femtosecond laser consists of a solid state neodymium (Nd):glass laser source and chirped pulse amplification to reach surgical energy levels. Pulses are generated at repetition rates of 3 to 5 kHz with each pulse of 500-femtosecond duration. The delivery system produces a beam focused to 3 to 5 μm size within the corneal stroma with each pulse estimated to remove 27 to 125 μm^3 of stromal tissue (a sphere of diameter 3 to 5 μm). Laser delivery occurs via a scanning spot with an accuracy of approximately 1 μm (35). To perform a lamellar cut, the laser spots have to be placed in a contiguous spiral or raster pattern in any plane provided that treatment is started at the deepest level. Static gas bubbles occlude delivery of energy to a depth greater than the initial spot location. At present, the system that has received Food and Drug Administration (FDA) approval, Intralase Pulsion FS, requires control of the focal plane via a suction ring, pressure of 35 mm Hg, and flat applanation contact lens to achieve a claimed depth accuracy of 10 μm (35).

Potential advantages of the femtosecond laser include reduced flap complication rates, increased consistency of flap thickness and diameter, reduction in suction pressure required, and flexibility of hinge creation. The potential disadvantages include the longer procedure/vacuum time and required interval for "bubble" dispersion prior to LASIK treatment.

Published clinical trials using femto-LASIK microkeratomes report a flap thickness of 159 $\pm$ 8.5 μm (with a target of 160 μm). Time taken for flap creation was approximately 1 minute with flaps requiring 500,000 to 800,000 spots, with a superior hinge created. The same study reported standard deviations of flap diameter of $\pm$0.1 mm for attempted 8.5- to 9.5-mm flap diameters. Target flap thickness achieved for an intended 160 μm thickness varied between $\pm$10 μm for an 8.5-mm-diameter flap and $\pm$13 μm for a 9.5-mm-diameter flap in porcine eyes (35).

In summary, the femtosecond laser appears to provide the means of providing accurate and reproducible lamellar incisions as well as further applications in corneal surgery (35). The proposed techniques of intrastromal refractive procedures require further investigation to determine both the feasible refractive treatment range and stability. Other applications of the femtosecond laser are discussed in Chapter 83.

EXCIMER LASER AND GUIDELINES FOR LASER SETTINGS

Although excimer lasers are capable of great accuracy, the demand for increasing accuracy with small scanning spot and variable spot lasers has increased the complexity of the software and hardware. As with any device, increased complexity is achieved with increased needs of both maintenance and calibration. In particular, the parameters that merit special attention include the fluence, beam homogeneity, beam size/ablation profile, and laser room environment.

Principles

The excimer laser utilizes a 193-nm ultraviolet (UV) wavelength produced by the dissociation of an excited dimer, consisting of argon and fluoride elements, to produce energy levels (6.4 eV) high enough to breakdown covalent carbon-carbon bonds (3.5 eV) (38). Pulses produced are of approximately 10-nsec duration with laser repetition rates of between 5 and 250 Hz. A detailed description of the history of the excimer laser is included in the Chapter 75.

The term *ablative photodecomposition* was first used by Srinivasan and Leigh (39) to describe molecular fragments being ejected from material irradiated by the 193-nm laser. Molecular fragments of approximately 10 to 20 carbon atoms are ejected in a plume lasting 3 to 15 μsec with initial velocities of approximately 400 m/sec in the first 5 to 15 nsec after a laser pulse (Fig. 76-7) (40,41). This wavelength was chosen for the lower energy densities required for molecular cleaving as well as for not displaying mutagenic or cataract forming behavior and minimal thermal effects, which is a concern with other UV wavelengths (42).

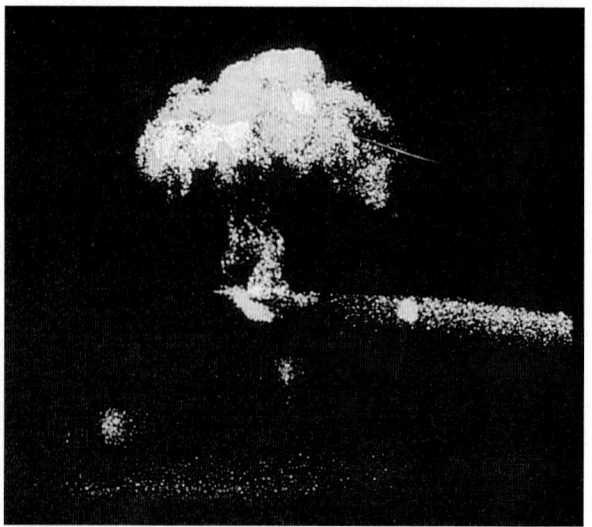

FIGURE 76-7. High-speed photography demonstrating the plume created by an excimer laser pulse. The picture demonstrates the air currents/vortices that occur. (From Ref. 41)

This direct breakage of chemical bonds by a high-energy laser has been termed *photochemical ablation* to differentiate longer wavelengths, which produce an increasing rise in local temperature or photothermal effect. At the 193-nm wavelength, high photon energy was thought to result in a purely photochemical process, with short pulses and low repetition rates also minimizing thermal side effects. Even so, Kerr-Muir et al. (43) reported the presence of a "pseudo-membrane" that formed adjacent to areas transected by the laser.

Thermal Loading

Thermal loading from the interaction of excimer laser with corneal tissue has been recognized to be dependent on fluence and repetition rate of the laser (44). More recently, the thermal effect of photorefractive keratectomy has been investigated in animal studies, showing a mean rise in corneal temperature of between 7° and 9°C for myopic ablations of ≤10 diopters (45,46). High-speed temperature analysis has shown a peak temperature of >100°C, which was reached at a fluence of 80 mJ/cm^2, increasing to 240°C with a fluence of 180 mJ/cm^2 (47). This is in direct contrast to a clinical study that has failed to observe any significant change in temperature of a scanning small-beam laser with either a sequential or randomized ablative pattern (48).

Pressure Waves and Endothelial Changes

Endothelial toxicity from the excimer laser radiation is probably negligible, as there is nearly complete absorption of radiation within 1 μm of the ablated tissue. Nevertheless, there has been a report of endothelial changes in rabbit corneas after surface ablation by the 193-nm laser, which may be due to high pressures transmitted to the endothelium (49,50). The process of molecular expulsion, as previously described by Puliafito et al. (41), generates reactive forces occurring within the cornea and eye (51,52). Pressure rises of up to 100 atmospheres amplitude has been reported in both cornea and anterior chamber by Gobbi et al. (52) and Krueger et al. (53). In the same study, Gobbi et al. also reported the bipolar nature of the pressure wave and reduction in the pressure amplitude measured at the retina, to about 10 atmosphere, by decreasing the spot diameter. A further study by Krueger et al. (54) reported the occurrence of a focus for the pressure amplitude at 5 mm in porcine eyes and estimated at 7 to 8 mm in two human eyes (Fig. 76-8). This effect was noted to be maximal for 6.0- and 7.5-mm beam diameters and less for a 4.5-mm beam, recording peak amplitudes of approximately 80 atmosphere. Beam size of 3.0- and 1.5-mm diameter failed to demonstrate this effect. The posterior surface of the cornea has been estimated to undergo stress wave amplitudes of ≤45 atm with a fluence of 180 mJ/cm^2 during excimer laser treatment.

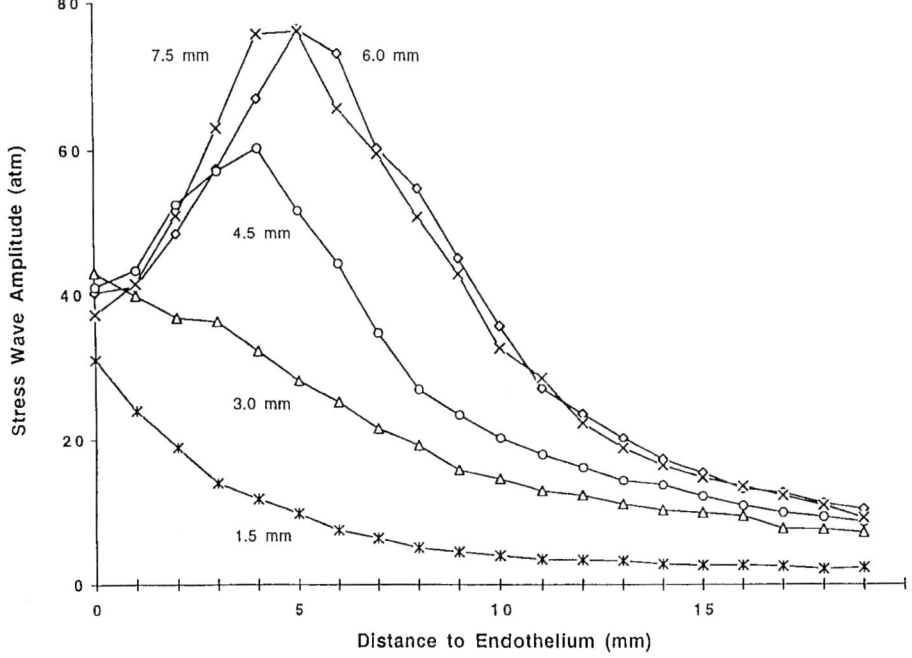

FIGURE 76-8. Graph depicting the pressure wave occurring with different ablation diameters. The pressure peak is focused at 5 to 6 mm posterior to the cornea, with the effect reducing when beam diameters are less than 4.5 mm. (From Krueger RR, et al. Stress wave amplitudes during laser surgery of the cornea. *Ophthalmology* 2001;108(6):1070–1074, with permission.)

The majority of studies on endothelial cell changes following both LASIK and PRK have not demonstrated significant changes after surgery when compared to the changes induced by contact lens wear (55–60). Although these reports do not show significant endothelial changes, there have been reports of changes occurring in both animal experiments and high myopes, and in association with tranquilizers (61–64). Acute endothelial changes following both PRK and LASIK have been reported, with transient endothelial cell morphology changes noted using broad-beam and variable-beam lasers (65,66).

Laser Fluence

Laser fluence is a measure of the energy density and is described as the amount of energy applied per unit area with each pulse. This is measured in millijoules per centimeter squared (mJ/cm²). The minimum fluence necessary for proper photoablation of the cornea is approximately 50 to 60 mJ/cm² (67,68). Laser fluence should be checked before every ablation, which is usually automatically performed in most lasers. Two factors that affect fluence are gas concentrations and voltage. A low fluence level is an indication that the gas concentrations should be raised to prevent inadequate tissue ablation and therefore undercorrections. Gas levels that are too high can cause higher fluence and overcorrections. Similarly, increasing or reducing voltage also increases or decreases fluence, respectively.

Beam Homogeneity

Beam homogeneity is a measure of the consistency of energy distribution applied over the ablation area. Poor homogeneity, especially in broad-beam lasers, can lead to irregular ablation and potential loss of best spectacle-corrected visual acuity. It is thought to be of less significance in small scanning spot lasers, as any inhomogeneity present would be spread out evenly over the treatment area. This assumption may have to be revised in view of the demand on consistency and accuracy of beam placement in custom ablation. In these lasers the delivery system becomes the critical factor rather than the homogeneity of the beam itself. Verification of beam homogeneity is essential and is accomplished by test ablations into appropriate substrate materials as provided by the laser manufacturer. Poor homogeneity on test ablation is usually secondary to deterioration of the laser optics or delivery system (Fig. 76-9). In this situation the procedure is canceled until the problem can be remedied.

Beam Size, Ablation Profile, and Repetition Rates

All the current laser systems in production utilize scanning beams of either fixed or variable size, in isolation or combi-

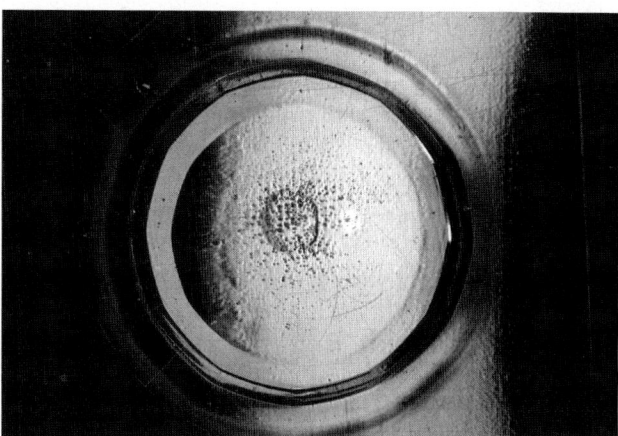

FIGURE 76-9. Test plate demonstrating poor homogeneity—central area of irregularity.

nation with another method of delivery, i.e., scanning slit. The smaller a beam size, the easier it is to control the homogeneity of the beam. The trade-offs for a smaller beam size include increased treatment time, corneal dehydration becoming a significant factor, and the effects on efficacy with small amounts of decentration (see Ocular Alignment and Eye-Tracking Systems section, later in this chapter).

With the onset of wavefront-adjusted ablation, attention has focused on the beam qualities, i.e., size and profile, required for such accurate treatment. Two theoretical studies of spot size and beam profile on aberration correction using numerical simulations showed that a top hat beam had an equivalent effect to a Gaussian beam with spot sizes of approximately 1.0 mm (11,12). With increasing beam size, ≥2.0 mm, the performance deteriorated with increased secondary aberrations. The paper concluded that beam sizes of ≤1.0 mm was adequate for correcting up to fourth-order Zernike terms with terms up to sixth-order requiring beams ≤0.6 mm diameter.

Ablation depth per laser pulse is dependent on radiant exposure with a threshold of approximately 50 mJ/cm² and with most current lasers operating at fluence values of 120 to 250 mJ/cm². The amount of tissue removed per pulse is dependent on fluence and beam profile (11). With current operating fluence values, ablation depths vary between 0.2 and 0.5 μm per pulse. Mrochen and Seiler (69) studied the effect of corneal curvature on ablation efficacy and reached the following conclusions:

1. Effective ablation depth decreases with increasing radius at the corneal surface.
2. Increasing fluence reduces this effect.
3. Decreasing corneal curvature results in an increased effect (Fig. 76-10).

Smaller spot sizes, understandably, require more pulses for a specified refractive correction, and thus an increase in the treatment time, which in turn may increase the likelihood

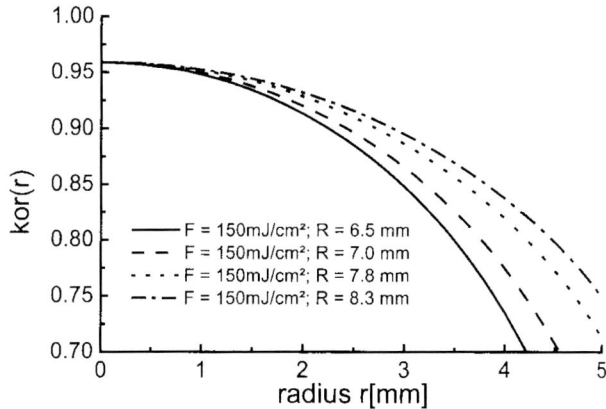

A

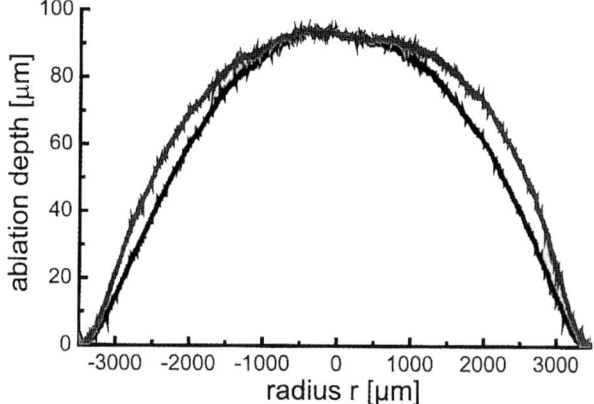

B

FIGURE 76-10. A: Graph demonstrating the relationship between corneal surface radii (r) and corneal curvature (R) on effective ablation depths (kor[r]) of laser pulses. **B:** Ablation profile for −6.00 D (optical zone 7.00 mm) with *(gray line)* and without *(black line)* taking the reflection losses into consideration. (From Mrochen M, Seiler T. Influence of corneal curvature on calculations of ablation patterns used in photorefractive laser surgery. *J Refract Surg* 2001;17:S584–S587, with permission.)

of corneal dehydration. Treatment time can be minimized by increasing laser repetition rate and increasing fluence. Laser repetition rate is limited by eye-tracking ability per laser as well as the possible effects of plume debris and thermal build up.

Laser Room Environment

The laser room environment is an important variable that must be controlled. The room should be kept cool for optimal laser performance. This varies from laser to laser, but a temperature of 18° to 24°C should be maintained. An ambient relative humidity between 40% and 50% is optimal and should be maintained as constant as possible. Humidity can significantly affect the ablation rate of corneal tissue, with overcorrections more likely in very dry conditions and undercorrections more likely in more humid conditions (70). The room should be kept free from particulate debris, which can adversely affect ablation regularity if deposited on the optical system of the laser and may also contribute to diffuse lamellar keratitis (71). This can be achieved with an active filtration system using a high-efficiency particulate air (HEPA) filter. These systems are capable of removing particles as small as 0.1 μm, including bacteria. The system should be in operation continuously, as shutdown periods allow particulate matter to coat the optics of the laser system.

Adjustments to Standard Laser Nomograms

Current excimer lasers have evolved through several generations and provide advanced features such as wider optical zones, multiple treatment zones, transition zones, and software to reduce surface irregularities such as central islands. However, each laser is used in different settings, and surgeons have individual variations in technique and operating environment. To allow for these differences, individual nomograms should be developed to improve the accuracy and predictability of treatments.

Among the factors that can contribute to the final visual and refractive outcome after LASIK are patient characteristics; preoperative refractive data; equipment (laser, keratome, wavefront analyzer, and operating room environment); surgical technique; and postoperative medications. All these factors may either be modified or taken into account by the surgeon (Table 76-2). Patient characteristics and preoperative-refractive data, especially patient age and amount of attempted refractive correction, are

TABLE 76-2. FACTORS TO CONSIDER WHEN PLANNING REFRACTIVE CORRECTION

Patient	Instrumentation	Surgical
Age	Laser design/manufacture	Ocular alignment
Refraction	Microkeratome type	Ocular surface
Corneal/ocular surface status, e.g., anterior basement membrane disease	Laser software	Flap thickness
	Laser calibration	Ablation zone size
	Wavefront analyser	Corneal hydration: wetting/drying, vacuum/forced air
	Topographer	Procedure time/flap exposure time
	Pachymetry	Postoperative medication
	Operating room environment: temperature, humidity, air quality, altitude	

examples of important factors, although not alterable, that must be taken into account by the surgeon. In terms of wavefront sensing, topography and pachymetry, different machines utilize different measuring techniques and resolutions, and may not be directly comparable in their results. Factors that can be influenced by the surgeon must be made as consistent as possible in order to achieve predictable results and allow accurate nomograms to be constructed (72).

OCULAR ALIGNMENT AND EYE-TRACKING SYSTEMS

With the development of scanning spot and variable spot laser systems, as well as the accuracy required to deliver wavefront adjusted treatments, the necessity of accurate ocular alignment has been recognized in order to fully utilize the potential of the excimer laser as a refractive tool (73).

Patient-controlled methods of ocular alignment rely on the patient to maintain proper head orientation and fixation on a fixation target. On their own, subjective methods are vulnerable to involuntary eye movements and to changes in the eye fixating. Using suction/fixation rings for the eye and head may introduce potential problems of corneal distortion, surgeon-induced decentration, and interruption of suction during the procedure (74). Eye tracking is an indirect surgeon-controlled technique that has the potential advantage of being completely independent of subjective influences.

Tracking Systems

The basic components of any tracking system consist of an image-acquiring sensor, microprocessor to compute the eye position, and a control system to move the laser beam appropriately, thereby maintaining alignment. The methods currently in use for image acquisition are either photoelectric or video-based. Photoelectric devices have the advantage of a high-frequency response but require pupil dilation and are unable to account for cyclotorsion directly. This deficiency can be remedied by rotating the treatment and aligning with ocular marks. Video-based systems require the image to be acquired and then processed/digitized, introducing delays affected by the video sampling rate with the advantage of not requiring pupil dilation. Methods of detecting cyclotorsion by iris recognition are currently under development by several manufacturers.

Latency and Random Eye Movements

During fixation, microsaccades and other eye movements are still present. These other movements include torsional changes secondary to the vestibular ocular reflex as well as involuntary optokinetic and vergence eye movements.

Random eye movements during fixation have amplitudes of 10 seconds to 10 minutes angular range ($\leq 450\ \mu$m) and peak velocities of 10 to 300 min/s (75).

The accuracy of laser delivery is dependent on tracking eye movements, the time delay between eye position recognition to delivering the laser pulse, latency, and the accuracy of the mirrors to deliver the laser to the designated position. Latency, which limits the accuracy of each laser pulse subject to the angular velocity of the eye movement in that interval, is mainly due to the mirror adjustment time and the electronic times required for image computing and laser pulse actuation. The mirror adjustment time is dependent on the speed of the mirror movement and the distance of travel between positions. Higher image sampling rates produce a theoretical advantage in the reduction of laser movement necessary between each image, which is only maximally realized if the latency is less than the interval between each image sampled, e.g., for a 200-Hz sampling, the latency has to be <5 msec.

An ideal tracking system, therefore, would have a high sampling rate greater than or equal to the laser ablation rate, with a minimum delay between the laser delivery and image capture, as well as the capability to compensate for cyclotorsional movements and accurate mirror movements.

Effects of Eye Tracking on Treatment Outcomes

Eye tracking does not necessarily improve centration, which is also dependent on patient fixation. Studies on video and photoelectric tracker guided scanning laser PRK demonstrated mean ablation decentration of 0.33 ± 0.32 mm (PRK), 0.35 ± 0.26 mm (LASIK), and 0.42 ± 0.28 mm (PRK), respectively, a figure similar to results from wide-beam systems (Fig. 76-11) (76,77). A study comparing centration with and without video-based tracking in LASIK patients showed no statistical difference in centration between the two groups (78).

Even an ablation decentration of less than 1.0 mm may result in increased ocular aberrations (9). Bueeler et al. (73), investigating alignment accuracy required for accurate wavefront guided surgery, showed that a 95% diffraction limit for a 3.0-mm pupil was achieved with a lateral alignment accuracy of 0.2 mm, but a 7.0-mm pupil would require an accuracy of ≤0.07 mm. A comparative study on the effects of video-based tracking reported visual acuity that was significantly better with less induced ocular aberrations in tracker-assisted eyes, with a reduction of both induced high- and low-order aberrations but no significant difference in refractive outcomes (79). Considering the theoretical limits of video tracking, two early studies comparing wavefront guided in one eye to standard LASIK in the fellow eye reported better corrected visual acuity with the wavefront group (3,4).

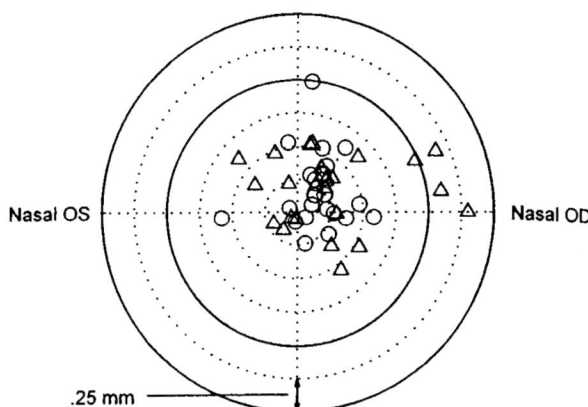

FIGURE 76-11. Surgeon's view of decentration of right eyes *(circles)* and left eyes *(triangles)* plotted as the distance from pupil center to ablation center in millimeters. Mean decentration ($\pm$ standard deviation) was 0.42 $\pm$ 0.28 mm (range 0.05 to 1.30 mm; *n* = 49) (OD, right eye; OS, left eye). (From Coorpender, et al. Corneal topography of small-beam tracking excimer laser photorefractive keratectomy. *J Cataract Refract Surg* 1999;25(5): 765–864, with permission.)

It therefore appears that although tracking may not improve centration with current technology, tracking-assisted ablations have been reported to demonstrate fewer induced aberrations by maximizing spot placement regularity. Future technology may improve registration of images between the wavefront capture device and the laser tracker device.

WAVEFRONT SENSING DEVICES

The method of ray tracing for measuring wavefront aberration was first described by Tscherning (80) and Hartmann (81) at the end of the 19th century. The basic principles of aberrometry can be traced to Scheiner, who described the Scheiner's disk in 1619. This was an opaque disk with two holes through which a subject would view a far distant object, e.g., a star, and therefore parallel rays of light. Any optical imperfections of the viewing eye would result in two images observed. It wasn't until the last half of the 20th century that wavefront aberration gradually entered into the field of interests of vision science with the developments of the Smirnov aberrometer and Shack's modification of a Hartmann screen, resulting in the first measurement of ocular aberrations in 1994 by Liang et al. (13) and others (82,83).

Basic Principles

In contrast to corneal topography, which measures the aberrations of the corneal surface in isolation, wavefront sensing is the measurement of the total refractive error of the eye. The commercial aberrometers in use today are all objective methods using image-sensing devices. They are based on the three main methods of wavefront

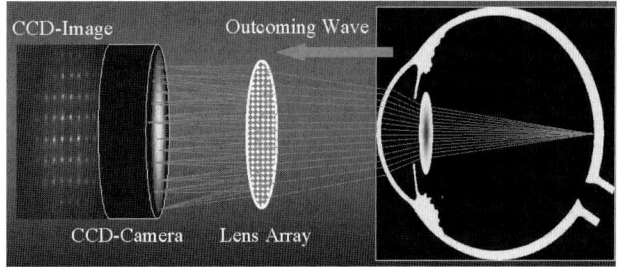

FIGURE 76-12. In a Hartmann shack aberrometer, the exiting light rays are passed through an array of lenslets to measure the wavefront emerging across the pupil. (Courtesy of John A. Vukich, M.D.)

sensing: out-going reflection (Shack-Hartmann), ray imaging (ray tracing/Tscherning), and in-going adjustable refractometry (spatially resolved refractometer). The Shack-Hartmann sensor utilizes approximately 200 spots that focus light, exiting the eye from a laser beam projected on the fovea, onto a detection array. Displacement of the aberrated spot is measured against the ideal, and the resulting wavefront is constructed (Fig. 76-12) (13). The ray tracing/Tscherning method involves projection of a grid (Tscherning) or sequential spots (Tracey ray tracing) on the retina, which is then recorded and compared to the ideal (Fig. 76-13) (84). In-going adjustable refractometry as described originally, was a subjective method, which via a technique of scanning slit retinoscopy has been developed into an objective test (85).

PRACTICAL ASPECTS

All three methods of wavefront sensing are currently employed in various commercially available aberrometers. Clinical comparison of the different sensors has not been studied to date, keeping in mind the different resolutions and algorithms in constructing the wavefront and the limitations of the individual methods used. In the Shack-Hartmann sensor, individual spot blurring due either to macro- or microaberrations are not taken into account. Macroaberrations occur when the wavefront is significantly curved over the flat sensing array, inducing a blurred spot, which is difficult to localize accurately, or possibly overlapping spots. Microaberrations are irregular and fine, causing blur rather than displacement of individual spots. The majority of sensing devices, therefore, may have limited abilities to measure gross aberrations, e.g., after penetrating keratoplasty. All devices are also sensitive to tear-film abnormalities, accommodation, pupil size, lenticular changes over time, and corneal changes over time or after surgery. The quality of each

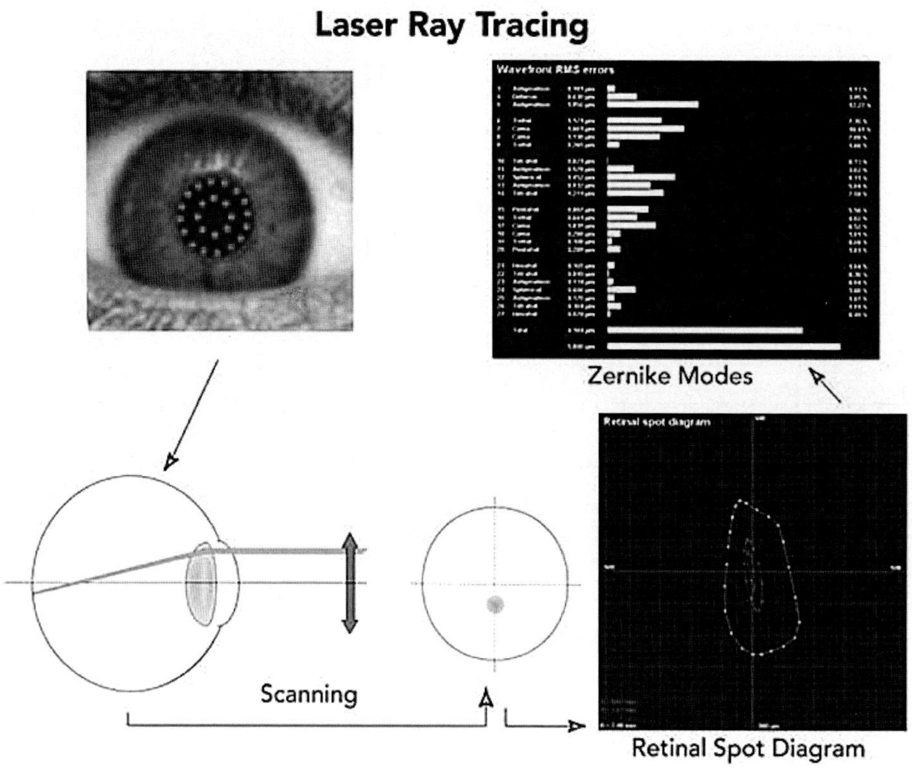

Laser Ray Tracing

FIGURE 76-13. Figure demonstrating the principal of ray tracing. (Courtesy of Tracey Technology.)

capture should be determined by examining the un-processed captured image.

Wavefront Terminology

The wavefront information collected is displayed as a wavefront refraction, in terms of conventional sphere and cylinder, as well as maps depicting total optical aberration, higher order aberration, and optical path difference—either as a wavefront error or refractive correction map, acuity map, point spread function, and a Zernike Coefficients table. Zernike polynomials are a form of mathematical functions, in turn dependent on functions of radius and meridian of a point in the pupil plane, used to describe fundamental shapes. An example of the shapes represented by the first six orders of Zernike polynomials is shown in Fig. 76-14.

The point spread function attempts to describe the effect of the visual aberrations on a point source of light. The magnification scale is very important in interpreting this map, and is displayed below the diagram. Zernike coefficients can be displayed in a Zernike coefficients table (Fig. 76-15). The Zernike coefficients can be displayed using standard or polar coordinates. Standard Zernike coordinates express the exam data using classical mathematical terms, whereas polar Zernike coordinates use vector combination to combine similar Zernike terms

to represent the optical properties obtained from the exam data.

The onset of wavefront sensing has introduced a new nomenclature to ophthalmologists similar to the introduction of corneal topography. Ophthalmologists will have to familiarize themselves with the systems that they acquire and remember that, just as in topography, the scales of each map must be considered.

Wavefront Ablation: Technological Requirements

From the earlier topics, the onset of wavefront sensing has led to an increased ability to discover and quantify the changes in aberrations that are caused by physiologic variations as well as refractive surgery. This in turn has led to a greater understanding of technological improvements necessary to achieve the goal of custom refractive surgery. These demands include accurate tracking with a small error, ability to utilize small beam spot sizes, and the development of flap creation or modulation of wound healing that will be as aberration neutral as possible.

At present, it is still undetermined as to whether all aberrations require treatment to achieve the best potential vision for patients. It appears that reducing aberrations to the fifth Zernike order results in objective and subjective improvements in vision (3,4,79).

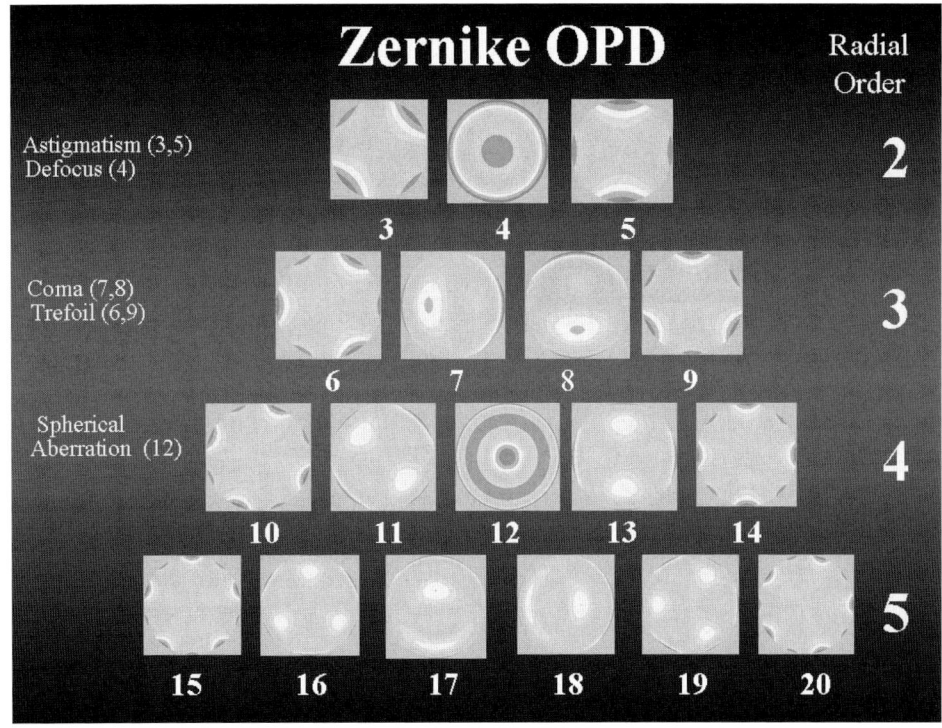

FIGURE 76-14. Color depiction of aberrations based on Zernike polynomial calculations.

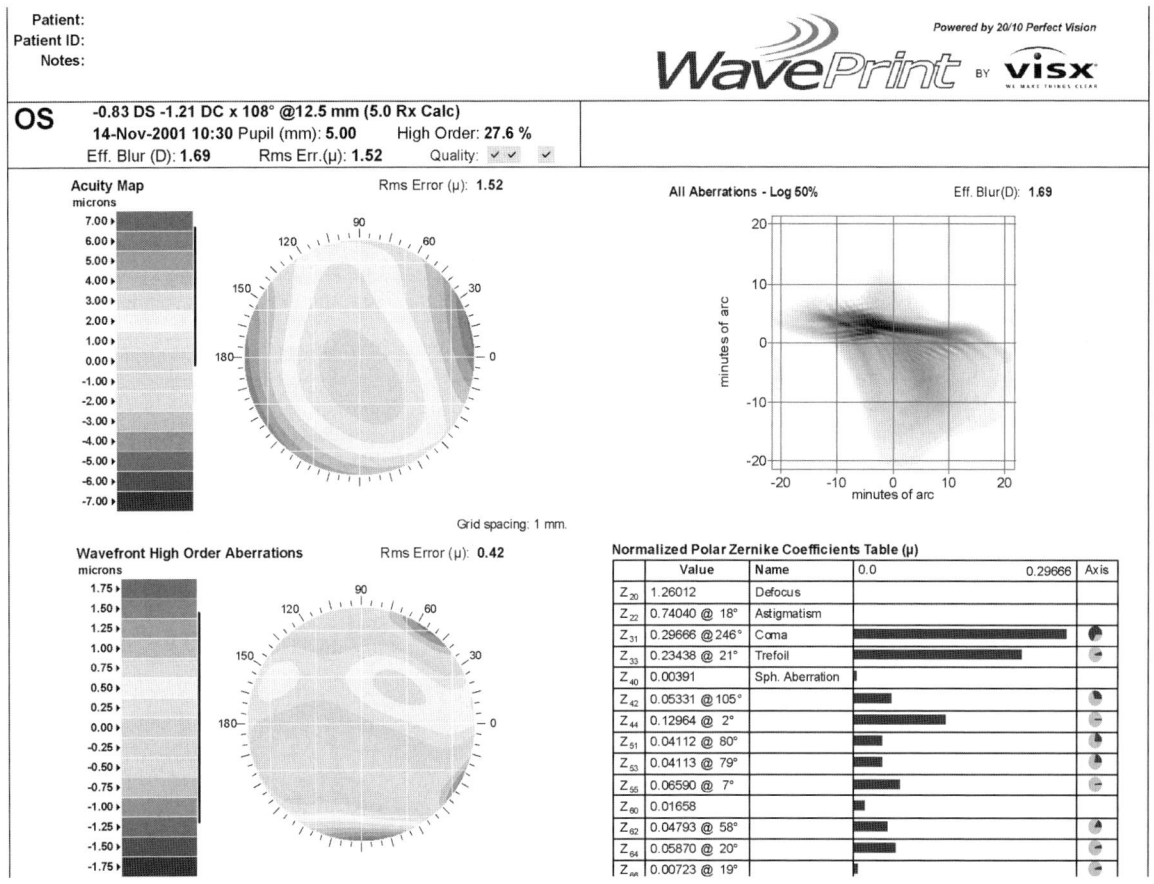

FIGURE 76-15. Wavefront analysis with the VISX WaveScan shows a sphere of −0.83 D and a cylinder of −1.21 D. The higher-order aberrations represent 27.6% of the total aberrations. Note the RMS value of 1.52 μm and the table of Zernike coefficients. The effective blur of this wavefront is 1.69 diopter *(top right of display)*.

CONCLUSION

LASIK has continued to be progressively safer and more effective with continuous advances in the field. The proper selection of microkeratome settings and development of personal laser nomograms are important elements of a successful LASIK procedure. The diligent attention to surgical details is necessary in order for physicians to optimally utilize the techniques of wavefront driven ablation. The availability of customized ablation has demanded further control of microkeratome and laser settings. This increase in the accuracy of laser ablation has stimulated the investigation of corneal structural changes and tissue remodeling after refractive surgery. The results of treatment are dependent on surgeons' understanding the nuances of utilizing their unique equipment for laser vision correction.

REFERENCES

1. Mrochen M, Kaemmerer M, Seiler T. Clinical results of wavefront-guided LASIK as 3 months after surgery. *J Cataract Refract Surg* 2001;27(1):201–207.
2. McDonald MB. Summit-Autonomous and CustomCornea laser in situ keratomileusis outcomes. *J Refract Surg* 2000;16(5):S617–S618.
3. Nuijts RMMA, Nabar VA, Hament WJ, et al. Wavefront-guided versus standard laser in situ keratomileusis to correct low to moderate myopia. *J Cataract Refract Surg* 2002;28(11):1907–1913.
4. Phusitphoykai N, Tungsiripat T, Siriboonkoom J, et al. Comparison of conventional versus wavefront-guided laser *in situ* keratomileusis in the same patient. *J Refract Surg* 2003;19(2):S217–S220.
5. Nagy ZZ, Palagyi-Deak I, Kovacs A, et al. First results with wavefront-guided photorefractive keratectomy for hyperopia. *J Refract Surg* 2002;18(5):S620–S623.
6. Nagy ZZ, Palagyi-Deak I, Keleman E, et al. Wavefront-guided photorefractive keratectomy for myopia and myopic astigmatism. *J Refract Surg* 2002;18(5):S615–S619.
7. Alessio G, Boscia F, La Tegola G, et al. Corneal interactive programmed topographic ablation customized photorefractive keratectomy for correction of postkeratoplasty astigmatism. *Ophthalmology* 2001;108(11):2029–2037.
8. Alessio G, Boscia F, La Tegola G, et al. Topography driven excimer laser for the retreatment of decentralized myopic photorefractive keratectomy. *Ophthalmology* 2001;108(9):1695–1703.
9. Mrochen M, Kaemmerer M, Mierdel P, et al. Increased higher-order optical aberrations after laser refractive surgery. *J Cataract Refract Surg* 2001;27(3):362–369.
10. Pallikaris IG, Kymionis GD, Panagopoulou SI, et al. Induced optical aberrations following formation of a laser *in situ* keratomileusis flap. *J Cataract Refract Surg* 2002;28(10):1737–1741.
11. Huang D, Arif M. Spot size and quality of scanning laser correction of higher-order wavefront aberrations. *J Cataract Refract Surg* 2002;28(3):407–416.
12. Guirao A, Williams DR, MacRae SM. Effect of beam size on the expected benefit of customized laser refractive surgery. *J Refract Surg* 2003;19(1):15–23.
13. Liang J, Grimm B, Goelz S, et al. Objective measurement of the wave aberrations of the human eye. *J Opt Soc Am A* 1994;11(7):1949–1957.
14. Roberts C. Future challenges to aberration-free ablative procedures. *J Refract Surg* 2000;16(5):S623–S629.
15. Oshika T, Klyce SD, Applegate RA, et al. Changes in corneal wavefront aberrations with aging. *Invest Ophthalmol Vis Sci* 1999;40:1351–1355.
16. Panagopoulou SI, Pallikaris IG. Wavefront customized ablations with the WASCA Ascelepsion Workstation. *J Refract Surg* 2003;17(5):S608–S612.
17. Barraquer JI. Keratomileusis. *Int Surg* 1967:48:103–117.
18. Argento C, Cosentino MJ, Valenzuela G. Influence of keratometry on the flap size. ASCRS Symposium on Cataract, IOL, and Refractive Surgery, San Diego, 1998, p. 119.
19. Choi YI, Park SJ, Song BJ. Corneal flap dimensions in laser *in situ* keratomileusis using the Innovatome automatic microkeratome. *Korean J Ophthalmol* 2000;14(1):7–11.
20. Yi WM, Joo CK. Corneal flap thickness in laser *in situ* keratomileusis using an SCMD manual microkeratome. *J Cataract Refract Surg* 1999;25(8):1087–1092.
21. Binder PS, Moore M, Lambert RW, Seagrist DM. Comparison of two microkeratome systems. *J Refract Surg* 1997;13(2):142–153.
22. D Huang, Sur S, Seffo F, et al. Surgically induced astigmatism after laser *in situ* keratomileusis. *J Refract Surg* 2000;16:515–518.
23. Donnenfield E, Solomon K, Perry HD, et al. Effect of hinge position on dry eye signs and symptoms following LASIK. *Ophthalmology* 2003;110(5):1023–1029.
24. Kumano Y, Matsui H, Zushi I, et al. Recovery of corneal sensation after myopic correction by laser *in situ* keratomileusis with a nasal or superior hinge. *J Cataract Refract Surg* 2003;29(4): 757–760.
25. Seiler T, Koufala K, Richter G. Iatrogenic keratectasia after laser *in situ* keratomileusis. *J Refract Surg* 1998;14:312–317.
26. Amoils SP, Deist MB, Gous P, et al. Iatrogenic keratectasia after laser *in situ* keratomileusis for less than −4.0 to −7.0 diopters of myopia. *J Cataract Refract Surg* 2000;26(7):967–977.
27. Munnerlyn CR, Koons SJ, Marshall J. Photorefractive keratectomy: a technique for laser refractive surgery. *J Cataract Refract Surg* 1988;14(1):46–52.
28. Behrens A, Seitz B, Langenbucher A, et al. Evaluation of corneal flap dimensions and cut quality using the Automated Corneal Shaper microkeratome. *J Refract Surg* 2000;16(1):83–89.
29. Gailitis RP, Lagzdins M. Factors that affect corneal flap thickness with the Hansatome microkeratome. *J Refract Surg* 2002;18(4):439–443.
30. Kim YH, Choi JS, Chun HJ, et al. Effect of resection velocity and suction ring on corneal flap formation in laser *in situ* keratomileusis. *J Cataract Refract Surg* 1999;25(11):1448–1455.
31. Hoffmann S, Krummenauer F, Tehrani M, et al. Impact of head advance and oscillation rate on the flap parameter: a comparison of two microkeratomes. *Graefes Arch Clin Exp Ophthalmol* 2003;241(2):149–153.
32. Yildirim R, Aras C, Ozdamar A, et al. Reproducibility of corneal flap thickness in laser *in situ* keratomileusis using the Hansatome microkeratome. *J Cataract Refract Surg* 2000;26(12): 1729–1732.
33. Spadea L, Cerrone L, Necozione S, et al. Flap measurements with the Hansatome microkeratome. *J Refract Surg* 2002;18(2):149–154.
34. Nordan LT, Slade SG, Baker RN, et al. Femtosecond laser flap creation for laser *in situ* keratomileusis: six month follow-up of initial U.S. clinic series. *J Refract Surg* 2003;19(1):8–14.
35. Ratkay-Traub I, Ferincz IE, Juhasz I, et al. First clinical results with the femtosecond neodymium-glass laser in refractive surgery. *J Refract Surg* 2003;19(2):94–103.
36. Kurtz RM, Liu X, Elner VM, et al. Photodisruption in the human cornea as a function of laser pulse width. *J Refract Surg* 1997;13(7):653–658.

37. Kurtz RM, Horvarth C, Liu HH, et al. Lamellar refractive surgery with scanned picosecond and femtosecond laser pulses. *J Refract Surg* 1998;14(5):541–548.

38. Srinivasan R. Kinetics of ablative photodecomposition of organic polymers in the far-ultraviolet (193 nm). *J Vac Sci Technol Bull* 1983;11:923.

39. Srinivasan R, Leigh WJ. Ablative photodecomposition on poly (ethylene terephthalate) films. *J Am Chem Soc* 1982;104:6784.

40. Kahle G, Stadter H, Seiler T, et al. Gas chromatograph/mass spectrometer analysis of excimer and erbium-YAG laser ablated human corneas. *Invest Ophthalmol Vis Sci* 1992;33(7):2180–2184.

41. Puliafito CA, Stern D, Krueger RR, et al. High-speed photography of excimer laser ablation of the cornea. *Arch Ophthalmol* 1987; 105(9):1255–1259.

42. Kochevar IE. Cytotoxicity and mutagenicity of excimer laser radiation. *Lasers Surg Med* 1989;9(5):440–445.

43. Kerr-Muir MG, Trokel SL, Marshall J, et al. Ultrastructural comparison of conventional surgical and argon fluoride excimer laser keratectomy. *Am J Ophthalmol* 1987;103(3 pt 2):448–453.

44. Bende T, Seiler T, Wollensak J. Side effects in excimer corneal surgery. Corneal thermal gradients. *Graefes Arch Clin Exp Ophthalmol* 1988;226(3):277–280.

45. Kitazawa Y, Tokoro T, Ito S, et al. The efficacy of cooling on excimer laser photorefractive keratectomy in the rabbit eye. *Surv Ophthalmol* 1997;42(11):S82–S88.

46. Maldonado-Codina C, Morgan PB, Efron N. Thermal consequence of photorefractive keratectomy. *Cornea* 2001;20(5): 509–515.

47. Ishihara M, Arai T, Sato S, et al. Measurement of the surface temperature of the cornea during ArF excimer laser ablation by thermal radiometry with a 15-nanosecond time response. *Lasers Surg Med* 2002;30(1):54–59.

48. Vetrugno M, Maino A, Valenzano E, et al. Corneal temperature changes during photorefractive keratectomy using the Laserscan 2000 flying spot laser. *J Refract Surg* 2001;17(4):454–459.

49. Hanna KD, Pouliquen Y, Waring GO 3rd, et al. Corneal stromal wound healing in rabbits after 193 nm excimer laser surface ablation. *Arch Ophthalmol* 1989;107(6):895–901.

50. Zabel R, Tuft S, Marshall J. Excimer photorefractive keratectomy: Endothelial morphology following area ablation of the cornea. *Invest Ophthalmol Vis Sci* 1988;29(suppl):390.

51. Srinivasan R, Dyer PE, Braren B. Far-ultraviolet laser ablation of the cornea: photoacoustic studies. *Lasers Surg Med* 1987;6(6): 514–519.

52. Gobbi PG, Carones F, Brancato R, et al. Acoustic transients following excimer laser ablation of the cornea. *Eur J Ophthalmol* 1995;5(4):275–276.

53. Krueger RR, Krasinski JS, Radzewicz C, et al. Photography of shockwaves during excimer laser ablation of the cornea. Effect of helium gas on propagation velocity. *Cornea* 1993;12(4): 300–334.

54. Krueger RR, Seiler T, Gruchman T, et al. Stress waves amplitude during laser surgery of the cornea. *Ophthalmology* 2001;108(6): 1070–1074.

55. Stulting RD, Thompson KP, Waring GO, et al. The effects of photorefractive keratectomy on the corneal endothelium. *Ophthalmology* 1996;103(9):1357–1365.

56. Carones F, Brancato R, Venturi E, et al. The corneal endothelium after myopic excimer laser photorefractive keratectomy. *Arch Ophthalmol* 1994;112(7):920–924.

57. Trocme SD, Mack KA, Gill KS, et al. Central and peripheral endothelial cell changes after excimer laser photorefractive keratectomy for myopia. *Arch Ophthalmol* 1996;114(8):925–928.

58. Jones SS, Azar RG, Cristol SM, et al. Effects of laser *in situ* keratomileusis (LASIK) on the corneal endothelium. *Am J Ophthalmol* 1998;125(4):465–471.

59. Perez-Santonja J, Sakla HF, Alio JL. Evaluation of endothelial changes one year after excimer laser *in situ* keratomileusis. *Arch Ophthalmol* 1997;115(7):841–846.

60. Perez-Santonja J, Sakla HF, Gobbi F, et al. Corneal endothelial changes after laser *in situ* keratomileusis. *J Cataract Refract Surg* 1997;23(2):177–183.

61. Dehm EJ, Puliafito CA, Adler CM, et al. Corneal endothelial injury in rabbits following excimer laser ablation at 193 and 248 nm. *Arch Ophthalmol* 1986;104(9):1364–1368.

62. Pallikaris IG, Siganos DS. Excimer laser *in situ* keratomileusis and photorefractive keratectomy for correction of high myopia. *J Refract Corneal Surg* 1994;10(5):498–510.

63. Lambert RW, Anderson JA, Heitzman J, et al. Excimer laser effects on human corneal endothelium. Modulation by serum factor(s). *Arch Ophthalmol* 1996;114(12):1499–1505.

64. Nakaya-Onishi M, Kiritoshi A, Hasegawa T, et al. Corneal endothelial cell loss after excimer laser keratectomy, associations with tranquilizers [letter]. *Arch Ophthalmol* 1996;114(10): 1282–1283.

65. Carones F, Brancato R, Venturi E, et al. The human corneal endothelium after myopic excimer laser photorefractive keratectomy. Immediate to one-month follow up. *Eur J Ophthalmol* 1995;5(4):204–213.

66. Kim T, Sorenson AL, Krishnasamy S, et al. Acute corneal endothelial changes after laser *in situ* keratomileusis. *Cornea* 2001; 20(6):597–602.

67. Krueger RR, Trokel SL. Quantification of corneal ablation by ultraviolet laser light. *Arch Ophthalmol* 1985;103(11):1741–1742.

68. Seiler T, McDonnell PJ. Excimer laser photorefractive keratectomy. *Surv Ophthalmol* 1995;40(2):89–118.

69. Mrochen M, Seiler T. Influence of corneal curvature on calculations of ablation patterns used in photorefractive laser surgery. *J Refract Surg* 2001;17(5):S584–S587.

70. de Souza IR, de Souza AP, de Queiroz AP, et al. Influence of temperature and humidity on laser *in situ* keratomileusis outcomes. *J Refract Surg* 2000;17(2 suppl):S202–204.

71. Anonymous. A mystery tale: the search for the cause of 100+ cases of diffuse lamellar keratitis. *J Refract Surg* 2002;18(5):551–554.

72. Sanchez-Thorin JC, Cope WT. Nomogram generation for keratomileusis: an introduction to multivariate analysis and neural nets. *Int Ophthalmol Clin* 1996;36(4):39–44.

73. Bueeler M, Mrochen M, Seiler T. Maximum permissible lateral decentration in aberration-sensing and wavefront-guided corneal ablation. *J Cataract Refract Surg* 2003;29(2):257–263.

74. Sher NA, Fundingsland BR, Bergin A, et al. The effects of various methods of eye immobilization on corneal topography. *J Refract Surg* 1996;12(4):467–471.

75. Huppertz M, Schmidt E, Teiwes W. Eye tracking and refractive surgery. In: MacRae SM, Krueger RR, Applegate RA eds. *Customized corneal ablation: the quest for supervision.* Thorofare, NJ: Slack, 2001:149–160.

76. Tsai YY, Lin JM. Ablation centration after active eye-tracker-assisted photorefractive keratectomy and laser *in situ* keratomileusis. *J Cataract Refract Surg* 2000;26(1):28–34.

77. Coorpender SJ, Klyce D, McDonald MB, et al. Corneal topography of small-beam tracking excimer laser photorefractive keratectomy. *J Cataract Refract Surg* 1999;25(5):765–684.

78. Pineros OE. Tracker-assisted versus manual ablation zone centration in laser *in situ* keratomileusis for myopia and astigmatism. *J Refract Surg* 2001;18(1):37–42.

79. Mrochen M, Eldine SM, Kaemmerer M, et al. Improvement in photorefractive corneal laser surgery results using an active eye-tracking system. *J Cataract Refract Surg* 2001;27(7): 1000–1006.

80. Tscherning M. Die monochromatischen Abberationen des menschlichen Auges. *Z Psychol Physiol Sinn* 1894;6:456–471.

81. Hartmann J. Bemerkungen ueber den Bau und die Justierung von Spektrographen. *Zeitschrift fuer Instumentenkunde* 1900;20:47.

82. Smirnov MS. Measurement of the wave aberration of the human eye. *Biofizika* 1961;6:687–703.

83. Shack RV, Platt BC. Production and use of a lenticular Hartmann screen. *J Opt Soc Am A* 1971;11:1949–1957.

84. Mierdel P, Wiegard W, Kinke HE, et al. Measuring device for determining monochromatic aberrations of the human eye. *Ophthalmologe* 1997;94(6):441–445.

85. He JC, Marces S, Webb RH, et al. Measurement of the wavefront aberration of the eye by a fast psychophysical procedure. *J Opt Soc Am A* 1998;15(9):2449–2456.

77

LASIK TECHNIQUES AND OUTCOMES

IOANNIS G. PALLIKARIS AND
GEORGE D. KYMIONIS

One of the fields that could characterize the last decade in ophthalmology is the evolution and advancement of refractive surgery. An important factor in the general acceptance of refractive surgery by patients and doctors was the introduction of laser *in-situ* keratomileusis (LASIK) (1,2). Quick visual rehabilitation, minimal postoperative discomfort, the ability to correct high degrees of ametropia, reduced risk of postoperative corneal haze, improved predictability, and stability are a few of the reasons for LASIK's popularity over other surgical refractive correction options. It has been estimated that every year approximately 1.5 million patients worldwide undergo LASIK. This chapter describes this technique that continues to evolve.

ESSENTIAL LASER PHYSICS FOR THE REFRACTIVE SURGEONS

Excimer lasers are gas lasers that emit powerful ultraviolet pulses lasting from a few to hundreds of nanoseconds. The usual active medium is a gas mixture containing a rare gas and a halogen, which are combined to form a short-lived rare-gas halide molecule. Clinical excimer lasers use argon and fluorine gases to generate ultraviolet light with a wavelength of 193 nm. The energy from this wavelength of light is high enough to break the molecular bonds in the cornea and remove tissue. The ablation results in submicron tissue removal with every laser pulse, with minimal to no damage to the remaining tissue.

Ablation Depth

An algorithm developed by Munnerlyn et al. (3) depicts the relationship between the refractive effect produced and the depth of ablation. The Munnerlyn formula was based on affecting a theoretical lenticular curve within polymethylmethacrylate (PMMA) model, refined through *in vivo* models. The essentials of the Munnerlyn formula are found in the following formula:

$$\text{Depth of ablation (micrometers)} = \frac{[\text{optical zone (mm)}^2 \times \text{diopters of correction (D)}]}{3}$$

The main principle to be drawn from the formula is that the depth of ablation increases with the square of the optical zone. A small increase in the optical zone results in a large increase in the amount of tissue ablated for any dioptric correction.

Optical Zone

An evolution of technique toward larger optical zones continues despite the resultant greater depth of ablation, increasing the risk of corneal ectasia. Larger optical zones have two primary benefits—reduced night glare and reduced regression of effect—leading to more stable high corrections.

Eye Tracking System

Active eye tracking means that the laser detects a change in the eye's location and moves the next laser pulse in an attempt to meet the change. Passive tracking, however, simply detects change and shuts down further laser pulsing when the change exceeds a predetermined distance.

Fluence

Fluence correlates the amount of tissue that is ablated with each pulse (millijoules/sq cm). A fluence test is performed prior to each surgery and is crucial for laser beam calibration, homogeneity and alignment.

Custom Ablation

The linking of the laser device to various instruments (such as topography, wavefront analyzers) allows for correction of irregular (eccentric) ablations and high-order aberrations.

Microkeratome: A Critical Element

Microkeratome is another issue that is critical to the LASIK technique. There are several characteristics that can describe a microkeratome. Some of them are the following:

- Function (automated or manual)
- Cutting mechanism (blade, water or laser beam)
- Oscillation rate (customizable, predetermined)
- Hinge position (nasal, superior, 360-degree placement)
- Disposability
- Visibility of the cornea during keratectomy
- Suction to create a lamellar corneal flap and ability to check the intraocular pressure (IOP) intraoperatively
- Complexity, service, and cost

An important issue for each microkeratome is the cutting flap thickness. A microkeratome that tends to cut thin flaps is more likely to produce buttonholes, whereas thick flaps leave a thinner residual corneal bed, which limits the amount of ablation that can be safely performed. The average flap thickness does not predictably follow the manufacturer's label due to instrument variability and other operative factors (preoperative corneal thickness and curvature, microkeratome oscillation rate, suction ring pressure) (4). Intraoperative pachymetry (pre- and intraoperative after the flap is lifted, to determine flap and residual corneal bed thickness after flap creation) and predicted stromal ablation (calculated from the nomograms of the laser device according to the attempted correction and optical zone size) are important factors in maximizing the safety of the procedure.

Each of these factors is important for the evaluation of a microkeratome, and, regrettably, there is no perfect microkeratome. A general rule is that the microkeratome that meets the needs of each surgeon is the best microkeratome.

PREOPERATIVE EVALUATION

Limitations and Contraindications of LASIK

Preoperative evaluation of candidate LASIK patients consists of a detailed ophthalmic examination, which includes a complete medical and ophthalmic history and an informed consent.

There are several reasons for not performing LASIK. These contraindications result from the accumulated experience with LASIK with retro- and prospective studies (5). Some of them are the following:

- The upper limit of attempted correction: There are many factors that could affect the accepted upper limit for LASIK; we cannot simplify and state a single accepted attempted correction in LASIK procedures. Several factors, such as attempted correction, flap thickness, pupil diameter, pre- and intraoperative (after the

flap's creation) corneal thickness, are some of the parameters that determine the attempted correction in each patient individually. But attempted myopic corrections of more than 10 D or predicted myopic post-LASIK topographic curvature readings of less than 32 D are unacceptable (even though the previous criteria are fulfilled) due to increased risk of postoperative ectasia, induced optical aberrations, the decrease in functional optical zone, and the induced multifocality of the post-LASIK cornea. All these induced alterations result in a decrease in safety and efficacy of the LASIK procedure. Furthermore, hyperopic corrections of more than 5 D have poor results due to lost lines of best corrected visual acuity (BCVA), increased induced optical aberrations, and high incidence of regression.

- Patient's personality, occupation, psychological condition (patients with high expectations of the surgery)
- Patients younger than 18 years old (or older than 50 years old especially with high ammetropies) or unstable refraction (more than 0.5 D of change over 1 year)
- Previous intraocular or corneal surgery in the eye to undergo LASIK
- Good uncorrected visual acuity
- Corneal warping due to contact lens (CL) (soft CL must be removed 3 weeks before surgery and rigid CL at least 2 months before surgery)
- Thin corneas (less than 500 μm) for myopic patients
- Corneal dystrophies (ectatic-epithelial-stromal)
- Active ocular infection
- Pupil diameter more than 8 mm
- The presence of cataract
- Monocular patients
- Glaucoma or glaucoma suspects
- Retinal diseases (macular degeneration, myopic maculopathy, retinal tears)
- Systemic diseases (diabetes mellitus, Sjögren's syndrome, rheumatoid arthritis, and collagen vascular disorders)
- Pregnancy-lactation

All these limitations are debatable and can be changed at any time as they correlate with the current status of research.

OPERATIVE TECHNIQUE

Although LASIK offers almost immediate visual correction, improved comfort and stability, and minimum wound healing complications compared to photorefractive keratectomy (PRK), it requires far more surgical skill, as it involves the use of both sophisticated and complicated microkeratome technology.

The technician and the surgeon should check the laser and the microkeratome before surgery. The surgeon should also confirm that the correct treatment data are entered into the laser computer. Both the surgeon and the technician should verify the patient's name, the pupil diameter (in scotopic conditions), the thickness of the central cornea, and the attempted correction.

An eyelid speculum is inserted in the operative eye, which has been anesthetized topically, and the fellow eye is covered. The cornea is marked with an instrument that can allow postoperative proper flap alignment. A suction ring is placed on the eye to achieve an adequate IOP for the creation of the cornea flap. There are several indications that suction is adequate for flap creation, such as pupil dilatation, contact applanation device, or the patient's decreased vision. Corneal lamellar dissection has a steep learning curve, with the potential for severe, vision-threatening complications. Newer microkeratomes have improved the safety and reliability of the procedure. After flap creation (some microkeratomes give surgeons the ability to choose the hinge position—superior, nasal, or oblique), the residual corneal bed stroma is examined for irregularities. The next steps include flap protection, intraoperative pachymetry, centration and ablation; all these steps should be done as quickly as possible to minimize the time of exposure of the stromal surface (avoiding stromal dehydration, which eventually leads to overcorrection and, in very rare conditions, to corneal perforation).

Centration of the laser beam is also crucial for a successful operation. For myopic eyes, the ablation beam is centered on the center of the pupil. It is centered slightly nasal to the corneal light reflex for hyperopic corrections.

The tracking system is activated during the beam centration. Small saccadic eye movements are acceptable, but the surgeon must stop the ablation if the eye starts drifting away from the fixation target. Once the ablation is completed, the corneal stromal bed is cleaned with a dry sponge. The flap is replaced onto the bed using a bent cannula while irrigation of the interface with balanced salt solution is performed to remove any remaining debris. This also facilitates the floating of the flap back into its original position. Aggressive irrigation should be avoided because it leads to flap edema, which increases the incidence of epithelial ingrowth (presence of an area of poor flap adherence). For proper flap alignment, the corneal marks should be properly aligned.

POSTOPERATIVE MANAGEMENT

The majority of LASIK patients require minimum postoperative follow-up and have excellent refractive results, even in the presence of minor flap complications. Severely complicated cases, however, require intensive monitoring of the eye's status.

The main goals of postoperative management include the proper flap alignment to the stromal bed, the recognition and management of complications, and the modulation of

refractive status. LASIK patients are typically examined 1 to 2 hours after the operation (to ensure that the flap is properly aligned), on the first postoperative day (if striae or other flap irregularities are evident, the flap should be lifted back and repositioned), and at 1, 3, 6, and 12 months postoperatively.

The postoperative regimen varies significantly between refractive surgeons, but in general it includes a topical combined antibiotic-steroid agent tapered for 15 days to prevent infection and control inflammation.

AVOIDANCE OF LASIK COMPLICATIONS

The widespread growth of LASIK has not resulted in notably serious complications. The few that have occurred, however, are of great importance when considering the elective nature of such a procedure and the ever-growing number of available alternatives (6–8). Among the many classifications of LASIK complications, the most popular is the one that lists complications in chronological order.

Intraoperative

Intraoperative complications include buttonholes, half flaps, irregular/thin flaps, total caps, epithelial defects, and overhydrated or dehydrated flaps (Fig. 77-1). Most, if not all, are the results of a poor surgical technique and are preventable (9). Some of the predisposing factors for improper keratectomy are extreme corneal keratometric values (corneas steeper than 46.00 D are more prone to buttonholed or centrally thinned flaps, whereas corneas flatter than 41 D are more prone to free caps), lack of synchronization between oscillatory blade and microkeratome movement,

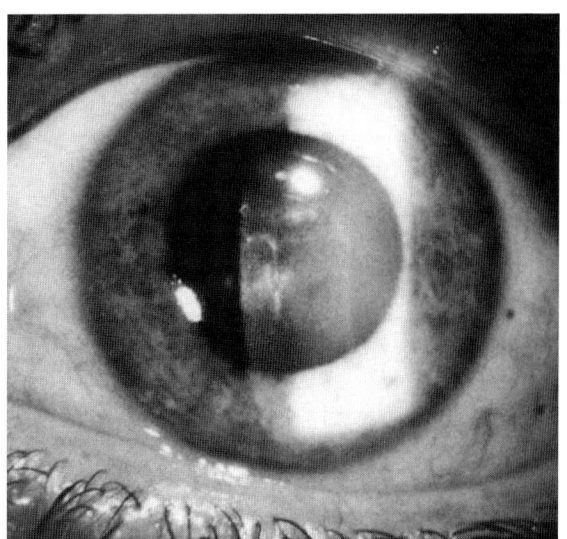

FIGURE 77-1. Slit-lamp photograph of a patient with post-LASIK buttonhole, showing a central irregular corneal scar.

irregular oscillation rate, poor suction, and defective microkeratome plates (7,8,10). Proper assembly of the microkeratome, marking of the cornea prior to the keratectomy, good exposure of the treated eye, customized microkeratome settings depending on the corneal keratometric readings (larger suction ring for flat corneas) as well as adequate suction during keratectomy (pressure above 80 mm Hg) are some of the details that are fundamental in order to eliminate these complications.

The operation should be aborted if serious intraoperative complications occur. A new LASIK should be attempted no sooner than 3 months. This interval is necessary to allow the flap to adhere strongly to the stromal bed. A deeper depth plate should be used for reoperation (180 or 200 μm). It may be safe to complete the operation in selected cases, for example, where a total cap seems regular and of reasonable thickness.

Early Postoperative

The majority of early postoperative complications present during the first week after LASIK. We discuss those that are most common.

Flap Striae

Small irregularities of the corneal surface are almost unavoidable after LASIK. Although extremely wrinkled or dislodged flaps are very rare, flap striae may complicate even the most uneventful operation. Thinner, larger flaps and high attempted corrections are some of the predisposing factors for surface wrinkling (Fig. 77-2).

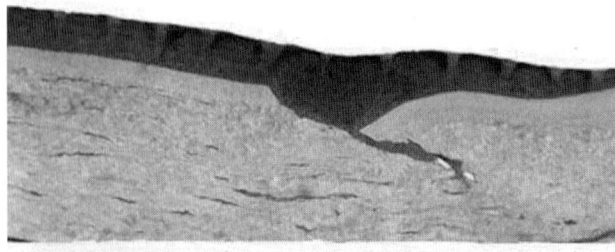

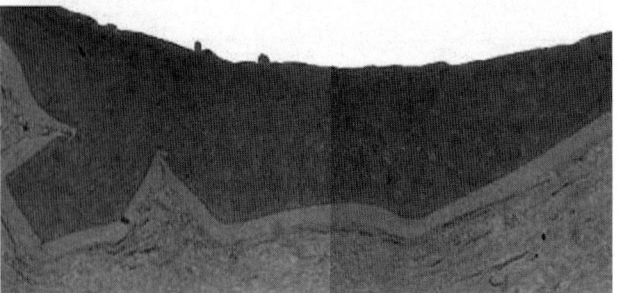

FIGURE 77-2. Histopathology of excised cornea reveals areas of epithelial ingrowth (*top*) and flap shrinking (*bottom*) (trichrome stain).

Striae are evident as soon as the first few hours after LASIK. Insignificant striae are asymptomatic, whereas significant ones cause irregular astigmatism with optical aberrations and BCVA loss in the presence of successful refractive outcome and regular topographic ablation pattern (11). Macrofolds (full-thickness flap tenting) are visualized by slit-lamp examination, whereas microfolds (wrinkles in Bowman's layer in the epithelial basement membrane) are visualized by retroillumination (12).

Flap striae are not a self-limiting condition. Significant striae (especially those that cross the visual axis) should be treated as soon as they are diagnosed, because with time they become embedded into the stromal bed and cause permanent damage to Bowman's membrane, with subsequent failure of any attempt to realign the flap. Several techniques have been described for management of flap striae (10,13). A technique that has worked well is the so-called flap ironing. During this procedure, the flap is reflected back and the stromal surface is hydrated with balanced salt solution (BSS) for about 30 seconds. The flap is then floated back into position. After irrigation is completed, ironing of the flap is done using a moistened sponge, starting from the hinge and pressing toward the opposite end of the flap (painting of the flap) while stretching it perpendicular to the striae. The flap is left for 5 minutes to attach to the bed. Hypertonic saline solution, 5%, may be applied to enhance striae treatment.

Infectious Keratitis

Keratitis is extremely rare after LASIK (0.1%), as the intact epithelium acts as a barrier to invasion of microorganisms (14,15). Conjunctival injection and moderate to severe pain that persists throughout the first postoperative day are the most common symptoms. Any corneal infiltrate associated with an epithelial defect after LASIK should be considered infective and should be treated aggressively. Patients with epithelial defects should be examined daily until reepithelialization, to detect early signs of bacterial keratitis. Proper draping of the operating eye and sterilization of the microkeratome and assisting instruments can minimize the risk of infection.

Diffuse Lamellar Keratitis (DLK)

Diffuse lamellar keratitis (a relatively infrequent complication) was first described in 1998 by Smith and Maloney (16). The reported incidence of this complication in the literature varies with the etiology and the severity of the complication from 0.2% in mild cases up to 30% in so-called epidemic DLK (17).

A classification in four stages, according to the severity and the evolution, has been described with clinical observation and confocal microscopy measurements (17–19). In stage I, granulocytes and mononuclear cells are localized at the peripheral flap (in the interface level). In stage II there is an additional involvement of the central cornea with linear acellular spindle-shaped bodies in the interface. In stage III there are sparse infiltrates in the anterior stroma and accumulation of decayed inflammatory cells in the central portion of the interface (spindle-shaped bodies and debris in confocal microscopy observation). Finally, in stage IV there are inflammatory cells, stromal and Bowman's folds, keratocyte activation in confocal microscopy, and flap melting, resulting in a decrease of flap thickness.

The exact cause and the ideal treatment of DLK have not been determined. The possibility of infection was excluded by negative culture (20). Contaminations of the interface during LASIK from soap, disinfectants, microkeratome blade debris, topical antiinflammatory nonsteroidal (AINS) agents and anesthetics, have been described (21). Late, recurrent or traumatic epithelial defect and erosion (22,23), meibomian gland secretion, and concomitant contact dermatitis (24) have also been blamed (25).

Early recognition of DLK is essential in order to optimize the treatment effect. Linebarger et al. (17) proposed guidelines for the management of DLK in correlation with the stage of this postLASIK complication. Intense topical corticosteroids (prednisolone 1%) must be administered every hour for moderate inflammation (stages I to II). In severe cases (stages III to IV) flap lift, irrigation, and scrape-off should be added. Close follow-up every day is necessary until decrease of inflammation.

Late Postoperative

Dry Eye

A frequent postLASIK complication (up to 30% to 40%) is dry-eye symptoms, especially in patients with preexisting dry eye (26). This postLASIK complication may be due to decreased corneal sensation with subsequent decreased blinking frequency and or to damage to the keratolimbal-area goblet cells from the suction ring. Perez-Santonja et al. (27) found that corneal sensitivity returned to preoperative levels 6 months after LASIK, whereas Chuck et al. (28) reported that corneal sensation tended to return to near baseline levels 3 weeks after surgery. In addition, a statistically significant correlation with attempted correction and reduction in corneal sensation has been proved (29). Frequent use of artificial tears and/or temporary punctal plugs has proved to be effective for the time period of post-LASIK dry-eye symptoms.

Epithelial Ingrowth (EI)

Accumulation of epithelial cells in the interface is the second most common LASIK complication after flap striae (Figs. 77-2 and 77-3). Although the overall incidence of this condition is approximately 14%, most EI is insignificant

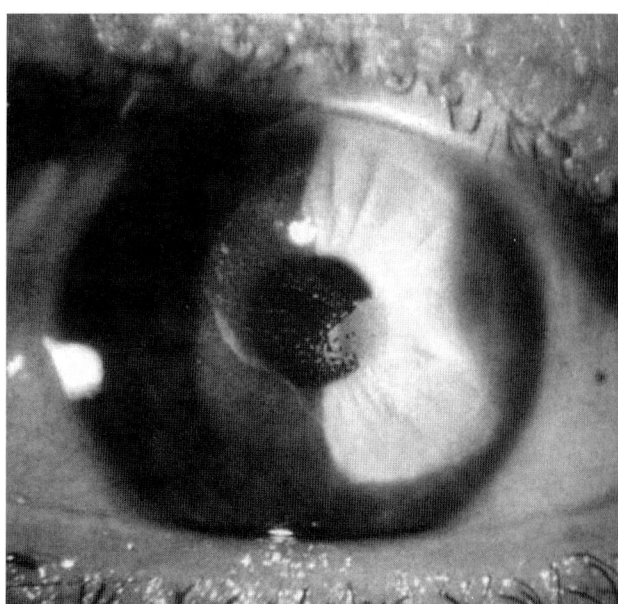

FIGURE 77-3. Central (into the visual axis) epithelial ingrowth with progressive flap melting.

and nonprogressive. However, cases with significant and progressive EI can eventuate in melting at the borders of the flap (by blocking aqueous diffusion and flap's nutrition or by producing proteolytic enzymes). The overall incidence of significant EI has been declining over the past 3 years, and this is mainly attributed to refinements in surgical techniques and improvements in microkeratome technology (30,31).

Possible risk factors for epithelial ingrowth include advanced age, anterior basement membrane dystrophy, history of recurrent epithelial erosions, ingrowth in the fellow eye, hyperopic LASIK correction, flap instability, edema, inflammation, dislocated flap, and reoperations. Epithelial defects at the time of surgery or loose epithelium (which caused an excessive hydration, resulting in poor adhesion of the flap) could be risk factors for subsequent epithelial ingrowth (31). The use of topical anesthetic should be limited to avoid corneal toxicity, whereas gentle handling of the flap can prevent accidental epithelial trauma. Very edematous flaps that are prone to displacement should be allowed to adhere to the stroma for a longer time at the end of the procedure.

Patients with minimal loss of BCVA and with stabilization of epithelial ingrowth dimensions do not need further intervention except follow-up. In cases of progression toward the visual axis (extend 2 mm beyond the flap edge), significant loss of BCVA, or induced flap irregularities that cause optical aberrations, surgical intervention is required. Gentle flap manipulations should be made to avoid any corneal epithelium trauma. The EI material is then scraped off from both the stromal bed and underneath the flap (Fig. 77-4). The interface is carefully irrigated; overhydration may hinder proper flap reattachment. The flap is then floated back into position and left to dry in room air for a few minutes.

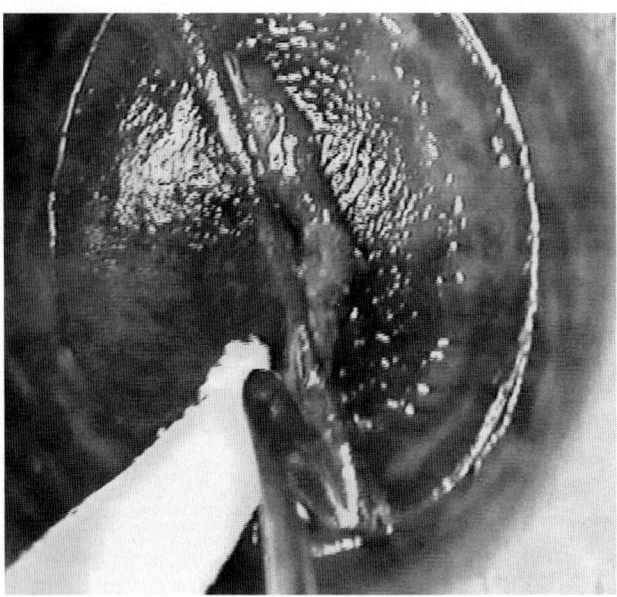

FIGURE 77-4. Flap lifting with epithelial removal in a patient with postLASIK epithelial ingrowth.

PostLASIK Corneal Ectasia

During the last 5 years there has been increasing concern about the occurrence of postoperative keratectasia. After LASIK, the cornea is structurally weakened, not only due to the laser central stromal ablation (depending on the attempted correction) but also from the creation of the flap itself. Since 1998, when Seiler et al. (32) published the first article regarding this complication, we have not elucidated the exact pathophysiology of this phenomenon, although several mechanisms and factors are proposed for contributing to this postLASIK complication (33,34).

Several studies reported that the amount of residual corneal thickness after ablation is crucial for the development of postLASIK ectasia. In clinical practice, we usually presume that 250 μm is safe. Seiler et al. (32) suggested this limit (250 μm) of the residual bed thickness to avoid ectasia after LASIK, whereas other studies found that even this limit is not safe to avoid postLASIK corneal ectasia (34,35).

Up to now, the therapeutic options for patients with post-LASIK ectasia were limited to spectacles and contact lenses (36) and in the advanced stages penetrating keratoplasty (PKP), whereas there are few publications in the literature regarding the management of patients with cornea ectasia after LASIK with Intacs all of which report encouraging results. Intacs seem to offer a minimally invasive alternative treatment for post-LASIK ectatic eyes, especially at the early stages of the disease, with fewer topographic irregularities (37,38).

Ablation-Related Complications

Ablation-related complications are a problem for both the patient and the surgeon (39). Each complicated case is a unique entity in terms of objective and subjective symptoms and should be treated as such.

An ablation is considered to be eccentric when the ablation center does not correspond to the center of the optical axis (40). This is a serious complication that needs to be treated, because it induces multifocality of the optical zone with inevitable visual problems. Small degrees of decentrations (eccentrations of 0.5 to 1 mm) could affect low-contrast visual acuity and induce wavefront higher order aberrations (41). But when a significant decentration (more than 1 mm) occurs, visual performance is highly compromised: symptoms such as glare, asymmetric halos (due to a prismatic effect which is more pronounced at night), and diplopia (mainly due to induced multifocality of the cornea) have been reported (42). In addition, an eccentric optical zone may produce ghost images, which further reduce visual acuity, particularly when the central zone of the uniform power is restricted to a small portion of the corneal surface.

There is a considerable variation in the incidence and the amount of eccentricity following LASIK, as has been shown in several studies (43). The amount of decentration is correlated with higher attempted correction and smaller ablation zones (44). Excimer laser systems utilizing mask techniques, such as hand-held rotating or erodible masks, or using smaller ablation zones are more liable to result in eccentric ablations. The incorporation of tracking systems in the excimer laser units had reduced the incidence of eccentricity (45). Despite this, several patients who have been treated with first- and second-generation laser systems require retreatment for correction of eccentric ablation. Furthermore, an active eye-tracking system alone cannot ensure proper centration. Additional factors such as learning curve and experience of the surgeons, saccadic movements, and patient-related factors such as cooperation, fixation, and misalignment of the patient's head relative to the laser could affect the ablation's centration (44).

Several topographically driven customized ablations are performed for corneal irregularity correction with varied results. The visual benefits of customized ablation include reduction in irregular astigmatism, improvement of visual quality, reduction of preoperative symptoms, and correction of lower-order aberrations. Knorz and Jendritza's (46) and Wiesinger-Jendritza et al. (47) report a high incidence of undercorrection and regression after topographically driven customized ablations, whereas other studies report satisfactory results (48,49).

Infrequent Complications

Diplopia After LASIK

Diplopia represents another postoperative complication with a low-reported incidence after LASIK (50). Kushner and Kowal (51) report that the etiology of diplopia was technical problems (scarring, small ablation zone, decentered treatment zone, astigmatism or power change, residual hyperopia in patients with accommodative esotropia, overcorrection), prior need of prism, aniseikonia, monovision, and incorrect targeted outcome.

Retinal Detachment After LASIK

There are few reports in the literature describing retinal detachment after LASIK. Arevalo et al. (52) report that the mean time of retinal detachment after LASIK was 16.3 months, whereas the frequency of rhegmatogenous retinal detachments after LASIK for the correction of myopia was 0.08%. Dilated indirect funduscopy with scleral depression and treatment of any retinal lesion predisposing to development of a rhegmatogenous retinal detachment, before LASIK surgery, is the best way to avoid such a complication (53,54).

PostLASIK Corneal Endothelium Damage

There are several contributory factors such as acoustic and shock waves during ablation, and increased IOP during flap creation in LASIK that could lead to corneal endothelial cell damage. Kim et al. (55) found that LASIK could affect the endothelial cell morphology temporarily, whereas Collins et al. (56) found that LASIK has no effect on central endothelial cell density 3 years after surgery. Vroman et al. (57) described endothelial corneal decompensation after LASIK in a patient with mild Fuchs' dystrophy, indicating that LASIK could affect endothelial cell function, especially in patients with defective endothelial cell function.

MANAGEMENT OF POSTLASIK PATIENTS

Intraocular Pressure (IOP) Measurements

Goldmann applanation tonometry is considered the gold standard for measuring IOP in a clinical setting. It is based on the modified Imbert-Fick law, which takes into account the corneal rigidity force, affected by central corneal thickness (CCT). The relationship between IOP and CCT is crucial for IOP measurements. Overestimation or underestimation of IOP affected by CCT could lead to a false diagnosis in eyes with normal IOP, ocular hypertension, primary open-angle glaucoma, or normal tension glaucoma. Several studies demonstrate that there is a correlation between the corneal thickness and IOP measurements, whereas other studies suggest that IOP measurements are in direct correlation with corneal curvature. LASIK affects both CCT and curvature, resulting in IOP alternations (58). Ehlers et al. (59) report a mean error of 5 mm Hg in the Goldmann tonometer for each 70-μm change in CCT, with a thinner cornea causing an underestimation, whereas other studies report a mean error of 3.5 mm Hg for a decrease in CCT of 70 μm and underestimation

or overestimation of the IOP by as much as 4.9 mm Hg or 6.8 mm Hg (60). Zadok et al. (61) found that there was a decrease in IOP after LASIK measured by central Goldmann applanation tonometry, whereas differences in pneumotonometry were less substantial, with greater reliability of pneumotonometry than Goldmann tonometry after LASIK.

Intraocular Lens Calculations

Intraocular lens power for cataract surgery in a patient who has had prior refractive surgery remains challenging. Several issues contribute to miscalculations of intraocular lens power after refractive surgery. The most important factors are the induced alterations in anterior and posterior corneal curvature and the effective index of refraction. These factors could lead to miscalculations of intraocular lens (IOL) power. Several indirect (clinical history method, contact lens overrefraction, intraoperative autorefraction, and vertexed IOL power method) and direct (linear regression models) methods of keratometric power estimation after refractive surgery have been developed (62).

LASIK RESULTS

For low to moderate myopia, results from studies have shown that LASIK is effective and predictable. For moderate to high myopia (>6 D), the results are more variable, given the wide range of preoperative myopia. The results are similar for treated eyes with low to moderate degrees of astigmatism (<2 D) (63). Hyperopic laser surgery still achieves only acceptable results and remains inaccurate and unstable (for moderate and high hyperopia), with significant regression, and shows more optical aberration and less satisfactory results than myopic surgery. Postoperative and final postoperative keratometric powers are reported as predictive factors for the final outcome in hyperopic LASIK treatments (64). Furthermore, the preoperative ametropia is strongly related to the final outcome, whereas various degrees of ametropia have been proposed as the upper limit (65–68). It seems that the alterations in ablation zone profiles and the differences in each laser nomogram that is used could affect the final outcome.

LASIK Versus PRK

Although the results of safety and efficacy studies for LASIK and for PRK are comparable, there are not enough prospective studies to compare the results of these techniques. Several studies report similar final visual acuity and refractive outcomes with both techniques (69), whereas LASIK offers more rapid visual recovery and stable refractive result than PRK (70,71). Van Gelder et al. (72) found that there is a tendency toward earlier visual rehabilitation after LASIK in comparison with PRK, although the final visual outcomes were comparable for mild to moderate myopia. It seems that both techniques have comparable results for low myopia patients, whereas in high myopia (over −6 D), LASIK technique seems to be superior than PRK.

LASIK Versus LASEK

Laser subepithelial keratomileusis (LASEK) was popularized in 1999 by Camellin (73). This technique is based on the creation of an epithelial flap after the instillation of an alcohol solution on the cornea. The epithelial flap is repositioned on the cornea after the ablation and is supposed to act as a therapeutic contact lens (74). Various concentrations of alcohol have been used for a different amount of time (20 seconds to 3 minutes) for the loosening of the epithelial layer (75,76). Stromal flap complications are eliminated in LASEK, so this technique can be performed in patients in whom LASIK may be contraindicated (thin, steep, flat corneas, high myopia). Prospective studies have shown that LASEK may have superior and comparable results to PRK and LASIK, respectively (77). The disadvantages of this technique in comparison with LASIK are the varying degrees of discomfort and blurry vision in the first postoperative days, mild recurrent erosion symptoms, and the need for more prolonged use of steroid eyedrops than in LASIK patients. Another crucial issue is the possible toxicity to the "epithelium–basement membrane" complex of alcohol used for the epithelial separation in the LASEK technique. A new method in which a mechanical epithelial flap separation is done without the need of alcohol has been developed at the University of Crete (called epi-LASIK, from the Greek word *epipolis*, which means superficial) with promising results. This technique has the advantages of LASEK without the risk of alcohol toxicity to the cornea. Preliminary histologic studies show that this technique is less invasive to the epithelial integrity as compared to the use of alcohol.

LASIK Versus Phakic Refractive Lens

LASIK has been used to treat high levels of refractive errors, but its predictability and stability decrease with the amount of the attempted correction. Large ablation depths also predispose the cornea to the risk of ectasia, which makes surgeons more conservative with extensive corrections (34,78). Furthermore, there is evidence that altering the shape of the cornea in extensive attempted corrections may result to poor quality of vision (79). Phakic intraocular lenses represent an evolving technique in the field of refractive surgery for the correction of moderate to high refractive errors (80). The implantation of a phakic intraocular lens does not affect the shape of the

cornea and induces minimal changes to the nature of the optical system. The technique has been proven to be stable and potentially reversible. Malecaze et al. (81) found that in moderate to high myopia, LASIK and the Artisan phakic intraocular lens seemed to produce a similar predictability, whereas the BCVA and subjective evaluation of quality of vision were better for the phakic intraocular lens group. Individual parameters of the cornea and the anterior chamber depth are two of the main factors that could affect the final choice.

Conventional Versus Wavefront-Guided LASIK

In the last couple of years wavefront aberrations from the research field have found their way to clinical interest in refractive surgery. In this concept, refractive corneal laser surgery focuses not only on the correction of spherocylindrical errors as the most apparent and disturbing optical aberrations of the human eye, but also on the correction of higher order aberrations as well. The expected benefits of custom ablation include the reduction in higher aberrations; improvement of visual quality (perhaps even a gain in BCVA); a reduction or no worsening for preoperative symptoms, such as halos and glare at night; and more accurate measurement and correction of lower-order aberrations.

Several studies have demonstrated that natural existing optical aberrations increase substantially after refractive surgery, suggesting a degradation of overall retinal image quality (82). Moreno-Barriuso et al. (83) found that LASIK increases the total wavefront error rool mean square (RMS), with the largest increase occurring in spherical aberrations, whereas other studies reported that only flap creation could affect the natural existing high-order aberrations (84). The naturally occurring higher order aberrations, combined with the aberrations induced by refractive surgery, can affect the visual performance after surgery. To avoid a loss of or achieve an increase in visual acuity, the use of individual ablation patterns, based on wavefront aberrations, has been introduced. The basic concept of wavefront-guided LASIK includes measurement of the wavefront aberrations with a wavefront analyzer and mathematical transfer of the measured wavefront aberrations into an adequate ablation pattern to be performed by a scanning-spot excimer laser.

Nuijts et al. (85) published encouraging results with wavefront-guided LASIK, whereas other studies did not show a statistically significant differences between wavefront and conventional LASIK (86). Mrochen et al. (87) found a statistically significant reduction in pre-LASIK higher-order RMS value in 22.5%, whereas on average, optical aberrations were increased by a factor of 1.44 after 3 months (one order of magnitude smaller than the factor in standard corneal laser surgery). Future prospective studies are needed in order to elucidate the impact of wavefront guided LASIK.

FUTURE PERSPECTIVES FOR LASIK: BEYOND LASIK

A decade after the introduction of the LASIK technique in refractive surgery, a number of issues have arisen. The technique has entered its maturity. The initial enthusiasm was replaced by a more conservative approach, which contributes to better patient selection and the reduction of intra- and postoperative complications. Even though these criteria limit the number of LASIK-candidate patients, they contribute to the reduction of postoperative complications, resulting in increased patient satisfaction and physician confidence.

Future challenges for the LASIK surgeons will be to minimize the side effects or complications of this technique (a new subspecialty in ophthalmology for the management of postLASIK complications could be the next step) and to customize the LASIK treatment for each patient individually. Furthermore, after LASIK the optical system is modified and a new optical system is created, through intervention in the cornea. Evaluation of this optical system still requires further studies.

Another important issue that correlates with the application of new technological evolutions of refractive surgery is that not all patients will benefit from these new technological advantages. Overenthusiasm and promises in the name of commercial goals could lead to dangerous consequences, not only for refractive surgery but also for our profession as ophthalmologists as well.

REFERENCES

1. Pallikaris IG, Papatzanaki ME, Siganos DS, et al. A corneal flap technique for laser *in situ* keratomileusis. Human studies. *Arch Ophthalmol* 1991;109(12):1699–1702.
2. Pallikaris IG, Papatzanaki ME, Stathi EZ, et al. Laser *in situ* keratomileusis. *Lasers Surg Med* 1990;10(5):463–468.
3. Munnerlyn CR, Koons SJ, Marshall J. Photorefractive keratectomy: a technique for laser refractive surgery. *J Cataract Refract Surg* 1998;14(1):46–52.
4. Yildrim R, Aras C, Ozdamar A, et al. Reproducibility of corneal flap thickness in laser *in situ* keratomileusis using the Hansatome microkeratome. *J Cataract Refract Surg* 2000;26(12):1729–1732.
5. Hori-Komai Y, Toda I, Asano-Kato N, et al. Reasons for not performing refractive surgery. *J Cataract Refract Surg* 2002;28(5):795–797.
6. Azar DT, Farah SG. Laser *in situ* keratomileusis versus photorefractive keratectomy: an update on indications and safety. *Ophthalmology* 1998;105(8):1357–1358.
7. Leung AT, Rao SK, Cheng AC, et al. Pathogenesis and management of laser *in situ* keratomileusis flap buttonhole. *J Cataract Refract Surg* 2000;26(3):358–362.
8. Farah SG, Azar DT, Gurdal C, et al. Laser *in situ* keratomileusis: literature review of a developing technique. *J Cataract Refract Surg* 1998;24(7):989–1006.
9. Pallikaris IG, Katsanevaki VJ, Panagopoulou SI. Laser *in situ* keratomileusis intraoperative complications using one type of microkeratome. *Ophthalmology* 2002;109(1):57–63.
10. Melki SA, Azar DT. LASIK complications: etiology, management, and prevention. *Surv Ophthalmol* 2001;46(2):95–116.
11. Carpel EF, Carlon KH, Shannon S. Folds and striae in laser *in situ* keratomileusis flaps. *J Refract Surg* 1999;15(6):687–690.
12. Rabinowitz YS, Rasheed K. Fluorescein test for the detection of striae in the corneal flap after laser *in situ* keratomileusis. *Am J Ophthalmol* 1999;127(6):717–718.
13. Probst LE, Machat J. Removal of flap striae following laser *in situ* keratomileusis. *J Cataract Refract Surg* 1998;24(2):153–155.
14. Lin RT, Maloney RK. Flap complications associated with lamellar refractive surgery. *Am J Ophthalmol* 1999;127(2):129–136.
15. Hovanesian JA, Faktorovich EG, Hoffbauer JD, et al. Bilateral bacterial keratitis after laser *in situ* keratomileusis in a patient with human immunodeficiency virus infection. *Arch Ophthalmol* 1999;117(7):968–970.
16. Smith RJ, Maloney RK. Diffuse lamellar keratitis. A new syndrome in lamellar refractive surgery. *Ophthalmology* 1998;105(9):1721–1726.
17. Linebarger EJ, Hardten DR, Lindstrom RL. Diffuse lamellar keratitis: diagnosis and management. *J Cataract Refract Surg* 2000;26(7):1072–1077.
18. Holland SP, Mathias RG, Morck DW, et al. Diffuse lamellar keratitis related to endotoxins released from sterilizer reservoir biofilms. *Ophthalmology* 2000;107(7):1227–1233.
19. Buhren J, Baumeister M, Cichocki M, et al. Confocal microscopic characteristics of stage I to 4 diffuse lamellar keratitis after laser *in situ* keratomileusis. *J Cataract Refract Surg* 2002;28(8):1390–1399.
20. Haw WW, Manche EE. Sterile peripheral keratitis following laser *in situ* keratomileusis. *J Refract Surg* 1999;15(1):61–63.
21. Kaufman SC. Post-LASIK interface keratitis, Sands of the Sahara syndrome, and microkeratome blades. *J Cataract Refract Surg* 1999;25(5):603–604.
22. Shah MN, Misra M, Wihelmus KR, et al. Diffuse lamellar keratitis associated with epithelial defects after laser *in situ* keratomileusis. *J Cataract Refract Surg* 2000;26(9):1312–1318.
23. Schwartz GS, Park DH, Schloff S, et al. Traumatic flap displacement and subsequent diffuse lamellar keratitis after laser *in situ* keratomileusis. *J Cataract Refract Surg* 2001;27(5):781–783.
24. Macaluso DC, Rich LF, MacRae S. Sterile interface keratitis after laser *in situ* keratomileusis: three episodes in one patient with concomitant contact dermatitis of the eyelids. *J Refract Surg* 1999;15(6):679–682.
25. Anonymous. A mysterious tale: the search for the cause of 100+ cases of diffuse lamellar keratitis. *J Refract Surg* 2002;18(5):551–554.
26. Todo I, Asano-Kato N, Hori-Komai Y, et al. Laser assisted *in situ* keratomileusis for patients with dry eye. *Arch Ophthalmol* 2002;120(8):1024–1028.
27. Perez-Santonja JJ, Sakla HF, Cardona C, et al. Corneal sensitivity after photorefractive keratectomy and laser *in situ* keratomileusis for low myopia. *Am J Ophthalmol* 1999;127(5):497–504.
28. Chuck RS, Quiros PA, Perez AC, et al. Corneal sensation after laser *in situ* keratomileusis. *J Cataract Refract Surg* 2000;26(3):337–339.
29. Kim WS, Kim JS. Change in corneal sensitivity following laser *in situ* keratomileusis. *J Cataract Refract Surg* 1999;25(3):368–373.
30. Asano-Kato N, Toda I, Hori-Komai Y, et al. Epithelial ingrowth after laser *in situ* keratomileusis: clinical features and possible mechanisms. *Am J Ophthalmol* 2002;134(6):801–807.

31. Wang MY, Maloney RK. Epithelial ingrowth after laser *in situ* keratomileusis. *Am J Ophthalmol* 2000;129(6):746–751.

32. Seiler T, Koufala K, Richter G. Iatrogenic keratectasia after laser *in situ* keratomileusis. *J Refract Surg* 1998;14(3):312–317.

33. Randleman JB, Russell B, Ward MA, et al. Risk factors and prognosis for corneal ectasia after LASIK. *Ophthalmology* 2003;110(2):267–275.

34. Pallikaris IG, Kymionis GD, Astyrakakis NI. Corneal ectasia induced by laser *in situ* keratomileusis. *J Cataract Refract Surg* 2001;27(11):1796–1802.

35. Joo CK, Kim TG. Corneal ectasia detected after laser *in situ* keratomileusis for correction of myopia. *J Cataract Refract Surg* 2000;26(2):292–295.

36. Eggink FAGJ, Houdijn Beekhuis WH. Contact lens fitting in a patient with keratectasia after laser *in situ* keratomileusis. *J Cataract Refract Surg* 2001;27(7):1119–1123.

37. Kymionis GD, Siganos C, Kounis G, et al. Management of post-LASIK corneal ectasia with Intacs. *Arch Ophthalmol* 2003;121(3):322–326.

38. Siganos C, Kymionis GD, Astyrakakis N, et al. Intrastromal corneal ring segments in patients with post-LASIK ectasia. *J Refract Surg* 2002;18(1):43–46.

39. Sugar A., Rapuano CJ, Culbertson WW, et al. Laser *in situ* keratomileusis for myopia and astigmatism: safety and efficacy: a report by the American Academy of Ophthalmology. *Ophthalmology* 2002;109(1):175–187.

40. Webber SK, McGhee NJ, Bryce IG. Decentration of photorefractive ablation zones after excimer laser surgery for myopia. *J Cataract Refract Surg* 1993;22(3):299–303.

41. Mrochen M, Kaemmerer M, Mierder P, et al. Increased higher-order optical aberrations after laser refractive surgery: a problem of subclinical decentration. *J Cataract Refract Surg* 2001;27(3):362–369.

42. Doane JF, Cavanaugh TB, Durrie DS, et al. Relation of visual symptoms to topographic ablation zone decentration after excimer laser PRK. *Ophthalmology* 1995;92(1):42–47.

43. Pallikaris IG, Siganos DS. Excimer laser *in situ* keratomileusis and photorefractive keratectomy for correction of high myopia. *J Refract Corneal Surg* 1994;10(5):498–510.

44. Tsai Y-Y, Lin J-M. Ablation centration after active eye-tracker-assisted photorefractive keratectomy and laser *in situ* keratomileusis. *J Cataract Refract Surg* 2000;26(1):28–34.

45. McDonald MB, Carr JD, Frantz JM, et al. Laser *in situ* keratomileusis for myopia up to −11 diopters with up to −5 diopters of astigmatism with the summit autonomous LADARVision excimer laser system. *Ophthalmology* 2001;108(2):309–316.

46. Knorz MC, Jendritza B. Topographically-guided laser *in situ* keratomileusis to treat corneal irregularities. *Ophthalmology* 2000;107(6):1138–1143.

47. Wiesinger-Jendritza B, Knorz MC, Hugger P, et al. Laser *in situ* keratomileusis assisted by corneal topography. *J Cataract Refract Surg* 1998;24(2):166–174.

48. Alessio G, Boscia F, La Tegola MG, et al. Topography-driven excimer laser for the retreatment of decentralized myopic photorefractive keratectomy. *Ophthalmology* 2001;108(9):1695–1703.

49. Alessio G, Boscia F, La Tegola MG, et al. Corneal interactive programmed topographic ablation customized photorefractive keratectomy for correction of postkeratoplasty astigmatism. *Ophthalmology* 2001;108(11):2029–2037.

50. Holland D, Amm M, de Decker W. Persisting diplopia after bilateral laser *in situ* keratomileusis. *J Cataract Refract Surg* 2000;26(10):1555–1557.

51. Kushner BJ, Kowal L. Diplopia after refractive surgery. Occurrence and prevention. *Arch Ophthalmol* 2003;121(3):315–321.

52. Arevalo JF, Ramirez E, Suarez E, et al. Retinal detachment in myopic eyes after laser *in situ* keratomileusis. *J Refract Surg* 2002;18(6):708–714.

53. Arevalo JF, Ramirez E, Suarez E, et al. Incidence of vitreo-retinal pathologic conditions 24 months after laser-assisted *in situ* keratomileusis (LASIK). *Ophthalmology* 2000;107(2):258–262.

54. Ruiz-Moreno JM, Perez-Santoja JJ, Alio JL. Retinal detachment in myopic eyes after laser *in situ* keratomileusis. *Am J Ophthalmol* 1999;128(5):588–594.

55. Kim T, Sorenson AL, Krishnasamy S, et al. Acute corneal endothelial changes after laser *in situ* keratomileusis. *Cornea* 2001; 20(6):597–602.

56. Collins MJ, Carr JD, Stulting RD, et al. Effects of laser *in situ* keratomileusis (LASIK) on the corneal endothelium 3 years postoperatively. *Am J Ophthalmol* 2001;131(1):1–6.

57. Vroman DT, Solomon KD, Holzer MP, et al. Endothelial decompensation after laser *in situ* keratomileusis. *J Cataract Refract Surg* 2002;28(11):2045–2049.

58. Argus WA. Ocular hypertension and central corneal thickness. *Ophthalmology* 1995;102(12):1810–1812.

59. Ehlers N, Bramsen T, Sperling S. Applanation tonometry and central corneal thickness. *Acta Ophthalmol* 1975;53(1):34–43.

60. Herndon LW, Choudhri SA, Cox T, et al. Central corneal thickness in normal glaucomatous, and ocular hypertensive eyes. *Arch Ophthalmol* 1997;115(9):1137–1141.

61. Zadok D, Tran DB, Twa M, et al. Pneumotonometry versus Goldmann after laser *in situ* keratomileusis for myopia. *J Cataract Refract Surg* 1999;25(10):1344–1348.

62. Hamilton DR, Hardten DR. Cataract surgery in patients with prior refractive surgery. *Curr Opin Ophthalmol* 2003;14(1): 44–53.

63. Sugar A, Rapuano CJ, Culbertson WW, et al. Laser *in situ* keratomileusis for myopia and astigmatism: safety and efficacy: a report by the American Academy of Ophthalmology. *Ophthalmology* 2002;109(1):175–187.

64. Rao SK, Cheng AC, Fan DSP, et al. Effect of preoperative keratometry on refractive outcomes after laser *in situ* keratomileusis. *J Cataract Refract Surg* 2001;27(2):297–302.

65. Arbelaez MC, Knorz MC. Laser in situ keratomileusis for hyperopia and hyperopic astigmatism. *J Refract Surg* 1999;15(4): 406–414.

66. Williams DK. One-year results of laser vision correction for low to moderate hyperopia. *Ophthalmology* 2000;107(1):72–75.

67. Sher NA. Hyperopic refractive surgery. *Curr Opin Ophthalmol* 2001;12(4):304–308.

68. Tabbara KF, El-Sheikh HF, Islam SM. Laser *in situ* keratomileusis for the correction of hyperopia from +0.5 to 11.50 diopters with the Keracor 117C laser. *J Refract Surg* 2001;17(2): 123–128.

69. Hersh PS, Brint SF, Maloney RK, et al. Photorefractive keratectomy versus laser *in situ* keratomileusis for moderate to high myopia: a randomized prospective study. *Ophthalmology* 1998;105(8):1512–1522; discussion 1522–1523.

70. El-Maghraby A, Salah T, Waring GO 3rd, et al. Randomized bilateral comparison of excimer laser *in situ* keratomileusis and photorefractive keratectomy for 2.50 to 8.00 diopters of myopia. *Ophthalmology* 1999;106(3):447–457.

71. el Danasoury MA, el Maghraby A, Klyce SD, et al. Comparison of photorefractive keratectomy with excimer laser *in situ* keratomileusis in correcting low myopia (from −2.00 to −5.50 diopters): a randomized study. *Ophthalmology* 1999;106(2): 411–421.

72. Van Gelder RN, Steger-May K, Yang SH, et al. Comparison of photorefractive keratectomy, astigmatic PRK, laser *in situ* keratomileusis, and astigmatic LASIK in the treatment of myopia. *J Cataract Refract Surg* 2002;28(3):462–476.

73. Camellin M. LASEK may offer the advantages of both LASIK and PRK. *Ocular Surgery News*, International edition, March 1999;28.

74. Lee JB, Seong GJ, Lee JH, et al. Comparison of laser epithelial keratomileusis and photorefractive keratectomy for low to moderate myopia. *J Cataract Refract Surg* 2001;27(4):565–570.

75. Carones F, Fiore T, Brancato R. Mechanical vs. alcohol epithelial removal during photorefractive keratectomy. *J Refract Surg* 1999;15(5):556–562.

76. Feit R, Taneri S, Azar DT, et al. LASEK results. *Ophthalmol Clin North Am* 2003;16(1):127–135.

77. Autrata R, Rehurek J. Laser-assisted subepithelial keratectomy for myopia: two-year follow-up (1). *J Cataract Refract Surg* 2003;29(4):661–668.

78. Perez-Santonja JJ, Bellot J, Claramonte P, et al. Laser *in situ* keratomileusis to correct high myopia. *J Cataract Refract Surg* 1997;23(3):372–385.

79. Applegate RA, Howland HC. Refractive surgery, optical aberrations, and visual performance. *J Refract Surg* 1997;13(3):295–299.

80. Gonvers M, Othenin-Girard P, Bornet C, et al. Implantable contact lens for moderate to high myopia. Short-term follow-up of 2 models. *J Cataract Refract Surg* 2001;27(3):380–388.

81. Malecaze FJ, Hulin H, Bierer P, et al. A randomized paired eye comparison of two techniques for treating moderately high myopia. LASIK and Artisan phakic lens. *Ophthalmology* 2002; 109(9):1622–1630.

82. Oshika T, Klyce SD, Applegate RA, et al. Comparison of corneal wavefront aberrations after photorefractive keratectomy and laser *in situ* keratomileusis. *Am J Ophthalmol* 1999;127(1):1–7.

83. Moreno-Barriuso E, Lloves JM, Marcos S, et al. Ocular aberrations before and after myopic corneal refractive surgery: Lasik-induced measured with Laser Ray Tracing. *Invest Ophthalmol Vis Sci* 2001;42(6):1396–1403.

84. Pallikaris IG, Kymionis GD, Panagopoulou S, et al. Induced optical aberrations following the formation of a LASIK flap. *J Cataract Refract Surg* 2002;28(10):1737–1741.

85. Nuijts RM, Nabar VA, Hament WJ, et al. Wavefront-guided versus standard laser *in situ* keratomileusis to correct low to moderate myopia. *J Cataract Refract Surg* 2002;28(11):1907–1913.

86. Phusitphoykai N, Tungsiripat, Siriboonkoom J, et al. Comparison of conventional versus wavefront-guided laser *in situ* keratomileusis in the same patient. *J Refract Surg* 2003;19(1):S217–220.

87. Mrochen M, Kaemmerer M, Seiler T. Clinical results of wavefront-guided laser *in situ* keratomileusis 3 months after surgery. *J Cataract Refract Surg* 2001;27(2):201–207.

LASIK OUTCOMES IN MYOPIA AND HYPEROPIA

DANIEL EPSTEIN

Laser *in-situ* keratomileusis (LASIK) took the ophthalmic world by storm in the second half of the 1990s and has since become by far the most widely performed corneal refractive procedure worldwide.

Arriving on the scene after several years of extensive experience with photorefractive keratectomy (PRK), it was obvious from the start that LASIK provided a much faster recovery of best spectacle-corrected visual acuity (BSCVA) than PRK. Ironically, this rapid visual rehabilitation has made it more difficult to obtain long-term follow-up on LASIK patients, because high levels of immediate satisfaction proved a disincentive for participation in prolonged studies. Accordingly, no 3-year or 5-year analyses of LASIK results can be found in the peer-reviewed literature.

As in all refractive surgery, the interpretation of reports on LASIK outcomes is somewhat tricky. For example, some patients may have a postoperative uncorrected visual acuity (UCVA) of 20/20 with a poor optical quality (e.g., ghosting), and others may have crisp 20/20 vision. But both types of patients are bundled together under the "20/20" rubric, and the reader is unable to obtain an accurate picture of the quality of the visual results.

Similarly, when reporting on postoperative lost lines of BSCVA, it is rarely made clear how rigorously visual acuity (VA) was registered preoperatively. If a patient is tested only to the level of 20/20 preoperatively, a 20/20 result postoperatively would indicate no loss of BSCVA. But most refractive surgery patients have a preoperative BSCVA of 20/16 to 20/14, and if the postoperative result is only 20/20, the failure to register the maximal preoperative VA would result in a misinterpretation of the safety of the procedure. In other words, even a 20/20 outcome may represent a loss of BSCVA.

A further unsatisfactory aspect is that low-contrast VA, which has been shown to decrease after corneal excimer surgery, is almost never reported in outcome papers.

Nevertheless, sufficient documentation is available to assess the outcomes of LASIK procedures over a wide range of refractive errors.

LOW TO MODERATE MYOPIA AND MYOPIC ASTIGMATISM

LASIK refractive and visual results in this category of patients are generally good to excellent even if the definition of low to moderate myopia is not identical in all studies (perceptions on this issue range from about -1 D to about -8 D). The cylinder component of the preoperative refraction is often identified only as a mean (no range); and an alarming number of studies fail to report vital preoperative or postoperative data. (Table 78-1 lists representative outcomes.)

These studies and numerous other publications (8–15) on patients with similar preoperative refractive errors collectively show that LASIK can effectively correct low to moderate myopia with or without a fair amount of astigmatism. As the procedure improved with the advent of better microkeratomes and lasers, investigators were able to focus on more ambitious results. Whereas an accuracy of ±1 D of emmetropia or aim and an UCVA $\geq20/40$ initially were considered acceptable treatment goals, the gold standard now requires that results be reported within 0.50 D of aim and that postoperative UCVA be stated in terms of $\geq20/20$.

Regression of effect after the correction of moderate myopia, a major reason for retreatments in the early days of LASIK (16,17), appears to have become much less of a problem, most likely because of improved ablation profiles. Although retreatments are still part and parcel of LASIK surgery, they are now usually used as enhancements in cases of undercorrection (18–20).

The American Academy of Ophthalmology (AAO) prepares Ophthalmic Technology Assessments (OTAs) to evaluate new and existing procedures, drugs, and diagnostic and screening tests. The goal of an OTA is to evaluate the peer-reviewed literature, and to distill what is well established about the technology. OTAs are submitted to the AAO's board of trustees for consideration as official academy statements.

TABLE 78-1. REPRESENTATIVE OUTCOMES OF MYOPIC LASIK STUDIES

Preop SE	Preop Cyl	Postop SE	Postop Cyl	±0.50D(%)	≥20/20(%)	Lost Lines (%)
−5.12 ± 0.81(1)		−0.42 ± 0.98		63	55.5	0†
−3.60 ± 1.27(2)	−1.01 ± 1.08	−0.12 ± 0.31	−0.19 ± 0.33	94	81	0†
−4.80 ± 1.60(3)		0.00 ± 0.60		73	67	6*
−2.90 ± 0.56(4)	NR	−0.41 ± 0.50	NR	NR	31	NR†
−4.90 ± 0.70(4)	NR	−0.67 ± 0.70	NR	NR	28	NR†
−3.77 ± 1.61(5)	−0.90 ± 0.43	0.00 ± 0.65	−0.28 ± 0.31	71.9	81.9	0†
−4.66 ± 2.21(6)	−1.16 ± 1.21	−0.02 ± 1.01	−0.50 ± 0.73	79.1	71.4	1.6*
−4.35 ± 2.11(7)		0.00 ± 0.21		92	83	0†

All preoperative and postoperative refractive values are means. SE, manifest refractive spherical equivalent; ±0.50D, within emmetropia or aim; ≥20/20, UCVA; lost lines, ≥2 lines of BSCVA; †, 6-month follow-up.*, 12-month follow-up; NR, not reported; ( ), reference.

The OTA on myopic LASIK, published in January 2002 (8), drew the following conclusion:

> For low to moderate myopia, the literature shows that LASIK is effective and predictable in terms of obtaining very good to excellent UCVA, and that it is safe in terms of minimal loss of BSCVA. For moderate to high myopia (6.00 D), the results are more variable. The results are similar for eyes with mild to moderate degrees of astigmatism (2.00 D). Serious adverse complications probably occur rarely; however, side effects such as dry eyes, nighttime star bursts, and reduced contrast sensitivity occur relatively frequently. There were insufficient data in prospective, comparative trials to describe the relative advantages and disadvantages of different lasers or nomograms.

Recently, a new dimension has been added to LASIK surgery: wavefront-guided LASIK. It is based on the concept of measuring the eye's aberrations with a wavefront analyzer (aberrometer) and mathematically transferring the measured wavefront aberrations into an ablation pattern to be performed by a scanning-spot excimer laser. The technique, which has been used mainly for the correction of myopia and myopic astigmatism, is still being developed and refined in clinical trials, and very few peer-reviewed papers have been published on the outcomes (21,22). Accordingly, it was deemed appropriate not to include these early results in this chapter.

HIGH MYOPIA

In the embryonic days of LASIK, the procedure was deemed suitable for the correction of myopia from −1 D to −30 D. However, it quickly became apparent that such a range was totally unrealistic, because the treatment of extreme myopia required the ablation of an extreme amount of stromal tissue. This resulted in an unphysiologically thin cornea, which in turn increased the risk for iatrogenically induced keratectasia, the most serious (noninfectious) complication of LASIK. When the initial excitement about LASIK's omnipotence died down, the consensus first settled on an upper limit of −15 D, then was lowered further to −10 D to −12 D.

Judging by practice patterns in 2003, there is a heavy bias toward abiding by a −8 D (possibly −10 D) limit for LASIK correction of myopia. This more conservative approach, actually returning to the traditional upper limits of PRK, reflects renewed awareness of the limitations of corneal refractive surgery. The only practical way of treating a very high myopia without causing excessive thinning of the cornea is to ablate a relatively small optical zone (ablation depth being proportional to optical zone diameter). However, a small optical zone tends to create major optical problems when the pupil dilates in mesopic illumination. As the pupil diameter exceeds the diameter of the optical zone, spherical aberration kicks in, and the patient complains of ghosting, halos, star bursts, and other optical disturbances. Patient dissatisfaction with such optical aberrations has brought the limits of LASIK down to the realm of the doable.

Table 78-2 presents the results of studies performed mainly before the dust settled with respect to reasonable limits for myopic LASIK. Several aspects distinguish these reports on high myopia from their counterparts on low to moderate myopia. First, the safety numbers reflect the

TABLE 78-2. RESULTS OF LASIK FOR HIGH MYOPIA

Preop SE	Preop Cyl	Postop SE	Postop Cyl	± 1 D(%)	≥20/25(%)	Lost Lines(%)
NR (−9 to −12) (26)	NR (0 to −3)	−0.14 ± 0.92	NR	79	58.7	5.1•□
NR (>−12 to −15) (26)	NR (0 to −3)	−0.31 ± 0.90	NR	77.1	42.9	5.8•□
−11.69 ± 1.46 (27)	1.66 ± 1.22	−0.37 ± 0.80	0.46 ± 0.53	84	~65	1.8*□
−13.24 ± 2.30 (28)	1.61 ± 0.80	−0.87 ± 0.80	0.41 ± 0.30	58.5	~46	12.2*□
−12.64 ± 2.16 (29)	NR	−1.78 ± 2.08	NR	64.6	~42	0†

All preoperative and postoperative refractive values are means, except when only ranges are supplied. SE, manifest refractive spherical equivalent; ± 1 D, within emmetropia or aim; ≥20/25, UCVA; lost lines, ≥ 2 lines of BSCVA; †, 6-month follow-up; •, 9-month follow-up; 12-month follow-up; □, including retreatments; NR, not reported; ( ), reference.

TABLE 78-3. REPRESENTATIVE OUTCOMES OF HYPEROPIC LASIK STUDIES

Preop SE	Postop SE	± 1 D(%)	≥20/20(%)	Lost Lines(%)
+2.35 ± 0.88 (34)	+0.08 ± 0.49	98	52	0*
+2.02 ± 0.51 (35)	+0.30 ± 0.71	88.9	42.2	0†□
+3.78 ± 0.57 (35)	+1.09 ± 0.92	51.8	25.9	1.4†□
+4.50 ± 1.73 (36)	+0.85 ± 1.74	74	52	5x
+2.16 ± 0.58 (37)	+0.41 ± 0.59	81.8	72.7(≥20/40)	0†
+4.88 ± 2.13 (32)	+0.30 ± 0.90	78(± 0.5D)	83(≥20/40)	0*
+2.56 ± 1.16 (31)	+0.05 ± NR	74.1(± 0.5D)	93.9(≥20/40)	3.4*

All preoperative and postoperative refractive values are means, except when only ranges are supplied. SE, manifest refractive spherical equivalent; ± 1 D, within emmetropia or aim; ≥20/20, UCVA; lost lines, ≥ 2 lines of BSCVA; †, 6-month follow-up; *, 12-month follow-up; x, 24-month follow-up; □, including retreatments; NR, not reported; ( ), reference.

much greater risk inherent in the treatment of high myopes. With up to 12.2% losing two or more lines of BSCVA (and with the Food and Drug Administration defining 5% as an upper acceptable limit), these results are much poorer than for the lower myopias.

Second, target UCVA and accuracy of outcome are less ambitious in high myopia treatments. Here results are stated within 1 D of aim instead of ±0.50 D as in low to moderate myopia, and postoperative UCVA reported in the range of 20/25 instead of 20/20. Because there is no general agreement on the use of the 20/25 level, the results of some studies have to be recalculated to 20/25 in order to be able to compare them with other published outcomes. Even given the less ambitious postoperative UCVA, fewer eyes attain that lower level. Only between 42.9% and about 65% of the high myopes reach 20/25 UCVA, whereas up to 83% of low to moderate myopes achieve 20/20. A further difference is that high myopia outcomes generally include retreatments (23–25).

The dream of successfully treating high myopia with LASIK dies hard. Studies on such procedures still appear occasionally, often rediscovering the significant optical disturbances that befall many of the patients postoperatively (29).

HYPEROPIA

Experience with hyperopic LASIK has been shorter and less extensive than with myopia. In addition, correcting hyperopia is more complicated than treating myopia, principally because it is much more difficult to steepen a cornea (as is the aim of the procedure in hyperopia) than to flatten it (as is done in myopia). The ablation pattern for the treatment of hyperopia is trickier to design. If the ablation results in high dioptric gradients between the central cornea and the periphery, patients may complain of optical aberrations. The hyperopic ablation profile also appears to induce a more aggressive postoperative healing response, which in turn can lead to a regression of the correction done in the first place. LASIK results of hyperopia reflect these realities and also explain why there is a general reluctance to correct high hyperopia with the excimer.

In this context high hyperopia is often defined as 4 D or higher, but it has been repeatedly shown that even corrections above 3 D may cause poorer predictability, unacceptable regression, and loss of BSCVA (30). Nevertheless, several recent studies, all with 1-year follow-ups, have argued that hyperopia up to 5 D (31) and even 6 D (32,33) can be treated safely and effectively. Differences in lasers (some are better in treating hyperopia, some in correcting myopia), and improvements in ablation profiles may explain the diverging views on the upper limits of hyperopic LASIK. (Table 78-3 lists representative outcomes.)

Nevertheless, in view of late regression surprises in the past, it may be wise to consider that studies with a maximum follow-up of 6 months do not necessarily reflect the final outcome.

REFERENCES

1. Maldonado-Bas A, Onnis R. Results of laser in situ keratomileusis in different degrees of myopia. *Ophthalmology* 1998;105:606–611.

2. Montes M, Chayet A, Gómez L, et al. Laser *in situ* keratomileusis for myopia of −1.50 to −6.00 diopters. *J Refract Surg* 1999;15:106–110.

3. El Maghraby A, Salah T, Waring GO, et al. Randomized bilateral comparison of excimer laser *in situ* keratomileusis and photorefractive keratectomy for 2.50 to 8.00 diopters of myopia. *Ophthalmology* 1999;106:447–457.

4. Reviglio VE, Luna JD, Rodríguez ML, et al. Laser *in situ* keratomileusis using the LaserSight 200 laser: results of 950 consecutive cases. *J Cataract Refract Surg* 1999;25:1062–1068.

5. Fernandez AP, Jaramillo J, Jaramillo M. Comparison of photorefractive keratectomy and laser *in situ* keratomileusis for myopia of −6D or less using the Nidek EC-5000 laser. *J Refract Surg* 2000;16:711–715.

6. Chitkara DK, Rosen E, Gore C, et al. Tracker-assisted laser *in situ* keratomileusis for myopia using the autonomous scanning and tracking laser. *Ophthalmology* 2002;109:965–972.

7. Nuijts RMMA, Nabar VA, Hament WJ, et al. Wavefront-guided versus standard laser *in situ* keratomileusis to correct low to moderate myopia. *J Cataract Refract Surg* 2002;28:1907–1913.

8. American Academy of Ophthalmology. Laser *in situ* keratomileusis for myopia and astigmatism: safety and efficacy. *Ophthalmology* 2002;109:175–187.

9. Balazsi G, Mullie M, Lasswell L, et al. Laser *in situ* keratomileusis with a scanning excimer laser for the correction of low to moderate myopia with and without astigmatism. *J Cataract Refract Surg* 2001;27:1942–1951.

10. El Danasoury MA, El Maghraby A, Klyce SD, et al. Comparison of photorefractive keratectomy with excimer laser *in situ* keratomileusis in correcting low myopia (from −2.00 to −5.50 diopters). *Ophthalmology* 1999;106:411–421.

11. Pop M, Payette Y. Photorefractive keratectomy versus laser *in situ* keratomileusis. *Ophthalmology* 2000;107:251–257.

12. Rashad KM. Laser *in situ* keratomileusis for myopic astigmatism. *J Refract Surg* 1999;15:653–660.

13. Reviglio VE, Bossana EL, Luna JD, et al. Laser *in situ* keratomileusis for myopia and hyperopia using the LaserSight 200 laser in 300 consecutive eyes. *J Refract Surg* 2000;16:716–723.

14. Tole DM, McCarty DJ, Couper T, et al. Comparison of laser *in situ* keratomileusis and photorefractive keratectomy for the correction of myopia of −6.00 diopters or less. *J Refract Surg* 2001;17:46–54.

15. Walker MB, Wilson SE. Recovery of uncorrected visual acuity after laser *in situ* keratomileusis or photorefractive keratectomy for low myopia. *Cornea* 2001;20:153–155.

16. Lyle WA, Jin GJC. Retreatment after initial laser *in situ* keratomileusis. *J Cataract Refract Surg* 2000;26:650–659.

17. Pérez-Santonja JJ, Ayala MJ, Sakla HF, et al. Retreatment after laser *in situ* keratomileusis. *Ophthalmology* 1999;106:21–28.

18. Mulhern MG, Condon PI, O'Keefe M. Myopic and hyperopic laser *in situ* keratomileusis retreatments. *J Cataract Refract Surg* 2001;27:1278–1287.

19. Patel NP, Clinch TE, Weis JR, et al. Comparison of visual results in initial and re-treatment laser *in situ* keratomileusis procedures for myopia and astigmatism. *Am J Ophthalmol* 2000;130:1–11.

20. Rashad KM. Laser in situ keratomileusis retreatment for residual myopia and astigmatism. *J Refract Surg* 2000;16:170–176.

21. Mrochen M, Kaemmerer M, Seiler T. Wavefront-guided laser *in situ* keratomileusis: early results in three eyes. *J Refract Surg* 2000;16:116–121.

22. Mrochen M, Kaemmerer M, Seiler T. Clinical results of wavefront-guided laser *in situ* keratomileusis 3 months after surgery. *J Cataract Refract Surg* 2001;27:201–207.

23. Brahma A, McGhee CNJ, Craig JP, et al. Safety and predictability of laser *in situ* keratomileusis enhancement by flap reel-evation in high myopia. *J Cataract Refract Surg* 2001;27:593–603.

24. Magallanes R, Shah S, Zadok D, et al. Stability after laser *in situ* keratomileusis in moderately and extremely myopic eyes. *J Cataract Refract Surg* 2001;27:1007–1012.

25. McDonald MB, Carr JD, Frantz JM, et al. Laser *in situ* keratomileusis for myopia up to −11 diopters with up to −5 diopters of astigmatism with the Summit Autonomous LADARVision excimer laser system. *Ophthalmology* 2001;108:309–316.

26. Kawesch GM, Kezirian GM. Laser *in situ* keratomileusis for high myopia with the VISX Star laser. *Ophthalmology* 2000;107:653–661.

27. Lyle WA, Jin GJC. Laser *in situ* keratomileusis with the VISX Star laser for myopia over −10.0 diopters. *J Cataract Refract Surg* 2001;27:1812–1822.

28. El Danasoury MA, El Maghraby A, Gamali TO. Comparison of iris-fixed Artisan lens implantation with excimer laser *in situ* keratomileusis in correcting myopia between −9.00 and −19.50 diopters. *Ophthalmology* 2002;109:955–964.

29. Dada T, Sudan R, Sinha R, et al. Results of laser *in situ* keratomileusis for myopia of −10 to −19 diopters with a Technolas 217 laser. *J Refract Surg* 2003;19:44–47.

30. Cobo-Soriano R, Llovet F, Gonzalez-Lopez F, et al. Factors that influence outcomes of hyperopic laser *in situ* keratomileusis. *J Cataract Refract Surg* 2002;28:1530–1538.

31. Salz JJ, Stevens CA, for the LADARVision LASIK hyperopia study group. LASIK correction of spherical hyperopia, hyperopic astigmatism and mixed astigmatism with the LADARVision excimer laser system. *Ophthalmology* 2002;109:1647–1657.

32. Ditzen K, Fiedler J, Pieger S. Laser *in situ* keratomileusis for hyperopia and hyperopic astigmatism using the Meditec MEL 70 spot scanner. *J Refract Surg* 2002;18:430–434.

33. Lian J, Ye W, Zhou D, et al. Laser *in situ* keratomileusis for correction of hyperopia and hyperopic astigmatism with the Technolas 117C. *J Refract Surg* 2002;18:435–438.

34. Jackson WB, Casson E, Hodge WG, et al. Laser vision correction for low hyperopia. *Ophthalmology* 1998;105:1727–1738.

35. Zadok D, Maskaleris G, Montes M, et al. Hyperopic laser *in situ* keratomileusis with the Nidek EC-5000 excimer laser. *Ophthalmology* 2000;107:1132–1137.

36. Esquenazi S, Mendoza A. Two-year follow-up of laser *in situ* keratomileusis for hyperopia. *J Refract Surg* 1999;15:648–652.

37. Pineda-Fernandez A, Rueda L, Huang D, et al. Laser *in situ* keratomileusis for hyperopia and hyperopic astigmatism with the Nidek EC-5000 excimer laser. *J Refract Surg* 2001;17:670–675.

LASIK OUTCOMES IN ASTIGMATISM

DAMIEN GATINEL AND THANH HOANG-XUAN

BACKGROUND

Compound astigmatism is the most common refractive error. Myopia is often associated with some degree of astigmatism in the general population. It is estimated that astigmatism of more than 0.50 diopters (D) is present in 44.4% of the population, and that 8.44% of these subjects have astigmatism of 1.50 D or more (1). Corneal incisions have been used to correct astigmatism for more than a century (2,3). In 1983, Trokel et al. (4) showed that smooth ablation of the cornea was feasible using a 193-nm excimer laser. In 1991, McDonnell et al. (5) used toric ablation to correct astigmatism by reshaping the anterior corneal surface. For more than a decade, excimer laser surgery has been the most predictive and safest technique to treat regular astigmatism. Currently, the most common surgical methods for correcting astigmatism are photoastigmatic refractive keratectomy (PARK) and laser *in-situ* keratomileusis (LASIK). LASIK provides better accuracy and higher patient satisfaction than PARK for the treatment of moderate to high astigmatism (6–8). However, in both cases the predictability of excimer laser surgery is lower for compound or pure astigmatism than for pure spherical myopic errors. This is partly due to the inherent remodeling imposed on the corneal surface by cylindrical profiles of ablation.

The profiles of ablation for conventional non-customized treatments do not take into account the higher-order optical aberrations of the human eye. Moreover, these treatments carry a risk of increasing higher-order aberrations such as coma and spherical aberration (9). Recently, wavefront sensors were introduced to quantify the overall optical aberration of the eye. The astigmatic refractive error can be isolated from a Taylor or Zernike polynomial expansion aimed at describing the wavefront error of the total eye over a circular pupil. It arises from the effects of second radial order and azimuthal frequency terms of the Zernike classification (10). New algorithms have been introduced for laser delivery systems, with the aim of correcting both low- and high-order optical aberrations, with encouraging early results.

This chapter focuses on the different strategies used to determine the profile of ablation, and on the particularities of the LASIK technique aimed at correcting pure, compound, and mixed regular astigmatism. The treatment of irregular and/or high-order astigmatism by means of customized ablation will not be discussed in detail.

DEFINITIONS: REGULAR ASTIGMATISM, IRREGULAR ASTIGMATISM, AND HIGH-ORDER ASTIGMATISM

The astigmatic error is a refractive error dependent on the meridian. It is usually due to one or more refracting surfaces—most commonly the anterior cornea, having a toroidal shape. In regular astigmatism, the principal meridians (maximum and minimum power) are perpendicular to each other, and the astigmatism is correctable with conventional spherocylindrical lenses or surgery.

When the principal meridians are not perpendicular to each other, the astigmatism is irregular. Computerized corneal topography has made an important contribution to the diagnosis of regular and irregular anterior corneal astigmatism.

In recent years interest has grown in measuring the optical aberrations of the human eye and changes induced by refractive surgery. The optical imperfections previously designated "irregular astigmatism" can now be more precisely characterized and quantified with novel approaches such as wavefront analysis. The variance of the normalized Zernike expansion is the tool most commonly used to describe and quantify optical aberrations in terms of wave-aberration coefficients. Each Zernike mode is defined by its radial order and azimuthal frequency, and is weighted by a coefficient. These coefficients correspond to the contribution of each mode to the total root mean square (RMS) wavefront error. Some Zernike modes (trefoil, quadrafoil, pentafoil, etc.) correspond to so-called high-order astigmatism. These modes have in common that their radial order is equal to their azimuthal frequency. Terms having an azimuthal frequency of 2 but a higher even radial order n are commonly referred to as "n-order" astigmatism. In normal patients, theory contribution to the degradation of the quality of vision is usually small relative to that induced by the conventional sphero-cylindrical refractive error, because of their small contribution to the total wavefront deviation. However, they may limit the vision of healthy eyes to less than retinal limits and, in some clinical circumstances (early keratoconus, corneal scarring, etc.), they may significantly affect visual acuity and overall quality of vision, especially in subjects with scotopic pupil.

PRINCIPLES OF CORRECTION OF REGULAR ASTIGMATISM

Regular astigmatism is mainly generated by excessive corneal toricity. Thereby, LASIK for astigmatism is a subtractive technique aimed at reducing this excessive toricity by etching from the corneal surface an adequate toric lenticule of corneal tissue of variable thickness. Corneal toricity can be suppressed by either flattening the steepest meridians to the curvature of the initially flatter meridian, or by "steepening" the flattest meridians to the curvature of the initially steeper meridian. Pure positive and negative cylindrical excimer laser treatments are based on the combination of three elementary profiles of ablation, as depicted in Fig. 79-1 and Table 79-1.

The treatment of astigmatism in LASIK requires proper alignment of the corneal surface relative to the delivery system, and smooth blending of the steep edges of variable depth induced at the periphery of the optical zone, in order to avoid undercorrection. These two major constraints may account for the high reported rate of undercorrection of the cylindrical component and overcorrection of the spherical component.

Some authors have drawn attention to the geometric particularities of astigmatic treatment, implying the need for a larger transition zone along the initially flatter meridian (11,12), minimization of the maximal depth of ablation, and comparison of different strategies for mixed and compound astigmatism (13). In a recent paper, we emphasized

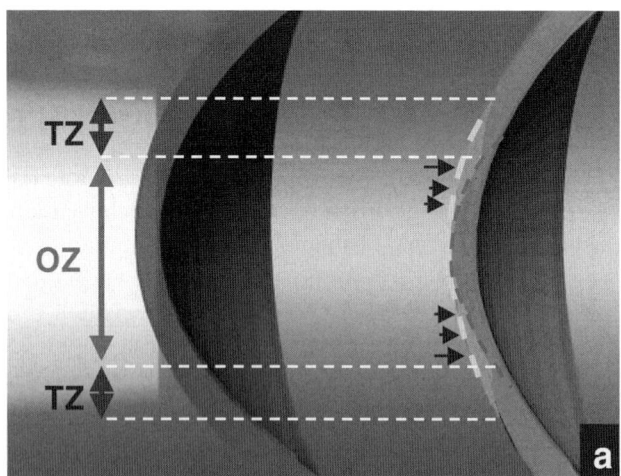

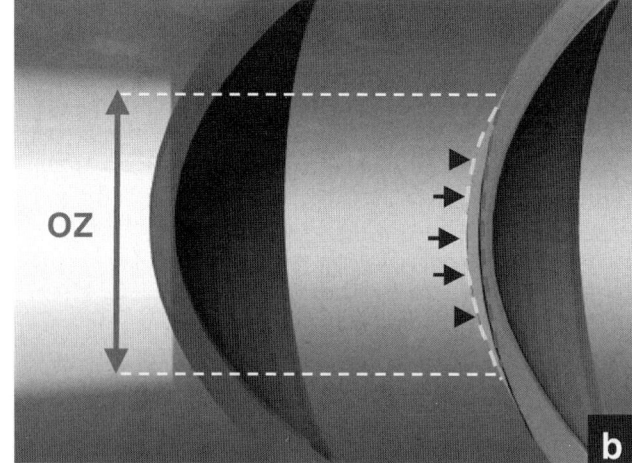

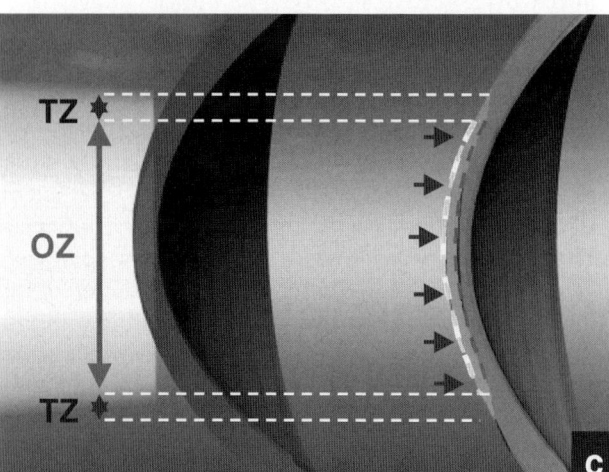

FIGURE 79-1. Schematic representation of the three elementary profiles of ablation used to establish the cylindrical profiles of ablation. Steepening of the meridians **(A)** is achieved in the pure positive cylindrical mode. Flattening **(B)** and plano ablation **(C)** are achieved in the pure negative cylindrical mode. (Artwork generated using computer-aided modeling)

TABLE 79-1. PRINCIPLES OF CORRECTION OF REGULAR ASTIGMATISM

	Steepening	Plano ablation	Flattening
Pure myopic astigmatism	No	Yes (steepest meridian)	Yes (all but one)
Pure hyperopic astigmatism	Yes (all but one)	No	No

the three-dimensional geometric features of the ablated lenticules of corneal tissue when correcting pure and compound astigmatism (14). We used computerized three-dimensional (3D) modeling to represent and compare the qualitative geometric characteristics of the different lenticules and ablation strategies. The surfaces of ablation were modeled as geometric primitives such as the sphere and the toroidal ellipsoid with which the Boolean operations were performed. To model the lenticules etched for pure cylindrical corrections, the initial corneal surface was modeled as a toroidal ellipsoid with two major apical radii of curvature along the principal meridians. For lenticules etched for pure spherical corrections, we modeled the initial surface as spherical. The final surface was always spherical. The principal radii of curvature of the initial and final surfaces were adjusted according to the nature of the ametropia (the radii of the initial surface being shorter for myopic lenticules and longer for hyperopic lenticules). The difference between each of the radii of curvature was exaggerated as compared to the surgical range so as to facilitate spatial visualization of the contour of the lenticules. Such an approach is useful to conceptualize the constraints of cylindrical treatments, to compare the depth and volume ablated in different strategies, and to anticipate some unpredicted effects. This approach is used in this chapter to illustrate the differences between strategies aimed at treating pure astigmatism and compound astigmatism.

Simple Astigmatism

Shape of the Ablated Lenticule in Pure Cylindrical Hyperopic Treatment

Cylindrical hyperopic ablation within the optical zone consists of ablating a lenticule with a concave shape along the initial flatter meridian, and of zero thickness along the opposite meridian, which has the same radius of curvature as the final surface (Fig. 79-2A). The maximal thickness of the cylindrical hyperopic lenticule is located at the edge of the optical zone, along the initial flatter meridian, and is identical to that of a spherical hyperopic lenticule for the same magnitude of treatment.

A transition zone is required to blend the edges of the treatment zone. To minimize the amount of tissue removed and to equalize the slope of the transition zone, the latter should be made elliptical, with maximal width along the initially flatter meridian (Fig. 79-2B) (11,12,15).

Shape of the Ablated Lenticule for Simple Myopic Astigmatism

Pure cylindrical myopic ablation consists of ablating a lenticule with a convex shape along the initial steeper meridian and with constant thickness along the initial flatter meridian, in order to preserve its curvature (Fig. 79-2C). Because of this latter constraint, the amount of the pure cylinder treatment is superior to the amount of the spherical treatment for a given degree of dioptric treatment. The maximal thickness of the myopic cylindrical ablated lenticule is located along the flatter meridian, and is identical to that of a spherical myopic lenticule for a given magnitude of treatment. This ablation pattern along the flat meridian is equivalent to that of a plano ablation, and explains the frequent unanticipated effects, from the optical and engineering perspectives, of negative cylindrical treatment, such as undercorrection and hyperopic shift (16). To minimize the intensity of these phenomena, the edges of the ablation over the optical zone have to be smoothed out evenly, by enlarging the transition along the initially flatter meridian, thus creating an elliptical perimeter for the total ablation zone (Fig. 79-2D).

Because the initially steeper principal meridian cannot be flattened selectively (this would imply plano ablation on the other principal meridian), the lenticule ablated for cylindrical myopic treatment can be considered as a combination of two successive treatments: cylindrical positive treatment of equal magnitude on the initially flatter meridian (to steepen its curvature until it equals that of the opposite principal meridian), followed by myopic spherical treatment of similar magnitude aiming to flatten both meridians (Fig. 79-3). The final surface is spherical, and its radius is equal to that of the initially flatter meridian. For example, a cylindrical treatment -1×180 degrees is equivalent in terms of the optical results and the amount of ablated tissue to the following sequential treatment: $+1 \times 90$ degrees and -1. This additive relation is useful to compare strategies used to treat compound and mixed astigmatism.

Mixed and Compound Astigmatism

Sequential Strategy

Conventional strategies used to correct compound myopic astigmatism are sequential: the spherical and cylindrical components of the refractive errors are treated successively, over a circular optical zone. Noncustom PARK or LASIK ablation of pure, compound, or mixed astigmatic refractive errors is based on paraxial models first described by Munnerlyn et al. (17). They generally employ one or more of four elementary treatments, namely spherical myopic, spherical hyperopic, cylindrical myopic, and cylindrical hyperopic. Thus, to achieve emmetropia, tissue photoablation within the optical zone must yield a single final apical corneal curvature. As refraction (as commonly measured in

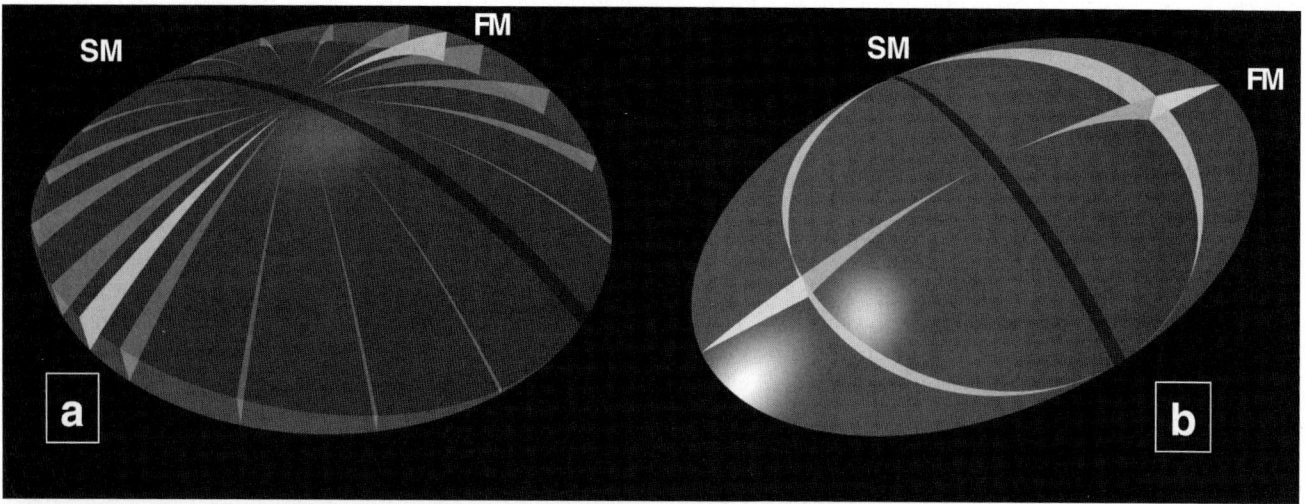

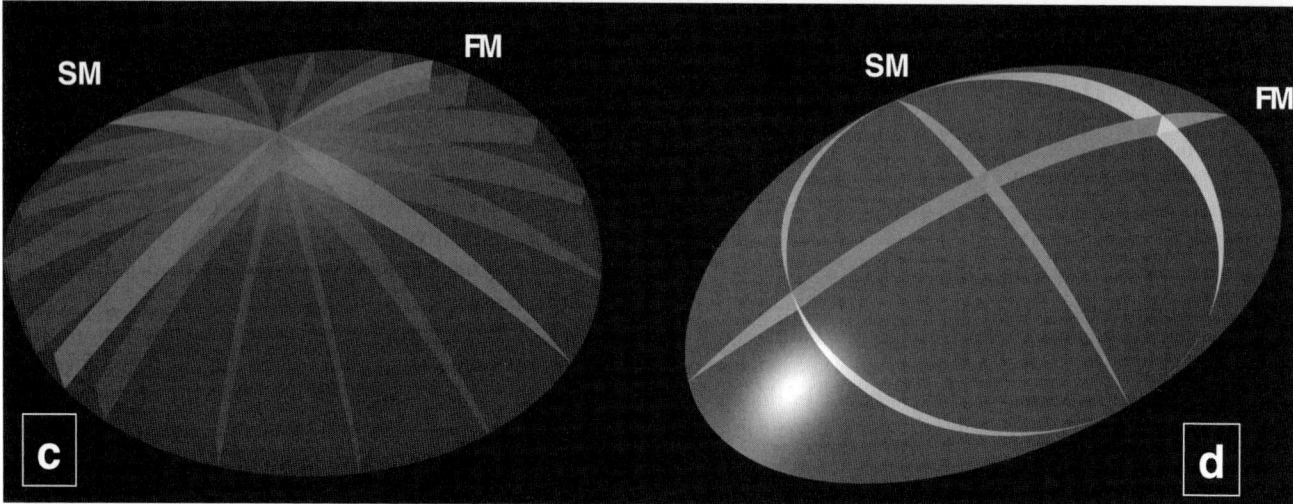

FIGURE 79-2. Schematic representation using three-dimensional computer modeling (Boolean operations) of the ablated lenticules etched for the positive cylinder treatment **(A,B)** and for the negative cylinder treatment **(C,D)**. The profile of ablation has been outlined over different meridians of the lenticules **(A,C)** (optical zone only). **B,D,** A lenticule corresponding to the tissue ablated for the realization of a transition zone of constant slope is added wherever an abrupt step is sculpted in the cornea at the outer perimeter of the optical zone. In both the negative and positive cylinder treatments, the peripheral depth is maximum along the initial flat meridian *(FM)*, and is null along the initial steep meridian *(SM)*. The transition zone is thus elliptical, having its widest diameter along the initial flatter meridian. (Artwork generated using computer-aided modeling)

clinical practice) is an arc-based mathematical expression limited to the principal major and minor axes, a compound astigmatic refractive error can be expressed by different equivalent expressions. Thus, various sequential treatment strategies for the correction of compound astigmatism have been proposed, consisting of a combination of spherical and cylindrical treatments, as follows:

- Ablating the cylinder along the flattest meridian, and then treating the residual spherical component (positive cylinder approach);
- Ablating the cylinder along the steepest meridian, and then treating the residual spherical component (negative cylinder approach);

- Ablating the total refractive error by two pure cylindrical ablations of opposite signs along the principal meridians (bitoric approach); and
- Ablating half the power of the cylinder along the steepest meridian, and the remaining half along the flattest meridian, before treating the residual spherical equivalent (cross cylinder approach).

These strategies have been employed to treat compound myopic, compound hyperopic and mixed astigmatism. Azar and Primack (13) have illustrated the use of these strategies in mixed and compound hyperopic astigmatism, and have shown that they may result in different amounts and depths of corneal tissue ablation. They found that

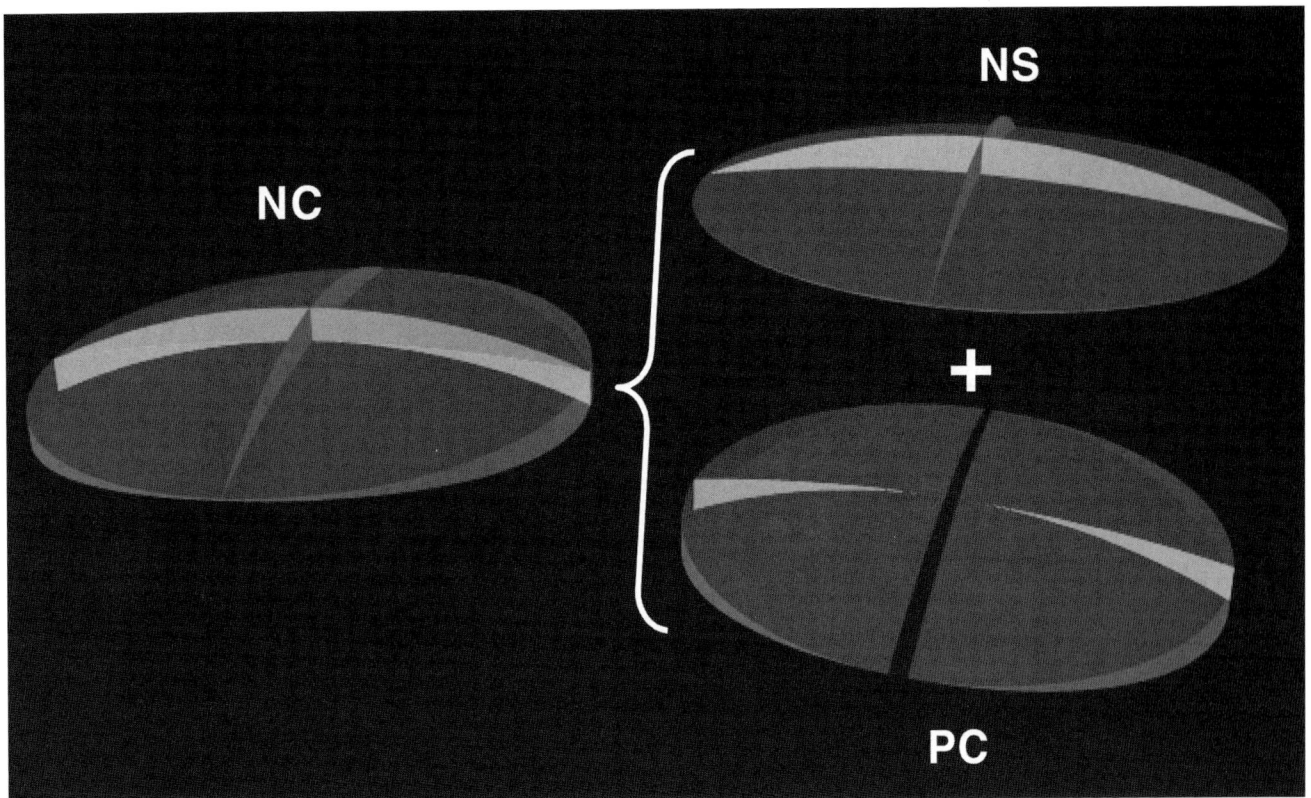

FIGURE 79-3. Decomposition of the lenticule corresponding to the volume ablated for the negative cylinder (*NC*) treatment into two lenticules, corresponding to the volume of a negative spherical and positive cylindrical volumes, respectively. For example, the negative cylinder treatment (−2 × 0 degrees) results in the same amount of ablated tissue that the following sequence: (−2 sphere) and (+2 × 90 degrees). (Artwork generated using computer-aided modeling)

strategies combining hyperopic spherical and myopic cylindrical corrections incur the greatest amount of corneal tissue ablation. The increasing number of reports of corneal ectasia following LASIK (18–23) suggests that strategies that remove the least corneal tissue should be preferred for the treatment of compound and mixed astigmatism. Azar et al. compared the theoretical ablation profiles and depths of tissue removal in the treatment of compound hyperopic astigmatism and mixed astigmatism, but did not offer a direct estimate of the difference in the amount of tissue ablation. Using Boolean operations, we designed a method to compare and illustrate the amount of tissue ablation incurred by different sequential strategies (14). This method confirmed the universal utility of combining plus cylindrical and negative or positive spherical ablations when treating any compound or mixed astigmatism while theoretically minimizing the volume of ablated corneal tissue (Figs. 79-4 and 79-5). Using this approach, the magnitude of astigmatism to correct is expressed in the positive cylinder format of the refraction. It implies variable steepening of the corneal surface, aimed at reducing or suppressing the toricity of the anterior corneal surface, followed by a pure positive or negative spherical treatment to correct for the remaining defocus.

Negative cylindrical approaches to compound hyperopic or mixed astigmatism result in additional tissue ablation, the amount of which results from the combination of the myopic spherical treatment in the flat meridian (which is part of the negative-cylindrical treatment) with a positive-spherical lenticule (in both meridians). This combination also occurs with the cross-cylindrical ablation strategy when it is used to correct mixed or compound hyperopic astigmatism. This strategy has been proposed to favor postoperative prolate asphericity and to reduce the overcorrection on nonprincipal meridians (24,25). In hyperopic astigmatism, the cross-cylinder technique may also reduce the increase in corneal eccentricity, leading to a more physiologic corneal shape (26).

For mixed astigmatism, the positive-cylindrical approach and bitoric ablation would theoretically incur the same minimum volume of tissue ablation. However, because of the global characteristics of the cylindrical profiles of ablation achieved with the newest delivery systems (wide elliptical transition zones), a bitoric strategy might be more practical to treat mixed astigmatism (27). The bitoric strategy has also been shown to reduce the hyperopic shift caused by the use of the negative cylindrical treatment, by ablating more selectively along the extremities of the flat

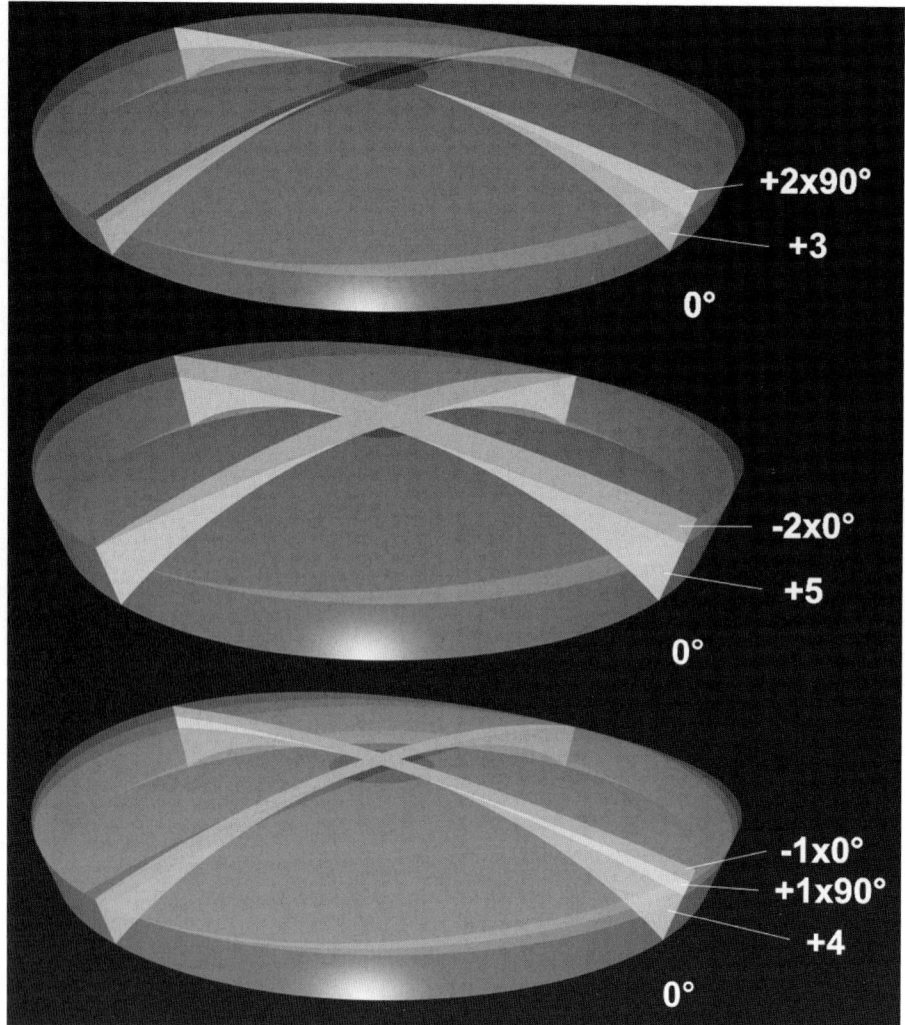

FIGURE 79-4. Comparison of the lenticules of corneal tissue ablated for the treatment of compound hyperopic astigmatism using different strategies: positive cylinder strategy **(top)**, negative cylinder **(middle)**, and cross-cylinder ablation **(bottom)**. The volume required for the transition zone is not represented. The optical zone is circular and identical for each of the cylindrical or spherical treatments. The positive cylinder strategy incurs the minimum of volume of ablated tissue. The negative cylinder strategy incurs the maximum of volume of ablated tissue. The positive cylinder approach spares the center of the ablation zone, as opposed to the negative cylinder and cross-cylinder strategies. (Artwork generated using computer-aided modeling)

meridian (positive cylindrical treatment), thus preventing the flattening of the latter and avoiding a shift of refraction toward hyperopia.

For compound myopic astigmatism (e.g., $-3 -2 \times 90$ degrees), all available sequential strategies would theoretically lead to the same amount of tissue ablation, because any negative cylindrical treatment (-2×90 degrees) can be split into a sequence combining a negative sphere (-2) and a pure cylindrical treatment ($+2 \times 180$ degrees) (14). Recombining the negative spherical components and the pure cylindrical treatment leads to the equivalent following refraction expressed in the positive-cylinder format -5 ($+2 \times 180$ degrees).

Elliptical Treatment for Compound Myopic Astigmatism

The sequential approach is not the only treatment for compound myopic astigmatism. By using a patented elliptical method, VISX software allows the full myopic and astigmatic correction to be sculpted into the cornea in one smooth ablation. This is made possible by the narrowing of the optical zone along the initially steeper meridians (Fig. 79-6). The treatment of compound myopic astigmatism aims both to suppress the toricity and to flatten the corneal anterior surface over the effective optical zone: in the elliptical modality, astigmatic and myopic correction is

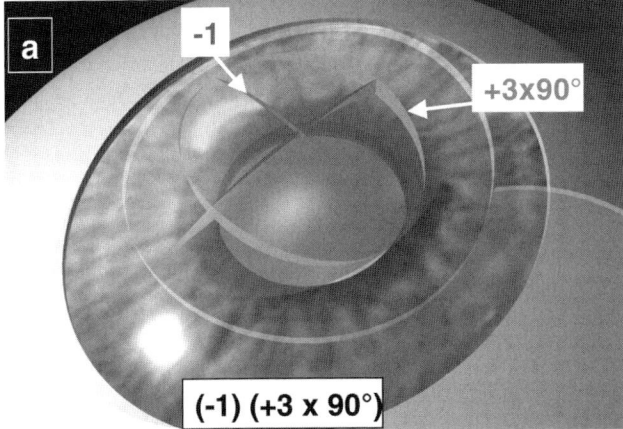

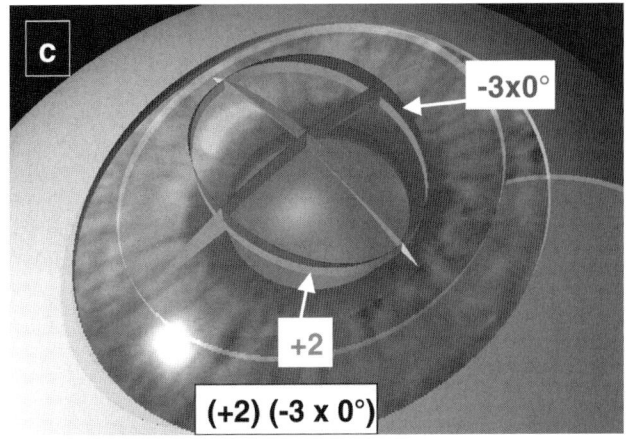

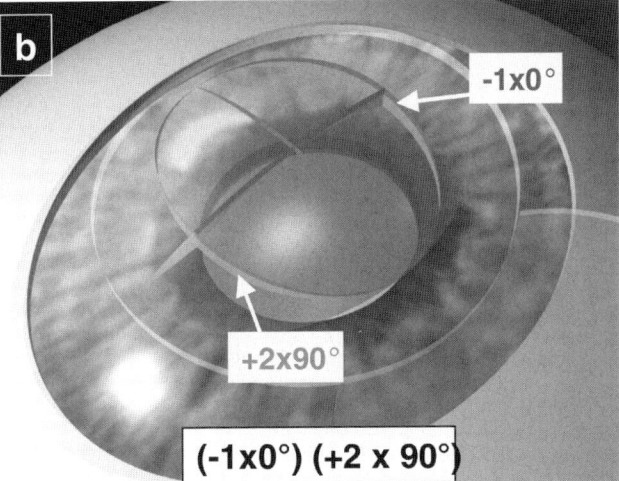

FIGURE 79-5. Schematic representation of the different strategies aimed at correcting mixed astigmatism with LASIK: positive cylinder strategy **(A)**, bitoric strategy **(B)**, and negative cylinder strategy **(C)**. The hinge of the flap is placed superiorly (90 degrees). The outer perimeter of the optical zone is circular and identical for each of the different treatment modes. The profile of ablation is along the outer perimeter and principal meridians of the photoablated lenticules corresponding to positive and negative cylinder treatments, respectively. The transition zone has the same slope for each of the depicted strategies. The deepest ablation is attained at the periphery of the optical zone along the initially flatter meridian. The transition zone has an elliptical perimeter, the widest diameter of which being located along the flatter meridian. The negative cylinder strategy **(C)** incurs the maximum amount of volume of ablated tissue and the deepest ablation. Because of this constraint, the transition zone has to be wider, and is necessarily extended along the vertical meridian to blend the abrupt step created by the delivery of the positive spherical treatment. The positive cylinder and cross-cylinder strategies incur the same amount of tissue ablation: due to the additive properties of the negative cylindrical treatment (see Fig. 79-3); the lenticule corresponding to the negative cylinder treatment (-1×0 degree) is equal to the sequential delivery: (-1 sphere) and ($+1 \times 90$ degree). (Artwork generated using computer-aided modeling)

achieved by varying the diameter in elliptical fashion, the narrowest diameter achieving the greatest flattening effect. The relative size of the major and minor axes of the elliptical cut depends on the ratio between the cylindrical and spherical magnitudes. A comparative clinical study has shown that the elliptical method leads to a significant improvement in the results in patients treated for myopic compound astigmatism (28). The elliptical method has several theoretical advantages, such as a reduction in the maximal depth of ablation and the induction of a natural transition zone with no steep edges. It implies, however, a reduction of the diameter of the optical zone along the initially steeper meridian, which could theoretically cause optical aberrations with pupil dilation in low-light conditions. Recently, a simplified formula was proposed to accurately approximate the volume of corneal tissue ablated within the optical zone during pure spherical corrections (29). However, no quantitative computations of the tissue removed during cylindrical corrections have yet been published.

TECHNICAL PARTICULARITIES OF LASIK TREATMENT OF ASTIGMATISM

The predictability of the LASIK technique is inferior when treating pure or compound astigmatism rather than pure spherical refractive errors. Centration and alignment are more critical, and corneal wound healing following correction of pure or compound astigmatic correction may be more complex than after correction of purely spherical myopic corrections. A residual refractive error after LASIK may indicate the need for an enhancement procedure, incurring additional cost and time, as well as specific and nonspecific risks associated with all surgical procedures.

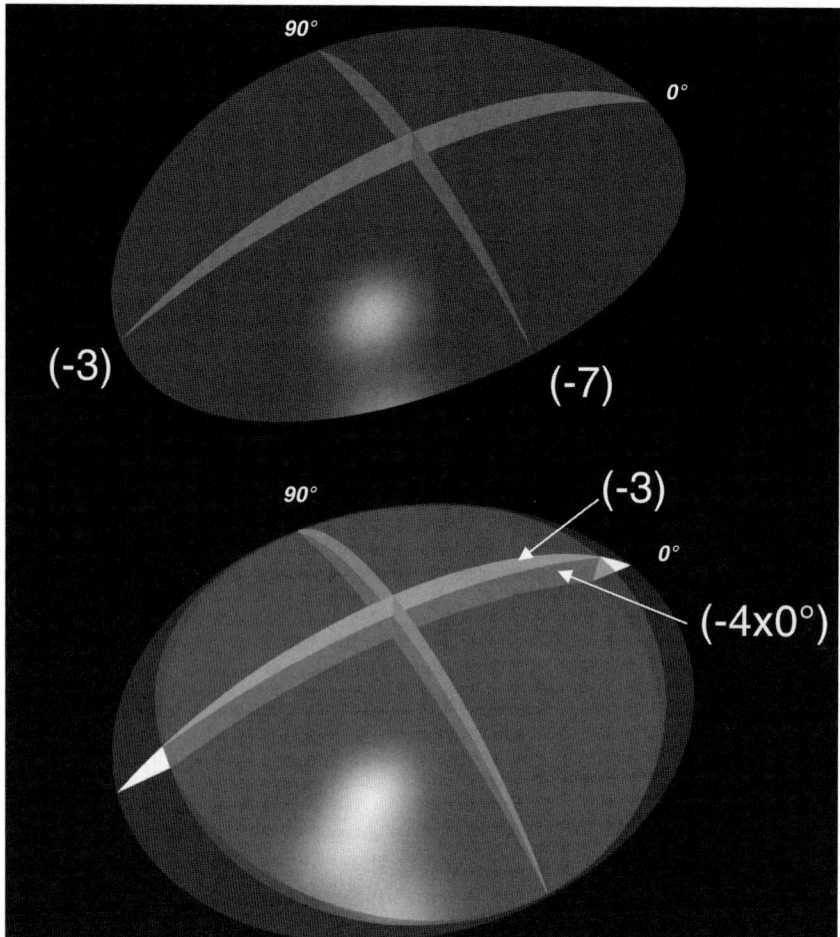

FIGURE 79-6. Comparison between the elliptical **(top)** and sequential **(bottom)** strategies to treat compound myopic astigmatism. In the elliptical strategy, the full correction is achieved by varying the width of the optical zone over the meridians to achieve the desired correction (maximum for the shortest, and minimum for the longest, respectively). In this example, it results in the narrowing of the vertical diameter of the optical zone, which provides a reduction in the maximal depth of ablation but may increase the incidence of night vision disturbances. In the elliptical strategy, there is no need of a transition zone, because the edge of the ablated lenticule has null thickness. In the sequential strategy, the realization of a transition zone is mandatory, to blend the abrupt edges caused by the negative cylinder treatment. (Artwork generated using computer-aided modeling)

To minimize the need for additional procedures and to optimize surgical outcomes of LASIK for astigmatism, the following tips are recommended:

Proper Preoperative Assessment

- The patient should be informed of the higher risk of refractive imprecision and postoperative visual disturbances such as halos and glare when the magnitude of the cylinder is high.
- Soft and rigid contact lenses should be removed at least 2 and 4 weeks before preoperative examination, respectively. In case of unstable refraction or corneal topography, it is recommended to repeat the examination after a few days.

Indications for the Treatment of Astigmatism

When the astigmatic component has a low and/or with-the-rule orientation, its inclusion in the photoablation planning should be discussed. If the best corrected visual acuities are identical with the spherical equivalent and the with spherocylindrical correction, the cylindrical component can be neglected and the correction of the spherical equivalent can be programmed.

Determination of the Magnitude and Axis of the Cylinder

Before treatment, the axis of the patient's manifest refraction cylinder and the corneal topography should be reviewed to ensure good correspondence. A significant discrepancy between the magnitude or axis of the cylinder as measured by objective, subjective refraction and/or the topographic cylinder requires recontrol of the refraction and investigations to rule out early keratoconus or contact lens-induced corneal warping. If the repeated measurements are reproducible and allow the patient to obtain a crisp 20/20 or more on manifest refraction, the cylinder treatment should be based on the manifest cylinder and axis.

Determination of the Profile of Ablation

To minimize biologic and biomechanical reactions of the cornea, and to avoid some corneal complications of LASIK such as corneal ectasia and regression, the choice of strategy should be guided by the minimal ablated volume of corneal tissue. This also reduces the duration of treatment, and facilitates the creation of the transition zone. These considerations depend on the possibilities offered by the delivery system, and may be influenced by encouraging results of particular strategies such as bitoric and cross-cylinder strategies in some situations.

Tips and Pitfalls in the Standard Astigmatic LASIK Technique

■ The refraction data entered in the laser software must be carefully checked to avoid mistakes, especially when transposing the refraction into different formats. Some delivery systems permit the dimensions of the ablation zone over the principal meridians to be adjusted; it can be advisable to slightly enlarge the optical zone and the transition zone along the initially flatter meridian.

■ Proper alignment of the patient's head and eyeball under the delivery system is critical to avoid cyclotorsion, which can lead to undercorrection and postoperative axis shift.

■ Limbal horizontal ink marks at the 6 and 3 o'clock meridians, made with the patient seated, can help to realign the eye under the laser microscope before ablation, and prevent cyclotorsion.

■ Optimal centration is mandatory to limit the risk of postoperative irregular astigmatism, especially with pure or compound hyperopic treatments. Some authors recommend centering the treatment on the pupillary center (52), whereas others use the corneal sighted light reflex, which best approximates the visual axis of the eye, especially for hyperopic correction (53).

■ Because of the elliptical shape of the overall ablation zone, the dimensions and hinge placement of the LASIK flap must be optimal. To minimize the risk of flap exposure to the laser beam, the hinge should be placed perpendicular to the initially flatter meridian (i.e., along the steeper meridian). Thus, the hinge should be positioned vertically for with-the-rule astigmatism, and horizontally for against-the-rule astigmatism.

■ The flap dimensions should be large enough to prevent exposure of the peripheral corneal epithelium to the laser and to limit the risk of postoperative complications such as irregular astigmatism or epithelial ingrowth. This is particularly important when hyperopic ablation profiles are used.

RESULTS OF LASIK TREATMENTS FOR ASTIGMATISM

Excimer laser treatment can be delivered with a variety of methods, including the scanning spot, the scanning slit or broad beam delivered through diaphragm and slit masks, and the ablatable mask (Fig. 79-N).

The treatment of myopic pure and compound astigmatism has been shown to be safe and effective for mild to moderate forms (30–32). However, a tendency to undercorrection and hyperopic shift of the cylindrical and spherical components was shown in a large retrospective analysis and in clinical studies with the NIDEK EC5000 scanning slit laser (16,33,34). This may be due to biologic and biomechanical responses of the cornea to the plano ablation along the flatter meridian. The use of cylindrical optical or elliptical ablation zones has been shown to provide better results in the treatment of myopic astigmatism (35). This may be related to the geometric optimization of the ablation on which these strategies are based. Various authors have proposed nomograms aimed at preventing the hyperopic shift of the refraction in pure myopic or compound myopic astigmatism with low sphere for the NIDEK EC5000 laser (27,33,34). Flying spot laser nomograms are proprietary, but refinements of the cylindrical profiles of ablation were likely made, based on similar early results.

The treatment of pure, compound hyperopic and mixed astigmatism has benefited from the implementation of the positive cylindrical profile of ablation, which steepens the flat meridian while leaving the steep meridian unablated (36–38). No shift in the spherical component of the refraction was observed with these treatments, possibly owing to the sparing of the center of the ablation zone and along the steepest meridian with the positive cylindrical correction. A tendency toward undercorrection, however, is observed, especially for high magnitudes of positive cylindrical treatment (33,34). This could be related to regression induced at the edge of the optical zone along the flatter meridian, despite the creation of a blend transitional zone (39). Encouraging results have been reported with the bitoric approach in mixed astigmatism (27,40).

LASIK retreatment of eyes with residual myopia and moderate astigmatism (up to −1.75D) can be achieved by lifting the flap and performing additional laser ablation, with good predictability and no significant complications (41). Customized photorefractive keratectomy has been proposed to improve best spectacle-corrected visual acuity and to minimize irregular astigmatism resulting from prior surgical procedures. LASIK for secondary hyperopia has been shown to provide satisfactory results for astigmatism from 0 to 2.75 D using the VISX star S2 and a nomogram adjusted for preoperative refraction, age, and prior refractive surgery (42). In selected post-radial keratectomy eyes with residual myopia and astigmatism, LASIK is an effective and safe procedure, improving patient satisfaction with overall vision(43). The predictability of LASIK correction of post-penetrating keratoplasty (PK) astigmatism is inferior to that of primary LASIK (44–50). The correction or reduction of the cylindrical component is more difficult to achieve than that of the spherical component. Because of the biomechanical properties of the grafted cornea, the cut of the flap without laser ablation can induce significant refractive and topographic changes, as shown by Busin et al. (51). These authors evaluated the effect of hinged lamellar keratotomy on refraction, vision, and corneal topography of postkeratoplasty eyes with high-degree astigmatism. At each postoperative examination time, there was a significant reduction in both average spherical equivalent and average absolute astigmatism relative to mean preoperative values. The main changes were seen as early as one day after surgery, but both progression and regression of the effect were documented at later postoperative examinations. In all patients, best spectacle-corrected acuity was maintained or improved after the procedure. Because hinged lamellar keratotomy improves the vision and refraction of postkeratoplasty eyes with high-degree astigmatism, it is sufficiently effective in some cases to make planned excimer laser treatment unnecessary.

Residual astigmatism is frequent after toric ablation, whereas induced astigmatism may occur after spherical ablation.

Poor patient alignment and irregular ablation can result in residual or induced astigmatism after LASIK (54). Decentration, flap irregularities, and central islands can induce irregular astigmatism (54,55). The diagnosis of postoperative astigmatism requires manifest and cycloplegic refraction, corneal topography, and wavefront analysis. Corneal topography is a major tool to distinguish between regular (uniform or bow-tie) and irregular patterns (central island, asymmetric bow-tie, peninsula, etc.). Refraction over hard contact lens can help to diagnose the presence of irregular astigmatism. Wavefront analysis has become a helpful tool to characterize and quantify the optical consequences of such irregular ablation and to correlate them with visual symptoms such as halo, glare, and monocular diplopia.

Because astigmatism has both magnitude and direction, changes after LASIK can be difficult to analyze. Various mathematical approaches, such as vector calculation, linear matrix, and polar coordinates, have been used to assess the spherical and astigmatism changes induced by LASIK. These methods are described in detail elsewhere (56–61).

Based on a retrospective analysis of 70 eyes that underwent spherical LASIK for myopia using a microkeratome

that creates a superior hinged flap (Hansatome, Bausch and Lomb, Irvine, CA), Huang et al. (62) found that surgery induced an average of 0.12 D with-the-rule astigmatism. This was attributed to the effects of the arcuate cut of the flap minus the effect of the hinge, where the absence of cut prevented the relaxation of the vertical meridian. Pallikaris et al. (63) recently showed that flap formation during LASIK can modify the eye's existing natural higher-order aberrations (especially spherical and coma-like aberrations along the axis of the flap's hinge), whereas visual acuity and refractive error remain unaffected. No significant modification of the astigmatic magnitude or axis was found using the authors' methodology.

CUSTOMIZED ABLATION FOR ASTIGMATISM

The advent of finely controlled excimer laser ablation may make it possible to correct directly some forms of corneal irregularity and irregular astigmatism with LASIK. Keratoconus is considered a contraindication to incisional refractive surgery such as radial keratotomy and LASIK, because of the corneal instability conferred by these procedures (64,65). To optimize visual function, both refractive and visual astigmatism must be considered, and vector analysis is helpful to address any discrepancy between these entities. However, noncustomized methods of excimer laser correction for corneal irregularity are based on partly empirical approaches and suffer from imprecision in establishing the profile of ablation and alignment (66,67). Alio et al. (68) produced a more regular corneal surface and improved best corrected visual acuity in patients with irregular astigmatism by using plano-scan excimer laser assisted with a viscous masking solution of 0.25% sodium hyaluronate. Videokeratoscopy-assisted techniques have given encouraging results in the treatment of irregular astigmatism. Examples of these techniques include Topolink (69), topography supported customized ablation (ToSCA) (70), and contoured ablation pattern (CAP) (71). Topolink has also been used to treat regular compound myopic astigmatism; LASIK based on corneal topography showed very high efficacy in low and moderate myopia with astigmatism, and maximal visual acuity was even improved in some cases. Precision was somewhat lower in high myopia with astigmatism (72).

LASIK guided by wavefront technology-linked techniques is a promising way of optimizing astigmatic treatments. By opening new vistas in the diagnosis and therapy of high-order optical aberrations of the human eye, this approach might refine the treatment of irregular astigmatism (73). However, results published in the peer-reviewed literature reveal that these treatments have not proven effective in reducing preexisting high-order aberrations (74,75), whereas a lower increase of postoperative high-order aberrations has been reported (76). Wavefront-guided LASIK also offers a new way of managing grossly decentered laser ablations. Unfortunately, some patients have aberrations too large for wavefront sensing or other clinical limitations such as a residual cornea too thin for further treatment (77). Optimized customized ablation patterns may further improve the visual results, by optimizing the geometry of the profiles of ablation and anticipating biomechanical and biologic reactions (78–80).

CONCLUSION

Approaches taking into account the geometric implications of astigmatic treatments have improved the predictability of the conventional LASIK procedure by identifying the best strategies to minimize the depth of ablation while increasing the tolerability of toric ablation using adapted blend zones. Better centration, together with topographic and wavefront-guided LASIK, may further improve the results of this procedure and provide better outcomes, especially for retreatment and irregular astigmatism.

REFERENCES

1. Guyton DL. Prescribing cylinders: the problem of distortion. *Surv Ophthalmol* 1977;22:177–188.
2. Troutman RC, Swinger C. Relaxing incision for control of postoperative astigmatism following keratoplasty. *Ophthalmic Surg* 1980;11:117–120.
3. Lindstrom RL, Lindquist TD. Correction of postoperative astigmatism. *Cornea* 1988;7:138–148.
4. Trokel SL, Srinivasan R, Braren B. Excimer laser surgery of the cornea. *Am J Ophthalmol* 1983;96:710–715.
5. McDonnell PJ, Moreira H, Garbus J, et al. Photorefractive keratectomy to creat toric ablations for correction of astigmatism. *Arch Ophthalmol* 1991;109:710–713.
6. Yan W, Kanxing Z, Tong Z, et al. Photoastigmatic refractive keratectomy of laser *in situ* keratomileusis for moderate and high myopic astigmatism. *J Refract Surg* 2000;16:S268–S271.
7. Yang SH, Van Gelder RN, Pepose JS. Astigmatic changes after excimer laser refractive surgery. *J Cataract Refract Surg* 2002;28:477–484.
8. Van Gelder RN, Steger-May K, Yang SH, et al. Comparison of photorefractive keratectomy, astigmatic PRK, laser *in situ* keratomileusis, and astigmatic LASIK in the treatment of myopia. *J Cataract Refract Surg* 2002;28:462–476.
9. Moreno-Barrisuso E, lloves JM, Marcos S, et al. Ocular aberrations before and after myopic corneal refractive surgery: LASIK induced changes measured with laser ray tracing. *Invest Ophthalmol Vis Sci* 2002;42:1396–1403.
10. Thibos LN, Applegate RA, Schwiegerling JT, et al., VSIA Standards Taskforce Members. Vision science and its applications. Standards for reporting the optical aberrations of eyes. *J Refract Surg* 2002;18:S652–660.
11. Macrae S. Excimer ablation design and elliptical transition zones. *J Cataract Refract Surg* 1999;25:1191–1197.
12. Gatinel D, Hoang-Xuan T. Modélisation tridimensionnelle et géométrie descriptive des profils de photoablation sphériques et cylindriques pures au laser excimer (French). *J Fr Ophtalmol* 2002;25:247–256.
13. Azar DT, Primack JD. Theoretical analysis of ablation depths and profiles in laser *in situ* keratomileusis for compound and mixed astigmatism. *J Cataract Refract Surg* 2000;26:1123–1136.
14. Gatinel D, Hoang-Xuan T, Azar DT. Three-dimensional representation and qualitative comparisons of the amount of tissue ablation to treat mixed and compound astigmatism. *J Cataract Refract Surg* 2002;28:2026–2034.
15. Gatinel D. Corneal surface profile after hyperopia surgery. In: Tsubota K, Wachler BSB, Azar DT, et al., eds. *Hyperopia and presbyopia.* New York: Marcel Dekker, 2003:141–150.
16. Huang D, Stulting RD, Carr JD, et al. Multiple regression and vector analyses of laser *in situ* keratomileusis for myopia and astigmatism. *J Refract Surg* 1999;15:538–549.
17. Munnerlyn CR, Koons SJ, Marshall J. Photorefractive keratotomy: a technique for laser refractive surgery. *J Cataract Refract Surg* 1988;14:46–52.
18. Seiler T, Koufala K, Richter G. Iatrogenic keratectasia after laser *in situ* keratomileusis. *J Refract Surg* 1998;14:312–317.
19. Joo CK, Kim TG. Corneal ectasia detected after laser *in situ* keratomileusis for correction of less than −12 diopters of myopia. *J Cataract Refract Surg* 2000;26:292–295.
20. McLeod SD, Kisla TA, Caro NC, et al. Iatrogenic keratoconus: Corneal ectasia following laser *in situ* keratomileusis. *Arch Ophthalmol* 2000;118:282–284.
21. Argento C, Cosentino MJ, Tytium A, et al. Corneal ectasia after laser *in situ* keratomileusis. *J Cataract Refract Surg* 2001;27:1440–1448.
22. Amoils SP, Deist MB, Gous P, et al. Iatrogenic keratectasia after laser *in situ* keratomileusis for less than −4.0 to −7.0 diopters of myopia. *J Cataract Refract Surg* 2000;26:967–977.
23. Pallikaris IG, Kymionis GD, Astyrakakis IN. Corneal ectasia induced by laser *in situ* keratomileusis. *J Cataract Refract Surg* 2001;27:1796–1802.
24. Vinciguerra P, Sborgia M, Epstein D, et al. Photorefractive keratectomy to correct myopic or hyperopic astigmatism with a cross-cylinder ablation. *J Refract Surg* 1999;15:S183–185.
25. Vinciguerra P, Camesasca FI. Cross cylinder ablation. In: MacRae SM, Krueger RR, Applegate RA, eds. *Customized corneal ablation: the quest for supervision.* Thorofare, NJ: Slack, 2001:319–327.
26. Vinciguerra P, Camesasca FI. Surgical treatment options for hyperopia and hyperopic astigmatism. In: Tsubota K, Wachler BSB, Azar DT, et al., eds. *Hyperopia and presbyopia.* New York: Marcel Dekker, 2003:69–82.
27. Chayet AS, Magallanes R, Montes M, et al. Laser *in situ* keratomileusis for simple myopic, mixed and simple myopic astigmatim. *J Refract Surg* 1998;14:S175–176.
28. Gallinaro C, Toulemont PJ, Cochener B, et al. Excimer laser photorefractive keratectomy to correct astigmatism. *J Cataract Refract Surg* 1996;22:557–563.
29. Gatinel D, Hoang-Xuan T, Azar DT. Volume estimation of excimer laser tissue ablation for correction of spherical myopia and hyperopia. *Invest Ophthalmol Vis Sci* 2002;43:1445–1449.
30. Shaikh NM, Manche EE. Laser *in situ* keratomileusis for myopia and compound myopic astigmatism using the Technolas 217 scanning-spot laser. *J Cataract Refract Surg* 2002;28:485–490.
31. Wang X, McCulley JP, Bowman W, et al. Results of combined myopic astigmatic LASIK treatment and retreatments. *CLAO J* 2002;28:55–60.
32. Yang CN, Shen EP, Hu FR. Laser *in situ* keratomileusis for the correction of myopia and myopic astigmatism. *J Cataract Refract Surg* 2001;27:1952–1960.
33. Rueda L, Pineda-Fernandez A, Huang D, et al. Laser *in situ* keratomileusis for mixed and simple myopic astigmatism with the Nidek EC-5000 laser. *J Refract Surg* 2002;18:234–238.
34. Payvar S, Hashemi H. Laser in situ keratomileusis for myopic astigmatism with the Nidek EC-5000 laser. *J Refract Surg* 2002;18:225–233.
35. Shah S, Smith RJ, Pieger S, et al. Effect of an elliptical optical zone on outcome of photoastigmatic refractive keratectomy. *J Refract Surg* 1999;15:S188–191.

36. Salz JJ, Stevens CA, LADARvision LASIK hyperopia study group. LASIK correction of spherical hyperopia, hyperopic astigmatism, and mixed astigmatism with the LADARvision excimer laser system. *Ophthalmology* 2002;109:1647–1656.

37. Lian J, Ye W, Zhou D, et al. Laser *in situ* keratomileusis for correction of hyperopia and hyperopic astigmatism with the Technolas 117C. *J Refract Surg* 2002;18:435–438.

38. Ditzen K, Fiedler J, Pieger S. Laser *in situ* keratomileusis for hyperopia and hyperopic astigmatism using the Meditec MEL 70 spot scanner. *J Refract Surg* 2002;18:430–434.

39. Ambrosio R, Wilson SE. Wound healing after hyperopic corneal surgery. Why there is greater regression in the treatment of hyperopia. In: Tsubota K, Wachler BSB, Azar DT, et al., eds. *Hyperopia and presbyopia.* New York: Marcel Dekker, 2003:173–187.

40. Lui MM, Silas MA, Aplebaum B, et al. Laser *in situ* keratomileusis with the Nidek EC-5000 excimer laser for astigmatism greater than 4.00 D. *J Refract Surg* 2002;18:S321–S322.

41. Rashad KM. Laser *in situ* keratomileusis retreatment for residual myopia and astigmatism. *J Refract Surg* 2000;16:170–176.

42. Lindstrom RL, Linebarger EJ, Hardten DR, et al. Early results of hyperopic and astigmatic laser *in situ* keratomileusis in eyes with secondary hyperopia. *Ophthalmology* 2000;107:1858–1863.

43. Shah SB, Lingua RW, Kim CH, et al. Laser *in situ* keratomileusis to correct residual myopia and astigmatism after radial keratotomy. *J Cataract Refract Surg* 2000;26:1152–1157.

44. Lima G da S, Moreira H, Wahab SA. Laser *in situ* keratomileusis to correct myopia, hypermetropia and astigmatism after penetrating keratoplasty for keratoconus: a series of 27 cases. *Can J Ophthalmol* 2001;36:391–396.

45. Donnenfeld ED, Kornstein HS, Amin A, et al. Laser *in situ* keratomileusis for correction of myopia and astigmatism after penetrating keratoplasty. *Ophthalmology* 1999;106:1966–1974.

46. Rashad KM. Laser *in situ* keratomileusis for correction of high astigmatism after penetrating keratoplasty. *J Refract Surg* 2000;16:701–710.

47. Nassaralla BR, Nassaralla JJ. Laser *in situ* keratomileusis after penetrating keratoplasty. *J Refract Surg* 2000;16:431–437.

48. Koay PY, McGhee CN, Weed KH, et al. Laser *in situ* keratomileusis for ametropia after penetrating keratoplasty. *J Refract Surg* 2000;16:140–147.

49. Arenas E, Maglione A. Laser *in situ* keratomileusis for astigmatism and myopia after penetrating keratoplasty. *J Refract Surg* 1997;13:27–32.

50. Webber SA, Lawless MA, Sutton GL, et al. LASIK for post penetrating keratoplasty astigmatism and myopia. *Br J Ophthalmol* 1999;83:1013–1018.

51. Busin M, Arffa RC, Zambianchi L, et al. Effect of hinged lamellar keratotomy on postkeratoplasty eyes. *Ophthalmology* 2001;108:1845–1851.

52. Uozoto H, Guyton DL. Centering corneal surgical procedures. *Am J Ophthalmol* 1987;103:264–275.

53. Pande M, Hillman JS. Optical zone centration after refractive surgery. Entrance pupil center, visual axis, coaxially sighted corneal reflex, or geometric corneal center? *Ophthalmology* 1993;100:1230–1237.

54. Melki SA, Azar DT. LASIK complications: etiology, management, and prevention. *Surv Ophthalmol* 2001;46:95–116.

55. Johnson JD, Azar DT. Surgically induced topographical abnormalities after LASIK: management of central islands, corneal ectasia, decentration, and irregular astigmatism. *Curr Opin Ophthalmol* 2001;12:309–317.

56. Alpins N. Astigmatism analysis by the Alpins method. *J Cataract Refract Surg* 2001;27:31–49.

57. Kaye SB, Patterson A. Analyzing refractive changes after anterior segment surgery. *J Cataract Refract Surg* 2001;27:50–60.

58. Holladay JT, Moran JR, Kezirian GM. Analysis of aggregate surgically induced refractive change, prediction error, and intraocular astigmatism. *J Cataract Refract Surg* 2001;27:61–79.

59. Thibos LN, Horner D. Power vector analysis of the optical outcome of refractive surgery. *J Cataract Refract Surg* 2001;27:80–85.

60. Naeser K, Hjortdal J. Polar value analysis of refractive data. *J Cataract Refract Surg* 2001;27:86–94.

61. Naeser K, Hjortdal J. Multivariate analysis of refractive data. *J Cataract Refract Surg* 2001;27:129–142.

62. Huang D, Sur S, Seffo F, et al. Surgically-induced astigmatism after laser *in situ* keratomileusis for spherical myopia. *J Refract Surg* 2000;16:515–518.

63. Pallikaris IG, Kymionis GD, Panagopoulou SI, et al. Induced optical aberrations following formation of a laser *in situ* keratomileusis flap. *J Cataract Refract Surg* 2002;28:1737–1741.

64. Colin J, Velou S. Current surgical options for keratoconus. *J Cataract Refract Surg* 2003;29:379–386.

65. Randleman JB, Russell B, Ward MA, et al. Risk factors and prognosis for corneal ectasia after LASIK. *Ophthalmology* 2003;110: 267–275.

66. Cheloudtchenko V, Kourenkov V, Fadeikina T. Correction of asymmetrical myopic astigmatism with laser *in situ* keratomileusis. *J Refract Surg* 1999;15:S192–S194.

67. Alio JL, Artola A, Rodriguez-Mier FA. Selective zonal ablations with excimer laser for correction of irregular astigmatism induced by refractive surgery. *Ophthalmology* 2000;107:662–673.

68. Alio JL, Belda JI, Shalaby AM. Correction of irregular astigmatism with excimer laser assisted by sodium hyaluronate. *Ophthalmology* 2001;108:1246–1260.

69. Knorz MC. TopoLink LASIK. *Int Ophthalmol Clin* 2000;40: 145–149.

70. Nagy ZZ. Laser *in situ* keratomileusis combined with topography-supported customized ablation after repeated penetrating keratoplasty. *J Cataract Refract Surg* 2003;29:792–794.

71. Tamayo Fernandez GE, Serrano MG. Early clinical experience using custom excimer laser ablations to treat irregular astigmatism. *J Cataract Refract Surg* 2000;26:1442–1450.

72. Knorz MC, Neuhann T. Correction of myopia and astigmatism using topography-assisted laser *in situ* keratomileusis (TopoLink LASIK). *Ophthalmologe* 2000;97:827–831.

73. Mrochen M, Seiler T. Fundamentals of wavefront-guided refractive corneal surgery. *Ophthalmologe* 2001;98:703–714.

74. Phusitphoykai N, Tungsiripat T, Siriboonkoom J, et al. Comparison of conventional versus wavefront-guided laser *in situ* keratomileusis in the same patient. *J Refract Surg* 2003;19:S217–S220.

75. Vongthongsri A, Phusitphoykai N, Naripthapan P. Comparison of wavefront-guided customized ablation versus conventional ablation in laser *in situ* keratomileusis. *J Refract Surg* 2002;18:S332–S335.

76. Panagopoulou SI, Pallikaris IG. Wavefront customized ablations with the WASCA Asclepion workstation. *J Refract Surg* 2001;17: S608–S612.

77. Mrochen M, Krueger RR, Bueeler M, et al. Aberration-sensing and wavefront-guided laser *in situ* keratomileusis: management of decentered ablation. *J Refract Surg* 2002;18:418–429.

78. Wu HK. Astigmatism and LASIK. *Curr Opin Ophthalmol* 2002;13:250–255.

79. Roberts C. Biomechanics of the cornea and wavefront-guided laser refractive surgery. *J Refract Surg* 2002;18:S589–S592.

80. Huang D, Tang M, Shekhar R. Mathematical model of corneal surface smoothing after laser refractive surgery. *Am J Ophthalmol* 2003;135:267–278.

LASIK COMBINED WITH OTHER PROCEDURES

**JONATHAN D. PRIMACK AND
DIMITRI T. AZAR**

The excimer laser revolutionized the field of refractive surgery and greatly facilitated its acceptance into mainstream ophthalmology. As techniques evolved, laser-assisted *in situ* keratomileusis (LASIK) replaced photorefractive keratectomy (PRK) as the procedure of choice given its lack of postoperative pain, quick visual rehabilitation, and ability to treat higher degrees of ametropia. LASIK has been shown to be a safe and efficacious technique for the correction of myopia, hyperopia, and astigmatism, but limitations exist (1–6). These limitations have inspired surgeons to combine LASIK with other ophthalmologic procedures for the correction of both naturally occurring and postsurgical refractive error.

Combining LASIK with other technologies appeals to the refractive surgeon for several reasons. First, it may allow for the successful treatment of high myopia and astigmatism beyond what is generally considered the safe range for LASIK [approximately 10 diopters (D) of myopia and 5 D of astigmatism]. Higher levels of myopia cannot be treated with deeper excimer laser ablations because a sufficient amount of corneal stromal tissue must remain to guard against potential keratectasia and refractive instability (7,8). Current recommendations suggest a minimal residual stromal bed thickness of approximately 250 μm. This precludes the application of highly myopic ablations, especially in those patients with thinner corneas. The residual myopia remaining after a maximal LASIK treatment could be corrected by combining LASIK with another refractive procedure that does not involve the removal of stromal tissue.

In eyes with moderate to high myopia and low pachymetry values, concerns over residual stromal bed thickness and potential iatrogenic keratectasia may preclude full LASIK correction or limit retreatment options should regression occur. These patients could also benefit from a combined approach that reduced ablation depth by redistributing part of the LASIK-dependent correction to another procedure. Reports of keratectasia occurring in patients with residual stromal beds greater than 250 μm suggests that less central stromal tissue removal may be safer (9–11). Additionally, decreasing the magnitude of refractive error to be corrected by LASIK may allow for the use of larger optical zones (OZs) with a smaller chance of subjective optical disturbances.

A last theoretical advantage of combining LASIK with another procedure is adjustability. If the additional technology is reversible or adjustable, it could allow for subsequent refractive changes desired by the patient.

COMBINATION OF LASIK WITH OTHER REFRACTIVE SURGERY TECHNIQUES

Combined LASIK and Incisional Keratotomy

Incisional keratotomy refers to procedures that decrease refractive error by means of almost full-thickness corneal incisions. Their effect is a function of incision length and OZ size. Examples include radial keratotomy (RK) and astigmatic or arcuate keratotomy (AK). These techniques are uncommonly performed today given the more predictable outcomes associated with excimer laser surgery (12).

There is one published report of RK enhancements after LASIK to treat residual myopia. Damiano and colleagues (13) reported on 60 eyes of 41 patients treated with combined RK and LASIK for a preoperative spherical equivalent (SE) -8.09 ± 2.60 D (range, -4 to -15.25 D). After the initial LASIK procedure, the SE decreased to -2.02 ± 1.02 D (range, -0.50 to -5.50 D). RK was chosen over LASIK retreatment for several reasons including a residual stromal bed of less than 250 μm, insufficient stromal thickness to safely correct the myopia with LASIK alone (planned procedure), and surgeon preference in the presence of a stromal bed thick enough to safely allow a full LASIK re-treatment. RK was performed using four, six, or eight centrifugal incisions with a 3- to 6-mm OZ. AK was performed if astigmatism greater than 1 D was observed. The mean time between LASIK and RK was 7.3 ± 6.5 months. After RK, the SE decreased to -0.43 ± 0.61 D (range, -2 to $+0.75$ D).

There are multiple theoretical concerns when performing incisional keratotomy on a postLASIK cornea. First, multiple incisions could potentially lead to epithelial ingrowth under the LASIK flap. Second, it may be difficult to predict the patient's response given the presence of a thinned cornea. Third, RK incisions could further weaken an already thinned cornea, resulting in iatrogenic keratectasia. Alternatively, a thinned cornea may develop pronounced flattening with a greater progressive hyperopic shift than has been observed with RK alone (14). Fourth, there may be a risk of the flap separating into fragments if the patient ever sustains corneal trauma or needs to have the flap relifted [i.e., for late diffuse lamellar keratitis (DLK)].

Damiano et al. (13) reported none of these complications after a mean follow-up time of 15.4 months. No eye lost two or more lines of best spectacle-corrected visual acuity (BSCVA), and all eyes had a BSCVA of 20/30 or better. Three patients with sufficient stromal bed thickness desired a LASIK enhancement after the RK procedure and this was performed uneventfully by lifting the original flap. All three eyes had an uncorrected visual acuity (UCVA) of 20/20 after the second LASIK treatment. Postoperative complications included mild glare and halos (23%), diurnal fluctuation (10%), and distorted vision (4%).

AK was most often used in conjunction with LASIK before the United States Food and Drug Administration (FDA) approved astigmatic excimer laser ablation corrections. Surgeons could perform AK to decrease a patient's astigmatism, followed by LASIK several months afterward to treat the residual spherical error. Some surgeons still combine AK with LASIK for select patients. These include individuals whose astigmatism exceeds that amount for which the laser is approved to correct and those patients with larger pupils who are at risk for optical aberrations with an excimer induced elliptical OZ.

Guell and Vazquez (15) described a staged procedure combining AK and LASIK to treat high astigmatism in 15 eyes. Thirteen of the eyes had naturally occurring astigmatism and two of the eyes had surgically induced astigmatism resulting from a phacoemulsification and a penetrating keratoplasty. AK was performed initially followed by LASIK 3 to 5 months later. The preoperative mean SE and the mean refractive astigmatism were -2.47 ± 3.69 D (range, -3.25 to $+1.50$ D) and -4.59 ± 1.66 D (range, -3.25 to -8 D), respectively. After both procedures, the mean cylinder power decreased to -1.21 ± 1.07 D and the mean SE measured -0.09 ± 1.50 D (12-month follow-up). One eye lost a line of best corrected visual acuity (BCVA) and two eyes gained one and two lines, respectively. No patients experienced epithelial ingrowth through the AK incision sites. No other complications occurred.

Limbal relaxing incisions (LRIs) to reduce astigmatism have also been reported in conjunction with LASIK (16). Unlike AK, LRIs are placed more peripherally near the limbus and are usually only 600 μm in depth. Their location places them outside of the lamellar corneal flap. LRIs are less effective than AK, but have the theoretical advantage of inducing less irregularity.

A role may exist for incisional keratometry after LASIK to treat topographic irregularities. Pulaski (17) reported both AK and combined AK/RK to treat asymmetrical steep islands in seven eyes after LASIK. Patients complained of poor UCVA and unwanted optical side effects. After undergoing the incisional secondary procedure, the SE decreased from -0.94 ± 0.48 D to -0.21 ± 0.12 D. Optical aberrations were reduced in all patients and the average UCVA improved from 20/40 to 20/25. Two patients experienced inferior steepening, and one microperforation occurred. No eyes lost two or more lines of BSCVA. The author suggested that this technique might be helpful in similar patients until topographically guided custom excimer laser ablations become available for the management of this problem.

The limited data available suggest that combined LASIK and AK/RK may be a safe procedure. Incisional keratotomy is an extraocular procedure (although microperforations can occur), it can be performed in an office or laser suite setting, and it does not further compromise corneal thickness. Additionally, accommodation is preserved. Disadvantages include its lack of predictability and stability, its inability to treat high myopia, the potential for flap complications, and its lack of adjustability and reversibility. We do not recommend performing RK primarily with a planned secondary LASIK treatment, given the above issues and the potential for healing problems and flap-related complications (18–20).

Combined LASIK and Phakic Intraocular Lenses

Phakic intraocular lenses (P-IOLs) are designed to correct high ametropia following surgical implantation anterior to the crystalline lens. P-IOLs may be angle fixated (e.g., Nuvita lens, Bausch & Lomb, Irvine, CA), iris fixated (e.g., Artisan lens, Ophtec B.V., Groningen, Netherlands), or located in the posterior chamber (e.g., STAAR lens, STAAR Surgical, Nidau, Switzerland). P-IOLs have been used for many years in Europe and South America. All models have undergone multiple design refinements to improve safety profiles, and several lenses are currently in FDA trials (21–23).

The practice of combining P-IOLs with LASIK is called *bioptics* and was first described by Zaldivar et al. (24). The concept's inspiration was the inability of P-IOLs alone to sufficiently correct very high degrees of myopia (greater than 15 to 20 D) and astigmation. A P-IOL thickens with increasing power; so concerns about lenticular or endothelial touch limit the lens' clinical utility. Decreasing the P-IOL OZ could mitigate this issue, but that could also result in glare or halos. The solution was bioptics—a P-IOL served to reduce the spherical error and a supplementary LASIK procedure corrected the residual sphere and astigmatism, thus extending the range of correction without compromising P-IOL OZ size (25,26).

Bioptics is a two-staged surgical procedure. Topical anesthesia may be used, but a retrobulbar block may be preferred to avoid inadvertent lenticular touch with eye movement. In the first stage, a hinged lamellar corneal flap is created using a microkeratome. The flap is inspected and refloated back into position without performing a laser ablation. The surgeon next fashions a scleral tunnel or clear corneal wound, the length of which is determined by the P-IOL size and material [i.e., foldable material vs. polymethylmethacrylate (PMMA)]. The next steps are determined by the intended location of the P-IOL. If the lens is to reside in the anterior chamber, acetylcholine is injected to induce miosis. This protects the crystalline lens from inadvertent contact and allows proper centering over the pupil. The anterior chamber is then filled with a viscoelastic agent. If the lens is to lie in the posterior chamber, the pupil is dilated preoperatively and viscoelastic is injected into the anterior chamber. Once a P-IOL is inserted into the anterior chamber, it must be manipulated into the proper orientation. Paracentesis sites may be helpful to allow for additional instruments. Depending on lens design, it may be tucked under the iris into the posterior chamber or manipulated so that the footplates reside in the angle or are enclaving iris tissue. If fixated in the posterior chamber, acetylcholine is injected to induce miosis and protect against P-IOL dislocation. If not performed preoperatively, a peripheral iridectomy should be created to prevent angle-closure glaucoma. Viscoelastic is then exchanged for balanced salt solution (BSS) and the incision may be sutured closed if necessary. Figure 80-1 illustrates these steps with the Artisan P-IOL. The target SE following P-IOL placement is low to moderate myopia.

The second stage of bioptics is the excimer laser ablation, which occurs 3 to 5 months later once the refraction has stabilized and all sutures have been removed (Fig. 80-2). The flap is relifted and the laser applied to treat the remaining refractive error. The flap is then refloated back onto the stromal bed.

Some authors have deferred creation of the LASIK flap until the second stage of the procedure (24), but theoretical safety concerns suggest that the surgical steps proceed in the aforementioned order. For instance, creating the LASIK flap prior to insertion of the P-IOL may prevent potential intraocular P-IOL movement during the microkeratome pass. This theoretically avoids P-IOL, endothelial touch in the case of anterior chamber lenses and P-IOL, and lenticular contact in the case of posterior chamber lenses. It may also preclude posterior chamber lenses from dislocating during the temporary mydriasis that occurs with suction ring application. The disadvantage

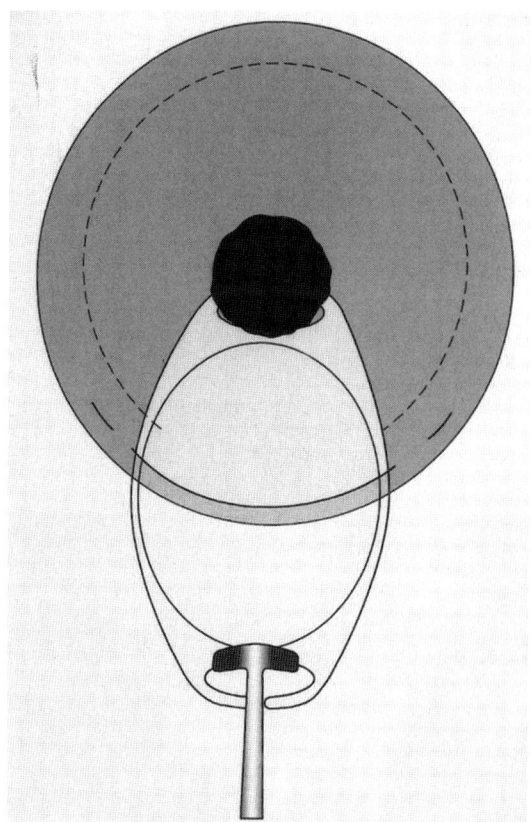

A

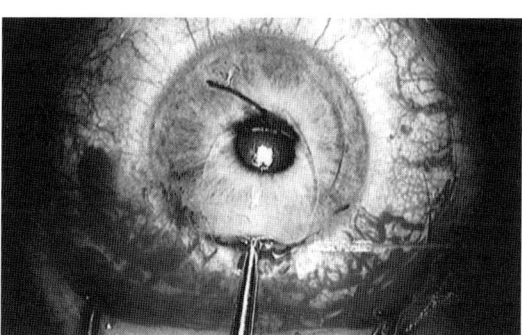

B

FIGURE 80-1. A,B: The first surgical stage of bioptics. A LASIK flap is created and refloated back into position without performing a laser ablation. A phakic intraocular lens (Artisan lens shown) is introduced into the anterior chamber and centered over the pupil. (From Guell JL, Vazquez M, Gris O. Adjustable refractive surgery: 6 mm artisan lens plus laser *in situ* keratomileusis for the correction of high myopia. *Ophthalmology* 2001;108: 945–952, with permission.)

of creating the LASIK flap during the first stage is the need to relift the flap for the second stage, which may increase the risk of epithelial ingrowth (28).

The suggested indications for bioptics include myopia greater than 15 to 18 D or myopia greater than 11 D with more than 1.50 to 2 D of astigmatism (24,29,30). A thorough preoperative examination is necessary including an evaluation of the corneal topography, corneal thickness,

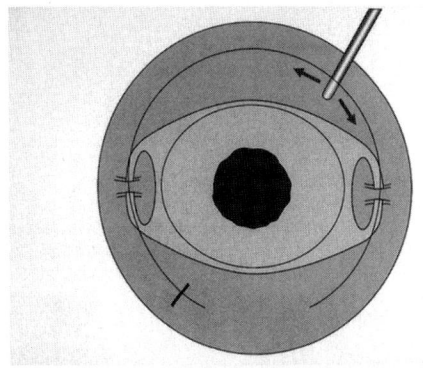

A

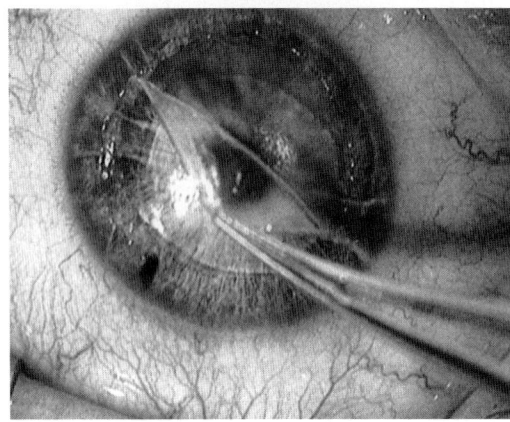

B

FIGURE 80-2. A–C: The second stage of bioptics. Months later, once the sutures have been removed and the refraction has stabilized, the flap is relifted and the LASIK ablation performed. (From Guell JL, Vazquez M, Gris O. Adjustable refractive surgery: 6 mm artisan lens plus laser *in situ* keratomileusis for the correction of high myopia. *Ophthalmology* 2001;108:945–952, with permission.)

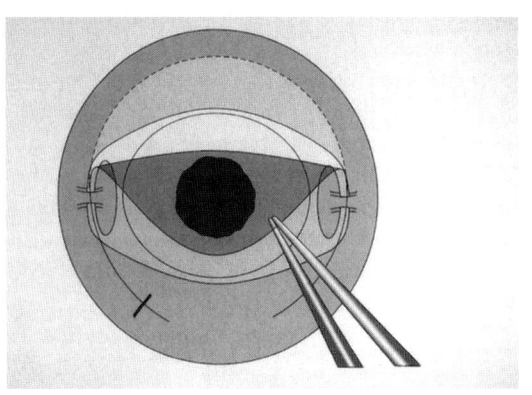

C

cycloplegic refraction, pupil size in scotopic conditions, anterior chamber depth, endothelial cell counts, and retinal periphery. Contraindications include a history of corneal irregularity (i.e., keratoconus), uveitis, glaucoma, shallow anterior chamber (for anterior chamber P-IOLs), low endothelial cell counts ($<$2,000 cells/mm^2), cataract, anterior

segment pathology, dry eye, unstable refraction, autoimmune disease, or uncontrolled systemic or eye disease.

The published results of bioptics are encouraging and Table 80-1 summarizes the available data. Zaldivar and coauthors (24) reported on 67 eyes that received a posterior chamber STAAR P-IOL followed by LASIK.

TABLE 80-1. SUMMARY OF VISUAL OUTCOMES FOLLOWING LASIK COMBINED WITH OTHER PROCEDURES

Technique	n	Preoperative mean SE (D)	% UCVA ≥ 20/40	% ± 1 D	Reference
LASIK and RK	54^	−8.09	94	NR	Damiano et al. [13]
LASIK and AK	15	−2.47	53.3	80	Guell et al. [15]
LASIK and Phakic IOL	411	−20.65	70	91	
	67	−23.00	69	85	Zaldivar et al. [24]
	26	−18.42	77	100	Guell et al. [30]
	37*	−17.97	89	97	Sanchez-Galeana et al. [31]
	281**	NR	67	NR	Zaldivar et al. [32]
LASIK and ICRS	2	−6.6	100	100	Primack and Azar [46]
Phacoemulsification and LASIK	34	+4.95	87	83	Pop et al. [52]
	22***	+5.22	82	95	Velarde et al. [54]
		−11.76			
	2	−15.50	100	100	Probst and Smith [53]
	64	NR	83	NR	Zaldivar et al. [32]

SE, Spherical Equivalent; D, Diopters; UCVA, Uncorrected Visual Acuity; NR, Not Reported;
RK, Radial Keratotomy; AK, Astigmatic Keratotomy; IOL, Intraocular lens;
ICRS; Intracorneal ring segments; ^, represents number of eyes corrected for distance;
*, Includes 28 LASIK and 9 PRK patients;
**, may include 67 patients from previously listed study;
***, number of patients myopic vs. hyperopic not reported.

The mean preoperative SE was -23 ± 3.60 D (range, -18.75 to -35 D). The mean SE decreased to -6.00 ± 2.80 D (range, -2 to -14.38 D) after implantation of the P-IOL. Mean SE after secondary LASIK (3 months follow-up) was -0.20 ± 0.90 D (range, $+1.75$ to -5.13 D). UCVA measured 20/40 or better in 46% of eyes. A gain of two or more lines of BSCVA was observed in 76% of eyes.

Guell et al. (29,30) reported their experience using the iris fixated Artisan P-IOL followed by LASIK 3 to 5 months later. The authors preliminarily reported on eight eyes, which was followed by a paper describing their results in 26 eyes. A -15 D PMMA lens with a 60-mm OZ was used in all patients. The mean preoperative SE measured -18.42 ± 2.73 D (range, -16 to -23.50 D) and, after bioptics, decreased to -0.38 ± 0.65 D (range, $+1$ to -1). After 24 months of follow-up, 100% of patients were ± 1 D of emmetropia and 77% of eyes had an UCVA of 20/40 or better. Endothelial cell counts decreased by a mean of 0.61% in the first year and 0.60% in the second year. It was unclear if this was the result of the Artisan lens or the operative procedure itself.

Sanchez-Galeana and coauthors (31) followed 37 eyes that received the STAAR posterior chamber P-IOL followed by either LASIK or PRK. The authors did not differentiate the results by type of surgery, but 28 of the eyes underwent LASIK. Mean follow-up time measured 8.1 months. Postoperatively, the mean SE decreased to -0.18 ± 0.53 D (range, -1 to $+1$) from a preoperative value of -17.97 ± 4.89 D (range, -9.75 to -28).

Zaldivar and colleagues (32) also reported on 281 patients with STAAR posterior chamber P-IOLs who subsequently underwent LASIK. Data regarding refractive error prior to P-IOL insertion was not provided. It is unclear if this publication included patients from a previous report (24). The mean SE prior to LASIK was -5.50 D (range, -1.37 to -16 D). One month after LASIK the mean SE decreased to -0.40 D. BSCVA measured 20/40 or better in 67% of eyes.

Bioptics offers several advantages over existing refractive surgery modalities. The most obvious is the ability to treat very high levels of myopia (approximately 25 to 30 D). The anticipated arrival of toric P-IOLs may also allow for concurrent correction of high astigmatism beyond what is currently treatable by LASIK alone (27). Another advantage of the procedure is adjustability. For instance, purposely undercorrected presbyopic patients may have their LASIK flap relifted and their myopia retreated should they later desire emmetropia. Alternatively, the P-IOL may be exchanged for one of a different power. The procedure also preserves accommodation, which is important in younger patients.

The potential disadvantages of bioptics include all of those inherent with P-IOLs and LASIK. The first is the inherent risk of endophthalmitis associated with intraocular surgery. One must also consider the risks of cataract forma-

tion and endothelial cell compromise that have plagued P-IOLs since their conception. Ongoing engineering refinements continue to address these issues; however, at the current time, no P-IOLs have attained FDA approval. Other known complications of P-IOLs include corneal edema, uveitis, glaucoma, decentration, retinal detachment, endophthalmitis, ischemic optic neuropathy, and pupil ovalization (33–36). Risks associated with LASIK include flap complications, overcorrection, undercorrection, irregular astigmatism, glare and halos, DLK, infection, dry eye, epithelial ingrowth, and loss of BSCVA. In the previously described reports, four patients with the STAAR posterior chamber P-IOL developed cataractous changes in the crystalline lens. LASIK complications included an incomplete flap, free caps, dry eye, flap striae, overcorrection, epithelial ingrowth, irregular stromal bed, traumatic flap dislocation, moderate glare and halos, DLK, and transient corneal edema. Two patients experienced macular hemorrhages thought to result from myopic degeneration and not from the surgical procedure (24,29–32). A theoretical disadvantage of bioptics is the creation of two new optical surfaces that could adversely influence optical aberrations. Interestingly, Guell et al. (30) found no difference in preoperative and postoperative assessments of contrast sensitivity. No aberrometry studies, however, have been performed on bioptics patients. More prospective studies are needed to assess its long-term safety.

Combined LASIK and Intracorneal Ring Segments

Intracorneal ring segments (ICRSs) consist of two 150-degree PMMA spacers that produce a hyperopic shift when implanted in the peripheral corneal stroma. The PMMA segments can correct up to 3 D of myopia by shortening the central corneal arc length. The commercially marketed form of ICRS is called Intacs (KeraVision, Inc., Fremont, CA) and is available in several widths (0.25, 0.30, and 0.35 mm). Segments of progressively greater girth produce more pronounced levels of correction (Table 80-2) (34–36). In phase III FDA trials, 99% of 90 patients with low myopia

TABLE 80-2. PREDICTED DIOPTRIC CORRECTION FOR INSTRASTROMAL RING SEGMENTS BY THICKNESS: REFINED NOMOGRAM_PHASE II STUDY RESULTS

Thickness (mm)	Predicted Average Correction (D)
0.25	-1.30
0.30	-2.00
0.35	-2.70
0.40	-3.40
0.45	-4.10

mm, Millimeters; D, Diopters (From Schanzlin DJ, Asbell PA, Burris TE, et al. The intrastromal corneal ring segments: phase II results for the correction of myopia. *Ophthalmology* 1997;104:1067–1078.)

TABLE 80-3. SURGICAL APPROACHES FOR COMBINED LASIK AND ICRS FOR HIGH MYOPIA

Method	Step 1_Form Stromal Channels and LASIK Flap	Step 2_Perform LASIK Ablation (% of maximally safe ablation)	Step 3_Place ICRS Segments into Channels	Expected Residual Error	Secondary Procedure (1-5 Weeks)
A	+	100	+	Minimal	Remove or Exchange ICRS
B	+	0	+	2–3 D less than preoperative refractive error	Perform LASIK Ablation
C	+	70–80	+	2–3 D	LASIK Ablation to correct residual error

LASIK, Laser in situ keratomileusis; ICRS, Intrastromal corneal ring segments; D, Diopters (Primack JD, Farah SG, Azar DT. LASIK and intrastromal corneal ring segments (ICRS). In: Azar DT, Koch DD, eds. *LASIK—fundamentals, surgical technique, and complications.* New York: Marcel Dekker, 2003:335–349.)

treated with Intacs had an UCVA of 20/40 or better and 92% of eyes were ±1 D of their intended correction (40). In April 1999, Intacs were FDA approved for the treatment of low myopia (1 to 3 D) with 1 D or less of astigmatism.

ICRSs possess specific qualities that make them a potentially valuable adjunct to LASIK (41). Specifically, the dissimilarity between the underlying mechanisms responsible for the induced corneal flattening suggests that the procedures can be additive. ICRS surgery does not remove central stromal tissue, so one could expect it to safely correct up to 3 D of residual myopia after a maximal LASIK treatment. Combining LASIK and ICRS implantation may provide a means to safely expand the range of high myopic correction without further compromising corneal thickness and stability. A second advantage is that the effect is adjustable and the final refractive result can be titrated by exchanging the ring segments (42). If the patient was dissatisfied, the segments could be removed altogether with an almost complete reversal of the refractive effect (37,40). Potentially, the refractive effect could be adjusted months to years postoperatively. A third advantage is that accommodation is preserved, which is important in younger patients. Additionally, the technique spares the visual axis of surgical manipulation. The PMMA segments are placed deep in the peripheral cornea and would not be expected to interfere with the centrally located corneal flap. ICRSs also maintain the natural prolate shape of the cornea, which may be associated with less optical aberrations than the oblate shaped cornea induced with excimer laser surgery (43–45). Finally, both LASIK and ICRS are extraocular procedures, so intraocular surgery and its attendant risks [e.g., retinal detachment (RD), endophthalmitis, uveitis, cataract, corneal edema, etc.] are avoided.

In patients with high myopia, LASIK and ICRS treatments may be performed as simultaneous or staged procedures. Table 80-3 describes three different surgical approaches (A to C) from which to choose when performing the techniques together. Figure 80-3 schematically illustrates method A. The implantation of ICRS may be performed in

a laser suite setting. Topical anesthetic drops and antibiotics are administered preoperatively. Peri- or retrobulbar anesthesia is unnecessary and could interfere with patient fixation if concomitant LASIK were also planned. Contraindications to the combined surgery include the standard contraindications to LASIK surgery.

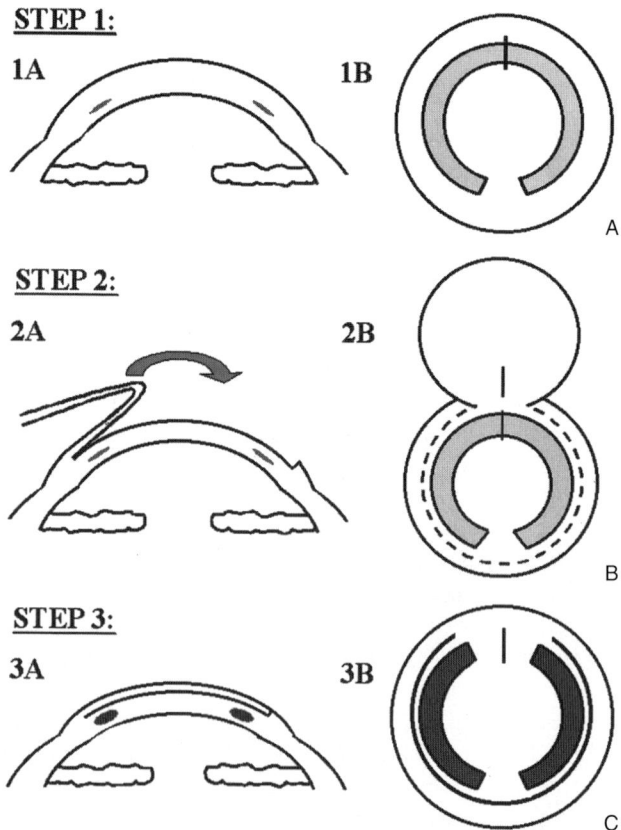

FIGURE 80-3. A-C: Surgical steps of combined LASIK and intracorneal ring segments (ICRS) procedure. Step 1: Creation of ICRS channels. Step 2: LASIK flap and excimer laser ablation. Step 3: Insertion of ICRS. (From Primack JD, Farah SG, Azar DT. LASIK and intrastromal corneal ring segments (ICRS). In: Azar DT, Koch DD, eds. *LASIK—fundamentals, surgical technique, and complications.* New York: Marcel Dekker, 2003:335–349, with permission.)

The surgical procedure is straightforward, but does require some unique instrumentation. The center of the cornea is located and an incision and placement marker (KeraVision, Inc., Fremont, CA) is applied to indicate where the PMMA inserts and superior, radial incision will ultimately lie. Ultrasonic pachymetry is performed at the 12 o'clock incision site and an approximately 1-mm incision of 68% corneal thickness is created with a calibrated diamond knife. A modified Suarez spreader may be used to perform a small lamellar dissection at the base of the incision, so as to create an entry pocket on either side. Next, a Vacuum Centering Guide (KeraVision, Inc., Fremont, CA) is positioned on the globe and stabilized under high suction. Specially designed dissectors measuring 0.9 mm are then introduced through the incision (clockwise and counterclockwise) to create stromal tunnels by blunt dissection. Ideally, the channels are located at two-thirds corneal depth. Suction is then released and the centering guide removed.

Once the channels have been created, a microkeratome is used to create a corneal flap. Based on the patient's intraoperative pachymetry value, the maximal excimer laser ablation considered to be safe is performed. Subsequently, the flap is refloated into place. Using forceps, the PMMA segments are introduced into the channels. In their final position, the segments are located 3 mm apart superiorly. If necessary, the flap could be refloated to eliminate any iatrogenically induced wrinkles. The incision site may be hydrated, or, alternatively, closed with 10-0 nylon sutures. Postoperatively, if the patient possesses mild ametropia or later desires undercorrection to ameliorate presbyopic symptoms, the ICRS may be removed or exchanged.

The presence of empty intralamellar channels in the corneal periphery should not interfere with performing LASIK. This becomes evident when one considers the spatial relationships between the channels, hinged corneal flap, and excimer laser OZ. The Intacs segments lie at two-thirds stromal depth, and have an inner diameter of 6.9 mm and an outer diameter of greater than 8 mm. A hinged corneal flap of 8.5 to 10 mm would cover the tunnels, but its anterior location would make intersection extremely unlikely. The flap could potentially incur a small, full-thickness defect where the microkeratome crosses the superior incision site, but that is of negligible clinical significance.

For illustrative purposes, let us consider a cornea with a peripheral thickness of 700 μm at the Intacs incision site and a central thickness of 550 μm. The empty tunnels (following dissection) are located 466 μm from the surface (two-thirds the depth of 700 μm). An 8.5-mm-wide flap measuring 160 μm thick would leave 306 μm of tissue that would have to be ablated from the stromal bed before the channels were penetrated (466 − 160 μm (flap) = 306 μm). This is a not a concern clinically for two reasons. First, most myopic excimer laser ablations have a 6.5-mm OZ that is central to the more peripherally located tunnels (inner diameter 6.9 mm). Second, if larger OZs were used, concerns over adequate residual central corneal thickness would preclude ablations deep enough to encounter the peripherally located tunnels.

Methods B and C (Table 80-3) are similar to method A except that the laser ablation is initially withheld or is partially performed, respectively. The remainder is completed later as a secondary procedure. An advantage of these techniques is that the surgeon can incorporate any ICRS-induced refractive changes (including astigmatism) into the final LASIK ablation.

Patients with a moderate degree of myopia could also benefit from combined LASIK and ICRS surgery (41). Up to 3 D of myopia could be treated with ICRS, sparing precious central stroma and improving corneal stability. Another advantage of this procedure is that surgeons could easily exchange ring segments with a resultant myopic shift if patients decided postoperatively that they wanted to become undercorrected to reduce presbyopic symptoms. If this change was dissatisfying, the ICRS could be reexchanged to restore the previous refraction.

As in the previous section, the surgeries could be performed simultaneously using multiple approaches (Table 80-4). In method A, a 70% to 80% LASIK ablation is performed (depending on intended final refraction) fol-

TABLE 80-4. SURGICAL APPROACHES FOR COMBINED LASIK AND ICRS FOR MODERATE MYOPIA

Method	Step 1_Form Stromal Channels and LASIK Flap	Step 2_Perform LASIK Ablation (% of maximally safe ablation)	Step 3_Place ICRS Segments into Channels	Expected Residual Error	Secondary Procedure (1-5 Weeks)
A	+	70–80	+	Minimal	ICRS Exchange or LASIK
B	+	0	+	3 D less than pre-operative refractive error	Perform LASIK Ablation for Remaining Myopia
C	+	70–80	−	2–3 D	ICRS placement

LASIK, Laser in situ keratomileusis; ICRS, Intrastromal corneal ring segments; D, Diopters (Primack JD, Farah SG, Azar DT. LASIK and intrastromal corneal ring segments (ICRS). In: Azar DT, Koch DD, eds. *LASIK—fundamentals, surgical technique, and complications.* New York: Marcel Dekker, 2003:335–349.)

lowed by ICRS implantation. Once the refraction has stabilized, either the ring segments can be exchanged or the LASIK treatment enhanced by relifting the flap. Alternatively, in method B, only the ICRSs are put into place initially. The LASIK ablation follows as a secondary procedure after the corneal curvature stabilizes. Another approach (method C) is to perform 70% to 80% of the LASIK ablation initially followed by ICRS implantation 1 week postoperatively to correct residual myopia. This technique may be less desirable as the ring segments may induce astigmatism that could require a third surgical visit for LASIK enhancement.

Primack and Azar (46) reported on two eyes that received combined LASIK and ICRS. Both patients were high myopes with low pachymetry values that precluded full treatment of their refractive error with LASIK. Preoperative examinations revealed no signs of keratoconus. The first patient had a preoperative refraction of -7 D and a corneal thickness of 490 μm. The patient underwent ICRS tunnel formation followed by a -4 D LASIK correction. A theoretical residual stromal bed thickness of 309 μm remained. Following the LASIK ablation, two 0.25-mm-wide PMMA channel inserts were placed into the stromal tunnels. A single 10-0 nylon suture was placed over the

ICRS incision and removed after 6 weeks. Three and a half months after surgery the UCVA was 20/30, and the BSCVA measured 20/25 with $+0.50 -1.75 \times 101$. The second patient had a preoperative refraction of $-9.25 -1 \times 180$ OD and an ultrasonic pachymetry measurement of 516 μm. Following ICRS tunnel formation, LASIK was performed for a correction of $-5.60 -1.25 \times 175$. A theoretical residual stromal bed thickness of 272 μm remained. Following the LASIK ablation, two 0.25-mm-wide PMMA channel inserts were placed into the stromal tunnels. A single 10-0 nylon suture was placed over the ICRS incision. Three weeks later the patient had an UCVA was 20/30 and a BSCVA of 20/20+, with $+0.75 -1.50 \times 80$. No complications occurred with either patient. Figure 80-4 illustrates the second patient's corneal topography following each step of the combined surgery.

Combined LASIK and ICRS surgery has some disadvantages and potential risks. A problem sometimes associated with ICRS surgery is corneal flattening in the meridian of the ICRS incision (against-the-rule astigmatic shift). In the two cases cited above, induced astigmatism was also against-the-rule. In patients with high myopia, it may be advantageous to initially perform 60% to 70% of the maximally safe LASIK ablation. This technique allows incorporating ICRS-induced

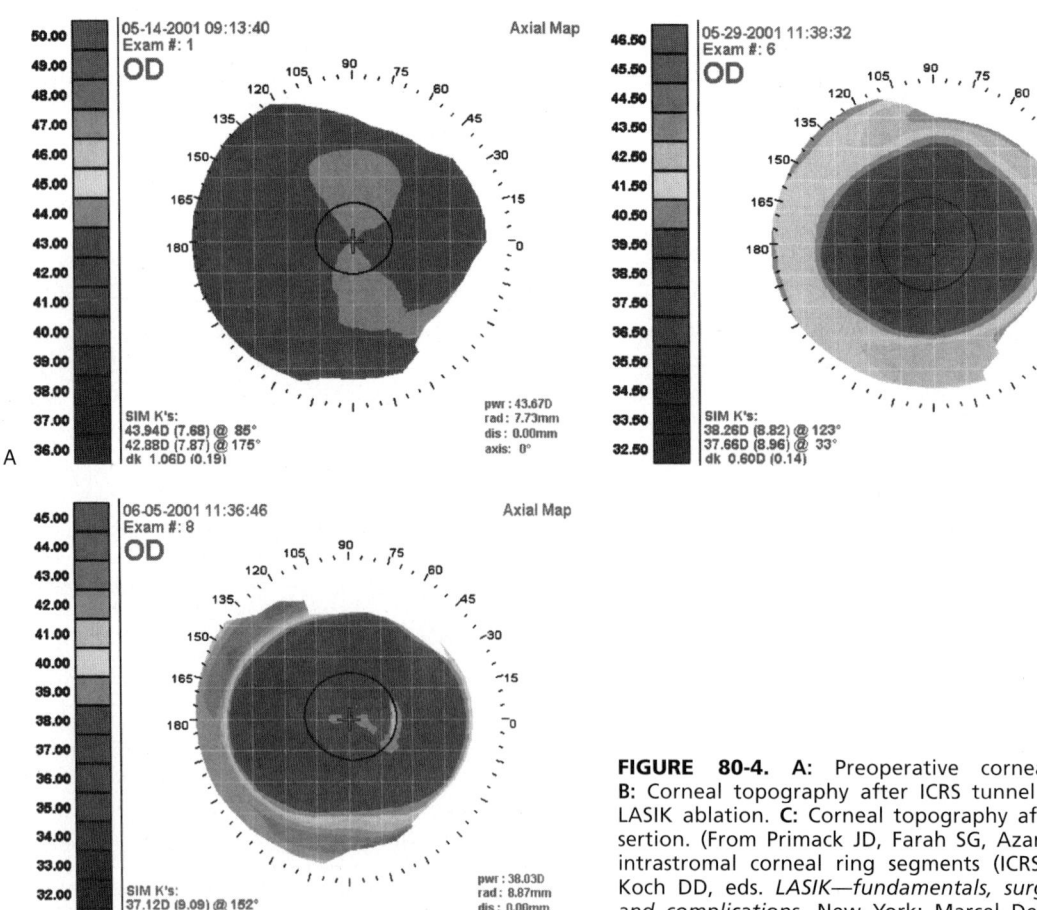

FIGURE 80-4. A: Preoperative corneal topography. **B:** Corneal topography after ICRS tunnel formation and LASIK ablation. **C:** Corneal topography after segment insertion. (From Primack JD, Farah SG, Azar DT. LASIK and intrastromal corneal ring segments (ICRS). In: Azar DT, Koch DD, eds. *LASIK—fundamentals, surgical technique, and complications.* New York: Marcel Dekker, 2003:335–349, with permission.)

refractive changes into a later LASIK re-treatment. It also helps avoid an ICRS-induced overcorrection that could result from a greater than expected flattening effect in a thinned stromal bed. Another potential problem is the ICRS incision site. Epithelial ingrowth could occur where it intersects the flap. Additionally, epithelial defects, which occur at the ICRS incision site, could cause DLK. In theory, encountering the stromal tunnels during the microkeratome pass or laser ablation is possible but unlikely. This could occur if the channels were dissected too superficially and with poor centration. Finally, patients with low pachymetry values and high myopia may not be good candidates for the procedure as concerns over residual corneal thickness may preclude LASIK ablations deep enough to provide good UCVA.

The opportunity to implant ICRS in an eye that has previously undergone LASIK may arise if the ablation was deep enough to preclude the safe application of further excimer laser. Patients corresponding to this profile usually include high myopes and patients with thin corneas. Potential candidates should understand that the hyperopic shift expected following ICRS would be no more than approximately 3 D.

It would seem that the technical challenge underlying ICRS implantation following LASIK would be to form the intralamellar channels without disturbing the corneal flap. As discussed earlier, this process requires a suction ring that theoretically could compromise the flap, resulting in wrinkles, dislocation, or potentially avulsion. Preliminary reports of this procedure, however, have been without complications. Fleming and Lovisolo (47) reported a patient who received ICRS 10 months following LASIK that left a residual SE of −3.375 D. Four months after ICRS placement, the patient had an UCVA of 20/20. No flap complications occurred. Lovisolo (48) also presented a series of 15 eyes at the American Society of Cataract and Refractive Surgery (ASCRS) 2000 meeting that underwent Intacs implantation following LASIK. Patients had received their LASIK 6 to 11 months previously and had residual myopia ranging from a SE of −2.75 to −4.75 D. Eight months following ICRS placement, all eyes had an UCVA of 20/25. Once again, no flap complications were observed. ICRS may be a safe procedure following LASIK if enough time is allowed between procedures to ensure adequate corneal flap healing.

Conversely, patients may develop refractive errors after the placement of ICRS. If, over time, a patient with Intacs develops additional nearsightedness, the PMMA spacers may be exchanged for a different thickness to treat up to 3 D of myopia. However, if the error exceeds −3 D or requires cylindrical correction, the patient must consider other refractive modalities. LASIK may be an appropriate option for treating such conditions.

The surgeon must anticipate the potential influence of ICRS when performing LASIK. ICRS and LASIK can coexist on the same cornea without interference; however, the presence of previously placed PMMA spacers could theoretically disrupt proper flap formation. The ICRS could cause tissue distortion that prevents adequate suction or tissue distribution during the microkeratome pass, resulting in an irregular stromal bed surface. At this time it is unclear what effect ICRSs have on LASIK flap formation and which approach is safer, as no reports have yet been published. To avoid potential problems, the surgeon may wish to preoperatively explant the ICRS and then perform LASIK. As discussed in the previous section, the excimer laser ablation should not penetrate deeply enough to affect the channels holding the Intacs segments. Once LASIK has been performed, subsequent changes in refraction could be addressed by simply relifting the flap and ablating further stromal tissue.

Combined LASIK and Phacoemulsification

Phacoemulsification is a minimally invasive intraocular surgery that removes the crystalline lens through a small limbal or corneal incision measuring 3 to 4 mm. Axial length, corneal curvature, and desired refractive outcome determine whether the patient is left aphakic or receives an intraocular lens (IOL). IOLs may be minus or plus powered and are sometimes "piggybacked" in order to correct high refractive errors. The success of the procedure is highly dependent on the accuracy of IOL calculation formulas. Although these usually generate accurate estimates of IOL power, undesirable refractive outcomes can occur, especially in patients with high degrees of preoperative ametropia where the formulas tend to be less accurate (49,50). Postoperatively, these patients may complain of poor UCVA from residual refractive error. This may be observed after clear lens extraction (CLE), a procedure in which a clear (noncataractous) crystalline lens is removed (with or without IOL placement) in order to treat high myopia or hyperopia. Historically, postoperative ametropia has been treated with IOL exchange or corrective lenses. Combining phacoemulsification and LASIK, however, provides the refractive surgeon with an improved ability to address residual postoperative refractive error following crystalline lens extraction (51).

The combined LASIK and phacoemulsification procedure is performed in a manner similar to bioptics. First, a hinged corneal flap is created with a microkeratome. After inspection, it is refloated into position without any laser treatment. CLE is performed several weeks later with a postoperative refractive goal of low myopia. After several months, once the refraction has stabilized and all sutures (if present) have been removed, the flap is relifted and the remaining refractive error treated by the LASIK ablation.

It is not absolutely necessary to create the corneal flap prior to CLE. Phacoemulsification wounds are very small and unlikely to compromise flap formation during the microkeratome pass, assuming the incision has had several months to heal. There is, however, a theoretical advantage.

Should the posterior capsule rupture during phacoemulsification necessitating a sulcus fixated posterior chamber IOL or an anterior chamber IOL, there may be concern over IOL displacement or IOL-endothelial touch during suction ring application. These concerns are negated with the suggested protocol. Interestingly, a study by Zaldivar et al. (32) included three pseudophakic patients who underwent LASIK after neodymium:yttrium-aluminum-garnet (Nd:YAG) capsulotomy. No complications were reported, but these patients all had posterior chamber IOLs with their haptics presumably fibrosed inside the capsular bag.

LASIK combined with phacoemulsification (whether for CLE or status postcataract extraction) appears to correct refractive error very well. Pop and coauthors (52) reviewed 34 eyes retreated with LASIK for residual refractive error following CLE for high hyperopia. The mean interval between CLE and LASIK was 69 ± 53 days (range, 30 to 272 days). Postoperatively, 86.9% of patients had an UCVA of 20/40 or better. Probst and Smith (53) reported on two eyes of one patient that underwent combined CLE and LASIK for high myopia. The mean SE decreased from a value of -15.50 D to -0.50 D and the final UCVA measured 20/25 OD and 20/20 OS. Vellarde et al. (54) performed CLE followed by LASIK on 22 eyes with moderate to high myopia and hyperopia. Twelve of the eyes had residual refractive error after phacoemulsification surgery and 10 eyes had both procedures planned preoperatively. The mean SE in the myopic group was -11.76 D and in the hyperopic group $+5.22$ D. After surgery, the combined mean SE was $+0.26$ D (range, -0.375 to $+1.50$ D). Zaldivar and colleagues (32) reported on 64 pseudophakic eyes that subsequently underwent LASIK for residual refractive error. The mean SE decreased from -2.61 D (range, $=0.50$ to -5.50 D) to -0.07 D.

"Pseudophakic" bioptics has several desirable qualities. First, phacoemulsification extends the corrective range of LASIK and does so in a way that spares corneal thickness and is potentially adjustable (IOL exchange). Viscoelastic agents, well-manufactured IOLs, and modern phacoemulsification units with advanced fluidics have increased the procedure's safety. Second, the procedure offers many of the advantages of bioptics without some of the safety concerns associated with P-IOLs. For instance, there is little concern over progressive endothelial cell loss, and cataractogenesis is no longer an issue. A major disadvantage of the combined procedure is loss of accommodation. Thus, it is usually reserved for patients in the presbyopic age range. The development of accommodating IOLs may eventually overcome this issue.

Three specific patient populations could benefit from combined phacoemulsification and LASIK. The first is those patients with high ametropias who are beyond the range of what can safely be corrected with LASIK alone. CLE could treat the majority of the correction, followed by LASIK. The second group is those patients who have unexpected postoperative refractive error secondary to either inaccurately performed IOL calculations or implantation of the incorrect IOL. The risks of another intraocular surgery to exchange the IOL could potentially be avoided by performing LASIK. The third group of patients is those who are unhappy after uneventful phacoemulsification due to mild to moderate residual refractive error and suboptimal UCVA.

The potential risks associated with combined surgery include all those associated with LASIK (discussed earlier) and phacoemulsification. The latter is an intraocular procedure that carries the risks of endophthalmitis and other sight-threatening complications. Intraoperative concerns include vitreous loss, retained lens fragments, and suprachoroidal hemorrhage. Postoperatively, patients can develop chronic cystoid macular edema or bullous keratopathy. Among the patients reported to have undergone both procedures, none experienced complications related to phacoemulsification. Several patients did develop opacification between piggybacked IOLs (52). Zaldivar and colleagues (32) reported several LASIK complications including an irregular stromal bed, corneal edema, DLK, flap striae, and dry eye. The authors found no increased incidence of complications in older patients.

The risk of retinal detachment is an important concern when performing phacoemulsification on a highly myopic eye. Colin and coauthors (55) observed an 8.1% incidence of retinal detachment over 7 years in high myopes (>-12 D) who had undergone CLE. The incidence was nearly double that estimated for persons with myopia greater than -10 D who did not undergo surgery. Preoperatively, a thorough dilated examination is necessary to evaluate and potentially treat peripheral retinal pathology. An additional risk of retinal detachment exists should the patient develop posterior capsular opacification (PCO) and require a Nd:YAG capsulotomy. These concerns have prevented CLE from becoming a routine option for the correction of high myopia.

CONCLUSION

LASIK, when combined with other procedures, may benefit high and moderate myopes. The combination of two procedures may be especially valuable for patients with relatively thin corneas. Early reports of combined surgeries are promising, but further studies are necessary to establish efficacy, stability, and safety of these surgical procedures.

REFERENCES

1. Lindstrom RL, Hardten DR, Chu YR. Laser *in situ* keratomileusis for the treatment of low, moderate, and high myopia. *Trans Am Ophthalmol Soc* 1997;95:285–296.
2. Kawesch GM, Kezirian GM. Laser *in situ* keratomileusis for high myopia with the VISX star laser. *Ophthalmology* 2000;107:653–661.
3. Knorz MC, Wiesinger B, Liermann A, et al. Laser *in situ*-keratomileusis for moderate and high myopia and myopic astigmatism. *Ophthalmology* 1998;105:932–940.

4. Sugar A, Rapuano CJ, Culbertson WW, et al. Laser *in situ* keratomileusis for myopia and astigmatism: safety and efficacy—a report by the American Academy of Ophthalmology. *Ophthalmology* 2002;109:175–187.

5. Chayet AS, Montes M, Gomez L, et al. Bitoric laser *in situ* keratomileusis for the correction of simple myopic and mixed astigmatism. *Ophthalmology* 2001;108:303–308.

6. Salz JJ, Stevens CA. LASIK correction of spherical hyperopia, hyperopic astigmatism, and mixed astigmatism with the LADARVision excimer laser system. *Ophthalmology* 2002;109:1647–1657.

7. McLeod SD, Kisla TA, Caro NC, et al. Iatrogenic keratoconus: corneal ectasia following laser *in situ* keratomileusis for myopia. *Arch Ophthalmol* 2000;118:282–284.

8. Wang Z, Chen J, Yang B. Posterior corneal surface topographic changes after laser *in situ* keratomileusis are related to residual corneal bed thickness. *Ophthalmology* 1999;106:406–410.

9. Pallikaris IG, Kymionis GD, Astyrakakis NI. Corneal ectasia induced by laser *in situ* keratomileusis. *J Cataract Refract Surg* 2001;27:1796–1802.

10. Amoils SP, Deist MB, Gous P, et al. Iatrogenic keratectasia after laser *in situ* keratomileusis for less than −4.0 to −7.0 diopters of myopia. *J Cataract Refract Surg* 2000;26:967–977.

11. Randleman JB, Russell B, Ward MA, et al. Risk factors and prognosis for corneal ectasia after LASIK. *Ophthalmology* 2003;110:267–275.

12. Choi DM, Thompson RW Jr, Price FW Jr. Incisional refractive surgery. *Curr Opin Ophthalmol* 2002;13:237–241.

13. Damiano RE, Kouyoumdjian GA, Forstot SL, et al. Combined laser *in situ* keratomileusis and radial keratotomy for the treatment of moderate to high myopia. *J Cataract Refract Surg* 2003;29:908–911.

14. Waring GO III, Lynn MJ, McDonnell PJ. Results of the prospective evaluation of radial keratotomy (PERK) study 10 years after surgery; the PERK study group. *Arch Ophthalmol* 1994;112:1298–1308.

15. Guell JL, Vazquez M. Correction of high astigmatism with astigmatic keratotomy combined with laser *in situ* keratomileusis. *J Cataract Refract Surg* 2000;26:960–966.

16. Nichamin LD. Combined technique: AK and LASIK [letter]. *J Cataract Refract Surg* 2001;27:648–650.

17. Pulaski JP. Arcuate keratotomy for asymmetrical steep islands after laser *in situ* keratomileusis and automated lamellar keratoplasty. *J Cataract Refract Surg* 2002;28:1424–1432.

18. Forseto AS, Nose RA, Francesconi CM, et al. Laser *in situ* keratomileusis for correction of secondary hyperopia after radial keratotomy. *Int Ophthalmol Clin* 2000;40:125–132.

19. Yong L, Chen G, Li W, et al. Laser *in situ* keratomileusis enhancement after radial keratotomy. *J Refract Surg* 2000;16:198–190.

20. Lyle WA, Jin GJC. Laser *in situ* keratomileusis for consecutive hyperopia after myopic LASIK and radial keratotomy. *J Cataract Refract Surg* 2003;29:879–888.

21. Maloney RK, Nguyen LH, John ME. Artisan phakic intraocular lens for myopia—short term results of a prospective, multicenter study. *Ophthalmology* 2002;109:1631–1641.

22. Implantable contact lens in treatment of myopia study group. U.S. food and drug administration clinical trial of the implantable contact lens for moderate to high myopia. *Ophthalmology* 2003;110:255–266.

23. Zaldivar R, Davidorf JM, Oscherow S. Posterior chamber intraocular lens for myopia −8 to −19 diopters. *J Refract Surg* 1998;14:294–305.

24. Zaldivar R, Davidorf J, Oscherow S, et al. Combined posterior chamber phakic intraocular lens and laser *in situ* keratomileusis: bioptics for extreme myopia. *J Refract Surg* 1999;15:299–308.

25. Guell JL. The adjustable refractive surgery concept [letter]. *J Refract Surg* 1998;14:271.

26. Guell J, Vazquez M. Bioptics. *Int Ophthalmol Clin* 2000;40:133–143.

27. Dick HB, Alio J, Bianchetti M, et al. Toric phakic intraocular lens: European multicenter study. *Ophthalmology* 2003;110:150–162.

28. Perez-Santonja JJ, Ayala MJ, Sakla HF, et al. Retreatment after laser *in situ* keratomileusis. *Ophthalmology* 1999;106:21–28.

29. Guell JL, Vazquez M, Gris O, et al. Combined surgery to correct high myopia: iris claw phakic intraocular lens and laser *in situ* keratomileusis. *J Refract Surg* 1999;15:529–537.

30. Guell JL, Vazquez M, Gris O. Adjustable refractive surgery: 6 mm artisan lens plus laser *in situ* keratomileusis for the correction of high myopia. *Ophthalmology* 2001;108:945–952.

31. Sanchez-Galeana CA, Smith RJ, Rodriguez X, et al. Laser *in situ* keratomileusis and photorefractive keratectomy for residual refractive error after phakic intraocular lens implantation. *J Refract Surg* 2001;17:299–304.

32. Zaldivar R, Oscherow S, Piezzi V. Bioptics in phakic and pseudophakic intraocular lens with the Nidek ec-5000 excimer laser. *J Refract Surg* 2002;18(suppl):S336–S339.

33. Trindade F, Pereira F. Cataract formation after posterior chamber phakic intraocular lens implantation. *J Cataract Refract Surg* 1998;24:1661–1663.

34. Alio JL, Hoz F, Perez-Santonja JJ, et al. Phakic anterior chamber lenses for the correction of myopia—a 7 year cumulative analysis of complications in 263 cases. *Ophthalmology* 1999;106:458–466.

35. Brauweiler PH, Wehler T, Busin M. High incidence of cataract formation after implantation of a silicone posterior chamber lens in phakic, highly myopic eyes. *Ophthalmology* 1999;106:1651–1655.

36. Jimenez-Alfaro I, Benitez del Castillo JM, Garcia-Feijoo J, et al. Safety of posterior chamber phakic intraocular lenses for the correction of high myopia—anterior segment changes after posterior chamber phakic intraocular lens implantation. *Ophthalmology* 2001;108:90–99.

37. Schanzlin DJ, Asbell PA, Burris TE, et al. The intrastromal corneal ring segments: phase II results for the correction of myopia. *Ophthalmology* 1997;104:1067–1078.

38. Burris TE, Ayer CT, Evensen DA, et al. Effects of intrastromal corneal rings size and thickness on corneal flattening in human eyes. *Refract Corneal Surg* 1991;7:46–50.

39. Burris TE, Baker PC, Ayer CT, et al. Flattening of central corneal curvature with intrastromal corneal rings of increasing thickness: an eye bank study. *J Cataract Refract Surg* 1993;19:182–187.

40. Twa MD, Karpecki PM, King BJ, et al. One year results from the phase III investigation of the keravision Intacs. *J Am Optom Assoc* 1999;70:515–524.

41. Primack JD, Farah SG, Azar DT. LASIK and intrastromal corneal ring segments (ICRS). In: Azar DT, Koch DD, eds. *LASIK—fundamentals, surgical technique, and complications.* New York: Marcel Dekker, 2003:335–349.

42. Asbell PA, Ucakhan OO, Durrie DS, et al. Adjustability of refractive effect for corneal ring segments. *J Refract Surg* 1999;15:627–631.

43. Linebarger EJ, Song D, Ruckhofer J, et al. Intacs: the intrastromal corneal ring. *Int Ophthalmol Clin* 2000;40:199–208.

44. Holmes-Higgin DK, Baker PC, Burris TE, et al. Characterization of the aspheric corneal surface with intrastromal corneal ring segments. *J Refract Surg* 1999;15:520–528.

45. Holmes-Higgin DK, Burris TE, Intacs Study Group. Corneal surface topography and associated visual performance with Intacs for myopia: phase III clinical trial results. *Ophthalmology* 2000;107:2061–2071.

46. Primack JD, Azar DT. Laser *in situ* keratomileusis and intrastromal corneal ring segments for high myopia—three step procedure. *J Cataract Refract Surg* 2003;29:869–874.

47. Fleming JF, Lovisolo CF. Intrastromal corneal ring segments in a patient with previous laser *in situ* keratomileusis. *J Refract Surg* 16:365–367, 2000.

48. Lovisolo CF. Intac ring segments and LASIK: better quality vision for high myopia; removal option for prepresbyopic patients (abstr). American Society of Cataract and Refractive Surgery (ASCRS) Meeting, abstract 763, 2000.

49. Kora Y, Koike M, Suzuki Y, et al. Errors in IOL power calculation for axial high myopia. *Ophthalmic Surg* 1991;22:78–81.

50. Holladay JT. Standardizing constants for ultrasonic biometry, keratometry, and intraocular lens calculations. *J Cataract Refract Surg* 1997;23:1356–1370.

51. Nichamin LD. Expanding the role of bioptics to the pseudophakic patient [letter]. *J Cataract Refract Surg* 2001;27:1343–1344.

52. Pop M, Payette Y, Amyot M. Clear lens extraction with intraocular lens followed by photorefractive keratectomy or laser *in situ* keratomileusis. *Ophthalmology* 2001;108:104–111.

53. Probst LE, Smith T. Combined refractive lensectomy and laser *in situ* keratomileusis to correct extreme myopia. *J Cataract Refract Surg* 2001;27:632–635.

54. Velarde JI, Anton PG, Valentin-Gamazo L. Intraocular lens implantation and laser *in situ* keratomileusis (bioptics) to correct high myopia and hyperopia with astigmatism. *J Refract Surg* 2001;17(suppl):S234–S237.

55. Colin J, Robinet A, Cochener B. Retinal detachment after clear lens extraction for high myopia: seven-year follow-up. *Ophthalmology* 1999;106:2281–2284.

WAVEFRONT-GUIDED CUSTOM LASIK AND LASEK: TECHNIQUES AND OUTCOMES

PATRICK C. YEH AND DIMITRI T. AZAR

The efficacy, predictability, and safety of using the excimer laser in the correction of refractive errors have been widely demonstrated and accepted (1–4). Optical engineers, physicists, and refractive surgeons continue to refine surgical techniques and break new ground in laser vision correction using novel technologies and new applications of previous innovations. Chief among them is the exponential progress in the fields of wavefront-guided and topography-guided custom corneal ablation, with the ultimate aim of sculpting an optically perfect eye in which the unaided postoperative visual acuity exceeds the preoperative spectacle corrected visual acuity.

The desire to eliminate optical aberrations has led to great interest in the pursuit of ocular wavefront-sensing and the coupling of the sensors to lasers to create wavefront-guided ablations. In contrast to corneal topography, which measures only the aberrations created by the corneal surface, wavefront sensing measures the aberrations of the entire optical system of the eye, including those resulting from the anterior surface of the cornea, as well as additional aberrations emanating from the posterior corneal surface and the lens.

The current status of custom cornea treatment is improvement of the quality of the image of a point object, or the point spread function (PSF) on the retina, primarily by reducing preexisting wavefront aberrations (5). As our understanding of the more visually significant surgically induced aberrations continues to increase, we may soon be able to correct them to achieve the so-called supervision with greater predictability.

In the 20th century, eye care professionals were able to reduce refractive errors with spectacles, contact lenses, intraocular lenses, and various refractive surgeries by successfully correcting the sphere and cylinder, which are lower-order aberrations (defocus and astigmatism, respectively). It was not until recently that we have the means of measuring and treating higher-order aberrations in a clinical setting. Other optical phenomena, such as the unavoidable effects of pupil-dependent diffraction that may limit sharpness of

retinal images, become the remaining optical limiting factors (6). Quantification of these phenomena may soon lead to development of newer diagnostic and therapeutic tools in the field of refractive surgery.

One obvious advantage of correcting the optical aberrations in the eye is the potential for creating an optically perfect retinal image. However, the complexity of the visual system, including the optics, photoreceptors, neuronal processing of visual signals, and the formation of the visual percept, creates upper limits to supernormal vision.

The visual acuity is limited by receptor diameter, receptor packing, as well as biologic variations. The neural retina does not have a uniform distribution of cones. The foveola has the highest packing density of cones and the highest spatial resolving capacity, and as such it is the area that provides the sharpest central vision. Cone density and spatial resolving ability decrease as the distance from the foveola increases. Within the foveola, the diameter of the cone photoreceptors also limits the retina's ability to sample the retinal image. For instance, if the eye's optics are corrected to such a degree as to allow the image of the letter "E" to fall on a single cone, the visual system cannot differentiate the "E" from a period (Fig. 81-1). This is an example of neuronal undersampling, which results in a phenomenon known as "aliasing" (5). For proper interpretation, the components of "E" must be imaged over a certain number of photoreceptors. Given the spacing of foveal cones, which is about 2 to 3 μm, the best achievable acuity for the normal eye is estimated to be 20/8 and 20/10 (75 cycle/degree and 60 cycle/degree), depending on pupil size (7,8). Furthermore, neural processing of visual signals and the formation of the visual percept may add more limitations to achieving perfect and useful vision. A perfect and useful vision requires proper functioning at all levels of this intricate visual system. The visual cortex cannot form a useful visual percept without a good retinal image. Likewise, an optically perfect retinal image cannot be turned into a useful vision without the capability of interpreting the image in proper context. Nonetheless, despite these well-known

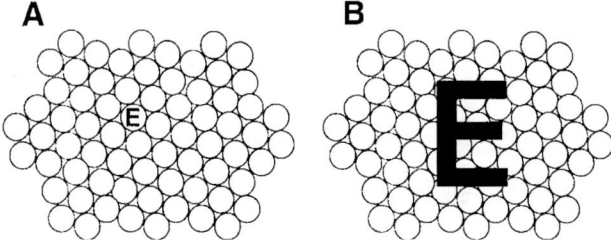

FIGURE 81-1. A, If the letter "E" falls within a single photoreceptor, then the visual system cannot differentiate the "E" from a period. **B,** The letter "E" must be sampled by enough photoreceptors to differentiate the letter's component parts. (From Applegate RA. Limits to vision: can we do better than nature? *J Refract Surg* 2000;16(suppl):S548, with permission.)

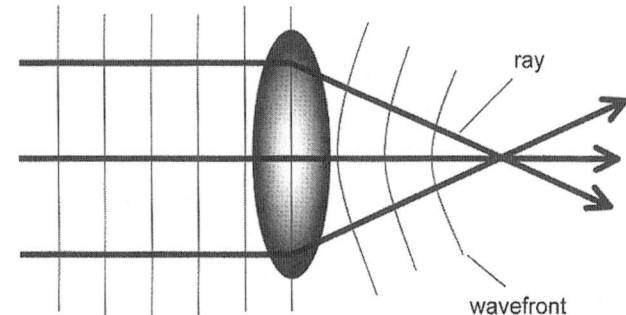

FIGURE 81-2. Optical system and wavefront. A wavefront is always perpendicular to the direction of the light rays. (From Maeda N. Wavefront technology in ophthalmology. *Curr Opin Ophthalmol* 2001;12:295, with permission.)

inherent challenges and limitations in pursuing superior clinical outcomes with customized corrections, removing higher-order aberrations in addition to defocus and astigmatism have been shown to improve retinal image contrast at each spatial frequency, resulting in better visual quality (9).

HISTORY, PRINCIPLES, AND METHODS OF WAVEFRONT ANALYSIS

Original applications of wavefront technology appeared as early as 1619, when Scheiner, a philosopher-astronomer, developed the Scheiner disk perforated with two pinholes to demonstrate the focusing ability of the human eye. Double retinal images of a single object are formed when an ametropic eye views through the Scheiner disc (10). Beginning with the development of an "aberroscope" by Tscherning (11) in 1894 wave aberration could be evaluated via a subjective method for the first time. Its principle was expanded by Hartmann and resulted in the development of Hartmann's wavefront sensor in 1900. Shack and Platt (12) in 1971 published the first work related to the foundation of wavefront technology and made modifications to the Hartmann's wavefront sensor. The result was known as the Hartmann-Shack aberrometer. By 1976 the principle of adaptive optics based on the Hartmann-Shack wavefront sensor was widely utilized in the field of astrophysics to enhance the images through ground-based telescope. In 1994 this technology was first adapted successfully to clinical ophthalmology by Liang et al. (13,14) in the measurement of the eye's wave aberration. In 1997 the technology was furthered in its application to allow accurate removal of those aberrations using a deformable mirror, or adaptive optics. As a result, high-resolution and noninvasive retinal imaging of microscopic structures the size of single photoreceptors in a living human retina was made possible for the first time (15,16). These experiments moved the center stage of wavefront sensing from astronomy to refractive surgery. Wavefront sensing has recently expanded its horizon of applications and permeated to other areas of interests and studies in ophthalmology, such as wavefront-aided

intraocular lens (IOL) design to reduce chromatic aberrations and improve contrast sensitivity (17).

What is a wavefront? In physical optics, light is considered as a wave that spreads in all directions; a wavefront is like a ripple that is in phase when a stone is thrown into a still pond. A wavefront describes light rays emanating from a source and represents an isochronous surface shape, that is, all the points along the rays that are in-phase (18) (Fig. 81-2). It measures the optical path in its entirety and is not limited to any given refractive surface. Thus, the wavefront describes the aggregate effects of the optical system of the whole eye as the light passes through every location of the pupil. In a "perfect" eye, the optical system of the eye does not induce any distortions in the wavefront from the image. The wavefront would exit the eye as a perfect plane that is perpendicular to the visual axis. On the other hand, when optical aberrations are present, as it is in all eyes (even in unoperated eyes), the wavefront would form an imperfect surface rather than a plane. Wavefront aberrations are defined as the deviation between the wavefront surface originating from a given optical system and the hypothetical wavefront plane originating from an ideal optical system. For a given eye, the shape of the wavefront is a fundamental and unique description of the optical quality of the whole eye (Fig. 81-3).

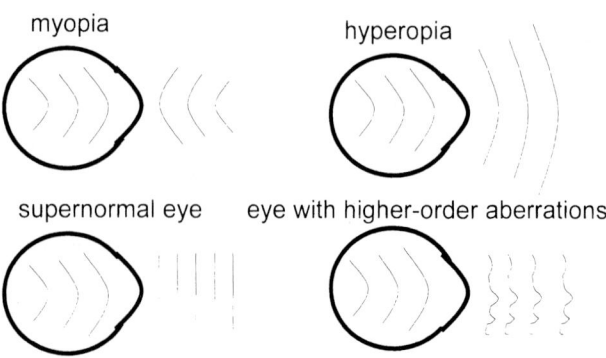

FIGURE 81-3. Schematic representation of refractive errors diagrams using wavefront. (From Maeda N. Wavefront technology in ophthalmology. *Curr Opin Ophthalmol* 2001;12:295, with permission.)

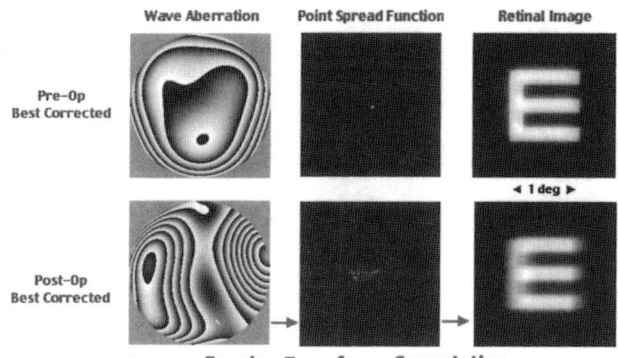

FIGURE 81-4. The retinal image can be simulated by computing the point-spread function. (From Applegate RA, Azar DT, Klyce SD, et al. Corneal topography vs. wavefront sensing. Rev Refract Surg 2002;10, with permission.)

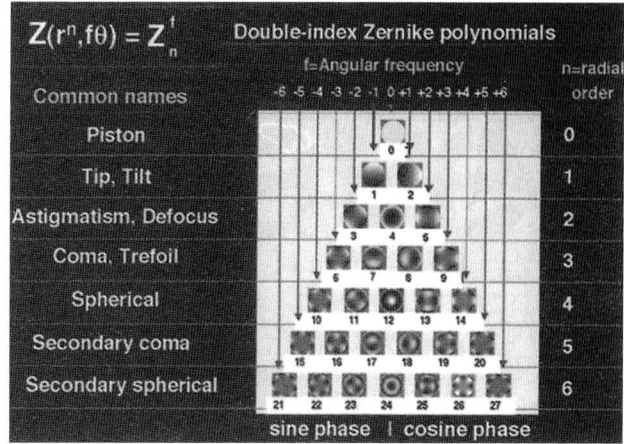

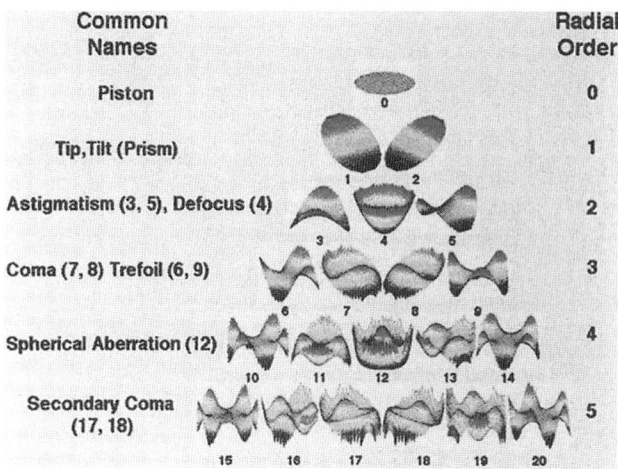

FIGURE 81-5. A, Two-dimensional pictorial representation of some of the Zernike polynomials. **B,** Three-dimensional pictorial representation. (From Wavefront sensors: the shape of things to come. *Rev Refract Surg* August 2001;14, with permission.)

Wavefront analysis assesses the optical quality of the eye by evaluating the shape of its wavefront. It expresses the deformity of wavefront shape in three-dimensional space. The unit used in wavefront analysis is micrometers or fractions of wavelengths, and is often displayed as the root mean square (RMS). Alternatively, the influence of aberration on retinal image quality can be simulated by computing the point-spread function (PSF) using the standard Fourier optics methods (Fig. 81-4).

Wavefront aberrations are usually expressed mathematically in polynomial expansions (18). In the first half of the last century, Zernike developed a set of polynomial equations and applied them for the analysis of wavefront properties of optical systems (19). Zernike decomposition breaks the wave aberration into its component aberrations. A multitude of optical aberrations exist and are usually grouped into two major categories: lower order and higher order aberrations. There are three components to the lower order aberration: zero order (a constant), first order (tilt or prism), and second order (defocus and astigmatism). Lower order aberrations can be corrected with glasses, contact lenses, and conventional laser surgery. Higher order aberrations are simply fit to a more complex wavefront shape. They represent smaller irregularities in the optical system of the eyes, representing about 17% of the total optical error in humans. Some of the more common higher order aberrations include third order (coma and trefoil), fourth order (spherical aberration and secondary astigmatism), fifth order (secondary coma), and sixth order (secondary spherical aberration) (Fig. 81-5). Polynomials can be expanded up to any arbitrary order if sufficient numbers of measurements for calculations are made. Using the Zernike coefficients of each term, monochromatic aberrations can be evaluated quantitatively. The understanding of the clinical significance of many of the higher order aberrations is still at its infantile stage. Although it has been recognized that spherical aberration and coma can result in reduced quality of vision, the effect of other higher aberrations is less well understood (9,14,19).

Despite differences in their operating principles, wavefront analyzers usually use ray-tracing methods to trace the path of multiple light rays through the individual eye to reconstruct the wavefront. In general, the wavefront sensors can be classified into three types: (1) in-going retinal imaging aberrometry, as in Tscherning and sequential retinal ray tracing method; (2) out-going wavefront aberrometry, as is used in the Hartmann-Shack aberrometer; and (3) in-going feedback aberrometry, as in skiascopy and spatially resolved refractometer.

Tscherning Aberrometry

Tscherning aberrometry can be traced back to 1890s when Tscherning (11) devised a subjective method of evaluating optical aberrations of the human eyes. More recently, this initially subjective method was converted into an objective means for measuring the optical aberrations. A collimated laser beam [frequency doubled neodymium:yttrium-aluminum-garnet (Nd:YAG) laser,

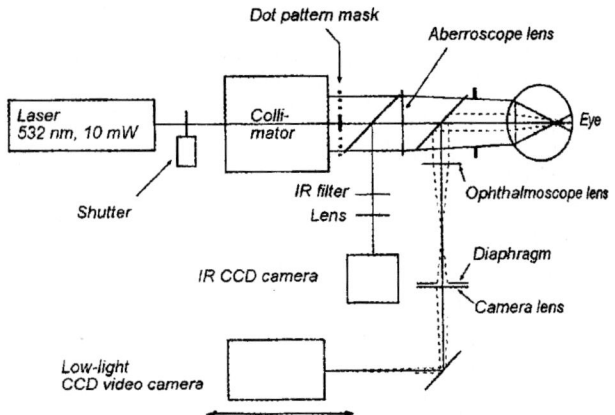

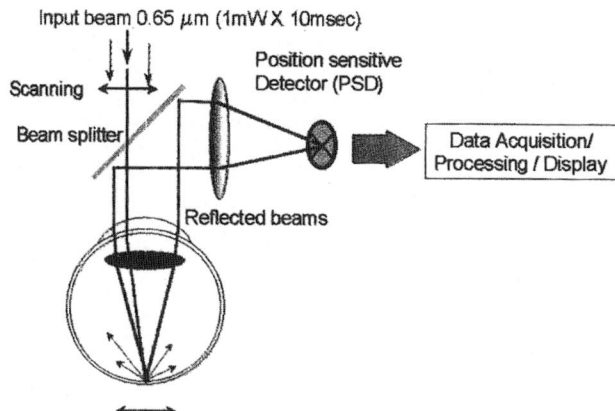

FIGURE 81-6. Schematic diagram of wavefront sensor based on the principles of Tscherning aberrometry. (From Mrochen M, Kaemmerer M, Mierdel P, et al. Principles of Tscherning aberrometry. *J Refract Surg* 2000;16(suppl):S570, with permission.)

FIGURE 81-7. Schematic diagram of Tracey. (From Clinical experience with the Tracey technology wavefront device. *J Refract Surg* 2000;16:S589, with permission).

wavelength 532 nm] was used to illuminate a mask with regular matrix pin holes creating 168 single light rays. These rays form a retinal spot grid pattern on the retina. By indirect ophthalmoscopy, a low-light charge-coupled-device (CCD) camera was used to detect the distortion on the retinal (Fig. 81-6). The aberrations were calculated based on the deviations from their ideal regular positions. The optical aberrations were computed from these values in the form of Zernike polynomials up to the eighth order (20). The wavefront diagnostic devices that utilize Tscherning's aberroscope include Allegretto Wavefront Analyzer (Wavelight) and ORK Wavefront Aberrometer (Schwind).

Sequential Ray Tracing Aberrometry

Ray tracing aberrometry uses measurement of the position of a thin laser beam (0.3 mm in diameter) projected onto the retina. The beam is directed into the eye parallel to the visual axis through various points of the pupil. To compensate for

saccadic eye movements during measurement, the scanning is performed within 10 to 20 msec. The measured location of each ray as it exits the eye is calculated against the known position, and the wave aberration function is described by Zernike polynomials (21). The Tracey Technology wavefront device is based on ray tracing aberrometry (Fig. 81-7).

Hartmann-Shack Aberrometry

A Hartmann-Shack aberrometer projects a laser light into the eye to illuminate a small spot on the retina. The probe light reflected from the fovea is imaged onto the Hartmann-Shack sensor, which consists of a matrix of small lenslets. These lenslets sample corresponding areas of the pupils and divide the wavefront into individual beams, producing multiple images of the same retinal spot of light to form a spot pattern that is focused onto a CCD camera. The deviation of each spot from its corresponding lenslet axis is used to calculate the aberrations (Fig. 81-8).

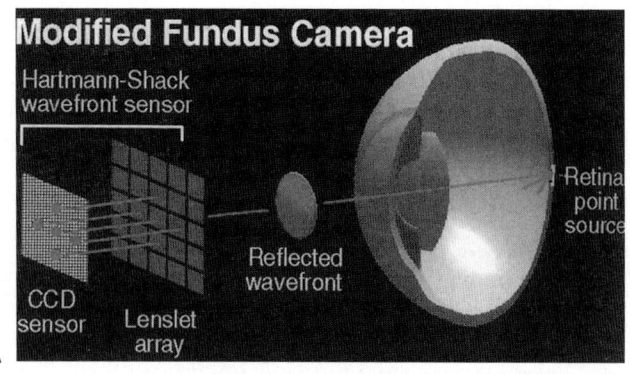

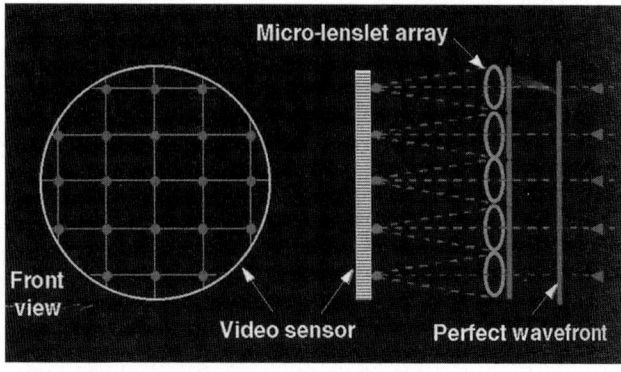

FIGURE 81-8. Hartmann-Shack aberrometer. **A,** The wavefront of the reflected retinal point source is sampled by an array of small lenses (the lenslets) in the aberrometer. **B,** The displacement of each spot from its calibrated position is a direct measure of the slope of the wavefront over the lenslet that formed a particular spot. (From Thibos LN. Principles of Hartmann-Shack aberrometry. *J Refract Surg* 2000;16(suppl);S564, with permission.)

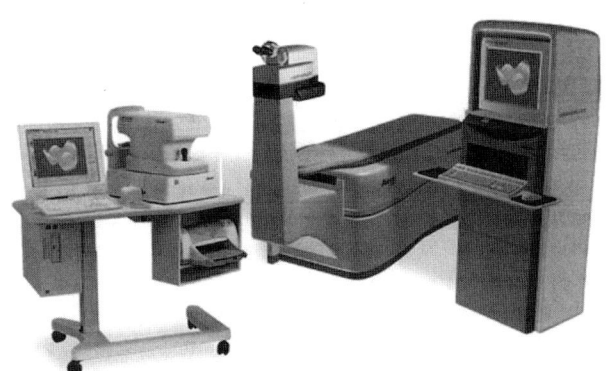

FIGURE 81-9. The LADARWave wavefront measuring device.

Mathematical integration of the deviation yields the shape of the aberrated wavefront, expressed in terms of Zernike polynomials (10). Wavefront devices that utilize the Hartmann-Shack technology include LADARWave (Alcon) (Fig. 81-9), WaveScan WaveFront (VISX) (Fig. 81-10), ZyWave (Bausch & Lomb), WASCA Wavefront Aberrometer (Asclepion-Meditec), and Quantum Light Wavefront Analyzer (Zeiss Humphrey Systems).

Dynamic Skiascopy

Using the principle of retinoscopy, skiascopy optical path detection projects a moving slit into the eye. The projecting system consists of an infrared light-emitting diode (LED) that emits light going through a chopper wheel with slit apertures, which is located between the LED and the projecting lens. The wheel rotates constantly at high speed (180 degrees in 0.4 second across both hemimeridians) to

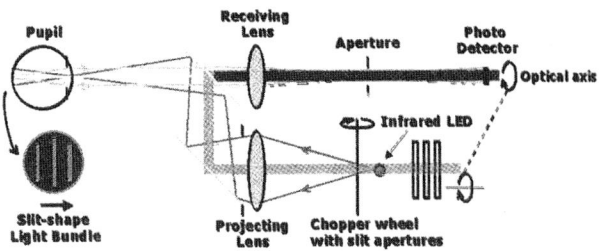

FIGURE 81-11. Schematic diagram of wavefront sensor based on the principles of dynamic skiascopy. (From MacRae SM, Fujieda M. Slit skiascopic-guided ablation using the Nidek laser. *J Refract Surg*, 2000;16:S576, with permission.)

scan the retina. The slit light rays are reflected back out of the eye through a receiving lens, an aperture stop, and photo detectors that receive the light signals. The relative motion of the slit's image is used to calculate the refractive error along each segment (22) (Fig. 81-11). The wavefront system based on skiascopy includes the OPD-scan (Nidek).

CUSTOMIZATION IN REFRACTIVE SURGERY

Several optical, anatomic, and functional parameters may influence the outcomes of custom LASIK and LASEK. Optical customization relies on accurate measurement of an optical aberration profile and its transfer to a reliable laser ablation system for the customized ablation with high fidelity. There are two approaches to optical customization in refractive surgery: corneal topography-guided and wavefront-guided ablation. Anatomic considerations include individual structural variations of the eye that are relevant to refractive surgery, such as corneal diameter and thickness, and pupil size under different lighting conditions. In general, these factors may influence the visual outcome to a lesser degree than the optical parameters. Nonetheless, anatomic factors such as the anterior chamber depth, axial length, and the lens shape may become incorporated into customized ablations in the future. Functional consideration may also influence the acceptance of customized corneal outcomes in a given patient, and thus should be considered in the surgical strategy. These include patients' individual needs, occupational and recreational alike, in addition to age, refraction, and psychophysiologic tolerance (e.g., monovision) (23).

CORNEAL TOPOGRAPHY-GUIDED ABLATION AND OUTCOMES

Computerized corneal topography has revolutionized the diagnosis and treatment of corneal diseases over the past decade. Its development has proven to be a valuable tool that allows refractive surgeons to more reliably assess

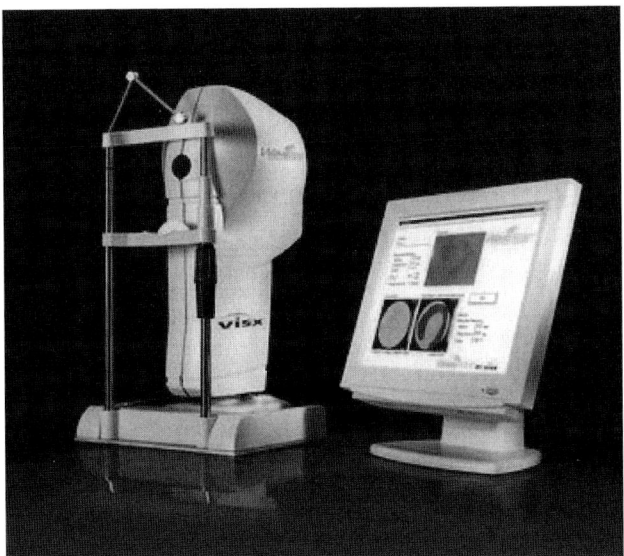

FIGURE 81-10. The WaveScan WaveFront System.

information about the anterior corneal surface. Linkage between corneal topography and the excimer laser may be useful in the treatment of surface irregularities of the cornea.

Although currently available corneal topographic systems allow detection of many corneal abnormalities, precise representations of corneal shape relative to the absolute contour of the surface are relatively lacking in the very center and far periphery of the cornea (24–28). This may be a limitation in linking the topography to ablation. Another limitation is that many patients may have optical aberrations that do not originate from the anterior surface of the cornea. A potential advantage of linking topography to ablation is that a "real-time" linkage, as opposed to "snapshot" linkage using a single preoperative topography, would allow second-to-second alteration in ablation as the corneal contour changes (29). However, there are many technical difficulties to this ideal, especially obtaining topography during ablation.

Corneal topography-guided ablation has been attempted to treat patients with irregular astigmatism, decentered ablations, and central islands. This approach is especially helpful when hard contact lens overrefraction prior to surgery can eliminate the associated adverse visual symptoms. Several studies have reported encouraging results (30–36). For instance, using software that allowed coupling of topography mapping system (Orbscan, Orbtek, Inc., Salt Lake City, UT) with a flying spot laser (Laserscan 2000, Lasersight, Orlando, FL), Alessio et al. (33) showed that the topography-linked excimer laser is a promising tool for correcting irregular astigmatism of various etiologies. In one study where 42 eyes were treated for hyperopic astigmatism and myopic astigmatism, 92.8% in the hyperopic group and 85.7% in the myopic group had an uncorrected visual acuity (UCVA) better than 20/40 (33). Twelve hyperopic eyes (42.8%) and five myopic eyes (35.7%) had a UCVA of 20/20. Only one eye lost one Snellen line of best corrected visual acuity (BCVA). All patients fell between 1 diopter (D) of attempted correction in spherical equivalent (SE). No decentration and/or haze were observed after treatment in any patient.

In another study, the efficacy for correction of decentration following myopic photorefractive keratectomy (PRK) was evaluated (34). All of the 32 eyes in the study had reduced BCVA and quality of vision secondary to irregular astigmatism following PRK because of decentered treatment of more than 1 mm. After retreatment, 90.6% had a UCVA superior to 20/40, of which 59.4% had a UCVA of 20/20. Twenty-two eyes (68.75%) were within 0.50 D of attempted correction in SE, and 28 eyes (87.5%) were within 1 D. No eye lost Snellen lines of BCVA, whereas 56.25% gained Snellen lines. At a 6-month follow-up visit, all eyes were stable within 1 D of the manifest refraction. In the authors' other study, topographically customized ablation was shown to be effective in treating 10 eyes with

irregular astigmatism after penetrating keratoplasty (PK) (35). Preoperatively, the SE ranged from +3.75 D to −19 D. Their results showed that after treatment, 70% had a UCVA better than 20/40, and 30% had a UCVA of 20/20. Five eyes (50%) were within 0.50 D of attempted correction in SE, and eight eyes (80%) were within 1 D. All eyes gained Snellen lines of BCVA, and there was no observed decentration or haze after treatment. In addition, halos and glare, which were present preoperatively in all patients, disappeared postoperatively in all patients.

In a study by Dausch et al. (32), topography-controlled PRK, using Orbscan II (Orbtek, Salt Lake, UT) and MEL-70 system (Asclepion Meditec, Jena, Germany), was also shown to be effective in improving refractive errors in eyes with corneal surface irregularities. In this study, 10 eyes were treated for irregular astigmatism secondary to idiopathic asymmetrical astigmatism, keratoconus, corneal scarring, decentration after myopic, and hyperopic PRK, and following PK. The treatment goal in the study was to obtain the BCVA that can be attained by wearing hard contact lenses. Six months after topography-controlled PRK, there was improvement in UCVA of two or more lines in five eyes and no change in the remaining five eyes. BCVA was improved in two eyes by two to three lines and nine eyes by one to three lines. One eye (postPK) remained unchanged, which was attributed to the development of central reticular haze 3 to 4 months postoperatively. The level of resolution and outcome in this study could have been limited by the larger laser spot size utilized (1.8 mm for MEL-70 versus 0.8 mm for Laserscan 2000).

Wiesinger-Jendritza et al. (30) also assessed the feasibility of LASIK assisted by corneal topography. In their study, LASIK was performed in 23 eyes for irregular astigmatism after PK, previous excimer laser surgery, or penetrating injury. Although mean postoperative UCVA improved to 20/50 from 20/80, there was no postoperative improvement in average spectacle-corrected visual acuity after topography-assisted LASIK. In addition, there was a high percentage of re-treatment for undercorrection (19.4%) and regression (14.3%) in the study. In this study, excimer ablation was based on preoperative corneal topography data (Corneal Analysis System, EyeSys Technologies) using a proprietary algorithm (Topographic Assist, Chiron Technolas). However, there was no direct link between the topography and the centration of the ablation. Of note is that the laser spot size was 2 mm.

Overall, the early results of corneal topography-guided ablation in treating corneal surface irregularities are encouraging, especially in patients suffering from irregular astigmatism following PK, previous corneal trauma, or refractive surgery. Despite these encouraging results, it is likely that this approach may be replaced by wavefront-guided treatment as the experience with and understanding of the latter technology increases.

WAVEFRONT-GUIDED ABLATION AND OUTCOMES

As of the end of 2003, there were three U.S. Food and Drug Administration (FDA)-approved wavefront-guided laser platforms available in the United States: LADARVision system by Alcon, VISX WaveScarn by VISX, and Technolas 217z Zyoptix System by Bausch & Lomb. All three systems are based on the same optical principles, namely the Hartmann-Shack principle, but they differ slightly in their range of capabilities to capture wavefronts in terms of maximum order of measured aberrations, range of sphere, and maximum cylinder and pupil size ranges.

The LADARVision platform using the LADARWave wavefront sensing device (CustomCornea LASIK) was approved by the FDA in October 2002 for customized wavefront-guided laser eye treatment of myopia up to -7 D and astigmatism up to -0.49 D. Because the FDA approval allowed a 1-D variation between manifest and wavefront refraction, wavefront refractive errors up to -7.99 D and up to -1.49 D of astigmatism was acceptable for treatment. LADARWave sensor is capable of measuring up to the eighth order of aberrations with a range of sphere between -15 and $+15$ D and a maximum cylinder of 8 D. Its allowed pupil size ranging from 2.5 to 10 mm, and a 3.5-mm pupil size is used for the phoropter predicted refraction.

A multicenter study was performed in the United States and Canada. The U.S. arm of the study began in October 1999 and the Canadian arm began in November 2000. Analyzed data from 426 myopic eyes of 264 patients were submitted to the FDA. The effectiveness cohort consisted of the 139 eyes treated for spherical myopia with less than -0.5 D of astigmatism. No nomogram adjustments were made in the trial, but ablation algorithm was refined and used to treat the last 141 myopic eyes to compensate for the spherical undercorrection of 0.25 to 0.5 D in the initial algorithm treatment cohort (37,38).

In their clinical trial, the preoperative spherical equivalents were about -3.5 D with cylinders up to -4 D in the initial group. In the algorithm-adjusted group, the preoperative spherical equivalents were about -3 D with cylinders up to -2.5 D. In the initial group, at 6 months 48% had 20/16 UCVA, 73% had 20/20 or better UCVA, and 88% had 20/25 or better UCVA. In the refined group, 63% achieved 20/16 UCVA, 88% had 20/20 or better UCVA, and 98% had 20/25 or better UCVA. The accuracy of the spherical equivalent within $\pm 0.5\%$ of the intended treatment improved from 69% in the initial group to 90% in the refined group. Overall, BCVA improved from 18% preoperatively to 39% postoperatively in patients with 20/12.5 vision, and improved from 86% to 92% in patients with 20/16 vision. For most patients, CustomCornea LASIK did not reduce higher-order aberrations from baseline levels prior to surgery. However, more patients treated with CustomCornea had

reductions in higher order aberrations from preoperatively to 6 months postoperatively as compared to the conventional treatment (38% versus 14%). The amount of postoperative higher order aberrations at 6 months was also significantly less for CustomCornea LASIK eyes than for the conventional LASIK eyes (20% vs. 82%). Regarding coma, 44% of the customized group had reduced coma compared with 33% of the conventionally treated group. Forty-six percent in the customized group had reduced spherical aberration compared with 12% of the conventional group. Data also showed that at 6 months 2.2% of CustomCornea LASIK patients gained with 0.7% lost contrast sensitivity under photopic conditions. Under mesopic conditions, 15.2% gained while 5.8% lost two levels.

In the study, one eye had a miscreated flap related to microkeratome. The eye, which later received conventional laser ablation, was not included in cohort analysis. Two eyes of the same patient experienced recalcitrant diffuse lamellar keratitis (DLK) with blepharitis. One eye developed horseshoe retinal tear that was unrelated to the device. Postoperatively, three eyes lost two lines of best spectacle-corrected visual acuity (BSCVA). There was one eye with BSCVA worse than 20/25. Overall, no eye lost more than two lines of BSCVA and no eye had a BSCVA worse than 20/40.

Since its FDA approval 1 year ago from the time of this writing, CustomCornea LASIK has also been used successfully by the authors. Our initial observations show that the correction of preexisting higher and lower order aberrations offers a potential advantage over conventional laser vision correction. The latter can produce excellent results, but for many patients customized ablations may deliver better results and improved quality of vision. Other clinical data and case reports of initial commercial experience with CustomCornea showed favorable results in improving contrast sensitivity and subjective visual quality (39–42). It has also been demonstrated to be an effective tool in treating abnormal eyes with clinically significant visual symptoms related to higher order aberrations to improve vision with reduction of aberrations, although slight overcorrections occurred (42). In one case report, CustomCornea was applied effectively, as an off-label use, to retreat two patients for previous LASIK and PRK, primarily for subjective quality of night vision complaints (41).

The VISX STAR S4 Excimer Laser System and WaveScan WaveFront System (VISX CustomVUE) was approved by the FDA in May 2003 to perform wavefront-guided LASIK for correction of myopia up to -6 D of manifest refraction spherical equivalent (MRSE) with astigmatism between 0 and -3 D. WaveScan system measures up to the sixth order of aberrations with a spherical ranges of -8 to $+6$ D and a maximum cylinder of 5 D. Its pupil size limits ranges from 3 to 6 mm.

In their multicenter clinical trial, a total of 351 eyes from 189 patients were enrolled. No nomogram adjustment was utilized in the trial, and all eyes were targeted for emmetropia

(43). Of all eyes treated, 318 eyes were evaluated for effectiveness. The preoperative average spherical refractive error was −3.6 ± 1.4 D (−0.75 to −7 D) with cylinder of +0.7 ± 0.7 D (0 to +3 D). The study showed that for UCVA at 6 months, 74% of eyes were 20/16 or better and 94% were 20/20 or better. At 6 months, 69% of eyes also had either the same or better postoperative UCVA compared to their preoperative BSCVA. The study also demonstrated postoperative stability with 97% of eyes changed ≤0.5 D between 3- and 6-month follow-up visits and 99% changed ≤1 D. A lower degree of postoperative higher order aberrations was observed in eyes that received custom wavefront treatments as opposed to the conventional treatments. Overall, at 6 months 71% of eyes had a decrease in coma, 92% in trefoil, and 76% in spherical aberration. This was manifested in improved subjective quality of vision with a decrease in halo and glare, as four times as many participants were very satisfied with their night vision after wavefront treatments compared to their night vision with their glasses or contact lenses.

Eight adverse events were reported. Two eyes experienced epithelial defect, which resolved without loss in BSCVA. Five eyes developed DLK. All five eyes had a UCVA of either 20/20 or better at 1 month, and all events resolved with no loss in lines of BSCVA. One eye had a partial LASIK flap, which was repositioned and no laser treatment applied. Manifest refraction was unchanged from baseline. At 3 months, there was a loss of two or more lines of best corrected vision in one of 239 astigmatic myopia eyes that can be obtained with spectacles. There was no loss of two or more lines of BCVA in 79 spherical myopia eyes. There was one of 239 astigmatic myopia eyes, none in the 79 spherical eyes, with BSCVA worse than 20/25. Overall, no eye lost more than two lines of BSCVA and no eye had a BSCVA worse than 20/40.

In October 2003, the Bausch & Lomb Technolas 217z Zyoptix System for performing wavefront-guided LASIK received approval from the FDA. The approved Zyoptix system has the widest treatment range available in the U.S., with correction of myopia up to −7 D, astigmatism up to −3 D, and MRSE equal to or less than −7.50 D. Its wavefront-sensing device, Zywave, has a maximum of the fifth order of measured aberrations. Similar to LADARWave, it has a range of sphere from −15 to +15 D and a maximum cylinder of 8 D. Its pupil size range is slightly smaller, from 2.5 to 8 mm.

Their U.S. multicenter clinical trial results included a cohort of 340 eyes–117 spherical eyes and 223 spherocylindrical eyes. All treated eyes were available for analysis of safety at 3 months, and all eyes were followed for 6 months. After surgery with the Zyoptix system, 99.4% (338/340) were corrected to 20/40 or better and 91.5% (311/340) were corrected to 20/20 or better visual acuity without spectacles or contact lenses; 70.3% of patients had unaided 20/16 vision. Overall, 60.4% had improvement in their BSCVA, whereas 78% had UCVA greater

than or equal to their preoperative BSCVA. Improvement in contrast sensitivity after surgery was found in 24.4% of subjects under photopic condition and 22.7% under mesopic condition. At the 6-month follow-up, more than 94% of subjects maintained or improved from their best-corrected vision. There was a loss of two or more lines of best corrected vision that can be obtained with spectacles in 1/223 astigmatic myopia eyes and in 1/117 spherical myopia eyes. There was no eye with astigmatic or spherical myopia with BSCVA worse than 20/25, if 20/20 or better preoperatively. During the course of study, no eye lost more than two lines of BSCVA and no eye had BSCVA worse than 20/40. Six months after surgery, 99.0% of subjects reported that they were satisfied with the results; 99.7% indicated improvement in quality of vision, of which more than 40% reported improvement in night vision while driving.

Using the Tscherning-type aberrometer linked to WaveLight Allegretto (WaveLight Laser Technologie AG, Ellangen, Germany) scanning spot excimer laser (1 mm spot size), Seiler's group (44) performed the first wavefront guided LASIK on three eyes of three patients in July 1999. At 1 month postoperatively, all three eyes gained up to two lines of BCVA improving to 20/10. Two eyes had 20/10 UCVA and one eye had 20/12.5 at 1 month. Moreover, the wavefront deviations were reduced by 27% by average compared to preoperative. The same team of investigators later reported another study of 1-month outcomes of wavefront-guided LASIK in 15 eyes (45). Best corrected visual acuity increased on average from 20/15 to 20/12. Four eyes (27%) achieved 20/10 or better vision. In their 3-month report on 35 patients with a mean preoperative spherical refraction of −4.8 D and a cylinder of −1.1 D, UCVA of 20/20 or better was achieved in 93.5% of eyes and of 20/10 or better in 16.0% (46). Although this procedure is effective for myopia and myopic astigmatism correction, this study also demonstrated less predictability in reducing higher order aberrations. Postoperative wavefront analyses revealed a reduction of high-order aberrations in 22.5% of eyes. However, on average, there was an increase of aberrations by a factor of 1.44 (pupil diameter 5 mm) after 3 months. Nonetheless, the increase factor is far less than that of conventional corneal laser surgery. For instances, for a 7-mm pupil, an increase factor ranging from 11 to 17.65 in total wave aberration was found following conventional PRK (47,48). Similar results were also reported by Oliver et al (49).

In a prospective study of customized LASIK using Nidek EC-5000 with OPD-scan, Vongthongsri et al. (50) applied custom ablation to one eye of each 11 patients and conventional ablation to the contralateral eye. Their results showed that the BCVA was the same 1 month after LASIK for both the conventional and custom ablation groups. There was also no statistically significant difference between preoperative and 1 month postoperative higher order aberrations between the study and control group. Gimbel and Stoll (51), on the other hand, reported good results in a case report in which Nidek EC-5000 with OPD-scan was used to perform customized segmental ablation to correct irregular astigmatism following LASIK with one enhancement. Preoperatively, despite a BCVA of 20/20 with $+1.25$ D sphere, the patient reported monocular diplopia with a film in front of the eye. At 1 month after custom ablation, the BCVA improved to 20/15 with $+0.75$ -0.75 $\times$ 075. The quality of vision was markedly improved, with the postoperative OPD-scan maps appearing more regular.

It is clear that the major limitation of wavefront-guided ablations, at least as of the time of this writing, is that this technology cannot predictably overcome the problem of surgically induced higher aberration when performing primary customized LASIK surgery. One approach that we have utilized was to perform customized LASEK surgery aiming at full correction. The assumption behind this approach is that the epithelial thickness after LASEK is approximately the same as that prior to surgery. However, there are no studies, to date, confirming the superiority of this approach over custom LASIK surgery. An alternative approach is to perform conventional or customized LASIK surgery aiming at intentional undercorrection in the range of -0.50 to -1.25 D, followed by wavefront-guided re-treatment 2 to 8 weeks after original procedure. The obvious limitation of this approach is the need for two surgical procedures and the possible increased risk of potential side effects.

FUTURE CHALLENGES FOR CUSTOM LASIK AND LASEK

Early clinical data suggest that wavefront technology produces better clinical outcomes than the conventional systems in a great proportion of eyes. Engineers and refractive surgeons continue to be faced with many challenges in customized laser refractive corrections. Patient variability exists as a direct result of differential corneal wound healing, flap effect, and biomechanical response. These factors invariably confound optimal customized treatment outcomes. Other important practical difficulties include inherent technical difficulties and limitations in accurately measuring ocular aberrations in a given eye, as well as precise centration to compensate for cyclotorsion during laser treatment. Moreover, the impact of optical aberrations on visual function remains unclear.

Wavefront technology characterizes optical quality in terms of the aberration map and retinal images. However, wavefront quantification of optical aberrations and their corrections may not correlate with vision quality and visual performance. Eyes are known to contain natural strategies, such as photopic response and the Stiles-Crawford effect, for reducing the degree of apparent degradation in image contrast caused by chromatic aberration (52). In photopic response, the cone receptor sensitivity peaks for green light and has decreased sensitivity for red and blue wavelengths. Chromatic aberration consequently is reduced by weighting the central portion of the visible spectrum more than the edges. The Stiles-Crawford effect occurs by virtue of the effective preference of the individual photoreceptors of the fovea for light entering through the center of the pupil relative to light entering through the edges of the pupil. As a result, the Stiles-Crawford effect decreases monochromatic aberrations by reducing retinal response to the more aberrated portions of the wavefront (53). Image quality is determined not only by the refractive properties of the eye, but also by their interaction with the cones' directional characteristics. Therefore, optical aberrations of the eye may not be of random errors. The monochromatic wave aberrations from imperfect optics may be the eye's defense against chromatic blur (54). It has been demonstrated that for a given RMS error, not all coefficients of the Zernicke polynomial induce equal decrease in high- and low-contrast sensitivity. Wavefront errors near the center of the Zernicke pyramid, such as coma and spherical aberration, have a more adverse effect on visual performance and visual acuity than those near the edge of the pyramid, such as trefoil and tetrafoil. Moreover, not every wavefront aberration is a hindrance to good vision; some wavefront aberrations may cancel each other out, resulting in a better image (Fig. 81-12) (55).

The potential inherent challenges of an accurate aberrometry arise from the fact that ocular aberrations are not constant; they are a dynamic phenomenon. The magnitude and pattern of aberrations, in particular spherical aberration and coma, vary with the state of accommodation (56–58). Even during microfluctuations around a fixed state of accommodation there is instability in the aberration within seconds or less (59). Optical aberrations are also dependent on the stability of the corneal tear film. Because of the higher refractive index of the tear relative to air, light rays that traverse an area of relatively thin tear film would propagate faster and arrive at the retina faster than those passing through an intact tear film. This effect on aberrations varies greatly between subjects and even between blinks in the same subject (60–62). Higher order aberrations also evolve and change with normal aging. Thus, longitudinal variability due to the changing internal optics of an aging eye may potentially compromise on the long-term outcomes of the permanent surgical corrections made at the present time (63–65).

The pupil controls the amount of light enters the visual system, and wavefront aberrations occur as a consequence of local deviations in the path of light entering the eye through different points in the pupil. The larger the pupil, the greater are the higher-order aberrations (66). Moreover, the location of the pupil center can change under photopic, mesopic, and pharmacologically dilated conditions (67). Although the changes in centration are typically slight, significant changes have been observed. In these instances, there could be

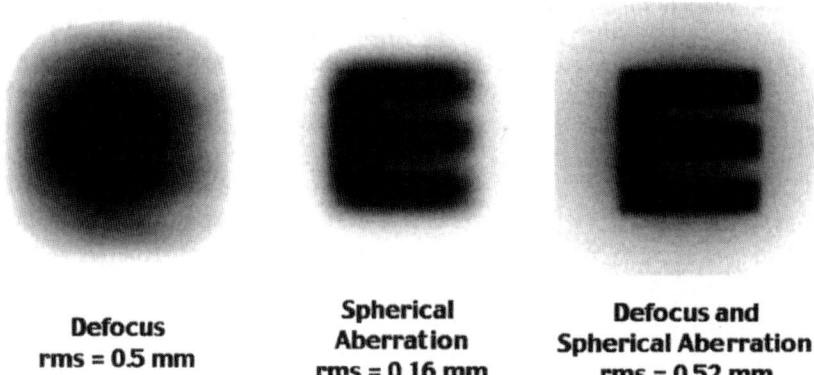

Defocus
rms = 0.5 mm

Spherical
Aberration
rms = 0.16 mm

Defocus and
Spherical Aberration
rms = 0.52 mm

FIGURE 81-12. The resulting retinal image blur produced by the aberration is not always predicted by the root mean square (RMS), or the square root of the sum of the squares of the deviation of the actual wavefront from the ideal wavefront. As seen in this example when defocus **(left)** and spherical aberration **(middle)** are combined, they tend to cancel each other out, producing an overall better image **(right)** even though this image has the greatest RMS wavefront error. (From Williams DR. What adaptive optics can do for the eye. *Rev Refract Surg* 2002:18, with permission.)

relatively large changes in the refractive state of the eye as the curvature of the cornea changes with location. Moreover, optic aberrations are of monochromatic and chromatic origins. Current wavefront aberration quantification is based on monochromatic systems. In our natural, polychromatic world, the optical quality and visual performance may be better predicted by polychromatic systems. However, chromatic aberrations cannot be corrected with current refractive surgical techniques because these errors are inherent to the properties of the optics, rather than its shape (6).

Perhaps the most perplexing variable in custom ablation is the biomechanical responses of the cornea following laser surgery. Wavefront custom ablation is based on the principles of adaptive optics from astronomy. However, the cornea is not like a piece of plastic or an optical element on which the exact ablation pattern can be reproduced to compensate for the ocular aberrations. Corneas respond biomechanically following laser ablation due to structural and shape change. There is a persistent increase in elevation, curvature, and pachymetry outside the ablation zone (67–70). This biomechanical effect over the entire cornea is independent of the ablation profile and induces aberrations. Factors such as corneal hydration and biologic variability in wound-healing process, stromal remodeling, and epithelial hyperplasia in eyes following laser surgery also play a very important role (71). Optical aberrations induced by the creation of a LASIK flap are believed to be a result of biomechanical changes in corneal asphericity and wound healing process (72,73). The outcomes of wavefront-guided ablation can thus be invariably compromised by these inherent biologic factors. Consequently, it has been suggested that surface ablation, in which the act of severing and removing cornea lamellae is avoided, may improve the success of wavefront-guided custom ablations.

At the time of this writing, clinical trials for CustomCornea PRK as well as treatment of higher amounts of astigmatism and hyperopia are still ongoing in the U.S.

In general, short-term outcomes of wavefront-guided custom ablation were promising but far from optimal. Many aspects of the technical challenges in accurate aberrometry, as well as the inability to predict and compensate for the biomechanical and biologic responses of the corneal tissue, limit our ability to produce customized ablations with high fidelity. Moreover, refractive changes associated with wound healing occur over time. Predictive value as to which eye would benefit more with wavefront treatment based on the preoperative higher order aberration still remains unknown. Until more research is done, unrealistic patient expectations should be avoided. Wavefront-guided custom ablation may offer the possibility of better quality vision with more accuracy then conventional LASIK. The ability to achieve "supernormal vision" with predictability and consistency, however, is not yet a reality.

Despite these difficulties, wavefront technology, in an unprecedented way, has altered the traditional paradigm of thinking with regard to refractive characteristics of the eye, and has completely transformed the approach to clinical treatment. Wavefront technology and its applications will continue to have an enormous impact on refractive surgery and ophthalmology as a whole. It has, without doubt, positioned itself at the forefront of ophthalmology.

REFERENCES

1. Hersh PS, Stulting RD, Steinert RF, et al. Results of phase III excimer laser photorefractive keratectomy for myopia. The Summit PRK Study Group. *Ophthalmology* 1997;104:1535–1553.

2. Knorz MC, Wiesinger B, Liermann A, et al. Laser *in situ* keratomileusis for moderate and high myopia and myopic astigmatism. *Ophthalmology* 1998;105:932–940.

3. Argento CJ, Cosentino MJ. Laser *in situ* keratomileusis for hyperopia. *J Cataract Refract Surg* 1998;24:1050–1058.

4. Waring GO III, Carr JD, Stulting RD, et al. Prospective randomized comparison of simultaneous and sequential bilateral laser *in situ* keratomileusis for the correction of myopia. *Ophthalmology* 1999; 106:732–738.

5. Liang J, Williams DR. Aberrations and retinal image quality of the normal human eye. *J Opt Soc Am A* 1997;14:2873–2883.

6. Thibos LN. The prospects for perfect vision. *J Refract Surg* 2000;16(suppl):S540–S546.

7. Applegate RA. Limits to vision: can we do better than nature? *J Refract Surg* 2000;16(suppl):S547–S551.

8. Campbell FW, Green DG. Optical and retinal factors affecting visual resolution. *J Physiol (London)* 1965;181:576–593.

9. Porter J, Guirao A, Cox IG, et al. A compact description of the eye's aberrations in a large population. In: *Vision science and its applications*. OSA Technical Digest. Washington DC: Optical Society of America; 2000:PD4-1–PD4-4.

10. Thibos LN. Principles of Hartmann-Shack aberrometry. *J Refract Surg* 2000;16(suppl);S563–S565.

11. Tscherning M. Die monochromatischen aberrationen des menschlichen auges. *A Psychol Physiol Sinne* 1894;6:456–471.

12. Shack RV, Platt BC. Production and use of a lenticular Hartmann screen. *J Opt Soc Am* 1971;61:656.

13. Liang J, Grimm B, Goelz S, et al. Objective measurement of the wave aberrations of the human eye using a Hartmann-Shack wavefront sensor. *J Opt Soc Am A* 1994;11:1949–1957.

14. Liang J, Williams DR. Aberrations and retinal image quality of the normal human eye. *J Opt Soc Am A* 1997;14:2873–2883.

15. Miller DT, Williams DR, Morris GM, et al. Images of cone photoreceptors in the living human eye. *Vis Res* 1996;36:1067–1079.

16. Liang J, Williams DR, Miller DT. Supernormal vision and high-resolution retinal imaging through adaptive optics. *J Opt Soc Am A* 1997;14:2882–2892.

17. Packer M, Fine IH, Hoffman RS, et al. Prospective randomized trial of an anterior surface modified prolate intraocular lens. *J Refract Surg* 2002;18:692–696.

18. Maeda N. Wavefront technology in ophthalmology. *Curr Opin Ophthalmol* 2001;12:294–299.

19. Howland HC, Howland B. A subjective method for the measurement of monochromatic aberrations of the eye. *J Opt Soc Am* 1977;67:1508–1518.

20. Mrochen M, Kaemmerer M, Mierdel P, et al. Principles of Tscherning aberrometry. *J Refract Surg* 2000;16(suppl):S570–S571.

21. Molebny VV, Panagopoulou SI, Molebny SV, et al. Principles of ray tracing aberrometry. *J Refract Surg* 2000;16:S572–S575.

22. MacRae SM, Fujeida M. Slit skiascopic-guided ablation using the Nidek laser. *J Refract Surg* 2000;16:S576–S580.

23. MacRae SM. Supernormal vision, hypervision, and customized corneal ablation. *J Cataract Refract Surg* 2000;26:154–157.

24. Pardhan S, Douthwaite WA. Comparison of videokeratoscope and autokeratometer measurements on ellipsoid surfaces and human corneas. *J Refract Surg* 1998;14:414–419.

25. Hilmantel G, Blunt RJ, Garrett BP, et al. Accuracy of the tomey topographic modeling system in measuring surface elevations of asymmetric objects. *Optom Vis Sci* 1999;76:108–114.

26. Schultze RL. Accuracy of corneal elevation with four corneal topography systems. *J Refract Surg* 1998;14:100–104.

27. Jeandervin M, Barr J. Comparison of repeat videokeratography: repeatability and accuracy. *Optom Vis Sci* 1998;75:663–669.

28. Belin MW, Ratliff CD. Evaluating data acquisition and smoothing functions of currently available videokeratoscopes. *J Cataract Refract Surg* 1996;22:421–426.

29. Wilson SE, Ambrosio R. Computerized corneal topography and its importance to wavefront technology. *Cornea* 2001;20:441–454.

30. Wiesinger-Jendritza B, Knorz M, Hugger P, et al. Laser *in situ* keratomileusis assisted by corneal topography. *J Cataract Refract Surg* 1998;24:166–174.

31. Knorz MC, Neuhann T. Treatment of myopia and myopic astigmatism by customized laser *in situ* keratomileusis based on corneal topography. *Ophthalmology* 2000;107:2072–2076.

32. Dausch D, Schroder E, Dausch S. Topography-controlled excimer laser photorefractive keratectomy. *J Refract Surg* 2000;16: 13–22.

33. Alessio G, Boscia F, La Tegola MG, et al. Topography-driven photorefractive keratectomy. *Ophthalmology* 2000;107:1578–1587.

34. Alessio G, Boscia F, La Tegola MG, et al. Topography-driven excimer laser for the retreatment of decentralized myopic photorefractive keratectomy. *Ophthalmology* 2001;108:1695–1703.

35. Alessio G, Boscia F, La Tegola MG, et al. Corneal interactive programmed topographic ablation customized photorefractive keratectomy for correction of postkeratoplasty astigmatism. *Ophthalmology* 2001;108:2029–2037.

36. Argento C, Cosentino MJ. Customized ablation for asymmetrical corneal astigmatism. *J Cataract Refract Surg* 2001;27:891–895.

37. Brint SF. Wavefront-guided myopic LASIK with CustomCornea. Paper presentation at annual meeting of the American Society of Cataract and Refractive Surgery, June 1–5, 2002, Philadelphia.

38. Alcon CustomCornea LASIK Physician's Booklet–Myopia. Alcon Laboratories, 2002.

39. Durrie DS. First 100 CustomCornea commercial eyes. *J Refract Surg* 2003;19:S687–690.

40. Lawless MA, Hodge C, Rogers CR, et al. Laser *in situ* keratomileusis with Alcon CustomCornea. *J Refract Surg* 2003;19:S691–S696.

41. Salz JJ. Wavefront-guided treatment for previous laser *in situ* keratomileusis and photorefractive keratectomy: case reports. *J Refract Surg* 2003;19:697–702.

42. Carones F, Vigo L, Scandola E. Wavefront-guided treatment of abnormal eyes using the LADARVision platform. *J Refract Surg* 2003;19:S703–708.

43. *Http://www.visx.com.*

44. Mrochen M, Kaemmerer M, Seiler T. Wavefront-guided laser *in situ* keratomileusis: early results in three eyes. *J Refract Surg* 2000; 16:116–120.

45. Seiler T, Mrochen M, Kaemmerer M. Operative correction of ocular aberrations to improve visual acuity. *J Refract Surg* 2000; 16:S619–S622.

46. Mrochen M, Kaemmerer M, Seiler T. Clinical results of wavefront-guided LASIK at 3 months after surgery. *J Cataract Refract Surg* 2001;27:201–207.

47. Seiler T, Kaemmerer M, Mierdel P, et al. Ocular optical aberrations after photorefractive keratectomy for myopia and myopic astigmatism. *Arch Ophthalmol* 2000;118:17–21.

48. Martinez CE, Applegate RA, Klyce SD, et al. Effect of papillary dilation on corneal optical aberrations after photorefractive keratectomy. *Arch Ophthalmol* 1998;116:1053–1062.

49. Oliver KM, Memenger RP, Corbett MC, et al. Corneal optical aberrations induced by photorefractive keratectomy. *J Refract Surg* 1997;13:246–254.

50. Vongthongsri A, Phusitphoykai N, Naripthapan P. Comparison of wavefront-guided customized ablation vs. conventional ablation in laser *in situ* keratomileusis. *J Refract Surg* 2002;18(suppl): S332–S335.

51. Gimbel HV, Stoll SB. Photorefractive Keratectomy with customized segmental ablation to correct irregular astigmatism after laser *in situ* keratomileusis. *J Refract Surg* 2001;17(suppl): S229–S232.

52. Schwiegerling J. Theoretical limits to visual performance. *Surv Ophthalmol* 2000;45:139–146.

53. Stiles WS, Crawford BH. The luminous efficiency of rays entering the eye pupil at different points. *Proc R Soc Lond B Biol Sci* 1933;112:428–450.

54. McLellan JS, Marcos S, Prieto PM, et al. Imperfect optics may be the eye's defense against chromatic blur. *Nature* 2002;417:174–176.

55. Applegate RA, Sarver EJ, Khemsara V. Are all aberrations equal? *J Refract Surg* 2002;18:S556–562.

56. Atchison DA, Collins MJ, Wildsoet CF, et al. Measurement of monochromatic ocular aberrations of human eyes as a function of accommodation by the Howland aberroscope technique. *Vision Res,* 1995;35:313–323.

57. Ninomiya S, Fujikado T, Kuroda T, et al. Changes of ocular aberration with accommodation. *Am J Ophthalmol* 2002;134:924–926.

58. Artal P, Fernandez EJ, Silvestre M. Are optical aberrations during accommodation a significant problem for refractive surgery? *J Refract Surg* 2002;18:S563–S566.

59. Hofer HJ, Artal P, Aragon JL, et al. Temporal characteristics of the eye's aberrations. *Invest Ophthalmol Vis Sci* 1999;40(suppl):S365.

60. Tutt RC, Begley CG, Bradley A, et al. The optical effects of tear film disruption. *Invest Ophthalmol Vis Sci* 1997;37(suppl):S152.

61. Thibos LN, Hong X. Clinical application of the Shack-Hartmann aberrometer. *Optom Vis Sci* 1999;76:817–825.

62. Thibos LN, Himebaugh N, Wright A, et al. Comparison of fluorescein, retro-illumination, and Shack-Hartmann wavefront sensing methods for monitoring tear film breakup. *Invest Ophthalmol Vis Sci* 2000;41(suppl):S65.

63. Berrio ME, Guirao A, Redondo M, et al. The contribution of the cornea and the internal ocular surfaces to the changes in the aberrations of the eye with age. *Invest Ophthalmol Vis Sci* 2000;41(suppl):S105.

64. Oshika T, Klyce SD, Applegate RA, et al. Changes in corneal wavefront aberrations with aging. *Invest Ophthalmol Vis Sci* 1999;40:1351–1355.

65. Marcos S. Changes in ocular aberrations with age. *J Refract Surg* 2002;18:S572–578.

66. Artal P, Navarro R. Monochromatic modulation transfer function of the human eye for different pupil diameters: an analytical expression. *J Opt Soc Am A* 1994;11:246–249.

67. Yang Y, Thompson K, Burns SA. Pupil location under mesopic, photopic, and pharmacologically dilated conditions. *Invest Ophthalmol Vis Sci* 2002;43:2508–2512.

68. Roberts C, Mahmoud A, Herderick EE, et al. Characterization of corneal curvature changes inside and outside the ablation zone in LASIK. *Invest Ophthalmol Vis Sci* 2000;41(suppl):S679.

69. Roberts C. The cornea is not a piece of plastic. *J Refract Surg* 2000;16:407–413.

70. Roberts C. Biomechanics of the cornea and wavefront-guided laser refractive surgery. *J Refract Surg* 2002;18:S589–592.

71. Wilson SE, Mohan RR, Hong JW, et al. The wound healing response after laser *in situ* keratomileusis and photorefractive keratectomy. *Arch Ophthalmol* 2001;119:889–896.

72. Pallikaris I, Kymionis GD, Panagopoulou S, et al. Induced optical aberrations following formation of a laser *in situ* keratomileusis flap. *J Cataract Refract Surg* 2002;28:1737–1741.

73. Schwiegerling J, Snyder RW, Lee JH. Wavefront and topography: keratome-induced corneal changes demonstrate that both are needed for custom ablation. *J Refract Surg* 2002;18:S584–588.

LASIK COMPLICATIONS: ETIOLOGY, PREVENTION, AND MANAGEMENT

NEDA SHAMIE, KOUROSH EGHBALI, AND PETER J. MCDONNELL

Laser *in-situ* keratomileusis (LASIK) has gained international popularity among ophthalmic surgeons and patients as the procedure of choice for refractive surgical correction of myopia and low to moderate degrees of hyperopia (1,2). Its popularity has surpassed that of photorefractive keratectomy (PRK) with its benefits including more rapid recovery of vision, less postoperative discomfort, and lower risk of postoperative stromal haze in high refractive corrections (3–5). This benefit lies in the creation of a corneal flap and maintaining the surface epithelial and Bowman's layers prior to laser ablation of the stromal bed in LASIK.

As with other refractive surgical procedures, LASIK may be associated with both intraoperative and postoperative complications. These include ablation-related complications, suboptimal refractive corrections, postoperative visual aberrations, and loss of best corrected visual acuity. With the creation of the corneal flap in LASIK, however, a new category of flap-related complications unique to corneal lamellar surgery may occur, including intraoperative flap complications such as free caps or buttonholes and postoperative complications such as flap striae and diffuse lamellar keratitis.

Complications occur infrequently, with skilled surgeons reporting a rate of 1% to 2% incidence of minor complications and 0.2% to 0.3% incidence of major sight-threatening complications (6–9). With experience we are recognizing preoperative patient-related factors that may increase the rate of known complications. By modifying the surgical technique, surgical parameters, and patient selection, a surgeon can decrease, but not eliminate, the incidence of complications and patient dissatisfaction. More importantly, a careful preoperative assessment and recognition of a high-risk patient can help counsel the patient appropriately to allow for a more informed consent and more realistic expectations. Although some complications can be avoided with careful planning and attention to detail, others are unavoidable. When complications do occur, early recognition of the problem with prompt management is key in restoring an optimal outcome.

INTRAOPERATIVE COMPLICATIONS

Poor Exposure

Inadequate globe exposure can prevent proper placement of the suction ring leading to inadequate suction and related flap complications. In addition, with poor exposure, a smooth passage of the microkeratome may not occur, leading to further intraoperative complications. This problem is one that can often be anticipated and prevented with proper preoperative evaluation. Inadequate exposure is related to orbital and facial anatomy in patients with a history of facial/orbital fractures, sunken or small eyes, prominent brows, or narrow palpebral fissures (10). A lid speculum with a posteriorly angulated hinge and a locking mechanism can improve the exposure in some patients. Also, careful draping and proper patient head positioning may help alleviate this problem (10). When necessary, the assistant may exert downward pressure on the lid speculum to proptose the eye during the microkeratome pass. Incomplete passes of the microkeratome due to interference from the drape, lids, or redundant conjunctiva can be prevented. Occasionally, the microkeratome pass can be performed without using a lid speculum, with tape used to isolate the lashes. In rare cases, some suggest doing a lateral canthotomy in patients with narrow palpebral fissures or a retrobulbar injection in patients with sunken eyes or prominent brows (6). Lastly, PRK should be considered in this challenging subset of patients.

Inadequate Suction

Inadequate suction or loss of suction can lead to serious problems during the microkeratome pass such as thin flaps, perforated flaps, or free caps (6,10). The proper placement of the suction ring requires adequate exposure and the surgeon's attention to detail. The surgeon and the technician must be familiar with the workings of the microkeratome and the suction mechanism. They may be falsely reassured by the readings on the suction console when in fact adequate

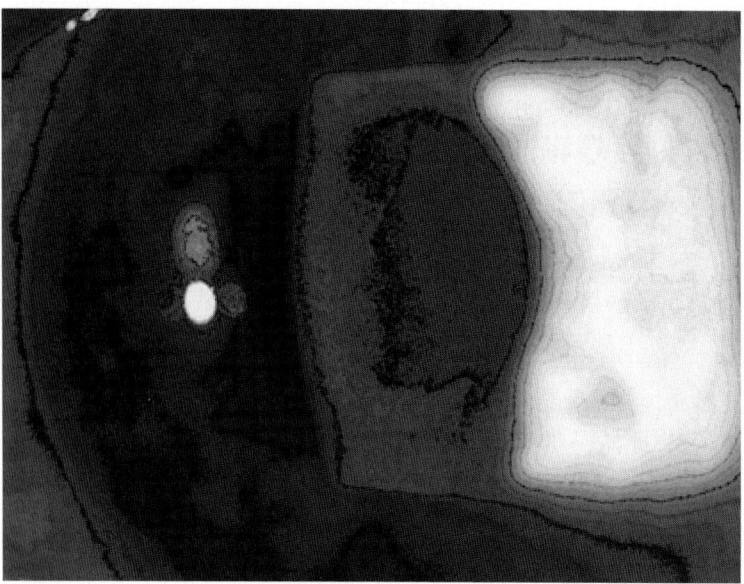

FIGURE 82-1. A central area of buttonhole is shown in this flap, which occurred as a result of a partial loss of suction during the microkeratome pass. (Courtesy of Farid Eghbali, O.D., with permission.)

suction has not been obtained. It is therefore advisable to look for the following signs indicating an intraocular pressure of at least 65 mm Hg: pupillary dilation, transient loss of the patient's vision, and sufficient intraocular pressure (IOP) measurement using a Barraquer tonometer or pneumotonometer (6,10).

Redundant conjunctiva or chemotic conjuctiva (as a result of repeated failed attempts of obtaining adequate suction) can result in pseudosuction as the conjunctiva obstructs the orifice of the suction ring. If redundant conjunctiva is noted, the redundancy can be decreased by expanding the lid speculum and stretching the conjunctiva. Rarely, a conjunctival peritomy needs to be done to place the suction ring directly onto bare sclera for adequate suction. When chemotic conjunctiva occurs iatrogenically, patience is often the best remedy. After 30 to 60 minutes, minor chemosis may resolve (6,10). A small incision in the conjunctiva may also allow drainage of the fluid, as can "milking" the fluid away from the limbus using a blunt instrument such as a Merocel sponge (10). The safest option remains delaying the surgery for several days.

Microkeratome-Related and Flap Complications

Thin Flaps and Buttonholes

Buttonhole flaps (Fig. 82-1) and especially thin flaps are among the more common LASIK flap-related intraoperative complications encountered, with incidence ranging from 0.1% to 0.2% depending on surgeon experience (11–16). In addition to surgical expertise, other factors that may affect the incidence of this complication include inadequate suction, corneal anatomy, and microkeratome malfunction or defect (17,18).

With loss of suction or with insufficiently elevated IOPs during the microkeratome pass, buckling of the central cornea may result in thin or perforated buttonhole flaps (Fig. 82-2). This problem can be minimized by assuring an IOP of at least 65 mm Hg using a Barraquer tonometer or pneumotonometer, verifying from the patient that the vision has dimmed or observing dilatation of the pupil intraoperatively after obtaining suction (18). Patients with excessive vitreous syneresis or history of vitrectomy may be at increased risk due

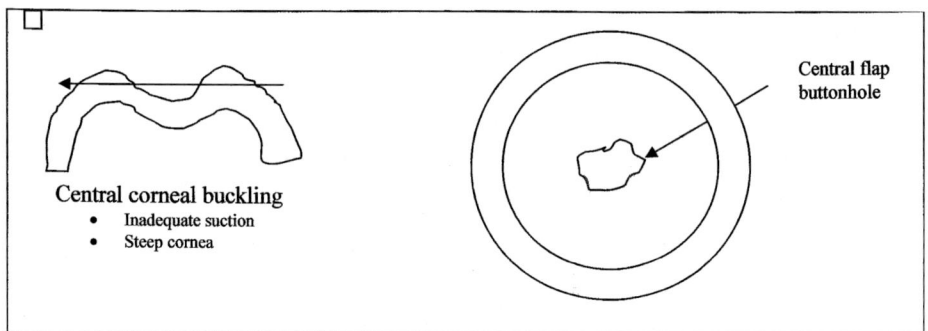

FIGURE 82-2. Central corneal buckling can occur in very steep corneas or when inadequate suction results in decreased intraocular pressure during the microkeratome pass. This can result in a thin or buttonhole flap.

to the difficulty of maintaining high enough IOPs using the suction ring and should be counseled appropriately (19).

Abnormally steep corneal curvature can also predispose a patient to intraoperative flap complications. Corneas steeper than 47 D or with irregular surface (i.e., history of previous penetrating keratoplasty or scleral buckle) may be at increased risk of developing buttonhole flaps or flaps with central thinning. As in the case of inadequate suction, this is thought to occur as a result of central corneal buckling during the microkeratome pass (Fig. 82-2) (19). The surgeon can opt to use a thicker plate and a smaller ring on these steeper corneas. Another option is to avoid the lamellar cut and proceed with PRK instead.

Probably the most avoidable factor that may predispose to this complication is microkeratome malfunction and poor blade quality (20). Meticulous attention to cleaning, assembly, and preoperative assessment of the blade and the microkeratome system can help minimize intraoperative complications. Additionally, avoidance of significant manual torque of the cornea during the microkeratome pass can also help avoid irregular and possibly perforated flaps (18).

In the case when a buttonhole flap is created, a consensus exists that the surgeon should not proceed with laser ablation of the stromal bed, and should instead replace the flap and abort further surgery until at least 3 months later, when a new, thicker flap can be recut (18,19). In the case when a thin flap without a buttonhole is created, the decision to abort further surgery is not as clear. Ablation can be safety done if the central flap appears to be of adequate thickness. Some have proposed converting to immediate transepithelial photorefractive keratectomy after repositioning the defective flap (21). The relative merits of this approach and the possibility of increased risk of haze with PRK in this setting are not yet completely understood. Of concern in the case of both buttonhole flaps and thin flaps is the increased risk of epithelial ingrowth (Fig. 82-3), irregular astigmatism, stromal scarring, and flap striae (17,18).

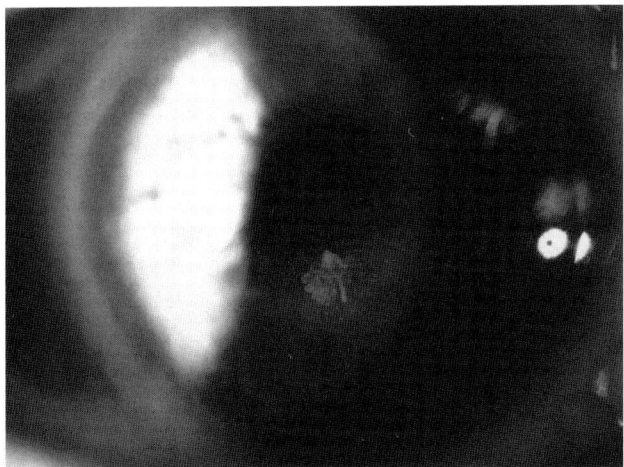

FIGURE 82-3. An area of epithelial ingrowth (inferiorly) starting from the edge of a buttonhole flap. (Courtesy of Farid Eghbali, O.D., with permission.)

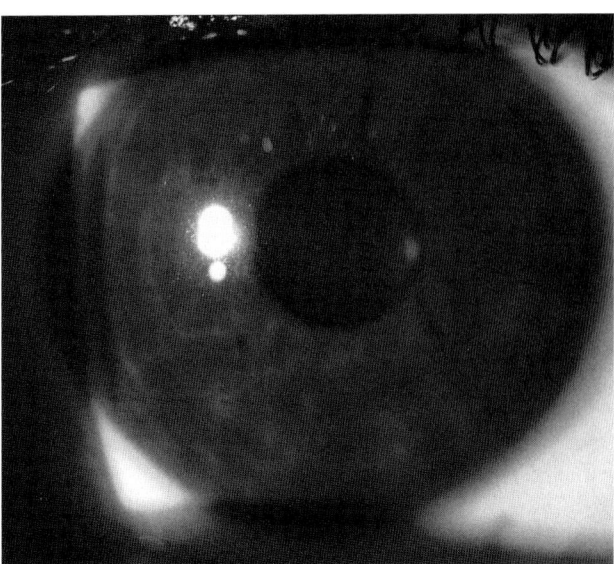

FIGURE 82-4. An incomplete flap due to inadequate suction causing an incomplete pass of the microkeratome. The edge of the flap is easily seen when one follows the outer edges of the fibrosed flap. (Courtesy of Farid Eghbali, O.D., with permission.)

Incomplete Flap

Incomplete primary cuts (Fig. 82-4) can occur as a result of a variety of causes interfering with a smooth and complete pass of the microkeratome. One of the most common causes is interference of the forward movement of the microkeratome by the speculum, eyelids, eyelashes, conjunctiva, or drapes. Additionally, electrical power outage, loss of suction, a problem with the gear mechanism, or premature release of the foot pedal can lead to shortened cuts. Other mechanical causes include improper assembly of the microkeratome system and salt crystal accumulation causing excess friction in the forward movement of the microkeratome through the suction ring slots (18,19).

Ensuring good exposure and proper maintenance, cleaning, and preoperative assembly of the microkeratome-suction ring system can reduce the incidence of incomplete flaps. In the case when an incomplete flap does occur, the burden is on the surgeon to decide whether or not to proceed with laser ablation. If the hinge is near but outside the outer diameter of the planned treatment zone, laser ablation can be performed. If the hinge is more central, most authors believe the flap should be repositioned and further surgery delayed until at least 3 months later when a LASIK flap recut can be safely performed (22,23). More importantly, the surgeon should avoid the temptation to manually complete the lamellar cut as this can lead to irregular astigmatism and scarring. If the etiology of the incomplete pass was due to anatomic reasons such as a narrow palpebral fissure, every effort should be made to prevent a repeat event, including possibly creating a lateral canthotomy (18,19). Photorefractive keratectomy should also be considered as an alternative in the case where the risk of flap complications is not thought to be preventable even at the later date.

Free Cap

Free caps or flaps with a 360-degree cut and no hinge are uncommon intraoperative complications and usually do not prevent an excellent surgical outcome (17,22). Possible causes are either mechanical or anatomic in nature. Careful attention needs to be paid to the assembly of the microkeratome/suction ring system to ensure sufficient advancement of the stopper or proper assembly of the blade and the microkeratome onto the track. Flat corneas less than 41 D of mean keratometry are at increased risk of developing free caps. With the larger flat corneas, an insufficient amount of cornea is presented to the microkeratome through the suction ring, which may result in a smaller diameter, free cap (18,19).

Prevention is the key to avoiding this as well as other intraoperative flap-related complications. Understanding the risk factors leading to this complication can help the surgeon in counseling the patient appropriately. If on preoperative evaluation the mean corneal curvature is found to be less than 41 D and the diameter is larger than 14.5 mm, the physician should counsel the patient about the increased risk of flap complications, use a larger suction ring, and consider PRK instead of LASIK (18).

If a free cap does occur, every effort should be made to maintain the orientation of the cap and to keep the cap protected. The cap could be kept covered in the microkeratome or placed in an antidesiccation chamber, epithelial side down, while the ablation is being performed. Upon completion of the ablation, the cap should be replaced onto the stromal bed in the correct orientation, taking advantage of corneal markings made prior to the microkeratome cut or repeat marks made upon realization that a free cap has been cut. Interface irrigation can be done with careful attention so as not to overly hydrate the cap. To ensure good adherence of the cap to the stromal bed, some recommend a prolonged drying time of at least 5 minutes prior to removing the lid speculum and allowing blinking. A striae test can help ensure good adherence as can making note of a symmetrically small gutter. Rarely is it necessary to suture the cap in place. Although the use of the bandage contact lens is controversial as some propose that it may result in dislodgment of the free cap, it may be helpful if disruption of the epithelium has occurred during the procedure (18,19).

Epithelial Defects

Epithelial defects can occur both preoperatively as well as intraoperatively. Patients with a history of dry eyes, basement membrane disorder, or recurrent erosions are at greatest risk for development of this complication. Some surgeons opt to test epithelial adherence in the preoperative evalua-

tion at the slit lamp using a dry cotton tip applied to the surface epithelium after instillation of topical anesthetic. If the patient is deemed to be at high risk due to epithelial surface disease, PRK may be offered as an option.

In preparation for the surgery, avoidance of excessive topical anesthetic eyedrops is necessary to reduce the risk of possible epithelial toxicity predisposing to sloughing. Intraoperatively, ensuring proper assembly of the microkeratome system, lubricating the surface of the cornea and the microkeratome tracks, and keeping the patient calm to avoid excessive movement of the eye can all help protect the epithelium. The use of toothed forceps in reflecting the flap, aggressive marking of the flap, or improper use of dry sponges on the corneal surface can also result in disruption of the surface epithelium.

If epithelium is disrupted during the surgery, every attempt should be made to smooth the epithelium back into its original position. This can be done using a cellulose sponge. If repositioning of the epithelium cannot be done in a way to ensure a smooth surface, the epithelial tags should be removed. Care must be taken to avoid introducing epithelial remnants under the flap. If severe epithelial disruption occurs, a loose fitting bandage contact lens can be used until the surface is fully epithelialized. Frequent topical nonsteroidal or steroidal eyedrop use should be avoided as these may delay epithelialization of the surface.

Intraoperative Bleeding

Many patients who are considering laser refractive surgery have been long-term contact lens users and may have related peripheral corneal neovascularization. This predisposes the patient to having intraoperative bleeding during the microkeratome pass (Fig. 82-5). Although not of great

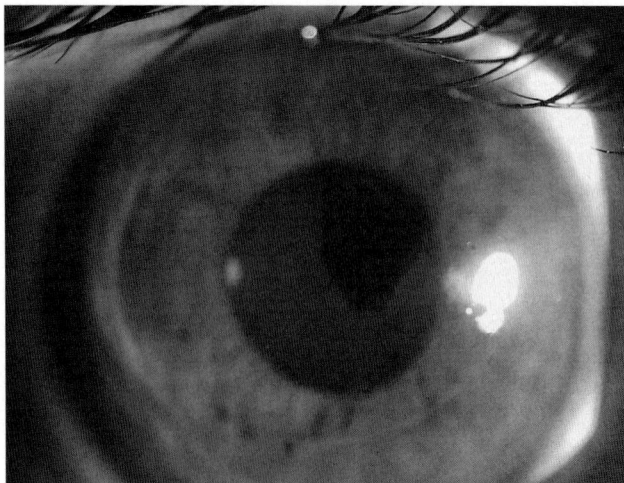

FIGURE 82-5. Interface blood under the flap minutes after the procedure. The source of the blood is the superior pannus as a result of extended soft contact lens wear. (Courtesy of Farid Eghbali, O.D., with permission.)

concern, intraoperative bleeding can be a nuisance during the surgery and can result in an increased risk of diffuse lamellar keratitis (DLK) or epithelial ingrowth, impede uniform stromal laser ablation, and possibly cause blood staining of the flap (18,24).

A thorough preoperative evaluation and attention to the presence of and location of a peripheral corneal pannus can help guide the surgeon in modifying the size of the flap or the location of the hinge to try to avoid this complication. Preoperative argon laser ablation of large peripheral vessels has been reported to close the vessels (18). Additionally, the use of topical brimonidine has been suggested to decrease the risk of subconjunctival hemorrhage, bleeding from the micropannus, and postoperative hyperemia (25).

Intraoperatively, if bleeding occurs, every effort should be made to first avoid extension of the blood into the interface. Prior to lifting the flap, a sponge soaked with 2.5% or 10% phenylephrine drops can be placed over the area of bleeding to vasoconstrict the vessels (2). Manual pressure can also be applied onto the suction ring for a short period of time to encourage coagulation of the vessel. A Gimbel-Chayet sponge may be used to prevent tracking of the blood into the interface or onto the stromal bed (19). If during the laser stromal bed ablation bleeding continues, laser treatment should be interrupted while the blood is wiped off of the bed. Intermittent irrigation may help minimize blood in the interface (19). Often flap replacement and interface irrigation tamponades any oozing vessels at the conclusion of the procedure (18,19). Given the need for more aggressive irrigation of the interface, readherence of the flap may be delayed and drying time should be increased. In the authors' experience, bleeding rarely prevents an excellent outcome.

Decentered Flap

Decentered flaps can occur as a result of surgeon decentration of the suction ring, globe torque, and loss of suction, lack of patient cooperation, and error in centering the optical axis. Often there is only a slight decentration of the flap, and laser ablation can safely be done if the ablation zone centered on the optical axis falls within the margins of the flap. When the decentration is to a degree that the surgeon cannot safely proceed with the laser ablation, the flap should be repositioned and the surgery postponed until 3 to 4 months later when a new flap can be recut (18).

Corneal Perforation

Corneal perforation is a devastating complication of LASIK that rarely occurs with the newer generation of microkeratome systems. It has been described in the context of improper microkeratome assembly with failure to properly place the depth plate into the microkeratome assembly. With meticulous assembly of the microkeratome system, as well as the current use of newer generation microkeratomes

with fewer components, this devastating complication is highly preventable (26,27).

If corneal perforation occurs during LASIK, sudden expulsion of the intraocular contents can take place as a result of markedly elevated IOP. Rapid response time in this setting is critical. Aqueous leakage, if recognized early, can prompt the surgeon to immediately stop the power and suction and, it is hoped, limit the ocular damage. In the event of perforation, the eye should be protected with a shield and the patient immediately transferred to the operating room to undergo anterior segment reconstruction with possible anterior vitrectomy, lensectomy with or without intraocular lens implantation, iridoplasty, corneal laceration repair, and possibly penetrating keratoplasty. A retinal specialist may be required, as these eyes often suffer vitreoretinal complications (18).

Laser Ablation-Related Complications

Central Islands

With newer software and with scanning beam and flying spot lasers, central islands occur infrequently. The occurrence of central islands in association with the earlier generation broad-beam lasers resulted in loss of best corrected visual acuity and poor visual quality (28). According to Kang et al. (29), the diagnosis of central islands is made based on topographic examination with a central area 2.5 mm or more in diameter of a higher refractive power of more than 1.5 D as compared to the midperiphery (Fig. 82-6). Patients present clinically with halos, glare, ghosting, and residual myopia. Most cases present within the first week after LASIK and more than 75% of cases persist more than 6 months (28). Excimer laser phototherapeutic keratectomy has been performed on the stromal bed in the persistent cases with some positive results but with unpredictability of the refractive outcome (28,30). A small-diameter shallow PRK can also be effective in managing these islands.

Decentered Ablation

Decentered ablation (Fig. 82-7) can result in postoperative irregular astigmatism, loss of best spectacle-corrected and uncorrected visual acuity, and visual aberrations (i.e., glare, halos, ghost images) (18). It can occur as a result of poor fixation by the patient or poor centration of the laser beam by the surgeon. Prior to initiating the laser ablation, the surgeon and the assistant should confirm proper patient head positioning. With reassurance and calm instruction of the patient throughout the laser ablation, the surgeon can guide good patient fixation. If the patient loses fixation, the surgeon must stop the ablation and continue only after adequate fixation is regained. Rarely a fixation ring is warranted. Mild to moderate amounts of decentration (up to 1 mm) are typically well tolerated. It is possible that eye-tracking systems will reduce

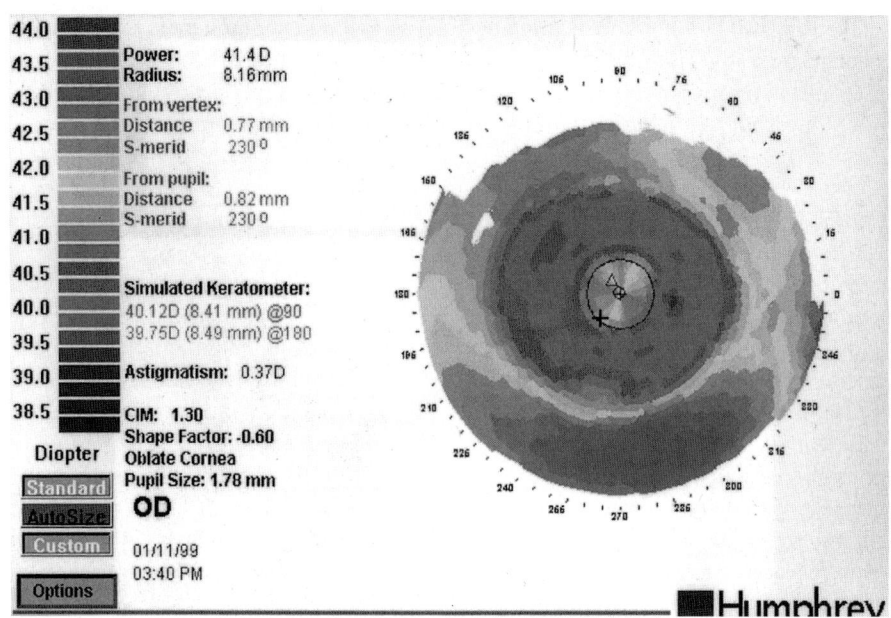

FIGURE 82-6. An axial map showing a central area of steepening adjacent to an area of flattening post myopic LASIK. This is known as a central island. (Courtesy of Farid Eghbali, O.D., with permission.)

the incidence of decentration, but most studies to date have not documented a lower risk of decentration with eye-tracking delivery systems (31,32).

Irregular Astigmatism

Irregular astigmatism is defined as one with an irregular topographic map (18). It can result from a decentered ablation, incorrect flap repositioning, epithelial ingrowth or interface debris, irregular or incomplete lamellar keratectomy, and preexisting irregular astigmatism. Usually minor postoperative irregular astigmatism resolves within several months and only 1% to 2% of patients develop enough irregular astigmatism to cause loss of vision (18). With irreversible irregular astigmatism, rigid gas-permeable contact lenses can be prescribed to obtain the best corrected visual acuity. The utility of wavefront-guided excimer lasers in treating postLASIK irregular astigmatism has not yet been

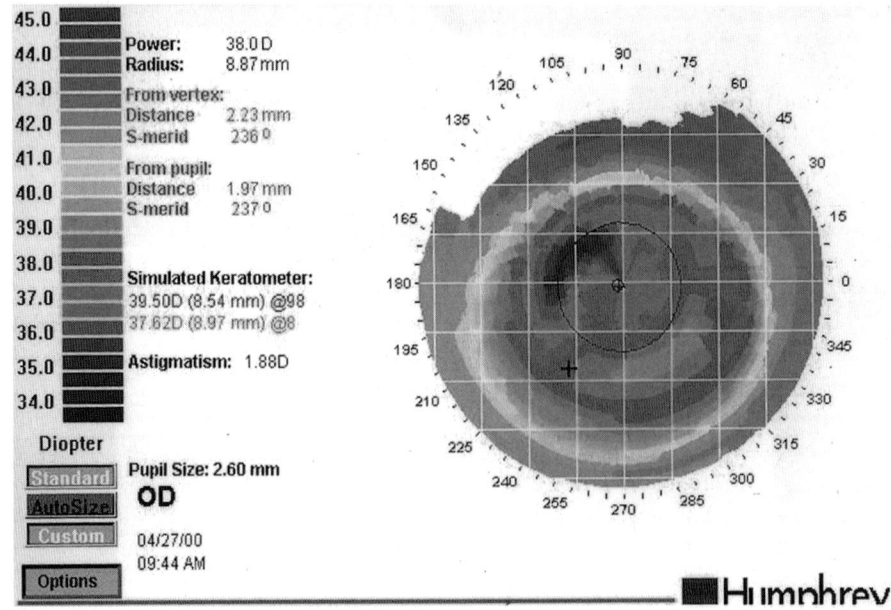

FIGURE 82-7. This topography map shows an ablation decentered inferiorly by approximately 1 mm. Each of the boxes on the map corresponds to 1 mm on the cornea. (Courtesy of Farid Eghbali, O.D., with permission.)

evaluated in the initial clinical trials, but may be an enticing option for this difficult to treat subset of patients.

Over- and Undercorrection

Residual refractive error may result from undercorrection, overcorrection, or regression with an overall re-treatment rate of 5.5% to 28% (33,34). Undercorrection or regression is seen more frequently especially after high myopic corrections. It may result from difficult preoperative refraction, unstable ametropia, or simply patient-specific factors affecting the healing process, and the expected results are based on population nomograms. Assuring a stable preoperative refraction can help decrease the chance of postoperative refractive surprises. This is especially true in patients who have a long history of contact lens use. The recommendation is for patients using soft contact lenses to discontinue use for at least 2 weeks and those using rigid gas permeable lenses to discontinue use for at least 3 to 4 weeks prior to a refractive surgery evaluation. This helps avoid instability of refractive error as a result of corneal warping. If there is any question, some recommend reevaluating in 1 month to prove a stable refractive error (within 0.50 D of sphere or cylinder and minimal change in axis) prior to proceeding.

Overcorrection occurs less frequently partly because surgeons often err on the side of undercorrection to avoid the risk of postoperative hyperopia in their myopic patients. At high altitudes with lower humidity levels in the laser room, the corneal stroma dehydrates, resulting in more tissue ablation for each laser spot delivered; this in turn results in overcorrection. Regardless of the cause, postoperative hyperopia as a result of overcorrection leads to more patient dissatisfaction and is more difficult to treat than residual postoperative myopia.

Regression results in unstable postoperative refractive outcome with continued loss of effect over several months. It is thought to occur as a result of epithelial hyperplasia and remodeling of the stroma in response to surgery (10). More regression is often noted with greater depth of ablation and smaller treatment zone. Usually stability is noted within 3 months after surgery for moderate refractive errors and within 6 months for high refractive errors (10). It is important not to confuse progressive keratectasia and related myopic shift with regression.

In the instance that postoperative refractive outcome is not ideal and is proven to have stabilized, the patient may opt to undergo an enhancement. The approach for the retreatment can follow either lifting the original lamellar flap or recutting a new flap. Most relift the original flap especially if done within 1 year of the original surgery, but recutting a flap, especially if a larger ablation zone is necessary, can offer a safe and effective alternative. Although studies have shown no statistically significant difference in complication rates between these two approaches, each incurs its own set of risks, which is outside the scope of this chapter.

POSTOPERATIVE COMPLICATIONS

Interface Debris

Nonorganic and organic materials can be introduced into the interface during LASIK. Talc from surgical gloves, lint from the drapes, metal shavings from microkeratome blades, and sponge fibers have all been described (35). Organic materials such as mucus or oil from the tear film are also commonly seen deposited in the interface (18,35). If the debris is noted during or immediately after the procedure, it probably should be immediately removed by irrigation of the interface. If noted on follow-up visits, interface debris such as mucus or tear film and even metal filings or sponge particles rarely cause inflammation, irregular astigmatism, or loss of best corrected or uncorrected visual acuity and need not be removed. Inorganic materials such as talc might result in inflammation and loss of best corrected visual acuity, and their removal should be contemplated (36). Regardless of the source of the debris, if there is loss of visual acuity or quality due to inflammation, irregular astigmatism, and flap irregularity deemed secondary to the debris, every attempt should be made to irrigate or if needed lift, irrigate, and reposition the flap. Of importance is the ability to differentiate debris from diffuse lamellar keratitis (DLK), infectious keratitis, or epithelial ingrowth, all of which require immediate attention and intervention as discussed further in this chapter.

Flap Displacement

Flap displacement is an immediate postoperative complication that normally occurs within 24 to 48 hours. The incidence ranges from 0.85% to 2.0% (8,15,37). The direction of the displacement is usually a function of the location of the hinge. For example, a nasal hinged flap often displaces inferiorly, whereas a superior hinged flap displaces laterally. The etiology of the displacement is mainly mechanical in nature. Eye rubbing, dry eyes, and hitting the flap with the tip of postoperative medication bottles are thought to account for mechanical shifting of the flap in some patients. Other causes include a poorly adherent flap due to poor endothelial pump function or excessive intraoperative stromal hydration. Delayed traumatic flap displacement has also been reported as late as 38 months after surgery (38). A review of the literature has demonstrated some unexpected causes such as accidental self-induced amputation of the flap or accidental trauma during sports (39–41).

Many surgeons evaluate the flap biomicroscopically immediately after surgery to ensure that the flap has not been displaced from blinking. Some surgeons recommend at least a 2-minute drying time at the conclusion of the surgery prior to removing the lid speculum to allow for flap adherence to the stromal bed, whereas others believe it is best to maintain a well-lubricated surface (18). Also, the use of an eye shield for three nights after the procedure results in a very low risk of inadvertent nocturnal flap displacement.

Flap displacement exposes an area of stroma that as a result can increase the chance of DLK, infectious keratitis, or epithelial ingrowth. It is therefore important to surgically reposition the flap promptly. Shifted or dislodged flaps can be managed by lifting the affected area, cleaning the epithelium or debris from the stromal bed, and refloating the flap into its correct position. If the repositioning is excessively delayed, the flap can become markedly edematous with a shrunken diameter, increasing the difficulty of repositioning and resulting in delayed adherence to the stromal bed and a large asymmetric gutter. Sutures may be needed to secure the flap in the correct alignment.

When a small flap displacement occurs, the rapid epithelial growth over the exposed stroma can sometimes confuse the diagnosis, mimicking flap striae. Careful slit-beam inspection of the gutter can help differentiate flap displacement from flap striae and guide the surgeon toward the correct management.

Corneal Neurotrophic Epitheliopathy and Dry-Eye Syndrome

Corneal sensation is mediated by axon terminals of the long ciliary nerves derived from the ophthalmic division of the trigeminal nerve (42). Large radial branches (stromal nerve roots) of the ciliary nerves penetrate the corneal domain from the limbus in the anterior third of the stromal depth, with most entering from the 3 and 9 o'clock meridia. As these nerves course to the center of the cornea, they branch horizontally and vertically, giving rise to the dense subepithelial plexus above Bowman's layer (42–45). Fibers from this plexus pass into the epithelium and form a network called the basal epithelial nerve plexus, from which intraepithelial nerve terminals emerge between the epithelial cells (46). When these stromal nerve roots are transected proximally, as occurs in the formation of the lamellar LASIK flap, the distal nerve endings degenerate and corneal sensation is lost (47–51). This has led to the term *postLASIK neurotrophic epitheliopathy*, describing a focal phenomenon in which central keratopathy occurs within the margins of the LASIK flap (52). This condition is thought to be due to alterations of the normal epithelial physiology as a result of a decreased blink reflex, tear flow, and local neuromodulatory factors (47,48,52–54).

PostLASIK dry eyes or neurotrophic epitheliopathy occurs in about 4% of patients; symptoms can last 6 months to 1 year, resulting in an accumulation of unhappy patients (52,55). The degree of neuropathy can be related to flap thickness (56), flap diameter, and depth of stromal ablation (55,57). Additionally, a number of anecdotal reports have shown a difference in postoperative corneal sensation with less neuropathy in cases where a nasal hinge instead of a superior hinge was created. Theoretically, a nasal hinge maintains a greater number of the stromal nerve roots, as the majority of these nerve roots have been shown to enter in the horizontal meridian (51). Additionally, PRK results in a shorter

period of corneal neuropathy as compared to LASIK, likely due to a more superficial ablation of the stroma (58,59). Finally, we have observed more rapid reinnervation of femtosecond laser cut flaps as compared to microkeratome flaps, possibly due to a more uniformly thin flap, smaller diameter flap for the same stromal bed area, or more vertically cut flap edge.

In summary, the phenomenon of postLASIK dry eyes is common and can result in temporary loss of best corrected and uncorrected visual acuity, irritation, and dissatisfaction. Patients with a history of dry eyes may have more prolonged symptoms but do not appear to be at increased risk of developing LASIK-related neurotrophic epitheliopathy (52). The surgeon, therefore, is faced with a condition that is often difficult to predict with very few preoperative clues to help guide prophylactic management or identification of high-risk patients.

The treatment is similar to that of dry-eye syndrome, with the understanding that the epitheliopathy in most cases resolves within 3 to 6 months. Therefore, reassurance of the patient is key. In addition, aggressive topical lubrication with nonpreserved lubricating eyedrops and punctual occlusion can be very helpful.

Diffuse Lamellar Keratitis

DLK, also known as sands of the Sahara, is a noninfectious diffuse inflammation at the level of the LASIK flap interface (60). DLK usually occurs between 1 and 7 days postoperatively, with a few case reports of delayed onset as long as 6 months after LASIK (61–66). The review of the literature reveals various degrees of clinical severity of inflammation, with an incidence of DLK ranging from 0.75% to 58.3% (67,68).

The clinical appearance of DLK, depending on its severity, is described as multiple small, flat infiltrates scattered diffusely under the flap's interface without extension posteriorly into the stroma or anteriorly into the flap. The diffuse granular powdery white appearance of these infiltrates is evocative of its nickname, "sands of the Sahara." However, the preferred term, *diffuse lamellar keratitis*, is more descriptive of not only the probable inflammatory nature but also the location of the infiltrates (60).

Although unclear, the etiology has been postulated to be an immune response to endogenous and exogenous factors. Some anecdotal reports have implicated interface debris, oils present on the microkeratome, bacterial exotoxins and endotoxins, detergents on instruments, and other environmental factors acting as chemotactic stimuli to leukocyte migrations into the interface (67,69–71). In several case series reporting on epidemics, bacterial endotoxins such as lipopolysaccharides from gram-negative bacteria and peptidoglycans of gram-positive bacteria were demonstrated in sterilizer reservoirs (71–73).

The symptoms of DLK reported by patients can be unrelated to the degree of inflammation and range from no

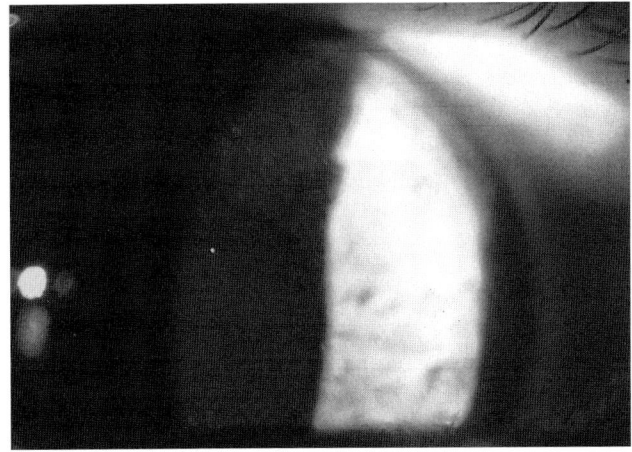

A

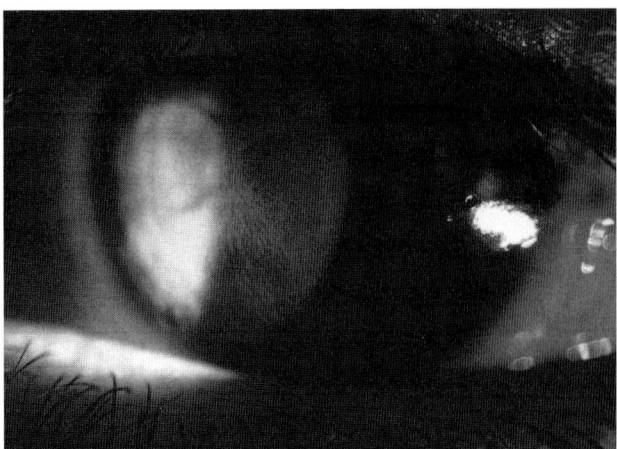

B

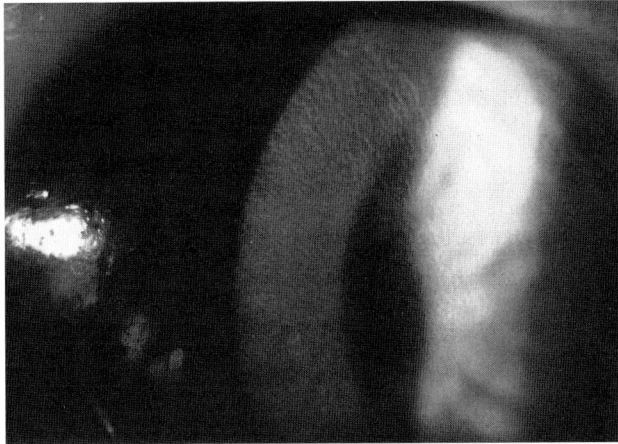

C

FIGURE 82-8. A, Grade 1 diffuse lamellar keratitis (DLK), consisting of mild small scattered infiltrates under the flap. **B,** Grade 2 DLK, consisting of moderate multiple small scattered infiltrates under the flap. **C,** Grade 3 DLK, consisting of severe multiple small scattered infiltrates under the flap. (Courtesy of Farid Eghbali, O.D., with permission.)

symptoms to severe photophobia, decreased vision, pain, redness, or tearing. DLK has been classified into different grades depending on clinical findings (Fig. 82-8) (74). Based on general convention of grading and ease of classification, the severity of DLK can be classified into four grades (Table 82-1). The purpose of this classification system is to help guide the clinician's treatment plan. For example, a more aggressive treatment is recommended when the clinician is faced with denser more centrally located, visually compromising infiltrates consistent with a grade 3.

The treatment of choice for this inflammatory condition varies among surgeons. Most authors recommend topical and, in some cases, oral steroids (75). In more severe presentations of DLK, the surgeon may consider lifting the flap and washing the interface in addition to increasing the steroid dosage. If management is delayed or the DLK progresses despite aggressive monitoring and treatment, flap melt and subsequent loss of best corrected visual acuity can occur (73).

A rare type of central necrotic lamellar inflammation that has been classified by some as type IV DLK is nonresponsive to steroids or flap lift and irrigation (Fig. 82-9) (76). The unique characteristic of this rare condition is central haze, thinning of the stroma, stromal wrinkles, and refractive hyperopic shift along with reduced best corrected vision. This

condition is usually self-limited without any medical or surgical intervention. The central haze tends to resolve, the condensed stroma will relax, and as a result the wrinkles will disappear. The resultant hyperopic shift will subsequently regress and the best corrected vision will improve. The above-mentioned changes tend to take place over many months. When the above physiologic and anatomic changes occur and the refraction and the best corrected vision remain stable, optical correction or laser enhancement can be indicated.

One of the challenges in the diagnosis of DLK is to differentiate it from other clinical conditions that may mimic DLK. The most commonly confused diagnosis is infectious keratitis, which if treated with steroids for presumed DLK can result in a devastating outcome (see Infectious Keratitis, below, for more detailed discussion). Aside from microbial keratitis, the differential diagnosis of DLK also includes interface debris, epithelial ingrowth, and interface heme.

Infectious Keratitis

Infectious keratitis is an uncommon but devastating complication of LASIK. The reported incidence ranges from 1 in 1,000 to 1 in 5,000 cases (77). This may be an underestimation, as many cases probably remain unreported. The

TABLE 82-1. DIFFUSE LAMELLAR KERATITIS (DLK) GRADING AND APPROPRIATE TREATMENT

Grade	Clinical Signs	Treatment
1	• White cells distributed in the periphery of the flap • No decrease in BCVA	• Topical prednisolone 1% every hour
2	• White cells distributed in the interface and crossing the visual axis • No decrease in BCVA • Minimal patient symptoms	• Topical prednisolone 1% every hour • May consider oral corticosteroids (prednisone 60 or 80 mg q.i.d.)
3	• White cells distributed throughout the interface • More dense accumulation of cells with areas of clumping • Decrease in BCVA • Patients may complain of haze and photophobia	• Topical prednisolone 1% every hour • Oral corticosteroids (prednisone 60 or 80 mg q.i.d.) • Consider lifting the flap for irrigation
4	• Scarring, edema, and large folds noted in the visual axis • Decrease in BCVA • Patients can be highly symptomatic • Hyperopic shift	• Consider treating as grade 3 if progressive changes are noted • Permanent scarring does not respond to even aggressive treatment • May improve over 6 to 12 months

BCVA, best corrected visual acuity.

creation of the LASIK lamellar flap poses an increased risk for this sight-threatening complication. The disruption of the normal corneal structure, loss of normal epithelial physiology, and possible introduction of infectious microbes under the flap through which antibiotic penetration may be limited all create an environment conducive to rapid growth of the infectious organisms. This risk is accentuated, as LASIK is currently done in an aseptic but unsterile setting; many components of the surgical instruments used in LASIK cannot be autoclaved (77). Other related risk factors include presence of blepharitis, long-term use of topical steroids, and persistent epithelial defects.

The clinical appearance of infectious keratitis post-LASIK can be varied based on the organism involved and patient-related factors (Fig. 82-10). Typically a white infiltrate emerges

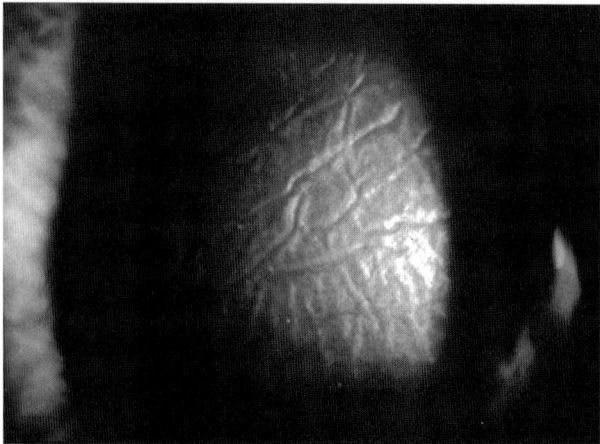

FIGURE 82-9. A rare case of central haze post-LASIK that has been graded by some as grade 4 DLK. The characteristics are well-defined dense central haze, wrinkles in the stroma, thinning of the cornea, and hyperopic shift. (Courtesy of Farid Eghbali, O.D.)

at the level of the interface with or without extension anteriorly or posteriorly into the stroma. There may be an overlying epithelial defect or surrounding stromal edema. In severe cases, flap dislodgment, severe anterior segment inflammation, and hypopyon may be noted. Satellite lesions can also be present and may warn of a possible fungal etiology. Often patients complain of decreased vision, irritation, pain, and redness.

Several anecdotal case reports and reports of outbreaks implicate atypical *Mycobacteria* as currently the most common pathogen involved in postLASIK keratitis (78–87). These organisms are omnipresent in soil, foodstuffs, and tap and laboratory water. They are common contaminants, as they can multiply rapidly in distilled water and can remain viable for up to a year despite exposure to chemical disinfectants such as chlorine (84,87). The clinical presentation of nontuberculous mycobacterial keratitis after LASIK is often confused with signs of DLK. Whereas topical corticosteroids improve the course of DLK, postoperative corticosteroids are thought to contribute to the proliferation of these organisms and worsening of the signs and symptoms (87–89). The diagnosis is often delayed due to the protracted and atypical presentation of the keratitis. Often after a delayed period of uncertainty about the pathogen involved, the diagnosis may be entertained as the distinctive focal infiltrates at the level of the interface described as "cracked windshield" in appearance develop (86). Currently, despite aggressive topical antibiotic treatment with often hourly regimens of very toxic antibiotics such as amikacin, clarithromycin, or imipenem in combination with each other or with ciprofloxacin and steroids, outcomes have been disappointing. Often due to high rates of resistance or poor penetration of these antibiotics through intact epithelium, many reported cases of atypical mycobacterial keratitis

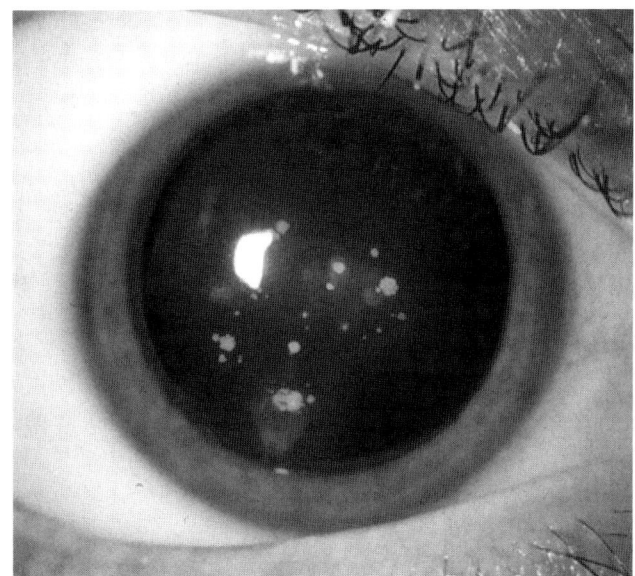

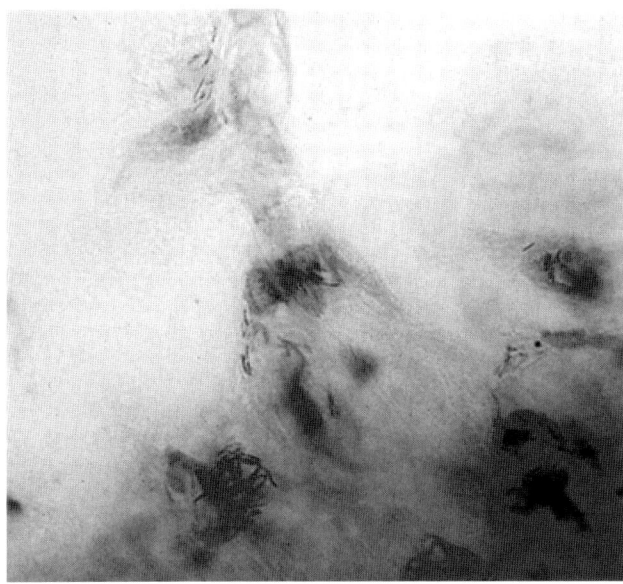

FIGURE 82-10. PostLASIK mycobacterial keratitis. **A:** The left eye of this patient who had undergone bilateral simultaneous LASIK using the same blade for the right and left eye developed multifocal coarse, granular stromal infiltrates involving the bed of the flap extending anteriorly into the stroma. **B:** Scraping of the plaquelike infiltrate disclosed acid-fast bacilli with the Ziehl-Nielson stain as shown. Cultures grew heavy nonTB mycobacteria later identified as *Mycobacterium chelonae* subspecies abscessus.

have resulted in severe stromal scarring, perforation, or need for flap amputation (77,85–88). In one case study, despite 8.4 weeks of topical clarithromycin and amikacin treatment every 2 hours, the flap had to be amputated and viable acid-fast bacilli could still be demonstrated in histologic sections (84).

Staphylococcus aureus is the next most commonly reported pathogen with *Streptococcus viridans*, coagulative-*negative Staphylococcus, Streptococcus pneumoniae*, fungus, and *Nocardia*

as less frequent causes of postLASIK infectious keratitis (77). Risk factors associated with staphylococcal keratitis include meibomian gland disease and blepharitis. With preoperative recognition of these risk factors and intervention with lid hygiene and possible oral doxycycline therapy, the risk of this dreaded complication may be significantly decreased. Unlike mycobacterial keratitis, staphylococcal keratitis is often associated with a more rapid response to therapy and a better outcome (77). This false sense of safety is not long lived due to the emergence of resistant strains to the currently used agents including second-generation fluoroquinolones. From 1993 to 1997, as much as 35% of *S. aureus* strains were shown to be resistant to currently available second- and third-generation fluoroquinolones (90).

Fourth-generation fluoroquinolones such as gatifloxacin and moxifloxacin have been developed to address this problem and have been the subject of many recent studies (91). In a rabbit model of postLASIK infectious keratitis using multidrug resistant strains of *S. aureus*, the 8-methoy fluoroquinolone gatifloxacin was found to be an effective prophylactic agent in preventing keratitis (91a). This was not the case in eyes treated prophylactically with ciprofloxacin or levofloxacin. With a similar animal model of *Mycobacteria chelonae* keratitis, gatifloxacin achieved complete eradication of the *M. chelonae* species after 3 weeks of therapy (submitted for publication).

In summary, early detection and aggressive management of any suspicious inflammation after LASIK often leads to more favorable outcomes. Superficial cultures should be attempted, but often when the overlying epithelium is intact, cultures remain negative. If so, the surgeon must consider lifting the flap and performing cultures and smears of the interface. This also allows for antibiotic irrigation of the bed and the flap, which has been found to result in improved results if done early (77). Due to the high incidence of atypical pathogens in the setting of postLASIK keratitis, cultures should be inoculated on blood, as well as chocolate, Sabouraud, and Lowenstein-Jensen agar. Also, in addition to Gram stain, Giemsa, Calcofluor white (for *Acanthamoeba*), and Ziehl-Neelsen (for acid-fast bacteria) stains should be considered. Initial treatment can include frequently dosed fluoroquinolone alone in less severe cases or in combination with fortified vancomycin or cefazolin in more vision-threatening cases (77). This treatment should be modified appropriately based on culture or smear results. Finally, with the emergence of more multidrug-resistant pathogens, clinicians can take advantage of newer generation antibiotics in treating this dreaded complication of LASIK.

Epithelial Ingrowth

Epithelial ingrowth is a rare complication of LASIK that presents clinically days to months after the procedure; the majority of the cases present within 2 months of surgery

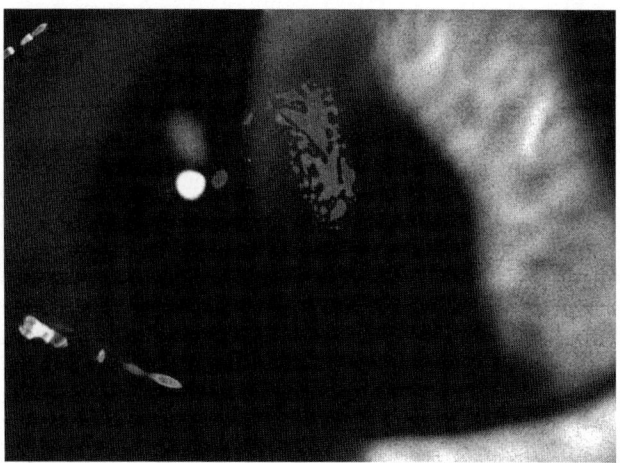

FIGURE 82-11. An area of epithelial ingrowth superiorly adjacent to the LASIK flap margin. The ingrowth ends at the demarcation line and not where the epithelial pearls end. (Courtesy of Farid Eghbali, O.D., with permission.)

(92,93). On slit-lamp examination, nests of epithelial cells may be found centrally as a result of intraoperative implantation of the epithelium under the flap or more commonly as whorl-like isthmus of cells extending centrally from the flap edge (Fig. 82-11) (94). Risk factors related to epithelial ingrowth include intraoperative flap complications such as buttonhole or epithelial defects (92,95); postoperative flap complications such as dislodged flap (36); large-diameter hyperopic treatments (36); interface debris, inflammation, or blood (92); and poor flap adhesion.

The clinical course of epithelial ingrowth is often unpredictable, but close follow-up is crucial. Usually the epithelial cells remain stable with no further expansion. In an interventional case series of eyes with epithelial ingrowth after LASIK, 90% of epithelial ingrowth either decreased or remained stable (92). Of concern are the few cases when the epithelial ingrowth expands and results in irregular astigmatism, loss of best corrected visual acuity, discomfort, and keratolysis or overlying stromal melt.

As is true for most postLASIK complications, prevention of epithelial ingrowth is preferable. Some advocate using a bandage contact lens in the setting when an intraoperative flap complication occurs or when an epithelial defect is present adjacent to the flap margin (92). In hyperopic treatments with a large ablation zone, the surgeon must ensure a large-diameter flap has been cut to minimize ablation beyond the edge of the lamellar bed. Prior to flap repositioning, any epithelial tags or debris should be cleared carefully.

If epithelial ingrowth is noted, close monitoring, especially early in the follow-up, is necessary to avoid the related complications. Flap lift and debridement of the epithelial cells from the stromal bed and the flap undersurface is warranted if the ingrowth is visually significant due to either its progression across the visual axis or

related irregular astigmatism. Also, some advocate debridement if the area of the ingrowth is greater than 2 mm as it may be related to a higher chance of keratolysis (94). Recurrence of the epithelial ingrowth after the first debridement may occur in 20% to 40% of eyes. Repeated lifting of the flap with scraping of the epithelium from the stromal bed and the flap undersurface may be sufficient. If a fistula is present at the edge of the LASIK flap, interrupted 10-0 nylon sutures placed at the originating site of the ingrowth will close the fistula and reduce the chance of recurrence (93). We recommend caution with use of adjunctive chemicals, like alcohol or mitomycin, due to reported complications.

Flap Fold, Striae, or Microstriae

Various terms have been used in the literature to describe flap wrinkles such as fold, striae, and microstriae, in descending order of clinical severity. The term *flap wrinkles* is used in this section as a general term to describe the characteristics, diagnosis, and management of this category of postLASIK complication. Some wrinkling of Bowman's layer is probably the rule rather than the exception after LASIK, as this is typically seen if surface epithelium is debrided in an eye that has had this surgery.

The etiology of flap wrinkles can be mechanical or anatomic in nature. The mechanical etiology of flap wrinkles is similar to the etiology of flap displacement; eye rubbing, dry eyes, and trauma to the flap can result in wrinkling of the flap. The anatomic nature of the flap wrinkles is simply based on the fact that after the laser photoablation there is more flap surface area relative to the underlying flattened stromal bed. In higher myopes, where more treatment is performed and as a result, a larger flap (in square area) needs to cover a smaller underlying stromal bed, there is a greater risk of developing flap wrinkles (96,97). These wrinkles can have a mud crack appearance with no or minimal effect on vision, and can be seen on the 1-day postoperative evaluation.

Flap wrinkles are best seen in direct retroillumination or indirect retroillumination via slit-lamp examination (Fig. 82-12A). It is often recommended to use fluorescein staining to detect wrinkles (Fig. 82-12B) (98). The areas of negative staining are peaks and the areas of positive pooling are the valleys of the wrinkles.

The treatment of flap wrinkles is the same as that of flap displacement, with the exception that the urgency in proceeding with lifting and repositioning the flap is greater in flap displacement. The determining factor for the decision to reposition the flap in the case of flap wrinkling is based on reduction of best corrected visual acuity and the patient's related symptoms. If an area of peripheral wrinkles is observed that does not affect vision, further intervention is not warranted as the risk of flap lift may exceed the benefit of eliminating the wrinkles.

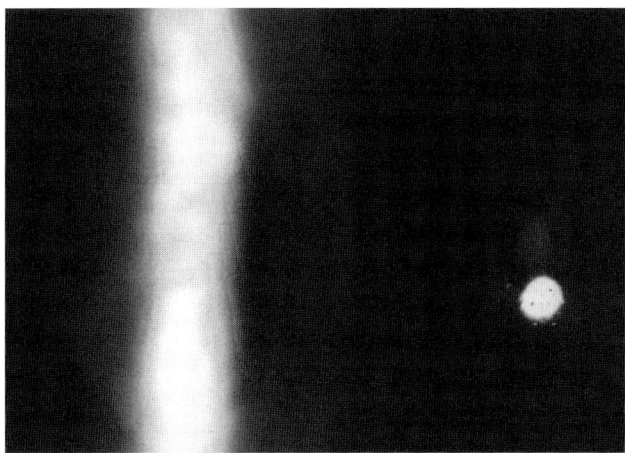
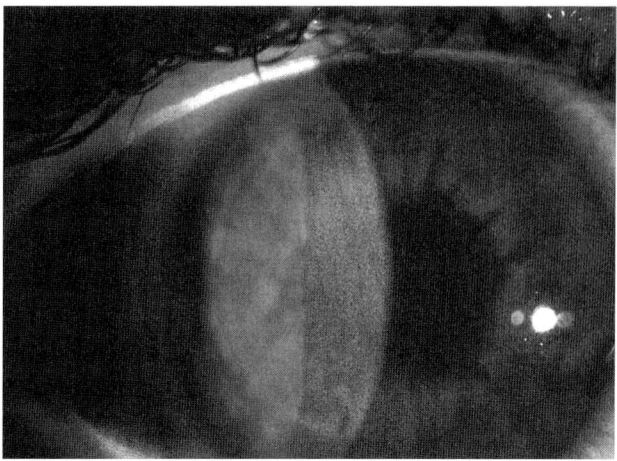

FIGURE 82-12. A, Vertical folds are visible in this flap on the 1 day postoperative LASIK. **B,** To differentiate this from flap stretch marks, sodium fluorescein can be used. Areas of negative staining designate elevated areas of the flap. (Courtesy of Farid Eghbali, O.D., with permission.)

When intervention is deemed appropriate, the flap should be lifted and refloated. Using the tips of a dry sponge, the flap can be stretched 90 degrees from the direction of the folds (99). This can be done either while the flap is lifted from its underside or after it has been repositioned and adhered onto the stromal bed (99,100). Hydration of the flap with hypotonic saline, sometimes in combination with central epithelial debridement, may be effective in reducing folds in Bowman's layer. If the wrinkles persist, one can consider suturing the flap edges (101). Lastly, phototherapeutic keratectomy of the superficial layer has been described as an option that is often successful (100,102). Such an ablation is often unnecessary and may lead to a shift in the refractive power of the cornea.

Interface Haze

Stromal haze is much less common after LASIK than after PRK. Normally, it is associated with treatment of very high refractive errors (18). There have also been a number of case reports describing severe stromal haze after LASIK retreatment for residual refractive error following PRK (103) or PRK re-treatment for residual refractive error following LASIK (104). Others have described a pattern of annular crystalline haze developing after hyperopic LASIK ablations (94). In the occasion that interface haze does occur, it usually responds favorably to a course of topical corticosteroids (94). More importantly the surgeon must differentiate true interface haze from the more commonly reported complications of LASIK such as DLK, interface debris, epithelial ingrowth, or infectious keratitis that can clinically mimic stromal haze.

Iatrogenic or Progressive Ectasia

Progressive corneal ectasia remains a concerning and often unpredictable complication of laser refractive surgery.

It occurs as a result of postoperative alterations in the corneal integrity and progressive thinning and steepening of the inferior cornea for reasons not yet fully understood (105). It is unclear if biomechanical changes in the cornea as a result of laser-induced proteolysis, a natural course of disease in patients with preoperative subclinical evidence of ectasia, or a combination of the two can explain the pathophysiology of this condition (106). This presents clinically as a progressive myopic shift, an increase in astigmatism, monocular diplopia or visual distortions, loss of uncorrected visual acuity, and often even loss of best spectacle-corrected visual acuity (94). The incidence has been reported to be 0.04% in a large case series, but this is thought to be an underestimation (107). Ectasia has been mostly reported in cases in which there was preoperative evidence of high myopia, keratoconus, or forme fruste keratoconus, although some patients have had no recognized risk factors (108–116). In addition, the differentiation of forme fruste keratoconus from mildly asymmetric astigmatism may be very difficult.

In high myopic patients, the risk is thought to be due to the increased depth of ablation required to treat the refractive error resulting in a substantially thinned stromal bed. The consensus among refractive surgeons is that the residual stromal bed thickness should be at least 250 μm (117) and in some reports 300 μm (118) to avoid this complication. It has been postulated that thinning of the load-bearing central cornea from a thickness of 500 to <250 μm mimics the loss of elasticity of the keratoconic cornea, resulting in an iatrogenic and possibly more rapidly progressive form of this keratectatic condition (113,119). Others argue that instead of an absolute thickness of 250 μm, the appropriate target should be to leave a residual stromal bed thickness equal to 50% of the preoperative corneal thickness. The burden is on the surgeon to estimate the amount of residual stromal bed thickness that may remain after the laser ablation. This of course is limited due to the inexactness of the predicted lamellar flap thickness, as often the same microkeratome can cut flaps with varying thickness depending on corneal anatomy and surgeon technique (120–122). The residual stromal bed thickness can be calculated by either subtracting the predicted flap thickness for the microkeratome used and the depth of ablation from the preoperative pachymetry reading or subtracting the predicted flap thickness from the postoperative pachymetry reading (107).

The presence of forme fruste keratoconus preoperatively is another risk factor for the development of progressive postLASIK keratectasia. Videokeratographic criteria to detect forme fruste keratoconus were first offered by Rabinowitz and McDonnell (123) in 1989. Central corneal keratometry readings of greater than 47.2 D, a quantitative measurement of inferosuperior asymmetry (I-S value) of greater than 1.40, and substantial asymmetry in central power between the right and left eyes seemed to separate normal from abnormal patients (123,124). The absolute numbers may vary by model and manufacturers of videokeratograph instruments, and other researchers have proposed alternative quantitative criteria.

The key in the management of postLASIK keratectasia is prevention. A thorough preoperative evaluation with strict attention to clinical as well as diagnostic criteria, which may point to a high-risk patient, can aid in the decision not to proceed with laser refractive surgery in this subgroup of patients. A red flag should be raised in any patient with a best spectacle-corrected vision of less than 20/20 with no other obvious medial opacities or macular disease. Significant irregular astigmatism with inferior steepening (Fig. 82-13) not attributable to contact lens-induced corneal warping or other corneal surface disease can be a sign of forme fruste keratoconus and should be further evaluated. An unstable preoperative refraction with progressive

astigmatic and myopic shift could also warn of progressive keratectasia. Finally, preoperative estimation of the residual stromal bed thickness that will remain after the attempted treatment should be done in every patient, especially those with high preoperative myopia, to ensure sufficient stromal thickness of at least 250 μm will remain.

If postoperative keratectasia does occur, conservative management with spectacles, soft contact lenses, or rigid gas-permeable contact lenses can often restore best corrected vision. In up to 30% of advanced cases, penetrating keratoplasty is needed for restoration of best corrected vision (107). The surgeon should also avoid mistaking progressive ectasia resulting in a myopic shift with regression of results. This can lead to unnecessary retreatments that aggravate the keratectasia (107).

RARE COMPLICATIONS OR COMORBIDITIES

Optic Nerve Damage/Progressive Visual Field Loss

Since the advent of LASIK, some investigators have been concerned about the possible effect the brief iatrogenic elevation of the intraocular pressure may have on the intraocular blood flow, the nerve fiber layer, and associated visual field loss. Although the length of pressure elevation in LASIK is of shorter duration as compared to high-resistance wind instrument playing or gravity inversion, both activities, in rare cases, have been associated with visual field loss; the magnitude of the IOP elevation is greater in LASIK that in these activities (125–128). It may be advisable to consider a certain subset of patients with compromised optic nerves related to advanced visual field deficits at high risk for developing further optic neuropathy as a result of the brief elevation in the IOP during LASIK. On the other hand, well-controlled glaucoma is not a contraindication for LASIK, but these patients should be informed about the possible risk of developing worsening optic neuropathy as a result of the procedure. Understanding this small but real risk of LASIK-induced optic neuropathy may influence their decision in considering other alternatives for laser vision correction such as PRK.

There have also been a series of case reports describing steroid-induced glaucoma after LASIK associated with fluid accumulation in the interface. The key features in the eyes described include a steroid-induced elevation in the IOP, interface fluid accumulation, and, if left unrecognized or untreated, progressive glaucomatous visual field loss (129). It has been postulated that as the IOP rises in the steroid-responsive patient, fluid permeates through the stroma and separates the interface and collects in this potential space (129). This is then complicated further by falsely low tonometry measurements as the pressure being measured is that of the fluid in the interface and not the

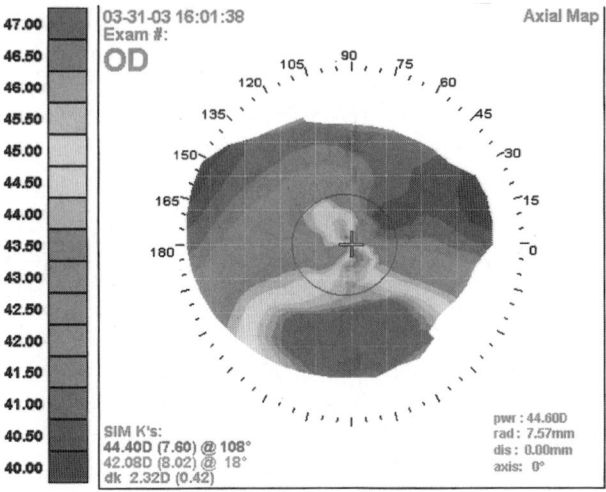

FIGURE 82-13. A typical topographic representation of a patient with irregular astigmatism with inferior steepening. This patient may be at increased risk of post-LASIK keratectasia, given the preoperative evidence of forme fruste keratoconus.

elevated IOP. Most cases were associated with DLK or epithelial ingrowth. It is unclear if the diagnosis of DLK was accurate or if the corneal edema and the presence of interface fluid associated with the steroid-induced elevated IOP mimicked the interface haze seen in DLK. Also the presence of epithelial ingrowth is not thought to be associated with interface fluid. It is possible, though, that the collection of the interface fluid elevates the edge of the flap and thus increases the likelihood of developing epithelial ingrowth (129). The management of this condition lies in its early detection. Unusually low postoperative IOP, the presence of interface fluid on biomicroscopic examination, and an atypical clinical course of DLK can guide the physician toward this diagnosis.

Of another concern in the subset of patients with glaucoma or ocular hypertension who desire to undergo laser refractive surgery is the effect the altered corneal structure has on IOP measurements or nerve fiber layer analysis using currently available diagnostic tools. It has been demonstrated that post-LASIK eyes have lowered measured IOP as compared to preoperative measurements, which may delay intervention and appropriate management of either known glaucoma or the onset of the disease (130–132). To complicate matters more, other glaucoma diagnostic and follow-up tools such as the scanning laser polarimeter used to measure the retinal nerve fiber layer also give inaccurate readings in the setting of an altered corneal architecture (133).

Given these considerations, LASIK can be offered to this high-risk subset of patients with some added caution. The patients need to be well informed of the possible increased risk related to their underlying eye condition but should be aware that glaucoma alone is not a contraindication to laser refractive surgery.

Vitreoretinal Complications

Retinal detachments are the most commonly reported vitreoretinal complication occurring after LASIK (15,134,135). Others have included simple retinal tears without a retinal detachment (134), subhyaloid hemorrhage (136), and macular hemorrhage from choroidal neovascular membranes or lacquer cracks (137). The difficulty in evaluating the causal relationship between LASIK and these vitreoretinal complications is that most of the reported patients who developed these complications had very high myopia and may have suffered from these vitreoretinal events as part of the natural history of their pathologic myopia. It is yet to be demonstrated that vitreoretinal problems occur with a frequency after LASIK that exceeds the baseline rate in these often highly myopic eyes. However, it is possible that the sudden change in the IOP during the prolonged suction and release of suction for creating the lamellar flap may result in a mechanical stretch in the vitreous base, which may put eyes with long axial lengths at a higher risk

of developing retinal tears or detachments, vitreous hemorrhages, and macular bleeds (135).

A thorough preoperative evaluation including a careful indirect ophthalmoscopic evaluation can help detect preoperative retinal tears, lattice changes, or choroidal neovascular membranes. The surgeon can then recommend a detailed retinal evaluation and management prior to even considering LASIK in this high-risk subset of patients.

Diabetes and LASIK

According to the National Institutes of Health (NIH), diabetes in the general U.S. population has reached a prevalence of 6.2%, and afflicts 8.6% of those over 20 years of age (138). Many of these patients are under the care of their ophthalmologist and inevitably many will inquire about laser refractive surgery. Well-controlled diabetes alone is not an absolute contraindication to laser refractive surgery, but the clinician must be aware of the potential increased risks associated with this comorbidity. Diabetes is often associated with abnormal epithelial surface physiology, with a degree of neurotrophic epitheliopathy, and with related poor wound healing. Fraunfelder and Rich (139) conducted a retrospective review of 30 eyes of diabetic patients who had undergone LASIK and compared the outcomes with a large group of age- and gender-matched control eyes that had undergone LASIK in the same period and at the same center. They found that in their group of well-controlled diabetic patients in otherwise good health the overall complication rate was 47% versus 6.9% in the control population. The complications were mostly related to corneal epithelial surface disease such as persistent punctate epitheliopathy and epithelial defects. This apparent high risk awaits confirmation in other prospective studies, and conflicts with the authors' personal experience.

An important red flag related to the diabetic patient seeking LASIK is brittle diabetes with poor blood sugar control. This can result in fluctuating refraction, more rapidly progressive cataracts, and diabetic retinopathy, all of which can affect the final outcome of LASIK and increase the risk of surgery.

In summary, with a very thorough preoperative evaluation and proper counseling, the refractive surgeon can safely proceed with LASIK in this subpopulation of patients if the diabetes has been well controlled and if no other related ocular abnormalities are present.

AIDS/HIV and LASIK

Posterior segment complications related to human immunodeficiency virus (HIV) and AIDS have been well described, but anterior-segment complications as a possible direct consequence of the underlying immunocompromised state are often overlooked (140). For example, infectious keratitis in patients with HIV has been described in the absence of reported predisposing factors such as contact lens wear or trauma, hinting at an increased risk simply due to the comorbid immunocompromised state (140). A case report described the occurrence of severe bilateral bacterial keratitis after LASIK in a patient with HIV (141). This patient developed a very rare complication of refractive surgery and suffered from a very poor outcome despite prompt recognition and immediate and very aggressive management of the infection. The authors postulated that the immunocompromised state possibly contributed to the patient's risk of acquiring the bilateral infection and bad outcome. In short, based on very limited number of reported cases, with caution and with proper counseling, LASIK probably can be safely offered to patients with immunocompromised states.

Of a different concern in this subpopulation of patients is the possible health hazard to the surgeon. The surgeon may be apprehensive about the possibility of virus transmission by the excimer laser plume during the vaporization of the corneal tissue. The possibility of infectious virus particles in laser plumes has been convincingly demonstrated with the treatment of viral plates with the carbon dioxide laser. The risk of viral aerosolization with the excimer laser plume, however, appears to be uncommon, based on laboratory experiments (142,143). This conclusion would of course be difficult to test in an *in vivo* setting and, as part of universal precautions, the surgeon may opt to use nonporous masks when operating on high-risk patients.

REFERENCES

1. Pallikaris IG, Papatzanaki ME, Siganos DS, et al. A corneal flap technique for laser *in situ* keratomileusis. Human studies. *Arch Ophthalmol* 1991;109:1699–1702.
2. Ibrahim O. Laser *in situ* keratomileusis for hyperopia and hyperopic astigmatism. *J Refract Surg* 1998;14:S179–S182.
3. Lee JB, Seong GJ, Lee JH, et al. Comparison of laser epithelial keratomileusis and photorefractive keratectomy for low to moderate myopia. *J Cataract Refract Surg* 2001;27(4):565–570.
4. Tole DM, McCarty DJ, Couper T, et al. Comparison of laser *in situ* keratomileusis and photorefractive keratectomy for the correction of myopia of −6.00 diopters or less. Melbourne Excimer Laser Group. *J Refract Surg* 2001;17(1):46–54.
5. Fernandez AP, Jaramillo J, Jaramillo M. Comparison of photorefractive keratectomy and laser *in situ* keratomileusis for myopia of −6 D or less using the Nidek EC-5000 laser. *J Refract Surg* 2000;16(6):711–715.
6. Gimbel HV, Penno EEA. *LASIK complications: prevention and management*, 2nd ed. Thorofare, NJ: Slack, 2001:261.
7. Gimbel HV, Penno EE, van Westenbrugge JA, et al. Incidence and management of intraoperative and early postoperative complications in 1000 consecutive laser *in situ* keratomileusis cases. *Ophthalmology* 1998;105(10):1839–1847; discussion 1847–1848.
8. Lin RT, Maloney RK. Flap complications associated with lamellar refractive surgery. *Am J Ophthalmol* 1999;127(2):129–136.
9. Wilson SE. LASIK: management of common complications. Laser *in situ* keratomileusis. *Cornea* 1998;17(5):459–467.
10. Buratto L, Brint SF. *LASIK: surgical techniques and complications*. Thorofare, NJ: Slack, 2000;ix, 608.
11. Pallikaris IG, Siganos DS. Laser *in situ* keratomileusis to treat myopia: early experience. *J Cataract Refract Surg* 1997;23(1):39–49.
12. Gimbel HV, Basti S, Kaye GB, et al. Experience during the learning curve of laser *in situ* keratomileusis. *J Cataract Refract Surg* 1996;22(5):542–550.
13. Bas AM, Onnis R. Excimer laser *in situ* keratomileusis for myopia. *J Refract Surg* 1995;11(3 suppl):S229–S233.
14. Marinho A, Pinto MC, Pinto R, et al. LASIK for high myopia: one year experience. *Ophthalmic Surg Lasers* 1996;27(5 suppl):S517–S520.
15. Stulting RD, Carr JD, Thompson KP, et al. Complications of laser *in situ* keratomileusis for the correction of myopia. *Ophthalmology* 1999;106(1):13–20.
16. Lindstrom RL, Hardten DR, Chu YR. Laser *in situ* keratomileusis (LASIK) for the treatment of low moderate, and high myopia. *Trans Am Ophthalmol Soc* 1997;95:285–306.
17. Jacobs JM, Taravella MJ. Incidence of intraoperative flap complications in laser *in situ* keratomileusis. *J Cataract Refract Surg* 2002;28(1):23–28.
18. Buratto L, Brint SF. Complications of LASIK. In: Brint SF, ed. *LASIK surgical techniques and complications*, 2nd ed. Thorofare, NJ: Slack, 2000.
19. Gimbel HV, Penno EA. Intraoperative Complications. In: Penno EA, ed. *LASIK complications: prevention and management*, 2nd ed. Thorofare, NJ: Slack, 2001.
20. Slade S. LASIK complications and their management: Free cap, thin and perforated corneal flaps. In: Machat JJ, ed. *Excimer laser refractive surgery: practice and principles*. Thorofare, NJ: Slack, 1996.
21. Jain VK, Abell TG, Bond WI, et al. Immediate transepithelial photorefractive keratectomy for treatment of laser *in situ* keratomileusis flap complications. *J Refract Surg* 2002;18(2):109–112.
22. Tham VM, Maloney RK. Microkeratome complications of laser *in situ* keratomileusis. *Ophthalmology* 2000;107(5):920–924.
23. Holland SP, Srivannaboon S, Reinstein DZ. Avoiding serious corneal complications of laser assisted *in situ* keratomileusis and photorefractive keratectomy. *Ophthalmology* 2000; 107(4): 640–652.
24. MacRae S, Macaluso DC, Rich LF. Sterile interface keratitis associated with micropannus hemorrhage after laser *in situ* keratomileusis. *J Cataract Refract Surg* 1999;25(12):1679–1681.
25. Norden RA. Effect of prophylactic brimonidine on bleeding complications and flap adherence after laser *in situ* keratomileusis. *J Refract Surg* 2002;18(4):468–471.
26. Joo CK, Kim TG. Corneal perforation during laser *in situ* keratomileusis. *J Cataract Refract Surg* 1999;25(8):1165–1167.
27. Chang SW, Ashraf FM, Azar DT. Wound healing patterns following perforation sustained during laser *in situ* keratomileusis. *J Formos Med Assoc* 2000;99(8):635–641.
28. Tsai YY, Lin JM. Natural history of central islands after laser *in situ* keratomileusis. *J Cataract Refract Surg* 2000;26(6): 853–858.
29. Kang SW, Chung ES, Kim WJ. Clinical analysis of central islands after laser *in situ* keratomileusis. *J Cataract Refract Surg* 2000;26(4):536–542.
30. Manche EE, Maloney RK, Smith RJ. Treatment of topographic central islands following refractive surgery. *J Cataract Refract Surg* 1998;24(4):464–470.
31. Tsai YY, Lin JM. Ablation centration after active eye-tracker-assisted photorefractive keratectomy and laser *in situ* keratomileusis. *J Cataract Refract Surg* 2000;26(1):28–34.
32. Taylor NM, Eikelboom RH, van Sarloos PP, et al. Determining the accuracy of an eye tracking system for laser refractive surgery. *J Refract Surg* 2000;16(5):S643–S646.

33. Lyle WA, Jin GJ. Retreatment after initial laser *in situ* keratomileusis. *J Cataract Refract Surg* 2000;26(5):650–659.

34. Febbraro JL, Buzard KA, Friedlander MH. Reoperations after myopic laser *in situ* keratomileusis. *J Cataract Refract Surg* 2000;26(1):41–48.

35. Hirst LW, Vandeleur KW Jr. Laser *in situ* keratomileusis interface deposits. *J Refract Surg* 1998;14(6):653–654.

36. Gimbel HV, Penno EA. Early Postoperative Complications. In: Penno EA, ed. *LASIK complications: prevention and management*, 2nd ed. Thorofare, NJ: Slack, 2001.

37. Lam DS, Leung AT, Wu JT, et al. Management of severe flap wrinkling or dislodgment after laser *in situ* keratomileusis. *J Cataract Refract Surg* 1999;25(11):1441–1447.

38. Iskander NG, Peters NT, Anderson Penno E, et al. Late traumatic flap dislocation after laser *in situ* keratomileusis. *J Cataract Refract Surg* 2001;27(7):1111–1114.

39. Tumbocon JA, Paul R, Slomovic A, et al. Late traumatic displacement of laser *in situ* keratomileusis flaps. *Cornea* 2003;22(1):66–69.

40. Melki SA, Talamo JH, Demetriades AM, et al. Late traumatic dislocation of laser *in situ* keratomileusis corneal flaps. *Ophthalmology* 2000;107(12):2136–2139.

41. Sridhar MS, Rapuano CJ, Cohen EJ. Accidental self-removal of a flap—a rare complication of laser *in situ* keratomileusis surgery. *Am J Ophthalmol* 2001;132(5):780–782.

42. Muller LJ, Vrensen GF, Pels L, et al. Architecture of human corneal nerves. *Invest Ophthalmol Vis Sci* 1997;38(5):985–894.

43. Mensher JH. Corneal nerves. *Surv Ophthalmol* 1974;19(1):1–18.

44. Muller LJ, Pels L, Vrensen GF. Ultrastructural organization of human corneal nerves. *Invest Ophthalmol Vis Sci* 1996; 37(4):476–488.

45. Ishida N, del Cerro M, Rao GN, et al. Corneal stromal innervation. A quantitative analysis of distribution. *Ophthalmic Res* 1984;16(3):139–144.

46. Schimmelpfennig B. Nerve structures in human central corneal epithelium. *Graefes Arch Clin Exp Ophthalmol* 1982;218(1):14–20.

47. Albietz JM, Lenton LM, McLennan SG. Effect of laser *in situ* keratomileusis for hyperopia on tear film and ocular surface. *J Refract Surg* 2002;18(2):113–123.

48. Battat L, Macri A, Dursun D, et al. Effects of laser *in situ* keratomileusis on tear production, clearance, and the ocular surface. *Ophthalmology* 2001;108(7):1230–1235.

49. Davidorf JM. LASIK and dry eye. *Ophthalmology* 2002; 109(11):1948–1949; author reply 1949.

50. Linna TU, Vesaluoma MH, Perez-Santonja JJ, et al. Effect of myopic LASIK on corneal sensitivity and morphology of subbasal nerves. *Invest Ophthalmol Vis Sci* 2000;41(2):393–397.

51. Linna TU, Perez-Santonja JJ, Tervo KM, et al. Recovery of corneal nerve morphology following laser *in situ* keratomileusis. *Exp Eye Res* 1998;66(6):755–763.

52. Wilson SE. Laser in situ keratomileusis-induced (presumed) neurotrophic epitheliopathy. *Ophthalmology* 2001;108(6):1082–1087.

53. You L, Kruse FE, Volcker HE. Neurotrophic factors in the human cornea. *Invest Ophthalmol Vis Sci* 2000;41(3):692–702.

54. Toda I, Asano-Kato N, Komai-Hori Y, et al. Dry eye after laser *in situ* keratomileusis. *Am J Ophthalmol* 2001;132(1):1–7.

55. Nassaralla BA, McLeod SD, Nassaralla JJ Jr. Effect of myopic LASIK on human corneal sensitivity. *Ophthalmology* 2003;110(3): 497–502.

56. Chang-Ling T, Vannas A, Holden BA, et al. Incision depth affects the recovery of corneal sensitivity and neural regeneration in the cat. *Invest Ophthalmol Vis Sci* 1990;31(8):1533–1541.

57. Kim WS, Kim JS. Change in corneal sensitivity following laser *in situ* keratomileusis. *J Cataract Refract Surg* 1999;25(3):368–373.

58. Tervo K, Latvala TM, Tervo TM. Recovery of corneal innervation following photorefractive keratoablation. *Arch Ophthalmol* 1994;112(11):1466–1470.

59. Perez-Santonja JJ, Sakla HF, Cardona C, et al. Corneal sensitivity after photorefractive keratectomy and laser *in situ* keratomileusis for low myopia. *Am J Ophthalmol* 1999;127(5):497–504.

60. Smith RJ, Maloney RK. Diffuse lamellar keratitis. A new syndrome in lamellar refractive surgery. *Ophthalmology* 1998; 105(9):1721–1726.

61. Chung MS, Pepose JS, El-Agha MS, et al. Confocal microscopic findings in a case of delayed-onset bilateral diffuse lamellar keratitis after laser *in situ* keratomileusis. *J Cataract Refract Surg* 2002;28(8):1467–1470.

62. Haw WW, Manche EE. Late onset diffuse lamellar keratitis associated with an epithelial defect in six eyes. *J Refract Surg* 2000; 16(6):744–748.

63. Yeoh J, Moshegov CN. Delayed diffuse lamellar keratitis after laser *in situ* keratomileusis. *Clin Exp Ophthalmol* 2001;29(6):435–437.

64. Weisenthal RW. Diffuse lamellar keratitis induced by trauma 6 months after laser *in situ* keratomileusis. *J Refract Surg* 2000; 16(6):749–751.

65. Chang-Godinich A, Steinert RF, Wu HK. Late occurrence of diffuse lamellar keratitis after laser *in situ* keratomileusis. *Arch Ophthalmol* 2001;119(7):1074–1076.

66. Aldave AJ, Hollander DA, Abbott RL. Late-onset traumatic flap dislocation and diffuse lamellar inflammation after laser *in situ* keratomileusis. *Cornea* 2002;21(6):604–607.

67. Yuhan KR, Nguyen L, Wachler BS. Role of instrument cleaning and maintenance in the development of diffuse lamellar keratitis. *Ophthalmology* 2002;109(2):400–404.

68. Johnson JD, Harissi-Dagher M, Pineda R, et al. Diffuse lamellar keratitis: incidence, associations, outcomes, and a new classification system. *J Cataract Refract Surg* 2001;27(10):1560–1566.

69. Samuel MA, Kaufman SC, Ahee JA, et al. Diffuse lamellar keratitis associated with carboxymethylcellulose sodium 1% after laser *in situ* keratomileusis. *J Cataract Refract Surg* 2002;28(8):1409–1411.

70. Nakano EM, Nakano K, Oliveira MC, et al. Cleaning solutions as a cause of diffuse lamellar keratitis. *J Refract Surg* 2002;18(3 suppl):S361–S363.

71. Peters NT, Iskander NG, Anderson Penno EE, et al. Diffuse lamellar keratitis: isolation of endotoxin and demonstration of the inflammatory potential in a rabbit laser *in situ* keratomileusis model. *J Cataract Refract Surg* 2001;27(6):917–923.

72. Holland SP, Mathias RG, Morck DW, et al. Diffuse lamellar keratitis related to endotoxins released from sterilizer reservoir biofilms. *Ophthalmology* 2000;107(7):1227–1233; discussion 1233–1234.

73. Wilson SE, Ambrosio R Jr. Sporadic diffuse lamellar keratitis (DLK) after LASIK. *Cornea* 2002;21(6):560–563.

74. Buhren J, Baumeister M, Cichocki M, et al. Confocal microscopic characteristics of stage 1 to 4 diffuse lamellar keratitis after laser *in situ* keratomileusis. *J Cataract Refract Surg* 2002;28(8):1390–1399.

75. MacRae SM, Rich LF, Macaluso DC. Treatment of interface keratitis with oral corticosteroids. *J Cataract Refract Surg* 2002; 28(3):454–461.

76. Parolini B, Marcon G, Panozzo GA. Central necrotic lamellar inflammation after laser *in situ* keratomileusis. *J Refract Surg* 2001;17(2):110–112.

77. Karp CL, Tuli SS, Yoo SH, et al. Infectious keratitis after LASIK. *Ophthalmology* 2003;110(3):503–510.

78. Freitas D, Alvarenga L, Sampaio J, et al. An outbreak of Mycobacterium chelonae infection after LASIK. *Ophthalmology* 2003;110(2):276–285.

79. Winthrop KL, Steinberg EB, Holmes G, et al. Epidemic and sporadic cases of nontuberculous mycobacterial keratitis associated with laser *in situ* keratomileusis. *Am J Ophthalmol* 2003; 135(2):223–224.

80. Fulcher SF, Fader RC, Rosa RH Jr, et al. Delayed-onset mycobacterial keratitis after LASIK. *Cornea* 2002;21(6):546–554.

81. Alvarenga L, Freitas D, Hofling-Lima AL, et al. Infectious post-LASIK crystalline keratopathy caused by nontuberculous mycobacteria. *Cornea* 2002;21(4):426–429.

82. Holmes GP, Bond GB, Fader RC, et al. A Cluster of cases of Mycobacterium szulgai keratitis that occurred after laser-assisted *in situ* keratomileusis. *Clin Infect Dis* 2002;34(8):1039–1046.

83. Seo KY, Lee JB, Lee K, et al. Non-tuberculous mycobacterial keratitis at the interface after laser *in situ* keratomileusis. *J Refract Surg* 2002;18(1):81–85.

84. Solomon A, Karp CL, Miller D, et al. Mycobacterium interface keratitis after laser *in situ* keratomileusis. *Ophthalmology* 2001;108(12):2201–2208.

85. Garg P, Bansal AK, Sharma S, et al. Bilateral infectious keratitis after laser *in situ* keratomileusis: a case report and review of the literature. *Ophthalmology* 2001;108(1):121–125.

86. Reviglio V, Rodriguez ML, Picotti GS, et al. Mycobacterium chelonae keratitis following laser *in situ* keratomileusis. *J Refract Surg* 1998;14(3):357–360.

87. Chandra NS, Torres MF, Winthrop KL, et al. Cluster of Mycobacterium chelonae keratitis cases following laser *in situ* keratomileusis. *Am J Ophthalmol* 2001;132(6):819–830.

88. Dugel PU, Holland GN, Brown HH, et al. Mycobacterium fortuitum keratitis. *Am J Ophthalmol* 1988;105(6):661–669.

89. Zimmerman LE, Turner L, McTigue JW. Mycobacterium fortuitum infection of the cornea. A report of to cases. *Arch Ophthalmol* 1969;82(5):596–601.

90. Goldstein MH, Kowalski RP, Gordon YJ. Emerging fluoroquinolone resistance in bacterial keratitis: a 5-year review. *Ophthalmology* 1999;106(7):1313–1318.

91. Smith A, Pennefather PM, Kaye SB, et al. Fluoroquinolones: place in ocular therapy. *Drugs* 2001;61(6):747–761.

91a. Tungsiripat T, Sarayba MA, Kaufman MB, et al. Fluoroquinolone therapy in multiple-drug resistant Staphylococcal keratitis after lamellar keratectomy in a rabbit model. *Am J Ophthalmol* 2003;*in press.*

92. Asano-Kato N, Toda I, Hori-Komai Y, et al. Epithelial ingrowth after laser *in situ* keratomileusis: clinical features and possible mechanisms. *Am J Ophthalmol* 2002; 134(6): 801–807.

93. Wang MY, Maloney RK. Epithelial ingrowth after laser *in situ* keratomileusis. *Am J Ophthalmol* 2000;129(6):746–751.

94. Gimbel HV, Penno EA. Late postoperative complications. In: Penno EA, ed. *LASIK complications: prevention and management,* 2nd ed. Thorofare, NJ: Slack, 2001.

95. Domniz Y, Comaish IF, Lawless MA, et al. Epithelial ingrowth: causes, prevention, and treatment in 5 cases. *J Cataract Refract Surg* 2001;27(11):1803–1811.

96. Carpel EF, Carlson KH, Shannon S. Fine lattice lines on the corneal surface after laser *in situ* keratomileusis (LASIK). *Am J Ophthalmol* 2000;129(3):379–380.

97. Charman WN. Mismatch between flap and stromal areas after laser *in situ* keratomileusis as source of flap striae. *J Cataract Refract Surg* 2002;28(12):2146–2152.

98. Rabinowitz YS, Rasheed K. Fluorescein test for the detection of striae in the corneal flap after laser *in situ* keratomileusis. *Am J Ophthalmol* 1999;127(6):717–718.

99. Probst LE, Machat J. Removal of flap striae following laser *in situ* keratomileusis. *J Cataract Refract Surg* 1998;24(2):153–155.

100. Hernandez-Matamoros J, Iradier MT, Moreno E. Treating folds and striae after laser *in situ* keratomileusis. *J Cataract Refract Surg* 2001;27(3):350–352.

101. Tehrani M, Dick HB. [Striae in the flap after laser *in situ* keratomileusis. Etiology, diagnosis and treatment]. *Ophthalmologe* 2002;99(8):645–650.

102. von Kulajta P, Stark WJ, O'Brien TP. Management of flap striae. *Int Ophthalmol Clin* 2000;40(3):87–92.

103. Artola A, Ayala MJ, Perez-Santonja JJ, et al. Haze after laser *in situ* keratomileusis in eyes with previous photorefractive keratectomy. *J Cataract Refract Surg* 2001;27(11):1880–1883.

104. Carones F, Vigo L, Carones AV, et al. Evaluation of photorefractive keratectomy retreatments after regressed myopic laser *in situ* keratomileusis. *Ophthalmology* 2001;108(10):1732–1737.

105. Koch DD. The riddle of iatrogenic keratectasia. *J Cataract Refract Surg* 1999;25(4):453–454.

106. Comaish IF, Lawless MA. Progressive post-LASIK keratectasia: biomechanical instability or chronic disease process? *J Cataract Refract Surg* 2002;28(12):2206–2213.

107. Randleman JB, Russell B, Ward MA, et al. Risk factors and prognosis for corneal ectasia after LASIK. *Ophthalmology* 2003;110(2):267–275.

108. Schmitt-Bernard CF, Lesage C, Arnaud B. Keratectasia induced by laser *in situ* keratomileusis in keratoconus. *J Refract Surg* 2000;16(3):368–370.

109. Amoils SP, Deist MB, Gous P, et al. Iatrogenic keratectasia after laser *in situ* keratomileusis for less than −4.0 to −7.0 diopters of myopia. *J Cataract Refract Surg* 2000;26(7):967–977.

110. Lafond G, Bazin R, Lajoie C. Bilateral severe keratoconus after laser *in situ* keratomileusis in a patient with forme fruste keratoconus. *J Cataract Refract Surg* 2001;27(7):1115–1118.

111. Geggel HS, Talley AR. Delayed onset keratectasia following laser *in situ* keratomileusis. *J Cataract Refract Surg* 1999;25(4):582–586.

112. McLeod SD, Kisla TA, Caro NC, et al. Iatrogenic keratoconus: corneal ectasia following laser *in situ* keratomileusis for myopia. *Arch Ophthalmol* 2000;118(2):282–284.

113. Seiler T, Koufala K, Richter G. Iatrogenic keratectasia after laser *in situ* keratomileusis. *J Refract Surg* 1998;14(3):312–317.

114. Seiler T, Quurke AW. Iatrogenic keratectasia after LASIK in a case of forme fruste keratoconus. *J Cataract Refract Surg* 1998;24(7):1007–1009.

115. Joo CK, Kim TG. Corneal ectasia detected after laser *in situ* keratomileusis for correction of less than -12 diopters of myopia. *J Cataract Refract Surg* 2000;26(2):292–295.

116. Argento C, Cosentino MJ, Tytiun A, et al. Corneal ectasia after laser *in situ* keratomileusis. *J Cataract Refract Surg* 2001; 27(9):1440–1448.

117. Machat JJ. *Excimer laser refractive surgery: practice and principles.* Thorofare, NJ: Slack, 1996:300.

118. Barraquer J. *Queratomileusis y Queratofaquia.* Bogota: Instituto Barraquer de America, 1980.

119. Andreassen TT, Simonsen AH, Oxlund H. Biomechanical properties of keratoconus and normal corneas. *Exp Eye Res* 1980;31(4):435–441.

120. Jacobs BJ, Deutsch TA, Rubenstein JB. Reproducibility of corneal flap thickness in LASIK. *Ophthalmic Surg Lasers* 1999;30(5):350–335.

121. Yildirim R, Aras C, Ozdamar A, et al. Reproducibility of corneal flap thickness in laser *in situ* keratomileusis using the Hansatome microkeratome. *J Cataract Refract Surg* 2000; 26(12):1729–1732.

122. Durairaj VD, Balentine J, Kouyoumdjian G, et al. The predictability of corneal flap thickness and tissue laser ablation in laser *in situ* keratomileusis. *Ophthalmology* 2000;107(12):2140–2143.

123. Rabinowitz YS, McDonnell PJ. Computer-assisted corneal topography in keratoconus. *Refract Corneal Surg* 1989;5(6):400–408.

124. Maeda N, Klyce SD, Smolek MK. Comparison of methods for detecting keratoconus using videokeratography. *Arch Ophthalmol* 1995;113(7):870–874.

125. Sanborn GE, Friberg TR, Allen R. Optic nerve dysfunction during gravity inversion. Visual field abnormalities. *Arch Ophthalmol* 1987;105(6):774–776.

126. Friberg TR, Sanborn G, Weinreb RN. Intraocular and episcleral venous pressure increase during inverted posture. *Am J Ophthalmol* 1987;103(4):523–526.

127. Schuman JS, Massicotte EC. Author's reply. *Ophthalmology* 2000;107(7):1221–1222.

128. Schuman JS, Massicotte EC, Connolly S, et al. Increased intraocular pressure and visual field defects in high resistance wind instrument players. *Ophthalmology* 2000;107(1):127–133.

129. Hamilton DR, Manche EE, Rich LF, et al. Steroid-induced glaucoma after laser *in situ* keratomileusis associated with interface fluid. *Ophthalmology* 2002;109(4):659–665.

130. Gimeno JA, Munoz LA, Valenzuela LA, et al. Influence of refraction on tonometric readings after photorefractive keratectomy and laser assisted *in situ* keratomileusis. *Cornea* 2000;19(4):512–516.

131. El Danasoury MA, El Maghraby A, Coorpender SJ. Change in intraocular pressure in myopic eyes measured with contact and non-contact tonometers after laser *in situ* keratomileusis. *J Refract Surg* 2001;17(2):97–104.

132. Park HJ, Uhm KB, Hong C. Reduction in intraocular pressure after laser *in situ* keratomileusis. *J Cataract Refract Surg* 2001;27(2):303–309.

133. Kook MS, Lee S, Tchah H, et al. Effect of laser *in situ* keratomileusis on retinal nerve fiber layer thickness measurements by scanning laser polarimetry. *J Cataract Refract Surg* 2002;28(4):670–675.

134. Arevalo JF, Ramirez E, Suarez E, et al. Incidence of vitreoretinal pathologic conditions within 24 months after laser *in situ* keratomileusis. *Ophthalmology* 2000;107(2):258–262.

135. Ozdamar A, Aras C, Sener B, et al. Bilateral retinal detachment associated with giant retinal tear after laser-assisted *in situ* keratomileusis. *Retina* 1998;18(2):176–177.

136. Mansour AM, Ojeimi GK. Premacular subhyaloid hemorrhage following laser *in situ* keratomileusis. *J Refract Surg* 2000; 16(3):371–372.

137. Ellies P, Le Rouic JF, Dighiero P, et al. Macular hemorrhage after LASIK for high myopia: a causal association? *J Cataract Refract Surg* 2001;27(7):966–967.

138. Hanson RL, Imperatore G, Bennett PH, et al. Components of the "metabolic syndrome" and incidence of type 2 diabetes. *Diabetes* 2002;51(10):3120–3127.

139. Fraunfelder FW, Rich LF. Laser-assisted *in situ* keratomileusis complications in diabetes mellitus. *Cornea* 2002;21(3):246–248.

140. Hemady RK. Microbial keratitis in patients infected with the human immunodeficiency virus. *Ophthalmology* 1995; 102(7):1026–1030.

141. Hovanesian JA, Faktorovich EG, Hoffbauer JD, et al. Bilateral bacterial keratitis after laser *in situ* keratomileusis in a patient with human immunodeficiency virus infection. *Arch Ophthalmol* 1999;117(7):968–970.

142. Hagen KB, Kettering JD, Aprecio RM, et al. Lack of virus transmission by the excimer laser plume. *Am J Ophthalmol* 1997;124:206–211.

143. Moreira LB, Sanchez D, Trousdale MD, et al. Aerosolization of infectious virus by excimer laser. *Am J Ophthalmol* 1997; 123:297–302.

ULTRASHORT PULSED LASERS IN CORNEAL APPLICATIONS

RONALD M. KURTZ, MELVIN A. SARAYBA, AND TIBOR JUHASZ

CORNEAL PHOTODISRUPTION

The mechanism of photodisruption in the cornea is similar to that in other materials, beginning with a process termed laser-induced optical breakdown (LIOB). In LIOB, a strongly focused, short-duration laser pulse generates a high-intensity electric field, leading to the formation of a mixture of free electrons and ions called a plasma (1). The plasma expands with supersonic velocity, rapidly cooling and displacing surrounding tissue (2–5). As the plasma expansion slows, the supersonic displacement front propagates through the tissue as a shock wave. The shock wave loses energy and velocity as it propagates, ultimately relaxing to an ordinary acoustic wave (6). Because adiabatic expansion of the plasma occurs on a time scale that is short in comparison to the time required for heat transfer, thermal effects are minimized or avoided. The cooling plasma vaporizes a small volume of corneal tissue, forming a cavitation bubble that consists mainly of CO_2, N_2, and H_2O (7).

The specific characteristics of photodisruption depend primarily on the pulse duration, pulse energy, and focusing geometry of a particular laser system. Until recently, ophthalmic photodisruption was limited to a few intraocular procedures, such as iridotomy and capsulotomy, due to the relatively large energies needed to initiate LIOB with available nanosecond pulse-duration neodymium:yttrium-aluminum-garnet (Nd:YAG) lasers (8). The resulting large shock waves and cavitation bubbles produce significant collateral tissue effects. Reducing either the focal spot size or the pulse duration of the laser decreases the threshold energy required for LIOB (2–6,9). Although a smaller spot size can be achieved with a large focusing angle, this makes scanning systems for delivery of pulses over large areas (such as the cornea) impractical. Alternatively, the laser pulse duration can be decreased from the nanosecond (10^{-9} sec) to the femtosecond regime (10^{-15} sec).

In contrast to the nanosecond systems, femtosecond laser photodisruption requires lower laser energy, minimizing collateral tissue effects that scale with energy. Photodisruptive shock wave size (radial propagation distance to decay to an acoustic wave) and cavitation size (maximum bubble radius) for pulses in the few hundred femtoseconds range are significantly smaller than those generated by picosecond (10^{-12} sec) and nanosecond pulses. The small amount of energy deposited in tissue and the rapid (faster than 1 μs) adiabatic plasma expansion prevent significant heat transfer to surrounding tissue. Narrow collateral tissue damage zones have been demonstrated in cadaver corneal tissue with femtosecond photodisruption (10,11).

The cornea presents an attractive target for femtosecond laser surgical applications because its superficial location and transparency make it easily accessible to femtosecond pulses with negligible nonlinear focusing effects. To be used for high-precision cutting applications, multiple laser pulses can be placed contiguously to create incision planes within the cornea in nearly any orientation (horizontal, vertical, or oblique; Fig. 83-1). The only limitation to creating arbitrary incision planes is that pulses must be delivered in a deep to superficial order, because the cavitations bubbles created can block the optical path to deeper tissue. Intersecting these resection planes can create complex shapes. The lack of vascular structures in the cornea is another benefit of working in this tissue, because photodisruptive lasers do not coagulate blood vessels.

COMMERCIAL SYSTEMS

The IntraLase FS (IntraLase Corp., Irvine, CA) is currently the only clinically available femtosecond laser surgical system. It consists of a high repetition rate (10–15 kilohertz), femtosecond laser source, and precision scanning delivery system that allows creation of uniform lamellar resections within a diameter of approximately 10 mm and to a depth of 500 μm (Fig. 83-2). To attain depth reproducibility in the 10 μm range, the system utilizes an applanation lens to temporarily flatten the anterior surface of the cornea. The surgeon first fixes the eye's position with a limbal suction

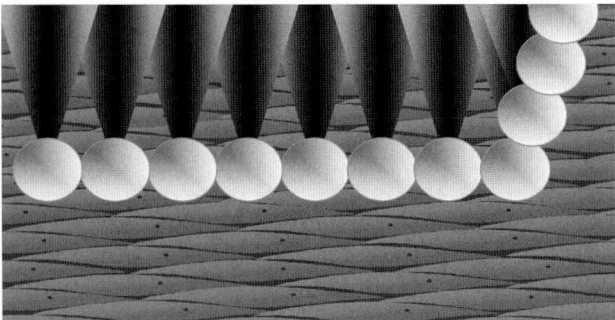

FIGURE 83-1. Laser pulses are delivered contiguously to create a resection. Orientation can be horizontal, vertical, or oblique.

ring and then places the applanating lens, securing it via an internal clamp. This process mechanically couples the eye to the beam delivery system, thereby maintaining a fixed reference distance from the laser's focusing objective (Fig. 83-3).

The IntraLase FS has received Food and Drug Administration (FDA) clearance for four surgical indications: creation of a hinged LASIK flap, anterior lamellar keratoplasty, channel formation for intracorneal ring segments, and *in-situ* keratomileusis for the correction of myopia. Several additional applications are under development, including posterior lamellar keratoplasty and so-called intrastromal refractive procedures.

CREATION OF LASIK FLAP

Rationale

LASIK's dominance in refractive surgery results from its rapid visual rehabilitation, minimal postoperative discomfort, and high predictability, all of which can be linked to creation of a corneal flap that avoids significant disturbance of the epithelial surface (11–13). Although primarily responsible for these advantages, the flap is also the main source of vision-threatening LASIK complications such as free caps; globe perforation; incomplete or irregular flaps; and thin, thick, and buttonhole flaps. Flap-related LASIK complications occur in as many as 8.8% of cases

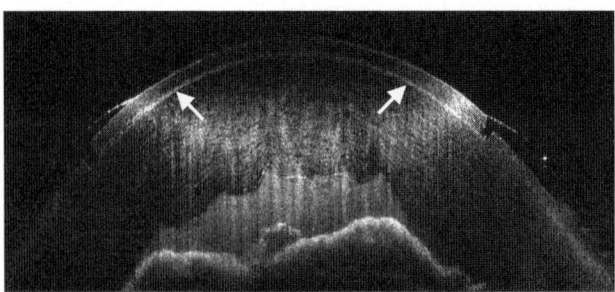

FIGURE 83-2. A uniform planar cut *(arrows)* with sharp edges is demonstrated on a cadaver eye using optical coherence tomography.

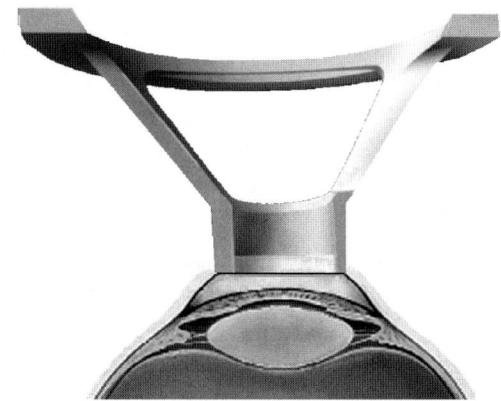

FIGURE 83-3. The applanating cone with a fixed distance from the laser head is coupled to the eye to assure depth accuracy.

(14–17). Even when performed without complication, mechanical flap creation has been associated with significantly nonuniform resections, which may influence refractive outcomes (18).

Femtosecond Laser Surgical Technique

A LASIK flap is created by scanning a pattern of laser pulses (approximately 500,000 to 800,000) at a desired depth parallel to the applanated corneal surface. After the resection plane is created, a side cut is made by advancing the laser toward the surface in a circular pattern. A hinge can be placed at any meridian by blocking the beam for a short time during each circle pass. When the laser reaches the surface, gas bubbles escape from the interface and the suction is released. The flap can then be elevated for excimer laser ablation, similar to traditional LASIK with the mechanical microkeratome. Both spiral (circular) and raster (X-Y) scan patterns (Figs. 83-4 and 83-5) can be used to create the planar cut. In addition, a reservoir (termed a "pocket") can be formed outside of the planar cut to create a drainage channel for cavitation bubbles, thereby reducing the spread of gas into the stroma. The most common method now used for flap creation utilizes the raster scan pattern and reservoir depicted in Fig. 83-6.

Early Clinical Studies

In cadaver eye studies (19), excellent reproducibility was identified for key flap parameters such as thickness (standard deviation 12 μm) and diameter (standard deviation 200 μm). Initial human flap resections performed in 46 eyes in 1999 and 2000 (19,20) demonstrated no significant intraoperative complications. Suction and/or applanation were lost during the procedure in several eyes; however, all such cases underwent a subsequent successful procedure on the same or next surgical day (within 24 hours). No postoperative inflammation, diffuse lamellar

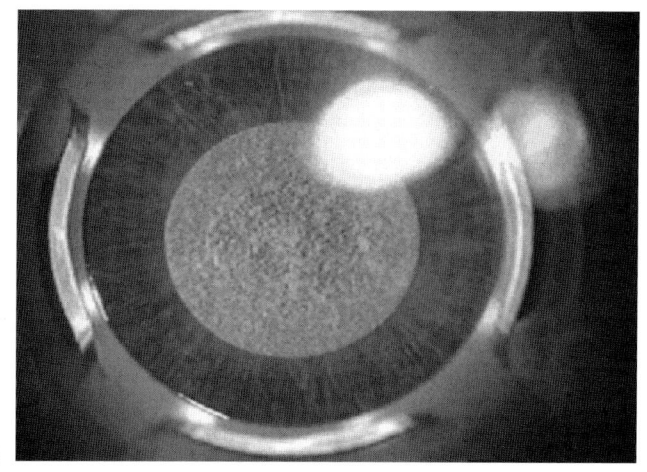
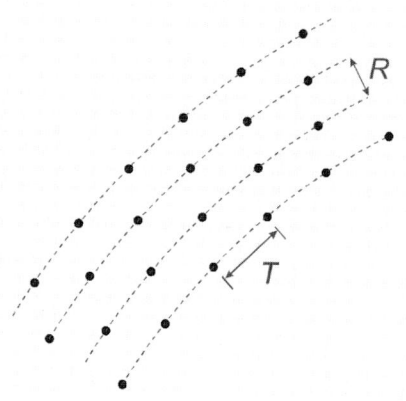

FIGURE 83-4. A: Lamellar resection is performed using a circular pattern. **B:** A schematic diagram of the pattern.

keratitis, or flap dislocations were observed and none of the eyes experienced a loss of more than one line of best spectacle-corrected visual acuity (BSCVA).

Initial U.S. Clinical Series

The initial U.S. clinical series was completed between June and October 2000 (21), with follow-up through 2001. A total of 208 procedures were performed by two surgeons using a first-generation femtosecond laser model to create the corneal flap and either a VISX S2 or Technolas 217 for excimer ablation. Complications included loss of suction in 4 eyes (1.9%), all of which were successfully completed after a delay of 5 to 45 minutes. Postoperative flap complications such as striae, dislocation/slippage, diffuse lamellar keratitis, and epithelial downgrowth were not seen in this series, and no change in the standard LASIK nomograms of each surgeon was required. All eyes in the low myopia group (less than −3 D) were within one diopter of emetropia, whereas 95% were within 0.5 D. All of the low myopia eyes achieved uncorrected visual acuity (UCVA) of 20/30 or better at 6 months, without benefit of any retreatments. For the moderate myopia group (−3 to −6 D), 96% were within one diopter of emetropia, whereas 96% achieved UCVA of 20/40 or better. In the high myopia group (greater than −6 D), 95% of eyes were within

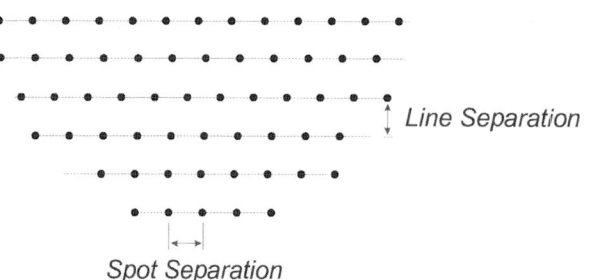

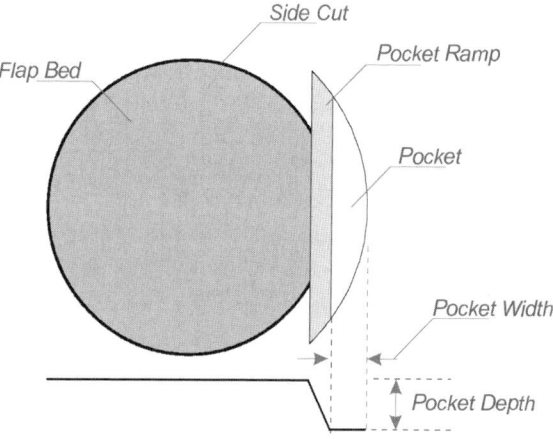

FIGURE 83-5. A: Lamellar resection is performed using a raster pattern. **B:** A schematic diagram of the pattern.

FIGURE 83-6. A schematic diagram of the raster pattern with a reservoir to eliminate the dispersion of deposited bubbles into the cornea.

one diopter of emetropia, whereas 92% achieved UCVA of 20/40 or better.

Clinical Experience Following U.S. Commercial Introduction

In the 2-year period since U.S. commercial introduction in early 2002, over 100,000 LASIK procedures have been completed using the IntraLase FS for flap creation at over 100 clinical sites. Several clinical reports have been made at national meetings and are beginning to appear in the literature. The following subsections summarize the clinical observations.

Flap Reproducibility

Binder (22,23) reported on the reproducibility of flap parameters, as well as the incidence of complications. He noted standard deviations for flap thickness from 12 to 18 μm and for flap diameter from 120 to 260 μm. Chayet (24a) also reported a standard deviation of approximately 15 μm in 30 eyes with an intended flap thickness of 130 μm. When compared to standard mechanical microkeratomes, this nearly twofold reduction in standard deviation reduces the upper range (two standard deviation level) of achieved flap thickness from approximately 60 μm greater than intended to less than 30 μm (24–29). Put another way, on average 1 in 40 blade flaps will be at least 60 μm greater than the mean flap thickness for a particular blade keratome, whereas only 1 in 4,000 flaps created with the femtosecond laser system reaches this level.

Flexibility of Flap Architecture

The femtosecond laser allows surgeons to customize flap thickness, diameter, hinge position, hinge angle, and side cut angle. The clinical advantages of particular flap architectures have yet to be evaluated comprehensively.

Induced Astigmatism

Several clinical reports have noted a reduction in induced astigmatism when compared with historical LASIK controls performed with standard keratomes (29a,29b,30). This observation was also made in a prospective randomized study comparing femtosecond laser and standard keratome flaps in fellow eyes in which the excimer ablation was delayed for 2 months (30a). Significantly more lower order aberrations, primarily induced cylinder, were noted in the standard keratome treated eyes, suggesting that differences in flap architecture (such as the full bed laser cut versus partial, mechanical cut) might be clinically relevant.

Epithelial Defects

There have been several reports of statistically significant lower rates of epithelial defects in initial case series of femtosecond laser cases than in the historical comparative LASIK population that used a mechanical keratome (30,30b,30c). The lack of moving parts over the surface of the cornea is the likely etiology of this difference.

Dry Eye

Approximately 4% of LASIK patients develop a prolonged dry eye syndrome that is now linked to the transection of corneal nerves and loss of superficial corneal innervation (31–34). Christenbury (30b) has reported significant differences in dry-eye complaints between patients undergoing standard LASIK and femtosecond laser procedures. In this retrospective review of 600 cases in each group, there was a reduction in dry-eye complaints from over 50% to 15% after conversion to the femtosecond laser system. In a prospective study of eight patients (16 eyes), one eye underwent corneal flap creation by a standard microkeratome, whereas the fellow eye underwent corneal flap creation by the femtosecond laser keratome. Intended flap thickness, hinge position, and flap diameter were matched to be similar. In all patients, corneal sensitivity (measured using a Cochet-Bonnet esthesiometer) was significantly more depressed within the margins of the standard microkeratome-created flap than one created by the femtosecond laser system, in which corneal sensitivity was nearly at normal levels. It was postulated that the femtosecond laser, due to its ability to create a uniformly thin and a precisely sized corneal flap, may transect peripheral corneal nerve fibers after they have undergone more branching or lost their nerve sheath, possibly decreasing dry-eye symptoms associated with standard LASIK in some patients.

Dislodged/Slipped Flaps

In data from a porcine eye model, increased flap thickness, side cut angle, and hinge angle were all associated with increased stability (greater force required to displace the flap). Despite these findings, several surgeons reported an increased risk of flap slippage if certain topical agents (such as phenylephrine) are used after the corneal flap is made (Will B, Binder P, personal communication). Entry of topical medications through the flap edge (where the epithelial barrier is broken) may cause endothelial dysfunction and loss of adherence.

Summary

Femtosecond laser flap creation is a promising technique that improves the accuracy and reproducibility of this first step in LASIK. The impact of these attributes (as well as its increased architectural flexibility) on the safety and effectiveness of the LASIK procedure continue to be evaluated.

OTHER CORNEAL SURGICAL APPLICATIONS

Anterior and Posterior Lamellar Keratoplasty

Potential clinical advantages of anterior lamellar keratoplasty over penetrating keratoplasty include no endothelial rejection risk, superior wound integrity, less stringent donor tissue requirements (use of donor corneas with poor-quality endothelium), and reduced incidence of high refractive errors and topographic distortion. The major disadvantages are the technical difficulty of the current manual procedure and reduced quality of vision, both of which have limited the number of annual lamellar procedures performed in the U.S. to less than a few thousand (35–38).

The availability of automated microkeratomes and the development of the artificial anterior chamber that can allow use of corneoscleral rim donor tissue have improved this procedure (39–44). Although easier to use, these automated devices still demonstrate poor cap thickness and diameter predictability, especially at greater depths (45), making it difficult to match the recipient bed with the donor tissue.

Although the femtosecond laser keratome would appear to offer better potential for matching host and donor resection dimensions, there have been few clinical reports of the procedure (45a). Importantly, a recent *ex vivo* study has shown that corneal opacities do not represent a significant limitation (45b). Deep lamellar resection could readily be created in cadaver corneas with significant (grade 4) chemically induced corneal opacity by altering the laser pulse energy and spot separation.

Femtosecond laser techniques analogous to mechanical procedures such as deep lamellar endokeratoplasty (46,47) are now being developed and tested. Potential advantages over current techniques include small wound size and reduced operative complexity.

Intracorneal Ring Segments Channel

Intracorneal ring segments (ICRS), an implantable device for the correction of low spherical myopia (48), has not gained widespread clinical acceptance since clearance by the FDA in 1996. More recent application to therapeutic applications, such as in keratoconus, has revived some interest in the technology (49). The femtosecond laser may reduce some of the complications and variations associated with traditional intercorneal ring segment (ICRS) implantation techniques (20). Because laser energy is delivered optically to a precise depth, using a precalibrated and preassembled disposable contact lens, tunnel resections and entry cuts may be highly reproducible, with essentially no risk of corneal perforation. The surgeon can select the meridional location of the entry cut, as well as its length, allowing implantation geometries different from the traditional nasal/temporal ring orientation (Fig. 83-7).

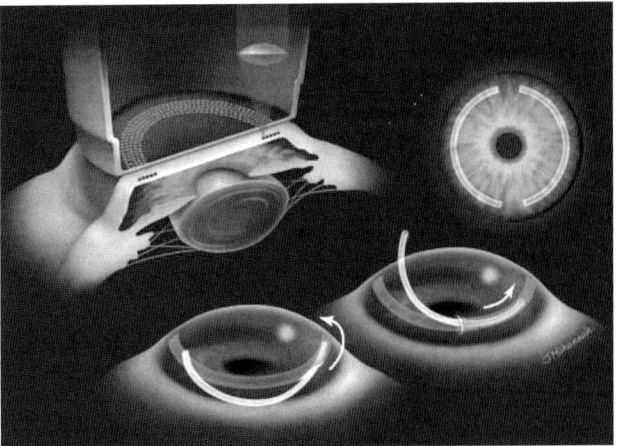

FIGURE 83-7. A schematic diagram of intracorneal ring segment (ICRS) channel creation using the femtosecond laser.

Stand-Alone Femtosecond Refractive Procedures

Two refractive procedures that utilize the femtosecond laser to remove corneal tissue and reshape the corneal surface continue to be investigated:

Femtosecond Laser Keratomileusis

A small clinical case series has been reported in which a lens-shaped stromal lenticule was outlined by the femtosecond laser and then manually removed via a laser created flap. Analogous to mechanically performed automated lamellar keratomileusis (ALK), this procedure resects both surfaces of the lenticule during the same applanation, greatly increasing its precision. In five amblyopic eyes undergoing femtosecond laser keratomileusis, mild corneal edema occurred during the first 2 postoperative days. Centration of the procedures was excellent and large myopic corrections were produced, with UCVA better than preoperative BSCVA in all patients. Corneal transparency was reported to be maintained, with good refractive stability (20).

Intrastromal Refractive Procedures

First proposed in the early 1990s with both the nanosecond Nd:YAG and the picosecond neodymium:yttrium-lithium-fluoride (Nd:YLF) lasers, this is a purely intrastromal refractive surgery that could eliminate the need for any incision or surface disruption of the cornea. However, in early picosecond laser myopic intrastromal clinical trials, refractive effects could not be reliably produced (50,51).

In vivo testing in rabbits of intrastromal femtosecond laser photodisruption was aimed at evaluating effects on corneal wound healing and transparency (52). No significant corneal or intraocular inflammation was seen on slit-lamp examination, despite the minimal use of topical antiinflammatories. Histologic results revealed eosinophilic staining in the areas treated, with surrounding areas of apoptosis, similar to reactions to excimer laser procedures. A recent report on procedures performed in partially sighted eyes to correct low hyperopia revealed that refractive results were stable by the first month, achieving a mean correction of +2 D. Additional human clinical trials are ongoing.

DISCUSSION

The femtosecond laser is a new, high-precision, programmable surgical tool that enables a number of currently available and future corneal procedures. Although it has been most extensively used to create LASIK flaps, a number of additional corneal applications are being developed and investigated. Its increasing dissemination should make it available for use by future generations of corneal surgeons.

REFERENCES

1. Bloembergen N. Laser-induced electric breakdown in Solids. *IEEE JQE* 1974;10:375–386.
2. Fujimoto JG, Lin WZ, Ippen EP, et al. Time-resolved studies of Nd:YAG laser-induced breakdown. *Invest Ophthalmol Vis Sci* 1985;26:1771–1777.
3. Zysset B, Fujimoto JG, Deutsch TF. Time resolved measurements of picosecond optical breakdown. *Appl Phys* 1989;B48:139–147.
4. Vogel A, Hentschel W, Holzfuss J, et al. Cavitation bubble dynamics and acoustic transient generation in ocular surgery with pulsed Nd:YAG laser. *Ophthalmology* 1986;93:1259–1269.
5. Glezer EN, Scaffer CB, Nishimura N, et al. Minimally disruptive laser induced breakdown in water. *Optics Letters* 1997;23:1817.
6. Vogel A, Schweiger P, Freiser A, et al. Intraocular Nd:YAG laser surgery: light-tissue interactions, damage-range and reduction of collateral effects. *IEEE JQE* 1990;26:2240–2260.
7. Habib MS, Speaker MG, Shnatter WF. Mass spectrometry analysis of the byproducts of intrastromal photorefractive keratectomy. *Ophthalmic Surg Lasers* 1995;26;481–483.
8. Steinert R, Puliafito C. *The Nd:YAG laser in ophthalmology.* Philadelphia: WB Saunders, 1985.
9. Kurtz RM, Liu X, Elner VM, et al. Plasma-mediated ablation in human cornea as a function of laser pulse width. *J Refract Surg* 1997;13:653–658.
10. Lubatschowski H, Maatz G, Heisterkamp A, et al. Application of ultrashort laser pulses for intrastromal refractive surgery. *Graefes Arch Clin Exp Ophthalmol* 2000;238:33–39.
11. El-Maghraby A, Salah T, Waring GO 3rd, et al. Randomized bilateral comparison of excimer laser *in situ* keratomileusis and photorefractive keratectomy for 2.50 to 8.00 diopters of myopia. *Ophthalmology* 1999;106:447–457.
12. Pallikaris IG, Siganos DS. Excimer laser *in situ* keratomileusis and photorefractive keratectomy for correction of high myopia. *J Refract Corneal Surg* 1994;10:498–510.
13. Sutton G, Kalski RS, Lawless MA, et al. Excimer retreatment for scarring and regression after photorefractive keratectomy for myopia. *Br J Ophthalmol* 1995;79:756–759.
14. Pallikaris IG, Siganos DS. Excimer laser *in situ* keratomileusis and photorefractive keratectomy for correction of high myopia. *J Refract Corneal Surg* 1994;10:498–510.
15. Azar DT, Farah SG. Laser *in situ* keratomileusis versus photorefractive keratectomy: an update on indications and safety. *Ophthalmology* 1998;105:1357–1358.
16. Carr J, Stulting R, Thompson K, et al. Laser *in situ* keratomileusis. *Refract Surg* 1997;10:533–542.
17. Lin RT, Maloney RK. Flap complications associated with lamellar refractive surgery. *Am J Ophthalmol* 1999;127:129–136.
18. Reinstein DZ, Silverman RH, Raevsky T, et al. Arc-scanning very high-frequency digital ultrasound for 3 D pachymetric mapping of the corneal epithelium and stroma in laser *in situ* keratomileusis. *J Refract Surg* 2000;16:414–430.
19. Ratkay I, Juhasz T, Kiss K, et al. Ultrashort pulsed laser surgery: initial application in LASIK. *Ophthalmol Clin North Am* 2001;14:347–355.
20. Ratkay-Traub I, Ferincz IE, Juhasz T, et al. First clinical results with the femtosecond neodynium-glass laser in refractive surgery. *J Refract Surg* 2003;19:94–103.
21. Nordan LT, Slade SG, Baker RN, et al. Femtosecond laser flap creation for laser *in situ* keratomileusis: six-month follow-up of initial US clinical series. *J Refract Surg* 2003;19:8–14.
22. Binder P. The femtosecond and the flap. *Rev Refract Surg* 2003;4:37–39.
23. Binder P. Flap dimensions created with the IntraLase pulsion laser. *J Cataract Refract Surg* 2003; *submitted.*
23a. Chayet A. Depth accuracy and advanced applications with IntraLASIK. Presented at the American Academy of Ophthalmology annual meeting, 2002.
24. Behrens A, Seitz B, Langenbucher A, et al. Evaluation of corneal flap dimensions and cut quality using the automated corneal shaper microkeratome. *J Refract Surg* 2000;16:83–89.
25. Behrens A, Langenbucher A, Kus M, et al. Experimental evaluation of two current-generation automated microkeratomes: Hansatome and Supratome. *Am J Ophthalmol* 2000;129:59–67.
26. Maldonado MJ, Ruiz-Oblitas L, Munuera JM, et al. Optical coherence tomography evaluation of the corneal cap and stromal bed features after laser *in situ* keratomileusis for high myopia and astigmatism. *Ophthalmology* 2000;107:81–87.
27. Jacobs BJ, Deutsch TA, Rubenstein JB. Reproducibility of corneal flap thickness in LASIK. *Ophthalmic Surg Lasers* 1999;30:350–353.
28. Yi W-M, Joo C-K. Corneal flap thickness in laser *in situ* keratomileusis using an SCMD manual microkeratome. *J Cataract Refract Surg* 1999;25:1087–1092.
29. Yildirim R, Aras C, Ozdamar A, et al. Reproducibility of corneal flap thickness in laser *in situ* keratomileusis using the Hansatome microkeratome. *J Cataract Refract Surg* 2000;26:1729–1732.
29a. Sloane H. Comparison of clinical outcomes of mechanical and IntraLase FS laser keratectomy. Presented at the American Society of Cataract and Refractive Surgery annual meeting, 2003.
29b. Neatrour P. IntraLASIK: comparison of outcomes after adding nomogram adjustment and tracking. Presented at the American Society of Cataract and Refractive Surgery annual meeting, 2003.
30. Kezirian G, Stoneciper K. Comparison of the IntraLase femtosecond laser and mechanical keratomes for LASIK. *J Cataract Refract Surg* 2004;30:804–811.
30a. Tran D. Understanding induced wavefront aberrations with LASIK flap technology. Presented at the American Society of Cataract and Refractive Surgery annual meeting, 2003.

30b. Christenbury. Clinical results of IntraLASIK versus Hansatome created flaps. Presented at the American Academy of Ophthalmology annual meeting, 2002.

30c. Binder P. Integration of femtosecond mode laser into a refractive practice. Presented at the American Society of Cataract and Refractive Surgery annual meeting, 2003.

31. Yu EY, Leung A, Rao S, et al. Effect of laser *in situ* keratomileusis on tear stability. *Ophthalmology* 2000;107:2131–2135.

32. Chuck RS, Quiros PA, Perez AC, et al. Corneal sensation after laser *in situ* keratomileusis. *J Cataract Refract Surg* 2000; 26:337–339.

33. Toda I, Asano-Kato N, Komai-Hori Y, et al. Dry eye after laser *in situ* keratomileusis. *Am J Ophthalmol* 2001;132:1–7.

34. Donnenfeld ED, Solomon K, Perry HD, et al. The effect of hinge position on corneal sensation and dry eye after LASIK. *Ophthalmology* 2003;110:1023–1030.

35. Huang SC, Wu SC, Wu WC, et al. Microbial keratitis—a late complication of penetrating keratoplasty. *Trans R Soc Trop Med Hyg* 2000;94:315–317.

36. Merchant A, Zacks CM, Wilhelmus K, et al. Candidal endophthalmitis after keratoplasty. *Cornea* 2001;20:226–229.

37. Everts RJ, Fowler WC, Chang DH, et al. Corneoscleral rim cultures: lack of utility and implications for clinical decision-making and infection prevention in the care of patients undergoing corneal transplantation. *Cornea* 2001;20:586–589.

38. Haring G, Behrendt S, Wiechens B, et al. Severe intra- and postoperative supra-choroid hemorrhage. Risk factors, therapy, results. *Ophthalmologe* 1999;96:822–828.

39. Melles GR, Lander F, Rietveld FJ, et al. A new surgical technique for deep stromal, anterior lamellar keratoplasty. *Br J Ophthalmol* 1999;83:327–333.

40. Hanna KD, David T, Besson J, et al. Lamellar keratoplasty with the Barraquer microkeratome. *Refract Corneal Surg* 1991; 7:177–181.

41. Haimovici R, Culbertson WW. Optical lamellar keratoplasty using the Barraquer microkeratome. *Refract Corneal Surg* 1991; 7:42–45.

42. Rasheed K, Rabinowitz YS. Superficial lamellar keratectomy using an automated microkeratome to excise corneal scarring caused by photorefractive keratectomy. *J Cataract Refract Surg* 1999;25:1184–1187.

43. Maguen E, Villaseñor RA, Ward DE, et al. A modified artificial anterior chamber for use in refractive keratoplasty. *Am J Ophthalmol* 1980;89:742–744.

44. Azar DT, Jain S, Sambursky R. A new surgical technique of microkeratome-assisted deep lamellar keratoplasty with a hinged flap. *Arch Ophthalmol* 2000;118:1112–1115.

45. Behrens A, Dolorico AM, Kara DT, et al. Precision and accuracy of an artificial anterior chamber system in obtaining corneal lenticules for lamellar keratoplasty. *J Cataract Refract Surg* 2001;27:1679–1687.

45a. Nordan L. The femtosecond laser. Presented at the American Academy of Ophthalmology annual meeting, 2001.

45b. Sarayba M. Lamellar keratectomy using IntraLase femtosecond laser in opaque corneas. Presented at the American Society of Cataract and Refractive Surgery annual meeting, 2003.

46. Melles GR, Lander F, Nieuwendaal C. Sutureless, posterior lamellar keratoplasty: a case report of a modified technique. *Cornea* 2002;21:325–327.

47. Terry MA, Ousley PJ. Replacing the endothelium without corneal surface incisions or sutures: the first United States clinical series using the deep lamellar endothelial keratoplasty procedure. *Ophthalmology* 2003;110:755–764; discussion 764.

48. Schanzlin DJ, Abbott RL, Asbell PA, et al. Two-year outcomes of intrastromal corneal ring segments for the correction of myopia. *Ophthalmology* 2001;108:1688–1694.

49. Colin J, Cochener B, Savary G, et al. INTACS inserts for treating keratoconus: one-year results. *Ophthalmology* 2001;108: 1409–1414.

50. Hu XH, Juhasz T. Experimental study of corneal ablation with picosecond laser pulses at 211 nm and 263 nm. *Lasers Surg Med* 1996;18:373–379.

51. Krueger RR, Juhasz T. The Nd:YLF picosecond laser in refractive surgery. *Ophthalmol Pract* 1998;16:73–83.

52. Sletten KR, Yen KG, Sayegh S, et al. An *in vivo* model of femtosecond laser intrastromal refractive surgery. *Ophthalmic Surg Laser* 1999;30:742–749.

INDEX

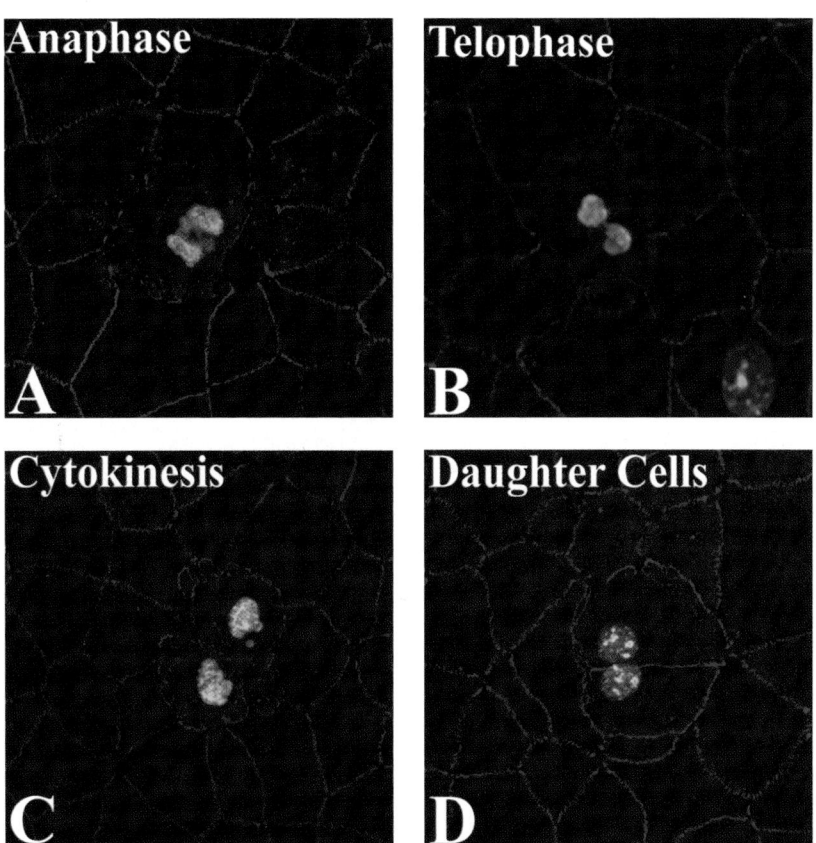

PLATE 1. Final stages of mitosis and daughter cell formation in *ex vivo* human corneal endothelium [after Joyce (108)]. Cornea from a 52-year-old donor was treated with ethylenediamine tetraacetic acid to break cell–cell contacts, followed by incubation for 48 hours in the presence of 10% serum. (Original magnification, ×600.)

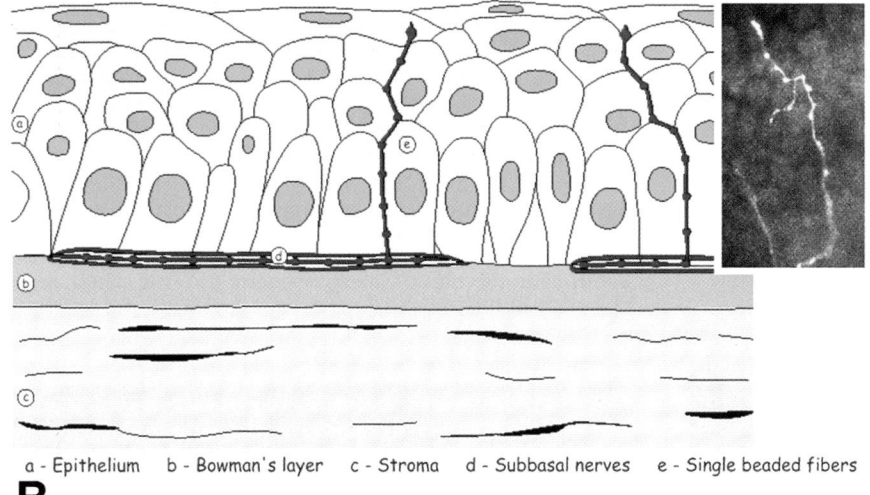

a - Epithelium   b - Bowman's layer   c - Stroma   d - Subbasal nerves   e - Single beaded fibers

PLATE 2. Diagram adapted from Müller et al. (107) of the corneal epithelium showing the nerve bundles (leashes) in the subbasal plexus (d). The bundle contains both beaded and straight fibers, but as demonstrated in the micrograph at right, which has been labeled with antibodies to substance P, only the beaded nerves turn to enter the epithelium, where they terminate in the apical layers of cells (Adapted from Müller LJ, Marfurt CF, Kruse F, et al. Corneal nerves: structure, contents and function. *Exp Eye Res* 2003;76:521—542.)

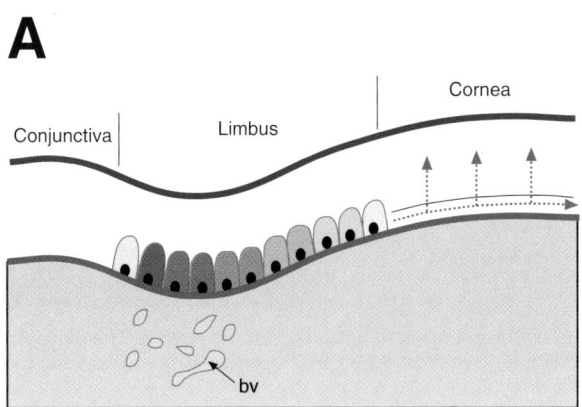

PLATE 3. Diagram demonstrating corneal stem cells in the limbal zone. A stem cell is indicated, along with a gradient of undifferentiated cells with some stem cell-like characteristics. Blood vessels (bv) are localized directly subjacent to the limbal basal cells. (Adapted from Zieske JD, Gipson IK. Agents that affect corneal wound healing: Modulation of structure and function. In: Albert DM, Jakobiec FA, eds. *Principles and practice of ophthalmology: basic sciences.* Philadelphia: WB Saunders, 1994: 1093–1099, and Schermer A, Galvin S, Sun TT. Differentiation-related expression of a major 64K corneal keratin in vivo and in culture suggests limbal location of corneal epithelial stem cells. *J Cell Biol* 1986; 103:49–62.)

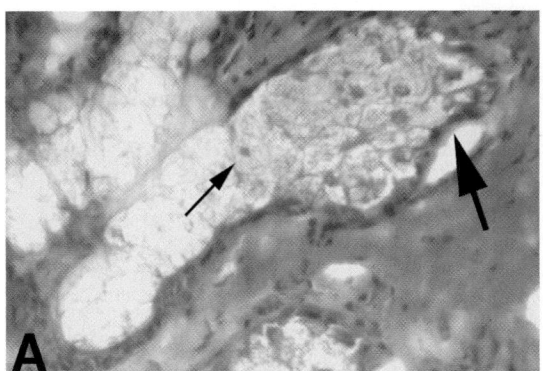

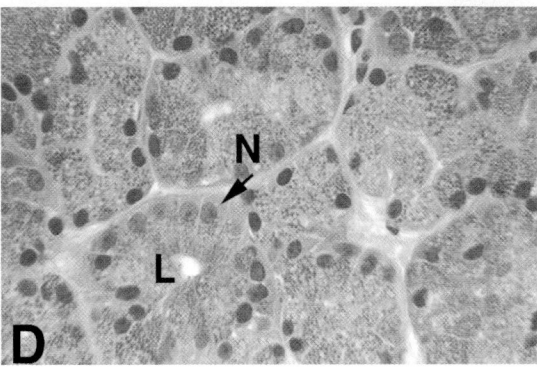

PLATE 4. A: Section through the acinus of a human meibomian gland stained with hematoxylin-eosin. A single layer of basal epithelial cells (*large arrow*) gives rise to more differentiated suprabasal cells containing lipid droplets. The superficial, inner layer of cells (*small arrow*) ruptures in a holocrine fashion releasing both the lipid secretion and cell debris. (Original magnification, ×350.) **D:** Light micrograph of a section of human lacrimal gland showing acinar morphology. Epithelial cells are arranged concentrically with the apical aspect of the plasma membrane toward the lumen (L) of the secretory tubule. Secretory granules fill the cell and displace the nucleus (N) basally. (Original magnification, ×350.)

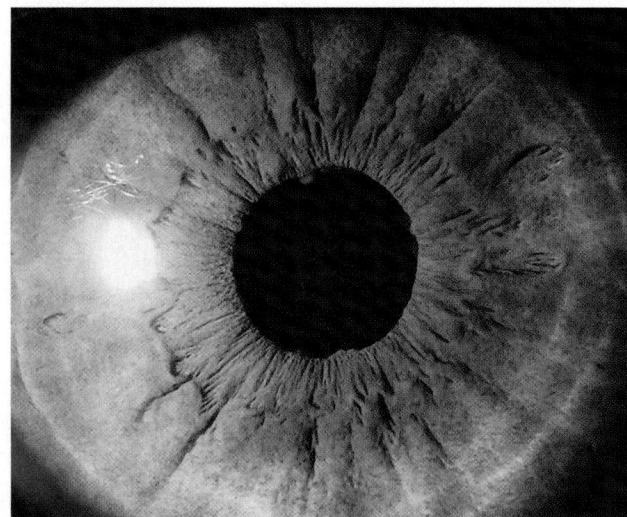

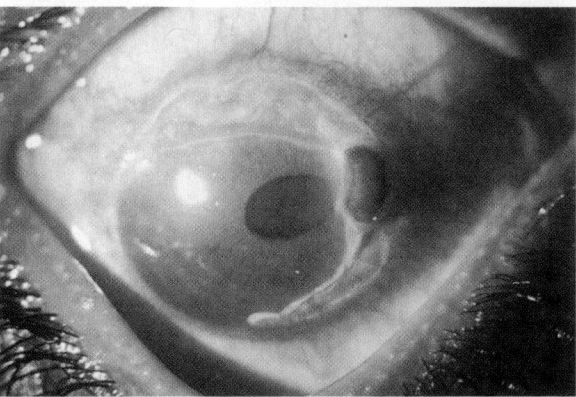

FPLATE 6. A. Tangential illumination with a broad beam of a normal iris. The observed shadows result from elevations on the iris surface. This technique can permit the examiner to determine whether an observed lesion is flat or elevated. **B.** Tangential illumination of an eye with Mooren's ulcer with perforation. The protruding iris casts a shadow, suggesting it is elevated above the plane of the cornea.

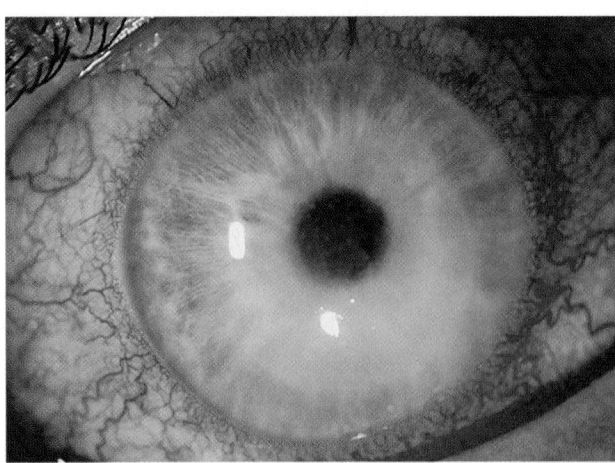

PLATE 5. Diffuse, broad-beam illumination of a patient with herpes simplex keratouveitis. The low magnification combined with diffuse illumination permits the examiner to comprehend the "big picture." In this case, this technique documents ciliary flush, keratic precipitates, and corneal edema.

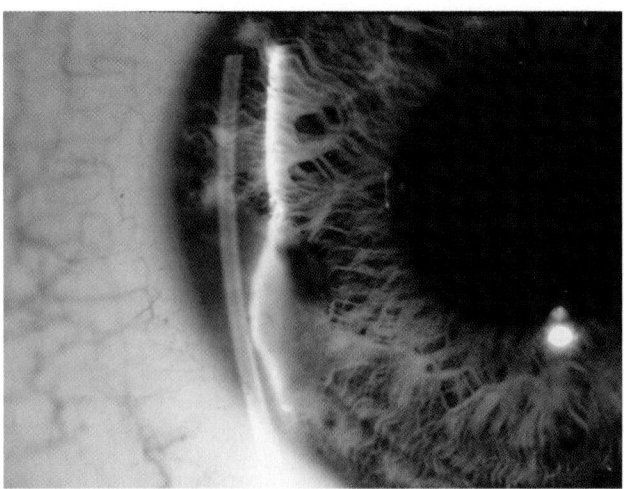

PLATE 7. Slit-beam examination of iris melanoma. The elevated lesion results in a light beam that appears to bend toward the examiner.

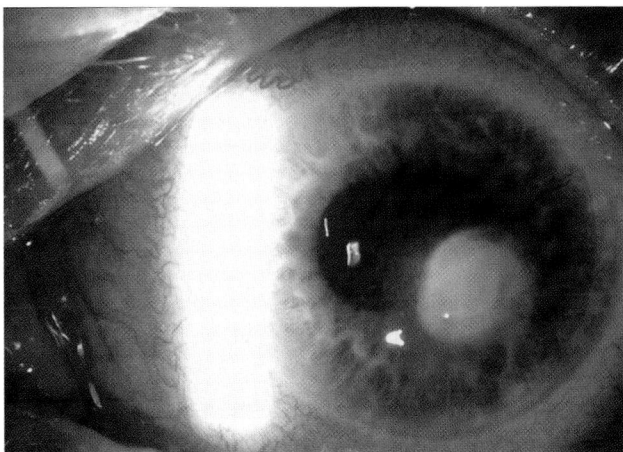

PLATE 8. Sclerotic scatter reveals diffuse stromal infiltrate surrounding a bacterial corneal ulcer.

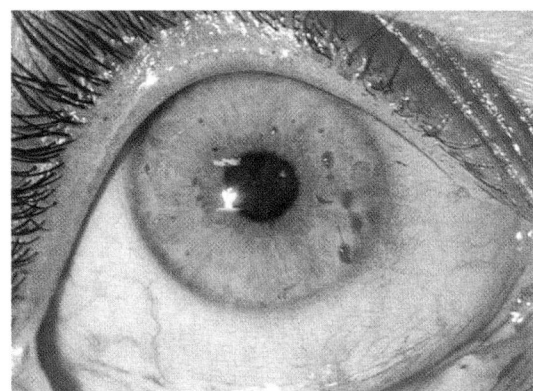

PLATE 11. Rose bengal staining of filamentary keratitis in severe dry eye. (See color figure.)

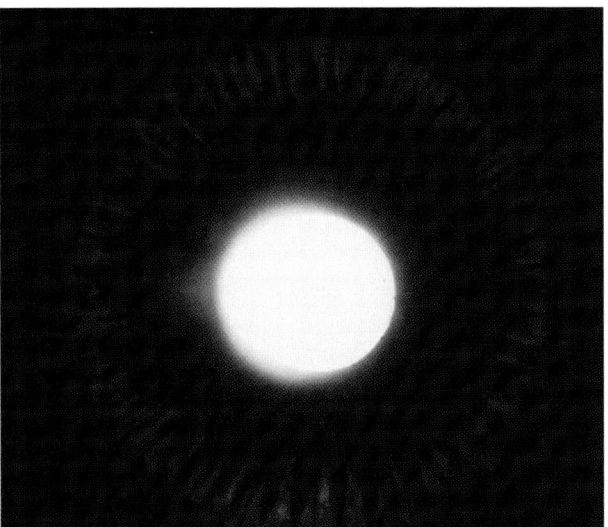

PLATE 9. Radial iris transillumination defects in pigment dispersion syndrome observed with retroillumination from the fundus.

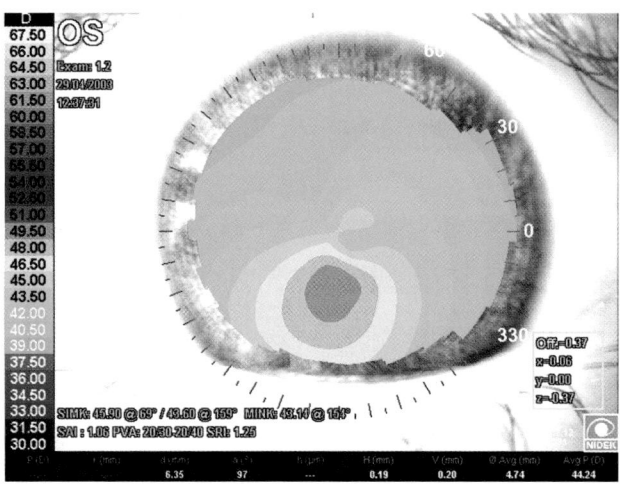

PLATE 12. Topographic example of clinical keratoconus.

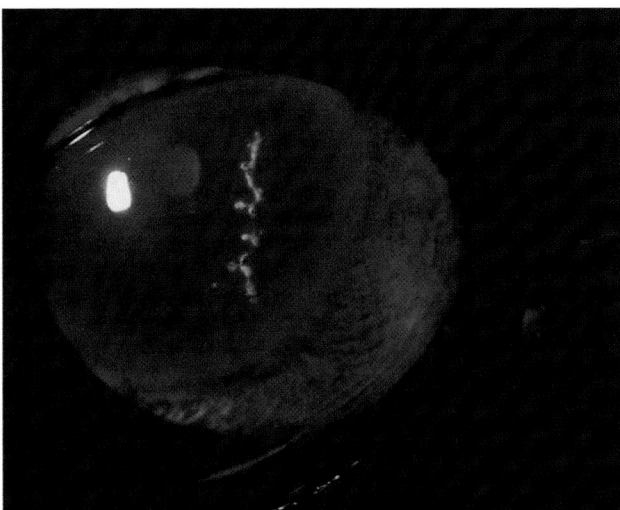

PLATE 10. Herpes simplex dendrite stained with fluorescein and observed with the cobalt blue filter. (See color figure.)

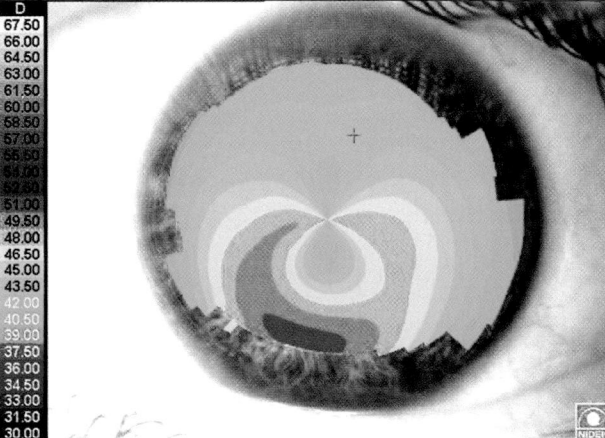

PLATE 13. Topographic example of pellucid marginal degeneration. Note the characteristic inferior arcuate steepening.

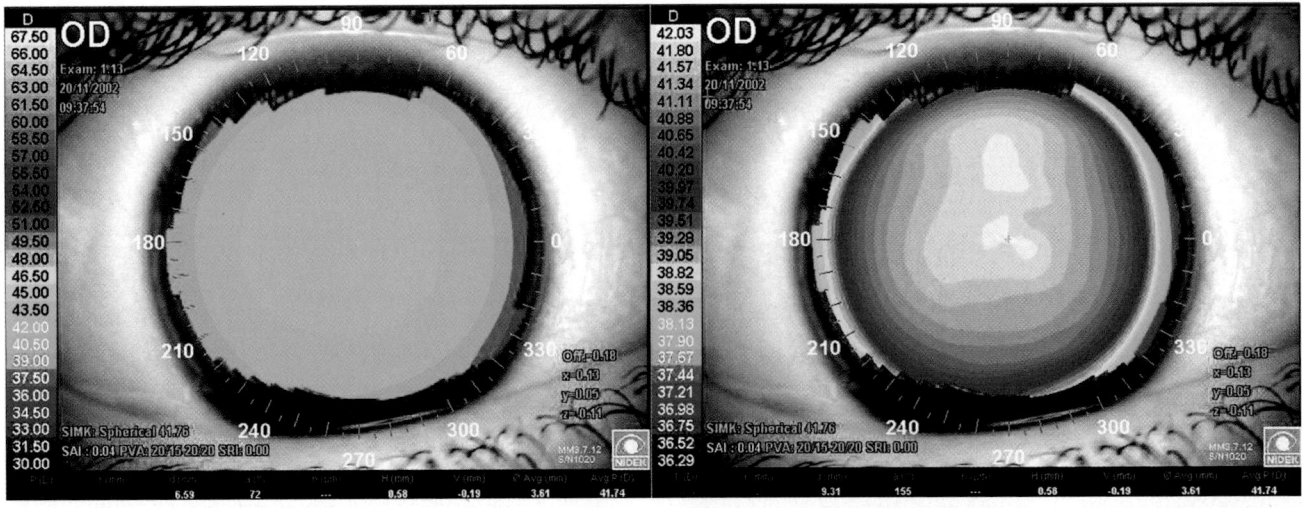

PLATE 14. Example of clinical keratoconus and its detection by two different methods.

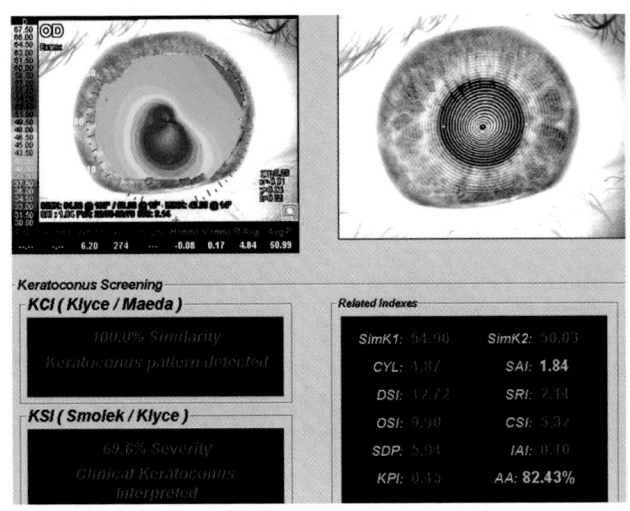

PLATE 15. Example of the problems encountered when adaptable scales are used. *Left*, A normal cornea displayed with the Smolek/Klyce scale. *Right*, The same cornea displayed with an adaptable scale, which makes it look erroneously problematic.

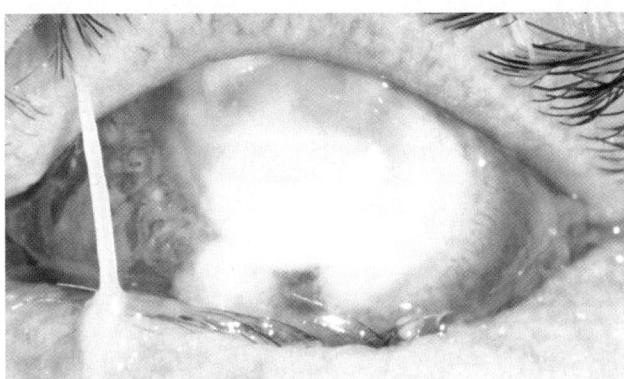

PLATE 17. Suppurative keratitis in a patient who had been wearing extended-wear soft contact lenses around the clock, and now has *Pseudomonas* keratitis with hypopyon.

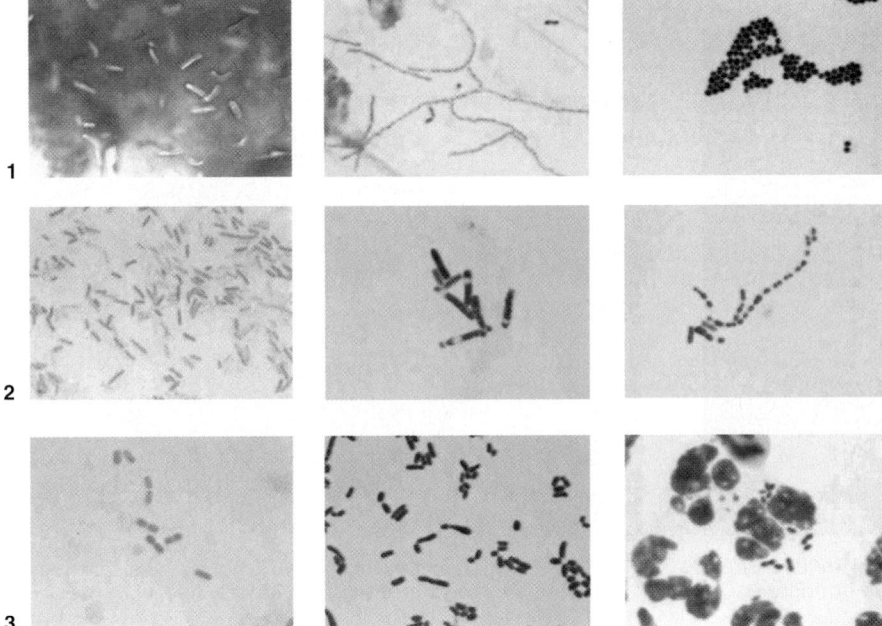

PLATE 16. Microphotographs of gram-positive (blue) and gram-negative (red) bacteria that infect the cornea. (Original magnification × 100, oil immersion; photographed by Lisa M. Karenchak.) *Row 1, left*: diplococci (*Streptococcus pneumoniae*); *row 1, middle*: pleomorphic rods (diphtheroids); *row 1, right*: diplobacilli (*Moraxella*). *Row 2, left*: chain of cocci (*Streptococcus*); *row 2, middle*: rods with endospores (*Bacillus*); *row 2, right*: rods (*Pseudomonas aeruginosa*). *Row 3, left*: grapelike clusters of cocci (*Staphylococcus aureus*); *row 3, middle*: thin filaments (*Actinomyces*); *row 3, right*: nonstaining ghost rods (*Mycobacterium chelonae*). (See color figure.)

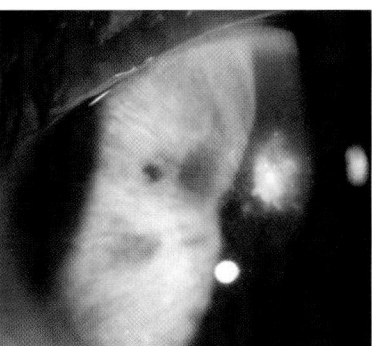

PLATE 18. Infection at the interface in a patient who previously had undergone laser *in situ* keratomileusis keratorefractive surgery.

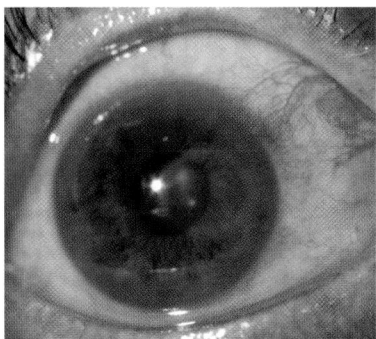

PLATE 19. Wessely ring, much as might be seen in an antigen–antibody reaction on an Ouchterlony plate (or "immune ring").

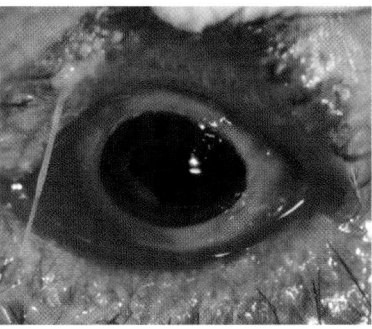

PLATE 20. Complete dissolution of the corneal stroma in a patient with *Pseudomonas* keratitis. The glistening light reflex is from Descemet's membrane.

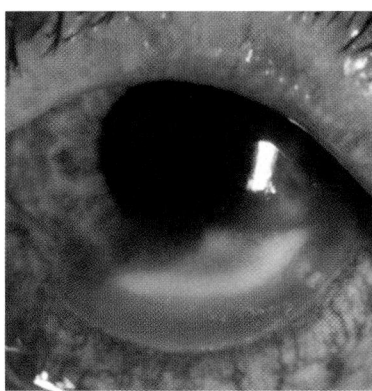

PLATE 21. *Moraxella* corneal ulcer, with an inflammatory infiltrate in an arcuate, scimitar pattern in the inferior aspect of the cornea.

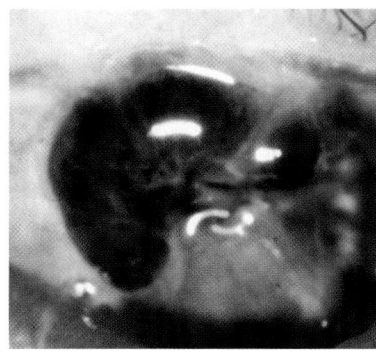

PLATE 22. Corneal ulcer with perforation in a patient with *Neisseria* gonococcus infection. The process began just 5 days earlier, illustrating the rapidity with which the process can progress, with dissolution of the corneal stroma.

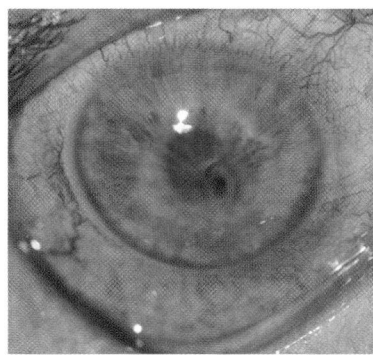

PLATE 23. Bacterial corneal ulcer with progression to perforation, with the perforation now plugged with iris.

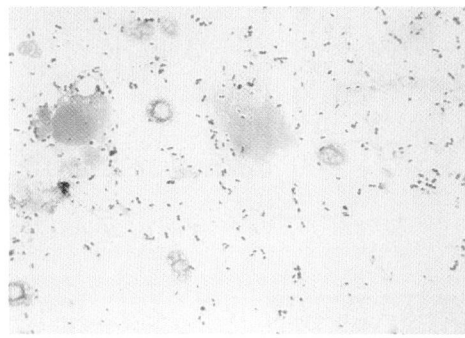

PLATE 24. Smear from corneal scraping taken from a patient with suppurative keratitis. Note the lancet-shaped diplococci, almost diagnostic of *Streptococcus pneumoniae*.

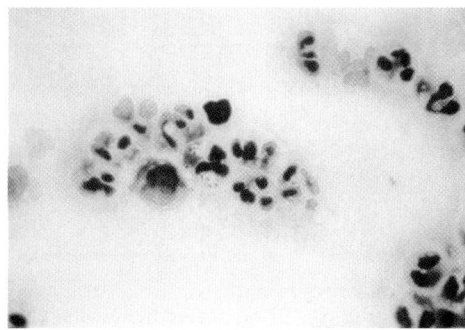

PLATE 25. A Gram-stained specimen similar to that shown in Fig. 48–14, although from a different patient, illustrating (with some difficulty) intracellular gram-negative diplococci, almost pathognomonic for *Neisseria* species.

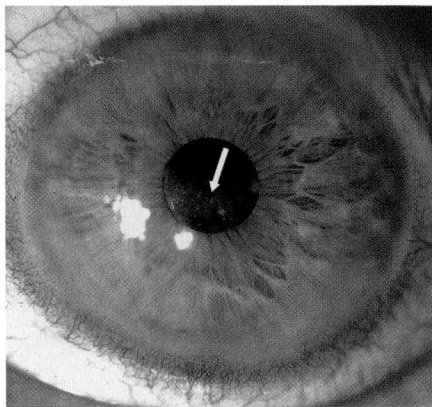

PLATE 26. Acute herpes simplex virus iritis with 360 degrees of limbal ciliary flush, keratic precipitates, and cells and flare in the anterior chamber.

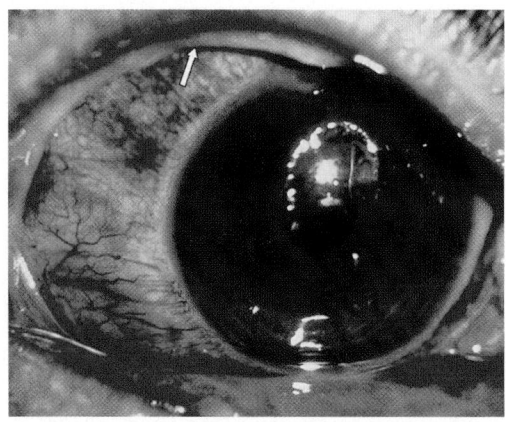

PLATE 29. Acute adenoviral blepharoconjunctivitis with diphtheric-like true membrane formation under the upper lid. Membrane is rubbing a mechanical epithelial defect into the corneal epithelium. A thin soft contact lens was placed to protect and heal the cornea until the membrane resolved.

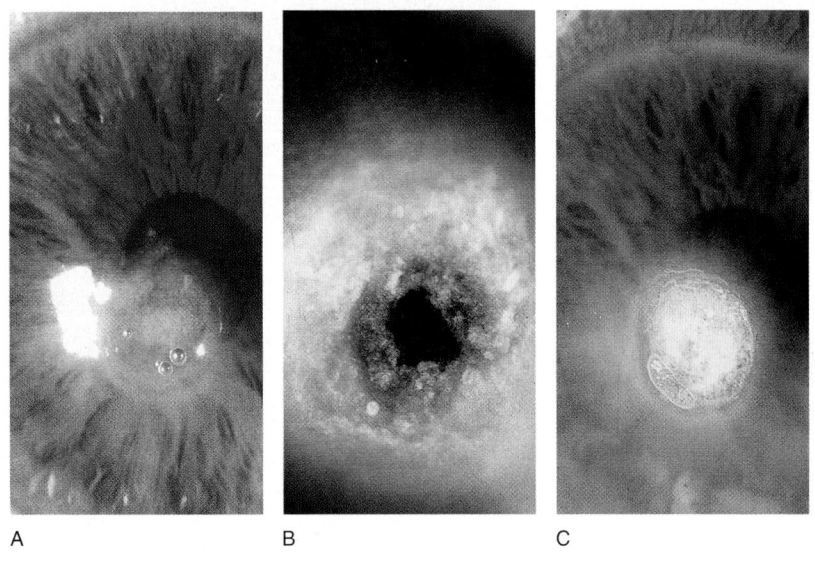

A   B   C

PLATE 27. A: Melting herpes simplex virus trophic ulcer neglected by patient. **B:** Ulcer ultimately perforated in the absence of treatment. Anterior chamber is flat. **C:** Perforation was sealed with cyanoacrylate tissue adhesive to reform the chamber. Unfortunately, the ulcer continued to melt, the glue dislodged, and emergency penetrating keratoplasty was performed.

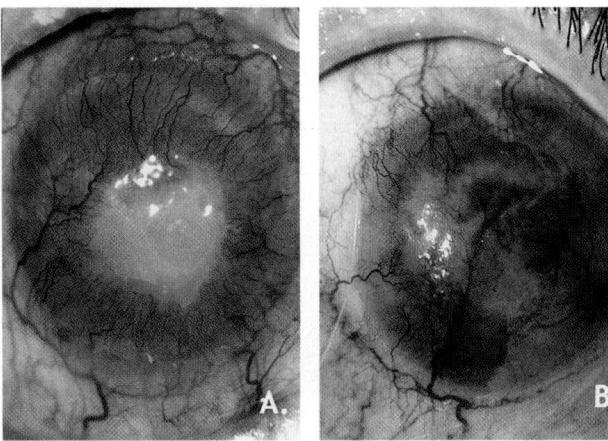

PLATE 28. A: Herpes zoster ophthalmicus soft trophic ulcer in anesthetic cornea gradually being healed by vascular pannus. **B:** Same eye 6 months after thin soft contact lens application, with pannus complete and inflammation resolving.

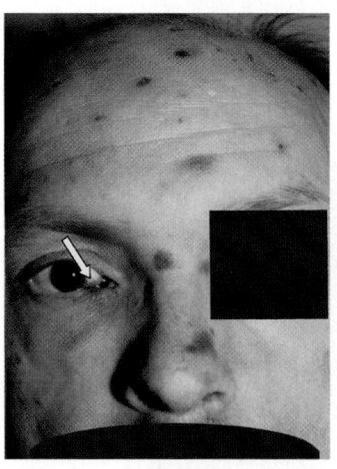

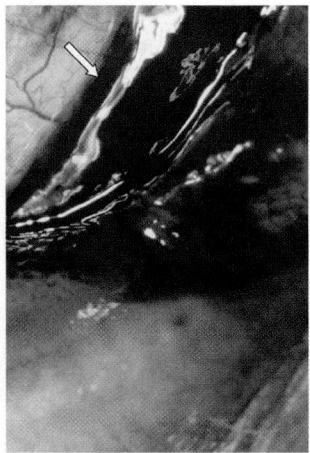

A   B

PLATE 30. A: Thirty-year-old human immunodeficiency virus– positive man with multiple Kaposi's sarcoma lesions scattered over his face and scalp. Medial canthal sarcoma (*arrow*) can be seen in the right eye. **B:** Close-up of medial canthal sarcoma in A showing lesion that resembles conjunctival lymphoma.

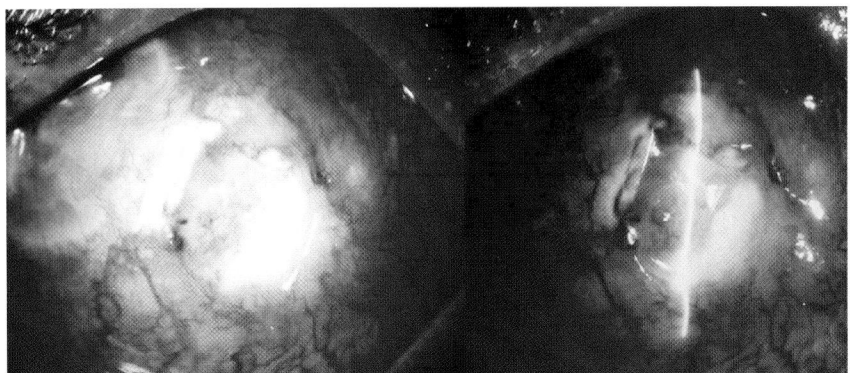

PLATE 31. Fungal scleritis caused by *Aspergillus flavus.* Note scleral necrosis with suppuration.

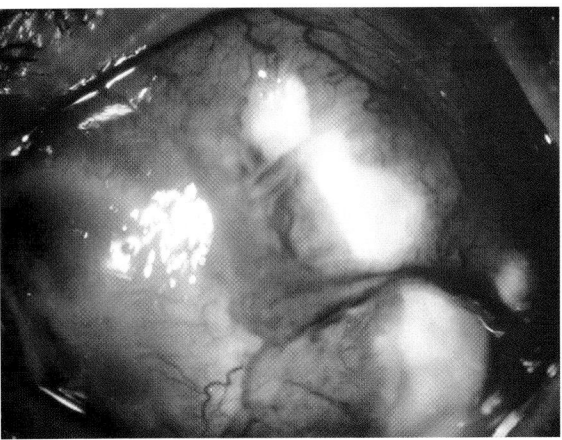

PLATE 32. Multifocal infiltrate in fungal scleritis.

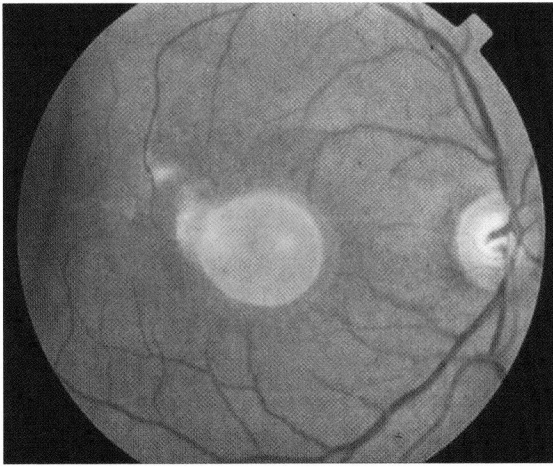

PLATE 33. Subretinal cyst in cysticercosis. (From Sharma T, Sinha S, Shah N, et al. Intraocular cysticercosis: clinical characteristics and visual outcome after vitreoretinal surgery. *Ophthalmology* 2003;110:996–1004, with permission.)

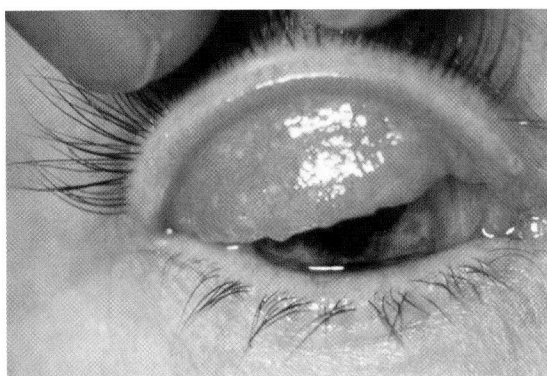

PLATE 34. Follicular conjunctivitis in trachoma.

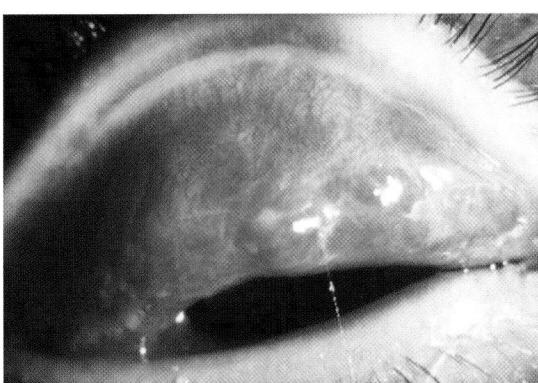

PLATE 35. Trachoma. Cicatrizing conjunctivitis.

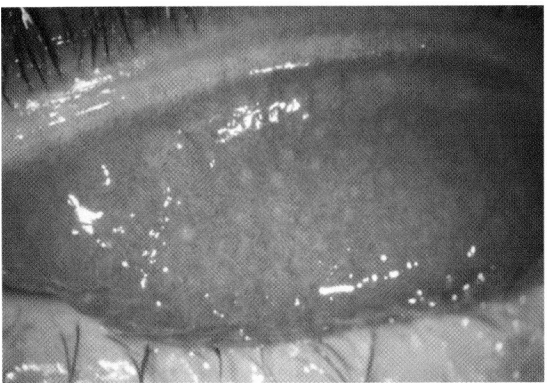

PLATE 36. Adult inclusion conjunctivitis. Follicular conjunctivitis localized to the inferior tarsal conjunctiva

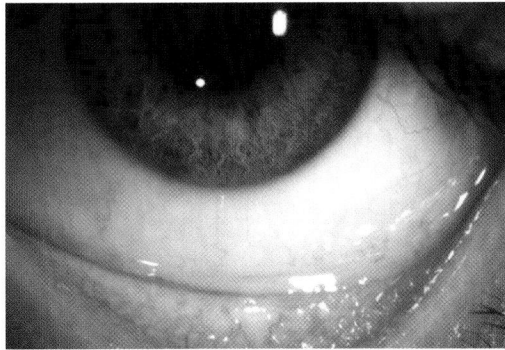

PLATE 37. Adult inclusion conjunctivitis. Follicular conjunctivitis of the upper tarsal conjunctiva.

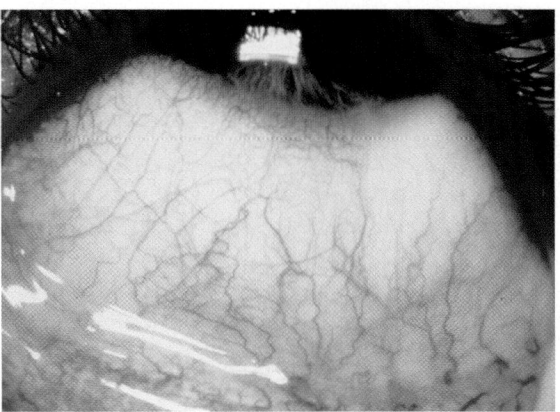

PLATE 38. Seasonal allergic conjunctivitis showing chemosis and hyperemia.

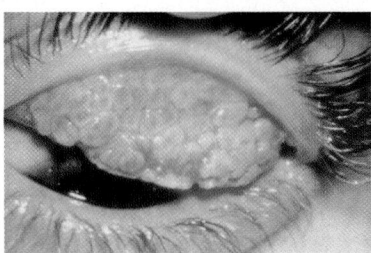

PLATE 39. Flat-topped giant papillae of vernal keratoconjunctivitis (VKC).

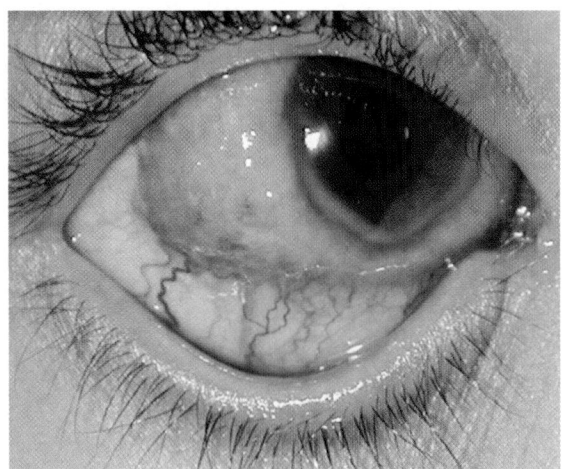

PLATE 40. Limbal vernal lesion.

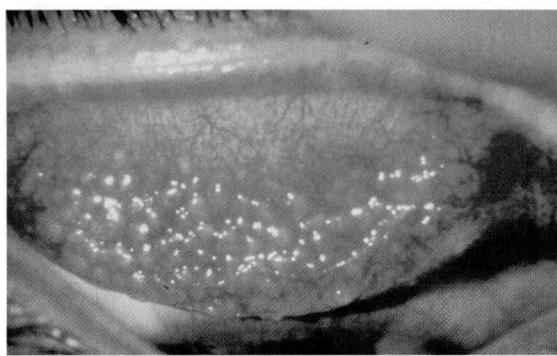

PLATE 41. Greater than 1.0-mm-diameter papilla of giant papillary conjunctivitis (GPC).

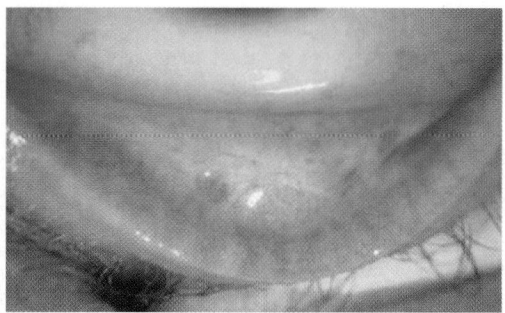

PLATE 42. Lacy white lines of subepithelial fibrosis, commonly perivascular in localization in the inferior fornix and tarsal conjunctiva, representing the earliest sign of cicatrization.

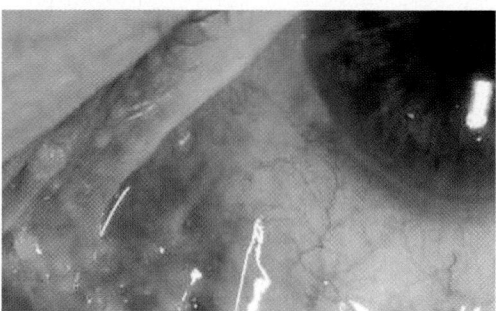

PLATE 43. Involvement of the medial canthus, leading to shallow canthal recess and conjunctival subepithelial fibrosis.

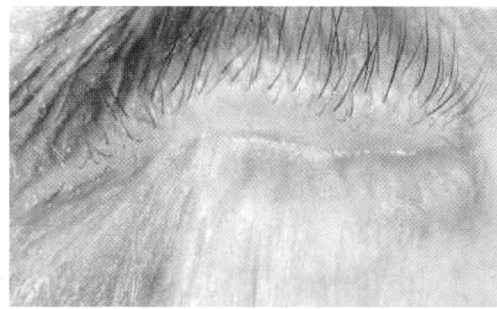

PLATE 44. Ankyloblepharon, total fusion of the eyelids to the bulbar conjunctiva and cornea.

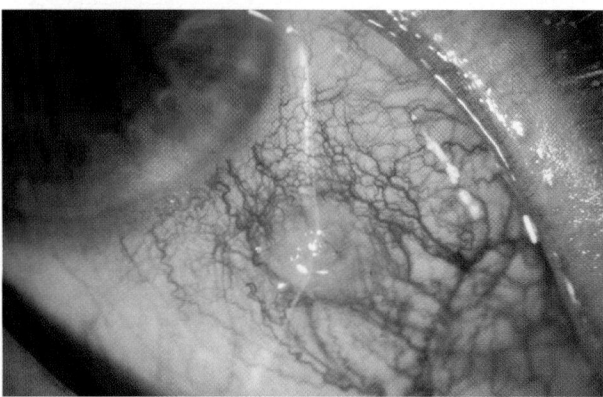

PLATE 45. Conjunctival phlyctenule in a patient. This amorphous, pink to gray nodule typically appears at or near the limbus with associated conjunctival injection. The lesion commonly ulcerates, as in this example, and reepithelializes over a period of 2 weeks. Symptoms are mild to moderate and include tearing, photophobia, burning, itching, and foreign-body sensation. (Courtesy of B. J. Mondino, M.D.)

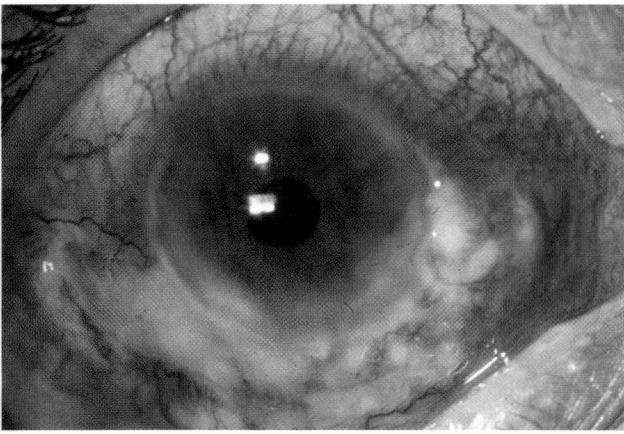

PLATE 46. Example of peripheral ulcerative keratitis (PUK) in a patient with Wegener's granulomatosis, with associated adjacent scleritis, obviously very different from the characteristics of Mooren's ulcer shown in Fig. 24–1.

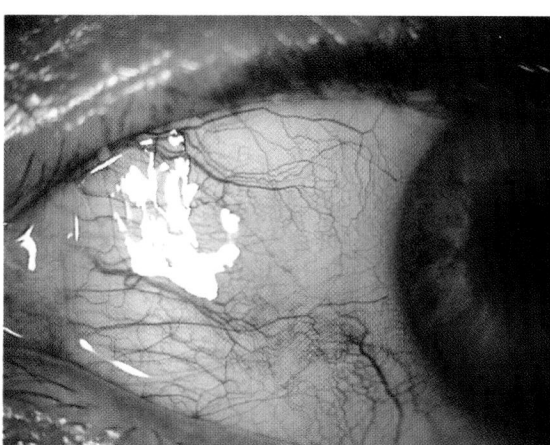

PLATE 49. Nodular episcleritis. Note the vascular dilatation of conjunctival plexus and superficial episcleral plexus and the presence of a localized nodule over the sclera. Congested vessels follow the usual radial pattern. The edema is localized in the episcleral tissue.

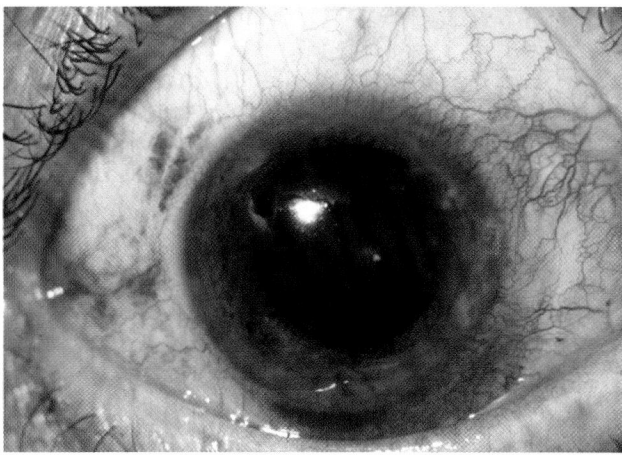

PLATE 47. Vascularized, thinned peripheral bed of previously ulcerating cornea in a patient with PUK caused by Mooren's ulcer; note the area at approximately 2 o'clock.

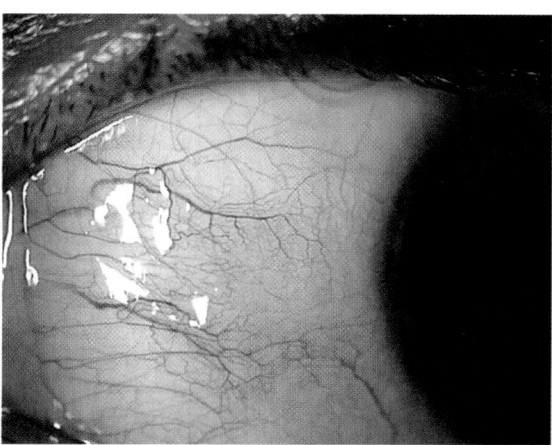

PLATE 50. Same eye as in Fig. 25-1 after topical application of 10% phenylephrine. The eye appears white since phenylephrine blanches the superficial episcleral plexus.

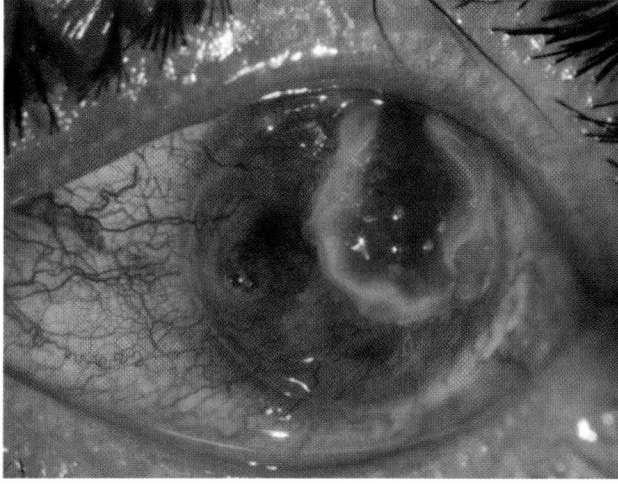

PLATE 48. A more advanced example of progressive Mooren's ulcer, with only a small residual area of remaining full-thickness cornea, with the infiltrated edge of the overhanging lip, and a vascularized, thinned residuum of cornea left in the wake of the advancing ulcer.

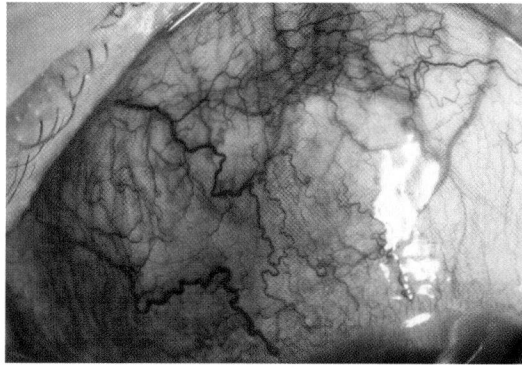

PLATE 51. Diffuse scleritis. Note the vascular dilatation of conjunctival, superficial episcleral, and deep episcleral plexuses. The edema is localized in the episcleral and scleral tissues.

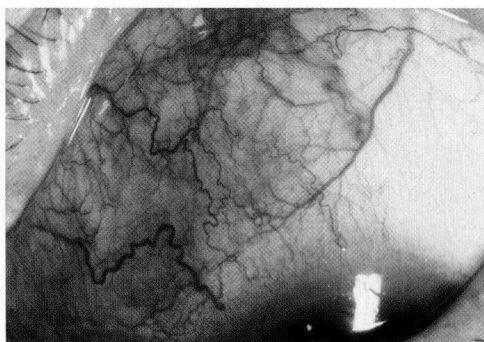

PLATE 52. Same eye as in Fig. 25-3 after topical application of 10% phenylephrine. The eye remains congested since phenylephrine only blanches the superficial episcleral plexus without any effect on the deep episcleral plexus.

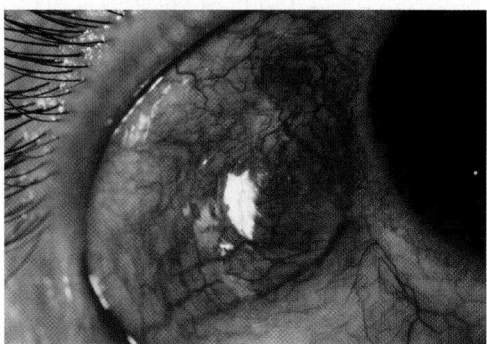

PLATE 53. Nodular scleritis. As part of the sclera, the nodule is immobile as one tries to palpate and move it.

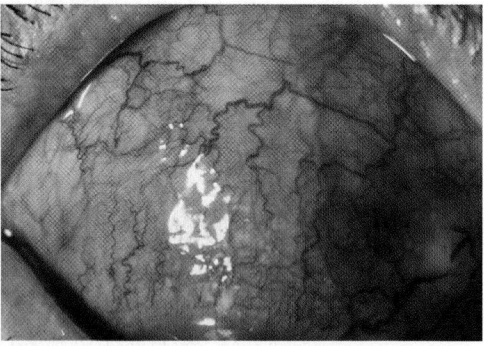

PLATE 54. Necrotizing scleritis. The damaged area becomes thinned and translucent and shows the underlying uvea.

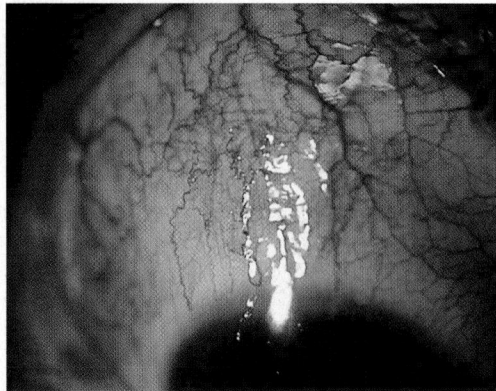

PLATE 55. Diffuse scleritis with uveitis and ocular hypertension. The detection of uveitis and ocular hypertension accompanying scleritis requires early and aggressive therapy to control the inflammatory processes.

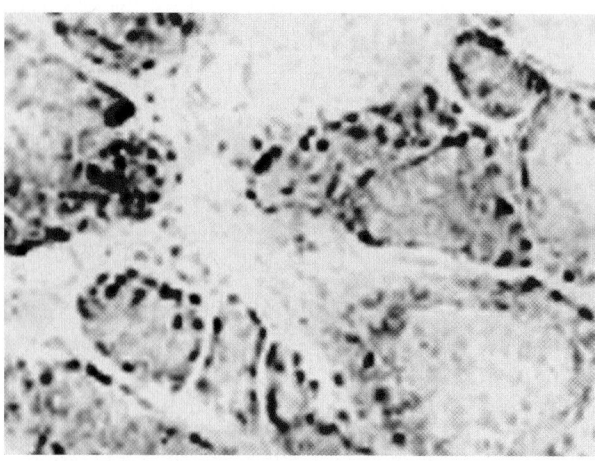

PLATE 56. Presence of androgen receptor protein in acinar cells of the rat meibomian gland. Immunoperoxidase microscopy of meibomian gland showing the location of androgen receptor protein in acinar cells. (From Sullivan DA, Sullivan BD, Ullman MD, et al. Androgen influence on the Meibomian gland. *Invest Ophthalmol Vis Sci* 2000;41:3732–3742.)

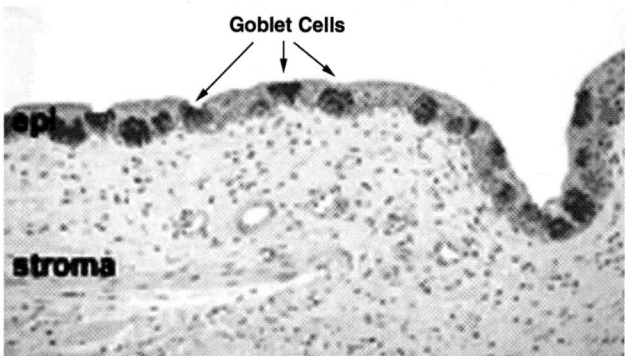

PLATE 57. Histochemical reactivity of conjunctiva to Alcian blue/periodic acid-Schiff's (AB/PAS) reagent. Secretory products present in goblet cells of the conjunctiva reacted positively to AB/PAS, indicating the presence of both acidic (blue) and neutral (pink) glycoconjugates associated with the cells. epi, epithelium. (Magnification ×200.) (From Shatos MA, Rios JD, Tepavcevic V, et al. Isolation, characterization, and propagation of rat conjunctival goblet cells in vitro. Invest Ophthalmol Vis Sci 2001;42:1455–1464.)

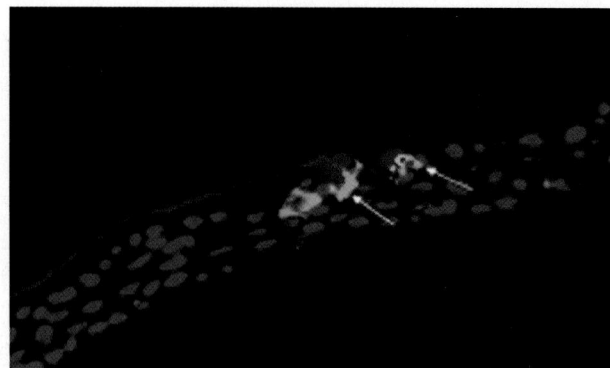

PLATE 58. Immunolocalization of VIP in human goblet cells. Cryosections from human conjunctival biopsy were labeled with an anti-VIP antibody (*green*) to indicated parasympathetic nerves; HPA, *Helix pomatia* agglutin, (*red*) to indicate location of goblet cells and DAPI 4',6-diamidino-z-phenylindole to indicate the nucleus of the cells. Parasympathetic nerves were detected coursing through the conjunctival epithelium and adjacent to or surrounding goblet cells (*arrows*). (Magnification ×380.) (From Rios JD, Forde K, Diebold Y, et al. Development of conjunctival goblet cells and their neuroreceptor subtype expression. *Invest Ophthalmol Vis Sci* 2000;41:2127–2137.)

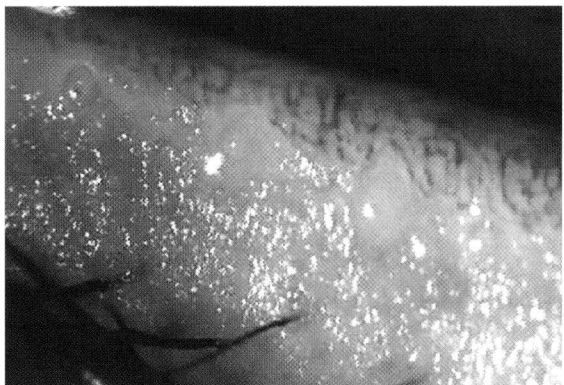

PLATE 59. Meibomian gland dysfunction. Thick turbid secretions expressed at the mouth of meibomian glands.

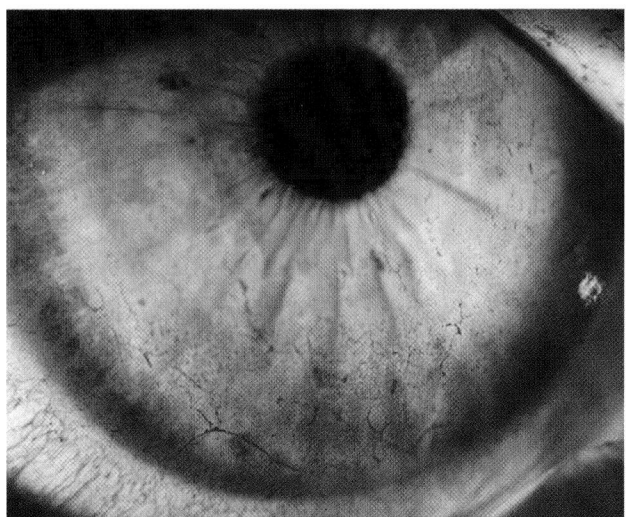

PLATE 60. Keratoconjunctivitis sicca with typical epithelial erosions showing a characteristic pattern of distribution.

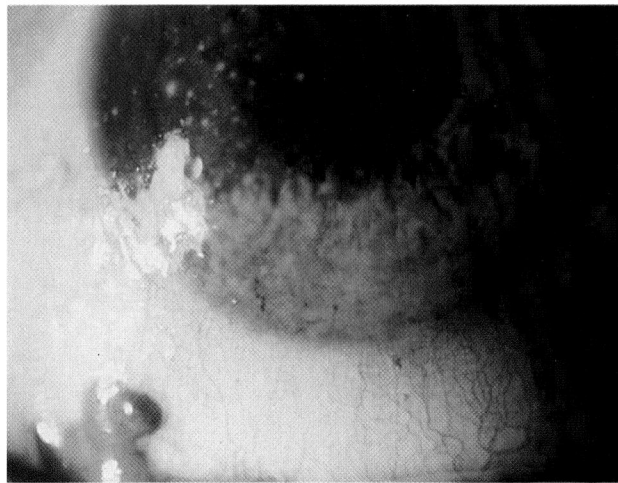

PLATE 61. Superficial punctate keratopathy showing the exposed interpalpebral area of ocular surface, in keratoconjunctivitis sicca.

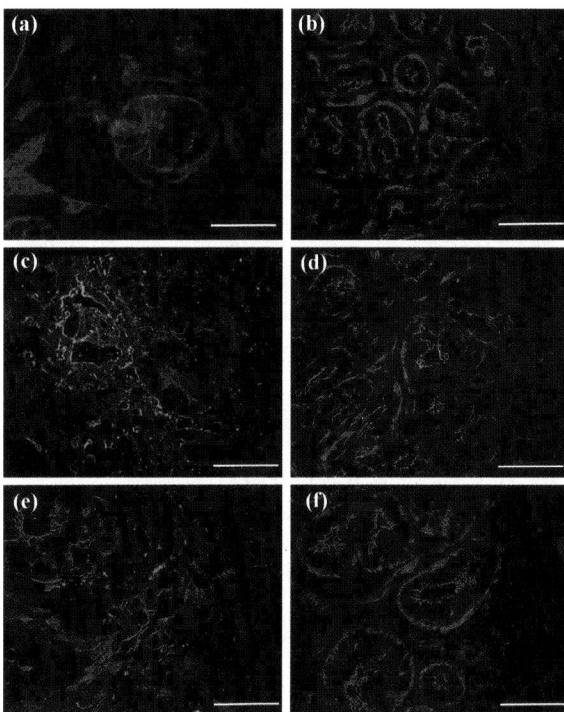

PLATE 62. Quantitative evaluation and evidence of apoptotic mechanisms in Sjögren's syndrome (SS): double staining of actin and Apo2.7, Fas, or FasL in lacrimal gland. **A,C,E:** Lacrimal glands from SS. **B,D,F:** Lacrimal glands from non-SS were stained with Apo2.7 **(A,B)**, Fas **(C,D)**, and FasL **(E,F)** antibody followed by rhodamine-phalloidin. Bars: 50 μm. **A:** SS lacrimal gland. Note the (+) acinar cells. **B:** Non-SS lacrimal gland. No acinar cells are stained with Apo2.7 antibody. **C:** SS lacrimal gland. Note the (+) acinar cells, **D:** Non-SS lacrimal gland. Some acinar cells are stained with Fas antibody. **E:** SS lacrimal gland. Note (+) staining of infiltrating lymphocytes. **F:** Non-SS lacrimal gland. FasL antibody did not stain any cells. (From Tsubota K, Fujita H, Tsuzaka K, et al. Quantitative analysis of lacrimal gland function, apoptotic figures, Fas and Fas ligand expression of lacrimal glands in dry eye patients. *Exp Eye Res* 2003; 76:233–240. Copyright 2003, with permission from Elsevier.)

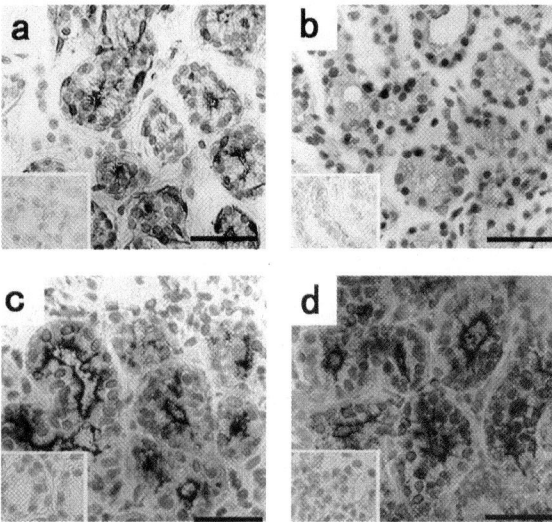

PLATE 63. Immunolocalization of AQP5 in lacrimal glands. **A:** Normal control. **B:** Sjögren's syndrome (SS). **C:** Non-SS patient. **D:** Mikulicz's disease. All samples labeled with antibodies to human AQP5 and visualized with peroxidase conjugated secondary antibodies. Insets are (−) controls. Bars: 50 μm. (From Tsubota K, Hirai S, King LS, et al. Defective cellular trafficking of lacrimal gland aquaporin-5 in Sjögren's syndrome. Lancet 2001; 357:688–689, with permission from Elsevier.)

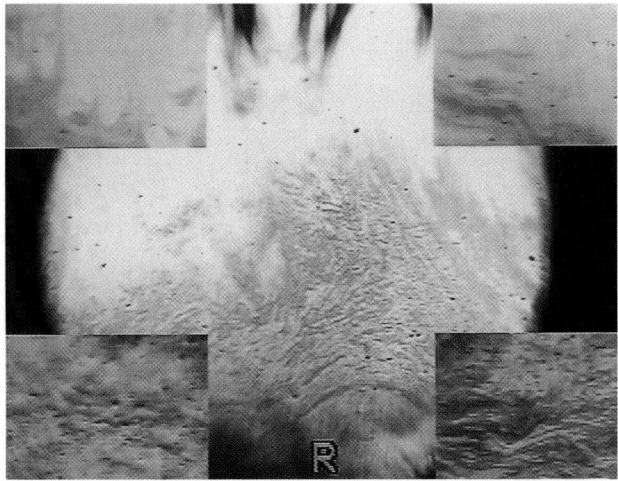

PLATE 64. Tear film lipid layer interferometry in a patient with secondary Sjögren's syndrome revealed an irregular corneal surface with interference colors and numerous black dry spots, indicating a grade 4 change. **Upper left insert:** Grade 2 change, indicated by nonuniform distribution and normal pattern. **Upper right insert:** Grade 3 change, seen as having nonuniform distribution, and low-grade dry eye change. **Lower left insert:** Grade 4 change, indicated by nonuniform distribution and moderate dry eye change. **Lower right insert:** Grade 5 change, indicated by partially exposed corneal surface and severe dry eye change.

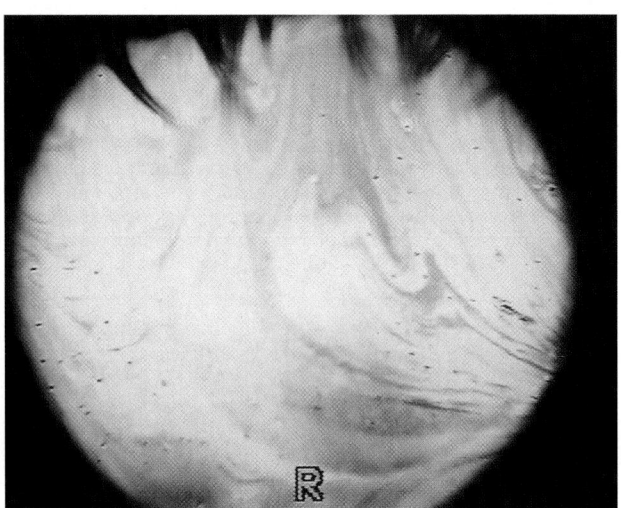

PLATE 65. Tear film lipid layer interferometry in the same patient as in Fig. 29-5 showed the disappearance of interference colors after 2 months of autologous serum treatment (grade 2 change).

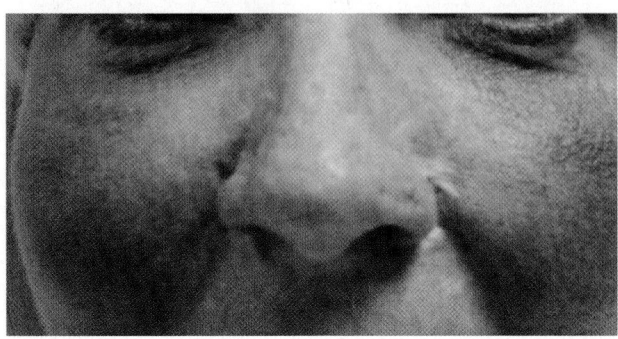

PLATE 66. Rosacea.

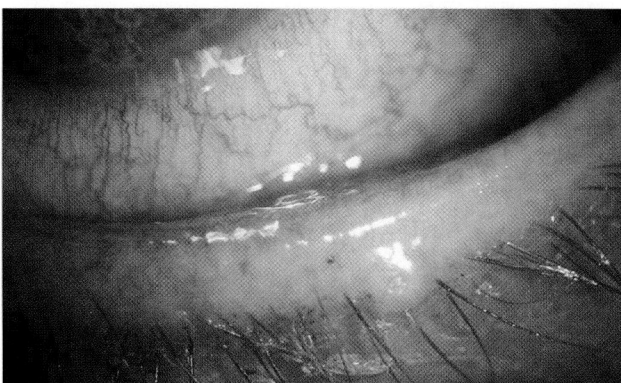

PLATE 67. Molluscum contagiosum.

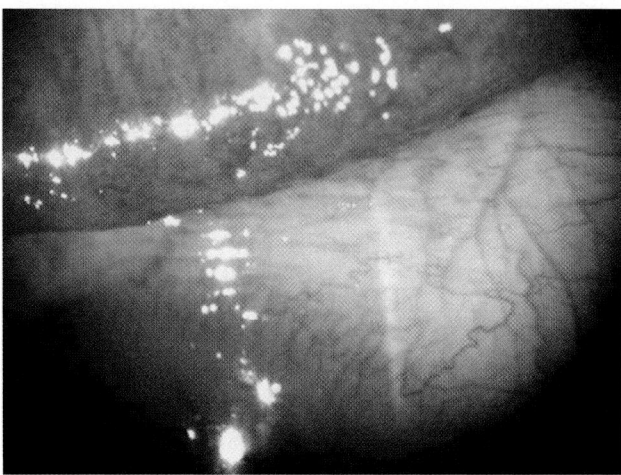

PLATE 68. On instilling a drop of lissamine green in superior limbic keratoconjunctivitis, papillary hypertrophy of the superior tarsal conjunctiva is better seen, as well as the horizontal folds of the superior bulbar conjunctiva due to the poor adherence of the latter to the sclera. Also note the lucid appearance of the edematous superior limbal conjunctiva.

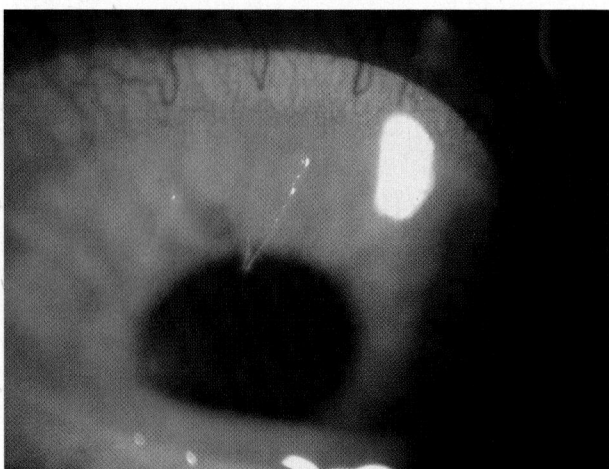

PLATE 69. Filaments at the upper cornea in superior limbic keratoconjunctivitis.

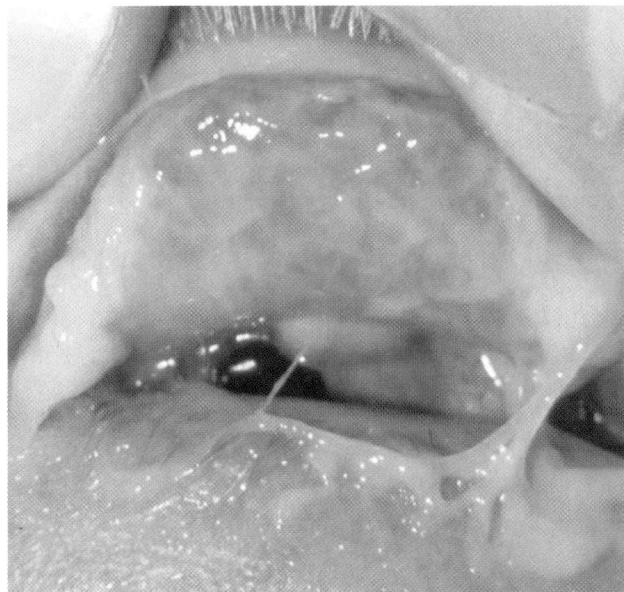

PLATE 70. Everted upper lid showing the thick pseudomembrane attached to the upper tarsal surface.

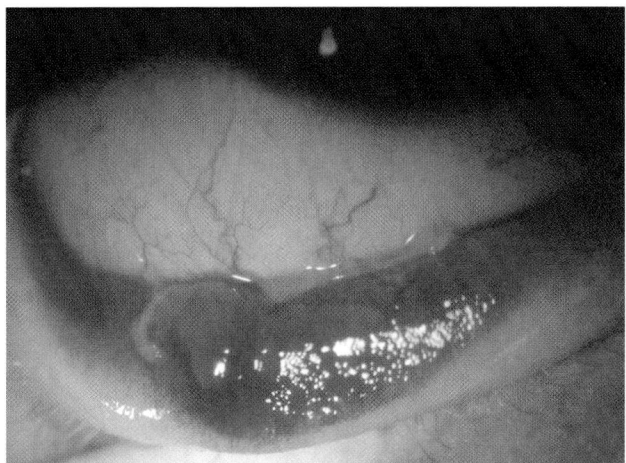

A

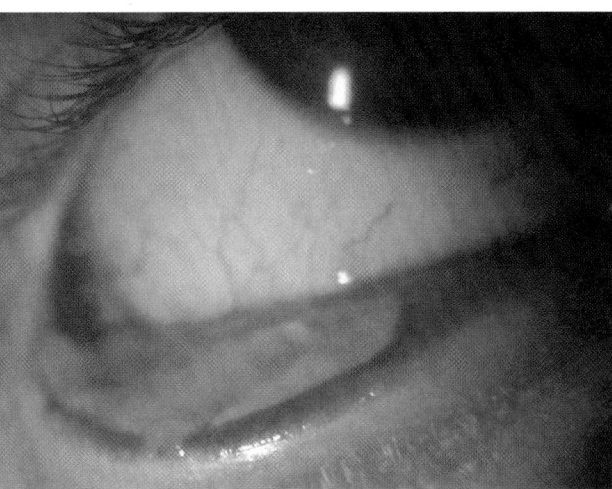

B

PLATE 72. A: Lesion involving inferior tarsal surface before surgical removal. **B:** Recurrence of lesion 10 days after surgical removal, applications of cryotherapy, and subconjunctival injection of Decadron followed by topical treatment with α-chymotrypsin, hyaluronidase, and cromolyn.

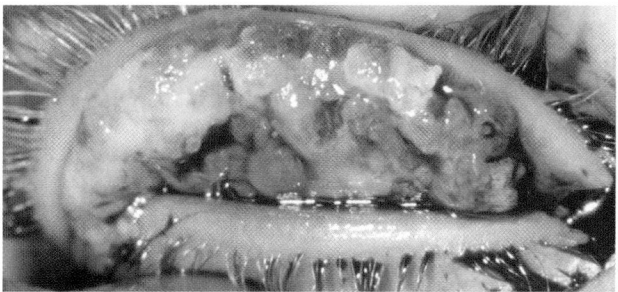

PLATE 71. Thick firm woody appearance of the superior tarsal surface.

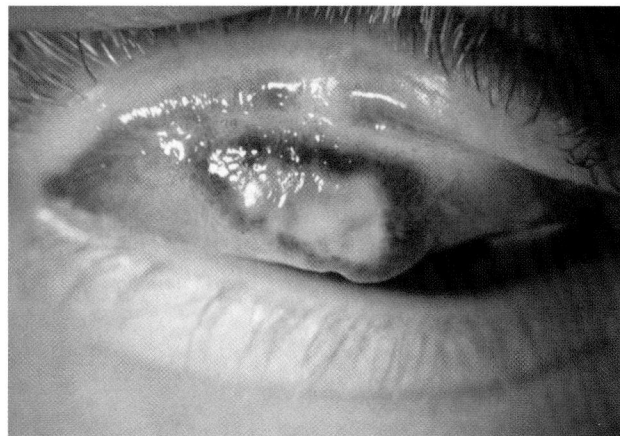

PLATE 73. Pedunculated lesion with flat, smooth, whitish surface.

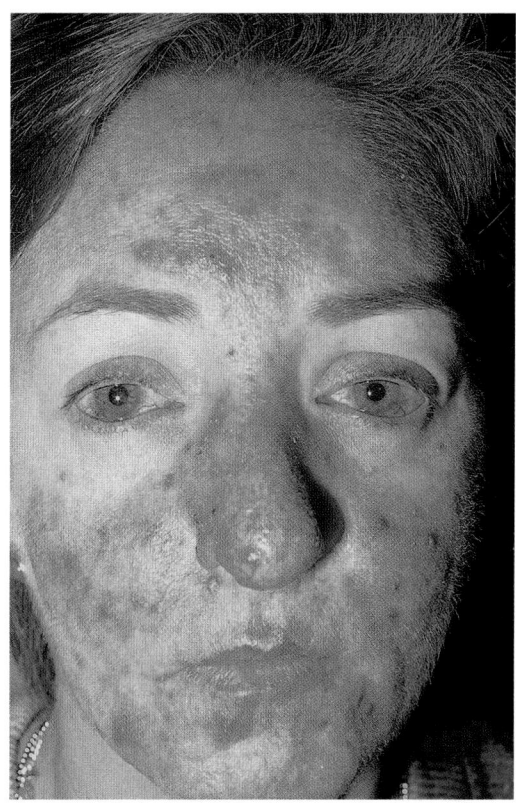

PLATE 74. Rosacea dermatitis. Note the typical features of facial rosacea which include (1) facial erythema, (2) papules and pustules, and (3) rhinophyma.

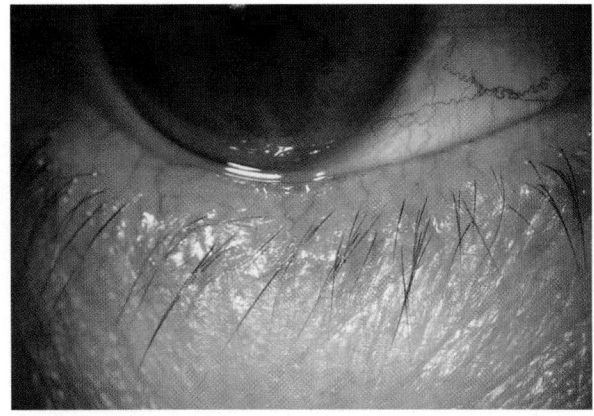

PLATE 75. Thickened, hyperemic, telangiectatic lid margin.

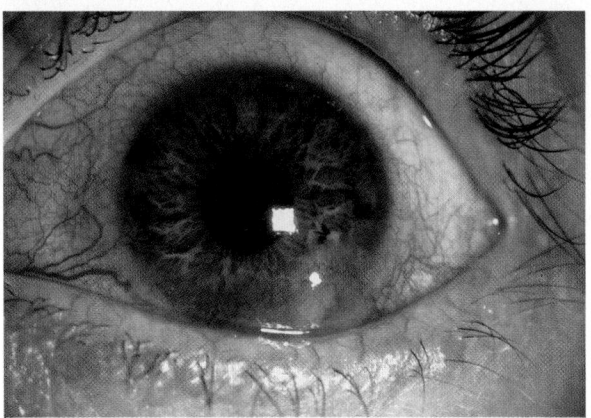

PLATE 76. Vascularized corneal nodular infiltrate seen crossing the inferior limbal margin. Note the extensive corneal neovascularization that is present.

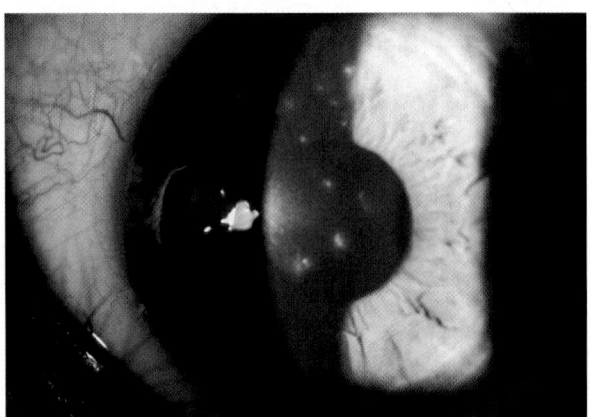

PLATE 77. Thygeson's superficial punctate keratitis (TSPK) corneal lesions evident on broad slit illumination.

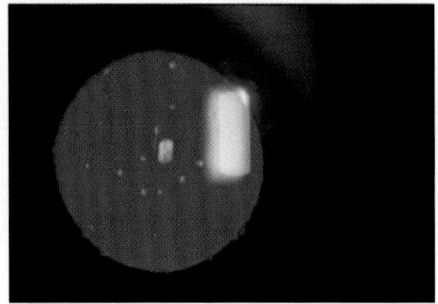

PLATE 78. TSPK corneal lesions apparent on retroillumination.

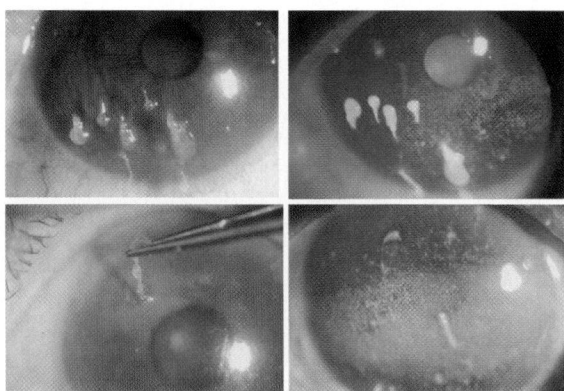

PLATE 79. Various types of filamentary keratitis.

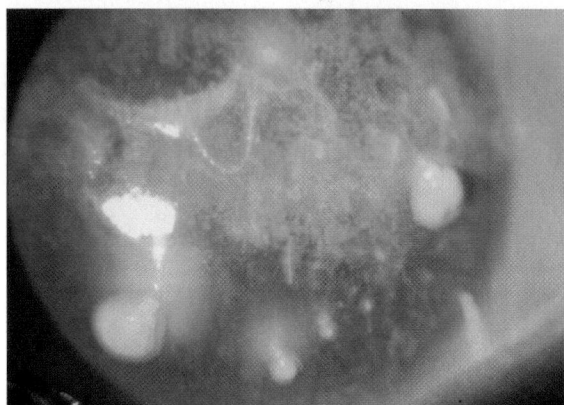

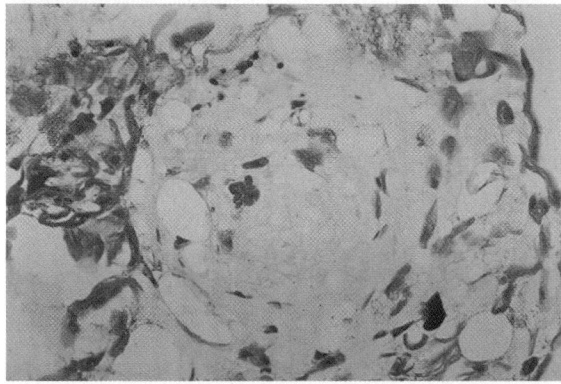

PLATE 80. The large filament (*top*) taken for histologic examination is composed of a central mucin core and degenerated epithelial cells surrounding the core (*bottom*).

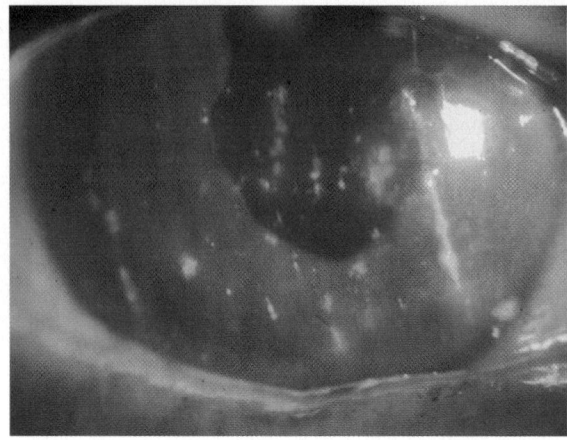

PLATE 81. Filamentary keratitis after cataract surgery.

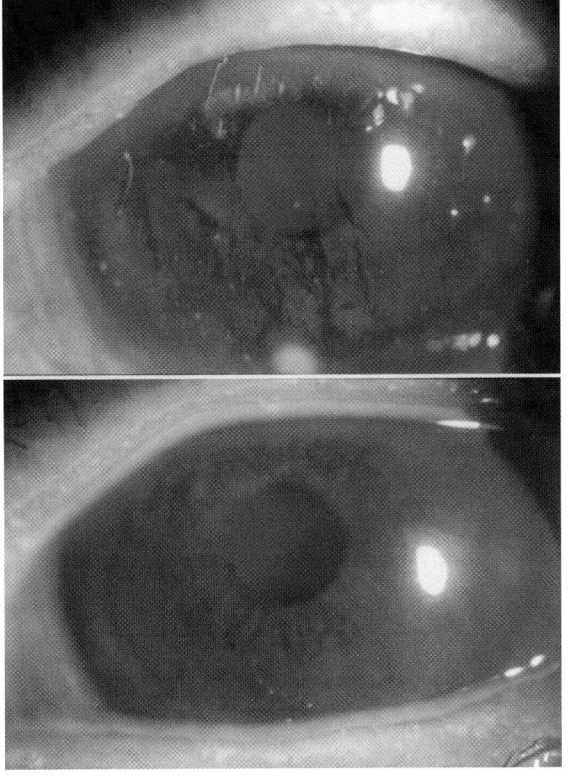

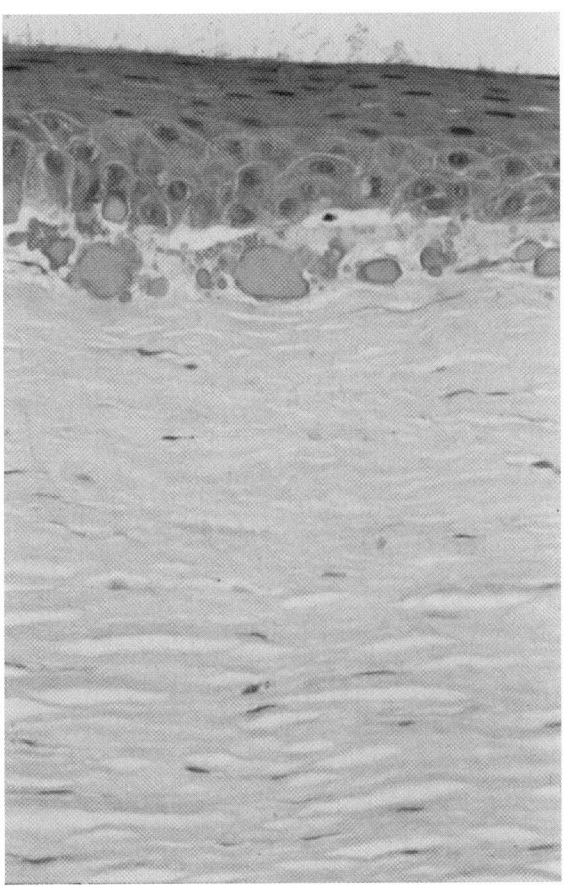

PLATE 82. Filamentary keratitis in tear-deficient dry eye (*top*). Filaments disappear after punctal occlusion to both the upper and lower puncta (*bottom*).

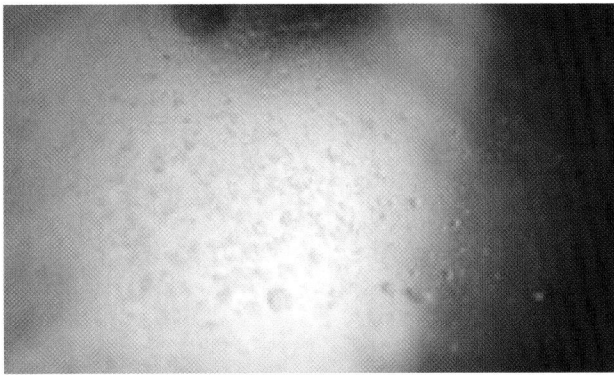

PLATE 83. Early clinical appearance of deposits of climatic keratopathy. (Courtesy of George Michelson, University Eye Clinic, Erlangen, Germany, from *Atlas of Ophthalmology*, online atlas: *atlasophthalmology.com*.)

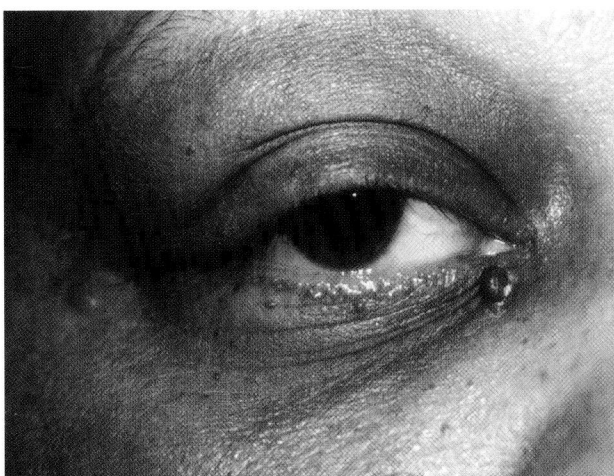

PLATE 85. Enlarged right lacrimal gland in a patient with chronic dacryoadenitis secondary to biopsy-proven sarcoidosis.

[image of hematoxylin and eosin section]

PLATE 84. Hematoxylin and eosin section of tissue showing hyaline deposits.

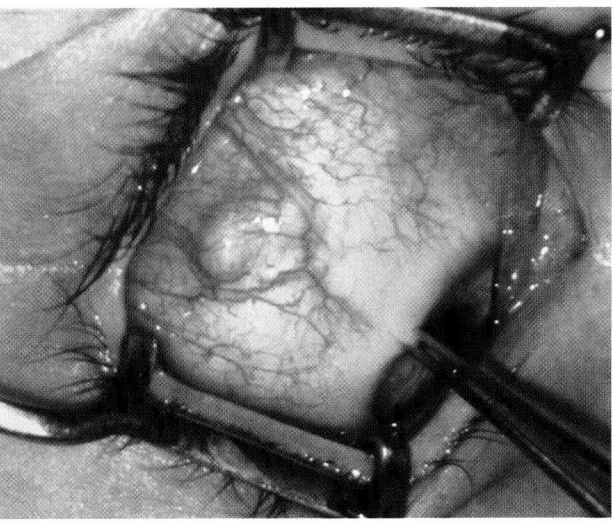

PLATE 86. Epibulbar osseous choristoma on bulbar conjunctiva superotemporally, presenting as a firm, palpable mass.

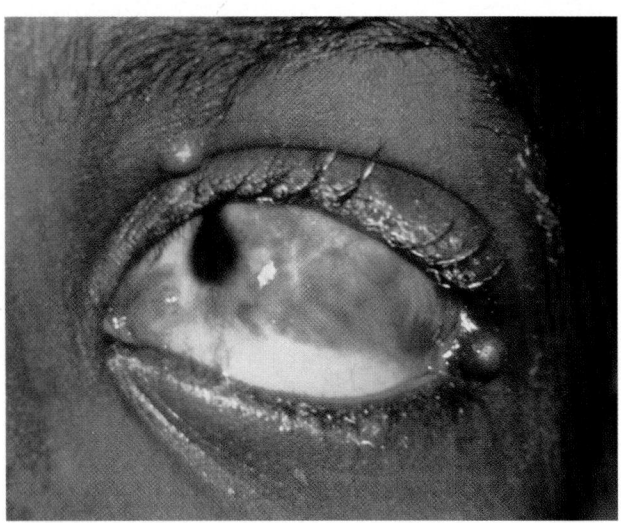

PLATE 87. Epibulbar complex choristoma that was found histopathologically to have cartilage and ectopic lacrimal gland.

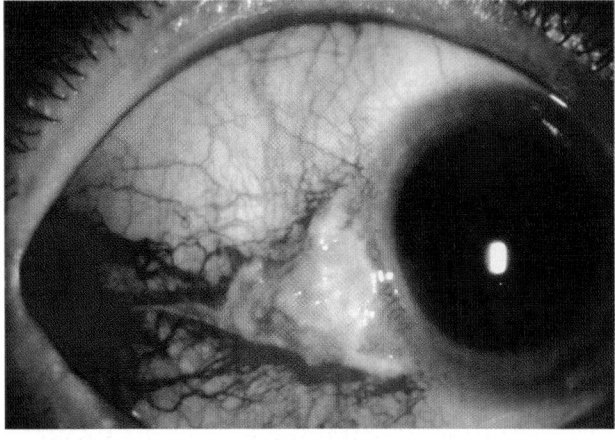

PLATE 88. Hereditary benign intraepithelial dyskeratosis in a young woman who was a descendent of a Haliwa Indian. The opposite eye had a similar lesion.

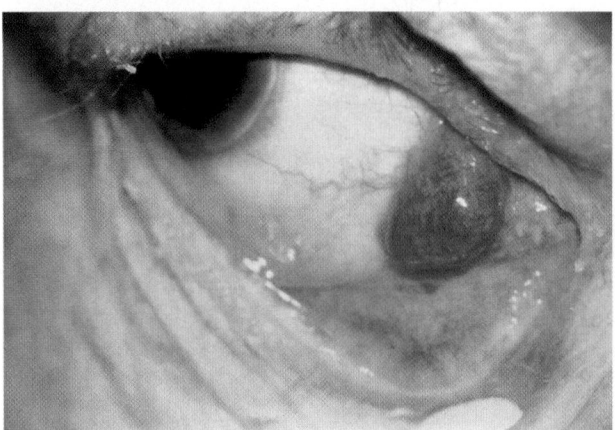

PLATE 89. Epibulbar inclusion cyst with thick mucous from conjunctival glands.

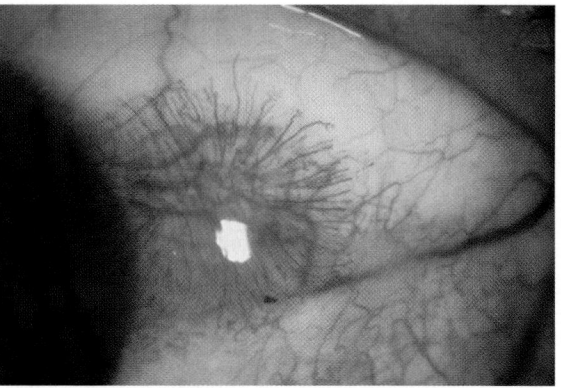

PLATE 90. Conjunctival intraepithelial neoplasia (CIN, carcinoma-in-situ) with corneal involvement, displaying leukoplakia on both the conjunctiva and cornea.

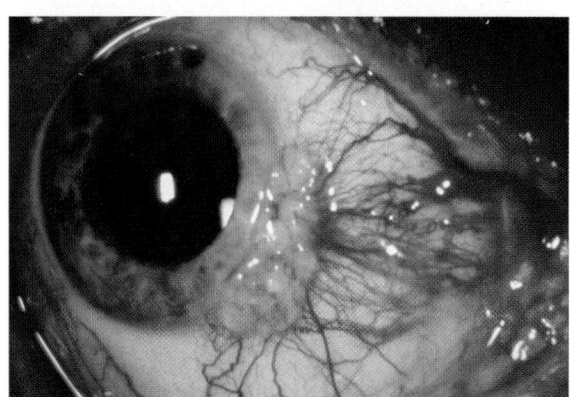

A

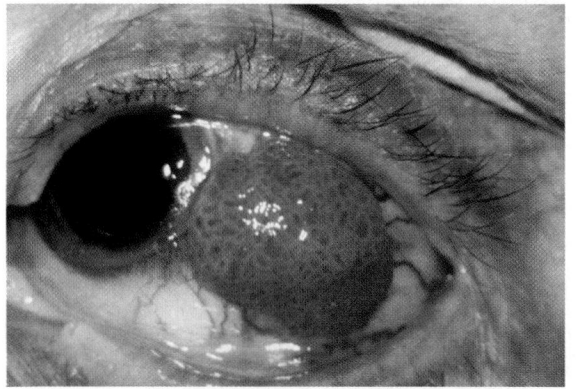

B

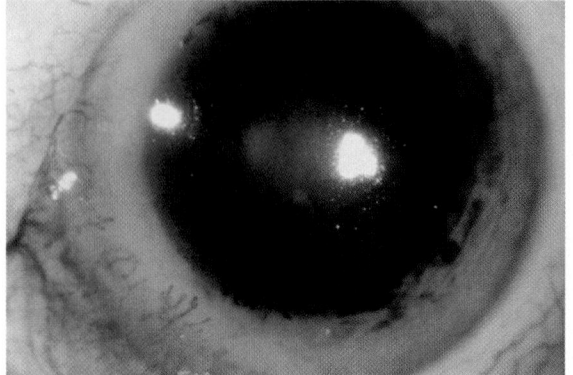

C

PLATE 91. Invasive squamous cell carcinoma of the conjunctiva. **A:** Gelatinous limbal squamous cell carcinoma. **B:** Nodular squamous cell carcinoma. **C:** Flat diffuse squamous cell carcinoma.

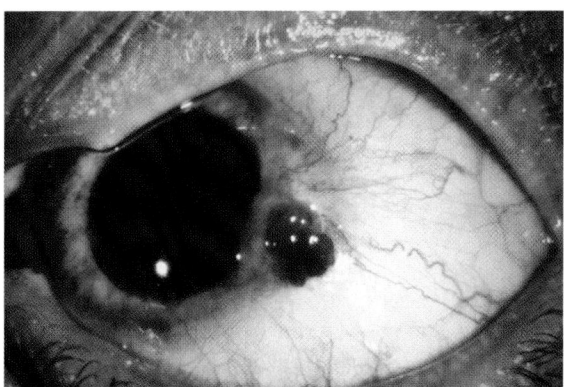

A

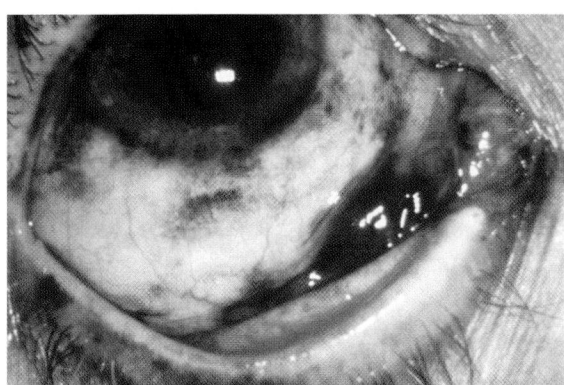

B

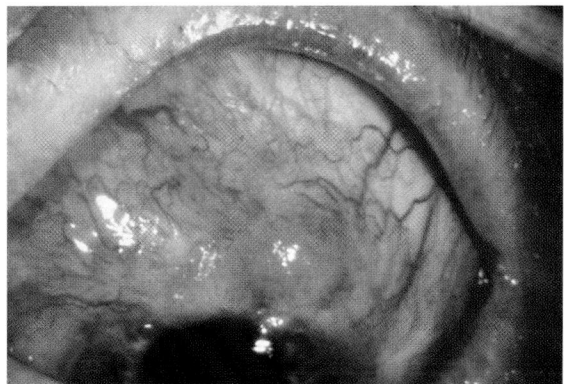

C

PLATE 92. Conjunctival melanoma. **A:** Pigmented melanoma that arose de novo. **B:** Pigmented melanoma that arose from primary acquired melanosis *(left arrow)*. Note the flat extension of the melanoma into the cornea. **C:** Nonpigmented melanoma, recurrent following previous excisions.

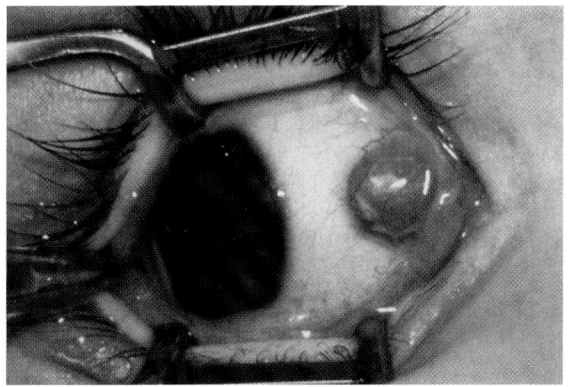

PLATE 93. Capillary hemangioma of the conjunctiva in a newborn infant.

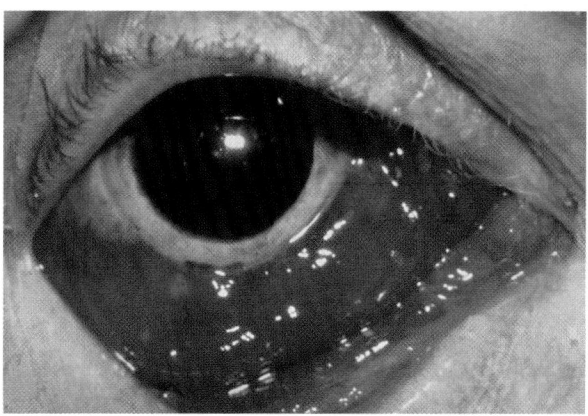

PLATE 94. Kaposi's sarcoma of the conjunctiva with typical surrounding hemorrhage.

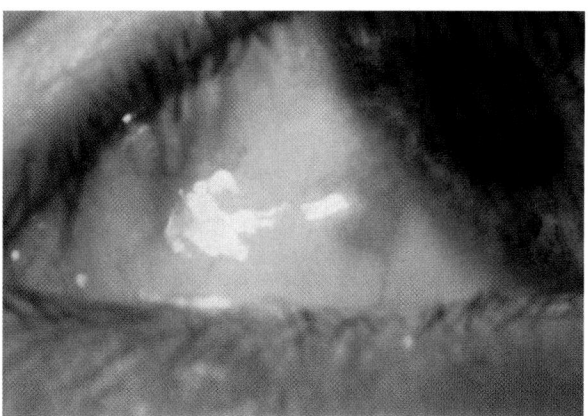

PLATE 95. Juvenile xanthogranuloma of the conjunctiva in a child.

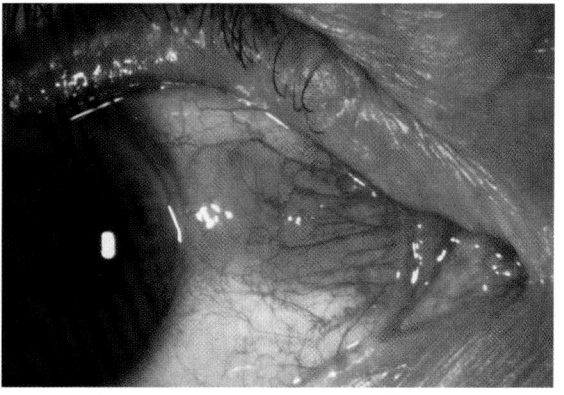

A

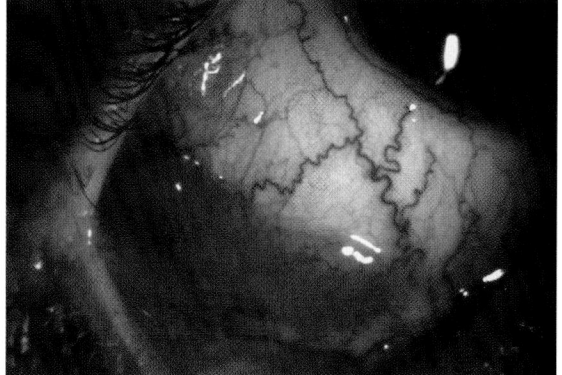

B

PLATE 96. Conjunctival lymphoma. **A:** Limbal tumor. **B:** Forniceal tumor.

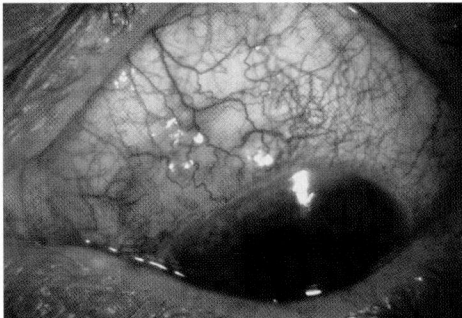

PLATE 97. Metastatic breast carcinoma to the conjunctiva.

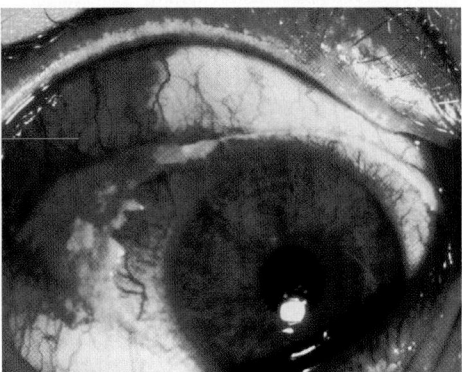

PLATE 98. Hereditary benign intraepithelial dyskeratosis (HBID). Raised, vascular hyperkeratotic lesion is located on the temporal interpalpebral conjunctiva. (Courtesy of the Armed Forces Institute of Pathology).

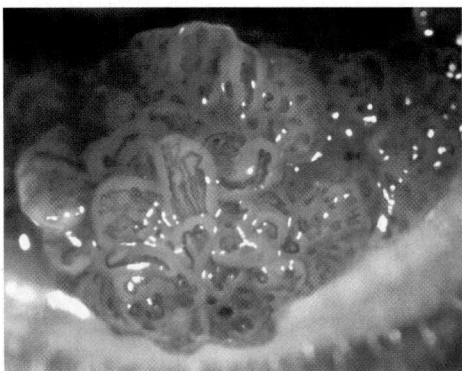

PLATE 99. Squamous papilloma. Exuberant proliferation of benign conjunctiva is present in the inferior fornix.

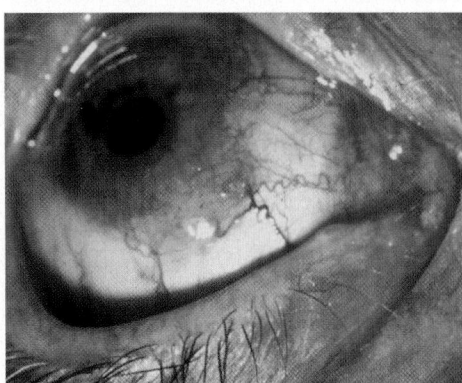

PLATE 100. Conjunctival intraepithelial neoplasia (CIN). A thickened, gelatinous lesion with increased vascularity is noted at the limbus. (Courtesy of the Armed Forces Institute of Pathology).

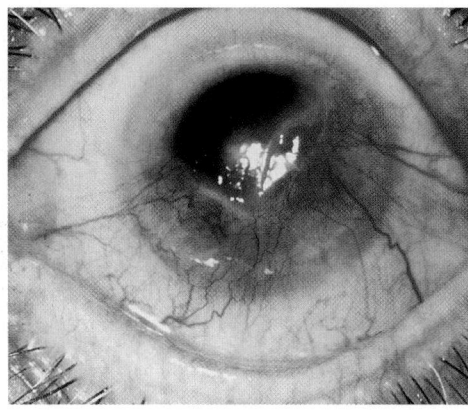

PLATE 101. CIN. Extension of translucent dysplastic epithelium into the cornea. This degree of limbal involvement causes limbal stem cell deficiency. (Courtesy of the Armed Forces Institute of Pathology).

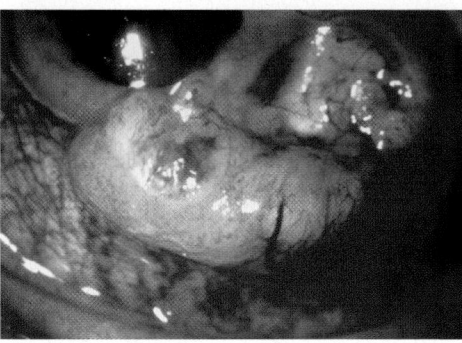

PLATE 102. Squamous cell carcinoma. A markedly thickened conjunctival tumor originates at the limbus. (Courtesy of the Armed Forces Institute of Pathology).

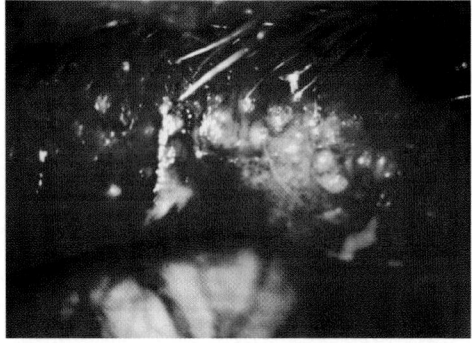

PLATE 103. Sebaceous carcinoma. The eyelid is thickened and inflamed. Sebaceous carcinoma is often mistaken for recurrent chalazion or chronic blepharitis.

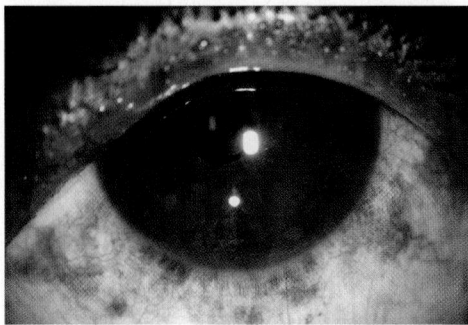

PLATE 104. Racial melanosis in a 45-year-old black woman with neurofibromatosis. Lisch nodules are an incidental finding.

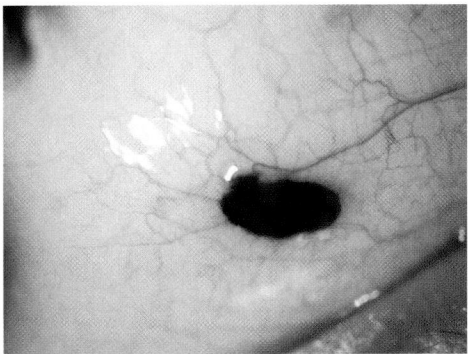

PLATE 105. Small localized pigmented conjunctival nevus in a 12-year-old boy.

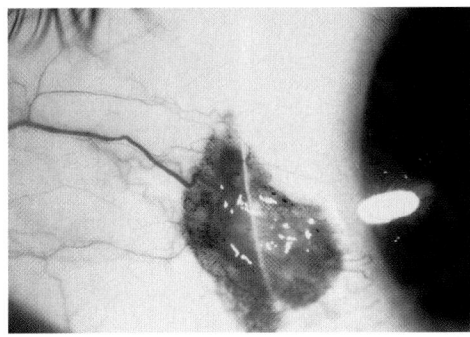

PLATE 106. Conjunctival nevus illustrating characteristic clear cysts. (Photo courtesy of Frederick A. Jakobiec, M.D.)

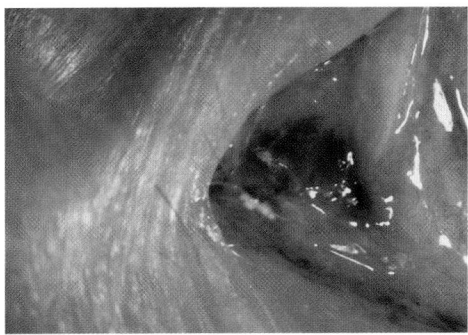

PLATE 107. Invasive malignant melanoma of the caruncle. The tumor is nodular and multifocal.

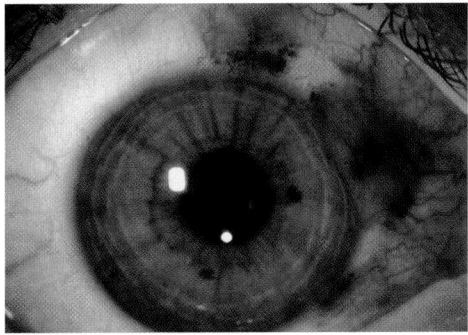

PLATE 108. Multifocal invasive conjunctival melanoma in a 23-year-old white woman. Note variations in pigment and prominent vasculature. Conjunctival melanomas are extremely rare in young adults.

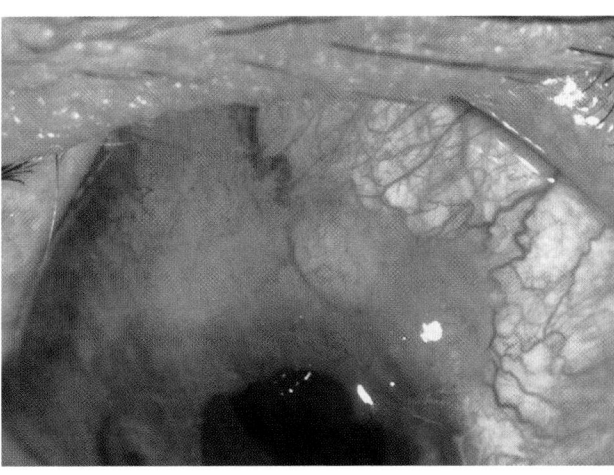

PLATE 109. Recurrent amelanotic malignant melanoma. The original tumor was pigmented. (Photo courtesy of Frederick A. Jakobiec, M.D.)

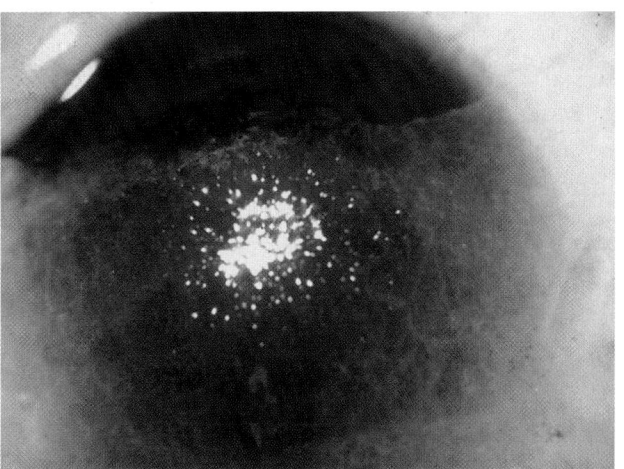

A

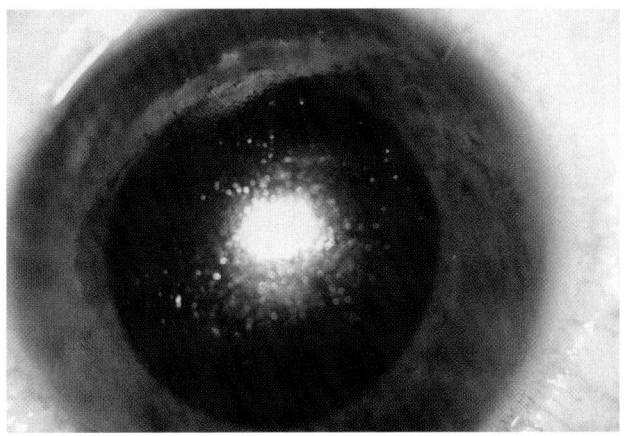

B

PLATE 110. A: Acid injury of the cornea and adjacent conjunctiva. Note the opalescent surface, a consequence of protein denaturation of the full thickness of the affected epithelium. **B:** Stripping off the cloudy epithelial layer uncovers the underlying crystal clear corneal stroma. Healing can take place without scarring or with very mild superficial nebulae.

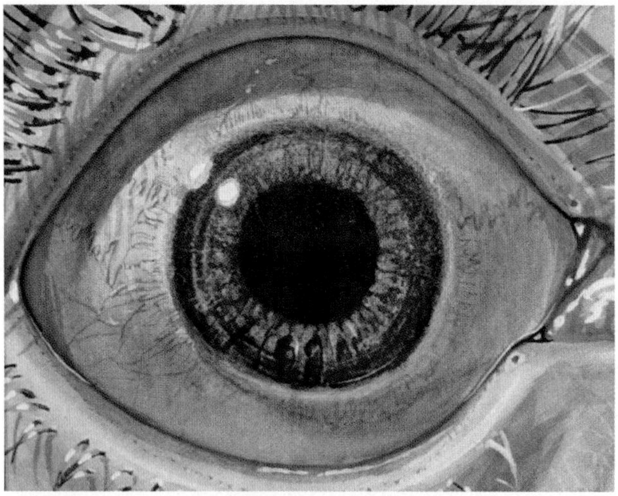

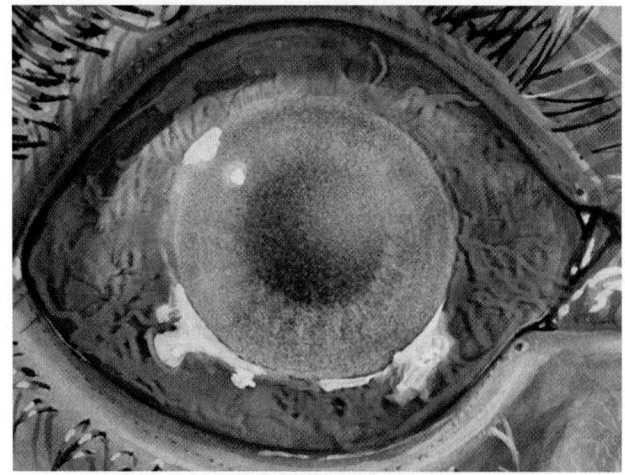

PLATE 111. Classification of alkali and very severe acid injuries of the eye. (Hughes classification modified by Pfister). Each painted illustration is accompanied by a photographic example. (From Pfister RR, Koski J: The pathophysiology and treatment of the alkali burned eye. *South Med J* 1982;75:417–422, with permission from *South Med J.*) **A:** Mild: corneal epithelial erosion, faint anterior stromal haziness, no ischemic necrosis of perilimbal conjunctiva and sclera. Prognosis: healing with little or no corneal scarring; visual loss usually no greater than one to two lines. **B:** Clinical photograph of mild alkali injury. **C:** Moderate: moderate corneal opacity, little or no significant ischemic necrosis of perilimbal conjunctiva. Prognosis: slow healing of epithelium with moderate scarring, peripheral corneal vascularization, and visual loss of two to seven lines. **D:** Clinical photograph of moderate alkali injury. **E:** Moderate to severe: corneal opacity blurring iris details, ischemic necrosis of conjunctiva limited to less than one third of perilimbal conjunctiva. Prognosis: prolonged corneal healing with significant corneal vascularization and scarring; vision usually limited to 20/200 or less.

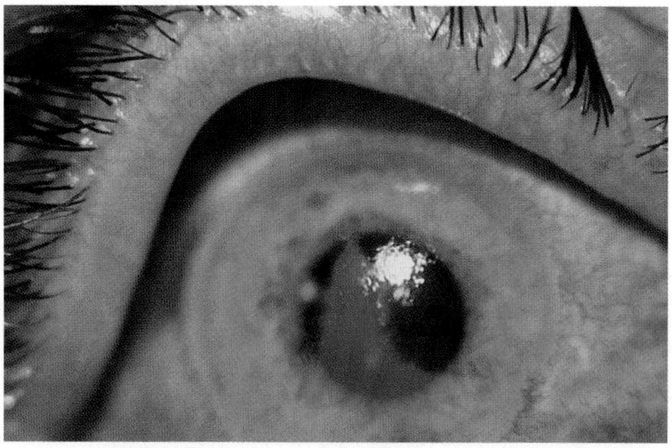

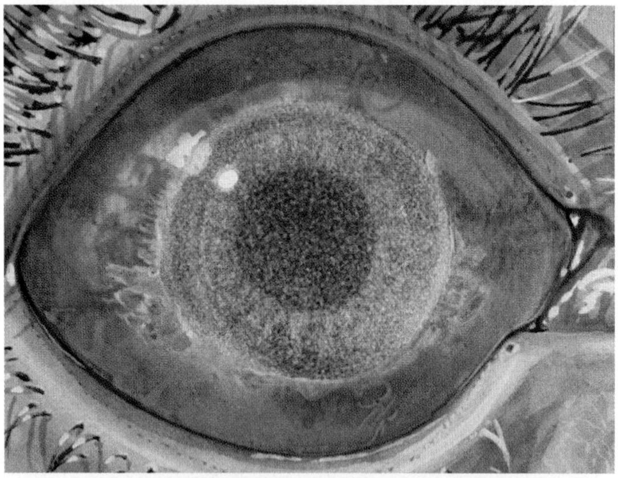

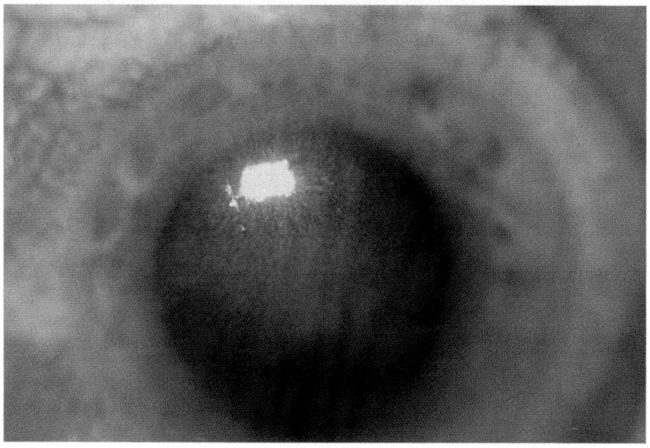

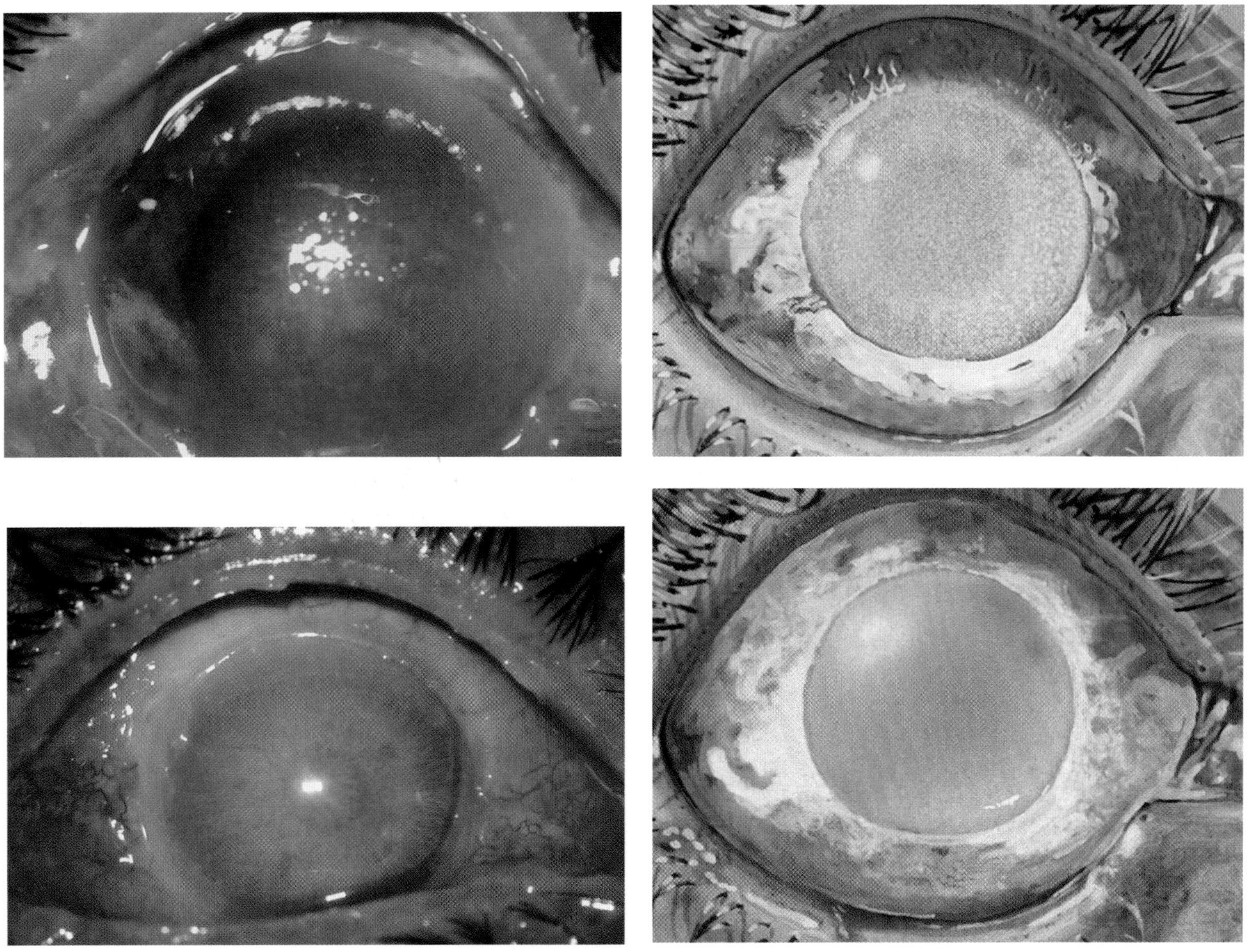

F

G

H

I

PLATE 111. *(Continued)* **F:** Clinical photograph of moderate to severe alkali injury. **G:** Severe: blurring of pupillary outline, ischemia of approximately one third to two thirds of perilimbal conjunctiva, cornea often marbleized. Prognosis: very prolonged corneal healing with inflammation and high incidence of corneal ulceration and perforation. In the best cases, there is severe corneal vascularization and scarring with counting fingers vision. **H:** Clinical photograph of severe alkali injury. **I:** Very severe: pupil not visible; greater than two-thirds ischemia of perilimbal conjunctiva, cornea often marbleized. Prognosis: very prolonged corneal healing with inflammation and high incidence of corneal ulceration and perforation. In the best cases, there is severe corneal vascularization and scarring with counting-fingers vision.

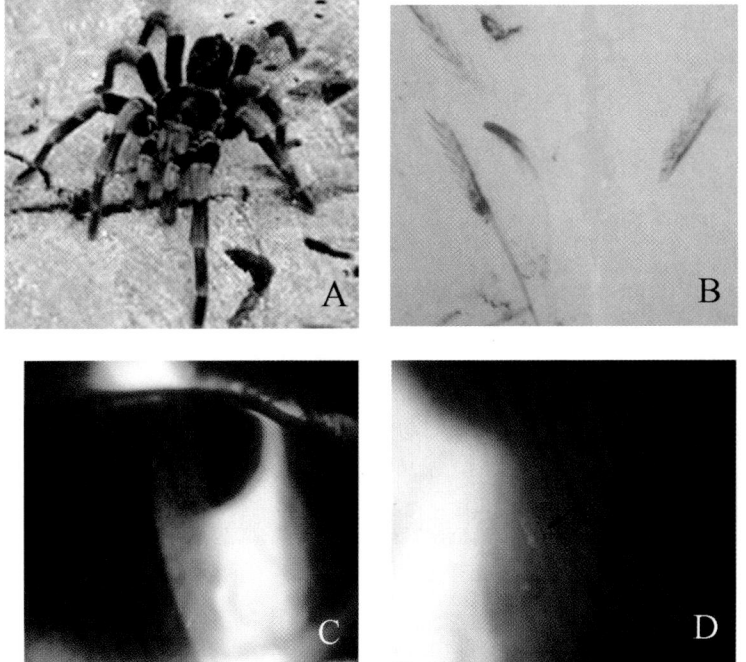

A

B

C

D

PLATE 112. Tarantula keratits. **A:** Tarantula spider. **B:** High magnification examination of the tarantula hairs. **C:** Corneal edema. **D:** Higher magnification of the cornea demonstrating embedded tarantula's hair *(arrow).*

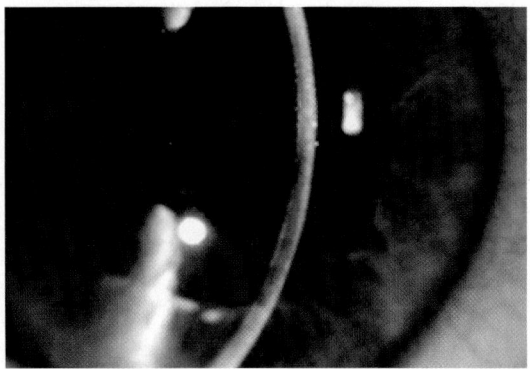

PLATE 113. Central corneal guttae without stromal thickening.

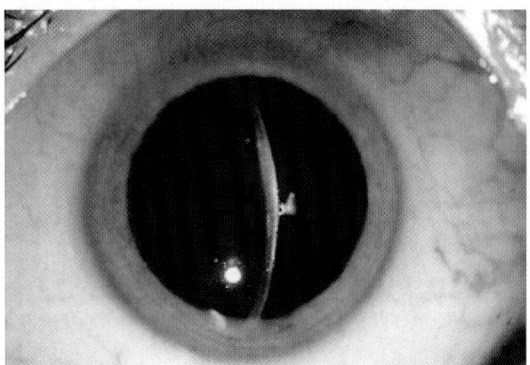

A

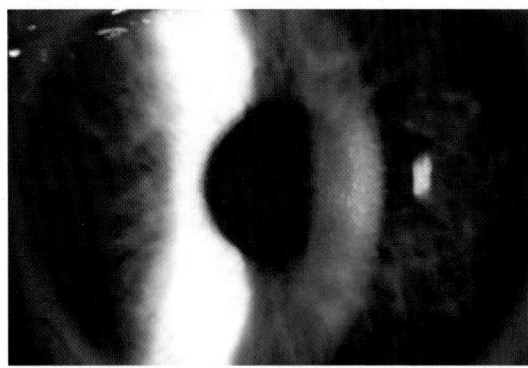

B

PLATE 114. A: Stage 2 Fuchs' endothelial dystrophy. Corneal guttae with pigmentary dusting create a beaten metal appearance. Note the stromal edema in central cornea; peripheral cornea is of normal thickness. **B:** Late stage 2 Fuchs' endothelial dystrophy. The cornea has diffuse stromal edema with haze. No epithelial edema is noted.

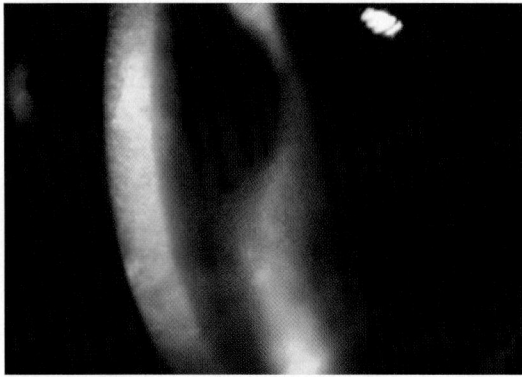

PLATE 115. Stage 3 Fuchs' endothelial dystrophy showing diffuse stromal and epithelial edema with microcystic changes.

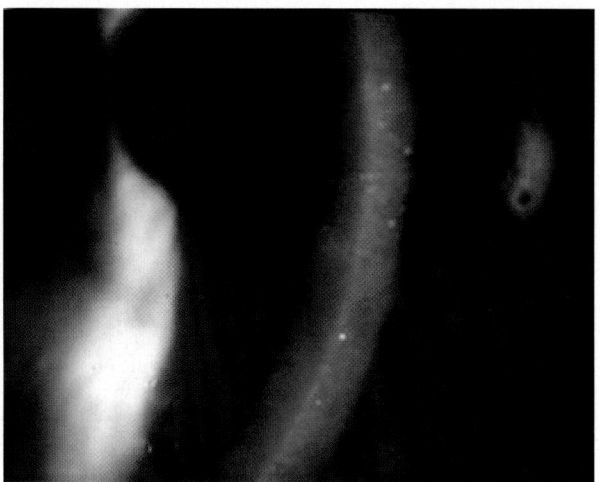

A

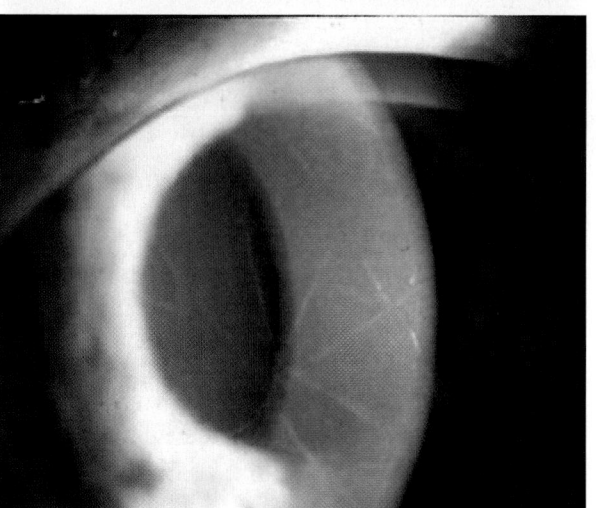

B

PLATE 116. A: Posterior polymorphous dystrophy (PPMD). Endothelial vesicular lesions with scalloped edges are seen in the paracentral cornea. (Photo courtesy of Claes H. Dohlman, M.D., with permission) **B:** PPMD. Irregular endothelial bands are present throughout the central cornea.

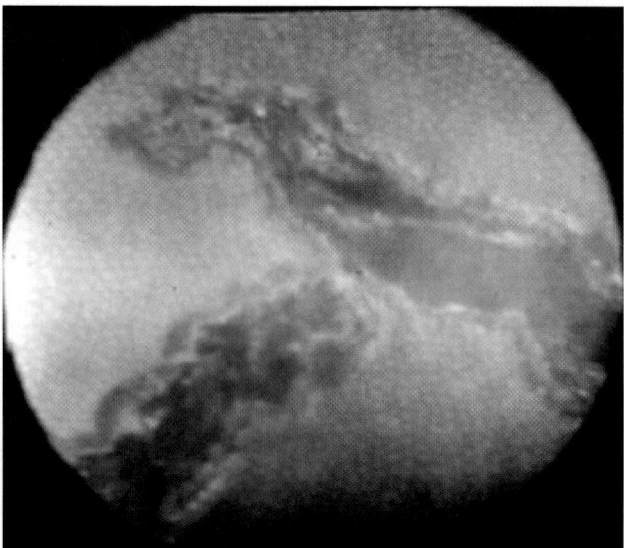

PLATE 117. Specular microscopy of PPMD. Grouped vesicles with indistinct borders coalesce to create black areas in the endothelial mosaic. The surrounding endothelium has a normal appearance. (Photo courtesy of Claes H. Dohlman, M.D., with permission.)

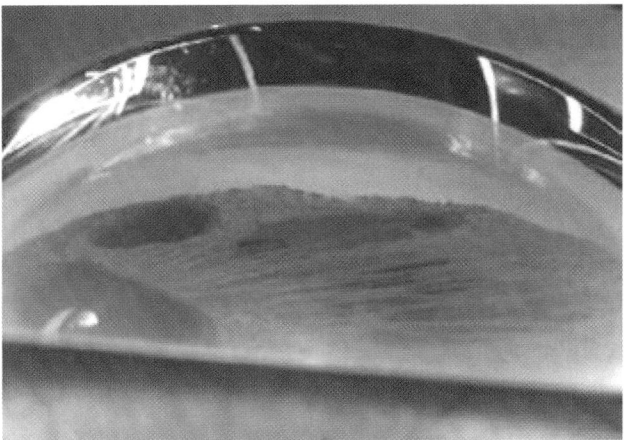

PLATE 118. Gonioscopic photograph of ICE syndrome shows extensive peripheral anterior synechiae associated with corectopia, ectropion uveae, iris stretching, and atrophy. Multiple iris holes are present.

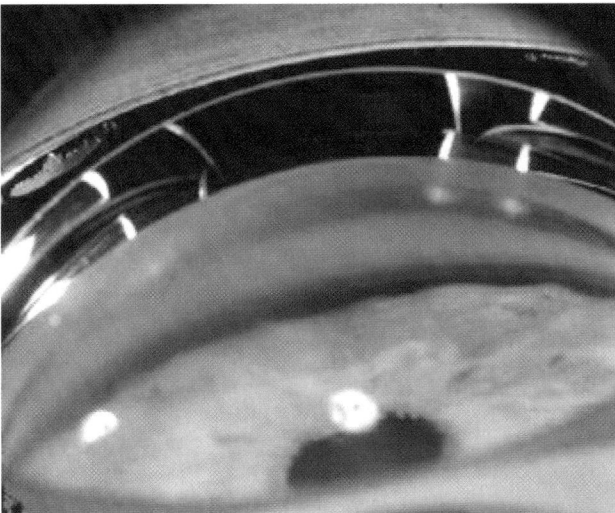

PLATE 119. Chandler's syndrome. Peripheral anterior synechiae are usually subtle and visible only with gonioscopy.

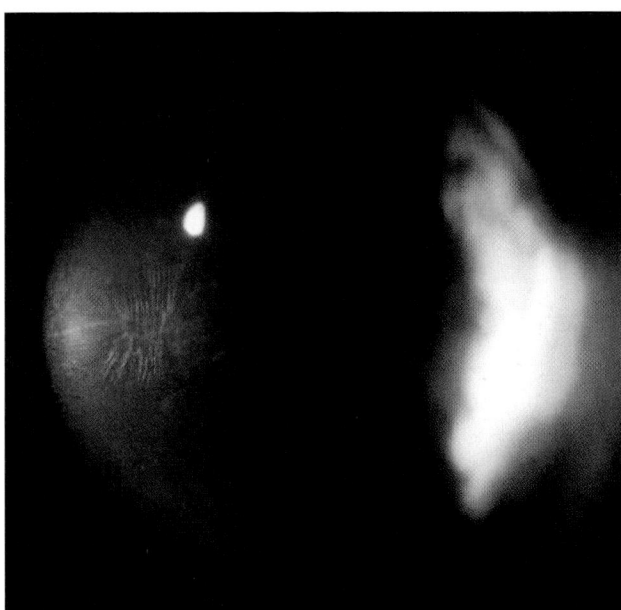

PLATE 121. Slit-lamp photograph demonstrating Vogt's striae at the level of Descemet's membrane.

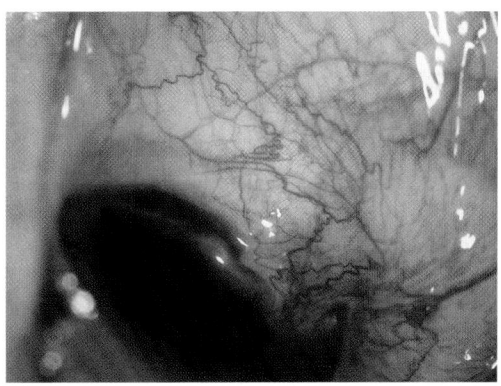

A

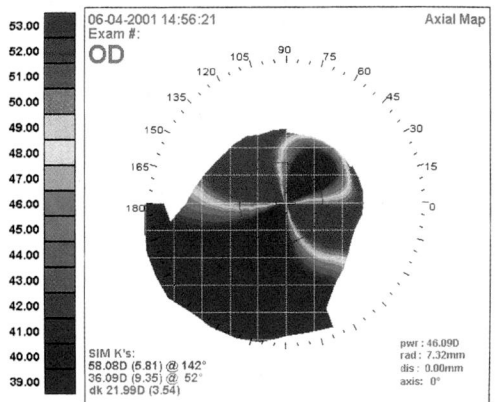

B

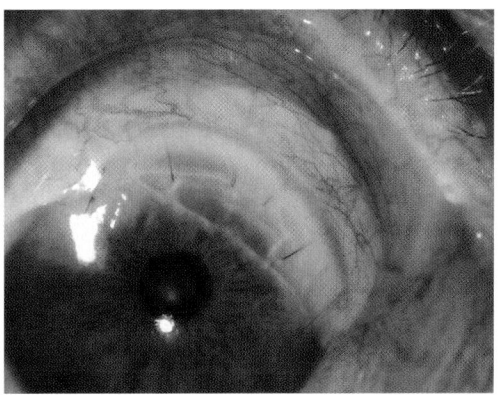

C

PLATE 120. A: A 70-year-old patient presented with a history of decreased visual acuity of the right eye since the age of 47. Examination of the cornea revealed extensive corneal thinning superiorly and an adjacent conjunctival cyst. **B:** Corneal topography of the cornea in Fig. 48-11A showed induced high oblique astigmatism. **C:** The patient underwent excision of the conjunctival cyst and tectonic corneal grafting to reinforce the eye.

PLATE 122. Magnified view of Vogt's striae or stress lines in the cornea.

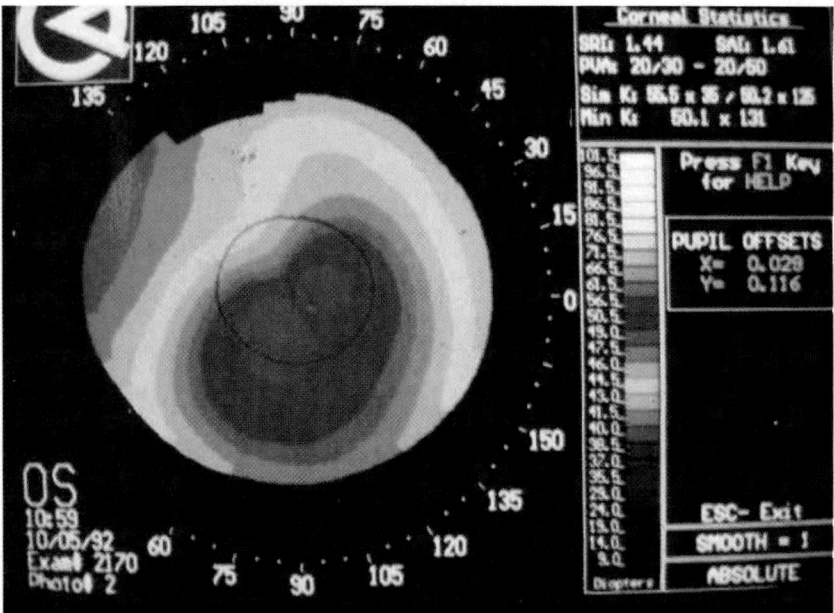

PLATE 123. Videokeratograph of an oval cone in keratoconus.

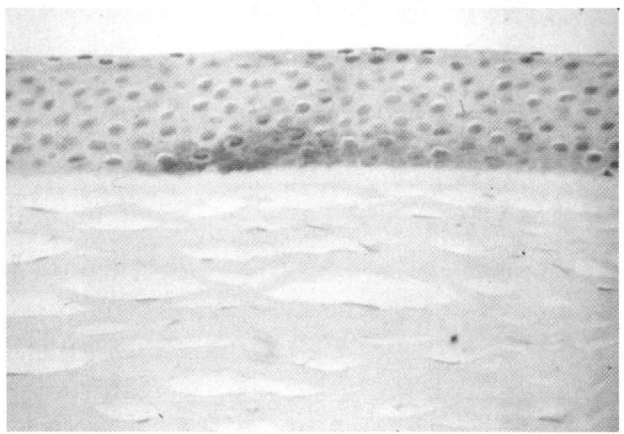

PLATE 124. Histopathologic micrograph illustrating iron deposition at the basal epithelial layer seen in keratoconus.

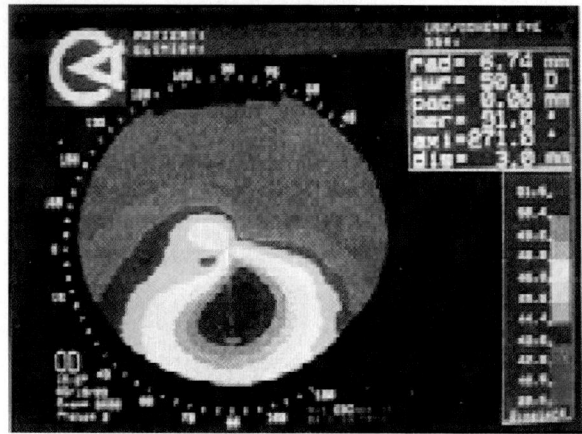

PLATE 125. Topographic phenotypic features of keratoconus and calculation of the I-S value (inferior-superior dioptric asymmetry).

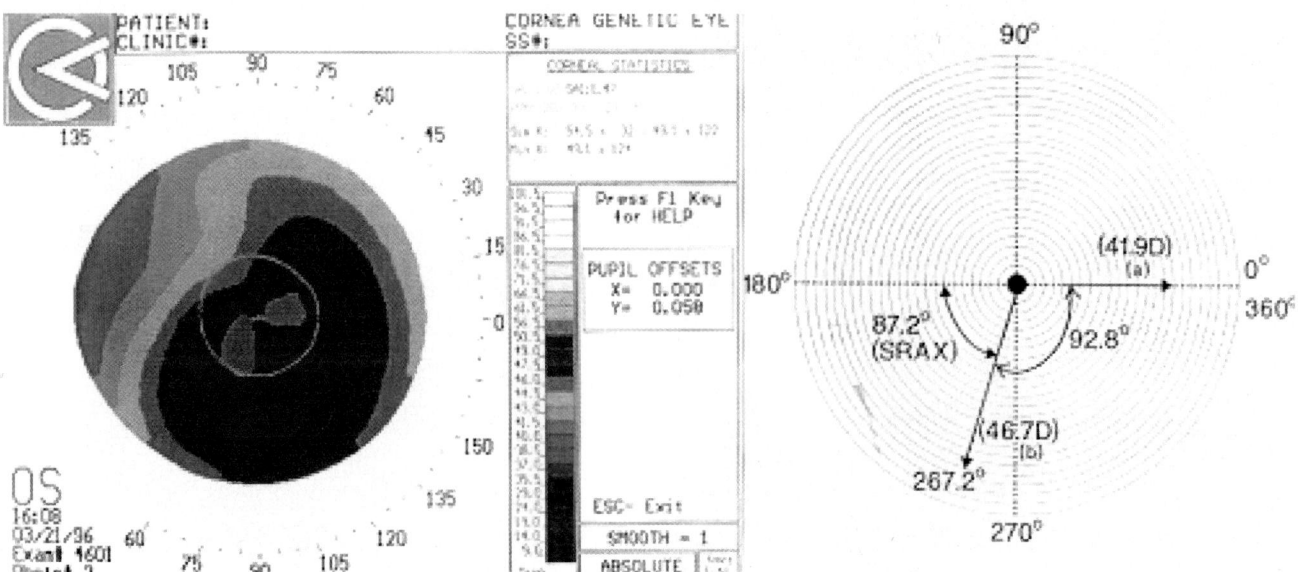

PLATE 126. Topographic phenotypic features of keratoconus and calculation of the SRAX index, used in calculating the KISA% index.

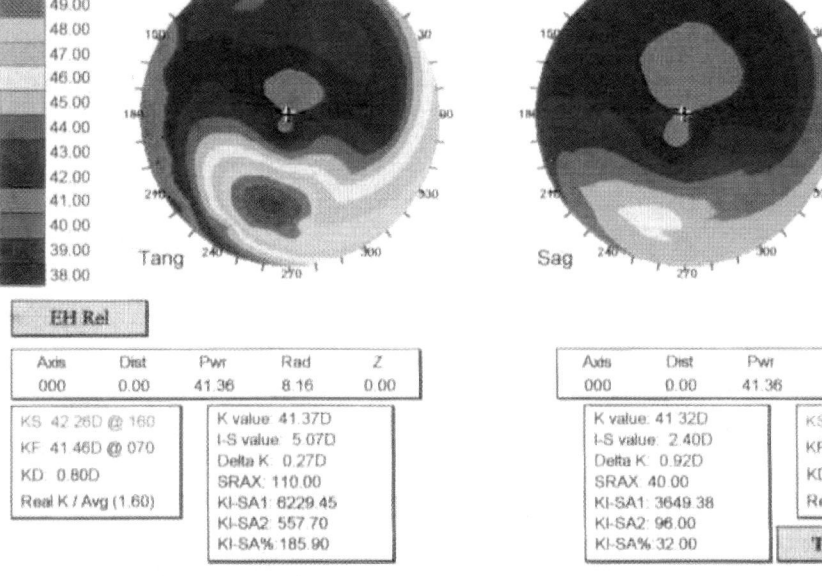

Axis	Dist	Pwr	Rad	Z
000	0.00	41.36	8.16	0.00

KS 42.26D @ 160	K value: 41.37D
KF 41.46D @ 070	I-S value: 5.07D
KD 0.80D	Delta K: 0.27D
Real K / Avg (1.60)	SRAX: 110.00
	KI-SA1: 6229.45
	KI-SA2: 557.70
	KI-SA%: 185.90

Axis	Dist	Pwr	Rad	Z
000	0.00	41.36	8.16	0.00

K value: 41.32D	KS 41.96D @ 170
I-S value: 2.40D	KF 40.97D @ 070
Delta K: 0.92D	KD 0.99D
SRAX: 40.00	Real K / Avg (1.60)
KI-SA1: 3649.38	
KI-SA2: 96.00	Tang. vs. Sag.
KI-SA%: 32.00	

PLATE 127. Calculation of the KISA% index, the K value, and I-S value in the fellow eye of a patient with keratoconus both in the sagittal and tangential mode, showing increased sensitivity of tangential topography for detecting keratoconus.

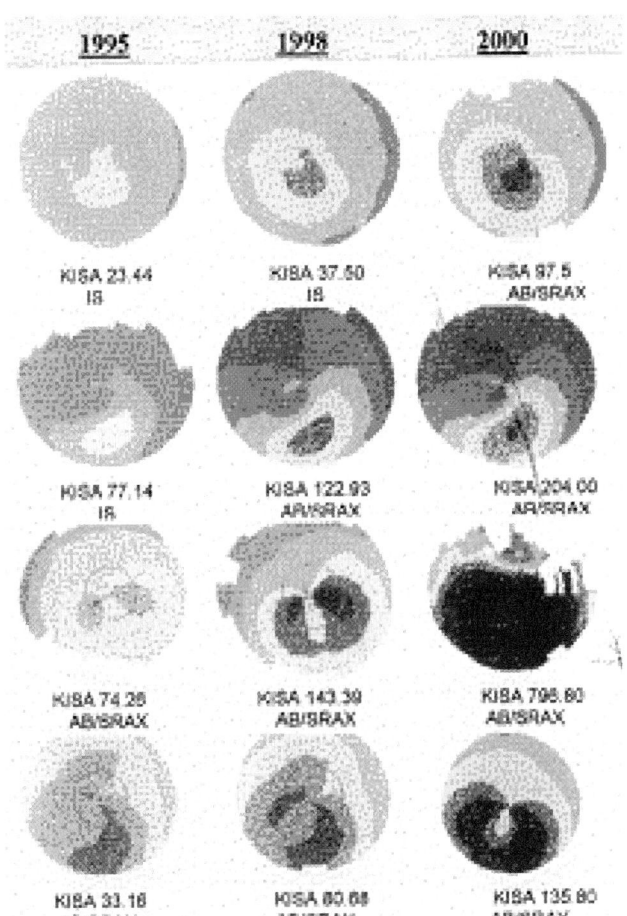

PLATE 128. Examples of eyes that progressed from normal and keratoconus suspect to keratoconus over time, illustrating accompanying pattern analyses and KISA% quantitative indices.

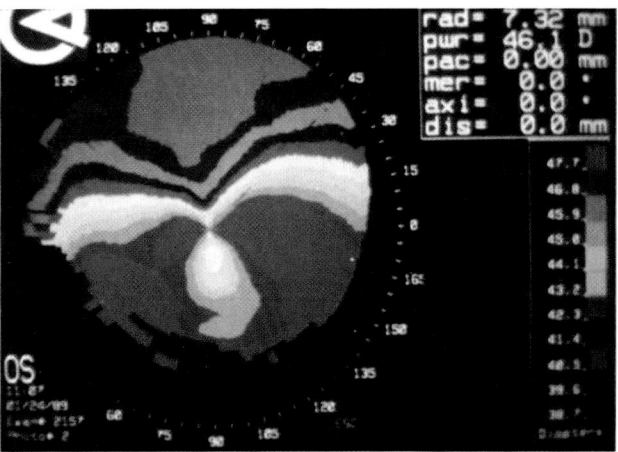

PLATE 129. Videokeratograph of pellucid marginal degeneration showing typical "crab claw" appearance and against-the-rule astigmatism.

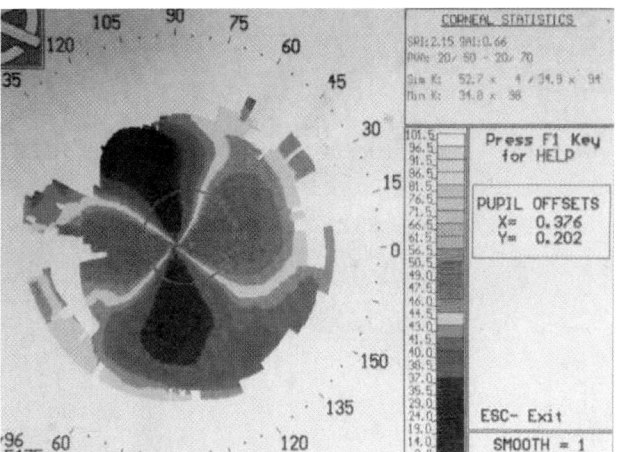

PLATE 130. Videokeratograph showing large amount of astigmatism following penetrating keratoplasty not correctable with glasses or contact lenses.

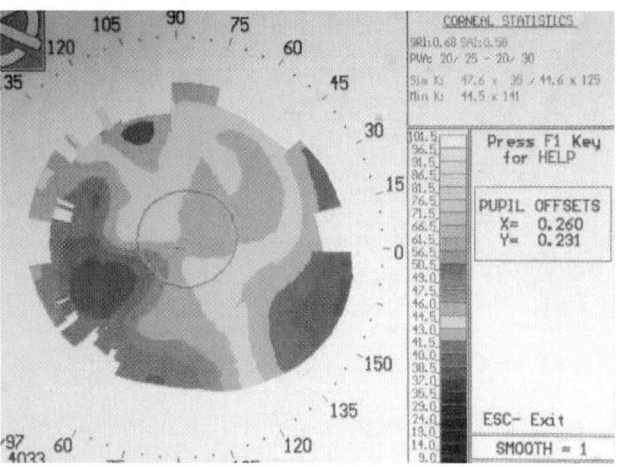

PLATE 131. Videokeratograph showing reduction of astigmatism following arcuate astigmatic keratotomy and compression sutures.

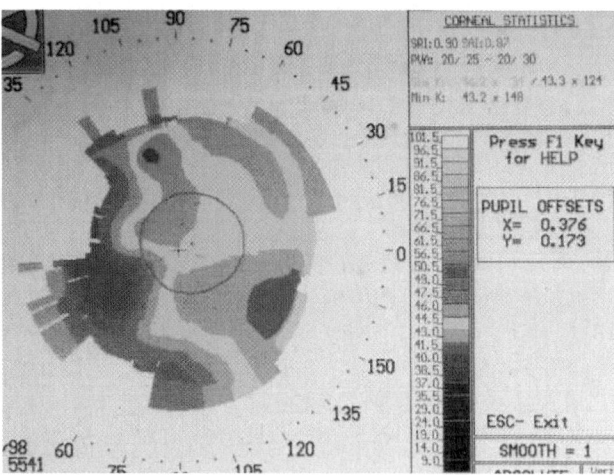

PLATE 132. Videokeratograph showing further reduction of astigmatism and myopia after LASIK; uncorrected vision of 20/30.

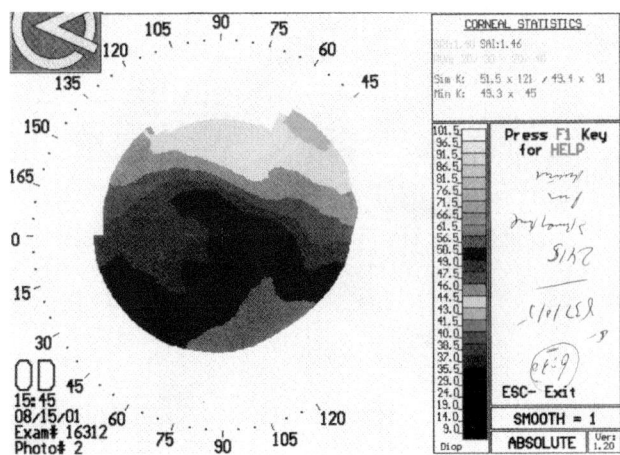

PLATE 133. Ectasia in a patient who had LASIK with undiagnosed early keratoconus.

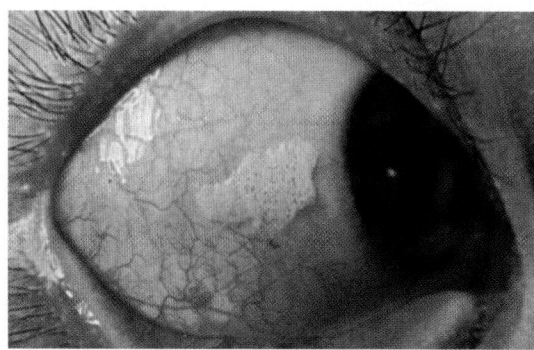

PLATE 134. Bitot's spot, a foamy, light-gray area of conjunctiva frequently found in vitamin A deficiency in humans. (From Sommer A. *Nutritional blindness: xerophthalmia and keratomalacia.* New York: Oxford University Press, 1982, with permission.)

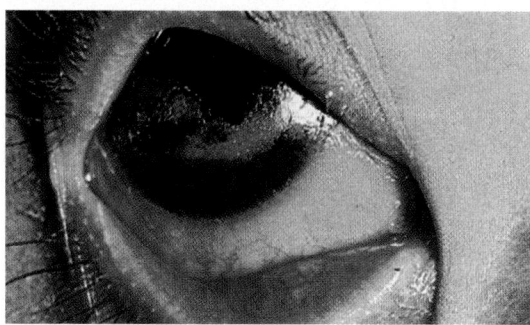

PLATE 135. Corneal xerosis. Keratinization and superficial punctate keratitis are characteristic of epithelial involvement in nutritional disease. (From Sommer A. *Field guide to the detection and control of xerophthalmia.* Geneva: World Health Organization, 1978, with permission.)

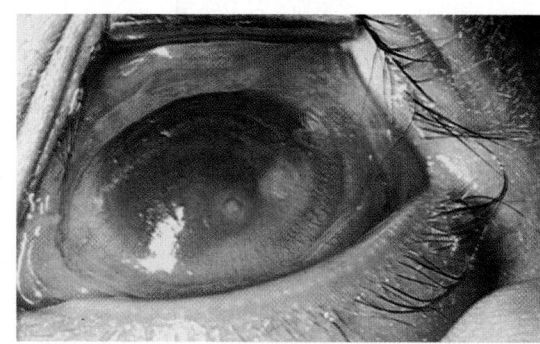

PLATE 136. Corneal ulceration with xerosis. (From Sommer A, Tjakrasudjatma S. Corneal xerophthalmia and keratomalacia. *Arch Ophthalmol* 1982;100:404, with permission.)

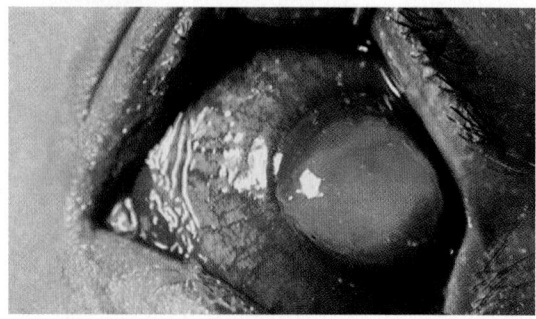

PLATE 137. Keratomalacia. Rapid melting of cornea accompanies advanced starvation in children. (From Sommer A. *Nutritional blindness: xerophthalmia and keratomalacia.* New York: Oxford University Press, 1982, with permission.)

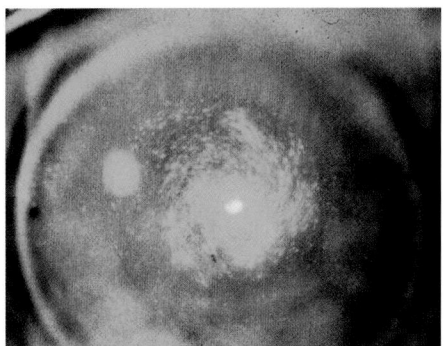

PLATE 138. Typical whorl-shaped staining pattern caused by contact lens apical compression.

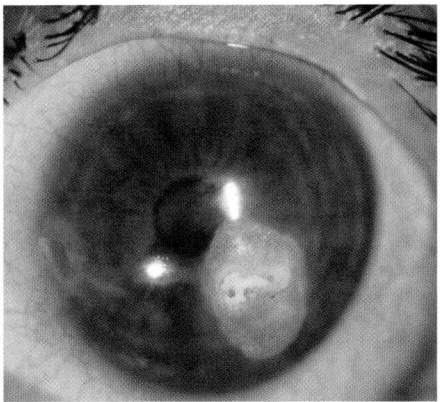

PLATE 139. Tissue adhesive on a paracentral corneal ulcer.

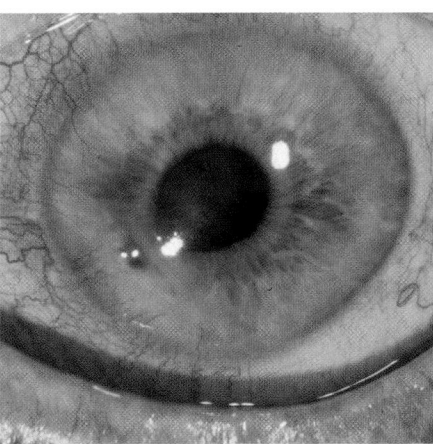

PLATE 140. Peripheral ulcerative sterile keratitis in an 84-year-old patient without an underlying immunologic disorder.

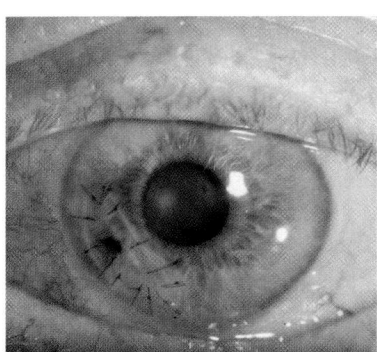

PLATE 141. Same patient as in Fig. 53-1. One month after tectonic keratoplasty and iridectomy.

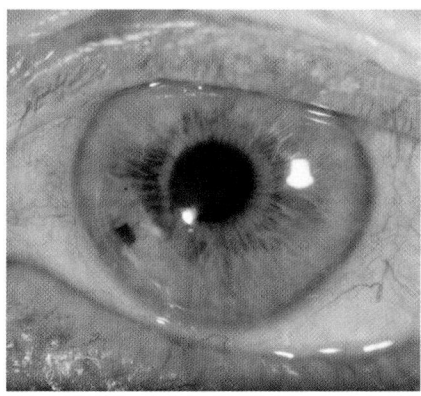

PLATE 142. Same patient as in Fig. 53-1. Three years after tectonic keratoplasty.

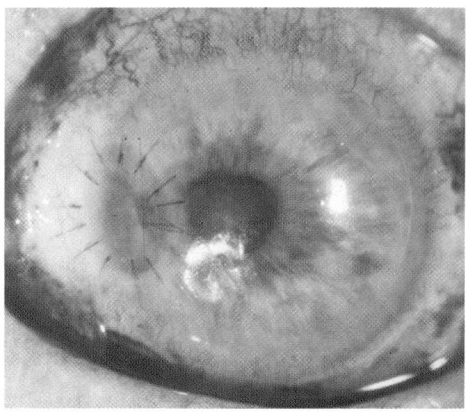

PLATE 143. Peripheral minikeratoplasty for perforated rheumatoid ulcer in a 75-year-old patient.

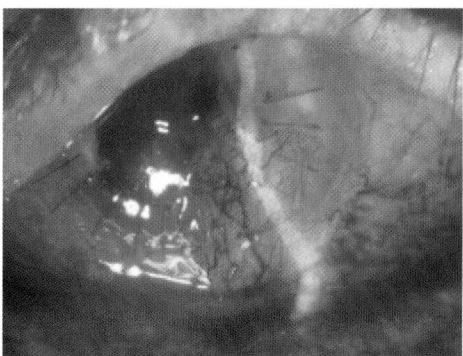

PLATE 144. Corneal graft melting in patient with rheumatoid arthritis treated succesfully with partial pedicle conjunctival flap.

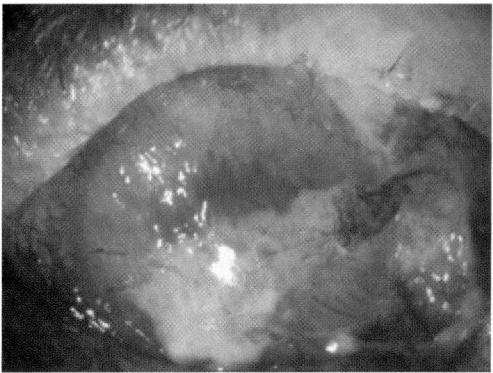

PLATE 145. Partial conjunctival flap necrosis in patient with ocular cicatricial pemphigoid 6 weeks after surgery.

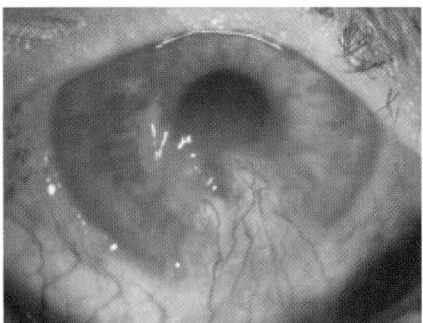

PLATE 146. Corneal melting on the central margin of partial conjunctival flap in patient with stromal herpetic keratitis.

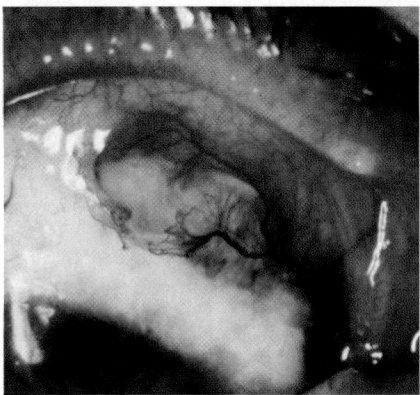

PLATE 147. Necrotizing scleritis with inflammation.

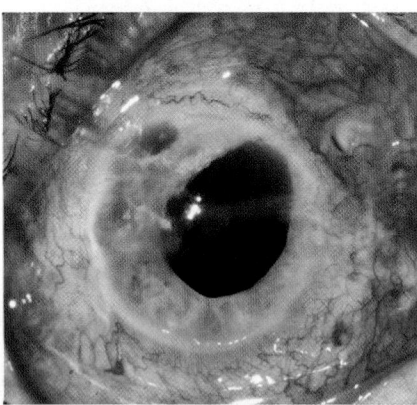

PLATE 148. Necrotizing scleritis with associated peripheral corneal ulceration.

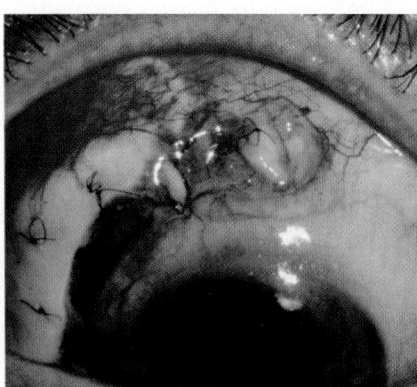

PLATE 149. Recurrence of necrotizing scleritis in a patient with rheumatoid arthritis who was not immunosuppressed, but whose necrotizing scleritis was simply treated with scleral grafting, a strategy guaranteed to have this outcome.

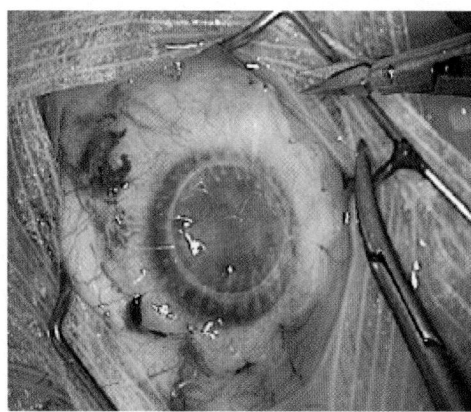

PLATE 150. Overlay amniotic membrane graft.

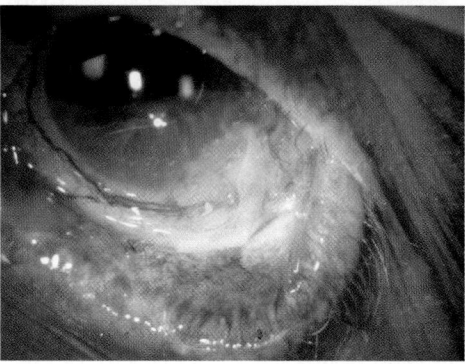

PLATE 151. Symblepharon in a patient with ocular cicatricial pemphigoid 1 month after conjunctival fornix reconstruction with amniotic membrane graft.

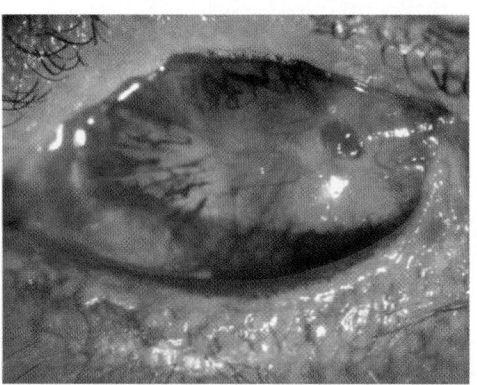

A

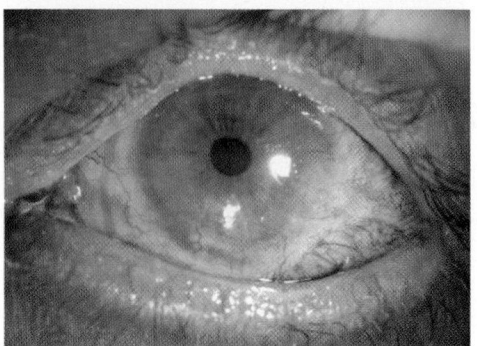

B

PLATE 152. A patient with history of toxic epidermal necrolysis before **(A)** and 6 months after **(B)** limbal stem cell allotransplantation.

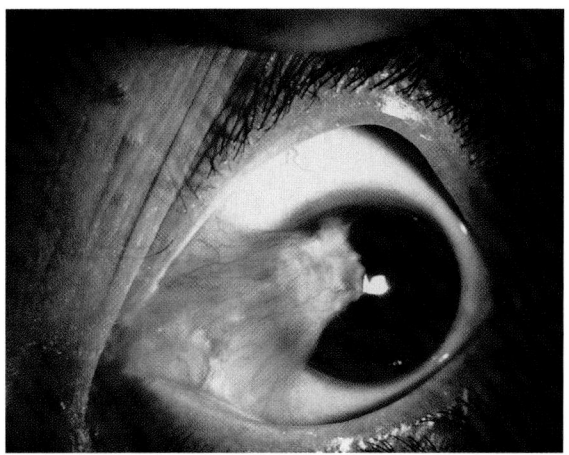

PLATE 153. Primary nasal pterygium growing into visual axis.

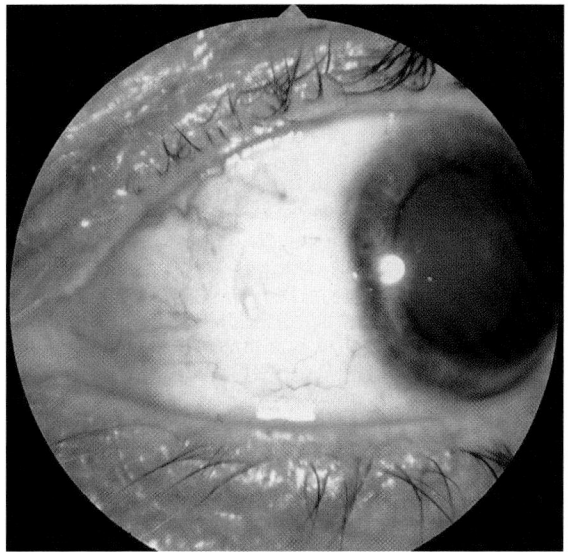

PLATE 154. Scleral thinning seen 2 years after beta irradiation of the bare sclera as adjunctive treatment after excision of a nasal pterygium. There are no signs of pterygium recurrence.

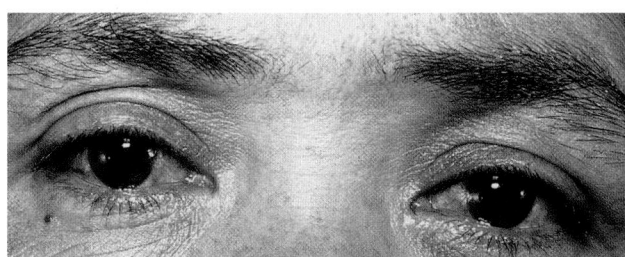

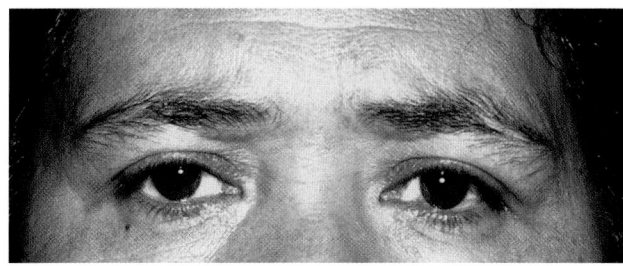

PLATE 155. A, Preoperative *primary* double pterygia in the right eye and a primary nasal pterygium in the left eye. **B,** Same patient without pterygium recurrence in either eye and excellent cosmetic results seen 2 years after surgery with adjunctive use of 0.4 mg/mL (0.04%) mitomycin C.

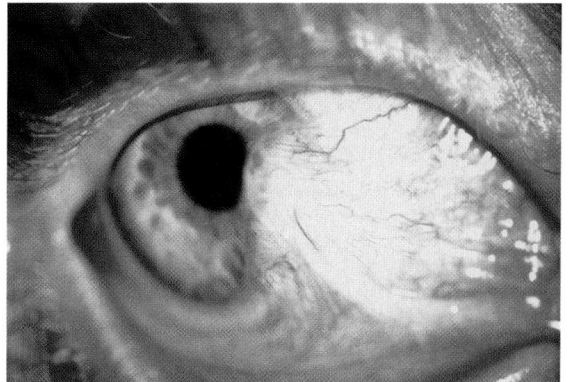

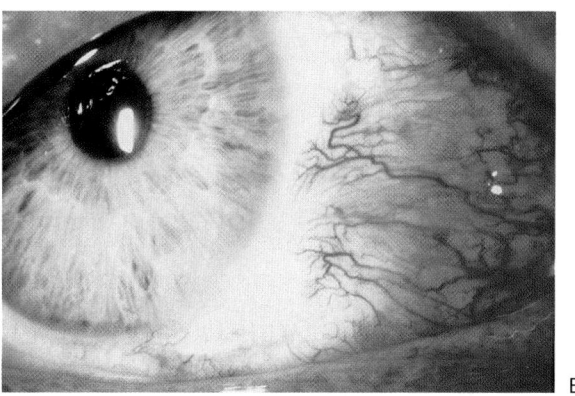

PLATE 156. A: Preoperative appearance of recurrent nasal pterygium that had been operated four times previously with conjunctival autografting. **B:** Same eye without any recurrence 9 months after pterygium excision and adjunctive use of 0.4 mg/mL (0.04%) mitomycin C.

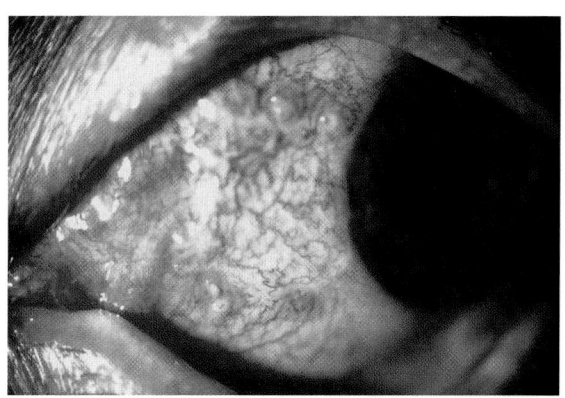

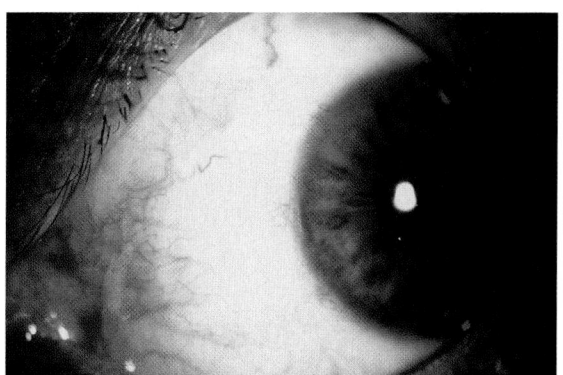

PLATE 157. A: Conjunctival autograft 2 weeks after primary nasal pterygium excision. **B:** Same eye with excellent results 1 year after conjunctival autografting.

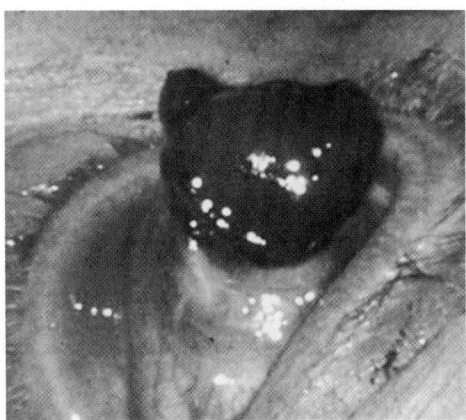

PLATE 158. Expulsive hemorrhage.

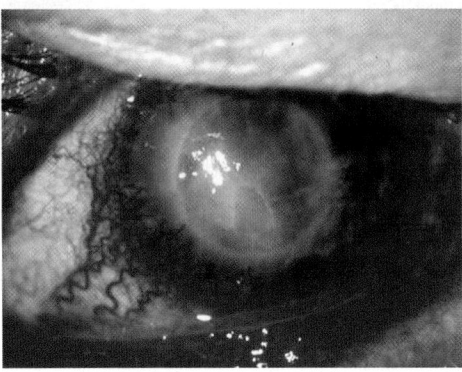

PLATE 159. A persistent epithelial defect.

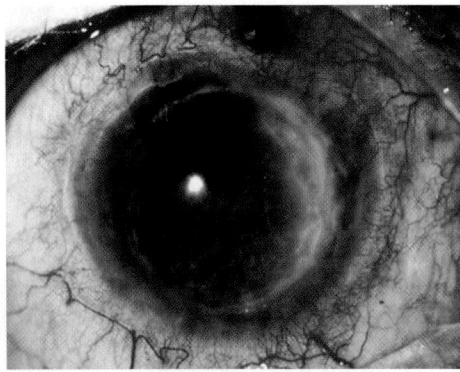

PLATE 160. Herpes simplex virus disease epithelial recurrence in graft.

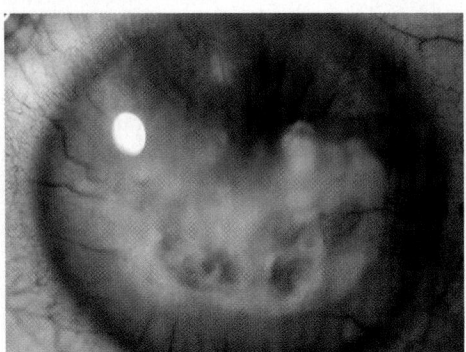

PLATE 161. Corneal leukoma secondary to herpes simplex virus infection, with marked neovascularization.

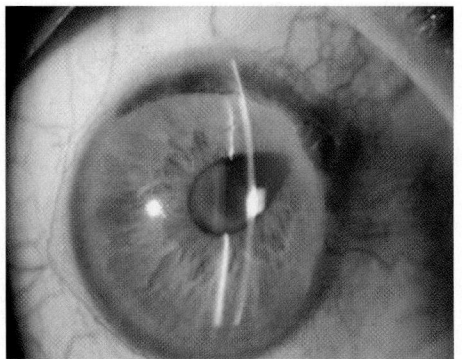

A

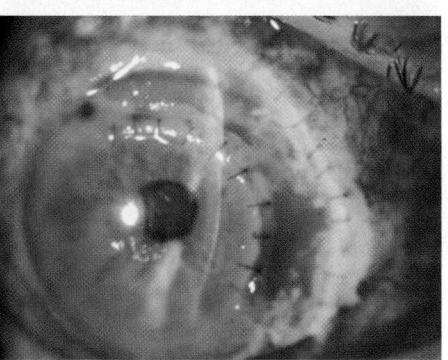

B

PLATE 162. Tectonic lamellar keratoplasty for the treatment of a perforated Terrien's marginal degeneration after trauma. **A:** Peripheral corneal perforation is shown with iris incarceration in the corneal wound and a peaked pupil. **B:** Corneal integrity is restored by a tectonic horseshoe-shaped lamellar graft. (Courtesy of Jeffrey D. Lanier, M.D., with permission)

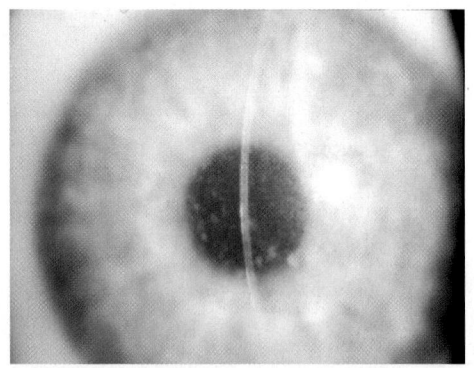

A

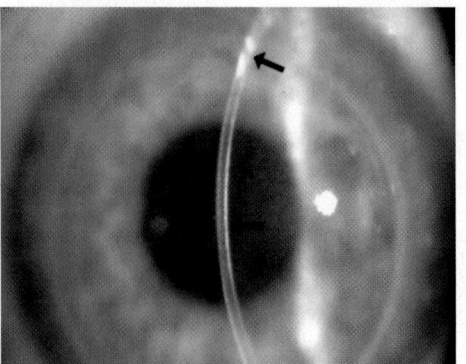

B

PLATE 163. Macular corneal dystrophy. **A:** Preoperative photograph showing diffuse stromal opacities consistent with macular dystrophy. **B:** Clear lamellar graft 3 months after surgery. *Top arrow* shows the perforation site, which required closure with a 10 nylon suture to complete the procedure. *Bottom arrow* shows slight interface haze, but patient has 20/25 acuity.

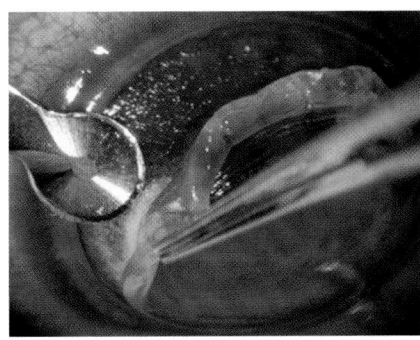

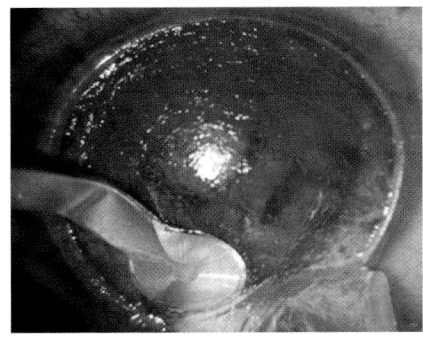

PLATE 164. Intraoperative lamellar keratectomy using Malbran's technique on a patient with advanced keratoconus. **A:** Peripheral lamellar dissection keeping blade slightly upward just anterior to white stromal fibers, which form when air enters the dissection plane. **C:** As the peripheral aspect of the inferior edge is reached, the microsurgical blade is used to complete the lamellar keratectomy. Note the glassy, smooth appearance of the central stromal bed, which was safely created without the use of the lamellar blade.

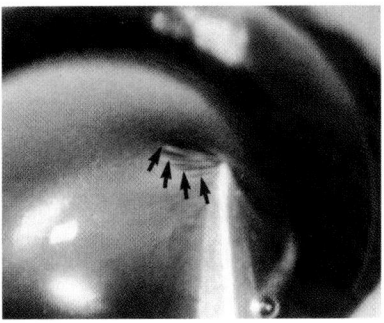

PLATE 165. Folding effect. Small folds (*arrows*) in the posterior corneal tissue are visible adjacent to the tip of a dissection blade that approaches the posterior corneal surface. (From Melles GRJ, Rietveld FJR, Beekhuis WH, et al. A technique to visualize corneal incision and lamellar dissection depth during surgery. *Cornea* 1999;18:80-86.)

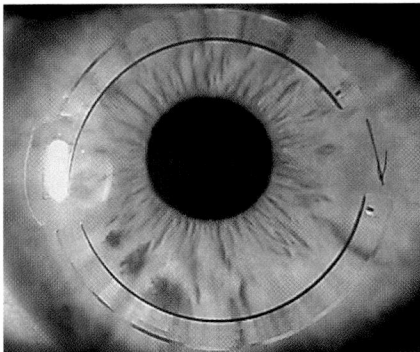

PLATE 167. Slit-lamp aspect of the keratoconic cornea after Intacs implantation.

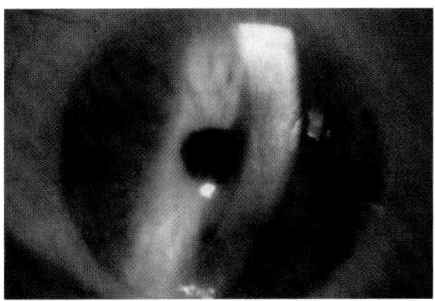

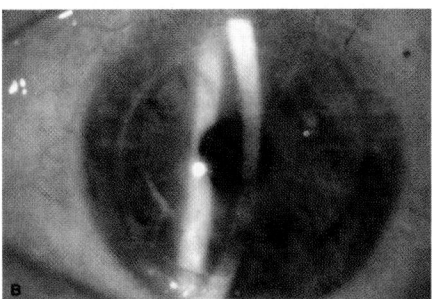

PLATE 166. A, Preoperative photograph of edematous cornea due to Fuchs' dystrophy. **B,** Postoperative photograph of grafted cornea after months. Note the clarity of the central grafted cornea and the persistent edema of the nongrafted peripheral cornea. (From Terry MA, Ousley PJ. Deep lamellar endothelial keratoplasty in the first United States patient: early clinical results. *Cornea* 2001;20:239-243.)

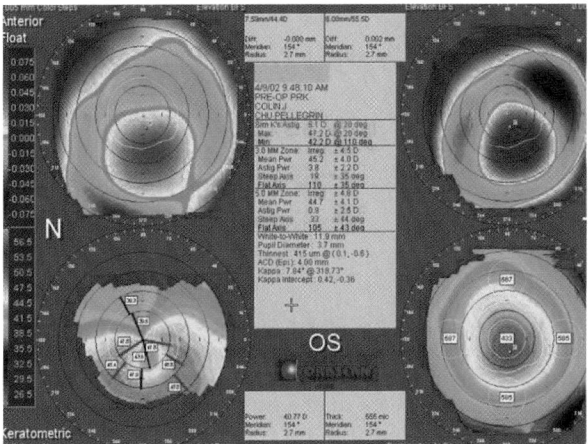

PLATE 168. Corneotopographic image of a keratoconus case before surgery.

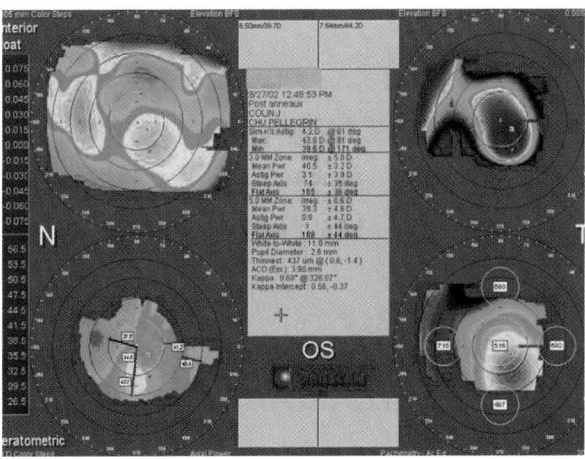

PLATE 169. Same eye as in Fig. 64-2 after Intacs implantation.

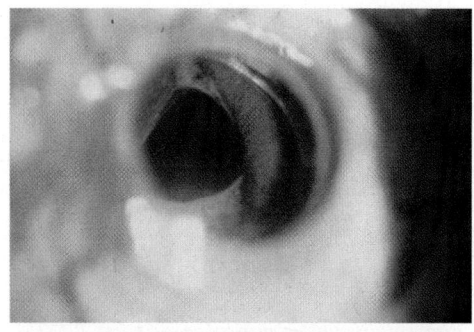
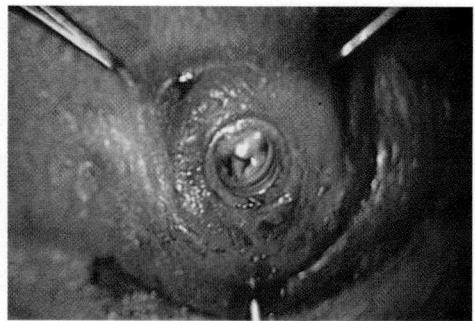
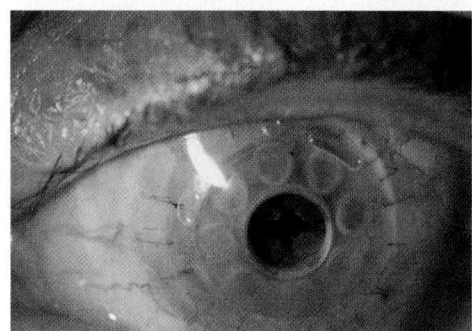
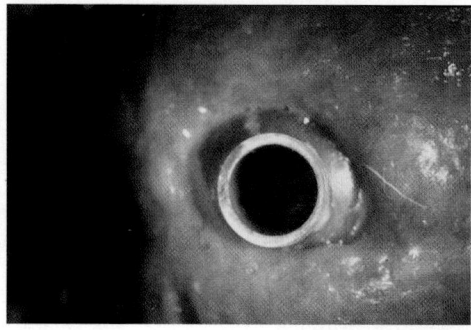

PLATE 170. *Upper left*: In cases with prolonged postoperative inflammation, a retroprosthesis membrane can form. If thin, it can be readily broken up with the YAG laser. *Upper right*: In more severely inflamed cases, laser treatment may be difficult. *Lower left*: If a thick membrane with blood vessels has formed, only a three-part membranectomy under pressure is effective (35). *Lower right*: Skin retraction around a type II nub is not uncommon and may require revision. Prophylactic antibiotics drops are effective in preventing infection.

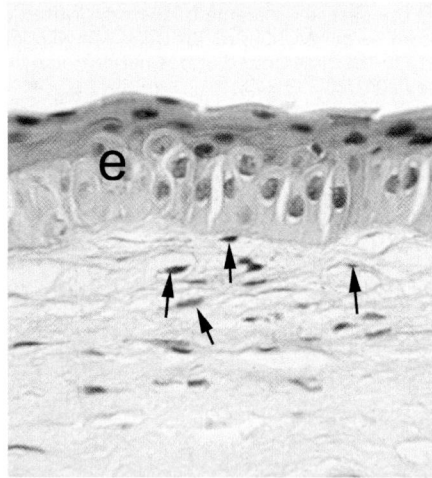

PLATE 171. Destruction of Bowman's layer in bullous keratopathy with chronic edema of the epithelium. Notice that Bowman's layer is no longer present and fibroblastic cells that are thought to be derived from keratocytes now lie immediately beneath the epithelium.

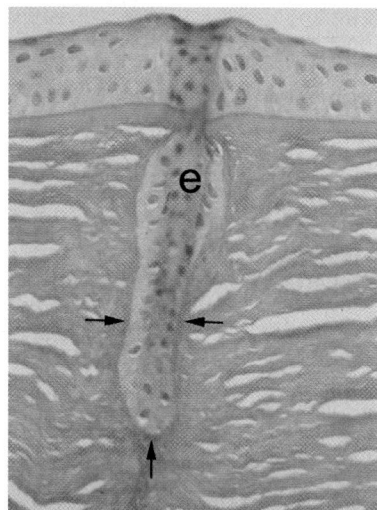

PLATE 172. Human cornea that had radial keratotomy many years before histologic analysis. Note retained epithelial plug (e) extending deep into the stroma. Also note the acellular Bowman's like layer (*arrows*) extending around the epithelial plug. This layer is likely derived and maintained through ongoing epithelial–stromal interactions (hematoxylin and eosin stain, original magnification ×250). (Courtesy of Perry S. Binder, with permission.)

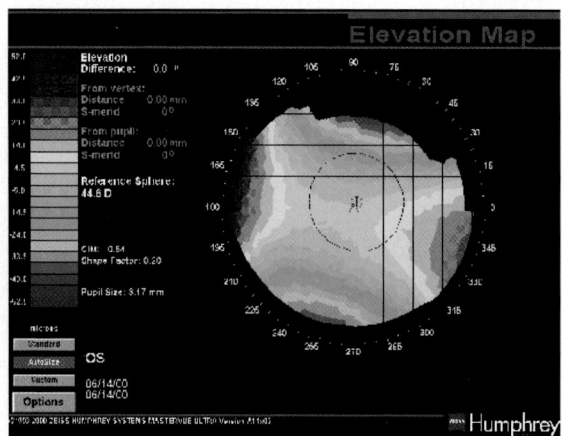

PLATE 173. Elevation map of a cornea with regular astigmatism. The elevated portion represents the flatter meridian of the cornea.

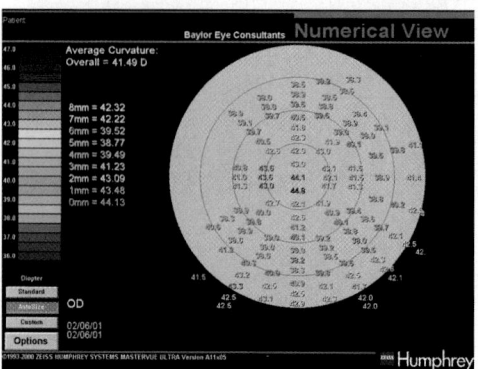

PLATE 174. Numeric display from Humphrey Atlas.

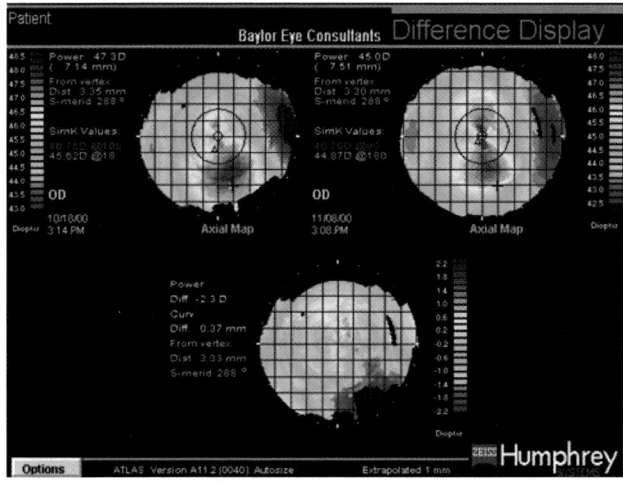

PLATE 175. Contact lens–induced corneal warpage (*upper left*) that reversed 1 month after discontinuation of contact lens wear (*upper right*). Difference map (*bottom*) shows the inferior flattening that occurred after contact lens wear was stopped.

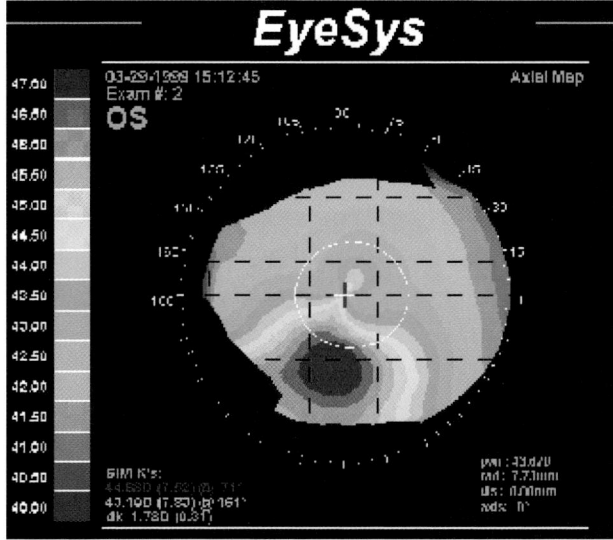

PLATE 176. Classic pattern of keratoconus as displayed on an axial radius of curvature map.

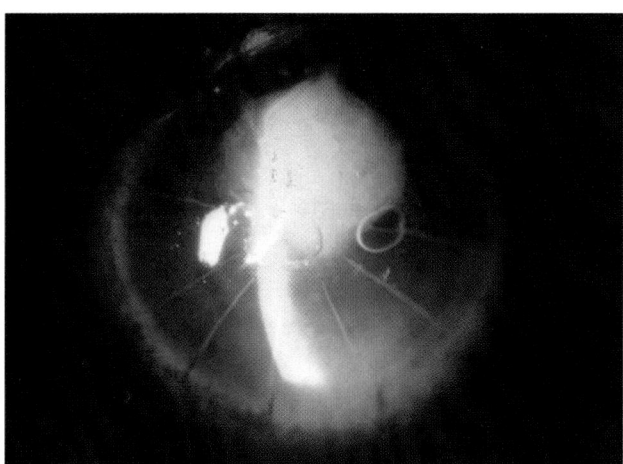

PLATE 177. Infectious keratitis. (Incisional keratotomy complication.)

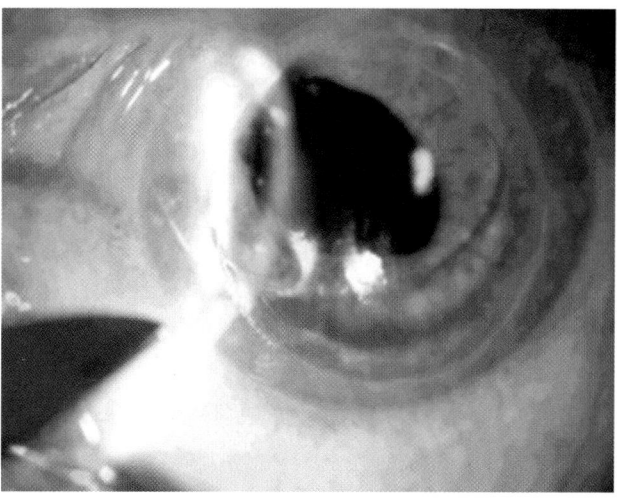

PLATE 178. A blade breaks down the scar at Bowman's layer to create a relaxing incision in the keratoplasty incision.

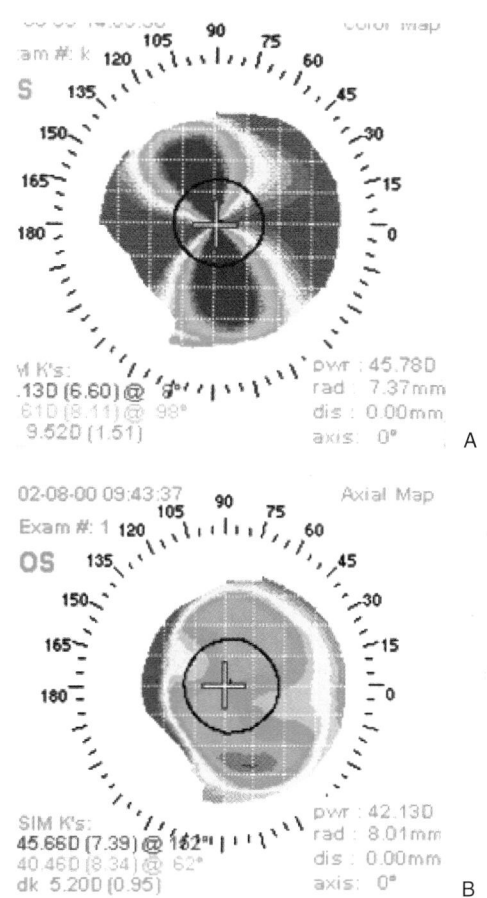

PLATE 179. Case 1. **A:** A high degree of astigmatism is present after keratoplasty with a regular pattern. **B:** After LASIK, a marked reduction in the astigmatism is evident.

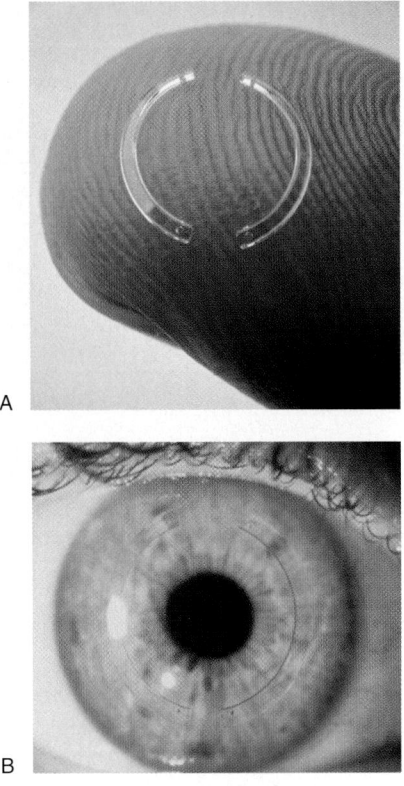

A

B

PLATE 180. Intrastromal corneal ring segment (Intacs) 150-degree segments for myopia *ex vivo* (**A**) and *in vivo* (**B**).

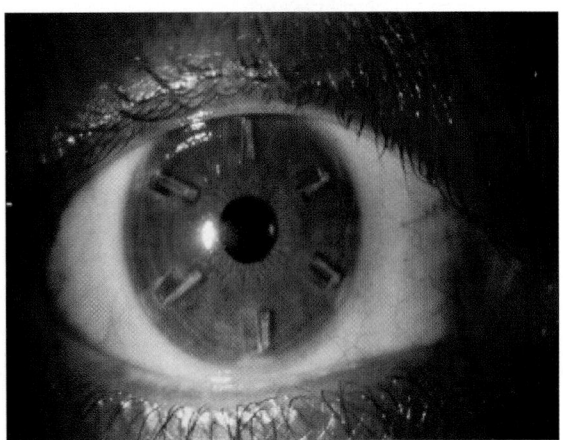

PLATE 181. Intacs segments for correction of hyperopia.

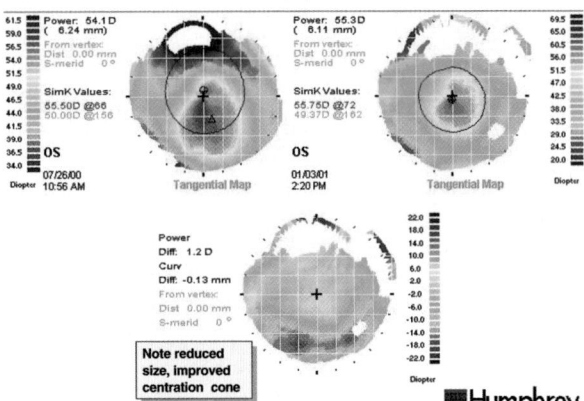

PLATE 182. Topographic effect of Intacs for Keratoconus.

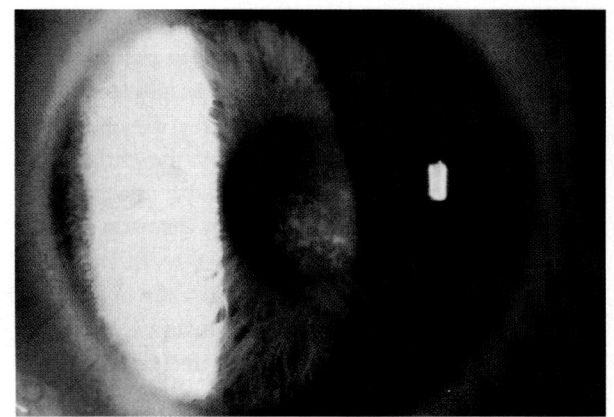

A

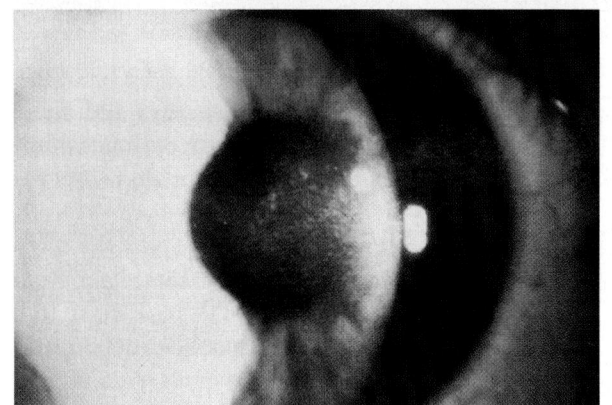

B

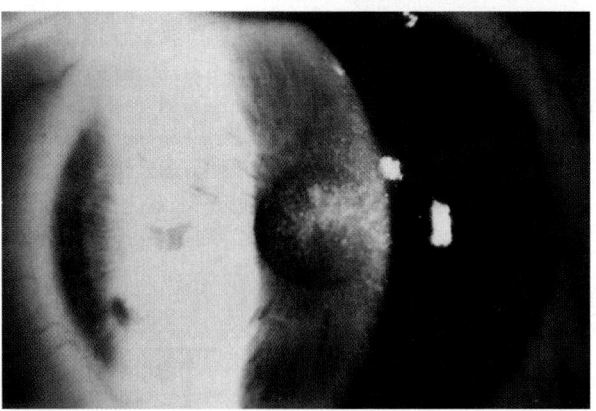

C

PLATE 183. Postoperative haze formation. Subepithelial haze may present by 1 month postoperatively, peak between 3 and 6 months, and gradually subside by 12 to 18 months. The slides represent trace (**A**), mild (**B**), and moderate haze (**C**). (From Thompson V, Seiler T. Excimer laser photorefractive keratectomy for myopia. In: Azar DT, ed. *Refractive surgery.* Stamford, CT: Appleton and Lange, 1997:427, with permission.)

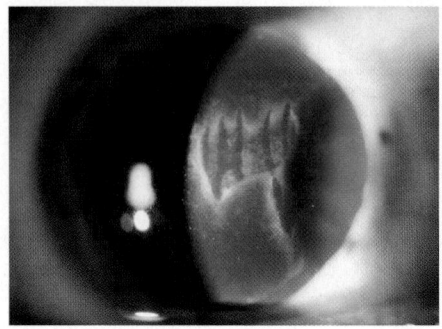

PLATE 184. Button-hole formation with secondary scarring.

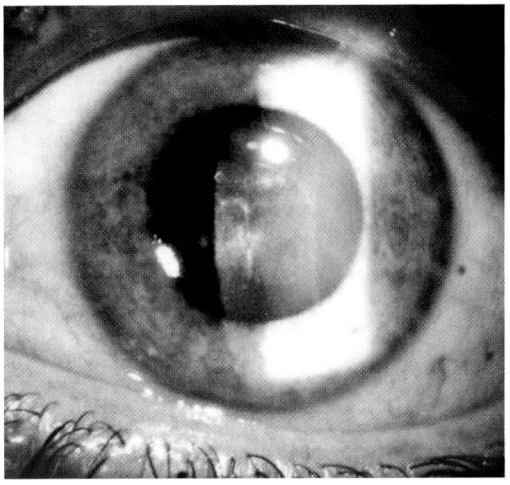

PLATE 185. Slit-lamp photograph of a patient with post-LASIK buttonhole, showing a central irregular corneal scar.

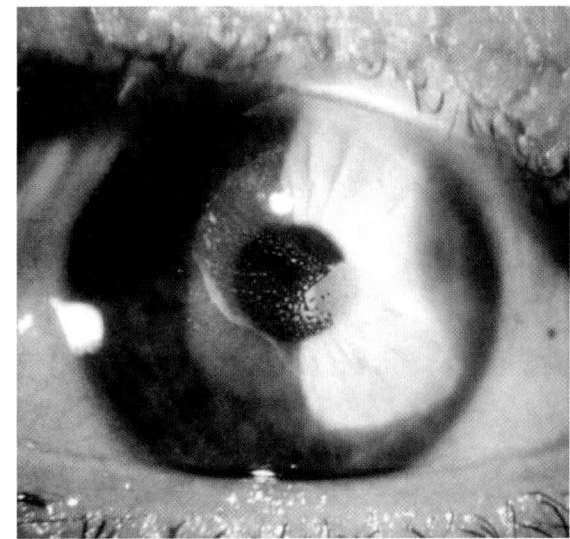

PLATE 186. Central (into the visual axis) epithelial ingrowth with progressive flap melting.

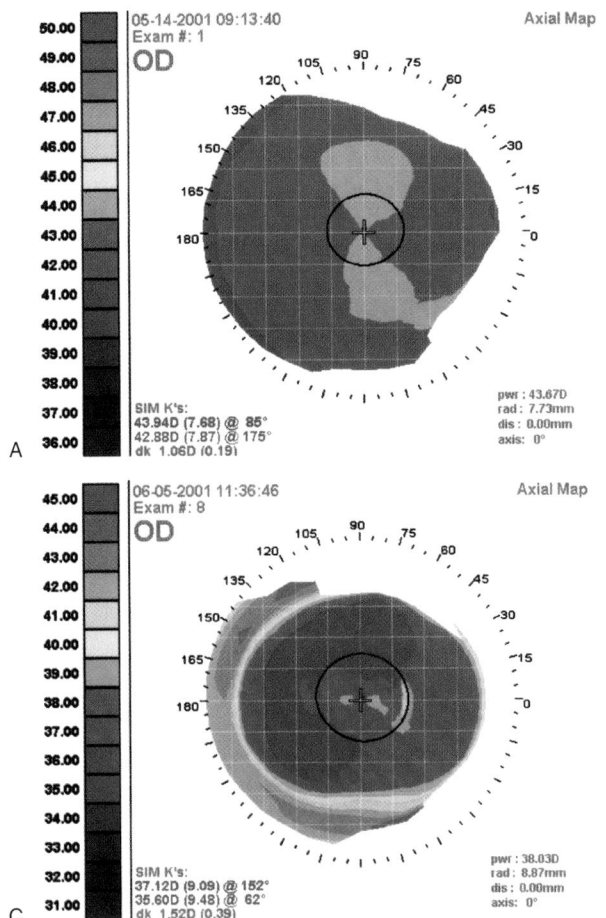

PLATE 187. A: Preoperative corneal topography. **B:** Corneal topography after ICRS tunnel formation and LASIK ablation. **C:** Corneal topography after segment insertion. (From Primack JD, Farah SG, Azar DT. LASIK and intrastromal corneal ring segments (ICRS). In: Azar DT, Koch DD, eds. *LASIK—fundamentals, surgical technique, and complications.* New York: Marcel Dekker, 2003:335– 349, with permission.)

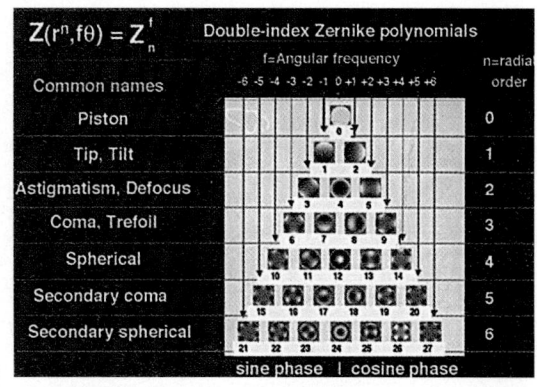

A

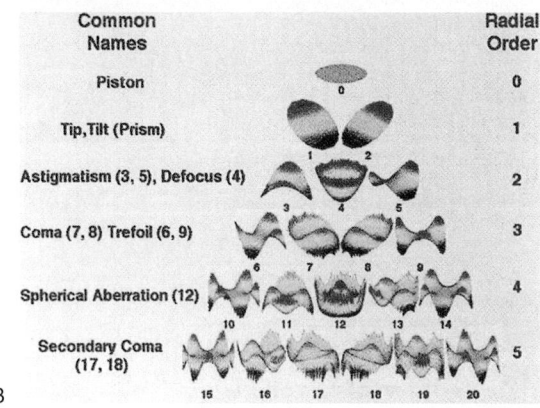

B

PLATE 188. A, Two-dimensional pictorial representation of some of the Zernike polynomials. **B,** Three-dimensional pictorial representation. (From Wavefront sensors: the shape of things to come. *Rev Refract Surg* August 2001;14, with permission.)

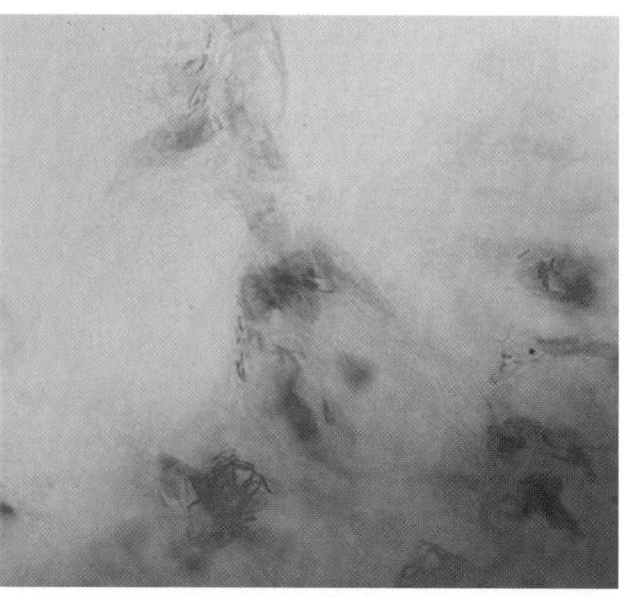

PLATE 189. PostLASIK mycobacterial keratitis. Scraping of the plaquelike infiltrate disclosed acid-fast bacilli with the Ziehl-Nielson stain as shown. Cultures grew heavy nonTB mycobacteria later identified as *Mycobacterium chelonae* subspecies abscessus.